MW00837202

*Goodman and Fuller's*

# PATHOLOGY

## Implications for the Physical Therapist

Fifth Edition

FIFTH EDITION

*Goodman and Fuller's*

# PATHOLOGY

## Implications for the Physical Therapist

Editors: **Catherine Cavallaro Goodman, MBA, PT and Kenda S. Fuller, PT**

Associate Editor: **Rolando T. Lazaro, PT, PhD, DPT, MS**
Associate Professor
College of Health and Human Services
California State University Sacramento
Sacramento, California
Medical Director: **Celeste Knight Peterson, MD**
Pelvic Health Consultant: **Elizabeth Shelly, PT, DPT, WCS, BCB PMD**

*Section Editors/ Reviewers/Assistants:*
SECTION 1: Introduction: **Charlene Marshall, BS, PTA**
SECTION 2: Clinical Medicine: **Rolando T. Lazaro, PT, PhD, DPT, MS**
Research Assistant: **Domenique (Nikki) Javier, PT, DPT**
SECTION 3: Pathology of the Musculoskeletal System: **Kevin Helgeson, DHSc, MS, PT**
Section Reviewer: **Coral Gubler, PT, PhD, MPT, MSS, ATC**
SECTION 4: Pathology of the Nervous System: **Karen L. McCulloch, PT, PhD, NCS**
SECTION 5: Important Resources: **Rolando T. Lazaro, PT, PhD, DPT, MS**

*Pharmacologic Consultant:*
**Sherrill J. Brown, DVM, PharmD, BCPS**
Director, Drug Information Service
Associate Professor, Pharmacy Practice
University of Montana Skaggs School of Pharmacy
Missoula, Montana

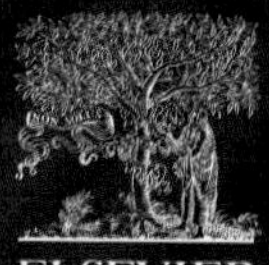

ELSEVIER

Elsevier
3251 Riverport Lane
St. Louis, Missouri 63043

GOODMAN AND FULLER'S PATHOLOGY: IMPLICATIONS
FOR THE PHYSICAL THERAPIST, FIFTH EDITION

ISBN: 978-0-323-67355-6

**Copyright © 2021 by Elsevier, Inc. All rights reserved.**

No part of this publication may be reproduced or transmitted in any form or by any means, electronic or mechanical, including photocopying, recording, or any information storage and retrieval system, without permission in writing from the publisher. Details on how to seek permission, further information about the Publisher's permissions policies and our arrangements with organizations such as the Copyright Clearance Center and the Copyright Licensing Agency, can be found at our website: www.elsevier.com/permissions.

This book and the individual contributions contained in it are protected under copyright by the Publisher (other than as may be noted herein).

**Notice**

Practitioners and researchers must always rely on their own experience and knowledge in evaluating and using any information, methods, compounds or experiments described herein. Because of rapid advances in the medical sciences, in particular, independent verification of diagnoses and drug dosages should be made. To the fullest extent of the law, no responsibility is assumed by Elsevier, authors, editors or contributors for any injury and/or damage to persons or property as a matter of products liability, negligence or otherwise, or from any use or operation of any methods, products, instructions, or ideas contained in the material herein.

Previous editions copyrighted 2015, 2009, 2003, and 1998.

**Library of Congress Control Number:** 2020932132

*Senior Content Strategist:* Lauren Willis
*Senior Content Development Manager:* Luke Held
*Senior Content Development Specialist:* Maria Broeker
*Publishing Services Manager:* Julie Eddy
*Senior Project Manager:* Rachel E. McMullen

Printed in India

Last digit is the print number: 9 8 7 6 5 4 3 2 1

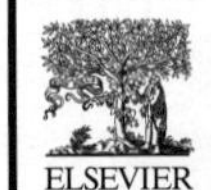

Working together
to grow libraries in
developing countries

www.elsevier.com • www.bookaid.org

# CONTRIBUTORS

**Jamila Aberdeen, PT, DPT, OCS, BSc (Hons)**
Physical Therapy Supervisor
Center for Rehabilitation
Children's Hospital of Philadelphia
Philadelphia, Pennsylvania

**Fabrisia Ambrosio, PhD, MPT**
Associate Professor
Physical Medicine & Rehabilitation
University of Pittsburgh;
Director of Rehabilitation
University of Pittsburgh Medical Center
Pittsburgh, Pennsylvania

**Heather L. Atkinson, PT, DPT, NCS**
Physical Therapist
Physical Therapy
The Children's Hospital of Philadelphia
Philadelphia, Pennsylvania

**Pamela Bartlo, PT, DPT, CCS**
Clinical Associate Professor
Physical Therapy
D'Youville College
Buffalo, New York

**Lori Thein Brody, PT, PhD, SCS, ATC**
Senior Clinical Specialist
Research Park Physical Therapy
UW Health
Madison, Wisconsin;
Professor
Health Sciences
Rocky Mountain University of Health Professions
Provo, Utah

**Teressa F. Brown, PT, DPT, PhD, OCS**
Dean and Program Director
School of Physical Therapy
Arkansas Colleges of Health Education
Fort Smith, Arkansas

**Annie Burke-Doe, PT, MPT, PhD**
Dean
Department of Physical Therapy
West Coast University
Los Angeles, California

**Michelle H. Cameron, MD, PT**
Associate Professor
Neurology
Oregon Health & Science University;
Acting Chief
Neurology
VA Portland Health Care System
Portland, Oregon

**Heather Campbell, PT, DPT, MA, OCS (Emerita)**
Affiliate Faculty
School of Physical Therapy
Rueckert-Hartman College for Health Professions, Regis University
Denver, Colorado

**Michael S. Castillo, PT, DPT, MHS, MPA, GCS, NCS**
Home Health Rehab Services Clinical Supervisor
Martinez Home Health
Kaiser Permanente
Martinez, California

**Joy Cohn, BSPT**
Physical Therapist
Penn Therapy and Fitness
Good Shepherd Penn Partners
Philadelphia, Pennsylvania

**Catherine L. Curtis, PT, EdD**
Assistant Professor
Physical Therapy
New York Medical College
Valhalla, New York

**Audrey C. Czejkowski, PT, DPT, NCS, MSCS**
Physical Therapist
Rehabilitation Services
UNC Health
Chapel Hill, North Carolina

**Erica DeMarch, MSPT**
Founder, CEO
Physical Therapy
Step and Connect
Denver, Colorado

**Jan Dommerholt, PT, DPT**
President/CEO
Physical Therapy
Bethesda Physiocare, Inc.;
President/CEO
Myopain Seminars, LLC
Bethesda, Maryland

**Lara A. Firrone, BS, PT, NCS**
Staff PT
Rehabilitation Services
Methodist LeBonheur Healthcare
Memphis, Tennessee

**Beth Anne Fisher, PT, DPT, CSCS, WHC**
Owner and Pelvic Health Physical Therapist
Physical Therapy
Womb Matters PLLC
Denver, Colorado

**Joseph Anthony Fraietta, PhD**
Assistant Professor
Microbiology
University of Pennsylvania
Philadelphia, Pennsylvania

**Karen A. Gibbs, PhD, DPT, MSPT, CWS**
Professor
Department of Physical Therapy
Texas State University
Round Rock, Texas

**Robyn Gisbert, PT, DPT**
Assistant Professor
University of Colorado School of Medicine
Physical Therapy Program
University of Colorado Anschutz Medical Campus
Aurora, Colorado

**Allan M. Glanzman, PT, DPT, PCS**
Clinical Specialist PT IV
Department of Physical Therapy
Children's Hospital of Philadelphia
Philadelphia, Pennsylvania

**Allon Goldberg, BSc, BSc Med (Hons), PhD**
Associate Dean for Research and Professional Development
College of Health Sciences
University of Michigan-Flint;
Professor of Physical Therapy
Physical Therapy Department
University of Michigan-Flint
Flint, Michigan

**Jared M. Gollie, PhD**
Director, Skeletal Muscle Laboratory
Research Service
Washington DC VA Medical Center;
Adjunct Faculty
Health, Human Function, and Rehabilitation Science
The George Washington University
Washington, District of Columbia;
Adjunct Assistant Professor
Rehabilitation Science
George Mason University
Fairfax, Virginia

**Ira Gorman, PT, PhD, MSPH**
Assistant Dean/Associate Professor
School of Physical Therapy
Regis University
Denver, Colorado

**Brittany N. Grant, BS**
Collegiate Cross Country Coach
Athletics
Whatcom Community College
Bellingham, Washington

**Catherine Hamilton, PT, DPT, MSCS**
Physical Therapist
Rehabilitation Therapies
UNC Health Care
Chapel Hill, North Carolina

**Ann Harrington, PT, DPT, PhD**
Research Scientist
Center for Rehabilitation
Children's Hospital of Philadelphia
Philadelphia, Pennsylvania;
Assistant Professor
Department of Physical Therapy
Arcadia University
Glenside, Pennsylvania

**John D. Heick, DPT, PhD, OCS, NCS, SCS**
Associate Professor
Department of Physical Therapy and Athletic Training
Northern Arizona University
Flagstaff, Arizona

**Kevin Helgeson, DHSc, MS, PT**
Professor
Physical Therapy
Rocky Mountain University of Health Professions
Provo, Utah

**Jeri B. Innis, MA, LPC, PT**
Owner
Innis Integrative Bodymind Therapy
Boulder, Colorado

**Dawn Kelly James, PT, DPT, DSc**
Associate Professor
Department of Physical Therapy
West Coast University
Los Angeles, California

**Kristen M. Johnson, PT, EdD, MS, NCS**
Associate Professor
Doctor of Physical Therapy
University of St. Augustine for Health Sciences
San Marcos, California;
Associate Professor, Neurologic Concentration Track Director
PhD in Health Sciences
Rocky Mountain University of Health Professions
Provo, Utah

**Brett Koermer, DPT, CCS**
Physical Therapist
Adult Inpatient Physical & Occupational Therapy
Duke University Hospital
Durham, North Carolina

**Michelle Laging, DPT, BLA**
Lead ACUTE Physical Therapist
ACUTE Center for Eating Disorder by Denver Health
Denver Health and Hospital Authority;
Founder & Physical Therapist
Movement is Medicine Physical Therapy and Wellness
Denver, Colorado

**Bonnie B. Lasinski, MA, PT, CI-CS, CLT-LANA**
Clinical Director—Retired
Lymphedema Therapy
Boris-Lasinski School—A Casley Smith US Affiliate
Pawleys Island. South Carolina

**Ian M. Leahy, PT, DPT, OCS, SCS, CSCS, FAAOMPT**
Physical Therapist
Sports Medicine and Performance
Children's Hospital of Philadelphia;
Adjunct Facutly
College of Health Professions
Thomas Jefferson University
Philadelphia, Pennsylvania;
Adjunct Faculty
Physical Therapy/Biokinesiology
University of Southern California
Los Angeles, California

**Jeannette Lee, PT, PhD**
Associate Professor
UCSF/SFSU Graduate Program in Physical Therapy
San Francisco State University
San Francisco, California

**Kimberly Levenhagen, PT, DPT, WCC, CLT, FNAP**
Associate Professor
Department of Physical Therapy and Athletic Training
Saint Louis University
St. Louis, Missouri

**Karen L. Litos, PT, DPT, WCS**
Clinic Owner
No Mom Left Behind PT, LLC
Okemos, Michigan

**Sean T. Lowers, PT, DPT, CCS**
Physical Therapist
Cardiopulmonary Rehab
Duke Health
Durham, North Carolina

**Charlene Marshall, BS, PTA**
Director of Rehabilitation
Aegis Therapies
Edgewater Haven Nursing Home
Port Edwards, Wisconsin

**Nathan Mayberry, PT, DPT, OCS, CSCS, CMTPT**
Instructor
Physical Therapy Continuing Education
Myopain Seminars
Bethesda, Maryland

**Karen L. McCulloch, PT, PhD, NCS**
Professor
Allied Health Sciences, Division of Physical Therapy
University of North Carolina at Chapel Hill
Chapel Hill, North Carolina

**Vicki Stemmons Mercer, PT, PhD**
Associate Professor
Division of Physical Therapy
University of North Carolina at Chapel Hill;
Director
Human Movement Science PhD Program
University of North Carolina at Chapel Hill
Chapel Hill, North Carolina

**Nicole A. Miranda, PT, DPT**
Affiliate Faculty
Doctor of Physical Therapy
Regis University
Denver. Colorado
Adjunct Faculty
Doctor of Physical Therapy
South College
Knoxville, Tennessee

**Heather L. Moky, PT, DPT**
Physical Therapy Specialist
Rehab, UIC/UI Health
Chicago, Illinois

**G. Stephen Morris, BS, MSPT, PhD, FACSM**
Distinguished Professor
Physical Therapy
Wingate University
Wingate, North Carolina

**Traci Norris, PT, DPT, GCS, CEEAA**
Rehabilitation Clinical Specialist
Department of Rehabilitation
Barnes-Jewish Hospital
St. Louis, Missouri

**Renee Ostertag, DPT, MPT, MPhysio**
Owner
Physical Therapy
Green Tree Mind, LLC
Denver, Colorado

**Lora Packel, PT, PhD**
Chair & Associate Professor
Department of Physical Therapy
University of the Sciences
Philadelphia, Pennsylvania

**Gina Pariser, PT, PhD**
Professor
Doctor of Physical Therapy
Bellarmine University
Louisville, Kentucky

**Celeste Knight Peterson, MD**
Doctor, Long-Term Care Group
Providence
Missoula, Montana

**Vance Pounders IV, MS, DPT**
College of Health Sciences
Tennessee State University
Nashville, Tennessee

**Megan M. Pribyl, PT, CMPT, CMTPT**
Rehabilitation Services
Olathe Health System
Olathe, Kansas;
Instructor/Course Developer
Herman & Wallace Pelvic Rehabilitation Institute
Seattle, Washington

**Edilberto Alcantara Raynes, MD, PhD**
Professor
Physical Therapy
Tennessee State University
Nashville, Tennessee

**Margaret E. Rinehart-Ayres, PT, PhD**
Consultant
Ambler, Pennsylvania

**Lynzie Schulte, PT, DPT**
Adjunct Faculty
Department of Physical Therapy
Clarkson University
Potsdam, New York

**Korre L. Scott, PT, DPT**
Physical Therapist
Rehabilitation Services
UNC Health Care
Chapel Hill, North Carolina

**Elizabeth Shelly, PT, DPT, WCS, BCB PMD**
Pelvic PT
Physical Therapy
Beth Shelly Physical Therapy
Moline, Illinois

**Irina V. Smirnova, MS (Hon), PhD**
Associate Professor; Director, PhD in Rehabilitation Science Program
Physical Therapy and Rehabilitation Science
University of Kansas Medical Center
Kansas City, Kansas

**Karen Snowden, PT, DPT, WCS**
Doctor of Physical Therapy
Rehabilitation Services
Lehigh Valley Health Network
Allentown, Pennsylvania

**MJ Strauhal, PT, DPT, BCB-PMD**
Clinical Advancement Program Lead- Pelvic Health
Rehabilitation Services Department
Providence St. Vincent Medical Center
Portland, Oregon

**Candy Tefertiller, PT, DPT, PhD, NCS**
Executive Director of Research and Evaluation
Craig Hospital;
TBI Model Systems Co-Project Director
Englewood, Colorado

**James Tompkins, PT, DPT**
Senior Director
Rehabilitation Services
Bayhealth
Dover, Delaware

**Chelsea R. Van Zytveld, PT, DPT**
Physical Therapist
Physical Therapy
South Valley Physical Therapy, P.C
Denver, Colorado

**Karen von Berg, PT, DPT**
Physical Therapist
Physical Medicine & Rehabilitation
The Johns Hopkins Hospital
Baltimore, Maryland

**Chris L. Wells, PhD, PT, ATC, CCS**
Cardiovascular & Pulmonary Clinical Specialist
Department of Rehabilitation Services
University of Maryland Medical Center;
Associate Professor, Adjunct II
Physical Therapy & Rehabilitation Science
University of Maryland, School of Medicine
Baltimore, Maryland

**Deborah M. Wendland, PT, DPT, PhD**
Associate Professor
Physical Therapy–College of Health Professions
Mercer University
Atlanta, Georgia

**Patricia A. Winkler, PT, DSc, NCS, (emeritus)**
Assisstant Professor (retired)
School of Physical Therapy
Regis University
Denver, Colorado

**April M. Xayavong, PT, DPT, CBIS**
Rehabilitation Services
UNC Health Care
Chapel Hill, North Carolina

## DEDICATION IN MEMORIAM

*To Margaret (Peg) Waltner who was our Developmental Editor extraordinare over the decades through multiple editions of all our published works with Elsevier. She taught us so much about the craft of book making and carried us through difficult moments and ongoing challenges. Many of the design elements that have become a permanent part of the text were her original ideas. She was a true artist in every sense of the word.*

*[August 18, 1946 – September 2, 2014].*

*And with extra special thanks to her "connected-at-the-hip" husband, partner, and right-hand man: Doug Waltner. His advice, counsel, and love are embedded in this text as well.*

# FOREWORD

An understanding of pathology is foundational to the decisions made by physical therapists. Knowledge of pathology provides the basis for understanding the health condition and is used throughout the decision-making process, informing screening and examination strategies, evaluation, and informing of prognosis for both activities and participation. This knowledge—along with knowledge of other concomitant conditions, personal, and environmental factors—assists the physical therapist in anticipating likely physiological responses to physical interventions. While pathology has long been part of the physical therapist's education and practice, the use of that information has evolved substantially over the past decades and will continue to evolve. The evolution to date is summarized, followed by emerging directions as we enter the third decade of the 21st century.

In the 1970s and early 1980s, pathology was part of the educational curriculum, though only loosely tied to clinical practice. By the 1990s, exploration was underway of implications of pathology for the physical therapist's practice. For example, the importance was recognized of the location of the lesion of a stroke in determining resulting impairments (e.g., consequences of a stroke differ substantially in the sensory versus the motor cortex) and the implication for differing physical intervention strategies. Knowledge of tissue healing was incorporated into decisions regarding mobilization of injured structures in musculoskeletal physical therapy. Timing related to injury and interpretation of the patient's pathologic state were recognized as critical factors in safely restoring tissue mobility without risk of contracture and loss of mobility (e.g., ACL repair).

As the physical therapist's scope of practice expanded to include more autonomy and professional responsibility, including direct access, physical therapists needed to effectively screen and triage patients, highlighting the importance of identifying "red flags" associated with pathological conditions. Physical therapists are now trained extensively to recognize signs and symptoms of pathological conditions that may warrant referral to a medical provider. For example, those who work with patients following joint replacement may be the first to recognize signs of potential DVTs or PEs, necessitating referral to a physician. The first edition of *Pathology, Implications for the Physical Therapist*, was published in 1995, bringing together this and relevant critical information related to pathology in context of physical therapist practice.

By the turn of the century, models of the disablement process had entered the lexicon of physical therapists, clearly outlining a link between pathology and disability. The second edition of the *Guide to Physical Therapy Practice* was released, incorporating the disablement framework as an organizing structure. Additional implications of pathology for physical therapist practice were highlighted. By the middle part of that decade there was greater appreciation of the bidirectional relationship between pathology and exercise. Not only was it important to consider how pathology influences or limits exercise, but the influence of exercise on attenuating progression of pathology was becoming apparent in conditions such as osteoarthritis and cardiovascular disorders. Early evidence from animal models suggested that exercise could potentially protect against the progression of chronic or progressive neurological conditions.

By 2007, physical therapists had begun to think beyond the disablement process, embracing the International Classification of Function (ICF). This framework, which was introduced in the third edition of *Pathology, Implications for the Physical Therapist*, focused broadly on the process by which pathological conditions influence a person's ability to function and participate in society. The ICF shifted emphasis from pathology as the main contributor to a person's difficulty with function, highlighting the important contributions of personal and environmental factors. Additionally, the ICF shifted from emphasizing what the person cannot do (i.e., functional limitation, disability) to what the person can do (i.e., activity, participation). Thus introduction of the ICF set the stage for a more holistic approach to physical therapists' strategies for intervention. For example, investigations were conducted examining relationships between exercise capacity and measures of cardiac performance and lung function in patients with heart failure and COPD. Findings demonstrated that exercise training has variable impact on classic measures of cardiac/pulmonary performance (e.g., ejection fraction, $FEV_1$), but has undeniable positive impact on skeletal muscle structure and function, which has been linked to improved exercise capacity and walking ability (activity limitations) as well as quality-of-life measures (participation).

The implications are just emerging of two important advances in the last two decades. First is recognition of the microbiome and its importance in pathology of numerous conditions. Second is epigenetics and its implications for personalized medicine. These two advances will have profound implications for pathology and physical therapist practice in the coming years.

By 2010, there was a growing appreciation of the effect of stress on the endocrine and sympathetic/parasympathetic systems. These systems are fundamental components of the hypothalamic–pituitary–adrenal axis (HPA axis), which is closely tied to the stress response and is central to the mind-body connection. The connection between mind and body has its roots in ancient times but was largely ignored in the West throughout much of the 18th and 19th centuries. Evidence began to emerge in the 1960s of the impact of stress on the immune system, leading to the emergence of meditation and related practices that were largely considered "cults" at that time. By the 1990s, these practices were part of what was considered "alternative medicine"; at the turn of the 21st century, they, along with spirituality, were often referred to in the context of "integrative medicine." Today, meditation, spirituality, mindfulness, and the mind-body connection have found a place in mainstream medicine. Indeed, during the past 20 years, evidence has been growing suggesting meditation and mindfulness can reduce stress and anxiety and improve well-being and happiness. Evidence also demonstrates that meditation has direct physiologic effects, including increasing cortical grey matter density in critical parts of the cortex, as well as telomere length. The potential impact on epigenetics is under investigation along with the psychological and physiological role of meditation in the treatment of a variety of chronic conditions. This focus, combined with an understanding of the impact of pathology on movement and participation, has the potential to augment the physical therapist's care of people who seek treatment.

In summary, the context in which knowledge of pathology is interpreted continues to evolve. As with each previous edition of *Pathology, Implications for the Physical Therapist,* the current edition has added content that encompasses some of the fundamental considerations related to the microbiome, epigenetics, spirituality, meditation, and the mind-body connection that relate directly to pathology and also to the implications for pathology on movement, activity, and participation.

**Margaret Schenkman, PT, PhD, FAPTA**
Professor
Physical Therapy Program
Department of Physical Medicine and Rehabilitation
University of Colorado Anschutz Medical Campus
Aurora, Colorado

# PREFACE

The time has come for us (Kenda and Catherine) to turn the reins of this text over to a new champion and a larger circle of leaders. Toward that end, we have selected Rolando T. Lazaro, PT, PhD, DPT as the new Associate Editor going forward for this 5th edition and beyond. Dr. Lazaro is an academician, researcher, and writer; he has extensive experience updating textbooks and guiding them through the long and detailed process of publishing. As Primary Editor of *Umphred's Neurological Rehabilitation* and coeditor of *Goodman and Snyder's Differential Diagnosis for Physical Therapists,* he now adds this text to his credit.

With the large amount of information available today in all disciplines and topics, we have also selected capable individuals to help us oversee and update specific sections.

Charlene Marshall, BS, PTA, editor of *Pathology for the Physical Therapist Assistant* as well as coauthor of *Recognizing and Reporting Red Flags for the Physical Therapist Assistant,* is the section leader for the Introductory portion (Chapters 1-6) of this edition.

Kevin Helgeson, DHSc, PT, MS remains at the helm of section three *Pathology of the Musculoskeletal System* (Chapters 22-27). He has been an important and integral part of this text for several editions now.

Elizabeth Shelly, PT, DPT, WCS, BCB PMD remains the content editor for Men's and Women's Health bringing all pertinent information in compliance with the APTA Pelvic Health following guidelines provided by *Women's Health Guidelines for First Professional Content in Women's Health.*

Karen L. McCulloch, PT, PhD, NCS has come on board to govern and guide Section four: *Pathology of the Nervous System* (Chapters 28-39). She was awarded her NCS in 1990 and the Service to the Section Award from the Academy of Neurology recognizing her many years of contribution. She has served as an editorial board member for the *Journal of Neurologic Physical Therapy.*

This text continues to benefit from the expertise and years of experience of our medical director, Celeste Knight Peterson, MD. Once again, Dr. Peterson took on the updating of medical material outside the scope of our knowledge base. She did so with an unerring ability to capture the details a physical therapist needs to know.

Over the years spanning the first four editions, students and clinicians have come to rely on this body of work to assist them in evaluating and treating a wide range of patients with varied diagnoses, impairments, and deficits. Here are some of their comments in support of this work.

*As a new graduate physical therapist, learning pathology has been crucial in giving me a deeper understanding of how a person's unique impairments and or condition impact my clinical reasoning and clinical decisions. Without understanding pathology, I cannot fully understand the "why" behind the examination items or the treatment strategies we learned about in school and use throughout practice.* [Racheal Eckert, PT, DPT Class of 2018]

*Almost every decision I make as a physical therapist is rooted in pathology. Pathology gives insight into not only a patient's condition, but also their prognosis and most effective plan of care. Beyond this knowledge is a more important understanding of pathologies relating the patient's entire being. Regulation of the sympathetic and parasympathetic systems often take precedence in my plan of care. Disruption in these systems will ultimately change the prognosis relating to the primary pathology if not addressed. It is this understanding of interaction of pathological systems and states of being that gives me the tools to best care for patients.* [Morgan Wilson, PT, DPT Class of 2016]

*As a physical therapist specializing in outpatient vestibular and neurological rehabilitation, my knowledge and understanding of pathology constantly affects my clinical decisions to provide effective care and helps me differentiate between potential conditions. It allows me to determine if a patient's symptoms are coming from a peripheral musculoskeletal or a neurological issue, central nervous system pathology, or from how sensory input is being centrally integrated. Knowing other body system pathologies like the cardiovascular and endocrine systems leads to appropriate referrals. A patient's autonomic nervous system and emotional state impacts symptoms and influences the ability to learn and engage in therapy. I frequently teach patients about the autonomic nervous system and integrate self-regulation strategies, meditation, and mindfulness into traditional therapy sessions. My knowledge and understanding about the mind-body connection has radically changed how I educate my patients about pain and dizziness.* [Chelsea R. Van Zytveld, PT, DPT Class of 2013]

Readers of this fifth edition will see that we are keeping the material fresh and up to date. You will see reflected throughout a concerted effort to incorporate new discoveries and findings in the science of epigenetics, quantum physics, mind-body connection, and consciousness-based energy medicine.

We have every confidence that Dr. Lazaro and this team of dedicated professionals will continue to guide physical therapy students, clinicians, and our profession forward into the exciting and challenging course health care will take into the 21st century.

**Catherine Cavallaro Goodman**

**Kenda S. Fuller**

# ACKNOWLEDGMENTS

As we (Kenda and Catherine) turn over this text to our Associate Editor, Rolando T. Lazaro, we want to acknowledge some important people who have been a very valuable part of this project. A textbook as large and as comprehensive as this 5th edition of *Pathology: Implications for the Physical Therapist* could not exist without the assistance, advice, support, and collaboration of many people over the many years represented by the first four editions.

Some of you helped develop the chapters early on and kept them up to date for many years. Your names remain associated with each edition you worked on. We regret that we are unable to list everyone in this space but we appreciate every word you wrote, every hour you spent giving this text the best of your expertise; we acknowledge and thank you sincerely.

We do want to give special thanks to several individuals. First: William G. (Bill) Boissonnault who was our original collaborator and co-author. Your vision for the project and help getting it off to its first start were invaluable and still remain woven into the very fabric of this textbook. We want to continue to acknowledge your contribution with gratitude. And to Michael B. Koopmeiners, MD who was our medical director and advisor for that first edition.

Next, Margaret Biblis, who was at that time, the acquisition editor at W.B. Saunders (now Elsevier). Margaret brought the project on board, kept us on track, and steered us through that first edition. She set us up with our wonderful Developmental Editor [for whom this text is dedicated] and guided us through the production process on the publishing side. Thank you, thank you(!), Margaret. Your support and belief in us and in the project never waivered through many challenges. We still raise a toast to you verbally whenever we recall the history of this project.

Finally and most importantly: Celeste Knight Peterson, MD, our long-standing medical director who always responded cheerfully and quickly to our requests and questions (many last minute). Dr. Peterson has consistently provided thorough reviews and updates of medical material throughout this text. What a gift you are to this work!

Contributors for this 5th edition are credited with each chapter or section they participated in, but we still want to acknowledge all the hard work, time, late nights, weekends, and vacations you spent completing the task of updating information and keeping the project on time. You are most valuable to this work, to our students, and to our profession as a whole. You are the best!

Now, we reserve the rest of this section for those individuals who provided support of another type whether that was networking to find contributors, researching topics or updating references, brainstorming ideas for content, and for some of you—standing by ready to assist as a contributor only to be let off the hook later due to page constraints. Thank you!

*Laurita M. Hack, Mary Lou Galantino, Margaret Plack, Barb Norton, William Santamore, Courtney Frankel, Rebecca H Crouch, Dianne Platz*

And finally, a salute to the many people (past, present, and future) at Elsevier who have made this work possible. To the "old guard" who, like us, have retired or moved on to other work: Sally Schrefer, Linda Duncan, Kathy Falk, Christy Hart, Jolynn Gower, and David Stein. And to our current Elsevier team: Elizabeth (Liz) Kilgore, Lauren Willis, Kelly Skelton, Rachel McMullen, and Maria Broeker.

**Catherine Cavallaro Goodman**

**Kenda S. Fuller**

**Rolando T. Lazaro**

# CONTENTS

SECTION 1 INTRODUCTION

# CHAPTER 1

# Introduction to Concepts of Pathology

CATHERINE CAVALLARO GOODMAN • KENDA S. FULLER • ALLON GOLDBERG • CATHERINE L. CURTIS • KAREN L. MCCULLOCH • KEVIN HELGESON • CHARLENE MARSHALL

## PATHOGENESIS OF DISEASE

*Pathology* is defined as the branch of medicine that investigates the essential nature of disease, especially changes in body tissues and organs that cause or are caused by disease.[77] *Clinical pathology* in medicine refers to pathology applied to the solution of clinical problems, especially the use of laboratory methods in clinical diagnosis. *Pathogenesis* is the development of unhealthy conditions or disease or, more specifically, the cellular events and reactions and other pathologic mechanisms that occur in the development of disease.

This text examines the pathogenesis of each disease or condition—that is, the progression of each pathologic condition on both its cellular level and its clinical presentation whenever signs and symptoms are manifested. Advances in medicine have resulted in a population with greater longevity but also with a more complex pathologic picture. Orthopedic and neurologic conditions are no longer present as singular phenomena; they often occur in a person with other medical pathology. We must be knowledgeable of the impact other conditions and diseases have on the individual's neuromusculoskeletal system and the steps necessary to provide safe, effective treatment.

For the physical therapist, clinical pathology has a different meaning regarding the effects of pathologic processes (i.e., disease) on the individual's functional abilities and limitations. The relationship between impairment and functional limitation is a key focus in therapy. How the person with the pathologic condition is able to participate in his or her family and community is paramount. Current clinical practice should include an emphasis on the person's activity level, participation, level of supports, and environment. Despite the disease process and related loss of function, the whole person must be considered.

## CONCEPTS OF HEALTH, ILLNESS, AND DISABILITY

### Health

Many people and organizations have attempted to define the concept of health. Since 1948, the World Health Organization (WHO)[115] has defined individual *health* as a state of complete physical, mental, and social well-being and not merely as the absence of disease or infirmity. Definitions that present health as an either/or circumstance, meaning an individual is either healthy or ill, is an outdated concept.

The idea of health status for a nation (e.g., the United States) is a description of the health of the total population using information that is representative of most people living in that country. However, it must be noted that our current epidemiologic system does not keep data on people who do not obtain treatment; no universal or uniform registry is available in the United States.

Health status of a nation can be measured by birth and death rates, life expectancy, quality of life, morbidity from specific diseases, risk factors, use of ambulatory care and inpatient care, accessibility of health personnel and facilities, financing of health care, health insurance coverage, and many other factors. The leading causes of death are often used to describe the health status of a nation. According to the annual report *Health, United States, 2017*, obesity, alcoholism, drug abuse, and tobacco use are health risk factors in the most common causes of morbidity and mortality.[55]

The health of an individual is more accurately viewed as a reflection of a person's biologic, psychologic, emotional, spiritual, and sociologic state. Health is a dynamic process that varies with changes in interactions between an individual and the internal and external environments, a concept discussed in greater detail in Chapter 2. New information about the role of epigenetics in the development of diseases is another factor in how health can become compromised by illness and disease. On the other hand, epigenetic modifications can also lead to new therapies for common diseases.[43]

### Illness

*Illness* is often defined as sickness or deviation from a healthy state; the term has a broader meaning than disease. *Disease* refers to a biologic or psychologic alteration that results in a malfunction of a body organ or system. The term *disease* is usually used to describe a biomedical condition that is substantiated by objective data such as elevated temperature or presence of infection (as demonstrated by positive blood cultures).

Illness is the perception and response of the person to not being well. Illness includes disturbances in normal human biologic function and personal, interpersonal, and cultural reactions to disease. Disease can occur in an individual without the person being aware of illness and without others perceiving illness. However, a person can feel very ill even though no obvious pathologic processes can be identified.

### Acute Illness

*Acute illness* usually refers to an illness or disease that has a relatively rapid onset and short duration; it is not synonymous with "severe." The condition often responds to a specific treatment and is usually self-limiting, although exceptions to this definition are numerous. If no complications occur, most acute illnesses end in a full recovery, and the individual returns to the previous level of functioning.

Subacute refers to how long a disease has been present, but there is no set time that divides subacute from the other time descriptions (i.e., acute and chronic). Subacute describes a time course that is between acute and chronic. A symptom that is subacute has been present for longer than a few days but less than several months. Chronic conditions sometimes flare up and may be referred to as acute or subacute depending on the time period.

Acute illnesses usually follow a specific sequence, or stages of illness, from onset through recovery. The first stage involves the experience of physical symptoms (e.g., pain, shortness of breath, fever); cognitive awareness (i.e., the symptoms are interpreted to have meaning); and an emotional response, often one of denial, fear, or anxiety.

Most people move from acute or subacute illness in a natural progression to the final stage of recovery or rehabilitation. During this stage, the individual begins to resume more normal activities and responsibilities. Individuals with long-term or chronic illnesses may require a longer period to adjust to new lifestyles.

There are some factors that contribute to how a condition transitions from an acute to a chronic phase. For example, chronic inflammation associated with diseases such as diabetes, cancer, and heart disease involves a "persistent injurious trigger that shifts homeostasis," or the body's capacity to self-correct.[69] Ideally, intervention to restore the body's ability to recover and restore fully begins at the start of the interruption of homeostasis, but the resiliency and ability of the human body to restore natural, healthy homeostasis at any point in the process can never be underestimated.

### Chronic Illness

*Chronic illness* describes illnesses that include one or more of the following characteristics: permanent impairment or disability, residual physical or cognitive disability, or the need for special rehabilitation and/or long-term medical management. As a result of the control of many infectious agents, the eradication of childhood diseases, and the current increasing age of the some population, chronic diseases now top the list as causes of morbidity and mortality in the United States (see Table 2.1).

Over the last century, a shift from infectious to noncommunicable chronic diseases such as heart disease, cancer, and diabetes has occurred. In the past, diseases such as stroke and diabetes contributed directly to mortality, but with today's medical treatment, life is extended albeit with the potential for decreased quality of life because of the long-term effects of these conditions and the medical treatment involved.

Chronic illnesses and conditions may fluctuate in intensity as acute exacerbations occur that cause physiologic instability and necessitate additional medical management (e.g., diabetes mellitus, fibromyalgia, rheumatoid arthritis, multiple sclerosis). A person who has exacerbations of chronic illness may progress through the stages of illness described in the previous section.

Many chronic illnesses are modifiable through changes in behavior and lifestyle, a concept that has grown in understanding through the more recent scientific study of epigenetics. Mindfulness, meditation, and prayer are proven ways to change the physiologic and biologic state of the body,[113,56,30,51] which will enhance lifestyle modifications made, such as increased physical activity and exercise and changes in diet and nutrition.

## Psychologic Aspects of Illness

One of the most important factors influencing psychologic reactions to illness is the premorbid (before illness) personality and psychologic profile of the affected person. The impact of abnormal neural wiring and firing associated with repeated negative thoughts may contribute to the progression of a psychologic disorder (e.g., be the same process by which change occurs when an individual's neurosis becomes psychosis).

For example, a person with a dependent-type personality may become very dependent, perhaps seeking unusually large amounts of advice or reassurance from the health care specialist or expecting attention beyond that required for the degree of illness present. A narcissistic (self-centered) person may be particularly concerned about the need to take medication or the loss of the ability to work. The stoic person (indifferent to or unaffected by pain) may have difficulty admitting to being sick at all.

Other factors that affect a person's psychologic reaction include the extent of the illness and the particular symptoms that develop. Extremely mild disease may have little effect, whereas completely unexpected and debilitating illness may be very distressing. A common reaction to any illness is fear or anxiety related to the loss of control over one's own body. Denial is an unconscious defense mechanism that allows a person to avoid painful reality as long as possible. Denial can be a natural part of the process of dealing with illness, which culminates in acceptance.

Noncompliance with treatment may have a psychologic basis, such as denial ("There is nothing wrong with me, so I do not need medical treatment."), but it may also occur as a result of previous experience. For example, noncompliance with prescribed corticosteroid therapy may be based on aversion to side effects experienced during use of this drug in a previous disease flare. With chronic autoimmune diseases (e.g., connective tissue diseases), denial may continue for years as a coping mechanism for the individual who continues to decline in physical functional capacity.

## Disability

### Physical Disability

Disability is a large public health problem in the United States, affecting more than 61 million Americans who report disabling conditions. In other words, more than 25% of the U.S. population (1 in 4 persons) currently lives with at least one disability.[89,17] Prevalence of disability is higher among women than men and is reported highest among people 65 years of age and older. One of the U.S. national health goals is to eliminate health disparities among different segments of the population including among people with disabilities.

The number of baby boomers (persons born between 1946 and 1964) reporting disabilities is expected to continue rising as increasing numbers enter the 65 years of age and older group, which has a much higher risk for disability. Almost half of all older adults (over age 65) self-report having a physical, sensory, mental, or learning disability of some kind. The added number of persons reporting disabilities will likely place more demands on the health care and public health systems. This trend will impact physical therapists directly, as there will be an increased need for additional health care providers trained in musculoskeletal conditions.[27]

### Cognitive Disability

Disabilities are not just limited to the physical body. Mental illnesses such as depression, alcoholism, schizophrenia, and cognitive impairments are seriously underestimated sources of disabilities in an estimated 18% of U.S. adults.[79] These conditions are often undiagnosed, and although physical therapists cannot diagnose these impairments, recognizing the deficits is important. Only cognitive disability is discussed in this section; common mental illnesses are discussed in Chapter 3.

Executive functions may be described as cortical functions involved in formulating goals and in planning, initiating, monitoring, and maintaining behavior.[20] Behavior is defined here in its broadest terms to include not only overt motor behavior but also affective and social behavior. A person with executive function deficits typically appears inert or apathetic. Clinically, these individuals typically have a right hemisphere lesion and apraxia, unilateral neglect, or both. When frontal lobe damage occurs, the effects of impaired executive functions may be inappropriately attributed to depression. Although the two may occur simultaneously, depression is usually characterized by a lack of energy, whereas impaired executive functions are demonstrated by a lack of involvement.

Complex problem solving may be described as the effective handling of new information. Impaired problem solving results in concrete thinking, inability to distinguish the relevant from the irrelevant, erroneous application of rules, and difficulty generalizing from one situation to another. For example, when a client learns how to accomplish wheelchair transfers and then generalizes that information to various settings (bed to chair, chair to toilet, chair to car, in hospital, at home), he or she is using new information in complex problem solving.

Information processing involves the speed with which information travels from one part of the brain to another and the amount of information assimilated at that speed. Whereas complex problem solving has to do with the orchestration of information, information processing involves the efficient transfer of information.

As a result of genetic, environmental, and educational factors, some people are more proficient processors than others. As a result of trauma, some people may lose processing ability and speed. Noise levels, external sensory stimulation (e.g., presence of other people and other activities), and presentation of more than one kind of information at a time (e.g., providing a written home program then discussing the time of the next appointment) are examples of distractions to people with reduced information-processing abilities.

Memory deficits result from a failure to store or retrieve information. Before it can be determined that the person is experiencing a memory lapse, it must be established that the material was learned in the first place. Memory problems typically are acquired rather than developmental. Depression may masquerade as memory loss, but the depressed person is usually less attentive or interactive with the environment and therefore registers (or learns) less. For example, a client may appear to be suffering from a memory dysfunction when, in fact, the decreased attention span is a result of depression that has reduced learning.

Learning disability occurs in a person with normal or near-normal intelligence as difficulty acquiring information in specific domains such as spelling, arithmetic, reading, and visual-spatial relationships. Therapists most commonly encounter learning disabilities manifested as noncompliance with written treatment programs, repeated tardiness for or absence from treatment sessions, and an overly anxious approach to the physical symptoms that have brought the client to the therapist in the first place.

### Disabilities Among Military Personnel and Veterans

According to the U.S. Census, there were 18.2 million military veterans in the United States in 2017. An estimated 3.8 million veterans have a service-connected disability rating, with the most typical injuries being traumatic brain injury, amputation, and posttraumatic stress disorder. Physical therapists see many combat-related disabilities among men and women in the military as well as in the civilian sector once they are discharged. This population has the added burden of increasing age while living with long-term disabilities that can include both physical and cognitive impairments.

**Note to Reader:** We acknowledge that this section regarding the members of our military is very brief. The information presented here does not do justice to the topic, but we would be remiss not to highlight it separately from the previous discussion of disabilities. The topic deserves much more discussion than this chapter allows.

## CLASSIFICATION OF HEALTH AND HEALTH-RELATED DOMAINS

### International Classification of Functioning, Disability, and Health

The American Physical Therapy Association (APTA) has joined the WHO, the World Confederation for Physical Therapy, the American Therapeutic Recreation Association, and other organizations in endorsing a model first established in 2001 called the *International Classification of Functioning, Disability, and Health,* or ICF framework. The ICF framework promotes international exchange using a common, consistent, and universal language to provide a platform for discussion of disability and related phenomena.[64] The ICF is presented as the international standard to describe and measure health, function, and ability (rather than disability) for individuals and populations. It can be used by all health care professionals, thus promoting interpersonal as well as intrapersonal communication across and among various disciplines. The ICF is a good framework for research from a global perspective—this one instrument can provide an international health information system. It will allow for research and clinical study describing function that can be combined and compared for better statistical significance and understanding.

The ICF takes a broad biopsychosocial view that looks beyond mortality and disease to focus on how people live with their conditions; this approach helps physical therapists more accurately identify and address the multiple factors that affect and contribute to an individual's recovery.[36,37,63-65,111] Whereas traditional health indicators are based on the mortality (i.e., death) rates of populations, the ICF shifts focus to "life" (i.e., how people live with their health conditions and how these conditions can be improved to achieve a productive, fulfilling life). The ICF model is an interactive, integrative, and universal model that focuses on human functioning, not pathology. Most notable in the current structure is the inclusion of epigenetic "host factors" (environmental and personal factors) that impact the behavior of the individual such as demographic background, physical and social environments, and psychologic status.

The ICF includes the following six components: (1) body structures/functions, (2) activities, (3) participation, (4) environmental factors, (5) personal factors, and (6) health conditions (Fig. 1.1). The full description of this model can be found at www.who.int/classifications/icf/en/.

**Note to Reader:** The ICF model briefly summarized here has been incorporated into this text whenever possible. There are numerous articles written for the physical therapist further discussing the use of the ICF that may aid you in applying the ICF to specific problems related to the human movement system.[4,5,91,40,64,95,96,29] Readers are encouraged to look at these publications; additional information can be found on the APTA website at http://www.apta.org/ICF/.

SPECIAL IMPLICATIONS FOR THE THERAPIST 1.1

### *Health, Illness, and Disability*

#### Incidence and Prevalence

When discussing various diseases, disorders, and conditions, incidence and prevalence may be reported. Incidence is the number of new cases of a condition in a specific period of time (e.g., 6 months or 1 year) in relation to the total number of people in the population who are "at risk" at the beginning of the period. Prevalence measures all cases of a condition (new and old) among people at risk for developing the condition. Measures of prevalence are made at one point in time (e.g., on a specific day).

#### Natural History

The natural history of a condition, disorder, or disease describes how it progresses over time. The natural history of some conditions, such as cancer, can be judged based on the stage of the tumor at the diagnosis and response to treatment. Scientists are actively engaged in identifying predictive factors that help tell what the prognosis and outcome might be. In medicine, predictive factors (both negative and positive) are the closest thing we have to a crystal ball.

Even with known predictive factors, the natural history is not always clear; predicting what is going to happen and when it is going to happen can have wide or narrow margins, depending on the condition. For example, individuals with some forms of muscular dystrophy have a more predictive natural history, whereas patterns of change for individuals with cerebral palsy may not be so easy to gauge, especially during the early years of growth and development.

The therapist must develop a plan of care keeping in mind the natural history of the condition and where the individual is in the life span or life stage. Some thought should be given to dovetailing our view of impairments, dysfunctions, and disabilities with the natural history of the disease, condition, or illness. This is particularly important when working with individuals who have long-term, degenerative, or progressive neurologic or chronic conditions.

Improvements in treatment for neurologic and other conditions previously leading to a premature death (e.g., cancer, cystic fibrosis, amyotrophic lateral sclerosis) are now extending the life expectancy for many individuals. Improved interventions bring new areas of focus such as quality-of-life issues. With some conditions (e.g., muscular dystrophy, cerebral palsy, cystic fibrosis, fetal alcohol syndrome), the artificial dichotomy of pediatric versus adult care is gradually being replaced by a lifestyle approach that takes into consideration what is known about the natural history of the condition. Many individuals with childhood-onset diseases now live well into adulthood. For these individuals, the original pathology or disease process has given way to secondary impairments. These secondary impairments create further limitations and issues as the person ages.

### Models of Health Care

Both the traditional medical model and the ICF framework are reflected in this text. Diagnosis and treatment of disease are presented from the medical model, along with assessment based on the ICF of the impact of acute and chronic conditions on the functioning of specific body systems (impairments) and basic human performance (functional limitations).

The ICF was developed to counter the medical model of pathology with its primary emphasis on diagnosis and treatment of disease by placing the focus on the functional consequences of disease. By using the ICF, physical therapists can describe the whole person, the changes that occur in the person's body, the person's ability to perform tasks, the person's social roles, and the environment that forms the context of that person's life. Using this model makes it possible to describe (rather than classify) individuals more accurately according to their functioning.

The reader will see terminology reflecting these two models, such as *etiology, pathogenesis, diagnosis,* and *prognosis* from the traditional medical model and *impairments, interventions, desired outcomes,* and *functional limitations* from the ICF model.

Using these tools and the definition of clinical pathology, we ask the following questions: *How does this particular disease or condition affect this person's functional abilities and functional outcome? What precautions should be taken when someone with this condition is exercising? Should vital signs be monitored during therapy for this disease? How will that information affect the plan of care or intervention?*

### Physical Disabilities

The WHO ICF framework stresses the importance of environment, including physical environment, attitudes of others, or policies enforced as barrier or facilitator in the daily activities of persons with disabilities. The extent to which environment affects the lives of people with disabilities may depend on the person's demographic characteristics (e.g., level of income, level of education, urban versus rural setting) and severity of disability.

Disabilities can be physical, sensory, mental, emotional, or learning. Environmental barriers related to disability can include restricted social activity, not knowing where or how to obtain disability resource information, needing home modifications but having no way to obtain them, having difficulty accessing a health care provider's office because of physical layout or location, and being treated unfairly at a health care provider's office.

There remains a need for environmental improvements to reduce social isolation and facilitate activities of daily living among persons with disabilities. Physical therapists can take an active and proactive role in educating the public and removing barriers. Therapists can help community leaders ensure that public places such as restaurants, stores, and movie theaters comply with the Americans With Disabilities Act.

Within our own clinical practice, we can modify our actions to meet the needs of persons with disabilities. For example, physical therapists should sit down when speaking with a client in a wheelchair and speak directly to the client rather than to the person with the client. If needed, extra time should be scheduled for clients who have trouble undressing or difficulty getting on and off the table.

When talking with someone who is hearing impaired, say the person's name first and get his or her attention before speaking. This can help you avoid repeating everything you say. You may or may not have to speak louder, but clearly enunciate your words when speaking to a person with a hearing loss.

The Americans With Disabilities Act of 1990 was designed to eliminate discrimination against people with disabilities, including discrimination in health care services. Although the Americans With Disabilities Act has improved health care access, barriers still exist for many people in receiving full age-appropriate primary care services. Individuals with disabilities, especially women age 65 and older with disabilities, often do not receive appropriate primary care. The more severe the disability, the less likely a person is to receive adequate care and undergo health screening. The physical therapist can be instrumental in assessing access of the disabled person to important screening and prevention services, advocate for the care of individuals with disabilities, encourage people with disabilities to become their own advocates for health care, and conduct research on people with disabilities.

Each individual client must be evaluated on the basis of the clinical presentation in conjunction with the underlying pathology. For example, a client with osteoporosis may require joint mobilization, but this technique must be modified for the presence of osteoporosis. A client with cardiac valvular disease may need a different exercise program than one prescribed for a healthy athlete. An adult with musculoskeletal symptoms of thoracic spine pain, muscle spasm, and loss of thoracic motion who has a primary medical diagnosis (e.g., posterior penetrating ulcer) will be unaffected by therapy techniques aimed at the human movement system.

### Cognitive Disability

Although physical therapists cannot diagnose cognitive deficits, the therapist's evaluation and clinical observations may help identify cognitive deficits that might interfere with treatment. Appropriate referral is always recommended when problems beyond our expertise are suspected.

There is a new prevalence of executive function impairments as a result of new information regarding the impact of multiple concussions on cognitive performance. Soldiers serving in combat zones or training to serve have a large incidence of blast injuries and concussions. In addition, athletes are being monitored for the effects of single concussion versus multiple concussions. These topics will be discussed in more depth in subsequent chapters related to neurologic pathologies.

Overall, a person with cognitive impairments requires adapted intervention and follow-up strategies. The treatment area may have to be modified to reduce noise, reduce lighting, and reduce the amount of activity so that the person can concentrate and improve. Home programs may need to be in an altered format and not exclusively written. Multisensory formatting such as audio recording, video recording, or many repetitions may need to be implemented to assist the client in succeeding with the home program.

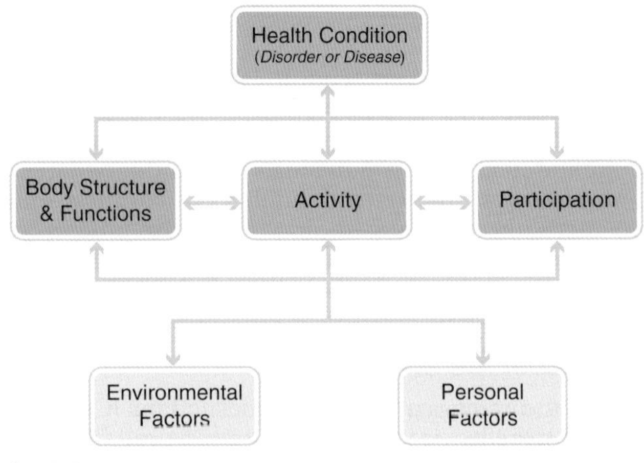


**Fig. 1.1**

**Structure of the International Classification of Functioning, Disability, and Health (ICF).** (From World Health Organization [WHO]. Available online: www.who.int/classifications/icf/en.)

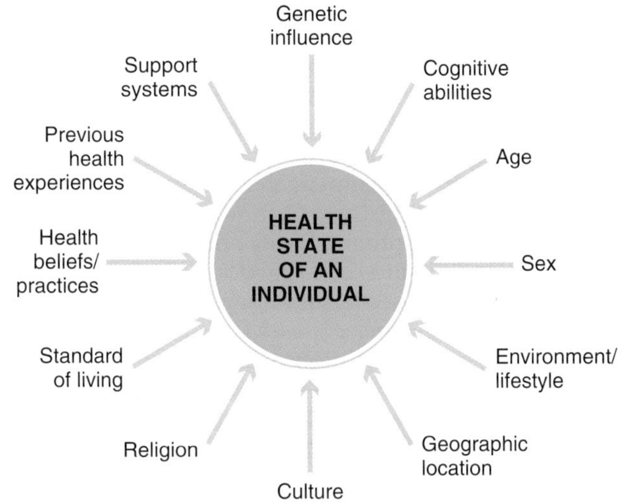


**Fig. 1.2**

**Multiple variables influence the health and illness of an individual.** (From Ignatavicius DD, Workman ML: *Medical-surgical nursing: patient centered collaborative care*, ed 8, Philadelphia, 2015, Saunders.)

## THEORIES OF HEALTH AND ILLNESS

It is no easy task to summarize the many theories developed over time as to the cause of illnesses. In fact, there are volumes of literature providing a historical summary for the interested reader.[88] From the Cartesian model to Louis Pasteur's germ theory to the present-day understanding of microbiomes in the gut and the gut–brain–immune system triad, it is safe to say we are still evolving in our understanding of health and illness. Modern technology has provided a much clearer inspection into the human body that is advancing our knowledge, understanding, and approach to health, illness, and disease.

### Evolving Models of Understanding

With each new discovery into the cause of illness and disease, scientists, researchers, and medical practitioners have adapted in finding unique and specific ways to treat affected individuals. History shows how we moved from model to model to explain the development of diseases (e.g., biomedical model, multicausal theories, homeostasis model, general adaptation theory, psychosocial theory, psychoneuroimmunologic theory, and theory of consciousness-based energy medicine).

With each updated model has come a greater understanding of cause-and-effect relationships, psychosocial components of disease (e.g., age, lifestyle, personality, compliance with treatment), and, as mentioned, epigenetics or the role of the internal and external environment in disrupting biologic and physiologic homeostasis. No one is dismissing the role of many additional factors associated with health and the development of illness (Fig. 1.2), but we are recognizing that these are only part of the overall process.

Injury occurs when the cells or tissues have been required to adapt beyond their limitations. Similar to a muscle that has exceeded its ability to stretch, has ruptured, and is no longer able to contract, cells can be irreparably damaged and unable to return to the original steady state. Illness is the result of an imbalance in the ability of the body (cell) to regulate the internal environment. The concept of "fight, flight, or freeze" to explain the body's reactions to emergencies was added to the homeostasis theory and continues to be used today to explain homeostasis as a dynamic equilibrium designed to maintain a steady state.

This theory suggests that stress causes disease by placing excessive demands on the body, which in turn produces high levels of adaptive hormones. In very simple terms, these hormones influence the inflammatory process and regulation of electrolyte and water metabolism, lowering the body's resistance to disease and contributing to organ damage. When stress is continuous and the hormones of stress remain elevated in the bloodstream for long periods of time, the adaptive capacity of the body may be exceeded, and disease (or even death) may result.

## More Recent Discoveries

The psychoneuroimmunology model, first described in the 1980s, created a major shift in our understanding of the development of human diseases. Psychoneuroimmunology is the study of the interactions among behavior and neural, endocrine, enteric, and immune system functions.

Illness was once thought of as the result of a breakdown within the immune system alone, but immune function is now recognized as the integrative defense mechanism of multiple systems. This theory outlined the influence of the nervous system on immune and inflammatory responses and how the immune system communicates with the neuroendocrine systems. This information remains relevant in understanding host defenses and injury/repair processes.

Further, the integration of the hypothalamic-pituitary-adrenal axis and the neuro-endocrine-enteric axis has a biologic basis first discovered in the late 1990s. Physiologically adaptive processes occur as a result of these biochemically based mind–body connections. Each thought and emotion is a message to the rest of the body, mediated by an intricate array of nerve signals, hormones, and various other bioactive substances driving the responses of these interactions.

Chemical messengers (e.g., peptides, neuropeptides, ligands, neurotransmitters) move through the bloodstream to every cell of the body. When these chemicals find body cells with receptors that attract them like magnets, they attach and make significant changes in that cell's (and all future daughter cells') DNA. These information molecules are the messengers the body uses to communicate between all the major body systems. For example, the digestive (enteric) system is now also considered a part of the neurologic system along with the brain, spinal cord, and peripheral nerves. These systems have the ability to communicate with the immune system via these peptides and can exchange information and influence one another's actions.

At the beginning of the 21st century, hundreds of mitochondrial DNA diseases were reported as a result of research led by Douglas Wallace, PhD, director of the Center for Mitochondrial and Epigenomic Medicine at Children's Hospital of Philadelphia Research Institute. Dr. Wallace has been at the forefront of study centered on mitochondrial DNA.

It is hypothesized that mitochondrial DNA genetic disorders starve the body's cells of energy, resulting in a wide range of conditions from autism to neurodegenerative diseases, autoimmune conditions, cancer, and other inflammatory-based conditions. As more and more mitochondrial DNA mutations occur over time, human capacity for repair, restoration, and homeostasis is eroded. This phenomenon may be the cause of reduced energy with aging and even aging itself. The results of this new information are contributing to how disease is viewed at the energetic level (rather than strictly at the biochemical level) and highlights the way energy will be investigated and used in developing prevention and treatment of diseases in the future.[36]

### Quantum Model of Health and Disease

Our current understanding is being revolutionized by the knowledge of how the principles of quantum physics influence function of the whole person. The Quantum Model of Health[34] and Disease directs us to see the human form as a dynamic and ever-changing energy field that creates, influences, and potentially enhances our health status.[74]

The quantum concept suggests that all cells at the smallest nanoparticle are in constant communication with all other energetic units. The effect of energy (electrical, vibrational, chemical, magnetic, thermal) moving through our bodies, cells, viscera, and systems creates change that can lower vibrational frequencies, contributing to cellular disharmony ultimately leading to "dis-ease" of the cells. Alternatively, this model suggests that energy at higher levels of coherence and synchronicity among all the cells, organs, and systems can improve a person's health. In fact, emerging evidence suggests this state can be created through thought alone.[32,33,35]

Neuroscientists and medical doctors have been informing the medical community of the importance of starting with this view of health, healing, and wholeness.[2,3] This approach has the potential to direct efforts in health care to find ways to enhance health with the goal of prevention of pathologic processes that result in illness and disease. Many believe that adopting a consciousness-based, energetic approach to pathology will change the face of health care, directing treatment in new ways in the coming years.[76]

### Consciousness-Based Health Care

Consciousness may be defined in a variety of ways, but in the simplest terms, it is the way that people perceive and shape their reality or, in other words, their sense of awareness or being. In the quantum model of reality, everything is interconnected. Experiencing that phenomenon in the human body reveals information and energy that is not limited by space and time. This model of health care allows for the inner wisdom of both patients and health care providers to be combined with scientific and technologic advances for the promotion of health and well-being.[25]

Some of the most influential figures in this area of research around consciousness and physical health and well-being include Christof Koch, at Allen Institute for Brain Science, Seattle, Washington; Giulio Tononi, at University of Wisconsin; Edgar Mitchell, former astronaut who co-founded the Institute of Noetic Sciences in 1971, Doc Lew Childre, Jr, founder of the Institute of HeartMath; and David Chalmers, professor at New York University. These scientists among many others worldwide are investigating what causes consciousness. Two theories of consciousness have been introduced: the *global workspace theory*[7] and the *integrated information theory*.[107] In particular, the search is for the neural correlates of consciousness; in other words, where and how does this sense of being we call consciousness originate (e.g., area of the brain, frequency of brain waves, switching mechanisms)?

Other well-known individuals (e.g., Bruce Lipton, Joe Dispenza, James Oschman) with extensive training and research in neuroscience have attempted to bring together evidence to provide an explanation for the consciousness-based energetic exchanges that take place in all therapies. Studies in biophysics have shown that fluctuations in the quantum properties of the body can affect regulatory control mechanisms. Altering these energetic fields to create cellular coherence (e.g., through mindfulness and meditation) has shown promising results.[32] This consciousness-based approach has at its core an understanding that consciousness (in the form of beliefs, feelings, emotions, expectations, and intention) plays a central role in maintaining and restoring health and well-being when it has been compromised.

## HEALTH PROMOTION AND DISEASE PREVENTION

Noncommunicable diseases, also called lifestyle or chronic diseases, are the major cause of morbidity and mortality in the United States and in most countries around the world. Noncommunicable diseases such as heart disease, stroke, cancer, diabetes, and lung disease negatively affect millions of people worldwide and cost billions of dollars annually in treatment and loss of productivity. Because these diseases are strongly associated with risk factors or behaviors such as physical inactivity, unhealthy diet, and tobacco use, they are largely preventable.

The medical system in the United States, however, continues to be oriented toward treating illness and disease, rather than prevention or wellness, and the incidence and prevalence of lifestyle diseases continue to grow. As a result, the WHO and the Centers for Disease Control and Prevention have labeled lifestyle diseases both epidemic and pandemic and have identified the need for the development of new solutions to address this growing problem.[49]

Physical therapists are in an ideal position to promote health and wellness. Physical therapists can reduce risk factors and prevent and treat noncommunicable diseases by providing patient and client education; prescribing physical activity and exercise; and performing noninvasive, hands-on interventions consistent with a biopsychosocial paradigm.[11]

### Health Promotion

Health promotion as a concept and as an active process is built on the principles of self-responsibility, nutritional awareness, stress reduction and management (including retraining the brain's wiring and firing), and physical activity and exercise. Health promotion is not limited to any particular age or level of ability but rather extends throughout the life span from before birth (e.g., prenatal care) through old age, including anyone with a disability of any kind.

Health promotion programs that encompass the entire life span are applicable to people of both genders and all socioeconomic and cultural backgrounds, to people who have no health problems, and to people with chronic illnesses and disabilities. Many types of health promotion programs exist including health screening, wellness, safety, stress management, and support groups for specific diseases.

### Disease Prevention

Preventing disease is more cost-effective than treating disease. Many new areas of study have developed as a result of this paradigm shift in focus from treatment to prevention. Scientists are revolutionizing the way we reduce inflammation and its effects, fight infection, manage chronic illness, and stay well. Physical therapists should be the practitioners of choice in this arena.

Preventive medicine as a branch of medicine is categorized as *primary, secondary,* or *tertiary.* Primary prevention is geared toward removing or reducing disease risk factors,[66] for example, through good nutrition, through maintaining adequate levels of calcium intake and regular exercise as a means of preventing osteoporosis and subsequent bone fractures, or by giving up (or not starting) tobacco use to reduce multiple causes of morbidity. Use of seat belts, use of helmets by motorcyclists and bicyclists, and immunizations are other examples of primary prevention strategies.

Secondary prevention techniques are designed to promote early detection of disease and to employ preventive measures to avoid further complications. Examples of secondary prevention include skin tests for tuberculosis and screening procedures such as mammography, colonoscopy, or routine cervical Pap smear.

Tertiary prevention measures are aimed at limiting the impact of established disease (e.g., radiation or chemotherapy to control localized cancer). Tertiary prevention involves rehabilitation. The goal of tertiary prevention is to return the person to the highest possible level of functioning and to prevent severe disabilities. Most adults with disabilities can participate in physical activity. Almost half of the 21 million adults with disabilities in the United States are sedentary and susceptible to chronic diseases that develop as a result of inactivity.[18]

SPECIAL IMPLICATIONS FOR THE THERAPIST 1.2

#### *Health Promotion and Disease Prevention*

The APTA Council on Prevention, Health Promotion, and Wellness in Physical Therapy was established in January 2018. The council is a community for physical therapists, physical therapist assistants, and students who are interested in incorporating prevention, health promotion, and wellness as an integral aspect of physical therapist practice, promoting and advocating for healthy lifestyles to reduce the burden of disease and disability on individuals and society. In collaboration with interprofessional teams, the goal is to contribute to improved health outcomes by focusing on the values of individuals and populations.

Physical and occupational therapists are being consulted earlier in the course of medical care to help prevent secondary complications of immobility. For example, in the acute care setting, decreasing mortality from critical illness has led to an increasing number of patients being discharged from the intensive care unit. These survivors of severe critical illness commonly have significant and prolonged neuromuscular complications that impair their physical function and quality of life after hospital discharge. The strong evidence that links functional abilities in the immediate post-hospitalization period to readmission risk outlines the role physical therapists play within care transition models. Physical therapists are uniquely qualified to assess physical function, which represents a strong independent risk factor for hospital readmission.

### The Therapist's Role in Primary, Secondary, and Tertiary Care

Prevention is not confined to a single form of presentation but rather takes one of three forms: primary, secondary, or tertiary. All individuals are included—even those who already have one or more primary disabilities.[41]

*Primary prevention* involves preventing disease in a susceptible or potentially susceptible population through general health promotion. Physical therapists are often called on to treat individuals with one or more chronic medical conditions, which are inherent causes of impairments, dysfunctions, and disabilities and increase the risk of other pathologic conditions. For example, diabetes is a cause of considerable dysfunction and disability as well as a risk factor for cardiopulmonary disease. Risk factor assessment should be part of the initial evaluation to determine appropriate intervention strategies focused on reducing or preventing the chance of progression to cardiopulmonary disease.[31]

Physical and occupational therapists are involved in primary prevention and wellness activities, screening programs, and the promotion of positive health behavior. These initiatives decrease costs by helping clients achieve and restore optimal functional capacity; minimize impairments, functional limitations, and disabilities related to congenital and acquired conditions; maintain health and thereby prevent further deterioration or future illness; and create appropriate environmental adaptations to enhance independent function.

Physical and occupational therapists also play major roles in *secondary* and *tertiary care.* Clients with musculoskeletal, neuromuscular, cardiopulmonary, or integumentary conditions are often treated initially by another health care practitioner and then referred to the therapist for secondary care. Therapists provide secondary care in a wide range of settings from hospitals to preschools.

*Tertiary care* is provided by therapists in highly specialized, complex, and technologically based settings (e.g., transplant services, burn units, emergency departments) or when supplying specialized services (e.g., to clients with spinal cord lesions or closed-head trauma) in response to requests for consultation made by other health care practitioners.

### Prescriptive Exercise in Health Promotion and Disease Prevention

The beneficial role of prescriptive exercise for health and disease has been documented many times and in many ways. When prescribed appropriately, exercise, including cardiovascular, endurance, and strength training, is effective for developing fitness and health, for increasing life expectancy, for prevention of injury and disease, and for rehabilitation of impairments and disabilities (see Appendix A and Box A.2).

Prescriptive exercise programs to develop and maintain a significant amount of muscle mass, endurance, and strength contribute to overall fitness and health. Exercise plays a significant role in reducing risk factors associated with disease states (e.g., osteoporosis, diabetes mellitus, heart disease), the risk of falls and associated injuries, and the morbidity associated with chronic disease.[91]

Physical therapist education reflects the need for skills to promote prevention to be included as a part of the standard curriculum. The study and understanding of basic mechanisms of disease physiology and pathokinesiology along with an understanding of the role of epigenetics (e.g., identification of lifestyle or risk factors) in health and disease are necessary for clinical practice. Many variables affect the relationships among pathology, impairments, and disability. Attention must be paid to the psychosocial, spiritual, educational, and environmental variables that can modify client outcomes.

## GENETIC ASPECTS OF HEALTH AND DISEASE

In 1953 Watson and Crick proposed the double helix structure of DNA.[112] The DNA molecule consists of a sugar-phosphate backbone, with 4 bases (adenine [A], thymine [T], guanine [G], cytosine [C]) attached to the sugar. The bases are paired with each other through hydrogen bonds such that A is paired with T and G is paired with C. The DNA molecule carries genetic instructions for all forms of life[81] with the sequence of the bases providing three-letter codons[82] for assembling amino acids and proteins. Genes are arranged on chromosomes and are the units of inheritance. Genes contain the information required to specify the traits (characteristics) of an individual.[83] Genes encode proteins,[80] such as enzymes, which are involved in cellular functions. The genome[84] consists of all of the DNA on the 23 chromosomes in the nucleus as well as the DNA on the circular chromosomes of the mitochondria. The entire genome consists of approximately 3.1 billion bases. A *genotype*[85] refers to the two alleles an individual carries at a specific location in a gene, whereas *phenotype*[86] refers to observable traits of the individual (e.g., height, presence or absence of disease).

### Genomic Variation

Humans exhibit a large amount of similarity in DNA sequences; differences in the DNA sequences between any two human genomes are estimated as less than 0.1% overall.[104] Sequence differences among individuals may be associated with health and disease. Locations in the genome where humans differ in their sequence are variations; different versions of these sequences are alleles.[42] Variation in the genome can be considered under three major categories: changes in single base pairs, insertions and deletions of a small or a large number of base pairs, and structural rearrangements on a chromosome.[21] These changes may have no effect on the health of the individual or may have significant health consequences.[21]

A *polymorphism* is a common variant that occurs at a frequency of greater than 1%.[21,52] Single nucleotide polymorphisms (SNPs) are single base variations commonly found in the human genome. SNPs as well as other longer DNA sequence variants may be associated with increased risk for common diseases. Conversely, some DNA variants may confer no added risk for disease.

*Mutations* are DNA sequence changes that are associated with pathology,[21] such as is found in Huntington disease (HD).[103] The mutation causing HD is an expanded CAG repeat sequence in the *IT15* gene (also known as *HTT* gene) on chromosome 4.[106] HD is a monogenic (single-gene) neurodegenerative disease with an autosomal dominant pattern of inheritance.[50] In contrast, many common complex conditions such as hypertriglyceridemia, which is associated with elevated risk for cardiovascular disease, are due to the interaction of multiple susceptibility genes and environmental factors.[73] A recent study showed that hypertriglyceridemia is primarily a polygenic disorder, with accumulation of common variants a predominant feature and a substantial number of individuals also carrying rare variants.[37]

In considering variation in the human genome, researchers have used genome-wide association studies (GWASs) in the search for genetic variants associated with many diseases such as coronary artery disease,[39] rheumatoid arthritis,[116] diabetes,[99] and stroke.[102] GWASs have provided valuable insights into the role of various proteins and biologic pathways involved in pathology.[21] Uncovering genetic variants associated with disease phenotypes elucidates cellular pathways involved in disease and may point to new treatment approaches.[70]

## Large-Scale Genomics Initiatives

The Human Genome Project (HGP) began in 1990 as a component of an international Human Genome Initiative to map and sequence the entire human genome, along with model organisms such as the mouse. The overarching goal of the initiative was to advance understanding of human genetics and the role of genes in health and disease. Five-year goals for the HGP were initially laid out in 1990 by the Human Genome Programs of the National Institutes of Health and the Department of Energy.[108]

Goals were outlined for specific activities to be achieved in the first 5 years in each of the following areas: (1) mapping and sequencing the human genome and genomes of model organisms such as the mouse; (2) development of informatics systems including software, algorithms, and analytic tools to support collection, storage, distribution, analysis, and interpretation of genomic information generated; (3) development of an understanding of the ethical, legal, and social implications of genomic information that would be generated from the HGP; (4) creating training programs for scientists from a diverse array of backgrounds including genetics, biology, chemistry, physics, engineering, and computer science to enable trained individuals to maximize the use of genomic products and data emanating from the HGP; (5) development and improvement of technology to support the needs of the HGP; (6) technology transfer and collaboration with industry to enhance medically useful applications. The goals were to be reviewed annually and updated with advances in technology.

Owing to advances in technology, in 1993 an even more ambitious approach was undertaken, and new but related goals were refined and extended through September 1998.[21] These goals included development of new technologies for rapid genotyping for medical research purposes, development of technology for high-throughput sequencing, development of efficient methods in identifying genes and incorporating them onto the maps being produced, enhanced emphasis on bioinformatics technologies, and emphasis on sequencing of mouse DNA and corresponding human DNA for regions of high biologic interest.

In 1998 new 5-year goals were presented, with the primary goal of completing the sequence of the human genome by 2003.[23] Goals included making the sequence publicly and freely available to all to maximize its use for the public good to improve human health. Attention also focused on developing technologies for identifying DNA sequence variation in the genome, particularly single base pair variations known as SNPs. In 2001 the International Human Genome Sequence Consortium reported a draft sequence covering the majority of the human genome including initial analyses.[62] At that time, it was thought there were about 30,000 to 40,000 protein-coding genes; we now know this number to be an overestimate. In 2003 the HGP was completed, a time in the history of our species referred to as the dawn of the genomic era.[22] In 2004 the International Human Genome Sequence Consortium published an accurate version of the vast majority of the entire human genome, reporting that our genome contains about 20,000 to 25,000 protein-coding genes.[61]

The completion of the human sequence laid the foundation for genomics as a central discipline of biomedical research.[62] New knowledge generated by the HGP laid the foundation for an enhanced understanding of the biology of disease. The fruits of the HGP provide us for the first time ever with a reference sequence of the nucleotides comprising the entire human genome. This has facilitated uncovering protein-coding regions of the genome as well as functionally important regions of noncoding DNA. It was recognized early on, even before completion of the HGP, that availability of the human sequence would bring opportunities to study genetic variation in our species by creating SNP maps.[100] The International Haplotype Map (HapMap) Projects provided scientists with a map of common variation in the genome in the form of SNPs,[58-60] while the 1000 Genomes Project uncovered a broad spectrum of human genetic variants including SNPs, insertions/deletions, and structural variants.[105] These large-scale genomics initiatives facilitate the study of genetic variation in relation to disease phenotypes, with GWASs uncovering many genetic variants associated with common diseases.

SPECIAL IMPLICATIONS FOR THE THERAPIST 1.3

## *Genomics for Rehabilitation Clinicians*

Advances in the medical and biologic sciences over the past 30 years have given health care clinicians including physical, occupational, and speech therapists unprecedented opportunities for management of many conditions. There is an increasing body of evidence that genetic factors are associated with disease risk, severity and progression of disease, and variation in response to exercise and rehabilitation programs.

### Genetic Factors in Disease Risk

Genetic factors are associated with risk for conditions and diseases encountered by rehabilitation clinicians. Family history studies indicate substantial familial risk for many conditions. Risk for incident stroke is increased threefold in offspring of individuals with stroke.[98] In a study of hypertensive individuals in a multiethnic population, a positive family history of cardiovascular disease was associated with risk for nonstroke cardiovascular disease as well as risk for stroke.[110] Individuals with Alzheimer disease or Parkinson disease had greater likelihood of a family history of Alzheimer disease or Parkinson disease, respectively, compared with control individuals.[94] There is an elevated risk of osteoarthritis in the same joint in siblings of individuals who underwent hip and knee replacement.[71,87] Numerous family history studies highlight familial aggregation of risk for disease, suggesting a genetic contribution to many common diseases.

Disease heritability studies point to a genetic contribution to risk for many diseases. Heritability is defined as the proportion of variation in the phenotype attributable to variation in genetic factors among individuals.[9,53] Heritability is typically computed by comparing trait occurrence in monozygotic and dizygotic twins, with trait variance being apportioned into genetic and environmental components.[101] Heritability can range from 0% (absence of a genetic influence) to 100% (completely influenced by genetic factors).

Heritability of Parkinson disease or parkinsonism was estimated as 40% based on longitudinal data from the Swedish Twin Registry.[114] Although twin studies are commonly used to estimate heritability, newer methodologies have emerged such as use of genetic variants from whole-genome datasets to estimate heritability.[13] Analysis of whole-genome array data estimated heritability for young-onset stroke (<55 years of age) as 42% and old-onset stroke (≥55 years of age) as 34%.[45] Heritability of osteoarthritis of the hip leading to hip replacement was 47% in a study of Danish twins,[100] while heritability of kyphosis based on Cobb angle was estimated to be 54% in the second- and third-generation offspring of the original Framingham Study cohort.[118]

Genetic variants are associated with risk for neurologic diseases including stroke, Alzheimer disease, Huntington disease, and Parkinson disease.[50] A population-based study of more than 306,000 participants showed that risk of incident stroke was 35% higher in individuals in the top third of polygenic risk scores (defined by 90 SNPs known to be associated with stroke) compared with participants in the lowest third.[97] Unfavorable lifestyle (defined as zero healthy lifestyle factors or one healthy lifestyle factor) was associated with elevated risk of incident stroke compared with a more favorable lifestyle (defined as three or four healthy lifestyle factors) independent of genetic risk (high risk, intermediate risk, low risk). These results suggest that even in individuals with a high genetic risk for stroke, lifestyle interventions and modifications may reduce risk of stroke.[67]

Similarly, genetic variants are associated with musculoskeletal conditions. A meta-analysis of GWASs ($N$ = 15,934) identified nine SNPs at eight genetic loci to be associated with hip joint shape, a risk factor for hip osteoarthritis and fracture,[8] whereas a case-control study identified associations between SNPs in the *COL11A1* and *ADAMTS5* genes (both expressed in the intervertebral disc) and lumbar disc degeneration in Chinese Han.[65] Genetic factors have also been associated with risk for rheumatoid arthritis in African American individuals.[72] Risk for many other conditions such as coronary artery disease, diabetes,[110,117] kidney disease,[57] and obesity[44] is associated with genetic variants.

### Genetic Factors in Severity and Progression of Disease

Genetic factors play a role in severity and progression of many diseases. A study of interleukin-1 gene polymorphisms and low back pain indicated that intensity of pain was associated with carriage of two specific interleukin-1 alleles in 131 middle-aged men from three diverse occupational groups (machine drivers, carpenters, and office workers).[101] Progression of knee osteoarthritis over 10 years (assessed as changes in Kellgren-Lawrence score, osteophyte grade, and joint space narrowing) has been associated with SNPs in four genes,[109] whereas in patients with low back pain, single nucleotide variants of genes in the aggrecan pathway are associated with severity of lumbar disc herniation.[92] Individuals with impaired glucose tolerance with the TT genotype of a polymorphism in the *TCF7L2* gene were more likely to progress from impaired glucose tolerance to diabetes than participants with the CC genotype.[45] In individuals with Huntington disease, longer CAG repeat length predicts earlier age at admission to a nursing home and earlier age at percutaneous endoscopic gastrostomy placement, suggesting that longer CAG repeat length is associated with a more rapid progression of Huntington disease.[75]

### Genetic Factors and Variation in Response to Exercise and Rehabilitation Programs

Evidence from studies of young and older adults as well as clinical populations indicates that genetic factors are associated with variation in response to programs of exercise and rehabilitation. An investigation of the role of the *ACE* gene on isometric strength of the quadriceps in untrained healthy men (18 to 30 years of age) showed that the response to 9 weeks of quadriceps isometric strength training was genotype-dependent. Participants with the ID and DD genotypes exhibited greater quadriceps strength gains compared with individuals with the II genotype (increases in quadriceps strength: ID, 17.6%; DD, 14.9%; II, 9.0%).[46] After an 18-month exercise program consisting of walking and resistance training three times per week for 1 hour per session in obese older adults, the *ACE* DD genotype group showed marked gains in quadriceps strength, in contrast to the II and ID genotype groups, both of which showed no improvement relative to control groups not engaging in exercise.[48]

The Val66Met *BDNF* polymorphism has been associated with variation in response to exercise and other interventions in healthy individuals as well as in individuals with neurologic disease such as stroke. In young adults, 30 minutes of finger exercise using the first dorsal interosseous was associated with increases in first dorsal interosseous motor map area in Val/Val participants, but not in Val/Met or Met/Met participants. Motor evoked potentials and map volume showed greater percentage increases in Val/Val participants compared with Val/Met or Met/Met participants, suggesting that response to motor training is associated with *BDNF* genotype.[68] These results may have implications for potential for recovery from neurologic disease, raising the possibility that individuals with the Met allele might respond less favorably than individuals with the Val/Val genotype to motor rehabilitation interventions.

In a study of recovery after acute stroke, individuals with the Met allele (individuals with Val/Met genotype or with Met/Met genotype) had higher modified Rankin Scale scores (greater disability) than individuals with the Val/Val genotype 3 months after discharge from a neurorehabilitation unit.[67] In contrast, a study of the relationship between the *BDNF* Val66Met polymorphism and 10 meter walk test in survivors of chronic stroke (6 months after stroke) showed that the *BDNF* Val66Met polymorphism was not associated with, or predictive of, performance on the 10 meter walk test in people in the chronic phase of poststroke recovery.[47] Participants in the Glycine Antagonist in Neuroprotection clinical trials with the ApoE ε4 genetic polymorphism exhibited poor recovery at 30 days after stroke and had a lower proportion of participants classified as minimal/no disability 3 months after stroke.[28]

### Applications for Clinical Practice

In this era of genomic medicine, we are witnessing the implementation and application of precision medicine in which prevention and intervention strategies are tailored to the individual based on analyses of genomic and cellular information as well as information about the individual's environment, activities, behavior, and social networks.[10,24] "Exercise genomics" in the form of personalized rehabilitation programs based on DNA sequence variation has been proposed and recommended.[15] The "science of the individual," as medical care has been described in this genomic era, captures an individual's unique genetic makeup, development, and experiences, all of which influence health and disease.[19] Technologies such as whole-genome sequencing, although currently not routinely used in clinical practice, are likely to be increasingly used to generate genomic information in clinical settings, particularly as sequencing costs decrease and individuals seek knowledge of disease risk and medication therapies based on genotypic information.[90]

Optimizing patient management based on whole-genome sequencing is occurring in clinical settings. A 40-year-old man with a family history of vascular disease and early sudden death underwent clinical assessment for coronary artery disease, screening for causes of sudden death, and genetic counseling.[6] Whole-genome sequencing and an integrated analysis of his complete genome with clinical findings were conducted. Risk analysis focused on variants for mendelian disorders, novel mutations, variants associated with pharmacotherapeutic responses, and SNPs associated with common diseases. The analyses highlighted elevated risk for myocardial infarction, type 2 diabetes, and certain cancers. Importantly, the patient had risk markers at the 9p21 locus, which has been associated with myocardial infarction.[16] He also had a copy of a rare variant of the *LPA* gene, which encodes the apolipoprotein A precursor and is associated with high plasma Lp(a) lipoprotein levels such as were observed in this individual. As the patient's genome included genetic variants predictive of a higher likelihood of a beneficial response to statins (including reduced risk for statin-associated myopathy), the physician recommended a lipid-lowering medication as a preventive option. As genetic information regarding risk for adverse events such as myocardial infarction becomes increasingly incorporated into clinical practice, health and wellness issues related to exercise and behavioral modifications will become increasingly important and relevant to the rehabilitation clinician.

Clinicians must be prepared to support patients on a number of issues related to genomics. Although genetic testing is typically conducted for patients with a family history of a particular disorder and who are considered at risk of carrying genetic variants for a particular condition, with reductions in the costs of whole-genome sequencing there is likely to be an increase in the use of this technology in clinical settings.

Clinicians should be aware of the psychological impact of this expanded form of testing, as whole-genome sequencing may uncover increased risk for serious and life-threatening diseases or conditions. The ethical, legal, and social implications of genomics, such as privacy and confidentiality, discrimination based on genetic factors, disclosure of findings in the context of participation in research studies, disclosure of findings that might affect family members, and concerns regarding direct-to-consumer genetic testing, are important for the clinician to understand and consider.[1,12,54,93] The 2008 Genetic Information Nondiscrimination Act and the 2010 Patient Protection and Affordable Care Act provide protection against discrimination based on genetic information in the workplace and when seeking insurance coverage.[78]

## REFERENCE

To enhance this text and add value for the reader, all references are included in the enhanced ebook on Student Consult that accompanies this textbook. The reader can view the reference source and access it online whenever possible.

# CHAPTER 2

# Epigenetics: Behavioral, Social, and Environmental Factors

CATHERINE CAVALLARO GOODMAN • KENDA S. FULLER • MEGAN M. PRIBYL (NUTRITION) • IRA GORMAN (OBESITY)

## EPIGENETICS: ROLE OF THE PHYSICAL THERAPIST IN THE CURRENT HEALTH CARE ENVIRONMENT

Many behavioral, social, and environmental factors influence health and may either enhance health or mitigate the effects of disease. In the current health care environment, these factors have significant effects on how physical therapists function as rehabilitation specialists. By focusing on improving physical function and performance of daily activities, the physical therapist can help reduce the impact of diseases and their effects on individuals. The role of these environmental factors on health and disease is a major focus of scientific investigation worldwide under a relatively new area of study called *epigenetics*. New information about the influence of epigenetics on health will be the focus of this chapter. The role of physical therapists will be to integrate this understanding and to develop appropriate treatments or interventions that can impact our patients and clients in positive ways.

### What Is Epigenetics?

Epigenetics is the study of how biologic (internal) and environmental (external) signals determine gene expression. Epigenetic signals can prompt changes in the number of methyl chemical groups attached to a gene, turning it on (upregulating) or off (downregulating).

Epigenetics describes heritable mechanisms that are reversible because they occur without any alteration of the underlying DNA sequence.[16] DNA is the blueprint that directs the gene to put together the building blocks that produce the functional molecules called proteins, and proteins are the basis for our human physiologic form and structure. The DNA (blueprint) does not turn itself on or off. Rather, the mind is considered the "master controller" of gene expression. In effect, the DNA is not changed—it is the *expression* of DNA and the subsequent *reading of* the gene that can be changed (altered or manipulated). This change occurs by becoming aware of (and subsequently changing) individual perceptions, beliefs, and attitudes as well as behaviors and lifestyle choices.[68,102,101] To state this in a slightly different way, we are not the victims of our heredity or destined to develop a particular disease or condition. In other words, having a genetic predisposition is not the single predictive factor of a certain outcome.

The term "epigenetics" was first coined by Waddington in the late 1930s.[162] Bruce Lipton, PhD, at the University of Wisconsin School of Medicine and later Stanford University School of Medicine, advanced the field of study in the early 1970s through his embryonic stem cell research, in which he repeatedly demonstrated that the environment in which cells live determines genetic activity.[100,99] Dr. Lipton simultaneously exposed (in vitro) groups of stem cells with identical genetic makeup to different compositions of culture medium. These identical stem cells then created different lines of cells (e.g., fat, muscle, bone). This discovery that cells adjust to their external environment (or change in response to the environment they are contained in) has been studied extensively since that time.[154,170]

This new information shifted the traditional biologic model of health and disease toward what is now referred to as "the new biology." Dr. Lipton's work challenged the accepted idea that we are victims of our heredity and have no more effective treatment for disease and other health conditions than pharmaceuticals and surgery. This was followed by the discovery that the placebo effect accounts for 30% to 60% of all healing responses to medical treatment.[95] Likewise, the nocebo effect (adverse effect of treatment from negative thinking) was shown to be equally powerful as a downward causation of attitudes and beliefs about health.[124,80,165]

Since then, epigenetics has become an entire field of research aimed at explaining changes in gene expression, transgenerational effects (i.e., epigenetic effects are effects that manifest in the first unexposed generation), and inherited expression states.[52] With the development of the Human Genome Project and subsequent discoveries, it became clear that only a small percentage of the world population is born with true genetic conditions (i.e., inherited genetic mutation). These are the conditions that are expressed at birth or shortly thereafter. The remaining

95% of people who develop such conditions acquire them through the influence of social determinants, lifestyle choices, and behaviors and the consequences of those behaviors, which constitute the main areas of study in epigenetics.[149] Only 5% to 10% of cases of cancer occur as the result of an inherited genetic mutation[118] and only when there is sufficient environmental stimuli to signal the expression of that genetic aberration. In other words, there is a clearer understanding now that cancer formation is determined by the environment in which those cells live and are expressed.[100]

Epigenetics directs us to look at ourselves within our environment and recognize how our internal and external environments impact and influence our health. By changing behaviors and mitigating the effects of stress we can potentially change the "readout" of the genes. When we change the learned subconscious routines and patterns of thoughts, feelings, and emotions, we can change the mind and behaviors that create the environment that predicts and determines our health outcome. It has been said then that we are "not doomed by our genes or hardwired to be a certain way or locked into a condition for the rest of our lives."[55]

Our goal in this chapter is to help physical therapists understand their own health as well as the health of their patients and clients in the context of these influences. The role of nutrition, mood, exercise, prolonged stress, resiliency, and coping will be examined in the context of epigenetic factors.[98,164]

## EPIGENETICS: PHYSICAL AND SOCIAL ENVIRONMENTS

There are different ways to divide and describe environmental epigenetic factors. Some of the publications in scientific and social literature divide these factors into internal versus external environment, whereas others focus on the physical environment and the social environment. The physical environment is often divided between the built environment (surroundings that support human activity, such as buildings and parks—spaces where people live, work, and recreate) and the natural (physical) environment (e.g., air, water, soil/rock, sun). The material in this section is a simplified compilation of both approaches that does not adequately cover all factors and variables but will provide an introduction to the topic.

The *internal environment* is the interaction of attitudes, thoughts, emotions, feelings, beliefs, and reactions or responses to events that directly affect our physiologic function. Within the internal environment, neural connections are activated. With repetition of thoughts, emotions, feelings, and events, the brain wires and fires a program that repeats itself over and over subconsciously, driving our actions and reactions. In essence, the way we think changes our physiologic and biologic function.

Automatic negative thoughts[2] are repetitive thoughts, images, and ideas that pop up in the brain automatically and alter the person's mood. Left unchallenged, they take over the person's thoughts and increase the levels of stress hormones circulating through the body, which lowers brain reserve, contributes to weight gain, and puts the affected individual at greater risk for age-related cognitive decline.[1,2]

Prolonged, chronic stress with elevated levels of cortisol and other stress hormones has been targeted as the most common factor in everything from the common cold to depression to heart disease. The stress hormone cortisol plays an important role in regulating multiple systems including the immune system. In the simplest of terms, when stress is ongoing, cells of the immune system become insensitive to cortisol, resulting in unchecked inflammation. Inflammation has been implicated as the major force in the development of many chronic conditions, diseases, and autoimmune disorders. Because of the significance of the stress phenomenon and the role of trauma in health, we have reformulated Chapter 3 of this text to explore the concepts of stress, resiliency, and trauma in our lives and the lives of our patients and clients.

Other physiologic maladaptations occur as a result of chronic, prolonged stress (e.g., joints stiffen, muscles tighten, fascia loses elasticity, nonefficient patterns of movement develop), resulting in further physiologic pathology. At the cellular level, this is reflected as greater disruption of vibrational energy and cellular coherence. The cells can wire and fire together with greater harmony and coherence, thereby promoting efficient physiologic function.[53,54] Or, as occurs more often, repeated unconscious thoughts, feelings, and emotions release corresponding neuropeptides and neurohormones, keeping the body in a constant state of sympathetic overdrive. These "molecules of emotion"[130] interrupt cellular communication signaling genes to upregulate or downregulate. The end result is cellular incoherence or "dis-ease" manifesting as a specific disease process (one that may be inherited but not yet expressed).

Based on this information, new therapies are emerging for many health problems and mental health disorders. For example, specific types of meditation and mindfulness practices[40,111,147,168] are being studied based on creating heart–brain coherence.[53,75,104,107] There is also a transcranial magnetic stimulation modality approved by the U.S. Food and Drug Administration used to treat depression and obsessive-compulsive disorder[34,48] with potential for treatment of other chronic conditions and chronic pain by modifying dysfunctional motor responses. The stimulation is designed to alter brain circuitry and modify repetitive patterns of neural firing. It is expected that this area of study (i.e., epigenetics) will grow rapidly with many changes anticipated in our understanding of the human body–mind connection and ways to approach healing outside the traditional health care or medical model.

**Note to Reader:** There is much controversy, concern, and debate among physical therapists over terms such as "consciousness" or "mindfulness" (sometimes referred to as metacognition).[87] There are some very useful resources for physical therapists to help us understand these terms, gain an appreciation for the current research results in this area, and learn how to employ the techniques in our practice. For further understanding of the concepts of consciousness or mindfulness, please refer to references and resources cited here.[38,111,128,168]

The *external environment* includes variables such as the air we breathe, water we drink, food we eat, and toxins in the environment. A person's social network, community, sense of purpose in life,[176] and spiritual beliefs are also considered significant contributors to a sense of well-being. These variables are believed to be linked to long-term physiologic benefits including overall longevity.[47,44] Alternatively, factors such as prolonged psychologic and emotional stress, feeling out of control, and social isolation may have a greater impact on health and longevity than previously recognized.

Over long periods of time, stimulus from the external environment, when combined with our thoughts and lifestyle choices, can contribute significantly to the body's biochemical responses. When these conditioned responses create dysregulation of the autonomic nervous system (again over time), there can be subsequent expression of inherited genetic traits that might not have otherwise been manifested.

The expanding influence of epigenetics in health care does not negate previously described models of health and health care. The interrelationships between individual-level characteristics and large-scale social forces remain important points to consider.

Various levels of influence that have an impact on health from the individual to the environment are shown in Fig. 2.1. This view greatly broadens the types of interventions that can improve health and helps us understand the role pathologic processes have at the cellular level as they interact with the environment to cause disease, impairment, functional limitations, and disability.

## EPIGENETIC FACTORS THAT INFLUENCE HEALTH

### Overview

According to the World Health Organization, the highest number of deaths are attributed to the risk factors of high blood pressure, tobacco use, high blood glucose, physical inactivity, overweight and obesity, and high cholesterol, in that order.[169] More than half of deaths from the leading causes in the United States (Table 2.1) are associated with behavioral and lifestyle factors such as diet, exercise, smoking, and substance abuse. These factors not only contribute to the number of deaths but also contribute significantly to disability and the burden of disease.

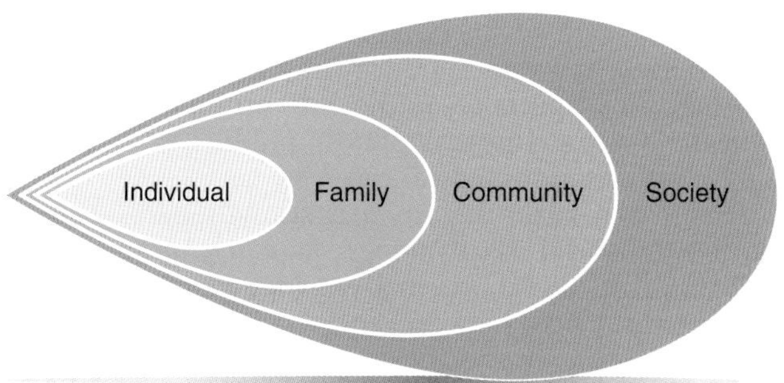


**Fig. 2.1**

**Social structures influencing the individual.** Aside from the pathology itself, many behavioral, social, and environmental factors influence health and may mitigate or enhance the effects of disease. The individual is influenced in various ways by family, community, and society. Each of these nested social structures influences the individual and can shape behavior including the ability to make health decisions, compliance with regimens, or even initial health choices. (Courtesy Ira Gorman, PT, MSPH, Department of Physical Therapy, Regis University, Denver, CO.)

More than any other intervention, changing behavior and lifestyle could help prevent death, enhance quality of life, and reduce the escalating costs of treating chronic illnesses. For example, although heart disease remains the number one cause of death in the U.S. adult population, the cardiac death rate has been reduced by 52% over the last 2 decades as a result of changes in diet and lifestyle.[112]

Many psychologic and behavioral risk factors in lifestyle affecting health status, health outcomes, and health care are considered individually modifiable. This chapter on epigenetics specifically examines selected lifestyle and behavioral factors that affect health and directly influence physical therapy practice. The list of risk factors is extensive and can include personal habits such as rest and sleep; diet and nutrition, including calcium, fat, and fiber intake; tobacco use; alcohol and other drug use; level of activity and exercise (fitness); trauma (domestic violence, adverse childhood experiences), stress, resilience, and coping ability; travel; environmental or occupational status; and high-risk sexual activity.

### Geographic Variations

The concept of "community" as it relates to where individuals live, work, and play geographically and the characteristics of that place has a definite impact on the status of people's health. Although somewhat controversial and highly debated, some of the most stressful U.S. cities and jobs have been identified. It is thought by experts that your zip code may determine your health just as much, if not more, as your family or personal health history.[69,89] Some published lists base their findings on cost of living, crime index, education, divorce, population density, unemployment, and average commuting time. Likewise, suggestions have been made regarding the least stressful locations and occupations.[10,30,43,88] Other factors such as urban pockets of minority groups (usually associated with increased levels of poverty), access to fresh fruits and vegetables (or lack thereof), and even local smoking ordinances also contribute to the geographic variations people experience that can impact their health.[127]

The geographic and political climates of countries also play a role in determining how people live and the health problems that commonly develop. A half-century ago, a few physicians cultivated an interest in diseases that seemed to have strict geographic boundaries. As a result, a discipline called *geographic pathology* developed. Geographic pathology was concerned with diseases endemic (present in a community at all times) to certain areas of the world, most often parasitic and infectious diseases that seemed unique to individual geographic regions. A component called *occupational disease* was added with the discovery that chemical agents are mediators of a variety of tissue changes and the recognition that many of these causative agents are environmental contaminants.

Table 2.1 Leading Causes of Death in the United States[a]

| Causes of Death in 1900 | Causes of Death in 2017 | Associated Lifestyle/Behaviors/Modifiable Risk Factors for Causes of Death in 2017 |
|---|---|---|
| Pneumonia, influenza | Heart disease | Tobacco use, poor diet, physical inactivity[5] |
| Tuberculosis | Cancer | Smoking, alcohol use, poor diet[3] |
| Heart disease | Unintentional injuries (accidents) | Motor vehicles |
| Diarrhea, enteritis | Chronic lower respiratory disease | Toxic agents (e.g., environmental pollutants) |
| Stroke | Stroke | Alcohol consumption, tobacco use, poor diet,[42] illegal drug use |
| | Alzheimer disease | Smoking, physical inactivity, depression, midlife hypertension, obesity[17] |
| | Diabetes | Obesity, physical activity, high blood pressure, abnormal cholesterol levels[4] |
| | Influenza and pneumonia | Microbial agents (e.g., influenza) |

[a]Listed in descending order of incidence; 10 leading causes of death accounted for 74% of all deaths in the United States. Causes may vary when evaluated by age (e.g., unintentional injuries and suicide account for more deaths in younger individuals, whereas chronic conditions are attributed more to deaths in older adults).

Data from National Center for Health Statistics. Death in the United States, 2017. Available at: http://www.cdc.gov/nchs/data/databriefs/db99.htm.

Disease caused by contaminants was included to constitute the field of *environmental pathology*. For further discussion, see Chapter 4.

One other issue related to geographic variations is the fact that treatment for a single medical condition can vary significantly from one geographic location to another. Rates and types of surgical procedures differ from one geographic location to another, depending on the prevailing health care system, physician and hospital preferences (notably not client preferences or needs), and where the physician was trained.[28,27,61,106,123]

## Socioeconomic Status

The most adverse influence on health is socioeconomic status, with a higher percentage of people in the low socioeconomic status group experiencing health-related problems than any other group. The percentage of people in the lowest income bracket reporting limitation in activity caused by chronic disease is three times that of people in the highest income bracket.[160] Lack of health insurance coverage and/or access to quality health care may result in delayed or postponed diagnosis and treatment of health problems.

Differences in attitudes toward health have been found to be greater between social classes than between races or ethnic groups. Ninety percent of all health care dollars is spent on extraordinary care in the last 2 to 3 years of life. This style of death-based medicine assigns the greatest financial and professional resources to treating the diseases of aging.[66]

People who are homeless or unsheltered have become one of the fastest-growing populations in need of health care in the United States. Traditionally, the homeless group consisted primarily of older, single men, often alcoholics, but now this group includes families and children who are runaways or adolescent throwaways. Declining public assistance, a shortage of affordable rental housing, and an increase in poverty are contributing factors to the rise in homelessness. Although estimates of homeless people vary, the National Coalition for the Homeless[119] reports that on any given night, 700,000 Americans are homeless, and up to 2 million homeless people are reported in a year's time. This number includes an estimated 100,000 children in the United States who are homeless; more than half are under age 5.

## Epigenetics: Health Disparities and Inequities

Health disparities have been defined as differences in individual or regional community health owing to lack of access, high cost, or other factors that create barriers to health services.[156] Although over the last 100 years health care has dramatically improved the life span and the quality of life for many people through advances in public health, medical discoveries, and technology, not every segment of the population has benefited equally from health care advances. Research indicates that health care in itself has accounted for only 7 of the 35 years of increased life expectancy in the 20th century. Most of the increase is due to improvement in public health and living conditions, not medical care.[109]

Health across the life span is strongly and adversely affected by social disadvantage. Research in epigenetics indicates that alterations in DNA methylation may provide a causal link between social adversity and health disparity.[121] Known social determinants of health such as air and water quality, access to green space or parks and recreational activities, and networks of family and community are just a few that are being reevaluated given the context of epigenetics. Other social factors such as socioeconomic status, access to health care, language differences, place of birth, residential segregation, and access to nutrition are being studied as potential epigenetic variables that help explain the disparities in health that result in higher morbidity and mortality rates among various groups of Americans.

## Epigenetics and Social Support

Social support and social networks as internal factors directly affect an individual's health status. *Social network* refers to the web of social relationships that link us together.[74,161] Health across the life span is strongly and adversely affected by social disadvantage.[32,166] Alterations in DNA methylation may provide a causal link between social adversity and health disparity. Likewise, accelerated loss of telomeres (the protective ends of chromosomes) is highly correlated with chronic stress, including social stress and aging, and may provide a link between adversity and some of the health problems associated with health disparities.[96,121]

The strength of weak ties (acquaintances) between people is as important as the strength of strong ties (close friends).[70] Social support and social networks are connected to physical and mental health including all-cause mortality,[25] cardiovascular disease,[90,125] stroke,[23,81] infectious disease[116] including the common cold, and HIV/AIDS.[92]

Berkman and Glass[24] describe the impact on health by social networks as being along a continuum of factors (e.g., cultural, socioeconomic, political, religious, geographic, psychologic). More specifically, poverty, discrimination, and conflict are social structural conditions that can exert a negative influence on health, whereas factors such as access to resources and material goods, close family ties, and help-seeking behaviors provide positive social support. The concept of epigenetics suggests that reducing social inequities and lack of support that keep people from experiencing optimal health and well-being may have a beneficial impact at the level of the genome.

## Environmental Barriers to Health Care

Although there are environmental exposures that lead to disease, the specific nature of the physical environment has an impact on health and disease outcomes. The environmental influences on eating, physical activity, and subsequent obesity have been reviewed in detail. These obesogenic environments strongly influence the behaviors of individuals and lead to an epigenetic effect.[91,97,132]

Eating behavior is affected by food supply trends, nutritional content of foods, larger portion sizes, availability of fast food items, and eating away from home regularly. Individuals are subjected to television advertising and media campaigns and are affected by pricing. Grocery store chains in high-income markets offer fewer energy-dense foods than stores in low-income markets, which further affects the income disparity in obesity.[97] Present trends in the reduction of physical activity because of increased screen time, increased automobile use, change in types of occupational activities, increase in availability of labor-saving devices, and reduced accessibility to parks and recreational space have caused the obesity epidemic to spread in all populations and demonstrate the need to intervene at the environmental level.

Simple environmental interventions such as placing music and artwork in stairwells have led to a 39% increase in stair use.[97] Architectural changes such as designing buildings with stairwells that are easier to access than elevators can make differences that would surpass the 100 kcal/day recommendation for daily activity.[77]

Pilot projects at some universities have been instigated to increase walking on campus. Signs and campus-wide competition encouraging increased walking as well as structural environmental changes such as changing the locations of various parking lots are strategies employed in this effort. The Community Preventive Services Task Force recommends built environment strategies that combine one or more interventions to improve pedestrian or bicycle transportation systems with one or more land use and environmental design interventions to increase physical activity.[46]

## Cultural Influences

Variations in lifestyle influencing clients' perceptions of health care may occur as a result of cultural, religious, socioeconomic, or even age factors. Although clinical manifestations of a disease or condition are essentially the same across cultures, how a person (or family member) responds or interprets the experience can vary. Epigenetics has opened focus on how cultural influences and the environment in which family members are raised may contribute to how genetic traits are stimulated to express the disease or condition carried by the gene.[172,173]

This phenomenon of response based on cultural influence is called *cultural relativity*—that is, behavior must be judged first in relation to the context of the culture in which it occurs. For example, some groups consider health as a function of luck (good or bad), whereas others see health problems as a punishment for bad behavior and good health as a reward for good behavior.

Cultural factors may also prevent illness. For example, people belonging to religious faiths that forbid drinking or smoking have lower cancer rates than the general population. Kosher laws protected Jews in the Middle Ages from pork-related diseases. Religious beliefs related to health must be recognized and respected. Research on the effects of religiosity as a predictor of outcome in a variety of disorders is beginning to draw definitive conclusions about the efficacy of prayer, religious practices and activities, and philosophic orientation toward health.[12,86,152] Research suggests that one of the principal reasons people are attracted to alternative medicine is that they find many of these therapies in keeping with their personal, cultural, or religious beliefs.[13]

### Beyond Cultural Competence: Transnational Competence

Cultural diversity, sensitivity, understanding, and acknowledgment and cultural competence have become familiar topics in the physical therapist's education. Likewise, some consideration of these topics has become a part of all U.S. medical schools. Given rapidly changing global demographics, changing patterns of immigration, and the associated health disparities, social science has moved beyond cultural competence to embrace *transnational competence*. Transnational competence teaches the health care professional how to address issues of physical and mental health along with experiences related to geographic dislocation and adaptation to unfamiliar settings.[84]

It is not enough to consider lists of ethnocultural characteristics and single-factor explanations such as health belief systems. Relevant links between health and post-migration stressors may include employment status and experiences, discrimination, insecurity of immigration status, or family fragmentation.[85] Transnational competence requires a multidimensional approach that takes into account the current era of globalization and migration and their impact on health beliefs, disparities, and diversity within ethnic groups.

### Adverse Childhood Experiences

There is a clear relationship between exposure to abuse or household dysfunction during childhood and multiple risk factors for several of the leading causes of death in adults.[9,56,60] Adverse experiences in childhood are linked to the development of problems later in life including alcohol and other drug use, drug and/or tobacco addiction, obesity, fibromyalgia, or other autoimmune disorders. Children who have been exposed to four or more adverse experiences in childhood are more likely to have attempted suicide and to have had multiple sex partners, increasing their risk of sexually transmitted diseases.

The increasing number of people diagnosed with the conditions *posttraumatic stress syndrome* (PTSD) and *complex PTSD* has come under scrutiny for underlying epigenetic factors.[150] It is estimated that 50% to 60% of the U.S. adult population will be exposed to at least one traumatic event in their lifetime, whereas the lifetime prevalence of PTSD is comparatively low, ranging from 7% to 30% depending on population and trauma type.[83] This difference suggests there are likely individual differences in response to trauma. Although there is some thought that PTSD "runs in families," these parent–offspring connections are complicated by shared genetic and environmental risk[150] and remain under investigation.

The somatic effects of these conditions among all age groups brings this topic into sharp focus for the physical therapist. An expanded discussion of the impact of adverse and traumatic experiences is provided in Chapter 3).

## Epigenetics: Variations in Client Populations

The observed epigenetic differences between people and populations can be caused by genetic or environmental variation or a combination of both. As presented in this chapter, DNA methylation is an epigenetic modification, influenced by both genetic and environmental variation, that plays a key role in transcriptional regulation. Although patterns of DNA methylation have been shown to differ between human populations, it remains to be determined how epigenetic diversity relates to the patterns of genetic and gene expression variation on a global scale. DNA methylation has been measured, analyzed, and compared in diverse human populations to provide a deeper understanding of worldwide patterns of human epigenetic diversity as well as initial estimates of the rate of epigenetic divergence in recent human evolution.[37]

In the broad perspective, it is recognized that humans have genetically adapted to different environments (e.g., climate, food sources available and nutrition, exposure to microbes and other pathogens).[136] When environments are dynamic (e.g., climate change effects), there may be an "epigenetic advantage" to phenotypic switching by epigenetic inheritance rather than by gene mutation. Epigenetic phenotype switching from an epigenetically modified phenotype back to the original phenotype may occur to help bridge periods of environmental stress.[33]

There are many ways to view, study, and understand epigenetics and its influence on health from a global down to a local perspective. The global research is mentioned to give the reader a sense of how the information about epigenetics is influencing many levels of research around the world. However, in this section, the most common variations (e.g., race and ethnicity, gender, demographics, aging) in *client* populations (as opposed to worldwide groups) are briefly discussed in relation to epigenetics and in the context of a physical therapist's clinical practice. Other important genetic and epigenetic variables (e.g., personality disorders, adverse childhood experiences, trauma, coping and resiliency) are presented in Chapter 3.

### Epigenetics: Race and Ethnicity

The use of the terms "race" and "ethnicity" is generally thought to have less scientific and biologic significance than sociologic and cultural importance. The American Sociological Association notes that race refers to physical differences that groups and cultures consider socially significant, while ethnicity refers to shared culture, such as language, ancestry, practices, and beliefs.[7]

In the past, it was believed that race or ethnic background predisposed people to certain diseases and chronic conditions. However, during the last 50 years, "race" has been scientifically disproved—that is, race is not a real, natural phenomenon. Data on human variation come from studies of genetic variation, which are clearly quantifiable and replicable. Genetic data show that no matter how racial groups are defined, two people from the same racial group are as different as two people from any two different racial groups.

Current rethinking of race is taking place in terms of epigenetics rather than genetics and may help explain the health disparities experienced by various groups (e.g., blacks, Hispanics, Native Americans, Alaskan Natives, Native Hawaiians, Pacific Islanders). These differences are thought to be the result of the complex interaction among genetic variations, environmental factors, and specific sociocultural and health behaviors. Efforts are underway between the U.S. Department of Health and Human Services Office of Minority Health and the Centers for Disease Control and Prevention to conduct interviews through the Behavioral Risk Factor Surveillance System to provide an improved understanding of the health status of various groups.[21] The American Sociological Association Section for Sociology of Race and Ethnic Minorities contains excellent information and resources for further study, including the official journal of the Section, *Sociology of Race and Ethnicity*.[8]

### Epigenetics: Gender

Increasingly, research efforts are finding that the differences between males and females go far beyond the reproductive organs to affect every physiologic function and organ in the body, including the aging process.

Gender-based biology has demonstrated major gender differences in such things as risk factors, response to medications, response to surgical procedures, and response to treatment. Striking physiologic differences exist between men and women, and notably, there is greater understanding now that gender is more than biological.[140] Apart from the biology and physiology of an individual, gender can be discussed in terms of a social construct defined as a person's own internal understanding of sexual identity.

Traditionally, it was believed that biologic differences between males and females contributed to sex differences in brain function and to many sex-specific illnesses and disorders and that such differences were largely due to hormonal regulation. However, now it is known that there are both genetic and epigenetic effects,[138] and gender goes beyond a binary distinction of male and female. Differences in patterns of disease based on gender may represent either environmental or genetic factors. Diseases with rates of occurrence that differ between men, women, transgender individuals, and individuals who identify themselves in other ways may reflect lifestyle or environmental differences or anatomic and hormonal differences.

The influence of sex differences on neural function is important; epigenetic mechanisms are also known to contribute to sex differences in neural gene expression and function.[138] Epigenetic changes in the nervous system induced by early life experience, hormonal exposure, trauma and injury, or learning and memory may differ in their effects in males and females. Steroid hormones exert epigenetic effects on the developing nervous system, resulting in sex differences in brain and behavior. Sex differences in the brain are largely determined by steroid hormone exposure during a perinatal sensitive period that alters subsequent hormonal and nonhormonal responses throughout the life span. Many steroid-induced epigenetic changes are restricted to a single life span, but there is evidence that endocrine-disrupting compounds can exert multigenerational effects (primary offspring and subsequent generations). The study of epigenetics of sex differences across the epigenome to fully understand sex differences in brain and behavior is a new area of study.[105]

**Epigenetics and the LGBTQQ Community.** The LGBTQQ (lesbian, gay, bisexual, transgender, queer, and questioning) population comprises a diverse community of all races, ethnicities, religions, and social classes with a wide range of different health concerns. According to information from HealthyPeople 2020: "sexual orientation and gender identity questions are not asked on most national or State surveys, making it difficult to estimate the number of LGBT individuals and their health needs."[73]

Research gathered for HealthyPeople 2020 suggests that LGBT individuals face health disparities linked to societal stigma, discrimination, and denial of their civil and human rights. Discrimination against LGBT persons has been associated with high rates of psychiatric disorders,[110] substance abuse,[76,78] and suicide.[141] Experiences of violence and victimization are frequent for LGBT individuals and have long-lasting effects on the individual and the community.[144] Personal, family, and social acceptance of sexual orientation and gender identity affects the mental health and personal safety of LGBT individuals.[73] More research is needed to document, understand, and address the environmental factors that contribute to health disparities in the LGBT community.[67]

### Demographics by Generation

Generational differences are seen among different age groups such as the Matures, also known as postwar/Depression-era (born from 1900 to 1946); the Baby Boomers (born from 1946 to 1964); the Generation X-ers (born from 1965 to 1979); the Millennials, also referred to as Generation Y (born from 1980 to 1999), Generation Z, or the Digital Natives (the first generation to grow up using technology as a way to communicate, study/educate, record personal/societal history, and understand and make global connections)[134]; and Homelanders, the name suggested for the youngest generation (other names suggested for this group include iGen or Generation Net, as they were born into the world integrated with technology and the Internet). Many people born before 1946 tend to assume a behavioral style that is passive in their own health and in receipt of health care by accepting whatever happens to them and whatever treatment is outlined. However, baby boomers have grown up questioning authority, and their offspring are even more likely to consider themselves consumers, asking for treatment rationales, seeking second opinions, and combining allopathic treatment with alternative/integrative approaches (e.g., naturopathy, aroma therapy, acupuncture, massage therapy, Reiki, BodyTalk, yoga, tai chi, qi gong).

There is also information to support the concept of transgenerational epigenetics, the idea that epigenetic modifications accumulated throughout the entire life span can cross the border of generations and be inherited by children or even grandchildren.[146] There is strong evidence that not only the inherited DNA itself but also the inherited epigenetic instructions contribute in regulating gene expression from generation to generation. In fact, research at the Max Planck Institute of Immunology and Epigenetics has shown there are biologic consequences of this inherited information.[79,175] These studies showed that humans inherit more than just genes from parents. We also get a "fine-tuned as well as important gene regulation machinery"[79] that can be influenced by our environment and individual lifestyle. Epigenetic memory is essential for the development and survival of the new generation; as the disruption of epigenetic mechanisms may cause diseases such as cancer, diabetes, and autoimmune disorders, these new findings will have implications for human health.[175]

## Epigenetics and Aging

Aging is a complex multifactorial biologic process characterized by a gradual decline of normal physiologic functions in a predictable pattern over time. Age often represents the accumulated effects of genetic and environmental factors over time, increasing our susceptibility to many diseases including cancer, metabolic disorders (e.g., obesity, diabetes), cardiovascular disorders, and neurodegenerative diseases.[117]

Senescence, the process or condition of growing old, may be the result of continuous cellular metabolism, cellular damage, and inefficient repair systems throughout the entire life span. Many of the factors that affect longevity act primarily through the modification of the epigenome. The unfolding of information on epigenetic influences over the aging process is changing our current understanding of aging. Studies show that progressive changes to epigenetic information accompany aging in both dividing and nondividing cells. Epigenetic changes during aging alter local accessibility to the genetic material, leading to aberrant gene expression, reactivation of transposable elements, and genomic instability.[126]

Epigenetic information can function in a transgenerational manner to influence the life span of the next generation; it is understood now that rather than being genetically predetermined, our life span is largely epigenetically determined.[126] Lifestyle factors and other environmental influences can alter our life span by changing the epigenetic information. The discovery of inhibitors of epigenetic enzymes that influence life span has provided a better understanding of the mechanisms involved in aging that might lead to ways of reversing disease and even reversing aging processes.[26] This same discovery has led to the development of epigenetic "therapies" such as an epigenetic diet and drugs for a variety of age-related diseases including specific types of cancer.[143,174]

Examples of environmentally induced damage include alterations to DNA; formation of free radicals from oxidative processes causing damage to tissues and cells; and increased cross-linking of tendon, bone, and muscle tissue, reducing tissue elasticity and obstructing the passage of nutrients and waste between cells. These concepts are discussed in greater detail in Chapter 6.[143,174]

An alternative explanation for the aging process is *programmed-based*, which presumes that aging is a genetically driven process and not primarily the result of ongoing and accumulated cellular or environmental processes. In other words, aging is regulated by a biologic clock. Changes in gene expression are either preprogrammed or derived from DNA structural changes and affect the systems responsible for maintenance, repair, and defenses.[35] Examples of the programmed-based explanation of aging include the *gene mutation theory*, the *genetic control theory*, and the *planned obsolescence theory*. Both damage-based and programmed-based theories acknowledge that aging is influenced to some degree by intrinsic and extrinsic factors. It is also possible that elements of both theoretic models apply.

A newer theory in the field of antiaging medicine is the *telomere* or *telomerase theory* of aging.[65] Telomeres are sequences of nucleic acids extending from the ends of chromosomes. The basis of this theory is that the shortening of telomeres in the process of DNA replication during cell division determines how long a cell functions and when cellular apoptosis occurs. Telomeres do not encode genes; their shortening changes gene expression, and changes in gene expression (not aging genes or genes that cause any disease or condition) are the real key to aging and age-related diseases.[64,65]

Telomeres act to maintain the integrity of our chromosomes by ensuring that the sequence lost during replication is a nonessential, noncoding sequence. However, every time our cells divide, telomeres are shortened. Once the safety margin provided by a telomere is consumed, gene coding regions of the chromosome are no longer protected during replication, leading to replicative senescence, progressive damage to the chromosome, and eventual cellular damage and cellular death associated with telomere shortening.[82]

The idea that both aging and age-related diseases are genetic is no longer valid. The notion of "aging genes" and "genes that cause Alzheimer disease" (or genes that cause any other condition) is obsolete. According to Michael B. Fossel, MD, PhD, the leading expert in understanding and explaining these concepts:

*Both aging and age-related diseases are not genetic, they are epigenetic. The difference between a typical young cell and a typical old cell is not genes, but gene expression. What makes a cell "old" is not gene damage or altered genes, but alterations in the way those genes are expressed. Aging—and age-related diseases—are not the result of one gene, nor the result of the change of expression in one gene, but rather the result of wholesale and subtle changes of expression in many genes, acting in concert. Nor do such epigenetic changes stop there. It isn't enough to focus on a single gene. As the telomere influences the expression of a few local genes, these in turn influence the expression of more distant genes, which in turn influence genes on other chromosomes. Moreover, there are interactional effects between such genes: for example, gene a1 may affect three other genes, but such "downstream" genes may well be influenced by other genes as well. To account for the broad changes, it is necessary to account for all the gene changes and account for the turnover rates as gene expression changes.*[64,65]

Researchers also found that the enzyme *telomerase* is a key factor in rebuilding the disappearing telomeres. Telomerase is found only in germ cells and cancer cells. Telomerase may be manipulating the biologic clock that controls the life span of dividing cells. Future development of telomerase inhibitors may be able to stop cancer cells from dividing. The hope is to convert them back into normal cells. The future focus of research will be on resetting gene expression by addressing the change in telomere lengths through this key enzyme.

## Centenarians and Supercentenarians

A dramatic extension of longevity has occurred in the last 100 years. In 1900, people older than age 65 constituted 4% of the U.S. population. By 1988, that proportion was up to 12.4%, and it is predicted that by 2025, one-third of all Americans will be age 65 or older, and 30% of the over 65 population will be nonwhite by 2050, representing an even greater cultural diversity among older people.[14]

The most rapid population increase in the past decade has been among people older than age 85 and the "oldest old" over 100 years of age (centenarians, those who live to the age of 109, and supercentenarians, those who live to the age of 110 or more).[113] More than half (62.5%) of the 53,364 centenarians alive at the 2010 census were age 100 or 101: 82.5% were white, 12.2% were black or African American, 5.8% were Hispanic, and 2.5% were Asian. Women outnumbered men in all ages and ethnic groups; there were 330 reported supercentenarians.[113]

This aging trend of the U.S. population is reflected in the kinds of clients and problems physical therapists will treat in the coming decades. Confusion; fractures and other injuries related to falls; strokes; infections; and effects of polypharmacy, inappropriate medications, and decline in drug clearance are just a few of the more common characteristic problems older adults face.

In terms of epigenetics, centenarians and supercentenarians are models of successful aging. The data suggest that this group of individuals inherited the right genetic variants from parents or acquired epigenetic variants through the environment. The study of epigenetic signatures of healthy aging is becoming an important area of research in an effort to identify the role of DNA methylation (remember this is an epigenetic modification that alters how DNA is read and expressed without altering the underlying sequence) in aging and understand how to manage this fine-tuning system.[72,135]

Analysis of DNA methylation can also provide information on biologic age, which is a measure of how well the body functions compared with the individual's chronologic age. As a biomarker of age, DNA methylation has been referred to as the "epigenetic clock."[155] For instance, people with fatty liver disease have a faster-ticking clock, whereas centenarians have a slower clock.[155] According to the concept of developmental plasticity, it may be that people with longevity have a more powerful "engine" shaped by evolution and that the environment, through epigenetics, is a component influencing outcome.[135]

The older adult can be assessed for modifiable epigenetic risk factors that contribute to functional decline. Slow gait, short-acting benzodiazepine use, depression, low exercise level, and obesity with its associated comorbidities are significant modifiable predictors of functional decline in both vigorous and basic activities. Weak grip predicts functional decline in vigorous activities, whereas long-acting benzodiazepine use and poor visual acuity predict decline in basic activities. Known nonmodifiable predictors of functional decline include age, education, medical comorbidity, cognitive function, smoking history, and presence of previous spine fracture.[148]

## EPIGENETICS AND LIFESTYLE CHOICES

Lifestyle choices regarding diet and exercise, tobacco use, alcohol and other drug use, exposure to trauma, or any combination of these (and other) extrinsic factors comprise the majority of triggers contributing to epigenetic-based changes in gene expression. These changes in gene expression along with telomere shortening can lead to an individual's decline in health or the development of chronic conditions, diseases, and illnesses.

The complexities of how lifestyle choices and experiences influence gene expression are not completely understood yet. A full discussion is beyond the scope of this text, but it is important for physical therapists (as part of the scientific and rehabilitation community) to be aware of these concepts and how they might impact their work in the prevention, treatment, and rehabilitation of clients and patients.

### Epigenetics and Nutrition

Of all the epigenetic environmental factors, diet and nutrition most likely top the list in terms of importance and impact on the gene. Further, nutrition has been identified by the APTA as a component of the professional scope of practice for physical therapists. The APTA identifies *the role of the physical therapist to screen for and provide information on diet and nutritional issues to patients, clients, and the community within the scope of physical therapist practice.*[122] However, each state has its own jurisdictional scope of physical therapy practice, so therapists must check their state practice act and state laws governing nutritional practice before introducing dietary guidelines and nutrition information.

It is well established that Americans rely heavily on industrially processed foods as a foundation of dietary intake. The acronym S.A.D. has been widely used to describe the standard American diet and its inclusion of processed foods including carbonated drinks, margarines and spreads, cookies, crackers, breakfast cereals, energy bars, energy drinks, prepared pies, pizzas, meat nuggets, and prepackaged or ready meals.[158]

These processed foods tend to be high in empty calories with an abundance of unhealthy fat; refined carbohydrates; salt; and chemicals such as pesticides, stabilizers, antibiotics, and preservatives. Such a diet is poor in fiber, micronutrients, and antioxidants and is proinflammatory.[157] Studies are confirming that industrialized food additives are not just "bad for us" but in fact damage the gut/intestinal lining by killing helpful gut bacteria and damaging intestinal wall integrity.[94]

This damage can lead to a phenomenon called *intestinal permeability*. If the intestinal barrier is damaged or inflamed, the selective sorting and absorption mediated by a complex gut-associated immune-regulated process becomes disrupted. Intestinal permeability allows any molecule passing through the intestine to permeate the gut, enter the bloodstream, and have access to the whole body circulation. This pathway of potential toxins can lead to a host of disturbances including systemic inflammation and blood–brain barrier disruption.[114]

Disruptions in gastrointestinal microbiotas can contribute to a broad range of physiologic effects including activation of the hypothalamic-pituitary-adrenal axis (stress response) and altered activity of neurotransmitter systems and immune function.[139] With the gut microbiota impacting the hypothalamic-pituitary-adrenal axis, the amygdala, and the vagus nerve, it is critical to recognize the scaffolding that supports this entire system: the enteric nervous system.

The enteric nervous system is a dense collection of 200 million to 600 million neurons in our gut commonly referred to as our "second brain." This second brain serves as a storage reservoir and production site of neurotransmitters.[159] While research into the role of the microbiota–tight junction–gut–brain axis in pain processing is in its infancy, preliminary insights are compelling. By direct or indirect routes through the gut mucosal system and its local immune system, microbial factors, cytokines, and gut hormones find their way to the brain, impacting cognition, emotion, mood, stress resilience, recovery, appetite, metabolic balance, and pain.[93] In other words, what we eat will sooner or later affect our brain and its processing, for better or for worse.

A thorough description of these foods is beyond the scope of this text. There are critical points of nutritional emphasis that are important for people with chronic disease. Richness and diversity in wholesome, properly prepared, nourishing foods, including cultured foods, are the pinnacle of a healthy microbiome and a nourished nervous system. Cultured foods, also known as probiotic foods, provide living organisms to the digestive tract to contribute to the microbiome and help it perform its numerous functions. Cultured foods include, but are not limited to, kefir, kombucha, and fermented vegetables such as kimchi or fermented sourkraut.[39]

Living organisms within the gastrointestinal tract thrive when the diet contains prebiotic foods.[36,41,120] Prebiotic foods include fruits, vegetables, herbs, and spices, which provide "food and fodder" or nondigestible fiber to these microorganisms, particularly in the colon.[45] Specifically, but not exclusively, pomegranate, raspberries, blackberries, and strawberries have been shown to modulate intestinal inflammation and help feed the gut microbiota.[19] A healthy gut also requires a healthy collagenous turnover of epithelial cells.[133] This process is supported by foods such as bone broth and gelatin from healthy animals eating traditional diets.[50,115] Especially during stress or illness states including chronic pain, the burden of digestion can be greatly eased by the inclusion of accessible protein.

Individual nutrients have also been studied for their role in pain conditions and are also tied to gut health. Studies show that individuals with chronic pain often have low vitamin D levels.[157] Vitamin $D_3$ supplementation alone has been shown to reduce pain symptoms.[51] A vitamin $D_3$ supplement of 2000 IU is generally regarded as safe and is a point of reference for clinicians. The best source of vitamin D is the action of sunlight on the skin in the presence of cholesterol. Vitamin $D_3$, magnesium, vitamin C, selenium, zinc, glutamine, omega-3 fatty acids, and B vitamins are beneficial nutrients that have been examined in the context of chronic conditions.[18,131,163]

It is well established that many factors in our modern lifestyles can harm the microbiota and intestinal barrier and are best avoided or kept to a minimum. Processed foods, alcohol, nonsteroidal antiinflammatory drugs, antibiotics, stress, sugar, and sugar substitutes all damage the microbiota. Processed foods typically contain food additives that have been shown to cause a marked reduction in microbial diversity and induce epithelial inflammation in the gut, leading to development of ulceration and inflammatory infiltrates.[19,49] Specific food additives including glucose, refined salt, organic solvents, microbial transglutaminase, and nanoparticles have similar effects.[94]

Glucose, or sugar, feeds harmful bacteria in the gut. Highly processed sugar or industrialized fructose, also known as high fructose corn syrup, has been linked to fructose-induced neurotransmitter changes in the central nervous system and more aggressive malignancy in cancer. High fructose corn syrup is also called "natural sweetener" on food labels.[171] Food processing has profound implications on chronic conditions through direct and harmful action on the gut.[57]

Gluten intake is a complex discussion. It is important to recognize that wheat varieties grown today are high in gluten content and are subject to drastic processing techniques, rendering ultraprocessed food products containing gluten very difficult to digest. This contributes to intestinal inflammation.[58] Further, gluten is a root cause of systemic inflammation. Gluten is linked to both local inflammation within the intestine and systemic inflammation because it stimulates additional molecular activity, leading to intestinal permeability. If gluten is consumed, it should be in moderation with consideration of preparation by soaking, sprouting, or sour fermenting the wheat grains before consumption, as it was typically prepared before industrialization.[59]

Advice on what to avoid is critically relevant in the discussion of food. It is important for physical therapists to relay the gut–brain–microbiota connection to patients in the context of why nutrition matters. It is also important to share that processed foods, and especially popular diet soda, truly harm the gut contributing to joint pain, fatigue, autoimmune disorders, and many other inflammation-based diseases such as diabetes, cancer, cardiovascular disease, and autoimmune conditions.[129,153]

These harmful foodstuffs can prevent healing in an individual with chronic disease and pain owing to the damaging effects on the microbiota and ensuing sequelae. In addition to encouraging patients to avoid or minimize processed foods, additives, and sweeteners, physical therapists can promote inclusion of richness and diversity available in real, wholesome, properly prepared nourishing foods. The rationale is to motivate patients to vary the foods they eat daily to increase micronutrient diversity and feed different classes of gut microbes.[15] In asking patients about foods they routinely eat, the physical therapist validates the importance of nutrition and acknowledges the concept that we can, through nutritious food, nourish the nervous system and build resilience to pain.

## Epigenetics and Obesity

Remembering that the mechanism of epigenetic regulation of gene expression is through DNA methylation, histone modifications, and the production of noncoding RNAs (microRNAs),[63] there is evidence to demonstrate that methylation levels can be influenced by dietary factors including consumption of monounsaturated and polyunsaturated fat. Environmental cues such as diet, exercise, and toxins or pathologic states such as oxidative stress, inflammation, and metabolic changes can directly affect the target gene through epigenetic influences and determine the final phenotype or, in these cases, the disease state.[97]

Because obesity is a multifactorial disease with complex interactions between lifestyle, environment, and genetics, an understanding of how genetic expression through environmental influence causes an individual to be susceptible to obesity is essential to develop effective prevention and treatment strategies.[145] Physical therapists are in a unique position to have a positive effect on the present obesity epidemic through improving physical activity, diet, and education. Rates of obesity have increased in adults during the last 30 years but have also increased dramatically in children, especially in the United States. In fact, some authors feel the current worldwide pandemic of obesity should be considered as a communicable versus a noncommunicable disease because it is a "socially contagious feature of globalization."[31]

The dramatic increase in obesity rates in the high-income world and across the United States affecting individuals of all ages and ethnic groups in the last half of the 20th century has raised questions of how a genome can change in a short period of time to predispose an entire world to obesity if indeed these are heritable changes. Recent and increasing evidence on animal and human studies support the involvement of epigenetic status of our genes in the obesity epidemic. Much evidence supports that environmental factors, such as lifestyle and nutrition, affect the epigenetic programming of parental gametes, the fetus, and early postnatal development, so that the epigenetic marks induced in utero and in early life could determine a significant increase in obesity (and in other complex diseases such as type 2 diabetes and cardiovascular disease) and could be transmitted transgenerationally.[103]

Obesity is of great concern because of the direct effects on mortality and morbidity and the impact on health care costs as a high disease burden. It is also linked to other costly chronic diseases such as insulin resistance, type 2 diabetes, fatty liver disease, endocrine and immune disorders, and cardiovascular disease.[22,62] Measures of obesity including body mass index, waist circumference, and waist-hip ratio show an estimate of heritability between 40% and 70%.[103] Early hypotheses of a mechanism of an evolutionary perspective for obesity centered on the complementary thrifty genotype and thrifty phenotype theories explain a fetal programming hypothesis.

## Epigenetics: Physical Activity and Exercise

The current literature clearly demonstrates that the epigenetic response is highly dynamic and influenced by different biologic and environmental factors including (and especially) physical activity and exercise. Physical activity and exercise can modulate gene expression through epigenetic alterations, although the type and duration of exercise eliciting specific epigenetic effects that can result in health benefits and prevent chronic diseases remains to be determined. Many epigenetic studies[167] involving physical activity and exercise interventions have shown clear benefit to chronic diseases such as metabolic syndrome, diabetes, cancer, cardiovascular disease, and neurodegenerative disease.[71,142]

One epigenetic-modifying factor is *regular and continuous* physical activity.[142] Efforts are ongoing to investigate the positive effects of regular physical activity and exercise on changes in histone proteins and gene expression as well as the effect of these exercises on the prevention of certain cancers and age-related illnesses. DNA methylation and the prevention of certain diseases such as cancer and respiratory diseases, caused by antioxidative interactions that occur more often in elderly individuals, have been studied.[142] For the physical therapist, this text includes a full section on Physical Activity and Exercise in Appendix.

## Epigenetics: Smoking, Tobacco Use, Alcohol, and Other Drugs

As discussed throughout this chapter, the expression of genes is directly related to lifestyle choices and the influences of the environment, both external and internal, including the use of substances such as tobacco, alcohol, and other drugs. More specific information regarding these behaviors and lifestyle choices is discussed in Chapter 3 as they relate to stress, trauma, and addictions.

SPECIAL IMPLICATIONS FOR THE THERAPIST 2.1

### *Epigenetics and the Role of the Physical Therapist*

**Current Health Care Environment**

Physical therapists have received recognition as essential health care professionals within the current health care delivery system. The APTA has provided a vision for physical therapists in society as partners in the national health agenda.[156] The physical therapist will be the recognized specialist in the human movement system. In this role, physical therapists provide primary care (including rehabilitation), primary and secondary prevention, and health promotion while also reducing the effects of disease to protect the physical health and mobility of the human movement system.[156]

Our practice as physical therapists takes us from birth to death through all health care settings (e.g., emergency departments, schools, home health, inpatient, outpatient, transitional unit, assisted living, long-term care, hospice). This includes preventing disease or injury at the community level, risk reduction at all life stages, preventing early disability, promoting the health and well-being of people with disabilities, and assisting children and adults who have comorbid health conditions. We must not be constrained to the traditional medical model with its emphasis on the diagnosis and treatment of disease or injury in an environment of episodic care but rather address the effects of disease or injury on the human movement system throughout life stages across the life span.[156]

The newest frontier of physical therapy is the field of epigenetics.[151] This will lead us to better understand the intricate cellular adaptations that the functional changes we observe in patients are predicated upon. It will allow us to target our exercise-based interventions that can cause gene expression at the epigenetic level leading to what will be known as *precision physical therapy*.[167] Similar to precision medicine that uses genotyping to optimize pharmaceutical treatment,[11] physical therapists will use exercise programs tailored to an individual's genotype to maximize the effectiveness of the intervention and prescribe the optimal treatment.[137] Physical therapy interventions include long-duration movement activities that have the specific type of environmental stimulus that causes epigenetic adaptations. Exercise is a systemic stressor that elicits epigenetic adaptations in different tissues including skeletal muscle and adipose tissue.[108] The physical therapist has a tremendous opportunity, from having an understanding of the interaction between exercise and epigenetic changes in a person, to provide effective management and prevention of chronic conditions such as diabetes and obesity.

### Adapting Treatment Intervention to the Individual

In the final decades leading to the 21st century, the demographics of the United States changed rapidly, bringing with them a better understanding of the biopsychosocial-spiritual variables that affect the episode of care seen in a physical therapist's practice, especially health care issues centered around minorities and economic variables. The physical therapist's role in education and prevention has never been more important as we come to understand the effect individual modifying (risk) factors have through epigenetics on pathology and recovery. Our role as prevention and rehabilitation specialists is more important than ever as the clear correlation has been made between modifiable epigenetic risk factors and results, especially in chronic diseases and disorders.

### Social, Psychologic, and Emotional Support

Social support may influence the prognosis of individuals with acute or chronic conditions. Understanding the importance of social support in the lives of our clients and patients encourages the development of new treatments or interventions that impact an individual's health. Physical therapists need information not only about the impact of pathology on individual health but also on the role of social and environmental factors that can lead to improved outcomes in our clients. Simple steps the therapist can take to become informed about a client or patient's social support can include:

- Assessing social support in the initial intake.
- Asking about social support components including family, partners, peers, religious or faith-based organizations, work, and culture.
- Becoming part of the social support network by providing education and prevention as well as direct delivery of health care.
- Acknowledging transgender status/gender identity and recognizing the impact of this factor on health and recovery.

### Cultural Awareness

Race/ethnicity, culture, and religion are important factors in an individual's response to pain, disability, and disease. It is essential to remember that people of any culture may deal with pain, impairment, movement dysfunctions, and disability differently than expected.

The culturally sensitive health professional must screen for cultural practices, such as fasting or the use of alternative remedies; document these practices; and communicate appropriate information to other members of the team providing care for that individual. This is especially important for the client who may have a medical condition (e.g., diabetes mellitus, hypertension) that could be compromised by these practices.

The APTA is committed to ensuring equality in physical therapy services through education of physical therapy professionals. This education focuses on increasing knowledge about the inequalities that currently exist in health care and in the education of culturally competent and transnational professionals who engage in evidence-based physical therapy that eliminates racial, ethnic, geographic, and socioeconomic health disparities.[6]

In any setting, it is important for therapists to be aware of their own attitudes and values regarding lifestyle choices; responses to pain, illness, and disability; and health practices. It may be beneficial to adapt the individual intervention program to ethnic practices and beliefs. Health care education may be most effective if provided without trying to change the individual's or family's long-standing beliefs. Knowing what is needed to effectively rehabilitate an individual does not ensure success unless care is provided within a cultural and socioeconomic framework acceptable to the individual or family.

Some cultures have a very conservative view of physical contact, requiring a modified approach to the hands-on or manual therapist. In all situations where control may be an issue, the rationale and specifics for direct intervention must be clearly communicated and acceptable to the client.

Illness, especially life-threatening illness, often results in feelings of loss of control. Control, modes of control (e.g., passive acceptance, positive yielding or acceptance, or assertive control), and the desire for control are considered important variables that may influence physiologic function and health outcomes. Balancing active and yielding control styles and matching control strategies to client control styles and preferences may lead to optimal psychosocial adjustment and quality of life in the face of life-threatening illnesses.[20,29]

Language barriers make health care literature unavailable to many individuals who do not speak English and who require an interpreter (often unavailable) or for whom English is a second language, especially if English is spoken but not read. Keeping an open mind, asking questions, and respecting cultural differences are other ways to improve health care quality and delivery among minority groups.

### Physical Activity and Exercise

As so well put in a recent publication for physical therapists: Physical therapists are ideally suited to contribute to the discovery of the dose-response relationship between exercise (e.g., dose, mode, duration) and a healthy epigenetic profile.[167] A new term, "precision physical therapy," is put forth as "a means by which physical therapists can capitalize on epigenetic discoveries to optimize exercise-based interventions."[167] The article by Woelfel and colleagues[167] summarizes research in this area and encourages physical therapists to be alert to new epigenetic knowledge that can enhance the specificity and efficacy of movement-based treatment.

## REFERENCES

To enhance this text and add value for the reader, all references are included in the enhanced ebook on Student Consult that accompanies this textbook. The reader can view the reference source and access it online whenever possible.

CHAPTER 3

# Physiologic Self-Regulation: The Intersection with Mental, Social, and Emotional Well-being

KENDA S. FULLER • RENEE OSTERTAG • BETH ANNE FISHER • MICHELLE LAGING • JERI B. INNIS • BRITTANY N. GRANT

*Cynics might dismiss the concept of sensitive practice, but reality tells us that only by listening to our clients can we know about them and their condition. The knowledgeable listener who can act on what the client says needs to couple that skill with keen observations of unspoken messages. All the while, the physical therapist must be wary about receiving messages never meant to be sent, messages that come from within the practitioner, born out of bias and personal agendas.*[428]

JULES ROTHSTEIN, PHD, PT, FAPTA

## PSYCHOLOGIC CONSIDERATIONS IN HEALTH CARE

### Overview

The cognitive, physical, psychologic, and spiritual systems are intricately intertwined and impact health status. Stress reactions reflect social and psychologic phenomena that influence both neurochemical and physiologic changes in the brain and body. Impact on the endocrine and immune systems are related to progressive deterioration of many systems, leading to persistent pain and chronic disease. When an individual has been exposed to trauma, the reactions are even greater, requiring specific interventions for management. Psychologic disorders can appear throughout the lifespan and create some of the greatest challenges for the individual and health care team.

The amount of time spent with clients provides opportunities for physical therapists to evaluate the vague symptoms that are the result of contributions from these areas, creating multifaceted problems.[434] Symptoms that are associated with psychologic phenomena will not resolve unless the underlying causes of the problems have attention. It is critical to recognize the need to work in concert with other health care professionals to adequately address rehabilitation of the whole person.

Individuals who have a history of psychologic trauma may have psychologic symptoms reactivated during health care encounters, even if their physical impairments are being appropriately addressed.[98,115,346,347] It is vital, as health care professionals, that we are sensitive to the effects of our care on the *whole* person. Attention to psychologic resources, personal beliefs, support systems, resiliency, self-efficacy, and spiritual reserves are critical to healing and enhanced outcomes.[396]

### Supporting Psychologic Healing

Physical therapists have a privileged opportunity to provide support on all levels of the human experience for their clients. Physical therapists often have more consistent interactions with their clients than other professionals on the health care team, and this frequency and consistency of interactions with clients can create a safe environment that allows clients to reach out to their PT for support as well as disclosing psychologic problems.

The physical therapist should be familiar with stress and psychologic management options to support interdisciplinary care and be able to apply some behavioral and learning techniques to facilitate improvement in physical function. Techniques from MI (motivational interviewing), CBT (cognitive behavioral therapy), ACT (acceptance commitment therapy), and NVC (non-violent communication) can be supportive to physical therapists in their work with clients.

PTs should also be aware of their own limitations of knowledge, skill, and comfort. It is critical to know when the psychologic needs of the patient are greater than what the PT can provide and must instead lead to referring the client to the appropriate mental health professional. The PT will also need to be skilled in how to manage destructive interactions. Stephen Kapman describes relational transactions by determining the role of victim, rescuer, and perpetrator,[233] which may shift throughout an experience. The skills necessary to understand and manage these situations can be developed through exploration and training. Therapists are encouraged to seek opportunities for such training throughout their careers.[450]

Barriers to healing include time constraints driven by financial and insurance restrictions, increasing paperwork and productivity requirements placed upon the health care practitioners within insurance systems. These pressures can reduce time available to listen and make personal connections with individual clients. They can also heighten stress, anxiety, and irritability, leading to burnout for the practitioner and reducing the capacity to connect with clients and other staff. Recognition of these challenges is important so that the clinician can take action to offset the burdens and barriers with appropriate self-care, boundaries, and self-regulation.

### Perception: Safety versus Threat

*Perception* is defined as the state of being or process of becoming aware of something through the senses. The five senses can be utilized to orient to the present environment and recognize that no danger is present, which promotes the engagement of the ventral vagal system and "safe circuitry." In individuals with a history of trauma and abandonment, their perceptual system biases toward using painful past learning experiences rather than the senses to orient to the present. Thus, their orientation is biased toward perceiving threat rather than safety.

David Butler encourages use of a simple and clinical definition. "We will have pain when our brains weigh the world, everything going on outside, inside, and makes a credible judgement that there's more danger than safety. Equally, we will not have pain, when our brains weigh the world and judge that there is more safety (out there, in here) than danger." He also goes on to say that danger and safety, hide in hard to find places.[337]

The more the therapist can be aware of and promote cues for safety while reducing and eliminating unnecessary clues for danger, the more there is contribution to the individual's healing, both physical and psychologic. Safety cues can be provided by regulating one's own nervous system, including calm breathing, genuine smiles, listening, and kind eye contact. Identifying unhelpful belief systems about pain and providing therapeutic neuroscience pain education[289] can eliminate unnecessary cues for danger.[250]

## Physiologic Connections for Psychologic Control

### Homeostasis

Equilibrium of the complex biological systems is the basis for homeostasis in the body and is essential for health, survival, and sense of safety. The cycles of our body are related to those of our planet and universe. Sleep-wake cycles match the oscillations of light and dark. Disorders of sleep-wake appear in many of the disorders described in this chapter. The hypothalamus-pituitary-adrenal axis (HPA) is implicated in stress and psychologic disorders. The generator of arousal is the amygdala as a part of the limbic system. Homeostasis is achieved through the response of the autonomic nervous system. The autonomic nervous system is regulated by the vagal nerve or the tenth cranial nerve. Integrated somatically, perceptually, and cognitively, it is a profound regulator of internal energy systems. Co-regulation is a part of mammalian physiology, enabling one mammal to help regulate the physiologic state of another mammal. In humans, cueing occurs during social engagement and provides signals of safety or threat. The social engagement system allows us to convey to another person the status of our physiologic state. The sense of safety activates the spontaneous features of the social engagement system. (A further description of brain function related to emotional instability is included in the Introduction to Central Nervous System Disorders).

Polyvagal theory, coined by Steven Porges, helps us understand that both branches of the vagal nerve calm the body, but they do so in different ways. Porges' research identified that the parasympathetic nervous system has two presentations that depend upon whether you feel safe or feel threatened. In times of safety, the parasympathetic nervous system facilitates rest, relaxation, and digestion. However, in times of threat, the parasympathetic nervous system has a defensive mode. Mammals have two vagal circuits; an evolutionarily older circuit called the dorsal vagal complex and a more recently evolved vagal circuit called the ventral vagal complex. The dorsal vagal complex connects to the organs underneath the diaphragm including the stomach, spleen, liver, kidneys, and small and large intestines. The ventral vagal social nervous system connects above the diaphragm to the heart, lungs, larynx, pharynx, inner ear, and the facial muscles around the mouth and eyes. The ventral vagal network supports health, growth, and restoration. This system is also associated with the phenomenon of fight or flight when there is a perceived harmful event, attack, or threat to survival. The sympathetic nervous activation of fight or flight includes the adrenal medulla producing a hormonal cascade that results in the secretion of catecholamines, including norepinephrine, epinephrine, and neurotransmitters dopamine, and serotonin. There are increases in hormones estrogen, testosterone, and cortisol. This prepares the body for fighting or fleeing and includes increased heart rate, increased use of metabolic energy sources, and dilation of blood vessels for muscular action. After the episode, the ventral system should return to the functions of homeostasis as described above. When the ventral vagus is really functioning at a high level and regulating well, then the sympathetics are merely part of the homeostatic processes. They support health, growth, and restoration. They also support non-defensive movement patterns.[401]

Relative danger and related anxiety, panic, and fear, are determined at the level of the amygdala. Closely linked to the hippocampus and other structures of the limbic lobe controlled by the prefrontal cortex, it is associated with the learning of fear, and activates autonomic responses. Many of the disorders described in this chapter have a component that reflects disordered processing of the amygdala. The phenomenon of freeze-or-faint occurs when the dorsal branch of the vagal nerve shuts down, resulting in abnormal sense of fatigued muscles and lightheadedness and potentially progressing to immobility or dissociation. In the face of threat, either real or imagined, engaging the social nervous system is a way to reestablish a sense of connection and safety. If a client is unable to create a safe relational bond, the evolutionarily older biobehavioral defense strategies can become activated. If the sympathetic system fails to eliminate the danger, or perception of danger, the dorsal defense system can become engaged for long periods of time. The goal of intervention is to keep the sympathetic and dorsal systems out of persistent and ineffective defensive roles.[273]

## Reward

Much of survival learning is based on internal reward systems. These reward systems are made up by the brain's neurotransmitters and neuropeptides and the areas of the body that make use of them. The reward that is provided by these neurotransmitters is pleasure. The primary pleasure center is in the basal ganglia and linked to dopamine. This can also play a role in the addiction and placebo effects. Dopamine is released during the use of amphetamines, nicotine, cocaine, and opiates. Sedative drugs such as alcohol, tranquilizers, and benzodiazepines act by mimicking the inhibitory neurotransmitter GABA. GABA inhibits arousal triggered by the amygdala. The addictive brain is constantly seeking means of calming or shutting down the amygdala to achieve stability and peace. Endorphins are hormones that act like opioids and narcotics. Deep relaxation, meditation, and acupuncture increase production, as does vigorous exercise (known as runner's high). They also can be induced by fight/flight or freeze for survival to reduce painful distraction in severe situations.

Oxytocin is another hormone released by the pituitary gland that provides a sensation of pleasure. Receptor sites are in the limbic brain, including the amygdala. Oxytocin is secreted during sexual arousal and in new mothers and has recently been found to be associated with grandmothering. Disruption of the various neurotransmitters that modulate the structures of the limbic lobe and basal ganglia is associated with emotions of pleasure, fear, and calm. Changes in these transmitter substances, or the inability to process them, affect social engagement and underlie the phenomenon of mental disturbances that effect behavior.[440]

## Right versus Left Hemispheres

The areas of the brain involved in receptive and expressive communication, contributing to one's perception of safety versus threat, are distributed across both hemispheres. The left hemisphere controls linguistic communication and analytical interpretation, whereas the right hemisphere is responsible for nonverbal receptive and expressive communications. Functions related to the right brain are described in Box 3.1. Both brain hemispheres work together to seek and verify consistency and accuracy of information and stimuli to determine if the individual is safe or in danger, either real or perceived. Traumatic experiences interrupt brain function and precipitate conflicting interpretation of sensory and cognitive input, priming it toward perceiving threat where there is no danger.

Maturation of the right brain in infancy is equated with the early development of self, which encompasses brain-mind-body. The right hemisphere of the brain, more than the left, develops vast connections with the emotion-processing limbic areas of the brain. These areas have a powerful influence on behavior and perception of safety versus threat. Nonverbal communication through facial expression, body language, and tone of voice relays the dominant message when communicating emotional messages.[447,449] These messages operate at a subconscious level and are derived from past experiences, deep emotions, and perceptions of both the sender and receiver. The brain is continuously utilizing these messages in the present. The receiver's brain generates a somatosensory representation of the sender's emotion during the interaction, with interpretation of the message determined by the perceived emotion.[448]

Emotional interpretations, such as impressions of joy, frustration, contentment, insecurity, confidence, fear, and peace, are often the first, strongest, and most lasting messages, no matter what words or ideas are verbalized. The right hemisphere of the brain is also responsible for processing stress and emotions and for learning how to compensate for negative or stressful experiences. Even positive events and experiences can be perceived as stressful but without negative responses.[450,451]

> **Box 3.1**
>
> **RIGHT BRAIN HEMISPHERE FUNCTION**
>
> The right hemisphere of the brain is *dominant* for:
>
> - Receiving, expressing, interpreting, and communicating emotional states (right hemisphere to right hemisphere)
> - Sending and receiving subconscious, nonverbal communication
> - Retaining the most deeply ingrained message (the nonverbal, which overrides the verbal message)
> - Registering emotional messages from the subconscious facial expression and tone of voice of the sender then generating a somatosensory bodily representation of how the sender feels about self (receiver) and about the emotional status of the sender
> - Primary-process cognition
> - Adapting to complex, internally contradictory information
> - Processing of "image thinking": simultaneous, multilevel incorporation of varied image messages and components
> - Processing of stress and negative emotions, utilizing negative environmental stimulus for error compensation
> - Storing emotions that are then expressed physically and nonverbally, mostly subconsciously, by the right hemisphere

## The Right Orbital Prefrontal Cortex

The importance of right brain function in the ability to experience joy and resolve emotional and psychologic conflicts can be understood in relation to the role of the right orbital prefrontal cortex (ROPC). The ROPC of the human brain develops between birth and 18 months of age. How much and how fast this area grows depends directly on the nature and quality of stimulation this area receives through interaction with a caregiver. Growth in the ROPC occurs when children receive nonverbal messages that they are safe, valued, and cared for through eye contact, voice tone, and touch, which become positive motivators for the child younger than 12 months old.[435,449,451]

There are normal growth spurts of the ROPC between birth and 18 months of age, with peaks at 3 months and 9 months of age; between 3 and 5 years of age with the peak at 4 years of age; between 7 and 10 years of age; at 15 years of age; and at the birth of the first child.[447] Biochemical changes during pregnancy prepare the mother's brain for ROPC growth. The last identified growth spurt of the ROPC occurs at the birth of the first grandchild.[447-449] Throughout life, the ROPC retains its ability to grow, and thus its ability to perceive safety and heal, to the same extent as from infancy. ROPC deficits can be restored in persons suffering previous developmental or trauma losses.[448,449] This is strong evidence that healing is possible and available for everyone.

From birth and throughout life, connection with other people or lack thereof impacts every aspect of our health, perspective, and functioning. Just as neglect and abuse interfere with normal development, nurture and relational joy promote healthy growth and development and a secure, resilient identity. Joy has been identified as a necessity for human development. Joy is relational and results in growth, perception of safety, and health beyond actual circumstances. Happiness is an emotion that is closely related but can be manipulated and governed by circumstances and by the person's will. Although some growth of the ROPC will occur with even minimal joyful experiences, the most favorable growth and healing of the ROPC occurs during frequent and consistent experiences of joy, reflected in genuine smiles. ROPC function is enhanced when the right hemisphere messages are congruent with the verbal left hemisphere content and when there is synchrony of communication. Brain scans confirm that the ROPC grows in response to joy, targeting the left eye.[447-449,548,549] In the absence of joyful stimulation, the ROPC will atrophy, and the full growth potential will not be achieved.

Humans mirror nonverbal interpersonal communication paths. For example, a child will mirror what the child receives nonverbally from interactions with older children and adults, and behavior is mimicked from that exposure.[447-449] The attitude and emotions of the sender, conveyed nonverbally, carry the deepest and most lasting message to the receiver. The healthier and more mature person can more accurately understand left and right hemisphere communications and resolve conflicting verbal and nonverbal messages while retaining a solid and consistent self-perception and response stability.[448,449] Tone of voice and facial expression messages are perceived much more quickly than verbal communication. Subconscious messages from facial expressions occur as fast as 40 milliseconds, or the time it takes for one brain cell to fire. The complete cycle of sent and received nonverbal messages occurs at six times per second.[447-449]

### Neuroplasticity

"Neurons that fire together wire together" is a way of saying neurons that engage together in the brain create increased strength of connectivity over time. Paired stimuli that are associated together is the basis for Pavlovian theory. Neighboring neurons respond preferentially to immediate time sequences of neighboring neurons, which creates an associative memory[369] set. Frontal cortical activity is engaged when making a conclusion in thought or when evoking a voluntary movement. Learning-driven changes in connections increase cell to cell cooperation, increasing reliability of response. The brain is changed by internal mental rehearsal in the same way and involves the same processes that control changes achieved through interactions with the external world. Memory[66] guides and controls most learning. Every moment of learning provides a moment of opportunity for the brain to stabilize and reduce the disruptive power of potentially interfering backgrounds or noise. Episodic memory is viewed as subject to lifelong transformations that are reflected in the neural substrates involved in mediation of the area. Episodic memory involves the hippocampus and is involved in perception, language, empathy, and problem solving.[336]

It is important to remember that brain plasticity can work in both directions. It is just as easy to generate negative changes as positive.[323] Interventions require feedback that drives improvement and allows the engagement of the desired neuron pools while at the same time working to extinguish the neuronal activity that leads to unwanted movements or thought. Resilience, mindfulness, and meditation as described below make use of positive neuroplasticity.

## Resilience

Hans Selye said, "It's not stress that kills us, it is our reaction to it." There are hot and cold reactors among us, related to an individual response to stress.[455] Resilience is the ability to bounce back to baseline when confronted with a difficult situation. It is the ability to maintain equilibrium under stress, and it is successful adaptation to persistent adversity. Dr. Mejia-Downs describes four components of resilience, which include positive affect, effective coping, purpose for living, and social support. *Positive affect* is the positive brain changes that occur with positive feelings.[315] Functional MRIs reflect activity in the structures of emotion when a person is thinking about positive experiences. *Effective coping* represents the ability to understand that if something can't be changed, one must accept that reality and cope with it. Energy is best spent working on acceptance of the circumstances. It is important to have a variety of coping strategies for different situations and to recognize when the current strategy is not successful and switch to another option that may bring success. This is called coping flexibility. Coping flexibility has an impact on the risk of depressive symptoms.[234]

*Purpose for living* is finding meaning in life. This has been shown to increase resilience. In addition, having a purpose improves the chance that you will make positive changes in your life. Identifying one's purpose in life can increase the ability to avoid illness.[485]

*Social support,* both perceived and actual, has been shown to be protective against stress. It also decreases the chance of developing depression and helps to recover from emotional trauma. Lower rates of morbidity from heart disease occur among the socially connected.[190] Resilience is something you can cultivate and enhance. Everyone has some level of resilience. Studies have determined that it is possible to learn how to bring it out, and that practice enhances the results.[425,533]

## PSYCHOLOGIC HEALING POTENTIAL

A study done in clients receiving psychotherapy demonstrates that occurrences that happen outside of therapy account for over 40% of positive outcomes.[114] In other words, 60% of outcomes can be influenced as a function of therapeutic factors. In the realm that the therapist can influence, 30% of improvement comes from therapeutic relationship, 15% comes from positive expectancy and hope, and 15% occurs through the model of intervention used incorporating specific techniques. In short, 75% of therapist influence comes from therapeutic alliance and hope, while 25% of patient outcomes relies on therapeutic model and techniques.[157]

The capacity to establish a strong therapeutic alliance, trust, and safety within the relational field with the patient covers 30% of positive outcomes. If there is hope and the expectation of success within the condition, that adds another 15%. If hope does not exist, education about the polyvagal theory and the autonomic nervous system would be part of an appropriate intervention.[402] The polyvagal theory, as discussed by Stephen Porges, provides strong scientific evidence that all individuals possess the mechanisms for healing. When the higher-brain structures perceive safety in the surrounding environment, they allow the brainstem to regulate the autonomic nervous system in a way that promotes health, growth, and restoration. In situations perceived as safe, the more primitive survival defense systems of sympathetic fight/flight and dorsal vagal shutdown work together with neocortical structures to engage the ventral vagal system to support healing, play, and social engagement.

Practitioners can be confident in creating hope and supporting positive expectancy by engaging concepts related to safe circuitry. This comes with the knowledge of the biological phenomenon of the immense internal healing capacity with which every individual is born. The therapist's words, actions, and physiology should reflect the understanding of these concepts. When therapists are connected to a felt sense of their own regulated nervous system, they powerfully tap into the co-regulatory potential of the ventral vagal system and its healing capacities, communicating it both verbally and nonverbally, and promoting safety, trust, and healing in the relational field.

### Phases of Healing

Most stress- and trauma-related pathologies can be managed because the brain has great potential for healing. Psychologic healing occurs when consistent messages are received and confirmed by both the cognitive (more logical) left hemisphere and the more emotional right hemisphere, along with the somatic, felt sense experience produced by the right hemisphere. The reconciliation between the two aspects of communication, learning, and emotional development may be unfamiliar and initially uncomfortable to the person who has lived with mixed messages and emotional, mental, and spiritual wounds for prolonged periods.

Healing often requires the assistance of a mental health provider who understands that the ability to tolerate disruption and uncertainty is fundamental to life, health, and growth and who can assist and mentor the individual in exploring that truth during treatment. Physical therapists may not have the full repertoire of psychologic treatment tools to enable psychologic healing, and referral to appropriate providers is an important step, especially because clients may not seek help on their own. However, reinforcement of psychologic strategies, consistent support and caring through a safe therapeutic relational field, cues for safety, hope, positive expectancy, avoidance of further stress, and reduction of cues for threat assist with alleviation or adaptation to physical diagnoses.

Dr. Judith Herman, psychiatrist and author of *Trauma and Recovery*, describes three phases of healing in trauma recovery. These phases will be described briefly, followed by relevant knowledge and tangible strategies for the physical therapist.[191]

#### Phase I: Safety and Stabilization

People in this stage feel unsafe in their bodies and relationships with others. Areas of their life feel unstable. They have difficulty regulating and soothing difficult emotions. Speaking about their experiences is emotionally overwhelming. Signs of autonomic dysregulation are present, such as overwhelming emotions, tears, high-pitched voice with fast pace, muscle tightness, increased pain, flat facial expressions, low monotonous vocal expression, decreased eye contact, or globalized low tone.

**Supporting Phase I: Guide for the Therapist.**

- Resolve any real tissue danger or pathology that are expressed through peripheral mechanisms of inflammatory, ischemic or peripheral neurogenic pain.
- Provide education that enables the individual to distinguish between real versus perceived threat.
- Develop a battery of regulation, relaxation, grounding, and containment skills.
- Stay regulated in your own system while clients talk about their experiences, especially if they are emotional. Your best support is to stay calm, relaxed, and listening—fixing, making it better, or finding the silver lining for them is ineffective and unhelpful. Say things like, "Wow, that must be so hard," "I can't even imagine what that must be like," or "I'm so sorry, that sounds really difficult."
- Offer frequent reminders of safety, subtly offered throughout the course of conversation. "There's nothing dangerous happening right now." "There's nothing unsafe in here right now."
- Orient to the present using the five senses rather than the post-traumatic brain, which orients to the present through a predictive model that is constantly predicting the immediate future based on painful past experiences.
- Encourage affirmations such as "you made it, you survived, it's over, you're here now." Allow 5 to 10 seconds for their attention to notice those words and what they feel like in the body.
- Orientation to the present and cues for safety are also helpful with a simple 3-2-1 exercise: have them look around the room and list 3 things they see, 2 things they hear, and 1 thing they touch.

### Phase II: Remembrance and Mourning

This stage shifts to processing the trauma by putting words and emotions to the experience and making meaning of it. This process is usually undertaken with a counselor or therapist in group and/or individual therapy. It might not be necessary to spend a lot of time in this phase, but it is important to continue to attend to safety and stability during this phase.

**Supporting Phase II: Guide for the Therapist.**

- Monitor and reinforce cues for safety.
- Recognize and bring attention to physiologic expressions of threat that may no longer be necessary. Encourage attention to cues for safety to encourage neuroplasticity in the direction of safety rather than unnecessary reinforcement of paired physiologic threat with movement.
- An important intervention PTs can apply here is inviting individual awareness of patients' physiology during vocalization of their story (of injury, surgery, accident, pain). Patients will often demonstrate signs of dysregulation as they recount their story, unconsciously reinforcing dysregulation circuitry to be paired up with the memories of events. Invite them to calm and settle their system before going on with their story to uncouple dysregulated physiology from the memory of trauma and pain.
- Questions of consent and permission such as, "Do I have your permission to ___________ (touch your arm, approach you, move your leg)?" "Does this _____ (exercise, movement, intervention) feel safe?" "Is it ok if I approach you?" provide new learning experiences and cues of safety.

### Phase III: Reconnection and Integration

In this phase, there must be a creation a new sense of self and a new future. This final task involves redefining oneself in the context of meaningful relationships. Through this process, the trauma no longer is a defining and organizing principle in someone's life. The trauma becomes integrated into their life story but is not the only story that defines them.

Consider how restoration of movement, activity participation, and function support the development of a new sense of self.

**Supporting Phase III: Guide for the Therapist.**

- Integrate, celebrate, savor positive and safe experiences. Five to10 seconds of focused attention is sufficient to reduce amygdala activity and enhance prefrontal cortex activity. Notice the good and pause to feel it throughout the day.
- Focus on meaningful goals and celebrate with the patient every step of success on their way towards restoration of movement and function.
- It can be easy to focus on the disability, pathology, and areas where there is lack, problems, or pain. Of equal importance is actively looking for, acknowledging, and encouraging recognition of small gains; where attention goes, neural firing flows and synaptic connections grow. If the gains and wins are not attended to, a chance for neural growth in the direction of safety, health, growth, and restoration is missed.

## Boundary Basics for the Provider

Personal boundaries are critical to a person's identity and function. Clients may come for therapy with their own unhealthy boundaries. It is important for the therapist to be clear in determining appropriate boundaries and expectations. Boundaries can be flexible or rigid, open like fences, or be solid like walls or versatile like a gate. Nature has provided us with a beautiful metaphor, that of a semi-permeable membrane. Whereas positive life experiences promote exploration and testing of boundaries, negative or painful life experiences cultivate avoidance behaviors, especially every real or perceived trauma-related boundary. As a health care provider, it is important to understand personal boundaries in relation to other people and the work as a therapist. Questions to ask oneself in order to discover this might include:

- Do I give more than I receive from others?
- Do I feel resentful often?
- Do I stay late at work regularly to get things done?
- Am I comfortable saying no or disappointing others when I have reached my limits?
- Do I know my limitations and honor them or often try to push past them in ways that leave me exhausted?

Although uncommon in the physical therapy realm, supervision and consultation groups are very common and often a requirement for maintaining licensure among our counseling, psychology, and spiritual director colleagues. These types of groups provide a safe place for providers to share their patient care challenges. Some groups are structured around having a more experienced facilitator, and others rely on a structure of peer-guided supervision, in which peers take turns sharing cases in different meetings. The suggested purpose of these groups is not centrally focused on getting technical feedback to solve a patient's clinical issue as much as it is for the clinician to share his or her feelings, triggers, and internal responses to the clinical situation being discussed. Participation in such a regular supervision or consultation group with peers is helpful for healthy accountability, support, and perspective. Role playing potentially difficult sessions with peers can be helpful at times. Practicing clear statements and interactions that convey empathy, clarity, confidence, boundary delineations, and decisiveness can support the challenged clinician. There is a difference between supporting a patient on the healing path and providing education and guidance versus attempting to rescue or fix them. It is emphasized that it is *their* path, not yours. Rescuing a patient is an overextension of the clinician's personal and professional boundary with a patient.

Healthy clinicians take the time to scrutinize themselves to determine positive and negative effects in caring for needy people. Healthy boundaries maintain an adult-to-adult equality in the relationship, prevent the provider from taking on unrealistic responsibility for outcomes, and keep the focus on the needs of the client. Practicing healthy personal boundaries is critical for the client as a model of safety, respect, and health. This allows the clinician to uphold ethical integrity and moral excellence. Establishing healthy boundaries allows others to know who you are and what to expect, facilitating a safe and trusting relationship.

Difficult or complex individuals can generate internal fears, insecurities, anger, or other emotions. Psychologic healing can be supported by the health care professional's ability to empathize with the person's distress and model appropriate management of stress. This requires the therapist to synchronize with the client visually, by vocal tone, and in body language.

People with harbored hurts tend to keep the darker emotions of anger, shame, and fear hidden and to avoid positive opportunities for secure connection with trust, joy, and helpful support. The function of these abnormal boundaries can be reversed during therapy to allow the client to maintain positive and healthy connections while keeping out negative, harmful elements. As health improves, personal boundaries help strengthen and magnify coping ability. The clinician is encouraged to clearly define the clinical relationship with the client, including goals, expectations, roles, policies, and options. The therapist is advised to follow established policies; do not pacify the client by changing the rules. If concessions are made within established policies and healthy boundaries, let the client know what concessions are available and clearly identify the sustaining or limiting parameters. Appeasing the client may give relief for the moment, but changing the policies can cause confusion and insecurity in the future.

**SPECIAL IMPLICATIONS FOR THE THERAPIST 3.1**

### Maintaining Healthy Boundaries

Participation in regular consultation groups with peers promotes healthy accountability, support, and perspective. These settings allow the therapist to practice clear statements and interactions that convey empathy, clarity, confidence, and decisiveness. The goal is to be objective, not defensive or emotion-laden. Responses to highly charged, emotional messages or phone calls should include the space to allow the clinician to choose a response rather than an unfiltered reaction. It can be helpful to seek counsel from peers, write out the chosen response, and offer options that are win-win. Documentation should be thorough with objective, nonjudgmental terms. The client, the client's family, lawyers, and other professionals will have access to your notes.[295]

Self-regulation includes the following:

- Maintaining a sense of one's own interoceptive processes allows for improved control of one's own physiologic state and how it impacts another's state.
- Develop awareness of when your brain is perceiving threat or safety, as well as the resultant physiologic expressions.
- Make frequent scans of the body every 5 to 20 minutes, notice what's tight, and relax your muscles, find your breath to practice and develop automatic self-regulation habits.

Verbal and nonverbal communication includes:

- Communicate consistent messages by ensuring that your body language, vocal cues, and physiology match verbal and cognitive educational, treatment, and self-care information.
- Reinforce verbal communication with written instructions. Having the client speak and/or write out their instructions reinforces their learning. Ask the client to review what was conveyed and exercise healthy boundaries.
- Reduce use of threatening language (i.e., bulging, degenerative, torn, ripped, worn, etc.). Consider how language is received by the brain—is it safe or a threat to the individual—and seek to find replacement words, as well as encouraging clients to consider the language they use verbally, as well as in their thinking.
- Listen without bias, encourage without coercion, offer options, and step back, allowing the individual to make the choice—good or bad.
- Monitor nonverbal body language, including tone, pitch, and speed of voice; posture; facial expressions; and environmental positioning, to ensure you are providing cues of safety to the client's nervous system, rather than threat.
- Listen attentively to the client and reflect feelings and circumstances.

### Patient-Sensitive and Trauma-Cognizant Approaches

A primary goal for a physical therapist working with anyone with a history of psychologic trauma is to encourage client control and responsibility in his or her own care.[115,443,545] Schachter et al.[115] have suggested nine principles of sensitive practice for individuals with a history of sexual abuse: respect, taking time, developing rapport, sharing information, sharing control, respecting boundaries, fostering mutual learning, understanding nonlinear healing, and demonstrating awareness of interpersonal violence. They provide more detail on specific suggestions to promote these principles gleaned from interviews with survivors of childhood sexual abuse. These include:

- Monitor the client for stress responses through attentive listening and observation.[115]
- Sensitive inquiry about discomfort is usually appreciated by everyone.[443]
- Work with the individual to identify and avoid triggers and hyperarousal, such as allowing the person to discontinue or change positions, treatment, and equipment.[115,443]
- Encourage clients to identify and exercise options and choices and to report what they are thinking and feeling.[115]
- If stress reactions are observed, direct questioning or redirecting attention may diffuse somatic responses.[115]
- Provide a safe environment by adjusting surrounding space and proximity to other clients (especially if opposite gender or specific characteristics trigger stress).[115,443]
- Offer a choice of gender of therapist, especially if the client has a history of abuse.[443]
- Provide positive feedback for achievement of psychologic and physical goals.
- Support the individual's coping strategies (developed with a psychology professional); for example, this may include cognitive reframing, conscious

attention to the present circumstances, breathing techniques.[115]

- Simple spirituality screening questions give the physical therapist information that can enhance client coping, trust, and hope and inform the physical therapist's plan of care.

Therapists should be mindful of their own facial expressions being conveyed to patients. The more that messages of joy and safety are conveyed, the greater the promotion of physical and psychologic pain reduction; conversely, the more messages of frustration, anger, and stress are conveyed, the greater the promotion of increased physical and psychologic pain. For both the client and the therapist, the goal of interactions is to avoid an immediate negative reaction by choosing to create a space between the stimulus and the response. It is in that space that there is power to choose the response. The response provides the opportunity for growth and freedom.

#### Meditation

Mindfulness meditation has been reported to produce positive effects on psychologic well-being that extend beyond the time the individual is formally meditating. Mindfulness is the opposite of mind chatter or intrusive thoughts. Meditation involves the development of awareness of present-moment experience with a compassionate, nonjudgmental stance.[230] This process is associated with a perceptual shift in which one's thoughts and feelings are recognized as events occurring in the broader field of awareness.[70] Given the importance of the regulation of emotions and cognition in healthy psychologic functioning, the morphologic changes in the brain likely contribute to the positive effects of mindfulness meditation. These structural changes in the particular brain network involved in the projection of oneself into another perspective may underlie this perceptual shift.[291] Functional MRIs show activation of the frontal lobes during meditation, an area that modulates the limbic process. Neuroscience mechanisms suggest that several brain networks are involved.[13] Heartfulness meditation is associated with significant decrease in burnout and improvement in emotional wellness in healthcare providers.[220]

### Breathing

Controlled breathing is associated with many of the interventions presented in this chapter and is the basis of meditative practices. The effect of breathing is amplified during exhalation and is attenuated during inhalation. Training for belly breathing or abdominal breathing allows access to increased ventral vagal flow. Many of the very powerful afferents related to breathing for the ventral vagal system are embedded in the diaphragm. Voluntary breathing patterns train individuals to push the diaphragm down and to extend the duration of exhalations compared to inhalations. Adding pursed lip or "voo" sounds helps to extend the exhalation and increases the soothing feeling of ventral vagal engagement. Breath work associated with mindful meditation affects homeostasis through a relationship between heart rate and breathing. During inhalation the heart rate increases; during exhalation, it decreases. This is known as heart rate variability or HRV. As the difference between the two numbers increases, there is a drive toward improved emotional and physical health. HRV can be monitored in the clinic, and clients can be trained to perform the measurement at home.

In his work, Porges adds another dimension, which is working with facial muscles. This is a part of what he calls the integrated social engagement system, giving sensory feedback to the brain stem area that regulates the ventral vagal nerve. It involves using laryngeal, pharyngeal, trigeminal, and facial muscles plus listening or being aware of the acoustic environment. In a hypervigilant state, hearing gets biased towards low-frequency and high-pitched sounds. It loses its acuity in the range of prosodic features of human voice. Addressing clients' needs in this arena can help overall function and social integration. Language can also be a powerful tool to trigger autonomic responses. Use of vocabulary during interventions is critical to enhanced engagement.

#### Exercise

It is well known that vigorous physical activity is related to lower stress levels, and exercise releases brain-derived neurotrophic factor (BDNF), a substance that improves brain health. Exercise increases the number of serotonin neurotransmitter receptors in the hippocampus via stimulation of neurogenesis. The release of endorphins during aerobic exercise and the reduction of cortisol levels in the bloodstream elevate mood, reduce pain, and mediate stress reactions. Many of the special implications for physical therapists in this chapter include the psychologic benefits of exercise.[417]

### Spiritual Development in the Health Care Profession

Spirituality can be defined as a dynamic and intrinsic aspect of humanity through which persons seek ultimate meaning, purpose, and transcendence and experience relationship to self, family, others, community, society, nature, and the significant or sacred. Spirituality is expressed through beliefs, values, traditions, and practices.[179] Spirituality can be viewed as one's search for ultimate purpose, meaning, and connection with the transcendent, or a larger sense of Oneness. Spirituality is also understood as that which makes a person thrive in his or her life. The concept of spirituality is found in all cultures and societies.

Spirituality is considered a larger umbrella under which religion exists as a part of some individuals' spiritual dimension of life. Religion may be defined as a way for a person to express their spirituality within a larger system or community. One might also observe that there are spiritual communities, whether formal or informal, that are not particularly religious in nature. Regardless, the core value of spirituality in our time is agreed upon to be a way of making meaning out of life for oneself and the world around us. This effort and activity of meaning-making, whether individually or within a group, is the way in which one finds the will, animating purpose, and vitality to be present in one's own life.

The impact of human spirituality and beliefs has come under closer scrutiny in research, secular publications, and clinical education. A national consensus conference developed spiritual care guidelines for interprofessional clinical spiritual care. These guidelines, as well as the educational advances, research, and ethical principles, have supported the developing field of spirituality and health.[410] Professional development now offers more ways to develop spirituality, especially as it relates to the health care professional's sense of calling to their profession, the basis of relationship-centered care, and the provision of compassionate care.[409] In addition, consensus also exists to support the role of all health care providers as spiritual care generalists in relationship to their patients, meaning that they have a front-line role in identifying, addressing, and referring out for the spiritual needs of their patients as appropriate to their level of skill and training.

Spirituality is recognized as a factor that contributes to health.[245,427] Studies show an association between religion or spirituality and health outcomes such as hypertension, lower fasting glucose levels, recovery from surgery, coping with illness, and the will to live.[201,245] Many studies demonstrate that spiritual practices or associations, specifically prayer, in the coping process of individuals with cancer, pain control, and other chronic conditions has been shown to decrease the medical costs associated with end-of-life care.[34,36,104,246] The relationship between religious activities and lowered blood pressure, improved mental health, and decreased depression in older adults also has been reported.[247,248,331]

Individuals whose spiritual needs are not met are less satisfied with their care.[30] Most people polled want a more holistic approach to health care, which includes conversation with their health care provider about spirituality, their faith, and their spiritual needs.[37] Some organizations, such as the National Cancer Institute, have published materials to help health care professionals learn how to talk about spiritual beliefs, values, and practices and their effect on health, illness, disease, and stress.[349,294] Spiritual care is not in any one provider's domain in our current model of health care. It is the responsibility of everyone on the health care team to listen to what is important to the individual, respect the individual's spiritual beliefs, and be able to communicate appropriately with the person as those issues and beliefs are shared. Health care providers can ask clients in a nonbiased, nonjudgmental way about their spirituality to encourage and support a more holistic approach to health and healing.[306,208]

The health care provider's openness and ability to address a client's spiritual issues as the client reveals such concerns or beliefs are essential to the health and healing of the whole person. Jensen and Mostrom conclude that a physical therapist's level of comfort in addressing the spiritual domain along with others is related to the physical therapist's own level of comfort with the spiritual domain.[223]

It is important for health care providers to be aware of their own spirituality, as well as personal historical biases if they exist from participating in a religious community, in order to be more fully present in a nonjudgmental way to the patient's perspective and values. Awareness of physiologic self-regulation as a part of one's spiritual biases is a critical component of effective intervention. Our physiology can express what we believe to be true of our own spirituality and therefore our ability to sit with clients as they express or struggle with their own spirituality. This might be experienced as a sense of internal peace within the nervous system, supporting a positive personal sense of one's spirituality, or on the other hand a sense of sympathetic arousal, such as irritation, anger, or sadness, more associated with a freeze response. Regardless, the important factor is to notice this energy within oneself in a nonjudgmental way and explore these physiologic expressions.

Often critical or life-threatening illness can threaten one's foundation, and particularly one's trust in a kind and loving transcendent being. A patient's expression of this struggle can touch on the practitioner's physiology, creating expressions of sympathetic or parasympathetic dysregulation. If the practitioner has not fully processed his or her own spiritual struggles with this topic, it will be more difficult for the practitioner to be fully present with the patient. This leads to a greater potential for the practitioner to experience a state of burnout. Spiritual support from chaplains, pastoral care professionals, or family members and friends, as well as personal spiritual beliefs, is an important component of hospital stays.[121]

Some individuals do not desire a spiritual interaction with their physicians.[121] Patients also may not want to discuss their spiritual needs and values with their provider for fear that the difference in beliefs may impact the relationship they have established with that provider. Obstacles to spiritual care interactions include the physician's own feeling of discomfort with engaging topics of spirituality and faith when their own belief is different from that of the patient. In the provider-patient relationship, there may be a perceived power inequity, making it difficult for a patient to feel safe in sharing a conversation about their spirituality.

### Spiritual Perceptions and Health

Spiritual distress can be defined as the impaired ability to experience and integrate meaning and purpose in life through connectedness with self, others, art, music, literature, nature, or a power greater than oneself. Spiritual distress is important to identify in patients because studies show that people with relatively higher levels of spiritual distress are more likely to have pain, more likely to be depressed, be at higher suicide risk, have higher levels of clinically impactful anxiety, and have a higher resting heart rate. Research indicates that spiritual struggles are associated with greater psychologic distress and diminished levels of well-being. Recognizing pastors, chaplains, pastoral care professionals, rabbis, priests, imams, spiritual directors, and other spiritual leaders as part of the interdisciplinary team should lead to appropriate referrals. The role of physical therapists as spiritual care generalists suggests that they be aware of these red flag situations to identify a patient's need for a specialist spiritual care provider.

How an individual perceives his or her condition determines response to a disease, illness, or other physical or mental health condition. Spiritual experiences, beliefs, and perspectives can have a powerful impact on an individual's understanding of his or her illness.[202] For example, in numerous studies, African American women identified the tremendous support spirituality provided in coping with breast cancer.[498] Religious convictions can affect an individual's scope of options and decision-making process.

Spiritual convictions may constitute a foundational need in health care or may cause a person to refuse procedures or treatment altogether. Individuals who identify themselves as Jehovah's Witnesses reject blood products due to religious beliefs. The lack of blood transfusions may affect the timing of mobilization in the postoperative physical therapy plan of care for a patient with a severely low hemoglobin count following a total knee replacement procedure.

Studies of both positive and negative coping strategies have found that religious or spiritual experience and practices extend the individual's coping resources and are associated with improvement in health care outcomes. People who perceive their suffering as punishment from a transcendent being, who have excessive guilt or anger about failed expectations, or who feel betrayed by their connection with a transcendent being experience more depression, a poorer quality of life, and greater callousness toward others. People who associate with a transcendent being who is friendly, kind, or loving may be more compelled to depend on this being for strength, guidance, and help and show less psychologic distress. In asking for forgiveness or by forgiving others, their spiritual beliefs provide strength and comfort beyond themselves.[387,408,495] Research examining the physiologic benefits of forgiveness among various faith traditions reports findings of association between forgiveness and cardiovascular health, stress levels, and improved overall health.[225,263,265,412]

A person who has experienced spiritual abuse might actively avoid anything with a religious or spiritual connotation. Knowing the pertinent history will allow the caregiver to gather information about words, expressions, and other triggers that might cause a negative reaction in the client. Likewise, providers who have experienced spiritual abuse in their own past would also benefit from being aware of their own triggers and identifying supports such as chaplains or counselors who can help them process these experiences.

Spiritual emptiness is considered the phenomenon of having no sense of available resource outside of self, and understandably leads to self-limited coping, strength, and potential. This is different from spiritual distress in that spiritual emptiness has a more futile quality of void about one's spirituality, as opposed to having an instability or shifting in beliefs brought on by dire life circumstances. If we believe there are no resources outside of ourselves, we tend to struggle under unrealistic expectations and pressures on self and others.

Shouldering responsibility for managing life and circumstances without a sense of any transcendent support can deplete and stress every system. Dependence on human fallibility, frailty, and limitation alone can result in exhaustion and pervasive feelings of burnout, depression, loneliness, hopelessness, and helplessness for some people.

Stress that is chosen, such as a desire to serve above and beyond, triumph over a challenge, or master new situations, can foster eustress, which is good, pleasant, or curative stress with optimal physiologic arousal. Eustress is not defined by the type of stressor but the perception of the situation as negative or threatening versus positive or challenging.[454,481,495]

Human history is full of accounts of people going through extreme, incomprehensible, life-threatening experiences or severe loss and finding the resolve to survive and the strength to endure through their faith and trust in a transcendent being. Healing, beyond medical understanding or imagination, termed *miracles* or *spontaneous healing* by both clients and health care providers, is attributed to prayer and supernatural intervention. Although the tangible, consistent differences between those who spontaneously heal and those who do not are still being sought, the impact of spirituality is being considered and studied.[178]

Spiritual health, for both patients and providers, fosters coping beyond normally accepted parameters by giving the following[245,408]:

- *Sense of control*: Faith and trust are choices. Making the choice to trust beyond logical understanding lessens a sense of helplessness, actively engages the person in self-awareness and assessment, and expands coping potential through the experience of empowerment.
- *Hope for restoration, for healing, for attaining goals, for a peaceful death*: People can find the ability to accept and deal with current conditions through belief in a transcendent being.
- *Acceptance*: Inconceivable stresses and demands can be tolerated when trust in a transcendent being gives meaning and purpose to life and suffering beyond understanding.
- *Strength and endurance*: A personal faith imparts peace beyond understanding or explanation, strength beyond self, and the ability to focus outwardly instead of being overwhelmed by internal suffering.[198]

Therapists are often patients themselves at one time or another, confronting the same spiritual challenges and stresses related to mortality and illness that their patients do. Therapists are encouraged to explore and attend to their own emotional, mental, physical, and spiritual condition.

Subsequently, physical therapists should be familiar with levels of spiritual distress. O'Brien identified seven levels of spiritual distress: spiritual pain, spiritual alienation, spiritual anxiety, spiritual guilt, spiritual anger, spiritual loss, and spiritual despair.[370]

- Spiritual pain may be expressed during routine conversation when clients disclose that normal spiritual support is not available because of decreased mobility or other pathology.
- Spiritual alienation is related to concerns about material resources, such as finances or care of a spouse or child.
- Spiritual anxiety reflects the individual's fear of judgment from members of the normal spiritual support group.
- Spiritual guilt is the fear that the situation is a result of one's poor choices.
- When people blame a transcendent being or situation, they are demonstrating spiritual anger.
- When people express that life no longer has meaning or they no longer feel supported by others, spiritual loss is present.
- Finally, the most severe form of spiritual distress is spiritual despair or loss of hope.

Once the status is determined and a healthy relationship between the therapist and client has been established, the therapist should be able to:

- Provide a safe environment by giving attention to the physical environment and to nonverbal messages.
- Listen attentively to the client, reflect feelings, and respond appropriately.
- Accept the individual as a person whether they agree or approve, verbally and nonverbally respecting and valuing the person as they partner in discovering truth and evaluating options.
- Recognize the signs of spiritual distress to determine if a client might benefit from interaction with a spiritual care specialist, such as a chaplain or clergy member.[25,34,134,300,404,408]
- Obtain a spiritual history, which is more extensive than a spiritual screen. This should also help to identify the client's need for avoidance of discussion of spiritual topics.
  - FICA Spiritual History Tool (It is recommended to obtain additional training as a spiritual care generalist to complete a spiritual history as opposed to a spiritual distress screen.)
  - NCCN Distress Thermometer from the National Comprehensive Cancer Network, Copywrite 2018.
- Honor spiritual practices, as appropriate.

**SPECIAL IMPLICATIONS FOR THE THERAPIST 3.2**

### *Practices to Foster Spiritual Awareness and Development*

Reflecting on the definitions of spirituality set forth prior, we can conclude that almost any personal practice that helps a practitioner to return to physiologic self-regulation, make meaning, and get in touch with a sense of thriving in life can be considered spiritual. As you reflect on your own experience of spirituality and the practices in life that help you to return to a sense of centeredness and balance, consider the following questions:

- What helps me to feel a sense of joy in my life?
- Why do I want to serve other people in my profession?
- What would I do in my spare time if I could do anything I wanted to do?
- How do I feel after doing _________? (activity): renewed, drained, calm, motivated
- If not positive feelings, what do I need to do to experience those feelings more often in my life?

Caring for self includes balancing your professional work with personal joys. While life often brings with it the fullness of family life, service obligations, and other duties, consider how you can consistently bring in any of the following activities that enliven your spiritual dimension. Remember, any activity that draws you into a sense of "flow" or losing sense of time and feeling joy, while not being detrimental to your body and well-being, can be considered a spiritual practice. Anything that contributes to your thriving counts. The following are only examples and not exhaustive:

- Reading a book for fun
- Yoga or other mindful movement practice
- Walking
- Artistic projects or music
- Meditation: mindfulness or transcendental
- Being out in nature
- Cooking a meal without rushing
- Journaling
- Engaging in unrushed moments with a family member or friend
- Play: with children, playful movement, using imagination

Practices that can help the provider within the work day to return a sense of physiologic calm, which in turn helps them to maintain a sense of meaning or purpose, may include such practices as:

- Heart-focused breathing
- Taking a deep three-dimensional breath (all three dimensions of the rib cage expand with inhalation and passively contract with exhalation) with the focus on the movement of air in and out of the body
- Doing a "body scan" for tight muscles in one's body, then focusing on one muscle to relax for a few seconds with breathing
- Using proprioception or interoception to sense the state of one's pelvic floor and associated gluteal muscles—take a moment to relax them
- Adopting a mantra or saying to return to between patients or in "down" moments; such as "I am supported in my work," or "I choose to be a conduit of service today," or "I choose to be grounded in joy in this moment."

Remember that returning to a sense of physiologic calm contributes to one's ability to connect with one's own sense of the transcendent, which allows a return to connections with the meaningful aspects of life. This is living out spirituality in everyday practice, even while accomplishing our work as health care providers.[519]

## PAIN PERCEPTION: THE LINK BETWEEN PSYCHOLOGIC AND PHYSICAL CONNECTIONS

### Overview

Pain has been defined as an unpleasant sensory and emotional experience associated with actual or potential tissue damage.[322] Pain is one of the most important functions of the nervous system and provides information about the presence or threat of injury. Pain is a complex perception and exists 100% of the time when the brain perceives greater credible evidence of danger than safety. Conversely, pain does not exist when the brain perceives greater credible evidence of safety than danger.[338] Pain can be thought about as a phenomenon that has a distinct feature separate from the physical response of nociception; it can develop into a feeling that compels us to protect a body part by our larger self that has agency over our body. Integral to this are the relationships between true danger to the body, nociception, and pain. These relationships are variable and progressively more tenuous as pain persists. The biopsychosocial model declares that pain involves the intricate, variable interaction of biologic factors (genetics, biochemical, etc.), psychologic factors (mood, personality, behavior, etc.), and social factors (cultural, familial, socioeconomic, medical, etc.). In other words, pain is complex, can be difficult, and requires time, effort, and serious work to understand.[339]

Chronic or persistent pain has been recognized as pain that persists past the normal time of tissue healing, thus lacking the acute warning function of physiologic nociception.[87] Persistent pain can occur with a wide variety of musculoskeletal, neurologic, endocrine, and oncologic diagnoses.[136] The progression of acute to chronic pain can result in more complex and devastating physical, psychologic, and socioeconomic sequelae than the original disease entity.[136] Box 3.2 lists the most common chronic pain conditions encountered by the physical therapist.

Persistent pain is associated with increased rates of depressive disorders[374] and suicidal tendencies.[416] The associated mental disorders may precede the pain disorder and possibly predispose the individual to it, co-occur with the pain, or result from the pain.[19]

Persistent pain disorders can occur at any age and are extremely common, with some estimating that approximately one third of adults in the United States are influenced by chronic pain, with 39.5 million adults who report daily pain.[403] Health economists have reported the annual cost of persistent pain in the United States is as high as $635 billion a year, which is more than the yearly costs for cancer, heart disease, and diabetes.[99]

Acute pain serves as a warning system and serves to protect from tissue damage. It follows a linear, predictable timeline for healing and carries the expectation of resolution. Chronic pain is less well-defined, follows an emergent unpredictable timeline for healing, is not protective, and does not serve a biologic purpose. Because it is difficult to treat and is more complex to resolve, the therapist should support both realistic and hopeful expectations.[290]

**Box 3.2**

**COMMON CHRONIC PAIN CONDITIONS**

- Arthritis
- Persistent neck/back pain
- Neuralgias
- Peripheral neuropathies
- Peripheral vascular disease
- Causalgia
- Chronic regional pain syndrome (formerly reflex sympathetic dystrophy)
- Hyperesthesia
- Myofascial pain syndrome
- Fibromyalgia syndrome
- Phantom limb pain
- Cancer
- Postoperative pain
- Spinal stenosis

### Risk Factors

Predisposition to pain is difficult to determine because so many factors come into play. In a systematic review of persistent pain following traumatic injury, predictive factors for persistent pain included symptoms of anxiety and depression, patients' perception that the injury was attributable to an external source meaning that the patient was not at fault, cognitive avoidance of distressing thoughts, alcohol consumption prior to the trauma, lower educational status, injury at work, eligibility for compensation, pain at initial assessment, and older age, all factors that may be a function of biologic and psychologic vulnerabilities.[426]

The extent of pain experiences follows the importance of the pain and the interpretation of the pain based on previous experience, beliefs, attitudes, and expectations. Available coping strategies affect the responses. Resultant behaviors are influenced by psychologic variables, such as pain catastrophizing that results in exaggerated negative attitude to a minimal physical event,[489] fear-avoidance behaviors,[269,271] and pain-related anxiety,[436,531] which can impact postsurgical and rehabilitation outcomes.[144] The greatest pain burden, persistent disability, and poorer treatment outcome can be linked to several factors: lower formal education levels, poorer self-rated health status, lower socioeconomic status, decreased self-efficacy, history of smoking, and depression.[59,123,278,386,394,429,520,553]

Among the most common general medical conditions associated with persistent pain are musculoskeletal conditions, typically disk herniation, osteoporosis, osteoarthritis or rheumatoid arthritis, myofascial syndromes, neuropathies associated with diabetic neuropathies, postherpetic neuralgia, and malignancies in which the tumor infiltrates nerves and bone.[19,288]

### Etiology and Pathogenesis

The neurophysiologic changes that occur in the presence of persistent pain are complex and prolonged neurochemical changes. This process includes increased sensitization of peripheral and central nociceptive pathways and changes in areas of sensory appreciation in the cortex. From the peripheral direction, noxious stimuli to dorsal horn neurons cause substance P and glutamate to produce cellular changes, which can enhance nociceptive transmission to the brain.

Sensitization of central pathways reflects changes in cortical sites that are involved in sensory discrimination, including the somatosensory cortex. Other sites can be affected that relate to motivation, such as the cingulate and insular cortices and amygdala. Abnormal sensitization in the prefrontal cortex can affect the planning of complex cognitive behaviors, personality expression, decision making, and moderating social behavior. This sensitization can spread its effects to the motor cortex and motor neurons, which changes the choices for movement.

Prolonged central sensitization or decreased threshold of neural excitability eventually requires lower or no external stimuli to be self-perpetuating. In addition to sustaining cellular changes in the spinal cord, individuals with persistent pain have a more complex brain response to additional pain experiences than people without persistent pain histories. Persistent pain can impair sleep, cognitive function, memory, mood, cardiovascular health, digestive health, endocrine function, inflammatory processes, and sexual function and influence every facet of an individual's social interactions.[136]

Persistent pain disorders can be psychologically based, the result of a general medical condition, or a mixture of both. Persistent pain may also be linked to psychologic trauma through memories of physical trauma, transference of psychologic distress, or by decreased immune responses and healing.[168,118] Psychologic history may be critical in the transition from acute to chronic pain and predictive of the development of chronic pain postoperatively.[135] An increasing number of studies now support the concept that spinal pain is commonly triggered by biopsychosocial factors that may influence prognosis,[363,490] transitioning from acute to persistent pain,[277] leading to development of disability.[203,289,316,490]

## Diagnosis and Clinical Manifestations

### Pain Mechanism Classification Systems

The clinical evaluation of pain currently involves identification or diagnosis of the primary disease/etiologic factors considered responsible for producing/initiating the pain; placing the individual within a pain mechanism category, and then identifying the anatomic distribution, quality, and intensity of pain. Classification systems and subgrouping leads to more effective and efficient interventions. Subgrouping patients assists clinicians in recognizing dominant psychologic and physiologic factors to aid in the interpretation of the patient's prognosis and selection of interventions and to maximize outcomes.[249]

*Nociceptive pain* is caused by an injury that stimulates pain receptors. This pain mechanism is related to neural tissue outside the dorsal and medullary horns, such as nerve root, trunk, and axon, and their connective tissues. Nociceptive pain is primarily due to nociceptor activation, further processed through the central nervous system (CNS), typically resulting in acute localized pain. Examples of stimuli that can sensitize nociceptors are in Box 3.3. Within the CNS, nociceptive signals are under constant modulation by cortical and brain-stem pathways, which can be facilitatory or inhibitory.

Box 3.3

**NOCICEPTORS ACTIVATED BY THE FOLLOWING CAN RESULT IN THE SENSATION OF PAIN**

Mechanical pressure
Heat or cold
Byproducts of inflammation
Hormones released at the site of tissue damage or infection
Release of bradykinins related to asthma and gut disorders
Cytokines such as interferon, interleukin, and tumor necrosis factors related to immune system function
Waste products (metabolites) produced during excessive muscular contraction including chloride, potassium, lactic acid, ATP, magnesium ($Mg^{2+}$), reactive oxygen species, and inorganic phosphate.

Box 3.4

**PAIN PERCEIVED BY THE CORTEX CAUSES CHANGES IN BEHAVIOR AND ANS RESPONSES**

- Posturing (guarding) in limbs due to muscle spasm
- Abnormal gait patterns
- Enhanced sympathetic activity resulting in sweating, rapid shallow breathing, increased heart rate and blood pressure
- Irritability and depressed mood
- Increased sensitivity to environmental stimuli

Emotional and sensory components of pain are also modulated at higher levels. The pain signals travel through the nervous system for recognition and response to an injury or the possibility for injury. As nociceptive pain develops, there is increased responsiveness and reduced threshold of nociceptive neurons in the periphery to the stimulation of their receptive fields. Neurons become more excitable or sensitized. Peripheral sensitization of nociceptive neurons can enhance or prolong the pain experience, even without sensitization of central neurons. As the response magnitude to noxious stimuli increases or the response threshold to noxious stimuli decreases, there can also be spontaneous activity and activation of silent nociceptors. Increases in receptive field size may also occur. Box 3.4 describes changes the therapist should consider as possible phenomena related to nociceptive changes.[292]

*Peripheral nociceptive inflammation* is related to excessive fluid that activates nociceptors that are thermal, mechanical, and chemical. This mechanism occurs at the neuron level (primary nociceptor) in response to specific irritation from inflammation and occurs in connective tissue in the periphery (muscle, ligament, bone, tendon, fascia, cartilage).

*Peripheral nociceptive ischemia* is related to insufficient blood flow and oxygen. It originates in target tissues as a result of mechanical and physiologic processes of injured tissues that stimulate high threshold primary afferent C and A-delta fibers. Tissues become more acidic, hypoxic, and rich in chemicals such as bradykinin, potassium ions, and prostaglandins. Essential circulation is deprived as a result of continuous stretching, compression, sustained positioning, or poor repair and remodeling phases of connective tissue healing.

*Nociplastic pain* arises from altered nociception despite no clear evidence of actual or threatened tissue damage causing the activation of peripheral nociceptors or evidence for disease or lesion of the somatosensory system causing the pain. Alterations of nociceptive processing within the CNS are suspected such as enhanced central excitability or diminished central inhibition. This has been referred to as central sensitization. Nociplastic pain is more persistent and widespread than nociceptive pain. Nociplastic pain can occur independently of peripheral nociceptor activity but can be concurrent with nociceptive pain. The patient's pain alarm system is in an overprotective mode.[85] The altered CNS circuitry and processing are dominated by the patient's thoughts, beliefs, fears, worries, and concerns related to the pain experience and the potential threat of the injury, unhealed tissue, or pathology. Pain education to reduce fears, unhelpful beliefs, and misconceptions should be the central focus in care.

*Neuropathic pain* is caused by a lesion or disease that changes the function of the somatosensory nervous system. Neuropathic and neurogenic pain result from alterations in nerve structure, function, and dynamics that cause neural dysfunction. It may also involve the nerve's interface with other tissues in its anatomic path, as in neural entrapment. Neuropathic pain is evidenced by positive neural symptoms such as tingling, burning, and dysesthesia, or negative neural symptoms such as loss of sensation. These symptoms can be evaluated using sensory testing or the painDETECT questionnaire.[147]

**Affective.** This pain mechanism involves central pathways and circuits and is related to negative emotions and their perception. Emotion or affect is a dimension of the pain experience, as well as a possible mechanism contributing to it. In other words, pain can manifest as the result of emotional turmoil or an unresolved emotional or social conflict. The way people think and feel has vast repercussions on brain processing, and growing evidence has shown that psychosomatic (mind-body) disorders may develop as a result of repressed negative emotions in the unconscious mind related to life pressures, childhood experiences, and relationships. A three-dimensional journal to track pain experiences is a helpful tool for patients to self-discover the triggers and alleviators in three dimensions of pain: mechanical/physical, emotional/mental, and social.

**Motor/Autonomic.** This pain mechanism involves pain related to various output systems of the brain. It involves the involuntary sympathetic and parasympathetic systems. Symptoms are heavily influenced by the somatic, motor, and autonomic nervous systems, as well as neuroendocrine and immune system symptoms. General malaise, lymphedema, spasticity, tone, and hypersensitivity are common symptoms when this pain mechanism is dominating.

There is still some discussion about how to label normal but less helpful psychologic reactions to injury compared to psychopathology such as depression and PTSD

**Fear-Avoidance Behavior.** Fear-avoidance behaviors can also be a part of disability from chronic pain. The Fear-Avoidance Model of Exaggerated Pain Perception was first introduced in the early 1980s.[248,468] The concept is based on studies that show a person's fear of pain (not physical impairments) is the most important factor in how he or she responds to low back pain.

Fear of pain commonly leads to avoiding physical or social activities. Screening for fear-avoidance behaviors can be done using the Fear-Avoidance Beliefs Questionnaire (FABQ).[532] Elevated fear-avoidance beliefs are indicative of someone who has been in the past considered a poor candidate for rehabilitation. However, it is now considered an indication for modified approaches that can be highly successful. Success is often heightened with collaboration with the pain-educated psychologist or behavioral counselor.

Fear of pain commonly leads to avoiding physical or social activities. When the client shows signs of fear-avoidance beliefs, then the therapist's management approach should include education that addresses the client's fear and avoidance behavior while considering a graded approach to therapeutic exercise.[158] It is important that education include the concept that persistent pain does not mean continued tissue injury is taking place.[544]

### Treatment

Pain mechanisms are used to describe factors that can contribute to the development, maintenance, or enhancement of pain. They can occur in a cyclical manner in reaction to the pain. It is important to remember that multiple pain mechanisms may occur simultaneously. Clinicians are encouraged to screen for signs of altered nociceptive function, thus improving diagnosis and treatment, because patients suffering from altered nociceptive function typically respond better to central than peripheral targeted therapies.[159]

A mechanism-based approach to pain management incorporates and builds on the biopsychosocial model by defining specific pathobiology in pain processing and pain-relevant psychologic factors. Movement disorders may reflect the pain mechanism. Mechanism-based evaluation of specific pain mechanisms leads to prescribing the appropriate treatments to target altered mechanisms. Pain processing physiology, as well as psychologic states, can vary within a single diagnosis. Education may be the most useful for those with maladaptive cognitions and behaviors associated with altered CNS processing. This educational model has been shown to increase central inhibition.[524]

### Prognosis

Pain neuroscience education for chronic musculoskeletal disorders is effective in reducing pain and improving patient knowledge of pain, improving function and lowering disability, reducing psychosocial factors, enhancing movement, and minimizing health care utilization. Pain levels in chronic pain sufferers have been demonstrated to drop an average of 3 points on the NPRS pain scale after one year with the use of pacing, graded exposure, exercise and pain neuroscience education.[271,468]

SPECIAL IMPLICATIONS FOR THE THERAPIST 3.3

## Intervention for Persistent or Chronic Pain Disorders

*The cornerstone of a unified approach to chronic pain syndrome is a comprehensive behavioral program. Whenever possible, the physical therapist should reinforce the behavioral approaches used by the other members of the team. Some of these goals are listed in Box 3.5.*

### Pain Neuroscience Education

The educational model of teaching people about pain biology and physiology is called therapeutic neuroscience education or pain neuroscience education. It aims to explain to patients the biologic and physiologic processes involved in a pain experience and, more importantly, defocus the issues associated with anatomic structures. Physical therapists demonstrate that pain education provides compelling evidence in reducing pain, disability, pain responses, and limitation of functional physical movement.[287,293,470,503]

A more extensive social history can be used to assess the client's recent life stressors and history of depression or drug or alcohol abuse. Pain may lead to inactivity and social isolation, which in turn can lead to additional depression and anxiety. Reduction in physical endurance results in fatigue and additional pain.

- The ACES study, Life Stress Indicators, and Yellow Flag Risk Form questionnaires are helpful outcome measurement tools to promote patient awareness and guide treatment plans.
- The FABQ[165,532] can be useful to indicate clients who have high fear avoidance and indicate the need to modify intervention choices and consider referral to a psychologist or behavioral counselor. The work subscale of the FABQ is the strongest predictor of work status. There is a greater likelihood of return-to-work for scores less than 30 and less likelihood of return-to-work or increased risk of prolonged work restrictions for scores greater than 34.[151]
- Screening for depression in patients with chronic pain related to musculoskeletal diagnoses can be conducted using a brief two-question screening tool using yes or no responses from the *Primary Care Evaluation of Mental Disorders Procedure*: (1) "During the past month, have you often been bothered by feeling down, depressed or hopeless?" (2) "During the past month, have you often been bothered by little interest or pleasure in doing things?"[177]
- Cognitive-behavioral interventions (CBT) are based on the concept that thoughts and perceptions influence behavior. Feeling distressed may distort one's perception of reality. CBT aims to identify harmful thoughts, assess whether they are an accurate depiction of reality, and if they are not, employ strategies to challenge and overcome them.
- Knowledge of progress in treatment is useful for clients and may prompt joint problem solving and education that will influence exploring pain behavior or other factors influencing the client's perceptions, including self-control and self-efficacy.[181,517]
- Regular exercise reduces central excitability and expression of excitatory neurotransmitters in spinal cord, brain stem, and cortical nociceptive sites. Regular exercise reduces glial cell activation, increases antiinflammatory cytokines, and decreases inflammatory cytokines in the spinal cord. Exercise improves depression, anxiety, pain catastrophizing, and fear of movement.[275] In people with diabetic neuropathy, increased growth of epidermal nerve fibers after a regular exercise program creates decreased pain and can be considered a disease-modifying treatment in neuropathic pain by enhancing healing of injured tissues. These concepts can be integrated into interventions appropriate for each level of pain mechanism.
- Pain Coping Skills Training can include
  - Deep breathing
  - Progressive muscle relaxation
  - Guided imagery
  - Pacing/activity-rest cycling
  - Pleasant/valued activities
  - Cognitive restructuring (balancing thoughts)
  - Mindfulness meditation
  - Movement therapy such as yoga and tai chi[343,446]
- Virtual Hope Box (2014 DoD Innovation Award) is an accessory to treatment (coping, relaxation, distraction, positive thinking)
- Graded motor imagery, right-left discrimination, mirror therapy, self-regulation strategies, and education regarding the polyvagal theory are useful treatment interventions.

Box 3.5

**BEHAVIORAL GOALS AND GUIDELINES FOR PERSISTENT OR CHRONIC PAIN**

- Identify and eliminate pain reinforcers.
- Decrease drug use.
- Use positive reinforcers that shift the focus from pain.
- Concentrate on abilities, not disabilities.
- Avoid the concept of cure; concentrate on control of pain and improved function.
- Avoid discussion of pain except as arranged by the team (e.g., only during monthly reevaluation, only with a designated team member).
- Use a home program to focus on function and functional outcome (e.g., self-help tasks within capabilities).
- The client should keep a log of accomplishments so that progress can be measured and remembered.
- Measure success by what the individual client can accomplish, not based on others' success or expectations.
- Take one day at a time. Direct energy toward solving today's problems rather than focusing on the future.
- Avoid negative reinforcers such as sympathy and attention to symptoms, especially pain.
- Encourage tolerance to increasing activity levels.
- Gradual progress is better than quick results with increased symptoms.
- Teach the client how and when to ask for and accept help when necessary. Do not offer help or yield to the demands of someone who does not need help.

# TRAUMA

## Overview

Trauma and psychologic contributors can cause extensive comorbidity for people treated by rehabilitation providers. Trauma can be defined as an overwhelming or life-threatening event either experienced or witnessed resulting in intense fear, helplessness, and horror. The physiologic responses to trauma known as fight-or-flight responses of the sympathetic nervous system and the freeze response of the dorsal vagal system of the parasympathetic nervous system are immediate, automatic, and appropriate responses to avoid danger or imminent harm. The emotional responses to the traumatic event and the resulting autonomic nervous system dysregulation are more complex and individual, with different coping responses that may be influenced by family history, genetic influences, and emotional development.

Trauma can include physical, sexual or emotional abuse, violent physical injury such as motor vehicle accidents (MVAs), injuries sustained during combat, assault, and medical interventions and surgeries. An unexpected event perceived as a threat (e.g., dog bite) can result in acute psychologic stress symptoms such as anxiety, dissociation (detachment of the mind from the emotional state or even the body), intense fear, helplessness or horror, reexperiencing the event and increased arousal.[20]

*Physical abuse* involves nonaccidental physical injury, which can range from superficial bruises and welts to broken bones, burns, serious internal injuries, and death. *Emotional and psychologic abuse* can result from acts or omissions that cause or could cause serious behavioral, cognitive, emotional, or mental disorders as a result of actions such as confinement or the constant use of verbally abusive language and criticism. *Sexual abuse* ranges from nontouching offenses, such as exhibitionism, to the contact offenses that include fondling, rape, molestation, or the forced use of a child or an adult in the production of pornographic materials. *Neglect* can involve the withholding of or failure to provide adequate food, shelter, clothing, hygiene, emotional support, medical care, or supervision needed for optimal health and well-being. Neglect also includes refusal of or delay in seeking health care, abandonment, inadequate supervision, and expulsion from home. *Stalking* involves repeated visual or physical proximity, nonconsensual communication, or verbal, written, or implied threats, or a combination thereof, that would cause a reasonable person fear.

Observation of physical trauma such as torture, disasters, or violent personal assaults[476] can result in the development of *acute stress disorder*, which is the appropriate diagnosis if the characteristic anxiety, dissociative, and other symptoms occur within 1 month of the trauma.[21] If these symptoms are still present beyond 4 weeks, the diagnosis changes to *post-traumatic stress disorder*.

Terrorist activities and the fear associated have negative effects on the general public. Just living in the approximate area of exposure can cause traumatic stress responses. The number of individuals suffering psychogenic illness could far exceed the number of actual casualties in a chemical, biologic, radiologic, or other life-threatening event.[335] Distress experienced in populations and social groups can persist for at least 18 months after an incident. It is critical to maintain open and consistent communication, personal involvement with those perceiving or recovering from trauma, and community support in trauma healing.[335]

Medical diagnostics and treatment have been directed toward physical causes often without adequate consideration of emotional and psychologic symptoms as primary diagnoses, secondary responses, or comorbid conditions. Psychologic diagnoses are also extremely important to consider for overall prognosis.[150,151,277,363] If medical and rehabilitation professionals ignore the psychologic elements of a person's diagnosis or the causative factors, outcomes are often adversely impacted.[363] Attention to psychologic resources, personal beliefs, support systems, resiliency, self-efficacy, and spiritual reserves are critical to healing and enhanced outcomes.

## Incidence

Family and interpersonal violence is the most common type of trauma. Table 3.1 reports incidence rates. Torture and war provide intense, repeated, and extremely

**Table 3.1** Incidence of Interpersonal Trauma

| Type of Trauma | Reported Incidence |
|---|---|
| Child Abuse | • A global meta-analysis concluded that 12.7% of the population reported that they had been victims of childhood sexual abuse: 18% females, 7.6% males.[484]<br>• In the United States, more than 740,000 children are treated in hospital departments as a result of violence each year.<br>• Youth violence resulted in more than 656,000 emergency room treatments in 2008 with nearly 6,000 homicides in 2007. |
| Adult/Elder Abuse | • 1-2 million adults older than age 65 yr are estimated to suffer abuse or neglect annually.<br>• Violence accounts for approximately 51,000 deaths in the United States annually. |
| Rape | • In a national survey of 9,684 adults, 10.6% female and 2.1% male respondents reported being raped at some stage in their lives, with 60%-70% of these individuals being raped before age 18,[49] while another survey reported as many as 17.6% of women and 3% of men reporting forcible rape.[509] |

Modified from Centers for Disease Control and Prevention (CDC). *Injury center: violence prevention.* Available online at http://www.cdc.gov/ViolencePrevention/; Stoltenborgh M: The neglect of child neglect: a meta-analytic review of the prevalence of neglect. *Soc Psychiatry Psychiatr Epidemiol* 48(3):345–355, 2013.

damaging stressors for those directly involved, for their families, and sometimes even for medical personnel who are called upon to assist with individuals who are being tortured.[83] Large numbers of refugees who now reside in the United States have experienced or witnessed torture to varying degrees.[167] They have also been exposed to death on a large scale, with high prevalence of major depressive disorders, post-traumatic stress disorder (PTSD), anxiety and panic attacks, as well as physical and psychologic pain.[167,242]

The trauma of war can affect not only the warriors, but also their partners and children. Trauma associated with war can cause problems with self-esteem, communication, sexuality, and parenting. A condition of hyperawareness or hyperarousal is common long after the euphoria of returning home has worn off. Adrenaline rushes from constantly being on alert in war zones do not just get turned off once the soldier is home or in a safe environment.

Combat trauma can lead to anxiety, depression, PTSD, addiction, and other forms of emotional and physical pain. The most common problems confronting families of combat veterans include addiction, emotional numbing, sexual difficulties, anger, family violence, and guilt. Healing the wounds of war is becoming the focus of new research and clinical attention.[297]

## Pathogenesis

Worry, fear of the unknown, and other anxieties are normal occurrences, which usually resolve. Empathetic support from caring people who listen, offer reassurance, and point out options for dealing with the event may help alleviate fear or anxiety.[458] In the presence of danger, fear is helpful for the purpose of initiating an appropriate short-term survival response, referred to as the sympathetic fight, flight, or freeze response already mentioned. Anxiety or fear of potential threat in the absence of real danger or for extensive time periods can cause damaging psychologic and physiologic patterns.

Animal studies confirm that in repeated experiences of overwhelming trauma, freezing becomes the default coping mechanism, even when other options for escape or defense are available. *Dissociation* (lapses in consciousness, decreased awareness of the surroundings, loss of memory, or occasionally loss of identity) is an extreme manifestation of the freeze response that occurs as a response to severe trauma.[344,441,443,522] The concept of dissociation is defined as *a detachment of the mind from the emotional state or body*. This condition can be as mild and fleeting as daydreaming, or it can be so severe that the personality is shattered into adaptive "parts" such as in dissociative identity disorder.

Living in the shadow of unresolved trauma and depending constantly on coping systems designed as temporary, short-term defenses for survival have implications for physical, emotional, mental, and spiritual health. Individuals with dysregulated responses to unresolved trauma (including dissociation) are often unaware of their fractured state until the coping mechanisms begin to break down and functioning becomes increasingly difficult.

There is also a negative impact on the brain and sympathetic nervous system as a result of the long-term effects of living in a constant state of anxiety and survival mode. Persistent fear and a sense of being unsafe, either perceived or real, has devastating effects on every aspect of health. The normal acute stress responses include activation of the hypothalamic-pituitary-adrenal system with release of cortisol, epinephrine, and norepinephrine, resulting in the fight-or-flight response.[163] The release of cortisol reduces metabolic activity and elevates blood glucose. After prolonged stress responses, the body responds by activating a negative control on the hypothalamic-pituitary-adrenal system to stop the acute responses when high levels of cortisol are present.[163,542] Persistent, long-term stress without resolution results in a down-regulated system with low cortisol levels and the possibility of decreased immune function. The physical effects of low cortisol are closely related to inadequate immune responses to microtrauma,[163] infection, or neoplasms.[168]

Impairments in the regulatory cycle of the hypothalamic-pituitary-adrenal system may correspond with physical pain, excessive fatigue, and tension with negative effects on the anatomy and function of the brain. Young children who experience abuse or neglect show abnormal cortisol levels, indicative of a dysregulated stress response. These changes often remain after the child has been removed to a safe, caring environment and are persistent in individuals who show clinical or subclinical symptoms of PTSD.[170,483]

Individuals with PTSD have also been shown to exhibit high levels of inflammatory cytokines partly attributed to low cortisol levels.[163,168] However, the opposite relationship has also been proposed whereby chronic inflammation results in changes in dopamine activity in the hippocampus and amygdala, contributing to fear responses and memory retrieval of trauma with similar symptoms to individuals with major depression.[163,168] Research continues to explore these relationships, as well as pharmacologic management, including serotonin uptake inhibitors and responses to hydrocortisone.

### Effects of Developmental Trauma on Brain Development: A-Type (Neglect) Trauma and B-Type (Abuse) Trauma

The terms *type A* and *type B* psychologic trauma have been used to describe *neglect* (type A) and *abuse* (type B). Type A trauma results from the absence of positive support for psychologic health and well-being, such as nurturing by and healthy bonding with parents. Physiologically, lack of early childhood support results in changes in the limbic and related areas of the brain where strong emotions are processed and stored. Type A traumas will present as painful feelings emerging when the wounded person realizes the impact of lack of nurturing in his or her own development.

Type B traumas are negative events that take place during childhood or adulthood. Dissociative coping mechanisms and barriers or distortions to memory are more likely to result from negative events. The harbored reactions, feelings, and beliefs related to the trauma stimulate a flight-or-fight fear reaction associated with sympathetic nervous system activation as well as a shutting-down response associated with the dorsal vagal system of the

**Table 3.2** Developmental Impact of Trauma

| Age | Normal Developmental Steps | Potential Tendencies and Traits |
|---|---|---|
| Birth to 3 years | • Caregivers meet needs in healthy ways (temperature, caring/protective touch)<br>• Caregiver relationships, faces and voice tones confirm personal value/belonging<br>• Child experiences safety; healthy conflict resolution and management of emotions is modeled by caregivers | • Fear and insecurity in relationships<br>• Manipulative, self-centered, isolated, or discontented personality<br>• Difficulty regulating emotions; emotional outbursts, worry, depression<br>• Narrow scope of emotional tolerance |
| 4 to 12 years | • Child learns to identify needs, ask and receive appropriately<br>• Child discovers and owns up to the consequences of own choices/behaviors<br>• Child sees benefit in doing tasks the child does not feel like doing<br>• Child experiences success exercising own talents and initiative | • Passive-aggressive; persistent frustration/disappointment when needs and expectations are not met<br>• Addictive; searching for satisfaction<br>• History of repeated failure; "stuck," undependable, focuses on comfort, daydream fantasies<br>• Unproductive goals and activities |
| 13 years to birth of first child | • Young adult cares for self and others<br>• Young adult able to tolerate and successfully manage difficult situations<br>• Young adult recognizes and owns effects of personal actions on self and others; able to contain self; avoids harm to others<br>• Young adult is able to maintain healthy relationships over time and distance | • Self-centered; difficult to be around<br>• Conforms to negative/destructive group activities<br>• Insensitive to others; defensive, controlling, harmful, victim mentality<br>• Shows excessive self-importance, loner |

*Note:* Failure to receive healthy nurture and instructions listed as part of Normal Developmental Steps can lead to unhealthy tendencies and traits listed.
Data from Wilder EJ: *The life model,* Pasadena, CA, 2004, Shepherd's House.

parasympathetic nervous system, influencing the ability to receive or express joy. Dissociative amnesia is the brain's coping mechanism for overwhelming, life-threatening trauma and can occur any time after infancy.[20,442]

Both type A and type B traumas increase the individual's conscious and unconscious need for self-protection, activating the sympathetic system and escalating adrenal activity. Self-perpetuation of mixed messages (the inability of the brain's two hemispheres to make sense of and resolve the explicit cognitive message and implicit sensory input) results in a persistent sense of helplessness. The conflicting and stressful input can cause sustained elevated cortisol levels, expressed physically as somatic pain and psychologically as emotional representations of the ongoing internal, mental conflict.

Mild-to-extreme incidents of sexual trauma and domestic violence are frequently well hidden. Often individuals do not disclose their history of abuse because of feelings of shame and guilt and fear of retribution.[180] The fear of not being believed, as well as implications for further violence or loss of support, also may result in not disclosing the trauma. The effects of trauma in early development on brain cognition and memory can destroy victim credibility and promote denial in the victim. Physicians and therapists who serve as entry points into the health care system need to be able to recognize signs of psychologic trauma presenting as primary diagnoses, secondary comorbidities, or somatic symptoms in order to be able to refer to mental health professionals and to adapt evaluation and treatment strategies.[115,196,276,444,443]

If the trauma is severe, the sense of self can be shattered, confounding identity and destroying the concept of personal boundaries. Childhood trauma disrupts the course of normal development and perpetuates brain dysregulation. Consistent character traits and functional difficulties can be traced from deficits in early development. Major deficits in any of the normal developmental steps can lead to the unhealthy tendencies and traits listed in Table 3.2.

## Diagnosis

### Identification and Disclosure of History of Trauma

Many physical, mental, and emotional pain and behavioral problems are common to abuse, and traumatic experience survivors often experience their problems as primarily somatic.[522] Because of dissociation, amnesia, and survival reactions at the time of trauma, the person may not have any conscious awareness of the abuse and trauma history until much later, especially if the trauma occurred during childhood.[523]

People suffering from unresolved trauma often work to cover their severe distrust of people and unfamiliar environments. Safety, real or perceived, is foreign and unidentifiable because of their history. The effects of past trauma can be expressed both physically and emotionally and are set off by normal daily events, especially medical treatment. Sensory information through sound, smell, taste, sight, touch, and position or movement that replicates the original trauma can elicit physical or emotional reactions, apparently unrelated to the current treatment focus or context.[441,443,444]

Medical offices may be associated with care following the trauma and can make even a person without a traumatic background feel uneasy or unsafe. The clinician

**Table 3.3** Signs of Unresolved Trauma

| Physical | Emotional | Behavioral | Mental |
|---|---|---|---|
| • Hypervigilance<br>• Cannot differentiate between healthy and unhealthy pain<br>• Joint and muscle pain<br>• Headaches, shoulder and neck pain, and tension-related problems<br>• Balance, vestibular problems, and dizziness<br>• Visual disturbances or loss<br>• Hearing loss and tinnitus<br>• Recurrent high blood pressure<br>• Gait abnormalities<br>• Paresis<br>• Disconnection from body<br>• Syndromes and diseases, such as:<br>  • Chronic fatigue syndrome<br>  • Fibromyalgia<br>  • Irritable bowel syndrome<br>  • Reactive bladder<br>  • Restless legs syndrome<br>  • Meniere disease<br>  • Lupus erythematosus<br>  • Multiple sclerosis<br>  • Autoimmune diseases<br>• Teeth clenching and bruxing (grinding)<br>• Digestive and intestinal problems<br>• Blood pressure problems, heart arrhythmias, chest pain<br>• Nervous tics, tremors<br>• Rashes, itching<br>• Exhaustion<br>• Allergies<br>• Insomnia<br>• Shortness of breath<br>• Diagnoses unresolved by medical tests and treatment; comorbidity | • Egocentric, self-blame ("I am the cause of everything that happens")<br>• Inability to tolerate feelings or conflicts<br>• Intense self-blame and feeling unworthy<br>• Staying stuck in victim or perpetrator roles<br>• Disconnection from feelings, emotions<br>• Feeling very isolated, alone, vulnerable<br>• Anxious, fearful, panic attacks—fear of the unknown, consistently anticipating the worst<br>• Depression, doubt, discouragement<br>• Paranoia, distrust<br>• Secrecy, guilt, shame<br>• Insecurity/poor self-worth<br>• Feeling out-of-control, overwhelmed, at the end of one's rope<br>• Sudden, exaggerated emotional reactions<br>• Flaring anger, rage, hatred; abusive talk/actions<br>• Quarreling, fighting, complaining, judging<br>• Nightmares, sleep disorders; flashbacks, "triggers"<br>• Bitterness, resentment, shame | • Cannot recognize, define, or emulate healthy behaviors, relationships<br>• Does not know what is "normal"<br>• Does not know how to model or live "normal"<br>• Child-like, unrefined, or harsh social skills<br>• Difficulty with relationships; unhealthy boundaries<br>• Self-injury, self-persecution/blame; destructive lifestyle<br>• Inappropriate threat/defense reactions<br>• Failure to own responsibility; victim mentality<br>• Greed, materialism<br>• Cheating; lying; stealing; apathy; laziness; procrastination<br>• Obsessive; impulse driven<br>• Disorganization, procrastination<br>• Difficulty keeping promises, appointments<br>• Reactive, inconsistent personality traits<br>• Reckless driving, accident prone<br>• Impatience, irritability, inappropriate social reactions<br>• Disorders in eating, sleeping, sexual desire<br>• Addictions—alcohol, drugs, sexual, smoking, food<br>• Inability to speak needs or feelings<br>• Withdrawn, isolated, loner<br>• Disorganized attachment patterns—clinging or avoidance behaviors<br>• Out-of-control, self-injurious, and/or suicidal behaviors and patterns | • Difficulty with problem solving and intentional focus<br>• Confusion, forgetfulness<br>• Difficulty saying "No" and/or making decisions<br>• Intrusive, negative, or destructive thoughts, images, feelings<br>• Failure to recognize and act on available options<br>• Identity confusion and deception; overriding focus on self |

Data compiled by Bonnie Yost; sources available on request.

may use hands-on techniques, such as pushing, pulling, stretching, compressing, touching, rubbing, and other sensory or sudden changes, that can impact a client with a history of abuse in a negative way. Persistence in cajoling, cheerleading, or demanding compliance meant as encouragement may further victimize the individual. In addition, default coping strategies surface repeatedly and reinforce the physical, emotional, and mental survival reactions as if past trauma was occurring in the present. This often presents as "freeze" reactions accompanied by shallow breathing or breath holding.

These triggers might be difficult for the physical therapist or client to identify without careful observation of body language, consistency of verbal responses, or through questioning.[115,443,444] The astute provider can look beyond the superficial and obvious symptoms to consider the contributions from all systems and underlying pathology. Dissociative changes are very subtle, allowing the survivor to conceal tremendous turmoil internally. Table 3.3 lists the most common signs and symptoms of unseen wounds and unresolved trauma; this list is not exhaustive, and there may be other symptoms experienced by some people. Sensitive observation, attentive listening, and appropriate questions help the clinician to grasp subtle changes that indicate client status.

SPECIAL IMPLICATIONS FOR THE THERAPIST 3.4

## *Trauma*

*Therapists frequently encounter people suffering from childhood and adult trauma. The APTA recommends that all physical therapists routinely ask their clients about the existence of abuse. Physical symptoms can be identified by the therapist during the evaluation and during the intervention process when body parts are exposed. Table 3.4 describes clinical manifestations of domestic violence.*

Literature suggests that asking direct, nonjudgmental questions about abuse can open the door, allowing clients an opportunity to disclose abuse and possibly seek help. To avoid offending clients, the physical therapist should explain that it is routine to ask all clients about domestic violence because it is so common. By doing so, the physical therapist communicates reassurance that abuse can happen to anyone and that the therapist is knowledgeable about how to address the situation. Evidence supports that most women in abusive relationships are in favor of being asked about abuse and might feel empowered to discuss the abuse if health care workers raise the issue in a sensitive physical manner. Health care professionals must be sensitive to the most wounded and complicated client to maximize the potential for whole-person healing. It is difficult to identify a perpetrator or survivor of abuse by outward appearances. Perpetrators are skilled at cover-up, and survivors cope through dissociation to look normal because of conditioned fear.

Many individuals with unresolved, unseen emotional and psychologic wounds do not know the reasons for their comorbid diagnoses; failed treatments; reactive, destructive lifestyles; and bankrupt relationships. They have survived by hiding their pain, disability, and terror from themselves and from others. Triggers, flashbacks, and nightmares often do not intrude into daily life until well into adulthood, when the survivor is unable to continue the exhausting cover-up, fear-based façade, and denial stemming from overwhelming shame and trauma. It is common to label clients with these behaviors as noncompliant or difficult, and they often move between care providers in their search for success.

Common health care practices often significantly hinder the recovery of abuse and trauma survivors. Medical practitioners are trained to take control and move through treatment within limited time allowances. Persistence in cajoling, cheerleading, or demanding compliance meant as encouragement may further victimize the individual.[240] Problems of this type in practice can be remedied, and significant improvements can be seen in client satisfaction and response when involved professionals understand the specific needs of the individual and the dynamics of the deeper heart-mind-body pathology.

### Screening, Observation, and Assessment

Observe the client for:

- Excessive tension, rapid breathing, and freeze patterns observed during positioning and hands-on activities
- Inappropriate responses to questions or evaluation techniques
- Excessive fear responses (body language, flinching, startling, or pulling away, facial expressions, declining treatment)
- Sudden fear, muscle guarding, sweating, or the need to move from a specific location
- Darting eye movements, sweating, or lack of conscious attention
- Treatment or touch results in excessive reports of pain or muscle spasms that are inconsistent with the area or the extent of pressure

Evaluation tools that may assist in identifying psychologic contributions:

- Questions on the intake evaluation related to abuse or emotional trauma[443]
- Sensitive open-ended questions to allow disclosure[443]
- Adverse Childhood Experiences (ACE) self-report questionnaire to screen for childhood adversity exposure[131]
- Tampa Kinesophobia Scale (>39 elevated score)[3,253,546,547]
- Pain catastrophizing scale (>20 elevated score)[3,546,547]
- Beck Depression Inventory (>13 elevated score)[54,182,547]
- PTSD Scale[141]
- Evaluation of inconsistencies between subjective reported pain or influence on function and observed functional capabilities
- Evaluation of progress and identification of:
  - Failure to progress
  - Difficulty complying with his or her independent self-care program
  - Belief that there is an answer to physical discomfort that will take away all the pain such as another health care provider opinion, explanations derived from MRI or other sophisticated testing, surgery or pharmaceutical management

*Strategies to enable disclosure or identify if referral to a psychologist is needed or modifications to physical therapy treatment are required include:*[443]

- Establish an environment of personal safety and trust.
- At the appropriate time, explain that sharing apparently unrelated reactions is important to successful intervention because thoughts, feelings, and sensations reveal factors contributing to the symptoms and may interfere with positive outcomes.
- Identify triggers that increase stress reactions through careful observation, discussion with the client and ongoing monitoring of both physiologic and psychologic responses.

*Referral for psychologic management includes identification of clients who might benefit from referral for psychologic services. This is an important element of evaluation with possible elements such as identification of "yellow flags," client-reported history of abuse or emotional trauma, identifying inconsistencies or exaggerated responses to physical diagnosis, fear-avoidance behaviors, or lack of progress.*[327] *It is important to inform the client of options in obtaining those services and the benefits of receiving such services. Have a prepared referral list with contact information for carefully screened interdisciplinary professionals. Having a list to consider can help smooth the client's transition in thinking about taking advantage of adjunct services.*[443]

*Documentation is a critical part of managing the care of the person with suspected abuse. Recorded descriptions should include the size, shape, color, and anatomic location of injuries, as well as the type of wound. If written permission can be obtained, photographs should be taken of bruises and injuries, with care to include the person's face in some of the pictures in case they are needed for evidence at criminal trials. Documentation created during several treatment sessions, especially if all observed information is objectively recorded on a body map, allows the physical therapist to create an ongoing record of injuries.*

*Documentation should also include any agencies that are contacted. It is essential, however, that physical therapists obtain permission from the individual before contacting anyone. Reports of abuse should include the client's own description of how the injuries occurred. If a person fears for his or her immediate safety, local law enforcement should be notified. The physical therapist should stay with the client until police arrive.*

## SPECIFIC PSYCHOLOGIC CONDITIONS

It is estimated that 1 in 17 persons experience a significant negative impact in their ability to participate fully in life roles because of a serious mental disorder. Men and women are equally likely to experience a mental health disorder. The *International Classification for Functioning, Disability, and Health*[559] addresses mental health disorders through coding the impact on body function, body structure, activities, and participation. It emphasizes the impact of personal characteristics, such as motivation, attention, and drive as well as environmental factors on both activities and participation in life roles.

Physical therapists will encounter clients who have a psychiatric comorbidity and therefore must understand the impact psychopathology has on a client, on interaction with the client, and on intervention, maximizing the individual's performance of activities and minimizing participation restrictions.[482] It is important to remember that clinical interactions can either exacerbate psychopathology or enhance healing as described above. In addition to the benefits of sensitive, insightful therapeutic care, knowing when and to whom a referral should be initiated is critical to a successful practice.

Physical therapists should be alert to symptoms that are physical, behavioral, and cognitive and/or language that may by symptomatic of a mental health disorder. Table 3.4 describes this phenomenon. Conditions most likely encountered in the provision of physical therapy services are included in this chapter. The World Health Organization's International Classification of Functioning, Disability and Health is endorsed by the American Physical Therapy Association (APTA).[17] The psychiatric disorders in this chapter can be found in the American Psychiatric Association taxonomy, the *Diagnostic and Statistical Manual of Mental Disorders, Fifth Edition* (DSM-5), which was published in 2013.[20] Updates are available at https://www.psychiatry.org/psychiatrists/practice/dsm/updates-to-dsm-5accessed February 2019. The *International Statistical Classification of Diseases and Related Health Problems (ICD)* is used internationally to categorize mental health disorders.

**Table 3.4** Clinical Manifestations of Domestic Violence

| All Populations | Child Abuse | Intimate Partner Violence | Elder Abuse |
|---|---|---|---|
| | **PHYSICAL MANIFESTATIONS** | | |
| Cuts, lacerations, puncture wounds, fractures<br>Bruise, welt, and wound patterns that resemble utensils, bite marks, cords, etc.<br>Any injury incompatible with history<br>Untreated injuries; delay in obtaining medical care<br>Burns from cigarettes, acids, friction from ropes or chains<br>Defensive pattern of injuries when the hands and arms are used to protect the face, head<br>Injuries in various stages of healing<br>Injuries to genitals and inner thighs from sexual abuse | Explanation of injuries incompatible with child's age, size, and developmental skills<br>History of frequent illness affecting the ears, throat, lungs, chest, and GI tract<br>Shaken baby syndrome—retinal hemorrhage, signs of TBI<br>Subdural hematoma; skull fracture in infants<br>Upper lip and frenulum injuries from forced feedings | Head, neck, and facial injuries; temporomandibular joint pain<br>Injuries in a central pattern that involves the breasts/chest, abdomen, and genital areas<br>TBI; mild TBI; postconcussive syndrome<br>Back, neck, and chest pain; abdominal and pelvic pain<br>Vague symptoms of pain; chronic pain<br>Posttraumatic distress symptoms<br>Frequent headaches; migraine headaches<br>Pregnancy complications | Soiled clothing or bed; fecal or urine smell; health or safety hazards in living environment<br>Absence of hair and/or hemorrhaging below scalp<br>Dehydration and/or malnourishment/weight loss without illness-related cause<br>Poor skin condition, poor skin hygiene, rashes, pressure ulcers<br>Marks around mouth indicating that the person has been gagged<br>Rope burns or abrasions on the wrists, ankles, torso, and neck from restraints<br>Inadequate clothing, heat, food |
| | **BEHAVIORAL MANIFESTATIONS** | | |
| Mood and appetite disturbances; eating disorders<br>Depression/suicidal tendencies<br>Sleep disturbances<br>Use of emergency departments for health care<br>Frequently missed/cancelled therapy/medical appointments | Neglect may result in head banging and rocking<br>Failure to thrive; developmental delays<br>Speech delays<br>Aversion to touch | Increased use of alcohol and drugs<br>Partner answers all questions; partner always present<br>Fatigue | Increased use of alcohol and drugs<br>Caregiver answers all questions; caregiver always present |

Courtesy Claudia B. Fenderson, PT, EdD, PCS, Mercy College, Dobbs Ferry, New York.

## Posttraumatic Stress Disorder

### Overview

PTSD is a traumatic stress disorder that can occur at any age, including childhood. PTSD can result from emotional, mental, spiritual, physical, or sexual trauma. Other traumatic events may include violent personal assault (sexual assault, physical attack, robbery, mugging); being kidnapped or taken hostage; torture; incarceration as a prisoner of war or in a concentration camp; natural or manmade disasters; experiencing a significant medical event (e.g., cardiac arrest and resuscitation); or being diagnosed with a life-threatening illness (e.g., cancer) or being treated in an intensive care unit for critical illness.[188,226]

The acute stress responses to a major stressor are triggered by reminders of the event, including flashbacks, intrusive thoughts and images, nightmares, hyperarousal, sleep disturbances, agitation, irritability, anger, and impulsiveness. Sensory hypoactivation may include numbing, withdrawal, avoidance, confusion, depression, and dissociation.[19,460]

### Risk Factors and Incidence

War, military combat, natural disasters, acts of terrorism (local and global), sexual and criminal assaults, and domestic violence have contributed to a rise in recognition of the prevalence of this condition. PTSD may occur as a result of an overwhelming personal experience of an actual or threatened death or serious injury; threat to one's physical integrity; or witnessing of an event that involves death, injury, or threat to someone else. The traumatic event does not have to be experienced directly. Health care workers dealing with the aftermath of violence or natural disasters have developed PTSD.[162] Despite the large number of individuals exposed to significant traumatic events, only a minority develop PTSD. Risk factors are the magnitude of the stress,[342] previous history of traumatization,[152] and presence of both physical and psychologic trauma.[460] Genetic predisposition may increase the vulnerability of individuals exposed to physical or psychologic trauma.[439,563,564] A high percentage of individuals with a history of childhood sexual abuse develop PTSD symptoms. Sexual assault is the most common precipitating cause reported by women with PTSD. Combat deployments are the most commonly identified etiology in men. Sleep disturbances can diminish resiliency and increase risk for PTSD.[379,452]

### Clinical Manifestations

The person with PTSD experiences persistent symptoms of anxiety, unwanted and distressing thoughts and nightmares, increased arousal, or hypervigilance not present before the trauma. Symptoms also may include difficulty falling or staying asleep, exaggerated startle response, or difficulty concentrating on or completing tasks. Children may also exhibit various physical symptoms such as headaches and stomach aches, bed wetting, or acting out the situation during play. Emotional numbing symptoms leave affected individuals unresponsive and unattached emotionally to other people.[116]

Symptoms of PTSD can be divided into three types: intrusion, avoidance, or arousal. *Intrusion* refers to reexperiencing the trauma in nightmares; daytime flashbacks; or unwanted memories, thoughts, images, or sensations. Triggers associated with the traumatic event reproduce excessive autonomic responses. Both young children and adults have dreams of the traumatic event that may evolve into generalized nightmares of monsters, of rescuing others, or of threats to self or others.

*Avoidance symptoms* are represented by social withdrawal and becoming numb to feelings of any kind, either positive or negative, avoiding stimuli that might trigger memories or experiences similar to the trauma. People who suffer from PTSD frequently say they cannot feel emotions, especially toward those to whom they are closest. As the avoidance continues, the person seems to be bored, cold, or preoccupied. Family members often feel rebuffed by the person because he or she lacks affection and acts mechanically.

Combat or military veterans with PTSD avoid accepting responsibility for others because they think they failed in the past to ensure the safety of people who did not survive the trauma. They feel guilt about surviving a disaster while others who may be friends or family did not. In combat veterans or survivors of civilian disasters, this guilt may be worse if they witnessed or participated in behavior that was necessary to survival but unacceptable to society.[525] Such guilt can deepen depression as the person begins to look on himself or herself as unworthy, a failure, or a person who violated his or her predisaster values.

*Arousal symptoms* are the final type of PTSD symptom. These symptoms, sometimes referred to as hyperarousal, put the person on guard and may lead to panic attacks. The persistence of a biologic alarm reaction is expressed in exaggerated startle reactions. They may feel sweaty, have trouble breathing, and may notice their heart rate increasing. They may feel dizzy or nauseated. Difficulty with relationships, insomnia, irritability, difficulty concentrating, and being easily startled are hallmark symptoms of PTSD. War veterans may revert to their war behavior, diving for cover when they hear a car backfire or firecrackers exploding.

Other symptoms include inappropriate responses triggered by sensory aspects associated with the initial trauma including more passive, fearful responses, and inappropriate cognitive or behavioral responses to perceived threats. Individuals with PTSD have problems with sustained attention and working memory when memories are intrusive. Persistent hypervigilance limits concentration and accompanies sleep distubances.[115,522] Increased pain responses or lower thresholds to pain[160] may be part of the inability to distinguish between relevant and irrelevant sensory stimuli and may be associated with pain experienced during the initial stressor.[522] There are also some occasions when the psychologic stress is misinterpreted as somatic complaints or somatization.[522]

There is a high rate of comorbid psychologic conditions such as anxiety disorders.[309] Other associated conditions can exist in those with PTSD, such as agoraphobia, OCD, social phobia, specific phobia, MDD, somatization disorder, and substance abuse disorders. Recent studies show a link between combat-related PTSD and heart attack in military veterans even when accounting for known cardiac risk factors.[200,259]

Substance use disorders can develop associated with anxiety, irritability, and depression. Alcohol use provides temporary relief of symptoms because drinking compensates for deficiencies in endorphin activity after a traumatic experience. Long-term success is unlikely unless the underlying PTSD is treated along with the alcohol and substance abuse.[368]

### Pathogenesis

There is less activity in the prefrontal cortex visible with functional magnetic imaging in individuals with PTSD.[204,462] Disturbances in self-referential or self-focus processing involve the medial prefrontal cortex and posterior cingulate in PTSD.[52] The prefrontal cortex is the area of the brain responsible for inhibition of emotions and repression of memories, as well as allowing verbal relay of the history (see section on ROPC and responses to trauma earlier in this chapter).[204]

The excessive and continuous fight-or-flight responses result in abnormal hypothalamic-pituitary-thyroid activity and maladaptive stress responses.[460] Adrenaline and norepinephrine in the brain stimulate the amygdala, which is the seat of emotional memories associated with threat.[393] In PTSD, the amygdala becomes overactive, causing the individual to be on high alert with disproportionate fear responses to ordinary circumstances that interfere with normal fear-memory function. Abnormalities in amygdala pathways can affect both the acquisition and expression of fear conditioning.[154] After endorphin levels gradually decrease, a period of endorphin withdrawal lasting from hours to days occurs, producing emotional distress and contributing to the symptoms of PTSD. Areas of the brain that normally balance the amygdala, such as the hippocampus, anterior cingulate cortex, prefrontal cortex, insula, and superior temporal and inferior frontal cortex, are smaller in size and do not function as well in people with PTSD.[60,418]

### MEDICAL MANAGEMENT

**DIAGNOSIS.** The diagnosis of PTSD is made if symptoms from each of the five DSM-5 categories of symptoms are experienced. Category A: history of significant physical or emotional trauma; category B: reexperiencing; category C: avoidance numbing; category D: negative alterations in thoughts and mood; and category E: hyperarousal.[21] The presence of both numbing and hyperarousal symptoms is relatively unique to PTSD.[115,529]

PTSD should be differentiated from an *adjustment disorder* which is usually a temporary phenomenon in response to a stressor such as a traumatic injury or medical condition that causes loss of wages or other impact on family structure. During the adjustment phase, the person gathers resources to maintain self-worth, acceptance, and ability to cope. The adjustment stage can become a maladjustment stage, with excessive fear, disbelief, anger, guilt, or depression. The individual remains hampered by the disease's real or perceived impairment. Chronic illnesses, such as chronic obstructive pulmonary disease or multiple sclerosis, are often associated with such an adjustment disorder.

**TREATMENT.** Pharmacologic interventions may include antidepressants, antianxiety medications, mood-stabilizing drugs, and antipsychotics when appropriate.[214] The long-term effects on the neural bases of memory with the use of β-adrenergic antagonists to prevent or erase pathologic emotional memories in the amygdala remain unknown at this time.[164]

Psychologically based treatment options have been cognitive in nature, including trauma-focused cognitive behavioral therapy[49] (CBT) based on neural patterning techniques,[84] progressive desensitization, cognitively based stress management techniques, hypnosis, and relaxation.[49] Both cognitive and somatically based approaches restore balance between the rational and emotional parts of the brain. Trauma memories are primarily processed and stored in the emotional parts of the brain, the limbic system. Disturbing thoughts arise in the cognitive centers. Disturbing body felt sensation of hyper- and hypoarousal arise from the limbic system center. To make changes in the post-traumatic reactions, the emotional brain needs to be accessed.

Eye movement desensitization and reprocessing (EMDR) is an effective form of psychotherapy for PTSD.[221,268,382] Exercise can create decreased anger levels, increased mental awareness, and increased energy levels in individuals with PTSD.[258,381]

**PROGNOSIS.** The symptoms of PTSD usually begin within six months of the traumatic event and resolve within 12 months. Persistence depends on many factors including personal resilience, secondary stresses, level of support, prior traumatic experiences, ongoing injury, and severity of the stressor. Prognosis also depends on how soon symptoms are recognized and diagnosed, allowing for immediate treatment.

## Anxiety Disorders

### Overview and Incidence

*Anxiety* is defined as a generalized excessive emotional state of fear and apprehension usually associated with a heightened state of physiologic arousal. The experience of anxiety is the common thread among the specific anxiety disorders.[19,23] See Table 3.5.

*Generalized anxiety disorder* is characterized by excessive and persistent worry and concern about everyday things (e.g., money, health, family), sometimes just worrying how to get through the day or night. Approximately 18.1% of the adults in the United States have an anxiety disorder in any given 12-month period, and 28.8% of adults will experience an anxiety disorder at least once during their life.[238] The most common anxiety disorders encountered in the therapy practice include general anxiety disorder, panic disorder, and specific phobias.

A *panic attack* is an acute onset of intense or excessive anxiety, fear, or discomfort that includes four or more of the symptoms in Box 3.6. Panic attacks typically occur without warning and can occur at any time, even during sleep. A panic attack may be a component of any of the anxiety disorders or may occur in the absence of an underlying anxiety disorder. A panic attack may occur comorbidly with medical conditions. Initial panic attacks may develop during a period of extreme stress or after surgery, a serious accident, illness, or childbirth. The premenstrual period is one of heightened vulnerability for women. Panic attacks occur at least once in approximately 3% of the population.[473] It is not uncommon for an individual experiencing a panic attack to believe that he or she is

**Table 3.5 Symptoms of Anxiety**

| Physical | Behavioral | Cognitive |
|---|---|---|
| • Increased sighing respiration<br>• Increased blood pressure<br>• Tachycardia<br>• Shortness of breath<br>• Dizziness<br>• Lump in throat<br>• Muscle tension<br>• Headaches<br>• Dry mouth<br>• Diarrhea<br>• Nausea<br>• Clammy hands<br>• Sweating or chills<br>• Pacing<br>• Chest pain[a] | • Hyperalertness<br>• Irritability<br>• Uncertainty<br>• Apprehensiveness<br>• Difficulty with memory or concentration<br>• Sleep disturbance | • Fear of losing one's mind<br>• Fear of losing control<br>• Sense of terror<br>• Fear of dying |

[a]Chest pain associated with anxiety accounts for more than half of all emergency room admissions for chest pain. The pain is substernal, a dull ache that does not radiate and is not aggravated by respiratory movements but is associated with hyperventilation and claustrophobia.

**Box 3.6**

**DIAGNOSTIC SYMPTOMS OF PANIC ATTACK[7]**

- Palpitations
- Pounding heart
- Tachycardia
- Sweating
- Trembling or shaking
- Perceived shortness of breath or choking
- Feeling heat or chills
- Cold, clammy feeling
- Chest tightness, pain, or discomfort
- Dizziness
- Light-headedness
- Unsteadiness
- Numbness or tingling
- Feeling detached, disconnected
- Nausea
- Diarrhea
- Fear of losing control, going crazy
- Fear of dying

Data from American Psychiatric Association. DSM-5 *Development: Panic Attack*. Retrieved from http://www.psych.org/practice/dsm and Mayo Clinic Staff: Panic attacks and panic disorder, 2013. Available at http://www.mayoclinic.com/health/panic-attacks/DS00338/DSECTION=symptoms.

having a heart attack and, consequently, go to a hospital emergency department.[5,405]

*Panic disorder* is an anxiety disorder in which the person experiences recurring panic attacks with no known precipitating event. Having experienced panic attacks, the person with panic disorder begins to become preoccupied with worry, fear, or dread about having another. The person may even begin to avoid situations in which a panic attack has occurred, hoping that the avoidance will prevent future attacks.

*Specific phobias* are manifested as persistent significant, irrational (or disproportionate) fear toward an object or specific situations that cause marked distress for the person. Common phobias involve heights, flying, storms, animals, enclosed spaces, and medically related situations that may be related to injections, blood, or just white coats. *Agoraphobia* occurs when anxiety prevents a person from participating in social/leisure/occupational roles because of fear of panicking in the situation. The "lived-world" of the person becomes smaller and smaller. Agoraphobia may be encountered in the home care setting.

### Etiology and Pathogenesis

The cause of panic attacks and anxiety disorders is not clear. Proposed factors that contribute to anxiety disorders include genetics, biologics, including neurocircuitry, neurotransmitters, and neuronal hormones.[55,195,478] Environmental factors related to family relationships, situations of abuse, and other stressors will enhance the genetic or biologic vulnerability.

The number of 5-$HT_{1A}$ serotonin receptors in the anterior cingulate, posterior cingulate, and the raphe nuclei is reduced in persons with panic disorder.[362] Efferent neurons from the raphe nuclei secrete serotonin throughout most of the brain as well as in the spinal cord. Other imaging studies have linked the prefrontal cortex and the amygdala with anxiety disorders.[298]

Increased pain perception including intensity, related activity limitations and participation restrictions, and health-related QOL are associated with anxiety.[35] The hippocampus and associated areas are active in the modulation of pain.[318] Increased activity in the entorhinal cortex of the hippocampus found during functional MRI studies is associated with induced anxiety resulting in decreased modulation of pain.[400] Autonomic nervous system function is disordered in panic disorder, with decreased sympathetic nervous system activity and poor heart rate variability.[308]

### Clinical Manifestations

The physical manifestations of a panic attack are identified in Box 3.6, and the symptoms of anxiety are outlined in Table 3.5. These represent the most common symptoms, but other manifestations of anxiety include irritability, difficulty with memory or concentration, uncertainty, hypervigilance to somatic symptoms, muscle tension, and headache. Symptoms range in severity; mild anxiety may cause minor activity limitations or participation restrictions, but severe anxiety can completely prohibit the ability to participate in social/occupational and leisure roles.

Panic disorder is characterized by periods of sudden, unprovoked, intense anxiety with associated physical symptoms lasting a few minutes up to 2 hours. Residual sore muscles and fatigue are a consistent finding after the panic attack. Recurrent panic attacks during sleep occur in approximately 30% of panic disorders. The person with sleep panic attacks awakens feeling fatigued, stiff, and sore. Persons with generalized anxiety disorder experience restlessness and muscle tension that can lead to body aches, headaches, procrastination, and delayed decision making in response to their worries.

Persons with anxiety disorders often feel frustrated and embarrassed that they cannot control their symptoms on their own. Anxiety can become self-generating because the symptoms reinforce the reaction, causing a spiral effect. Stimulants, such as caffeine, cocaine, or other stimulant drugs; medications containing caffeine; or stimulants used in treating asthma can trigger anxiety disorders.

## MEDICAL MANAGEMENT

**DIAGNOSIS.** A physical exam is performed to rule out predisposing medical conditions. DSM-5 criteria include symptoms that must be present for at least 1 month for a diagnosis of panic disorder, and the excessive worry associated with generalized anxiety disorder must be present for at least 3 months.

**TREATMENT.** A combination of pharmacologic and psychotherapy interventions is most effective for the various anxiety disorders.[188,304,359,459,535] The goal of therapeutic intervention is to manage or relieve levels of anxiety and prevent panic attacks or minimize the impact and duration of a panic attack.

Two types of psychoactive medications are typically used, in various combinations, depending on the type and severity of the anxiety disorder. Antidepressants (SSRIs, SNRIs) primarily increase the availability of serotonin. Antianxiety medications and benzodiazepines help control the symptoms of a panic attack and have various pharmacokinetic characteristics.

The same interventions suggested in management of persistent pain are effective with anxiety and panic. (See Special Implications for the Physical Therapist Intervention for Persistent or Chronic Pain Disorders.) CBT is a particularly effective psychotherapeutic intervention. CBT focuses on the way the person thinks, reducing "cognitive chatter," and how the person responds to the person's own thoughts.

**PROGNOSIS.** The prognosis is quite good for most individuals with anxiety disorders because CBT and psychopharmacologic interventions are very effective alone or in combination.[188,459,535] Generalized anxiety disorder can lead to significant sleep disorders, gastrointestinal conditions, persistent headaches, and bruxism (teeth grinding). Specific phobias can lead to activity limitations and participation restrictions, for example, avoiding medical care, social situations, driving out of the way to avoid a bridge. Agoraphobia may become so severe that the individual can no longer leave the house or, in the worst case, a specific room in the home. Depression, suicidal thoughts, and substance use disorders are serious potential complications of poorly managed anxiety disorders.

**SPECIAL IMPLICATIONS FOR THE THERAPIST 3.5**

### *Anxiety Disorders*

A client explained how panic disorder impacts her ability to participate in therapy: "First, what if I have a panic attack while I am at therapy? The therapist will think I am crazy, or stupid—that I should be able to control this. This fear frequently makes me want to cancel my appointment. Then I worry about doing my exercises. When I have a panic attack, my heart beats fast and pounds in my chest. What if exercising increases my heart rate and that triggers a panic attack? I can't let that happen. What if I can't tell the difference between a panic attack and a heart attack or a stroke? I've been to the emergency room several times already. One of these times, it really might be a heart attack.... How will I know? How will I know when to say something?"

Identifying symptomology that points toward anxiety or panic during the examination or intervention is critical. The therapist must differentiate between a hypoglycemic episode, a panic attack, and a true cardiac event. A hypoglycemic episode will resolve quickly in response to ingestion of orange juice or similar source of sugar. During a panic attack, symptoms decrease if the person walks around and talks it out. If it is a true cardiac event, symptoms will increase with increased activity. If a client experiences an initial panic attack during a therapy session, referral to a physician or mental health professional is appropriate.

Hyperventilation can be modulated through breath awareness, and retraining may be helpful.[119] Clients may be hypervigilant of their vital and other somatic signs and symptoms during therapy. Redirection of the client's focus may decrease anxiety. Some individuals, including children, may have "white coat" phobias. Not wearing a lab coat and making the therapeutic environment welcoming and less clinical may help with this specific phobia.

Preparatory information decreases pain perception by suppressing hippocampal activity[35,400] and can help clients whose perception of pain intensity becomes magnified by anxiety or depression.

#### Anxiety and Exercise

Regular aerobic exercise and/or resistance training is a direct intervention for anxiety disorders, especially generalized anxiety disorder.[29,193,219,437] Combining physical therapy with behavioral therapy or appropriate medications can often accelerate both the physical and psychologic rehabilitation process.[219] New approaches to anxiety disorders developed by the HeartMath Institute focus on interrupting the brain patterns and changing the individual's biochemistry and neural patterning.[84,213] Physical therapists may have a role in helping affected individuals establish new neural connections.

When working with an individual with an anxiety disorder, physical therapists must remain alert to the possibility of suicide. Screening for suicide potential consists of asking a few questions (see Box 3.19). Suspicion of either suicide or alcohol abuse should be reported to the case manager, counselor, or physician (see Suicidal Behavior Disorder). The Generalized Anxiety Disorder-7 is also a useful screening tool for anxiety that can be used by therapists.[477] A high score on the Generalized Anxiety Disorder-7 should be reported to the case manager, counselor, or physician.

## Depressive Disorders

### Overview and Incidence

Major depressive disorder (MDD) occurs when an individual experiences one or more major depressive episodes. MDD interferes with the individual's ability to perform activities and may prevent participation in social or occupational roles. Depression is the most commonly seen mood disorder within a therapy practice. Depression is more than two times more prevalent in young women than men during the ages of 14 to 25 years old; this ratio decreases with age, but women continue to have increased prevalence.[8]

### Etiology and Pathogenesis

Predisposing factors for the development of depression may be genetic, familial, biologic, or psychosocial or may be related to extensive medical or surgical conditions. Genetic predisposition for depression when combined with psychosocial stressors may exacerbate symptoms. Psychosocial factors include psychologic trauma (e.g., childhood sexual abuse), significant life events (e.g., death of a loved one, divorce, childbirth),[45] or chronic stress. Psychosocial stressors may play a more significant role in the precipitation of the first or second episodes of MDD but less of a role in subsequent episodes.

Psychoneuroimmunology points toward links among neural activity, the endocrine system, and altered immune responses in people with depressive disorders, including connections among stress, depression, and inflammatory pathways. At the cellular level, T-lymphocytes are critical in the susceptibility or resilience to major depressive disorder. The role of hypothalamic-pituitary-adrenal (HPA) axis–mediated interactions between the serotonin regulation pathway and the stress response pathway is under investigation. The depression-associated inflammatory networks often have overlaps with physical disorders including asthma, rheumatoid arthritis, cardiovascular diseases, obesity, cancer, and neurodegenerative diseases.[561] This may be the mechanism related to persistent chronic sympathetic system stimulation such as during repeated abuse.

Neurotransmitters, particularly norepinephrine, dopamine, and serotonin, play a role in depression. These neurotransmitters are either produced in inadequate amounts or the receptor sites are not functioning properly. Chemical precursors (molecules from which neurotransmitters are built) may be in short supply. Molecules that facilitate the production of neurotransmitters, such as specific enzymes, may also be in short supply.

Brain abnormalities have been identified in persons with depression including abnormal electroencephalograms and MRIs.[260] MRI studies indicate that lesions of the striato-pallido-thalamocortical pathways are evident in older adults diagnosed with vascular depression, which is correlated with vascular disease.[9,38,424] It appears to be a biologic rather than chemical alteration rather resulting in small infarcts (lacunes) observed in the basal ganglia representing cerebral ischemia or silent strokes.[256]

*Major depressive disorder with seasonal pattern* is a variation of MDD commonly referred to as *seasonal affective disorder* (*SAD*). SAD has a consistent pattern of depressive symptoms that occur with the advent of colder weather and fewer hours of daylight and dissipate as daylight hours increase in the spring. SAD is most prevalent in geographic areas north of 40 degrees latitude. Interestingly, Native Alaskans are less likely to have SAD than people who move there from some other geographic location. Women are affected by SAD three times more often than men. With shorter days and less exposure to sunlight, the body produces more melatonin, a hormone secreted by the pineal gland that is made almost exclusively at night to help us sleep and may help to synchronize other circadian rhythms.[541] It is possible that some people with SAD do not produce more melatonin but are hypersensitive to the hormone.

*Depressive disorder associated with another medical condition* is biologically based and associated with other physical illness. Chronic general medical conditions are a risk factor for more persistent depressive episodes. Structural changes in the brain associated with disease such as multiple sclerosis or brain trauma can cause depressive reactions, either on a short-term or recurring basis. This is described in the chapters related to the specific disorder in this text.

Depression in children and adolescents is of significant concern, both in the present and the lifelong impact of the disorder.[326] The lifetime prevalence of depressive disorders in 13- to 18-year-olds is 11.2%.[321] Children and adolescents with depression often present differently than adults and may have difficulty expressing their feelings. Hallmarks of adolescent depression may include helplessness, anger, aggressiveness, withdrawal, avoiding friends and classmates, apathy, low self-esteem, and resistance to authority. There may be reluctance to go to school, decreased performance at school, and risky behaviors, including sex and drug use.

Depression in older adults is difficult to identify because they typically present as medically complex. Occasions for bereavement are more frequent with aging; depression may be misidentified as normal grieving. Depression in older adults may manifest itself in difficulty concentrating and marked forgetfulness, which may be mistaken as symptoms of dementia. Depression in older adults is often a cause of sleep disturbances. Older adults with depression are often reluctant to talk about how they feel.

### Clinical Manifestations

MDD can occur as a single, isolated episode that lasts weeks to months or intermittently throughout a person's life. Severely depressed mood and loss of interest in usually pleasurable activities are the hallmarks of MDD described in Box 3.7.

Box 3.7

**CLINICAL MANIFESTATIONS OF BIPOLAR DISORDER**

***Manic Episode***
**Mood Changes**

- Excessive high or euphoric feelings
- Irritable, agitated, uncomfortable

**Behavior Changes**

- Increased energy, activity, restlessness, racing thoughts, and rapid talking
- Decreased need for sleep
- Unrealistic beliefs in one's abilities and powers
- Distractibility and restlessness
- Uncharacteristically poor judgment
- Impulsivity
- Increased high-risk or pleasurable activities: sex, shopping, drug abuse
- Denial that anything is wrong

***Depressive Episode***
**Mood Changes**

- Depressed mood (sad, empty, lack of hope, pessimism)
- Loss of interest or pleasure in almost all ordinary activities, including sex (anhedonia)

**Behavior Changes**

- Decreased energy, feeling fatigued, or being slowed down
- Feelings of guilt, worthlessness, or helplessness
- Difficulty concentrating, remembering, making decisions, initiating activities
- Irritability
- Sleep disturbances (insomnia or hypersomnia)
- Change in appetite and weight (unintentional loss or gain)
- Change in activity level (lethargic or restlessness)
- Chronic pain or other persistent bodily symptoms that are not caused by physical disease
- Thoughts of death or suicide; suicide attempts

From National Institute of Mental Health (NIMH): What are the symptoms of bipolar disorder? 2013. Available at http://www.nimh.nih.gov/health/publications/bipolar-disorder/what-are-the-symptoms-of-bipolar-disorder.shtml.

More than 95% of depressed people report having decreased energy, even for minor daily tasks; 90% report having problems with concentration and memory. The inability to accomplish new or challenging activities often restricts participation in social/occupational roles.[96]

People with MDD may present with somatic complaints, most commonly headache, gastrointestinal disturbances, or unexplained pain. Other complaints are included in Box 3.8. Medical disorders can be the trigger for MDD and are listed in Box 3.9.

Depressed individuals also present with irritability, brooding, and obsessive rumination and report anxiety, phobias, excessive worry over physical health, and pain. Depression is also associated with elevated heart rate and reduced heart rate variability, which are known risk factors for cardiac disease.[73,479]

Depression is strongly correlated with increased severity of chronic musculoskeletal pain. Almost 80% of depressed people report problems with sleep, including early morning and frequent nocturnal awakenings. Sleep abnormalities associated with depression[260] include

Box 3.8

**SOMATIC SYMPTOMS ASSOCIATED WITH MAJOR DEPRESSIVE DISORDERS[4]**

- Fatigue
- Sleep disturbance
- Weakness
- Headaches
- Back pain
- Joint pain (arthralgia)
- Muscle pain (myalgia)
- Chest pain
- Dizziness
- Palpitations
- Excess perspiration
- Rapid breathing
- Dry mouth or excessive salivation
- Dry skin
- Blurred vision
- Tinnitus
- Flushing
- Slurred speech
- Confusion
- Sexual dysfunction
- Amenorrhea, polymenorrhea
- Difficulty with urination
- Digestive problems, constipation

Data from Tykeem A, Gandhi P: The importance of somatic symptoms in depression in primary care. *Prim Care Companion J Clin Psychiatry* 7(4):167–176, 2005.

decreased rapid eye movement (REM) latency (the time between falling asleep and the first REM period), longer first REM period, less continuous sleep, and early morning awakenings.

Other mental disorders often occur with MDD such as substance-related disorders, panic disorder, obsessive-compulsive disorder, generalized anxiety disorder, PTSD, anorexia nervosa, bulimia nervosa, and borderline personality disorder. Decreased health-related QOL and participation restrictions in social/occupational roles are consistently reported.[35] Individuals who have both medical conditions and depression tend to have more severe physical and mental impairments, leading to greater activity limitations and participation restrictions as well as increased health care cost.[75]

## MEDICAL MANAGEMENT

**DIAGNOSIS.** The DSM-5 outlines the following criterion to make a diagnosis of depression. The individual must be experiencing five or more symptoms during the same 2-week period, and at least one of the symptoms should be either depressed mood or loss of interest or pleasure. To receive a diagnosis of depression, these symptoms must cause the individual clinically significant distress or impairment in social, occupational, or other important areas of functioning. The symptoms must also not be a result of substance abuse or another medical condition.

The latest edition of the DSM-5 added two specifiers to further classify diagnoses: *with mixed features*, which allows for the presence of manic symptoms as part of the depression diagnosis in patients who do not meet the full criteria for a manic episode. *With anxious distress* is diagnosed

Box 3.9

**MEDICAL AND SURGICAL CONDITIONS COMMONLY ASSOCIATED WITH DEPRESSION**

***Cardiovascular***

- Atherosclerosis
- Hypertension
- Myocardial infarction
- Angioplasty or bypass surgery

***Central Nervous System***

- Parkinson disease
- Huntington disease
- Cerebral arteriosclerosis
- Cerebrovascular accident/stroke
- Alzheimer disease
- Temporal lobe epilepsy
- Postconcussion injury
- Multiple sclerosis
- Miscellaneous focal lesions

***Endocrine, Metabolic***

- Hyperthyroidism
- Hypothyroidism
- Addison disease
- Cushing disease
- Hypoglycemia
- Hyperglycemia
- Hyperparathyroidism
- Hyponatremia
- Diabetes mellitus
- Pregnancy (postpartum)

***Viral***

- Acquired immunodeficiency syndrome
- Hepatitis
- Pneumonia
- Influenza

***Nutritional***

- Folic acid deficiency
- Vitamin $B_6$ deficiency
- Vitamin $B_{12}$ deficiency
- Anemia

***Immune***

- Fibromyalgia
- Chronic fatigue syndrome
- Systemic lupus erythematosus
- Sjögren syndrome
- Rheumatoid arthritis
- Immunosuppression

***Cancer***

- Pancreatic
- Bronchogenic
- Renal
- Ovarian

***Miscellaneous***

- Pancreatitis
- Sarcoidosis
- Syphilis
- Porphyria

Box 3.10

**DRUGS COMMONLY ASSOCIATED WITH DEPRESSION**

***Psychoactive Agents***

- Amphetamines
- Cocaine
- Benzodiazepines
- Barbiturates
- Neuroleptics

***Antihypertensive Drugs***

- β-Blockers, especially propranolol (Inderal)
- $\alpha_2$-Adrenergic antagonists
- Methyldopa (Aldomet)
- Hydralazine (Apresoline)

***Analgesics***

- Salicylates
- Propoxyphene (Darvon, Darvocet-N)
- Pentazocine (Talwin)
- Morphine
- Meperidine (Demerol)

***Cardiovascular Drugs***

- Digoxin (Lanoxin)
- Procainamide (Pronestyl)
- Disopyramide (Norpace)

***Anticonvulsants***

- Phenytoin (Dilantin)
- Phenobarbital

***Hormonal Agents***

- Corticosteroids
- Oral contraceptives
- Anabolic steroids

***Miscellaneous***

- Alcohol, illicit drugs
- Histamine $H_2$ receptor antagonists, especially cimetidine (Tagamet)
- Metoclopramide (Reglan)
- Levodopa
- Nonsteroidal antiinflammatory drugs
- Antineoplastic agents
- Disulfiram (Antabuse)
- Cytokines (interferons)

when anxiety coexists in patients that may affect prognosis, treatment options, and the patient's response to them. Clinicians will need to assess if the individual experiencing depression also presents with anxious distress.

The diagnosis of MDD requires the individual to have five or more of the criteria of a major depressive episode within a 2-week period, which significantly restricts participation in social/occupational roles. There can be no history of a manic or hypomanic episode. The health care provider will use the history, laboratory findings, and physical examination to determine whether the MDD is independent of or is associated with a medical or surgical condition.

MDD is considered a risk factor for cardiac morbidity and mortality. Vascular depression accounts for 30% to 40% of all depression in people older than age 65 years. Depression may occur as a result of medications listed in Box 3.10, especially sedatives, hypnotics, cardiac drugs, antihypertensives, and steroids, alcohol and cocaine. Exposure to heavy metals or toxins found in gasoline, paint, organophosphate insecticides, nerve gas, carbon monoxide, and carbon dioxide can trigger depression.[26]

**TREATMENT.** There are three primary interventions for the treatment of depressive disorders: psychotropic medications, psychologic/psychosocial interventions, and electroconvulsive therapy (ECT). These may be used individually or in combination. Psychotropic medications used to treat depression may also reduce cardiac disease.[521]

There are six primary categories of antidepressant medications.[302,357] Mechanisms of action vary between classes, as do the type, number, and severity of side effects. Many of these drugs take 4 to 6 weeks to reach therapeutic levels. A serious concern with antidepressants is the potential increased risk of suicide, particularly in children, adolescents, and young adults; this may also be a concern in older adults.[98] Other side effects are listed in Box 3.11.

*Selective serotonin reuptake inhibitors* (SSRIs) inhibit the reabsorption of the neurotransmitter serotonin, making serotonin more available for postsynaptic receptors with a resultant elevation of mood. *Serotonin and*

Box 3.11

**SIDE EFFECTS OF ANTIPSYCHOTIC MEDICATIONS**

***Dopaminergic Side Effects***

- Pseudoparkinsonism
  - Cogwheel rigidity
  - Shuffling gait
  - Parkinsonian tremor
  - Masked facies
- Acute dystonias, such as opisthotonus, torticollis, and laryngospasm, which may cause acute airway obstruction
- Increased prolactin secretion that may lead to galactorrhea
- Akathisia—subjective or observable restlessness ("Thorazine shuffle")
- Tardive dyskinesia, tardive dystonia
- Neuroleptic malignant syndrome (NMS)

***Anticholinergic Side Effects***

- Dry mouth
- Blurred vision
- Constipation that may lead to adynamic ileus
- Urinary hesitancy or obstruction
- Memory and concentration difficulties, up to frank delirium

***α-Adrenergic Blockade***

- Hypotension; orthostatic hypotension

***Antihistaminergic Side Effects***

- Sedation, drowsiness
- Weight gain

***Others***

- Agranulocytosis
- Electrocardiogram (ECG) changes (prolonged QT interval)
- Elevated liver function tests
- Elevated creatine phosphokinase
- Fetal toxicity
- Photosensitivity
- Pigmentary retinopathy
- Seizures (decreased seizure threshold)
- Sexual dysfunction (erectile problems, impotency, delayed, absent, or retrograde ejaculation, priapism)
- Skin rashes

Data from Jacobson JL: *Psychiatric secrets*, ed 2, St. Louis, Hanley and Belfus, 2001.

*norepinephrine reuptake inhibitors* (SNRIs) work like the SSRIs except that they effectively increase the availability of both neurotransmitters simultaneously. *Norepinephrine and dopamine reuptake inhibitors* effectively increase the availability of the two neurotransmitters without impacting the availability of serotonin. Norepinephrine and dopamine reuptake inhibitors are one of the few classes of antidepressants that do not have sexual side effects. *Tricyclic antidepressants* (TCAs) is an older class of drugs, but the outcomes on depression are generally as effective as the newer classes. However, the side effects are often much less tolerable. TCAs block absorption of serotonin and norepinephrine but are less focused because they also affect other neurotransmitters. TCAs sometimes work when the newer drugs do not. Ketamine has shown promise in quickly reducing symptoms in patients with treatment resistant depression and bipolar depression. Using ketamine may be helpful for patients that have exhausted other therapeutic options.[169]

Transcranial magnetic stimulation, or TMS, is a noninvasive form of brain stimulation. TMS doesn't require anesthesia, and it is generally exceptionally well tolerated as compared to the side effects often seen with medications and ECT. Approximately 50% to 60% of people with depression who have tried and failed to receive benefit from medications experience a clinically meaningful response with TMS. About one third of these individuals experience a full remission, meaning that their symptoms go away completely, but this is not permanent. Most TMS patients feel better for many months after treatment stops, with the average length of response being a little more than a year.[281]

Psychosocial interventions for depressive disorders include various types of psychologic therapies. Cognitive behavioral therapy (CBT) changes the focus of thought patterns, or "cognitive chatter," to more positive thoughts. As thought patterns become more positive, the individual begins to perceive their environment and those they interact with more positively. Problem solving and concentration may also improve. Interpersonal therapy focuses on enabling the person to develop better communication and interpersonal skills.[356]

Electroconvulsive therapy (ECT), formerly known as electroshock therapy, is an intervention in which electrical currents are passed through the brain. Theories on how ECT works are speculative, but relief is usually immediate, including in severe cases of depressive disorders.[383] Side effects include memory loss and confusion, usually short-lived. It is a painless and safe procedure used for depressed people with dementia who do not improve with antidepressant therapy[414] or who are severely suicidal, self-mutilating, catatonic, or unable to eat or function. Repetitive transmagnetic cranial stimulation may have the same effect as ECT.[100,127]

Vagal nerve stimulation, originally used to control epilepsy, has been used with severe depression that is intervention-resistant in 30% to 44% of cases. Vagal nerve stimulation changes the concentration of neurotransmitters in the cerebrospinal fluid or their metabolites (e.g., γ-aminobutyric acid [GABA]).[432] The device, implanted under the clavicle with direct attachment to the vagus nerve, sends electrical pulses to the brain and improves mood.

Interventions for SAD include phototherapy, psychologic therapy, and drugs related to serotonin levels.[176] Negative air ionization, which acts by liberating charged particles in the sleep environment, has also become effective in treatment of SAD.[176] Light therapy is often the first line of treatment for SAD.[258,501] The light system uses white fluorescent light (10,000 lux) with a diffusing screen that filters out ultraviolet rays that can cause eye damage and skin cancer. Light therapy begins in the fall and is done in the early morning for 30 minutes. The light must reach the retina, or it will not produce any results. A *dawn simulator* uses a bedside timer to gradually increase the bedroom light in the morning to create an artificial early dawn.[16,258,501]

**PROGNOSIS.** Recurrent MDD is a chronic relapsing disorder associated with high morbidity and mortality; the severity of the initial depressive episode appears to predict persistence.[474] Adolescent-onset depressive disorder may carry an increased risk for poor outcome.[543] Researchers are investigating whether treating depression will improve medical prognosis in people who have a depressive disorder and a history of coronary artery disease or who have suffered an acute myocardial infarction.[74]

Up to 15% of people diagnosed with MDD die by suicide. Epidemiologic evidence also suggests a fourfold increase in death rates in people with MDD who are older than age 55 years. In fact, adults older than age 65 years, particularly those with major depression, are at a higher risk for suicide than any other age group.[433] Depression affects an estimated 15 to 19% of Americans ages 65 years and older living in a variety of settings, yet the illness often goes unrecognized and untreated.[68] People with depression admitted to nursing homes may have a markedly increased likelihood of death in the first year.[2,430,431,471]

**SPECIAL IMPLICATIONS FOR THE THERAPIST 3.6**

### *Depressive Disorders*

*When depression is noted, it should be included as a condition in the care plan; the team can then develop strategies to help the person. A client who is not progressing in rehabilitation and who is moderately or severely depressed but not receiving intervention for the depression may need to delay rehabilitation until the depression is under control. Under these circumstances, the therapist should not hesitate to refer a client for evaluation and treatment.*

Because of the rapport developed early in the client–therapist relationship, the therapist may identify early signs of depression separate to or in conjunction with a response to a medical condition. If the therapist suspects the possibility of depression, baseline information can be obtained and provided to the physician when referring that client. Screening tests, such as the Beck Depression Index (BDI),[44] the McGill Pain Questionnaire,[317] the Multidimensional Pain Inventory (MDI),[27] and the Geriatric Depression Scale,[565] are noninvasive, easy to administer, and do not require interpretation outside the scope of a therapist's practice. It is recommended that routine screening for depression and anxiety be included in the examination for all clients. Asking for permission to discuss symptoms of depression with the referring practitioner or other appropriate health care professional is recommended; in the case of a minor, parental consent may be needed.

Lack of motivation, lack of interest in participation, and nonadherence during therapy with minimal or no adherence in following a home program may be indicative of depression. The depressed client may cry easily, and often for no apparent reason. Depression may also lead to anger, which is observed as outbursts of hostility, attempts to sabotage treatment efforts, or blaming the worksite, employer, significant other, or the therapist for the injury. Situations can be handled by offering compassionate listening and reassurance. Once the client has felt heard and understood, the therapist can redirect attention toward the instructions, activity, or other more positive topics.

People with depression commonly have global memory loss, whereas dementia results in loss of recent memory but retention of detail. Osteoporosis related to increased stress hormone cortisol causes risk for fracture in older people, so fracture prevention should be considered.[325] Depression and anxiety have also been associated with slowed wound healing, also potentially attributed to elevated cortisol levels.[90,529]

The previously described techniques that drive toward positive neuroplasticity such as mindful meditation can be combined using the polyvagal theory in interventions.[126,237] Exercise including yoga and tai chi is effective, and both mild and aerobic exercise five to six times a week should be considered. Outdoor activities are encouraged because being in nature and in natural light make positive changes in brain activity.

For the client taking TCAs, heart rate during peak exercise should be monitored because the anticholinergic effect of these medications significantly increases heart rate. Drugs used to treat depressive disorders may cause other side effects as a result of increased norepinephrine levels such as dry mouth, blurred vision, urinary retention, constipation, and palpitations (see Table 3.6).

Orthostatic hypotension can be the source of dizziness and fainting, increasing the risk of falls and accidents, especially in older adults. Older adults taking TCAs are at greater risk for heat stroke as a consequence of decreased ability to adjust easily to ambient air temperatures, which may affect their exercise program or pool therapy. The therapist should always encourage the client to report any breakthrough symptoms and side effects to the prescribing physician.

Withdrawal from antidepressants must be monitored by the physician, because tapering of the dosage is required to prevent withdrawal symptoms. If the physical therapist is aware that the client has decided to discontinue use of these medications without physician approval, appropriate counsel should be offered. The therapist may be the first to recognize withdrawal signs and symptoms such as nausea, vomiting, dizziness, poor balance, tremors, twitching, paresthesia, fatigue, and lethargy as a complication of SSRI withdrawal. The therapist should communicate the findings with the physician or other appropriate provider.

## Obsessive-Compulsive Disorder

### Overview and Incidence

Obsessive-compulsive disorder (OCD) is characterized by constantly recurring thoughts such as fear of exposure to germs, repetitive actions such as washing the hands hundreds of times a day, repeated checking such as repeatedly checking door locks, and nervous rituals such as opening and closing a door a certain number of times before entering or leaving a room.[10,385] The client has no control over the thoughts, and their uncontrolled presence results in anxiety. The compulsive behaviors are an attempt to manage the anxiety related to the obsessions. A person is not considered to have a disorder unless the obsessive and compulsive behaviors are extreme enough to interfere with daily activities. Major depression is present in

**Table 3.6** Side Effects of Antidepressants

| Drug Class | Tricyclic Antidepressants (TCA) | Selective Serotonin Reuptake Inhibitors (SSRIs) | Monamine Oxidase (MAO) Inhibitors |
|---|---|---|---|
| Examples: | • Amitriptyline (Elavil/Endep)<br>• Amoxapine (Asendin)<br>• Desipramine (Norpramin, Pertofrane)<br>• Doxepin (Adapin, Sinequan)<br>• Imipramine (Janimine, Tofranil) | • Citalopram (Celexa)<br>• Fluoxetine (Prozac)<br>• Fluvoxamine (Luvox)<br>• Paroxetine (Paxil)<br>• Sertraline (Zoloft) | • Phenelzine (Nardil)<br>• Tranylcypromine (Parnate)<br>• Selegiline (Deprenyl) |
| Function: | Increase norepinephrine and serotonin levels | Block reuptake of serotonin, resulting in higher circulating levels of active serotonin | Inactivate MAO, the enzyme responsible for degradation of norepinephrine and serotonin |
| Effects: | • Anticholinergic effects<br>  • Dry mouth<br>  • Blurred vision<br>  • Nausea, vomiting<br>  • Abdominal bloating<br>  • Constipation<br>  • Confusion (older adults)<br>• Heart arrhythmia<br>• Tachycardia<br>• Orthostatic hypotension<br>  • Low blood pressure or sudden drop<br>  • Dizziness<br>  • Weakness<br>• Sedation/drowsiness<br>• Sleep disturbance/nightmares<br>• Sexual dysfunction<br>• Weight gain<br>• Fine tremor (older adults)<br>• Skin rash/photosensitivity | • Nervousness/jitteriness<br>• Gastrointestinal distress<br>  • Appetite loss<br>  • Nausea<br>  • Diarrhea<br>• Headache<br>• Insomnia/sleep disturbance<br>• Sexual dysfunction | • Hypertensive crisis<br>• Postural hypotension<br>• Insomnia<br>• Headache<br>• Anemia<br>• Hyperreflexia<br>• Muscle weakness, tremors<br>• Syndrome of inappropriate antidiuretic hormone (SIADH)-like syndrome<br>• Sexual dysfunction<br>• Gastrointestinal disturbance |

two-thirds of cases of OCD, making it a notable comorbidity. 19 years is the mean age of onset.[238,272]

### Etiology and Pathogenesis

OCD is linked to genetic, neurobiologic, and environmental factors. Family history and significant stressful events may trigger OCD, younger age of onset within family history increases individual risk. A proposed model for OCD suggests that genetic vulnerability to environmental stressors may result in modification of gene expression within neurotransmitter systems. This, in turn, results in changes to brain circuitry and function. Serotonin regulation appears to be abnormal given the selective response to serotonergic medication. Recent research also demonstrates the role of glutamate, dopamine, and possibly other neurochemicals. Structural brain changes in orbital-frontal lobes and the basal ganglia have been seen. Studies involving the gene BTBD3 show evidence of modulation of behavior in OCD, and there appears to be a link to the hippocampus.[392]

### Clinical Manifestations

Obsessions tend to be centered on fear of exposure to germs and may be manifested by repetitive hand washing, refusing to touch certain objects or shake hands, and refusal to eat at a potluck. Order and symmetry might manifest by continually lining up objects, performing tasks in a specific order, or repeatedly checking a door to see if it is locked. Most clients do not mention the symptoms or the disorder unless questioned. People with OCD should not be confused with a much larger group of individuals who are sometimes considered compulsive because they hold themselves to a high standard of performance in their work and even in their recreational activities.

## MEDICAL MANAGEMENT

DIAGNOSIS. Diagnosis is made according to the criteria established in the DSM-5 based on observation, history, and interview. The diagnosis includes presence of obsessions, compulsions, or both. Obsessions are defined by recurrent and persistent thoughts, urges, or images that are experienced, at some time during the disturbance, as intrusive and unwanted, and that in most individuals cause marked anxiety or distress. The individual attempts to ignore or suppress such thoughts, urges, or images or to neutralize them with some other thought or action.[24]

Compulsions are defined by repetitive behaviors that the individual feels driven to perform in response to an obsession or according to rules that must be applied rigidly. The behaviors or mental acts are aimed at preventing or reducing anxiety or preventing some dreaded event or situation. The acts are not connected with the phenomenon they are designed to neutralize or prevent. Diagnosis should specify if there is good or fair insight, meaning that the individual recognizes that obsessive-compulsive disorder beliefs may or may not be true. When poor insight is specified, the individual thinks obsessive-compulsive disorder beliefs are probably true. Absent insight/delusional beliefs reflect that the individual is completely convinced that obsessive-compulsive disorder beliefs are true. Tic-related behavior is associated with history of a tic disorder. The obsessive-compulsive symptoms must not be attributable to the physiologic effects of a substance (e.g., a drug of abuse, a medication) or another medical condition. The disturbance is not better explained by the symptoms of another mental disorder.

OCD has now been grouped with other components. Body dysmorphic disorder is a preoccupation with perceived defects or flaws in physical appearance. Individuals seek care from dermatologists and cosmetic surgeons to address perceived defects. This is most often seen during adolescence. Excoriation or skin-picking disorder results in skin lesions, more common in females starting at the beginning of puberty. Trichotillomania is a hair-pulling disorder.[132] Hoarding disorder is persistent difficulty discarding or parting with possessions, creating accumulation of possessions to a degree that the space where possessions accumulate cannot be used as intended.

**TREATMENT.** The interventional approach for persons with OCD is multimodal, with both pharmacologic and psychotherapy interventions. CBT is the usual psychologic approach. Antidepressants (SSRIs and SNRIs) and antianxiety medications are the drugs of choice. It may take up to 3 months for the medications to have a therapeutic effect.[380] Transmagnetic stimulation can be effective.[12]

**PROGNOSIS.** OCD is a chronic condition, but symptoms may ebb and flow over time. OCD is one of the most common causes of severe participation restriction in a mental health condition. MDD may be linked to OCD through the prefrontal cortex and is present in approximately two-thirds of people with OCD.

**SPECIAL IMPLICATIONS FOR THE THERAPIST 3.7**

*Obsessive-Compulsive and Related Disorders*

Clients with obsessive-compulsive tendencies must be given specific guidelines for any home program prescribed. Specific limits for numbers of repetitions must be provided, including the strict admonishment to avoid checking or forcing through their pain or loss of motion to see if any improvement has occurred. Changes in therapy schedules, sequence of interventions or individuals providing therapeutic interventions, may induce significant stress in clients with OCD. Similarly, people with OCD may be reluctant to touch equipment, sit or lie on mats, and so on. Using linens on large surfaces and having a container of antiseptic wipes and easy access to a sink with soap and water may facilitate the flow of the therapy session.

## Somatic Symptom Disorders

### Overview and Incidence

Somatic symptom disorder (SSD) is characterized by somatic symptoms that are either very distressing or result in significant disruption of functioning, as well as excessive and disproportionate thoughts, feelings, and behaviors regarding those symptoms.[262]

The prevalence of somatic symptom disorder in the general population is estimated up to 7%, making this one of the most common categories of patient concerns in the primary care setting. An estimated 20% to 25% of patients who present with acute somatic symptoms go on to develop a chronic somatic illness.[480] These disorders can begin in childhood, adolescence, or adulthood. Females tend to present with somatic symptom disorder more often than males.[189]

### Etiology Risk Factors and Pathogenesis

Somatic symptoms may result from a heightened awareness of certain bodily sensations, combined with a tendency to interpret these sensations as indicative of a medical illness. Risk factors for chronic and severe somatic symptoms include childhood neglect, sexual abuse, chaotic lifestyle, and a history of alcohol and substance abuse. In addition, somatic symptom disorder has been associated with personality disorders.[97] Psychosocial stressors and culture affect how patients present, with significantly higher rates of unemployment and impaired occupational functioning in individuals with somatic symptom disorder. When psychiatric symptoms are stigmatized by cultures, there may be an increase in somatization. Symptoms of somatic symptom disorders are consistent with unresolved trauma, conflict, or stress and can coexist with a concurrent physical illness, emphasizing the need for ongoing evaluation. There is evidence of a biologic component related to either an inflammatory or an immune process or some combination of both.

### Clinical Manifestations

The essential markers for SSDs are the absence or inadequacy of physical findings, insatiable complaints, excessive social and occupational consequences, preoccupation with problems, and lack of obvious secondary or material gain. The person with a somatoform disorder often presents with vague pain complaints that ultimately cannot be cured or successfully managed. In the case of conversion disorder, the person demonstrates a deficit in voluntary sensory or motor function that cannot be explained by a known organic etiology. The most common symptoms are neurologic with paralysis, blindness, loss of sensation or loss of voice, hearing, or smell. Symptoms are unconscious, meaning the individual is unaware that the problem has a psychologic, emotional, or stress-induced etiology.[106]

## MEDICAL MANAGEMENT

**DIAGNOSIS.** Somatic symptom disorder can result in unnecessary testing and treatment. Concern with physical symptoms can manifest as one or more somatic symptoms that result in excessive thoughts, feelings, or behaviors related to those symptoms and that are distressing or result in significant disruption of daily life.[415] Criteria include significant thoughts about the seriousness of the symptoms, a high level of anxiety about the symptoms, or excessive energy spent with regard to symptomatic concern. Diagnosis should *specify* if symptoms are present with **predominant pain**. **Persistent** is described as a persistent course characterized by severe symptoms, marked impairment, and duration of more than 6 months. Symptoms are considered **mild** if only one of the symptoms is present, **moderate** if two or more of the symptoms are present, and **severe** if two or more symptoms are present, plus there are multiple somatic complaints or one very severe somatic symptom. Characteristics of the subclasses of somatic symptom disorder are described in Table 3.7.

**TREATMENT AND PROGNOSIS.** Psychotherapy and CBT used in conjunction with antidepressants seems to be the most effective treatment.[138,257,491,551,558]

**Table 3.7** Somatic Symptom Disorders

| Disorder | Presentation |
|---|---|
| Somatic Symptom Disorder | • One or more distressing somatic symptoms[a]<br>• Preoccupation with symptoms: thoughts, feelings, behaviors<br>• Associated with increased anxiety related to the physical symptoms<br>• Chronic |
| Illness Anxiety Disorder | • Somatic symptoms only mild or nonexistent<br>• Preoccupation with the fear of having or the idea that one has a serious disease<br>• Constantly scanning or checking for symptoms<br>• Chronic |
| Conversion Disorder | • Unexplained symptoms affecting voluntary motor or sensory functions<br>• Symptoms are not indicative of known neurologic or medical condition<br>• Significant activity limitations and decreased participation in social/occupational roles |
| Psychologic Factors Affecting Medical Conditions | • Diagnosed with a medical condition<br>• Psychologic/behavioral factors: (1) correlate with onset, exacerbation, or prolongation of condition, (2) interfere with treatment, (3) contribute to additional health risks, (4) impact the pathophysiology, worsening the condition |
| Factitious Disorder | • Intentionally fake physical or psychologic signs/symptoms; inflict injury<br>• Tell others that they have impairments, activity limitations, disability<br>• No apparent reward for initiating or continuing the behavior<br>• Can be related to self or to another by proxy |

[a]Digestive; pain in back, extremities, head, chest; dizziness, fatigue, sleep disturbances.
Data from American Psychiatric Association (APA), DSM-5 Development, Somatic Symptom Disorders, http://www.psych.org/practice/dsm. Accessed February 28, 2019.

Persons with SSDs often seek treatment from several physicians concurrently, which may lead to complicated and sometimes hazardous polypharmacy. The therapist is encouraged to maintain close communication with the physician(s) if the client appears to have multiple medications prescribed from multiple physicians or if evidence of substance use, intoxication, or withdrawal exists.

Frequent use of medications may lead to side effects and substance-related disorders. Tricyclic antidepressants appear to have more success than selective serotonin reuptake inhibitors.

Conversion disorder is often of short duration, and hospitalized individuals have remission within 2 weeks in most cases. A good prognosis for conversion is associated with acute onset; presence of clearly identifiable stress at the time of onset; a short interval between onset and the initiation of treatment; above-average intelligence; and symptoms of paralysis, aphonia, and blindness. Poor prognostic indicators include symptoms of tremors and seizures. The course of factitious disorder may be limited to one or more brief episodes, but it is more often of a chronic nature with a lifelong pattern of hospitalization.

SPECIAL IMPLICATIONS FOR THE THERAPIST 3.8

### *Somatic Symptom Disorders*

It is often challenging for a physical therapist to work with persons with SSDs because it can be frustrating to not be able to identify a cause or make sense of the presenting symptoms. The provider should accept and treat highly involved clients in the same way as any other client while establishing healthy boundaries, letting time and confirming evidence, or lack thereof, provide client feedback and treatment direction.

After the client–provider relationship is established, a discussion of the confirming or contradictory evidence, along with the client's needs and perspectives, can occur. Such a discussion can help give clients an explanatory model that focuses on processes and functioning rather than on structural or biomedical abnormalities. It is better to stay supportive and conservative, and treat only what is objectively found and not what is subjectively reported.[557] Table 3.8 lists possible clinical strategies for physical therapists.

Factitious disorder involves a client who falsifies signs or symptoms through self-injury and ingestion of substances that will create symptoms. There often is no apparent direct gain for this behavior. When a person has factitious disorder by proxy, the parent fosters a close relationship with the medical team and pushes for findings not supported by the physical examination or laboratory tests of the child. The perpetrator may even convince the therapy staff of the need for support in obtaining invasive diagnostic procedures.

The health care professional should be observant of a parent with little formal education or training who has extensive knowledge of the child's medical condition, a history of repeated hospitalizations or trips to the emergency department accompanied by an apparent lack of concern on the part of the parent, inconsistent medical history, and clinical presentation that does not fit the history or neuromuscular/musculoskeletal patterns. There should be concern if the child's condition develops only when left alone with the parent in question.

Because these are also red flags for child abuse or ritual abuse, any of these findings requires a consultation with the physician and a competent counselor. The child will rarely verbally report or confirm experiences of abuse out of fear, but careful observation of body language, facial expression, physical condition, and discerning palpation will allow the body to speak. If time and red flags lead the clinician to suspect abuse, it is wise to confer with the appropriate health care providers.

**Table 3.8** Clinical Strategies for Persons with Somatic Symptom Disorders

| Do... | Don't... |
|---|---|
| • Assess regularly<br>• Keep accurate records of all physical findings<br>• Assess and focus on physical needs of the client<br>• Remain professional<br>• Document objectively and unemotionally<br>• Demand regular improvement and set criteria early in treatment for what improvement looks like<br>• Focus on a client's strengths<br>• Focus on what you can change (e.g., stiffness) and avoid what you cannot (e.g., nausea)<br>• Mention progress often<br>• Praise strengths<br>• Remember pain cannot be measured directly, focus on the indirect effects of pain<br>• Utilize a multidisciplinary approach<br>• Stay upbeat<br>• Downplay any undue attention to the actual area of disfigurement<br>• Gently confront inconsistencies<br>• Refer appropriately | • Tell the client that it is in his or her "head," even if you are right<br>• Confront the obvious contradictions<br>• Become more than a physical therapist<br>• Get angry with your client<br>• Have the client talk about his/her feelings about the body part in question<br>• Tell the client that he/she is being unreasonable<br>• Say, "I know how you feel"<br>• Try to be a friend<br>• Take the client's responses or behaviors personally<br>• Allow emotions to creep into your documentation |

Modified from Woltersdorf MA: Hidden disorders: psychologic barriers to treatment success, *PT Mag* 3(12):58–66, 1995.

## Malingering

### Overview

The DSM-5 describes malingering as the intentional production of false or grossly exaggerated physical or psychologic problems, further stating that malingering is not a mental disorder but is, instead, a condition that may be a focus of clinical attention. Listed under a general heading of *Nonadherence to Medical Treatment*, Malingering is defined as an intentional production of grossly exaggerated or feigned symptoms motivated by an external incentive, such as obtaining financial compensation or evading criminal prosecution. To determine that a patient is malingering, the following conditions must be met: symptoms are feigned or grossly exaggerated, excessive symptom production must be with intention to deceive, and the symptom production is motivated by an external incentive. Malingering should be suspected in the medicolegal context, when there is discrepancy between self-report and medical findings, when there is poor patient cooperation, and with antisocial personality disorder. These conditions are included to potentially aid clinicians in flagging cases in which malingering should be considered, but it is important to be aware that these supportive features cannot determine malingering.[567]

Both malingering and factitious disorders involve feigning of physical or psychologic illness. The motivation for feigning associated with factitious disorders is a desire to assume the sick role rather than an obvious external incentive such as disability payments. In malingering, external incentive should be tangible, usually related to work or criminal justice, while a patient with factitious disorder who repeatedly injects insulin to induce hypoglycemia may jeopardize his or her own well-being—a high personal cost just to assume the sick role.[56]

### MEDICAL MANAGEMENT AND DIAGNOSIS

Instruments intended to assess malingering are typically designed to minimize the number of false diagnoses of malingering on the principle that a false diagnosis is more harmful than a missed diagnosis. Therefore, some individuals who are malingering may evade detection with psychologic testing alone, and clinicians should integrate all available data, with test results viewed as one piece of that data set. Also, specific malingering tests may not differentiate a factitious disorder presentation from malingering, so the use of clinical judgment about motivations for feigning is necessary.

A health care provider cannot rely on any single test to determine malingering, and symptoms of unresolved trauma can easily be confused with malingering tendencies, especially early on. It is important to document completely and to compare and triangulate data collected at different times and settings with other members of the health care team. The physical therapist may see that pain patterns and activity limitations observed during treatment either change or disappear outside of the clinical setting as the client arrives or leaves the clinic or is seen outside of the professional relationship. Observations regarding effort, motivation, and inconsistent behavior offer valuable feedback.

If the physician has ruled out the possibility of an underlying systemic disorder accounting for the client's clinical manifestations, then the best approach is to discuss the therapist's concerns with the client over the lack of effort or inconsistent findings that have no apparent clinical meaning and consider referral to a competent counselor. The therapist should avoid confrontation or directly labeling the person as a malingerer but remain focused on objective data and function. The therapist may need to make the difficult decision to terminate the episode of care after carefully considering all evidence. If a clinician chooses to speak directly to the client regarding evidence of feigning to further the assessment or to give the client a chance to explain discrepancies, the following may be helpful, known as ABCS: Avoid accusations of lying; Beware of countertransference; Clarification, not confrontation; Security measures. Security is included because some malingerers may respond by escalating their behavior to justify their self-reports and become physically aggressive or induce self-injury.

The therapist should not conclude too quickly that the person is malingering because systemic disorders, complex medical conditions, and unresolved trauma can masquerade as neuromusculoskeletal pathology and can present with apparent mismatching or disproportionate symptoms for the injury or pathology.

## Feeding and Eating Disorders

### Overview

Feeding and eating disorders are persistent disturbances of eating or eating-related behavior that result in the altered consumption or absorption of food and that significantly impair physical health or psychosocial functioning. American Psychiatric Association's DSM-5 diagnostic criteria include pica, rumination disorder, avoidant/restrictive food intake disorder, anorexia nervosa, bulimia nervosa, and binge-eating disorders.[365]

The term *disordered eating* refers to a spectrum of subclinical abnormal or atypical eating patterns that are often episodic in nature, typically engaged in before or during stressful events or during major athletic competitions.[445,494] Disordered eating is more discreet and difficult to recognize than eating disorders because it encompasses a wide spectrum of eating patterns that may not necessarily be perceived as abnormal behaviors and may not be regularly or consistently practiced daily. Examples of disordered eating include the restriction or elimination of certain foods from one's diet, for example, eliminating fats or carbohydrates.

Other disordered eating behaviors may include general caloric restriction, compulsive dieting or fasting, poor food selections, and the use of laxatives, diuretics, or diet pills for the purpose of losing weight or increasing lean body mass.[445,494] Individuals who adopt vegetarian (and vegan) diets for the sole purpose of losing weight or becoming lean may also practice behaviors that fall under the classification of disordered eating. Often the rationale for adopting the behavior, rather than the behavior itself, may be the delineating factor between normal behavior and a pathological response.

Disordered eating is often considered benign to the health of an individual because it may not inevitably affect one's long-term health or ability to function in society. In children, adolescents, and some genetically susceptible individuals, however, disordered eating may be a risk factor for the development of a clinical eating disorder.

While there is no DSM category specific to orthorexia, the obsessional preoccupation with eating "healthy foods," focusing on concerns regarding the quality and composition of meals with rigid avoidance of foods believed to be "unhealthy" may be considered within the avoidant/restrictive food intake disorder (ARFID).

Pica is the persistent eating of nonnutritive, nonfood substances over a period of at least one month. Rumination disorder is characterized by the repeated regurgitation of food over a period of at least one month, and regurgitated food may be rechewed, reswallowed, or spit out.

It has been suggested recently by the International Olympic Committee that the term relative energy deficiency in sport (RED-S) be introduced. The syndrome of RED-S refers to impaired physiologic functioning caused by relative energy deficiency and includes, but is not limited to, impairments of metabolic rate, menstrual function, bone health, immunity, protein synthesis, and cardiovascular health. The etiological factor of this syndrome is low energy availability (LEA). A consensus on the use of this term is still being discussed.[340]

According to the National Eating Disorders Association, the prevalence of feeding and eating disorders in the United States is more than 10 million.[351] Feeding and eating disorders have the highest mortality rate of any mental illness at 12 times higher than that of young women in the general public and affect approximately 1% of college-aged women.[28,206]

### Etiology and Risk Factors

The etiology of eating disorders is unknown, although development of an eating disorder is likely some combination of biologic, psychologic, genetic, and sociocultural factors. Typically, an underlying dissatisfaction with body image exists that is based on the faulty belief that weight, shape, or thinness is the primary source of self-worth and value.

Relevant risk factors include personality traits or disorders such as perfectionism, rigidity, and risk aversion. Dieting and family history of eating disorders, social pressure such as military personnel obligated to adhere to certain weight requirements, elite athletic performance, or activities valuing thinness such as dancing, gymnastics, modeling, and acting are also common risk factors. Homosexual men tend to be more dissatisfied with their body image and may be at greater risk for symptoms of eating disorders compared to heterosexual men.[231]

A personal or family history of obesity, drug or alcohol abuse, depression, or sexual abuse or other forms of trauma are additional risk factors for this type of disorder.[86,142] Family issues such as separation, divorce, parental/guardian overinvolvement, or abandonment are risk factors for eating disorders.[251] Critical comments about eating from teacher/coach/siblings and a history of depression have also been reported as potent risk factors.[216]

Disordered eating can occur in male and female individuals alike. Any factor that causes a person to restrict dietary intake or exercise for prolonged periods of time could be considered a risk factor for disordered eating and low energy availability, whether the behavior is intentional or not. Gender differences in body composition and societal influences and expectations regarding body image may explain why women may be more susceptible to disordered eating than men. Risk factors for disordered eating may go unrecognized because these practices are often considered to be acceptable and harmless.

Up to 20% of women with type 1 diabetes mellitus have an eating disorder; this, in turn, predisposes them to further complications with glucose control. The treatment of diabetes mellitus greatly emphasizes weight control, dietary habits, and food. This focus, combined with stress, poor self-esteem, and altered body image that can result from any chronic illness, contributes to the risk of eating disorders in this population. In addition, these individuals may discover that they can lose weight through excessive urination, noting that by skipping insulin injections, hyperglycemia can be induced.[312] This practice leads to a higher mortality rate for individuals who have anorexia nervosa coupled with type 1 diabetes mellitus and is commonly referred to as diabulimia.[80,366]

## Pathogenesis and Clinical Manifestations

*Low energy availability* drives the pathology associated with eating disorders and disordered eating. Energy availability is defined as dietary energy intake minus exercise energy expenditure and represents the amount of energy or calories that are available for essential metabolic bodily functions. Hormonal changes likely occur to conserve energy for more important bodily functions or to use the body's energy reserves for vital processes. In women, low energy availability as a result of disordered eating can affect normal menstrual cycle function because it inhibits hormonal release in the hypothalamus, pituitary gland, and ovaries.[284]

Disruption of systems can include the hypothalamic-pituitary-gonadal axis, alterations in thyroid function, changes in appetite-regulating hormones (decreased leptin and oxytocin, increased ghrelin, peptide YY and adiponectin), decreases in insulin and insulin-like growth factor 1 (IGF-1), increased growth hormone (GH) resistance, and elevations in cortisol.[10]

Initially, gonadotropin-releasing hormone (GnRH) from the hypothalamus gets suppressed,[283,445,538] which normally triggers the release of luteinizing hormone (LH) and follicle-stimulating hormone from the pituitary gland.[65,445,538] When GnRH release is inhibited, normal pulses of LH and follicle-stimulating hormone may be disrupted or reduced, causing amenorrhea or irregular menstrual cycles.[283] Leptin, a hormone secreted by adipocytes, plays a role in the process because it regulates basal metabolic rate, and critical thresholds of leptin (1.85 mg) are required to maintain normal menstrual cycles.

Hypothalamic dysfunction results in the reduction of normal LH pulses, causing inadequate release of estrogen and progesterone by the ovaries (hypoestrogenemia), which can lead to menstrual cycles that occur at intervals longer than 35 days (oligomenorrhea) or a loss of menstruation (hypothalamic amenorrhea).[264,285,420]

Estrogen plays an important and complicated role in the physiology of BMD and bone formation. Estrogen inhibits bone remodeling and bone resorption, which then increases and enhances bone formation. Low estrogen levels may also cause impaired endothelial cell function and impaired arterial dilation, precursors to cardiovascular disease.[211]

The degree of disruption of reproductive function and the effect on bone health as a result of low energy availability depends on the severity of GnRH and estrogen deficiencies.[65] It has been determined that the amount of energy that needs to be available to maintain energy balance in young adults is about 45 kcal/kg of fat-free body mass per day (kcal/kgFFM/day).[282] In women, this is the amount of dietary energy that must remain, after exercise expenditure has been accounted for, to allow normal menstrual function to occur.

Low energy availability as a result of disordered eating can impede the development of peak bone mass, skeletal growth, and maturation when it occurs during adolescence and young adulthood. The risk for stress fractures increases during dietary insufficiency when calcium and vitamin D intake falls below normal levels.[173,342] Women who become amenorrheic as a result of disordered eating and who have not been treated within the first year the condition manifests (when bone loss is most rapid), and those who do not reach normal age levels of bone mineral density when menses resume, may be most susceptible to developing osteoporosis in the future.[109,110,235]

Specific changes in men are not completely understood; however, reduced leutinizing hormone (LH) pulsatility and amplitude have been described in a case series of male marathon runners, a population at high risk for LEA.[47] Other studies, primarily in endurance male athlete populations, have shown reductions in testosterone and inconsistent findings in differences in basal LH parameters.[307] More research related to LEA in males is warranted.[244]

### MEDICAL MANAGEMENT

**DIAGNOSIS.** A common tool to aid diagnosis is the investigator-based interview Eating Disorder Examination (EDE) and the questionnaire EDE-Q.[128,222,328] The Eating Disorders Inventory (EDI-3) consists of 91 items organized into 12 primary scales: Drive for Thinness, Bulimia, Body Dissatisfaction, Low Self-Esteem, Personal Alienation, Interpersonal Insecurity, Interpersonal Alienation, Interoceptive Deficits, Emotional Dysregulation, Perfectionism, Asceticism, and Maturity Fears. It yields six composites: one that is eating-disorder specific, the Eating Disorder Risk, and five that are general integrative psychologic constructs: Ineffectiveness, Interpersonal Problems, Affective Problems, Overcontrol, and General Psychologic Maladjustment.[550]

Other self-report eating disorder questionnaires are also available based on population (males vs. females, adolescents vs. adults, acute vs. chronic condition). For those individuals admitted to local emergency departments, the SCOFF Questionnaire may be helpful for screening and is relatively quick to administer.[107] The Clinical Impairment Assessment appears to provide valid and reliable results when used with individuals who are at high risk for eating disorders.[527] Various laboratory tests may be performed to evaluate hormone levels in men and women, and imaging studies may include a dual-energy x-ray absorptiometry scan to evaluate bone density.

Feeding and eating disorders are often accompanied by additional associated psychiatric disorders.[272]

Table 3.9 Diagnostic Criteria for Eating Disorders

| Anorexia Nervosa | Bulimia Nervosa | Binge-eating Disorder |
|---|---|---|
| • Body weight 15% below expected weight for age and height; less than minimally normal<br>• Intense fear of weight gain; refusal to maintain or gain weight<br>• Inaccurate perception of own body size, weight, or shape | • Recurrent binge eating (at least once/ week for at least 3 months)<br>• Recurrent purging, excessive exercise, or fasting (at least twice/week for 3 months)<br>• Excessive concern about body weight or shape<br>• Absence of anorexia nervosa | • Recurrent binge eating (at least once/ week for 3 months)<br>• At least 3 of these behavioral symptoms:<br>  • Eating rapidly<br>  • Eating alone or in secret<br>  • Eating until bloated or full<br>  • Eating when not hungry<br>  • Feeling shame, guilt, or disgusted after binging<br>• Absence of anorexia nervosa |

*Binging* is defined as eating large amounts of food at one time or over a short period of time.
Data from Hoffman L: *Eating disorders*, Bethesda, MD, 1993, National Institutes of Health, NIH Publication No. 93-3477, and the American Psychiatric Association: *Diagnostic and statistical manual of mental Disorders, ed 5* (DSM-5), Washington, DC, 2013, American Psychiatric Association, Available at http://www.psych.org/practice/dsm. Accessed February 28, 2019.

Concomitant psychiatric disorders may include mood disorders such as major depression or bipolar disorder, anxiety disorders, obsessive compulsive disorders, alcohol/drug abuse, and personality disorders.[312]

Avoidant/restrictive food intake disorder (ARFID) is a broad category manifested by persistent failure to meet appropriate nutritional and energy needs. ARFID is associated with one or more of the following: significant weight loss, significant nutritional deficit, dependence on enteral feeding or oral nutritional supplements, and impaired psychosocial functioning. Table 3.9 provides the diagnostic criteria for eating disorders.

TREATMENT. Prevention, early detection, and early treatment are critical in the management of eating disorders. Education efforts should be focused on students in early middle school or junior high because of the rapid bone formation during puberty and the increased role of hormones on health that will continue for the rest of their lives. Targeting preventive interventions when there are high weight and shape concerns, a history of critical comments about eating, weight, and shape, and a history of depression may reduce the risk for eating disorders.[295]

The prevention of eating disorders in at-risk college-age women has been demonstrated using an eight-week Internet-based cognitive behavioral psychosocial intervention. Women with high weight and shape concerns participated with follow-up for three years with appropriate weight reduction and decreased risk for eating disorders.[216,499] Other online family-based programs for adolescents have provided easily accessible, brief programs when therapist support is minimal or unavailable.[228]

PROGNOSIS. The role of pharmacology has increased in the treatment of eating disorders with the availability of antidepressants such as SSRIs and SNRIs. These medications help control depression, anxiety, and compulsive behaviors (especially around food and exercise) so that behavioral, cognitive, and family therapy can be more effective.

Seventy percent of people with eating disorders can be cured. However, it may take years, and the chance of relapse on the road to recovery is as high as 30%, but the overall prognosis is better than for individuals with bulimia nervosa.[102,203]

### Anorexia Nervosa, Subtypes of Restricting and Binge-Eating/Purging (AN-R and AN-BP)

**Overview.** Anorexia nervosa is a broad term to describe self-induced malnutrition. Restricting anorectics typically restrict calorie intake by eating small, insufficient portions of food and/or engage in excessive exercise. It is the restriction of energy intake relative to requirements that leads to significantly low body weight while there is an intense fear of gaining weight or becoming fat. There is a disturbance in the way in which one's body weight or shape is experienced. It is characterized by severe weight loss in the absence of obvious physical cause and is attributed to emotions such as anxiety, irritation, anger, fear, and desire for control. Individuals with this disorder often have distorted thinking that includes a fear of becoming obese despite progressive weight loss and body dysmorphia, or the perception that the body is fat when it is underweight.

Anorexia nervosa can be further delineated into restricting or binge-eating/purging subtypes. The restricting subtype is defined by weight loss accomplishment through dieting, fasting, and/or excessive exercise. The binge-eating/purging subtype is defined by recurrent episodes of binge-eating or purging behaviors and is characterized by recurrent episodes of eating larger amounts of food and having a decreased sense of control over eating during these episodes followed by compensatory behaviors of self-induced vomiting, laxative abuse, or excessive exercise to prevent weight gain. These individuals are typically able to maintain 85% or greater ideal body weight.

Anorexia nervosa, in general, has been characteristically observed in adolescent and young adult females from middle- and upper-class families, often at or near the onset of menstruation (menarche), but this has spread to include younger girls, older women (midlife and beyond),[570] boys, and all economic classes. Experts are exploring the genes that control hormone production as a potential underlying factor in the development of anorexia.

Regardless of subtype, the effects of starvation have psychologic, emotional, and physical sequelae. Severe medical complications may even lead to death.

**Etiology and Risk Factors.** Higher levels of homocysteine are found in females with anorexia nervosa compared to women with bulimia nervosa or healthy controls. Homocysteine can induce neuronal cell death, leading to brain atrophy, and is linked with depressive disorders and this finding has potential significance, remaining a topic of further investigation.[148,149] Anorexia nervosa may have a genetic component with the possibility of an inherited biologic basis.[33,64] Although rare in the general population, approximately 2 in 1000, a person with a family history of anorexia nervosa has a 1 in 30 chance of developing it. In addition, a biologic twin has a 50% increased risk of developing anorexia nervosa when the twin sibling carries the diagnosis.[469]

The biologic basis for anorexia nervosa suggests that individuals who lose too much weight may trigger adaptive survival mechanisms when in starvation conditions. Denial of starvation, hyperactivity, and food restriction may be characteristic of ancestral nomadic foragers leaving depleted environments. Genetically susceptible individuals may trigger these adaptations when they lose too much weight.[94,174]

**Clinical Manifestations.** Besides the denial of appetite and refusal to eat accompanied by weight loss, other signs and symptoms may occur as a result of starvation, vomiting, and chronic laxative or diuretic abuse (Box 3.12). These practices also lead to alternating periods of dehydration and "rebound" which is excessive water retention observed as swelling or edema in the abdomen, fingers, ankles, or face. Specifically, swelling of the parotid glands, known as sialadenosis, typically occurs approximately three days after the cessation of vomiting and laxative abuse. Normalization of food intake and discontinuation of the purging practices will gradually reduce the wide swings in water balance. However, this perception of weight gain, although not a true weight increase, often causes such alarm in the individual that they resort to their behaviors, and the body is denied the opportunity to return to normal.[155,514] Box 3.13 provides a comprehensive list of behavioral symptoms associated with these disorders.

*Refeeding syndrome* often manifests as the accumulation of edema and occurs with the reintroduction of food, typically in the form of carbohydrates. It is more common for individuals who have lost more than 30% of their ideal body weight.[312] The complexity of this process is still being studied, but the physical therapist should be aware that these individuals will be at high risk for muscle breakdown, respiratory failure, and cardiac failure.

Starvation seriously affects growth and compromises cardiac functioning. Altered cardiac function, which generally includes bradycardia and hypotension, may result in life-threatening arrhythmias when combined with electrolyte disturbances. Mitral valve prolapse may occur secondary to starvation-induced decrease in left ventricular volume. Brain scans are abnormal in more than half of all anorexia nervosa cases and in some cases of bulimia nervosa. In both disorders, this condition appears to reverse itself with renourishment.[511] Loss of body fat results in cessation of menstrual cycle known as amenorrhea, cold intolerance known as hypothermia, and the subsequent development of fine hair known as lanugo that is often encountered on newborn infants.

**Box 3.12**

**PHYSICAL COMPLICATIONS OF EATING DISORDERS**

- Electrolyte disturbances
- Edema and dehydration

Cardiac abnormalities
  - Bradycardia
  - Tachycardia
  - Hypotension
  - Ventricular arrhythmias
  - Mitral valve prolapse
  - Cardiomyopathy (ipecac use)
  - Cardiac failure
- Kidney dysfunction
- Hematologic disorders
  - Leukopenia (low white blood cell count)
  - Anemia (low iron count)
  - Thrombocytopenia (less common, low platelet count)
- Neurologic abnormalities
  - Cerebral atrophy (apathy, poor concentration, poor recall or memory)
  - Seizures
  - Muscular spasms (tetany)
  - Peripheral paresthesia
- Endocrine dysfunction
  - Cold intolerance, hypothermia
  - Hair loss, growth of lanugo (fine hair)
  - Dry, yellow skin
  - Brittle nails
  - Constipation
  - Fatigue
  - Diabetes insipidus
  - Menstrual dysfunction (amenorrhea)
  - Reproductive dysfunction (delayed sexual development, infertility, prenatal complications)
  - Osteopenia, osteoporosis
  - Sleep disturbance
- Musculoskeletal impairments
- Proximal muscle weakness (ipecac use)
  - Abnormal muscle biopsy
  - Abnormal electromyography
  - Gait disturbance
- Bone fractures (associated with osteopenia/osteoporosis)
- Gastrointestinal disturbances
  - Hypertrophy of salivary glands/facial swelling
  - Atrophy of small and large intestine musculature (causes delayed emptying and bloating, reflux)
- Esophagitis
  - Abdominal pain/bloating
  - Diarrhea/constipation
  - Rectal bleeding
- Dental deterioration/discoloration
- Finger clubbing
- Anemia
- Emotional/psychologic disturbance
  - Depression
  - Anxiety
  - Irritability
  - Mood swings
  - Personality changes

There are other serious sequelae associated with malnutrition due to anorexia and bulimia nervosa. Skeletal myopathy can be seen in these disorders. The typical presentation is proximal muscle weakness from extreme weight loss and may have a metabolic basis. Fortunately,

Box 3.13

**COMMON BEHAVIORAL SYMPTOMS OF EATING DISORDERS[9]**

- Excessive weight loss in relatively short period of time
- Continuation of dieting although bone-thin
- Dissatisfaction with appearance; belief that body is fat even though severely underweight
- Unusual interest in food and development of strange eating rituals
- Eating in secret
- Obsession with exercise
- Serious depression
- Binging (consumption of large amounts of food)
- Vomiting or use of drugs to stimulate vomiting, bowel movements, and urination
- Binging but no noticeable weight gain
- Disappearance into bathroom for long periods of time to induce vomiting
- Abuse of alcohol or other drugs
- Self-esteem based on weight and shape

From National Institutes of Mental Health (NIMH), *Eating disorders*, 2013. Available online at http://www.nimh.nih.gov./index.shtml Accessed Jan 20, 2019.

this type of metabolic myopathy resolves with improved nutrition.[310] Bone density is also decreased in women with anorexia and bulimia nervosa, possibly resulting from estrogen deficiency, low intake of nutrients, low body weight, early onset and long duration of amenorrhea, low calcium intake, reduced physical activity, and hypercortisolism. Impaired muscular forces inhibit the normal cycle of bone resorption and bone formation. This type of reduced bone density is associated with a significantly increased risk of fracture even at a young age.[171]

## MEDICAL MANAGEMENT

TREATMENT. Nutritional rehabilitation and weight restoration can be challenging and take several months to years. Treatment may include behavior therapy, demand feeding, behavioral contracts, psychotherapy, family therapy, nutritional counseling, and correction of nutritional status.

Hospitalization is indicated if the body weight or body mass index (BMI) drops below a certain minimum (e.g., less than 16 BMI for adults), electrolyte abnormalities are present, treatment-resistant binging occurs, or vomiting or laxative abuse persists.[26] It is imperative that the physical therapist be persistent in checking vital signs throughout activity episodes and communicate consistently with the multidisciplinary team to determine appropriate activity levels during this stage of recovery to address the possibility of starvation-induced cardiac failure.[140]

Weight restoration in premenopausal females is the safest therapy, with the goal of spontaneous resumption of menses.[108] It is important to understand that even with full disease recovery, bone mineral density does not completely normalize. Calcium and vitamin D supplementation should be optimized. For those individuals with a lower bone mineral density score than is expected for their age and having a high fracture risk, transdermal estrogen with oral progesterone, bisphosphonates, or teriparatide may be considered as pharmacologic management. For males, denosumab or testosterone may be trialed but have not been tested specifically in this population. It is agreed that early diagnosis and treatment of anorexia nervosa are essential to prevent initial weight loss and subsequent loss of bone.[313]

***Prognosis.*** The prognosis for individuals diagnosed with anorexia nervosa is very poor. This illness carries a significant risk of suicide.[251] Although 84% of affected individuals achieve a partial recovery at some point in the course of the illness, the rate of sustained full recovery is approximately 33%.[194] A poorer prognosis for recovery exists for those who have been repeatedly hospitalized for treatment, have a later age of onset for the disorder, or have had a longer duration of illness.[140]

### Bulimia Nervosa (BN)

OVERVIEW. Bulimia nervosa is characterized by episodic binge eating followed by purging behavior such as self-induced vomiting, fasting, laxative and diuretic abuse, and excessive exercising. Individuals with this disorder are typically able to maintain weight greater than 85% of ideal body weight. Before the 1970s, this disorder was relatively uncommon, but since that time, its incidence has increased to exceed that of anorexia nervosa.

**Etiology and Risk Factors.** Low tryptophan levels are involved in reduced production of serotonin, neurologic dysfunction, and seizure. Disturbance in the appetite and satiety center of the hypothalamus is associated. This disorder is perpetuated by the vicious cycle of depression, followed by overeating to feel better, followed by purging or fasting with exercise to maintain normal weight, and then followed by a subsequent bout of depression to refuel the process.[251]

Risk factors are the same as for anorexia nervosa. The individual with bulimia has a preoccupying pathologic fear of becoming overweight despite being within normal weight standards. The individual is usually aware that the eating pattern is abnormal, and self-recrimination is frequent.

**Clinical Manifestations.** Unlike individuals with anorexia nervosa, who restrict food as a means of gaining control over problems, people with bulimia nervosa react to distress by the binge-purge cycle.[464] For many people with bulimia nervosa, the binge-purge cycle is initiated by a period of starving or extreme dieting and excessive exercise to lose weight. Periods of normal eating may occur, but the pattern of fasting or binging with compensatory behaviors will resume at some point in time.

The person with bulimia nervosa may appear to be of normal weight or even overweight. The effects of bulimia nervosa are related to self-induced vomiting in anorexia nervosa binge-eating/purge subtype: erosion of the tooth enamel and subsequent dental decay, irritation of the throat and esophagus, fluid and electrolyte imbalances, and rectal bleeding associated with laxative abuse.

## MEDICAL MANAGEMENT

DIAGNOSIS AND TREATMENT AND PROGNOSIS. Physical findings, laboratory testing such as electrolyte abnormalities, and increased serum amylase levels lead diagnosis. Cognitive behavioral therapy (CBT) is the psychosocial treatment of choice for people with bulimia nervosa.[18] Interventions may include interpersonal therapy, group therapy, antidepressants, and nutritional counseling. The prognosis for bulimia nervosa is much better than for individuals with anorexia nervosa. Full recovery is possible for those individuals who seek treatment.[194]

### Binge-Eating Disorder (BED)

**Overview.** Binging, or *compulsive overeating*, is consuming an unusual amount of food in a discrete period, usually within any 2-hour period, feeling out of control of the quantity consumed or being unable to stop consumption. This can be a normal consequence of restrictive eating or dieting.

Usually, the individual is waiting too long between meals and snacks, avoiding certain types of food (usually considered high in calories and/or fat), or is not obtaining the necessary caloric or nutrient needs. A fear of weight gain underlies this disorder; however, purging via the use of laxatives or induced vomiting is not typical.

Binge eating is considered a core feature of bulimia nervosa but what differs in this disorder is that the individual does not engage in compensatory behaviors such as vomiting, diuretics, laxatives, or fasting. Binge eating is also frequently observed in obesity. It differs from overeating by normal individuals in that during binge eating, the food is eaten more rapidly than normal, the person eats until uncomfortably full, eats large amounts when not feeling physically hungry, and experiences feelings of disgust and shame by how much has been eaten. Guilt and depression are often part of the behavioral characteristics.[411]

### Etiology and Risk Factors

Binge-eating disorder may be a familial disorder caused in part by factors distinct from other familial factors typically seen in obesity. BED-specific familial factors may independently increase the risk of obesity, especially severe obesity. In other words, BED may be a distinct behavioral pattern with a familial etiology.[207] This emerging disorder is designated in the DSM-5 as a condition requiring further study.

### Clinical Manifestations

Binge eating results in abdominal distention and discomfort or pain until relieved by fasting. Obesity is more commonly associated with BED than with purging or non-purging bulimia nervosa.[411] Persons with BED represent a substantial number of people in weight-loss programs.[102,103] Nighttime eating often accompanies BED but is still considered by many experts as a separate eating disorder. Nighttime eating disorder may be an eating, sleep, and mood disorder with distinctive behavioral characteristics.[486]

Other symptoms may include mood changes, secretiveness, impulsive behaviors, sleep difficulties, and obsession with food and exercise (see Boxes 3.12 and 3.13). SAD (major depressive disorder with seasonal pattern) is associated with bulimia nervosa. This connection is likely a result of a common neurobiologic abnormality in the serotonergic dysfunction common to these disorders.[161]

## MEDICAL MANAGEMENT

**DIAGNOSIS, TREATMENT, AND PROGNOSIS.** Surveys for eating disorders such as the Eating Disorder Inventory,[156] Binge Eating Scale,[166] or Eating Disorder Examination[129] may be used to confirm the diagnosis. Treatment includes psychotherapy, family therapy, and self-help groups. Pharmacotherapy may include SSRIs such as Prozac, Zoloft, Luvox, Celexa, and Paxil. Treating BED with antidepressant drugs to increase serotonin levels may decrease the number of binge episodes and ease the associated depression.

BED is treated with CBT in a self-help format. This method of treatment has been shown to be the most effective for this disorder, including individuals who are obese in addition to having BED.[552] Goals of treatment include cessation of binge eating and improvement of eating-related concerns about weight and shape, weight loss, or prevention of further weight gain. Improvement of physical health is paramount.[102] Treatment can be successful, but recovery is often a long process with a high risk of relapse. Family-based approaches are possibly the most effective; the Maudsley method, a family-based approach, boasts an 80% recovery rate with no further treatment required after only 20 sessions over a six-month period.[53,270,422,513]

### Orthorexia

**Overview.** Orthorexia nervosa describes a pathologic obsession with proper nutrition that is characterized by a restrictive diet, ritualized patterns of eating, and rigid avoidance of foods believed to be unhealthy or impure. Although prompted by a desire to achieve optimum health, orthorexia may lead to nutritional deficiencies, medical complications, and poor quality of life.

Orthorexia nervosa, literally meaning *proper appetite*, is a pathologic fixation with healthy food described as a disease disguised as a virtue. Symptoms overlap between orthorexia and anorexia nervosa, obsessive-compulsive disorder (OCD), obsessive-compulsive personality disorder (OCPD), somatic symptom disorder, illness anxiety disorder, and psychotic spectrum disorders. Neuropsychologic data suggest that orthorexic symptoms are independently associated with key facets of executive dysfunction for which some of these conditions already overlap.[255,466]

Meals are often consumed alone, and for women at least, this is more often associated with a slimming diet and attempts to lose weight. Orthorexic individuals are at risk for social isolation, as they may believe that they can only maintain healthy eating while alone and in control of the environment. This can also manifest as moral superiority about their food habits such that they do not wish to interact with others who are unlike them.[296] Less data exists about orthorexia than the other disorders described. There has been an increased focus on eating healthy in the general population; therefore it is essential to conduct further research to determine the characteristics of high-risk groups.[376]

**Etiology, Risk Factors, and Prevalence.** The fixation on food quality, a combination of the nutritional value of food and its perceived purity, is prompted by a desire to maximize one's own physical health and well-being rather than religious beliefs or concerns for sustainable agriculture, environmental protection, or animal welfare. Such preoccupation with health from food may elicit eating patterns that are especially complex. Rules such as which foods can be combined at one sitting or at certain times of day or beliefs that maximal digestion of one food type occurs a certain amount of time after ingestion of another food type can create challenges to scheduling meals and activity.

Epidemiologic studies have not shown a clear gender, age, educational, or body type bias. It may be the case that individuals who are focused on nutrition and health for their career or leisure such as performing arts and athletics may be at an increased risk for developing orthorexia.[6,57] These individuals may have greater insights and concern regarding health and nutrition and may feel pressure to be role models.[453] Tendencies toward perfectionism may further increase the risk.[243]

**Diagnosis.** Orthorexia nervosa diagnostic criteria have been proposed by Moroze et al. as obsessional preoccupation with eating healthy foods, with excessive focus on concerns regarding the quality and composition of meals including two or more of the following:

- Consuming a nutritionally unbalanced diet owing to preoccupying beliefs about food purity."
- Preoccupation and worries about eating impure or unhealthy foods and of the effect of food quality and composition on physical or emotional health or both.
- Rigid avoidance of foods believed by the patient to be "unhealthy," which may include foods containing any fat, preservatives, food additives, animal products, or other ingredients considered by the subject to be unhealthy.
- For individuals who are not food professionals, excessive amounts of time (e.g., 3 or more hours per day) spent reading about, acquiring, and preparing specific types of foods based on their perceived quality and composition.
- Guilty feelings and worries after transgressions in which "unhealthy" or "impure" foods are consumed.
- Intolerance to others' food beliefs.
- Spending excessive amounts of money relative to one's income on foods because of their perceived quality and composition.

The obsessional preoccupation becomes impaired by either of the following:

- Impairment of physical health owing to nutritional imbalances (e.g., developing malnutrition because of an unbalanced diet).
- Severe distress or impairment of social, academic, or vocational functioning owing to obsessional thoughts and behaviors focusing on patient's beliefs about "healthy" eating.

It is critical to determine that the disturbance is not merely an exacerbation of the symptoms of another disorder such as obsessive-compulsive disorder or of schizophrenia or another psychotic disorder. The behavior is not better accounted for by the exclusive observation of organized orthodox religious food observance or when concerns with specialized food requirements are in relation to professionally diagnosed food allergies or medical conditions requiring a special diet.[334]

**Clinical Manifestations.** Orthorexia may cause nutritional deficiencies due to omission of entire food groups and may cause some of the same medical complications that are associated with anorexia: osteopenia, anemia, hyponatremia, metabolic acidosis, pancytopenia, testosterone deficiency, and bradycardia.[388] There can be intense frustration when these food-related practices are disrupted or when food purity appears to be compromised. Like the other eating disorders, guilt and self-loathing is activated when there are perceived food transgressions. Worry about imperfection and nonoptimal health sustains the behavior. Dietary violations may lead to even stricter diets or fasts.

**Treatment.** A multidisciplinary team that includes physicians, psychotherapists, and dieticians is appropriate to combine medication, cognitive behavioral therapy, and psychoeducation. Significant weight loss and malnourishment may require specific inpatient care experienced in refeeding syndrome. Useful medications include serotonin reuptake inhibitors which are frequently prescribed for both anorexia and OCD.[467] Antipsychotics may decrease the obsessive nature of food-related thinking. Orthorexic individuals may decline use of pharmaceuticals because of the synthetic nature of medications. Habit reversal training and cognitive restructuring can counteract distortions surrounding food, eating, and health, as well as associated problematic traits such as perfectionism. Various forms of relaxation training may assist with anxiety and other manifestations of health anxiety.[487,457] Behavior modification strategies may be useful to expand clients' food repertoire, increase socialization during meals, and diversify leisure activities to include nonfood themes.[1]

**SPECIAL IMPLICATIONS FOR THE THERAPIST 3.9**

### *Eating Disorders*

Individuals with eating disorders may be relatively open about severely restrictive dieting, but they are usually less likely to spontaneously offer information about purging or the use of exercise to compensate for eating. Denial of the illness is quite common among individuals with eating disorders, and interview techniques to obtain information are often unsuccessful. The therapist should be aware there are other less-common eating issues that have not been discussed in this chapter, including selective eating, restrictive food refusal, appetite loss secondary to depression, and pervasive refusal syndrome.

Establishing a strong therapeutic relationship characterized by genuineness, acceptance, honesty, and warmth is a prerequisite to eliciting accurate information. The therapist should be aware that individuals with eating disorders may be very resistant or ambivalent about seeking counseling, nutritional guidance, or direct intervention of any kind.

Therapists who work with individuals who demonstrate the behaviors that reflect an altered sense of body image can help promote acceptance of a healthy body image. The National Eating Disorders Association (NEDA) provides helpful tips for health care professionals discussing body image.[352,461] For example, the therapist can help affected individuals do the following:

- Remember that treatment requires a receptive client as well as a competent provider. Meeting the individual where the individual is, listening carefully and skillfully, appropriately interviewing while attending to both verbal and nonverbal cues, and seeking to identify the underlying needs of the client are the first priorities.
- Using worksheets and self-awareness techniques that allow the client to realize and accept healthy truth is most helpful for lasting improvement. We can tell the client what the realities are, but until that individual is able to receive our suggestions and make the concepts their own, professional advice is useless and sometimes increases guilt or shame.
- Recognize that bodies come in all different sizes and shapes. Everyone is unique; accept your own individuality. There is no one "right" body size.
- Look critically at messages from the media and our culture that emphasize a certain body type as ideal. Do not set obtaining a perfect body as a goal.
- Remember that body size, shape, or weight does not determine value, intelligence, or identity. Identify other unique qualities to develop or enhance such as sensitivity, cooperation, caring, patience, empathy, or being artistic or musical.
- Be aware of negative self-talk and substitute positive inner dialogue. For example, if you start giving yourself a message like, "I look gross," substitute a positive affirmation, "I accept myself the way I am," or "I'm a worthwhile person, no matter what I look like."
- Learn how to express yourself by developing meaningful relationships, learning how to solve problems, establishing goals, and contributing to life. View exercise and balanced eating as aspects of your overall approach to a life that emphasizes self-care.

Routine screening for eating disorder risk factors will increase early detection. Appropriate evaluation and intervention can help decrease the consequences of eating disorders.

### Anorexia

It is important for the therapist to be aware of the physical side effects of previously diagnosed anorexia nervosa. Rehabilitation may be required for the person with anorexia nervosa to regain muscle mass lost as a result of low-calorie diets, malnutrition, binging, and purging. These individuals may present with difficulty participating in their activities of daily living and require appropriate intervention to re-integrate these skills. Key strategies for physical therapist intervention include vigilant medical monitoring in the early stages of nutritional rehabilitation, creation of movement programs to return to independent functioning in all activities of daily living, appropriately crafted interventions with an awareness of potential exercise misuse, and consistent communication with a multidisciplinary team.[141] Furthermore, it is imperative to engage in authentic discussions with the individual being treated, to maintain appropriate boundaries, and to address situations about exercise abuse that may be uncomfortable for both participants.

The physical therapist should establish regular consultation with the individual's dietitian and/or primary care physician to ensure appropriate weight restoration during the physical therapy episode of care. Appropriate nutrition is the precursor for regular physical therapy care and lays the foundation to optimize muscle function. It is impossible to improve decreased bone mineral density without weight gain and supplementation. Weight restoration does not always improve bone density and, even with full disease recovery, bone mineral density may not completely normalize.

Weight is not a necessary value for each physical therapy encounter; however, it is important to confirm that the individual is consistently meeting prescribed calorie intake requirements and demonstrating appropriate weight trends. This may best be accomplished through monitoring vital signs with every session and communicating with the individual's care team. Strategies such as using a food log done directly with the client may overemphasize food intake. Evidence suggests that use of an exercise log or contracts may be beneficial to promote adherence to exercise prescription and allow individuals to integrate exercise as a tool for healthy living.[93] If the physical therapist determines at any time during the episode of care that the individual demonstrates inadequate food intake, their appearance changes in an unhealthy manner, or new complaints surface regarding pain or symptoms such as dizziness, lightheadedness, near falls, or generalized numbness and tingling, the session should be stopped and the physician contacted. The physical therapy episode of care should not resume until the individual has followed up with his or her medical team and the physician has given clearance for the individual to resume physical therapy treatment.

Vital sign instability can be severe, including orthostatic hypotension, irregular and decreased pulse, and bradycardia and hypothermia, all of which can result in cardiac arrest. Heart rate must be monitored and maintained within safe limits during exercise for all individuals affected by this disorder. Exertional tachycardia, a disproportional increase in heart rate with simple motions such as sit-to-stand, is often observed in individuals admitted to medical stabilization units. In addition, profound heart abnormalities have been observed during exercise and can be associated with sudden death.

Electrolyte imbalance and dehydration, fatigue, muscle weakness, and muscle cramping are physical complications associated with starvation, self-induced vomiting, and laxative abuse. Poor nutritional status and dehydration also contribute to easy bruising and poor wound healing. The individual should also be monitored for lower extremity edema and cardiac abnormalities due to refeeding syndrome, as discussed earlier, as these complications may require further attention if severe.

Posture is often poor because of the loss of upper body muscle mass. In addition, skin integrity may be compromised with higher risk for developing pressure sores, especially in those who present with severe malnutrition in tandem with functional mobility deficits. Exercise tolerance may be low and endurance reduced significantly as a result of malnutrition. Individuals may resist exercise or may engage in excessive exercise to burn caloric intake, cope with their feelings, or as punishment.

Individuals with anorexia nervosa demonstrate decreased bone mass when compared with healthy controls in 90% of cases. Weight-bearing exercises provided at the proper time, with proper instruction, and of proper intensity may be indicated. It is important to note that timing is key, as it has been found that exercises that excessively load the body while still recovering may adversely affect bone mass.[539]

### Bulimia

Bulimia nervosa contributes to problems associated with fluid depletion and temperature regulation. For people who use vomiting to purge and abuse laxatives or diuretics, significant dehydration and potassium loss are quite frequent. The immediate outcome of such behavior is usually muscle cramping, including irregular heartbeat as the heart muscle cramps; fatigue; and low blood pressure on standing.

In such situations, the physical therapist should mediate intervention until electrolyte levels are within normal limits and encourage fluid intake and reduced activity level. In the more extreme condition, motor incoordination, confusion, and disorientation may be observed, requiring medical attention.

Most deadly among the forms of purging is the abuse of ipecac, an emetic (syrup that induces vomiting) used to treat poison victims. Many people who try it once find it so unpleasant that they avoid further use, but repeated use of ipecac can cause toxic levels in the body, producing myopathy with arm or leg weakness or affecting the heart and causing sudden death.

### Exercise and Eating Disorders

A medical provider must assess when an individual is safe to exercise no matter what the weight or BMI.[192] Guidelines are individualized. Some treatment teams use the 10th percentile for children and adolescents and a BMI of 18 kg/m$^2$ for adults; others use a BMI of 19 or return of menses as a guideline to participation in exercise. Clients with BMIs lower than 18 may require the expertise of a physical therapist because of a lack of functional independence or the presence of postural instability. These impairments are typically observed in cases of severe weakness associated with the advanced starvation process. In these cases, physical therapy intervention should be initiated slowly, with close monitoring of vital signs and a de-emphasis on typical exercise perceptions.[140]

Education should include appropriate technique, type, and frequency of appropriate and healthy amounts of exercise. The importance of reconnecting with the body through movement while allowing oneself to move for the joy of it should be underscored.

When considering the plan of care, it is vital to be aware of the tendency for individuals with eating disorders to use exercise as a means of controlling calorie consumption. The therapist can guide the client in avoiding excessive exercise, which is defined as exercise that is accompanied by intense guilt when it is postponed or exercise solely to burn calories and influence weight or shape. Addressing dysfunctional exercise behavior is both part of prevention and intervention for eating disorders.[329]

Communication with the client's psychotherapist is critical to integrate concepts from psychotherapeutic treatment into the physical therapy plan. After entering a recovery program or during hospitalization, a graduated exercise program should be introduced when clinically safe. Exercise programs should be adjusted for bone density and cardiac status, and laboratory values must be monitored for signs of dehydration, low white blood cell count, or anemia.

### Screening

The therapist can be instrumental in screening for undiagnosed eating disorders, especially among preadolescents, adolescents, and young adults. Physical therapists may use tools such as the SCOFF questionnaire to screen clients suspected to demonstrate signs consistent with an eating disorder.[332] The therapist may notice the presence of a painless swelling of the salivary glands and accompanying facial swelling during a head and neck examination. Although this finding may require further examination by a physician for other causes, it can be associated with bulimia nervosa or anorexia nervosa binge-eating/purging subtype, as the parotid glands tend to swell two to three days after an episode of vomiting activity is discontinued.[312]

A musculoskeletal problem can be an indication of an eating disorder. Overuse injuries, such as shin splints, tendinitis, stress fractures, or hip or back pain, can occur from excessive exercise; the individual may continue to exercise despite fatigue, weakness, and pain. The therapist can assess exercise habits of clients with the following list of questions[361]:

- Do you force yourself to exercise, even if you don't feel well?
- Do you prefer to exercise rather than being with friends?
- Do you become very upset if you miss a workout? Or what happens if you miss a workout?
- Do you base the amount of exercise on how much you eat?
- Do you have trouble sitting still because you think you're not burning calories?
- Do you worry that you'll gain weight if you skip exercising for a day?
- What is your motivation for exercise?
- Do you enjoy the exercise in which you partake?

Furthermore, use of the Compulsive Exercise Test (CET) may provide further information about exercise compulsion.[324] In addition to observation of clinical manifestations, the therapist can identify the presence of risk factors and ask screening questions presented elsewhere.[165] Early detection and prompt referral are essential. A behavioral approach to function and exercise is listed in Box 3.14.

Pauline Powers and Ron Thompson's book *The Exercise Balance*[406] and a chapter on "Normalizing Exercise" in Herrin and Matsumoto's *The Parent's Guide to Eating Disorders*[192] (website, http://www.marciaherrin.com Accessed March 1, 2019) provide information on eating disorders.

Box 3.14

**BEHAVIORAL GOALS AND GUIDELINES FOR EATING DISORDERS**

- Obtain an accurate exercise history.
- Determine the person's target heart rate and teach how and why it is important to monitor heart rate during exercise.
- Develop a well-rounded program of exercise, including stretching exercises, breathing techniques, light weights for upper-extremity toning, aerobic exercise, and cool down.
- Convey to the person that the treatment or exercise plan is to help and protect the person's overall health status and is not meant to control the person.
- Instruct each person on how to determine the appropriate frequency, intensity, and duration of each component of exercise. Monitor daily and weekly amounts of exercise using a chart or written record, and use this tool to help the person develop a consistent and appropriate level of exercise.
- Make clear upper limits on number of repetitions and/or sets, since a tendency to overexercise exists.
- Encourage the client whenever possible to make decisions about the treatment plan; this will help provide a sense of control and increase self-confidence.
- Discern the person's attitude toward exercise and consistently encourage recognition of exercise as part of the overall health plan, not just as a means of losing weight.
- Exercise is only one tool for stress relief; encourage each individual to develop alternative ways of expressing feelings.
- Modifying thought patterns and changing behavior is a slow process. Encouragement and support are essential. Reinforce even small steps and successes.
- Watch for signs of dissociation (e.g., glazed look or faraway expression) and assist the person to remain aware of the effect of exercise on the physical body; paying attention to the physical discomfort helps prevent working through fatigue, striving for the runner's high, overexercising, and overuse injuries.
- Avoid making value judgments about the client's body or physical condition. When the client makes comments such as "I lost/gained a pound this week" or "I cannot believe how fat my arms are," do not react or judge by saying, "You are not supposed to be weighing yourself" or "You are not fat at all!" Seek professional guidance to handle such situations.

Box 3.15

**DISORDERED EATING AND FEMALE ATHLETE TRIAD**

***Risk Factors for Female Athlete Triad***

- Poor body image
- Intensive exercise training schedule
- Perceptions of competition, performance, and success
- Eating disorder with negative energy balance
- Loss of menstrual cycle or delay of starting
- Family dysfunction such as depression, alcoholism, abuse
- Personal traumatic life event

***Clinical Manifestations***

- Osteoporosis/osteopenia
- Amenorrhea/suppressed luteal phase
- Anorexia/eating disorders/negative energy balance
- Common components
  - Negative energy balance—calorie intake less than calorie output
  - External and internal pressure lead to disordered eating
  - Often resulting in lean body fat below 12%
  - Decreased estrogen occurs
  - Leading to amenorrhea and eventually osteoporosis
- Further resulting in:
  - Increased illness—calcium imbalance with cardiac effect
  - Increased injury
  - Longer recovery times
  - Decreased performance

Data from Papanek PE. The female athlete triad: an emerging role for physical therapists. *J Orthop Sports Phys Ther* 33:594–614, 2003. Compiled by and courtesy of Beth Shelly, PT, DPT, WCS, BCB-PMD.

### Low Energy Availability in Athletes

**Definition and Overview.** The female athlete triad is a syndrome that has been observed in female athletes who present with three interrelated components characterized by relative dysfunction in energy availability (with or without disordered eating), menstrual function, and bone mineral density (BMD).[280] Low energy stores increase an athlete's risk of developing the remaining components of the triad.[299,506]

**Prevalence.** Most of the available data has focused on disordered eating, eating disorders,[42,67,371,421,472,493] or menstrual dysfunction[16,41,285,286,420] in female athletes.[41,420] Athletes participating in lean-type sports such as elite distance running, gymnastics, dance, and equestrian riding have been shown to demonstrate up to 60% prevalence of low energy availability with the potential to develop the other components.[494]

Disordered eating has been reported to be more prevalent in athletes who were told that they were overweight by their coach and were unsupervised when dieting to lose weight.[445] More recently, female high school athletes who reported disordered eating were found to be more than twice as likely to suffer a musculoskeletal injury compared to those reporting normal eating behaviors; those who already had a history of prior injury were five times as likely to sustain an injury during the season in which they practiced their sport.[419,507] Understanding this risk may be critical to engaging the athlete in self-management.

**Risk Factors and Clinical Manifestations.** In athletes, high levels of competition anxiety can be associated with disordered eating, which may be influenced by the level of sport in which an athlete plays, the importance of the competition, and how the athlete perceives success. The expectations of coaches, peers, or parents; future scholarships; and public recognition in addition to how winning or losing impacts their self-esteem can be significant factors.[493] Risk factors that should be screened include a history of menstrual irregularity, stress fracture, dieting, and overtraining as well as personality factors such as perfectionism and obsessiveness. Preparticipation examinations for female athletes should include these considerations. An athlete with no history of stress injury is considered low risk; athletes with increasing risk factors may need to be restricted from sport participation.[101] Box 3.15 describes the phenomenon related to disordered eating and the female athlete triad.

## MEDICAL MANAGEMENT

**DIAGNOSIS.** DEXA is the diagnostic modality of choice for evaluation of BMD. When interpreting BMD from a DEXA scan of a premenopausal female athlete aged ≥20 years, the Z-score of the hip and a PA radiographic view of the lumbar spine should be used. In adolescents and children, a PA radiographic view of the spine and total body less the head are the preferred methods for evaluating BMD.[504] If a female athlete has a history of stress fractures or stress reactions, further investigation of low BMD is suggested.

**TREATMENT.** Any athlete with signs suggesting the triad should be questioned and educated regarding the components and potential health risks of this condition. The cascade of events that can result from low energy availability can be managed through adequate screening and early intervention using a multidisciplinary team approach.[537]

Screening begins with a thorough physical examination that includes age, sex, height, weight, vital signs (pulse, blood pressure), BMI, a history of physical activity and nutrition diary, a history of musculoskeletal injury and particularly stress fractures, and a detailed menstrual history. Screening exams can be performed during annual health checkups for children and adolescents involved in team sports, or it can conveniently be administered during preparticipation sport physical examinations.[14,360] It is also prudent to screen for other factors that may accelerate bone loss, including corticosteroid use, regular alcohol consumption, cigarette smoking, protein deficiency, and hyperthyroidism.

Coaches, athletic trainers, and health care providers should also be educated about the female athlete triad to detect and recognize its components before athletes reach the pathologic end of the spectrum. When disordered eating is associated with sport performance and a desire to achieve or maintain physical leanness, physical therapists, certified athletic trainers, and coaches can work together in recognizing the athletes who display unhealthy behaviors and attitudes toward training. Modifications in exercise routines and referral to the appropriate nutritionist or dietitian should be made to assist them in increasing dietary intake by making healthy choices. Athletes who understand the importance of optimal energy availability in relationship to performance and injury are more likely to make the appropriate changes to avoid both bone and reproductive pathologies. By preventing premature bone loss in young female athletes, future fragility fractures can be decreased.

Exercise and adequate nutrition are important for treatment and prevention of low BMD. Weight-bearing and dynamic exercises have a positive effect on bone formation and BMD, especially in premenopausal females. In the female athlete, menstrual function should be evaluated and must be corrected if it is abnormal, because estrogen plays a direct role in bone health and remodeling. Increasing energy availability is the mainstay of treatment for amenorrhea.

A common practice has been to place amenorrheic women, especially athletes, on oral contraceptives (OCP) to provide estrogen replacement in hopes of protecting against bone loss and/or stress fracture. However, there is emerging evidence that this practice is not beneficial and may even lead to harm. OCPs should not be used as a first-line treatment to halt additional bone loss but may play a role in the overall management.

The amenorrhea that occurs within the spectrum of the female athlete triad is referred to as functional hypothalamic amenorrhea. It is an adaptive mechanism that reduces a woman's fertility when the body perceives that there is inadequate energy to support the substrate, let alone a fetus. Although this may seem beneficial to many athletes, as they may not be seeking pregnancy, the adverse effects of this hormonal disruption are manifested in negative impacts on bone health. It is likely that combined OCP containing only estrogen and progesterone cannot overcome the alterations in hormone levels associated with low energy availability, including decreased total triiodothyronine, leptin, insulin, insulin-like growth factors, glucose, luteinizing hormone pulsatility, and follicle-stimulating hormone, as well as an increase in growth hormone and cortisol as noted above.[111]

Not only are OCP unable to counter the impact these hormone alterations have on bone health; they may contribute, in fact, to worsening bone health. Exogenous estrogen replacement in young athletes may lead to premature closure of growth plates, and early OCP use has been associated with lower BMD in the spine and femoral neck among female distance runners.[183]

An athlete's general health and any medical complications that exist from disordered eating are typically monitored by a physician. A registered dietitian, preferably one who specializes in sport nutrition, can address individual nutritional needs by reviewing a nutritional diary and exercise and training habits to identify who may be at risk for low energy availability and to determine if there is disordered eating. Food logs can provide a record of nutritional inadequacies and triggers leading to disordered eating and can help monitor positive changes and progress that occur with healthy eating behaviors.

The role of a registered dietitian is to ensure that daily energy intake from calories and nutrients is appropriately matched with daily energy expenditure including calories burned during exercise.[112] Athletes may have normal BMI but do not match food intake to energy expenditure.

The goal is to increase caloric intake above 30-kcalkg-1 fat-free mass (FFM); some would recommend upward of 45-kcalkgj-1 FFM to produce changes in bone mineral density. What this translates into practically is approximately 1,912 cal for a 110-lb female distance runner with 15% body fat (110 lb 0.85 = 93.5-lb FFM Y 42.5-kg FFM 45-kcalkg-1 FFM = 1,912 kcal). Assuming she was continuing to train throughout this recovery period, adding additional calories to cover exercise-related expenditures would be required to replace the deficit (~100 kcalmile-1).[89]

Standards on minimal healthy weights established by the Centers for Disease Control and Prevention indicate that in adults (older than 20 years), a BMI less than 18.5 is classified as being underweight.[14,77] For children and teens up to age 20 years age-specific BMI values are used; values that are less than the fifth percentile of the normal BMI range for that age are considered underweight.[14,77] Caution should be exercised when using body composition measurements to establish weight management goals for this population because body composition changes during normal pubertal growth and maturation can be significant and can considerably affect BMI values.[43]

Even though nutritional education is first and foremost in addressing the physical effects that can result from disordered eating, modifying and treating the emotional thought processes, fears, and concerns that trigger the behaviors may require concurrent psychologic counseling by a licensed mental health expert. The goals of such an intervention would be to identify the psychologic barriers that preclude healthy eating patterns and to provide support to increase the likelihood that permanent attitudinal and behavioral changes are made.

***Prognosis.*** Research indicates that the prognosis for low energy availability and disordered eating is good with early intervention. Harmful long-term effects of the condition can be avoided or prevented.[113,252,537]

SPECIAL IMPLICATIONS FOR THE THERAPIST 3.10

### *Low Energy Availability and the Female Athlete Triad*

Physical therapists play an important part of the multidisciplinary team that not only screens and treats clients with disordered eating but, most importantly, can act to prevent complications that exist as a result of the condition. They can be indirectly involved in recognizing warning signs that indicate disordered eating and make the appropriate referral so that early intervention can begin. Physical therapists are well equipped to examine, correct, and modify training errors and recovery from exercise that may lead to overuse injury. When a history of musculoskeletal injury is present, physical therapists are an important part of the team in treating musculoskeletal and biomechanical faults responsible for injury, as well as providing tools for preventing future injury.

Each team member involved in the care of the individual with disordered eating should be responsible for knowing when to treat and when to refer the individual to another team member or health professional when intervention is out of the scope of their knowledge base. Referring an individual to an appropriate health care professional requires having knowledge and awareness of the condition, as well as good communication skills, so they can best serve the individual with disordered eating.

Preparticipation physical examinations provide an excellent opportunity for assessing current and previous activity levels, menstrual history, and identifying and treating musculoskeletal and biomechanical faults.[14,266] In the clinic, when treating physically active children and young adults, physical therapists should routinely assess daily activity patterns both during formal training and on the athlete's own time, modifying activities to prevent injury. Any signs that indicate nutritional needs are not being met, such as excessive fatigue, preoccupation with weight or food, history of stress fractures, should raise a red flag.

Table 3.10 includes some guidelines of what questions to ask when assessing disordered eating and the potential consequences that can occur as a result of this condition.[266] Because disordered eating behaviors are not easily admitted to, especially if there is a belief that negative consequences may result if the behaviors are exposed, menstrual history at least provides an indication for young women that disordered eating or an eating disorder may exist. Menstrual dysfunction can be caused by other factors besides disordered eating, so it is important that other causes for the dysfunction are first ruled out by a qualified endocrinologist. Girls not menstruating after age 16 years should be referred for medical evaluation, including baseline screening for osteoporosis.

During stages of rehabilitation of an injury, a physical therapist's expertise can be used to determine whether the selection of exercise is appropriate to the stage of tissue healing, particularly when stress fractures are present. An exercise program should be carefully modified to minimize risk rather than having the individual limit or stop activity, which often leads to frustration, depression, and noncompliance that may trigger disordered eating. Young female athletes with unexplained pain should be screened for fracture and possible onset of osteoporosis.

When determining the appropriateness of an exercise, the desired effect on bone should be considered. Choice of weight training versus weight-bearing exercise or alternating both should be determined by the goals set for that individual in the rehabilitation process. Educating and helping an individual understand that incorporating days of recovery from exercise and complying with dietary recommendations enhances mental and physical performance will drive successful behavioral changes. When suspicious of disordered eating in athletes, education should extend to coaches, parents, and teammates[205] so that normal and realistic body images and healthy habits become a part of everyone's knowledge and awareness.

## Sleep–Wake Disorders

### Overview

The body has an internal timing system called the circadian system that regulates daily behavior and bodily functions through cycles called circadian rhythms. Circadian rhythms influence things such as sleeping and eating patterns, body temperature, and the production of certain hormones. These rhythms repeat approximately every 24 hours. A particular part of the brain called the suprachiasmatic nucleus generates circadian rhythms. Exposure to light also affects the timing of the rhythms. Normally, circadian rhythms are in sync with the surrounding environment, which helps people stay awake during the daytime and fall asleep at night. Circadian rhythm sleep–wake disorders occur when the synchronization between circadian rhythms and the external environment is lost or when the circadian system itself is dysfunctional.

**Table 3.10 Questions a Physical Therapist May Ask Clients to Screen for Disordered Eating and Complications Related to Disordered Eating**

**Disordered Eating**

1. What is your present weight?
2. Are you happy with your weight?
3. How much would you like to weigh?
4. Are you trying to lose weight?
5. In the last year, what was your highest weight? Lowest weight?
6. Has anyone recommended you change your weight or eating habits?
7. Do you lose weight regularly to meet weight requirements for your sport?
8. At what weight do you intend to compete?
9. Do you limit or carefully control what you eat?
10. Have you ever tried diet pills, sitting in a sauna, diuretics, laxatives, vomiting, or similar techniques to lose weight?
11. Have you ever been diagnosed with anorexia, bulimia, or another type of eating disorder?

**Menstrual Disorders**

1. Have you ever had a menstrual period?
2. How old were you when you had your first period?
3. How many periods have you had in the last 12 months?
4. How much time do you usually have from the start of one period to the start of another?
5. What was the longest time between periods in the last year?
6. Do you take birth control pills or any form of estrogen replacement?

**Osteoporosis**

1. Have you had any broken or fractured bones?
2. Have you ever had a stress fracture? If so, how many, when, and where in your body?
3. Have you ever had a bone density test?
4. Is there a history of osteoporosis in your family?
5. Do you take calcium, vitamin D, or other supplements for bone health?

From Sundgot-Borgen J: Disordered eating. In Ireland ML, Nattiv A, eds: *The Female Athlete*, Philadelphia, Saunders, 2002:242–243.

There are at 12 sleep disorders identified in the DSM-5, including insomnia, sleep apnea, and restless legs syndrome. Sleep deprivation can impact most, if not all body functions. Elimination of neurotoxic waste, tissue healing, and cardiovascular and metabolic mechanisms are affected by loss of sleep.[465] Neuroplasticity and neuroprotection are influenced by sleep, as disturbances can lead to glial overactivation which leads to a neuroinflammatory state and creates higher levels of BDNF, IL-1β, TNF-α leading to increased excitability of the CNS.[367] Sleep–wake disorders can lead to learning and memory problems and decreased eye–hand coordination.[560]

Heightened perception of pain has now been established as a side effect of lack of sleep.[384] There is evidence that a sleep-deprived driver may be more impaired by alcohol than when adequately rested.[184]

## Etiology and Pathogenesis

Sleep abnormalities are consistently associated with depression, including decreased REM latency (the time between falling asleep and the first REM period), longer first REM period, less continuous sleep, and early morning awakenings. Animal studies show that many antidepressants can reset the internal clock. Depression may cause alterations in REM sleep. As many as 40% of people with depression have insomnia. Posttraumatic stress disorder (PTSD) can produce vivid and terrifying nightmares. Anxiety disorders predispose to insomnia. The most common of these are generalized anxiety disorder, panic disorder, and anxiety disorders not otherwise specified. Thought disorders and misperception of sleep state are other potential states that cause insomnia. Psychotropic medications, such as antidepressants, may interfere with normal REM sleep patterns. Rebound insomnia from benzodiazepines or other hypnotic agents is common.

Chronic medical conditions often have characteristic alpha brain-wave activity that intrudes into the deeper stages of sleep. This activity can readily be seen on the EEG. Individuals with insomnia often have some degree of sleep-state misperception, wherein they perceive and believe that they achieve significantly less sleep than they actually get.

## Diagnosis

Tools to determine the level of sleep–wake disorder include the Insomnia Severity Index (ISI). The Insomnia Severity Index has seven questions. The seven answers are added up to get a total score, which is then matched into the following categories: 0–7 = No clinically significant insomnia; 8–14 = Subthreshold insomnia; 15–21 = Clinical insomnia (moderate severity); 22–28 = Clinical insomnia (severe).[40] The Sleep Hygiene system consists of 13 items scored on a 5-point Likert scale from 0 or Never to 4 or Always. Higher scores indicate more maladaptive sleep hygiene.[456]

CBT, either alone or in combination with medication can improve sleep latency, time awake after sleep onset, and sleep efficiency during initial therapy. Long-term outcome was optimized when medication was discontinued during maintenance CBT.[333]

Melatonin is a hormone produced by the body that regulates sleep–wake cycles, and melatonin supplements may be used in some situations to help align the body's circadian rhythms with the outside environment.[569] Many medications have been developed to either promote wakefulness or facilitate sleep.

Substances such as alcohol, nicotine, and caffeine should be avoided in a person with sleep–wake disorder. Alcohol creates the illusion of good sleep, but it adversely affects sleep architecture. Nicotine and caffeine are stimulating and should be avoided in the second half of the day, from late afternoon on. Consumption of tryptophan-containing foods like milk may help induce sleep.

Strenuous exercise during the day may promote better sleep, but this same exercise during the 3 hours before bedtime can cause initial insomnia. Stimulating activities should be avoided 3 hours before bedtime. Watching television or late-night use of electronic devices should also be avoided.

## Prognosis

Chronic insomnia is associated with an increased risk of depression and accompanying danger of suicide, anxiety, excess disability, reduced quality of life, and increased use of health care resources.

Mood and anxiety disorders may develop from untreated sleep disturbances. Medical literature supports the theory that these brain-based mental status changes are risk factors for morbidity and mortality from a host of medical conditions such as cardiovascular disease.

## Substance Use Disorders

### Overview

Understanding and treating addiction is best done through the complex and interdependent relationship of genetic, environmental, social, and psychologic factors, using the epigenetic model discussed in Chapter 2. We are the product of our biology, our environment, our life experiences, our exposure to psychologic and physical traumas, adverse childhood experiences, the influence of poverty, and acts of prejudice and discrimination, to name just a few. We are influenced by our perceptions, thoughts, and beliefs. These influences increase our vulnerability and require resourcefulness to offset the expression of addictions.

Our biology provides us with genetic material. According to our genetics, a person can inherit genetic code that may predispose them to a vulnerability to addiction. Just because a person carries the genetic code vulnerability to addiction does not mean that person will experience addiction. Whether this gene gets expressed, turned off, or remains dormant is explained by epigenetics. Certain life experiences can cause genes to be silenced or expressed over time. These influences are everywhere. The expression of genes is directly related to the influences of the environment, both external and internal environments.

*Substance Use Disorders* indicate that the person has continued use/abuse of a substance for 12 or more months. The DSM-5 establishes nine types of Substance-Related Disorders, which will be addressed individually below. With all substances, addiction is related to the pathologic set of behaviors related to the use that leads to abuse. These behaviors are summarized into categories. *Impaired Control* is identified by taking the substance in larger amounts or for longer than intended with unsuccessful attempts to cut down or stop using the substance related to uncontrolled cravings and urges.

*Social Impairment* is spending a lot of time getting, using, and recovering from use of the substance, problems at work, home, or school because of substance use, and continuing to use, even when it causes problems in relationships and giving up important social, occupational, or recreational activities because of substance use.

*Risky Use* includes using substances repetitively, with knowledge that it is dangerous, and continuing to use, despite physical or psychologic problem worsened by the substance and using the substance in unsafe environments.

*Pharmacologic* concerns include developing tolerance to the substance, thus needing more of the substance to create effect and withdrawal symptoms that are relieved by taking more of the substance.

A person needs to meet at least two of these criteria to be diagnosed with a substance-use disorder. The severity of addiction is determined by the number of criteria met. If a person is experiencing withdrawal symptoms at the time they are being evaluated for treatment, they will be diagnosed with both substance use and substance withdrawal.[186]

*Substance Intoxication* refers to the single use of substantial quantities of the substance resulting in significant impairment of psychologic status and/or behavior that restricts participation in social/occupational/leisure roles combined with additional specific signs and symptoms

*Substance Withdrawal* is the pattern of physical responses severe enough to create restrictions in participation when regular drug use is discontinued. The onset of withdrawal signs and symptoms may occur within minutes or after a few days when a physically dependent person abruptly stops consumption. Withdrawal can cause emotional, psychologic, and/or physical distress and, with certain substances, can be so severe that it results in death (see Table 3.11).

### Etiology and Pathogenesis

Dopamine, a neurotransmitter, plays a pivotal role in substance dependence by activating mesolimbic pathways (nucleus accumbens, amygdala, hippocampus, prefrontal cortex) in the brain that register feelings of arousal, reward, and satisfaction—the so-called reward pathway.[88] For people who become drug dependent, the pathway becomes more deeply ingrained with each use and becomes linked with cues evoking drug use, such as smells, location, paraphernalia, or certain companions. When a person who is substance dependent encounters a use-associated cue, a spontaneous and overwhelming desire for the substance occurs, triggered by a dopamine release in the brain. Stimulation of the mesolimbic dopamine reward pathway may induce neuroplastic changes in the prefrontal-striatal networks, impairing impulse control, further augmenting the addictive behavior and increasing the likelihood of relapse or recidivism.[82]

Two neurotransmitters, GABA (inhibitory) and glutamate (excitatory), are implicated in addictive behavior. Various substances impact the availability of these neurotransmitters, explaining the psychotropic effects of certain classes of drugs. Alcohol increases GABA activity and decreases glutamate activity, resulting in sedative effects on the brain, leading to feelings of pleasure, calmness, or sleepiness. Sedatives increase the GABA availability, while caffeine inhibits GABA and increases glutamate and phencyclidine (PCP) and other stimulants increase glutamate availability.

### Diagnosis

Diagnosis of substance use and addictive disorders is made primarily through examination, particularly a thorough history, identification of the various signs and symptoms of substance use, intoxication, and withdrawal. Appropriate questionnaires should be used in addition to the history. The DSM-5[20] delineates the criteria that must be met to diagnose the individual disorders. A thorough physical examination is also required to rule out medical conditions that may mimic substance use, to measure levels of substances in the body, and to identify comorbid medical conditions. In older adults, slowed response, hypersomnia, and increasing confusion sometimes thought

**Table 3.11** Specific Effects of Substance Use, Intoxication, and Withdrawal

| Substance | Behavioral or Psychologic Impairments that Impact Activities and Participation in Social, Leisure, or Occupational Roles | Intoxication/Adverse Effects | Signs and Symptoms of Withdrawal |
|---|---|---|---|
| **Alcohol** (wine, beer, liquor) | • Inappropriate sexual behavior<br>• Mood lability<br>• Impaired judgment | • Slurred speech<br>• Incoordination<br>• Unsteady gait<br>• Nystagmus<br>• Impaired attention<br>• Impaired memory<br>• Stupor or coma | • Hyperactive SNS*<br>• Tachycardia<br>• Sweating<br>• Hand tremor<br>• Insomnia<br>• Nausea/vomiting<br>• Hallucinations<br>• Psychomotor agitation<br>• Anxiety<br>• Generalized tonic-clonic seizures |
| **Caffeine** (some soda pops, energy drinks, coffee, black tea, chocolate, some over-the-counter medications) | | • Restlessness<br>• Irritability<br>• Nervousness<br>• Excitement<br>• Headache<br>• Insomnia<br>• Flushed<br>• Diuresis<br>• GI disturbance<br>• Muscle twitching, tension<br>• Rambling flow of thought/speech<br>• Tachycardia/arrhythmia<br>• Periods of inexhaustibility, sleep disturbances<br>• Psychomotor agitation<br>• Enhances pain perception | • Headache<br>• Marked fatigue or drowsiness<br>• Dysphoric mood, depressed mood, irritability<br>• Difficulty concentrating<br>• Flu-like symptoms, nausea, vomiting, muscle pain/stiffness |
| **Cannabis** marijuana (pot, weed), THC, hashish | • Impaired motor coordination<br>• Euphoria<br>• Anxiety<br>• Sensation of slowed time<br>• Relaxed inhibitions<br>• Impaired judgment<br>• Paranoia, social withdrawal | • Red sclera<br>• Increased appetite<br>• Dry mouth<br>• Tachycardia | • Irritability, anger or aggression<br>• Nervousness or anxiety<br>• Sleep difficulty<br>• Decreased appetite or weight loss<br>• Restlessness<br>• Depressed mood<br>• Sweating<br>• Chills<br>• Headache |
| **Hallucinogens** LSD, PCP, peyote, psilocybin (mushrooms, "schrooms," "rooms") | • Marked anxiety or depression<br>• Ideas of reference<br>• Paranoid ideation<br>• Impaired judgment | • Pupillary dilation<br>• Tachycardia<br>• Sweating<br>• Blurring of vision<br>• Tremors<br>• Incoordination | • Persisting perception disorder<br>• Continued signs/symptoms of intoxication |
| **Inhalants** (gasoline, nitrous oxide, nitrite gases, aerosols) | • Belligerence<br>• Assaultiveness<br>• Apathy<br>• Impaired judgment | • Dizziness<br>• Nystagmus<br>• Incoordination<br>• Slurred speech<br>• Unsteady gait<br>• Lethargy<br>• Depressed reflexes<br>• Psychomotor retardation<br>• Tremor<br>• Generalized muscle weakness<br>• Blurred vision or diplopia<br>• Stupor or coma<br>• Euphoria | |

Continued

Table 3.11 Specific Effects of Substance Use, Intoxication, and Withdrawal—cont'd

| Substance | Behavioral or Psychologic Impairments that Impact Activities and Participation in Social, Leisure, or Occupational Roles | Intoxication/Adverse Effects | Signs and Symptoms of Withdrawal |
|---|---|---|---|
| **Opioids** (morphine, Demerol, Dilaudid, Vicodin, codeine) | • Euphoria<br>• Psychomotor agitation/retardation<br>• Impaired judgment | Pupil constriction plus 1 or more:<br>• Drowsiness or coma<br>• Slurred speech<br>• Impairment in attention or memory | • Dysphoric mood<br>• Nausea/vomiting<br>• Muscle aches<br>• Lacrimation or rhinorrhea<br>• Pupil dilation, piloerection, sweating<br>• Diarrhea<br>• Yawning<br>• Fever<br>• Insomnia |
| **Sedatives/Hypnotics** Benzodiazepines (Xanax, Valium), barbiturates (Seconal), heroin | • Inappropriate sexual behavior<br>• Mood lability<br>• Impaired judgment | • Slurred speech<br>• Incoordination<br>• Unsteady gait<br>• Nystagmus<br>• Impairment in cognition (e.g., attention, memory)<br>• Stupor or coma<br>• Death (overdose) | • Autonomic hyperactivity (sweating, HR > 100)<br>• Hand tremor<br>• Insomnia<br>• Nausea or vomiting<br>• Hallucinations (visual, tactile, auditory)<br>• Psychomotor agitation<br>• Anxiety<br>• Grand mal seizures |
| **Stimulants** amphetamines ("speed"), cocaine (crack), methamphetamine, ecstasy | • Euphoria or affective blunting<br>• Hypervigilance<br>• Anxiety<br>• Tension<br>• Interpersonal sensitivity | • Tachycardia or bradycardia<br>• Pupillary dilation<br>• Elevated or lowered blood pressure<br>• Increased pulse rate<br>• Perspiration or chills<br>• Nausea or vomiting<br>• Weight loss<br>• Psychomotor agitation/hallucinations<br>• Muscle weakness<br>• Respiratory depression<br>• Chest pain<br>• Arrhythmias<br>• Confusion<br>• Seizures<br>• Dyskinesias<br>• Dystonias<br>• Coma<br>• Death (overdose) | • Dysphoric<br>• Fatigue<br>• Vivid, unpleasant dreams<br>• Insomnia or hypersomnia<br>• Increased appetite<br>• Psychomotor retardation or agitation |
| **Tobacco** (cigarettes, cigars, chewing or spit tobacco, pipe tobacco) | | • Increased risk of heart disease, respiratory disease, and many types of cancer<br>• Poor wound healing<br>• Back pain, spinal disk disease<br>• Osteoporosis | • Irritability, frustration, or anger<br>• Anxiety<br>• Difficulty concentrating<br>• Increased appetite or weight gain<br>• Restlessness<br>• Depressed mood<br>• Insomnia |

to relate to aging may be symptoms of toxic drug levels. Signs and symptoms of withdrawal may not be readily diagnosed in older adults.

### Treatment

Substance abuse can be characterized as a psychologic condition, a medical condition, or a combination of both. From a substance recovery perspective, a biopsychosocial approach is most common and effective. Interventions include education, counseling, CBT, behavior modification, and for many substances, pharmacologic help. Success depends on the individual's desire to correct the problem and adherence with treatment regimens.

A mindfulness-based intervention called *urge surging* has been developed for calming, curbing, or extinguishing cravings. This behavioral approach relies on the idea that urges for addictive substances or activities rarely last very long and can be used to deal with the internal struggle that feeds cravings. This approach may not initially reduce urges but may change the response to such thoughts.[58]

More specific information about this technique is available online at: http://www.mindfulness.org.au/urge-surfing-relapse-prevention/ accessed December 12, 2018.

Prevention is the key to any successful substance abuse program. The American Medical Association has released guidelines recommending that all people older than age 60 years be screened and treated for substance abuse problems.

## Prognosis

Substance abuse is associated with child and spousal abuse; sexually transmitted diseases, including HIV infection; teen pregnancy; school failure; motor vehicle crashes; mental health conditions; escalation of health care costs; low worker productivity; and homelessness. Individual characteristics, length and severity of use, and support networks all impact the prognosis.

## Alcohol Use Disorders

Alcoholism is the most common drug abuse problem in the United States, affecting more than 15 million Americans, including the adolescent and aging populations. The frequency of binge drinking, defined as five or more drinks at a time for men or four or more drinks for women on an occasion during the past 30 days,[78] among college students has increased dramatically in the last decade with an increase in the number of alcohol-related injuries, property damage, and disruption.[78,203] Excessive alcohol consumption kills approximately 75,000 people each year in the United States.[512] Alcohol-related deaths outnumber deaths related to other drugs 4 to 1, and alcohol is a factor in more than half of all domestic violence and sexual assault cases.[353]

Alcoholism is extremely prevalent yet underdiagnosed among adults with symptomatic terminal cancer.[22] Binge drinking has also been identified as a risk factor for all strokes.[492] Alcohol withdrawal usually begins 3 to 36 hours after the last drink and may be accompanied by behavioral manifestations or physiologic complications such as electrolyte disorders, dehydration, polyneuropathy, or myopathy.[130] Research provides evidence of a genetic predisposition in alcohol.[407] Stress, depression, peer pressure, anxiety, and mental illness, such as schizophrenia, PTSD, antisocial personality disorder, and borderline personality disorder, increase the risk of addiction.

Early-age-onset alcohol use disorder involves multiple phenotypes including biochemical, physiologic, and psychologic, which interacts with the environment beginning at conception. Alterations in biobehavioral phenotypes have been linked with substance use, first as difficult or abnormal temperament in infancy, progressing to conduct disorder in childhood and culminating in early adolescence substance abuse, becoming severe by young adulthood.[497,536] Protein kinase C-epsilon (PKC-ε) has been implicated in both nicotine and alcohol addictions. PKC-ε may impact the reward system by signaling α(6)-containing nicotine receptors, reducing dopamine release in the nucleus accumbens (part of the brain's pleasure center).[267] Inhibiting this enzyme may remove the rewarding effects of alcohol.[199]

Women feel the effects of alcohol sooner and more intensely than do men. Women produce substantially less of the gastric enzyme alcohol dehydrogenase, which breaks down ethanol in the stomach. As a result, women absorb 75% more alcohol into the bloodstream. Women (and older adults of either gender) have less water in their tissues than men of comparable height and build. Because alcohol is soluble in water, it tends to dissolve more slowly, resulting in longer-lasting intoxication after fewer drinks.

Individuals with alcohol use disorder are likely to drink in one of three patterns: regular binge drinking, consistent heavy drinking, or occasional heavy binge drinking interspersed with periods of no drinking. Drowsiness, perceptual changes, and motor impairments including decreased balance, coordination, reaction, and movement time are responsible for increased incidence of MVAs (40% of all MVAs) and a large percentage of accidents that occur on the job.[232] Restricting participation in social/occupational/leisure roles is associated with the effects of alcohol abuse.

Individuals with more advanced physiologic effects of chronic alcohol abuse may be impaired cognitively from Wernicke-Korsakoff syndrome. Wernicke-Korsakoff syndrome is a well-described syndrome of neurologic and cognitive problems that comprises both Wernicke encephalopathy and Korsakoff syndrome. When Wernicke encephalopathy is undiagnosed or inadequately treated, it can progress to Korsakoff syndrome or dementia.[508]

Treatment may be one-to-one or in a group setting. Twelve-step programs (e.g., AA, Celebrate Recovery), which combine a social and spiritual approach, seem to be effective for many.[133] Other psychosocial approaches include cognitive behavior and motivational enhancement therapies. Pharmacologic interventions include SSRIs,[397] naltrexone and nalmefene, which block opioid receptors thus diminishing the pleasurable effects, in turn decreasing cravings.[34,330] Antabuse causes nausea when alcohol is consumed.[301] Detoxification may take 2 to 7 days depending on severity of use.[555]

Treatment for alcohol abuse is a life-long process, either as an active alcoholic (currently drinking) or a recovering alcoholic (currently not drinking). The prognosis is good for those in whom a biopsychosocial approach aligns with their values and personality.[261,502,571]

The most severe consequence associated with alcohol use during pregnancy is fetal alcohol syndrome. Destruction of neurons in the developing human brain leads to reduced brain mass and associated dysfunction.[212]

## Caffeine Use Disorders

Caffeine is the most common behaviorally active drug that can result in physical dependence. The most common source of dietary caffeine is coffee, with average consumption around 200 mg/day, soda pop, and energy drinks.

Caffeine inhibits GABA and increases glutamate, resulting in a stimulatory effect. Caffeine acts as an inhibitory neurotransmitter and reduces inhibitory function, thereby creating an excitatory response. It can enhance cognition, learning, and memory in the short term but have detrimental effects long term.[423] The positive effects are being examined relative to diseases such as Alzheimer and Parkinson diseases, among others.

Functional MRI studies indicate that caffeine increases responses in the bilateral medial frontopolar cortex (BA 10) and the right anterior cingulate cortex (BA 32), brain structures associated with executive function and attention during working memory.[164] An abrupt decrease in caffeine may cause withdrawal symptoms, such as headaches, fatigue, irritability, and difficulty focusing on tasks.

### Cannabis Use Disorders

In 2015, about 4 million people in the United States met diagnostic criteria for a substance use disorder based on cannabis use.[76] Marijuana has been used medically to treat nausea associated with chemotherapy and for persons with intractable pain. Recent data suggest that 30% of those who use marijuana may have some degree of marijuana use disorder.[187] People who begin using marijuana before the age of 18 are four to seven times more likely to develop a marijuana use disorder than adults.[554]

People who use marijuana and carry a specific variant of the AKT1 gene, which codes for an enzyme that affects dopamine signaling in the striatum of the basal ganglia and associated with production ofdopamine, are at increased risk of developing psychosis. The risk of psychosis among those with this variant was seven times higher for those who used marijuana daily compared with those who did not use or used it infrequently.[105]

The psychoactive compound in cannabis-related substances is Δ9-THC (Δ9-tetrahydrocannabinol). Δ9-THC acts as a cannabinoid (CB1) receptor agonist, impacting motor activity, pain, affective state, and appetite.[390] Δ9-THC stimulates the dopamine reward system via the CB1 receptors. Evidence indicates that the interaction of Δ9-THC with A2A adenosine receptors contributes to physical dependence, tolerance, and motivation in mice.[475] The effects of cannabis derivatives usually last a few hours. As a result of a long half-life and the development of tolerance, less of the drug is needed to produce the same effects. The agent persists in the body as an active metabolite for as long as 8 days after use. Dysfunction in the hippocampus can lead to impaired memory.[319] Heavy marijuana use in youth has also been linked to increased risk for developing mental illness and poorer cognitive functioning.[314,463]

Cumulative lifetime exposure to marijuana is associated with lower scores on a test of verbal memory but may not affect other cognitive abilities such as processing speed or executive function. A large longitudinal study in New Zealand found that persistent marijuana use disorder with frequent use starting in adolescence was associated with a loss of an average of 6 or up to 8 IQ points measured in mid-adulthood. Significantly, in that study, those who used marijuana heavily as teenagers and quit using as adults did not recover the lost IQ points.[32,215] There is growing concern that the increased potency of legal and available edibles is leading to higher levels of exposure.

There are no FDA-approved medications for the treatment of marijuana use disorder, but research is active in this area. Because sleep problems feature prominently in marijuana withdrawal, some studies are examining the effectiveness of medications that aid in sleep. Medications that have shown promise in early studies or small clinical trials include the sleep aids, antianxiety/antistress medication. Antiepileptics such as gabapentine may improve sleep and executive function. The nutritional supplement N-acetylcysteine and chemicals called FAAH inhibitors may reduce withdrawal by inhibiting the breakdown of the body's own cannabinoids. Future directions include the study of substances called allosteric modulators that interact with cannabinoid receptors to inhibit THC's rewarding effects. As in other substance-related disorders a biopsychosocial approach may be most effective. Many users of cannabis quit of their own accord after a period of experimentation.

### Hallucinogenic Use Disorders

Hallucinogens (psychedelic drugs) are a chemically diverse group of drugs that affect the thought processes, perceptions of the physical world, and sense of time passing. Hallucinogens can be plant based, but the most common use is related to those that are produced synthetically. The best-known hallucinogens are lysergic acid diethylamide (LSD), mescaline, psilocybin, and MDMA (ecstasy).

These drugs bind with one type of serotonin receptor (5-$HT_2$) in the brain. Serotonin is a neurotransmitter that facilitates transmission of nerve impulses in the brain and is associated with feelings of well-being, as well as many physiologic responses.[364] When a hallucinogenic compound binds with serotonin receptors, serotonin is blocked from those receptor sites, and nerve transmission is altered, creating an increase in unattached serotonin in the brain. The result is a distortion of the senses of sight, sound, and touch, disorientation in time and space, and alterations of mood.

Hallucinogens distort the perception of reality. In the case of hallucinogen intoxication, there remains an awareness that these changes in perception are caused by the hallucinogen. This differs from hallucinations, which are imagined visions or sounds (e.g., hearing voices). Hallucinogens alter the perception of something that is physically present. A face may appear to be melting, or colors may become brighter or moving. Sounds may be "seen" rather than heard. More than with other drugs, the mental state of the hallucinogen user and the environment in which the drug is taken influence the experience a user has.

To be diagnosed as a psychiatric disorder, flashbacks must cause significant distress or interfere with daily life activities. They can come on suddenly with no warning or be triggered by specific environments. Flashbacks may include emotional symptoms, seeing colors, geometric forms, or, most commonly, persistence of trails of light across the visual field. Many individuals use hallucinogenic drugs as a temporary experiment, often stopping after having a negative experience.[500]

### Inhalant-Related Disorders

The number of possible inhalants makes it impossible to pinpoint a pathogenic action. The variety of substances that may be inhaled is large—paint, gasoline, glue, nail polish, hair spray, lighter fluid, and more. Inhalants are more likely to be used by children and teens than any other groups.

Inhalants can alter brain chemistry and may induce lifelong damage to the nervous system. Some inhaled gases can replace oxygen in the lungs and result in *Sudden Sniffing Death.* Use is often temporary, but death can occur the first time an inhalant is used.

### Opioid Use Disorders

The prescribing of opioids has increased significantly in the last 3 decades and now is considered a crisis in the United States. This reflects addictive use and does not correlate to the incidence or magnitude of pain conditions. The United States constitutes only 4.6% of the world population; however, it consumes 80% of the world's opioid supply and 99% of the world's hydrocodone supply. Preoccupation with acquiring the drug causes individuals to seek ongoing and possibly unnecessary medical care.[373]

Opioid dependence and withdrawal symptoms originate from the locus ceruleus (LC) of the brain stem. Neurons in the LC produce a chemical, noradrenaline (NA), and distribute it to other parts of the brain, where it stimulates wakefulness, breathing, blood pressure, and general alertness, among other functions. When opioid molecules link to mu receptors on brain cells in the LC, they suppress the neurons' release of NA, resulting in drowsiness, slowed respiration, and low blood pressure, causing the familiar effects of opioid intoxication. With repeated exposure to opioids, however, the LC neurons adjust by increasing their level of activity. With continued use of opioids, the suppressive impact is offset by heightened activity in the LC. Then when opioids are not available to suppress the LC brain cells' heightened activity, the LC neurons release excessive amounts of NA, triggering jitters, anxiety, muscle cramps, and diarrhea.[254] This creates the physiologic need to replace the opioid activity in the brain, leading to addictive, drug-seeking behaviors.

According to DSM-5, opioid intoxication is significant problematic behavioral or psychologic changes that develop during or shortly after opioid administration. For example, initial euphoria followed by symptoms of depression and anxiety such as apathy, dysphoria, psychomotor agitation or retardation and impaired judgment. Pupillary constriction, drowsiness, slurred speech, and signs of anxiety are seen after use. The diagnostic feature of substance/medication-induced depressive disorder include the symptoms of a depressive disorder associated with the administration of a substance. The depressive symptoms must persist beyond the expected length of physiologic effects, intoxication, or withdrawal period.

Opioids depress central nervous system activity, creating decreased respirations, lowered heart rate, and loss of consciousness. When opioids are taken together with other drugs that depress central nervous system activity, such as benzodiazepines, there are often serious and fatal results. Anxiolytics like benzodiazepines are often prescribed to treat anxiety and depression, often despite the history of chronic opioid use. Benzodiazepines significantly exacerbate both opioid-induced depression and anxiety.

DSM-5 classifies major depressive disorder as a prominent and persistent depressed mood causing clinically significant distress or impairment in social, occupational or other important areas of functioning that is not attributable to the psychologic effects of a substance or another medical condition. Benzodiazepines are substantially involved in opioid deaths. In 2011 more than 30% of opioid overdose deaths involved benzodiazepines.[81] This problem is exacerbated by the fact that opioids are prescribed by primary care physicians and surgeons, whereas antianxiety and antidepressants are typically prescribed by psychiatrists.[227]

Tolerance to opioids develops quickly, and withdrawal symptoms are difficult and can be fatal. Discontinuation of severe opioid use may take multiple days and often is done cold-turkey in a medically supervised inpatient facility.

## Sedatives, Hypnotics, or Anxiolytic Use-Related Disorders

Sedatives, hypnotics, and anxiolytics (SHA) are prescribed for physical and psychologic medical conditions. These substances reduce arousal and stimulation of the brain, creating an experience of calm or sedation, sleep, respiratory depression, or coma. This class of substances includes all prescription sleeping medications and almost all prescription antianxiety medications, or tranquilizers. Sedative-, hypnotic-, or anxiolytic- (SHA-) related disorders include SHA intoxication, SHA use disorder, and SHA withdrawal.

Prolonged use can be addictive for some people. Symptoms may include sudden changes in mood, impaired judgment, inappropriate sexual or aggressive behavior, slurred speech, lack of coordination, unsteady walk, repetitive, uncontrolled eye movements, impaired attention and memory, and stupor or coma. Memory problems are common following SHA intoxication. People may not recall anything that happened while under the influence of the substance. The pathogenesis of sedatives mimics alcohol. Sedatives increase the availability of the neurotransmitter GABA, resulting in a generalized sedative effect on the brain.

SHA intoxication is diagnosed when recent exposure to these substances causes significant problematic behavioral or psychologic changes. Diagnosis for SHA-use disorder requires that the individual has been taking these medications in larger amounts or over more time than was originally intended or over 12 months. There must be a strong craving or urge to use sedatives, hypnotics, or anxiolytics, despite having a strong desire to decrease or stop use. There is increased time recovering from the effects of the medication, continuing use when problems are caused by these drugs in major areas of life or under hazardous conditions. There is an increased need for higher doses of the medication for intoxication or desired effect. People experiencing SHA withdrawal may experience sweating, increased heart rate, hand tremor, insomnia, nausea or vomiting, visual, tactile, or auditory hallucinations, anxiety, and/or seizures.

Recovery from SHA use disorder involves a one-month period of abstinence, along with behavioral counseling that includes instruction on stress management, relaxation, and coping techniques. Medication may be used to reduce withdrawal symptoms and help maintain abstinence. Self-help groups such as 12-step programs and other types of recovery programs can provide long-term support and help prevent relapse. These drugs have also been linked to problems with memory and depression, and some are under investigation for increasing the risk of dementia.[48] Withdrawal from sedatives can be complicated by the *kindling* phenomenon. This is a neurologic condition in which withdrawal symptoms magnify with each subsequent withdrawal attempt and can become very severe, including seizures.

### Stimulant-Related Disorders

Stimulants include drugs such as amphetamines, methamphetamine, and cocaine. They increase energy, attention, and alertness but also cause increased respiration and heart rate. Stimulants may be prescribed to treat obesity, attention-deficit/hyperactivity disorder, narcolepsy, and depression. Use disorders may include prescription drugs that were initially legitimately prescribed. Illicit drugs include cocaine and methamphetamine, which is also known as speed or crystal when it is swallowed or sniffed, crank when it is injected, and ice or glass when it is smoked. Addiction is often immediate with the first methamphetamine use. Stimulant drugs are classified as controlled substances because they have high potential for addiction and abuse. Stimulant-related disorders include stimulant intoxication, stimulant use disorder, and stimulant withdrawal. Stimulants increase the availability of the neurotransmitter glutamate in the brain, resulting in excitation and increased activity. Many stimulants mimic monoamine neurotransmitters (e.g., dopamine, norepinephrine), enhancing the influence of dopamine on the dopamine reward system. Methamphetamine has toxic effects on dopamine axon terminals.

Manifestations of stimulant use disorder include taking stimulants in larger amounts or over more time than was originally intended; having a strong craving or urge to use stimulants; having a strong desire to cut down on stimulant; use making unsuccessful efforts to stop; spending a lot of time obtaining, using, or recovering from the effects of stimulants; and continuing to use stimulants despite the drug causing problems in major areas of life or despite its being physically hazardous. Increased amounts of the stimulant to become intoxicated or reach the desired effect and experiencing withdrawal symptoms when the stimulant use is discontinued is a sign of disorder. Stimulant use disorder may be diagnosed when the use of an amphetamine-type substance, cocaine, or other stimulant leads to significant impairment or distress within a 12-month period.

Stimulant intoxication is diagnosed when recent exposure to a stimulant causes significant problematic behavioral or psychologic changes, such as excessive euphoria, hypervigilance, anger, interpersonal sensitivity, auditory hallucinations, paranoid thoughts, and/or repetitive movement. Physical symptoms may include abnormally fast or slow heartbeat, dilation of the pupils, elevated or lowered blood pressure, sweating or chills, nausea or vomiting, weight loss, and/or muscle weakness.

Stimulant addiction treatment involves nonconfrontational behavioral counseling that provides general information about the addiction process and specifics about the individual treatment plan. Counseling may be offered to family and significant others for general treatment information and their own self-help purposes. In addition to initial individual counseling, a treatment plan for stimulant-related disorder usually includes setting up abstinence goals, attending group therapy, encouraging family support, and establishing long-term support and follow-up.

Withdrawal symptoms, though generally not as severe as with other substances, include fatigue, vivid, unpleasant dreams, insomnia or hypersomnia, and/or abnormally slow heartbeat. These symptoms typically develop within a few hours to several days after stimulant use has stopped. Drug craving and an inability to feel pleasure (anhedonia) may also be present. Hypothermia and convulsions can result in death.

### Tobacco-Use Disorders

Tobacco use is a global problem with the development and marketing of e-cigarettes, "heat-not-burn" tobacco, and dissolvable tobacco. There are over 5 million tobacco-related deaths per year globally—almost twice that for alcohol and illicit drugs combined. This number could grow to 1 billion people in this century, with most deaths occurring in poorer countries. Tobacco use is up to three times more prevalent among individuals with other psychiatric disorders, including anxiety, attention-deficit, mood, and other substance use disorders. Smoking rates in this vulnerable population remain high despite the general trend for decreasing smoking rates in the United States as a whole.[572]

Vaping, the use of e-cigarettes, increased 78% among high schoolers from 2017 to 2018. This epidemic is setting the stage for another generation of Americans addicted to tobacco products and ultimately more tobacco-caused death and disease. According to the American Lung Association, the amount of nicotine in one cartridge is more than an entire pack of cigarettes, and e-cigarettes contain known carcinogens.

Tobacco is one of the most addictive agents, with even greater development of dependence than cocaine and heroin. The active substance in tobacco products is nicotine, a mild stimulant. Nicotine causes release of dopamine and upregulation of receptors, creating sensations of pleasure, appetite reduction, and reduction in anxiety. Nicotine's short half-life of 1 to 2 hours leads to withdrawal symptoms of irritability, frustration, anxiety, difficulty concentrating, restlessness, depressed mood, insomnia, increased appetite, weight gain, and cravings. In the lung, smoking slows fibroblast proliferation and makes fibroblasts less mobile, leading to slower repair of injured lung tissue.[345]

Smoking also has a well-known negative effect on wound healing, bone graft incorporation, and pain reduction.[185] Persons who smoke have an increased risk of lung cancer, chronic obstructive pulmonary disease (emphysema), and bronchial conditions as the result of the tar in cigarette smoke. Carbon monoxide in the smoke increases the risk of cardiovascular disease.

The presence of certain genes may predispose individuals to both alcohol dependence and habitual tobacco use.[172] Smoking exposure during pregnancy is a risk factor for premature birth, growth retardation, and adverse long-term neurobehavioral effects. Nicotine is metabolized more quickly in pregnant women, easily passes the placental barrier, and accumulates in breast milk. The effects of prenatal exposure to nicotine are less well known, but there is emerging evidence that prenatal nicotine exposure is associated with premature birth, stillbirth, and abnormal brain development.[51]

Smokeless (chew) tobacco can lead to nicotine addiction, and long-term use can lead to health problems including periodontal disease. Chronic use of any tobacco products can lead to cancer and cerebrovascular and cardiovascular disease as long-term consequences. There is a known link between active smoking and cervical cancer; a similar association likely exists between passive smoke exposure and cervical carcinogenesis.[516]

The Surgeon General's report on the consequences of involuntary exposure to tobacco smoke reports the following major conclusions[71]:

- Secondhand smoke causes premature death in children and adults who do not smoke.
- Children exposed to secondhand smoke are at an increased risk for sudden infant death syndrome, acute respiratory infections, ear problems, anxiety and depression,[39] and more-severe asthma.
- Exposure of adults to secondhand smoke has immediate adverse effects on the cardiovascular system and causes coronary heart disease and lung cancer.

**Diagnosis.** Nicotine addiction requires daily use of tobacco products to maintain nicotine levels in the brain, primarily to avoid withdrawal but also to modulate mood. Regular tobacco users exhibit altered levels of stress, arousal, and impulsivity.[46] Nicotine dependence is the single most common psychiatric diagnosis in the United States. Substance abuse, major depression, and anxiety disorders are the most prevalent psychiatric comorbid conditions associated with nicotine dependence.

Of the estimated 48 million adult smokers in the United States, approximately 16 million people attempt to stop smoking cigarettes for at least 24 hours annually; another 2 to 3 million attempt to stop but cannot abstain for 24 hours. CBT and pharmacologic interventions for any tobacco addiction, including smokeless tobacco, increase the success rates.[117] However, 1.2 million people stop smoking each year, often without the behavioral and pharmacologic aids.

There are many FDA-approved medications for smoking cessation, including two non-nicotine replacement pill options of bupropion and varenicline and nicotine-replacement therapies (NRT). NRT patches, gum, lozenges, inhaler, and nasal spray are available.[31] Many factors influence the amount of nicotine replacement that might be needed to manage or change behaviors. Choice of medication depends on history, patient input, cost, previous attempts, and severity of dependence/withdrawal and breakthrough symptoms.

The use of tobacco products continues to be the single most preventable cause of disease and death in the United States. Smoking results in more deaths each year in the United States than AIDS, alcohol, cocaine, heroin, homicide, suicide, motor vehicle crashes, and fires combined.

Smoking harms nearly every organ of the body, damaging the smoker's overall health even when it does not cause a specific illness.[72] Smoking has been linked conclusively to acute myeloid leukemia and cancers of the cervix, kidney, pancreas, and stomach. Smoking is known to cause elevated blood pressure, pneumonia, abdominal aortic aneurysm, cataracts, and periodontitis. Smokers are at an increased risk of developing diabetes, heart disease,[145] major depression,[241] and suicide.[61] Smokers may be at increased risk of low back pain.[11] as nicotine has been linked with accelerated disk degeneration.

SPECIAL IMPLICATIONS FOR THE THERAPIST 3.11

### *Substance Use and Addictive Disorders*

Primary intervention in these disorders is essential. Many people who seek medical attention for seemingly unrelated conditions fail to disclose their use of alcohol or other drugs. Low screening rates among excessive drinkers may be more a matter of missed screening opportunities.

As part of the assessment process, therapists using a systems approach can screen for these disorders by asking about the use of prescribed drugs, nonprescription drugs, and self-prescribed drugs such as nicotine, caffeine, and alcohol or other drugs. Recognition of the problem is crucial to successful management. The therapist must be able to recognize impairments of the cognitive and motor systems associated with these disorders.

The behavioral impact of substance use disorder can be identified by asking one or more of the following questions:

- When is it that you feel you need these substances?
- How do these activities help you?
- Are you concerned about your dependence?
- Do you have a pattern of cutting back or stopping the use of alcohol, cigarettes/tobacco, sleeping aids, or other substance but then restarting it?
- Have you been concerned, or has anyone around you raised concern about your use of these substances?

An appropriate final question may be "Because it is important to the results of your treatment, do you take (use) any drugs or substances that you have not told me about yet?"

The National Council on Alcoholism and Drug Dependence has a self-test available for assessing the signs of alcoholism. If the client reports the use of substances, the therapist may want to ask whether the person has discussed this with his or her physician or other health care personnel. Encourage the client to seek medical attention, or inform the individual that this will be addressed as a medical problem in your communication with the physician.

In the acute care setting, it is estimated that one in five patients suffers from an alcohol use disorder and may be at risk for the adverse effects of alcohol withdrawal, a potentially life-threatening condition.[389] Signs and symptoms of alcohol withdrawal syndrome, such as hand tremors, headaches, palpitations, diaphoresis, anxiety, insomnia, motor hyperactivity, nausea or vomiting, and transient hallucinations or illusions, can be easy to miss or attribute to adverse effects of medications.[95,120,530]

More than half of all people with spinal cord injury or TBI incurred their disabilities while under the influence of drugs or alcohol; some studies report as much as 80%. It is estimated that two-thirds of people with disabilities who abuse drugs and/or alcohol did so before their injury and may return to substance use afterward to cope with life changes caused by the disability. Medical professionals should also be observant for excessive sleeping and unusual symptoms, such as muscular inflammation and myopathies, which can occur with the use of street drugs.

The Clinical Institute Withdrawal of Alcohol Scale (CIWA)[488] is an assessment tool used to monitor alcohol withdrawal symptoms. Although it is used primarily to determine the need for medication, it can provide the therapist with an indication of stability level when determining patient safety before initiating physical therapy. The assessment requires about 5 minutes to administer and is available online with no copyright restrictions. A CIWA score greater than zero suggests the individual is still detoxing and therefore will still need some time. If the score equals zero, then physical therapy intervention may be appropriate to address any residual impairments.

The therapist should be aware of potential hazards of treating anyone who appears to have been consuming alcohol before coming to the treatment session. If the physical therapist suspects the client may be consuming alcohol in excessive amounts, remember that certain medications, both prescribed and nonprescription, have the potential for adverse reactions when taken with alcohol. Many of these adverse interactions can have a serious, negative impact on the physical therapy plan of care. Many medications, both prescription and nonprescription, contain significant percentages of alcohol. Some of the medications physical therapy clients may be taking (and their interaction with alcohol) are listed in Box 3.16.[518]

### Tobacco

Smoking exacerbates circulatory problems, leading to foot amputation in people with diabetes. This population generally has a lower oxygen supply to the lower extremities because they are subject to advanced atherosclerosis. The detrimental effects of cigarette smoking on wound healing, ability to cope with pain, and peripheral circulation are well documented. Heavy smoking is commonly associated with chronic alcohol abuse, and both addictions have a negative influence on bone formation, probably the result of defective osteoblastosis.

The relationship between smoking and pain has also been documented, including an association with the incidence and prevalence of back pain in all ages. A link between smoking and back pain in occupations requiring physical exertion was also established, possibly as a result of smoking-related reduced-oxygen perfusion and malnutrition of tissues in or around the spine, causing these tissues to respond inefficiently to mechanical stresses.[125]

The effects of tobacco use (see Table 3.11) have a direct impact on the client's ability to exercise and must be considered when starting a treatment intervention or exercise program. Smokers are more likely than nonsmokers to suffer fractures, sprains, and other physical injuries even at an early age; these detrimental effects of smoking on injuries appear to persist at least several weeks after cessation of smoking. Adverse effects of tobacco need to be considered and discussed with women who are pregnant. Many lifestyle improvements occur when a woman and her family are expecting a child. Taking the time to educate your prenatal clients about the negative effects of smoking on fetal development, pain tolerance in labor/delivery, healing postpartum, and potential harm to her own body and family can have a significant positive impact.[566]

In addition to the overall effects of nicotine, inhaled nicotine has additional pulmonary effects. The combination of smoking and coffee ingestion raises the blood pressure of hypertensive clients about 15/33 mm Hg for as long as 2 hours,[146] requiring careful monitoring of vital signs during exercise.

## Smoking Cessation

Health care providers should offer culturally appropriate or tailored interventions for all populations, as it has been reported that receiving advice to quit for some cultural groups may clash with their beliefs. The APTA endorsed the Agency for Healthcare Policy and Research's *Clinical Practice Smoking Cessation Guideline*. This has been superseded by an updated Tobacco Cessation Guideline released by the Public Health Service.[139]

The guidelines recommend that every client who smokes or uses tobacco products should be advised on the known dangers of tobacco use and increased success of smoking cessation programs.

When the client has trust in a therapist, it allows the opportunity for supportive education. Brief advice has been shown to have a positive impact on attempts to quit and actual cessation.[569] Explaining some of the immediate and long-term benefits of smoking cessation may be helpful (Table 3.12), as well as discussing the effects of tobacco on the integumentary, musculoskeletal, and neuromuscular systems. Because there is an increase in use of e-cigarettes, it should be addressed in that population. *A Youth Tobacco Cessation Guideline*[79] and *Role of the Physical Therapist in Smoking Cessation*[398] have also been published to help guide physical therapists in this type of counseling.

Whenever possible, clients who smoke should be encouraged to stop smoking or at least reduce tobacco use before surgery and when recovering from wounds, pressure ulcers, or injuries resulting from trauma (including surgery) or disease.

### Injection Drug Use

Injection drug use is associated with a high rate of skin and soft tissue infections from the use of unsterile intravenous and subcutaneous injection (skin popping). This factor, combined with the presence of pathogenic microorganisms on the skin, results in a wide range of clinical problems from simple cellulitis and abscess to life-threatening necrotizing fasciitis and septic thrombophlebitis.

The clinical appearance of the skin is often atypical and subtle because of longstanding damage to the skin and to venous and lymphatic systems, resulting in underlying lymphedema, hyperpigmentation, scarring, and regional lymphadenopathy. The therapist may observe redness, warmth, and tenderness of inguinal or axillary lymph nodes. Skin ulcers resulting from skin popping consisting of low-grade foreign-body granulomatous inflammation and necrosis are common and easily become superinfected (coinfected with more than one virus at a time), requiring local wound care and occasionally requiring skin grafting.

## Personality Disorders

### Overview and Incidence

Personality is the way of thinking, feeling, and behaving that makes a person different from other people. An individual's personality is influenced by experiences, environment, and inherited characteristics. A person's personality typically stays the same over time. Personality disorders are distinct and separate from personality types. Some personality types may not blend well together and therefore create conflicts. Personality disorders are long-term patterns of behavior and inner experiences that differ significantly from what is expected. Personality disorders affect at least two of these areas: thinking about oneself and others, responding emotionally, relating to other people, and controlling one's own behavior.[305,375]

Personality disorders tend to appear in adolescence or early adulthood, continue over many years, and cause a great deal of distress. They can cause enormous conflict with other people, cause relationships to fail or prevent them from developing in the first place, interfere with the ability to function appropriately in social situations, and get in the way of reaching life goals. The prevalence of personality disorders is 9% of the US population.

### Diagnosis

Often these personality disorders become apparent during interaction with the patient. Box 3.17 describes some common behaviors that may indicate the need for further identification and referral.

### Etiology and Pathogenesis

Many of the personality disorders are thought to be learned behaviors in response to dysfunctional family relationships and/or childhood trauma, including sexual and physical abuse, particularly in borderline personality disorder, narcissistic personality disorder, and avoidant personality disorder.[438] There is some evidence that narcissistic personality disorder may be found more often in older individuals, in men, and in individualistic societies.[143] Borderline personality disorder may be the result of type A and type B traumas (discussed earlier in this chapter, "Effects of Trauma on Brain Development"), especially when occurring in childhood; 80% of physically and sexually abused victims demonstrate borderline personality symptoms.

One model of borderline personality disorder[311] presents this disorder as a result of dissociation and a lack of sense of self involving developmental, neurobiological, and behavioral factors. The Meares model emphasizes failure of synthesis among the elements of psychic life and points to the need for both personal and social development, integration of unconscious traumatic memory, affect regulation, and restoration of the self.[311]

Genetics may be a factor in borderline personality disorder.[279,528] Biologic factors have also been implicated in various personality disorders. There appears to be decreased gray matter in the prefrontal cortex and the right superior temporal gyrus and decreased size of the amygdala and hippocampus associated with some disorders.[540,562]

Persons with borderline personality disorder often have cognitive-perceptual impairments, suggesting a central nervous system component. Obsessive-compulsive personality disorder may have similar central nervous system involvement and may be on a continuum presenting as obsessive-compulsive disorder.[137]

### MEDICAL MANAGEMENT

**TREATMENT.** There are no medications specifically to treat personality disorders. However, medications such as antidepressants, antianxiety medication, or mood stabilizing medication may be helpful in treating some symptoms. More severe or longer-lasting symptoms may require a team approach involving a primary care doctor, psychiatrist, psychologist, social worker. and family members.

Medical management of personality disorders requires a collaborative alliance between the health care provider and the client that makes restoration of function (rather than elimination of symptoms) the goal of treatment. The type of treatment will depend on the specific personality disorder, how severe it is, and the individual's circumstances.

The National Alliance on Mental Illness (NAMI) lists several types of psychotherapy that may be useful for treating personality disorders including psychoanalytic/psychodynamic therapy oriented toward gaining insight and knowledge about the disorder and what is contributing to symptoms with discussion about thoughts, feelings and behaviors. Psychotherapy can help a person understand the effects of their behavior on others and learn to manage or cope with symptoms and to reduce behaviors causing problems with functioning and relationships.

Dialectical behavior therapy helps the individual learn to regulate emotions, tolerate distress, self-manage, and be more effective with other people. Increasing skills use can be a mechanism of change for suicidal behavior, depression, and anger control.

Cognitive behavioral therapy (CBT) helps the individual recognize negative thoughts and learn effective coping strategies. Psychoeducation involves teaching the individual and family members about the illness, treatment, and ways of coping. Mentalization-based therapy (MBT) teaches people to notice internal states and to develop empathy for others.

**PROGNOSIS.** The natural course of personality disorders varies, but each tends to be stable across time and context. Impact on activities and participation in social/leisure and occupational roles varies with the severity and type of personality disorder. Borderline personality disorder and antisocial behavior disorder are particularly difficult to treat. Depression is associated with several personality

Box 3.16

## INTERACTION OF ALCOHOL WITH PRESCRIPTION AND NONPRESCRIPTION DRUGS

Many medications, both prescription and nonprescription, have the potential for adverse reactions when taken with alcohol. Age is an additional risk factor, as older adults are more likely to mix alcohol and other drugs.

Some of the more common medications physical therapy clients may be taking (and their interaction with alcohol) are presented here. With many new drugs developed each year, it is difficult to make sure a list of this type is always current. Individuals can and should always consult with their physician or pharmacist for any specific medications prescribed.

**Analgesics** (e.g., aspirin [Percodan], acetaminophen [Darvocet, Datril, Tylenol] propoxyphene [Darvon]):

- May result in increased alcohol intoxication, excessive sedation, stomach and intestinal bleeding, also increased susceptibility to liver damage from acetaminophen. Affected individuals may fall asleep during treatment or have balance problems as a result of the apparent increased intoxication.
- Aspirin may increase the bioavailability of alcohol, increasing the effects of the alcohol. Chronic alcoholic ingestion activates enzymes that transform acetaminophen into liver-damaging chemicals. Even small amounts of acetaminophen with varying amounts of alcohol can have this harmful effect.

**Antianxiety** (e.g., benzodiazepines):

- Benzodiazepines are often used to treat anxiety and insomnia. The sedative effect of these medications is enhanced by alcohol ingestion. Severe drowsiness can result in household accidents and MVAs. Older adults often have an increased response to these drugs and can experience impaired driving ability, breathing difficulties, and depressed cardiac function.

**Antibiotics** (e.g., furazolidone [Furoxone], griseofulvin [Grisactin], metronidazole [Flagyl], quinacrine [Atabrine]):

- The client may experience nausea, headache, possible convulsions, or respiratory paralysis. Some of these medications are rendered less effective by chronic alcohol use.
- The availability of antitubercular drugs such as isoniazid and rifampin used together to treat tuberculosis is decreased with alcohol consumption. The effectiveness of the medication is reduced. Older adults and homeless alcoholics are especially at risk for both tuberculosis and chronic use of alcohol.

**Anticoagulants** (e.g., warfarin [Coumadin], heparin):

- Acute alcohol consumption enhances anticoagulation, increasing the person's risk for life-threatening hemorrhages. The therapist must be alert to the effects of increased anticoagulation, such as easy bruising, bleeding from any opening, and joint bleeds. Physical therapy interventions, such as soft tissue mobilization, can result in more hemorrhage or bruising, and excessive bleeding may occur with sharp debridement.

**Antidepressants** (e.g., amitriptyline, doxepin, sertraline [Zoloft], paroxetine [Paxil], mirtazapine [Remeron], citalopram [Celexa], bupropion [Wellbutrin]):

- There are many commonly used psychiatric drugs affected by the ingestion of alcohol. Metabolism of these drugs is generally (but not always) delayed by alcohol. Alcohol increases the sedative effects of tricyclic antidepressants.
- Tyramine, a chemical found in some beers and wine, interacts with some antidepressants (e.g., monoamine oxidase inhibitors) to cause dangerously elevated blood pressure.
- The combination of alcohol and amitriptyline results in a marked increase in body sway. The interaction between alcohol and antidepressants also is noted for adverse effects on psychomotor skills. The combination of alcohol and psychiatric drugs is often reported as a cause of death in accidental or nonaccidental (suicide) deaths.

**Antidiabetics** (e.g., metformin [Glucophage], tolbutamide [Orinase]):

- When oral hypoglycemic drugs used to help lower blood sugar levels are taken concurrent with alcohol consumption, increased antidiabetic effect or excessive low blood sugars may occur. Acute alcohol consumption prolongs, and chronic alcohol use decreases, the availability of Orinase. Alcohol also interacts with some oral hypoglycemics, causing nausea and headache.
- The individual whose plan of care includes more vigorous physical activity may experience problems related to low blood sugar.

**Antihistamines** (e.g., all nonprescription asthma, hay fever, and cold remedies and nasal decongestants; acetaminophen [Actifed, Benadryl], carbinoxamine [Dimetane], dimenhydrinate [Dramamine], orphenadrine [Norflex], hydroxyzine [Vistaril]):

- When taken concurrent with alcohol consumption, the individual may experience increased interference with the central nervous system, increased sedation, reduced alertness, dizziness, or increased danger when operating machinery or autos, thus resulting in potential difficulties during an intervention session requiring alertness or fine motor skill.

**Antihypertensives** (e.g., methyldopa [Aldomet], chlorothiazide [Diuril], propranolol [Inderal], furosemide [Lasix], reserpine [Serpasil]):

- When taken concurrently with alcohol, increased blood pressure, orthostatic hypotension, or lowered effectiveness of some of these medications may occur. The client whose plan of care includes more vigorous physical activity may readily experience problems normally associated with uncontrolled hypertension or lose consciousness while standing.

**Antipsychotics** (e.g., chlorpromazine [Thorazine]):

- Drugs used to diminish psychotic symptoms such as delusions and hallucinations can cause breathing problems, impaired, coordination, and liver damage when combined with alcohol.

**Antispasmodics/Muscle Relaxants** (e.g., cyclobenzaprine [Flexeril], diazepam [Valium], methocarbamol [Robaxin]):

- When taken concurrently with alcohol, muscle relaxants can cause increased drowsiness, blurred vision, rapid pulse, excessive sedation, or mental confusion. Physical therapy interventions that require alertness and cooperation on the part of the patient or client may be compromised.

**Cardiovascular** (e.g., nitroglycerin for angina and many antihypertension medications):

- Alcohol consumption with many of the medications prescribed to treat cardiac and vascular problems can cause orthostatic hypotension accompanied by dizziness and fainting. Chronic alcohol use decreases the availability of some drugs (e.g., propranolol [Inderal]) used to treat high blood pressure. Monitoring vital signs is important.

**Narcotic Pain Relievers** (e.g., meperidine [Demerol], propoxyphene [Darvon], morphine and morphine derivatives, codeine, oxycodone [OxyContin]):

- When taken concurrent with alcohol consumption, dangerous depression of autonomic nervous system, increased intoxication, or excessive sedation may occur. Use of thermal agents may be contraindicated because of the potential for enhanced anesthetic effects of alcohol and excessive sedation.
- Coingestion of alcohol and long-acting opioids for chronic pain relief can accelerate release of the extended-release capsules. This effect is called *dose dumping* and has resulted in removal of some drugs from the market. Serious side effects, such as respiratory depression, coma, and even death, have been reported and remain potential problems when alcohol is combined with other slow-release morphine-based opioids.

From DiPiro JT, Talbert RL, Yee GC, et al, editors: *Pharmacotherapy. A pathophysiologic approach*, ed 8, New York, 2011, McGraw Hill; Brunton LL, Chabner BA, Knollmann BC, editors: *Goodman & Gilman's the pharmacological basis of therapeutics*, ed 12, New York, 2011, McGraw Hill; Micromedex Healthcare Series [Internet database]. Greenwood Village, CO, Thomson Reuters (Healthcare), updated periodically; From Drug Facts and Comparisons. *Facts & comparisons eAnswers* [online], 2012. Available from Wolters Kluwer Health, Inc.

**Table 3.12** Benefits of Smoking Cessation

| Time Since Last Cigarette | Benefit |
|---|---|
| 20 min | Vital signs return to person's baseline normal level (blood pressure, pulse, temperature) |
| 8 h | Oxygen levels increase; carbon monoxide levels decrease |
| 1 day | Risk of myocardial infarction (heart attack) decreases |
| 2 days | Increased ability to smell and taste; nerve endings begin repair |
| 2 wk to 3 mo | Improved circulation and lung function; reduced shortness of breath, improved exercise capacity |
| 1-9 mo | Cilia in lungs regenerate, improving movement of secretions; reduced coughing and sinus congestion; decreased fatigue and increased energy levels |
| 1 y | Risk of coronary heart disease reduced to one-half that of a smoker |
| 5 y | Risk of lung cancer reduced by 50%; reduced risk of cerebrovascular accident (stroke); risk of oropharyngeal cancer (mouth, throat) reduced to one-half that of a smoker |
| 10 y | Lung cancer death rate corresponds to nonsmoker's rate; risk of other tobacco-related cancers reduced |
| 15 y | Risk of coronary heart disease equals that of a nonsmoker |

Data from American Cancer Society, 2013 (http://www.cancer.org/).

**Box 3.17**

**BEHAVIORS THAT CAN BE IDENTIFIED DURING INTERVENTIONS THAT MAY INDICATE A POSSIBLE PERSONALITY DISORDER**

- A person with *schizotypal personality disorder* may have odd beliefs, peculiar behavior, and speech.
  - They may have difficulty forming relationships.
  - Distorted thinking and eccentric behavior may be evident during interactions, and they may display excessive social anxiety.
- People with *paranoid personality disorder* often assume people will harm or deceive them and don't confide in others or become close to them.
  - The therapist may observe pervasive distrust of other people, concerns about being deceived or exploited by others, or angry outbursts if they think they have been deceived.
- A person with *schizoid personality disorder* typically does not seek close relationships, chooses to be alone, and seems to not care about praise or criticism from others.
  - The therapist may note that the patient seems preoccupied with introspection and fantasy.
- A person with *borderline personality disorder* may go to great lengths to avoid being abandoned, display inappropriate intense anger, or describe ongoing feelings of emptiness.
  - They may demonstrate poor self-image, report instability in interpersonal relationships, and demonstrate intense emotions and appear impulsive.
  - They may have a history of repeated suicide attempts.
- People with *histrionic personality disorder* may be uncomfortable when they are not the center of attention and may use physical appearance to draw attention to themselves.
  - The therapist may become aware of socially inappropriate attention seeking behavior and mood swings that represent the failure to be the center of attention.
- A person with *narcissistic personality disorder* may have a grandiose sense of self-importance, a sense of entitlement, and readily take advantage of others while showing lack of empathy.
  - They appear self-centered, have a constant need for admiration, and display an exaggerated self-image.
- *Antisocial personality disorder* will appear at an earlier age than the other disorders and reflect disregard for rules and social norms.
  - The person may be deceptive or impulsive, often violating the rights of others.
- People with *dependent personality disorder* may have difficulty making daily decisions without reassurance from others or may feel uncomfortable or helpless when alone because of fear of inability to take care of themselves.
  - They will describe a fear of being alone, request more help than necessary, and appear submissive and clingy.
- A person with *obsessive-compulsive personality* disorder may be overly focused on details or schedules, work excessively (not allowing time for leisure or friends), or may be inflexible in their morality and values.
  - This can be seen in a preoccupation with orderliness, perfection, and control of relationships. This does not fit the same category as obsessive-compulsive disorder (OCD).
- *Avoidant personality disorder* can also show up during childhood and may be described as extreme shyness.
  - They may describe themselves as not being good enough or socially inept.
  - They seem to be preoccupied with being criticized or rejected.

These "red flags" should prompt the therapist to seek the opinion of a professional who is familiar with personality disorders, as described in the American Psychiatric Association's 2013 publication *Diagnostic and Statistical Manual of Mental Disorders, Fifth Edition (DSM-5).*

disorders and persons with borderline personality disorder are more likely to attempt suicide.[251]

SPECIAL IMPLICATIONS FOR THE THERAPIST 3.12

### *Personality Disorders*

Personality disorders cannot be "fixed" but rather should be approached by the therapist with an eye toward the therapist's own personal health while providing sensitive care and accepting the client without bias or resistance. This can be accomplished through self-awareness and understanding of the disorder involved. The healthy, sensitive, and insightful therapist who offers consistent professional help in the therapist's area of expertise will fare well. Progressively, the client learns from the clinician's ability to appropriately respond to emotional changes while upholding healthy boundaries. The therapist should be familiar with specific strategies for dealing with personality disorders.[556]

People with borderline personality disorder have stormy and unpredictable ways of relating to other people. This behavior covers up poor self-esteem and feelings of anger and of not deserving anything good. Borderline personality disorder impacts the person's ways of thinking, feeling, and behaving, which causes many problems, socially and medically. BPD can impact medical care in the following ways:

- Passive-aggressive behaviors (the clinician is great/awful)
- Playing one caregiver against another and manipulating to prevent accountability
- Poor compliance in self-care and appointment times
- As people reconnect with feelings, expect to see an increased urgency to regress in cognitive, emotional, and behavioral areas
- Misunderstanding of instructions, relationships, boundaries
- Prolonged treatment time required because of nonphysical triggering and the development of extensive, subtle physical symptoms
- Self-persecution and egocentric perspective ("I caused it, it's my fault")
- Insurance challenges as a result of complexity of diagnoses/failed care

Healing is accomplished as the healthy clinician works with the individual diagnosed with borderline personality disorder in the same way as with any other person suffering from brain injury. As the caregiver practices sensitive care, within individual client tolerances, and remains true to self through whatever the client presents, the individual with BPD benefits from consistent right and left hemisphere messages from the healthy provider.[447,548,549]

## Bipolar and Related Disorders

### Overview and Incidence

*Bipolar I, Bipolar II* and *Cyclothymic Disorders* are characterized by cyclical mood swings between depressed episodes and manic or hypomanic episodes. A *Manic Episode* manifests as a rapid elevation of mood, which severely disrupts the ability to perform activities and restricts participation in social/occupational roles. A *Hypomanic Episode* is a less-severe elevation in mood with less disruption in function. *Depressed Episodes* also vary in severity and can include a major depressive disorder (MDD). Bipolar I is the most severe form, with mood shifting between manic and MDD. Bipolar II is less disruptive, with mood swings between hypomania and MDD. Cyclothymic disorder is the least-severe form with mood swings that are not extreme. Prevalence of the bipolar disorders is estimated at 1.0% (bipolar I), 1.1% (bipolar II), and 2.4% (cyclothymic), or 3.5% of the adult population.[63,197,320] Onset of bipolar disorders is usually in the 20s.

### Etiology and Pathogenesis

Genetic-based pathogenesis is suspected for bipolar disorder based on a clear familial pattern and chromosomal linkage studies. Evidence exists that the key gene involved in the transmission of bipolar disease is X-linked. Studies show genetic variation changes the expression of the SNAP25 protein in the brain, which may impact information processing between brain regions involved in regulating emotions. Consistent with this idea, the variant was associated with larger amygdala volume and altered prefrontal-limbic connectivity.[218] Late-onset of a bipolar disorder is often associated with another medical condition, for example, hyperthyroidism.[348] Mania is linked to excessive levels of norepinephrine and dopamine.

### Clinical Manifestations

Clinical manifestations of Bipolar and Related Disorders are listed in Box 3.7. Mania is characterized by abnormal and persistent euphoria and/or irritability, grandiose thoughts, decreased need for sleep, increased energy and activity, racing thoughts, rapid speech, and increased risk taking. Mania severely limits activities and participation in social/occupational roles.[355] Bipolar I is characterized by mood swings between manic and depressive episodes. Bipolar II is characterized by distinct periods of depression and hypomania, and periods of depression tend to last longer than the hypomania.

The bipolar disorders are characterized by cyclical mood swings that may last from days to months, switching back and forth quickly or with normal periods in between. Heightened creativity and creative talent are sometimes associated with all phases of bipolar disorder.

## MEDICAL MANAGEMENT

**DIAGNOSIS.** Bipolar I disorder is characterized by the occurrence of 1 or more manic or mixed episodes (the manic episode may have been preceded by and may be followed by hypomanic or major depressive episodes, but these are not required for diagnosis). There is a distinct period of abnormally and persistently elevated, expansive, or irritable mood, and increased goal-directed activity or energy lasting 1 week or more, and any duration if hospitalization is necessary. It must be present most of the day, nearly every day.

During the mood disturbance and increased energy or activity, ≥3 (or 4 if irritable mood only) of the following are present: inflated self-esteem or grandiosity, decreased need for sleep, pressured speech, racing thoughts or flight of ideas, distractibility, increased activity with excessive pleasurable or risky components. This should reflect marked impairment not due to a substance or medical condition. The occurrence should not cause functional impairment, necessitate hospitalization, or reflect other psychotic features.

Bipolar II disorder is considered when there is lack of a full manic episode but at least 1 hypomanic episode and at least 1 major depressive episode. It would include a distinct period of abnormal and persistent elevated, expansive, or irritable moods with increased goal-directed activity or energy lasting 4 hours but less than 7 days. This activity should be clearly different from usual nondepressed mood and present most of the day, nearly every day. During the hypomanic episode, symptoms reflect the manic phase of the bipolar 1 disorder, and the episode is an unequivocal change in functioning, uncharacteristic of person, and observable by others. It is not severe enough to cause marked impairment. It is not due to substance or medical condition, and no psychosis (if present, then this is mania by definition).

There must be five or more of the following symptoms present during the same 2-week period (during the major depressive episode) and represent a change from previous functioning. At least one of the symptoms is either depressed mood or loss of interest or pleasure and can also include significant weight loss when not dieting or weight gain which can be associated with persistent decrease or increase in appetite. Insomnia or hypersomnia, psychomotor agitation or retardation, fatigue, or loss of energy can indicate an episode. Included as well are feelings of worthlessness or excessive or inappropriate guilt (which may be delusional), diminished ability to think or concentrate, indecisiveness, recurrent thoughts of death (not just fear of dying), recurrent suicidal ideation with or without a specific plan. The behaviors cause functional impairment (e.g., social, occupational) and are not better explained by substance misuse, medication side effects, or other psychiatric or somatic medical conditions.

*Substance/medication-induced bipolar and related disorder* can be considered when there is prominent and persistent disturbance of mood characterized by elevated, expansive, or irritable mood with or without depressed mood that develops during substance intoxication or withdrawal, and the substance/medication is capable of producing disturbance of mood.

**TREATMENT.** A multimodal approach is often used to manage bipolar disorders. Mood-stabilizing drugs such as lithium or depakote are often the first drug of choice. Antipsychotics and antidepressants are often used in conjunction with a mood stabilizer.[355] Some people prefer to experience the extremes of this disorder so as to avoid losing the creative edge that can occur when the medication balances mood swings. Group, family, and individual psychotherapy, educational approaches, and behavior modification are common interventions. Some programs advocate a predetermined plan of action to put in place when warning signs of mania develop.

**PROGNOSIS.** Bipolar and Related Disorders are chronic with recurring episodes, often separated by symptom-free periods of time. Insight can be impaired with 55% of individuals diagnosed with bipolar denying any psychiatric problems.[395] Bipolar disorder is frequently accompanied by alcoholism and/or other drug abuse. It is not clear if alcohol is a trigger for bipolar episodes or if the individual is using alcohol to self-medicate. Comorbidity of alcohol abuse with bipolar disorder often delays early diagnosis, especially when alcohol abuse has been the primary focus of intervention. Other comorbidities may also exist (e.g., migraine headaches, asthma, anxiety and panic attacks, allergies, eating disorders).[69,122]

**SPECIAL IMPLICATIONS FOR THE THERAPIST 3.13**

### *Schizophrenia Spectrum and Other Psychotic Disorders; Bipolar and Related Disorders*

The role of the physical therapist in providing multidisciplinary care for people with schizophrenia spectrum and other psychotic disorders is not clearly differentiated, but efforts have been made to identify the value added by physical therapy.[526] Aerobic exercise can improve the severities of symptoms on the negative and general psychopathology scales in individuals with schizophrenia being treated with antipsychotics.[534] Integration of yoga, breathing techniques, and progressive muscle relaxation is appropriate for management of psychiatric symptoms and distress. Studies are linking improved short-term memory.[239]

#### Adverse Effects of Medications

Antipsychotic medications are used to treat psychotic symptoms, including hallucinations, delusions, paranoia, combativeness, agitation and hostility, insomnia, catatonia, hyperactivity, bizarre psychomotor behaviors, and poor grooming and self-care.[217] Antipsychotics are often used in long-term care settings to help normalize disturbances of thought. They do not cure psychosis associated with acute mania and schizophrenia but help manage signs and symptoms. Some can control fluency of ideas and language and alleviate the diminished ability to concentrate, express emotions, pursue goal-directed activity, and experience pleasure.[50]

The therapist must be aware of anyone taking these medications because of the potential adverse side effects. Increased levels of serotonin may affect regulation and release of antidiuretic hormone, requiring close monitoring for dehydration; watch for headache, increased confusion, loss of appetite, and muscle cramps.

There may be movement disorders commonly observed with their use. Dystonias, sustained abnormal postures, and disruption of movement caused by muscle tone alterations can develop within 5 days of administration. Other common extrapyramidal effects may include restlessness, anxiety, or pacing (akathisia) and Parkinson-like symptoms. Long-term use of antipsychotics can result in permanent involuntary choreoathetoid muscle movements of the face, jaw, tongue, and extremities.

## Schizophrenia Spectrum and Other Psychotic Disorders

### Overview and Incidence

Schizophrenia is often characterized by periodic exacerbations of symptoms, referred to as an active phase. This is preceded by a prodromal phase in which behavior declines and the person begins to withdraw from reality. The active phase is followed by a residual phase, with behaviors not unlike the prodromal phase.[350] In a 12-month period, the prevalence of schizophrenia in adults is 1.1% in the United States.[354] The age of onset often is in the late teens or early 20s; women are generally diagnosed less frequently and at an older age than men.[496]

Subtypes can be identified as follows: *Schizotypal personality disorder* exhibits personality characteristics that create difficulty with interpersonal relationships.

*Delusional Disorder* is a form of psychosis where the main symptom is delusions—the inability to shake untrue beliefs and creating unbelievable scenarios. Most delusions involve the belief of potential harm as described below in *Schizophrenia*. These delusions may be a heightened exaggeration of reality or just a false belief. A distinguishing characteristic of individuals suffering from this condition is that among other things, there is no bizarre behavior. It is not apparent that someone is suffering from this condition if it weren't for the delusions.

*Brief Psychotic Disorder* is a short-term occurrence of schizophrenia, where there is a sudden onset of symptoms that only persist for less than one month. The causes of these brief stints of psychosis include an obvious stressor (e.g., death of a loved one, trauma from natural disasters), no apparent stressor (i.e., the symptoms come on due to no obvious reaction to a disturbing event), and postpartum psychosis—occurring in women within 4 weeks of giving birth. During this brief episode of psychosis, hallucinations, delusions, and cognitive deficits are common. It is unknown what causes brief psychotic disorder to affect certain individuals, but certain genetic and environment factors have been examined, including predisposition to develop mood disorders and psychoses within the family history.

*Schizophreniform Disorder* is another short-form occurrence of full-blown schizophrenia, where the affected individual experiences distorted thinking, emotional reactions, and perceptions of reality. Though the symptoms of schizophreniform disorder and general schizophrenia overlap, the major difference is the length of duration. When symptoms last for more than six months, it is likely converted to a diagnosis of schizophrenia.

*Schizoaffective Disorder* is a disorder that combines symptoms of schizophrenia with a mood disorder, likely either major depression or bipolar disorder. This type of schizophrenia is chronic and appears in intermittent episodes. Mood or affective symptoms occur at the same time as the schizophrenic symptoms and the schizophrenic symptoms often stay put after the mood symptoms disperse. Common symptoms of schizoaffective disorder include depression, mania, and classic schizophrenia.

*Schizophrenia* is the most common type of schizophrenia, characterized by psychosis misaligned with reality. Common paranoid delusions include coworkers, spouses, the government, and neighbors believed to be in a plot to cause harm. There is often a belief that there is an intent to spy, poison, kill, or make life miserable. Paranoid schizophrenia has a severe impact on relationships, believing that it is the people closest to the person that are likely to cause harm. Paranoid delusions may be accompanied by hallucinations including voices that are insulting or prompting inappropriate behavior.

*Shared Psychotic Disorder*, also known as "folie a deux" (the folly of two), is a rare form of psychosis where an otherwise healthy individual begins to adopt the psychotic beliefs/delusions of someone suffering from schizophrenia.

### Etiology and Pathogenesis

There is evidence of a genetic predisposition for schizophrenia. First-degree relatives have a 10-times higher risk; a child who has two parents diagnosed with schizophrenia has a 40% risk of developing the disease.[236] However, it is thought that psychosocial stressors may be required in addition to the genetic predisposition to trigger active symptoms as well as exacerbate symptoms. The expression and function of risk genes during brain development is the focus of investigation.[91,209,210] Research implicates the neurotransmitter dopamine, particularly in the prefrontal cortex, as a contributing factor.[341] Imaging studies have identified changes in brain structure including changes in connectivity and decreased gray matter volume in the superior and middle temporal gyri and anterior cingulate, among other areas.[515]

### Clinical Manifestations

Schizophrenia is sometimes characterized by periods when the symptoms are less severe, but people with schizophrenia rarely recover completely. Periodic outbreaks of psychotic symptoms such as hallucinations and delusions are common. Hallucinations are most commonly auditory or visual, and delusions may vary in type. Symptoms will be persistent in approximately 50% of individuals. The DSM 5 includes associated behaviors that include disturbed sleep pattern, dysphoric mood, depression, anxiety, anger, and phobias. Depersonalization with detachment or feeling of disconnect from self, derealization, a feeling that surrounding aren't real, cognitive deficits impacting language, processing, executive function, and/or memory are common. There is a lack of insight into disorder, with social cognition deficits with activity associated with hostility and aggression. Inappropriate affect with laughing in the absence of a stimulus can be another component that disrupts social interactions.

Cognitive impairments caused by the disorder may persist when other symptoms are in remission. Schizophrenia is associated with social and occupational dysfunction. Completing education and maintaining employment are negatively impacted by symptoms of the illness, and most individuals diagnosed with schizophrenia are employed at a lower level than their parents. Many have few or limited social relationships outside of their immediate family.

## MEDICAL MANAGEMENT

**DIAGNOSIS.** The DSM 5 defines the diagnosis of schizophrenia as two or more of the following for a one-month or greater period and must include one of the following: delusions, hallucinations, disorganized speech, grossly disorganized or catatonic behavior along with diminished emotional expression. Impairment is seen in one of the major areas of functioning for a significant time since the onset of the disturbance: work, interpersonal relations, or self-care. Signs of the disorder must last for a continuous period of at least 6 months. This six-month period must include at least one month of symptoms (or less if treated) included in the active phase and may include periods of residual symptoms. During residual periods, only negative symptoms may be present.

The diagnosis is determined when schizoaffective disorder and bipolar or depressive disorder with psychotic features have been ruled out; there is no evidence that depressive or manic episodes occurred concurrently with active phase symptoms or have been present for only minor times during the active and residual phases of the illness. It should be established that the disturbance is not caused by the effects of a substance or another medical condition. If there is a history of autism spectrum disorder or a communication disorder with childhood onset, the diagnosis of schizophrenia is only made if prominent delusions or hallucinations, along with other symptoms, are present for at least one month.

**TREATMENT.** A multimodal approach is used in the treatment of an individual with schizophrenia. Antipsychotics are the most common form of treatment for individuals with schizophrenia. They significantly reduce positive symptoms by impacting the neurotransmitter systems. The goal of treatment with antipsychotic medications is to effectively manage signs and symptoms at the lowest possible dose determined by trying different drugs, different doses, or combinations over time to achieve the desired result. Other medications also may help, such as antidepressants or antianxiety drugs. It can take several weeks to notice an improvement in symptoms.

Because medications for schizophrenia can cause serious side effects, people with schizophrenia may be reluctant to take them. Willingness to cooperate with treatment may affect drug choice. For example, someone who is resistant to taking medication consistently may need to be given injections instead of taking a pill.

First-generation antipsychotics have frequent and potentially significant neurologic side effects, including the possibility of developing a movement disorder (tardive dyskinesia) that may or may not be reversible. First-generation antipsychotics include chlorpromazine, fluphenazine, haloperidol, and perphenazine. These antipsychotics are often cheaper than second-generation antipsychotics, especially the generic versions, which can be an important consideration when long-term treatment is necessary. Drugs considered second-generation medications are preferred because they pose a lower risk of serious side effects than do first-generation antipsychotics. Once psychosis recedes, in addition to medication, psychologic and social (psychosocial) interventions are initiated.

Psychotherapy may help to normalize thought patterns. Also, learning to cope with stress and identify early warning signs of relapse can help people with schizophrenia manage their illness. Social skills training focuses on improving communication and social interactions and improving the ability to participate in daily activities. Family therapy provides support and education to families dealing with schizophrenia. Vocational rehabilitation and supported employment can help to prepare for, find, and keep jobs.

Most individuals with schizophrenia require some form of daily living support. Many communities have programs to help people with schizophrenia with jobs, housing, self-help groups, and crisis situations. A case manager or someone on the treatment team can help find resources. With appropriate treatment, most people with schizophrenia can manage their illness. During periods of crisis or times of severe symptoms, hospitalization may be necessary to ensure safety, proper nutrition, adequate sleep, and basic hygiene. For adults with schizophrenia who do not respond to drug therapy, electroconvulsive therapy (ECT) may be considered. ECT may be helpful for someone who also has depression. See section on depression above.

**PROGNOSIS.** Long-term outlook represents 33% to 50% of individuals showing good outcomes.[124,224] Environmental barriers and facilitators, as well as personal factors, including family support, age, gender, education, and financial status, impact long-term outcomes. In addition, there are multiple subtypes of schizophrenia. After a first schizophrenic episode, only 14% to 20% of individuals will recover completely.

The prevalence of cardiovascular disease in persons with schizophrenia is above average. Up to 6% of people with schizophrenia die by suicide, about 20% make suicide attempts on more than one occasion, and many more have significant suicidal thoughts. Suicidal behavior can be in response to hallucinations, and suicide risk remains high over the life span of individuals with schizophrenia.[413]

## Suicidal Behavior Disorder

### Overview and Incidence

Suicidal behavior takes over a million lives worldwide every year. Nonfatal suicidal behavior is estimated to be 25 to 50 times more common. Suicidal behavior often occurs in the context of psychiatric conditions but not exclusively. In the US, about 10% of people who die by suicide have no identifiable mental disorder. Even among the psychiatric conditions associated with high risk for suicidal behavior, most patients do not attempt suicide. Suicidal behavior does not appear to be an intrinsic dimension of any specific psychiatric disorder.[377]

### Etiology, Pathogenesis, and Risk Factors

Defective transmission of serotonin is related to elevated 5-HT1A autoreceptors in the dorsal raphe nucleus of depressed suicide victims, which leads to decreased serotonin firing and can predict more lethal suicidal behavior.[378] The HPA axis has also been heavily researched in relation to suicide related to its role in the stress-response system. There appears to be an association between cortisol and suicide attempts that may be related to age. Higher levels of cortisol are related to individuals under 40 years old compared with lower levels in those over 40.[372]

Disturbances in cytokine levels have also been associated with suicidality. Elevated pro-inflammatory IL-6

Box 3.18

**RISK FACTORS FOR SUICIDE**

- Past history of attempted suicide
- Suicidal ideation, talking about suicide, determining a suicide method
- Mood disorders or mental illness:
  - Clinical depression, especially manic-depressive illness
  - Schizophrenia
  - Personality disorders, especially borderline and antisocial
- Chronic alcohol and drug abuse
- Comorbidities (chronic pain and nonpsychiatric conditions)
- Circumstantial risk factors: stressful life events
- Exposure to suicide or suicidal behavior, especially in adolescents and young adults
- Genetic predisposition/family history of suicidal behaviors
- Decreased levels of serotonin
- Availability of firearms (most common method of completed suicide)
- Gender (males are 5 times more likely to commit suicide)
- Age (younger than age 40 years or older than age 65 years; risk increases 5× in white males older than age 80 years)

Data from the American Foundation for Suicide Prevention, New York, 2013 (http://www.afsp.org; [888] 333-AFSP).

levels have been found postmortem in the brain and blood after suicide, compared to individuals without suicidality or healthy controls. Microgliosis, another indicator of neuroinflammation, has also been associated with suicide.[510] In one study, a higher proportion of activated microglia and perivascular macrophage density was observed in the dorsal anterior cingulate white matter of postmortem brain samples from suicide deaths compared with matched non-suicide deaths.[153]

The kynurenine pathway, the main metabolic pathway for the degradation of tryptophan, has appeared in the suicide literature. Quinolinic acid (QUIN), one of the main metabolites, is considered neurotoxic due to its activation of N-methyl-d-aspartate (NMDA) receptors, as well as the increased release of glutamate and inhibition of glutamate uptake, leading to glutamatergic neurotransmission overactivation. Another important metabolite, kynurenic acid (KYNA), is a neuroprotective, anticonvulsive, and antioxidant substance that acts mainly through NMDA, alpha-amino3-hydroxy-5-methyl-4-isoxazolepropionic acid (AMPA), and kainate receptors antagonism.[62]

People who are both impulsive or aggressive and depressed have a much higher likelihood of attempting suicide. Half of all successful suicide victims were described by family or friends as being depressed or suffering some other mental health problem just before their death.[391] Suicidal mass murders currently on the rise in the United States are theorized to be part of a suicide wish on the part of the perpetrator.[274] Box 3.18 defines risk factors for suicide.

Psychoactive drugs, specifically antidepressants, may increase the risk of suicide, particularly in adolescents and young adults.[175] Males are five times more likely to take their own lives, and suicide rates are highest for people younger than age 25 years and for white men older than age 80 years. Chronic medical illness in older adults has been linked with increased rates of suicide. The risk is greatly increased in individuals with multiple illnesses.[229]

Diseases of the nervous system such as multiple sclerosis, Huntington disease, brain and spinal cord injury, and seizure disorders carry increased risk. Malignant neoplasms, HIV/AIDS, peptic ulcer disease, and chronic obstructive pulmonary disease create increased attempts, especially in men. Suicide is greater with significant pain and progressing functional impairment.

Older adults do not necessarily attempt suicide more often than younger people. Instead, they are more likely to succeed and are less likely to tell anyone their intentions. Older adults living alone are less likely to be found in time to be saved. Risk factors for children include the loss or death of a family member or close friend, traumatic experiences such as physical or sexual abuse, and being bullied.[303]

## MEDICAL MANAGEMENT

**DIAGNOSIS AND TREATMENT.** Patients with suicidal thoughts, plans, or behaviors should generally be treated in the setting that is least restrictive yet most likely to be safe and effective. Treatment settings and conditions include a continuum of possible levels of care, from involuntary inpatient hospitalization through partial hospital and intensive outpatient programs to occasional ambulatory visits. Choice of specific treatment setting depends on the estimate of the patient's current suicide risk and potential for dangerousness to others. Other issues include medical and psychiatric comorbidity, strength and availability of a psychosocial support network, and the ability to provide adequate self-care, along with the ability to provide reliable feedback and cooperation with treatment. The benefits of intensive interventions such as hospitalization must be weighed against their possible negative effects related to employment, financial, and other stressors along with social stigma. If suicidal ideation is present the specific plans or steps that have been taken toward enacting those plans need to be immediately addressed.

Major depression can be treated via counseling and trauma/stress resolution and/or pharmacologically, although it is often undertreated, even in the presence of a history of suicide attempt. Some suicide attempts may be preventable if depression is diagnosed early and treated adequately. The need for psychoeducation among health professionals and the public is evident.[557]

SPECIAL IMPLICATIONS FOR THE THERAPIST 3.14

### *Suicide*

All suicidal thoughts and acts must be taken seriously and responded to appropriately. Three-fourths of all suicide victims give some warning of their intentions to a friend or family member. Many older adults who commit suicide have contact with a health care professional in the month before killing themselves.[519] Box 3.19 includes questions appropriate to ask clients if the health care providers have a suspicion of pending suicide or suicidal thoughts.

Observe for changes in client mood such as calmness or tranquility in a formerly hostile, angry, or depressed client. Such a behavior change may be a prelude to a suicidal event. Comments such as, "I won't be seeing you again," or "My family would be better off without me" may be a form of suicidal communication.

Developing a contract with the client and identifying when and who should be contacted, as well as the consequences of breaching the contract, may be helpful to the caring relationship and to treatment success.

The following are common behaviors that indicate suicide risk:

- Past attempts
- Disrupted sleep patterns
- Increased anxiety and agitation
- Outbursts of rage or low frustration tolerance
- Risk-taking behavior
- Increased alcohol or drug use
- Sudden mood change for the better
- Any talk or indication of suicidal ideation or intent, planning, or actual actions taken to procure a means[399]

The Joint Commission has provided these resources as a part of its reviews:

- Zero Suicide Toolkit, from the Suicide Prevention Resource Center and the National Action Alliance for Suicide Prevention
- ED-SAFE Materials, from the Emergency Medicine Network Caring for Adult Patients with Suicide Risk—A Consensus Guide for Emergency Departments
- Quick Guide for Clinicians, from the Suicide Prevention Resource Center
- Means Matter website, from the Harvard T.H. Chan School of Public Health Mental Health Environment of Care Checklist
- SAFE-T Pocket Card for Clinicians—Five-step evaluation and triage for suicide assessment
- Suicide Prevention Clinical Workforce: Guidelines for Training from the Clinical Workforce Preparedness Task Force of the National Action Alliance for Suicide Prevention
- VA/DoD Clinical Practice Guideline for Assessment and Management of Patients at Risk for Suicide, from the Department of Veterans Affairs, Department of Defense, June 2013.

Age-appropriate tools to screen for depression are available. For example, the Center for the Advancement of Children's Mental Health at Columbia University has developed a Youth Depression Screening test.[92] The Geriatric Depression Scale can be used with older adults. It should be noted that for now the accuracy of methods to screen for high risk of suicide is unknown. Likewise, few studies have shown that screening reduces suicide attempts or mortality rates from suicide. More research is needed in this area.[518]

Focus on suicide prevention has increased in the last 10 years. The National Institute of Mental Health[358] and the American Foundation for Suicide Prevention[15] have a major focus on education, research, and health information related to depression and suicide. Other organizations with a focus on suicide prevention target specific groups.[505]

People who are suicidal may also be manipulative; therefore, all health care providers need to be aware of and manage their own feelings while empathizing with the client's point of view. When in doubt, report concerns to the appropriate resource.

The physical therapist should chart accurately anything the client says or does that might suggest a suicide threat. It is better to meet the required standard of care and err on the side of caution through documentation and the referral process.

In an acute crisis, do not leave the person alone. In addition, remove all potential objects that could be used for suicide. Get the person to the nearest emergency department—call 911 if necessary. A national suicide resource is available by calling 800-SUICIDE (800-784-2433) or 800-273-TALK (800-273-8255) while waiting for transportation or to talk to a counselor.

Box 3.19

**QPR FOR SUICIDE PREVENTION**

**Q**—Question the person about suicide. Do you have thoughts of suicide? *If yes*, do you have a suicide plan in mind? Tell me about your plan.

Indirect questions:

- Are you unhappy enough to wish you were dead?
- Do you wish you could go to sleep and never wake up?
- Have you ever wanted to stop living?
- Do you feel your life is no longer worth living?

**P**—Persuade the person to get help. Listen carefully. Offer to help by making a referral or accompany the person to get help.

**R**—Refer for help. Contact the individual's physician, minister, rabbi, counselor, tribal leader, or call 1-800-SUICIDE (1-800-784-2433) for assistance in finding local agencies or services in your area.

PLEASE NOTE: QPR is not intended as a form of counseling or prevention. It is a screening and prevention tool to help assess warning signs of suicide and potentially prevent a successful suicide. Asking questions about suicide does NOT increase the risk of suicide attempts or success.

## ACKNOWLEDGMENT

The authors would like to thank Brittany Grant for her assistance with this chapter, specifically for her special focus on the Athlete with Relative Energy Deficiency in Sport (RED-S) and Low Energy Availability and the Female Athlete Triad. She introduced orthorexia nervosa as category of eating disorder that physical therapists should recognize.

### REFERENCES

To enhance this text and add value for the reader, all references are included in the enhanced ebook on Student Consult that accompanies this textbook. The reader can view the reference source and access it online whenever possible.

# CHAPTER 4

# Environmental and Occupational Medicine

LYNZIE SCHULTE

## INTRODUCTION

*Environmental medicine* is a broad term used to describe how disease correlates to the environment. These environments include home, work, school, and community and involve exposure to environmental hazards within food, water, air, drugs, and soil. The basic understanding is that whatever people may eat, drink, or be exposed to has an effect on their health. Environmental medicine encompasses occupational medicine, a specialty involving the health of workers and workplaces. Once known as *industrial medicine,* occupational medicine can be considered a special form of environmental medicine and will be discussed throughout this chapter.

The Merriam-Webster dictionary defines the term *environment* as "the complex of physical, chemical, and biotic factors (such as climate, soil, and living things) that act upon an organism or an ecological community and ultimately determine its form and survival."[83a] Intrinsic factors include the genetic makeup of the host, medical history, and current state of health. Cell injury and resultant disease result from interplay of the environment and intrinsic factors when the defenses of the host are overcome. Whether in the home, workplace, school, or community, chemical, physical, biologic, psychosocial, and traumatic hazards exist.

The focus of environmental medicine tends to be on chemical and physical hazards in the environment. Many diseases, disorders, and defects (contact dermatitis, obstructive lung disease, nephropathy, neuropathy, autoimmune disorders, various cancers, and birth defects are some examples) occur when the body is exposed to some agent or stressor in the environment. Psychosocial hazards have become more relevant as researchers examine the effects these hazards can have on a person's health. Climate change has become a global concern, with research focused on both its direct and indirect impact on a person's health.

### Molecular Epidemiology

Another area of research called *molecular epidemiology* is aimed at identifying interactions between genetics and the environment and how these can influence individual susceptibility to disease. Completed in 2003, the Human Genome Project aimed to identify and map all of the genes of the human genome. This 13-year international project funded by the U.S. National Institutes of Health has increased genetic and population-based association studies focused on identifying underlying susceptibility genes and contributions from gene–environment interactions to common complex diseases. The National Human Genome Research Institute is developing a 2020 vision for future genome research to positively impact the lives of the human population.

Exposure to environmental contaminants, including hydrocarbons and tobacco smoke, can now be measured using biomarkers such as metabolites in urine, chromosomal aberrations, mutations in specific genes, or DNA. Biomonitoring is able to measure chemicals within people by testing small amounts of bodily substances such as blood, urine, breast milk, and saliva. With this type of measuring available, nutrition of the population can be assessed, exposure to toxic levels of chemicals can be monitored, and environmental actions and policies can be researched for effects on population health.

Epidemiologic studies support the use of chromosomal breakage as a relevant biomarker of neurodegenerative disorders, cancer, diabetes, cardiovascular diseases, and inflammatory diseases, as well as aging.[217] For example, particulate air pollution can cause damage to DNA, and eating fruits and vegetables or ingesting antioxidants may be able to reduce the breakage and initiate repair.[143]

### Regulation of Environmental Health Care

Multiple agencies exist for the investigation and regulation of environmental health care. The National Institute for Occupational Safety and Health (NIOSH) is the federal research agency through the U.S. Centers for Disease Control and Prevention (CDC). Its goals include conducting research, providing recommendations, and collaborating globally to reduce worker illnesses, increase worker safety, and improve worker health. The Occupational Safety and Health Administration (OSHA) is the primary regulatory agency that determines which of the standards proposed by NIOSH are adopted and enforced.

NIOSH and OSHA were created from the Occupational Safety and Health Act of 1970, with its primary purpose to protect employees from working in environments with recognized hazards. NIOSH does not have legal authority to adopt or enforce regulations, whereas OSHA standards are law throughout the United States; OSHA compliance officers can inspect the workplace at any time to determine the status of health and safety.

The mission of the U.S. Environmental Protection Agency (EPA) is to protect human health and the environment. The agency develops and writes regulations based on environmental laws passed in Congress and then enforces those regulations. The EPA performs both human health risk assessments and ecologic risk assessments to aid in determining health effects on humans from exposure to environmental hazards. This is useful for regulating new chemicals by determining how much harm is acceptable to human health, animals, or the environment. For example, risk assessment can determine how much hormone or pesticide residue is allowed in food, how much of a toxic substance can be discharged into a river, and how much pollutant can be released as automobile exhaust. Risk managers use this information to determine what type of current or future consequence there will be from human or ecologic exposure. Their role is to protect humans and the environment from risky exposures. It is worth noting that assessments looking at whether the hazard is even necessary, as opposed to how much is safe, would likely be beneficial to reduce negative effects on humans and the environment.

## ENVIRONMENTAL MEDICINE

### Overview

Environmental medicine takes into account risk factors in the environment and human health and how they interact with one another. In 2017, close to 2.8 million nonfatal workplace injuries and illnesses were reported in the private sector of the United States, making the incidence rate 28 cases per 1000 full-time workers.[40] This is about 45,000 fewer incidences compared with 2016. The number of workers who had days away from work due to these injuries, however, remained around the same when comparing years. The median number of days away from work (8 days/case) also remained unchanged.[40] Overexertion and body reaction were the most common events that resulted in injury and illness, with strains, sprains, and tears being the most commonly reported injuries.

Health care and social services had the highest number of nonfatal workplace injuries and illnesses in 2017, totaling around 1 in 5 of the reported cases. The number of nonfatal occupational injuries and illness resulting from exposure to a harmful substance or environment was 37,110 in 2017.[42] The total number of fatal work injuries in the United States in 2016 was 5190, and this was the first time since 2008 that fatalities were over 5000 cases. The most common cause of workplace fatality involved roadway incidents, with 1252 cases; the second most common involved injuries by persons or animals. Falls, slips, or trips accounted for 849 deaths from work injuries in 2016, and exposure to harmful substances or environments (including electricity, temperature extremes, harmful substances, use of drugs/alcohol, and inhalation of harmful substances) accounted for 518 deaths in 2016.[41]

Worldwide, it is estimated that there were 2.78 million deaths attributed to work, using data from 2014 and 2015. Mortality from work-related disease accounted for 86.3% of those deaths, whereas fatal accidents accounted for 13.7%. The top three diseases that make up more than 75% of total work-related mortality are circulatory diseases, malignant neoplasms, and respiratory diseases.

In the United States, there were a total of 302,837 work-related mortality incidents in 2015, with workers affected by malignant neoplasms (42%), circulatory diseases (28%), respiratory diseases (12%), occupational injuries (8%), neuropsychiatric conditions (4%), communicable diseases (4%), digestive diseases (1%), and genitourinary diseases (1%).[107] Because of the difficulty of diagnosis and the likelihood that occupational illness claims will be disputed by employers, these figures are most likely gross underestimates of the true incidence of environmentally induced illnesses.

Noncommunicable diseases from environmental factors account for 12.6 million deaths per year worldwide. The World Health Organization (WHO) estimated 6 million deaths in 2012 from heart disease, stroke, lung disease, and cancers that were due to ambient (outdoor) and household (indoor) air pollution.[66]

An estimated 23% of preventable illnesses worldwide and 16% of preventable illnesses in the United States can be attributed to poor environmental quality.[308] In 2016 the United States had a mortality rate attributed to household and ambient air pollution of 13.3 per 100,000 population, while deaths across the globe totaled 7 million.[309] It is estimated that by 2060, air pollution will cost 1% gross domestic product (around 2.6 trillion U.S. dollars annually) based on days away from work, medical bills, and reduced agriculture output.[189] It is clear, based on the trends, that without action to improve environmental quality, premature death will continue to increase. The Clean Air Act of 1970, which was last amended in 1990, requires the EPA to set National Ambient Air Quality Standards (NAAQS) for pollutants considered harmful to public health and the environment.

This Act established two types of national air quality standards. *Primary standards* set limits to protect public health, including the health of sensitive subgroups such as children, older adults, and anyone with conditions such as asthma or chronic obstructive pulmonary disease. *Secondary standards* set limits to protect public welfare, crops, vegetation, and buildings. The six criteria of pollutants that are reviewed include carbon monoxide (CO), ozone, lead, nitrogen dioxide, particulate matter, and sulfur dioxide.[277] As the EPA sets new NAAQS or revises existing standards, the Agency then needs to determine how and if the standards are being met. Areas that exceed the EPA national standards are termed attainment areas, areas that do not meet the standards are termed nonattainment areas, and areas that the EPA cannot determine if standards are met are termed unclassifiable. Once classifications are obtained, local and state government need to determine how they will achieve or maintain the EPA NAAQS.[276]

### Effects of Environmental Contaminants on Children

Children are more likely to be adversely affected by environmental contaminants than adults, owing to their immature nervous, respiratory, digestive, reproductive, and immune systems. Compared with adults, children eat more food, drink more fluid, and breathe more air in proportion to their body weight. They absorb a greater proportion of substances through their intestinal tract and lungs and detoxify and excrete toxins differently than adults. Children are outdoors more often, engage in hand-to-mouth activity, and often play in the dirt or on the floor or carpet, which places them closer to the source of many pollutants. Studies are looking at exposure of children from disadvantaged, low-income neighborhoods and have found that these children are at the high end of exposure to environmental contaminants compared with national averages. These contaminants include pesticides, metals, tobacco smoke, and other chemicals.[233]

In 1997 a Presidential Executive Order was signed to protect children from environmental health and safety risks. This requires federal agencies to make it a high priority to identify and assess environmental factors that affect children disproportionally, as well as make sure programming, policies, and activities address these disproportions.[204] This Executive Order has guided the EPA in its establishment of the Office of Children's Health Protection. Its goals are to reduce negative environmental impacts on children through policies, rules, enforcement, and research; protect children with safe chemical management; and assist community-based programming to eliminate threats to children's health.[273]

Polybrominated diphenyl ethers (PBDEs) are flame retardants that have been added to a multitude of products to reduce flammability. PBDEs are also recognized as a neurotoxin. PBDEs do not chemically bind to products they are intended for; therefore leaching of the chemical occurs very easily. In the United States, 97% of the population has detectable levels in their blood. There are more than 200 different formulas of PBDEs; the pentaBDE and octaBDE mixtures have not been manufactured or imported in the United States since 2004, and the decaBDE mixture was phased out in 2013. PBDEs are still concerning, as there are products still in circulation in the United States, and there are still some PBDE products imported. PBDEs have been found in breast milk samples from around the world, including both the northern and southern hemispheres, indicating this chemical has become a worldwide pollutant.

A study looking at new mothers found a significant decline in PBDE and polychlorinated biphenyl levels in breast milk since the PBDE bans took place.[106] Studies have also looked at prenatal and postnatal effects of PBDEs and found long-lasting neurologic abnormalities that alter motor activity, cognition, and behavior.[289] It was found that PBDEs affect fertility in women, resulting in a decreased fecundability (the probability that conception will occur in a given population of couples during a specific time period) and increased time to conceive for women who had increased levels of PBDEs.[109,119,236,259,317]

Bisphenol A (BPA) is a chemical that is widely used in the production of polycarbonate plastics and epoxy resins. They have been used in food and drink packaging including baby bottles, water bottles, safety equipment, and medical devices, as well as food cans, bottle tops, and water supply pipes. BPA is poorly soluble in water and can leach out of materials readily, especially if put through repeated wear and tear and heating. In their 2003–2004 National Health and Nutrition Examination Survey, the CDC found that of 2517 urine samples gathered, 93% of them had detectable levels of BPA.[178] Studies have looked at prenatal, postnatal, and fetal levels of BPA. In 2005, the Environmental Working Group (EWG), a nonprofit organization that focuses on protecting human health and the environment, looked at 10 umbilical cord samples from babies born in U.S. hospitals and found 287 industrial chemicals and pollutants. The blood contained pesticides; chemicals from nonstick cooking pans and plastic wrap; long-banned polychlorinated biphenyls; and wastes from burning, gasoline, and garbage.[114] The EWG found 9 out of 10 umbilical cords from minority infants born between 2007 and 2008 contained BPA, which was only 1 of the 232 industrial compounds and pollutants identified.[84]

A study completed in 2018 looked at BPA exposure levels in various bodily fluids and tissues of pregnant women and examined fetus and infant exposures to BPA, based on those levels. The highest concentration of BPA was found in the neonatal urine, followed by maternal urine, cord serum, maternal serum, breast milk, and the placenta.[138] Uncertainty remains regarding BPA, including its use in various products and its effects on the population throughout the life span. The National Children's Study was established in 2000, which examined the effects of environmental influences on the health and development of more than 100,000 children across the United States from birth to age 21. Its main goal was to improve the health and well-being of children; however, in December 2014, the National Children's Study was canceled. A study that could have advanced pediatric disease research and connected exposures to diseases later in life barely got off the ground before numerous factors shut it down.[176,186] Ways to prevent exposure to BPA include the following:[176]

- Do not microwave polycarbonate plastic food containers.
- Be aware that plastic recyclable containers with codes 3 or 7 may be made with BPA.
- Reduce use of canned foods.
- Use glass, porcelain, or stainless steel containers, especially with hot items.
- Use BPA-free baby bottles and children's cups.

## Etiologic Factors

Chemical (organic and inorganic), physical, and biologic agents that can be considered environmental hazards are numerous (Box 4.1). Despite the many restrictions on industries placed by the EPA, according to the Toxic Release Inventory (TRI), the increased number of polluters in the United States (and worldwide) and under-reporting practices have resulted in the release of more toxic chemicals into the environment each year. The TRI is a publicly available EPA database that contains information on more than 650 toxic chemical releases and other waste management activities reported annually by

Box 4.1

**ENVIRONMENTAL HAZARDOUS AGENTS**

***Chemical Agents***

- Pollution or occupational exposure
  - Air (carbon monoxide, smog, radon, acid rain, tobacco smoke, household cleaning products, sick building syndrome; see text for others)
  - Water (industrial chemicals, pesticides, disease)
  - Food (pesticide residues, hormone residues, irradiation, genetic modification, food additives, preservatives)
  - Soil contamination
- Asbestos
- Manmade minerals
- Aging PVC (e.g., dolls, toys)
- Fire and pyrolysis products
- Heavy metals
- Waste
  - Solid waste
  - Hazardous waste
  - Incinerator waste
  - Medical/infectious waste

***Physical Agents***

- Electromagnetic fields
- Vibration
- Heat stress
- High-altitude and aerospace medicine
- Mechanical factors
  - Cumulative or repetitive trauma
  - Accidents/injury
- Noise

***Biologic Agents***

- Bacteria
- Viruses
- Allergens
- Fungi (molds)
- Parasites

***Epigenetic Factors (see Chapter 2)***
***Psychologic and Physical Health (see Chapter 3)***

*PVC*, Polyvinyl chloride.

some industry groups as well as federal facilities.[267] These agents, combined with psychosocial factors, can lower the body's resistance, making a person more susceptible to infectious diseases.

## Chemical Agents

Chemical agents can be classified by use (e.g., agricultural chemicals, automotive products, pharmaceutical agents, cleaning agents, paints, dyes, explosives); mechanism of action (e.g., enzyme disruption, metabolic poison, irritants, free radical formation); and target organs (e.g., neurotoxins, hepatotoxins, cardiotoxins). Although many toxic effects can occur, they can be broken down into three main categories: local acute effects, systemic effects, and idiosyncratic (unpredictable) effects.

**Air Pollution.** Many investigations of home and workplace environments have clearly documented the role of air pollutants in causing health complaints and disease. Although exposure to air pollution is classified separately as indoor and outdoor, the concept of total personal exposure, whether exposure occurs in the home, in the office, outdoors, in a car, in a movie theater, and so on, is relevant to every individual. Anecdotal evidence and statistical studies have made a correlation between pollution and a variety of diseases, particularly asthma, heart disease, respiratory disorders, and cancer, as well as damage to the brain, nervous system, liver, and kidneys. Short-term effects of air pollution can cause eye, nose, and throat irritation; upper respiratory infections; headaches; nausea; and allergic reactions.

People considered especially susceptible to air pollution include elderly adults; infants and young children; pregnant women; cigarette smokers (and those exposed to secondhand smoke); and people with heart disease, asthma, or lung disease, including chronic obstructive pulmonary disease, emphysema, or chronic bronchitis. Pollution from coal-fired plants in the United States results in 13,000 premature deaths, 20,000 heart attacks, and hundreds of thousands of asthma attacks annually. The cost of these health impacts exceeds $100 billion each year.[64] Carbon dioxide ($CO_2$) emissions from coal-fired plants has been almost cut in half since 2010, with many power plant owners closing or with plans to close.

In 2015 the Clean Power Plan was passed, which would cut greenhouse gas emissions from power plants 32% by 2030. The federal government gave states targets to reduce emissions and encouraged closure of coal-fired power plants. A new rule was passed in 2018 called the Affordable Clean Energy Rule, which would allow states to set targets themselves; instead of encouraging closure of coal-fired power plants, it encouraged them to increase their efficiency. The EPA has analyzed the rule and is concerned about the negative impact on human health, as they anticipate an increased level of emissions of certain pollutants, causing increased morbidity and mortality rates. Improvements in federal and state policies to address air pollution and increased use of clean energy will have immediate and long-lasting positive effects on population health. Long-term exposure to particulate matter and nitrogen oxides at levels consistent with NAAQS have been shown to age blood vessels prematurely and lead to a rapid buildup of calcium in the coronary artery.[135]

Increased rates of heart attacks and other cardiovascular events are reported, with increased exposure to air pollution for individuals with known heart and blood vessel disease. Fine particulate matter that travels directly into the bloodstream, constricting arteries, is considered to be the mechanism for this effect.[35,36] It has been found that there is an increase in hospital admissions for cardiovascular diagnoses on the days there is an increase in elemental carbon in the air and an increase in admissions for respiratory diagnoses on the days there is an increase in organic carbon matter in the air. This increase in air pollution containing elemental carbon and organic carbon matter comes primarily from vehicle emissions, diesel, and wood burning.[199] Evidence is emerging that shows additional relationships between particulate matter; pollution; and other noncommunicable diseases, including diabetes, decreased cognitive function, attention-deficit/hyperactivity disorder, autism, and neurodegenerative disease, including dementia. Further research is needed to identify a possible link between air pollution and sudden infant death syndrome.[14,135,197]

**Table 4.1** New Air Quality Index[a]

| Air Quality Index Levels of Health Concern | Numeric Value | Meaning |
|---|---|---|
| Good | 0–50 | Air quality is considered satisfactory, and air pollution poses little or no risk. |
| Moderate | 51–100 | Air quality is acceptable; however, for some pollutants, there may be a moderate health concern for a very small number of people who are unusually sensitive to air pollution. |
| Unhealthy for sensitive groups | 101–150 | Members of sensitive groups may experience health effects. The general public is not likely to be affected. |
| Unhealthy | 151–200 | Everyone may begin to experience health effects; members of sensitive groups may experience more serious health effects. |
| Very unhealthy | 201–300 | Health alert; everyone may experience more serious health effects. |
| Hazardous | >300 | Health warnings of emergency conditions. The entire population is more likely to be affected. |

[a]The air quality index shows how clean or polluted the air is in a specific geographic area. The higher the index number, the greater the level of air pollution and the greater the health concern. The index number is based on the number of harmful particles in the air on any specific day (or time). You can access this information at https://airnow.gov. AirNow also has a Facebook page (https://www.facebook.com/airnow) and Twitter handle (@AirNow) as well as free Apps for iPhone and Android to monitor air quality.

From AirNow: Today's AQI forecast. Available at: https://airnow.gov.

***Indoor Air Pollution.*** Sources of indoor air pollution include tobacco smoke; fireplaces; space heaters; stoves; pilot lights; gas ranges; mothballs; cleaning fluids; glues; photocopiers; formaldehyde in foam, glues, plywood, particleboard, carpet backing, and fabrics; and infectious and allergic agents such as dust mites, cockroaches, bacteria, fungi, viruses, and pollen. Worldwide, over 3 billion people use open fires and rudimentary stoves for cooking food and heating their home. The use of wood, dung, agricultural waste, and coal increases the particulate matter and toxins within the home and contributes to the 3.8 million deaths associated with household air pollution annually. In 50% of cases, death from pneumonia in children younger than age 5 is due to household air pollution.[187,306]

Construction and architectural modifications introduced in the 1970s as a result of the worldwide energy crisis have resulted in better insulated and tighter buildings, with reduced ventilation. Illnesses that develop from indoor air pollution in tight, energy-efficient homes and buildings with poor ventilation and reduced air-exchange rates are known as *sick building syndrome* or *building-related illness*. The EPA has created an Indoor AirPLUS program to help home builders distinguish themselves as being able to offer a home with improved air quality.

*Radon*, a product of the breakdown of radium, poses an environmental risk because of its carcinogenic (especially lung cancer) properties. It is the leading cause of lung cancer in nonsmokers and is estimated to cause around 21,000 lung cancer deaths each year, with 2900 of those deaths in people who never smoked.[265,274] Radon comes from the natural breakdown of uranium in soil, rock, and water and can be found all over the United States. Exposure is predominantly naturally occurring rather than generated by human polluters and occurs in poorly ventilated homes in the form of an odorless gas that seeps through cracks in the foundation. Tobacco smoke multiplies the risk of concurrent exposure to radon; for example, with a radon level of 4 pCi/L, the lifetime risk of radon-induced lung cancer death for a nonsmoker is 7 per 1000, whereas a smoker's risk is 62 per 1000.[55,136,139]

***Outdoor Air Pollution.*** The Air Quality Index (AQI) reports daily air quality on a scale of 0 to 500. The higher the number, the more pollutants that are present in the air, resulting in higher risk of health problems arising (Table 4.1). The national air quality standard for pollutants has a value of 100, which is the level the EPA has set to protect public health. When the AQI is below 100, air quality is satisfactory, and when the AQI is above 100, air quality is unhealthy. The EPA calculates the AQI based on four major air pollutants: ground-level ozone, particulate matter, CO, and sulfur dioxide. Nitrogen dioxide is currently under review for the national air quality standard.

As part of the Clean Air Act of 1990, the EPA set air quality standards to protect sensitive population groups from outdoor air pollutants. Each decade, Healthy People sets goals to improve the health of Americans by establishing science-based objectives. These are 10-year objectives meant to increase length of life and quality of life by promoting good health. For Healthy People 2020, the AQI objective was to reduce the number of days the AQI exceeded 100. The baseline in the years 2006–2008 was 8.488 billion people days when the AQI was more than100. The objective for Healthy People 2020 was to decrease this number to 7.638 billion people days. Between the baseline data in 2006–2008 and 2014–2016, the number of days decreased by 49% to 4.327 billion people days when the AQI was more than 100, exceeding the target objective for 2020.[190]

It is known that plants remove $CO_2$ through photosynthesis, break down volatile organic compounds, and can sequester particulate matter. Research is demonstrating that the use of biofiltration technology to clean up airborne waste is effective and could have the potential to reduce the amount of overall toxicity and airborne carcinogens.[95,121,122]

*CO*, an odorless, tasteless, and colorless gas, is a common environmental pollutant from automobile exhaust emissions, the use of liquefied petroleum gas–powered forklifts in inadequately ventilated warehouses and production facilities, fires, and home heating systems. A total of 2244 deaths occurred between 2010 and 2015 from unintentional CO poisoning. The total number of unintentional deaths in 2015 was 393, with 36% of those deaths occurring between December and February.[57] CO is a leading cause of poisoning in the United States, resulting in over 15,000 visits to the emergency department annually for nonfire unintentional CO poisoning, with close to 1300 persons being admitted to the hospital annually. Most of the hospital cases involve older people (45 to 64 years old) living in the South or Midwest. CO poisoning is preventable with education on proper use of household fuel devices and installation of CO monitors.[246]

CO is commonly recognized for its toxicologic characteristics, especially central nervous system (CNS) and cardiovascular effects. CO combines 240 times more quickly with hemoglobin (or myoglobin affecting muscles) than oxygen, so when $CO_2$ is bound to hemoglobin, its oxygen-carrying capacity is decreased. In the presence of CO, oxygen is not released normally by the blood, resulting in tissue hypoxia.

Tissue hypoxia has serious functional consequences for organ systems that require a continuous supply of oxygen, such as the brain and the heart. Exposure to CO causes impaired visual acuity, headache, nausea, vomiting, fatigue, seizures, behavioral change, and ataxia. In addition, when tissue partial pressure of oxygen is low, CO binds to intracellular hemoproteins such as myoglobin, inhibiting their function and thereby affecting muscle function.

Other air pollutants include *smog*, a combination of smoke and fog that develops when vehicle emissions and exhaust fumes containing nitrous oxides and hydrocarbons are photochemically oxidized. Ozone and nitrogen, the components of smog, result from the action of sunlight on the products of vehicular internal combustion engines. Both of these by-products are toxic to the respiratory tract, damaging ciliated endothelial cells lining bronchioles and impairing the mucociliary clearance mechanism.

There is new green technology aimed at reducing smog with various materials, including honeycomb-shaped tiles coated with titanium dioxide and concrete with titanium dioxide mixed together. Chemical reactions occur when sunlight hits the tiles, resulting in smog-eating technology. These technologies are being used on roof tiles, building walls, and sidewalks. The EPA found that over 1 year, a 2000-square-foot roof with these tiles would destroy as much nitrogen oxide as produced by a car driven 10,800 miles.

Growing evidence from around the world shows that the harmful effects of smog extend even to the unborn in utero. More than a dozen peer-reviewed studies in the United States, Brazil, Europe, Mexico, South Korea, and Taiwan have linked smog to low birth weight, premature births, stillbirths, and infant deaths. Research has found that children exposed in utero to higher levels of ambient pollution during the third trimester are 60% more likely to have raised systolic blood pressure during childhood compared with children exposed to low levels. Exposure to mothers before pregnancy was not associated with raised blood pressure in their children, showing how important in utero exposure to air quality is to newborn health.[210,315]

*Acid rain* is an air pollutant caused by the interaction of sulfur dioxide and nitrogen oxides in the atmosphere that form fine sulfate and nitrate particles. Although natural sources such as volcanoes and decaying vegetation can lead to acid rain, the main source of acid rain comes from the burning of fossil fuels. The sulfur dioxide and nitrogen dioxide interaction is then transported by wind currents over long distances through the air. It is damaging to lakes, streams, and forests, as well as all of the plants and animals that live there. In the United States, the northeast is the most often affected, owing to the dense populations, large number of cities, and concentration of power and industrial plants. It can damage the surfaces of buildings and deteriorate statues and other structures. Human health is not affected by acid rain; in fact, walking in acid rain and swimming in lakes affected by acid rain does not cause any more harm than normal rain or lake water. Sulfur dioxide and nitrogen dioxide that cause acid rain, along with sulfate and nitrate particles, can be harmful to human cardiopulmonary health when inhaled.

A study that looked at the trends and effects of acid rain between 1984 and 2009 found that sulfite emissions dropped more than 50% and nitrate emissions dropped more than 30% over that time frame. Researchers believe this is due in part by the Clean Air Act of 1990 amendments that regulated emissions of these gases, which, when mixed with rain water, become sulfuric and nitric acid.[279] Improvements can be seen in nature, including clearer waterways and top soil layers, fish in lakes that were once empty of fish, and revival of the red spruce in the Northeastern United States.[132]

**Water Pollution.** Water pollution in the form of contamination of drinking water by toxic chemicals has become widely recognized as a public health issue since the late 1970s. Increased monitoring since then has shown that many pesticides and industrial chemicals can be detected in drinking water. The EPA, in conjunction with public health officials and the drinking water industry (e.g., Partnership for Safe Water), has worked diligently to survey and reduce water-borne disease outbreaks, chemical contamination from leached industrial waste chemicals, and toxins released into recreational and drinking water.[22] The Safe Drinking Water Act is a federal law passed in 1974 aimed at protecting public drinking supplies throughout the United States.

The EPA and states, tribes, public water systems, and certified laboratories work in partnership to provide safe drinking water. The EPA, states, and tribes ensure public drinking water meets federal standards through regular monitoring and reporting. A private source of water (e.g., cistern or well water) does not come under this type of protection. Every 6 years, the EPA is required to review these regulations (termed Six-Year Review) and determine if any revision is needed based on new information on health effects, treatment technologies, occurrence and exposure, and other factors to protect the health of the population. Regulations look at inorganic chemicals, organic chemicals, disinfectants and disinfection by-products, and microbiologic contaminants. The EPA provides the names of contaminants, Maximum Contaminant Level, health effects of the contaminant, and monitoring requirements for the contaminant.

There are secondary standards (guidelines, which are unenforceable by law) for contaminants in water that may cause cosmetic or aesthetic effects on individuals. Examples of secondary standards include contaminants such as copper, fluoride, iron, and pH levels. The EPA includes future potential regulations, which are reviews and proposals outside of the Six-Year Review.[2] The Flint Water Crisis began in 2014 with violations of *Escherichia coli* and total coliform levels. This was due to the city of Flint, Michigan, deciding to make changes to the way it delivered drinking water to its residents. In 1967 Flint began purchasing wholesale treated water because of a growing population. To save on costs in 2012 the city passed a resolution to allow mixing of the wholesale treated water with Flint River water. In 2013 the city continued their cost-reducing measure and looked at a new supplier of treated water. The city decided to wait for the new pipeline to be formed by the supplier that would bring water in from Lake Huron. In the interim, water was used straight from the Flint River and treated at the city's own facility. The Flint River water quality was poor as a result of industries and municipalities performing unregulated discharges into the river, and this was now the water the residents in Flint were receiving in their homes, workplaces, and schools. The Michigan Department of Environmental Quality notified Flint of violating the Safe Drinking Water Act. As water samples continued to be tested, lead was found in Flint homes at levels exceeding the maximum contaminant level of 15 µg set by the EPA. Blood levels tested by a local pediatrician showed blood lead levels in the children of Flint had increased by a factor of around 2.5. Morbidity and mortality have been reported in connection to this water crisis, including cases of legionellosis. The EPA, with recommendations from the National Drinking Water Advisory Committee, is revising the lead and copper rules based on what has been learned from the Flint water crisis.[158]

Some subgroups of people may be more vulnerable to contaminants in drinking water than the general population. Immunocompromised individuals, such as patients with cancer who are undergoing treatment, organ transplant recipients, people with HIV/AIDS or other immune system disorders, some older adults, and infants are at increased risk from infections.

Disinfection with chlorine is the most common method to ensure drinking water safety in the United States. A dramatic decline in water-borne diseases such as cholera and typhoid fever occurs when water systems are disinfected this way. One potential downside of this disinfectant treatment is the increased genotoxicity that occurs with water treatment. The disinfection by-products that are created when chlorine and other disinfectants react with organic matter in the water are being investigated for their effects on the population. A study looking at detection of a cholesterol-lowering drug in U.S. wastewater found that water chlorination may increase the toxicity of pharmaceutically active compounds in surface water.[39]

Other forms of water pollution include combined sewer overflows (sewage and stormwater runoff released into water bodies) and release of treated sewage offshore into deep waters via outfalls (long undersea pipelines). Research has found an uptick in emergency department visits for gastrointestinal illness with heavy rainfall in areas that use combined sewer overflows, linking the possibility of drinking water contamination in those areas.[124] With outfalls, wastewater is filtered and processed, but many contaminants, including estrogenic compounds and human pharmaceutical drugs, remain and settle into ocean sediment where they are consumed by bottom-feeding organisms that become food for other ocean life. Evidence of abnormalities in animals and fish exposed to sewage and industrial contaminants has been reported, but the effect on overall health and abundance of fish populations and the rest of the marine ecosystem remains unknown.[147,260]

**Food.** Food as a pollutant is one of the major environmental agents to which people are exposed. In many documented cases, reversible and irreversible human and ecologic damage has occurred as a result of pollution-induced food contamination. As scientific and epidemiologic information accumulates, society is questioning to what degree these technologies and by-products contribute to the steadily rising incidence of certain cancers, autoimmune and other chronic diseases, birth defects, autism, learning disorders, and other health problems for which the cause is not well understood.

***Pesticides, Insecticides, and Herbicides.*** Pesticide, insecticide, and herbicide residues in food; hormone residues; food irradiation (a method of preservation and protection from microbial contamination); genetically modified foods; and food additives and preservatives are major consumer concerns. The EPA sets limits on how much of a pesticide may be used on food while growing and processing it, as well as how much may remain on food purchased by consumers. In 2015 the EPA revised the Worker Protection Standard to reduce the risk of pesticide poisoning and injury to over 2 million agricultural workers and pesticide handlers who work in the agricultural industry. Annual training, access to certain chemical information, and other worker protection requirements are some of the updates to the Worker Protection Standard. This EPA regulation does not necessarily apply to farm owners and their immediate family, who are exempt from many of the regulations, but it is aimed at providing more protection for agricultural workers.

The U.S. Department of Agriculture monitors the chemicals in the food supply via the Pesticide Data Program, which works with the EPA to monitor pesticide residues in food. In 2016 the program found pesticide residue on 70% of conventionally grown (nonorganic) produce samples; however, only 0.46% of those residues exceeded the tolerance levels set by the EPA.[270] The EWG takes the information from the Pesticide Data Program and creates Dirty Dozen and Clean Fifteen lists to help educate people about the foods most and least affected by pesticides. In 2018 the cleanest foods (Clean Fifteen) in order included avocados, sweet corn, pineapple, cabbages, onions, frozen sweet peas, papayas, asparagus, mangoes, eggplants, honeydew melons, kiwi, cantaloupe, cauliflower, and broccoli. In the same year, the most pesticide residue (Dirty Dozen) was found in order in strawberries, spinach, nectarines, apples, grapes, peaches, cherries, pears, tomatoes, celery, potatoes, and sweet bell peppers.[65,79]

Pesticide and herbicide exposure can cause many different health effects, from acute problems such as dermatitis, asthma exacerbations, and gastroenteritis to chronic problems such as chronic obstructive pulmonary disease, chronic bronchitis, and cancer.[153,223] There is evidence to suggest that increased pesticide exposure can cause birth defects, fetal death, and neurodevelopmental disorders.[127,222] Researchers have been looking at the possible association of pesticide exposure with neurodevelopment disorders such as attention-deficit disorder, with or without hyperactivity and autism spectrum disorder. Current evidence shows that pesticide exposure at low levels that do not garner acute toxicity may be one of the causes of attention-deficit/hyperactivity disorder and autism spectrum disorder.[211] Among people most in danger from pesticide exposure are farmers and agricultural workers. Many studies of these groups have shown an increase in soft tissue sarcomas, presumably from herbicide exposure.[99] There are higher rates of prostate cancer, ovarian cancer, and skin cancer in this population. There is growing evidence linking pesticide exposure as a key contributor to rising cancer rates in the general population. School-aged children are at increased risk for acute illnesses from repellants and pesticides applied within school grounds, pesticide drift exposure from farmland, and pesticide use at parks.[9] Studies have shown that girls exposed to dichlorodiphenyltrichloroethane before puberty are five times more likely to develop breast cancer during middle age, and dichlorodiphenyltrichloroethane exposure in the womb increased risk of breast cancer by four times.[67,68]

Childhood leukemia, non-Hodgkin lymphoma, and Hodgkin lymphoma have been linked with the use of home and pet insecticides, garden fungicides, and, to a lesser degree, herbicides during pregnancy and early childhood.[218] Acute lymphoblastic leukemia rates have been found to be increased in boys with maternal use of insecticides inside the home 1 year before pregnancy, during pregnancy, and while breastfeeding. Acute lymphoblastic leukemia rates were found to be increased in boys and girls with frequent maternal use of insecticides inside the home or if there were pesticide applications on farms near the home.[118] The treatment of pediculosis (lice) with an insecticidal shampoo may be associated with an increased risk of childhood leukemia.[166] Lindane, an insecticide used to treat head lice and scabies since the 1950s, is known to cause neurotoxic effects and bone marrow suppression, even when used as prescribed. It is not considered an acceptable therapy for head lice, with multiple advisories regarding the side effects from the EPA and U.S. Food and Drug Administration (FDA). The WHO has labeled lindane as a probable carcinogen. In 2002 California banned pharmaceutical use of lindane, and in 2009 the American Academy of Pediatrics stopped recommending the product; however, it is still available to be prescribed, and the FDA has rejected attempts to ban lindane lice and scabies treatments from the U.S. market.[73]

There are over 1055 active ingredients registered as pesticides, which can create thousands of pesticide products. These products can accomplish many things, including weed prevention and elimination of troublesome rodents or insects. They are intended to provide efficient solutions to these problems, which tend to require increased time and resources when treated organically. The many health problems associated with pesticide exposure are overwhelming. It will be important to address their continued use and develop alternative organic methods that will reduce morbidity and mortality in the population. States are trying out the idea of creating buffer zones around schools in agricultural areas to protect children from potential adverse effects of pesticide exposure. Although this would not account for prenatal exposure and there still may be drift of pesticides from the farms, it would be a positive step in reducing childhood exposure.[105]

**Contaminated Soil.** Contaminated soil is often the main source of chemical exposure for humans, and an active interchange of chemicals occurs between soil and water, air, and food. Direct contact with soil and ingestion of soil are important exposure pathways, and inhalation of volatile compounds or dust must also be considered. The movement of contaminants through soil is very complex, some moving rapidly and others slowly, eventually reaching and contaminating surface or ground water on which people rely for drinking and other purposes.

**Asbestos.** Asbestos continues to be a significant occupational hazard, with the WHO estimating 125 million people around the world being exposed to asbestos annually in the workplace. It is a known carcinogen, with evidence showing its causal relationship to mesothelioma and other cancers of the lung, larynx, and ovary. The International Labour Organization estimates 107,000 workers die each year from a disease related to asbestos. It was not until the late 1960s and early 1970s that the public was made aware of the health hazards of products that contained asbestos, ranging from automotive brake linings to building insulation and hundreds of other items. Long latency (exposure occurring 30 or more years ago continues to affect former workers) and long-term, low-level exposure to the presence of indoor asbestos remain risk factors.

Commercial use of asbestos has decreased dramatically. An asbestos ban has been put in place in 55 countries; however, China, Russia, India, Canada, and the United States continue production and import of asbestos products.[161,303] See Chapter 15 for a discussion of asbestosis.

**Other Chemical Compounds.** Polyvinyl chloride (PVC), a type of plastic made flexible through the addition of chemicals called phthalates, is used in a variety of products from pipes to flooring and toys to school supplies. PVC is also found in medical products, such as saline bags that store medical solutions, blister packs, medical shrink wrap, and intravenous (IV) lines. Concern exists over the possibility of chemical plasticizers leaching into long-term IV solutions used in certain patient populations, including patients on dialysis, patients with hemophilia, and neonates exposed at critical points in development.

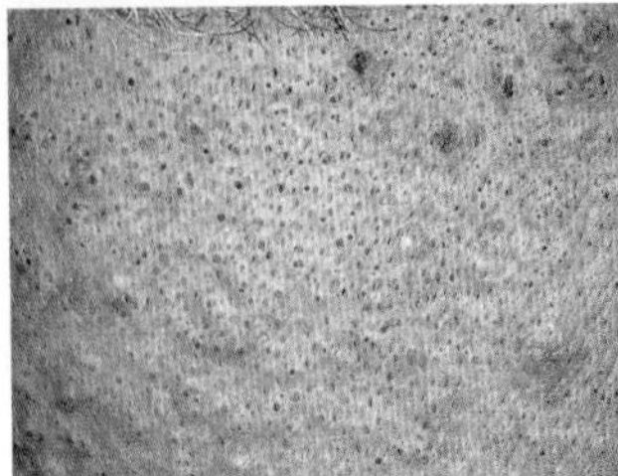
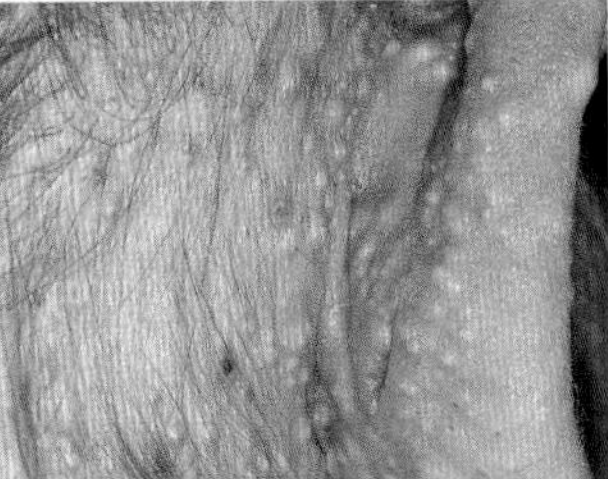

**Figure 4.1**

**Chloracne.** (From Bolognia JL, Jorizzo JL, Rapini RP: *Dermatology*, St. Louis, 2003, Mosby.)

PVC production includes three main chemical processes: chlorine gas converts to ethylene dichloride (which the EPA lists as a probable carcinogen), which then converts to vinyl chloride (which the EPA, WHO, and U.S. Department of Health and Human Services have listed as a known carcinogen). Vinyl chloride exposure has been shown to increase the risk of a rare liver cancer. OSHA has regulated workplace exposure to vinyl chloride since 1974. The by-products of PVC manufacturing and disposal include organochlorines and dioxins; both are classified as persistent organic pollutants, and both are included in the United Nations "dirty dozen" list of most harmful chemicals known to science. Organochlorines have been shown to cause major health problems, including endocrine dysfunction, developmental impairment, birth defects, reproductive dysfunction, infertility, immunosuppression, and cancer. Dioxins have been shown to cause cancer, birth defects, immune system dysfunction, reproductive system dysfunction, and decreased intelligence.[81]

Additionally, measured changes in the acidity of IV solutions in PVC packaging have been reported.[248] The observed toxicities of these chemicals have resulted in the request for PVC-free medical devices and reduction of environmental contamination with these compounds to the lowest level possible.[137,258] High levels of dioxin exposure are associated with chloracne (Fig. 4.1), a distinctive form of acne, and with porphyria cutanea tarda (Fig. 4.2). Numerous health care institutions in the United States no longer purchase medical equipment made with PVC.

In March 2015 the EPA finalized new national emission standards for new and existing PVC production facilities. The changes to the rules decreased the levels of allowable PVC emissions compared with the 2012 final ruling to improve air quality and health.[88,266]

Perfluorooctanoic acid (PFOA), a chemical compound used to manufacture Teflon-coated cookware and Gore-Tex waterproof material, has been detected in 98% of the U.S. population in low-level amounts. PFOA never breaks down in the environment, so it will always be around. Research has found that PFOA causes a modest increase in cholesterol and uric acid, with higher levels increasing risk of chronic kidney disease. Researchers are looking into the effects on thyroid function, cancers, diabetes, sexual reproduction, and fetal development.[201,247] PFOA has been linked to testicular, liver, and pancreatic cancer in animals.[44,130,193] Drinking water is the major source of exposure to PFOA. In May 2016, the EPA established drinking water health advisories of 70 parts per trillion for combined concentration of PFOA and perfluorooctane sulfonate. Several states have drinking water guidelines for PFOA and perfluorooctane sulfonate. The EPA, WHO, and other agencies have labeled PFOA as a confirmed animal carcinogen and a possible human carcinogen.[278]

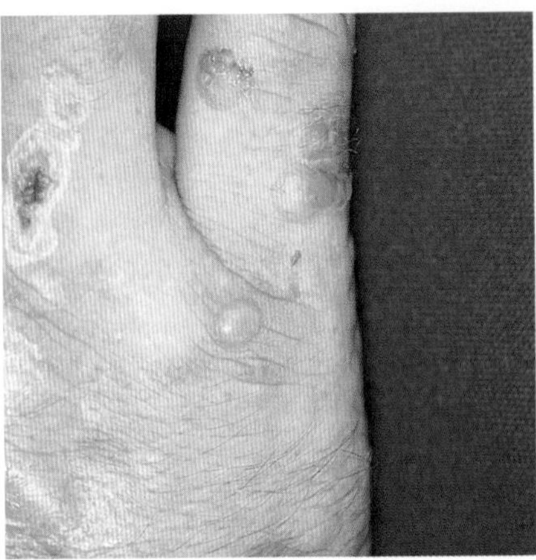

**Figure 4.2**

**Porphyria cutanea tarda.** Erosion, crusting, and vesicles on the dorsum of the hand in an individual with porphyria cutanea tarda. (From Goldman L: *Cecil textbook of medicine*, ed 22, Philadelphia, 2004, Saunders.)

**Fire and Pyrolysis.** Pyrolysis, or incomplete combustion, of wood releases many highly toxic compounds that can react with other organic substances to produce new toxic and irritant chemicals. Incomplete combustion and firefighting water produce highly acidic aerosols. Smoldering or partially controlled fires release many toxic products. Death can occur as a result of smoke inhalation and myocardial infarction. In fact, the number one cause of on-the-job deaths for firefighters is sudden cardiac death.[242,244] See Occupational Burns later in chapter.

Pyrolysis has been studied regarding its benefits, such as utilization as a fuel. Scrap tires can be reprocessed into activated carbon, carbon black, Boudouard carbon, and fuel gas.[304] The Department of Agriculture performs biomass pyrolysis research, with the objectives to develop a pyrolysis process for commercial production of pyrolysis oil, upgrade it into fuels, and make it scalable.[269]

**Waste.** Waste from solid, hazardous, and incinerator by-products is not likely to be encountered directly in a therapy practice. However, the effects of exposure to medical/infectious waste may be more problematic. Standard precautions for handling all medical/infectious waste are available (see Chapter 8).

## Heavy Metals

Heavy metals, such as lead, arsenic, and mercury, actually fall under the chemical agents category but are mentioned separately because of their former prevalence and uniqueness as classic occupational and environmental hazards. In the early 1990s, environmental concerns shifted attention away from lead, mercury, arsenic, and asbestos exposure despite continued high production volume chemical development, toxicology testing, and issues centered around environmental justice.[140]

More recent findings from the EPA TRI have resulted in a resurgence of interest and research in this area. In 2015 TRI findings reported managing 27.24 billion lb of toxic chemicals in on-site and off-site production waste. While 44% of the waste was recycled, 32% was treated, and 11% was energy recovered; 13% or 3.36 billion lb of that waste was disposed of or released by other means into the environment.[85]

**Lead Poisoning.** A normal blood lead level is 0. No safe blood lead levels have been identified for children. Reference levels for children are 5 μg/dL, which identifies their blood lead levels as much higher than most children. An elevated blood lead level in adults is defined as concentrations greater than 5 μg/dL, a change implemented by NIOSH in 2015 from the prior 10 μg/dL limit. Before 2010 the adult referenced limit was a blood lead level of 25 μg/dL. OSHA prohibits workers with levels greater than 50 μg/dL (or higher for construction workers and 60 μg/dL or higher for general industry workers) from returning to the workplace where lead is present. Workers are permitted to return to work when their blood lead level is less than 40 μg/dL.[10] The National Health and Nutrition Examination Survey found that in the years 2009–2010, the average blood lead levels of all adults in the United States was 1.2 μg/dL.[58]

Lead poisoning has declined in the United States as a result of federal initiatives to end the use of lead in numerous readily available products, such as gasoline, lead solder in the seams of food cans, lead-based paints, and plumbing in homes. Data from 1994–2009 collected by the CDC showed that in 1994 there were 14 per 100,000 employed adults who have blood lead levels ≥25 μg/dL, whereas in 2009 this dropped to 6.3 per 100,000.[50] In 2010 when NIOSH changed the elevated blood lead levels to 10 μg/dL, there were 26.6 adults per 100,000 with an elevated lead level, which decreased to 19.1 adults per 100,000 in 2014.[51,59]

The Institute for Health Metrics and Evaluation estimated that long-term health effects of lead exposure accounted for 540,000 deaths worldwide in 2016. They estimated that more than 60% of idiopathic developmental intellectual disability worldwide was due to lead exposure. Lead exposure was linked to ischemic heart disease and stroke, each accounting for 3% of worldwide occurrence.[307]

***Children.*** Lead is particularly toxic to infants and children for several reasons, including (1) the blood-brain barrier is immature before the age of 3, allowing lead to enter the brain more readily; (2) ingested lead has a 40% bioavailability in children, compared with 10% in adults; and (3) the behavioral hand-to-mouth habits of children. Apparent toxicity in children is not usually demonstrated until the blood serum lead levels exceed 10 μg/dL.

In the United States there are more than 500,000 children between the ages of 1 and 5 years who have blood lead levels >5 μg/dL.[53] Lead absorption relies on several factors, including method of exposure; size of particles; and nutritional status, health, and age of a person. Smaller sized particles can have higher absorption rates compared with larger particles; and there is less absorption when the stomach is full from a meal, compared with an empty stomach.[7]

After lead is absorbed, it enters the bloodstream and attaches to proteins in the blood, which then carry it to various organs and tissues throughout the body. In adults, more than 90% of the total body stores of lead are found in the teeth and bone, and in children around 73% of stores are found in bone. Differences between lead accumulation in bones of children and adults include higher accumulation in cortical bone in children and accumulation in both cortical and trabecular bone in adults. Lead accumulation in dense bones of adults accounts for around 70% of the total lead burden in a person's body.[16,21] Lead can adversely affect many organ systems, including the CNS and the gastrointestinal, hematopoietic, reproductive, and renal systems. The body is able to rid itself of lead through the urinary and gastrointestinal tracts, but most people are unable to get rid of as much lead as they take in.

Health effects in infants born to women with moderately elevated blood lead levels include preterm birth, decreased gestational maturity, lower birth weight, reduced postnatal growth, increased incidence of minor congenital anomalies, and early neurologic or neurobehavioral deficits. It is unclear how long these neurologic effects persist, but some evidence suggests a link between prenatal elevated lead levels and decreased intelligence in children up to age 7 years.[45]

There is no safe blood lead concentration, and levels as low as 5 μg/dL in children may be associated with decreased intelligence, learning problems, and behavioral disorders. Higher accumulations of lead in children is associated with IQ deficits; antisocial behaviors; slowed growth; decreased competency in verbal performance and auditory processing; impaired hearing; and medical issues, including anemia, hypertension, renal impairment, immunotoxicity, and damage to the reproductive organs. Extremely high levels of exposure can cause coma, convulsions, or death, and if the child survives, he or she may have cognitive and behavioral disorders.[48,212,232,307]

**Arsenic.** Arsenic is a naturally occurring metal-like element found in the earth's crust. The two forms of arsenic, organic and inorganic, are found in water, air, soil, and food. Inorganic arsenic has been shown to be a human carcinogen and is a global concern, owing to its leaching into groundwater that is used for human consumption. Arsenic can be found in its organic form in animals, most notably fish and shellfish, but is less harmful than inorganic arsenic. Drinking contaminated water, eating food prepared with contaminated water, and irrigation of crops with contaminated water are the major avenues whereby arsenic gets into the body, but it can be breathed in as a dust or leached through the skin as well. Although considered toxic, arsenic has been used for thousands of years in traditional Chinese medicine to treat major illness. In certain individuals with acute promyelocytic leukemia, a single dose of arsenic trioxide has been found to be a more effective treatment with fewer side effects, compared with other medications.[83,198]

The EPA standard for arsenic in drinking water is 10 parts per billion, which was adopted in 2001, changing the previous standard of 50 parts per billion. Arsenic binds to tissue proteins and is concentrated in the liver, skin, kidney, nervous system, and bone, with bone being affected to a lesser extent than with lead. Typically arsenic is excreted in the urine within 1 week of exposure, with any remaining arsenic mostly found in the hair, nails, and skin.

Initial symptoms of acute arsenic poisoning may include severe burning of the mouth and throat, abdominal pain, nausea, vomiting, and diarrhea followed by numbness, tingling, hypotension, muscle spasms, and even death. With chronic inorganic arsenic poisoning, the first signs are typically seen in the skin, with small dark spots appearing on the trunk, neck, face, arms, and legs. Then the palms of the hands and soles of the feet develop cornlike growths.[262]

Long-term ingestion of inorganic arsenic can lead to other health problems, including cardiomyopathy, developmental effects, diabetes, jaundice, renal impairment, red cell hemolysis, ventricular arrhythmias, coma, seizures, and intestinal hemorrhage. Painful dysesthesia in the hands and feet, bone marrow depression, transverse white striae of the nails, altered mentation, and occasionally garlicky perspiration odor may occur. Arsenic has been linked to increased infant mortality; increased young adult mortality; and decreased cognitive development, intelligence, and memory.[305]

Cancers of the skin, kidney, bladder, and lungs have been associated with arsenic poisoning, but the mechanisms responsible for arsenic carcinogenesis have not been established. Increasing evidence indicates that arsenic acts at the level of tumor promotion by modulating the signaling pathways responsible for cell growth.[239,292] The risk of arsenic-induced cancer is associated with 20 or 30 years of drinking polluted water, not from a brief or occupational exposure. Research has been done in the United States looking at the effects on population health since the federal regulation for arsenic in drinking water changed to 10 parts per billion in 2001. There was a 17% decrease in arsenic found in urine of subjects who used public water (but not private wells) between 2003 and 2014. Researchers were able to estimate that this reduced exposure to arsenic would reduce yearly lung and bladder cancer cases by 200 to 900 or would reduce yearly skin cancer cases by 50.[185] Research such as this is important in demonstrating the positive impact of federal drinking water regulations on preventing disease and protecting human health.

**Mercury.** Mercury is a chemical that has the symbol Hg on the periodic table of elements. It is a naturally occurring element found in nature and can be dangerous when ingested, inhaled, or absorbed through the skin. Mercury is a hard shiny, silver metal that is liquid at room temperature and turns to a colorless, odorless gas once it is heated. Methylmercury is the most common organic mercury compound in nature and is created when bacteria interacts with mercury. Methylmercury is more toxic to humans because it is more easily absorbed into the body. Current research has found no safe level of methylmercury in the blood.

*Sources of Mercury.* Mercury is found in the earth's crust and can be found in many rocks, including coal. In the United States more than 40% of mercury emissions in the air are from coal-burning power plants. Common products that may contain mercury include thermometers, switches, fluorescent light bulbs, and dental amalgam (silver) fillings. Phasing out these mercury-containing products has already become a national trend.

Inorganic mercury compounds form when mercury combines with another element such as oxygen or sulfur. It takes the form of mercury salts, which are generally white powders or crystals. In the United States these are used in some industries and to make other chemicals. It can be found in some skin lotions and creams manufactured outside the United States. It is important to read the ingredients in these products and discontinue use if any contain mercury, calomel, mercury chloride, mercuric, or mercurio.

Harmful mercury vapors can be transferred to water and soil, where they can be introduced into the food chain. Although eating contaminated fish is the leading cause of mercury accumulation in humans, elevated levels of emissions from coal-burning power plants and petroleum refineries, mining-related wastes, and the improper disposal of mercury products have resulted in increased mercury in the environment, with the trickle-down effects on fish; larger fish have higher concentrations of mercury (Fig. 4.3).

In January 2017 the EPA and FDA issued updated consumer advice about mercury in fish intended for women of childbearing age, especially women who are pregnant or breastfeeding, and for parents with small children. There are more chemicals used in health care facilities than any other facilities with some medical supplies containing mercury. In 1997, medical waste incinerators were one of the main contributors to mercury air release, which raised concern, and the EPA created regulations for emissions from these incinerators. These regulations have been updated over the years; the 2013 update to emission guidelines for hospital and infectious waste incinerators included an 89% reduction in mercury emissions. In 2012 the Healthier Hospitals Initiative began, which is a national campaign to implement a new approach to improve environmental health and sustainability in health care facilities. The Healthier Hospitals Safer Chemicals Challenge includes achieving mercury-free status by developing and implementing a mercury elimination plan.[110]

*Clinical Manifestations (Mercury Exposure).* Exposures to women of childbearing age, pregnant and nursing women, and children younger than age 15 are of great concern because of the susceptibility of these groups and resultant adverse effects. The National Health and Nutrition Examination Survey has been reporting levels of blood mercury in eligible participants who are 1 year old and older since 2003. Non-Hispanic black women had the highest levels of blood mercury, followed by non-Hispanic whites and then Mexican Americans. Fetuses are most susceptible to developmental effects on their growing CNS, and in 2000 the National Research Council of the National Academy of Sciences found that 85 μg/L in cord blood was associated with neurodevelopmental effects. Research in New York City found decreased IQ scores in toddlers whose mothers had higher levels of mercury in cord blood.[294] Research conducted in Massachusetts found that higher mercury blood levels during the second trimester of pregnancy resulted in decreased cognitive development in 3-year olds.[191]

## Advice About Eating Fish

### What Pregnant Women & Parents Should Know

Fish and other protein-rich foods have nutrients that can help your child's growth and development.

**For women of childbearing age (about 16-49 years old), especially pregnant and breastfeeding women, and for parents and caregivers of young children.**

- *Eat 2 to 3 servings of fish a week from the "Best Choices" list OR 1 serving from the "Good Choices" list.*
- *Eat a variety of fish.*
- *Serve 1 to 2 servings of fish a week to children, starting at age 2.*
- *If you eat fish caught by family or friends, check for fish advisories. If there is no advisory, eat only one serving and no other fish that week.**

**Use this chart!**

You can use this chart to help you choose which fish to eat, and how often to eat them, based on their mercury levels. The "Best Choices" have the lowest levels of mercury.

**What is a serving?**

**To find out, use the palm of your hand!**

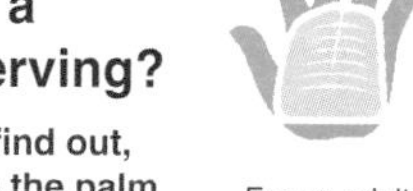

For an adult
4 ounces

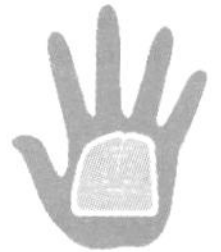

For children, ages 4 to 7
2 ounces

**Best Choices** EAT 2 TO 3 SERVINGS A WEEK

| | | |
|---|---|---|
| Anchovy | Herring | Scallop |
| Atlantic croaker | Lobster, American and spiny | Shad |
| Atlantic mackerel | Mullet | Shrimp |
| Black sea bass | Oyster | Skate |
| Butterfish | Pacific chub mackerel | Smelt |
| Catfish | Perch, freshwater and ocean | Sole |
| Clam | Pickerel | Squid |
| Cod | Plaice | Tilapia |
| Crab | Pollock | Trout, freshwater |
| Crawfish | Salmon | Tuna, canned light (includes skipjack) |
| Flounder | Sardine | Whitefish |
| Haddock | | Whiting |
| Hake | | |

OR

**Good Choices** EAT 1 SERVING A WEEK

| | | |
|---|---|---|
| Bluefish | Monkfish | Tilefish (Atlantic Ocean) |
| Buffalofish | Rockfish | Tuna, albacore/ white tuna, canned and fresh/frozen |
| Carp | Sablefish | Tuna, yellowfin |
| Chilean sea bass/ Patagonian toothfish | Sheepshead | Weakfish/seatrout |
| Grouper | Snapper | White croaker/ Pacific croaker |
| Halibut | Spanish mackerel | |
| Mahi mahi/ dolphinfish | Striped bass (ocean) | |

**Choices to Avoid** HIGHEST MERCURY LEVELS

| | | |
|---|---|---|
| King mackerel | Shark | Tilefish (Gulf of Mexico) |
| Marlin | Swordfish | Tuna, bigeye |
| Orange roughy | | |

*Some fish caught by family and friends, such as larger carp, catfish, trout and perch, are more likely to have fish advisories due to mercury or other contaminants. State advisories will tell you how often you can safely eat those fish.

www.FDA.gov/fishadvice
www.EPA.gov/fishadvice

EPA United States Environmental Protection Agency — FDA U.S. FOOD & DRUG ADMINISTRATION

THIS ADVICE REFERS TO FISH AND SHELLFISH COLLECTIVELY AS "FISH." / ADVICE UPDATED JANUARY 2017

**Figure 4.3**

**Advice about eating fish during pregnancy.** (From United States Environmental Protection Agency. 2017 EPA-FDA Advice About Eating Fish and Shellfish. Last updated January 2017. Available at: www.epa.gov/fishadvice or www.fda.gov/fishadvice. Accessed May 29, 2019.)

Mercury is a neurotoxin that can cause various symptoms in individuals with exposure. Symptoms depend on several factors, including what type of mercury, how much mercury, how old the person is, how long the exposure lasts, how the person is exposed, and the health status of the person. Exposure to hazardous levels of mercury can cause permanent neurologic heart and kidney impairment. Neurologic or neurodegenerative diseases, cerebral palsy, seizures, memory loss, learning disabilities, cognitive and other developmental delays, autoimmune disorders, mental health disorders, and birth defects are among the many conditions associated with mercury exposure.[301] There have been inconclusive findings regarding cancer risk from elemental mercury; researchers are now looking at the possibility of mercury toxicity acting as a promoter of cancer.[314] The EPA has labeled inorganic mercury and methyl mercury a Group C, possible human carcinogen. More research is needed to understand mercury and its possible carcinogenic role.

Vaccines commonly given to children before 2001 contained a preservative (Thimerosal) that contained mercury. There were concerns raised over the total number of vaccinations given to children during the first 6 months of life that could lead to toxic levels of mercury. There was some suspicion that increased rates of autism could be the result of mercury poisoning from vaccines, but this has not been proved conclusively. A 2011 study comparing urinary mercury between children with autism and control children showed no statistical differences in levels of urinary mercury levels even when controlled for age, gender, and amalgam fillings.[310]

Acute exposure to high levels of elemental mercury results in CNS effects such as tremors, mood changes, and slowed sensory and motor nerve function. Chronic exposure can cause CNS effects such as increased excitability, irritability, and tremors, as well as a chronic personality disorder called the Mad Hatter syndrome, characterized by unusual shyness, labile affect, and decline in intellect. Acute exposure to inorganic mercury orally may result in nausea, vomiting, and severe abdominal pain. Kidney damage is a major effect from chronic exposure to inorganic mercury. Acute exposures to very high

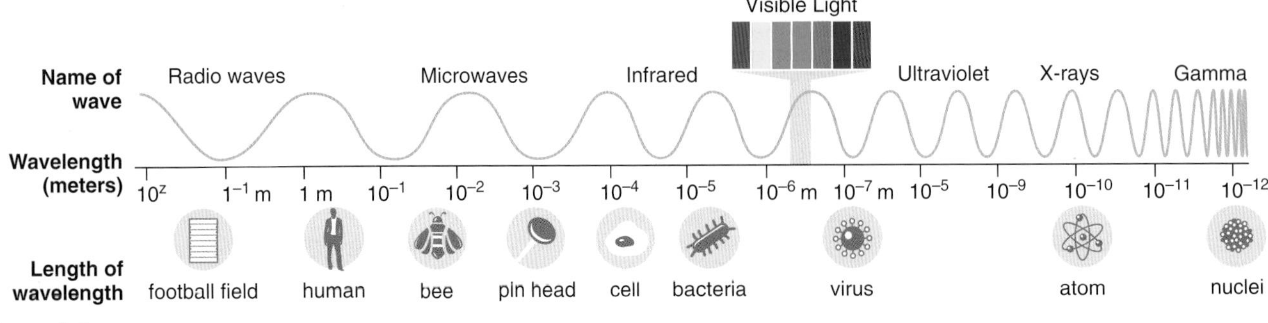


**Figure 4.4**

**Electromagnetic spectrum.** Different types of electromagnetic radiation have different frequency or wavelengths. Radio waves, television waves, and microwaves all are types of electromagnetic waves. The electromagnetic spectrum includes, from longest wavelength to shortest, radio waves, microwaves, infrared, optical, ultraviolet, x-rays, and gamma rays. Waves in the electromagnetic spectrum vary in size from very long radio waves the size of buildings to very short gamma rays smaller than the size of the nucleus of an atom. The frequency is the rate at which the electromagnetic field goes through one complete oscillation (cycle) and is usually given in Hertz (Hz), where 1 Hz is one cycle per second. As the frequency rises, the wavelength gets shorter.

levels of methylmercury can result in CNS effects such as blindness, deafness, and impaired consciousness levels. Chronic exposure may lead to paresthesia, blurred vision, malaise, speech difficulties, and constriction of the visual field.[8]

***Mercury Regulation.*** In 2005 the EPA took its first step toward reducing mercury pollution from coal-fired power plants with the Clean Air Mercury Rule, designed to reduce mercury emissions by 70% over the next 20 years. In December 2011, the EPA announced the Mercury and Air Toxics Standards (MATS), the first national standard to protect families from power plant emissions. The EPA estimated that in 2016 the health benefits of these changes would be between $37 billion and $90 billion and would avoid 4200 to 11,000 premature deaths, 2800 cases of chronic bronchitis, 4700 heart attacks, 130,000 cases of aggravated asthma, 5700 hospital and emergency department visits, 6300 cases of acute bronchitis, 140,000 cases of respiratory symptoms, 540,000 days of missed work, and 3.2 million days when people restrict their activities.[275]

A second phase of the Clean Air Mercury Rule was due in 2018, which would place a second cap on coal-fired power plants, further reducing emissions to 15 tons. Instead of initiating the second phase, updates to the proposed rules and changes to MATS by the EPA continue to occur as the current White House administration directs the Agency to investigate all of the costs and benefits of MATS. A proposal by the EPA on December 28, 2018, stated that although emission standards and other requirements of the MATS rule would remain, it is not "appropriate and necessary" to regulate hazardous air pollutants from power plants. Proposals and changes such as this make monitoring both positive and negative changes to environmental hazard regulations by the government important to follow.

## Physical Agents

**Electromagnetic Radiation.** The long-term effects of exposure to electromagnetic radiation or electromagnetic fields (EMFs) including radiofrequency and microwave, ultraviolet light, x-ray, and gamma rays remain under intense scrutiny (Fig. 4.4). Ionizing radiation is the result of electromagnetic waves entering the body and acting on neutral atoms or molecules with sufficient force to remove electrons, creating an ion. The most common sources of ionizing radiation exposure in humans are accidental environmental exposure and medical, therapeutic, or diagnostic irradiation.

All living material is vulnerable to ionization by high-energy radiation because the disruption of atoms joined into molecules producing ions and free radicals can result in further biochemical damage, including somatic effects such as cell death and genetic effects such as reproductive effects and cancer. Radiation-induced changes can cause genetic mutations and structural rearrangements in chromosomes that can be transmitted from generation to generation.[27,261]

Exposure to nonionizing radiation (i.e., the electromagnetic wave does not have enough energy to strip an atom of its electron) occurs most commonly as a result of the use of a wide variety of industrial and electronic devices. Nonionizing, human-made devices can be either extremely low-frequency EMFs or radiofrequency radiation. Extremely low-frequency devices can include electrical wiring, lamps, shavers, hair dryers, and power lines. Common radiofrequency radiation sources include radio and television signals, magnetic resonance imaging (MRI) scanners, microwaves, television and computer screens, digital gas and electric meters, Wi-Fi access points, routers, cordless phones including their base, smartphones, tablets, and Bluetooth devices. Most exposures to electromagnetic interference are transient and pose no threat to people with pacemakers and implantable cardioverter defibrillators; however, MRI and prolonged exposure to EMFs are contraindicated in people with pacemakers.[202]

There are increasing numbers of people with chronic illness and disease without specific symptoms, making it challenging for health care providers to identify causes of disease. Looking at EMF exposure of individuals to possibly account for these nonspecific cases is gaining more support. Symptoms of prolonged EMF exposure include headaches, decreased concentration, poor sleep, depression, fatigue, low energy, and flu-like symptoms. Symptoms are typically intermittent but over time increase in frequency and severity. Treatment strategies include reducing EMF exposure to allow the body to recover, as well as supporting homeostasis efforts to protect against disease.

There has been considerable speculation around the world that long-term exposure to EMFs is correlated with the development of breast cancer; leukemia; miscarriage; and neurodegenerative diseases such as Alzheimer disease, Parkinson disease, and amyotrophic lateral sclerosis (ALS).[123] One study completed in Denmark found no increased risk for developing dementia, Parkinson disease, multiple sclerosis, and motor neuron disease in people living close to powerless and no increased risk of Alzheimer disease for people living within 50 meters of a power line.[96] Another study found that occupational exposure to relatively high levels of extremely low-frequency EMFs was significantly associated with increased risk of ALS in pooled studies and case-control studies, but not in cohort studies.[316] The unexplained high incidence of breast cancer in industrialized nations is suspected to be linked to electric power generation and consumption. The proposed biologic mechanism is the inhibition of melatonin caused by the products of electric power generation, EMFs, and light at night, but this has not been proved, and further investigation is warranted.[78,162,188] One study that looked at more than 29,000 cases of breast cancer demonstrated no increased risk of developing breast cancer related to distance lived from power lines. This was also true for leukemia, brain or CNS cancers, and malignant melanoma.[82] A meta-analysis performed in 2000 looking at extremely low-frequency EMF exposure and breast cancer risk found no significant association between extremely low-frequency EMF exposure and breast cancer risk in women.[62]

Most studies have shown no statistically significant increase in brain or CNS cancers related to cellular telephone usage. Three large studies have been conducted looking at brain cancer and tumors in cell phone users: the Interphone study, the Danish cohort study, and the Million Women Study. The Interphone study was conducted by researchers across 13 countries with multiple publications coming from the data obtained from questionnaires completed by participants. There was no statistically significant increase in brain or CNS cancers related to higher cell phone use. One study found a modest increase in risk of glioma in people with the highest amount of cell phone use; however, the investigators deemed it inconclusive. They also found that intracranial distribution of tumors within the brain correlated with self-reported location of phone use; however, the researchers could not draw firm conclusions about cause and effect for this finding.

Another study using data from European countries in the Interphone study showed increased risk of acoustic neuroma in individuals who used cell phones for more than 10 years.[49,256,206,227] The Danish study looked at more than 258,000 cell phone subscribers in Denmark with incidence of brain tumor. They found no association between cell phone use and incidence of glioma, meningioma, or acoustic neuroma, even after more than 13 years of cell phone use.[97,125,228]

The Million Women study was performed in the United Kingdom and gathered data from completed questionnaires. This study found no association between self-reported cell phone use and increased risk of glioma, meningioma, or non-CNS tumors.[26] Concerns that cell phone radiation is linked to tumors of the head and neck (including brain and salivary gland tumors) or causes a variety of serious problems (e.g., genetic damage, pacemaker or implantable cardioverter defibrillator disruption, interference with heart/lung monitors, or compromise to the blood-brain barrier) have not been substantiated.[260] Long-term studies of longer induction periods, especially for slow-growing tumors with neuronal features, conclude that the data do not support the hypothesis that cell phone use is related to an increased risk of brain tumors.[144,214,229]

In 2011 the WHO and International Agency for Research on Cancer (IARC) classified radiofrequency EMFs as *possibly carcinogenic to humans* (2B classification) based on an increased risk for glioma associated with cell phone use. The evidence was shown to be limited among users of cells phones for glioma and acoustic neuroma and was shown to be inadequate to draw conclusions for other cancers.

Research has been completed looking at the radiofrequency electromagnetic radiation of cell phone use and its effects on sperm. A systematic review and meta-analysis completed in 2014 found reduced sperm motility and viability in cell phone users. Effects on sperm concentration were found to be unclear, with variations from study to study.[1] Lynch and colleagues[150] found that women trying to get pregnant were more successful if their α-amylase levels in their saliva were lower. Higher levels of this enzyme led to a 29% lower probability of pregnancy. The α-amylase enzyme has been found to be higher among individuals living within 100 meters of cell phone towers, resulting in increased EMF exposure.[150] Research looking at the effects of radiofrequency exposure on the ovaries of mice is limited at this time. Research on the effects of radiofrequency exposure during pregnancy is also limited.[5,6,298]

A previous concern that living in close proximity to power lines was correlated to cancer has not been proved,[31,241] and reports linking video display terminals to miscarriages have not been substantiated.[89] Studies have looked at exposure to magnetic fields during pregnancy. One study found strong evidence that prenatal maximum magnetic field exposure above a certain level (possibly 16 mG) may be associated with miscarriage risk.[142] Another study found that women who were exposed to higher magnetic field levels had 2.72 times risk of miscarrying compared with women with lower exposure levels.[141]

**Vibration.** Vibration is divided into two types: whole-body vibration (WBV) and hand-arm vibration. Truck, tractor, bus, and boat drivers; helicopter pilots; heavy equipment operators; miners; and others are at increased risk for WBV. Major clinical concerns of WBV exposure are chronic back pain and degenerative disk diseases, sciatica, visual and vestibular changes, and circulatory and digestive system disorders.[29,43,104,168] The risk for increased spinal loading and physiologic changes associated with WBV can be reduced by vibration damping, good ergonomic design, reducing exposure, and reducing other risks such as lifting.[203]

Vibration-induced white finger disease is the most common example of an occupational injury caused by vibration of the hands. This condition occurs secondary to the use of hand tools, such as power saws, grinders, sanders, pneumatic drills, and jackhammers, and other equipment used in construction, foundry work, machining, and mining.

WBV is used as a neuromuscular training method for a range of individuals from athletes to geriatric clients. WBV has been found to increase the mechanical power output of muscles and improve neuromuscular efficiency in athletes and can increase walking speed, step length, and single-leg stand time in geriatric clients. Research on WBV therapy as a treatment for osteoporosis is ongoing. Positive results have been found for improving strength and balance, reducing fall risk and thus lowering risk of fractures, with very little information on potential harms of WBV. However, there are safety concerns including possible long-term harm. Further research to define the role of WBV in osteoporosis management is needed.[33,86,94,128,167,194,209,299,312]

**Heat Stress.** Heat stress exceeding human tolerance can result in heat-related disorders (e.g., exertional heat stroke, exhaustion, cramps, dehydration, prickly heat) and heat illnesses (e.g., chronic heat exhaustion, reduced heat tolerance, anhidrotic heat exhaustion, exertional hyponatremia), some of which are fatal. Heat illness is more likely in hot, humid weather but can occur in the absence of hot and humid conditions.

Between 1999 and 2010, there were 8081 deaths in the United States related to heat, with 69% of the deaths in men and 36% in adults older than 65 years old. The most common states where heat-related deaths occur are Arizona, Texas, and California, which account for 43% of the total. Heat-related deaths occur more often in urban areas (81%) and occur mainly during warm weather months between May and September (94% of total deaths). Hyperthermia contributed to 2298 of the total deaths related to heat, with more than half (1595 deaths) having a cardiovascular condition as the underlying cause of death.[77,93,131]

***Heat-Related Illness.*** Hispanic people who are not U.S. citizens are at increased risk for heat-related deaths compared with U.S. citizens, with greater than 2% of total deaths in Hispanic non–U.S. citizens being related to heat compared with 0.02% of total deaths in U.S. citizens. Of deaths in Hispanic non–U.S. citizens related to heat, 75.4% were in adults 18 to 44 years old, whereas U.S. citizens in that age range accounted only for 20.7% of deaths related to heat. Almost 20% of extreme heat exposure in this population occurs on farms. These numbers show the disparities in the non–U.S. citizen population and the importance of further research identifying the risk factors and limitations in resources within this population.[254]

Groups at higher risk of heat stress, including illness and mortality, include older adults aged 65 and over; children younger than 4; and people with chronic medical conditions, including obesity, diabetes, and heart disease. Participating in strenuous activity during hot weather can cause heat illnesses in people at any age. Other activities that result in increased risk for heat illness include drinking alcohol and taking medications that decrease the body's ability to thermoregulate. Individuals receiving medications that interfere with salt and water balance are at increased risk for heat-related illness and death. Therapists should be aware of diuretics, anticholinergic agents, and tranquilizers that impair sweating, as well as antidepressants, such as tricyclic antidepressants, that affect the body's ability to respond to temperature changes.

The signs and symptoms of exertional heat illnesses may vary from person to person but often include thirst, sweating, transient muscle cramps, fatigue, dizziness or lightheadedness, and dehydration (Table 4.2). Headache, nausea, loss of appetite, decreased urine output, chills, weakness, pallor, or cool and clammy skin may occur, especially with exercise (heat) exhaustion.

Disorientation, staggering, seizures, loss of consciousness (coma), or emotional instability (even hysteria) can occur with exertional heat stroke. Exertional hyponatremia is characterized by increased core body temperature, low blood sodium level, progressive headache, confusion, lethargy, significant mental compromise, seizures, swelling of the hands and feet, and coma.[30,61]

**High Altitude.** A high-altitude environment (8000 to 14,000 feet) is characterized by atmosphere with decreasing partial pressure of oxygen and decreasing temperature. The drop in barometric pressure causes a decrease in partial pressure of oxygen along every point in the oxygen transport chain, from initial oxygen intake to the cellular mitochondria. Hypoxia (reduced availability of oxygen to the body) appears to be the underlying cause of most of the physiologic changes of elevated altitude.

Acute altitude sickness includes *acute mountain sickness (AMS), high-altitude pulmonary edema (HAPE),* and *high-altitude cerebral edema (HACE)*. These three represent a continuum of disease, but each has different symptom complexes, pathogenesis, and slightly different treatment interventions.

AMS usually occurs in unacclimated individuals within 4 to 12 hours of arriving at the new altitude, with the most common symptom being headache; other symptoms include nausea, fatigue, dizziness, and insomnia. Antiemetics and analgesics are the first line of defense with AMS. Treating dehydration with fluids and adding acetazolamide and dexamethasone may help with more severe symptoms. Descending from the high altitude is recommended for individuals whose symptoms do not resolve using the above-mentioned measures.

With HAPE, fluid accumulates in the lungs when the arteries become constricted because of a lack of oxygen and the decrease in air pressure. It normally occurs within 1 to 5 days after arrival at altitudes more than 8000 to 10,000 feet. Early symptoms include fatigue, breathlessness at rest, mild cough, chest tightness, and reduced exercise performance. Worsening cough and dyspnea, orthopnea, gurgling in the chest, pink frothy sputum, cyanosis, tachypnea, tachycardia, chest tightness, and drowsiness all are signs that the condition is worsening. Treatment includes accessing a health care facility for management with supplemental oxygen and close observation. If this is not feasible, descending to a lower

**Table 4.2** Clinical Manifestations of Exertional Heat Illnesses

| Heat Illness | Risk Event | Signs and Symptoms | Intervention |
|---|---|---|---|
| Dehydration | Fluids are not maintained or replenished | Dry mouth; thirst; irritability; headache; dizziness; cramps; fatigue; decreased athletic performance | Move to a cool environment; rehydration |
| Heat cramps | Intense exercise; fluid deficiencies; electrolyte imbalance | Intense muscle pain; prolonged muscle contraction | Rehydration; replace sodium if needed; light activity (stretching, slow walking); massage; relaxation |
| Heat syncope | Exposure to high environmental temperatures; first 5 days of acclimatization; prolonged standing | Orthostatic dizziness; dizziness or fainting; tunnel vision; pallor; sweaty skin; decreased pulse rate | Move to cool (shaded) area; adequate hydration; modified activity levels until acclimatized; elevate legs above level of heart; instruct person to increase venous return before standing (e.g., ankle pumps, arms over head, change positions slowly) |
| Heat exhaustion | Hot, humid conditions (e.g., indoor pool, sauna or hot tub, outdoor weather) | Unable to continue exercise or activity; unable to sustain cardiac output; loss of coordination; dizziness or fainting; profuse sweating; headache; nausea and vomiting; diarrhea; muscle cramps | Move to cooler environment; remove excess clothing; recline and elevate legs above heart; cool with fans, ice towels, or ice bags; rehydration if possible (no nausea or vomiting) |
| Exertional heat stroke | Temperature regulation system is overwhelmed by excessive heat production or inhibited heat loss in challenging environmental conditions | Elevated core body temperature (>40°C/104°F); tachycardia; hypotension; vomiting; sweating or dry skin; altered mental status; seizures; coma; death | Whole body cooling (e.g., immersion); monitor body temperature recovery every 5–10 minutes; avoid overcooling; medical referral if physician is not on-site |

Data from Centers for Disease Control and Prevention (CDC): Extreme heat: a prevention guide to promote your personal health and safety. Available at: https://stacks.cdc.gov/view/cdc/7023. Accessed January 22, 2019.

elevation and treatment with supplemental oxygen or portable hyperbaric chamber and a pulmonary vasodilator is recommended. Preferred pharmaceutical management is nifedipine.

HACE produces brain swelling severe enough to interfere with brain function. The affected individual may experience confusion, inability to think or concentrate, confusion, and truncal ataxia. Vision can become blurred if bleeding occurs from blood vessels at the back of the eye. With onset of neurologic symptoms, immediate descent is warranted. Supplemental oxygen or a portable hyperbaric chamber is recommended for treatment if quick descent is not possible. Pharmaceutical management includes administration of dexamethasone until the person has descended or symptoms resolve. HACE can lead to coma without treatment and usually leads to death, commonly within 24 hours.

Differential diagnosis for AMS, HAPE, and HACE includes exhaustion, hypothermia, hyponatremia, migraine, dehydration, infection, $CO_2$ poisoning, drug and alcohol intoxication, hypoglycemia or hyperglycemia, transient ischemic attack, stroke, and acute psychosis.

Strategies to prevent altitude sickness include slow ascents, pre-acclimatization, avoiding overexertion, and avoiding excessive alcohol and opiate consumption. Pharmacologic prophylaxis may be used for prevention of acute altitude illness but is not necessary in all persons; use is based on the planned trip itinerary and the individual prior performance at high altitude. Acetazolamide and dexamethasone have been shown to be useful to prevent AMS, and nifedipine, tadalafil, and salmeterol have been successful in preventing HAPE.[149]

## Risk Factors

Environmental pathogenesis requires an understanding of latency, the concept that a hazardous or toxic agent may initiate a series of internal reactions that do not manifest as overt disease for many years or even decades as the body strives to maintain a state of optimal health or homeostasis. Exposures to any of the agents discussed in the previous section on etiology are in fact risk factors. Many additional factors such as route of exposure (e.g., inhalation, ingestion, or absorption through the skin), magnitude or concentration (dose) of exposure, duration (e.g., minutes, hours, days, lifetime), and frequency (e.g., seasonal, daily, weekly, or monthly) contribute to the development of progressive and overt disease.

Likewise, personal factors that vary from one person to another may affect pathogenesis and must be considered. These include age, gender, ethnicity, nutritional status, personal habits and lifestyle, genetic makeup and host susceptibility, and the strength of individual defense mechanisms. The host–agent–environment interactions are immensely complex and poorly understood at this time.

## Pathogenesis

Once a hazardous substance is released into the environment, it may be transported and transformed in a variety of complex ways. For example, a chemical may be modified by the environment before entering the body; transformed by chemical or biochemical processes; or undergo vaporization, diffusion, dilution, or concentration by physical or biologic processes. Plants and animals may accumulate small doses of a chemical agent and bioconcentrate them to the degree that they become hazardous when consumed by humans.

All cells respond to a variety of different adverse environmental stimuli with a cellular defense response now commonly referred to as the *stress response*. Molecules released by the cells in response to stress (e.g., hyperthermic shock, radiation, toxins, or viral infections) are called *heat shock* or *stress proteins*. Increased levels of these proteins after a cellular injury from any of the environmental hazardous agents seem to act as molecular chaperones that facilitate the synthesis and assembly of new reparative proteins.

Cell stress proteins within the cardiovascular system have been shown to be cardioprotective; however, they may have other roles. The three cardiovascular functions being studied are the stress proteins maintaining normal homeostatic cardiovascular signals, the stress proteins working as antiinflammatory cells that inhibit cardiovascular pathology, and the stress proteins working as proinflammatory cells that promote cardiovascular pathology.[112] Stress proteins may be influential in certain immunologic responses and may be a requirement for cells to recover from a metabolic insult.[87] Research looking at the role of stress proteins is ongoing and has found that heat shock proteins increase the level of maturation and expression of cells and can regulate cell differentiation and proliferation both physiologically and pathologically.[4]

Immunologists have discovered a possible connection between stress proteins and autoimmune disease, which may lead to preparations of specific protective vaccines.[63,300] Research is being done on the role of heat shock proteins in chronic inflammatory diseases such as multiple sclerosis. Although the results are controversial, the research shows that cells release heat shock proteins that trigger proinflammatory and immunoregulatory responses. If these heat shock proteins can be overexpressed, it may be an option for treatment.[154,171]

Chronic exposure to air particulate matter leads to inflammation and oxidative stress, precursors to pulmonary and cardiovascular diseases and cancer.[75,208] Exposure to environmental pollutants has been linked with oxidative DNA damage in humans.[115,240] Exposures are genotoxic and interfere with DNA repair and inhibit the cellular apoptosis needed to prevent cancer. Biomonitoring studies show that DNA damage is influenced by a variety of lifestyle and environmental exposures, including exercise, air pollution, sunlight, diet, and the chemical and physical agents discussed in this chapter.[28,169,252]

## Clinical Manifestations

An environmental illness may manifest in a variety of ways. The illness may manifest as a newly developed clinical syndrome or an aggravation or change in a preexisting condition. Local toxicities from exposure to environmental agents, such as ocular damage, mucous membrane complaints (eye, nose, and throat irritation), chemical burns to skin, noise-induced hearing loss, and vestibular disorders, can occur. Systemic toxicities can involve any organ system (Table 4.3). The clinical syndrome may mimic a wide range of psychiatric, metabolic, nutritional, inflammatory, and degenerative diseases.

Beginning in the 1950s an allergist named Theron G. Randolph documented observations of people who got sick from low-level exposure (lower than the recommended thresholds) to environmental substances. *Multiple chemical sensitivity (MCS)*, also termed idiopathic environmental intolerance, is a complex disease that is difficult to diagnose. Although research pertaining to MCS has been done, none of the results have provided definitive diagnostic criteria.

There are four stages to this syndrome, with varying symptoms in each stage:

Stage 0: Tolerance—normal adaptation to the environment unless limits for certain hazardous substances are exceeded

Stage 1: Sensitization—irritation of the skin, eyes, or respiratory tract; fatigue; muscle and joint pain; headache; nausea; tachycardia; balance problems

Stage 2: Inflammation—chronic inflammation in different body tissues, organs, and systems; development of dermatitis, vasculitis, arthritis, colitis, asthma

Stage 3: Deterioration—chronic inflammation causing damage to body tissues, organs, and systems; could affect the CNS, kidneys, liver, lungs, immune system; diagnoses of lupus, ischemia, cancer, psychiatric syndromes, heart failure

The two scientific approaches to MCS include toxicologic and psychiatry/psychosomatic. The toxicologic approach follows the above stages and is recognized by ecologists (scientists who study the relationship between organisms and their environment). The psychiatry/psychosomatic approach looks at the psyche of the individual and finds a self-induced cause of the symptoms, not something that is brought on by reactions to a reduced chemical exposure.[216]

The EPA and the Americans With Disabilities Act in the United States have recognized MCS as a pathology, the International Classification of Diseases contains codes for this diagnosis. However, MCS is not internationally accepted, owing to differing opinions among researchers and scientists across the globe. Additional research is needed to identify strong evidence to properly identify and treat MCS. Until then, the entire concept continues to ignite considerable controversy in the fields of medicine, toxicology, immunology, allergy, psychology, and neuropsychology.[134]

### Neurotoxicity

Of particular interest to the therapist may be the effects of hazardous or toxic agents on the nervous system. Neurologic symptoms are common presenting symptoms in people seen by occupational and environmental health professionals. Confusion and other cognitive difficulties, headaches, fatigue, dizziness, limb paresthesias, and abnormal gait patterns are often experienced, but these are nonspecific and seldom point to a single disease or cause.

**Table 4.3** Systemic Manifestations of Toxicity

| Systems | Clinical Manifestations |
|---|---|
| Optic | Optic nephropathy<br>Optic neuritis<br>Optic atrophy |
| Integument | Atopic dermatitis<br>Urticaria<br>Pain, itching, erythema<br>Pustules, papules<br>Chemical burns |
| Cardiovascular | Cardiac arrhythmia<br>Coronary artery disease<br>Hypertension<br>Myocardial injury<br>Nonatheromatous ischemic heart disease<br>Peripheral arterial occlusive disease |
| Respiratory system | Airway inflammation and hyperreactivity<br>Bronchitis<br>Asthma<br>Hypersensitivity pneumonitis<br>Pneumoconiosis<br>Interstitial fibrosis<br>Asbestosis<br>Silicosis<br>Granuloma formation<br>Diffuse alveolar damage |
| GI tract | Cancer |
| Liver | Acute or subacute hepatocellular injury<br>Cirrhosis<br>Angiosarcoma<br>Carcinoma<br>Hepatitis |
| Kidney and urinary tract | Acute renal disease<br>Chronic renal failure<br>Tubulointerstitial nephritis<br>Nephrotic syndrome<br>Rapidly progressive glomerulonephritis |
| Central nervous system | Sensorimotor polyneuropathies (mild to severe systemic weakness)<br>Muscular fasciculations and weakness<br>Reduced or absent reflexes<br>Cranial neuropathy<br>Prominent autonomic dysfunction<br>Encephalopathy<br>Cerebellar ataxia |
| Hematopoietic system | Aplastic anemia<br>Hemolytic anemia<br>Myelodysplastic syndromes<br>Multiple myeloma<br>Toxic thrombocytopenia<br>Porphyria |
| Immune system | Allergic disease<br>Allergic rhinitis<br>Bronchial asthma<br>GI allergy (food)<br>Anaphylaxis<br>Autoimmune diseases<br>Neoplasia |
| Reproductive system | Menstrual disorders<br>Altered fertility or infertility<br>Spontaneous abortion or stillbirth<br>Birth defects, low birth weight<br>Cancer<br>Reduced libido or impotence<br>Altered or reduced sperm production<br>Premature menopause |

*GI*, Gastrointestinal.

Many toxins manifest as a nonspecific syndrome of distal sensorimotor impairment that is indistinguishable from the neuropathy caused by common systemic diseases (e.g., diabetes mellitus, vitamin $B_6$ deficiency, alcoholism, or uremia). Toxins, such as lead, have a striking predilection for motor fibers and usually produce minimal sensory symptoms.

Neurologic symptoms that appear immediately after acute exposure are usually a result of the physiologic effects of the specific (usually chemical) agent. These symptoms subside with cessation of exposure and elimination of the compound from the body. By contrast, delayed neurologic disorders are generally a result of pathologic alterations of the nervous system.

Symptoms appear in a subacute manner over days or weeks after short-term exposure. In the case of long-term exposure, symptoms may appear insidiously and progress over many weeks or months. Recovery can be expected after cessation of exposure, but recovery is slow and depends on the extent of neuronal damage, the half-life of the chemical (i.e., continued exposure until the drug is out of the system), and the adverse effects of chelates used in the chemotherapy of metal poisoning.

Neurotoxicants do not cause focal (asymmetric) neurologic syndrome. Neurotoxins reach the nervous system by the systemic route and cause neurologic symptoms and deficits in a diffuse and symmetric manner, resulting in polyneuropathy. Significant asymmetry in the presentation, such as weakness or numbness affecting one limb or one side of the body, is not likely to be attributed to neurotoxicity. Although the effects of neurotoxins are symmetric, neurons from different parts of the nervous system react differently to the agent.

Toxic polyneuropathy affects the distal limbs first, reflecting the greater vulnerability of the longest nerve axons. Sensory disturbances are usually reported as a tingling or burning sensation distributed in a stocking-and-glove pattern. The toes and the feet are affected first, with hand symptoms rarely present during the early stage. Involvement of the motor nerve fibers, if present, manifests first as bilateral atrophy and weakness of the intrinsic foot and hand muscles. More severe cases may manifest with footdrop or wristdrop, reflecting degeneration of motor axons to the lower leg and forearm muscles.

Neuropathic pain is commonly encountered in people with peripheral neuropathies, regardless of the cause. In other words, pain patterns associated with chemically induced peripheral neuropathies do not differ significantly from the clinical picture of pain associated with neuropathy of other causes. Often this pain bears little relationship to the severity of neuropathy and may intensify during a period of recovery, or it may remit paradoxically as the neuropathy progresses, often with further loss of sensation. Pain is not a reliable indicator of neurologic progression or recovery.

## MEDICAL MANAGEMENT

Clinical assessment may include assessing the details of exposure and correlating them with the medical condition. Various testing procedures may be developed on the basis of the historical information provided by the client. The clinical presentation, environmental history, and results of laboratory tests assist the physician in demonstrating a correlation between exposure and the clinical manifestations. Nerve conduction velocity studies and electromyography are the primary tools for the laboratory evaluation of neuromuscular disorders. A toxic polyneuropathy is characterized by a diffuse and relatively symmetric pattern of nerve conduction velocity abnormalities.

Removal from exposure and decontamination of the exposed victim are essential in the treatment of exposure-linked toxicity. Specific intervention protocols depend on the agent involved (e.g., pesticide poisoning requires symptom-specific therapy, such as IV anticonvulsants to halt a seizure; antihistamines are used for allergic reactions), the particular organ system involved, and the presenting pathologic condition.

SPECIAL IMPLICATIONS FOR THE THERAPIST 4.1

## *Environmental Medicine*

### Environmental Hazards

Given the context of industrial, occupational, and environmental medicine and the single overriding factor of latency, health care professionals must view each client's health status holistically, as a composite of the individual's total life experience. Whenever symptoms present in the absence of a clearly identifiable history or cause, the client's past medical history must be carefully reviewed.

An environmental and occupational history includes dates of employment, a list of current and longest-held jobs, average hours worked per week, exposure to potential hazards in the workplace, common illnesses in coworkers, and personal protective equipment worn (or not worn) on the job. When taking an exposure history, health care providers can use the mnemonic $CH^2OPD^2$ (Community, Home, Hobbies, Occupation, Personal habits, Diet, Drugs) as a tool to identify an individual's history of exposures to potentially toxic environmental contaminants.[157] Specific questions for the therapist to ask are available.[101,157] A sample of a thorough exposure history form using the above-mentioned mnemonic is available at http://www.eha-ab.ca/acfp/docs/taking-an-exposure-history.pdf.

Each geographic area has its own specific environmental and occupational concerns. The therapist must find out about specific local exposures and community concerns. Overall, the chronic exposure to chemically based products and pesticides has escalated the incidence of environmental allergies and cases of MCS. Frequently, these conditions present in a physical therapy setting with nonspecific neurologic and/or musculoskeletal manifestations.

The therapist must be aware that chemically induced illnesses may manifest as generalized muscle rigidity, peripheral neuropathy, or neurocognitive impairment as a result of neurotoxicity. Any unexplained muscle weakness and atrophy, sensory loss, depressed or absent deep tendon reflexes, memory loss, delirium, ataxia, or global change in muscle tone should raise a red flag for possible chemical etiology.[196]

### Air Pollution

Vigorous exercise outdoors, which increases the dose of pollution delivered to the respiratory tract, should be avoided during periods of ambient air pollution.[92,221] Health care providers can reasonably advise all clients, especially clients with respiratory disorders, as well as athletes in training,[205] to stay indoors during pollution episodes.

Respiratory protective equipment has been developed for use in the workplace to minimize exposure to toxic gases and airborne particles. Many of these devices, particularly those likely to be most effective, add to the work of breathing and are not well tolerated by some people, especially people with respiratory disease. The major limitation of respiratory protective equipment is that the anticipated protection is achieved only if the equipment fits properly. Much remains unknown about the efficacy of respiratory protective equipment, and concerns have been raised about the risk of dangerous $CO_2$ accumulation within the device, proper fit and inward leakage, resistance to airflow as the filter load increases, and individual breathing rates and filter replacement schedules. Research to answer these questions is necessary before specific recommendations can be made for the general population, as well as for individuals with known respiratory disease.

### Carbon Monoxide

Anyone with lung injury or reduced lung capacity may have a reduced ability to diffuse CO when it is encountered. Individuals with low lung volumes for any reason (e.g., restrictive lung disease, sickle cell anemia, or lobectomy) who try to exercise may be at risk for CO poisoning under conditions a healthy individual would be able to tolerate.[116]

The main symptoms of CO poisoning are dizziness, headache, nausea, weakness, and tachypnea, followed at higher amounts by loss of consciousness, coma, convulsions, and death. As CO binds to hemoglobin, it forms carboxyhemoglobin (COHb).[72,102,130,238] Up to one-third of individuals with moderate-to-severe CO poisoning will present with a myocardial injury. This is due to the reduced capacity of the blood to deliver oxygen to the tissues. Higher levels of COHb exposure are associated with short- and long-term development of myocardial infarctions and can also lead to left ventricular dysfunction, myocardial ischemia, cardiac dysfunction, atrial and venous thrombosis, and cardiac arrhythmias.

Acute myonecrosis (death of individual muscle fibers) has been associated with CO poisoning. Clinical studies of people with heart disease have been carried out to evaluate the effects of CO exposure on exercise capacity. During exercise, people with coronary artery disease experience a decreased time to occurrence of myocardial ischemia when exposed to CO compared with healthy subjects.[3,11]

CO poisoning can cause long-term neurocognitive affects relating to brain injury with symptoms of impaired memory, cognitive dysfunction, depression, anxiety, vestibular compromise, and motor deficits.

These symptoms are typically seen within 6 weeks, followed by gradual improvements over several months; some of the neurocognitive effects are irreversible. Risk factors for this delayed neurologic compromise include age older than 36 years and more than 24-hour duration of CO exposure (chronic low levels of CO exposure could also cause these neurologic symptoms).[200,215]

Prevention of CO poisoning is important to reduce the incidence, and it is important to educate the public on signs and symptoms of CO poisoning. Initial treatment following CO poisoning includes removing the person from the source of CO, initiating cardiac pulmonary resuscitation if the person is not breathing and has no pulse, and initiating 100% inspired oxygen via a tight-fitting mask. Hospitalization normally is needed when COHb levels in normal healthy individuals are greater than 25%, greater than 15% in individuals with heart or lung disease, and greater than 10% in pregnant women. Hyperbaric oxygen and normobaric oxygen therapy both increase the partial pressure of oxygen in the alveoli, which increases the CO dissociation from hemoglobin, but this equipment is limited among health care facilities. Unfortunately, these nonpharmacologic options have not demonstrated improved neurocognitive outcomes, but additional research is needed.[38] Extracorporeal membrane oxygenation is an invasive option for severe cases that can provide immediate improvement in oxygenation, reduction of COHb, and reversal of cardiovascular compromise. Although there are no pharmacologic antidotes to CO poisoning, drug therapies are being used and researched to improve outcomes in individuals affected by it.[215]

### Lead

The brain is the target of lead toxicity in children, but adults usually present with manifestations of peripheral neuropathy. Typically the radial and peroneal nerves are affected, resulting in wristdrop and footdrop, respectively. Anyone presenting with vague or nonspecific symptoms of myalgias, paresthesias, arthralgias accompanied by fatigue, irritability, lethargy, abdominal discomfort, poor concentration, headaches, tremors, and known risk factors may have lead poisoning.

Pica (compulsive chewing on nonnutritive objects such as dirt, paint, plaster, or clay) observed in children, may be associated with lead toxicity and must be evaluated. Lead anemia and lead nephropathy may also occur (see Neurotoxicity later). For more information, contact the National Lead Information Center Clearinghouse at (800) 424-5323.

### Vibration

Equipment and tools can be modified to reduce some of the dangerous levels of vibration. Seat upgrades have been found to help reduce vibration by up to 60% on large equipment that workers drive.[70] Using antivibration gloves, taping handles with vibration-dampening tape, maintaining and balancing hand tools regularly, and using lower-vibration tools can also help decrease vibration. When vibration increases, muscles tend to tighten, and the tighter the grip on the equipment, the more vibration gets transmitted to hands and arms.

### Heat Stress

Even with a heat illness prevention plan that includes medical screening, acclimatization, conditioning, environmental monitoring, and suitable practice adjustments for the athlete, heat illness can and does occur. Monitoring vital signs in anyone at risk will help identify early signs of heat exhaustion (e.g., weak, rapid pulse; elevated body temperature; shallow, fast breathing; changes in blood pressure).

Observe for or ask about heat rash, a red cluster of pimples or small blisters on the neck and upper chest, in the groin, under the breasts, or in the elbow creases. The therapist must be prepared to respond quickly to alleviate symptoms and minimize morbidity and mortality.[30]

Exercise-associated muscle (heat) cramps represent a condition that manifests during or after intense exercise sessions as an acute, painful, involuntary muscle contraction. Muscle cramps and distal extremity edema, dehydration, and electrolyte imbalance are the most commonly observed phenomena associated with heat stress in a therapy practice. The implications surrounding these adverse effects are discussed fully in Chapter 5.

For athletes with spinal cord injuries, regulating heart rate, circulating blood volume, production of sweat, and transferring heat to the surface varies with the level and severity of the spinal cord lesion. The therapist must monitor these athletes closely for heat-related problems and be prepared to provide more fluids; lighter clothing; or cooling of the trunk, legs, and head.[30]

Individuals who experience heat stroke may have compromised heat tolerance for up to a year or more. For an athlete, this can affect training and competition. Gradual return to sports is advised, with close monitoring during exercise. The National Athletic Trainers' Association (NATA) guidelines for heat acclimatization for athletes include recommendations for athletes affected by heat stress returning to their sport available at www.nata.org/health-issues/heat-acclimatization. Older athletes have a decreased ability to maintain an adequate plasma volume during exercise, which may put them at risk for dehydration. Regular fluid intake is essential to avoid hyperthermia. The older athlete may need cardiovascular stress testing before participating in sports or strenuous activities in hot environments.[30]

The NATA published a position statement on exertional heat illnesses with recommendations for the prevention, recognition, and treatment of exertional heat illnesses.[30] The NATA also formed the Inter-Association Task Force on Exertional Heat Illnesses with representation from 18 leading medical, nutritional, and sports medicine–related organizations. This group has provided a consensus statement on exertional heat illnesses that contains additional information to increase safety and performance in individuals participating in physical activity in warm and hot weather.[175]

### High Altitude

Many issues related to altitude change (e.g., effects on fetal size and development, ultraviolet intensity with increases in altitude, sympathetic nervous system changes during acclimatization, air pollution at higher elevations, physiologic changes and pathologic conditions occurring in military and aerospace personnel) are being researched and reported in the literature. These are beyond the scope of this text. Implications here are confined to the more common issues in a therapy practice related to exercise capacity. Chronic exposure to high altitude is known to result in changes in the mechanisms regulating oxygen delivery to the contracting muscles, but the underlying cause of changes in exercise capacity associated with high altitude is not completely understood.[103]

The primary effect of altitude on exercise capacity is through effects on the cardiovascular system, with decreased maximum oxygen consumption, increased ventilation, increased cardiac output, increased red cell mass, increased blood oxygen-carrying capacity. and many other changes at the cellular levels. Increased blood pressure, increased resting and exercise heart rate, and increased minute ventilation also occur. Owing to hypoxia in the alveoli and hypoxemia in the arteries, higher altitudes cause increased pulmonary vascular resistance and pulmonary artery pressure. Studies of oxygen saturation during submaximal exercise in natives of high-altitude areas compared with individuals born at sea level and acclimated to high altitudes suggest that oxygen saturation during exercise may be influenced by adaptation during growth and development and larger lung volume and pulmonary diffusion capacity for oxygen in the native high-altitude population.[37]

With continued exposure to increased altitude, exercise capacity does seem to improve, but it never reaches that attained by the native population at sea level.[226] People with congestive heart failure, ischemic heart disease, systemic arterial hypertension, and cerebrovascular conditions are more likely to be symptomatic at high altitudes. Malignant cardiac arrhythmias have not been found to increase and implanted devices have not been shown to be affected by high-altitude exposure. Supplemental oxygen should be used with individuals with functional pulmonary hypertension (who are on a vasodilator) at high altitudes, owing to effects of hypoxia.

People with congenital heart defects including right-to-left shunts and cyanotic heart conditions may develop more severe hypoxemia, but research has shown that the increase in cardiac output and increased hematocrit at higher altitudes allow for the needed oxygen delivery throughout the body.[117,170,195] With carbohydrate loading at high altitudes, it has been found that athletes have a reduced rate of perceived exertion and improved physical performance. This was found to be especially true during prolonged and high-intensity exercise tasks.[192]

Mild sensory neuropathy may also occur at high altitudes, both as part of the burning feet–burning hands syndrome associated with chronic mountain sickness and as a separate entity among control groups studied. This condition resolves with a low-altitude sojourn (even for high-altitude natives), suggesting that a mechanism of altered axonal transport may be involved. Additionally, reduced thickness of microvessels observed implies that adaptive structural changes to hypobaric hypoxia may occur in peripheral nerves and are similar to changes reported in other tissues of high-altitude natives.[257]

#### Neurotoxicity

Neurologic recovery is facilitated by the plasticity of the nervous system. Peripheral sensory and motor nerve fibers have a remarkable capacity to regenerate after removal of the neurotoxin. Although the neurons in the CNS lack the ability to multiply, the surviving neurons may eventually take over the function of degenerated neurons and partially restore neurologic function. Physical and occupational therapy is beneficial during the recovery time to facilitate this process. When given sufficient time (18 to 24 months), partial clinical improvement is demonstrable in the majority of cases.

*Coasting* is the phenomenon of continuing clinical progression of neurologic deficits after removal of the offending toxin. Weakness or sensory deficits of these neuropathies often worsen for 4 to 5 months after cessation of exposure, reflecting the delayed neuronal death or degeneration induced by the toxin.

Litigation and other potential sources of secondary gains often complicate environmental or occupational exposures that result in neurologic disorders. Psychologic factors may have profound effects on the client's perception of neurologic symptoms, even in people with genuine organic disease. Emotional issues must be recognized and addressed throughout the rehabilitation process.

## OCCUPATIONAL INJURIES AND DISEASES

### Overview

Each year, millions of the estimated 140 million U.S. workers are injured on the job or become ill from exposure to hazards at work. These work-related injuries and illnesses result in substantial human and economic costs for workers, employers, and society. In 2017, 47.2 million injuries occurred, with estimates of direct and indirect costs of work-related injuries and illnesses of approximately $1034.6 billion. Although this cost is high, OSHA rates of injury were 2.8 per 100 full-time workers in 2017, which marks the 5th consecutive year of a decreased incidence rate.[180]

Computers and other timesaving devices have resulted in less physically demanding jobs, but new physical challenges and risk of impairments occur from incorrect ergonomics and prolonged (static) postures and positions, as well as repetitive motions. Injuries can occur in sedentary workers who go out on the weekend (or on an occasional basis during free time) and participate in sports or other strenuous physical activities (these individuals are termed "weekend warriors"). Overuse injuries and muscle strains are common, especially in middle-aged and older adults. Activities such as gardening, hiking, or making household repairs can be more strenuous than they seem in these age groups.[126]

## Risk Factors for Occupational Injury

Risk factors for musculoskeletal occupational injury have been identified by OSHA. If workers are exposed to two or more of these factors (Box 4.2) during their shift, they are at increased risk and require preventive intervention. In April 2000, Congress adopted the Senior Citizens' Freedom to Work Act that allows retired seniors to continue working without losing their Social Security benefits. Older workers have increased rates of injury and disease, requiring more time away from work and resulting in increased costs.

As the workforce ages, changes will need to be made to prevent injury, improve well-being, and increase worker abilities. Reducing sitting time and increasing physical activity during the working years, as well as making ergonomic adjustments, will be important as individuals work past the retirement age of 65.[152]

Other risk factors in the general population may include psychosocial stress, gender, and personality. For example, psychosocial stress increases the physical demands of lifting for people with certain personality traits, making those people more susceptible to spine-loading increases and suspected low back disorder risk.[156]

People who work in nursing homes, including nurses, aides, and therapists, will come across frequent heavy lifting and repositioning of residents that may exceed their capacity. In 2016 the rate of injury within nursing and residential care facilities was 13.7 per 100 full-time workers, the highest rate of all industries. Hospitals

Box 4.2

**RISK FACTORS FOR OCCUPATIONAL INJURY**

***Worker Characteristics***

- Age
- Psychosocial stress
- Gender
- Personality
- Physical fitness, including aerobic capacity, endurance, strength, flexibility, range of motion
- Health status, including lifestyle and presence of pregnancy or diseases, such as chronic fatigue, fibromyalgia, Raynaud phenomenon, diabetes, arthritis, coronary artery disease
- Individual anatomy and physiology (e.g., body capacity versus job requirements, tissue resilience, functional reach)
- Work experience and training

***Occupational Risk Groups***

- Manufacturing (e.g., assembly line work, meat packing, automobile plants)
- Health care workers, especially in hospitals and nursing and personal care facilities
- Lumber and building material retailing
- Trucking (over the road) and ground courier (e.g., United Parcel Service, Federal Express)
- Sawmills, planing mills, millwork
- Construction
- Computer operators (keyboarding)
- Crude petroleum and natural gas extraction
- Retail store clerks and cashiers, especially grocery stores
- Musicians
- Agriculture production
- Beauty salons

***Work Site Factors***

- Lighting, temperature, noise
- Poor workstation ergonomics
- Poor ergonomic practices; inadequate injury prevention training
- Vibration
- Overtime, irregular shifts, length of workday; recovery time between shifts
- Infrequent or no breaks during work shift
- Continuing to work when injured or hurt (voluntarily or involuntarily)

***Task-Specific Factors***

- Performance of the same motions or motion pattern every few seconds for more than 2 hours at a time (repetition)
- Fixed or awkward work postures for more than a total of 2 hours (e.g., overhead work, twisted or bent back, bent wrist, kneeling, stooping, or squatting)
- Use of vibrating or impact tools or equipment for more than a total of 2 hours
- Unassisted manual lifting, lowering, or carrying of anything weighing more than 25 lb more than once during the work shift
- Piece rate or machine-paced work for more than 4 hours at a time
- Using hands/arms instead of available tool(s)
- Improper positioning or use of tools
- Static or awkward postures
- Contact stress (placing the body against a hard or sharp edge)
- Computer keyboard usage more than 15 hours/week

***For the Health Care Worker***

- Performing manual orthopedic techniques
- Assisting clients during transfers and gait training activities
- Working with confused or agitated clients
- Unanticipated sudden movements or falls by client
- Treating a large number of clients in 1 day
- Rehabilitation, acute care, long-term care facilities
- Working with patients with TBI, SCI, or stroke (high physical demands)

From Milhem M, Kalichman L, Ezra D, Alperovitch-Najenson D. Work-related musculoskeletal disorders among physical therapists: A comprehensive narrative review. *International Journal of Occupational Medicine and Environmental Health* 29(5):735-747, 2016.
*SCI*, Spinal cord injury; *TBI*, traumatic brain injury.

injuries totaled 8.2 per 100 full-time workers that same year.[271] Not only do proper body mechanics need to be learned by those working with the patients, but these workers also need to have proper equipment to protect them. This can include mechanical lifts, stand lifts, transfer boards, slide boards, various types of beds and chairs, and gait belts, as well as making sure that adaptive equipment is safe, not broken, and appropriate for each individual.[69] This can also apply to therapists treating clients in the acute rehabilitation setting, the acute care setting, the skilled nursing setting, and the home health care setting.[54]

Thomas R. Waters spent most of his career at NIOSH developing a lifting equation to address musculoskeletal injuries in the workplace. The original NIOSH lifting equation was published in 1981 with a revision published in 1993. There has been ongoing research regarding the use and accuracy of this tool, which is utilized worldwide. A review of the literature has suggested that there is a relationship between the lifting index/composite lifting index (which is an estimate of the physical stress associated with a particular manual lifting task) and low back pain outcomes, but further research is needed.[148,295,296]

It is typical in the United States for mothers and pregnant women to work outside the home. In 2017, 75.7% of mothers with children ages 6 to 17 and 65.1% of mothers with children younger than age 6 were employed. More than 50% of pregnant women work full time, with 82% of them working to within 1 month of giving birth and over 70% of them returning within 6 months after giving birth. The United States is the only developed country that does not have a national paid maternity (or parental) leave, which leads to issues with job protection, health insurance, and wages. Physicians and therapists are vital in prenatal and postpartum care of women to help them safely work.[219]

Recommendations for pregnant workers in physically demanding jobs vary, likely owing to limited training and limited research on guidelines. Research has found a relationship between heavy lifting and increased risk of preterm birth; as the cumulative daily load increases, so does preterm birth risk.[219] Evidence has also shown a small increased risk for lower birth weight, as well as miscarriage, in relationship to heavy physical work including lifting.[151]

Aside from risks of lifting, pregnancies can cause additional musculoskeletal injuries, especially secondary to the increased joint laxity that occurs during pregnancy. Low back pain occurs in up to two-thirds of women during pregnancy, and pelvic pain occurs in about 20% of women during pregnancy.[151] Combine these typical musculoskeletal injuries with a physically demanding job, and the pregnant woman is at increased risk for additional health effects. Although guidelines for lifting were published by the American Medical Association and by NIOSH in the 1980s and 1990s, neither of these sets of guidelines fully encompassed the physiologic and physical changes associated with pregnancy. Provisional guidelines were developed for uncomplicated pregnancies in 2013 following an extensive review of the literature. Owing to the increasing number of women working during and after pregnancy, additional research is warranted, especially for high-repetition lifting during pregnancy and for lifting postpartum (Fig. 4.5).[151]

Research continues to be done on lifting techniques. Studies have looked at the recommended weight limits for lifting and holding limbs in the orthopedic setting,[297] as well as safe patient handling in the orthopedic setting.[231] Research is also looking at various lifting devices and the amount of force required for operating them,[207] as well as the effectiveness of curriculum in schools that target safe handling and movement of people.[181] This needs to be a continued area of focus to provide quality patient and client care in each setting, with decreased risk for injury.[181,207,231,297]

## Ergonomics

Derived from the Greek terms *ergon*, meaning work, and *nomos*, meaning law, *ergonomics* is the study of work and of the relationship between humans and their working and physical environment. Over the last 2 decades, ergonomics has become a branch of industrial engineering that seeks to maximize productivity by minimizing worker discomfort and fatigue. Ergonomics is the science of fitting the task or the job to the worker.

Ergonomics is an interdisciplinary field of study that integrates engineering, medicine, and physical and behavioral management sciences and addresses issues arising from the interaction of humans in an increasingly technologic society. As a field of study, ergonomics deals with job design, work performance, health and safety, stress, posture, body mechanics, biomechanics, anthropometry (measurement of body size, weight, and proportions in relation to the task requirements), manual material handling, equipment design, quality control, environment, workers' education and training, and employment testing.

The goal is to provide an environment that allows the individual to adequately absorb and dissipate forces placed on the body. Fitting the work to the worker makes it possible to enhance productivity while controlling errors and reducing musculoskeletal strain and fatigue. Ergonomics reduces risk factors known to contribute to occupational ergonomic-related injuries.

Humans have limitations arising from factors such as gender differences; differences in size, weight, and body proportions; aging; physical fitness and lifestyle choices; diet; stress; and pain and injury. Our abilities (and limitations), combined with the necessary acquired skills, determine how well we perform our daily tasks. Ergonomics helps people recognize their abilities and limitations for safe and effective performance within the environment. Work environments are often designed without adequate consideration for the people who will use them. Inadequate workplace design can contribute to stress, injury, pain, job-related impairments, disabilities, and subsequent lost productivity. If products are designed without considering the human factor, health and safety hazards can occur.

A substantial body of validated scientific research and other evidence (epidemiologic, biomechanical, and pathophysiologic studies) supports the positive outcomes of ergonomic programs.[174] The evidence strongly supports two basic conclusions: (1) a consistent

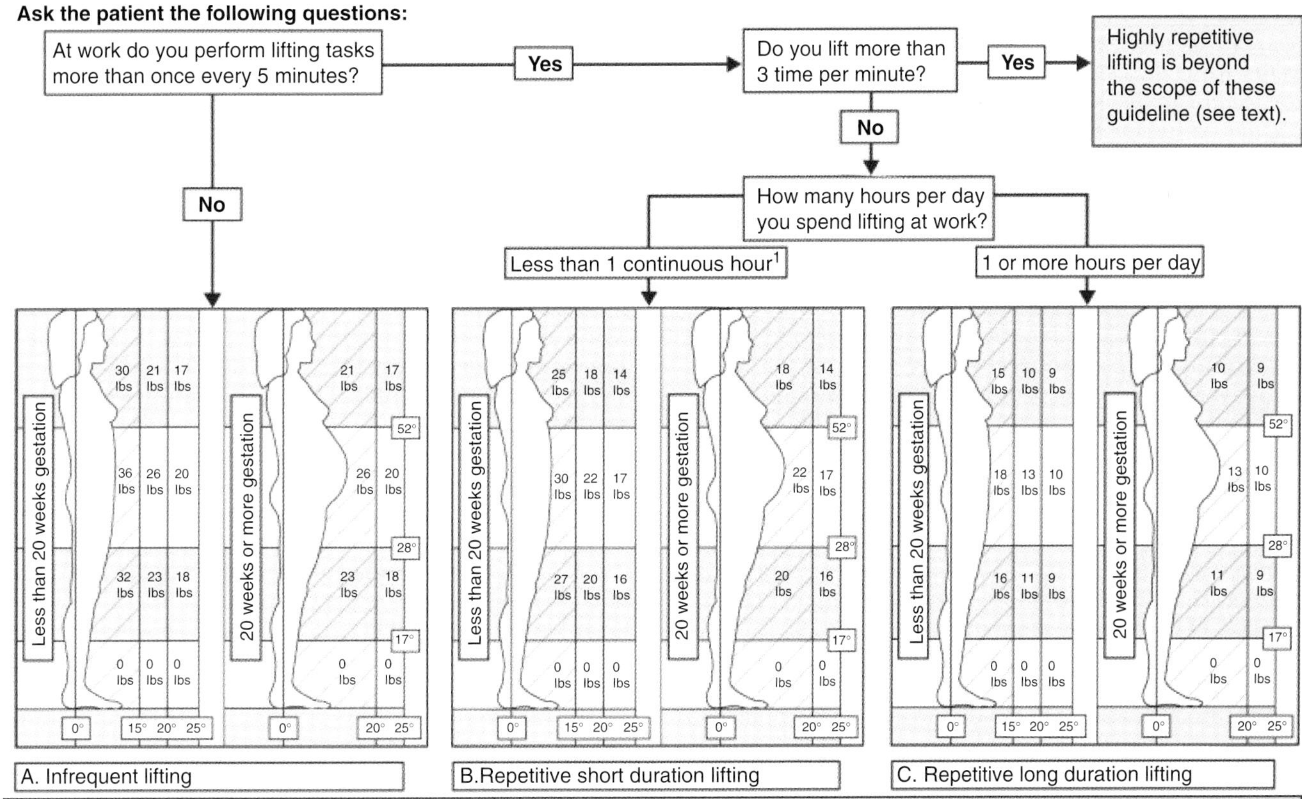


**Instruction for using graphic A,B or C:**

1) Select the left figure if gestation < 20 weeks;select the right figure if gestation ≥ 20 weeks.
2) Ask the patient to demonstrate the lifting motions to determine the lifting height from the floor and the distance in front of the body.
3) Select the numerical weight limit values along the entire path the object would travel. If the object crosses more than one weight limit category, select the lowest weight limit.
4) The number selected in step 3 above is the Recommended Weight Limit (RWL) for the gestation period.

*[1]Repetitive short duration lifting (Graphic B) can encompass multiple hours of lifting per day;however,each continuous lifting period should be less than one hour and followed by a minimum of one hour of non-lifting activity before the next continuous lifting period is initiated.*

**Figure 4.5**

**Clinical guidelines for occupational lifting in pregnancy.** (From MacDonald LA, et al: Clinical guidelines for occupational lifting in pregnancy: Evidence summary and provisional recommendations. *Am J Obstet Gynecol* 209:80–88, 2013.)

relationship exists between musculoskeletal disorders (MSDs) and certain workplace factors, especially at higher exposure levels, and (2) specific ergonomic interventions (e.g., proper equipment, postural education, and use of correct body mechanics) can reduce these injuries and illnesses.

Physical therapists and other specialists with a background in anatomy, physiology, kinesiology, pathology, and ergonomics can become certified in ergonomics through various institutions. They use knowledge of the relationship between pathology and work to match the demands of the job to the capacity of the worker. They analyze the person performing the work and the setting in which they work to make positive ergonomic changes. Concentrating on improved safety focuses on physiologic improvement, which in turn increases productivity.

The following list includes resources to learn more about ergonomic programs and interventions, continuing education with a focus on ergonomics, professional certifications in ergonomics, and networking opportunities for individuals interested in ergonomics.

1. American Physical Therapy Association (APTA) Orthopaedic Section Occupational Health Special Interest Group https://www.orthopt.org/content/special-interest-groups/occupational-health
2. Board of Certification in Professional Ergonomics (http://www.bcpe.org)
3. Ergoweb (http://www.ergoweb.com)
4. International Ergonomics Association (http://www.iea.cc)
5. IMPACC
6. Oxford Research Institute (http://www.oxfordresearch.org)
7. CDC NIOSH (www.cdc.gov/niosh/topics/ergonomics)

## Musculoskeletal Disorders

The U.S. Bureau of Labor Statistics defines MSDs as follows:

*[I]nclude cases where the nature of the injury or illness is pinched nerve; herniated disc; meniscus tear; sprains, strains, tears; hernia (traumatic and nontraumatic); pain, swelling,*

*and numbness; carpal or tarsal tunnel syndrome; Raynaud's syndrome or phenomenon; musculoskeletal system and connective tissue diseases and disorders, when the event or exposure leading to the injury or illness is overexertion and bodily reaction, unspecified; overexertion involving outside sources; repetitive motion involving microtasks; other and multiple exertions or bodily reactions; and rubbed, abraded, or jarred by vibration."*[272]

In 2015, MSDs accounted for 31% of all work-related injuries and illnesses.[287] MSDs do not include injuries resulting from slips, trips, falls, or accidents. The disorder must be directly related to the employee's job and specifically connected to activities that form the core or a significant part of the job (e.g., a poultry processor might report tendinitis, but a back injury while occasionally changing the water bottle on a water cooler would not be covered).

The most frequent workers with work-related MSDs include laborers; freight, stock, and material movers; nursing assistants; and heavy and tractor trailer truck drivers. Workers with sprains, strains, or tears required a median of 12 days to return to work, compared with 8 days for all types of work injuries and illnesses.[287]

### Etiology and Risk Factors

Risk factors for MSDs are divided into four major categories: genetic, morphologic, biomechanical, and psychosocial. Among the various biomechanical risk factors, exposure to repetitive, static, and vibratory activities is known to result in MSDs.[133] Differences in physical, occupational, and physiologic factors may contribute to MSDs.

Men are more likely to have a work-related MSD (35.9 per 10,000 full-time workers, compared with women at 27.4 per 10,000 full-time workers), and workers in the 45- to 54-year-old age group have the highest number of days away from work.[286] In 2015 workers with carpal tunnel syndrome (CTS) had the second most missed days of work (after workers with fractures), with a median of 28 days until return to work.[286] In addition to workers who spend hours at the computer, CTS has been reported in meat packers, assembly line workers, retail clerks scanning labels, jackhammer operators, athletes, physical and occupational therapists, and homemakers. In both genders, CTS can be associated with other medical conditions, such as thyroid problems, liver disease, multiple myeloma, and diabetes, as well as with other MSDs that may or may not be work-related. For all work-related CTS, poor worksite design, poor posture and body mechanics, and industrial equipment and computers that take out the automatic pauses of work must be evaluated as possible contributors. An in-depth discussion of CTS is presented in Chapter 39.

### Pathogenesis

The exact pathomechanisms of MSDs remain obscure because of the difficulty of analyzing tissues of individuals in the early stages of work-related MSDs. A systematic literature review completed in 2015 found an interdependence between force and repetition related to MSD risk. Low-force repetitive tasks have shown a modest risk for MSDs, whereas high-force repetitive tasks have shown a rapid increase in risk.[100] Tissue injury caused by repeated motion may involve an inflammatory response, but why one worker develops symptoms while others doing the same task do not remains unknown and a topic of discussion and study. The relationship between cellular responses to these activities, number of strains, and inflammatory response is under investigation. Research regarding psychosocial factors found that low job satisfaction, low social support, and monotonous work increased risk for new-onset widespread pain.[108] Additionally, poor working conditions (physical and psychosocial factors) have been found to be strongly associated with high levels of musculoskeletal pain.[183] The role of epigenetics is also being considered[17,18,245] and may play an important role in preventing and treating work-related MSDs.[12,15,255]

A systematic review of the literature looking at work-related MSDs found the following risk factors with reasonable evidence of a causal relationship for the development of MSDs: heavy physical work, smoking, high body mass index, high psychosocial work demands, and presence of comorbidities. The most common biomechanical risk factors with reasonable evidence of a causal relationship for the development of work-related MSDs include excessive repetition, awkward postures, and heavy lifting.[74]

The development of MSDs is likely multifactorial, with variations in individual tissue tolerances. Each individual may have his or her own threshold below which tissue integrity is preserved and above which injury results. It is possible that the combined and/or accumulative effects of risk factors for MSDs can exceed tissue tolerance capacity and cause injury. When continued task performance is superimposed on injured and inflamed tissues, a cycle of injury, inflammation, and motor dysfunction occurs.[19,20]

MSDs in the lumbar spine may have a different mechanism. Static lumbar loading applied to ligaments results in creep (e.g., stretch of viscoelastic tissue over time that is not fully restored immediately after load removal). In theory, ligaments that remain stretched beyond their resting length may result in increased laxity of intervertebral joints and risk of instability and injury. In the spine, ligaments have a secondary role in maintaining intervertebral stability.[243]

Static lumbar flexion under constant load results in long-lasting viscoelastic creep that does not fully recover after 7 hours of rest. The creep developed gives rise to a neuromuscular disorder with reduced reflexive muscle activity, muscle spasms during flexion, and hyperexcitability of muscle activity during rest that may last 24 hours or more. The viscoelastic creep and associated neuromuscular disorder can occur even with low loads, which may help explain how cumulative low back problems develop.[243]

### Clinical Manifestations

Workers with MSDs, especially upper extremity MSDs, may experience decreased grip strength and range of motion, impaired muscle function, and inability to complete activities of daily living. Symptoms are persistent (although intermittent; they return and progress over time) and most commonly include pain (e.g., headache, neck, back, shoulder, wrist, hip, knee); burning sensation, numbness, and/or tingling (hands or feet); Raynaud

Box 4.3

**COMMON WORK-RELATED MUSCULOSKELETAL DISORDERS**

- Carpal tunnel syndrome
- Carpet layer's knee
- Cubital tunnel syndrome
- de Quervain disease
- Epicondylitis (medial or lateral tennis elbow)
- Focal hand dystonia
- Hand-arm vibration syndrome
- Herniated spinal disc
- Pronator syndrome
- Radial tunnel syndrome
- Raynaud phenomenon
- Rotator cuff syndrome
- Sciatica
- Tendinitis (shoulder, elbow, wrist)
- Tenosynovitis (finger flexors or extensors; trigger finger)
- Tension neck syndrome, thoracic outlet syndrome, cervical radiculopathy
- Thoracic outlet syndrome
- Ulnar nerve syndrome

phenomenon; and myalgias and arthralgias with spasm, stiffness, swelling, or inflammation. Common MSDs and upper extremity MSDs are listed in Box 4.3.

A predictable sequence of events leads to MSDs of a repetitive nature or disorders caused by static postures (e.g., some tasks such as prolonged writing or typing at a keyboard require cocontraction of the agonists and antagonists). Fatigue and the inability to recover from fatigue brought on by additional hours and pressured deadlines combined with emotional stress and improper posture, improper use of tools, or an ergonomically inadequate workstation result in muscle soreness. Over time and without intervention or a change in the contributing factors, the body strains to keep up and pain develops, followed by injury or trauma.

**SPECIAL IMPLICATIONS FOR THE THERAPIST 4.2**

### *Occupational Injuries and Diseases*

OSHA has created a comprehensive plan called Ergonomics for the Prevention of Musculoskeletal Disorders: Guidelines for Nursing Homes,[287] designed to reduce ergonomic injuries through the development of guidelines, enforcement measures, workplace outreach, and research. OSHA researched nursing and personal care facilities with high injury and illness rates, focusing on specific hazards that account for the majority of staff injuries and illnesses. Those hazards include ergonomics (primarily back injuries from patient handling); bloodborne pathogens/tuberculosis; and slips, trips, and falls. The OSHA recommendations include minimizing and eliminating manual lifting of residents and having employers implement an effective ergonomics process that includes management support, involvement of employees, identification of problems, and implementation of solutions, as well as addressing reports of injuries, providing training, and evaluating ergonomic efforts.[287]

Therapists can have an important role in the development of health and safety programs that will accurately assess hazards in the workplace and reduce the risk of musculoskeletal injuries, amputations, and illnesses. For all clients with MSDs, questions related to occupation and exposure to toxins (such as chemicals or gases) should be included during physical therapy assessments because well-defined physical and health problems occur in people engaging in specific occupations.[184] Agricultural workers who come to a physical therapist for an MSD are commonly exposed to pesticide, and office workers who report asthma and sick building syndrome may seek the skills of a physical therapist for an MSD.

#### Ergonomics

The therapist can have a significant role in the prevention (e.g., worksite analysis and workstation redesign) and rehabilitation of occupational injuries. The role of ergonomics in injury management includes a prompt and safe return to work, cost savings, and prevention of injuries or reduction of injury progression or recurrence. There is evidence that combined workstation stretching exercises and ergonomic modifications can reduce musculoskeletal discomfort for workers sitting in front of a computer or other video display terminal.[89,155,164,235]

When conducting a job analysis, the therapist evaluates job duties and environmental factors that put physical stress on the worker; stressors most typically include force (any weight that is lifted, pushed, or carried), repetition, and posture. The therapist will assess the amount of force needed to produce the necessary work, the number of repetitions, and the postural tolerances required by the job.

These variables are evaluated for both newly developing programs or job tasks and in industrial rehabilitation programs for cases of work conditioning and work hardening. The APTA defines work conditioning as "an intensive, work-related, goal-oriented program designed specifically to restore systemic neuromusculoskeletal functions, motor function, range of motion, and cardiovascular/pulmonary functions. It is meant to restore physical capacity and function to enable the worker to return to work."[13a] The APTA defines work hardening as "a highly structured, goal-oriented, individualized intervention program designed to return a worker to work. They are multidisciplinary, use real/simulated work activities designed to restore physical, behavioral, and vocational functions. Work hardening addresses the issues of productivity, safety, physical tolerance and worker behaviors."[13a]

The main goal of these programs is to return injured or disabled workers to work or to improve the work status of the worker. The focus is on simulating the worker's job tasks in a safe and supervised location. Throughout the program, there is focus on psychological, physical, and emotional tolerance, as well as improving endurance.[160,225] The Orthopedic Section within the APTA has advanced work rehabilitation guidelines for occupational health physical therapy, including work conditioning and work hardening programs.[13]

### Silver Collar Workers

The growing silver collar workforce (adults of the baby boomer generation working past the age of 65) may represent a unique risk factor because aging is associated with a progressive decrement in various components of physical work capacity, including aerobic power and capacity, muscular strength and endurance, flexibility and coordination, and tolerance of thermal stress.[237] Aging may thus contribute to additional workplace injuries and accidents.

The Bureau of Labor Statistics has shown that the rate of older workers continues to climb. In 2010, 19% of workers were 55 and older, in 2015 this number increased to 22.6%, and it is estimated to reach 24.8% by 2024.[60] Therapists need to modify traditional intervention strategies for prevention and treatment of injuries in the silver collar workforce.[213]

The NIOSH Office for Total Worker Health includes policies, programs, and practices to protect workers from injuries and health hazards on the worksite and promote prevention efforts to improve worker well-being. The Office for Total Worker Health is the host of the National Center for Productive Aging and Work. This center focuses on four attributes of productive aging: (1) a life span perspective, (2) a comprehensive and integrated framework, (3) outcomes that recognize the priorities of both workers and organizations, and (4) a supportive work culture for multigenerational issues. Assessing work environments to prevent injuries and reduce risks, promoting health and maintaining health over time, career-specific training, and determining physical demands and ways to reduce them are being looked at by NIOSH to develop a good model for the aging workforce.[60]

Therapists can assist industries and job sites to adapt job duties to accommodate for age-related conditions such as reduced muscle strength and motion. Providing ergonomically correct worksites and work areas, implementing diagnostic and training programs for prevention of specific injuries and disease, and instituting wellness programs to include home- or gym-based exercise programs and organized stretch/walk breaks will help keep all employees, particularly elderly employees, in good health and injury-free.[23]

### Physical Therapists With Work-Related Symptoms

Physical therapists are predisposed to work-related MSDs resulting from manual therapies, lifting and transfers, and repetitive motions performed throughout treatment and interventions with patients and clients. Researchers have demonstrated that knowledge of ergonomics, injury, and intervention strategies is not associated with a reduced risk of injury among therapists.[71,113] For example, maintaining good body mechanics is not always protective when a client is starting to fall and pulls the therapist down. Lifting with sudden maximal effort, bending and twisting, repetitious movement, awkward postures maintained for a prolonged period of time, and using high levels of force are correlated with work-related injuries among therapists.[32,113]

Activities in specific practice areas have been associated with increased therapist injuries. These areas include performing functional activities with patients in acute care, preventing patient falls in skilled nursing facilities, and working on motor vehicle activities with individuals in home care.[76] Therapists working in rehabilitation units with patients who have brain injuries, stroke, and spinal cord injuries with high physical demands are at increased risk of work-related injuries. Clients who are less mobile in long-term care facilities, skilled nursing facilities, or acute care often put the greatest demands on therapists.[290]

Other risk factors include heavy client loads, working with combative clients, increased number of hours performing manual therapy, and injuries that occur outside the workplace that are not treated or healed before returning to work. Manual therapy and transfers/lifts have been associated with 54% of all physical and occupational therapy injuries.[76] The cultural context in which therapists work might contribute to work-related MSDs. For example, the need to demonstrate hard work and care for patients and clients along with the need to appear knowledgeable and skilled by remaining injury-free may increase risk for therapists. The therapist may put the needs of the patient or client first, subsequently sustaining an injury. The therapist also may fail to report the injury to avoid being perceived as incompetent. There is also a tendency for therapists to try to manage their own condition, which can lead to delays in recovery.[72]

Studies have suggested that inexperienced therapists are at greatest risk compared with seasoned therapists (more than 50% have their first injury as a student or in their first 5 years of practice) or a mean age of 27.6 years.[37] Other studies have found that older and younger therapists have similar work-related MSDs but that older therapists had more severe pain and were more likely to change jobs because of their injury.[129] It has been reported that 1 in 6 physical therapists change their work setting or leave the profession because of a work-related MSD; 57% to 88% of physical therapists will have a work-related MSD.[46]

Studies have found that the most frequently injured body part of a physical therapist is the low back, followed by the upper back, hand, and wrist. Settings with the highest number of work-related MSDs are the school system and private practice.[46] One study has also found that male therapists were more likely (63%) to have a work-related MSD than female therapists (37%).[234]

Therapists are encouraged to maintain good body mechanics, change position often, ask for help, and report injuries when they occur. Using gait belts for patient transfers, using appropriate adaptive equipment such as a walker for ambulation, having a wheelchair behind a client who is unsteady, using parallel bars for gait training, and using mechanical aids such as Hoyer lifts or stand lifts is advised when appropriate for patient and therapist safety and injury prevention. The therapist should seek care and modify work or take time off when necessary. It is not a good idea to try to work through the injury.[290]

## Occupational Burns

Of the more than 1 million firefighters employed in the United States, almost 350,000 are career firefighters, with the rest being volunteer firefighters. Firefighter deaths while on duty are due to various causes, including training, on-scene fire, after an incident, and others.[280] Number of deaths have declined since the 1970s and 1980s with the mandatory use of gloves, self-contained breathing apparatus, and full personal protective clothing. Firefighting is a physically demanding job, with overexertion and stress accounting for 52 deaths from heart attacks and strokes in 2017.[268,288,280]

Aside from the acute injurious effects of fire, clinicians must be alert to the pathophysiologic changes associated with exposure to heat and smoke and to the chronic physical and psychologic sequelae (Table 4.4). In addition to the management of burns and trauma, it is necessary to evaluate clients for all acute systemic effects of exposure to smoke, heat, or toxic substances; recognize toxic effects that may be obscured by more serious traumatic effects; be alert for delayed consequences; and recognize acute and chronic exposure and health effects as a result of toxic chemicals in smoke, especially among firefighters.

**Table 4.4** Types of Fire-and-Rescue–Related Acute and Chronic Injury

| Acute | Chronic |
|---|---|
| Lacerations, contusions | Chronic cardiovascular disease |
| Falls (including on-site and from moving apparatus) | Chronic respiratory disease |
| Burns (superficial, deep, internal) | Noise-induced hearing loss |
| Dermal reactions to toxicants | Posttraumatic stress disorder |
| Eye irritation, injuries, and burns | Physical disability |
| Smoke inhalation | Hepatitis C |
| Sore throat, hoarseness, cough | |
| Exacerbated asthma | |
| Dyspnea, tachypnea, wheezing | |
| Headaches | |
| Cyanosis | |
| Cardiovascular strain | |
| Musculoskeletal trauma | |
| Heat stress and fatigue | |
| Neuropsychiatric effects | |
| Renal damage | |
| Death (motor vehicle accidents, falls, asphyxiation, burns) | |

Modified from National Institute for Occupational Safety and Health (NIOSH) and Centers for Disease Control and Prevention: Fire fighter fatality investigation and prevention. Last reviewed April 3, 2018. Available at: http://www.cdc.gov/niosh/fire/. Accessed January 22, 2019.

## Occupational Pulmonary Diseases

Materials inhaled in the workplace can lead to all the major chronic lung diseases except those resulting from vascular disease. Exposure in office buildings and hospitals is now included as a known workplace-related cause of disease. As new industries are developed, new problems are reported. For example, obstructive lung disease has been reported in workers in the microwave popcorn and flavor manufacturing industry who have not been adequately protected from chemical exposures.[159]

Identifying the source of illness is important because it can lead to cure and prevention for others.[25] Disorders caused by chemical agents are classified as (1) pneumoconiosis, (2) hypersensitivity pneumonitis, (3) obstructive airway disorders, (4) toxic lung injury, (5) lung cancer, and (6) pleural diseases. These conditions are discussed more fully in Chapter 15.

Asbestos and other silicates, such as kaolin, mica, and vermiculite, can cause *pneumoconiosis*. Asbestos-induced diseases cause lung inflammation and fibrosis as a result of activation of alveolar macrophages. Coal workers' pneumoconiosis is another parenchymal lung disease caused by inhalation of coal dust.

*Hypersensitivity pneumonitis* has many other names, such as extrinsic allergic alveolitis, farmer's lung, mushroom picker's disease, humidifier or air conditioner lung, bird breeder's or bird fancier's lung, and detergent worker's lung, and is characterized by a granulomatous inflammatory reaction in the pulmonary alveolar and interstitial spaces. Silicosis is a parenchymal toxic lung disease caused by inhalation of crystalline silica, a component of rock and sand. Workers at risk include miners, tunnelers, quarry workers, stonecutters, sandblasters, foundry workers, glass blowers, and ceramic workers.

The pathogenesis of these occupational lung diseases varies among different pneumoconioses, but the bottom line is that cilia and mucus-secreting cells are absent in the small bronchioles and alveoli. Thus the body depends on macrophages to remove any of the tiny particles that lodge in these areas. The macrophages then carry the particles to the mucociliary elevator or dump them into the lymphatics. The process is often sabotaged because substances, such as silica dust, can destroy the macrophages. In the process, substances are released that trigger inflammation and pulmonary fibrosis.

Exposure to allergens and irritants has resulted in the recognition of a new disease called *work-related (or occupational) upper airway disease* or *united airway disease.* Although not life threatening, this disease has been reported to cause affected individuals to experience reduced quality of life. Occupational allergens identified are many and varied, including plants (e.g., tobacco leaf dust, grapes, asparagus, or flowers), insects (e.g., bees or locusts), powder paints, and others.[291]

Health problems caused by these irritants range from runny nose to full-blown allergic rhinitis. Up to 40% of individuals in the workplace with allergic rhinitis also have asthma, and 92% of workers with occupational asthma report symptoms of occupational rhinitis. The link between rhinitis and asthma is the presence of inflammation of the nasal and bronchial mucosae. The incidence of having both occupational asthma and rhinitis is highest for farmers and woodworkers.[172,173,291]

Occupational asthma is asthma that is attributable to or is made worse by environmental exposures (e.g., inhaled gases, dusts, fumes, or vapors) in the workplace. The air in health care institutions may contain irritating and sensitizing chemicals and particles that can aggravate asthma (Box 4.4).

Box 4.4

**ASTHMA-TRIGGERING SUBSTANCES IN THE HEALTH CARE SETTING[a]**

- Latex (primarily latex gloves)
- Glutaraldehyde (sensitizing agent used in cold sterilization)
- Ammonia and chlorine (cleaning and disinfecting solutions)
- Antimicrobial pesticides (sterilizers, disinfectants, sanitizers)
- Dust and irritating particles in the air (construction and remodeling projects)
- Mold and fungus (carpeting, ceiling tiles exposed to water)
- Perfumes, scented personal care products worn by clients/patients, coworkers, visitors
- Pharmaceutical drugs (e.g., psyllium, rifampin, penicillin, tetracycline)
- Formaldehyde used in specimen preparation
- Diacetyl (ingredient in artificial butter and other flavoring)

[a]Includes hospitals, medical and dental clinics, nursing and personal-care facilities, and other facilities such as dialysis centers, specialty outpatient facilities, and medical laboratories.

Data from Bain EI: Perils in the air: avoiding occupational asthma triggers in the workplace, *Am J Nurs* 100:88, 2000; and Centers for Disease Control and Prevention (CDC): Acute antimicrobial pesticide-related illnesses among workers in health care facilities—California, Louisiana, Michigan, and Texas, 2002–2007. *MMWR Morb Mortal Wkly Rep.* 59:551–556, 2010.

About 15% of all adults with asthma have occupational asthma. Occupational asthma has become the most prevalent occupational lung disease in developed countries, is more common than is generally recognized, and can be severe and disabling. The reactions can be immediate or delayed, sometimes hours after leaving the workplace. More than 250 substances have been identified to cause asthma or to exacerbate work-related asthma. The key approaches to controlling occupational asthma include preventing the disease by reducing or eliminating allergens and irritants, detecting asthma early in the disease process, and avoiding making the symptoms worse by repetitive exposure or additional exposures to other harmful substances.[98]

OSHA requires employers to provide a safe and healthy work environment free from recognized hazards. In addition, the Americans With Disabilities Act of 1990 requires employers to accommodate workers with asthma. Suspected episodes of occupational asthma should be documented, including symptoms, suspected exposures, visits to health services, and similar symptoms reported by other employees. Many effective and appropriate substitutions and controls are available that can be incorporated to eliminate or prevent airborne and topical exposures.[17]

## Occupational Cancer

In 2017 the IARC listed 47 of the 120 group I carcinogens as occupational, with contact occurring most likely at the workplace.[146] This is an increase since 2004 when only 28 were identified and it is more than likely an underestimation of the carcinogens present in the workplace. Substances used in workplaces and workplace conditions have only been studied to a small degree.[251] It is estimated that over 650,000 deaths are caused by occupational cancers each year globally, with occupational exposures accounting for 5.3% to 8.4% of all cancers. Lung cancer accounts for 54% to 75% of occupational cancer, with asbestos being the prime culprit (55% to 85% of occupational lung cancer cases).[253] Each year, it is estimated that there are 20,000 cancer deaths and 40,000 new cases of cancer in the United States that are attributed to occupation (Table 4.5). Studies continue to provide evidence that cancer in humans has environmental causes. Examples include exposure to arsenic being associated with increased risk of skin, urinary bladder, and respiratory tract cancers; chronic exposure to ultraviolet light being associated with skin cancers; vinyl chloride being associated with liver cancer; dry cleaning solvents being associated with kidney and liver cancer and non-Hodgkin lymphoma; and ionizing radiation (including radon) being associated with increased risk of leukemia, lung cancer, and breast cancer (with susceptibility greater for women with certain breast cancer gene mutations).[90,120,249,250,313] In 2013, outdoor air pollution was classified as a carcinogen by the IARC, based on research showing it causes lung cancer and an increased risk of bladder cancer.[145] Research is ongoing to assess combined epigenetic and environmental contributions to risk.[80,111,224]

Alteration or mutation in the genetic material (DNA) may occur as a result of exposure to carcinogenic chemical, radiation, or oxidation. Human DNA repair systems have evolved at the cellular level to maintain genome integrity. DNA repair research is a rapidly growing field; Tomas Lindahl, Paul Modrich, and Aziz Sancar received the 2015 Nobel Prize in Chemistry for their work on how cells conduct DNA repair and protect genetic information.[24] Both experimental animal models of cancer and the study of human cancers with known causes have revealed the existence of a significant interval between first exposure to the responsible agent and the first manifestation of a tumor. This period is referred to as the *induction period, latency period,* or *induction-latency period.*

For humans, the length of the induction-latency period varies from a minimum of 4 to 6 years for radiation-induced leukemias to 40 or more years for some cases of asbestos-induced mesotheliomas. For most tumors, the interval ranges from 12 to 25 years; such a long period may easily obscure the relationship between a remote exposure and a newly discovered tumor.

Therapeutic cancer vaccines have been shown to have a clinical benefit. Longer survival, not eradication of cancer, has been found to be the main outcome, owing to suboptimal vaccine design and the immunosuppressive environment in which cancer resides. Some human oncogenic viruses include Epstein-Barr virus, human T-cell lymphotropic virus type I, hepatitis B virus, hepatitis C virus, human papillomavirus, Kaposi sarcoma-associated herpes virus, and Merkel cell polyomavirus. These viruses are associated with diseases, including cancers, that have specific therapeutic vaccine targets to treat them. It should be understood that cancer vaccines need to be used in combination treatments to block immunosuppressive activity at the cellular level within the cancerous environment.[165] Continued work on the design of powerful cancer vaccines is needed so that individuals with a high environmental risk of developing cancer may benefit from this type of immune stimulation.[91] Individual

Table 4.5 Cancer Sites Associated With Occupational Exposure

| Cancer Site | Examples of High-Risk Substances | Examples of High-Risk Processes, Industries and Occupations With Increased Risks |
|---|---|---|
| Bladder (urinary) | Aromatic amines [e.g., 4,4′-methylenebis(2-chloroaniline) (MOCA), para-chloroaniline, 2,6-dimethylaniline (2,6-xylidine)]; arsenic and inorganic arsenic compounds; benzidine and benzidine-based dyes; benzo[a] pyrene; coal tars and pitches; diesel engine exhaust; tetrachloroethylene; ortho-toluidine | Barbers; cable makers; calendar operatives; chemical/petroleum workers; coke production; dry cleaners; firefighters; gas-retort house workers; hairdressers; machinists; manufacturing of aluminum, magenta, auramine, *p*-chloro-*o*-toluidine, pigment chromate, textiles, and dyes; miners; painters; pipefitters; plumbers; rubber production; sheet metal workers; synthetic latex production; tire curing |
| Bone | Ionizing radiation | — |
| Brain and central nervous system | Ionizing radiation | — |
| Breast | Ethylene oxide; ionizing radiation; polychorinated biphenyls | Shift work that involves circadian disruption |
| Colon and rectum | Asbestos; ionizing radiation | — |
| Esophagus | Ionizing radiation | Dry cleaning; rubber production industry |
| Eye | — | Welding; solar radiation |
| Kidney | Arsenic and inorganic arsenic compounds; cadmium and cadmium compounds; perfluorooctanoic acid; trichloroethylene | Printing processes |
| Larynx | Acid mists, strong inorganic; asbestos | Insulation material production (pipes, sheeting, textiles, clothes, masks, asbestos cement products); insulators and pipe coverers; isopropanol manufacture (strong-acid process); rubber production industry; shipyard and dockyard workers |
| Leukemia and/or lymphoma | Benzene; 1,3-butadiene; diazinon; formaldehyde; ethylene oxide; lindane; ionizing radiation; malathion; methylene chloride; styrene; trichloroethylene | Boot and shoe manufacturing and repair; firefighters; painting; petroleum refining; rubber industry |
| Liver and bile duct | Arsenic and inorganic arsenic compounds; 1,2-dichloropropane, methylene chloride; ionizing radiation; occupational infections with hepatitis B and C; polychlorinated biphenyls (PCBs); trichloroethylene | Health care workers; smelting of ores containing arsenic; vinyl chloride production; wood preservation |
| Lung | Arsenic and arsenic compounds; asbestos; benzo[a]pyrene; beryllium; 1,3-butadiene; cadmium and cadmium compounds; chromium (hexavalent) compounds; coal tars and pitches; diesel engine exhaust; epichlorohydrin; fibrous silicon carbide; ionizing radiation; mineral oils (untreated and mildly treated); nickel and nickel compounds; radon; silica (crystalline); soots; strong inorganic acid mists containing sulfuric acid; talc containing asbestiform fibers; 2,3,7,8-tetrachlorodibenzo-*p*-dioxin (TCDD); tobacco smoke—involuntary (passive) smoking | Aluminum production; asphalt workers; coal gasification; copper smelting; hematite mining (underground) with radon exposure; iron and steel founding; isopropanol manufacture (strong acid process); painters; printing processes; roofers; rubber production; uranium mining; vineyard workers; welding fumes |
| Mesothelioma | Asbestos; talc containing asbestiform fibers | Blasters; boilermakers; bricklayers; construction workers; drillers; electricians; machinists; mechanics; miners; pipefitters; plumbers; sheet metal workers; shipbuilding workers; welders |
| Nasal cavities and paranasal sinuses | Chromium (hexavalent) compounds; formaldehyde; selected nickel compounds including combinations of nickel oxides and sulfides in the nickel refining industry; wood dust | Boot and shoe manufacturing and repair; carpenters; furniture and cabinet making; isopropanol manufacture (strong acid process); miners; plumbers; pulp and paper mill workers; textile workers; welders |
| Nasopharynx | Formaldehyde; wood dust | Embalmers; formaldehyde production; laboratory workers; medical personnel; plywood production/particle-board production |
| Ovary | Asbestos; ionizing radiation | — |

Continued

**Table 4.5** Cancer Sites Associated With Occupational Exposure—cont'd

| Cancer Site | Examples of High-Risk Substances | Examples of High-Risk Processes, Industries and Occupations With Increased Risks |
|---|---|---|
| Prostate | Arsenic and inorganic arsenic compounds; cadmium and cadmium compounds; ionizing radiation; malathion | Rubber production industry |
| Skin | Arsenic and inorganic arsenic compounds; coal tar distillation; creosotes; mineral oils (untreated and mildly treated); polycyclic aromatic hydrocarbons (PAHs) such as benzo[a]pyrene, benz[a]anthracene, and dibenz[a,h]anthracene; shale oils or shale-derived lubricants; solar radiation; soots | Coal gasification; coke production; outdoor workers; petroleum refining; vineyard workers |
| Stomach | Asbestos; lead compounds, inorganic; ionizing radiation | Asbestos mining; insulation material production (pipes, sheeting, textiles, clothes, masks, asbestos cement products); insulators and pipe coverers; rubber production industry; shipyard and dockyard workers |

Modified from Canadian Centre for Occupational Health and Safety: OSH Answers Fact Sheet. Last updated October 3, 2016. Available at: https://www.ccohs.ca/oshanswers/diseases/carcinogen_site.html. Accessed January 22, 2019.

cancers and their treatment are discussed in organ-specific chapters in this text (see also Chapter 9).

## Occupational Infections

Occupational infections are diseases caused by work-associated exposure to microbial agents, including bacteria, viruses, fungi, and protozoa. Occupational infections are distinguished by the fact that some aspect of the work involves contact with a biologically active organism. Occupational infection can occur after contact with infected people, as in the case of health care workers; infected animal or human tissue, secretions, or excretions, as in laboratory workers; asymptomatic or unknown contagious humans, as happens during business travel; or infected animals, as in agriculture (e.g., brucellosis).

Physical therapists should be aware of all types of occupational infections in order to treat anyone who may have signs and symptoms of an occupational infection. Therapists also need to be aware of the occupational infections they may come across during a workday. Common occupational infections therapists may encounter include hepatitis, HIV/AIDS, herpes simplex and herpes zoster (shingles), methicillin-resistant *Staphylococcus aureus, Clostridium difficile,* influenza, H1N1 (swine flu), and tuberculosis.

## Occupational Skin Disorders

Occupational skin diseases are one of the most common types of occupational disease in the United States, especially among agriculture and manufacturing workers. It is likely that many cases of work-related skin disorders are underreported because it is often not a life-threatening condition and is never diagnosed or treated. Other industries commonly affected include food service, cosmetology, cleaning, painting, mechanics, printing/lithography, and construction.

The most common forms of occupational skin diseases include irritant contact dermatitis, allergic contact dermatitis, skin cancers, skin infections, skin injuries, and miscellaneous skin diseases. Dermatoses are more prevalent in some states, such as California and Florida. Contact dermatitis from plants, particularly in combination with sunlight, and chemicals, such as pesticides or fertilizers, is common among agricultural workers. Contact dermatitis (acute, chronic, or allergic) is the most common occupational skin disorder, with an estimated annual cost to treat that exceeds $1 billion; other types include contact urticaria, psoriasis, scleroderma, vitiligo (areas of depigmentation), chloracne (see Fig. 4.1), actinic skin damage known as farmer's skin or sailor's skin, cutaneous malignancy, and cutaneous infections.

There are four different causes of occupational skin diseases: chemical agents, mechanical trauma, physical agents, and biologic agents. Chemical agents are the most common cause and can be divided into primary irritants, which act directly on the skin, and sensitizers, which react with repeated exposure. Physical agents include extreme temperature and radiation; mechanical trauma includes friction, pressure, abrasions, lacerations, and contusions; and biologic agents include parasites, microorganisms, plants, and other animal materials.

Skin cancer is an important occupational illness and is most often the result of excessive exposure to ultraviolet light; farmers, fishermen, roofers, and road workers who continuously work in the sun are at greatest risk.[56] For further discussion of specific skin disorders, see Chapter 10.

### Rubber Latex Allergy

The incidence of natural rubber latex allergy (LA) has dramatically increased; not only among the general population but also among health care workers, the latter because of repeated contact as a result of standard precautions and subsequent increased occupational exposure. Although government agencies limit the number of approved latex products, most finished products do not label whether they contain latex or not, thus making latex products difficult to identify. The global prevalence of LA in health care workers is 9.7% compared with 4.3% in the general population.[311] Certain high-risk groups for LA are listed in Box 4.5.

This occupational sensitivity to natural rubber latex (NRL) (i.e., latex proteins and in some cases the associated cornstarch glove powder serves as a carrier for the allergenic proteins from the NRL) has resulted in the following three types of reactions:

- Immediate hypersensitivity (type I hypersensitivity; IgE-mediated) with urticaria (hives), watery eyes, rhinitis, respiratory distress, and asthma or skin rash, which can spread from the hands, up the arms, and to the face (it can also cause swelling of the lips, eyes, ears, and larynx [laryngeal edema can prevent the person from speaking])
- Irritation or irritant contact dermatitis manifested as dry, crusty, hard bumps; sores; and horizontal cracks on the skin (Fig. 4.6)
- Mild-to-severe allergic contact dermatitis (delayed type IV hypersensitivity; cell-mediated) (Fig. 4.7)

The first two reactions are related to mechanical and chemical exposure, whereas LA is caused by sensitization to the proteins in NRL. These responses occur when items containing latex touch the skin, mucous membranes (eyes, mouth, nose, genitals, bladder, or rectum), or open areas.

Latex exposure has become one of the leading causes of occupational asthma. Once sensitized, some health care workers are at risk for severe systemic allergic reactions, which can be fatal in some cases. In susceptible individuals, airways react to low levels of a variety of sensitizers and irritants in the environment. The two major routes of exposure include dermal exposure and inhalation exposure. The elimination of wearing latex gloves has been successful in reducing the rate of latex sensitization 16-fold. Complete elimination has not occurred because latex allergens are airborne and can be carried in dust through air ducts.[293]

Latex-induced rhinitis and occupational asthma are forms of occupational illness secondary to airborne latex allergens in operating rooms, intensive care units, and dental suites. A patient with LA should be treated as the first case of the day, whether in the operating room or in a therapy department, to avoid latex in the air and to avoid introducing any latex from clothes or materials from previous contacts.

**Box 4.5**

**RISK FACTORS FOR LATEX ALLERGY**

Repeated or frequent exposure to latex products via one or more of the following:

- Repeat or frequent catheterization or other urologic procedures
- Occupation
  - Health care workers (dentists, nurses, surgeons, laboratory or operating room technicians, therapists, especially wound care specialists)
  - Rubber or latex industry workers
  - Doll manufacturing workers
  - Occupation requiring gloves (hair stylist, food handler, gardener or greenhouse worker, housekeeper)
- Immunocompromised individuals
- Individuals with spina bifida or myelomeningocele
- Spinal cord injury (presence of indwelling urinary catheter)
- History of multiple surgeries
- Individuals (including children) receiving home mechanical ventilation
- Personal or family history of eczema, asthma, or atopy (allergies) including food allergies[a]

[a]Cross-reactivity can occur between latex and some plant-derived foods including avocado, kiwi fruit, papayas, chestnuts, brazil nuts, tomatoes, and bananas. This latex-fruit syndrome may be due to the latex proteins being structurally homologous with other plant proteins.

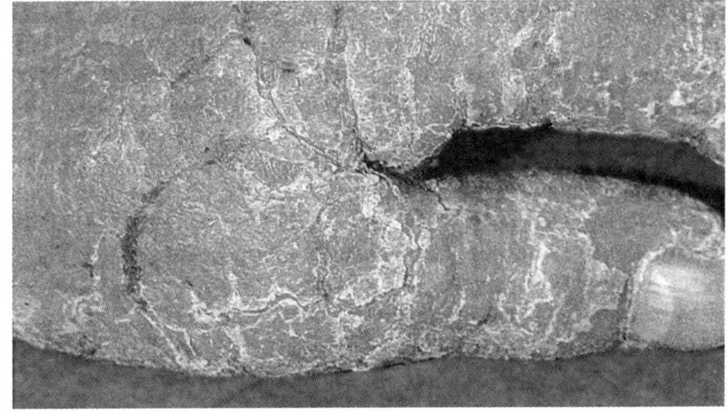

**Figure 4.6**

**Rubber glove dermatitis.** (From Baxter PJ, et al: *Hunter's diseases of occupations*, ed 9, CRC Press, 2000.)

**SPECIAL IMPLICATIONS FOR THE THERAPIST 4.3**

## *Rubber Latex Allergy*

In the hospital setting or therapy clinic, latex is not only in the disposable gloves but also can be found in stethoscopes, blood pressure cuffs, syringes, electrode pads, exercise bands, mats, and rubber balls. Other products that often have latex include spatulas, balloons, swimming goggles, condoms, mouse pads, rubber bands, erasers, and expandable fabrics.

All clients should be screened for known LA or risk factors on admission. It is not enough to ask if someone is allergic to latex; risk factors and medical history must be assessed. This is especially important because anaphylaxis could be the first sign of LA.

A health care worker with a known sensitivity should wear a medical alert bracelet, and the individual should have auto-injectable epinephrine (EpiPen) for use if another reaction occurs. A person experiencing the first reaction should not ignore the symptoms; further episodes must be avoided by developing a latex-safe environment and using latex-free products.

All patients with myelomeningocele should be treated as if LA is present. The therapist, family members, and caregivers must avoid using toys, feeding utensils, pacifiers, nipples, or other items made of latex that the infant or child might put in the mouth. Clothes and shoes with elastic anywhere must be avoided. Parents must be advised to read all labels and avoid all items

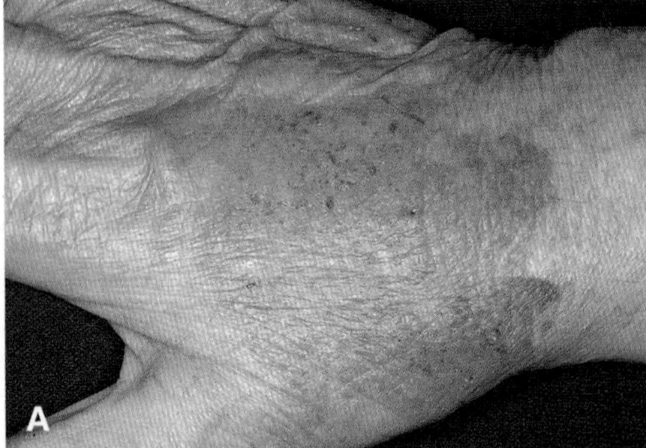


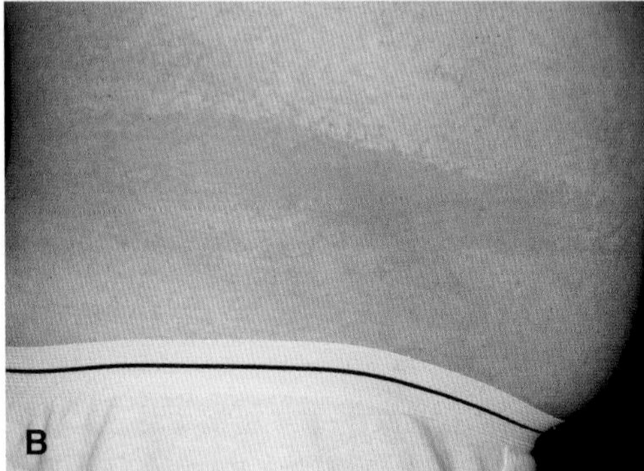


**Figure 4.7**

**Latex allergy dermatitis.** (A) Latex glove allergy should be suspected in health care workers who present with eczema, blistering, or skin peeling anywhere on the hands. (B) Allergy to the rubber band of underwear. Washing clothes with bleach may make the rubber allergenic. Similar skin reactions can be seen in women across the midback under the bra strap (not shown). (From Habif TP: *Clinical dermatology*, ed 4, St. Louis, 2004, Mosby.)

containing latex. If no indication of latex content is evident, the manufacturer should be contacted for verification before purchase or use of the item.

Handwashing before donning and after removing gloves must be carried out at all times, with special care given to using a pH-balanced soap and rinsing well to remove all residue. All medical products containing NRL that could come in contact with clients must be labeled. Keep in mind that many latex-free supplies have packaging that contains latex (glue), and the workers in the production or packaging of these products may have worn latex gloves.

No latex balloons or toys containing latex should be allowed in health care facilities; crash carts should be latex free. Personnel in the therapy department must be aware of the many items in the department that contain latex and replace these with latex-free products or a latex-free barrier (Table 4.6). Almost all equipment, supplies, and personal protective equipment are available in latex-free form, although not by all manufacturers. Complete guidelines for prevention and protection are available through the American Nurses Association at (800) 274-4ANA.

Several potential sources of powder-free, natural hypoallergenic latex gloves may be tolerated by latex-sensitive individuals, but no single replacement glove has been found for all people with latex sensitivity. Cotton

**Table 4.6** Potential Sources of Latex in a Rehabilitation Department[a]

| Item | Replacement Item |
|---|---|
| **Personal Protective Equipment** | |
| Gloves (sterile and nonsterile) | Nitrile, neoprene, or thermoplastic elastomer examination gloves |
| Goggles | |
| Hair covers | |
| Respirators | |
| Rubber aprons | |
| Shoe covers | |
| Surgical masks | |
| **Equipment/Supplies** | |
| Bandages | |
| Casting material | |
| Compression sleeves/garments | |
| Crash cart | |
| Crutch and walker handgrips | Cover with stockinette |
| Crutch axillary pads | Cover with stockinette |
| Dressings | |
| Elastic netting | Band Net Latex Free (Western Medical, Ltd.)<br>Stretch Net: Latex Safe (DeRoyal)<br>The Net Works (Wells Lamont Medical) |
| Electrode pads, especially disposable TENS | |
| Exercise balls | Cover ball with a towel |
| Exercise bands | Use the following latex-free brands:<br>REP Band (Magister Corporation)<br>Theraband Latex Free<br>Latex-free CANDO exercise band (SPRI)<br>Use free weights that are not covered with materials containing latex |
| Exercise mats | |
| Foam rubber lining splints, braces, mattresses and inside pillows | Cover with sheet or blanket |
| Mini-trampoline | Line with cloth, felt |
| Positioning supports and pads of foam rubber without complete coverings | Cover with stockinette |
| Reflex hammer | Cover with latex-free plastic bag |
| Rubber bands | String, paper clips |
| Shoe orthotics | |
| Stethoscope tubing | Cover with gauze or premade cover |
| Sphygmomanometer | Cover cuff or extremity with gauze |
| Tape (all kinds) | Cover skin first with gauze; tape over gauze |
| Toys; toys made from latex gloves | Toys made without latex |
| Vascular stockings | |
| Wheelchair cushions | Cover with cloth |
| Wheelchair tires | Propel with leather or cloth gloves |

[a]Many manufacturers now make latex-free items. Any medical supply with latex must be so marked.
*TENS*, Transcutaneous electrical nerve stimulation.
Courtesy Harriett B. Loehne, PT, DPT, CWS, FCCWS.

liners or barrier creams can be effective interventions. Vinyl gloves are generally less protective than latex and more be prone to tearing. Some of the new synthetic materials, such as nitrile, neoprene, and thermoplastic elastomer, offer equal or superior barrier protection and durability and are a reasonable alternative to latex or vinyl, offer better protection than latex when handling lipid-soluble substances and chemicals, and are reasonably priced.[220]

However, similar to latex, synthetic glove products can cause allergic reactions because they may contain chemical additives similar to those found in latex and both are manufactured using the same process, called vulcanization. Additionally, synthetic gloves provide a poorer fit than their latex counterpart and come with environmental concerns (e.g., the production and disposal of vinyl gloves releases toxic substances such as dioxins into the environment). Be alert for reactions to neoprene and spandex, as some people with LA are also sensitive to these materials. Therapists working with individuals to control lymphedema must be aware of all materials in compressive garments and monitor for sensitivities and reaction.

## Military-Related Diseases

Military personnel are exposed to a wide range of chemical, physical, and environmental hazards during military service. Examples include Agent Orange, an herbicide used during the Vietnam War; radiation exposure from participation in radiation-risk activities such as Hiroshima and Nagasaki; uranium exposure from military tank armor and bullets; chromium exposure from contaminated sodium dichromate dust; polychlorinated biphenyl exposure from coolant and insulating fluid; burn pits for waste disposal at military sites; and sulfur fire that released large amounts of sulfur dioxide into the air in Iraq.

Seven diseases (asthma, laryngitis, chronic bronchitis, emphysema, and three eye ailments) have been identified by the Department of Veterans Affairs for compensation as a result of exposure to toxic chemicals during World War II. The Department of Veterans Affairs has added Parkinson disease, ischemic heart disease, and B-cell leukemias to the disorders it automatically considers to be service connected. For a full list of the diseases that may qualify a Vietnam veteran (or that veteran's spouse or widow) for disability compensation and Department of Veterans Affairs health care, go to https://www.publichealth.va.gov/exposures/index.asp.

Posttraumatic stress disorder (PTSD) is a type of anxiety disorder found among individuals who have seen or experienced a traumatic event that involved the threat of injury or death. Military personnel are at higher risk than the general population for this disorder because of the nature of their work. Veterans' groups have introduced the idea that this condition is more accurately called *posttraumatic stress* (without the *disorder* because the stress responses to conditions soldiers are exposed to are normal, not disordered).

### Agent Orange

The Department of Veterans Affairs recognizes some cancers and other health problems associated with exposure to Agent Orange or other herbicides during military service. Survivors of the Vietnam War who served between January 1962 and May 1975 are presumed to have been exposed to dioxin (2,3,7,8-tetrachlorodibenzo-*p*-dioxin) contained in the herbicide mixture Agent Orange (sprayed from the air, by boat, and on the ground in Vietnam to defoliate jungles where the enemies were hiding). These veterans are known to be at risk for numerous diseases including diabetes, AL amyloidosis, chronic B-cell leukemias, chloracne, Hodgkin disease, ischemic heart disease, multiple myeloma, non-Hodgkin lymphoma, Parkinson disease, peripheral neuropathy, porphyria cutanea tarda, prostate cancer, respiratory cancers, and soft tissue sarcomas. The risk for other types of cancer has never been conclusively proven, but as Vietnam veterans continue to age, additional research will yield more information about cancer risk.[99,264]

There has been concern about the reproductive effects of Agent Orange, such as birth defects in the children of exposed veterans. Neural tube defects, neurotoxicity, neuropsychiatric dysfunction, deficits in motor function, and peripheral neuropathy may be linked to Agent Orange exposure, but considerable uncertainty exists about these associations.[99] The Department of Veterans Affairs has recognized spina bifida as being associated with exposure of veterans to Agent Orange or other herbicide between the aforementioned specific dates during the Vietnam War.

### Gulf War Illness

**Overview.** Once a hotly debated topic, Gulf War illness (GWI) has more scientific research indicating that it is real and a result of neurotoxic exposures during Gulf War deployment. This disorder, once termed Gulf War syndrome, affected many Gulf War veterans with symptoms including fatigue, widespread pain, cognitive/memory problems, skin rashes, gastrointestinal difficulties, and respiratory difficulties. Not all Gulf War veterans were affected; 25% to 30% deployed soldiers had GWI, and those that were affected did not have exactly the same symptoms.[182,302]

**Incidence and Clinical Manifestations.** The Gulf War Research Panel has found that one in four of the 697,000 U.S. veterans of the 1991 Gulf War have GWI.[34] CDC data show that GWI affects 27% of veterans compared with 2% of nonveterans. The first neurologic disorder identified as occurring at increased rates in Gulf War veterans was ALS. This was found to span for only the first 10 years after the war and was related to specific locations. Increased death rates owing to brain cancers have also been identified in Gulf War veterans, possibly secondary to exposure to nerve gas agents. Other diagnoses that were increased in Gulf War veterans compared with nondeployed control subjects include repeated seizures, neuralgia, neuritis, stroke, migraine headaches (64% were diagnosed), and chronic fatigue syndrome. The rate of diagnosis of PTSD in veterans with GWI was 25% to 32% compared with 3% to 6% in other Gulf War veterans, with severity of PTSD being related to poorer physical health after deployment. Research has also found that exposure to war casualties leads to increased mental health decline, and combat exposure was related to PTSD, depressive symptoms, and alcohol abuse.[182,302]

**Etiologic Factors.** The focus of GWI research has turned to chemical exposures for etiology, owing to the nervous system symptoms in Gulf War veterans, with psychiatric rationales being ruled out. Many neurotoxicants were used in the Gulf War, including organophosphates, carbamates, and other pesticides; sarin/cyclosarin nerve agents; and pyridostigmine bromide medications for use as a prophylaxis against chemical warfare attacks. There have been different definitions for this illness, including chronic multisymptom illness, the Kansas GWI definition, the Haley syndrome criteria, and various adaptations to each. Each of these definitions has strengths and weaknesses, and it is important for future research to develop a consensus on a GWI definition for improved understanding of the disease.[302]

**Pathogenesis.** Imaging and electroencephalography studies have shown structural and electrical abnormalities within the CNS of veterans with GWI. Neuroimaging has shown reduced volumes in white and gray matter on MRI of symptomatic Gulf War veterans, as well as reduced signaling in the thalamus, caudate, hippocampus, globus pallidus, and putamen.[302]

## MEDICAL MANAGEMENT

No specific intervention beyond management and symptomatic measures exists. Understanding the entire spectrum of illnesses from chronic fatigue syndrome to fibromyalgia to ALS to GWI in light of treatment must be the means to developing multidisciplinary treatment programs for affected people that includes allopathic, naturopathic, and alternative treatment. Additional research is needed to understand the mechanism and etiology of health disparities in Gulf War veterans. This can lead to prevention of similar health effects in future military deployments, as well as aid in the development of new treatments for GWI, related neurologic dysfunction, and treatment of workers in other occupations with similar chemical exposures for which there is no treatment yet.[302]

### Posttraumatic Stress Disorder

**Overview.** PTSD can occur at any age and can affect a variety of individuals, including war veterans, children, and people who have experienced traumatic events (e.g. physical or sexual assault, abuse, accident, disaster). About 6 of every 10 men and 5 of every 10 women experience at least one trauma in their lives.[281]

**Incidence.** The National Center for PTSD has found that 7 to 8 out of 100 people will experience PTSD in their lifetime. Women are more likely than men to experience PTSD, with 10 of every 100 women developing PTSD in their lifetime compared with about 4 of every 100 men.[281] The Military Health System recorded over 38,000 military personnel that were diagnosed with PTSD and depression between 2013 and 2014.[263] Rates of PTSD occurring in military veterans varies based on service area. Of the most recent veterans from Operations Enduring Freedom and Iraqi Freedom, 11% to 20% have PTSD each year.[230] In comparison, Gulf War (Desert Storm) veterans have annual PTSD rates of 12%, and it is estimated that 30% of Vietnam War veterans will have PTSD in their lifetime.[282]

**Clinical Manifestations.** There are no diagnostic tests for PTSD; diagnosis is based on symptoms. For PTSD diagnosis, the symptoms are present for at least 30 days. If the time period is shorter, acute stress disorder may be diagnosed. Mental health examinations, physical examinations, and blood tests are done to rule out other illnesses that can appear similar to PTSD.

A PTSD diagnosis must include at least one reexperiencing symptom (flashbacks, bad dreams, frightening thoughts), at least one avoidance symptom (staying away from places, events, or objects that are reminders of the traumatic experience; avoiding thoughts or feelings related to the traumatic event), at least two arousal and reactivity symptoms (being easily startled, feeling tense, having difficulty sleeping, having angry outbursts), and at least two cognition and mood symptoms (trouble remembering key features of the traumatic event, negative thoughts about self or the world, distorted feelings such as guilt or blame, loss of interest in enjoyable activities). Older children and teens with PTSD will have similar symptoms to adults; however, children younger than 6 years old will present with different symptoms, including wetting the bed (when already potty trained), forgetting how to or being able to talk, acting out the scary events during playtime, and being abnormally clingy with a parent or other adult.[179]

**Pathogenesis.** The cause of PTSD is unknown. It is a combination of psychological, epigenetic, physical, and social factors and the body's response to stress. Experiences that place individuals at increased risk for PTSD include living through dangerous events/trauma, getting injured, seeing another person get injured or die, childhood trauma, feeling helpless, having little or no social support after a traumatic event, dealing with extra stress after a traumatic event (e.g., loss of a loved one, pain/injury, loss of job/home), and having a history of mental illness or substance abuse. People with a reduced risk of developing PTSD include individuals who seek out support from other people, find a support group, learn to feel good about their own actions, have positive coping strategies, and are able to act and respond effectively, even with feelings of fear.[179] For further discussion of PTSD, resiliency, and coping, see Chapter 3.

## MEDICAL MANAGEMENT

Trauma-focused therapy has been found to be the most effective type of talk therapy for treatment of PTSD. Current research supports three different types. Typically an individual will meet with a therapist once a week to work on skills to manage PTSD symptoms, using these talk therapy strategies. Each of the three research-supported treatments uses various techniques to assist with processing the traumatic experience. Prolonged exposure involves talking about the trauma and doing things that have been avoided because of the trauma in order to gain control by facing negative feelings. Cognitive processing therapy involves talking about the negative thoughts surrounding the trauma, reframing them, and doing writing assignments. Eye movement desensitization and reprocessing involves the individual replaying the trauma in his or her head while focusing on back-and-forth movement, light, or sounds; this has been shown to help process the trauma and sense of it.[285]

Pharmacologic therapy is another option, with recommendations following along the same line as treatment for depression and anxiety. Currently there are four antidepressant medications found most effective for treating PTSD, including sertraline, paroxetine, fluoxetine, and venlafaxine.[283] Benzodiazepines, typically used to reduce anxiety and improve sleep, are not recommended for individuals with PTSD. These medications provide short-term relief from stress, but individuals can become dependent on them, feeling as though they need the medication to get through stressful situations. They are unable to learn to manage their stress, making it harder to recover from PTSD.[284]

It is important to watch for other problems developing in this population, including alcohol or substance abuse, depression, suicidal thoughts or plans, and other medical conditions related to these problems. It is advised for people with PTSD to have a good social support system. This can include family, friends, and/or group therapy. A combination of pharmacotherapy and psychotherapy may help people recover from PTSD more effectively than just one type of therapy.

## REFERENCES

To enhance this text and add value for the reader, all references are included in the enhanced ebook on Student Consult that accompanies this textbook. The reader can view the reference source and access it online whenever possible.

# CHAPTER 5

# Problems Affecting Multiple Systems

CELESTE KNIGHT PETERSON • LARA A. FIRRONE

Many conditions and diseases seen in the rehabilitation setting can affect multiple organs or systems (Box 5.1). With the kinds of multiple comorbidities and system impairments encountered in the health care arena, the therapist must go beyond a systems approach and use a biopsychosocial-spiritual approach to client management. Chronic diseases and multiple system impairments require such an approach because risk factors correlate with health outcome; early intervention and intervention results are correlated with improved outcome.

Individual modifying (risk) factors, such as lifestyle variables and environment, affect pathology and modify how a person responds to health, illness, and disease. For example, adverse drug events are correlated with increasing age and obesity, whereas fitness level has a profound impact on recovery from injury, anesthesia, and illness.

Additionally, a single injury, disease, or pathologic condition can predispose a person to associated secondary illnesses. For example, the victim of a motor vehicle accident suffered a traumatic brain injury and concomitant pelvic fracture then developed pneumonia and pulmonary compromise, subsequently experiencing a myocardial infarction.

This type of clinical scenario involving multiple organs and comorbidities is not uncommon. Also consider the medically complex person who needs a splint. The therapist must first review laboratory values to determine albumin levels (nutritional status) and platelet levels (potential for bleeding), perform a skin assessment, and consult with both nursing staff and the nutritionist before providing an external device that could create skin breakdown and add to an already complex case.

Although medical conditions encountered in the clinic or home health care setting are discussed individually in the appropriate chapter, the health care provider must understand the systemic and local effects of such disorders. This chapter provides a brief listing of the systemic effects of commonly encountered pathologic conditions and a basic presentation of acid–base and fluid and electrolyte imbalances. The scope of this text does not allow for an in-depth discussion of each condition or disease and its related multiple systemic effects.

## SYSTEMIC EFFECTS OF PATHOLOGY

### Systemic Effects of Acute Inflammation

Acute inflammation can be described as the initial response of tissue to injury, particularly bacterial infections and necrosis, involving vascular and cellular responses. Local signs of inflammation (e.g., redness, warmth, swelling, pain, and loss of function) are commonly observed in the therapy setting. Local inflammation can lead to abscesses when excessive suppuration (formation of pus) occurs.

Systemic effects of acute inflammation include fever, tachycardia, and a hypermetabolic state. These effects produce characteristic changes in the blood, such as elevated serum protein levels (C-reactive protein, serum amyloid A, complement, and coagulation factors) and an elevated white blood count (leukocytosis).[403]

### Systemic Effects of Chronic Inflammation

Chronic inflammation is the result of persistent injury, repeated episodes of acute inflammation, infection, cell-mediated immune responses, and foreign body reactions. The tissue response to injury is characterized by accumulation of lymphocytes, plasma cells, and macrophages (mononuclear inflammatory cells) and production of fibrous connective tissue (fibrosis). Fibroblasts and small blood vessels, along with collagen fibers synthesized by fibroblasts, constitute fibrosis. Grossly, fibrotic tissue is light gray and has a dense, firm texture that causes contraction of the normal tissue.

The associated fibrosis may cause progressive tissue damage and loss of function. Systemic effects of chronic inflammation may include low-grade fever, malaise, weight loss, anemia, fatigue, leukocytosis, and lymphocytosis (caused by viral infection). Inflammation is reflected by an increased erythrocyte sedimentation rate. In general, as the disease improves, the erythrocyte sedimentation rate decreases.

Box 5.1
**CONDITIONS THAT AFFECT MULTIPLE SYSTEMS**

- Autoimmune disorders
- Burns
- Cancer
- Cystic fibrosis
- Congestive heart failure (CHF)
- Connective tissue diseases:
  - Rheumatoid arthritis
  - Progressive systemic sclerosis (scleroderma)
  - Polymyositis
  - Sjögren syndrome
  - Systemic lupus erythematosus
  - Polyarteritis nodosa
- Endocrine disorders (e.g., diabetes, thyroid disorders)
- Environmental and occupational diseases
- Genetic diseases
- Infections (e.g., tuberculosis, human immunodeficiency virus [HIV])
- Malnutrition or other nutritional imbalance
- Metabolic disorders
- Multiple organ dysfunction syndrome (MODS)
- Renal failure (chronic)
- Sarcoidosis
- Shock
- Trauma
- Vasculitis

## Systemic Factors Influencing Healing

In addition to local factors that affect healing (e.g., infection, blood supply, extent of necrosis, presence of foreign bodies, protection from further trauma or movement), a variety of systemic factors influence healing as well. Systemic factors may include general nutritional status, especially protein and vitamin C; psychologic well-being; presence of cardiovascular disease, cancer, hematologic disorders (e.g., neutropenia), systemic infections, and diabetes mellitus; and whether the person is undergoing corticosteroid or immunosuppressive therapy.[234]

Healing in specific organs varies according to the underlying cause and site of the injury. For example, myocardial infarctions heal by scarring, and the heart may be weakened. A cerebrovascular accident, or stroke, may cause permanent disability, and healing occurs by the formation of glial tissue (e.g., astrocytes, oligodendrocytes, and microglia) rather than by collagenous scar formation; this process is called *gliosis*.

In other organs, effective tissue regeneration depends primarily on the site of injury. Necrosis of only parenchymal (functional visceral) cells with retention of the existing stroma (framework or structural tissue) may permit regeneration and restoration of normal anatomy, whereas necrosis that involves the mesenchymal framework (connective tissue, including blood and blood vessels) usually results in scar formation (e.g., as in hepatic cirrhosis).

## Consequences of Immunodeficiency

Immunodeficiency diseases are caused by congenital (primary) or acquired (secondary) failure of one or more functions of the immune system, predisposing the affected individual to infections that a noncompromised immune system could resist. The therapist is more likely to encounter individuals with acquired (rather than congenital) immunodeficiency from nonspecific causes, such as those that occur with viral and other infections; malnutrition; alcoholism; aging; autoimmune diseases; diabetes mellitus; cancer, particularly myeloma, lymphoma, and leukemia; chronic diseases; steroid therapy; cancer chemotherapy; and radiation therapy.[127]

Predisposition to opportunistic infections, resulting in clinical manifestations of those infections, is the primary consequence of immunodeficiency. Selective B-cell deficiencies predispose an individual to bacterial infections. T-cell deficiencies predispose to viral and fungal infections. Combined deficiencies, including AIDS, are particularly severe because they predispose to many kinds of viral, bacterial, and fungal infections.

## Systemic Effects of Neoplasm

Malignant tumors, by their destructive nature of uncontrolled cell proliferation and spread, produce many local and systemic effects. Locally, the rapid growth of the tumor encroaches on healthy tissue, causing destruction, necrosis, ulceration, compression, obstruction, and hemorrhage.

Pain may or may not occur, depending on how close tumor cells, swelling, or hemorrhage occurs to the nerve cells. This process also occurs locally at metastatic sites. Pain may occur as a late symptom as a result of infiltration, compression, or destruction of nerve tissue. Secondary infections often occur as a result of the host's decreased immunity and can lead to death.[433]

A person with a malignant neoplasm often presents with systemic symptoms, such as gradual or rapid weight loss, muscular weakness, anorexia, anemia, and coagulation disorders (granulocyte and platelet abnormalities). Continued spread of the cancer may lead to bone erosion or liver, gastrointestinal (GI), pulmonary, or vascular obstruction. Other vital organs may be affected; increased intracranial pressure in the brain by tumor cells can cause partial paralysis and eventual coma. Hemorrhage caused by direct invasion or necrosis in any body part leads to further anemia or even death if the necrosis is severe.

Advanced cancers produce cachexia (wasting) as a result of tissue destruction and the body's nutrients being used by the malignant cells for further growth. Multiple mechanisms may be involved in this process, including release of cytokines such as tumor necrosis factor (also called *cachectin*).

Paraneoplastic syndromes are produced by hormonal mechanisms rather than by direct tumor invasion. For example, hypercalcemia can be caused in cases of lung cancer by the secretion of a peptide with parathyroid hormone, and polycythemia can result from the secretion of erythropoietin by renal cell carcinoma. Neuromuscular disorders, such as Eaton-Lambert syndrome, polymyositis/dermatomyositis, and hypertrophic pulmonary osteoarthropathy, are other examples of paraneoplastic syndromes that can occur as a systemic effect of neoplasm.

SPECIAL IMPLICATIONS FOR THE THERAPIST 5-1

### *Systemic Effects of Pathology*[102,103]

Medical advances, the aging of America, the increasing number of people with multisystem problems, and the expanding scope of the therapist's practice require that the therapist anticipate, assess, and manage the manifestations of disease and pathology. Physical and occupational therapists are primary health care professionals who focus on maximizing functional capacity and physical independence by optimizing healthy active lifestyles and community-based living.

*Interventions to maximize oxygen transport (e.g., mobilization, positioning, breathing control, and exercise) should be an important focus, even in people who are acutely and critically ill. Enhancing oxygen transport centrally and peripherally improves the body's ability to respond to stress. At the same time, many therapy interventions elicit an exercise stimulus that stresses an already strained oxygen transport system. Exercise is now recognized as a prescriptive intervention in pathology that has indications, contraindications, and side effects. These factors necessitate careful and close monitoring of cardiopulmonary status, especially in the person with multisystem involvement.*

*Hematologic abnormalities require that the results of the client's blood analysis and clotting factors be monitored so that therapy intervention can be modified to minimize risks. Individualized treatment programs are developed for each person addressing the special needs of that client and the family, responding to physical, psychologic, emotional, and spiritual needs. The reader is encouraged to review an excellent article103 for an additional in-depth discussion of specific implications for physical therapy management in systemic disease.*

## ADVERSE DRUG EVENTS

Drugs were once developed through a hit-or-miss process in which researchers would identify a compound and test it in cells and animals to determine its effect on disease. When a compound appeared to be successful, it was often tested in humans, with little knowledge of how it worked or what side effects it might have. Today, biochemists know much more about disease processes and work at the molecular level, designing drugs to interact with specific molecules. Disease-modifying antirheumatic drugs, selective estrogen receptor modulators (SERMs), and monoclonal antibodies are examples of such"designer drugs."

Drugs in the future will have greater molecular specificity, possibly with the ability to accommodate for gender, age, and genetic differences between individuals. Despite these advances, reactions are still a significant problem in the health care industry today.

### Definition and Overview

In 2010, as part of the Patient Protection and Affordable Care Act, the government developed an action plan, including incentive programs, to prevent and reduce the number of adverse drug events.[392] *Adverse drug events* (ADEs) are defined as injury, physical and/or mental, caused from the use of a medication. ADEs include medication errors, adverse drug reactions, allergic drug reactions, and overdoses. ADEs may be classified as preventable or nonpreventable. Medication errors are errors made in the process of giving a medication that may or may not cause harm. They may occur during the process of prescribing, dispensing, or administering a drug. Adverse drug reactions (ADRs) relate to the properties of the drug itself and effects from the medication at normal dosages. Potential ADEs are often referred to as "near misses" and are medication errors that do not cause harm to the client or are caught by staff prior to giving a medication. Most ADEs are medication reactions or side effects. A *drug–drug* interaction occurs when medications interact unfavorably, possibly adding to the pharmacologic effects. A *drug–disease* interaction occurs when a medication causes an existing disease to worsen. *Side effects* are usually defined as predictable pharmacologic effects that occur within therapeutic dose ranges and are undesirable in the given therapeutic situation. Overdosage toxicity is the predictable toxic effect that occurs with dosages in excess of the therapeutic range for a particular person.

ADEs may be dose-related (predictable drug injury) or non–dose-related (unpredictable or idiosyncratic drug injury). Dose-related effects may include drug toxicity from overdose, variations in pharmaceutical preparations, preexisting liver disease, presence of comorbidities such as renal or heart failure, or drug interactions. Non–dose-related effects may occur as a result of hypersensitivity, resulting in acute anaphylaxis or delayed hypersensitivity or other nonimmunologic idiosyncratic reactions, according to individual susceptibility.

### Incidence

ADEs have been declared a national public health problem with more than 1.3 million emergency department (ED) visits (or a prevalence of 4 ED visits per 1000 people) and 350,000 hospitalizations required for further treatment after the emergency visit.[67,349] The annual incidence of death caused by ADEs is estimated to be between 0.08/100,000 and 0.12/100,000 people.[350] According to one study of primary care outpatients, ADEs were common and often preventable (25%).[147]

Adults older than age 65 years are twice as likely to go to an emergency department because of an ADE and are almost seven times more likely to experience an ADE requiring hospitalization than a younger person.[54-56] Older adults often take multiple medications, increasing the possibility of a detrimental interaction. Death rates secondary to an ADE are also highest in people older than age 55 years, with the greatest risk in those older than 75 years.[350] The Centers for Disease Control and Prevention report inappropriate medications are prescribed to older adults in about 1 of every 12 visits (8%) and most of the hospitalizations are due to just a few medications, such as anticoagulants, diabetic medications, antibiotics, and opioids.[66,163]

Inappropriate use of pain medications has led to a national crisis. The opioid epidemic in America led to a declaration of a public health emergency in 2017 and strategies to combat it.[215] Over 11.4 million people misuse prescription opioids, with more than 130 people dying each day from an opioid-related drug overdose.[266,422,329] Care should always be taken to prescribe only the needed dose and type of medication to match pain relief goals. Many states have prescription drug monitoring programs to aid in this effort.

ADEs can occur in any type of medical setting—inpatient[79] (ICU, emergency department, operating room), outpatient, chemotherapy clinics,[146] and long-term care facilities. Most occur at points of transition in medical care, such as hospital admission and discharge or transfer to an extended care facility.[43,218] Efforts have been made to reconcile all medications between institutions and levels of care.[382]

## Etiologic and Risk Factors

Definite risk factors for experiencing a serious ADE can include age (older than age 75 years, younger children),[377] gender, polypharmacy, ethnicity, concomitant alcohol consumption, new drugs, dosages, concomitant use of herbal compounds,[95] duration of treatment, noncompliance (e.g., unintentional repeated dosage) and presence of underlying conditions (e.g., hepatic or renal insufficiency).[77,84]

Of all the risk factors, age has the most prevalent effect in the aging American population.[226] Factors that contribute to ADEs in older people include age-related physiologic changes, a greater degree of frailty, an increased number of underlying diseases, and the presence of polypharmacy.[222,247] Age-related physiologic changes affect the distribution of drugs. A decrease in lean body mass and an increase in the proportion of body fat results in a decrease in body water. As a result, water-soluble drugs (e.g., morphine) have a lower volume of distribution that speeds up onset of action and raises peak concentration. High peak concentrations are associated with increased toxicity.

On the other hand, lipid-soluble drugs, such as benzodiazepines, are distributed more widely, have a prolonged half-life, and accumulate with repeated dosing.[226] Many drugs are protein bound and the portion not bound is referred to as "free" and elicits the effects. Many elderly people have low albumin stores, thus increasing the proportion of the drug that is free and active. This leads to higher toxicity, particularly with drugs such as ibuprofen and phenytoin.[226]

Aging adults are also at risk for drug accumulation because of changes in both metabolism and elimination. With advanced age, functional liver tissue diminishes and hepatic blood flow decreases. Consequently, the capacity of the liver to break down and convert drugs and their metabolites declines. This may be exacerbated by other changes, such as age-related reduction in renal mass and blood flow, the accompanying decline in glomerular filtration and tubular reabsorption rates, and other conditions such as dehydration, cancer, heart failure, and cirrhosis.

Another common problem seen in the elderly with polypharmacy is the interaction of multiple medications with cytochrome P450 (which metabolizes drugs). For example, haloperidol inhibits cytochrome P450, thereby slowing down the metabolism of amitriptyline and leading to increased anticholinergic effects and risk for injury.[226] Interactions between drugs that inhibit cytochrome P450 should be carefully monitored.

There are also changes in the sensitivity of the cardiovascular system with age. For example, with the addition of β-adrenergic agonists and antagonists, there is less responsiveness of the cardiovascular system and orthostatic events increase.[122] Box 5.2 lists the drugs most commonly associated with ADEs in the aging.

Cardiac or pulmonary toxicity may occur as a result of irradiation and immunosuppressive drugs given to prepare recipients for organ transplantation or for treatment of cancer. Box 5.3 lists some of the more common specific target organs and effects.

### Box 5.2

**DRUGS THAT ARE COMMONLY ASSOCIATED WITH ADVERSE DRUG REACTIONS IN THE AGING**

- Anticholinergics
- Antidiarrheals
- Antihistamines (first-generation)
- Antiplatelets
- Benzodiazepines (anxiolytics)
- β-Blockers
- Calcium-channel blockers
- Corticosteroids (systemic)
- Digoxin
- Diuretics
- Hypoglycemics (e.g., sulfonylureas, insulin)
- Muscle relaxants
- Neuroleptics
- Nonsteroidal antiinflammatory drugs (NSAIDs)
- Opioids
- Tricyclic antidepressants
- Vasodilators (e.g., nitrates)
- Warfarin

Based on data from Fick DM, Cooper JW, Wade WE, et al: Updating the Beers criteria for potentially inappropriate medication use in older adults: results of a US consensus panel of experts. *Arch Intern Med* 163(22):2716–2724, 2003; Thomsen LA, Winterstein AG, Søndergaard B, et al: Systematic review of the incidence and characteristics of preventable adverse drug events in ambulatory care. *Ann Pharmacother* 41(9):1411–1426, 2007; Gallagher P, O'Mahony D. STOPP (Screening Tool of Older Persons' potentially inappropriate Prescriptions): application to acutely ill elderly patients and comparison with Beers' criteria. *Age Ageing* 37(6):673–679, 2008; Budnitz DS, Lovegrove MC, Shehab N, Richards CL: Emergency hospitalizations for adverse drug events in older Americans. *N Engl J Med* 365:2002–2012, 2011; Budnitz DS, Shehab N, Kegler SR, Richards CL: Medication use leading to emergency department visits for adverse drug events in older adults. *Ann Intern Med* 147:755–765, 2007.

## Clinical Manifestations

Rashes, fever, and jaundice are common signs of drug toxicity. Adverse skin (cutaneous) reactions include erythema, discoloration, itching, burning, urticaria, eczema, acne, alopecia, blisters, or purpura (Fig. 5.1). Onset may be within minutes to hours to days. Signs and symptoms suggestive of a mild reaction include anxiety, dizziness, headache, nasal congestion, shakiness, and brief vomiting. Persons with a moderate drug reaction may present with abdominal cramps, dyspnea, hypertension or hypotension, palpitations, tachycardia, and persistent vomiting. Severe reactions can include arrhythmia, seizures, laryngeal edema, profound hypotension, pulmonary edema, and cardiopulmonary arrest. Arthralgias and myalgias may present in mild or moderate reactions.

Older adults may develop ADEs that are clearly different from those seen in younger persons, such as cognitive and functional decline (Box 5.4).[226] The therapist should be aware of increased bruising indicative of warfarin toxicity or nausea/vomiting with/without cardiac manifestations suggestive of digitalis toxicity. Elevated levels of both medications can be life threatening. Early symptoms of salicylate intoxication include tinnitus, disequilibrium, drowsiness, and a moderate delirium.

The long-term use of neuroleptic drugs, particularly older types (typical, first generation) such as haloperidol, can cause motor tics called *tardive dyskinesia*. Repetitive, involuntary, purposeless movements characterize tardive dyskinesia. The client may demonstrate repetitive grimacing, tongue protrusion, lip smacking, puckering and pursing, and rapid eye blinking. Rapid movements of the arms, legs, and trunk may also occur. Involuntary movements of the fingers may give the person the appearance of playing an invisible guitar or piano.

## MEDICAL MANAGEMENT

Differentiating an ADE from underlying disease requires a thorough history, especially when a symptom appears 1 to 2 months after a medication regimen has been started. Monitoring blood cell counts, liver enzymes, electrolytes, blood urea nitrogen (BUN), and creatinine is indicated for certain drugs. Cardiotropic drugs can cause arrhythmias that require electrocardiogram monitoring. With dose-related ADEs, dose modification is usually all that is required, whereas with non–dose-related ADEs, the drug therapy is usually stopped and reexposure avoided.

The federal initiative Partnership for Patients has a goal to reduce the number of preventable rehospitalizations by 20%, and the reduction of ADEs is a key focus of the partnership.[213] Hospitals, clinics, nursing facilities, pharmacies, etc., are expected to evaluate their prescribing, testing, and follow-up methods in order to reduce ADEs.

SPECIAL IMPLICATIONS FOR THE THERAPIST 5-2

### *Adverse Drug Events*

Many people treated by physical therapists today have a pharmacologic profile. It is not unusual to find out during the client interview that the person is taking many different prescription or nonprescription medications. Often there is an equally long list of nutritional aids, supplements, herbs, or vitamins, sometimes referred to as nutraceuticals. Adults age 65 years or older commonly have complicated medication regimens that may result in ADEs. Age-related physiologic changes result in altered pharmacokinetic and pharmacodynamic response to medications that contribute to adverse responses.[139]

*Knowing when a person is having an ADE to medication or supplements versus experiencing symptoms of disease or illness is not always easily distinguished. Knowing about potential drug effects and using a drug guide to look up potential side effects is a good place to start.*

*Client/patient education is important. The therapist can remind his or her clients to take their medication as prescribed and to report any unusual signs and symptoms to their doctor, physician's assistant, or nurse practitioner. Encourage your clients to keep follow-up appointments with the health care professional who prescribed the drug and to make sure that person knows all drugs and supplements currently being taken.*

*If the therapist suspects drug- or nutraceutical-related signs or symptoms, several observations can be made and reported to the physician, such as correlation between the time medication is taken and length of time before signs and symptoms appear (or increase). Additionally, family members can be asked to observe whether the signs or symptoms increase after each dosage. Documentation of observed or reported behavior or signs and symptoms and the date first observed is important. Make note of the client's clinical condition and your interventions. Follow your facility's policies for notification of suspected ADE.*

*Interpretation of drug-related or disease-induced signs and symptoms is beyond the scope of a therapist's practice, but the therapist can identify when these clinical manifestations are interfering with rehabilitation and make the necessary referral for evaluation. Any time a client has reached a plateau or has demonstrated poor potential for improvement, the therapist should consider that these responses may be a result of an ADE.*

*Any signs of tardive dyskinesia should be reported to the physician. There is no standard treatment for tardive dyskinesia. The first step is generally to stop or minimize the use of the neuroleptic drug. This may not be possible for anyone with a severe underlying condition. Replacing the neuroleptic drug with substitute drugs may help some people. Other drugs, such as benzodiazepines, adrenergic antagonists, and dopamine agonists, may also be beneficial.*

*Symptoms of tardive dyskinesia may continue even after the person has stopped taking the drugs (usually neuroleptics). Some symptoms may improve and/or disappear over time with proper medical management.*

#### Exercise and Drugs

Exercise can produce dramatic changes in the way drugs are absorbed, distributed, localized, metabolized, and excreted in the body (pharmacokinetics). The magnitude of these changes is dependent on the characteristics of each drug (e.g., route of administration, chemical properties) and exercise-related factors (e.g., exercise intensity, mode, and duration).

*A single exercise session can cause sudden changes in pharmacokinetics that may have an immediate impact on people who exercise during therapy. Exercise training can also produce changes in pharmacokinetics, but these tend to occur over a longer period and cause a slower and fairly predictable change in a person's response to certain medications.*

*Drugs that are administered locally by transdermal techniques or by subcutaneous or intramuscular injection may have altered or increased absorption in the presence of exercise, local heat, or massage of the administration site. Diuretics, herbal products, nonsteroidal antiinflammatory drugs, statins, and insulin medications are some of the more common medications that can affect physiologic function during exercise, causing a wide range of potential adverse effects.*

*In addition, allergic and potentially fatal anaphylactic drug reactions are mediated by exercise. The therapist should always consider the possibility that anyone in therapy taking drugs may have an altered response to those drugs as a result of interventions used in therapy.343 The possibility of drug–exercise interactions requires careful and consistent monitoring of vital signs.*

Box 5.3

## TARGET ORGANS AND EFFECTS OF ADVERSE DRUG EVENTS

### Heart

- Arrhythmia
  - Adenosine
  - Flecainide
  - Propafenone
  - Digoxin
  - Procainamide
- Cardiomyopathy
  - Adriamycin
  - Antipsychotics
  - Anthracyclines (i.e., doxorubicin, daunorubicin, epirubicin)
  - Trastuzumab
- Myocardial infarction/acute coronary syndrome
  - Oral contraceptives
  - Selective cox-2 inhibitors (NSAIDs)
  - Abacavir
  - Didanosine
- Orthostatic hypotension
  - Atypical antipsychotics
  - Antihypertensives
  1. Calcium-channel blockers
  2. Centrally acting α-adrenergic agonists
  3. Peripheral α-blockers
  4. β-Adrenergic blockers
  5. Peripherally acting vasodilators
  6. Diuretics

### Lung

- Interstitial lung disease/pulmonary fibrosis
  - Methotrexate
  - Cyclophosphamide
  - Amiodarone
  - Tamoxifen
  - Bleomycin
- Asthma/bronchospasms
  - Aspirin
  - NSAIDs
  - Sulfites
  - Acetaminophen

### Gastrointestinal Tract

- Gastritis and peptic ulcer
  - Aspirin
  - NSAIDs
  - Bisphosphonates
  - Potassium chloride
- Gingival hyperplasia
  - Phenytoin
  - Cyclosporine
  - Nifedipine
  - Verapamil
- Pseudomembranous colitis
  - Broad-spectrum antibiotics
- Hepatic and cholestatic disease
  - Tacrine
  - Nucleoside reverse transcriptase inhibitors
  - Isoniazid
  - Protease inhibitors
  - Amiodarone
  - Quinidine
  - Rifampin
  - Dapsone
  - Leflunomide

### Fetal Injury

- Phocomelia
  - Thalidomide
- Vaginal carcinoma
  - Diethylstilbestrol
- Discoloration of teeth
  - Tetracyclines
  - Minocycline
  - Ciprofloxacin
- Multiple congenital anomalies
  - Disulfiram
  - Estrogens
  - Progestins
  - Human chorionic gonadotropin
  - Antineoplastic agents
  - Phenytoin
  - Warfarin
  - Isotretinoin

### Kidneys

- Acute interstitial nephritis
  - Rifampin
  - Lithium
  - NSAIDs
  - β-Lactam antibiotics
- Acute tubular necrosis
  - Aminoglycosides
  - Amphotericin B
  - Radiocontrast media
  - Cisplatin
- Nephrolithiasis
  - Indinavir
  - Topiramate
  - Sulfonamides
- Glomerulonephritis
  - Allopurinol
  - Lithium
  - NSAIDs

### Endocrine System

- Adrenocortical atrophy
  - Corticosteroids
- Hypothyroidism
  - Amiodarone
  - Interferon-α and -β
  - Lithium
  - Thalidomide
- • Hyperthyroidism
  - Amiodarone
  - Interferon-β

### Skeletal System

- Osteoporosis/osteomalacia
- Corticosteroids
- Antineoplastic agents
- Aromatase inhibitors
- Methotrexate
- Heparin

### Nervous System

- Seizures
  - Tramadol
  - Propofol
  - Bupropion
  - Tricyclic antidepressants
  - Cyclosporine
- Movement disorders
  - Droperidol
  - Metoclopramide
  - Prochlorperazine
  - First-generation antipsychotics
  - Atypical antipsychotics
- Peripheral neuropathy
  - Leflunomide
  - Didanosine
  - Stavudine
  - Carboplatin
  - Cisplatin
  - Vincristine
- Delirium
  - Opioids
  - Clozapine
  - Valproic acid
  - Lithium
  - Digoxin
- Depression
  - Phenobarbital
  - Primidone
  - Interferon-α and -β
  - Gonadotropin-releasing hormone agonists
  - Triptans
  - Corticosteroids
- Anxiety
  - Amphetamines
  - Antipsychotics
  - Bupropion
  - Caffeine
  - Dopamine agonists and antagonists
  - Theophylline

### Blood and Bone Marrow

- Anemias
  - Penicillins
  - Cephalosporins
  - Methyldopa
  - Antimalarial drugs
  - Sulfonamides
  - Nitrofurantoin
  - Methotrexate
  - Phenytoin
  - Antineoplastic agents
- Thrombocytopenia
  - Abciximab
  - Heparin
  - Valproate
  - NSAIDs
- Deep vein thrombosis
  - Heparin

Box 5.3

**TARGET ORGANS AND EFFECTS OF ADVERSE DRUG EVENTS**

- Erythropoietin
- Estrogen-containing hormones
- Raloxifene
- Tamoxifen
- Anastrozole
- Megestrol
- Contrast agents

***Skin***

- Allergies, pseudoallergies
  - Radiocontrast media
  - Angiotensin-converting enzyme inhibitors
  - Heparin
  - Penicillins
  - Omalizumab
  - Cephalosporins
- Photosensitivity
  - Voriconazole
  - Methotrexate
  - Diclofenac
  - Ibuprofen
  - Amiodarone
- Alopecia
  - Anticonvulsants
  - Chemotherapy agents
  - Immunosuppressants
  - Interferons
  - Retinoids
- Hirsutism
  - Cyclosporin
  - Danazol
  - Testosterone

***Ears, Nose, and Throat***

- Ototoxicity
  - Carboplatin
  - Cisplatin
  - Doxycycline
  - Gentamicin
  - Interferon
  - Minocycline
  - Neomycin
  - Tobramycin

***Eyes***

- Severe visual disturbances
  - Amiodarone
  - Clomiphene
  - Digitalis
  - Isotretinoin
  - NSAIDs, nonsteroidal antiinflammatory drugs

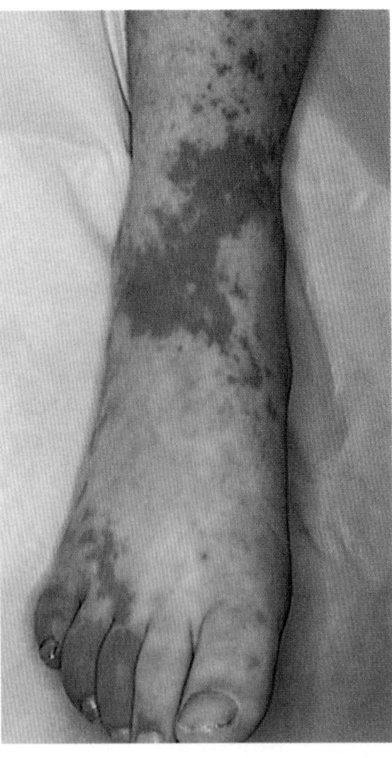

**Figure 5.1**

**Purpura.** Hemorrhaging into the tissues, particularly beneath the skin or mucous membranes, producing raised or flat ecchymoses or petechiae. Seen most often in a physical therapy practice as a result of thrombocytopenia (e.g., drug-reaction or medication-induced, especially nonsteroidal antiinflammatory drugs, methotrexate, Coumadin or warfarin; radiation- or chemotherapy-induced); also occurs in older adults as blood leaks from capillaries in response to minor trauma. (From Hurwitz S: *Clinical pediatric dermatology: a textbook of skin disorders of childhood and adolescence*, ed 2, Philadelphia, 1993, Saunders.)

Box 5.4

**COMMON SIGNS AND SYMPTOMS OF ADVERSE DRUG REACTIONS IN THE AGING**

- Dry mouth
- Dyspepsia
- Restlessness
- Orthostatic hypotension (dizziness, weakness, decreased blood pressure, falls)
- Depression
- Dehydration
- Confusion, delirium
- Impaired memory or concentration
- Nausea
- Loss of appetite
- Constipation
- Incontinence
- Extrapyramidal syndromes (e.g., parkinsonism, tardive dyskinesia)
- Fatigue, weakness
- Sedation

# SPECIFIC DRUG CATEGORIES

## Nonsteroidal Antiinflammatory Drugs

Nonsteroidal antiinflammatory drugs (NSAIDs) are a heterogeneous group of approximately 20 drugs in 6 classes that reduce inflammation, provide pain relief, and reduce fever. NSAIDs are commonly used postoperatively for discomfort; for painful musculoskeletal conditions, especially among the older adult population[98]; and in the treatment of inflammatory rheumatic diseases.

These medications may consist of nonprescription preparations, such as acetylsalicylic acid or aspirin; other salicylates; ibuprofen (e.g., Advil, Motrin), naproxen

(Aleve); or prescription drugs (Table 5.1). Because of their extensive clinical uses, over 43 million people regularly use aspirin and more than 29 million people regularly take NSAIDs in the United States.[442] Because these medications are used for diseases that frequently affect the elderly, over 14 million people over the age of 45 use an NSAID routinely.

### Mechanism of Action

The primary mechanism of action of NSAIDs involves inhibiting the production of prostaglandins, prostacyclin, and thromboxanes from arachidonic acid by reversibly or irreversibly binding to the enzyme cyclooxygenase (COX). There are two principal forms of COX: COX-1 and COX-2. Among the classes, NSAIDS exhibit variability in their binding to COX, both 1 and 2 isoforms. COX-1 is found in most cells. It is responsible for regulating normal cell function and contributes to gastric cytoprotection, kidney function, vascular homeostasis, platelet aggregation, and the production of prostacyclin. COX-2 may be present in cells under normal conditions but is also an inducible enzyme and is produced when cytokines and other proinflammatory factors are present because of fever, inflammation, or pain. It is typically found only in the brain, kidney and bone.[117] NSAIDS, as well as glucocorticoids, inhibit COX-2.

NSAIDS also have effects other than inhibiting COX (aspirin's antiinflammatory effect is only through prostaglandin formation inhibition). These medications are able to insert into cell membranes and may interrupt cellular functions, such as not allowing arachidonate into the cell. They interfere with neutrophil functions as well, including inhibiting adherence to vascular endothelial cells, the process that initiates neutrophil response to infection.

NSAIDs are reversible platelet inhibitors resulting in antiplatelet activity. Aspirin is the most powerful agent because it irreversibly binds to platelets. A single dose of aspirin impairs clot formation for 5 to 7 days, and two aspirin can double bleeding time. These characteristics of acetylsalicylic acid also make it an important drug in the treatment of coronary artery disease, myocardial infarctions, and stroke.

Prostaglandins, created during inflammation, are also potent inhibitors of apoptosis (programmed cell death). NSAIDS are able to return cells to normal cell cycles through inhibiting prostaglandin formation and may reduce the risk for certain cancers.[238] NSAIDS, through their inhibition of COX-2, may suppress tumor initiation and progression. Although NSAIDS, including aspirin, appear to decrease the risk of colorectal cancer, patient selection, doses, and duration of treatment are questions that still need more definitive answers.[68,118,238]

### Adverse Effects

Although the incidence of serious side effects from using NSAIDs is rather low, the widespread use of readily available nonprescription NSAIDs results in a substantial number of people being adversely affected, particularly in the elderly.[282,431] NSAIDs cause 21% of all ADEs in the United States and are a frequent cause of hospital admissions.[187] The use of NSAIDs is associated with a wide spectrum of potential clinical toxicities (Table 5.2), but serious side effects are most often seen with the GI tract, kidneys, and cardiovascular system.

**Table 5-1** Nonsteroidal Antiinflammatory Drugs*

| Generic | Common Brand Names |
|---|---|
| **Nonprescription** | |
| Aspirin | Ascriptin,[a] Bayer,[a] Bufferin,[a] Ecotrin[a] |
| Ibuprofen | Advil, Midol, Motrin |
| Naproxen | Aleve, Midol Extended Relief |
| **Prescription Traditional COX-inhibitors** | |
| Diclofenac | Cataflam, Flector, Voltaren |
| Diflunisal | Dolobid |
| Etodolac | Lodine |
| Fenoprofen | Nalfon |
| Flurbiprofen | Ansaid |
| Ibuprofen | IBU-Tab |
| Indomethacin | Indocin |
| Ketoprofen | Orudis |
| Ketorolac | Toradol |
| Meclofenamate | Meclomen |
| Mefenamic acid | Ponstel |
| Meloxicam | Mobic |
| Nabumetone | Relafen |
| Naproxen | Anaprox, Naprelan, Naprosyn |
| Oxaprozin | Daypro |
| Piroxicam | Feldene |
| Sulindac | Clinoril |
| Tolmetin | Tolectin |
| **Prescription COX-2 Selective Inhibitors** | |
| Celecoxib | Celebrex |

[a]These all have additives to minimize GI side effects but are known as aspirin products. Many nonselective (standard) NSAIDs are available nonprescription at a lower dosage (e.g., 200 mg) and by prescription at a higher dosage (e.g., 500 mg).

Courtesy Tanner Higginbotham, PharmD. Drug Information Specialist, University of Montana Skaggs School of Pharmacy, Department of Pharmacy Practice, Missoula, Montana.

**Gastrointestinal System.** Many NSAIDs are nonselective and inhibit both COX-1 and COX-2. However, because COX-1 is involved with prostacyclin formation, which normally protects the stomach, NSAIDs have been designed to selectively inhibit COX-2 in attempts to reduce unwanted GI side effects. NSAIDs can cause GI symptoms ranging from mild dyspepsia to more serious complications, such as GI bleeding, ulceration, and perforation. These serious side effects may occur without previous symptoms (e.g., dyspepsia) and are particularly more likely to occur in persons taking higher doses, in older adults (>60 years), people with a previous history of GI bleeding, individuals taking anticoagulants, SSRIs, antiplatelet agents (i.e., clopidogrel) or glucocorticoids, and with chronic use.[149,193]

Medications should be considered for prophylactic use in clients requiring NSAID treatment (e.g., osteoarthritis or rheumatoid arthritis [RA]), such as proton pump inhibitors and misoprostol, which have been shown to reduce the development of symptomatic ulcers.[137,168,333] COX-2 inhibitors have shown a reduction in GI-related toxicities, but their connection to cardiovascular events has led to their careful use.[380]

**Table 5-2** Possible Systemic Effects of Nonsteroidal Antiinflammatory Drugs

| Site | Sign/Symptom |
|---|---|
| Gastrointestinal | Abdominal pain<br>Anorexia<br>Gastroesophageal reflux<br>Gastric ulcers<br>GI hemorrhage and perforation<br>GI obstruction<br>Nausea<br>Diarrhea |
| Hepatic | Jaundice<br>Transaminase elevation |
| Renal | Sodium and water retention<br>Hypertension (particularly in clients with hypertension)<br>Hyperkalemia<br>Renal insufficiency<br>• Papillary necrosis<br>• Nephrotic syndrome<br>• Interstitial nephritis<br>Renal dysgenesis (infants of mothers given NSAIDs during third trimester)<br>Decreased urate excretion (especially with ASA) |
| Hematologic | Thrombocytopenia<br>Anemia<br>Prolonged bleeding time<br>Increased risk of hemorrhage |
| Cardiovascular | Blunt action of cardiovascular drugs (e.g., diuretics, ACE inhibitors, β-blockers)<br>Hyper- or hypotension<br>Congestive heart failure (for those on diuretics or otherwise volume depleted)<br>Edema (exacerbation of CHF)<br>Prèmature closure of ductus arteriosus<br>Myocardial infarction<br>Stroke<br>Thrombosis |
| Cutaneous | Rashes<br>Pruritus<br>Flushing<br>Urticaria (hives), angioedema<br>Sweating |
| Respiratory | Bronchospasm—ASA sensitive asthma<br>Rhinitis |
| Central nervous system | Headache<br>Vertigo<br>Dizziness, lightheadedness<br>Drowsiness<br>Aseptic meningitis—rarely seen with ibuprofen therapy<br>Tinnitus<br>Hyperventilation (salicylates)<br>Confusion (elderly treated with ASA, indomethacin, ibuprofen) |
| Ophthalmologic | Blurred vision, decreased acuity<br>Scotomata |
| Other | Anaphylaxis<br>Shock<br>Prolongation of gestation<br>Labor inhibition |

*ACE*, Angiotensin-converting enzyme; *ASA*, aspirin; *CHF*, congestive heart failure; *NSAIDs*, nonsteroidal antiinflammatory drugs.
From Grosser T, Smyth E, FitzGerald GA. Anti-inflammatory, antipyretic, and analgesic agents; pharmacotherapy of gout. In: Brunton LL, Chabner BA, Knollmann BC, eds: *Goodman & Gilman's the pharmacological basis of therapeutics*, ed 12, New York, 2011, McGraw Hill, pp. 959–1004.

Although the stomach has received most of the attention for GI-related NSAID toxicities, the small intestine can sustain damage as well. Approximately 55% to 75% of asymptomatic NSAID users have evidence of injury to the small bowel.[142,240] Erosions, ulcers, and strictures[439] from chronic NSAID use have been documented. These intestinal types of lesions may also be potentiated by the concomitant use of a PPI.[35,68]

**Renal System.** Kidney toxicities caused by NSAIDS are less common than GI or cardiovascular. However, approximately 1% to 5% of people taking an NSAID will experience a kidney-related toxicity.[419] In the kidney, COX-dependent prostaglandins are involved with renin release, sodium excretion, and maintenance of renal blood flow, especially during times of volume contraction. When NSAIDs block the production of prostaglandins, conditions or medications that create a low volume state (and decrease renal perfusion) increase the risk for kidney injury. Some of these conditions include heart failure, nephrotic syndrome, liver failure, or those clients taking angiotensin-converting enzyme inhibitors (ACEI) or angiotensin receptor blockers (ARBs).[22] Inhibition of COX enzymes leads to hyperkalemia, a result of the suppression of the renin-aldosterone system; sodium retention, with resulting edema; and decreased glomerular filtration rate (GFR), hypertension, and acute kidney injury.[71,406] To varying degrees, all NSAIDs can cause sodium retention and edema in susceptible people. NSAIDs may also cause acid–base disorders and electrolyte abnormalities, as well as acute interstitial nephritis (immune-related inflammation with associated injury) and papillary necrosis (necrosis of the kidney due to ischemia). NSAIDs should be avoided in clients at risk for kidney injury. Since elderly clients often have several comorbidities, care should be taken when prescribing NSAIDs to older clients.[393,207]

**Cardiovascular System.** In 2004 and 2005, rofecoxib and valdecoxib (selective COX-2 inhibitors) were taken off the market due to increased cardiovascular events.[429] However, studies confirm that both nonselective and COX-2 selective NSAIDs increase the risk for serious adverse cardiovascular events, such as myocardial infarction (MI), stroke, and cardiovascular death.[52,141,142,148,164] Other adverse clinical outcomes include atrial fibrillation, venous thromboembolism, and heart failure.[335,394] These risks persist with continued use.[290]

The mechanism for cardiovascular injury is most likely multifactorial. NSAIDs are known to inhibit the enzyme COX-2 and the production of prostacyclin (vasodilator and platelet function inhibitor) by vascular endothelial cells. There is, however, not a significant concomitant inhibition of thromboxane A2 (a vasoconstrictor and platelet agonist), which leads to a prothombotic state and increased risk for stroke and MI. Additional side effects that contribute to cardiac injury include increased blood pressure, fluid retention, and induction of reactive oxygen species.[153,389]

NSAIDs are also known to interact with hypertension medications, particularly angiotensin-converting enzyme inhibitors, angiotensin receptor blockers, and β-blockers, thereby modestly increasing blood pressure.[411,420] Careful monitoring is required of older adults taking NSAIDs in both the short and long term.

### Risk Factors

When prescribing NSAIDs, consideration of side effects must be taken into account, individualizing treatment according to risk factors the client may have.[3,334,390,431] Risk factors associated with increased toxicities include advanced age, higher doses, increased frequency, volume depletion, concurrent use of corticosteroids, SSRIs, anticoagulants, previous history of GI bleed or ulcer, or serious comorbidities.[72,334] NSAID-induced cardiovascular event risks are higher in persons with established cardiovascular disease. For individuals already taking aspirin, the addition of an NSAID increases the risk of GI bleeding.

## Immunosuppressive Agents

Immunosuppressive agents are used traditionally and most frequently in organ and bone marrow transplantation. These medications have also been found to be helpful in treating other diseases, such as autoimmune diseases, but because of their significant toxicities are only indicated for serious, debilitating, and nonresponding disease.

Immunosuppressive agents for transplantation are used to initially induce immunosuppression (induction therapy), maintain immunosuppression (maintenance therapy), or treat acute rejection. The period of time with the highest risk for acute rejection begins right

**SPECIAL IMPLICATIONS FOR THE THERAPIST 5-3**

### *Nonsteroidal Antiinflammatory Drugs*

The therapist is advised to observe for any side effects or adverse reactions to NSAIDs, especially among older adults; those taking high doses of NSAIDs for long periods (e.g., for RA); those with peptic ulcers, renal or hepatic disease, CHF, or hypertension; and those treated with anticoagulants. NSAIDs have antiplatelet effects that can be synergistic with the anticoagulant effects of drugs such as warfarin (Coumadin). Easy bruising and bleeding under the skin may be early signs of hemorrhage.

*Ulcer presentation without pain occurs more often in older adults and in those taking NSAIDs. Often, people who take prescription NSAIDs also take Advil or aspirin. Combining these medications or combining these medications with drinking alcohol increases the risk for development of peptic ulcer disease. Any client with GI symptoms should report these to their physician.*

*Musculoskeletal symptoms may recur after discontinuing NSAIDs because of the pain-relieving effects of antiinflammatory agents and the fact that they do not prevent tissue injury or affect the underlying disease process.*[254]

*Depending on the therapy intervention planned, the therapist may schedule the client according to the timing of the medication dosage. For example, with a chronic condition such as adhesive capsulitis, the goal may be to increase joint accessory motion, which requires more vigorous joint mobilization techniques. Relieving local painful symptoms may help the client remain relaxed during mobilization procedures.*

*When pain can be predicted (i.e., pain is brought on by treatment intervention), the drug's peak effect should be timed to coincide with the painful event. For nonopioids, such as NSAIDs, the peak effect occurs approximately 2 hours after oral administration. However, in a condition such as shoulder impingement syndrome, teaching the client proper positioning and functional movement to avoid painful impingement may require treatment without the maximal benefit of medication. The therapy session could be scheduled for a time just before the next scheduled dosage.*

*NSAIDs produce modest increases in blood pressure, averaging 5 mm Hg, and should be avoided in people who have borderline blood pressures or are hypertensive. All NSAIDs are renal vasoconstrictors with the potential of increasing blood pressure, resulting in increased fluid retention, especially lower-extremity edema. NSAIDs also reduce the antihypertensive effects of β-blockers and angiotensin-converting enzyme inhibitors and should generally be avoided in people receiving these cardiac medications. Interaction between most NSAIDs and loop and thiazide diuretics reduces the effects of the diuretic and may lead to a worsening of CHF in a person predisposed to this condition.*

*It is important to check blood pressure the first few weeks of therapy and to periodically check thereafter to identify any adverse blood pressure response to the combination of NSAIDs, antihypertensive agents, and activity. In addition, NSAIDs may increase serum potassium and lithium levels. Indomethacin may increase the plasma concentration of digoxin, requiring close monitoring of digoxin levels.*

after surgery and continues for 3 to 6 months. Induction therapy refers to intense immunosuppressive treatments started after surgery to reduce the risk of acute rejection. This may involve the use of anti-thymocyte polyclonal antibodies and IL-2 receptor antagonists. Maintenance therapy refers to the agents required throughout a person's lifetime to prevent both acute and chronic rejection. Agents typically utilized include glucocorticoids, a calcineurin inhibitor, an antiproliferative agent, and an antimetabolite drug. Acute rejection (either T-cell mediated or antibody mediated) can be treated with corticosteroids and/or by increasing the dosage of maintenance drugs, among other therapies.

Many of the newer drugs used for immunosuppression are monoclonal antibodies. *Monoclonal antibodies* are designed to target a specific antigen that is required for graft rejection. Muromonab-CD3, one of the first monoclonal antibodies approved, had significant side effects and marketing was discontinued in 2010 because of the availability of other effective, but less toxic, drugs. Numerous monoclonal antibodies are currently approved for many types of disease, such as RA, Crohn disease, hematologic cancers, and dermatologic diseases.

**Drug Classes and Mechanisms of Action.** Immunosuppressive drugs fall into multiple classes depending on their mechanisms of action.[428] The main types of immunosuppressives are: (1) T cell–directed agents (e.g., calcineurin inhibitors), (2) B cell–directed agents (e.g., Rituximab), (3) agents that target cytokines (e.g., corticosteroids, Basiliximab), (4) immunosuppressive agents with multiple cellular targets (e.g., antiproliferative and antimetabolite agents, Sirolimus, Alemtuzumab, azathioprine and micophenolate), and (5) pooled polyclonal antibodies.

Drugs that affect T cells include *calcineurin* drugs (target signal 1) and agents that block signal 2. T cells play a key role in graft rejection, so one method of reducing rejection is to block T-cell activation. The calcineurin agents inhibit transcription of genes required for further T-cell activation, or the first signal. Well-known examples of this class of medication are cyclosporine and tacrolimus. Careful drug monitoring is required for cyclosporine and tacrolimus because toxicities are often dosage dependent. These drugs lead to vasoconstriction, which increases blood pressure and reduces blood flow to the kidney. Once a T cell has been activated and an effective immune response has begun, there is normally a downregulation of T cells in order to hold the response in check.[428] New hybrid protein medications imitate this downregulation process or affect the second signal in T cell response, such as Belatacept.

Another group of immunosuppressant medications function by altering B-cell maturation and differentiation. Rituximab is a monoclonal antibody and an example of an agent that blocks CD20. CD20 is a transmembrane protein that is responsible for B-cell differentiation. People are at risk for reactivation of hepatitis B.[243] Belimumab inhibits B-cell maturation, whereas Eculizumab interferes in the proinflammatory role of complement, thus diminishing neutrophil function.[363]

Several immunosuppressive agents act by inhibiting various cytokines. Cytokines are released by cells in order to regulate the immune response. Corticosteroids are the oldest and most common immunosuppressant in this category. Corticosteroids inhibit all cytokine transcription, making it very nonspecific in its inhibition. Because of the global suppression of the immune system and possibility for severe side effects, most transplant recipients are tapered off of corticosteroids over the first year following transplantation.[432] Basiliximab is a specific monoclonal antibody that inhibits IL-2 binding (IL-2 receptor antagonist).[246] After T cells respond to signals 1 and 2, binding of IL-2 leads to T-cell proliferation. Basiliximab blocks this proliferation. Tocilizumab inhibits IL-6 and is being studied for various roles in preventing transplant rejection.[73]

Many of the drugs used for immunosuppression have multiple cellular targets. Alemtuzumab binds CD52, found on both T and B cells. Antiproliferative agents, such as Sirolimus and Everolimus, inhibit the mTOR pathway. This pathway is utilized to signal cell progression and proliferation in lymphocytes, as well as multiple other cell types. Azathioprine (AZA) and its metabolites are purine analogs that interfere with purine synthesis and the synthesis of DNA and RNA. It also halts cell cycle progression. Mycophenolate inhibits the enzyme IMPDH, which is required for purine and DNA synthesis. Mycophenolate (MMF) is the most commonly used antimetabolite in transplant medicine. It has been found to have less toxicity than mTOR inhibitors and better efficacy than AZA for prevention of rejection. Due to differing side effects (people treated with MMF had more tissue-invasive CMV), use of drugs should be tailored to the client.[212,407]

The last class of immunosuppressants is *polyclonal antibodies,* which are given as a prophylaxis for early rejection (desensitization) or can by used in induction of immunosuppression.[415] Unlike monoclonal antibody medications, which are targeted against a specific antigen involved in rejection, polyclonal antibody agents are directed against multiple antigens. Examples of this class of agents are intravenous Ig (IVIG), antithymocyte globulin-rabbit (thymoglobulin) and Fresenius antithymocyte globulin (ATG).[152,169] Thymoglobulin is made by immunizing rabbits with human thymocytes. ATG is created by immunizing rabbits with lymphocytes from a T cell leukemia cell line. IgG is separated out from the sera and then purified. Many of the IgG immunoglobulins are anti-T cell, leading to a depletion of T cells; however they are nonspecific and may react with other cell types.

### Adverse Effects

All immunosuppressants have adverse side effects, some of the most serious being an elevated risk of infection[94,131,132] and transplant-related malignancies.[413] However, some immunosuppressants may actually decrease the incidence of malignancy, such as the proliferation signal inhibitors sirolimus and everolimus.[62] Adverse effects related to immunosuppression are often the most serious consequences of transplantation. Most immunosuppressive agents render transplant recipients prone to infection, particularly cytomegalovirus. There is also an increased risk of developing fungal (especially *Candida* species) and bacterial infections. Viruses, such as herpes simplex virus and varicella zoster, may disseminate or reactivate.

An increase in certain kinds of malignancy occurs with long-term use of immunosuppressants, including lymphoma and other lymphoproliferative malignancies and nonmelanoma skin cancers.[180,305] Host and graft survival are improving, making infection and cancer more relevant complications. Newer protocols are being developed to reduce the risk for infection and cancer.[69]

The goal of therapy is to provide an adequate balance of immunosuppression so that transplant clients do not experience rejection, while endeavoring to minimize side effects. Drugs are administered at the lowest possible doses while still maintaining adequate immunosuppression. Individual medical factors often determine the choice of immunosuppressive agent. For example, clients who have hypertension or hyperlipidemia may be given tacrolimus instead of cyclosporine. Usually, intensive immunosuppression is required only during the first few weeks after organ transplantation or during rejection crises. Subsequently, the immune system accommodates the graft and can be maintained with relatively small doses of immunosuppressive drugs, with fewer adverse effects. Table 5.3 provides a summary of drug-related adverse effects of immunosuppressive agents.

**SPECIAL IMPLICATIONS FOR THE THERAPIST 5-4**

*Immunosuppressants*

Careful handwashing is essential before contact with any client who is immunosuppressed. If the therapist has a known infectious or contagious condition, the therapist should *not* work with the immunosuppressed client. Both client and therapist can wear a mask in the presence of an upper respiratory infection.

*Peripheral neuropathies and subsequent functional impairment can be addressed by the therapist while the client waits for resolution of these side effects. Upper-extremity splinting (e.g., cockup splint for the hand) may be appropriate, or an ankle-foot orthosis to prevent falls and assist in continued and safe ambulation may be provided.[59] Delayed response in the fingers and toes to temperature may require education to prevent injuries.*

## Corticosteroids

Corticosteroids are naturally occurring hormones produced by the adrenal cortex. These hormones are steroid-based, with similar chemical structures but quite different physiologic effects. Generally, they are divided into *glucocorticoids* (cortisol), which mainly affect carbohydrate and protein metabolism; and *mineralocorticoids* (aldosterone), which regulate electrolyte and water metabolism. Many corticoidsteroid hormones can be synthesized for clinical use. Box 5.5 contains a list of commonly prescribed synthetic corticosteroids.

Glucocorticoids are used to decrease inflammation in a broad range of local or systemic conditions, for immunosuppression (see"Immunosuppressive Agents" above), and as an essential replacement steroid for adrenal insufficiency.

Therapists most often see people who have received prolonged, systemic glucocorticoid therapy in the treatment of cancer, transplantation, autoimmune disorders, and respiratory diseases (e.g., asthma). Mineralocorticoids are given for adrenal insufficiency or adrenogenital syndrome.

Generally, glucocorticoids cause fluid imbalances, and mineralocorticoids cause electrolyte imbalances. However, mineralocorticoids are used less frequently. Most adverse effects seen by the clinical therapist will be related to glucocorticosteroids.

### Adverse Effects of Glucocorticoids

Glucocorticoids have multiple actions; they exert both antiinflammatory and immunosuppressive properties. However, long-term use of glucocorticoids to sustain disease benefits is accompanied by an increased risk of side effects and adrenal suppression. Fortunately, glucocorticoids for treatment of most illnesses are used for a limited time along with disease-modifying medications, whereas long-term use is only necessary for adrenal insufficiency and a few other diseases (e.g., inhaled steroids for asthma).

Glucocorticoids affect many functions of the body, especially in persons taking long-term steroids. Therapists should be familiar with common adverse effects, such as change in sleep and mood, GI irritation, hyperglycemia, bone loss, and fluid retention (Table 5.4); side effects are related to dose and duration of treatment.[111,190] Each synthetic glucocorticoid varies in its bioavailability and its ability to bind to cell receptors and regulate gene expression.[320] The most serious side effect of steroid use is increased susceptibility to infection and the masking of inflammatory symptoms from infection or intraabdominal complications.

**Mood.** Most clients taking glucocorticoids notice a change in mood, behavior, or sleep. Individuals often describe a nervous or "jittery" feeling. Symptoms may range from mild anxiety and hypomania to confusion or psychosis. People receiving longer courses of glucocorticoids can also experience depression. Changes are typically noted 5 to 14 days after glucocorticoid therapy begins; improvement is seen with withdrawal of the medication.

**Effects on Skin and Connective Tissue.** Effects on the skin and connective tissue include thinning of the

**Table 5-3** Major Immunosuppressive Agents and Adverse Effects[a]

| Agent | FDA-labeled Indications for Use | Adverse Effects |
|---|---|---|
| Antithymocyte globulin (rabbit [thymoglobulin], | Renal transplant (acute rejection and induction) | Fever, hypertension, peripheral edema, tachycardia, hypotension, hyperkalemia, shivering, leukopenia, thrombocytopenia, anaphylaxis, cytokine release syndrome |
| Azathioprine (Imuran) | Renal transplant<br>Rheumatoid arthritis | Opportunistic infections, leukopenia, thrombocytopenia, anemia, nausea, vomiting, hepatotoxicity, myalgias, malignancy, infection |
| Basiliximab (Simulect) | Renal transplant | Nausea/vomiting, hyperglycemia, asthenia, insomnia, hypertension, peripheral edema, anemia, dysuria, candidiasis, cough, cytomegalovirus infection, fever, headache, hypersensitivity reactions |
| Corticosteroids (see Box 5-3) | Transplant<br>Various inflammatory conditions<br>Neoplasms<br>Autoimmune diseases | Hypertension, atrophy of skin, fluid retention, decreased body growth, hypernatremia, opportunistic infections, osteoporosis, depression, Cushing syndrome, hyperglycemia, adrenocortical insufficiency, cataract, glaucoma, pulmonary tuberculosis |
| Cyclosporine (Sandimmune, Neoral) | Renal, cardiac, hepatic transplant | Opportunistic infections, renal disease, hypertension, malignant neoplasms (lymphoma and skin cancers), hirsutism, hyperglycemia, headache, electrolyte abnormalities |
| Intravenous immune globulin (IVIG) | Immunodeficiency,<br>Infections, Autoimmune/inflammatory conditions, | Hypotension, thromboembolic events (MI, stroke, VTE), headache, acute kidney injury, hyponatremia, diarrhea, nausea/vomiting, flushing, pruritus, muscle pain, fatigue, fever, tachycardia, hemolytic anemia, rarely anaphylaxis. Can impair response to live vaccines. |
| Mycophenolate mofetil (CellCept)<br>Mycophenolate sodium (Myfortic), enteric coated for delayed release | Renal, cardiac, and hepatic transplant | Opportunistic infections, leukopenia, gastrointestinal complaints (diarrhea, nausea, dyspepsia), elevated transaminases. Possible association with Progressive Multifocal Leukoencephalopathy (PML). |
| Sirolimus (Rapamune) | Renal transplant | Opportunistic infection, malignant neoplasms, gastrointestinal complaints (diarrhea and nausea), elevation of liver enzymes, decrease in platelets and leukocytes, epistaxis, blood pressure changes, headaches, hypertriglyceridemia |
| Tacrolimus (Prograf) | Hepatic, cardiac, and renal transplant | Opportunistic infections, renal disease, hypertension, malignant neoplasms, hyperglycemia, neurotoxicity (tremor, headaches, sensory changes), hirsutism, pulmonary symptoms (dyspnea), gastrointestinal complaints (nausea, vomiting, abdominal pain) |

[a]All immunosuppressive agents increase the incidence of infection and may increase the potential for malignancies (posttransplantation lymphoproliferative disease, skin malignancies).

**Box 5.5**

**COMMONLY PRESCRIBED CORTICOSTEROIDS**

- Betamethasone (Celestone; Diprolene)
- Beclomethasone (Qvar [inhaler])
- Budesonide (Symbicort [combination product inhaler])
- Cortisone (Cortone)
- Desoximetasone (Topicort)
- Dexamethasone (Decadron; Dexameth; Dexone;)
- Fludrocortisone (Florinef)
- Fluticasone (Flonase [nasal spray]; Advair [inhaler])
- Hydrocortisone (Solu-Cortef; Cortef; Hydrocortone)
- Methylprednisolone (Medrol; Solu-Medrol; Depo-Medrol; A-Methapred)
- Prednisolone (Pediapred; Delta-Cortef; Prelone)
- Prednisone (Deltasone; Liquid Pred)
- Triamcinolone (Aristocort; Kenacort; Kenalog; Nasacort AQ [nasal spray])

subcutaneous tissue, accompanied by splitting of elastic fibers with resultant red or purple striae (stretch marks). Ecchymoses (bruising) and petechiae are caused by decreased vascular strength.

Glucocorticoids alter the response of connective tissue to injury by inhibiting collagen synthesis,[78] which is why these agents are used to suppress manifestations of collagen diseases. Clients who are taking steroids experience delayed wound healing with decreased wound strength, inhibited tissue contraction for wound closure, and impeded epithelization.

**Cardiovascular Effects.** Corticosteroids are related to increased fluid retention, hypertension and atherosclerotic disease. As with other effects of glucocorticoids, cardiovascular effects are dose-dependent and, for individuals receiving low doses, these effects are less noticeable. Fluid retention may be a factor in disease exacerbation in people with heart failure or kidney disease. Worsening

**Table 5-4** Possible Adverse Effects of Prolonged Systemic Corticosteroids

| System | Symptom |
|---|---|
| Metabolic | Increases glucose/protein metabolism |
| | Stimulates appetite |
| | Weight gain with truncal obesity |
| | Hypokalemia |
| | Suppresses hypothalamic-pituitary-adrenal axis |
| Endocrine | Delays puberty |
| | Reduces estrogen and testosterone production |
| | Menstrual irregularities and amenorrhea |
| | Hyperglycemia |
| | Insulin resistance |
| | Diabetes |
| | Cushing syndrome (hypercortisolism) |
| Cardiovascular | Dyslipidemia |
| | Increases blood pressure |
| | Fluid retention/edema |
| | Capillary fragility |
| | Heart failure |
| | Ischemic heart disease |
| Immune | Increases risk of opportunistic infections |
| | Activates latent viruses |
| | Masks infection |
| Musculoskeletal | Increases muscle catabolism (degenerative myopathy, muscle wasting) |
| | Retards bone growth |
| | Tendon rupture |
| | Osteoporosis |
| | Osteonecrosis, avascular necrosis of femoral head |
| | Bone fractures |
| Gastrointestinal | Peptic ulcer disease |
| | Gastrointestinal bleeding |
| | Gastritis |
| | Pancreatitis |
| | Nausea |
| Nervous | *Central:* Changes behavior (insomnia, euphoria, nervousness) |
| | Psychosis, depression |
| | Changes cognition, mood, and memory |
| | Cerebral atrophy |
| | Pseudotumor cerebri |
| | *Autonomic:* Autonomic nervous system dysfunction |
| | *Peripheral:* Peripheral neuropathy |
| Ophthalmologic | Cataracts |
| | Glaucoma |
| Integumentary | Acne |
| | Striae (stretch marks) |
| | Bruising, petechiae |
| | Dermal thinning |
| | Delays wound healing |
| | Hirsutism |
| | Facial erythema |
| | Increases sweating |

Based on data from Moghadam-Kia S, Werth VP: Prevention and treatment of systemic glucocorticoid side effects, *Int J Dermatol* 49(3):239–248, 2010; Stanbury RM, Graham EM: Systemic corticosteroid therapy—side effects and their management, *Br J Ophthalmol* 82(6):704–708, 1998; Barnes PJ: Pulmonary pharmacology. In Brunton LL, Chabner BA, Knollmann BC, editors: *Goodman & Gilman's the pharmacological basis of therapeutics,* ed 12, New York, 2011, McGraw Hill, pp. 1031–1066; Cannon GW: Immunosuppressing drugs including corticosteroids. In Goldman L, Shafer AI, Arend WP, et al, editors: *Goldman's Cecil medicine,* ed 24, New York, 2012, Elsevier, pp. 159–165.

of high blood pressure is typically seen at high instead of low doses. Persons with inflammatory disease, such as RA, that require glucocorticoids may have increased rates of myocardial infarction, heart failure, and stroke.[17,358]

**Steroid-Induced Myopathy.** In high doses, glucocorticoids can cause muscle weakness and atrophy called *steroid-induced myopathy.* Glucocorticoids reduce protein synthesis (mediated by a reduction of growth factors), while increasing muscle catabolism (by increasing the expression of genes involved with atrophy). This results in muscle wasting and atrophy severe enough to interfere with daily function and activities.[304]

**Table 5-5 Functional Classifications of Corticosteroid-Induced Myopathy**

| Level | Function |
|---|---|
| Advanced | Person has difficulty climbing stairs |
| High | Person cannot rise from a chair |
| Intermediate | Person cannot walk without assistance |
| Low | Person cannot elevate extremities or move in bed |

Modified from Askari A, Vignos PJ, Moskoweitz RW: Steroid myopathy in connective tissue disease, *Am J Med* 61:485–492, 1976.

Steroid-induced myopathy is insidious, appearing as painless proximal weakness, in both the upper and lower extremities, weeks to months after the initiation of treatment. There is no special or definitive test to make the diagnosis of myopathy, and the diagnosis is one of exclusion. Electromyograms and muscle enzymes are often normal, and muscle biopsies are nonspecific.

Clients present with bilateral atrophy and weakness of proximal muscles; the pelvis, hips, and thighs are typically affected first. Upper limb muscles can be affected; occasionally distal limb muscles are involved. The diaphragm may also be involved, which results in difficulty breathing, especially in people with underlying pulmonary disease. Physical therapy intervention may be helpful in counteracting this glucocorticoid-induced muscle dysfunction.[221]

Recovery from chronic myopathy (with cessation of drug) is possible with reduction or discontinuation of the drug. Improvement is most often seen after 3-4 weeks, but may take months up to 1 to 2 years.[304] Prognosis depends on the underlying diagnosis before treatment with corticosteroids (e.g., organ transplantation requiring long-term administration of glucocorticoids) but nearly all recover with discontinuation of glucocorticoids. Four functional classifications of muscle weakness can occur in people with steroid-induced myopathy (Table 5.5).

**Effect on Growth and Bone.** Long-term use of glucocorticoids in children causes apoptosis of the chondrocytes at the epiphyseal plate, leading to growth retardation.[113] Although there is an increase in bone synthesis once the drug is discontinued, full height may not be achieved.[398] In adults, prolonged use of glucocorticoids inhibits bone mineralization, induces apoptosis of osteoblasts, and encourages osteoclastic activity.[51] There is also decreased GI calcium absorption and increased calcium excretion by the kidneys, leading to elevated serum PTH levels, also increasing bone resorption. These combined changes result in osteoporosis.[78,230,421] Strategies should be in place before extended therapy of glucocorticoids (greater than 3 months) to avoid bone loss.[53,325] Bone fractures from glucocorticoid use are seen at higher bone mineral densities (BMD) than fractures from postmenopausal osteoporosis.

Long-term exposure to corticosteroids increases the risk of avascular necrosis, which often requires orthopedic intervention (e.g., total hip replacement). Glucocorticosteroids are also associated with an increase in the prevalence of vertebral fracture compared with individuals who are not treated with corticosteroids.[159,228]

**Hyperglycemia.** Elevated blood glucose due to corticosteroids is a frequently encountered problem. Total dose and duration of therapy are predictors for the development of hyperglycemia.[83] Glucocorticoids produce hyperglycemia through increasing insulin resistance by interfering with signaling cascades. They may also reduce the production of insulin by promoting apoptosis of pancreatic beta cells. Because of the insulin resistance, the liver is not as sensitive to the presence of insulin and continues gluconeogenesis despite elevated blood glucose levels. Fat and muscle cells also exhibit insulin resistance and do not readily take up glucose.[220] Individuals already requiring oral diabetic agents or insulin frequently need an increase in their dosage and uncommonly induce diabetes mellitus.[372] Persons at risk for diabetes (e.g., glucose intolerance) may require a diabetic agent.[378] Glucose monitoring is essential. New therapies may be available to prevent the development of steroid-induced hyperglycemia.[401]

**Other Side Effects.** For clients with asthma, long-term treatment with inhaled glucocorticoids is common. Glucocorticoids decrease inflammation and aid in counteracting the vasodilation caused by $\beta_2$ agonists. Researchers initially hoped that the inhaled delivery of the glucocorticoids would eliminate or significantly reduce the side effects of the glucocorticoids; but bone loss and other adverse effects remain problematic in people with asthma or chronic obstructive pulmonary disease (COPD) using inhaled steroids.[93,192,208]

The GI effects of steroids are fewer than with NSAIDs, yet they are known to cause gastritis, esophageal irritation, GI bleeding, and, less commonly, peptic ulcers. Many clients take both glucocorticoids and NSAIDs, increasing their risk for adverse GI events (e.g., ulcer with perforation). For these individuals, a GI protective agent (e.g., proton pump inhibitor or misoprostol) may be beneficial.

Glucocorticoids are also known to cause cataracts, typically in the posterior subcapsular area. Cataract formation is dependent on dose and duration of use. They typically develop bilaterally but slowly.[199] Development of glaucoma is also related to glucocorticoid use. Clients with a history of glaucoma and taking glucocorticoids long term may have an increase in pressure while taking glucocorticoids, making pressure checks advisable.

Because glucocorticoids cause adrenal suppression, withdrawal must be slow and tapered to allow for endogenous hormones to be produced by the adrenal cortex. Severe adrenal insufficiency may follow sudden withdrawal of the medication, particularly in the presence of infection or other stress. The person may experience vomiting, orthostatic hypotension, hypoglycemia, restlessness, arthralgia, anorexia, malaise, and fatigue.

### Performance-Enhancing Drugs and Anabolic–Androgenic Steroids

Performance-enhancing drugs (PEDs) are any drug used by athletes and nonathletes to improve athletic ability and performance and/or appearance. These typically include androgens, such as testosterone, anabolic–androgenic steroids, androgen precursors, and selective androgen receptor modulators (SARMS). Other drugs such as human chorionic gonadotropin and antiestrogens (e.g., tamoxifen, raloxifene) lead to an increase in testosterone levels. One of the more commonly used PEDs is anabolic–androgenic steroids (AASs). Anabolic–androgenic, anabolic steroids, or "roids," are synthetic derivatives of the hormone testosterone. They are most commonly used in a nonmedical setting to develop secondary male characteristics (androgenic function) and to build muscle tissue (anabolic function).[36-38] The use of anabolic steroids to enhance physical performance by athletes has been declared illegal by all national and international athletic committees. Even so, an estimated 3 to 4 million individuals in the United States alone are current or past nonmedical users of AASs and over 1 million have experienced dependence.[101,311] Administration of these compounds can be orally, transdermally, or by IM injection, with IM injection the most common route.

In 2006, 500 AAS users who frequented AAS internet sites were questioned about their habits. Ninety-nine percent stated they most frequently injected the steroids and 13% used unsafe needle practices.[300]

**Users.** Most users begin in their 20s, with only 22% starting before the age of 20.[311] Studies indicate that adolescent AAS[214] users are significantly more likely to be males and to use other illicit drugs, alcohol, and tobacco.[16] AAS users of all ages are more likely to use illicit drugs and alcohol than those who do not use AAS.[112] Previously, more athletes were found to use AAS than nonathletes to enhance their sport. However, now the majority of AAS users are nonathlete weight lifters who want to enhance their masculine appearance. A broader spectrum of users is also found among professionals working in military, law enforcement, and casual fitness enthusiasts.[13,64,205]

The use of this type of steroid is illegal and potentially unsafe, unless given under the direction of a licensed physician; most of these drugs cannot even be prescribed legally but are still obtained from the internet, other athletes, physicians, and coaches.

Athletes tend to take doses that are 10, 100, or even 1000 times larger than the doses prescribed for medical purposes. Users exhibit various patterns in taking AAS. They may escalate the dosage prior to a competition, a technique known as *pyramiding*, or combine 2 or more different steroids or drugs, called *stacking*. They then taper the dose down or even stop using AAS for a time, termed *off-cycle*, in order to avoid detection and recover from side effects. Human growth hormone, diuretics, IGF-1, and blood boosters (such as erythropoietin) have been used alone and in combination with anabolic steroids to further enhance athletic performance.[50] Many users attempt to mask side effects with other drugs.

**Adverse Effects.** Nearly all users of AAS report side effects; some side effects are reversible with cessation of the drugs, while others may be permanent. The most common include mood disorders (e.g., mania, hypomania, and depression), excessive muscle bulk, severe acne, and aggression (Fig. 5.2).[283,310] Individuals may also develop dyslipidemia, with an increase in low-density lipoproteins and a decrease in high-density lipoproteins, complicating atherosclerosis and coronary artery disease.[13] The development of thrombosis (i.e., venous thromboembolism, stroke, retinal vein occlusion) is also seen in persons taking AAS.[235,310] Gynecomastia is frequently present due to high levels of peripheral testosterone that is converted

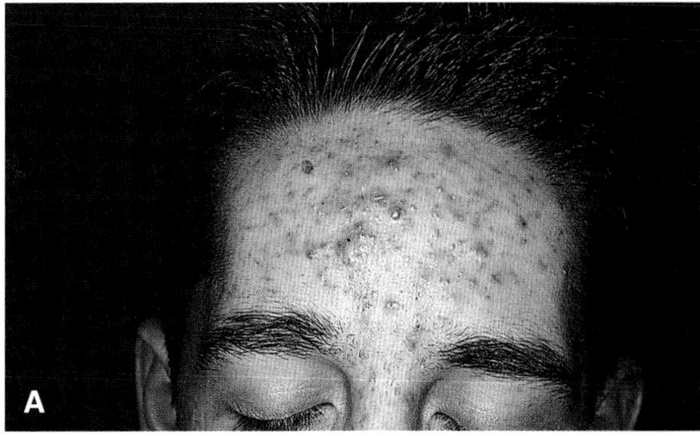


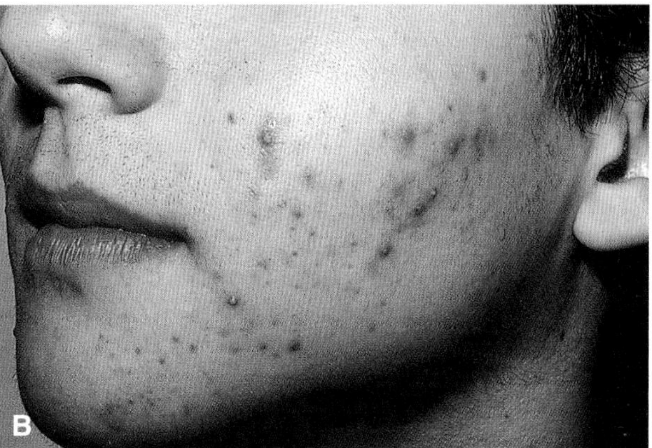


**Figure 5.2**

**Acne vulgaris on the forehead (A) and lower face (B) associated with the use of anabolic steroids.** It is considered an abnormal response to normal levels of the male hormone testosterone. The face, chest, back, shoulders, and upper arms are especially affected. There are many other causes of this form of acne; its presence does not necessarily mean the individual is using anabolic steroids. (From Callen JP: *Color atlas of dermatology*, ed 2, Philadelphia, 2000, WB Saunders.)

to estradiol. Elevated levels of serum testosterone suppress the secretion of gonadotropin, causing small testes, decreased spermatogenesis, and infertility.[115]

Misuse of supraphysiologic doses of AAS for nonmedical reasons has been linked with serious side effects, such as hypertension, left ventricular hypertrophy, myocardial ischemia, polycythemia, cardiac conduction abnormalities, and rarely peliosis hepatis (liver tissue is replaced by hemorrhagic cysts), hepatocellular carcinoma, and sudden and premature death.[2,14,109,170,224,256,338]

Users of anabolic steroids may experience an increased susceptibility to tendon strains and injuries, especially biceps and patellar tendons, because muscle size and strength increase at a rate far greater than tendon and connective tissue strength.[204] Adolescent steroid use may lead to accelerated maturation and premature epiphyseal closure.[371]

Shared use of multidose vials, dividing drugs using syringes, and increased sexual risk-taking behavior are risk factors associated with AAS use and are potential routes for HIV and hepatitis infection.[249] Contaminated vials or improper injection technique also lead to abscesses at injection sites.

**Therapeutic Use.** There are, however, legitimate medical uses for anabolic steroids that have come about as a result of physiologic evidence that anabolic steroids prevent loss of lean body mass. Oxandrolone, a synthetically derived testosterone, is approved as an adjuvant therapy to promote weight gain after weight loss secondary to chronic infections (HIV wasting), severe trauma (severe burns),[313] Turner syndrome,[140,332] and extensive surgery.

Another anabolic steroid with a practical use is oxymetholone. It is indicated for the adjuvant treatment of anemia secondary to a lack of red blood cell production such as occurs in Fanconi anemia. Because of the side effects and drug interactions, these agents should be used with caution.

SPECIAL IMPLICATIONS FOR THE THERAPIST 5-5

## *Corticosteroids*

### Inflammation and Infection

In the rehabilitation setting, large doses of steroids are administered early in the treatment of traumatic brain injury and in some spinal cord–injured clients to control cerebral or spinal cord edema. Suppression of the inflammatory reaction in people who are given large doses of steroids may be so complete as to mask the clinical signs and symptoms of major diseases, intraabdominal complications, or spread of infection (blocking of inflammatory mediators). In the orthopedic population, local symptoms of pain or discomfort are also masked, so the therapist must exercise caution during evaluation or treatment to avoid exacerbating the underlying inflammatory process.

*Increased susceptibility to the infections associated with impaired cellular immunity and the decreased rate of recovery from infection associated with corticosteroid use requires careful infection control. Special care should be taken to avoid exposing immunosuppressed clients to infection, and everyone in contact with that person should follow strict handwashing policies.*

*Some facilities recommend that people with a white blood cell count of less than 1000 mm³ or a neutrophil count of less than 500 mm³ wear a protective mask. Therapists should ensure that anyone who is immunosuppressed is provided with equipment that has been disinfected according to standard precautions.*

*If back pain occurs in a person who is receiving corticosteroids, diagnostic measures should be undertaken to rule out osteoporosis or compression fracture.*

### Intensive Care Setting

Although clients in the intensive care unit (ICU) are often treated with steroids for various serious illnesses, the use of these medications may increase the risk for complications, such as infection, impaired wound healing, ICU-acquired paresis (ICUAP) or muscle weakness,[100] or death. Individuals who develop ICUAP have been found to require mechanical ventilation for a longer period of time compared to those without ICUAP, supporting clinical observations that clients treated with glucocorticoids often experience difficulty weaning from the ventilator or clearing lung secretions.

*Glucocorticoids (methylprednisolone) do not improve persistent acute respiratory distress syndrome, and if begun 2 weeks after the initial episode, may increase the risk for death.*[121] *Glucocorticoids, however, may be of benefit to clients with COPD requiring mechanical ventilation.*[280] *Studies are ongoing to determine the most efficacious use of glucocorticoids in this fragile population.*

### Intraarticular Injections

Occasionally, intraarticular injections of corticosteroids are necessary to control acute pain in a joint that is not responding to oral analgesics, particularly if an effusion is present. Such injections can provide short-term relief and improve the client's mobility and function.[202] The rationale for use in the joint is to suppress the synovitis because no evidence currently indicates that intraarticular injections retard the progression of erosive disease. Intraarticular injections must be carefully selected, and no single joint should have more than three or four injections before other procedures are pursued.[274]

*Most steroid injections are accompanied by an anesthetizing agent, such as lidocaine or bupivacaine, which usually provides immediate pain relief, although the antiinflammatory effect may require 2 to 3 days. During this time, the client should be advised to continue using proper supportive positioning and avoid movements that would otherwise aggravate the previous symptoms.*

*Some controversy remains as to whether the person can bear weight on the joint for several days after the injection; a less conservative approach permits nonstrenuous activity. Vigorous exercise may speed resorption of the steroid from the joint and reduce the intended effect. Intraarticular injection of corticosteroids may also result in pigment changes that are most noticeable among dark-skinned people.*

### Exercise and Steroids

The harmful side effects of glucocorticoids can be delayed or reduced in their severity by physical activity, regular exercise (aerobic or fitness), strength training, and proper nutrition. Unfortunately, these clients are often too sick to engage in exercise at all, much less at a level of intensity that would reverse myopathy. When possible, the therapist can help emphasize the importance of exercise, especially activities that produce significant stress on the weight-bearing joints (e.g., walking; jogging is not usually recommended), to decrease the calcium loss from long bones that is attributable to prolonged steroid use. It is essential to consult with the client's physician before initiating aerobic exercise.

*Glucocorticoid-induced changes in body composition in heart transplant recipients occur early after transplantation. However, 6 months of specific exercise training restores fat-free mass to levels greater than before transplantation and dramatically increases skeletal muscle strength. Resistance exercise, as part of a strategy to prevent steroid-induced myopathy, should be initiated early after transplantation.*[48]

*Strength training or stair exercise is one way to maintain the large muscle groups of the legs, which are most affected by the muscle-wasting properties of corticosteroids. The treatment plan should also include closed-chained exercises to prevent shearing forces across joint lines and to allow for normal joint loading, prevention of vertebral compression fractures, and education about proper body mechanics during functional activities.*[374]

*Client education on the importance of proper footwear and choice of exercise surfaces is important for the individual receiving long-term corticosteroid therapy. For the person who is at risk for avascular necrosis of the femoral head, exercising the surrounding joint musculature in a non–weight-bearing position may be required.*

### Monitoring Vital Signs

Long-term use of corticosteroids may result in electrolyte imbalances (e.g., hypokalemia, hypocalcemia, metabolic alkalosis, sodium and fluid retention, edema, and hypertension), which necessitates monitoring of vital signs during aerobic activity because of the demand placed on the cardiovascular system in conjunction with these adverse effects.

*Many glucocorticoids have mineralocorticoid activity as well. This causes sodium and fluid retention and enhanced angiotensin II activity, leading to hypertension. Careful monitoring of blood pressure should be performed in clients with previously existing high blood pressure, as glucocorticoid administration may require an increase in the dosage of antihypertensives.*

*Increased fluid retention may also lead to an exacerbation of CHF in susceptible people; monitoring for signs and symptoms of heart failure is important. Clients may develop hypokalemia secondary to potassium loss from the kidneys; individuals with a history of hypokalemia or taking diuretics benefit from monitoring of blood chemistries.*

### Steroids, Nutrition, and Stress

People taking steroids may be advised to increase their dietary intake of calcium and vitamin D to counteract the loss of calcium in the urine.[303] Clients may also require a medication to decrease the loss of bone, such as a bisphosphonate. Protein intake is recommended for muscle growth to offset steroid-induced catabolism. Individuals may also require potassium supplementation because of increased potassium loss in the urine.

*Corticosteroids stimulate gluconeogenesis and interfere with the action of insulin in peripheral cells, which may result in glucose intolerance or diabetes mellitus or may aggravate existing conditions in diabetes. Regular blood glucose monitoring is recommended to detect steroid-induced diabetes mellitus.*

*Some facilities establish exercise protocols based on blood glucose levels. Exercise is not recommended for people with blood glucose levels greater than 300 mg/dL without ketosis or greater than 250 mg/dL with ketosis.*[11]

*Clients taking glucocorticoids long-term for Addison disease or RA may need to increase the required dosage during medically stressful situations, particularly with infections or surgery. Temporary mineralocorticoid dosage increases may also be indicated if the client receiving replacement mineralocorticoid experiences profuse diaphoresis for any reason (strenuous physical exertion, heat spells, or fever).*[133] *Either of these situations requires physician evaluation.*

### Psychologic Considerations

Corticosteroid use can result in a range of mood changes from irritability, euphoria, and nervousness to more serious depression and psychosis. Insomnia is often also a reported problem during corticosteroid therapy. The intensity of changes in mood may depend on the dosage administered, the sensitivity of the individual, and the underlying personality. When intense changes are observed, the physician should be notified so that an adjustment in dosage can be made.

*Chronic corticosteroid use may alter a person's body image because of changes in adipose tissue distribution, thinning of skin, and development of stretch marks. The classic characteristics of a cushingoid appearance may develop, including a moon-shaped face; enlargement of the supraclavicular and cervicodorsal fat pads (buffalo hump); and truncal obesity.*

*Some people may be extremely self-conscious about these cosmetic changes, and others may be emotionally devastated by them; caution is required in discussing assessment findings with the client. These cosmetic changes do reverse when the drug is discontinued slowly.*

*The therapist needs to be aware of the affected individual's coping abilities. Treatment intervention can include educating the individual about traditional stress-management techniques. Therapists can facilitate psychosocial support by contacting social work and clinical nurse specialists to integrate programs such as survivorship support groups and image consultants.*

### Anabolic Steroids[209]

Therapists working with athletes, especially adolescent athletes, may observe signs and symptoms of (nonmedical, illegal) anabolic steroid use, including rapid weight gain (10-15 lb in 3 weeks); elevated blood pressure and associated peripheral edema; acne on the face, upper back, and chest; alterations in body composition with marked muscular hypertrophy; and disproportionate development of the upper torso, along with stretch marks around the back and chest. After prolonged anabolic steroid use, jaundice may develop.

*Therapists working with adolescents may see cases of recurrent tendon or muscle strain. Soft tissues working under the strain of added muscle bulk and body mass take longer than expected for physiologic healing to occur. Reinjury is not uncommon under these conditions.*

*Other signs of steroid use include needle marks in the large muscle groups, development of male pattern baldness, and gynecomastia (breast enlargement). Abscesses from injection use may also develop. Among females, secondary male characteristics may develop, such as a deeper voice, breast atrophy, and abnormal facial and body hair.*

*Irreversible sterility can occur (females being affected more than males), and menstrual irregularities may develop in women.*

*Changes in personality may occur; the user may become more aggressive or experience mood swings and psychologic delusions (e.g., believe he or she is indestructible). "Roid rages," sometimes referred to as steroid psychosis and characterized by sudden outbursts of uncontrolled emotion, may be observed. Severe depression is one of the signs of withdrawal from steroids. Withdrawal from AAS is a risk factor for suicide.*

*Despite the side effects of AAS use, steroid users are not readily apparent. The therapist who suspects an athlete may be using anabolic steroids should report findings to the physician and consider approaching that person to discuss the situation. The U.S. Olympic Committee provides a toll-free hotline ([800] 233-0393) for questions on steroids, medications, and prohibited substances. The U.S. Antidoping Agency also offers an online drug reference at http://www.usantidoping.org.*

*Testing for elevated blood pressure may provide an opportunity for evaluation of anabolic steroid use. Information as to the long-term adverse effects of anabolic steroids should be provided as part of the education process for all athletes. The therapist or trainer can provide healthy and safe strength training, stressing the importance of nutrition and proper weight-training techniques.*

## RADIATION INJURIES

### Definition and Overview

Radiation therapy, or radiotherapy, is the treatment of disease (usually cancer) by delivery of radiation to a particular area of the body. Radiation therapy is one of the major treatment modalities for cancer and is used in approximately 50% of all cases of cancer.[25] Radiotherapy is used in the local control phase of treatment but has both direct and indirect toxicities associated with its use. Radiation reactions and injuries are the harmful effects (acute, delayed, or chronic) to body tissues through exposure to ionizing radiation.

Today, a pencil-thin beam of radiation can be targeted to deliver extremely high doses of radiation to within millimeters of a cancer site. Advanced computer technology creates a three-dimensional model of the tumor to allow target mapping. Careful preplanning and delivery of targeted, modulated radiation doses have contributed to a reduced number of radiation side effects.

### Etiologic and Risk Factors

Risk factors for developing radiation toxicities arising from therapeutic radiation are often multifactorial, depending on the organ radiated, individual variations and tolerance, tumor type, volume radiated, and fraction size (Table 5.6).

People may also be exposed to radiation found in the environment, such as radon in their homes, or when rare nuclear events release large amounts of radioactivity, exposing people to total-body irradiation. Bone marrow transplant clients may receive total-body irradiation as a preparative regimen.

Medical radiation, or the amount of radiation received during a medical scan, carries a small risk for malignancy. Each test varies in the amount of radiation, with CT angiograms and nuclear imaging/cardiac stress tests among the tests with higher average effective doses of radiation. In 2009, Brigham and Women's Hospital determined that the risk of developing cancer from medical radiation was 0.7% over the normal lifetime risk for developing cancer. For people who received multiple CT scans, this risk increased to 2.7% to 12%.[357] People who have received radiation therapy for cancer can be at risk for a second malignancy, which often is not apparent for 10 to 15 years following the completion of therapy.[373]

**Table 5-6** Factors Contributing to Radiation Toxicity

| | | ENTEROCOLITIS | | |
|---|---|---|---|---|
| **Neurotoxicity** | **Dermatitis** | **Acute** | **Chronic** | **Pulmonary** |
| • High total dose<br>• High fractionation dose<br>• Large field size<br>• Increased edema<br>• Age less than 12 years and greater than 60 years<br>• Concurrent chemotherapy<br>• Presence of underlying diseases which affect the vasculature (diabetes, hypertension)<br>• Stereotactic surgery and interstitial brachytherapy | • Total dose/volume irradiated<br>• Fractionation dose<br>• Surface area exposed | • Large volume irradiated<br>• High total dose<br>• High fractionation dose<br>• Receiving concurrent chemotherapy | • Older age<br>• Received postoperative radiation<br>• Presence of collagen vascular disease<br>• Received concurrent chemotherapy<br>• Poor radiation technique | • Older age<br>• Lower performance status<br>• Lower baseline pulmonary function<br>• Large volume treated |

Based on data from Cross NE, Glantz MJ: Neurologic complications of radiation therapy. *Neurol Clin* 21(1):249–277, 2003; Hymes SR, Strom EA, Fife C: Radiation dermatitis: clinical presentation, pathophysiology, and treatment 2006. *J Am Acad Dermatol* 54(1):28–46, 2006; Nguyen NP, Antoine JE. Radiation enteritis. In Feldman M, Friedman LA, Sleisenger MH: *Sleisenger & Fordtran's gastrointestinal and liver disease: pathophysiology, diagnosis, management*, ed 7, Philadelphia, 2002, Saunders; Machtay M: Pulmonary complications of anticancer treatment. In Abeloff MD, Armitage JO, Niederhuber JE, Kastan MB, McKenna WG, editors, *Clinical oncology*, ed 3, New York, 2004, Churchill-Livingstone.

## Pathogenesis

Radiation therapy uses high-energy ionizing radiation to ionize atoms in DNA and break both atomic and molecular bonds, particularly causing breaks in the double-stranded helix. While normal, healthy cells are able to repair the damage (they exhibit a redundancy in repair mechanisms), malignant cells often lack the mechanisms of repair, leading to cell death and necrosis. Although cells in all phases of the cell cycle can be damaged by radiation, cells in $G_2$ and M phases have the greatest sensitivity to radiation, making rapidly dividing cells most likely to be damaged.

Ionizing radiation also indirectly causes damage through the production of free radicals, which leads to membrane damage and breakdown of structural and enzymatic proteins, resulting in cell death.[26] Often arterioles supplying oxygenated blood are damaged, resulting in inadequate nutritional supply, leading to ischemia and death of the irradiated tissues. The damage to nucleic acids may result in gene mutations, possibly leading to neoplasia years later. Normal cells and their progeny, not adjacent to tumor cells or in the treatment field, may also experience damage due to signals transmitted from cells directly irradiated. This has been termed the *bystander effect*. This is believed to occur due to signaling cascades and cytokine-mediated cellular toxicity, as well as cell-to-cell communication.[26,27]

## Clinical Manifestations and Medical Management

The clinical manifestations of radiation, similar to risk factors associated with radiation therapy, depend on individual variations, location and type of tumor, radiation volume and fraction dose, and organ system involved. Although newer techniques allow for organ shielding and lower volumes and fraction doses, radiation therapy continues to cause symptoms and injuries.

Each organ has its own tolerance to radiation, therefore injuries vary between organ systems. Yet there are some general principles that encompass radiation therapy injuries. Most organ systems exhibit both acute injuries that occur within 30 days of irradiation and delayed injuries that occur more than 30 days later (Table 5.7). Acute injuries are frequently self-limiting, whereas delayed effects are often irreversible and difficult to treat. Acute symptoms may delay further radiation treatments because of damage to GI mucosa, bone marrow, and other vital tissues.

**Table 5-7** Immediate and Delayed Effects of Ionizing Radiation[a]

| System Affected | Immediate | Delayed Effect |
|---|---|---|
| Musculoskeletal | | Soft tissue (collagen) fibrosis, contracture, atrophy<br>Orthopedic deformity |
| Neuromuscular | Fatigue<br>Decreased appetite<br>Subtle changes in behavior and cognition<br>Short-term memory loss<br>Ataxia (subacute) | Myelopathy (spinal cord dysfunction)<br>Cerebral injury, neurocognitive deficits<br>Radionecrosis (headache, changes in personality, seizures)<br>Plexopathy (brachial, lumbosacral, or pelvic plexus)<br>Gait abnormalities |
| Cardiovascular/ pulmonary | Fatigue, decreased endurance<br>Radiation pneumonitis | Radiation fibrosis (lung)<br>Cardiotoxicity<br>Coronary artery disease<br>Myocardial ischemia/infarction<br>Pericarditis<br>Lymphedema |
| Integumentary | Erythema<br>Edema<br>Dryness, itching<br>Epilation or hair loss (alopecia)<br>Destruction of nails<br>Epidermolysis (loose skin)<br>Delayed wound healing | Skin scarring, delayed wound healing, contracture<br>Telangiectasia (vascular lesion)<br>Malignancy (basal cell, squamous cell, melanoma) |
| Other | Gastrointestinal: anorexia, nausea, dysphagia; vomiting, diarrhea, xerostomia (dry mouth); stomatitis (inflammation of mouth mucosa); esophagitis; intestinal stenosis<br>Renal/urologic: urinary dysfunction | Bone marrow suppression (anemia, infection, bleeding)<br>Cataracts<br>Endocrine dysfunction (cranial radiation) including amenorrhea, menopause, infertility, decreased libido<br>Hepatitis<br>Nephritis, renal insufficiency<br>Malignancy<br>Skin cancer<br>Leukemia<br>Lung cancer<br>Thyroid cancer<br>Breast cancer |

[a]Some of the delayed effects of radiation (e.g., cerebral injury, pericarditis, pulmonary fibrosis, hepatitis, nephritis, GI disturbances) may be signs of recurring cancer. The physician should be notified of any new symptoms, change in symptoms, or increase in symptoms.

Management of acute injuries is often treated symptomatically with red blood cells and platelet transfusions, antibiotics, fluid and electrolyte maintenance, and other supportive medical measures as needed. With prognosis poor in many cases of delayed radiation complications, more effort is being placed on prevention. Clinicians have been attempting to optimize the therapeutic ratio, or the risk/benefit, in order to achieve tumor control with minimal effects to normal tissue. Modifications are made when chemotherapy is used in conjunction with radiation.

Because there are unique or specific injuries to different organ systems, the following section specifies toxicities, clinical manifestations, and treatment pertaining to different organ systems. Toxicities can lead to dosage limitations of radiation and reduce therapeutic choices and overall effectiveness of therapy.

### Radiation Esophagitis and Enterocolitis

The esophagus is a centrally located organ in the mediastinum and is often involved in the radiation fields under treatment for lung cancer. An acute reaction may occur within 2 to 3 weeks after the initiation of radiation therapy, manifested by abnormal peristalsis activity, odynophagia (pain with swallowing), and dysphagia (difficulty swallowing). Resolution of symptoms typically occurs 1 to 3 weeks after completion of radiotherapy. Late esophagitis is a result of inflammation and fibrosis of tissue, causing stricture and fistula formation. Dilation and surgical repair may be necessary.[418]

Radiation to the stomach leads to loss of chief and parietal cells, gastric acid production, inflammation, and edema. Continued radiation treatments can cause erosions and ulcers. Nausea and vomiting can begin within 24 hours of the initial treatment and up to one-half of people will develop emesis after 2 to 3 weeks of treatments. These symptoms usually abate, in 1 to 2 weeks, once treatments have completed. Late complications include antral stenosis, due to fibrosis, or gastric ulcers (about 5 months following completion of therapy). Stomach cells are less able to tolerate radiation if clients are receiving concomitant chemotherapy consisting of a taxane agent, epidermal growth factor, or tyrosine kinase inhibitors.

As in other organs receiving radiation, the small intestine exhibits both acute and chronic symptoms from radiation treatment. Acutely, the rapidly dividing stem cells located in the crypts of Lieberkühn are induced into apoptosis, or programmed cellular death, no longer able to replace mucosal cells lost due to radiation. Within a few weeks, leukocytes infiltrate the mucosa with formation of abscesses in the crypts. Increasing edema from cytokines, signaling cascades, and lymphatic blockage leads to small blood vessel occlusion and ischemia. These changes are referred to as acute radiation enteritis or more accurately *radiation enteropathy* or *radiation mucositis*, reducing the surface area required for nutrient absorption and leading to dehydration and malnutrition. The colon typically is more resistant to radiation; however, symptoms often overlap. Injury to the colon is termed *radiation colitis*.

Typical acute symptoms include diarrhea, anorexia, abdominal cramping/pain, bloating, and nausea/vomiting. Intestinal motility also changes. Acute symptoms become most pronounced around the third week of treatment and most resolve within 2 weeks to 3 months following treatment.

Dehydration may require hospitalization and a break in the radiation schedule, but is usually not life-threatening. Concurrent chemotherapy causes an increase in cellular damage when compared to radiation alone, with resulting neutropenia leading to serious infections and sepsis.[167] Mucosal damage can lead to ulceration with subsequent perforation or formation of fistulas with abscesses.

With healing, the intestinal wall can become thickened and fibrotic, leading to chronic radiation enteritis associated with narrowing of the lumen, formation of strictures or even bowel obstruction. The incidence of chronic radiation enteritis is unknown and probably underreported but may occur in up to 15% of cases involving the intestines. Common symptoms include postprandial pain, nausea, weight loss, diarrhea, and malabsorption of nutrients. Bacterial overgrowth and bleeding are also seen. If the terminal ileum is included in the radiation field, there may be a reduction in the absorption of $B_{12}$ and bile acids, leading to $B_{12}$ deficiency and steatorrhea/diarrhea, respectively. Breakdown of lactose is often impaired with development of flatulence, diarrhea, and bacterial overgrowth. Symptoms typically occur 18 months to 6 years after treatment.[361] Unlike acute radiation symptoms, chronic symptoms often require treatment or surgery, with more serious outcomes.

### Radiation Heart Disease

Complications from radiation injury to the heart are delayed and seen following treatment. Although newer techniques and lower doses of radiation have led to a reduction in cardiotoxicity, complications from incidental radiation to the heart for treatment of breast, Hodgkin lymphoma, and other malignancies still remains a leading cause of morbidity and mortality.[344,443] The risk of having a cardiovascular event (e.g., myocardial infarction, ischemic heart disease) related to radiation therapy is elevated by 5 years after treatment completion and continues for up to 20 years.[96] Although the absolute risk for experiencing a cardiovascular event following radiation is small, preexisting cardiac disease risk factors, such as smoking, hypertension, and hyperlipidemia, may increase the risk.[96] Increasing size of radiation field and total dosage of radiation also affect the risk. Radiation to the chest can cause coronary heart disease, cardiomyopathy, valvular dysfunction, conduction abnormalities, and pericarditis. Heart failure caused by diastolic dysfunction is more common than systolic dysfunction. Significant valvular disease can be seen affecting aortic, mitral, and tricuspid valves. Bradycardia, various degrees of heart block, and sinus node dysfunction are some of the arrhythmias noted following radiation. Care must be taken when individuals are treated concomitantly with chemotherapy agents with known cardiotoxicities, such as an anthracycline or trastuzumab.

### Radiation Lung Disease

The lung is a radiosensitive organ that can be affected by radiation therapy. Risk factors for the development of pulmonary toxicity include the method of irradiation, volume of lung radiated, the dose and fraction rate of therapy, concurrent chemotherapy, and presence of underlying lung disease (e.g., prior thoracic radiation, COPD, smoking history, interstitial lung disease).[70] The incidence of toxicity is principally determined by the regimen utilized and percentage of lung volume irradiated.[23]

Radiation-induced lung injury (RILI) presents in typically two phases—acutely, known as radiation pneumonitis, and a chronic phase termed radiation fibrosis; although the symptoms often overlap. *Radiation pneumonitis* is caused by significant interstitial inflammation creating a reduction of gas exchange. The hallmark of this toxicity is symptoms disproportionate to other findings, including appearance on radiographs. It usually occurs 1 to 3 months (range: 1 to 6 months) after completion of radiotherapy and typically resolves within 6 to 12 months.

Symptoms range from a dry cough with dyspnea on exertion to severe cough and dyspnea at rest. Fever is noticed more commonly in radiation pneumonitis than chronic fibrosis. Chest pain is seen not only with radiation pneumonitis, but also with esophageal pathology, rib fracture or pleuritis. Hypoxia is common, but clients rarely develop acute respiratory distress requiring intubation and ventilation. Multiple grading systems have been published, particularly for research, to assess and quantify symptoms of radiation pneumonitis.

Making the diagnosis of radiation pneumonitis can be difficult because individuals with malignancy are also susceptible to thromboembolic disease, infection, and extension of tumor. Preexisting lung disease compounds this difficulty. Newer immunotherapies utilized for lung cancer can also cause pneumonitis.[276] Imaging studies (CT scans), bronchoscopy, and pulmonary function tests aid in delineating the diagnosis. Glucocorticoids are often used to treat symptomatic disease. Other supportive care includes supplemental oxygen, antitussive therapy, antibiotics, and treatment for any underlying lung disease. Ongoing studies and research are exploring better methods of reducing RILI.[198]

*Pulmonary radiation fibrosis* may occur 6 to 12 months (or even years) after radiation therapy. Radiation fibrosis is caused by cytokines and chronic inflammatory signaling. It is progressive, and symptoms may develop slowly. Only supportive therapy is available, such as oxygen supplementation, bronchodilators, and treating infection. Corticosteroids have no value, but studies are ongoing to find preventive measures.[198]

Other radiation-induced pulmonary problems include formation of bronchopleural fistulas, pneumothorax, hemoptysis, and bronchial stenosis.

### Radiation Dermatitis

Damage to the skin is one of the more common side effects of radiation because it is involved in most therapies, despite tumor location. Up to 95% of people receiving RT will experience injury to the skin.[355] Although most injury to the skin is reversible, severe reactions can cause delay in therapy or a change in dosing. The cutaneous effects of radiation can be separated into acute and chronic. Most of the acute changes occur secondary to the destruction of keratinocytes, melanocytes, sebaceous glands, and hair follicles. Microvascular injury leads to ischemia and necrosis. Continued radiation promotes release of cytokines and activation of inflammatory signaling, which can stimulate fibrosis and chronic inflammation.

The National Cancer Institute has provided guidelines for grading acute cutaneous damage to the skin after radiation ranging from mild (grade 1) to severe (grade 3-4).[86] A collection of photographs has also been published to aid in bringing consistency to staging.[440] Common clinical manifestations include erythema, dry desquamation, moist desquamation, and necrosis. Grade 1 reactions resemble sunburn and are accompanied by hair loss, dry desquamation, pruritus, and blanchable erythema (Fig. 5.3). Treatment is supportive, including keeping the area clean using warm water and mild soap and use of hydrophilic moisturizers or low-potency steroids. Loose fitting clothes should be worn to avoid friction with damaged skin.

Grade 2 reactions produce persistent erythema or patchy moist desquamation in the folds and creases of the skin, often associated with pain and edema. Bullae may form, rupture, and become superinfected. These changes present 2 to 4 weeks into therapy and peak 1 to 2 weeks after treatment completion. Resolution of symptoms occurs within 2 to 4 weeks following treatment. Confluent, moist desquamation of the skin with pitting edema characterizes grade 3 reactions. Compared to grade 2 reactions, the edematous erythema of grade 3 is not confined to the skin folds. Treatment for stages 2 and 3 include prevention/treatment of infection and the use of dressings, such as hydrocolloid or foam bandages, over skin that is sloughing. Pain control is important and, with high stages of injury, may be resistant to opioids.

Grade 4 reactions (rare) are severe, with skin necrosis or ulceration of full-dermis thickness associated with bleeding. Pain can be severe. Treatment requires a multidisciplinary approach. Infrequently, grade 4 reactions do not heal and progress into consequential late effects, eliciting fibrosis, with breakdown of necrotic tissue, ulceration, and exposure of underlying structures such as bone. These injuries are difficult to heal because much of the tissue is avascular secondary to radiation.

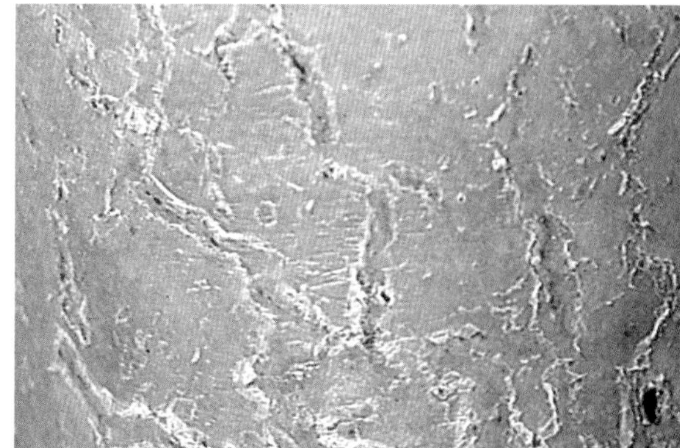

**Figure 5.3**

**Dry desquamation with scaling associated with radiation.** (From Habif TP: *Clinical dermatology*, ed 4, Edinburgh, 2004, Mosby.)

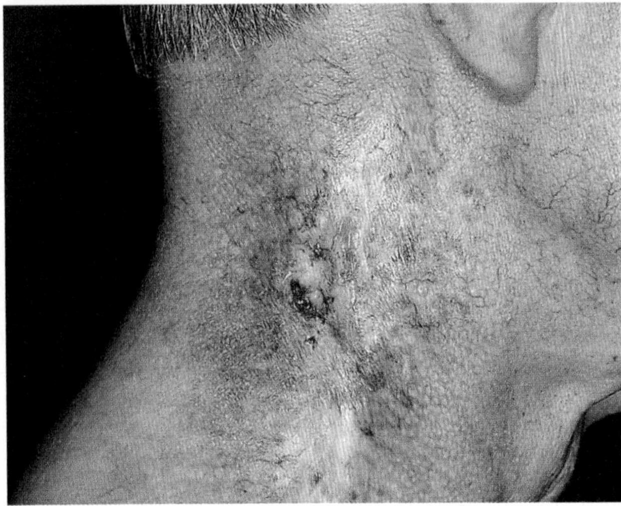

**Figure 5.4**

**Radiation dermatitis.** Acute or chronic inflammation of the skin caused by exposure to ionizing radiation (radiation therapy for cancer). Symptoms may include redness, blistering, and sloughing of the skin. The condition can progress to scarring, fibrosis, and atrophy as shown here. (From Callen JP: *Color atlas of dermatology*, ed 2, Philadelphia, 2000, WB Saunders.)

Chronic radiation-induced effects develop after 90 days following radiation. Symptoms may present months to years after treatment. Repeated doses of radiation without sufficient time between doses to repair can lead to significant cutaneous injury. This injury is often manifested by atrophic skin, telangiectasia, hyperpigmentation, and hypopigmentation. Sebaceous glands, hair follicles, and nails may be permanently affected. Fibrosis of the dermis accompanied by absorption of collagen creates contracted, atrophic skin, which is susceptible to tearing and ulceration (Fig. 5.4). An abnormal proliferation of arteriole cells may occur, causing thrombosis of the vessels, which combined with fibrosis, inhibits healing and predisposes ulcers to infection. These complex ulcers are painful and difficult to heal.

Diligence is required to keep fibrotic tissue intact. Active and passive range-of-motion exercises are important to retain mobility and reduce contractures. The drug pentoxifylline, lasers, and hyperbaric oxygen therapy (HBOT) have been used to treat radiation-induced fibrosis, although evidence is lacking.[49,359,430]

Another type of radiation-induced reaction is *radiation recall*. Radiation recall reactions (Fig. 5.5) are inflammatory reactions that occur in a previously irradiated site after the administration of various chemotherapeutic drugs (e.g., dactinomycin, doxorubicin, bleomycin, gemcitabine, and paclitaxel), newer therapies (e.g., trastuzumab and bevacizumab), antiinflammatory drugs, lipid lowering agents, or antibiotics.[58,206] The reaction is characterized by a "recalling" of inflammation in the entire skin region previously exposed to radiation therapy. Symptoms include erythema, pruritus, dry desquamation, and edema. Treatment consists of topical or systemic corticosteroids, antiinflammatory agents, and discontinuation of the offending drug. Clients should avoid sun exposure and using tanning beds.

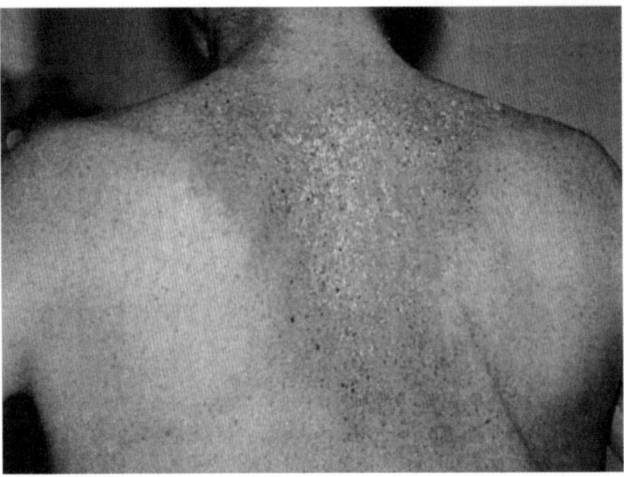

**Figure 5.5**

**Radiation recall.** This person had small cell cancer of the lung treated with radiation. Cytoxan treatment some months later elicited erythema and desquamation within the portal of radiation. This lesion is in the healing phase. (From Abeloff MD: *Clinical oncology*, ed 3, Philadelphia, 2004, Churchill Livingstone.)

Recall may occur in the skin, mucous membranes, lungs, central nervous system (CNS), esophagus, and GI tract, although the skin is most frequently involved.[58] Months, and even years, may pass from the time of the initial radiation therapy to the onset of this reaction. More significant reactions display moist desquamation with blister formation and may even progress to full dermis necrosis and ulceration.

### Effects of Radiation on Connective Tissue

Radiation therapy is well known to cause significant long-term or chronic effects on connective tissue. Acute irradiation toxicity is less likely because connective tissue has a slower turnover rate and striated muscle tolerates relatively high doses of radiation. Late changes, such as fibrosis, atrophy, and contraction of tissue, can occur to any area irradiated but especially to collagen tissue.

In growing bones and limbs, irradiation can cause profound and irreversible changes resulting in limb-length discrepancies and scoliosis requiring orthopedic surgical correction. Radiation-induced osteoporosis may lead to pathologic fractures. For example, women who have received radiation for pelvic tumors have a 65% increased incidence of hip fracture 5 years after completing therapy.[30,424] Osteoblasts are relatively more sensitive to injury as compared to osteoclasts, leaving bone hypocellular; yet osteoclasts acutely experience activation and increase in numbers.[295,424] The vasculature is also affected. Initially there is edema and loss of endothelial cells in the vascular channels of the bone marrow, which are later replaced by sclerotic connective tissue. Later there is fibrosis within the blood vessel walls, leading to thickening and occlusion of the blood vessel.[424] Bone mass and quality are reduced, resulting in radiation-induced osteoporosis.

Fibrosis of connective tissue can result in edema, decreased range of motion, and functional impairment. Radiation of the pelvic cavity often causes dense pelvic adhesions that may cause painful motion restrictions and more rarely, plexopathy. Subsequently, these effects lead to soft tissue fibrosis, resulting in decreased range of motion, pain, and, in some cases, lymphedema.

Postoperative radiation is a strong risk factor for the development of lymphedema, increasing the incidence, in some cases, tenfold.[18,306] Many malignancies require lymph node dissection and removal, compounding the problem of lymphedema. The mechanisms for the development of lymphedema following postoperative radiation are unknown. It may be due to destruction or dysfunction of lymphatic channels.[18] Another cause may be related to the formation of fibrosis. Although lymphatic vessels maintain their structural integrity after being irradiated, fibrosis occurs in the surrounding tissue. This effect can inhibit normal growth of lymphatic vessels into healing tissues and delay lymphatic proliferation in response to inflammation. These types of effects can be minimized by sparing lymphatics/lymph nodes from the radiation portal and reducting the number of lymph nodes removed (e.g., using sentinel lymph node biopsy), but presently, from 7% to 38% of breast cancer survivors in the United States develop lymphedema sometime in their lifetime.[165,294,345]

It is important to remember that lymphedema may not be a side effect of radiation but rather a sign of advanced progressive metastases associated with cancer recurrence. Lymphedema can develop when lymphatic overload contributes to systemic congestion; a medical differential diagnosis is required. Currently, physical therapy and supportive measures are the mainstay of therapy.

### Effects of Radiation on the Nervous System

Radiation therapy is used to treat primary or metastatic malignancies of the brain and nervous system. Neurotoxicity related to radiation increases as the volume of nervous tissue being irradiated increases and the total dose and fraction size increase.[90] Toxicities also develop due to varying individual reactions; complications are more likely to happen to the young (less than 5 years old) or the elderly, or with concomitant or subsequent chemotherapy.

Clinical manifestations of nervous system radiation toxicity can be separated into three categories: acute, early-delayed, and late. Neurologic symptoms relating to acute and early-delayed complications are most often self-limiting, requiring only supportive measures. The chronic or late complications are more often severe and progressive.

**Acute Symptoms.** Acute symptoms generally occur during the period of treatment and up to 6 weeks following completion. The most common symptom is progressive and sometimes debilitating fatigue. Symptoms begin about 2 weeks into therapy and peak near the end of treatment, slowly resolving over weeks to months. Other clinical manifestations of cranial irradiation may include lethargy, nausea/vomiting, headaches, short-term memory difficulties, and subtle changes in behavior and cognition. General symptoms that may occur during brain irradiation include decreased appetite, dry skin, hearing loss, hair loss, and uncommonly, decreased salivation (parotitis). Swelling due to radiation may initially worsen symptoms associated with the tumor by increasing the mass effect of the tumor. Clients infrequently develop hydrocephalus accompanied by ataxia and incontinence.[383] Rarely, radiation may lead to acute encephalopathy, particularly when larger amounts of brain tissue are irradiated. Acute radiation encephalopathy, probably related to disruption of the blood-brain barrier and cerebral edema, is manifested by headache, nausea and vomiting, lethargy, seizures, new focal deficits, and mental status changes. Due to the use of modern techniques, the incidence has significantly decreased, although it can be life-threatening in clients that do develop this complication.

**Early-delayed Symptoms.** Early-delayed symptoms are noted 1 to 6 months after the completion of therapy. Many people continue to feel fatigue and decreased stamina. Difficulty with memory may persist for months following treatment, but these changes are typically reversible and improve within one year. Some clients may also experience a delay in worsening symptoms due to radiation-induced edema that mimic initial tumor symptoms with associated headache and focal neurologic signs. If treatment included the cervical spine (and to a lesser degree the thoracic), clients may experience radiation myelopathy, a tingling, shocklike sensation passing down the arm or trunk when the neck is flexed (Lhermitte sign). This sign occurs in up to 29% of clients receiving mantle radiation therapy for lymphoma.[438] Newer methods of irradiation (IMRT) have reduced exposure of the cervical spinal cord and reduced the incidence of Lhermitte sign in people receiving radiation for head and neck cancer to 3.9%.[261] Symptoms are usually self-limiting and appear about 3 months after treatment. Irradiation of the brainstem may cause ataxia, nystagmus, and dysarthria. Occasionally, a transient brachial plexopathy occurs, causing paresthesias and muscle weakness, which improves over time.

*Pseudoprogression* is a phenomenon described particularly in individuals with gliomas treated with temozolomide and external beam irradiation to the brain. Postradiation MRI demonstrates increased uptake, suggesting tumor progression but not actual increase in tumor size.[301] This is most likely due to edema surrounding the tumor and interruption of myelin synthesis. The person may be asymptomatic or have mild symptoms similar to initial tumor symptoms; these symptoms are transient and improve without treatment.[301]

**Late Complications.** Even though many of the acute and early-delayed complications of radiation are self-limiting or mild, late complications can be more serious and do not appear for 6 months to years after therapy. For example, when exposed to radiation, cerebral vasculature, both small[328] and large, may be damaged, leading to coronary artery disease, transient ischemic attacks, stroke, or myocardial infarction. Other late effects are described as follows and in Table 5.7.

***Radionecrosis.*** One of the best-described complications of cerebral radiotherapy is delayed cerebral radionecrosis. This typically occurs 1 to 3 years after completion of therapy (although it may appear up to 10 years later).[367] Higher fraction and total doses, larger treatment volumes, and concurrent chemotherapy or radiation sensitizers increase the risk for radionecrosis. Radiation not only destroys neurologic cells and their precursors, it also affects the vasculature. Disruption and inflammation of vessels leads to a breakdown in the blood-brain barrier, with subsequent fibrosis and thickening of some vessels while others dilate. The development of fibrosis in smaller vessels occludes the lumen, resulting in local necrosis and demyelination of surrounding nerve tissue. Vascular endothelial growth factor (VEGF) and other inflammatory mediators may play a role in the development of radionecrosis. Radionecrosis occurs at the site of the tumor or adjacent to the tumor, typically areas that have received the highest dose. Symptoms are dictated by the location of the necrosis and can include headache, changes in cognition and personality, focal neurologic deficits, and seizures. Radionecrosis is often self-limiting, but symptoms can be treated with glucocorticoids to aid in the reduction of edema. Bevacizumab (an antibody that binds VEGF) may also be beneficial for certain people.[232,331] Infrequently surgery may be required to remove necrotic tissue to reduce mass effect or laser interstitial thermal therapy may be utilized.[6]

Another serious long-term complication of radiotherapy of the brain is the development of tumors, including meningiomas, gliomas, lymphomas, fibrosarcomas, and malignant schwannomas. These tumors are often aggressive and difficult to cure.

Up to 80% of individuals who receive radiation that includes the pituitary or hypothalamus develop endocrinopathies. Abnormalities in growth hormone, gonadotropins, thyrotropin, prolactin and adrenocorticotropin may be seen.[15] Hyperprolactinemia commonly occurs and can resolve spontaneously.[90] Ototoxicity (tinnitus and high-frequency hearing loss), optic neuropathy (visual impairments), xerophthalmia (dry eyes), and cataracts are other late complications of radiation.

***Myelopathy.*** Radiotherapy of the spinal cord may cause a radiation-induced myelopathy, which is evident by the appearance of Lhermitte sign. This is clinically manifested by a tingling, shocklike sensation passing down the arm or trunk when the neck is flexed and is felt to be secondary to demyelination of the nerves. It appears in about 10% of individuals who receive radiation to the spine and is seen 2 to 6 months after treatment completion.[231] It is typically transient and does not progress to chronic symptoms.

Chronic progressive myelopathy presents as paresis and numbness 6 to 12 months following treatment. Unlike acute myelopathy, these symptoms may be progressive and are usually not reversible. Signs may include lower extremity weakness, hyperreflexia, foot drop, complete paresis below the damaged area of the spinal cord, or the Brown-Séquard syndrome. Sphincter dysfunction may be involved. Increased incidence is seen in clients who receive higher total and fraction doses of radiation and larger fields of treatment. There is no standard treatment, although glucocorticoids and bevacizumab are often utilized.[232] The Brown-Séquard syndrome is a rare disorder that presents with muscle weakness on one side of the body and loss of sensation on the opposite side. Lower motor neuron syndrome is uncommonly seen after pelvic radiation (originally seen after treatment for testicular cancer). Clients develop muscle weakness with atrophy of muscles, fasciculations, and areflexia. Sensory examination remains unchanged. This syndrome can progress over years before reaching a plateau.

***Plexopathy.*** The brachial and lumbar plexuses may also be injured by radiation treatment, with symptoms presenting from 10 months up to 20 years following therapy.[21,196] The incidence of brachial plexopathy after radiation therapy has been reduced significantly with improved treatment.[12] Today, the overall incidence of plexopathies is approximately 2% to 5% of clients who receive radiation in the brachial and lumbar plexuses[196] and as little as 0.5% in women receiving radiation for breast cancer.[105]

Clinical manifestations of radiation-induced brachial plexopathy include paresthesias, with progressive motor deficits, muscle atrophy, fasciculation, decreased tendon reflexes, and pain.[60,160] Rarely, clients may lose hand function or develop arm paralysis, with associated loss of sensation.[21,126] Lumbar plexopathy is also possible when the pelvic area is irradiated and appears to be secondary to the development of fibrosis around the nerve trunks, ischemia to the nerves, and direct toxicity to nerve axons. Symptoms include paresthesias, hypoesthesia, progressive weakness, decreased reflexes, and pain. Plexopathies can be caused by cancer recurrence rather than the effects of irradiation and must be evaluated.

Currently, no curative treatment is available for either brachial or lumbar plexopathies, although therapeutic interventions can achieve significant pain control and improve strength and function in the affected limb.[166] Clients benefit from a multidisciplinary team approach. Pain can be treated with tricyclic antidepressants, serotonin-norepinephrine reuptake inhibitors, membrane stabilizers (e.g., gabapentin), tramadol, or nerve blocks.[105] Neurolysis surgery to release fibrotic entrapment of the plexus provides only short-term improvement.[161]

Loss of neural mobility from radiation fibrosis can be addressed using neural mobility assessment and treatment techniques.[370] Treating all tissues of the radiated field (skin, muscle, joint mobility), along with neural mobilization, addresses the big picture rather than just focusing on the loss of nerve gliding. Caution should be used to avoid stretching the nerve tissue in the acute phase until the individual demonstrates symptom stability and nonirritation of the nerve(s) in question. The therapist can begin with restoration of the glide component without reaching end ranges and without using overpressure until the individual responses can be monitored and treatment advanced accordingly.

**SPECIAL IMPLICATIONS FOR THE THERAPIST 5-6**

## *Radiation*

### Radiation Hazard for Health Care Professionals

People who receive external radiation do not give off radiation to those who come in contact with them. Likewise, patients coming to physical therapy after a nuclear medicine scan pose no hazard to the therapist. Internal implants can present some hazards to others as long as the implant is in place. Pregnant staff members should avoid all contact with the internally radiated client. Radiation from internal implants (brachytherapy) is usually exhausted after 12 months.

*When administering direct care, staff members should plan interventions so that each task can be accomplished as quickly as possible. Because distance provides some protection, it is advisable to use positions that place the staff person as far away from the radioactive implant as possible. For example, if the implant is in the pelvis, the caregiver might stand at the head or foot, not the side, of the bed.*

*The use of protective lead aprons or portable shields may be recommended according to the hospital protocol. Each staff member is encouraged to know and follow the recommended policies and procedures for the given institution. A film badge or ring badge worn on the outside of any protective devices or clothing of the caregiver records the cumulative dose of radiation received and is used to monitor exposure over a period. When removed, this badge should be stored in a location where no additional radiation exists.*

*Some sources of radiation (e.g., iodine-131, phosphorus-32) are excreted in body fluids (e.g., urine, sweat, tears, or saliva) for several days after administration to the client. Detectable radioactivity is emitted for up to 3 days after a bone or thyroid scan; up to 51 days for cardiac scans; and up to 95 days after iodine therapy. These clients are placed in strict radioactive isolation during hospitalization and treatment. All articles used by the client, such as urinals, toothpicks, tissues, and bed linens, are considered as a possible radiation hazard. Disposal of all such items should follow hospital protocol. Good quality examination gloves made of latex or a strong synthetic material (not vinyl) are adequate for general care, although the use of 2 sets of gloves is recommended when in direct contact with body fluids deemed radioactive.*[434]

*Careful removal and disposal of any personal protective equipment worn by the therapist must be done according to radiation safety instructions posted. Thorough handwashing after glove removal is essential.*[434]

### Postradiation Therapy

For the client who is in the process of receiving external radiation therapy, handwashing before treating the client is essential to protect him or her from infection. Skin care precautions include the following:

- Avoid topical use of alcohol or other drying agents, lotions, gels, oils, or salves; creams and gels on the skin can potentiate the received skin dosage and lead to increased adverse effects; do not wash away markings for the target area.
- Avoid positions in which the client is lying on the target area.
- Avoid exposure to direct sunlight, heat lamps, or other sources of heat, including thermal modalities.
- Avoid friction to the tissue in the radiation field (i.e., by direct manipulation of the tissue or application of compression in or near affected skin, until acute effects of radiation have resolved).
- Delayed wound healing associated with radiotherapy requires assessment early on of other factors that impair wound healing, such as smoking or tobacco use, poor nutrition, weight loss before the start of treatment, and infection.[317]

*Radiation to the low back may cause nausea, vomiting, or diarrhea because the lower digestive tract is exposed to the radiation.*[265] *Radiation of the pelvic cavity often causes dense pelvic adhesions that can cause painful motion restrictions. The therapist's role in the postradiation treatment of these clients is to increase range of motion and provide stretching exercises. Early intervention by the therapist is essential to prevent or minimize restrictive scarring through instruction in effective, focused, and efficient flexibility exercises for long-term use.*

*Some effects of radiation on the nervous system can develop years after treatment. Radiation plexopathy can develop many years after exposure to the radiation doses used 20 or 30 years ago. Pain relief has been achieved with surgical release of the nerves from surrounding soft tissue, but improvement in sensation or motor function may not be seen in chronic cases or in situations of delayed diagnosis. With early diagnosis of radiation-induced neuropathies, new disease-modifying treatments may improve outcomes in the future.*[316]

*The therapist should be aware of anyone at risk for seizures, observe for any signs of seizure activity, and take appropriate actions to ensure client safety. Anyone with neurologic signs or symptoms of unknown cause must be questioned about past medical history (cancer, heart disease) and the possibility of prior radiation treatment, keeping in mind that progressive disease or a vascular event can also cause an acute or subacute neurologic event. The physician must rule out cancer recurrence in anyone with a previous history of cancer and evaluate for the presence of some other cause of new onset neurologic signs and symptoms.*

### Postradiation Infection

Signs and symptoms of infection are often absent because the immunosuppressed person cannot mount an adequate inflammatory response. Fever may be the first and only sign of infection. Swelling, redness, and pus may be absent in infected tissue. The therapist must observe very carefully for any sign of infection, anemia, or bleeding, and other signs of thrombocytopenia and refer the individual immediately for physician assessment/treatment the same day.

### Radiation Therapy and Exercise

Radiation and chemotherapy can cause permanent scar formation in the lungs and heart tissues, whereas drug-induced cardiomyopathies can contribute to limitations in cardiovascular function.

*Both of these variables require monitoring of vital signs when working with people who are recovering or in remission from cancer treatments. Clients should be taught to monitor their own vital signs, including pulse rate, respiratory rate, perceived exertion rate, which is not to exceed 15 to 17 for moderate-intensity training or submaximal testing, and observe for early signs of cardiopulmonary complications of cancer treatments, such as dyspnea, pallor, excessive perspiration, or fatigue during exercise.*

*Low- to moderate-intensity aerobic exercise (e.g., self-paced walking) during the weeks of radiation treatment can help manage treatment-related symptoms by improving physical function and lowering reported levels of fatigue, anxiety, depression, and sleep disturbance.*[253,339] *Patients must be educated that avoidance of exercise due to fatigue can increase their fatigue and deconditioning and adoption of a daily "dose" of activity as prescribed can be beneficial in both the short and long term. An American College of Sports Medicine roundtable publication stated: "The advice to 'avoid inactivity,' even in cancer patients with existing disease or undergoing difficult treatments, is likely helpful."*[336] *Excellent guidelines for many cancer diagnoses and safe prescription of exercise are included.*

*A successful aerobic training protocol for a client with cancer should include client education, an exercise evaluation, and an individualized exercise prescription. Ideally, these components of cancer treatment should begin when the person receives the diagnosis. Current guidelines recommend that clients should be advised not to exercise within 2 hours of chemotherapy or radiation therapy because increases in circulation may increase the effects of the treatments.*[151] *Guidelines for choosing an exercise test and prescribing an exercise prescription are available.*[10,116]

### Radiation and Soft Tissue

Direct treatment of the radiated tissue is not advised during the acute inflammatory phase other than to teach gentle global flexibility for the general area and discuss simple skin care (which the radiation oncology nurses have usually covered well). Postirradiated tissue can tear when stretching. Therapist and client must directly observe for blanching of the skin during exercise and avoid stretching beyond that point.

*Soft tissue mobilization can be performed carefully and judiciously around the immobile area. Direct tissue work over the irradiated area must be postponed until after the subacute phase of healing (usually after four months). Active range of motion for generalized tissue mobility is the therapist's first-line approach, with maximum respect for irradiated tissue. Remember to teach diaphragmatic breathing during all activities. This is particularly true for the individual who has had surgery/irradiation to the chest wall as ipsilateral rib excursion is often reduced because of scarring and soft tissue fibrosis. Active motion to the end range as a means of stretching the soft tissues must be continued for at least 18 to 24 months postirradiation because the fibrotic process continues for that amount of time or longer (up to 5 years).*

*With irradiated tissue, assessment should include the borders of the irradiated field (seen clearly in Fig. 5.6, A and B as a result of the erythema) but often must be found by exploration for the reference tattoos, the temperature of the tissue to touch, the mobility of the tissue (adherent to underlying structures versus mobile), the presence of telangiectasia (dilated capillary beds at surface of skin, reflecting damage to the autonomic innervation causing permanent vasodilation in that region), and blanching of the tissue to light touch (a sign of acute inflammation still resolving).*

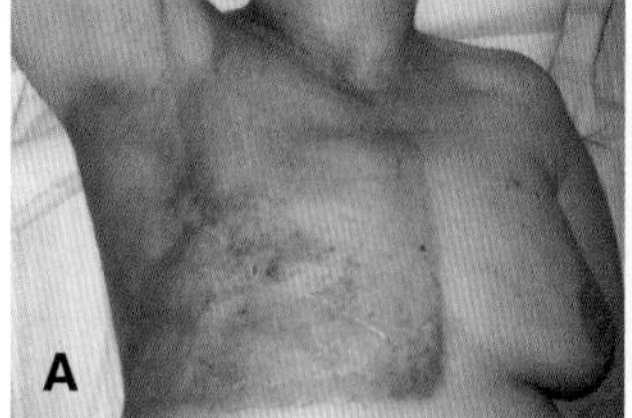


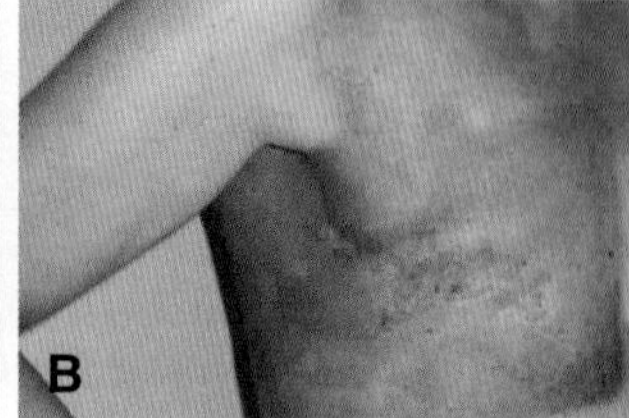


**Figure 5.6**

**Overview of skin changes from radiation therapy.** Note the scar/incision site and boundaries or borders between radiated and nonradiated tissue. **A,** Individual nearing the end of her radiation treatment postmastectomy for breast cancer. There is mild-to-moderate erythema, with some dry desquamations (skin toxicity also known as *radiation dermatitis*) for which the individual has received topical skin care products for self-application. Areas of redness show "hot" or radiated tissue; areas of brown skin show healing following damage from radiation. Note that the more red the tissue (just like a sunburn on steroids) the more fragile and damaged the skin and underlying tissue. No visible wet desquamations, which would usually cause the radiation oncologist to put a temporary hold on treatment. These side effects usually appear after about 4 to 5 weeks of radiation. Although there is no visible sign of chest lymphedema, it is important to know that there is a risk of lymphedema for the entire quadrant (not just the upper extremity). With irradiated tissue, assessment should include the borders of the irradiated field (in these photos very obvious because of the erythema, but often must be found by exploration for the reference tattoos), the temperature of the tissue to touch, the mobility of the tissue (adherent to underlying structures versus mobile), the presence of telangiectasia (dilated capillary beds at surface of skin reflecting damage to the autonomic innervation causing permanent vasodilation in that region), and blanching of the tissue to light touch (a sign of acute inflammation still resolving). **B,** Close-up view of same individual postmastectomy during radiation treatment. **A** and **B,** Courtesy Catherine C. Goodman. Used with permission.

*Once the area no longer blanches with light palpation, then the therapist can begin to apply gentle compression, with frequent checks for irritation due to almost certain decreased sensation in the field. Generalized flexibility exercises can be progressed at this time. There is reduced vascularity and sensation so the tissue is at increased risk for injury and reduced capacity to heal; for these reasons, the application of deep tissue techniques to free soft tissue if fixed to underlying structures is not advised at any time. Additionally, increased erythema created by deep techniques may be the inciting event for a lymphedema in this "at risk" tissue.*

## CHEMOTHERAPY

Over 650,000 individuals each year receive chemotherapy.[317] Systemic chemotherapy plays a major role in the management of the 60% of malignancies that are not curable by regional modalities. As with radiation therapy, chemotherapy acts by interfering with cellular function and division. Chemotherapy may be used to cure cancer, to palliate or stabilize disease as preliminary therapy before bone marrow transplantation, or as adjuvant therapy.

In contrast to most cells in the body, tumor cells undergo frequent cell division, leading to an accumulation

## A THERAPIST'S THOUGHTS*

### *Adjuvant Therapies: Radiation*

**Note to Reader:** It is difficult to discuss separate effects of adjuvant therapies (radiation therapy vs. chemotherapy) when so many individuals receive both. Comments here are directed toward radiation therapy, although many of the concepts apply to all people who have been treated for cancer with adjuvant therapy; see also discussion of Adjuvant Therapies: Chemotherapy in the next section below in this chapter.

There were an estimated 13.7 million cancer survivors in the United States in 2012 and that number was expected to rise dramatically in the coming years as mortality from a cancer diagnosis continues to trend downward.[9] This means that there is a high likelihood that an individual seeking physical therapy evaluation and treatment may have a history of cancer with adjuvant treatment such as radiation or chemotherapy. In particular, the therapist's understanding of the tissue and sensory changes associated with previous cancer treatment is critical for patients seeking physical therapy for pain or other musculoskeletal problems.

**Evaluation**

Eliciting a complete past medical history is essential because people often fail to mention previous cancer diagnoses! Careful inspection of scars on the abdomen and trunk will often lead to additions to the history obtained on an intake form. Many people understandably avoid the emotions/reminder associated with a previous cancer diagnosis.

General sensory testing for protective sensation, balance, and proprioception are indicated with a history of radiation (and chemotherapy). Careful examination of the individual who has received radiation treatment is necessary to find boundaries of a previous field of radiation; look for tattoos, skin mobility, surgical scars, sensory changes, temperature, and color. Specific signs associated with radiation changes may include:

- Telangiectasia—seen usually in areas of thinner skin such as the axilla and trunk.
- Collateral veins—seen in unusual areas such as the chest wall; these can represent collateralization of the venous circulation caused by obstruction from deep radiation fibrosis, tumor, or previous deep venous thrombosis (DVT) and always require a physician clearance prior to treatment.
- Lymphedema—assess for lymphedema but keep in mind that a significant swelling of rapid onset or progression (days to weeks) in the proximal aspect of a limb associated with complaints of neurogenic pain is almost *never* a benign presentation and requires a physician's assessment. This clinical presentation is often a sign of recurrence of a cancer—even if the person has been previously treated for lymphedema of this same region (see Chapter 13, The Lymphatic System). Patients with cancer are at increased risk for DVT, which also suggests that physician evaluation is needed when this type of change develops.

**Treatment Planning**

The use of modalities is a standard treatment option in treating many musculoskeletal conditions; however, the use of modalities in the region of previous tumor growth/irradiation/surgery requires very careful consideration. It is important to keep in mind that impaired sensation and circulation, acute inflammation, loss of skin integrity, and acute DVT are common occurrences in this population with exposure to adjuvant therapies. Additionally, there are several risks associated with use of these interventions including possible stimulation of tumor growth/metastasis, increased blood flow allowing potentiation of active chemotherapy or radiation, and increased tissue injury.

Tissue fibrosis is often a significant factor in limitations of active range of motion seen in this population long term. Deep tissue mobilizations in regions of tissues adherent to the underlying structures is not recommended because of the risk of tissue damage in avascular structures, including underlying bone (ribs in particular). However, careful consideration of the layers of musculoskeletal tissue in an irradiated region can lead to the development of focused flexibility exercises to address rib cage, spinal, scapular, and extremity mobility. Instruction in self-mobilization with visual monitoring of the tissue via use of a mirror or direct visualization can assist a patient in maintaining mobility in tissue less amenable to exercise (e.g., the breast).

The emphasis in this population must be on the development of a long-term home exercise program, which is focused in effect and time needed for execution. This is critical given the extended timeframe for tissue remodeling in irradiated tissue and the prolonged nature of the effects of radiation and chemotherapy with regards to cancer fatigue. Flexibility exercises that incorporate multiplanar and multijoint motions are preferable. Practical suggestions as to how to incorporate the needed exercise into daily activities (e.g., while showering) can be very effective in encouraging long-term adherence.

Discomfort and reduced tissue flexibility in a region treated with radiation often leads a patient to consider applying superficial heat to the affected region. Patients must be educated as to the risk of application of superficial heat to tissues that have been exposed to radiation even in the distant past. The tissue is relatively avascular/insensate, leading to a greater risk of thermal injury with increased scarring and extended time to heal. Additionally, local heating of the tissues may trigger lymphedema in a region at risk.

of cells that are cytologically and histologically defective. Cellular processes needed to support this increased cell division, such as DNA synthesis, DNA repair, DNA replication, and RNA transcription, are themselves accelerated. The principal goal of chemotherapy is to destroy malignant cells, with the least harm to normal cells or the host. Although most chemotherapeutic agents are nonspecific and therefore affect both malignant and normal cells, newer medications that target cancer specific abnormalities and immunotherapies are being developed and utilized in cancer treatment.

## Characteristics and Categories of Chemotherapeutic Drugs

Most chemotherapeutic agents are given systemically, meaning they are able to affect the entire body to reach cells in the primary tumor, as well as cancerous cells that may have metastasized. Drugs may be given orally, intramuscularly, intravenously, subcutaneously, and in special cases intrathecally (injected into the spinal fluid), or intraperitoneally (administered into the peritoneum). Most are given intravenously.

Normal cells most at risk for damage by nonspecific chemotherapeutic agents are those that normally have high mitotic rates, such as mucosal cells of the gastrointestinal tract, cells found in the skin, bone marrow cells, and cells involved in hair growth. However, virtually every organ in the body can be affected by these drugs; for this reason, chemotherapy is often accompanied by multisystem problems and complications.

Several major categories of systemic chemotherapeutic agents are recognized, each of which interferes in some manner with cell processes or growth (Table 5.8). *Alkylating agents* were among the first chemotherapy agents employed and are some of the most commonly used chemotherapy drugs today. These agents inhibit cell division by acting directly on DNA; they are able to insert themselves into DNA strands, creating cross-linking of DNA, abnormal base pairing, and breaks in DNA strands. Side effects include bone marrow toxicities, hair loss, GI toxicity, and some increased risk for secondary malignancies (such as bladder cancer from the use of cyclophosphamide and lymphoproliferative cancers). The platinum-based drugs are significantly emetogenic (causing nausea and vomiting), with nephrotoxicity, ototoxicity, and neurotoxicity.

Drugs known as *antimetabolites* are structurally similar to the purine and pyrimidine bases that form the backbone of each DNA strand. These drugs act either by being incorporated into the DNA strand, leading to the synthesis of a defective DNA strand, or by inhibiting enzymes necessary for DNA and RNA replication, as well as protein synthesis. Bone marrow suppression, hepatic dysfunction, and GI toxicities are among the more common side effects seen.

Several chemotherapeutic agents are referred to as *antitumor antibiotics*. These compounds are incorporated into the DNA strand, preventing the synthesis of DNA and to a lesser degree RNA and protein synthesis. They may also induce the formation of free radicals, leading to DNA strand breakage. Pulmonary toxicity is the most severe toxic effect (bleomycin), but GI toxicities and bone marrow suppression are the most common.

Another class of chemotherapy drugs inhibits the enzyme topoisomerase (some inhibit type I while others inhibit type II). Topoisomerase catalyzes the cutting and re-ligating of DNA strands during the unwinding/rewinding process of DNA replication. Topoisomerase inhibitors render the cell unable to replicate. The subclass anthracyclines carry a significant cardiotoxicity, and heart function must be monitored.

A variety of *plant alkaloids* are effective in treating cancers, due to their interference with the formation of the mitotic spindle, preventing the division of cells. They are also known as *mitotic inhibitors* because the cell is arrested in metaphase. Subclasses include the vinca alkaloids and taxanes. The problematic toxicity with vincristine is neurotoxicity.

Although nonspecific chemotherapy drugs remain the mainstay of chemotherapy, drugs targeting critical biochemical pathways unique to tumor cells have become available. One class of antineoplastic agents includes those that inhibit tyrosine kinases. These drugs prevent the phosphorylation and activation of proteins by the class of enzymes known as tyrosine kinases. This leads to dysfunction of the cell and eventually cell death. TKIs have proven to be very effective in treating chronic myeloid leukemia by blocking the BCR-ABL1 pathway (an abnormal fusion gene).[417] They are also used for renal cell carcinoma, hepatocellular carcinoma, and small cell lung cancer, among others.

Other targeted therapies include monoclonal antibodies, which are designed to bind to specific proteins. Angiogenesis inhibitors, for example, were designed to bind and neutralize vascular endothelial growth factor (VEGF) in order to block signaling between cancer cells. Normally as cells grow in a tumor, the cells in the center eventually require a better blood supply, and send out a message for new growth of blood vessel tissue. Blocking of VEGF not only inhibits neovascularization, but also "normalizes" the process, by allowing poorly formed vessels to be reabsorbed, with improvement of existing blood flow.[197] This may explain why VEGF inhibitors, such as bevacizumab, work better with standard chemotherapy; they allow better blood flow and delivery of systemic chemotherapy.[318]

Trastuzumab and pertuzumab, anti-HER2 monoclonal antibodies, are used with traditional chemotherapy to treat some women with breast cancer. Approximately 15% of individuals with invasive breast cancer have increased expression of the human epidermal growth factor receptor (HER2), resulting in aggressive tumors and poor prognosis.[277] These monoclonal antibodies specifically target HER2 receptors and in doing so, increase the likelihood of tumor regression in select individuals. These targeted therapies do not randomly attack rapidly dividing cells, so they generally cause fewer side effects than do traditional chemotherapy drugs.

### Chemoprevention

Breast cancer prevention is a public health focus. Although mammography, screening MRI, and surgery are available to aid in prevention, chemoprevention drugs are available to reduce the risk of developing invasive breast cancer in women at high risk (5-year risk greater than 1.67%; can use the Gail Model Risk Assessment Tool to determine risk at https://bcrisktool.cancer.gov). Chemoprevention is also indicated for those with atypical hyperplasia or lobular carcinoma in situ. The best known of these drugs are those developed to reduce the reoccurrence of breast cancer in women who had tumors responsive to estrogen (or estrogen receptor positive tumors). Tamoxifen and raloxifene are selective estrogen receptor modifiers (SERMs). SERMs block the ability of estrogen to stimulate tumor growth in estrogen positive tumors. Tamoxifen is indicated for use in premenopausal and postmenopausal[91,130] women, whereas raloxifene is only used in postmenopausal women.[270] Tamoxifen is also utilized in the treatment of breast cancer and may be slightly better at reducing the risk of invasive breast cancer.[271,405]

The side effects of these medications include hot flashes; hypertension; increased thromboembolic events; peripheral edema; vaginal bleeding, atrophy, and dryness; depression; fatigue; and nausea. Women taking tamoxifen had an increased incidence of thromboembolic events,

**Table 5-8** Major Toxicities Commonly Associated with Cancer Chemotherapeutic Agents

| Chemotherapy Agents | Major Toxicities |
|---|---|
| **Alkylating Agents** | |
| Busulfan | Myelosuppression,[a] nausea/vomiting |
| Lomustine | Myelosuppression, nephrotoxicity |
| Carmustine | Myelosuppression, nephrotoxicity |
| Chlorambucil | Myelosuppression |
| Cyclophosphamide | Hemorrhagic cystitis, myelosuppression, nausea/vomiting |
| Ifosfamide | Neurotoxicity, myelosuppression, nephrotoxicity, hemorrhagic cystitis |
| Bendamustine | Myelosuppression, mucositis |
| Temozolomide | Myelosuppression, liver toxicity, nausea/vomiting |
| Dacarbazine | Myelosuppression, liver toxicity, nausea/vomiting |
| Cisplatin | Neurotoxicity, peripheral neuropathy, nephrotoxicity, ototoxicity, nausea/vomiting |
| Carboplatin | Myelosuppression |
| Oxaliplatin | Peripheral neuropathy, nausea and vomiting |
| **Antimetabolites** | |
| Pemetrexed | Mucositis, myelosuppression, nausea/vomiting |
| Methotrexate | Mucositis, hepatotoxicity, myelosuppression, neurotoxicity, nephrotoxicity |
| Thioguanine | Myelosuppression, hepatotoxicity |
| Mercaptopurine (6-MP) | Myelosuppression, hepatotoxicity |
| Capecitabine | Myelosuppression, hand-foot syndrome, diarrhea |
| 5-Fluorouracil (5-FU) | Mucositis, diarrhea, myelosuppression |
| Cytarabine | Myelosuppression, hepatotoxicity, neurotoxicity, nausea/vomiting |
| Gemcitabine | Myelosuppression, hepatotoxicity, neurotoxicity, nausea/vomiting |
| Decitabine | Myelosuppression |
| Azacytidine | Myelosuppression |
| Fludarabine | Myelosuppression, immunosuppression |
| Cladribine | Immunosuppression |
| Pentostatin | Immunosuppression |
| **Topoisomerase Inhibitors** | |
| Teniposide | Myelosuppression |
| Etoposide | Myelosuppression |
| Doxorubicin | Cardiotoxicity, alopecia |
| Daunorubicin | Myelosuppression, cardiotoxicity |
| Idarubicin | Myelosuppression, cardiotoxicity |
| Epirubicin | Myelosuppression, cardiotoxicity |
| Mitoxantrone | Myelosuppression, cardiotoxicity, mucositis |
| Topotecan | Myelosuppression, diarrhea |
| Irinotecan | Diarrhea, myelosuppression |
| **Antitumor Antibiotics** | |
| Mitomycin | Myelosuppression, reversible and nonreversible pulmonary fibrosis, nausea/vomiting |
| Bleomycin | Dermal toxicities, reversible and nonreversible pulmonary fibrosis, nausea/vomiting |
| Hydroxyurea | Myelosuppression, interstitial pneumonitis |
| L-Asparaginase | Hypersensitivity reactions, protein synthesis inhibition |
| Actinomycin D | Fatigue, peripheral neuropathy, bone marrow suppression, nausea/vomiting, secondary malignancies, hepatic dysfunction |
| Vorinostat | Fatigue, nausea, diarrhea, thrombocytopenia, QT prolongation |
| **Mitotic Inhibitors** | |
| Vinblastine | Myelosuppression, neurotoxicity |
| Vincristine | Neurotoxicity |
| Vinorelbine | Myelosuppression |
| Paclitaxel | Myelosuppression, neurotoxicity |
| Docetaxel | Myelosuppression, edema |
| Estramustine | Myelosuppression, estrogenic side effects |
| Ixabepilone | Myelosuppression, neurotoxicity |
| **Monoclonal Antibodies** | |
| Rituximab (CD20) | Infusion-related toxicity, B-cell depletion, neutropenia |
| Ibritumomab tiuxetan (CD20) | Hematologic toxicity, myelodysplasia |
| Tositumomab (CD20) | Hematologic toxicity, myelodysplasia |

*Continued*

**Table 5-8** Major Toxicities Commonly Associated with Cancer Chemotherapeutic Agents—cont'd

| Chemotherapy Agents | Major Toxicities |
|---|---|
| Alemtuzumab (CD52) | Infusion-related toxicity, T-cell depletion, myelosuppression |
| Cetuximab (EGFR) | Infusion-related toxicity, skin rash |
| Panitumumab (EGFR) | Infusion-related toxicity, skin rash |
| Bevacizumab (VEGF) | Hypertension, bleeding, thrombotic events |
| Trastuzumab (HER-2) | Cardiomyopathy, infusion-related reactions, myelosuppression |
| **Tyrosine Kinase Inhibitors** | |
| Erlotinib (EGFR) | Rash, diarrhea, interstitial lung disease |
| Lapatinib | Diarrhea, hepatotoxicity, rash, QT prolongation |
| Sorafenib (broad inhibition of multiple kinases) | Diarrhea, fatigue, rash, hand-foot syndrome |
| Sunitinib (broad inhibition of multiple tyrosine kinases) | Diarrhea, fatigue, rash, congestive heart failure |
| Imatinib | Diarrhea, nausea/vomiting, edema, hepatotoxicity, myelosuppression |
| Dasatinib | Diarrhea, nausea/vomiting, edema, hepatotoxicity, myelosuppression, pleural effusions |
| Nilotinib | Diarrhea, nausea/vomiting, edema, hepatotoxicity, myelosuppression, QT prolongation |
| **Miscellaneous** | |
| Bortezomib (inhibits proteasomes) | Myelosuppression, fatigue, peripheral neuropathy |
| Temsirolimus (inhibits mTOR) | Rash, mucositis, myelosuppression, fatigue, pulmonary infiltrates |
| Everolimus (inhibits mTOR) | Rash, mucositis, myelosuppression, fatigue, pulmonary infiltrates |
| Thalidomide (multiple mechanisms, antiangiogenic) | Sedation, constipation, peripheral neuropathy, thromboembolic events |
| Lenalidomide (multiple mechanisms) | Myelosuppression, hepatotoxicity, renal dysfunction, thromboembolic events |
| Retinoids (decrease cell proliferation and induces differentiation) | Dry skin, cheilitis, retinoic acid syndrome |
| Interferons (multiple actions) | Flu-like symptoms, depression, anxiety, myelosuppression |
| Interleukin-2 (Aldesleukin) | Capillary leak syndrome, arrhythmia, rash |
| Denileukin Diftitox | Hypersensitivity reaction, capillary leak syndrome |

[a]Myelosuppression: bone marrow suppression resulting in anemia, leucopenia, and/or thrombocytopenia.

*CD20*, B-lymphocyte antigen CD20 (used to treat B cell diseases); *CD52*, found on mature immune cells (not stem cells), used to treat B cell chronic lymphocytic leukemia; *EGFR*, epidermal growth factor receptor; *VEGF*, vascular endothelial growth factor; *HER*, also a human epidermal growth factor receptor; types 1 and 2; *mTOR*, a serine/threonine-protein kinase (regulates proteins through phosphorylation and affects signaling pathways).

Data from DiPiro JT, Talbert RL, Yee GC, et al, editors. *Pharmacotherapy. A pathophysiologic approach*, ed 8, New York, 2011, McGraw Hill; and Brunton LL, Chabner BA, Knollmann BC, editors. *Goodman & Gilman's the pharmacological basis of therapeutics*, ed 12, New York, 2011, McGraw Hill.

cataracts, and endometrial cancer, as compared to placebo and raloxifene, especially in older women. Overall incidence of adverse events is low. Compared with women receiving placebo, overall quality of life was not significantly different.[99] Raloxifene also increases bone density (the purpose for its original development). SERMs are able to reduce the risk of developing breast cancer by 7 to 9 women per 1000 cases and are given for 5 years. The protective effect against estrogen receptor-positive invasive breast cancer continues after the cessation of tamoxifen.[91]

An additional class of drugs that can be considered as an alternative to SERMs (for women unable to use or tolerate SERMs) for chemoprevention of breast cancer, although not currently approved as such, are *aromatase inhibitors*, such as exemestane and anastrozole.[92] Aromatase inhibitors block an enzyme called aromatase, which changes androgens produced by the adrenal gland in postmenopausal women into estrogen.[404]

Women taking these medications also have a lower risk of blood clots and endometrial cancer as compared to individuals on tamoxifen, but aromatase inhibitor drugs are associated with decreased bone density and a significant percentage of women reporting symptoms of arthralgia or myalgia. The arthralgias involve multiple joints and are reported most often as morning stiffness/pain that diminishes as the day progresses with increased activity. Approximately 25% of women taking anastrozole in one trial reported joint symptoms. A significant number of women with joint symptoms (46%) have reported that a preexisting joint problem was made worse, but in the rest the arthralgia/myalgia symptoms were of new onset.[385]

Symptoms occurred usually within the first 2 years of taking the drugs and were reported to have resolved in 50% of affected individuals within 6 months and in 75% within 18 months. However, there is a high rate of nonadherence with reported rates of 31% to 73% of women having discontinued treatment before completing 5 years of therapy,[262] so the full impact of these medications and their associated side effects (such as arthralgias and myalgias) may be underestimated. General recommendations for symptom management include exercise, weight management, and nonsteroidal medications.[427]

## Adverse Effects of Chemotherapy

Many chemotherapy agents have unique, dose-limiting toxicities. Chemotherapy drugs are used in combination for their specific actions on cells and care is taken not to use agents with significant overlapping toxicities. Table 5.8 outlines the short- and long-term toxicities of commonly used chemotherapy drugs.

Most chemotherapeutic agents have the propensity to cause nausea and vomiting with the administration of the drug, and mucositis, diarrhea, myelosuppression, and alopecia often occur after treatment. Many cause sterility and are toxic to a fetus.

### Alopecia

Alopecia (hair loss) is the most noticeable cutaneous side effect of chemotherapy and often the most distressing because it has a profound social and psychologic impact on the individual. Actively growing hair, or hair in the anagen phase, is the most rapidly proliferating cell population in the human body and therefore very susceptible to the effects of systemic chemotherapeutic agents.

Depending upon which drugs and doses are used, clients may experience varying amounts of hair loss, ranging from thinning of hair to complete loss of hair, including eyelashes, eyebrows, and body hair. Hair loss typically occurs within 1 to 3 weeks after the initiation of chemotherapy. Hair loss is usually temporary, with regrowth of hair 2 to 3 months after termination of treatment (treatment with docetaxel may cause permanent alopecia). Full hair restoration may require 1 to 2 years and may be accompanied by changes in hair color, texture, and type.[176] Clients should be encouraged to prepare for hair loss and given treatment options.[437] Standard advice includes use of a gentle shampoo, wearing scarves, shaving the head, or purchasing a wig.

The scalp may be tender and require special care such as routine application of sunscreen and keeping warm. The application of 2% minoxidil has limited data, but may shorten the time to maximal regrowth.[437]

Although no treatment has been found to be completely effective at reducing hair loss, scalp hypothermia has been shown to provide a varying benefit for people receiving chemotherapy for solid tumors, especially breast cancer.[264,330,397] This treatment consists of placing a cooling device (DigniCap or Paxman) on the scalp during chemotherapy infusion. Overall, only 50% of people who utilize scalp hypothermia retain 50% of their hair and many people are not candidates for this type of treatment. [216,264,330,352] Side effects include feeling uncomfortably cold, dry skin, and headaches.

### Gastrointestinal Toxicity

Chemotherapy drugs cause the most damage to cells that are rapidly growing. Although this is the means by which eradication of tumor cells occurs, these cytotoxins also affect cells that normally divide quickly, such as cells of the oral cavity and GI tract. This damage leads to mucositis, which is defined as ulcerations or damage of the mucous cells lining the GI tract because of cytotoxic cancer chemotherapy and/or radiation.[375] Clinical symptoms include abdominal pain, bloating, nausea/vomiting, diarrhea, and constipation. These side effects are the most common reasons to reduce doses of chemotherapy drugs, delay treatment, or stop treatment.[252] Cytotoxic agents and radiation each have their own potential for causing mucositis and in varying degrees. Mucositis occurs in approximately 20% to 40% of persons receiving chemotherapy and 80% of all those receiving high-dose chemotherapy preparatory for stem-cell transplantation.[219] Current treatment for mucositis is supportive and based on symptom and pain control.[219]

Chemotherapy drugs have a varying ability to cause nausea/vomiting, known as emetogenic potential. High-dose platinum-based agents are among the most strongly emetogenic drugs. Chemotherapy-induced nausea and vomiting (CINV) can be acute or delayed. Acute CINV typically occurs 1 to 2 hours after the administration of the agent, with the effects peaking at 4 to 10 hours after administration and lasting approximately 12 to 24 hours.

Risk factors for CINV include chemotherapy agent used, sex (women affected more frequently than men), age (younger clients), and a previous history of nausea/vomiting with previous chemotherapy, among others. Potential medical complications of chemotherapy-induced emesis include dehydration, electrolyte and acid–base disturbances, and anorexia with accompanying weight loss. Prophylaxis is the best treatment strategy and a variety of antiemetic drugs are currently available to be given prior to treatment and after a treatment.[135,177,267]

Other agents, such as platinum-based agents (i.e., oxaliplatin, cisplatin), are known to cause delayed nausea and vomiting, with symptoms occurring 1 to 5 days after drug administration. Some people suffer nausea and vomiting before drug administration, apparently in anticipation of becoming sick. Acute nausea and vomiting is usually the most severe, whereas the course of delayed nausea and vomiting can be prolonged, leading to dehydration and poor nutrition.

The mechanisms responsible for acute and delayed CINV are varied and not completely understood, and different drugs may cause nausea by utilizing different pathways.[178,200] Chemotherapy agents are felt to induce the release of neurotransmitters (such as serotonin) from enterochromaffin cells in the small intestine. These neurotransmitters bind to receptors on afferent nerve fibers that then activate the brainstem centers. These centers then signal vomiting via the vagus nerve. This model demonstrates the usefulness of serotonin receptor antagonists in acute CINV. Acute emesis appears to be peripherally initiated, but delayed emesis appears to involve a central pathway. This pathway utilizes other neurotransmitters such as substance P and is best treated with neurokinin-1 (NK-1) receptor antagonists, which block substance P. New antiemetics are being developed that are able to block specific neurotransmitters in order to treat CINV.

Constipation and diarrhea are common side effects of chemotherapy that significantly impact the physical and emotional well-being of clients receiving cancer treatment. Constipation is most frequently a consequence of pain medication and inadequate fluid intake. Fecal impactions can be uncomfortable and cause significant morbidity, particularly in the elderly, and clients should be educated and frequently questioned regarding bowel habits in order to avoid complications. Fecal incontinence may be an undisclosed problem. Clients may develop severe diarrhea associated with chemotherapy drugs, particularly with fluoropyrimidines and irinotecan. These and other agents can cause dehydration and life-threatening conditions such as severe acid–base disturbances, requiring hospitalization. Tyrosine kinase inhibitors are also recognized for inducing diarrhea. Chemotherapy-related diarrhea can develop due to secretion of electrolytes (secretory diarrhea), increased osmotic substances in the lumen (osmotic diarrhea), or due to changes in intestinal motility. *Clostridioides difficile*–associated colitis is also a cause for diarrhea and needs to be distinguished from chemotherapy-induced diarrhea. Research is evaluating the gastrointestinal enteric nervous system to aid in treating/preventing chemotherapy-induced diarrhea and constipation.[123]

One rare but life-threatening side effect of intensive chemotherapy is neutropenic enterocolitis,[155] reportedly caused by breakdown of gut defensive mechanisms leading to an invasion of microorganisms and necrosis of bowel. Clinical signs/symptoms include diarrhea, fever, neutropenia, and abdominal pain. Early diagnosis and intervention are keys to successful treatment.[272]

### Myelosuppression

Myelosuppression, defined as the inhibition of bone marrow cells resulting in fewer red cells, white cells, and platelets, is a frequent side effect of many cancer treatments. Myelosuppression often results in anemia, infections, and bleeding, as a result of a reduced number of cells. A reduction of white cells, referred to as leukopenia, or more specifically neutropenia (reduced number of neutrophils), is a major dose-limiting toxicity of cancer treatment and often delays further treatment, possibly compromising outcomes. It is also one of the most serious adverse effects of chemotherapy resulting in significant morbidity, mortality, and cost. Prolonged neutropenia can result in severe, life-threatening infections, requiring prolonged hospital stays and aggressive antibiotic therapy.

Neutropenia (absolute neutrophil count [ANC] less than 1500) increases the risk for infection, and fever with neutropenia is common. *Neutropenic fever* or *febrile neutropenia* is defined as a fever (temperature of 100.4 °F sustained for an hour or one temperature of 101 °F) accompanied by an ANC less than 500 (severe neutropenia).[138] Over 80% of people with hematologic malignancies receiving chemotherapy will develop a neutropenic fever, while it occurs in only 10% to 50% of people with solid tumors.[138] Depending on the expected duration and severity of neutropenia, clients may be at high risk or low risk for complications. Scoring systems are available to aid in determination of risk (e.g., Multinational Association for Supportive Care in Cancer [MASCC]). People at high risk are expected to be severely neutropenic for 7 days or longer and have higher risk scores, while those at low risk are neutropenic for less than 7 days with lower risk scores. Because of the lack of white blood cells, the cause of fever may be bacterial, fungal, or viral. With prolonged neutropenia, fungal infections become more likely (particularly persons who have undergone myeloablative therapy). A source is found in only 20% to 30% of neutropenic fevers,[138] with bacteria ranking as the most common cause. Gram-positive bacteria are seen most often,[182] with *Staphylococcus epidermidis* the most common organism. Gram-negative organisms are the cause of the most serious infections, with a higher mortality (mortality of Gram-positive bacteremia is about 5% while Gram-negative bacteremia mortality is 18%).[138] Unfortunately, the incidence of antibiotic resistant infections continues to rise.

Individuals who develop neutropenic infections are treated initially with antibiotics, with coverage broadening and the addition of antifungals as neutropenia and fever persist.[138,229,379] Antivirals can be used as prophylactic agents or treatment of known viruses. Colony-stimulating factors (CSFs) that stimulate the proliferation and differentiation of hematopoietic progenitor cells are used only prophylactically.[138]

Although erythropoietin analogues increase red blood cell synthesis and reduce anemia, questions have arisen over adverse outcomes (thromboembolism and increased mortality) in certain cancer patient populations, and administration has become more targeted.[293,324] Administration of blood products, such as blood and platelet transfusions, helps alleviate adverse effects and symptoms.[124]

### Fatigue

It has been estimated that between 70% and 100% of all individuals with cancer will experience cancer-related fatigue.[136,181] Cancer-related fatigue may be defined as a persistent, distressing, subjective sense of physical, emotional, and/or cognitive tiredness related to cancer or cancer treatment that is not relieved by rest and is disproportional with recent activity; it also significantly interferes with a person's ability to perform daily tasks.[33,45] Although most people will experience fatigue during treatment (chemotherapy, postsurgery, or postradiation), upwards of 35% still experience fatigue 24 months after completing therapy.[46,342]

Fatigue often peaks within a few days after receiving cyclic chemotherapy then declines until the next treatment cycle. Fatigue significantly reduces quality of life. It is generally agreed that fatigue has multiple cancer-related or treatment-induced causes that can be described as being either physiologic or psychologic. Physiologic causes of fatigue include underlying cancer; cancer treatment; anemia; infection; accompanying pulmonary, hepatic, cardiac, and renal disorders; sleep disorders; poorly controlled pain; lack of exercise, hormonal changes, and malnutrition. Psychologic causes of fatigue include anxiety disorders, depressive disorders, and cognitive losses that include decreased attention span and concentration.[314]

All clients with cancer should be screened for cancer-related fatigue at the initial visit, at each chemotherapy visit, at the end of treatment, and during follow-up care.[45] Because cancer-related fatigue is multifactorial, multidimensional interventions involving both physical and psychologic components are required to successfully treat it.[33,402,416]

**Cardiotoxicity.** Over the last 20 years, therapies for cancer have improved, and more people are surviving cancer. However, aggressive therapies have led to more toxicities, with resulting long-term effects, including toxicities of the heart.[250] Many classic chemotherapy agents and targeted therapies used to treat cancer affect the cardiovascular system.[7] Combining chemotherapy and other agents with cardiotoxic effects or with radiation often amplifies cardiovascular injury.

Each agent used in treating cancer varies in its capacity to cause cardiac damage. Cardiotoxicity may be revealed as a cardiomyopathy manifested as heart failure, with a reduced left ventricular ejection fraction (HFrEF), arrhythmias, myocarditis, myocardial ischemia or infarction, and pericarditis.[7,340] All clients who are to receive chemotherapy agents with known cardiotoxicities should undergo a baseline evaluation of heart function prior to treatment. Individuals with heart abnormalities prior to therapy should receive an alternative agent without cardiotoxicities.

The mechanisms of cardiovascular injury are complex, and most drugs have more than one means of causing injury. The following is a brief summary of some of the more common cardiotoxic drugs; for more details see Table 5.8 for a list of chemotherapy toxicities.

The most common chemotherapy drug class to cause significant cardiotoxicity is the anthracyclines (such as doxorubicin, daunorubicin, and idarubicin). Mitoxantrone, an anthraquinone, is frequently implicated as a cardiotoxic agent as well. These medications can cause HFrEF. The toxicity is cumulative and dose-dependent.[351] Clients receiving these drugs can experience cardiac complications up to 10 years posttreatment.[285] Mitoxantrone is also known to cause arrhythmias during infusion.

Antimetabolite therapies (such as cytarabine) can induce cardiac ischemia and pericarditis. Cardiac ischemia (myocardial necrosis) with resultant myocardial infarction can be seen with the use of fluoropyrimidines, such as 5-fluorouracil.[7] Antimicrotubular agents, such as the vinca alkaloids (particularly vinblastine), can cause hypertension, cardiac ischemia (and infarction), and thromboembolic events. Alkylating agents are associated with acute cardiomyopathy and arrhythmias. Myocardial ischemia and infarction and coronary artery disease has been seen in people receiving antitumor antibiotics, especially bleomycin.

Newer treatments also have significant toxicities. Trastuzumab, a monoclonal antibody to the HER-2 receptor, is associated with the risk of developing cardiac dysfunction, which increases substantially when this drug is used in combination with anthracyclines or cyclophosphamide.[134,154,340] Arrhythmias are seen with histone deacetylase inhibitors; protein kinase inhibitors (tyrosine kinase inhibitors [TKI])[4,292] such as nilotinib [368]; and taxanes. Myocardial necrosis with resulting HFrEF is noted in the use of sunitinib and other multitargeted kinase inhibitors[97] that target vascular endothelial growth factor; alemtuzumab, a CD52 monoclonal antibody; and taxanes in combination with anthracyclines. Bosutinib and IL-2 both increase edema and can lead to pericardial effusions. Antiangiogenic agents[183,244] and proteasome inhibitors (bortezomib)[171] can cause HFrEF, myocardial ischemia/infarction, and cardiac arrest.

High-dose regimens and the total dose per course increase the likelihood of developing cardiac disease. Cessation of the drug will often decrease symptoms. Complicating risk factors for the development of cardiovascular injury caused by drugs include dose, infusion rate, younger and advanced age, exposure to mediastinal radiation, previous heart disease, and hypertension.

Clients with risk factors or who are to receive agents known to cause cardiotoxicities are monitored carefully. Risk factors should be optimized prior to receiving therapy such as manage hypertension; treat coronary artery disease; clients should stop smoking; lose weight (if needed); and maintain an exercise program. They may receive cardioprotective medications, liposomal-based formulation of an anthracycline,[322] serial echocardiograms[291] or multiple gated acquisition scans to evaluate heart function, or blood tests evaluating troponin levels, looking for myocardial damage.[309] More accurate biomarkers are needed in order to find cardiovascular injury earlier.

Dexrazoxane, a cardiotoxicity preventive medication, has been shown to slow or reduce the effects of anthracyclines,[191] although due to uncertainty concerning the drug's effect on cancer, it is restricted to treating women with metastatic breast cancer who have received doxorubicin in the past and require doxorubicin again. ACE inhibitors/ARBs and beta-blocker medications are beneficial in the treatment of HFrEF; however it is uncertain if these medications provide protection from anthracycline therapy.[44] Statins are currently being evaluated as a cardioprotective agent.[1]

### Pulmonary Toxicity

Pulmonary toxicity as a result of cancer treatments is relatively common, affecting 20% to 30% of people receiving chemotherapy.[108,143] Many classes of chemotherapy agents are known to have pulmonary toxicities that range from bronchospasm to pneumonitis to acute lung injury.[396]The most common classical chemotherapy drugs to induce pulmonary toxicities are bleomycin and mitomycin. Newer agents have also been connected with pulmonary toxicities, such as rituximab, bevacizumab, and erlotinib.[259] Unfortunately, it is often difficult to determine if disease complications or drugs are causing pulmonary disorders.[396] Clients with a history of underlying pulmonary disease are monitored to minimize any further pulmonary decline, and chemotherapy agents are carefully chosen.

Risk of pulmonary toxicity is increased with advancing age, tobacco use, concomitant irradiation, and accumulated dose. For those clients with previous unrelated pulmonary disease, the development of pulmonary pneumonitis or fibrosis may be life-threatening. Symptoms of lung toxicity typically occur within a few months of starting treatment,[396] although fibrosis, seen with nitrosoureas and bleomycin, can occur years after completion of treatment.[286] Lung injury due to chemotherapy agents typically leads to discontinuation of the medication and may affect treatment prognosis.

### Renal Toxicity (Nephrotoxicity)

Many chemotherapy agents, antibiotics, and other drugs used in cancer treatment are metabolized and excreted by the kidneys, making the renal system prone to injury or exacerbating underlying disease. Renal abnormalities are one of the most commonly encountered problems associated with cancer therapy, which may alter dosing or require a change in therapy. Renal impairment can be manifested as a range of abnormalities spanning from an asymptomatic increase in BUN and creatinine on laboratory tests, to more serious disorders, such as acute and chronic kidney injury. In one study, the risk of developing acute kidney injury (AKI) at one and five years from cancer diagnosis was approximately 18% and 27% respectively.[75] AKI occurred most commonly in people with kidney cancer, liver cancer, and multiple myeloma. About 5% of these clients with AKI required dialysis within one year of developing AKI (renal replacement therapy). Many people already have chronic kidney injury (CKI) prior to treatment, and CKD and end stage renal disease are both risks for developing cancer, such as renal cancer and urothelial cancers.[236]

As with other systems affected by chemotherapy, clients with underlying kidney disease require special care and monitoring to maintain kidney function. The classical chemotherapy agents that are most often related to renal injury include cisplatin, methotrexate, and the alkylating class of drugs. Cyclophosphamide and ifosfamide are particularly known to cause hemorrhagic cystitis. The metabolite created from these agents (acrolein) irritates the bladder, causing bleeding and pain. Mesna (2-mercaptoethanesulfonate) can be administered with the drug in order to reduce the risk of hemorrhagic cystitis by binding acrolein and forming an inactive compound that is excreted. Targeted therapies and immunotherapies are also known to cause AKI, such as tyrosine kinase inhibitors, rituximab, anti-VEGF agents, and ipilimumab.

A serious complication of chemotherapy that has significant adverse effects on the kidneys is tumor lysis syndrome (TLS). Tumor lysis syndrome is considered an oncologic emergency and occurs when cytotoxic drugs destroy malignant cells, releasing large amounts of intracellular ions and metabolic byproducts into the bloodstream (e.g., potassium, phosphate, and uric acid). The kidneys are unable to tolerate the sudden load, producing hyperkalemia, hyperuricemia, and hyperphosphatemia. Hypocalcemia subsequently develops due to hyperphosphatemia. Damage occurs to the kidneys when crystals form from these compounds, leading to inflammation, obstruction, and eventually decrease in the glomerular filtration rate (GFR). This can be life-threatening, leading to cardiac dysrhythmias and renal failure.

Clients who have renal insufficiency before treatment, large tumors, or rapidly dividing tumors that are sensitive to chemotherapy, such as acute leukemias and some lymphomas, are at highest risk for this syndrome. Treatment consists of early recognition, hydration, close monitoring, and treatment of metabolic abnormalities. The medications allopurinol and rasburicase are used prophylactically to reduce the risk of hyperuricemia, and rasburicase is used to treat (if not given prophylactically) hyperuricemia associated with tumor lysis syndrome.[120]

Thrombotic microangiopathy (TMA) is an uncommon but serious disorder caused by vessel damage and occlusion of small blood vessels by platelet microthrombi. TMA can occur due to cancer, as well as secondary to specific drugs, such as VEGF inhibitors (bevacizumab) and gemcitabine. Clinical manifestations include microangiopathic hemolytic anemia, thrombocytopenia, and organ injury (including AKI). Gemcitabine is associated with an immune reaction to the drug that injures small vessels, causing acute onset kidney disease that may lead to CKI with hypertension.VEGF inhibitors are associated with dose- and time-dependent injury that appears slowly, resulting in kidney injury and hypertension.[150]

### Hepatic Toxicity

Multiple chemotherapy agents are known to cause acute or chronic liver injury, which can be compounded by other hepatotoxic drugs or radiation. Damage to the liver can also change the metabolism of other chemotherapy drugs or medications used for other purposes, increasing toxicities. Preexisting viral hepatitis can be exacerbated by chemotherapy. Classic chemotherapy drugs that are known to cause hepatotoxicity include methotrexate, l-asparaginase, carmustine, mercaptopurine, dacarbazine, etoposide, gemcitabine, fluorouracil (5-FU), irinotecan, cisplatin, oxaliplatin, and capecitabine (see Table 5.8).[319] Ipilimumab, pembrolizumab, gemtuzumab, and nivolumab are a few newer antineoplastic agents that are also associated with hepatotoxicity. For clients with preexisting liver injury, dose modifications or careful selection of agents is needed to avoid further damage and systemic toxicities. Drug-induced liver injury is frequently responsible for altering or interrupting treatment plans.[19]

Several patterns of injury occur due to chemotherapy drugs, including steatosis, chemotherapy-induced steatohepatitis, noncirrhotic portal hypertension,[189] and sinusoidal injury. Approximately 85% of people receiving chemotherapy develop steatosis, which is the synthesis of fatty acids and retention of lipids in hepatocytes.[319] This can be problematic in that hepatocytes with a high lipid content may be more prone to injury from subsequent treatment.[76] Steatohepatitis, inflammation and injury of hepatocytes, although less common, is more serious than steatosis because it can progress to irreversible fibrosis and cirrhosis. Sinusoidal injury may range from sinusoid dilation to obstruction.

Sinusoidal obstruction syndrome (SOS) (previously termed venoocclusive disease) is typically seen in clients receiving high-dose chemotherapy in preparation for bone marrow transplant and has also been linked to the use of oxaliplatin in colorectal liver metastases.[119] Damage to endothelial cells of the central veins by toxic agents produces congestion with progressive hemorrhagic necrosis of centrolobular hepatocytes. Later there is deposition of fibrin in the vessel walls, causing a nonthrombotic occlusion of the terminal hepatic venules.[319] In its severe form, SOS is usually fatal. Prevention of SOS consists of minimizing risk factors, and use of prophylactic ursodiol (a bile acid).[201] Bevacizumab may help reduce the incidence of SOS, although it is associated with other significant side effects (such as stroke and thromboembolic events).[119] Clients who may receive therapy utilizing a drug known to cause liver injury should also avoid hepatotoxic agents such as alcohol and acetaminophen.

Chemotherapy is also frequently given prior to surgery for metastatic colorectal cancer to the liver, in order to shrink the size of tumor(s). The damage caused by chemotherapy often leaves the liver with little reserve to tolerate surgery,[326] poor regeneration ability, and injury to the biliary tree, and postsurgical outcomes are accompanied by complications such as intraoperative bleeding and increased postoperative infections.[210]

### Neuropathies

Many chemotherapeutic agents adversely affect the nervous system either peripherally or centrally, depending on the pharmacologic properties of the class of chemotherapy drug. Chemotherapy-induced peripheral neuropathy (CIPN), a toxicity-related injury of peripheral neurons, is commonly observed in several classes of chemotherapy agents—microtubule targeting agents (i.e., taxanes and vinca-alkaloids), heavy metal compounds (i.e., platinum compounds), and some biologic agents (i.e., bortezomib, thalidomide) (see Table 5.8 for a specific list).

Although the mechanism of injury is not fully understood, these drugs tend to be found in higher concentration in the dorsal root ganglion, where sensory nerve cell bodies are found, compared to ventral horn cell bodies of motor neurons.[307,387,435] In addition, it has been documented that clients with CIPN have a dying back of sensory neurons[57,225] more than motor neurons. These observations are consistent with the predominately sensory symptoms experienced by clients. However, some clients also experience motor and autonomic symptoms.

CIPN symptoms can develop within hours after an infusion or may not appear for several days to weeks after treatment has stopped. Although most symptoms will improve or resolve, some clients report their symptoms persist for years after completing treatment.[321] Clients will often describe numbness, tingling (paresthesias/dysesthesias), or burning of their hands or feet, that will progress in a distal to proximal pattern as the neuropathy becomes more severe.

Other common impairments include diminished or absent deep tendon reflexes, increased vibration and touch thresholds, hyperalgesia, allodynia, and reduced sural and peroneal nerve conduction amplitudes. In cases where motor neuropathy occurs, clients will present with weakness and/or cramping of distal muscles in the hands and feet; and in the rare case of autonomic neuropathy, orthostatic hypotension, constipation, and dysfunction of sexual organs and urinary bladder may be reported.

The severity of neuropathy is related to several factors, including cumulative dose, coexisting peripheral neuropathy, and combination therapy of several neurotoxic chemotherapy agents.[425] As a result of impairment to peripheral nerve function, clients may experience deficits in the activity and participation realm, such as decreased balance, gait instability, and decreased fine motor coordination.[114,387,426]

Oncology physicians and nurses monitor their patients for the development and severity of CIPN. Physical therapists can also assess CIPN severity, but often are more concerned with the functional implications of the neuropathy as it progresses (see tools used by the physical therapist in the "Special Implications: Chemotherapy/Neuropathy" section of this chapter). The most commonly used method by physicians is the CTCAE version 4.0.[395] There are two scales, one for sensory symptoms and one for motor symptoms. In grade 1 neuropathy, clients are asymptomatic for motor symptoms, and/or present with loss of deep tendon reflexes or paresthesias. In grade 2, clients experience moderate symptoms that limit instrumental activities of daily living. In grade 3, symptoms are severe and limit self-care activities of daily living. And in grade 4, symptoms are life-threatening. Many physicians will not change drug dose or drug type unless the client experiences a severe, grade 3 or 4, neuropathy. However, it is becoming recognized by the medical community that a prospective surveillance model for CIPN that includes early intervention for symptoms and mobility-related limitations, such as a referral for physical therapy, will help minimize acute and long-term morbidity associated with CIPN.[369]

Central nervous system toxicity may present as an acute or delayed complication from some chemotherapy drugs. Impairments can manifest as a range of problems, including neurovascular complications, headaches, focal neurologic deficits, generalized neurologic decline with cognitive impairment, seizure activity, spinal cord damage with myelopathy, cortical atrophy, and white matter abnormalities. The mode of administration (intrathecal versus intravenous) and cumulative dose impacts the severity of toxicity.

Alkylating agents, such as cisplatin or ifosfamide, are known to be neurotoxic. Like many other chemotherapy-related impairments, symptoms may be transient or chronic in nature.[110,273] Antimetabolites, such as methotrexate, cytarabine, and gemcitabine also cause neurotoxicity. Methotrexate, in particular, may cause acute (within hours of administration) symptoms, including headache, neck pain, nausea/vomiting, fever, and photophobia as the result of an aseptic meningitis. Subacutely (within 2 weeks of a dose),[65] recipients may develop acute stroke-like symptoms with focal weakness/seizures or myelopathy-like symptoms with bladder dysfunction, back pain, or local limb weakness.

Chemotherapy-related cognitive impairment, sometimes referred to as "chemobrain," continues to be a controversial topic in oncology care. The subjective and objective measures vary, making it difficult to have a clear definition of this phenomenon. Regardless, many clients will report changes to their attention, memory, or other cognitive function (e.g., learning and speed of processing information) during or after chemotherapy treatment. Individuals treated with high-dose protocols or increased number of cycles of chemotherapy are more likely to complain of impairment.[250] There are several measurement tools available to the therapist to document these changes.[157] A case study series has shown that complementary therapies, such as yoga, may be beneficial for this problem.[145] Referral for speech or occupational therapy for cognitive retraining may also be helpful.

## Adverse Effects of Hematopoietic Cell Transplantation

See Chapter 21 for full discussion of the adverse effects of hematopoietic cell transplantation.

SPECIAL IMPLICATIONS FOR THE THERAPIST 5-7

## *Chemotherapy*

### Chemotherapy Hazard for Health Care Professionals

Questions are often raised by therapists working directly with clients during chemotherapy or during the period shortly after infusion. Are contact precautions required? Is there any evidence to support this practice? The general consensus of clinical oncology specialists is that although chemotherapy is excreted through the person's body fluids (urine, feces, saliva, vomit, blood), very few agents are secreted through sweat glands and/or skin, and only in high doses, such as in transplant settings. Two drugs known to exit the body via sweat are thiotepa (Thioplex) and cyclophosphamide (Cytoxan).[239,347] Gloves for skin-to-skin contact during and within 24 hours of infusion of these medications may be advised. Otherwise contact precautions are not required in most facilities while working with patients on chemotherapy. Until there is evidence to support this policy, some health care professionals are choosing to wear gloves as a contact precautionary measure.

**Note to Reader:** When we asked our PharmD consultant to research this topic for us, here's what he reported: "This has been a frustrating search for me. Unfortunately, I cannot find any good references that support using gloves when in contact with a chemotherapy patient's sweat. I've found some general recommendations that suggest using gloves for 48 hours after chemotherapy when in contact with a chemotherapy patient's body fluids. But again, no good supporting evidence. I think the recommendations in this section are accurate and safe. The following are links to some information describing this same precaution:"

- American Cancer Society (ACS). Understanding chemotherapy: a guide for patients and families. Available online at http://www.cancer.org/treatment/treatmentsandsideeffects/treatmenttypes/chemotherapy/understandingchemotherapyaguideforpatientsandfamilies/understanding-chemotherapy-chemo-safety-for-those-around-me
- St. Jude Children's Research Hospital. Patient medications: cyclophosphamide. Available online at: http://www.stjude.org/SJFile/cyclophosphamide.pdf
- St. Jude Children's Research Hospital. Patient medications: thiotepa. Available online at: http://www.stjude.org/SJFile/thiotepa.pdf

### Chemotherapy-Related Considerations for the Client

The period during chemotherapy administration is critical for each client, who may be susceptible to spontaneous hemorrhage and infection. Anyone receiving chemotherapeutic drugs is at increased risk of acquiring an infection because these drugs often reduce white blood cell numbers; almost one-third of all chemotherapy patients are impacted by febrile or severe neutropenia, most commonly in the first cycle.[89,237] Because neutropenia can occur with a normal white blood cell count, the number of absolute neutrophil count is often used as a measure of neutropenia. An absolute neutrophil count of less than 1500 cells/mm$^3$ defines neutropenia.

*The usual precautions for infection control must be strictly adhered to, including proper hand hygiene and the usual precautions for thrombocytopenia. The importance of strict handwashing technique with an antiseptic solution cannot be overemphasized.*

*The therapist should be alert to any sign of infection and report any potential site of infection, such as mucosal ulceration or skin abrasion or tear. Check skin for petechiae, ecchymoses, cellulitis, and secondary infection.*

*Myelosuppression or bone marrow suppression is the most frequent side effect of many chemotherapeutic drugs. These drugs can cause the circulating numbers of one or more of the mature red blood cells to fall to dangerous levels. Significantly decreased hemoglobin, hematocrit, and red blood cell numbers can compromise an individual's ability to engage in physical activity.*

*Drug-induced mood changes ranging from feelings of well-being and euphoria to depression and irritability may occur; depression and irritability may also be associated with the cancer. Knowing these and other potential side effects of medications used in the treatment of cancer can help the therapist better understand client reactions during rehabilitation or therapy intervention. Collectively, the therapist should do the following:*

- Be aware of the possibility of myelosuppression in the person on chemotherapy drugs.
- Monitor the hematology values in these individuals.
- Be aware of the signs and symptoms of the major side effects of myelosuppression (e.g., anemia, infection, and bleeding).
- Treat clients appropriately within the context of the limitations and risks represented by myelosuppression.

*As part of the cancer care team, the therapist should keep abreast of reliable up-to-date information about treatment. The American Cancer Society publishes educational materials such as Understanding Chemotherapy: A Guide for Patients and Families. These types of introductory materials may help the therapist come to a better understanding of the patient's own early experiences and questions. Educational materials are usually provided free. Contact the local American Cancer Society office; if there is no local or district office, contact the national organization (www.cancer.org or (800) ACS-2345).*

### Late Effects of Chemotherapy

It is important for the therapist to realize that the adverse effects of many chemotherapeutic agents may not appear for many years after treatment has been completed. For example, bleomycin can cause significant pulmonary fibrosis, resulting in decreased pulmonary function; Adriamycin can cause significant cardiac damage 5 to 20 years after treatment; and growth hormone deficiency is the most common endocrinopathy after cranial radiation for brain tumor.

*Survivors face an increased risk of morbidity, mortality, and diminished quality of life associated with cancer treatment. Risk is further modified by the survivor's genetics, lifestyle habits, and comorbid health conditions. The Childhood Cancer Survivor Study provides much information on survivorship, occupational outcomes, health-related quality of life issues, long-term complications, and the underutilization of physical therapy among cancer survivors.*[211,255,287]

*Because a therapist is less likely to see individuals receiving these drugs acutely, the greater concern is for the cardiac and other organ damage, which manifests itself months to years after the cancer treatment has ended. Survivors of childhood and adolescent cancer are one of the higher risk populations seen. The curative therapy administered for the cancer also affects growing and developing tissues.*[287]

*Careful history taking is important in gaining this information. The therapist must be aware of this because it may explain the symptoms the therapist is evaluating or create comorbid conditions that impact the plan of care.*

### Neuropathy

CIPN is a toxic neuropathy that may cause sensory, motor or autonomic nervous system impairments (see Table 5.8 for a list of neurotoxic drugs). Sensory symptoms often predominate and include numbness, tingling, and burning of the hands and feet and may progress in a proximal pattern. Motor symptoms include weakness and/or cramping of distal muscles. Autonomic symptoms of orthostatic hypotension, constipation and dysfunction of sexual organs and urinary bladder may also be observed.

*There are many methods to measure the severity of CIPN, including symptom-based questionnaires like the chemotherapy-induced peripheral neuropathy assessment scale,*[386] *touch thresholds using Semmes Weinstein monofilaments, or quantitative vibration thresholds. Many feel that it is best to use a polymodal test, such as a modified or reduced total neuropathy scale, to capture sensory, motor, large and small fiber impairments in one test. These reduced scales have shown high reliability to the gold standard Total Neuropathy Scale, but because they exclude nerve conduction testing, they are more clinically feasible.*[156,157,356,409]

*The severity of CIPN and which types of nerves have been impaired will impact the therapist's treatment plan. If the client has impaired protective sensation, then education in proper foot wear and how to protect him- or herself from cuts or burns is warranted. In the case of hypersensitivity to cold (seen acutely after oxaliplatin therapy) or touch, therapists can use sensory reeducation and desensitization techniques to minimize pain. Weakness of ankle or hand muscles would necessitate a strengthening program. If the weakness is severe, an ankle–foot orthotic for foot drop or adaptive equipment to assist weak hand muscles in activity of daily living tasks may be helpful.*

*The therapist will want to assess balance in all individuals taking neurotoxic chemotherapy, because even low scores on the modified total neuropathy scale, indicating a mild neuropathy, have been associated with significant balance impairments.*[410] *Breast cancer survivors, even up to 2 years out from completing their chemotherapy, have been documented to report falls and balance problems.*[179,426] *When developing a balance intervention, the therapist should consider strengthening exercises, as well as static and dynamic skill practice with various sensory challenges (i.e., eyes open, eyes closed, on foam, with head shakes).*[408] *The therapist may also recommend an assistive device in cases of severe balance problems.*

*Finally, if the therapist recommends aerobic exercise for other impairments, such as cancer-related fatigue, then several CIPN impairments may need to be considered. If the client is unsteady with walking, then it may be better to recommend biking or swimming. The therapist will need to monitor for abnormal heart rate and blood pressure responses in clients with autonomic peripheral neuropathy.*

### Chemotherapy and Exercise

For a discussion of chemotherapy and exercise, see "Cancer, Physical Activity, and Exercise Training" in Chapter 9.

# SPECIFIC DISORDERS AFFECTING MULTIPLE SYSTEMS

## Vasculitic Syndromes

*Vasculitis* is a term that applies to a diverse group of diseases characterized by inflammation in blood vessel walls that causes narrowing, blockage, aneurysm formation, or rupture. Vasculitis is classified according to the size of the vessel affected (i.e., large-vessel, medium-vessel, and small-vessel vasculitis). The primary forms of vasculitis encountered in a therapy practice include: giant cell (temporal) arteritis, polymyalgia rheumatic (not a vasculitis but often accompanies giant cell arteritis), and Takayasu arteritis (large-vessel disease); polyarteritis nodosa and Kawasaki disease (medium-vessel disease); and granulomatosis with polyangiitis (formerly known as Wegener granulomatosis) (small-vessel disease) and IgA vasculitis (formerly known as Henoch-Schönlein purpura) (immune complex-mediated vasculitis).

Large-vessel disease often produces headache, aching in the shoulders/neck/hip, limb claudication, hypertension, aortic dilation, and bruits. Vasculitis of the medium vessels causes cutaneous nodules (Fig. 5.7), edema or erythema of the digits, coronary aneurysms, mononeuritis multiplex, and abdominal pain. Sinusitis, palpable purpura, glomerulonephritis (renal disease), and alveolar hemorrhage (pulmonary disease) can be seen in disease affecting small vessels.

Most clients with vasculitis will exhibit constitutional symptoms such as fever, arthralgias, arthritis, weight loss, and malaise.[365] Vasculitis may occur as a primary disease (as described above) or as a secondary manifestation of other illnesses such as autoimmune diseases (RA or

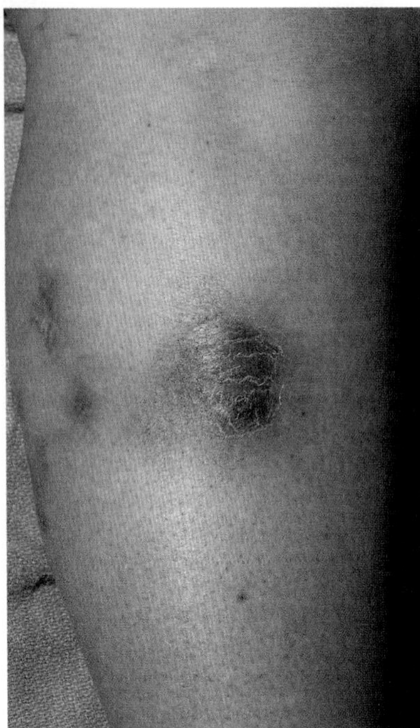

**Figure 5.7**

**Nodular vasculitis caused by inflammation of the medium blood vessels.** From James W, et al: *Andrews' diseases of the skin: Clinical dermatology*, ed 13, St. Louis, 2020, Elsevier.

systemic lupus erythematosus), infection (hepatitis B), malignancy (hairy cell leukemia), or as a drug-induced illness (hydralazine).

## Rheumatoid Arthritis

See the complete discussion of RA in Chapter 27.

RA is best known as a progressive, autoimmune disease affecting the synovial tissue and joints. Yet RA has many extraarticular manifestations involving bone, muscle, eyes, lung, heart, and the skin.[85] The presence and severity of extraarticular manifestations generally depends on the duration and severity of the RA, with increased risk seen in people with rheumatoid factor, anti-citrullinated peptide antibodies (ACPA), and individuals that smoke. The most frequent skin manifestation is the rheumatoid nodule. These are most commonly found subcutaneously on extensor surfaces, such as the forearm (olecranon region), or pressure points, such as the sacrum in immobile clients, but have been noted in the lung.

Other extraarticular conditions that can occur with RA include vasculitis, lung involvement, bone marrow involvement (anemia/thrombocytopenia), and osteopenia/osteoporosis. *Rheumatoid vasculitis* has become much less frequent over the last decade, probably because of disease-modifying agents, yet it remains the most feared complication of RA, with considerable morbidity and mortality. Vasculitis is more common in men and usually develops in persons with the most significant active disease (deforming arthritis and high rheumatoid factor titers).

Clinical features of systemic rheumatoid vasculitis are diverse because the disease affects both large and small vessels throughout the body. The most common findings are cutaneous lesions such as nail-edge infarctions, purpura (see Fig. 5.1), and skin ulcers (e.g., pyoderma gangrenosum). Skin ulcers usually develop suddenly as deep, punched-out lesions at sites that are unusual for venous ulceration, such as the dorsum of the foot or the upper calf.

Neurologic manifestations of RA present most commonly as either a mild distal sensory neuropathy (paresthesia or numbness) or as a severe sensorimotor neuropathy, such as wrist or foot drop (mononeuritis multiplex), as seen with RA vasculitis. Carpel tunnel syndrome is the most common neurologic manifestation of extraarticular RA. Involvement of the central nervous system is rare.

People with RA have a higher risk of developing coronary artery disease, heart failure, and atrial fibrillation.[144,391] Cardiovascular disease is one of the leading causes of death in people with RA. Affected individuals may already have traditional risk factors for heart disease, which are then superimposed with chronic inflammation from RA.[281] Aggressive treatment of RA has been shown to decrease the development of heart disease.[248] Lung involvement may be manifested as pulmonary effusions or interstitial lung disease. Infarction of the intestine may occur, requiring bowel resection.

Dry eyes are a common manifestation affecting 10% to 20% of clients with RA. Episcleritis and scleritis are uncommonly encountered (less than 5%).

Systemic manifestations of rheumatoid vasculitis may include unexplained weight loss, anorexia, and malaise. Malaise may be related to the release of cytokines (substances released by lymphocytes with various immunologic functions) and may be accompanied by fatigue, low-grade fever, and night sweats. Individuals with severe RA who experience any of these symptoms should be referred to the physician for further evaluation. Clients with multiple manifestations of vasculitis have a poor prognosis and require aggressive treatment.

Anemia secondary to RA is usually mild with normocytic/normochromic features and is proportional to the disease severity. More than three-fourths of people with RA and anemia have anemia of chronic disease; one-quarter will respond to iron supplementation. In addition, either group may have superimposed $B_{12}$ or folate deficiency.[302] If an individual with RA is noted to have iron deficiency, sources of bleeding must be explored, such as GI bleeding from therapy with NSAIDs. Anemia with a hemoglobin value less than 10 is rarely associated with RA and should be investigated aggressively for another cause. The therapist should follow special precautions related to anemia until the disease is under control.

Thrombocytosis is frequently seen in clients with RA, particularly in people who have extraarticular manifestations and severe disease. Felty syndrome is an uncommon but serious manifestation of severe RA. Clients exhibit splenomegaly, thrombocytosis, and neutropenia and are at risk for infection, skin ulcerations, and other complications.

Osteopenia and osteoporosis may result from postmenopausal bone loss, treatment with glucocorticoids, or general immobility, but it may also be an inherent part of

RA. Because most clients with RA may have all these risk factors for bone loss, they should be aggressively treated to reduce bone loss. With longstanding disease, osteoporosis may become generalized and can lead to fractures after minimal stress, particularly the fibula.

## Systemic Lupus Erythematosus

Lupus erythematosus is an autoimmune disease that appears in two forms: discoid lupus erythematosus, which affects only the skin, and systemic lupus erythematosus (SLE), which affects both the skin and multiple organ systems. SLE most commonly causes rashes of the skin; polyarthalgia, polyarthritis, and myalgias; and nonscarring alopecia. The most serious complications affect the heart (pericarditis, endocarditis, myocarditis, coronary artery disease), kidneys (nephritis and nephrosis), CNS (vasculitis associated transverse myelitis, aseptic meningitis, stroke, seizure, encephalitis), and the lungs (pleuritis). SLE also affects the bone marrow, leading to anemia, thrombocytopenia, and leukopenia. Gastrointestinal manifestations are often underrecognized and undiagnosed. SLE clients have a higher risk of developing a malignancy, such as non-Hodgkin lymphoma. Like RA, SLE is characterized by recurring remissions and exacerbations. Morbidity and mortality are increasingly related to side effects from medications (infection, malignancy) and long-term organ damage from severe disease (chronic kidney disease, cardiac, or neurologic complications). SLE is also an independent risk factor for cardiovascular disease.

## Systemic Sclerosis

Scleroderma or systemic sclerosis (SSc) is a generalized connective tissue disorder of unknown etiology characterized by immune dysregulation (autoantibody production), microangiopathy (vasculitis and obstruction of small vessels), and fibrosis of skin and internal organs. It may also affect the heart, lungs, kidneys, GI tract, and musculoskeletal system.

Although there are many subgroups termed *scleroderma* (scleroderma-like), it is often categorized into three main subgroups to help clinically prognosticate: limited and diffuse cutaneous scleroderma and systemic sclerosis sine scleroderma (ssSSc). Limited cutaneous scleroderma (lcSSc) is characterized by skin thickening that typically does not progress proximal to the elbows and knees (although the face and neck may be involved). A subset of clients with lcSSc demonstrates a syndrome known as the CREST syndrome (Calcinosis, Raynaud phenomenon, Esophageal dysmotility, Sclerodactyly, and Telangiectasia).

Diffuse cutaneous scleroderma (dcSSc) extends proximally to the elbows and knees, including the chest, abdomen, upper arms, and shoulders. Clients with dcSSc are more likely to develop rapid progression of their disease with internal organ injury secondary to ischemia and fibrosis, whereas ssSSc is characterized by fibrosis of internal organs without the presence of skin manifestations.

There is significant variability of symptoms and organ involvement between clients. It affects women more than men, especially between ages 35 and 50 years. Better therapy for specific complications (such as scleroderma renal crisis, pulmonary hypertension) has developed with immune suppression recommended for fibrosis of the skin and lung.[24,107] Significant research into immunosuppressive therapy, antifibrotic therapies, and other investigational studies are ongoing.[24] (See Chapter 10 for discussion of this condition.)

## Tuberculosis

Tuberculosis (TB) is an acute or chronic infection caused by *Mycobacterium tuberculosis,* an acid-fast staining bacillus. Although the primary infection site is the lung, mycobacteria, through hematogenous dissemination, can spread to other parts of the body; this is referred to as *extrapulmonary TB.* Extrapulmonary TB is present in about 30% of active TB cases but is often present without symptomatic lung disease or abnormalities on chest radiographs. The extrapulmonary sites may include the renal system, skeletal system (osteomyelitis; vertebral TB is known as *Pott disease*), GI tract, meninges (tuberculous meningitis), pericardium, peritoneum, lymph system, and genitourinary system. Extrapulmonary TB occurs with increased frequency in people with HIV infection. Clinical suspicion, physical exam, and testing aid in the diagnosis of extrapulmonary TB. Testing may include histologic examination and nucleic acid amplification test (NAAT) on tissue obtained in extrapulmonary sites.[233] (See Chapter 15 for more on pulmonary TB; see Chapter 25 for more on tuberculous spondylitis [Pott disease]).

## Sarcoidosis

Sarcoidosis is a multisystem disorder characterized by the formation of noncaseating granulomas, defined as a core of monocyte-derived epithelioid cells and multinucleated giant cells interspersed with or surrounded by lymphocytes. These granulomas may develop in any organ but often are noted in multiple organs at once, including the lungs (90% of clients with sarcoidosis will have lung involvement), skin, heart, lymph nodes, kidney, musculoskeletal system, CNS, or eyes.

Presenting symptoms of sarcoidosis can often be confused with other inflammatory or infectious processes that form granulomas, making the diagnosis difficult and usually requiring a biopsy.[28,376,39] Sarcoidosis involvement of the skin and eye occurs more commonly among women, whereas men have a higher incidence of heart involvement.[203]

There is significant morbidity and mortality associated with this multisystem disease. Treatment for inflammatory disease consists of glucocorticoids, DMARDS, and TNF-alpha inhibitors.[28,29,423] Most deaths are related to disease involvement of the heart or lung.

## Sepsis

### Overview

Sepsis is a systemic syndrome that affects all ages, is found in communities, hospitals, and extended-care facilities, and involves all medical specialties. It is a significant public health issue costing over $24 billion dollars in hospital costs alone in 2013.[388] Sepsis is the most costly hospital condition, with costs rising as the severity of sepsis increases. This not only increases the length of hospital stay, it can also leave lasting physical and psychological effects on individuals. Efforts are being made for earlier recognition of sepsis in order to provide timely, appropriate care to avoid septic shock. The 2016 SCCM/ESICM Third International Consensus Conference on sepsis (Sepsis-3) redefined sepsis as "a life-threatening organ dysfunction caused by a deregulated host response to infection." Septic shock was similarly redefined as a "subset of sepsis in which underlying circulatory and cellular/metabolic abnormalities are profound enough to substantially increase mortality."[346,354] Criteria for septic shock included hypotension requiring vasopressor therapy to keep the mean arterial blood pressure greater than 65 mm Hg and a serum lactate level greater than 2 mmol/L after adequate hydration.[346] Unlike sepsis, *bacteremia* is defined only as the presence of bacteria in the blood. Previously, criteria were formulated to distinguish the presence and degree of severity of sepsis, termed *systemic inflammatory response syndrome* (SIRS). This has been replaced by the use of the qSOFA (Quick Sequential (Sepsis-Related) Organ Failure Assessment) scoring system. This system utilizes readily available clinical information to quickly identify organ dysfunction due to sepsis, including altered level of consciousness, systolic blood pressure less than 100 mm Hg, and a respiratory rate greater than 22 rpm. The Sepsis-3 definitions are not entirely accepted by all and some continue to use older definitions of SIRS, severe sepsis, and septic shock.

### Incidence and Risk Factors

The incidence of sepsis in the United States has been increasing, while the mortality rate has decreased. Sepsis is relatively common, with almost a million cases per year with an overall mortality of 12.5%.[297] Risk factors include advanced age, the presence of comorbidities (such as COPD, CHF, diabetes mellitus, and cancer),[241,242] bacteremia, previous hospitalization, immunosuppression, ICU admission, a hospital-associated infection, and community acquired pneumonia. Not all people with sepsis have bacteremia, although most people with positive blood cultures develop sepsis or septic shock. Sepsis in the elderly often presents atypically and is difficult to diagnose.[82]

### Pathogenesis

Infectious organisms are composed of foreign molecules termed *pathogen-associated molecular patterns*, which are recognized by the immune system as foreign, triggering both immunologic and inflammatory pathways. *Damage-associated molecular patterns* are the noninfectious molecules that are released after cellular injury of the host (i.e., trauma) and can also induce the immune response. Pathogen-associated molecular patterns are recognized by proteins called *pattern-recognition proteins* that can be found in cell membranes (transmembrane) or cytosol, or can be secreted.

Once pattern-recognition proteins are activated, various pathways are triggered, leading to the release of proinflammary cytokines and the recruitment of leukocytes and other cells. Fungi, viruses, and parasites also activate pattern-recognition proteins, but the process isn't as well characterized as it is for bacteria.

Primary mediators then induce the release of secondary mediators that amplify the inflammation process. Endothelial cells become damaged from the presence of leukocyte adhesion molecules on the surface that recruit neutrophils and other immune cells to the site of the infection.[80] This further drives the inflammatory response. The coagulation system is also activated, with an increase in proinflammatory and procoagulant tissue factors. The complement pathway is stimulated with cross-talking with the immune system.[362] Some bacteria produce and secrete toxins, or exotoxins, which are taken into cells and significantly change cellular function, often leading to cell injury and death.

Normally the immune response is balanced between proinflammatory (such as tumor necrosis factor and interleukin-1) and antiinflammatory mediators and remains in the area of the infection. However, under certain conditions, the inflammatory response becomes systemic, where the response is uncontrolled, unregulated, and self-sustaining. Alterations in multiple systems lead to sepsis. Changes in cellular metabolism and mitochondrial dysfunction lead to localized hypoxemia. Cytokines affect endothelial cells, which causes alterations in blood flow and contributes to shunting of blood and changes in oxygen utilization. Capillaries also become "leaky," allowing extravasation of fluid outside the vessels into surrounding tissues. Some cells undergo early apoptosis (lymphocyte number is reduced) while apoptosis of neutrophils is delayed. Bacterial components can stimulate coagulation, causing consumption of coagulation proteins and platelets (thrombosis) then resulting in bleeding when coagulation components are consumed (disseminated intravascular coagulation [DIC]). Other immune pathways are suppressed (reprogramming of antigen-presenting cells) (see Chapter 6).[362,399] Sepsis progresses to septic shock (and possibly multiple organ failure) when the proinflammatory process is not controlled.

### Clinical Manifestations

Signs and symptoms related to sepsis frequently depend upon the location of the infection, which are seen in conjunction with the generalized signs of fever, tachycardia, and tachypnea. If the infection begins in the lungs, shortness of breath, productive cough, and chest pain accompanied with an elevated white blood count, hypoxia, and low oxygen saturations may be present. A GI infection may exhibit nausea/vomiting, diarrhea, ileus, and/or abdominal pain.

As sepsis worsens, people may demonstrate signs of shock, such as hypotension, cool or mottled skin, and evidence of tissue hypoperfusion and organ dysfunction. This may include decreased urine output, acute kidney injury (AKI), and altered mental status, particularly in the elderly. The blood pH may reveal acidosis, and kidney function tests may show an increased BUN/creatinine. Leukocytosis may be evident, although in older people the WBC may be low. Many diseases clinically appear similar to sepsis and a complete evaluation must be pursued.

### MEDICAL MANAGEMENT

**DIAGNOSIS, TREATMENT, AND PROGNOSIS.** There is no ideal biomarker for sepsis, although lactate, C-reactive protein (CRP), and procalcitonin (PCT) are utilized in context of the clinical situation to add information. PCT and CRP are often elevated with the initial proinflammatory stage of sepsis. Elevated lactate is indicative of tissue hypoxia and may portend more severe disease and organ dysfunction.[323] Imaging is obtained according to clinical evaluation or to locate a site of infection (i.e., chest CT for symptoms of hypoxia and cough.)

Mild cases of sepsis can often be managed outside the ICU and are treated with fluids, supplemental oxygen, and antibiotics according to the source of infection. Septic shock requires emergent recognition and treatment.[441] Cultures should be obtained and then combined, and broad-spectrum antibiotics should be administered within the first hour of recognition of sepsis (if infective organism is unknown). Hypotension requires aggressive fluid resuscitation, using crystalloid with the addition of vasopressors if hypotension persists despite adequate fluid replacement.

People with septic shock often require early intubation to reduce the work of breathing and to protect the airway if there is an altered level of consciousness. Insulin should be utilized once serum glucoses reach over 180 mg/dl. The administration of steroids remains controversial and can be given for refractory septic shock after fluid resuscitation and vasopressors fail.[106]

Prognosis depends upon age, underlying conditions, presence of immunocompromise, delay in diagnosis, and the type of organism responsible for the infection. Overall mortality rate is around 12.5% but increases to 34% in cases involving septic shock.[297]

## The Medically Complex Patient: Critical Illness

Lara A. Firrone, PT, NCS

**Note to Reader:** The December 2012 issue of the *Journal of the American Physical Therapy Association* (Vol. 92, No. 12) features a special series on rehabilitation for people with critical illness. The publication is an excellent compilation of information about this condition for the physical therapist.

### Overview

To a certain extent, people admitted to the hospital are there because they are sick, and it is assumed that those in the ICU must be the sickest. One factor to consider is that the ICU contributes to that sickness. Some patients in the ICU can develop severe ICU-related complications.[436] It seems to be more so with those who have required prolonged mechanical ventilation (depending on the setting, that could be as few as 3 days or many more).[40,222,444] It can also be those who develop sepsis or multiple system organ dysfunction. There is a debate about individuals who have been on high doses of corticosteroids and neuromuscular blocking agents and their frequency of developing lasting complications.[104,299] The short-term issues range from difficulty or failure to wean from the ventilator to severe muscle weakness and loss of muscle function; many face chronic disability.

Of the individuals in the ICU who require advanced life support, there are those who handle it well; 75% are weaned from the ventilator on the first try. Once off ventilation, that patient can make a recovery that leads to discharge from the hospital. Unfortunately, others struggle and develop complications when they fail to wean, which can impact all systems in the body, from cardiovascular and respiratory to neuromuscular, as well as the more difficult to identify (e.g., psychologic and social).[175,279]

As the medically complex patient who has been sedated becomes more stable, the medical staff (e.g., physicians, nurses, and occasionally the respiratory therapists) may begin to realize that the patient is functionally impaired or that the medical issues present on admission are much worse now. This group of symptoms or conditions can go by many names. Terms like ICU-acquired weakness (ICU-AW), critical illness polyneuropathy (CIP or CIPN), critical illness myopathy or neuromyopathy (CIM), ICU-acquired paresis, and others are used interchangeably.

These are all ways of saying that there has been an impact on nerves and/or muscles to the point that movement and function reach critical levels of impairment. In other words, the impact reaches a level that becomes clinically demonstrable and lasting and is out of proportion to the patient's preadmission baseline, considering the primary medical problem. There is also being added into this mix the use of "postintensive care syndrome" to cover those patients who leave the ICU and hospital with lasting deficits.[125]

### Incidence

Incidence of critical illness is compounded by how the disorder is defined, what diagnostic tools and tests are used, and when those diagnostic measures are initiated and repeated. Studies report incidence in a range from 25% to 58%.[100,268,364] Some studies that had more restricted criteria for their cohorts and the reported incidence rate for neurologic and muscular deficits rise even higher, from 50% up to 100%.[278,341]

### Etiology and Risk Factors

The cause or etiology of these deficits in strength and sensation is still under debate and research. Part of the problem is related to the fact that there may be more than one type of illness being grouped together. For example, in one study patients were excluded if they were older than 75 years or younger than 18 years, if they had diabetes or renal problems, a stroke or spinal cord injury or prior neuropathy, cancer, or certain infections. This same study started with 490 survivors of the ICU, and 102 were excluded because of the criteria described. So essentially, 20% had some kind of weakness, but they were not going to call it ICU-AW because it may have had another cause. Other studies have tried to link the weakness to the use of certain drugs (e.g., corticosteroids, insulin)[100,172,188,263,364] or the diagnosis of sepsis or hyperglycemia,[173,364] the use of sedative or paralytics, and orders for strict bedrest, but nothing conclusive has been shown.[32,88,110,136]

With the debate about the cause, there is also some question as to risk factors. From a practical standpoint, the more systems involved and the more medical support the person needs (especially if it is invasive, like intubation or dialysis) the greater the risk that the patient will develop measurable weakness, with a drop in functional performance compared to the prehospitalization baseline. Sepsis, SIRS, and multiorgan failure are risk factors for CIP and CIM.[222]

As noted above, the more problems the individual develops, the less likely a formal diagnosis of ICU-AW (or CIP, or CIM, etc.) will be made. If the individual happened to have had a stroke in the past, then some might call it a decompensation due to the stress of the current illness. Or perhaps there was a previous history of polio, so the diagnosis becomes postpolio; for multiple sclerosis, it might be presumed to be an exacerbation.

### Pathogenesis

CIP and CIM are not isolated events; they are an integral part of the process leading to multiorgan dysfunction and failure. Peripheral nerves and muscle (excitable tissues) are key targets, and are probably damaged by a combination of ischemic and toxic means.[128,353] Therefore, shared microcirculatory, cellular, and metabolic pathophysiologic mechanisms are likely.

When considering a body that is affected by illness like multiple organ involvement and sepsis, there should be an awareness of the changes the body undergoes on the physical and chemical level and the system level. The nerves can be damaged by the impaired delivery of oxygen and nutrition on a cellular level. But this alteration is also directly linked to the person's whole-body medical status. Impaired glucose metabolism (hyperglycemia) can affect microcirculation to peripheral nerves, and cytokines can be toxic to the tissues. Prolonged disuse of muscle with muscle wasting (prominent features of sepsis) can be linked to increased muscle protein breakdown that may contribute to the myopathic symptoms seen in these individuals.[61]

During critical illness, microcirculation is impaired throughout the body (ischemic hypoxia). Mitochondrial function is impaired with reduced adenosine triphosphate biosynthesis, energy generation, and use (cytopathic hypoxia), which is thought to be a cause of cellular and organ dysfunction in critical illness. For more details of the proposed pathophysiologic mechanisms, as well as electrophysiologic and histologic features of CIP and CIM, the reader is referred to any of the recent studies referenced in this section, especially Latronico and Bolton[222] and Nordon-Craft et al.[278]

Diaphragmatic weakness, injury, and atrophy develop rapidly during mechanical ventilation (especially when combined with sedation),[284] and the scale of damage is significantly correlated with the duration of this medical treatment.[195] Subsequent weakness of the diaphragm makes breathing harder, thus contributing even more to the affected individual's immobility.

The therapist must always keep in mind that skeletal muscle immobility can contribute substantially to muscle wasting, even in the absence of systemic inflammatory changes.[284] Muscle atrophy begins within hours of bed rest or deep sedation, and even healthy people can have large loss of muscle mass and strength within 10 days of bed rest, particularly from the lower limbs.[217] Bower[47] does an excellent job detailing how the body declines and changes as a result of extended inactivity.

### Clinical Manifestations

Muscle weakness is the hallmark finding of this condition; onset of clinical signs can be rapid. This is first generally observed when the individual fails to wean from the ventilator. Then when the sedation is lifted, other areas of motor weakness become apparent; sensation can also be impaired. Although a patient may demonstrate elements of delirium or impaired consciousness, these are usually related to effects of medication or coma or a separate pathology (e.g., stroke, septic encephalopathy).

Most affected individuals will demonstrate both sensory and motor impairments. Weakness and sensory loss is symmetric, somewhat more distal than proximal for CIP affecting limb and respiratory muscles. Facial muscles are not usually affected.[222]

For primary myopathy associated with CIM, muscle weakness and atrophy are usually symmetric and more proximal, but without sensory impairments. There can be flaccid limbs, and deep tendon reflexes may be reduced. Some individuals have difficulty coughing and clearing and may speak in a hoarse voice.[87,222]

Differentiating CIP from CIM can be difficult in the ICU setting; if the individual makes a favorable recovery, it is likely because that individual had CIM alone versus CIP alone.[341] Practically speaking, the average therapist is going to see patients with combined damage.

## MEDICAL MANAGEMENT

**DIAGNOSIS.** Difficulty weaning an individual who has been critically ill from mechanical ventilation and that is unexplained by increased respiratory or cardiac load, metabolic disturbances, nutritional deficiencies, delirium, or other medical condition points to the possible diagnosis of CIM and/or CIP.[40] CIP/CIM is suspected when there is weakness and/or flaccid limbs or what little limb movement the patient initially shows does not improve over time. Diagnosis relies on clinical presentation and physical examination findings, testing that can include radiologic, electrophysiologic, or laboratory services, and potentially tissue studies.[87]

Muscle strength can be tested using the Medical Research Council (MRC) scale. The MRC can be found at www.medicalcriteria.com, as well as on the official MRC website (www.mrc.ac.uk). Instructions, as well as reliability and validity information, are provided. For an excellent summary of the MRC, see Confer et al.[87] The MRC composite score examines the results from three muscle groups from each limb.

Nerve function can also be examined, but the type of testing depends on the resources available. Some patients in some facilities may be tested with monofilaments or the more complete nerve conduction and electromyography tests. Simple light touch may be all that is done because of concerns for infection and overall infection control issues. Swelling and skin integrity issues may limit the validity of any of the tests used. Noninvasive testing of reflexes like deep tendon reflexes may be performed.

Respiratory muscle strength can be tested by measurement of the maximal inspiratory and expiratory pressures and vital capacity. Low scores on these measures are correlated with limb muscle weakness[221,223] associated with delayed extubation, prolonged ventilation, and unplanned readmission to the ICU.

Imaging studies may include a CT or MRI of the head and spine to rule out other conditions. The same guidelines are used when determining the need for a lumbar puncture. Unfortunately there is no simple blood test that is definitive for this condition. The medical differential diagnosis is more a process of elimination and a bit of presuming it is present, with treatment accordingly.

**PREVENTION.** Ideally the health care team works to prevent this condition from developing in the first place. The medical team can adjust some of the drugs on board and can attempt strict control of the blood glucose to reduce the hyperglycemic effects, as well as stabilizing the individual's electrolytes and ensuring there is adequate nutrition provided. The attempt should be made to wean the patient from the use of ventilator support as quickly as possible. The primary cause or initial presenting diagnosis should be addressed as quickly as possible; however, as previously noted, the various types of critical illness weakness can be difficult to diagnose and differentiate from other diseases. Thus a person with multiorgan failure may have so many issues that weakness is the least of the team's concerns as they work to keep the individual alive. There may come a time when everyone gets the preventative care regardless.

**TREATMENT.** Medical treatment is very limited and more of a management approach than a medical cure. There is no one drug or combination of drugs that will reverse the weakness and/or sensation losses. Once the condition is recognized, the health care team continues to provide the same care used for prevention. Gaining adequate glycemic control, getting the patient off the ventilator as quickly as possible, and reducing the use of medications that may be toxic are the best ways to prevent this condition from progressing.

**PROGNOSIS.** When looking at survival with CIM, CIP, and ICU-AW, the more severe the case, the more it can be anticipated that there will be a poor prognosis for full recovery; muscle weakness has been linked with increased mortality.[8]

Studies show that up to two-thirds of the people in the ICU will develop one of the disorders, and of those, 23% die in the hospital and another 33% die within 6 months after hospital discharge.[348] Many who have this disorder do not make it home. If discharged from the hospital with an opportunity to stay at home, they can exceed the care the family can provide and end up in community placement, either skilled or intermediate. Unfortunately, many families may see this occur in a relatively short period of time.

Investigations show there is a favorable chance for a return to functional independence in the long term, but only in those affected individuals who are young (the average reported age was 56 years) and for those who have no concomitant diseases.[284,341] Survivors of critical illness conditions may demonstrate significant residual disability.[194] Muscle weakness can persist months and even years with serious exercise limitations.[175]

There is growing evidence of additional changes in the quality of life for a survivor. Cognitive impairments, delirium, and inability to return to work or be active at a community level have been observed and reported.[184] According to Nordon-Craft et al,[278] these physical and psychologic and social limitations are now being quantified by tools like the 6-Minute Walk Test, 36-Item Short Form Health Survey, and RAND 36-Item Health Survey.

Cox et al[88] reported at 1 year posthospitalization that only 9% of the patients were alive and functionally independent (out of the 56% that survived the hospitalization), whereas 61% of the survivors needed daily assistance. The societal impact was significant, with 84% of caregivers having to alter or quit their job to accommodate the care the affected family member needed. There was also a very poor prognosis for emotional recovery for the person who survived, as well as for the caregivers regardless of the patient's survival.

SPECIAL IMPLICATIONS FOR THE THERAPIST 5-8

## *The Medically Complex Patient: Critical Illness*

The role of the therapist is both in prevention and treatment of the deconditioning and respiratory conditions that can occur in critically ill individuals. Reductions in functional performance, exercise or respiratory capacity, and quality of life are indicators that rehabilitation following a stay in the ICU should be recommended.[174]

*Recent evidence suggests that early rehabilitation can be safely and effectively implemented in the ICU to maintain patients' physical function, provided that patients are given an appropriate amount of sedation.[222] The therapist's focus is most often directed toward the functional limitations, reduced respiratory capacity, decreased cardiac reserve, and other limitations imposed by the physiologic deficiencies. The therapist also has an important role in providing emotional support and facilitating communication with patient, family, and staff.*

*More information and details of treatment protocols specific to the physical therapist are being investigated and researched and will be available in the literature at the time of this publication.[288] This adds to the studies that are already published, including targeted activity and exercise with the appropriate mode and at the recommended intensity.[123,162,296,327] Considerations for when to move a critically ill individual versus the risk of immobility, safety concerns, and approaches to acutely ill, cooperative but also sometimes uncooperative patients are discussed.[162] Some protocols might be difficult to reproduce, depending on constraints based on a particular facility's staffing, funding, and philosophy.*

### Review of Systems

The principal of "Keep it Simple" seems impossible when there are so many factors to consider. However, approaching any patient requires that the therapist look at all the systems, make appropriate assessments, and devise a plan of care that addresses those deficits. There are always more factors to consider when working with patients in a critical care unit.

*The therapist must step back and look at the big picture: Is there just a single organ involvement or multiple organ systems impaired? For example, did the patient have a car accident with some broken limbs or did he or she have a heart attack and was otherwise healthy prior to admission? Or, as the case seems to be more and more, were there multiple comorbidities and then an acute event that sent them over the edge? For instance, there may be the patient with diabetes who came in for an amputation, got into some kidney trouble, ending up on dialysis, and then had a stroke and respiratory failure that required mechanical ventilation.*

*Once the number of systems or organs that are involved is known, then the therapist can start looking at the clinical manifestations and see if any signs and symptoms present are related to the known issues or if there might be another medical condition playing a part. Sometimes a therapist can identify an underlying or new problem and alert the team and participate in active management before permanent issues arise.*

### The Role of Early Mobilization

The benefit of early mobilization has been well-documented.[20,41,88,257,258,269,298,308,327,337] More and more studies are being done that support getting the patient up and moving as quickly as possible. Early mobilization can decrease the length of stay in an ICU, as well as aid the person who is difficult to wean. PTs have an active role in the initiation of an early mobilization program. Starting strengthening and mobilization as early as clinically indicated and feasible may be the most valuable thing for anyone at risk for these disorders. There is a flip side to this as noted by Berney and Haines,[34] regarding the benefit from continuing the care started in the ICU to the outpatient setting, but they also note that maintaining compliance over the long term can be difficult.

## A THERAPIST'S THOUGHTS*

***Early Mobilization***

Physical therapists may not know that they have had experience with this condition. Some medical records do not include it in the problem (diagnosis) list, despite the fact that they might have 20 or more diseases and as many medications. It might be that a therapist treated patients when on a rotation in the ICU of an acute care setting. However, as the studies showed, there are survivors of the various ICU-related disorders, and they frequently do not go home but end up in inpatient rehab, extended acute care, or long-term care facilities.

When seen in the ICU, the environment can be challenging, especially as these individuals tend to be more complex and more fragile. The patient's diagnosis or multiple diseases the patient is facing can be strongly impacted by the environment, the critical care that the patient requires, and by real-world problems like staffing and equipment. Clinical manifestations of ICU-AW will necessitate longer term physical therapy intervention; this can be very challenging when in alternative care settings (i.e., outside the ICU).

And as the saying goes "the times, they are 'a changing'"—in health care that seems particularly true. Clinicians are seeing overall larger, more obese, and sicker patients than ever before. When I started work as a therapist almost 20 years ago, a 300-pound patient was considered large. Today, individuals this size are more the average; I regularly see people in the very severely obese category (Obese Class 3 body mass index: over 40; largest man I ever walked was more than 800 lb and the largest patient I ever treated approached 1200 lb).

Diseases once thought to be the hallmark of old age are striking much younger people. Patients with stroke are now regularly in their 20s and 30s, and the patients who are older than 70 years are seeing more devastating effects. Staff on the various medical and rehab teams are also seeing newer complications that their predecessors never had to deal with, such as superbug infections, multiple organ failure, and newer disorders that are just now being recognized. It is also the case for comorbidities, that is, patient diagnoses now routinely include 20 to 30 medical diagnoses instead of the 2 to 5 when I started. Coronary artery disease CHF, diabetes mellitus, hypertension, hypercholesterolemia, peripheral vascular disease, gastroesophageal reflux disease, cardiovascular accident, and COPD are almost standard in my ICU patients, except the occasional frank trauma who was otherwise fit. This doesn't even include their past and current list of surgical and invasive procedures, which can number in the dozens (or more).

Some facilities are not staffed to permit the type of evidence-based best care described in the literature. A hospital may not be able to have a therapist be in the ICU throughout the day. Having adequate staffing allows the timing of interventions for the most opportune moment. Knowing when a patient is going to get a "sedation vacation" allows the therapist to see the patient in a more active state and better assess their actual deficits. It would also allow active movement, which is key to regaining muscular function. Another consideration might be seen as the opposite line of thought by having the therapist provide range of motion and stretching at a time when the patient is sedated; this schedule permits the sedation vacation to be used for active weaning from the ventilator. The question becomes how to most effectively use the patient's available energy, apply it first to strengthen the limbs or to the lungs?

Other barriers to consider when mobilizing patients include the actual equipment and hospital policy. Some facilities do not permit mobilizing with an endotracheal tube in place or only if certain staff members are present (e.g., a respiratory therapist must be present in the event of accidental extubation). Practical matters can be additional speed bumps, like the fact that the patient is being taken to tests or having bedside procedures. This may mean that having daily and lengthy physical therapy sessions is more difficult to reproduce consistently. But that does not necessarily mean it should not be tried.

In an ideal world, ICUs would be staffed with a therapist similarly to the way nursing is staffed, with one therapist covering a small number of patients. The rehab staff would have access to appropriate and necessary equipment. For example, the availability of tilt tables with

## A THERAPIST'S THOUGHTS*—cont'd

### Early Mobilization

a sliding mechanism that permits gradual body weight tasks such as a modified squat at a 45-degree angle would be very helpful. As the patient improves, the angle can be increased to increase the patient's work load until the point that they are ready to step off the end. Some ICUs have a modified walker with the ability to support the patient and a portable vent, along with all the IV pumps and equipment that is attached to the patient. This setup would leave the therapist's hands free to assist the patient. Other useful tools include weights and resistance bands that meet infection control policies and interactive games like the Wii for individuals who are restricted to the bed for other reasons.

For those who are in less-well-funded facilities, it means being more creative. If the tilt table is too big to put next to the patient's bed to permit transfers and there are no power outlets that can power it in the hall where there might be more space, then the therapist can direct intervention toward gradually raising the head of the bed. This approach will improve patient tolerance to a more upright position. Pulmonary hygiene will be part of the plan of care until the patient can tolerate a functional supine-to-sit transition on the side of the bed. Marching in place at the side of the bed is suggested when there are not additional staff members to permit walking in the hallway, for instance when nursing and respiratory staff are on transport with another patient. Manual resistance can replace bands and weights when the patient is in isolation.

An area that rehab staff can also impact with very little cost but show a big payoff is in communicating with the patient and the family. Therapists are at the bedside longer than most of the other professionals. RNs come to give a med and then leave. RT might apply a treatment to the vent and the return to draw an arterial blood gas. These take a few minutes. Doing exercises and giving appropriate rest breaks and mobilizing out-of-bed takes time. The return on that time can be increased considerably by using those extra minutes to answer questions and give additional information, and later alert staff to any deficits that other team members may need to address.

Rehab staff can provide honest assessments of functional tasks that a patient and family member can relate to more than numbers from lab values. When a patient becomes visibly fatigued with 5 minutes of static sitting, the physical therapist can point out that it might take 10 minutes to eat a small meal, which is a vital dynamic task. In this way, the therapist can demonstrate more clearly how far the patient has to improve to accomplish this basic task. Or when the family says the patient must be able to be left alone for 4 hours while a caregiver works a part-time job, the therapist can use this guideline to create appropriate goals and outcome measures.

In conclusion, patients can be very sick; some are more complicated than others. Sometimes the therapy staff is working with a known diagnosis, and other times we are dealing with the unknown. As long as the therapist looks at the whole patient and an attempt is made to address all of that patient's needs, then an appropriate plan of care can be developed. The focus is on returning the individual to his or her highest level of function and, hopefully, preparing the individual for the day when discharge from the ICU is possible (and eventually return to home or transition to another facility from the hospital).

## Multiple Organ Dysfunction Syndrome (MODS)

### Overview

Care of critically ill people has progressed significantly during the last 50 years. Substantial advances have been made in the care of shock, acute kidney injury, acute brain injury, and acute respiratory failure, with more people surviving these conditions.

However, despite these advances, progressive deterioration of organ function may occur in people who are critically ill or injured. People often die of complications of disease rather than from the disease itself. MODS is often the final complication of a critical illness; it is one of the most common causes of death in the ICU.

### Definition and Etiologic and Risk Factors

MODS, also called *multiple organ failure syndrome*, is the progressive failure (over more than 24 hours) of two or more organ systems after a severe illness or injury.[158,414] It is more common in older adults and pediatric ICU infants.[414] Although sepsis and septic shock from infection are the most common causes, infection is not required for its development. MODS also can be primary (the original insult can be directly linked to MODS) or secondary, where MODS is a result of the person's response to the insult. It may be triggered by acute respiratory distress syndrome; severe inflammatory processes (e.g., pancreatitis, vasculitis); other types of shock; and traumatic injury (e.g., burns or surgery). MODS carries a high mortality rate that increases with each organ that fails.

Several scoring systems have been developed, such as the Sequential Organ Failure Assessment (SOFA) or the Logistic Organ Dysfunction System, which correlate with mortality.[227,251] Sepsis, septic shock, and MODS are a result of excessive activation of inflammatory pathways and form a spectrum of disease.

After an initial insult or injury, other factors can increase the risk of developing MODS, including inadequate or delayed resuscitation, sepsis, age (old and very young), hypoxemia, immunosuppression, acute leukemia, alcoholism, diabetes, surgical complications (infection), bowel infarction, or the previous existence of organ dysfunction (e.g., renal insufficiency).[414]

### Pathogenesis

Although MODS may be a final common pathway in critical illnesses, actual causes and cellular changes leading to MODS are not completely understood. Most likely multiple mechanisms and factors are responsible or contribute to the development of MODS. The pathophysiology is similar to septic shock and may be considered as a continuum of that inflammatory process (see the section on pathophysiology of sepsis).

Macrophages are activated either due to the presence of damage-associated molecular patterns (proteins from damaged tissue) or pathogen-associated molecular patterns (microbial proteins) and release proinflammatory cytokines. These cytokines recruit leukocytes into the affected area and begin a series of signals that result in the phagocytosis of bacterial proteins (if present) and begin the process of removing damaged tissue and repairing. Primary mediators stimulate release of other cytokines. Typically this inflammatory process is balanced and regulated by antiinflammatory mediators. However, if there is dysregulation of this process, favoring inflammation with continued elevated levels of cytokines, cellular alterations continue. This may include changes in cellular metabolism and mitochondrial function; apoptosis; and coagulation pathways.[400] Inflammation becomes uncontrolled and self-sustaining. Endothelial cells may be chronically activated, leading to thrombotic microangiopathy, and the immune system becomes unable to appropriately respond or aid in tissue repair, often refered to as *immunoparalysis*.[63,186,360]

This uncontrolled hyperinflammation and hypercoagulation leads to the development of edema, cardiovascular instability, endothelial damage, and clotting abnormalities.

At the same time, initial oxygen consumption demand increases due to oxygen requirements at the cellular level. Blood flow and oxygen consumption are mismatched because of a decrease in oxygen delivery to the cells caused by maldistribution of blood flow, myocardial depression, and a hypermetabolic state. The end result is abnormal cellular respiration and function (tissue hypoxia with cellular acidosis and death), resulting in the multiple organ dysfunction characteristic of MODS.[298]

### Clinical Manifestations

After the precipitating event, clients often present with fever, tachycardia, dyspnea, and altered mental status. Sepsis and septic shock become apparent, with evidence of tissue hypoxia including hypotension, cool skin, and decreased urine output (acute kidney injury). Changes in laboratory values may include an increase in BUN/creatinine, elevated lactate, leukocytosis, thrombocytopenia, low blood pH (acidosis), and elevated procalcitonin (see Chapter 15).

The circulatory system experiences dysregulation with resulting hypotension. The heart demonstrates both systolic and diastolic dysfunction, leading to low cardiac output. Endothelial cells of small blood vessels are affected, resulting in microvascular permeability and local edema. Ischemia and inflammation are responsible for CNS manifestations. Protein metabolism is also affected, and amino acids derived from skeletal muscle, connective tissue, and intestinal viscera become an important energy source. The result is a significant loss of lean body mass. Continued hypoxia on the cellular level and the organ level both contribute to large-volume cellular damage to organs with eventual failure.

### MEDICAL MANAGEMENT

Early detection and supportive therapy are essential for MODS because no specific medical treatment exists for this condition. Therapy is similar to treatment for septic shock. Pharmacologic treatment may include antibiotics to treat infection; adequate fluid replacement; vasopressors to counteract myocardial depression and hypotension; and supplemental oxygen and ventilation to reduce the work of breathing and keep oxygen saturation levels at or above 90%. Nutritional support is also provided.

MODS is the major cause of death (usually occurring between days 21 and 28) after septic, traumatic, and burn injuries. If the affected individual's condition has not improved by the end of the third week, survival is unlikely. The mortality rate of MODS is 60% to 90% and approaches 100% if three or more organs are involved, sepsis is present, and the individual is older than 65 years.

**SPECIAL IMPLICATIONS FOR THE THERAPIST 5-9**

***Multiple Organ Dysfunction Syndrome***

Only the critical care or burn unit therapist will encounter the client with MODS/SIRS. The hypermetabolism associated with this condition is accompanied by protein catabolism, primarily of skeletal muscle and visceral organs. Lean body mass can be significantly depleted in 7 to 10 days, necessitating skin precautions and skin care.

## FLUID AND ELECTROLYTE IMBALANCES

Observing clinical manifestations of fluid or electrolyte imbalances may be an important aspect of client care, especially in the acute care and home health care settings. Identifying clients at risk for such imbalances is the first step toward early detection.

The causes of fluid and electrolyte imbalance are many and varied and include disease processes, injury, medications, medical treatment, dietary restrictions, and imbalance of fluid intake with fluid output.[384] The most common causes of fluid and electrolyte imbalances in a therapy practice include burns, surgery, diabetes mellitus, malignancy, alcoholism, and the various factors affecting the aging adult population (Box 5.6).

The normal homeostatic processes of fluid and electrolyte balance are briefly presented here.

### Aging and Fluid and Electrolyte Balance

The volume and distribution of body fluids composed of water, electrolytes, and nonelectrolytes vary with age, gender, body weight, and amount of adipose tissue. Throughout life, a slow decline occurs in lean body or fat-free mass, with a corresponding decline in the volume of body fluids. Only 45% to 50% of the body weight of aging adults is water compared with 55% to 60% in younger adults. This decrease represents a net loss of muscle mass and a reduced ratio of lean body weight to total body weight and places older people at greater risk for water-deficit states.

There are also changes in the kidney that further potentiate the risk for fluid and electrolyte disturbances. With increasing age, there is a decrease in renal mass and GFR. This, in turn, may lead to the inability of the aging kidney to excrete free water in the face of fluid excess, causing hyponatremia.

Box 5.6

**FACTORS AFFECTING FLUID AND ELECTROLYTE BALANCE IN THE AGING**

- Acute illness (fever, diarrhea, vomiting)
- Bowel cleansing for GI diagnostic testing
- Change in mental status
- Constipation
- Decreased thirst mechanism
- Difficulty swallowing
- Excessive sodium intake:
  - Diet
  - Sodium bicarbonate antacids (e.g., Alka-Seltzer)
  - Water supply or water softener
  - Decreased taste sensation (increased salt intake)
- Excessive calcium intake:
  - Alkaline antacids
- Immobility
- Laxatives (habitual use for constipation)
- Medications:
  - Antiparkinsonian drugs
  - Diuretics
  - Propranolol
  - Tamoxifen (breast cancer therapy)
- Sodium-restricted diet
- Urinary incontinence (voluntary fluid restriction)

Yet hypernatremia can also be problematic in the aging adult secondary to a defect in the ability of the kidney to concentrate urine combined with a decreased thirst despite dehydration, often seen with age. Although these changes are seen in normal aging, factors that depress the sensorium in the frail and sick elderly (stroke and medications) further complicate hypernatremia by suppressing the natural compensatory mechanism for fluid intake.

Infection, dementia, neurologic disorders, and other systemic illnesses can decrease the release of arginine vasopressin, further placing older adults at high risk for dehydration.[74] Renin and aldosterone decrease with age, accompanied by a blunted response to aldosterone. These changes can lead to hyperkalemia, particularly if other factors are present, such as the use of potassium-sparing diuretics.

## Fluid Imbalances

### Overview

Approximately 45% to 60% of the adult human body is composed of water, which contains the electrolytes that are essential to human life (see "Electrolyte Imbalances" below). This life-sustaining fluid is found within various body compartments, including the intracellular (within cells) and extracellular compartments. The extracellular compartment can be subdivided into the interstitial (fluid that surrounds the cells), intravascular (within blood vessels), and transcellular compartments.

Fluid in the transcellular compartment is present in the body but is separated from body tissues by a layer of epithelial cells. This fluid includes digestive fluids, water, and solutes in the renal tubules and bladder, intraocular fluid, joint-space fluid, and cerebrospinal fluid. The fluid in the interstitial and intravascular compartments comprises approximately one-third the total body fluid, called the *extracellular fluid* (ECF). Fluid found inside the cells, called the *intracellular fluid* (ICF), accounts for the remaining two-thirds of total body fluid.

The cell membrane is water permeable with equal concentrations of dissolved particles on each side of the membrane, maintaining equal volumes of ECF and ICF and preventing passive shifts of water. Passive shifts occur only if an inequality occurs on either side of the membrane in the concentration of solutes that cannot permeate the membrane. For example, water will move from one compartment to another if there is a change in sodium ion concentration.

The following five types of fluid imbalances may occur:

1. ECF volume deficit
2. ECF volume excess
3. ECF volume shift
4. ICF volume excess
5. ICF volume deficit

A simpler approach to this subject is to view fluid shifts in terms of intravascular or extravascular movement. Movement from the vascular space to the extravascular areas and vice versa takes place easily and is the first mechanism of extracellular movement.

The material in this section is presented on the bases of three broad categories: fluid deficit, fluid excess, and fluid shift (see Chapter 13).

### Etiologic Factors and Pathogenesis

Maintaining constant internal conditions (homeostasis) requires the proper balance between the volume and distribution of ECF and ICF to provide nutrition to the cells, allow excretion of waste products, and promote production of energy and other cell functions. Maintenance of this balance depends on the differences in the concentrations of ICF and ECF fluids, the permeability of the membranes, and the effect of the electrolytes in the fluids.

A fluid imbalance occurs when either the ICF or ECF gains or loses body fluids or electrolytes, causing a fluid deficit or a fluid excess. Sodium is the major ion that influences water retention and water loss. A deficit of total-body fluid occurs with either an excessive loss of body water/fluids or an inadequate compensatory intake. The result is an insufficient fluid volume to meet the needs of the cells. It is manifested by dehydration (Box 5.7), hypovolemia, such as blood or plasma loss, or both. Severe fluid volume deficit can cause vascular collapse and shock.

An *excess* of water occurs when an overabundance of water is in the interstitial fluid spaces or body cavities (edema) or within the blood vessels (hypervolemia). This may occur as a consequence of an inability to excrete excess fluid, as with renal disease, or an inability of the heart to move fluid/blood from the venous system to the arterial system, as with HF. A *fluid shift* occurs when vascular fluid moves to interstitial or intracellular spaces or interstitial or ICF moves to vascular fluid space.

Loss of intravascular fluid that shifts into a third space (tissues, peritoneal cavity or pleural cavity) and is not in equilibrium with extracellular fluid is referred to as *third-space fluid*. Third-space fluid is commonly seen in a therapy practice as a result of bleeding, such as seen with a hip fracture where blood is lost into the tissue adjacent to the fracture, depleting the intravascular fluid. It is also noted due to altered capillary permeability secondary to

Box 5.7

**CLINICAL MANIFESTATIONS OF DEHYDRATION**

- Absent perspiration, tearing, and salivation
- Body temperature (subnormal or elevated)
- Confusion
- Disorientation; comatose; seizures
- Dizziness when standing
- Dry, brittle hair
- Dry mucous membranes, furrowed tongue
- Headache
- Incoordination
- Irritability
- Lethargy
- Postural hypotension
- Rapid pulse
- Rapid respirations
- Skin changes:
    - Color: gray
    - Temperature: cold
    - Turgor: poor
    - Feel: warm, dry if mild; cool, clammy if severe
- Sunken eye
- Sunken fontanel (children)

tissue injury or inflammation, such as with severe pancreatitis or major surgery. Fluid and protein may leak from the intravascular space to the interstitial space. Third spacing is commonly seen in liver disease. Decreased serum protein (hypoalbuminemia) associated with liver disease and states of malnutrition results in third-space fluid accumulation in the abdomen because there is a higher concentration of protein outside the vascular system (in the peritoneal space) than inside the vascular system and fluid shifts to a space with a higher protein concentration.

Other areas, called *potential spaces* (normally not fluid-filled), can fill with fluid in the presence of inflammation or fluid imbalances. Examples of potential spaces include the peritoneal cavity (e.g., ascites) and the pleural cavity (e.g., pleural effusion).

### Clinical Manifestations

*Fluid volume deficit* (FVD) is most often accompanied by symptoms of decreased vascular volume, such as decreased blood pressure, increased pulse, oliguria, and orthostatic hypotension. FVD can occur from loss of blood (whether obvious hemorrhage or occult GI bleeding), loss of plasma (burns or peritonitis), or loss of body fluids (diarrhea, vomiting, diaphoresis, or lack of fluid intake), resulting in dehydration. The affected individual experiences symptoms of thirst, weakness, dizziness, decreased urine output, weight loss, and altered levels of consciousness (i.e., confusion). Significant decreases in systolic blood pressure (less than 70 mm Hg) result in symptoms of shock and require immediate medical treatment and possibly life-sustaining emergency management.

*Fluid volume excess* is primarily characterized by weight gain and edema of the extremities. With intravascular fluid volume excess, other clinical manifestations include dyspnea, engorged neck veins, and a bounding pulse. In the early stages, the person may not exhibit any of these symptoms.

*Fluid shift* from the vascular to the extravascular spaces (e.g., burns or peritonitis) is manifested by signs and symptoms similar to FVD and shock, including skin pallor, cool extremities, weak and rapid pulse, hypotension, oliguria, and decreased levels of consciousness. When the fluid returns to the blood vessels, such as following major surgery, the clinical manifestations are similar to those of fluid overload, such as bounding pulse and engorgement of peripheral and jugular veins.

## MEDICAL MANAGEMENT

The ECF is the only fluid compartment that can be readily monitored; clinically, the status of ICF is inferred from analysis of plasma and the condition of the person. A fluid balance record ("ins and outs") is kept on any individual who is susceptible to or already experiencing a disturbance in the balance of body fluids. In addition, medical evaluation of clinical signs and laboratory tests are helpful in the assessment of a person's hydration status. Laboratory tests may include serum osmolality, sodium, hematocrit, and BUN/creatinine measurements.

Serum osmolality measures the concentration of particles in the plasma portion of the blood. Osmolality increases with dehydration and decreases with overhydration. Serum sodium is an index of water deficit or excess; a decrease in sodium (hyponatremia) demonstrates an excess of water in relation to sodium. This may occur with an inability to excrete water, as seen with kidney disease or the release of antidiuretic hormone (ADH) or the increased secretion of sodium. An elevated level of sodium in the blood (hypernatremia) would indicate that the loss of water from the body has exceeded the loss of sodium such as occurs in gastrointestinal tract loss (e.g., vomiting), uncontrolled diabetes insipidus, or inability to respond to thirst. Hematocrit increases with dehydration and decreases with excess fluid. BUN serves as an index of kidney excretory function; BUN increases with dehydration and decreases with overhydration.

Treatment is directed to the underlying cause; in the case of FVD, the aim is to improve hydration status. This may be accomplished through replacement of fluids and/or electrolytes by oral or IV means.

SPECIAL IMPLICATIONS FOR THE THERAPIST 5-10

### *Fluid Imbalances*

#### Monitoring Fluid Balance

Fluid balance is so critical to physical well-being and cardiopulmonary sufficiency that fluid input and output records are often maintained at bedside. The therapist may be involved in maintaining these records, which also include fluid volume lost in wound drainage, GI output, and fluids aspirated from any body cavity. Body weight may increase by several pounds before edema is apparent. The dependent areas manifest the first signs of fluid excess. Individuals on bed rest show sacral swelling; people who can sit on the edge of the bed or in a chair for prolonged periods tend to show swelling of the feet and hands.

*Water and fluids should be offered often to older adults and clients with debilitating diseases to prevent body fluid loss and hypernatremia. However, increasing fluid intake in clients with CHF or severe renal disease is usually contraindicated.*

*Caffeinated fluids and alcohol can increase water loss, thereby increasing the serum sodium level; these beverages should be avoided to prevent fluid loss as a consequence of this diuretic effect. Water is the preferred fluid for hydration except in athletic or marathon race situations, which require replacement of electrolytes.*[129]

*Thirst is not always a reliable signal for fluid intake or even dehydration. A person may not feel "thirsty" until the body reaches a dangerous point of fluid loss. Therapists and clients should both be encouraged to keep water and clear fluids on hand and drink on a schedule rather than wait until they feel thirsty. Many people confuse thirst for hunger and eat instead of drinking when the thirst mechanism does kick in.*

*Urine is a good gauge of adequate hydration. A low volume of dark or highly concentrated urine is a yellow flag. When accompanied by other signs of dehydration (e.g., dry mouth, irritability, constipation, fatigue, or muscle weakness), it becomes a red flag.*

### Dehydration

Healthy older adults can become at risk for dehydration for many physiologic and psychosocial reasons. Older individuals have an impaired thirst response to dehydration; abnormal circadian rhythm of AVP leads to nocturia and increased fluid loss. Other contributing medical factors include diabetes, urinary tract infections, renal failure, and medications such as diuretics.[260]

*Psychosocial factors also play a key role in the development of dehydration in the older age group. Isolation, depression, and confusion are associated with reduced oral intake and impaired fluid status and can make dehydration worse.*[260]

*Dehydration (water deficit) degrades endurance exercise performance, and physical work capacity is diminished even at marginal levels of dehydration (defined clinically as a 1% loss of body weight through fluid loss). Alterations in $VO_2max$ (aerobic capacity) occur with a 2% or more deficit in body water loss. Greater body water deficits are associated with progressively larger reductions in physical work capacity.*

*Dehydration results in larger reductions in physical work capacity in a hot environment (e.g., aquatic or outdoor setting) for individuals in any age group, as compared with a thermally neutral environment. Prolonged exercise that places large demands on aerobic metabolism is more likely to be adversely affected by dehydration than is short-term exercise.*[31]

*Core body temperature increases predictably as the percentage of dehydration increases. The heart rate increases about 6 beats/min for each 1% increase in dehydration. This is not true for older adults, who may have limited rate changes with increased activity.*

*Older individuals are especially at risk for negative sequelae associated with dehydration. Hospitalization for dehydration is common and mortality is high. Almost 50% of Medicare patients who are hospitalized with dehydration die within a year of admission.*[260,412]

*Anyone with hypovolemia cannot compensate as easily with an increased heart rate like younger people can, so shock is more difficult to treat. In addition, aging individuals are often being treated with cardiac medications, such as β-blockers or digoxin that block or inhibit a rapid heart rate and limit rate changes with increased activity. Heart transplant recipients also have a unique situation because the heart has been denervated.*

*Individuals exercising in the heat, including aquatic exercise, should be encouraged to drink water in excess of normally desired amounts. When exercise is expected to cause an increase of more than 2% in dehydration, target heart rate modifications are necessary.*[245]

*Severe losses of water and solutes can lead to hypovolemic shock. It is important for the therapist to be aware of possible fluid losses or water shifts in any client who is already compromised by advanced age or by the presence of an ileostomy or tracheostomy, resulting in a continuous loss of fluid.*

*Dehydration may contribute to underlying disabilities caused by orthostatic hypotension and dizziness. It may result in symptoms such as confusion and weakness that can interfere with rehabilitation outcomes, especially after orthopedic surgery.*[260]

*Because the response to fluid loss is highly individual, it is important to recognize the early clinical symptoms of fluid loss (see Box 5.7) and to carefully monitor clients who are at risk (e.g., observe for symptoms and monitor vital signs). People at risk for profound and potentially fatal FVD, as in severe and extensive burns, should be assessed frequently and regularly for mental acuity and orientation to person, place, and time.*

### Skin Care

Careful handling of edematous tissue is essential to maintaining the integrity of the skin, which is stretched beyond its normal limits and has a limited blood supply. Turning and repositioning the client must be done gently to avoid friction. A break in or abrasion of edematous skin can readily develop into a pressure ulcer.

*Client education may be necessary in the proper application and use of antiembolism stockings or other appropriate compression garments, lower-extremity elevation, and the need for regular exercise. Clients should be cautioned to avoid crossing the legs, putting pillows under the knees, or otherwise creating pressure against the blood vessels.*[275]

## Electrolyte Imbalances

### Overview

Electrolytes are chemical substances that separate into electrically charged particles, called *ions*, in solution. The electrolytes that consist of positively charged ions, or *cations*, are sodium ($Na^+$), potassium ($K^+$), calcium ($Ca^{2+}$), and magnesium ($Mg^{2+}$). Those that consist of negatively charged ions, or *anions*, are chloride ($Cl-$); bicarbonate ($HCO_3-$); and phosphate ($PO_4^{3}-$).

Concentration gradients of sodium and potassium across the cell membrane produce the membrane potential and provide the means by which electrochemical impulses are transmitted in nerve and muscle fibers.

*Sodium* affects the osmolality of blood and therefore influences blood volume and pressure and the retention or loss of interstitial fluid. Sodium imbalance affects the osmolality of the ECF and is often associated with fluid volume imbalances.

Adequate *potassium* is necessary to maintain function of sodium–potassium membrane pumps, which are essential for the normal muscle contraction–relaxation sequence. Imbalances in potassium affect muscular activities, notably those of the heart, intestines, and respiratory tract, and neural stimulation of the skeletal muscles.

*Calcium* influences the permeability of cell membranes and thereby regulates neuromuscular activity. Calcium plays a role in the electrical excitation of cardiac cells and in the mechanical contraction of the myocardial and vascular smooth muscle cells. An imbalance in calcium concentrations affects skeletal muscle, bones, kidneys, and the GI tract. Conditions that can cause movement of calcium from the bones into the ECF (e.g., bone tumors, multiple fractures, hormone imbalances, or osteoporosis) can cause hypercalcemia. (Table 5.9 lists other causes of hypocalcemia or hypercalcemia.)

*Magnesium*, an important intracellular activator for more than 300 enzymatic processes, exerts physiologic effects on the nervous system that resemble the effects of calcium. Two-thirds of the body's magnesium is found in the bones; most of the rest is located in the ECF, including the vascular compartment and interstitial spaces. As a result, the normal serum magnesium concentration is relatively low.

Magnesium plays a role in maintaining the correct level of electrical excitability in the nerves and muscle cells by acting directly on the myoneural junction. Magnesium depresses acetylcholine release at synaptic junctions. Magnesium influences cardiovascular function because of its vasodilatory effect.[315]

Neuromuscular irritability results from hypomagnesemia (e.g., malnutrition from poor diet, chronic alcohol abuse, diuretic use [renal loss of magnesium], or prolonged diarrhea with impaired intestinal absorption of magnesium), and magnesium excess (rare but occurs with renal failure or the overuse of magnesium-containing antacids) causes neuromuscular depression affecting the musculoskeletal and cardiac systems.[5]

**Table 5-9 Causes of Electrolyte Imbalances**

| | Risk Factors for Imbalance |
|---|---|
| **Potassium** | |
| Hypokalemia | Dietary deficiency (rare) |
| | Intestinal or urinary losses as a result of diarrhea or vomiting (anorexia, dehydration), drainage from fistulas, overuse of gastric suction |
| | Trauma (injury, burns, surgery): damaged cells release potassium, are excreted in urine |
| | Medications such as potassium-wasting diuretics, steroids, insulin, penicillin derivatives, amphotericin B |
| | Metabolic alkalosis |
| | Cushing syndrome, severe magnesium deficiency |
| | Hyperaldosteronism |
| | Integumentary loss (sweating) |
| | Type 2 renal tubular acidosis |
| | Diabetic ketoacidosis |
| Hyperkalemia | Conditions that alter kidney function or decrease its ability to excrete potassium (chronic renal disease or renal failure) |
| | Intestinal obstruction that prevents elimination of potassium in the feces |
| | Addison disease |
| | Chronic heparin therapy, lead poisoning, insulin deficit, NSAIDs, ACE inhibitors, cyclosporine |
| | Trauma: crush injuries, burns |
| | Metabolic acidosis |
| | Rhabdomyolysis |
| | Tumor lysis syndrome |
| | Hyperglycemia |
| | Digitalis toxicity |
| | Hypoaldosteronism |
| **Sodium** | |
| Hyponatremia | Inadequate sodium intake (low-sodium diets) |
| | Excessive intake or retention of water (kidney failure and heart failure) |
| | Excessive water loss and electrolytes (vomiting, excessive perspiration, tap-water enemas, suctioning, use of diuretics, diarrhea) |
| | Loss of bile (high in sodium) as a result of fistulas, drainage, GI surgery, and suction |
| | Trauma (loss of sodium through burn wounds, wound drainage from surgery) |
| | IV fluids that do not contain electrolytes |
| | Adrenal gland insufficiency (Addison disease) or hypoaldosteronism |
| | Cirrhosis of the liver with ascites |
| | SIADH: brain tumor, cerebrovascular accident, pulmonary disease, neoplasm with ADH production, medications, pain, nausea |
| | Hypothyroidism |
| | Nephrotic syndrome |

*Continued*

**Table 5-9** Causes of Electrolyte Imbalances—cont'd

| | Risk Factors for Imbalance |
|---|---|
| Hypernatremia | Decreased water intake (comatose, mentally confused, or debilitated client)<br>Water loss (excessive sweating, osmotic diarrhea), fever, heat exposure, burns<br>Hyperglycemia<br>Excess adrenocortical hormones (Cushing syndrome)<br>IV administration of high-protein, hyperosmotic tube feedings and diuretics<br>Diabetes insipidus<br>Central: loss of neurohypophysis from trauma, surgery, neoplasm, CVA, infection<br>Nephrogenic: renal resistance to ADH drugs (lithium), hypercalcemia papillary necrosis, pregnancy |
| **Calcium** | |
| Hypocalcemia | Inadequate dietary intake of calcium and inadequate exposure to sunlight (Vitamin D) necessary for calcium use (especially older adults)<br>Impaired absorption of calcium and Vitamin D from intestinal tract (severe diarrhea, overuse of laxatives, and enemas containing phosphates; phosphorous tends to be more readily absorbed from the intestinal tract than calcium and suppresses calcium retention in the body)<br>Hypoparathyroidism (injury, disease, surgery)<br>Severe infections or burns<br>Overcorrection of acidosis<br>Pancreatic insufficiency<br>Renal failure<br>Hypomagnesemia (especially with alcoholism)<br>Medications—anticonvulsive medications |
| Hypercalcemia | Hyperparathyroidism, hyperthyroidism, adrenal insufficiency<br>Multiple fractures<br>Excess intake of calcium (excessive antacids), excess intake of vitamin D, milk alkali syndrome<br>Osteoporosis, immobility, multiple myeloma<br>Thiazide diuretics<br>Sarcoidosis<br>Tumors which secrete PTH (bone, lung, stomach, and kidney)<br>Multiple endocrine neoplasia tumors (types I and II) |
| **Magnesium** | |
| Hypomagnesemia | Decreased magnesium intake or absorption (chronic malnutrition, chronic diarrhea, bowel resection with ileostomy or colostomy, chronic alcoholism, prolonged gastric suction, acute pancreatitis, biliary or intestinal fistula)<br>Excessive loss of magnesium (diabetic ketoacidosis, severe dehydration, hyperaldosteronism and hypoparathyroidism)<br>Vitamin D deficiency<br>Impaired renal absorption<br>Parenteral nutrition/enteral feeding with inadequate magnesium replacement<br>Acute tubular necrosis<br>Medications: diuretics, cisplatin, foscarnet, cyclosporine, amphotericin B, some proton pump inhibitors<br>Hyperthyroidism<br>Metabolic acidosis<br>SIADH<br>Pregnancy |
| Hypermagnesemia | Chronic renal failure or renal insufficiency[a]<br>Overuse of antacids and laxatives containing magnesium<br>Severe dehydration (resulting oliguria can cause magnesium retention)<br>Overcorrection of hypomagnesemia<br>Diabetic ketoacidosis<br>Tumor lysis syndrome<br>Near-drowning (aspiration of sea water)<br>Intestinal obstruction<br>Trauma, burns<br>Hypothyroidism<br>Addison disease (adrenal insufficiency)<br>Shock, sepsis |

[a]Hypermagnesemia is much less common than hypomagnesemia because normally functioning kidneys easily excrete magnesium.
*ACE*, Angiotensin-converting enzyme; *ADH*, antidiuretic hormone; *CVA*, cardiovascular accident; *GI*, gastrointestinal; *IV*, intravenous; *NSAIDs*, nonsteroidal antiinflammatory drugs; *SIADH*, syndrome of inappropriate antidiuretic hormone.
Data from Porth CM. *Essentials of pathophysiology*, ed 3, Philadelphia, 2011, Lippincott Williams & Wilkins.

### Etiologic and Risk Factors

An electrolyte imbalance exists when the serum concentration of an electrolyte is either too high or too low. Stability of the electrolyte balance depends not only on adequate intake, distribution, and excretion of the electrolyte, but is often tightly connected to and dependent on fluid balance, particularly sodium. Many conditions can interfere with these processes and result in an imbalance (see Table 5.9). For example, cell death (from ischemia, chemotherapy, trauma) results in the release of electrolytes such as potassium, calcium, phosphate, and magnesium. Medications (i.e., diuretics) lead to an excessive excretion of electrolytes, and diseases (i.e., renal failure) interfere with the excretion of electrolytes. Often, as with sodium, the laboratory value may appear too high or too low, yet the total amount of sodium is normal; it is frequently an imbalance in fluid that alters the concentration of sodium.

### Clinical Manifestations

In a therapy practice, paresthesias, muscle weakness, muscle wasting, muscle tetany, and bone pain are the most likely symptoms first observed with electrolyte imbalances (Table 5.10) (see "Clinical Manifestations" under "Common Causes of Fluid and Electrolyte Imbalances" below).

## MEDICAL MANAGEMENT

Potassium, calcium, sodium, and chloride can be measured in plasma. Intracellular levels of electrolytes cannot be measured; consequently, all values for electrolytes are expressed as serum values. Serum values for electrolytes are given as milliequivalents per liter (mEq/L) or milligrams per deciliter (mg/dL). As with fluid imbalances, the underlying cause of electrolyte imbalances must be determined and corrected. Electrolyte supplementation, when needed, can be given orally or intravenously.

**SPECIAL IMPLICATIONS FOR THE THERAPIST 5-11**

### *Electrolyte Imbalances*

With appropriate medical therapy, cardiac, muscular, and neurologic manifestations associated with electrolyte imbalances can be corrected. Delayed medical treatment may result in irreversible damage or death. That is why continual assessment for signs and symptoms of electrolyte imbalance must be ongoing, and changes need to be reported immediately. Observing for accompanying signs and symptoms of fluid and electrolyte imbalances will help promote safe and effective exercise for anyone with the potential for these disorders.

*Encourage adherence to a sodium-restricted diet when prescribed. The use of nonprescription medications for people on a sodium-restricted diet should be approved by the physician. Encourage activity and alternate with rest periods. Monitor for worsening of the underlying cause of fluid or electrolyte imbalance and report significant findings to the nurse or physician.*

*If dyspnea and orthopnea are present, teach the client to use a semi-Fowler position (head elevated 18 to 20 inches from horizontal with knees flexed) to promote lung expansion. Frequent position changes are important in the presence of edema; edematous tissue is more prone to skin breakdown than normal tissue.*

#### Hypokalemia

Older adults have frequent problems with hypokalemia most often associated with the use of diuretics. Decreased potassium levels can result in fatigue, muscle cramping, and cardiac dysrhythmias, usually manifested by an irregular pulse rate or complaints of dizziness and/or palpitations. Fatigue and muscle cramping increase the chance of musculoskeletal injury.

#### Hypomagnesemia

Monitor carefully any individual being medically treated for hypomagnesemia because administration of magnesium for hypomagnesemia can result in hypermagnesemia and signs and symptoms associated with magnesium toxicity (e.g., loss of deep tendon reflexes).

#### Hypermagnesemia

For hospitalized patients with severe hypermagnesemia (usually secondary to renal failure), monitor vital signs carefully and initiate safety precautions as appropriate. Watch for hypotension, bradycardia, and respiratory depression. Assess neuromuscular function and level of consciousness regularly. Frequently, individuals with hypermagnesemia are restricted from mobility activities (sitting up, ambulating) without supervision.

#### Postoperative Electrolyte Imbalances

Electrolyte imbalances associated with complex spinal surgeries have been reported in more than 40% of all cases.[366] It is believed that this figure has previously been underreported and thanks to a spinal specific tool used to report and classify severity of complications, this information has come to light. Therapists in the acute care setting and early outpatient rehab for these individuals should keep this in mind and monitor closely for electrolyte disturbances. Again, early recognition and intervention may reduce morbidity and mortality.[336]

## Common Causes of Fluid and Electrolyte Imbalances

### Overview

A brief description of the common causes of fluid and electrolyte imbalances and overall clinical picture encountered in a therapy practice is included here. Burns, surgery, and trauma may result in a fluid volume shift from the vascular spaces to the interstitial spaces. Tissue injury causes the release of histamine and bradykinin, which increases capillary permeability, allowing fluid, protein, and other solutes to shift into the interstitial spaces.[81]

In the case of burns, the fluid shifts out of the vessels into the injured tissue spaces, as well as into the normal (unburned) tissue. This causes severe swelling of these tissues and a significant loss of fluid volume from the vascular space, which results in hypovolemia. Severe

**Table 5-10** Clinical Features of Various Electrolyte Imbalances

| | SYSTEM DYSFUNCTION | |
|---|---|---|
| **Potassium Imbalance** | | |
| | **Hypokalemia** | **Hyperkalemia** |
| Cardiovascular | Dizziness, hypotension, arrhythmias, electrocardiogram (ECG) changes, cardiac arrest (with serum potassium levels 2.5 mEq/L) | Tachycardia and later bradycardia, ECG changes, cardiac arrest (with levels >7.0 mEq/L) |
| Gastrointestinal (GI) | Nausea and vomiting, anorexia, constipation, abdominal distention, paralytic ileus or decreased peristalsis | Nausea, diarrhea, abdominal cramps |
| Musculoskeletal | Muscle weakness and fatigue, leg cramps | Muscle weakness, flaccid paralysis |
| Genitourinary | Polyuria | Oliguria, anuria |
| Central nervous system (CNS) | Malaise, irritability, confusion, mental depression, speech changes, decreased reflexes, pulmonary hyperventilation | Areflexia progressing to weakness, numbness, tingling, and flaccid paralysis |
| Acid–base balance | Metabolic alkalosis | Metabolic acidosis |
| **Calcium Imbalance** | | |
| | **Hypocalcemia** | **Hypercalcemia** |
| CNS | Anxiety, irritability, twitching around mouth, laryngospasm, seizures, Chvostek sign, apathy, irritability, confusion | Drowsiness, lethargy, headaches, depression, or Trousseau sign |
| Musculoskeletal | Paresthesia (tingling and numbness of the fingers), tetany or painful tonic muscle spasms, facial spasms, abdominal cramps, muscle cramps, spasmodic contractions | Weakness, muscle flaccidity, bone pain, pathologic fractures |
| Cardiovascular | Arrhythmias, hypotension | Signs of heart block, cardiac arrest in systole, hypertension |
| GI | Increased GI motility, diarrhea from dehydration | Anorexia, nausea, vomiting, constipation, dehydration, polyuria, prerenal azotemia |
| **Sodium Imbalance** | | |
| | **Hyponatremia** | **Hypernatremia** |
| CNS | Anxiety, headaches, muscle twitching and weakness, confusion, seizures | Agitation, restlessness, seizures, ataxia, confusion |
| Cardiovascular | Hypotension; tachycardia; with severe deficit, vasomotor collapse, thready pulse | Hypertension, tachycardia, pitting edema, excessive weight gain |
| GI | Nausea, vomiting, abdominal cramps | Rough, dry tongue; intense thirst; severe hypotension |
| Genitourinary | Oliguria or anuria | Oliguria |
| Respiratory | Cyanosis with severe deficiency | Dyspnea, respiratory arrest, and death (from dramatic rise in osmatic pressure) |
| Cutaneous | Cold clammy skin, decreased skin turgor | Flushed skin; dry, sticky mucous membranes |
| **Magnesium Imbalance** | | |
| | **Hypomagnesemia** | **Hypermagnesemia** |
| Neuromuscular | Muscle tremors and weakness; athetoid movements Hyperirritability, tetany, leg and foot cramps, Chvostek sign (facial muscle spasms induced by tapping the branches of the facial nerve) | Diminished reflexes, muscle weakness, flaccid paralysis, respiratory muscle paralysis that may cause respiratory impairment and even respiratory arrest |
| CNS | Confusion, apathy, depression, delusions, hallucinations, psychosis, seizures | Drowsiness, flushing, lethargy, confusion, diminished sensorium |
| Cardiovascular | Arrhythmias (ventricular tachycardia, ventricular fibrillation), vasomotor changes (vasodilation and hypotension), occasionally hypertension | Bradycardia, weak pulse, hypotension, heart block, cardiac arrest |

hypovolemia can result in shock, vascular collapse, and death. In the case of major tissue damage, potassium is also released from the damaged tissue cells and can enter the vascular fluids, causing hyperkalemia.

In an attempt to treat shock, large quantities of fluid are administered intravenously to maintain blood pressure, cardiac output, and renal function. After 24 to 72 hours, capillary permeability is usually restored and fluid begins to leave the tissue spaces and shift back into the vascular space. If renal function is not adequate, the accumulation of fluid used for treatment and fluid returning from the tissue spaces into the vascular space can cause fluid volume overload. Fluid overload can then lead to HF and pulmonary edema.

*Diabetes mellitus* (type 1) may result in a condition called *diabetic ketoacidosis*, which is caused by a lack of insulin. This leads to hyperglycemia, polyuria, and an overproduction of ketones that results in metabolic acidosis. Hyperglycemia draws ICF into the intravascular compartment (fluid shift), causing an intracellular dehydration; it also leads to an osmotic diuresis with not only loss of fluid, but also loss of electrolytes (potassium, sodium, and phosphate). Although many clients present with a laboratory value consistent with hyperkalemia (a result of metabolic acidosis), once adequate fluid has been restored it is evident that there is actually hypokalemia, which, unless treated immediately, can cause life-threatening cardiac dysrhythmias. The sodium value must be "corrected" for the amount of hyperglycemia. If the corrected sodium is elevated, then one-half isotonic saline is administered.

Hyponatremia is one of the most common electrolyte imbalances affecting hospitalized patients. Hyponatremia is typically caused by an increase in water with normal sodium stores (increased extracellular volume) and is most frequently seen as a result of HF, renal failure (nephrotic syndrome), or liver disease (ascites). Treatment is to manage the underlying condition along with fluid restriction.

Hyponatremia may also be seen when extracellular volumes are normal, but sodium is elevated. This is typically secondary to the syndrome of inappropriate antidiuretic hormone, but may also be a result of severe hypothyroidism or water intoxication (psychogenic polydipsia). Tumors and pulmonary and CNS disorders often inappropriately produce antidiuretic hormone (ADH), which is not regulated by normal suppression feedback loops; consequently, the ectopic hormone continues to be released by the tumor, often causing serious electrolyte imbalances. One example of this phenomenon is the ectopic production of ADH by lung carcinomas, resulting in hyponatremia.

A more local effect of malignancy occurs when metastases to the skeletal system produce hypercalcemia from the osteolysis of bone. The treatment of malignancies also can create fluid and electrolyte imbalances such as occur with hormonal treatment for breast cancer (e.g., tamoxifen can cause hypercalcemia). Hyponatremia and hypokalemia may also result from nausea and vomiting caused by chemotherapy. Certain chemotherapeutic drugs (e.g., vincristine and cyclophosphamide) are associated with syndrome of inappropriate antidiuretic hormone, causing hyponatremia.

*Alcohol withdrawal* and *eating disorders* are also associated with physiologic changes that can include electrolyte imbalances.

Hypernatremia may be seen with severe systemic disease (i.e., sepsis, surgery), volume loss without adequate water replacement (i.e., diarrhea or osmotic diuresis), or impaired sensorium or physical disability that prevents access to water. Diabetes insipidus also leads to hypernatremia because of a lack of ADH or resistance to ADH.

Hyperkalemia can be life-threatening. Mild hyperkalemia may be a consequence of improper potassium supplementation; moderate to severe hyperkalemia can be seen with renal failure, acidosis (i.e., diabetic ketoacidosis), digitalis toxicity, rhabdomyolysis, and insulin deficiency.

Box 5.8

**CLINICAL MANIFESTATIONS OF FLUID/ELECTROLYTE IMBALANCE**

***Skin Changes***

- Poor skin turgor
- Changes in skin temperature

***Neuromuscular Irritability***

- Muscle fatigue
- Muscle twitching
- Muscle cramping
- Tetany

***CNS Involvement***

- Changes in deep tendon reflexes
- Seizures
- Depression
- Memory impairment
- Delusions
- Hallucinations

***Edema***

- Changes in vital signs:
  - Tachycardia
  - Postural hypotension
  - Altered respirations

Hypokalemia may result from diarrhea, vomiting, acute leukemia, magnesium deficiency, diabetic ketoacidosis, and diuretics.

## Clinical Manifestations

The effects of a fluid or electrolyte imbalance are not isolated to a particular organ or system (Box 5.8). Symptoms most commonly observed by the therapist may include skin changes, neuromuscular irritability (muscle fatigue, twitching, cramping, or tetany), CNS involvement, edema, and changes in vital signs, especially tachycardia and postural (orthostatic) hypotension.

*Skin changes* include changes in skin turgor and alterations in skin temperature. In a healthy individual, pinched skin will immediately fall back to its normal position when released, a measure of skin turgor. In a person with FVD, such as dehydration, the skin flattens more slowly after the pinch is released and may even remain elevated for several seconds, referred to as *tenting* of tissue (Fig. 5.8). Tissue turgor can vary with age, nutritional state, race, and complexion, and must be accompanied by other signs of FVD to be considered meaningful.

Skin turgor may be more difficult to assess in older adults because of reduced skin elasticity compared with that of younger clients. Skin temperature may become warm and flushed as a result of vasodilation (e.g., in metabolic acidosis) or pale and cool because of peripheral vasoconstriction compensating for hypovolemia.

*Neuromuscular irritability* can occur as a result of imbalances in calcium, magnesium, potassium, and sodium. Specific signs of neuromuscular involvement associated with these imbalances occur because of increased neural excitability, specifically increased acetylcholine action at the nerve ending, resulting in lowering of the threshold of the muscle membrane.

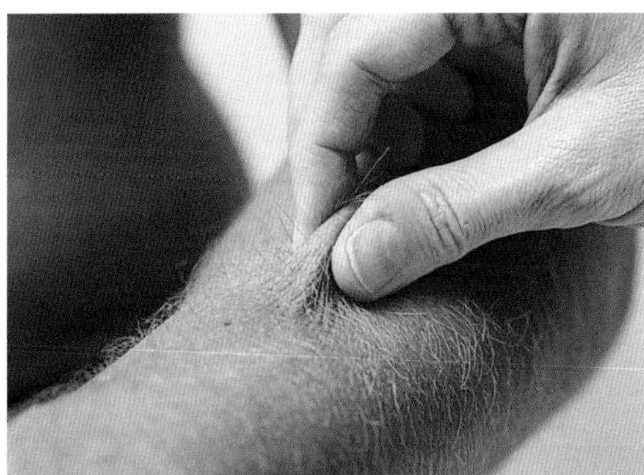

**Figure 5.8**

**Testing skin turgor (normal resiliency of a pinched fold of skin).** Turgor is measured by the time it takes for the skin and underlying tissue to return to its original contour after being pinched up. If the skin remains elevated (i.e., tented) for more than 3 seconds, turgor is decreased. Normal turgor is indicated by a return to baseline contour within 3 seconds when the skin is mobile and elastic. Turgor decreases with age as the skin loses elasticity; testing turgor of some older persons on the forearm (the standard site for testing) is less valid because of decreased skin elasticity in this area. From Ball JW, Dains JE, Flynn JA, et al: *Seidel's guide to physical examination,* ed 9, St Louis, 2019, Elsevier.

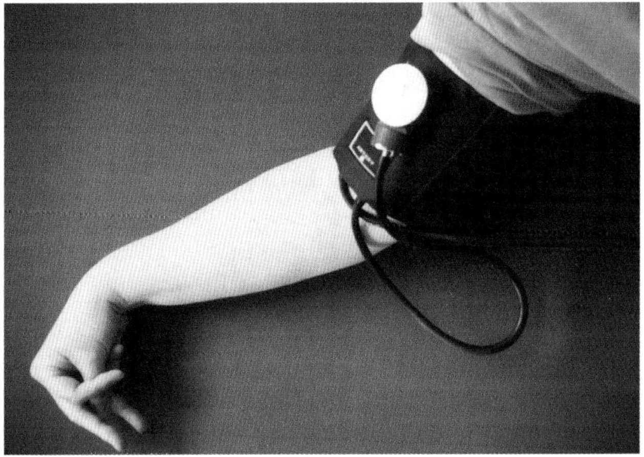

**Figure 5.9**

**Carpopedal attitude of the hand, a form of latent tetany associated with hypocalcemia, is called the *Trousseau sign.*** This can be tested for by inflating a blood pressure cuff on the upper arm to a level between diastolic and systolic blood pressure and maintaining this inflation for 3 minutes. A positive test results in the carpal spasm shown here. (From Ignatavicius DD, Workman ML: *Medical-surgical nursing: critical thinking for collaborative care,* ed 5, Philadelphia, 2006, WB Saunders.)

*Tetany* (continuous muscle spasm) is the most characteristic manifestation of hypocalcemia. The affected person may report a sensation of tingling around the mouth (circumoral paresthesia) and in the hands and feet, and spasms of the muscles of the extremities and face. Less-overt signs (latent tetany) can be elicited through the Trousseau sign (Fig. 5.9), the Chvostek sign (Fig. 5.10), and changes in deep tendon reflexes (DTRs) (Table 5.11). Many other factors can produce abnormalities in DTRs, requiring the therapist to evaluate altered DTRs in light of other clinical signs and client history.

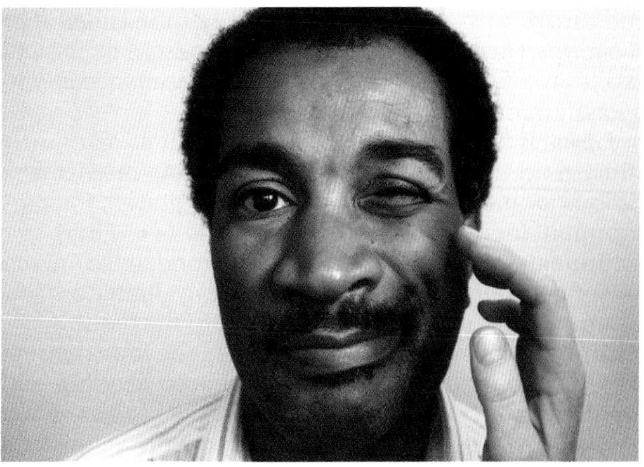

**Figure 5.10**

**To check for the *Chvostek sign,* tap the facial nerve above the mandibular angle, adjacent to the ear lobe.** A facial muscle spasm that causes the person's eye and upper lip to twitch, as shown, confirms tetany. (From Ignatavicius DD, Workman ML: *Medical-surgical nursing: critical thinking for collaborative care,* ed 5, Philadelphia, 2006, WB Saunders.)

**Table 5-11** Changes in Deep Tendon Reflexes Associated with Fluid and Electrolyte Imbalance

| Increased (Hyperactive) | Decreased (Hypoactive) |
|---|---|
| Hypocalcemia | Hypercalcemia |
| Hypomagnesemia | Hypermagnesemia |
| Hypernatremia | Hyponatremia |
| Hyperkalemia[a] | Hyperkalemia |
| Alkalosis | Acidosis |

[a]Generally hyperkalemia is accompanied by decreased or absent deep tendon reflexes (DTRs); some sources do report hyperactive DTRs with hyperkalemia. In the clinical situation, DTRs are never used to determine a potassium imbalance. They are a warning sign for the therapist to assess the client further and report all pertinent findings.

*Nervous system* involvement may occur in the peripheral system (hyperkalemia) or the CNS (hypocalcemia, hypercalcemia, hyponatremia, and hypernatremia). CNS manifestations of hypocalcemia may include seizures, irritability, depression, memory impairment, delusions, and hallucinations. In chronic hypocalcemia, the skin may be dry and scaling, the nails brittle, and the hair is dry and falls out easily.

Signs and symptoms of hyponatremia include headaches, confusion, lethargy, muscle weakness, tremors, gait disturbances, and nausea/vomiting. People with severe acute hyponatremia may progress from confusion to coma and respiratory arrest. People with chronic hyponatremia often have fewer symptoms because their hyponatremia has progressed slowly.

*Hypokalemia* seen in a therapy practice can be accompanied by muscular weakness. The weakness is initially most prominent in the legs, especially the quadriceps; it extends to the trunk and arms, with involvement of the respiratory muscles soon after.[289] Severe hypokalemia can cause paralysis, gastrointestinal ileus, respiratory failure, and cardiac arrhythmias. Finally, a condition called *rhabdomyolysis* (disintegration of striated muscle fibers with excretion of myoglobin in the urine) can occur with potassium or phosphorus depletion.

*Edema* is defined as an excessive accumulation of interstitial fluid. Many disease processes result in edema in various locations of the body. Because of gravity, the most common location is the lower extremities. Fluid may accumulate in the ankles and legs secondary to incompetent veins or from a lack of protein in the blood (low albumin), leading to a shift of fluid into the tissues.

Another common cause of edema in the lower extremities is HF. Because the heart is unable to keep up with the demand of pumping blood from the venous system to the arterial system, fluid backs up in the venous system, causing an increase in pressure and shifting of fluid into the tissue. There is also less fluid entering the kidneys, resulting in oliguria. Fluid may also accumulate in the interstitial tissues and airspaces of the lung leading to pulmonary edema.

Clinical symptoms are indicative of the underlying process. Edema of the lower extremities may be the only symptom if incompetent veins are the only cause. If fluid retention, as a result of HF, renal failure, or liver disease, is the cause, symptoms often include shortness of breath, orthopnea, increased respiratory rate, distended neck veins (observed best when the individual's head is elevated 45 degrees), weight gain, and pitting edema of the lower extremities (Fig. 5.11). Laboratory findings may be abnormal (e.g., electrolytes, serum creatinine, BUN, and hemoglobin).

*Vital sign changes*, including pulse, respirations, and blood pressure, may signal early development of fluid volume changes. Decreased blood pressure and tachycardia are usually the first signs of the decreased vascular volume associated with FVD, as the heart pumps faster to compensate for the decreased plasma volume. Irregular pulse rates and dysrhythmias may also be associated with magnesium, potassium, or calcium imbalances.

Orthostatic hypotension is another sign of volume depletion (hypovolemia). Moving from a supine to standing position causes an abrupt drop in venous return, which is normally compensated for by sympathetically mediated cardiovascular adjustments. For example, in the healthy individual, increased peripheral resistance and increased heart rate maintain cardiac output. Blood pressure is unaffected or characterized by a small decrease in systolic pressure, and the diastolic pressure may actually rise a few millimeters of mercury (mm Hg).

In contrast, for the person with FVD, systolic pressure may fall 20 mm Hg or more, accompanied by an increase in the pulse rate greater than 15 beats/min.[185] The decreased volume results in compensatory increases in pulse rate as the heart attempts to increase output in the face of decreased stroke volume.

As fluid volume depletion worsens, blood pressure becomes low in all positions from loss of compensatory mechanisms and autonomic insufficiency. Conditions such as diabetes, associated with autonomic neuropathy, and Parkinson disease, can also produce orthostatic blood pressure and pulse changes (see "Orthostatic Hypotension" in Chapter 12).

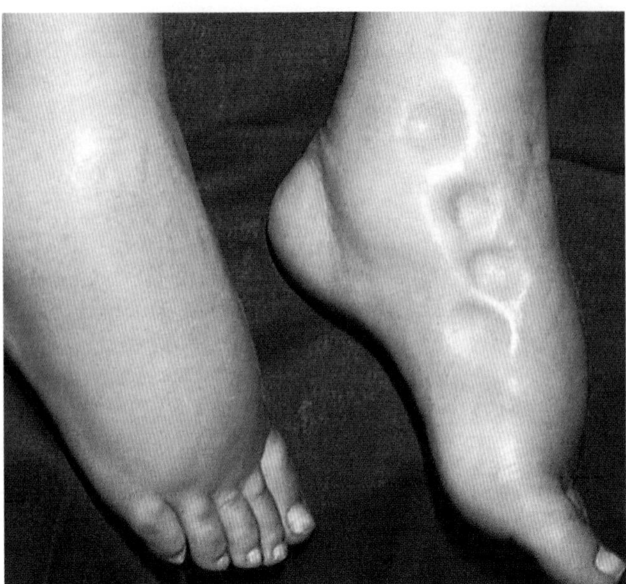

**Figure 5.11**

Severe, dependent, pitting edema occurs with some systemic diseases, such as congestive heart failure and hepatic cirrhosis. Note the finger-shaped depressions that do not refill after pressure has been exerted by the examiner. (From Bloom A, Ireland J: *Color atlas of diabetes*, ed 2, St Louis, 1992, Mosby.)

SPECIAL IMPLICATIONS FOR THE THERAPIST 5-12

### *Assessment of Fluid and Electrolyte Imbalance*

Assessment of fluid and electrolyte balance is based on both subjective and objective findings (Table 5.12). At the bedside or in the home health care setting, the therapist must be alert to complaints of headache, thirst, and nausea and changes in dyspnea, skin turgor, and muscle strength. More objective assessment of fluid and electrolyte balance is based on fluid intake, output, and body weight. (See "Special Implications for the Therapist: Fluid Imbalances and Electrolyte Imbalances" above.)

## ACID–BASE IMBALANCES

### Overview

The normal function of body cells to maintain homeostasis depends on regulation of hydrogen ion concentration ($H^+$) so that $H^+$ levels remain within very narrow limits. Acid–base imbalances occur when these limits are exceeded and are recognized clinically as abnormalities of serum pH (i.e., the measure of acidity or alkalinity of blood). Normal serum pH is 7.35 to 7.45. Cell function is seriously impaired when pH falls to 7.2 or lower or rises to 7.55 or higher (see "Laboratory Values" in Chapter 40).

Three physiologic systems act interdependently to maintain normal serum pH: immediate buffering of excess acid or base by the *blood buffer systems*, excretion of acid by the *lungs* (occurs within minutes to hours), and excretion of acid or reclamation of base by the *kidneys* (occurs within 24 to 48 hours). The four general classes of acid–base imbalance are respiratory acidosis, respiratory

**Table 5-12** Assessment of Fluid and Electrolyte Imbalance

| Area | Fluid Excess/Electrolyte Imbalance | Fluid Loss/Electrolyte Imbalance |
|---|---|---|
| Head and neck | Distended neck veins, facial edema | Thirst, dry mucous membranes |
| Extremities | Dependent pitting, edema, discomfort from weight of bed covers | Muscle weakness, tingling, tetany |
| Skin | Warm, moist; taut, cool feeling when edematous | Dry, decreased turgor |
| Respiration | Dyspnea, orthopnea, productive cough, moist breath | Changes in rate and depth of breathing sounds |
| Circulation | Hypertension, distended neck veins, atrial arrhythmias | Pulse rate irregularities, arrhythmia, postural hypotension, tachycardia |
| Abdomen | Increased girth, fluid wave | Abdominal cramps |

Modified from Briggs J, Drabek C: Fluid and electrolyte imbalance. In Phipps WJ, Sands J, Marek J, editors: *Medical-surgical nursing: concepts and clinical practice*, ed 6, St Louis, 1999, Mosby.

alkalosis, metabolic acidosis, and metabolic alkalosis. Table 5.13 summarizes these four imbalances.

*Acidosis* (metabolic or respiratory) refers to any pathologic process causing a relative excess of acid in the body (pH less than 7.35). This can occur as a result of accumulation of acid or depletion of the alkaline reserve (bicarbonate content, $HCO_3-$) in the blood and body tissues.

*Acidemia* refers to excess acid in the blood and does not necessarily confirm an underlying pathologic process. The same distinction may be made between the terms *alkalosis* and *alkalemia;* alkalosis indicates a primary condition resulting in excess base in the body. Although efforts have been made to standardize acid–base terminology, these terms are often used interchangeably.

### Incidence

The incidence of acid–base imbalances in hospital settings is high. Acid–base imbalances are often related to respiratory and/or metabolic problems typical of the critically ill or injured individual. Some people have more than one acid–base imbalance at the same time.

### Clinical Manifestations

Table.13 is a guide to the clinical presentation of acid–base imbalances. Besides the major distinguishing characteristics of acid–base imbalance described in this chapter, potassium excess (hyperkalemia) is associated with both respiratory and metabolic acidosis, and neuromuscular hyperexcitability is associated with both respiratory and metabolic alkalosis.

### MEDICAL MANAGEMENT

**DIAGNOSIS.** Pulse oximetry is used most often to measure oxygen saturation, yet it does not provide needed information regarding the effectiveness of ventilation or the pH of the blood. A more comprehensive procedure is the arterial blood gas test. This measurement is important in the diagnosis and treatment of ventilation, oxygen transport, and acid–base problems. The test measures the amount of dissolved oxygen and carbon dioxide in arterial blood and indicates acid–base status by measurement of the arterial blood pH. The pH is inversely proportional to the hydrogen ion concentration ($H^+$) in the blood. Therefore, as the hydrogen ion concentration ($H^+$) increases (acidosis), the pH decreases; as the hydrogen ion concentration ($H^+$) decreases (alkalosis), the pH increases.

The $PCO_2$ is a measure of the *partial pressure of carbon dioxide* in the blood. $PCO_2$ is termed the *respiratory component* in acid–base measurement because the carbon dioxide level is primarily regulated by the lungs. As the carbon dioxide level increases, the pH decreases (respiratory acidosis); as the carbon dioxide level decreases, the pH increases (respiratory alkalosis).

**TREATMENT.** Treatment in acid–base imbalances is directed toward the underlying cause and correction of any coexisting electrolyte imbalance. For example, respiratory infections contributing to ventilatory failure (respiratory acidosis) are managed with appropriate antibiotic therapy, pulmonary hygiene, oxygen support, and possibly, continuous mechanical ventilation. Use of pharmaceutical agents that depress the respiratory control center is minimized. Dialysis may be indicated in renal failure (metabolic acidosis) or overdose of toxins.

## Respiratory Acidosis

Respiratory acidosis is nearly always a result of hypoventilation and subsequent retention of $CO_2$ (hypercapnia). In a therapy setting, respiratory acidosis is most commonly observed in the population with pulmonary disease or obstruction (COPD, asthma, pneumonia, pulmonary edema, interstitial lung disease); depressed CNS (drugs, infection, or brain injury), or whenever the diaphragm is impaired (e.g., Guillain-Barré syndrome, myasthenia gravis, or chest wall deformities); secondary to burns; and as a result of lesions of the CNS (e.g., tumor, stroke, or muscular dystrophy).

The respiratory system has an important role in maintaining acid–base equilibrium. In response to an increase in the hydrogen ion concentration in body fluids, the respiratory rate increases, causing more $CO_2$ to be released from the lung.

Respiratory acidosis can be acute because of a sudden failure in ventilation, or chronic, as with long-term pulmonary disease (e.g., COPD). Acutely, excess $CO_2$ is buffered when it unites with water to form hydrogen ions and bicarbonate, decreasing the blood pH. After 3 to 5 days, the kidneys begin to excrete more acid and retain more bicarbonate to correct the acid imbalance.

*Chronic* respiratory acidosis results from gradual and irreversible loss of ventilatory function. The kidneys attempt to compensate by retaining bicarbonate and thereby maintaining a pH within tolerable limits. However, if even a minor respiratory infection develops, the person is subjected to a rapidly developing state of acute acidosis because the lungs remove only a limited amount of carbon dioxide.

### Clinical Manifestations

Acute respiratory acidosis is often accompanied with hypoxemia, compounding symptoms. Symptoms are principally CNS related. Effects range from restlessness and anxiety to sleepiness, confusion, a fine or flapping tremor or coma. The person may report headaches, blurred vision, and shortness of breath with retraction and use of accessory muscles. On examination, DTRs may be depressed. This disorder may also cause cardiovascular abnormalities such as tachycardia, atrial and ventricular arrhythmias, and in severe acidosis, hypotension with decreased cardiac output. Clients with chronic respiratory acidosis manifest more mild symptoms, such as memory loss, restlessness, and irritability.

## Respiratory Alkalosis

Respiratory alkalosis, the opposite of respiratory acidosis, occurs as a result of a loss of acid (hypocapnia) without compensation due to increased ventilation (hyperventilation).

Conditions associated with respiratory alkalosis fall into the following two categories:

1. *Pulmonary*, caused by hypoxemia in early stage pulmonary problems (e.g., pulmonary edema, pulmonary embolism, pneumonia, and acute asthma) and by overuse of a mechanical ventilator.
2. *Nonpulmonary*, which includes anxiety, pain, fever, high environmental temperature, pregnancy, drug toxicities (salicylates, theophylline), CNS disease (brainstem tumors, infection), high altitude, and hyperthyroidism (see Table 5.13).

Acute respiratory alkalosis leads to an increase in blood pH, which is compensated with the diffusion of hydrogen ions from intracellular storage that combine with bicarbonate to regenerate $CO_2$. The kidneys are able to further compensate by excreting bicarbonate after 2 to 3 days. Hyperventilation and the subsequent respiratory alkalosis is a common finding in ICU patients.

### Clinical Manifestations

The cardinal sign of respiratory alkalosis is deep, rapid breathing, possibly exceeding 40 breaths/min (much like the Kussmaul respirations that characterize diabetic acidosis) (see Table 5.13). Such hyperventilation usually leads to CNS and neuromuscular disturbances such as dizziness, light-headedness, and confusion (caused by below-normal $CO_2$ levels that decrease cerebral blood flow); inability to concentrate; tingling and numbness of the extremities and around the mouth; blurred vision; diaphoresis; dry mouth; muscle cramps; carpopedal (wrist and foot) spasms; twitching (possibly progressing to tetany); and muscle weakness. Severe respiratory alkalosis may cause cardiac arrhythmias, seizures, and syncope.

## Metabolic Acidosis

Metabolic acidosis is an accumulation of acids or a deficit of bases in the blood. This type of acidosis can occur with an acid gain (e.g., ketones with diabetic ketoacidosis, lactic acid with hypoxia, toxins such as ethylene glycol, and renal failure) or bicarbonate loss (e.g., diarrhea).

Metabolic acidosis can be divided into two categories: (1) metabolic acidosis with an anion gap and (2) metabolic acidosis with a normal anion gap. An anion gap is based on the principle of electrical neutrality in the body (i.e., cations should equal anions). The anion gap can be estimated from the equation: anion gap = sodium − (chloride + bicarbonate). A normal anion gap is positive (sodium constitutes over 90% of cations), usually $12 \pm 4$ (some labs may use $7 \pm 4$).

However, if the anion gap is elevated, there are unmeasured (and unaccountable) anionic molecules present in the blood. The osmolal gap can also be calculated (expected osmolality − calculated osmolality), which demonstrates the presence of low-molecular-weight substances seen in toxic overdoses. Table 5.13 lists specific etiologic factors. Metabolic acidosis with an elevated anion gap can be caused by toxic ingestions (methanol, ethylene glycol, isoniazid, iron, ethanol, salicylates, propylene glycol), uremia, diabetic ketoacidosis, lactic acidosis (metformin, propofol), and starvation.

*Ketoacidosis*, a major cause of metabolic acidosis, occurs when insufficient insulin for the amount of glucose results in increased breakdown of fat (lipolysis). This accelerated fat breakdown produces ketones and other acids. Although the body attempts to neutralize these increased acids, the plasma bicarbonate ($HCO_3-$) is depleted.

In the case of uremia associated with *renal failure*, the failing kidney is not able to excrete acid (unable to excrete ammonium and phosphoric acid). Hydrogen ions are buffered by bicarbonate in the extracellular fluids, but eventually this is not enough to keep the pH in the normal range. *Lactic acidosis* is the most common cause of metabolic acidosis in the hospital. It occurs when the production of lactic acid is greater than the removal of lactic acid, which is typically associated with hypoxemia. The body is usually able to utilize lactic acid through metabolism in the liver; however with some diseases, the body is unable to utilize lactic acid as quickly as it is produced, perhaps due to decreased hepatic perfusion. Other causes for developing lactic acidosis include excessive exercise, generalized seizures, cardiopulmonary failure, shock, acute pulmonary edema, carbon monoxide poisoning, smoke inhalation, sepsis, trauma, adverse reactions to medications (metformin) or toxins, alcohol abuse, liver disease, cancer, and HIV infection.

Alcoholic ketoacidosis occurs when a person abruptly stops drinking alcohol and has prolonged vomiting associated with a background of fasting or starvation. This most often occurs in adults with alcoholism, although it can be seen in younger binge drinkers. Because of a low nutritional state, insulin production is reduced while other counterregulatory hormones are increased. Lipolysis is upregulated with release of fatty acids, which are then oxidized to ketone bodies by the liver.

Metabolic acidosis with a normal anion gap is caused by a loss of bicarbonate from GI sources such as diarrhea,[289] loss of bicarbonate from the kidney (type 2 renal tubular acidosis [RTA]), or inability of the kidney to excrete acid (type 1 and 4 RTAs, chronic kidney disease). Typically with acidosis, the kidney increases excretion of acid in the form of ammonium (ammonia + $H^+$ creates ammonium). Because this is difficult to measure, the urine anion gap approximates the amount of acid being excreted.

The urine anion gap is calculated by the following equation:

Urine Anion Gap = (Urine Sodium + Urine Potassium) - Urine Chloride

If the anion gap is negative, the kidney is able to excrete acid and is not the cause. A positive urine anion gap suggests a distal renal tubular acidosis. The presence of hypokalemia or hyperkalemia further aids in differentiating between the types of RTAs. Type 1 is associated with hypokalemia, whereas type 4 is associated with hyperkalemia. Type 2 manifests with loss of bicarbonate and other compounds such as glucose, phosphate, and amino acids. Hypokalemia may also be present.

#### Clinical Manifestations

The symptoms of metabolic acidosis can include rapid breathing, tachycardia, decreased appetite, weakness, malaise, nausea, vomiting, diarrhea, and headache (see Table 5.13). If the acidosis is severe, myocardial depression and hypotension can occur. Compensatory hyperventilation may occur as a result of stimulation of the hypothalamus as the body attempts to rid itself of excess $CO_2$. As the acid level goes up, these symptoms progress to stupor, unconsciousness, coma, and death.

Some causes of metabolic acidosis have symptoms that may be present and point to the diagnosis. Diabetics with ketoacidosis may have breath with a fruity odor in the presence of ketone production. Methanol ingestion produces visual changes, whereas salicylate overdose leads to tinnitus and vertigo.

### Metabolic Alkalosis

Metabolic alkalosis occurs when either an abnormal loss of acid or excess accumulation of bicarbonate occurs. There are two phases: a generation phase (where bicarbonate accumulates) and a maintenance phase (where the kidneys are unable to effectively excrete excess bicarbonate). Generation of excess bicarbonate typically occurs due to a GI loss of acid as seen in vomiting, or the kidney (due to volume depletion, the kidney retains bicarbonate). Volume contraction, chloride depletion, decreased glomerular filtration, and hypokalemia contribute to maintenance of metabolic alkalosis. Conditions that may cause metabolic alkalosis include volume loss; vomiting; postoperative loss of acid through gastric suctioning; and use of diuretics. Bulimia with vomiting and diuretic abuse associated with an eating disorder are notable causes, particularly in the young. Table 5.13 lists other causes. Urine chloride often aids in determining the cause and therefore the treatment.

#### Clinical Manifestations

Signs and symptoms occur as the body attempts to correct the acid–base imbalance, primarily through hypoventilation. Respirations are shallow and slow as the lungs attempt to compensate by building up carbonic acid stores. Clients with severe metabolic alkalosis develop hypokalemia and hypocalcemia. Clinical manifestations may be mild at first, with muscle weakness, irritability, confusion, and muscle twitching (see Table 5.13). If untreated, the condition progresses and the person may become comatose, with possible seizures, cardiac arrhythmias, and respiratory paralysis.

**Table 5-13** Overview of Acid–Base Imbalances

| Mechanism | Etiologic Factors | Clinical Manifestations | Treatment |
|---|---|---|---|
| **Respiratory Acidosis** | | | |
| Hypoventilation | Acute respiratory failure COPD<br>Neuromuscular disease<br>• Guillain-Barré<br>• Myasthenia gravis<br>Respiratory center depression<br>Drugs<br>• Barbiturates<br>• Sedatives<br>• Narcotics<br>• Anesthetic<br>CNS lesions<br>Tumor<br>Stroke<br>Inadequate mechanical ventilation | Hypercapnia, restlessness, disorientation, confusion, sleepiness, visual disturbances, headache, flushing, dyspnea, cyanosis, decreased deep tendon reflexes, hyperkalemia, palpitation, pH <7.35, $PaCO_2$ >45 mm Hg | Treatment underlying cause; support ventilation; correct electrolyte imbalance |
| Excess carbon dioxide production | Hypermetabolism<br>Sepsis<br>Burns | | |

*Continued*

**Table 5-13** Overview of Acid–Base Imbalances—cont'd

| Mechanism | Etiologic Factors | Clinical Manifestations | Treatment |
|---|---|---|---|
| **Respiratory Alkalosis** | | | |
| Hyperventilation | Hypoxemia<br>Pulmonary embolus<br>High altitude<br>Impaired lung expansion<br>Pulmonary fibrosis<br>Ascites<br>Scoliosis<br>Pregnancy[a]<br>Congestive heart failure<br>Stimulation of respiratory center<br>Anxiety hyperventilation<br>Encephalitis/meningitis (hepatic failure)<br>Salicylates (aspirin overdose)<br>Theophylline<br>CNS trauma<br>CNS tumor<br>Excessive exercise<br>Extreme stress<br>Severe pain<br>Mechanical overventilation | Tachypnea, hypocapnia, dizziness, difficulty concentrating, numbness and tingling, blurred vision, diaphoresis, dry mouth, muscle cramps, carpopedal spasm, muscle twitching and weakness, hyperreflexia, arrhythmias pH >7.45, $PaCO_2$ <35 mm Hg, hypokalemia, hypocalcemia (see Table 5.10) | Treat underlying cause; increase carbon dioxide retention (rebreathing, sedation) |
| **Metabolic Acidosis** | | | |
| Acid excess | Renal failure (acid retention)<br>Diabetic or alcoholic ketoacidosis<br>Lactic acidosis (see text)<br>Starvation and fasting<br>Ingested toxins<br>• Aspirin<br>• Antifreeze<br>• Cyanide<br>• Iron | Hyperventilation (compensatory), muscular twitching, weakness, malaise, nausea, vomiting, diarrhea, headache, hyperkalemia (cardiac arrhythmias), pH <7.35, $HCO_3-$, <22 mm mEq/L, $PaCO_2$ normal (35-45 mm Hg) or slightly decreased, coma (death) | Treat underlying cause, correct electrolyte imbalance; $NaCO_3$ for severe acidosis (pH <7.2) |
| Base deficit | Severe diarrhea ($HCO_3-$ loss)<br>Renal failure (inability to reabsorb $HCO_3-$) | | |
| **Metabolic Alkalosis** | | | |
| Fixed acid loss (with base excess) | Hypokalemia<br>Diuretic therapy<br>Steroids<br>Vomiting<br>Nasogastric suctioning | Hypoventilation (compensatory): dysrhythmias, nausea, prolonged vomiting, diarrhea, confusion, irritability, agitation, restlessness, muscle twitching, cramping, hypotonia, weakness, Trousseau sign, paresthesias, seizures, coma, hypokalemia, pH >7.45, $PaCO_2$ normal (35-45 mm Hg) or slightly increased | Treat underlying cause; administer potassium chloride |
| Excessive $HCO_3-$ intake | Peptic ulcer<br>• Milk-alkali syndrome<br>• Excessive intake of antacids<br>Overcorrection of acidosis<br>Massive blood transfusion | Hypochloremia | |
| Excessive $HCO_3-$ resorption | Hyperaldosteronism<br>Cushing disease | | |

[a]In the third trimester of pregnancy, the hormone progesterone also stimulates respiration.
*COPD*, Chronic obstructive pulmonary disease; *$HCO_3-$*, bicarbonate ion; *$NaCO_3$*, sodium bicarbonate; *$PaCO_2$*, partial pressure of carbon dioxide.

## Aging and Acid–Base Regulation

Acid–base disturbances are common in the elderly and frequently determine outcome and prognosis.[381] The normal aging process results in changes in the lung, such as decreased ventilatory capacity and loss of alveolar surface area for gas exchange; thus older adults are prone to respiratory acidosis caused by hypoventilation and to respiratory alkalosis caused by hypoxemia and subsequent hyperventilation. Older adults are often taking multiple medications for hypertension (diuretics) or cardiovascular disease that may contribute to hypokalemia and metabolic alkalosis. Respiratory compensation in these conditions can be compromised because of the structural and functional changes mentioned. Respiratory alkalosis may be the result of hyperventilation caused by anxiety, CNS infection/infarction, pulmonary embolism, or pulmonary edema.

Several alterations in the kidney of the elderly lead to an inability to compensate for acid–base changes in order to maintain homeostasis. There is a decline in the GFR and capacity to excrete an acid load, resulting in a chronic, low-level metabolic acidosis. Complications may include nephrolithiasis, bone demineralization, and muscle wasting. Aldosterone is less effective in older adults, as is ammonia buffering. These changes limit renal compensation for respiratory imbalances and place the individual at higher risk for metabolic imbalance.[384]

**SPECIAL IMPLICATIONS FOR THE THERAPIST 5-13**

### *Acid–Base Imbalances*

The therapist must observe clients at risk for acid–base imbalance for any early symptoms. This is especially true for people with known pulmonary, cardiovascular, or renal disease; clients in a hypermetabolic state, such as occurs in fever, sepsis, or burns; clients receiving total parenteral nutrition or enteral tube feedings that are high in carbohydrates; mechanically ventilated clients; clients with insulin-dependent diabetes; older clients whose age-related decreases in respiratory and renal function may limit their ability to compensate for acid–base disturbances; and clients with vomiting, diarrhea, or enteric drainage. Specific reference values in acid–base disorders are listed in Table 5.13.

*Client and family education in the prevention of acute episodes of metabolic acidosis, particularly diabetic ketoacidosis, is essential. A fruity breath odor from rising acid levels (acetone) may be detected by the therapist treating someone who has uncontrolled diabetes.*

*The therapist should not hesitate to ask the client about this breath odor, as immediate medical intervention is required for diabetic ketoacidosis. Dehydration occurs rapidly as a result of severe hyperglycemia. A rising pulse rate and a drop in blood pressure are critical (and often late) indicators of a fluid volume deficit caused by dehydration.*

*Safety measures to avoid injury during involuntary muscular contractions are the same as for convulsions or epileptic seizures. Vigorous restraint can cause orthopedic injuries as the muscles contract strongly against resistance. Placing padding to protect the person is a key to prevention of injury.*

*Measures that facilitate breathing are essential to client care during respiratory acidosis. Frequent turning, coughing, and deep breathing exercises to encourage oxygen–carbon dioxide exchange are beneficial. Postural drainage, unless contraindicated by the client's condition, may be effective in promoting adequate ventilation.*

*In the case of respiratory hyperventilation, rebreathing* $CO_2$ *in a paper sack is helpful, as well as encouraging the individual to hold the breath. Oxygen may be given to reduce respiratory effort and the resultant blowing off of* $CO_2$ *by the person who has anoxia caused by pulmonary infection or CHF. Individuals with COPD may retain* $CO_2$*; the use of oxygen is contraindicated in these clients because it can further depress the respiratory drive, causing death.*

*Any client receiving diuretic therapy must be monitored for signs of potassium depletion (e.g., postural hypotension, muscle weakness, and fatigue; see Table 5.10) and alkalosis (see Table 5.13). Decreased respiratory rate may be an indication of compensation by the lungs, but the physician must make this assessment. Signs of neural irritability, such as the Trousseau sign (see Fig. 5.8), may be seen when taking blood pressure measurements, and they are helpful in detecting early stages of tetany caused by calcium deficiency.*

## REFERENCES

To enhance this text and add value for the reader, all references are included in the enhanced ebook on Student Consult that accompanies this textbook. The reader can view the reference source and access it online whenever possible.

# CHAPTER 6

# Injury, Inflammation, Healing, and Repair[a]

ANNIE BURKE-DOE • TERESSA F. BROWN • DAWN KELLY JAMES • ROLANDO T. LAZARO

## OVERVIEW

*Pathology* is defined as the structural and functional changes in the body caused by disease or trauma. Understanding the normal structure and function of the tissues is required before the discussion of pathology.

The organization of the material presented in this chapter parallels the processes underlying pathology—that is, cell injury and the factors causing this injury, inflammation as a secondary response to cell injury, and tissue healing and repair, which are essential components to return the tissue to optimal function. Fig. 6.1 illustrates the possible cellular responses to stress and injury and serves as a roadmap for our discussion in this chapter. A thorough understanding of the concepts that underpin cellular injury, inflammation, healing, and repair provides a solid foundation to facilitate comprehension of the other topics presented in this text.

## CELL INJURY

### Introduction

The structural and functional changes produced by pathology start with injury to the cells that make up the tissues. Mild injury produced by stressors leads to sublethal alterations of the affected cells that may be reversible, whereas moderate or severe injury leads to lethal alterations that are likely irreversible and can lead to cell death. We start by discussing the most common causes of cellular injury.

### Causes of Cell (Tissue) Injury

Cells may be damaged by a variety of factors. The most important causes are listed in Box 6.1. As mentioned earlier, cell injury may be reversible or irreversible. Whether the injury is reversible depends on the cell's ability to withstand the derangement of homeostatic mechanisms and its adaptability (i.e., ability to return to a state of homeostasis). Reversing the injury and achieving homeostasis are determined by a combination of factors including the mechanism of injury, the length of time the injury is present without intervention, and the severity of the injury.

#### Ischemia

At the tissue or organ level, ischemia occurs when the blood flow is insufficient to maintain cell homeostasis and metabolic function. This can be due to a reduction in flow or an increase in metabolism of the tissue beyond the capability of the arterial vascular system. Insufficient blood flow results in partial (hypoxia) or total (anoxia) reduction in oxygen supply, decreased delivery of nutrients, and decreased removal of waste products from the tissue. The lack of oxygen leads to loss of aerobic metabolism. The resulting reduction in adenosine triphosphate (ATP) synthesis leads to accumulation of ions and fluid intracellularly. The cells swell, and their function is compromised. This concept is discussed further in Reversible Cell Injury later in this chapter.

Hypoxia or anoxia may occur under many circumstances including obstruction of the respiratory tree (e.g., suffocation secondary to drowning), inadequate transport of oxygen across the respiratory surfaces (e.g., pneumonia), inadequate transport of oxygen in the blood (e.g., anemia), or an inability of the cell to use oxygen for cellular respiration (e.g., carbon monoxide poisoning).[132] Ischemia is usually the result of arterial lumen obstruction and narrowing caused by atherosclerosis and/or an intravascular clot called a *thrombus*. Ischemia resulting in myocardial infarction (MI) or stroke (lack of blood flow to the heart or brain, respectively) can cause death of tissue (necrosis) and accounts for two of the three leading causes of mortality in industrialized nations.[254]

#### Infectious Agents

Infectious agents such as bacteria, viruses, mycoplasmas, fungi, rickettsiae, protozoa, prions, and helminths (see Chapter 8), may also cause cell injury or death. Bacterial and viral agents are responsible for most infections.

Bacterial infections cause cell injury primarily by invading tissue and releasing exotoxins and endotoxins that can cause cell lysis and degradation of extracellular matrix and aid in the spread of the infection. Injury can also result from the inflammatory/immunologic reactions induced by bacteria in the host. For example, exotoxins may be released by clostridial organisms that cause gas gangrene, tetanus, and botulism.

[a]The authors acknowledge the contributions of Rolando T. Lazaro in the fourth edition of this text.

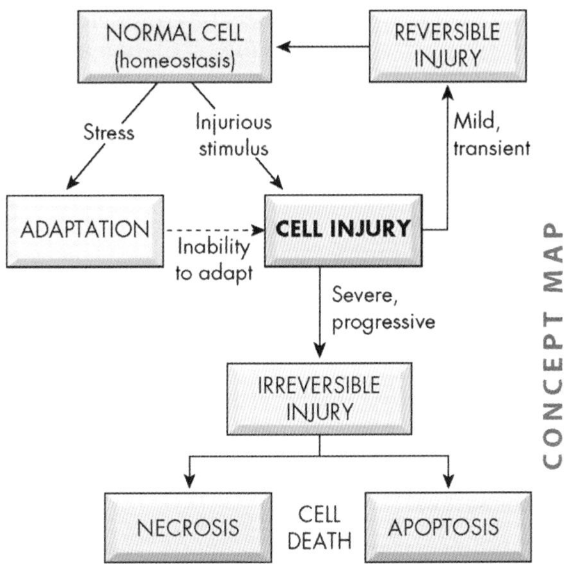


**Figure 6.1**

**Cellular response to stress and injurious stimuli.** (From Kumar V, et al: *Robbins and Cotran pathologic basis of disease*, ed 8, Philadelphia, 2010, Saunders.)

Box 6.1

**CAUSES OF CELL INJURY**

- Ischemia (lack of blood supply)
- Infectious agents
- Immune reactions
- Genetic factors
- Nutritional factors
- Physical factors
- Chemical factors

*Clostridium tetani,* for example, releases an exotoxin that is preferentially absorbed by the alpha motor neurons and delivered into the central nervous system (CNS). Once inside the CNS, the exotoxin crosses the synapse of the anterior horn cell and interferes with release of inhibitory neurotransmitters. This disruption of homeostasis eventually causes the activation of motor neurons that in turn cause involuntary muscular contractions (tetanus).

When microorganisms or their toxins are present in the blood, a condition called *sepsis* can occur (see further discussion in Chapter 5). Endotoxins released from gram-negative bacteria induce the synthesis of cytokines (extracts of normal leukocytes such as tumor necrosis factor [TNF] and interleukins [ILs]) that are responsible for many of the systemic manifestations of sepsis (Box 6.2). In sepsis, endothelial cell damage, loss of plasma volume, and maldistribution of blood flow result in hypovolemia. Cardiovascular collapse may ensue and lead to a condition called *septic shock*. The detection of an infectious agent initiates an inflammatory reaction designed to contain and inactivate the pathogen, but the magnitude of this defensive response by the host may also cause cellular or tissue destruction in the infected area.

Box 6.2

**ACTIONS OF CYTOKINES: INTERLEUKIN-1 AND TUMOR NECROSIS FACTOR**

***Local***

- Stimulates leukocyte adhesion to endothelium
- Modulates the coagulation cascade
- Stimulates production and/or secretion of inflammatory mediators (including interleukin-1 itself)
- Activates fibroblasts, chondrocytes, osteoclasts

***Systemic***

*Metabolic*

- Induces fever
- Increases body metabolism
- Decreases appetite
- Induces sleep
- Induces adrenocorticotropic hormone release to secrete corticosteroids
- Nonspecific resistance to infection

*Hemodynamic*

- Causes hypotension
- Hypovolemia (sepsis)

*Hematologic*

- Changes blood chemistry (see text)
- Activates endothelial, macrophage, and resting T cells
- Increases neutrophils in circulation
- Decreases lymphocytes in circulation
- Stimulates synthesis of collagen and collagenases

Viruses kill cells by one of two mechanisms (Fig. 6.2) and are the consequence of complete redirection of the cell's biosynthesis toward viral replication. The first is a direct cytopathic effect usually found with RNA viruses. These viruses kill from within by disturbing various cellular processes or by disrupting the integrity of the nucleus and/or plasma membrane.

The second mechanism is an indirect cytopathic effect mediated by immune mechanisms. In this process, virally encoded proteins become inserted into the plasma membrane of the host cell (forming a channel) and alter the permeability of the cell membrane to ions. The resulting loss of the ionic barrier leads to cell swelling and death. DNA viruses also kill cells through an indirect cytopathic effect by integrating themselves into the cellular genome. These viruses encode the production of foreign proteins, which are exposed on the cell surface and recognized by the body's immune cells. Immunocompetent cells such as T lymphocytes recognize these virally encoded proteins inserted into the plasma membrane of host cells and attack and destroy the infected cell. When the immune system is compromised or if the number of invading microorganisms overwhelms the immune system, disease (and the symptoms of illness) occurs (see further discussion in Chapter 7).

## Immune Reactions

Although the immune system normally functions in defense against foreign antigens, sometimes the system becomes

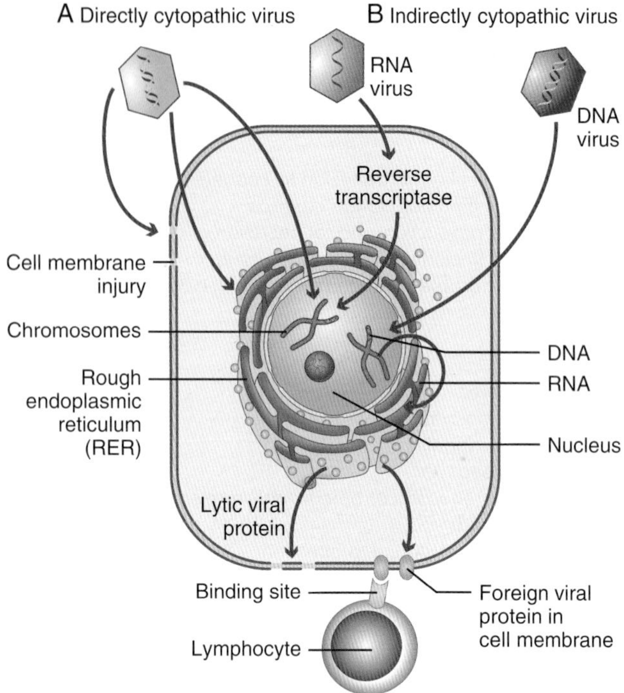


**Figure 6.2**

**Mechanisms of cell destruction by viruses.** (A) Direct cytopathic effect: RNA virus inserts itself in a receptor on the cell membrane and is brought into the cell. The RNA virus is altered into DNA by reverse transcriptase. The DNA within the nucleus of the cell forms various types of RNA that allow for protein synthesis in the rough endoplasmic reticulum *(RER)*. The protein formed inserts itself into the cell membrane, forming a channel that allows ions and extracellular fluid to enter, leading to cell lysis (directly killing the cell). (B) Indirect cytopathic effect mediated by immune mechanisms: DNA virus inserts itself in a receptor on the cell membrane and is brought into the cell. The DNA virus within the nucleus of the cell forms various types of RNA that allow for protein synthesis in the RER. This foreign viral protein inserts into the cell membrane and becomes a neoantigen. This neoantigen will be recognized by the T lymphocytes that will react to and kill (indirectly) the infected cell. (From Damjanov I: *Pathology for the health-related professions*, ed 4, St. Louis, 2012, Elsevier.)

overzealous in its activity, leading to hypersensitivities ranging from a mild allergy to life-threatening anaphylactic reactions or autoimmune (attacking oneself) disorders. The mechanisms by which the immune system can lead to cell injury or death include antibody attachment, complement activation, and activation of the inflammatory cells (e.g., neutrophils, macrophages, T and B lymphocytes, mast cells, and basophils). See Chapter 7 for a complete discussion of the immune system and its function.

Cell injury and disease can be caused by the immune system in numerous ways. For example, allergies are caused by the presence of high numbers of a specific antibody, immunoglobulin E (IgE), on the surface of specialized cells (mast cells and basophils, which release histamine), resulting in mild, moderate, or severe allergic reactions. Examples of mild reactions include runny nose and watery eyes caused by a mild allergic response.

Moderate reactions include severe hypoxia caused by asthmatic bronchoconstriction. Severe reactions can result in a potentially life-threatening circulatory collapse seen in anaphylaxis (a whole-body allergic reaction). The presence of what would normally be considered optimal ratios of antigen to antibody in the circulation may lead to damage of filtration in the kidney because of excess deposition of antigen-antibody complexes in the glomeruli.

Cross-reactivity between foreign and host antigens is another immune mechanism that can compromise the body. For example, cross-reaction between streptococcal and myocardial antigens can occur in rheumatic fever and result in injury of cardiac valves. Alternatively, the chronic persistence of a foreign antigen by a foreign body or microorganism that cannot be cleared by the body may lead to a specific type of chronic inflammatory reaction called a *granuloma* (e.g., tuberculosis). Finally, sensitization to endogenous antigens can lead to type 1 diabetes mellitus caused by destruction of islet cells by T lymphocytes sensitized by islet antigens released during an antecedent viral infection.[238]

## Chemical Factors

Toxic substances cause chemical injury. These substances can be divided into two categories: substances that can injure cells directly and substances that require metabolic transformation into the toxic agent. Examples of chemicals that injure cells directly are heavy metals, such as mercury, that bind to and disrupt critical membrane proteins and several toxins and drugs, such as alkylating agents, used in chemotherapy.

Alkylating agents, such as nitrogen mustards, induce cross-linking of DNA and inactivation of other essential cellular constituents. Carbon tetrachloride and acetaminophen are examples of inert substances that must be metabolized to reactive intermediates to cause cell injury. Taken in large amounts, most medications can be toxic, and many are lethal. Suicide by drug overdose is a common example of drug-induced chemical toxicity.

**Free Radical Formation.** An important mechanism of cell injury and disease is the production of reactive oxygen species (ROS), sometimes referred to as the formation of *free radicals*. Free radicals are an integral part of metabolism and are formed continuously in the body. They can exert positive effects (e.g., on the immune system) or negative effects (e.g., lipid, protein, or DNA oxidation). A variety of normal and pathologic reactions can lead to the activation of oxygen by the sequential addition or subtraction, respectively, of one electron at a time (Fig. 6.3).

For example, the body's natural process of using oxygen and food to produce energy can create free radicals as a by-product of these functions. These unpaired electrons are reactive and commonly bind to oxygen for stabilization. The oxygen then binds to hydrogen for stabilization. This series of reactions generated by normal cellular metabolism results in a phenomenon referred to as *oxygen toxicity* and yields superoxide ($O_2^-$), hydrogen peroxide ($H_2O_2$), and hydroxyl radical ($OH^-$). These forms of reactive oxygen are referred to as *oxygen radicals*, which are toxic to cells.

The cellular enzymes always scavenging the body to protect cells from this type of injury normally inactivate these radicals and convert the free radical back to usable oxygen. Some unstable oxygen molecules (i.e., free radicals) enable the body to fight inflammation, kill bacteria, and help regulate the autonomic nervous system.

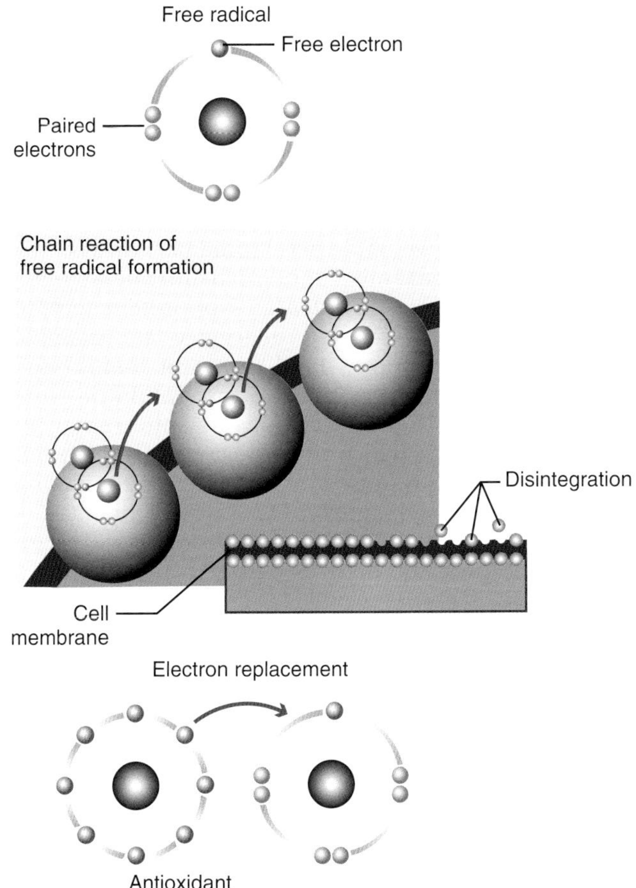


**Figure 6.3**

**The oxidative process and formation of free radicals.** Normal metabolic processes and a variety of other extrinsic factors such as pollution, poor nutrition, and exposure to toxic chemicals can result in the formation of free radicals when normal oxygen atoms lose one of their four paired electrons. The resulting unstable atom attempts to replace the missing electron by "stealing" an electron from a healthy cell, creating another unstable atom (free radical) and setting off a chain reaction referred to as oxidation. Oxidation as a by-product of metabolism damages cell membranes, leading to intrinsic cellular damage, a part of the normal aging process. Free radical damage (oxidation) is believed to alter the way cells encode genetic information in the DNA and may contribute to various diseases and disorders. Antioxidant molecules freely give up an electron to stabilize the oxygen atom without becoming unstable and without initiating a chain reaction.

However, if produced in excess amounts (a situation referred to as *oxidative stress*), these radicals can become the mechanism of cell injury and subsequent cell death. Free radicals have been considered central to the damaging effects that can lead to conditions such as heart disease, cerebrovascular disease, diabetes mellitus, cataracts, Parkinson disease, Alzheimer disease, premature aging, and cancer.[224] In fact, research has shown that oxidative stresses caused by ROS are factors in more than 90% of lifestyle-related diseases.[99,164]

ROS or free radical formation occurs as a result of many events such as prolonged exercise; exposure to high levels of oxygen, irradiation, ultraviolet or fluorescent light, pollutants, tobacco smoke, and pesticides (airborne or in food); drug overdose; heat stress; and reperfusion injury that is induced by the restoration of normal blood flow after a period of ischemia such as occurs during organ transplantation or after MI. Free radical toxicity may also be the underlying cause of degeneration of neurons located in the *substantia nigra,* leading to the loss of dopamine necessary for the normal control[224] of movements that produces the abnormal movements seen in Parkinson disease.[208]

**Antioxidants.** Oxygen-like atoms are the most likely source of free radicals in the human body; the use of oxygen as a life-supporting mechanism means oxidative stress is an inescapable part of the human biologic system. The simultaneous presence of antioxidants is an adaptive response to help the body ward off the potentially harmful effects of oxygen and its derivatives including free radicals.[256]

Antioxidants neutralize the extra free radicals and keep them from taking electrons from other molecules that would otherwise result in cellular and DNA damage. A variety of enzymatic and nonenzymatic defense mechanisms are present within cells to perform the function of antioxidants detoxifying ROS and protecting the cells from this type of injury. These are called *endogenous antioxidants*. Researchers are finding a variety of uses for natural antioxidants in combating the effects of aging and disease.

There are also *exogenous antioxidants* that can be obtained from outside the body through diet. Vitamin C, vitamin E, and beta carotene are three important exogenous antioxidants. More than 200 antioxidants have been identified in food or plant substances. For example, the Age-Related Eye Disease Study (AREDS) study concluded that high doses of antioxidants such as vitamins C and E, beta carotene, and copper significantly slow the progression of age-related macular degeneration. Researchers postulated that the antioxidants bind with the free radicals that are produced following the absorption of light in the retina.[4,9] Lycopene, the compound that makes tomatoes red, is a potent antioxidant that may be potentially effective in promoting prostate health.[93,136]

Multiple trials are ongoing to investigate oxidation and its effect on cellular injury, aging, and disease (e.g., cancer, heart disease, and cataracts) and the use of antioxidants found naturally in food and plants to combat oxidative stress, thereby preventing or possibly modifying diseases at the cellular level. Animal and human studies have confirmed that regular, moderate physical activity and exercise strengthen the antioxidant defense system, whereas intense or prolonged, strenuous exercise (especially in a person who has a sedentary lifestyle) leads to oxidative stress and may be potentially harmful.[71,75,96,101,189]

**Nitric Oxide.** The nitric oxide (NO) molecule is composed of one nitrogen atom and one oxygen atom. It is present in all mammals including humans and is one of the few gaseous signaling molecules known. NO should not be confused with nitrous oxide ($N_2O$), a general anesthetic, or with nitrogen dioxide ($NO_2$), which is a poisonous air pollutant.

The NO molecule is a free radical, which is relevant to understanding its high reactivity. NO is recognized as an important modulator of an enormous number of physiologic responses. Reduced NO bioavailability that is a result of oxidative stress seems to be a common molecular disorder causing many pathologic effects within the body. For example, decreased NO bioavailability is associated with risk factors for cardiovascular disease.[69,86]

NO assists in long-term memory. It also influences neuronal transmission by increasing the permeability of nerve endings, making acetylcholine transfer across the synapses easier. NO alters the ability of the gastrointestinal (GI) mucosa to resist injury induced by toxins, thereby influencing the immune system. NO inhibits virally induced cytokine and chemokine production, possibly combating the common cold.[191] It also stimulates collagen synthesis for wound healing, modulates fracture healing, and is useful in the treatment of tendinopathy.[178,179,195]

NO is an antilipid that provides a nonstick coating to the lining of blood vessels. This helps explain how NO might prevent heart attacks and strokes and why nitroglycerin works—nitroglycerin is converted to NO inside vascular tissue, where it relaxes smooth muscle in arteries and causes blood vessels to dilate. It also controls platelet function by preventing platelets from clumping together, thus preventing the formation of blood clots.

**Exercise and Free Radicals.** Physical activity and exercise can have positive or negative effects on oxidative stress depending on training load, training specificity, and basal level of training. Oxidative stress seems to be involved in muscular fatigue and overtraining.[83] Excessive exercise has been shown to induce DNA damage in peripheral leukocytes. Exhaustion of the leukocyte ROS may reduce the body's ability to combat microbial invasions (i.e., infections) before the system has been restored.[175] In contrast, moderate stress in the form of regular exercise training may have protective effects against exercise-induced DNA damage.[202]

Current evidence supports improved NO bioavailability with exercise training. Upregulation of endogenous antioxidant defense systems and complex regulation of repair systems are seen in response to training and exercise.[43] Upregulation of antioxidants and modulation of the repair response may be mechanisms by which exercise can influence our health in a positive way.[80] Regular, long-term aerobic exercise has been shown to reduce migraine pain severity, frequency, and duration, possibly a result of increased NO production.[172]

Researchers are studying the effect of NO on free radicals that cannot be stabilized or removed. Studies show that NO appears to play a role in exercise-induced dilation of blood vessels supplying cardiac and skeletal muscle. Exercise training enhances NO-mediated vasodilation. The exact mechanism is not clear yet, but a growing number of studies suggest that exercise training, perhaps via increased capacity for NO formation, retards atherosclerosis.[153] There is also accumulating evidence that NO is involved in skeletal muscle glucose uptake during exercise.[154,174]

### Genetic Factors

Genetic alterations lead to cellular injury or death via three primary means: (1) alterations in the structure or number of chromosomes that induce multiple abnormalities, (2) single mutations of genes that cause changes in the amount or functions of proteins, and (3) multiple gene mutations that interact with environmental factors to cause multifactorial disorders. These genetic alterations can be severe enough to cause fetal death in utero, resulting in spontaneous abortion. Some may cause congenital malformations, whereas others do not manifest pathologic alterations until midlife such as Huntington chorea. Down syndrome is an example of an alteration in the number of chromosomes that results in multiple abnormalities. This condition, caused by the abnormal presence of a third chromosome in the 21st pair, includes cardiac malformations, increased susceptibility to severe infections, cognitive and developmental delays, and increased risk of leukemia[152] and Alzheimer dementia.[53]

Sickle cell anemia, low-density lipoprotein receptor deficiency, and α-antitrypsin deficiency are examples of single gene mutations. In the case of α-antitrypsin deficiency, the deficiency in a protease inhibitor causes enhanced degradation of elastic tissue surrounding the alveoli of the lungs, which in turn leads to emphysema. Examples of diseases caused by multiple gene mutations include hypertension and type 2 diabetes mellitus. In type 2 diabetes, obesity and other environmental factors induce the expression of the diabetic genetic trait.

### Mechanical Factors

The *physical stress theory* may help explain mechanical factors influencing tissue adaptation and injury. The physical stress theory proposes that changes in the relative level of physical stress cause a predictable adaptive response in all biologic tissue. Typical tissue response to physical stress includes decreased stress tolerance (e.g., atrophy), maintenance, increased stress tolerance (e.g., hypertrophy), injury, and death.[170] Conversely, a decrease in mechanical stress may also be detrimental, particularly as it relates to bone health.[10]

Failure of a tissue occurs when the applied load exceeds the failure tolerance of the tissue. Soft tissues are influenced by the history of recent physical stresses so that the accumulation of individual stresses can cause injury. Characteristics of the load such as rate, compression, and forces (e.g., torsion, shear), along with the properties of the affected tissue, determine the type and extent of tissue damage. The time elapsed since injury and the extent of tissue damage determine the inflammatory response.[21]

With repetitive and/or forceful tasks, the initiating stimuli for inflammatory responses include repeated overstretch, compression, friction, and anoxia. These insults lead to mechanical injury of cellular membranes and intracellular structures and a localized release of proteins such as collagen, fibronectin, and cytokines.[21]

A single high load or stress from a traumatic fall, car accident, or other traumatic event can cause significant injury. Bones can fracture and ligaments can rupture from one episode of high-magnitude force. These tissues could also fail from repeated bouts of moderate-magnitude loads. Stress fractures or stress reactions in the bones could result from repeated episodes of moderate-magnitude force,[114] whereas slow degradation of tissue tolerance can occur in workers lifting heavy boxes repeatedly. Decreasing tissue tolerance may explain why there are no active acute inflammatory indicators in tendons associated with chronic tendinopathy.[88] Instead, antiinflammatory mediators and fibrotic proliferation are observed, suggesting the acute inflammatory phase has resolved. Conditions such as tennis elbow and golfer's elbow are recognized in many cases as a noninflammatory condition occurring after an inflammatory episode.[14,21,78,79]

In fact, research is ongoing to find ways to reinitiate the inflammatory cascade and promote healing in an otherwise degenerative process.[68] Low loads sustained over a long period of time, such as workers who remain in a fixed, flexed posture for prolonged periods of time, can also result in tissue injury because of decreased tissue tolerance.[170]

Altering mechanical stress (either increasing or decreasing forces) can be used to benefit individuals under varying circumstances. For example, reducing mechanical stress by offloading or pressure reduction is a concept used for healing ulcers and preventing their recurrence.

Controlled increase in physical stress is the underlying principle of progressive resistive exercise used to cause muscle fibers to hypertrophy and thereby able to withstand and generate greater force. Moreover, higher-than-normal levels of physical stress can promote remodeling in bone. Musculoskeletal tissues subjected to higher-than-normal levels of stress become more tolerant to subsequent physical stresses and are more resistant to injury.[170]

### Nutritional Factors

Imbalances in essential nutrients can lead to cell injury or cell death. For example, deficiencies of essential amino acids interfere with protein synthesis. Synthesis of proteins is required to replace cell proteins lost through normal catabolism, through growth, and in preparation for cell replication. Cell replication is essential for the healing processes after cell injury and the replacement of cells lost through normal turnover.

The consequence of protein malnutrition is a condition called *kwashiorkor;* marasmus, another form of malnutrition, is a consequence of generalized dietary deficiency. These two diseases are still leading causes of death in impoverished countries. In many industrialized countries, excessive nutrient intake leads to obesity and its many complications.

Nutritional imbalance can also occur as a result of abnormal levels of either vitamins or minerals. These nutrients function as cofactors for biosynthetic reactions or are essential components of proteins or membranes; their deficiency usually affects selected cells or tissues. For example, a deficiency of iron leads to anemia, and the presence of excessive amounts of iron in the tissues can cause damage by the formation of free radicals.

### Physical Factors

Trauma and physical agents can lead to cell injury and/or death. Blunt trauma resulting from motor vehicle accidents is a leading cause of death in the United States.[149] Massive brain contusions, injury to internal organs and soft tissues, and blood loss may lead to immediate mortality. Survivors may die later of infections and multiple organ failure. Repair of injuries to soft tissue, skeletal and muscular systems, and internal organs often requires prolonged periods of physical rehabilitation. Penetrating trauma inflicted by a variety of weapons can result in multiple complications.

Cells may be damaged by extremes of physical agents such as temperature, radiation, and electricity. Generalized increases in body temperature (hyperthermia) or reduction in body temperature (hypothermia) can lead to cell injury; high or low tissue temperatures can cause tissue injury or death. With increased temperature, the resulting morbidity and mortality are dependent on the severity of the burn and the total surface area that was burned. Markedly reduced temperatures may induce the freezing of tissue (frostbite). Ice crystals in cellular tissue rupture the cell membrane, which leads to cell death.

Irradiation for the treatment of cancer can cause injury of susceptible normal cells. Ionizing radiation causes radiolysis of water and the production of hydroxyl radicals. These radicals will lead to membrane damage and breakdown of structural and enzymatic proteins that result in cell death. Often, arterioles that supply oxygenated blood are damaged by ionizing radiation, resulting in inadequate nutritional supply, leading to ischemia and death of the irradiated tissues. Irradiation also causes damage to nucleic acids and may result in gene mutations, possibly leading to neoplasia years later.

### Psychosocial Factors

Psychosocial factors can have an impact on tissue adaptation, especially as related to tissue injury.[155] Psychosocial factors (e.g., fear, tension, or anxiety) may influence individual threshold values for tissue adaptation and injury. Many studies have investigated the role of mechanical and psychosocial factors in the onset of musculoskeletal (and other regional) acute and chronic pain. For example, people who are only occasionally or never satisfied in their work settings or who describe their work as "monotonous" have a higher risk of injury than people who are somewhat or completely satisfied with support from supervisors and colleagues.[31,103,104,171]

## CELLULAR AGING

Aging and age-related changes can significantly influence homeostasis and the recovery process. The ability of a cell to resist microorganisms or to recover from injury or inflammation depends in part on the underlying state or health of the cells. Age-related changes at the cellular level are present but remain difficult to measure or quantify; researchers are working toward finding satisfactory biomarkers of aging at the cellular level. Age-associated deterioration in cells leads to tissue or organ deficiencies and ultimately to the expression of aging or disease.

Various components of cells (e.g., mitochondria, ribosomes, or cell membrane) are subject to changes associated with aging. Mitochondrial DNA is considered a prime target for age-related changes. DNA must replicate and maintain itself to preserve the primary genetic message. This takes place through division, which can result in alterations of the genetic code by anything that can damage DNA (e.g., physical, chemical, or biologic factors; spontaneous mutations of genes; exposure to radiation). Anything that can alter the information content of the cell can cause changes in function and affect the ability of the cell to maintain homeostasis.

The presence of a component called *lipofuscin* is the most well-described age-associated change in the subcellular structure (lysosomes) of postmitotic cells. Lipofuscin is an aging-pigment granule that is found in high concentrations in old cells. The explanation for the increase of lipofuscin with age and the effects of these intracellular deposits on function remains under investigation. It is suspected that pressure from this pigmented lipid on the cell nucleus may interfere with cellular function.[197,205]

## Theories of Cellular Aging

With aging, the cells demonstrate deceased capacity to respond to stress, resulting in a progressive decline in homeostatic balance and possibly leading to pathology.[246] More than 300 theories exist to explain the aging phenomenon from a cellular level. Many of these theories originate from the study of changes that accumulate with time. In organs such as the heart and brain composed of cells that cannot regenerate, the *wear-and-tear theory* may account for the decline in function of these organs. Other factors may also play a role such as the influence of genetics suggested by the genetic hypothesis that aging is a genetically predetermined process.

The *free radical theory* of aging is the most popular and widely tested and is based on the chemical nature and wide presence of free radicals causing DNA damage and cellular oxidative stress as it relates to the aging process (see Chemical Factors under Mechanisms of Cell Injury earlier).

The discovery of the telomeres, the structure at the end of chromosomes, has added the *telomere aging clock theory* for the molecular mechanisms that lead to senescence. This theory suggests that the telomere acts as a molecular clock signaling the onset of cell senescence. Normal human cells will not divide forever but eventually enter a viable nondividing state (senescence). The progressive accumulation of senescent cells contributes to, but does not exclusively cause, the aging process. Cell senescence acts as an anticancer mechanism to control the potential for cellular proliferation (see further discussion in Chapter 9).[2,118,237] Because of the close association between telomere dysfunction and malignancy, both pathologists and clinicians expect this molecule to be a useful malignancy marker.

The epigenetic clock theory is based on changes to the structure of DNA that affects patterns of gene expression without modifying the primary nucleotide sequence. Methylation of cytosine residues within CpG dinucleotides (5-methyl-cytosine) is one of several known epigenetic changes that characterizes CpG sites and/or genomic regions that become either hypermethylated or hypomethylated with increasing age, suggesting a role for DNA methylation in biological aging.[112]

Pathologic changes associated with aging vary from individual to individual but usually consist of reduced functional reserve caused by atrophy of tissues or organs. Resistance to infection declines with age, and pathologic processes such as atherosclerosis result in increased cardiovascular and cerebrovascular injuries or death.

Of particular value to physical therapists is the ability of our interventions to influence some of the processes that may lead to cellular aging. For example, studies have shown that considerable potential exists for improving aerobic capacity by training. This observation has cellular implications, as mitochondria of cardiac and skeletal muscle cells improve function under appropriate training conditions.[38] Moreover, changes in diet and exercise or treatment with hormones or compounds such as antioxidants (see Fig. 6.3) are able to modify damage by ROS, which may allow the body to reestablish cellular norms.

# TYPES OF CELL INJURY

Alteration in a cell's functional environment, either acute or chronic, produces a stress to the cell's ability to attain or maintain homeostasis. The extent to which the cell is able to alter mechanisms and regain homeostasis in the altered environment is considered an adaptation by the cells or tissues. When the cell is unable to adapt, injury can occur. A *reversible cell injury* occurs if the stress is sufficiently small in magnitude or short enough in duration that the cell is able to recover homeostasis after removal of the stress. If the injurious or stressful stimulus is of sufficient magnitude or duration or if the cell is unable to adapt, *irreversible cell injury* occurs (see Fig. 6.1).

## Reversible Cell Injury

Cells react to injurious stimuli by changing their steady state to continue to function in a hazardous environment. Reversible (sublethal) injury caused by any of the mechanisms of cell injury listed in Box 6.1 is a transient impairment in the cell's normal structure or function. Normal cell structure and function can return after removal of the stressor or injurious stimulus (Fig. 6.4).

Acute reversible injury causes an impairment of ion homeostasis within the cell and leads to increased intracellular levels of sodium and calcium. An influx of interstitial fluid into the cell accompanies these ionic shifts and causes increased cell volume (swelling). Swelling occurs within the cytosol (liquid medium of the cytoplasm) and within organelles such as mitochondria and the endoplasmic reticulum. Swollen mitochondria generate less energy. Thus instead of oxidative ATP production, the cell reverts to less efficient anaerobic glycolysis, which results in excessive production of lactic acid. The pH of the cell becomes acidic, which slows down the cell metabolism, resulting in further cellular damage. The injured cell forms plasma membrane *blebs* that can seal off and detach from the cell surface. In severely injured cells, ribosomes detach from the rough endoplasmic reticulum, and a decrease in the number of polysomes occurs. These changes lead to reduced protein synthesis by the affected cells, and the cycle of damage can continue.

However, if the cell nucleus remains undamaged and the energy source is restored or the toxic injury is neutralized, the cell is able to recover and pump the ions and excess fluid back out. The swelling disappears, and the cell is returned to the original steady state, constituting a reversible cell injury.

### Cellular Adaptations in Chronic Cell Injury

When a sublethal stress remains present over a period of time, stable alterations (adaptations) take place within the affected cells, tissues, and organs. Adaptation enables the cells to function in an altered environment and thereby avoid injury. Characteristics of cell adaptation such as change in size, number, or function increase the cell's ability to survive; these changes are also potentially reversible. In many, but not all, cases, these changes benefit the function of the parent organ or structure within which the cell resides. Common cellular adaptations include atrophy, hypertrophy, hyperplasia, metaplasia, and dysplasia (Fig. 6.5).

*Atrophy* is a reduction in cell and organ size. Atrophy can occur with vascular insufficiency, reduction in hormone levels, malnutrition, immobilization, pain that limits movement and function, and chronic inflammation.

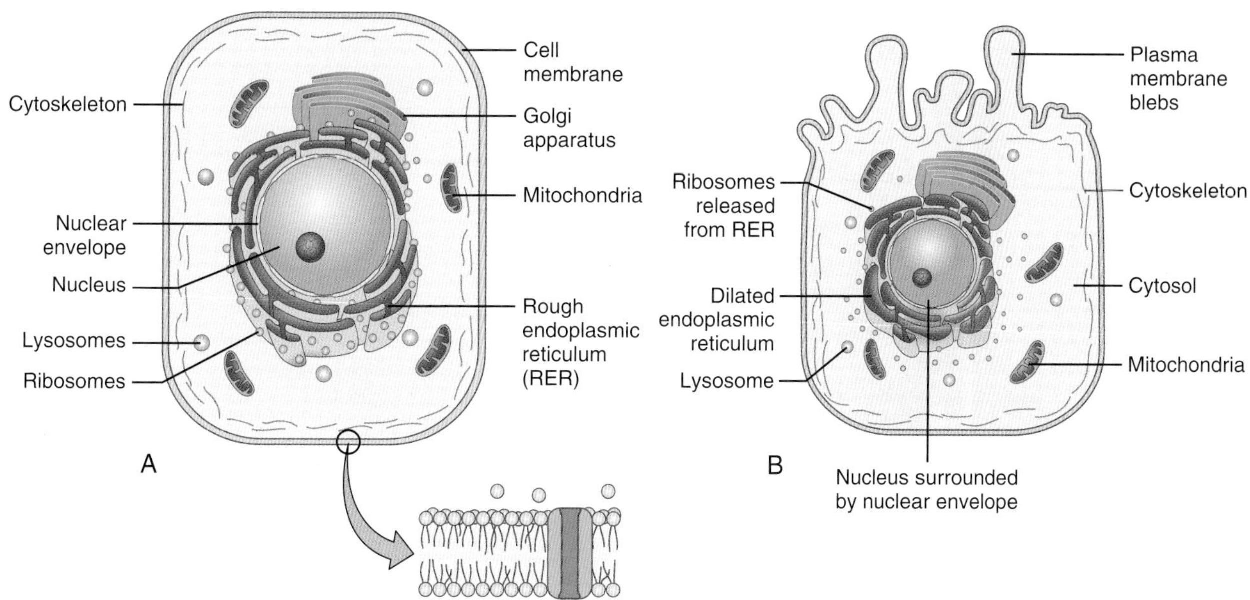


**Figure 6.4**

(A) Normal cell with its organelles. (B) Reversible cell injury with cellular swelling, accumulation of fluid in endoplasmic reticulum, and release of ribosomes and formation of membrane blebs. (Courtesy S.H. Tepper, PhD, PT.)

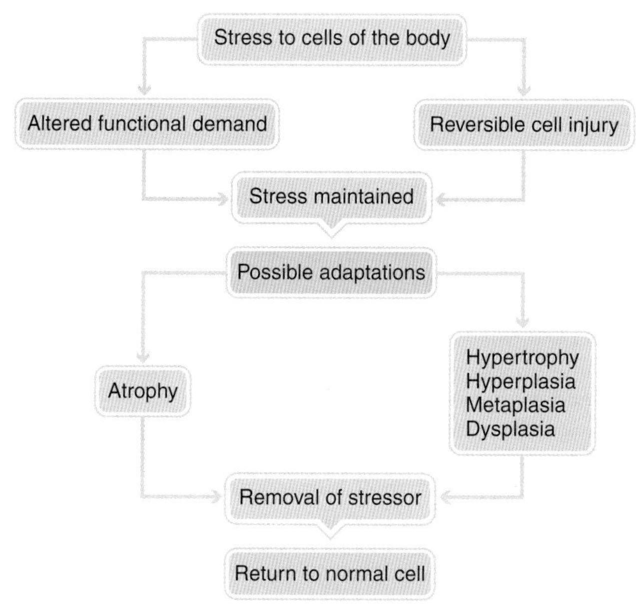


**Figure 6.5**

**Cellular adaptations and reversible cell injury in response to stress.** When the body is under persistent stress leading to either reversible cell injury or altered functional demand, the tissues adapt. Adaptations could include atrophy, hypertrophy, hyperplasia, metaplasia, or dysplasia. All of these changes are reversible with removal of the stressor. (Courtesy S.H. Tepper, PhD, PT.)

Bone loss, muscle wasting, and brain cell loss (Fig. 6.6) are examples of either tissue or organ atrophy associated with aging. Pathologic atrophy occurs as a consequence of cell injury due to ischemia, inadequate nutrition, or physical factors previously mentioned (see previous section Causes of Cell [Tissue] Injury). For example, ischemia of the viscera results in atrophied organs; cancer or malnutrition can result in cachexia, a general wasting of the body; and spinal cord injury results in atrophy of the affected muscles.

*Hypertrophy* is an increase in the size of the cell and organ. Hypertrophy can occur when increased functional demands are placed on the cells, tissue, or organs and with increased hormonal input (e.g., exercise stress can induce skeletal muscle hypertrophy). Pure hypertrophy occurs only in the heart and striated muscles because these organs consist of cells that cannot divide. Hypertrophy of the heart is a common pathologic finding that occurs as an adaptation of heart muscle to an increased workload. Specifically, hypertrophy of the left ventricle is a typical complication of hypertension. Increased blood pressure requires that the heart produce more force to eject the blood. The additional force is produced by hypertrophy of muscle fibers in the left ventricle.

*Hyperplasia* is an increase in the number of cells, leading to increased organ size. In tissues consisting of cells that are capable of dividing, the presence of excessive functional demands can cause a consequent increase in cell number. Pure hyperplasia typically occurs because of hormonal stimulation (e.g., prolonged estrogen exposure causes the endometrium of the uterus to become thick) or chronic stimulation (e.g., persistent pressure on the skin induces hyperplasia and the formation of a callus). Some hyperplasia has no discernible cause and may represent early neoplasia. Hypertrophy and hyperplasia often occur together such as in the case of prostate enlargement and obstruction of the urethra and bladder. The result is an increase in size and number of smooth muscle cells in the wall of the urinary bladder.

*Metaplasia* is a change in cell morphology and function resulting from the conversion of one adult cell type into another. For example, in smokers, portions of the respiratory tract change from ciliated pseudostratified columnar epithelium into stratified squamous epithelium, leading to a thickening of the respiratory epithelium and loss of the functional clearance of mucus and debris along the respiratory tree.

*Dysplasia* is an increase in cell numbers that is accompanied by altered cell morphology and loss of histologic organization. Considered to be a preneoplastic alteration,

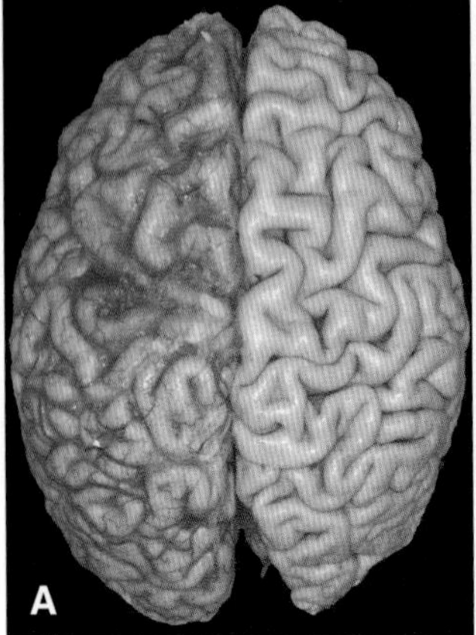


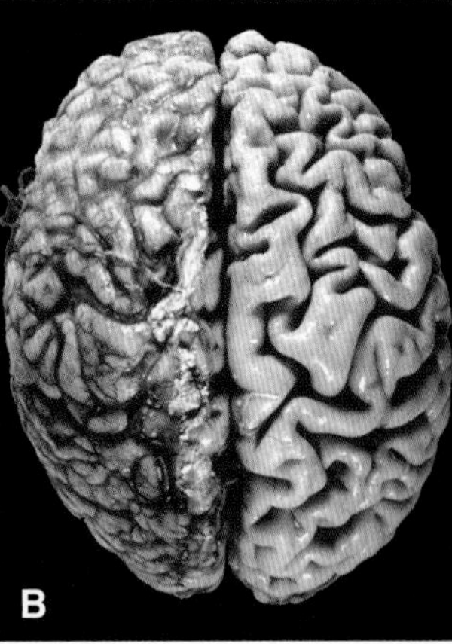


**Figure 6.6**

**Atrophy.** (A) Normal brain of a young adult. (B) Atrophy of the brain in an 82-year-old man with atherosclerotic cerebrovascular disease, resulting in reduced blood supply. Note that loss of brain substance narrows the gyri and widens the sulci. The meninges have been stripped from the right half of each specimen to reveal the surface of the brain. (From Kumar V, et al: *Robbins and Cotran pathologic basis of disease*, ed 8, Philadelphia, 2010, Saunders.)

dysplasia can be found in areas that are chronically injured and undergoing hyperplasia or metaplasia.

### Intracellular Accumulations or Storage

Intracellular accumulations are increases in the storage of lipids, proteins, carbohydrates, or pigments within the cell that occur as a result of an overload of various metabolites or exogenous material. These accumulations can also be caused by metabolic disturbances altering cell function. For example, when the liver is sublethally injured, lipid (triglyceride) accumulates within the hepatocyte. This lipid accumulation occurs when a reduction in protein synthesis occurs as a result of disaggregation of the ribosomes from the rough endoplasmic reticulum as previously discussed. Hepatocytes normally produce endogenous lipoproteins. With sublethal damage to hepatocytes (e.g., due to alcohol abuse), a lack of protein shell formation occurs so that lipoproteins cannot be packaged and transported to the plasma. As a result, lipids remain within the hepatocyte, causing the characteristic "fatty liver" found in alcoholics.

## Irreversible Cell Injury

Irreversible cell injury is synonymous with cell death. Cell death occurs as a result of *apoptosis* or *necrosis*.[126] Table 6.1 summarizes the features of apoptosis and necrosis, whereas Fig. 6.7 illustrates the changes in the cellular structure during these two processes.

Apoptosis, or programmed cell death, is a genetically mediated and managed process that causes cells to die. This type of cell death is generally physiologic but could also be pathologic. Apoptosis begins with either an activation of a trigger or stimulus or the suppression of a specific agent that then allows the process of cell death to occur. It is typically not associated with an inflammatory response.

The active process of degradation of dead cells is called *necrosis*. Necrosis is the end point of a pathologic process that results in lethal, irreversible cell injury. Hallmarks of lethally injured cells include alterations in the cell nucleus, mitochondria, and lysosomes and the rupture of the cell membrane (see Fig. 6.7).

**Table 6.1** Comparison of Apoptosis and Necrosis

| Feature | Necrosis | Apoptosis |
|---|---|---|
| Cell size | Enlarged (swelling) | Reduced (shrinkage) |
| Nucleus | Pyknosis → karyorrhexis → karyolysis | Fragmentation into nucleosome-size fragments |
| Plasma membrane | Disrupted | Intact; altered structure, especially orientation of lipids |
| Cellular contents | Enzymatic digestion; may leak out of cell | Intact; may be released into apoptotic bodies |
| Adjacent inflammation | Frequent | No |
| Physiologic or pathologic role | Invariably pathologic (culmination of irreversible cell injury) | Often physiologic, means of eliminating unwanted cells; may be pathologic after some forms of cell injury, especially DNA damage |

From Kumar V, et al: *Robbins and Cotran pathologic basis of disease*, ed 8, Philadelphia, 2010, Saunders.

Damage to the cell nucleus can manifest in three forms: pyknosis, karyorrhexis, and karyolysis. Nuclei undergo clumping or pyknosis, which is a degeneration of the cell as the nucleus shrinks in size and the chromatin condenses to a solid mass. The pyknotic nuclei can fragment, a process termed *karyorrhexis,* or it can undergo dissolution (karyolysis).

Mitochondria lose their membrane potential and become unable to synthesize ATP, leaving the cell without the necessary energy production for cell function. Morphologically, irreversibly injured mitochondria appear swollen, contain large lipid-protein aggregates called *flocculent densities,* and may also contain dense crystalline deposits of calcium (Fig. 6.8).

After cell death, lysosomes release their digestive enzymes within the cytoplasm of the cell, initiating enzymatic degradation of all cellular constituents, a process that may be aided by enzymes released from inflammatory cells. Enzymes help dissolve the dead tissue, making it easier for phagocytic cells to remove the dead tissue in preparation for healing by repair (laying down of a collagenous tissue scar) or regeneration (regrowth of parenchymal tissue). Dead cells release their contents into the extracellular fluid, eventually making their way into the circulation, where they can be measured as clinically useful signs of cell injury. For example, levels of aspartate aminotransferase, creatine kinase (CK), and lactate dehydrogenase are typically elevated in the serum of people with myocardial infarct or viral hepatitis.

### Types of Necrosis

The process of necrosis begins with the dissolution of irreversibly injured cells within living tissue. Removal

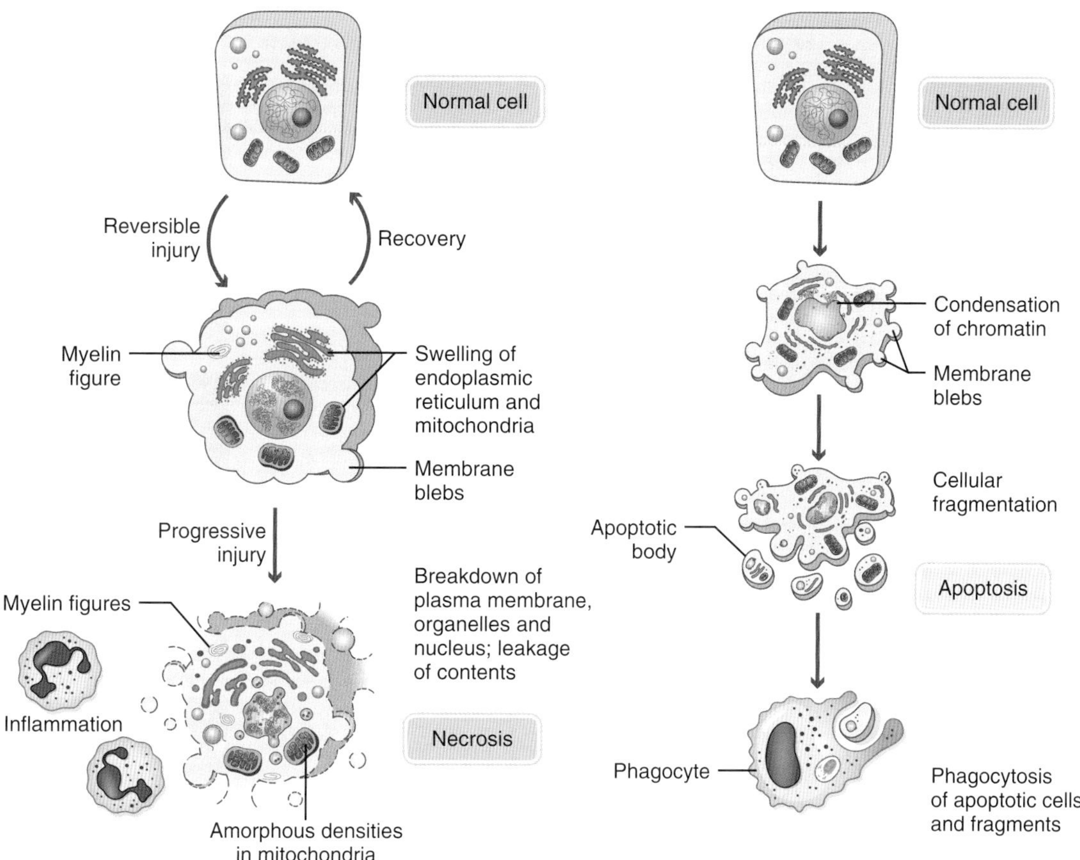


**Figure 6.7**

**Schematic illustration of the morphologic changes in cell injury culminating in necrosis or apoptosis.** (From Kumar V, et al: *Robbins and Cotran pathologic basis of disease*, ed 8, Philadelphia, 2010, Saunders.)

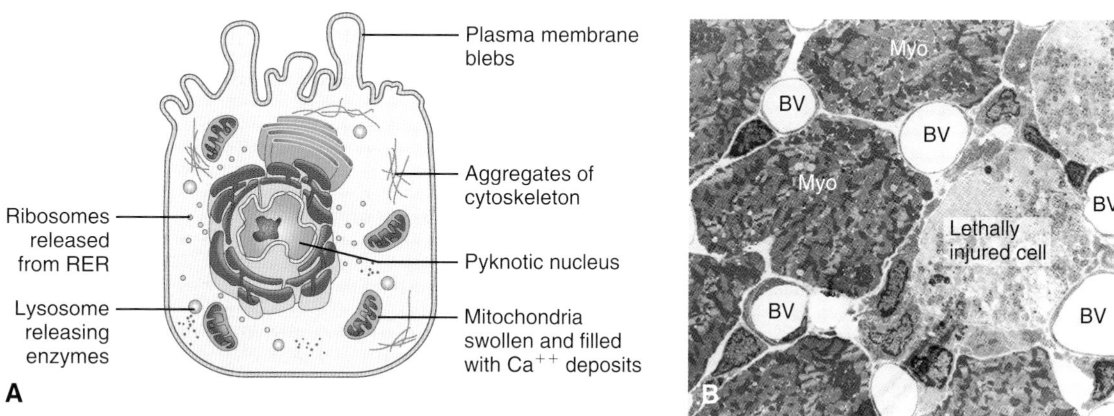


**Figure 6.8**

**Irreversible cell injury: ultrastructural alterations in an irreversibly killed cell.** (A) Mitochondria are nonfunctional and filled with flocculent densities (particles suspended together in a cluster). Lysosomes are releasing their digestive enzymes. The nucleus is condensing upon itself (pyknosis). Membrane breakdown allows intracellular enzymes to be released into the interstitial area. (B) Electron micrograph of lethally injured cardiomyocytes next to healthy viable cardiomyocytes. Note lethally injured cells to the right of the healthy viable cardiomyocytes are swollen, mitochondria are filled with flocculent densities, there is a loss of myofilaments, and mononuclear phagocytic cells are beginning to remove these dead cells. *BV,* Blood vessel; *Myo,* healthy viable cardiomyocytes. Original magnification ×1500. (A, Courtesy S.H. Tepper, PhD, PT; B, From Tepper SH, Anderson PA, Mergner WJ: Recovery of the heart following focal injury induced by dietary restriction of potassium. *Pathol Res Pract* 186:265–285, 1990.)

**Table 6.2** Types of Necrosis

| Type | Cause | Effects | Area of Involvement | Example |
|---|---|---|---|---|
| Coagulative | Ischemia (lack of blood supply | Cell membrane is preserved; nucleus undergoes pyknosis and karolysis (dissolution); organelles dissolve | Solid internal organs (e.g., heart, liver, kidneys) | Wedge-shaped kidney infarct |
| Caseous ("cheesy") | *Mycobacterium tuberculosis* (TB); seen with other fungal infections | Cell membrane is destroyed; debris appears cheeselike and does not disappear by lysis but persists indefinitely; damaged area is walled off in a fibrous calcified area, forming a granuloma | Lungs, bronchopulmonary lymph nodes, skeletal bone (extrapulmonary TB) | Tuberculosis of the lung, with yellow-white and cheesy debris. |
| Liquefactive | Pyogenic bacteria (e.g., *Staphylococcus aureus*) | Death of neurons releases lysosomes that liquefy the area, leaving pockets of liquid and cellular debris (abscess of fluid-filled cavity); shapeless, amorphous debris remains | Brain tissue (e.g., brain infarct); skin, wound, joint infections | Infarct of the brain, showing dissolution of the tissue |
| Fatty necrosis | Acute pancreatitis, abdominal trauma | Formation of calcium soaps by the release of pancreatic lipases | Abdominal area | White, chalky deposits indicating fatty necrosis in the mesentery |
| Fibrinoid | Trauma in blood vessel wall | Plasma proteins accumulate; cellular debris and serum proteins form pink deposits | Blood vessels (tunica media, smooth muscle cells) | Fibrinoid necrosis in an artery |

*TB*, Tuberculosis.
Photographs from Kumar V, et al: *Robbins and Cotran pathologic basis of disease*, ed 8, Philadelphia, 2010, Saunders.

of this dead tissue is essential for healing to take place. Histologically, several different types of necrosis are recognized (Table 6.2), with some additional subcategories.

Gangrene is a negative sequela of necrosis. Gangrene caused by bacterial infection and associated with tissue ischemia (peripheral vascular disease) may form coagulative necrosis (dry gangrene) or liquefactive necrosis (wet gangrene). The fermentation reactions caused by certain bacterial pathogens may cause the formation of gas bubbles in the infected tissue. In muscle necrosis, one of the causative agents is *Clostridium perfringens*. The term used to describe this condition is clostridial myonecrosis or gas gangrene (see Chapter 8).

SPECIAL IMPLICATIONS FOR THE THERAPIST 6.1

### *Cell Injury: Multiple Cell Injuries*

The concepts discussed in this first section on cell (tissue) injury are essential for understanding the pathogenesis of a variety of acute illnesses and injuries the therapist may see in any clinical setting. Often, multiple episodes of care with complex cases involving comorbidities occur in clinical practice. For example, the victim of a motor vehicle accident experiencing a traumatic brain injury (TBI) and concomitant pelvic fracture may develop pneumonia and pulmonary compromise and subsequently experience MI. The therapy staff following this client throughout the continuum of care—from the intensive care unit through rehabilitation to a home health service setting and possibly as an outpatient—can better meet the needs of such an individual during the healing process by understanding these concepts of injury and recovery.

TBI could occur during motor vehicle accidents. With direct trauma to the head, primary and secondary injury can lethally damage the brain tissue. Primary injury to the brain may occur in the following areas: (1) local brain damage occurs at the site where the brain impacts the skull (coup injury) and the site opposite impact (contrecoup injury); (2) polar brain damage occurs at the tips (poles) of the frontal, temporal, and occipital lobes and the undersurface of the frontal and temporal lobes when the brain moves inside the skull; (3) diffuse axonal injury occurs throughout the subcortical white matter (and brainstem if the magnitude of force is great enough) with sufficient shear force to injure axons. The extent of primary damage to the brain depends on the nature, direction, and magnitude of the forces applied to the skull.

Secondary injury is usually the result of hypoxic-ischemic injury caused by cerebral edema. Because the soft and pliable brain is enclosed within the rigid skull, abnormal brain fluid dynamics caused by cerebral edema result in increased intracranial pressure (ICP). Signs and symptoms of increased ICP include headache, loss of sense of smell, and altered level of consciousness. Even a mild increase in ICP is sufficient to cause death of neural tissue caused by inadequate perfusion. Moderate and severe increases in ICP can cause brain tissue to shift position or herniate from one chamber into another and may also cause compression of neural structures. Intracranial hematomas (epidural, subdural, and intracerebral) are another source of secondary brain damage.

Passive imaging techniques (e.g., computed tomography and magnetic resonance imaging) are useful to visualize the structural changes that occur with TBI. Active imaging techniques (e.g., electroencephalogram, positron emission tomography, diffusion tensor imaging, and evoked potentials) are useful to visualize physiologic changes that occur with TBI.

Open wounds and fractures are common sequelae associated with motor vehicle accidents. In this case example, the pelvic fracture resulted from the mechanical force distributed through the pelvis during a motor vehicle accident. Fractures are often diagnosed by radiograph. When a bone is fractured, its normal blood supply is disrupted. Osteocytes (bone cells) die from the trauma and the resulting ischemia. Bone macrophages remove the dead bone cells and damaged bone.

A precursor fibrocartilaginous growth of tissue occurs before the laying down of primary bone, eventually followed by the laying down and remodeling on normal adult bone. This process from fracture to full restoration of the bone takes weeks to months, depending on the type of fracture, location, vascular supply, health, and age of the individual. See further discussion of bone fractures in Chapter 27.

In this example, if the myocardium is subjected to ischemia for a sufficient duration, the myocytes become irreversibly injured. A cascade of physiologic and anatomic changes leads to the death of myocardial cells. Coagulative necrosis ensues, followed by acute inflammation, and finally repair by scar tissue formation (Fig. 6.9).

Coagulative necrosis begins with the release of lysosomal enzymes that cause dissolution of the normal structural relationships found within myocytes. The dead cells attract acute inflammatory cells that phagocytize the necrotic debris and release growth factors. The growth factors initiate the proliferation of blood vessels (angiogenesis) and fibroblasts, resulting in the eventual production of a collagenous scar.

Signs and symptoms correlate with the different stages of lethal cell injury and differ according to the organ or structures involved. During acute MI, the individual often experiences angina, shortness of breath, sweating, and nausea. These symptoms of physiologic stress are caused by the release of histamines, bradykinins, and prostaglandins such as substance P from the lethally injured myocytes.

An electrocardiogram reveals ST segment elevation and Q waves over the affected area. The person is also at an increased risk for life-threatening dysrhythmias due to the loss of electrical conductivity of lethally injured myocytes and disrupted conductivity (irritability) of the adjacent cells. If a significant percentage of the myocardium is infarcted, cardiogenic shock or congestive heart failure may ensue.

Cytoplasmic enzymes or proteins (e.g., myocardial isoenzyme of creatine kinase [CK-MB]) are released from the dead cells. Normally the plasmalemma is impermeable to these large molecules and contains them within the confines of the cytoplasm. After lethal injury, the plasmalemma is broken down by the actions of phospholipases, and these molecules are released from inside the cell. A number of cytoplasmic proteins are released into the interstitial area and are taken up by adjacent lymphatic vessels and finally enter the bloodstream. Lactate dehydrogenase, CK-MB, and troponin are clinically relevant for diagnosis and assessment of the severity of MI.

The therapist must understand the process of injury and repair to the brain, pelvic bones, and myocardium (or other involved organs and structures), as appropriate client care is determined by the different stages of this process. For example, recovery from TBI tends to follow the progression outlined by the Rancho Los Amigos Levels of Cognitive Function (LOCF).

In general, intervention is directed by the person's current LOCF level. During LOCF levels I to III, primary goals involve increasing tolerance of activities including intervention, tolerating upright posture, and increasing interaction with the environment. During levels IV to VI, the emphasis shifts to increasing physical and cognitive endurance. During levels VII and VIII, intervention focuses on the skills necessary to reenter the community.

After fracture of bone, a period of immobilization usually occurs to remove longitudinal stress. This period allows for the phagocytic removal of necrotic bone tissue and the initial deposition of the fibrocartilaginous callus. As the fracture heals, as revealed by radiograph, gradual progression of stress is applied. Mobilization of this individual will occur depending on the type of fixation used on the pelvis. For example, if an external fixation is applied for fracture stabilization, mobilization can occur almost immediately within tolerance of the person's symptoms.

The highest risk of death during the first hours after MI stems from dysrhythmias. Rupture of the myocardium is possible during days 3 through 10 after a transmural MI (from outside epicardium to inside endocardium). The risk of these events dictates that exercise during this time must not subject damaged cells to excessive stress. Proper mobilization of the individual soon after infarction may decrease the likelihood of succumbing to the negative effects of bed rest but may be complicated by variables such as pelvic fracture, pneumonia, and the TBI in this case.

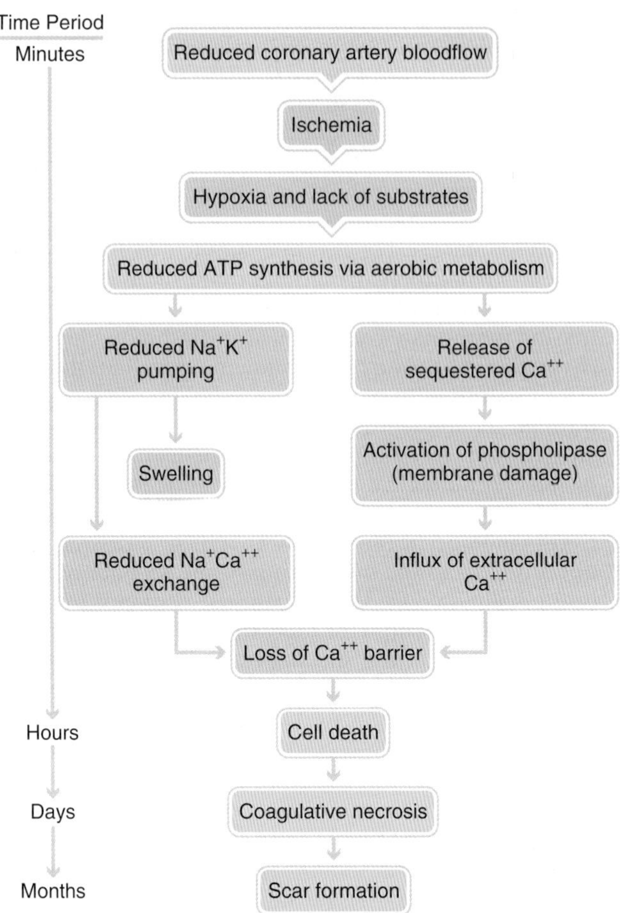


**Figure 6.9**

**Pathogenesis of myocardial infarction.** With reduction in coronary artery blood flow caused by thrombus formation, ischemia results in reduction of aerobic metabolism. Irreversible cell injury occurs, followed by necrosis of the heart tissue. Release of intracellular enzymes (myocardial isoenzyme of creatine kinase, troponin) from the dead heart tissue serve as biochemical markers in the early diagnosis of myocardial infarction. In the following weeks, healing occurs by repair, the formation of a connective tissue scar. *ATP,* Adenosine triphosphate. (Courtesy S.H. Tepper, PhD, PT.)

# INFLAMMATION

## Overview and Definition

After cell injury, the body reacts by initiating the process of inflammation. The amount, type, and severity of the inflammatory reaction are dependent on the amount, type, and severity of the injury. As part of the healing process, the inflammatory process is responsible for the removal of the injurious agent, removal of cellular debris, and initiation of the healing process. The healing process occurs to allow restoration of structure and function whenever possible.

Inflammation serves a vital role in host defense against pathogens and in response to cell injury. The inflammatory process provides us with the capability to both get rid of the initial cause of cell injury (trauma, bacteria, and toxins) and the consequences of such an injury (damaged cells and tissue). It proceeds as a complex set of overlapping reactions of vascular and cellular responses. Each reaction serves a specific purpose and is necessary as the body responds to tissue injury or damage.

There are several mechanisms by which injury can cause inflammation and the vascular and cellular reactions it triggers. If microbes are introduced, they can stimulate potent inflammatory cells,[201] particularly innate immune cells such as neutrophils (white blood cells [WBCs]) and macrophages (phagocytes).[49] Traumatic stimulation of mast cells and nerves can also lead to the release of proinflammatory mediators (histamine, serotonin, prostaglandins, and leukotrienes).[12,221] If trauma causes bleeding, hemostatic mechanisms (platelets and clotting) that are triggered can also generate inflammatory mediators.[128,135] Additionally, cell death is a universal and potent stimulator of sterile inflammation (inflammation in the absence of microorganisms).[49,201] These[82] soluble factors produced by cells and plasma proteins can initiate and amplify the response as well as determine the pattern, severity, and clinical and pathologic manifestations.[138]

The termination of inflammation occurs when the injurious agent is removed. The reaction resolves quickly because cytokines are broken down and dissipated, and leukocytes have short life spans in the tissues. Additionally, antiinflammatory mechanisms are activated that serve to control the response and prevent it from causing excessive damage to the host.[138]

The inflammatory process is closely intertwined with the process of repair and stimulates the necessary response to try to heal the damaged tissue. Repair begins during inflammation but reaches completion usually

**Table 6.3** Four Cardinal Signs/Symptoms of Inflammation

| Sign | Precipitating Events |
|---|---|
| Erythema | Vasodilation and increased blood flow |
| Heat | Vasodilation and increased blood flow |
| Edema | Fluid and cells leaking from local blood vessels into the extravascular spaces |
| Pain | Direct trauma; chemical mediation by bradykinins, histamines, serotonin; internal pressure secondary to edema; swelling of the nerve endings |

after the injurious influence has been neutralized. The process of healing occurs by regeneration (regrowth of original tissue) or by repair (formation of a connective tissue scar) or, most commonly, by a combination of these two processes.

Normally, inflammation has a protective role and is generally beneficial to the body. However, inflammation, whether in the acute or chronic stage (and with all of its components), can be detrimental and has the potential of causing damage (and even death) to adjacent healthy tissue.

The degree and persistence of the inflammatory response is a major factor in the outcome of the repair process. Complete regeneration and repair without scar can be expected if the inflammation is minimal and there are no complicating factors. However, if the inflammation is chronic and persistent and comorbidities, risk factors, and complications are present, resulting chronic wounds could be expected.

Inflammation has been linked with many other conditions in the absence of infection[49] (e.g., Alzheimer disease, atherosclerosis, cancer, diabetes, insulin resistance syndrome, and obesity). The focus of this chapter is inflammation in relation to the musculoskeletal system.

## Acute Versus Chronic Inflammation

Inflammation of sudden onset and short duration is referred to as *acute inflammation;* the main characteristics are exudation of fluid and plasma proteins (edema) and the migration of leukocytes, predominately neutrophils (called polymorphonuclear leukocytes).[138] Inflammation that does not resolve but persists over time is called *chronic inflammation* and is associated with the presence of lymphocytes and macrophages, the proliferation of blood vessels and fibrosis, and tissue destruction.[138]

In the *acute inflammation* stage, the inflammatory stimulus acts on blood cells and plasma constituents to deliver leukocytes and plasma proteins to sites of infection and tissue injury. Acute inflammatory reactions can be triggered by many stimuli such as infections, tissue necrosis, foreign bodies, and immune reactions. All inflammatory reactions share the same basic features, although different stimuli may induce reactions with some distinctive characteristics.[138] The clinical manifestations of inflammatory reaction are redness, swelling, increased temperature, pain, and decreased function of the affected site (Table 6.3). Arteriolar vasodilation gives rise to the redness and heat. The exudation and leukocyte infiltration give rise to the swelling. Pain and loss of function occur as a result of the increased pressure from the edema on the peripheral nerves[21] (Fig. 6.10).

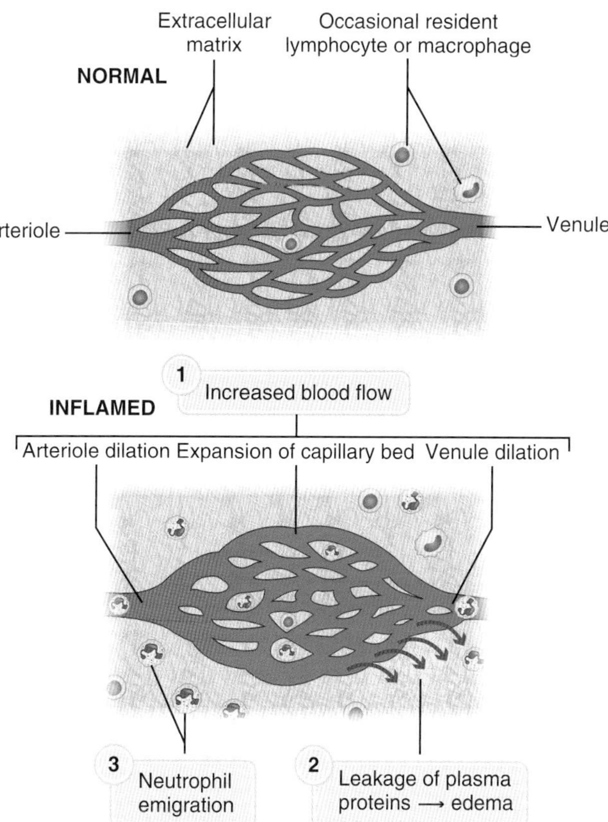


**Figure 6.10**

**Major local manifestations of acute inflammation compared with normal.** (1) Vascular dilation and increased blood flow (causing erythema and warmth); (2) extravasation and extravascular deposition of plasma fluid and proteins (edema); (3) leukocyte emigration and accumulation in the site of injury. (From Kumar V, et al: *Robbins and Cotran pathologic basis of disease*, ed 8, Philadelphia, 2010, Saunders.)

Once the injurious agent is removed, acute inflammation subsides. If little necrosis is present and replacement of lost parenchymal cells is possible, restitution of normal structure and function of the tissue occurs.

*Chronic inflammation* may occur in the presence of extensive necrosis or if regeneration of parenchymal cells is not possible (e.g., heart, CNS, or peripheral nervous system cells). The inflammatory reaction may also become chronic if the underlying cause is not addressed and the injurious agent persists for a prolonged period. Repeated episodes of acute inflammation in the same tissue over time or low-grade, persistent immune reactions can also result in a chronic inflammatory response (Fig. 6.11).

The hallmark of chronic inflammation in a tissue is the accumulation of macrophages, lymphocytes, and plasma cells (Fig. 6.12). The macrophage accumulation is the result of chemotaxis (locomotion or movement) of monocytes (precursors to macrophages) to the area of injury. Macrophages modulate lymphocyte functions and promote growth of endothelial cells and fibroblasts by the release of growth factors. Eosinophils may also be present, particularly if allergic reactions or parasite invasions are involved.

Granulation tissue made up of proliferating endothelial cells and fibroblasts is also seen in areas of chronic

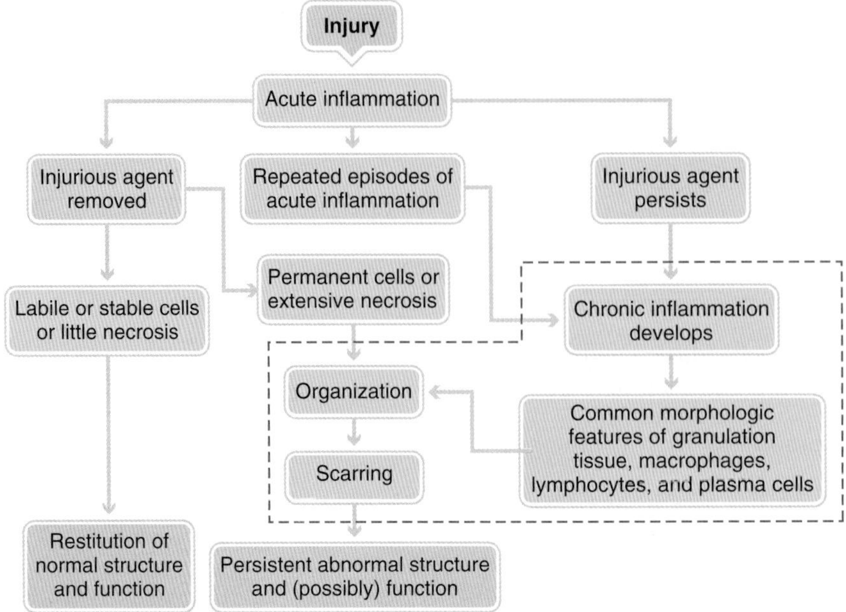


**Figure 6.11**

**Overview after tissue injury: acute inflammation, chronic inflammation, and the likely healing process.** (Courtesy S.H. Tepper, PhD, PT.)

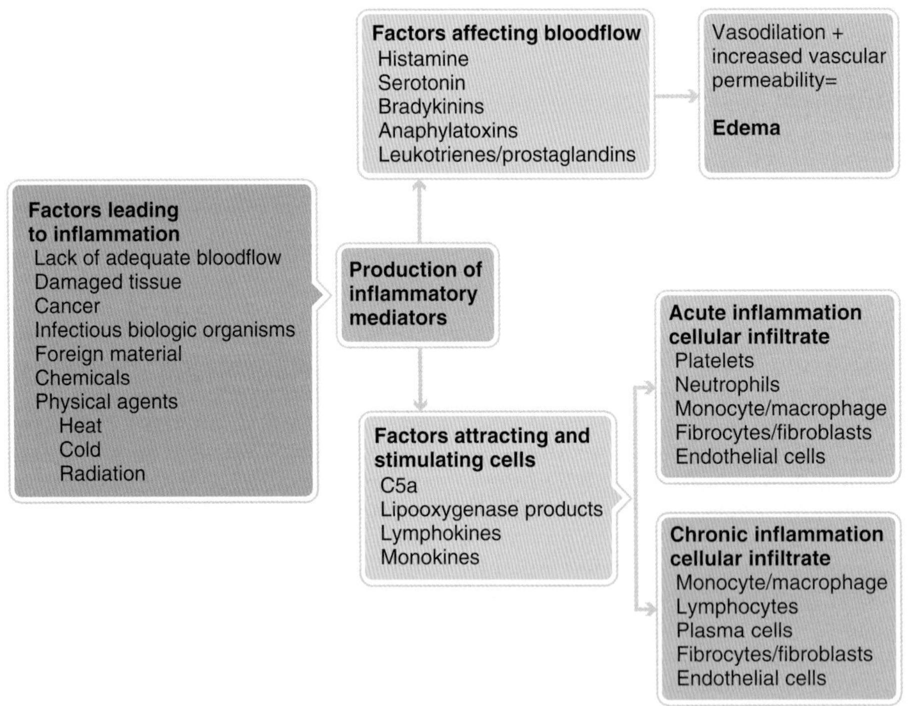


**Figure 6.12**

**Contributing factors and components of inflammation.** Note the vascular alterations associated with factors affecting blood flow (vasoactive mediators) leading to edema and the factors attracting and stimulating cellular alterations (chemotactic factors) resulting in acute (and sometimes) chronic inflammation. (Courtesy S.H. Tepper, PhD, PT.)

inflammation. Granulation tissue can be seen in well-healing, open wounds. Inspection of the wound site reveals red "beefy" tissue with pinpoint red dots (new capillaries) and a granular surface composed of newly formed collagen.

Certain diseases cause the formation of a specific type of chronic inflammation called a *granuloma*. The granuloma is a microscopic (less than 2 mm in diameter) aggregate of macrophages often surrounded by lymphocytes. Most of the macrophages are flattened and epithelioid in appearance,

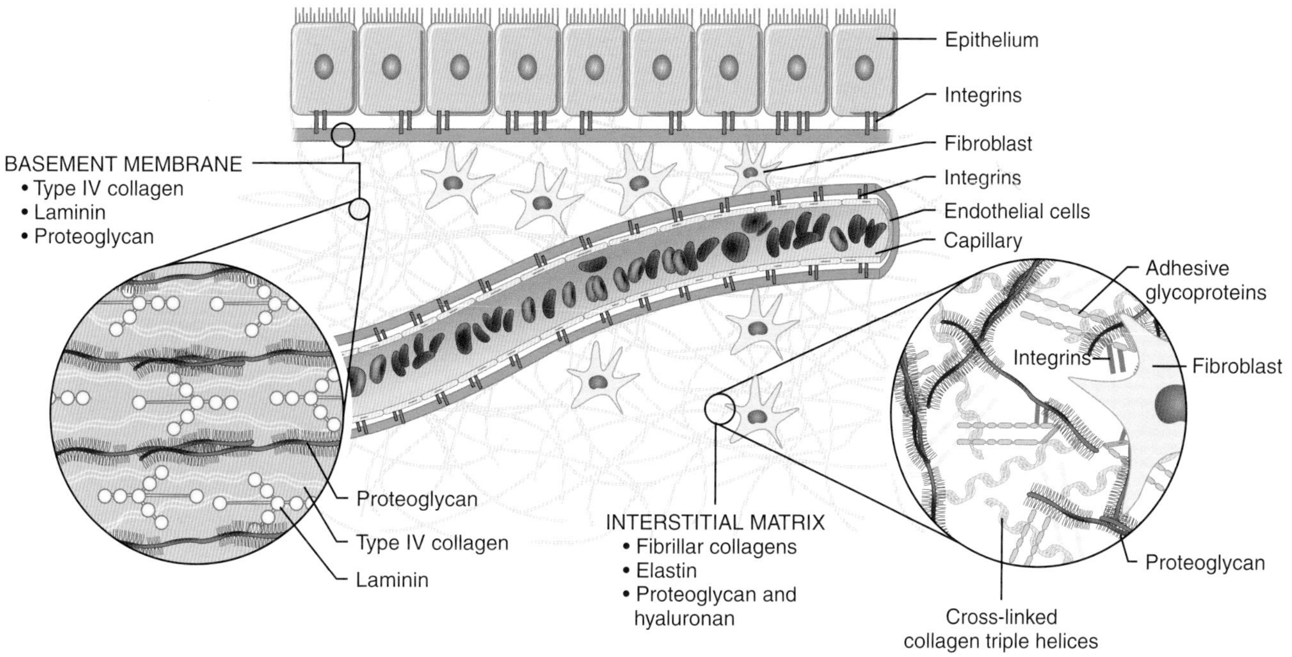


**Figure 6.13**

**Main components of the extracellular matrix (ECM) including collagens, proteoglycans, and adhesive glycoproteins.** Both epithelial and mesenchymal cells (e.g., fibroblasts) interact with ECM via integrins. Basement membranes and interstitial ECM have different architecture and general composition, although there is some overlap in their constituents. For the sake of simplification, many ECM components (e.g., elastin, fibrillin, hyaluronan, and syndecan) are not included. (From Kumar V, et al: *Robbins and Cotran pathologic basis of disease*, ed 8, Philadelphia, 2010, Saunders.)

and some may fuse together, giving rise to large cells with multiple nuclei (Langerhans and foreign body giant cells).

The presence of granulomatous inflammation is clinically important because it aids in the diagnosis of the injurious stimulus. Tuberculosis, a disease caused by *Mycobacterium tuberculosis,* classically causes granulomas or tubercles with a central focus of caseous necrosis. The presence of a foreign body (e.g., a suture) is another common cause of granulomatous inflammation.

Chronic inflammation can contribute to the healing of injured tissue but usually without a full return of function. The proliferation of endothelial cells reconstitutes the vasculature in the injured tissue, whereas proliferation of fibroblasts and the production of collagens and proteoglycans (polymers that form the gel between collagen fibrils) reconstitute the extracellular matrix (Fig. 6.13). Together, these constituents make up the granulation tissue and lead to the formation of a connective tissue scar. This process is regulated by growth factors derived from macrophages, platelets, and plasma.

## Components of the Inflammatory Reaction

### Vascular Alterations

Acute inflammation can last from a few minutes (e.g., redness and swelling from scratching your skin) to a few days (e.g., after an open cut on the finger), during which time a series of vascular events occurs. The goal of the series of vascular changes is to increase the movement of plasma proteins and circulating cells out of the intravascular space and into the site of injury. The escape of fluid, protein, and blood from the vasculature system into tissue or body cavities is known as *exudation.*[48] Exudate is an extravascular fluid that contains a high protein concentration and cellular debris (phagocytic cells) and has a high specific gravity.[138] Exudation occurs when an increase in capillary permeability allows proteinaceous fluid and/or cells to leak out primarily through openings created between adjacent endothelial cells in the capillaries or venules (Fig. 6.14).[48,138] Various types of exudate are evident in the tissue, depending on the stage of inflammation and its cause (Table 6.4). In contrast, a *transudate* is a fluid with low protein content, little or no cellular material, and low specific gravity. It is essentially an ultrafiltrate of blood plasma that results from osmotic or hydrostatic imbalance in a vessel without an increase of vascular permeability (e.g., left ventricular failure, cirrhosis, and nephrosis).[18] When fluid transudates or leaks from blood vessels and accumulates inside an anatomic space, such as the pleural, pericardial, or peritoneal cavities or the joint space, these accumulations are called effusions. *Effusion* is a more general term referring to the escape of a fluid and can be either a transudate or an exudate.

Removal of the fluid for analysis is required when differentiating between transudates and exudates and helps establish a specific diagnosis. Sometimes exudates are described by visual appearance (e.g., serosanguineous exudate, a fluid containing erythrocytes, or red blood cells [RBCs]).

Although nerve reflexes at the site of injury can cause immediate vasoconstriction,[67] the rapid response of chemical mediators results in the characteristics of acute inflammation, as follows: (1) vasodilation, one of the earliest manifestations, causing increased blood flow with resultant heat and redness (erythema); (2) increased capillary permeability, which permits the passage of plasma

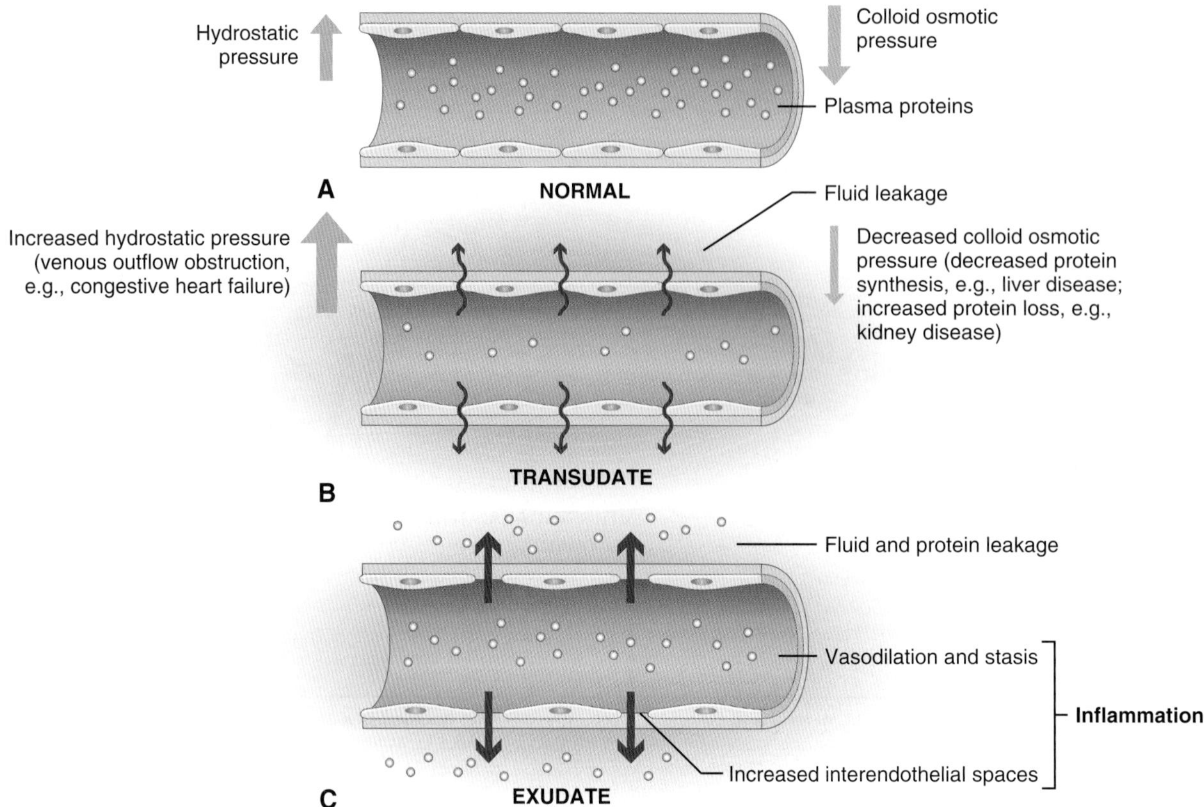


**Figure 6.14**

**Formation of transudates and exudates.** (A) Normal hydrostatic pressure *(blue arrows)* is about 32 mm Hg at the arterial end of a capillary bed and 12 mm Hg at the venous end; the mean colloid osmotic pressure of tissues is approximately 25 mm Hg, which is equal to the mean capillary pressure. Therefore the net flow of fluid across the vascular bed is almost nil. (B) A transudate is formed when fluid leaks out because of increased hydrostatic pressure or decreased osmotic pressure. (C) An exudate is formed in inflammation because vascular permeability increases as a result of increased interendothelial spaces. (From Kumar V, et al: *Robbins and Cotran pathologic basis of disease*, ed 8, Philadelphia, 2010, Saunders.)

**Table 6.4** Inflammatory Exudates

| Type | Appearance | Significance |
|---|---|---|
| Hemorrhagic; sanguineous | Bright red or bloody; presence of RBCs | Small amounts expected after surgery or trauma; large amounts may indicate hemorrhage; sudden large amounts of dark, red blood may indicate a draining hematoma |
| Serosanguineous | Blood-tinged yellow or pink; presence of RBCs | Expected for 48–72 hours after injury or trauma to the microvasculature; a sudden increase may precede wound dehiscence (rupture or separation) |
| Serous | Thin, clear yellow or straw-colored; contains albumin and immunoglobulins | Occurs in the early stages of most inflammations; common with blisters, joint effusion with rheumatoid arthritis, viral infections (e.g., skin vesicles caused by herpesvirus); expected for up to 1 week after trauma or surgery; a sudden increase may indicate a draining seroma (pocket of serum within tissue or organ) |
| Purulent | Viscous, cloudy, pus; cellular debris from necrotic cells and dying neutrophils (PMN leukocytes) | Usually caused by pus-forming bacteria (streptococci, staphylococci) and indicates infection; may drain suddenly from an abscess (boil) |
| Catarrhal | Thin, clear mucus | Seen with inflammatory process within mucous membranes (e.g., upper respiratory infection) |

*PMN*, Polymorphonuclear; *RBCs*, red blood cells.
Modified from Black J: Wound healing. In Black JM, Matassarin-Jacobs E, editors: *Luckmann and Sorensen's medical-surgical nursing*, ed 8, Philadelphia, 2009, Saunders.

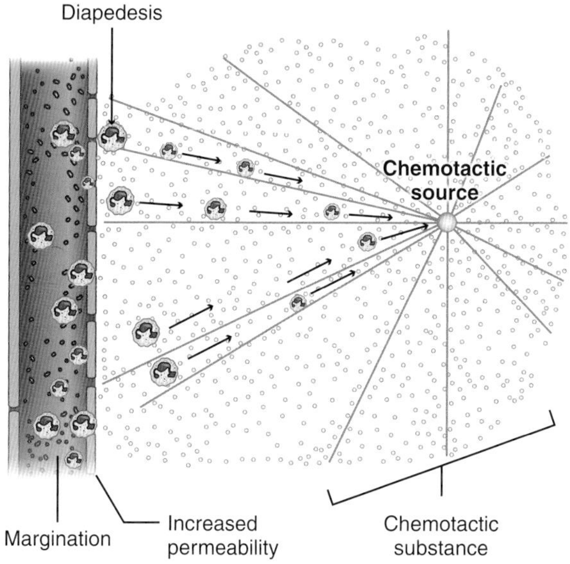


**Figure 6.15**

**Many different chemical substances in the tissues cause both neutrophils and macrophages to move through the capillary pores in a process called *diapedesis* and toward the area of tissue damage by chemotaxis.** Chemotaxis depends on the concentration gradient of the chemotactic substance. The concentration is greatest near the source, which directs the unidirectional movement of the white blood cells. Chemotaxis is effective up to 100 μm away from an inflamed tissue. Because almost no tissue area is more than 50 μm away from a capillary, the chemotactic signal can easily move vast numbers of white blood cells from the capillaries into the inflamed area. (From Hall JE, Guyton AC: *Textbook of medical physiology*, ed 12, Philadelphia, 2011, Saunders.)

proteins and leukocytes into the extravascular space, causing edema; (3) loss of fluid due to increased vessel permeability that leads to slower blood flow, a higher concentration of RBCs in small vessels, and increased viscosity of the blood; (4) clotting of the fluid in the interstitial spaces because of increased fibrinogen and other proteins to wall off the invader; and (5) migration of leukocytes from the microcirculation, their accumulation in the focus of injury, and their activation to eliminate the offending agent, resulting in swelling of the tissues.

## Leukocyte Accumulations

An important consequence of the exudation of protein and fluid from the vasculature is the engorgement of vessels with blood cells. This causes a slowing or cessation of blood flow in the affected vessels, a phenomenon called *stasis*.[138] During stasis, the leukocytes (WBCs) accumulate and adhere to the endothelial cells of blood vessel walls at the site of injury in a process called *margination*. Inflammatory mediators cause an increased expression of specific glycoproteins called *adhesion molecules* on the surface membrane of leukocytes and endothelial cells. These adhesion glycoproteins, by adhering to each other, function as receptors and counterreceptors. The adhesion glycoproteins are the glue that binds the leukocytes to each other and to the endothelium of venules and capillaries.

The binding of leukocytes to receptors on endothelial cells of venules is the first step in the migration of leukocytes from the vasculature to the interstitial tissues. This process initiates the circulation of leukocytes through the extravascular space in normal conditions and the infiltration of leukocytes into the site of inflammation.

In the next stage, the leukocytes actively migrate out of the vessels, passing through the vascular walls without damaging the blood vessels and entering the interstitial space in a process called *diapedesis*, or oozing (Fig. 6.15). The continued migration of leukocytes in interstitial space is directed by a chemical trail created by a concentration gradient of one of many possible attractants. The attractants are called *chemotactic agents*, and the process of locomotion is called *chemotaxis*. In other words, leukocytes are attracted to and accumulate at the site of an inflammatory reaction in response to a chemical stimulus.

The presence of leukocyte accumulations in tissue or fluid specimens is diagnostic of an inflammatory process. The predominant cell type found in a specimen identifies the type of inflammation and/or its duration and original stimulus. Typically during acute inflammation, neutrophils predominate (neutrophilia). Neutrophils inhibit bacterial growth by releasing lactoferrin, a protein that binds with iron, thus preventing microorganisms from using iron for growth and development. Neutrophils also demonstrate direct cytotoxic activity toward viruses, fungi, and bacteria by releasing defensins, which are peptides with natural antibiotic activity.

If the inflammatory stimulus subsides, the neutrophils rapidly die out because their life span (after extrusion from the circulation) is approximately 24 hours; they are replaced by monocytic/macrophage cells responsible for cleaning up the cellular debris left after neutrophils have done their job. Certain inflammatory stimuli can induce a sustained neutrophil response (e.g., first defense against pyogenic bacteria), a predominantly lymphocytic response (e.g., fight tumor cells or respond to viruses), or an eosinophilic response (e.g., plays a role in asthma and allergies or attacks parasites).

In addition to the types of WBCs present, the total and differential counts of the leukocytes in the circulating blood are very important diagnostic tools. An increased number of circulating leukocytes (leukocytosis) is often an indication of an active inflammatory reaction (typically to an infection or tissue injury). A decreased WBC count (leukopenia) can, for example, be seen in certain types of infections and is an indicator of grave prognosis in severe systemic infections (sepsis).

The main function of the leukocytes recruited to the affected tissue is to remove or eliminate the injurious stimulus. Leukocytes achieve this function by releasing enzymes and toxic substances that kill, inactivate, and degrade microbial agents, foreign antigens, or necrotic tissue. Leukocytes also take up these materials by phagocytosis and release growth factors necessary for healing or regeneration (see section on phagocytosis later).

In addition to the role played by blood vessels in inflammation, a contribution is made from a system of thin-walled channels formed by endothelial cells with loose junctions. These channels are called the *lymphatics* and ultimately drain into the subclavian vein via the thoracic duct. These channels in physiologic conditions help drain fluid and protein from the interstitium, thereby reducing edema. They also serve as a conduit for the removal of certain leukocytes and inflammatory stimuli.[194]

**Table 6.5 Mediators of Inflammation**

| Cell-Derived Sources | Plasma Cell–Derived Sources |
|---|---|
| Circulating platelets (platelet-activating factor, histamine, serotonin)<br>Tissue mast cells (histamine)<br>Basophils (histamine)<br>Polymorphonuclear leukocytes (neutrophils)<br>Endothelial cells<br>Monocytes/macrophages<br>Injured tissue itself<br>Arachidonic acid derivatives (prostaglandins, leukotrienes)<br>Cytokines (TNF, IL-1) | Blood coagulation cascade<br>Fibrinolytic system<br>Kinin enzymatic system: bradykinin, Hageman factor<br>Complement system: C3a, C3b, C5a, C5b<br>Membrane attack complex |

*IL-1*, Interleukin-1; *TNF*, tumor necrosis factor.

The movement of the phagocytic cells into the lymphatic vessels allows presentation of the engulfed material to immunocompetent cells located in the lymph nodes. Hyperplasia of immunocompetent cells (T and B lymphocytes) in the lymph nodes leads to an enlargement of the nodes called *lymphadenopathy*. During the process of removing infectious agents, lymphatics and their lymph nodes may become actively inflamed. Clinically, the inflamed lymphatics may appear as red streaks under the epidermis and may be painful to palpation; this condition is called *lymphangitis*.

**Chemical Mediators of Inflammation.** A large number of chemical mediators are responsible for the vascular and leukocyte responses generated by the cells involved in an acute inflammatory response. These mediators are either released from inflammatory cells (cell-derived) or generated by the action of plasma protease (plasma-derived). Mediators of inflammation are multifunctional and have numerous effects on blood vessels, inflammatory cells, and other cells in the body. Some of their primary effects in the inflammatory response include vasodilation or vasoconstriction, modulation of vascular permeability, activation of inflammatory cells, chemotaxis, cytotoxicity, degradation of tissue, pain, and fever. These mediators include histamine, serotonin, bradykinin, the complement system, platelet-activating factors, arachidonic acid derivatives (e.g., prostaglandins, leukotrienes), and cytokines (Table 6.5).

**Histamine.** Histamine is synthesized and stored in granules (for quick availability and release) of mast cells, basophils, and platelets. Histamine causes endothelial contraction, leading to the formation of gaps, which increase blood vessel permeability and allow fluids and blood cells to exit into the interstitial spaces (vascular leak). Histamine's effect occurs quickly but is short-lived because it is inactivated in less than 30 minutes. Histamine is also a potent vasodilator and bronchoconstrictor. Serotonin is another mediator released from platelets. It induces vasoconstriction, but its effect is usually overridden by the vasodilator action of histamine.

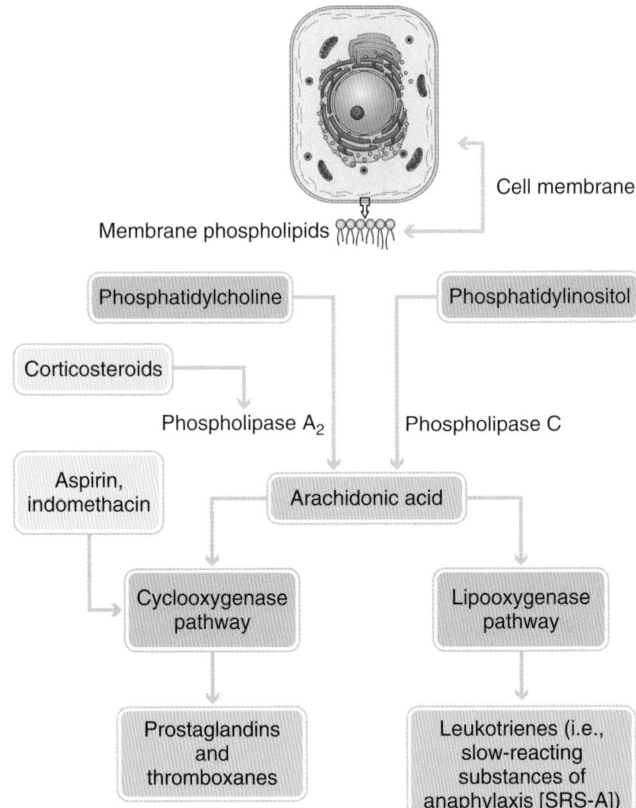


**Figure 6.16**

**Production of prostaglandins and leukotrienes from damaged cell membranes.** Note sites for pharmacologic (aspirin and prednisone) interventions. (Courtesy S.H. Tepper, PhD, PT.)

**Platelet-Activating Factor.** Leukocytes and other cells on stimulation also synthesize three classes of inflammatory mediators that are derived from phospholipids (the major lipids present in cell membranes). The first of these mediators is an acetylated lysophospholipid named *platelet-activating factor* (PAF). The other two classes of mediators are derived from a fatty acid (arachidonic acid) of membrane phospholipids and are called *prostaglandins* and *leukotrienes*. All three of these lipid mediators have potent and wide-ranging inflammatory activities. In addition, these mediators have hormone-like functions that modulate physiologic responses and induce pathology in a variety of organ systems.

PAF was so named because it was first found to induce platelet activation and secretion. PAF is now known to be a potent activator of cells, such as smooth muscle cells, endothelial cells, and leukocytes, by receptor binding and intracellular signaling mechanisms. As a consequence, PAF can induce the aggregation of leukocytes and leukocyte infiltration in tissues and can profoundly affect vasomotor tone and permeability.[216] PAF can potentiate (increase or strengthen) the activity of other inflammatory mediators.

**Arachidonic Acid Derivatives.** The synthesis of prostaglandins and leukotrienes begins with the cleavage (splitting) of arachidonic acid from membrane phospholipids by the action of the phospholipase (Fig. 6.16). Once this step is completed, either a cyclooxygenase enzyme or a lipoxygenase enzyme further metabolizes the arachidonic acid. The cyclooxygenase pathway leads to the production of several types of prostaglandins that modulate vasomotor tone and platelet aggregation (e.g., thromboxane is a strong platelet aggregator and vasoconstrictor, whereas prostacyclin [also known as $PGI_2$] is a strong platelet inhibitor and vasodilator). Clinically, prostaglandins are also important because they are mediators of the fever and pain responses associated with inflammation.[173]

The lipoxygenase pathway leads to the production of leukotrienes. Leukotrienes occur naturally in leukocytes and produce allergic and inflammatory reactions similar to those of histamine. They are extremely potent mediators of immediate hypersensitivity reactions and inflammation, producing smooth muscle contraction, especially bronchoconstriction; increased vascular permeability; and migration of leukocytes to areas of inflammation. They are thought to play a role in the development of allergic and autoimmune diseases such as asthma and rheumatoid arthritis. Certain leukotrienes (C4, D4, and E4) are collectively known as a slow-reacting substance of anaphylaxis (SRS-A), which is the name that was given when their potent bronchoconstrictor activity was discovered; they also cause leakage of fluid and proteins from the microvasculature.

The importance of the arachidonic acid metabolites in the inflammatory process is made evident by the excellent clinical response to treatment of acute and chronic inflammatory conditions with drugs that block the production of arachidonic acid (corticosteroids) or inhibit the enzyme and block the production of prostaglandins and cyclooxygenase (nonsteroidal antiinflammatory drugs [NSAIDs] such as aspirin or newer cyclooxygenase-2 inhibitors). These antiinflammatory medications are commonly used for people with somatic pain or inflammatory conditions, especially rheumatoid arthritis.

**Cytokines.** Leukocytes also produce polypeptide substances called *cytokines* (see Chapter 7) that have a wide range of inflammatory actions affecting either the cytokine-producing cells themselves (autocrine effects) or adjacent cells (paracrine effects). Cytokines also have a number of systemic "hormonal" inflammatory effects.

Two important cytokines with overlapping functions are IL-1 and TNF. As many as 15 ILs[5] are now identified. Most ILs direct other cells to divide and differentiate, each IL acting on a particular group of cells that have receptors specific for that IL. TNF is thought to be capable of inducing most of the actions of IL-1, with the exception of activation of lymphocytes.

IL-1 has a number of local actions that promote the inflammatory reaction and a number of systemic actions that induce metabolic, hemodynamic, and hematologic alterations (see Box 6.2). These alterations are discussed in some detail because of their importance in the clinical and laboratory diagnosis of inflammation. IL-1 causes fever by increasing the production of prostaglandins in the hypothalamus and thereby resetting the threshold of temperature-sensitive neurons.

Fever in turn raises the systemic metabolism and increases the systemic consumption of oxygen by approximately 10% for each 1 °C of body temperature elevation. As a result, a decrease in systemic vascular resistance occurs, thereby producing hypotension and an increase in cardiac output to increase the flow of blood and the delivery of oxygen to various organs. These hemodynamic changes are characteristic of severe systemic infections and a febrile condition.

IL-1 also causes characteristic changes in blood chemistry. Albumin and transferrin levels are decreased, while levels of coagulation factors complement components, C-reactive protein, and serum amyloid A increase. These changes occur because IL-1 alters the rate of synthesis of these proteins by the liver. IL-1 also increases the number of neutrophils and decreases the number of lymphocytes in the circulation.

**Blood Coagulation, Fibrinolytic, and Complement Systems.** Plasma proteins produce chemical inflammatory mediators by the enzymatic activity of proteases on plasma proteins. Plasma proteases are enzymes that act as a catalyst in the breakdown of proteins. These plasma protein systems are the blood coagulation and fibrinolytic, kinin enzymatic, and complement systems.

All of these systems can become activated by contact with by-products of cell injury or foreign materials. Examples include contact with components of denuded vascular endothelial cells revealing their underlying basement membrane, which occurs with trauma to the vessel wall and contact with bacterial endotoxins. The key plasma protein in the activation sequence of these systems is clotting factor XII, also known as *Hageman factor*.

The blood coagulation system (Fig. 6.17) is formed in part by plasma proteins. The design is to bandage injuries with clots (coagulation), then disassemble (lyse) the clots when the job is done. The system protects against both hemorrhage and catastrophic clotting. To maintain homeostasis, these two processes must remain in balance.

Platelets circulating throughout the bloodstream are always ready to seal any damage to blood vessels with a hemostatic plug. When there is no need for the platelets, the smooth vascular walls prevent platelets from adhering and aggregating. At the same time, endothelial cells in the walls of the blood vessels make tissue plasminogen activator to prevent fibrin deposits from forming and for breaking down existing clots.

More specifically, when injury or bleeding occurs, a series of enzymes is activated sequentially to generate the enzyme thrombin, which converts the plasma protein fibrinogen to fibrin, the essential component of a blood clot. Fibrin forms a meshwork at bleeding sites to stop the bleeding and trap exudate, microorganisms, and foreign materials and keep this content contained in an area where eventually the greatest number of phagocytes will be found. This localizing effect prevents the spread of infection to other sites and begins the process of healing and tissue repair.

The fibrinolytic system (designed to dissolve these clots) is activated by the conversion of plasminogen to the enzyme plasmin (also known as *fibrinolysin,* which means "to loosen"). Plasmin splits or divides fibrin and lyses the blood clots. Both the coagulation and the fibrinolytic systems are activated in inflammation and function together in a system of checks and balances to preserve vascular function.

The products of fibrin degradation are chemotactic for leukocytes and increase vascular permeability. The kinin enzymatic system is also activated by Hageman factor and functions to produce bradykinin. Bradykinin is a mediator that causes dilation and leakage of blood vessels and induces pain.

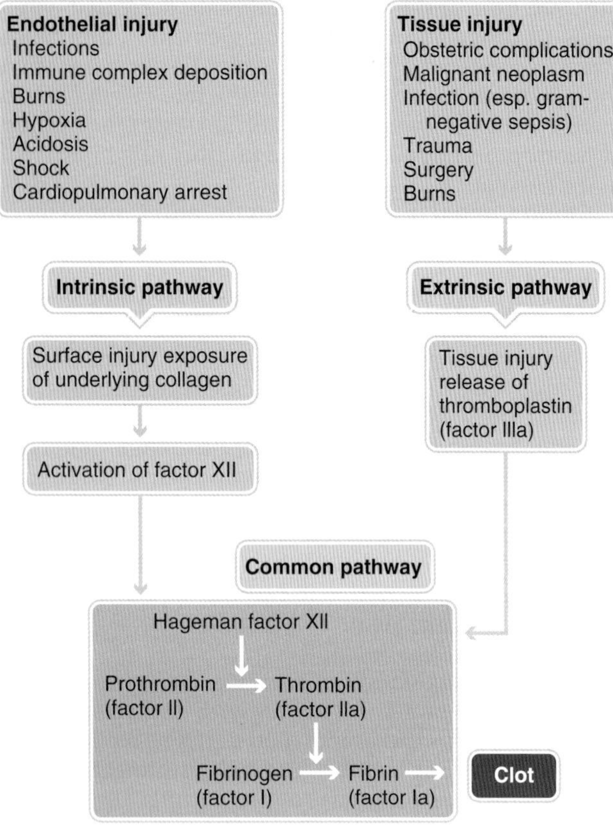


**Figure 6.17**

**Clinical causes of the activation of a clotting cascade, intrinsic and extrinsic pathways of activation, and the mechanism by which both pathways lead to the formation of fibrin threads, or clot.** In the chain reaction, inactive proenzymes (represented by Roman numerals) are converted into active enzymes (represented by Roman numerals followed by the letter "a"). The clotting cascade can follow two pathways: intrinsic and extrinsic. The intrinsic pathway is activated within the vascular compartment. The extrinsic pathway is activated outside the vascular compartment, when blood comes in contact with any tissue other than blood vessels. In the case of internal bleeding, both pathways are activated. (Courtesy S.H. Tepper, PhD, PT, material revised.)

The complement system is composed of a group of plasma proteins that normally lie dormant in the blood, interstitial fluid, and mucosal surfaces. Then, through a series of enzymatic reactions, several plasma protein fragments (C3a, C3b, C5a, and C5b) are formed that are potent inflammatory mediators. These components are also active in immunologic processes. In the nomenclature used for the complement system, each complement component (C) is designated by a number (1 through 9). The individual subunits that make up each component are designated by a letter. For example, the first component of complement is designated C1. C1 is made up of three subunits that are designated C1q, C1r, and C1s. The protein fragments that are generated from the proteolytic degradation of complement components are also identified by a letter (a, b).

The complement system is activated by microorganisms or antigen-antibody complexes, causing four events to occur that promote inflammation: (1) vasodilation of the capillaries, which increases blood flow to the area, (2) facilitation of leukocyte migration into the area by chemotaxis, (3) opsonization (coating) of the surfaces of microbes to make them vulnerable to phagocytosis, and (4) formation of a membrane attack complex (MAC).

Complement activation can follow one of two pathways, the classic or the alternative pathway; each pathway produces the same active complement components. The products of the complement system bind to particles of foreign material, microorganisms, or other antigens, coating them to make them vulnerable to phagocytosis by leukocytes, a process called *opsonization*. Activation of the complement cascade by either pathway also results in the formation of the MAC. The MAC is inserted in cell membranes of the microorganism, where it creates an opening (pore or channel) in the cell membrane, leading to influx of sodium and extracellular fluid, eventually leading to its lysis (Fig. 6.18). For example, in hemolytic anemia, MAC bores holes in the cell membrane of RBCs, causing their destruction.

The plasma protease systems (blood coagulation, fibrinolytic, kinin enzymatic, and complement systems) are interconnected at several steps. This arrangement serves to amplify the stimulus for the inflammatory reaction as a balance mechanism. For example, the activation of the plasma protein Hageman factor can initiate both the coagulation system (blood clotting) and the kinin system (produces bradykinin causing dilation and vascular leakage).

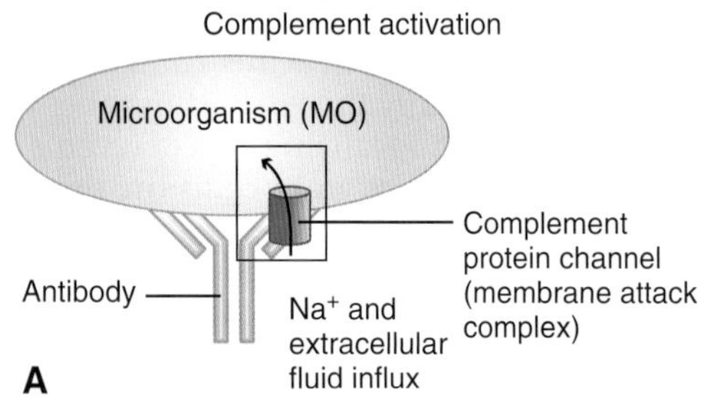


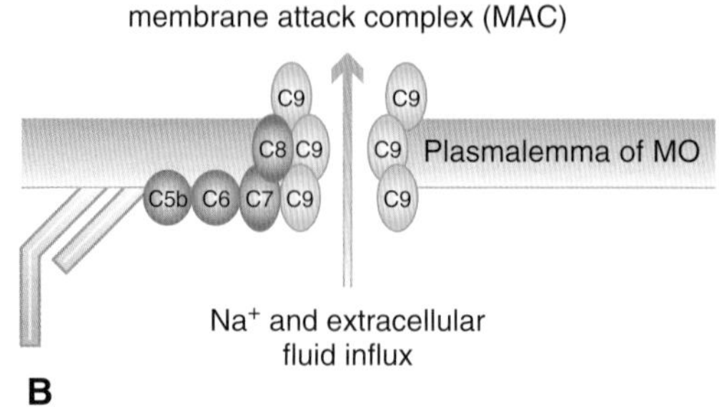


**Figure 6.18**

(A) When an antibody attaches to an antigen (foreign protein) on a microorganism *(MO)*, the antibody-antigen stimulates plasma-derived complement proteins to attach and form the membrane attack complex *(MAC)*. (B) This MAC forms a channel through the membrane of the invading cell and allows ions and extracellular fluid to enter, causing cytolysis (death of the MO). (Courtesy S.H. Tepper, PhD, PT.)

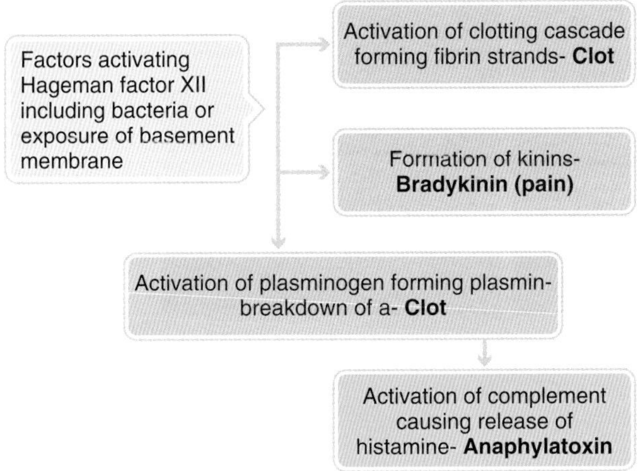


**Figure 6.19**

**Clot formation.** The mechanisms for activating both the intrinsic and the extrinsic pathways for clot formation. Either of the above pathways leads to activation of Hageman factor XII, which results in the formation of a fibrin clot. (Courtesy S.H. Tepper, PhD, PT.)

The kinin system can in turn activate the fibrinolytic system by producing plasmin (splits or divides fibrin and lyses blood clots). Plasmin then can activate the complement system and further amplify these protease loops by activating Hageman factor, once again starting the cycle (Fig. 6.19).

**Phagocytosis.** One of the most important functions of the inflammatory reaction is to inactivate and remove the inflammatory stimulus and to begin the process of healing. The process of ingestion (phagocytosis) of microorganisms, other foreign substances, necrotic cells, and connective tissue constituents by specialized cells (phagocytes) is important in achieving this goal. As mentioned earlier, the chemical mediators attract the phagocytic cells to the area for removal of the dead tissue or microorganisms. After ingestion by phagocytic cells, microorganisms are killed or inactivated, and necrotic debris is removed to allow tissue healing to proceed.

The most important phagocytes involved in the inflammatory and healing reactions are neutrophils, monocytes, or, when found in tissues of the body, macrophages. Macrophages have different names depending on their location (e.g., histiocytes in the skin, osteoclasts in bone, and microglial cells in the CNS).

The mechanism of phagocytosis is well understood. Phagocytosis is facilitated by the coating (opsonization) of particles to be ingested by IgG antibody or by the C3b component of complement. These opsonins bind to specific receptor sites located on the cell surface of neutrophils and macrophages. This receptor binding initiates a process of transmembrane signaling, allowing calcium influx that activates cytoskeletal proteins within the cell. These cytoskeletal structures allow the movement of cell membranes that is necessary for phagocytosis.

The internalization of the opsonized particle begins by the enfolding of the cell surface membrane (Figs. 6.20 and 6.21). The membrane folds surround the particle to be ingested and seal it within a pouch that separates it from the cell surface and becomes an intracellular vacuole called the *phagosome*. The phagosomes fuse with lysosomes (containing digestive materials and bactericidal components) and acquire enzymes and other substances

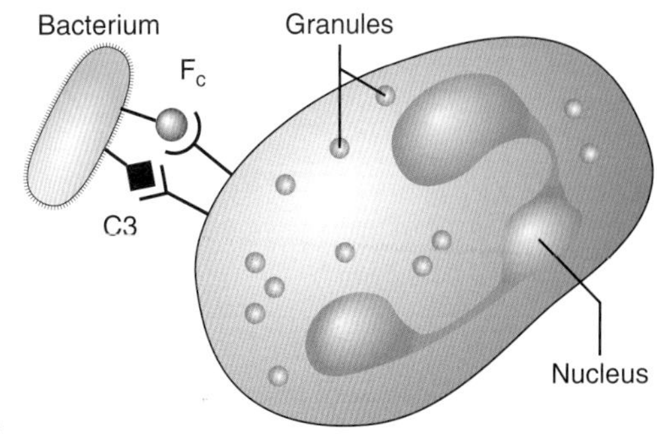


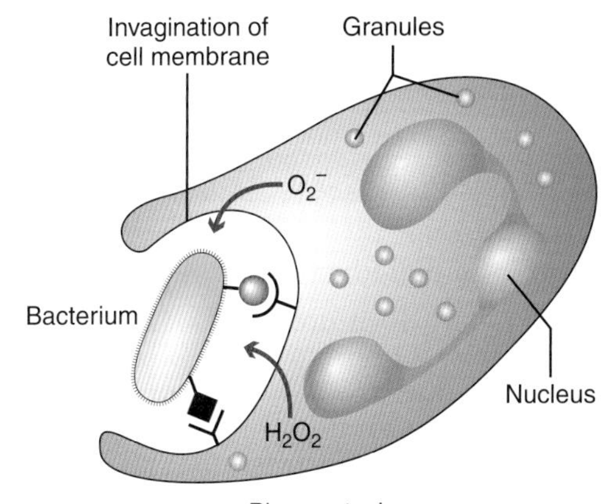


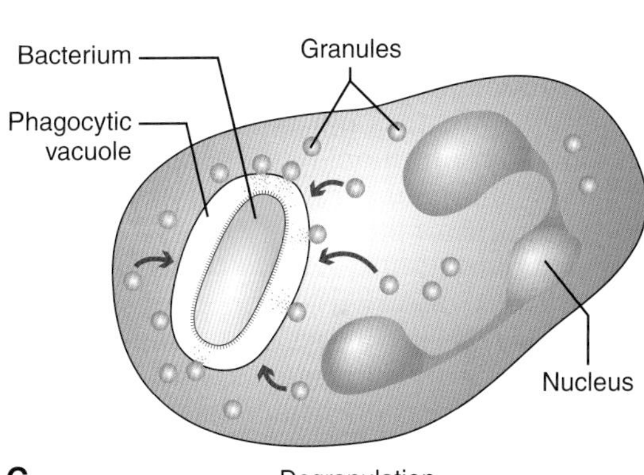


**Figure 6.20**

**Phagocytosis of bacteria.** (A) The bacterium that was opsonized (coated with IgG and complement [C3]) binds to the Fc and complement receptors on the surface of the leukocytes. (B) Engulfment of the bacterium into an invagination of surface membrane is associated with an oxygen burst and formation of oxygen radicals that are bactericidal and thus kill the bacterium. (C) Inclusion of the bacterium into a phagocytic vacuole is associated with the fusion of the vacuole with lysosomes and specific granules of the leukocyte. The contents of the lysosomes and specific granules are bactericidal and contribute to final inactivation and degradation of the bacterium. The cytoplasm of the leukocyte becomes devoid of granules in a process referred to as degranulation of leukocytes. (From Damjanov I: *Pathology for the health-related professions*, ed 4, St. Louis, 2012, Elsevier.)

that allow the killing and degradation of microorganisms and other ingested materials. Many neutrophils (e.g., polymorphonuclear neutrophils) die in their battle with bacteria. Dead and dying leukocytes, mixed with tissue debris and lytic enzymes, form a viscous yellow fluid known as *pus*. Inflammations identified by their pus formations are called *purulent* or *suppurative* (see Table 6.4).

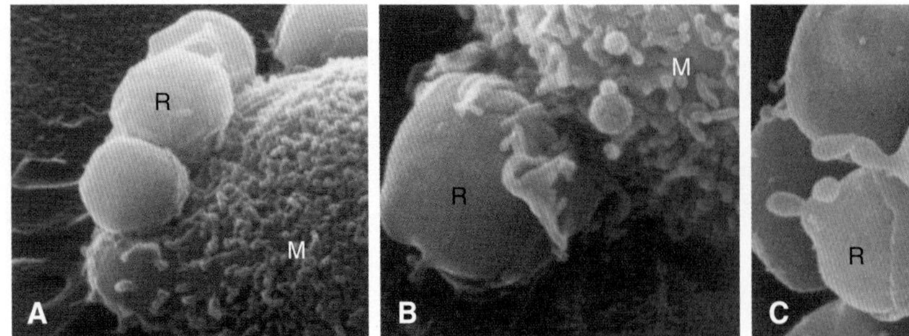


**Figure 6.21**

**Phagocytosis.** This series of scanning electron micrographs shows the progressive steps in phagocytosis of damaged red blood cells (RBCs) by a macrophage. (A) RBCs *(R)* attach to the macrophage *(M)*. (B) Plasma membrane of the macrophage begins to enclose the RBC. (C) The RBCs are almost totally ingested by the macrophage. (Courtesy Emma Shelton.)

SPECIAL IMPLICATIONS FOR THE THERAPIST 6.2

## *Inflammation*

### Clinical Example: Rheumatoid Arthritis

Inflammation, which involves all of the processes described in this section, is a normal, healthy response to tissue injury, but it can also damage adjacent healthy tissue. Chronic activation of inflammatory cells can cause tissue injury such as occurs with rheumatoid arthritis. The role of the therapist is important in supporting the healing process and, when appropriate, to limit inflammation and its consequences. The therapist must remember that finding and correcting the cause of inflammation is the goal, not just addressing the inflammatory process. Poor lifestyle choices including poor nutrition, improper posture and body mechanics, and poor breathing habits can contribute to the chronicity of this condition.

Rheumatoid arthritis illustrates how the inflammatory mediators discussed are activated and how this process leads to clinical manifestations observed in a therapy practice. Inflammatory activity can be detected by the erythrocyte sedimentation rate. The therapist can review laboratory values to assess systemic factors; in general, as the inflammation improves, the erythrocyte sedimentation rate decreases. Systemic effects of acute and chronic inflammation are discussed in Chapter 5.

The majority of people with rheumatoid arthritis produce rheumatoid factor, an antibody that is made against the person's own antibodies of the IgG class. In this case, the IgG antibody actually functions as an antigen (Ag) capable of inducing an immune response.

This antibody-to-antibody attachment can occur in the joint space where it leads to the formation of large antibody-antigen aggregates. Antibody-antigen complexes stimulate complement activation by the classic pathway and the formation of the strongly chemotactic cleavage products C3a and C5a. These products attract neutrophils, which then release free radicals (see Fig. 6.3) and enzymes that degrade the joint cartilage, prostaglandins, and leukotrienes that amplify the inflammatory reaction. The antibody-antigen complex is phagocytosed by synovial-lining cells that are stimulated to release collagen-degrading enzymes, prostaglandins, and IL-1.

Lymphocytes contribute to the acute reaction by the production of rheumatoid factor and are responsible for the evolution of a chronic inflammatory reaction by producing cytokines that attract and activate macrophages. The macrophages produce cytokines such as IL-1 that further amplify the inflammatory reaction by attracting more neutrophils and lymphocytes and by stimulating the synthesis and release from fibroblasts, chondrocytes, and osteoclasts of enzymes that degrade cartilage and bone.

Clinically, the joints affected by the inflammatory process appear red and swollen and are painful; a low-grade fever may also be present. A prominent symptom is joint stiffness that is relieved by activity. With disease progression, damage to the joints occurs; with loss of cartilage, narrowing of the joint space occurs, and resorption of bone is evident on radiograph. These changes are associated with a decrease in the range of motion of the affected joints. In later stages, obvious joint deformities develop that are accompanied by muscle wasting. Antiinflammatory agents, such as aspirin and corticosteroids and disease-modifying antirheumatic drugs, are effective in providing symptomatic relief and in slowing the progression of the disease.

The inflammatory process associated with rheumatoid arthritis may also affect other organ systems. Foci of chronic inflammation can develop in muscles, tendons, blood vessels, nerves, and various organs of the body (e.g., heart and lungs). In the skin, these foci cause the deposition of connective tissue called *subcutaneous nodules*.

In the inflammatory phase of the condition, physical therapy may be beneficial for pain control, preservation of available motion, and protection of joint retardation or atrophy. The therapist should avoid exercises that will cause compression and irritation of the joints, potentially prolonging the inflammatory process. At this stage, limitation of joint motion is primarily due to joint swelling; therefore stretching exercises may overstretch the tissues and cause joint hypermobility when the swelling subsides. Furthermore, because osteoporosis and ligamentous laxity are potential side effects of steroid medication, the bones and joints must be protected from excessive loads.[134]

During the remission phase of the condition, there is strong evidence that exercise of various modes and intensities is effective in improving the functional performance of patients with rheumatoid arthritis.[159] The therapist must still exercise extreme care when performing stretching exercises, as the previous active inflammatory process might have caused some damage to joints, capsules, ligaments, and tendons,[134] and stretching, especially if done vigorously, might further damage these structures.

### Diet and Inflammation

Physical therapists also have responsibility in wellness and health promotion as well as prevention and risk reduction. Part of that responsibility is giving advice to the affected individual on how to improve health by considering changes that affect modifiable risk factors.

There has been an abundance of recent evidence about inflammatory markers and their relationship to various diseases, especially coronary artery disease and diabetes mellitus, both among the top 10 causes of mortality in the United States.[165] A number of other diseases are inflammatory in nature, including asthma,[228] rheumatoid arthritis,[26,144] and inflammatory bowel disease[58,106] as well as other chronic diseases including obesity[26,250] and cancer.[95] Many dietary components are thought to influence various elements of inflammation and therefore play a role in predisposing individuals to inflammatory conditions.

Additionally, altering nutrition to produce antiinflammatory effects may be beneficial in the therapy of such conditions. Dietary changes over the last 30 years including (1) increased consumption of refined carbohydrates, (2) increased consumption of refined vegetable oils rich in omega-6 fatty acids, and (3) decreased consumption of long-chain omega-3 fatty acids are known to produce inflammation and its clinical biomarkers of inflammation.[207]

Clinical biomarkers of inflammation are used to study the effect of dietary components on development of inflammatory conditions as well as treatment and prevention. C-reactive protein, which is an acute phase reactant protein, is a common clinical biomarker of cardiac-related inflammation[117,196] and a general marker of inflammation. Other common clinical indicators of inflammation include high erythrocyte sedimentation rate, high WBC count, and low albumin level.[144] However, these tests are nonspecific, meaning an abnormal result might result from a condition unrelated to inflammation. Various cytokines and adhesion molecules are not commonly used clinically because they do not identify the source of inflammation.[30,130,206]

Diseases or conditions with a well-recognized inflammatory component are often treated with general or specific antiinflammatory pharmaceuticals.[42] Antiinflammatory nutrition is the understanding of how individual nutrients affect the same molecular targets affected by pharmacologic drugs.[207] Identification of dietary changes that may decrease inflammation may improve function and reduce need for medications in some cases.[151]

### Exercise and Inflammation

Animal and human studies have found that various forms of physical activity decrease both acute and chronic inflammation, as measured by reductions in C-reactive protein and certain proinflammatory cytokines.[77,253] Additionally, regular physical activity is important in reducing one's risk for obesity and chronic diseases associated with inflammation.[39] However, excessive exercise can increase systemic inflammation and suppress immune function. For example, overtraining syndrome in athletes is associated with systemic inflammation and suppressed immune function.[11] The mechanisms of exercise-associated muscle damage and the initiation of the inflammatory cytokine cascade are further discussed in Chapter 7 (see Exercise and the Immune System).

## TISSUE HEALING

The process of tissue healing begins soon after tissue injury or death and occurs either by regeneration (regrowth of original tissue) or by repair (formation of a connective tissue scar). The inflammatory cells that are recruited from the blood circulation begin the healing process by breaking down and removing the necrotic tissue. This is accomplished primarily by phagocytes that secrete degradative enzymes and also phagocytose the cellular debris, connective tissue fragments, and plasma proteins present in the dead tissue (Fig. 6.22).

The healing process is complex and influenced by many components such as fibronectin, proteoglycans and elastin, collagen, and parenchymal and endothelial cells. In addition, there is a wide range of factors that affect tissue healing and must be taken into account during recovery and rehabilitation. Both the components and the factors that affect tissue healing are presented in this section, followed by a discussion of the multiphasic process of tissue healing and recovery.

### Components of Tissue Healing

#### Fibronectin

Fibronectin has numerous functions in wound healing, the most important of which are the formation of scaffold, the provision of tensile strength, and the ability to "glue" other substances and cells together. It is one of the earliest proteins to provide the structural support that stabilizes the healing tissue. Plasma proteins that leak from inflamed vessels are the first source of fibronectin for the healing tissue. Plasma-derived fibronectin binds to and stabilizes fibrin, a protein that makes up the blood clots that are present in the injured tissue.

Fibronectin binds together several types of proteins present in the extracellular matrix and can also bind to debris such as DNA material derived from necrotic cells, thereby acting as an opsonin (molecule that acts as a binding enhancer to facilitate phagocytosis) during the breakdown of necrotic tissue. Fibronectin is also responsible for attracting fibroblasts and macrophages by chemotaxis to the healing tissue. The stimulated fibroblasts in turn secrete more fibronectin. Fibronectin binds to

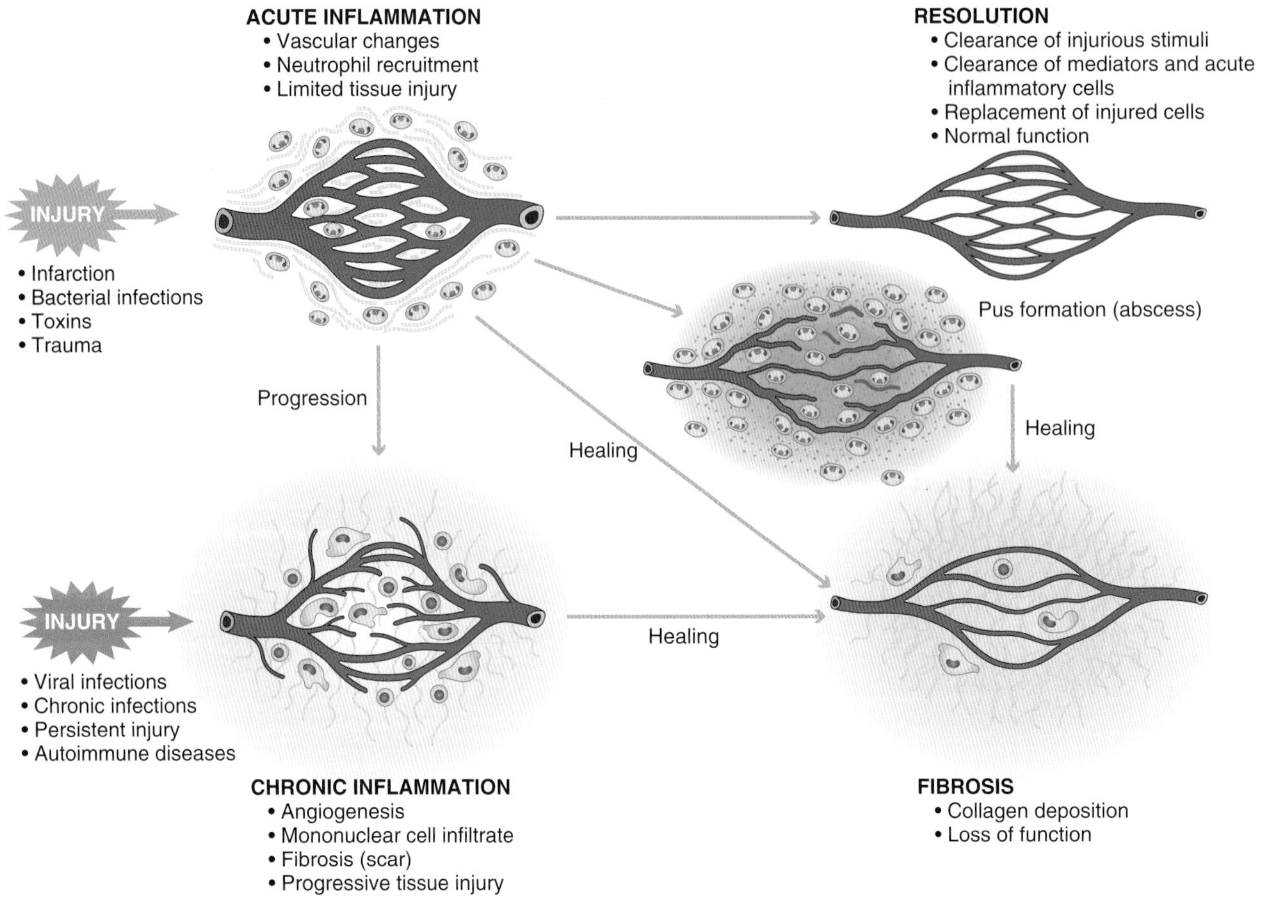


**Figure 6.22**

**Outcomes of acute inflammation: resolution, healing by fibrosis, or chronic inflammation.** Components of the various reactions and their functional outcomes are listed. (From Kumar V, et al: *Robbins and Cotran pathologic basis of disease*, ed 8, Philadelphia, 2010, Saunders.)

proteoglycans and collagens, and this binding further stabilizes the healing tissue.

The importance of fibronectin can be seen as researchers seek to explain the lack of a functional healing response in the anterior cruciate ligament (ACL) after injury.[148] Studies focusing on the signaling pathways and on binding to fibronectin for specific tissues such as the ACL may yield improved prevention and intervention strategies in the future.[157,233]

## Proteoglycans and Elastin

Proteoglycans, proteins containing carbohydrate chains and sugars, are secreted in abundance by fibroblasts early during the tissue repair reaction. Proteoglycans bind to fibronectin and to collagen and help stabilize the tissue that is undergoing repair. Proteoglycans also retain water and aid in the hydration of the tissue being repaired. Once the tissue is healed, proteoglycans contribute to the organization and stability of collagen and create an electrical charge that gives basement membranes the property of functioning like molecular sieves. Fibroblasts also synthesize and secrete elastin, a protein that becomes cross-linked to form fibrils or long sheets that provide tissues with elasticity.

## Collagen

Collagen is the most important protein to provide structural support and tensile strength for almost all tissues and organs of the body. The different types of collagen give stability to healing tissue; the word *collagen* is derived from Greek and means "glue producer." Collagen is a fibrous protein molecule consisting of three chains of amino acid coiled around each other in a triple helix (Fig. 6.23). Improved technology has made it possible to identify collagen types and measure protein turnover. It is the most abundant protein in the body; at least 28 collagen types have been identified.[98,161]

We know that exercise is a potent stimulus for protein synthesis in skeletal muscle. Collagen in the extracellular matrix of muscle and tendon is also sensitive to mechanical stimuli. Collagen does not appear to be nutritionally sensitive, which may contribute to the loss of muscle during aging. It is possible that the tissue is unable to respond adequately to increased availability of nutrients.[240]

**Organization of Collagen.** Each collagen type has a specialized function (Table 6.6). The amino acid makeup of the collagen molecule and the manner in which the molecules are assembled together vary for each one of the collagen types. The differences in organization and

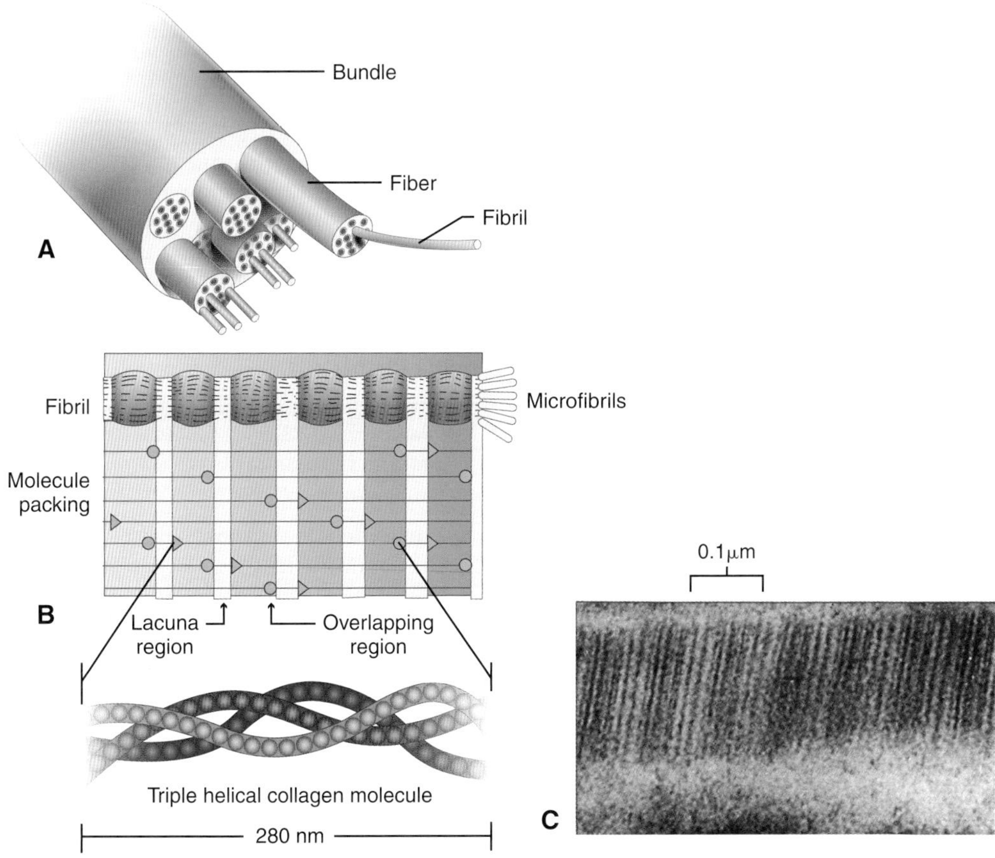


**Figure 6.23**

**Structure of collagen.** (A) The collagen fiber is composed of fibrils, each of which is composed of microfibrils. (B) The molecule itself consists of three polypeptide chains called alpha chains that wrap around each other in a triple helix. The helix is made possible because each third amino acid in the polypeptide chain is glycine. The molecules are quarter-staggered one to another, which ensures that no weak points occur across the fibril to prevent overload and slippage. (C) Visualized by transmission electron microscopy, the individual collagen fibrils are seen to have two orders of banding. The larger bands result from the gaps between the individual molecules of collagen, which then overlap the adjacent molecules to form a strong bond. (From Bullough PG: *Bullough and Vigorita's orthopaedic pathology*, ed 3, St. Louis, MO, 1997, Mosby.)

composition account for the structural properties of each collagen type. For example, collagen organized in unidirectional or parallel bundles contributes to the strength of tendons. Collagen is the principal extracellular component of normal tendon.

Collagen in random arrangement provides flexibility of the skin and rigidity of bone. When organized at right angles, collagen allows transmission of light in the cornea and vitreous. Collagen laid down in a tubular fashion contributes to the elasticity of the blood vessels.

Some collagen molecules are assembled into progressively thicker and stronger filamentous structures, allowing the molecules to become cross-linked. These cross-links impart tensile strength to collagen fibers and prevent slippage of molecules past one another when under tension. The structural stability of the extracellular matrix is primarily a consequence of collagen and the extent of cross-linking.[51]

**Types of Collagen.** Type I collagen, the most common form, is assembled as a thick bundle that is structurally very strong and can be found in all body tissues, where it forms bundles together with other collagen types. Type I collagen is the main component of mature scars and is also predominant in strong tissues such as tendons and bones.

Type II collagen is assembled into thin supporting filaments and is the predominant collagen type found in cartilaginous tissue and the physis (growth plate).[20] Type II fibers of the external annulus have a half-life of about 3 months. This allows maintenance of the nutritive exchanges between degenerative external annulus and any healthy remaining tissue, possibly delaying or avoiding further degeneration.[125,241]

Type III collagen is assembled into thin filaments that make tissues strong but supple and elastic.[223] It contains interchain disulfide bonds or bridges not found in type I or II and is the collagen type first deposited in wound healing (i.e., fresh scars). This type of highly soluble collagen accounts in part for the plasticity of skin and blood vessels. Overexposure to the sun speeds up the breakdown of collagen and elastin, two proteins that give skin its strength and resilience, thus contributing to the development of skin wrinkling.

Type III collagen is more prevalent in newborns; with each passing decade, collagen-producing cells make less of the soluble collagen and progressively convert to synthesizing an insoluble, more stable type I collagen. The changing ratio of collagen types I and III throughout the

**Table 6.6 Types of Collagen**

| Type | Location |
|---|---|
| I | Predominant structural collagen of the body; constitutes 80%–85% of dermal collagen; prominent in mature scars, tendon, bone, and dentin; joints; labrum (capsular side) |
| II | Predominant component of physis (growth plate) and hyaline cartilage (e.g., outer ear, end of nose, joint); not present in skin; found in nucleus pulposus external annulus; labrum (capsular side) |
| III | Prominent in vascular and visceral structures (e.g., blood vessels, GI tract, liver, uterus) but absent in bone and tendon; constitutes 15%–20% of dermal collagen; abundant in embryonic tissues; first collagen deposited in wound healing (granulation tissue) |
| IV | Found in basement membranes (base of epithelial, endothelial, and mesenchymal cells found in developing fetus); glomeruli of kidney nephron |
| V | Present in most tissues but never as a major component; prominent in fetal membrane, cornea, and heart valve; minor component of skin; synovial membranes |
| VI | Prevalent in most connective tissues |
| VII | May be involved in matrix and bone disorders, anchoring filaments of lymphatic vessels and at dermal-epidermal junctions |
| VIII | Secreted by rapidly proliferating cells; found in basement membranes; may provide a molecular bridge between different types of matrix molecules |
| IX | Minor component in hyaline cartilage; vitreous humor (fluid of the eye); also found in the physis (growth plate) |
| X | Formed only in the epiphyseal growth plate cartilage; may have a role in angiogenesis; may be involved in matrix and bone disorders |
| XI | Hyaline cartilage; physis |
| XII | Embryonic skin and tendon; periodontal ligament |
| XIII | Endothelial cells |
| XIV | Fetal skin and tendons; similar to type I |
| XV–XXVII | Identified but not clearly understood |

*GI*, Gastrointestinal.

body is so reliable that chronologic age can be determined by analyzing the collagen type III content of a skin sample.[18]

During the initial stages of tissue repair, fibroblasts secrete large amounts of type III collagen, which provides support for the developing capillaries. Within a few days after the tissue injury, type III collagen is degraded by enzymes secreted by fibroblasts and other cells and is replaced by newly synthesized type I collagen. Type I collagen enhances wound tensile strength and is the main component of the scar tissue that remains after repair is completed. Type IV collagen is not assembled into fibers. Together with other proteins, it forms the basement membrane to which epithelial, endothelial, and certain mesenchymal cells are anchored.

Mutations in the genes for collagen cause a wide spectrum of diseases of bone, cartilage, and blood vessels, including osteogenesis imperfecta; various chondrodysplasias; Alport syndrome; Ehlers-Danlos syndrome; and, more rarely, some forms of osteoporosis, osteoarthritis, and familial aneurysms. Scientists are finding that aberrant collagen cross-linking and increased collagen synthesis are present in some malignancies,[28,32] whereas the presence of free radical scavengers inhibits the rate of collagen formation.[160]

When either collagen or elastin becomes resorbed, elements are released into blood and concentrate in urine. Determining the presence of these components in tissues and body fluids provides important markers in the clinical investigation of various diseases.[214] Methods to quantify the number of collagen cross-links in tissue are also being further developed at this time.[27,129,184,213,239]

**SPECIAL IMPLICATIONS FOR THE THERAPIST 6.3**

## *Tissue Healing (Part 1)*

### Collagen

Much debate has been directed toward the role of the therapist in using myofascial and soft tissue mobilization techniques (including deep/cross-friction massage) to change collagen structures and improve mobility, increase joint range of motion, or alter scar tissue. Whether these techniques can break the collagen cross-links and allow slippage to lengthen or realign the collagen fibers continues under investigation at this time.[20,23,203,204,235] The use of instrument-assisted cross-friction massage on animal ligaments has been shown to increase strength and stiffness, while improving the ability of the soft tissue to absorb energy compared with untreated (acute) ligament injuries. Electron microscopy images demonstrated improved collagen fiber bundle formation and orientation with the scar region in injured ligaments treated with cross-fiber massage.[147] Human studies evaluating the effectiveness of friction massage (whether instrument assisted or not) in improving physical impairments and function have generated mixed results. Most studies have investigated the effectiveness of friction massage in combination with other interventions; therefore its therapeutic value as an individual treatment remains to be confirmed.[29,35,124,146] It has been found that regular mobility of affected tissues helps maintain lubrication and critical fiber distance.[6] Immobilization is associated with excessive deposition of connective tissue in associated areas. This is accompanied by a loss of water and subsequent dehydration. The result is an increase in intermolecular cross-linking, which further restricts normal connective tissue flexibility and extensibility.[54]

Another topic that has elicited considerable attention is the use of manual or movement techniques to elicit a corresponding change to the myofascial structures. It is possible that some of divergent points of view can be attributed to varying definitions of fascia[139] and therefore conflicting expert opinions about its function and relevance. More studies are needed to conclusively determine the efficacy of these techniques in decreasing pain, improving muscular and connective tissue extensibility, and facilitating performance of activity.

Related to this topic is the increasing attention to the concept of *tensegrity* as a framework to understand how the human body is structured and organized and how physical movement, whether self-generated or provided by an external force (as in manual therapy or soft tissue mobilization techniques), affects biochemistry of the cells and physiology of the tissues.[116] This framework posits that the human body is in itself a transegrity structure, with compression structures (primarily the skeletal system) providing strength and stability, while a network of fascia, tendons, and muscles provides the tension force that is transmitted through the body, thereby resulting in movement. Transegrity also highlights the interconnectedness of the components of the system, such that a dysfunction in one component affects the entire structure. Examples of therapeutic approaches such as myofascial release, Rolfing, and other bodywork techniques are based on the concept of biotransegrity. Research, at both the basic and clinical science levels, is ongoing and will deepen our understanding of the importance of this emerging viewpoint in facilitating movement and function.

### Therapeutic Ultrasound in Tissue Healing

The use of ultrasound to increase collagen tissue extensibility, increase enzymatic activity at the site of wound healing, absorb joint adhesions, and reduce fibrous tissue volume and density in scar tissue has been widely accepted, although some of these effects have to be definitively proven. Ultrasound has been shown to facilitate the development of stronger and better-aligned scar tissue[44]; studies have been published that examined the ability of ultrasound to heat human tendon and muscle.[45,66] Ultrasound as a therapeutic intervention in the treatment of human tendinopathy remains under investigation.[7,57,92,115,195,200,244,247]

In the physiologic response of injury or wound healing, the key to growth or replacement tissue at sites of injury is stimulation of protein synthesis in fibroblasts. Exposure of injured tissue to ultrasound at clinically practical doses seems to provide this stimulation.[252] The pulsed mode of ultrasound is used to achieve its nonthermal effects. It is thought that these nonthermal effects include cellular diffusion, membrane permeability, and fibroblastic activities such as protein synthesis, which speeds up tissue regeneration during the proliferative phase.[45,123] Pulsed ultrasound at the lower ranges of intensity may be used during the acute phase to stimulate the release of vasodilator amine histamine from mast cells.[84]

Continuous ultrasound during the first week of wound healing may hinder repair because the consequent heating of the tissues will exacerbate the inflammatory response. After 3 weeks, collagen synthesis continues to occur for remodeling during the subacute stage of healing, and ultrasound can be used as an adjunct to other interventions to promote this collagen synthesis[192] and to minimize adhesions. Reducing adhesions occurs by raising the tissue temperature to increase viscoelastic properties during the proliferation to remodeling stage.[66,73] It has been reported that ultrasound, laser, and a combination of ultrasound and laser all are equally as effective in facilitating tendon healing.[7,63]

Ultrasound aids in reabsorption of joint adhesions by depolymerization of mucopolysaccharides, mucoproteins, or glycoproteins and may reduce the viscosity of hyaluronic acid in joints, thereby reducing joint adhesions. In terms of mature scar tissue, the mechanical effects of ultrasound disrupt the glucoside bonds forming scar tissue, which could assist in the remodeling process.[177] Tight capsular tissue and tendon can also obtain increased extensibility when ultrasound is properly applied and followed immediately by slow, static stretching. Proper dosing of the ultrasound treatment is critically important to achieve the necessary tissue temperature rise to alter the viscoelastic properties of the connective tissue.[66] This must be immediately followed by a slow, controlled stretching and then active motion through the full available range of motion to assist in restoring mobility in tissue and between the tissue interfaces.[45,107] The stretch must be held until the collagen reaches a deformation phase. Without these follow-up techniques, the bond will re-form in its original position.[215]

The therapist is advised to make careful assessment of the phase of injury and clinical results in the use of ultrasound and discontinue its use if there are increases in pain or edema or decreases in range of motion or function. When using ultrasound, it is very important to select the appropriate treatment parameters including the mode (pulsed or continuous), intensity, and duration based on the stage of tissue healing and treatment goals.

## Factors That Affect Tissue Healing

Many variables regulate or affect the healing process and facilitate, inhibit, or delay wound healing (Box 6.3). Because local blood supply is vital to the delivery of the materials necessary for wound healing, factors that impede local circulation or depletion of the necessary materials could delay rehabilitation. Certain tissues (e.g., tendons, ligaments, cartilage, disc) have a decreased blood supply; thus the healing process may require additional time.

### Growth Factors

The cells involved in the tissue repair response produce proteins called *growth factors* that regulate a number of cellular reactions involved in healing. Growth factors regulate cell proliferation, differentiation, and migration; biosynthesis and degradation of proteins; and angiogenesis. Through all of these varying functions, growth factors integrate the inflammatory events with the reparative processes. When these complex mechanisms are disturbed, the result can be delayed healing and an inferior scar (hypotrophic) or elevated levels of growth factor, resulting in hypertrophic scarring such as occurs after a burn injury or in the formation of keloids.[234]

Growth factors act by binding to receptors on the plasma membranes of specific cells and have a stimulatory or inhibitory effect on these cells. This binding initiates a process of transmembrane signaling that results in the phosphorylation of proteins (the process of attaching a phosphate group to the protein). These steps lead to the activation of gene expression and DNA synthesis in the cell.

The signals that turn on proliferation of normal cells and cause tissue healing are also responsible for turning

Box 6.3

**FACTORS INFLUENCING HEALING**

- Physiologic variables (e.g., age, growth factors, vascular sufficiency)
- General health of the individual; immunocompetency; psychologic/emotional/spiritual well-being
- Presence of comorbidities (examples):
  - Diabetes mellitus
  - Decreased oxygen perfusion (e.g., COPD, CHF, CAD, pneumonia)
  - Hematologic disorders (e.g., neutropenia)
  - Cancer (local and systemic effects)
  - Incontinence
  - Alzheimer disease
  - Neurologic impairment
  - Immobility
- Tobacco, alcohol, caffeine, other substance use/abuse
- Nutrition
- Local or systemic infection; presence of foreign bodies
- Type of tissue
- Medical treatment (e.g., prednisone, chemotherapy, radiation therapy)

*CAD*, Coronary artery disease; *CHF*, chronic heart failure; *COPD*, chronic obstructive pulmonary disease.

on proliferation of cancer cells. With continued growth of neoplastic cells, a neoplasm or tumor may develop. The significant difference between the healing process and cancer is that the growth of the cancer cells goes on unchecked. These analogies have led to the designation of cancers as wounds that do not heal.

Platelets, endothelial cells, fibroblasts, macrophages, and cytokines are important sources of growth factors. Two important growth factors are platelet-derived growth factor, which activates fibroblasts and macrophages, and fibroblast growth factor, which stimulates endothelial cells to form new blood vessels. An example of a growth factor that inhibits cell growth and inactivates macrophages is transforming growth factor β.

Recombinant human platelet-derived growth factor BB (becaplermin) is a growth factor approved by the U.S. Food and Drug Administration that has been proven to be effective in facilitating the healing of lower extremity ulcers of people with diabetes.[22,219] This is available in a gel form and applied to wounds usually once daily, with the wound being dressed after application.[50,62] Another growth factor, granulocyte colony-stimulating factor, has been shown to reduce the need for amputation and decrease length of hospitalization stay in patients with diabetic foot ulcer when used as an adjunct to usual wound care. Granulocyte colony-stimulating factor acts by facilitating the release of neutrophil endothelial progenitor cells, resulting in improved neutrophil function.[55]

Researchers continue to explore the most appropriate medium to effectively deliver these growth factors to the wound bed. Currently several of these wound dressings are already approved by the Food and Drug Administration, whereas others are still being investigated.[62] Platelet-rich plasma is also being used successfully for the treatment of tendon, ligament, muscle, and cartilage injuries and early osteoarthritis. The presence of critical growth factors and signaling molecules (e.g., cytokines, fibrinogen) in platelets that govern and regulate the tissue-healing process speeds up the healing process through the inflammatory, reparative, and remodeling phases.[52,185]

Finally, cytokines such as IL-1, IL-2, IL-15, and TNF can also regulate some aspects of the healing response. Some ILs have been identified as T-cell growth factors with proinflammatory properties or the transforming growth factor associated with hypertrophic scarring. Further studies are necessary to clarify the mechanism of cytokine release in normal postoperative wounds before therapeutic use can be developed.[110]

### Nutrition

Nutrition is an important factor influencing healing. Adequate nutritional intake is necessary to support the active metabolism of cells involved in repair. Trauma, including surgery, infections, or large draining wounds, often increases the systemic rate of protein catabolism (loss), which further limits the body's ability to synthesize proteins required for healing. Inadequate intake of specific nutritional factors can specifically affect collagen production and remodeling and increase risk for infection.[218]

Zinc is essential for the activity of enzymes that degrade collagen and enzymes that are responsible ultimately for the induction of protein synthesis. Zinc deficiency therefore impairs healing. People with cancer often manifest delayed healing because of poor nutritional status associated with the cancer process or medical treatment (e.g., chemotherapy); particularly notable is the poor healing in tissues that have been subjected to radiation therapy.

### Other Factors

Other factors that influence healing include vascular supply, presence of infection, immune reaction, client age, and presence of other medical conditions, referred to as *comorbidities*. Healing is often adversely affected in people who smoke, who are immunosuppressed, or who have other compromising medical conditions. For example, incontinence, peripheral vascular disease, confusion associated with dementia or Alzheimer disease, or other neurologic impairment can contribute to delayed wound healing.

Diseases associated with decreased oxygen (tissue) perfusion (e.g., anemia, congestive heart failure, chronic obstructive pulmonary disease, or diabetes mellitus) can also delay healing. Diabetes mellitus is associated with poor healing; one of the causes appears to be impaired function of phagocytic cells, and another is a defect in granulation tissue formation.[76,140]

Medications can directly affect healing, especially the prolonged use of corticosteroids or undergoing chemotherapy or radiation treatment. Anyone taking prednisone or other corticosteroids may be at risk, as steroids are well known to impair the healing process by inhibiting the inflammatory response necessary for tissue regeneration or repair.

An adequate vascular supply is critical to provide oxygen and nutrients to support healing. Vascular insufficiency, particularly in the lower limbs, is an important cause of slow-healing or nonhealing wounds. When blood return is not normal, a buildup of fluid can occur, reducing the body's ability to supply nutrients and oxygen to the wound site.

Infection interferes with healing by inciting a severe and prolonged inflammatory reaction that can increase tissue damage. Certain microorganisms can also release toxins that directly cause tissue necrosis and lysis. Foreign bodies may retard healing by inducing a chronic inflammatory reaction, by interfering with closure of a tissue defect, and by providing a site protected from leukocytes and antibiotics where bacteria can multiply.

It may be necessary to offload weight-bearing surfaces to relieve pressure on the wound and surrounding area. Immobility, lack of desire to exercise or follow a plan of care, and refusal to change dietary or other lifestyle behaviors contributing to poor wound healing must also be considered.

Healing may be delayed or inhibited for individuals who are in a constant state of survival or sympathetic nervous system stimulation. When the sympathetic nervous system is locked in a hyperactive mode, exaggerated responses to relatively minor stimuli cause the body to work against itself for healing and recovery.

## SPECIAL IMPLICATIONS FOR THE THERAPIST 6.4

### *Tissue Healing (Part 2)*

#### Healing in Relation to Chronic Tissue Injury

The therapist is often involved with individuals who have chronic tissue injury, often caused by stresses of moderate magnitude that are repeated many times a day. Injuries from this mechanism range from cervical and back pain to patellofemoral dysfunction, tendinopathies, impingement syndromes, stress fractures, and carpal tunnel syndrome.[170] The therapist must identify and modify all factors that may contribute to excessive stress on injured tissues. This includes movement and alignment (e.g., motor control, posture, and muscle length), extrinsic factors (e.g., footwear, gravity, and ergonomic environment), psychosocial factors, medications, age, obesity, or other comorbidities.[170]

After sources of excessive stress have been addressed, injured tissues are still less tolerant of stress than before the injury. Once pain and inflammation have subsided, previously injured tissue must be exposed gradually to higher levels of physical stress. This progression will help restore the tissues' ability to tolerate greater levels of stress. Once healing occurs and tissue integrity is restored, activity tolerance can be increased.[170]

Mueller and Maluf[170] offer a good example of how to think about our clients in this way. An older adult has asked the therapist to help her stand independently from a sitting position. The examining therapist identifies the primary modifiable factors limiting this activity as being lower extremity muscle atrophy resulting in poor force production, decreased ankle dorsiflexion, poor motor control (movement and alignment factors), and a low seat surface (extrinsic factor).

A plan of care that considers her age as an important physiologic factor includes a progressive resistive exercise program for lower extremity extensor muscles with at least 70% of maximum effort, two to three times a week, to increase muscle force production. At the same time, the client is instructed in stretching exercises to increase ankle range of motion and appropriate movement strategies with good alignment to practice going from a seated to a standing position. Finally, the client is advised to use a higher chair to lower muscle force needed to meet her goal of independently standing from a seated position.[170]

#### Delayed Wound Healing

Understanding the interaction of the wound, wound microorganisms, and the immune response is central to developing successful therapeutic interventions for wound care and management. This chapter has carefully explained how wounding of normal tissue initiates an inflammatory response that ordinarily contributes to the healing process orchestrated by specific and nonspecific immune responses. Inflammatory cells provide growth factors and stimulate the deposition of matrix proteins and phagocytose debris. However, the maturation and resolution of a wound may be complicated by the presence of microorganisms. The effects of microorganisms on oxygen consumption and pH or toxin production may interrupt the natural course of wound healing.

Numerous other factors may delay or inhibit wound healing (see Box 6.3). Because local blood supply is vital to the delivery of the materials necessary for wound healing, factors that impede local circulation or a depletion of the necessary materials could delay rehabilitation. The healing process may even be longer for certain tissues that have a decreased blood supply, such as tendons, cartilage, and discs.

It is also important for therapists to thoroughly screen a client's medical history for the presence of conditions such as diabetes, chemical dependency (e.g., alcoholism), and cigarette smoking, because these factors could delay healing and recovery. Finally, local infection delays healing. If an abscess is present, the expected fever, chills, and sweats associated with infection may not be present in someone who is taking steroid medications. A sudden worsening of symptoms; the presence of a hot, acutely inflamed joint; or the onset of fever should warn the therapist that something more serious may exist. In general, the more compromised the host, the greater the chance of a slow or incomplete recovery.

The wound may not progress from the acute phase but may become a nonhealing chronic or recalcitrant wound as long as the antigens from microorganisms or underlying pathology remain, leading to wound infection. Even so, most chronic wounds progress toward healing, depending on the wound care strategy employed.[230] For example, a venous leg ulcer will heal once the proper compression and support have been provided to counteract the underlying venous hypertension and appropriate wound care has been provided. Similarly, diabetic neuropathic foot ulcers do not heal until the disordered glucose metabolism is controlled, adequacy of the vascular supply is ensured, and causative pressure on the foot is offloaded.

Successful healing of chronic wounds involves intervention to address the underlying causes and clinical wound management that provides an environment to tip the balance in favor of healing.[61] The therapist is more likely to select appropriate intervention measures if the evaluation and assessment process takes into consideration the physiology of tissue repair along with the many factors that can affect wound healing. Investigating the status of these other factors (e.g., nutritional status; mobility status; turning schedule for immobile individuals; continence status; use of substances such as tobacco, alcohol, or caffeine; and medication schedule) requires collaboration with other health care specialists and with the family.[225]

Laboratory values such as prealbumin levels indicating nutritional status in the previous 48 hours may be helpful. Glucose levels, hemoglobin, and hematocrit provide the therapist with necessary information to monitor wound healing when setting up and carrying out an appropriate intervention plan.

Specific techniques for wound management are beyond the scope of this text. The reader is referred to other texts for this information.

## PHASES OF HEALING

Acute wounds caused by trauma or surgery usually heal according to a well-defined process that has the following four phases that overlap each other and can take months to years to complete[16,248]:

- Hemostasis and degeneration
- Inflammation
- Proliferation and migration
- Remodeling and maturation

### Hemostasis and Degeneration

When tissue injury occurs, hemostasis is the first step. Hemostasis occurs immediately after an acute injury as the body tries to stop the bleeding by initiating coagulation. Blood fills the gap, and the coagulation cascade commences immediately, clumping platelets together to form a loose clot. Platelets release bioactive proteins that act as chemical messengers including growth factors that summon inflammatory cells to the wounded tissue. Growth factors stimulate proliferation and migration of epithelial cells, fibroblasts, and vascular endothelial cells. Growth factors also regulate the differentiation of cells such as expression of extracellular matrix proteins.[16]

The inflammatory process described in detail in the next section begins right away, bringing fluid to the area to dilute harmful substances and support infection-fighting and scavenger cells (neutrophils and macrophages). Some sources describe this first phase as degeneration and inflammation.

The degeneration phase is characterized by the formation of a hematoma, necrosis of dead cells, and, as mentioned, the start of the inflammatory cell response. After the removal of the dead tissue, the healing process undertakes the repair of the tissue defect that remains. Tissue repair begins within 24 hours of the injury with the migration of fibroblasts from the margins of the viable tissue to the defect caused by the injury. The fibroblasts proliferate and synthesize and secrete proteins such as fibronectin, various proteoglycans and elastin, and several types of collagen. The function of these proteins is to reconstitute the extracellular matrix and provide a scaffolding-like framework for the developing endothelial and parenchymal cells.

At this point, proliferation and migration occur as epidermal skin cells in the top layer move down the sides of the wound to help fill in the gap. Fibroblasts move in from the dermis, and new blood vessels form to create granulation tissue, which later becomes scar tissue. The next phase of remodeling eventually progresses into the final maturation phase as the regenerated tissue reorganizes into healthy scar tissue.

But we have just jumped ahead to tell you the "rest of the story" by discussing proliferation and migration before describing the inflammatory process. Because the phases of tissue healing overlap, it is difficult to describe the process from start to finish without interrupting the discussion.

### Inflammation

This phase of healing has been discussed in detail in the previous section of this chapter. To review, remember that inflammation serves a vital role in the healing process. Inflammation has both protective and curative features. Every step serves a specific purpose and is necessary as the body responds to tissue injury or damage. The ultimate goal of the inflammatory process is to replace injured tissue with healthy regenerated tissue, a fibrous scar, or both.[21]

The inflammatory phase begins once the blood clot forms. Vasodilation and increased capillary permeability activate the movement of various cells, such as polymorphonuclear leukocytes and macrophages, to the wound site. These cells destroy bacteria, release proteases such as elastase and collagenase, and secrete additional growth factors.

Growth factors, cytokines, and chemokines are the key molecular bioregulators of the inflammatory phase of tissue healing. The functions of these three bioregulators overlap considerably. About 5 days after injury, fibroblasts, epithelial cells, and vascular endothelial cells move into the wound to form granulation tissue. This newly developing tissue is not strong, so there is a higher risk of wound dehiscence during this time.[16]

In contrast to cell injury, which occurs at the level of single cells, inflammation is the coordinated reaction of body tissues to cell injury and cell death that involves vascular, humoral, neurologic, and cellular responses. Regardless of the type of cell injury or death, the inflammatory response follows a basically similar pattern. As a result of all of these factors, inflammation occurs only in living organisms.

The functions of the inflammatory reaction are to inactivate the injurious agent, to break down and remove the dead cells, and to initiate the healing of tissue. The key components of the inflammatory reaction are as follows:

- Blood vessels
- Circulating blood cells
- Connective or interstitial tissue cells (fibroblasts, mast cells, and resident macrophages)
- Chemical mediators derived from inflammatory cells or plasma cells
- Specific extracellular matrix constituents, primarily collagen and basement membranes

Basement membranes are thin, sheetlike structures deposited by endothelial cells (cells that line the heart, blood vessels, lymph vessels, and serous body cavities) and epithelial cells (cells that cover the body and viscera) but are also found surrounding nerve and muscle cells. They provide mechanical support for resident cells and function as a scaffold for accurate regeneration of preexisting structures of tissue. Basement membrane tissue also serves as a semipermeable filtration barrier for macromolecules in organs such as the kidney and the placenta and acts as regulators of cell attachment, migration, and differentiation. The major constituents are collagen type IV and proteoglycans.

## Proliferation and Migration Phase

Within 2 days after a skin wound or injury, endothelial cells from viable blood vessels near the edge of the necrotic tissue begin to proliferate. The purpose of the endothelial cell proliferation is to establish a vascular network that can transport oxygen and nutrients and support the metabolism of the healing tissue. The endothelial cells bud out from the vessels and form new capillary channels that merge with each other as they develop and grow toward the tissue defect caused by the injury. This process of formation of new blood vessels is called *neovascularization* or *angiogenesis*.

The rich network of developing blood vessels with its connective tissue matrix can be seen with the naked eye in healing wounds. As described previously, the appearance of a reddish granular layer of tissue was therefore given the name "granulation tissue." Histologically the main cellular components of granulation tissue are the endothelial cells and the fibroblasts, although some inflammatory cells are also commonly present.

Initially the newly formed vessels are leaky, and this leak contributes to the edematous appearance of tissue undergoing repair. As tissue healing is completed, blood flow to the newly formed vasculature shuts down, and the nonfunctional vessels are degraded, leaving few blood vessels in mature scar tissue.

Tissue gaps are replaced during the proliferation phase when the number of inflammatory cells decreases, and fibroblasts, endothelial cells, and keratinocytes take over synthesis of growth factors. The result is the continued promotion of cell migration, proliferation, and formation of new capillaries and synthesis of extracellular matrix components.[16] The next step is the removal of damaged matrix as new matrix builds up to fill the wound. The wound initially fills with provisional wound matrix, which consists primarily of fibrin and fibronectin. As fibroblasts are drawn into the matrix, they synthesize new collagen, elastin, and proteoglycan molecules, which cross-link the collagen of the matrix and produce the initial scar.[16]

Damaged proteins in the matrix have to be removed before the newly synthesized matrix components can be properly integrated. This process is facilitated by proteases secreted by neutrophils, macrophages, fibroblasts, epithelial cells, and endothelial cells. Epithelial cells are at the front of the wound edge, traveling across the highly vascularized extracellular matrix, forming granulation tissue to re-form the epidermal layer. This process can take several weeks.[16]

## Remodeling and Maturation Phase

In the maturation phase of healing, the scar tissue is reduced and remodeled, leaving tissue smoother, stronger, less dense, and less red in color (in fair-skinned individuals) as the concentration of blood vessels in the area decreases. In all skin colors, the scar tissue becomes more like the natural skin tones of the person. The density of fibroblasts and capillaries needed in the early phase of healing but no longer needed now declines, primarily through apoptosis or programmed cell death. The remodeling phase can take years as the skin first produces collagen fibers, which are broken down and rearranged to withstand stress. Over time, scar tissue grows stronger, relaxes, and then lightens.

### Tissue Contraction and Contracture

As the healing process proceeds, the newly formed extracellular matrix draws together, causing shrinkage (contraction) of the healing tissue. In this manner, the size of the tissue defect caused by the injury is diminished. Some fibroblasts within the healing tissue differentiate and acquire some of the morphologic and functional characteristics of smooth muscle cells (myocytes). These specialized fibroblasts are called *myofibroblasts*. Myofibroblasts contain abundant contractile proteins and apparently contract and contribute to the shrinkage of the healing tissue.

Tissue contraction is a normal process that contributes to tissue repair by approximating the margins of the healing tissue and speeding up the closure of wounds. In some cases, excessive shrinkage of the healing tissue occurs, in addition to the pulling of the deeper tissue to approximate the healing site.[70] This condition is called *contracture*. Contracture is an undesirable outcome of healing because it can limit mobility and organ function and can be disfiguring. For example, people with severe burns often develop skin contractures because of the process of hypertrophic scarring that can result in significant movement impairments and subsequent disability.

Contracted tissue with excessive arthrofibrosis can occur in the joints (most often the shoulder and knee) after either injury or surgery. Postoperative or posttraumatic arthrofibrosis is characterized by local or global periarticular scarring that can restrict, and in some cases a thickened, fibrotic capsule inhibits motion. Arthrofibrosis can be caused by a variety of factors including prolonged immobilization, infection, or graft malposition after ligament reconstruction (e.g., ACL reconstruction).[162]

There is anecdotal evidence suggesting that immature scar tissue can be successfully treated conservatively (e.g., analgesia and antiinflammatory medications, early motion, bracing, strengthening, electrical stimulation, or manual therapy techniques). However, a recent systematic review reported weak evidence regarding the use of soft tissue mobilization in scar management.[211]

Exactly when scar tissue becomes mature is variable and remains a topic of debate. Some estimate an open window of 3 to 4 months, after which time interventions such as surgical manipulation (open or arthroscopic) or manipulation under anesthesia may be performed. In a systematic review, these three methods resulted in increases in knee range of motion in patients with arthrofibrosis following total knee replacement.[91] It should be noted, however, that forceful manipulation of the stiff joint can create excessive joint compression, leading to articular cartilage damage and even fracture.[163]

### Tissue Regeneration

Within a few hours after lethal injury to skin, epithelial cells, the viable cells that surround the necrotic tissue, detach from their extracellular matrix anchorage sites and separate from the other epithelial cells. The remaining epithelial cells flatten out to cover the area left bare by the necrotic cells. These epithelial cells also divide and migrate into the tissue using the extracellular matrix support provided by the proteins secreted by the fibroblasts. This process of replacement of dead parenchymal cells by new cells is called *regeneration*. Regeneration is a very desirable healing process because it restores normal tissue structure and function. In most cases, healing of tissue is achieved by both cell regeneration and replacement by connective tissue (scarring) called *repair*. In the case of skin, for example, this type of healing occurs after wounds that involve both the epidermis and the dermis. In some instances, tissue healing occurs almost exclusively by the progress of regeneration (regrowth of original tissue).

Regeneration can occur only if the parenchymal cells can undergo mitosis. Cells are classified as *permanent, stable,* and *labile* based on their ability to divide. Regeneration does not occur in permanent tissues that cannot divide (e.g., cardiac myocytes or central or peripheral neurons); they are long-lived and irreplaceable. Regeneration also can occur only in labile or stable tissues and only if the inflammatory reaction that follows injury is short-lived and does not disrupt the basement membranes, other extracellular components, and vascular structures of labile or stable parenchymal cells. Labile cells such as epithelial cells of the skin and GI system and bone marrow divide continuously. Hematopoietic (blood cell–forming) stem cells continuously divide, giving rise to specialized cells such as erythrocytes and neutrophils with finite life spans.

Under these conditions, the regenerating parenchymal cells can use the existing connective tissue scaffolding to reconstitute the normal structure and function of the organ. This type of tissue healing can be seen after superficial mechanical injury to epithelia. An example is a superficial abrasion of the skin that causes only necrosis of the epidermis. In this case, regeneration occurs with little or no scarring.

Stable cells such as hepatocytes, skeletal muscle fibers, and kidney cells normally do not divide but can be induced to undergo mitosis by an appropriate stimulus. For example, if a portion of the liver is removed by surgery or if liver cells are killed by a viral infection (hepatitis), the remaining hepatocytes divide and sometimes can fully replace the missing liver tissue.

Studies have revealed some capability of neurons to regenerate (neurogenesis) but only in certain areas of the brain (e.g., hippocampus, olfactory bulb, and subventricular zone).[34,56] The reasons for the restriction of neurogenesis to a few regions of the brain in mammals compared with a more widespread neurogenesis in other vertebrates remain unknown.[176,182] It may be that neuronal stem cells persist in these areas throughout the life span, but why they do not persist in all areas is still a mystery.[12] What we do know is that neural stem cells residing in specific niches are able to proliferate and differentiate, giving rise to migrating neuroblasts, which in turn mature into functional neurons. These new neurons integrate into the existing circuits and contribute to the structural plasticity of certain brain areas.[181]

Scientific evidence suggests that the process could become more general under pathologic conditions. For example, adult neurogenesis increases under acute and chronic brain diseases. Neuronal precursors are directed to the lesions, where they contribute to tissue repair. Investigations are underway to find ways to manipulate and direct the neurogenic process toward the amelioration of neurodegenerative diseases.[1,97,183,229]

### Tissue Repair (Formation of Scar Tissue)

Skin has the remarkable ability to heal, often without scarring. Growth factors, blood components, and epithelial (skin) cells mobilize to seal off wounds and protect the body. Scarring does not occur unless the cut, incision, damage, or trauma extends beneath the surface layer (epidermis).

Tissue repair, including the formation of a connective tissue scar, requires removal of the connective tissue matrix. Without this matrix, labile cells do not regenerate, or else they regenerate in an incomplete fashion. Therefore the structural integrity of the parenchymal tissue depends on the formation of this connective tissue scar (dense, irregular laying down of collagen). In many cases, however, healing of tissue is achieved by both cell regeneration and replacement by connective tissue (which is what constitutes scarring). In the case of skin, for example, both types of healing occur in wounds that involve both the epidermis and the dermis.

Minimizing tissue scarring is important not only for cosmetic reasons, as is the case in skin, but also because excessive scarring can interfere with organ function. Very large tissue defects may require the use of grafts or flaps of tissue to achieve optimal healing. It is possible to minimize scarring by surgical obliteration of the tissue defect caused by injury and cell necrosis. For example, treatment of skin wounds begins with careful cleansing of the wound to remove foreign materials and bacterial contamination, which interfere with healing. This is followed by débridement to remove nonviable tissue that normally would be broken down by the inflammatory reaction.

Careful attention to hemostasis minimizes the deposition of blood into the wound. During closure, the wound margins are closely apposed under the right amount of tension by surgical sutures. A clean, closed wound is free of infectious and other foreign material, fibrin, and necrotic debris. As a result, the duration and intensity of the inflammatory reaction are minimized. Little granulation tissue forms, and the epithelial cell surface is readily reconstituted.

The healing that occurs in the type of wound described is called *primary union* or *healing by first intention* and results in a small scar (Fig. 6.24). In the presence of large tissue defects or infections and in other conditions where surgical closure is not possible or desirable, healing occurs by secondary union. In this situation, the time required for healing is longer and the amount of scarring is greater. There is a distinction between closure and healing; the wound or skin may close, but healing takes much longer, as much as 2 years in some situations.

Even after wound closure is complete, degradation and resynthesis of collagen continue. This is a response at least in part to shifts in the stress forces to which the

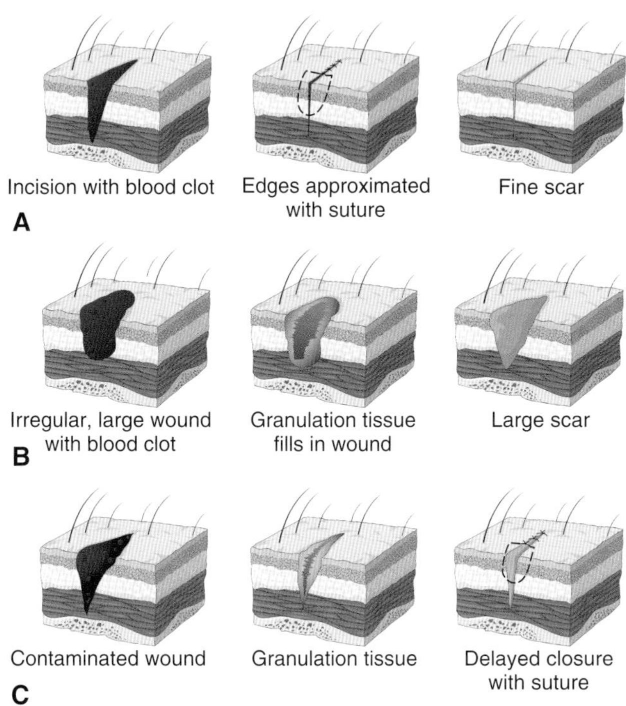


**Figure 6.24**

(A) Healing by primary intention is the initial union of the edges of a wound, progressing to complete healing without granulation. (B) Healing by secondary intention is wound closure in which the edges are separated, granulation tissue develops to fill the gap, and epithelium grows in over the granulations, producing a scar. (C) Healing by tertiary intention is wound closure in which granulation tissue fills the gap between the edges of the wound, with epithelium growing over the granulation at a slower rate and producing a larger scar than results from healing from second intention. Suppuration is also usually found in tertiary wound closure. (From Lewis SL, Heitkemper MM, Dirksen SR: *Medical surgical nursing: assessment and management of surgical problems*, ed 8, St. Louis, 2011, Mosby.)

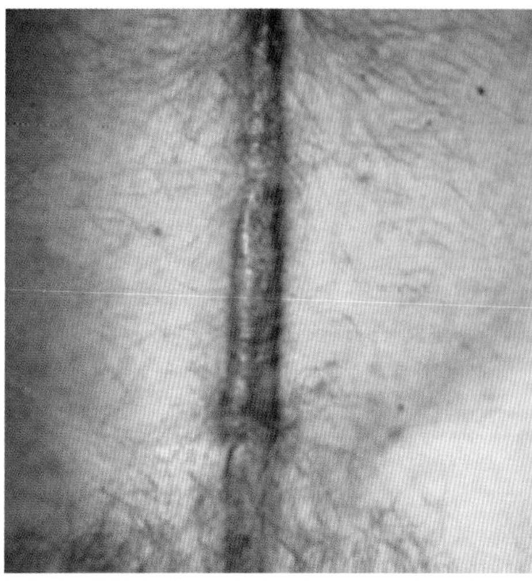

**Figure 6.25**

**Keloid (hypertrophic) scar composed predominantly of type III collagen, rather than type I collagen.** Keloids result from defective remodeling of scar tissue and the persistence of type III collagen, which is typical of immature scar. Epidermis is elevated by excess scar tissue, which may continue to increase long after healing occurs, and looks smooth, rubbery, and clawlike. Young women, black people, and people of Mediterranean descent are particularly susceptible to keloid formation. (From Rakel RE: *Textbook of family medicine*, ed 7, Philadelphia, 2007, Saunders.)

tissue is subjected. Cross-linking of collagen fibers continues for a period of several weeks, providing progressive strengthening of scar tissue. However, even under optimal conditions, the repaired tissue never fully regains its original stability. In the case of skin, a fully mature fibrous scar requires 12 to 18 months and is about 20% to 30% weaker than normal skin.

In some people, especially people of African or Asian descent, there is an inherited tendency to produce excessive amounts of collagen during the healing process, causing large amounts of collagen arranged in thick bundles to accumulate in the tissue. These collagenous masses are called *keloids* and can be seen protruding from the skin surface (Fig. 6.25). Keloids are more than just raised, hypertrophic scar tissue. Both keloid and hypertrophic scar tissue result from excess collagen formation, but hypertrophic scars generally calm down in 12 to 24 months, whereas keloids tend to grow larger and appear worse, often invading surrounding tissue.

Several methods are used to treat keloids, although none of them are 100% successful. Surgical keloid excision, form pressure garments, radiation therapy, laser therapy, and pharmacologic interventions have some reported success.[242,250] Necrosis of heart tissue (myocardial infarct) results in a fibrous scar because cardiac myocytes do not replicate to any great extent. Outcomes that can result from tissue repair in various tissues and conditions are summarized in Fig. 6.11. The CNS differs in its healing process because neurons are permanent cells and do not replicate.

After tissue necrosis, neither regeneration nor tissue scarring occurs. No fibroblasts are present in the brain parenchyma, and no collagen is produced. After a brain infarct (stroke), the inflammatory cells arrive from the blood circulation and clear away the necrotic tissue, leaving behind an empty cavity (cyst). Specialized CNS cells called *astrocytes (glial cells)* proliferate, forming dense aggregates around the necrotic area called *glial scars* or *gliosis*.

### Special Mention: Chronic Wounds

When a wound fails to heal normally, reepithelialization and closure do not occur. Chronic wounds can occur when the wrong biochemicals are present in the wrong amounts at the wrong times and fail to function effectively. There may be a deficiency in endogenous growth factors, which have the primary role of stimulating cell migration, proliferation, and extracellular matrix deposition. Chronic wounds remain in the inflammatory and proliferative phases.[72] Understanding the normal repair process and factors that affect tissue healing can help guide the therapist in removing barriers to healing. Preparing the wound bed appropriately changes the wound's biochemical environment back to an acute wound, thus reinitiating the healing cascade.

SPECIAL IMPLICATIONS FOR THE THERAPIST 6.5

### *Tissue Healing (Part 3)*

**Healing of Scar Tissue**

The clinical implications of tissue repair can be seen in the example presented earlier in this chapter (see "Special Implications for the Therapist 6.3: Collagen"). In this example, after a transmural MI, a symptom-limited stress test will usually be given after phase II of cardiac rehabilitation, around 8 to 12 weeks after MI. With understanding of the material presented in this chapter, one can see the logical explanation.

As mentioned previously, the damaged human heart muscle is not capable of regeneration.[74] Healing of the myocardium occurs primarily through the process of tissue repair and requires 8 to 12 weeks to form a dense connective tissue scar. This dense scar allows for structural integrity and force transduction of the viable myocardium, leading to a complete heart contraction. Because the connective tissue scar is not contractile, this area of the heart will never return to full function. Of great importance is the fact that after MI, a person's aerobic fitness can improve (or exceed) to the level before his or her premorbid state with proper exercise. Studies have shown that regular exercise that includes aerobic conditioning improves quality of life and tolerance to activities and results in the improvement of modifiable risk factors in individuals who have had a previous MI.[90]

# TISSUE REPAIR

## Introduction

The intent of the repair process is to attempt to restore the healing injured tissue to its optimal function. Healing and repair are intricately connected. Throughout this chapter, examples of cell types and healing processes within various organs and systems of the body have been discussed. Some organs are composed of cells that cannot regenerate (e.g., heart, CNS, or peripheral nervous system cells), whereas other organs such as the liver and epithelial cells of the integumentary and GI systems can replace missing tissue through cell division (mitosis). Some cells such as skeletal muscle cells and renal cells do not divide but can be induced to undergo mitosis. The extent to which cells can regenerate depends on the type of cell (e.g., permanent, stable, labile), the cell's ability to divide, the type of damage incurred (e.g., lethal, sublethal), and other factors discussed (e.g., nutrition, age, immunocompetency, vascular supply, or presence of microorganisms leading to infection).

Also, it is important to note that advances in the fields of biotechnology and biomaterials are providing new techniques for regeneration or repair of tissue lost to injury, disease, or aging. Bioengineered tissues including skin, bone, articular cartilage, ligaments, and tendons are under investigation for clinical use.[13,119,145]

Using an example of a person with TBI who also experiences MI, healing of brain and myocardial tissue was discussed earlier in this chapter (see "Special Implications for the Therapist 6.1: Cell Injury"). In this final section, only tissues not specifically included in the main body of this chapter are discussed further.

## Lung

After lethal injury to alveolar cells (type I and II pneumocytes), regeneration can occur only when the basement membrane remains intact. After the phagocytic removal of the necrotic cells, adjacent living epithelial cells migrate onto the remaining basement membrane and differentiate into type II pneumocytes (cells that primarily produce surfactant). Eventually, some of these cells differentiate into type I pneumocytes (cells that permit gas exchange), and full lung function is restored. If the damage to the lung disrupts the basement membrane, healing must be achieved by repair, which is characterized by fibrosis and scar formation—epithelial cells that may be dysfunctional.[24] Also, certain injurious agents such as inhalation of asbestos can trigger the formation of scar tissue, leading to restrictive lung disease.

## Digestive Tract

The healthy gut is lined with multiple rows of villi structures. These finger-like projections are responsible for nutrient absorption and the production of digestive enzymes. Gut cells grow single file from the base of the villi up toward the top. They slough off into the intestinal tract and pass out of the body every 5 days or so. Damaged or injured cells are constantly leaving, whereas healthy cells renew the GI environment. It takes about 3 to 4 weeks for a complete turnover of all gut cells throughout the digestive tract.

Because two-thirds of all immune system function and 90% of serotonin function take place in the gut, healing the gut can assist in bringing both of these functions back into balance. Serotonin is needed to produce melatonin, which is an essential component for good, restful sleep; the proper amount of circulating and functioning serotonin is also needed to stabilize mood.[60]

## Peripheral Nerves

When a nerve is cut, the peripheral portion rapidly undergoes myelin degeneration and axonal fragmentation. The lipid debris is removed by macrophages mobilized from the surrounding tissues in a process referred to as *wallerian degeneration*. Within 24 hours of section, new axonal sprouts from the central stump are observed with proliferation of Schwann cells from both the central and the peripheral stumps.

Careful microsurgical approximation of the nerve may result in reinnervation, especially those with gaps less than 3 mm.[59] The most important factor in achieving successful nerve regeneration after repair is the maintenance of the neurotubules (basement membrane and connective tissue endoneurium), along which the new axonal sprouts can pass.[40]

## Skeletal Muscle

Skeletal muscle is composed of contractile and connective tissue elements. Actin and myosin myofilaments make up the sarcomere units of muscle fibers. Each individual myofiber is surrounded by a delicate sheath called the *endomysium* (basement membrane) and then arranged in bundles. Satellite cells surround the muscle fibers and are important for tissue regeneration following injury. The greater the degree of muscle injury, the larger the amount of connective tissue that is disrupted.[36]

Contrary to widespread belief, muscle tissue can regenerate, but the restoration of normal structure and function is strongly dependent on the type of injury sustained. In *severe infections*, the muscle fibers may be extensively destroyed. However, the sarcolemmal sheaths (basement membrane and connective tissue endomysium) usually remain intact, and rapid regeneration of muscle cells within the sheaths occurs so that the function of the muscle may be completely restored.

After *transection of a muscle*, muscle fibers may regenerate either by growth from undamaged stumps or by growth of new, independent fibers.[40] Again, this type of regeneration after lethal cell injury to skeletal muscle fibers is possible when the basement membrane remains intact through mitotic division of satellite cells. Satellite cells play an integral role in normal development of skeletal muscle and are essential to the repair of injured muscle by serving as a source of myoblasts for fiber regeneration. These proliferating satellite cells support the process of regeneration either by combining with other myogenic cells causing the development of new fibers or by fusing with remaining muscle fibers.[232]

*A muscle that is contused* or *strained* has the capability to repair itself, but the period of recovery is markedly prolonged and results in strength losses. At the conclusion of the healing process, the repaired site shows a high rate of reinjury.[46,113] Recovery is largely dependent on the severity of the injury but follows the same phases of degeneration, inflammation, regeneration, and fibrosis described in this chapter.

As with all healing, muscle fiber injury is regenerated or repaired through a consistent sequence of events that go into motion as soon as an injury occurs. Hemostasis with hematoma formation and inflammation overlap in the first phase, starting in the first 24 to 48 hours after injury. This phase is followed by phagocytosis with the removal of detritus, activation of satellite cells, and subsequent myofiber regeneration. This second phase can last 6 to 8 weeks after injury. The final phase involves tissue remodeling. This phase is characterized by complete reorganization and maturation of the regenerated muscle.[47,113,143]

With death of the muscle cell and ensuing necrosis, chemotactic agents attract macrophages within the basement membrane confines to engulf the remnants of the dead cell. Macrophages release growth factors, stimulating the division of the satellite cells. These cells migrate to the central region and begin to differentiate into expressing the usual characteristics of a skeletal muscle fiber. This healing process can occur after lethal cell injury (e.g., muscular dystrophy) when the connective tissue matrix (primarily basement membrane) is disrupted and regeneration is attempted. However, disruption of basement membrane leaves the satellite cells no place to set up and multiply.

The end result is that the muscle tissue heals by forming a connective tissue scar (i.e., repair). This at least maintains the structural integrity of the tissue but not the complete functional capability. This type of healing of muscle (repair versus regeneration) could occur after the trauma of a motor vehicle accident or a knife wound.

The complete recovery of injured skeletal muscle appears to be further hindered by fibrosis, which begins during the second week after muscle injury. The formed scar tissue that replaces the damaged muscle fibers is disorganized and therefore has decreased ability to withstand tensile forces. The result is that these repaired muscles have a higher risk of injury.[142]

## Bone

Bone is composed of two types of tissue: cortical and cancellous (trabecular). Cortical bone accounts for approximately 80% of skeletal tissue. It is the tough outer layer of bone, is densely packed, and surrounds trabecular or cancellous bone. The remaining 20% is cancellous bone, which consists of spongy, intermeshing thin plates (trabeculae) that are in contact with the bone marrow. Bone has two surfaces, referred to as *periosteal* (external) and *endosteal* (internal).

Loss of bone occurs when there is an imbalance between destruction and production of bone cells or when there is a defective mineralization of bone matrix. An increase in osteoclasts or failure of osteoblasts to assemble can result in bone resorption faster than bone is being built up.

A variety of conditions can affect bone and require a reparative process, including fracture, infection, inflammation (e.g., tuberculosis or sarcoidosis), metabolic disturbances (e.g., Paget disease, osteoporosis, or osteogenesis imperfecta), tumors, response to implanted prostheses, bone infarction, and any other systemic diseases that have skeletal manifestations (e.g., sickle cell disease, amyloidosis, or hemochromatosis). For a discussion of these specific conditions and their impact on bone, the reader is referred to each individual chapter that includes those diseases. Only the bone response to injury and the reparative process (specifically fracture) will be discussed in this chapter.

### Fracture Healing and Repair

Fracture repair is a healing process by regeneration and remodeling (i.e., without a scar) and with the potential for a return of optimal function in many cases. After an uncomplicated fracture, bone heals in similar overlapping phases previously discussed in this chapter (Fig. 6.26). At the moment bone injury occurs, secondary to fracture, tiny blood vessels through the haversian systems are torn at the fracture site. A brief period of local internal bleeding occurs, resulting in a hematoma around the fracture site called a fracture hematoma. Bleeding from

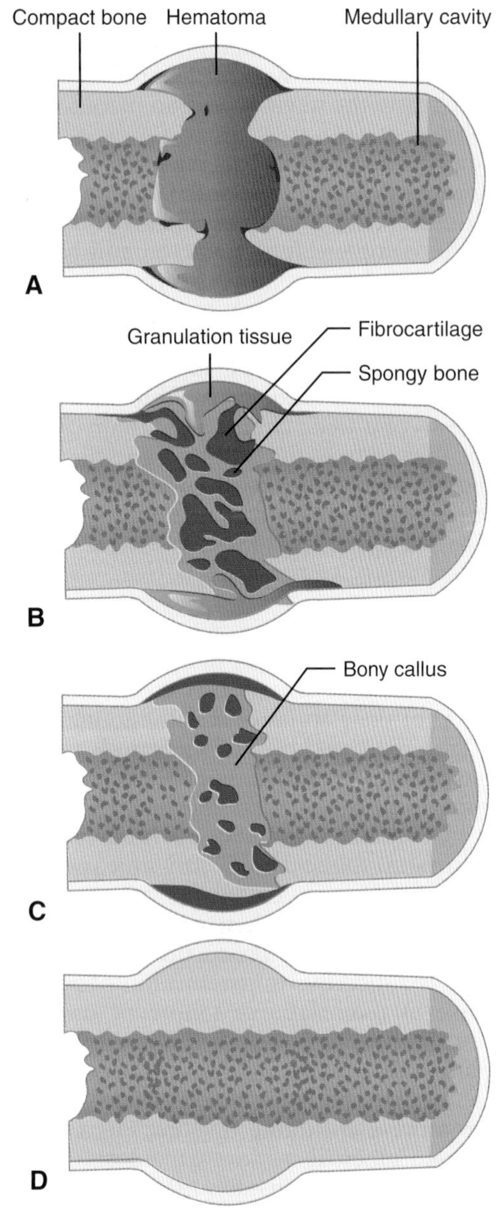


**Figure 6.26**

**Fracture healing occurs in overlapping stages or phases.** (A) Immediate vascular response with hematoma formation and inflammatory response. (B) Granulation tissue and fibrocartilage formation during early reparative phase. (C) Fibrocartilaginous union (soft callus) is replaced by a fibro-osseous union (bony callus). (D) Remodeling phase with complete restoration of the medullary canal. (From Damjanov I: *Pathology for the health-related professions*, ed 4, St. Louis, 2012, Elsevier.)

the fracture site delivers fibroblasts, platelets, and osteoprogenitor cells, which secrete numerous growth factors and cytokines. They stimulate transformation of the initial hematoma into a more organized granulation tissue, eventually promoting callus formation.

The *inflammatory phase* occurs as inflammatory cells arrive at the injured site, accompanied by the vascular response and cellular proliferation. Clinical evidence of this phase includes pain, swelling, and heat.

Clotting factors from the blood initiate the formation of a fibrin meshwork. This meshwork is the scaffolding for the ingrowth of fibroblasts and capillary buds around and between the bony ends. By the end of the first week, phagocytic cells have removed most of the hematoma, and neovascularization and initial fibrosis are occurring.

The *reparative phase* begins during the next few weeks and includes the formation of the soft callus seen on radiographs about 2 weeks after the injury, which is eventually replaced by a hard callus. During this phase, osteoclasts (bone macrophages) clear away the necrotic bone while the periosteum and endosteum regenerate and begin to differentiate into formation of hyaline cartilage (soft callus) and primary bony spicules (hard callus). Bone growth factors including bone morphogenetic proteins, fibroblast growth factor, insulin-like growth factors, platelet-derived growth factor, transforming growth factor β, and vascular endothelial growth factor are major components of the fracture healing (reparative) phase.[65]

Once the callus is sufficient to immobilize the fracture site, repair occurs between the fractured cortical and medullary bones when the fibrocartilaginous union (soft callus) is replaced by a fibro-osseous union (hard callus). The process is called enchondral ossification. Delayed union and nonunion fractures result from errors in this phase of bone healing. The completion of the reparative phase (usually occurring between 6 and 12 weeks) is indicated by fracture stability. Radiographically, the fracture line begins to disappear.[111]

The *remodeling phase* begins with clinical and radiographic union (no movement occurs at the fracture site) and persists until the bone is returned to normal, including restoration of the medullary canal. During this phase, which may take months to years, the immature, disorganized woven bone is replaced with a mature organized lamellar bone that adds further stability to the fracture site. The excessive bony callus is resorbed, and the bone remodels in response to the mechanical stresses placed on it.

In the normal adult skeleton, approximately 10% to 30% of the bone is replaced or remodeled to replace microfractures from stress and maintain mineral balance. Bone remodeling is carried out by bone cells, including osteoblasts, osteoclasts, and osteocytes. Osteoblasts produce the bone matrix and initial bone mineralization, while osteoclasts resorb bone. Osteocytes detect local mechanical loading and send signals to the surface osteoblasts to initiate bone remodeling.[8]

The time for overall bone healing varies depending on the bone involved, the fracture site and type, treatment required (e.g., immobilization versus surgical repair, the need for bone grafting or use of bone graft substitutes), degree of soft tissue injury, treatment complications, and other factors mentioned previously (e.g., age, vascular supply, nutritional status, or immunocompetency). New biotechnologies have resulted in new approaches to facilitate repair in cases of insufficient bone regeneration.[64,243] The physical therapist should be aware of how these new approaches affect rehabilitation management. Specific types of fractures, their treatment, and special implications for the therapist are discussed in greater detail in Chapter 27.

## Tendons and Ligaments

Tendons and ligaments are dense bands of fibrous connective tissue composed of 78% water, 20% collagen, and 2% glycosaminoglycans. This composition allows them to sustain high unidirectional tensile loads, transfer forces, provide strong flexible support, and help the tissue respond to normal loads while resisting excessive mechanical or shearing forces and deformation. The viscoelastic characteristics of these tissues make them capable of undergoing deformation under tensile or compressive force yet still capable of returning to their original state after removal of the force. Both are made up of parallel fibers of type I collagen produced by fibroblasts/fibrocytes, glycosaminoglycans/proteoglycans, a small vascular supply, and sensory innervation. The mechanical properties of tendons and ligaments are dependent not only on the architecture and properties of the collagen fibers but also on the proportion of elastin that these structures contain (e.g., minimal elastin in tendons and ligaments of the extremities, substantial elastin in the ligamentum flavum). Also, thicker tendons with higher collagen content have more tensile strength.

### Tendon Injury and Healing

It has been reported that when forces are applied rapidly and obliquely, tendons have the highest risk for rupture. Another significant risk for tendon rupture is the presence of degenerative changes in the tendon itself because tensile strength is decreased under degenerative conditions.[210]

In the case of acute injury and tendon rupture, tendons may heal either as a result of proliferation of the tenoblasts from the cut ends of the tendon or more likely as a result of vascular ingrowth and proliferation of fibroblasts derived from the surrounding tissues that were injured at the time of the tendon injury. Because the surrounding tissues contribute so much to the healing of a tendon, adhesions are very common. With rupture of the Achilles tendon, rotator cuff tendons, or cruciate ligaments, functional restoration requires surgical repair to appose and suture the cut ends.[40]

The healing and reparative processes progress through the same three overlapping phases as other tissues: hemostasis and inflammation, cellular proliferation and matrix deposition, and long-term remodeling. Hemostasis begins immediately, followed by the inflammatory process, which begins during the first 72 hours (3 to 5 days) after injury and/or surgical intervention.

*Hemostasis* occurs as platelets from blood plasma enter the tear to initiate clot formation. Fibrin and fibronectin form cross-links with collagen fibers to form a fragile bond, which helps reduce hemorrhage. The activity of phagocytic cells clears away the debris in the area from damaged and devitalized tissue. Chemotactic mediators attract inflammatory WBCs to the area, including polymorphonuclear leukocytes and monocytes.

The *inflammatory phase* overlaps and transforms into the *proliferative phase,* which usually occurs 2 to 3 weeks after tendon injury or repair but can begin as early as 48 hours after injury.[41] Granulation tissue is formed by the migration and proliferation of fibroblasts and vascular buds from the surrounding connective tissue. Capillary sprouts grow out of blood vessels around the edges of the wound-forming loops by joining with each other or with capillaries already carrying blood. The new blood vessels enhance delivery of nutrients to the healing tissue. While this is occurring, the fibroblasts are secreting soluble type III collagen molecules, which form fibrils. A new extracellular matrix is formed. In this step, the original fibrin clot and scaffolding are replaced with more permanent repair tissue.

Approximately 2 weeks into the healing process, the collagen fibrils are oriented and rearranged into thick bundles, providing the tissue with greater strength. During this period, the affected area remains immobilized to relieve stress from the healing tissue and prevent rupture recurrence. The lack of stress causes the newly forming collagen to be deposited in random alignment without the formation of cross-links. The immature collagen is randomly oriented and has limited strength.

Now the transition from the proliferative phase to the *maturation phase* takes place. The maturation and remodeling phase begins around week 3 after the initial injury. The immature type III collagen is replaced by mature type I collagen; the latter aligns along tensile forces. The collagen is continually remodeled until permanent repair tissue is formed that is oriented along the lines of stress and organized to provide increasing resistance to stretch and tearing.[233] On the basis of animal models, we know that tendon healing takes at least 12 to 16 weeks to reach a level at which the tendon can be stressed.[163]

When the healing tissue has achieved adequate integrity, motion is permitted once again. The remodeling collagen then aligns to the lines of stress produced by the motion, thereby permitting the healed tendons and ligaments to provide support in line with the stress. Realignment of collagen to its usual parallel arrangement also permits the restoration of full, normal range of motion after repair. The tensile strength of lacerated and repaired tendons was only 40% to 60% of healthy intact tendon.[102] Human tendons and ligaments regain normal strength in 40 to 50 weeks postoperatively; this means that even as long as a year after injury, the tendon or ligament may not have achieved premorbid tensile strength.

Although the process of healing is by repair (formation of a connective tissue scar), this constitutes regeneration because tendons and ligaments are originally composed of connective tissue. However, the scar tissue is weaker and larger and has compromised biomechanical integrity with an increased amount of minor collagens (types III, V, and VI), decreased collagen cross-links, and an increased amount of glycosaminoglycans.[108] These changes lead to impaired function, increased risk of reinjury, and increased risk of osteoarthritis.

Healing of intrasynovial tendon injuries is complicated by the formation of adhesions between the tendon and surrounding synovial sheath. It has been postulated that adhesions result from the infiltration of tenocytes from the surrounding tissue to the site of the injured tendon, thereby attaching to the site.[210] In hand injuries, range of motion can be limited because adhesions disrupt normal tendon gliding. Adhesions account for about one-fourth of fair to poor functional outcomes following tendon repairs.[251]

*Tendinopathy,* a term used to denote clinical conditions with pain and pathologic changes, includes both tendinitis (implying an inflammatory process) and tendinosis, a degenerative process with little or no inflammation but histopathologic changes in the collagen matrix. Overuse and chronic overload with repetitive microtrauma are the most common etiologic risk factors.[210]

Chronic tendon disorders are usually caused by overuse. There are many theories to explain the exact mechanism by which tendons are injured under conditions of overuse (e.g., mechanical or overload theory, neural theory, vascular insufficiency theory, and exercise-induced hyperthermia theory).[195] Clearly, load applied has a major effect on location of tendon injuries. Older age, female sex with hormone fluctuations, and decreased joint motion and tendon/muscular flexibility seem to contribute to the problem.[195] Achilles tendon ruptures have been reported with the use of a particular family of antibiotics (quinolones) and with prolonged use of steroids. Running or training on concrete surfaces will also increase the risk of tendon problems, especially of the patellar (knee) tendon.

### Ligament Injury and Healing

Sprains and tears of the tendinous or ligamentous structures around a joint can be caused by abnormal or excessive joint motion. These injuries can be classified as first-, second-, or third-degree injuries, depending on the changes in structural or biomechanical integrity (ranging from injury of a few fibers without loss of integrity to a complete tear).

Common sites for this type of injury include the ankle, knee, and fingers, with clinical manifestations of local pain, edema, increased local tissue temperature, ecchymosis, hypermobility or instability, and loss of motion and/or function. After injury, if the therapist notes quick onset of joint effusion, and the joint feels hot to the touch with extremely painful and limited movement, the joint needs to be examined by a physician to rule out hemarthrosis.

In many extraarticular ligaments (e.g., medial collateral ligament [MCL]), healing occurs by the same basic phases described in the previous section (i.e., hemorrhage, inflammation, repair, and remodeling). However, there is variation in the manner in which ligaments heal; some intraarticular ligaments (e.g., ACL) have a poor healing response. After the ligament ruptures, the thin synovial sheath is disrupted and blood dissipates, preventing clot and hematoma formation. Healing cannot take place without a foundation for repair or localization of chemotactic cytokines and growth factors.[186]

Studies have revealed that after injuries, ligament tissues such as the ACL release large amounts of matrix metalloproteinases. These enzymes have a devastating effect on the healing process of the injured ligaments. Matrix metalloproteinases are critically involved in the extracellular matrix turnover, which may help explain one of the reasons repair of the injured ACL is minimal. In addition, matrix metalloproteinase activity is less in the MCL, which may account for the difference in healing capacities between the MCL and the ACL.[227]

The remodeling phase of ligament healing consists of a continuous cycle of collagen synthesis and degradation with the intent of generating a ligament that is as close to normal as possible. This process can take months to years, and evidence exists that the replacement tissue is similar to scar tissue and does not have the histologic and biomechanical properties of a normal ligament.[105]

Moreover, the quality of the repaired tissue has been found to also depend on the load and stresses subjected to the ligament during the healing process. On one hand, returning to aggressive high-impact sports activities too soon in the healing process will subject the ligament to excessive amounts of load and stress, thereby risking ligament failure. On the other hand, too little load and stress brought about by prolonged immobilization will result in a very inferior ligament and delayed healing process. Immobilization during the healing phase leads to significant decreases in failure load at 6 to 14 weeks after ligament injury. Joint laxity is a clinical problem brought about by an inferior ligament healing process and increases the risk of reinjury to the structure. These findings reinforce the clinical importance of early mobilization in ligament injuries.[167,231]

Another potential hindrance to healing is the use of NSAIDs. Animal studies demonstrated decreases in load to failure in healing ligaments when NSAIDs were used in the first 2 weeks following injury.[245] As mentioned earlier, an important component of healing is the initiation of the inflammation process mediated by prostaglandins. Therefore as NSAID use blocks the production of prostaglandins, the healing process is impaired. It is thus recommended that individuals use NSAIDs judiciously during the healing process.[105]

## Cartilage Injury and Healing

Several forms of cartilage are recognized. Articular cartilage is found at the ends of the bones; fibrocartilage is found in the menisci of the knee, at the annulus fibrosus, at the insertions of the ligaments and tendons into the bone, and on the inner side of tendons as they angle around pulleys (e.g., at the malleoli); and elastic cartilage is found in the ligamentum flavum, external ear, and epiglottis (Table 6.7).

Articular cartilage has many individual zones that make up the whole (Fig. 6.27). It is composed of hyaline cartilage made up of water (75%), chondrocytes, type II collagen (20%), and glycosaminoglycans/proteoglycans (5%). It is aneural, avascular, and alymphatic and does not appear to regenerate well after adolescence, most likely because of its avascularity and low cell-to-matrix ratio. Proteoglycan, produced by the chondrocytes and secreted into the matrix, is responsible for the compressive strength of cartilage. It binds growth factors and traps and holds water used to regulate matrix hydration.

Ideal conditions for healing of articular cartilage require a source of cells, provision of matrix, removal of stress concentration, and intact subchondral bone plate with some mechanical stimulation. Following cartilage injury, the normal inflammatory process that involves the migration of repair cells to the site is impeded because the articular cartilage lacks the vascularization to bring these cells to the area.[166] Therefore in adults without intervention, the healing of articular cartilage occurs by fibrous

**Table 6.7** Types of Cartilage

| Types of Cartilage | Location |
|---|---|
| Articular (hyaline) | Joint surfaces; bone apophyses; epiphyseal plates; costal cartilage (ribs); fetal skeleton |
| Fibrocartilage | Tendon and ligament insertion; meniscus; disc |
| Elastic | Trachea (epiglottis); earlobe; ligamentum flavum |
| Fibroelastic | Meniscus |

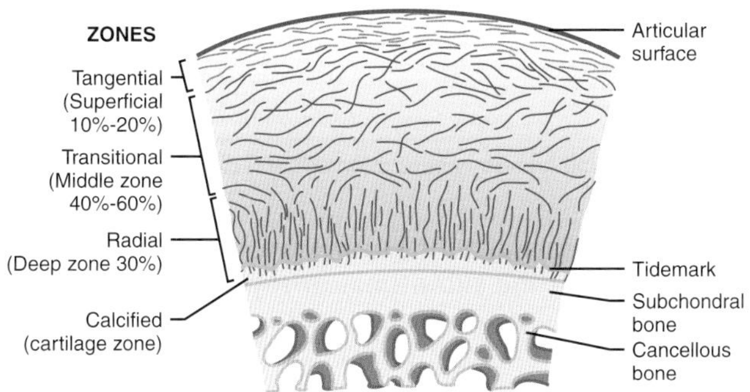


**Figure 6.27**

**Zones of cellular distribution in adult articular cartilage.** The superficial tangential zone comprises type II collagen fibers that are oriented tangentially to the surface, providing the greatest ability to resist shear stresses. The transitional (middle) zone is composed primarily of proteoglycans, but collagen fibers present are arranged obliquely to provide a transition between the shearing forces of the surface layer and the compression forces in the cartilage layer. The radial (deep) zone includes collagen fibers that are attached vertically (radial) into the tidemark; this zone distributes loads and resists compression. The tidemark zone is located in the calcified zone. The tidemark is the line that straddles the boundary between calcified and uncalcified cartilage; it separates hyaline cartilage from subchondral bone. The calcified zone is a layer just above subchondral bone containing type X collagen. Subchondral bone and cancellous bone are the final two zones.

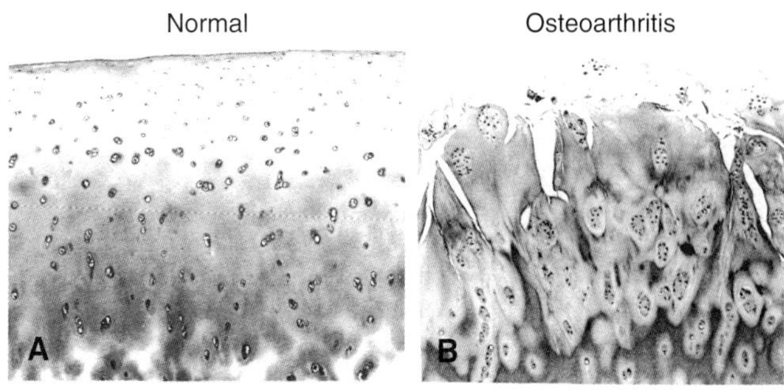


**Figure 6.28**

**Histologic sections of normal (A) and osteoarthritic (B) articular cartilage obtained from the femoral head.** The osteoarthritic cartilage demonstrates surface irregularities, with clefts to the radial zone and cloning of chondrocytes. (From Harris ED: *Kelley's textbook of rheumatology*, ed 7, Philadelphia, 2005, Saunders.)

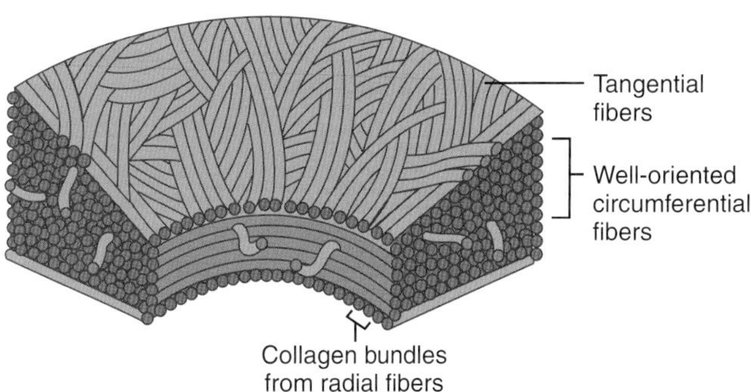


**Figure 6.29**

**Diagrammatic representation of the distribution of collagen fibers in the meniscus of a knee.** Collagen is oriented throughout the connective tissues in such a way as to maximally resist the forces placed on these tissues. Most of the type I collagen fibers in the meniscus are circumferentially arranged, with a few fibers on or near the tibial surface placed in a radial pattern. This structural arrangement enables the meniscus to resist the lateral spread that occurs during high compressive loads generated during weight bearing. Longitudinally arranged collagen fibers facilitate shock absorption and sustain the tension generated between the anterior and posterior attachments. (From Bullough PG: *Bullough and Vigorita's orthopaedic pathology*, ed 3, St. Louis, 1997, Mosby.)

scar tissue or fails to heal at all. This replacement tissue does not function as well as the original, and the adjacent joint surface can be affected.

Fibrous scarring of the articular cartilage leads to local degenerative arthritis (Fig. 6.28). This is the reason several treatment approaches designed to repair cartilage healing induce the formation of precursor cells to the injured area to assist healing. For example, microfracture techniques to enhance chondral resurfacing have made it possible to stimulate the formation of a durable repair cartilage cap over the lesion, thereby facilitating cartilage healing and repair.[193,217,222]

## Menisci (Knee)

The menisci are fibrocartilaginous structures consisting of cartilage bundles composed mainly of collagen, although proteins such as elastin and proteoglycan are also present. The amount of proteoglycan increases dramatically in the injured, degenerate meniscus. Water accounts for 70% of meniscal composition, contributing to the meniscal function of joint lubrication. Water in the menisci also provides resistance to compressive loads. Collagen constitutes up to 70% of the dry weight; 90% of it is type I collagen fibers, with types II, III, V, and VI present in much smaller amounts.[100] In young individuals, the menisci are usually white, translucent, and supple on palpation. In older individuals, the menisci lose their translucency, become more opaque and yellow in color, and become less supple.

The cells of the meniscus sometimes are called fibrochondrocytes because of their appearance and the fact that they synthesize a fibrocartilaginous matrix. The principal orientation of collagen fibers in the menisci is circumferential, designed to disperse compressive load, resist shear, aid in shock absorption, and withstand the circumferential tension within the meniscus during normal loading (Fig. 6.29). A few small, radially oriented fibers present on the tibial surface probably act as ties to resist lateral splitting of the menisci from undue compression.

At birth, the entire meniscus is vascular; by age 9 months, the inner one-third has become avascular. By

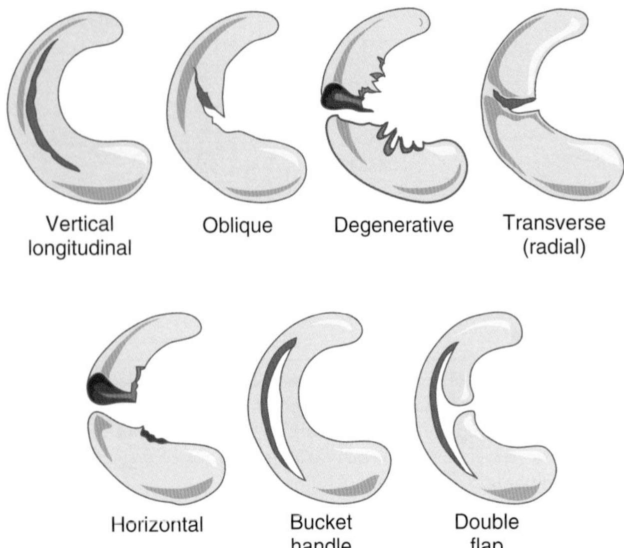


**Figure 6.30**

**Classification of most common meniscal tears.**

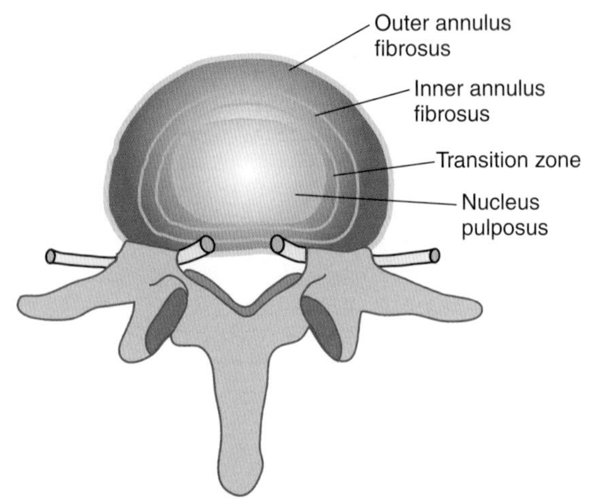


**Figure 6.31**

**Zones of the adult human lumbar intervertebral disc.**

adulthood, only the outer 10% to 30% of vascularity remains, with blood supplied via the perimeniscal capillary plexus off the superior and inferior medial and lateral genicular arteries.[209] Blood supply to the meniscus flows from the peripheral to the central meniscus principally through diffusion or mechanical pumping (movement).[13,190]

Meniscal tears heal by migration of cells from the synovial membrane adjacent to the meniscus. The remodeling events of the healing process remain unknown. Healing of meniscal tears may be inhibited based on the location of the tear; less vascular locations have less vigorous healing capability.

Similarly, nerve fibers originating in the perimeniscal tissues radiate into the outer one-third of the menisci. Nerves in the densely populated anterior and posterior horns play a proprioceptive role in protecting the joint through reflexive neuromuscular control of joint motion and loading.[94,100]

Injury and degeneration leading to laceration are the two most common causes of symptoms that require surgical intervention.[40] The presence of clinical symptoms of pain, swelling, locking and catching, and loss of motion often requires surgical intervention. Proper management depends on the type of tear and its location (Fig. 6.30).[100] Meniscectomies cause alterations in the biomechanical functioning of the menisci, causing alterations in the normal loading mechanism of the joint and ultimately increasing the risk for development of osteoarthritis.

## Synovial Membrane

The synovial membrane lines the inner surface of the joint capsule and all other intraarticular structures (e.g., subcutaneous and subtendinous bursae sacs, tendon sheaths), with the exception of articular cartilage and the meniscus. Synovial membrane consists of two components: the intimal (cellular layer or synoviocytes) layer next to the joint space and the subintimal or supportive layer made of fibrous and adipose tissue.

The synovial membrane has three principal functions: secretion of synovial fluid hyaluronate, phagocytosis of waste material, and regulation of the movement of solutes, electrolytes, and proteins from the capillaries into the synovial fluid. This latter function provides a regulatory mechanism for maintenance of the matrix through various chemical mediators such as ILs.

Injury to any of the joint structures affects the synovium and results in hemorrhage, hypertrophy, and hyperplasia of the synovial lining cells and mild chronic inflammation.[40] In the case of prolonged, chronic synovitis, such as occurs in hemophilia, abnormal synovial fluid, joint immobilization, and fibrous adhesions, a progressive destructive condition in the joint can result.

Any type of immobilization leads to contraction of the capsule. Loss of glycosaminoglycans with the associated water loss further increases capsule stiffness and results in decreased joint motion. The synovial membrane lining the inside of the capsule hypertrophies and forms adhesions between itself and the adjacent articular cartilage.[168]

## Disc and Disc Degeneration

The intervertebral disc sits between each pair of vertebrae and is made of connective tissue (collagen fibers) that helps the disc withstand tension and pressure (Fig. 6.31). The disc is made of three zones: (1) the outer annulus fibrosus, a lamellated ring of alternately obliquely oriented, densely packed type I collagen fibers that insert onto the vertebral bodies; (2) the fibrocartilaginous inner annulus fibrosus, consisting of a type II collagen fibrous matrix; and (3) the viscoelastic central nucleus pulposus with type II collagen fibers along with various mucopolysaccharides and a high concentration of proteoglycans.[15] This composition supports the high water content of the nucleus, which behaves biomechanically as a fluid cushion that transmits loading forces to the outer annulus fibrosus as well as to the vertebral endplate.[188]

The nucleus is held in place by the *annulus,* a series of strong ligament rings surrounding it. The annulus is primarily composed of type I collagen arranged in multiple concentric layers. This fiber arrangement allows the annulus to resist tensile, radial, and torsional forces. With acute trauma or degenerative changes and microtrauma over time, the fibers of the annulus may be disrupted.[188] The blood supply of the normal disc is restricted to the peripheral outer annulus. The blood vessels of the vertebral body lie directly against the endplates but do not enter the disc itself. The nutrition of the more centrally located disc cells is derived from diffusional and convection transport of nutrients and wastes through the porous solid matrix.[15] The metabolism of the avascular disc is so slow that the turnover of proteoglycans takes 20 years.[226]

Although the nucleus has no nerve supply, the outer third of the annulus is innervated, receiving supply from both the sinuvertebral nerve, which innervates the posterior and posterolateral regions, and the gray ramus, which is distributed primarily anteriorly and laterally. More recent studies have confirmed that the annulus is a source of pain in people with chronic low back pain.[220]

### Aging and Disc Degeneration

Our intervertebral discs change with age and demonstrate degenerative changes relatively early in life because of their large size and poor vascular supply. Cell senescence in the disc has been linked with degenerative disease, with more senescence of cells in the nucleus pulposus compared with the annulus fibrosus in individuals with herniated discs.[199]

Disc degeneration follows a predictable pattern. First, the nucleus in the center of the disc begins to lose its ability to absorb water. This occurs as a result of a decrease in cell density in the disc that is accompanied by a reduction in synthesis of cartilage-specific extracellular matrix components such as type II collagen.[89]

As the proteoglycan content of the disc decreases, a loss of water-binding capacity by the disc matrix occurs, and the disc becomes dehydrated. Then the nucleus becomes thick and fibrous so that it looks much the same as the annulus. As a result, the nucleus is not able to absorb shock as well. Routine stress and strain begin to take a toll on the structures of the spine. Tears called *fissures* form around the annulus. In addition to these, continued compressive forces to the spine due to inactivity, weight gain, poor posture, and poor tone of the muscles supporting the spine further slow the ability of the disc to heal.[220] As the disc weakens, it starts to collapse, and the bones of the spine compress.

Along with the pathology of degeneration, changes in the extracellular matrix content affecting collagen fibers can reduce the load-bearing capacity of the disc. Calcification of the vertebral endplates is another factor thought to contribute to disc degeneration. Alterations in permeability adversely affect chondrocyte metabolism. The passage of nutrients and waste products across the endplate depends on fluid flowing into the disc during the night while we rest and flowing out during the day when we move about.[89]

Injury to the disc (herniation) is more likely in the morning soon after waking, when the nucleus pulposus is maximally hydrated after a prolonged period of rest. Vigorous early morning activities increase the vertical load beyond the strength of the collagen in the annulus. Other proposed risk factors for lumbar disc herniation include lifting heavy loads, torsional stress, strenuous physical activity, and occupational driving of motor vehicles.[3,15]

Conditions such as a major back injury or fracture can affect how the spine works, making the changes occur even faster. Daily wear and tear and certain types of vibration can also speed up degeneration in the spine. In addition, strong evidence suggests that smoking speeds up degeneration of the spine. Scientists have also found links among family members, showing that genetics play a role in how fast these changes occur.

**SPECIAL IMPLICATIONS FOR THE THERAPIST 6.6**

### *Specific Tissue or Organ Repair*

Therapists have an important role in the rehabilitation of acute injuries. Certain components of the inflammatory process must be controlled quickly for recovery to proceed. For example, if edema is a component of a joint injury, it must be controlled as quickly as possible. Studies have demonstrated that joint edema can inhibit or hinder local muscle activity, which could result in altered joint mechanics and further irritation.[85] The anticipated goals are to facilitate healing of the injured structure and maintain the normal function of noninjured tissue and body regions. The overall goal of the rehabilitation program is to return the person to normal activity as soon as possible, yet not so fast that irritation and further inflammation of the injured area occur. A fine line exists between maximizing activity and overdoing the activity to the point of injury aggravation.

Client education is essential regarding the injured individual's role in facilitating tissue healing. Adherence to weight-bearing guidelines, avoiding aggravating movements, applying ice appropriately, and performing the prescribed exercises are key to the recovery process.

Recent studies have further clarified the role of exercises prescribed by physical therapists in the promotion of tissue repair from a cellular standpoi nt.[131,137,141] The mechanical loading brought about by appropriate exercise prescription produces a consequent cellular response that promotes changes in the tissue structure. This process, called *mechanotransduction,* has been shown in many studies to promote healing of tendon, muscle, articular cartilage, and bone. For example, physical loads brought about by shear or compressive forces during exercise perturb the cells. This physical perturbation results in a variety of intracellular and intercellular chemical signals. In muscles and tendons, these chemical signals could result in the upregulation of growth factors that facilitate healing and repair. Loading of mechanosensitive cells in the articular cartilage (chondrocytes) and bone (osteocytes) has also been postulated to promote tissue growth via the same processes.[131] The concept of transegrity and mechanotransduction (transegrity is discussed earlier in the text) could also explain the positive effects of other physical therapy interventions such as soft tissue mobilization.[116,212]

Lastly, advances in the fields of biotechnology and biomaterials are providing new techniques for regeneration or repair of tissue lost to injury, disease, or aging. Bioengineered tissues including skin, bone, articular cartilage, ligaments, and tendons are under investigation for clinical use.[119,120]

### Prevention

Appropriate rehabilitation is necessary for soft tissue injuries, especially severe muscle strains and frank rupture of any tendon or muscle. Return to full activity, especially high-impact sports, can (and often does) result in recurrence of injury. Injury prevention should include addressing issues such as muscle fatigue, weakness, and lack of flexibility. Stronger muscles are better able to absorb energy and thereby limit the magnitude of tissue stretch. In other words, muscle strengthening is an important way to avoid muscle strain. The value of stretching before activity continues to be a controversial topic. Although some studies have shown that a warm-up program that includes stretching may reduce strain injuries, more studies are needed to confirm this relationship.[156]

### Rehabilitation of Repaired Soft Tissues

Careful monitoring of the timeline for tissue recovery, observing presenting signs and symptoms, and monitoring response to specific activities, movements, and treatments could guide the therapist in deciding when and how to progress intervention and activity level. The type of tissue involved also makes a difference because tendon tear/repair requires a period of rest to avoid disrupting the healing process and subsequent reinjury, whereas prolonged rest and immobilization after muscle strain can result in unwanted consequences such as stiffness. This monitoring can also be taught so the client understands the limits of his or her condition.

The process is somewhat more difficult with acute back or neck injuries than with peripheral injuries. Owing to the depth of the tissues of the spine, increased temperature and erythema are not always present or palpable if present. It is important for the therapist to pay close attention to the degree of pain, changes in movement limitation, and possible presence of protective muscle tone in deciding when the program can be progressed.

If the repair process involves sutures, the therapist must remember that as a general guideline for tissue healing, during the inflammatory phase after injury or surgery (first 3 to 5 days), the ability of the soft tissue (e.g., tendon, ligament, or muscle) to hold sutures is at an all-time low. Protected rest is imperative during this stage. The next stage involves gradually increasing tensile force on the healing tissue. An incremental approach that is slow enough to allow and promote the stages of proliferation, maturation, and fiber realignment while at the same time being mindful of the deleterious effects of inactivity (such as the development of adhesions, stiffness, or muscle atrophy) is important to optimize the healing process and return the individual to optimal function at the soonest possible time.

### Tendon or Muscle Rupture

During the proliferative phase (usually 5 to 28 days after tendon injury/repair), controlled passive movement is allowed. The repaired tissue is kept protected to avoid excessive force. Passive range of motion is continued as healing progresses and until the tissue moves into the remodeling phase of healing (around 4 to 8 weeks after injury/repair). Aggressive early motion that stresses the repair and exceeds the mechanical strength of the repair should be avoided. During the early weeks of the remodeling phase, the force required to rupture a lacerated and repaired tendon can be less than the force generated by a maximum muscle contraction. These findings suggest that maximum muscle contraction forces should be avoided for at least 8 weeks after tendon repair; the therapist can expect to see significant tendon weakness for a considerable period afterward.[41]

Active range of motion is then initiated with controlled movements (e.g., gravity-eliminated positions). The idea is to prevent excessive resistance from the weight of the limb while still working on gradually increasing the force of the muscle contraction. As the repair strengthens, the therapist can allow increased muscle force through increased antigravity movements.[41]

Resistance with weights, rubber tubing, elastic bands, and so on is not started until at least 8 weeks after the repair. Once again, resistance is increased progressively (between 8 and 12 weeks). At the end of 12 weeks, if there have been no complications (e.g., infection, wound dehiscence) and there are no comorbidities to delay healing (e.g., tobacco use, diabetes, peripheral vascular disease), full force muscle contraction can be tolerated.

In terms of the muscle, surgical repair of a complete muscle tear has its own protocol. Clinicians must be aware that muscle repair is difficult, as the muscle fibers do not hold sutures well.[36] More importantly, guidelines for nonsurgical and postoperative rehabilitation for ligament, tendon, and muscle tear/repair vary based on geographic regions and physician preferences and protocols and are reported widely in the literature. The plan of care should always be based on an understanding of the healing stages of injured tissue. As mentioned previously, the goal is to restore motion and strength without subjecting the healing tissue to excessive forces that may hinder healing or rupture the repair.

Health promotion, injury prevention, and risk reduction are important roles of the physical therapist. Clinicians have the responsibility of educating patients on risk factors that predispose an individual to soft tissue injuries to prevent the onset of injuries or recurrence of the condition if an injury is sustained.

### Muscle Injury

Muscle injuries including contusion, strain, and laceration are common injuries, occurring particularly in sports; about 90% of all muscle injuries are either contusions or strains. A muscle *contusion* occurs when the muscle is subject to a sudden, heavy compressive force such as a direct blow to the muscle. Muscle *strains* occur when excessive tensile force leads to overstraining of the myofibers.[122] This is more likely to occur during eccentric contraction when the muscle is lengthening because tension is greater than the muscle's resistance to stretch; the resultant forces are large. Muscles that cross two joints (e.g., hamstrings or gastrocnemius) are especially vulnerable to stretch injury because they are simultaneously affected by angular positions and velocities of the adjacent joints.[36]

The most common site of strain injury is the myotendinous junction, a region of highly folded basement membranes between the end of the muscle fiber and the tendon. These involutions maximize surface area for force transmission. The transition from compliant muscle fibers to relatively noncompliant tendon may account for the vulnerability of the myotendinous junction. If the force of stretch on a muscle is too great to be resisted by the contractile unit, resistance shifts from the contractile unit to the connective tissues. Pathogenic stretch (passive or active) that is beyond the threshold length of the entire musculotendinous unit can result in disruption at the myotendinous junction. Complete tears do occur but less often than muscle strain.[36]

Recovery from severe muscle strain may begin with a short period of immobilization and application of appropriate electrotherapeutic and physical agents to provide pain relief and protect the tissue during the initial phase of healing. Immobilization followed by mobilization of muscle may help muscle fiber regeneration and fiber orientation with reduced scar formation.[121,127] As soon as pain and swelling subside, a program can be initiated to recover range of motion, strength, and endurance. Return to sports is considered safe when there is 80% return of strength compared with the noninvolved side.[133]

### Modalities

Physical therapy modalities such as thermotherapy (application of heat and cold) and electrical modalities such as transcutaneous electrical nerve stimulation, iontophoresis, and ultrasound may be used to manage pain and limited motion, but their impact on the underlying tear and healing tissue is not fully known. In his text, Belanger[25] clearly articulates the evidence behind the use of these modalities according to the phases of tissue healing. The reader is advised to consult this text for an in-depth discussion of the evidence. As an example, although there is evidence supporting the use of cryotherapy in minimizing wound bleeding, it must be applied immediately after the injury for it to be effective.[25] Also, cryotherapy when applied within the first 24 to 48 hours of the injury is effective in reducing the consequent tissue damage following the inflammatory process.[25] Several modalities may be used to promote the development of new blood vessels, repair cells in the proliferative stage, and enhance remodeling with the intent of optimizing functional gains in the maturation phase. Examples of these modalities have been included in the respective sections that discuss the healing process for each type of tissue.

### Motor Control and Muscle Inhibition

As mentioned previously, injury to the muscle and the consequent repair and healing process causes alterations in movement patterns. Chronic pain could be a complication of the healing process and may also be a factor in abnormal movement. Neurophysiologic adaptation to chronic pain appears to result in changes in motor control and muscle recruitment strategies. Recent research has also documented the role of cortical reorganization in abnormal movement patterns related to chronic pain following a musculoskeletal injury.[169] Physical therapy interventions that are aimed at altering these abnormal cortical representations may be beneficial for individuals with chronic pain and abnormal motor control. New information regarding muscle injury and repair, pain, and movement mirrors this complex relationship and highlights the interaction of multiple body systems in the production of movement.[109]

### Medications

A significant percentage of people coming to outpatient therapy clinics are taking salicylates or NSAIDs.[33] These medications can play a key role in recovery from an acute injury, facilitating the therapist's role and clinical decision making. The common clinical practice to administer NSAIDs should be limited to early symptom control during the early phases of tissue healing. Prolonged NSAID use may be counterproductive for the biologic healing process, because complete tissue recovery involves delicate and finely coordinated elements of cellular and metabolic inflammatory reactions, which can be interrupted by NSAIDs.[158,180] Moreover, because NSAIDs also help control pain, patients may put more strain on the injured tissue (because of lack of pain), thereby exacerbating the injury and delaying the healing process.[245]

Considering the widespread use of salicylates and NSAIDs, therapists must also be aware of potential side effects that would warrant communication with a physician. Irritation of the GI system is the most common potential side effect. The risk of developing peptic ulcer disease increases significantly if someone is taking more than one of these types of drugs. This pattern of drug use exists in the therapy population, in which significant numbers of subjects are taking one or more over-the-counter antiinflammatory agents along with a prescribed NSAID.[32]

### Tissue Response to Immobilization or Decline in Joint Mobility

In addition to having an important role in the rehabilitation of acute injuries, therapists often deal with clinical problems secondary to the effects of immobilization. Although not traumatic in the classic sense, immobilization of a limb or joint can result in significant impairment and activity limitations.

Immobilization takes a variety of forms including bed rest, casting or splinting of a body part, and non–weight-bearing status of a lower extremity. On a tissue level, significant changes can occur with immobilization (Table 6.8). Besides the inert joint structures, changes also occur in muscle, particularly a loss of strength. Such changes can occur without injury, which magnifies the importance of maintaining function in noninjured tissue and body areas. A rehabilitation program should be designed to address the needs of each of the tissues.

As previously mentioned, prolonged immobilization negatively impacts tendon and ligament healing. During immobilization, the lack of strain and loading on these tissues will cause corresponding decreases in the cross-sectional area and strength of these tissues, resulting in joint hypermobility and laxity. With restoration of loading and movement, these deleterious effects are reversed.[255] The therapist must therefore initiate mobilization activities as soon as safely possible to counter these negative effects.

The use of orthotic devices such as braces has been a common intervention to prevent reinjury of individuals who have either deficient or reconstructed ligaments. Although results of studies on the use of knee bracing to prevent ligament injuries have been mixed, there is some evidence that knee bracing provides 20% to 30% greater ligament protection,[198] increased strain relief for the MCL, increased knee stiffness, and perception of the ability of the brace to protect and/or affect performance.[37]

**Table 6.8** Effects of Prolonged Immobilization

| Tissue | Results of Immobilization |
|---|---|
| Muscle | Atrophy; decreased strength; contracture; reduced capillary-to-muscle fiber ratio; reduced mitochondrial density; reduced endurance |
| Bone | Generalized osteopenia of cancellous and cortical bone |
| Tendons and ligaments | Disorganization of parallel arrays of fibrils and cells; increased deformation with a standard load or compressive force |
| Ligament insertion site | Destruction of ligament fibers attaching to bone; reduced load to failure |
| Cartilage | Adherence of fibrofatty connective tissue to cartilage surfaces; loss of cartilage thickness; pressure necrosis at points of contact where compression has been applied |
| Synovium | Proliferation of fibrofatty connective tissue into joint space |

Continued

### Stiffness

Muscle stiffness is a common problem with advancing age. As humans get older, the elasticity of muscle decreases, owing to connective tissue changes involving the musculotendinous unit. Small amounts of fibrinogen (produced in the liver and normally converted to fibrin to serve as a clotting factor) leak from the vasculature into the intracellular spaces, adhering to cellular structures. The resulting microfibrinous adhesions among the cells of muscle and fascia cause increased muscular stiffness. Activity and movement normally break these adhesions; however, with the aging process, production of fewer and less efficient macrophages combined with immobility for any reason result in reduced lysis of these adhesions.[187]

Other possible causes of aggravated stiffness include increased collagen fibers from reduced collagen turnover, increased cross-links of aged collagen fibers, changes in the mechanical properties of connective tissues, and structural and functional changes in the collagen protein. Stiffness related to impairments in tissue extensibility may respond well to a regimen of application of heat[87] followed by low-load, long-duration stretching.[81] Age-related muscular stiffness could be improved by increased physical activity and movement. A general conditioning program for the older adult will not only result in improved mobility and decrease muscular pain but also improve cardiovascular performance and overall health.

### Deep Venous Thrombosis

While initiating rehabilitation after immobilization, the therapist must remain vigilant for the possible presence of deep vein thrombosis (DVT). A potential complication of DVT is pulmonary embolus, which represents one of the leading causes of morbidity and mortality and is reported to account for 10% of hospital deaths.[150] Although a large percentage of clients with DVT are asymptomatic, severe local pain and edema, fever, chills, and malaise all are possible manifestations. The types of immobilization that carry the risk of DVT include bed rest; a limb being placed in a cast or splint; and non–weight-bearing status following a lower extremity injury, a surgical procedure, or a long car or plane ride. In terms of interventions for DVT, studies have shown that early mobilization does not increase the risk of developing pulmonary embolism[236] in people with DVT.

### Special Note on Regenerative Rehabilitation

There has been an increased focus on the implications of advances in regenerative medicine in physical therapy. Regenerative medicine is an emerging medical practice area that seeks to identify approaches that could potentially replace, repair, or regenerate organs and tissues. These new treatments further deepen our understanding of alternative repair and healing mechanisms in human tissues and organs. Within the PT profession, the FiRST Initiative (Frontiers in Rehabilitation Science and Technology) seeks to clarify the role of regenerative rehabilitation in optimizing movement and function in individuals. For further information, please see the article by Wolf[249] and the proceedings of the FiRST Initiative lecture series during the American Physical Therapy Association (APTA) 2014 NEXT Conference. The APTA website also provides an overview of genetics in physical therapy (http://www.apta.org/genetics/). This webpage contains additional links pertaining to regenerative rehabilitation.

**Table 6.8** Effects of Prolonged Immobilization—cont'd

| Tissue | Results of Immobilization |
|---|---|
| Menisci | Adhesions of synovium villi; decreased synovial intima length; decreased synovial fluid hyaluronan concentrations; decreased synovial intima macrophages |
| Joint | *0–12 weeks:* Impaired range of motion; increased intraarticular pressure during movements; decreased filling volume of joint cavity<br>*After 12 weeks:* Force required for the first flexion-extension cycle is increased more than 12-fold |
| Heart | Reduced strength of contraction (SV); reduced maximal cardiac output; reduced endurance; increased work of the heart for a submaximal load |
| Lung | Reduced airway clearance of mucus; increased likelihood of pneumonia; reduced maximal ventilatory volume |
| Blood | Reduced hematocrit and plasma volume; reduced endurance and temperature regulation |

*SV*, Stroke volume.

## REFERENCES

To enhance this text and add value for the reader, all references are included in the enhanced ebook on Student Consult that accompanies this textbook. The reader can view the reference source and access it online whenever possible.

CHAPTER 7

# The Immune System

EDILBERTO ALCANTARA RAYNES • VANCE POUNDERS IV

## FOUNDATIONS OF THE IMMUNE SYSTEM

### Cells of the Immune System

The immune system is comprised of a number of cells. These groups of cells belong to three broad groups: the innate immune system, the adaptive immune system, or a combination of both systems. The innate immune system includes monocytes, neutrophils, eosinophils, basophils, mast cells, and natural killer cells. The adaptive immune system includes B and T cells or lymphocytes. The T cells of the adaptive immune system can be further divided into helper T cells and cytotoxic T cells. Finally, the immune system has macrophages and dendritic cells that play a role in both the innate and adaptive immune system. In the succeeding sections, the different cells of the immune system are discussed.

### Hematopoietic Stem Cells

In order to understand how the cells of the immune system work, one must understand their lineage. The erythrocytes, leukocytes, and thrombocytes are collectively termed formed elements of the blood system. These formed elements are all differentiated from a common lineage, the hematopoietic stem cell. Although these formed elements are extensively discussed in the Hematologic System (Chapter 14), it is worth recalling some of the formed elements that participate in the immune system.

The hematologic stem cell produces myeloid stem cells and lymphoid stem cells. The myeloid stem cells further differentiate into myeloblasts, which eventually mature into basophils, eosinophils, and neutrophils. On the other hand, the lymphoid stem cells differentiate into lymphoblasts and eventually mature into either B or T lymphocytes or cells (Fig 7.1).

#### Neutrophils

Neutrophils are small, short-lived cells produced in bone marrow and are the predominant leukocytes of the peripheral blood. Neutrophils are also referred to as polymorphonuclear cells (PMNs) due to their segmented nucleus, which has three to five lobes. They increase dramatically in number in response to infection and inflammation. Neutrophils can be classified as both phagocytes and granulocytes. During phagocytosis, bacteria and debris are engulfed and digested by certain molecules contained within the neutrophils.

Primary granules of neutrophils possess myeloperoxidase and cationic proteins, whereas their secondary granules contain lysozyme and lactoferrin. Although these factors allow neutrophils to effectively kill invading pathogens or threats, damage is sometimes done to host tissues in the process. Neutrophils die after phagocytosis; the accumulation of dead neutrophils and phagocytosed bacteria contributes to the formation of pus. Importantly, neutrophils are the first cells to arrive at sites during acute inflammation and constitute a major line of defense against pus-forming bacteria such as *Neisseria, Staphylococcus,* and *Streptococcus.*

#### Monocytes and Macrophages

Monocytes are large, long-lived cells with a bilobed nucleus that originate in bone marrow. Monocytes circulate in the blood; when they migrate into tissues in response to infection and inflammation, they mature into residing *macrophages*, which means "large eaters."

After neutrophils kill the invading organism and the process of phagocytosis begins, macrophages appear to "filter" the debris produced by the neutrophils and kill any damaged, but not dead, bacteria or bacteria that are too large for neutrophils to eliminate. Phagocytosis of bacteria by neutrophils and macrophages depends on cell-surface receptors, including scavenger receptors, mannose receptors on macrophages, and receptors for complement components.

Macrophages also play an important role in removing other cells such as aged red blood cells or dead neutrophils. Macrophages ingest bacteria and are able to digest bacteria into components. After ingestion, they take and place a peptide (antigen) on their major histocompatibility complex (MHC) class II complex, essentially expressing the bacteria they ingested. T helper cells (CD4+) then read this complex and respond accordingly. Further information on MHC is discussed in another section of the chapter.

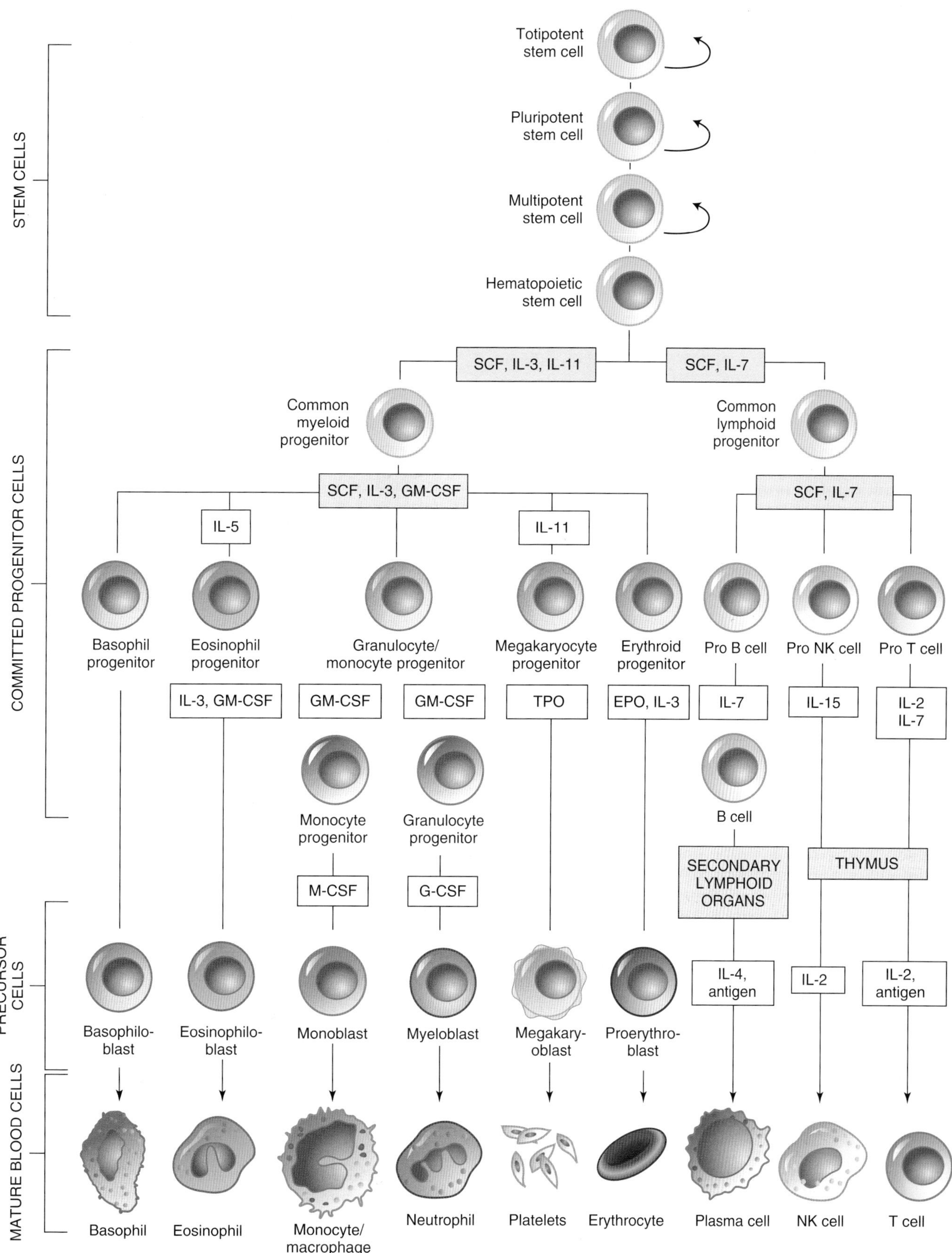


**Figure 7.1**

**Differentiation of hematopoietic cells.** (From McCance KL, Huether SE: *Pathophysiology: the biologic basis for disease in adults and children*, ed 8, St Louis, MO: Elsevier, 2019.)

### Eosinophils

*Eosinophils* are the next group of leukocytes that participate in innate immunity. Eosinophils are derived from bone marrow and are involved in both allergic responses and parasitic infections. When invading organisms are too large for neutrophils and macrophages to eliminate, eosinophils surround the pathogen and release the contents of their granules to induce membrane damage and subsequent death. The granules contain histamine, heparin, and cytokines. Histamine is an important vasodilator, heparin acts as an anticoagulant, and cytokines have a role in inflammatory reactions.

### Basophils and Mast Cells

*Basophils* are granulocytes that circulate in peripheral blood and release active substances from their cytoplasmic granules, which play a major role in certain allergic responses. Basophils and mast cells are located close to blood vessels throughout the body and have similar functional characteristics.

*Mast cells* possess granules containing histamine and other molecules that dilate blood vessels when released. Antihistamines function by neutralizing the histamines and reducing this type of excessive immune (allergic) response. These cells are derived from stem cells and are released into the blood in an undifferentiated form. They differentiate when they enter tissues and are usually found in small numbers in the connective tissue of organs. In addition to playing a major role in allergy and anaphylaxis, they participate in wound healing and are important for defense against invading pathogens.

Basophils and mast cells increase the blood supply in the area where a pathogen is located. This increase in circulation helps to recruit more phagocytes to the site of infection. Increased circulation is typically accompanied by the feeling of congestion during an allergic reaction.

### Erythrocytes and Thrombocytes

Erythrocytes and thrombocytes (also called platelets) have an important role in the immune system. Platelets are important for thrombosis and hemostasis, and they have surface receptors that interact with bacteria.[77] Overall, the responsibility of the erythrocytes and platelets is movement and removal of antigens, antibodies, and portions of the complement system.

### Lymphocytes (B and T Lymphocytes)

Lymphocytes are key cells that play an important role in adaptive immunity. The two broad groups of lymphocytes are T lymphocytes and B lymphocytes. B lymphocytes are cells that mature in the bone marrow and produce antibodies in reaction to antigens. The antibodies of B cells have the ability to neutralize invading pathogens. T lymphocytes are produced in the bone marrow but mature in the thymus and consist of two types: helper T cells and cytotoxic T cells.

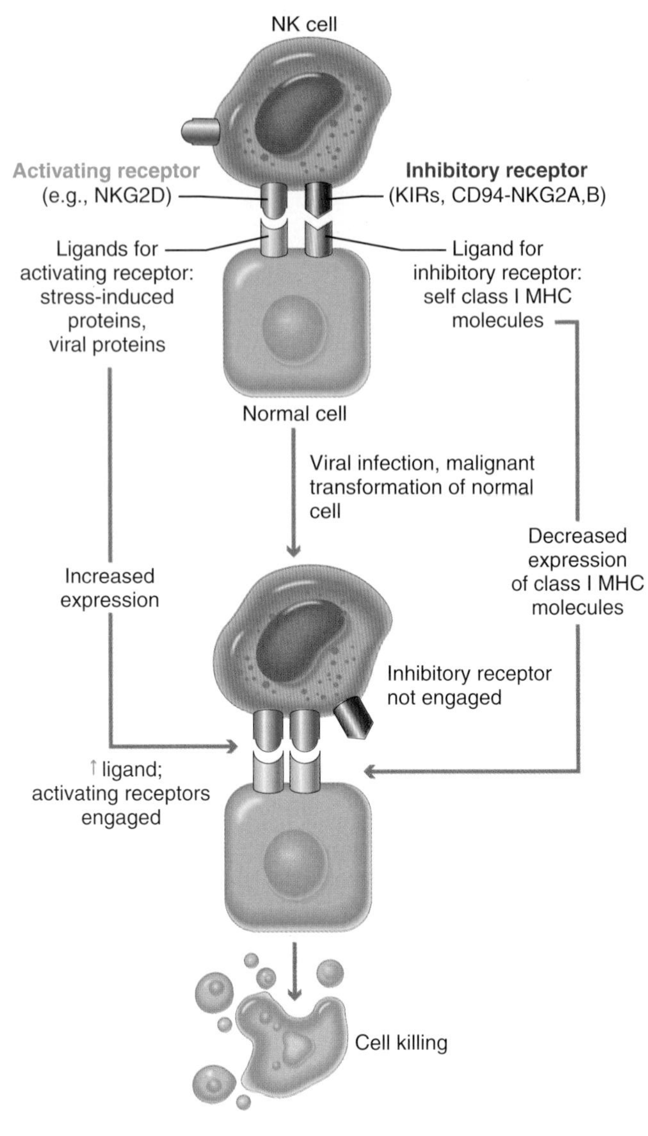


**Figure 7.2**

**Schematic of NK cell receptors and cell killing.** NK cells express activating and inhibitory receptors; some examples of each are indicated. Normal cells are not killed because inhibitory signals from normal major histocompatibility complex class I molecules override activating signals. In tumor cells or virus-infected cells, there is increased expression of ligands for activating receptors and reduced expression or alteration of major histocompatibility complex molecules, which interrupts the inhibitory signals, allowing activation of NK cells and lysis of target cells. (Reprinted from Kumar V: *Robbins and Cotran: pathologic basis of disease,* ed 8, Philadelphia, 2009, WB Saunders.)

## Natural Killer Cells

Natural killer (NK) cells are large, granular lymphocytes that are distinct from T cells and B cells. Mature populations of NK cells found in the blood and spleen are localized to infected tissues in response to inflammatory cytokines. The function of NK cells is to kill cells infected with viruses and other intracellular pathogens, as well as tumor cells. Unlike T cells and B cells, NK cells do not express antigen-specific receptors. Instead, NK cells express activating and inhibitory receptors on their surfaces that interact with ligands on the target cell. Effector functions associated with NK cells include cytotoxicity and cytokine production[153] (Fig. 7.2). When activated, proteins contained within the cytoplasmic granules of NK cells are released onto the surface of a cellular target. These granules create pores in the plasma membrane of the infected cell, allowing other proteins to enter and activating a programmed death cascade. NK cells also collaborate with the adaptive immune system in the process of antibody-dependent cellular cytotoxicity (ADCC).

Cytokines such as TNFα and IFNγ produced by NK cells are important for the recruitment and activation of macrophages that are able to phagocytose and kill pathogenic microbes, as well as secrete additional cytokines, chemokines, and antimicrobial effector molecules. The cytokine milieu produced early during infection is extremely important for the initiation of adaptive immunity and greatly influences the nature of these responses.

## Mononuclear Phagocytes and Granulocytes

*Phagocytes* participate in innate immunity by readily ingesting pathogens, such as bacteria or fungi, and killing them in order to protect the body against infection. The two principal families of phagocytes are *neutrophils* (a component of granulocytes) and *monocytes* (a component of nongranulocytes). Both neutrophils and monocytes are leukocytes. Granulocytes are short-lived (2–3 days) compared to monocytes and macrophages, which may persist for months or years.

Neutrophils, eosinophils, basophils, and monocytes are classified as phagocytic leukocytes that function in innate immunity. A large decrease in the absolute numbers of these cells in the blood is the principal cause of susceptibility to infection in people treated with intensive radiotherapy or chemotherapy. These treatments suppress the bone marrow, resulting in deficiencies of these phagocytic cells. It is important to know if clients are receiving any type of treatment that could lower their immune system response.

## Antigen Presenting Cells

There are three major antigen presenting cells (APCs), namely: macrophages, dendritic cells, and B cells. Their purpose is to display an antigen to a T cell in order to activate it. This enables the body to see and react to antigens that the body is exposed to.

### Macrophages

Macrophages ingest bacteria and are able to digest the bacteria into components. They then take and place a peptide (antigen) on their MHC class II complex. Essentially, they express the bacteria that they ingested. T helper cells (CD4+) recognize this complex and respond accordingly.

### Dendritic Cells

These cells are called "dendritic" because they possess projections that give them a dendrite-like appearance. Their purpose is to capture protein antigens and present them to T cells. These types of APCs are typically found in areas exposed to the external environment. These cells also present the antigen on an MHC class II complex and are recognized by T Helper cells (CD4+).

### B Cells

As discussed previously, B cells are important in the antibody mediated immune system or the humoral immunity. These cells also use MHC class II complex and present the antigen to T helper cells (CD4+) but through receptor-mediated endocytosis instead of through phagocytosis.

### The Major Histocompatibility Complex

Parallel to the discussion on APCs, major histocompatibility complex (MHC) molecules are membrane proteins that function to present antigenic peptides for recognition by T cells. MHC molecules were first identified as transplantation antigens because immunologic reactions against antiserum or skin grafts were traced to MHC differences between donors and recipients. In cases of graft rejection, the T cells of the recipient recognize the donor's MHC/peptide complexes as foreign antigens. Conversely, graft-versus-host disease occurs when the T cells from donor tissue mount immune responses against the host MHC/peptide. It is now known that the principal function of MHC molecules is to present peptides derived from protein antigens to T cells possessing distinct specificity for a particular epitope.

The MHC locus is a collection of genes that are present in all mammals. MHC proteins found in humans are known as human leukocyte antigens (HLAs) because of the discovery that these molecules could be identified with specific antibodies. The linked genes of the HLA loci are located on the short arm of chromosome 6. Because of their close proximity, these genes are typically inherited as a group or block known as a *haplotype*. The MHC genes are highly polymorphic, meaning that there are alternative forms of genes or alleles that exist among different people in a particular population.

The three polymorphic MHC class I genes in humans, designated HLA-A, HLA-B, and HLA-C, encode antigen presentation complexes that are expressed on almost all nucleated cells. Because each individual inherits one set of paternal genes and another set of maternal genes, each cell can express six different MHC class I molecules. Unlike MHC class I and class II genes, MHC class III genes do not encode antigen presentation complexes; but rather, secreted proteins associated with immune processes, including complement system, soluble serum protein, and tumor necrosis factors.

Certain MHC alleles have been associated with a statistically significant increase in the incidence of autoimmune diseases. Although these diseases occur more frequently among persons who express a particular MHC/HLA, no HLA allele is associated with disease in 100% of the cases. Therefore, MHC/HLA is likely to be only one of the contributing factors involved in disease development. Finally, Class I and class II MHC molecules are very similar in terms of molecular structure. Both MHC class I and class II molecules possess four immunoglobulin domains and a peptide binding groove that is large enough to accommodate small antigenic peptides (Fig. 7.3).

There are two major antigen-processing pathways: the endogenous (cytosolic) pathway and the exogenous (endocytic) pathway. The endogenous pathway generally presents antigens from cytosolic sources, whereas the exogenous pathway presents antigens from the

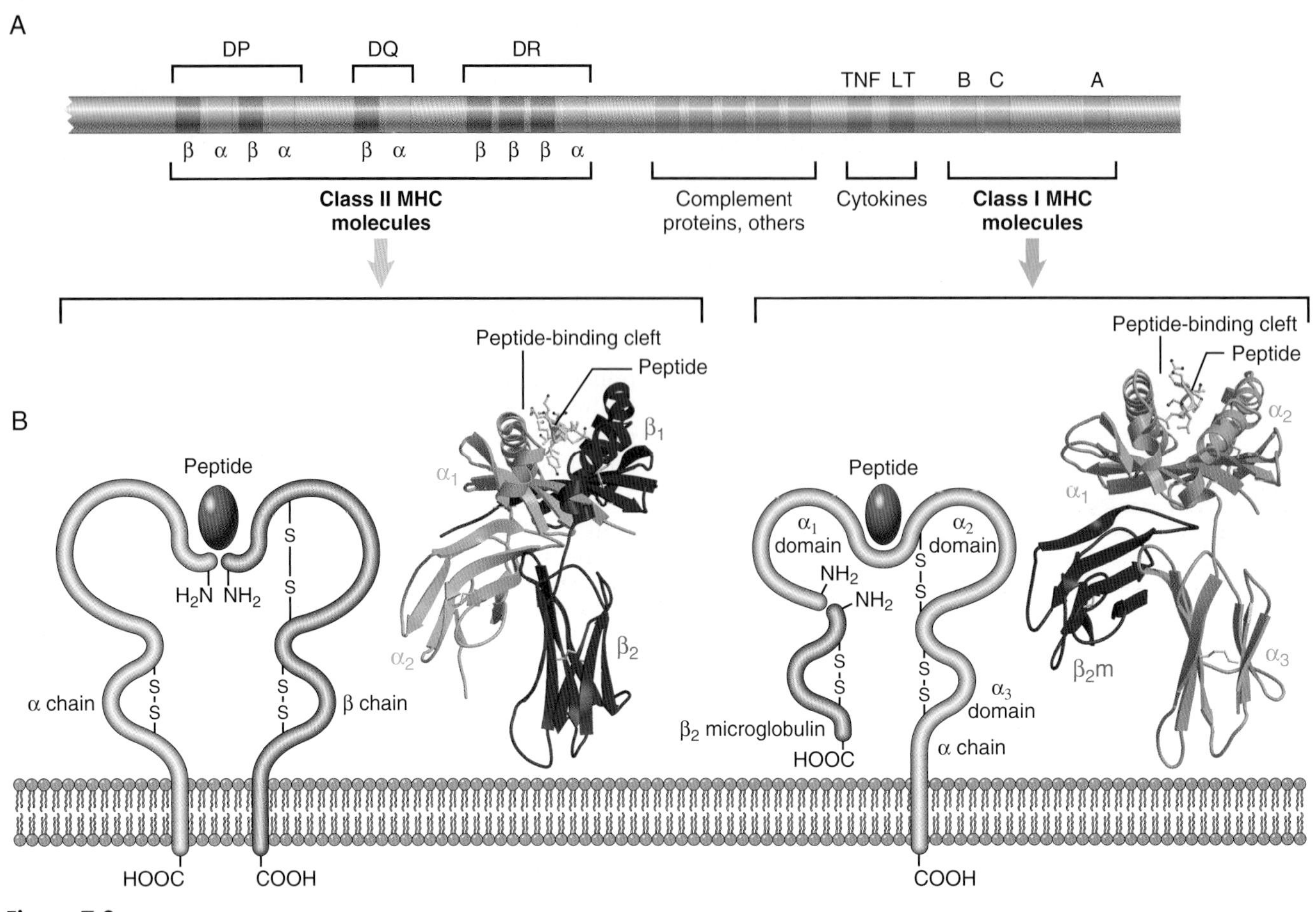


**Figure 7.3**

**The human leukocyte antigen (HLA) complex and the structure of HLA molecules.** (From Kumar V, Abbas AK, Aster JC: *Robbins basic pathology*, ed 10, Philadelphia, 2018, Elsevier. Crystal structures are courtesy of Dr. P. Bjorkman, California Institute of Technology, Pasadena, California.)

extracellular environment. The separation of antigens by source allows for different classes of T cells to recognize antigens from different compartments. In this way, different classes of T cells can respond to both extracellular and intracellular invaders, resulting in a more effectively targeted cellular immune response.

**Major Histocompatibility Class I.** MHC class I molecules are capable of binding constituents of proteins that have been synthesized in the cellular cytoplasm. In theory, any protein (self, viral, bacterial, tumor, etc.) that was generated in cytoplasm of a cell could be expressed on an MHC class I molecule. In this pathway, endogenous antigen (e.g., protein synthesized by a virus replicating within a cell) is broken down in the cytoplasm by a degradation "machine" known as the proteasome. The digested cytosolic protein constituents are then transported into the rough endoplasmic reticulum by the *transporter associated with antigen processing (TAP)*. The MHC class I presentation complex is then loaded with peptide and moves from the rough endoplasmic reticulum through the Golgi apparatus to the plasma membrane. If the protein fragment is distinguished as non-self, the peptide/MHC complex present on the surface of the cell is recognized by cytotoxic CD8+ T cells. Once activated through their T-cell receptor (TCR), the cytotoxic T lymphocytes (CTLs) will destroy the cell presenting foreign antigen.[144]

**Major Histocompatibility Class II.** MHC class II molecules can bind fragments of proteins that have been phagocytized, pinocytosed, or endocytosed from the extracellular environment. Following internalization into the cell, foreign proteins move into intracellular vesicles known as endosomes or phagosomes, which may fuse with lysosomes. Ultimately, these degraded enzymes produce peptide fragments. The peptides then move to the plasma membrane. If the antigenic peptide is distinguished as non-self, this complex on the cellular surface can be recognized by helper CD4+ T cells. Once activated through antigen receptors, CD4+ T cells will produce cytokines that regulate both cellular and humoral immunity.[144]

# HUMAN DEFENSE MECHANISMS

## Types of Immunity

To combat a potential threat, the body uses two major immune responses: innate (natural or nonspecific immunity) and adaptive immunity (acquired or specific immunity) (Fig. 7.4). Innate immunity consists of molecular and cellular defense mechanisms that are present prior to exposure to a threat and function as a first line of defense. If the innate immune response

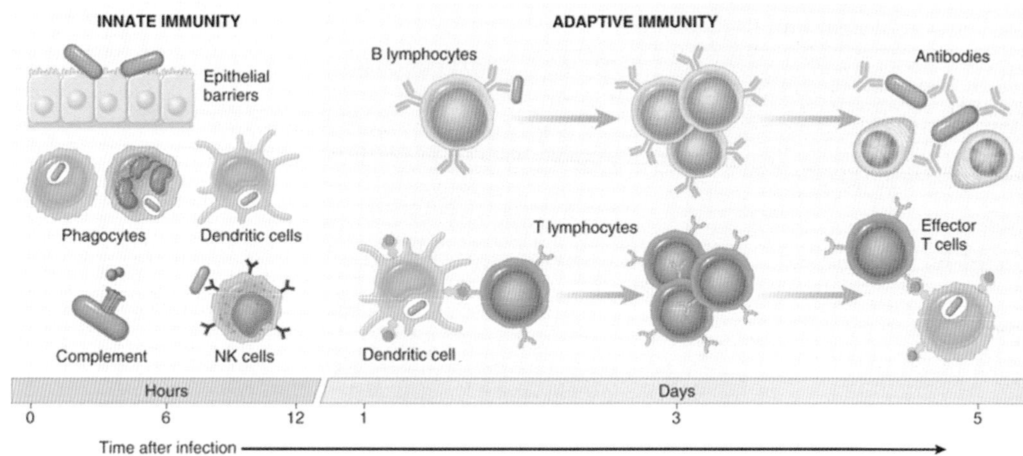


**Figure 7.4**

**The principal mechanisms of innate and adaptive immunity and their development over time.** Physical mechanisms (e.g., epithelial barriers) prevent initial microbial colonization. If the invading microbe breaches this first line of defense, nonspecific innate immune mechanisms (e.g., phagocytes, NK cells, and the complement system) function to eliminate the pathogen. When innate immunity fails to prevent the spread of infection, adaptive immunity serves as a specific and comprehensive third line of defense. The adaptive immune response takes time to develop and is mediated by lymphocytes and their products. The kinetics of these responses may differ, depending on the type of infection. (Reprinted from Kumar V: *Robbins and Cotran: pathologic basis of disease,* ed 8, Philadelphia, 2009, WB Saunders.)

**Table 7.1** Types of Acquired Immunity

| Type of Acquired Immunity[a] | Method Acquired | Length of Resistance |
|---|---|---|
| **Active** | | |
| Natural | Natural contact and infection with the antigen (environmental exposure) | Usually permanent but may be temporary |
| Artificial | Inoculation of antigen (vaccination) | Usually permanent but may be temporary (occasional exceptions) |
| **Passive** | | |
| Natural | Natural contact with antibody transplacentally (mother to fetus) or through colostrum and breast milk | Temporary |
| Artificial | Inoculation of antibody or antitoxin; immune serum globulin | Temporary |

[a]Active immunity occurs when a person produces his or her own antibodies to the infecting organism; passive immunity occurs when the antibody is formed in another host and transferred to an individual.

fails to control and eliminate the pathogen, the adaptive immune response is activated and begins a few days following the initial infection. Moreover, the adaptive immune system can be further classified into humoral and cell-mediated. See Tables 7.1 and 7.2 for an overview of the immune system and its response and on types of acquired immunity.

## The First Line of Defense

### Innate Immunity

*Innate immunity* acts as the body's first line of defense to prevent the entry of pathogens and is capable of resolving most threats. The innate immune system is comprised of early host defense mechanisms that can limit the spread of infection and, in some cases, eliminate the invading pathogen, mediate the initiation and development of adaptive immunity that is pathogen-specific and work in concert with adaptive immune responses to effectively clear a microbial threat.

Certain innate immune defenses are broadly effective against a diverse array of insults, whereas other components are most effective against certain classes of pathogens (e.g., viruses, bacteria, fungi, or parasites). Innate immune system components include external defenses that are present at the site of infection (e.g., physical, mechanical, chemical, and biochemical barriers) and internal defenses (cellular and soluble components). A diverse array of threats that an individual may encounter in his or her lifetime is dealt with by the innate arm of the immune system through recognition molecules that identify patterns common to many different types of pathogens. Therefore, although the innate immune system responds to common features of multiple threats, it has a limited number of specificities. Furthermore, it does not remember the interaction with a specific invader for help during potential future encounters.

### External Defenses

The first line of defense includes the physical, chemical, and mechanical barriers that act nonspecifically and provide protection against all invaders. The purpose of this first line is to limit the ability of an organism to penetrate the host. These physical barriers include the skin and mucus. The next barrier present is the mechanical barrier, which consists of peristalsis, coughing, and sneezing. Finally, the

**Table 7.2** The Immune System and Its Response

| | ADAPTIVE IMMUNITY | |
|---|---|---|
| **Innate Immunity** | **Humoral** | **Cell-Mediated** |
| Nonspecific interaction with different antigens; lacks immunologic memory | Specific interaction with different antigens | Specific interaction with different antigens |
| **Exterior defenses:** | | |
| Skin, mucosa, secretions, nasal hair, ear wax | Mediated by antibody, present as serum globulins | Mediated by T lymphocytes |
| **Phagocytes (leukocytes):** | | |
| Neutrophils (polymorphonuclear neutrophils)<br>Monocytes/macrophages<br>Eosinophils<br>Basophils<br>Mast cells and platelets (inflammation) | Antibodies are produced by plasma cells (differentiated form of B lymphocytes) | Secretion of cytokines<br>Production of helper T cells ($CD4^+$), cytotoxic T cells ($CD8^+$) and regulatory/ suppressor T cells ($CD4^+CD25^+$) |
| **Soluble mediators:**<br>Complement and interferons; see Table 6.5<br>Natural killer cells or large granular lymphocytes | Primary and secondary (memory) antibody response | Primary and secondary (memory) T-cell response |

body has chemical barriers found in the stomach (hydrochloric acid), cerumen, tears, and saliva. Both the tears and saliva contain lysosomes that have degradation enzymes to break down cell walls of microorganisms (Fig. 7.5).

### Internal Defenses

The innate immune system is comprised of many different internal defenses that can be classified as soluble factors (e.g., complement system, cytokines, chemokines, acute phase proteins) and cellular components (neutrophils, monocytes/macrophages, natural killer cells). Cell membrane–bound receptors can also be utilized as effectors (able to neutralize or eliminate the threat). Unlike the finely tuned specificity of adaptive immunity, innate immune system components recognize repeating patterns of molecular structure that are common to certain classes of pathogens. These pathogen-associated molecular patterns (PAMPs) are of limited variability and usually part of structures that are essential to the invading pathogen (e.g., double- and single-stranded viral RNA, endotoxin of Gram-negative bacteria, peptidoglycan in bacterial cell wall, terminal mannose residues of bacterial and viral surface components).[24,269]

The interaction of innate pattern recognition receptors (e.g., Toll-like receptors) with their cognate PAMPs may result in phagocytosis and killing of the pathogen and/or recruitment of immune cells to the site of infection. Upon detection of PAMPs by soluble or membrane-bound pattern recognition receptors, certain immunologic response modifiers are produced that act locally, whereas others travel through the bloodstream and function at distant target sites. These effector molecules may serve to restrict proliferation of the pathogen, recruit and activate additional immune cells to the site of infection, and/or facilitate the development of an adaptive immune response.

Examples of these immune mediators include *cytokines* (soluble proteins or glycoproteins synthesized by a variety of cells that can modify cellular behavior) and *chemokines* (small cytokines that can induce chemotactic migration of leukocytes and enhance inflammation). Local actions of cytokines and chemokines include increased vascular permeability, activation of vascular epithelial tissue, changes in blood flow and white blood cell (leukocyte) migration patterns, and the generation of a chemotactic gradient of leukocytes to the site of inflammation.

Type I interferons (IFN$\alpha$ and IFN$\beta$) are cytokines produced by cells infected with viruses early in infection (usually a few hours), and these cytokines limit the spread of the infection by protecting surrounding (uninfected) cells. Interferons also inhibit tumor growth. Most cells in the body express receptors for type I interferons that, upon ligation by IFN$\alpha/\beta$, signal the host cell to activate or increase the synthesis of large sets of proteins. Although responses may differ depending on the cell type, the result is resistance to viral replication in all cells and the initiation of effector responses to destroy virally infected cells.

**Acute-Phase Response.** An acute-phase response occurs when high levels of proinflammatory cytokines (e.g., interleukin [IL]-1, IL-6, tumor necrosis factor [TNF]$\alpha$) are produced. Systemic effects of proinflammatory cytokines include fever, occlusion of blood vessels, leukocytosis, mobilization of energy from muscle and fat stores, and increased production of acute phase proteins, such as fibrinogen (factor I). Mannose-binding protein and C-reactive protein are other acute-phase proteins that participate in activation of the lectin-associated complement pathway.

## The Second Line of Defense: The Inflammatory Response

Inflammation is a process that requires interplay between cells and tissues. The inflammatory response is important for not only microorganism destruction but also tissue repair and healing. The major components of the inflammatory

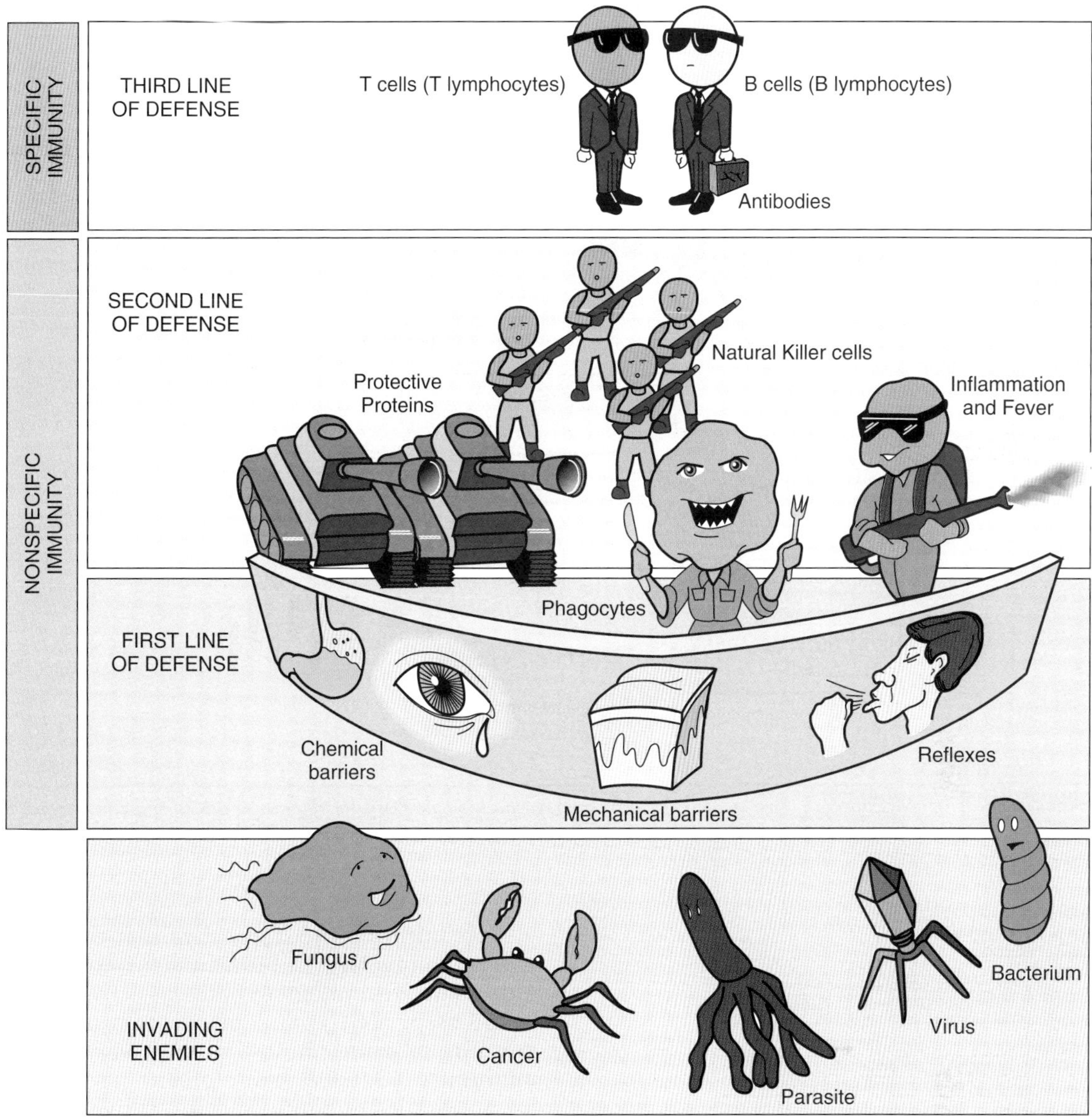


**Figure 7.5**

**Visualization of the body's external defenses.** (From Herlihy BL, Maebius NK: *The human body in health and illness*, ed 1, Philadelphia, 2000, WB Saunders.)

response are the vascular response, the plasma protein system, the complement system (Fig. 7.6), the kinin system (Fig. 7.7), and the clotting system (Fig. 7.8). This chapter briefly discusses the vascular response and the complement system.

## Vascular Response

Injury or infection can activate inflammation in the vascular system. Once this system is activated, a sequence of events is initiated. First, vasodilation occurs to increase blood flow and decrease blood velocity. Accompanied with vasodilation is increased permeability, allowing leakage of fluids and cells. White blood cells begin to accumulate and stick to vessel walls. Eventually, they will migrate across the vessel walls into the tissue, a process known as diapedesis. This mechanism was previously discussed in Chapter 6, but the way it works with the immune system was not clearly identified. This process of increased cellular debris and fluid eventually drains through the lymphatic systems. The lymphatic vessels are an important part of adaptive immunity. After an infection, residual cellular components passing through the lymph nodes help mature the B and T cells of the adaptive immune system.[133]

## The Plasma Protein Systems

There are three important plasma protein systems: the complement, clotting, and kinin systems. These proteins are normally found inactive in the blood. The process of inflammation has the ability to activate these proteins to cause a cascade of events. The clotting and kinin systems were previously discussed in Chapter 6.

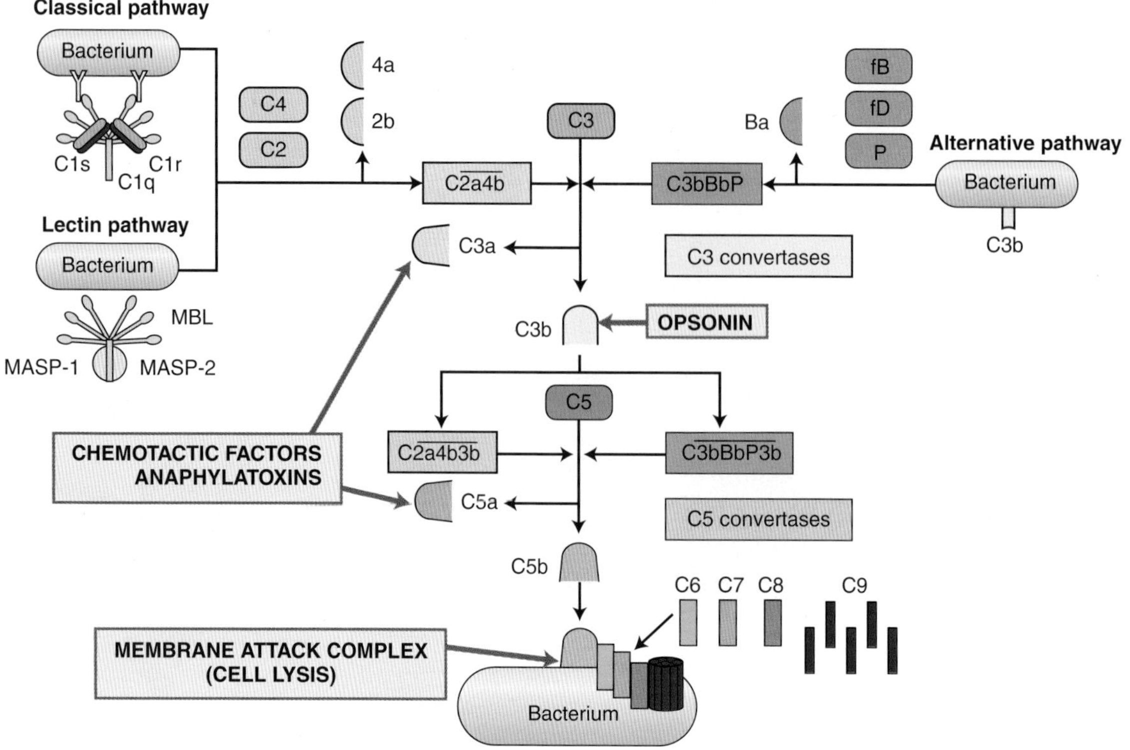


**Figure 7.6**

**The complement system.** (From McCance KL, Huether SE: *Pathophysiology: the biologic basis for disease in adults and children*, ed 8, St Louis, 2019, Elsevier.)

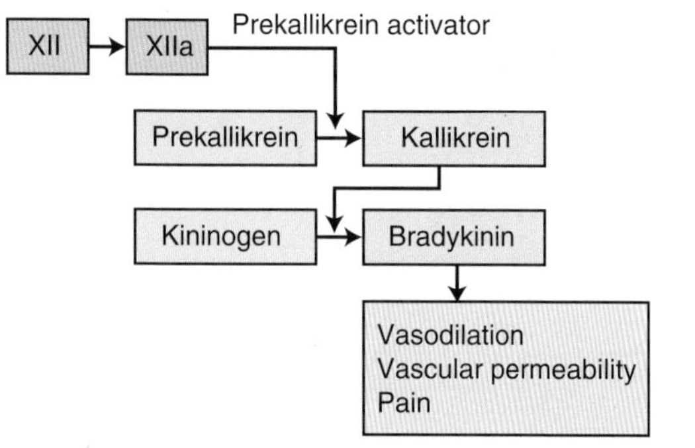


**Figure 7.7**

**The kinin system.** (From McCance KL, Huether SE: *Pathophysiology: the biologic basis for disease in adults and children*, ed 8, St Louis, 2019, Elsevier.)

### Complement System

The complement system consists of more than 30 proteins that are key components of the acute inflammatory response. When activated, these proteins interact in a cascade-like process and aggregate to damage the membranes of microbial cells, resulting in death by lysis. The complement system also possesses serum glycoproteins that, upon activation, aid in phagocytosis of the target (opsonization; see further discussion in Chapter 6). Another role of complement in the inflammatory response is to promote the clearance of immune complexes that are formed by the specific binding of an antibody to a soluble antigen.

It is important to appreciate that the complement system is involved in both innate immune responses (alternative complement pathway activated by PAMPs; lectin-associated complement pathway activated by binding of acute phase proteins) as well as adaptive immunity (classical complement pathway activated by antibodies bound to specific antigens of a particular threat).

## The Third Line of Defense: The Specific Immune System

### Adaptive Immunity

*Adaptive immunity* is characterized by specificity and memory. The goal of this comprehensive line of defense is to specifically recognize the threat, promote an effective immune response, destroy/remove the invading pathogen, and establish long-term memory.

Adaptive immunity results when a pathogen gains entry into the body and a specific response is elicited against the invader. This type of immunity requires preactivation (days to weeks for a full effect). The adaptive immune system is activated if a threat is present at a high enough level for a prolonged period of time (activation threshold). Adaptive immunity continually "develops" throughout life following exposure to a particular threat and has memory so that when the same disease-causing microorganism is encountered again, the body can respond even more rapidly and with a heightened immune response.

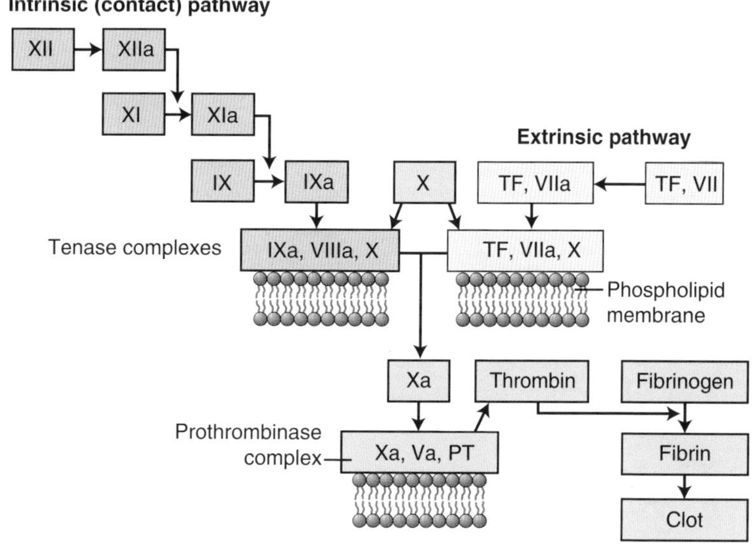


**Figure 7.8**

**The clotting system.** (From McCance KL, Huether SE: *Pathophysiology: the biologic basis for disease in adults and children,* ed 8, St Louis, 2019, Elsevier.)

The two components of adaptive immunity include the humoral immunity and cell-mediated immunity (see Table 7.2 and Fig. 7.9). Furthermore, the adaptive immune responses can occur as a result of active or passive immunity. Active immunity includes natural immunity and artificial immunity. Artificial immunity is intended or deliberate, and passive immunity is the transfer of antibodies or sensitized cells to another (Table 7.1).

*Active immunity* refers to protection acquired by introduction (either naturally from environmental exposure or artificially by vaccination) of an antigen (any molecule that binds specifically to an antibody or T-cell receptor) into a responsive host.

The concept of vaccination is based on the fact that deliberate exposure to a harmless version or component of a pathogen generates immunologic memory but not disease induced by the infectious agent itself. In this way, the immune system is primed to mount a secondary immune response with strong and immediate protection should the pathogenic version of the microorganism be encountered in the future.[74] Some of the most promising prophylactic and therapeutic vaccine strategies are currently being investigated for malaria, cancer, HIV, asthma, influenza, diabetes, hepatitis C, dengue, and many other diseases.

*Passive acquired immunity* occurs when immune products such as antibodies or sensitized lymphocytes produced by an immune person are transferred to a nonimmune individual (see Table 7.1). For example, the transplacental transfer of antibodies from mother to fetus, the transfer of antibodies to an infant through breast milk, or the administration of immune serum globulin ($\gamma$-globulin) provides immediate protection but does not result in the formation of memory cells and therefore provides only temporary immunity.

**Antigens and Antibodies.** The adaptive immune response involves recognizing components with a higher degree of specificity than the detection mechanisms of innate immunity, which distinguish features common to groups of foreign molecules. The antibody and T-cell receptor are the unique molecules of the adaptive immune system that recognize specific antigenic determinants or *epitopes*. An epitope is an immunologically active site on an antigen that binds to a T-cell receptor or to an antibody (Fig 7.10).

***Antigens.*** Bacteria, viruses, parasites, foreign tissues, and large proteins possess constituents that are defined as antigenic because they can interact specifically with antigen receptors (i.e., T-cell receptors and/or antibodies). Although molecules may be antigenic, some may not necessarily induce a specific immune response. In other words, they do not possess immunogenicity.

There are several factors that may influence the immunogenicity of a particular antigen. These include the following: degree of foreignness, structural and chemical complexity, molecular size, genetic makeup of the host, mode of administration (such as route, dose, and timing), and any substance that enhances specific responses elicited by an immunogen.[104] For example, an adjuvant is an immunostimulatory substance that is frequently included in vaccine preparations and serves to increase the response to a vaccine.

***Antibodies.*** Antibodies are produced by B cells and consist of two identical heavy (H) chains and two identical light (L) chains. The heavy chain possesses four or five immunoglobulin domains. Each light chain is bound to a heavy chain. These polypeptides are held together by intra-/interchain disulfide bonds, hydrophobic bonds, as well as electrostatic interactions to form heterodimers.

In its simplest form, an antibody resembles a Y-shaped molecule with two antigen-binding sites. The fragment antigen-binding (Fab fragment) is the portion of an antibody that binds to antigens. Aminoterminal ends of the light or heavy chain possess a high degree of variation among antibodies with different antigen specificities,

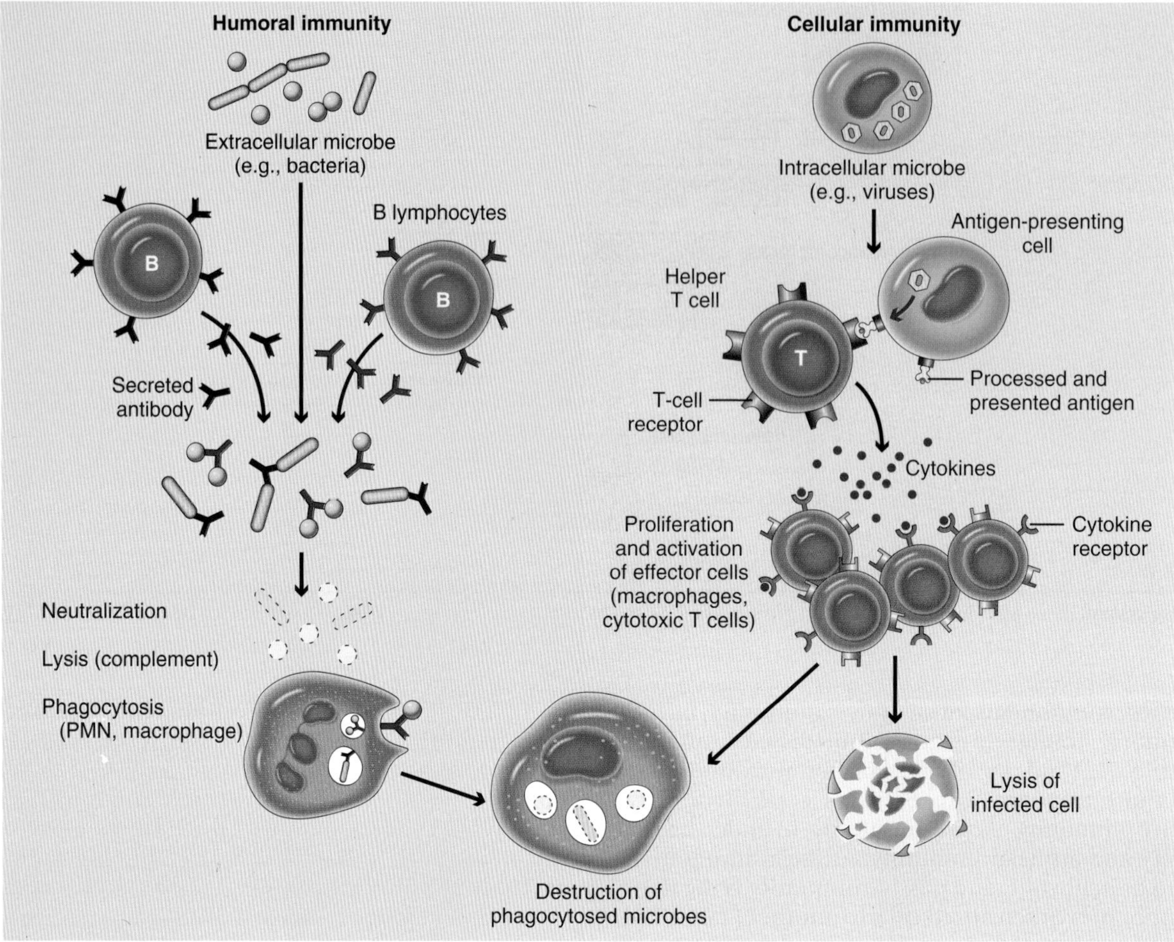

**Figure 7.9**

**Humoral and cell-mediated immunity.** Different types of lymphocytes detect distinct types of antigens. B cells recognize soluble or cell-surface antigens and differentiate into antibody-producing cells. Effector functions of B lymphocytes include neutralization of the microbe, complement activation, and phagocytosis. T cells recognize processed antigens that are displayed in the context of MHC molecules on the surfaces of antigen-presenting cells. Helper T cells secrete cytokines that elicit various mechanisms of immunity and inflammation. Cytotoxic T cells kill infected cells expressing processed microbial antigen. (Reprinted from Kumar V: *Robbins and Cotran: pathologic basis of disease*, ed 8, Philadelphia, 2009, WB Saunders.)

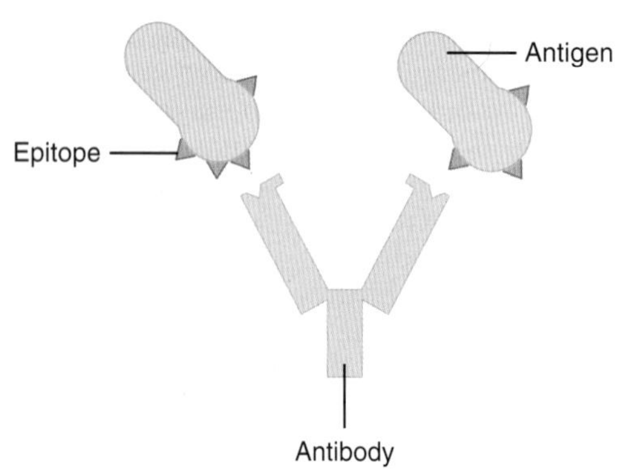


**Figure 7.10**

**Antibodies bond to epitopes.** Epitopes protrude from the surface of an antigen and combine with the appropriate binding site of an antibody. For small antigens, the binding site on the antibody may be a pocket or cleft, but in most cases it more closely resembles an undulating surface.[213] (Reprinted from Black JM, Hawks JH, Keene AM: *Medical-surgical nursing: clinical management for positive outcomes*, ed 7, Philadelphia, 2005, WB Saunders.)

and are thus designated as variable (**V**) regions (**V**$_H$ for the heavy chain and **V**$_L$ for the light chain). Sequence variation in **V**$_H$ and **V**$_L$ confers the antigen specificity of an antibody. Hypervariable regions within **V**$_H$ and **V**$_L$, known as complementarity-determining regions, constitute the antigen binding site of the molecule. Differences in specificity between antibodies are usually found in these areas (Fig. 7.11).

In contrast, other regions of an antibody that do not contain antigen binding sites and are relatively invariant within an immunoglobulin (Ig) class are known as constant regions (designated C$_L$ for the light chain and C$_H$**1**, C$_H$**2**, C$_H$**3**, C$_H$**4** for the heavy chain). The region between the C$_H$**1** and C$_H$**2** regions is known as the *hinge region* and allows for flexibility between the two Fab arms of the *antibody* molecule. The heavy chain determines the type (isotype/class) of the antibody (IgM, IgG, IgE, IgA, or IgD). Each constant region of the immunoglobulin heavy chain is encoded by a gene segment that corresponds to a lowercase Greek letter: μ (mu) encodes IgM, γ (gamma)

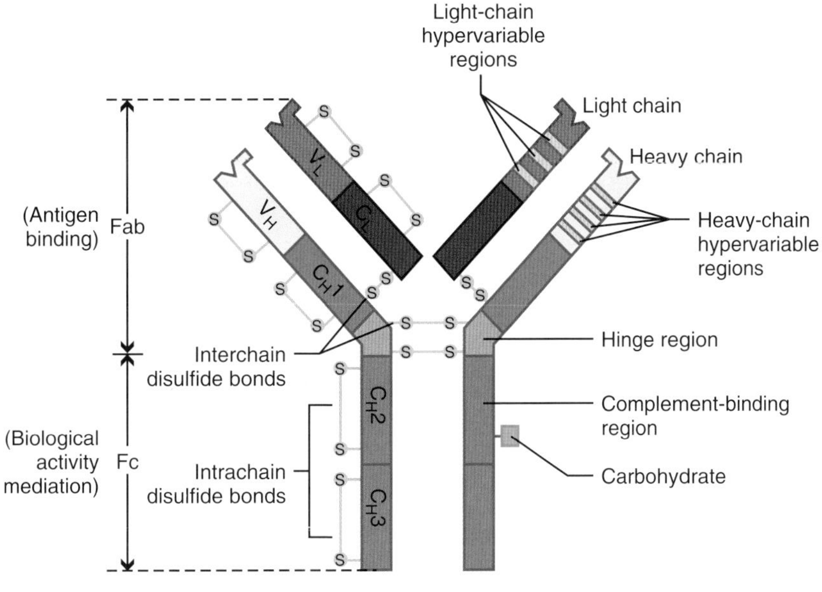


**Figure 7.11**

**Chain and domain structure of an immunoglobulin (Ig) molecule with hypervariable regions within variable regions of both H and L chains.** Fab and Fc refer to fragments of the IgG molecule formed by protein cleavage. The former contains the VH and CH1 H chain regions and intact L chain; the latter consists of the CH2 and CH3 regions of two H chains linked to one another by disulfide bonds. (From Wasserman RL, Capra JD: Immunoglobulin. In Horowitz MI, Pigman W [eds]: *The glycoconjugates*, New York, 1977, Academic Press, pp. 323–348, with permission.)

Box 7.1

**MAJOR FUNCTIONS OF IMMUNOGLOBULINS**[a]

- Immunoglobulins directly attack antigens, destroying or neutralizing them through the processes of agglutination, precipitating the toxins out of solution, neutralizing antigenic substances, and lysing the organism's cell wall.
- Immunoglobulins activate the complement system.
- Immunoglobulins activate anaphylaxis by releasing histamine in tissue and blood.
- Immunoglobulins stimulate antibody-mediated hypersensitivity.

[a]Globulins with antibody activity are referred to as *immunoglobulins*.
From Firestein GS: *Kelley's textbook of rheumatology*, ed 9, Philadelphia, 2012, WB Saunders.

encodes IgG, ε (epsilon) encodes IgE, α (alpha) encodes IgA, and δ (delta) encodes IgD.

The gene segments within the heavy chain are exchanged by isotype switching, which allows the antibody to change its effector characteristics and distribution. The heavy chain also contains the Fc ("fragment, crystallizable") portion of the antibody that possesses binding sites for the C1q complement protein and Fc receptors expressed on macrophages, lymphocytes, and other accessory cells. There are two light-chain types, kappa (κ) and lambda (λ), and a B cell expresses either κ or λ but never both. These peptides are encoded by one of two genes at different chromosomal loci and can be associated with any heavy chain isotype.[91]

Immunoglobulins. Each immunoglobulin isotype possesses unique biochemical properties. Box 7.1 lists the major functions of immunoglobulins. *IgM* is an antibody produced by and expressed on the surface of a B cell. It is the first secreted antibody and is predominant in a primary or initial immune response. As a monomer, it can function as a B-cell receptor (BCR) on B cells that have not encountered antigen (naïve B cells). Pentameric forms of IgM are found in the blood; because of its large size, it is almost exclusively localized in the intravascular compartment. IgM is most efficient at activation of the classical complement pathway, and its other effector functions include agglutination and neutralization of foreign invaders.

*IgG* is the major antibacterial and antiviral antibody in the blood and is carried by plasma into tissues. It is the major immunoglobulin synthesized during a secondary immune response (after IgM initially responds to foreign pathogens), conferring long-term immunity. IgG can activate complement via the classical pathway, promote phagocytosis (opsonization) of pathogens, and neutralize them. IgG can also cross the placenta and provide passive protection against infections in newborns during the first months of life.

*IgA* is found in serum and secretions. Secretory IgA defends external body surfaces, is the predominant immunoglobulin on mucous membrane surfaces, and is found in secretions such as saliva, breast milk (colostrum), urine, seminal fluid, tears, nasal fluids, and respiratory, gastrointestinal (GI), and urogenital secretions. IgA binds to pathogens and prevents their adherence to mucosal surfaces and colonization at the site of entry.

*IgE* is present at very low levels in the blood and is predominantly found bound to high-affinity receptors on mast cells and basophils. This immunoglobulin serves as a primary factor in the elimination of helminthic parasites, such as roundworms. *IgE* also functions during allergic reactions by triggering the degranulation of mast cells and basophils, resulting in histamine release in association with allergies, anaphylaxis, extrinsic asthma, and urticaria (hives). This response of *IgE* is a normal reaction but becomes excessive in people with allergies.

*IgD* is found at low levels in the blood. Its primary function is to serve as an antigen receptor on mature naïve B cells.

Antigen Sequestration, Presentation, and Recognition in Adaptive Immunity. The elicitation of antigen-specific adaptive immune responses poses a very interesting challenge for the immune system: that is, tailoring individual responses against the limitless multitude of threats. Because interactions between antigens and their receptors are highly specific, millions of receptors are required for effective immune surveillance. The solution to this dilemma was revealed when it was discovered that virtually every characterized antibody molecule had a unique molecular signature in its variable region.

Through gene rearrangement processes, the genes that encode the BCR undergo permanent changes in DNA sequence during B-cell development to create millions of unique antigen receptors. Thus, the generation of immunoglobulin diversity occurs through the process of gene rearrangement. In addition, different forms of antibodies are created by RNA processing.[176] The result is the generation of $10^9$ to $10^{11}$ different immunoglobulins. Accordingly, the DNA in a mature B cell is unique from every other cell, including B cells, unless the daughter cell was derived from the same original clone.

The generation of a diverse T-cell repertoire depends upon rearrangement of genes that comprise the variable region of the T-cell receptor (TCR) ($10^7$-$10^{10}$ unique TCRs are generated). More information about organization and rearrangement of BCR and TCR genes is available.[40,70] It should be noted that the genes encoding TCRs and immunoglobulins are different and are present on different chromosomes. Furthermore, variable regions of certain immunoglobulin genes rearrange only in B cells, whereas TCR gene arrangement occurs only in T cells.

B cells and T cells detect different types of antigens.[229] In addition to existing in a secreted form, antibodies may serve as membrane-bound antigen receptors on the surface of a B cell. TCRs exist only as membrane-bound antigen receptors of T cells. The BCR recognizes three-dimensional epitopes of macromolecules including nucleic acids, proteins, carbohydrates, lipids, and small chemical groups. Soluble or membrane-bound antigens in a native or denatured form can directly bind/crosslink the BCR.[229] For the antigens to be recognized, they must be accessible to the BCR. By contrast, the TCR recognizes constituents of protein antigens (peptides) that are presented (bound) by a major histocompatibility complex (MHC) on host cells. The TCR cannot detect free antigens (e.g., virus particles) that are not processed and presented in the context of an MHC. Thus, T-cell recognition depends on detection of both self-MHC and peptide antigen (MHC-restricted antigen recognition).

Antigen receptors are composed of unique recognition domains that will differ between lymphocytes, as well as nonvariable regions that are necessary for structural maintenance and effector function. These invariant domains are relatively conserved among all antigen-specific immune cell clones. For example, the chains of the TCR possess one variable (V) region and one constant (C) region. The variable regions of certain TCR subunits contact the MHC and antigen complex.[8] Similar to antibodies, areas of hypervariability or complementarity-determining regions within the V region vary greatly between different TCRs. Although the TCR and BCR can recognize antigens, the receptors themselves cannot transmit signals within the cell. For this reason, antigen receptors are linked to conserved molecules that function to transmit intracellular activation signals. Therefore, the recognition of a specific antigen and the resulting targeted response involves specific molecules (the receptors), and conserved sets of molecules that maintain the structure of the complex or facilitate signal transduction.

Importantly, the signaling that is mediated by antigen receptors requires the aggregation or crosslinking of two or more receptors through association with adjacent antigenic molecules. When this receptor triggering takes place, enzymes localize to signaling portions of the receptor complexes within the cell cytoplasm and initiate the phosphorylation of downstream proteins. These phosphorylation events activate a number of complex signaling pathways that ultimately result in the synthesis of molecules responsible for mediating immune responses. More information about the processes of T and B lymphocyte signaling and activation is available.[1]

## Adaptive Immune Responses

Adaptive responses involve the proliferation of antigen-specific B and T cells, which occur when the surface receptors of these cells bind to antigen and initiate immune responses.

The two types of adaptive immune responses are *cell mediated* (also referred to as T-cell immunity) and *humoral* (also called B-cell immunity) (Fig. 7.9). Although these two responses are often discussed separately, they work together; failure of one can alter the effectiveness of the other. Even though these two branches of adaptive immunity overlap and interact considerably, the distinction is useful when attempting to understand how the immune system is activated.

### Cell-Mediated Immunity

Cell-mediated immunity is the arm of the adaptive immune response that protects the host against infection by intracellular pathogens. The principal function of T cells is the destruction of microbes that are able to survive in the cytoplasm or phagocytic vesicles of infected cells. Cell-mediated immune responses can sometimes be harmful to the host, as they are responsible for the rejection of transplanted tissue and certain autoimmune diseases.

T-cell development begins when a progenitor cell from the bone marrow migrates to the thymus gland, which is a primary lymphoid organ. Immature T cells enter the cortex of the thymus and mature as they travel toward the medulla. While in the thymus, T cells encounter both soluble and membrane-bound components that direct their development. Rearrangement of TCR genes occurs in the thymus, and this determines the antigen specificity of the cells.

After the TCR is expressed, both CD4 and CD8 will be coexpressed to produce double- positive cells. During this stage, positive selection occurs to ensure that the T cell can identify peptides restricted by the MHC of the host. Negative selection also takes place to delete cells that recognize "self" peptides of the host.

This selection process is a form of *immunologic tolerance* in which the immune system is rendered nonreactive to self. Failure of negative selection will lead to autoimmune disease in which T cells recognize and react against "self" antigens presented by "self" MHC. It should be noted that mechanisms of peripheral tolerance exist to suppress autoreactive lymphocytes that have escaped selection in the central lymphoid organs. Peripheral tolerance may involve regulatory T cells ($T_{regs}$) (also known as suppressor T cells), which are discussed later in this section.

Mature naïve T cells exit the thymus and migrate through the peripheral blood to secondary lymphoid organs, such as the lymph nodes and spleen, where they encounter antigens and exert appropriate effector functions.[306]

T cells recirculate through the peripheral lymphoid organs on a constant basis in search of nonself antigens. Although naïve T cells can recognize foreign antigens, they are unable to produce the effector responses that are capable of eliminating a particular threat. For T cells to mount effector responses, they must first be stimulated through antigen recognition and then differentiate.

Antigen-presenting cells, such as dendritic cells and macrophages, phagocytose antigens in the tissue and transport them to the draining lymph nodes. *Dendritic cells* are the most potent antigen-presenting cells of the immune system and are thus crucial in the initiation of these primary immune responses. The antigens are processed and presented to naïve T cells in the context of MHC molecules. Naïve T cells sample various MHC/peptide antigen combinations through low-affinity interactions mediated by cellular adhesion molecules. If the antigen is not present, they detach and move on to another cell.

Upon activation, a rapid proliferation of antigen-specific cells occurs (clonal expansion). Some of the naïve T cells will become effectors that remain in the lymph node and eliminate the pathogen, whereas others will provide signals to aid other immune cells in generating responses against the pathogen (e.g., production of antibodies by B cells). Other effector cells will exit the lymph nodes and migrate to the site of infection to eradicate the threat. Furthermore, some of the T cells that have proliferated in response to antigenic stimulation will become long-lived memory T cells that can persist for months or even years.

When the host is reexposed to an antigen, a secondary immune response is generated in which memory T cells rapidly differentiate into effectors that can respond more rapidly and with heightened immune responses, resulting in pathogen clearance. This phenomenon, known as *immunologic memory*, is the basis for vaccination. Following removal of a pathogen by effector T cells, the antigenic stimulus is eliminated, and the immune system returns to its basal state.[306]

Cytotoxic T lymphocytes (CTLs) are effector cells that can kill other cells (Fig. 7.12). These lymphocytes are critical players in immune responses against intracellular threats such as viruses, abnormal/cancer cells, and intracellular bacteria. CTLs recognize and destroy infected cells or "nonself" cells (e.g., rejection of transplanted tissue). CTLs are primarily CD8+ T lymphocytes and thus MHC class I restricted. CTLs play a critical role in controlling viral infections by directly killing virally infected cells and producing cytokines such as IFN$\gamma$ that inhibit viral replication.

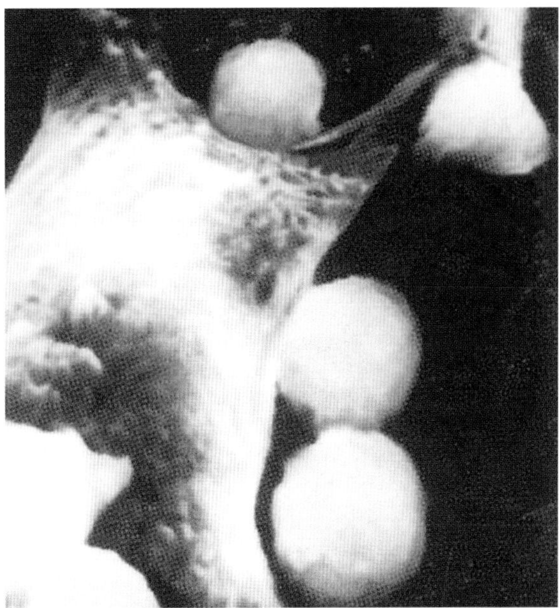

**Figure 7.12**

**T cells.** The blue spheres seen in this scanning electron microscope view are T cells attacking a much larger cancer cell. T cells are a significant part of our defense against cancer and other types of foreign cells. (Courtesy James T. Barrett.)

CTLs kill their target cells by inducing programmed cell death (apoptosis). Naïve CD8+ T cells (CTL precursors) differentiate into effector cytotoxic CD8+ T cells by a number of mechanisms that can be either independent or dependent on CD4+ T cells. During CD4+ T cell independent differentiation, dendritic cells stimulate naïve CD8+ T cells through their TCR by an MHC class I/antigen and a costimulatory signal. When CD4+ T cells provide help, they recognize antigen on the same target cell and induce upregulated expression of costimulatory molecules on antigen-presenting cells and produce IL-2 that serve as a growth factor for the CD8+ T cells.

As discussed, when memory $CD8^+$ T cells encounter their antigen, they rapidly proliferate and develop into effector cytotoxic cells. Memory T cells produce their own IL-2 and do not require costimulation (i.e., "signal 2") to proliferate and become effectors. When the TCR is triggered on a CTL, granules containing perforin (forms pores in the membrane of the target cell) and granzyme (proteolytic enzyme that activates the apoptotic program) are released onto the target cell, resulting in its destruction.[236]

CD4+ T lymphocytes are helper T cells that promote immunity against both intracellular and extracellular pathogens. It is important to appreciate that most threats are extracellular at some point (e.g., viruses). CD4+ T cells produce different cytokines that modulate the immune

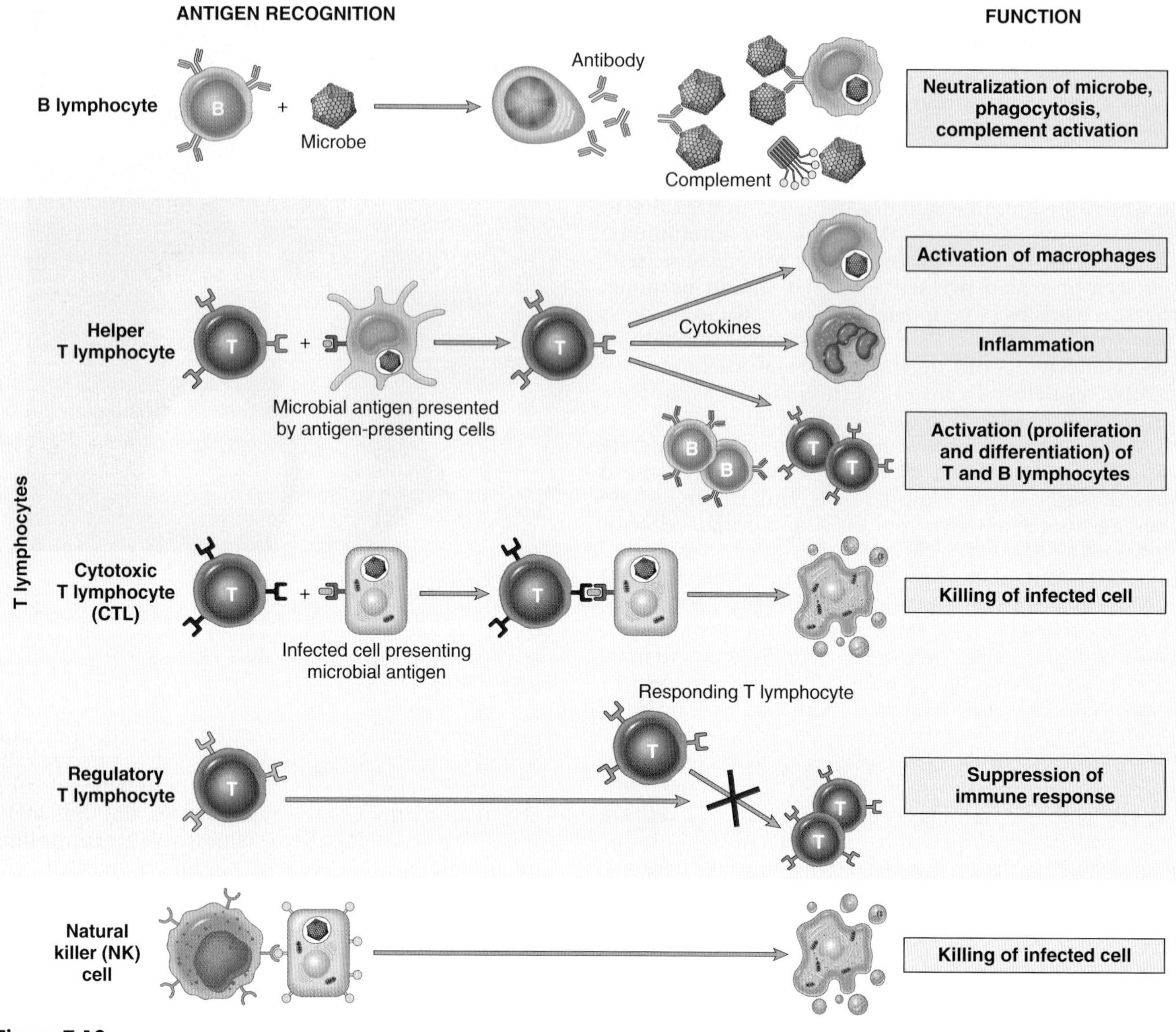


**Figure 7.13**

**Summary of antigen recognition of B cells, T cells, and NK cells.** (From Kumar V, Abbas AK, Aster JC: (2018). *Robbins basic pathology*, Philadelphia, 2018, Elsevier.)

system and help it to mount effective responses against foreign invaders. Some of these functions include: (1) helping B cells augment the production of antibodies, (2) activating macrophages and helping them to destroy bacterial pathogens, (3) helping CTLs to proliferate and destroy virally infected cells, (4) helping NK cells kill infected cells, (5) neutrophil recruitment, and (6) downregulation of the adaptive immune response. As discussed later in this chapter, HIV infection results in the gradual decline of CD4+ T cells, rendering the host susceptible to a multitude of infectious agents.[231]

The adaptive immune system also consists of $T_{regs}$ that prevent inappropriate responses against "self" antigens of the host or commensal microorganisms. $T_{regs}$ accomplish this through the generation of inhibitory cytokines such as IL-10 and transforming growth factor (TGF)-β. $T_{regs}$ are characterized as expressing both CD4 and high levels of CD25 (the α-subunit of the IL-2 receptor) and by the production of IL-10 and TGFβ. $T_{regs}$ are generated when naïve CD4+ T cells are stimulated by dendritic cells that are producing high levels of TGFβ but none of the other cytokines involved in helper T-cell differentiation.[279] See Fig. 7.13 for a summary of antigen recognition of B cells, T cells, and NK cells.

## Humoral Immunity

The humoral immune response is mediated by antibodies present in different body fluids or secretions, such as saliva, blood, or vaginal secretions. Antibodies produced by B lymphocytes are very effective against organisms that are free floating in the body and thus can be easily accessed and neutralized. B cells develop in the bone marrow and migrate to secondary lymphoid organs such as the spleen and lymph nodes. Membrane-bound antibodies on the surface of a B cell bind to immunogens present at these sites, which signals the cell to become activated. The B cell then proliferates and differentiates into plasma cells, which produce soluble antibodies and memory B cells. All of the daughter cells and antibodies that are generated by plasma cells have the same antigenic specificity as the surface receptor of the parent B cell. The secreted antibody or immunoglobulin binds to antigens and triggers one or more effector functions in order to eliminate a particular threat.

B lymphocytes originate from pluripotent stem cells in the bone marrow (Fig. 7.14). The development of a B cell is independent of antigen and occurs as the result of interactions with bone marrow stromal cells, which produce a microenvironment that is conducive to early growth and differentiation. Once committed to the B lineage, cells progress through a series of developmental stages that are defined by the status of immunoglobulin heavy and light chain genes. If gene rearrangement is successful, an immature B cell will form that possesses an antigen receptor in the form of a cell membrane–bound IgM that interacts with its environment.[108]

For a B-cell response to be effective, it must establish and maintain a diverse array of B-cell clones that can react to foreign antigens, but not "self" antigens. Immature B cells exit the bone marrow and recirculate through the circulatory and lymphatic systems in order to sample antigens. Upon migration into secondary lymphoid organs such as the spleen, lymph nodes, bone marrow, and mucosal-associated lymphoid tissues, they receive critical survival signals. At this stage, immature B cells express IgD on the cell surface and become mature B cells. Naïve B cells express BCRs of the IgM and IgD isotypes. The IgM and IgD molecules expressed on the same cell have the same V region and therefore the same antigenic specificity. These cells are now prepared to be activated by antigen.[1]

B cells encounter antigens that crosslink the BCR and activate them. Like naïve T cells, B cells require a second signal for proliferation. This signal can come from helper T cells or from innate immune components such as complement proteins. In an antigen-dependent fashion, activated B cells divide, differentiate, and begin producing antibodies in secreted rather than membrane-bound form. The first isotype created is IgM.

Helper T cells aid B cells by increasing proliferation, antibody production, affinity maturation, and isotype switching. *Affinity maturation* results in an increased affinity of antibodies for protein antigens during progression of a humoral response. The reader should recall that after isotype switching occurs, the resultant antibody will possess specificity and affinity for the same antigens but can now interact with different effector molecules.[34] Following an initial encounter with an antigen, some activated B cells do not differentiate into plasma cells but instead become memory cells. Memory B cells are long-lived and remain in the circulation until they reencounter a particular antigen. When this takes place, memory B cells generate a secondary antibody response by differentiating into plasma cells (Fig. 7.15).

## SUMMARY OF THE IMMUNE SYSTEM

The immune system has evolved to protect multicellular organisms from a vast array of threats. Immunology is the study of how the immune system works and the consequences of its dysfunction. Through past and present research on various immune response mechanisms, ways in which the immune system can be manipulated to benefit the host are being discovered. The principal function of the immune system is to eliminate infectious agents and abnormal "self" components (e.g., cancer cells) without attacking the body's own tissues. The immune

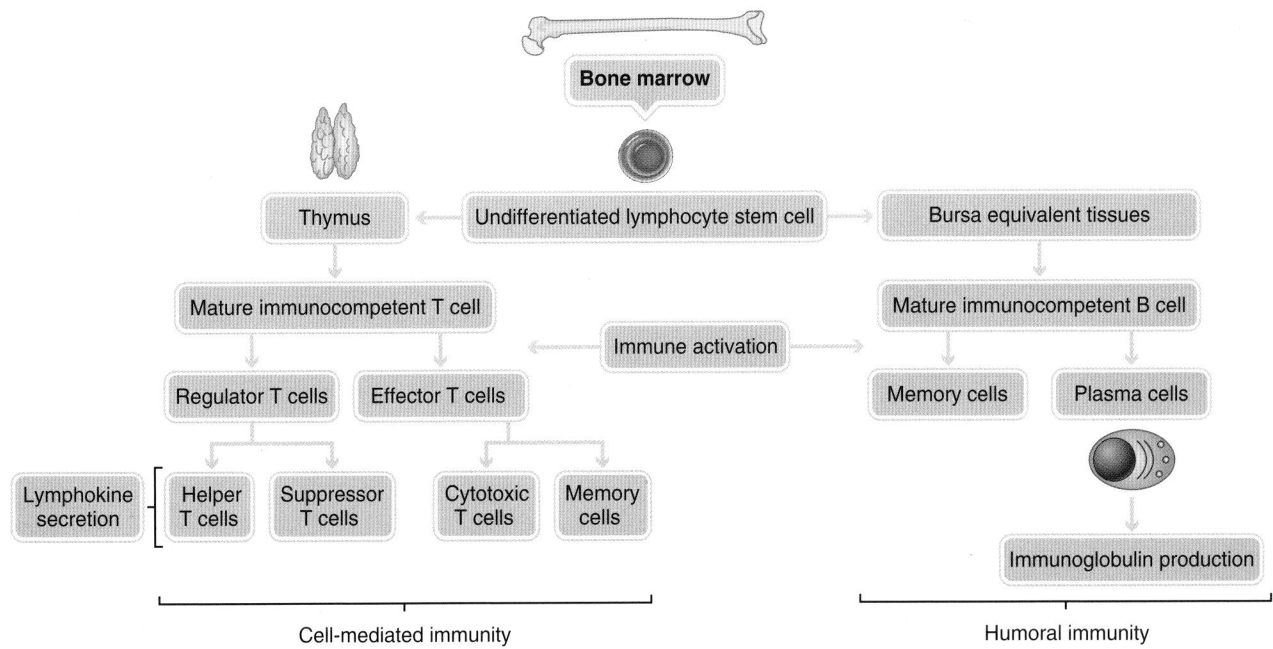


**Figure 7.14**

**The pathway of lymphocyte maturation.** Undifferentiated lymphocyte stem cells are derived from the bone marrow. B cells reach maturity within the bone marrow, but T cells must travel to the thymus to complete their development. Activation of either T or B cells by antigens leads to proliferation of immune cells that mediate either cell-mediated immunity or humoral immunity, respectively. (Reprinted from Black JM, Matassarin-Jacobs E, editors: *Medical-surgical nursing: clinical management for continuity of care*, ed 5, Philadelphia, 1997, WB Saunders, p. 597.)

system must maintain a state of balance such that when an external or internal threat is encountered, an appropriate response is generated to control the invader, and the system returns to equilibrium. This encounter with a particular insult educates the immune system to produce memory so that upon reencountering a foreign invader, it reacts more rapidly and with a stronger response.

Most pathogens are encountered after they are inhaled or ingested. Antigens entering the body through mucosal surfaces activate cells in the mucosa-associated lymphoid tissues, including the tonsils, adenoids, and Peyer patches.[75]

Keep in mind that the innate immunity and adaptive immunity systems function in concert (Fig. 7.9). Within the adaptive immune system, humoral immunity and cellular immunity are working simultaneously, such that a variety of immune responses can occur when a pathogen attempts to invade the body. The first line of defense consists of exterior barriers that prevent microbial colonization and host invasion. If the pathogen manages to cross these barriers, the innate immune system is equipped to detect it through a limited repertoire of molecules that recognize motifs, which are common to many different pathogens. If innate immunity fails to eliminate the pathogen, the adaptive immune response provides a comprehensive third line of defense to clear the threat and prevent reinvention or recurrence of illness.

## Phases of the Immune Response

The phases of an immune response are as follows: (1) *Recognition phase* during which innate immune receptors bind to common molecular motifs on pathogens or antibodies that are bound to the invader. Adaptive immune recognition involves highly specific antigen receptors. (2) *Amplification phase* involving complement cascades, production of soluble factors (e.g., acute phase proteins, cytokines) and the recruitment of an army of cells (e.g., neutrophils) in the case of innate immunity. Amplification of adaptive immunity requires the proliferation of lymphocytes (T or B cells) and the differentiation of these cells into effectors. One antigen-activated lymphocyte replicates into an army of clones that all express the same antigen receptor. (3) *Effector phase* that results in removal of antigens by a number of different mechanisms (e.g., neutralization, lysis, phagocytosis, direct killing by cytotoxic T cells). (4) *Termination phase* that dampens the immune system after the antigen has been cleared. This phase is critical for the prevention of excessive responses that may harm the host (e.g., tissue damage). (5) *Memory* involving the generation of long-lived T and B lymphocytes. These types of cells have a lower threshold for activation and will react more quickly and in an amplified fashion. It should be appreciated that although memory is maintained by adaptive immunity, it functionally involves both innate and adaptive responses. Figs. 7.15 and 7.16 illustrate the phases of humoral immunity and cell-mediated immunity.

Dysfunction of the immune system can contribute to a variety of diseases. For example, two general types of genetic alterations could lead to immunologic abnormalities: mutations that inactivate the receptors or signaling molecules involved in innate immune recognition and

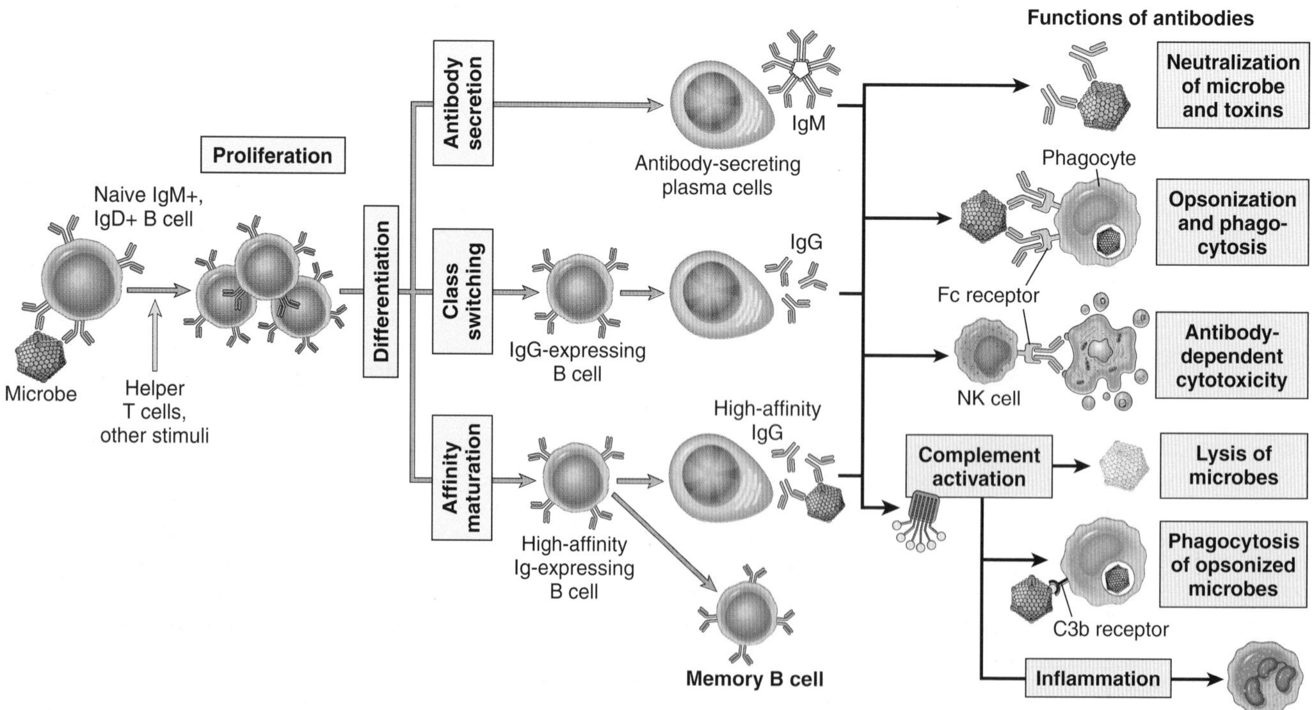


**Figure 7.15**

Naïve B lymphocytes when exposed to antigens and influenced by T helper cells (CD4), transcription factors, and cytokines are activated and begin proliferation. Once they have begun proliferating, they undergo different forms of differentiation: either antibody secretion, class switching, or affinity maturation. These forms of differentiation give them different effector functions and creation of long-lived memory B cells. (From Kumar V, Abbas AK, Aster JC: *Robbins basic pathology*, ed 10, Philadelphia, 2018, Elsevier.)

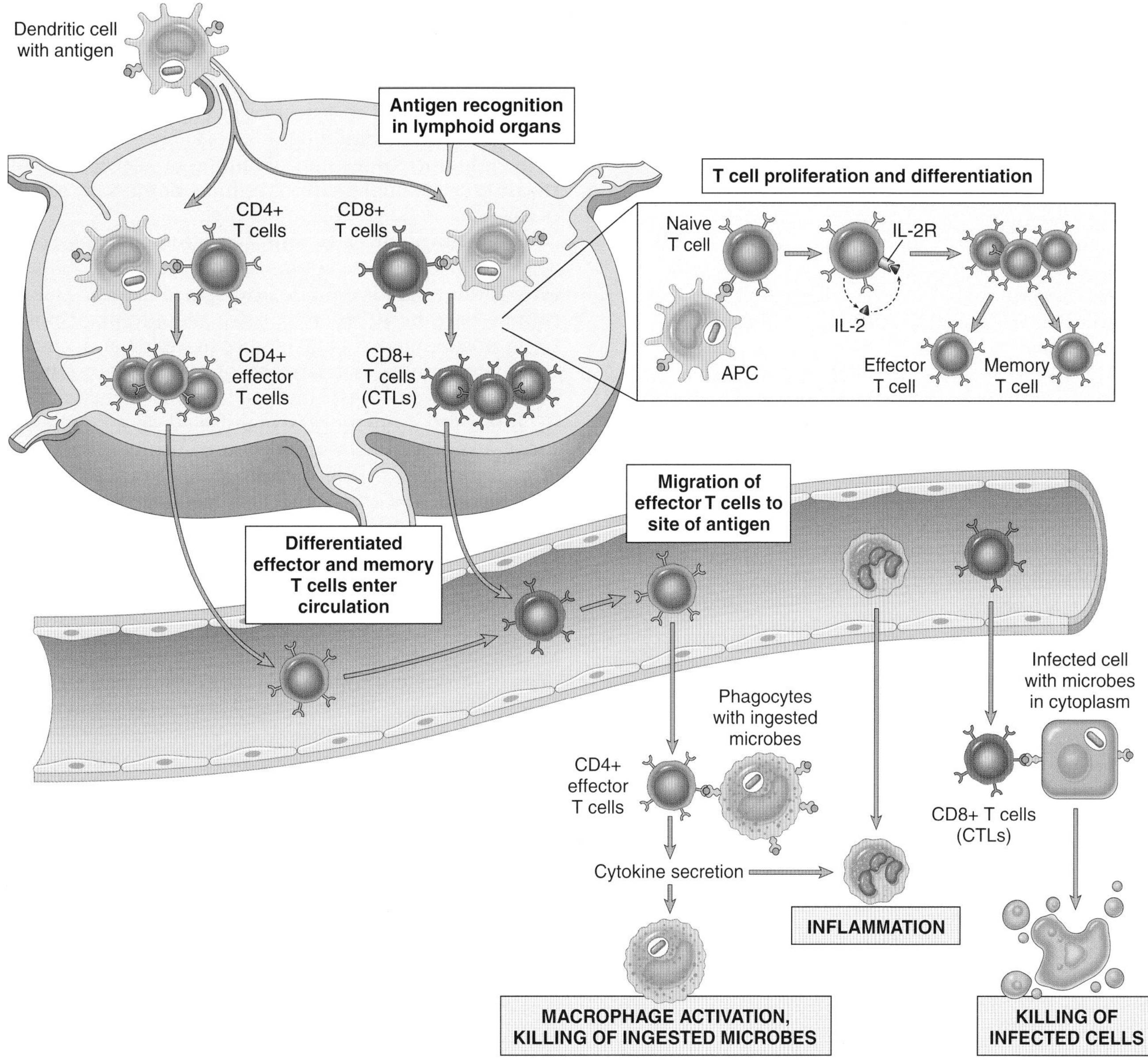


**Figure 7.16**

Dendritic cells (DCs) are antigen presenting cells (APCs), the main function of which is to process and present antigens to T cells. The DC enters the lymph node and initiate activation of naïve T lymphocytes via MHC. Activation of T cells causes proliferation and differentiation of both CD4+ and CD8+ T cells. (From Kumar V, Abbas AK, Aster JC: *Robbins basic pathology*, ed 10, Philadelphia, 2018, Elsevier.)

mutations that render them active all of the time. The first type of mutation can result in various types of immunodeficiencies. Further discussions on immunodeficiencies can be found later in the chapter. The second type of mutation can trigger aberrant immune responses and contribute to a variety of conditions with inflammatory components (e.g., asthma, allergy, arthritis, autoimmune diseases).[180] Some autoimmune diseases are explored later in the chapter.

## FACTORS AFFECTING IMMUNITY

In addition to the effects of aging, other factors can affect the immune system. These factors may include: nutrition, environmental pollution and exposure to chemicals that influence the host defense, prior or ongoing trauma or illnesses, medications, splenectomy (removal of the spleen), influences of the enteric, endocrine, and neurochemical systems, stress, and psychosocial-spiritual well-being and socioeconomic status.

Box 7.2 lists these factors and clinical conditions that contribute to an immunocompromised state. Sleep deprivation also has important effects, similar to stress, on the immune system by reducing cellular immunity.[17,227] Some factors, such as the iatrogenically introduced interventions listed and sexual practices, do not alter the immune system directly but increase a person's exposure to pathogens.

New information is being discovered about the sensory functions of the intestine and how neural, hormonal, and immune signals interact. Representatives of all the major categories of immune cells are found in the gut or can be rapidly recruited from the circulation in response to an inflammatory

Box 7.2

**FACTORS AFFECTING IMMUNITY**

***Factors That Alter the Immune System***

- Aging
- Sex and hormonal influences
- Nutrition/malnutrition
- Environmental pollution
- Exposure to toxic chemicals
- Trauma
- Burns
- Sleep disturbance
- Presence of concurrent illnesses and diseases:
  - Malignancy
  - Diabetes mellitus
  - Chronic renal failure
  - HIV infection
- Medications, immunosuppressive drugs
- Hospitalization, surgery, general anesthesia
- Splenectomy
- Stress, psychospiritual well-being, socioeconomic status

***Factors That Increase Exposure to Pathogens***

- Iatrogenic
  - Urinary catheters
  - Nasogastric tubes
  - Endotracheal tubes
  - Chest tubes
  - Peripherally inserted central catheter (PICC line)
  - Intracranial pressure monitor
  - External fixation devices
  - Implanted prostheses
- Sexual practices

stimulus. The gut immune system has 70% to 80% of the body's immune cells, and the protective blocking action of the secretory response in the gut is crucial to the integrity of the GI tract immune function and host defense.[21]

*Nutritional status* can have a profound effect on immune function. Nutrients have fundamental and regulatory influences on the immune response of the GI tract and, therefore, on host defense. Reduction of normal bacteria in the gut after antibiotic treatment or in the presence of infection may interfere with the nutrients available for immune function in the GI tract. In their review of literature on the gut–brain axis and mood disorder, Liu and Zhu found evidence linking the association of intestinal microbiota with the neuro-endocrine-immune pathways and mood disorders.[160]

Severe deficits in calories, protein intake, or vitamins such as vitamin A or vitamin E can lead to deficiencies in T-cell function and numbers. Deficient zinc intake can profoundly depress both T- and B-cell function. Zinc is required as a cofactor for at least 70 different enzymes, some of which are found in lymphocytes and are necessary for their function.

Secondary zinc deficiencies may be associated with malabsorption syndrome, chronic renal disease, chronic diarrhea, or burns or severe psoriasis (loss of zinc through the skin). Dietary changes may alter aspects of immunity, although research in this area is ongoing. Additionally, morbid obesity may alter the immune system by creating a vulnerability to certain diseases, including cancer.

Some *medications* (e.g., cancer chemotherapeutic agents) profoundly suppress blood cell formation in the bone marrow. Other drugs (e.g., analgesics, antithyroid medications, antiseizure, antihistamines, antimicrobial agents, and tranquilizers) induce immunologic responses that destroy mature granulocytes. Although chemotherapy could lead to a decrease of almost all measured immune cells, Schmidt and associates[241] argued that, with endurance or resistance training in individuals with breast cancer, suppression of cellular immunity may not occur.

Many drugs affect B- and T-cell function, especially against antigens that require the interaction of helper T cells and B cells for antibody production. These complications have been observed since the advent of potent immunosuppressive (e.g., corticosteroids) and chemotherapeutic drugs as treatment of people with autoimmune diseases, transplants, or cancer. Depression of B- and T-cell formation is manifested as a progressive increase in infections with opportunistic microorganisms (e.g., *Pneumocystis carinii*, cytomegalovirus (CMV), *Candida albicans*, and other fungi).

*Surgery* and *anesthesia* can suppress both T- and B-cell function for up to 1 month postoperatively.[169] Because of the invasive nature of any surgical procedure, and because defects in immunity have been described in most major illnesses, it is logical to assume that the majority of hospitalized surgical clients are immunocompromised to some degree. Hogan and colleagues (2011) conducted an extensive review on the mechanisms of how surgery can induce immunosuppression. Surgery to remove the spleen results in a depressed humoral response against encapsulated bacteria, especially *Streptococcus pneumoniae, Haemophilus influenzae, Staphylococcus aureus*, the group A streptococci, and *Neisseria meningitidis*.

*Burns* cause increased susceptibility to severe bacterial infections as a result of decreased external defenses (intact skin), neutrophil function, decreased complement levels, decreased cell-mediated immunity, and decreased primary humoral responses. Blood serum from clients with burns contains nonspecific immunosuppressive factors that suppress all immune responses, regardless of the antigen involved.

The relationship between *stress, psychosocial-spiritual well-being*, and *socioeconomic status* and susceptibility to disease through depressed immune function has become an area of intense research interest. In the past, there have been anecdotal reports of increased incidence of infection, diseases, and malignancy associated with periods of both intense and relatively minor stress.

## EXERCISE IMMUNOLOGY

Exercise immunology is important for two major reasons. First, exercise can regulate the ability of the immune system to initiate a response against pathogens. Second, the immune system is important in inflammation, healing, and repair. The effect of physical activity and exercise (aerobic, endurance, and resistance) on the immune and neuroimmune systems has been a growing area of research interest.[281] A brief summary of the results is presented here, but a more detailed accounting of exercise and the immune system and future direction for studies is available.[115,160,191,203,241,281] For example, Liu and Zhu argued the link of neuro-endocrine-immune pathways with mood disorders.[160]

Depending on the intensity, activity or exercise can enhance or suppress immune function. In essence, the immune system is enhanced during moderate exercise. Moreover, regular, moderate physical activity can prevent the neuroendocrine and detrimental immunologic effects of stress.[89]

In contrast to the beneficial effects of moderate exercise on the immune system, strenuous or intense exercise or long-duration exercise such as marathon running is followed by impairment of the immune system. Intense exercise can suppress the concentration of lymphocytes, suppress NK cell activity, and leave the host open to microbial agents, especially viruses that can invade during this open window of opportunity, and may lead to infections.

Extreme and long-duration strenuous exercise appears to lead to deleterious oxidation of cellular macromolecules. The oxidation of DNA is important because the oxidative modifications of DNA bases are mutagenic and have been implicated in a variety of diseases, including aging and cancer.[214]

### Effect on Neutrophils and Macrophages

Exercise triggers a rise in blood levels of PMNs and stimulates phagocytic activity of neutrophils and macrophages. The exercise-evoked increase in the PMN count is greater if the exercise has an eccentric component, such as downhill running. If the exercise goes beyond 30 minutes, a second, or delayed, rise in PMNs occurs over the next 2 to 4 hours while the exerciser is at rest.

This delayed rise in PMNs is probably the result of cortisol, which spurs release of PMNs from the bone marrow and hinders the exit of PMNs from the bloodstream.[178] After brief, gentle exercise, the PMN count soon returns to baseline, but after prolonged, strenuous exercise, this return to normal may take 24 hours or longer.[81]

In many instances, exercise enhances macrophage function and can increase antitumor activity in mice, but many questions still remain regarding the mechanism(s) by which short- or long-term exercise affects macrophage function.[298]

### Effect on Natural Killer Cells

Most researchers agree that the number of NK cells and the function or activity of these cells in the blood increase during and immediately after exercise of various types, duration, and intensity.[224,249,303] Promoting the natural cytotoxicity of NK cells, referred to as *NK enhancement*, is temporary and seems to be the result of a surge in epinephrine levels and from cytokines released during exercise.[282] NK enhancement by exercise occurs in everyone regardless of sex, age, or level of fitness training; however, once a person is accustomed to a given exercise level, the NK enhancement falls off, suggesting it is a response not to exercise per se but to physiologic stress.

After intense exercise of long duration, the concentration of NK cells and NK cytolytic activity declines below preexercise values. Maximal reduction in NK cell concentrations and lower NK cell activity occurs 2 to 4 hours after exercise.[203] Although this depression in NK cell count seems too brief to have major practical importance for health, there may be a cumulative adverse effect in athletes who induce these changes several times per week.[246]

### Effect on Inflammatory Response

Regular moderate exercise as well as resistance training and long-lasting endurance exercise is known to induce proinflammatory cytokines.[10,92,268,281] Brisk exercise (even brief, heavy exertion such as maximal bicycle ergometry for 30 or 60 seconds) increases the white blood cell count in proportion to the effort.[106,190] This exercise-induced increase in white blood cells (including lymphocytes and NK cells) is largely the result of the mechanical effects of an increased cardiac output and the physiologic effects of a surge in serum epinephrine concentration. Lymphocytes may be recruited to the circulation from other tissue pools during exercise (e.g., the spleen, lymph nodes, or GI tract). The number of cells that enter the circulation is determined by the intensity of the stimulus.[203]

The number of lymphocytes in circulation increases during exercise but decreases below the normal levels for several hours after intense exercise. Decreased numbers of lymphocytes are associated with decreased lymphocyte responsiveness and antibody response to several antigens after intense exercise.[128]

Strenuous or high-intensity exercise, defined as exercising at a minimum of 80% of maximal oxygen consumption ($VO_2max$), can suppress immune function and damage enough tissue to evoke the *acute-phase response* in human beings.[202,304] This complex cascade of reactions can modulate immune defense by activating complement and spurring the release of TNF, INFs, ILs, and other cytokines.

Plasma IL-6 increases in an exponential fashion with exercise (without muscle damage) and is related to exercise intensity, duration, the mass of muscle recruited, and endurance capacity. The antiinflammatory effects of IL-6 are demonstrated by the fact that IL-6 stimulates the production of antiinflammatory cytokines IL-1ra and IL-10.[208] The possibility exists that, with regular exercise, antiinflammatory effects of an acute bout of exercise will protect against chronic systemic low-grade inflammation. This long-term effect of exercise may be ascribed to the antiinflammatory response elicited by a short-term bout of exercise, which is partly mediated by muscle-derived IL-6.[208]

### Exercise, Aging, and Apoptosis

Aging is associated with a decline in the normal functioning of the immune system that is described by the term *immunosenescence*. Habitual exercise is capable of regulating the immune system and delaying the onset of immunosenescence.[245] Regular exercise is associated with enhanced responses to vaccinations, lower numbers of exhausted/senescent T cells, increased T-cell proliferative capacity, lower circulatory levels of inflammatory cytokines, increased neutrophil phagocytic activity, lowered inflammatory response to bacterial challenge, greater NK cell cytotoxic activity, and longer leukocyte telomere lengths in aging humans.[28,80,139,252]

The role of apoptosis, or programmed cell death, in exercise is the focus of much research in the area of exercise science. Some exercise conditions have been shown to delay apoptosis.[185] Accelerated apoptosis has been documented to occur in a variety of disease states, such as AIDS and Alzheimer disease, and in the aging heart. In striking contrast, failure to activate this genetically regulated cell death may result in cancer and certain viral infections. It is surmised that exercise may delay apoptosis, and separately, exercise-induced apoptosis is a normal regulatory process that removes certain damaged cells without a pronounced inflammatory response, thereby ensuring optimal body function.[185,187,206,210]

## Exercise, Overtraining, and the Immune System

Research indicates that moderate exercise can have a positive effect on the immune system regulation.[33] The degree of strenuousness in physical activity depends on a myriad of factors. These factors include but are not limited to: current level of fitness, recovery (short and long term), presence of pathogens, and nutrition. In evaluating the different factors associated with overtraining, it is thought that people who are overtrained are more susceptible to infections or dysfunction with inflammation and healing.[243] Bell and Ingle[16] conducted a systematic review on the effect overtraining had on the immune system. Their research found that the immune cells most altered by overtraining were neutrophils. All other cells and markers show little to no difference. Overall, the research is still inconclusive as to not only how but if overtraining leads to dysfunctions in the immune system. Further research will be needed in order to elicit any involvement between overtraining and the immune system.

SPECIAL IMPLICATIONS FOR THE THERAPIST 7.1

### *Exercise Immunology*

Physical therapists use exercise in the treatment of people of all ages with a variety of clinical problems, thereby influencing immune function. Exercise as a means of preventing illness and attaining a healthy lifestyle and as an intervention tool in immunodeficiency states is becoming a larger part of preventive services. Research in the area of exercise immunology is growing. Keeping abreast of research results is the first step to examining the clinical implications in this area.[281]

Aged adults constitute a growing and important consumer group of therapy services. Because immune function declines with advancing age, it is important that we understand the effects of exercise on immune function. Very few absolute guidelines have been developed; it seems intense or strenuous exercise may be detrimental to the immune system, whereas a lifetime of moderate exercise and physical activity enhances immune function. Further research is needed to clarify or modify this guideline.

It takes 6 to 24 hours for the immune system to recover from the acute effects of severe exercise. Each individual client must be evaluated after exercise to determine the perceived intensity of the exercise or intervention session. For example, in the deconditioned older adult with compromised cardiopulmonary function, reduced oxygen transport, and impaired mobility, ambulating from the bed to the bathroom may be perceived by their body as strenuous exercise.

Although intense exercise causes suppression of immune parameters in young subjects, data from aged animals[128,129] and human beings[130] show that intense exercise has no detrimental effect on immune function or rate of infections in older adults. Thus, relatively intense exercise programs may be prescribed that could maximize cardiopulmonary and musculoskeletal function without impairing immune function in frail, elderly people.[281]

Nevertheless, intense exercise during an infectious episode should be avoided. For anyone, especially competitive athletes, who wonders whether to exercise in the presence of an acute viral or bacterial infection (e.g., when manifesting constitutional symptoms), a "neck check" should be conducted. If the symptoms are located above the neck, such as a stuffy or runny nose, sneezing, or a scratchy throat, exercise should be performed cautiously through the scheduled workout at half speed. If after 10 minutes the symptoms are alleviated, the workout can be finished with the usual amount of frequency, intensity, and duration.

If instead the symptoms are worse and the head is pounding or throbbing with every footstep, the exercise program should be stopped, and the person should rest. If a fever or symptoms below the neck are evident, such as aching muscles, a hacking cough, diarrhea, or vomiting, exercise should not be initiated.[81] (See the specific exercise guidelines for the person with HIV in Special Implications 7.3 in this chapter.)

# IMMUNODEFICIENCY DISEASES

The etiopathologic mechanisms of immune deficiency diseases may occur as a result of either primary or secondary causes. The primary cause is due to inherited defects in the genesis of the immune system. On the other hand, secondary causes include many factors such as infection, aging, malnutrition, chemotherapy, autoimmune disorders, or immunosuppression. People who suffer from immune deficiency manifest with high predilection to infections and cancer. For example, individuals who may have defective immunoglobulins, complement, or phagocytosis greatly suffer from on-and-off infections with pyogenic bacteria. On the other hand, individuals who may have defective cell-mediated immunity are susceptible to infections caused by viruses, fungi, and intracellular bacteria. In the next section, the discussion is divided into primary immune deficiencies and secondary immune deficiencies.

## Primary Immune Deficiencies

With the development of gene discovery, the International Union of Immunological Societies (IUIS) Expert committee convened to discuss and update the classification of primary immunodeficiency diseases (PID). Al-Herz and associates published a report on the updated classification of PID.[7] The updated classification was designed to assist in establishing the diagnosis for individuals with these diseases.

Most of the primary immune deficiencies are genetically determined and are either innate host defense or adaptive immunity, which can be humoral or cellular.

The deficiencies are the consequences of a single gene defect, characterized as mutations that are sporadic rather than inherited. Sporadic means that the defect occurred before birth, but the clinical manifestations occur either early or late depending on the disease Fig. 7.17. Several researchers conducted epidemiologic studies to support the genetic mechanisms of PID.[147,159,168]

## Genetic Deficiencies of Components of Innate Immunity

**Complement Proteins.** As mentioned earlier, complement proteins have dual roles in inflammatory and immunologic responses. C3, a hereditary deficiency of complement component, plays a crucial role in both classical and alternative pathways. The defect results in increased vulnerability to pyogenic bacteria. On the other hand, patients who have inherited deficiencies of C1q, C2, and C4 are not susceptible to infections but are instead at higher risk of immune complex mediated diseases such as systemic lupus erythematosus (SLE) due to impaired clearance of apoptotic cells or antigen-antibody complexes in the blood circulation.[146]

In regard to the late components of the classical component pathway, patients who have deficiencies in C5-C8 have a propensity to recurrent infections by *Neisseria* (either gonococci or meningococci) but not by other microbes. The lack of regulatory C1 inhibitors causes continuous C1 activation, with the generation of downstream vasoactive 3 complement mediators. The result is hereditary angioedema, which is manifested by recurrent episodes of localized edema in the skin and/or mucous membranes.[20,146,177]

**Phagocytes.** Congenital defects in phagocytes include chronic granulomatous disease, leukocyte adhesion deficiencies, Chediak-Higashi syndrome, C3 receptor deficiency, severe congenital neutropenias, and chronic granulomatous disease. Generally, phagocytosis is accompanied by bacterial opsonization with IgG or C3b, which was discussed in the chapter on Cellular Injury and Inflammation (Chapter 6). Disorders of phagocytes result in recurrent infections with encapsulated bacteria, which are linked with antibody and complement deficiencies.[7,20,67,127,146,147,159,168,177,182,196,197,198,219,290,300]

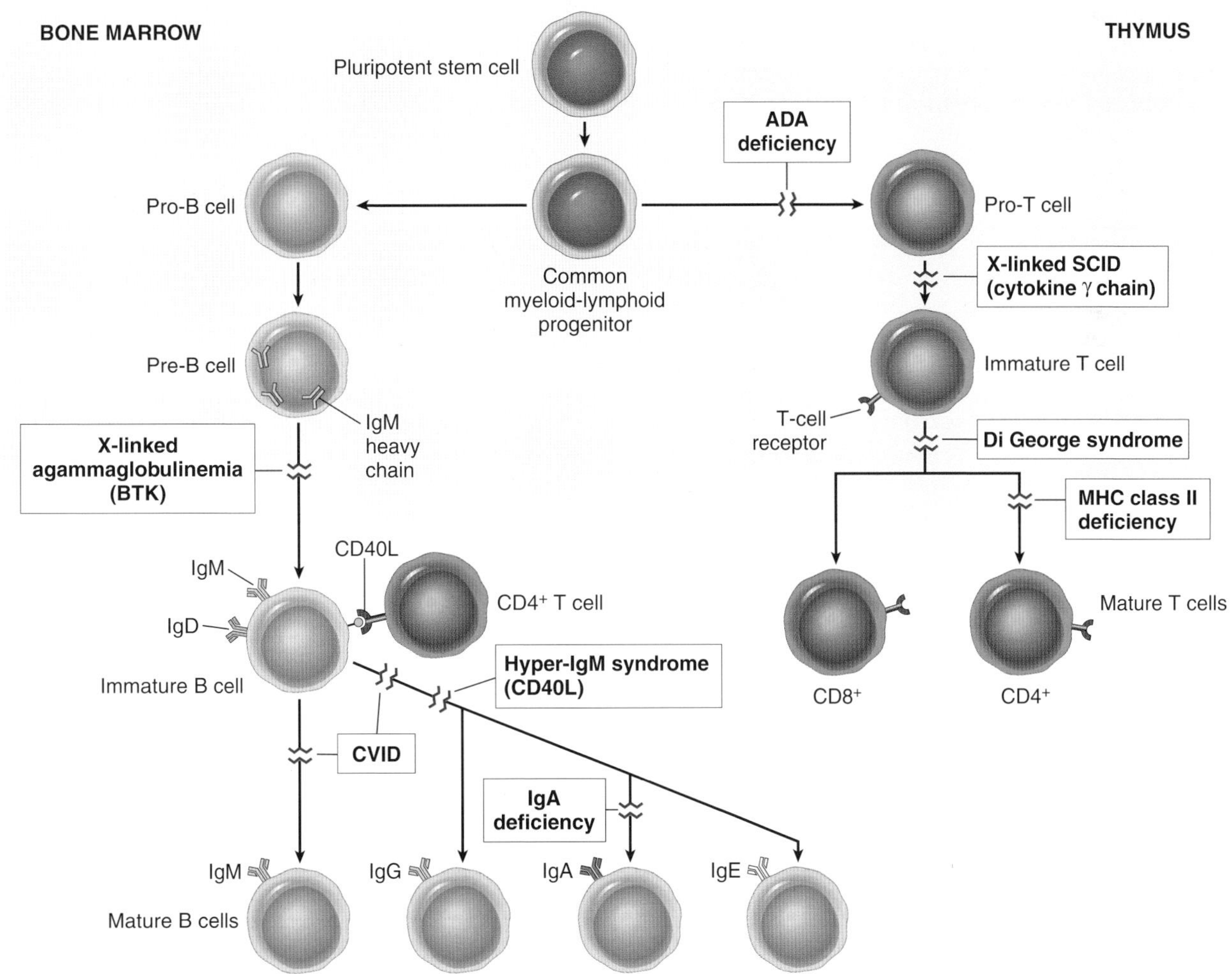


**Figure 7.17**

**Primary immune deficiency diseases.** Primary immune deficiencies from both the bone marrow and thymus are depicted above. Deficiencies are shown as breaks in the lymphocyte development and the altered genes. Knowledge of which pathway and where in the continuum it is affected helps understand the presentation of each deficiency. (From Kumar V, Abbas AK, Aster JC: *Robbins basic pathology*, ed 10, Philadelphia, 2018, Elsevier.)

## Secondary Immune Deficiencies

Secondary immune deficiencies are frequently encountered in people with pre-existing conditions such as malnutrition, infection, cancer, renal disease, or sarcoidosis. Chinen and Shearer[56] argued that primary immune deficiencies are less common than secondary, or acquired, immune and inflammatory deficiencies. The discussion on Acquired Immunodeficiency Syndrome is the focus of discussion in secondary immune deficiencies.

### Acquired Immunodeficiency Syndrome (AIDS)

The discussion of acquired immunodeficiency syndrome (AIDS) is included in this chapter because the disease causes massive destruction of the immune system, which consequently leads to an increased vulnerability to other infections and diseases. To better understand the disease processes of AIDS, a description of the etiologic agent is necessary. The syndrome is caused by a virus called the human immunodeficiency virus (HIV). HIV is notoriously capable of infecting and debilitating the immune system; HIV selectively attacks and incapacitates the CD4 molecule of the immune system, leading to depletion of helper/inducer T lymphocytes.

**Incidence and Prevalence.** According to HIV.gov, HIV,[276] the etiologic agent of AIDS, is still the most disturbing public health threat. Globally, there are approximately 36.9 million people suffering from HIV/AIDS. Of the current statistics, children less than 15 years old represent 1.8 million. These children were born from mothers who were positive with HIV during pregnancy, childbirth, or breastfeeding.[170,276] The majority of this population come from sub-Saharan Africa. Of importance, 75% of people afflicted with HIV worldwide are aware of the HIV status in 2017; 25% of people living with HIV still require further HIV testing services. The majority of people diagnosed with HIV come from low- and middle-income countries. For instance, 53% of people with HIV are from eastern and southern Africa; 16% in western and central Africa; 14% in Asia and the Pacific; and 2.2 million in Western and Central Europe and North America.[50,53,276] Despite the alarming statistics, there has been an increase in accessibility to HIV treatment. In 2010, there were only 8 million people who had access, but this number has progressively increased to 23.3 million in 2016 and further increased by 1.6 million in 2017. Fig. 7.18 shows the worldwide prevalence of HIV among adults 15 to 47 years in 2017.[299]

In the United States, more than 1.1 million people are currently living with HIV, but only 1 in 7 of them are unaware of their HIV status.[276] In 2015, approximately 38,500 Americans were newly infected with HIV. Gay, bisexual, and other men who have sex with men (MSM) remain the highest vulnerable group of new HIV infections. However, there has been an 8% decline in the estimated number of annual HIV infections from 2010 to 2015. In 2015, the Centers for Disease Control and Prevention (CDC) estimated that 1.1 million people (aged 13 and older) in the United States were living with HIV. However, almost 15% of these had not been diagnosed.[49,53,276]

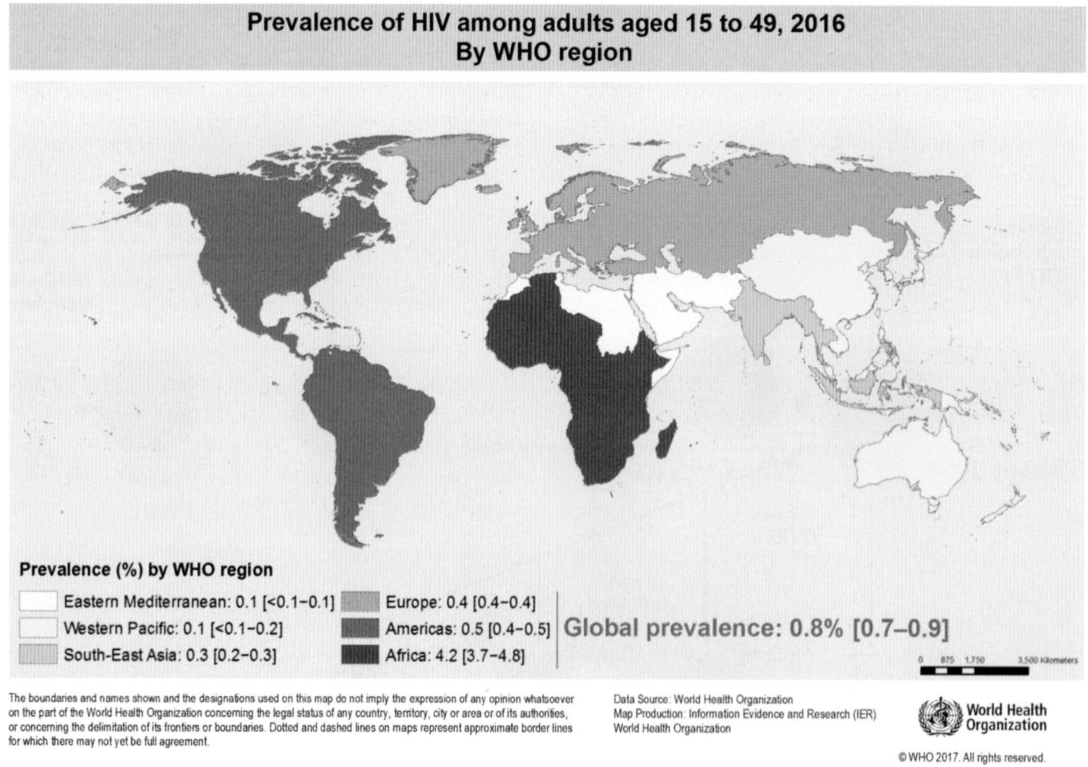


**Figure 7.18**

**Worldwide prevalence of HIV among adults 15-47 years in 2018.** Global number of men, women, and children living with, newly infected, and related deaths. (From World Health Organization: *Global Health Observatory data: HIV/AIDS*, 2018. Retrieved from https://www.who.int/gho/hiv/en/.)

In the United States, the greatest impact of the epidemic is among men who have sex with men (MSM) and injection-drug users (IDUs). In 2017, adult and adolescent transmission of HIV in the United States was attributed to MSM in 61% of cases, IDU in 8% of cases, MSM+IDU in 3% of cases, and heterosexual sex in 28% of cases. Infection rates are higher in racial/ethnic minority groups such as blacks and Hispanics.[53,276] Increases have been observed in the number of cases attributed to heterosexual transmission among minority women and women older than 50 years.[50] Fig. 7.19 is an infographic of HIV incidence and prevalence in the United States from 2010 to 2015.

Since 2010, the annual number of HIV infections has decreased among women but remained stable among males. In 2015, the rate for males (24.1) was 4.8 times the rate for females (5.0). In the same year of comparison (2010), the annual number of HIV infections in 2015 decreased among African Americans and persons of multiple races. But the annual number of infections in 2010 and 2015 remained stable for Asians, Hispanics/Latinos, and Caucasians. In 2015, the highest rate was for African Americans (49.5), followed by the rate for persons of multiple races (25.2).[49] The annual number of HIV infections in 2015, compared with 2010, decreased among persons aged 13 to 24, 35 to 44, and 45 to 54 but increased among persons aged 25 to 34. The number of infections in 2010 and 2015 remained stable among persons more than 55 years old. In 2015, the rate was highest for persons aged 25 to 34 (31.3), followed by the rate for persons aged 13 to 24 years (18.3).[49]

**The Virus.** HIV is a ribonucleic acid (RNA) virus, also known as retrovirus. Through the process of transcription, the cells make proteins using the deoxyribonucleic acid (DNA) as a template in order to make another nucleic acid called ribonucleic acid (RNA). The presence of retroviruses is necessary to carry out transcription in reverse. These viruses contain the reverse transcriptase enzyme that transcribes the viral RNA into DNA so that the DNA can be inserted into the genome of the host cell. Finally, the virus is able to multiply inside the cell by synthesizing viral RNA and proteins.[177,257,276]

The HIV genome has a dense cylindrical core that contains two identical RNA genomes and the virus-encoded enzymes, which are reverse transcriptase, protease, and integrase. These virus-encoded enzymes are used mainly for efficient replication. The core is surrounded by a lipid bilayer envelope containing the glycoprotein spikes.[85,257]

There are two major strains of HIV. HIV-1 causes the global epidemic because it is more readily transmitted than the other strain (HIV-2). In a review on HIV-1 and HIV-2, Nyamweya and associates[195] conducted extensive epidemiologic comparisons between these two viruses. Table 7.3 illustrates the differences between HIV-1 and HIV-2.

**Transmission.** There are three main avenues for HIV transmission: (a) contaminated blood, (b) sexual activity (anal, vaginal, very rarely oral), and (c) maternal to child (either through pregnancy, during delivery, or breastfeeding).[257] Transmission of HIV occurs by exchange of body fluids such as blood and semen and is associated with high-risk behaviors.[51] High-risk behaviors include unprotected anal, vaginal, and oral sex, including having six or more sexual partners in the past year, sexual activity with someone known to carry HIV, or IV drug use. HIV is not transmitted by fomites (e.g., coffee cups, drinking fountains, or telephone receivers) or casual household or social contact. Cases of HIV transmission from bone or tendon allograft are possible but are generally preventable via donor screening and testing of allograft material.[121] Intravenous drug users (IDU) continue to play a key role in the HIV epidemic.[82,260]

Transmission of HIV varies by gender. In 2010, 77% of male HIV infections were related to MSM, 7% were related to IDU, and 12% of the infections resulted from heterosexual sex. In the same year in females, 86% of HIV infections were related to heterosexual sex and 14% resulted from IDU.[305] A woman is twice as likely as a man to contract HIV infection during vaginal intercourse, and the presence of other STDs greatly increases the likelihood of acquiring or transmitting HIV infection. The rates of gonorrhea and syphilis are higher among women of color, especially between the ages of 15 and 24 years.[45]

In the United States, MSM has been the most common mode of HIV transmission, followed by IDU and heterosexual contact. To avoid social isolation, discrimination, or verbal or physical abuse, many MSM, especially young and minority MSM, do not disclose their sexual orientation.[305]

**HIV Life Cycle.** There are two main reasons to learn and understand the HIV life cycle: (a) tracing the pathogenicity and infectivity of the virus and (b) mapping the possible sites of therapeutic interventions, specifically the HIV-1 strain. Fig. 7.20 shows the seven stages of HIV life cycle: (a) binding, (b) fusion, (c) reverse transcription, (d) integration, (e) replication, (f) assembly, and (g) budding. Using the machinery of the CD4 cells, HIV is able to multiply and spread throughout the body leading into its virulence and pathogenicity. Hence, the virus attacks, kills, and destroys the CD4 (the white blood cell). In turn, the role of the immune system—to protect the body from infection and other forms of opportunistic infections—is compromised.

**Pathogenesis.** Untreated HIV infection eventually leads to profound pathology through destruction of CD4+ cells, other immune cells, or neuroglial cells, or indirectly through the secondary effects of immunosuppression. The natural history of HIV disease begins with infection by the HIV retrovirus, detectable only by laboratory tests. This retrovirus predominantly infects human T4 (helper) lymphocytes (also known as CD4 cells). CD4 cells are major regulators of the immune response, and HIV destroys or inactivates them. Macrophages, B cells, dendritic cells, and microglial cells are also infected (Fig. 7.21).

Once HIV enters the body, CD4 cells and macrophages serve as receptors for the HIV retrovirus, allowing direct passage of the infection into other target cells in the GI tract, uterus/cervix, and neuroglia. After attaching to and fusing with a cell, the HIV *virion* injects the core proteins and the two strands of viral RNA into the cell.

HIV virions contain enzymes including reverse transcriptase, integrase, and protease. All are required for successful reproduction. Before viral replication can occur in

# HIV Incidence and Prevalence Report*

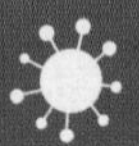

The CDC can determine the **burden of HIV** in the U.S. by using **three different measures.**

| **HIV Incidence** in 2016 | **HIV Prevalence** in 2016 | **HIV Diagnoses**† in 2017 |
|---|---|---|
| **38,700**** | **1.1 M**** | **38,739***** |
| The estimated number of **new HIV infections** in a year | The estimated number of all people with **diagnosed or undiagnosed** HIV infections at a point in time | The number of **HIV diagnoses** reported for a year |

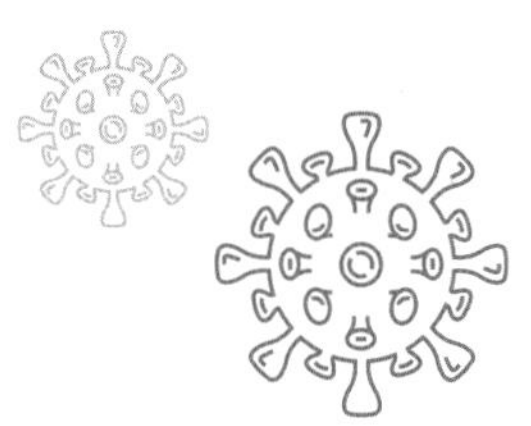

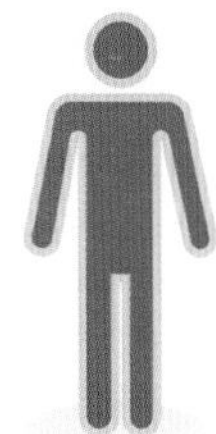

**1** in **7** **did not know** they were infected

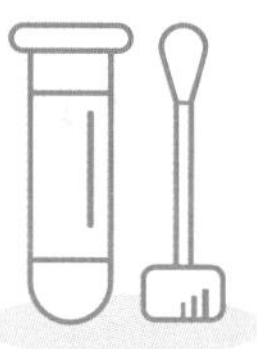

** U.S. only ***U.S. and 6 dependent areas †https://www.cdc.gov/hiv/pdf/library/reports/surveillance/cdc-hiv-surveillance-report-2017-vol-29.pdf

## Annual New Infections (Incidence) 2010-2016

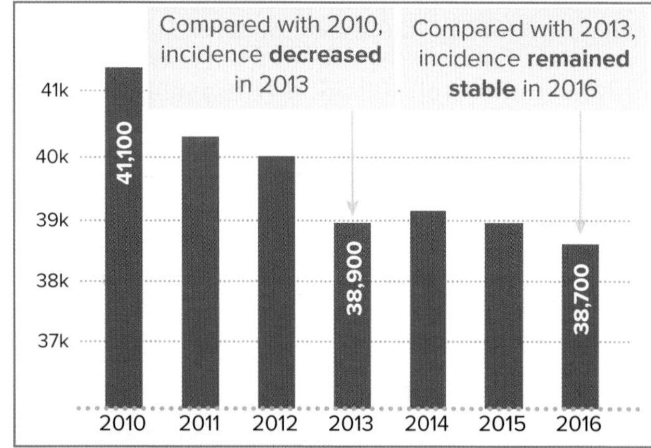


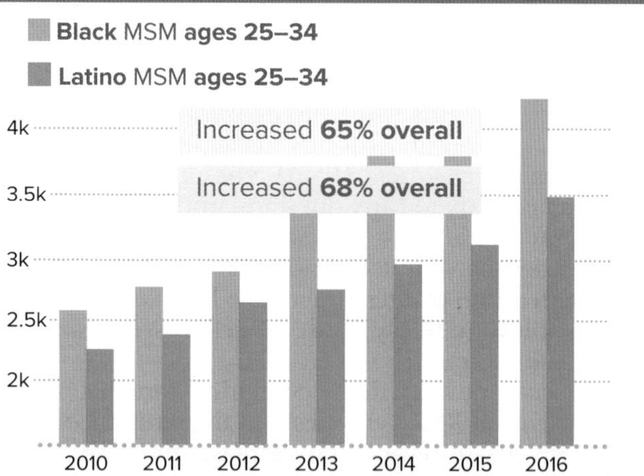


## Men who have Sex with Men (MSM) represented 68% of new infections in 2016

| White MSM | Black/African American MSM | HIspanic/Latino MSM |
|---|---|---|
| Down 16% | stable | up 30% |

National Center for HIV/AIDS, Viral Hepatitis, STD, and TB Prevention
Division of HIV/AIDS Prevention

CDC

* Centers for Disease Control and Prevention. Estimated HIV incidence and prevalence in the United States, 2010–2016. HIV Surveillance Supplemental Report 2019;24(No. 1). http://www.cdc.gov/hiv/library/reports/hiv-surveillance.html. Published February 2019.

**Figure 7.19**

**Estimated HIV incidence and prevalence in the United States, 2010–2015.** (From Centers of Disease Control: *Estimated HIV incidence and prevalence in the United States, 2010–2015.* https://www.cdc.gov/hiv/pdf/library/reports/surveillance/cdc-hiv-incidence-infographic-vol24-1.pdf.)

## Persons with HIV (Prevalence)

In 2016, **only 86%** of people with HIV **had a diagnosed infection**

**162,500 people** still **did not know they were infected**

## Undiagnosed HIV Infections

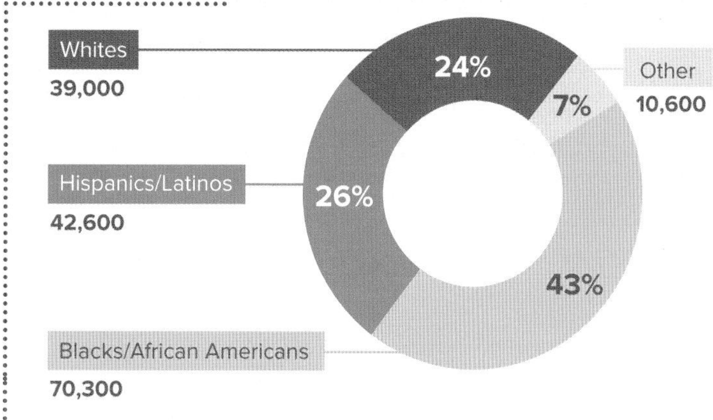


## Persons Who Inject Drugs (PWID)

5% of HIV infections in the U.S. are among **PWID**

Infections **decreased by 34% among all women** with an infection attributed to injection drug use 2010–2016

## Opioid Crisis

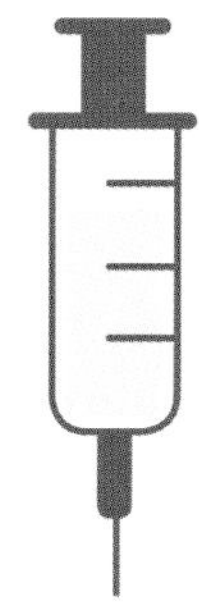

While HIV infections from injection drug use have **steadily declined,** the **nation's opioid crisis threatens this progress.**

## The South

In 2016:

**51%** of **annual** HIV infections

**45%** of **persons living with** HIV infections

**50%** of **undiagnosed** HIV infections

Southern states account for **38%** of the US population but bear the highest burden of HIV infection

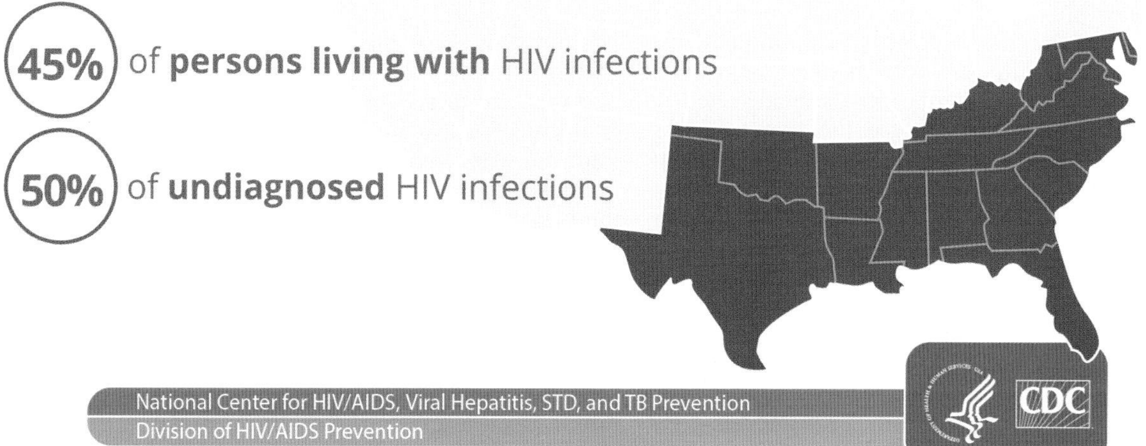


**Figure 7.19 cont'd**

**Table 7.3** Comparison of HIV-1 and HIV-2

| Parameter | HIV-1 | HIV-2 |
|---|---|---|
| Location | Worldwide and more common strain | Predominantly found in West Africa |
| Progression of viral strain | The viral strain progresses rapidly and worst. | The viral strain less likely to progress. For those people infected remain lifelong non-progressors. Hence, progression of viral strain is slower. |
| Immune system status | Average level of immune system activation is higher. | Average level of immune system activation is lower. |
| CD4 count | Lower CD4 counts than HIV- 2 | Higher CD4 counts than HIV-1 |
| Viral load | The plasma viral loads are higher. | The plasma viral loads are lower. |

Data from: Nyamweya S, Hegedus A, Jaye A, et al: Comparing HIV-1 and HIV-2 infection: Lessons from viral immunopathogenesis. *Rev Med Virol* 2013. https://doi.org/10.1002/rmv.1739.

the host cell, reverse transcriptase enables the copying of all the genetic information from the HIV RNA strand to make viral DNA. Once the viral genome is transcribed, integrase enables it to be integrated into the host's DNA and duplicated many times. Final assembly of new HIV virion particles is enabled by protease.

Replication of the virus can cause cell death, although the person remains asymptomatic for a period of time. Seroconversion refers to the emergence of HIV antibodies in the bloodstream (i.e., the person becomes positive for HIV antibodies) and usually takes place 3 to 6 weeks after infection; however, it can take up to 6 months for seroconversion to occur. Thus, an antibody test used for screening will yield a negative result for a period of time after exposure. During this pre-seroconversion period, contagion is possible because of the viral loads being high immediately after acute infection. After seroconversion, less virus is found in the blood; but HIV antibodies can be detected.

During asymptomatic HIV disease, the virus migrates from the serum into the tissues to infect CD4 cells in lymph tissue. The virus continues to kill the CD4 cells in the lymph nodes, although the CD4 count remains above 500 cells/mm$^3$.

As CD4 cells in lymph nodes are depleted, the virus once again enters the blood to infect any remaining lymphocytes and clinically apparent disease, known as symptomatic HIV disease, emerges. By the time this happens, the immune system has been compromised and is ineffective and unable to mount a specific immune response to these virions. The immune system dysfunction places the individual at risk for opportunistic diseases.

The decline in CD4 cells results in progressive loss of immune system function and the development of a wide variety of clinical signs and symptoms (see Table 7.4). In this symptomatic phase, CD4 count ranges between 200 and 500 cells/mm$^3$.

When the CD4 count declines less than 200 cells/mm$^3$ and/or when an AIDS defining illness (opportunistic infection), wasting, or dementia occurs, the person is classified as having advanced HIV disease, or AIDS. Immunocompromised and elevated viral load occur during the advanced stage and are associated with the development of opportunistic infections (Fig. 7.22).

This infectious process and subsequent immunosuppression may result in one or more of the following: immunodeficiency with opportunistic infections and unusual malignancies; autoimmune conditions such as rheumatoid arthritis, lymphoid interstitial pneumonitis, hypergammaglobulinemia, and production of autoimmune antibodies; or neurologic dysfunction, including HIV-associated dementia, HIV encephalopathy, and peripheral neuropathies.

HIV has an extremely high mutation rate even within a single individual, producing competing strains of the same virus that fight for survival against the weapons produced by the immune system and contribute to the development of resistance to antiretroviral medications.

**Clinical Manifestations.** HIV infection manifests itself in many different ways (Table 7.4) and differs between the adult and pediatric populations. Great variation exists among individuals as to the amount of time that passes between acute HIV infection, the appearance of symptoms, the diagnosis of AIDS, and death. The clinical picture of an individual with HIV varies on the spectrum of infection based on what stage is present. The stages of infection vary from acute to asymptomatic to symptomatic. Each stage of infection somehow correlates with the level of the CD4 counts.

***Acute Infection.*** One to 6 weeks after an exposure and acute infection with HIV, the person may experience a transient period of flu-like symptoms and lymphadenopathy. Viral loads are typically high after an acute infection; however, antibody tests used the screen for HIV disease will remain negative until the point of seroconversion.

***Asymptomatic HIV Disease (CD4 Count of 500 Cells/mm$^3$ or More).*** During the asymptomatic stage, the person demonstrates a positive antibody test for HIV but remains asymptomatic, for a period that can range between 1 and 20 years. At this stage of infection, the infected person is clinically healthy and capable of normal daily activities, normal work habits, and unrestricted level and duration of exercise. However, fatigue and generalized lymphadenopathy with swollen and firm lymph glands may be observed during this stage.

***Symptomatic HIV Disease (CD4 Count Between 200 and 500 Cells/mm$^3$).*** As the infection progresses and the immune system becomes increasingly more compromised, a variety of symptoms may develop, including persistent generalized adenopathy, nonspecific symptoms (such as diarrhea, weight loss, fatigue, night sweats, and fever), or neurologic symptoms resulting from HIV encephalopathy. The length of this phase is variable. If untreated, the person will eventually progress to advanced HIV disease.

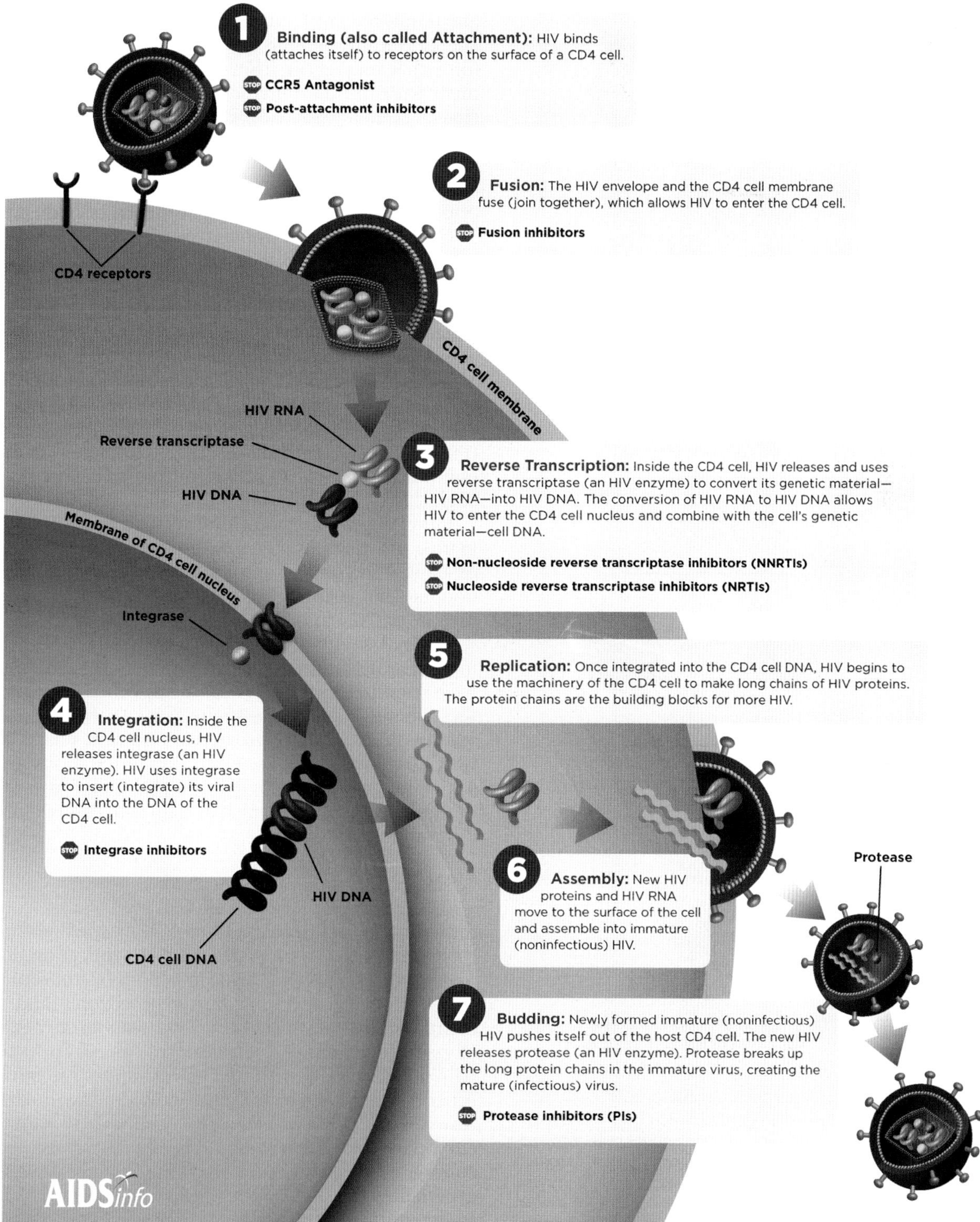


**Figure 7.20**

**Seven stages of the HIV life cycle.** (From US Department of Health and Human Services: *The HIV Life Cycle. US Department of Health and Human Services AIDS Info*. From https://aidsinfo.nih.gov/understanding-hiv-aids/fact-sheets/19/73/the-hiv-life-cycle.)

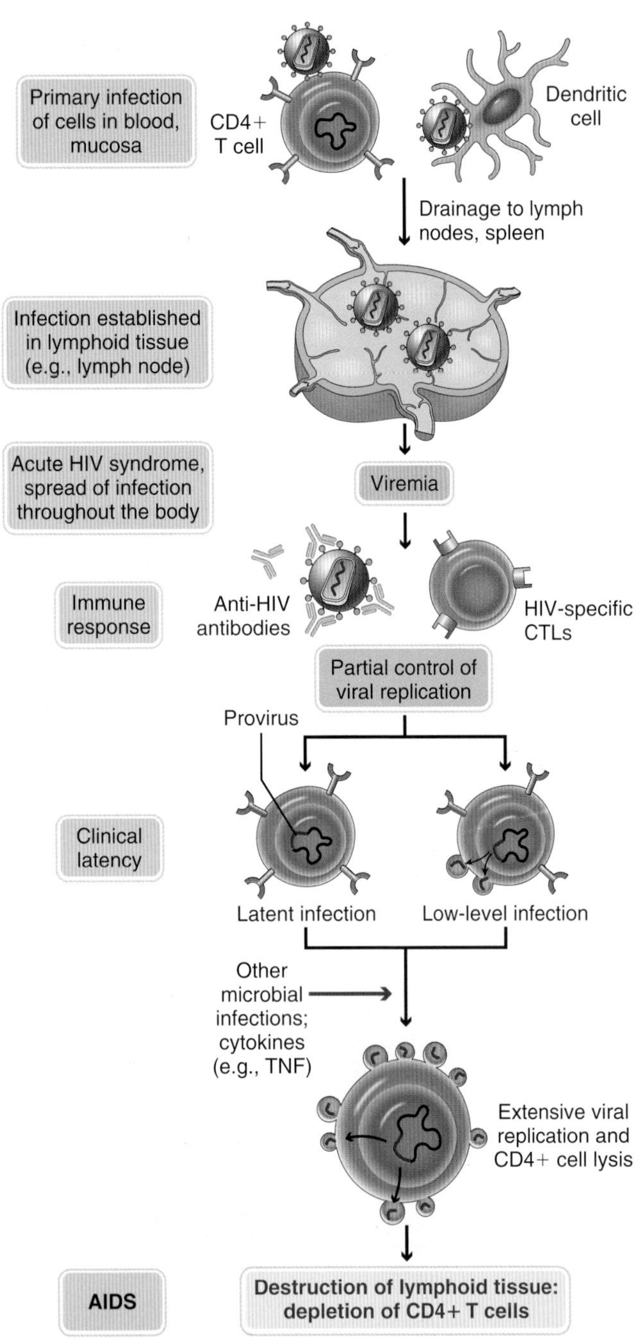


**Figure 7.21**

**Pathogenesis of HIV-1 infection.** Initially, HIV-1 infects T cells and macrophages directly or is carried to these cells by Langerhans cells. Viral replication in the regional lymph nodes leads to viremia and widespread seeding of lymphoid tissue. The viremia is controlled by the host immune response (not shown), and the patient then enters a phase of clinical latency. During this phase, viral replication in both T cells and macrophages continues unabated, but there is some immune containment of virus (not illustrated). A gradual erosion of CD4+ cells by productive infection (or other mechanisms, not shown) continues. Ultimately, CD4+ cell numbers decline, and the patient develops clinical symptoms of full-blown AIDS. Macrophages are also parasitized by the virus early; they are not lysed by HIV-1, and they may transport the virus to tissues, particularly the brain. (Reprinted from Kumar V: *Robbins and Cotran: pathologic basis of disease,* ed 8, Philadelphia, 2009, WB Saunders.)

***Advanced HIV Disease (AIDS) (CD4 Count of 200 Cells/mm$^3$ or Less, and/or Occurrence of an AIDS-defining Illness [Opportunistic Infection], Wasting, or Dementia).*** The neurologic manifestations of advanced HIV disease are numerous and can involve the central, peripheral, and autonomic nervous systems. In addition to the symptoms that may occur from opportunistic diseases, treatment with multiple medications can cause adverse side effects, sometimes creating a confusing clinical picture. The immune system dysfunction, as evidenced by a precariously low CD4 counts, places the person at risk for an opportunistic infection (such as *P. carinii* pneumonia, cytomegalovirus [CMV], toxoplasmosis) or malignancy.

CMV can cause peripheral neuropathy and HIV retinitis (with possible blindness). *P. carinii* pneumonia is a fungal infection of the lungs that causes symptoms such as dyspnea on exertion, chest discomfort, nonproductive cough, and weight loss. Toxoplasmosis is a parasitic disease that affects the central nervous system (CNS).

Dermatologic conditions are common in individuals with advanced HIV disease and can be extensive, including malignancies, bacterial, viral, or fungal infections (Fig.7.23), and reactions to drug treatment. Cutaneous manifestations of HIV can present as dry flaking skin, telangiectasias, and thinning of the skin (and hair).

Other dermatologic conditions such as seborrheic dermatitis, psoriasis, Reiter syndrome, acquired ichthyosis, or Kaposi sarcoma may occur. Kaposi sarcoma (purple nodular skin lesions) predominantly affects homosexual men (Figs. 7.24 and 7.25).

***Other Associated Clinical Manifestations.*** The following associated clinical features of individuals with HIV have relevance in the physical therapy practice. Note that these manifestations are sequelae of HIV disease as the severity of the disease progresses and as it relates to the lymphocyte count. These clinical manifestations are presented below into organ systems and into constellations of signs and symptoms such as pain syndromes and lipodystrophic syndromes.

### *Neurologic Manifestations*

Pain Syndromes in Individuals with HIV Disease. Pain syndromes seen in individuals with HIV are divided into three groups: pain associated with HIV infection, immunosuppression, opportunistic infections or comorbidities; pain caused by HIV diagnostic procedures and treatment; and pain unrelated to HIV disease or its treatment (e.g., diabetic neuropathy, discogenic pain). For example, pain is associated with extensive Kaposi sarcoma and other dermatologic conditions. Individuals with HIV disease may experience headache, abdominal pain,[179,238] chest pain, and arthralgias and myalgias. Namisango and colleagues[186] conducted a multicenter study on the pain experienced by ambulatory individuals with HIV/AIDS to determine the intensity and prevalence of pain. They found that patients who were in clinical stage 4, according to the World Health Organization clinical staging, have a high risk of experiencing severe pain, and higher CD4 T-cell count was associated with lower risk of experiencing severe pain. They recommended strengthening the quality of pain management especially to these ambulatory patients.

**Table 7.4** Clinical Manifestations of HIV Disease

| Musculoskeletal | Neurologic/Neuromuscular | Cardiopulmonary | Integumentary | Other |
|---|---|---|---|---|
| Myalgia/arthralgia<br>Rheumatologic manifestations:<br>• Inflammatory joint disorders (e.g., Reiter syndrome, reactive arthritis, psoriatic arthritis)<br>• Myositis/ pyomyositis<br>• Connective tissue disease<br>Avascular necrosis (osteonecrosis)<br>Musculoskeletal pain syndrome/HIV wasting syndrome<br>Myopathy (disease or drug-induced)<br>Pelvic pain (e.g., pelvic inflammatory disease)<br>Extrapulmonary tuberculosis<br>Delayed healing (can lead to sepsis and death)<br>Myositis ossificans | HIV encephalitis:<br>• Gait disturbance<br>• Intention tremor<br>• Delayed release of reflexes | Dyspnea, especially on exertion<br>Nonproductive cough<br>Hypoxia<br>Symptoms associated with opportunistic infections of the pulmonary system<br>Pericardial effusion<br>Cardiomyopathy<br>Endocarditis<br>Vasculitis | Alopecia (hair loss)<br>Basal cell carcinoma<br>Kaposi sarcoma<br>Mucocutaneous ulcers<br>Rash<br>Urticaria (diffuse skin reaction, wheals)<br>Delayed wound healing | Constitutional symptoms:<br>• Flu-like symptoms<br>• Fever, sore throat<br>• Generalized adenopathy<br>• Weight loss<br>• Lethargy, fatigue<br>• Night sweats, fevers |
| | HIV-associated dementia:<br>• *Behavioral*: apathy, lethargy, social withdrawal, irritability, depression<br>• *Cognitive:* memory impairment, confusion, disorientation<br>• *Motor*: ataxia, leg weakness with gait disturbances, loss of fine motor coordination, incontinence, paraplegia (advanced stage)<br>Guillain-Barré syndrome<br>Headache, seizures (toxoplasmosis)<br>HIV myelitis (osteomyelitis)<br>Radiculopathy | | | Opportunistic infections:<br>• Cytomegalovirus<br>• Bacterial pneumonia<br>• Tuberculosis<br>• Toxoplasmosis<br>• *Pneumocystis carinii*<br>• Sinusitis<br>• Vaginal infection<br>Malignancy (most common)<br>• Non-Hodgkin lymphoma<br>• Kaposi sarcoma<br>• Cervical cancer<br>GI disturbance, including wasting syndrome<br>Lymphedema<br>Lipodystrophy<br>Renal (kidney) failure<br>Hepatic (liver) failure<br>Oral thrush<br>Gingivitis<br>Visual disturbance<br>HIV-related psychiatric disorders |
| | Peripheral neuropathy:<br>• Pain (burning tingling<br>• Sensory loss<br>• Secondary motor deficits, gait disturbances<br>Brachial neuropathy<br>Vacuolar spinal myelopathy | | | |

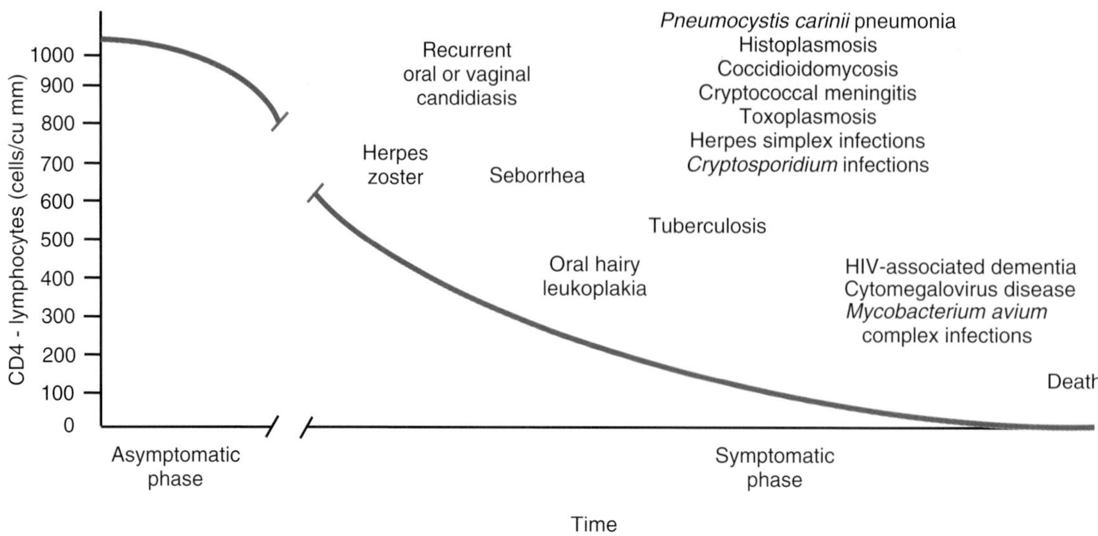


**Figure 7.22**

**Complications of HIV disease as related to lymphocyte count.**

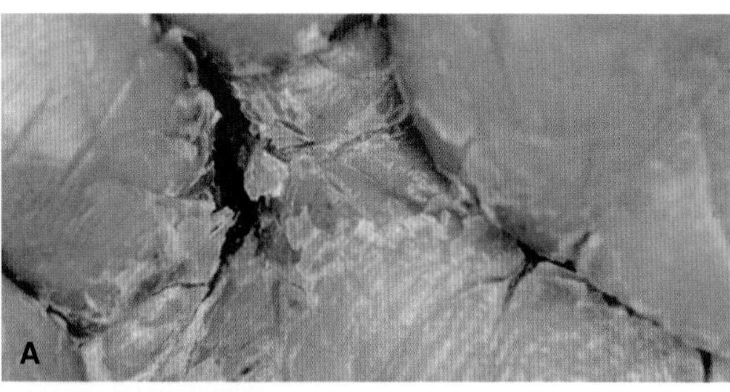


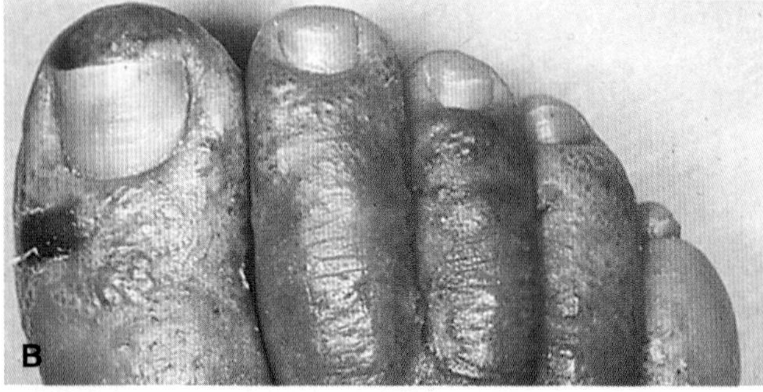


**Figure 7.23**

**Tinea pedis.** (A) Fungal infections, such as tinea pedis (also known as athlete's foot), often begin between the toes and extend to the surface of the toes and foot. Red, itching skin may begin to peel or cause foot odor. (B) The condition can progress, as shown here. Skin changes can become even more severe, with complete destruction of the nail beds (not shown). (A, Reprinted from Seidel H: *Mosby's guide to physical examination*, ed 5, St Louis, 2003, Mosby. B, Reprinted from Cohen J, Powderly WG: *Infectious diseases*, ed 2, St Louis, 2004, Mosby.)

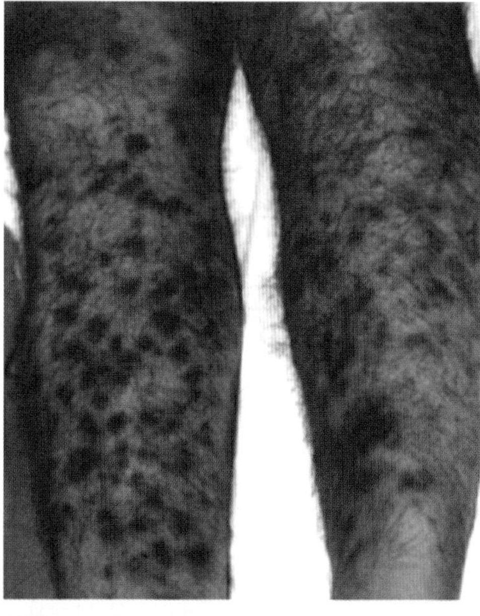

**Figure 7.24**

Kaposi sarcoma is not limited to the upper body; it can also appear in the lower quadrant. (Courtesy Julie Hobbs, Kingwood Medical Center, Kingwood, TX.)

Peripheral Neuropathies. A form of peripheral neuropathy known as *distal sensory polyneuropathy* (DSP) is the most common neurologic cause of pain in HIV disease, affecting one-third of individuals with AIDS.[278] The risk factors associated with DSP include: (a) advanced stages of HIV disease; (b) low CD4 lymphocyte count; and (c) higher plasma HIV-1 viral load.[102] Several studies have explored the association of the level of viral load of individuals with HIV in regard to symptomatology related to neuropathic pain in DSP.[55,250,253,254]

Symptoms of peripheral neuropathies, as well as pain and symptoms of musculoskeletal disorders, occur most often in advanced stages of HIV disease but can occur earlier and may be the presenting manifestation. Neuropathic conditions in individuals with HIV may develop as a result of neurotoxic antiretroviral medications, chronic HIV infection, vitamin deficiencies resulting from poor nutrition, metabolic abnormalities, and opportunistic infections such as CMV.[175,242]

Peripheral neuropathies affect a large portion of people with AIDS. Although DSP is the most common form,

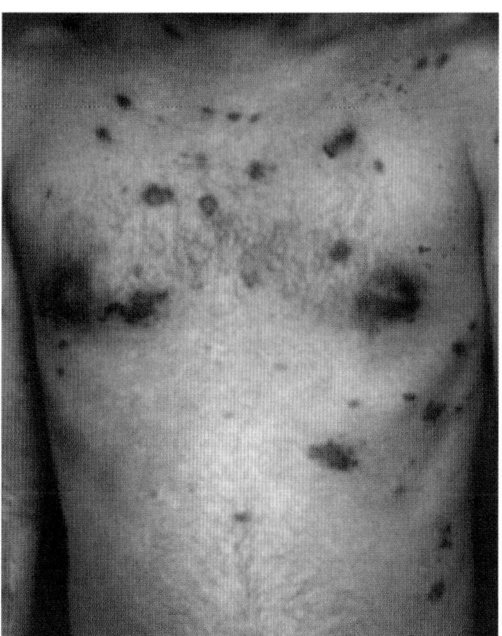

**Figure 7.25**

**Kaposi sarcoma.** There is a reduced incidence of Kaposi sarcoma in the HIV population because of better treatment, so fewer people progress this far in the disease. With better treatment have come fewer complications. Kaposi sarcoma appears primarily in the upper body, sometimes starting as a bulbous lesion on the end of the nose but also involving the face, chest, and lymph nodes. (Courtesy Julie Hobbs, Mayo Clinic, Rochester, Minnesota.)

other peripheral neuropathies may occur, and other parts of the body may be affected such as the face or trunk. DSP symptoms present in a stocking-glove distribution, with the feet and legs more commonly affected than the hands and arms. Involvement of the upper extremities is less common and often occurs much later in the disease process.

Symptoms of DSP include sensory disturbances (paresthesias, numbness), impaired sensation (vibration, pain, light touch, temperature), burning pain, allodynia, hyperalgesia, leg cramping, weakness in intrinsic foot muscles (in advanced cases), sleep disturbances, difficulty with activities of daily living, and impaired balance.[242]

**Neuromusculoskeletal Diseases.** AIDS is associated with *neuromusculoskeletal diseases* such as osteomyelitis, bacterial myositis, and infectious (reactive) arthritis. Osteonecrosis, osteopenia, and osteoporosis are increasingly observed in clients who have been living with HIV disease for long periods. Avascular necrosis (osteonecrosis) of the femoral head(s) has been reported with the use of antiretroviral therapy containing protease inhibitors.[174] The increased incidence of osteonecrosis in HIV/AIDS may be a result of the use of protease inhibitors or possibly as a result of an increased frequency of risk factors previously associated with osteonecrosis, such as hyperlipidemia, corticosteroid use, alcohol abuse, and hypercoagulability.[11,174]

Some *musculoskeletal pain syndromes* seen in individuals with HIV disease may be associated with *HIV wasting syndrome*. HIV wasting is characterized by a disproportionate loss of metabolically active tissue, specifically body cell mass (i.e., tissue involved with glucose oxidation, protein synthesis, and immune system function). These conditions occur secondary to low food intake, altered metabolism, and poor nutrient absorption with manifestations such as extreme weight loss, chronic diarrhea, unexplained weakness, fever, and malnutrition.[84,134,194]

*HIV-associated myopathy* presents with a progressive weakness in the proximal limb and trunk muscles. The weakness is symmetrical and often involves the muscles of the face and neck. This type of myopathy may occur in individuals with HIV at every stage of illness. Muscle biopsies have shown necrosis of muscle fibers with and without inflammatory infiltrates.[88]

**Rheumatologic Diseases.** Rheumatologic manifestations may be transient, subtle, or severe and appear more often as HIV disease progresses. HIV-related arthritis does not necessarily respond to conventional medications. Arthritis may precede or accompany seroconversion. Polymyositis involves bilaterally symmetrical proximal muscle weakness.[88,142]

**Cardiopulmonary Diseases.** Cardiopulmonary diseases continue to be an important cause of illness and death in people with HIV. Bacterial pneumonia, bronchitis, tuberculosis (pulmonary and extrapulmonary), and CMV are common opportunistic diseases in individuals with HIV/AIDS. Emphysema, asthma, and pulmonary hypertension are also observed in this population. Cardiac involvement (heart and blood vessels) occurs as a result of a combination of the HIV infection, medical management, and secondary opportunistic infections. Both HIV infection and HAART can cause changes in lipid and glucose metabolism as well as elevation of blood pressure, promoting the development of atherosclerosis.[27,172,277]

Cardiovascular diseases have become a major cause of mortality among individuals with HIV who respond well to antiretroviral therapy. Myocardial infarction, cardiomyopathy, pericardial effusion, and pericarditis are some other cardiovascular conditions that occur as a result of HIV and/or its treatment.[151]

**Lipodystrophic Syndrome.** Lipodystrophic syndrome, a syndrome of defective fat metabolism, dyslipidemia, and insulin resistance, manifests as central fat accumulation (Fig. 7.26) with visceral fat deposition documented by computed tomographic scans. It is a common problem that may occur soon after starting HAART.[262] Loss of fat occurs in the arms, legs, or face with concomitant fat deposits in the abdomen, breasts (men and women), and back of the neck.[274]

**AIDS-Related Lymphoma.** AIDS-related lymphomas, including Burkitt lymphoma,[103] non-Hodgkin lymphoma, Hodgkin lymphoma, and other more uncommon types (e.g., primary effusion lymphoma), are more likely to occur in individuals with HIV compared to the general population. AIDS-related lymphomas are now the second most common cancer associated with HIV after Kaposi sarcoma and increase with time after infection.[15,132,283] The incidence of non-Hodgkin lymphoma appears to be declining with the use of HAART, whereas the incidence of Hodgkin lymphoma may actually have increased in individuals with HIV.[65] AIDS-related lymphoma can occur at any CD4+ level, but the risk is increased with declining CD4+ lymphocyte counts.[35] The course of disease is often aggressive, with

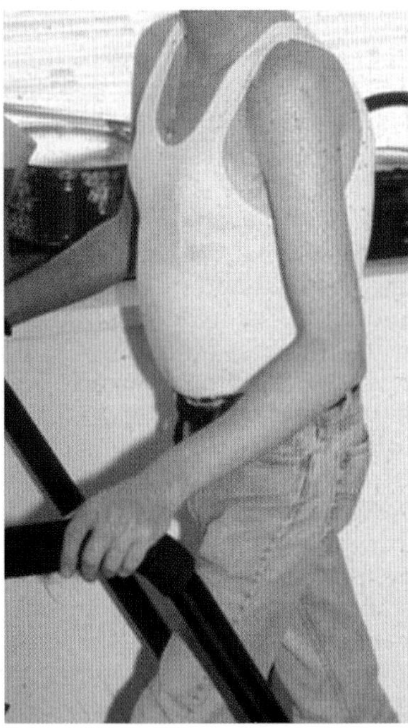

**Figure 7.26**

**Lipodystrophic syndrome (LDS) in clients with HIV/AIDS has become more prevalent as a result of HAART treatment.** LDS with cardiac complications from hyperlipidemia affects men and women, with fat deposits in the upper body and breasts contributing to body image problems, emotional trauma, and cardiac involvement. Additional fat deposits in the upper thoracic area and abdomen with loss in the extremities are seen in this client with AIDS. (Courtesy Julie Hobbs, Mayo Clinic, Rochester, Minnesota.)

extranodal metastases involving unusual sites such as the jaw, heart, body cavities, gallbladder, skin, and soft tissues.[47]

## Medical Management

**Prevention.** Education regarding sexual activity and IDU has been the main emphasis of public health prevention programs. The CDC's overarching HIV prevention goal is to reduce the number of new HIV infections and to eliminate racial and ethnic disparities by promoting HIV counseling, testing, and referral and by encouraging HIV prevention among persons living with HIV and those at high risk for contracting the virus.[47] Socioeconomic factors (e.g., high rates of poverty and unemployment, lack of access to health care) are associated with high rates of HIV risk behaviors among minority MSM and are barriers to accessing HIV testing, diagnosis, and treatment. Reaching minority MSM who may not identify themselves as homosexual or bisexual with prevention messages remains a challenge.

The CDC now recommends routine HIV testing for all individuals between the ages of 13 and 64 years, with annual testing for those in high-risk groups. The CDC also recommends routine HIV testing of all pregnant women and routine screening of any infant whose mother was not screened.[31,124] Routine screening, along with partner notification and availability of sustained treatment for infected individuals, contributes to prevention of transmission. Increased availability and use of simple, rapid HIV tests and at-home HIV tests may help overcome some of the traditional barriers to early diagnosis and treatment of infected persons.

**Box 7.3**

### RISK REDUCTION BEHAVIORS FOR THE PREVENTION OF HIV TRANSMISSION

***Obtain testing for HIV[a] if any of the following is true:***

- You received blood or blood products before 1985.
- You have (or have had) sex, especially if with multiple partners.
- You inject drugs and share needles.
- You have sexual intercourse (vaginal, anal, or oral) with someone else who injects drugs and shares needles.
- You have sex without a condom ("rubber") with someone who has HIV.
- You share used needles for tattooing or body piercing.

***Protect yourself during sexual activities as follows:***

- Abstinence or a monogamous relationship (sex with only one partner; both partners must be HIV free) is the only known prevention for the transmission of HIV.
- Use latex glove when inserting finger(s) into vagina or rectum.
- Use a new condom each time you have oral, anal, or vaginal sex.
- Latex or polyurethane is best, because HIV can pass through lambskin or natural condoms.
- Do not use outdated condoms (check expiration date).
- Use the new condom with each sexual act from beginning to end (i.e., put on the condom before genital contact with partner and when the penis is erect; hold the condom firmly against base of penis during withdrawal; withdraw penis while still erect).
- Use water-based lubricants (e.g., KY jelly), *not* oils, lotions, or Vaseline that can cause a condom to tear or break.
- Ensure that no air is trapped in tip of condom.

***Protect yourself as follows if you use drugs:***

- Never share drug needles or "works."
- Participate in clinic needle exchange programs or clean drug needles with 100% bleach, leave 30 seconds, repeat three times, and then rinse three times with water between uses.
- Mixing sex, drugs, and alcohol increases your risk. If you are drunk or high, it is harder to make good decisions about sexual practices.

***Protect yourself as follows if you are pregnant:***

- You can pass on HIV to your unborn child during pregnancy, birth, or breastfeeding. If you are pregnant and you have engaged in HIV risk behaviors, obtain HIV testing and appropriate treatment if you test positive for HIV.
- Medications taken during pregnancy can reduce your risk of HIV transmission to the fetus during pregnancy.

[a]A simple blood test (some centers offer a saliva test) can determine HIV infection 6 months after exposure. This test can be obtained anonymously (without giving out your name) and is free or low cost in most states. Contact your local Health Department.

Data from Centers for Disease Control and Prevention (CDC) (http://www.cdc.gov/hiv/prevention/programs/pwp/risk.html). Accessed 7/6/2014.

Behavior intervention, the primary prevention tool, includes school-based programs, peer-to-peer interventions, strategies that limit needle sharing, parent-to-child communication, client-centered counseling, and personalized risk-reduction strategies (Box 7.3). The introduction of routine counseling, voluntary testing for women with HIV, and providing zidovudine (commonly known as *AZT*) antiretroviral drugs to infected pregnant women and their infants have dramatically reduced mother-to-child transmission rates.[41,47]

Effective behavior change programs need to address possible behavioral disinhibition (i.e., continuing or returning to high-risk behaviors when one feels protected) among persons who receive preventative interventions. Prevention counseling that addresses safe sex, reducing the number of sex partners, and using condoms correctly and consistently, and other reproductive health needs (e.g., STD treatment and family planning) must be incorporated alongside any other potential prevention interventions such as preexposure prophylaxis.[47]

Restricting sex to partners of the same serostatus does not protect against transmission of other STDs or the possibility of HIV coinfection or superinfection (resistance to two or more classes of antiretroviral drugs) unless condoms are used correctly and consistently.[122] Controlling the AIDS epidemic requires sustained prevention programs in all affected communities, particularly programs targeting MSM, sexually active individuals with multiple partners, IDUs, and minorities.

Even though potent antiviral treatment can eradicate HIV from the blood, these drugs cannot completely eliminate the virus from the body, especially in semen. Although antiretroviral therapy reduces shedding of HIV in semen, thereby reducing HIV transmissibility, a substantial portion of people with HIV may still be infectious and may have drug-resistant strains of the virus.[14] Safe sex practices should continue to be reinforced in all people with HIV.

Researchers are working to find a topical inhibition strategy that would prevent sexual HIV-1 transmission by using a microbicide that can target a diversity of HIV-1 strains without causing mucosal inflammation in the lining of the vagina and have a minimum of adverse side effects, all while maintaining effectiveness for prolonged periods.[221] For individuals with HIV disease, prevention of other infections is important. For example, *P. carinii* pneumonia prophylaxis can be achieved with drugs such as Bactrim. *Mycobacterium tuberculosis* has a higher prevalence in the HIV population. It is communicable, preventable, and treatable. One in three adults with HIV disease is coinfected with *M. tuberculosis*. Tuberculin skin testing should be available and routinely offered to individuals at HIV testing sites. Guidelines for the prevention of other opportunistic infections in people with HIV are now available.[46,131]

**Diagnosis.** Early diagnosis is important for effective treatment to be initiated in a timely manner. Sex partners should be notified of their risk of HIV and the subsequent need for HIV testing. In their most recent publication, Branson and colleagues[30] from the Office of Centers for Disease Control and Prevention updated the recommendations on the laboratory testing for the diagnosis of HIV infection. The algorithm presented here illustrates steps in the laboratory testing. The testing commences with detection of the immunoassays of the two strains of HIV, HIV-1 and HIV-2, antibodies combined with testing for HIV-1 p24 antigen. If all specimens reacted on the initial assays, then a supplemental testing is done to differentiate HIV-1 from HIV-2 antibodies. Next, if the specimens are reactive to the initial immunoassay and nonreactive on the antibody differentiation assay, then testing proceeds to HIV-1 nucleic acid testing for resolution.

The Centers for Disease Control and Prevention[42] recommends three types of HIV diagnostic tests: nucleic acid tests (NAT), antigen/antibody tests, and antibody tests. NATs search for the virus in the blood. Laboratory testing used previously to diagnosis HIV-1 infection such as HIV-1 Western blot and HIV-1 IFA were removed from the algorithm above. If individuals test positive to the above algorithm, supplemental laboratory testing is required (e.g., HIV-1 viral load, CD4 T-lymphocyte determination, and antiretroviral resistance assay). This is done for several reasons: (a) to confirm infection with HIV-1; (b) to determine the stage of HIV disease; and (c) to guide the appropriate antiretroviral drug therapy.[199]

**Treatment.** There are three important facts to note concerning HIV treatment: (a) HIV medications cannot cure the etiologic agent; they can promote healthier lives and prolong the lives of people with HIV; (b) combinations of medicines are taken to prevent HIV from advancing to AIDS; and (c) the medicines can reduce the risk of transmissibility to other people; however, safe sex (use of condoms and barriers) is still highly recommended.[275]

Highly active antiretroviral therapy (HAART) is the recommended treatment for individuals with HIV. The Food and Drug Administration (FDA) has approved HIV medicines that are categorized into different drug classes. The drug classes are: nucleoside reverse transcriptase inhibitors (NRTIs), nonnucleoside reverse transcriptase inhibitors (NNRTIs), protease inhibitors (PIs), fusion inhibitors, CCR5 antagonists, integrase inhibitors, postattachment inhibitors, and pharmacokinetic enhancers.[86,275] It is worth recalling the life cycle of HIV, because the drug classes are mapped out accordingly. For details of the FDA-approved HIV medicines, go to the following link: https://www.fda.gov/ForPatients/Illness/HIVAIDS/Treatment/ucm118915.htm. The initial regimen for individuals who are HIV positive includes three HIV medicines from at least two different classes.

Despite the FDA-approved HIV medicines, there are investigational drugs being tested to treat or prevent HIV infection. These investigational drugs are not approved by the FDA and are not approved for general consumption or for sale within the United States. Additionally, there are drugs that are in clinical trials to treat HIV-related opportunistic infections. These opportunistic infections are infection-related cancer and/or infections that are more severe in destroying the immune systems of people with healthy immune systems.[275]

***Vaccines in HIV.*** There are two types of HIV vaccines: therapeutic HIV vaccine and preventive HIV vaccine.[275] The therapeutic HIV vaccine is geared toward improving the immune system of individuals with HIV. This type of vaccine slows the progression of HIV to AIDS, keeping the person who is HIV positive at undetectable levels without requiring the use of HAART. This vaccine may reduce the likelihood of transmitting HIV to others. Currently, there is no approved therapeutic HIV vaccine; clinical trials are in progress. On the other hand, the preventive HIV vaccine is administered to people who have not contracted HIV with the aim of HIV prevention. As with therapeutic HIV vaccine, there is currently no FDA-approved preventive HIV vaccine; this is still under investigation.

SPECIAL IMPLICATIONS FOR THE THERAPIST 7.2

### *Infection Control in Immune Deficiencies*

Although infection control strategies, such as handwashing, standard precautions, and disinfection, are important for all people treated in the health care system, they are especially critical for people whose immune systems are altered by primary immunodeficiency disorders, secondary immunodeficiency disorders, and HIV infection.

It is important that health care providers are aware of altered defense mechanisms, infectious agents, reservoirs, and modes of transmission and employ infection control strategies to prevent infection in this population (Fig. 7.27).

Pulmonary complications are common among the immunocompromised, accompanied by poor cough reflexes, an inability to cough effectively, and susceptibility to pulmonary and other opportunistic infections. Additionally, these individuals are often debilitated and easily fatigued. Frequent mobilization and body positioning enhance gas exchange and promote comfort while maintaining strength.[73]

SPECIAL IMPLICATIONS FOR THE THERAPIST 7.3

### *Human Immunodeficiency Virus Disease*

With advances in treatment, improved care, and longer survival, therapists can expect to see increasing numbers of people in their practices who may have HIV. Maximal effectiveness from physical therapy requires a therapist who is knowledgeable about HIV disease and the rehabilitation issues surrounding individuals with HIV disease.[237] It is possible for individuals with HIV to come to a therapy practice undiagnosed or unwilling to disclose their HIV status. Women who have been raped have an increased risk of HIV transmission and may not report this information.

Consideration of HIV status should be integrated into history and/or medical screening. For example, anyone presenting with musculoskeletal or neuromuscular symptoms of unknown origin, with or without constitutional symptoms, should be interviewed more specifically about medical history, including whether they have had a HIV test (especially if the person is in a high-risk group). This may potentially lead to medical referral, diagnosis, and appropriate therapy. Providing a discreet and nonjudgmental environment with assurance of confidentiality while emphasizing the importance of disclosing accurate risk information may help facilitate risk disclosure. Clients at any stage of HIV disease may need psychosocial support to deal with depression, anxiety, or emotional problems that may develop. Thus, screening for depression and anxiety is essential; referral for further treatment may be indicated.[136]

Therapists have a role in osteoporosis education, prevention, and screening. Risk factor assessment is advised for anyone with HIV infection. Anyone at high risk for osteopenia or osteoporosis should be referred for dual x-ray absorptiometry measurement of bone mineral density. Clients should be encouraged to minimize risk for developing osteoporosis with dietary calcium and vitamin D intake, maintaining a normal body mass index, avoiding tobacco and alcohol abuse, and maintaining a long-term weight-bearing exercise program.[222]

#### Prevention of Transmission in the Health Care and Athletic Settings

In all health care settings, standard precautions (e.g., using barriers for working with any liquid that comes from another person, excluding sweat, should be observed to prevent the transmission of any bloodborne pathogens. Box 7.4 includes specific recommendations for health care professionals working with clients with HIV. Individuals with advanced HIV disease are likely to be immunodeficient, and every precaution must be taken to prevent infection for that person.

The risk of transmission of the virus from client to health care worker is exceedingly small. Sources of HIV that may pose a risk of transmission through these routes include blood, visibly bloody fluids, tissues, and other body fluids, including semen; vaginal secretions; and cerebrospinal, synovial, pleural, peritoneal, pericardial, and amniotic fluids. In addition, any direct cutaneous or mucosal contact, without barrier protection to concentrated HIV in a research laboratory or production facility is considered to be an exposure.[171]

#### Postexposure Prophylaxis

Postexposure prophylaxis (PEP) is used to prevent HIV infection after occupational exposure, unsafe sex with an infected partner, sexual assault, or high-risk IDU.[181,200] Occupational exposure should be considered an urgent medical concern requiring timely postexposure management.[44] Health care providers with occupational exposure to HIV should receive follow-up counseling, postexposure testing, and medical evaluation regardless of whether they receive PEP treatment.

PEP consists of a 28-day course of HAART and must be initiated as quickly as possible (within hours) after exposure. The antiretroviral medications may help to diminish or end viral replication, thereby reducing the viral inoculum to a more potentially manageable target for the host's defenses. Determining level of risk and appropriateness of drug selection should be conducted as soon as possible after an exposure has occurred.

Exposed health care providers are advised to use precautions to prevent secondary transmission, especially during the first 6 to 12 weeks postexposure (e.g., avoid blood or tissue donations, breastfeeding, or pregnancy). Other guidelines for HIV PEP are available.[181,200,44]

### Guidelines for Health Care Workers with HIV

According to the Center for HIV Law & Policy:

> States differ slightly in their guidelines on restrictions on an HIV-positive HCW's [health care worker's] practice and on patient notification. Regarding restrictions on an HCW's practice, all states agree that infection alone is not a basis for imposing restrictions and each employ some form of committee or expert review panel to make the decision regarding use of restrictions. Some states require that HIV-positive HCWs cease performing invasive procedures until they have sought the advice of the panel. Other states, however, make the decision to seek the advice of the panel more voluntary. Most states provide for continued review and/or supervision following the imposition of any restrictions. Regarding patient notification, many states leave that decision to the review committee to make on a case-by-case basis, while others require the consent of the patient before the HCW can participate in an invasive procedure.[272]

### HIV and Rehabilitative Therapy

Today, chronic conditions such as cardiovascular disease related to lipodystrophic syndrome and rheumatologic and musculoskeletal conditions are much more common in those with HIV. Therefore, physical therapists are generally focused on assisting the individual with the management of specific impairments and functional limitations related to chronic HIV infection, its comorbidities, and/or opportunistic infections when they arise.

The individual with HIV disease may demonstrate clinical manifestations of overlapping pathologic processes and disabilities that need appropriate rehabilitation intervention. For example, the CNS can be the site of more than one opportunistic disease process simultaneously,[101] or the individual may sustain a stroke in addition to having an already existing peripheral neuropathy or other neuromusculoskeletal manifestations. The therapist may be involved in wound intervention when integumentary impairment is caused by HIV opportunistic infections, while providing intervention to relieve problems associated with rheumatologic dysfunctions.[237]

Physical therapists need to consider physical fitness, quality-of-life issues, work, activities of daily living, and community management skills such as access to transportation, socialization opportunities, shopping, banking, ability to negotiate health care and insurance systems[101] and participation in church, synagogue, or other spiritual networks. Home programs must be simple and easily incorporated into the patient's lifestyle.

Often individuals with AIDS are overwhelmed by the disease process, the complicated treatment, the multiple health care appointments, and scheduling to manage all of these tasks. Adding an exercise program may result in frustration and noncompliance unless the person can see a clear benefit and way to manage yet another aspect of the treatment program.

For individuals with CNS involvement, rehabilitation therapy may help the client optimize functional ability. These clients may respond to an eclectic blend of rehabilitation strategies such as those for other individuals who have CNS involvement as a result of stroke or head injury.[135]

Distal sensory peripheral neuropathy is one of the most common causes of pain in people with chronic HIV disease. It may be related to certain drugs used to treat HIV or related to effects of the chronicity of the infection.[98] The use of conventional transcutaneous electrical nerve stimulation may be helpful in addressing peripheral pain in HIV-related peripheral neuropathies; there is no known evidence that this modality is contraindicated but studies are needed to verify its true benefit. Joint and soft tissue mobilization, stretching, gait and balance training, and desensitization techniques can be very effective. The alternative use of microcurrent electroacupuncture has been reported to reduce pain, improve functional status, and increase perceived strength. Discussion of the possible mechanisms for these effects is available.[98]

The presence of peripheral neuropathies may also signal nutritional deficiencies requiring nutritional counseling. This is especially true for the client who has the wasting syndrome that often accompanies advanced HIV disease. In addition, without proper nutrition, therapy involving balance training, extremity strengthening and stretching, and motor skills may be limited in benefit.

Diminished sensory information associated with peripheral neuropathies of the lower extremities makes balance and gait control more difficult. Clients with HIV disease may have balance deficits at lower movement speeds compared to healthy adults. Motor slowness is associated with both neuropathy and myopathy.[163] Formulating a rehabilitation approach must be based on the underlying neurophysiologic deficit(s) present.[99] Other guidelines for management of the lower extremity complications, balance, and postural derangements associated with distal symmetrical polyneuropathy are available.[100,244]

For individuals with acute inflammatory myopathy, exercise is generally contraindicated until the inflammatory condition is managed medically. For many other musculoskeletal conditions, progressive resistance training with weights, elastic bands, or tubing to strengthen specific muscles may be beneficial.

Improper body mechanics, poor postural alignment and postural instability, balance and gait problems, and other biomechanical changes may occur in the person who has developed muscle weakness and fatigue from progression of the disease process, malnutrition, or the wasting syndrome. Postural awareness, stretching and strengthening of specific muscles, and attention to nutrition may be part of the treatment plan.

Cardiopulmonary complications (see Table 7.4) in advanced stages of HIV disease contribute to morbidity and mortality. Oxygen transport mechanisms can be adversely affected. Muscle and joint mobilization techniques and breathing exercises are essential for the person who has been immobilized for any length of time as a result of respiratory or other disease involvement. Cardiac rehabilitation principles should be applied as needed for individuals with specific cardiopulmonary conditions such as myocardial infarction, pericardial effusion, or myocarditis.

#### Exercise and HIV Disease

##### *Early Asymptomatic Stage of HIV Disease*

Exercise is considered safe for people with HIV and an important way to increase the CD4 cells at earlier stages of the disease, possibly delaying symptoms while increasing muscle strength and size. During asymptomatic stages of HIV disease, metabolic parameters are within normal limits, with no limitations placed on the individual. Individuals with asymptomatic HIV disease should be encouraged to exercise regularly, including both aerobic and resistance exercise components.[138]

The effect of HIV and its treatment with protease inhibitors on exercise and activity tolerance has been reported. Physical activity intolerance resulting in functional limitations may be caused by diminished aerobic capacity (decreased peak $VO_2$) far below that occurring as a result of physiologic deconditioning alone. Individuals who receive HAART may have a reduced ability to extract and use oxygen from the muscle during exercise, limiting their ability to increase the intensity of activity.[38]

*Symptomatic and Advanced Stages of HIV Disease*

During symptomatic and advanced stages of HIV disease, functional capacity is reduced, requiring more individualized exercise prescription and lower intensities.[156] Neurologic dysfunction and deconditioning are common. Regular physical activity and exercise are just as important in this group but are more difficult and symptom limited. Among people with HIV disease who have known cardiovascular disease, pulmonary limitations, or muscle dysfunction, exercise prescription should address impairments and limitations. Collaboration with the physician to determine any contraindications for exercise is advised.

Strenuous or exhaustive exercise training is not recommended; aerobic exercise at moderate levels of intensity is suggested with medical clearance.[267] Constant or interval aerobic exercise for at least 20 minutes, at least three times per week for 4 weeks, may lead to improved cardiopulmonary fitness and improved psychologic status, with an accompanying maintenance of immunologic function.[192] Supervised aerobic exercise training safely decreases fatigue, weight, body mass index, fat, and central fat in HIV-1–infected individuals. It may not affect dyspnea.[255]

Clients with advanced disease may be at greater risk for exercise-related injuries due to chronic myopathic and neuropathic tissue changes. Recovery periods after exercise may be prolonged. Response to exercise should be carefully monitored.[138]

Individuals with acute inflammatory myopathy or myositis should not perform strenuous or resisted exercises until creatine phosphokinase levels normalize. Bouts of acute inflammatory arthralgia may require periods of joint protection and relative rest as well as medical management.[138]

Exercise has beneficial effects for those with AIDS-related wasting syndrome. Progressive resistance exercise can increase lean body mass significantly.[232,234]

The role of exercise in the treatment of lipodystrophic syndrome is important[26] and has been shown to have potential in normalizing insulin resistance, to be effective in managing metabolic abnormalities without causing further side effects,[66] and to reduce trunk fat mass.[233] Short-term intervention of aerobic exercise combined with a low-lipid diet can increase functional capacity but may not change plasma lipid levels.[271]

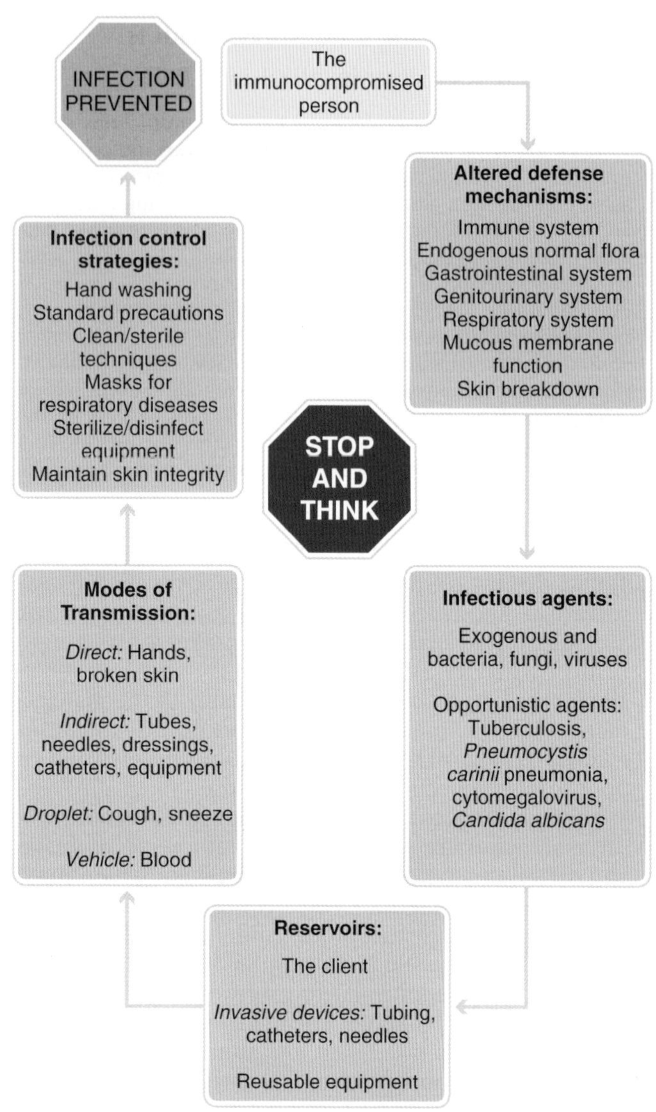


**Figure 7.27**

Factors affecting the immunocompromised person, leading to the selection of the correct infection control strategies to prevent infectious complications. (Courtesy Julie Hobbs, Mayo Clinic, Rochester, Minnesota.)

**Box 7.4**

**STANDARD HIV PRECAUTIONS FOR HEALTH CARE WORKERS**

- Use protective barriers (gloves, eye shields, gowns) when handling blood, body fluids, and infectious fluids.
- Wash hands, skin, and mucous membranes immediately and thoroughly if contaminated by blood or other body fluids.
- Prevent needle or scalpel sticks.
- Ventilation devices are available for resuscitation.
- Any health care worker with open wounds or skin lesions should not treat clients or handle equipment until the lesion(s) heals.
- Pregnant health care workers should take extra precautions. See Appendix A for additional information.
- Occupational exposure to HIV should be followed immediately by evaluation of exposure source and postexposure prophylaxis.

From Centers for Disease Control and Prevention (CDC): *Occupational HIV transmission and prevention among health care workers*, 2011. Available online at: http://www.cdc.gov/hiv/resources/factsheets/hcwprev.htm.

## Chronic Fatigue and Immune Dysfunction Syndrome

### Overview

Chronic fatigue and immune dysfunction syndrome, chronic fatigue syndrome (CFS), chronic Epstein-Barr virus, myalgic encephalomyelitis, and neuromyasthenia all denote a highly publicized but not new illness. The Centers for Disease Control and Prevention[48] uses CFS interchangeably with myalgic encephalitis (ME). The name *chronic fatigue syndrome* indicates that this illness is not a single disease but the result of a combination of factors. Furthermore, it is a subset of *chronic fatigue*, a broader category defined as unexplained fatigue of greater than or equal to 6 months' duration. This distinction is made to facilitate epidemiologic studies of populations with prolonged fatigue and chronic fatigue.

### Incidence and Risk Factors

The 2015 report from the Institute of Medicine indicated 836,000 to 2.3 million Americans are afflicted with ME/CFS, but 90% of them have not been diagnosed. The economic impact is estimated to be $17 to $24 billion of medical costs and loss of income. 48 Two U.S. community-based CFS studies found prevalence among adults of 0.23% and 0.42%; the rates were higher in women, members of minority groups, and people with lower educational attainment and occupational status.[125,230]

People of every age, gender, ethnicity, and socioeconomic group can have CFS. Demographic data show that in most studies, 75% or more of people with CFS are female. The mean age at onset of CFS is between 29 and 35 years. The mean illness duration ranges from 3 to 9 years.[39] Although CFS is much less common in children than in adults, children can develop the illness, particularly during the teen years.

### Etiologic Factors and Pathogenesis

Many studies have investigated the etiology and pathogenesis of CFS.[150] More than half of the CFS studies between 1980 and 1995 concentrated on the physical etiology of CFS, with a slight shift toward psychologic and psychiatric research in the next few years.[62]

Many somatic and psychosocial hypotheses on the etiology of CFS have been explored. Explanations for CFS were sought in viral infections, immune dysfunction, neuroendocrine responses, dysfunction of the CNS, muscle structure, exercise capacity, sleep patterns, genetic constitution, personality, and (neuro)psychologic processes.

Although several studies found abnormalities, only a few were diagnosed in large groups of people with CFS and were independently confirmed in well-controlled studies, an exception being the subtle changes in the hypothalamopituitary–adrenal axis.

Neuroendocrine challenge tests have found a lower-than-normal cortisol response to increased corticotrophin concentrations and upregulation of the serotonergic system. Studies of neuroendocrine function in individuals with CFS have found no evidence for uniform dysfunction of the hypothalamopituitary–adrenal axis or stress hormones.[64] Increasing evidence points to acquired neuroendocrine dysregulations in people with CFS.[97]

However, abnormalities of the neuroendocrine system and CNS alone are not sufficient to explain the symptoms of CFS. More complex interactions between regulating systems are assumed to be at work and seem to involve the CNS, the immune system, and the hormonal regulation system. The etiology and pathogenesis are generally thought to be multifactorial.[54,63]

Personality and lifestyle are presumed to influence vulnerability to CFS. Personality characteristics of neuroticism and introversion have been reported as risk factors for the disorder.[220]

Inactivity in childhood and inactivity after infectious mononucleosis have been found to increase the risk of CFS in adults.[279,287] Acute physical or psychologic stress can trigger the onset of CFS.

Three quarters of the individuals with this disorder have reported an infection, such as a cold, flu-like illness, or infectious mononucleosis, as the trigger,[72,239] and high rates of chronic fatigue after Q fever and Lyme disease have been found.[161] Finally, serious life events, such as the loss of a loved one or a job, and other stressful situations have been found to precipitate the disorder.[110,273]

### Clinical Manifestations

At illness onset, the most commonly reported CFS symptoms are sore throat, fever, muscle pain, and muscle weakness. As the illness progresses, muscle pain and forgetfulness increase along with prolonged (lasting more than 6 months), often overwhelming fatigue that is exacerbated by minimal physical activity.

Neurally mediated hypotension, caused by disturbances in the autonomic regulation of blood pressure and pulse, is common in people with CFS. This condition is characterized by lowered blood pressure and heart rate accompanied by lightheadedness, visual dimming, or slow response to verbal stimuli. Many people with neurally mediated hypotension experience lightheadedness or worsening fatigue as they stand for prolonged periods or when in warm places (e.g., hot shower, sauna, indoor pool environment).

The severity of CFS varies from person to person, with some people able to maintain fairly active lives. By definition, CFS significantly limits work, school, and family activities.

Although symptoms vary from person to person in number, type, and severity, all individuals with CFS are functionally impaired to some degree. CDC studies show that CFS can be as disabling as multiple sclerosis (MS), lupus, rheumatoid arthritis, heart disease, end-stage renal disease, chronic obstructive pulmonary disease, and similar chronic conditions.

CFS often follows a cyclical course, alternating between periods of illness and relative well-being. Some people experience partial or complete remission of symptoms during the course of the illness, but symptoms often reoccur.

This pattern of remission and relapse makes CFS especially hard for clients and their health care professionals to manage. People who are in remission may be tempted

Box 7.5

**ME/CFS DIAGNOSTIC CRITERIA**

Diagnosis requires that the patient have the following three symptoms:

1. A substantial reduction or impairment in the ability to engage in pre-illness levels of occupational, educational, social, or personal activities that persists for more than 6 months and is accompanied by fatigue, which is often profound, is of new or definite onset (not lifelong), is not the result of ongoing excessive exertion, and is not substantially alleviated by rest, and
2. Postexertional malaise[a], and
3. Unrefreshing sleep[a]

At least one of the two following manifestations is also required:

1. Cognitive impairment[a] or
2. Orthostatic intolerance

[a]Frequency and severity of symptoms should be assessed. The diagnosis of ME/CFS should be questioned if patients do not have these symptoms at least half of the time with moderate, substantial, or severe intensity.

From Institute of Medicine of the National Academies, Proposed Diagnostic Criteria for ME/CFS, http://www.nationalacademies.org/hmd/~/media/Files/Report%20Files/2015/MECFS/MECFS_ProposedDiagnosticCriteria. Accessed August 13, 2019.

to overdo activities when they are feeling better, which can exacerbate symptoms and fatigue and cause a relapse. In fact, postexertional malaise is a hallmark of the illness.[43]

### Medical Management

**Diagnosis.** There are no physical signs or diagnostic laboratory tests that help identify CFS. People who suffer from the symptoms of CFS must be carefully evaluated by a physician, since many treatable medical and psychiatric conditions are hard to distinguish from CFS.

Common conditions that should be ruled out through a careful medical history and appropriate testing include mononucleosis, Lyme disease, thyroid conditions, diabetes, MS, various cancers, depression, and bipolar disorder. Box 7.5 lists the proposed diagnostic criteria for ME/CFS by the Institute of Medicine.

**Treatment.** Because there is no known cure for CFS, treatment is aimed at symptom relief and improved function. A combination of drug and nondrug therapies is usually recommended. No single therapy exists that helps all individuals with CFS.

Lifestyle changes, including prevention of overexertion, reduced stress, dietary restrictions, gentle stretching, and nutritional supplementation, are frequently recommended in addition to drug therapies used to treat sleep disturbances, pain, and other specific symptoms.

Carefully supervised physical therapy may be part of treatment for CFS. However, symptoms can be exacerbated by overly ambitious physical activity. A very moderate approach to exercise and activity management is recommended to avoid overactivity and to prevent deconditioning.[43] Systematic reviews have investigated the effectiveness of several CFS treatments, and cognitive behavior therapy and graded exercise therapy are the only interventions found to be beneficial.[218,228,288]

**Prognosis.** CFS affects each individual differently. Some people with CFS remain homebound and others regain the ability to resume work and other activities, despite experiencing symptoms.

The CDC's research shows that those who have CFS for 2 years or less are more likely to improve. It remains unknown if early intervention is responsible for this more favorable outcome; the longer a person is ill before diagnosis, the more complicated the course of the illness appears to be.

Recovery rates for CFS are unclear. Improvement rates varied from 8% to 63%, with a median of 40% of clients improving during follow-up. Full recovery from CFS may be rare, with an average of only 5% to 10% sustaining total remission.[43]

SPECIAL IMPLICATIONS FOR THE THERAPIST 7.4

## *Chronic Fatigue Syndrome*

The client with CFS is treated following guidelines and protocols for autoimmune disorders such as fibromyalgia (see "Fibromyalgia" in this chapter). Pacing, energy conservation, stress management, and balancing life activities are extremely helpful in preventing worsening of fatigue and maintaining an even flow of energy from day to day. Support groups may be beneficial in providing emotional and psychologic support and in helping the individual keep up with the latest research results and progress in medical intervention.

### Exercise and Chronic Fatigue Syndrome

Carefully controlled and graded exercise is the center of effective intervention for CFS.[94,95,205,215] Many affected individuals fear a relapse and avoid physical activity and exercise, but deconditioning and muscle atrophy increase fatigue and worsen other symptoms.

The physical therapist can be very instrumental in providing a prescriptive program of regular, moderate exercise to avoid deconditioning while advising against overexertion during periods of remission. During the acute onset or during flare-ups, people with CFS are unable to sustain physical activity or exercise. Beginning with low-level, intermittent physical activity throughout the day to accumulate 30 minutes of exercise has been shown to be effective without exacerbating symptoms.[59]

People with CFS may have a significantly reduced exercise capacity. Always assess for conditioning before initiating even a simple exercise program with anyone who has had CFS longer than 6 months. Athletes and sports participants may require special help to develop a progressive exercise regimen. Impairments of peak aerobic power and muscle strength may occur with self-imposed or physician-imposed inactivity.[247]

Although abnormal lung function or low concentration of oxygen with accompanying dyspnea or shortness of breath is not a clinical feature of this disease, anyone who is severely deconditioned and attempts light exercise may experience dyspnea. Reaching age-predicted target heart rates may be limited by autonomic disturbances.[71] It may be better to begin a strengthening program before challenging the cardiovascular system.

The therapist must evaluate for altered breathing patterns, components of poor posture, and inefficient or biomechanically faulty movement patterns contributing to pain. Addressing these areas is an important part of the rehabilitation process.

Stretching, strengthening, and cardiovascular training are essential aspects of therapy. Like people with fibromyalgia, those diagnosed with CFS must progress slowly and avoid overexertion, since they often do not have the internal mechanism to alert them to stop an activity.

Soft tissue and joint mobilization combined with stretching are important components of intervention, especially in the presence of postural components or faulty mechanics. Prolonged inactivity, rest in poorly supported positions for long periods, and assuming postures dictated by pain can contribute to muscle shortening (see "Modalities and Fibromyalgia" in this chapter).

Over time, some individuals can be progressed to graded aerobic exercise therapy (some can begin at this level depending on the individual clinical presentation). Continuous exercise must be started at a short duration appropriate to the client's baseline ability. A more specific description of how to deliver a graded exercise therapy program to people with CFS is available.[93] This is significantly more effective than just stretching and relaxation exercises.[94,285]

### Monitoring Vital Signs

Assessment of vital signs in adults with CFS may demonstrate very large fluctuations in pulse rate and blood pressure, which are not consistent with the person's position or movement. Whereas the blood pressure and pulse rate normally show a slight increase as a physiologic response to a change in position from sitting to standing, orthostatic hypotension is marked in the CFS population. Vital signs may stay the same or even decrease, resulting in dizziness, lightheadedness, or loss of balance. The symptoms may result in decreased self-confidence in the ability to pursue activities.

During the initiation of an exercise program, it is advised to monitor blood pressure, rate of perceived exertion, heart rate, and respiratory rate for any signs of physiologic distress. Although the rate of perceived exertion may not change during the exercise session, the individual may perceive fatigue as worse after initiating exercise. If this increase in fatigue does not exceed 1 unit on a scale of 1 to 5 from the baseline level established before exercise, symptom exacerbation following exercise can potentially be avoided.[59]

## HYPERSENSITIVITY DISORDERS

Although the immune system protects the host against foreign agents or infectious organisms, it can cause tissue damage when it responds incorrectly. The inaccurate responses are attributable to overexpression to a substance or hypersensitivity reactions, reacting to the host's own cells (autoimmunity), transfusion or transplantation reactions (alloimmunity), or inadequacy to protect the host (immunodeficiency).

The hypersensitivity disorders are categorized into four types of immune mechanisms: Type I hypersensitivity reactions or immunoglobulin E (IgE)-mediated or immediate-type, Type II hypersensitivity reactions or cytotoxic reactions to self-antigens or tissue-specific type reactions, Type III hypersensitivity reactions or immune complex-mediated reactions, and Type IV hypersensitivity reactions or cell-mediated or delayed-type reactions (Table 7.5). Table 7.6 summarizes the clinical manifestations of the hypersensitivity disorders.

### Type I (IgE-mediated or Immediate Type) Hypersensitivity

Type I reaction involves an IgE-mediated antibody that is formed from a CD4 Th2 cell-dependent mechanism that binds with receptors on mast cells and basophils. This binding is referred to as cytophilic antibody. Upon binding, it activates a series of reactions (Fig. 7.28). For example, when a person has been exposed to an allergen that provokes IgE, that person becomes sensitized. Subsequent exposures to that allergen then cause immediate hypersensitivity reactions. With repeated exposures to the antigen, recruitment of additional IgE antibody occurs rather than other types of immunoglobulins in the form of IgM or IgG. In order to activate the mast cell or basophil, the antigen crosslinks to more than one IgE antibody molecule.

Mast cells and basophils are not only activated by antibodies but are also activated by other agents, including complement-derived anaphylatoxic peptides, C3a, and C5a. Granules from mast cells and inflammatory mediators are then released. For instance, the biogenic amine histamine is released that induces constriction of vascular and nonvascular smooth muscles, causing vasodilation and increasing venule permeability. This is mediated by an H1 type of receptor. This mechanism results in early manifestations of immediate hypersensitivity reactions (e.g., in the lungs as bronchoconstriction of the airways, and in the skin as wheal and flare).

Other preformed products are released from the cells including heparin, chemotactic factors, proteases, and eosinophil chemotactic factors. Cytokines such as IL-1, IL-3, IL-4, IL-5, IL-6, tumor necrosis factor (TNF), and others are also synthesized and secreted by mast cells. This event occurs during the latter part of the immediate hypersensitivity reactions, which last 2 to 24 hours.

Several inflammatory mediators are also synthesized and released upon activation of the cells. These include the products of the arachidonic acid pathway: cyclooxygenase (prostaglandins $D_2$, $E_2$, $F_2$, and thromboxane) and lipoxygenase (leukotrienes $B_4$, $C_4$, and $E_4$). The products of this pathway are responsible for smooth muscle contraction, vasodilation, and edema. Specifically, what were previously called slow reacting substances or SRSAs (leukotrienes $C_4$, $D_4$, and $E_4$) are responsible for the delayed bronchoconstriction during anaphylaxis. Additionally, platelet-activating factor (PAF) is synthesized by mast cells. PAF is a potent platelet aggregator and is responsible for the release of vasoactive amines from platelets.

**Table 7.5** Immunologic Mechanisms of Tissue Destruction

| Type | Name | Rate of Development | Class of Antibody Involved | Principal Effect or Cells Involved | Complement Participation | Examples of Disorders |
|---|---|---|---|---|---|---|
| I | IgE-mediated reaction | Immediate | IgE | Mast cells | No | Seasonal allergic rhinitis |
| II | Tissue- specific reaction | Immediate | IgG<br>IgM | Macrophages in tissues | Frequently | Autoimmune thrombocytopenic purpura, Graves disease, autoimmune hemolytic anemia |
| III | Immune complex-mediated reaction | Immediate | IgG<br>IgM | Neutrophils | Yes | Systemic lupus erythematosus |
| IV | Cell-mediated reaction | Delayed | None | Lymphocytes, macrophages | No | Contact sensitivity to poison ivy and metals (jewelry) |

From McCance KL, Huether SE: *Pathophysiology: the biologic basis for disease in adults and children*, ed 7, St Louis, 2014, Mosby.

**Table 7.6** Clinical Manifestations of Hypersensitivity Disorders

| Type I | Type II | Type III | Type IV |
|---|---|---|---|
| Varies according to the allergies present<br>Classic symptoms:<br>• Wheezing<br>• Hypotension<br>• Swelling<br>• Urticaria<br>• Rhinorrhea<br>Anaphylaxis | *General:* malaise, weakness<br>*Dermal:* hives, erythema<br>*Respiratory:* sneezing, rhinorrhea, dyspnea<br>*Upper airway:* hoarseness, stridor; tongue and pharyngeal edema<br>*Lower airway:* dyspnea, bronchospasm, asthma (air trap-ping), chest tightness, wheezing<br>*Gastrointestinal:* increased peristalsis, vomiting, dysphagia, nausea, abdominal cramps, diarrhea<br>*Cardiovascular:* tachycardia, palpitations, hypotension, cardiac arrest<br>*Central nervous system:* anxiety, seizures | Headache<br>Back (flank) pain<br>Chest pain similar to angina<br>Nausea and vomiting<br>Tachycardia<br>Hypotension<br>Hematuria<br>Urticaria | Fever<br>Arthralgias<br>Lymphadenopathy<br>Urticaria<br>Anemia |

## Type II (Tissue-Specific) Hypersensitivity

Type II hypersensitivity reaction is also called tissue-specific hypersensitivity. In contrast with Type I, IgG and IgM antibodies are involved rather than the IgE. There is a specific cell or tissue targeted to produce an immunologic response. Aside from the major histocompatibility locus antigens (HLAs), other tissue-specific antigens are involved, since these types of antigens are expressed on plasma membranes. The symptomatology of type II hypersensitivity reactions depends on what organ or tissue expresses the particular antigen. For instance, when an antigen such as drugs or their metabolites binds to erythrocytes, bleeding manifestations may occur due to osmotic lysis of the erythrocytes.

To better understand type II hypersensitivity reactions, there are five mechanisms by which this type can affect cells (Fig. 7.29). These five mechanisms have the same initiation process—the antibody binds to tissue-specific antigens or antigens that have bound to certain tissues. In the *first mechanism*, lysis of cells occurs due to antibody (IgG or IgM) response and activation of the complement cascade via the classical pathway. The membrane attack complex (MAC) consisting of C5-9 facilitates destruction of the cell membrane, which eventually causes lysis of the cells. This mechanism is seen with autoimmune hemolytic anemia where erythrocytes are destroyed by complement-mediated lysis or as a consequence of ABO incompatibility transfusion reactions, termed alloimmune reaction.

The *second mechanism* involves phagocytosis and antibody, where the antibody may cause destruction of the cell via phagocytosis by macrophage. The IgG as well as the C3b of the complement system are opsonins, binding to the receptors on the macrophage followed by phagocytosis. For example, the antibodies against antigens of the erythrocytes of the Rh system coat those cells resulting in removal by phagocytosis in the spleen rather than by complement-mediated lysis (Fig. 7.29 B).

The *third mechanism* involves interaction of antibody and complement, which may attract the polymorphonuclear cells or neutrophils. The antigen is expressed either on the vessel wall or as soluble antigens in the circulation when released from cells within the body, from infectious agents, or from medications. As the antibody stimulates the complement cascade, the chemotactic for neutrophils (C3a and C5a) is released, and the complement component C3b is deposited within the tissues. The neutrophils bind for the Fc receptors of the antibody or for C3b with the intent to phagocytose the tissue, but phagocytosis is not completed due to the large size of the tissue. Despite the incompleteness of the phagocytosis, the polymorphonuclear cells are able to release their

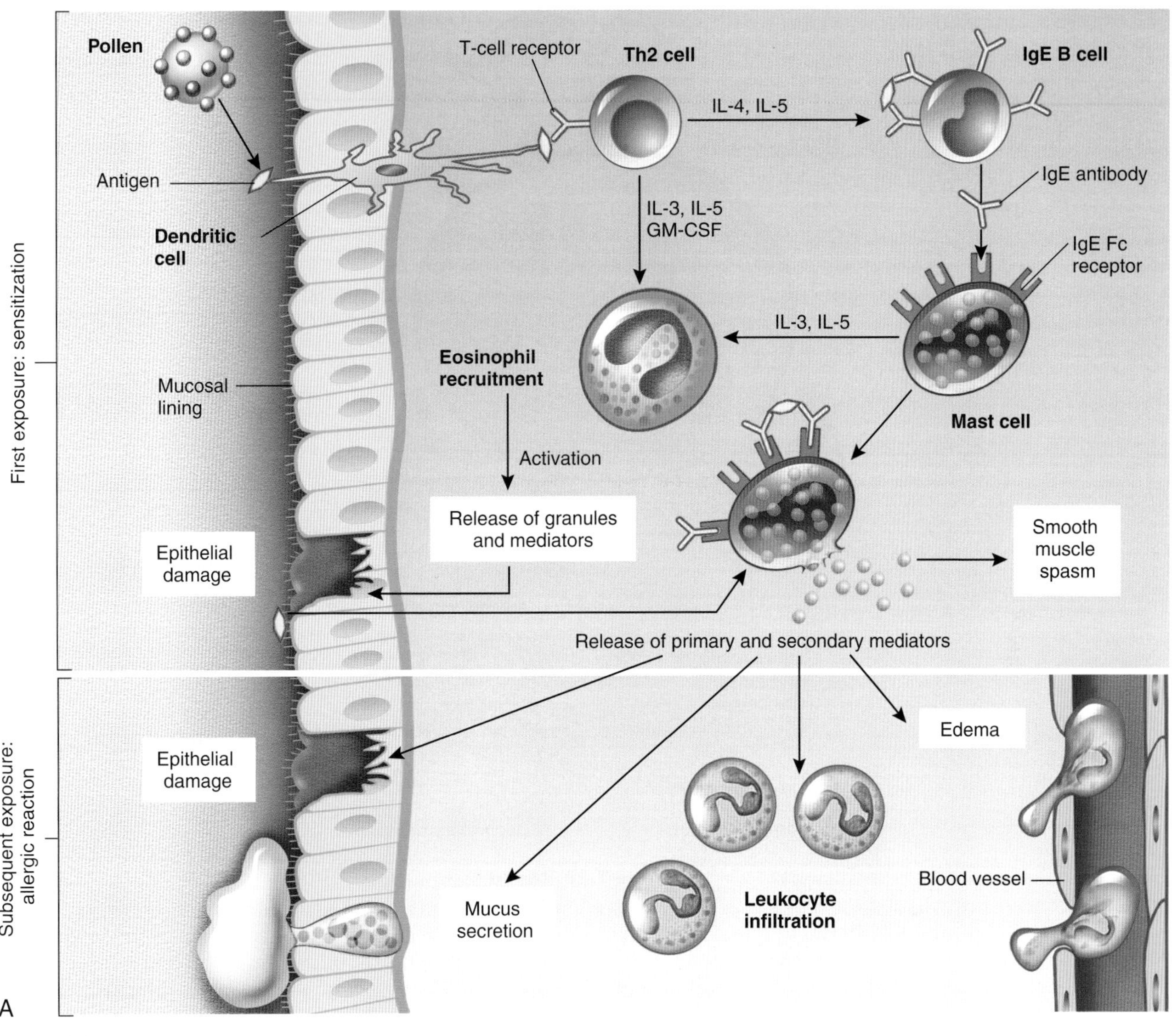


**Figure 7.28**

**(A and B) Mechanism of type I IgE-mediated reactions.** (From: McCance KL, Huether SE: *Pathophysiology: the biologic basis for disease in adults and children*, ed 8, St Louis, 2019, Elsevier.)

granules to the healthy tissue and release their toxic oxygen reactive species, thereby damaging the tissue (Fig. 7.29 C).

The *fourth mechanism* involves the antibody-dependent cell-mediated toxicity (ADCC). The cells involved in this mechanism are the natural killer cells (or NK cells), which are non–antigen-specific cells. As recognized by the Fc receptors on the NK cells, the antibody on the target cell releases toxic substances causing destruction of the target cell (Fig. 7.29 D).

The *fifth mechanism* is unique because it does not involve destruction of the target cell but rather facilitates malfunction of the cell. The antibody reacts with its own antireceptor antibody on the target cell surface, altering and modulating the functions of the receptor either by blocking the interaction with its normal ligands, by displacing the ligand, or by destroying the receptor. A good example of this mechanism is myasthenia gravis, where antibody to acetylcholine receptor prevents acetylcholine neurotransmitter from attaching to its own acetylcholine receptor on the motor end plates of skeletal muscles, thereby inhibiting neuromuscular transmission and causing asthenia (from a Greek word *asthenia* meaning weakness) of the skeletal muscles (Fig. 7.29 D).

To summarize the different mechanisms involved in Type II hypersensitivity, Table 7.7 provides the disease, target antigen, mechanisms, and clinicopathologic manifestations.

## Type III (Immune Complex–Mediated) Hypersensitivity

In the type III hypersensitivity reaction, the antigen-antibody immune complexes are formed in the circulation and are deposited in the vessels and in the extravascular tissues (Fig. 7.30); hence the term immune complex–mediated. The specific antibodies involved in type III are IgG, IgM, and occasionally IgA. The kidneys, joints, skin, and blood vessels are the most common tissues affected.

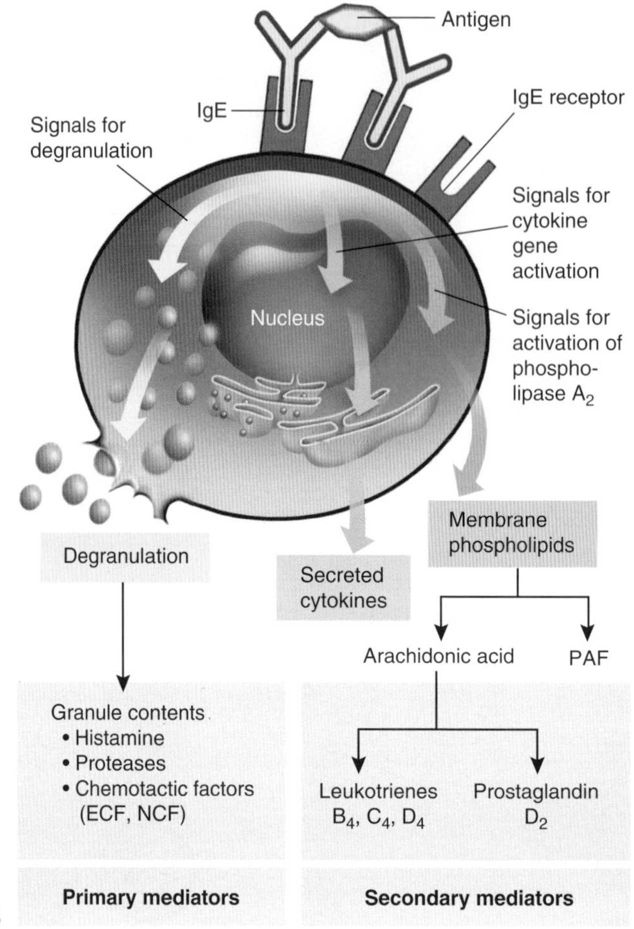


**Figure 7.28, cont'd**

There is some commonality between type II and type III hypersensitivity reactions in regard to involvement and deposition of antigen-antibody complexes in the tissues. The main difference between these two types lies in the process of how the immune complexes are deposited in the tissues. For instance, type II hypersensitivity antibody binds to the antigen located on the cell surface. On the other hand, in type III reactions, once the antibody binds to the soluble antigens, they are released into the circulation either in the blood or body fluids. The antibody-antigen complex is then deposited in the tissues. Although the type III reaction is tissue specific, it is not organ specific.

The deleterious effects of the immune complex deposits are due to activation of the complement system, specifically the chemotactic factors for neutrophils. Once activated, the neutrophils bind to the antibody and C3b, which in turn phagocytizes the immune complexes. Lysosomal enzymes are then released, causing tissue damage. Additionally, the tissue damaging mediators such as proteases and reactive oxygen species are released. Oftentimes, the process of phagocytosis is unsuccessful because the immune complexes are bound to large areas of tissue. For example, small-size immune complexes are filtered through the kidneys without any pathologic consequences such as inflammation. The intermediate-size immune complexes most likely will be deposited in the tissues causing deleterious effects in certain target tissues, such as inflammation in the kidneys (as in the case of glomerulonephritis), in the blood vessels (as in the case of vasculitis), or in the joints (as in the case of various arthritides or degenerative joint diseases). The large-size immune complexes are quickly released into the circulation by tissue macrophages.

There are some human diseases that are affected by the immune complex–mediated reactions. These include: Henoch-Schönlein purpura (a disease where IgA deposits are found at the blood vessels); cryoglobulinemic vasculitis associated with hepatitis C infection, and systemic lupus erythematosus (SLE), in which anti–double-stranded DNA is demonstrated in the vasculitic lesions. A separate discussion of SLE is provided later. Some immune complex diseases do not cause tissue injury but are detected only in the plasma. In instances where vascular permeability occurred, localization of circulating immune complexes may be determined. Examples include autoimmune diseases of connective tissue (e.g., SLE and rheumatoid arthritis), other types of vasculitis, and many selections of glomerulonephritis.

There are two paradigms of type III hypersensitivity reactions that facilitate understanding of diseases associated with this type of reactions. The first is serum sickness, which represents systemic manifestations of type III. Serum sickness was first described as a result of administration of foreign serum that comes from a horse, which contained antibody against tetanus toxin.[212] Currently, serum sickness can result from increased frequency of administration of drugs. Serum

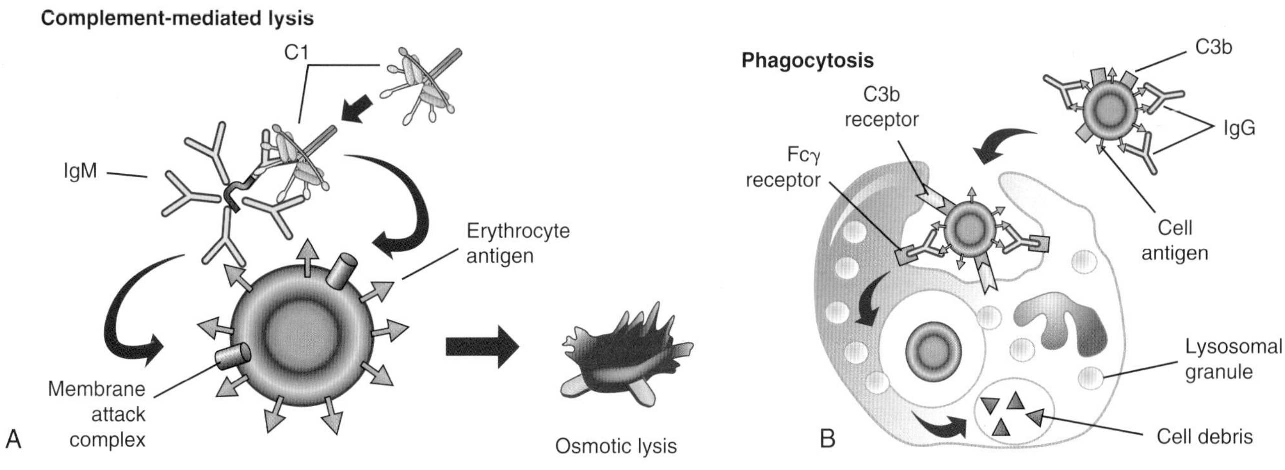


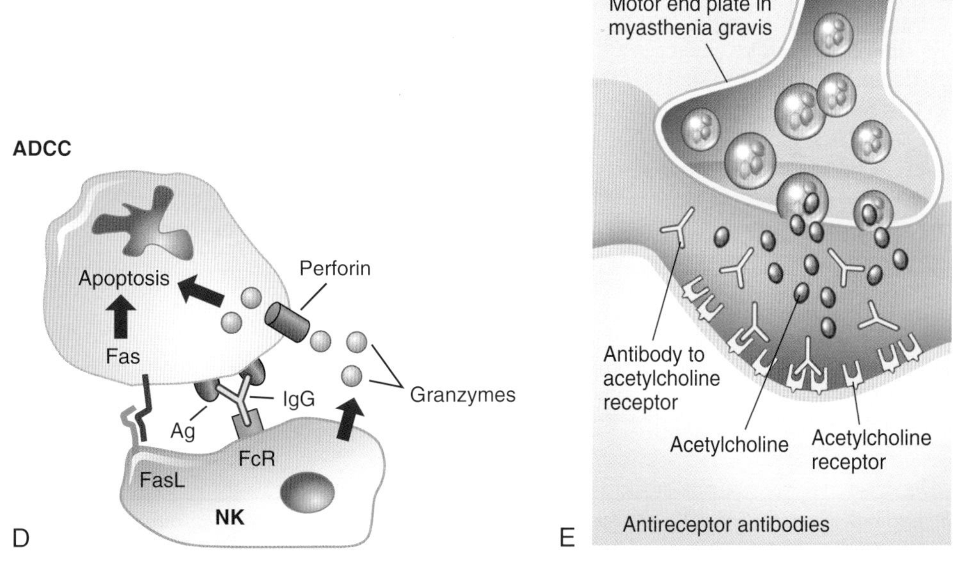


**Figure 7.29**

**Mechanisms of type II tissue-specific reactions.** (From McCance KL, Huether SE: *Pathophysiology: the biologic basis for disease in adults and children*, ed 8, St Louis, 2019, Elsevier.)

**Table 7.7** Examples of Antibody-Mediated Diseases (Type II Hypersensitivity)

| Disease | Target Antigen | Mechanisms of Disease | Clinicopathologic Manifestations |
|---|---|---|---|
| Autoimmune hemolytic anemia | Red cell membrane proteins (Rh blood group antigens, I antigen) | Opsonization and phagocytosis of erythrocytes | Hemolysis, anemia |
| Autoimmune thrombocytopenic purpura | Platelet membrane proteins (GpIIb/IIIa integrin) | Opsonization and phagocytosis of platelets | Bleeding |
| Pemphigus vulgaris | Proteins in intercellular junctions of epidermal cells (epidermal desmoglein) | Antibody-mediated activation of proteases, disruption of intercellular adhesions | Skin vesicles (bullae) |
| Vasculitis caused by ANCA | Neutrophil granule proteins, presumably released from activated neutrophils | Neutrophil degranulation and inflammation | Vasculitis |
| Goodpasture syndrome | Noncollagenous protein (NC1) in basement membranes of kidney glomeruli and lung alveoli | Complement- and Fc receptor-mediated inflammation | Nephritis, lung hemorrhage |
| Acute rheumatic fever | Streptococcal cell wall antigen; antibody cross-reacts with myocardial antigen | Inflammation, macrophage activation | Myocarditis |
| Myasthenia gravis | Acetylcholine receptor | Antibody inhibits acetylcholine binding, down-modulates receptors | Muscle weakness, paralysis |
| Graves disease (hyperthyroidism) | TSH receptor | Antibody-mediated stimulation of TSH receptors | Hyperthyroidism |
| Insulin-resistant diabetes | Insulin receptor | Antibody inhibits binding of insulin | Hyperglycemia, ketoacidosis |
| Pernicious anemia | Intrinsic factor of gastric parietal cells | Neutralization of intrinsic factor, decreased absorption of vitamin $B_{12}$ | Abnormal myelopoiesis, anemia |

*ANCA*, Antineutrophil cytoplasmic antibodies; *TSH*, thyroid-stimulating hormone.
From Kumar V, Abbas AK, Aster JC: Robbins basic pathology, ed 9, Philadelphia, 2013, WB Saunders.

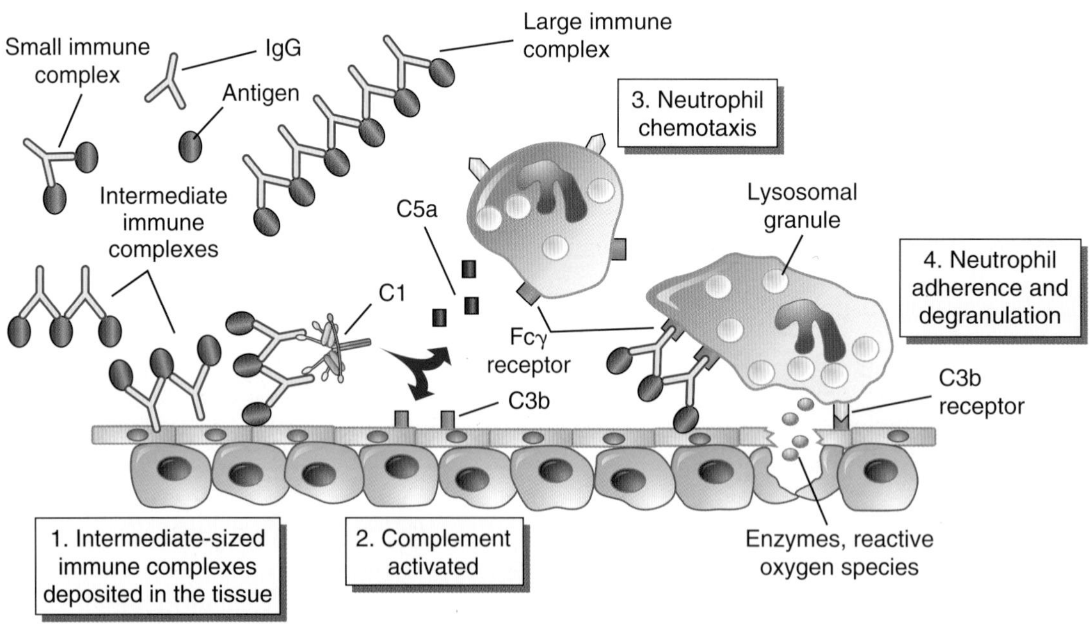


**Figure 7.30**

**Mechanisms of type III reactions.** (From McCance KL, Huether SE: *Pathophysiology: the biologic basis for disease in adults and children,* ed 8, St Louis, 2019, Elsevier.)

sickness reactions are due to the formation of immune complexes in the blood and their deposition into the tissues such as kidneys, blood vessels, and joints. The affected individual exhibits fever, lymphadenopathy, rash, and pain at the sites of inflammation. Raynaud phenomenon is a form of serum sickness. It is caused by cold temperature–dependent deposition of immune complexes in the capillary beds leading to blood vessel spasms, consequently blocking the blood supply to the tips of fingers, toes, nose, and ears. The affected individual manifests numbness and localized pallor to the

**Table 7.8** Examples of Immune Complex-Mediated Diseases

| Disease | Antigen Involved | Clinicopathologic Manifestations |
|---|---|---|
| Systemic lupus erythematosus | Nuclear antigens | Nephritis, skin lesions, arthritis, others |
| Poststreptococcal glomerulonephritis | Streptococcal cell wall antigen(s): may be "planted" in glomerular basement membrane | Nephritis |
| Polyarteritis nodosa | Hepatitis B virus antigens in some cases | Systemic vasculitis |
| Reactive arthritis | Bacterial antigens (e.g., *Yersinia)* | Acute arthritis |
| Serum sickness | Various proteins (e.g., foreign serum protein such as horse antithymocyte globulin) | Arthritis, vasculitis, nephritis |
| Arthus reaction (experimental) | Various foreign proteins | Cutaneous vasculitis |

From Kumar V, Abbas AK, Aster JC: *Robbins basic pathology*, ed 9, Philadelphia, 2013, WB Saunders.

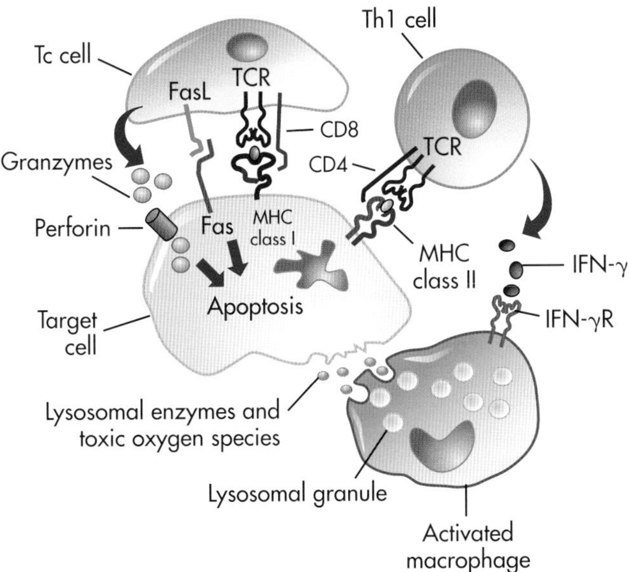


**Figure 7.31**

Mechanisms of type IV, cell-mediated reactions. (From McCance KL, Huether SE: *Pathophysiology: the biologic basis for disease in adults and children*, ed 8, St Louis, 2019, Elsevier.)

affected tissue, which in turn lead to cyanosis and eventual gangrene if the blood circulation is not restored.

The second exemplary paradigm of type III hypersensitivity reaction is the so-called Arthus reaction. In contrast with serum sickness, Arthus reaction is more localized or cutaneous. It is caused by repeated exposure to an antigen that interacts with preformed antibodies and immune complex deposition in the walls of local blood vessels. The symptomatology of Arthus reaction commences within 1 hour of exposure and peaks between 6 and 12 hours. A typical local inflammatory reaction occurs with accumulation of neutrophils, increased vascular permeability, edema formation, hemorrhage, clotting, and tissue damage (Table 7.8).

## Type IV (Cell-Mediated Immunity) Hypersensitivity

A distinct characteristic of type IV hypersensitivity reaction is the presence of T lymphocyte–mediated reactions rather than the involvement of antibodies, which occurs in types I, II, and III hypersensitivity reactions. The mechanisms of type IV reaction arise as either cytotoxic T lymphocyte (Tc cells) or lymphokine-producing Th1 and Th17 cells. As the name implies, Tc cells kill and destroy the target cells, whereas Th1 and Th17 cells generate cytokines, especially interferon gamma (IFN-γ), which activate macrophages. The activated macrophages attach to the targets and release cytolytic enzymes as well as reactive oxygen intermediates, which facilitate tissue destruction (Fig. 7.31).

Type IV is also called delayed type hypersensitivity reaction, which occurs in contact dermatitis after sensitization to an allergen in the form of cosmetics, topical medications, adhesives, poison ivy, latex sensitivity, or the response to a tuberculin skin test present 48 to 72 hours after the test. A classic example of type IV hypersensitivity reactions occurs either during graft rejection or allergic reactions (Table 7.9).

SPECIAL IMPLICATIONS FOR THE THERAPIST 7.5

### *Hypersensitivity Disorders*

Immediate action is required for any client experiencing a type I hypersensitivity reaction or anaphylaxis. When a severe reaction occurs, the health care professional must call for emergency assistance.

Type IV reactions may occur in response to lanolin added to lotions, ultrasound gels, or other preparations used in massage or soft tissue mobilization, requiring careful observation of all people for delayed skin reactions to any of these substances.

With the first exposure, no reaction necessarily occurs, but antigens are formed, and on subsequent exposures, hypersensitivity reactions are triggered. Anyone with known hypersensitivity should have a small area of skin tested before use of large amounts of topical agents in the therapy setting. Careful observation throughout treatment is recommended.

Beginning in the 1980s, the use of latex gloves to protect health care workers against exposure to blood and body fluids increased. Since then, the number of reported cases of latex sensitivity has increased. Reactions to latex range from contact dermatitis (type IV hypersensitivity) to anaphylactic shock (type I hypersensitivity).

Therapists who are allergic to latex should avoid contact with latex gloves and other products that contain latex. Use of low-powder, powder-free, and nonlatex gloves provides therapists with a strategy for preventing exposure to latex allergens.[162]

**Table 7.9** T-Cell Mediated Diseases (Type IV Hypersensitivity)[a]

| Disease | Specificity of Pathogenic T Cells | Principal Mechanisms Tissue Injury | Clinicopathologic of Manifestations |
|---|---|---|---|
| Rheumatoid arthritis | Collagen?; citrullinated self proteins? | Inflammation mediated by $T_H17$ (and $T_H1$?) cytokines; role of antibodies and immune complexes? | Chronic arthritis with inflammation, destruction of articular cartilage and bone |
| Multiple sclerosis | Protein antigens in myelin (e.g., myelin basic protein) | Inflammation mediated by $T_H1$ and $T_H17$ cytokines, myelin destruction by activated macrophages | Demyelination in CNS with perivascular inflammation; paralysis, ocular lesions |
| Type II diabetes mellitus | Antigens of pancreatic islet β cells (insulin, glutamic acid decarboxylase, others) | T cell-mediated inflammation, destruction of islet cells by CTLs | Insulitis (chronic inflammation in islets), destruction of β cells; diabetes |
| Hashimoto thyroiditis | Thyroglobulin, other thyroid proteins | Inflammation, CTL-mediated killing of thyroid epithelial cells | Hypothyroidism |
| Inflammatory bowel disease | Enteric bacteria; self antigens? | Inflammation mediated mainly by $T_H17$ cytokines | Chronic intestinal inflammation, ulceration, obstruction |
| Autoimmune myocarditis | Myosin heavy chain protein | CTL-mediated killing of myocardial cells; inflammation mediated by $T_H1$ cytokines | Cardiomyopathy |
| Contact sensitivity | Various environmental chemicals (e.g., urushiol from poison ivy or poison oak) | Inflammation mediated by $T_H1$ (and $T_H17$?) cytokines | Epidermal necrosis, dermal inflammation with skin rash and blisters |

[a]Examples of human T cell-mediated diseases are listed. In many cases, the specificity of the T cells and the mechanisms of tissue injury are inferred on the basis of similarity to experimental animal models of the diseases.

*CNS*, Central nervous system; *CTL*, cytotoxic T lymphocyte.

From Kumar V, Abbas AK, Aster JC: *Robbins basic pathology*, ed 9, Philadelphia, 2013, WB Saunders.

## AUTOIMMUNE DISEASES

### Overview

Autoimmune diseases fall into a category of conditions in which the cause involves immune mechanisms directed against self-antigens. More specifically, the body fails to distinguish self from nonself, causing the immune system to direct immune responses against normal (self) tissue and become self-destructive.

More than 56 autoimmune diseases have been identified, affecting everything from skin and joints to vital organs. Autoimmune diseases can be viewed as a spectrum of disorders, some of which are systemic and others of which involve a single organ. Table 7.10 lists a portion of the known diseases most likely to be seen in a rehabilitation setting.

**Table 7.10** Autoimmune Diseases

| Organ-Specific | Systemic |
|---|---|
| Addison disease | Amyloidosis |
| Crohn disease | Ankylosing spondylitis |
| Chronic active hepatitis | Mixed connective tissue disease |
| Diabetes mellitus | Multiple sclerosis |
| Giant cell arteritis | Myasthenia gravis |
| Hemolytic anemia | Polymyalgia rheumatic |
| Idiopathic thrombocytopenic purpura | Progressive systemic sclerosis (scleroderma) |
| Polymyositis/dermatomyositis | Psoriasis (psoriatic arthritis) |
| Postviral encephalomyelitis | Reiter syndrome |
| Primary biliary cirrhosis | Rheumatoid arthritis |
| Thyroiditis | Sarcoidosis |
| Graves disease | Sjögren syndrome |
| Hashimoto disease | Systemic lupus erythematosus |
| Ulcerative colitis | |

At one end of the continuum are organ-specific diseases, in which localized tissue damage occurs, resulting from the presence of specific autoantibodies. An example is Hashimoto disease of the thyroid, characterized by a specific lesion in the thyroid gland with production of antibodies with absolute specificity for certain thyroid constituents.

In the middle of the continuum are disorders in which the lesion tends to be localized in one organ, but the antibodies are not organ specific. An example is primary biliary cirrhosis, in which inflammatory cell infiltration of the small bile ductule occurs, but the serum antibodies are not specific to liver cells.

At the other end of the spectrum are non–organ-specific diseases, in which lesions and antibodies are widespread throughout the body and not limited to one target organ. SLE is an example of this type of autoimmune disease. Identification of ANAs that attack the nucleic acids (DNA and RNA) and other components of the body's own tissues established SLE as an autoimmune disease.

Fibromyalgia, CFS, and SLE are discussed in this chapter. Other individual autoimmune disorders are discussed separately in chapters associated with the type of disorder and the specific effects.

## Etiologic and Risk Factors

Although the autoimmune disorders are regarded as acquired diseases, their causes often cannot be determined. Autoimmunity is thought to result from a combination of factors, including genetic, hormonal (women are affected more often than men by autoimmune diseases), and environmental influences (e.g., exposure to chemicals, other toxins, or sunlight and drugs that may destroy suppressor T cells).

Although no single gene has been identified as responsible for autoimmune diseases, clusters of genes seem to increase susceptibility. In most autoimmune disorders, a known or suspected genetic susceptibility is evident, and certain HLA types show increased risk, such as ankylosing spondylitis with HLA-B27.

The influence of hormonal factors is confusing as some autoimmune diseases occur among women in their 20s and 30s, when estrogen is high, and others develop after menopause or before puberty, when estrogen levels are low. During pregnancy, many women with rheumatoid arthritis or MS experience complete remission, whereas pregnant women with SLE often experience exacerbations.

Other factors implicated in the development of immunologic abnormalities resulting in autoimmune disorders include viruses, stress, cross-reactive antibodies, and various autoimmune diseases occurring in women who have had silicone gel breast implants. This organ-specific autoimmune disease is associated with musculoskeletal problems.

It is important to understand that autoimmunity indicates loss of self-tolerance. Prior to discussing the pathogenesis, it is crucial to learn more about the mechanisms of normal immunologic tolerance.

## Immunologic Tolerance

*Immunologic tolerance* refers to the unresponsiveness of certain antigens induced by their exposure to lymphocytes. Self-tolerance refers to lack of recognition and responsiveness to one's own tissue antigens. There are several mechanisms that explain how the body prevents self-reactivity and inhibits certain immune reactions from attacking against one's own antigens. Both central and peripheral tolerance can explain these mechanisms (Fig. 7.32). Central tolerance refers to the loss of self-reactive T and B lymphocytes, which leads to immature lymphocytes that recognize self-antigens during their maturation in central (generative) lymphoid organs. T cells originate from thymus, whereas B cells originate from bone marrow. As illustrated, the immature lymphocytes are killed by apoptosis; for instance, in the B-cell lineage, switching occurs between self-reactive lymphocytes and the new antigen receptors, which are not self-reactive (Fig. 7.32).

On the other hand, in peripheral tolerance, the mature lymphocytes that recognize self-antigens become either anergic (i.e., functionally inactive) or suppressed by regulatory T cells or undergo apoptosis.

## Pathogenesis

How does autoimmunity occur? From the preceding discussion on self-tolerance and the development of autoimmunity, the mechanisms of autoimmunity can be associated with gene susceptibilities and epigenetic changes in tissue (e.g., due to injuries or infections that alter the recognition of self-antigens) (Fig. 7.33).

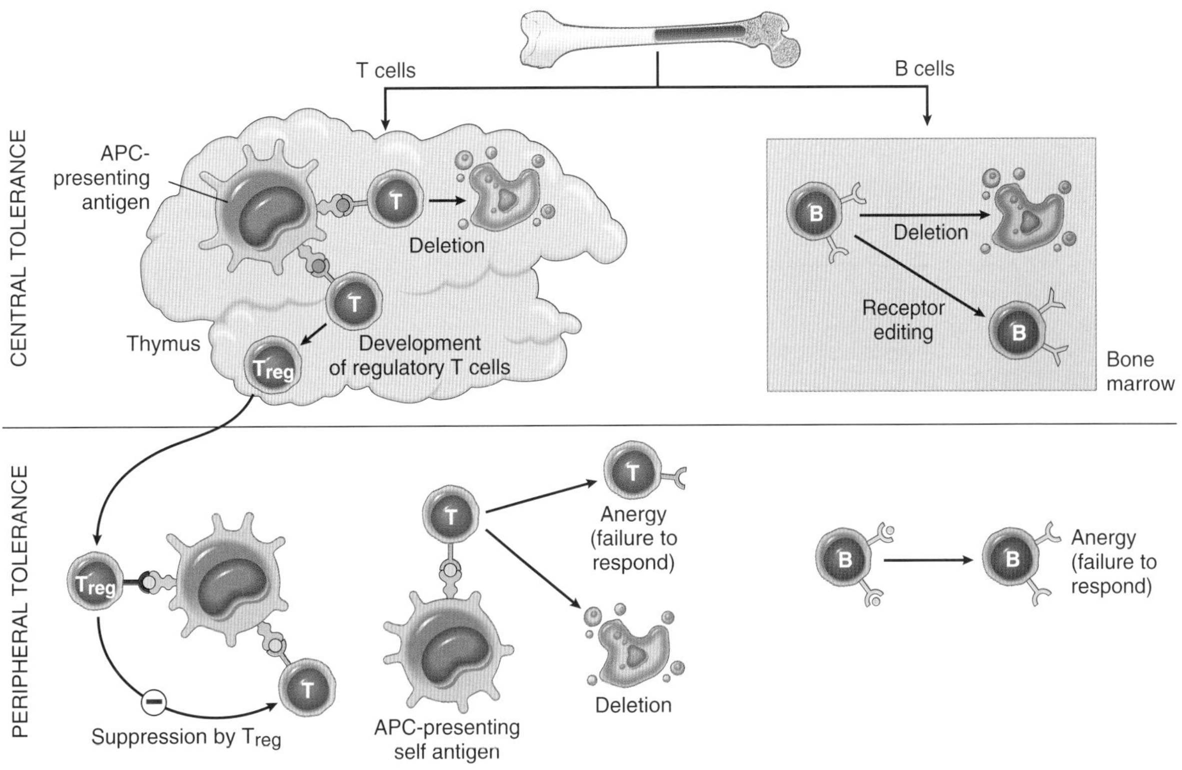


**Figure 7.32**

**The principal mechanisms of central and peripheral self-tolerance in CD4f T-cells.** (From Kumar V, Abbas AK, Aster JC: *Robbins basic pathology*, ed 10, Philadelphia, 2018, WB Saunders.)

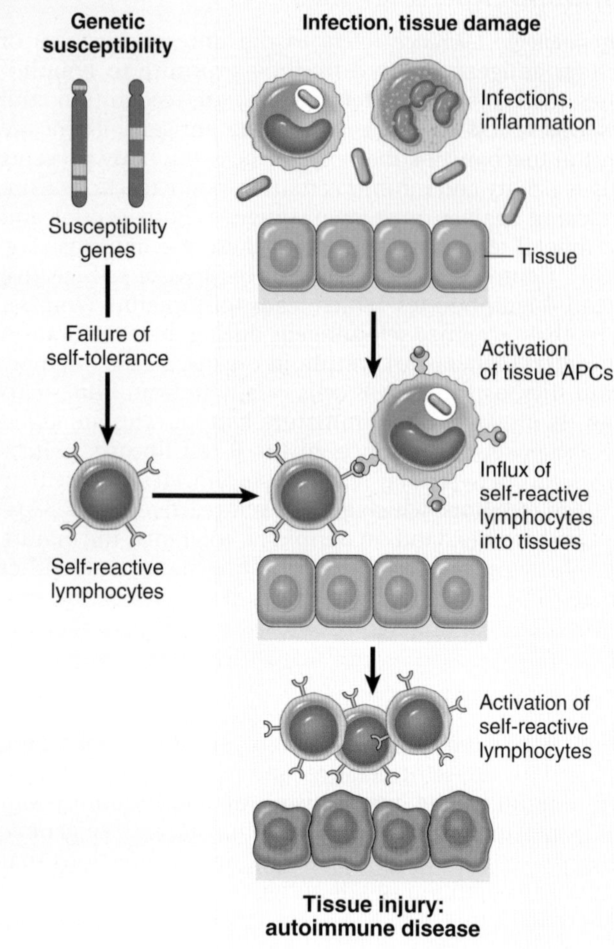


**Figure 7.33**

**Pathogenesis of autoimmunity.** (From Kumar V, Abbas AK, Aster JC: *Robbins basic pathology*, ed 9, Philadelphia, 2013, WB Saunders.)

## Gene Susceptibility in Autoimmunity

Some autoimmune diseases affect a single organ (e.g., pancreas in type I diabetes), whereas others affect a large system or more than one system (e.g., multiple sclerosis [MS]). In some cases, the autoimmune process overstimulates organ function as in Graves disease, in which excess thyroid hormone is produced.

Gene-mapping studies have demonstrated that allergy and autoimmunity must involve not only the recognition of antigen by T cells but also the immunoregulatory effects of cytokines, inhibitory receptors, and survival factors. Linkage analysis of human genome has revealed candidate loci for susceptibility to MS, type I diabetes, SLE, and Crohn disease, but as discussed in Chapter 2, there are a multitude of epigenetic (internal and external) environmental factors that contribute to whether (and when) the gene is expressed.

Other autoimmune diseases are associated with the HLA locus, specifically class II alleles such as HLA-DR,-DQ. For instance, rheumatoid arthritis is linked with HLA-DR4, ankylosing spondylitis with HLA-B27, type I diabetes mellitus with HLA-DR3, HLA-DR4, or HLA-DR3/DR4, and other diseases (Table 7.11).

**Table 7.11** Association of HLA with Disease

| Disease | HLA Allele | Odds Ratio[a] |
|---|---|---|
| Rheumatoid arthritis (anti-CCP Ab–positive)+ | DRB1 | 4-12 |
| Type 1 diabetes | DRB1*0301-DQA1*0501-DQB1*0201 haplotype | 4 |
| | DRB1*0401-DQA1*0301-DQB1*0302 haplotype | 8 |
| | DRB1*0301/0401 haplotype heterozygotes | 35 |
| Multiple sclerosis | DRB1*1501 | 3 |
| Systemic lupus erythematosus | DRB1*0301 | 2 |
| | DRB1*1501 | 1.3 |
| Ankylosing spondylitis | B*27 (mainly B*2705 and B*2702) | 100-200 |
| Celiac disease | DQA1*0501-DQB1*0201 haplotype | 7 |

[a]The *odds ratio* (also called *relative risk)* is the approximate value of the increased risk of the disease associated with the inheritance of particular HLA alleles. The data are from European-derived populations.

*Anti-CCP Ab*, Antibodies directed against cyclic citrullinated peptides. Data are from patients who tested positive for these antibodies in serum.

Table courtesy of Dr. Michelle Fernando, Imperial College London.

## Infections, Tissue Injury, and Autoimmunity

Certain bacteria, mycoplasmas, and viruses can trigger autoimmunity by several mechanisms. In the concept of molecular mimicry, viruses and microbes (such as *Klebsiella*) share cross-reacting epitopes with self-antigens where microbial antigens tend to attack self-tissues. This is illustrated by the type II hypersensitivity reaction (antibody-mediated diseases) as seen in rheumatic heart disease (i.e., immune response against streptococci cross-reacts with cardiac antigens).

Some microbial infections with tissue necrosis and inflammation can induce upregulation of costimulatory molecules on resting APCs in tissue that initiates T-cell energy and subsequent T-cell activation–induced death. Local tissue injury altered by infections and other triggers causes the release of self-antigens and autoimmune responses.

# Systemic Lupus Erythematosus

## Definition and Overview

Lupus erythematosus, sometimes referred to as *lupus*, is a chronic inflammatory autoimmune disorder that appears in several forms, including *discoid lupus erythematosus (DLE)*, which affects only the skin (usually face, neck, scalp) (see Chapter 10), and *SLE*, which can affect any organ or system of the body.

The clinical picture of SLE presents on a continuum with different combinations of organ system involvement. The most common of these presentations are latent lupus, drug-induced lupus, antiphospholipid antibody syndrome, and late-stage lupus. *Latent lupus* describes a constellation of features suggestive of SLE but does not qualify as classic SLE. Many people with latent lupus persist with their clinical presentation of signs and symptoms over many years without ever developing classic SLE.

*Drug-induced lupus* may be diagnosed in people without prior history suggestive of SLE in whom the clinical and serologic manifestations of SLE develop while the person is taking a drug (most often hydralazine used to treat hypertension or procainamide used to treat arrhythmia). The symptoms cease when the drug is stopped, with gradual resolution of serologic abnormalities.

*Antiphospholipid antibody syndrome* describes the association between arterial and venous thrombosis, recurrent fetal loss, and immune thrombocytopenia with a variety of antibodies directed against cellular phospholipid (lipids in cell membranes containing phosphorus) components. This syndrome may be part of the clinical manifestations seen in SLE, or it may occur as a primary form without other clinical features of lupus.

*Late-stage lupus* is defined as chronic disease duration of greater than 5 years. In such cases, morbidity and mortality are affected by long-term complications of SLE that result either from the disease itself or as a consequence of its therapy. These late complications may include end-stage renal disease, atherosclerosis, pulmonary emboli, and avascular necrosis. In late-stage lupus, when no evidence of active disease exists and the client is on low-dose or no corticosteroids, cognitive disabilities are a common manifestation.

### Incidence

SLE is primarily a disease of young women; it is rarely found in older people. It usually develops in young women of childbearing years, but many men and children also develop lupus. Lupus is three times more common in African American women than in white women, and is also more common in women of Hispanic, Asian, and Native American descent.

SLE also appears in the first-degree relatives of individuals with lupus more often than it does in the general population, which indicates a strong hereditary component. Most cases of SLE occur sporadically, indicating that both genetic and environmental factors play a role in the development of the disease.

### Etiologic and Risk Factors

The cause of SLE remains unknown, but evidence points to interrelated immunologic, environmental, hormonal, and genetic factors. With its periods of intermittent exacerbations and flare-ups, the theory of a latent virus infection (e.g., Epstein-Barr virus), which occasionally switches to lytic cycle, also makes sense.[79]

But whether SLE represents a single pathologic entity with variable expression or a group of related conditions remains unknown. Immune dysregulation in the form of autoimmunity is thought to be the prime causative mechanism. SLE shows a strong familial link, with a much higher frequency among first-degree relatives. Evidence for genetic susceptibility is present, and linkage studies in conjunction with genome scans may delineate this more specifically in the future.[301]

Genetically determined immune abnormalities may be triggered by both exogenous and endogenous factors. Although the predisposition to disease is hereditary, it is likely to involve different sets of genes in different individuals. As the human genome becomes more extensively mapped, a susceptibility gene may be found, although it remains possible that the differences in disease course among ethnic groups relate solely to their environment and other social factors.

Other factors predisposing to SLE may include physical or mental stress, which can provoke neuroendocrine changes affecting immune cell function; streptococcal or viral infections; exposure to sunlight or ultraviolet light, which can cause inflammation and tissue damage; immunization; pregnancy; and abnormal estrogen metabolism.

Whether pregnancy induces lupus flare-ups has not been established; existing data suggest both that it does and does not. More studies are needed to further determine the effects of pregnancy on this condition.

A higher incidence of SLE exacerbation occurs among women taking even low-dose estrogen contraceptives. Because an increased risk of thrombosis is possible in young women with SLE, estrogen-containing contraceptives are avoided or used at the lowest effective dose.

No evidence exists that postmenopausal estrogen replacement therapy is associated with SLE flare-ups, and because women in this age range are at increased risk for coronary artery disease and osteoporosis, estrogen replacement therapy can be taken. For all women with SLE who have been treated with cyclophosphamide, an increased risk of gynecologic malignancy is evident.[209]

The role of the Epstein-Barr virus as a possible risk factor for SLE remains under investigation.[79,123,164,235] SLE may also be triggered or aggravated by treatment with certain drugs (e.g., quinidine, hydralazine, anticonvulsants, penicillins, sulfa drugs, and oral contraceptives), which could modify both cellular responsiveness and immunogenicity of self-antigens.

### Pathogenesis

Three main mechanisms are implicated in the development of lupus: autoantibodies, vascular abnormalities, and inflammatory mediators. The central immunologic disturbance in SLE is autoantibody production (e.g., antineuronal, antiribosomal P, antiphospholipid). The body produces antibodies against its own cells and antigens. Deposition of the combined antigen-antibody complexes at various tissue sites can suppress the body's normal immunity and damage tissues.

In fact, one significant feature of SLE is the ability to produce antibodies against many different tissue components such as red blood cells, neutrophils, platelets, lymphocytes, or almost any organ or tissue in the body. This wide range of antigenic targets has resulted in SLE being classified as a disease of generalized autoimmunity. Given the clinical diversity of SLE, the disease may be mediated by more than one autoantibody system and several immunopathogenic mechanisms.

Specific pathologic findings are organ dependent; for example, repeat biopsies of the kidney show inflammation; cellular proliferation; basement membrane abnormalities; and immune complex deposition comprised of IgM, IgG, and IgA.

Skin lesions demonstrate inflammation and degeneration at the dermal-epidermal junction, with the basal layer being the primary site of injury. Other organ systems affected by SLE are usually studied only at autopsy. Although these tissues may show nonspecific inflammation or vessel abnormalities, pathologic findings are sometimes minimal, suggesting a mechanism other than inflammation as the cause of organ damage or dysfunction.

## Clinical Manifestations

Generally, SLE is more severe than discoid lupus, and no two people with SLE will have identical symptoms. For some people, only the skin and joints will be involved. For others, joints, lungs, kidneys, blood, or other organs and/or tissues may be affected.

**Musculoskeletal.** Arthralgias and arthritis constitute the most common presenting manifestations of SLE, but the onset of SLE may be acute or insidious and may produce no characteristic clinical pattern. Other early symptoms may include fever, weight loss, malaise, and fatigue.

Acute arthritis can involve any joint but typically affects the small joints of the hands, wrists, and knees. It may be migratory or chronic; most cases are symmetrical, but asymmetrical polyarthritis is not uncommon.

Unlike rheumatoid arthritis, the arthritis of SLE is not usually erosive or destructive of bone, and symptoms are not usually severe enough to cause joint deformities, but pain can cause temporary functional impairment. When deformities do occur, ulnar deviation, swan-neck deformity, or fixed subluxations of the fingers often occur as well. Tenosynovitis and tendon ruptures may occur.

**Cutaneous and Membranous Lesions.** The skin rash occurs most commonly in areas exposed to sunlight (ultraviolet rays) and may be exacerbated by the use of cosmetic products containing alpha hydroxy acids. The classic butterfly rash over the nose and cheeks is common (Fig. 7.34).

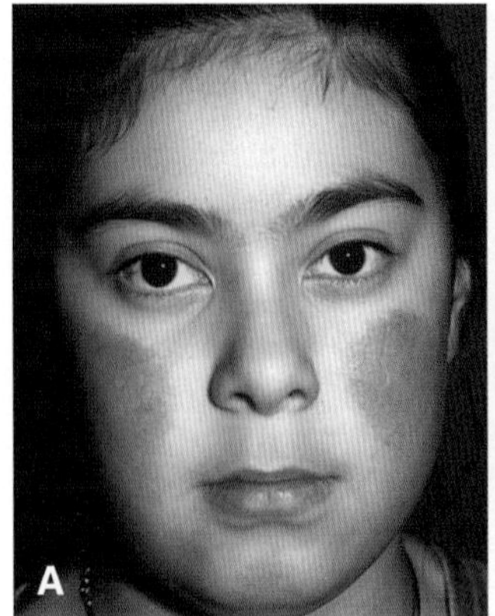


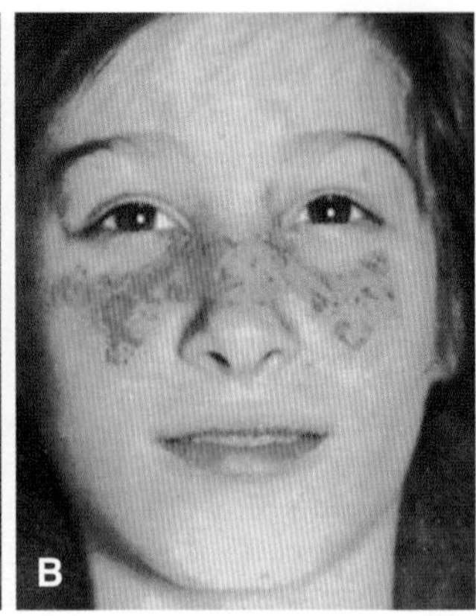


**Figure 7.34**

**The butterfly rash of SLE.** The rash can vary from an erythematous blush (A) to thickened epidermis to scaly patches (B). (Reprinted from Kliegman R, et al: *Nelson textbook of pediatrics,* ed 19, Philadelphia, 2011, WB Saunders.)

Discoid lesions associated with discoid lupus erythematosus are raised, red, scaling plaques with follicular plugging and central atrophy. This raised edging and sunken center give them a coinlike appearance.

Vasculitis (inflammation of cutaneous blood vessels) involving small- and medium-size vessels may cause other skin lesions, including infarctive lesions of the digits (Fig. 7.35), splinter hemorrhages, necrotic leg ulcers, or digital gangrene. Raynaud phenomenon occurs in approximately 20% of people.

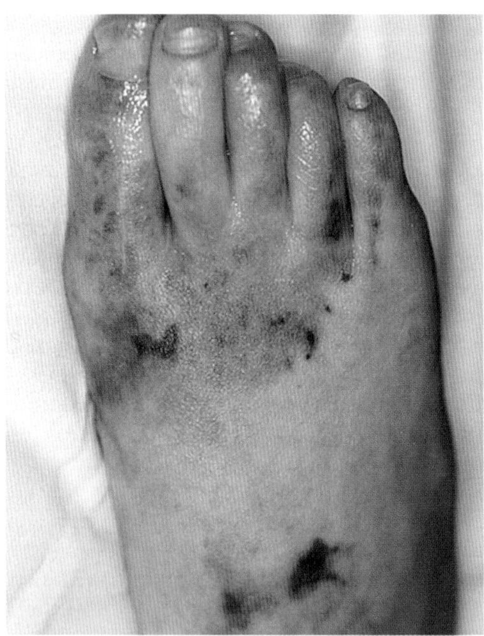

**Figure 7.35**

**A 12-year-old girl with SLE and antiphospholipid antibodies with painful cutaneous vasculitis of the right foot.** Arterial thrombosis documented by angiography resulted in cyanosis of the large toe. Symptoms resolved with treatment with heparin and corticosteroids. (Reprinted from Kliegman R, et al: *Nelson textbook of pediatrics,* ed 19, Philadelphia, 2011, WB Saunders.)

Diffuse or patchy alopecia (hair loss) may be temporary, with hair regrowth once the disease is under control. Permanent hair loss can occur from the extensive scarring of discoid lesions. Painless ulcers of the mucous membranes are common involving the mouth, vagina, and nasal septum.

**Cardiopulmonary System.** Signs of cardiopulmonary abnormalities may develop as immune complexes are deposited in the pericardial and pleural spaces, (e.g., pleuritis, pericarditis, and dyspnea). Myocarditis, endocarditis, tachycardia, and pneumonitis (acute or chronic) may also occur. Pulmonary hypertension and congestive heart failure are less common and usually secondary to a combination of factors. Anyone with SLE with the antiphospholipid antibody syndrome is at a high risk of thrombosis.

**Central Nervous System.** A significant number of people with SLE will have CNS involvement at some point in their illness, sometimes referred to as *neuropsychiatric manifestations*. Clinical manifestations may be related to specific autoantibodies that react with nervous system antigens and/or cytokine-mediated brain inflammation and include headaches, irritability, and depression (most commonly).

Emotional instability, psychosis, seizures, cerebrovascular accidents, cranial neuropathy, peripheral neuropathy, and organic brain syndrome can also occur. Return to the previous level of intellectual function may follow remission of the neuropsychiatric flare, or permanent cognitive impairment may occur.

The pattern of cognitive dysfunction is diverse; intensity can vary within the same person and can be affected by mood.[188] The person may have difficulties with verbal memory, attention, language skills (verbal fluency, productivity), and psychomotor speed. Progressive cognitive impairment, sometimes subtle and sometimes obvious, may develop even in the absence of clinically diagnosed episodes of neuropsychiatric disease.[76] People with SLE may or may not have other signs of lupus when they experience neurologic symptoms.

**Renal System.** Approximately 50% of individuals with SLE have renal disease (e.g., glomerulonephritis), usually from deposition of immune complexes and resultant inflammation and tissue damage.

**Other Systems.** Anemia from decreased erythrocytes is a common finding, with associated amenorrhea (cessation of menstrual flow) among women. Sometimes the spleen and cervical, axillary, and inguinal nodes are enlarged; hepatitis may also develop. Nausea, vomiting, diarrhea, and abdominal pain may occur with GI involvement. All symptoms mentioned in this section can occur at the onset or at any time during the course of lupus. Nearly all people with SLE experience fluctuations in disease activity with exacerbations and remissions.

### Medical Management

**Prevention.** There is no known way to prevent SLE, but preventive measures can reduce the risk of flare-ups. For photosensitive people, avoidance of (excessive) sun exposure and/or the regular application of sunscreen usually prevents rashes. Regular exercise helps prevent muscle weakness and fatigue. Immunization protects against specific infections.

Support groups, counseling, and reliance on family members, friends, and health care professionals can help alleviate the effects of stress. Lifestyle choices and personal behavior, such as smoking, excessive consumption of alcohol, too much or too little of prescribed medication, or postponing regular medical checkups, are very important for people with SLE.[149]

**Diagnosis.** Diagnosis of SLE is difficult since it often mimics other diseases. The symptoms are vague, varying greatly from individual to individual. The diagnosis and subclassification of SLE is based on a combination of clinical findings and laboratory evidence, including pattern of organ involvement.

The Systemic Lupus International Collaborating Clinics (SLICC) group revised and validated the American College of Rheumatology (ACR) SLE classification criteria in 2012. Based on those revised criteria, the diagnosis of SLE depends on the affected person having one clinical item/criterion and one immunologic criterion of biopsy-proven lupus nephritis in the presence of ANAs (anti-nuclear antibodies) or anti–double-stranded DNA antibodies.

The clinical criteria include: acute or chronic cutaneous lupus, oral ulcers, nonscarring alopecia, synovitis involving two or more joints or tenderness in two or more joints and at least 30 minutes of morning stiffness, serositis (pleurisy, pericardial pain), renal involvement, neurologic manifestations, hemolytic anemia, leucopenia, and thrombocytopenia.

The immunologic criteria are evaluated through laboratory studies, including levels of ANA, anti–double-stranded DNA antibody, anti-Sm antiphospholipid antibody, and low complement. Due to the changes in immunologic criteria, the new criterion for ANA requires a precise ELISA assay cut-off. Additionally, two biomarkers have been added to the immunologic criteria: anti-B2 glycoprotein 1 and low complement, both of which play a role in the pathogenesis of SLE.[301a]

**Table 7.12 Neuropsychiatric Syndromes in Systemic Lupus Erythematosus**

| Central Nervous System | Peripheral Nervous System |
|---|---|
| Aseptic meningitis | Acute inflammatory demyelinating polyradiculoneuropathy |
| Cerebrovascular disease | Guillain-Barre syndrome |
| Demyelinating syndrome | Autonomic disorder |
| Headache (including migraine and benign intracranial hypertension) | Mononeuropathy, single/multiplex |
| Movement disorder (chorea) | Myasthenia gravis |
| Myelopathy | Cranial neuropathy |
| Seizure disorders | Plexopathy |
| Acute confusional state | Polyneuropathy |
| Anxiety disorder | |
| Cognitive dysfunction | |
| Mood disorder | |
| Psychosis | |

From Yu C, Gershwin MES, Chang C: Diagnostic criteria for systemic lupus erythematosus: A critical review, *J Autoimmunity* 2014. https://doi.org/10.1016/j.jaut.2014.01.004.

With the involvement of CNS as manifestation of SLE, the ACR created a case definition of neuropsychiatric SLE based on a population-based study. Table 7.12 lists the neuropsychiatric syndromes observed in SLE.

**Treatment.** The objectives of medical intervention are to control disease activity, prevent damage from disease, and prevent flare-ups that can cause further damage. At the present time, pharmacologic interventions are the primary means of accomplishing these goals and must be customized for each individual to accomplish the treatment goals and spare the person adverse effects of the medications.[96]

Mild symptoms can be managed with nonsteroidal antiinflammatory drugs to relieve muscle and joint pain while reducing tissue inflammation. Corticosteroid-sparing agents (e.g., methotrexate) used earlier preserve bone and offer protection from premature cardiovascular disease. Anticoagulants for individuals who have antiphospholipid antibody syndrome and coagulopathies ensure a more favorable outcome.

Antimalarial agents (e.g., chloroquine [Aralen], hydroxychloroquine [Plaquenil]) are useful against the dermatologic, arthritic, and renal symptoms of this disease. Immunomodulating drugs (e.g., azathioprine [Imuran], cyclophosphamide [Cytoxan]) are immunosuppressive drugs used to suppress inflammation and subsequently the immune system. These are used only with active disease, especially with severe kidney involvement. Corticosteroids and cytotoxic drugs are given in more severe disease that has not responded to these other types of drug therapy.

Biologic immune-targeted treatments such as B-cell–targeted therapy, cytokine blockade, and peptide-based treatments are being developed based on current understanding of the dysregulated immunologic pathways involved in SLE pathogenesis.[25] Stem cell transplantation for severe SLE remains under investigation; early results have not been favorable.[173]

**Prognosis.** The prognosis improves with early detection and intervention that prevents organ damage and improves life expectancy. The overall reduction in the use of large doses of corticosteroids over the past 2 decades has significantly reduced morbidity and mortality rates.

People with SLE have an increased prevalence of valvular and atherosclerotic heart disease, apparently because of factors related to the disease itself and to drug therapy necessary in severe cases. Symptomatic large-vessel occlusive disease in SLE, occurring several years after the diagnosis of the disease, is associated with a relatively poor short-term outcome. There is an increased risk of certain cancers in SLE; the risk appears to be most heightened for lymphoma.[22]

Prognosis is less favorable for those who develop cardiovascular, renal, or neurologic complications or severe bacterial infections. High stress, poor social support, and psychologic distress are modifiable factors associated with health outcomes for people with SLE.[78,282]

SPECIAL IMPLICATIONS FOR THE THERAPIST 7.6

### *Systemic Lupus Erythematosus*

Physical and occupational therapy intervention can be important components of the overall treatment plan for lupus. Recurrence of disease can be managed with carefully controlled and sometimes restricted activities. After an exacerbation, gradual resumption of activities must be balanced by maximum rest periods, usually 8 to 10 hours of sleep a night and several rest periods during the day.

Most of the principles and reference materials outlined in the following section on fibromyalgia also apply to SLE. Management of joint involvement follows protocols for rheumatoid arthritis (see "Special Implications for the Therapist: Rheumatoid Arthritis" in Chapter 27). Clients with skin lesions should be examined thoroughly at each visit. The therapist can be instrumental in teaching and assisting with skin care and prevention of skin breakdown.

Functional limitations among people with SLE vary according to the type and degree of the disease. Generalized fatigue, defined as "the inclination to rest, even though pain and weakness are not limiting factors," is a common problem and can be very debilitating, especially for those individuals with both SLE and fibromyalgia.[5]

The therapist can be very instrumental in teaching clients how to avoid lupus flares by spacing activities and conserving energy, following a prescriptive exercise plan, avoiding excessive bed rest, and protecting joints. Excessive bed rest can worsen fatigue, promote muscle disuse and atrophy, and promote osteoporosis. Prescriptive exercise should strengthen the muscles and improve endurance while avoiding undue stress on inflamed joints. Patient education should include identifying triggers (e.g., too much work, not enough rest, emotional stress, poor diet, ultraviolet light exposure) and self-monitoring for the earliest signs of a flare-up. The person with SLE must limit exposure to direct sunlight (and take sun exposure precautions), fluorescent light, halogen lamps, overhead lights, computer screens, and photocopiers at home, in public, and at work.

Attention to socioeconomic factors is important because women of color are disproportionately affected by this autoimmune disease and may not receive the full care needed to manage a chronic condition of this type. Working with other members of the health care community, especially social workers, can be very helpful in meeting the goals and needs of these individuals.[114]

Septic arthritis or osteonecrosis may develop as a complication of SLE or its treatment (e.g., steroid medications). Septic arthritis is uncommon in SLE, but it should be suspected when one joint is inflamed out of proportion to the others. People with SLE may develop a drug-related myopathy secondary to corticosteroids or as a complication of antimalarials (see "Corticosteroid Myopathy" in Chapter 5).

Anyone taking corticosteroids or immunosuppressants must be monitored carefully for signs of infection, especially people at heightened risk of infection such as those with renal failure, cardiac valvular abnormalities, or ulcerative skin lesions. (See specific side effects and "Special Implications for the Therapist 5.5: Corticosteroids" in Chapter 5). The client should contact the physician if a fever or any other new symptoms develop. The therapist can provide osteoporosis prevention and intervention management.

High-dose oral corticosteroid treatment remains the major predisposing cause of avascular necrosis in SLE and other autoimmune disorders. The most common site is the femoral head of the hip; less commonly, the femoral condyle of the knee is affected. Although the condition may be bilateral, it most often presents with an insidious onset of unilateral hip or knee pain that is worse with ambulating but often present at rest. Symptoms are progressive over weeks to months.

Observe carefully for any sign of renal involvement such as weight gain, edema, or hypertension. Take seizure precautions if there are signs of neurologic involvement. The therapist may recognize signs of cognitive dysfunction or decline, either directly observed in the client or by family report. These manifestations should be reported to the physician for consideration in evaluating medications. If Raynaud phenomenon is present, teach the client to warm and protect the hands and feet.

A discussion of pregnancy and SLE is beyond the scope of this text but may be of importance to the therapist involved in women's health issues. More detailed information is available elsewhere.[37,184,201,225,226,256,266]

## Fibromyalgia

### Definition and Overview

Fibromyalgia or fibromyalgia syndrome (FMS), formerly mislabeled or misdiagnosed as fibrocytis, fibromyositis, myofascial pain, CFS, or SLE, is a chronic muscle pain syndrome. Fibromyalgia is defined as chronic widespread pain with allodynia or hyperalgesia to pressure pain and is classified as one of the largest groups of soft tissue pain syndromes (not a disease).[4] Simply stated, it is a disorder of pain processing (i.e., abnormal pain modulation with hypersensitivity to painful stimuli and reduced pain inhibition).[265]

Sometimes FMS occurs as a result of some other medical condition. For example, individuals with inflammatory conditions (e.g., rheumatoid arthritis, polymyalgia rheumatic, SLE), metabolic dysfunction (e.g., thyroid problems), or cancer often develop a type of FMS referred to as *reactive* fibromyalgia. It is important to identify whether or not the FMS is *primary* (the main problem) or *secondary/reactive* (caused by other problems).

Fibromyalgia has been differentiated from myofascial pain (see "Myofascial Pain Syndrome" in Chapter 27) in that fibromyalgia is considered a systemic problem involving biochemical, neuroendocrine, and physiologic abnormalities, with widespread multiple tender points as one of the key symptoms. Myofascial pain is a localized condition specific to a muscle and may involve as few as one or as many as several areas with characteristic trigger points that are painful and refer pain to other areas when pressure is applied.

The person with myofascial pain syndrome does not exhibit other associated constitutional or systemic signs or symptoms unless palpation elicits a painful enough response to elicit an autonomic nervous system response with nausea and/or vomiting, increased blood pressure, and increased pulse.

It has been proposed that fibromyalgia and CFS are two names for the same syndrome, with CFS being an early form of FMS, but at present, CFS is thought to differ by the greater degree of fatigue. People with fibromyalgia tend to experience more pain. In contrast to CFS, fibromyalgia is associated with a variety of initiating or perpetuating factors such as psychologically distressing events, primary sleep disorders, inflammatory rheumatic arthritis, and acute febrile illness.

Fibromyalgia and CFS have similar disordered sleep physiology, and evidence suggests a reciprocal relationship of the immune and sleep–wake systems. Interference with either system has effects on the other and will be accompanied by the symptoms of CFS.[183] A significant number of people with FMS meet the criteria for CFS and vice versa.

### Incidence

Fibromyalgia occurs in more than 6 million Americans. It has now surpassed rheumatoid arthritis as the most common musculoskeletal disorder in the United States.[154] Women are affected more often than men (90% are women), with symptoms appearing between the ages of 20 and 55 years, although it has been diagnosed in children as young as 6 years and adults as old as 85 years.

### Risk Factors

Risk factors or triggering events for the onset of fibromyalgia may include prolonged anxiety and emotional stress, trauma (e.g., motor vehicle accident, work injury, surgery), rapid steroid withdrawal, hypothyroidism, and viral and nonviral infections. Exposure to tobacco products has been suggested as a possible risk factor for the development of fibromyalgia, but this has not been investigated fully or proven.[286]

Fibromyalgia may also develop with no obvious precipitating events or illnesses. It is more prevalent in minimally to moderately physically fit persons and is not usually found in highly trained athletes. Anxiety, depression, and posttraumatic stress disorder (perhaps associated with physical and/or sexual abuse in childhood and adulthood)[111,259] also seem to be linked with FMS.[29] Having a bipolar illness increases the risk of developing FMS dramatically.[280]

### Etiologic Factors

Research is now ongoing to determine the cause of fibromyalgia; most likely the initiation of this condition is multifactorial (Fig. 7.36). Possible etiologic theories include diet; viral origin; sleep disorder; occupational, seasonal, or environmental influences; and adverse childhood experiences, including sexual abuse. Psychologic and cognitive/behavioral factors seem to cooccur with FMS including psychiatric disorders such as major depression, anxiety disorders, personality disorders, altered pain perception, and catastrophizing.[289]

Familial aggregation of fibromyalgia and a reduced pain threshold in first-degree female relatives of affected individuals (even in family members without obvious clinical symptoms) provides evidence of fibromyalgia as a heritable disorder. Clear genetic markers have not been identified; candidate genes linked to fibromyalgia support a genetic (biologic) basis for this condition in some people.[155] How much is genetic influence and how much can be attributed to shared environment remains unknown at this time.[3,23]

### Pathogenesis

Its pathogenesis is not entirely understood, although it is currently thought to be the result of a CNS malfunction that increases pain transmission and perception[4] accompanied by ineffective pain inhibition.[265] Fibromyalgia syndrome is currently perceived by rheumatologists and pain physicians alike as representing the classic condition of central sensitization.[2] Accumulating evidence suggests the underlying cause of fibromyalgia pain results from abnormal pain processing particularly in the CNS rather than from dysfunction in peripheral tissues where pain is perceived.[207]

Previous theories that abnormalities of the hypothalamic–pituitary–adrenal axis were the cause of FMS have been set aside, as only a small subset of individuals demonstrate these abnormalities as a precipitating factor. There is no doubt the hypothalamic–pituitary–adrenal axis is involved, but it looks more like the onset of fibromyalgia may bring about disturbances in the regulatory systems of the body, not the other way around.[289]

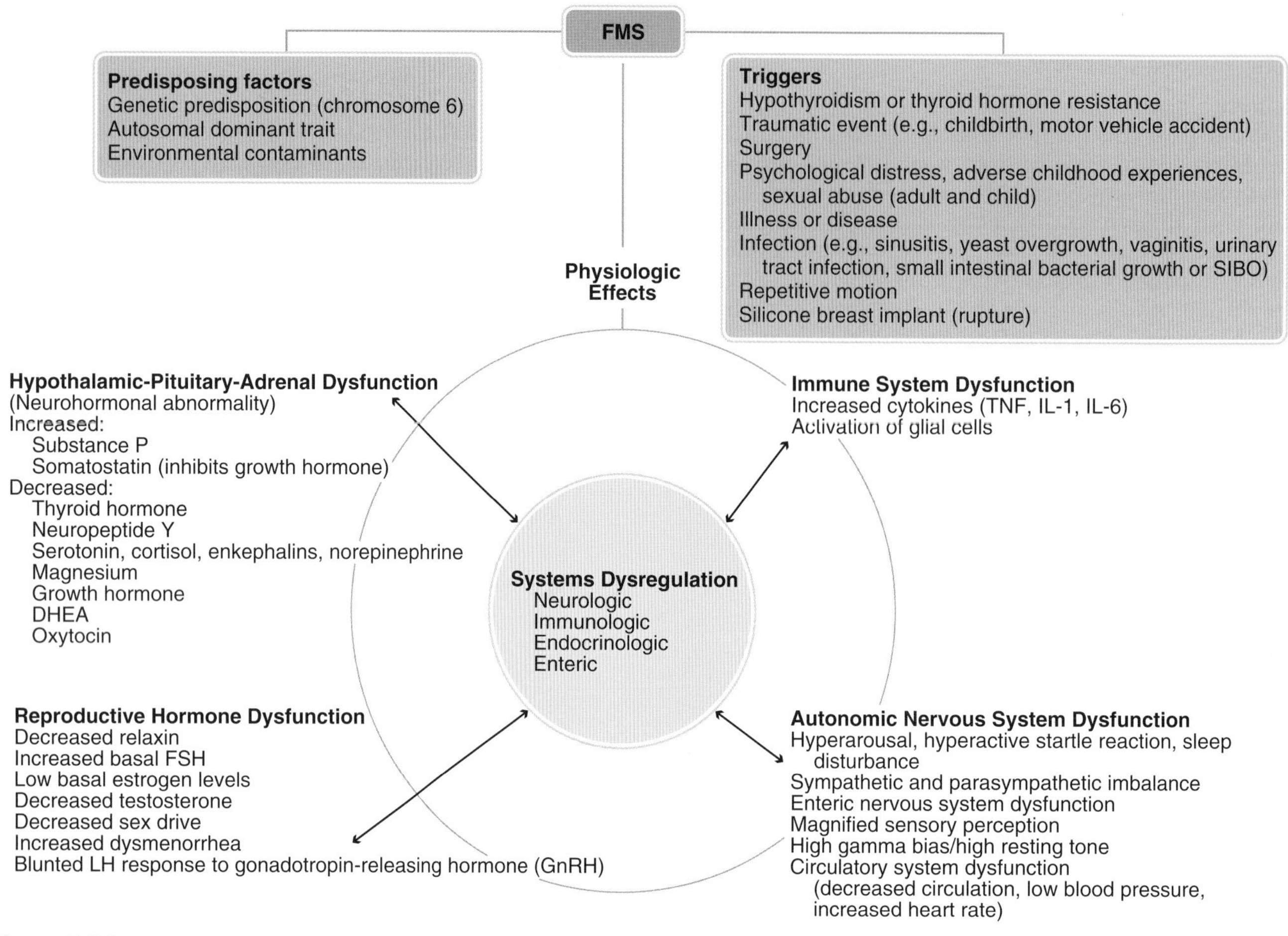


**Figure 7.36**

**Multifactorial causes of FMS.** There are many hypotheses and models of how multiple factors contribute to the development of FMS. This model represents data thus far to support FMS as a biologic (organic) disorder caused by neurohormonal dysfunction of the autonomic nervous system. The physiologic effects of four primary systems' dysfunction are listed.

**Autonomic Nervous System.** Many researchers have shown that people with fibromyalgia have an autonomic nervous system with a hyperactive sympathetic branch and an underactive parasympathetic branch. The activity of the skeletal muscles, heart, stomach, intestines, blood vessels, and sweat glands during daily stress tends to be excessive in fibromyalgia. These organs overactivate, resulting in the heart beating faster, the stomach secreting excessive digestive juices and contracting erratically, the smooth muscles of the intestines and bowel contracting abnormally, breathing becoming rapid and shallow, and blood vessels constricting, which decreases blood flow to body parts. In FMS, the nervous system's ability to modulate and return to normal is fragile and lacks the subtle ability to respond quickly; responses are more exaggerated and the return to normal takes more time.[119,303]

The enteric system (autonomic nervous control of the digestive system) is often significantly disrupted in fibromyalgia. Digestion is often compromised, and the absorption of nutrients into the bloodstream (where they can be used by the body for cell function) is often inadequate for healthy daily function. The enteric system's interaction with other systems (e.g., brain, immune system) links effects of nutritional deficits to other functions as well.[119]

Sleep disturbances may contribute to fibromyalgia symptoms; researchers are investigating alterations of the neuroimmunoendocrine systems that accompany disordered sleep physiology, resulting in the nonrestorative sleep, pain, fatigue, and cognitive and mood symptoms that people with fibromyalgia (and CFS) experience.[216]

People affected do not enter restorative sleep (phase IV sleep) or rapid eye movement sleep. Deficiency of non–rapid eye movement sleep also contributes to sleep disturbance by reducing the amount of time the muscles enter a state of resting muscle tone. Eighty percent of the body's growth hormone is secreted by the pituitary gland (under hypothalamic control) during deep sleep, and it is crucial for normal muscle metabolism and tissue repair. Substantial nighttime decreases in growth hormone have been reported in FMS.[150]

These types of sleep disturbances are not unique to fibromyalgia but have been observed in many people with rheumatoid arthritis, osteoarthritis, and other painful rheumatic diseases.

**Immune System.** Finally, a model for pathologic pain syndromes (such as FMS and CFS) has been formulated based on pain facilitatory effects produced by the immune system. Immune cells, activated in response to infection,

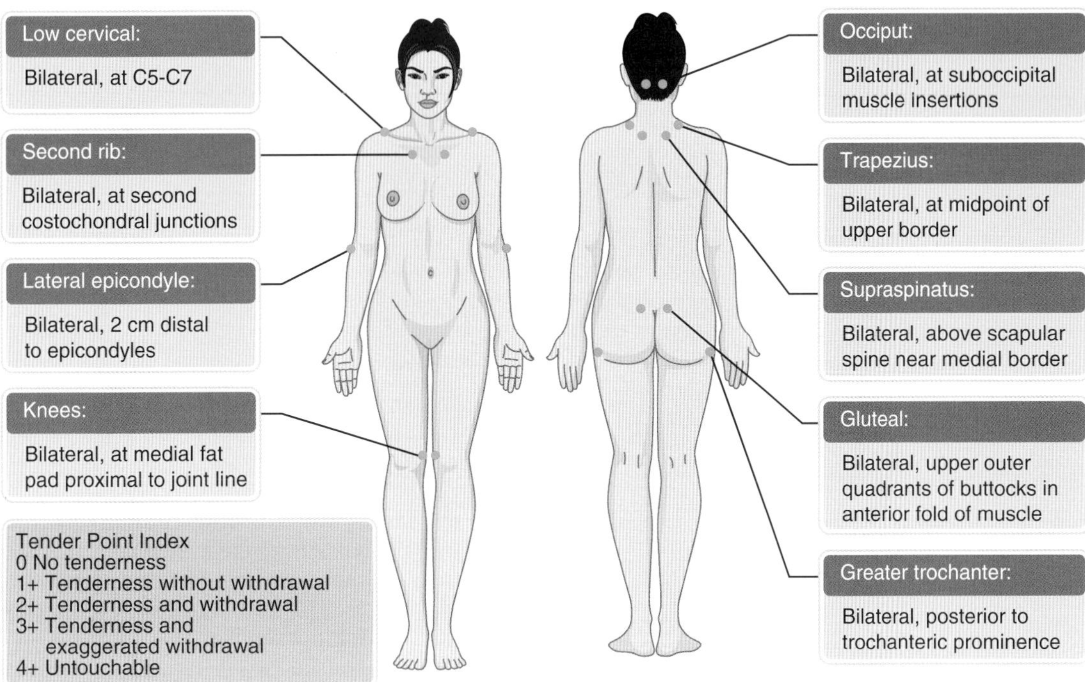


**Figure 7.37**

**Anatomic locations of tender points associated with fibromyalgia.** According to the literature, digital palpation should be performed with an approximate force of 4 kg (enough pressure to indent a tennis ball), but clinical practice suggests much less pressure is required to elicit a painful response. For a tender point to be considered positive, the subject must state that the palpation was "painful." A reply of "tender" is not considered a positive response. Counting the number of points as part of the clinical diagnosis of FMS has been discounted[204]; however, the presence of multiple tender points is still a key feature of FMS. (Reprinted from Goodman CC, Hieck J, Lazaro R: *Differential diagnosis for physical therapists: screening for referral,* ed 6, Philadelphia, 2017, WB Saunders.)

inflammation, or trauma, release proinflammatory cytokines that signal the CNS to release glia within the brain and spinal cord. Pain has been classically viewed as being mediated solely by neurons, but the discovery that spinal cord glia (microglia and astrocytes) amplify pain has changed this view.

When glial cells become activated by sensory signals arriving from the periphery, they can release a variety of substances known to be involved in chronic pain (e.g., nerve growth factor, excitatory amino acids, nitric oxide), and they can also control the release of neurotransmitters (e.g., substance P).

Once activated, such as when viruses and bacteria enter the CNS, glial cells cause prolonged release of proinflammatory cytokines (e.g., TNF, IL-1, IL-6), creating an exaggerated pain state. Glia may be the key driving force for the pain created by tissue inflammation and nerve injury, since they increase the release of pain transmitters and cytokines from the neurons in the surrounding area, and they are connected to large networks that allow activation of glia at distant sites.

This pain model emphasizes again the need for anyone with FMS to minimize pain-generating aggravators such as infectious agents, trauma, and inflammation (including dietary) or other triggers (Fig. 7.37).[284]

**Clinical Manifestations.** The major symptom of fibromyalgia is muscle pain, often described as aching or burning, a "migraine headache of the muscles." Diffuse pain or tender points are present on both sides of the body in many muscle groups (not just the 18 points originally suggested).

Sleep disturbances result in fatigue and exhaustion, even after a night's sleep. Men with fibromyalgia typically have fewer symptoms and milder tender points (less "hurt all over" reports), less fatigue, and fewer incidences of irritable bowel syndrome compared with women who have FMS.[4]

Other symptoms or associated problems occur with a high frequency (Table 7.13), sometimes more incapacitating than the pain and tender points. Symptoms are often exacerbated by stress; overloading physical activity, including overstretching; damp or chilly weather; heat exposure or humidity; sudden change in barometric pressure; trauma, or another illness.

People with fibromyalgia who are aerobically fit manifest fewer symptoms than those who remain physically deconditioned and aerobically unfit. Individuals with FMS display alterations in heat, cold, and mechanical sensitivity.[32] Biofeedback specialists have shown that blood circulation to the affected areas is often significantly decreased while at rest, and a noticeable decrease in circulation occurs with changes in barometric pressure.

During exercise, when circulation should normally increase to muscles and the brain, in fibromyalgia, the opposite happens, and circulation is decreased significantly.[119] Real-time ultrasonography has confirmed the lower magnitude of muscle vascularity following dynamic and during static exercise. The immediate flow response to muscular activity was lower in magnitude and of a shorter duration in people with fibromyalgia compared to healthy controls.[83]

**Table 7.13** Clinical Manifestations of Fibromyalgia

| Sign/Symptom | Incidence (%)[a] |
|---|---|
| Muscle pain (myalgia), tender points | 99 |
| Visual problems (e.g., blurring, double vision, bouncing images) | 95 |
| Mental and physical fatigue | 85 |
| Morning stiffness (persists >30 min) | 75 |
| Mitral valve prolapse | 75 |
| Global anxiety | 72 |
| Cognitive (memory) problems (e.g., decreased attention span, impaired short-term memory, decreased concentration, increased distractibility) | 71 |
| Irritable bowel syndrome | 70 |
| Headaches | 70 |
| Sicca syndrome (dry eyes/mouth) | 63 |
| Hypersensitivity to noise, odors, heat, or cold (cold intolerance) | 50-60 |
| Inflammatory bowel disease (Crohn disease, ulcerative colitis) | 50-60 |
| Constipation (decreased intestinal motility) | 59 |
| Sleep disturbance/morning fatigue | 57 |
| Dizziness or faintness going from sit to stand | 57 |
| Paresthesias | 50 |
| Swollen feeling (joint or soft tissues) | 50 |
| Muscle spasms or nodules | 50 |
| Reactive hypoglycemia (e.g., weakness, irritability, disorientation) | 45-50 |
| Pelvic pain | 43 |
| Irritable bladder syndrome, female urethral syndrome | 40 |
| Hypotension (low blood pressure, elevated heart rate); neurally mediated hypotension or vasopressor syncope | 40 |
| Raynaud phenomenon | 38 |
| Respiratory dysfunction (e.g., dyspnea, erratic breathing patterns during exertion) | 33 |
| Lack of libido | 33 |
| Restless leg syndrome, nocturnal myoclonus, periodic leg movement disorder | 30-60 |
| Diaphoresis (unexplained sweating) | 30 |
| Auditory problems | 30 |
| Temporomandibular dysfunction | 25 |
| Depression | 20 |
| Allergies | Unknown |
| Skin discoloration | Unknown |
| Sciatica | Unknown |

[a]These figures were compiled from a variety of sources but represent a fairly accurate clinical perspective.

Data from Solano C: Autonomic dysfunction in fibromyalgia assessed by the Composite Autonomic Symptoms Scale (COMPASS), *J Clin Rheumatol* 15(4): 179-176, 2009.

The diaphragm is significantly affected in fibromyalgia to the point that it ceases to function as the major breathing muscle, and accessory muscles of the neck and upper chest take over. This overwork results in tender points or tightness of the neck and chest muscles.

In general, the level of muscular activity in fibromyalgia is high, even when the body is sitting or reclining. During daily activities such as cleaning, cooking, typing, and even socializing, the muscles used for these activities are at a higher level of activity than the muscles of a normal person doing the same tasks.

When the activity is over and the person with fibromyalgia is resting, those same muscles continue to repeat the activity over and over at a lower intensity so that no outward movement is apparent. At the same time, increased pain sensation after repeated exposure to a stimulus creates central sensitization. This phenomenon, called the "wind-up response," combined with increased central pain processing, may lower tender point thresholds and result in prolonged after-sensations.[289]

### Medical Management

**Diagnosis.** No definitive test is currently available to determine the presence of fibromyalgia, and usually the organs involved are not the cause but merely the messenger of a problem originating elsewhere in the body. Research underway to find biomarkers for CFS and fibromyalgia has discovered increases in the expression of sensory, adrenergic, and immune genes not found in normal subjects. These changes were only observed after sustained moderate exercise.[158]

The ACR has used two criteria for a medical diagnosis of FMS: (1) widespread (four-quadrant) pain both above and below the waist present for at least 3 months and (2) subjective report of pain when pressure is applied to 11 of the 18 common FMS tender points on the body (see Fig. 7.37).

Subjective assessment of tender points can be elicited by the use of an instrument called a *dolorimeter*, which distributes pressure equally over a discrete point. With a dolorimeter, the pressure required to produce pain in a given area can be recorded.

Controversy also exists regarding current use of the ACR's criteria for tender point count in clinical diagnosis of FMS. In fact, the original author of the ACR criteria has suggested that counting the tender points was "perhaps a mistake" and has advised against using it in clinical practice as the only means of diagnosis.[292,295]

A somatic symptom scale (SSS) was subsequently developed and validated by Wolfe to help differentiate FMS from other rheumatologic conditions (e.g., SLE or polymyalgia rheumatica) with similar widespread pain.[293,294]

Since that time, Wolfe and associates have proposed new diagnostic criteria, which the ACR has adopted.[292,296] The new tool focuses on measuring symptom severity rather than relying on the tender point examination. The new criteria use a clinician-queried checklist of painful sites and a symptom severity scale that focuses on fatigue, cognitive dysfunction, and sleep disturbance. Tender point assessment still has value; people with fewer than 11 of the 18 tender points included in the ACR classification criteria may still be diagnosed with fibromyalgia if they have other clinical features consistent with fibromyalgia.[23,137] Overall, the most effective way to diagnose fibromyalgia is by using the widespread pain index (WPI) and somatic symptom scale (SSS). Current research is looking at primary and secondary fibromyalgia.[297] This research can help distinguish how fibromyalgia works with other pathologies.

Often, the diagnosis is determined as a process of elimination by ruling out other conditions based on

Box 7.6

**DIFFERENTIAL DIAGNOSIS OF FIBROMYALGIA**

***Endocrine Disorders***

- Hypothyroidism
- Hypopituitary
- Hyperparathyroidism
- Growth hormone deficiency
- Diabetes mellitus
- Adrenal insufficiency
- Pregnancy
- Menopause
- Menstrual disorders

***Illness***

- Rheumatoid arthritis
- Systemic lupus erythematosus
- Sjögren syndrome
- Polymyositis/dermatomyositis
- Polymyalgia rheumatica/giant cell arteritis
- Metabolic myopathy (e.g., alcohol)
- Metastatic cancer
- Chronic fatigue syndrome

***Infection/Inflammation***

- Subacute bacterial endocarditis
- Lyme disease
- Hepatitis C
- AIDS
- Chronic syphilis
- Tuberculosis

***Other***

- Temporomandibular joint dysfunction
- Disk disease
- Myofascial pain syndrome
- Silicone breast implant
- Neurosis (depression/anxiety)
- Substance abuse
- Malnutrition
- Allergies (including food intolerances)

Data from Cleveland Clinic: *Current clinical medicine*, ed 2, Philadelphia, 2011, WB Saunders.

clinical presentation and past medical history (Box 7.6). In addition to the presence of tender points, skin fold tenderness, increased reactive skin hyperemia, and low tissue compliance (in the trapezius and paraspinal regions) provide further diagnostic information.

No special laboratory or radiologic testing is necessary for making a diagnosis of FMS; routine testing for rheumatoid factor or ANAs is not recommended. Although routine inexpensive tests, including complete blood count, basic chemistry (blood urea nitrogen, creatinine, hepatic enzymes, serum calcium), and thyroid function, should be undertaken (if not done in the past year), any other test to rule out other conditions, unless clinically indicated (by both symptoms and physical examination), is a waste of time and resources.

A routine complete blood count test may demonstrate anemia caused by medications or another disease, which may contribute to fatigue, and cytopenia; a baseline chemistry test is useful in monitoring various medication side effects. Because spinal pain in FMS and pain caused by pathologic changes in the spine (e.g., osteoarthritis and osteopenia with vertebral compression fracture) cannot always be distinguished clinically, a spinal x-ray may be necessary for a middle-aged or older adult, especially considering other risk factors for these conditions. It is important not to miss these diagnoses, because the management approach is likely to be different from FMS alone. A sleep study should be considered only when history suggests a primary sleep disorder.[302]

Albrecht et al. theorize glial activation in the brain as being not only a possible cause but also a way to screen for fibromyalgia.[6] As such, the results of this study suggest that it may be useful to use positron emission tomography (PET) to screen for increases of TSPO, a translocator protein found in the mitochondrial membrane of microglia and astrocytes. This protein is expressed in low levels in individuals who do not have CNS disorders. High levels of this protein indicate an inflammatory response. The researchers hypothesized that TSPO binding in the brain would be elevated in individuals with fibromyalgia when compared to a control group. A PET scan was performed to measure brain glial activation in all participants. The results of their study demonstrated an increase in glial cell activation in the cortex. The conclusion of their research suggests that a possible treatment for FMS using glial cell modulation. Further research is needed due to the small sample size of this study.[6]

**Treatment.** Effective treatment of the widespread pain of FMS, attributed mainly to an increase in the processing and handling of pain by the CNS, must be directed toward function of the CNS.[2] Current clinical practice guidelines of several American and European medical societies recommend a multimodal, holistic, and multidisciplinary[12,109,240] approach, including education and support, stress management, nutrition and lifestyle training (e.g., coping strategies, applying work simplification and ergonomic principles, and cognitive-behavioral therapy), medications (e.g., antidepressants,[112] muscle relaxants, analgesics, and anticonvulsants), local modalities and techniques for muscle pain (e.g., relaxation techniques, biofeedback, physiologic quieting, or soft tissue techniques, electrotherapy), and conditioning and aerobic exercise.

Cognitive behavioral therapy, especially combined with exercise, is strongly recommended.[109,143] This approach is aimed at altering sensory, affective, cognitive, and behavioral aspects of chronic pain (e.g., pain severity, emotional distress, depression, anxiety, pain behavior) and is effective over a long period, even when the disease process cannot be controlled and symptoms worsen. Based on current evidence, a stepwise program emphasizing education, certain medications, exercise, cognitive therapy, or all four should be recommended.[289]

Other treatment such as acupuncture, herbal or vitamin supplements, chiropractic, hypnotherapy, and meditative movement therapy (e.g., qi gong, tai chi, yoga) often provides palliative relief from symptoms and depression severity for varying periods of time.[68,152] Like most interventions, no single intervention is effective all the time, and the person with FMS may cycle through various treatment approaches over time.

**Prognosis.** Many people with mild symptoms are managed without a specialist and have an expected good long-term outcome, but most people experience persistent symptoms of fibromyalgia for many years or a lifetime. Good therapy must be instituted early in the client's course if there is to be any chance of achieving substantial improvement or a remission.

SPECIAL IMPLICATIONS FOR THE THERAPIST 7.7

### *Fibromyalgia*

Therapists are often the first to recognize the history and clinical manifestations suggestive of fibromyalgia and request medical diagnosis and intervention. The Composite Autonomic Symptoms Scale (COMPASS) can be used to document symptoms produced by abnormal function of the autonomic nervous system.[258]

Efforts to assess the accuracy of thumb nail-bed blanching as a means of determining the presence of tender points suggest that the therapist can quickly learn to use the 4 kg/cm$^2$ of force required to administer a tender point examination (manual tender point survey).[4] Nail-bed blanching refers to the definition of a tender point being one that is painful when 4 kg of pressure is applied (the amount of pressure needed to blanch the examiner's thumbnail when palpating the palm of the examiner's own hand).

Accurate assessment allows the therapist to establish a baseline sensitivity to aid in determining progress and direct intervention.[57] Specific procedures for identifying and palpating each site are available.[145,264] A complete compendium of blank assessment forms and information on how to obtain assessment instruments for FMS are also available.[119,167]

Rehabilitative therapy is an important component in managing fibromyalgia. Many people with FMS have undergone unnecessary exploratory or corrective surgery and have residual functional limitations. Chronic musculoskeletal conditions that are sources of noxious neural input to the CNS often involve the shoulder(s) and spine.

Therapy is helpful first in directing individuals to reach goals of lessening pain and fatigue and eliminating sleep disturbance. Outcomes can be measured in a variety of ways, not only by reduction in tender points but also by global scores of pain, fatigue, sleep, reduction of other distressing symptoms, improved quality of life, reduced visits to the physician, reduction or elimination of medications, increased sexual activity, improved work performance, and so on.

Therapists should listen for reports of adverse effects from pharmaceuticals used to treat FMS. The tricyclic antidepressants (such as amitriptyline) and the serotonin noradrenaline (norepinephrine) reuptake inhibitors (e.g., duloxetine and milnacipran) are first-line options for the treatment of individuals diagnosed with FMS. There is evidence that a small number of people experience substantial symptom relief with no or minor adverse effects from these medications. At the same time, a large number of people stop taking them because of intolerable adverse effects or they only get a small amount of relief from symptoms, which do not outweigh the adverse effects.[112]

Many people with FMS have been told they must "learn to live with it." A more positive approach is to suggest working together to learn how to move forward with FMS, respecting limitations but not being controlled by them. The therapist can be very instrumental in guiding that person to understand how to manage this condition. Prevention programs for osteoporosis and falls related to low blood pressure are additional services the therapist can provide.

Strategies for work modification and applying ergonomic techniques to increase efficiency and decrease pain are important interventions. A chronic pain program may be appropriate. The reader is referred to more specific literature for treatment regimens, self-stabilizing techniques, and therapy protocols for this condition.[1,52,119,223]

#### Monitoring Vital Signs

Monitoring tests provide an indication of the present physiologic status but cannot predict future status, so regular monitoring is necessary. Depending on the current status, the individual may have to self-monitor every 2 hours, whereas others are able to maintain a balance by monitoring twice daily or less often. For most people with FMS, the sensory system and the autonomic nervous system (ANS) are overactive. Monitoring tests are a helpful tool in developing techniques to quiet these hypersensitivities and achieve a state of physiologic quiet.[119]

Blood pressure and heart rate are indicators of cardiac and circulatory system function and should be monitored. Most people with FMS have low blood pressure and usually an elevated pulse rate even at rest (some individuals have a slow pulse). Hypotension in people with FMS is now referred to as *neurogenic hypotension*. It has been suggested that thyroid hormone regulation will normalize the heart rate and contractility and often normalizes the blood pressure.[165]

For some individuals with a hypoglycemic component, blood glucose assessment may be necessary. Hand temperature is one indicator of ANS function and can be easily assessed using a handheld biofeedback device (e.g., PhysioQ)[211] designed to measure hand temperature. This tool along with a program of physiologic quieting provides a mean of modulating the ANS, improving circulation, and reducing pain levels. The therapist can monitor medical and physical therapy intervention outcomes by assessing vital signs and documenting results.

#### Modalities and Fibromyalgia

There is still conflicting evidence on which types of modalities provides the best therapeutic response. A number of physical therapy interventions with thermal or mechanical properties have been studied in regards to FMS. These interventions include cryotherapy, moist heat, massage, manual therapy, soft tissue treatment, electrical stimulation, ultrasound, and low level laser. These treatments require more research to test efficacy but show promising results with decreased pain and improved FIQ scores.[116]

The use of noninvasive cranial electrotherapy stimulation (sending mini currents of electricity through the brain) for the treatment of refractory pain associated with FMS is under investigation.[193] Limited study shows that this treatment intervention can provide a significant improvement in tender point scores and in self-rated scores of general pain level, along with dramatic gains in six stress-related psychologic test measures.[141,157]

Ultrasound can be an effective therapeutic modality for the treatment of pain in people with FMS when combined with connective tissue manipulation and high-voltage pulsed galvanic stimulation.[58] Also, pulsed ultrasound has been shown to be effective in treatment of pain in FMS as combined therapy with interferential current.[9]

There are some reports on the use of ultrasound as an effective therapeutic modality for its thermal effects and for the treatment of myofascial trigger points often present in people with FMS. Continuous ultrasound is preferable to pulsed ultrasound and should be combined with a complete trigger point protocol.[270] The intensity must be reduced from standard settings to accommodate hypersensitivity in most people with FMS. Specific positions, tissue effects, intervention techniques, and treatment parameters are available.[117,118]

Again, additional steps must be taught to sustain pain relief, for example, using biofeedback or physiologic quieting[119] to avoid contracting the involved muscle; gentle, slow stretching combined with moist heat several times each day; appropriate changes in work style, patterns of movement, or postures; and nonprescription analgesics such as ibuprofen or naproxen (when approved by the physician).[118]

Soft tissue techniques may correct the neurocirculatory abnormality and thereby reduce or eliminate the nociceptive signal transmission from the muscle. The result should be to relieve pain and improve tender point index scores or other FMS pain scores assessed.

Given the proposed mechanism of muscle pain (hyperresponsive myofascial mechanoreceptors/impaired CNS pain-inhibiting system), soft tissue techniques must be applied gently and slowly to increase circulation while avoiding an increase in nociceptive signal transmission. With the typical FMS client, posttreatment discomfort can be avoided by keeping the discomfort level during treatment between 1 and 5 on a self-assessment scale of 1 to 10. Cross-friction massage is not advised.[165]

### Exercise and Fibromyalgia

The primary nonpharmacologic modality in the management of FMS is prescriptive exercise. low- to moderate-intensity aerobic exercise and strength training are strongly recommended.[36,291] Improvement in both subjective pain and objective measurement has been demonstrated with cardiovascular fitness training or simple flexibility training.[120,289] Increases in β-endorphin, adrenocorticotropic hormone, and cortisol levels in response to exercise at aerobic levels (i.e., 60% of maximal oxygen consumption) also have been shown in this population.[189]

Aerobic exercise also contributes by increasing the metabolic rate of the lean tissues for those individuals with a thyroid component.[248] Resistance exercise contributes to the increase in metabolism by increasing lean tissue mass, which has a higher metabolic rate than fat tissue.[217] Resistance exercise can reduce acute pain perception in women with fibromyalgia if they are able to exercise at a workload level high enough to reach the threshold necessary to trigger this response.[140] Well-managed prescriptive exercise regimens improve sleep and result in a decrease in pain and fatigue.[61]

Only general concepts are included in this text; other texts are available for specific exercise regimens.[18,105,119] Aerobic and strength training exercises can improve FIQ score and decrease pain,[261] but as with the use of medications that may mask the symptoms rather than treat the underlying cause, these treatments are often more effective if taken in conjunction with exercise, stretching, and stress management.[23]

Combining self-care and management strategies with an exercise program helps the individual reach the goals of optimal function and fitness while maintaining decreased pain and fatigue and increasing endurance for daily activities. A number of excellent self-care books are available for consumers.[54,69] Gentle stretching exercises performed routinely throughout the day may reduce fatigue. The Fibromyalgia Impact Questionnaire can be used to measure changes in pain, fatigue, stiffness, and other measures of functional performance.[87,90,263] A cardiopulmonary fitness component should be included at whatever level the individual presents with at the time of assessment.

Sometimes the person's condition is so acute that exercise is not tolerated immediately. This is often the reason for using modalities in the early stage of therapy. Exercising too soon and committing to too much can set the person back considerably, but at the same time, the therapist must keep in mind the long-term goal to increase strength and improve aerobic fitness.

Aquatic therapy is an ideal way to begin conditioning, especially for individuals with FMS who have injuries, are overweight, or are sensitive to axial load. Aquatic therapy provides low-load progressive exercises, gradually increasing strength and endurance while improving overall cardiovascular fitness.[13,107] Ideal pool temperature is between 28.9° C (84° F) and 32.2° C (90° F) (compared with 27.8° C [82° F] to 28.9° C [84° F] for the general population and 32.2° C [90° F] to 34.4° C [94° F] for people with arthritic conditions).[148]

As with all exercise programs with this population (whether aquatic or other therapy), people with fibromyalgia fatigue quickly and may have a low tolerance for exertion. The key is to avoid activating the peripheral sensory mechanisms in order to avoid increasing pain postexercise.

The person with FMS will respond to stimuli that would not ordinarily be perceived as painful (referred to as *allodynia*). This requires short exercise sessions, according to individual tolerance using the rate of perceived exertion, that are possibly even only 3 to 5 minutes at first.

The client is encouraged to increase exercise duration in small daily increments, sometimes only by seconds or minutes. Reaching a goal of 30 minutes of daily exercise may take weeks to months; some individuals are only able to tolerate one to three daily exercise cycles, each lasting only 5 to 10 minutes, but this will produce beneficial effects.

The individual with FMS must be taught to set aside the philosophy of "no pain, no gain" and to avoid "pushing through the pain." In the normal individual, growth hormone is increased with exercise, but this does not happen in the person with FMS.

Rather, as a result of ANS dysfunction, reduced microcirculation (capillary flow and other small vessels that supply muscles) causes microtrauma in muscles with vigorous, strenuous, or excessive exercise. The resulting postexertional muscle pain or discomfort aggravates the abnormal pain filter experienced by this population. All causes of increased pain should be minimized, reduced, or eliminated.[19]

Poor compliance is common when the use of muscle relaxants, sedatives, or other medications reduces desire or drive to exercise. Symptoms of pain and fatigue increase during exercise, resulting in limited compliance and limited long-term benefits. The therapist can explain that pain may result in part from muscle spasm and reduced blood flow to muscles, both of which can be aided by persistence in managing exercise.

Using training intensity as a measure of improvement may be helpful. Before performing the physical activity or exercise, compute the maximum heart rate (MHR = 220 − Age). During the activity/exercise, take the pulse and record this for later calculations.

Once the activity/exercise is completed, compute the intensity of work ($I_W$): $I_W$ = Pulse/MHR. Multiply $I_W$ by the number of minutes exercised to determine the training index (TI): TI = $I_W$ × number of minutes. Keep track of the TI for each activity/exercise session and total them up for 1 week. Track this value over time to assess improved outcomes.[60]

People with fibromyalgia are also more vulnerable to overuse syndromes than are people with normal muscle histology, requiring a slower, longer rehabilitation process. This may not be activity induced as once thought but rather may occur as a result of sarcolemmal abnormality.[126] At present, until more is known and understood about this phenomenon, whenever possible an aerobic exercise routine should become a part of the client's life before individual muscle group strengthening is started.

Additionally, trigger points, a separate entity from tender points, must be detected and eliminated before initiating exercise using those muscles. Specific assessment and intervention for trigger point therapy is available,[52,113,251] but it should be noted that trigger points are treatment resistant in some individuals with inadequate thyroid hormone at the cellular level. For these individuals, treatment of the underlying hypothyroidism and/or thyroid resistance is essential first.166

# ISOIMMUNE DISEASE

## Organ and Tissue Transplantation

With recent advances in technology and immunology, organ and tissue transplantation is becoming commonplace. In fact, transplantation of almost any tissue is feasible, but the clinical use of transplantation to remedy disease is still limited for many organ systems because of the rejection reaction. Transplant rejection, an isoimmune phenomenon, occurs in response to transplantation because the body usually recognizes the donor tissue as nonself and attempts to destroy the tissue shortly after transplantation.

In all cases of graft rejection, the cause is incompatibility of cell surface antigens. The rejection of foreign or transplanted tissue occurs because the recipient's immune system recognizes that the surface HLA proteins of the donor's tissue are different from the recipient's.

For this reason, HLA matching of donor and recipient greatly enhances the probability of graft acceptance. Certain antigens are more important than others for a successful transplant, including ABO and Rh antigens present on red blood cells and histocompatibility antigens, and most importantly, the HLA. As expected, a better chance of graft acceptance is evident with syngeneic or autologous transplants because the cell surface antigens are identical.

### REFERENCES

To enhance this text and add value for the reader, all references are included in the enhanced ebook on Student Consult that accompanies this textbook. The reader can view the reference source and access it online whenever possible.

CHAPTER 8

# Infectious Disease

KIMBERLY LEVENHAGEN • CELESTE KNIGHT PETERSON

Although human beings are continually exposed to a vast array of microorganisms in the environment, only a small proportion of those microbes are capable of interacting with the human host in such a way that infection and disease result. With the steady advances being made in medicine, people are living longer, but infection is still a frequent cause of hospital admission and remains an important cause of death, especially in the aging and immunocompromised population.

Organized efforts to immunize all children lowered the incidence of vaccine-preventable diseases such as measles, mumps, rubella, diphtheria, tetanus, poliomyelitis, chickenpox (varicella), human papillomavirus (HPV), influenza, and hepatitis A and B. Additionally, the widespread availability and use of antibiotics has successfully treated tuberculosis, syphilis, gonorrhea, bacterial meningitis, scarlet fever, and rheumatic fever. However, there is growing concern over the resistance of parents to vaccinating their children, creating an environment that allows for the return of diseases thought to be in the past.[51,246] New infectious agents are also appearing. For example, *Legionella*, human immunodeficiency virus (HIV), norovirus, Ebola, antibiotic-resistant organisms, avian flu, and a resurgence of tuberculosis have returned focus to the prevention and treatment of infectious diseases. Although a number of new infectious diseases have appeared in recent years, a worldwide resurgence of long-standing diseases once thought to be well controlled has occurred. Among infectious diseases globally, *Mycobacterium tuberculosis* is one of the world's leading causes of death in adults, killing approximately 1.3 million people in 2017.[141] Organisms travel on the shoes of tourists, in the ballast of cargo ships, within the confines of jetliners, and in the blood of human beings.

When natural systems are weakened or altered by ecologic stresses (e.g., pollution, habitat destruction, weather disasters, climate change, famine), they become more vulnerable to damage or destruction by invading organisms, which can result in the spread of infection. Opportunistic organisms take advantage of the weakened defenses. Infectious diseases have the ability to spread more rapidly throughout the world than in the past, facilitated by a combination of environmental disruption and increasing human mobility.

At the same time, infectious agents are suspected in disorders such as cancer (liver and cervical), gastric and duodenal ulcers, heart disease, neurologic diseases, and autoimmune diseases.[173,181] In addition, an area of major public health concern is the continued emergence of antibiotic-resistant microorganisms that appear in health care facilities and communities.

Infectious pathogens (a pathogen is any microorganism that has the capacity to cause disease) almost invariably mutate, leading to eventual resistance to antibiotics/antivirals and other treatments. This is compounded by the misuse and overuse of antibiotics in treatment of infections or potential infections. Other variables include large numbers of children in daycare facilities; a sicker population base when hospitalized (therefore more susceptible to infection); crowding of prisons, military facilities, or multifamily dwellings; and the reliance of modern agriculture on antibiotics to boost growth and limit disease among animals. Poor immunologic resistance (e.g., in premature infants; aging adults; and individuals with debilitating disease, burns, or wounds) is a contributing factor in the rapid and progressive spread of human bacterial infections.

The resistant organisms spread quickly and easily when inadequate precautions are taken to prevent transmission (e.g., poor use of hand hygiene and transmission-based precautions). (The U.S. Centers for Disease Control and Prevention [CDC] uses the term *hand hygiene* to include gloves, rubbing alcohol, and non–alcohol-based cleansers). The presence of these multidrug-resistant organisms in health care facilities limits the number of effective antimicrobials available for treatment. In 2013 the CDC reported *Clostridioides difficile* (formerly *Clostridium difficile*) as the most common heath care–associated infection (HAI) in the United States.[78] The CDC identified *C. difficile* as an urgent threat requiring increased education and prevention strategies. In 2011 more than 29,000 people died within 30 days of the initial diagnosis with 80% of people who died older than age 65.[217] Additionally, the CDC identified carbapenem-resistant *Klebsiella* strains as an urgent threat owing to increasing incidence and associated mortality secondary to bloodstream infections.[78]

As a result of surveillance and education, more common resistant bacteria such as methicillin-resistant *Staphylococcus aureus* (MRSA), vancomycin-resistant enterococci (VRE), *Pseudomonas aeruginosa,* and multidrug-resistant *M. tuberculosis* are declining in incidence, but a resurgence in incidence is possible if prevention strategies do not continue.[78,231]

All health care professionals must maintain a vigilant attitude toward preventing infectious disease. This requires an understanding of the infectious process, the chain of transmission, and selected aspects of control. In this chapter, a basic understanding of these concepts is provided along with a discussion of a few infectious diseases. Other pertinent infectious diseases are presented in appropriate chapters according to the primary clinical pathology (such as pneumonia in Chapter 15 and bacterial meningitis in Chapter 29).

## SIGNS AND SYMPTOMS OF INFECTIOUS DISEASES

Clinical manifestations of infectious disease are many and varied depending on the etiologic agent (e.g., viruses, bacteria) (see Types of Organisms later) and the system affected (e.g., respiratory, central nervous system [CNS], gastrointestinal [GI], genitourinary).

Systemic symptoms of infectious disease include fever and chills, sweating, malaise, nausea, and vomiting. Changes in blood composition may occur, such as an increased number of leukocytes or a change in the types of leukocytes. Older adults may experience a change in mentation (e.g., confusion, memory loss, difficulty concentrating). When observing any person for early signs of infection, the therapist will most likely see one or only a few symptoms (Box 8.1).

A change in body temperature is a characteristic systemic symptom of infectious disease, but fever may accompany noninfectious causes such as inflammatory, neoplastic, and immunologically mediated diseases (Box 8.2). *Fever,* a sustained temperature above normal, can be caused by abnormalities of the hypothalamus, brain tumors, dehydration, or toxic substances affecting the temperature-regulating center of the hypothalamus. Certain protein substances and toxins can cause the set-point of the hypothalamic thermostat to rise. This results in activation of the hypothalamus to conserve heat and increase heat production. Substances that cause these effects are called *pyrogens.*

In infectious disease, the endotoxins of some bacteria and the extracts of normal leukocytes (cytokines) are pyrogenic. They act to raise the thermostat in the hypothalamus, thus raising the body temperature. Fever patterns may differ depending on the specific infectious disease present and occur clinically on a continuum, from fever associated with an acute illness lasting 7 to 10 days, to sepsis and ongoing infection lasting longer than 10 days, to fever of unknown origin associated with a possible infectious origin lasting at least 3 weeks.

Fever patterns can include *intermittent fever* (temperature returns to normal at least once every 24 hours), which is usually associated with sepsis, abscesses, and infective endocarditis; *remittent fever* (temperature fluctuates but does not return to normal), associated with viral upper respiratory infection, *Legionella,* and *Mycoplasma* infections; *sustained* or *continuous fever* (temperature remains above normal with minimal variations); and *recurrent* or *relapsing*

**Box 8.1**

**SIGNS AND SYMPTOMS OF INFECTIOUS DISEASE**

- Fever, chills, malaise (most common early symptoms)
- Enlarged lymph nodes

***Integument***

- Purulent drainage from abscess, open wound, or skin lesion
- Skin rash, red streaks
- Bleeding from gums or into joints; joint effusion or erythema

***Cardiovascular***

- Petechial lesions
- Tachycardia (see Aneurysm and Thrombophlebitis in Chapter 12)
- Hypotension
- Change in pulse rate (may increase or decrease depending on type of infection)

***Central Nervous System***

- Altered level of consciousness, confusion, seizures
- Headache
- Photophobia
- Memory loss
- Stiff neck, myalgia

***Gastrointestinal***

- Nausea
- Vomiting
- Diarrhea

***Genitourinary***

- Dysuria or flank pain
- Hematuria
- Oliguria
- Urgency, frequency

***Upper Respiratory***

- Tachypnea
- Cough
- Dyspnea
- Hoarseness
- Sore throat
- Nasal drainage
- Sputum production
- Oxygen desaturation
- Decreased exercise tolerance
- Prolonged ventilatory support

***In the Older Adult***

Signs and symptoms may be subtle and atypical:

- Change in mental status
- Subnormal body temperature
- Bradycardia or tachycardia
- Fatigue (or increased fatigue)
- Lethargy
- Decreased appetite

*fever* (episodic fevers lasting 1 to 3 days with 1 or more days of normal temperatures between episodes).

Other causes of fever include neoplasms (lymphoma and leukemia are the most common); autoimmune disorders (systemic lupus erythematosus and polyarteritis nodosa); and miscellaneous diseases including temporal arteritis, thromboembolic disease, alcoholic hepatitis, and drug-induced fever, among others.

A general guideline, the 39°C (102°F) rule, divides conditions into two groups: conditions that do not cause temperature elevations exceeding 39°C (102°F) and those that regularly exceed 39°C (102°F). Table 8.1 reflects hospital data; the outpatient population is more likely to experience fever accompanied by generalized arthralgias and myalgias associated with a self-limiting illness or fever with localized symptoms such as a sore throat, cough, or right lower quadrant pain, as occurs with bacterial infection. Temperature elevation to 40°C (104°F) may cause delirium and seizures, particularly in children. An extremely high fever may damage cells irreversibly.

It is important to note that some people with serious infection do not initially develop fever but instead become *tachypneic* (rapid breathing), become *confused*, or develop *hypotension*. Most often this situation occurs in older adults, individuals with an HAI, or immunocompromised persons.

Inflammation and its exudates may remain localized, permeate the tissue, or spread throughout the body via the blood or lymph. For example, an *abscess* begins as a localized infection with inflammation and purulent exudate. Leukocytes form a wall around the organisms. The abscess deepens as more leukocytes are drawn into the area, more organisms are killed, and more necrotic tissue is dissolved. The exudate may eventually be autolyzed and resorbed by the body, in which case the inflammation and infection are resolved. Rupture of the abscess and drainage into other tissues can spread the infection to other areas of the body.

For example, infectious abdominal disorders (e.g., diverticulitis, appendicitis), tuberculosis of the spine, pelvic inflammatory disease, vertebral osteomyelitis, septic arthritis of the sacroiliac joint, and tumor of the thigh can result in abscess formation in the space between the posterior peritoneum and the psoas and iliac fascia. A psoas abscess is usually confined within the psoas fascia, but occasionally, because of anatomic relationships, infection extends to the buttock, hip, or upper thigh.

**Box 8.2**

**COMMON INFECTIOUS AND NONINFECTIOUS CAUSES OF FEVER IN THE HOSPITALIZED PERSON**

***Infectious*[a]**

- Urinary tract infection
- Respiratory tract infection
- Catheter-related infection
- Surgical wound infection
- Infected pressure injuries
- Other (less common): colitis, peritonitis, meningitis

***Noninfectious (Injured or Abnormal Cells Incite Production of Pyrogens)***

- Drug reaction
- Pulmonary emboli
- Neoplasm
- Tissue necrosis (e.g., stroke, myocardial infarction)
- Autoimmune diseases

[a]The most common infectious causes are urinary tract infections, bacteremia, and pneumonia. Medical charting often lists "primary bloodstream infection," which includes catheter line–associated bloodstream infections (instead of recording the condition as bacteremia, septicemia, or catheter line–associated infection).

Data from Bor DH: Fever in hospitalized medical patients: characteristics and significance. *J Gen Intern Med* 3:119–125, 1988.

**Table 8.1** Most Common Causes of Prolonged Fever[a]

| Conditions in Which Fever Generally Does Not Exceed 39°C (102°F) | Conditions in Which Fever Regularly Exceeds 39°C (102°F) |
|---|---|
| Catheter-associated bacteriuria | Malignant hyperthermia (secondary to anesthesia) |
| Atelectasis | Transfusion reactions |
| Phlebitis | Urosepsis |
| Pulmonary emboli | IV line sepsis |
| Dehydration | Prosthetic valve endocarditis |
| Pancreatitis | Intraabdominal or pelvic peritonitis or abscess |
| Myocardial infarction | *Clostridioides difficile* colitis |
| Uncomplicated wound infections | Procedure-related bacteremia |
| Any malignancy | Health care–associated pneumonia |
| Cytomegalovirus | Drug fever |
| Hepatitis | HIV infection |
| Infectious mononucleosis (Epstein-Barr virus) | Heat stroke |
| Subacute bacterial endocarditis | Acute bacterial endocarditis |
| Tuberculosis | Tuberculosis (usually disseminated or extrapulmonary) |
| | Lymphoma |
| | Metastasizing carcinoma to liver or central nervous system |

[a]The evaluation of fever magnitude with the 39°C (102°F) rule is most often done in the acute care setting. This is a general guideline that must be taken into consideration with other presenting factors.

*IV*, Intravenous.

Such an abscess causes true musculoskeletal symptoms of back pain, pain referred to the hip or knee, and limited range of hip motion from an underlying systemic cause. Flexion contracture of the hip (positive Thomas test) may develop from reflex spasm, and extension of the thigh is very painful; hip abduction and adduction evoke minimal discomfort. An unexplained limp may be the initial symptom, an important clinical clue when taking a history. Lower abdominal pain develops days to weeks later, and the person becomes acutely ill with a high fever.

*Rash* with fever can result from an infectious process caused by any microbe that has successfully penetrated the stratum corneum and multiplied locally. Skin rashes may also occur with infection elsewhere in the body unrelated to local skin disease (e.g., scarlet fever caused by streptococci, also called *scarlatina*).

The most common types of skin lesions associated with infectious disease are maculopapular eruptions (e.g., classic childhood viral illnesses such as measles, rubella, roseola, fifth disease), nodular lesions (e.g., *Streptococcus, Pseudomonas*), diffuse erythema (e.g., scarlet fever, toxic shock syndrome), vesiculobullous eruptions (e.g., varicella, herpes zoster), and petechial purpuric eruptions (e.g., Epstein-Barr virus [EBV] and cytomegalovirus [CMV]). Specific types of skin lesions are discussed in Chapter 10.

*Red streaks* may develop from an infection site in the direction of regional lymph nodes, known as acute lymphangitis. Lymphangitis usually occurs as a result of group A streptococci (GAS) entering the lymphatic channels from an abrasion or local trauma, wound, or infection. The red streak may be obvious, or it may be faint and easily overlooked, especially in dark-skinned people. As bacteria travel to the lymph nodes, septicemia, or bacteria in the bloodstream, may result, leading to rapid systemic deterioration. Involved nodes are usually tender and enlarged (greater than 3 cm).

*Inflamed lymph nodes* can be associated with other infectious diseases and may be palpated by the therapist, especially in cervical, axillary, or inguinal areas when presenting musculoskeletal symptoms are evident in those areas. For example, intraoral infection may cause an inflamed cervical node, leading to spasm of the sternocleidomastoid muscle, causing neck pain. Palpation may appear to aggravate a primary spasm as if originating in the muscle, when in fact a lymph node under the muscle is the source of the symptom.

In acute infections, nodes are tender, asymmetric, and enlarged. The overlying skin may be erythematous (red) and warm. Unilaterally warm, tender, enlarged, and fluctuant lymph nodes sometimes associated with elevated body temperature may be caused by pyogenic infections and require medical referral.

Supraclavicular and inguinal nodes are also common metastatic sites for cancer. Nodes involved with metastatic cancer are usually hard and fixed to the underlying tissue. Any suspicious lymph node (e.g., changes in size greater than 1 cm, changes in shape such as matted together, or changes in consistency such as rubbery) or the presence of painless, enlarged lymph nodes must be evaluated by a physician.

*Joint effusion*, usually of one joint (monarticular), associated with infectious arthritis can occur as a result of bacterial, mycobacterial, fungal, or viral etiologic agents. Streptococcal bacteremia from any cause can result in suppurative arthritis (inflammation with pus formation).

## AGING AND INFECTIOUS DISEASES

As a group, older adults (those older than 65 years of age) are more susceptible to infectious diseases and experience increased morbidity and mortality compared with younger people; this is especially noted in frail and debilitated older adults. This increased susceptibility is most likely multifactorial, encompassing changes in immune function,[92,257] called immunosenescence, as well as comorbidities such as diabetes, chronic obstructive pulmonary disease, vascular disease, malnutrition, and renal failure.[137]

The immune system is complex and requires well-orchestrated adaptability and responsiveness.[152] To aid in this interplay, each person exhibits both innate and adaptable immunity. Innate immunity refers to responses a person is born with such as skin barriers, mucous membranes, macrophages, neutrophils, natural killer cells, and complement proteins. With aging, there are modest changes in innate responses. Some innate responses decrease, while others are heightened, leading to a low-grade, chronic inflammatory state.[344] For instance, the function and number of macrophages decrease with age, while neutrophil number remains stable and natural killer cells increase with aging.

While changes in innate immunity are modest, adaptive immunity, relating to T and B cells, undergoes a more significant change with aging. As the thymus ages and involutes, there is a decrease in the number of naïve T cells released. The diversity of T-cell subsets is then reduced as well as the capacity to proliferate and signal other cells. This leads to difficulty in responding to new antigens, especially viruses, and to stimulating B cells to proliferate and produce antibodies. T regulatory cells normally regulate the immune system, keeping it in check. After the age of 50, there is a reduction in the function of these cells, leading to the inability to regulate inflammatory, tumor, and autoimmune responses. There is also a reduction in hematopoietic tissue with aging, reducing the number of B cells that leave the bone marrow,[131] although no decrease in the total level of immunoglobulins produced by B cells is noted. Naïve B cells produce immunoglobulin M (IgM). After exposure to an antigen (infectious organism or vaccine), naïve B cells convert to specific, antigen-related B cells, producing IgA, IgG, or IgE. With age, the amount of specific immunoglobulins decreases,[215] and there is a reduction in the diversity of B cells (not as many B cells that are specific for certain antigens). Memory B and T cells are another layer of protection offered by the adaptive immune system. These cells are retained to react more quickly to antigens they have already seen and to which they have previously responded. With fewer cells being released (both T and B cells), the body depends on older memory cells to reexpand and proliferate to respond to a previously known antigen. Older memory cells function well with aging,[161] whereas newer cells respond less vigorously to an antigen.[407] However, each time a T cell divides, there is a shortening of the telomeres on the DNA, until there is a critical reduction in length of the telomeres that causes an arrest in proliferation.[228] This contributes to the inability of memory T cells to continue to respond. Viral infections such as CMV and EBV can chronically stimulate T cells and lead to premature cessation of proliferation and responsiveness.[100]

Diminished cell-mediated immunity results in the reactivation of dormant infections such as herpes zoster and tuberculosis as well as a decreased response to vaccines.[152] Although elderly people may have a decreased response to new vaccines, techniques are being evaluated to improve this response, such as increasing the vaccine dose, providing routine boosters (second responses are more robust than primary responses), using specific adjuvants (molecules or proteins that can accelerate or enhance response to the antigen),[367] timing of vaccination,[224] and determining which vaccine and mode of administration elderly individuals respond to best.[408]

Extrinsic factors apart from the immune system can lead to increased susceptibility to infection in an older adult. Atrophic skin is more easily damaged, decreased cough and gag reflexes make it more difficult to control secretions, and decreased bronchiolar elasticity and mucociliary activity contribute to the development of pneumonia.

Denture-associated infections may occur in up to 60% of older adults who wear dentures. Predisposing factors include flaccid, sagging cheeks; deepened labial angles constantly moistened by saliva; and ill-fitting dentures, often worn for a considerable time without replacement or repair. These age-related changes compromise individuals' first line of defenses, leaving them at increased risk for infection.

Many types of infections are seen in aging adults, but early recognition of infection in an older adult is difficult because people underreport symptoms; the presentation is often vague, blunted, or atypical; and symptoms are difficult to assess. An older adult may be unable to describe the present illness or past history or list the medications being taken. A complete physical examination may be difficult because of the person's uncooperativeness, cognitive impairment, neurologic deficits, or physical impairments. Pain may be poorly localized or absent, or it may be confused with preexisting conditions, such as in septic arthritis in a client with degenerative joint disease.

Another important reason infection may be difficult to recognize in older adults is the presence of implanted devices. Elderly adults are more likely to have an implanted device such as joint prostheses, pacemakers, defibrillators, peripherally inserted central catheter lines, stents, and grafts. Implanted devices can develop a biofilm, which consists of organisms surrounded by a self-produced protective layer of polysaccharides, proteins, nucleic acids, and lipids that adhere to the synthetic device.[129] Frequently there is no overt initial response, and the infection subtly grows.

The aging person can have more serious infections with little or no fever because of an impaired thermoregulatory system or the masking effects of drugs such as aspirin, other antiinflammatory drugs, and corticosteroids. Fever in older people may not be high enough to cause concern because the basal body temperature is low. A lower threshold for infection should be used (e.g., oral temperature of 37.2°C [99°F] or 37.8°C [100°F]), especially if the person is taking a medication that masks fever. Watch for (or ask family about) any recent episodes of confusion, memory loss, or other change in mental status; these may be the first symptoms of infection.[122]

The absence of the febrile response in an older adult with a serious infection is a grave sign. Acute infections in the older adult may cause delirium or a sudden change in mental status. Chronic infections of the lungs, bone, skin, kidneys, and CNS may cause mental status changes perceived as dementia.

Many frail elderly adults are in acute- or extended-care settings and are therefore more likely to be exposed to health care–associated pathogens such as *C. difficile*, gram-negative bacilli, *S. aureus*, and VRE.

## INFECTIOUS DISEASES

### Definition and Overview

Infection is a process in which an organism establishes a parasitic relationship with its host. This invasion and multiplication of microorganisms produces an immune response and subsequent signs and symptoms. Such reproduction injures the host by causing cellular damage from microorganism-producing toxins or intracellular multiplication or by competing with the host's metabolism.

The host's immune response may compound the tissue damage; such damage may be localized (e.g., as in infected pressure injuries) or systemic. However, in some instances, microorganisms may be present in the tissues of the host and yet not cause symptomatic disease. This process is called *colonization of organisms*. A person with colonization may be a carrier and transmit the organisms to others but does not have detectable symptoms of infection unless or until the immune system is weakened or compromised.

The development of an infection begins with transmission of an infectious organism (agent, pathogen) and depends on a complex interaction of the pathogen, an environment conducive to transmission of the organism, and the susceptibility of the human host. Even after successful transmission of a pathogen, the host may experience more than one possible outcome.

The pathogen may merely contaminate the body surface and be destroyed by first-line defenses such as intact skin or mucous membranes that prevent further invasion, or a subclinical infection may occur in which no apparent symptoms are evident other than an identifiable immune response of the host. A rise in the titer of antibody directed against the infecting agent is often the only detectable response. Antibiotic treatment is not necessary, although infection control procedures remain in force to prevent spreading the bacteria to others.

A third possible outcome is the development of a clinically apparent infection in which the host–parasite interaction causes obvious injury and is accompanied by one or more clinical symptoms. This outcome is called *infectious disease* and ranges in severity from mild to fatal depending on the organism and the response and underlying health of the host.

The period between the pathogen entering the host and the appearance of clinical symptoms is called the *incubation period*. This period may last a few days to several months, depending on the causative organism and type of disease. Disease symptoms herald the end of the incubation period. A *latent* infection occurs after a microorganism has replicated but remains dormant or inactive in the host, sometimes for years (e.g., tuberculosis, herpes zoster). The host may harbor a pathogen in sufficient quantities to be shed at any time after latency and toward the end of the incubation period. This time period when an organism can be shed is called the *period of communicability*.

From this concept of communicability, communicable diseases can be defined as any disease whereby the causative agent may pass or be carried from one person to another directly or indirectly. It usually precedes symptoms and continues through part or all of clinical disease, sometimes extending to convalescence; however, it is important to note that an asymptomatic host can still transmit a pathogen. The communicable period, similar to the incubation period and mode of transmission, varies with different pathogens and different diseases.

## Types of Organisms

A great variety of microorganisms are responsible for infectious diseases, including viruses, mycoplasmas, bacteria, rickettsiae, chlamydiae, protozoa, fungi (yeasts and molds), helminths (e.g., tapeworms), mycobacteria, and prions. All microorganisms can be distinguished by certain intrinsic properties such as shape, size, structure, chemical composition, antigenic makeup, growth requirements, ability to produce toxins, and ability to remain alive (viability) under adverse conditions (e.g., drying, sunlight, or heat).

These properties provide the basis for identification and classification of the organisms. Knowledge of the properties permits diagnosis of a specific pathogen in specimens of body fluids, secretions, or exudates. All these properties are important to consider when looking for ways to interfere with the mechanisms of transmission.

*Viruses* are subcellular organisms made up of only an RNA or a DNA nucleus covered with proteins. They are the smallest known organisms, visible only through an electron microscope. Viruses are completely dependent on host cells and cannot replicate unless they invade a host cell and stimulate it to participate in the formation of additional virus particles.

The hundreds of viruses that infect human beings are classified according to their size, shape (spherical, rod shaped, or cubic), host, genome, or means of transmission (respiratory, fecal-oral, or sexual). Viruses are not susceptible to antibiotics. However, antiviral medications can mitigate (moderate) the course of the viral illness. For example, acyclovir, an antiviral medication used for herpesvirus, interferes with DNA synthesis, causing decreased viral replication and decreasing the time of lesional healing.

*Mycoplasmas* are unusual, self-replicating bacteria that have no cell wall components and very small genomes. For this reason, antibiotics that are active against bacterial cell walls have no effect on mycoplasmas. At the present time, mycoplasmas remain sensitive to some antibiotics. They require a strict dependence on the host for nutrition and sustenance and are able to pass through many bacteria-retaining filters or barriers because they are very small.

*Bacteria* are single-celled microorganisms with well-defined cell walls that can grow independently on artificial media without the need for other cells. Bacteria can be classified according to shape. Spherical bacterial cells are called *cocci,* rod-shaped bacteria are called *bacilli,* and spiral-shaped bacteria are called *spirilla* or *spirochetes.*

Bacteria can also be classified according to their response to staining (gram-positive, gram-negative, or acid-fast), motility (motile or nonmotile), tendency toward capsulation (encapsulated or nonencapsulated), and capacity to form spores (sporulating or nonsporulating) (Fig. 8.1).

Bacteria can also be classified according to whether oxygen is needed to replicate and develop (aerobic) or whether they can sustain life in an oxygen-poor (anaerobic) environment. Normal human flora is primarily anaerobic, and disease can be produced when these normal organisms are displaced from their usual tissue sites (e.g., mouth, skin, large bowel, female genital tract) into other tissues or closed body spaces. Other common anaerobic organisms include spore-forming bacilli such as *Clostridium botulinum, Clostridium tetani,* or *C. difficile* that thrive in a strictly anaerobic environment.

*Rickettsiae* are primarily animal pathogens that typically produce disease in human beings through the bite of an insect vector such as a tick, flea, louse, or mite. They are small, gram-negative obligate intracellular organisms that often cause life-threatening infections. Similar to viruses, these microorganisms require a host for replication. Three categories of the family Rickettsiaceae are *Rickettsia, Coxiella,* and *Bartonella.*

*Chlamydiae* are smaller than rickettsiae and bacteria but larger than viruses. They too depend on host cells for replication, but unlike viruses, they always contain both DNA and RNA and are susceptible to antibiotics.

*Protozoa* have a single-cell unit or a group of nondifferentiated cells loosely held together and not forming tissues. They have cell membranes rather than cell walls, and their nuclei are surrounded by nuclear membranes. Larger parasites include roundworms and flatworms.

*Fungi* are unicellular to filamentous organisms possessing hyphae (filamentous outgrowths) surrounded by cell walls and containing nuclei (eukaryocyte). Fungi show relatively little cellular specialization and occur as yeasts (single-cell, oval-shaped organisms) or molds (organisms with branching filaments). Depending on the environment, some fungi may occur in both forms. Fungal diseases in human beings are called *mycoses.*

*Prions* are proteinaceous, infectious particles consisting of proteins but without nucleic acids. These particles are transmitted from animals to human beings and are

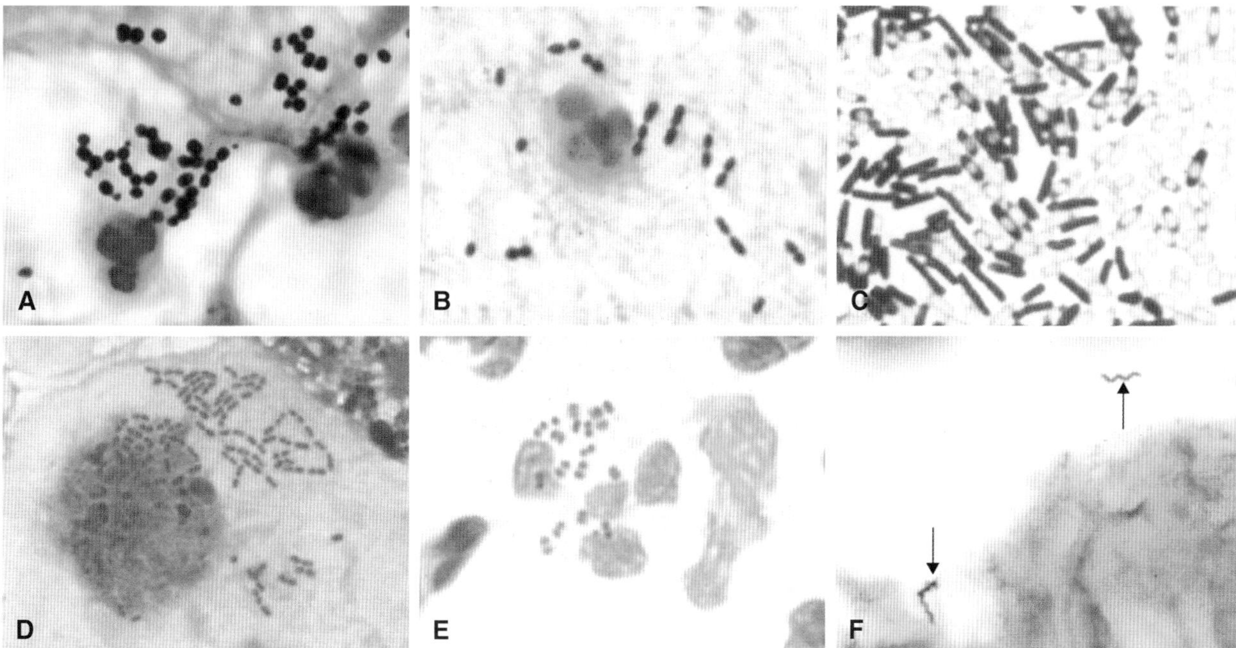


**Figure 8.1**

**A variety of bacterial morphology.** (A) Gram stain of sputum from a person with pneumonia. There are gram-positive cocci in clusters *(Staphylococcus aureus)* with degenerating neutrophils. (B) Gram stain of sputum from an individual with pneumonia. Gram-positive elongated cocci in pairs and short chains *(Streptococcus pneumoniae)* and a neutrophil are seen. (C) Gram stain of *Clostridium sordellii* grown in culture. A mixture of gram-positive and gram-negative rods, many of which have subterminal spores (clear areas), are present. *Clostridium* species often stain as both positive and negative on Gram stain, although they are true gram-positive bacteria. (D) Gram stain of a bronchoalveolar lavage specimen showing gram-negative intracellular rods typical of Enterobacteriaceae such as *Klebsiella pneumoniae* and *Escherichia coli.* (E) Gram stain of urethral discharge from a person with gonorrhea. Many gram-negative diplococci *(Neisseria gonorrhoeae)* are present within a neutrophil. (F) Silver stain of brain tissue from a person with Lyme disease meningoencephalitis. Two helical spirochetes *(Borrelia burgdorferi)* are indicated by *arrows.* The panels are at different magnifications. (A–C, From Kumar V, Abbas AK, Fausto N: *Robbins and Cotran pathologic basis of disease*, ed 7, Philadelphia, 2005, Saunders, courtesy Dr. Kenneth Van Horn. D, Courtesy Karen Krisher, Wayne State University, Detroit MI.)

characterized by a long latent interval in the host. When reactivated, they cause rapidly progressive, deteriorating disease in the host known as prion disease or transmissible spongiform encephalopathy such as Creutzfeldt-Jakob disease, kuru, and variant Creutzfeldt-Jakob disease (linked to bovine spongiform encephalopathy, or mad cow disease).[175]

## Chain of Transmission

Infection begins with transmission of a pathogen to the host. Successful transmission depends on a pathogenic agent, a reservoir, a portal of exit from the reservoir, a mode (mechanism) of transmission, a portal of entry into the host, and a susceptible host. This sequence of events is called the *chain of transmission* (Table 8.2).

*HAIs* (formerly known as nosocomial infections) are infections that develop in hospitalized persons or persons admitted to a health care facility that were not present before admission. In the United States, about 1 in every 31 people who are hospitalized will contract an HAI. Much has been done to reduce this number, and in 2015 a hospitalized person was 16% less likely to develop an HAI than in 2011.[233] Between 2015 and 2016 there was a 2% to 11% decrease in specific HAIs nationally.[45,61] Transmission can be through any of the possible routes discussed in this section. HAIs result in prolongation of hospital stays, increase in cost of care, and significant morbidity and mortality. In 2015 the CDC reported 687,000 HAIs occurred in U.S. hospitals and more than 72,000 deaths associated with an HAI.[45] Most were caused by pneumonia, GI tract infection (with *C. difficile* accounting for the majority of cases), and surgical site infections (SSIs).[232]

In general, HAIs continue to be related to frequent use of invasive devices for monitoring or therapy, more colonization and infection by multidrug-resistant organisms, and greater debilitation and severity of illness of hospitalized clients who acquire these infections. The increased use of invasive and surgical procedures, immunosuppressants, and antibiotics and the lack of hand hygiene predispose people to such infections and superinfections. At the same time, the growing number of personnel who come into contact with the client makes the risk of exposure greater.

Prevention is of critical importance in controlling HAIs. The concept of Standard Precautions emphasizes that all clients must be treated as though each one has a potential bloodborne, transmissible disease; thus all body secretions are handled with care to prevent disease. Hand hygiene has been cited as the easiest and most effective means of preventing HAIs and must be done routinely, even when gloves are used.[348] See further discussion under Control of Transmission later.

**Table 8.2** Chain of Transmission of Infectious Disease

| Transmission | Chain Factors |
|---|---|
| Pathogen or agent | Viruses, mycoplasmas, bacteria, rickettsiae, chlamydiae, protozoa, fungi, prions, helminths |
| Reservoir | Humans (clinical cases, subclinical cases, and carriers)<br>Animal, arthropod, plant, soil, food, organic substance |
| Portal of exit | Genitourinary tract, gastrointestinal tract, respiratory tract, oral cavity, open lesion, blood, vaginal secretions, semen, tears, excretions (urine, feces) |
| Transmission | Contact (direct or indirect)<br>Airborne (float on air currents and remain suspended for hours; small particles)<br>Droplet (fall out within 3 feet of source; large particles)<br>Vehicle (through a common source such as water or food)<br>Vector-borne (carried by insects or animals) |
| Modes of entry | Ingestion, inhalation, percutaneous injection, transplacental entry, mucous membranes |
| Susceptible host | Specific immune reactions<br>Nonspecific body defenses<br>Host characteristics: age, sex, ethnic group, heredity, behaviors<br>Environmental and general health status |

## Pathogens

Humans coexist with many microorganisms in complex, mutually beneficial relationships. Even so, many organisms are parasitic, maintaining themselves at the expense of their host. Some parasites arouse a pathologic response in the host and are called *pathogens* or *pathogenic agents*. A *pathogen* was defined at the beginning of this chapter as any microorganism that has the capacity to cause disease. As such, pathogens are ineffective parasites because they stimulate a disease response, which may harm the host and eventually kill the pathogen.

The ability of a pathogen to stimulate an immune response in the host (antigenicity) varies greatly among organisms, depending on the site of invasion, the number of pathogenic organisms, and the dissemination of organisms in the body. The immune status of a person plays the largest role in determining the risk for infection and the ability of the host to combat organisms that have gained entry.

The mode of action of a pathogen refers to how the organism produces a pathologic process. Great variation exists among the various pathogens. Some intracellular pathogens such as viruses invade cells and interfere with cellular metabolism, growth, and replication, whereas others invade and cause hyperplasia and cell death. Yet other organisms, such as the influenza virus, have the potential to alter their antigenic characteristics. This virus is capable of extensive gene rearrangements, resulting in significant changes in surface antigen structure. This ability allows new strains to evade host antibody responses directed at earlier strains.

Some viruses (e.g., all members of the herpesvirus group) cause a persistent latent infection that can be reactivated in certain circumstances. HIV causes immunosuppression by destroying helper T lymphocytes. Some pathogens such as the tetanus bacillus produce a toxin that interferes with intercellular responses. Some bacteria such as diphtheria and tetanus secrete water-soluble antigenic exotoxins that are quickly disseminated in the blood, causing potentially severe systemic and neurologic manifestations. Larger parasites such as roundworms cause anemia and interfere with the function of the GI system.

The characteristics of the organism and the susceptibility of the host influence the likelihood of a pathogen producing infectious disease and the type of disease produced. Not all pathogens have an equal probability of inducing disease in the same host population. *Principal* pathogens regularly cause disease in people with apparently intact defense systems.

*Opportunistic* pathogens do not cause disease in people with intact host defense systems but can clearly cause devastating disease in many hospitalized and immunocompromised clients. Organisms that may be harmless members of normal flora in healthy people may act as virulent invaders in people with severe defects in host defense mechanisms.

*Pathogenicity*, the ability of the organism to induce disease, depends on the organism's speed of reproduction in the host, the extent of damage it causes to tissues, and the strength of any toxin released by the pathogen. *Virulence* refers to the potency of the pathogen in producing severe disease and is measured by the case fatality rate (i.e., the number of people who die of the disease divided by the number of people who have the disease). Virulence provides a quantitative measure of pathogenicity. The amount and destructive potential of released toxin are closely related to virulence.

## Reservoir

A reservoir is an environment in which an organism can live and multiply, such as an animal, plant, soil, food, or other organic substance or combination of substances. The reservoir provides the essentials for survival of the organism at specific stages in its life cycle. Some parasites have more than one reservoir, such as the yellow fever virus, which can maintain life in human beings and other animals. Some parasites require more than one reservoir at different growth stages, and still others, such as most sexually transmitted organisms, require only a human reservoir.

Human and animal reservoirs can be symptomatic or asymptomatic carriers of the pathogen. A carrier maintains an environment that promotes growth, multiplication, and shedding of the parasite without exhibiting signs of disease. Hepatitis is a common example of this carrier state in human beings.

## Portal of Exit

The portal of exit is the place from which the parasite leaves the reservoir. In general, this is the site of growth of the organism and corresponds to the system of entry into the next host. For example, the portal of exit for GI parasites is usually the feces, and the portal of entry into a new host is the mouth. Exceptions to the case include hookworm eggs, which are shed in the feces but enter through the skin of a person walking barefoot in soil containing hatched eggs.

Common portals of exit include secretions and fluids (e.g., respiratory secretions, blood, vaginal secretions, semen, tears), excretions such as urine and feces, open lesions, and exudates such as pus from an open wound or ulcer. Some organisms, such as HIV, have more than one portal of exit. Knowledge of the portal of exit is essential for preventing transmission of a pathogen.

## Mode of Transmission

For infection to be transmitted, the invading organism must be transported from the infected source to a susceptible host. Microorganisms are transmitted by several possible routes, and the same microorganism can travel by more than one route. The five main routes of transmission are contact, airborne, droplet, vehicle, and vector-borne.

*Contact transmission* occurs directly or indirectly. Direct contact is the direct transfer of microorganisms that come into physical contact by either skin-to-skin contact or mucous membrane–to–mucous membrane contact (e.g., sexual contact, biting, touching, kissing).

Indirect contact involves transfer of microorganisms from a source to a host by passive transfer from an inanimate, intermediate object, called a *fomite*. Inanimate objects can include items such as the telephone, sphygmomanometer, bedside rails, tray tables, countertops, and other items that come into direct contact with the infected person. To highlight the importance of consistent hand hygiene and environmental cleaning across all facilities, the CDC has provided guidelines for inpatient, outpatient, and long-term care facilities.[348] In addition, The Joint Commission, which publishes its specific national initiatives to improve patient safety, has extended patient safety goal 7 to include long-term care facilities.[186]

An example of indirect transmission is transfer of HIV from a contaminated source to a host through a needlestick. Another example of indirect contact includes fecal-oral transmission by the ingestion of enteric pathogens from food prepared by a person who does not wash his or her hands.[348]

*Airborne transmission* occurs when disease-causing organisms are so small (less than 5 μm) that they are capable of floating on air currents within a room and remain suspended in the air for several hours. They are often propelled from the respiratory tract through coughing or sneezing. A host then inhales the particles directly into the respiratory tract (e.g., tuberculosis, chickenpox, rubeola measles).

*Droplet transmission* is different from airborne transmission because droplets are larger particles (greater than 5 μm) than airborne particles, and they do not remain suspended in air but fall out within 3 feet of the source. They are produced when a person coughs or sneezes and then travel only a short distance. A common example of droplet-spread infection is influenza. People who are in closest proximity to the infected source have the highest risk for infection.

*Vehicle transmission* occurs when infectious organisms (e.g., salmonellosis) are transmitted through a common source (e.g., contaminated food, water, and intravenous [IV] fluid) to many potential susceptible hosts.

*Vector-borne transmission* of infectious organisms involves insects and/or animals that act as intermediaries between two or more hosts. Lyme disease and Rocky Mountain spotted fever are examples of vector-borne diseases. Lyme disease will be discussed in this chapter, but refer to Chapter 29 for more information regarding mosquito-borne Zika and West Nile viruses.

## Portal of Entry

A pathogen may enter a new host by ingestion (GI tract), inhalation (respiratory tract), or bites or injury of the skin. Microbes commonly enter through contact with mucous membranes and, less frequently, transplacentally. Infectious diseases vary as to the number of organisms and the duration of exposure required to start the infectious process in a new host.

## Host Susceptibility

Each person has his or her own susceptibility to infectious disease, and this susceptibility can vary throughout time. A susceptible host has personal characteristics and behaviors that increase the probability of an infectious disease developing.

Biologic and personal characteristics such as age, sex, ethnicity, and heredity influence this probability. General health and nutritional status, hormonal balance, and the presence of concurrent disease also play a role. Likewise, living conditions and personal behaviors such as drug use, diet, hygiene, and sexual practices influence the risk of exposure to pathogens and resistance once exposed.

Older adults in hospitals and long-term care facilities are already susceptible hosts, especially if poorly nourished. Immunosuppressive agents and corticosteroids decrease the body's ability to resist infection. Inadequate or absent hand hygiene or other breaches of aseptic technique result in transmission of microorganisms from health care workers (HCWs) to clients/patients.

Surfaces of equipment can become contaminated and then spread microorganisms that cause infection. Incorrect isolation procedures such as leaving doors open to rooms in which airborne precautions are in effect or not using masks and gowns increase the risk of transmitting organisms that cause HAIs.

The presence of underlying medical disorders (e.g., malignancy, diabetes, renal failure, AIDS, and cirrhosis) decreases T cell– and B cell–mediated immune function. Breaches of body integrity such as nasogastric and chest tubes, intubation, urinary catheters, and IV devices impair the body's defense mechanisms, decreasing the ability of the integumentary, GI, genitourinary, and respiratory systems to resist invasion by microorganisms.

### Lines of Defense

Susceptibility is also influenced by the presence of anatomic and physiologic defenses, sometimes called *lines of defense*. The *first-line defenses* are external, such as intact skin and mucous membranes; oil and perspiration on skin; cilia in respiratory passages; gag and coughing reflexes; peristalsis in the GI tract; and the flushing action of tears, saliva, and mucus.

These first-line defenses act to inhibit invasion of pathogens and remove them before they have an opportunity to multiply. The chemical composition of body secretions such as tears and sweat, together with the pH of saliva, vaginal secretions, urine, and digestive juices, further prevents or inhibits growth of organisms. Compromise in any of these natural defenses increases host susceptibility to pathogen invasion.

Another important first-line defense is the normal flora of microorganisms that inhabit the skin and mucous membranes in the oral cavity, GI tract, and vagina. These organisms occur naturally and usually coexist with their host in a mutually beneficial relationship. Through a mechanism called *microbial antagonism*, they control the replication of potential pathogens.

The importance of this mechanism is evident when it is disturbed, as happens when extensive antibiotic therapy destroys normal flora in the oral or vaginal cavity, resulting in *Candida albicans*, an overgrowth of yeast. Some normal flora can become pathogenic under specific conditions such as immunosuppression or displacement of the pathogen to another area of the body. Displacement of normal flora is a common cause of HAIs. This can occur when *Escherichia coli*, ordinarily normal flora in the GI tract, invade the urinary tract. Invasive procedures increase the risk of displacing these organisms.

The *second-line defense*, the inflammatory process, and the *third-line defense*, the immune response, share several physiologic components. These include the lymphatic system; leukocytes; and a multitude of chemicals, proteins, and enzymes that facilitate the internal defenses.

Once a microorganism penetrates the first line of defense, the inflammatory response is initiated. Inflammation is a local reaction to cell injury of any type whether from physical, chemical, or thermal damage or microbial invasion. As a response to microbial injury, inflammation is aimed at preventing further invasion by walling off, destroying, or neutralizing the invading organism.

The early inflammatory response is protective, but it can continue for sustained periods in some infections, leading to granuloma formation. The production of new leukocytes may be stimulated for weeks or months and is reflected in an elevated white blood cell count. However, sustained inflammation can become chronic and result in destruction of healthy tissues. Extensive necrosis from persistent inflammation can increase tissue susceptibility to the infectious agent or provide an ideal setting for invasion by other pathogens.

The first- and second-line defenses are nonspecific; that is, they operate against all infectious agents in the same way. In contrast, the immune system responds in a specific manner to individual pathogens as long as the organism has antigenic characteristics. In general, antigens are proteins, large polysaccharides, or large lipoprotein complexes that stimulate an immune response.

Not all microorganisms are antigenic, but some are bound by complement or other host-produced substances to form an antigen that elicits an immune response. An immune response is triggered after foreign materials have been cleared from an area of inflammation. For specific details regarding cell-mediated versus humoral immune responses, see Chapter 7.

### Control of Transmission

Much can be done to prevent transmission of infectious diseases, including education for everyone (including clients and families); the use of barriers and isolation; comprehensive immunizations including the required immunization of travelers to or emigrants from endemic areas; drug prophylaxis; improved nutrition, living conditions, and sanitation; avoiding risk-taking behaviors; and correction of environmental factors. Breaking the transmission chain at any of these links can help control transmission of infectious diseases. The link most amenable to control varies with the characteristics of the organism, its reservoirs, the type of pathologic response it produces, and the available technology for control. The general goal is to break the chain at the most cost-effective point or points—that is, the point at which the greatest number of people can be protected with available technology and the least amount of resources.

*Isolation and barriers* can be used to prevent the transmission of microorganisms from infected or colonized people to other unaffected people. In hospital or institutional settings, the purpose of isolating individuals or residents is to prevent the transmission of colonized or infectious microorganisms among clients, visitors, and HCWs.

The CDC and the Hospital Infection Control Practices Advisory Committee continues to update the 2007 isolation guidelines based on emerging evidence.[348] For example, the newer guidelines provide updated information regarding Ebola virus, mumps, and measles. The guidelines outline a two-tiered approach with specific recommendations categorized as Standard Precautions or Transmission-Based Precautions.

*Standard Precautions* assume any person may be contagious. These precautions continue to be the foundation for preventing the transmission of infectious organisms and include hand hygiene, wearing personal protective equipment, and respiratory hygiene/cough etiquette. Box 8.3 presents a list of what is considered infectious and safe waste. Boxes 8.4 and 8.5 present hand hygiene indications and technique.

Standard Precautions apply to all clients, whereas Transmission-Based Precautions apply to anyone with documented or suspected infection or colonization with highly transmissible or epidemiologically important organisms that require additional precautions (i.e., in addition to Standard Precautions) to prevent transmission.

**Box 8.3**

**INFECTIOUS AND SAFE MEDICAL WASTE**

| Infectious Waste | Safe Waste |
|---|---|
| Blood and components | Cotton balls, Band-Aids |
| All disposable sharps (used or unused) | Gloves (latex and latex-free), masks, or other personal protective devices |
| Urine, stool, or emesis if visibly contaminated with blood | Nasal secretions |
| Vaginal secretions | Sputum |
| Semen | Feces |
| Cerebrospinal fluid | Urine |
| Synovial fluid | Vomitus |
| Pericardial fluid (mediastinal tubes) | Tears |
| Amniotic fluid | Sweat |

Regulation of medical waste disposal is primarily regulated at the state level. To determine the laws that apply in your state, go to U.S. Environmental Protection Agency: http://www.epa.gov/osw/nonhaz/industrial/medical/programs.htm. Click on your state for information about your state medical waste regulations and programs.

**Box 8.4**

**INDICATIONS FOR HAND HYGIENE AND HAND ANTISEPSIS[a]**

Handwashing with soap (microbial or non-antimicrobial) and water:

- When hands are visibly soiled with blood or body fluid
- Before eating
- After using the restroom
- If proven or suspected exposure to *Bacillus anthracis* or *Clostridioides difficile*
  Decontaminate hands with alcohol-based rub:
- After exposure to body fluids or excretions but hands not visibly soiled
- After having direct contact with a client
- Before and after putting on gloves for client care
- Before and after putting on gloves for a nonsurgical procedure
- After contact with intact client skin
- After attending to a contaminated body site and before moving to a clean body site on the same client
- After contact with objects in client area

[a]For visual orientation to handwashing, see the World Health Organization's poster: How to Handwash. Available online at http://www.who.int/gpsc/5may/How_To_HandWash_Poster.pdf. Video presentations in multiple languages are also available at http://www.who.int/gpsc/5may/hand_hygiene_video/en/.

Data from Boyce JM, Pittet D; Healthcare Infection Control Practices Advisory Committee; HICPAC/SHEA/APIC/IDSA Hand Hygiene Task Force: Guideline for hand hygiene in health-care settings. Recommendations of the Healthcare Infection Control Practices Advisory Committee and the HICPAC/SHEA/APIC/IDSA Hand Hygiene Task Force. Society for Healthcare Epidemiology of America/Association for Professionals in Infection Control/Infectious Diseases Society of America. *MMWR Recomm Rep* 51(RR-16):1–45, 2002. Available at http://www.cdc.gov/mmwr/PDF/rr/rr5116.pdf.

**Box 8.5**

**PROPER HAND-HYGIENE TECHNIQUE**

***Alcohol-Based Rubs***

Using alcohol-based hand rubs may reduce contamination better than soap and water. Apply product in the palm of the hand and rub hands together, remembering to cover all areas of the hands, including the back of the hands and webs of the fingers, until dry.

***Washing Hands With Soap and Water***

Wet hands before beginning then add soap. Rub hands together vigorously for at least 15 to 20 seconds, covering all areas of the hands and fingers. Rinse soap from hands and dry completely with a disposable towel. Turn the water off using the towel. Avoid hot water, as this may increase the risk for dermatitis.

***Special Considerations***

- Jewelry may sequester gram-negative organisms, but more studies are needed to determine if this translates to increased transmission of the organisms.
- Artificial nails or extenders can harbor high concentrations of coagulase-negative staphylococci and gram-negative rods. Although more studies are needed to determine if artificial nails increase the likelihood of transmitting organisms, the Centers for Disease Control and Prevention (CDC) recommends that artificial nails or extenders not be worn when in contact with clients at high risk for infection (https://www.cdc.gov/mmwr/PDF/rr/rr5116.pdf).
- Wear gloves as a standard precaution if you have contact risk with blood, body fluids, mucous membranes, nonintact skin, or environmental surfaces.
- For therapists in outpatient settings, the CDC developed guidelines for infection control.[43] This is especially helpful when your facility does not have an infectious disease department.

For more information on hand hygiene and infection control, visit the websites for the Centers for Disease Control and Prevention (CDC) (https://www.cdc.gov/handhygiene/index.html), the World Health Organization (http://www.who.int/gpsc/5may/tools/9789241597906/en/), and the Association for Professionals in Infection Control and Epidemiology (https://apic.org/Resources/Topic-specific-infection-prevention/hand-hygiene).

Data from Boyce JM, Pittet D; Healthcare Infection Control Practices Advisory Committee; HICPAC/SHEA/APIC/IDSA Hand Hygiene Task Force: Guideline for hand hygiene in health-care settings. Recommendations of the Healthcare Infection Control Practices Advisory Committee and the HICPAC/SHEA/APIC/IDSA Hand Hygiene Task Force. Society for Healthcare Epidemiology of America/Association for Professionals in Infection Control/Infectious Diseases Society of America. *MMWR Recomm Rep* 51(RR-16):1–45, 2002. Available at http://www.cdc.gov/mmwr/PDF/rr/rr5116.pdf.

*Transmission-Based Precautions* are defined accor ing to the major modes of transmission of infecti agents (contact, airborne, and droplet) in the h care setting (Table 8.3). Specific guidelines hav published according to the type of infection (i multidrug-resistant organisms) and conditio

**Table 8.3 Type of Transmission-Based Precautions and Prevention Guidelines[a]**

| Type of Precaution | Type of Microorganism | Measures Taken |
|---|---|---|
| Standard Precautions | Bloodborne pathogens; applies to all clients | • Perform hand hygiene<br>• Use PPE whenever possible exposure to pathogen<br>• Perform cough etiquette/respiratory hygiene<br>• Clean patient care area and equipment with EPA-registered disinfectant<br>• Handle laundry carefully<br>• Ensure proper handling of sharp objects |
| Airborne Precautions | Microorganism transmitted by small particle residue; can suspend in the air and be dispersed by air currents (i.e., coughing, sneezing, talking)<br>*Examples:*<br>• Measles (rubeola)<br>• *Mycobacterium tuberculosis* (MDRT)<br>• Varicella (chickenpox)<br>• Zoster (disseminated shingles) | • Private room with monitored airborne infection isolation room<br>• ROOM DOOR CLOSED and client in room<br>• PPE when entering room including a fit-tested NIOSH-approved respirator<br>• Restrict entry of certain susceptible people (immunosuppressed, pregnant women) when rubella or varicella is suspected or known<br>• Limited transport of client from room (only when essential); place surgical mask on restricted individual transported and observe Respiratory Hygiene/Cough Etiquette |
| Droplet precautions | Microorganisms transmitted by large particle droplets about 3 feet from the source; generated by sneezing, coughing, talking or during procedures<br>*Examples:*<br>• Invasive *Haemophilus influenzae* type B including meningitis, pneumonia, epiglottis, sepsis<br>• Invasive *Neisseria meningitidis*<br>• Diphtheria, pertussis<br>• *Mycoplasma pneumoniae*<br>• Pneumonia plaque<br>• Streptococcal pharyngitis, pneumonia, or scarlet fever in infants and young children<br>• Adenovirus<br>• Influenza, RSV<br>• Mumps, rubella<br>• Parvovirus B19 | • Private room or house with others with same infection<br>• Door may remain open<br>• Use PPE, don mask on entry into patient room or space<br>• Limit client transport to only when necessary; place surgical mask on client when transported and follow Respiratory Hygiene/Cough Etiquette |
| Contact precautions | Microorganisms that can be transmitted by direct contact with client (hand/skin-to-skin contact) or indirect contact (touching environmental surfaces or client/care items)<br>*Examples:*<br>• Gastrointestinal, respiratory, skin or wound infections<br>• Multidrug-resistant bacteria (MRSA, VRE)<br>• Enteric infections (low infectious dose or prolonged environmental survival, *Clostridioides difficile*)<br>• Diapered or incontinent clients (enterohemorrhagic *Escherichia coli; Shigella;* hepatitis A; rotavirus)<br>*In infants and young children:*<br>• RSV<br>• Parainfluenza virus<br>• Enteroviral infections<br>• Highly contagious skin infections or those that may occur on dry skin<br>• Diphtheria; herpes simplex virus; impetigo; noncontained abscesses, cellulitis, or decubiti; pediculosis; scabies; herpes zoster (disseminated)<br>• Viral/hemorrhagic conjunctivitis<br>• Viral hemorrhagic infections (e.g., Ebola) | • Private room<br>• Don PPE including gown and gloves on entry and for all interactions<br>• Change gloves after having contact with infective material that may contain high concentrations of microorganism (e.g., fecal material, wound drainage)<br>• Remove gown and gloves before leaving the client environment and wash hands immediately with antimicrobial soap (if *C. difficile* infection or hands are visibly soiled) or waterless antiseptic<br>• After removing gloves and washing hands, DO NOT TOUCH potentially contaminated surfaces or materials<br>• Limit transport of person from room<br>• Dedicate use of noncritical client care items to only this person (e.g., stethoscope)<br>• Disinfect equipment and frequently touched surfaces with approved disinfectant before using with other clients |

[a]See section in the "2007 Guideline for Isolation Precautions: Preventing Transmission of Infectious Agents in Health Care Settings" document[348] pertaining to risk in ambulatory care centers. The delineation of the different facilities in this document confirms the need to keep in mind the importance of appropriate environmental cleaning and hand hygiene in all settings.

*EPA*, Environmental Protection Agency; *MDRT*, multidrug-resistant tuberculosis; *MRSA*, methicillin-resistant *Staphylococcus aureus*; *NIOSH*, National Institute for Occupational Safety and Health; PPE, personal protective equipment; RSV, respiratory syncytial virus; VRE; vancomycin-resistant enterococci.

be found at https://www.cdc.gov/infectioncontrol/pdf/guidelines/isolation-guidelines.pdf. These precautions are in addition to Standard Precautions.

*Immunizations* have become a mainstay for curtailing, if not eliminating, infectious diseases. The World Health Organization has estimated that globally, more children are being immunized than ever before, but 1.5 million more lives could be saved by the expanded use of vaccines.[411] Immunizations, by decreasing host susceptibility, can now control many diseases, including diphtheria, tetanus, pertussis, measles, mumps, rubella, some forms of meningitis, poliomyelitis, hepatitis A and B, pneumococcal pneumonia, influenza (certain strains), and rabies.

Each year the CDC issues updated information based on the recommendations of the Advisory Committee on Immunization Practices (ACIP) on the vaccine and antiviral agents available for controlling influenza during the current influenza season.[150] Vaccines contain either live but attenuated (altered) microbes or killed microbes; these actively induce immunity to diseases by stimulating white cells to produce antibodies. When a virus or bacteria invades the body, antibodies are produced and attach to specific proteins on the virus or bacteria. Other immune defenses are then stimulated to destroy it.

Another mode of providing immunity to certain organisms is to manufacture specific immune globulins, rather than stimulate the production of antibodies. Immune globulins are previously formed antibodies from hyperimmunized donors or pooled plasma and provide temporary passive immunity (they bind to the virus or bacterium, which then stimulate destruction). Passive immunization is generally used when active immunization is life threatening or when complete protection requires both active and passive immunization (e.g., immune globulins used for hepatitis B or for tetanus.

Side effects to immunization can occur, but the incidence of significant adverse effects of immunization among human beings remains very small. The potential increase in susceptibility to influenza and death from respiratory illness in high-risk people (e.g., those with rheumatoid arthritis, the aging adult, and chronically ill or immunosuppressed individuals) suggests that the influenza and pneumococcal vaccines should include these groups in standard immunization programs.

*Prophylactic antibiotic therapy* may prevent certain infections and is usually reserved for people at high risk of exposure to dangerous infections or adverse outcomes (e.g., *Pneumocystis jirovecii* pneumonia in clients with HIV/AIDS, postexposure of HCWs to percutaneous contamination from individuals with HIV, preoperatively before joint replacement surgery).[6] Prophylactic antibiotics may also be beneficial following the removal of a urinary catheter after abdominal surgery to avoid urinary tract infections.[237]

*Improved nutrition, living conditions,* and *sanitation* through the use of hand hygiene, disinfection, and sterilization can inactivate multidrug resistant organisms such as *S. aureus, C. difficile,* and carbapenem-resistant Enterobacteriaceae (CRE).

*Correction of environmental factors,* particularly water treatment, food and milk safety programs, and control of animals, vectors, rodents, sewage, and solid wastes, can best eradicate nonhuman environments (reservoirs) and thus control pathogens.

Other prevention methods in this category include proper handling and disposal of secretions, excretions, and exudates; isolation of infected clients (doors must remain closed, especially in airborne infection isolation rooms); and quarantine of contacts. Even though many pathogens can be transmitted through fomites, routine environmental cultures are not required, since many organisms are present normally. If present and no one is infected, these pathogens are not considered a functional problem. The CDC offers guidelines for preferred methods for cleaning, disinfection, and sterilization of patient care medical devices and environmental surfaces. This includes durable medical equipment and hydrotherapy and therapeutic pools.[320]

The CDC has recommended specific transmission precautions[348] based on knowledge of the transmission chain for individual infections. The precautions were designed to prevent transmission of pathogens among hospitalized people, HCWs, and visitors (see Table 8.3). Specific recommendations have been made for individual diseases.[348]

**SPECIAL IMPLICATIONS FOR THE THERAPIST 8.1**

### *Control of Transmission*

The impact of infections cannot be underestimated in a physical therapy practice or rehabilitation setting. Infections, and especially HAIs, decrease patients' endurance and delay recovery and progression toward discharge or transfer to a more independent setting. We must do everything we can to halt the spread of organisms that can cause or contribute to infections leading to morbidity and mortality at all levels of care.

The CDC has set up guidelines for the care of all clients regarding precautions against the transmission of infectious disease. These should be used with all clients regardless of their disease status. All blood and body fluids are potentially infectious and should be handled as such (see Box 8.3).

All clients receiving therapy (and thus in contact with HCWs) may be asymptomatic hosts during the period of communicability. The careful use of precautionary measures severely limits the transmission of any disease. Keep in mind risk factors that make people more susceptible to infections (any opening in the skin from wounds, pressure injuries, surgical incisions; diabetes mellitus or even elevated blood glucose levels; bowel or bladder incontinence following spinal surgery) and include appropriate preventive measures in the plan of care.[283]

Each hospital has transmission-based precautions organized according to categories of transmission routes to prevent the spread of infectious disease to others. Every HCW must be familiar with these procedures and follow them carefully. Whereas previous focus has been on the hospital setting, recently the CDC published guidelines for infection prevention in the general outpatient setting, outpatient oncology setting,[47,48] as well as

Continued

nursing homes and assisted living[355] facilities in order to further reduce morbidity and mortality statistics. Transmission-based precautions and prevention guidelines are provided in Table 8.3.

The CDC and the Advisory Committee on Immunization Practices (ACIP) recommend all health care providers become involved in ensuring that individuals are fully immunized regardless of whether they provide vaccinations. Health care professionals who do not provide vaccination such as physical therapists should routinely assess vaccination status, recommend the needed vaccines, and make appropriate referrals. The CDC provides resources for health care providers regarding vaccine-specific recommendations as well as immunization schedules and guidelines. In addition, the CDC offers communication strategies for discussing vaccines with individuals.[76,80,267]

HCWs should be concerned about improving their own resistance and decreasing their susceptibility to infectious diseases. Maintaining an adequate immunization status is one approach. Every HCW should be adequately immunized against influenza, hepatitis B, measles, mumps, rubella, polio, tetanus, diphtheria, and varicella. Table 8.4 lists the most recent CDC recommendations for immunization of HCWs. A complete schedule of recommended adult immunizations is available.[56]

## Health Care–Associated Infections

Therapists can help prevent transmission of HAIs from themselves to others, from client to client, and from client to self by following Standard Precautions and recommendations presented in Box 8.6 and Table 8.5. HAIs include central line–associated bloodstream infections (CLABSIs), catheter-associated urinary tract infections (CAUTIs), ventilator-associated pneumonia (VAP), and SSIs.

**Central Line–Associated Bloodstream Infections.** The use of central venous catheters is an integral part of modern health care, allowing for the administration of IV fluids, blood products, medications, and parenteral nutrition as well as providing access for hemodialysis and hemodynamic monitoring. The use of central venous catheters is associated with the risk of bloodstream infection caused by microorganisms that colonize the external surface of the device or the fluid pathway when the device is inserted or manipulated after insertion. CLABSIs are associated with increased morbidity, mortality, and health care costs.[256] It is now recognized that CLABSIs are largely preventable when evidence-based guidelines are followed for the insertion and maintenance of central venous catheters.[383]

As part of an effort to address preventable infections, the Society for Healthcare Epidemiology of America, the Infectious Diseases Society of America), the American Hospital Association, the Association for Professionals in Infection Control and Epidemiology, and The Joint Commission collaborated to publish the most current, evidence-based guidance for the prevention of CLABSIs. Mortality for CLABSIs is as high as 25% in the United States.[383]

Although this is more of a nursing-directed prevention program, therapists must be aware of the potential for central or peripheral line infections and remain vigilant in assessing dressing integrity anywhere near these lines and assist in maintaining entry points that are waterproof and shielded from the external

**Table 8.4** Centers for Disease Control and Prevention (CDC) Recommendations for Immunization of Health Care Workers (HCWs)[a]

| Vaccine | Schedule |
|---|---|
| Hepatitis B | Recombinant vaccine (IM) given in a 3-dose series; obtain anti-HBs serologic testing 1–2 months after last dose |
| Influenza | Annual influenza vaccination is recommended for all persons aged 6 months and older who have no medical contraindications; therefore, vaccination of all HCWs who have no contraindications is recommended |
| Measles, mumps, rubella (MMR) | For anyone born in 1957 or later without serologic evidence of immunity or prior vaccination (adults born before 1957 generally are considered immune); contraindicated in pregnancy |
| Varicella-zoster virus (chickenpox) | HCWs who have no serologic proof of immunity, prior vaccination, or history of chickenpox (2 doses of varicella vaccine, 4 weeks apart); contraindicated in pregnancy |
| Tetanus and diphtheria (Td) | Recommended for all adults with booster every 10 years; tetanus prophylaxis advised for HCWs in wound management; advised after needlestick injury. ACIP recommendations for Tdap (combined tetanus, diphtheria, and pertussis vaccine) in adults and HCWs were released in 2011[b] |
| Meningococcal | Not recommended routinely for all HCWs; recommended for HCWs in direct contact with respiratory secretions from infected persons without proper use of precautions; microbiologists who are routinely exposed to *Neisseria meningitidis*; postexposure prophylaxis advised (1 dose) |
| Bacille Calmette-Guérin (BCG) | Not used in United States as prophylaxis; foreign-born HCWs who have received this vaccine outside the United States must be aware that it does *not* provide lifelong immunity |

[a]HCWs should consult with their physicians for individual recommendations based on medical and other indications.

[b]Updated recommendations for use of tetanus toxoid, reduced diphtheria toxoid, and acellular pertussis (Tdap) vaccine from the Advisory Committee on Immunization Practices, 2010. *MMWR Morb Mortal Wkly Rep* 60(1):13–15, 2011. For more complete information, visit the Immunization Action Coalition (IAC) website: http://www.immunize.org/; check for updates here: http://www.immunize.org/new/.

*ACIP*, Advisory Committee on Immunization Practices; *IM*, intramuscular.

Data from Shefer A, et al: Immunization of health-care personnel: recommendations of the Advisory Committee On Immunization Practices (ACIP). *MMWR Recomm Rep* 60(RR07):1–45, 2011. Updated 2017. Available at: https://www.cdc.gov/mmwr/pdf/rr/rr6007.pdf. Accessed February 14, 2019.[345]

Box 8.6

**TIPS FOR PREVENTING INFECTION**

***Chest Tube***

- Prevent chest tube from kinking by carefully coiling the tubing on top of the bed and securing it to the bed linen (usually according to nursing protocol), leaving room for the person to turn.

***Tracheostomy***

- Maintain the head of bed at 30°; this helps minimize the risk of hospital-acquired pneumonia.
- Contact with secretions occurs with a tracheostomy; follow Standard Precautions. When direct contact is made and potential splash secondary to expelled secretions occurs, gown, mask, protective face wear, and gloves are needed.

***Urinary Catheter***

- Follow Standard Precautions for hand hygiene.
- Do not allow the drainage bag spigot to come in contact with a contaminated surface.
- When the drainage tubing becomes disconnected, do not touch the ends of the tubing or catheter. Contact the nursing staff for reconnecting.
- Before turning, moving, or transferring a catheterized person, locate the proximal end of the tubing and either clamp it to the person's gown or hold it to allow necessary slack during movement. This will help prevent the catheter from accidentally and traumatically being pulled out.
- Whenever possible, avoid raising the drainage bag above the level of the person's bladder.
- If it becomes necessary to raise the bag during transfers, clamp the tubing, but avoid prolonged clamping or kinking of the tubing (except during bladder conditioning).
- Avoid allowing large loops of tubing to dangle from the bedside, wheelchair, or walker.
- Drain all urine from tubing into the bag before the person exercises or ambulates.

***Intravenous Devices***

- If you have exudative lesions or weeping dermatitis, refrain from all direct contact with intravenous (IV) or invasive equipment until the condition resolves.
- Notify the nursing staff of any suspicious observations such as if the IV device is not dripping at a steady rate (either none at all or flowing very fast), if the IV bag is empty, or if blood is flowing from insertion of the IV catheter tip into the person's body out into the IV line.

***Nasogastric and Feeding Tubes***

- Care must be taken to avoid excessive movement or pulling and tugging of these tubes.
- Wash your hands before and after touching the entry point of the tube into the body.

***Hydrotherapy***[338]

- Hydrotherapy for wound care (pulsatile lavage with suction) should be performed in a private treatment room with all walls and doors closed.
- Proper personal protective equipment must be worn when treating the client and/or cleaning hydrotherapy equipment.
- Whirlpool equipment and surrounding area should be cleaned before and after treatment following manufacturer guidelines and using a disinfectant registered by the Environmental Protection Agency.

environment. It is truly a team effort to keep patients safe and infection-free.[143] Hand hygiene remains an integral part of team effort to prevent all infections including CLABSIs.

**Catheter-Associated Urinary Tract Infections.** Urinary tract infections are the most common HAI with 70% to 80% of these infections due to indwelling urethral catheters.[406] A biofilm develops around the indwelling catheter resulting in bacteriuria during catheterization.[273] The morbidity associated with a single episode of catheterization is limited, but the risk increases with higher frequency of catheter use during hospitalization. In 2011 CAUTI rates in adult intensive care units (ICUs) ranged from 1.2 to 4.5 per urinary catheter days.[63] As with all HAIs, prevention is the key. Hand hygiene is imperative when mobilizing patients with urinary catheterization and ensuring there are no kinks in the tubing that would obstruct urine flow.

**Ventilator-Associated Pneumonia.** In 2012 the CDC further defined ventilator-associated events to better capture VAPs,[202] as mechanical ventilation can result in other serious complications. VAPs are defined as a pneumonia that occurs 48 to 72 hours after endotracheal intubation with the signs and symptoms of infection, Gram stain–positive purulent pulmonary secretions, and quantitative growth of a pathogenic organism.[202] Approximately 5% to 10% of patients develop pneumonia as a result of mechanical ventilation.[232] Strategies to reduce VAP involve a multidisciplinary team using the best evidence-based practice regarding hand hygiene, standard and isolation practices, and environmental cleaning. There is good evidence to support facilitation of an early mobility program to reduce the average duration of mechanical ventilation[171,269,335] and reduce mortality. In addition, therapists can minimize the risk of aspiration by ensuring the head of the bed is elevated to 30° to 45°.[25]

**Surgical Site Infections.** SSI accounts for 20% of all HAIs, making it the most common and costly HAI.[199,219] There is strong evidence to support education about modifiable risk factors such as glucose control, obesity, and smoking to reduce SSI incidence. Other strategies to implement include hand hygiene, cleaning environmental surfaces with a disinfectant registered by the Environmental Protection Agency, and education regarding incisional care.[12]

## SPECIFIC INFECTIOUS DISEASES

Most infections are confined to specific organ systems. In this book, many of the important infectious disease entities are discussed in the specific chapter dealing with

**Table 8.5** Summary of Important Recommendations and Work Restrictions for Personnel With Infectious Diseases

| Disease/Problem | Work Restriction | Duration |
|---|---|---|
| Conjunctivitis | Restrict from client contact and contact with the client's environment | Until discharge ceases |
| Cytomegalovirus infections | No restriction | |
| Diarrheal diseases | | |
| Acute stage (diarrhea with other symptoms) | Restrict from client contact, contact with the client's environment, or food handling | Until symptoms resolve |
| Convalescent stage, *Salmonella* | Restrict from care of high-risk clients | Until symptoms resolve; consult with local and state health authorities regarding need for negative stool cultures |
| Diphtheria | Exclude from duty | Until antimicrobial therapy completed and 2 cultures obtained ≥24 hours apart are negative |
| Ebola | Exclude from duty while determining exposure and monitoring for symptoms such as fever | 21 days after exposure |
| Enteroviral infections | Restrict from care of infants, neonates, and immunocompromised persons and from their environment | Until symptoms resolve |
| Hepatitis A | Restrict from client contact, contact with client's environment, and food handling; use proper handwashing | Until 7 days after onset of jaundice |
| Hepatitis B | | |
| Personnel with acute or chronic hepatitis B surface antigenemia who do not perform exposure-prone procedures | No restriction,[a] refer to state regulations; Standard Precautions should always be observed | |
| Personnel with acute or chronic hepatitis B antigenemia who perform exposure-prone procedures | Do not perform exposure-prone invasive procedures until counsel from an expert review panel has been sought; panel should review and recommend procedures the worker can perform, taking into account specific procedure and skill and technique of worker; refer to state regulations | Until hepatitis B e antigen (a marker of a high titer of virus) is negative |
| Hepatitis C | No recommendation | |
| Herpes simplex | | |
| Genital | No restriction | |
| Hands (herpetic whitlow) | Restrict from client contact and contact with client's environment | Until lesions heal |
| Orofacial | Evaluate for need to restrict from care of high-risk clients | |
| HIV | Do not perform exposure-prone invasive procedures until counsel from an expert review panel has been sought; panel should review and recommend procedures the worker can perform, taking into account specific procedure and skill and technique of the worker; Standard Precautions should always be observed; refer to state regulations | |
| Measles | | |
| Active | Exclude from duty | Until 7 days after rash appears |
| Postexposure (susceptible) | Exclude from duty | From 5th day after first exposure through 21st day after last exposure and/or 4 days after rash appears |
| Meningococcal infections | Exclude from duty | Until 24 hours after start of effective therapy |
| Mumps | | |
| Active | Exclude from duty | Until 5 days[348] after onset of parotitis |
| Postexposure (susceptible personnel) | Exclude from duty | From 12th day after first exposure through 26th day after last exposure or until 9 days after onset of parotitis |
| Pediculosis | Restrict from duty | Until treated and observed to be free of adult and immature lice |
| Pertussis | | |
| Active | Exclude from duty | From beginning of catarrhal stage through 3rd week after onset of paroxysms or until 5 days after start of effective antimicrobial therapy |

**Table 8.5** Summary of Important Recommendations and Work Restrictions for Personnel With Infectious Diseases—cont'd

| Disease/Problem | Work Restriction | Duration |
|---|---|---|
| Postexposure (asymptomatic personnel) | No restriction, prophylaxis recommended | |
| Postexposure (symptomatic personnel) | Exclude from duty | Until 5 days after start of effective antimicrobial therapy |
| Rubella | | |
| Active | Exclude from duty | Until 5 days after rash appears |
| Postexposure (susceptible personnel) | Exclude from duty | From 7th day after first exposure through 21st day after last exposure |
| Scabies | Restrict from client contact | Until cleared by medical evaluation |
| *Staphylococcus aureus* infection | | |
| Active, draining skin lesions | Restrict from contact with client and client's environment or food handling | Until lesions have resolved |
| Carrier state | No restriction, unless personnel are epidemiologically linked to transmission of the organism | |
| Streptococcal infection, group A | Restrict from client care, contact with client's environment or food handling | Until 24 hours after adequate treatment started |
| Tuberculosis | | |
| Active disease | Exclude from duty | Until proved noninfectious |
| PPD converter | No restriction if not an active case and if cleared medically | |
| Varicella | | |
| Active | Exclude from duty | Until all lesions dry and crust |
| Postexposure (susceptible personnel) | Exclude from duty | From 10th day after first exposure through 21st day (28th day if VZIG given) after last exposure |
| Viral respiratory infections, acute febrile | Consider excluding from the care of high-risk clients[b] or contact with their environment during community outbreak of RSV influenza | Until acute symptoms resolve |
| Zoster | | |
| Localized in healthy person | Cover lesions; restrict from care of high-risk clients[c] | Until lesions dry and crust |
| Generalized or localized immunosuppressed person | Restrict from client contact | Until lesions dry and crust |
| Postexposure (susceptible personnel) | Restrict from client contact | From 10th day after first exposure through 21st day (28th day if VZIG given) after last exposure or, if varicella occurs, until all lesions dry and crust |

[a]Unless epidemiologically linked to transmission of infection.
[b]High-risk patients defined by the Advisory Committee of Immunization Practices for complications of influenza.
[c]Those susceptible to varicella and who are at increased risk of complications of varicella such as neonates and immunocompromised persons of any age.
*PPD,* Purified protein derivative; *RSV,* respiratory syncytial virus; *VZIG,* varicella-zoster immunoglobulin.
Modified from Centers for Disease Control and Prevention. Infection Control in Healthcare Personnel: *Infrastructure and Routine Practices for Occupational Infection Prevention and Control Services.* 2019. (https://www.cdc.gov/infectioncontrol/guidelines/healthcare-personnel/index.html).

the affected anatomic area. Only the most commonly encountered infectious problems not covered elsewhere are included in this chapter.

## Bacterial Infections

### Enterobacteriaceae

The Enterobacteriaceae family of gram-negative bacteria includes *Klebsiella, E. coli, Proteus, Serratia,* and *Yersinia,* many of which cause significant disease. This group is typically found in the GI tract of humans, although the oropharynx can also be colonized. These species are also the most commonly isolated gram-negative bacteria in the hospital setting. These bacteria cause a wide range of infections, including wound, respiratory, bloodstream, and urinary tract infections.

Similar to other bacteria such as *S. aureus,* this family continues to develop resistance to multiple classes of antimicrobials. This resistance is mediated through specific enzymes that are produced by the bacteria, such as one of the metallo-beta-lactamases (MBLs, metallo referring to the requirement of zinc) or *K. pneumoniae* carbapenemase (KPC) among the more clinically important. One of the more resistant MBLs is the New Delhi MLB-1, with susceptibility to only two antibiotics—colistin and tigecycline. These enzymes are able to break down most antibiotics traditionally used for this class of bacteria, particularly cephalosporins, including third- and fourth-generation cephalosporins, aztreonam, and extended-spectrum penicillins (termed extended-spectrum β-lactamases). Because this resistance is conferred by plasmid, resistance to aminoglycosides, trimethoprim-sulfamethoxazole, and fluoroquinolone drugs is frequently included. Organisms exhibiting this extended spectrum of resistance were often then treated with "last resort" carbapenems, such as imipenem. However, CRE bacteria or carbapenemase-producing Enterobacteriaceae (see Fig. 8.1) exhibit resistance to carbapenems and, although uncommon, are causing increasing cases of infections in acute care settings. In 2013 the CDC recognized CRE as one of the three most urgent antibacterial resistance threats in the United States.[75] Imipenem and other drugs in the carbapenem class are now restricted in use to avoid widespread bacterial resistance.

Currently, KPC is the most commonly encountered carbapenemase in the United States. It may be found in any of the Enterobacteriaceae including *E. coli* and *P. aeruginosa*. KPC is resistant to almost all available antimicrobial agents, and no one drug regimen is proven to be more effective than another. Treatment for serious infections should be determined in conjunction with an infectious disease expert in multidrug resistance and based on susceptibility profiles of the organism. Serious infections caused by carbapenemase-producing bacteria are associated with high rates of morbidity and mortality.[238,272,313,329,356] People at risk include severely ill, neutropenic, or immunosuppressed individuals; organ transplant recipients; persons exposed to mechanical ventilation, indwelling arterial or central venous catheters, or urinary catheters; and persons who have experienced trauma. There is concern that increasing human air travel and migration will allow strains of these bacteria to disseminate worldwide.[276,403]

All individuals with CRE are managed by using (and reinforcing the use of) meticulous hand hygiene and contact precautions, including environmental cleaning and disinfecting with appropriate cleaners. Aggressive detection and control strategies are employed to prevent the spread of KPC and MBLs as a public health threat regarding antimicrobial resistance among gram-negative bacteria. The Agency of Healthcare Research and Quality, World Health Organization, and CDC provide updates and toolkits for acute-care hospitals and long-term care facilities to prevent and control transmission but are not intended for ambulatory care facilities at this time.[40,49,154]

### *Clostridioides* (Formerly *Clostridium*) *difficile* Infections

**Overview.** *C. difficile*[214] is an important public health issue as the most common cause of health care–associated diarrhea worldwide. In 2013 the CDC placed *C. difficile* infections (CDI) as one of the three most urgent threats to public health.[75] Once thought to be associated only with antibiotic use in medical settings, it is now also detected in healthy persons in the community without a history of antibiotic exposure. *C. difficile* is an anaerobic, spore-forming bacillus that can cause symptoms ranging from mild diarrhea to severe colonic inflammation leading to death. It is the only anaerobe that poses a health care–associated risk. CDIs are most often recognized among residents of long-term care facilities or persons in acute care or short-stay hospitals because of the high rates of antibiotic use.

**Incidence.** CDI rates continue to increase sharply in the United States and Canada and show no sign of decline. In 2011 the estimated number of CDIs in the United States was 453,000, with the highest rates reported in whites, females, and adults age 65 years or older. Between the years 1996–2009, the incidence of CDI rates in persons older than age 65 years increased 200%. About half of CDIs are acquired in the community, with greater than 80% of these people reporting visiting a doctor's or dentist's office before developing diarrhea.[217] In approximately 5% of cases, there is no known previous health care or antibiotic exposure. Colonization without symptoms is seen in more than 20% of people hospitalized and is an important source of transmission.[109] The reason for rising rates of CDIs has been ascribed to the appearance of hypervirulent strains, misuses of antibiotics, and an increase in the number of susceptible people (e.g., people with immune deficiency, advanced age, etc.). The severity of disease has also increased with higher rates of morbidity and mortality.

**Etiology, Transmission, and Risk Factors.** *C. difficile* is a bacterium that is commonly present in the everyday environment in natural water sources, soil, and animal and human feces. Because *C. difficile* exists in a hardy spore form, it is able to survive for weeks or months. Disease is thought to develop once these spores are picked up and inadvertently ingested (fecal-oral route).

Typically, healthy people do not develop symptoms because of the high numbers of normal bacteria in the intestine. Susceptible persons often have decreased levels of normal flora as a consequence of antibiotic treatment, which allows *C. difficile* to spread quickly. Contamination of the patient care environment also plays an important role. Spores have been found on cart handles, bedrails, bedside tables, toilets, sinks, stethoscopes, thermometers, telephones, and remote controls.[108]

Data on risk factors for developing CDI are conflicting relating to whether it is the initial infection, a recurrence, hospital acquired, or community acquired.[119] The most significant risk factors include age (65 years and older), use of antibiotics (even many months before symptoms), recent hospitalization, residence in a long-term care facility, serious underlying illness, immunosuppression, or a previous diagnosis with CDI.[119,136] Almost all classes of antibiotics are associated with CDIs; however, the most common antibiotics include fluoroquinolones, cephalosporins, clindamycin, and penicillins.[136,353]

Factors that disrupt the intestinal mucosa also increase the likelihood of developing a CDI such as chemotherapy, GI surgery, enteral feeding, inflammatory bowel disease, and decreased gastric acidity from the use of proton pump inhibitors and $H_2$ blockers.[119,136,180] Recurrent CDI is seen more frequently in persons who require ongoing antibiotics while being treated for CDI, have an elevated creatinine level, are older than 65 years, have significant comorbid disease, and lack an immune response to *C. difficile* toxins.[101]

**Pathogenesis.** Disease itself is secondary to an overgrowth of *C. difficile* organisms and the release of toxins (A and B and binary toxin) produced by *C. difficile*.

Antibiotics most likely suppress the normal GI microbiota, allowing for overgrowth of *C. difficile* organisms. Although *C. difficile* is rarely invasive, toxins produced by the bacteria are transported into intestinal cells. These toxins lead to a dysregulation of the cytoskeleton and disrupt the tight junctions, causing ulceration of the cells. Levels of toxins reflect the severity of the clinical disease.[5] Toxin A leads to intestinal fluid secretion and mucosal injury, whereas both A and B promote the migration of neutrophils.[207] Toxin B is significantly more virulent than toxin A. The NAP1/B1/027 strain produces a binary toxin and, when seen in an epidemic setting, has a lower cure rate and increased recurrence with more severe disease.[305,337]

**Clinical Manifestations.** The clinical presentation of CDI is varied but is typically recognized by persistent diarrhea associated with antibiotic use in conjunction with abdominal cramping and tenderness. Although loose stools are frequently associated with antibiotic use without infection, CDI is noted by watery diarrhea three or more times a day for 24 hours. Fever and an elevated white blood count are often not present in mild to moderate infections. Severe disease can be manifested by fever, abdominal pain, ileus, toxic megacolon, perforation, and sepsis. When initially evaluating a person with CDI, it is helpful to stratify care by presenting signs and symptoms. People with leukocytosis (greater than 15,000/μL), elevated creatinine, age greater than 60, elevated temperature, and low serum albumin are more likely to have a complicated and more severe course requiring a higher level of care.[98,119]

## MEDICAL MANAGEMENT

**DIAGNOSIS AND TREATMENT.** CDI should be suspected in people with more than three loose stools in 24 hours with associated risk factors. The laboratory routinely rejects formed stools. For clients with an ileus, a rectal swab for toxin assay or *C. difficile* culture (although this takes time) is recommended. The diagnosis is made through the detection of either the *C. difficile* toxin or the *C. difficile* Toxin B gene in stool. Of note, *C. difficile* toxin degrades at room temperature after 2 hours. Stool samples that are delayed in getting to the laboratory should be kept at 4 °C. A positive laboratory result of the Toxin B gene is indicative of the presence of *C. difficile* but not necessarily symptomatic infection (colonization versus CDI). The two available tests are an enzyme immunoassay (EIA) for glutamate dehydrogenase antigen and toxins A and B and nucleic acid amplification test (NAAT). If EIA is positive for both the antigen and the toxins, CDI is diagnosed. If one is positive and the other negative, NAAT can be used. CDI is present if NAAT is positive. If NAAT is negative, the person is presumed not to have CDI. Some clinicians use only NAAT, which is more sensitive but may lead to overdiagnosis and overtreatment (colonization versus infection).[245,277,295] Computed tomography of the abdomen is helpful in diagnosing severe manifestations of CDI. Colonoscopy identifying pseudomembranous lesions (present in severe disease) may help identify difficult-to-diagnose cases but is not recommended for diagnostic purposes.

Treatment can be divided into several categories: initial infection, recurrent infection, severe disease, and fulminant disease. Standard treatment consists of prompt discontinuation of the antibiotic agent; if an antibiotic is required for treatment of concomitant disease, this often leads to prolonged diarrhea, treatment failure, and higher risk for recurrent CDI.[260] An assessment of the severity of disease should be done for placement in the appropriate level of care (see Clinical Manifestations). For an initial episode, clients found to be positive for CDI should receive oral vancomycin or fidaxomicin.[245] Fidaxomicin has a lower recurrence rate but is more expensive than vancomycin.[245,260] Metronidazole can be used if neither vancomycin nor fidaxomicin is available.

Relapse is common, occurring in approximately 20% to 35% of patients. Of these, approximately 45% have only a single recurrence, whereas the remaining 55% have two or more relapses. This is often caused by persistence of spores rather than drug resistance. Retreatment of the relapse is again based on severity, although second relapses are often treated with the same medications as initially used, either oral vancomycin (in a pulse-tapered fashion) or fidaxomicin; metronidazole should not be used. If metronidazole or fidaxomicin was the initial agent, oral vancomycin would be the appropriate drug. For the second or greater recurrence, treatments include prolonged oral vancomycin (pulse-tapered), fidaxomicin, or oral vancomycin followed by rifaximin.[245] For clients who develop three episodes (initial episode plus two recurrences), fecal microbiota transplantation (FMT) is advocated. This procedure involves the placement of processed stool from a healthy donor into the colon of the person with CDI. Although multiple studies have shown improved outcomes in people who have undergone FMT,[193,397] there are several practical limitations.[172] These include the potential of transferring other infectious agents (such as norovirus), choice of appropriate donors, and logistics needed to make FMT widely available.

Clients with severe or fulminant CDI require higher levels of care and close monitoring for complications such as toxic megacolon, perforation, and necrotizing colitis. Severe and fulminant CDIs are often associated with an ileus (partial or complete), slowing down the transit of oral medication into the colon. In these situations, a vancomycin enema, given via a rectal tube, should be considered. Oral vancomycin or fidaxomicin is the initial treatment, and IV metronidazole is added if ileus is present. Early surgical consultation should be obtained if serum lactate increases to 2.2 mmol/L or greater, there is no clinical improvement, or toxic megacolon or peritoneal signs develop, with colectomy (subtotal or total) as a management option. FMT is also an alternative treatment, although data are lacking.[170]

Probiotics have been advocated to repopulate the intestine with normal gut bacteria. Currently the evidence is inconclusive as to the benefit in reducing CDI recurrences, particularly owing to a lack of consistency between the various products.[291]

**PREVENTION.** Prevention of this HAI is imperative to reduce patient morbidity and mortality and reduce health care costs associated with infection control, medication, and excess hospital days. As CDI is by and large an HAI, most prevention and control efforts take place in the health care setting. Proven strategies include hand hygiene, environmental disinfection, barrier precautions, and antimicrobial stewardship.[30,107,245]

Proper handwashing, requiring 1 to 2 minutes of washing followed by proper hand drying to remove spores, is the most effective prevention. Only chlorine-based disinfectants and high-concentration vaporized hydrogen peroxide are able to kill spores. Of note, alcohol-based hand products are not sporicidal and are ineffective in removing spores from the hands.[378] Sporicidal wipes that may reduce the transmission of *C. difficile* are now available.[107,227,245]

Contact precautions are recommended to prevent the transmission of *C. difficile* in the health care setting consisting of using private rooms or rooms shared by patients with CDI, using gloves and gowns for all contact, and using disposable equipment or cleaning equipment between use with each patient.[245] Bundles (grouping together practices rather than performing each separately) can also control infection rates in hospitals.[35,263]

Preventing oral ingestion of the *C. difficile* organism is important whenever suction devices are used in the oral cavity. A strong correlation has been noted between VAP rates and CDI rates in critical care patients, emphasizing again the importance of cleanliness of anything introduced into an individual's mouth and stomach.

A significant means of reducing risk is through the careful use of antimicrobial drugs. Both hospital and outpatient settings have antibiotic stewardship programs that improve outcomes while reducing unintended consequences.[18] These programs also aid in the reduction of CDI.[107,234] For clients who require antibiotics for a concomitant infection, prophylactic vancomycin may be of benefit to prevent another CDI.[42] Probiotics have been looked to as a means of preventing CDI; however, they have not been shown to be of benefit for primary prevention of CDI.[7] Bezlotoxumab, a monoclonal antibody approved in 2016 for the secondary prevention of CDI in people at high risk for recurrence, is a new modality of treatment still awaiting data to determine its best usage.[139]

**SPECIAL IMPLICATIONS FOR THE THERAPIST 8.2**

### *Clostridioides difficile*

With CDI rates increasing along with the strain's pathogenicity, therapists have an important role in taking measures to reduce transmission, thus potentially preventing the severity of the disease among persons at increased risk (e.g., older adults, immunocompromised individuals).

Keep in mind that anyone who has had a history of *C. difficile* is also at increased risk for relapse or recurrence. Half of all individuals experiencing a relapse of *C. difficile* within 2 months of the primary infection are likely infected with a new strain. In these cases, disease control practices are key to preventing recurrence.

Appropriate measures include adequate hand hygiene with soap and water before and after contact. Spores are resistant to alcohol, so alcohol-based hand rubs are not considered adequate when the disease is in a spore state; most *C. difficile* organisms released during disease outbreaks are in the vegetative form and can be killed by alcohol.[244] Without knowing the exact state of the condition, it is difficult to know when alcohol-based products will be effective.

One other important step the therapist can take to help prevent reinfection is to ensure the environment around the affected individual is clean.[321] Only a few disinfectants (e.g., bleach) are capable of killing the spore-forming organism that causes *C. difficile,* but sanitizers potent enough to kill these organisms damage equipment and surfaces.[68,321] The CDC and American College of Gastroenterology update guidelines for preferred cleaning, disinfection, and sterilization methods as new evidence emerges.[68,321,377]

## Staphylococcal Infections

**Overview and Incidence.** Staphylococci bacteria are among the most common bacterial pathogens normally residing on the skin. Although there are more than 40 species of staphylococci, only a few are clinically relevant, particularly *S. aureus*. They are hardy and able to survive on inanimate objects for an extended period. *S. aureus* is responsible for about 100,000 invasive infections with approximately 19,000 deaths each year.[201]

*S. aureus* can demonstrate a wide variety of clinical manifestations; it can colonize normal skin and mucous membranes, or if allowed into the bloodstream or other tissues, it can cause serious infections. *S. aureus* isolates can be divided into various categories, based on their molecular and clinical characteristics. *Staphylococcus* species can be described as coagulase positive or negative (able to convert fibrinogen to fibrin). *S. aureus* is typically coagulase positive, whereas *Staphylococcus epidermidis* and *Staphylococcus saprophyticus* are coagulase negative. Methicillin-susceptible *S. aureus* indicates the strain is sensitive to most beta-lactam antibiotics; MRSA signifies that the isolate is resistant to beta-lactam antibiotics including cephalosporins and penicillins. MRSA isolates can be further distinguished as community-acquired MRSA (CA-MRSA) and health care–associated MRSA (HA-MRSA). HA-MRSA can be further subdivided into health care–associated hospital onset and health care–associated community onset.

CA-MRSA is defined as cases where the client has not had contact with the health care system within the 12 months before diagnosis. HA-MRSA with hospital onset refers to cases where the symptoms and diagnosis were made more than 48 hours after hospitalization. HA-MRSA with community onset refers to cases that are diagnosed in the community but within 12 months of exposure to the health care system. However, with more cases of CA-MRSA introduced to hospitals, the line of distinction is beginning to blur, with CA-MRSA endemic in some hospitals.[94,200,297,306,312] Some clinicians find this classification clinically unhelpful and consider MRSA as health care related but no longer confined to acute care settings.[201]

*S. aureus* is a significant health problem both in the hospital (as a major source of HAIs) and in the community. MRSA continues to be ranked by the CDC as one of the serious threats to public health.[44]

**Risk Factors.** *S. aureus* spreads by direct contact with colonized surfaces (e.g., towels, razors, equipment) or people (typically skin-to-skin) or inhalation of infected droplets. People at risk for CA-MRSA outbreaks are those living in close quarters such as households, military personnel, jail detainees, children in daycare and daycare workers, and athletes.[62,102,158,192,341] Other risk factors in developing MRSA infection include HIV infection, injection drug use, and prior antibiotic use.[177,241] Risk factors for HA-MRSA include recent hospitalization or admission to a medical or long-term care facility, recent surgery, hemodialysis, and having an indwelling device such as a urinary catheter.

The most common location of human colonization of *S. aureus* is the nares (almost 30% of people have it in their nostrils),[145] although the skin, axilla, groin, intestines, perineum, vagina, and oropharynx can also be colonized. Infections occur more frequently in individuals who are colonized than those who are not (typically with their own colonized strain). Therefore colonization is a significant risk factor for developing a *S. aureus* infection.[274,306,323] Transient contamination of HCWs' hands can also transmit the bacteria to clients and is an important cause of spreading bacteria in health care settings.[90]

Predisposing factors are multiple and varied depending on disease location (Table 8.6). Individuals more likely to develop a *Staphylococcus* infection from damaged skin after surgery or burn injury; individuals with diabetes (from needlesticks, decreased leukocyte function)[296]; anyone who is neutropenic (neutrophils dangerously low); and anyone with prosthetics, chronic skin disease, rheumatoid arthritis, catheters, or on corticosteroid therapy (unable to control local infections sufficiently).

**Pathogenesis.** *S. aureus* cannot invade through intact skin or mucous membranes; infection usually begins

**Table 8.6** Staphylococcal Infections

| Type | Predisposing Factors |
|---|---|
| Bacteremia | Infected surgical wounds<br>Abscesses<br>Infected intravenous or intraarterial catheter sites; catheter tips<br>Infected vascular grafts or prostheses<br>Infected pressure ulcers<br>Osteomyelitis (see further details below in this table)<br>Injection drug abuse<br>Source unknown (primary bacteremia)<br>Cellulitis<br>Burns<br>Immunosuppression<br>Debilitating diseases (e.g., diabetes, renal failure)<br>Infective endocarditis<br>Cancer (leukemia) or neutropenia after chemotherapy or radiation |
| Pneumonia | Immunodeficiency (especially older adults and children [age 2 years])<br>Chronic lung disease and cystic fibrosis<br>Malignancy<br>Antibiotics that kill normal respiratory flora but spare *Staphylococcus aureus*<br>Viral respiratory infections, especially influenza<br>Bloodborne bacteria spread to the lungs from primary sites of infections (e.g., heart valves, abscesses, pulmonary emboli)<br>Recent bronchial or endotracheal suctioning or intubation |
| Enterocolitis | Broad-spectrum antibiotics as prophylaxis for bowel surgery or treatment of hepatic coma<br>Elderly; newborn infants (associated with staphylococcal skin lesions) |
| Osteomyelitis | Hematogenous organisms (bloodborne)<br>Skin trauma<br>Infection spreading from adjacent joint or other infected tissues<br>*S. aureus* bacteremia<br>Orthopedic surgery or trauma<br>Cardiothoracic surgery<br>Usually occurs in growing bones, especially femur and tibia of children <12 years old<br>Male sex |
| Food poisoning | Contaminated food |
| Skin infections | Decreased immunity<br>Burns or pressure injuries<br>Decreased blood flow<br>Skin contamination from nasal discharge<br>Foreign bodies<br>Underlying skin diseases such as eczema and acne<br>Common in persons with poor hygiene living in crowded quarters |

with inoculation of the organism through damaged skin. Once inside the body, the organism is a virulent pathogen, secreting membrane-damaging enzymes and toxins that cause harm to host tissues.

Staphylococci stimulate a significant host immune response, recruiting neutrophils and forming a suppurative or pustular local response. If the bacteria are then able to evade local host defenses, they can spread via the bloodstream to almost any location in the body. The bones, joints, kidneys, lungs, and heart valves are the most common sites of *S. aureus* infections. *Staphylococcus* species are frequently involved in sustaining chronic infections (particularly bones and prosthetic devices) because of their ability to create a biofilm.[243] A biofilm forms when foreign material becomes coated with a layer of collagen, fibrinogen, fibronectin, and other proteins. Staphylococcal bacteria then attach to these proteins, either through hydrophobic interactions or through specific adhesins. These organisms produce an extracellular matrix that surrounds the adhered bacteria, which is resistant to antimicrobials and host defense systems.[138,195] Biofilms are also a source of spreading free-floating bacteria into the bloodstream and are able to infect another site. (See Chapter 25 for a complete discussion of this topic.)

Another method *S. aureus* uses to evade antibiotics is through genes that impart resistance. The *mec* gene is required for methicillin resistance in MRSA.[286] Laboratory tests are able to detect this gene to identify MRSA more rapidly.[252]

**Clinical Manifestations.** *S. aureus* can cause a broad spectrum of disease ranging from mild skin infections to life-threatening disease and can be implicated in almost every type of infection. CA-MRSA has a predilection for causing skin and soft tissue infections, characteristically inducing a suppurative response with abscess formation. The abscesses range in size from microscopic to lesions several centimeters in diameter filled with pus and bacteria (Fig. 8.2).

*S. aureus* may invade superficially, causing impetigo or infection of the epidermis or infection of the superficial dermis (called folliculitis), or even deeper in the dermis, creating a furuncle, carbuncle, or abscess. Infection of skin in intertriginous areas (e.g., armpits, groin, under breasts) is referred to as hidradenitis suppurativa. Cellulitis occurs when the bacteria invade into the subcutaneous tissues (see Cellulitis in Chapter 10). Scalded skin syndrome is typically seen in infants with exfoliation of skin secondary to staphylococcal-produced toxins. Symptoms of skin and soft tissue infections caused by *S. aureus* include erythema, pain, fevers, and abscess formation.

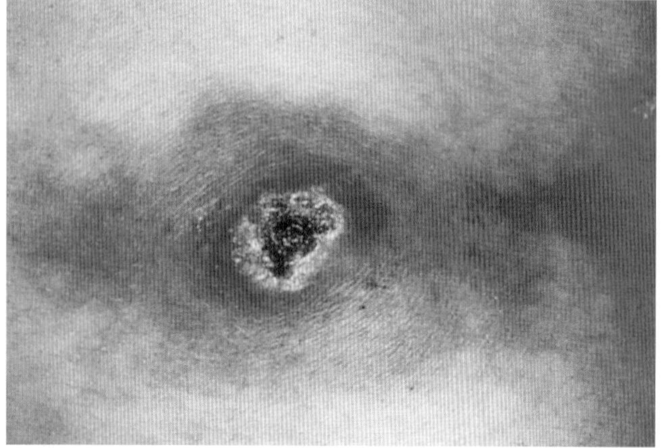

**Figure 8.2**

***Staphylococcus* skin abscess.** (From Braverman IM: *Skin signs of systemic disease*, ed 3, Philadelphia, 1998, Saunders.)

Consumption of toxins produced by staphylococcal species in contaminated food is a common cause of food poisoning, producing nausea, vomiting, abdominal cramping, and diarrhea within 1 to 6 hours of ingestion.

HA-MRSA is often associated with more severe, invasive infections including bacteremia, endocarditis, infection of cardiac prosthetic devices, septicemia and surgical incision infections, osteomyelitis, prosthetic joint infections, septic arthritis, and pneumonia. *S. aureus* is one of the most common causes of both community-acquired and hospital-acquired bacteremia. Clients with bacteremia may have associated hypotension and fever. Bacteremia may occur secondary to another infection (such as from the skin) or may lead to an infection in a site that was previously uninfected.

*S. aureus* is the most common cause of endocarditis, where bacteria seed and grow (forming vegetations) on heart valves, both prosthetic and damaged native valves. The bacteria produce enzymes that can break down tissue, further damaging the valve. Abscesses can form around the valve, and vegetations can break off with embolization to the brain, kidneys, spleen, and other parts of the body, creating metastatic abscesses. Clinical manifestations include a new murmur (from malfunctioning of the valve) and fevers (often fluctuating). Emboli to the brain and congestive heart failure are complications that cause most of the morbidity and mortality associated with endocarditis.[253] Because *S. aureus* thrives on prosthetic devices (see Pathogenesis), it may also infect other cardiac devices, such as implantable cardioverter defibrillators and permanent pacemakers.

Sepsis and toxic shock syndrome are caused from the production of toxins by bacteria, most commonly *S. aureus* or GAS, in skin wounds or surgical wounds or due to superabsorbent tampons. Symptoms include fever, GI and flu-like symptoms, confusion, and rash, similar to a sunburn. Later symptoms include hypotension and sepsis, which is out of proportion to the appearance of the wound infection.

*S. aureus* is the most common bacteria causing osteomyelitis, prosthetic joint infections, and septic arthritis.[390] Osteomyelitis can occur by hematogenous spread or from an infection near the bone (such as a paravertebral abscess infecting the vertebra). The primary symptoms are fever, tenderness, and pain of the bone. There may also be loss in range of motion, swelling, or erythema of the skin. Prosthetic joints may become infected at the time of surgery or be seeded hematogenously. (See Chapter 25 for a complete discussion of this topic.)

Native joints may also become infected (septic arthritis), typically by hematogenous spread. Similar to osteomyelitis, common symptoms include pain, reduced range of motion, fever, warmth, erythema, and tenderness of the joint.

Pneumonia may also be caused by *S. aureus*,[339] especially when associated with clients who are colonized and then intubated or are injection drug users. Symptoms are similar to pneumonias caused by other organisms and include shortness of breath, productive cough, fever, and chest pain.

## MEDICAL MANAGEMENT

**DIAGNOSIS, TREATMENT, AND PROGNOSIS.** Gram stain and culture of the organism from the infected site, blood, or other fluid is usually diagnostic; antibiotic sensitivity testing is important. Rapid culture methods and molecular techniques are available to identify *S. aureus* and MRSA quickly, making it possible to start treating MRSA infections within 24 hours. Because coagulase-negative staphylococci are ubiquitously found on the skin and are a common contaminant, the isolation of coagulase-negative staphylococci does not always indicate infection.

Isolation of *S. aureus* in blood cultures usually confirms bacteremia. Several positive blood cultures can be diagnostic of endocarditis in the presence of a new murmur or echocardiogram, demonstrating valvular vegetations.

CA-MRSA often retains susceptibility to some oral medications such as trimethoprim-sulfamethoxazole, tetracyclines, and clindamycin, which may be used for minor soft tissue and skin infections. Not all purulent soft tissue infections require antibiotics. For small abscesses (less than 5 cm) without associated systemic symptoms (i.e., fever, tachycardia, or blood pressure instability), incision and drainage may suffice. For moderate to severe invasive infections with systemic symptoms, hospitalization with IV antibiotic treatment (typically vancomycin) is warranted with appropriate incision and drainage.[93] Treatment of HA-MRSA often requires IV treatment with vancomycin or daptomycin.[222] Vancomycin is often used before daptomycin owing to more clinical experience available with vancomycin and decreased cost. Some strains of MRSA respond only minimally to vancomycin. In this situation, daptomycin is the drug of choice.[258] Newer drugs are becoming available for the treatment of MRSA including telavancin, ceftaroline, oritavancin, dalbavancin, and delafloxacin; more research and U.S. Food and Drug Administration approval are required for these drugs.

Prevention still remains key to reducing the number of HA-MRSA cases. The Veterans Administration implemented a bundling system to significantly decrease HA-MRSA infections by 62%. This consisted of universal admission surveillance, contact precautions, hand hygiene, and a change in institutional culture.[179] They found an admission colonization rate of 13.6%. Evidence suggests that applying a bundled intervention including both nasal decolonization and glycopeptide prophylaxis for MRSA carriers may decrease rates of SSIs caused by *S. aureus*.[336] Various countries have used different strategies to control and manage MRSA infections. Currently the United States has one of the highest prevalence rates of MRSA, although the incidence has been decreasing in recent years. Universal basic techniques include careful hand hygiene and adherence to contact precautions (i.e., gowns and gloves) with clients known to have MRSA. Debate continues concerning universal screening surveillance when clients are admitted to a medical facility, and studies are needed to determine effectiveness and cost-effectiveness of this approach.[39] One study demonstrated that active surveillance led to discontinuation of contact precautions sooner in clients treated for MRSA, thus reducing cost.[346] Decolonization is another method employed to reduce the spread of MRSA; however, more recent data suggest that it is not consistently effective in eliminating MRSA colonization, and resistance develops to the agents used for decolonization.[16] It may be appropriate in the ICU setting or outbreaks. Other effective measures include meticulous environmental cleaning of surfaces (MRSA is susceptible to most hospital disinfectants)[39] and appropriate use of antibiotics (antibiotic stewardship).

Prognosis is good with treatment, although antibiotic-resistant strains are increasingly associated with increased morbidity and mortality. Infective endocarditis with *S. aureus* remains a serious life-threatening illness, with 20% to 25% mortality.[404] Visceral abscesses, bacteremia, and septicemia are potentially lethal illnesses.

SPECIAL IMPLICATIONS FOR THE THERAPIST 8.3

### *Staphylococcal Infections*

Some organisms such as *S. aureus* (and streptococci) are considered resident organisms because they are not easily removed by scrubbing and often can be cultured from the skin of HCWs. Many HCWs carry *S. aureus* without sequelae and shed organisms into nonintact skin areas of susceptible hosts, causing infections.

For the most part, good handwashing[71] with soap or an alcohol-based rub is adequate in the therapy or home setting, but therapists need to consistently educate family members and caregivers about infection control through proper hand hygiene and environmental management.

Antimicrobial soaps that contain chemicals to kill transient and some resident organisms may be recommended, although debate continues over questions of long-term resistance. The choice of using an antimicrobial soap or plain soap is usually based on the need to reduce and maintain minimal counts of resident organisms and to mechanically remove transient organisms such as *Pseudomonas, E. coli, Salmonella,* or *Shigella*.

When working with people who are infected with drug-resistant,[349] gram-positive cocci such as MRSA or vancomycin-resistant enterococci, antimicrobial soap may be recommended because some studies show that these organisms persist on hands until an antimicrobial product is used.[146,348] In 2014, Yokoe and colleagues[426] rated strategies to prevent HAI based on the quality of the evidence. Most strategies including hand hygiene were rated medium to low, with universal decolonization of ICUs having a high level of evidence in preventing MRSA infections.

Some questions have been raised regarding isolation procedures for methicillin- or vancomycin-resistant clients who have been discharged from an isolation setting as an inpatient but are now returning to therapy as an outpatient. A study by Kim and associates[196] reported multidrug-resistant organisms on equipment such as tables, ultrasound transducer heads, hot packs, and therapeutic balls in physical therapy clinics, indicating the importance of environmental cleaning between clients. Therefore outpatient therapists should be aware of environmental cleaning requirements to prevent risk of transmission. Anyone with an active, resistant infection should not be discharged from an inpatient setting. However, if such a case is encountered, the therapist must remember that these organisms are spread by contact. Symptoms may improve, but the patient is still colonized for days to months, placing the caregiver and others at risk. Therefore the same germicidal cleaning measures used in a hospital or institutional setting are required. The CDC has published several guidelines for outpatient settings.[48,321,349]

All equipment that comes in direct contact[338] with a draining area needs to be cleaned with an approved germicidal before and after use. Isolation (e.g., private room or separate area of the gym or clinic) is not required. The American Physical Therapy Association (APTA) directs physical therapists to the CDC for guidelines on environmental cleaning, including outpatient settings,[9] hydrotherapy, and aquatic programs. The recommendations state that clients with MRSA may attend therapy programs provided that the area of colonization can be contained. If it is in a wound, the drainage must be contained within the dressing without evidence of breakthrough.

### Streptococcal Infections

Streptococci are gram-positive bacteria (take up crystal-violet stain) in pairs or chains. They are classified by their colony morphology, their ability to cause hemolysis, biochemical reactions (they do not have the enzyme catalase), and their serologic characteristics. Streptococci are divided into groups depending on their ability to cause hemolysis: (1) β-hemolytic streptococci cause complete hemolysis, (2) α-hemolytic streptococci cause incomplete hemolysis, and (3) γ-hemolytic streptococci cause no hemolysis. They are also classified from A to V by the antigens they present in their cell wall. Only group A has virulence factors that allow for significant invasive disease.

**Group A Streptococci.** *Streptococcus pyogenes,* the prototype of GAS, is one of the most common bacterial pathogens of humans of any age. It causes many diseases of diverse organ systems, ranging from skin infections to acute self-limited pharyngitis to postinfectious syndromes of rheumatic fever and poststreptococcal glomerulonephritis (Box 8.7).

GAS is typically transmitted via contact with respiratory droplets, although other, less common mechanisms have been identified, such as foodborne transmission. In health care settings, personnel may spread GAS after contact with clients who have infected secretions or may become infected themselves. The infected person can subsequently develop a variety of GAS-related illnesses (e.g., toxic shock–like syndrome, cellulitis, and pharyngitis).

HCWs who are GAS carriers have infrequently been linked to sporadic outbreaks of SSI, postpartum infection, or burn wound infection and to foodborne transmission of GAS causing pharyngitis. Adherence to Standard Precautions or other Transmission-Based Precautions can prevent health care–associated transmission of GAS to personnel. Restriction from client care activities and food handling is indicated for personnel with GAS (see Table 8.5).

Signs, symptoms, and complications of GAS depend on the location of the infection.

**Streptococcal Pharyngitis.** Streptococcal pharyngitis, commonly known as *strep throat,* occurs most commonly in children accounting for 15% to 30% of all sore throats in children and occurs in only 5% to 15% of adults.[205,347] The infection occurs most commonly from October to April in children ages 5 to 10 years, but a recent increase has occurred among adults ages 30 to 50 years. This organism often colonizes in throats of people with no symptoms; up to 20% of schoolchildren may be carriers.[342] Symptoms usually have an abrupt onset.

Diagnosis is made through physical examination and laboratory testing.[347] Although many criteria have been developed to aid in the decision to test for GAS, none have specificity or sensitivity in children. However, if a child (typically school age) has the following symptoms without typical viral symptoms, their likelihood of having GAS increases to greater than 50%: (1) scarlatiniform rash, (2) palatal petechiae, (3) tonsillar enlargement, (4) vomiting, and (5) tender cervical nodes.[343] Affected children may have symptoms too mild for diagnosis. Children younger than age 3 years rarely develop acute rheumatic fever and uncommonly develop GAS pharyngitis except if they have older siblings who are concomitantly infected. These children often have atypical symptoms (e.g., nasal congestion, low-grade fever). The Centor criteria were developed to aid in the diagnosis of GAS for adults and include (1) fever, (2) absence of cough, (3) tonsillar exudates, and (4) tender anterior

Box 8.7

**STREPTOCOCCAL INFECTIONS**

**Streptococcus pyogenes *(Group A Streptococci)***

*Suppurative*

- Streptococcal pharyngitis
- Scarlet fever (scarlatina)
- Impetigo (streptococcal pyoderma)
- Streptococcal gangrene (necrotizing fasciitis)
- Streptococcal cellulitis
- Streptococcal myositis
- Puerperal sepsis (following vaginal delivery or abortion)
- Toxic shock syndrome
- Pneumonia (rare)

*Nonsuppurative*

- Rheumatic fever
- Acute poststreptococcal glomerulonephritis

**Streptococcus agalactiae *(Group B Streptococci)***

- Neonatal streptococcal infections
- Adult group B streptococcal infection

***Streptococcus pneumoniae***

- Pneumococcal pneumonia
- Otitis media
- Meningitis
- Endocarditis

cervical lymphadenopathy. However, similar to children, the positive predictive value is low, and the criteria are more helpful in determining people who do not have GAS. Clients who exhibit fewer than three of the Centor criteria most likely do not have GAS and do not require further testing. Clients who have three or more criteria should be tested for GAS.[124]

Diagnosis is usually by rapid antigen detection test (RADT), which has a specificity of greater than 95% and sensitivity of 85% to 95%. Negative RADTs in children should be followed with a throat culture, although adults do not routinely need a throat culture for a negative RADT. RADT is unable to distinguish between active streptococcal infection and people who carry streptococci and are infected with a virus. Molecular assays (polymerase chain reaction [PCR]–based) are also available with high sensitivity and specificity, but they are not universally available, and the cost is higher. Treatment is with antibiotics to avoid poststreptococcal syndromes. A positive test for *Streptococcus* should be obtained before treatment to avoid overuse of antibiotics.

Complications have been significantly reduced with the advent of antibiotics but may include otitis media, sinusitis, peritonsillar or retropharyngeal abscess, necrotizing fasciitis (NF), bacteremia, endocarditis, meningitis, pneumonia, and osteomyelitis. Poststreptococcal sequelae include acute rheumatic fever, acute glomerulonephritis, reactive arthritis, and pediatric autoimmune neuropsychiatric disorders associated with streptococcus.

**Scarlet Fever.** Scarlet fever usually follows untreated streptococcal pharyngitis but may also occur after wound infections. It is a delayed-type skin reactivity to the pyrogenic exotoxins produced by S. *pyogenes* and is most common in children ages 2 to 10 years. *S. pyogenes* is acquired by inhalation or direct contact with oral secretions.

Scarlet fever manifests with sore throat, fever, strawberry tongue (white-coated tongue with prominent red papillae), and a fine erythematous rash that blanches on pressure and has been described as feeling like sandpaper. The white coat on the tongue disappears, leaving a red, "beefy" tongue. The rash first appears on the groin and armpits then quickly spreads to the trunk and then to the extremities, sparing the soles and palms. The rash fades over a week, and after 6 to 9 days there is a general desquamation of the skin, which can last for weeks. Because of the availability of antibiotics, severe disease and complications are rarely seen. Complications and disease may include high fever, hypotension, arthritis, and jaundice. Rare poststreptococcal complications are acute rheumatic fever and acute poststreptococcal glomerulonephritis.

**Impetigo.** Impetigo is included here so the reader may appreciate that it is principally caused by GAS, although other streptococcal or staphylococcal species may be involved. See Chapter 10 for a complete discussion of this condition. Colonization with GAS most often precedes the skin lesions, so good hygiene is essential.

**Streptococcal Cellulitis.** Streptococcal cellulitis, an acute spreading inflammation of the deep dermis and subcutaneous tissues, usually results from infection of burns, wounds, or other breaks in the skin, although in some cases no entry site is noted. *Streptococcus* is the most common cause of cellulitis, typically from GAS or *S. pyogenes*. Recurrent episodes of cellulitis may occur in extremities in which lymphatic drainage has been impaired (e.g., post–axillary node dissection, site of saphenous vein harvest) or chronic fungal infections (particularly of the feet) serve as a reservoir.

The skin is painful, warm, and swollen with accompanying erythema. Superficial bullae may form. Systemic symptoms such as fever and chills are often associated with the skin infection. Cellulitis can rapidly spread or involve bacteremia or lymphangitis. Lymphangitis is readily recognized by the presence of red, tender, linear streaks directed toward enlarged, tender regional lymph nodes. It is accompanied by systemic symptoms such as chills, fever, malaise, and headache (see Cellulitis in Chapter 10 and Lymphangitis in Chapter 13). Other complications include endocarditis, osteomyelitis, sepsis, and toxic shock syndrome.[303]

**Erysipelas.** This skin infection is a type of cellulitis typically seen in young children or older adults. It is caused by GAS and involves the upper dermis and superficial lymphatics. The skin is painful, very red, shiny, and swollen in appearance (Fig. 8.3) (elevated above the surrounding normal skin). This type of cellulitis develops

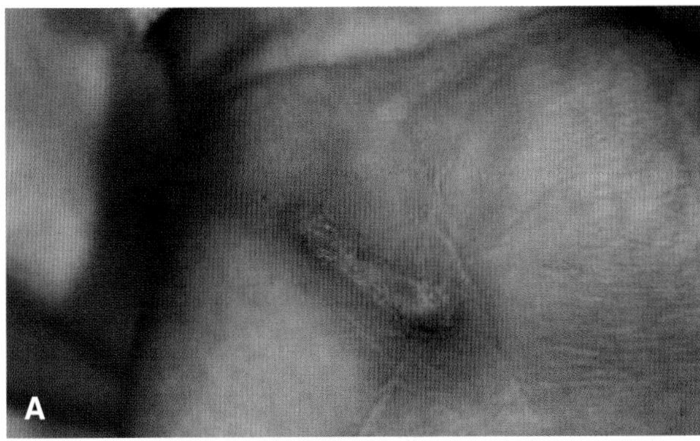


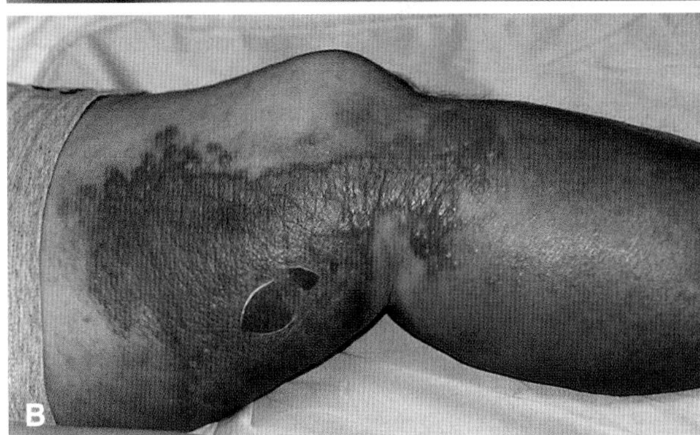


**Figure 8.3**

**Cellulitis and lymphangitis.** (A) Infection in a wound is usually caused by streptococcal bacteria but often in combination with *Staphylococcus*. Infection can be local without streaking (cellulitis), local infection with streaking toward the heart (lymphangitis or blood poisoning), or pus forming (boil or abscess). This boy stuck a needle into a burn blister on his palm the previous day. Note the redness and the streaking. B, Erysipelas, a type of cellulitis, is more of a clinical diagnosis describing an infectious skin condition characterized by sharp, elevated, demarcated borders; redness; swelling; vesicles; bullae; fever; pain; and lymphadenopathy. Erysipelas affects the face and legs most often. It is almost always caused by group A streptococci, but can be caused by *Staphylococcus*. (A, Courtesy Bruce Argyle, Utah Mountain Biking, http://www.utahmountainbiking.com/firstaid/infect.htm. B, From Black JM, Hawks JH: *Medical-surgical nursing: clinical management for positive outcomes*, ed 7, Philadelphia, 2006, Saunders.)

over a few hours; vesicles and bullae may form in the affected areas after 2 to 3 days. Severely infected skin may have petechiae and bruising; unlike cellulitis, erysipelas is nonpurulent. The margins between normal and infected skin are well demarcated. Systemic symptoms such as fever, chills, malaise, and headache are common.

The most common area affected is the legs (almost always unilateral), followed by the face, although erysipelas can occur anywhere. Antibiotics that cover GAS are the treatment of choice but may need to be broadened to include staphylococcal species.

**Streptococcal Toxic Shock Syndrome.** Streptococcal toxic shock syndrome (STSS) is any invasive streptococcal infection that leads to shock and organ failure, although most are GAS (yet most GAS are not invasive). Streptococcal species involved in STSS typically carry virulence factors, allowing for aggressive, penetrating behavior.[85] Most cases are sporadic, although reports of transmission from equipment or another infected person have been published.[22] It may occur in persons of any age, and most are healthy individuals.

STSS is a complication of many subtypes of invasive streptococcal infections such as streptococcal NF, postpartum infection, and joint infection. *Streptococcus* enters the body via the vagina, pharynx, mucosa, and skin (trauma) or during a surgical procedure, although a source is not identified in many cases. Viruses such as varicella and influenza provide a means for *Streptococcus* to enter the skin. *Streptococcus* pharyngitis rarely leads to STSS.

Once the microbe has entered the body, it may be able to penetrate into deeper tissue and the bloodstream secondary to an existing injury or wound or invade intact tissue. Superantigenic pyrogenic exotoxins (such as NADase) are produced, activating the immune system and causing the release of large amounts of inflammatory cytokines. This leads to capillary leak, tissue damage and shock, and organ failure.

Initial symptoms (24 to 48 hours) may resemble influenza including fever, chills, myalgias, nausea, and vomiting. For individuals who subsequently develop NF, pain is typically the first symptom. Systemic symptoms include tachycardia, persistent fever, and tachypnea; these symptoms are followed by sudden shock exhibited by hypotension (often unresponsive to aggressive therapy), delirium, and evidence of organ failure (i.e., renal and liver impairment, coagulopathy, respiratory distress syndrome). Treatment consists of locating the source of the infection, surgical débridement, supportive measures, and IV antibiotics.

**Streptococcal Necrotizing Fasciitis.** NF (also called necrotizing soft tissue infections) is a rare but serious infection that is typically caused by either polymicrobial (type I) or monomicrobial (type II) infections. Most monomicrobial infections are due to GAS. Type II infections can occur in people of any age and without any underlying illness. NF progresses rapidly along fascial planes, usually in the legs, causing severe tissue damage secondary to virulence factors as it spreads and destroys whatever soft tissue is in its path (fat, muscle, nerves, connective tissue).

NF can occur following a serious injury or in a surgical wound, but also with something as simple as a rug burn, punch on the arm, paper cut, insect bite, or muscle strain. NF is a rare but serious complication of chickenpox lesions and should be suspected in children with progressive pain, fever, and lethargy.[412]

NF may be difficult to diagnose initially. Pain (usually disproportionate to the appearance) and fever are present, but the overlying skin often is without abnormalities. In approximately 50% of all type II NF cases, a precipitating lesion is not found, and NF most likely results from hematogenous spread or blunt trauma.[370]

The infection spreads rapidly (within hours), causing edema and tenderness. Changes later occur in the skin as thrombosis of blood vessels occurs. Loss of sensation due to damage of superficial nerves may be a clue to ongoing destruction. The skin turns a dark red color with accompanying induration. Between 3 and 5 days, bullae form and fill with dark fluid. Later the skin becomes friable and turns a maroon or black color consistent with ischemia.[370]

Affected individuals commonly experience toxic shock syndrome with hypotension, nausea, vomiting, and delirium. There is often renal and hepatic compromise as well as pulmonary infiltrates, leading to respiratory distress. Mortality rate is high, with 14% to 34% of persons with a type II NF infection dying.[270] The mortality rate is highest among blacks, Hispanics, American Indians, and people with comorbidities of diabetes mellitus and obesity.[13]

Immediate surgery with aggressive débridement of all necrotic tissue along with appropriate broad-spectrum IV antibiotics is essential to save muscles and limbs. Gram stain and culture of the site is essential to identify the organism and antimicrobial susceptibility. Multiple procedures and serial débridement may be necessary with secondary closure, as the demarcation line of infection is difficult to identify.[369]

**Streptococcal Necrotizing Myositis.** Streptococcal necrotizing myositis is a rare but potentially life-threatening entity characterized by severe pain and inflammation in the infected muscle with few abnormalities of overlying skin. Typically blunt, nonpenetrating trauma or hematologic seeding of bacteria to the muscle leads to the infection.[304] Most often, one muscle group is affected, usually in the lower extremity. Streptococcal necrotizing myositis is fulminant with systemic symptoms, STSS, high fever, bacteremia, and a high mortality rate (80%).[373]

Clinical features of myositis and NF often overlap and are distinguished at surgery and by biopsy.[3] Therapy includes aggressive surgical débridement and IV antibiotics (see Myositis in Chapter 25 and Streptococcal Necrotizing Fasciitis earlier in this chapter).

**Puerperal Sepsis.** Puerperal sepsis follows abortion or normal delivery when streptococci colonizing the woman or transmitted from medical personnel invade the endometrium and surrounding structures, lymphatics, and bloodstream.[358] Women present with fever and abdominal pain; hypotension may develop as a sign of STSS. The resulting endometritis and septicemia may be complicated by pelvic cellulitis, septic pelvic thrombophlebitis, peritonitis, or pelvic abscess. Before the antibiotic era and the benefits of handwashing between clients were known, this disease was more common and associated with a high mortality rate.

SPECIAL IMPLICATIONS FOR THE THERAPIST 8.4

*Streptococcal Infections*

Health care personnel can transmit and acquire streptococcal infections. Guidelines for preventing transmission must be followed at all times (see Boxes 8.4 and 8.5).

**Group B Streptococci.** Group B streptococci (GBS), the most common being *Streptococcus agalactiae,* are implicated in infections in pregnant women, neonates, and nonpregnant adults. GBS colonize the GI and vaginal tracts of up to 40% of pregnant women.[308] The bacteria can then be transmitted during labor to the neonate by spreading up into the amniotic fluid with the rupture of membranes (or sometimes with intact membranes) or as the neonate moves through the birth canal. In an effort to decrease the number of neonatal GBS infections, guidelines were established in 2002 and updated in 2010 for universal screening at 35 to 37 weeks of gestation for maternal GBS colonization.[398] Women with positive cultures are given prophylactic intrapartum antibiotics. A vaccine is under development that would reduce the number of women and infants exposed to antibiotics.[221] GBS can cause peripartum infections in women, such as bacteremia, puerperal sepsis, urinary tract infections, and upper genital tract infections including endometritis or chorioamnionitis. Rarely, resulting bacteremia can lead to endocarditis or meningitis. Appropriate antibiotics are required for treatment.

GBS is the leading cause of neonatal pneumonia, meningitis, and sepsis. The incidence of early-onset disease has decreased over the last decade as a result of universal screening of pregnant women and intrapartum antibiotic prophylaxis.[69,115,289] Neonatal GBS continues to occur and has plateaued.[302] About 50% of cases involve preterm neonates,[396] who have a higher mortality than term neonates.[67]

Neonates who develop early-onset infections (birth to 1 week) present with hypotension, pneumonia (and respiratory distress), bacteremia, or meningitis. Symptoms typically occur within the first 24 hours of birth. Late-onset disease (1 week to 3 months) is acquired either at birth or from contact with the infected mother or other personnel. These neonates demonstrate fever, bacteremia, and meningitis; they are less likely to develop shock compared with neonates with early-onset disease.

Owing to the decreased incidence of GBS in neonates and pregnant women, adults (men and nonpregnant women) now comprise the majority of cases (approximately three-quarters) of GBS infections.[352] Risks for developing GBS infections are most noted in elderly adults and residents of nursing facilities and clients with HIV, obesity, or a chronic disease such as diabetes.[116,168,289,294]

The most common infections in adults are skin and soft tissue infections, primary bacteremia, and pneumonia. Other infections include urinary tract infections, upper respiratory tract infections, septic arthritis, osteomyelitis, endocarditis, and meningitis. Adults are more likely to die of GBS infections than neonates, with a mortality rate between 15% and 38% depending on the location of the infection.[281,332] Mortality increases with age and presence of underlying disease.[116]

Box 8.8

**RISK FACTORS FOR PNEUMOCOCCAL DISEASE**

Age
- Children aged younger than 2 years
- Adults aged 65 years or older

Recent episode of influenza or viral respiratory infection
Chronic illness
- Diabetes mellitus
- Heart disease
- Pulmonary disease
- Renal disease
- Liver disease

Immunosuppression/unable to make antibodies
- HIV
- Multiple myeloma
- Leukemia
- Lymphoma
- Hodgkin disease
- Transplant recipients
- Chronic use of corticosteroids

Smoking
Neurologic impairment (cerebrospinal fluid leak)
History of alcoholism
Asplenia (absent, removed, or nonfunctioning spleen)
Crowding or close contact with infected persons (shelters, nursing homes, prisons, military camps, daycare centers)

**Streptococcus pneumoniae**

***Etiologic and Risk Factors.*** *Streptococcus pneumoniae* can colonize the upper respiratory tract and nasopharynx and lead to both invasive disease (i.e., meningitis and bacteremia) and noninvasive disease (i.e., pneumonia, otitis media, and sinusitis). When *S. pneumoniae* causes pneumonia, it is often referred to as pneumococcal pneumonia. Transmission from person to person is by direct contact or inhalation of droplets of respiratory secretions. Children younger than 2 years of age, adults older than 65 years, and people with underlying medical conditions have the highest risk of developing an invasive *S. pneumoniae* infection.[210,259] Pneumococcal pneumonia often follows influenza or viral respiratory infections.[37] *S. pneumoniae* is the most common cause of meningitis in adults, infants, and toddlers. Head trauma, cerebrospinal fluid leaks, otitis media, and sinusitis may precede pneumococcal meningitis, creating an extension of disease or opportunity for direct infection. Pneumonia may lead to bacteremia with subsequent seeding of the meninges (Box 8.8). As a result of the availability of vaccines (see Medical Management), the morbidity and mortality caused by this organism are significantly reduced.[147,254] However, it continues to be responsible for greater than 800,000 deaths worldwide in children younger than age 5 years.[279] In the United States, *S. pneumoniae* causes more than 500,000 cases of pneumonia and more than 30,000 cases of invasive disease, with about 3500 deaths.[57,66,123]

*Clinical Manifestations.* *S. pneumoniae* continues to be one of the most common causes for community-acquired pneumonia.[262] Clinical manifestations of pneumonia include acute onset of fever, chills, pleuritis with pleuritic chest pain, and dyspnea. A productive cough or purulent sputum that may be blood tinged is typically present. Because pneumococcal disease occurs most commonly in the very young and the very old, the presenting features will vary. Older adults may have only a slight cough or delirium but lack a fever or elevated white blood count. An elevated respiratory rate is frequently present. Increased morbidity and mortality are associated with a lack of fever and hypothermia. Complications from pneumococcal pneumonia may include empyema (approximately 5% to 12% of cases),[38] bacteremia, sepsis, or meningitis.

The most common severe complication of pneumococcal bacteremia is meningitis. Infection of the meninges (meningitis) stimulates a robust inflammation, leading to increased intracranial pressure and brain edema with headache and nausea/vomiting, mental status changes, stiff neck, and fever. The disease progresses rapidly over 24 to 48 hours, and mortality rates are 20% to 30%, even with appropriate treatment.[333] Rare complications of *S. pneumoniae* include pericarditis, endocarditis, peritonitis, and septic arthritis.

## MEDICAL MANAGEMENT

**DIAGNOSIS, TREATMENT, AND PREVENTION.** Diagnosis of pneumococcal disease is by laboratory examination of sputum (pneumonia), cerebrospinal fluid (meningitis), or blood (bacteremia) with Gram stain and culture of the organism. Up to 20% to 25% of blood cultures are positive in clients with pneumococcal pneumonia.[324] For rapid detection, the urine can be tested for pneumococcal urinary antigens, which are positive in 87% of people with pneumococcal bacteremia and 64% in persons without bacteremia.[156,355] Chest x-ray and chest computed tomography identify location and extent of pneumonia. Treatment is with antibiotics that are effective against local pneumococcal strains and takes into consideration resistance patterns in the community.

Immunization for pneumococcal disease is available and is recommended in specific circumstances as defined by the CDC. In 2010 a 13-valent pneumococcal polysaccharide conjugate vaccine (PCV13) became available for young children and infants.[278] This vaccine also eliminates colonization of the nasopharynx of serotypes included in the vaccine, thereby reducing the spreading of *S. pneumoniae* to others (the herd effect). Currently the 23-valent pneumococcal polysaccharide vaccine (PPSV23) is available for adults and is not recommended for children younger than 2 years of age.[389] PPSV23 is recommended for adults with heart disease, lung disease, liver disease, alcohol use disorder, and diabetes mellitus and for smokers. Both PCV13 and PPSV23 should be administered sequentially (PCV13 before PPSV23) to all adults age 65 years and older and to individuals 19 to 64 years old with defined conditions, such as immunocompromise, HIV, asplenia, chronic renal failure, nephrotic syndrome, malignancy, cochlear implant, or cerebrospinal fluid leak.[77,389] With the introduction and implementation of vaccine programs, rates for hospitalization and clinic visits for infections relating to *S. pneumoniae* have significantly decreased.[278]

Overall, the rate of antibiotic-resistant invasive pneumococcal infections has decreased for all ages[184] with the expanded valence vaccines (more serotypes are covered). Prudent use of antibiotics will aid in decreasing the presence of drug-resistant species.

### Clostridial Myonecrosis (Gas Gangrene)

*Definition and Overview.* Clostridial myonecrosis is a severe, life-threatening muscle infection caused by anaerobic bacteria, typically from the genus *Clostridium,* that progressively invade healthy tissue and cause muscle destruction. Clostridial myonecrosis may develop from trauma or spontaneously. Trauma-related gas gangrene (70% of gas gangrene cases) is most often caused by *Clostridium perfringens,* whereas spontaneous gas gangrene is frequently due to *Clostridium septicum*. Deep, penetrating trauma, such as seen with knife or gunshot wounds or with crushing injuries, not only introduces the bacteria into the wound but also disrupts the vascular supply, producing an anaerobic environment that is optimal for the proliferation of *C. perfringens. C. perfringens* accounts for 80% of trauma-related gas gangrene.[4] Clostridial gas gangrene is also associated with abortion, intrauterine fetal demise, prolonged rupture of membranes, retained placenta, bowel or biliary tract surgery, and compound fractures.

Spontaneous clostridial myonecrosis usually occurs secondary to hematogenous spread from the GI tract (seen in persons with malignancy or intestinal tract abnormalities).[372] In contrast to *C. perfringens, C. septicum* does not require anaerobic conditions to proliferate. The GI tract allows the bacteria to enter the bloodstream and seed healthy muscle.

*Pathogenesis.* Both *C. perfringens* and *C. septicum* produce toxins that facilitate the destruction of healthy muscle tissue. *C. perfringens* produces alpha and theta toxins, although the alpha toxin is primarily responsible for tissue necrosis. Alpha toxin leads to the aggregation of platelets and the adherence of polymorphonuclear neutrophils (PMNs) to endovascular cells, causing occlusion and thrombosis of blood vessels, further reducing blood supply to the injured area. PMNs are also prevented from entering the infected site, creating the characteristic lack of pus or inflammation in the necrotic muscle. The few PMNs that are able to cross into the infected tissue are destroyed by both alpha and theta toxins. Alpha toxin suppresses myocardial activity, while theta toxin reduces vascular resistance, leading to hypotension and shock.

*C. septicum* produces multiple toxins, including alpha, beta, gamma, and delta toxins. In contrast to the alpha toxin for *C. perfringens,* the mechanism for the alpha toxin produced by *C. septicum* is unknown.

*Clinical Manifestations.* The incubation period for *Clostridium* averages 24 hours (range from 6 hours to 3 days). Sudden, severe pain (often out of proportion to examination findings) occurring at the site of the wound is an early symptom of gas gangrene. The pain is thought to be secondary to ischemia produced by the bacteria toxins. The area is tender and edematous. The skin darkens because of hemorrhage and cutaneous necrosis. The lesion develops a thick discharge with a foul odor and may contain gas bubbles. Crepitation may be felt on palpation of the skin from the gas bubbles in muscles and subcutaneous tissue and when present is the most specific sign.

True gas gangrene produces myositis and anaerobic cellulitis, affecting only soft tissue. The skin over the wound may rupture, revealing dark red or black necrotic muscle tissue accompanied by a foul-smelling watery or frothy discharge. Associated symptoms may include fever, sweating, and disproportionate tachycardia followed by hemolytic anemia (from toxins), septic shock, liver necrosis, and renal failure (caused by hypotension, myoglobinuria, and hemoglobinuria). Details on any of these conditions can be found in individual chapters (see Index).

## MEDICAL MANAGEMENT

**DIAGNOSIS, TREATMENT, AND PROGNOSIS.** Radiographs may demonstrate evidence of gas formation, although gas may not be seen in early stages, whereas computed tomography or magnetic resonance imaging may show infection along fascial planes. Diagnosis is made through demonstration of the characteristic gram-positive rods. These bacteria can be detected and cultured from blood or tissue. If a Gram stain is performed directly from tissue, the organism may appear both gram-positive and gram-negative. If localized in the blood or culture media from tissue, it will stain as gram-positive. Biopsy of necrotic muscle tissue microscopically shows muscle that is devoid of inflammatory cells, and during surgical evaluation, the muscle does not bleed.

Early, immediate intervention is necessary (diagnostic tests should not delay surgery) with surgical débridement and excision of necrotic tissue. Delay of more than 12 hours is associated with an increase in mortality.[4] Broad-spectrum antibiotics are administered (until specific culture and sensitivities are available), but if significant gangrene develops, amputation may be necessary. Hyperbaric oxygen therapy following surgery is controversial. Mortality can be very high, often depending on the location of the infection (extremities are easier to débride than the trunk or internal organs). People who present with shock have the highest mortality, ranging up to 40%.[189,204,369,371]

### SPECIAL IMPLICATIONS FOR THE THERAPIST 8.5

### *Gas Gangrene*

Careful observation may result in early diagnosis. With any postoperative or posttraumatic injury, look for signs of ischemia such as cool skin, pallor or cyanosis, sudden severe pain, sudden edema, and loss of pulses in the involved limb. Record carefully and immediately report these findings to the medical staff because this is a serious infection that may lead to amputation of a limb or death. Throughout this illness, adequate fluid replacement is essential as well as assessing pulmonary and cardiac functions often. The primary treatments for gas gangrene include débridement and antibiotics. Although there is limited high-quality evidence, additional treatments may include hyperbaric oxygen therapy.[422]

Special care to prevent skin breakdown is important, and meticulous wound care following surgery is imperative. To prevent gas gangrene, routinely take precautions to render all wound sites unsuitable for growth of *Clostridia* by attempting to keep granulation tissue viable; adequate débridement is imperative to reduce anaerobic growth conditions. Notify the physician immediately of any devitalized tissue. Position the client to facilitate drainage.

Psychologic support is critical, as these clients can remain alert until death, knowing that death is imminent and unavoidable. The therapist must be prepared for the foul odor from the wound and prepare the client emotionally for the large wound after surgical excision. Wound care may require sterile procedures to prevent spread of bacteria. It is important to be aware of facility policies when disposing of drainage material and dressings in single leak-resistant plastic bags of adequate tensile strength and using hypochlorite-based products for disinfecting the environmental surface.[338] No special cleaning measures are required after the client is discharged.

### Pseudomonas

**Overview.** *P. aeruginosa* is a major opportunistic pathogen and one of the most common hospital-acquired (particularly ICU) and nursing home–acquired pathogens. *Pseudomonas* is uncommon in community-acquired infections and healthy individuals but can manifest as a skin rash or ear infection in children after exposure to inadequately chlorinated pools and hot tubs.[153] The organism is ubiquitous in nature and infrequently colonizes humans (upper respiratory tract), but it can cause disease, particularly in the hospital environment, where it is associated with pneumonia,[134] wound infections, urinary tract infection, and bacteremia/sepsis in individuals who are immunocompromised.

Burns, urinary catheterization, cystic fibrosis, chronic lung diseases, ventilator use, neutropenia associated with chemotherapy, and diabetes all predispose to infections with *P. aeruginosa*.[409] It thrives on moist environmental surfaces, making swimming pools, whirlpool tubs, respiratory therapy equipment, sinks, flowers, endoscopes, bronchoscopes, and cleaning solutions prime targets for growth.[134]

This organism produces several virulence factors and is intrinsically antibiotic resistant. Spread of the organism in a health care setting is by contact, typically from a reservoir as described earlier. HCWs have been known to pass the organism on their hands or under fingernails.[29]

**Pathogenesis.** *P. aeruginosa* is a versatile bacterium that relies on complex signaling pathways and release of toxins to produce acute or chronic disease or simply colonize a tissue. *P. aeruginosa* produces an array of proteins, which allow it to attach to, invade, and destroy host tissues while avoiding host inflammatory and immune defenses. Injury to epithelial cells uncovers surface molecules that serve as binding sites for *P. aeruginosa*. The organism releases extracellular enzymes or toxins, which facilitate tissue invasion and are partially responsible for the necrotizing lesions associated with *Pseudomonas* infections. This pathogen can also invade blood vessel walls and produce systemic pathologic effects through endotoxin and several systemically active exotoxins.[118]

Successful colonization with evasion of host immunologic defenses may be due to the ability of the organism to downregulate the production of toxins and selection for bacteria without genes for flagellum or pili, which are highly immunogenic. Many strains of this pathogen produce a proteoglycan that surrounds the bacteria (i.e., a biofilm), protecting them from mucociliary action, complement, and phagocytes.[240,242]

**Clinical Manifestations.** Signs and symptoms of *Pseudomonas* infection vary with the site of infection and the state of host defenses. If the host has the capacity to respond to the invading bacteria with neutrophils, an acute inflammatory response results.

The *Pseudomonas* organism often invades small arteries and veins, producing vascular thrombosis and hemorrhagic necrosis, particularly in the lungs and skin. Blood vessel invasion predisposes to bacteremia, dissemination, and sepsis. This bacterium causes infections of the respiratory tract (pneumonia), bloodstream, CNS, skin (Fig. 8.4) and soft tissues, bone and joints, and other parts of the body.

***Respiratory Tract Infections.*** Pneumonia caused by *P. aeruginosa* is one of the most common causes of health care–acquired pneumonia.[134] Of all sites that may become infected with *P. aeruginosa,* lung infections with associated bacteremia carry the highest mortality.[134] Lung infections occur as three principle syndromes: (1) in persons with chronic lung disease such as cystic fibrosis or chronic obstructive pulmonary disease; (2) hospital-acquired, typically in the ICU and ventilator-associated[405]; and (3) secondary to a bacteremia that spread to the lungs,[209] often seen in neutropenic individuals.[134] With the advent of antiretroviral therapy (ART) for the treatment of HIV, pneumonia caused by *P. aeruginosa* in people with HIV has significantly decreased.[280,376]

The signs and symptoms of pneumonia caused by *Pseudomonas* are typical of pneumonias seen with other organisms, such as dyspnea, fever, productive purulent cough, low oxygenation, elevated white cell count, and delirium. Clients on ventilator support may experience reduced performance, necessitating higher oxygenation requirements and ventilator settings. In the lungs, infection with *P. aeruginosa* causes necrosis of tissue and hemorrhaging. Radiographic features are variable and similar to other causes of pneumonia. Diagnosis may be challenging, as most blood cultures (except in clients with concomitant bacteremia) are negative. Patients with endotracheal tubes and clients with underlying chronic lung disease can also be colonized without a true infection, adding to the diagnostic difficulty. Isolation of the organism, either blood or sputum culture, makes the diagnosis. Bronchoalveolar lavage is most sensitive for the diagnosis.[391]

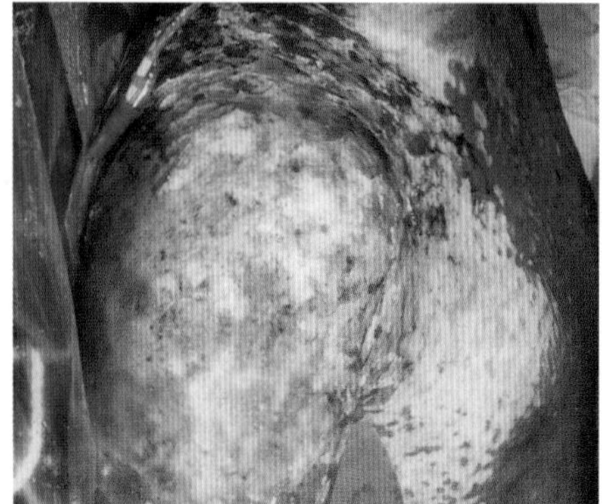

**Figure 8.4**

***Pseudomonas.*** Blue-green color in a burn wound indicates infection by *P. aeruginosa.* (Reprinted from Gould BE: *Pathophysiology for the health professions*, ed 3, Philadelphia, 2006, Saunders, courtesy Judy Knighton, Ross Tilley Burn Center, Sunnybrook and Women's College Health Center, Toronto, Ontario, Canada.)

Although on the decline,[88] *P aeruginosa* is the most common organism isolated in adults with cystic fibrosis.[326] It is also the most common cause of respiratory failure and a majority of deaths.[220] *P. aeruginosa* is acquired in early childhood in children with cystic fibrosis. Initially the *P. aeruginosa* does not produce a mucoid (exopolysaccharide/alginate) protection and is susceptible to antibiotics and phagocytosis. However, with time, strains mutate and are able to create a mucoid barrier, which is not as amenable to antibiotics or the host's immune system. Over time there is chronic progression of symptoms with acute exacerbations of disease. Clients typically experience mucous plugging and airway inflammation that leads to a chronic inflammatory reaction with lung damage and fibrosis. Current efforts are underway to eradicate the organism early before the mucoid phase.[255]

***Bacteremia.*** *Pseudomonas* bacteremia typically occurs in persons with significant underlying conditions (approximately 90%) such as cancer, diabetes, renal failure, congestive heart failure, immune system deficiencies, or posttransplant. It is an important cause of serious, life-threatening bloodstream infections in clients with neutropenia and burns. *P. aeruginosa* bacteremia is usually acquired in the hospital and may be primary (no identifiable source, which occurs in 40% of cases)[382] or secondary to a focal infected site (e.g., skin, lungs, pancreatobiliary tract, intravascular source, indwelling catheters, GI or urinary tracts).[20,399]

As with other *Pseudomonas* infections, bacteremia is rapidly progressive without treatment, with high morbidity and mortality rates. Clients experience fever, tachypnea, tachycardia, hypotension, and delirium, which can lead to renal failure, acute respiratory distress syndrome, and death. Rarely characteristic lesions of *Pseudomonas* bacteremia, *ecthyma gangrenosum,* develop on the skin. These vesicles form following perivascular invasion of arteries and veins and are initially hemorrhagic with progressive necrosis and ulceration. They occur as single lesions or in small groups. Endocarditis from *P. aeruginosa* is uncommon, but when it occurs, it is most often secondary to IV drug use and/or prosthetic heart valves or pacemakers. The tricuspid valve is typically involved if IV drug use is the source of the bacteria, and endocarditis manifests with symptoms related to infective emboli to the lungs such as coughing (may have hemoptysis), fever, tachypnea, and chest pain.

***Central Nervous System Infections.*** *Pseudomonas* infections of the CNS including meningitis or abscess formation in or around the brain are rare and typically involve people with serious underlying illness. Infection may result from extension from a contiguous structure such as the ear, mastoid, or paranasal sinus; direct inoculation into the subarachnoid space or brain by means of head trauma or neurosurgical procedures (intraventricular shunts); or bacteremic spread from a distant site of infection such as the urinary tract, lung, or endocardium.

The clinical manifestations of *Pseudomonas* meningitis are similar to manifestations of other forms of bacterial meningitis (see Chapter 29) such as fever, headache, stiff neck, nausea, and confusion. The onset of disease may be acute and occur suddenly or may be more gradual and insidious. Symptoms of a brain abscess vary depending on the location but often include headache, mental status changes, fever, seizures, nausea/vomiting (from increased pressure), muscle weakness, and dysarthria.

***Skin and Soft Tissue Infections.*** *Pseudomonas* disease of the skin and mucous membranes can result from primary or metastatic foci of infections. Common predisposing factors for primary skin and soft tissue infections are a breakdown in the integument, especially resulting from surgery, burns, trauma, and pressure injuries; whirlpool use; and chemotherapy-induced neutropenia. *P. aeruginosa* is the most common organism isolated in infections from piercing through cartilage.[357]

The wound is hemorrhagic and necrotic but rarely has the characteristic fruity odor (sweet, grapelike odor) with a blue-green exudate that forms a crust on wounds (see Fig. 8.4). *Pseudomonas* bacteremia may produce distinctive skin lesions known as *ecthyma gangrenosum,* as described previously under Bacteremia.

*Pseudomonas* burn wound infection is a dreaded complication of extensive full thickness burns and is characterized by multifocal black or dark brown discoloration of the burn eschar; degeneration of the underlying granulation tissue with rapid eschar separation and hemorrhage into subcutaneous tissue; edema, hemorrhage, and necrosis of adjacent healthy tissue; and erythematous nodular lesions on unburned skin.

Systemic manifestations may include fever, disorientation, hypotension, oliguria (low output of urine), ileus, or leukopenia. The diagnosis is made through a quantitative culture of a skin biopsy of the burn site or adjacent skin. Because *P. aeruginosa* colonizes burn sites, growth of $10^5$ colonies or greater is indicative of infection. A significant number of *P. aeruginosa* burn infections exhibit antibiotic resistance requiring careful selection of antibiotics, typically two, until culture information with antibiotic sensitivities is available.[130] Treatment also necessitates aggressive surgical débridement of necrotic tissue and infected eschar. If the bacteria spread into the bloodstream causing bacteremia and sepsis, mortality can be high. Early recognition accompanied by early treatment is key to a better prognosis.[282]

***Bone and Joint Infections.*** *Pseudomonas* infections of the bones and joints are not as common as *S. aureus,* coagulase-negative staphylococcus, or beta-hemolytic streptococcus. However, *P. aeruginosa* infections of the bone and joints result from hematogenous spread from other sites or extension from contiguous sites of infection. Contiguous infections are usually related to penetrating trauma, surgery, or overlying soft tissue infections. Bone and joint infections may occur following complex fractures, particularly fractures requiring open reduction and internal fixation. Prosthetic joints may be seeded hematologically or at the time of implantation surgery and are difficult to cure. Early, delayed, or late symptoms may occur, depending on when the joint was seeded. Early to delayed symptoms include erythema surrounding the surgical site, joint pain, fever, edema, drainage, or necrosis at the surgical site. Persistent wound drainage, acute onset of pain (after the joint has been functioning well), and chronic pain are often seen in late infections. IV drug users may contaminate drugs or water with *Pseudomonas,* which often seeds the sternoclavicular, sacroiliac, or other atypical joints.[318]

*P. aeruginosa* is the most common cause of osteochondritis of the foot following a puncture wound, particularly if the person is wearing a tennis shoe.[127,182] Infection involves the cartilage of the small joints and the bones of the foot. Typically the person experiences early improvement in pain and swelling following a puncture wound only to have the symptoms recur or worsen several days to months later.

The average duration of symptoms before diagnosis is several weeks; fever and other systemic signs are usually absent. An area of superficial cellulitis is evident on the plantar surface of the foot, or there may merely be tenderness to deep palpation.

Bloodborne *Pseudomonas,* from IV drug use or pelvic surgery, appears to have a predilection for fibrocartilaginous joints such as the symphysis pubis.[317] Vertebral osteomyelitis caused by *P. aeruginosa* is occasionally associated with complicated urinary tract infections and genitourinary surgery or instrumentation. This disease occurs most often in older adults and involves the lumbosacral spine. Physical signs include local tenderness and decreased range of motion in the spine; fever and other systemic symptoms are relatively uncommon. Mild neurologic deficits may be present (see further discussion in Chapter 27).

**Other *Pseudomonas* Infections.** *Pseudomonas* is the most common cause of simple external otitis (swimmer's ear) and the most common bacteria to cause chronic suppurative otitis media. *P. aeruginosa* is the most common cause of bacterial keratitis (infection of the cornea) in contact lens users, particularly in users of extended-wear lenses. Infection of the cornea can lead to corneal ulcers that progress rapidly associated with complications such as corneal perforation, anterior chamber involvement, and endophthalmitis. *P. aeruginosa* is the most common cause of health care–associated urinary tract infections often arising from urinary catheters, instrumentation, or surgery. The prostate or kidney stones may harbor the bacteria, resulting in recurrent infections.

## MEDICAL MANAGEMENT

DIAGNOSIS, TREATMENT, AND PROGNOSIS. Diagnosis requires isolation of the *Pseudomonas* organism in blood, cerebrospinal fluid, urine, exudates, or tissue. *P. aeruginosa* infections are among the most aggressive human bacterial infections, often progressing rapidly to sepsis, especially in people with poor immunologic resistance (e.g., premature infants; aging adults; and persons with debilitating disease, burns, or wounds). Septicemic *Pseudomonas* infections are associated with a high mortality rate.[382]

Antibiotic therapy should be initiated immediately because of the virulent nature of the bacteria. Owing to significant drug resistance,[298] presumed *Pseudomonas* infections are treated empirically with two antipseudomonal drugs (different classes) until culture susceptibility is available.[20] Antibiotic de-escalation with monotherapy can be employed once culture data are available for most cases except for infections in people who are high risk (immunosuppressed) and/or in whom infection is severe (e.g., bacteremia and endocarditis).[20,185]

In local *Pseudomonas* infections, treatment is usually successful, and complications are rare. Medical management is directed according to the site of infection and may include antibiotics, surgery with aggressive débridement, pulmonary therapy, respiratory assistance if necessary, and other supportive measures dictated by the presence of septic shock and other complications. Prompt removal of infected devices and catheters is indicated. Novel methods are under development including new antipseudomonal drugs and devices.[417]

SPECIAL IMPLICATIONS FOR THE THERAPIST 8.6

### *Pseudomonas Infections*

Reservoirs for *P. aeruginosa* are most often medical equipment or moist areas in the health care setting such as sinks, pools, and whirlpools.[153,157] In addition, aerolization generated from showers, faucets, and pulsatile lavage can result in exposure to the organism.[338] The source of some outbreaks has been traced to HCWs' hands or nails.[111,132] *P. aeruginosa* can be removed from the skin by following proper hand hygiene guidelines, which prevents further spread of the organism.[71,187,330]

Proper cleaning of any equipment in contact with mucous membranes or a moist environment is absolutely critical.[265] Health care facilities should maintain stringent cleaning and disinfection practices in accordance with the manufacturer's instructions and current evidence. Some facilities have adopted tub liners to minimize environmental contamination, but this should not change the importance of disinfection. A risk-benefit analysis should be considered for using hydrotherapy as well as exploring alternative aseptic techniques for wound management.[338] For example, all immunocompromised clients should be protected from exposure to this infection.

## Viral Infections

### Bloodborne Viral Pathogens

The bloodborne viruses that most endanger HCWs are the bloodborne pathogens hepatitis B virus (HBV), hepatitis C virus (HCV), and HIV. In 1991 the U.S. Congress passed the Bloodborne Pathogens Standard, amended in accordance with the Needlestick Safety and Prevention Act of 2000, prepared by the Occupational Safety and Health Administration and written to help eliminate or minimize occupational exposure to HBV, HCV, HIV, and other bloodborne pathogens.

The guidelines are based on the use of Standard Precautions, including appropriate hand hygiene and barrier precautions to reduce contact with body fluids potentially contaminated by these viruses. The use of safety devices and techniques to reduce the handling of sharp instruments can help in the reduction of significant contact with body fluids, particularly blood or blood-containing fluids.[338]

SPECIAL IMPLICATIONS FOR THE THERAPIST 8.7

### *Bloodborne Viral Pathogens*

Bloodborne viral pathogens are mentioned here to help the reader appreciate the big picture of patient problems. Taking a moment to recognize that hepatitis and HIV are transmitted through blood and blood products renews our understanding of why Standard Precautions are so important in preventing the transmission of these pathogens. In addition, many individuals are asymptomatic in the early stages and therefore go undiagnosed. An in-depth discussion of hepatitis can be found in Chapter 17; HIV is discussed in Chapter 7.

### Herpesviruses

**Overview and Definition.** The term *herpes* is derived from the Greek word *herpein*, which means "to creep." The word refers to the tendency for this type of viral infection to become chronic, latent, and recurrent. The known human herpesviruses (HHVs) are divided by genomic and biologic behavior into eight types (Box 8.9).

All herpesviruses are morphologically similar, but the biologic and epidemiologic features of each are distinct. Subclinical primary infection with the herpesviruses is more common than clinically symptomatic illness, and each type then persists in a latent state for the rest of the life of the host.

With the herpes simplex virus (HSV) and varicella-zoster virus (VZV), the virus remains latent in sensory ganglia, and on reactivation, lesions appear in the distal sensory nerve distribution. Virus reactivation in immunocompromised hosts may lead to widespread lesions in affected organs such as the viscera or the CNS.

Severe or fatal illness may occur in infants and immunocompromised individuals. Association with malignancies includes EBV with Burkett lymphoma and nasopharyngeal carcinoma and HHV-8 with Kaposi sarcoma and body cavity lymphoma.[81,385]

**Herpes Simplex Viruses Types 1 and 2.** See Table 8.7.

***Incidence, Etiologic Factors, and Risk Factors.*** Approximately 70% of Americans older than 14 years harbor HSV-1, which is usually responsible for cold sores. Herpes type 2 is one of the most common sexually transmitted diseases (STDs) in the world and the principal cause

Box 8.9

**TYPES OF HERPESVIRUSES**

| | |
|---|---|
| Herpes simplex virus (HSV) | Type 1 |
| Herpes simplex virus (HSV) | Type 2 |
| Varicella-zoster virus (VZV) | Type 3 |
| Epstein-Barr infectious mononucleosis virus (EBV) | Type 4 |
| Cytomegalovirus (CMV) | Type 5 |
| Roseola (exanthema subitum) human herpesvirus (HHV) | Type 6 HHV |
| Herpesvirus serologically associated with roseola (HHV) | Type 7 HHV |
| Human herpesvirus associated with Kaposi sarcoma (HHV) | Type 8 sarcoma |

of genital ulcers and genital herpes. It was estimated by the CDC in 2016 that 47.8% of the population has HSV-1 and 11.9% are infected with HSV-2. More than 50 million people are living with HSV-2.[31] However, the majority of initial cases go unrecognized (81%).[248]

Both strains can infect any visceral organ or mucocutaneous site, and HSV-1 can be transmitted to the genital area during oral sex.[322] HSV creates a significant health risk, as infection with HSV-2 can increase the risk of acquiring HIV infection by at least twofold.[133] Seroprevalence for both viruses increases with age and with sexual activity for HSV-2.

Intermittent, asymptomatic shedding is common and is the typical time of transmission, usually during the period immediately preceding appearance of sores. Sexual contact during asymptomatic periods is less likely to result in transmission of the virus than when sores are present. However, because people with genital herpes are more likely to engage in sexual contact when they are free of sores, the rate of asymptomatic transmission is still significant.

Infants born to women with genital herpes can be infected with HSV when they pass through an infected birth canal. The virus can also be passed to other regions of the body by direct contact, particularly in people who are immunosuppressed (e.g., older adults, transplant recipients, people with cancer undergoing chemotherapy, and anyone with HIV or other conditions that weaken the immune system).

## Pathogenesis

Even though HSV-1 and -2 are the two most closely related herpesviruses and share antigenic cross-reactivity, these two agents are genetically and serologically distinct and produce different clinical symptoms. HSV-1 and -2 primarily affect the oral mucocutaneous (cold sores and mouth sores) and genital (genital herpes) areas, respectively. Primary infection occurs through a break in the mucous membranes of the mouth, throat, eye, or genitals or via minor abrasions in the skin. Initial infection can be asymptomatic, although minor localized vesicular lesions may be evident.

Local multiplication occurs, followed by viremia and systemic infection with a subsequent lifelong latent infection and periodic reactivation of the virus. During primary infection, the virus enters peripheral sensory nerves and migrates along axons to sensory nerve ganglia in the CNS, allowing the virus to escape immune detection and response.

During latent infection of nerve cells, viral DNA is maintained and not integrated into surrounding cellular structures, thus maintaining true latency. Various disturbances such as physical or psychologic stress can disrupt the delicate balance of latency, and reactivation of the latent virus occurs. The virus travels back down sensory nerves to the surface of the body and replicates, forming new lesions. Although painful, most recurrent infections resolve spontaneously, recurring at a later time.

***Clinical Manifestations.*** Primary HSV-1 (first episode) typically affects the mouth and oral cavity, causing vesicles in the mouth, in the throat, and around the lips. Vesicles typically open to form moist ulcers after several days. Systemic symptoms can accompany the lesions such as fever, myalgias, and malaise. Symptoms and lesions resolve within 3 to 14 days.

Primary infection is often asymptomatic. Recurrences are usually milder, involve fewer lesions, are of shorter duration, and in immunocompetent hosts are usually confined to the lips (herpes labialis). Recurrent genital HSV-1 is milder and less frequent than HSV-2. Recurrences are most commonly induced by stress, fever, sunlight, infection, or other factors.

HSV-2 is most often acquired through sexual contact. Primary HSV-2 causes vesicles to form on the mucosal and cutaneous surfaces of the genital area. Lesions are usually painful, small, grouped, and vesicular, with possible burning and itching. The blister-like lesions break and weep after a few days, leaving ulcer-like sores that usually crust over and heal in 1 to 3 weeks.

Genital ulcers may occur on the genital area, cervix, buttocks, rectum, urethra, or bladder, causing vaginal and urethral discharge, dysuria, cervicitis, proctitis, and tender inguinal adenopathy. Systemic symptoms occasionally noted include headache, malaise, myalgias, and fever. Primary infection is often asymptomatic. Genital HSV-2 reactivation may be associated with a prodrome such as tingling or pain.

First symptomatic episodes may not be the initial infection. Known as nonprimary infections, individuals may have been previously exposed to HSV-1 and produced antibodies but not developed symptoms until exposed to HSV-2 or vice versa. In these cases, the initial symptomatic nonprimary infection has fewer symptoms and complications compared with a first episode without previous exposure.

HSV can be responsible for other infections. Viral meningitis from HSV is caused by inflammation of the meninges surrounding the brain. This occurs more commonly from HSV-2 than HSV-1. Aseptic meningitis may develop 3 to 12 days following the appearance of lesions but may also occur without skin lesions. Typical symptoms are headache, nausea, stiff neck, and fever. Meningitis may develop concomitant with the primary infection or recurrent episodes. Because of the latent nature of HSV-2, episodes of recurrent meningitis also occur.[26] The prognosis is good for immunocompetent hosts.

**Table 8.7** Most Common Sexually Transmitted Infections

| Infection | Incidence | Transmission | Clinical Manifestations | Treatment[a] |
|---|---|---|---|---|
| Human papillomavirus (HPV) (genital warts) | 14 million new cases/year | Unprotected sexual contact (including oral sex; condoms do not provide 100% protection, as virus can be spread by contact with an infected part of the genitals not covered by a condom); vertical transmission from mother to newborn with vaginal delivery (rare) | Often asymptomatic; warts on the vulva, anal region, vagina, cervix, mouth, penis, scrotum, or groin: 1–6 months after sexual contact with infected person; can also cause oropharyngeal cancer; *in women:* abnormal Pap smear; HPV can cause cervical cancer | Usually is cleared by immune system (90% within 2 years). When it is not, no treatment exists for the virus, but symptoms can be treated. Warts can be removed using topically applied chemicals, cryotherapy, or surgical therapies. Recurrence is not uncommon. |
| *Chlamydia* | >1.7 million new cases/year | Unprotected vaginal or anal intercourse, oral sex; infection transmitted from infected mother to infant during delivery | *In men:* none or urethritis with discharge or burning with urination<br>*In women:* commonly none or vaginal discharge or pain with urination; can cause PID with fever, abdominal pain, and pain with intercourse; infertility if untreated; eye infections and respiratory tract infections in newborn | Can be cured with antibiotics. Partner must be treated as well. PID may require additional treatment. |
| Herpes simplex virus type 2 (genital herpes) | >700,000 new cases/year | Oral, genital, or anal sex; kissing or touching an infected area where there is a break in the skin; can be spread by asymptomatic person; transmission from mother to child during vaginal birth | None or vesicular (blister-like) lesions on genitals, vagina, cervix, anal region, mouth, or throat; can cause serious complications if untreated | Cannot be cured, but healing can be accelerated and recurrence of outbreaks can be reduced with antivirals. Partner must be informed. |
| Gonorrhea (the "clap") | >500,000 new cases/year | Unprotected oral, vaginal, or anal sex; transmission to baby during delivery | *In men:* urethritis with discharge, frequent urge to urinate and pain during urination; may be asymptomatic<br>*In women:* none or slight vaginal discharge and difficulty or pain during urination; pelvic pain; vaginal bleeding between periods; PID<br>*Both:* arthritis (if untreated) | Most cases can be cured with antibiotics (third-generation cephalosporins), although strains are resistant to fluoroquinolones and are becoming resistant to available cephalosporins. |
| Hepatitis B | 20,000 (estimated) new cases/year (significant decrease since vaccination of children began) | Infected blood; sexual contact; occupational needlesticks; sharing needles; baby infected during delivery | May be asymptomatic; jaundice, arthralgias, dark urine, anorexia, nausea, abdominal pain, cirrhosis, liver failure, liver cancer, clay-colored stools, fever | Can be prevented with hepatitis B vaccine. In unvaccinated people, hepatitis B immune globulin and hepatitis B vaccine given as postexposure prophylaxis; interferon and antiviral agents are used, but relapse on cessation of treatment is common. |
| Syphilis (primary) | >30,000 new cases/year (primary and secondary combined); | Unprotected sexual contact (vaginal, oral, anal); sexual contact with exudates of skin and mucous membranes of infected person; transplacental infection of fetus if mother is infected; can be transmitted through blood transfusions | Painless papule or chancre at site of infection (genitals, mouth) occurring 3–8 weeks after infection; lymphadenopathy | Can be cured with antibiotics in primary, secondary, and latent stages. Late-stage disease may cause irreversible damage to brain, nerves, heart, blood vessels, eyes, liver, bones, joints. |

*Continued*

**Table 8.7** Most Common Sexually Transmitted Infections—cont'd

| Infection | Incidence | Transmission | Clinical Manifestations | Treatment[a] |
|---|---|---|---|---|
| Syphilis (secondary) | See Syphilis (primary) above | Progression of untreated primary-stage syphilis (spirochetes spread throughout body) | Can be asymptomatic; flu-like symptoms, lymphadenopathy, mucocutaneous lesions (chancres) and rash (maculopapular) occurring 6–12 weeks to 1–2 years after infection (but has a wide range of clinical symptoms, e.g., fatigue, fever, headache, myalgia, sore throat, weight loss); can cause fetus to abort in untreated pregnant women | |
| Syphilis (latent) | | Can still transmit disease to others | Test positive but no symptoms of clinically active disease | |
| Syphilis (late; can occur up to 20 years after second stage) | | Progression of untreated primary, then secondary syphilis | Cardiovascular and central nervous system damage (e.g., ataxia, paresis, paresthesias, dementia, visual loss) | |
| HIV/AIDS | >39,000 new cases/year; majority of transmissions caused by sexual contact (men who have sex with men) | Exposure to blood/blood products; exposure to body fluids (blood, semen, vaginal secretions, breast milk); sexual contact; shared needles in injection drug users; transmission from mother to child during vaginal delivery or breastfeeding | Widespread illness because of immune system decline; may not develop symptoms for ≥10 years after infection | Cannot be cured, but combined antiviral therapy can significantly prolong life for many people |

[a]All sexually transmitted diseases can be prevented by sexual abstinence and mutually monogamous sex between two uninfected partners.
*PID*, Pelvic inflammatory disease.
Data from Braxton J, Davis D, Emerson B, et al: Centers for Disease Control and Prevention. Sexually Transmitted Disease Surveillance 2017. Division of STD Prevention, September 2018. Atlanta, 2018, U.S. Department of Health and Human Services; McQuillan G, Kruszon-Moran D, Flagg EW, et al: Prevalence of herpes simplex virus type 1 and type 2 in persons aged 14–49: United States, 2015–2016. NCHS Data Brief, No. 304. Hyattsville, MD, 2018, National Center for Health Statistics; Workowski K, Bolan G: Sexually transmitted diseases treatment guidelines, 2015. *MMWR Morb Mortal Wkly Rep* 64:1–140, 2015.

Herpes encephalitis (an infection of the brain tissue), although rare, is a more serious infection and carries a 70% mortality without treatment.[218,393] It is almost exclusively caused by HSV-1, although HSV-2 can be the cause in neonates. In children and young adults, primary infection is the main cause. Adults may have reactivation as the principal source.

Presenting symptoms include fever, headache, behavioral and speech disturbances, and seizures. Abnormalities caused by HSV can be seen on magnetic resonance imaging. Encephalitis carries high morbidity and mortality rates, and permanent neurologic sequelae often result despite treatment.[393]

Neonatal herpes simplex encephalitis is a devastating infection of the fetus, typically from primary HSV-2 (30% of cases are HSV-1). The majority (70%) of infants born with this rare infection were born to mothers who did not manifest symptoms of the infection.[26,292]

The risk of the fetus of acquiring HSV from a primary maternal infection is approximately 30% to 50%[26,34] but much lower in mothers with a prenatal history of recurrent HSV-2 (17%). The most severe complications of neonatal HSV infection are dissemination and CNS involvement. Neonatal herpes may also occur from unknown shedding in the mother's genital tract at the time of delivery. Cesarean section reduces the risk of neonatal herpes in mothers known to be shedding the virus.[34,410]

Herpetic keratitis (ulceration of the cornea from infection) is one of the most common causes for corneal blindness in the United States. Onset is acute, accompanied by blurred vision, conjunctivitis, and pain. Despite treatment, recurrences are common and cause scarring, making this a chronic disease. Severe scarring is an indication for corneal grafting.

Herpetic whitlows (herpetic infection of the fingers) can result from inoculation of the finger from a herpes lesion (Fig. 8.5). Before implementation of standard glove precautions, herpetic whitlow was most often seen in HCWs. In children, herpetic whitlow is typically caused by HSV-1, whereas HSV-2 is implicated in cases involving adults.[418]

HSV can also disseminate to visceral organs, causing severe consequences such as hepatitis, thrombocytopenia,

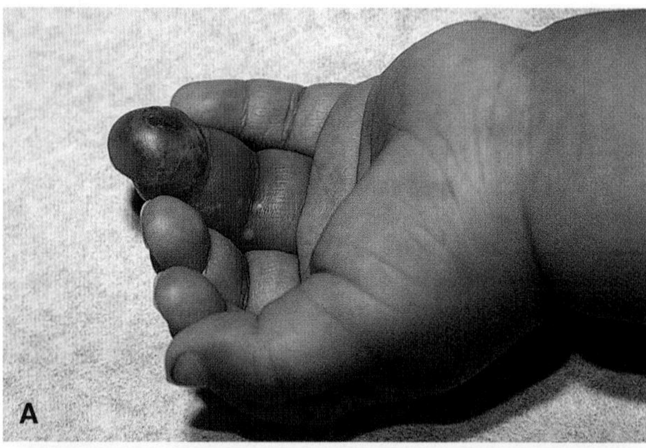


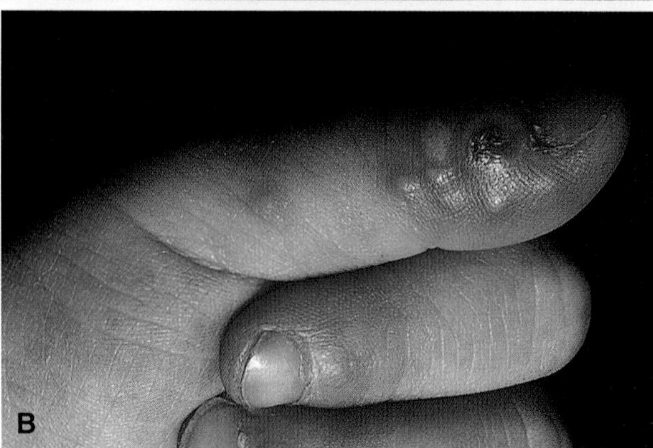


**Figure 8.5**

**Herpetic whitlow.** Herpetic whitlow is an intense, painful infection of the hand involving one or more fingers and typically affecting the terminal phalanx. Herpes simplex virus type 1 (HSV-1) is the cause in approximately 60% of cases of herpetic whitlow, and HSV-2 is the cause in the remaining 40%. (A) Herpes simplex infection of the finger in a child. (B) Herpetic whitlow of the thumb in an adult. (From Callen JP: *Color atlas of dermatology*, ed 2, Philadelphia, 2000, WB Saunders.)

arthritis, and pneumonitis. Disseminated infection typically occurs in pregnant women (primary genital HSV) or immunocompromised persons (primary or recurrent HSV). HSV esophagitis is seen in immunocompromised hosts but rarely noted in immunocompetent persons.

## MEDICAL MANAGEMENT

DIAGNOSIS, TREATMENT, AND PREVENTION. Clinical diagnosis of herpes is often insensitive. Up to 30% of first-episode genital herpes cases are caused by HSV-1, which has a low recurrence rate compared with HSV-2, making distinction between the two types important.

Viral culture has been the standard laboratory test for identifying HSV. However, the sensitivity is only 50%. Real-time PCR is more sensitive and is the test of choice for cerebrospinal fluid.[415] PCR is also useful in detecting asymptomatic shedding, particularly in the case of discordant couples. The sample must be collected during the first few days the lesion is present for the results to be accurate. Direct fluorescence antibody and serology are alternative tests.

Although elusive, research continues to develop an HSV vaccine.[83] Although no immunization against HSV infection is available, antiviral drugs can be used to treat initial cases, reduce the frequency and degree of viral shedding, and suppress recurrences.

The CDC has released recommendations and guidelines for the treatment of HSV-2. Acyclovir, famciclovir, and valacyclovir are approved for treatment and suppression of HSV-2,[414] although famciclovir may be somewhat less effective in controlling asymptomatic shedding. Individuals should consider long-term suppressive therapy if they have more than six recurrences per year. Clients may also elect episodic treatment over suppression. HSV suppressive therapy in people with HIV does not decrease the risk of transmission of HIV or HSV-2.[52] Acyclovir is used for neurologic complications of HSV, and penciclovir is approved for the treatment of cold sores.

These medications do not eradicate the virus, and once they are discontinued, there is no change in frequency, duration, or severity of recurrences. In recent years, mutations have led to the development of acyclovir-resistant HSV. This should be suspected when the diagnosis is certain but there is no clinical response.[310] Foscarnet is the drug of choice in this situation.

Counseling regarding transmission and education on how to recognize symptoms and defer sex are essential in preventing new cases. Daily suppressive use of valacyclovir along with safe sex can reduce transmission of HSV-2.[87] Proper use of condoms can also reduce the risk of acquiring HSV-2.[401] This is particularly helpful for couples in which one is seropositive and the other is seronegative for HSV.

SPECIAL IMPLICATIONS FOR THE THERAPIST 8.8

### *Herpes Simplex Virus*

Recurrent disease is best treated with acyclovir, and recurrent genital disease requires barrier precautions during sexual activity in addition to medication. Although herpes simplex is contagious, health care–associated transmission is rare. However, it has been reported in some high-risk areas, such as nurseries, ICUs, burn units, and other areas where immunocompromised individuals might be placed.

Transmission of HSV occurs primarily through contact with lesions or with virus-containing secretions such as saliva, vaginal secretions, or amniotic fluid. Exposed areas of skin, particularly when minor cuts, abrasions, or other skin lesions are present, are the most likely sites of viral entry. The incubation period of HSV is 2 to 14 days.

HCWs may acquire a herpetic infection of the fingers (herpetic whitlow or paronychia) from exposure to contaminated oral secretions. Such exposures are a distinct risk for HCWs who have direct contact with either oral or respiratory secretions from clients.

HCWs can protect themselves from acquiring HSV by adhering to Standard Precautions including hand hygiene before and after all client contact and by the use of appropriate barriers such as gloves to prevent direct hand contact with the lesion. HCWs should be excluded from work when active lesions are present (e.g., herpetic whitlow) and return to work only when lesions are dry and crusted (healed) (see Table 8.5).[348] No reports are evident that HCWs with genital HSV infections have transmitted HSV to clients, so no work restriction for people with HSV-2 is indicated.[394]

During the prodromal stage of herpes simplex, the levator scapulae becomes vulnerable to activation of its trigger points by mechanical stresses that are usually well within its tolerance. However, stiff neck syndrome can develop 1 or 2 days before the fully developed symptoms of herpes simplex.[351]

Careful questioning regarding previous history of herpes, presence of prodromal symptoms, and observation for the development of a new outbreak of sores during the episode of care will help the therapist in making an accurate assessment of the client's presentation.

### Varicella-Zoster Virus (Herpesvirus Type 3)

***Incidence.*** VZV is known to cause *chickenpox* and *shingles*. Before the availability of the varicella vaccine, primary or first-infection VZV accounted for about 3 to 4 million cases of chickenpox per year in the United States.[58] With the implementation of a varicella vaccine program in 1996, the incidence of varicella decreased by greater than 90% by 2005.[155] Postvaccination data show a significant decline in incidence, hospitalizations, and death from varicella, particularly since the addition of a routine second dose.[226,236]

One in three people will develop the secondary, or reactivation, form of VZV in their lifetime, resulting in herpes zoster, or shingles.[163] Approximately 1.2 million cases of shingles occur in the United States every year and cause significant pain and disability.[423] The risk of developing shingles starts to increase around age 50 years. Individuals who are immunocompromised (e.g., individuals with HIV infection, receiving chemotherapy, receiving corticosteroid therapy, or with cancer) are also at increased risk. Young adults such as college students living in dormitories are at increased risk for VZV as either chickenpox (first time) or shingles (recurrence).

***Pathogenesis.*** Similar to other herpesviruses, VZV has the capacity to persist in the body (dorsal root ganglia next to the spinal cord) following an initial infection of chickenpox. VZV is acquired from contact with infected airborne droplets (from coughing or sneezing) into the respiratory tract or by direct contact with vesicular fluid to mucous membranes or eye. The virus enters lymphoid tissue and is taken up by T lymphocytes. The virus then downregulates the major histocompatibility complex and interferon response genes of the T cells to partially evade the host's immune system. VZV DNA can be found in T lymphocytes 11 to 14 days before the rash appears. Subsequently the virus is able to spread throughout the body in the blood (viremia), occurring 6 to 8 days before the appearance of skin lesions. Once the virus spreads to the skin, forming vesicles, replication of the virus continues; however, the virus is no longer in cells. VZV is then able to infect nerve endings and move along retrograde to the regional ganglia. Infection of the nerves may also occur during the viremia.[206] The host's cell-mediated immunity is eventually able to clear the virus from the body except in the dorsal root ganglia and keep it in check. While latent in the ganglia, only a few viral genes are transcribed, and typically entire infectious viruses are not identified.[99] The exact mechanism for reactivation of VZV remains unknown, although it is related to the host's cell-mediated immune system. It is thought that if a compromise to immunity occurs, there is no longer a check on the latent virus. Replication proceeds with antegrade infection of the nerves, resulting in new skin lesions.[99] The nerves exhibit severe inflammation with associated hemorrhagic necrosis of nerve cells, leading to the characteristic pain. Viral infection of the skin and mucosa produces vesicles filled with high titers of infectious virus, which, when broken, then shed more viruses. The incubation period is 14 to 16 days from exposure with a range of 10 to 21 days.[53] This may be prolonged in immunocompromised persons, and individuals can be contagious 1 or 2 days before the appearance of the rash. Individuals remain contagious until the lesions have crusted.

***Clinical Manifestations.*** Disease manifestations are either chickenpox (varicella) or shingles (herpes zoster). Primary VZV is virtually always symptomatic. Second episodes of chickenpox are uncommon unless the child is younger than 1 year at the time of the first episode. A mild prodrome consisting of headache, photophobia, and malaise may precede the onset of the rash in adults, whereas in children the rash is often the first sign of disease.

The rash is classically described as a "dewdrop on a rose petal," with a vesicle on an erythematous base. The lesions begin as macules that quickly progress to papules, vesicles, and then pustules before crusting. VZV usually appears first on the scalp and moves to the trunk and then the extremities. Successive crops appear over several days, with lesions present in several stages of evolution at any one time.

The generalized pattern of eruption without specific dermatome distribution distinguishes varicella from herpes zoster (Fig. 8.6). Shingles in an adult manifests as blister-like lesions that erupt unilaterally along a specific dermatome supplied by a dorsal root ganglia. The highest concentration of lesions on the trunk corresponds with dermatomes from T3 to L3 (Fig. 8.7). Pain and itching are common symptoms during the eruption of the vesicles.

Complications of varicella occur more often in adults, infants, and immunocompromised persons. Adults are more likely to develop pneumonitis and CNS involvement (cerebellar ataxia and encephalitis) than are healthy children. Immunocompromised people, especially those with leukemia or lymphoma who are receiving continuous chemotherapy, can develop disseminated disease with severe visceral involvement, including pneumonitis and encephalitis. The most common complication in persons with VZV is secondary bacterial skin infections.

When contracted during the first or second trimesters of pregnancy, varicella carries a low risk of congenital malformations. However, if a mother develops varicella within 5 days before delivery to 2 days after delivery, the newborn is at risk of serious disseminated disease.

Shingles also can lead to chronic, often debilitating nerve pain called *postherpetic neuralgia* (PHN), defined as pain lasting 90 days after the onset of skin lesions that may continue months to years. It often results in significant morbidity and reduction in quality of life. The risk of developing PHN with each episode of zoster is 10% to 15%.[106]

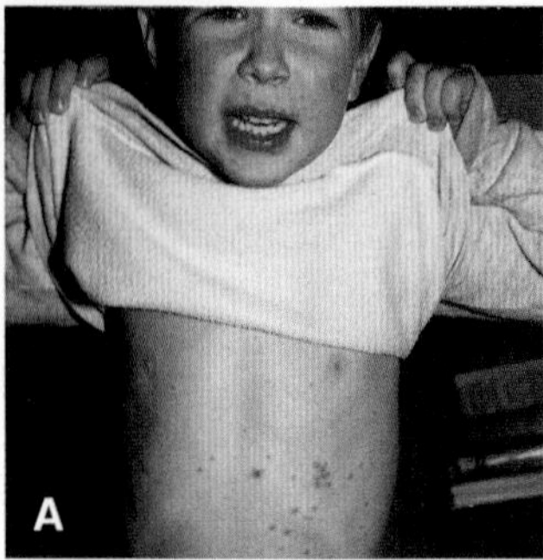


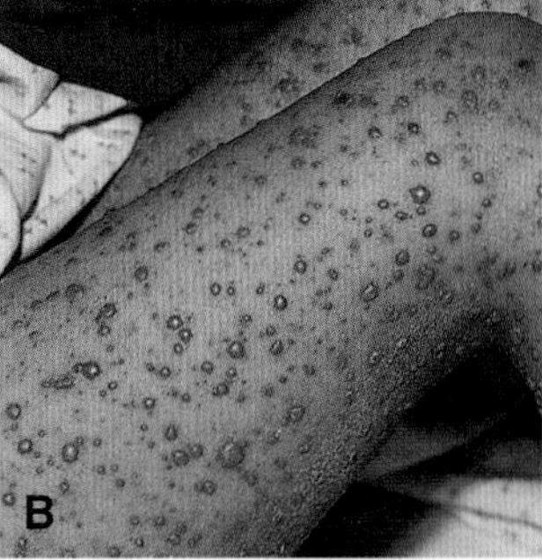


**Figure 8.6**

**Varicella (chickenpox).** (A) Early onset of varicella (chickenpox) in a young child. Painful itching can cause severe distress. Note the lesions on the face and trunk. (B) Varicella (chickenpox) with the more characteristic rash classically described as a "dewdrop on a rose petal," with a vesicle on an erythematous base. (A, Courtesy Catherine Goodman. B, From Callen JP: *Color atlas of dermatology*, ed 2, Philadelphia, 2000, Saunders.)

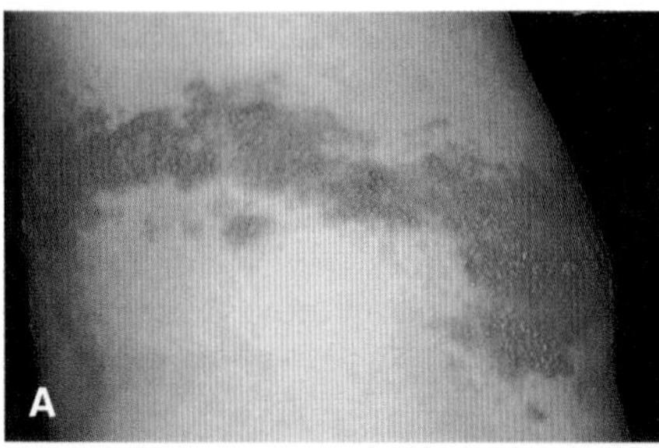


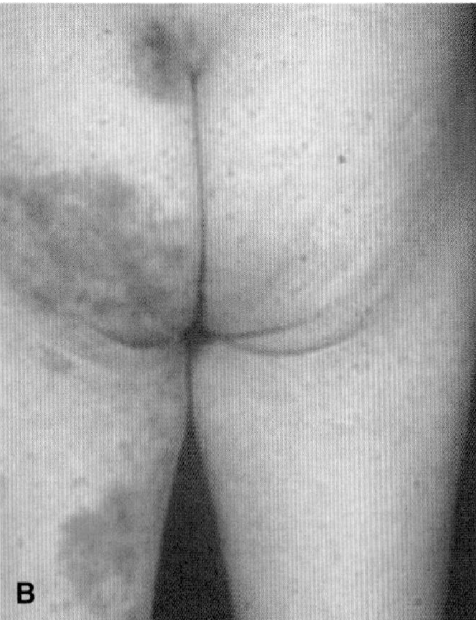


**Figure 8.7**

**Herpes zoster (shingles).** Small grouped vesicles occur along the cutaneous sensory nerve, forming pustules that crust over. Reactivation of varicella-zoster virus, the dormant chickenpox virus, is the underlying cause of this condition. A, Commonly seen on the trunk, these outbreaks can occur anywhere along the dermatome of the affected nerve. B, Lesions appear unilaterally and do not cross the midline. Usually external, these lesions can occur internally as well. Pain is often severe and can become chronic, a condition called *postherpetic neuralgia*. (A, From Hurwitz S: *Clinical pediatric dermatology: a textbook of skin disorders of childhood and adolescence*, ed 2, Philadelphia, 1993, Saunders. B, Courtesy Mary Lou Galantino, Richard Stockton College of New Jersey, Pomona, NJ.)

Pain, hyperalgesia, and allodynia are typical of PHN. Examples of allodynia include pain from the touch of clothing (touch allodynia) or pain that occurs from a draft of warm or cold air on the skin (thermal allodynia). The pain may be constant or intermittent and vary from light burning to a deep visceral sensation. The cause of PHN is not fully understood. Scarring and degenerative changes involving the nerve trunks, ganglia, and skin may be important factors. The incidence of scarring and hyperpigmentation is much higher in older adults. For individuals who develop shingles, factors that predict the severity and occurrence of PHN include the severity of pain both before and after onset of the rash, the extent of the rash, advancing age, and immunosuppression.[188]

Occasionally herpes zoster involves the cranial nerves, especially the trigeminal and geniculate ganglia or the oculomotor nerve. Geniculate zoster may cause vesicle formation in the external auditory canal, ipsilateral facial palsy, and ear pain (Ramsay Hunt syndrome). Trigeminal ganglion involvement, herpes zoster ophthalmicus, causes eye pain and possibly corneal and scleral damage with loss of vision. Herpes zoster ophthalmicus is considered a medical emergency. All persons with VZV near the eye should be evaluated by an ophthalmologist.

In rare cases, herpes zoster leads to generalized CNS infection (e.g., encephalitis, aseptic meningitis), muscle atrophy, motor paralysis (usually transient), acute transverse myelitis, and ascending myelitis. Generalized infection may cause acute retention of urine and unilateral paralysis of the diaphragm. Severely immunocompromised people can experience dissemination of the virus with skin (lesions not in the same or adjacent dermatome) and visceral (e.g., pneumonia, encephalitis, hepatitis) involvement.

## MEDICAL MANAGEMENT

**DIAGNOSIS AND TREATMENT.** Diagnosis is usually made based on clinical symptoms (widespread vesicles in chickenpox and clustered vesicles in a dermatomal pattern in shingles); however, with the advent of the varicella vaccine, the number of atypical cases has increased, making laboratory diagnosis more relevant. Fluid from a vesicle may be stained and viewed under a microscope to identify multinucleated giant cells. Real-time PCR assay can identify VZV virus rapidly and with high sensitivity from several sources, including skin lesions, cerebrospinal, bronchoalveolar lavage, and blood. This test also identifies vaccine-modified infection.[162] Direct fluorescent antibody staining is also available, but sensitivity is limited by the quality of the specimen. Serology (checking for IgG antibodies to VZV) is used to determine the immunity status of a person to VZV.

Treatment for varicella (chickenpox) is not curative. Most immunocompetent children do not require more than supportive care to relieve symptoms while waiting for the immune system to clear the virus (although it remains dormant in the dorsal root ganglia). Resting at home is recommended until the fever has gone down, and the skin should be kept clean to avoid secondary bacterial contamination. Itching can be relieved with oral antihistamines, topical calamine lotion, and other skin-soothing lotions and baths.

Antiviral medications are used to treat individuals at high risk for complications of varicella including unvaccinated adolescents, adults, pregnant women, and people who are immunocompromised (i.e., receiving high-dose corticosteroids) or have chronic skin or pulmonary disease.[197] Oral antiviral medications, acyclovir and valacyclovir, are used for immunocompetent children without complications; acyclovir, valacyclovir, and famciclovir may be given to immunocompetent adults without evidence of complications. IV acyclovir is typically administered to children and adults who are hospitalized with complications. Higher doses of acyclovir are required to treat VZV than HSV. Antiviral therapy may reduce the risk and severity of complications and decrease the time to resolution of symptoms. If antiviral medication is used, it should be started within 24 hours of the appearance of the rash.[402] Recovery from varicella infection usually results in lifetime immunity.

Individuals who are hospitalized are admitted to an airborne infection isolation room, and HCWs don respirators before entering the room. Susceptible HCWs are restricted from entering the room. Additionally, HCWs should adhere to Standard Precautions and contact isolation precautions due to draining skin lesions and have dedicated equipment to minimize transmission.[348]

For the treatment of zoster (shingles), the CDC recommends antiviral therapy (valacyclovir, famciclovir, or acyclovir) for persons older than 50 years who have moderate or severe pain, moderate or severe rash, or involvement of nontruncal dermatomes (particularly near the eye). Pregnant women are treated with acyclovir. Antiviral therapy reduces the number of days new lesions appear, reduces the severity and duration of pain associated with the acute rash, reduces shedding and transmission of the virus, and may reduce the risk for PHN.[113] People who develop shingles should begin antiviral therapy within 72 hours of the appearance of the rash (preferably when the pain begins). For clients presenting with new lesions more than 72 hours after the first lesions appeared, antiviral therapy should be offered, as this represents ongoing viral replication. There is most likely little benefit to giving antivirals if the lesions are crusted. Individuals with complicated VZV (e.g., encephalitis, disseminated disease, retinal necrosis) should be hospitalized and receive IV acyclovir. All immunocompromised people should receive antiviral therapy. Pain due to acute neuritis can be treated with acetaminophen, nonsteroidal antiinflammatory drugs, or stronger analgesics. Secondary bacterial infections of lesions are treated with antibacterial ointment or oral antibiotics if severe. There is no evidence that gabapentin, tricyclic antidepressants, or corticosteroids are beneficial in the acute treatment of VZV.[112,165] Glucocorticoids may be helpful in certain acute instances such as acute retinal necrosis. People with zoster can transmit the virus to people who have not had varicella and so should avoid exposing unvaccinated or immunocompromised people or pregnant women. The rash should be covered and appropriate hand hygiene used until the lesions have crusted.

Treatment for PHN can be complex, with various trials of medications needed to find the treatment that provides the best relief. Gabapentin, serotonin-norepinephrine reuptake inhibitors, and tricyclic antidepressants are first-line treatments.[125] Nonopioid analgesics, capsaicin cream, or topical lidocaine may also be beneficial.[125,167] PHN can be a chronic problem, and more research is needed to determine the best treatments.[125]

For individuals who are exposed, but are without immunity, to varicella, the varicella vaccine can be used up to 3 days after exposure (particularly in outbreaks) to aid in modifying symptoms or preventing the infection.[60] For individuals at high risk for severe complications and for whom the vaccine is contraindicated (e.g., immunocompromised persons, pregnant women who lack immunity to VZV, neonates), postexposure prophylaxis can include VariZIG (a varicella zoster immune globulin).[59,66]

**PREVENTION.** The varicella vaccine (Varivax) is recommended for all children age 12 months or older, with a second dose between ages 4 and 6 years.[236] It should be administered as a routine vaccination for those who do not have evidence of immunity (children, adolescents, adults), especially in persons who have close contact with individuals at high risk for severe disease and complications. Adults who are at high risk for exposure and transmission should receive the vaccine if not already immune (such as teachers of young children, child care employees, and residents and staff at medical facilities).

It is recommended that all children who have not developed immunity by the age of 13 years should be vaccinated. Most adolescents who do not have a history of varicella do not require preimmunization testing for immunity because most have not been exposed to the wild-type virus. However, individuals born before 1980 or in another country may have been exposed and should receive prevaccination serology testing to determine if they have already had the disease and do not require the vaccine. The varicella vaccine is also available with the measles, mumps, and rubella (MMR) vaccine (ProQuad).

Because the vaccine is a live attenuated vaccine, it is contraindicated in pregnant women and in women who may become pregnant within 4 weeks of receiving the vaccine; guidelines are available for individuals with HIV and other individuals who are immunocompromised.[236,319] People who are severely immunocompromised and receive the vaccine can develop disseminated disease.

The vaccine provides long-lasting (but not lifelong) immunity, with a 90% efficacy rate in preventing primary varicella infection and a 99% efficacy in preventing severe varicella disease.[236] Vaccine breakthrough cases are common but mild, and people typically present with fewer lesions (usually fewer than 50) and lack systemic symptoms (such as fever).[236]

A shingles vaccine is now available, called Shingrix, and is recommended by the CDC for individuals 50 years of age and older.[55] It is a non-live recombinant vaccine supplied with an adjuvant (to increase immune reaction). It is more than 90% effective in preventing shingles and PHN, which is an improvement over the older vaccine, Zostavax. Protection remains above 85% for at least the first 4 years, even in people older than 70 years.[91] Two doses are required at an interval of 2 to 6 months. The principal side effect is soreness of the injection site, although flu-like symptoms are also common.

**PROGNOSIS.** Overall prognosis is good unless the infection spreads to the brain (rare). Most people recover completely, with the possible exception of scarring and, with corneal damage, visual impairment. One of the most significant complications associated with VZV is PHN. Occasionally, intractable pain associated with PHN may persist for months or years. PHN pain can be very difficult to treat, but many options are available. Signs of the disorder in immunocompetent persons resolve within a month, but the area that was affected may be partly insensitive or show postinfectious skin changes. Studies are lacking on recurrent zoster, although it is thought that one episode of zoster is not protective against a second. Recurrent zoster is more common in immunocompromised people.[424]

SPECIAL IMPLICATIONS FOR THE THERAPIST 8.9

### *Varicella-Zoster Virus*

Varicella is highly contagious. The period of communicability extends from 1 to 2 days before the onset of the rash through the first 4 to 5 days or until all lesions have formed crusts. Immunocompromised individuals with progressive varicella are probably contagious during the entire period new lesions continue to appear.

Any patient or client suspected of having herpes zoster (shingles) requires immediate medical attention. Reports of prodromal pain, symptoms, or onset of rash are red flags to warrant immediate diagnosis and early treatment. Early intervention can reduce morbidity.

Because airborne transmission of VZV occurs, affected individuals in a hospital setting should be isolated in airborne infection isolation rooms until crusts have dried.

HCWs who take care of VZV clients should use contact precautions, including careful use of barriers such as gloves, gowns, and masks whenever in contact with active lesions. If serologic immunity of the HCW cannot be verified, varicella vaccine is recommended (see Table 8.4).

Health care–associated transmission of VZV is well known. Sources for exposure include clients or residents, HCWs, and visitors including children, with either varicella or zoster.

The CDC has set up guidelines for the care of all clients regarding precautions for the transmission of infectious skin diseases (see Table 8.5). These Standard Precautions should be used with all clients regardless of their disease status.

All skin lesions are considered potentially infectious and should be handled as such. The careful use of these precautionary measures severely limits the transmission of any disease. In addition, each hospital has isolation precautions organized according to categories of disease to prevent the spread of infectious disease to others. Every health care professional must be familiar with these procedures and follow them carefully. See also the section on Isolation Procedures in Table 8.3.

Neither heat nor ultrasound should be used on a person with shingles, because these modalities can increase the severity of the person's symptoms. For a person with severe herpetic pain, relaxation techniques may be useful. In the case of unresolved PHN, the individual may benefit from a program of chronic pain management including iontophoresis and transepidermal nerve stimulation.[203,285]

#### For the Therapist

Adults with shingles are infectious to persons who have not had chickenpox, and the person with shingles can develop shingles more than one time. To develop shingles, it is necessary to have been exposed to chickenpox and harbor the virus in your nervous system.[266] For this reason, therapists who have never had chickenpox should receive the vaccination; complications and morbidity associated with adult onset of varicella warrant this precaution. It is generally advisable to allow only HCWs who are immune to varicella to take care of clients with VZV.

Any female therapist who is pregnant or planning a pregnancy should be tested for immune status if unsure about her previous history of varicella. This is especially important because transmissibility of the virus occurs 2 to 3 days before symptoms develop; immunocompromised clients with shingles are probably contagious during the entire period new lesions are appearing until all lesions are crusted over.

This means that anyone receiving intervention by a therapist may be an asymptomatic host during the period of communicability; exposure to self and further transmission to others can occur without the therapist's awareness.

Susceptible HCWs with significant exposure to varicella should be relieved from direct client contact from day 10 to day 21 after exposure. If HCWs develop chickenpox, varicella lesions must (see Table 8.5) be crusted before they return to direct client contact.

Because of the possibility of transmission to and development of severe illness in high-risk clients, HCWs with localized zoster should not take care of such clients until all lesions are dry and crusted. However, they may take care of others if they cover their lesions.

When vaccinated HCWs are exposed to varicella, serologic testing for antibodies may be done, and exclusion from duty can occur if they are seronegative or develop varicella symptoms. Varicella-zoster immunoglobulin and acyclovir are not routinely recommended after exposure for healthy HCWs (exceptions may be made for pregnant or immunocompromised HCWs).[211]

### Infectious Mononucleosis (Herpesvirus Type 4)

***Overview.*** Infectious mononucleosis is a clinical syndrome most commonly associated with EBV, a member of the herpesvirus family. Although it may be seen at any age, it primarily affects young adults and children. In children, it is usually so mild that the symptoms are attributed to nonspecific illnesses.

Once thought to have an association with chronic fatigue syndrome (CFS), it now seems clear that no one infectious agent causes myalgic encephalomyelitis/CFS. The CDC conducted a four-city surveillance to determine if an infectious etiology for CFS existed and found no one organism was responsible.[74] It may be that CFS has multiple causes with the same end point (see Chronic Fatigue and Immune Dysfunction Syndrome in Chapter 7).[300]

***Incidence, Etiologic Factors, and Risk Factors.*** Infection with EBV is common in the United States, with 95% of people between the ages of 35 and 40 years having been infected.[230] When an adolescent or young adult becomes infected with EBV, 30% to 50% of the time, they will develop the symptoms of infectious mononucleosis. Both genders are affected equally. Incidence varies seasonally among college students but not among the general population. The reservoir of EBV is limited to human beings, and transmission is through contact with oral secretions, blood, or transplanted organs infected with the virus.[392] Because people shed EBV in the saliva during the acute infection and for an indefinite period afterward, it is sometimes called the "kissing disease."[386]

***Pathogenesis and Clinical Manifestations.*** EBV causes lymphoid proliferation in the blood, lymph nodes, and spleen. Characteristically the virus produces fever, sore throat, and tender cervical lymphadenopathy; headache, malaise, and abdominal pain (from splenic enlargement or hepatitis) may also be present. The incubation period is about 4 to 6 weeks.

Temperature fluctuations occur throughout the day, peaking in the evening. There is often an increase in the white blood cell count, with an elevation in atypical lymphocytes. Hepatomegaly (accompanied by elevated liver enzymes), palatal petechiae, and splenomegaly are clinically detectable in 15% to 65% of cases, although most affected persons have splenomegaly on ultrasound. The spleen may enlarge to two to three times its normal size, causing left upper quadrant pain with possible referral to the left shoulder and left upper trapezius region. Although uncommon, affected individuals are at risk for splenic rupture (occurring in approximately 1% of cases), and care should be taken to avoid trauma.

Both the peripheral nervous system and the CNS can be involved (1% to 5% of cases), producing neurologic abnormalities including Guillain-Barré syndrome, encephalitis, aseptic meningitis, peripheral neuritis, and optic neuritis. Although typically mild, the most common complications are hematologic (25% to 50%) and include hemolytic anemia, aplastic anemia, thrombocytopenia, and thrombotic thrombocytopenic purpura.[230] Symptoms subside about 6 to 10 days after onset of the disease but may persist for weeks. Symptoms from EBV-related infectious mononucleosis rarely last longer than 4 months.

## MEDICAL MANAGEMENT

**DIAGNOSIS, TREATMENT, AND PROGNOSIS.** Diagnosis is based on clinical examination, laboratory tests, and a positive heterophil (Monospot) test. In clients with acute EBV, there are generally 10% atypical lymphocytes on the peripheral blood smear. Heterophil antibodies (a group of IgM antibodies, which cause agglutination of sheep red blood cells) are negative in 25% of people during the first week of acute infection and in 5% to 10% in the second week.[114] In children younger than 4 years, the heterophil test is positive in only 25% to 75% of cases. Once antibodies are present, they may persist for up to a year.[230] If a definitive diagnosis is required, tests specific for EBV (IgM and IgG antibodies for portions of the virus) are available.[380]

EBV is a transforming virus and may have a pathogenic role in causation of cancers such as Burkitt lymphoma, nasopharyngeal carcinoma, Hodgkin disease,[169,383] and lymphoproliferative disorders in immunosuppressed and posttransplant clients.[250,315,385] Oral hairy leukoplakia, Hodgkin lymphoma, and non-Hodgkin lymphoma are diseases that are linked with EBV in HIV-positive individuals.[178,239,268]

There may be an association between infectious mononucleosis and the subsequent development of multiple sclerosis for both adults and children, although no definitive link to EBV has been demonstrated.[41,229,325,350,381]

The prognosis is excellent with rest and supportive care. Clinical symptoms typically improve within a month, although the fatigue and lymphadenopathy may persist longer. Most people are back to normal activities within 2 to 3 months.[17] Return to contact sports decisions should be individualized owing to the variability in the disease. Evidence varies as well, with some studies reporting return to unrestricted play at 28 days and others at 8 weeks.[19,23]

No other specific interventions appear to alter or shorten the disease process, although studies have evaluated antiviral medications and corticosteroids.[311] Larger trials are needed to determine if either of these treatments is beneficial, particularly in clients with immunodeficiencies or severe complications. If given ampicillin, clients often develop a maculopapular rash. Because the virus can live indefinitely in B lymphocytes and the oropharynx, reactivation of the virus frequently occurs. The virus is commonly found in the saliva, although most often without symptoms.

**SPECIAL IMPLICATIONS FOR THE THERAPIST 8.10**

### *Infectious Mononucleosis*

Infectious mononucleosis is probably contagious from before symptoms develop to until the fever subsides and the oral and pharyngeal lesions disappear. Although infectious mononucleosis appears to be only mildly contagious, adherence to standard precautions, especially good hand hygiene and avoidance of shared dishware or food items with other people, is essential in preventing the HCW from contracting this condition.

A person with infectious mononucleosis should be cautioned against engaging in excessive activity, especially contact sports, which could result in splenic rupture or lowered resistance to infection. Usually this guideline is appropriate for a period of at least 1 month.

Any sign of splenic rupture (e.g., abdominal or upper quadrant pain, Kehr sign, sudden left shoulder pain, or shock) requires immediate medical evaluation. Any soft tissue mobilization or myofascial techniques necessary in the left upper quadrant, especially up and under the rib cage, must take into consideration the enlarged liver and/or spleen; indirect techniques away from the spleen are indicated.

In rare cases, mononucleosis impairs the CNS. Any change in neurologic status must be evaluated and reported to the physician. Changes in respiration or signs and symptoms of airway obstruction may require emergency intervention.

### Cytomegalovirus (Herpesvirus Type 5)

*Overview and Incidence.* CMV (herpesvirus type 5) is a commonly occurring DNA herpesvirus. It increases in frequency with age. In the United States, 36% of children 6 to 11 years old have the virus, while CMV was detected in 91% of people over the age of 80.[360]

For the majority of people who are infected with the virus after birth, there are few symptoms or complications. However, for unborn babies or immunocompromised people (posttransplant or with HIV disease), the consequences can be severe or life threatening. In the literature, a distinction is made between CMV infection, both primary and recurrent infection (reactivation or infection with a new strain), and CMV disease. Infection signifies a positive laboratory result, whereas disease refers to an infection with associated symptoms.[223]

*Etiologic and Risk Factors.* CMV is transmitted by human contact with infected secretions such as urine, saliva, breast milk, feces, blood, semen, and vaginal and cervical secretions. It may also be transmitted through the placenta. The virus can be acquired from transplanted organs and, rarely, via blood transfusions. As with other herpesviruses, CMV can remain dormant to evade detection and persists in multiple organs. There is frequent intermittent reactivation with asymptomatic shedding of virus, while new and different strains may cause another infection.

*Pathogenesis and Clinical Manifestations.* CMV has been found in lymphocytes or mononuclear cells, which may then carry the virus to other parts of the body. CMV usually does not cause symptoms unless the host's immune system is not able to eliminate the virus and a high viral load is achieved in the blood.[148] In the immunocompromised host, the virus can replicate, causing disease in the lungs (CMV pneumonitis), liver (CMV hepatitis), GI tract (CMV gastroenteritis), eyes (CMV retinitis), and CNS, where it produces inflammatory reactions. Complications include diffuse interstitial pneumonitis, leading to respiratory distress syndrome, hepatitis, GI ulcerations and bleeding, vision loss, and loss of transplanted organs.

In healthy adolescents or adults, the infection is usually asymptomatic or manifests as an infectious mononucleosis–like illness with a self-limiting course of fever and mild hepatitis. In contrast to infectious mononucleosis from EBV, CMV causes less pharyngitis or adenopathy.

In approximately 2% of women who have their first or primary infection during pregnancy, 30% to 40% of the fetuses become infected.[194,425] The fetus may also become infected from reactivation of the maternal virus or maternal infection by another CMV strain. The course of the illness for the fetus ranges from mild splenomegaly or hepatitis to disseminated disease. About 1% of seropositive mothers before pregnancy will deliver a baby with congenital CMV. Sensorineural hearing loss (SNHL) is a common finding in children with congenital CMV, seen in one-third to one-half of symptomatic babies.[142] Children born with CMV hearing loss often acquire the virus from a maternal reactivation of the virus.[96] SNHL may occur in isolation or with other sequelae. Sequelae are more severe when the infection occurs early in pregnancy. Often prenatal ultrasound is suggestive of CMV disease, and diagnosis and management may begin before birth. Approximately 10% of infected babies are born with acute symptoms such as jaundice, hepatosplenomegaly, microcephaly, and small size for gestational age.[28] About 8% to 10% of symptomatic babies have severe disease, with mortality as high as 30%.[225] Approximately 5% to 15% of congenitally infected babies born without initial symptoms will go on to develop later sequelae.[425] Approximately 90% of babies born with CMV do not have symptoms, although 10% to 15% will later develop SNHL. Of babies born with symptoms, 78% may later develop complications such as seizures, visual impairment, dental problems, intellectual disability, cerebral palsy, and delayed psychomotor development; although SNHL is the most common manifestation.[105]

In immunosuppressed people, particularly transplant recipients and persons with HIV, various manifestations of disease develop with CMV infection. Transplant recipients who are at greatest risk for severe disease are those who are negative for CMV but receive a donor-positive organ/tissue. Fever, splenomegaly, hepatitis, pneumonitis, esophagitis, gastritis, colitis, meningioencephalitis, or retinitis may occur in individuals who are immunocompromised.

CMV is also associated with an increase in risk of infection by other viruses and bacteria.[128,166] The specific transplanted organ is particularly susceptible to disease (e.g., hepatitis in liver transplants). Transplant recipients are most at risk the first 100 days following transplantation (see Chapter 21). With improved treatment of HIV using ART, CMV retinitis has significantly decreased but remains an important cause of blindness in advanced HIV disease.

## MEDICAL MANAGEMENT

**DIAGNOSIS, TREATMENT, AND PROGNOSIS.** Diagnosis of an acute infection is made by real-time PCR (viral load testing), serology (e.g., enzyme-linked immunosorbent assay [ELISA]), antigen-detection tests, or shell viral culture. Real-time PCR quantifies CMV DNA and is used to diagnose and monitor disease progression or response.[307] Serology tests identify the presence of antibodies to CMV. IgM usually indicates an acute or recent infection. However, CMV IgM antibodies can persist in the blood for several months and so may not provide an accurate assessment of the timing of infection, particularly if an earlier sample is not available for comparison. Another indication of recent infection is noted when two different samples, drawn at least 2 to 4 weeks apart, demonstrate at least a 4-fold increase in titers of IgG antibodies. IgG antibodies typically do not appear until 2 to 3 weeks after the onset of symptoms and persist throughout life. Serology is also helpful in determining appropriateness of donor tissue for people who have not been exposed to CMV. Antigenemia assays are able to detect CMV proteins in the blood, and the quantity correlates to the risk of developing active CMV disease.

Because most people infected with CMV are asymptomatic or display nonspecific and self-limiting symptoms, treatment is not required. In immunocompromised clients, pharmacologic treatment, such as ganciclovir and valganciclovir, has proven effective. These agents are also used prophylactically (to prevent infection) or preemptively (such as a seropositive person on immunosuppressants) in clients receiving a transplant.[284]

The prognosis for people with transplanted organs or who are immunocompromised can be associated with poor outcome, as they may have fatal disseminated infections with multiple organ involvement.[128,413] People with HIV and reactivated CMV disease benefit from ART, which may aid the immune system in recovering enough to suppress the virus, making anti-CMV treatment unnecessary.[97,176]

Infants who are born with severe symptoms related to CMV infection may be treated with ganciclovir or valganciclovir, with treatment response monitored through quantitative viral load. Infants with congenital CMV should have their hearing and vision checked regularly.

Vaccines and new antiviral medications are currently in development.[11,82]

SPECIAL IMPLICATIONS FOR THE THERAPIST 8.11

### *Cytomegalovirus*

Other practice patterns depend on organ systems involved and clinical presentation. The two principal reservoirs of CMV in health care institutions are (1) infants and young children and (2) immunocompromised individuals. However, HCWs who provide care to these high-risk populations have a rate of primary CMV that is no higher than among personnel without such client contact.

CMV transmission appears to occur directly either through close, intimate contact with contaminated secretions or through excretions, especially saliva or urine.[89,90] Transmission by the hands of HCWs or individuals with the virus has also been suggested. The incubation period for person-to-person transmission is not known. Although CMV can survive on environmental surfaces or objects for only a very short time, there is some evidence of fomite transmission.[10,374] There is some evidence to suggest there is an occupational risk of transmission to daycare employees via environmental surfaces at daycare facilities.[187a]

Pregnant women and immunosuppressed people should avoid exposure to confirmed or suspected CMV infection. Pregnant women or women of childbearing age need to be counseled regarding the risks and prevention of transmission of CMV, but no data show that HCWs can be protected from infection by transfer to areas with less contact with individuals with a CMV diagnosis. Work restrictions for HCWs who contract CMV are not necessary, as the risk of transmission of CMV can be reduced by careful adherence to hand hygiene and standard precautions.[393a]

Clients with CMV infection should be encouraged to wash their hands thoroughly and frequently to prevent spreading it. It is especially important to impress this on young children. As difficult as it may be, the child should not be allowed to kiss others, and parents and others should also avoid kissing the affected child.

**HERPESVIRUSES TYPES 6, 7, AND 8.** HHV-6 was first isolated from people with lymphoproliferative disorders and was originally called human B-cell lymphotropic virus; the name was changed once the virus was characterized.[1] Two distinct species exist, HHV-6A and HHV-6B, although HHV-6B is responsible for the majority of clinical illness, both primary infection and reactivation. It is the principal cause of exanthema subitum (roseola infantum, or sixth disease). Primary HHV-6 is common in children, with 77% to 90% infected by the age of 2 years.[427] Although classically described as 3 to 5 days of high fever followed by a macular rash on the neck and trunk (roseola), children more commonly develop a fever, fussiness, diarrhea, and rash.[427] Most children are symptomatic with the primary infection.[427] It is rarely contracted as a primary infection as adults, but reactivation of the virus is associated with immunocompromised states such as HIV, transplant recipients, and lymphoma. It is associated with graft rejection,[213] encephalitis, pneumonitis, hepatitis, and bone marrow suppression in transplant recipients.[104,395] Both HHV-6 and HHV-7 reactivation have been implicated in the exacerbation of multiple sclerosis.[275]

HHV-7 is a T-cell lymphotropic virus that is biologically similar to HHV-6. HHV-7 does not appear to be as clinically significant as other herpesviruses, although it may at times explain a "recurrent" case of roseola. HHV-8 is associated with Kaposi sarcoma in AIDS and other immune-related diseases (e.g., primary effusion lymphoma). (See Kaposi Sarcoma in Chapter 10.)

### Viral Respiratory Infections

Viral respiratory infections (e.g., influenza, respiratory syncytial virus [RSV]) are common problems in health care settings. Many viral pathogens can cause respiratory infections, but influenza and RSV are associated with significant morbidity and mortality rates.

**Influenza.** Each year in the United States, influenza viruses cause serious illness and even death, especially in young children, persons with chronic diseases, immunocompromised adults, and frail elderly adults. During the 2017–2018 flu season, the CDC estimated there were more than 49 million cases with 960,000 hospitalizations and 96,000 deaths.[79] During a given influenza season, the incidence of infection ranges from 3% to 11%.[388] Influenza is caused by influenza virus A or B and occurs in epidemics between late fall and early spring. Influenza A is subdivided and numbered according to two surface proteins: H (hemagglutinin) and N (neuraminidase). There are 18 different H type proteins and 11 N type proteins. Influenza B is subdivided by strain.

In recent years, two influenza A viruses emerged that have caused significant morbidity and mortality worldwide. In 2005 an avian influenza A virus made the news for its ability to cause severe symptoms with fatal outcomes in humans. The subtype is H5N1 and was originally identified in Asia. In 2009 the subtype H1N1 (previously seen in swine) led to a pandemic outbreak of influenza. The complication rate reported in the normally healthy age range of 19 to 64 years was greater than typically seen.

The mode of transmission is from person to person by inhalation of aerosolized virus (sneezing, coughing into the air) or by direct contact. Health care–associated transmission of influenza has been reported in acute and long-term health care facilities and has occurred from clients to HCWs, from HCWs to clients, and among HCWs. The incubation period is usually 1 to 4 days (average of 2 days).

Influenza types A and B resemble other respiratory illnesses such as parainfluenza, RSV, rhinovirus, *Mycoplasma pneumoniae,* and adenovirus. The onset of symptoms is usually abrupt, with high fever, chills, malaise, muscular aching (myalgia), headache, sore throat, nasal congestion, and nonproductive cough. The fever lasts about 1 to 7 days (usually 3 to 5 days). Children often present with nausea, vomiting, and otitis media. The infection can progress rapidly in the first few days, causing pneumonia and respiratory failure, predominantly in high-risk groups. Secondary bacterial pneumonia may also develop, usually 5 to 10 days after the onset of viral symptoms, particularly in older adults.

## MEDICAL MANAGEMENT

**PREVENTION.** In 2010 the ACIP recommended that all persons 6 months old and older should be vaccinated.[65] Vaccination is the most effective means of preventing influenza and its complications. In HCWs, vaccination has shown a total reduction in mortality in clients in long-term care facilities,[299] whereas vaccinations given during an epidemic reduce the risks for pneumonia, hospitalization, and death in elderly persons.[151]

The influenza virus is able to mutate at a remarkable rate; for this reason, a new vaccine is made each year to better match existing strains. It requires approximately 6 months to manufacture a vaccine from the time of selection of the strains thought most likely to affect the population to final production.

Two types of vaccines are available. One is the inactivated influenza vaccine (IIV), available in a standard dose trivalent, high-dose trivalent (Fluzone High-Dose), adjuvanted trivalent (elicits a greater immune response), or quadrivalent (Flucelvax) form. An IIV that uses a jet injector (Afluria) is available for persons who are needle phobic. The standard dose trivalent and quadrivalent IIV vaccines can be used in all adults including adults with immunosuppression, adults with chronic disease, and women who are pregnant. It is also recommended for children 6 months and older. Adults older than 65 should receive the high-dose trivalent vaccine. The quadrivalent live attenuated influenza vaccine now includes a better strain to H1N1 and is again recommended for use.[150] It is administered intranasally and may be used for healthy nonpregnant persons ages 2 to 49 years (FluMist).[149] Because the safety and effectiveness of live attenuated influenza vaccine in persons with underlying medical conditions has not been established, it is recommended that these people continue to be vaccinated with only inactivated influenza vaccine.[149] The quadrivalent vaccines are recommended over the trivalent when possible.

Oseltamivir and zanamivir are recommended for prevention and postexposure prophylaxis in persons at high risk for complications (see Treatment) and residents in long-term care facilities.[86] Antivirals should not be used in place of the vaccine but can be used in conjunction during outbreaks, particularly in high-risk people, such as in long-term care facilities. If unvaccinated individuals at high risk for influenza complications are exposed to influenza (i.e., close contact with a person during their most infectious period, which is 1 day before fever until 24 hours after fever breaks), they should receive chemoprophylaxis within 48 hours of the exposure and also receive the vaccine. Healthy unvaccinated individuals and HCWs can receive postexposure prophylaxis if they will be in close contact with a person who is at high risk of complications.[164]

**DIAGNOSIS.** During an outbreak, influenza in individuals who are not at high risk for complications can be diagnosed clinically. However, clients with increased risk for complications, particularly if the results change management, should be tested. The virus may be isolated from nasopharyngeal aspirate, nasopharyngeal or nasal swabs, or throat swabs (highest to lowest yield of virus). The two tests available are a rapid antigen detection test (ELISA or immunofluorescent assay [IFA]) or molecular assay (conventional reverse transcriptase PCR). Molecular assay tests have a higher sensitivity and are preferred over rapid antigen detection tests, if available. Owing to the lower sensitivity (i.e., false negatives are more common than false positives), a negative result on a rapid detection test should have clinical correlation, and if the likelihood is high that the person has influenza, he or she should be treated or a molecular assay test should be considered.

**TREATMENT.** Treatment should be given to people with suspected or confirmed influenza with severe disease, particularly persons requiring hospitalization; persons at high risk for complications of influenza; children younger than 1 year of age; and persons with influenza caused by H1N1, influenza A H3N2, influenza B, or influenza A with unknown subtype. Duration of symptoms can be reduced by one-half day to 3 days when treatment is initiated within 48 hours of disease presentation.[33,73,126] There is controversy about whether antiviral therapy reduces the severity, complications, or risk of complications of influenza.[103,183] Groups of people thought to be at high risk for influenza complications include nursing home residents, adults 65 years old or older, pregnant women and women up to 2 weeks postpartum, Native Americans, individuals with morbid obesity, and individuals with chronic medical diseases.[61] Treatment should not be delayed for people with significant symptoms until diagnostic tests are available. Adults who are not in a high-risk category do not require testing or treatment, but if they present to medical care within 48 hours of symptoms, antiviral therapy is a consideration. If presenting greater than 48 hours of symptoms, they should not be treated because it most likely will not be beneficial.

There are currently several licensed medications available for the treatment of influenza that fall into three classes: neuraminidase inhibitors (e.g., oseltamivir, zanamivir, and peramivir), influenza cap-dependent endonuclease (e.g., baloxavir), and the adamantanes (e.g., amantadine and rimantadine). The newest is baloxavir, which inhibits the initiation of messenger RNA synthesis. It was approved in the United States in October 2018 for children 12 years and older and adults. Similar to oseltamivir, it reduces time to symptom alleviation compared with placebo. Dosing is easy, requiring only one weight-based dose compared with oseltamivir, which is dosed over 5 days.

Resistance to these antivirals does occur, and providers should be aware of local and state surveillance data for oseltamivir resistance. Amantadine is effective only against influenza A, and there are high rates of resistance. Oseltamivir is typically used for treatment of uncomplicated and severe cases of influenza and for prophylaxis; peramivir is given intravenously for uncomplicated influenza and can be used, although not approved, for severe cases. Zanamivir and baloxavir are used for treatment of uncomplicated influenza. The CDC monitors and recommends specific, effective treatment for each season.

Many people with influenza prefer to rest in bed; analgesics and a cough medicine mixture are often used. Droplet precautions (see Table 8.3) are imperative for all diagnosed and suspected cases of influenza. Antibacterial antibiotics are used only for treatment of bacterial complications.

**PROGNOSIS.** The duration of uncomplicated illness is 3 to 7 days, and the prognosis is usually very good in previously healthy people. Most fatalities related to influenza are caused by bacterial and viral pneumonia in high-risk groups.[384]

**RESPIRATORY SYNCYTIAL VIRUS.** RSV is the leading cause of lower respiratory tract infections in children worldwide.[265] In the United States approximately 57,000 hospitalizations are related to RSV among children younger than 5 years old, and 2.1 million outpatient visits occur in children younger than age 5 years.[159] Most children are infected by the time they are 2 years old. More than 170,000 elderly people are hospitalized each year for RSV, with 14,000 deaths reported.[120]

In adults and older children, reinfection is common and manifests as mild upper respiratory tract infection and tracheobronchitis. Serious pulmonary RSV infections have been described in older and immunocompromised individuals, and there is a high mortality rate in bone marrow and solid organ transplant recipients. In addition, infants with congenital heart disease, patients in ICUs, individuals with cystic fibrosis, and older adults are at high risk for serious and complicated RSV. Other high-risk groups include premature infants, children with Down syndrome, people with underlying lung disease, and infants younger than 6 months of age.

Annual epidemics occur in fall, winter, and spring, although there is geographic variation. The incubation period is 3 to 8 days. Inoculation occurs through the eyes or nose and rarely the mouth.

Health care–associated transmission of RSV occurs among clients, visitors, and HCWs. RSV is present in large numbers in the respiratory secretions of children with symptomatic RSV infections. It can be transmitted through large droplets (aerosolized spread has also been implicated[208]) during close contact with such individuals or indirectly by hands or fomites that are contaminated with RSV. Hands can become contaminated through touching or handling of fomites or respiratory secretions and can transmit RSV by touching the nose or eyes.

Usually people shed the virus for 3 to 8 days, but young infants may shed the virus for 3 to 4 weeks. Symptoms of RSV can be similar to symptoms of other common respiratory pathogens such as influenza, including fever, cough, rhinorrhea, tachypnea, and wheezing. Hyperinflated lungs, decreased gas exchange, and increased work of breathing are also often present. Sinusitis and otitis media are common complications. Severe symptoms include pneumonia, acute respiratory failure, and apnea.

Rapid diagnosis of RSV may be made by viral antigen identification of nasal washings using an ELISA or IFA; this test is sensitive in children but less so in older children or adults. Culture of nasopharyngeal secretions gives a definitive diagnosis but requires 4 to 15 days. Real-time PCR assays for RNA of the virus are becoming more available and are more sensitive in adults.

Treatment consists of hydration, humidification of inspired air, and ventilatory support as needed. Corticosteroids and bronchodilators may be beneficial in treating adults and older children but are not recommended for children. Aerosolized ribavirin (an antiviral agent) has been found to be beneficial in treating adults who have undergone hematopoietic cell transplant.[400] It is approved by the Food and Drug Administration for the treatment of RSV in children, but close monitoring must be provided, and its use is not routinely recommended. Pregnant women should avoid ribavirin exposure, as it may be associated with fetal malformation, although this is uncertain.[314]

Providing passive immunity with monoclonal antibodies does not provide benefit in treating hospitalized infants and young children.[135] Palivizumab (a humanized monoclonal antibody) has been approved for prevention of serious lower respiratory tract illness in infants and young children who are at high risk of serious RSV,[174] but it is expensive and must be administered intramuscularly on a monthly basis during the RSV season.

Avoidance of exposure to tobacco smoke, cold air, and air pollutants is also beneficial to long-term recovery from RSV bronchiolitis. A number of vaccines to prevent this infection are currently being studied, but because the immune response is neither durable nor complete, it has been a difficult task.

SPECIAL IMPLICATIONS FOR THE THERAPIST 8.12

## *Viral Respiratory Infections*

### Influenza

HCWs must follow the guidelines in Tables 8.3 and 8.5 regarding prevention of transmission of influenza for both themselves and their clients. Recommendations for immunization must be reviewed and acted on individually. Because immunization for influenza does not provide immunity for the entire year or for all strains of influenza, common sense must prevail in the case of an HCW who suspects he or she has early signs and symptoms of influenza.

An early diagnosis can result in the use of antivirals to minimize intensity and duration of symptoms, especially in people at high risk for complications. HCWs must be aware of their responsibility to avoid transmission of infectious diseases such as influenza and either use personal protective equipment or practice self-isolation by staying home. This is especially important for the therapist in a setting with elderly, immunocompromised, or chronically ill individuals.

Influenza can cause substantial morbidity and mortality among persons age 65 years and older and among adults age 50 years and older who have chronic illnesses. Anyone in these two groups is vulnerable to the serious complications of influenza. Routine influenza vaccination is associated with reductions in influenza-associated and all-cause mortality during influenza season.[14,274] Despite the benefits of vaccination, utilization remains below target rates. Therapists can be instrumental in reducing morbidity and mortality rates by encouraging clients to get a flu shot each year and by getting one themselves.

**Special Focus: COVID-19:** At the time of publication of this textbook, the Covid-19 pandemic has been raging around the world. We acknowledge that the information presented here is preliminary and much more data will become available, changing some of the presented material.

***Overview***

On December 31, 2019, The World Health Organization (WHO) was informed of a cluster of cases of severe pneumonia in the city of Wuhan, Hubei province in China. It was determined that this illness was caused by a novel coronavirus that carried a higher mortality rate than the previous severe acute respiratory coronavirus (SARS-CoV-1) or influenza viruses. The WHO termed the virus SARS-CoV-2 or Covid-19. Covid-19 is an enveloped, single-strand RNA virus thought to be related to coronaviruses found in bats. This is a new virus which people have not "seen" before nor have immunity against.

***Etiologic and Risk Factors***

The virus is principally spread through droplets that can be directly inhaled following coughing, sneezing, or even talking. The virus may also be spread through contact and aerosolization. SARS-CoV-2 can remain viable on surfaces for an extended period of time–stainless steel and plastic can harbor the virus for up to 3 days while it only remains on paper for approximately 24 hours.[395a,415b] Covid-19 can also be aerosolized through devices, such as CPAP, and procedures, including bronchoscopy and intubation. In a research environment, studies have demonstrated that the virus can remain in the air for several hours, although the duration in real time is not known. The virus has an incubation period of 2-12 days, with the median time to symptom development of 6.4 days. Unlike the SARS-CoV-1 virus where viral loads were highest after developing symptoms, viral loads for Covid-19 are high beginning the day before development of symptoms, making the spread of the virus more rapid. Even people who are initially asymptomatic or have very mild symptoms can shed virus and contribute to the spread of the disease.[16b,219a,428]

People at highest risk for severe morbidity and mortality include those over the age of 65, people with underlying medical problems, such as cardiac disease (2.5% to 15%), hypertension (15% to 30%), immunosuppression, COPD, asthma, cancer and diabetes.[82b,152a,404a] Covid-19 also affects younger people. Of total hospitalizations, about 20% are between the ages of 20-44. This age group also accounts for 12% of ICU admissions. Children appear to be less affected by the virus but may remain a source of infection to others.

***Pathophysiology***

SARS-CoV-2 is believed to exploit the same mechanism to enter cells as SARS-CoV-1, by utilizing the ACE2 receptor.[170a] Following infection with Covid-19, there is a downregulation of ACE2 and activation of the renin-angiotensin system (RAS). Activation of the RAS leads to excessive neutrophil migration, increased vascular permeability with resultant pulmonary edema and acute respiratory distress syndrome (ARDS).[154a] Severe disease is often accompanied by elevated levels of IL-6 in what is termed a "cytokine storm." People infected with Covid-19 demonstrate elevated levels of angiotensin II which correlates to lung injury and viral load.[222a]

There is debate of whether angiotensin-converting enzyme inhibitors (ACEIs)/angiotensin receptor blockers (ARBs), play a role in the ability of the virus to enter target cells and mediate severity of the disease or if they act to ameliorate the pathologic process caused by the virus.[154a] ACEIs and ARBs upregulate ACE2 expression as well as block ACE-1 and angiotensin II type 1 receptor, which could increase the number of receptors (ACE2) available to the virus to gain entry into cells. Yet ACEIs/ARBs may also reduce lung and heart injury by inactivating the renin-angiotensin system.

***Clinical Manifestations***

The majority of people (80%) infected with Covid-19 do not require hospitalization and many exhibit few symptoms (paucisymptomatic). Some remain asymptomatic. This latter group many not know they are infectious and inadvertently spread the virus.

Infection with Covid-19 can lead to a range of symptoms, from mild to severe. The most common symptoms are fever, muscle aches, fatigue, shortness of breath, and dry cough. Other symptoms include sore throat, loss of taste/smell, and gastrointestinal symptoms such as nausea, vomiting, and/or diarrhea.

Approximately 20% will require hospitalization. In susceptible people, severe infections and cytokine release syndrome ("cytokine storm") may develop 5 to 10 days after becoming symptomatic. This is characterized by high fever, hypoxemia, and elevated IL-6 levels. Between 17% to 29% of people with Covid-19 related pneumonia develops acute respiratory distress syndrome (ARDS). In Washington state, about 85% of people who developed severe illness had an underlying comorbidity.[12a] Early studies from Wuhan, China, show that neurological manifestations may occur in >30% of hospitalized patients with Covid-19, including acute stroke and impaired consciousness.[235a]

Complications occur such as a high tendency for deep-venous thrombosis (DVT) and pulmonary embolism (PE), cardiomyopathy, and rarely encephalitis.

***Diagnosis***

There are currently multiple tests available for the diagnosis of Covid-19 through both local health departments and private labs; however, the supply has been limited and the CDC has created criteria for which patients can be tested. Confirmatory testing is by polymerase chain reaction tests (PCR), that are able to detect viral particles from a nasopharyngeal swab. Rapid molecular tests are also becoming available. Sensitivity of PCR tests are unknown but may be as low as 70%, requiring multiple tests for persons highly suspected of the infection but with negative initial results. Serologic tests are also available that detect IgM or IgG antibodies to the virus. Sensitivity appears to be highest after 7 days, making these tests more useful later into the illness. PCR testing may be most useful initially, with serology becoming more meaningful with time. Serologic testing, however, is currently not validated for diagnosing initial infection nor indicative of protective immunity.

Imaging is abnormal in most people needing hospitalization. Chest CT may initially show a ground-glass appearance that may progress into areas of consolidation and then the development of ARDS. Radiographic findings typically peak by day 10 and begin to resolve after 14 days. Even though CT may demonstrate changes prior to symptoms, the diagnosis should appropriately be made through PCR testing.

***Treatment***

There is currently no known optimal treatment for this novel virus and most care is supportive. Since the majority of people only develop minor symptoms, those with mild symptoms or a positive test for Covid-19 should self-quarantine for 14 days and seek medical attention with worsening symptoms. Many state governments have asked/required general residents to shelter-in-place and to practice social distancing (6 feet) when out in public (the distance droplets are believed to travel from an infected person). Countries have closed borders and imposed travel bans. Social distancing

*Continued*

and shelter-in-place orders have been felt to reduce the number of cases and deaths related to Covid-19, as well as reduce the number of people who would acutely need medical care at one time. Thereby "flattening the curve" (number of patients versus available hospital beds/ventilators) and not overwhelming the medical system. Masks are universally recommended for use in public.

Many types of medications are under investigation and trials ongoing for the treatment of Covid-19, including testing new antivirals, such as remdesivir and EIDD-2803[345a]; some antiviral drugs have already been shown to be ineffective, such as the antivirals Lopinavir and ritonavir. The medications hydroxychloroquine and azithromycin have been touted as beneficial; however, small studies demonstrate little benefit, particularly considering toxicities/side effects of these drugs .[82a,255a] Immunomodulators that inhibit the inflammatory cytokine overexpression, such as IL-6 inhibitor Tocilizumab, are also being actively investigated.

The FDA has approved serum with neutralizing antibodies obtained from convalesced patients for emergency use (severe illness or immediately life-threatening symptoms).[345b] Phase I trials for a vaccine have begun.[415a]

***Prognosis***

The majority of people (about 80%) who become infected with Covid-19 will recover and not require hospitalization, while 20% will need hospital care. Currently, in the United States, infection with SARS-CoV-2 carries a 2% to 4% mortality rate, which is about 6 to 10 times higher than influenza. In Washington state, the mortality of patients requiring ICU care was 67%. Elderly people are more likely to die, with a 10% to 27% mortality rate in people older than 85 years.[51a] Other countries have experienced higher rates, such as Spain, Italy and France (up to 13%). Some countries have much lower rates but this is most likely due to testing. Germany and South Korea, for example, have been able to perform testing on a large scale, including symptomatic, paucisymptomatic, and asymptomatic people. They are able to include asymptomatic or paucisymptomatic people in their total number of infected, resulting in a lower mortality rate. The United States has not had readily available testing.

For those that recover, there may be lasting effects, principally in the heart and lungs. Cardiomyopathy was noted in 33% of people who required ICU care in Washington state.[12a] ARDS may lead to life-long exercise limitations and neuropsychological disorders.

***Information Pertinent to Physical Therapy[174a]***

The American Physical Therapy Association (APTA)and the World Confederation for Physical Therapy (WCPT) have compiled resources related to Covid-19 that is pertinent to the physical therapy profession. Please refer to their respective websites for details. At this time, the key concepts include reducing facility risk by limiting visitors and screening each person for Covid-19 symptoms prior to entering the facility. Protection of healthcare workers (HCWs) and patients includes hand hygiene, correctly donning and doffing personal protective equipment (PPE), adhering to standard and transmission based precautions, and minimizing exposure through telemedicine or collaboration with the healthcare team. Hand hygiene should be performed before and after donning and doffing PPE using 60% to 90% alcohol based hand rub or 20 seconds of handwashing. HCWs should wear a facemask at all times in the healthcare facility for protection and as source control. When entering the room of an individual with Covid-19 the HCW should don a respirator, gown, gloves, and eye protection. Collaboration with the healthcare team minimizes the number of people entering the room of an individual with Covid-19 and therefore reduces HCWs as vectors. At this time, physical therapists are prioritizing individuals with Covid-19 to avoid contamination of clothing, skin, and the environment.[382a] To minimize risk and exposure to the at-risk population, physical therapists are utilizing telemedicine for subjective interviews and screenings. As with all HCWs at risk of exposure, physical therapists should monitor for signs and symptoms of Covid-19 and stay at home if signs and symptoms develop.

## Miscellaneous Infectious Diseases

### Lyme Disease

**Definition and Overview.** Lyme disease is an infectious multisystemic disorder caused by three closely related tickborne spirochete species, *Borrelia burgdorferi, Borrelia afzelii,* and *Borrelia garinii*. In the United States, most cases of Lyme disease are caused by *B. burgdorferi*. In Europe and Asia, it is most often caused by *Borrelia afzelii* and *Borrelia garinii*.

Lyme disease was first recognized in 1976 when a group of children in Lyme, Connecticut, developed an unusual type of arthritis and a bull's-eye rash.[363] Some of these children also had a history of tick bites. It was not until 1982 that the organism was recovered from affected individuals and tick vectors established the relationship between the spirochete and the infection.[36]

In the United States the disease is transmitted to human beings only by certain ticks of the *Ixodes* species: *Ixodes scapularis* (formerly called *Ixodes dammini*), known as the deer or black-legged tick in the Northeast (from Massachusetts to Maryland) and North Central United States (Wisconsin and Minnesota), and *Ixodes pacificus,* the Western black-legged tick found on the western coast of northern California and Oregon. The ticks are extremely small, measuring approximately 1 to 2 mm.

**Incidence.** Lyme disease has become the most prevalent vector-borne infectious disease in the United States.[261,316] During the years 2004–2016, the annual reports of vector-borne diseases in the United States doubled from 22,000 cases in 2004 to more than 48,000 cases in 2016. Of these, Lyme disease accounted for 82%.[316] This increased frequency is most likely multifactorial, a result of a heightened awareness of the illness in endemic areas, global travel, climate warming (the ticks have expanded their habitat west and south), and an expansion of the animal reservoir habitat.

Most cases (almost 90%) have been reported from the Mid-Atlantic, Northeast, and North Central regions of the United States. In 2017 the CDC confirmed more than 29,000 cases of Lyme disease in the United States, with numbers continuing to rise. Children between the ages of 5 and 14 years and adults over 40 were most often infected.[2] Lyme disease is often seen in the late spring and summer months in the United States when the tick nymphs are most active and human outdoor activities are greatest.

**Pathogenesis.** *I. scapularis* exists in larval, nymphal, and adult stages. Larvae contract *B. burgdorferi* by feeding on infected rodents (white-footed mouse or other small rodents). The larva then molts into a nymph the following spring. The infection is spread to other mammals (rodent or humans) when the nymph seeks a blood meal. Once fed, the nymph molts into an adult in the fall. The host of the adult is the white-tailed deer during the colder months, which is required for the survival of the tick but not the survival of the spirochete. The female adult eventually falls onto the forest floor sometime in the autumn or winter but does not lay eggs until the spring, beginning the 2-year cycle again. Ticks that are seeking a blood meal wait on the underside of shrubs or grass. They are able to sense warmth and carbon dioxide and latch onto animals and humans as they walk past.

Human beings generally acquire the infection from nymphs when they attach to the skin to feed (adults are larger and usually unable to escape detection for greater than 36 hours). The tick becomes engorged with blood and turns a grayish color. The ticks require at least 36 hours or more (up to 72 hours) of feeding before the spirochetes move from the midgut to the salivary glands and are then injected into the host.[110] More commonly, however, the tick falls off or is removed before the bacteria are injected into the host's bloodstream.

After incubating for 3 to 32 days, the spirochetes cause an inflammatory response, resulting in characteristic skin lesions at the site of the tick bite (see Clinical Manifestations). The bacteria then disseminate to other organs via the bloodstream or lymphatic system if not treated.

The human host activates an immune response, producing cytokines and antibodies against the bacteria. Despite the host's response and if untreated, *B. burgdorferi* can survive in certain areas of the body by genetically adapting and inhibiting host immune responses.[290,366,387,421]

Human vertical transmission—that is, infected mother to child in utero—can occur and is more likely when the mother is infected in the first trimester. The incidence of transmission is believed to be quite low. Studies have demonstrated no congenital or adverse fetal outcomes through perinatal transmission of *B. burgdorferi*.[375]

**Clinical Manifestations.** Lyme disease manifests a broad array of signs and symptoms. Symptoms vary widely and may not develop for as long as 1 month after a bite; in some cases, symptoms do not develop at all. Clinical manifestations of the infection typically occur in three stages, but some may overlap.

*Stage 1, the early, localized stage,* usually occurs within 5 to 14 days (less than 1 month) following a tick bite. Approximately 80% of affected individuals will have a red, slowly expanding rash called *erythema migrans* that develops central clearing or a bull's eye appearance (Fig. 8.8).[365] Not all people with the disease develop the telltale rash, and because early symptoms are often mild, some people may remain undiagnosed and untreated. Erythema migrans resolves spontaneously without treatment within an average of 4 weeks. Flu-like symptoms suggestive of early dissemination such as fatigue, chills, fever, headache, lethargy, myalgias, and arthralgias may also develop early in the course of the infection and may be the presenting symptoms for anyone without a rash.

*Stage 2, early, disseminated infection,* particularly involves the skin, nervous system, heart, and joints. Skin manifestations include multiple, smaller erythema migrans, similar to the original rash, occurring days to weeks after infection.

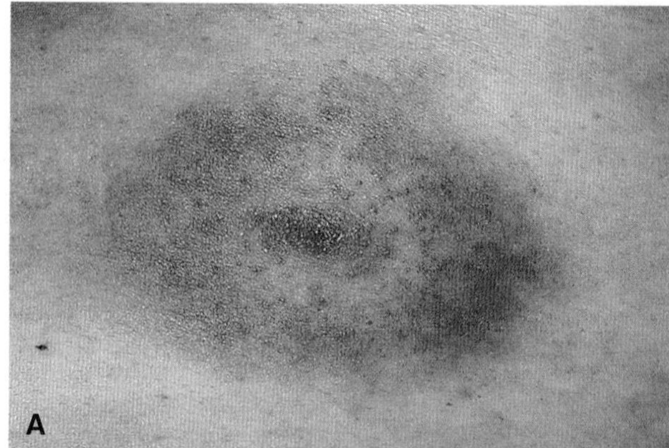


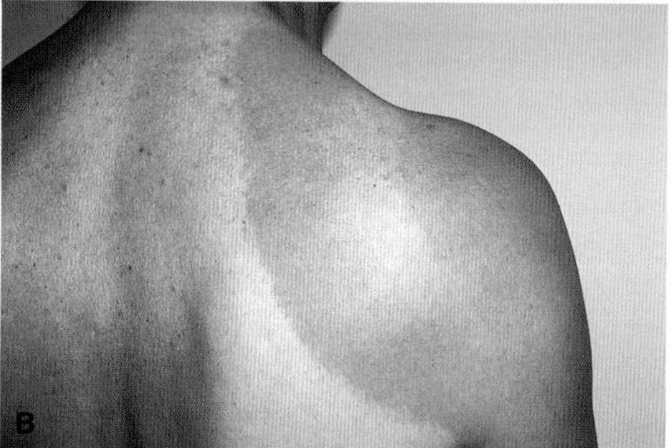


**Figure 8.8**

**Examples of erythema migrans associated with Lyme disease.** (A) Many sources describe a characteristic bull's-eye rash with Lyme disease. (B) However, a wide range of skin reactions, known as erythema migrans, is possible with Lyme disease, as shown. Some skin rashes may be so minor as to be ignored or go unnoticed by the affected individual. (A, From Swartz MH: *Textbook of physical diagnosis: history and examination*, ed 4, Philadelphia, 2002, Saunders. B, From Mandel GL: *Principles and practice of infectious diseases*, ed 6, Edinburgh, 2005, Churchill Livingstone.)

**Box 8.10**

**NEUROLOGIC MANIFESTATIONS OF LYME DISEASE**

Facial nerve palsy (Bell's palsy)

Cognitive impairment (e.g., forgetfulness, decreased concentration, personality changes)

Inflammation of the brain, spinal cord, or nerves
- Cranial neuritis
- Encephalitis
- Encephalomyelitis
- Encephalopathy
- Meningitis
- Radiculoneuropathies

Neurologic symptoms, beginning weeks to months after the initial infection, may be the first to arise and occur in 15% of all cases, most commonly manifested as aseptic meningitis with mild headache, stiff neck, and difficulty with mentation; cranial neuropathies, particularly Bell's palsy (involvement of cranial nerve VII); and radiculopathies (Box 8.10).[160] The classic triad is lymphocytic meningitis, facial nerve palsy, and radiculoneuritis, although they may occur alone. Even if untreated, neurologic symptoms may improve or resolve.

Some people (approximately 5%) experience cardiac signs and symptoms. The most common are conduction abnormalities (usually atrioventricular block) and dysrhythmias, which can result in irregular, rapid, or slowed pulses; dizziness; fainting; chest pain; and shortness of breath. Symptoms typically resolve after several days to weeks. Myocarditis is less commonly seen.[293] Clients may also experience migratory arthralgias, but not arthritis, during this stage. It is typically of a relapsing/remitting pattern. Migratory musculoskeletal pain in joints, bursae, tendons, muscle, and bone may occur in one or a few locations at a time, often lasting days to weeks in a given location.

*Stage 3, late persistent infection,* may become apparent months to years after the initial infection and typically involves the joints and nervous system. In the United States approximately 60% of individuals left untreated develop stage 3 joint symptoms characterized by intermittent or chronic monarticular (one joint) or oligoarticular (affecting only a few joints) arthritis.[364] This arthritis is associated with marked swelling, especially in the large joints, such as the knees (Fig. 8.9). Joint pain is typically not severe and related to effusion size; systemic symptoms are minor. Rarely, affected individuals may go on to develop erosions or permanent joint abnormalities.

Early treatment can prevent the development of arthritis. If untreated, approximately 80% develop joint involvement.[364] Treatment aids in the resolution of symptoms and prevents recurrences and damage to joints.[362] Several months of antibiotics may be required before there is complete resolution of symptoms.

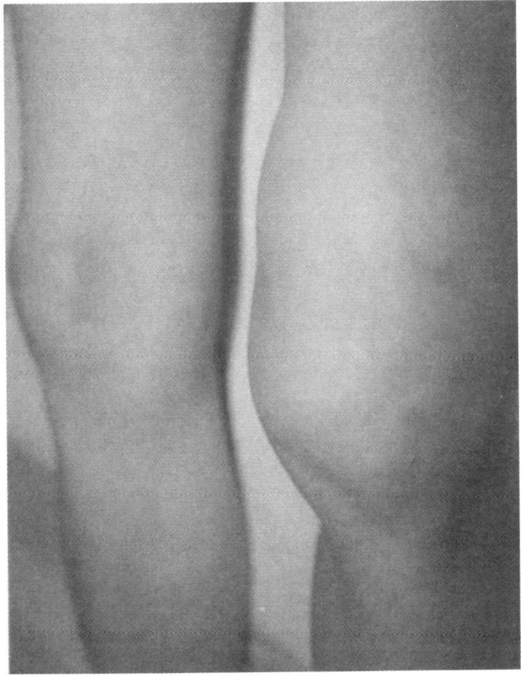

**Figure 8.9**

**Swollen knee of a youth with Lyme arthritis.** (Reprinted from National Institutes of Health: *Lyme disease: the facts, the challenge*, NIH publication no. 92-3193, Bethesda, MD, 1992, U.S. Department of Health and Human Services, p. 12.)

The manifestations of late-onset neurologic disease is different from early, disseminated disease, consisting of a chronic, axonal polyneuropathy with spinal radicular pain or distal paresthesias, associated with minor cognitive slowing or memory difficulties.

**Postinfection Syndromes.** Several syndromes have been reported describing persistent symptoms despite antibiotic treatment. One such syndrome, called post–Lyme disease syndrome, resembles fibromyalgia. Affected individuals describe disabling fatigue, headache, diffuse muscle or joint pain, cognitive difficulties, and sleep abnormalities. The Infectious Diseases Society of America has formalized criteria for this syndrome including history of prior Lyme disease treated with an acceptable antibiotic regimen with resolution or stabilization of symptoms; presentation of new symptoms within 6 months of the initial infection and persisting for 6 months after completion of antibiotics.[416] Approximately 5% to 15% of people meet the criteria for post–Lyme disease syndrome.[121] Most people with these symptoms improve slowly over 6 months to 1 year.

*Chronic Lyme disease* is a term used by some patient advocacy groups describing not only post–Lyme disease syndrome but also other symptoms, often related to fibromyalgia or other illness. Most evidence demonstrates that the diagnosis of Lyme disease is appropriate for only a minority of patients in whom it is suspected.[212,261] In studies that followed patients with an accurate diagnosis of Lyme disease, few went on to demonstrate chronic syndrome complaints. There is no current evidence to support the use of repeat antibiotic treatment for continuing symptoms.[24] Of persons with documented, treated disease, it is hypothesized that the bacteria may trigger a neurohormonal or immunologic process that causes symptoms despite eradication of the spirochete.[301] Although evidence of the spirochete exists in the synovial fluid before treatment, posttreatment joint fluid is often negative for infection. This may be immune rather than infection related.[361]

## MEDICAL MANAGEMENT

**PREVENTION.** Prevention is the key to avoiding Lyme disease.[261] Lyme disease is most common during the late spring and summer months in the United States, when nymphal ticks are most active and human populations are frequently outdoors and most exposed. People who live or work in residential areas surrounded by woods or overgrown brush infested by ticks and rodents or live in the endemic geographic areas are at risk. People who participate in outdoor recreational activities in tick habitat are also at risk for Lyme disease. Current prevention research includes developing better insect repellents, such as nootkatone; the use of permethrin-treated clothing as a method of repelling ticks[117]; use of bait boxes that treat rodents for ticks[334]; and the development of an oral rodent vaccine against the spirochete.[144]

Prophylactic treatment is controversial, but a single dose of doxycycline for ticks that have been attached to the skin for between 36 and 72 hours may be helpful.[264,416] Treatment must begin within 72 hours of tick removal. Box 8.11 provides specific strategies available for Lyme disease prevention.

Box 8.11

**PREVENTION OF LYME DISEASE**

These precautions are provided for people living in tick-infested areas:

- Avoid tick-infested areas, especially in May, June, and July (check with local health departments or park services for the seasonal and geographic distribution in your area).
- Walk along cleared or paved surfaces rather than through tall grass or wooded areas.
- Wear long-sleeved shirts, long pants tucked into socks, and closed shoes (no part of foot exposed).
- Wear light-colored clothing to make it easy to detect ticks.
- Always check for ticks after being outdoors. If ticks are removed within 36 hours of attachment, the risk of infection decreases significantly.
- Shower as soon as possible after being outdoors. Ticks take several hours to attach themselves to the skin and can be washed away first.
- Wash clothing worn outdoors immediately and use a dryer (heat kills the ticks). If no access to laundry facilities is available, the clothing should not be stored in the bedroom, or if camping, the clothing should not be stored in the same area where people are sleeping.
- If bitten by a tick, remove the tick immediately by grasping it as close to the skin as possible with tweezers and tugging gently. Do not twist or turn the tweezers; pull straight away from the skin. Do not use petroleum jelly, fingernail polish, or a hot match to remove ticks.
- To lessen the chance of contact with the bacterium, do not crush the tick's body or handle the tick with bare hands. Clean the bite area thoroughly with soap and water, then swab the area with an antiseptic to prevent bacterial infection.
- Whenever possible, save the tick in a glass jar for identification should symptoms develop.
- If living in an area in which deer ticks are common, keep the weeds and grass around the house mowed. Consider using wood chips where lawns meet forested areas. Ticks are less able to survive in a dry environment.
- Use flea and tick collars on pets; brush and examine them carefully after they have been outdoors. People can use insecticides such as permethrin or insect repellents containing diethyltoluamide (DEET).[a]

[a]The use of such chemicals may be objectionable to some people because they may cause neurotoxicity in children. Alternative methods are available.

**DIAGNOSIS.** Persons with the typical erythema migrans do not require testing, and it is not recommended. There are no consistently reliable tests for early disease, as antibodies are not present for 1 to 2 weeks following infection.

For clients who have had symptoms longer than a few weeks, the CDC suggests a two-step process in diagnosing Lyme disease.[64] The first step is to test the blood for antibodies to the spirochete. This is done with a sensitive EIA (ELISA) or IFA. If this test is positive or equivocal, a Western immunoblot should be performed to confirm the diagnosis. If the Western blot is negative, the person does not have the disease, while a positive result demonstrates the person has been exposed to *B. burgdorferi*. If the Western blot for IgM is positive and symptoms have been present for more than 6 to 8 weeks, and the IgG is negative, the positive IgM most likely represents a false positive.[340]

Positive serologic tests do not necessarily indicate acute infection. Antibodies (IgG) can be present for years after successful treatment[190] and are not indicative of an infection causing the current symptoms. Symptoms, physical examination, and history along with serological testing help make the proper diagnosis. No direct test can indicate whether living *Borrelia* are present in the blood. There is some concern and controversy over the use of inappropriate tests for the diagnosis of Lyme disease such as culture methods, urine antigen testing, PCR on inappropriate specimens, and lymphocyte transformation tests. The CDC has issued a direct warning against using any "unapproved" tests.[54] Care must also be taken not to overdiagnose. Often serum antibody tests are done for "screening" purposes when clients have nonspecific symptoms. In this case, a false-positive result could lead to unnecessary treatment with antibiotics[365] and an incorrect diagnosis.

**TREATMENT.** Early Lyme disease is treated with oral antibiotics, typically doxycycline, amoxicillin, or cefuroxime. Antibiotics are given for 14 days. Clients may experience worsening of symptoms within the first day of treatment. If third-degree heart block develops, IV antibiotics are given for 14 to 28 days along with admission for cardiac monitoring and possible temporary pacemaker placement. Neurologic symptoms are treated for 14 to 28 days, most often with oral antibiotics, although encephalitis typically requires IV treatment.[160] People with late neurologic findings are treated with IV antibiotics for 28 days. Lyme arthritis can be treated with oral or IV antibiotics, depending on the severity of symptoms, although oral therapy is easier and often equally effective. Treatment is typically for 28 days.[416] For anyone with continued arthritis despite recommended treatment, another round of treatment may be given. If the person had partial resolution, oral antibiotics can be used. If there was no improvement, IV antibiotics should be administered for 28 days. If symptoms persist despite the second treatment, data do not support the continued use of antibiotics.[416] Nonsteroidal medications, disease-modifying antirheumatic drugs, and arthroscopic synovectomy have been used as alternatives to treat arthritis, although studies are lacking for these approaches.[301]

**PROGNOSIS.** For most people, Lyme disease is curable with standard antibiotic therapy at any stage, and the effects of Lyme disease resolve completely within a few weeks or months of treatment. Nonspecific symptoms such as fatigue and muscle and joint pain may persist for weeks to months but do not necessarily indicate failure of treatment. For a minority of clients who continue to experience symptoms 6 months following treatment, efforts should be made to determine if they have continued infection, inflammation resulting from infection (postinfection), or another disease.[261] No natural immunity develops from exposure to Lyme disease, and anyone can be reinfected. Although Lyme disease is rarely fatal, heart complications may cause life-threatening cardiac arrhythmias.

SPECIAL IMPLICATIONS FOR THE THERAPIST 8.13

### *Lyme Disease*

Chronic arthritis is the most widely recognized result of untreated Lyme disease in the United States. In contrast to other forms of rheumatoid arthritis, Lyme arthritis does not affect the joints bilaterally, although both sides may be affected alternately.

The condition has been called chronic because episodes can last months, occurring intermittently over a period of 1 to 3 years. Permanent joint damage and cartilage destruction can occur if excessive use occurs during the inflammatory period. Range-of-motion and strengthening exercises are important but must be carried out carefully and without overexertion.

Nervous system abnormalities can develop weeks, months, or years following an untreated infection. These symptoms often last for weeks or months and may recur. The therapist may treat such a client at any time during the course of symptomatic presentation.

For anyone with known Lyme disease, frequent assessment of the person's neurologic function and level of consciousness is important. Any signs of cardiac abnormality or increased intracranial pressure and cranial nerve involvement (e.g., ptosis, strabismus, diplopia) must be reported to the physician immediately. Both upper and lower extremity peripheral nerve impairments can occur and are managed as any neuropathy from other causes.

It has been hypothesized that people who present with symptoms of multiple sclerosis but respond to antibiotics may have been bitten by ticks years ago. Along the same lines, the question has been raised whether Lyme disease triggers fibromyalgia, as symptoms consistent with fibromyalgia and chronic fatigue syndrome develop in individuals with clear-cut Lyme disease, even after adequate treatment. To date, no biologic relationship has been proven between these conditions and Lyme disease.[251]

## Sexually Transmitted Diseases

HIV/AIDS is discussed in Chapter 7, but it is mentioned here to remind us that it is an infectious disease with a specific chain of transmission and control of transmission as discussed in this chapter.

**Overview and Incidence.** STDs are a variety of clinical syndromes caused by pathogens that can be acquired and transmitted through sexual activity. Each year about 20 million Americans contract an STD. There has been a steady and steep increase in the number of STDs in the United States since 2013.[32] In 2017 a record number of 2,295,739 cases were reported. Currently the STDs that require reporting to the CDC include syphilis, gonorrhea, chancroid, and chlamydia. Accurate data are often difficult to obtain because of underreporting. It is likely that the incidence of STDs is underreported for several reasons. Not all STDs have symptoms, and infected persons may not seek medical attention. There also continues to be significant social stigma related to STDs, which may lead individuals to postpone or avoid seeking treatment. Physicians may fail to report STD cases to local health departments despite being mandated to do so. Physicians also rely on individuals to notify their sexual partners, who may or may not be tested and/or treated. A lack of free screening or reimbursement for screening may also be a contributing factor as well as limited government resources.

Syphilis was once thought to be trending toward elimination, but the incidence has steadily increased. The diagnosis of primary and secondary syphilis increased 76% between 2013 and 2017.[32] In 2017 more than 26,000 cases were diagnosed. The majority of cases were in men (88% of cases) and men who have sex with men (68% of cases). The largest increase was in newborns (up 44% from 2016). The incidence of gonorrhea continues to rise in the United States (increased 75% since 2009 and 18% from 2016), and chlamydia and HPV remain significant health problems. Chlamydia is the most common bacterial STD in the United States, with more than 1.7 million cases reported to the CDC in 2017, a 22% increase from 2013.[32] About two-thirds of cases are in young women between the ages of 15 and 24. It is estimated that the actual number of people infected (not just reported cases) is approximately 2.8 million annually. Untreated chlamydia and gonorrhea can progress to pelvic inflammatory disease, infertility, ectopic pregnancy, and chronic pelvic pain.[379]

HPV, a collection of more than 100 serotypes that can infect the genital area, infects more than 14 million men and women per year.[46] Specific serotypes of HPV (e.g., 16 and 18) can cause cervical cancer in women and are linked with oral squamous cell carcinoma.[328] The national oral infection incidence is high at 6.9% of the population.[140] Other serotypes (e.g., 6 and 11) can cause genital warts.

Although the number of seropositive HSV-2 cases has been trending down, it is a chronic disease, and most cases remain undiagnosed.[247] It is estimated that more than 50 million people carry the HSV-2 virus.[420]

STDs are spread primarily through sexual contact, but some cases may also be spread by sharing infected needles or by transmission from mother to child during vaginal childbirth. Many STDs are easily treated and cured, but others remain chronic. More than 50 different STDs have been described; only the most common ones are included here (see Table 8.7).

**Risk Factors.** All groups of people are potentially at risk for STDs, but women, teens, men who have sex with men, and minorities have been disproportionately affected. Although 25% of all STDs occur in people younger than 25 years, numerous surveys of healthy adults verify that older people are sexually active and less likely to practice safe sex. Direct contact with an infectious lesion is the main risk factor.

Other risk factors include multiple sex partners, persons who initiate sex early in adolescence, a partner with a known risk factor, persons residing in detention facilities, men having sex with men, obstacles in obtaining health care, a history of a blood transfusion between 1977 and 1984, failure to use a condom (or use it properly) during sexual intercourse, and sharing needles during illicit drug use. The presence of STDs is a risk factor itself for facilitating the transmission of HIV. In fact, persons with an STD are three to five times more likely than a person without an STD to sexually acquire HIV.[133]

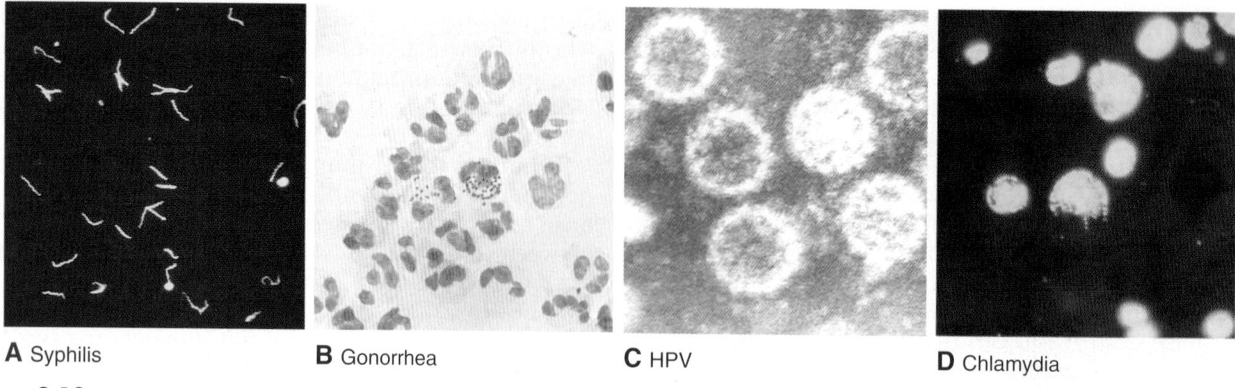


**Figure 8.10**

**Sexually transmitted infections.** (A) Syphilis mimics so many diseases it is called "the great imitator." Dark-field microscopy shows several spirochetes in scrapings from the base of a syphilitic chancre. (B) Gonorrhea, called the "preventer of life," can cause sterility. Gram-stained smear of urethral discharge shows intracellular gram-negative diplococci characteristic of gonorrhea. (C) Human papillomavirus (HPV) is the most common cause of cervical and other reproductive cancers. D, Chlamydia is the most common sexually transmitted disease reported in the United States. (A, From Kumar V, Abbas AK, Fausto N: *Robbins and Cotran pathologic basis of disease*, ed 7, Philadelphia, 2005, Saunders, courtesy Paul Southern, Department of Pathology, University of Texas Southwestern Medical School, Dallas, TX. B, From Mandell GL: *Principles and practice of infectious diseases*, ed 6, Philadelphia, 2005, Churchill Livingstone. C, From Kumar V, Abbas AK, Fausto N: *Robbins and Cotran pathologic basis of disease*, ed 7, Philadelphia, 2005, Saunders, courtesy Ian Frazer, Princess Alexandra Hospital, University of Queensland, Australia. D, From Mandell GL: *Principles and practice of infectious diseases*, ed 6, Philadelphia, 2005, Churchill Livingstone, courtesy Robert Suchland, Seattle, WA.)

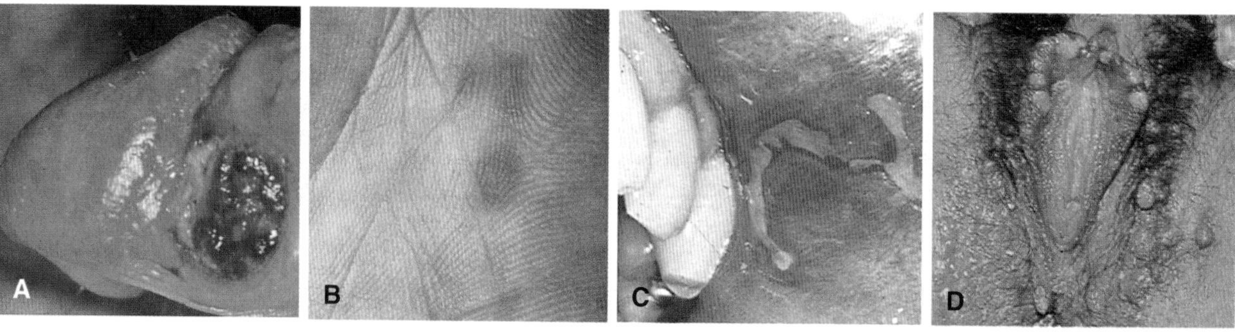


**Figure 8.11**

**Clinical manifestations of syphilis.** Many sexually transmitted infections manifest with lesions of the skin and/or genitals. Each one manifests differently based on the stage of the disease. (A) Chancre in primary syphilis on the penis. (B) Palmar lesions of a coppery color in secondary syphilis. (C) Mucous patch of the mouth in secondary syphilis. (D) Genital lesions called condylomata lata in a female patient (secondary syphilis). (A, C, and D, From Forbes CD, Jackson WF: *Color atlas and text of clinical medicine*, London, 2003, Mosby. B, From Habif TP: *Skin disease: diagnosis and treatment*, St. Louis, 2001, Mosby.)

**Pathogenesis and Clinical Manifestations.** STDs are caused by bacteria, viruses, and occasionally parasites and may have a considerable latency period when the infectious organism lies dormant before triggering symptomatic presentation (Fig. 8.10).

Clinical manifestations vary according to the STD present (Figs. 8.11 and 8.12; see also Table 8.7). STDs may be completely asymptomatic and therefore are less likely to be diagnosed until serious problems develop. Complications of STDs are often more severe and more frequent among women than men. Once infected, women are more susceptible to reproductive cancers, infertility, and contracting other STDs including HIV.

## MEDICAL MANAGEMENT

A brief summary of these key points is provided; for details, the reader is referred to the CDC's updated treatment guideline.[414]

**PREVENTION.** Prevention is the most important key to managing STDs. The CDC has identified five principal strategies for the prevention of STDs: (1) education and counseling of persons at risk on ways to avoid STDs through changes in sexual behaviors and use of recommended prevention services; (2) identification of asymptomatically infected persons and of symptomatic persons unlikely to seek diagnostic and treatment services; (3) effective diagnosis, treatment, and counseling of infected persons; (4) evaluation, treatment, and counseling of sex partners of persons who are infected with an STD; and (5) preexposure vaccination of persons at risk for vaccine-preventable STDs.[414]

Primary prevention of STDs begins with changing the sexual behaviors that place persons at risk for infection. The only prevention that is 100% effective is abstinence from oral, vaginal, and anal sex or to be in a mutually monogamous sexual relationship (single partner) with an uninfected partner.

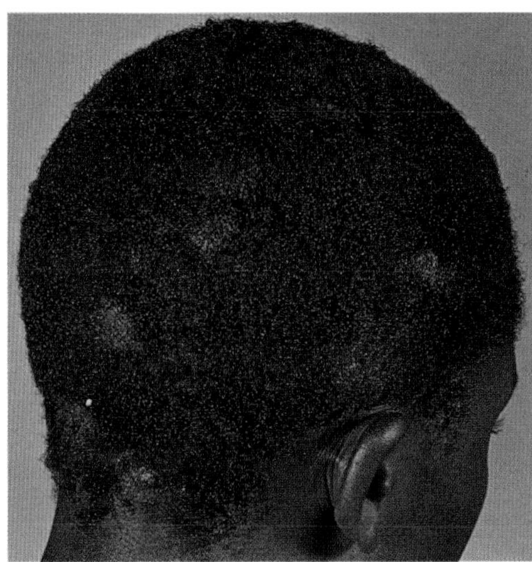

**Figure 8.12**

**Alopecia of the scalp (balding) associated with secondary syphilis.** This is a temporary, irregular presentation of alopecia sometimes referred to as moth-eaten alopecia. (From Habif TP: *Clinical dermatology*, ed 4, St. Louis, Mosby, courtesy Subhash K. Hira.)

For people who are sexually active, condoms, consistently and properly used, are able to reduce the transmission of STDs spread by mucosal fluid (e.g., gonorrhea, chlamydia, and HIV). However, condoms do not cover all surfaces and only protect the skin they cover and are therefore less likely to protect against diseases acquired from skin-to-skin contact such as syphilis, HPV, and HSV. Genital warts caused by HPV are contagious; avoid touching them. Spermicides with nonoxynol-9 are not effective against gonorrhea, chlamydia, or HIV infection; the CDC does not recommend the use of nonoxynol-9 with or without condoms for STD or HIV protection.[414]

To prevent transmission of STDs to newborns, pregnant women should have blood tests for syphilis, HBV, and HIV. Early syphilis, if untreated in pregnant women, can cause fetal death, particularly seen after 20 weeks. All pregnant women should be routinely tested for hepatitis B surface antigen during the first trimester, even if they have been previously vaccinated or tested.[394]

A vaccine is available to protect people, especially women of childbearing age, against HBV (see Table 8.4). Pregnant women should also be routinely tested for chlamydia, and women at high risk should be tested for gonorrhea and hepatitis C. Pregnant women with recurrent genital herpes and open sores benefit from cesarean section delivery to protect the child.[359,414]

Drug users, especially injection drug users, can prevent transmission of disease best by discontinuing drug use. However, in most cases, this is not immediately realistic. Programs have been set up to help reduce needle sharing by providing needle exchange centers and street education programs aimed at teaching more sterile practices.

Preexposure vaccination is one of the most effective methods for preventing transmission of some STDs. Two HPV vaccines are available for females age 9 to 26 years to prevent cervical precancer and cancer: the quadrivalent HPV vaccine, which protects against HPV types 6, 11, 16, and 18, and the 9-valent HPV vaccine (Gardasil 9), which provides protection not only against the quadrivalent but also includes five other types.[288] Gardasil is recommended for young men and women because it also prevents genital warts. The CDC recommends two doses of the HPV vaccine for all children at age 11 or 12 years with catch-up vaccination through age 26 for women and men who have sex with men and age 21 for men.[414] Details regarding HPV vaccination are available at https://www.cdc.gov/hpv/parents/vaccine.html.

**SCREENING, DIAGNOSIS, TREATMENT, AND PROGNOSIS.** STDs can often be identified by the clinical manifestations, but many individuals remain asymptomatic. Various tests are available to aid in diagnosis. The U.S. Preventive Services Task Force recommends annual screening for chlamydia of all sexually active adolescents and women 24 years or younger and older women with risk factors (new sex partner or multiple sex partners) as well as pregnant women.[216] NAATs use swabs from urogenital sites, including urine, and the same swab can be used to test for gonorrhea.[271] Posttest counseling remains an important key in treatment and prevention.

Treatment includes antibiotics and referral of all sexual contacts for testing and treatment from at least 60 days before symptoms or date of diagnosis. Follow-up testing is not recommended except in pregnant women.[271,414]

Certain HPV serotypes have been found to cause cervical cancer in women. Because there is currently no cure for the virus itself, prevention with immunizations and testing for precancerous and cervical cancer are the most appropriate management strategies. Recommendations for screening for cervical cancer have been published (see Table 20.2). Symptoms such as genital warts are treated with topically applied chemicals, cryotherapy, or surgical removal.

Although HPV is most often acquired in younger women, older women continue to be at risk, so testing should take into consideration risk factors. Various immunoassays, serologic techniques, and culture methods are used to diagnose HIV, syphilis, gonorrhea, herpes, and other STDs.

HSV is a lifelong disease, and only symptoms are managed. Antibiotics can cure some STDs (see Table 8.7), although some may be drug resistant. Currently there is concern that gonorrhea, known to be resistant to fluoroquinolones, may become resistant to the only effective antibiotics, third-generation cephalosporins.[27,198] Limiting the number of sexual partners, practicing abstinence, and practicing safe sex (proper use of condoms) are recommended to prevent the transmission of disease. Intercourse during an active infection dramatically increases the risk of transmitting STDs and sexually transmitted infections.

When working with clients with active disease, following contact precautions, frequent hand hygiene, and avoiding touching the affected areas are essential practices. Vaccines are now available for HBV and HPV[414]; vaccines against HIV and herpes are under investigation.[331]

The prognosis varies with each STD, but with treatment symptoms can be minimized and complications can be prevented. Without treatment, serious complications can occur such as infertility, chronic pelvic pain, ectopic pregnancy and miscarriage, cardiovascular disease, CNS impairment, blindness, cervical cancer, and death.

SPECIAL IMPLICATIONS FOR THE THERAPIST 8.14

### *Sexually Transmitted Diseases and Infections*

Any therapist treating men or women with clinical presentation of pelvic, buttock, hip, or groin pain of apparent unknown cause must be prepared to ask the client about past history of STDs and sexually transmitted infections, sexual activity, changes in sexual function, and presence of urogenital signs or symptoms (e.g., discharge from penis or vagina, painful urination, difficulty initiating or continuing a stream of urine). As clinical presentation of pelvic, buttock, hip, or groin pain may be the client's initial symptoms of an STD, the therapist may need to obtain a sexual health history in a nonjudgmental manner to assess risk. The Five P's is one approach to obtaining a sexual history concerning five key areas: Partners, Prevention of pregnancy, Protection from STDs, Practices, and Past history of STDs. Any suspicion that the clinical manifestations may be correlated to an STD must be further evaluated by a physician. A document from the CDC provides treatment guidelines for STDs along with guidelines for gathering information for client education regarding prevention and protection that may be of interest to the therapist.[70,414]

## Infections in Drug Users

Drug use in the United States continues to be a significant health problem, with 10.6% of people older than 12 years of age using illicit drugs each month during 2016.[72] Serious illnesses such as HIV and hepatitis are transmitted with injection drug use.

Drug users have a higher incidence of bacterial infections because of the various drugs used, the route and sites of administration, and preparation of the drug. Each of these factors determines risk for infection and the likelihood of specific bacterial infections.[419]

IV use of black-tar heroin causes sclerosis of the veins and leads to skin popping, or injecting the drug subcutaneously.[327] Continued injection into the same site creates a necrotic environment suitable for clostridial germination and toxin production.[95] NF with toxic shock syndrome can result from the spread of a clostridial infection.[4]

Drug users, particularly IV drug users, vary the site of administration. Local abscess formation or infections from hematogenous seeding are seen in unusual places because of the site of injection (the femoral vein, or "groin hit," and the neck, or "pocket shot"). Osteomyelitis may develop in the sternoclavicular, sacroiliac, or vertebral spine. Septic arthritis is often seen in the knees.[8]

Environmental factors frequently contribute to infections. Some users may lick the skin or needle before injecting, leading to polymicrobial infections. Others crush tablets between their teeth or blow clots out of needles before reusing. Sharing of needles and paraphernalia is also common. Because of these habits, drug users are more likely to develop certain types of bacterial infections with specific organisms.

The four types of infections most often seen are of the skin or soft tissue, endovascular infections, respiratory infections, and musculoskeletal infections.[191] *S. aureus* and streptococcal species (flora from the user's skin) are the most common pathogens in drug-related infections.[8] Drug users are more likely to be colonized with MRSA in the nares and skin than non–drug users; this most likely occurs because of tissue damage from inhaling or injecting drugs.[21]

Abscess formation is common. More serious infections such as endocarditis, septic thrombophlebitis, mycotic aneurysms, and sepsis occur from hematogenous spread of organisms. In injection drug users, *S. aureus* is the most common organism causing endocarditis. Although polymicrobial endocarditis is rare, it is most often seen in injection drug users. Complications of endocarditis include brain, lung, and splenic abscesses.

Drug users are more likely to develop a respiratory tract infection compared with non–drug users, and respiratory infections, particularly pneumonia, are the most common infection in drug users.[249] Smoking cocaine also leads to direct damage of the lung, causing disease such as interstitial fibrosis, pulmonary hypertension, and alveolar hemorrhage.[309] Damage to cells from inhaling drugs and chronic cigarette use (many drug users also smoke) may lead to inability to clear secretions. Aspiration may occur because of decreased mental alertness. Sharing of paraphernalia also increases the risk for infectious diseases.[235] People may also present with severe respiratory distress associated with noncardiogenic pulmonary edema related to heroin overdose.[368]

Clients with HIV may present with atypical features and radiographs, so a good history and physical examination are important. Pulmonary tuberculosis (and drug-resistant tuberculosis) is encountered more frequently in drug users who practice "shotgunning" (inhaling cocaine and blowing smoke into the mouth of another person),[287] live in crowded spaces, or have HIV.

Musculoskeletal infections may occur in unusual places, as discussed earlier. Flora from the skin is the most common pathogen, although polymicrobial infections are seen, especially if saliva contaminates the skin, drugs, or needles. The infection may be subtle, with mild fever and pain.

SPECIAL IMPLICATIONS FOR THE THERAPIST 8.15

### *Infections in Drug Addicts*

See Special Implications for the Therapist 3.12: Substance Use and Addictive Disorders in Chapter 3.

Being aware of the signs of substance abuse or drug addiction and the patterns of infection associated with drug addiction may assist the therapist in recognizing early signs of infection requiring medical evaluation and treatment.

Any therapist involved in wound care management, needle electromyography, or other high-risk practice techniques who has not already been immunized against HBV should be vaccinated. Because of the high risk of infection with bloodborne pathogens such as HIV, HBV, HCV, and CA-MRSA with open wounds in these individuals, environmental surfaces in the area of treatment need to be cleaned by U.S. Environmental Protection Agency–approved products, and HCWs should perform Standard Precautions.

## REFERENCES

To enhance this text and add value for the reader, all references are included in the enhanced ebook on Student Consult that accompanies this textbook. The reader can view the reference source and access it online whenever possible.

CHAPTER 9

# Oncology

JEANNETTE LEE • JOSEPH ANTHONY FRAIETTA (CANCER AND THE IMMUNE SYSTEM) • MICHELLE H. CAMERON (PHYSICAL AGENTS)

*Cancer* is a term that refers to a large group of diseases characterized by uncontrolled cell proliferation and spread of abnormal cells.[273] Other terms used interchangeably for cancer are *malignant neoplasm, tumor, malignancy,* and *carcinoma*. According to the American Cancer Society (ACS), about 5% to 10% of all cancers are genetic, whereas 90% to 95%[18] are related to other (often modifiable) factors. Only oncologic concepts are presented in this chapter; individual cancers are discussed in the chapters devoted to the affected system. Because cancer and cancer treatment can affect multiple systems, the reader is encouraged to read this chapter along with Chapter 5 for a more complete understanding of the potentially wide-ranging systemic effects of cancer.

## DEFINITIONS

### Differentiation

Normal tissue contains cells of uniform size, shape, maturity, and nuclear structure. Differentiation is the process by which normal cells undergo physical and structural changes as they develop to form different tissues of the body. Differentiated cells specialize in different physiologic functions.

In malignant cells, differentiation is altered and may be lost completely, so that the malignant cell may not be recognizable in relationship to its parent cell. When a tumor has completely lost identity with the parent tissue, it is considered to be undifferentiated (anaplastic). In this case it may become difficult or impossible to identify the tissue of origin of the malignant cell. In general, the less differentiated a tumor becomes, the faster metastasis (spread) occurs, and the worse the prognosis is.

### Dysplasia

A variety of other tissue changes can occur in the body. Some of these changes are benign, whereas others denote a malignant or premalignant state. *Dysplasia* is a general term that indicates a disorganization of cells in which an adult cell varies from its normal size, shape, or organization. This is often caused by chronic irritation, such as is seen with changes in cervical (uterine) epithelium as a result of long-standing irritation of the cervix. Dysplasia may reverse itself or may progress to cancer.

### Metaplasia

Metaplasia is the first level of dysplasia (early dysplasia). It is a reversible and benign but abnormal change in which one adult cell changes from one type to another. For example, the most common type of epithelial metaplasia is the change of columnar epithelium of the respiratory tract to squamous epithelium.

Another example of metaplasia is Barrett esophagus (also called Barrett syndrome), in which the squamous epithelium of the esophagus is replaced by the glandular epithelium of the stomach. Although metaplasia usually gives rise to an orderly arrangement of cells, it may sometimes produce disorderly cellular patterns (i.e., cells varying in size, shape, and orientation to one another). Anaplasia (loss of cellular differentiation) is the most advanced form of metaplasia and is considered the hallmark feature of malignant disease.

### Hyperplasia

Hyperplasia refers to increased number of cells in tissue, resulting in increased tissue mass. This type of change can be a normal consequence of physiologic alterations (physiologic hyperplasia) such as increased breast mass during pregnancy, wound healing, or bone callus formation. Neoplastic hyperplasia, however, is the increase in cell mass due to tumor formation and is an abnormal process. The presence of hyperplastic tissue increases the risk of later development of breast cancer, as well as other solid tumor cancers.[301]

### Tumors

Tumors, or neoplasms, are defined as abnormal new growth of tissue that serves no useful purpose and may harm the host organism by competing for vital blood supply and nutrients. These new growths may be benign or malignant (see following discussion of classification) and primary or secondary.

A primary tumor arises from cells that are normally local to the given structure, whereas a secondary tumor arises from cells that have metastasized from another part of the body. For example, a primary neoplasm of bone arises from within the bone structure itself, whereas a secondary neoplasm occurs in bone as a result of metastasized cancer cells from another (primary) site.

**Table 9.1** Classification of Neoplasms by Cell Type of Origin

| Tissue of Origin | Benign | Malignant |
|---|---|---|
| **Epithelial Tissue** | | |
| Surface epithelium (skin) and mucous membrane | Papilloma | Squamous cell, basal cell, and transitional cell carcinoma |
| Epithelial lining of glands or ducts | Adenoma | Adenocarcinoma |
| Pigmented cells (melanocytes of basal layer) | Nevus (mole) | Malignant melanoma |
| **Connective Tissue and Muscle** | | |
| Fibrous tissue | Fibroma | Fibrosarcoma |
| Adipose | Lipoma | Liposarcoma |
| Cartilage | Chondroma | Chondrosarcoma |
| Bone | Osteoma | Osteosarcoma |
| Blood vessels | Hemangioma | Hemangiosarcoma |
| Smooth muscle | Leiomyoma | Leiomyosarcoma |
| Striated muscle | Rhabdomyoma | Rhabdomyosarcoma |
| **Nerve Tissue** | | |
| Nerve cells | Neuroma | |
| Glia | | Glioma or neuroglioma |
| Ganglion cells | Ganglioneuroma | Neuroblastoma |
| Nerve sheaths | Neurilemoma | Neurilemic sarcoma |
| Meninges | Meningioma | Meningeal sarcoma |
| Retina | | Retinoblastoma |
| **Lymphoid Tissue** | | |
| Lymph nodes | | Lymphoma |
| Spleen | | |
| Intestinal lining | | |
| **Hematopoietic Tissue** | | |
| Bone marrow | | Leukemias, myelodysplasia, and myeloproliferative syndromes |
| Plasma cells | | Multiple myeloma |

Carcinoma in situ refers to a localized, preinvasive, and possibly premalignant tumor of epithelial tissue. At this stage of dysplasia, these tumors are contained within the host organ and have not broken through basement membrane. In situ tumors commonly occur in the cervix, bladder, skin, oral cavity, esophagus, bronchus, and breast. Carcinoma in situ that affects glandular epithelium occurs most commonly in the cervix, breast, stomach, endometrium, large bowel, and prostate gland (prostatic intraepithelial neoplasia). The time period between advent of cell dysplasia and invasion beyond local tissue is variable for different cancers.

## CLASSIFICATIONS OF NEOPLASM

A neoplasm (new growth) can be classified on the basis of cell type, tissue of origin, degree of differentiation, anatomic site, or whether it is benign or malignant.

A benign growth is usually considered relatively harmless and does not spread to or invade other tissue. Certain benign growths, recognized clinically as tumors, are not truly neoplastic but rather represent overgrowth of normal tissue elements (e.g., vocal cord polyps, skin tags, hyperplastic polyps of the colon). However, benign growths can become large enough to distend, compress, or obstruct normal tissues and impair normal body functions, as in the case of benign central nervous system (CNS) tumors. These tumors can cause disability as well as death.

Tumors (benign or malignant) are classified by cell type and are named according to the tissue from which they arise (Table 9.1). The five major classifications of normal body tissue are epithelial, connective and muscle, nerve, lymphoid, and hematopoietic tissue. Not all tissue types fit into one of these five categories, thus requiring a miscellaneous category for other tissues (not included in Table 9.1), such as the tissues of the reproductive glands, placenta, and thymus.

*Epithelium* covers all external body surfaces and lines all internal spaces, organs, and cavities. The skin, mucous membranes, gastrointestinal tract, and lining of the bladder are examples of epithelial tissue. The functions of epithelial tissues are to protect, excrete, and absorb. Cancers originating in epithelial tissue (endodermal origin) are called carcinomas. A common example of a tumor derived from glandular tissues is called an *adenocarcinoma*. Carcinomas represent the most common solid tumors prevalent in adults.

*Connective tissue* consists of elastic, fibrous, and collagenous tissues, such as bone, cartilage, and fat. Cancers originating in connective tissue and muscle (mesenchymal origin) are called *sarcomas*. Sarcomas are relatively rare tumors and are generally classified as either soft tissue sarcomas (e.g., rhabdomyosarcoma: striated muscle) or osteosarcomas (Ewing bone sarcoma). Further, osteosarcoma is generally diagnosed in children or adolescents, whereas soft tissue sarcomas are predominantly identified in adults.

Nerve tissue includes the brain, spinal cord, and nerves and consists of neurons, nerve fibers, dendrites, and supporting tissue composed of glial cells. Tumors arising in *nerve tissue* are named for the type of cell involved. For example, tumors arising from astrocytes, a type of glial cell thought to form the blood-brain barrier, are called *astrocytomas*. Tumors arising in nerve tissue are often benign, but because of their critical location they are more likely to be harmful than benign tumors in other sites.

Malignancies originating in *lymphoid tissues* are called *lymphomas*. Lymphomas can arise in many parts of the body, wherever lymphoid tissue is present. The most common sites of lymphoid malignancies are the lymph nodes and spleen. However, lymphomas can appear in other parts of the body, such as the skin, CNS, stomach, small bowel, bone, and tonsils.[301]

*Hematopoietic* malignancies include leukemias, multiple myeloma, myelodysplasia, and myeloproliferative syndromes.

Eponyms are used to describe the tumors as either benign or malignant, depending on the cell of origin. For example, a neoplastic lesion of adipose tissue (fat) if benign would be described as a lipoma, and a malignant lesion would be identified as a liposarcoma (see Table 9.1).

Box 9.1
**TNM STAGING SYSTEM**

***T: Primary Tumor***

| | |
|---|---|
| $T_X$ | Primary tumor cannot be assessed |
| $T_0$ | No evidence of primary tumor |
| $T_{IS}$ | Carcinoma in situ (confined to site of origin) |
| $T_1$, $T_2$, $T_3$, $T_4$ | Progressive increase in tumor size and involvement locally |

***N: Regional Lymph Nodes***

| | |
|---|---|
| $N_X$ | Nodes cannot be assessed |
| $N_0$ | No metastasis to regional lymph nodes |
| $N_1$, $N_2$, $N_3$ | Increasing degrees of involvement of regional lymph nodes |

***M: Distant Metastasis***

| | |
|---|---|
| $M_X$ | Presence of distant metastasis cannot be assessed |
| $M_0$ | No distant metastasis |
| $M_1$ | Distant metastasis |

*Note:* Extension of primary tumor directly into lymph nodes is considered metastasis to lymph nodes. Metastasis to a lymph node beyond the regional ones is considered distant metastasis.

(From National Cancer Institute. Cancer Staging. Available at: https://www.cancer.gov/about-cancer/diagnosis-staging/staging. Accessed November 20, 2018.)

## Staging and Grading

Staging is the process of describing the extent of disease at the time of diagnosis to aid treatment planning, predict clinical outcome (prognosis), and compare the results of different treatment approaches. The stage of disease at the time of diagnosis reflects the rate of growth, the extent of the neoplasm, and the prognosis. A simplified way to stage cancer is as follows:

- Stage 0: Carcinoma in situ (premalignant, preinvasive)
- Stage I: Early stage, cancer is usually localized to primary organ
- Stage II: Increased risk of regional spread because of tumor size or grade
- Stage III: Local cancer has spread regionally but may not be disseminated to distant regions
- Stage IV: Cancer has spread and disseminated to distant sites

In some cases, cancer may be staged as II or III depending on the spread of the specific type of cancer. For example, in Hodgkin disease, stage II indicates lymph nodes are affected on one side of the diaphragm. Stage III indicates affected lymph nodes above and below the diaphragm.[185,349]

### Systems of Staging

Staging systems are specific for each type of cancer. The TNM (tumor, node, metastases) system is used most often for solid tumors and has been adapted for other types of tumor. In the TNM classification scheme, tumors are staged according to the following basic components (Box 9.1):

- Tumor (*T*) refers to the size of primary tumor and carries a number from 0 to 4.
- Node (*N*) represents regional lymph node involvement; also ranked from 0 to 4.
- Metastasis (*M*) is zero (0) if no metastasis has occurred or 1 if metastases are present.

Numbers are used with each component to denote extent of involvement; for example, T0 indicates undetectable, and T1, T2, T3, and T4 indicate a progressive increase in size or involvement.

Some cancers do not have a staging system (e.g., brain cancer), and some can be staged using more than one system. The Union for International Cancer Control (UICC) is the universally accepted staging system, which incorporates the TNM classification of malignant tumors; the American Joint Committee on Cancer (AJCC) *AJCC Cancer Staging Manual, Eighth Edition,* released in 2017, is the current reference used by most institutions.[23,110] The National Cancer Institute (NCI) also provides detailed information about staging.[301]

It is important to understand that the TNM staging system is an anatomic staging system that describes the anatomic extent of the primary tumor, as well as the involvement of regional lymph nodes and distant metastases. In the TNM system, clinical stage is denoted by a small "c" (e.g., cT2N1M0), or pathologic stage is indicated by a small "p" (e.g., pT2N0). Clinical staging is based on clinical examination and testing of the individual before definitive treatment and is the stage of disease generally presented at tumor boards. The pathologic stage is determined by direct examination of the tumor by the pathologist once it has been removed and is considered a more accurate reflection of the tumor and its spread. Not all tumors are resected or excised, so pathologic staging is not always available.

Pathologic staging presented during tumor boards after resection of the tumor may alter the original clinical stage of the disease, allowing for a more accurate assessment of extent or degree of malignancy. Such information is critical to the oncologist in the determination of the best treatment intervention based on current clinical practice guidelines.

Conversely, pathologic staging may underestimate the true stage for individuals who received adjuvant treatment (radiation or chemotherapy) before surgery. Errors in the preparation or examination of tissue examined may result in false-positive or false-negative findings, resulting in misstaging and possibly altering diagnosis and treatment.

Staging as a process continues to evolve with new, more precise levels of screening sensitivity and specificity. Molecular screening for the presence of markers characteristic of some diseases will enable more accurate staging and treatment planning and monitoring of the effectiveness of targeted therapies.[349]

Revisions to the TNM staging system are made as understanding of the natural history of tumors at various sites improves with advancing technology. Beyond the TNM UICC systems, other staging systems are used in certain cases. For example, cervical cancer is staged using the International Federation of Gynecology and Obstetrics (FIGO) system of staging, which is based on clinical examination rather than surgical findings. Lymphomas are staged using Ann Arbor staging (Box 9.2).

**Immune Classification.** As mentioned above, tumor staging (AJCC/UICC TNM classification) summarizes

**Box 9.2**

**ANN ARBOR STAGING**

Ann Arbor staging is used for lymphomas (Hodgkin disease and non-Hodgkin lymphoma).

**Stage I:** Local cancer in one area, such as one lymph node and the local surrounding area; usually there are no other systemic or clinical symptoms

**Stage II:** Cancer is located in two separate regions on one side of the diaphragm (above or below the diaphragm); two separate regions refers to an affected lymph node or organ within the lymphatic system and a second affected area

**Stage III:** Cancer has spread to both sides of the diaphragm (above and below); includes one organ or area near the lymph nodes or the spleen

**Stage IV:** Diffuse or disseminated spread to one or more extralymphatic organs or area near the lymph nodes or the spleen; liver, bone marrow, or nodular involvement of the lungs is possible

Letters such as *A, B, E,* and *X* may be used to modify or append the stage:

*A* = absence of constitutional symptoms

*B* = presence of constitutional symptoms

*E* = extranodal (not in the lymph nodes or has spread from the lymph nodes to adjacent tissue)

X = used to describe mass larger than 10 cm or mediastinum wider than one-third of the chest on a chest x-ray

From Niederhuber J, Armitage J, Doroshow J, et al. *Abeloff's clinical oncology*, ed 5. Philadelphia, 2013, Saunders.

data on tumor burden (T), presence of cancer cells in draining and regional lymph nodes (N), and evidence for metastases (M). However, this classification provides limited prognostic information in estimating the outcome in cancer and does not predict response to therapy.

Cancer outcomes can vary significantly among individuals within the same stage. Cancer development may be controlled by the host's immune system, which points to the importance of including immunologic biomarkers for the prediction of prognosis and response to therapy. Data collected from large cohorts of human cancers have shown that the immune classification has a prognostic value that may be superior to the AJCC/UICC TNM classification. Efforts are under way to begin incorporating immune scoring as a prognostic factor and to introduce this parameter as a marker to classify cancers as part of the routine diagnostic and prognostic assessment of tumors.[124,125,201] The Immunoscore measures the density of 2 T lymphocyte populations in the center and periphery of the tumor, with a score ranging from 0 (I0) to 4 (I4), denoting low to high densities of both cell types in both regions.[124]

### Grading

Grading of tumor tissue is done by the pathologist using different grading for different types of tumors. For example, the Bloom-Richardson (or Nottingham) scale is used in breast cancer, the Gleason score is used in prostate cancer, and the Fuhrman scale is used in grading cancers of the kidney. Each grading method may use a different numerical score or scale, but generally the lower the value, the lower the tumor grade and the better differentiation of tissue within the tumor. A highly scored/scaled tumor is considered a high-grade tumor with poor cellular differentiation and a tendency to metastasize early.

Grading provides a measure of the anaplasia or differentiation of the tissue of the tumor. Additional important information includes the size, shape, and rate of nuclear division (mitosis) within the specimen; these factors further define the aggressiveness of the tumor.

In general, grading is classified into three categories: low, intermediate, and high. Low-grade tumors have better predictive and prognostic clinical outcomes compared with high-grade tumors. Grading of the tumor specimen when considered with anatomic staging (local, regional, and distant involvement) is critical in effective treatment planning, surveillance, and prognosis.

## INCIDENCE

Estimates of worldwide incidence, mortality, and prevalence of 36 types of cancers are available from the International Agency for Research on Cancer (IARC). Geographic variations between 20 large areas (185 countries) of the world are studied. The most recent report published in 2018 identified an 18.1 million incidence of new cases and 9.6 million deaths. Rates of survivorship in developing countries are less than one-half of the rates of developed countries because of late diagnosis and lack of availability of care. Additional international variation is due to exposure to known or suspected risk factors related to lifestyle or environment. The IARC has been researching and providing a database of global cancer estimates (GLOBOCAN) for the last 40 years.[51,177]

The most commonly diagnosed cancers are lung, prostate, breast, and colorectal; the most prevalent cancer in the world is lung cancer, and it accounts for the greatest number of cancer deaths worldwide.[51] In the United States the ACS publishes annual cancer statistics and estimates cancer trends (Table 9.2). Each year the ACS calculates estimates of the number of new cancer cases and expected cancer deaths in the United States and compiles the most recent data on cancer incidence, mortality, and survival.[12,355]

Based on statistical estimates, in 2019 the ACS predicted about 1.76 million new cases of invasive cancer in the United States and approximately 606,880 cancer-related deaths. This figure does not include most skin cancers (e.g., basal cell carcinomas, squamous cell carcinomas), which are believed to affect more than 4 million people per year.[12,355]

It is estimated that at least one in three people will be diagnosed with some form of invasive cancer in their lifetime and three of five people will be cured and/or survive 5 years after cancer treatment. However, cancer is still the second leading cause of death in the United States, exceeded only by heart disease. Poor health and nutrition habits, continued smoking, ozone destruction, and a long-term lack of exercise among many people continue to be discussed as contributors to the overall rise of this disease.[329]

**Table 9.2** Estimated New Cancer Cases and Cancer Deaths in 2018 in the United States (Percent Distribution of Sites by Gender)

| ESTIMATED NEW CASES | | | |
|---|---|---|---|
| MALES | | FEMALES | |
| **Type of Cancer** | **Number (%)** | **Type of Cancer** | **Number (%)** |
| Prostate | 174,650 (20) | Breast | 268,600 (30) |
| Lung and bronchus | 116,440 (13) | Lung and bronchus | 111,710 (13) |
| Colon and rectum | 78,500 (9) | Colon and rectum | 67,100 (8) |
| Urinary bladder | 61,700 (7) | Uterine corpus | 61,880 (7) |
| Melanoma of the skin | 57,220 (7) | Melanoma of the skin | 39,260 (4) |
| Kidney and renal pelvis | 44,120 (5) | Thyroid | 37,810 (4) |
| Non-Hodgkin lymphoma | 41,090 (5) | Non-Hodgkin lymphoma | 33,110 (4) |
| Oral cavity and pharynx | 38,140 (4) | Kidney and renal pelvis | 29,700 (3) |
| Leukemia | 35,920 (4) | Pancreas | 26,830 (3) |
| Pancreas | 29,940 (3) | Leukemia | 25,860 (3) |
| *All sites* | *870,970 (100)* | *All sites* | *891,480 (100)* |

| ESTIMATED DEATHS | | | |
|---|---|---|---|
| MALES | | FEMALES | |
| **Type of Cancer** | **Number (%)** | **Type of Cancer** | **Number (%)** |
| Lung and bronchus | 76,650 (24) | Lung and bronchus | 66,020 (23) |
| Prostate | 31,620 (10) | Breast | 41,760 (15) |
| Colon and rectum | 27,640 (9) | Colon and rectum | 23,380 (8) |
| Pancreas | 23,800 (7) | Pancreas | 21,950 (8) |
| Liver and intrahepatic bile duct | 21,600 (7) | Ovary | 13,980 (5) |
| Leukemia | 13,150 (4) | Uterine corpus | 12,160 (4) |
| Esophagus | 13,020 (4) | Liver and intrahepatic bile duct | 10,180 (4) |
| Urinary bladder | 12,870 (4) | Leukemia | 9690 (3) |
| Non-Hodgkin lymphoma | 11,510 (4) | Non-Hodgkin lymphoma | 8460 (3) |
| Brain and other nervous system | 9910 (3) | Brain and other nervous system | 7850 (3) |
| *All sites* | *321,670 (100)* | *All sites* | *285,210 (100)* |

From Siegel RL, Miller KD, Jemal A: Cancer statistics, 2019. *CA Cancer J Clin* 69:7–34, 2019.

The NCI established the Surveillance, Epidemiology, and End Results (SEER) program in 1973 as a way to report population-based data of site-specific incidences and outcomes of cancer. Estimates of new cancer cases are based on data collected and analyzed from 20 population-based registry sites. These sites serve as a representative sample of the general and minority-based population. The estimation of new cancer cases occurring annually is estimated using complex statistical measures.[71,425] Age-adjusted mortality rates are more accurate and are based on certificates of death as recorded by individual states. These statistics are reported on an annual basis through the National Vital Statistics Reporting Unit of the National Center for Health Statistics, part of the Centers for Disease Control and Prevention (CDC).[263]

Additional information related to the incidence of cancer in the U.S. population is available at the following website: https://surveillance.cancer.gov/statistics/types/incidence.html.

## Trends in Cancer Incidence and Survival

### Incidence

Overall incidence of cancer peaked in the early 1990s and has declined in the last decade by an average of 1.1% annually, with a 1.5% decline in cancer death rates. In 2003 and 2004 the rate of decline doubled to 2% per year, largely attributed to cessation of smoking among men, which had peaked in the mid-1960s. The latest decline in cancer deaths occurred across all four major cancer types (lung, colon and rectal, prostate, and breast; lung cancer deaths in women stayed relatively constant).

Targeted cancer therapies (i.e., drugs that seek out and selectively destroy cancer cells, leaving most normal cells unharmed) promise to reduce adverse events and improve these statistics in the coming years.[349] Cancer prevention strategies (e.g., smoking cessation, regular physical activity, and maintaining a healthy weight) may reduce the incidence of cancer occurrence and recurrence.[21,30,158]

### Survivorship

At the same time, survival rates for cancer are on the rise, increasing from 50% to approximately 67% over the last 30 years. A cancer survivor has been defined by the ACS as *any person who has been diagnosed with cancer, from the time of diagnosis through the balance of life,*[253] with three distinct phases associated with cancer survival: (1) the time from diagnosis through the end of initial treatment, (2) the transition from treatment to extended survival, and (3) long-term survival. It is estimated that there will be nearly

16.9 million American cancer survivors as of January 2019. Further, it is estimated that the number of survivors will increase to almost 22 million by 2029.[15] Male cancer survivors most commonly have diagnoses of prostate cancer (45%), colorectal cancer (10%), and melanoma. Female cancer survivors most commonly have diagnoses of breast cancer (44%), uterine cancer (9%), and colorectal cancer (9%).[253]

Currently, more focus and attention are being given to survivors and their unique health needs. The Institute of Medicine defines the essential needs of care of cancer survivors as follows:[157]

- Prevention and detection of new cancers and recurrent cancer
- Surveillance for cancer spread, recurrence, or second cancers
- Intervention for consequences of cancer and its treatment
- Coordination between specialists and primary care providers to ensure that all of the survivor's health needs are met

Consequences of cancer, and especially cancer treatment, are wide ranging and often include medical problems such as lymphedema and sexual dysfunction, symptoms such as pain and fatigue, psychologic distress experienced by both cancer survivors and their caregivers, and concerns related to employment and insurance. Coordination of care for survivors should include health promotion, immunizations, screening for both cancer and noncancerous conditions, and the care of concurrent conditions).[157]

The ACS regularly publishes a report in conjunction with the NCI dedicated to cancer survivorship titled *Cancer Treatment and Survivorship: Facts and Figures*.[11] This document provides survivorship statistics; descriptions of common adverse effects of treatment; and issues related to quality of life (QOL), long-term and late effects, risk of recurrence, and healthy behaviors. This document, based on SEER statistics, provides the basis and rationale for the importance of rehabilitation in the continuum of care and medical management of survivors of cancer.

### Gender-Based Incidence and Mortality

Among men, the most commonly diagnosed cancers are predicted to be cancers of the prostate, lung and bronchus, and colon/rectum. Among women, the three most commonly diagnosed cancers are expected to be cancers of the breast, lung and bronchus, and colon/rectum.

The largest decreases in deaths occurred among men (especially among black men), who bear the heaviest overall cancer burden and colorectal cancer burden in particular. Officials have attributed the steady downward trend to improved vigilance among Americans, who are benefiting from early screening and advances in treatment as well as smoking less, improving their diets, and exercising more. However, the U.S. population is aging, and cancer rates increase with age.[293]

For the period 1999–2015, overall cancer incidence declined about 2% per year in men and was stable in women. In the same period, average death rates per year decreased 1.8% in men and 1.4% in women.[293] Breast cancer alone accounted for approximately 266,120 new cancer cases in women in 2018 compared with 182,460 in 2008, but with mortality rates in the same period staying relatively similar.[83] The relative decline in rates of breast cancer deaths has been attributed in part to increased mammography but also to more aggressive therapy; overall decline in deaths among women may also be the result of the recent decrease in hormone replacement therapy.

Likewise, improved screening, detection, and treatment of prostate cancer have resulted in a decline in the death rate associated with this type of cancer. About a dozen cancers continue to increase in incidence or mortality, including melanoma, non-Hodgkin lymphoma, thyroid cancer, esophageal cancer, breast cancer (increased incidence but decreased mortality), and lung cancer in women.

## ETIOLOGY

The cause of cancer varies, and causative agents are generally subdivided into two categories: those of endogenous (genetic) origin and those of exogenous (environmental or external) origin. It is likely that most cancers develop as a result of multiple environmental, viral, and genetic factors working together to disrupt the immune system, along with failure of an aging immune system to recognize and scavenge cells that have become less differentiated.

Certain cancers show a familial pattern, giving people a hereditary predisposition to cancer. The most common cancers showing a familial pattern include prostate, breast, ovarian, and colon cancers. One of the potential objectives of the Human Genome Project completed in 2003 was to begin investigating and cataloguing genes that might be associated with various cancers. Such information would assist in identifying high-risk individuals for screening and early detection. Examples of such genetic testing include *BRCA1* and *BRCA2* genes for breast cancer. These genes belong to a family of cancer suppressor genes for which mutation (if inherited) significantly increases the lifetime risk of breast and/or ovarian cancer.

The ACS estimates that 50% of all cancers are caused by one or more of nearly 500 different cancer-causing agents (e.g., tobacco use, viruses, chemical agents, physical agents, drugs, alcohol, hormones).[210] Etiologic agents capable of initiating the malignant transformation of a cell (i.e., carcinogenesis) are called *carcinogens*. The study of *viruses* as carcinogens is one of the most rapidly advancing areas in cancer research today.

There is now evidence that viruses play a role in the pathogenesis of cervical carcinomas, some hepatomas, Burkitt lymphomas, nasopharyngeal carcinomas, adult T-cell leukemias, and, indirectly, many Kaposi sarcomas. Viruses such as HIV, the causative agent of AIDS, weaken cell-mediated immunity, resulting in malignancies.

*Chemical agents* (e.g., tar, soot, asphalt, dyes, hydrocarbons, oils, nickel, or arsenics) and *physical agents* (e.g., radiation or asbestos) may cause cancer after close and prolonged contact with these agents. Most people affected by chemical agents are industrial workers. Radiation exposure is usually from natural sources, especially ultraviolet radiation from the sun, which can cause changes in DNA structure that lead to malignant transformation. Notable exceptions include history of radiation treatment for acne, thymus, or thyroid

Box 9.3

**CANCER RISK FACTORS**

Advancing age
Previous cancer
Lifestyle or personal behaviors
  Tobacco use
  Diet and nutrition (high fat, low fiber)
  Obesity/type 2 diabetes
  Alcohol use
  Sexual and reproductive behaviors
  Physical inactivity
Exposure to viruses
  Human papillomavirus
  Epstein-Barr virus
  Hepatitis B virus
  Hepatitis C virus
  Helicobacter pylori
  Herpesvirus 8
Exposure to hormones (e.g., estrogen, testosterone)
Geographic location and environmental variables
Previous cancer treatment (e.g., radiotherapy)
Gender
Ethnicity
Socioeconomic status
Occupation
Heredity (family history of cancer)
Presence of precancerous lesions, polyps, or other
Stress
Inflammatory bowel disease

conditions. Basal and squamous cell carcinomas and malignant melanoma are linked to ultraviolet exposure.

Some *drugs*, such as cancer chemotherapeutic agents, are in themselves carcinogenic. Cytotoxic drugs, including steroids, decrease antibody production and destroy circulating lymphocytes. Clients with cancer who are treated with chemotherapy are at risk for future development of leukemia and other cancers.

*Hormones* have been linked to tumor development and growth, such as estrogen stimulating the growth of the endometrial lining, which over time becomes anaplastic. Other types of cancer occurring in target or hormone-responsive tissues include ovary and prostate cancers.

Excessive *alcohol* consumption is associated with cancer of the mouth, pharynx, larynx, esophagus, breast, and pancreas. It can also indirectly contribute to liver cancer (i.e., alcohol causes liver cirrhosis, which is associated with cancer).

The reader is directed to the following website for additional information on causes of cancer and risk factors for the development of cancer: https://www.cancer.gov/about-cancer/causes-prevention.

## RISK FACTORS

Advancing age is one of the most significant risk factors for cancer. In addition to age and the carcinogens described earlier in Etiology, predisposing factors influence the host's susceptibility to various etiologic agents (Box 9.3), which are discussed further in the next section.

Nine modifiable risk factors are responsible for more than one-third of cancer deaths *worldwide* (tobacco, alcohol, obesity/excess body weight, inactivity, diet/nutrition, unsafe sex, urban air pollution, indoor smoke from household fuels, or contaminated injections in health care settings). Of these, smoking, obesity/excess body weight, and alcohol consumption are the most damaging, accounting for nearly 33% of all cancer cases and 39.5% of cancer deaths in the United States. This means that even without the potential benefits of early detection and treatment, approximately two-fifths of cancer deaths are preventable.[87,181]

Experimental and epidemiologic evidence has established an association between at least eight viruses and various cancer sites. Tobacco and diet have also been linked to various cancers. Some risk factors are interactive and become exponential rather than additive (e.g., alcohol and smoking for oropharyngeal cancers).

There is no evidence to support popular theories that some people are more likely to develop cancer because of specific personality traits, such as anger, frustration, sexual repression, or conflicted parent–child relationship. Additionally, cancer survival is not predicted by personality type, including neuroticism, extroversion, or low self-esteem.[43,148,269]

### Heredity

Cancer is a disease of genes, which are vulnerable to mutation, especially over the course of a long human life span. However, evidence shows that only a small proportion of cancers (5% to 10%) linked to a single gene are inherited. It is abundantly clear that the incidence of all the common cancers in humans is determined by various controllable external factors, making cancer in large part a preventable disease.[413]

Evidence showing that patterns of cancer are altered by environmental factors rather than being genetically determined come from studies describing changes in the rates of different cancers in genetically identical populations that migrate from their native countries to other countries. Changes in the rates of the most common cancers (e.g., stomach, colorectal, breast, prostate) are significant after only one or two generations.[413]

### Aging

Age older than 50 years (some experts say age older than 40) is a significant risk factor for the development of cancer, but cancer is not an inevitable consequence of aging. The association of cancer and aging is becoming more common because of the aging of the general population. According to SEER report for the period 2005–2009, the median age for all races and gender at time of primary diagnosis is approximately 66 years. The median age is expected to increase over the next several decades.[293]

The risk of multiple diseases (comorbidity) also increases with age, creating limitations in the life expectancy of individual aging adults and enhancing the likelihood of treatment complications. Older people may be more susceptible to cancer simply because they have been exposed to carcinogens longer than younger people.

The effects of age on immune function and host defense are being studied to determine what the association is between cancer and age.

Factors such as accumulated nonlethal damage to DNA by free radicals, increased proinflammatory factors, and age-associated declines in DNA repair are important.[394] Mutations in cancer-causing structures, such as telomeres (a region of DNA at the end of chromosomes), DNA repair aberrations, and dysregulation of important hormonal and immune modulators, all are being reported as potential reasons for the increasing incidence of cancer in older adults.[161,346,361]

Clues about the life span of a cell and about aging in general are emerging from research on telomeres. In normal cells the telomere shortens each time a cell divides. Telomeres provide chromosomal stability by protecting the ends from degradation and recombination. A minimal telomere length is needed to maintain tissue homeostasis.[347]

The cell dies when the telomere becomes so short that it can no longer divide. An important enzyme, telomerase, helps keep normally dividing cells healthy by rebuilding the telomeres. Telomerase normally shuts down when cells are mature, but in cancer the enzyme enables cancer cells to grow with unlimited cell divisions. Telomerase is active in up to 85% of all human cancers.[182,346,347] See also Cellular Aging in Chapter 6. This understanding has led to discoveries regarding the life span of human cells, their relationship to aging, and the development of many illnesses associated with aging, such as cancer. It has been reported that normal cells do not divide indefinitely during the life span of a human because of a phenomenon called the *Hayflick limit* and a stopping process or permanent growth arrest called *cellular senescence*.

The Hayflick limit was discovered by Leonard Hayflick in 1965.[150] Hayflick observed that cells dividing in cell culture divided about 50 times before dying. As cells approach this limit, they show more signs of old age. For most differentiated cells, the limit to the number of times a cell divides has been determined in all cell types. The human limit is around 52, but there is some variation from cell type to cell type and, more significantly, from organism type to organism type (e.g., mice and humans). This limit has been linked to the shortening of telomeres and is thought to be one of the causes of aging. Telomeres may act as cellular clocks that control aging. This is called the *telomere theory of aging*. If the shortening of telomeres can be slowed or prevented, life expectancy may be extended but perhaps at a higher risk of tumorigenesis.[35]

Many in vitro and in vivo studies support the idea that telomere length is strongly correlated with life span. Longer telomeres have been associated with shorter life span (e.g., mice have very long telomeres and a short life span; the opposite is true for humans). Telomeres shorten progressively with each cell division; when a critical telomere length (Hayflick limit) is reached, the cells undergo senescence and subsequently apoptosis (programmed cell death).[347]

An alternative view is the *theory of dysfunctional senescence*. Some researchers have proposed that failure of cells or tissues to enter into cellular senescence occurs as a result of defects in genomic maintenance mechanisms after years of mutation and leads to cancer.[61,303] In other words, cellular senescence may reduce cancer mortality rather than promote it late in life, thus positively contributing to longevity in organisms with renewable tissues.[27]

Cancer cells constitute one exception to the limits on cell division. It is thought that the Hayflick limit exists principally to help prevent cancer. If a cell becomes cancerous and the Hayflick limit is approaching, the cell will be able to divide only a limited number of times before it dies. Once it reaches this limiting number of divisions, the formed tumor will no longer be able to reproduce and the cells will die off.

Cancer cells that have found ways around the Hayflick limit are referred to as immortal. Such immortal cells may still die, but the group of immortalized cells produced from cell division of an immortal cell has no limit as to how many times cell division might take place. Telomeres in immortal cells are maintained by telomerase. Regardless of telomere length, if telomerase is active, telomeres can be maintained at a sufficient length to ensure cell survival.[156] This presents a unique challenge in preventing and killing cancer cells. Creating telomerase inhibitors may possibly produce a means of supporting anticancer activity.

People age 65 years and older have a risk of cancer development much greater than younger persons, and some cancers in the older adult population seem to be biologically different from cancers in younger people. For example, the poor prognosis for older adults with acute leukemia is not just a result of poor tolerance of aggressive chemotherapy but is more likely associated with cytogenetic resistance to chemotherapy.[173]

All the cancers with the highest incidence affect older adults in larger numbers. In both men and women older than 65 years, cancers of the colon/rectum, stomach, pancreas, and bladder accounted for two-thirds to three-fourths of the total number of these malignancies. More than 65% of lung cancers and 50% of non-Hodgkin lymphomas occur in older men and women; 77% of cases of prostate cancer occur in men older than 65; and 48% of cases of breast cancer and 46% of cases of ovarian cancer occur in women older than 65.[376] Moreover, older adults with cancer continue to be underrepresented in clinical trials. Many available clinical trials often do not include end points pertinent to the older adult population such as preservation of function, cognition, and independence.[105]

As previously mentioned, malignancies of the lung, colon/rectum, breast, and prostate account for the highest number of cancer deaths in the United States. Malignancies of the pancreas, stomach, ovary, and bladder and non-Hodgkin lymphomas are also a major cause of cancer deaths. For each of these cancers, more than one-half of the cancer deaths occur in persons older than 65 years.[401]

## Lifestyle

Lifestyle choices or personal behaviors such as tobacco use, diet and nutrition, alcohol use, and sexual and reproductive behavior are cited as risk factors for the development of cancer. Lifestyle-related risk factors for cancer combined with cancer-causing substances in the environment and the presence of genes that increase the risk of cancer account for 70% of the total risk for developing cancer.

### Tobacco

Both epidemiologic and experimental data support the conclusion that tobacco (including smokeless tobacco) is carcinogenic and remains the most important cause of cancer. Tobacco use accounts for approximately 30% of cancer deaths, with lung cancer now the leading cancer causing deaths in both genders. Cigarette smoking is related to nearly 90% of all lung cancers, and accumulating evidence suggests that cigarette smoking increases the incidence of cancer of the bladder; the pancreas; and, to a lesser extent, the kidney, larynx, oral cavity, and esophagus.

### Diet and Nutrition

The major role of diet and nutrition in cancer risk is well established.[9,10,53,374] It is estimated that approximately one-third of cancer mortality in developing countries may result from dietary causes.[20,210,405] The reader is encouraged to read an excellent summary by Kushi and colleagues[210] on the role of nutrition (including the role of specific food items, additives, contaminants, dietary supplements, sweeteners/substitutes, spices, and antioxidants) and physical activity available at https://onlinelibrary.wiley.com/doi/full/10.3322/caac.20140.

Consumption of a poor diet may blunt the immune system's natural defense mechanisms against genetic damage caused by long-term exposure to an environmental carcinogen. Diet and nutrition can directly influence various hormonal factors affecting growth and differentiation in the carcinogenic process. A healthful diet is thought to act, at least in part, to detoxify carcinogens and to inhibit certain processes in carcinogenesis, particularly at the stage of growth and spread. Diet and nutrition can influence these processes (positively or negatively) by providing bioactive compounds to specific tissues via the circulatory system or by modulating hormone levels.

Differences in certain dietary patterns among populations explain a proportion of cancers. These dietary patterns, in combination with physical inactivity, contribute to obesity and metabolic consequences such as increased levels of growth factor, insulin, estrogen, and possibly testosterone. Studies propose that elevated serum insulin levels (insulin resistance) may be a risk factor for postmenopausal breast cancer. These hormones tend to promote cellular growth; high levels of circulating insulin increase the availability of insulin-like growth factors (IGFs) promoting cell growth and reproduction, including cells with damaged DNA that can develop into cancer.[189,190] New evidence suggests that a diet high in proinflammatory elements such as saturated fatty acids or *N*-nitroso compounds, among others, can increase the risk of cancer.[270] A history of obesity and/or type 2 diabetes is a risk factor for breast, prostate, pancreatic, and colorectal cancer.[93,219,223,304] Excess weight also contributes to cancers of the uterus, kidney, esophagus, pancreas, and gallbladder and less commonly to leukemia, multiple myeloma, and non-Hodgkin lymphoma.[323,324] Fat (adipose tissue) as an endocrine gland and its role in cancer is discussed in Chapter 11.

Clients are often highly motivated to improve nutrition and begin an exercise program after receiving a diagnosis of cancer. The ACS continues to publish and update best clinical practices related to optimal nutrition and physical activity during and after cancer treatment.[17,330] In the absence of scientific evidence that diet, nutrition, and physical activity[30] can prevent cancer recurrence, reasonable conclusions are offered.[210]

Cancer and cancer treatment can cause profound metabolic and physiologic alterations affecting the body's needs for adequate nutritional intake. Gastrointestinal side effects of treatment can lead to loss of appetite and weight loss accompanied by malnutrition. All the major treatment modalities (e.g., surgery, chemotherapy, radiation) can adversely impact how the body digests, absorbs, and uses food. Preserving lean body mass is an important goal of nutritional care for survivors, especially during active cancer treatment.[339]

The use of nutritional supplements and antioxidants remains controversial. Until more evidence is available that suggests more benefit than harm, the American Institute for Cancer Research suggests it is prudent for cancer survivors receiving chemotherapy or radiation therapy to avoid exceeding more than 100% of the daily value for antioxidant-type vitamins during the treatment phase.[212]

### Alcohol

Alcohol consumption has been linked to increased rates of cancer of the mouth, pharynx, larynx, esophagus, liver, breast, and probably colon. In people with a diagnosis of cancer, alcohol intake could also affect the risk for new primary cancers of these sites. Alcohol intake can increase the circulating levels of estrogens, theoretically increasing the risk for breast cancer and/or recurrence.[213,231]

With tobacco use, alcohol interacts with smoke synergistically, increasing the risk of malignant tumors by acting as a solvent for the carcinogenic smoke products and thus increasing the absorption of carcinogens. Evidence is suggestive in associating alcohol consumption and cancers of the colon, pancreas, breast, bladder, and head and neck.

### Sexual and Reproductive Behaviors

Sexual and reproductive behaviors are linked to the risk of developing various cancers. For example, the risk of developing cervical cancer is linked with early sexual intercourse and multiple partners. Pregnancy and childbearing seem to be protective against cancers of the endometrium, ovary, and breast. Prolonged lactation may also have a significant impact on the reduction of breast cancer risk by reducing the cumulative exposure of breast tissue to estrogen.[78] Other risk factors for breast cancer are discussed in Chapter 20.

### Hormonal Exposure

Hormonal exposure is a factor for women. For example, prolonged exposure to estrogen (e.g., early onset of menses, menopause after age 50, nulliparity or no children, having first child after age 30, never breastfed children, or use of first-generation oral contraceptives before 1975) is a risk factor for estrogen-sensitive breast cancer.

Prolonged use of estrogen hormone replacement therapy for relief of menopausal symptoms has been linked with increased rates of breast cancer. Data from the Women's Health Initiative resulted in a halt to the routine use of estrogen and progestin in combination (Prempro) in 2002 and estrogen alone (Premarin) in 2004. When compared with a placebo group, it was clear that hormone users were experiencing more breast cancer, heart disease, stroke, and blood clots. Estrogen showed some benefit, but it was not enough to outweigh the risks.[239]

Growth factors such as insulin-like growth factor 1 (IGF-1) and hormones such as estrogen and testosterone are considered risk factors linked with cancers other than breast and prostate (e.g., lung, endometrial, colon). A growing body of literature indicates that besides its essential role in growth and development, growth hormone may play a role in the development and progression of cancer.[24,77] Complex links between excess body weight, the insulin-IGF axis, and cancer suggest molecular mechanisms are present that lead to increased availability of IGF-1, providing a cellular environment that favors tumor formation.[123] Growth factor signaling pathways appear to be upregulated in hormone-resistant tumors and interact with estrogen receptor signaling, which remains functional even after long-term endocrine deprivation. Intensive research efforts to develop antitumor agents that inhibit IGF signaling in human tumors are under way, with mixed results. A need has been identified to develop biomarkers, gain a clearer understanding of insulin receptor function, and find ways to combine treatment regimens that are safe and effective while yielding positive outcomes [24,420]

## Geographic Location and Environmental Variables

The incidence of different types of cancer varies geographically. People living in rural areas are less likely to use preventive screening services or to exercise regularly. Colon cancer is more prevalent in urban than in rural areas, but in rural areas, especially among farmers, skin cancer is more common. Availability of specialty care is a possible contributing issue for this group of people.

The greater susceptibility of certain geographic areas within the United States is probably related to exposure to different carcinogens.[274] The increased incidence of cancer found in urban areas may be related to the increased pool of minorities, increased poverty represented in this group, local smoking ordinances, and diet (e.g., cost and availability of fresh fruits and vegetables).[422]

Occupational or environmental exposure to chemicals (e.g., herbicides, insecticides, dyes), fibers (e.g., asbestos), radon, and air pollution is a risk factor for lung and hematologic cancers. Researchers are investigating the possible causal relationship between environmental exposure and the increased incidence of childhood cancers. The U.S. Environmental Protection Agency has identified the carcinogenic effects from hazardous exposures. Heritable genetic and chromosomal mutations caused by environmental or occupational exposures to agents (e.g., chemicals, radiation) can be passed on to the next generation.

According to the seventh report on the Biological Effects of Ionizing Radiation (BEIR VII) issued by the National Academy of Science, exposure to even low-dose imaging radiology (including computed tomography [CT] scans) can result in the development of malignancy. Exposure to medical x-rays is linked with leukemia, thyroid cancer, and breast cancer. There is a 1 in 1000 chance of developing cancer from a single CT scan of the chest, abdomen, or pelvis. The latency period is 2 to 5 years for leukemias and 10 to 30 years for solid tumors.[284]

## Ethnicity

Despite advances in cancer diagnosis, treatment, and survival, racial and ethnic minorities suffer disproportionately from cancer. Differences among ethnic groups represent a challenge to understand the reasons and an opportunity to reduce illness and death while improving survival rates. Diagnosis at more advanced stages with lower survival rates at each stage of diagnosis is evident in African Americans compared with whites.

Poverty has emerged as a significant factor influencing poor cancer outcomes for all races, especially among minorities.[46,307] Inequities in insurance status adversely affect low-income families, preventing individual members from obtaining screening, access to quality care, or the entire range of cancer care available.[359] Other barriers to adequate screening and treatment include cultural issues regarding testing and treatment, fear, and scarcity of or difficulty with transportation.[309]

### African Americans

In particular, racial disparities exist between whites and other groups, especially African Americans. Overall, incidence and mortality from cancer is about 14% higher in African Americans compared with whites; this disparity in incidence and mortality is much larger for people younger than age 65 years than for people age 65 and older, likely in part due to health care access for older adults through Medicare.[12,208,355] Studies have shown that equal treatment yields equal outcomes among individuals with equal disease,[149,373,406] although there are also data suggesting that even when other factors are equivalent, racial and ethnic minorities tend to receive lower-quality care than whites.[204] At the present time, this increased incidence is attributed to preventable risk factors such as the absence of early screening, delayed diagnosis, and smoking and diet. Although the number of African American men who smoke is decreasing and tobacco-related cancers are declining, the incidence of lung cancer and other smoking-related diseases still remains high, possibly because black men tend to smoke cigarettes with a higher tar and nicotine content. The incidence rates of prostate cancer (the most commonly diagnosed cancer among African American men) are more than 50% higher than rates of prostate cancer compared with other ethnic groups.[99]

Lung cancer is the leading cause of cancer death among both African American men and women. African American men are 20% more likely to die of lung cancer than white men.[12,355] Breast cancer is the second leading cause of death for African American women. The number of

African American women of all ages who have died of breast cancer in the last 10 years is about 40% higher compared with non-Hispanic white women. Colorectal cancer has increased in both African American men and women. Black women are twice as likely to develop cervical cancer and nearly three times as likely to die of cervical cancer as other women. Finally, African American men have a 60% higher incidence rate of prostate cancer than white men in the United States and the highest rate worldwide, even though the mortality rates have decreased faster among blacks compared with whites in recent years.[12,355]

Some specific forms of cancer affect other ethnic groups at rates higher than the national average (e.g., stomach and liver cancers among Asian American populations and colorectal cancer among Alaska Natives). African Americans have a lower incidence of bladder cancer but higher mortality rates compared with other ethnic groups.[396] The incidence of and mortality rates for esophageal cancer are twice as high for African Americans compared with whites.[31]

### Hispanics/Latinos

Hispanic/Latino people originate from 23 different countries, with a wide range of diversity. Racial variations exist in tumor growth, susceptibility, and treatment response. For example, Hispanic/Latino populations have different drug resistance gene expression than non-Hispanic/Latino whites.[14,252]

Hispanics have lower incidence and death rates than non-Hispanic whites for all cancers combined, but the risk increases with the duration of U.S. residence. Cancer is the leading cause of death among U.S. Hispanics.[252] The association between infectious agents (e.g., hepatitis B virus [HBV], *Helicobacter pylori*) and cancer may account for higher rates of stomach, liver, uterine cervix, and gallbladder cancers, but lower screening rates, differences in lifestyle and dietary patterns, and genetic factors are highly prevalent risk factors.[252] Readers interested in an update on cancer statistics for Hispanics/Latinos can find this information online at https://www.cancer.org/research/cancer-facts-statistics/hispanics-latinos-facts-figures.html.[14]

### Asian Americans

Asian Americans have a unique situation in that they are the only racial/ethnic group to experience cancer as the leading cause of death, with proportionately more cancer of infectious origin (e.g., human papillomavirus (HPV)–induced cervical cancer, HBV-induced liver cancer, and stomach cancer) than any other minority group. Cultural barriers to intervention exist, such as overcoming resistance to physician visits, reducing tobacco use, and increasing exercise.[378]

The Office of Minority Health and Health Equity of the CDC is the leading federal agency charged with identifying the national impact of disparity in cancer diagnosis and treatment among various ethnic groups in the United States. The organization also describes specific research programs designed to investigate various contributing factors associated with cancer types and ethnic populations. The following website provides a summary of their findings and activities: https://www.cdc.gov/minorityhealth/index.html.

Public Law 106-525, enacted by Congress in November 2000, created a federal definition, authority, and commitment to the study and investigation of survivorship among minorities and health disparity in the United States.[176] Partnerships between the federal government and other agencies and the private sector have begun to address many of these socioeconomic and accessibility issues as well.[291]

In addition, the Patient Protection and Affordable Care Act (Public Law 111-148 and 111-152), federal legislation signed into law in 2010 and upheld by the Supreme Court in 2012, provided the authority for preventive screening for certain cancers (breast, cervical, and colorectal). It also provided insurance coverage for people with a preexisting chronic condition such as cancer, traditionally denied in the past. Elements of the law were incorporated over the last few years until 2020.

## Precancerous Lesions

Precancerous lesions and some benign tumors may undergo later transformation into cancerous lesions and tumors. Common precancerous lesions include pigmented moles, burn scars, senile keratosis, leukoplakia, and benign adenomas or polyps of the colon or stomach. All such lesions need to be examined periodically for signs of changes.

## Stress

Support continues to grow for links between biobehavioral and psychologic factors such as stress, depression, and social isolation and the progression (but not necessarily the initiation) of cancer.[259] Depression is a disorder of both immune suppression and immune activation. Markers of impaired cellular immunity (decreased natural killer [NK] cell cytotoxicity) and inflammation (elevated interleukin [IL]-6, tumor necrosis factor alpha [TNF-α], and C-reactive protein) have been associated with depression, suggesting the potential for a direct relationship between depression and cancer.[44,45] Chronic inflammation (with or without accompanying depression) may also be implicated in the progression of cancer.

The interaction between stromal cells (connective tissue cells of any organ) and tumor cells is known to play a major role in cancer growth and progression. Here again, the influence of stress hormones comes into action, as the crosstalk between tumor and stromal cells changes signaling pathways contributing to disease progression.

Research with animal models (animals with a disease that is similar to or the same as a disease in humans) suggests that the body's neuroendocrine response (release of hormones into the blood in response to stimulation of the nervous system) can directly alter important processes in cells that help protect against the formation of cancer, such as DNA repair and the regulation of cell growth.[235] Although substantial evidence supports a positive effect of psychosocial interventions on QOL in cancer, the clinical evidence for efficacy of stress-modulating psychosocial interventions in slowing cancer progression remains inconclusive, and the biobehavioral mechanisms that might explain such effects are still being investigated.[236]

The possibility that psychologic interventions and social support may enhance immune function and survival is under further investigation.[237] Proponents of psychooncology[298] (psychoneuroimmunology and cancer) suggest that advances in mind–body medicine research combined with healthy nutrition and lifestyle choices can have a significant impact on health, health maintenance, disease, and disease prevention, including cancer.[26]

Additional information about stress can be found on the National Institute of Mental Health (NIMH) website at https://www.nimh.nih.gov/index.shtml. The NIMH, a part of the National Institutes of Health (NIH), provides national leadership in the study of mental and behavioral disorders, including the causes and effects of psychologic stress.

## PATHOGENESIS

Early in the study of cancer, the concept that neoplasia originates in a single cell by acquired genetic change was proposed, and it remains the view of cancer pathogenesis most supported by experimental evidence. This hypothesis, called the *somatic mutation theory,* was first substantiated when investigations of tumors confirmed that tumor cells are characterized by numerical and structural chromosomal abnormalities.

The discovery that chromosomal aberration is one of the basic mechanisms of tumor cell proliferation laid the foundation of modern cancer cytogenetics (study of chromosomes in cancer). Chromosomal changes can include addition or deletion of entire chromosomes (numerical changes) or translocations, deletions, inversions, and insertions of parts of chromosomes (structural changes). Translocations occur when two or more chromosomes exchange material and are common in leukemias and sarcomas. Deletions or losses of chromosomal material are common in epithelial adenocarcinomas of the large bowel, lung, breast, and prostate. Chromosomal deletions may lead to neoplastic development when a tumor suppressor gene is lost. Chromosomal inversions and insertions are less common but still cause abnormal juxtaposition (side-by-side placement) of genetic material.

At first the question arose: Are acquired chromosomal abnormalities the cause of the neoplastic changes in cells or merely the result of the neoplastic state? Chromosomal banding techniques developed in the 1970s have allowed precise identification of chromosomal changes. This information, along with molecular genetics techniques developed during the 1980s, has enabled researchers to investigate this question by examining tumor cells at the level of individual genes.

From these studies, two functionally different classes of cancer-relevant genes have been detected: (1) the dominant oncogenes and (2) the recessive tumor suppressor genes. Oncogenes and tumor suppressor genes are present in all cells. In their normal, nonmutated form, they contribute to the regulation of cell division and death. The activation of oncogenes along with the inactivation of tumor suppressor genes is an important driver of cancer progression.

### Current Theory of Oncogenesis

The study of viruses in tumors has led researchers to discover small segments of genetic DNA called *oncogenes.* Oncogenes, also called *cancer-causing genes,* have the ability to transform normal cells into malignant cells, independently or incorporated with a virus. More than 100 oncogenes have been identified. *Protooncogenes* are the normal, nonmutated form of an oncogene that aid in regulating biologic functions such as cell division in normal cells. Oncogenes are thought to be the abnormal counterparts of protooncogenes.

Oncogenes may be activated by carcinogens, at which point they alter the regulation of growth in the cell. Oncogenes force a cell to grow even when its surroundings contain none of the cues that normally provoke growth. Oncogenes are hyperactivated versions of normal cellular growth-promoting genes. By releasing strong, unrelenting growth-stimulating signals into a cell, oncogenes can drive cell growth ceaselessly.

Researchers have also discovered a group of regulatory genes, first called *antioncogenes* and now called *tumor suppressor genes,* that have the opposite effect of oncogenes. When activated, tumor suppressor genes can regulate growth and inhibit carcinogenesis. Tumor suppressor genes (e.g., *p53* or telomeres) are the "brakes" to the "stuck accelerator" of the activated oncogene. When defects in the oncogene occur simultaneously with inactivation of growth-suppressing genes, aggressive cell proliferation takes place with the creation of certain types of tumor cells.

Exactly how chromosomal changes contribute to the malignant process remains unclear. Chromosomal rearrangements may lead to oncogene activation, either by a regulatory change causing increased production of normal oncogene-encoded peptides or by creating a deranged oncogene template that codes for an abnormal protein product.

Another proposed mechanism suggests that chromosomal changes inactivate a tumor suppressor gene through chromosomal deletion. Loss of tumor suppressor genes is suspected because chromosomal regions found to be consistently missing in tumor cells have been observed in carcinomas of the lung, breast, bladder, and kidney.

The *p53* gene appears to trigger programmed cell death (apoptosis) as a way of regulating uncontrolled cellular proliferation. The p53 protein is activated by cellular stresses that could facilitate tumor development, such as hypoxia, lack of nucleotides, or DNA damage. Mutations in the *p53* tumor suppressor gene result in loss of the ability of the gene protein to bind with DNA and act as a suppressor for the division of that cell.[327] When the p53 pathway has been altered by cancer, the mutated protein product cannot protect the genome. Mutations accumulate and produce resistance to chemotherapy and radiation therapy.

Additionally, researchers have demonstrated that cancer cells develop multiple mechanisms of their own to evade apoptosis. Cancer cells can inactivate proapoptotic factors or upregulate antiapoptotic factors. Strategies to induce apoptosis specifically in tumor cells are currently under investigation. One proapoptotic protein that has been shown to induce apoptosis in a wide variety of tumor cells is a member of the TNF superfamily called *TNF-related apoptosis-inducing ligand* (TRAIL).[70,187]

Another genetic suppressor of cell growth and division also plays a part in the aging process. As cells divide and grow older, there is continuous progressive shortening of the end portions of the chromosomes or telomeres of those cells. Studies of human fibroblasts and other human tissues have shown a very close association between the development of cancer and the overproduction of the enzyme telomerase. When this enzyme is present, it prevents the telomeres from shortening, thus lengthening the life span of the cell indefinitely. Telomerase has been found to be present in more than 85% of human cancer cells but is absent in most normal human tissues.[332]

Recurrent or persistent inflammation may induce, promote, or influence susceptibility to carcinogenesis by causing DNA damage, inciting tissue reparative proliferation, and/or creating an environment (soil) rich with cytokines and growth factors. Chronic inflammation and the metabolic products of phagocytosis are often accompanied by the excessive formation of reactive oxygen and nitrogen that are potentially damaging to DNA, lipoproteins, and cell membranes.[375]

Although much remains to be learned about the cascade of genetic changes for every kind of cancer, increasing understanding may suggest a means for interrupting the genetic events leading to cancer and for diagnosing the early stages of tumorigenesis. Current research continues to focus on the following major areas of biologic study:

- Regulation of cellular proliferation and expression of oncogenes and tumor suppressor genes
- Telomere length and telomerase
- Free radical–induced DNA damage and regulation of apoptosis
- Immune function and response (e.g., senescence, surveillance, enhancement)
- Cellular, metabolic, and humoral factors associated with the chronic inflammatory process[375]

## Cancer Stem Cell Hypothesis

Cancer stem cells have been identified in certain types of cancers such as leukemia, giving support to the idea that not all cancer cells are the same and leading to the development of the *cancer stem cell hypothesis*.

The cancer stem cell hypothesis predicts that there are different functional and morphologic cancer cells within a single tumor and a hierarchical order in which the abnormal stem cells form and feed a cancer. Emerging evidence indicates that these cells are also resistant to chemotherapy and radiation therapy because their DNA repair mechanisms are more highly developed. Targeting and eliminating the tumor-initiating stem cells may be a more efficient and direct way to eradicate cancer without killing fast-growing normal cells. This information, first reported more than a decade ago, set off a new direction in cancer research.[91,272,352]

## Tumor Biochemistry and Pathogenesis

Carcinogenesis is the process by which a normal cell undergoes malignant transformation. It is usually a multistep process, involving progressive changes after genetic damage to or alteration of cellular DNA through the development of hyperplasia, metaplasia, dysplasia, carcinoma in situ, invasive carcinoma, and metastatic carcinoma in that order.[391] These discrete stages in tumor development suggest that a single altered gene suffices only to push a cell part of the way down the path to actual malignancy. The process is completed when multiple, successive changes occur in distinct cellular genes, including activation or overexpression of oncogenes and loss or mutation of tumor suppressor genes.

The number of genetic events required for conversion of normal cells to malignant cells is still debated, but at least in the case of many solid tumors (e.g., colon carcinomas), this number may be as high as seven or eight. This high number of genetic events may imply that genetic instability occurs during cancer progression.[79,392] This requirement for multiple changes creates an important protective mechanism against cancer.

If a small number of genetic changes sufficed to transform a normal cell into a malignant one, multiple tumors would develop easily. These multiple barriers, along with the normal circuitry inside cells, ensure that only the rare cell will sustain the requisite number of changes for making a cancer cell.

However, cancer has developed multiple methods centering on genetic mutation to promote self-survival and perpetuation. The pliability of cancer cells to mutate in several different phenotypes in an attempt to find one that will survive and colonize at a metastatic site makes finding effective treatment difficult at best. The next section on Cancer and the Immune System will further demonstrate the complexity of carcinogenesis and give the reader an understanding of current treatment focus through translational medicine.

## Cancer and the Immune System

Joseph A. Fraietta

There is a considerable amount of clinical and scientific evidence to suggest that the human body responds immunologically to tumors. More than a century ago, it was first conceived that a primary function of the immune system is to prevent an "overwhelming frequency" of carcinomas.[111] In 1957 emerging discoveries on immune control of neoplastic disease were incorporated into the formal hypothesis of cancer *immunosurveillance*, which states that the immune system is continuously searching out and destroying potentially cancerous cells before they become harmful tumors.[56] These transformed cells are thought to constantly arise during the life span of the host.

### Immunosurveillance

The phenomenon of immunosurveillance is supported by the following observations: (1) a higher incidence of cancer after immunosuppression or in immunodeficiency,[127,305] (2) infiltration of tumors by lymphocytes and macrophages (i.e., positive correlation between the extent of in situ lymphocyte infiltration in tumors and patient survival rates),[109] (3) lymphocyte proliferation in response to tumors, (4) regression of metastases after ablation of the primary tumor, and (5) immune-mediated spontaneous regression of human tumors (especially in malignant melanoma, but also in neuroblastoma and other tumors).[335] Although the theory of cancer immunosurveillance has been challenged, a large amount of current data obtained by many independent researchers supports the basic principles of this concept that an unmanipulated immune system detects and eliminates primary tumors and this is heavily dependent on lymphocytes and the various factors they produce.[109]

Interestingly, experimental evidence suggests that inactivation of an oncogene with therapeutic agents (i.e., curing the oncogene addiction) leads to regression of tumors in immunocompetent hosts, but this effect is only transient in immunodeficient hosts.[319,397] Despite the fact that the immune system reacts against tumors, these immune responses may be associated with tumor inhibition but not elimination. Furthermore, recognition of tumor antigens by the immune system may result in tolerance rather than activation of a response. The fact that tumors arise in otherwise healthy individuals suggests that antitumor immunity is often insufficient and easily overwhelmed by a rapidly proliferating malignancy. For this reason, researchers have endeavored to identify and characterize various types of tumor antigens against which immune responses are elicited and continue to explore how immunity against cancer can be bolstered to benefit the patient.

### Tumor-Specific Antigens

A key feature of cancer immunology is the interaction between the immune system of the tumor-bearing individual and a constantly changing source of foreign molecules (tumor antigens). Tumor-specific antigens (TSAs) are tumor antigens that are uniquely expressed by tumor cells and are not expressed by normal cells. TSAs are often referred to as *neoantigens* or "new antigens" that may exist in the nucleus, cytoplasm, or cell membrane and may be excreted from the cell. Altered proteins are the result of gene mutations that give rise to new peptides (mutant peptides). If a portion of these peptides can be loaded onto major histocompatibility complexes (MHCs), the immune system will recognize a TSA as foreign.

*Fusion proteins* are a type of TSA that can be generated by translocations in which part of one gene moves to a different chromosome and recombines with another gene (e.g., BCR/ABL). The joining part of the two genes produces a new sequence because it spans the genes and is translated into a protein that does not normally exist. In addition to translocations and recombination, fusion proteins can be generated by deletions that resulted in joining of two or more genes that originally coded for separate proteins.

TSAs can also consist of *viral proteins* that are component proteins or new enzymes that aid in the replication of the virus. Tumor viruses can induce benign or malignant proliferation of the cells that they infect. The resultant tumors express viral antigens—these are not host proteins or unique in some way; they are simply viral proteins. Viral constituents found in tumors form a major part of the evidence that establishes a causal link between viruses and human cancers (e.g., HPV E6 and E7 proteins) (Fig. 9.1).[337]

### Tumor-Associated Antigens

Tumor-associated antigens (TAAs) are antigens that are expressed by tumors and normal cells. These tumor antigens are expressed at higher levels on tumors relative to normal cells or are expressed at different stages of development or differentiation. *Oncospermatogonal antigens* or cancer-testis antigens are expressed in spermatocytes and cancer cells, but not normal cells of the tissue of tumor origin (non–lineage-specific expression). For example, melanoma antigen–encoding gene (MAGE-1) is a normal testicular protein that is expressed by melanoma cells.[59] *Differentiation antigens* are TAAs that are expressed on a tumor and are also expressed at some stage of differentiation of nonmalignant cells of the tumor's cell lineage (lineage-specific antigens). Melanocyte differentiation antigens (e.g., MART-1/Melan-A) are antigens that are expressed by melanomas as well as by normal melanocytes. A normal melanocyte will express the antigen during its development and differentiation, and tumor cells will reexpress the antigen.[166] Prostate-specific antigen (PSA) is another common differentiation antigen.

In some cases, overexpression of a normal protein/antigen constitutes a TAA. For example, the epidermal growth factor (EGF) receptor is typically found on epithelial cells, as well as other cell types. Certain adenocarcinomas are characterized by EGF receptor expression that is manyfold higher than levels found on normal cells. In this way, the tumor is expressing a growth factor at very high levels and can detect it and continue to proliferate. Overexpression of EGF receptor can be exploited for therapeutic purposes (e.g., anti-EGF receptor and anti-HER-2 receptor antibodies are used to treat breast cancer).[248,344]

*Clonal antigens* are a very unique type of TAA. These antigens are expressed by a small clonal population of normal cells (i.e., idiotypes on B cells). Each B cell has a unique B-cell receptor, immunoglobulin, on its surface that will bind to a particular antigen. The B-cell receptor repertoire is created by different combinations of gene rearrangements to obtain unique V regions. In certain B-cell cancers such as leukemia and lymphoma, one B cell expands (i.e., the tumor is coming from one B cell), and all the B cells from that tumor express the same immunoglobulin sequence (i.e., idiotype). Therefore the V regions of the immunoglobulins on all the B cells from the tumor are identical. In that sense, a unique tumor antigen is created because the tumor expresses one immunoglobulin, and the rest of the healthy B cells in the body express different immunoglobulin sequences. Idiotypes can be exploited for cancer immunotherapy (e.g., antiidiotypic antibodies), but this type of antibody-based immune manipulation can be costly and laborious because it has to be customized on an individual patient basis.[134]

*Oncofetal antigens* are TAAs that are expressed by tumor cells, but not normally by nonmalignant adult cells. Genetic derangement in cancer causes certain tumors to reexpress antigens that are present only during fetal development and are not supposed to be expressed in adult tissues.[400] Carcinoembryonic antigen (CEA) is an antigen with expression that is normally produced only during the development of a fetus during the first two trimesters of gestation; it is usually not present in the blood of healthy adults. CEA is expressed by colon carcinoma

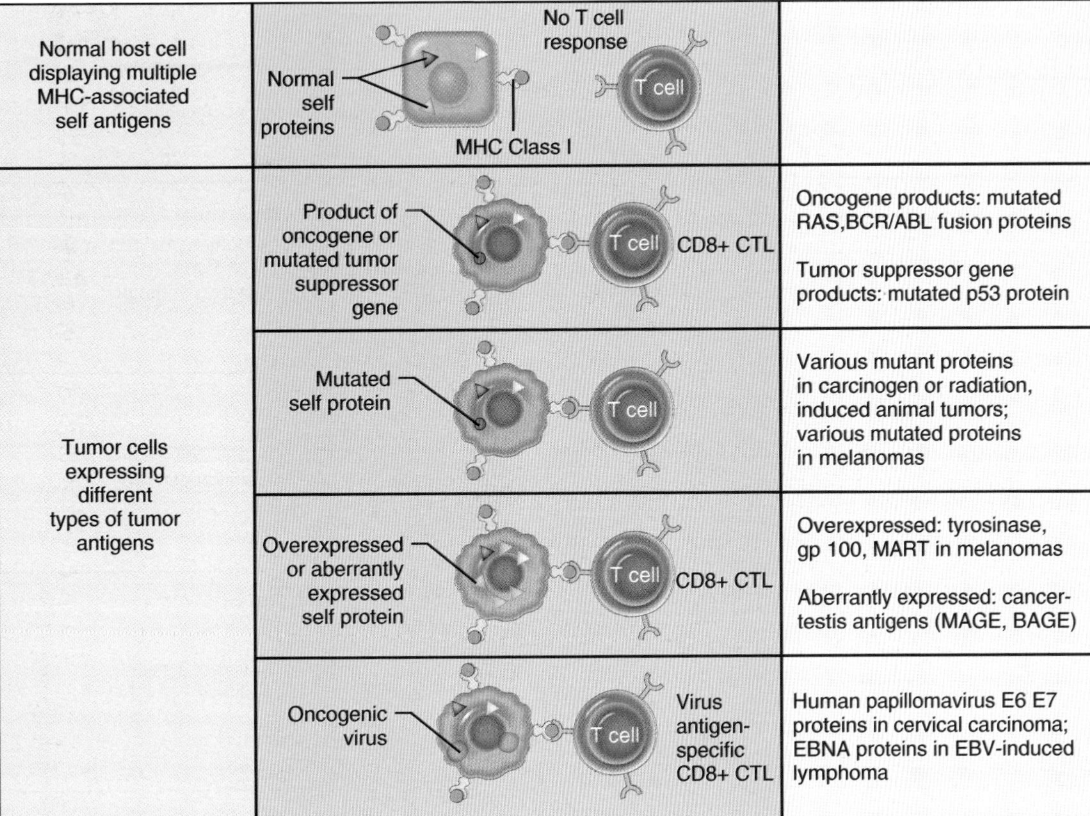


**Figure 9.1**

**T cells recognize different types of tumor antigens.** Tumor antigens that are recognized by antigen-specific T lymphocytes may be tumor-specific neoantigens (e.g., mutated forms of normal host proteins, viral proteins). T cells can also recognize tumor-associated antigens that are expressed at higher levels on tumors compared with normal cells or are expressed at different stages of development/differentiation. *EBV,* Epstein-Barr virus; *MHC,* major histocompatibility complex.

cells and may also be present in people with cancer of the pancreas, breast, ovary, or lung. Alpha fetoprotein is another oncofetal protein that is expressed by fetal liver and yolk sac cells and is also found on tumors of the liver and testis.

## Major Immune Responses Against Tumors

Major immune responses elicited against tumors that have been described in humans and animal models involve both innate and adaptive immunity. Innate immune responses against tumors may include NK cells that directly kill cancer cells without any previous exposure to the tumor. NK cells are activated by a balance of activating and inhibitory receptors. MHC class I is a ligand for an inhibitory receptor, and without inhibitory signals, NK cells are activated against tumor cells that have decreased MHC expression. Once contact with the tumor cell has been made, the NK cell releases soluble cytotoxic factors such as perforin, proteases, nucleases, and TNF-α. NK cells also have an Fc receptor (CD16) that binds to antibody-coated tumor cells and triggers antibody-dependent cell-mediated cytotoxicity.

Macrophages can function as effectors (antibody-dependent cell-mediated cytotoxicity, cytokine release, TNF-α production) that kill tumor cells. This activity does not require tumor antigen recognition directly. Macrophages do not recognize a specific tumor antigen, but similar to NK cells, they can distinguish normal cells from cancer cells. Detection by macrophages may involve phospholipids that are expressed ectopically in the membrane of a malignant cell. These innate immune cells generate many different antitumor products including hydrolytic enzymes, interferon (IFN)-α, TNF-α, hydrogen peroxide, and nitric oxide. As a bridge between innate and adaptive immune responses, it should be noted that tumor antigen–specific CD4+ T cells and B cells are required for antibody production and cytokine (i.e., IFN-α; TNF-α) activation of macrophages.

Complement-dependent cytotoxicity against tumor cells can be mediated by antibodies (e.g., immunoglobulin M [IgM]). On binding of antibody to the surface of a tumor cell, the classic complement pathway is activated, leading to the destruction of the tumor target via opsonization and intracellular destruction or exocytosis of lysosomal contents to destroy the cancer cell.

Adaptive immune responses against tumors include specific cytotoxic CD8+ T cells (cytotoxic T lymphocytes) that recognize tumor antigens and lyse tumor cells. These cells are the major immunologic barrier against tumors. Tumor-specific CD4+ T cells also play a critical role in adaptive immunity against cancer by helping to induce CD8+ T cells

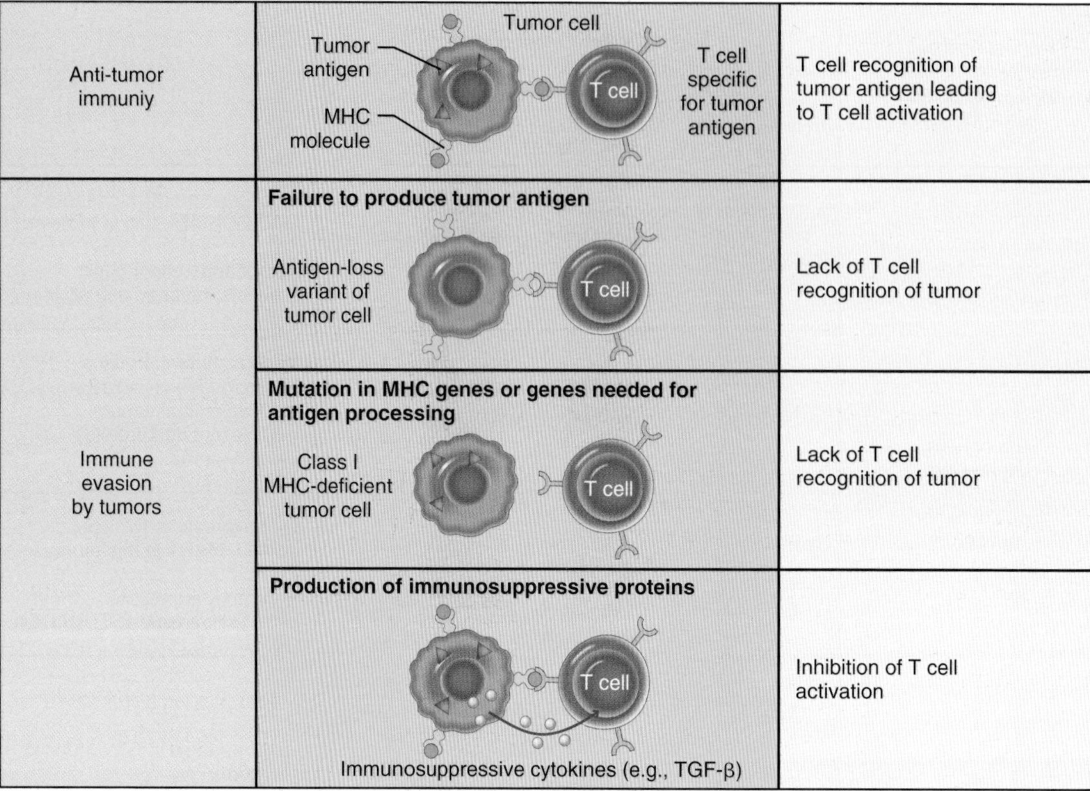


**Figure 9.2**

**Mechanisms of immune evasion by tumors.** T cell-mediated antitumor immunity develops upon recognition of a cognate tumor antigen and lymphocyte activation. Tumor cells have the capacity to evade immune responses by losing expression of antigens or MHC molecules or via the elaboration of immunosuppressive factors. *MHC,* Major histocompatibility complex; *TGF-β,* transforming growth factor beta.

as well as B cells. In addition, CD4+ T cells secrete cytokines that increase MHC expression, activate macrophages, and so on. The B-cell response against tumors is manifested by the formation of specific antibodies to tumor antigens that may mediate antibody-dependent cell-mediated cytotoxicity.[390]

Tumor progression results in the remodeling of surrounding stroma and deformation of tissue, leading to local damage and elicitation of the aforementioned immune responses. Proinflammatory factors released by damaged tissue include IL-1, IL-6, and TNF-α, and these factors aid in the recruitment of NK cells, T cells, and macrophages. IFN-γ produced by NK cells and T cells activates macrophages, making them potent killers. Necrotic cells at the center of a tumor may serve as a fodder for antigen-presenting cells, such as dendritic cells (DCs). DCs phagocytose tumor debris and migrate to the draining lymph nodes. Antigen is presented to CD4+ T cells in the context of MHC class II and to CD8+ T cells in the context of MHC class I. Activated CD4+ T cells and CD8+ T cells migrate to the tumor and differentiate into effector cells. CD4+ T cells are differentiated by the cytokine milieu into different helper T ($T_H$) cell subsets that aid other immune cells in mediating tumor clearance. CD8+ T cells acquire cytotoxic function. This is enhanced by $T_H1$ production of IFN-γ. In addition to helping B cells to produce antibodies, $T_H2$ cells may induce potent antitumor immune responses through IL-4–induced activation of NK cells.[36,202]

### Tumor Evasion Strategies

Despite the fact that immunity is mounted against neoantigens or antigens that are inappropriately expressed, one may ask why these responses are often insufficient to clear tumors. In other words, why does cancer develop in an immunocompetent individual? As it turns out, the immune system faces a daunting challenge of eliminating malignancies that are proliferating at such a rapid rate that immune defenses are simply overtaken. In addition, many tumor antigens are weak immunogens, perhaps because they vary only slightly from self-antigens.

Tumors have also evolved to evade innate and adaptive immune responses.[416] This is known as *immune escape* and can occur through many different mechanisms (Fig. 9.2) including the following:

1. *Loss of immunogenicity.* In the same way that virus infection induces MHC class I downregulation, selection of tumor cell variants with low levels of MHC class I occurs, and this prevents the induction of NK cells and cytotoxic CD8+ T cells. Tumors will also mutate antigenic peptides so that they cannot be loaded onto the class I MHC and be presented to CD8+ T cells. It should be appreciated that tumors are not professional antigen-presenting cells. T cells require two signals for activation—signal I through the T-cell receptor and signal II, which is costimulation. Even if the tumor cell presents antigen to T cells, it does not express

costimulatory molecules (e.g., B7-1) that could bind to CD28 on the T cell. In this situation, the tumor cell may be providing signal I, but not signal II, and that often leads to *tolerance* of T cells.[240] In addition, some tumors downregulate adhesion molecules such as intercellular adhesion molecule 1. In order for a CD8+ T cell to kill its target, it needs to bind, and tumors evolve to express very low levels of adhesion molecules. As a result, the cytotoxic T cell cannot make good contact with the tumor cell and undergo the remaining steps of triggering its killing mechanism.

2. *Antigenic modulation* refers to the loss of a surface antigen. When this occurs, tumor antigens are internalized or downregulated so that antibodies cannot bind.
3. *Induction of immune suppression*. Tumors produce a variety of suppressive factors that inhibit T cells directly and downmodulate the function of antigen-presenting cells such as DCs that infiltrate the tumor. These antigen-presenting cells pick up antigen from dying tumor cells to present to T cells. Immunosuppressive cytokines such as transforming growth factor beta and IL-10 will keep DCs in an immature state and also inhibit T-cell activation and proliferation.
4. *Prevention of NK- and T-cell activation*: Because MHC class I is downregulated on tumor cells, one may expect NK cells to effectively kill them. However, tumors have evolved strategies to avoid triggering of NK cell–activating receptors. For example, MHC class I chain-related molecule (MIC) is a stress protein that is upregulated on the surfaces of stressed cells such as rapidly proliferating tumor cells. Some tumors actually cleave MIC off of their surface; tumor-derived soluble MIC can downregulate the expression of activating receptors on NK cells and T cells.[188,418]

**Note to Reader:** This section on cancer immunotherapy is a complement to both the Pathogenesis and the Medical Management of Cancer: Immunotherapy sections of this chapter. It is presented here (rather than placing it all in the section on treatment) to aid the reader in better understanding current efforts to translate biologic research into more effective clinical treatment. You will find additional information on immunotherapy in Medical Management of Cancer later.

### Cancer Immunotherapy

Immunotherapy of cancer encompasses strategies aimed at boosting immune responses against tumors through the administration of immunomodulatory factors (e.g., cytokines, adjuvants) or more specific approaches such as monoclonal antibodies (mAbs) directed against a particular tumor antigen. Cytokines such as IFN-α, IFN-β, IFN-γ, IL-2, IL-4, IL-6, IL-12, and TNF have been used alone or in combination to bolster immune responses against cancer.[221] Similarly, a variety of adjuvants, such as attenuated strains of *Mycobacterium bovis* (bacillus Calmette-Guérin), VNP20009 (a derivative strain of *Salmonella typhimurium*), and other small molecule compounds, have been used to augment antitumor immunity by activating macrophages to generate various cytokines, increase MHC class II expression, upregulate costimulatory molecules (e.g., B7), inhibit cell differentiation, or serve as a vector for preferentially delivering cytotoxic peptides.

**Antibody-Based Therapy.** If the tumor antigen is known, mAbs can be administered that are "naked" or conjugated with agents that increase their efficacy. If a patient is injected with mAbs against a tumor antigen, NK cells can bind through their Fc receptors and get triggered to kill the tumor cell.

Complement may also play a role in the destruction of tumor cells following the binding of antibodies. In addition, mAbs can induce apoptosis of certain malignant cells (i.e., by cross-linking of surface immunoglobulin or CD20) or block or downregulate a receptor for a tumor growth factor (e.g., EGF receptor and HER-2 receptor blockade). mAbs are often coupled to immunotoxins (e.g., ricin) or to radionuclides to concentrate the substance/radiation at the tumor site, while sparing healthy tissues.[185]

A clever antitumor immunotherapy strategy involves the engineering of *bispecific antibodies* in which the binding sites of the immunoglobulin recognize different targets. For example, these antibodies have been used to simultaneously target tumor cells and CD3. Thus this type of bispecific antibody not only brings the T cells and tumor cells into proximity but also triggers the T cells for activation. In this way, recognition of the tumor is not antigen-specific because the T-cell receptor does not recognize a tumor antigen, but CD3 is cross-linked so that the T cell is activated and can kill the tumor.[85]

**Adoptive Cell Therapy.** The transfusion of immune cells, also known as adoptive cell therapy or cellular adoptive immunotherapy, has demonstrated efficacy for the treatment of cancer and chronic infections. Adoptive cell therapy for cancer may include the isolation of T cells from within or around a tumor (tumor-infiltrating lymphocytes) and ex vivo expansion of these cells with IL-2, followed by infusion back into the patient. This provides for superenrichment of cytotoxic T cells that may possess improved homing ability to the tumor site.[334] A similar adoptive cell therapeutic strategy involves the generation of lymphokine activated killer cells by culturing peripheral blood cells with growth factors. Lymphokine activated killer cells consist mainly of nonspecific, activated CD16+ CD3− NK cells.[139]

Chimeric antigen receptor (CAR) T cells are engineered T cells where T cells taken from a patient's blood are altered in a laboratory with the addition of the gene for a special receptor that attaches to a specific protein, antigen, or tumor cells. These reengineered cells are then grown in large numbers in the laboratory and reinfused into the patient. Thus a patient's T cells can be directed against virtually any tumor antigen.[334] Clinical trials on the use of CAR T cells have reported successes in blood cancers such as acute lymphocytic leukemia (ALL) and lymphoma.[285,377] One advantage of CAR T cells is their ability to potentially expand and persist longer in the patient's circulation.

**Cancer Vaccines.** See further discussion of cancer vaccines in Medical Management of Cancer later. Cancer vaccines are available either to treat individuals with an existing malignancy (*therapeutic* vaccines) or to prevent the development of cancer (*prophylactic* vaccines). In the context of therapeutic vaccines, when the tumor antigen has been identified, autologous antigen-presenting cells such as DCs can be isolated from the patient, loaded with the tumor antigen, and then reinfused into the patient with the hope of stimulating anticancer immunity. Viral vectors (e.g., adenovirus) can also be engineered to encode a particular tumor antigen. Because viruses strongly activate antigen-presenting cells, the immune system can be "tricked" so that there is enhanced presentation of tumor antigen, resulting in a more potent response.[215]

Although still largely experimental, DNA vaccines allow for tumor antigens to be encoded along with cytokines and perhaps costimulatory molecules so that T cells can be activated to inhibit tumor growth.[419] In addition, autologous tumor cells can be isolated from the patient and manipulated to express costimulatory molecules to activate T cells in the host.[106] Tumor cells can also be engineered to express granulocyte-macrophage colony-stimulating factor (GM-CSF), and when reinfused into the patient, these cells will facilitate the activation and differentiation of antigen-presenting cells to enhance presentation of tumor antigen to T cells.

Another useful strategy that can be employed when the tumor antigen is unknown is to immunize patients with cancer with autologous tumor-derived heat shock proteins. Heat shock proteins are chaperones that pick up antigenic peptides and shuttle them to MHC class I and class II. The rationale behind this strategy is that if heat shock proteins are isolated from a tumor, they should be loaded with immunogenic peptides from the cancer cells.[69]

The major challenge involved with developing prophylactic cancer vaccines is identifying a tumor antigen to immunize individuals against. This is further complicated by the tremendous amount of heterogeneity observed in human cancers. However, there are some conditions such as viral infections with which tumors are known to be associated. Therefore if a population is immunized against certain oncogenic viruses, it will be protected against the future development of tumors induced by these viruses (e.g., HPV or HBV). It should be noted that although these vaccines constitute very effective preventive strategies, they target viral and not tumor antigens.

## INVASION AND METASTASES

Malignant tumors differ from benign tumors in their ability to metastasize or spread from the primary site to other locations in the body. Metastasis occurs when cells break away from the primary tumor, travel through the body via the blood or lymphatic system, and become trapped in the capillaries of organs. From there, they infiltrate the organ tissue and grow into new tumor deposits. Cancer can also spread to adjacent structures and penetrate body cavities by direct extension. For example, ovarian tumors frequently shed cells into the peritoneal cavity where they grow to cover the surface of abdominal organs and cause ascites.

Patterns of metastasis differ from cancer to cancer. Although there is no clear explanation of the exact mechanism of metastasis, certain cancers tend to spread to specific organs or sites in the body in a predictable manner (Table 9.3). The five most common sites of metastasis are the lymph nodes, liver, lung, bone, and brain. The spread of cancer may be influenced by a variety of host factors such as the aging or dysfunctional immune system, increasing age, hormonal environment, pregnancy, and stress. Factors that may slow the spread of metastasis include radiation, chemotherapy, anticoagulants, steroids, and other antiangiogenic agents.

### Seed Versus Soil Theory of Metastasis

Some cancers favor certain sites of metastasis over others so that metastases occur only if the cancer cell (the seed) finds a favorable microenvironment at the site of the host (the soil). Certain tumor cells seem to have specific affinity for certain organs. The idea that metastasis is organ specific was proposed in 1889 by Stephen Paget, an English surgeon who first published the seed versus soil hypothesis to explain the pattern of metastasis.

Studies in the 1990s showed that there is "cross-talk" between metastatic cells and the organ microenvironment. Host cells secrete growth factors that prompt tumor cell replication and allow the tumor to take over the homeostatic mechanisms of the host. Angiogenesis, the process by which blood vessels from preexisting vessels grow into the solid tumor, is one way that tumor cells take over homeostatic mechanisms for their own gain.[369]

Traditional cancer treatment targets the seed, whereas today's research also focuses on approaches that target the soil, making the sites of metastasis unsuitable for the growth of cancer cells. There are many challenges in preventing metastasis because the microenvironments of metastasis sites can be very different. For example, lung cancer that spreads to the femur can behave very differently from lung cancer that spreads to the spine. Treatment that is optimal in the primary organ may not work in the metastatic sites.[299]

Animal studies and computational modeling have shown that the surgical removal of a primary tumor can result in the rapid growth of previously dormant metastatic cells. Additional challenges to preventing metastases are possible if this phenomenon occurs in humans.[60,95]

### Incidence of Metastasis

Approximately 30% of clients with newly diagnosed cancers have clinically detectable metastases. At least 30% to 40% of the remaining clients who are clinically free of metastases harbor occult (hidden) metastases. Most people have multiple sites of metastatic disease, not all of which manifest at any one time. The formation of metastatic colonies is a continuous process, starting early in the growth of the primary tumor and increasing with time.

Even metastases have the potential to metastasize; the presence of large, identifiable metastases in a given organ can be accompanied by a greater number of micrometastases that have been disseminated more recently from the primary tumor or the metastasis. The size variation in metastases and the dispersed anatomic location of metastases can make complete surgical removal of disease impossible, limiting the effective concentration of anticancer drugs that can be delivered only to tumor cells in metastatic colonies.

**Table 9.3** Pathways of Cancer Metastases

| Primary Cancer | Mode of Dissemination | Location of Primary Metastases |
|---|---|---|
| Breast | Lymphatics | Bone (shoulder, hips, sacrum, ribs, vertebrae); CNS (brain, spinal fluid, brachial plexus) |
| | Blood (vascular or hematogenous) | Lung, pleural cavity, liver, bone |
| Bone | Blood | Lungs, liver, bone, then CNS |
| Cervical (cervix) | Local extension and lymphatics | Retroperitoneal lymph nodes, bladder, rectum; paracervical, parametrial lymphatics |
| | Blood | CNS (brain), lungs, bones, liver |
| Chordoma | Direct extension | Neighboring soft tissues, spine |
| | Blood | Liver, lungs, heart, brain, spine |
| | Lymphatics | Lymph nodes, peritoneum |
| Colorectal | Direct extension | Bone (vertebrae, hip, sacrum) |
| | Peritoneal seeding | Peritoneum |
| | Blood | Liver, lung |
| Ewing sarcoma | Blood | Lung, bone, bone marrow |
| Giant cell tumor of bone | Blood | Lung |
| Kidney | Lymph | Pelvis, groin |
| | Blood | Lungs, pleural cavity, bone, liver, brain |
| Leukemia | | Does not really "metastasize" because it is present throughout the body and therefore causes symptoms throughout body |
| Liver | Blood | CNS (brain) |
| Lung (bronchogenic sarcoma) | Blood | CNS (brain, spinal cord) |
| | Blood | Bone (ribs, sacrum, vertebrae) |
| | Direct extension, lymphatics | Mediastinum (tissue and organs between the sternum and vertebrae such as the heart, blood vessels, trachea, esophagus, thymus, lymph nodes) |
| Lung (apical or Pancoast tumors) | Direct extension | Eighth cervical and first and second thoracic nerves within brachial plexus |
| | Blood | CNS (brain, spinal cord), bone |
| Lung (small cell) | Blood | CNS (brain, spinal fluid) |
| Lymphomas | Blood | CNS (spinal cord, spinal fluid), bone |
| | Lymphatics | Can occur anywhere, including skin and visceral organs, especially liver |
| Malignant melanoma | No typical pattern | Metastases can occur anywhere, including skin and subcutaneous tissue; lungs; CNS (brain, spinal fluid); liver; GI tract; bone |
| Multiple myeloma | Blood | Bone (sacrum) |
| Nonmelanoma skin cancer | Usually remain local without metastases; local invasion | Bones underlying involved skin; brain |
| Osteogenic sarcoma (osteosarcoma) | Blood | Lungs, CNS (brain) |
| | Lymphatics | Lymph nodes, lungs, bone, kidneys |
| Ovarian | Direct extension into abdominal cavity | Nearby organs (bladder, colon, rectum, uterus, fallopian tubes); spread beyond abdomen is rare |
| | Lymphatics, peritoneal fluid through the abdomen | Liver, lungs; regional and distant |
| Pancreatic | Blood | Liver |
| Prostate | Lymphatics | Pelvic, sacrum, and vertebral bones, sacral plexus |
| | | Bladder, rectum |
| | | Distant organs (lung, liver, brain) |
| Soft tissue sarcoma | Blood; lymphatics (rare) | Lung (first) but also bone, brain, liver, soft tissue (distant) |
| Spinal cord | Local invasion; dissemination through the intervertebral foramina | CNS (brain, spinal cord) |
| Stomach, gastric | Blood | Liver, vertebrae, abdominal cavity (intraperitoneum) |
| | Local invasion | |
| Testes | Local invasion | Bone (pelvis, lumbar spine, hip) |
| | Blood, lymphatics | Lung |
| Thyroid | Direct extension | Bone; nearby tissues of neck |
| | Lymphatics | Regional lymph nodes (neck, upper chest, mediastinum) |
| | Blood | Distant (lung, bone, brain) |

*CNS*, Central nervous system; *GI*, gastrointestinal.

From Goodman CC, Heick J, Lazaro RT: *differential diagnosis for physical therapists: Screening for referral*, ed 6, Philadelphia, 2018; Saunders.

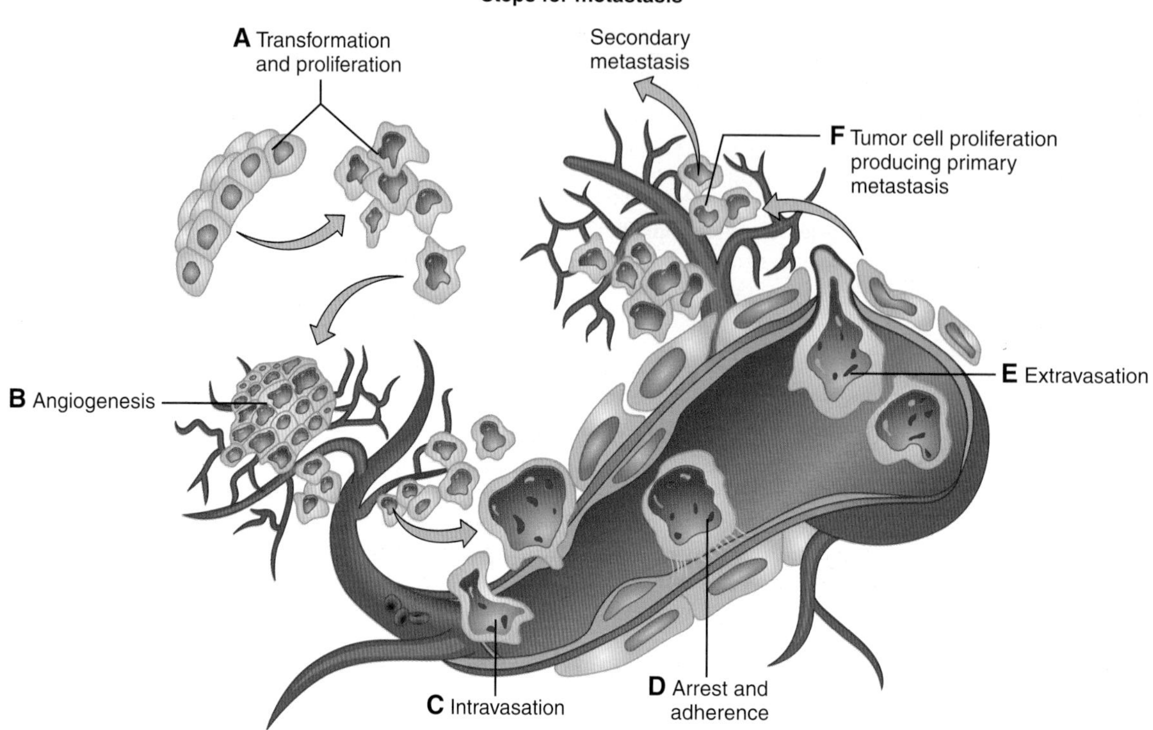


**Figure 9.3**

**Major mechanisms of metastases.** To metastasize, tumor cells must gain several unique biologic properties such as invasive growth (A), induction of vascular growth (B), vascular invasion (C), adherence to endothelial cells or thrombosis of peripheral sinusoids (D), continuation of invasive growth with extravasation (E), and formation of primary and secondary metastatic foci (F). Not all tumor cells develop all the properties shown here; some cell clones may subspecialize and just create angiogenesis; others may invade and move on. (From Dorfman HD, Czerniak B: *Bone tumors*, St. Louis, 1998, Mosby.)

## Mechanisms of Metastasis

For rapidly growing tumors, millions of tumor cells are shed into the vascular system each day. Only a very small percentage of circulating tumor cells initiate metastatic colonies because most cells that have invaded the bloodstream are quickly eliminated. Classic isotope studies have shown that 99% of circulating potentially tumorigenic cells are killed by blood vessel turbulence within 24 hours.[117,133,382] Metastases of the remaining 1% require a good deal of coordination between the cancer cells and the body (Fig. 9.3).

The greater the number of invasive tumor cells in the bloodstream, the greater the probability that some cells will survive to form metastases. Metastasis is more likely to occur via the veins as opposed to the arteries because the cancer cannot break through the arterial wall. The major challenge in treating cancer is not eradicating the primary tumor because surgery or radiation is effective in these early cases. Eradicating metastases, often already present at the time of diagnosis, is the key factor to cancer cure.

A complicated series of tumor–host interactions resulting in a metastatic colony is called the *metastatic cascade* and is similar for all tumor cells. Once a primary tumor is initiated and starts to move by local invasion, blood vessels from preexisting vessels grow into the solid tumor, a process called *tumor angiogenesis* (see Fig. 9.3). As a normal physiologic process, angiogenesis is crucial to tissue growth, repair, and maintenance.

The ability of a tumor to grow beyond a very small mass (1 to 2 mm) depends on its ability to gain access to an adequate supply of blood and in some cases (e.g., breast and prostate) the presence of hormonal factors. The supply of blood allows the tumor to obtain essential nutrients such as oxygen and to eliminate metabolic waste products such as carbon dioxide and acids. The blood supply to tumors is provided by growth of new capillaries and larger vessels into the tumor mass from the blood supply of adjacent normal tissues.

The normal process of angiogenesis begins with the formation of endothelial cell sprouts, followed by proliferation and migration of neighboring endothelial cells along the preformed extensions. The initiating event and mechanism of sprouting are unknown; in apoptotic cells, endothelial cell sprouting occurs via electrostatic signaling. Negatively charged membrane surfaces in apoptotic cells initiate the formation of directional endothelial cell sprouts that extend toward the dying cells.[124]

Tumor-derived proteins called *angiogenesis* or *angiogenic factors* also facilitate the use of nearby blood vessels from normal tissues and promote the growth of new blood vessels into the malignant tissue.[65] The actual factors involved in tumor angiogenesis are very complex, but two cytokines have been identified as primary stimulators of vascular proliferation.

Both vascular endothelial growth factor and fibroblast growth factor stimulate proliferation of vascular cells and even allow the newly formed blood vessels to be easily invaded by the cancer cells that are closely adjacent to them.[290] Increased tumor contact with the circulatory system provides tumors with a mechanism to enter the general circulation and colonize at distant sites. Resection without clear margins has the potential to provide remaining tumor cells with a means of metastasizing as new blood vessels form during the healing process. Antiangiogenic therapy shows promise as a strategy for cancer treatment (see Medical Management of Cancer).

Tumors generally lack a well-formed lymphatic network, so communication of tumor cells with lymphatic channels occurs only at the tumor periphery and not within the tumor mass. Lymphatic dissemination and hematogenous dissemination occur in parallel. Tumors excrete acid-like enzymes that dissolve the basement membrane and break through to the lymphatics. Cancer cells can enter the bloodstream where lymph nodes drain into veins (e.g., lymphatic intersection with the subclavian vein).

Some controversy exists with regard to the role/risk of needle biopsy and/or aspiration cytology and the risk for cancer recurrence and/or metastasis. Recurrence along the surgical pathway has been reported for some tumors.[352] It is hypothesized that this recurrence is the result of intraoperative seeding. Poorly planned biopsies or incomplete tumor resection increases the risk of local recurrence and metastasis. The biopsy tract should be excised when complete tumor removal occurs.

## Clinical Manifestations of Metastasis

Metastatic spread usually occurs within 3 to 5 years after initial diagnosis and treatment of malignancy, although some low-grade lesions can reappear 15 to 20 years later. It is therefore very important to conduct a thorough past medical history as part of any client interview. As mentioned before, metastases occur most commonly to areas of the body that provide an environment rich in nutrition to the colonized tumor cells, such as the lung, brain, liver, and bone; metastases can be found in other areas as well (e.g., lymph nodes, skin, ovaries, adrenal glands).

### Pulmonary System (Lungs)

Pulmonary metastases are the most common of all metastatic tumors because venous drainage of most areas of the body is through the superior and inferior venae cavae into the heart, making the lungs the first organ to filter malignant cells. Parenchymal metastases are asymptomatic until tumor cells have obstructed bronchi, resulting in pulmonary symptoms, or until tumor cells have expanded and reached the parietal pleura where pain fibers are stimulated.

A dry, persistent cough is often the first symptom of pulmonary metastases. Pleural pain can indicate pleural invasion, and shortness of breath (dyspnea) usually occurs in the presence of a malignant pleural effusion. If hemoptysis occurs, there is usually bronchial tissue invasion either by a primary lung malignancy or metastatic disease.[320]

### Hepatic System (Liver)

Liver metastases are among the most ominous signs of advanced cancer. The liver filters blood coming in from the gastrointestinal tract, making it a primary metastatic site for tumors of the stomach, colorectum, and pancreas. Symptoms include abdominal and/or right upper quadrant pain, general malaise and fatigue, anorexia, early satiety and weight loss, and sometimes low-grade fevers.

### Skeletal System (Bone)

Bone is one of the three most favored sites of solid tumor metastasis, indicating that the bone microenvironment provides fertile ground for the growth of many tumors. Although lung, breast, and prostate are the three primary sites responsible for most metastatic bone disease,[94,404] tumors of the thyroid and kidney, lymphoma, and melanoma can also metastasize to the skeletal system.

Bone metastases may be the osteolytic type, marked by areas of decreased bone density, or osteoblastic, appearing as areas of dense scarring and increased bone density. Osteolytic metastases occur predominately from lung, kidney, and thyroid cancer. Breast is primarily osteolytic but can be osteoblastic, and prostate is usually, but not always, osteoblastic. The axial skeleton is most commonly involved, with spread to the spine, pelvis, ribs, proximal femora, proximal humeri, and skull.[238]

The primary symptom associated with bone metastases is pain. Pain is usually deep and worsened by activity, especially weight bearing. Spinal metastases manifest with pain, neurologic symptoms, and instability.[240] Disabling pathologic fractures, especially of the vertebral bodies and proximal ends of the long bones, may occur in up to one-half of people with osteolytic metastases and are sometimes one of the first signs of a malignant process.[140] Blastic lesions often result in an elevated serum alkaline phosphatase, whereas lytic lesions may not.[227]

Hypercalcemia (abnormally high concentration of blood calcium) is a frequent complication of neoplastic disease and is associated with bone metastases, particularly osteolytic lesions as a result of increased bone resorption. The presence of tumor cells in the bone disturbs the balance between new bone formation and bone resorption, resulting in abnormal bone remodeling.

Carcinoma cells secrete a variety of factors that stimulate tumor growth as well as osteoclast recruitment and activation. Osteoclasts are bone cells that break down bone tissue. Although more than 80% of people with hypercalcemia have bony metastases, the severity of the hypercalcemia does not correlate with the extent of the bone disease.[343]

Assessment of risk for fracture in individuals with known metastasis to bone is often determined using a scoring system published by Mirels in 1989.[255] The total score is based on the location of the lesion, degree of pain, type of lesion, and percentage of cortex involved. The higher the score (maximum of 12), the higher the risk for fracture.

Hydration and administration of oral or intravenous bisphosphonates (e.g., alendronate [Fosamax], risedronate [Actonel], ibandronate [Boniva], zoledronate [Zometa]) are the mainstays of current treatment and have contributed to the decrease in the frequency of hypercalcemia and to minimizing or preventing bone loss. Bisphosphonates prevent thinning of the bone by inhibiting osteoclast function, thereby inhibiting bone resorption. There is no life-prolonging benefit with bisphosphonates, but there is a substantial reduction of morbidity (e.g., decreased pain, prevention of fracture and/or deformity) associated with bone metastases and improved QOL.[226,381,412]

### Central Nervous System

**Brain.** Many primary tumors may lead to CNS metastases. Lung carcinomas account for approximately one-half of all metastatic brain lesions. Breast carcinoma and malignant melanoma also commonly metastasize to the brain. Metastatic disease in the brain is life threatening and emotionally debilitating. Metastatic brain tumors can increase intracranial pressure, obstruct the normal flow of cerebrospinal fluid, change mentation and contribute to cognitive impairment, and reduce sensory and motor function. The management of cognitive impairments is important, and the therapist can use the same strategies employed for people with traumatic brain injury

Clinical manifestations of brain metastases depend on the location, either in the brain or outside the brain in the bony cranium exerting compression externally. The therapist can look at CT scan results, see the location of pathologic conditions, and correlate these to signs and symptoms observed clinically. Primary tumors of the CNS rarely develop metastases outside the CNS despite the highly invasive capacity of these tumors. Microscopically, some CNS (brain) tumor cells (astrocytomas) may spread widely within the CNS but rarely metastasize outside it.

Tumor cells traveling from the lung via the pulmonary veins and carotid artery can result in metastases to the CNS. Lung cancer is the most common primary tumor to metastasize to the brain. In fact, about 10% of patients with lung cancer present with brain metastases at the time of their initial diagnosis.[8]

**Spinal Cord.** Metastatic involvement of the vertebrae may result in epidural spinal (usually anterior) cord compression. In addition, severe, destructive osteolytic lesions can lead to fracture and fragility of one or more vertebral bodies. In such cases, compression of the cord occurs as a result of the subsequent deformity.[237] Spinal cord and nerve root compression cause either insidious or rapid loss of neurologic function. This compression phenomenon occurs in approximately 5% of people with systemic cancer and is most often caused by carcinoma of the lung, breast, prostate, or kidney. Lymphoma and multiple myeloma may also result in spinal cord and nerve root compression.

The earliest neurologic symptoms include gradual onset of distal weakness and sensory changes, including numbness, paresthesias, and coldness. The incidence of permanent motor dysfunction has markedly decreased in the past 2 decades because of earlier diagnosis and treatment.[226] A client who presents with spinal cord symptoms caused by metastatic epidural disease and resultant compression may have only transient symptoms with proper medical treatment. More than 95% of people with spinal cord compression complain of progressive central or radicular back pain often aggravated by recumbency, weight bearing, sneezing, coughing, or Valsalva maneuver. Sitting often relieves pain. Later symptoms may include a major change or loss of bowel or bladder function, which is considered by many a serious condition requiring immediate assessment for possible spinal stabilization.

**Lymphatic System.** Previous cancer-related surgery or adverse effects involving radiation fibrosis can affect the lymph nodes and may result in dysfunction of the lymphatic system, manifesting as lymphedema. It has a wide range of onset from weeks to years from the initial insult to the lymphatic system. The therapist may be the first health care professional to recognize subtle abnormalities or changes in the extremities.

## Diagnosis of Metastasis

Metastases usually reproduce the cellular structure of the primary growth well enough to enable a pathologist to determine the site of the primary tumor. For example, bone metastases from a carcinoma of the thyroid not only exhibit a microscopic structure similar to the original tumor but also may produce thyroid hormone. Sometimes symptoms of a cancer will occur in the metastatic site rather than the site of origin (primary site). If the primary tumor cannot be found, the malignant tissue is called *carcinoma of unknown primary*. Special histologic stains can be done on the unknown tissue and compared with slides of a previous malignancy to determine similarity.

## Cancer Recurrence

Disease-free survival describes the time between diagnosis and recurrence or relapse. Recurrences may be local, regional, disseminated, or a combination of these. The most important predictors of recurrent cancer are the stage at the time of initial therapy and histologic findings. Recurrence of cancer may be first recognized by the return of systemic symptoms associated with paraneoplastic phenomena. The metabolic or toxic effects of the syndrome (e.g., hypercalcemia or hyponatremia) may constitute a more urgent life-threatening condition than the underlying cancer.

# CLINICAL MANIFESTATIONS

## Local and Systemic Effects

In their earliest stages, most cancers are asymptomatic but are treatable if found. Primary site cancers cause certain symptoms that are recognizable causes for suspicion or concern. For example, endometrial cancer causes abnormal bleeding so often that it is usually detected in its early stages. Laryngeal cancer causes hoarseness, which is also an early sign. Conversely, lung cancer is usually quite extensive before it causes enough symptoms to warrant investigation; similarly, breast cancer or tumors deep to the chest wall may also be difficult to palpate and therefore not detected early. Current imaging techniques, including CT, magnetic resonance imaging (MRI), and positron emission tomography allow for early detection and therapeutic intervention.

As cancer progresses, symptoms characteristic of the involved organ or tissue may develop. With advanced cancer, nausea, vomiting, and retching accompanied by anorexia and subsequent weight loss are common as a result of the malignant process and its treatment. Nausea, vomiting, and retching are especially prevalent in association with lung carcinoma, renal carcinoma, and pancreatic carcinoma.

Anorexia has been attributed to tumor production of TNF, which is a polypeptide protein (a cytokine) also called *cachectin*. TNFs are thought to play an important role in mediating inflammation and cytotoxic reactions (along with ILs). TNFs produce necrosis of tumor cells by eliminating the blood supply to these growths. Small amounts of TNF are beneficial in promoting wound healing and preventing tumors, but uncontrolled production is accompanied by symptoms of fever, weight loss, and tissue damage that can cause more problems than the benefits provided.

Cancer-related anorexia/cachexia is a complex phenomenon in which metabolic abnormalities, proinflammatory cytokines produced by the host immune system, circulating tumor-derived catabolic factors, decreased food intake, and possibly other unknown factors all contribute. Profound muscle loss is prominent in cancer-related anorexia/cachexia syndrome as a result of decreased protein synthesis and abnormal muscle proteolysis.

Later, rapid growth of the tumor encroaches on healthy tissue, causing destruction, necrosis, ulceration, and hemorrhage, resulting in many local and systemic effects. Pain may occur as a late symptom caused by infiltration, compression, or destruction of nerves. With advanced or stage IV cancer, the host presents systemically with muscular weakness, anemia, and coagulation disorders, such as granulocyte and platelet abnormalities.

Pyrexia or fever may be seen with cancer in the absence of infection and is produced either by white blood cells inducing a pyrogen (an agent that causes fever) or by direct tumor production of a pyrogen. Continued spread of the cancer may lead to gastrointestinal, pulmonary, or vascular obstruction. Secondary infections frequently occur as a result of the host's decreased immunity and can lead to death.

Other vital organs may be affected, such as the brain, in which increased intracranial pressure by tumor cells can cause strokelike symptoms. In addition to the local effects of tumor growth, cancer can produce systemic signs and symptoms that are not direct effects of either the tumor or its metastases (e.g., paraneoplastic syndromes and fever with renal cancer).

## Cancer Pain

### Overview

One of the most common symptoms of cancer is pain, affecting 35% to 70% of clients in earlier stages and 60% to 90% of clients in later stages of the disease. It is estimated that 1.1 million Americans experience cancer-related pain annually.[160,383] Stated another way, pain occurs in approximately one-quarter of adults with newly diagnosed malignancies, one-third of individuals undergoing treatment, and three-quarters of all people with advanced disease.[160]

Depression and anxiety may increase the person's perception of pain or may be the result of the cancer pain. Symptoms often go unreported or underreported because clients are reluctant to take the pain medication prescribed. An unfounded fear of tolerance, addiction, or adverse effects from pain medication may result in underreporting of painful symptoms, with subsequent inadequate cancer pain control and unnecessary pain-induced loss of function. Likewise, physicians may hesitate to provide adequate pain medications based on this misconception of client addiction.

**Table 9.4** Common Patterns of Pain Referral

| Pain Mechanism | Lesion Site | Referral Site |
|---|---|---|
| Somatic | C7, T1-5 vertebrae | Interscapular area, posterior shoulder |
| | Shoulder | Neck, upper back |
| | L1, L2 vertebrae | Sacroiliac joint and hip |
| | Hip joint | SI and knee |
| | Pharynx | Ipsilateral ear |
| | TMJ | Head, neck, heart |
| Visceral | Diaphragmatic irritation | Shoulder, lumbar spine |
| | Heart | Shoulder, neck, upper back, TMJ |
| | Urothelial tract | Back, inguinal region, anterior thigh, and genitalia |
| | Pancreas, liver, spleen, gallbladder | Shoulder, midthoracic, or low back |
| | Peritoneal or abdominal cavity (inflammatory or infectious process) | Hip pain from abscess of psoas or obturator muscle |
| Neuropathic | Nerve or plexus | Anywhere in distribution of a peripheral nerve |
| | Nerve root | Anywhere in corresponding dermatome |
| | CNS | Anywhere in region of body innervated by damaged structure |

*CNS*, Central nervous system; *SI*, sacroiliac; *TMJ*, temporomandibular joint.
From Goodman CC, Heick J, Lazaro RT: *Differential diagnosis for physical therapists: Screening for referral*, ed 6, Philadelphia, 2018; Saunders.

### Etiology and Pathogenesis

The cause of cancer pain is multifaceted, and the characteristics of the pain depend on the tissue structure, as well as on the mechanisms involved (Table 9.4). Some pain is caused by pressure on nerves or by the displacement of nerves. Microscopic infiltration of nerves by tumor cells can result in continuous, sharp, stabbing pain generally following the pattern of nerve distribution. Ischemic pain (throbbing) may also result from interference with blood supply or from blockage within hollow organs.

A common cause of cancer pain is metastasis of cancer to bone. Lung, breast, prostate, thyroid, and the lymphatics are the primary sites responsible for most metastatic bone disease. Bone metastasis results in increased release of prostaglandins and cytokines and subsequent bone destruction caused by breakdown and resorption. Bone pain may be mild to intense. Movement, weight bearing, and ambulation exacerbate painful symptoms from bone destruction. Pathologic

**Table 9.5** Side Effects of Cancer Treatment

| Surgery | Radiation | Chemotherapy | Biotherapy | Hormonal Therapy | Transplant (Bone Marrow, Stem Cell) |
|---|---|---|---|---|---|
| Fatigue<br>Disfigurement<br>Loss of function<br>Infection<br>Increased pain<br>Deformity<br>Bleeding, hemorrhage<br>Scar tissue<br>Fibrosis | Fatigue<br>Radiation sickness<br>Immunosuppression<br>Decreased platelets<br>Decreased white blood cells<br>Infection<br>Fibrosis<br>Radiation recall<br>Mucositis<br>Diarrhea<br>Edema<br>Hair loss<br>Ulceration, delayed wound healing<br>CNS/PNS effects<br>Malignancy | Fatigue<br>GI effects<br>Anorexia<br>Nausea<br>Vomiting<br>Constipation<br>Anxiety and depression<br>Fluid/electrolyte imbalance from GI effects<br>Hepatotoxicity<br>Hemorrhage<br>Bone marrow suppression<br>Anemia<br>Leukopenia (infection)<br>Neutropenia<br>Decreased bone density with ovarian failure<br>Muscle weakness<br>Joint pain<br>Skin rashes<br>Neuropathies<br>Hair loss<br>Sterilization<br>Stomatitis, mucositis (oral, rectal, vaginal)<br>Sexual dysfunction<br>Weight gain or loss | Fever<br>Chills<br>Nausea<br>Vomiting<br>Anorexia<br>Fatigue<br>Fluid retention<br>CNS effects<br>Slowed thinking<br>Memory problems<br>Inflammatory reactions at injection sites<br>Anemia<br>Leukopenia<br>Altered taste sensation<br>Targeted therapies:<br>Skin rash<br>Paronychia<br>Diarrhea<br>Hypertension<br>Thrombus formation<br>Prolonged bleeding<br>Renal toxicity<br>Infusion reaction (fever, chills, shortness of breath, chest pain, back pain, flushing, changes in heart rate and blood pressure)<br>Mouth sores | Hypertension<br>Steroid-induced diabetes<br>Myopathy (steroid-induced)<br>Weight gain<br>Hot flashes<br>Erectile dysfunction<br>Decreased libido<br>Vaginal dryness<br>Joint symptoms (arthralgia, arthritis) | Severe bone marrow suppression<br>Mucositis<br>Nausea and vomiting<br>Graft-versus-host disease (allogeneic graft only)<br>Delayed wound healing<br>Venoocclusive disease<br>Infertility<br>Cataract formation<br>Thyroid dysfunction<br>Growth hormone deficiency<br>Osteoporosis<br>Secondary malignancy |

*CNS*, Central nervous system; *GI*, gastrointestinal; *PNS*, peripheral nervous system.

fractures with resultant muscle spasms can develop; in the case of vertebral involvement, nerve pain may also occur.

Pain may also result from diagnostic or therapeutic procedures such as surgery, radiation therapy, or chemotherapy (e.g., mucositis, stomatitis, esophageal inflammation, localized skin burns) (Table 9.5).

## Clinical Manifestations

Signs and symptoms accompanying mild-to-moderate superficial pain may include hypertension, tachycardia, and tachypnea (rapid, shallow breathing) as the result of a sympathetic nervous system response. In severe or visceral pain, a parasympathetic nervous system response is more characteristic, with hypotension, bradycardia, nausea, vomiting, tachypnea, weakness, or fainting.

Spinal cord compression from metastases may manifest as radicular back pain, leg weakness, and change or loss of bowel or bladder control. Back pain may precede the development of neurologic signs and symptoms. The presence of jaundice in association with an atypical presentation of back pain may indicate hepatobiliary obstruction and/or liver metastasis. Signs of nerve root compression may be the first indication of a cancer, in particular, lymphoma or multiple myeloma or cancer of the lung, breast, prostate, or kidney. Other neurologic or musculoskeletal manifestations of neoplasm are discussed in Paraneoplastic Syndromes later.

Immobility and inflammation can lead to pain. Inflammation with its accompanying symptoms of redness, edema, pain, heat, and loss of function may progress to infection, necrosis, and sloughing of tissue. If the inflammatory process alone is present, the pain is characterized by tenderness. Pain may be excruciating in the presence of tissue necrosis and sloughing.

## Pain Control

Pain management and control may depend on the underlying etiology. For example, epidural metastases with impending spinal cord compression may require treatment with steroids, radiation, chemotherapy, or neurosurgery. Abdominal pain caused by obstruction of the hollow organs may require surgical intervention. Other modalities, including integrative, psychologic, or rehabilitative strategies may also be considered when available, desired by the patient, and consistent with the goals of care.[314]

Treatment approaches depend on whether the individual is experiencing acute or chronic pain. The hope is to begin by gaining control of the pain during the acute phase and then to sustain that pain relief while minimizing side effects.

Pain should be screened, assessed, and managed according to clinical practice guidelines. Clinical practice guidelines for the treatment of cancer-related pain in adults outlining the process of screening, evaluation, and intervention have been published by the National Comprehensive Cancer Network (NCCN).[278] A similar clinical practice guideline is available from the NCCN for pediatric cancer pain,[279] and another is available for older adult cancer pain.[281]

Before starting therapy, the physician determines the underlying pain mechanism and diagnoses the pain syndrome. Pain control measures used include opioid and nonopioid analgesics; chemotherapy or radiation therapy or both; surgery; nerve blocks; or other, more invasive pain control measures such as intraspinal, rhizotomy, or cordotomy. Drugs such as bisphosphonates have been useful in the treatment of refractory bone pain.[276]

**Opioids.** Appropriate opioid selection may be difficult and depends on the individual's pain intensity and any current analgesic therapy. Morphine, hydromorphone, fentanyl, and oxycodone are commonly used opioids in the United States. A balance between analgesia and side effects might be achieved by changing to an equivalent dose of an alternative opioid. This approach, known as *opioid rotation,* is now a widely accepted technique used to address poorly responsive pain.[278]

Several methods of continuous infusion that are widely used in clinical practice include around the clock, as needed, and patient-controlled analgesia (PCA). Around-the-clock dosing is provided to patients with chronic pain for continuous pain relief. A rescue dose should be provided as a subsequent treatment for individuals receiving these controlled-release medications. Rescue doses of short-acting opioids should be provided for pain that is not relieved by sustained/controlled-release opioids.

Opioids administered on an as-needed basis are for individuals who have intermittent pain with pain-free intervals. The as-needed method is also used when rapid dose escalation is required.

The PCA technique allows a person to control a device that delivers a bolus of analgesic on demand (according to and limited by parameters set by a physician). This system permits the person to self-administer a premeasured dose of analgesic by pressing a button that activates a pump syringe containing the analgesic. Small intermittent doses of the analgesic administered via intravenous line maintain blood levels that ensure comfort and minimize the risk of oversedation. Clinical studies report that people using PCA effectively maintain comfort without oversedation and use less drug than the amount normally given by intramuscular injection.

**Nonpharmacologics.** Nonpharmacologic modalities such as massage, simple touch, acupuncture, imagery/hypnosis, reflexology, relaxation training, and other forms of complementary therapies, are recognized as part of integrative oncology used to manage procedural pain and distress and improve mood even among children, especially when fear, anxiety, and tension heighten pain perception.

Whereas severe cancer pain is treated pharmaceutically, mild-to-moderate joint and muscle pain can be addressed by the rehabilitation professional. Pain elimination through the use of medication may not be possible without accompanying severe loss of function, which is an undesirable outcome.

**Massage.** Massage therapy is increasingly used for pain and symptom relief in individuals with cancer,[222] though there is some debate about its safety in individuals with lymphedema or who are at risk for developing lymphedema.[330] A review of data included in the *Cochrane Database of Systematic Reviews* suggests that conventional care for people with cancer can safely incorporate massage therapy, although individuals with cancer may be at higher risk for adverse events. There is no evidence that massage therapy can spread cancer, although direct pressure over a tumor is usually discouraged.

The strongest evidence for the benefits of massage is reduction of stress and anxiety. Research regarding the use of massage for pain control and management of other symptoms is promising. Massage therapists may advocate the use of massage to reduce constipation, improve immune system function, help promote postoperative wound healing, and reduce scar tissue formation, as well as to help release metabolic waste by improving circulation. Published trials for these indications have not been widely reported.[47,350]

Modifications to massage (e.g., lighten pressure or avoid deep tissue massage) may be necessary to prevent potential harm, such as bleeding, fracture, or increased pain, when individuals with cancer receiving massage have a coagulation disorder (low platelet count or when receiving warfarin/heparin/aspirin therapy). Similar precautions are required for anyone with cancer metastases to the bones. Massage should be avoided over open or healing wounds or radiation dermatitis.[47,350]

### Physical Agents

Evidence from human clinical trials is not available to guide the use of physical agents in patients with cancer. This is largely because, given concerns raised by basic science and animal studies, such trials cannot be conducted ethically. Therefore guidance on the use of physical agents in patients with cancer is based on our current understanding of the likely risks and benefits of such intervention.

Various forms of electric, electromagnetic, and other biophysical energy sources have beneficial physiologic effects on tissue and therefore the potential to relieve some of the symptoms associated with cancer, but these modalities are not expected or intended to treat the cancer. Because physical modalities can alter cell membrane permeability and alter transmembrane potentials, potentially triggering tissue growth and development, there is concern that this could also promote cancer growth and metastasis.

Recommendations regarding the use of ultrasound and transcutaneous electrical stimulation for the treatment of pain associated with cancer and/or with cancer treatment remain equivocal.[171,232] The application of therapeutic ultrasound, particularly continuous ultrasound, or electrical stimulation over tumors is contraindicated because animal studies support that these interventions can accelerate tumor growth and metastasis.[113] Studies in mice and rats have shown that applying continuous ultrasound over a malignant tumor is associated with accelerated tumor growth, metastasis, and recurrence, likely because of increased blood supply to the area.[92,162,224,242,353]

Although in general low-level laser therapy is also not recommended over malignant tumors because animal studies have found that this can increase tumor growth,[234] treatment with a specific low-level laser therapy device with fixed treatment parameters is approved by the Food and Drug Administration (FDA) for the treatment of breast cancer–related lymphedema because of its association with reduced volume and pain in this disorder. Although the mechanisms underlying this effect are uncertain, it is thought that the laser promotes photochemical reactions at the cellular level that increase shoulder motion and scar mobility, while also reducing limb volume of the affected arm, extracellular fluid, and tissue hardness.[a]

**A THERAPIST'S THOUGHTS[a]**

***Modalities for the Patient With Cancer***

Many noninvasive physical agents, including thermotherapy, electrical stimulation, diathermy, lasers and light, and ultrasound are often considered for pain management; however, because all of these agents may increase circulation and promote cell function, growth, and replication, their use in individuals with cancer or a history of cancer is controversial. There are no studies in humans evaluating the effects of these physical agents on tumor growth or metastasis, as given the concern for potential adverse effects, such studies would be hard to conduct from an ethical standpoint. The few studies demonstrating increased rates of tumor growth and metastasis with the application of therapeutic ultrasound in animals support this concern.[353,354]

There is very limited evidence regarding the use of modalities at a site distant from the primary location of the cancer, although the mechanism of action of most physical agents suggests that their use may be safe if the agents are not used over an area where cancer is present. Because of the nature of cancer to metastasize to other areas, the clinician cannot know with certainty where the cancer is or is not. Therefore some clinicians avoid the use of physical agents in any location in patients for 5 years after they are known to have had cancer. Although this approach has appeal because many cancers do not recur beyond 5 years, given the variability in recurrence patterns for different malignancies, it is recommended that the clinician discuss the potential risks and benefits of using a physical agent in anyone with a history of cancer at any time in their life.

One exception commonly made to the contraindication for using physical agents in patients with a history of cancer is during hospice or palliative care where the priority is patient comfort and QOL over survival. In such circumstances, physical agents may provide pain relief with fewer and less severe side effects than medications and are sometimes used in place of, to supplement, or to allow lower doses of analgesic medications. One of the challenges in the use of physical agents in patients with cancer is that the level of risk or harm is really unknown—does the potential harm outweigh whatever immediate benefits the patient might get from use of the physical agent? It behooves the physical therapist to engage in open dialogue with patients to inform them about physical agents as a potential treatment modality for cancer-related symptoms.

[a]Michelle H. Cameron, MD, PT, OCS

[a]References 5,34,41,42,66,103,126,198,206,217,228,243,297,and 364.

**Neuropathic Pain.** People with cancer may also experience pain because of nerve damage. This damage can be caused directly by tumor invasion or indirectly as a side effect of cytotoxic drug therapy (e.g., taxanes or platinum agents). The treatment of neuropathic pain remains a dilemma because conventional analgesic drugs do not always provide relief.

Recommended treatment for neuropathic pain includes infrared light therapy (Anodyne), antidepressant drugs (e.g., amitriptyline), antiepileptics (e.g., carbamazepine and gabapentin), and steroids (e.g., methylprednisolone and dexamethasone). Pain relief is usually not immediate, and the drugs must be taken continuously; thus side effects such as sedation and bone marrow depression can be additional problems.[101,276] Many people seek alternative therapies such as Reiki, acupuncture, BodyTalk, touch therapy, and craniosacral therapy for relief from neuropathies.

Management of pain in people with cancer who live in long-term care facilities remains an ongoing concern. Consistent, daily pain is prevalent among nursing home residents with cancer and is frequently untreated or undertreated, particularly among older and minority clients.[193] For individuals with difficult-to-control chronic pain, complementary therapies can help even if it is only to reduce the level of analgesics required to maintain pain control.

## Cancer-Related Fatigue

Much has been written about cancer-related fatigue (CRF) and its impact on clients. CRF is a distressing, persistent, and subjective sense of tiredness or exhaustion related to cancer or cancer treatment that is not proportional to recent activity and interferes with usual functioning.[280] CRF syndrome is a collection of symptoms with multiple characteristics and problems. Fatigue is a nearly universal symptom in all people receiving chemotherapy, radiotherapy, and treatment with biologic response modifiers; reduced physical performance and fatigue are universal after stem cell/bone marrow transplantation.

Up to 30% of cancer survivors report a loss of energy for years after cessation of treatment. For many people with cancer, fatigue is severe and imposes limitations on normal daily activities.[165] Many people's perceptions are that fatigue is more distressing than pain or nausea and vomiting, which can be managed with medication for most clients.

Fatigue should be screened for, assessed, and managed according to clinical practice guidelines that have been published for CRF.[280] All individuals should be screened for fatigue at their initial visit, at regular intervals during and after cancer treatment, and as clinically indicated. Fatigue should be recognized, evaluated, monitored, documented, and treated promptly for all age groups at all stages of disease during and after treatment. Clients and their families should be informed that management of fatigue is an integral part of survivorship.[280]

Using a numeric rating scale, fatigue can be rated as mild (1–3), moderate (4–6), or severe (7–10).[254,395] Children can be asked whether they are "tired" or "not tired." Fatigue that causes distress or interferes with daily activities or functioning should be treated according to its severity and the presence of other treatable factors known to contribute to fatigue (e.g., pain, emotional distress, sleep disturbance, anemia, nutritional deficits, deconditioning, and comorbidities).

Clients should be reassured that treatment-related fatigue is not necessarily an indicator of disease progression. It may be the result of anemia, deconditioning, or the presence of certain cytokines (e.g., IL-1, IL-6, or TNF-α). There may be contributing psychosocial factors such as anxiety, depression, and disrupted sleep pattern.

Despite the prevalence of CRF, the exact mechanisms involved in its pathophysiology are unknown. Abnormal accumulation of muscle metabolites, production of cytokines, changes in neuromuscular function, abnormalities in adenosine triphosphate synthesis, serotonin dysregulation, and vagal afferent activation are just a few of the proposed theories. Comorbidities such as cardiopulmonary impairments may put an individual at greater risk for fatigue.[280]

Likewise, the cause of fatigue in individuals who are disease-free after treatment is unclear and likely multifactorial. Higher serum markers such as IL-1 receptor antagonist and soluble TNF receptor type II and lower cortisol levels have been observed in fatigued cancer survivors compared with nonfatigued survivors. Significantly higher levels of circulating T lymphocytes have also been observed in fatigued survivors. These findings together point to a chronic inflammatory process involving T cells as a possible fatigue-inducing mechanism.[280]

Additional clinical practice recommendations published by the NCCN on adolescent, young adult, and senior adult oncology care are available from the NCCN website.[281,282]

## Paraneoplastic Syndromes

### Overview and Definition

In addition to the local effects of tumor growth, cancer can produce systemic signs and symptoms that are not direct effects of either the tumor or its metastases. When tumors produce signs and symptoms at a site distant from the tumor or its metastasized sites, these remote effects of malignancy are collectively referred to as *paraneoplastic syndromes*.

Although malignant cells frequently lose the function, appearance, and properties associated with normal cells of the tissue of origin, they can acquire in some cases new cellular functions uncharacteristic of the originating tissue. Many of these syndromes involve ectopic hormone production by tumor cells or the secretion of biochemically active substances that cause metabolic abnormalities. For example, tumors in nonendocrine tissues sometimes acquire the ability to produce and secrete hormones that are distributed by the circulation and act on target organs at a site other than the location of the tumor. The most common hormone-secreting tumor associated with paraneoplastic syndromes is small cell cancer of the lung, which can produce adrenocorticotropic hormone in amounts sufficient to cause Cushing syndrome.

Malignancy is often associated with a wide variety of musculoskeletal disorders, which may be the presenting symptoms of an occult tumor. Although musculoskeletal symptoms often result from direct invasion by the malignancy or its metastases into bone, joints, or soft tissue, they may also occur without invasion as a result of the paraneoplastic disorders, including well-recognized syndromes as well as less well-defined disorders referred to as *cancer arthritis*.[368,426]

### Incidence

Previously, paraneoplastic syndromes occurred in about 10% to 20% of all clients with cancer, but this figure may be increasing because of greater physician awareness and the availability of serodiagnostic tests for some syndromes. Neurologic paraneoplastic syndromes are rare, occurring in 1% to 2% of people with malignancy, but physical therapists are often treating these individuals because of the neuromuscular and musculoskeletal manifestations.

### Etiology and Pathogenesis

The causes of paraneoplastic syndromes are not well understood, but the following four groups of mechanisms and their effects have been identified:

- A variety of vasoactive tumor products (e.g., serotonin, histamine, catecholamines, prostaglandins, and vasoactive peptides), which usually occur in the small bowel and less commonly in the lung or stomach
- The destruction of normal tissues by tumor such as occurs when osteolytic skeletal metastases cause hypercalcemia
- Unknown mechanisms such as unidentified tumor products or circulating immune complexes stimulated by the tumor (e.g., osteoarthropathy as a result of bronchogenic carcinoma)
- Autoantibodies (antibodies directed against the host's tissue); for example, cancer cells produce antibodies that impair presynaptic calcium channel activity, hindering the release of the neurotransmitter acetylcholine, resulting in muscle weakness

There is increasing evidence that many neurologic paraneoplastic syndromes appear to be an immune reaction against antigens shared by the cancer and the nervous system. The immune response is triggered by and directed against the tumor, which then cross-reacts with protein expressed by the peripheral nervous system or CNS. Consequently, any part of the nervous system can be affected.[50,233,192]

### Clinical Manifestations

Paraneoplastic syndromes are of considerable clinical importance because they may accompany relatively limited neoplastic growth and provide an early clue to the presence of certain types of cancer. Nonspecific symptoms such as skin changes, neurologic changes, anorexia, malaise, diarrhea, weight loss, and fever may be the first clinical manifestations of a paraneoplastic syndrome. Even these types of nonspecific symptoms occur as a result of the production of specific biochemical products by the tumor itself.

Paraneoplastic syndromes with musculoskeletal manifestations are listed in Table 9.6. Gradual, progressive muscle weakness may develop over a period of weeks to months. The proximal muscles (especially of the pelvic girdle) are most likely to be involved; the weakness does

**Table 9.6** Paraneoplastic Syndromes: Rheumatologic Associations and Clinical Features

| Malignancy | Rheumatologic Associations | Clinical Features |
|---|---|---|
| Lung cancer, particularly small cell lung cancer | Lambert-Eaton myasthenic syndrome | Proximal leg weakness |
| Lymphoproliferative disease (leukemia) | Vasculitis | Necrotizing vasculitis |
| Plasma cell dyscrasia | Cryoglobulinemia | Vasculitis, Raynaud disease, arthralgia, neurologic symptoms |
| Hodgkin disease | Immune complex disease | Nephrotic syndrome |
| Ovarian cancer | Complex regional pain syndrome | Palmar fasciitis and polyarthritis |
| Carcinoid syndrome | Scleroderma | Scleroderma-like changes: anterior tibia |
| Colon cancer | Pyogenic arthritis | Enteric bacteria cultured from joint |
| Mesenchymal tumors | Osteogenic osteomalacia | Bone pain, stress fractures |
| Renal cell cancer | Severe Raynaud phenomenon | Digital necrosis (and other tumors) |
| Pancreatic cancer | Panniculitis | Subcutaneous nodules, especially males |

stabilize. Reflexes of the involved extremities are present but diminished. Proximal leg weakness seen in Lambert-Eaton myasthenic syndrome is most often associated with small cell carcinoma of the lung. Diagnosis is made by needle electromyography and has a characteristic "dive bomber" sound on insertion of the needle into a muscle. Additional blood studies assist in further diagnosis and differentiation from myasthenia gravis, a related disorder.

Muscular, neurologic, and cutaneous disorders associated with malignancy are presented in Table 9.7. Many of these conditions can occur in association with or in the absence of underlying malignant disease. The appearance of any of these conditions requires a full medical evaluation but does not guarantee that a tumor will be found. Early tumor recognition, before metastasis occurs, may improve survival rates. Myositis may precede, follow, or arise concurrently with the malignancy and tends to occur most often in older people. Paraneoplastic dermatoses are a large group of paraneoplastic syndromes that may be associated with an internal malignancy.[356]

**Carcinoma Polyarthritis.** There may be rheumatologic symptoms referred to as *carcinoma polyarthritis*. This condition can be differentiated from rheumatoid arthritis by the presence of asymmetric joint involvement, involvement of primarily the lower extremity

**Table 9.7** Muscular, Neurologic, and Cutaneous Disorders Associated With Malignancy

| Muscular/Neurologic | Cutaneous |
|---|---|
| Amyloidosis | Acanthosis (diffuse thickening) |
| Amyotrophic lateral sclerosis | Dermatomyositis |
| Polymyositis | Extramammary Paget disease |
| Lambert-Eaton myasthenic syndrome | Nigricans (blackish discoloration; changes in skin pigmentation |
| Myasthenia gravis | Pemphigus vulgaris (water blisters) |
| Metabolic myopathies | Pruritus (itching) |
| Primary neuropathic diseases | Pyoderma gangrenosum (eruption of skin ulcers) |
| Type II muscle atrophy | Reactive erythemas (skin redness) |

Data from Hashefi M: Rheumatologic manifestations of malignancy. *Clin Geriatr Med* 33:73–86, 2017; Gilkeson GS, Caldwell DS: Rheumatologic associations with malignancy. *J Musculoskelet Med* 7:70, 1990; and Cohen PR: Cutaneous paraneoplastic syndromes. *Am Fam Physician* 50:1273–1282, 1994.

(although symmetric involvement of the hands has been reported),[370,426] explosive onset, older age at onset, and the presence of malignancy and arthritis together. Neurologic paraneoplastic syndromes are of unknown cause and include subacute cerebellar degeneration, amyotrophic lateral sclerosis, sensory or sensorimotor peripheral neuropathy, Guillain-Barré syndrome, myasthenia gravis, and Lambert-Eaton myasthenic syndrome.

**Stiff-Person Syndrome.** Isolated cases of paraneoplastic stiff-person syndrome have been reported in association with small cell lung cancer, colon cancer, thymoma (thymus), melanoma, breast adenocarcinoma, and graft-versus-host disease.[28,183,287,311,363] Women are affected twice as often as men, most likely because of the association with breast cancer. Paraneoplastic stiff-person syndrome is characterized by progressive symptoms of neuropathy or myelopathy with increased muscle tone and rigidity in the spine and lower extremities, especially the ankle dorsiflexors with loss of ankle motion.[40,155]

The disease may take years to manifest, but in some individuals, symptoms develop over a period of weeks. The first symptom may be a persistent progressive stiffening of the back or leg that is triggered by sudden noise, touch, or fatigue or made worse by stress such as time pressure (e.g., hurrying to cross a street). Stiffness progresses to hypertonia and spasm and then severe, painful rigidity, postural abnormalities, and musculoskeletal deformities. Walking becomes difficult, and the individual is at increased risk for unprotected falls (i.e., they fall like a tin soldier). Symptoms are greatly relieved during sleep.

Although rare, this condition has been encountered by therapists in an oncology practice.[154] Stiff-person syndrome is normally associated with a viral cause such as meningitis or encephalitis, but in the case of cancer-induced stiff-person syndrome, it is chemically induced by the tumor, classifying it as a paraneoplastic syndrome.[185] It is seen more often in clients with a history of diabetes and other autoimmune diseases (e.g., hyperthyroidism, hypothyroidism, or anemia).[40]

Diagnosis of stiff-person syndrome is made by physical examination and immunocytochemistry methods demonstrating the presence of anti–glutamic acid decarboxylase autoantibodies in the blood. Diagnosis may be confirmed by a positive response to medications used to treat this condition (e.g., benzodiazepines).

Physical therapy may have a role in the management of this disease,[154,191,315] as these patients/clients need to be taught how to properly stretch and maintain joint mobility as a lifelong commitment. Physical therapy interventions may include ultrasound, soft tissue mobilizations, manual stretching, and exercise. The therapist may need to assess for home adaptations, orthoses, and the need for durable medical equipment.[154]

#### MEDICAL MANAGEMENT

**DIAGNOSIS, TREATMENT, AND PROGNOSIS.** Serodiagnostic tests are available for some paraneoplastic syndromes, and characteristic abnormalities on MRI have been identified in association with neurologic paraneoplastic syndromes. Biochemical markers in urine provide specific monitoring of the response of bone metastases to treatment. This early diagnosis of paraneoplastic syndromes provides for prevention of tumor progression and subsequent problems, such as bone pain, fracture, and hypercalcemia. In the case of cancer polyarthritis, the absence of rheumatoid nodules, absence of rheumatoid factor, and absence of family history of rheumatoid disease help in the diagnostic process.

Paraneoplastic syndromes usually parallel the course of the disease. Treatment of the tumor leads to regression of the syndrome (especially the cutaneous dermatoses). In some cases the condition is related more to the amount of antibody present rather than the amount of tumor volume. Some cutaneous paraneoplastic syndromes will respond to specific measures, such as systemic corticosteroid therapy, but for the most part successful resolution requires eradication of the underlying malignancy.

## MEDICAL MANAGEMENT OF CANCER

### Prevention and Survivorship

The goal of *Healthy People 2020* is to reduce the number of new cancer cases, as well as illness, disability, and death caused by cancer.[380] There are 20 specific objectives listed under cancer in the *Healthy People 2020* summary of objectives. Two objectives specifically target survivorship and QOL:

- C-13: Increase the proportion of cancer survivors who are living years or longer after diagnosis
  Target: 71.7%; baseline: 65.2% of persons with cancer were living 5 years or longer after diagnosis in 2007.
- C-14 (Developmental): Increase mental and physical health-related QOL of cancer survivors.

Evidence suggests that several types of cancer can be prevented and that the prospects for surviving cancer continue to improve. The ACS estimates that one-half of all cancer deaths in the United States could be prevented if Americans adopted a healthier lifestyle and made better use of available screening tests.[312]

The ability to reduce cancer death rates depends in part on the existence and application of various types of resources. *First,* the means to provide culturally and linguistically appropriate information on prevention, early detection, and treatment to the public and to health care professionals are essential. *Second,* mechanisms or systems must exist for providing people with access to state-of-the-art preventive services and treatment. *Third,* a mechanism for maintaining continued research progress and for fostering new research is essential. Personalized prevention may become a tool in the future thanks to desktop oncology in the postgenome era of research.

*Desktop oncology* refers to the genomics data produced by high technology. Desktop oncology provides knowledge on demand to anyone regarding cancer-related biomarkers. Combining genetic screening for cancer predisposition in the general population and selecting individualized targeted chemoprevention may dramatically improve cancer rates in the future.[195,379]

#### Primary Prevention

Prevention is the first key to the *management* of cancer. Epigenetics may be the first step in the *prevention* of cancer. Primary prevention may include *screening* to identify high-risk people and subsequent reduction or elimination of modifiable risk factors (e.g., tobacco use, diet high in unsaturated fats and low in fiber, and sun or radiation exposure). Physical activity and weight control also can contribute to cancer prevention.

*Epigenetics* is a relatively new science that has brought to light the control we have as individuals on whether or not cancer develops in our bodies. Epigenetics is the study of long-lasting changes in gene *function or expression* that do not necessarily involve changes in gene *structure*. Scientists are beginning to understand through the study of epigenetics how nutrients and certain drugs can change the way cells age, reproduce, and ultimately die. Epigenetics addresses ways we can block the formation and progression of cancer cells through nutrigenomics and chemoprevention.

**Nutrigenomics.** Nutrigenomics is a relatively new field seeking to identify ways to prevent cancer through the impact of nutrition on gene structure and stability. Research is focusing on the impact of food, nutrition, obesity, and physical activity on the cancer process as the genetic message in the DNA code is translated into RNA and then into protein synthesis, leading to metabolic processes.[230,385] Gene sequencing and function, as well as changes in DNA sequence and modulation of oxidative stress in response to foods and beverages, are an area of current and future research focus in nutrigenomics.

Studying older adults who do not develop cancer may help identify the genetic changes associated with age-resistant protective mechanisms. Genetic information that can be used to improve disease prevention strategies is emerging for many cancers and may provide the foundation for improved effectiveness in clinical and preventive medicine services.

Even though we know that healthy everyday choices can reduce our chances of getting cancer, it is recognized that in the current American cultural environment, it is difficult for many people to make healthy choices. Far too often the unhealthy choice is the choice that is more convenient, more affordable, or more socially accepted. For readers who are interested in more information in this area, the *Policy and Action for Cancer Prevention* examines the factors—economic, environmental, and social—that influence what we eat and how much we move. The results of studies that have been designed to change our behaviors and thus our risk of cancer are available.[414]

**Chemoprevention.** Chemoprevention, the use of agents to inhibit and reverse cancer, has focused on diet-derived agents. Chemoprevention is effective in inhibiting the onset of cancer by eliminating premalignant cells and blocking the progression of normal cells into invasive tumors in experimental animal models. The transferability of similar results to humans remains under investigation.[184,249]

More than 40 promising agents and agent combinations (e.g., green and black tea phenols, lycopene, soy isoflavones, vitamins D and E, selenium, and calcium) are being evaluated clinically as chemopreventive agents for major cancer targets, including breast, prostate, colon, and lung cancer.[22,200,220] In addition, low-dose aspirin intake and nonsteroidal antiinflammatory drug intake have shown promising results in the prevention of gastrointestinal, endometrial, pancreatic, and other cancers. Chemoprevention is intended to stop a cancer before it ever reaches a size that could alter the body's homeostasis, cause symptoms, or be detected.

**Cancer Vaccine.** See previous discussion of cancer vaccines in Pathogenesis. Two types of *cancer vaccine* (prophylactic and therapeutic) are being investigated in clinical studies, although currently no known specific immunization prevents cancer in general. Currently, there are two vaccines against infectious agents being used in clinical practice for the prevention of cancer: the vaccine against HBV and the vaccine against HPV.[37] With therapeutic vaccines, the person's own tumor cells are obtained during surgery, irradiated to inactivate them, and then reinfused. This stimulates the immune system to react and make antibodies against these specific cells. The vaccine specifically evokes the activity of immune-surveillance cells to find the specified cancer cells and send killer T cells to directly target and destroy tumors in all vaccine recipients. Immunologic memory can be created so that if the cancer recurs, the immune system will respond before it becomes widespread.[143,411] A vaccine given on an outpatient basis would be less dangerous than surgery and less toxic than other cancer treatments such as chemotherapy and radiation therapy. Right now, efforts to develop such vaccines have been hampered by the fact that cancer cells seem to have the ability to evade immune-surveillance cells (see Tumor Evasion Strategies).

### Secondary Prevention

Secondary prevention aimed at preventing morbidity and mortality uses screening, early detection,[203] and prompt treatment. The ACS recommendations for early detection of cancer in average-risk, asymptomatic individuals, including cancer site (breast, cervix, colorectal, endometrial, prostate), population to be screened, recommended test or procedure, and frequency of testing are available online at https://onlinelibrary.wiley.com/doi/full/10.3322/caac.21446.[362] Some drugs, such as tamoxifen (Nolvadex, Soltamox), are used in both primary and secondary prevention of breast cancer. Tamoxifen has been approved by the FDA as a preventive agent in women who have a high risk for possible development of breast cancer.[96] Results of the large International Breast Cancer Intervention Study (IBIS) trials showed that women treated with 5 years of tamoxifen had a 29% reduction in the risk of developing any type of breast cancer compared with placebo-treated control subjects. Tamoxifen also had a protective effect several years after cessation of treatment.[84]

Multifactor risk reduction is an important part of secondary prevention for people with cancer at risk for recurrence. This is especially true because the adverse effect of several risk factors is cumulative, and many risk factors are interrelated.

#### A THERAPIST'S THOUGHTS[a]

***Screening Recommendations***

Recommendations for screening, including who to screen, when to screen, and frequency of screening, are published by different organizations and are not always consistent from group to group. Groups engaged in education, research, and recommendations include the U.S. Preventive Services Task Force (USPSTF), ACS, NCI, American Society of Clinical Oncology, NCCN, and IARC. Reports by various consumer and professional organizations advising changes to cancer screening frequency and importance have been controversially received among professional provider groups.

The USPSTF, although sponsored by the federal government, serves as an independent advisory group and submits reports with recommendations based on literature and evidence reviewed. The reports and guidelines can be accessed at https://www.uspreventiveservicestaskforce.org/Page/Name/recommendations. These recommendations are not considered official statements or positions of the U.S. Public Health Service or the U.S. Department of Health and Human Services. The Agency for Healthcare Research and Quality also publishes evidence-based reports that can be found at https://www.ahrq.gov/professionals/clinicians-providers/guidelines-recommendations/index.html.

The ACS recently published a review of current guidelines and issues in cancer screening.[364] This comprehensive document provides a history of past updates; recommendations for early detection by site, population test, and frequency; and reviews of prevalence of cancer screening in the United States by test, race, health insurance, and educational level.

In past editions of this text, we have tried to provide the therapist with a summary of the most current and appropriate screening guidelines. However, with recent changes and variations in guidelines, it seems more prudent to provide you, the reader, with information that will allow you to stay as current as possible with each individual type of cancer. In this way, you can adopt whatever screening or intervention is appropriate for your personal and/or practice situation.

Keep in mind that political and economic influences on health care policy provided by organizations such as the U.S. Department of Human Health Services and the Centers for Medicare and Medicaid Services affecting third-party payers will influence coverage for various screenings and treatments. Ultimately, these forces may direct clinical practice rather than evidence-based findings.

[a]Charles L. McGarvey, PT, MS, DPT, FAPTA

### Tertiary Prevention

Tertiary prevention focuses on managing symptoms, limiting complications, and preventing disability associated with cancer or its treatment.

## Diagnosis

Medical history and physical examination are usually followed by more specific diagnostic procedures. Useful tests for early detection and staging of tumors include laboratory values, radiography, endoscopy, isotope scan, CT scan, mammography, MRI, and biopsy. Advances in nuclear medicine have made it possible to examine images of organs, structures, and physiologic or pathologic processes and detect the distribution of radiopharmaceuticals according to their uptake and metabolism.

### Tissue Biopsy

Biopsy of tissue samples is an important diagnostic tool in the study of tumors. Tissue for biopsy may be taken by curettage (Papanicolaou [Pap] smear), fluid aspiration (pleural effusion, lumbar puncture, or spinal tap), fine-needle aspiration (breast or thyroid), dermal punch (skin or mouth), endoscopy (rectal polyps), or open surgical excision (visceral tumors and nodes).

An incisional biopsy or *open biopsy* consists of making an incision and removing a portion of the abnormal tissue. An incisional biopsy takes a slice or wedge of the lesion but does not attempt to remove the entire pathologic structure. The amount removed depends on the abnormality, but it is usually a piece of tissue about 1 inch in diameter.

An excisional biopsy (sometimes referred to as lumpectomy) consists of making an incision to excise all gross, abnormal tissue that is either visually apparent or identified using a needle placed to localize the lesion. Needle localization employs either ultrasound or MRI to accurately place a thin wire as a marker for the surgeon to locate and excise the specimen. The size of the specimen removed depends on the abnormality and the judgment of the surgeon to ensure a negative or clean margin as assessed under the microscope by a pathologist. If the specimen contains tumor cells within the margin, a reexcision by the surgeon is usually performed to obtain a negative margin before proceeding with other adjuvant therapies.

*Core needle biopsy* (sometimes referred to as Tru-Cut needle biopsy) uses a large-diameter needle to take a core or plug of tissue. Core needle biopsies can be accomplished directly by employing a manual approach to remove a single or multiple specimens from the organ. For example, the surgeon uses ultrasound or fluoroscopy in conducting a biopsy of the prostate gland for diagnosis and staging. Multiple samples of a specimen can also be removed indirectly by using computers and automation such as in the case of stereotactic biopsy of the breast.

*Stereotactic (mammotome) biopsy* of the breast uses digital x-rays of the breast taken from two angles to locate the abnormality seen on the mammogram. A computer then calculates the proper angle and depth of insertion of a core biopsy needle. This needle is inserted into the breast, using local anesthesia, and multiple (a dozen or more) core specimens are removed. Each core is about 2 mm by 15 mm long. These cores are then sent to the pathologist for diagnosis. As described previously, a second type of stereotactic procedure places a wire into the exact location of an abnormality within the breast. Ultrasound or mammography is used to find the lesion. The surgeon uses the wire to relocate the abnormality within the breast during an open biopsy. The procedure for placing the wire is the same as for taking a core biopsy, but a thin needle is used instead of a core biopsy needle. Once the needle is in place, a thin wire is inserted through the needle, and the needle is removed.

*Sentinel lymph node (SLN) biopsy* has become a standard diagnostic procedure to assess lymph node status of various tumors (e.g., breast, melanoma, endometrial, valvular, or head and neck) and to assess staging. A blue dye is injected around the cancerous tumor (or the biopsy site if the tumor has been removed). The dye flows through the ducts, and the first nodes it reaches are identified as the SLNs. An incision is made over the nodes, and the blue-stained SLNs (usually one to three in number) are removed and analyzed. The removal of more than three SLNs is considered to be a lower-level axillary dissection. Complications of SLN biopsy include allergic reaction to the blue dye (<1%), pneumothorax from unintended opening of the parietal pleura, sensory or motor nerve injury (small risk), lymphedema, surgical site infections (<1%), and seromas (10%).[153,403]

Information on the lymphatic drainage from the cancer can have a direct impact on surgery. SLN biopsy has reduced the number of unnecessary axillary dissections in breast cancer. The status of axillary nodes is the most important prognostic factor in breast cancer and in determining medical management. Studies comparing patients with SLN metastasis of breast cancer showed that the use of SLN biopsy alone compared with axillary lymph node dissection did not result in poorer survival for patients who underwent SLN biopsy alone.[131,421]

### Biologic Tumor Markers

Tumor markers, substances produced and secreted by tumor cells, may be found in the blood serum. The level of tumor marker seems to correlate with the extent of disease. A tumor marker is not diagnostic itself but can signal malignancies. CEA is one tumor marker that may indicate malignancy of the large bowel, stomach, pancreas, lungs, and breasts. CEA and other serum titers, such as CA-125 (ovarian), CA-27-29 (breast), and PSA, may be valuable during therapeutic intervention (adjuvant therapy) to evaluate the extent of response and detect tumor recurrence.

Other tumor markers found in the blood (no more specific than CEA) include alpha-fetoprotein, a fetal antigen uncommon in adults and suggestive of testicular cancer. $\beta_2$-microglobulin is used in the monitoring of lymphomas, and lactic dehydrogenase is particularly elevated in fast-growing malignancies. Human chorionic gonadotropin ($\beta$ subunit) may indicate testicular cancer or choriocarcinoma. PSA helps evaluate prostatic cancer. Because of the lack of specificity of the markers individually (except PSA), test panels are used more frequently rather than just individual tumor marker evaluations.[267,306]

Several research institutes have developed an mAb that identifies breast cancer and other cancer cells. The mAb is used to devise a simple blood test for use in diagnosis and monitoring treatment of breast and ovarian cancer and, more recently, colon cancer. Combining the breast cancer antibody with nuclear medicine scanning techniques will provide a noninvasive means of determining lymphatic spread and guide surgeons in determining the extent of surgery required.[25,424]

### Molecular Profiling

Molecular profiling using specific cancer biomarkers provides additional information for the oncologist in determining aggressiveness of the tumor, potential response to treatment, and prediction of risk for cancer diagnosis with a family. Such tests are classified as follows:

- Immunohistochemistry, which identifies the presence of specific proteins at the cellular level.
- Gene expression by microarray provides an illustration of the signal status of particular genes. These tests can predict fairly accurately what certain tumors may respond to certain interventions, such as chemotherapy. Research has shown that tumors, similar to any other living tissue, contain genetic information that can be read with increasing accuracy. The goal is to analyze the genetic makeup of the tumor and then choose the specific treatment most likely to be effective given that gene profile, while avoiding exposing the person to toxic therapies that might not be helpful or necessary. Two gene-profiling tests—Oncotype DX (21 genes) and Mammaprint (70 genes)—are currently available for breast cancer; others are being evaluated or developed for non-Hodgkin lymphoma, head and neck cancer, prostate cancer, kidney cancer, melanoma, and ovarian cancer. The FDA has approved FoundationOne CDx (324 genes), a genomic profiling test, to identify genetic alterations that may also aid in the selection of appropriate targeted therapies for specific cancers.[275]
- Fluorescence in situ hybridization is a technique used by pathologists to identify genes with multiple copies or arrangements.
- DNA sequencing via polymerase chain reaction is able to identify mutation in selected genes.

## Primary Antineoplastic Treatment Modalities

Changes in the health care system have shifted much of cancer care to the ambulatory and home settings. The medical management of cancer may be curative (i.e., with the intent to cure) or palliative (i.e., provides symptomatic relief but does not cure). Major therapies of curative cancer treatment at this time include surgery, radiation, chemotherapy, immunotherapy (or molecularly based therapy), antiangiogenesis therapy, and hormonal therapy.

Historically the sequence of treatment of solid tumors would begin with surgery to remove the primary tumor burden, followed by adjuvant therapies (chemotherapy and radiation therapy) to obtain local regional or systemic control and possibly finally long-term (5 years or greater) hormonal treatment. However, studies have indicated excellent results of neoadjuvant (before definitive surgical intervention) treatment with chemotherapy or radiotherapy to shrink the primary tumor or provide local or systemic control. As such, the decision to initiate neoadjuvant versus adjuvant therapies is based on the size, extent of involved tissue, and often the stage or grade of the tumor as assessed by multiple professionals and discussed at the cancer staging conference.

Following such analysis by the oncologists, a balanced discussion of the findings and recommendation of the group is conducted with the patient/family, and a mutually agreeable plan of care intended to result in ablation of primary disease and the highest-level control for future recurrence or metastasis is instituted. The desired outcome of such antineoplastic treatment is complete remission of disease.

Effective cancer treatment requires an understanding of the biology of metastasis and how tumor cells interact with the microenvironment of different organs to design effective therapies.[214] Each of the curative therapies described here may be used alone or in combination, depending on the type, stage, localization, and responsiveness of the tumor and on limitations imposed by the person's clinical status.

The administration of repeated or cyclic chemotherapy and/or radiation is designed to interrupt cell proliferation (the cell growth cycle) (see Fig. 9.3). Significant advances in altering the molecular biology and cellular signaling mechanisms that trigger or foster carcinogenesis are now being translated into treatment that will target cancer cells without affecting normal, healthy cells. With improved cancer targets, it may be possible to end the repeated doses of chemotherapeutic agents.[74,163,174,271,286]

### Cell Proliferation

One round of cell division requires duplication of DNA during the S phase and proper segregation of duplicated chromosomes during mitosis (M phase) (Fig. 9.4). $G_0$ cells are the resting cells, temporarily out of the proliferative cycle; when stimulated by growth factors and/or hormones, these cells move into the $G_1$ phase and begin to multiply. $G_1$ is a postmitotic period of growth and preparation of the chromosomes for replication. This is a checkpoint to stop the cell cycle if the DNA is damaged. In this phase the cell can either repair the DNA or undergo apoptosis. DNA repair is aided by retinoids/vitamin A, vitamin D, folate, coenzyme Q10, and selenium. The S phase represents the synthesis of DNA.

$G_2$ is the premitotic period and the last step in the mitotic cycle followed by mitosis (M), when cell division takes place. $G_2$ is another checkpoint when the cell cycle can be stopped if DNA is damaged or unreplicated, in which case repair or apoptosis occurs. During the M phase, there is a check to ensure each daughter cell gets the correct DNA. The end result of one full cycle is the formation of two identical ($G_0$) daughter cells. Most organ cells that are hormonally linked take approximately 19 to 33 days to complete one full cycle. Chemotherapy eliminates up to 95% of cancerous cells in the body; this is called the kill rate. Not all cancer cells will be eradicated; the immune system may be able to eliminate the remaining cells, but not always.

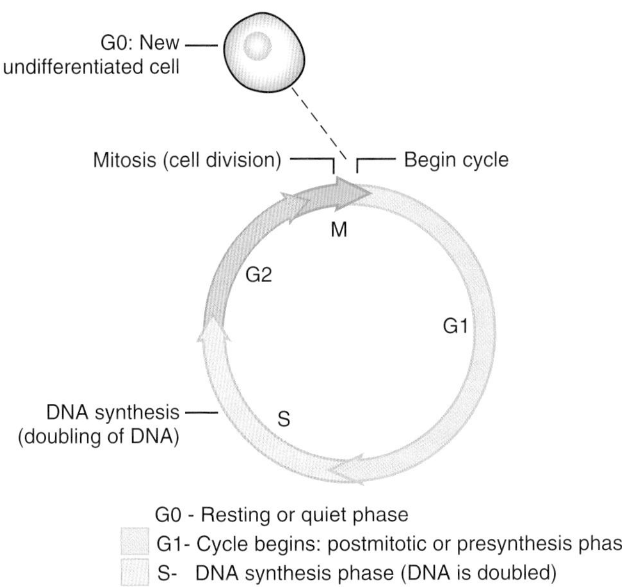


**Figure 9.4**

**Cell cycle.** $G_0$ phase represents the resting phase of cell proliferation. $G_1$ phase is the growth and preparation of the chromosomes for replication. S phase is the synthesis of DNA. $G_2$ phase is the preparation of the cell for division. Finally, *M* phase represents mitosis (cell division). The final result of the cell cycle is the production of two identical daughter cells. (See text for complete description of the cell cycle in relation to chemotherapy and radiation therapy.) (Modified from Niederhuber J, Armitage J, Doroshow J, et al: *Abeloff's clinical oncology*, ed 5, Philadelphia, 2013, Saunders.)

Adjuvant treatment, such as chemotherapy and radiation therapy, is administered in repeated doses over time in an attempt to kill cells in the most susceptible phases. For example, chemotherapy is most effective during DNA synthesis and mitosis. Cells are most sensitive to radiation therapy in the $G_2$ phase. A certain percentage of cells will be unaffected because they are in the $G_0$ or resting phase. Cells in the $G_0$ phase are undifferentiated or stem (mesenchymal) cells waiting until called on by the body to serve a particular (differentiated) need. Stem cells in the $G_0$ phase are resistant to chemotherapy and radiation therapy, and they may be the reason chemotherapy and radiation therapies are not 100% effective modalities in the ablation of microcirculation of tumor cells. The repeated or cyclic treatment is designed to catch $G_0$ cells later in the growth cycle.

Researchers are looking for ways to selectively target (and kill) cancer stem cells, but because not all cancers (e.g., pancreatic cancer) contain stem cells, there are ongoing attempts to answer the question of whether cancer stem cells are the result of a cancer or the cause of it.[180,313]

## Surgery

Surgery, once a mainstay of cancer treatment, is now used most often in combination with other therapies. Surgery may be used curatively for tumor biopsy and tumor removal or palliatively to relieve pain, correct obstruction, or alleviate pressure. Surgery can be curative in persons with localized cancer, but a large percentage of clients have evidence of micrometastases at the time of diagnosis, requiring surgery in combination with other treatment modalities to achieve better response rates. Adjuvant therapy used after surgery eradicates any residual cells.

Surgical oncologists are beginning to employ new technologies to assist in access to tumors with minimal time and tissue disruption and impact on other normal organs. Such newer methods employ the use of robotics (e.g., da Vinci surgical system), which allow for percutaneous entry into body cavities and removal of primary tumor without open surgical procedures.

## Irradiation Therapy

Irradiation therapy, also known as radiotherapy, plays a vital role in the multimodal treatment of cancer. It is used to destroy the dividing cancer cells by destroying hydrogen bonds between DNA strands within the cancer cells, while damaging resting normal cells as little as possible. Advances in radiotherapy have primarily involved improvements in dose delivery and the use of CyberKnife, a relatively new technology that incorporates robotic and precision mapping and treatment of nonoperable tumors. The focus of future treatment is on combining radiotherapy with targeted therapies such as angiogenesis inhibitors, as well as incorporating more refined imaging modalities to deliver more accurate doses to the tumor while sparing healthy tissues.[33]

Radiation consists of two types: ionizing radiation and particle radiation. Both types have the cellular DNA as their target; however, particle radiation produces less skin damage. The goal is to ablate as many cancer cells as possible while simultaneously sparing surrounding normal tissues. Radiation is given over a period of weeks to capture cells at each stage of the cell cycle. Radiation is particularly effective at the end of the $G_2$ phase (see Fig. 9.4) when the cells are most susceptible to radiation.

Radiation treatment approaches include external-beam radiation and intracavitary and interstitial implants. Radiation may be used preoperatively to shrink a tumor, making it operable, while preventing further spread of the disease during surgery. After the surgical wound heals, postoperative doses prevent residual cancer cells from multiplying or metastasizing.

Radiotherapy may be delivered externally or internally, depending on the type and extent of the tumor, by (1) external beam (teletherapy), (2) sealed source (brachytherapy), and (3) unsealed source (systemic therapy). When the distance between the radiation source and the target is short, the term *brachytherapy* is used. Brachytherapy allows for a rapid falloff in dose away from the target volume. When the radiation source is at a distance from the target, the term *teletherapy* is used. Teletherapy allows for a more uniform dose across the target volume.

X-rays generated by linear accelerators and gamma rays generated by radioactive isotopes (e.g., cobalt-60, radium-226, or cesium-137) are referred to as *sealed source* radiation therapies (or brachytherapy). This form of radiation is used for the treatment of visceral tumors because the rays penetrate to great depths before reaching full intensity and thereby spare the skin from toxic effects.

Modern radiology has advanced to include site-specific techniques that take into account complex tissue contours and irregular shapes, visceral movement, digestion, and the effect of respiration on the lungs when the lungs are the target organ.

A newer delivery procedure known as intensity-modulated radiation therapy (IMRT) allows for very precise delivery of radiation dose with less exposure to surrounding normal tissue. Interventional radiology comprises newer technologies, including brachytherapy, accelerated partial breast irradiation, radiofrequency ablation, and radiopharmaceutical therapy.

Radiofrequency ablation and stereotactic body radiotherapy (also known as stereotactic ablative radiation therapy) represent two forms of thermal ablation. IMRT allows for sculpting the radiation field and dose to match the area being irradiated. Computer optimization techniques help determine the distribution of beam intensities across a treatment volume. Improving accuracy and treatment time is also possible with RapidArc radiotherapy, an image-guided IMRT that is eight times faster than conventional or IMRT machines. The same number of treatments is required as for traditional radiotherapy but sessions are 5 to 10 minutes instead of 15 to 30 minutes, with tighter margins around a smaller targeted treatment area. The hope is for fewer side effects, less damage to surrounding healthy tissue, improved QOL, and cost-effectiveness.[175] The equipment rotates 360 degrees around the person, delivering a precisely sculpted three-dimensional dose during one revolution of the machine.[177,372]

Radiofrequency ablation involves the insertion of a needle electrode through the skin and underlying soft tissues and into the tumor. Retractable tines are deployed, and radiofrequency excitation generates a zone of heat that destroys the tumor. Stereotactic body radiotherapy treatments combine potent dose fractionation and target tumors with real-time image guidance, thereby limiting number of exposures to radiation (and reducing the number of treatments).[205] Evidence for the use of stereotactic ablative radiotherapy in individuals who are medically inoperable is emerging.[155,341]

Radiopharmaceutical therapy involves the use of radioactive elements and radioactive isotopes. Isotopes implanted in the tumor or a body cavity by external-beam sources are delivered in the form of electromagnetic waves (e.g., x-rays or gamma rays) or as streams of particles (e.g., electrons). Strontium and yttrium-aluminum-garnet lasers have been administered for the palliation of bone pain related to metastatic bone disease in both prostate cancer and breast cancer.[118,142] Electron beam irradiation is most useful in the treatment of superficial tumors because energy is deposited at the skin and quickly dissipates, sparing the deeper tissues from toxic effects.

Normal and malignant cells respond to radiation differently, depending on blood supply, oxygen saturation, previous irradiation, and immune status. Cells most affected by chemotherapy and radiation have the greatest oxygenation and are the fast-producing cells (e.g., hair, skin). In general, normal cells recover from radiation faster than malignant cells; damaged cancer cells cannot self-repair. Success of the treatment and damage to normal tissue also vary with the intensity of the radiation.

Standard radiation fractionation is a course of 1.8 to 2.0 Gy per day in single daily doses. Accelerated or hypofractionation refers to delivering the same total dose over a shortened treatment time (one or just a few treatment sessions). Hyperfractionation refers to the same total delivered dose over the same treatment time but in an increased number of fractions; in other words, smaller fractions are delivered more often than once a day. Although a large single dose of radiation has greater cellular effects than fractions of the same amount delivered sequentially, a protracted schedule may allow time for normal tissue to recover in the intervals between individual sublethal doses.[58]

Challenges with radiation treatment still remain because of the inability to identify microscopic disease with accuracy. Immobilizing people and keeping them completely still for the duration of treatment is also difficult. Weight loss associated with treatment alters body geometry, requiring further corrections in dosimetry.

The next step in radiation oncology is to account for physiologic movements during irradiation. This may be accomplished with adaptive radiation with daily modulation of prescription and delivery using real-time imaging called four-dimensional conformal radiation therapy.[58]

**Proton Therapy.** Proton therapy is also a newer area in radiation oncology. Highly targeted proton beam therapy, available in advanced medical centers (27 in the United States as of November 2018),[302] may replace RT (if something even better does not come along first). Proton therapy is able to destroy tumor DNA so completely that the repair mechanisms are ineffective. Proton beam therapy is most useful when the tumor is close to nerves, blood vessels, the eyes, or vital organs. The beam acts like a smart weapon as it is able to locate the tumor using precise coordinates obtained from CT and/or MRI scans. Computer programs can design a course of radiation that conforms to the silhouette of the tumor.

### Chemotherapy

Chemotherapy includes a wide array of chemical agents to destroy cancer cells. It is particularly useful in the treatment of widespread or metastatic disease, whereas radiation is more useful for treatment of localized lesions. Chemotherapy is used in eradicating residual disease, as well as inducing long remissions and cures, especially in children with childhood leukemia and adults with Hodgkin disease or testicular cancer. Several major chemotherapeutic agents are listed in Table 9.8.

Chemotherapy (and radiotherapy) kills most of the billion or more cells in each cubic centimeter of tumor tissue. However, cytotoxic therapies do not always eradicate every tumor cell for several reasons. In contrast to normal cells, cancer cells are genetically unstable and replicate inaccurately. As the tumor grows, multiple subpopulations of cells with different biologic characteristics develop. Some of the cells will be resistant to treatment. After the treatment-sensitive cells are eliminated, the resistant cells may divide rapidly, recreating a tumor that is now resistant to the therapy.[7]

Almost all chemotherapy agents kill cancer cells by affecting DNA synthesis or function, a process that occurs through the cell cycle. Each drug varies in the way this

**Table 9.8** Major Chemotherapeutic Agents

| Class and Agent | Mechanism of Action | Indications for Use |
|---|---|---|
| **Alkylating Agents** | | |
| Busulfan<br>Carmustine<br>Chlorambucil<br>Cyclophosphamide<br>Dacarbazine | Bind to DNA and prevent DNA replication | Acute and chronic leukemias, Hodgkin and non-Hodgkin lymphomas, brain tumors, breast cancer, and melanomas |
| **Heavy Metal Compounds** | | |
| Cisplatin<br>Carboplatin<br>Oxaliplatin | Bind to DNA, distorting the DNA structure and causing cellular damage | Breast, bladder, testicular, colon, and ovarian cancers |
| **Antimetabolites** | | |
| Cytarabine<br>Decitabine<br>Fluorouracil (5-FU)<br>Methotrexate<br>Mercaptopurine (6-MP) | Block cell growth by interfering with DNA, RNA, and nucleic acid synthesis | Acute and chronic leukemias; non-Hodgkin lymphoma; and breast, colon, rectum, pancreatic, lung, head and neck, and stomach cancers |
| **Topoisomerase Inhibitors** | | |
| Teniposide<br>Doxorubicin<br>Daunorubicin<br>Topotecan | Inhibit actions of enzymes responsible for maintaining DNA structure (topoisomerases) | Acute leukemias; Hodgkin disease; and bone, thyroid, lung, breast, gastric, ovarian, cervical, and bladder cancers |
| **Microtubule-Targeting Agents** | | |
| Vinblastine<br>Vincristine<br>Paclitaxel | Disrupt cellular mitosis by inhibiting microtubule assembly or disassembly | Acute leukemias; Hodgkin and non-Hodgkin lymphomas; and breast, ovarian, lung, and testicular cancers |
| **Agents That Target Cell Surface Glycoproteins, Growth Factor Receptors, and Ligands** | | |
| Rituximab<br>Ibritumomab tiuxetan<br>Cetuximab<br>Trastuzumab<br>Erlotinib<br>Bevacizumab<br>Sunitinib | Bind to targets on or in cancer cells and transmit intracellular signals resulting in cell death, deliver chemotherapeutic agents to the disease site, or prevent cell growth and proliferation | Chronic leukemias; Hodgkin and non-Hodgkin lymphomas; and colorectal, gastric, breast, lung, pancreatic, renal, and head and neck cancers |
| **Other Biologic Agents** | | |
| Interferons<br>Interleukin-2 | Increase proliferation and activity of immune cells that destroy cancer cells without harming normal cells | Leukemias, melanomas, non-Hodgkin lymphoma, and renal cancer |

Data from American Cancer Society: Types of chemotherapy drugs. How chemotherapy works. Available at: https://www.cancer.org/treatment/treatments-and-side-effects/treatment-types/chemotherapy/how-chemotherapy-drugs-work.html. Accessed December 3, 2018; pharmacotherapy update: DiPiro JT, Talbert RL, Yee GC, et al: *Pharmacotherapy: A pathophysiologic approach*, ed 8, New York, 2011, McGraw-Hill; and Brunton LL, Chabner BA, Knollmann BC: *Goodman and Gilman's the pharmacological basis of therapeutics*, ed 12, New York, 2011, McGraw-Hill.

occurs within the cell cycle. Chemotherapy interferes with the synthesis or function of nucleic acid targeting cells in the growth phase and therefore does not kill all cells (e.g., 5% are in the quiet or quiescent phase and are unaffected by chemotherapy) (see Fig. 9.4).

Combination therapies are often used because some drugs work better during different cell cycles. For example, antimetabolites are most effective during the presynaptic ($G_1$) phase, whereas alkylating agents target cells during the synthesis of DNA (S phase) and the postsynthesis ($G_2$) phase. Treatment is designed to capture cell cycles at different phases for optimum cell death.[167]

Chemotherapeutic drugs can be given orally, subcutaneously, intramuscularly, intravenously, intracavitarily (into a body cavity such as the thoracic, abdominal, or pelvic cavity), intrathecally (through the sheath of a structure, such as through the sheath of the spinal cord into the subarachnoid space), and by arterial infusion, depending on the drug and its pharmacologic action and on tumor location. Administration in any form is usually intermittent to allow for bone marrow recovery between doses.

Traditional chemotherapies and newer targeted agents are known to cause neurologic symptoms that can impact QOL.[218] Not all chemotherapy recipients develop problems with cognitive or mental function, but if it does happen, the effects can last several years. MRI scans of brain structures have shown temporary shrinkage in the brain structures that are responsible for cognition and awareness. Shrinkage may be a possible physiologic explanation for chemotherapy-related cognitive difficulties.[244]

**Mediating the Effects of Chemotherapy.** Colony-stimulating factors (CSFs) may be used to support the person with low blood counts related to chemotherapy. CSFs function primarily as hematopoietic growth factors, guiding the division and differentiation of bone marrow stem cells. They also influence the functioning of mature lymphocytes, monocytes, macrophages, and neutrophils.

Currently, erythropoietin, human granulocyte colony-stimulating factor (G-CSF), GM-CSF, and thrombopoietin and various ILs are being used for chemotherapy-induced pancytopenia (deficiency of all cellular components of blood). Erythropoietin is used to treat anemia by stimulating bone marrow production of red blood cells. ILs are a large group of cytokines sometimes called *lymphokines* when produced by the T lymphocytes or *monokines* when produced by mononuclear phagocytes. ILs have a variety of effects, but most direct other cells to divide and differentiate. Both G-CSF and GM-CSF are very useful in protecting individuals from prolonged neutrophil nadirs (lowest points after neutrophil count has been depressed by chemotherapy). Recombinant thrombopoietin (oprelvekin) has shown promise in promoting elevation in platelet counts.[212] There is evidence that GM-CSF, administered by a variety of different routes, may have antitumor effects, although results from larger trials have been inconsistent, and further research continues into how best to harness its antitumor activities.[197]

## Immunotherapy

See also Cancer Immunotherapy earlier. *Immunotherapy* (also known as biologic therapy or biotherapy) relies on biologic response modifiers to change or modify the relationship between the tumor and host by strengthening the host's biologic response to tumor cells. Much of the work related to biologic response modifiers is still considered experimental, so the availability of this type of treatment varies regionally within the United States.

Agents include IFNs, which have a direct antitumor effect, and IL-2, one type of cytokine, a protein released by macrophages to trigger the immune response.[89] In addition to their desired immune effects, IFNs cause a number of significant toxicities, including constitutional, hematologic, hepatic, and prominent effects on the nervous system, especially depression.[310]

**Hematopoietic Cell Transplantation.** Hematopoietic cell transplantation, including bone marrow transplantation, is used for cancers that are responsive to high doses of chemotherapy or radiation. These high doses kill cancer cells but are also toxic to bone marrow; hematopoietic cell transplantation provides a method for rescuing people from bone marrow destruction while allowing higher doses of chemotherapy for a better antitumor result.

Bone marrow transplantation was a technique developed to restore the marrow to people who had lethal injury to that site because of bone marrow failure, destruction of bone marrow by disease, or intensive chemical or radiation exposure. At first, the source of the transplant was the marrow cells of a healthy donor who had the same tissue type (human leukocyte antigen; markers on the white blood cells) as the recipient (usually a sibling or close family relative). Now donor programs have been established to identify unrelated donors who have a matching human leukocyte antigen.

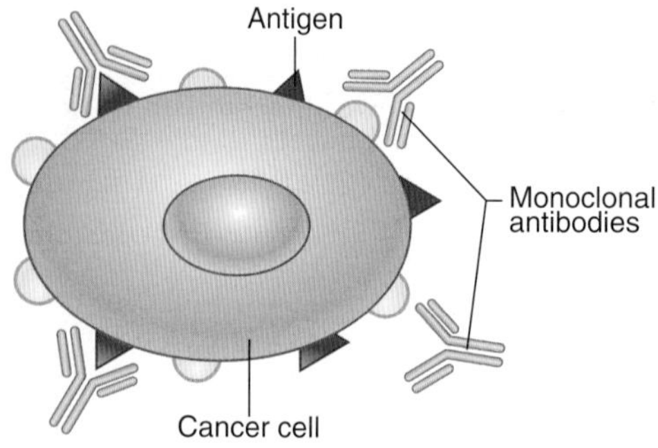


**Figure 9.5**

**Mechanism of action of monoclonal antibodies (mAbs).** mAbs are large, complex, Y-shaped molecules that bind to specific antigens on the surface of some cells. The mAb is like a key, and the antigen is the lock. When they fit together, the cancer cell is destroyed. Binding of extracellular receptor results in signals that block intracellular signaling, inducing cellular lysis and apoptosis (death).

The transplant product is a very small fraction of the marrow cells called *stem cells*. These cells occur in the bone marrow and circulate in the blood and can be harvested from the blood of a donor by treating the donor with an agent or agents (e.g., G-CSF) that cause a release of larger numbers of stem cells into the blood and collect them by hemapheresis. Because blood (peripheral site) as well as marrow is a good source of cells for transplantation, the term *hematopoietic cell transplantation* has replaced the general term for these procedures.

**Targeted Therapy.** Targeted therapy, or "smart drugs," is a form of immunotherapy and includes two broad groups: mAbs and small molecules (e.g., tyrosine kinase enzyme). By interfering with the pathway by which a normal cell becomes a cancer cell, targeted therapies are intended to spare surrounding healthy cells compared with treatment with radiation or chemotherapy (Fig. 9.5).[294,393,402]

Small molecules block enzymes and receptors involved in cancer cell growth and proliferation. mAb therapy uses specifically designed antibodies made by a pharmaceutical company instead of antibodies produced by a person's own immune system. These antibodies are biologic therapies that act specifically against a particular antigen. They can also be bound with radioisotopes and injected into the body to detect cancer by attaching to tumor cells. The antibody may not actually kill target cells, but rather it marks the cells so that other components in the immune system attack it or initiate a signaling mechanism that leads to the self-destruction of the target cell.[381] mAbs have been developed to help combat specific cancers including colorectal cancer and some forms of non-Hodgkin lymphoma.

Research is ongoing to use these antibodies as a means of destroying specific cancer cells without disturbing healthy cells. Rituximab (Rituxan), trastuzumab (Herceptin), bevacizumab (Avastin), alemtuzumab (CamPath), and cetuximab (Erbitux) are a few of the mAbs currently in use for cancer treatment (e.g., lymphoma, breast, colorectal, chronic leukemia, and head and neck cancer).

Bevacizumab, formerly known as anti–vascular endothelial growth factor, is an antibody used in combination with chemotherapy in the treatment of colon, lung, and breast cancer. This antibody binds to vascular endothelial growth factor made by the tumor cells and prevents it from forming new blood vessels to supply the tumor cells.

Rituximab is used primarily in the treatment of non-Hodgkin lymphoma. Rituximab binds to lymphoid cells in the thymus, spleen, lymph nodes, and peripheral blood to lyse and destroy specific immune target cells.

Trastuzumab is used in the treatment of metastatic breast cancer in women who have overexpression of the HER2 protein. It binds with this protein and inhibits proliferation of cells with this protein and mediates an antibody-mediated destruction of the cancer cells that have HER2 receptor overexpression.[241] Both agents are usually used in combination with or in addition to other chemotherapeutic agents for treatment.

Not all people respond to mAbs, presumably because of differences in the receptors being targeted. Molecular testing will have to become part of designer biologic therapy in which drugs are chosen on an individual basis after genetic profiling and immunoassay. Antibodies also function as carriers of cytotoxic substances, such as radioisotopes, drugs, and toxins, making them a key focus area of cancer research currently.[381]

### Antiangiogenic Therapy

Antiangiogenic therapy shows promise as a means of blocking the formation of new blood vessels supplying cancer cells but remains limited in use and under investigation.[186,386] Research has shown that the one common area of vulnerability of all cells in any phase of growth is the nonnegotiable need for oxygen. Tumor cells cannot survive without oxygen and other nutrients transported by the blood. In fact, tumor cells cannot survive at distances greater than 150 μm from a blood vessel.[121]

Antiangiogenic therapy may be able to put a stop to pathologic angiogenesis, the process by which a malignant tumor develops new vessels and is the primary means by which cancer cells spread. Antiangiogenesis factors, their receptors, and the signaling pathways that govern angiogenesis in solid tumors have been discovered. Treatment with antiangiogenesis factors (e.g., endostatin, angiostatin, or calpastatin) approved for use in the United States focuses on blocking the general process of tumor growth by cutting off their blood supply rather than on the destruction of an already formed cancerous mass.[318] Scientists expect that combinations of angiogenesis inhibitors or broad-spectrum angiogenesis inhibitors will be needed for long-term use in cancer if tumor cells have or develop multiple molecular signaling pathways, a characteristic called *redundancy*.[120]

In the future, antiangiogenic agents may be used as maintenance therapy to control cancer much the same way that medications are used to control hypertension or hyperlipidemia. It is expected that different mutations in cancer will require individualized therapy based on current knowledge of specific tumors, their patterns of resistance, and response to angiogenesis inhibitors.[388]

The NCI has produced a fact sheet addressing the most common questions and concerns regarding the use of antiangiogentic agents in the treatment of cancer. The reader can view the following website for additional information and references: https://www.cancer.gov/about-cancer/treatment/types/immunotherapy/angiogenesis-inhibitors-fact-sheet.

### Hormonal Therapy

Hormonal therapy is used for certain types of cancer shown to be affected by specific hormones. For example, tamoxifen, an antiestrogen hormonal agent, is used in breast cancer to block estrogen receptors in breast tumor cells that require estrogen to thrive.

The luteinizing hormone–releasing hormone leuprolide is now used to treat prostate cancer. With long-term use, this hormone inhibits testosterone release and tumor growth. Goserelin acetate (Zoladex) is another hormone used in prostate cancer that is a synthetic form of luteinizing hormone–releasing hormone. Goserelin acetate inhibits pituitary gonadotropic secretion, thus decreasing serum testosterone levels.[409]

Other cancers such as myelodysplasia and hematologic malignancies (e.g., lymphoma, myeloma, leukemia) can be treated effectively in older adults, although advanced age does present many challenges.

The future of oncologic care may rest on the model of individualized (tailored/targeted) therapy based on a pretreatment assessment of each individual's organ reserves, physical condition, and cognitive function. Identifying predictive factors of successful outcome will help assess who could benefit from more aggressive treatment and have the greatest chance for successful outcomes.[132] When curative measures are no longer possible or available, palliative treatment may include radiation, chemotherapy, physical therapy (e.g., physical agents, exercise, positioning, relaxation techniques, biofeedback, or manual therapy), medications, acupuncture, chiropractic care, alternative medicine (e.g., homeopathic and naturopathic treatment), and hospice care.

### Complementary and Alternative (Integrative) Medicine

Many people are seeking help in the cure and palliation of cancer through complementary and alternative medicine (CAM) therapies, sometimes referred to as integrative medicine, energy medicine, or bioenergetics (the field of biochemistry concerned with energy flow through living systems). Some examples of these modalities include acupuncture, Reiki, BodyTalk, hypnosis, mind–body techniques, massage, music, Tai Chi, qi gong, yoga, meditation, and other methods to improve physical and mental well-being. Conventional treatments do not always relieve symptoms of pain, fatigue, anxiety, and mood disturbance. Some people cannot tolerate the side effects of conventional treatment. CAM has gained the attention of consumers and caused concern among of providers of conventional or standard medical therapy.

The ACS has information on complementary and alternative methods used in cancer on its website (https://www.cancer.org/treatment/treatments-and-side-effects/complementary-and-alternative-medicine/complementary-and-alternative-methods-and-cancer.html).[16] The NCI has established a department (Office of Cancer Complementary and Alternative Medicine) specifically directed toward the research of integrative medicine (https://cam.cancer.gov//). The NIH has also established the National Center for Complementary and Integrative Health (https://nccih.nih.gov/). Major research institutions and universities are beginning to investigate the effectiveness of these types of interventions for cancer (e.g., Society for Integrative Oncology sponsored by the New York Academy of Medicine, Cochrane CAM Field—University of Maryland School of Medicine). A new movement toward integrative medicine combining the best of complementary modalities with mainstream conventional therapies has been launched. Several texts on this topic are available for physical therapists.[90,100]

## Prognosis

Previously, a cancer diagnosis was often a death sentence; survivors referred to themselves as "victims." However, cancer is no longer considered a death sentence, and many survivors return to the mainstream of family life, community activities, and work. Medical treatment is often provided in outpatient settings, making it possible to work during treatment, though not without some return-to-work issues (e.g., decreased physical functioning, fatigue, lack of workplace support), for many individuals.[138,245,399]

In general, improved survival rates occur with screening and early detection/treatment, especially for cancers that have a highly effective treatment. Prognosis is influenced by the type of cancer; the stage and grade of disease at diagnosis; the availability of effective treatment; the response to treatment; and other factors related to lifestyle such as smoking, alcohol consumption, diet, nutrition, and exercise. Despite advances in early diagnosis, surgical techniques, systemic therapies, and patient care, a major cause of death resulting from cancer is development of metastases that are resistant to therapy.[423]

The prognosis is poor for anyone with advanced, disseminated cancer. Researchers continue to search for the mechanisms responsible for cancer metastases and chemotherapeutic failure and develop new strategies to circumvent drug resistance. In general, the earlier cancers are found, the simpler treatment may be, and the greater likelihood of a cure.

There are many different terms used to describe treatment outcomes, such as *disease-free survival, event-free survival, progression-free survival, complete response, stable disease, near-complete response, partial response,* and *progressive disease*.[112] The term *no evidence of disease* may be used when all signs of the disease have disappeared after treatment but before the end of 5 years occurs and there are no signs of the disease using current tests. If the response is maintained for a long period, the term *durable remission* may be used. A person who is alive and without evidence of disease for at least 5 years after diagnosis is considered cured. The terms *survival* and *cure* do not always portray the functional status of a cancer survivor. Many people considered cured are left with physical limitations and movement dysfunctions that interfere with their daily lives.

Even without complete remission, cancer can be controlled to provide longer survival time and improved QOL, but these factors are not reflected in survival rates. Cancer statistics reported usually include a lag time so that rates may not reflect the most recent treatment advances. Survival rates for many cancers have increased from 1960 to the present, but not all cancers have been characterized by this increase. For example, while survival rates for Hodgkin disease and prostate, testicular, and bladder cancers have increased by at least 25%, the survival rates for cancers of the oral cavity and pharynx, liver, pancreas, esophagus, and colon have decreased or increased less than 5% during the same period.

A significantly lower survival rate in African American men for most cancer classifications has been noted. This difference may be due to a variety of factors including limited access to health care, little or no insurance, lack of a primary health care provider, limited knowledge of the benefits of early diagnosis and treatment, and greater exposure to carcinogens. Central to these social forces is access to health care, including prevention, information, early detection, and quality treatment.[206]

In terminally ill individuals, rates of change are more important indicators of survival than absolute measures. Using a modified Barthel Index composed of 10 activities of daily living, each with five levels of dependency (maximum score more than 100 points), can provide important predictions about length of time until death. One-half individuals with advanced cancer who lose 10 or more points per week die within 2 weeks, and three-fourths are dead at 3 weeks. In contrast, 50% of all individuals without declines in score survive for 2 months or more. This may be a useful tool for planning and end-of-life issues in a hospice setting.[38]

## Clinical Prediction of Outcomes

New approaches to prognostication are being used and/or developed. These techniques focus on the tumor itself or on the body's immune response to the tumor. For example, a test that focuses on the tumor to predict response to adjuvant chemotherapy is the Oncotype DX test for women with breast cancer. This test uses a core sample of the tumor to analyze gene mutations and can predict who would benefit from adjuvant chemotherapy in addition to estrogen-inhibiting drugs.

A test that looks more at the body's response to treatment is the Immunoscore. The Immunoscore approach provides a prediction of clinical outcome through histopathologic evaluation of tissue samples obtained during surgical resection of the tumor.[125] This technique measures cytotoxic T lymphocytes that infiltrate the tumor; the more T lymphocytes present, the stronger the immune response against the tumor. The Immunoscore measures markers of tumor-infiltrating T lymphocytes. Clinical trials have established that patients identified as being positive for CD3 and CD8 (showing an immune response against the tumor) have a better prognosis than patients who test negative for these markers.[125,147]

Two instruments are commonly used by providers to assess the functional level of newly diagnosed cases of cancer, the Karnofsky Performance Scale[338] and the Eastern Cooperative Oncology Group Performance Status.[296] The Karnofsky Performance Scale is an older scale that uses a score of 100 to 0 (normal to dead) to score function, and the newer Eastern Cooperative Oncology Group Performance Status uses a 0-to-4 scale (normal, unrestricted activity, bedridden, fully dependent).

Selected older adults with cancer can benefit from intensive care. Age is associated with higher mortality, especially for adults older than age 60 years and when combined with multiple comorbidities.[133] A comprehensive geriatric assessment can be helpful in identifying individuals likely to benefit from cytotoxic treatment. Therapies may be adjusted based on renal and cardiac function. Cardiac toxicity and neurotoxicity are common in persons aged 65 years and older.[345]

## SPECIAL IMPLICATIONS FOR THE THERAPIST 9.1

### *Oncology/Cancer*

#### The Role of the Physical Therapist in Cancer Treatment

> We must expand our paradigm thinking from treating "post-op" to treating from diagnosis to survivorship.
>
> Leslie J. Waltke, PT[392]

The therapist should be involved in all phases of care including prevention, restoration, support, and palliative care. Prevention lessens the impact of anticipated disability through education and training. Restorative care focuses on restoring physical function as much as possible. Supportive care assists in coping with the condition while maintaining maximal functional capacity. Palliative care provides comfort during function and activities of daily living to minimize dependence while offering emotional support.[295]

Many individuals with cancer would benefit from consultation with a physical therapist during the early stages of their cancer treatment. Treatment for cancer has improved over the past 20 years but often results in functional deficits caused by fibrosis, tissue or segmental bone resection, or joint or limb amputation.

There are site-specific cancer issues (e.g., cognitive impairment with brain tumors) and postsurgical problems (e.g., limited motion, soreness, disuse, pain, fatigue, sensory loss, weakness, deep venous thrombosis and emboli, lymphedema, or sleep disturbance). There are side effects of radiotherapy, chemotherapy, and bone marrow or stem cell transplantation. Any of these problems may require physical therapy intervention and education.[297]

The therapist is not just treating the disease but also the effects of medical intervention; medical oncologists must be encouraged to refer based on treatment effects, not type of disease.[391] Treatment can result in severe disfigurement; cancer is the major cause of amputation in children. Weakness, fatigue, inflexibility, osteoporosis, risk of falls, altered or diminished breathing patterns, and lymphedema are just a few of the challenges faced by many cancer clients—no matter what kind of cancer they have.

Therapists need to advocate as a group that appropriate oncology patients see a physical therapist—for example, targeting individuals ahead of time for immediate postoperative or post–lymph node dissection consultation. Automatic referral to a physical therapist once a diagnosis of cancer has been made is preferred over waiting until radiation-induced fibrosis causes disabling contractures or until lymphedema has caused significant swelling. More evidence is needed to identify people at risk for poor outcomes that could be improved with physical therapy and predictive factors supporting the need for physical therapy intervention.

As medical innovations help people with cancer live longer, there has been a shift in the way we approach cancer treatment. Shifting from the search for a cure to managing the disease as a chronic condition necessitates a more comprehensive and integrated management approach from diagnosis through survivorship.[328] There is greater emphasis on maximizing function and improving QOL, with a more holistic approach throughout the various phases of intervention and management.

Psychosocial/spiritual issues (e.g., loss, grief, and anger) and client diversity (e.g., life span, socioeconomic class, cultural beliefs, and ethnicity) require consideration in planning an effective therapeutic approach.[297] The client's psychosocial/spiritual status and cultural beliefs can be a driving factor in successful outcomes. Engaging the individual and caregivers in regular and honest discussion, listening to concerns or feelings, and sharing rehabilitation needs to set mutually achievable goals will enhance outcomes.[257]

#### Benign Tumors

The therapist may be asked by clients to examine unusual skin lesions or aberrant tissue, such as unusual moles, ganglion, fibromas, or lipomas. A general screening examination is required, with history, age, and risk factors taken into consideration. The ABCDE (asymmetry, border, color, diameter, evolving) skin cancer screening examination can be employed, with documentation of findings for any skin changes.

Benign fatty (lipoma) or fibrous tumors (fibroma) commonly located in the subcutaneous tissues can be located anywhere in the body. Lipomas are found most often in locations where fat accumulates, such as the abdomen, thighs, upper arms, back, and breast. These masses are usually round or oval in shape, soft, lumpy, and easily moveable. They may be small (pea-size) or as large as 3 to 4 inches across. Palpation reveals defined borders and a mass that is not fixed but moves readily with pressure along the edge.

These benign tumors are usually painless but can be tender when palpated. Many people who discover the lump are understandably concerned about cancer. Any suspicious integumentary or soft tissue mass must be evaluated medically, especially in a client with any additional risk factors. Only a pathologist can diagnose or rule out these types of lesions.

## Side Effects of Cancer Treatment

Although it may seem to make more sense to include a discussion of the side effects of cancer treatment in this chapter, we have opted to place that topic in Chapter 5 to emphasize the point that the long-term effects of cancer treatment are often problems that affect multiple systems. The therapist must take this approach when planning intervention and offering patient/client education.

With improved survival rates, we expect to see more delayed reactions and long-term sequelae to today's cancer treatment modalities. With improved survival and longevity, we may also see an increased prevalence of cancer recurrence in the future. This may mean worsening of symptoms such as peripheral neuropathy or lymphedema from second and third rounds of treatment. In time, with the identification of genetic traits of cancer, treatment may become more targeted to the cancer cells and less toxic to healthy cells and tissue, eventually reducing and maybe even eliminating side effects experienced by many cancer survivors today.

Table 9.5 compares the potential side effects associated with the major treatment modalities discussed in this section. See Chapter 5 for discussion of the intended and adverse systemic effects of chemotherapy agents, radiation sickness, radiation recall, CNS effects of immunosuppression, and steroid-induced myopathy.

The NIH MedLine Plus has an online repository for cancer drug information, including common side effects.[108] The NCCN offers a number of clinical practice guidelines for cancer in general and for specific types of cancer.[277] The NCI offers suggestions for optimizing the preservation of fertility for men and women during and after cancer therapy.[276]

Each individual will experience and report discomfort in a slightly different way. The occurrence of symptoms is a stressor of its own, sometimes initiating a response of fear behaviors and distress. The idea of symptom distress as an additional side effect of cancer treatment is a fairly new concept.[72,135] Individual perception of symptoms includes whether the person notices a change in how he or she usually feels or behaves; the intensity of the symptoms; and the impact of both the presence and the intensity of symptoms on daily activities, function, and QOL. Response to symptom distress includes physiologic, psychologic, sociocultural, and behavioral components. The therapist may have a role in helping people assess their symptoms and amount of distress associated with symptoms, helping them to monitor their own level of health.[216]

The most common and often distressing side effect of cancer and cancer-related treatment is fatigue. The therapist can be very instrumental in offering information and ideas about energy conservation (Box 9.4). The therapist can help the client set priorities, pace and delegate activities and responsibilities, and provide labor-saving devices and ideas. Scheduling activities at times of peak energy is important, along with a structured daily routine that focuses on one activity at a time. The importance of socializing, relaxing, and finding quiet moments of pleasure cannot be emphasized enough. The therapist may also be involved in relaxation and stress management, with referral for nutrition consultation, sleep therapy, and depression when indicated.[280]

**Box 9.4**

**TIPS FOR ENERGY CONSERVATION**

- Energy conservation is an organized procedure for finding ways to reduce the amount of effort and energy needed to accomplish a given task. By reducing the amount of energy needed to accomplish a task, more energy is available.
- Applying principles of energy conservation requires self-examination and assessment of habits and priorities. Making these types of changes requires patience but can result in continued activity over a longer period of time.
- Schedule the most strenuous activities during periods of highest energy.

Before starting any activity, analyze the task and answer the following questions:

- Is the task necessary?
- Can it be eliminated or combined?
- Am I doing this out of habit?
- Can it be simplified by combining or eliminating steps?
- Can a larger job be divided into smaller tasks?
- Are there any assistive devices, small appliances, or tools that could make the task easier?
- Can this be done by someone else?

Alternate more strenuous tasks with easier ones (e.g., heavy, light, heavy, light).

Plan frequent rest periods, sit down, or take naps as needed. A slow steady rate of activity with short rests in between is advised; working to the point of fatigue should be avoided.

Cluster activities so that it is not necessary to make frequent trips or walk long distances at home, school, or work.

Avoid or keep to a minimum stair climbing.

Keep certain tasks, such as driving, shopping, and housekeeping, to a minimum. Delegate as many responsibilities and jobs as possible.

Sit down to perform activities of daily living (e.g., tooth brushing, hair combing) or household tasks, including meal preparation.

Avoid sitting on low or soft furniture that requires more energy expenditure to get up again. Store items where they are easy to reach (neither too low requiring stooping nor too high to retrieve).

Encourage children to climb up on your lap or into a chair rather than lifting them up.

Minimize carrying objects; use a wheeled cart to carry things whenever possible.

Modify your living space to include grab rails in the bathroom, elevated toilet seat, and chairs placed appropriately throughout to provide rest steps.

Data from Eaton LH, Tipton JM: *Putting evidence into practice: improving oncology patient outcomes*. Pittsburgh, 2009, Oncology Nursing Society; National Comprehensive Cancer Network (NCCN): *NCCN guidelines for cancer-related fatigue*. Version 2, 2018. February 20, 2018.

Exercise to improve functional capacity, increase activity tolerance, manage stress, and improve mood is an integral part of fatigue management. See the in-depth discussion in Cancer, Physical Activity, and Exercise Training.

## Physical Therapist's Evaluation

In a physical therapy practice, anyone with a history of cancer, known cancer risk factors, and/or older than age 40 should be screened for red flags suggestive of cancer.

The therapist is a key professional in offering education for risk factor modification and cancer prevention. For an individual with a current diagnosis of cancer, an overall health assessment is important in providing the optimal exercise program. Physical examination will include observation, inspection, auscultation, percussion, palpation, and special tests. Guidelines for physical assessment, review of systems, and visceral assessment by physical therapists are available.[136] Gilchrist[129] suggests rehabilitation protocols during medical intervention with consideration for the specific cancer treatment.

The clinical behavior of the majority of musculoskeletal tumors is such that the symptoms are shared with a wide range of nontumorous orthopedic disorders. Pain, swelling, and local heat accompanying musculoskeletal tumors are also common to inflammatory conditions. In addition, the most likely sites of musculoskeletal tumors are regions frequently involved in sports injuries.[86]

Cardiovascular and pulmonary tests and measures including heart rate; breath sounds and respiratory rate, pattern, and quality; blood pressure; aerobic capacity test (e.g., 6-minute walk test); and pulse oximetry establish a baseline when developing an exercise program. This is especially important with the aging demographics of cancer survivors. The older people are when diagnosed with cancer, the greater the likelihood of other problems being present such as heart disease, hypertension, stroke, diabetes, and osteoporosis.

Observe for and document any cluster of signs and symptoms for accompanying health conditions or comorbidities from cancer or cancer treatment such as hypoxia, decreased peripheral vascular supply, deep vein thrombosis, hypercalcemia, fluid or electrolyte imbalances, anemia, hypertension, integumentary changes, and infection.

Integumentary, neuromuscular, musculoskeletal, and neurologic assessment should include, but is not limited to, skin characteristics and condition (including lymph node palpation); anthropometrics (e.g., limb length, limb girth, and body composition); functional strength testing; range of motion; flexibility; arousal, attention, and orientation tests; cranial and peripheral nerve integrity; motor function (e.g., dexterity, coordination, voluntary postures, and movement patterns); deep tendon and postural reflexes; and sensory testing (e.g., light touch, sharp/dull, temperature, deep pressure, proprioception, vibration, and stereognosis).[136]

The risk of falling is one of the more serious sequelae of both the local effects of cancer and the systemic consequences of cancer treatment. Weakness, pain, fatigue, orthostatic hypotension, peripheral neuropathy, decreased bone density (osteoporosis), and diminished flexibility, in various combinations, may result in falls. Some individuals will fail to inform their oncologist of debilitating peripheral neuropathies for fear of having their treatment delayed or prolonged.

The therapist can be very instrumental in patient/client education about the need to report side effects so the oncologist can evaluate dosage and treatment regimen. Anyone with neuropathies is at increased risk of falling; anyone with metastasized cancer to the spine or long bones may fracture these bones in a fall (or fall because of pathologic fractures), which can result in a serious, long-term disability.

Fall prevention and education are important aspects of the rehabilitation or exercise program. Assessment of the home environment is essential in providing a fall prevention program. In addition, the therapist must evaluate each client individually, possibly selecting an assistive device in appropriate cases. A walker with auto-stop wheels in the front may be a safer choice for some people than a standard walker or regular front wheel walker. A wheelchair may be necessary for someone who experiences dizziness, weakness, fatigue, or signs of disorientation.

Higher incidences of osteoporosis and osteopenia are found in individuals with cancer, especially women taking aromatase inhibitors such as exemestane or anastrozole for the primary prevention of breast cancer[146] or with chemotherapy-induced ovarian failure.[387] Men with prostate cancer on androgen deprivation therapy are also more likely to develop osteoporosis.[88] Management of long-term bone health is an important aspect of comprehensive cancer care.[137]

### Precautions

Patients with cancer are immunocompromised and immunodeficient and therefore at risk for various viral, bacterial, and fungal infections, but with preventive measures the possibility of such complications can be reduced. The therapist must practice standard precautions carefully to help the individual undergoing cancer treatment avoid infection. Closely monitoring blood counts (and other laboratory values) and vital signs and observing for signs of infection, bleeding, or arrhythmias are important.

The therapist should contact the physician when the client exhibits fever or cluster of constitutional symptoms, unusual fatigue or tiredness, irregular heart beat or palpitations, chest pain, unusual bleeding, or night pain (see complete list in Box 9.5). Radiated tissue must be treated with care to avoid local trauma; extreme temperatures must be avoided; management of lymphedema may be required.

Many people undergoing cancer treatment are using complementary and alternative herbs or supplements to mitigate side effects of cancer treatment. These herbs or supplements can have an adverse effect when combined with radiation or chemotherapy. If the client perceives disapproval, this information may not be relayed to the appropriate health care professional. By being open and nonjudgmental and inviting more discussion about the use of these substances, the therapist may be able to bring to light potential risks involved. The client should be advised that most herbal or natural supplements and complementary interventions are designed to support, not replace, more traditional medical interventions that have been proved effective.

There are many areas of question for therapists treating clients with a current or past history of cancer. Clinical research in this area is sorely needed. In the absence of evidence-based practice, we must fall back on clinical decision making based on what evidence is available, an understanding of the pathophysiology involved, and common sense in pursuing what is considered "best practice." Toward that end, any therapist working with this population group may want to take advantage of the collective ideas and suggestions made

Box 9.5

**SYMPTOMATIC PRECAUTIONS DURING EXERCISE TESTING OR TRAINING**

Anyone with cancer experiencing any of the following (especially brought on or exacerbated by exercise) should contact his or her physician.

- Fever
- Extreme or unusual tiredness or fatigue
- Unusual muscular weakness
- Irregular heartbeat, chest palpitations, or chest pain
- Sudden onset of dyspnea
- Leg pain or cramps
- Unusual joint pain
- Recent or new-onset back, neck, or bone pain
- Unusual bruising, nosebleeds, or bleeding from any other body opening
- Sudden onset of nausea during exercise
- Rapid weight gain or weight loss
- Severe diarrhea or vomiting
- Disorientation, confusion, dizziness, or light-headedness
- Blurred vision or other visual disturbances
- Skin pallor or unusual skin rash
- Night pain

Data from Schmitz KH, Courneya KS, Matthews C, et al. American College of Sports Medicine roundtable on exercise guidelines for cancer survivors. *Med Sci Sports Exerc* 42:1409–1426, 2010; and Drouin J, Pfalzer LA: Cancer and exercise. National Center on Health, Physical Activity, and Disability. 2012. Available at: https://www.nchpad.org/163/1255/Cancer~and~Exercise. Accessed November 20, 2018.

available through the American Physical Therapy Association (APTA) Academy of Oncologic Physical Therapy list serve, an excellent resource for asking questions of therapists actively engaged in the treatment of patients/clients with cancer. The Academy of Oncologic Physical Therapy also publishes an excellent peer-reviewed journal with relevant articles written by physical therapists and other health professionals in the field.

### Oncologic Emergencies

Oncology patients/clients can present complex challenges for the physical therapist. Treatment regimens and their potential side effects top the list of important considerations during the physical therapist's intervention. Early recognition of potential emergencies such as superior vena cava syndrome, tumor lysis syndrome (TLS), emergent spinal cord compression, severe thrombocytosis, and other conditions is extremely important in reducing morbidity and mortality.[371]

Most of these conditions are uncommon or rare, making knowledge of them even more important so the therapist does not miss early clinical manifestations. Each one is typically associated with a particular type of cancer; knowing the patterns of potentially serious problems linked with individual cancers can help the therapist conduct surveillance with appropriate clients. For example, superior vena cava syndrome associated with small cell lung cancer and lymphoma is caused by mediastinal metastasis and central lung lesions compressing the superior vena cava. Presentation of superior vena cava syndrome is insidious, with dilated neck veins and facial and arm lymphedema. Treatment may be palliative if the malignancy causing the compressive force is not curable; curative chemotherapy for lymphoma is the exception.[371]

*Tumor lysis syndrome* (TLS) refers to a constellation of metabolic disturbances that occur often in high-grade non-Hodgkin lymphoma after initiation of cancer treatment. TLS occurs in people with myeloproliferative disorders, such as acute leukemia and high-grade lymphoma, when chemotherapy causes lysis of a massive number of cells in a short period of time. The malignant cells die and release their contents into the bloodstream. Acute renal failure may occur from the inability to clear the rapid deposition of potassium, phosphate, and uric acid from the cell lysis.[168,371]

Symptoms of TLS are most common 6 to 72 hours after chemotherapy begins and reflect the severity of the underlying metabolic abnormalities. TLS may become clinically apparent in only a small number of affected individuals. The therapist may hear reports of and observe muscle weakness, spasm, and cramping from TLS. Rapidly increasing uric acid levels may lead to arthralgia and renal colic. Neurologic signs and symptoms can include paresthesia and paralysis (hyperkalemia); seizures, tetany, and lethargy (hyperphosphatemia); lethargy, malaise, sleepiness, and seizures (hyperuricemia); and paresthesia, tetany, confusion, delirium, and hallucinations (hypocalcemia).[168]

In addition, the therapist must monitor for cardiovascular effects such as arrhythmias, abnormal changes in blood pressure, and tachycardia during activity. Symptoms associated with volume overload may develop (e.g., dyspnea, pulmonary crackles, edema, hypertension). Accompanying gastrointestinal signs and symptoms can include anorexia, nausea, vomiting, diarrhea, hyperactive bowel sounds, and abdominal pain, bloating, or cramps. Electrolyte imbalances can trigger the clotting cascade, leading to disseminated intravascular coagulation. Any of these sequelae can be fatal. Early reporting of symptoms can prevent dangerous complications from this condition.

*Spinal cord compression* affects up to 30% of individuals with disseminated cancer from lung, breast, prostate, multiple myeloma, and colon. The thoracic spine is targeted most often, followed by the lumbosacral region. Back pain, muscle weakness, gait changes, or other signs and symptoms of cord compression may develop slowly or may progress rapidly; prognosis is better with slow onset.

The therapist should conduct surveillance examinations of serial muscle testing to detect decline in motor function potentially associated with spinal cord compression for individuals undergoing treatment for any of the cancers listed. A stable spine is essential before progressing to out-of-bed activities; surgical stabilization or use of an orthosis or brace may be needed.[371]

Many individuals undergoing treatment for cancer are *thrombocytopenic* (low platelet levels). Severe thrombocytopenia (the definition of "severe" may vary from institution to institution but generally is noted as less than 20,000 cells/mm$^3$; some institutions use 5000 cells/mm$^3$) increases the risk of spontaneous bleeding (e.g., intracranial, intramuscular, or joint bleeds). The therapist may be instrumental in preventing intracranial bleeds and falls for anyone with this complication.

### Sexual Issues

Sexual dysfunction is a frequent side effect of cancer treatment, especially for adults with cancer of the reproductive organs (e.g., breast, prostate, testicle, ovary, and uterus) and Hodgkin disease. The most common problems include loss of desire for sexual activity, erectile dysfunction in men, interrupted childbearing and/or infertility,[63] and dyspareunia in women. In contrast to many other physiologic side effects, sexual problems do not tend to resolve within the first year or two of disease-free survival but can persist for a long time.[251,342]

Physical therapists are often in a unique position to assist people with sexual concerns because of their repeated close contact with the affected individual. Sexual function is an important aspect of QOL and requires a brief assessment. It is often helpful to have a physical therapist who specializes in pelvic floor dysfunction and sexuality issues.[141,333] A therapist who is comfortable and knowledgeable in discussing sexual issues may be able to provide more focused assistance to the individual who is trying to adjust to changes in sexual style and practices as a result of the illness. Understanding the range of values and sexual history that clients (and possibly their partners) bring to the clinical situation and respecting appropriate provider–client boundaries are important.[32] More information on this topic is available.[32,196,321]

### Palliative and Hospice Care

> Palliative care is an approach that improves the quality of life of patients and their families facing the problem associated with life-threatening or serious illnesses, through the prevention and relief of suffering by means of early identification and impeccable assessment and treatment of pain and other problems, physical, psychosocial and spiritual.
>
> World Health Organization[415]

When curative measures have been exhausted and a cure is no longer possible or available, symptom management or palliative care may be offered regardless of how long the individual lives. The goals are to prevent symptoms; side effects caused by treatment of the disease; and psychologic, social, and spiritual problems related to the disease or its treatment. When prevention is not possible, treatment becomes the intervention.[57,282]

The CARING criteria are a practical tool to help identify individuals who may benefit from a palliative approach with end-of-life discussions and aggressive symptom management. The criteria are simple items easily identified on hospital admission and include the following:[119]

**C:** Primary diagnosis of *Cancer* (especially if cancer has metastasized)
**A:** Two or more hospital *Admissions* for a chronic illness in the last 12 months
**R:** *Resident* in a nursing home
**I:** *ICU* admission with multiple organ failure (MOF)
**N:** *Noncancer* hospice (meeting two or more of the National Hospice and Palliative Care Organization's
**G:** *Guidelines*)

Scoring for risk of death is as follows:

| | |
|---|---|
| Low: | <5 |
| Medium: | 5–12 |
| High: | ≥13 |

This set of screening criteria is highly predictive of death within 1 year in a hospitalized population. Even if the person ends up with a better result than predicted, there is no harm in instituting palliative care. The client ends up with a completed advance directive and is less likely to experience untreated pain. When death is imminent, hospice, defined as support and care given for people in the last phase of an incurable disease so they may live as fully and comfortably as possible,[283] may be provided in a free-standing hospice center, hospice hospital unit, or long-term care facility or at home. At the center of hospice and palliative care is the belief that everyone has the right to die pain-free and with dignity and that families should receive the necessary support to allow this to occur.

Though the terms *end of life, terminally ill,* and *terminal condition* are commonly used within the palliative and hospice care realm, these terms are inconsistently defined.[169] The International Association of Hospice and Palliative Care uses this definition of terminal condition: "a progressive condition that has no cure and that can be reasonably expected to cause the death of a person within a foreseeable future." This is inclusive of malignant and nonmalignant conditions.[178]

Although the cost of hospice may be covered by private insurance or by the client/family out-of-pocket, Medicare has three key eligibility criteria as follows: (1) the patient's physician and the hospice medical director use their best clinical judgment to certify that the patient is terminally ill with a life expectancy of 6 months or less if the disease runs its normal course, (2) the patient signs a statement choosing to receive hospice care rather than curative treatments for his/her illness, and (3) the patient enrolls in a Medicare-approved hospice program.[114]

Palliative care for a terminally ill person is aimed at improving the QOL of both the individual and family members. The primary goal is to decrease the physical and psychologic suffering of the individual while providing spiritual and emotional support. Every effort is made to help the individual achieve as full a life as possible, with minimal pain, discomfort, and restriction. Many medications, especially morphine, are used for pain control. Emphasis of hospice care is on emotional and psychologic support for the client and the family, focusing on death as a natural end to life.[282]

Physical therapy may enhance the QOL of individuals receiving palliative care, as well as dying individuals receiving hospice care. Disability in individuals with advanced cancer often results from bed rest, deconditioning, and neurologic and musculoskeletal complications of cancer or cancer treatment. Weakness, pain, fatigue, and dyspnea are common symptoms.

Physical therapy intervention aims to improve level of function and comfort of the patient and ensure patient and caregiver safety. Physical function and independence should be maintained as long as possible to improve QOL and reduce the burden of care for the caregivers.[317] Pain management and relief, positioning to prevent pressure ulcers and aid breathing, endurance training and energy conservation, home modification, and family education are just a few of the services the physical therapist can offer hospice clients and families. The therapist is an important team member in helping clients remain functional and retain dignity and control at the end of life.[326]

Currently, most studies examining the benefits of physical therapy in end-of-life and palliative care are small, quantitative, or observational, with few randomized trials. However, these studies show benefit in using physical therapy in end-of-life and palliative care settings in improving the physical, social, and emotional well-being of patients with life-threatening conditions, even those at the end of life.[319] Further evidence-based research may help expand reimbursement under Medicare to include physical therapy as a core service.[328] Therapists working with hospice programs are encouraged to attend interdisciplinary team meetings whenever possible—even if reimbursement for the time is not possible or the therapist has not been specifically invited or included. Discussing and demonstrating ways in which the physical therapist can benefit clients, while acknowledging the costs (and cost savings), can help advance the overall work of physical therapists in hospice care.[328]

For physical therapists interested or involved in palliative and/or hospice care, there is an APTA Academy of Oncologic Physical Therapy–sponsored special interest group (SIG) available for support and information: Hospice and Palliative Care SIG. The Hospice and Palliative Care SIG can help therapists who have a common interest in the treatment of life-limiting conditions meet, confer, and promote these interests.

**Radiation Hazard for the Health Care Worker**

Implant radiation therapy requires personal radiation protection for all staff members who come in contact with the client (this topic is discussed in Radiation Hazard for Health Care Professionals in Chapter 5).

## CANCER, PHYSICAL ACTIVITY, AND EXERCISE TRAINING

Lisa VanHoose, PhD, PT, CLT-LANA

In the last decade the body of knowledge focused on the relationship between exercise and cancer has exponentially increased. As with the prevention and management of heart disease, obesity, osteoporosis, and diabetes, exercise plays an important role in cancer prevention and ameliorating the side effects of cancer treatment and promoting improved health among cancer survivors. The various modes of exercise have resulted in clinical and statistical heterogeneity in the literature. Modes of exercise include aerobic, resistive, flexibility, balance training, and conditioning or any combination of these forms. Studies using a normal, healthy adult population have indicated that each type of exercise has its own physiologic and psychologic benefits, and researchers are currently investigating the effects in individuals with cancer.

Not all cancers are alike or affect the body in the same way. Exercise benefits may vary based on cancer type, stage, treatment, side effects of treatment, and other extraneous factors. Exercise appears to be safe, but long-term outcomes have not been reported. Some types of exercise such as aggressive weight and aerobic training have been shown to be detrimental to the immune system, and this must be considered when developing a physical therapy care plan. Therapists working with oncology patients are encouraged to evaluate the literature to find the best choice of prescriptive exercise for a specific cancer. Because of the various cancer types and the breadth of literature, only a composite summary is provided in this chapter.

### Exercise as a Cancer Prevention Strategy

Physical activity is defined as body movement caused by skeletal muscle contraction that results in quantifiable energy expenditure. Exercise is distinguished from other types of physical activity by the fact that the intensity, duration, and frequency of the activity are specifically designed to improve physical fitness. Intensity of exercise is commonly stratified based on heart rate, with 40% to 49% of maximum heart rate (MHR) defined as low. Activities that are part of one's daily routine are typically of low intensity and duration. Both epidemiologic and laboratory data indicate that physical activity of at least a moderate level may affect cancer risk.[30,258] Moderate intensity is defined as 50% to 69% of MHR, and activities include, but are not limited to, walking, dancing, volleyball, and golfing. Fast bicycling, jogging, and similar activities increase the heart rate to 70% or greater of the MHR.[1,152] However, therapists should be aware that the MHR equation, 220 − age, does not account for differences in resting heart rate. The Karvonen formula is a better method, although it is slightly more complicated. The Karvonen formula uses the MHR and heart rate reserve in calculating target heart rates or classifying the intensity of a task.[194,250]

Being sedentary is a risk factor for several of the most common types of cancer (e.g., breast and colon). A role for physical activity and exercise in specifically reducing cancer risk has been shown for several types of cancer including breast, colorectal cancer, liver, and lung cancers, with more equivocal evidence for others, such as melanoma and prostate cancer.[261] The mode and dosage of exercise needed to prevent cancer are debatable. Therapeutic responsiveness is currently based on cancer type, stage of disease, or treatment.[170] The ACS advises moderate habitual physical activity as a potentially protective measure against certain types of neoplasms, particularly tumors of the breast, colon, kidney, lung, pancreas, prostate, and the female reproductive tract.[211] The Women's Health Initiative reported that 1.25 to 2.5 hours per week of brisk walking lowered breast cancer risk by 18% in women.[247] Moderate-intensity physical activity should be performed for 30 minutes or longer at least 5 days a week.[1] The ACS recommendations are in line with the American Heart Association and American Diabetes

Box 9.6

**SPECIFIC EXERCISE PRECAUTIONS FOR CANCER SURVIVORS**

- Survivors with severe anemia may need to delay exercise; medical evaluation is required.
- Survivors with compromised immune function or who have had bone marrow transplantation should avoid public gyms and other public places until white blood cell counts return to safe levels; this could take up to 1 year or longer.
- Severe fatigue can keep an individual from doing any exercise; daily stretching is advised, and even 5-minute increments of mild activity (e.g., walking, Sit and Be Fit exercises) should be encouraged.
- Avoid exposure of irradiated skin to chlorine (e.g., swimming pools) until medically approved.
- Survivors with indwelling catheters must observe additional precautions: avoid water or other microbial exposures that can lead to infection; avoid resistance training of muscles that can dislodge the catheter.
- Recumbent stationary biking may be a better option than walking on a treadmill for individuals with significant peripheral neuropathies or gait disturbances.

Data from Rock CL: Nutrition and physical activity guidelines for cancer survivors. *CA Cancer J Clin* 62:243–274, 2012; and Schmitz KH, Courneya KS, Matthews C, et al. American College of Sports Medicine roundtable on exercise guidelines for cancer survivors. *Med Sci Sports Exerc* 42:1409–1426, 2010.

Association, recommending at least 30 to 60 minutes of moderate to vigorous physical activity at least 5 days per week to reduce the risk of cancer, cardiovascular disease, and diabetes.[211]

Research is elucidating the protective mechanisms of exercise. Exercise-induced changes in the activity of macrophages, NK cells, lymphokine-activated killer cells, neutrophils, and regulating cytokines suggest that immunomodulation may contribute to the protective value of exercise.[52,164]

At the present time, cytokine modulation with exercise is receiving considerable research attention. Researchers theorize that exercise can regulate production of certain hormones, which when unregulated, may spur tumor growth.[388] Also, exercise may enhance host defense against the tumor.[389] Exercise also improves energy balance, which increases one's ability to maintain a healthy weight. Being overweight or obese increases the risk of various cancers,[39,209,316,322] possibly because of inflammation and abnormalities in immune function[97] and hormone metabolism. Exercise can normalize many of these functions with appropriate dosing.

## Exercise for Cancer Survivors

The diagnosis of cancer begins the survivorship continuum from diagnosis to end of life. Exercise programs appear to have a beneficial influence throughout the continuum and especially during the early stages of the disease. However, survivors tend to decrease levels of physical activity and exercise at diagnosis, during treatment, and/or after completion of their treatment, especially if they were sedentary before their cancer diagnosis.[116,179] Low-intensity exercise can seem like high intensity for these individuals. In addition, some cancer therapies reduce exercise capacity because of cardiopulmonary, neurologic, and musculoskeletal impairments.

Therefore the type, frequency, duration, and intensity of exercise should be individualized on the basis of the survivor's age, previous fitness level, type of cancer and cancer treatment, and presence of any additional comorbidities. Some specific guidelines are available in Box 9.6. The American College of Sports Medicine (ACSM) has recommended that survivors follow the same exercise as the general population (150 minutes of moderate-level physical activity) with slow progression of resistance exercise.

Survivors should be educated to understand that any exercise has a linear benefit, with increasing health benefit with higher volume of physical activity. However, individuals should be cautioned that extremely high levels of exercise might increase the risk for infections and exercise-related injuries.[289] With almost 16 million Americans alive today who have experienced cancer,[13] it is important to develop interventions to enhance immune function and prevent or minimize muscle wasting, thus counteracting the detrimental physiologic effects of cancer and chemotherapy and maintaining QOL after cancer diagnosis.

Physical activity and exercise training are interventions that address a broad range of QOL issues including physical (e.g., muscular strength, body composition, nausea, and fatigue), functional (e.g., functional capacity), psychologic (e.g., coping and mood changes), spiritual, emotional, and social well-being.[130] Studies examining the therapeutic value of exercise for people with various cancers during primary cancer treatment suggest that exercise is safe and feasible, improving physical functioning and other aspects of QOL, regardless of cancer stage or treatment status.[55,102,207,351,370]

## Screening and Assessment

Medical screening should be conducted with all clients before their participation in an exercise program, particularly for exercise of more vigorous intensity.[19,410] This type of screening is especially important for people with cancer who receive various levels of treatment that can affect the physiologic response to exercise. For example, fatigue is a common symptom of nearly every form of cancer treatment.

The therapist will need to take a detailed history of treatment administered to date, examine laboratory results, and distinguish between fatigue from deconditioning and fatigue from medical interventions to determine the most effective and efficient approach to rehabilitation. The medical history should also identify conditions that may or may not be related to cancer and its treatment such as hypertension, diabetes, coronary artery disease, and preexisting orthopedic conditions. The person's current physical condition, condition before disease onset, age, and living environment are also important variables.[407,412] Based on a 2012 study in the *Physical Therapy Journal*, most clinicians rely heavily on the patient/client assessment for exercise prescription and progression.[144] Therefore a thorough assessment is crucial, and multiple assessment tools are available to aid the physical therapist.

A self-reporting survey instrument called the Cancer Rehabilitation Evaluation System (formerly called the Cancer Inventory of Problem Situations) is a useful tool for evaluating rehabilitation needs and interventions. The 36-Item Short Form Health Survey has been validated in multiple cancer populations and allows the therapist to assess disease burden.[261,308,325] Another tool commonly reported in the literature is the Functional Assessment of Chronic Illness Therapy surveys. Instruments are available for several cancer types and evaluate physical, social, functional, and emotional well-being.[49,68,417]

The therapist must understand the stages of the disease and know the type and timing of the medical interventions, especially radiation and chemotherapy treatment. The body's physiologic response to these agents (e.g., fatigue, neuropathy, or "chemo brain" or "chemo fog") may alter the normal training response and affect tolerance for exercise and compliance with exercise programs. Cognitive rehabilitation techniques may be useful to improve patient/client compliance, function, and QOL.[73,360]

Cardiac dysfunction can result in left ventricular failure, cardiomyopathy, and/or congestive heart failure months to years after chemotherapy. These conditions may impact the client's ability to exercise. Signs and symptoms of subclinical cardiac conditions may develop with the initiation of an exercise program. Careful history taking and clinical assessment may result in early detection and intervention, potentially reducing morbidity.

Auscultation to screen for abnormal lung or heart sounds is important to identify any precautions or contraindications to exercise. The individual is not likely to be able to sustain exercise levels if there are any physiologic abnormalities present. Medical consultation may be required before initiating or continuing a training program when high-risk medical conditions are identified by the physical therapist.

Older adults, especially older adults with bone disease or significant comorbidities and impairments such as arthritis or peripheral neuropathies, will need an assessment of balance, strength, and coordination to remain safe from falls and injuries during exercise.

## Monitoring Vital Signs

Monitoring physiologic responses to exercise is important in the immunosuppressed population. Baseline testing is important to determine safe guidelines and to provide a starting place against which to measure improvement and to identify the individual's functional exercise level. A hypertensive response to exercise is common among individuals with cancer and undergoing cancer treatment. Starting an aerobic training program is not advised if such a response is observed during preexercise testing.

Exercise intensity determined by training heart rate may be difficult because some people have inappropriate heart responses to exercise and large physiologic changes on a day-to-day basis from disease and treatment (e.g., changes in medications). Exercise intensity can be guided by heart rate ranges based on oxygen consumption or metabolic equivalent (MET) levels. The therapist can use test results to prescribe a program starting at approximately 60% of the individual's maximum level (moderate intensity). The therapist is advised to use prior exercise levels, prior exercise capabilities, baseline function, and individual abilities even when using the predictive formula because each client may respond differently (unpredictably).

The therapist (or client) should always monitor oxygen saturation with pulse oximetry and evaluate heart rate (for arrhythmias), pulse rate, breathing frequency, and blood pressure before, during, and after the treatment session. Borg Scale for Rating of Perceived Exertion (RPE) or other scales can be used to determine level of symptom distress or severity. RPE is also used when the client is taking cardiac medications that blunt heart rate response to exercise or when other conditions and comorbidities are present that may prevent the use of target heart rate formulas.

Watch closely for early signs (dyspnea, pallor, sweating, and fatigue) of cardiopulmonary complications of cancer treatment. Monitoring vital signs helps the therapist recognize early when an individual is reaching his or her tolerance level. The therapist must keep in mind the need to balance activities that push the heart rate up with energy conservation so the individual can remain functional for the rest of the day. The activity level of someone with anemia also may require adjustment. This client may have elevated pulse and respiratory rates due to hypoxia, with increased cardiac output resulting from the body's effort to maintain an adequate oxygen supply.

## Prescriptive Exercise

Types, limitations, and precautions of exercise intervention in the treatment of cancer are being studied. The programs studied vary in length from 6 weeks for individuals who undergoing radiation therapy to 6 months for individuals receiving chemotherapy and the entire duration of bone marrow transplantation. Exercise interventions vary somewhat, but most include progressive programs of 15- to 30-minute sessions, 3 to 5 days a week, at an intensity equal to 60% to 80% of MHR (RPE 11 to 14). A perceived exertion of no greater than 12 may be used as a guide when exercise testing is not possible. Although variations will occur in research and clinical protocols, the ACSM has recommended the FITT principles for clinical exercise prescription.[19] The acronym FITT stands for frequency, intensity, time, and type of exercise. The goal is that exercise promotes fitness, under the FITT principle, with improvements in cardiorespiratory and muscular function, flexibility, and body composition.

The frequency and duration/time of exercise are determined by the clinical status of the person. If weight training is prescribed, high-repetition, low-weight circuit programs are recommended that do not exceed RPE of 14.[225] Other clinical tools for monitoring and more specific guidelines for exercise are available.[81,264,266,336]

Clinical observations and case studies have reported that individuals who exercised more than 60 minutes per day were more likely to report higher levels of fatigue, suggesting a maximum effective dose for individuals receiving adjuvant chemotherapy. Moderate levels of exercise may enhance immunity, and vigorous activity may impair the immune response and increase fatigue symptoms or susceptibility to infections.[357] No serious adverse events were reported in any of the studies, although anyone in the high-risk category with serious comorbidities was excluded, and most exercise programs were flexible and symptom-limited.

The reported outcomes of these and other studies show that exercise has a powerful effect on CRF, with fatigue levels reported as 40% to 50% lower in exercising participants. Exercise reduces fatigue and emotional distress and improves QOL.[75,268] Without exception, all of these studies showed lower levels of fatigue and emotional distress as well as decreased sleep disturbance (if this was studied as an outcome) in people who exercised during treatment compared with control subjects or with baseline scores in single-group designs. A summary of the studies on exercise and CRF is included in the NCCN guidelines for CRF.[280]

Not all people with cancer are able to participate in aerobic exercise. People who ambulate less than 50% of the time, those confined to bed, and those who fatigue with mild exertion may not be candidates for aerobic exercise.[408] Range-of-motion and gentle resistive work may be appropriate until tolerance for activity improves. Energy-conservation techniques and work simplification (see Box 9.4) may be necessary for a person with chronic fatigue and for individuals whose functional status is declining. Therapeutic exercise should be scheduled during periods when the person has the highest level of energy.

Interval exercise or a bedside exercise program may be preferred at first. Interval exercise may be the only treatment possible in this circumstance. This is performed during frequent but shorter sessions throughout the day, with work-rest intervals beginning at the person's level of tolerance. This may be no more than 1 minute of exercise activity followed by 1 minute of rest, then 1 minute of exercise, and so on. As the person's endurance level increases, the duration of work may be increased and the interval of rest decreased.

Generalized weakness associated with cancer treatment can be more debilitating than the disease itself. Whenever possible, exercise including strength training and cardiovascular training is an essential component for many people with cancer. Improving strength and endurance aids in countering the effects of the disease and the effects of medical interventions. Increased physical activity may increase the homeostatic sleep drive to increase sleep quality and quantity and may help relieve CRF.[269]

### Exercise for Cancer-Related Fatigue

CRF is common and disabling for up to 100% of survivors undergoing chemotherapy and/or radiation.[62,364,398]CRF has been defined as a "distressing, persistent, subjective sense of physical, emotional, and/or cognitive tiredness or exhaustion related to cancer and/or cancer treatment that is not proportional to recent activity and interferes with usual functioning."[280] People receiving cancer treatment are often advised to rest after chemotherapy, but aerobic exercise and physical activity have been shown to help improve energy level and stamina, reduce fatigue, reduce nausea, increase muscle mass, and increase daily activities without increasing fatigue.

Approximately 30% of survivors will continue to report fatigue as a barrier to function after treatment, persisting for months and even years after the end of cancer treatment.[62,80,128]The use of exercise as an intervention for CRF has been proven as an effective strategy.[199] A 2012 Cochrane Summary indicated that exercise can attenuate fatigue throughout the cancer continuum. However, the authors stated that the type and intensity of exercise varied and additional research is needed to determine the most effective dosage. Traditional (e.g., walking or aerobics) and alternative (e.g., Tai Chi, dance, or yoga) forms of exercise are being investigated.[48,67,246,331,365,366]

Much of the exercise-related research is focused on breast cancer.[82,201] However, aerobic exercise after bone marrow transplantation[145,384] and exercise during treatment of cancers such as multiple myeloma, solid tumors, and lymphoma have been studied, with the majority of results having positive impact on many physical and psychosocial outcomes.

Clients receiving chemotherapy and radiation therapy experiencing CRF who are already participating in an exercise program may need to exercise temporarily at a lower intensity and progress at a slower pace; the goal is to remain as active as possible. For sedentary individuals, low-intensity activities such as stretching and brief, slow walks can be implemented initially and slowly advanced.[280]

However, it can be difficult to convince someone who is extremely tired (and especially individuals who did not exercise before cancer diagnosis) that exercise will improve his or her symptoms. The therapist may have to begin with discussions over a period of time about the importance of exercise and the pathophysiology of CRF.

The NCI has provided and frequently updates its Fatigue PDQ, which can be used for patient education. This is especially important if the person is significantly deconditioned. The therapist can begin with an assessment of previous exercise or activity patterns. Ask the following questions:

- Can you do your normal daily activities?
- Can you participate in a formal or informal exercise program?
- What is your normal amount and frequency of exercise?
- Have you had to modify or change your exercise level or other activity patterns since the development of fatigue?

Symptoms of fatigue, headache, and lethargy begin in most people when hemoglobin falls below 12 g/dL. Mild-to-moderate graded exercise is possible for many people at this level. Symptoms may become more pronounced when hemoglobin decreases to less than 10 g/dL, reducing exercise capacity.

Exercise is not always possible for most people when the hemoglobin level is 8 g/dL or less. Hemoglobin levels should be maintained around 12 g/dL during the administration of chemotherapy, as this has been shown to be related to overall survival and QOL gain.[29,122,262] However, protocols vary from institution to institution and

**Box 9.7**

**PRECAUTIONS TO AEROBIC EXERCISE IN CHEMOTHERAPY CLIENTS[a]**

| | | |
|---|---|---|
| Platelet count | <50,000/μL | With severe thrombocytopenia (<20,000/μL), consider a symptom-based approach for activity and fall risk awareness, may need to collaborate with interprofessional team for transfusion needs |
| Hemoglobin | <10 g/dL | If <8 g/dL, consider symptom-based approach for activity, may need to collaborate with interprofessional team for transfusion needs |
| White blood cell count | <3000/μL; 10,000/μL with fever (no exercise) | Symptom-based approach |
| Absolute neutrophil count | <2500/μL | If absolute neutrophil count is <1000/μL, infection risk; may need to collaborate with interprofessional team for transfusion needs |

[a]Single threshold values are not usually clinically relevant but rather provide a general guideline. Physical therapists should not rely exclusively on a single laboratory value. For example, hemoglobin levels have the most variability from client to client; protocols can vary from center to center and even from physician to physician. These general guidelines are for use as precautions to aerobic exercise. What constitutes aerobic can also vary from individual to individual and requires monitoring of vital signs and/or the use of rate of perceived exertion (Borg scale).

Data from Winningham ML, MacVicar MG, Burke CA: Exercise for cancer patients: guidelines and precautions. *Phys Sportsmed* 14:125–134, 1986. Please keep in mind that Winningham levels often cited may be considered quite conservative in today's oncologic practice, as these values were set by a research council more than 25 years ago. At that time there were more unknowns and greater concern for mortality compared with today's more evidence-based, aggressive approaches.[2,367]

even from one physician to another within the same facility. Bloodless medicine has made it possible for clients to tolerate lower hemoglobin levels previously thought unacceptable without compromising oxygen delivery.

The National Center on Health, Physical Activity, and Disability guidelines on Cancer and Exercise[64] and the ACSM guidelines for termination of testing or training may also be consulted. People with cancer are advised to contact their physician if any of the abnormal responses listed in Box 9.5 develop.

### Exercise During and After Radiation Therapy or Chemotherapy

Bone marrow suppression is a common and serious side effect of many chemotherapeutic agents and can be a side effect of radiation therapy in some instances, such as when radiation dosage exceeded 50 Gy in the past or currently when high levels of radiation are used to prevent death despite potential radiotherapy toxicities later. Therefore it is extremely important to take a client history of current or past radiation therapy dosages and to monitor the hematologic values in clients receiving these treatment modalities.

The therapist must review these values before any type of vigorous exercise or activity is initiated. Previous recommendations based on expert opinion of not exercising within 2 hours of treatment[409] for fear of attenuating the effectiveness of treatment and increasing risk of side effects have gone out of favor, as these fears have not proven true over the years. In fact, an argument might be made about the potential to enhance treatment effectiveness via increasing blood flow and drug delivery to the tumor site. Moderate-intensity aerobic exercise (walking for 20 to 45 minutes, three to five times per week at 50% to 70% of measured MHRs during 7 weeks of radiation) has been shown to maintain erythrocyte levels during radiation treatment (of breast cancer).[107]

Exercise may foster an individual's sense of wellness and increase the body's ability to recover from the effects of chemotherapy.[172,265] Exercise and physical activity can also improve mood and reduce anxiety and mental stress for people undergoing chemotherapy. Independence and QOL improve as functional ability improves.[54,115,256,271] A helpful guideline to indicate when aerobic exercise is contraindicated (or when reevaluation of the exercise program is indicated) in chemotherapy clients is provided in Box 9.7. Keep in mind these values are primarily educated estimates based on clinical consensus; further research and stronger evidence are needed to support these values.

### Exercise and Bone Metastases

See Special Implications for the Therapist: Metastatic Tumors in Chapter 26.

### Exercise and Lymphedema

In the past, therapists were cautioned to carefully design a program that did not cause or exacerbate cancer-related complications such as lymphedema. It was advised that repetitive or strenuous exercise of any type would increase the production of lymph fluid, and lymphedema would be the result because lymph nodes were removed during surgery, damaged by radiation therapy, or invaded by the tumor, leaving scar tissue that prevented normal lymph drainage. In fact, it is now known that exercise, graded appropriately, activates muscle groups and joints in the affected extremity, increases lymph flow, is safe for patients at risk for lymphedema, and does not exacerbate lymphedema in those who have been diagnosed with the condition.[260,358] Resistance training has not been shown to adversely affect lymphedema. It is important that exercise training should start supervised, at a low dose, and progressed according to symptomatic responses.[340]

Combining a specific exercise program for each individual with the use of sufficient compression will facilitate the process of decongestion by using the natural pumping effect of the muscles to increase lymph flow while preventing limb refilling. Most clinicians experienced in lymphedema treatment agree on basic guidelines for exercise. See further discussion in Chapter 13.

### Exercise and Advanced Cancer

With improved detection and treatment, more and more people are living with cancer as a controllable chronic disease or in advanced stages of cancer. Although the body of knowledge is evolving, and there is evidence that exercise is safe and has a positive impact on many physical and psychologic measures among these individuals,[104,159] there is insufficient research on exercise in such individuals to make specific recommendations for physical activity and exercise. In such cases, therapists are advised to prescribe exercise based on individual needs and abilities.

General training precautions for warm-up and cooldown should be followed while monitoring for abnormal heart rate or blood pressure responses and observing each individual for pathologic symptomatic responses (e.g., hypertension, chest pain, onset of wheezing, claudication or leg cramps, shortness of breath, and dizziness or fainting). Clients should be encouraged to remain adequately hydrated at all times unless medically directed otherwise.

Compromised skeletal integrity, especially in the presence of muscle wasting, increases the risk of fracture and may prevent weight-bearing activities. Aerobic exercise may have to begin with non–weight-bearing exercise such as cycling, rowing, or swimming (for clients who are not immunocompromised or neutropenic), with a gradual return to weight-bearing activities when possible to prevent loss of bone density. For people with severe muscle weakness or at risk for pathologic fractures, seated exercises, low-impact exercises, or symptom-limited exercises may be better tolerated.[151,348] Exercise has been suggested to improve fatigue in advanced disease,[105] and therapists should also consider the psychosocial benefits of group exercise.[4,300]

## CHILDHOOD CANCER

### Incidence and Overview

Among children (birth to 14 years of age) in the United States, cancer is the second most common cause of death. Each year, cancer is diagnosed in approximately 11,000 children.[355] With advances in treatment and care, the death rate has decreased more than 50% from 1975 to 2015, with 83.4% of children surviving 5 years or more after cancer diagnosis compared with 58% in the mid-1970s. Currently it is estimated that there are more than 400,000 survivors of childhood and adolescent cancer (diagnosed between the ages of 0 and 19 years) in the United States.[292]

Treatment-related deaths have declined as a result of advances in clinical supportive care (e.g., antibiotic therapy, indwelling venous access lines, blood products, and enteral and parenteral nutrition) that maximize the benefits and minimize the side effects of cancer therapy.

The types of cancers that occur in children vary greatly from those seen in adults. Leukemias, particularly ALL; lymphomas, particularly non-Hodgkin lymphoma (almost half of all childhood cancers involve the blood or blood-forming organs); brain and other nervous system tumors; and soft tissue sarcomas are the most common pediatric malignancies, whereas adenocarcinomas (e.g., lung, breast, or colorectal) are more common in adults.[355]

Other differences that must be taken into account when treating a child with cancer include the stage of growth and development, stage of psychosocial and cognitive development, and emotional response of the child to the illness and its treatment. The immaturity of the child's organ systems often has important treatment implications.

### Types of Childhood Cancers

The most common pediatric malignancies are ALL, non-Hodgkin lymphoma, Hodgkin disease, and primary CNS tumors. Neuroblastoma, Wilms (kidney) tumor, rhabdomyosarcoma, and retinoblastomas are the most common types of solid tumors that occur in children.

ALL, the most common childhood malignancy, accounts for almost one-third of all pediatric cancers. White boys are affected most often. Although the exact cause is unknown, radiation, chromosomal abnormalities, viruses, and congenital immunodeficiencies all have been associated with an increased incidence of leukemia.

Wilms tumor, a malignancy that may affect one or both kidneys, occurs in children younger than 14 years of age and is slightly more prevalent in girls than boys. Epidemiologic research suggests an increased incidence in children of men exposed to lead or hydrocarbons. An association between Wilms tumor and chromosomal abnormalities has been established, specifically deletion of a suppressor gene located on the short arm of chromosome. This chromosomal anomaly is an autosomal dominant trait, and evaluation of other family members is required.

Neuroblastoma is the most common extracranial solid tumor in children and the most commonly diagnosed neoplasm during the first year of life. In rare cases, it can be detected via ultrasound before birth. Approximately 800 new cases are diagnosed annually in the United States, and the incidence is higher among whites than nonwhites. Neuroblastoma can originate anywhere along the sympathetic nervous system, but more than half of the tumors occur in the retroperitoneal area and manifest as an abdominal mass. Other common sites include the posterior mediastinum, pelvis, and neck. If the bone marrow is involved, bone pain may occur.

Rhabdomyosarcoma is the most common soft tissue sarcoma in children. This tumor, which is more prevalent in boys than girls, originates from the same embryonic cells that give rise to striated muscle. The peak incidence is between 2 and 5 years of age, and a second peak occurs between 15 and 19 years of age. Survival rates are much improved with early detection and treatment. The most common tumor sites include the head and neck, genitourinary tract, and extremities. Rhabdomyosarcoma of the head and neck can lead to CNS involvement, including cranial nerve palsies, meningeal symptoms, and respiratory paralysis.

Other common cancers seen in children are bone cancers, both osteogenic and Ewing sarcomas (see Chapter 26), and brain tumors (see Chapter 30).

## Late Effects and Prognosis

As advances in cancer therapy improve, the prognosis of children with malignancies continues to improve. Over the past half century there have been significant improvements in the 5-year survival rate for many childhood cancers, especially ALL and acute myeloid leukemia, non-Hodgkin lymphoma, and Wilms tumor. With increasing survival rates, there is a growing concern about the late effects of disease and treatment.

The term *late effects* refers to the damaging effects of surgery, radiation, and chemotherapy on nonmalignant tissues, as well as to the social, emotional, and economic consequences of survival. These effects can appear months to years after treatment and can range in severity from subclinical to clinical to life threatening. Not all children experience such effects, but those who do often appear in the rehabilitation setting.

Late effects have been identified in almost every organ system. Treatment involving the CNS can cause deficits in cognition, intelligence, hearing, and vision. Treatment involving the CNS, head and neck, or gonads can cause endocrine abnormalities, such as short stature, hypothyroidism, or delayed secondary sexual development. Children treated with anthracyclines (e.g., doxorubicin [Adriamycin]) are at risk for development of cardiomyopathies, especially with increasing cumulative doses.[229]

Surgery and radiation involving the musculoskeletal system have been associated with defects such as kyphosis, scoliosis, and spinal shortening. Finally, a child who has received radiation or chemotherapy has a 10-fold greater chance of developing a second malignancy than a child who has never had cancer.[76]

## REFERENCES

To enhance this text and add value for the reader, all references are included in the enhanced ebook on Student Consult that accompanies this textbook. The reader can view the reference source and access it online whenever possible.

# CHAPTER 10

# The Integumentary System

KAREN A. GIBBS • DEBORAH M. WENDLAND

The integumentary system is an essential component of physical therapist practice. The *Guide to Physical Therapist Practice* includes the integumentary system and addresses wound prevention as well as superficial, partial-thickness, and full-thickness skin involvement secondary to injury.[28] Practitioners must also identify and treat common skin lesions and conditions secondary to allergy, pathology of disease, and sequelae of clinical medicine.

Skin is the largest body organ, constituting 15% to 20% of the body weight.[112] It differs anatomically and physiologically in different areas of the body, but the overall primary function of the skin is to protect underlying structures from external injury and harmful substances. Skin serves as a physical and chemical protective barrier, acts as insulation, contributes to sensory perception, assists with fluid balance and temperature regulation, absorbs ultraviolet (UV) radiation, metabolizes vitamin D, and synthesizes epidermal lipids.[112] Primary anatomic structures and layers of the skin are presented in Fig. 10.1 and Table 10.1.

## SKIN LESIONS

Skin lesions can result from a wide variety of etiologic factors (Box 10.1). Lesions of the skin or skin manifestations of systemic disorders can be classified as *primary* or *secondary* lesions.

A primary lesion is the first lesion to appear on the skin and has a visually recognizable structure (e.g., macule, papule, plaque, nodule, tumor, wheal, vesicle, pustule). When changes occur in a primary lesion (e.g., scale, crust, thickening, erosion, ulcer, scar, excoriation, fissure, atrophy), it becomes a secondary lesion. These changes may result from many factors, including scratching, rubbing, medication, natural disease progression, or processes of healing.

Birthmarks, commonly caused by a nevus (pl., nevi), may involve an overgrowth of one or more of the normal components of skin, such as pigment cells, blood vessels, and lymph vessels. Birthmarks may be classified as pigment (e.g., café au lait spot, Mongolian spot), vascular (e.g., port-wine stain, strawberry hemangioma), epidermal (e.g., epidermal nevus, nevus sebaceous), or connective tissue (e.g., juvenile elastoma, collagenoma) birthmarks.[13]

Most birthmarks do not require treatment. However, the presence of six or more café au lait spots more than 5 cm in length requires medical investigation, as these may be diagnostic of neurofibromatosis or Albright syndrome.[102] Mongolian spots (blue-black macules) can easily be mistaken for a large bruise by uninformed individuals; therefore complete history and physical examination of the skin may be necessary. Vascular birthmarks may be removed with laser therapy for cosmetic reasons.

## SIGNS AND SYMPTOMS OF SKIN DISEASE

*Pruritus* (itching) is one of the most common manifestations of dermatologic disease and can be a symptom of underlying systemic disease in individuals with generalized itching, especially among chronically ill and older people.[184,191] Xerosis (dry, rough skin) is the most common cause of pruritus.[184] Scratching to the point of skin injury impairs the skin's protective barrier and can result in increased inflammation, infection, and scarring. Many systemic disorders may cause pruritus, most commonly diabetes mellitus, drug hypersensitivity, and hyperthyroidism (Box 10.2).[184]

*Urticaria*, or hives, is a vascular skin reaction marked by smooth, slightly elevated patches (wheals)[176] that are redder or paler than surrounding skin and are often accompanied by severe itching. Eruptions are usually an allergic response to drugs or infection and rarely last longer than 2 days. However, urticaria may exist in a chronic form, lasting more than 6 weeks and, in rare cases, months to years.[247,266]

*Rash* is a generalized term for an eruption on the skin, most often on the face, trunk, axilla, and groin, and is often accompanied by itching. A rash can manifest as a continuum from erythema to macular lesions to a raised papular appearance. Eruptions typically occur as a secondary response to a primary agent, such as sun exposure, allergens, irritants, medications, or in association with systemic disease.

Common examples include rash associated with prolonged exposure to urine or feces (diaper rash or incontinence-associated dermatitis [IAD]),[185] drug rash,[44] heat rash, and butterfly rash associated with lupus. Rash appearing on the breast, especially on the areola or nipple, with or without symptoms of itching, soreness, or burning, may be a sign of Paget disease of the nipple, a rare form of breast cancer. Individuals with this rash should be referred for follow-up with a qualified health care professional.[136]

*Blisters* (vesicle or bulla) are fluid-containing elevated skin lesions with serous or bloody contents. Blisters may be primarily associated with genetic or autoimmune diseases or may be secondary to viral or bacterial skin infections (e.g., herpes simplex, impetigo), direct skin injury (e.g., burns, ischemia, pressure, dermatitis), or drug administration (e.g., penicillamine, captopril).[44] Blisters associated with an underlying neoplasm, called *paraneoplastic pemphigus,* may be the first sign of underlying malignancy.[255]

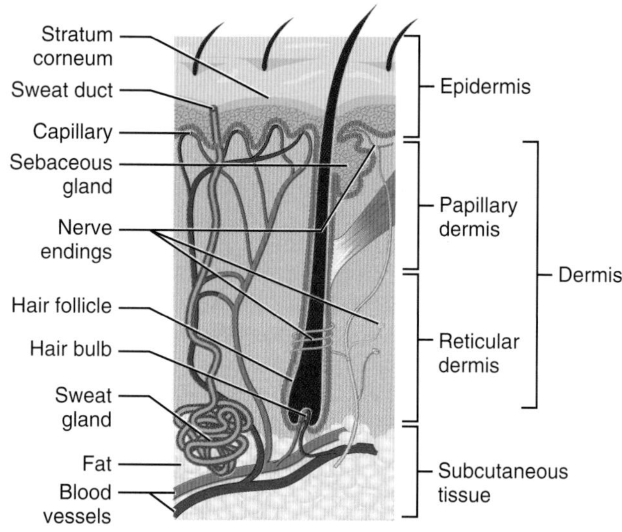


**Figure. 10.1**

**Overall skin structure.**

*Xeroderma* is a mild form of ichthyosis (excessive dryness) of the skin characterized by dry, rough discolorations with scaly desquamation (shedding of the epithelium in small sheets). This problem is exacerbated by drying skin cleansers or soaps, contact with disinfectants or solvents, and dry climates.

Unusual spots, rashes, moles, cysts, fibromas, nodules, edema, and/or changes in nail beds will likely be observed by therapists, as virtually everyone experiences some sort of skin issue at some point in their lives (Box 10.3). Any unusual spot that has appeared recently or changed since initial appearance should be examined by a qualified health care provider. On the legs, varicosities and signs of poor venous return may be indicated by changes in skin pigmentation, turgor, and texture. Lower extremity edema can be a sign of multiple systemic conditions, including heart, kidney, or liver disease.

SPECIAL IMPLICATIONS FOR THE THERAPIST 10.1

### *Skin Lesions*

The therapist must remain alert to skin changes that might indicate the onset or progression of a systemic condition or the presence of skin cancer. Any time a patient reports signs or symptoms of skin lesions, evaluation and documentation are warranted, and referral may be required. It is best to use proper lighting, measurement tools, and photography to aid clinical assessment.

**Table 10.1** Skin Structure

| Layer | Structure[a] | Function |
|---|---|---|
| Epidermis | Stratum corneum | Protection (from trauma, microbes); barrier (prevents fluid, electrolyte, and chemical loss) |
| | Keratinocytes (squamous cells) | Synthesis of keratin (skin protein) |
| | Langerhans cells | Antigen presentation; immune response |
| | Basal cells | Epidermal reproduction |
| Dermis | Collagen, reticulum, elastin | Skin proteins; skin texture |
| | Fibroblasts | Collagen synthesis for skin strength and wound healing |
| | Macrophages | Phagocytosis of foreign substances; initiates inflammation and repair |
| | Mast cells | Provide histamine for vasodilation and chemotactic factors for inflammatory responses |
| | Lymphatic glands | Removal of microbes and excess interstitial fluids; provide lymphatic drainage |
| | Blood vessels | Provide metabolic skin requirements; thermoregulation |
| | Nerve fibers | Perception of heat, cold, pain, itching |
| Epidermal appendages | Eccrine unit | Thermoregulation by perspiration |
| | Apocrine unit | Production of apocrine sweat |
| | Hair follicles | Production of hair; cavity enclosing hair |
| | Nails | Protection; mechanical assistance |
| | Sebaceous glands | Produce sebum (oil to lubricate skin) |
| Subcutaneous tissue | Adipose (fat) | Energy storage and balance; trauma absorption |

[a]Understanding the structure of the integument is important in wound management. Knowing why a wound closes the way it does is an essential assessment tool.

Modified from Nicol NH: Structure and function: assessment of clients with integumentary disorders. In Black JM, Matassarin-Jacobs E, editors. *Medical surgical nursing*, ed 5, Philadelphia, 1997, Saunders, p 2176.

**Box 10.1**

**CAUSES OF SKIN LESIONS (NOT INCLUSIVE)**

- Hereditary factors
- Physical trauma (e.g., pressure, laceration)
- Systemic origin (e.g., diseases with a cutaneous manifestation; vascular insufficiency, diabetes mellitus)
- Burns (thermal, electrical, chemical, inhalation)
- Dehisced surgical wounds
- Neoplasm (paraneoplastic syndrome)
- Reaction to radiotherapy
- Contact with infective organisms
- Reaction to medication
- Contact with injurious agents (e.g., chemical toxins)
- Reaction to allergens

**Box 10.2**

**SYSTEMIC CAUSES OF PRURITUS (NOT INCLUSIVE)**

- Candidiasis (systemic, intestinal)
- Solid tumor malignancies
- Diabetes mellitus
- Drug hypersensitivity
- Hyperthyroidism
- Intestinal parasites
- Iron deficiency anemia
- Leukemia
- Liver disease
- Lymphomas
- Polycythemia rubra vera
- Renal disease

Certain skin lesions should be examined by a qualified health care provider because of their premalignant status (e.g., actinic keratosis; slightly raised, red, scaly papules; and sebaceous cysts). A seborrheic keratosis is a common benign skin tumor that may mimic more serious lesions and may bleed when irritated by friction.[223] If these nonmalignant tumors develop in areas associated with high friction, they can easily be removed by a qualified health care provider.

In the case of pruritus, regardless of the cause, the therapist can offer practical suggestions to help soothe skin, ease itching, and prevent skin damage (Box 10.4). Bullous skin lesions are associated with risk of exposure to pathogens comparable to those in blood, and therefore adherence to Standard Precautions while treating anyone with skin lesions or burns is required.

When examining and documenting the presence of a skin disorder, note the location, size, irregularities in color, temperature, moisture, ulceration, texture, thickness, mobility, edema, turgor, odor, and tenderness (Box 10.5). If more than one lesion is present, note the pattern of distribution (localized, isolated, regional, general, universal). Document whether lesions are unilateral or bilateral, symmetric or asymmetric, and/or clustered or linear, especially if they occur as a result of contact with clothing, jewelry, or other objects.

**Box 10.3**

**SIGNS AND SYMPTOMS OF SKIN DISORDERS (NOT INCLUSIVE)**

- Pruritus
- Urticaria
- Rash
- Blisters
- Xerosis (dry skin)
- Unusual spots, moles, nodules, cysts
- Edema
- Changes in appearance of nails
- Changes in skin pigmentation, turgor, texture

Blisters may be associated with a variety of skin conditions, such as frostbite, dermatitis, burns, pressure, or malignancy or may occur as a side effect of medications. Blisters that are infected or located over joints and limiting motion should be débrided. Exceptions to this are hemorrhagic frostbite blisters[160,179] and stable noninfected arterial and heel blisters, which should be left in place and monitored for signs of infection or deep injury.[98,210] Small flat blisters with a known uncomplicated etiology may remain intact if quick fluid reabsorption is expected. In burn injuries, blisters are typically débrided based on size, location, severity of the heat source, risk of infection, and overall patient status.[132] Débridement of blisters in burn injuries, when appropriate, allows for direct examination, evaluation, and treatment of underlying injured tissues.

Although an intact blister is theoretically sterile, unintentional opening or tearing can introduce bacteria under the dead epidermal layer where coagulated blister fluid provides an ideal medium for bacterial growth. Blister fluid can also be detrimental, as it contains chemical factors that increase local vasoconstriction and inflammation and can retard normal fibrinolysis.[195]

Special skin care when working with older adults is very important. Avoiding shear and friction during treatment and repositioning is essential to avoid skin tears. Extreme caution is also necessary when using electrical or thermal modalities (heat or cold). Decreased circulation, reduced subcutaneous adipose tissue, and altered metabolism create a situation where initial skin resistance to electricity and poor dissipation of heat or cold can lead to tissue damage. Using appropriate skin moisturizers and nonadherent wound dressings and avoiding adhesives are also important steps in protecting the skin of older patients.

### Laboratory Values

Many factors affect the progression of a skin lesion to an open wound and the individual's subsequent ability to heal, including tobacco use, psychosocial status (e.g., comatose, homeless), and nutritional status. Laboratory values such as prealbumin (to indicate nutritional status) and glucose, hemoglobin, and hematocrit (to monitor wound healing) provide the therapist with necessary information for developing and implementing a safe and effective intervention plan.

**Box 10.4**

**SKIN CARE STRATEGIES**

***Reduce Pruritus***

- Avoid scratching.
- Keep fingernails trimmed short to prevent damage in case of unconscious or nighttime scratching.
- Bathe with nondrying, unscented soap or other agent when indicated.
- Use soothing bath products such as Aveeno oatmeal, mineral oil, or cottonseed oil added to warm, not hot, bath water.
- Systemic sclerosis: Apply cooling agents such as menthol or camphor (e.g., contained in Sarna lotion) to the affected areas.
- Psoriasis: Try skin preparations such as creams containing capsaicin, chaparral, or aloe (some advocate the use of pure aloe). Do not apply hot pepper creams on broken skin.
- Discuss with a physician the possible use of an alpha hydroxy acid product or other prescription cream containing urea to dissolve the outer layer of skin and remove dead scales.
- Second-rinse clothing and bedding to remove residual laundry soap; avoid use of fabric softeners.
- Wear open-weave, loose-fitting, cotton-blend fabrics to allow air to circulate and minimize perspiration, thereby reducing the risk of pruritus; avoid rough, wool, or tightly woven fabrics.
- Avoid temperature extremes that can trigger itching secondary to vasodilation and increased cutaneous blood flow. Avoid hot water (baths or hot tubs) for the same reason.
- Take antihistamines to reduce itching according to physician recommendation.
- Shower or bathe with mild soap immediately after swimming to remove residual chlorine or chemicals from the skin.

***Reduce Inflammation***

- Apply topical steroids (lotion, solution, gel, cream, or ointment) to affected areas as directed. Topical steroids are used to reduce skin inflammation, relieve itching, and control flare-ups of dermatitis and psoriasis. The proper preparation depends on the location and severity of the lesions and should not be applied to normal skin.
- Apply tar preparations (lotion, solution, gel, cream, ointment, or shampoo) to affected skin as directed. (Some tar preparations can be added to bath water.) The antiinflammatory properties of tars are not as fast-acting as topical steroids, but the effect is longer-lasting with fewer side effects.
- Tar preparations should not be used on acutely inflamed skin, as this may cause burning or irritation.

***Maintain Skin Hydration***

- Bathing has been discouraged because of its alleged drying effect, but some skin care professionals advocate the use of soaks in a warm (not hot) bath for 15 to 20 minutes, suggesting that soaking for 15 to 20 minutes allows the stratum corneum to become saturated with water.
- Other skin care professionals recommend only showers or brief baths.
- Both groups agree that drying of the skin is the result of failure to immediately apply the appropriate occlusive moisture, thereby allowing evaporation to occur. Avoid vigorous or brisk towel drying, as this removes more water from the skin and increases vasodilation; gently and quickly pat dry. Immediately (within 2 to 4 minutes) apply an appropriate emollient or prescribed topical agent after bathing.

***Avoid Sun (Light) Exposure***

- Wear sun-protective clothing with tightly woven material covering as much of the body as possible (e.g., long sleeves, long pants, neckline with a collar, hat with broad brim, UVA/UVB-protective sunglasses).
- Avoiding sitting near a window for prolonged periods of time.
- Avoid outdoor activities during peak sunlight hours (10:00 a.m. to 4:00 p.m. in most time zones but may vary geographically). Limit sun exposure during nonpeak hours.
- Avoid fluorescent lighting or reflected sunlight.
- Wear sunscreen daily year-round, even on cloudy days.
- Apply sunscreen 20 to 30 minutes before sun exposure to ensure maximum absorption. Sunscreen preparations must provide a minimum UVB sun protective factor (SPF) of 30 plus a UVA sunscreen for anyone with a current skin condition or who is at risk for skin cancer. A sunscreen of SPF 15 is considered adequate for others not meeting this criterion.
- Reapply sunscreen every 2 hours if swimming, exposed to wind, or perspiring. Sunscreens are not recommended for infants younger than 6 months of age. Infants of this age should be kept out of direct sunlight.
- Do not increase sun exposure because of sunscreen use. High SPF has been shown to lead to increased time spent in the sun by 25%.

## AGING AND THE INTEGUMENTARY SYSTEM

Skin undergoes numerous changes throughout the life span. Beginning at birth, skin is a dynamic organ. While variable across individuals, adaptation and change occur in infancy that affect skin acidification, barrier function, and hydration, bringing levels similar to that of an adult.[94,146,251] Obvious changes also occur during puberty and again during older adulthood. Hormone changes during puberty stimulate the maturation of hair follicles, sebaceous glands, and apocrine and eccrine sweat glands in certain body areas.[47] Mild acne, perspiration and body odor, freckles (promoted by sun exposure), and pigmented nevi (moles) commonly occur.

During adolescence and adulthood, the use of birth control pills or pregnancy may result in temporary changes in hair growth patterns or hyperpigmentation of the cheeks and forehead known as *melasma* or *pregnancy mask*.[95] Other hormonal abnormalities may result in excessive facial and body hair in women (androgen-related)[125,148] and male-pattern baldness (alopecia) in men.[264]

The skin exhibits changes that denote the onset of senescence (the process or condition of growing old). These changes are due to the aging process itself (intrinsic aging) and to extrinsic aging. Extrinsic aging is dominated by the cumulative effects of exposure to sunlight (photoaging) and, to a lesser degree, to factors such as cigarette smoking[239] (via smoke toxicity, vasoconstriction, and

**Box 10.5**

**DOCUMENTATION OF SKIN LESIONS**

***Characteristics***

- Size (measure all dimensions)
- Shape or configuration
- Color
- Temperature
- Tenderness, pain, or pruritus
- Texture
- Mobility; skin turgor
- Elevation (height) or depression
- Pedunculation (stemlike connections)

***Exudates***

- Color
- Odor
- Amount
- Consistency

***Pattern of Arrangement***

- Annular (rings)
- Grouped
- Linear
- Arciform (bow-shaped)
- Diffuse

***Location and Distribution***

- Generalized, localized, or universal
- Region of the body; unilateral or bilateral; symmetric or asymmetric
- Patterns (dermatomal, flexor or extensor, random, related to clothing lines or jewelry)
- Discrete or confluent (running together)

Modified from Hill MJ: *Skin disorders*, St. Louis, 1994, Mosby, p 18.

**Table 10.2** Effects of Aging on the Skin

| Structural | Functional |
|---|---|
| **Epidermis** | |
| Flattening of the dermal–epidermal junction | Decreased ability to resist friction and shear forces |
| Changes in basal cells | Decreased inflammatory responsiveness |
| Decreased number of Langerhans cells | Decreased immunologic responsiveness; increased risk of skin cancer; increased sensitivity to allergens |
| Decreased number of melanocytes | Impaired wound healing; loss of photoprotection with increased risk of skin cancer |
| **Dermis** | |
| Decreased dermal thickness; degeneration of elastin fibers | Decreased elasticity; increased wrinkling, slow wound healing, less scar tissue (cosmetic benefit) |
| Decreased vascularization | Decreased vitamin D production; slow wound healing |
| **Appendages** | |
| Decreased number and distorted structure of sweat glands | Decreased eccrine sweating; altered skin thermoregulation |
| Decreased number and distorted structure of specialized nerve endings | Impaired sensory perception; increased pain threshold |
| Decreased hair bulb melanocytes and decreased number of hair follicles | Change in hair color (gray, white); hair loss |

mechanical facial expressions).[46] As aging occurs, both structural and functional changes occur in the skin (Table 10.2),[38,239] resulting clinically in diminished pain perception, increased vulnerability to injury and irritants, decreased vascularity, decreased rate of epidermal turnover, and decreased capacity for healing.[239] Skin tear prevention strategies are particularly critical to consider (e.g., fingernail length maintenance [caregiver and patient]), avoidance of adhesives, caution with patient mobility) to mitigate skin tear risk.[38]

Visible indications of skin changes associated with aging include gray hair, balding and loss of secondary sexual hair, and increased facial hair. For women, excessive facial hair may occur along the upper lip and around the chin. Women may also experience balding after menopause. Men frequently develop increased facial hair in the nares, eyebrows, and helix of the ear.[239]

Other common age-related integumentary changes include lax skin, vascular changes (e.g., decreased elasticity of blood vessel walls, angiomas) (Fig. 10.2), dermal or epidermal degenerative changes, and wrinkling.[194,239] Wrinkling signifies loss of elastin fibers, weakened collagen, and decreased subcutaneous fat and is accelerated by above-noted extrinsic factors.[194,239]

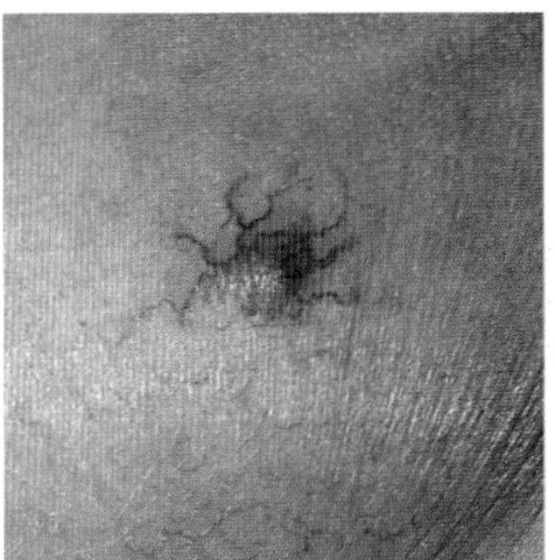
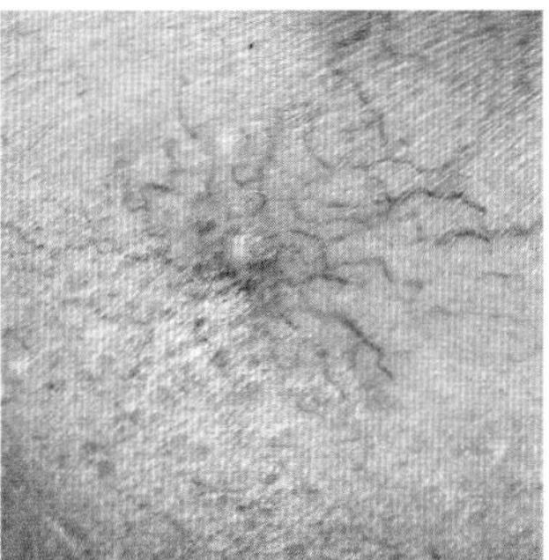

**Figure. 10.2**

**Spider angioma.** Spider angioma (arterial spider, spider telangiectasia, vascular spider) is so called because it consists of a central arteriole with numerous radiating small vessels resembling a spider's legs (ranging from pinhead size to 0.5 cm in diameter). Common sites are the necklace area, face, forearms, and dorsum of the hand. These lesions may be associated with rosacea, basal cell carcinoma, systemic sclerosis, pregnancy, liver disease, or estrogen therapy or may occur by themselves. (From Habif T: *Clinical dermatology*, ed 4, St. Louis, 2004, Mosby, Figs. 23.20, 23.21, p 830.)

With aging, blood vessels within the dermis are reduced in number, and the walls are thinned. This compromises blood flow and manifests as pale skin with impaired capacity to thermoregulate, a possible contributing factor to the increased susceptibility of older individuals to hypothermia and hyperthermia. Many other benign changes may occur, including seborrheic keratoses (brown/black wartlike growths), lentigines (liver spots, unrelated to the liver and secondary to sun exposure), and skin tags (small flesh-colored papules).

A primary factor in the loss of protective functions of the skin is the diminished barrier function of the stratum corneum (outermost layer of the epidermis) (see Fig. 10.1). As this layer becomes thinner, the skin becomes translucent and paper-thin, reacting more readily to minor changes in humidity, temperature, and other irritants. There are also fewer melanocytes, resulting in decreased protection against UV radiation.[239] A significant decrease in the number of Langerhans cells occurs with aging so that by the time a person reaches age 70, only half the number of Langerhans cells remains compared with early adulthood. A reduction in Langerhans cells represents a loss of immune surveillance and an increased risk of skin cancer.[133]

The epidermis is also one of the body's principal suppliers of vitamin D, which is produced when the hormone, 7-dehydrocholesterol, is exposed to sunlight. As people age, levels of this hormone decrease, which contributes to vitamin D deficiency. Vitamin D deficiency plays a role in bone mass and thus is linked to osteoporosis.[161]

It is generally agreed that one of the most significant contributors to skin disorders, diseases, and aging is oxidative damage that occurs to the skin as a result of environmental exposures and endogenous (within the skin itself) factors.[239] The skin is rich in lipids, proteins, and DNA, all of which are extremely sensitive to the oxidation process. Scientists are developing methods of decreasing protein cross-linking and accelerating increased collagen to slow down and aid in reversing the oxidation process.

Skin changes at the end of life may occur unrelated to quality of care. Changes may occur as part of the dying process when skin, similar to other organs, becomes dysfunctional and shuts down.[209]

**SPECIAL IMPLICATIONS FOR THE THERAPIST 10.2**

### *Aging and the Integumentary System*

The therapist must remain alert to changes in skin, as age-associated blunting of vascular and immune responses may produce subtle findings in older adults compared with younger patients with similar disorders. Vascular changes may also affect thermoregulation and wound healing, requiring careful consideration when planning therapy intervention.

Additionally, loss of collagen increases susceptibility of skin trauma owing to shearing forces and increases the risk of pressure injuries.[38] Wound healing is impaired in intrinsically aged skin compared with young skin in that the rate of healing is appreciably slower,[194] but paradoxically the resultant scar is usually more cosmetically acceptable.

Skin diseases and symptoms caused by skin disorders are also exceedingly common among older people. Although these disorders are not usually life threatening, they provoke anxiety and psychologic distress. Owing to the nature of skin exposure common in physical therapy, it is not uncommon for the therapist to be the first health care professional to observe a skin lesion.

It is important to ask about physical findings in other parts of the body (e.g., patient may not mention genital lesions, may be unaware of the significance of other symptoms). All dermatologic lesions must be examined by a qualified health care provider, and anyone with evidence of sun damage should have a full skin examination annually.

**A THERAPIST'S THOUGHTS[a]**

Older adults may present with intrinsic, extrinsic, and iatrogenic factors that may impact wound healing. It is best to consider a collaborative health care team approach to address modifiable factors in older adults. Research has shown a strong direct and indirect relationship between psychologic stress and wound healing. Psychologic stress may impair cellular immunity. Therefore the practitioner should mitigate stress for optimal wound healing.

[a]Alan Chong W. Lee, PT, PhD, DPT, CWS, GCS

## COMMON SKIN DISORDERS

### Atopic Dermatitis

#### Definition and Incidence

Atopic dermatitis (AD) is a chronic or relapsing inflammatory skin disease characterized by pruritus.[87,162,193] AD is among the most common types of eczema, often already present during the first year of life and affecting up to 30% of children.[32,62] In a longitudinal study of 7157 patients, investigators showed that AD symptoms frequently persist into adulthood.[164] AD is one manifestation of atopy that often appears before the development of allergic rhinitis or asthma.[32] The word *atopic* refers to a group of three associated allergic disorders: asthma, allergic rhinitis (hay fever), and AD.[162] Patients with AD often have a personal or family history of allergic disorders, including food allergies.[32]

#### Etiologic and Risk Factors and Pathogenesis

The cause and pathology of AD are multifaceted and include genetic, immunologic, and environmental factors. Two risk factors that have been linked to the development of AD are family history and aberrant skin barrier gene coding (filaggrin mutation).[32,162] It is unclear if inflammation exacerbates dysfunction with the skin barrier or if a problem with the skin barrier causes immune dysregulation.[211] Stress and emotional problems can worsen AD but do not cause it. Other triggers may include animal dander and the use of alkaline soaps or other products that alter the skin pH.[162] AD is often associated with increased levels of serum immunoglobulin E and with sensitization to food allergens.[87] Some foods may be responsible for exacerbations of skin inflammation, but

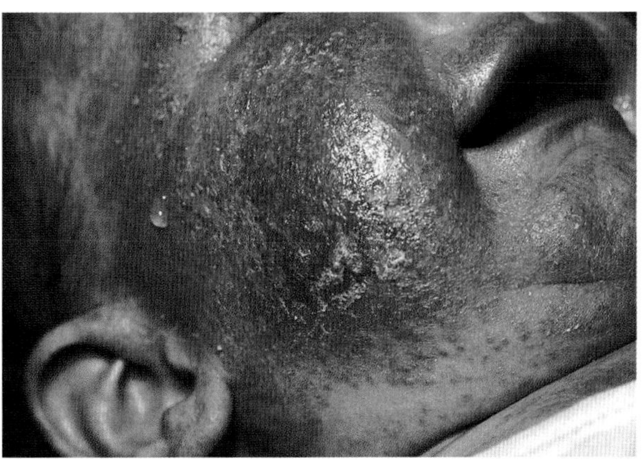

**Figure. 10.3**

**Infantile atopic dermatitis with oozing and crusting lesions.** (From Paller A, Mancini A: *Hurwitz clinical pediatric dermatology: a textbook of skin disorders of childhood and adolescence*, ed 3, Philadelphia, 2006, Saunders.)

their pathogenic role must be clinically assessed before an avoidance diet is recommended solely by allergy testing.[87] Xerosis (abnormal dryness) associated with AD is usually worse during periods of low humidity and over the winter months in northern latitudes.

Pathologic findings may be a result of the dry skin rather than the cause of the drying effects of this condition. Compared with normal skin, dry skin associated with AD has a reduced water-binding capacity, a higher transepidermal water loss, and a decreased water content.[193] Rubbing and scratching of itchy skin are responsible for many of the clinical changes seen in the skin, specifically lichenification.[32] Hands frequently in and out of water make the condition worse.

### Clinical Manifestations

For many, AD begins during infancy in the form of a red, oozing, crusting rash classified as acute dermatitis that typically spares the diaper area (Fig. 10.3).[32] As the child grows, the chronic form of dermatitis results in skin that is dry, thickened, and brownish gray in color (lichenified).[32] The rash tends to become localized to the large folds of the extremities as the person becomes older. It is found mainly on flexor surfaces, such as the anterior neck, sides of the face, eyelids, and dorsal surface of the hands and feet. Hand and foot dermatitis can become a significant problem for some people.

Xerosis and pruritus are the major symptoms of AD and cause the greatest morbidity, with severely excoriated lesions, infection, and scarring.[32,87] Sleep is often negatively affected.[88] Viral, bacterial, and fungal secondary skin infections may cause further skin changes. *Staphylococcus aureus* is the most common bacterial infection, resulting in extensive crusting with serous weeping, folliculitis (inflammation of hair follicles), pyoderma (pus), and furunculosis (boils).[32]

## MEDICAL MANAGEMENT

**DIAGNOSIS, TREATMENT, AND PROGNOSIS.** Although no cure exists, the burden of AD can be reduced through medical management and patient/caregiver education. Each patient should be evaluated individually owing to symptomatic variability of the disease. The goal of medical intervention is to break the inflammatory cycle that causes excess drying, cracking, itching, and scratching.[87,193] Topicals and systemic medications (e.g., antibiotics, antihistamines, antimicrobials, corticosteroids, immunosuppressants, nonsteroidals)[162] may be helpful, as well as adjuvant therapies (UV irradiation). *S. aureus*, known to colonize the skin of people with AD, may exacerbate skin lesions and needs to be treated with antibiotics. Superinfection with disease exacerbation is also treated with antimicrobial medications.[87,150,152]

Education is focused on controlling or minimizing triggers and skin care.[212] Personal hygiene, daily moisturizing of the skin, and avoidance of irritants is paramount. Dietary recommendations should be specific and given only in cases of diagnosed food allergy. A new addendum to guidelines includes early introduction to foods with peanuts as appropriate to prevent peanut allergy.[87] Allergen-specific immunotherapy to aeroallergens may be useful in selected cases. In the case of stress-induced exacerbations, behavioral counseling may be helpful.[150,152] Advancing knowledge of the disease process will continue to result in new local and systemic treatments. Updated guidelines for the treatment of this condition are available[87,150,152,193] and should be discussed with a qualified health care provider.

**SPECIAL IMPLICATIONS FOR THE THERAPIST 10.3**

### *Atopic Dermatitis*

The therapist may be instrumental in providing education that allows the patient to avoid factors that precipitate or exacerbate inflammation and prevent or limit flare-ups. Daily care (hydration and lubrication) of the skin is vital, and applications (two or three times daily) of moisturizers that occlude the skin to prevent evaporation and retain moisture should be recommended.

Creams or ointments containing petrolatum may be used (see Contact Dermatitis for sensitivity to lanolin); those that contain urea or lactic acid improve the binding of water in the skin and prevent evaporation. In the case of skin redness, the skin lesion must be identified first because of possible fungal origin requiring an antifungal preparation. Understanding the individual disease pattern and identifying exacerbating factors are crucial to effective management. Older patients should be encouraged to bathe with tepid water, using a nondrying, unscented soap or other agent when indicated. Moisturizers should be applied to the body soon after bathing. All patients should be encouraged not to overbathe.[87]

Dermatitis must be considered a precaution, if not a contraindication, to some treatment modalities used by therapists. The use of water, alcohol, or any topical agents containing alcohol should be avoided. Topical agents, such as ultrasound gel and mobilization creams, must be used carefully, observing for any skin reaction. A nonreactive response does not guarantee the patient will not react when such agents are subsequently applied in future interventions. Caution and careful observation are encouraged.

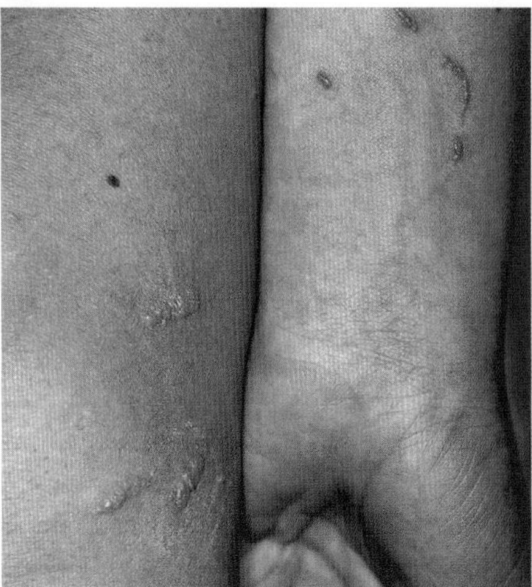

**Figure. 10.4**

**Primary contact dermatitis, a local inflammatory reaction, can occur in response to an irritant in the environment or an allergy.** Characteristic location of lesions often gives a clue to the cause. Erythema occurs first, followed by swelling, wheals or urticaria, or maculopapular vesicles accompanied by intense pruritus. The example shown here is a result of contact with poison ivy. (From Paller A, Mancini A: *Hurwitz clinical pediatric dermatology: A textbook of skin disorders of childhood and adolescence*, ed 3, Philadelphia, 2006, Saunders.)

## Contact Dermatitis

### Etiologic Factors, Incidence, and Pathogenesis

Contact dermatitis can be an acute or chronic skin inflammation caused by exposure to an external agent, that may act as an irritant or allergen. The offender could be a chemical, mechanical, physical, or biologic agent, including topical medications,[177] fragrance,[134] common items (e.g., silicone cell phone covers), or medical devices (e.g., insulin pumps).[118,256] Contact dermatitis is one of the most common environmental skin diseases and can occur at any age. However, as people age, acute dermatitis can occur because of skin and immune changes related to age.[55] Common allergens include nickel (found in jewelry),[134] wool fats (particularly lanolin found in moisturizers and skin creams), rubber additives, topical antibiotics (neomycin, bacitracin),[134,177] and topical anesthetics such as benzocaine or lidocaine.[65,177] Corticosteroids, often used to treat contact dermatitis, may also cause it.[177] Dermatitis of unknown cause is more commonly diagnosed in older people.

A small percentage of the population is allergic to silicone. The therapist might see this reaction in a sensitized person with an amputation using a silicone prosthetic liner, a patient using silicone-based wound dressings, or in a person using silicone sheets for scar reduction after a burn injury. Other silicone-related contact dermatitis cases have also been reported.[188,200,256]

### Clinical Manifestations

Intense pruritus, erythema (redness), and edema of the skin can occur 1 to 2 days after exposure in previously sensitized persons. Clinical manifestations begin at the site of exposure but can extend to more distant sites. These conditions may progress to vesiculation, oozing (watery discharges), crusting, and scaling (Fig. 10.4). If symptoms persist, the skin becomes thickened, with prominent skin markings and pigmentation changes. Older people can have a less pronounced inflammatory response to irritants compared with younger persons and may have delayed symptoms.

### MEDICAL MANAGEMENT

**DIAGNOSIS, TREATMENT, AND PROGNOSIS.** If contact dermatitis is suspected, the patient should be referred to a qualified health care provider. Acute lesions usually resolve in 3 weeks; chronic lesions persist until the causative agent has been removed. A detailed history and careful examination frequently are all that are needed to make the diagnosis.[134] Patch testing may be performed for the identification of the causative agent.[131] However, with aging, there are more instances where there is increased sensitivity on patch testing without clinical symptoms. This may show development of tolerance.[168]

Primary treatment is removal of the offending agent; treatment of the skin is secondary and similar to treatment for AD.[134] If known allergens are unavoidable, therapies to suppress the immune system may be beneficial.[16]

SPECIAL IMPLICATIONS FOR THE THERAPIST 10.4

### *Contact Dermatitis*

The therapist should always consider the patient's reaction to external substances, particularly when creams, topical agents, or solutions are used. Various modalities used within the profession may involve causative substances (e.g., whirlpool additives, ultrasound gels, self-sticking electrode pads).[65,177] The patient's skin must be examined before and after intervention for the appearance of adverse reactions. The patient should be instructed to report any discomfort or unusual findings during or after treatment to the therapist.

The person with contact dermatitis associated with the use of a silicone sleeve or prosthetic device liner should be cautioned about the use of soaps that do not include a rinsing agent, as residue on the skin combined with device friction can result in skin irritation or breakdown. In this case, the therapist may suggest the use of alcohol-based lubricants, soap-free cleansing agents, and petroleum-based ointments that can be applied to the limb before donning the liner. Water-based ointments should be avoided when using urethane liners because these can cause the normally tacky urethane to adhere to the skin so that when the liner is removed, bits of skin may be pulled off. Alcohol-based lubricants or soaps should also be avoided with urethane products because these components act as a solvent on urethane and can increase adherence.[26]

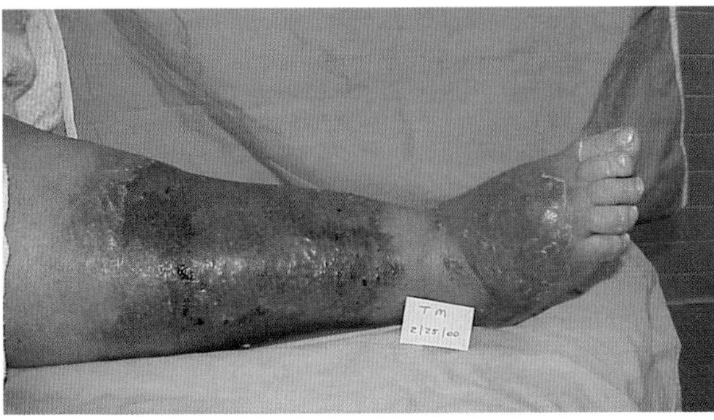

**Figure. 10.5**

**Stasis dermatitis secondary to venous insufficiency.** Hemosiderin staining (dark pigmentation) indicative of venous insufficiency is evident. Staining is caused by leakage of hemosiderin (an iron-rich pigment, the product of red cell hemolysis) as a result of blood that cannot return because of valvular incompetence. (Courtesy Harriett B. Loehne, PT, DPT, CWS, FACCWS. Used with permission.)

## Eczema and Dermatitis

### Definition and Overview

*Eczema* and *dermatitis* are often used interchangeably to describe a group of disorders with a characteristic appearance. Eczema (dermatitis) is a superficial itchy inflammation of the skin caused by irritant exposure (irritant dermatitis), allergic sensitization or delayed hypersensitivity (allergic or atopic dermatitis), or genetically determined idiopathic factors. Other types of dermatitis include seborrheic (scalp), nummular (discoid), and stasis dermatitis. Up to 40% of people with eczema have other atopic conditions such as food hypersensitivities, allergic rhinitis, and asthma.[58]

Eczema (dermatitis) is often characterized by periods of remittance and relapse[58] with three primary stages (acute, subacute, and chronic) that may manifest separately or coexist. *Acute dermatitis* is characterized by extensive erosions with serous exudate or intensely pruritic erythematous papules and vesicles.[165] *Subacute dermatitis* is characterized by erythematous, excoriated (scratched, abraded), scaling papules or plaques grouped or scattered over erythematous skin. Often the scaling is so fine and diffuse the skin appears to have a silvery sheen. *Chronic dermatitis* is characterized by thickened skin with increased skin marking (lichenification) secondary to rubbing and scratching; excoriated papules, fibrotic papules, and nodules (prurigo nodularis); and postinflammatory hyperpigmentation and hypopigmentation.[165]

### Incidence and Etiologic Factors

Dermatitis is a common skin disorder in children as well as older adults. It may be caused by hypoproteinemia, venous insufficiency, allergens, irritants, or underlying malignancy (e.g., leukemia, lymphoma). Because older people often take multiple medications, dermatitis from drug interaction can occur.[44] The normal aging process, including flattened epidermal–dermal junctions and thinning of the dermis, results in skin fragility and contributes to the development of skin tears and dermatitis.[194]

## Stasis Dermatitis

Stasis dermatitis is the development of erythematous itchy plaques that may open to form shallow ulcers on the lower legs. This form of dermatitis is one of several skin manifestations caused by underlying venous hypertension and resultant venous insufficiency (Fig. 10.5).[213,227] Increased venous pressure occurs with venous obstruction or when damaged/incompetent valves inside the veins permit retrograde venous flow, allowing for insufficient return of venous blood.[210,227] High venous pressure pushes red blood cells, proteins, and other cells normally retained within the vessel into the interstitial space, resulting in extravascular inflammation, increased tissue edema, and impaired tissue diffusion rates. Stasis dermatitis results when the local tissue environment is insufficient to maintain the health and viability of the skin. A history of varicose veins (indicative of high venous pressure), deep vein thrombosis (which can damage venous valves), and/or loss of the calf muscle pump may also be present.

Treatment of stasis dermatitis is aimed toward reducing venous hypertension. Compression is the gold standard for treating chronic venous insufficiency and includes the use of multilayer compression wraps and sleeves, pneumatic compression, and stockings.[213,227] Gait training and exercise are vital, as muscular contract–relax cycles act as a physical pump to assist with venous return. Medications that alter vessel tone and permeability, as well as laser ablation and minimally invasive surgical procedures to remove damaged veins, are other treatment options.[227]

## Environmental Dermatoses

Common environmental skin diseases seen in physical therapy practice include irritant and allergic dermatitis, acne lesions, pigmentary changes (hyperpigmentation, hypopigmentation, absence of pigmentation), photosensitivity reactions, systemic sclerosis (SSc), infectious disorders, and cutaneous malignancy. Each of these environmentally induced skin conditions is discussed later in this chapter.

## Rosacea

Rosacea is a common chronic facial disorder of middle-aged and older people. While it is most commonly seen in individuals with fair skin, rosacea has been diagnosed in patients with varying degrees of skin tone, including those of Asian and African descent.[8,97] Although rosacea is a form of acne, it is differentiated by age, the presence of a large vascular component (erythema, telangiectasis, flushing), and usually the absence of comedones.[97] No known cause or factor has been identified to explain the pathogenesis of this disorder.[37] It is currently considered a condition with vascular and inflammatory components in the presence of an altered innate immune response.[73,89]

Clinically the cheeks, nose, and chin (sometimes the entire face) may have a persistent rosy appearance marked by reddened skin.[144] Other symptoms may include pustules, papules, burning or stinging, episodic flushing, and facial edema.[97] Changes in body and/or environmental temperatures, UV radiation exposure, and spicy foods can trigger flare-ups.[224,253] The condition may worsen over time, resulting in lasting redness, pimples, telangiectasias, and/or nasal hypertrophy (rhinophyma). It is not uncommon to have associated ophthalmic disease including blepharitis and keratitis.

Medical management aimed at the inflammatory papules, pustules, and surrounding erythema may include topical and/or systemic therapies that act as immunomodulators to restore cutaneous homeostasis.[89] Laser and other light-based interventions are also beneficial in decreasing the erythematous discoloration and presence of telangiectasia common in rosacea.[144]

### Incontinence-Associated Dermatitis

Incontinence-associated dermatitis (IAD) describes skin damage resulting from chronic urine or feces exposure.[42] As such, IAD commonly occurs in the perineum between the anus and external genitalia but can extend to encompass much broader areas of skin. By definition, IAD is clinically and pathologically distinct from intertriginous dermatitis (dermatitis of the skin folds) and other types of moisture-associated skin breakdown from saliva, wound drainage, or perspiration.[108]

While there is a clear link between IAD and pressure injuries, IAD is not caused by pressure, and therefore differential diagnosis between the two is vital, as prevention and treatment for each condition are vastly different. Understanding that IAD injuries are not necessarily located over bony prominences and rarely cause full-thickness skin injury unless there is an infection can assist in accurate diagnosis.

IAD is characterized by pink or red discoloration with erythema and may or may not manifest with erosion of skin and maceration. Burning, itching, and/or tingling may occur. Associated skin changes in individuals with dark skin tones may appear yellow, dark red, purple, or white.[42,43]

Research supports the use of a skin care regimen based on principles of gentle cleansing and moisturizing, use of skin protectants, and limiting friction and shear during transfers and bed mobility.[42,43] Clinical experience also supports (1) application of an antifungal ointment or cream (powder is *not* recommended) in patients with evidence of cutaneous candidiasis, (2) briefless policy with urinary or fecal incontinence, and (3) highly selective use of a mild topical antiinflammatory product in selected cases.[109] Use of disposable briefs can cause worsening of the condition; the use of high-grade moisture-wicking underpads often provide a better option. Frequent monitoring is required to ensure the patient is kept clean and dry.

**SPECIAL IMPLICATIONS FOR THE THERAPIST 10.5**

*Incontinence-Associated Dermatitis*

Early assessment and recognition of skin changes (e.g., color, induration, tenderness) is important so that the plan of care includes appropriate interventions to minimize and prevent worsening (tissue weeping, infection, skin denudement). The Kennedy and Lutz skin assessment tool can be used to classify IAD,[141] and the Incontinence-Associated Dermatitis Intervention Tool (IADIT) can help guide nursing and physical therapy staff in providing skin care. More recent best practice principles recommend using the IAD Severity Categorisation Tool,[42] which presents categories to help guide clinical decision making. Experts agree that evidence is lacking to provide specific products and protocols in the prevention and treatment of this condition, but efforts have been made to provide health care providers with consensus statements and best practice recommendations.[42,85,109]

Differentiating IAD from pressure injuries is important in providing appropriate problem-specific care. Individuals with IAD may not need position changes or pressure redistribution devices (e.g., specialty mattress) saving time and reducing costs. It is important to remember, however, that excess moisture puts the patient at high risk for developing pressure injuries.

## SKIN INFECTIONS

Many bacterial, viral, fungal, and other parasitic skin infections encountered by the therapist are not the primary focus of intervention but rather occur in people who are hospitalized or being treated for other conditions. Many of these skin disorders are contagious (Table 10.3) and require careful handling by all health care professionals to avoid contracting and/or spreading the infection.

Sources of infection differ depending on the disease and mode of transmission. Predisposing factors to skin infections include decreased resistance, dehydrated skin, burns or pressure injuries, decreased perfusion, contamination from nasal discharge, poor hygiene, and crowded living conditions. Shaving body hair in preparation for the application of biophysical agents or adhesives can create microscopic nicks in the skin, which may allow bacteria and other surface pathogens to enter the body. Body hair should be cut or clipped to prevent skin damage and minimize the risk of skin infection.[259,260] Only the most common skin infections encountered in the therapy or rehabilitation setting are discussed further in this section.

### Bacterial Infections

Normal skin harbors a variety of bacterial flora, including major pathogenic varieties of staphylococci and streptococci. Pathogenicity depends on the invasiveness and virulence of the specific bacteria, skin integrity, and state of the immune and cellular defenses of the host. Openings in the skin (e.g., abrasions, scratches, punctures), especially on the hands, can be portals of entry for bacteria.

Individuals who are immunocompromised owing to acquired or inherited immunodeficiency or who are receiving immunosuppressive therapy have an increased risk of developing bacterial infections. Individuals with generalized malignancy (e.g., leukemia, lymphoma) and in poor general health are also at increased risk. Some conditions (e.g., impetigo) are easily spread by self-inoculation; therefore the affected person must be cautioned to avoid touching the involved area. Squeezing follicular

**Table 10.3** Infections of the Skin

| Type of Infection | Transmission |
|---|---|
| **Bacterial** | |
| Impetigo contagiosa | Contagious |
| Pyoderma | Contagious |
| Folliculitis (pimple, boil) | Contagious; minimal chance of spread |
| Cellulitis | Contagious[a] |
| **Viral** | |
| Verrucae (warts) | Contagious; self-inoculable[b] |
| Verruca plantaris (plantar wart) | Contagious; self-inoculable[b] |
| **Herpes simplex** | |
| Type 1: cold sore, fever blister | Contagious |
| Type 2: genital lesion | Contagious |
| Varicella-zoster virus (herpes zoster; shingles) | Contagious; chickenpox can occur in anyone with insufficient immunity |
| **Fungal** | |
| Tinea corporis (ringworm) | Person-to-person<br>Animal-to-person<br>Inanimate object–to–person |
| Tinea capitis (scalp) | Person-to-person<br>Animal-to-person |
| Tinea cruris (jock itch) | Person-to-person |
| Tinea pedis (athlete's foot) | Transmission to other people rare |
| Candidiasis | Person-to-person; transmitted during birth from mother to neonate |
| **Other** | |
| Scabies | Person-to-person; transmitted during birth from mother to neonate |
| Lice | Inanimate object–to–person<br>Same as scabies |

[a]Technically, cellulitis is contagious, but from a practical point of view the chances of transmission are very low and would require a susceptible host, for example, an open cut on the therapist's hand coming in contact with blood or pus from the patient's open wound.

[b]Capable of spreading infection to other locations on one's own body by scratching.

lesions may also spread infection, and all open wounds should be covered with an appropriate dressing to minimize exposure. All these factors emphasize the importance of careful, diligent handwashing and cleanliness by patients, caregivers, and health care professionals to prevent the spread of infection.

### Impetigo

**Definition and Overview.** Impetigo is a highly contagious superficial skin infection commonly caused by staphylococci or streptococci. It is most commonly found in infants, young children (i.e., 2 to 6 years of age), or older adults and occurs most often during hot, humid weather. Predisposing factors include close contact in schools, overcrowded living quarters, poor skin hygiene, anemia, malnutrition, and minor skin trauma.[91] Impetigo can be spread by direct contact or environmental contamination and often occurs as a secondary infection in conditions characterized by breaks in the skin (e.g., eczema, herpes zoster, mosquito bites).[114]

**Clinical Manifestations.** Small erythematous macules (flat spots) rapidly develop into erosive papular lesions or vesicles (small blisters) that become pustular (pus-filled). A less common presentation comprises a few isolated bullae. When vesicles break, the classic honey-colored crust develops from oozing lesions.[91] Itching is common, and scratching can spread the infection. Lesions frequently affect the face and extremities and typically close within 2 to 3 weeks without scarring.[114] Fever, pain, and cellulitis are uncommon in impetigo and if present may suggest another diagnosis or a more serious (methicillin-resistant *S. aureus*) or subcutaneous tissue infection.[91] If the infection is extensive, malaise, fever, and lymphadenopathy may be present.

## MEDICAL MANAGEMENT

Impetigo is generally considered a self-limiting infection; however, topical and/or systemic antibiotics covering both staphylococcal and streptococcal species are commonly used to hasten resolution. Rare complications of impetigo include cellulitis, septicemia, and poststreptococcal glomerulonephritis.[114]

### Cellulitis

Cellulitis is a rapidly spreading bacterial infection of the skin and subcutaneous tissue. *Streptococcus* and *Staphylococcus* species are the usual cause of this infection in adults,[228] and *Haemophilus influenzae* type b is the usual cause in children,[207] although other pathogens may be responsible. Symptoms of cellulitis include pain, advancing erythema, local edema, elevated temperature of affected skin, fever, chills, and malaise. Because cellulitis is not a reportable disease, the exact prevalence is uncertain. However, cellulitis is a relatively common infection affecting all racial and ethnic groups.

People at increased risk for cellulitis include older adults and immunocompromised individuals (e.g., owing to diabetes, malnutrition, chemotherapy, autoimmune diseases, steroid or immunosuppressant medications). Other predisposing factors include venous insufficiency, thrombophlebitis, obesity, edema, surgery, and substance abuse. Cutaneous inflammation, skin irritation, and open wounds (e.g., tinea, eczema, burns, trauma, bug bites) also increase the risk of developing cellulitis.[228]

While cellulitis may occur under the skin anywhere in the body, it most commonly affects the extremities and may be recurrent in cases of impaired lymphatic drainage (e.g., after axillary lymph node dissection, site of saphenous vein harvest). Repeated episodes of cellulitis may also occur because the initial infection was "controlled" but did not adequately resolve. Bilateral extremity presentation is rare, and other systemic etiologies should be considered in this instance.[228]

Cellulitis usually occurs in the loose tissue beneath the skin, but it may also occur in deeper tissues beneath mucous membranes or around muscle bundles. For example, facial cellulitis may involve the cheek or periorbital or orbital tissues and may extend into the neck,[71] and pelvic cellulitis may involve deep muscles within the pelvis.[155] Erysipelas is similar to cellulitis in appearance but instead affects the superficial dermis.[52] It is characterized by sharply defined, red patches of skin that are painful and hot to the touch. Red streaks extending from the patch indicate lymph vessels have been infected.

Intravenous antibiotic infusion is the primary treatment for cellulitis, but oral antibiotics can be effective if the infection is detected early. Individuals susceptible to recurrent cellulitis may have a prescription for oral antibiotics on hand that can be filled at the first sign of infection. The therapist should draw around the edges of erythematous areas and take photos to monitor progression. Signs of progression and/or new onset of constitutional symptoms (especially fever) require immediate medical referral for antibiotic therapy. Good nutrition and hydration are advised to help fight infection, repair tissue, and remove bacteria and their by-products. Extensive cellulitis requires surgical débridement of necrotic tissue. Lymphangitis may occur if cellulitis is untreated, and gangrene, metastatic abscesses, and sepsis can result.

## Viral Infections

Viruses are intracellular parasites that produce their effect by using intracellular substances of host cells. In a viral infection, epidermal cells react with inflammation and vesiculation (as in herpes zoster) or by proliferating to form growths (warts).

### Herpes Zoster

See discussion in Chapter 8.

### Warts (Verrucae)

Warts are common, benign viral infections of the skin and adjacent mucous membranes caused by human papillomaviruses.[157] Transmission is probably through direct contact, but self-inoculation is possible.

Warts may appear singly or as multiple lesions, with thick white surfaces containing many pointed projections. Clinical manifestations depend on the type of wart and its location. The most common wart, verruca vulgaris, appears as a rough, elevated, round surface most frequently on the extremities, especially the hands and fingers. Plantar warts are slightly elevated or flat and may occur singly or in large clusters *(mosaic warts)* at pressure points of the feet.

#### MEDICAL MANAGEMENT

**DIAGNOSIS.** Diagnosis is usually made by visual examination. Plantar warts can be differentiated from neuropathic ulcers, corns, and calluses by certain distinguishing features. Plantar warts obliterate natural lines of the skin, may contain red or black capillary dots that are easily discernible if the surface of the wart is shaved down with a scalpel, and are painful with pressure.[115] Both plantar warts and corns have a soft, pulpy core surrounded by a thick callous ring.

**TREATMENT.** Some warts respond to simple treatment, and some disappear spontaneously. The specific choice of treatment is influenced by the location, size, and number of warts; presence of secondary infection; amount of tenderness on palpation; age and gender of the patient; history of previous treatment; and individual choice and compliance. Topical over-the-counter salicylic acid preparations may be used to induce peeling of the skin.[115] Electrodesiccation and curettage of warts are widely used. Other methods of removal include surgical, cryotherapy, laser, chemical cautery, oral medications, and immunotherapy.[104,202] Recurrence rates can be high. As many of these techniques result in tissue trauma, the risk of scarring can complicate removal from the face, neck, and hands.

## Fungal Infections (Dermatophytoses)

Fungal infections such as ringworm are caused by a group of fungi that invade the stratum corneum, hair, and nails. These are superficial infections that live on, not in, the skin and are confined to the dead keratin layers, unable to survive in the deeper skin layers. Because keratin is being shed (desquamated) constantly, fungi must multiply at a rate that equals that of keratin production; otherwise the organisms would be shed along with desquamating skin cells. Fungal infections spread without treatment. Once a diagnosis is made, several over-the-counter and prescription-strength antifungal treatments are available. In cases of extensive infections, underlying immunosuppressive conditions should be explored.[240]

### Ringworm (Tinea Corporis)

Dermatophytoses, or fungal infections of the hair, skin, or nails, are designated by the Latin word *tinea*, with further designation related to the affected area of the body (see Table 10.3). Tinea corporis (ringworm) has no association with worms but is marked by the formation of ring-shaped pigmented patches covered with vesicles or scales that often become itchy (Fig. 10.6). As the ring expands outward, central clearing may occur.[240] Transmission occurs directly through close contact with infected persons or

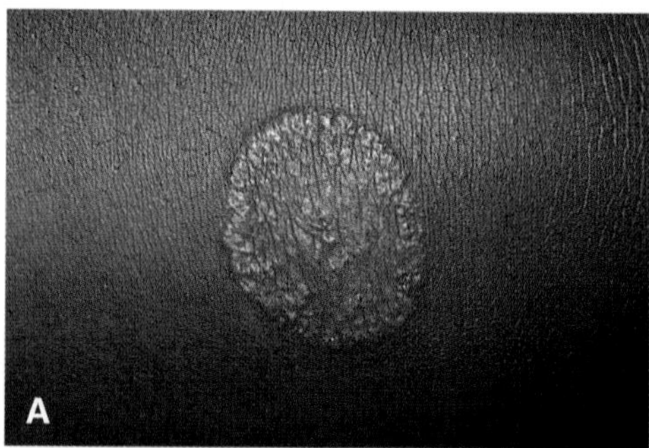


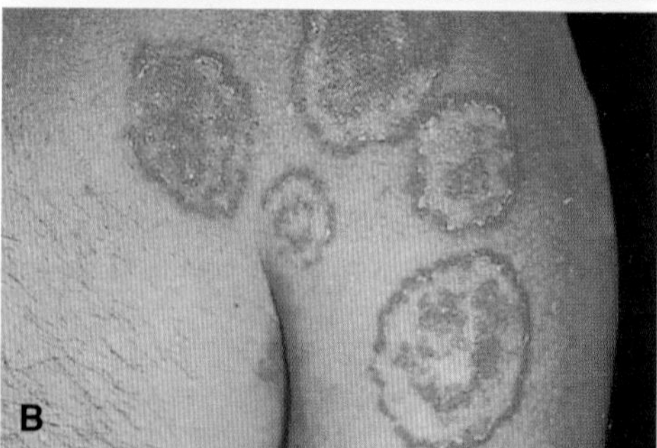


**Figure. 10.6**

**Tinea corporis (ringworm).** (A) Scales forming circular lesions with clear centers characteristic of tinea corporis. (B) Most adults and children present with multiple lesions that are hyperpigmented in individuals with light skin and depigmented in individuals with dark skin. Lesions occur most often on the face, chest, abdomen, and dorsal surface of the arms. (A, From Zitelli BJ, Davis HW: *Atlas of pediatric physical diagnosis*, St. Louis, 2002, Mosby. B, From Habif T: *Clinical dermatology*, ed 4, St. Louis, 2004, Elsevier.)

animals or indirectly through contact with contaminated objects such as shoes, towels, or shower stalls. Lesions can worsen in warm, moist environments.[182]

Formal diagnosis can be made through laboratory examination of the affected skin. Treatment for tinea corporis requires maintaining clean, dry skin and applying antifungal powder or topical agent as prescribed. Oral medications (e.g., terbinafine, griseofulvin, itraconazole) may be prescribed for patients with widespread involvement and may require closer monitoring for adverse side effects compared with topical treatments.[240]

### Athlete's Foot (Tinea Pedis)

Tinea pedis (athlete's foot) causes erythema, skin peeling, and pruritus between the toes that may spread from the interdigital spaces to the plantar surface of the foot. Severe infection may result in inflammation with severe itching and pain with walking. Some individuals may develop a strong foot odor.[182] Clean, dry socks and adequate footwear (i.e., well-ventilated, properly fitting) are important. After washing the feet and drying thoroughly between the toes, antifungal cream or powder (the latter to absorb perspiration and prevent excoriation) can be applied. If symptomatic treatment including topical preparations does not eradicate the problem, systemic treatment with oral antifungals may be required.[182]

### Yeast (Candidiasis)

Yeast infections (candidiasis) result from overpopulation of normally occurring yeast in chronically wet or moist areas.[222] As such, yeast infections related to the skin are frequently a complication of moisture-associated skin damage (MASD) owing to wound exudate, urine, stool, and/or perspiration. MASD can be found in periwound skin, in peristomal skin, in skin folds, and with IAD. Yeast infections usually appear as a bright red rash with tiny macules and papules, but they also can appear scaly.[120]

**SPECIAL IMPLICATIONS FOR THE THERAPIST 10.6**

*Fungal Infections*

Fungal infections require hygienic measures common to all infectious conditions. Affected persons should not share hair care products (e.g., combs, brushes, headbands), clothes, or other articles that have been in proximity of the infected area. Affected persons must use their own towels and linens.

**Ringworm**

Because ringworm can be acquired by animal-to-human transmission (see Table 10.3), all household pets should be examined for the presence of ringworm. Other sources of infection include seats with headrests (e.g., theater seats, seats on public transportation, other shared public seats).

**Athlete's Foot**

Although some may consider this condition a nuisance that does not require medical attention, it can be an entry point for bacterial infections, especially in older adults. Keeping athlete's foot under control can prevent progression to bacterial infection or cellulitis in the feet and legs and is especially important in patients with diabetes.

**Yeast**

Individuals who take immunosuppressive medications or have immune system disorders such as diabetes or cancer are at higher risk for developing yeast infections secondary to MASD. Over-the-counter antifungal ointments are available, as well as an antimicrobial silver-infused fabric, InterDry (Coloplast), for skin folds. Powder is not recommended because of clumping and possible allergic reaction. It is important to note that not all yeast infections remain superficial. Invasive yeast infections reaching the bloodstream and internal organs with potential serious complications are beyond the scope of this chapter.[222]

## Other Parasitic Infections

Some parasitic infections of the skin are caused by insects. Contact with insects that puncture the skin for the purpose of sucking blood, injecting venom, or laying eggs is relatively common. Substances deposited by insects are considered foreign to the host and may create an allergic sensitivity resulting in pruritus, urticaria, or systemic reactions of a greater or lesser degree depending on host sensitivity.

### Scabies

**Definition.** Scabies is a highly contagious skin eruption caused by a mite, *Sarcoptes scabiei*. The female mite burrows into the skin and deposits eggs that hatch into larvae in a few days.[49,235] Scabies is a common public health problem, with an estimated prevalence of 130 million cases worldwide.[258]

Scabies is easily transmitted by skin-to-skin contact or by contact with contaminated objects (linens or shared inanimate objects). Mites can spread rapidly between members of the same household, in nursing homes, or in institutions. The inflammatory response and itching do not occur until approximately 2 to 6 weeks after initial contact, often facilitating widespread transmission before awareness and diagnosis.[235]

**Clinical Manifestations.** Symptoms include intense pruritus (worse at night), excoriated skin, and one or more burrows, which is a linear ridge with a vesicle at one end. The mite is usually found in the burrow, commonly in the interdigital web spaces, flexor aspects of the wrist, axillae, waistline, nipples in females, genitalia in males, and umbilicus.[235,258] Intense scratching can lead to severe excoriation and secondary bacterial infection. Itching can become generalized secondary to sensitization.

#### MEDICAL MANAGEMENT

**DIAGNOSIS AND TREATMENT.** The mite can be excavated from one end of a burrow with a needle or scalpel blade and examined under a microscope. In long-standing cases, a mite may not be found. At that point, treatment is based on a presumptive diagnosis.

Traditional treatment is a scabicide, usually a lotion or cream containing permethrin or lindane, applied to the entire body from the neck down.[63] Permethrin is generally the treatment of choice for head lice and scabies because of its residual effect and because toxicity and absorption are minimal. Oral medications are available for individuals allergic to or who do not respond well to topical treatments.[63]

SPECIAL IMPLICATIONS FOR THE THERAPIST 10.7

### *Scabies*

If a hospitalized patient has scabies, prevent transmission by practicing good handwashing and by wearing gloves and gown when in close contact. Observe wound and skin precautions for 24 hours after treatment of scabies. Gas-autoclave blood pressure cuffs or other equipment used with the affected person before using them on others. If the person is treated outside the hospital room (e.g., plinth, treatment mat), the area must be thoroughly disinfected after each session.

In using a scabicide, the patient must understand that *no* area can be missed. After 24 hours, the affected person should bathe. All bed linens and clothes must be laundered in hot water or dry-cleaned. Other household members and people in close contact with the affected person should also be treated. A second application of the scabicide may need to be applied 7 days later. Itching may persist for 2 to 4 weeks after treatment, owing to hypersensitivity.[235] Widespread bacterial infections require additional treatment with systemic antibiotics.

## Pediculosis (Lousiness)

Pediculosis is an infestation by *Pediculus humanus*, a common parasite infecting the head, body, and genital area. Transmission is from one person to another, primarily through head-to-head contact or shared personal items such as combs, lockers, clothes, or furniture. Lice are not carried or transmitted by pets. Anyone can get pediculosis regardless of age, socioeconomic status, or status of personal cleanliness. Young children are easily infected secondary to close contact with playmates. People who live in overcrowded surroundings and older adults who depend on others for care or who live in nursing homes are also at increased risk. Severe itching accompanied by secondary eczematous changes develops, and small grayish or white nits (eggs) are usually seen attached to the base of hair shafts.

*Pediculus corporis,* the body or clothes louse, produces intense itching, which in turn results in severe excoriations from scratching and possible secondary bacterial infections. Lice or nits are generally found in the seams of the affected individual's clothing.

*Pediculus pubis (Phthirus pubis)*, the pubic or crab louse, is usually transmitted by sexual contact but can be transferred on clothing or towels. Lice and nits are usually found at the base of pubic hairs. Sometimes dark brown particles (louse excreta) may be seen on underclothes.

### MEDICAL MANAGEMENT

Traditional treatment has been with the appropriate disinfectant solution (e.g., shampoo or soap containing permethrin) specific to the type of louse present. Head lice has now become so common that topical treatments can be purchased as over-the-counter kits. As with scabies, oral-dose therapy can also be used in case of allergy or severe infestations (see Scabies).

SPECIAL IMPLICATIONS FOR THE THERAPIST 10.8

### *Pediculosis*

The therapist should wear gloves while carefully inspecting the head of any child or adult who scratches excessively. Look for bite marks, redness, and nits or movement that indicates a louse. If exposure to lice occurs, treatment for the individual as well as the therapist may be required, depending on exposure level. It is important to note that shampoos for lice are insecticides, so only people with confirmed head lice should be treated.[187]

Combs and brushes should be sanitized or replaced, and bed linen and clothing should be dry-cleaned or machine washed using hot water. Pillows, stuffed animals, rugs, upholstered furniture, and similar objects that come in close contact with the affected person must be vacuumed or cleaned thoroughly with hot water.[174] Items not easily cleaned can be stored in a sealed plastic bag for 2 weeks until lice have been killed.

# SKIN CANCER

The American Cancer Society (ACS) reports skin cancer as the most common form of cancer in the United States, with approximately 5.4 million nonmelanoma (i.e., basal and squamous cell) skin cancers diagnosed annually. There is no evidence that this epidemic has peaked.[20,23,24,186]

Solar radiation (exposure to midrange-wavelength ultraviolet B [UVB] radiation) is believed to be the major risk factor in developing skin cancer. It has been documented that protection from the sun, especially during the first 2 decades of life, significantly reduces the risk of skin cancer.[243] The melanoma rate is rising most rapidly in persons younger than 40 years of age and is now one of the most common cancers in women between 25 and 29 years of age.[243] Current predictions estimate greater than 91,000 new cases of melanoma and greater than 9000 melanoma deaths annually in the United States.[21] While people with light skin are at the highest risk of developing skin cancer, individuals with darker skin tones are not without risk. Darker skin may mask subtle color changes in skin, making early detection more difficult. In fact, skin cancers in individuals with dark skin tend to be more advanced at the time of discovery owing to lack of early screening and delayed diagnosis.[3] As such, it is important that health care practitioners provide appropriate screening and education to patients of *all* skin colors.

In this chapter, skin cancer is discussed in three broad categories: benign, premalignant, and malignant (Box 10.6). Malignant lesions of the skin are considered as either melanoma or nonmelanoma. Kaposi sarcoma (KS), which occurs in the skin, is not included in these categories and is discussed separately.

Benign skin lesions, such as seborrheic keratosis or nevi (moles), rarely undergo transition to melanoma and do not usually require treatment.[26] Although most moles remain as benign skin lesions, when malignant melanoma does occur, it often arises from a preexisting mole

**Box 10.6**

**TYPES OF SKIN CANCER**

| Benign | Premalignant | Nonmelanoma | Melanoma |
|---|---|---|---|
| Seborrheic keratosis<br>Nevi | Actinic keratosis<br>Bowen disease | Basal cell carcinoma<br>Squamous cell carcinoma | Superficial spreading melanoma<br>Nodular melanoma<br>Lentigo maligna melanoma<br>Acral lentiginous melanoma |

derived from pigment cells (melanocytes) of the skin. Malignant melanoma is the most serious form of skin cancer, resulting in early metastasis and possible death.

Precancerous lesions, such as actinic keratosis or Bowen disease (BD), may potentially progress to malignancy and must be carefully evaluated. The most common types of nonmelanoma skin cancer are basal cell carcinoma (BCC) and squamous cell carcinoma (SCC). These carcinomas occur twice as often in Caucasian men as in Caucasian women, with incidence increasing steadily with age.

## Benign Lesions

### Seborrheic Keratosis

Seborrheic keratosis is a benign neoplasm formed through proliferation of keratinocytes. These lesions occur most frequently after middle age on the chest, back, and face. Lesions also often appear following hormonal therapy or inflammatory dermatoses.[57] Areas are waxy, smooth, or raised lesions that vary in color from flesh tones to dark brown or black and may have a "stuck-on" appearance.[68,72] Size varies from barely palpable to large verrucous (wart-like) plaques. These tumors are usually left untreated unless itchy or painful. Cryotherapy with liquid nitrogen is a typical treatment when intervention is warranted.

### Nevi (Moles)

Nevi are benign pigmented or nonpigmented skin tumors forming from aggregations of melanocytes beginning early in life. Most are brown, black, or flesh-colored and may appear on any part of the skin. They vary in size and thickness, occurring in groups or singly.[22] Nevi seldom undergo transition to malignant melanoma, but when malignant melanoma does occur, it often arises from a preexisting mole. Therefore, individuals with many moles are at increased risk.[22] The chances of cancerous transformation are also increased when moles are exposed to constant irritation. Any change in size, color, or texture of a mole; bleeding; or excessive itching should be reported to a qualified health care provider.

## Premalignant Lesions

There are two common premalignant skin lesions: actinic keratosis and BD.

### Actinic Keratosis

Actinic keratosis *(solar keratosis)* is a skin neoplasm resulting from many years of exposure to the sun's UV rays. Damage from overexposure results in abnormal cell growth, causing a well-defined, crusty, or sandpaper-like patch or bump on chronically sun-exposed areas of the body (e.g., face, ears, lower lip, bald scalp, dorsa of hands/forearms).[30]

The base of these lesions may be light or dark; tan, pink, red, or a combination of these; or the same color as the skin. The scale or crust is horny, dry, and rough, making them recognized more by touch than sight. Occasional itching or tenderness may occur. Lesions tend to develop slowly, reaching 3 to 6 mm in size, but they may also spontaneously resolve.[48] The number of lesions that develop is directly related to heredity and lifetime sun exposure.

Actinic keratosis is most common in light-skinned individuals with blue, gray, or green eyes and red or blonde hair.[25,48,214] It is important that this condition be diagnosed properly because it is often difficult to distinguish a large or hypertrophic actinic keratosis from a SCC. A biopsy may be indicated. There is a known risk of malignant degeneration and subsequent metastatic potential in neglected lesions.

Treatment protocol is based on the nature and number of lesions as well as the age and health of the affected person. Common treatment options include single-dose freezing with liquid nitrogen (cryotherapy), curettage, electrodesiccation, or application of prescribed topical creams, gels, or solutions over the course of several weeks.[25] Fractional carbon dioxide laser resurfacing and other forms of photodynamic therapy where topical agents are applied and then activated by an agent-specific light source (i.e., red or blue laser, sunlight) are additional treatment options.[12,190,198] However, not all keratoses need to be removed.

People of fair complexion should be advised to avoid sun exposure (see Box 10.4) and use a high sun protection factor (at least 30 SPF) sunscreen 30 to 60 minutes before going outside.[5,19,35] People with darker skin have less risk of developing skin cancer owing to exposure, but they can still be affected and should take precautions. Fabric with a tight weave, such as cotton, is suggested, along with the use of a hat and sunglasses to protect the face and eyes. Sunscreens are generally not recommended for infants younger than 6 months of age; infants should be kept out of the sun or shaded from it.[17]

### Bowen Disease

BD is a nonmelanoma group of skin cancers typically associated with prolonged sun exposure, chemical exposure (e.g., arsenic), or human papillomavirus infection. Lesions manifest as persistent black, brown, or reddish brown scaly plaques with well-defined margins. BD is diagnosed most frequently in fair-skinned men older than age 50.[123,265] Treatment options are similar to those for actinic keratosis. Although rare, BD lesions have the potential to become invasive and metastasize[123,145]; therefore follow-up with a qualified health care provider is recommended.

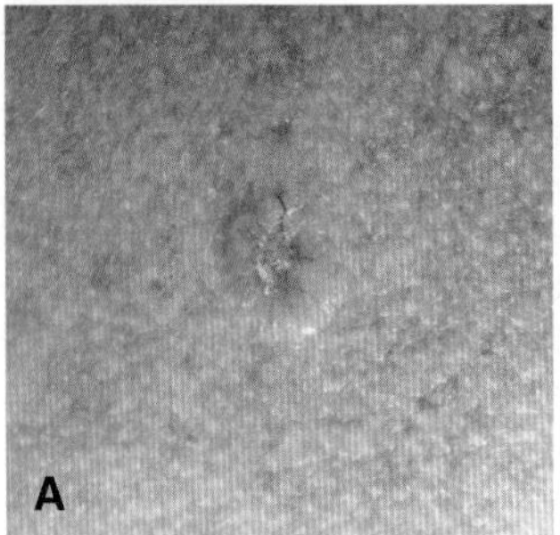


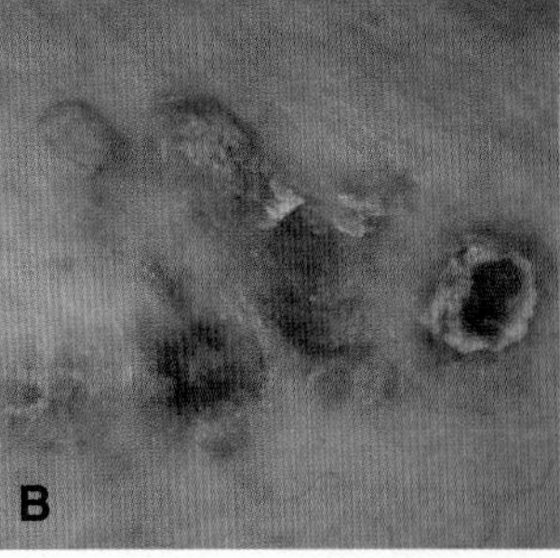


**Figure. 10.7**

**Basal cell carcinoma.** (A) Skin cancer in the form of basal cell carcinoma can appear as a shiny, pearly, or translucent pink, red, or white bump. There may be a rolled border with an indented center. (B) This type of skin cancer may also manifest as a red patch, a crusty open wound that will not heal, or a scarlike area. (A, From Lookingbill D, Marks J: *Principles of dermatology*, ed 3, Philadelphia, 2000, Saunders. B, From Townsend C, et al: *Sabiston textbook of surgery*, ed 17, Philadelphia, 2004, Saunders.)

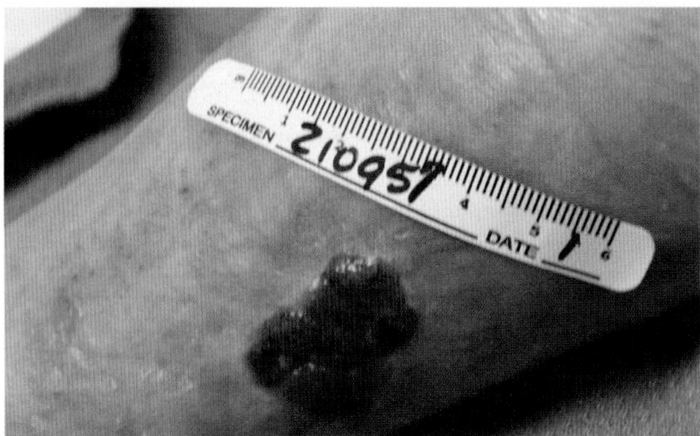


**Figure. 10.8**

**Chronic venous ulcer.** Basal cell carcinoma can also mimic a chronic venous ulcer, potentially causing a delay in diagnosis. Biopsy is required to make the definitive medical diagnosis. (Courtesy Harriett B. Loehne, PT, DPT, CWS, FACCWS. Used with permission.)

## Malignant Nonmelanoma Carcinomas

### Basal Cell Carcinoma

**Definition and Overview.** BCC is a slow-growing surface epithelial skin tumor originating from undifferentiated basal cells contained in the epidermis. This type of nonmelanoma carcinoma rarely metastasizes beyond the skin and does not invade blood or lymph vessels. However, early diagnosis and treatment by a qualified health care provider is important. If left untreated, BCC can cause significant local skin destruction and may invade local subcutaneous soft tissue and bone resulting in significant disfigurement and scarring.

**Incidence.** Of all types of cancer, BCC is the most common, and incidence rates continue to rise each year.[20,35,186] Historically this tumor rarely appeared before age 40 and was more prevalent in blond, fair-skinned men. However, increased incidence in younger adults and women is now well documented[69,135,263] and linked to increased and early-age exposure to UV radiation via outdoor activities and indoor tanning (e.g., tanning beds, lamps, booths).[92,135,186,263] An estimated 2000 people in the United States die each year of BCCs and SCCs.[20]

**Etiologic and Risk Factors.** Sun exposure is the most common cause of BCC. People with light skin have a higher risk of developing BCC compared with people with darker skin, as they have less natural protection from the sun, owing to comparatively less melanocyte activity and production of melanin.[3] For Caucasians, the lifetime risk of developing BCC is between 23% and 39%.[35,169] Other risk factors include immunosuppression (e.g., via organ transplant, HIV, long-term corticosteroid use),[18] advanced age (owing to cumulative sun exposure over time), and exposure to certain chemicals (e.g., arsenic, coal tar). Anyone, regardless of skin color, who has had one BCC is at increased risk of developing others, and recurrence of previously treated lesions is possible.[18]

**Pathogenesis.** Current research links the development of BCC closely with UV radiation exposure that results in DNA signaling pathway mutations, gene deactivation, and dysregulation of certain proteins in the skin.[3,35,186] Aberrant cell signaling and mutation is thought to be a factor in the initiation of most BCC tumors. Genetic alterations also play a role in BCC, as in the case of autosomally inherited basal cell nevus syndrome. An understanding of altered cell structure and function associated with environmental insults (e.g., UV radiation) and altered immune function provides a good link between BCC and other known risk factors.

**Clinical Manifestations.** BCC (Fig. 10.7) typically has a pearly or ivory appearance, has rolled edges, and is slightly elevated above the skin with small blood vessels on the surface (telangiectasia) (see Fig. 10.3). In early stages, it may appear as a small pink or red flat area on the skin.[149] Lesions can also appear similar to BD or chronic venous ulcer (Fig. 10.8) or may mimic SCC. The nodule is usually painless and slowly increases in size and may ulcerate centrally. More than 65% of BCCs are found on the head and neck. Other common locations are the trunk, forearms, and upper back and chest.

### MEDICAL MANAGEMENT

DIAGNOSIS AND TREATMENT. Diagnosis by clinical examination must be confirmed via biopsy and histologic study. Treatment depends on the size, location, and depth of the lesion and may include curettage and electrodesiccation, chemotherapy, surgical excision, cryotherapy, radiation, topical agents (e.g., imiquimod), and photodynamic therapy. BCC tumors form extensions that invade surrounding tissue beyond visible margins; therefore it is recommended that any type of removal demonstrate at least a 4-mm margin of normal skin.[50]

Surgical excision is the primary method of removal for BCC tumors. Most tumors, unless extensive, are removed in outpatient physician offices. Mohs micrographic surgery is the gold standard treatment, in which the specimen is excised, frozen, and examined for positive margins while the patient waits, thus immediately ensuring clean margins.[50] Radiation can be used if surgery is not an option and is delivered in multiple treatments over several weeks, depending on tumor size. Cure rates are lower with radiation compared with surgical excision and may

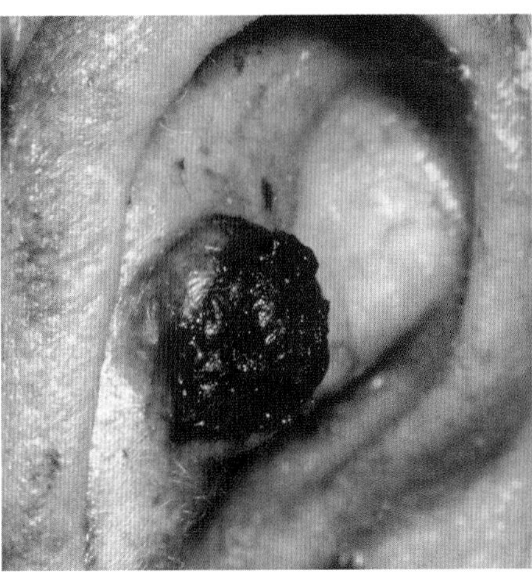

**Figure. 10.9**

**Squamous cell carcinoma.** Squamous cell carcinoma can take the form of a persistent, scaly, red patch that sometimes crusts or bleeds or an open wound that does not heal. This type of skin cancer may also manifest as a raised or wartlike growth that may bleed. (From Goldman L: *Cecil textbook of medicine*, ed 22, Philadelphia, 2004, Saunders.)

result in skin irritation, fibrosis, and discoloration.[50] Photodynamic therapy is also an option for small shallow tumors, especially in areas of skin where cosmesis is important.[203] Chemopreventive agents such as retinoids and certain nonsteroidal antiinflammatory drugs have shown promise as agents for long-term use that can both treat and prevent BCC.[237] If BCC is identified and treated early, local excision or nonexcisional destruction is usually curative.

PROGNOSIS. If untreated, BCC tumors slowly invade surrounding tissues over months and years, destroying skin, bone, and cartilage. As they are frequently located in sun-exposed areas, such as the face, ears, and neck, tissue destruction can lead to significant scarring and disfigurement without early intervention. Individuals who have had a BCC are at a higher risk of developing other BCC tumors and malignant melanoma. For these reasons, education of the patient and family regarding routine skin examinations performed at home and annually by a qualified health care professional is important.

## Squamous Cell Carcinoma

**Definition and Overview.** SCC is the second most common type of skin cancer.[6] It is a tumor of the epidermal keratinocytes that occurs most frequently in light-skinned individuals in sun-damaged skin areas, such as the ears, face, lips and mouth, back of the arm, and dorsa of the hands (Fig. 10.9).[6] While SCC occurs less commonly in people with darker skin tones, these individuals are still at risk with the lower extremities, head, neck, scalp, and areas not usually exposed to UV radiation being the most commonly affected.[3]

SCC in situ refers to tumors that are usually confined to the epidermis but may extend into the dermis. Invasive SCC is more aggressive and may invade deeper tissues. Whereas metastasis of BCC is rare, SCC has the potential to metastasize. Biopsy, ultrasound, computed tomography (CT), and magnetic resonance imaging (MRI) are used to determine the extent of spread.[226] Invasive SCC with deep tissue involvement and distant metastasis beyond the integumentary system is beyond the scope of this chapter.

**Incidence.** As with BCC, SCC incidence rates continue to rise. It is estimated that a minimum of 200,000 to 400,000 new SCC diagnoses occur annually in the United States.[6,137,138] SCC represents 20% to 50% of all skin cancers, affecting men more frequently than women.[189]

**Etiologic and Risk Factors.** UV radiation exposure, especially in childhood, is the most significant risk factor for developing SCC. Other significant risk factors include age and immunosuppression (e.g., via organ transplant, HIV, long-term corticosteroid use).[6,17] SCC also shares many risk factors associated with BCC (see Basal Cell Carcinoma).

Metastasis for SCC is estimated to be about 4%[6]; however, having multiple or high-risk factors can significantly increase the likelihood of spread.[101] High-level risk factors for metastasis include poorly defined tumor margins, deep extension through skin and subcutaneous fat, tumor diameter larger than 2 cm, perineural invasion, and recurrence in an area previously treated for SCC.[137,232]

**Pathogenesis.** Damage of cellular DNA by UV radiation and the resulting cell mutation and protein dysregulation continues to be one of the most significant causes of skin cancer. Disruptions of tumor suppressor genes and the normal process of apoptosis (programmed cell death) allow abnormal cell growth and expansion.[18,189] Both UVB and UVA rays also have direct and indirect effects on the cutaneous immune system, lowering the skin's cell-mediated immunity, which is another factor in carcinogenesis.

**Clinical Manifestations.** As previously indicated, a large majority of SCC tumors occur in the head and neck region, so new or unusual manifestations on the skin in these areas should be closely examined. Squamous cell lesions can sometimes be more difficult to characterize than BCC tumors because poorly defined margins tend to blend with surrounding skin. An SCC tumor may manifest as an ulcer, a flat red area, a cutaneous horn, an indurated plaque, or a nodule. It may be red to flesh-colored and surrounded by scaly tissue. Dermatoscopic examination may show vascular structures in dotted or curved hairpin-shaped patterns.[189] Whereas the tumors are normally slow growing, patients who are immunocompromised may experience faster tumor growth.[189]

Usually lesions on unexposed skin tend to be more invasive and more likely to metastasize, with the exception of lesions on the lower lip and ears.[3,189] These sites tend to metastasize early, beginning with the process of induration and inflammation of the lesion. Metastasis can occur to the regional lymph nodes, producing characteristic systemic symptoms of pain, malaise, fatigue, weakness, and anorexia.[252] An often benign form of skin cancer, keratoacanthoma, can be mistaken for some forms of SCC. A keratoacanthoma typically manifests as a round, well-demarcated nodule with central ulceration. These tumors often regress and spontaneously resolve but may first demonstrate rapid growth and become fairly large, with some reaching up to 20 cm.[154] Differentiation between keratoacanthoma and SCC is best determined through biopsy.

Malignant transformation of any chronic wound can occur (Fig. 10.10). SCC and BCC are two common types of nonmelanoma cutaneous cancers that may arise from chronic wound tissue or mature scar (especially mature burn scar).[31] A lesion with this etiology is referred to as a *Marjolin ulcer*. Theories for cancerous transformation include chronic inflammation and dysregulation of cell activation and reproduction.[31] A biopsy should be performed by a qualified health care provider when a chronic wound fails to show signs of improvement or manifests with abnormal or unusual appearing tissue.

**A THERAPIST'S THOUGHTS[a]**

**Chronic Wounds**

Therapists should consider recommending a biopsy for any chronic wound that does not progress toward healing with advanced wound management interventions.

[a]Harriett B. Loehne, PT, DPT, CWS, FACCWS

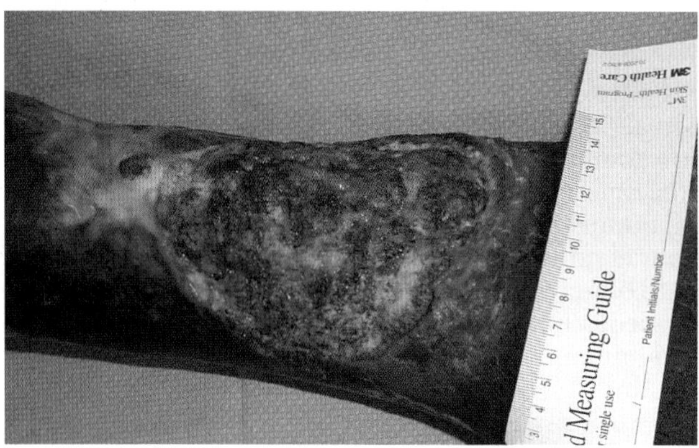


**Figure. 10.10**

**Marjolin ulcer.** This lesion constitutes a Marjolin ulcer. The patient had a history of venous ulcers and had been treated for many months by home health services with no improvement. She was seen at a wound management clinic. A biopsy was done immediately with a fresh-frozen section, and a diagnosis of Marjolin ulcer was made. The cancer had metastasized to the bone and a below-knee amputation was required. It was never clear whether the cancer began in a new ulcer or in scar tissue from a previous ulcer. (Courtesy Harriett B. Loehne, PT, DPT, CWS, FACCWS. Used with permission.)

## MEDICAL MANAGEMENT

**DIAGNOSIS, TREATMENT, AND PROGNOSIS.** An excisional biopsy provides definitive diagnosis and staging of SCC. Other laboratory tests may be appropriate depending on the presence of systemic symptoms. The size, shape, location, and invasiveness of a squamous cell tumor and condition of the underlying tissue, as well as patient status and preference, determine the best treatment method (see Basal Cell Carcinoma). Topical therapies used for BCC are not generally supported for treatment of SCC. Rather, surgical excision with a 4- to 6-mm clear skin margin is considered the most effective intervention.[6] A deeply invasive tumor may require a combination of techniques and widening of the surgical excision. Patients with terminal conditions or multiple comorbidities may opt for minimally invasive, less painful treatment options despite lower cure rates or may choose to have their skin cancer observed or monitored without direct intervention. Generally, early detection and treatment are positive factors for decreased risk of metastasis. Less favorable prognoses are associated with above-noted high-risk factors and the presence of multiple tumors and tumors manifesting in scar tissue.[6]

## Malignant Melanoma

### Definition and Overview

Malignant melanoma is a neoplasm of the skin originating from melanocytes or cells.[122] Melanomas occur most frequently on sun-exposed skin but can be found in the oral cavity, esophagus, anal canal, vagina, meninges, or eye. The clinical varieties of cutaneous melanoma are categorized into four types (Fig. 10.11)[26,248,216].

1. *Superficial spreading melanoma* is the most common type of melanoma, accounting for approximately 70% of all cutaneous melanomas. These tumors most often manifest on the upper back and trunk in men and the upper back and legs in women, but they can occur anywhere on the body. Melanoma can originate from a preexisting mole or new lesion and typically manifests as a brown or black raised patch with an irregular border and may include variable pigmentation (red, white, blue). It is usually asymptomatic and typically diagnosed in younger individuals.

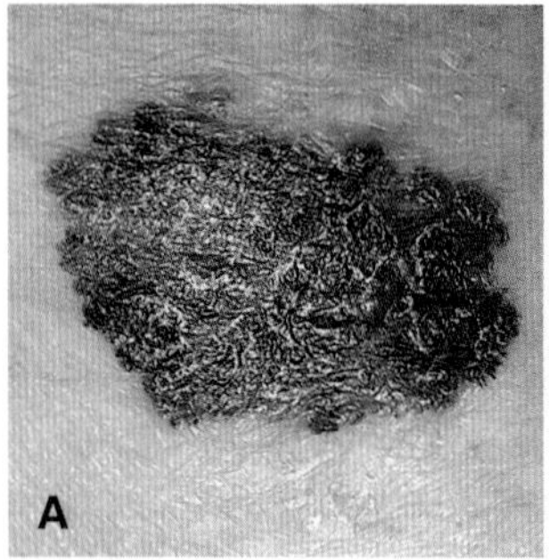

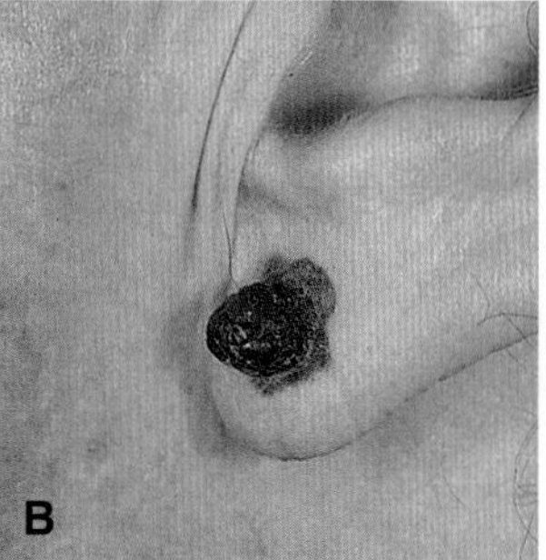

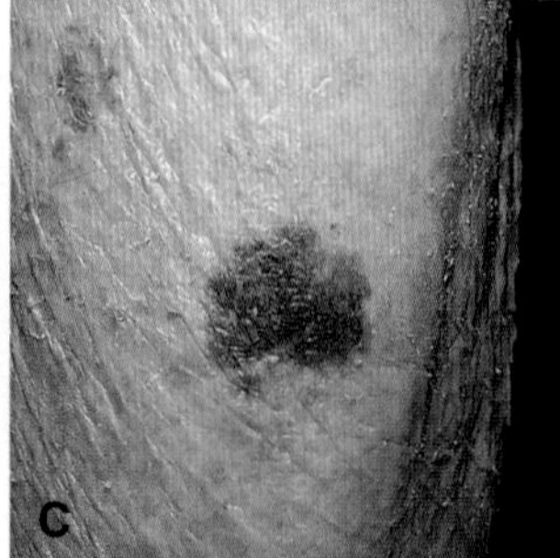

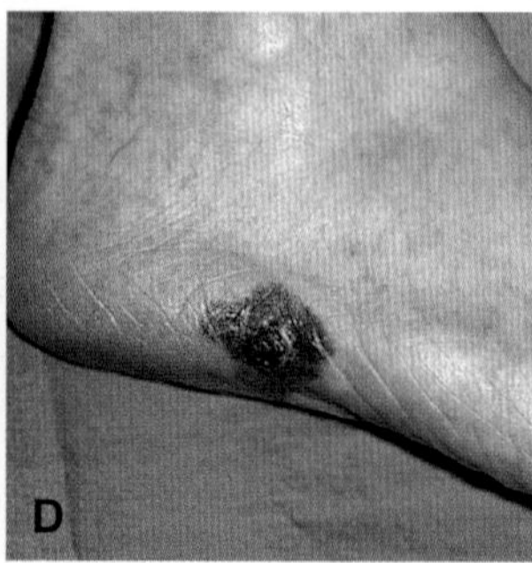


**Figure. 10.11**

(A) Superficial spreading melanoma. An irregular margin with multiple colors of black, blue, pale red, and white may be seen. (B) Nodular lesion of melanoma. This lesion developed on top of a benign compound nevus. (C) Lentigo maligna. If left alone, progression to lentigo maligna melanoma occurs. (D) Acral lentiginous melanoma. This brown-to-black, flat lesion has irregular borders and variable pigmentation. (From Callen JP, et al: *Color atlas of dermatology*, ed 2, Philadelphia, 2000, Saunders. D, Courtesy Dr. Neil A. Fenske, Tampa, FL.)

2. *Lentigo maligna melanoma* is a less common (approximately 10%) tumor occurring predominantly on sun-exposed areas, such as the head, neck, arm, and upper back or trunk in adults 50 to 80 years old. These lesions remain fairly superficial for some time and may appear as a flat or raised area of discoloration (tan, brown, or dark brown) with irregular borders. As lesions enlarge, they can show more variation in pigment. Approximately one-third develop into malignant melanoma and therefore require careful monitoring.
3. *Acral lentiginous melanoma* tends to appear on the palms of the hands, under the fingernails, or on the soles of the feet. Usually dark brown or black in color, this type of melanoma is most common in people with darker skin tones (African or Asian descent). It tends to grow on the epidermis for some time and is typically diagnosed once it becomes more advanced, as a result of delayed detection. This type of skin cancer accounts for approximately 5% of cutaneous melanomas.
4. *Nodular melanoma* is the most aggressive form of melanoma and can be found on any part of the body, with no specific site preference. Men 60 years of age and older are affected more frequently than women. It is often described as a small, suddenly appearing but quickly enlarging bump or papule. Most are black in color, but some may appear white, gray, tan, brown, blue, red, or normal skin tone. This type accounts for approximately 10% to 15% of cutaneous melanomas and is known to invade the dermis with early metastasis.

### Incidence

Worldwide there are approximately 287,000 new cases of melanoma annually and more than 60,000 deaths.[56] The United States accounts for greater than 90,000 of the new cases and just over 9000 annual deaths.[21,149] Incidence of invasive melanoma increases approximately 4% to 6% each year in the United States. Men have a higher incidence than women,[56] accounting for approximately 60% of newly diagnosed cases. The most common age for melanoma diagnosis is 63; however, it is not unusual for melanoma to occur in adults younger than 30. Caucasians have a 2.6% lifetime risk of having melanoma (1 in 38 people) compared with a 0.1% lifetime risk in African Americans (1 in 1000) and 0.58% in Hispanics (1 in 172).[21]

### Etiologic and Risk Factors

As UV radiation exposure is the primary risk factor for developing melanoma, people with fair complexions (i.e., light skin, green or blue eyes, blonde or red hair) who freckle or sunburn easily have a higher risk. Individuals with multiple or abnormal moles, past history of BCC or SCC, or a positive family history of melanoma are also at high risk. Increased exposure to UV radiation likely explains the increased incidence of melanoma in younger women.[21] The use of tanning devices is considered a significant risk factor for the development of skin cancer, with increases of 75% when indoor tanning starts before age 35.[217] In fact, individuals in their 20s who use indoor tanning have six times greater risk of developing melanoma than individuals who do not.[218] The greater the frequency and intensity of exposure, the greater the risk. Box 10.7 lists additional risk factors.

Melanomas appear to be more prevalent among people with fair skin who work indoors and take short vacations with intense sun exposure compared with people with chronic sun exposure. Easier and less expensive access to air travel (especially to warm, sunny destinations) has been reported as having a strong relationship with increased melanoma risk.[4] Airline pilots have also been shown to have a higher risk of developing both BCC and melanoma, in part owing to increased exposure to cosmic radiation.[110] The risk of developing melanoma increases in families with a previous melanoma diagnosis or with *atypical mole syndrome* (abnormally high numbers of normal and atypical moles that are 5 mm or larger in diameter).[119,219]

To reduce risk for and prevent the incidence of skin cancer, the U.S. Preventive Services Task Force recommends advising children, adolescents, and young adults between the ages of 10 and 24 with fair skin to minimize UV radiation exposure.[242] Parents are advised to keep infants and very young children out of direct sunlight.

### Pathogenesis

See Pathogenesis under Squamous Cell Carcinoma. The majority of malignant melanomas appear to be associated with intensity rather than duration of sun exposure; that is, most people who develop melanoma work indoors and have intense but limited exposure to the sun on weekends or during vacations. This accounts for the incidence of melanoma on skin that is covered most of the year.

### Clinical Manifestations

As previously described, melanoma can appear anywhere on the body, not just in sun-exposed areas. Common sites are the head, neck, trunk, and legs. Up to 70% arise from

**Box 10.7**

**RISK FACTORS FOR THE DEVELOPMENT OF MELANOMA[a]**

- Personal (previous) or family history of melanoma
- Fair skin; light hair; blue or green eyes
- Presence of marked freckling on the upper back; dysplastic nevi (moles); congenital melanocytic nevi
- Ultraviolet radiation exposure
  - History of three or more blistering sunburns before age 20 years
  - History of 3 or more years of an outdoor summer job during adolescence
  - Exposure to tanning devices
- Immune suppression (e.g., medications, organ transplant recipients)
- Genetic disorder: xeroderma pigmentosum
- Age: older adults or individuals younger than 30; melanoma that runs in families may occur at a younger age
- Being male (higher incidence in males, but varies by age group)

[a] Several risk factors that alone or in combination increase the risk of developing melanoma.

Data from American Cancer Society: *Melanoma Skin Cancer*. Last revised May 20, 2016. Available at: https://www.cancer.org/cancer/melanoma-skin-cancer/causes-risks-prevention/risk-factors.html.

a preexisting nevus. Any change in a skin lesion or nevus (increased size or elevation; bleeding; soreness or inflammation; changes in color, pigmentation, or texture) must be examined for melanoma (Fig. 10.12).

## MEDICAL MANAGEMENT

**DIAGNOSIS.** Early recognition of cutaneous melanomas can have a major impact on the surgical cure. The ACS suggests a monthly self-examination for people at high risk.[22] A biopsy with histologic examination of any suspicious lesion is recommended as the initial step in differential diagnosis.[229]

Melanoma skin cancer is staged according to depth of skin penetration (Breslow depth), appearance, and degree of tumor ulceration.[143,215] The Breslow method measures the thickness of the melanoma in millimeters; the thinner the melanoma, the better the prognosis. Generally, nonulcerated melanomas less than 0.8 mm in depth have less risk of metastatic spread.[229] Depending on the depth of tumor invasion and risk of metastatic spread, laboratory studies, radiography, ultrasound, bone scintigraphy, CT, and MRI may be performed for baseline evaluation and surveillance.[229]

**TREATMENT.** The treatment of choice for cutaneous melanoma is surgical excision. General recommendations for excision call for removal of tissue 1 to 2 cm around the melanoma tumor, although more invasive tumors may require deeper resection. Sentinel node biopsy may be recommended for tumors as thin as 0.8 mm. Node status is the best overall predictor for recurrence and survival. For cosmesis, Mohs micrographic surgery may be appropriate for melanomas on the face, ears, and scalp.[229]

Topical therapies for superficial melanoma are available (e.g., imiquimod cream 5%) when first-line surgical intervention is not possible. When topical therapies are used, there is a risk of undertreating the disease, and closer surveillance is required.[229] Some oral chemotherapy and immunotherapy treatments are also available when surgery is not an option, but these are associated with systemic side effects that must be monitored and managed (e.g., skin toxicity, hypopigmentation, pruritus, hyperkeratosis, SCC, severe photosensitivity).[229]

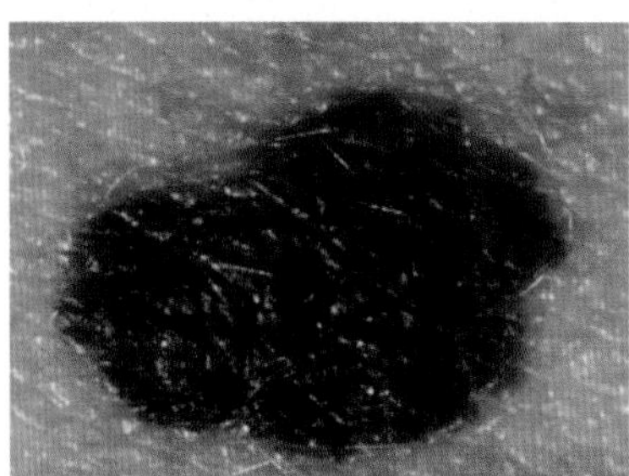

**Figure. 10.12**

**Malignant melanoma.** Warning signs of malignant melanoma include asymmetry, irregular border, two or more shades of color, and diameter as outlined in Box 10.8. Any other changes in moles or skin lesions (e.g., itchiness, tenderness, swelling, redness, softening, or hardening) should be evaluated by a qualified health care professional. (From Goldman L: *Cecil textbook of medicine*, ed 22, Philadelphia, 2004, Saunders.)

After tumor removal, the frequency of follow-up surveillance varies depending on multiple factors, including the patient's health status, family history, and location and thickness of the excised tumor. General recommendations call for reexamination every 6 to 12 months for the first 1 to 2 years. Annual skin examinations thereafter are recommended for life.[229] Treatment of metastatic melanoma is beyond the scope of this chapter.

**PROGNOSIS.** Malignant melanoma is a more serious problem than other types of skin cancer because it can spread quickly and insidiously, becoming life threatening at an earlier stage of development. It is, however, essentially 100% curable if detected early. Lack of awareness and early screening for melanoma in people with dark skin can delay diagnosis and treatment, resulting in a more serious prognosis in this population.[76]

The prognosis for all types of melanoma depends primarily on tumor thickness and depth of invasion.[171] More superficial and thinner tumors have a better prognosis. For example, stage I nonulcerated melanoma tumors less than 0.8 mm deep have an excellent prognosis (5-year survival rate is 97%). As tumor depth increases, prognosis declines, with average 5-year survival rates for stage IV melanoma of 15% to 20%.[21,26] Metastatic melanoma has a very poor prognosis, with a median survival of less than 1 year.[230] Education on the effects of UV radiation exposure and typical signs and symptoms combined with routine skin screenings can dramatically reduce the incidence and recurrence of skin cancer.

**SPECIAL IMPLICATIONS FOR THE THERAPIST 10.9**

### *Malignant Melanoma*

During observation and inspection of all colors of skin, the therapist should be alert to potential signs of skin cancer. Abnormal spots or lesions, especially in sun-exposed areas, that are rough in texture, persistently present, and bleed with minimal friction should be thoroughly examined. It is important to keep in mind, however, that a seborrheic keratosis commonly bleeds and once diagnosed, bleeding should not cause undue alarm. Likewise, therapists should not become overly concerned about small pink spots on a patient's skin, as other common skin conditions (e.g., eczema, psoriasis, seborrheic dermatitis) are prevalent.

As discussed in the text, *any* change in a wart or mole (color, size, shape, texture, ulceration, bleeding, itching) should be inspected by a qualified health care provider. The Skin Cancer Foundation advocates the use of the ABCDE method and ugly duckling sign for early detection of melanoma and dysplastic (abnormal in size or shape) moles (Box 10.8).[130,220]

Other signs and symptoms that may be important include irritation and itching; tenderness, soreness, or new moles developing around a questionable mole; a mole that looks different from the others (ugly duckling sign); or a wound that does not progress toward healing within 6 weeks. For any patient with a previous history of skin cancer, the need for continued close follow-up to detect recurrence should be emphasized. Education on the effects of UV radiation and taking precautions (Box 10.9) can dramatically reduce the incidence of skin cancer.

If surgery is required, the therapist may be involved with wound management that may involve care of a skin graft and associated donor site. Donor sites may be as painful as the tumor excision site and just as much at risk for infection. Standard Precautions are essential for postoperative patients. If lymphadenectomy is performed, the therapist may be involved in minimizing lymphedema or treating residual lymphedema.

For patients with terminal disease, hospice care will likely include pain control and management. It is important that pain medications be delivered on a schedule that significantly decreases or prevents pain. At this point, decisions regarding wound management are often palliative.

## Kaposi Sarcoma

### Definition and Overview

KS is a connective tissue malignancy that manifests as a skin or mucous membrane disorder. There are four types of KS: classic, endemic, iatrogenic, and epidemic.[205] *Classic KS* occurs predominately in older Eastern European or Mediterranean men, whereas *endemic KS*, or African KS, occurs in younger individuals of African descent. *Iatrogenic KS* is typically associated with organ transplantation. *Epidemic* KS occurs in individuals with HIV; the sudden emergence of this malignancy in the Western world is directly related to AIDS-associated immunodeficiency.

### Etiologic Factors, Incidence, and Risk Factors

KS typically manifests as a skin or mucous membrane disorder most frequently in individuals who are immunocompromised. It represents approximately 2% of cancers worldwide and 1 of every 200 cancers in the United States in patients with transplants.[205] As a result of the AIDS explosion in the 1990s, the incidence of KS in the United States increased from a ratio of 2:1,000,000 to 47:1,000,000. With appropriate treatment, the ratio has decreased to 6:1,000,000, with approximately 2500 KS cases each year.[205]

Risk factors associated with the four types of KS include genetic predisposition (classic and endemic), sexual activity with persons with AIDS and/or their sexual partners (epidemic), being male, and use of immunosuppressants (iatrogenic and epidemic).[205]

### Pathogenesis

KS is an angioproliferative tumor caused by the KS-associated herpesvirus.[205] It has a range of clinical presentation from inactive skin disorder to severe widespread involvement extending to the viscera.[199] Certain coexisting factors are involved in KS pathogenesis, including genetic predisposition, various environmental factors, and local (e.g., lymph congestion) and systemic (e.g., organ transplant, chemical exposure, immunomodulatory medications such as quinine) immunodeficiency.[199]

### Clinical Manifestations

Classic KS occurs commonly on the lower extremities. Affected areas are red, purple, or dark blue macules (Fig. 10.13) that slowly enlarge to become nodules or ulcers. Itching and pain in lesions that impinge on nerves or organs may occur. As the sarcoma progresses, lymphatic obstruction may result in edema, and lesions may spread by metastasis through the upper body to the face and oral mucosa.

In contrast to classic forms of the disease, epidemic KS is a multicentric entity that appears on the upper body (including face, chest, and neck) but can occur on the legs (Fig. 10.14). Early lesions are light pink and can easily be mistaken for bruises or nevi and be ignored.

### MEDICAL MANAGEMENT

**DIAGNOSIS, TREATMENT, AND PROGNOSIS.** Diagnosis is made by linking patient history with diagnostic findings. Diagnostics may include various laboratory tests and HIV screening; skin biopsy; radiography, MRI, or CT for

**Box 10.8**

**ABCDE METHOD OF EARLY MELANOMA DETECTION**

A Asymmetry: uneven edges, lopsided in shape, one half unlike the other
B Border: irregularity, irregular edges scalloped or poorly defined edges
C Color variability: black, shades of brown, red, white, pink, occasionally blue
D Diameter: larger than a pencil eraser (>6 mm)
E Evolution or change; one mole looks different from all the others on an individual (often referred to as the ugly duckling sign); mole changes, itches, or bleeds

**Box 10.9**

**SUNAWARE GUIDELINES FOR PREVENTION OF SKIN CANCER**

Teach everyone to decrease their risk of skin cancer using the AWARE acronym:

A Avoid unprotected exposure to sunlight, seek shade, never indoor tan
W Wear sun protective clothing including long-sleeve shirts, pants, wide-brimmed hat and sunglasses year-round
A Apply sunscreen with a sunburn protection factor (SPF) of 30 or greater to all exposed skin; reapply every 2 hours, especially if exposed to wind, water, or perspiration
R Routinely examine your whole body for changes in skin and have a health care provider evaluate any skin changes
E Educate your family and community; protect babies from day 1, and begin education early with young children

*Note:* The AWARE acronym is based on the advice given by countless organizations, including the Skin Cancer Foundation, World Health Organization, American Academy of Dermatology, Environmental Protection Agency, American Cancer Society, and Children's Melanoma Prevention Foundation.

Data from Children's Melanoma Prevention Foundation, SunAWARE 2018, Norwell, MA. For more information, see http://www.melanomaprevention.org.

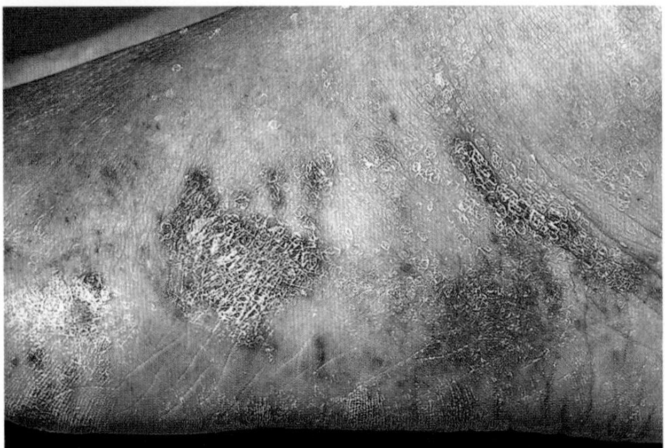

**Figure. 10.13**

**Classic Kaposi sarcoma is present as typical nodular lesions on this ankle and foot.** (From Kumar V, Abbas AK, Fausto M: *Robbins and Cotran pathologic basis of disease*, ed 7, Philadelphia, 2005, Saunders.)

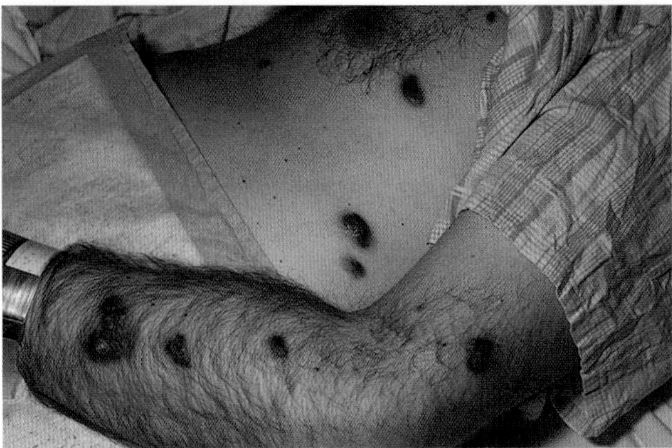

**Figure. 10.14**

**Epidemic Kaposi sarcoma in the plaque stage.** Evolving lesions develop into raised papules or thickened plaques that are oval in shape and vary in color from red to brown. (From Swartz MH: *Textbook of physical diagnosis*, ed 6, Philadelphia, 2009, Saunders.)

infiltrates; and Doppler studies.[205] Nonblanching large dermatologic manifestations of KS can be alarming, but visceral involvement associated with epidemic KS, the most aggressive type of KS, is the most life threatening.

Chemotherapy, surgical excision, and radiation are typical interventions for classic KS. Iatrogenic KS is treated similarly with the inclusion of limiting or eliminating the immunosuppressive factor where possible. Treatment for endemic KS is much the same and varies depending on availability. The standard treatment for epidemic KS is highly active antiretroviral therapy, which may be combined with chemotherapy and other drugs depending on the level of involvement or complicating factors. Local surgical therapy, laser therapy, or cryotherapy may be prescribed.[205] See discussion of AIDS in Chapter 7.

SPECIAL IMPLICATIONS FOR THE THERAPIST 10.10

*Kaposi Sarcoma*

Prevention of skin breakdown and wound management are the usual focus of intervention. Standard Precautions should be followed to prevent infection from being transmitted to the patient. Patients receiving radiation therapy must keep irradiated skin dry to avoid possible breakdown and subsequent infection.

# SKIN DISORDERS ASSOCIATED WITH IMMUNE DYSFUNCTION

## Psoriasis

### Definition and Prevalence

Psoriasis is a chronic, genetic, recurrent inflammatory but noninfectious dermatosis characterized by well-defined erythematous plaques covered with a silvery scale (Fig. 10.15). There are several types of psoriasis, including plaque, guttate, erythrodermic, and pustular.

Psoriasis occurs equally in both genders and can occur at any point across the life span. Once present, psoriasis becomes a chronic condition that may be remitting/recurring. While worldwide data show prevalence ranges

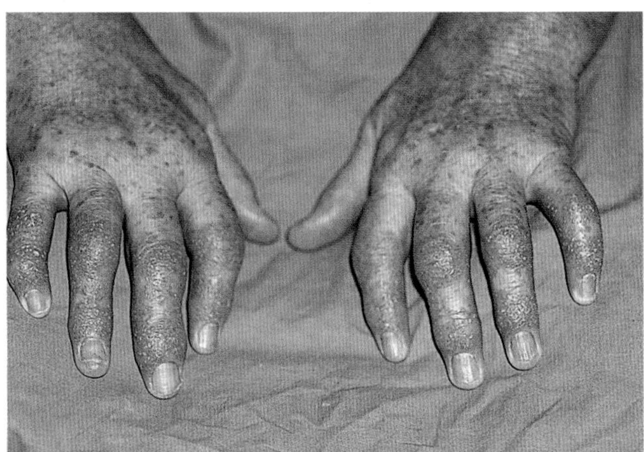

**Figure. 10.15**

Deforming arthritis of the hands in a person with psoriasis (psoriatic arthritis). (From Callen JP, et al: *Color atlas of dermatology*, ed 2, Philadelphia, 2000, Saunders.)

from less than 1% to 11.43%, reporting is largely of cases of European descent.[168]

### Etiologic and Risk Factors

Psoriasis is multifactorial and thought to be genetically linked with multigene involvement and is characterized by immune system dysregulation.[113,116] Triggers of the disease are not well understood but may include infection, prescription drug use, stress, excessive alcohol use, smoking, and injury to the skin.[64,116] Epigenetic factors may influence disease progression. Related disease susceptibility includes rheumatoid arthritis, Crohn's disease, multiple sclerosis, metabolic disorders, and cancer.[113,116]

### Pathogenesis

Normally, the life cycle of a skin cell is 26 to 28 days: 14 days to move from the basal layer to the stratum corneum and 14 days of normal wear and tear before the cell is sloughed off. In contrast, the turnover time of psoriatic skin is 3 to 4 days. This shortened cycle does not allow time for the cell to mature; thus cells stick and build up on the skin, resulting in a thick and flaky stratum corneum, which in turn produces the cardinal manifestations of psoriasis. A second component in the pathogenesis of psoriasis is an immune system reaction resulting in high levels of IL-17, which produces inflammation affecting the keratinocytes. Epidermal changes (e.g., proliferation, hyperplasia) are produced along with leukocyte recruitment.[116] These changes result in the typical presentation of psoriasis.

### Clinical Manifestations

Psoriasis appears as erythematous papules and plaques covered with silvery scales. Lesions typically have a predilection for the scalp, chest, nails, extensor surfaces, groin, skin folds, lower back, and buttocks.[53] Occurrence may vary from a solitary lesion to countless patches covering large areas of the body in a symmetric pattern.[53] Two distinguishing features are the tendency for this condition to recur and to persist.

Flare-ups are more common in winter, with increased skin dryness and decreased sunlight.[53] The severity of psoriasis varies over time, and exacerbations and remissions often correlate with stress and mental outlook. The most common subjective complaint is itching. Pain from dry, cracked, encrusted lesions can also occur. Psoriasis may spread to the fingernails, producing small indentations and yellow or brown discoloration. In severe cases the accumulation of thick, crumbly debris under the nail causes it to separate from the nail bed (nail dystrophy).[53]

As many as 30% of people with psoriasis (usually moderate to severe disease) develop arthritic symptoms referred to as psoriatic arthritis.[53] Psoriatic arthritis usually affects one or more joints of the fingers or toes or sometimes the sacroiliac joints. These patients report morning stiffness lasting more than 30 minutes. Early screening for psoriatic arthritis is important and allows for early treatment.[53]

## MEDICAL MANAGEMENT

**DIAGNOSIS.** Diagnosis depends on patient history, clinical presentation, and rarely skin biopsy to identify psoriatic changes in the skin.[53] Psoriasis must be distinguished from eczema, seborrheic dermatitis, and lichen-like papules.[53] The Psoriasis Area and Severity Index is used to quantify the extent of the disease.[51,53]

**TREATMENT.** In the absence of a cure, the goal of treatment is to maximize remission and minimize outbreaks. Therapy is highly individualized and often determined by trial and error, considering patient response. Psoriasis does not spread. Moreover, early treatment does not prevent the condition from progressing.

New options exist that adequately suppress the disease process and help provide better control of psoriasis through a combination of therapies. In 70% to 80% of cases of mild to moderate disease, the disease is controlled using topical treatment. In cases in which greater control is required, additional treatment may also include phototherapy (e.g., UVB), photochemotherapy, systemic therapy (e.g., methotrexate, cyclosporine), or biologics.[53,126]

Topical treatment of psoriasis is usually the first line of therapy with therapeutic agents, including tar derivatives, corticosteroids, and vitamin D analogues.[126] Topicals come in many forms, including ointments, sprays, foams, and gels.[126] Formulation, ease of use, acceptability of cosmesis, and patient preference are important for clinical choice and efficacy.[126] Corticosteroids are commonly prescribed for psoriasis, but long-term use can result in skin atrophy.[53]

Exposure to UV light (phototherapy), such as UVB or natural sunlight, acts as a local immunosuppressant and inhibits epidermal proliferation.[167] UVB is often combined with topical or oral medication (e.g., psoralens, methotrexate, or retinoids). Though phototherapy can increase the efficacy of treatment, it is time-consuming and can be associated with skin cancer.[53]

Methotrexate may be used to inhibit the rapid reproduction of keratinocytes in psoriasis. It also has an immunosuppressant effect, tempering the inflammatory response. Cyclosporine, also an immunosuppressant, has been approved as a psoriasis treatment. Drugs classed as biologics may also be beneficial. Many immunosuppressive medications used to treat psoriasis have potentially serious side effects and must be monitored closely.

**PROGNOSIS.** Psoriasis usually recurs at intervals and lasts for increasingly longer periods, but treatment typically brings relief during flare-ups. Spontaneous cure is uncommon, and the risk of infection is high. Individuals with psoriasis who are HIV positive are at a higher risk for infection.[77]

**SPECIAL IMPLICATIONS FOR THE THERAPIST 10.11**

### *Psoriasis*

Physical therapy and occupational therapy are key components in the treatment of moderate to severe psoriasis, with desired outcomes based on minimizing functional limitations. Consensus guidelines for the management of psoriasis including phototherapy protocols are available.

Patient instruction and direct intervention to provide skin care should emphasize the following: (1) steroid cream application must be in a thin film, gently rubbed into the skin until completely absorbed; (2) all topical medications, especially those containing anthralin and tar, should be applied with a downward motion to avoid rubbing them into hair follicles, causing inflammation (folliculitis); (3) medication should be applied only to the affected lesions, avoiding contact with normal surrounding skin; and (4) gloves must be worn when applying topical agents because anthralin stains and injures the skin.

After application the treated area should be dusted with powder to prevent anthralin from transferring onto clothes. Mineral oil followed by soap and water can be used to remove anthralin. A soft brush can be used to remove the scales, but vigorous rubbing should be avoided.

Any side effects must be reported immediately, especially allergic reactions; atrophy and acne from steroids; and burning, itching, and nausea. Squamous cell epithelioma may develop from psoralens combined with UVA (PUVA) treatment. Methotrexate may cause hepatic or bone marrow toxicity and may also be teratogenic, so it is not used for women who are pregnant, trying to become pregnant, or breastfeeding.

Other immunosuppressants when used over a long period have a cumulative effect and therefore the potential to cause serious side effects such as poor wound healing, high blood pressure, kidney damage, cancer, and many other complications. Additionally, relaxation and stress management techniques should be routinely employed to help prevent flare-ups.

**Psoriatic Arthritis**

Clinically, psoriatic arthritis differs from rheumatoid arthritis by the more frequent involvement of the distal interphalangeal joints, asymmetric distribution of affected joints, presence of spondyloarthropathy (including the presence of both sacroiliitis and spondylitis), and characteristic extraarticular features (e.g., psoriatic skin lesions, iritis, mouth ulcers, urethritis, colitis, aortic valve disease). Joints are less tender in psoriatic arthritis, which may lead to underestimation of the degree of inflammation. Pain and stiffness of inflamed joints are usually increased by prolonged immobility and alleviated by physical activity. Evidence of inflammation is pain on stressing the joint, tenderness at the joint line, and the presence of effusion.

**Psychologic Considerations**

Psoriasis can result in psychologic issues related to the appearance of skin lesions and fear of being contagious. It is important that patients understand psoriasis is not contagious, and flare-ups can be controlled or limited with medical treatment.[53] Stress management (e.g., relaxation techniques, group counseling, and medical management) may help prevent recurrences and improve patient outcomes.[77,111]

## Lupus Erythematosus

Lupus erythematosus (LE) is a chronic inflammatory disorder of the connective tissues.[100] It appears in several forms, including cutaneous LE primarily affecting the skin and systemic lupus erythematosus (SLE), which affects multiple organ systems (including the skin) with considerably more morbidity and associated mortality. The characteristic rash of lupus is red, hence the term *erythematosus*.[106]

### Cutaneous Lupus Erythematosus

**Overview and Incidence.** The subsets of LE involving the skin include chronic cutaneous LE, acute cutaneous LE, and subacute cutaneous LE.[180] Only the skin-related components of LE are discussed in this chapter. See also Systemic Lupus Erythematosus in Chapter 7.

Chronic cutaneous LE, formerly called discoid lupus, is marked by chronic skin eruptions on sun-exposed skin that can lead to scarring and disfigurement if untreated.[100] It occurs in 6% to 10% of people with SLE.[100] Acute cutaneous LE occurs in about 50% of patients who have SLE and includes both malar erythema (butterfly rash) and widespread erythema, as well as bullous lesions.[180] Association with systemic disease is highest in this subset of LE with virtually all patients meeting the American College of Rheumatology criteria for SLE. Subacute cutaneous LE is marked by recurrent lesions that are typically symmetrically distributed on sun-exposed skin. These lesions do not technically form scars; however, they may result in pigmentation changes or telangiectasia. Lesions rarely occur on the center of the face or over the knuckles.[180]

Cutaneous LE incidence increases with age and has been reported highest between the ages of 60 and 69.[129] It occurs more frequently in women than men, with a 10:1 ratio compared with systemic LE, which has a 3:1 female/male occurrence ratio.[129]

**Etiologic and Risk Factors and Pathogenesis.** The exact cause of cutaneous LE is not clear, but evidence suggests an abnormal response to apoptosis of keratinocytes. Tissue damage occurs at the epidermal–dermal junction, owing to faulty responses of the innate and adaptive immune systems.[147] Interrelated immunologic, environmental, hormonal, and genetic factors may trigger the immune response.[147] Smoking may increase the likelihood of worsening lupus, and patients may experience decreased responsiveness to antimalarials, which are sometimes used to treat the disease.[147]

Other risk factors for cutaneous LE include exposure to sunlight. It is thought that UV light can trigger an autoimmune state in the skin, causing a proinflammatory environment that initiates the autoimmune component of lupus pathogenesis.[147]

**Clinical Manifestations.** Discoid lesions (in chronic cutaneous LE) can develop from the rash often associated with lupus and become raised red, smooth plaques with follicular plugging and central atrophy. The raised edges and sunken centers give them a coinlike (discoid) appearance (Fig. 10.16).[100] Although these lesions can appear anywhere on the body, they usually erupt on the face, scalp, ears, neck, and arms or any part of the body that is exposed to sunlight.[180] Lesions more typical of systemic lupus are shown in Fig. 10.17.

With cutaneous LE, hair tends to become brittle, and scalp lesions can cause localized alopecia. Facial plaques sometimes assume the classic butterfly pattern, with lesions appearing on the cheeks and bridge of the nose. The rash may vary in severity from a sunburned appearance to discoid lesions. These lesions can occur in the absence of other lupus-related symptoms and tend to leave hypopigmented and hyperpigmented scars that can become a cosmetic concern.[106,180]

The most recognized skin manifestation of SLE (acute cutaneous LE) is the classic butterfly rash over the nose, cheeks, and forehead commonly precipitated by exposure to sunlight (UV rays). This classic rash occurs in a large percentage of affected people, but rash can occur on the scalp, neck, upper chest, shoulders, extensor surface of the arms, and dorsa of the hands.[106,180] Resolution of rashes may occur spontaneously or slowly over time, with lingering altered pigmentation.[180]

Other skin manifestations may point to the presence of vasculitis (inflammation of cutaneous blood vessels) leading to infarctive lesions in the digits, necrotic leg ulcers, or digital gangrene. Acute cutaneous LE is usually accompanied by other symptoms of SLE[180] that are beyond the scope of this chapter (see also Systemic Lupus Erythematosus in Chapter 7).

## MEDICAL MANAGEMENT

**DIAGNOSIS AND TREATMENT.** Patient history and appearance of the rash itself are diagnostic, but skin biopsy of the discoid lesions may be performed. The Cutaneous Lupus Erythematosus Disease Area and Severity Index (CLASI) is used to assess disease activity levels.[100]

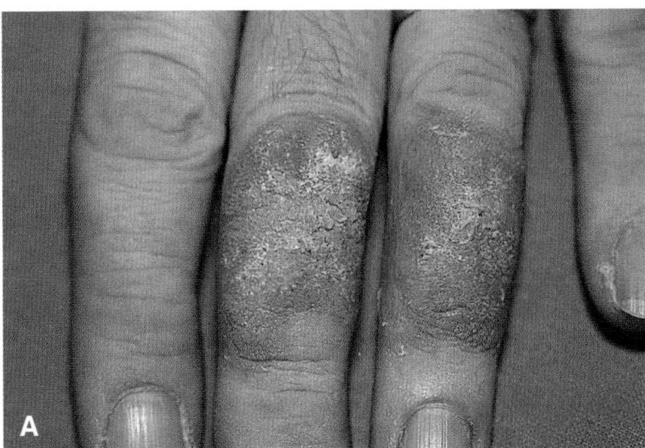


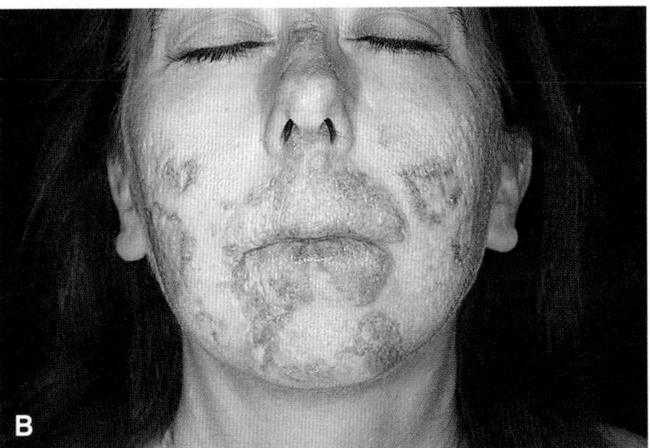


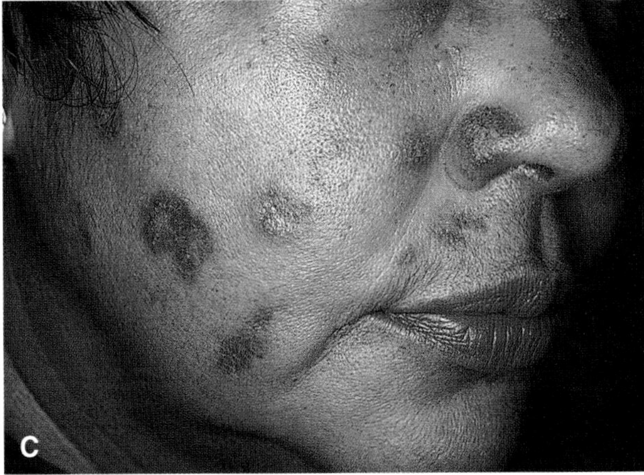


**Figure. 10.16**

**Discoid lupus erythematosus.** Skin changes associated with discoid lupus erythematosus can manifest in a variety of ways. (A) Hypertrophic discoid lupus erythematosus with prominent adherent scale. (B) Round or oval cutaneous lesions can occur on the face or other parts of the body. (C) Round or oval cutaneous lesions as they appear on a dark-skinned individual. (From Callen JP, et al: *Color atlas of dermatology*, ed 2, Philadelphia, 2000, Saunders.)

Patients with any form of cutaneous lupus should avoid prolonged sun exposure (especially during peak hours) and wear protective clothing, use sunscreen, and take actions to avoid sun exposure (see Box 10.4).[100] Any changes in the lesions should be reported to a qualified health care professional.

Drug treatment consists of topical, intralesional, or oral medications.[100] Corticosteroids are often used as first-line topical treatment. If corticosteroids are

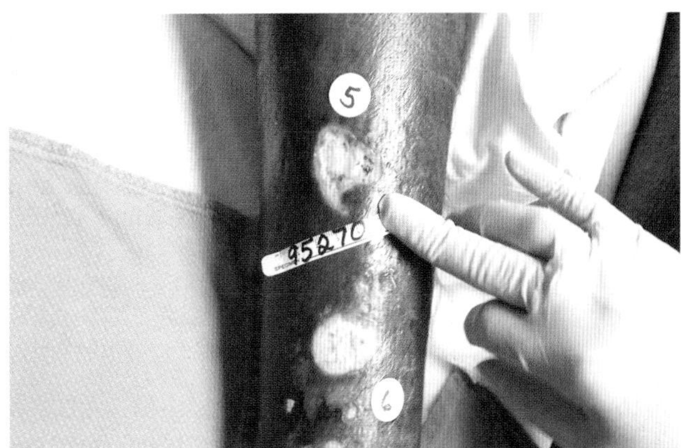

**Figure. 10.17**

**Lesions typical of systemic lupus erythematosus found on the lower extremities.** The lesions are ulcerated, punched-out wounds with necrotic bases. Discoid lupus lesions (see Fig. 10.16) are usually found on the face and scalp and are raised, flat, coin-shaped wounds. (Courtesy Harriett B. Loehne, PT, DPT, CWS, FACCWS. Used with permission.)

inappropriate, calcineurin inhibitors and/or a physical modality such as laser may also be used.[100] When topical or intralesional treatments fail, systemic treatments are chosen, starting with antimalarials. Other systemic treatments may follow (e.g., methotrexate, vitamin A analogues, biologics).[100]

Lesions may resolve spontaneously in affected individuals or may cause hypopigmentation or hyperpigmentation, atrophy, and scarring. Discoid lesions are not life threatening (unless accompanied by complications of SLE) but are associated with psychologic distress and altered quality of life.

**PROGNOSIS.** In general the prognosis of cutaneous LE is better than that of SLE. Over time, 5% to 10% of patients with chronic cutaneous LE progress to SLE. Of patients with subacute cutaneous LE, 50% to 60% may need immunosuppressant treatment for systemic manifestations. More active cutaneous LE may be indicated by the presence of photosensitivity, hair loss, Raynaud phenomenon, and oral ulcers. Monitoring is important to detect early progression of the disease.[231]

**SPECIAL IMPLICATIONS FOR THE THERAPIST 10.12**

### *Cutaneous Lupus Erythematosus*

Patients with LE with skin involvement require careful assessment, supportive measures, and emotional support. Skin lesions should be checked thoroughly at each visit. The patient should be urged to get plenty of rest, follow energy conservation guidelines, and practice good nutrition.

The therapist can be instrumental in teaching and assisting with skin care, prevention of skin breakdown, range-of-motion (ROM) exercises, prevention of orthopedic deformities, ergonomic and postural training, and relief of joint pain associated with SLE. Persons with LE exposed to the long-term effects of corticosteroids should be followed carefully.

## Systemic Sclerosis

### Definition and Overview

Systemic sclerosis (SSc), previously called scleroderma, is an autoimmune disease that affects connective tissues, causing fibrosis of the skin, joints, blood vessels, and internal organs. This chronic disease is classified according to the degree and extent of skin thickening.[40]

There are two distinct subtypes: SSc and localized SSc. SSc can take one of three forms: limited SSc, diffuse SSc, and an overlap form with either diffuse or limited skin thickening.[79]

Limited SSc was previously known as the *CREST syndrome* from its manifestations (*c*alcinosis, *R*aynaud phenomenon, *e*sophageal dysmotility, *s*clerodactyly, *t*elangiectasia). Persons with this form of SSc have a much lower incidence of serious internal organ involvement, although pulmonary hypertension and esophageal disease are not uncommon. Skin thickening is limited to the extremities distal to the elbows and knees.[40]

The diffuse form is far more debilitating, with skin thickening at the extremities in general and more severe organ involvement.[40] Organ damage can affect the heart, gastrointestinal tract, lungs, and kidneys.[80] Diffuse SSc is characterized by involvement of all body parts, including skin. Disease progression varies based in part on the timing of onset and extent of involvement.[7,33,121,127,163] Severity not only depends on the extent of involvement but also on the number of organs affected. Organ involvement in the first few years of diagnosis suggests more severe involvement.[81]

Localized SSc primarily affects the skin in one or many different areas without visceral organ involvement[153] and should not be confused with limited SSc. Classification of localized SSc includes limited, generalized, linear, deep, and mixed. The limited form is the most common, with its plaque formation (morphea).[153] Morphea is characterized by hard oval-shaped patches on the skin, generally on the trunk. These patches are usually white with a surrounding purple ring.[153] The generalized form is characterized by affecting at least three places, which tend to be on the trunk or thighs. Rarely, larger areas may be involved in a more disabling form (pansclerotic morphea).[153] The linear form refers to SSc with a bandlike lesion that occurs on the arms, legs, and forehead. Underlying bones and muscles may also be affected, resulting in mobility deficits.[153] One specific form of this is en coup de sabre, which involves the scalp (resulting in alopecia) and may involve the central nervous system.[153] The least common form is the deep form, in which deeper connective tissues are affected, including muscle, adipose, and fascia.[153] Finally in the mixed form, more than one subtype of localized SSc could be present.[153]

### Incidence and Prevalence

Incidence of SSc varies widely according to region. Worldwide, incidence ranges from 3.7 to 43 per 1 million.[40] In the United States, incidence has been reported to be between 13.9 and 21 per 1 million.[40] U.S. prevalence was reported from 276 to 659 per 1 million.[40]

### Etiologic and Risk Factors

SSc is an autoimmune disease that may be described as having dysfunctional connective tissue repair following injury. [80]Susceptibility to developing SSc may have genetic and environmental links.[80]

Environmental triggers that seem to put one at risk for SSc include exposure to silica, particularly for men.[40] While cigarette smoking has not been shown to increase risk for SSc, it may affect the severity of the disease.[40] Other chemicals have been linked to SSc, and for this reason, chemical exposure may be relevant in certain cases.[80]

SSc affects women more than men[40] with male-to-female ratios between 1:3.6 and 1:4.2.[29] Most commonly, onset occurs between the ages of 20 and 50 years, and age of onset seems to have an effect on the clinical presentation.[7] Early onset is more often linked to disease manifestations that include esophageal involvement and myositis, whereas individuals with late onset are less likely to have digital ulcers and more likely to have cardiac or pulmonary complications.[7,121,163]

For women considering pregnancy, it is important to consider possible ramifications of SSc. In general, people with SSc appear to have normal fertility without an increased incidence of miscarriage compared with the general population; however, they are more at risk for preterm delivery.[238] For women earlier in the disease process or at higher risk, delay of pregnancy is encouraged until the disease is inactive. While pregnancy does not seem to increase renal complications, kidney function should be monitored,[238] and pregnancy should be avoided in the presence of disease-related organ insufficiency (e.g., pulmonary hypertension).[238] In pregnant women with SSc, delivery room environment (i.e., warm temperature) should be considered.[238]

### Pathogenesis

Pathogenesis involves multiple types of cells and their processes.[80] While the early disease process may show vascular and immune components, progression is diverse owing to disease complexity.[80] As an understanding of the pathogenesis becomes clearer, so too do the targeted approaches to treatment.[80] Likewise, as screening and treatment improve, survival rate also improves.[40,80]

Widespread small vessel vasculopathy and fibrosis set SSc apart from other connective tissue diseases. SSc is a disease affecting the immune system in which damage to the microvasculature causes an immune response (e.g., production of autoantibodies and cytokines/chemokines that promote inflammation and fibrosis).[40] Dysregulation of the repair process of connective tissue is likely part of the pathophysiology.[80] This disease is marked by excessive collagen deposition in the intima of blood vessels, the pericapillary space, and the interstitium of the skin, resulting in scarring and fibrosis.[36,40] This distinguishes SSc from other autoimmune disorders.

Vasoconstriction in small vessels eventually leads to narrowing of the vessels and a lack of blood supply. The consequence of intermittent ischemia followed by reperfusion causes increased production of reactive oxygen species and further damage. Damaged endothelial cells cause local inflammation, including antiendothelial antibodies. This may lead to apoptosis and defective angiogenesis. Microangiopathy is thought to be related to the organ involvement seen in SSc.[36] The immune system also contributes to the disease process, and autoantibodies may be linked to the type of disease or organ damage present.[36,82]

### Clinical Manifestations

Initially, bilateral nonpitting edema is present in the fingers and hands and rarely in the feet. Edema can progress to the forearms, arms, upper chest, abdomen, back, and face. After a few weeks to several months, edema is replaced by thick, hardened skin. Peripheral nervous system involvement affects nerve terminals, reducing sensory fibers in affected skin. Neuropeptides released by sensory nerve endings are reduced, resulting in vasoconstriction in the skin.

**Integument.** Initial edema is replaced by skin that becomes tight, smooth, and waxy or shiny and seems bound down to underlying structures. Accompanying changes include a loss of normal skin folds, decreased flexibility, and skin hyperpigmentation and hypopigmentation. Facial skin may also become tight and inelastic, and the face can take on a stretched, masklike appearance, with thin lips and a pinched nose.[82]

Actual atrophy of skin may occur, particularly over joints at sites of flexion contractures, such as the proximal interphalangeal joints and elbows. Flexion contractures are especially severe in people with diffuse SSc.

Thinning of the skin contributes to the development of ulcerations at the sites of joint contractures. Pitting ulcers can also occur at the tips of the fingers.[82] Skin softening and return to normal may occur to some extent. Improvement typically begins centrally so that the last areas to become classically involved are the first to show this regression.

Subcutaneous calcification (calcinosis), a late-developing complication, is considerably more frequent in limited SSc. These calcifications vary in size from tiny deposits to large masses ulcerating the overlying skin. Sites of trauma are often affected, such as the fingers, forearms, elbows, and knees.[82]

**Raynaud Phenomenon.** Although SSc affects people differently (Box 10.10), a common first symptom is Raynaud phenomenon, appearing almost universally (95%) in cases of SSc.[7,82] Raynaud phenomenon is characterized by sudden blanching, cyanosis, and erythema of the fingers and toes as the walls of blood vessels supplying the hands and feet become narrowed. Closure of the muscular digital arteries, precapillary arterioles, and arteriovenous shunts of the skin causes the hands and/or feet to become white, numb, and then bluish in color as blood flow remains blocked. When the spasm eases and blood flow returns, rewarming occurs, and the fingers and/or toes become red and painful. This cycle is typically initiated in response to stress or exposure to cold.

**Neuromusculoskeletal System.** Most people with diffuse SSc have disuse atrophy of muscle because of limited joint motion secondary to skin, joint, or tendon involvement. A small percentage of people may have overlapping syndromes and demonstrate marked weakness and inflammatory myopathy indistinguishable from polymyositis or dermatomyositis.[82]

Box 10.10

**CHARACTERISTICS LIKELY TO BE SEEN IN CLIENTS WITH SYSTEMIC SCLEROSIS EARLY AND LATE IN THE DISEASE COURSE**

***Early (≤5 years)***

*Limited Disease*

- Rapidly progressive
  - Renal crisis (5%)
  - Interstitial lung disease (severe in 10%–15%)
- Slowly progressive
  - Raynaud phenomenon
  - Cutaneous ulceration
  - Esophageal dysmotility

*Diffuse Disease*

- Rapidly progressive
  - Skin thickening
  - Heart involvement (severe in 10%–15%)
  - Interstitial lung disease (severe in 15%)
  - Renal crisis (15%–20%)
  - Contractures, joint pain
  - Cutaneous ulcerations
  - Esophageal dysmotility
  - Gastrointestinal complications

***Late (>5 years)***

*Limited Disease*

- Slowly progressive
  - Raynaud phenomenon
  - Cutaneous ulcerations
  - Esophageal dysmotility
  - Gastrointestinal complications
- Very late
  - Pulmonary artery hypertension
  - Biliary cirrhosis

*Diffuse Disease*

- Improvement
  - Skin thickening
  - Musculoskeletal pain
- Slowly progressive
  - Heart, lung, kidney involvement
  - Raynaud phenomenon
  - Esophageal dysmotility
  - Gastrointestinal complications

Modified from Clements PJ: Systemic sclerosis: natural history and management strategies. *J Musculoskelet Med* 11:43–50, 1994.

Joint involvement is common and may include arthralgia affecting the wrist and hand as well as the ankles and knees.[82] Arthritic changes are not usually erosive.[82] Tendon friction rubs are more typically seen in diffuse SSc. Some individuals develop myositis or erosive arthropathy that complicates the joint retraction induced by skin fibrosis. Peripheral neuromuscular changes (e.g., carpal tunnel syndrome) may also occur.[82]

**Viscera.** Gastrointestinal motility dysfunction affects the esophagus and anorectal regions, causing frequent reflux, heartburn, dysphagia, and bloating after meals. Other effects include abdominal distention, diarrhea, constipation, and malodorous floating stools.

In advanced disease, cardiac and pulmonary fibrosis develops.[82] Cardiac involvement can be manifested as myocardial or pericardial disease, conduction system disease, or arrhythmias.[82] Pulmonary involvement is characterized by pulmonary arterial hypertension and pulmonary vascular disease. Pulmonary fibrosis may or may not be present. Pulmonary involvement can also manifest with interstitial lung disease.[82] There is a reduced occurrence of kidney involvement and SSc renal crisis because of the common prescription of angiotensin-converting enzyme inhibitors.[79,80]

**Other Symptoms.** Many adults with SSc report other symptoms, such as major depression, anxiety, sexual dysfunction, trigeminal neuralgia, hypothyroidism, dental involvement, and corneal tears.

## MEDICAL MANAGEMENT

**DIAGNOSIS.** Early diagnosis and accurate staging of visceral involvement are fundamental for appropriate management and therapeutic approach to this disease. However, diagnosis can be delayed because there is no single laboratory test diagnostic for SSc. Rather the diagnosis is based on classification criteria set by the American College of Rheumatology/European League Against Rheumatism, which include skin thickening on the fingers (with scores assigned based on presentation), lesions on the fingertips, telangiectasia, pulmonary arterial hypertension, interstitial lung disease, Raynaud phenomenon, and the presence of autoantibodies (e.g., anti–RNA polymerase III, anti–topoisomerase I, anti-centromere).[82]

Laboratory tests are performed to assess disease criteria and to rule out other disease processes. Various other tests may be used to screen for organ involvement (e.g., high-resolution CT to assess for interstitial lung disease).[82]

Early detection of organ involvement is critical because current treatments are most effective when started early. While the specific course the disease will take is unknown, some biomarkers are associated with risk of complication. For example, the presence of anti–RNA polymerase III antibodies is associated with a higher risk for renal crisis.[206]

**TREATMENT.** At the present time there is no cure for SSc. A global vision of SSc is necessary for this multisystem disease, and each treatment program is individualized to manage the specific disease process. Treatment is based on patient symptoms and depends on the organs that are involved. Whether the disease is limited or diffuse, vascular complications should be addressed (e.g., vasodilator prescription).[79] Follow-up and monitoring for complications related to organ involvement including regular blood pressure assessment is critical.[79]

When organ involvement occurs, it often develops early in the disease course and requires aggressive management. The treatment program depends on the organs involved but may include medications (e.g., immunosuppressants, vasodilators, antimetabolites, proton pump inhibitors, antiinflammatories), exercises, joint protection techniques, skin protection techniques, and stress management.[79,80,152] The therapist has an important role in designing a program to mitigate risks to mobility through exercise and joint protection techniques. Therapists can also contribute to skin protection for the patient and stress management.

Guidelines are available to assist health care providers in the management of SSc.[79,152] Manifestations of SSc in the skin have been managed successfully with immunomodulating agents. Methotrexate has been studied and shown to improve skin manifestations.[152] Skin moisturizers are important, and antihistamines may be used to address pruritus.[79] Therapists are well positioned to manage the associated pain and joint dysfunction with exercise and joint protection strategies.[80] All providers need to be aware of the organ systems that are typically involved so that each can contribute to early detection.[79] It is especially important for therapists to monitor vital signs with activity.

**PROGNOSIS.** Prognosis has improved with early detection of organ involvement and subsequent management, including advances in pharmacologic intervention.[150] Mortality is most often related to cardiac, pulmonary, and renal organ involvement.[150] For renal crisis, early treatment at a specialty center using angiotensin-converting enzyme inhibitors markedly decreases mortality rate.[206] Similarly, early treatment for interstitial lung disease improves outcomes.

Children with a diagnosis of SSc have a 98% 10-year survival rate. Once these children reach adulthood, prevalence of organ involvement is similar to disease with adult onset.[158] While most (approximately 80%) patients with SSc have lung fibrosis or interstitial lung disease, it becomes progressive only about 25% of the time. After early onset of interstitial lung disease, SSc usually becomes stable about 5 years after diagnosis.[80]

# Polymyositis and Dermatomyositis

## Definition and Overview

Polymyositis and dermatomyositis are idiopathic inflammatory diseases of muscle. They often progress slowly with frequent exacerbations and remissions and are characterized by symmetric and progressive proximal weakness. Weakness is most prevalent in the pelvis, neck, and pharynx. Patients may also present

SPECIAL IMPLICATIONS FOR THE THERAPIST 10.13

## *Systemic Sclerosis*

### Skin (Pruritus and Ulcers)

Itching can be a major problem in this condition, and excoriation from scratching can cause open wounds susceptible to infection. The therapist can offer simple suggestions to soothe skin, ease itching, and prevent skin damage (see Box 10.4). Local management of digital tip ulcers may include advanced dressings to promote wound healing and protect against trauma and infection. Guidelines suggest the use of an oral vasodilator and method for analgesia. Sildenafil is suggested before prostanoids or bosentan.[79] Any infection should be quickly addressed.[79] It is important to recognize that patients may have concerns regarding cosmesis following depigmentation or other skin changes.

### Muscle

Myositis is treated with corticosteroids and sometimes requires the addition of immunosuppressive drugs, whereas fibrotic myopathy (fibrotic tissue laid down within the muscle) is best managed with strengthening and ROM exercises. The efficacy of using soft tissue mobilization or similar techniques has not been investigated. Caution must be used when attempting such treatment because the skin of these patients can be heavily sclerosed and sensitive to pressure. Aquatic therapy is often an excellent choice of exercise.

### Joints and Tendons

Joint and tendon sheath involvement is common and may be treated successfully with nonsteroidal antiinflammatory drugs (NSAIDs). In early diffuse SSc, tenosynovitis can be very painful and can limit joint movement. In addition to NSAIDs, early aggressive therapy is important in preventing or minimizing contractures.

For patients with SSc, regular exercise will assist with keeping the skin and joints flexible, maintaining better blood flow, and preventing contractures. Active and passive stretching exercises are necessary, but difficult in the presence of extreme pain.

Analgesia is required to optimize participation in an exercise program. Protecting swollen and painful joints from stresses and strains is also an important factor. This may require teaching joint protection to carry out activities of daily living while minimizing strain on the joints.

Lightweight splints may be necessary to provide joint protection, with regular close monitoring of integumentary integrity. Dynamic splinting has not been found to be effective in preventing flexion contractures. Carpal tunnel syndrome, which often occurs before the diagnosis of SSc, usually responds well to conservative treatment without requiring surgery.

### Exercise

Practice patterns in this area vary depending on the form of cardiovascular or pulmonary involvement. When cardiopulmonary involvement occurs, intervention must take into consideration effects of this disease on the individual's activity and lifestyle. The patient's primary diagnosis and primary intervention may be integument or orthopedic-related, but functional limitations may be present secondary to systemic involvement (e.g., decreased aerobic capacity, endurance, overall general physical condition secondary to cardiovascular and/or pulmonary involvement).

### Psychologic Considerations

Individuals with early diffuse SSc with or without organ involvement are often anxious because their bodies are changing rapidly and in unexpected ways. They may not understand the grave nature of the disease.

Individuals with diffuse SSc are at greatest risk for early visceral disease and early mortality, and education about the disease is important, as is identifying where patients are in the natural history of SSc. Patients should be encouraged to monitor blood pressure at home at least three times per week, as this is the best method of screening for acute hypertension. Blood pressure screening should be included in physical therapy sessions as well.

with gastrointestinal symptoms, ventilation symptoms (e.g., shortness of breath), and skin changes (e.g., heliotrope rash, Gottron papules) accompanied by pruritus.[93,234]

### Incidence

Polymyositis and dermatomyositis are not very common, with incidence rates of 6 to 10 persons per 1 million reported.[45,84] Peak incidence is reported in the 50 to 59 age group for dermatomyositis and in the 60 to 69 age group for polymyositis.[84] Prevalence has been reported between 8 and 22 per 100,000[45,84] with more women affected than men.[208]

### Etiologic Factors

The cause of these conditions remains unknown, although there appears to be some autoimmune mechanism that may be triggered by environmental and genetic factors.[93] T cells inappropriately recognize muscle fiber antigens as foreign and attack muscle tissue. Autoantibodies are present in most cases.[93] Polymyositis and dermatomyositis may be drug induced, possibly triggered by a virus, or associated with other disorders as listed in Box 10.11.

### Pathogenesis

If these conditions are caused by an autoimmune reaction, diffuse or focal muscle fiber degeneration is followed by regeneration of muscle cells, producing remission. Muscle biopsy reveals focal or diffuse inflammatory infiltrates consisting primarily of lymphocytes and macrophages surrounding muscle fibers and small blood vessels. Muscle cells show evidence of degeneration and regeneration, and

Box 10.11

**TYPES OF INFLAMMATORY MYOPATHIES[a]**

- Primary idiopathic polymyositis
- Primary idiopathic dermatomyositis
- Dermatomyositis or polymyositis associated with malignancy (lung, breast, ovarian, gastric, colon)
- Juvenile polymyositis or dermatomyositis
- Polymyositis associated with other connective tissue diseases (overlap)
  - Sjögren syndrome
  - Mixed connective tissue disease
  - Rheumatoid arthritis
  - Systemic lupus erythematosus
  - Systemic sclerosis

[a]Listed in descending order of frequency. Primary idiopathic polymyositis and dermatomyositis account for nearly three-fourths of all cases.

fiber atrophy is most severe at the periphery of the muscle bundle. Extensive interstitial fibrosis and fatty replacement are common in long-standing cases. With chronic disease, individuals also display a lower proportion of slow-twitch muscle fibers and a higher proportion of fast-twitch fibers on biopsy.

### Clinical Manifestations

Symmetric proximal muscle weakness is the dominant feature of these diseases, although it is variable in onset, progression, and severity. In some people, symptoms appear suddenly, progress rapidly, and quickly result in a bedridden state, sometimes requiring ventilatory assistance and tube feeding.

More typically, malaise and weight loss develop insidiously over months or even years, with some patients either unable to identify the onset of the disease or unaware of the developing gradual disability. Fatigue, rather than weakness, is a commonly reported symptom, but close questioning usually reveals functional losses that indicate weakness as well. Pain is not a key feature of these diseases in adults, although aching muscles are not uncommon. Muscle wasting is observed in long-standing or severe cases.

Cardiac involvement is not uncommon and contributes significantly to mortality. Cardiac abnormalities have been reported in 75% of patients with polymyositis or dermatomyositis.[83] These abnormalities include arrhythmias, congestive heart failure, conduction defects, ventricular dysfunction, and pericarditis.[83]

Pulmonary disease (progressive pulmonary fibrosis) can result from weakness of the respiratory muscles, intrinsic lung pathologic conditions, or aspiration. Dysphagia is more common with disease progression.[84]

**Polymyositis.** Polymyositis begins acutely or insidiously, with muscle weakness, tenderness, and discomfort. The proximal muscles of the shoulder and pelvic girdle are affected more often than distal muscles and usually in a symmetric pattern.[93]

Early signs of proximal muscle weakness in upper and lower extremities may include impaired functional status, such as difficulty climbing stairs, getting up from a chair, reaching into an overhead cupboard, combing hair, or lifting the head from a pillow; difficulty with balance; or a tendency to fall, often resulting in fracture. As muscle weakness advances, muscular effects may include decreased deep tendon reflexes, contractures, arthralgias, arthritis, an inability to move against resistance (e.g., pushing open a heavy door, opening a car door), proximal dysphagia (difficulty swallowing), and dysphonia (difficulty speaking).[93]

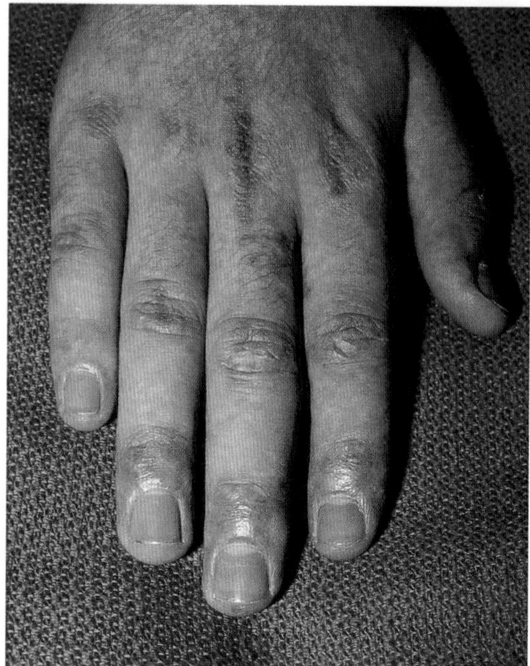

**Figure. 10.18**

**Gottron papules or Gottron sign.** Typical lesions over bony prominences on the extensor surfaces of the hand. (Courtesy, Joseph Jorizzo, MD: From Bolognia JL, Jorizzo JL, Rapini RP (Eds.). *Dermatology*, ed 2, Philadelphia, 2007, Elsevier.)

**Dermatomyositis.** When a rash is associated with polymyositis, it is referred to as *dermatomyositis.*[84] A characteristic purplish rash appears on the eyelids (heliotrope erythema), accompanied by periorbital edema (puffy eyelids).[93] The rash may progress to the anterior neck, upper chest and back, shoulders, and arms and may appear around the nail beds. Gottron papules (red or violet, smooth or scaly patches) may appear on the knuckles, elbows, knees, or medial malleoli (Fig. 10.18).[93] Rashes are typically pruritic.[93]

Although the disease usually begins with erythema and swelling of the face and eyelids, cutaneous manifestations can develop concomitantly or afterward, with proximal muscle weakness at the shoulders, pelvis, ventilator muscles, and pharyngeal muscles.[93] The cutaneous lesions of dermatomyositis are nearly always present by the time proximal muscle weakness manifests.

## MEDICAL MANAGEMENT

DIAGNOSIS. The diagnosis of myositis is often difficult because it closely resembles several other diseases, and the pathologic manifestation can be localized, sometimes resulting in nondiagnostic biopsies. The physician must first rule out internal malignancy with appropriate medical testing.

The presence of progressive symmetric weakness is a hallmark diagnostic finding.[93,234] Laboratory studies to evaluate muscle enzymes, biopsy to assess muscle fibers, and electromyography to measure the electrical activity of the muscles all are necessary to properly diagnose myositis.[93]

Most patients with these diseases have an elevated creatine kinase level at presentation. The creatine kinase level represents striated muscle involvement, although in patients with chronic disease, creatine kinase may be of the cardiac MB isotype. MRI can reveal muscle inflammation and may help to select the site on which to do a biopsy in difficult cases.[93]

**TREATMENT.** Treatment is individualized and includes medication, exercise, and careful monitoring for and prevention of complications.[93] Daily high-dose oral corticosteroid therapy is the usual initial pharmacologic treatment for polymyositis and dermatomyositis.[93] Steroids reduce inflammation, shorten the time to normalization of muscle enzymes, and reduce morbidity. Patients who do not respond well to steroids or who are unable to tolerate the high dosage may be treated with immunosuppressive drugs (e.g., azathioprine, methotrexate).[93] Physical therapy is critical for individualized exercise prescription (see Special Implications for the Therapist 10.14).[10,93] Individuals with skin involvement will need to avoid sun exposure and follow SunAWARE guidelines (see Box 10.9).

**PROGNOSIS.** The prognosis in adults varies depending on age and progression of the disease. Five-year survival rates have been reported as 77% with 62% 10-year survival.[208] While 5-year survival was about the same regardless of sex, at 10 years, survival rate in men was 18% versus 73% in women.[208]

Generally, prognosis is worse with visceral organ involvement, and death results from associated malignancy, respiratory disease, or heart failure.[93] Side effects of therapy (corticosteroids, immunosuppressants) contribute to long-term morbidity. The prognosis for children is guarded if the disease is left untreated, as it progresses rapidly to disabling contractures and muscular atrophy.

SPECIAL IMPLICATIONS FOR THE THERAPIST 10.14

*Polymyositis and Dermatomyositis*

The abrupt onset of any of the cutaneous lesions associated with polymyositis and dermatomyositis could also be a sign of underlying malignancy, particularly genitourinary or gastrointestinal. Differential diagnosis requires medical evaluation before proceeding with therapy intervention.

The therapist plays a pivotal role in the management of myositis. Manual muscle testing and tests of functional ability are useful in following disease progression and therapeutic response over a long period. Therapists may use the *Myositis Damage Index,* a tool that assesses damage in adults who have idiopathic inflammatory myopathy.

Exercise is a safe way to mitigate negative ramifications commonly seen in people with inflammatory myopathies.[10,11,236] Individualized exercise programs incorporating both resistance training and aerobic exercise have been shown to improve muscle strength and function.[10,93,236] While there is evidence that beginning exercise early after diagnosis is safe, it has not shown a significant short-term difference in muscle performance. However, individuals with early exercise did have higher function and were more active.[10] Exercise has been found to not only facilitate muscle development but also to suppress muscle inflammatory response.[172] Intense exercise can even reduce disease activity in patients with established inflammatory myositis while improving function.[10] Current studies are examining the effects of early intensive exercise for inflammatory myositis treatment.[10] Exercise sufficient to at least maintain function is tolerated by most patients; it is unclear whether the addition of medication will support exercise for patients with low tolerance.[10] Therapists treating individuals with this condition will want to stay abreast of any new developments in this area when creating a plan of care.

Preservation of functional mobility and activities of daily living skills including hand strength is important. Consistent follow-up and assessment is also important to modify exercise prescription in response to the patient's ability and response to exercise (e.g., fatigue, pain).[10]

Long-term use of steroids lowers resistance to infection, may induce diabetes, causes myopathy and/or neuropathy, and is associated with loss of potassium in the urine and gastric irritation. If side effects are marked, advise the patient to consult with his or her primary health care provider.

# THERMAL INJURIES

## Cold Injuries

Cold injuries result from overexposure to cold air or water and occur in two major forms: localized injuries (e.g., frostbite) and systemic injuries (e.g., hypothermia). Untreated or improperly treated frostbite can lead to gangrene and may necessitate amputation, requiring therapy and rehabilitation. Hypothermia is a medical emergency and is not within the scope of this chapter.

### Incidence, Etiology, and Risk Factors

Cold injuries, once almost exclusively a military problem, are becoming more prevalent among the general population. Frostbite results from prolonged exposure to subfreezing temperatures.[54] Data from the National Burn Repository and National Trauma Data Bank demonstrate frostbite injury to be more common in males, with the most common location for injury being the lower extremities. On average, approximately 100 patients are admitted to U.S. hospitals with frostbite injury each year.[178] The risk of serious cold injury is increased by lack of insulating body fat, advanced age, homelessness, drug or alcohol use, various peripheral vascular vasoconstrictive diseases, diabetes, altered mental status, and unplanned circumstances leading to cold exposure without adequate protective clothing.[204] There have also been reports of frostbite injuries resulting from inappropriate use and application of cryotherapy.[54,59,107]

### Pathogenesis and Clinical Manifestations

Cold-induced injuries can be local or systemic. Severe cold affects all organ systems, especially the central nervous and cardiovascular systems. Many biologic reactions and pathways become distorted or slowed with low core temperatures, resulting in slowed nerve conduction and muscle contraction and weakness. Reduced ability for physical activity in this instance can contribute to injury.

Typically an initial vasoconstriction in the skin offers some protection when core temperature drops. *Frostnip* is described as a temporary nondamaging, superficial cold injury marked by intense vasoconstriction secondary to exposure to cold. It usually occurs at the nose, cheeks, and/or ears.[166]

Continued exposure to cold to the point of tissue freezing results in intracellular and extracellular ice crystal formation. Ice crystals rupture cellular membranes, interrupt enzyme and metabolic pathways, and cause intracellular dehydration. Local cycles of vasoconstriction and dilation as the body attempts to preserve affected tissues results in blood coagulation and further tissue ischemia. Inflammatory mediators such as thromboxanes and prostaglandins increase edema. Together, these processes result in tissue death.[54]

Frostbite may be superficial or deep. Superficial frostbite affects the skin and subcutaneous tissue, especially of the face, ears, extremities, and other exposed body areas. Although it may go unnoticed at first, after return to a warm place, frostbite produces burning, tingling, numbness, swelling, and a mottled blue-gray skin color.

Deep frostbite extends beyond subcutaneous tissue to structures such as bone, tendon, and muscle[204] and usually affects the hands and/or feet. The skin becomes white until it has thawed and then turns purplish blue. Hemorrhagic blisters may form.[166] Deep frostbite produces pain, tissue necrosis, and gangrene (Fig. 10.19).

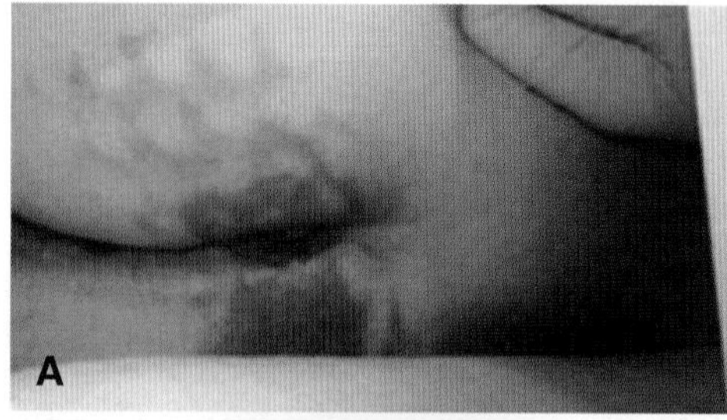


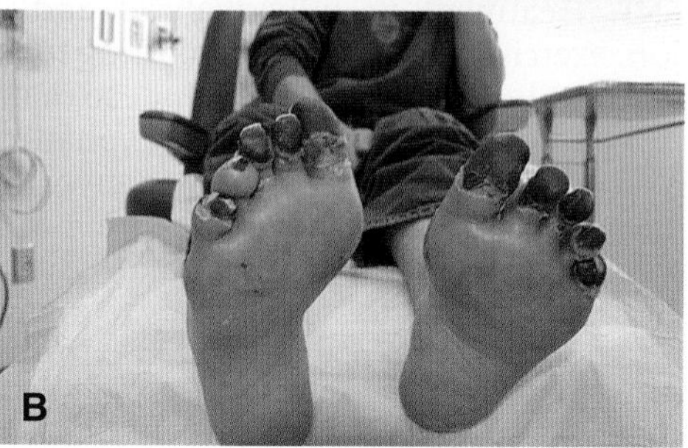


**Figure. 10.19**

**Frostbite.** (A) Frostbite injury on the buttocks caused by prolonged use of a cooling pad. (B) Frostbite injury of the toes. Blackened areas show tissue necrosis and gangrene. (A, Courtesy of Stephanie Woelfel, PT, DPT, CWS, FACCWS, Keck Medical Center of the University of Southern California, Los Angeles, CA. Used with permission. B, From Jurkovich GJ: Environmental cold-induced injury. *Surg Clin North Am* 87:247–267, 2007, Figure 3.)

## MEDICAL MANAGEMENT

**DIAGNOSIS AND TREATMENT.** Diagnosis is usually made based on history and clinical presentation, although the true extent of injury may be revealed only once the tissue is fully rewarmed.[204] Initial intervention should focus on managing hypothermia, preventing mechanical injury, and rapid rewarming.[166] Rewarming should not be performed when there is risk of refreezing, as this causes more severe injury.

Typical rewarming includes submerging affected body parts in 102 °F to 108 °F circulating water for approximately 15 to 30 minutes.[166,204] Rubbing or massage of injured areas is contraindicated, owing to the high risk of causing further damage. Intravenous and/or oral pain medication is delivered during the rewarming process along with ibuprofen for inflammation. Oral or intravenous fluids for general hydration are important to prevent hypovolemia and offset increased blood viscosity.[166]

Tetanus update is also recommended in situations where immunization records are unknown.[204] Prophylactic antibiotics may or may not be administered, depending on overall patient status. In the case of deep frostbite, medications to prevent thrombosis (i.e., vasodilators, anticoagulants) may be prescribed within the first 24 hours of thawing.[204] If present, hemorrhagic blisters are initially left intact, as they represent deeper tissue involvement.[166]

Proper positioning to minimize edema and avoidance of weight bearing is advised. Superficial frostbite areas may be treated topically with aloe vera cream.[166] Dry gauze is placed between toes and fingers to prevent maceration, and gentle nonadhesive foam dressings may be applied to absorb drainage and provide protection. Any circumferential gauze should be wrapped loosely to prevent compression. A bed cradle may be necessary to keep the weight of bedcovers off the affected part or parts. As smoking causes systemic vasoconstriction and slows healing, the patient should be advised to refrain from smoking at least during the recovery period.

In the case of a developing compartment syndrome, a fasciotomy may be performed to increase circulation by lowering edematous tissue pressure.[54] If gangrene occurs, amputation may be necessary. X-rays, MRI, electrocardiography, and/or angiography may be performed to assess blood flow, cardiac arrhythmias, and the presence of gas in soft tissues.[204]

**PROGNOSIS.** The prognosis depends more on duration of freezing than on the actual temperature. The longer tissues remain frozen, the more cell death and tissue damage will occur.[173] Complicating factors such as compartment syndrome,[54] necrosis, or gangrene further reduce the chances of a favorable outcome. Amputation of gangrenous areas is not uncommon. Rapid, controlled rewarming and treatment of frostbite improves the opportunity for a positive outcome. Long-term effects may include increased sensitivity to cold and chronic pain in affected areas.[204]

SPECIAL IMPLICATIONS FOR THE THERAPIST 10.15

## *Cold Injuries*

Local cold injury subsequent to prolonged environmental exposures may not be seen in a therapy practice until complications such as necrosis and gangrene occur. Intervention at this point may include patient and caregiver education regarding the process of autoamputation, protection and offloading of the affected area, and monitoring for signs and symptoms of infection. Postamputation care to maximize return to function may also be needed, depending on injury location and extent of the amputation.

Use of cryotherapy by the therapist as a modality among the general population can result in a cold injury with localized tissue damage requiring documentation (e.g., incident report) and possible medical evaluation and treatment (see Fig. 10.19A). Massage may cause further tissue damage and should not be carried out until local tissue has healed.

# Burns

## Definition and Overview

Injuries that result from direct contact with or exposure to any thermal, chemical, electrical, or radiation source are termed *burns*. Burn injuries occur when energy from a heat source is transferred to the tissues of the body. The resulting depth of injury is a function of temperature or source of energy (e.g., radiation) and duration of exposure.

Burn severity is determined by the depth of the burn injury and the total body surface area (TBSA) involved in the burn. Other factors that influence severity include burn location, age of the patient, general health status, risk of infection, and presence of inhalation injury.[75,128] Burn depth is classified based on the layer of skin damage (Fig. 10.20). Most burn wounds that require medical intervention are a combination of partial- and full-thickness injury.

Burn size or TBSA is determined by one of two techniques: the Wallace rule of nines (Fig. 10.21) or the Lund and Browder method (Figs. 10.22 and 10.23). The rule of nines chart divides the body into distinct anatomic

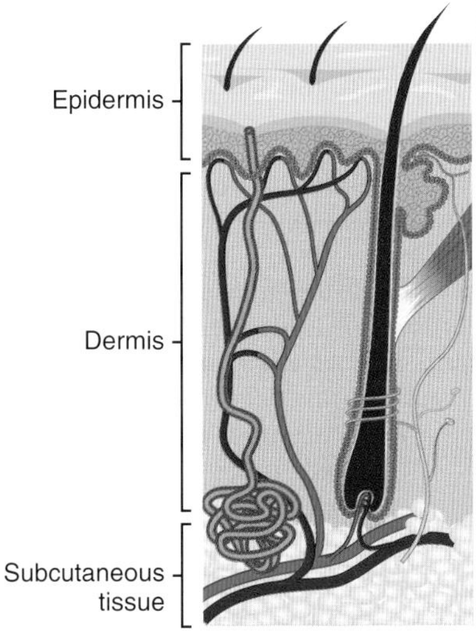

| | CAUSE | APPEARANCE | SENSATION | COURSE |
|---|---|---|---|---|
| Epidermis — SUPERFICIAL BURN, First-degree burn | Sunburn<br>Ultraviolet exposure<br>Brief exposure to flash, flame, or hot liquids | Mild to severe erythema; skin blanches with pressure; dry, no blisters; edema variable amount | Painful<br>Hyperesthetic<br>Tingling<br>Pain eased by cooling | Discomfort lasts about 48 hours<br>Desquamation in 3-7 days |
| Dermis — PARTIAL-THICKNESS BURN, Second-degree burn | Superficial: Scalding liquids, semiliquids (oil, tar), or solids<br>Deep: Immersion scald, flame | Large thick-walled blisters covering extensive area (vesiculation)<br>Edema; mottled red base; broken epidermis; wet, shiny, weeping surface | Painful<br>Sensitive to cold air | Superficial partial-thickness burn heals in 14-21 days<br>Deep partial-thickness burn requires 21-28 days for healing<br>Healing rate varies with burn depth and presence or absence of infection |
| Subcutaneous tissue — FULL-THICKNESS BURN, Third-degree or fourth-degree burn | Prolonged exposure to: Chemical, electrical, flame, scalding liquids, steam | Variable (e.g., deep red, black, white, brown)<br>Dry surface<br>Edema<br>Fat exposed<br>Tissue disrupted | Little or no pain<br>Insensate | Full-thickness dead skin suppurates and liquefies after 2-3 weeks<br>Spontaneous healing may be impossible but small areas may be left alone to form scarring without grafting (called secondary intent)<br>Requires removal of eschar and subsequent split- or full-thickness skin grafting<br>Hypertrophic scarring and wound contractures likely to develop without preventive measures |

**Figure. 10.20**

**Burn injury classification according to depth of injury.** *Partial-thickness* burns involve loss of epidermis and a portion of the dermis. As regenerative elements reside within the dermis, these injuries can heal by epithelialization. Deeper partial-thickness burns may scar. In *full-thickness* burns the entire epidermis and dermis are destroyed; healing occurs via granulation, contraction, and scar. Unless extremely small, many full-thickness burns require a skin graft.

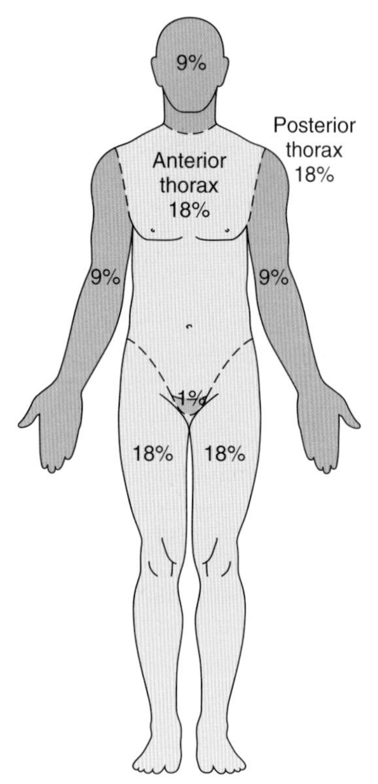


**Figure. 10.21**

The rule of nines provides a quick method for estimating the extent, or total body surface area, of a burn injury.

sections, each of which represents 9% or a multiple of 9% of the TBSA.[233] This chart is easy and quick to use in calculating TBSA. The Lund and Browder method modifies TBSA percentages to compensate for variation in body surface area among different age groups. While the Lund and Browder method offers a higher degree of accuracy, it can be more time-consuming to use. As both tools provide reasonably accurate estimates of TBSA, either may be used clinically.[233]

## Incidence

In the United States, approximately 40,000 burn-related hospitalizations occur each year. Of patients admitted to burn centers, 68% are male. Data from the National Burn Registry indicate accidents occurring at home account for 73% of all burn unit admissions.[14,15] Children are especially vulnerable, with accidental burns being the eighth most common cause of death in children younger than 1 year.[156] For children aged 5 to 9, burns are the third most common cause of death.[156]

## Etiologic Factors

Burn injuries are categorized according to their mechanism of injury: thermal, chemical, electrical, or radiation.[75,74] *Thermal* burns are caused by exposure to or contact with sources such as flame, hot liquid, steam, hot smoke, semisolids (tar), or hot objects. Thermal burns account for approximately 75% (43% flame or fire; 34% scalding) of all burn center admissions.[16]

Burns due to friction are generally considered and treated as thermal burns.[105] Examples include rope burns and carpet burns. The term *road rash* is often used when describing friction burns acquired when skin is scraped across pavement, such as with motorcycle or cycling accidents.

*Chemical* burns are caused by tissue contact with or ingestion, inhalation, or injection of strong acids, alkalis, or organic compounds. Chemical burns can result from contact with certain household cleaning agents and various chemicals used in industry, agriculture, and the military.

*Electrical* burns are caused by heat that is generated by electrical energy as it passes through the body. Electrical burns can result from contact with exposed or faulty electrical wiring, high-voltage power lines, or lightning.

*Radiation* burns are caused by exposure to a radioactive source. These types of injuries have been associated with the use of ionizing radiation in industry or with therapeutic radiation sources in medicine. A sunburn from prolonged exposure to UV rays is also considered a type of radiation burn.

## Risk Factors

Risk factors for burn injury include age, lack of smoke detectors, psychomotor disorders (e.g., impaired judgment, impaired mobility, drug or alcohol use), smoking, rural location, low socioeconomic status, occupation, and fireworks.[257] Children have higher risk, owing to inadequate supervision and abuse with scald injuries being the most prevalent. Individuals with seizure disorders (e.g., epilepsy) also experience higher risk of thermal burns related to falling onto hot surfaces or scald injuries.[192,244]

## Pathogenesis

Exposure to excessive heat results in denaturation of proteins, water vaporization, and cutaneous blood vessel thrombosis in affected areas.[74]

**Cutaneous Burns.** The pathophysiologic changes that occur immediately following a cutaneous burn injury depend on the extent and size of the burn. For smaller burns the body's initial inflammatory response to injury is localized to the injured area. With more extensive burns (15% or more TBSA),[74] the inflammatory response can be significant, and the effects can be systemic, potentially affecting all major systems of the body.[159] The systems more obviously affected include the cardiovascular, renal, gastrointestinal, immune, and respiratory systems.

*Cardiovascular* changes occur immediately following a burn injury as vasoactive substances (i.e., catecholamines, histamine, serotonin, leukotrienes, and prostaglandins) are released from injured tissue, causing an increase in capillary permeability.[74,75] Extensive burns result in generalized body edema in both burned and nonburned tissues and a decrease in circulating intravascular blood volume. Heart rate increases in response to catecholamine release and hypovolemia, but overall cardiac output falls. If the intravascular space is not replenished with intravenous fluids, hypovolemic (burn) shock and death may result.[74,75] Within 18 to 36 hours after the burn with appropriate care and fluid resuscitation, capillary permeability begins to decrease and continues a slow return to normal over several weeks following the injury. Cardiac

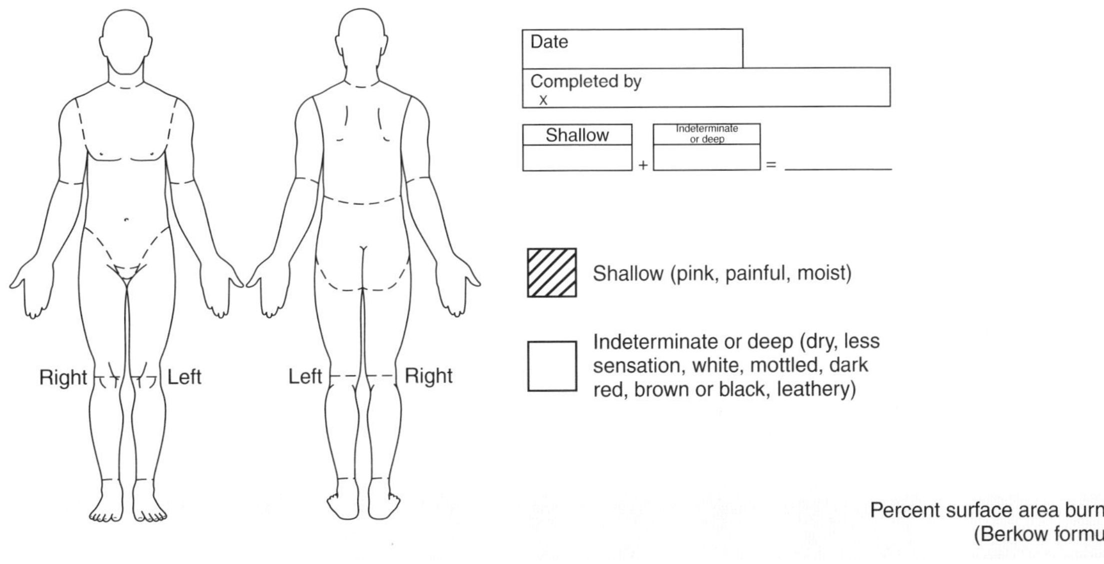


| Area | 1 Year | 1 to 4 Years | 5 to 9 Years | 10 to 14 Years | 15 to 18 Years | Adult | Shallow | Indeterminate or deep |
|---|---|---|---|---|---|---|---|---|
| Head | 19 | 17 | 13 | 11 | 9 | 7 | | |
| Neck | 2 | 2 | 2 | 2 | 2 | 2 | | |
| Ant. trunk | 13 | 13 | 13 | 13 | 13 | 13 | | |
| Post. trunk | 13 | 13 | 13 | 13 | 13 | 13 | | |
| R. buttock | 2½ | 2½ | 2½ | 2½ | 2½ | 2½ | | |
| L. buttock | 2½ | 2½ | 2½ | 2½ | 2½ | 2½ | | |
| Genitalia | 1 | 1 | 1 | 1 | 1 | 1 | | |
| R. U. arm | 4 | 4 | 4 | 4 | 4 | 4 | | |
| L. U. arm | 4 | 4 | 4 | 4 | 4 | 4 | | |
| R. L. arm | 3 | 3 | 3 | 3 | 3 | 3 | | |
| L. L. arm | 3 | 3 | 3 | 3 | 3 | 3 | | |
| R. hand | 2½ | 2½ | 2½ | 2½ | 2½ | 2½ | | |
| L. hand | 2½ | 2½ | 2½ | 2½ | 2½ | 2½ | | |
| R. thigh | 5½ | 6½ | 8 | 8½ | 9 | 9½ | | |
| L. thigh | 5½ | 6½ | 8 | 8½ | 9 | 9½ | | |
| R. leg | 5 | 5 | 5½ | 6 | 6½ | 7 | | |
| L. leg | 5 | 5 | 5½ | 6 | 6½ | 7 | | |
| R. foot | 3½ | 3½ | 3½ | 3½ | 3½ | 3½ | | |
| L. foot | 3½ | 3½ | 3½ | 3½ | 3½ | 3½ | | |
| Total | | | | | | | | |

**Figure. 10.22**

Sample chart for recording the extent and depth of a burn injury using the Lund and Browder formula.

output returns to normal and then increases approximately 24 hours after the injury to meet the increased metabolic needs of the body. The body begins to resorb the edema and excretes the excess fluid over the ensuing days and weeks.

The *renal* and *gastrointestinal systems* are affected as the body responds initially by shunting blood from the kidneys and intestines leading to oliguria (decreased urine output) and intestinal dysfunction[74] in patients with burns of greater than 25% TBSA. *Immune system* function is depressed, resulting in the patient becoming immunosuppressed, increasing the risk of infection and life-threatening sepsis.[74,75] The *respiratory system* may respond with pulmonary artery hypertension and decreased lung compliance even when there has been no inhalation injury.

**Smoke Inhalation.** Smoke inhalation injury may occur secondary to inhalation of carbon monoxide, poisoning resulting from inhalation of toxins contained in smoke, and/or thermal burns to the pulmonary airways. Signs that a smoke inhalation injury may have occurred include singed nasal hair or eyebrows; facial edema; burns on the upper chest, face, and neck; soot in the mouth; or carbonaceous sputum.[74]

**Electrical and Chemical Burns.** In electrical burns, heat is generated as the electricity travels through the body, resulting in internal tissue damage and potential multisystem injury.[221] Entrance wounds tend to be smaller compared with larger, more explosive exit wounds.

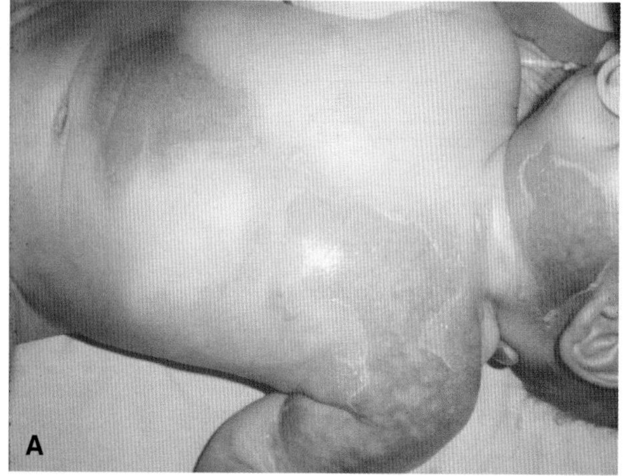


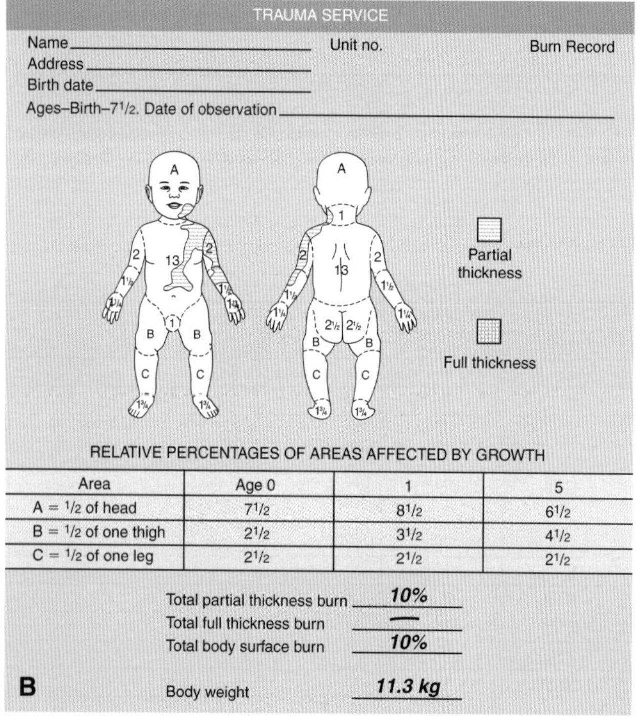

TRAUMA SERVICE

Name ______ Unit no. Burn Record

Address ______

Birth date ______

Ages–Birth–7½. Date of observation ______

Partial thickness

Full thickness

RELATIVE PERCENTAGES OF AREAS AFFECTED BY GROWTH

| Area | Age 0 | 1 | 5 |
|---|---|---|---|
| A = ½ of head | 7½ | 8½ | 6½ |
| B = ½ of one thigh | 2½ | 3½ | 4½ |
| C = ½ of one leg | 2½ | 2½ | 2½ |

Total partial thickness burn 10%

Total full thickness burn —

Total body surface burn 10%

B

Body weight 11.3 kg

**Figure. 10.23**

(A) Pediatric scald burn. (B) Corresponding Lund and Browder chart. (Courtesy Katherine S. Biggs, PT, Yale New Haven Hospital, New Haven, CT.)

Cutaneous burn injuries associated with electrical burns may be negligible, whereas soft tissue and muscle damage can be extensive, particularly in high-voltage electrical injuries. Voltage, type of current (direct or alternating), contact site, and duration of contact are important factors in the amount and type of damage sustained. Alternating current is more dangerous than direct current and is more often associated with cardiopulmonary arrest, ventricular fibrillation, and tetanic muscle contractions, which can prolong contact with the electrical source.[74,96] A single, forceful contraction occurs with direct current and typically pushes the person away from the source.[96]

Other significant injuries such as respiratory distress, fractures, spinal cord injury, or traumatic brain injury may occur. It is also possible for electrical sources to ignite the person's clothes, causing thermal burns.[96]

Chemical burns may be deep, as they often continue to burn until neutralized. Alkaline chemicals tend to result in deeper burn injuries, as contact causes liquefactive necrosis of tissues, allowing the agent to penetrate deeper into the body. Acids usually result in comparatively less extensive burns compared with alkalis. Acidic chemicals cause protein coagulation as they degrade tissue, forming a layer of coagulum that can prevent deeper penetration.[74] Chemical burns can also be associated with systemic toxicity from cutaneous agent absorption; see Environmental and Occupational Medicine in Chapter 4 for more details.

### Clinical Manifestations

Appearance, sensation, and course of injury of superficial, partial-thickness, and full-thickness burns are outlined in Fig. 10.20. Burn location influences injury severity in that burns on certain areas of the body are commonly associated with specific complications. For example, burns of the head, neck, and anterior chest have a higher risk of associated pulmonary and/or respiratory complications.

Burns involving the face may have associated corneal abrasions. Burns of the hands (Fig. 10.24) and joints can result in permanent physical and vocational disability, requiring extensive therapy and rehabilitation. Circumferential burns may produce a tourniquet-like effect and lead to compartment syndrome or total occlusion of circulation (Fig. 10.25).

In full-thickness burns, nerve endings are destroyed, rendering these specific burned areas of skin painless. However, most full-thickness burns occur in conjunction with surrounding superficial and partial-thickness injuries in which nerve endings are intact and exposed, so all areas of a burn injury should be carefully checked for sensation. Excised eschar (nonviable tissue) and fresh donor sites can directly expose nerve fibers and can be extremely painful. As peripheral nerves regenerate, painful sensation returns, creating increased pain with healing for some patients.

The clinical course for a patient with a major burn admitted to a burn unit can be divided into three overlapping phases: emergent, acute, and rehabilitative.[60] The *emergent phase* begins at the time of injury and includes fluid resuscitation (based on the Parkland formula), ventilatory management, assessment of the extent of the burn, and early wound management. This phase concludes when large shifts in fluid decrease and capillary permeability is restored.

In the *acute phase,* intervention is focused on management of the burn wounds and infection prevention. Débridement and skin grafting may be part of this phase. The goal of the *rehabilitation phase* is return to maximal independence and function. This phase coincides with the acute phase, as prescribed rehabilitation (e.g., stretching, strengthening, functional mobility) is initiated early in the course of most burns and lasts well beyond the period of hospitalization.[60]

Infection is the most common and life-threatening complication of burn injuries.[60,75] Burn wound infections can be classified on the basis of the causative organism,

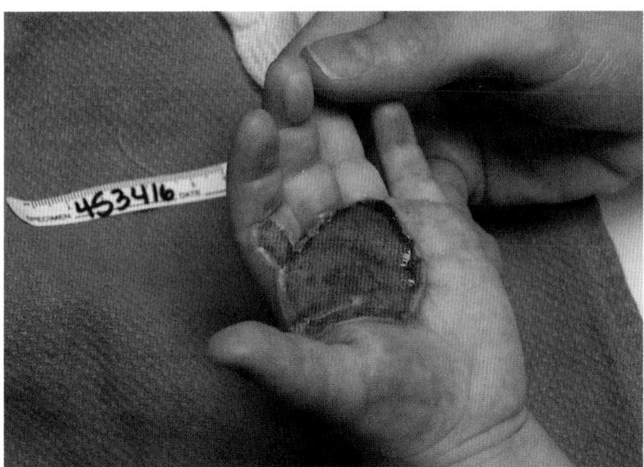


**Figure. 10.24**

**Pediatric hand burn.** This 2-year-old girl grabbed a hot iron, sustaining a partial-thickness burn to her hand. An intact blister remains on her middle finger. (Courtesy Harriett B. Loehne, PT, DPT, CWS, FACCWS. Used with permission.)

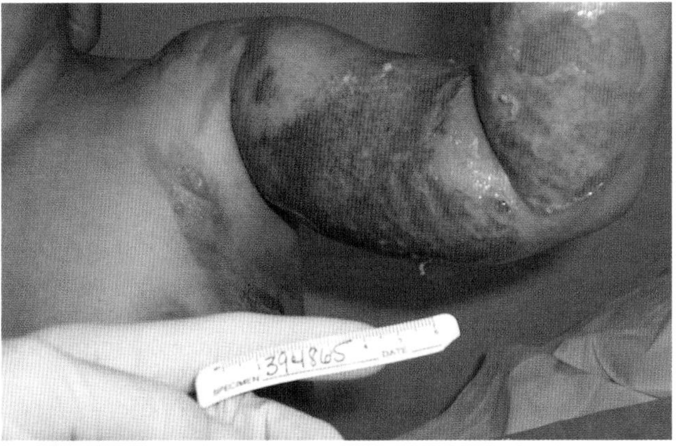


**Figure. 10.25**

**Circumferential burns of extremities may produce a tourniquet-like effect and lead to total occlusion of circulation.** This 3-year-old child reached into a microwave oven and spilled macaroni in boiling water, resulting in a partial-thickness scald burn. (Courtesy Harriett B. Loehne, PT, DPT, CWS, FACCWS. Used with permission.)

the depth of invasion, and the tissue response. Individuals with extensive burns and in whom wound closure is difficult to achieve are at the greatest risk for infection and other complications.

Inhalation injury is a major complicating factor and increases the risk of mortality owing to respiratory failure, pneumonia, and sepsis.[67] The multiple organ system response that occurs following a burn injury may result in multiple organ dysfunction syndrome and death (see Chapter 5).

Hypertrophic scarring is a second complication of burn injuries, and although not life threatening, it is associated with considerable morbidity and potential lifelong disfigurement. Less severe burns that reepithelialize within 2 to 3 weeks are not as prone to hypertrophic scarring, as closing within this time frame usually indicates partial-thickness injury. Children and individuals of African descent are at greatest risk for hypertrophic scarring, presumably because of the abundance of collagen in these populations. Aging white adults with wrinkled, loose skin have less hypertrophic scarring because of the absence of collagen.[61]

## MEDICAL MANAGEMENT

TREATMENT. The therapist may be involved in wound management for minor burns consisting of irrigation; removal of any damaging agents (e.g., chemicals, tar); débridement of nonviable tissue; application of topical antimicrobial creams, ointments, or dressings; and bandaging. Compression may also be applied. Blister management usually includes débridement of the blister (see Special Implications for the Therapist 10.1: Skin Lesions). Instructions for home care may include wound cleansing and dressing application, observation for clinical manifestations of infection, active ROM exercises to maintain normal joint function, and compression and positioning to decrease edema. All these components help achieve faster wound closure, decrease pain, and decrease the risk and severity of scar formation.

Treatment of major burns includes lifesaving measures (ABCs: *a*irway, *b*reathing, *c*irculation) immediately after the injury, followed by restorative care (e.g., infection control, wound management, skin grafts, pain management) during the acute phase. Physical therapists are closely involved early in the acute phase of recovery to maximize functional recovery and cosmetic outcome.

Therapeutic wound management interventions for the therapist in outpatient and inpatient settings include the following: irrigation; débridement; application of advanced wound dressings; stabilization of skin grafts to prevent shearing and edema; positioning and splinting for scar, contracture, and edema prevention and management; exercise; and ambulation and functional mobility.[75] Elasticized garments help reduce scar hypertrophy and may be worn for up to 2 years after deep burn injuries.

Bioengineered temporary biologic dressings may be used to minimize fluid and protein loss from the burn surface, prevent infection, and reduce pain. Types of temporary grafts include *allografts* (homografts), which are usually cadaver skin; *xenografts* (heterografts), which are typically pigskin; and *biosynthetic grafts,* which are a combination of collagen and synthetics.

To treat a full-thickness burn and permanently close the burn injury, an *autograft* (the person's own skin) is often used. A transplanted, full-thickness skin graft can be used over areas where appearance or joint movement is important. Split-thickness grafts that are meshed (fenestrated) allow a section of skin to be expanded up to three times its original size, providing for the creation of smaller partial-thickness donor-site injuries. Nonimmunogenic cultured epidermal grafts can be used to assist in coverage of large surface area injuries.[60] See also Skin Transplantation in Chapter 21.

PROGNOSIS. Overall, burn injury morbidity and mortality rates over the last decade have improved for all age groups as a result of advances in burn care and reduced infection with the use of effective topical antimicrobials and early burn excision.[86,225] Some evidence also shows that patients admitted to burn units are presenting with decreased size and severity of burns.[225]

TBSA, age, and inhalation injury are three classic determinants of burn mortality.[90,225] Factors such as obesity, alcoholism, and cardiac disorders that impair peripheral circulation (e.g., peripheral vascular disease) further complicate burn recovery and increase mortality rates in adults.

SPECIAL IMPLICATIONS FOR THE THERAPIST 10.16

### *Burns*

With the understanding that the risk of burns is highest for individuals at the extremes of age (the very young and the very old), education regarding prevention of burn accidents is especially important in these populations.[86,90] Reviewing simple cooking precautions may be helpful. For example: do not leave burners in use unattended, do not use high heat, do not wear clothing with loose sleeves or belts (especially bathrobes), use front burners when appropriate, and avoid leaning over hot front burners when using back burners. When small children are present, parents should use back burners to keep small hands from grasping hot cooking pots and pans, as this can lead to hand burns and scald injuries.

In large TBSA burns, the therapist will direct treatment intervention to encourage deep breathing and facilitate lung expansion; promote wound healing; reduce dependent edema formation and promote venous return; prevent or minimize deformities and hypertrophic scarring; increase ROM, strength, and function; increase independence in daily activities and self-care; and encourage emotional and psychologic well-being. Specific compression, lymphatic movement, débridement, and wound management procedures are beyond the scope of this text.

Throughout the acute and rehabilitation phases of burn care, the therapist must remain alert to the development of medical complications such as ileus, gastric ulcers, respiratory distress, infection, and impaired circulation. Monitoring vital signs (e.g., heart rate, blood pressure, oxygen saturation levels) helps guide the therapist in how much activity the patient with burns can tolerate. See Table 10.4 for additional medical complicating factors in adults with burn injuries.

Laboratory values will show changes when the body is challenged by burn injury, especially a full-thickness burn injury. It is important for the therapist to review laboratory values before interventions so that appropriate treatment plan adjustments can be made. Patients with burns with acute renal failure and abnormal sodium, potassium, chloride, and magnesium values are candidates for hemodialysis. Abnormal blood urea nitrogen can indicate decreased renal function or fluid intake. Wounds will not heal optimally without addressing protein status (prealbumin) and glucose levels, which can be affected by a catabolic, postburn state.

Regular inspection of the burn wound must be performed and any change in appearance reported. The amount of body surface area exposed at any one time during wound care should be minimized to prevent hypothermia, as increased amounts of body heat are lost through areas of compromised skin.

Patients with burn injuries are at high risk of infection because of the loss of skin barrier and inherent impaired immune response. Infection control techniques must be practiced carefully at all times. Skin donor sites require the same care and precautions as other partial-thickness wounds to promote healing and prevent infection.

Arrange any therapy likely to elicit a painful response to coincide with medications (allow 30 minutes for oral, 10 minutes for intramuscular, and 3 to 5 minutes for intravenous administration). Combining relaxation techniques, music therapy, distraction, and other techniques for pain modulation may be helpful.

Burned areas must be maintained in positions of physiologic function within the limits imposed by associated injuries, grafting, and other therapeutic devices (see Table 10.5 for positioning recommendations). Burned areas are prone to develop contractures requiring close assessment of ROM and muscle strength. Encourage active ROM exercises at least every 2 hours while the patient is awake unless this is contraindicated by recent grafting. Prolonged stretching is sometimes combined with splinting or orthoses to maintain motion. Provide honest, positive reinforcement throughout intervention, being aware that each individual will progress through the stages of denial, grief, and acceptance of injury and recovery differently.

Patients with less severe burns (and patients discharged from inpatient status) require much of the same care, including appropriate management of the open burn wounds, infection control, and stretching and exercise. As patients seen in outpatient settings typically perform more self-care, they require additional education and training to promote full closure and optimal results. During the rehabilitation phase, chronic pain protocols may be helpful.

## MISCELLANEOUS INTEGUMENTARY DISORDERS

### Integumentary Ulcers

Integumentary ulcers can be caused by a variety of underlying disorders, including neuropathy, vascular insufficiency, radiation, SSc, vasculitis, and prolonged pressure. Integumentary ulcers are discussed in individual sections according to pathogenesis (e.g., diabetic ulcers [see Diabetes Mellitus in Chapter 11], arterial insufficiency ulcers [see Peripheral Vascular Disease in Chapter 12]).

**Table 10.4** Assessing Medical Complications in the Burn-Injured Adult

| System | Complications |
|---|---|
| Urinary | Visible red or dark brown urine (catheter) |
| Respiratory | Signs of respiratory distress<br>Restlessness<br>Confusion<br>Labored breathing<br>Tachypnea (>24 respirations/min)<br>Dyspnea<br>$PaO_2$ <90 mm Hg; $O_2$ <95% |
| Peripheral vascular | Pulses absent on palpation<br>Capillary refill (unburned area) >2 s<br>Numbness or tingling<br>Increased pain with active range of motion exercises<br>Increased edema, changes in skin color |
| Infection | Discoloration of wound, periwound erythema, increased drainage, odor, delayed closure<br>Headache, chills, anorexia, nausea<br>Increased pain<br>Change in vital signs<br>Paralytic ileus, confusion, restlessness, hallucinations |
| Gastrointestinal | Paralytic ileus (painful, distended abdomen)<br>Stress-induced gastric ulcer (epigastric pain, abdominal distention, anorexia, nausea) |

## Pressure Injuries

### Definition and Overview

A pressure injury (formerly called *pressure ulcer, decubitus ulcer, bed sore*) is a lesion caused by unrelieved pressure, resulting in damage to underlying tissue. A person's general health and nutrition, skin perfusion, and microclimate (temperature and moisture) all can affect the ability of the skin to tolerate pressure.[175] Pressure injuries usually occur over bony prominences, such as the heels, sacrum, ischial tuberosities, greater trochanters, elbows, and scapula or under medical devices.[175] Pressure injuries are staged to classify the degree of tissue damage observed (Figs. 10.26 and 10.27; Box 10.12).[175]

In 1975 a landmark article was published describing a method of classifying pressure ulcers, according to extent of soft tissue damage.[207a] Over time the classification system for staging pressure injuries has been modified and developed into the current staging system that is reflective of the range of skin pigmentation (see Fig. 10.26). When the National Pressure Ulcer Advisory Panel (name changed to National Pressure Injury Advisory Panel (NPIAP) in 2019) completed the latest staging update in 2016, the terminology changed from pressure ulcer to pressure injury. The revised staging terms are now validated with photographs.[175] While some publications

**Table 10.5** Therapeutic Positioning for the Burn-Injured Patient

| Burned Area | Therapeutic Position | Positioning Techniques |
|---|---|---|
| **Neck** | | |
| Anterior | Extension | No pillow; small towel roll beneath cervical spine to promote neck extension |
| Circumferential | Neutral toward extension | No pillow |
| Posterior or asymmetric | Neutral | No pillow |
| Shoulder, axilla | Arm abduction to 90–110 degrees | Splinting; arms positioned away from body and supported on arm troughs; elbow splint |
| Elbow | Arm extension | Elbow splint; elbow positioned in extension with slight bend at elbow (≤10 degrees of elbow flexion)<br>Arms supported on arm troughs with forearm in slight pronation |
| **Hand** | | |
| Wrist | Wrist extension | Hand splint |
| MCP joints | MCP flexion at 90 degrees | Hand splint |
| PIP/DIP joints | PIP/DIP extension | Hand splint |
| Thumb | Thumb abduction | Hand splint with thumb abduction |
| Web spaces | Finger abduction | Web spacers of gauze, foam, or thermoplastics to decrease webbing formation |
| Hip | Hip extension | Supine with the head of bed flat and legs extended<br>Trochanter roll to maintain neutral rotation (toes pointing toward ceiling)<br>Prone positioning |
| Knee | Knee extension | Supine with knees extended and toes pointing toward ceiling<br>Prone with feet extended over end of mattress<br>Sitting with legs extended and elevated<br>Knee splint |
| Ankle | Neutral | Padded footboard<br>Ankle-positioning devices (avoid position of ankle inversion or eversion)<br>Suspend heels (lying and sitting) to prevent pressure injury |

*MCP*, Metacarpophalangeal; *PIP/DIP*, proximal interphalangeal or distal interphalangeal.

Modified from Carrougher GJ, Sandidge C: Management of clients with burn injury. In Black JM, Hawks JH, editors: *Medical-surgical nursing: Clinical management for positive outcomes*, ed 8, Philadelphia, 2008, Saunders, p 1262.

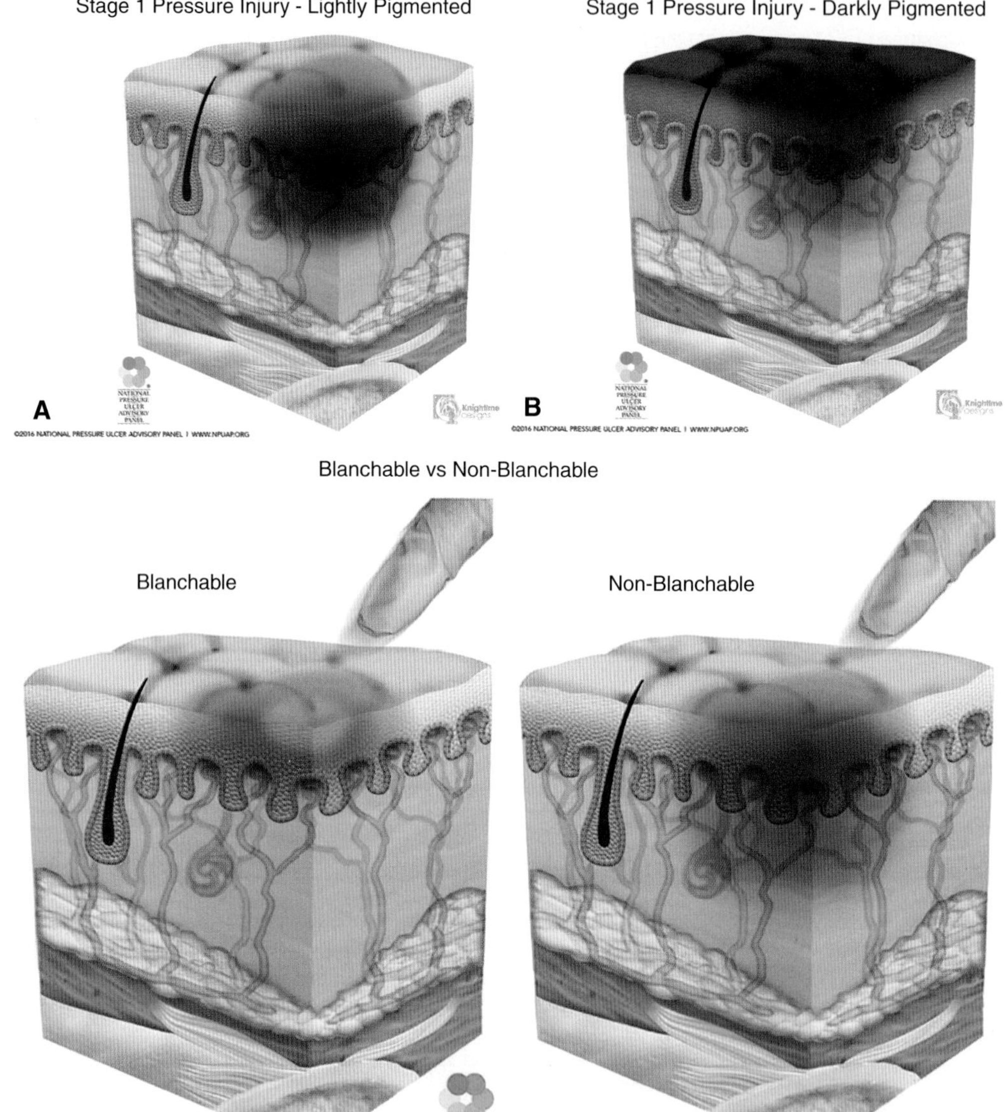


**Figure. 10.26**

**Staging pressure injuries is based on the depth and type of tissue damage.** This system was developed by the National Pressure Injury Advisory Panel. (See also Box 10.12). (A) Stage 1 pressure injury, lightly pigmented. (B) Stage 1 pressure injury, darkly pigmented. (C) Blanchable versus nonblanchable.

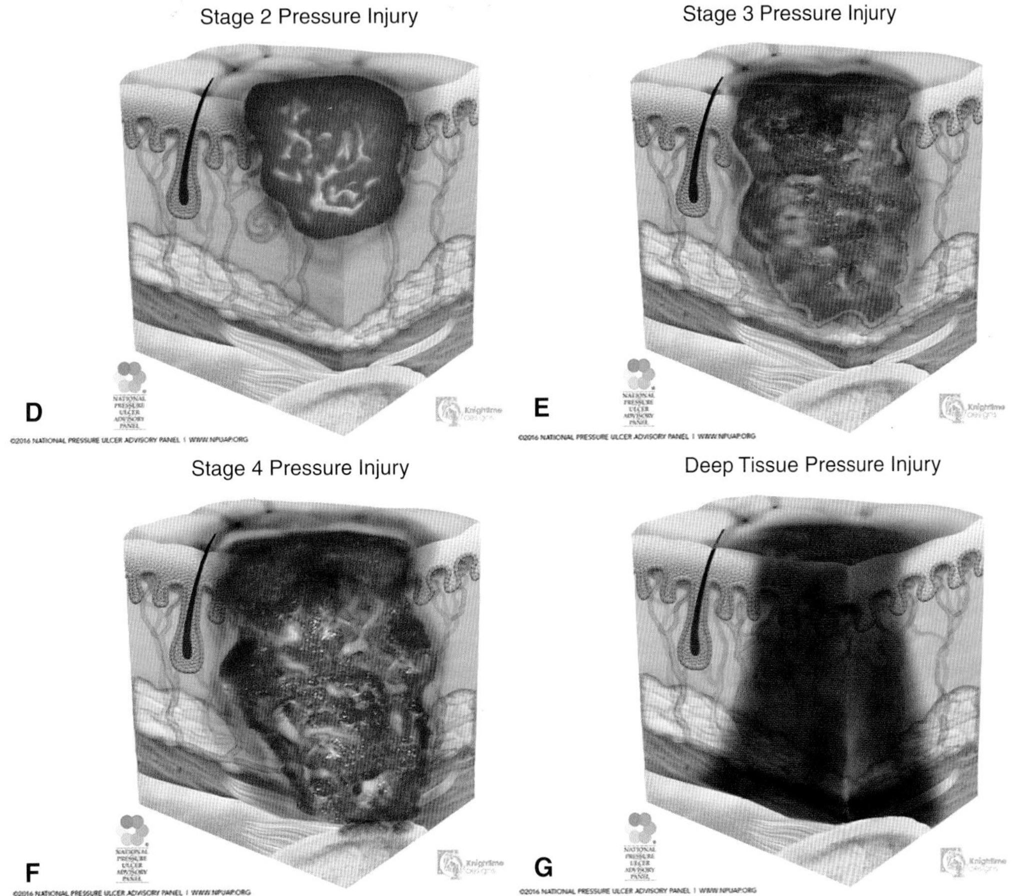


**Figure. 10.26—cont'd**

(D) Stage 2 pressure injury. (E) Stage 3 pressure injury. (F) Stage 4 pressure injury. (G) Deep tissue pressure injury. (From National Pressure Ulcer Advisory Panel (NPUAP), https://www.npuap.org/resources/educational-and-clinical-resources/npuap-pressure-injury-stages/. Reprinted with permission from the NPUAP.)

retain the use of "pressure ulcer," for the sake of clarity, the new terminology will be used in this chapter (see Box 10.12).

Wounds cannot be back-staged. Once a pressure injury is designated as stage 2, 3, or 4, it will retain this original classification until it has resolved. As the lesion fills with granulation tissue and closes via epithelialization, graft, or flap, it should be documented as a *healing* stage 2, 3, or 4 (still using the original deepest level documented).

It should be noted that this staging classification is for pressure injuries only. Other types of ulcers such as vascular (arterial, venous) are designated partial or full thickness. Neuropathic ulcers may be classified using the Wagner system (Table 10.6)[170,249] or SINBAD score.[140] The term *neuropathic ulcer* is used interchangeably with *diabetic ulcer,* but a diabetic ulcer is really a neuropathic ulcer in someone with diabetes. Neuropathic ulcers can occur in anyone with loss of sensation (e.g., alcoholic neuropathy, peripheral neuropathy).[34,254,261]

## Incidence and Prevalence

While incidence rates vary widely across clinical settings, more than 2.5 million patients in acute care hospitals are estimated to experience a pressure injury each year.[117] More attention is now directed toward pressure injury prevention, in part because the Centers for Medicare and Medicaid Services discontinued payment for hospital-acquired pressure injuries beginning in 2008. The International Pressure Ulcer Prevalence Survey reported that overall pressure injury prevalence decreased about 4%

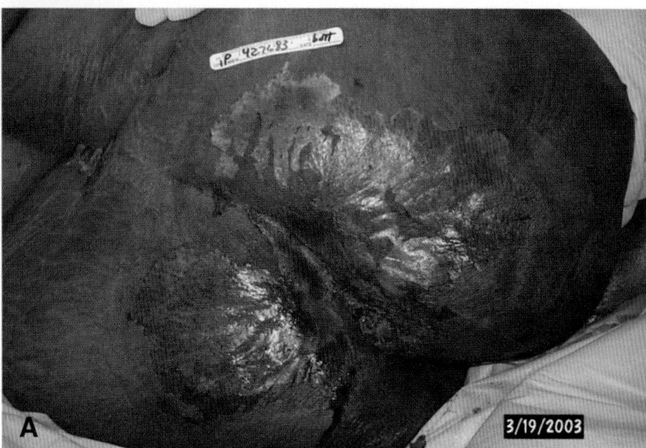


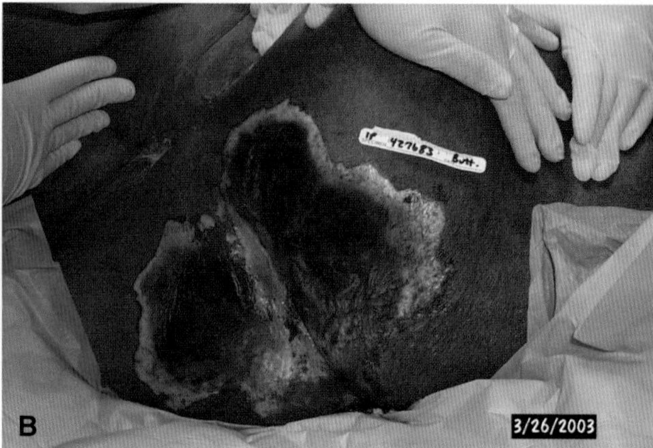


**Figure. 10.27**

**Deep tissue pressure injury (DTPI).** A DTPI manifests suddenly as a discolored or bruised-appearing area that quickly progresses to a deep wound regardless of any intervention. Because the skin is the largest organ in the body, necrosis of the skin will occur when circulation is significantly impaired. (A) The DTPI was discovered when an unstable patient in the intensive care unit was finally able to be turned over after 2 days. He had kidney failure, was on a ventilator, and had tenuous blood pressure. The wound appeared as a discolored area with intact skin (formerly required to be staged as a stage I pressure injury). (B) One week later it was solid eschar, which required sharp débridement because of purulent drainage at the margins and was necrosed to bone. The patient died several days later. (Courtesy Harriett B. Loehne, PT, DPT, CWS, FACCWS. Used with permission.)

Box 10.12

## STAGES OF PRESSURE INJURIES

***Stage 1. Pressure Injury: Nonblanchable Erythema of Intact Skin***

Intact skin with a localized area of nonblanchable erythema, which may appear differently in darkly pigmented skin. The presence of blanchable erythema or changes in sensation, temperature, or firmness may precede visual changes. Color changes do not include purple or maroon discoloration; these may indicate deep tissue pressure injury.

***Stage 2. Pressure Injury: Partial-Thickness Skin Loss With Exposed Dermis***

Partial-thickness loss of skin with exposed dermis. The wound bed is viable, pink or red, and moist and may also appear as an intact or ruptured serum-filled blister. Adipose (fat) is not visible and deeper tissues are not visible. Granulation tissue, slough, and eschar are not present. These injuries commonly result from adverse microclimate and shear in the skin over the pelvis and shear in the heel. This stage should not be used to describe moisture-associated skin damage, including incontinence-associated dermatitis, intertriginous dermatitis, medical adhesive–related skin injury, or traumatic wounds (skin tears, burns, abrasions).

***Stage 3. Pressure Injury: Full-Thickness Skin Loss***

Full-thickness loss of skin, in which adipose (fat) is visible in the ulcer and granulation tissue and epibole (rolled wound edges) are often present. Slough and/or eschar may be visible. The depth of tissue damage varies by anatomic location; areas of significant adiposity can develop deep wounds. Undermining and tunneling may occur. Fascia, muscle, tendon, ligament, cartilage, and/or bone are not exposed. If slough or eschar obscures the extent of tissue loss, this is an unstageable pressure injury.

***Stage 4. Pressure Injury: Full-Thickness Skin and Tissue Loss***

Full-thickness skin and tissue loss with exposed or directly palpable fascia, muscle, tendon, ligament, cartilage, or bone in the ulcer. Slough and/or eschar may be visible. Epibole (rolled edges), undermining, and/or tunneling often occur. Depth varies by anatomic location. If slough or eschar obscures the extent of tissue loss, this is an unstageable pressure injury.

***Unstageable Pressure Injury: Obscured Full-Thickness Skin and Tissue Loss***

Full-thickness skin and tissue loss in which the extent of tissue damage within the ulcer cannot be confirmed because it is obscured by slough or eschar. If slough or eschar is removed, a stage 3 or stage 4 pressure injury will be revealed. Stable eschar (i.e., dry, adherent, intact without erythema or fluctuance) on the heel or ischemic limb should not be softened or removed.

***Deep Tissue Pressure Injury: Persistent Nonblanchable Deep Red, Maroon, or Purple Discoloration***

Intact or nonintact skin with localized area of persistent nonblanchable deep red, maroon, or purple discoloration or epidermal separation revealing a dark wound bed or blood-filled blister. Pain and temperature change often precede skin color changes. Discoloration may appear differently in darkly pigmented skin. This injury results from intense and/or prolonged pressure and shear forces at the bone–muscle interface. The wound may evolve rapidly to reveal the actual extent of tissue injury or may resolve without tissue loss. If necrotic tissue, subcutaneous tissue, granulation tissue, fascia, muscle, or other underlying structures are visible, this indicates a full-thickness pressure injury (unstageable, stage 3 or stage 4). Do not use deep tissue pressure injury to describe vascular, traumatic, neuropathic, or dermatologic conditions.

Reprinted with permission from National Pressure Ulcer Advisory Panel. Available at: https://www.npuap.org/resources/educational-and-clinical-resources/npuap-pressure-injury-stages/. Accessed March 3, 2019.

**Table 10.6** Wagner Ulcer Grade Classification

| Grade | Characteristics |
|---|---|
| 0 | Preulcerative lesions; healed ulcers; presence of bony deformity |
| 1 | Superficial ulcer without subcutaneous tissue involvement |
| 2 | Penetration through subcutaneous tissue; may expose bone, tendon, ligament, or joint capsule |
| 3 | Osteitis, abscess, or osteomyelitis |
| 4 | Gangrene of digit |
| 5 | Gangrene of foot requiring disarticulation |

[a]This classification scheme for ulceration is used for neuropathic ulcers and does not represent pressure ulcers.

Data from Wagner REW: The dysvascular foot: a system for diagnosis and treatment. *Foot Ankle* 2:64–122, 1981.

between 2006 and 2015.[246] Despite this decrease, pressure injuries are still considered fairly common, occur at relatively high rates, and are typically connected to other problems within health care settings. The development of pressure injuries has been connected to quality of care in inpatient, outpatient, and home care settings. Pressure injuries related to medical device use account for almost one-third of hospital-acquired pressure injuries.[117]

### Etiologic and Risk Factors

Pressure injuries are caused by unrelieved pressure that can result in damaged skin, muscle, and underlying tissue usually located over bony prominences. The two primary causative factors for the development of pressure injuries are interface pressure (externally) and pressure with shearing forces.

Risk factors for pressure injury include mobility and activity limitations, impaired circulation, skin moisture, age, nutrition, and general health status.[70] Patients in critical care have similar risk factors along with additional factors (e.g., vasopressor infusion) that have been shown to be independent predictors of pressure injury.[9]

Pressure contributes to other types of ulcers (e.g., arterial, venous, neuropathic), and likewise, the underlying cause of the other types of ulcers can contribute to the development of pressure injuries. However, pressure injuries are a separate entity from other types of ulcers.

Intrinsic factors most commonly associated with pressure injury development include decreased sensation, impaired mobility or activity levels, incontinence, diaphoresis, impaired nutritional status, and altered levels of consciousness or cognition. Extrinsic factors include pressure, shear, friction, and moisture.[70,262]

Bedbound and chairbound patients and patients with impaired ability to reposition themselves should be assessed for additional factors (e.g., above-noted pressure injury risk factors) that increase the risk of developing pressure injuries. For these and other people at risk, a systemic risk assessment evaluating both sensation and physiologic risk of pressure injuries can be made using a validated risk assessment tool such as the Braden Scale (Fig. 10.28)[151,183] or the Norton Scale.[66,181]

Nutritional factors may include malnutrition, which may take the form of inadequate intake owing to a condition, disease, or underlying complicating factor, including difficulty with absorption of nutrients.[39] Because malnutrition is associated with poor health outcomes including impaired healing,[39] it is important to consider laboratory values that suggest nutritional compromise. Clinically significant malnutrition that impairs wound healing includes serum albumin less than 3.5 g/dL and serum prealbumin less than 19 mg/dL.

Prealbumin measurement, which determines protein over the previous 48 hours rather than over the previous 3 weeks as with serum albumin measurement, is a better indicator of the patient's current nutritional status. It is considered the gold standard for monitoring nutritional change, allowing for appropriate modification of interventions.

Nutrition screening can be an appropriate means to facilitate effective intervention to improve healing and mitigate cost of care.[39] Validated screenings, including some as short as 3 questions (Malnutrition Screening Tool), can be used by any trained health care provider to trigger the need for referral for specific nutrition care.[39] These referrals can facilitate improved healing and decreased length of stay.[39]

### Pathogenesis

Pressure is the external factor causing ischemia and tissue necrosis. Continuous pressure on soft tissues between bony prominences and hard or unyielding surfaces compresses capillaries and occludes blood flow. Transcutaneous partial pressure of oxygen is indicative of oxygen delivery relative to tissue need and provides information regarding local circulation.[124,201]

The local pressure may be exceeded when compression is applied to tissue, resulting in diminished vascular supply and lymph drainage in the area. The addition of shear forces can contribute to blood vessel damage, further injuring the integument.[124]

A brief period of rebound capillary dilation (called *reactive hyperemia*) occurs when pressure is relieved, and no tissue damage develops as long as the ischemia was for only a short time. If pressure is not relieved, endothelial cells lining the capillaries become disrupted by platelet aggregation, blood flow is occluded, and the surrounding tissue becomes necrotic.[124] Necrotic tissue predisposes bacterial invasion and subsequent infection, preventing healthy granulation. Muscle tissue is also negatively affected by excessive pressure loading (Fig. 10.29).[124]

In the case of neuropathic ulcers associated with diabetes, the primary pathogenesis is the absence of protective sensation combined with high pressure. The absence of

| Sensory Perception | Moisture | Activity | Mobility | Nutrition | Friction & Shear |
|---|---|---|---|---|---|
| **1. Completely Limited:** Unresponsive (does not moan, flinch or grasp) to painful stimuli, due to diminished level of consciousness or sedation. OR Limited ability to feel pain over most of body surface | **1. Consistently Moist:** Skin is kept moist almost constantly by perspiration, urine, etc. Dampness is detected every time patient is moved or turned. | **1. Bedfast:** Confined to bed. | **1. Completely Immobile:** Does not make even slight changes in body or extremity position without assistance. | **1. Very Poor:** Never eats a complete meal. Rarely eats more than 1/3 of any food offered. Eats 2 servings or less of protein (meat or dairy products) per day. Takes fluid poorly. Does not take liquid dietary supplement. OR Is NPO and/or maintained in clear liquids or IV's for more than 5 day. | **1. Problem:** Requires moderate to maximum assistance in moving. Complete lifting without sliding against sheets is impossible. Frequently slides down in bed or chair, requiring frequent repositioning with maximum assistance. Spasticity, contractures or agitation leads to almost constant friction. |
| **2. Very Limited:** Responds only to painful stimuli. Cannot communicate discomfort except by moaning or restlessness. OR Has a sensory impairment, which limits the ability to feel pain or discomfort over 1/2 of body. | **2. Very Moist:** Skin is often but not always moist. Linen must be changed at least once a shift. | **2. Chairfast:** Ability to walk severely limited or non-existent. Cannot bear own weight and/or must be assisted into chair or wheelchair. | **2. Very Limited:** Makes occasional slight changes in body or extremity position but unable to make frequent or slight changes independently. | **2. Probably Inadequate:** Rarely eats a complete meal and generally eats only about 1/2 of any food offered. Protein intake includes only 3 servings of meat or dairy products per day. Occasionally will take a supplement. OR Receives less than optimum amount of liquid diet or tube feeding. | **2. Potential Problem:** Moves feebly or requires minimum assistance. During a move skin probably slides to some extent against sheets, chair, restraints or other devices. Maintains relatively good position in chair or bed most of the time, but occasionally slides down. |
| **3. Slightly Limited:** Responds to verbal commands, but cannot always communicate discomfort or need to be turned. OR Has some sensory impairment, which limits ability to feel pain or discomfort in 1 or 2 extremities. | **3. Occasionally Moist:** Skin is occasionally moist, requiring an extra linen change approximately once a day. | **3. Walks Occasionally:** Walks occasionally during day, but for very short distances, with or without assistance. Spends majority of each shift in bed or chair. | **3. Slightly Limited:** Makes frequent though slight changes in body or extremity position independently. | **3. Adequate:** Eats over half of most meals. Eats a total of 4 protein (meat, dairy products) each day. Occasionally will refuse a meal, but will usually take a supplement if offered. OR TPN regimen, which probably meets most of nutritional needs. | **3. No Apparent Problem:** Moves in bed and chair independently and has sufficient muscle strength to lift up completely during move. Maintains good position in bed or chair at all times. |
| **4. No Impairment:** Responds to verbal commands. Has no sensory deficit, which would limit ability to feel or voice pain or discomfort. | **4. Rarely Moist:** Skin is usually dry, linen only requires changing at routine intervals. | **4. Walks Frequently:** Walks outside the room at least twice a day and inside the room at least once every 2 hours during waking hours. | **4. No Limitations:** Makes major and frequent changes in position without assistance. | **4. Excellent:** Eats most of every meal. Never refuses a meal. Usually eats a total of 4 or more servings of meat and dairy products. Occasionally eats between meals. Does not require supplementation. | |

*Used with Permission.*

If total is ≤ 18 and/or wound is present, initiate pressure ulcer prevention and/or wound treatment orders.

Total Score:____________

Identify Integumentary Integrity by placing appropriate letters on figure.

Key: ❑ ≤ 18: at risk for pressure ulcers ❑ 15–18: low risk ❑ 13–14: moderate risk ❑ 10–12: high risk ❑ < –9: Very high risk

## ❑ Skin Intact

E - Ecchymosis
L - Laceration
A - Abrasion
U - Ulcer
RH - Rash
I - Incision
Er - Erythema
O - Open Wound
B - Blister
PU - Pressure Ulcer
S - Scars (past 2 years)

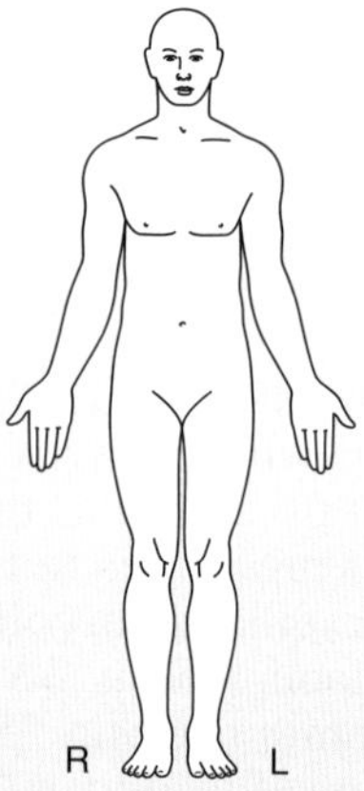

R L
Front

❑ IV Access

❑ Permanent Cath

Completed by:____________

____________
Therapist's Signature

____________
Date Time

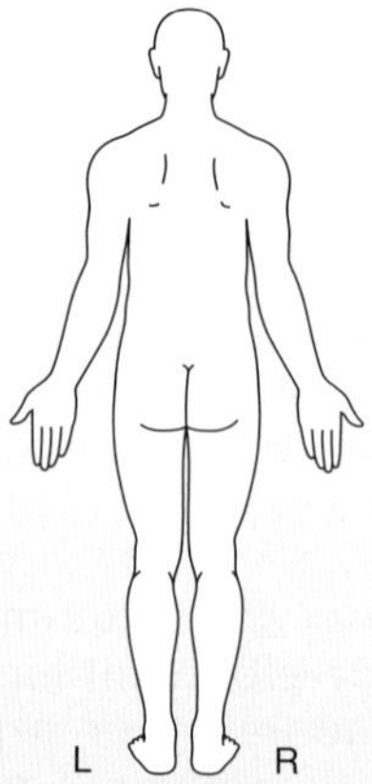

L R
Back

**Figure. 10.28**

**The Braden Scale for predicting injury risk.** *Note:* The question is often asked: Is there a score that should trigger a physical therapy consultation? We asked our panel of experts and received the following response: *It is advised that at all facilities (acute, inpatient rehab, swing bed, nursing home) every patient/resident should be scored on the Braden Scale. If a person scores <18, he/she should be placed on protocol orders for pressure injury prevention. The same is true if there is a wound or pressure injury, regardless of the Braden score. There should be a place on the protocol sheet to order physical therapy for wound management as well as a consult for mobility, strengthening, etc. All physicians approve, and the nurse can place the order ASAP; the physician later signs it.* (Used with permission of Braden B. Frantz R: Selecting a tool to measure skin integrity. In Stromberg M, editor: *Instruments for clinical nursing research*, ed 2, Norwalk, CT, 1997, Appleton-Lange Publishing Co.)

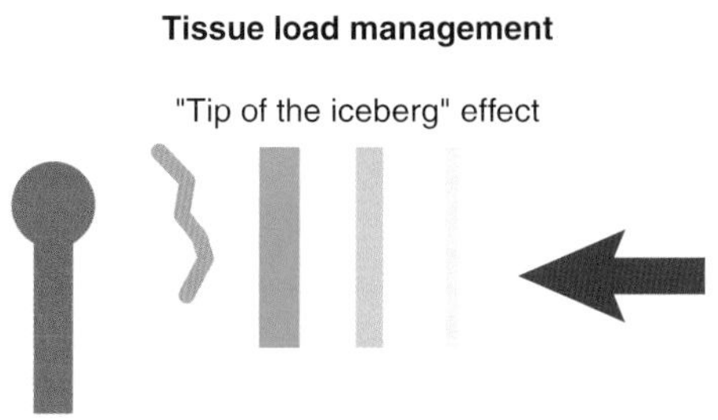

Tissue load management

"Tip of the iceberg" effect

**Figure. 10.29**

**Evolving stages of a stage 4 pressure injury.** This diagram represents a trochanter partially surrounded by tendon, with subcutaneous, dermis, and epidermis layers *(vertical lines left to right)*. As pressure occurs from the outside *(arrow)*, the tendon becomes ischemic first, and then the subcutaneous layer is affected because it is less vascular than the dermis. The last tissue to become ischemic is the epidermis. The observer would initially identify the epidermal tissue change as a stage 1 pressure injury. Initially the ischemic inner tissue layers would not be known. Only as the necrosis moves superficially will the full impact of tissue damage become observable, identifying the area as a stage 4 pressure injury with extensive damage to the bone. (Courtesy Karen Kendall, PT, CWS, Medical Center for Continuing Education, Holiday, FL.)

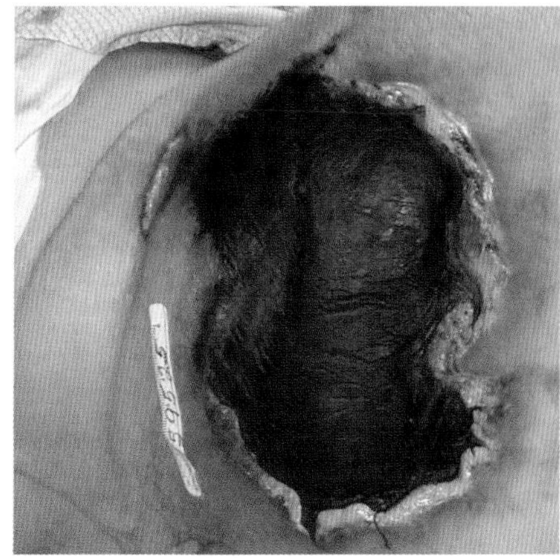

**Figure. 10.30**

**Unstageable (because of eschar) trochanteric pressure injury.** (Courtesy Harriett B. Loehne, PT, DPT, CWS, FACCWS. Used with permission.)

protective sensation indicates a high risk for pressure injuries on the plantar surface of the feet.

## Clinical Manifestations

Pressure injuries usually occur over bony prominences and often manifest with a circular pattern shaped like an inverted volcano, with the greatest tissue ischemia at the apex next to the bone. They may also assume the shape of objects causing the pressure such as tubing or clamps (medical device–related ulcers).[175] Elongated or irregular patterns indicate additional shearing forces or other contributing factors.[124]

Sacral ulcers are often large, undermined wounds and extend to the bone because the tissue mass over the sacrum is thin and erodes easily. Pressure injuries are manifested at the surface as the deeper tissues die so that a stage 1 ulcer can progress to stage 3 or 4 quickly and without further injury.[124]

As with other wound types, pressure injuries (Fig. 10.30) can be described, measured, and categorized with respect to surface area, exudate, and type of visible tissue. Therapists may also use the Pressure Ulcer Scale for Healing (PUSH) tool (available from the NPIAP at https://npiap.com/page/PUSHTool) to assess and document pressure injuries. When present, infection can be localized and self-limiting or can progress to sepsis. Proteolytic enzymes from bacteria and macrophages dissolve necrotic tissues, which can result in a foul-smelling discharge that appears to be, but is not, pus.

Necrotic tissue is insensate, but surrounding tissue can be painful in individuals with normal sensation. Positioning is the first step so that pressure is relieved completely or redistributed as much as possible.[175] Wound management interventions can be ameliorated by premedication with timing appropriate to the method of delivery.

Trauma to the tissues produces an acute inflammatory response with hyperemia, fever, and increased white blood cell count. However, many patients may not initiate a significant acute inflammatory response in cases where heavy bioburden from large amounts of necrotic tissue result in unresolved chronic inflammation. Patients who are immunosuppressed or who have diabetes mellitus are often unable to mount a sufficient inflammatory response to start the healing cascade and thus are at greater risk for infection.

## MEDICAL MANAGEMENT

**DIAGNOSIS.** Prevention is key (Box 10.13) starting with assessment of individuals at high risk for the development of pressure injuries. In fact, risk prediction should be an ongoing assessment carried out by all health care professionals. In addition to the Braden Scale (see Fig. 10.28), laboratory data on hemoglobin, hematocrit, prealbumin, total protein, and lymphocytes should be assessed by all involved health care providers. These values can be helpful for accurate assessment of general health and nutrition and can provide insight into pressure injury risk.[175]

The diagnosis of a pressure injury is made by looking at the location of the wound, the type of tissue response, and the overall patient status. The pressure injury is then staged using the NPIAP pressure injury stages (see Box 10.12 and Fig. 10.26).[175] If there is evidence of infection (e.g., erythema, heat, swelling, pain, purulence, delayed healing, foul odor),[99] viable tissue should be cultured after the wound has been irrigated with isotonic saline and débrided of necrotic tissue.

Sensitivity testing of cultured tissue to identify infecting organisms and to help determine appropriate topical or systemic antibiotics may be needed. Systemic antibiotics should be used in the presence of clinical findings positive for systemic infection (e.g., blood cultures, cellulitis, sepsis).[175]

**TREATMENT.** Eliminating or limiting associated risk factors as much as possible is the first step in preventing the occurrence of pressure injuries.[175] Monitoring devices have been shown to be helpful in reducing incidence of pressure injuries.[250] Preventing shear and friction forces requires education of the patient and primary caregivers. Should skin breakdown occur, intervention is focused on resolution of the causative pressure and good wound care techniques to promote a clean, moist wound healing environment.

Topical antimicrobials (e.g., cadexomer iodine, honey, silver) can be effective in local infections to control bacterial concentration. Topical antibiotic ointments (e.g., neomycin and bacitracin) should be selected with careful consideration, as they have been increasingly linked with allergic reactions.[78,177,241]

Some physicians continue to advocate the initial use of wet-to-dry dressing for débridement (application of open wet dressing, allowing it to dry on the ulcer, and mechanically débriding exudate by removal of the dressing). Because there is a risk of removing viable tissue, damaging new granulation tissue, bleeding, and causing significant pain with this procedure, it is not acceptable for débridement if any viable tissue is evident and should be used only rarely. Other methods of débridement that are safe and more efficacious are available. Wet-to-dry is not permissible as a dressing change order, only for débridement.

The use of antiseptics such as hydrogen peroxide or povidone-iodine is not recommended because these are cytotoxic and can be damaging to granulation tissue. Hyperbaric oxygen therapy has not been approved for pressure injuries except when osteomyelitis is present that has failed systemic antibiotic treatment or there are complications from a flap or graft.

Successful healing requires continued adequate redistribution of pressure (e.g., turning, positioning, support surfaces including sitting)[124] and absence of infection. The presence of necrotic tissue in a wound may provide an optimal environment for bacteria to grow, hence the importance of removing necrotic material from a wound as rapidly as possible.[175]

Therapeutic interventions may include pulsed lavage with suction (PLWS) (Fig. 10.31), negative pressure wound therapy, electrical stimulation, ultrasound, débridement (autolytic, enzymatic, mechanical, sharp, biologic), or any combination of these. An appropriate wound dressing is then applied to provide an optimal wound environment.[175]

In stage 3 pressure injuries, undamaged tissue near the wound can be rotated to cover the ulcer. In stage 4 pressure injuries, musculoskeletal flaps (a single unit of skin with its underlying muscle and vasculature) as well as a variety of other skin-grafting techniques may be used effectively to close the wound.[175]

Bioactive human dermal tissue capable of interacting with the wound bed is available commercially for use in pressure and neuropathic ulcer wound management. These skin substitutes derived from living human tissue (human fibroblasts) represent an important advance in the treatment of burns and skin ulcers, including neuropathic foot ulcers, venous ulcers, and pressure injuries.

**PROGNOSIS.** Most patients have multiple complicating medical factors that contribute to poor wound closure, and each responds differently to treatment. The wound should heal successfully, provided there is no infection, pressure has been removed or redistributed, and there is good perfusion, adequate nutrition, and well-managed overall health. The absence of any of these factors alters the prognosis negatively and complicates the course of care.

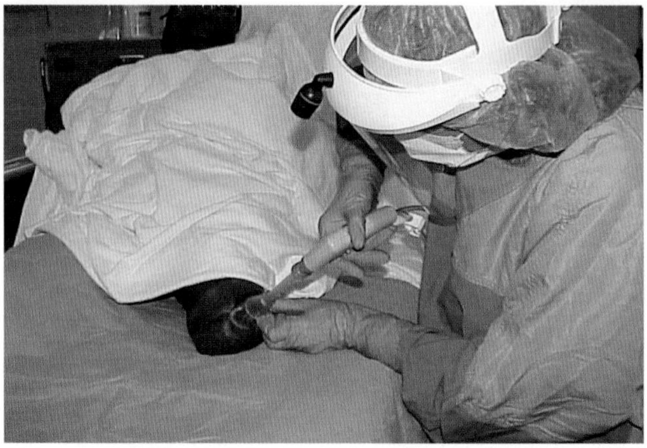

**Figure. 10.31**

**Personal protective equipment worn during treatment with pulsed lavage with suction.** (Courtesy Harriett B. Loehne, PT, DPT, CWS, FACCWS. Used with permission.)

## SPECIAL IMPLICATIONS FOR THE THERAPIST 10.17

### *Pressure Injuries*

The therapist plays a pivotal role in the prevention and management of pressure injuries. The therapist is an expert not only in the delivery of therapeutic modalities, but also in sharp débridement; dressing selection; education of patient, caregiver, and staff; positioning; management of tissue load (mechanical factors acting on the tissues); and patient mobility. Each of these are essential to the success of the intervention.

High-risk patients should be identified using the Braden Scale (see Fig. 10.28), but all patients in the health care delivery system should be evaluated for risk levels and reassessed at least every month for changes in status (or when there is a change in medical status).

Anyone with a history of previous pressure injury is considered a high-risk patient requiring a prevention protocol. Acute care patients should be reassessed daily, on transfer to another unit/floor, and with changes in medical status.

The high-risk patient will need frequent position changes (e.g., every 2 hours in bed, at least every hour while sitting, every 15 minutes if the patient can move independently).[124] For repositioning, use all turning surfaces, positioning the patient at a 30-degree oblique angle when sidelying.[124] While the suggested timing for turning is commonplace, repositioning is highly individualized based on general health, functional level, tissue tolerance, and the surface (Fig. 10.32).[124] Health care providers must always assess each patient individually to establish safe and effective turning schedules.

Elevate the head of the bed to no greater than 30 degrees when the patient is supine; if the head of the bed is elevated beyond 30 degrees (e.g., for eating, watching television, nursing care, therapy intervention), the duration of this position needs to be limited to minimize both pressure and shear forces. A trapeze bar, turning sheet, or transfer board can be used to prevent shearing injury to the skin during movement or position change. Frequent shifting of body weight prevents ischemia by redistributing the weight and allowing blood to circulate.[175]

Static or dynamic pressure-redistribution devices using air, gel, water, foam, or other substances are commercially available, but the therapist must be aware that the material covering these devices can also create heat and friction, contributing to pressure injury. Redistribution of skin pressure must be accompanied by adequate fluid and nutrition intake (see also Box 10.13). Doughnut cushions should never be used, as they can cause tissue ischemia and new pressure injuries.[175]

The patient who is incontinent presents an additional challenge to keeping the skin clean and dry. Stool and/or urine becomes an irritant and places the patient at additional risk for skin breakdown. Contamination of an existing wound by perspiration, urine, or feces is also a concern for patients who are incontinent and immobile.[124,175] Products for urinary and/or fecal incontinence are available to help prevent skin breakdown, including skin barriers, ointments, and fecal incontinence systems.[175]

Cleaning should be carried out using a mild agent that minimizes skin irritation and dryness. Avoid soaps, alcohol-based products that can cause vasoconstriction, tincture of benzoin (may cause painful erosions), and hexachlorophene (may irritate the central nervous system). During cleaning or wound care, the force and friction applied to the skin should be minimized. Use of disposable, no-rinse perineal cloths impregnated with a barrier ingredient is ideal.

Anyone performing PLWS (see Fig. 10.31) must be aware of the potential for aerosolization of microorganisms from the wound. Therapists and patients should wear appropriate personal protective equipment to limit contact with infectious agents during PLWS treatments. To prevent possible exposure of other patients, PLWS should be performed in a private room or in a treatment room with walls and doors that close, not curtains. In 2004 and 2005 the U.S. Food and Drug Administration and Centers for Disease Control and Prevention made recommendations for infection control that included the aforementioned plus covering of exposed supplies, patient items in the room, and open areas not being treated (e.g., tubes, ports). Also consider masking the patient. Observe Standard Precautions, discard suction canister or liner after each treatment, and dispose of single-use-only items. After treatment, disinfect all surfaces thoroughly.

Therapists are advised to use irrigation pressures between 4 and 15 psi.[175] All wound management PLWS products provide a psi of 15 or less. The use of whirlpools for wound cleansing and débridement is no longer recommended for open wounds.[1,27] Unknown psi, multiple known contraindications and precautions associated with whirlpools, need for cytotoxic additives, risk of cross-contamination, and cost and space issues as well as well-documented benefits of negative pressure tissue stimulation have resulted in PLWS essentially replacing the whirlpool as a primary method of nonselective mechanical débridement.

## Pigmentary Disorders

### Definition and Overview

Skin color or pigmentation is determined by the deposition of melanin, a dark polymer found in the skin as well as in the hair, ciliary body, choroid of the eye, pigment layer of the retina, and certain nerve cells. Melanin is formed in the melanocytes in the basal layer of the epidermis and is regulated (dispersion and aggregation) through the release of melatonin, a pineal hormone.

*Hyperpigmentation* is abnormally increased pigmentation resulting from increased melanin production. *Hypopigmentation* is abnormally decreased pigmentation resulting from decreased melanin production.

Pigmentary disorders (either hyperpigmentation or hypopigmentation) may be primary or secondary. Primary pigmentary disorders are direct changes in pigmentation (not resulting from skin damage or another skin condition). Secondary pigmentary changes occur as a result of damage to the skin: such as irritation; allergy; infection; excoriation; burns; or dermatologic therapy including curettage, dermabrasion, chemical peels, or freezing with liquid nitrogen.

### Etiologic and Risk Factors

The formation and deposition of melanin can be affected by external influences, such as exposure to heat, trauma, solar or ionizing radiation, heavy metals, and changes in oxygen potential. These influences can result in hyperpigmentation and/or hypopigmentation. Local trauma may destroy melanocytes temporarily or permanently, causing areas of hypopigmentation that may or may not be surrounded by areas of hyperpigmentation.

Other pigmentary disorders may occur from exposure to exogenous pigments, such as carotene, certain metals, and tattooing inks. Carotenemia occurs as a result of

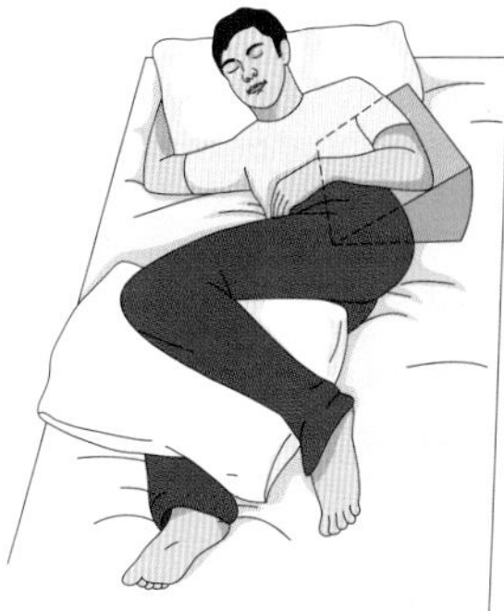

**Figure. 10.32**

**Following the rule of 30s.** Positioning example in which 30 degree sidelying position is preferred over direct (90 degree) sidelying and the bed is kept as flat as possible. (© Pressure Ulcer Prevention Points. Courtesy National Pressure Ulcer Advisory Panel, 2019 Guidelines.)

excessive carotene in the blood, usually from ingesting certain foods (e.g., carrots, yellow fruit, egg yolk). It may also occur in diabetes mellitus and in hypothyroidism. Exposure to metals such as silver can cause argyria, a poisoning marked by a permanent ashen gray discoloration of the skin, conjunctivae, and internal organs. Gold, when given long-term for rheumatoid arthritis, can also cause pigmentary changes.

## Clinical Manifestations

**Hyperpigmentation..** Primary disorders in the hyperpigmentation category include pigmented nevi, Mongolian spots, juvenile freckles (ephelides), lentigines (also called *liver spots*) from sun exposure, café au lait spots associated with neurofibromatosis, and hypermelanosis caused by increased melanocyte-stimulating hormone (e.g., Addison disease).

Secondary hyperpigmentation most commonly occurs after another dermatologic condition such as acne (e.g., postinflammatory hyperpigmentation seen in dark-skinned people). *Melasma,* a patterned hyperpigmentation of the face, can occur as a result of steroid hormones, estrogens, and progesterones such as occurs during pregnancy and in women taking oral contraceptives.[2] Secondary hyperpigmentation may also develop as a phototoxic reaction to medications, oils in perfumes, and chemicals in the rinds of limes and other citrus fruits and celery.

**Hypopigmentation and Depigmentation..** The disorder most commonly seen by a therapist in the hypopigmentation/depigmentation category is vitiligo. Vitiligo is a skin disorder affecting between 0.5% and 2% of the general population.[197] In this autoimmune disease process, melanocytes are destroyed, resulting in areas of skin and hair follicle depigmentation (Fig. 10.33).[197] The process may start when melanocytes are stressed and trigger the innate immune system.[197] This condition is associated with increased rates of diseases, such as thyroid disease, pernicious anemia, diabetes mellitus, Addison disease, and rheumatoid arthritis.[197] Stable versus active lesions may be clinically

**Box 10.13**

**GUIDELINES FOR PREVENTION OF PRESSURE ULCERS IN ADULTS**

- All clients at risk should have a systematic skin inspection at least once each day, paying particular attention to the bony prominences. Results of skin inspection should be documented (see Box 10.5).
- Cleanse skin at the time of soiling and at routine intervals. Individualize the frequency of skin cleaning according to need and client preference. Avoid hot water, and use a mild cleaning agent that minimizes irritation and dryness of the skin. During the cleaning or wound care process, minimize the force and friction applied to the skin. The use of disposable perineal cloths impregnated with dimethicone is ideal.
- Minimize environmental factors leading to skin drying such as low humidity (<40%) and exposure to cold. Treat dry skin with moisturizers.
- Do *not* perform massage over reddened areas. Perform indirect soft tissue mobilization techniques or massage of the tissue around and toward the area with caution.
- Minimize skin injury caused by friction and shear forces through proper positioning, transferring, and turning techniques. Reduce friction injuries by the use of moisturizers, skin sealants, and protective padding.
- Maintain current activity level, mobility, and range of motion. Evaluate the potential for improving the person's mobility and activity status, and institute rehabilitation efforts.
- Monitor and document interventions and outcomes.
- If prealbumin is abnormal (<20 mg/dL), request laboratory to assess prealbumin levels one to two times weekly and have dietitian follow to optimize nutrition.
- Reposition any person in bed who is assessed to be at risk of developing pressure ulcers at least every 2 hours if consistent with overall treatment goals.
- For persons in bed, use positioning devices such as pillows or foam wedges to keep bony prominences (e.g., knees, ankles) from direct contact with one another.
- Provide persons in bed who are completely immobile with devices that completely relieve pressure on the heels (e.g., *float* the heels).
- Do not use doughnut-type devices.
- When sidelying position is used in bed, avoid positioning directly on the greater trochanter. A 30-degree tilt is efficacious.
- Maintain the head of the bed at the lowest degree of elevation (30-degree lateral incline; see Fig. 10.32) consistent with medical conditions and other restrictions except at mealtimes. Limit the amount of time the head of the bed is elevated.
- Use lifting devices such as a trapeze, hydraulic lift, transfer board, or linen to move (rather than drag) persons who cannot assist during transfers and position changes.
- Place any person assessed to be at risk of developing pressure ulcers when lying in bed on a pressure-redistribution surface, such as foam, low air loss, or gel mattress.
- Avoid uninterrupted sitting in any chair or wheelchair for any person at risk of developing a pressure ulcer. Reposition the person, shifting the points under pressure at least every hour, or put him or her back in bed if consistent with overall management goals. Persons who are able should be taught to shift weight every 15 minutes.
- For chair-bound persons, use a pressure-redistribution device. Do not use doughnut-type devices.

Modified from Panel on the Prediction and Prevention of Pressure Ulcers in Adults: *Pressure ulcers in adults: Prediction and prevention.* Clinical practice guidelines. CPR publication no. 92-0050, Rockville, MD, 1992, Agency for Health Care Policy and Research, U.S. Public Health Service; and European Pressure Ulcer Advisory Panel, National Pressure Injury Advisory Panel and Pan Pacific Pressure Injury Alliance. Prevention and Treatment of Pressure Ulcers/Injuries: Clinical Practice Guidelines. The International Guideline. Emily Haesler (Ed.). EPUAP/NPIAP/PPPIA: 2019.

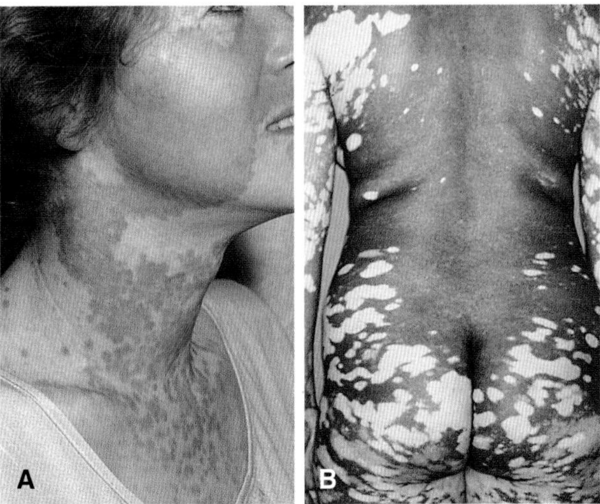


**Figure. 10.33**

***Vitiligo* is a term derived from the Greek word for "calf," used to describe patches of light skin caused by loss of epidermal melanocytes.** (A) Note the patchy loss of pigment on the face, trunk, and axilla. (B) This condition can affect any part of the face, hands, or body and can be very disfiguring, especially in dark-skinned individuals. (From Swartz MH: *Textbook of physical diagnosis*, ed 6, Philadelphia, 2009, Saunders.)

recognized by sharply or poorly defined borders.[46] Treatment may include topical creams, phototherapy, PUVA, narrowband UVB, oral immunosuppression, or even surgical techniques.[196]

## Blistering Diseases

### Definition, Incidence, and Etiologic Factors

Occasionally in a therapy practice blistering diseases may be seen that are severe enough to warrant localized treatment intervention (wound management). Blisters occur on skin and mucous membranes in the condition called *pemphigus*, which is an uncommon intraepidermal blistering disease in which the epidermal cells separate from one another. This disease occurs almost exclusively in middle-aged or older adults of all races and ethnic groups.[41,142]

The exact cause of blistering diseases is unknown, but they may occur as a secondary event associated with viral or bacterial infections of the skin, local injury, or certain drugs (see Skin Lesions in this chapter).[44] In other diseases, blistering of the skin occurs as a primary autoimmune event characterized by the presence of autoantibodies directed against specific adhesion molecules of the skin and mucous membranes.

Paraneoplastic pemphigus, an autoantibody-mediated mucocutaneous disease associated with underlying neoplasm, has a presentation that is heterogeneic and may include polymorphic lesions, lichenoid exanthema, and erythema multiforme.[41,139] This form of pemphigus has a poor prognosis, owing to underlying malignancy.[139]

### Clinical Manifestations

Blistering diseases are characterized by the formation of flaccid bullae or blisters. These bullae appear spontaneously, often on the oral mucous membranes or scalp, and are relatively asymptomatic. Erosions and crusts may develop over blisters.[41,139]

### MEDICAL MANAGEMENT

Medical management may include hospitalization (bed rest, intravenous antibiotics and feedings) when the disease is severe. For others, treatment may be with corticosteroids and local measures. The course of this disorder tends to be chronic in most people, and high-dose corticosteroids can mask the signs and symptoms of infection. If untreated, this condition is usually fatal within 2 months to 5 years as a result of infection. In the case of paraneoplastic pemphigus, early diagnosis and treatment of the underlying neoplasm is imperative.

## Cutaneous Sarcoidosis

Sarcoidosis is a multisystem disorder characterized by the formation of nonnecrotizing granulomas, inflammatory lesions containing mononuclear phagocytes usually surrounded by a rim of lymphocytes. These granulomas may develop in the lungs, liver, bones, or eyes and may be accompanied by skin lesions.[245]

Subcutaneous nodules around the knee and elbow joints may occur in association with pulmonary or cardiac involvement and resolve in response to systemic corticosteroids. In the United States, sarcoidosis occurs predominantly among African Americans[103] and affects twice as many women as men. Acute sarcoidosis usually resolves within 2 years. Chronic, progressive sarcoidosis, which is uncommon, is associated with pulmonary fibrosis and progressive pulmonary disability.[103]

### REFERENCES

To enhance this text and add value for the reader, all references are included in the enhanced ebook on Student Consult that accompanies this textbook. The reader can view the reference source and access it online whenever possible.

CHAPTER 11

# The Endocrine and Metabolic Systems

ANNIE BURKE-DOE • GINA PARISER • KRISTEN M. JOHNSON • TERESSA F. BROWN • IRA GORMAN

## ENDOCRINE SYSTEM

The endocrine system is composed of various glands located throughout the body (Fig. 11.1). These glands are capable of synthesis and release of special chemical messengers called *hormones,* which are transported by the bloodstream to the cells and organs on which they have a specific regulatory effect (Table 11.1). The endocrine system and the nervous system control and integrate body function to maintain homeostasis. Whereas the nervous system sends its messages along nerve fibers, eliciting swift and selective neural responses, the endocrine system sends its messages in the form of hormones via the bloodstream.

Hormonal effects have a slower onset than neural effects, but they maintain a longer duration of action. The actions of the endocrine system may be localized to one area or generalized to all the cells of the body.[223] The endocrine system has the following five general functions:

1. Differentiation of the reproductive and central nervous system of the developing fetus.
2. Stimulation of sequential growth and development during childhood and adolescence.
3. Coordination of the male and female reproductive systems.
4. Maintenance of optimal internal environment throughout the life span.
5. Initiation of corrective and adaptive responses when emergency demands occur.[298]

The endocrine system meets the nervous system at the hypothalamic–pituitary interface. The hypothalamus, the main integrative center for the endocrine and autonomic nervous systems, controls the function of endocrine organs by neural and hormonal pathways. Although the communicative and integrative roles of the endocrine and nervous systems are similar, the precise ways in which each system functions differ.

### Hypothalamic Control

Neural pathways connect the hypothalamus to the posterior pituitary (or neurohypophysis), providing the hypothalamus direct control over both the anterior and posterior portions of the pituitary gland (Fig. 11.2). Disorders of the hypothalamic–pituitary axis are manifested clinically, usually either by syndromes of hormone excess or deficiency or by visual impairment from optic nerve compression because of the location of the hypothalamus and pituitary.

Neural stimulation to the posterior pituitary provokes the secretion of two effector hormones: antidiuretic hormone (ADH) and oxytocin. The hypothalamus also exerts hormonal control at the anterior pituitary through releasing and inhibiting factors. Hypothalamic hormones stimulate the pituitary to release tropic (stimulating) hormones, such as adrenocorticotropic hormone (ACTH), thyroid-stimulating hormone (TSH), luteinizing hormone (LH), and follicle-stimulating hormone (FSH) (see Fig. 11.2). At the same time, effector hormones, such as growth hormone (GH) and prolactin, are released or inhibited, affecting the adrenal cortex, thyroid, and gonads. Endocrine pathology develops as a result of dysfunction of releasing tropic or effector hormones or when defects occur in the target tissue.

In addition to hormonal and neural controls, a negative feedback system regulates the endocrine system. The mechanism may be simple or complex. Simple feedback occurs when the level of one substance regulates the secretion of a hormone. For example, low serum calcium levels stimulate parathyroid hormone (PTH) secretion; high serum calcium levels inhibit it. Complex feedback loops occur through the hypothalamic–pituitary–target organ axis. For example, after an injury or major stress, secretion of the hypothalamic corticotropin-releasing hormone (CRH) releases pituitary ACTH, which in turn stimulates adrenal cortisol secretion. Subsequently, a rise in serum cortisol inhibits ACTH by decreasing CRH secretion (see Fig. 11.2).[493]

Steroid therapy disrupts the hypothalamic–pituitary–adrenal (HPA) axis by suppressing hypothalamic–pituitary secretion. Such treatment is necessary for some conditions, but problems can occur when there is too rapid or abrupt of a withdrawal of exogenous steroid. The result can be life-threatening adrenal insufficiency, because the HPA axis does not have enough time to recover sufficiently to stimulate cortisol secretion.

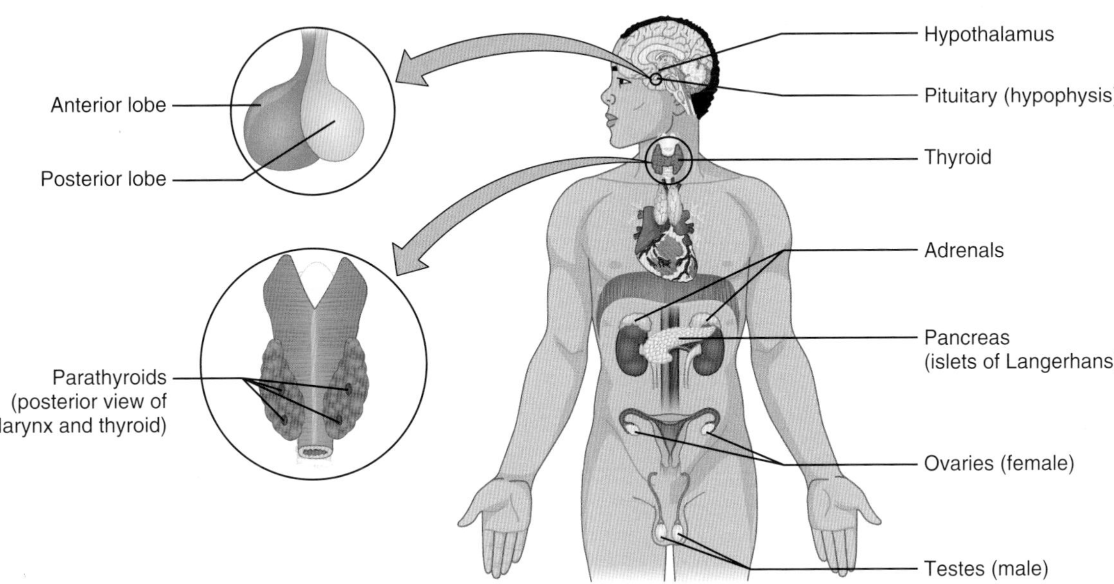


**Figure 11.1**

**Endocrine glands; adipose not shown.**

**Table 11.1** Endocrine Glands: Secretion, Target, and Action

| Gland | Hormone | Target | Basic Action |
|---|---|---|---|
| Pineal | Melatonin | Melanocyte | Antioxidant, causes drowsiness, helps regulate sleep–wake cycle |
| **Pituitary** | | | |
| Anterior lobe | Somatotropin (growth hormone [GH]) | Bones, muscles, organs | Stimulates growth and cell reproduction, releases insulin-like growth factor 1 from liver, retention of nitrogen to promote protein anabolism |
| | Thyroid-stimulating hormone (TSH) | Thyroid | Promotes secretory activity ($T_3$ and $T_4$) |
| | Follicle-stimulating hormone (FSH) | Ovaries, seminiferous tubules | Promotes development of ovarian follicle, secretion of estrogen (females), and maturation of sperm (males) |
| | Luteinizing hormone | Follicle, intestinal cell | Promotes ovulation and formation of corpus luteum, secretion of progesterone, and secretion of testosterone |
| | Prolactin (PRL; luteotropic hormone) | Corpus luteum, breast | Maintains corpus luteum and progesterone secretion; stimulates milk production; sexual gratification after sexual activity |
| | Adrenocorticotropic hormone (ACTH) | Adrenal cortex | Stimulates secretory activity, synthesis of corticosteroids |
| | Lipotropin (LPH) | Corticotropes (cells in anterior pituitary) | Breaks down fat (lipolysis); stimulates melanin production |
| | Melanocyte-stimulating hormone (MSH) | Melanotrope (cells in anterior pituitary) | Produces melanin in skin and hair |
| Posterior lobe | Antidiuretic hormone (ADH; vasopressin) | Distal tubules of kidney | Reabsorption of water (retention in kidneys), vasoconstriction, release ACTH in anterior pituitary |
| | Oxytocin (OXT) | Uterus | Stimulates contraction (cervix, vagina, orgasm), releases breast milk, regulates circadian rhythm (body temperature, sleep–wake cycle, activity level) |
| Thyroid | Thyroxine (T4) and Triiodothyronine (T3) | Widespread (heart, muscle, liver) | Regulate oxidation of body cells and growth metabolism, influence gluconeogenesis, mobilization of fats, and exchange of water, electrolytes, and protein synthesis, increase basal metabolic rate and sensitivity to catecholamines |

*Continued*

**Table 11.1 Endocrine Glands: Secretion, Target, and Action—cont'd**

| Gland | Hormone | Target | Basic Action |
|---|---|---|---|
| | Calcitonin | Skeleton | Calcium and phosphorus metabolism; construct bone, reduce serum calcium |
| Parathyroids | Parathyroid hormone (PTH) | Bone, kidney, intestinal tract | Essential for calcium and phosphorus metabolism and calcification of bone |
| **Adrenal** | | | |
| Cortex | Mineralocorticoids (aldosterone) | Widespread, primarily kidney | Maintains fluid/electrolyte balance; reabsorbs sodium chloride; secretes potassium |
| | Glucocorticoids (cortisol) | Widespread | Concerned with food metabolism and body response to stress; preserves carbohydrates and mobilizes amino acids; promotes gluconeogenesis; suppresses inflammation and immune function |
| | Sex hormone (testosterone, estrogen, progesterone) | Gonads | Ability to influence secondary sex characteristics |
| Medulla | Epinephrine (adrenaline) | Widespread | Fight-or-flight response[164]; cardiac; myocardial stimulation, increased heart rate, dysrhythmias; vasoconstriction with increased blood pressure; increased blood glucose via glycolysis; stimulates ACTH production |
| | Norepinephrine | Widespread | Vasoconstriction; other effects similar to epinephrine (see above) |
| Pancreas | Insulin | Widespread | Increased utilization of carbohydrate, decreased blood glucose |
| | Glucagon | Widespread | Hyperglycemic factor; increases blood glucose via glycogenolysis |
| | Amylin | Pancreatic beta cells | Slows down gastric emptying, inhibits digestive function and food intake |
| **Gonads** | | | |
| Ovaries | Estrogen | Widespread | Secondary sex characteristic; maturation and sexual function; multiple other functions affecting muscle, blood vessels, bone, platelets and coagulation, GI function, lung function |
| | Progesterone | Uterus, breast | Preparation for and maintenance of pregnancy |
| Testes | Testosterone (androgen) | Widespread | Secondary sex characteristics; maturation and normal sex function |
| Ovaries/Testes | Inhibin | Anterior pituitary | Inhibits production of FSH |
| Adipose tissue | Adiponectin leptin (LEP) Angiotensin | Widespread | Controls metabolism, hunger, and vasoconstriction |

When considering each patient/client's current health and pathology and when reading lab values, it is important to know basic hormone functions or effects that may have an impact on therapy treatment. Over 50 different hormones have been identified, but only those most common to therapy clients are included here.

## Hormonal Effects

In response to the hypothalamus, the *posterior pituitary* secretes oxytocin and ADH. Oxytocin stimulates contraction of the uterus and is responsible for the milk letdown reflex in lactating women. ADH controls the concentration of body fluids by alteration of the permeability of the kidney's distal convoluted tubules and collecting ducts to conserve water. The secretion of ADH depends on plasma volume and osmolality as monitored by hypothalamic neurons. Circulatory shock and severe hemorrhage are the most powerful stimulators of ADH; other stimulators include pain, emotional stress, trauma, morphine, tranquilizers, certain anesthetics, and positive-pressure breathing.

The *anterior pituitary* secretes prolactin, which stimulates milk production, and human GH (HGH), which affects most body tissues. HGH stimulates growth by increasing protein synthesis and fat mobilization and by decreasing carbohydrate utilization. Hyposecretion of HGH results in dwarfism; hypersecretion causes gigantism in children and acromegaly in adults.

The *thyroid gland* secretes the iodinated thyroid hormones thyroxine ($T_4$) and triiodothyronine ($T_3$). Thyroid hormones, necessary for normal growth and development, act on many tissues to regulate our basal metabolism (i.e., the rate at which we convert food and oxygen into energy) and to increase metabolic activity and protein synthesis. $T_4$ is more abundant in the bloodstream than $T_3$, but $T_3$ is more active in directing the production of proteins vital to cell function.

Thyroid hormones influence renal development, kidney structure, renal hemodynamics, GFR, the function of

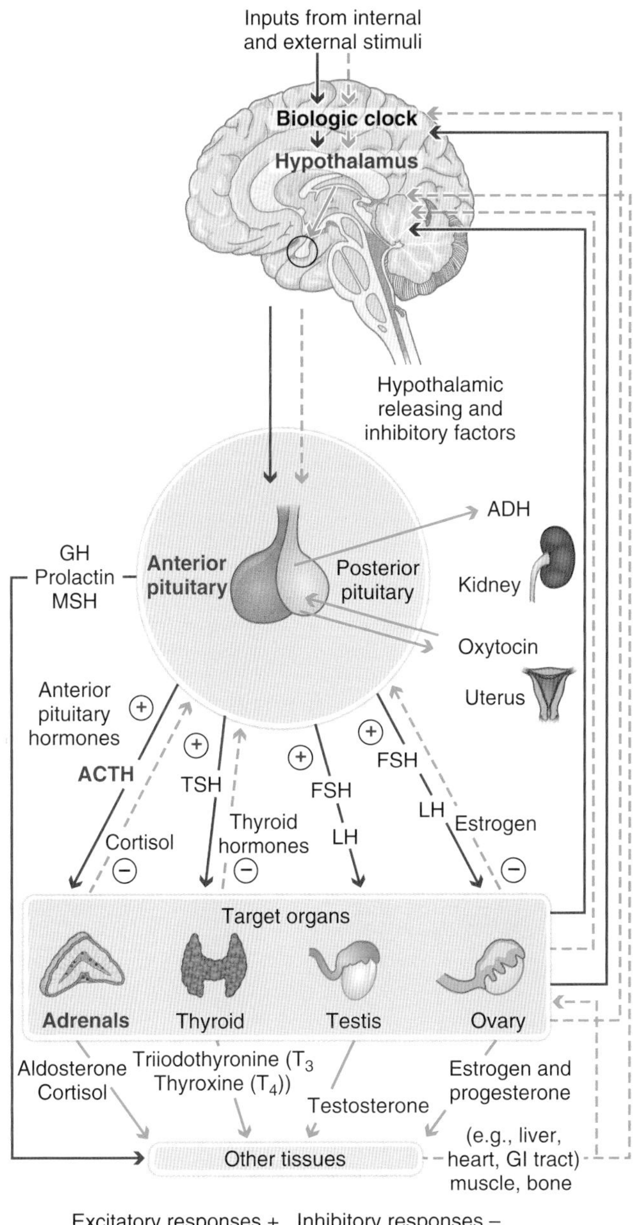


**Figure 11.2**

**Control of the endocrine system by the nervous system.** One example of the complex feedback loops described in the text is highlighted here. The hypothalamus controls the pituitary gland through releasing and inhibiting factors. The anterior lobe of the pituitary gland then releases tropic (stimulating) hormones that act on target glands (thyroid, adrenals, gonads). Endocrine pathology occurs when dysfunction occurs in releasing, tropic, or effector hormones, or when defects occur in the target tissue.

many transport systems along the nephron, and sodium and water homeostasis. These effects of thyroid hormone are in part due to direct renal actions and in part are mediated by cardiovascular and systemic hemodynamic effects that influence kidney function. Consequently, individuals with hypothyroidism or hyperthyroidism may experience clinically important alterations in kidney function.[291,122]

Deficiency of thyroid hormone causes varying degrees of hypothyroidism, from a mild, clinically insignificant form to the life-threatening extreme, myxedema coma. Congenital, autoimmune and iatrogenic hypothyroidism are conditions identified in the pediatric population.

Hypersecretion of thyroid hormone causes hyperthyroidism and, in extreme cases, thyrotoxic crisis. Excessive secretion of TSH from the pituitary gland causes thyroid gland hyperplasia, resulting in goiter in chronic iodine deficiency states. Other causes of goiter are discussed in this chapter.

The *parathyroid glands* secrete PTH, which regulates calcium and phosphate metabolism. PTH elevates serum calcium levels by stimulating resorption of calcium and phosphate from bone, reabsorption of calcium and excretion of phosphate by the kidneys, and by combined action with vitamin D, absorption of calcium and phosphate from the gastrointestinal (GI) tract.

Hyperparathyroidism results in hypercalcemia; hypoparathyroidism causes hypocalcemia. Altered calcium levels also may result from nonendocrine causes such as metastatic bone disease. Pathologic changes in calcium affecting bone bring these conditions to the therapist's attention.

The *endocrine pancreas* produces glucagon from the alpha cells and insulin from the beta cells. Glucagon, the hormone of the fasting state, releases stored glucose to raise the blood glucose level. Insulin, the hormone of the nourished state, facilitates glucose transport, promotes glucose storage, stimulates protein synthesis, and enhances free fatty acid uptake and storage. Insulin deficiency causes diabetes mellitus (DM); insulin excess can be exogenous (i.e., a person with diabetes may receive more insulin than is required) or insulin excess may result from a tumor of the beta cells called *insulinoma.* Whatever the cause of excess insulin, hypoglycemia (abnormally low level of glucose in the blood) is the result.

The *adrenal cortex* secretes mineralocorticoids, glucocorticoids, and sex steroids. Aldosterone, a mineralocorticoid, regulates the reabsorption of sodium and the excretion of potassium by the kidneys and is involved intimately in the regulation of blood pressure. An excess of aldosterone (aldosteronism) can result primarily from hyperplasia or from adrenal adenoma or secondarily from many conditions, such as congestive heart failure or cirrhosis. The *adrenal medulla* is an aggregate of nervous tissue that produces the catecholamines epinephrine and norepinephrine, which are involved in the fight-or-flight response.

The *testes* and *ovaries* are also endocrine glands responsible for synthesizing and secreting hormones.

*Adipose tissue* can be classified as an endocrine gland because it secretes several hormones responsible for metabolism, hunger, vasoconstriction, and cellular growth and development. The concept of adipose tissue as an endocrine organ is quite new, and it is clear that molecules secreted into the bloodstream by fat, such as adiponectin and leptin, act on target organs at distant sites.

## Endocrine Pathology

Dysfunctions of the endocrine system are classified as hypofunction and hyperfunction. The source of hypofunction and hyperfunction may be inflammation or tumor

**Table 11.2** Physiologic Effects of Cortisol

| Functions Affected | Physiologic Effects |
|---|---|
| Protein metabolism | Increases protein synthesis in the liver and depresses protein synthesis in muscle, lymphoid tissue, adipose tissue, skin, and bone; increases plasma level of amino acids |
| Carbohydrate and lipid metabolism | Diminishes peripheral uptake and utilization of glucose; increases output of glucose from the liver; enhances the elevation of blood glucose promoted by other hormones |
| Lipid metabolism | Breakdown of fat in the extremities (lipolysis) and produces/deposits fat in the face and trunk (lipogenesis) |
| Inflammatory effects | Decreases circulating eosinophils, lymphocytes, and monocytes; increases release of polymorphonuclear leukocytes from the bone marrow; decreases accumulation of leukocytes at the site of inflammation; delays healing; essential for vasoconstrictive action of norepinephrine |
| Digestive function | Promotes gastric secretion |
| Urinary function | Enhances urinary excretion |
| Connective tissue function | Decreases proliferation of fibroblasts in connective tissue (and thus delays healing) |
| Muscle function | Maintains normal contractility and maximal work output for skeletal and cardiac muscle |
| Bone function | Decreases bone formation |
| Vascular system and myocardial function | Maintains normal blood pressure; permits increased responsiveness of arterioles to the constrictive action of adrenergic stimulation; optimizes myocardial performance |
| Central nervous system function | Modulates perceptual and emotional functioning (mechanism unknown); essential for normal arousal and initiation of activity |

originating in the hypothalamus, the pituitary gland, or in other endocrine glands. Inflammation may be acute or subacute but is usually chronic, which results in glandular hypofunction. Chronic endocrine abnormalities (e.g., deficiencies of cortisol, thyroid hormone, or insulin) are common health problems requiring lifelong hormone replacement for survival. Rarely, some endocrine gland tumors result in ectopic hormone production and may affect the musculoskeletal system.

Ectopic hormone production is the production and secretion of hormones or hormone-like substances from a source other than the normal source of the hormone. For example, some endocrine gland tumors can metastasize and produce excess hormone from new tumor sites (e.g., some types of thyroid, parathyroid, and adrenal cancers). Some nonendocrine cancers, particularly certain lung cancers, can secrete ACTH and GH.

## Neuroendocrine Response to Stress

The concept that stress of any kind (emotional, physical, psychological, or spiritual) may influence immunity, and resistance to disease has been the foundation for psychoneuroimmunology for many years.[112] The endocrine system, together with the immune system and the nervous system, mounts an integrated response to stressors; this is the subject of many past and current studies. Only a brief review of the neuroendocrine response to stress contributing to disease is presented in this section.

Hormones of the neuroendocrine system affect components of the immune system,[82,105] and mediators produced by immune components regulate the neuroendocrine response. The sympathetic nervous system is aroused during the stress response and causes the medulla of the adrenal gland to release catecholamines, such as epinephrine, norepinephrine, and dopamine, into the bloodstream. Simultaneously, the pituitary gland releases a variety of hormones, including ADH (from the posterior pituitary gland), prolactin, GH, and ACTH from the anterior pituitary gland.

### Catecholamines

Catecholamines are organic compounds that play an important role in the body's physiologic response to stress. Their release at sympathetic nerve endings increases the rate and force of muscular contraction of the heart, thereby increasing cardiac output; constricts peripheral blood vessels, resulting in elevated blood pressure; elevates blood glucose levels by hepatic and skeletal glycogenolysis; and promotes an increase in blood lipids by increasing the catabolism (breakdown) of fats.

Glycogenesis is the splitting of glycogen, a starch stored primarily in the liver but also in the muscles, yielding glucose. The well-known metabolic effects of adrenal catecholamines prepare the body to take physical action in the fight-or-flight phenomenon. Stressors commonly associated with catecholamine release include exercise, thermal changes, and acute emotional states.

### Cortisol

Cortisol is the principal glucocorticoid hormone released from the adrenal cortex and is also known as *hydrocortisone* when synthesized pharmaceutically. Cortisol has multiple functions (Table 11.2), but it primarily regulates the metabolism of proteins, carbohydrates, and lipids to cause an elevation in blood glucose level. These effects on glucose level and fat metabolism result in increased blood glucose and plasma lipid levels and promote the formation of ketone bodies when insulin secretion is insufficient.

Cortisol is essential to norepinephrine-induced vasoconstriction and other physiologic phenomena necessary for survival under stress. The production of glucose promoted by cortisol provides a source of energy for body tissues (nerve cells in particular), and the pooling of amino acids from catabolized proteins may ensure amino acid availability for protein synthesis at sites where replacement is critical, such as muscle or cells of damaged tissue.

Another effect of cortisol is that of dampening the body's inflammatory response to invasion by foreign agents. This anti-inflammatory protective mechanism helps preserve the integrity of body cells at the site of the inflammatory response and provides the basis for the major therapeutic use of this steroid. Cortisol also inhibits fibroblast proliferation and function at the site of an inflammatory response and accounts for the poor wound healing, increased susceptibility to infection, and decreased inflammatory response often seen in individuals with chronic glucocorticoid excess. Whether cortisol-induced effects are adaptive or destructive depends on the subsequent concentration and length of cortisol exposure.

### Other Hormones

Other hormones, such as endorphins, GH, prolactin, and testosterone, may be released as part of the response to stressful stimuli. *Endorphins*, a term derived from *endogenous* and *morphine*, are a group of opiate-like peptides produced naturally by the body at neural synapses in the central nervous system. These hormones serve to modulate the transmission of pain perceptions by raising the pain threshold and producing sedation and euphoria.

As its name implies, *growth hormone* stimulates and controls the rate of skeletal and visceral growth by directly influencing protein, carbohydrate, and lipid metabolism. GH levels increase in the blood after a variety of physically or psychologically stressful stimuli such as surgery, fever, physical exercise, or the anticipation of exhausting exercise, cardiac catheterization, electroshock therapy, or gastroscopy.[292]

*Prolactin* stimulates the growth of breast tissue and sustains milk production in postpartum mammals. Prolactin levels in plasma increase with a variety of stressful stimuli, including such procedures as gastroscopy, proctoscopy, pelvic examination, and surgery, but they show little change after exercise. *Testosterone*, a hormone that regulates male secondary sex characteristics and sex drive (libido), decreases after stressful stimuli such as anesthesia, surgery, marathon running, and acute illness (e.g., respiratory failure, burns, or congestive heart failure). Decreased testosterone during these circumstances restrains growth and reproduction to preserve energy for protective responses.[292]

## Aging and the Endocrine System[145,229]

The exact effects of aging on the endocrine system are not clear. In particular, the question of whether changes in endocrine function are a cause of aging or a natural consequence of aging remains unresolved. The endocrine system has not been implicated as the direct cause of aging. Coexisting age-related variables, such as acute and chronic nonendocrine disease, use of medications, alterations in diet, changes in body composition and weight, and changes in sleep–wake cycle affecting the endocrine system, confuse the picture. Additionally, epigenetic studies suggest that heritable but reversible changes in gene function without changes in nucleotide sequence links genetics and environment in shaping endocrine function.[499] Further studies are linking environmental endocrine-disrupting chemicals (EDCs) to health and disease etiology.[142,54,175] The mechanisms underlying EDC actions and how exposures in animals and humans—especially during development—may lay the foundations for disease later in life.[175]

New epigenetic studies to evaluate the regulation of the endocrine system are predicted to yield important information in the next decade.

Age-associated declines in physiologic performance of the endocrine system are well documented, and it is accepted that the basis of this decline is a *failure of homeostasis*. The conventional view is that "normal" aging changes predispose to age-related disease and contribute to the poor recovery of aging adults after illness or severe stresses such as surgery. Equilibrium concentrations of the principal hormones necessary to maintain homeostasis are not necessarily altered with age, but what may differ as we get older is the way we achieve equilibrium hormone levels, which points to changes in regulatory control.

Collectively, available clinical data suggest a general model of early neuroendocrine aging in the human (both males and females) with variable but predictable disruption in the time-delayed feedback and feedforward interconnections among neuroendocrine glands.[455] Thus with advancing age, significant alterations in hormone production, metabolism, and action are found.

The continuum of the age-related changes is highly variable and sex dependent. Whereas only subtle changes occur in the pituitary, adrenal, and thyroid function, changes in glucose homeostasis, reproductive function, and calcium metabolism are more apparent. The role of the thyroid gland in the metabolism of the healthy older person remains unclear. No major defects are apparent in healthy individuals; however, during episodes of ill health, the thyroid's ability to maintain homeostasis is often limited.[145]

Aging is associated with a higher incidence of disorders or diseases of the endocrine system, including type 2 DM, hypothyroidism, and an increased incidence of atypical endocrine diseases during later life. Cellular damage associated with aging, genetically programmed cell change, and chronic wear and tear may contribute to endocrine gland dysfunction or alterations in responsiveness of target organs (as a result of changes with aging and disease, the target organs may lose their ability to respond to hormones).

Other endocrine changes that may be associated with aging and especially contribute to the age-associated failure in homeostasis include the *neuroendocrine theory of aging*. This theory attempts to explain the altered biologic activity of hormones, altered circulating levels of hormones, altered secretory responses of endocrine glands, altered metabolism of hormones, and loss of circadian control of hormone release. These changes are postulated to occur as a result of a genetic program encoded in the brain and then controlled and relayed to peripheral tissues through hormonal and neural agents.[298] This theory suggests that cells are programmed to function only for a given time.

Menopause as a result of programmed changes in the reproductive system is an example of this theory. Changes in the neuroendocrine system because of the loss of ovarian function at menopause have an important biologic role for women in the control of reproductive and nonreproductive functions and regulate mood, memory, cognition, behavior, immune function, the locomotor system, and cardiovascular functions.[363] It is thought that the temporal patterns of neural signals are altered during middle age, leading to cessation of reproductive cycles, and that the complex interplay of ovarian and hypothalamic/pituitary pacemakers becomes increasingly dysfunctional with aging, ultimately resulting in menopause.[363]

The relationship between aging and the structure and function of the endocrine system cannot be separated from the changes in the immune system and the central nervous system (CNS). Evidence is increasing in support of an immune–neuroendocrine homeostatic network in humans, with the thymus gland playing a key role in the immunoregulation of the nervous and endocrine systems. The early onset of thymus involution may act as a triggering event that initiates the gradual decline in endocrine homeostasis, resulting in the aging process.[176]

Additionally, as the nervous system ages, a progressive reduction takes place in the body's capacity to maintain homeostasis in the face of environmental stress. The overall effect of the changes in aging in the neuroendocrine system is a progressive resistance to the inhibitory feedback of the end-organ hormonal secretion (see Fig. 11.2). Thus, although the initial response to a stressful stimulus may be appropriate, as the body ages, the response is more likely to be persistent and ultimately inappropriate or even harmful.[128]

### Anatomic Changes with Aging

The *pituitary gland* undergoes both anatomic and histologic changes associated with aging. By age 80 years, the weight of the anterior pituitary lobe (adenohypophysis) is reduced approximately 75% from its peak during young adulthood. The blood supply is reduced, and a higher incidence of adenomas and cysts is described during later life.

The *thyroid gland* becomes relatively smaller and fibrotic, and its position becomes lower-lying and retrosternal with age. As with the pituitary gland, blood supply to the thyroid gland is decreased. Secretion of thyroid hormones may diminish with age.

The *parathyroid gland* demonstrates tissue changes with advancing age, but no major change is apparent in PTH levels. Hyperparathyroidism occurs primarily in persons older than 50 years and most commonly results from a single adenoma. It occasionally occurs with multiple adenomas or hyperplasia of two or more parathyroid glands. It is rarely caused by parathyroid carcinoma.

The *adrenal glands* have more fibrous tissue with aging, but because of compensatory feedback mechanisms, no relative alteration is apparent in functional cortisol levels. The most common cause of hypercortisolism occurs with the use of corticosteroids for medical conditions. As previously mentioned, because steroid use can suppress the pituitary–adrenal axis, adrenal insufficiency can occur after discontinuation of steroid therapy.

Changes in the *reproductive glands* have been shown clearly to have physiologic effects, most notably on the cardiovascular system and the skeleton (ovary) and muscle mass and libido (testis).[335]

### Hormonal Changes with Aging

The female reproductive system undergoes changes as part of the normal aging process. Menopause leads to changes in the genitourinary tract and accelerates the loss of minerals from bone and leads to an alteration in the lipid composition in the mature woman. Male hormones have been linked to preservation of bone and muscle mass and to an increased tendency toward developing certain diseases (e.g., benign prostatic hypertrophy or liver disease) during later life.

Loss of body hair, changes in the skin's collagen content and thickness, an increase in the percentage of body fat, a decrease in lean body mass, a decrease in bone mass, and a decrease in protein synthesis are signs of endocrinopathy that may be associated with decreased GH levels.[229] With the decline of GH secretion, sleep cycles are disrupted, and the potential for sequelae associated with sleep deprivation (e.g., depression, fibromyalgia) is now recognized.[448]

As mentioned, interactions between the endocrine and immune systems also influence the aging process. Declining hormonal levels are accompanied by increased activity of tumor-suppressor genes in the aging population unless these genes have been mutated so that suppressor function is lost. In fact, the most common somatic mutation of human cancers is the loss of tumor suppressor genes as a result of exposures to a lifetime of mutagens. In the presence of decreased hormonal levels, loss of tumor suppressor genes accounts for the increased probability of tumors with advancing age, again demonstrating the link between the endocrine and immune systems.[229]

All of these changes have an increasing effect on humans because the average life span has increased, meaning a greater part of women's lives will be lived in an hypoestrogenic state. Men and women alike will experience a decline in GH secretion, increased exposure to mutagens, and a greater possibility of the loss of tumor suppressor genes.[363]

## Musculoskeletal Signs and Symptoms of Endocrine Disease

Signs and symptoms of endocrine pathology vary, depending on the gland affected and whether the pathology is as a result of an excess (hyperfunction) or insufficiency (hypofunction) of hormonal secretions.[171,172] In a therapy setting, the most common signs and symptoms associated with endocrine pathology observed in the musculoskeletal system are presented here.

Growth and development of connective tissue structures are influenced strongly and sometimes controlled by various hormones and metabolic processes. When

**Table 11.3** Signs and Symptoms of Endocrine Dysfunction

| Neuromusculoskeletal | Systemic |
|---|---|
| Rheumatic-like signs and symptoms | Excessive or delayed growth |
| Muscle weakness | Polydipsia |
| Muscle atrophy | Polyuria |
| Myalgia | Mental changes (nervousness, confusion, depression) |
| Fatigue | Changes in hair (quality and distribution) |
| Carpal tunnel syndrome | Changes in skin pigmentation |
| Synovial fluid changes | Changes in distribution of body fat |
| Periarthritis | Changes in vital signs (elevated body temperature, pulse rate, increased blood pressure) |
| Adhesive capsulitis (diabetes mellitus) | Heart palpitations |
| Chondrocalcinosis | Increased perspiration |
| Spondyloarthropathy | Kussmaul respirations (deep, rapid breathing) |
| Diffuse idiopathic skeletal hyperostosis (DISH) | Dehydration or excessive retention of body water |
| Osteoarthritis | |
| Osteoporosis | |
| Osteonecrosis | |
| Hand stiffness | |
| Arthralgia | |
| Pseudogout | |

these processes are altered, structural and functional changes can occur in various connective tissues, producing musculoskeletal signs and symptoms in addition to other systemic signs and symptoms of endocrine dysfunction (Table 11.3).

The therapist must be aware that clients with an underlying but undiagnosed endocrine disorder may present initially with a musculoskeletal problem and that clients with established endocrine disorders are not cured by hormonal replacement or suppression. Rather, they may develop progression of musculoskeletal impairment in response to hormone fluctuations.

*Rheumatoid arthritis* can be an indicator of an underlying endocrine disease. Early rheumatic symptoms, such as myalgias and arthralgias, are seen commonly with several endocrine diseases. DM is associated with a variety of rheumatic syndromes such as the stiff-hand syndrome and limited joint motion syndrome. Although rheumatic symptoms can appear suddenly in people with an endocrine disorder, an insidious onset is much more common.

*Muscle weakness, atrophy, myalgia,* and *fatigue* that persist despite rest may be early manifestations of thyroid or parathyroid disease, acromegaly, diabetes, Cushing syndrome, or osteomalacia. In endocrine disease, most proximal muscle weakness is usually painless and may be unrelated to either the severity or the duration of the underlying disease. However, when true demonstrative weakness occurs (particularly in hyperthyroidism and hyperparathyroid disease), proximal muscle weakness is related to the severity and duration of the underlying endocrine problem. Any compromise of muscle energy metabolism aggravates and perpetuates trigger points such as are associated with myofascial pain syndrome or tender points in muscle associated with fibromyalgia syndrome.

*Carpal tunnel syndrome* (CTS) resulting from median nerve impairment at the wrist is a common finding in people with certain endocrine and metabolic conditions such as acromegaly, diabetes, pregnancy, and hypothyroidism. Any increase in the volume of contents of the carpal tunnel impinges on the median nerve (e.g., neoplasm, calcium, gouty tophi deposits, edema, or tenosynovitis).

In endocrine disorders, CTS is frequently bilateral, which is one characteristic that may distinguish it from overuse syndromes and other causes of CTS. Unreported tarsal tunnel syndrome may also occur, another distinguishing characteristic of an underlying systemic origin of symptoms when present along with CTS.

Tenosynovitis (inflammation of the tendon sheaths) occurs with some infectious processes and many musculoskeletal conditions.[334] Fluid infiltrating the tunnel may soften the transverse carpal ligament, which can make the bony arch flatten and compress the nerve.[169] Thickening of the transverse carpal ligament also may occur with systemic disorders such as acromegaly or myxedema.

CTS in persons with diabetes represents one form of diabetic neuropathy caused by ischemia-related microvascular damage of the median nerve. This ischemia then causes increased sensitivity to even minor pressure exerted in the carpal tunnel area.[207] Vitamin $B_6$ deficiency, repetitive activities, and obesity may also be factors in the development of CTS for the person with diabetes.[9,130]

CTS occurring during pregnancy may be caused by extra fluid and/or fat, diabetes (gestational or previously diagnosed), vitamin deficiencies, or other causes unrelated to the pregnancy itself (e.g., rheumatoid arthritis or job-related biomechanical stress). The fact that many women develop CTS at or near menopause may suggest that the soft tissues about the wrist may be affected in some way by hormones.[91]

*Periarthritis* (inflammation of periarticular structures including the tendons, ligaments, and joint capsule) and *calcific tendinitis* occur most often in the shoulders of people who have endocrine disease. *Chondrocalcinosis* is the deposition of calcium salts in the joint cartilage; when accompanied by attacks of gout-like symptoms, it is called *pseudogout.* In 5% to 10% of people with chondrocalcinosis, an associated underlying endocrine or metabolic disease occurs such as hypothyroidism, hyperparathyroidism, or acromegaly.[152,158] People diagnosed with fibromyalgia also may have altered thyroid function[277] and present with shoulder impingement secondary to chondrocalcinosis.

*Spondyloarthropathy* (disease of joints of the spine) and *osteoarthritis* occur in individuals with various endocrine or metabolic diseases, including hemochromatosis (disorder of iron metabolism with excess deposition in the tissues; also known as *bronze diabetes* and *iron storage disease*), ochronosis (metabolic disorder caused by alkali deposits, resulting in discoloration of body tissues), acromegaly, and DM.

*Hand stiffness,* hand pain, and arthralgias of the small joints of the hand may occur with endocrine and metabolic diseases. Flexor tenosynovitis with stiffness is a common finding in persons with hypothyroidism. This condition often accompanies CTS.[275]

**SPECIAL IMPLICATIONS FOR THE THERAPIST 11.1**

### *Overview of Endocrine and Metabolic Disease*

Disorders of the endocrine and metabolic systems may present with recognizable clinical signs and symptoms (see Table 11.3). Clients with a variety of endocrine and metabolic disorders report symptoms of fatigue, muscle weakness, and occasionally muscle or bone pain. Painless muscle weakness associated with endocrine and metabolic disorders usually involves proximal muscle groups. This muscle weakness and other symptoms, such as periarthritis and calcific tendinitis, may respond to treatment of the underlying endocrine pathology.

In most cases, the person who has received a diagnosis of an endocrine or metabolic disorder has undergone a combination of clinical and laboratory tests. This person may be in the care of a therapist for some other unrelated musculoskeletal problem that can be affected by symptoms associated with hormone imbalances.

Other clinical presentations of musculoskeletal symptoms, such as CTS, rheumatoid arthritis, or adhesive capsulitis, may be referred to the therapist without accurate diagnosis of the underlying endocrine pathology. The therapist always must remain alert to the client's report of systemic signs and symptoms (usually a constellation of symptoms, rather than an isolated few) preceding, accompanying, or developing along with the current musculoskeletal problems.

Additionally, the lack of progress in therapy should signal to the therapist the possibility of a systemic origin of musculoskeletal symptoms. Failure to recognize a metabolic cause of symptoms may result in prolonged, ineffective therapy; visits to a variety of therapists; and occasionally, one or more unsuccessful surgical procedures.

Any client who is taking diuretics must be monitored for signs or symptoms of potassium depletion or fluid dehydration before initiating exercise and then throughout the duration of exercise. Cortisol suppresses the body's inflammatory response, masking early signs of infection. Any unexplained fever without other symptoms in the immunocompromised client must be reported to the physician.

## SPECIFIC ENDOCRINE DISORDERS

### Pituitary Gland

The pituitary gland, or hypophysis, is a small (1 cm in diameter), oval gland located at the base of the skull in an indentation of the sphenoid bone directly posterior to the sphenoid sinus (see Figs. 11.1 and 11.2). It is often referred to as the *master gland* because of its role in regulating other endocrine glands. It is joined to the hypothalamus by the pituitary stalk (neurohypophyseal tract) and is influenced by the hypothalamus through releasing and inhibiting factors. The pituitary consists of two parts: the anterior pituitary (adenohypophysis) and the posterior pituitary (neurohypophysis) lobes. The anterior pituitary secretes six different hormones (ACTH, TSH, LH, FSH, HGH, and prolactin) (see Fig. 11.2).

The posterior pituitary is a downward offshoot of the hypothalamus and contains many nerve fibers; it produces no hormones of its own. The hormones ADH (also called *vasopressin*) and oxytocin are produced in the hypothalamus and then stored and released by the posterior pituitary. These hormones pass down nerve fibers from the hypothalamus through the pituitary stalk to nerve endings in the posterior pituitary; they accumulate in the posterior pituitary during less active periods of the body. Transmitter substances, such as acetylcholine and norepinephrine, are thought to activate release of these substances by the posterior pituitary gland when they are stimulated by nerve impulses from the hypothalamus.[292]

#### Anterior Lobe Disorders

Disorders of the pituitary gland occur most frequently in the anterior lobe, most often caused by tumors, pituitary infarction, genetic disorders, and trauma. The three principal pathologic consequences of pituitary disorders are hyperpituitarism, hypopituitarism, and local compression of brain tissue by expanding tumor masses.[47]

**Hyperpituitarism**

***Overview.*** Hyperpituitarism is an oversecretion of one or more of the hormones secreted by the pituitary gland, especially GH, resulting in acromegaly or gigantism. It is caused primarily by a hormone-secreting pituitary tumor, typically a benign adenoma. Other syndromes associated with hyperpituitarism include Cushing disease, amenorrhea, and hyperthyroidism.

Cushing disease is one form of Cushing syndrome and results from oversecretion of ACTH by a pituitary tumor, which in turn results in oversecretion of adrenocortical hormones. Pituitary tumors produce both systemic effects and local manifestations.

Systemic effects include the following:

1. Excessive or abnormal growth patterns, resulting from overproduction of growth hormone.
2. Hyperprolactinemia (increased prolactin secretion), resulting in amenorrhea, galactorrhea (spontaneous milk flow in women without nursing), and gynecomastia and impotence in men.
3. Overstimulation of one or more of the target glands, resulting in the release of excessive adrenocortical, thyroid, or sex hormones.

Local pituitary tumors produce symptoms as the growing mass expands within the bony cranium. Local manifestations may include visual field abnormalities (pressure on the optic chiasma where the optic nerve crosses over), headaches, and somnolence (sleepiness).

***Gigantism and Acromegaly.*** Gigantism, an overgrowth of the long bones, and acromegaly, increased bone thickness and hypertrophy of the soft tissues, result from GH-secreting adenomas of the anterior pituitary gland. Although GH-producing tumors that cause these conditions are rare, they are the second most common type of hyperpituitarism. Gigantism develops in children before the age when the epiphyses of the bones close; people who develop gigantism may grow to a height of 9 feet. Gigantism develops abruptly, whereas acromegaly develops slowly.

Acromegaly is a disease of adults and develops after closure of the epiphyses; the bones most affected are those of the face, jaw, hands, and feet. In adults, acromegaly occurs equally among men and women and usually between ages 30 and 50 years.[47] Both conditions are characterized by the same skeletal abnormalities because hypersecretion of GH produces cartilaginous and connective tissue overgrowth, resulting in coarsened facial features; protrusion of the jaw (prognathism); thickened ears, nose, and tongue; and broad hands, with spade-like fingers (Fig. 11.3).

In gigantism, as the tumor enlarges and invades normal tissue, target organ functions are impaired by the loss of other tropic (stimulating) hormones such as TSH, LH, FSH, and ACTH. Clients with acromegaly may experience local manifestations, such as headache, diplopia, blindness, and lethargy, as the tumor compresses brain tissue.

Acromegaly-induced myopathy with muscle weakness and reduced exercise tolerance may be more common than previously appreciated. The pathologic or physiologic reason for this weakness has not been determined. Alterations in muscle size and strength in individuals with acromegaly are an accepted association and may be multifactorial in origin. It could be the result of a combination of the direct effects of growth hormone on muscle, the metabolic and mechanical neuropathies present with the condition, the mechanical disadvantage occurring as a result of joint hypermobility, or restriction caused by articular changes and periarticular bone remodeling.[300]

### MEDICAL MANAGEMENT

**DIAGNOSIS, TREATMENT, AND PROGNOSIS.** Increased mortality is linked with elevated GH and/or the target growth factor called insulin-like growth factor I (IGF-I).[139] Timely diagnosis and appropriate treatment are imperative in reducing this potentially disabling chronic and progressive condition.[139] Uncontrolled GH and IGF-I may accelerate the rate of bone turnover; in a small number of people, this long-term exposure may predispose the individual to malignant bone tumor.[269] Long-term follow-up of disease activity and comorbidities is recommended, with management rather than cure being the primary goal.[138] Quality of life is often below reference values for the normal population of the same age.[469] Diagnosis is established by documenting autonomous GH hypersecretion and by imaging of the pituitary gland. Pituitary tumors are treated usually by surgical removal, drug therapy, and/or external beam radiation therapy.

Drugs are now available that effectively normalize levels of growth hormone and prolactin and decrease pituitary tumor size.[138] Drug therapy has replaced surgery in most cases of prolactin-secreting adenomas, but surgery is still the treatment of choice for pituitary adenomas that cause acromegaly.

Some drug or radiation therapy may be required if levels of GH remain high after surgery. Radiation therapy is also useful when surgery is not curative.[325] Frequently, after pituitary surgery, pituitary function is lost, and at that time, treatment with thyroid, cortisone, and hormone replacement may be necessary.

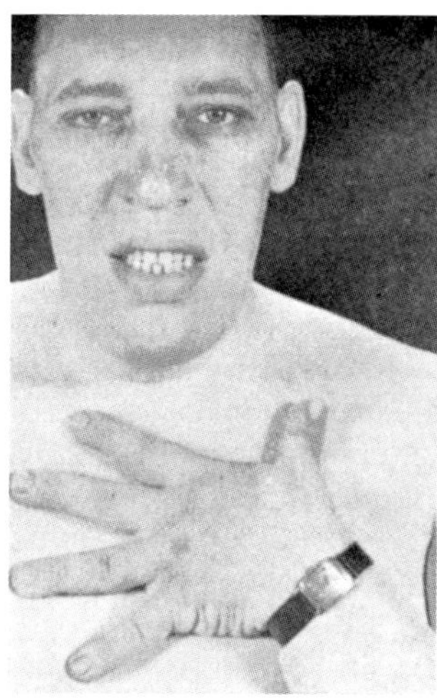

**Figure 11.3**

**Acromegaly (hyperpituitarism).** Acromegaly occurs as a result of excessive secretion of growth hormone after normal completion of body growth. The resulting overgrowth of bone in the face, head, and hands is pictured here. (From Jarvis C: *Physical examination and health assessment*, Philadelphia, 1992, WB Saunders.)

**SPECIAL IMPLICATIONS FOR THE THERAPIST 11.2**

*Hyperpituitarism*

**Postoperative Care**

Ambulation and exercise are encouraged within the first 24 hours after surgery. Coughing, sneezing, and blowing the nose are contraindicated after surgery, but deep breathing exercises are encouraged. Postoperatively, vital signs and neurologic status must be closely monitored. Any alteration in level of consciousness or visual acuity, falling pulse rate, or rising blood pressure may signal an increase in intracranial pressure resulting from intracranial bleeding or cerebral edema and must be reported immediately. Observe for signs of meningitis (e.g., severe headache, irritability, or nuchal [back of the neck] rigidity), a potential complication of surgery.

The nursing staff members monitor blood glucose levels often because GH levels fall rapidly after surgery, removing an insulin-antagonist effect in many people and possibly precipitating hypoglycemia (low blood glucose level). The therapist is advised to consult with nursing staff to determine the possible need for blood glucose monitoring during or after exercise. The therapist should be familiar with signs and symptoms and special implications of hypoglycemia.

Tumors causing visual changes may require the therapist to consciously remain within the client's visual field. Unexpected mood changes can occur, requiring patience and understanding on the part of health care workers. Although surgical removal of the tumor and/or pituitary gland prevents permanent soft tissue deformities, bone changes already present do not change.

### Orthopedic Considerations

Skeletal manifestations, such as arthritis of the hands and osteoarthritis of the spine, may develop with these conditions. Osteophyte formation and widening of the joint space as a result of increased cartilage thickening may be seen on x-rays. In late-stage disease, joint spaces become narrowed, and chondrocalcinosis occasionally may be present. CTS is seen in up to 50% of people with acromegaly and is thought to be caused by intrinsic and extrinsic factors (e.g., compression of the median nerve at the wrist from soft tissue hypertrophy, bony overgrowth, and hypertrophy of the median nerve).[301]

About half of individuals with acromegaly have thoracic and/or lumbar back pain. X-ray studies demonstrate increased intervertebral disk spaces and large osteophytes along the anterior longitudinal ligament. The therapist may be called on to provide a program that promotes maximum joint mobility, muscle strength, and functional skills. Assistance with activities of daily living may be an important aspect of intervention. Home health staff should assess the home to remove any obstacles and recommend necessary adaptive equipment or assistive devices.

## Acromegaly

Anyone with acromegaly should be screened for weakness, changes in joint mobility, and poor exercise tolerance. Skeletal abnormalities associated with acromegaly are usually irreversible. Joint symptoms are controlled with aggressive medical intervention with surgery, pharmacologic treatment, and in some cases, pituitary irradiation trying to normalize hormonal levels.[2] Improvement of joint pain, crepitus, and range of motion has been reported with the somatostatin analogues (drug therapy).[437] The role of physical therapy intervention in acromegaly has not been documented or validated.

Medical evaluation is necessary to rule out systemic causes of muscle weakness such as diabetes or thyroid or adrenal disorders.[261] The therapist should refer clients with acromegaly who exhibit unusual muscle weakness for a complete workup for neuropathies and inflammatory myopathies to rule out any underlying causes that can be treated. Individuals with diabetes who have persistently elevated serum creatine kinase levels should be evaluated for acromegaly.[300]

### Hypopituitarism

Hypopituitarism (also *panhypopituitarism* and *dwarfism*) results from decreased or absent hormonal secretion by the anterior pituitary gland. Panhypopituitarism refers to a generalized condition caused by partial or total failure of all six of the anterior pituitary's vital hormones (ACTH, TSH, LH, FSH, HGH, and prolactin).

Hypopituitarism and panhypopituitarism are rare disorders that occur as a result of the following:

1. Hypophysectomy (removal or destruction of the pituitary by surgery, irradiation, or chemical agents).
2. Nonsecreting pituitary tumors.
3. Postpartum hemorrhage (the fall in blood pressure and subsequent hypoxia after delivery causes necrosis of the gland).
4. Reversible functional disorders (such as starvation, anorexia nervosa, severe anemia, and GI tract disorders).

Clinical manifestations are dependent on the age at onset and the hormones affected (Box 11.1). More than 75% of the pituitary must be obliterated by tumors or thromboses before symptoms develop. Specific disorders resulting from pituitary hyposecretion include *GH deficiency*, with subsequent short stature, delayed growth, and delayed puberty; *secondary adrenocortical insufficiency* from diminished synthesis of ACTH by the pituitary gland, which in turn causes diminished secretion of adrenocortical hormones by the adrenal cortex; *hypothyroidism* (thyroid hormone is dependent on TSH secreted by the pituitary); and *sexual and reproductive disorders* from deficiencies of the gonadotropins (LH and FSH).

Treatment for hypopituitarism involves removal (if possible) of the causative factor, such as tumors, and lifetime replacement of the missing hormones.[290]

**Box 11.1**

**CLINICAL MANIFESTATIONS OF HYPOPITUITARISM**

***Growth hormone deficiency***

- Short stature
- Delayed growth
- Delayed puberty

***Adrenocortical insufficiency***

- Hypoglycemia
- Anorexia
- Nausea
- Abdominal pain
- Orthostatic hypotension

***Hypothyroidism (see also)***

- Fatigue
- Lethargy
- Sensitivity to cold
- Menstrual disturbances

***Gonadal failure***

- Secondary amenorrhea
- Impotence
- Infertility
- Decreased libido
- Absent secondary sex characteristics (children)

***Neurologic signs (produced by tumors)***

- Headache
- Bilateral temporal hemianopia
- Loss of visual acuity
- Blindness

**SPECIAL IMPLICATIONS FOR THE THERAPIST 11.3**

*Hypopituitarism*

Although rarely encountered in a therapy setting, the client with hypopituitarism may report symptoms associated with hormonal deficiencies until hormone replacement therapy is complete. The therapist may observe weakness, fatigue, lethargy, apathy, and orthostatic hypotension.

Infection prevention requires meticulous skin care. Impaired peripheral vision associated with bilateral hemianopia (blindness in half of the visual field) requires special consideration. The therapist must be certain to stand where the affected individual can see others and to move slowly in and out of the client's visual field.

Box 11.2

**CAUSES OF DIABETES INSIPIDUS**

- Intracranial or pituitary neoplasm
- Metastatic lesions (e.g., breast or lung cancer)
- Surgical hypophysectomy or other neurosurgery
- Skull fracture or head trauma (damages the neurohypophyseal structures)
- Infection (e.g., meningitis, encephalitis)
- Granulomatous disease
- Vascular lesions (e.g., aneurysm)
- Idiopathic
- Anorexia
- Autoimmune; heredity
- Drugs or medications (causing nephrogenic diabetes insipidus)
  - Lithium (most common)
  - Alcohol
  - Amphotericin B
  - Foscarnet
  - Aminoglycosides
  - Some chemotherapeutic agents

Data from pharmacotherapy update: Tisdale JE, Miller DA, eds: *Drug-induced diseases*, ed 2, Bethesda, MD, 2010, American Society of Health-System Pharmacists.

### Posterior Lobe Disorders

***Diabetes Insipidus.*** Diabetes insipidus, a rare disorder, involves a physiologic imbalance of water secondary to ADH deficiency or inaction. Injury or loss of function of the hypothalamus, the neurohypophyseal tract, or the posterior pituitary gland can result in diabetes insipidus (Box 11.2).

Because the major functions of ADH are to promote water resorption by the kidney and to control the osmotic pressure of the extracellular fluid, when ADH production decreases, the kidney tubules fail to resorb water. The end result is excretion of large amounts of dilute urine. Unlike urine in DM, which contains large amounts of glucose, urine in diabetes insipidus is dilute and contains no glucose. Other clinical manifestations include polydipsia (excessive thirst), nocturia (excessive urination at night), and dehydration (e.g., poor tissue turgor, dry mucous membranes, constipation, muscle weakness, dizziness, and hypotension). Fatigue and irritability may develop secondary to sleep disruption and in association with nocturia.

If a person is conscious and able to respond appropriately to the thirst mechanism, hydration can be maintained. However, if a person is unconscious or confused and unable to take in necessary fluids to compensate for fluid loss, rapid dehydration, shock, and death can occur. Treatment is usually exogenous replacement of ADH with vasopressin or a synthetic derivative, such as Pitressin, along with administration of diuretics. When this condition is caused by tumor, resection of the tumor can effect a cure.

SPECIAL IMPLICATIONS FOR THE THERAPIST 11.4

## *Diabetes Insipidus*

The therapist must be alert for possible serious side effects of any type of ADH administration. ADH stimulates smooth muscle contraction of the vascular system (causing increased blood pressure), the GI tract (causing diarrhea), and the coronary arteries (causing angina or myocardial infarction).[207]

Increases in blood pressure can cause additional serious problems in some people, particularly those with hypertension or coronary artery disease (CAD) and cerebrovascular disease. Additionally, after receiving vasopressin, clients must be assessed for signs and symptoms of water intoxication, which can lead to fluid overload (pulmonary crackles), cerebral edema, and seizures.

**Syndrome of Inappropriate Antidiuretic Hormone Secretion.** Syndrome of inappropriate ADH (SIADH) is a disorder associated with excessive release of ADH, which disturbs fluid and electrolyte balance, resulting in a water imbalance. SIADH has a wide variety of causes, including pituitary damage resulting from infection or trauma, but the most common cause is ectopic ADH production by malignancies (e.g., oat-cell lung, pancreatic, brain, or prostate cancer; Hodgkin disease; thymoma).[370]

Tumors can cause unregulated production of ADH, leading to severe hyponatremia (sodium depletion, less than 115 mEq/L) with resultant lethargy, nausea, anorexia, and generalized weakness. Mild hyponatremia (125–130 mEq/L) causes increased thirst, muscle cramps, and lethargy. Rapid onset of SIADH can result in coma, convulsions, or death.[430] SIADH can be triggered by the stress of surgery or many systemic disorders and response to certain medications, including chemotherapy medications such as vincristine and cyclophosphamide[353,430] (Box 11.3).

SIADH is the opposite of diabetes insipidus, so treatment of diabetes insipidus with vasopressin can lead to SIADH if excessive amounts are administered. In SIADH, instead of large fluid losses, water intoxication occurs as a result of fluid retention. Under normal circumstances, ADH regulates serum osmolality. Serum osmolality is a measure of the number of dissolved particles per unit of water in serum. In a solution, the fewer the particles of solute in proportion to the number of units of water (solvent), the less concentrated the solution. A low serum osmolality indicates a higher-than-usual amount of water in relation to the amount of particles dissolved in it.

In other words, serum osmolality provides a measure of hydration of cells. For example, a low serum osmolality accompanies overhydration (i.e., edema); an increased serum osmolality is present in a state of fluid volume deficit. Osmolality is proportional with dilutional or depletional states (true for water and sodium). The normal value for serum osmolality is 280 to 300 mOsm/kg of water.[85] When serum osmolality falls, a feedback mechanism causes inhibition of ADH, which promotes increased water excretion by the kidneys to raise serum osmolality to normal. When this feedback mechanism fails and ADH levels are sustained, fluid retention results. Ultimately, serum sodium levels fall, resulting in hyponatremia and water intoxication.[207]

Although fluid retention is the primary symptom, edema is rare unless water overload exceeds 4 L; much of

Box 11.3

**CAUSES OF SYNDROME OF INAPPROPRIATE ANTIDIURETIC HORMONE SECRETION (SIADH)**

- Oat cell carcinoma (accounts for 80% of cases)
- Pulmonary disorders
  - Pneumonia
  - Tuberculosis
  - Lung abscess
  - Mechanical ventilation (e.g., positive pressure)
- Central nervous system disorders
  - Brain tumor or abscess
  - Cerebrovascular accident
  - Head injury
  - Guillain-Barré syndrome
  - Systemic lupus erythematosus
- Other neoplasms (e.g., pancreatic or prostatic cancer, Hodgkin disease, thymoma)
- Infection
- Stress (e.g., surgery) or trauma
- Medications with the strongest association with SIADH:
  - Selective serotonin reuptake inhibitors (SSRIs)
  - Serotonin-norepinephrine reuptake inhibitors
  - Chemotherapeutic agents (e.g., vinca alkaloids, cisplatin, cyclophosphamide)
  - Carbamazepine
  - Oxcarbazepine
- Myxedema
- Psychosis
- Porphyria

Data from pharmacotherapy update: Tisdale JE, Miller DA, eds: *Drug-induced diseases*, ed 2, Bethesda, MD, 2010, American Society of Health-System Pharmacists.

the free water excess is within cellular boundaries. Neurologic and neuromuscular signs and symptoms predominate and are directly related to the swelling of brain tissue and to sodium changes within neuromuscular tissues. CNS dysfunction, characterized by alterations in level of consciousness, seizures, and coma, can occur when serum sodium falls to 120 mEq/L or less. Hyponatremia can result in diminished GI function; this problem is complicated further by the need for fluid restriction.

Correction of life-threatening sodium imbalance is the first aim of treatment, followed by correction of the underlying cause. If SIADH is caused by malignancy, success in alleviating water retention may be obtained by surgical resection, irradiation, or chemotherapy. Otherwise, treatment for SIADH is symptomatic and includes restriction of water intake, careful replacement of sodium chloride, and administration of diuretics. Other pharmaceuticals (e.g., demeclocycline and tetracycline or lithium) also may be used to block the renal response to ADH.

SPECIAL IMPLICATIONS FOR THE THERAPIST 11.5

### *Syndrome of Inappropriate Antidiuretic Hormone Secretion*

Anyone at risk for SIADH (see conditions listed in Box 11.3) should be monitored for sudden weight gain or fluid retention and changes in urination and fluid intake. Monitoring vital signs, oxygen saturation, and cardiac rhythm are important.

Throughout therapy, the client's cardiovascular status should be assessed regularly so that any unusual alterations can be noted immediately. Observe for headache, lethargy, muscle cramps, restlessness, altered mental status, irritability, convulsions, or weight gain without visible edema (≥2 lb a day).

Continued need for sodium and fluid restrictions may be necessary for the person discharged to home or who is in a facility other than the acute care setting (hospital). People with unresolved SIADH should avoid the use of aspirin or nonsteroidal antiinflammatory agents (NSAIDs) without a physician's approval, because these drugs can increase hyponatremia.

The role of the physical therapist has not been clearly defined for people with this condition. Clients with mild or moderate SIADH may benefit from physical therapy for intervention to improve mobility and prevent deconditioning, which can lead to further functional improvement and quality of life. Each client must be evaluated individually to determine the most appropriate plan of care, ranging from bed mobility and transfers to range of motion to a program of strengthening and conditioning.[430]

In the acute care setting, fluid restrictions must be noted and followed. This may require some coordination and scheduling for anyone who may need water in association with his or her exercise program. Individuals on fluid restriction must also be monitored for urinary output. Physical therapists should coordinate with nursing staff to monitor fluid intake and output.[430] Any change in mental status, motor coordination, or energy level should be recorded and reported for consideration by the medical and nursing staff.[38,251,392,447]

## Thyroid Gland

The thyroid gland is located in the anterior portion of the lower neck, below the larynx, on both sides of and anterior to the trachea (see Fig. 11.1). The primary hormones produced by the thyroid are thyroxine ($T_4$), triiodothyronine ($T_3$), and calcitonin. Both $T_3$ and $T_4$ regulate the metabolic rate of the body and increase protein synthesis. Calcitonin has a weak physiologic effect on calcium and phosphorus balance in the body. Thyroid function is regulated by the hypothalamus and pituitary feedback controls and by an intrinsic regulator mechanism within the gland.[184]

Both thyroid hormones travel from the thyroid via the bloodstream to distant parts of the body, including the brain, heart, liver, kidneys, bones, and skin, where they activate genes that regulate body functions. When the hypothalamus senses that circulating levels have dropped, it signals the pituitary gland, which sends TSH to the thyroid to trigger the release of thyroid hormones.

Disorders of the thyroid gland may be functional abnormalities, leading to hyperfunction or hypofunction of the gland or anatomic abnormalities such as thyroiditis, goiter, and tumor. Enlargement of the thyroid gland or neoplasm may or may not be associated with abnormalities of hormone secretion.

Susceptibility to thyroid disease is largely determined by the interaction of genetic makeup, age, and sex. Approximately 27 million Americans have been diagnosed with thyroid disease; many other people are undiagnosed because the signs and symptoms are so nonspecific. The risk of thyroid disease increases with age but is difficult to detect in adults older than age 60 because it typically masquerades as other illnesses such as heart disease, depression, or dementia. Women, particularly those with a family history of thyroid disease, are much more likely to have thyroid pathology than men. Although most thyroid conditions cannot be prevented, they respond well to treatment.

Thyroid hormone acts on nearly all body tissues, so excessive or deficient secretion affects various body systems. Alterations in thyroid function produce changes in nails, hair, skin, eyes, GI tract, respiratory tract, heart and blood vessels, nervous tissue, bone, and muscle.[184]

Women may notice disturbances in mood and in menstrual cycles. Menstrual irregularity, worsening premenstrual syndrome (PMS), new onset of depression later in life, postpartum depression (after pregnancy/birth), anxiety syndromes, and excessive fatigue have been reported by many women with thyroid dysfunction.

Both hyperthyroidism and hypothyroidism can adversely affect cardiac function. Sustained tachycardia in hyperthyroidism and sustained bradycardia with cardiac enlargement in hypothyroidism can result in cardiac failure. Both conditions affect the general rate of metabolism, the muscular system, the nervous system, the GI system, and, as mentioned, the cardiovascular system.

### Hyperthyroidism

**Definition and Overview.** Hyperthyroidism is an excessive secretion of thyroid hormone, sometimes referred to as *thyrotoxicosis*, a term used to describe the clinical manifestations that occur when the body tissues are stimulated by increased thyroid hormone. Excessive thyroid hormone creates a generalized elevation of body metabolism, the effects of which are manifested in almost every system.

The most common form of hyperthyroidism is the autoimmune condition known as Graves disease, which increases $T_4$ production and accounts for 85% of cases of hyperthyroidism. Like most thyroid conditions, hyperthyroidism affects women more than men (4:1), especially women between ages 20 and 40 years.

Rarely, a person with inadequately treated hyperthyroidism may experience what is called a *thyroid storm*. This potentially fatal condition is an acute episode of thyroid overactivity characterized by high fever, severe tachycardia, delirium, dehydration, and extreme irritability or agitation. Stress occurring in the presence of undiagnosed or untreated hyperthyroidism may precipitate such an event. Stressors may include surgery, infection, toxemia of pregnancy, labor and delivery, diabetic ketoacidosis (DKA), myocardial infarction, pulmonary embolus, and medication overdose.

**Etiologic and Risk Factors.** Hyperthyroidism may result from both immunologic and genetic factors. Graves disease, the most common form of hyperthyroidism, is most likely autoimmune in development, and although it is more common in women with family histories of thyroid abnormalities, major risk factors have not been identified. In addition, autoimmune hyperthyroid disease is present in people with other immune-related disorders such as Sjögren syndrome,[246] rheumatoid arthritis, and psoriatic arthritis.[295]

Hyperthyroidism also may be caused by the overfunction of the entire gland, such as in Graves disease, or less commonly, by hyperfunctioning of a single adenoma or multiple toxic nodules. Rarely, overtreatment of myxedema associated with hypothyroidism (see next section) may result in hyperthyroidism, and more rarely, thyroid cancer can cause glandular hyperfunction.

**Pathogenesis.** About 95% of people with Graves disease have circulating autoantibodies called thyroid-stimulating immunoglobulins (TSIs) that react against thyroglobulin (precursor for thyroid hormones). These autoantibodies may be the result of a defect in suppressor T-lymphocyte function that allows formation of TSIs. Evidently, TSIs in the serum of hyperthyroid Graves clients are autoantibodies that react against a component of the thyroid cell membranes, stimulating enlargement of the thyroid gland and secretion of excess thyroid hormone.

Because the action of thyroid hormone on the body is stimulatory, hypermetabolism results with increased sympathetic nervous system activity. The excessive amounts of thyroid hormone stimulate the cardiac system and increase the number of β-adrenergic receptors throughout the body. This excess thyroid hormone secretion, coupled with the increased secretion of catecholamines, leads to tachycardia, increased stroke volume, and increased peripheral blood flow. The increased metabolism also leads to a negative nitrogen balance, lipid depletion, and a resultant state of nutritional deficiency.

**Clinical Manifestations.** Because hyperthyroidism is caused by an excess secretion of thyroid hormone, the clinical picture of Graves disease is in many ways the opposite of that of hypothyroidism. The classic symptoms of Graves disease are mild symmetric enlargement of the thyroid (goiter), nervousness, heat intolerance, weight loss despite increased appetite, sweating, diarrhea, tremor, and palpitations. Hyperthyroidism may induce atrial fibrillation, precipitate congestive heart failure, and increase the risk of underlying CAD for myocardial infarction.

Exophthalmos (abnormal protrusion of the eyes) (Fig. 11.4) is considered most characteristic but is absent in many people with hyperthyroidism and may exacerbate after adequate treatment of the hyperthyroid state. Changes, such as swelling behind the eyes, are mediated by autoimmune production of antibodies to soft tissues (particularly the fibroblasts). Highly specialized ophthalmic surgery (surgical decompression) may be effective for correcting the severe exophthalmos when vision is impaired. Retroorbital radiation has also been shown to be effective.[258,467]

Many other symptoms are commonly present because this condition affects many body systems (Table 11.4). As mentioned, complications, such as thyroid storm and heart disease, can occur. Emotions are adversely affected by the increased metabolic activity within the body. Moods may be cyclic, ranging from mild euphoria to

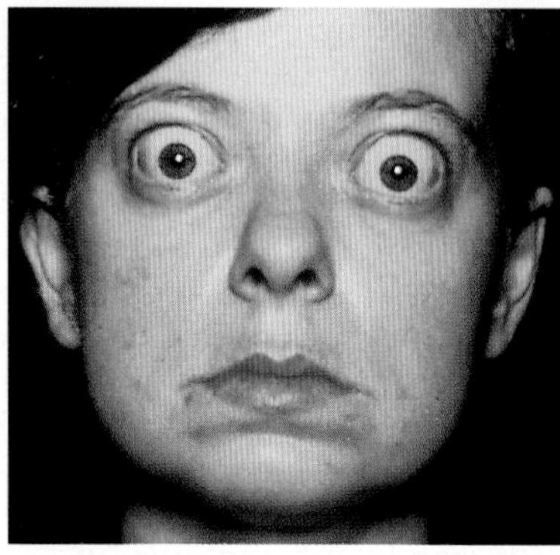

**Figure 11.4**

**Exophthalmos, or protruding eyes.** This is a forward displacement of the eyeballs associated with thyroid disease. Because the eyes are surrounded by unyielding bone, fluid accumulation in the fat pads and muscles behind the eyeballs causes protruding eyes and a fixed stare. Without treatment of the underlying cause, the client with severe exophthalmos may be unable to close the eyelids and may develop corneal ulceration or infection, eventually resulting in loss of vision. Note the lid lag; the upper eyelid rests well above the limbus (edge of the cornea where it joins the sclera), and white sclera is visible. This is evident when the person moves the eyes from up to down. Physical therapy is not recommended in these cases until after the endocrine problem is resolved. Then therapeutic intervention with ultrasound, joint mobilization, stretching, and strengthening may be indicated to treat any residual dysfunction. (From Seidel H, et al: *Mosby's guide to physical examination*, ed 3, St Louis, 1995, Mosby.)

extreme hyperactivity or delirium and depression, which may persist even after successful treatment of hyperthyroidism.[66] Excessive hyperactivity may be associated with extreme fatigue.

Hyperthyroidism in older adults is notorious for presenting with atypical or minimal symptoms.[52,540] Signs and symptoms are not the usual ones and may be attributed to aging. Many older people actually appear apathetic instead of hyperactive. Cardiovascular abnormalities, as described previously, are much more common in older adults.

***Neuromuscular Manifestations.*** Chronic periarthritis also is associated with hyperthyroidism. Inflammation that involves the periarticular structures, including the tendons, ligaments, and joint capsule, is termed *periarthritis.* This syndrome is characterized by pain and reduced range of motion. Calcification, whether periarticular or tendinous, may be seen on x-ray studies. Both periarthritis and calcific tendinitis can occur most often in the shoulder in clients who have undiagnosed, untreated, or inadequately treated endocrine disease. The involvement can be unilateral or bilateral and can worsen progressively to become adhesive capsulitis, or frozen shoulder. Acute calcific tendinitis of the wrist also has been described in such clients. Although antiinflammatory agents may be needed for acute symptoms, chronic periarthritis usually responds to treatment of the underlying hyperthyroidism.

**Table 11.4** Systemic Manifestations of Hyperthyroidism

| CNS effects | Cardiovascular and Pulmonary Effects | Musculoskeletal Effects | Integumentary Effects | Ocular Effects | Gastrointestinal Effects | Genitourinary Effects |
|---|---|---|---|---|---|---|
| Tremors<br>Hyperkinesis (abnormally increased motor function or activity)<br>Nervousness, irritability<br>Emotional lability<br>Weakness and muscle atrophy<br>Increased deep tendon reflexes<br>Fatigue | Increased pulse rate/ tachycardia/ palpitations<br>Increased cardiac output<br>Increased blood volume<br>Arrhythmias (especially atrial fibrillation)<br>Weakness of respiratory muscles (breathlessness, hypoventilation)<br>Increased respiratory rate<br>Low blood pressure<br>Heart failure | Muscle weakness and fatigue<br>Muscle atrophy<br>Chronic periarthritis<br>Myasthenia gravis | Capillary dilation (warm, flushed, moist skin)<br>Heat intolerance<br>Onycholysis (separation of the fingernail from the nail bed)<br>Easily broken hair and increased hair loss<br>Hard, purple area over the anterior surface of the tibia with itching, erythema, and occasionally pain | Exophthalmos<br>Weakness of the extraocular muscles (poor convergence, poor upward gaze)<br>Sensitivity to light<br>Spasm and retraction of the upper eyelids (bulging eyes), lid tremor | Hypermetabolism (increased appetite with weight loss)<br>Increased peristalsis<br>Increased frequency of bowel movements<br>Diarrhea, nausea, and vomiting<br>Dysphagia | Polyuria (frequent urination)<br>Amenorrhea (absence of menses)<br>Female infertility<br>Increased risk of spontaneous miscarriage (first trimester)<br>Gynecomastia (males) |

Modified from Goodman CC, Heick J, Lazaro R: *Differential diagnosis for physical therapists:screening for referral*, ed 6, Philadelphia, 2017, Saunders.

Proximal muscle weakness (most marked in the pelvic girdle and thigh muscles) accompanied by muscle atrophy, known as *myopathy*, can occur in cases of undiagnosed, untreated, or inadequately treated hyperthyroidism. The therapist may first notice problems with coordination or balance or notice weakness of the legs, causing a client difficulty in ambulating, rising from a chair, or climbing stairs.[136,380]

Respiratory muscle weakness can present as dyspnea. The pathogenesis of the weakness is still a subject of controversy; muscle strength seems to return to normal in 6 to 8 weeks after medical treatment, with a slower resolution of muscle wasting. In severe cases, normal strength may not be restored for months.

The incidence of myasthenia gravis, which is also an antibody immune disease, is increased in clients with hyperthyroidism, which in turn can aggravate muscle weakness. If the hyperthyroidism is corrected, improvement of the myasthenia gravis usually follows.

Sudden, periodic paralysis while at rest characterized by recurrent episodes of motor weakness of variable intensity can occur in a selective population (more common among people of Asian origin). This phenomenon is precipitated by intracellular shifts of potassium triggered by thyroid overactivity and hyperinsulinemia after ingestion of carbohydrates and increased physical activity. Administration of potassium is required to prevent life-threatening arrhythmias.[320,361]

## MEDICAL MANAGEMENT

**PREVENTION.** There is no way to prevent Graves disease. Early screening can help determine if someone is at risk. Two simple blood tests can be conducted, one to measure TSH and the second for antithyroid antibodies. Testing should be done by age 40 years (or perhaps earlier for women who intend to get pregnant), especially in the presence of a positive family history.

**DIAGNOSIS.** Diagnosis is based on clinical history, physical presentation, examination findings, and laboratory test results. Hyperthyroidism is almost always associated with suppressed TSH. The very rare exception is that of a TSH-secreting pituitary adenoma. In very mild hyperthyroidism, the $T_4$ would be normal, but the measurement of $T_3$ usually would be elevated or at the upper range of normal. This is called *$T_3$ toxicosis* and almost always precedes Graves disease.

Diagnostic tests, such as radioactive iodine uptake, can confirm the presence of hyperthyroidism and differentiate among causes of hyperthyroidism.[85] Radioactive iodine uptake studies are elevated in Graves disease and nodular thyrotoxicosis but are very low or negative in thyroiditis-caused hyperthyroidism. TSI is positive in almost all people with Graves disease. It is essential to distinguish hyperthyroidism caused by Graves disease and nodular thyrotoxicosis from thyroiditis because the treatment for each is different.[486]

**TREATMENT.** The three major forms of therapy are antithyroid medication, radioactive iodine (RAI), and surgery. Most endocrine specialists would now recommend radioactive iodine as first-line therapy in anyone older than 18 years of age who is not pregnant. Some physicians treat as young as the age of 12 years because long-term studies have shown no increased incidence of thyroid cancer or leukemia in people receiving such treatment.[457]

Iodine-131 therapy takes several months before it is effective, so adrenergic-blocking agents are sometimes given in the interim to control the activity of the sympathetic nervous system. Once the RAI is administered, the iodine concentrates in the thyroid gland, disrupting hormone synthesis. Typically, everyone who receives RAI becomes hypothyroid and requires thyroid hormone replacement for the rest of their lives. Almost everyone treated with radioactive iodine is hypothyroid during the first year of therapy but eventually normalizes with replacement therapy.

Use of antithyroid drugs (propylthiouracil and methimazole) is also effective and is the usual choice of therapy during pregnancy and for children under the age of 12 years. Side effects from drug treatment include rheumatoid-like arthritis and agranulocytosis (serious and potentially fatal) and usually resolve after 10 days of discontinuing the drug. About half of the people treated with antithyroid drugs have a later recurrence of hyperthyroid activity. Again, adrenergic-blocking agents may be used with these drugs.[467]

Partial or subtotal thyroidectomy is an effective way to treat hyperthyroidism caused by Graves disease and single or multinodular thyrotoxicosis. The ideal surgical treatment leaves a small portion of the functioning thyroid gland to avoid permanent hormone replacement. Surgical treatment is effective in most cases, although surgical complications can develop such as vocal cord paralysis (resulting from laryngeal nerve damage) or hypoparathyroidism leading to hypocalcemia (resulting from inadvertent removal of parathyroid gland tissue).[47]

**PROGNOSIS.** Antithyroid drugs may be tapered and discontinued if remission is possible. Remission rates are higher in people with mild degrees of hyperthyroidism, small goiters, and for those who are diagnosed early. Even with remission, lifelong follow-up is recommended because many remissions are not permanent. Relapses are most likely to occur in the postpartum period.[486]

After radioiodine treatment, regular lifelong medical supervision is required. Frequently, hypothyroidism develops even as long as 1 to 3 years after treatment. Exophthalmos may not be reversed by intervention. In severe cases, the person may be unable to close the eyelids and must have the lids taped shut to protect the eyes. Without intervention, severe exophthalmos can progress to corneal ulceration or infection and loss of vision.

**SPECIAL IMPLICATIONS FOR THE THERAPIST 11.6**

### *Hyperthyroidism*

Any time a therapist examines a client's neck and finds unusual swelling, enlargement with or without symptoms of pain, tenderness, hoarseness, or dysphagia (difficulty swallowing), a medical referral is required. For the client requiring lifelong thyroid hormone replacement therapy, nervousness and palpitations may develop with overdosage. A small number of people experience fever, rash, and arthralgias as side effects of antithyroid drugs. The physician should be notified of these or any other unusual symptoms, because it may be possible to use an alternative drug.

### Monitoring Vital Signs

Monitoring vital signs is important to assess cardiac function if the involved person is an older adult,[52,440] has CAD, or presents with symptoms of dyspnea, fatigue, tachycardia, and/or arrhythmia. If the heart rate is more than 100 beats/min, check the blood pressure and pulse rate and rhythm frequently. The person with dyspnea is most comfortable sitting upright or in a high Fowler position (head of the bed raised 18 to 20 inches above a level position with the knees elevated).

Because clients with Graves disease may suffer from heat intolerance, they should avoid exercise in a hot aquatic or pool physical therapy setting. Exercise in a warm pool would be safe and would not be contraindicated as long as the person's temperature is monitored. True heat intolerance usually is associated with severe hyperthyroid states, such as thyroid storm, and probably would not occur in a nonhospitalized individual.

### Postoperative Care

Postoperatively, observe for signs of hypoparathyroidism (muscular twitching, tetany, numbness and tingling around the mouth, fingertips, or toes), a complication that results from the accidental removal of the parathyroid glands during surgery. Symptoms can develop 1 to 7 days after surgery.

Any health care worker in contact with clients who have undergone radioiodine therapy must follow necessary precautions (see Chapter 5). Saliva is radioactive for 24 hours after iodine-131 therapy; health care professionals in contact with clients while they are coughing or expectorating must take precautions.

### Side Effects of Radioiodine Therapy

Radioiodine therapy has few immediate side effects. Rarely, anterior neck tenderness may develop 7 to 10 days after therapy, consistent with radiation-induced thyroiditis.[388] The potential exists for worsening hyperthyroidism soon after radioiodine therapy, secondary to inflammation and release of stored thyroid in the bloodstream. Older adults and anyone with cardiac disease usually are pretreated with antithyroid agents before receiving radioiodine to prevent this occurrence.

The major adverse reaction from radioiodine is iatrogenic hypothyroidism. This development is so characteristic that it is considered an inevitable consequence of therapy rather than a side effect. Hypothyroidism develops in at least 50% of all cases treated with radioiodine therapy within the first year after therapy, with a gradual increased incidence thereafter. This complication necessitates lifelong follow-up with close monitoring of thyroid function.

### Hyperthyroidism and Exercise

Hyperthyroidism is associated with exercise intolerance and reduced exercise capacity, although the exact relationship is unknown. Cardiac output is either normal or enhanced (e.g., increased heart rate) during exercise in the hyperthyroid state and blood flow to muscles is augmented during submaximal exercise. However, proximal muscle weakness with accompanying myopathy is characteristic in individuals with Graves disease and may affect exercise capability.

Impaired cardiopulmonary function (more noticeable in older people with hyperthyroidism) also may affect exercise capacity. Thyrotoxicosis can aggravate preexisting heart disease; lead to atrial fibrillation, congestive heart failure, and worsening angina pectoris; and increase the risk for myocardial infarction. These factors must be considered in the overall discussion and planning of any exercise program for clients who are hyperthyroid.

Fatigue as a result of the hypermetabolic state and rapid depletion of nutrients may affect exercise capacity.[133] Using perceived exertion or exercise tolerance as a guide, exercise parameters (frequency, intensity, duration) remain the same for the person treated for hyperthyroidism as for anyone who does not have this condition. However, the therapist must remain alert for signs of subclinical hyperthyroidism (especially reduced $VO_2$max and other signs of impaired exercise performance) in the person receiving long-term TSH-suppressive therapy. These manifestations improve or disappear after careful tailoring of the medications.[304]

### Ultrasound and Iontophoresis

The benefit of physical therapy intervention in the treatment of endocrine-induced calcific tendinitis has not been proved. Some experts advocate waiting until after the endocrine problem is resolved before initiating a plan of care. Therapeutic intervention with ultrasound, joint mobilization, stretching, and strengthening may be indicated to treat any residual dysfunction.

The limited research published on the subject of ultrasound in treating calcific tendinitis suggests that pulsed ultrasound, applied for 15 minutes at 2.5 $W/cm^2$ and at a frequency of 0.89 MHz, is associated with short-term clinical improvement in adults with calcific tendinitis when compared with sham treatment over a 6-week period of time. Decreased pain and improvement in quality of life were reported.[126,226]

Using acetic acid iontophoresis[226] to promote a chemical reaction in which insoluble calcium carbonate molecules combine with acetic acid to form calcium acetate, which is more soluble and therefore more easily dissolved within tendons and other soft tissues than calcium carbonate, has not been proved effective.[89,90,471] This intervention does not appear to be effective in accelerating resorption of calcific lesions in tendons.[343] More study is needed to determine if duration of treatment makes a difference.

## Hypothyroidism

**Definition and Etiologic Factor.** Hypothyroidism (hypofunction) refers to a deficiency of thyroid hormone in the adult that results in a generalized slowed body metabolism; it is the most common disorder of thyroid function in the United States and Canada. More than 50% of cases occur in families in which thyroid disease is present.

**Table 11.5** Causes of Hypothyroidism

| Primary | Secondary |
|---|---|
| Congenital defects | Pituitary tumor |
| Loss of thyroid tissue | Pituitary insufficiency |
| Radioiodine treatment of hyperthyroidism | Postpartum necrosis of the pituitary (Sheehan syndrome) |
| Surgical removal | |
| Radiation treatment for Hodgkin disease, lymphomas, cancer of the head and neck | |
| Defective hormone synthesis | |
| Chronic autoimmune thyroiditis (Hashimoto disease) | |
| Iodine deficiency | |
| Medications<br>• Lithium<br>• Interferon alpha and beta<br>• Interleukin<br>• Pharmaceutical overcorrection of hyperthyroidism<br>• Amiodarone (rarely used) | |

Data from Tisdale JE, Miller DA, eds: *Drug-induced diseases*, ed 2, Bethesda, MD, 2010, American Society of Health-System Pharmacists.

Like diabetes, hypothyroidism can be categorized as type I (hormone deficient) and type II (hormone resistant). The condition has traditionally been classified as either primary or secondary. *Type I/primary hypothyroidism* occurs as a result of reduced functional thyroid tissue mass or impaired hormonal synthesis or release. *Type II/secondary hypothyroidism* accounts for a small percentage of all cases of hypothyroidism and occurs as a result of inadequate stimulation of the gland because of pituitary or hypothalamic disease (failure to produce TSH and TRH, respectively) (Table 11.5).

In the United States and Canada, this disease commonly is caused by congenital autoimmune thyroiditis, thyroid ablation via surgery or RAI therapy, or medication with thiouracil or lithium; rarely, it is a result of subacute thyroiditis, iodine deficiency, dietary factors, congenital abnormalities in iodination, or pituitary failure.[257,485]

**Incidence.** Hypothyroidism is about four times more prevalent in women than in men. Although hypothyroidism may be congenital and therefore present at birth, the highest incidence is between ages 30 and 60 years. More than 95% of all people with hypothyroidism have the primary form of the disease.[207]

**Pathogenesis.** In type I/primary hypothyroidism, the loss of thyroid tissue leads to decreased secretion of thyroid hormone. In response to a decrease in thyroid hormone, TSH secretion is increased from the anterior pituitary gland as the body attempts to stimulate increased production of thyroid hormone. In the normal body, when hormone levels rise sufficiently, the pituitary slows TSH production. With hypothyroidism, the thyroid gland does not respond fully to TSH, so not enough $T_3$ and $T_4$ reach the body organs, and body functions begin to slow. Whenever the body perceives an inadequate amount of thyroid hormone, the pituitary releases more and more TSH in an effort to stimulate thyroid hormone production. The result is an elevated TSH level in the blood when thyroid function is low.

Decreased levels of thyroid hormone lead to an overall slowing of the basal metabolic rate. This slowing of all body processes leads to bradycardia, decreased GI tract motility, slowed neurologic functioning, a decrease in body heat production, and achlorhydria (absence of hydrochloric acid from gastric juice). Lipid metabolism also is altered by hypothyroidism, with a resultant increase in serum cholesterol and triglyceride levels and a concomitant increase in arteriosclerosis and coronary heart disease. Thyroid hormones also play a role in the production of red blood cells, with the potential for the development of anemia.

Type II/secondary hypothyroidism is most commonly the result of failure of the pituitary gland to synthesize and release adequate amounts of TSH.

**Clinical Manifestations.** As with all disorders affecting the thyroid and parathyroid glands, clinical signs and symptoms associated with hypothyroidism affect many systems of the body (Table 11.6). Typically, the early clinical features of hypothyroidism are vague and ordinary, so they escape detection (e.g., fatigue, mild sensitivity to cold, mild weight gain resulting from fluid retention [10-15 lb], forgetfulness, depression, and dry skin or hair).

As the disorder progresses, myxedema and its associated signs and symptoms appear. Myxedema is a result of an alteration in the composition of the dermis and other tissues, causing connective tissues to be separated by increased amounts of mucopolysaccharides and proteins. This mucopolysaccharide-protein complex binds with water, causing a nonpitting, boggy edema, especially around the eyes, hands, feet, and in the supraclavicular fossae. Thickening of the tongue, laryngeal and pharyngeal structures, hoarseness, and slurred speech occur as a result of myxedema.[485]

Other clinical manifestations associated with hypothyroidism may include decreasing mental stability; dry, flaky, inelastic skin; dry, sparse hair; hoarseness; upper eyelid droop; and thick, brittle nails. Cardiovascular involvement leads to decreased cardiac output, slow pulse rate, and signs of poor peripheral circulation. Other possible effects of hypothyroid function are anorexia, abdominal distention, menorrhagia, decreased libido, infertility, ataxia, intention tremor, and nystagmus.

*Neuromuscular symptoms* are among the most frequent manifestations of hypothyroidism seen in a therapy practice. Flexor tenosynovitis with stiffness can accompany CTS in persons with hypothyroidism. CTS arising from myxedematous tissue in the carpal tunnel area can develop before other signs of hypothyroidism become evident. Most people with CTS associated with hypothyroidism do not require surgical treatment because symptoms of median nerve compression respond to thyroid replacement.

A wide spectrum of rheumatic symptoms occurs in people with hypothyroidism. A subset of fibromyalgia with muscle aches and tender points may be seen early; replacement therapy with thyroid hormone eliminates the symptoms, which aids in the diagnosis of the underlying cause of this form of fibromyalgia. Most cases of

**Table 11.6** Systemic Manifestations of Hypothyroidism

| CNS Effects | Musculoskeletal Effects | Cardiovascular Effects | Hematologic Effects | Respiratory Effects | Integumentary Effects | Gastrointestinal Effects | Genitourinary Effects |
|---|---|---|---|---|---|---|---|
| Slowed speech and hoarseness<br>Slow mental function (loss of interest in daily activities, poor short-term memory)<br>Fatigue and increased sleep<br>Headache<br>Cerebellar ataxia<br>Anxiety, depression | Proximal muscle weakness<br>Myalgias<br>Trigger points<br>Stiffness<br>Carpal tunnel syndrome<br>Prolonged deep tendon reflexes (especially Achilles)<br>Subjective report of paresthesias without supportive objective findings<br>Muscular and joint edema<br>Back pain<br>Increased bone density<br>Decreased bone formation and resorption | Bradycardia<br>Congestive heart failure<br>Poor peripheral circulation (pallor, cold skin, intolerance to cold, hypertension)<br>Severe atherosclerosis; hyperlipidemia<br>Angina<br>Elevated blood pressure<br>Cardiomyopathy | Anemia<br>Easy bruising | Dyspnea<br>Respiratory muscle weakness | Myxedema (periorbital and peripheral)<br>Thickened, cool, and dry skin<br>Scaly skin (especially elbows and knees)<br>Carotenosis (yellowing of the skin)<br>Coarse, thinning hair<br>Intolerance to cold<br>Nonpitting edema of hands and feet<br>Poor wound healing<br>Thin, brittle nails | Anorexia<br>Constipation<br>Weight gain disproportionate to caloric intake<br>Decreased protein metabolism (retarded skeletal and soft tissue growth)<br>Delayed glucose uptake<br>Decreased glucose absorption | Infertility<br>Menstrual irregularity, bleeding (menorrhagia) |

Modified from Goodman CC, Heick J, Lazaro R: *Differential diagnosis for therapists: screening for referral*, ed 6, Philadelphia, 2017, Saunders.

fibromyalgia fall into the type II (hormone-resistant) category. It is likely acquired as a result of mutated receptors.[162]

An inflammatory arthritis indistinguishable from rheumatoid arthritis may be seen. The arthritis predominantly involves the small joints of the hands and apparently differs from the viscous noninflammatory effusions observed in large joints of individuals with hypothyroidism. In general, the arthritis resolves with normalization of the thyroid hormone levels.[230,285]

Proximal muscle weakness can occur in persons with hypothyroidism, sometimes accompanied by pain. Trigger points are frequently detected on examination, and diffuse muscle tenderness may be the major finding. Muscle weakness is not always related to either the severity or the duration of hypothyroidism; it can be present several months before a medical diagnosis of hypothyroidism is made. Deep tendon reflexes show delayed relaxation time (i.e., prolonged reflexes), especially in the Achilles tendon.[136]

## MEDICAL MANAGEMENT

**DIAGNOSIS.** A substantial delay in diagnosis resulting from the vague onset of symptoms is not uncommon. Specific testing of TSH levels is the most sensitive indicator of primary hypothyroidism. TSH levels are always elevated in primary hypothyroidism. $T_3$ (triiodothyronine) levels do not change dramatically, even in severe hypothyroidism. $T_4$ (thyroxine) levels, however, decrease gradually until they are well below normal in advanced hypothyroidism.

Serum cholesterol, alkaline phosphatase, and triglyceride levels also can be significantly elevated in the presence of hypothyroidism. In addition, the presence of antithyroid antibodies documents the existence of autoimmune thyroiditis resulting in progressive destruction of thyroid tissue by circulating antithyroid antibodies.[253,254,500]

**TREATMENT.** The goals of treatment for hypothyroidism are to correct thyroid hormone deficiency, reverse symptoms, and prevent further cardiac and arterial damage. If treatment with lifelong administration of synthetic thyroid hormone preparations is begun soon after symptoms appear, recovery may be complete. There is some controversy over whether mild hypothyroidism (defined by an elevated serum TSH level with a normal free thyroxine level) should be routinely screened, identified, and treated. Treatment is safe and effective, but the question is whether the clinical consequences are enough to justify screening and therapy.[254]

Proponents of early detection and treatment argue that they lower the risk of atherosclerotic cardiovascular disease (CVD) and prevent progression to overt hypothyroidism, especially in adults who are 65 or older. Older people with underlying heart disease (particularly underlying CAD) can be started on very low doses of thyroxine gradually increased in dosage to ultimately return the TSH to within the normal range. Cardiac complications can occur, including angina severe enough that intervention may be required. Only small doses should be initiated in anyone with preexisting heart problems.

Sometimes, individuals with diagnosed hypothyroidism and taking thyroid medication (e.g., Synthroid, Levothroid, Levoxyl, or Euthyrox) to regulate symptoms will have "normal" levels of TSH when tested but still experience lingering symptoms of the condition. Because there is a broad range of "normal," it is not always possible to find the exact dosage required for each individual.

Some physicians are reluctant to increase thyroid medication because of possible adverse side effects such as atrial fibrillation or osteoporosis. In some cases, a regimen of $T_4$ along with $T_3$ (Cytomel) works well along with lifestyle changes such as regular exercise and a healthy diet for gastrointestinal and other breakthrough symptoms.

**Note to Reader** Although we present the standard medical practice here, you should be aware that some physicians and other health care professionals have published alternative opinions and recommend a slightly different approach.[367,373] For example: *Although many endocrinologists continue to debate the appropriate levels of TSH to use as boundaries for normal limits, we think that using TSH to assess thyroid function is counterproductive, particularly in those patients attempting to lose weight. From the published literature and our own clinical experience, we have come to understand that the set point for metabolism is adjusted downward in the hypocaloric state. The decrease in metabolism is often referred to as part of the "famine response." This metabolic response has been documented in several major vertebrate classes, demonstrating its widespread importance in nature. In our current environment, the famine response limits the patient's ability to lose weight while consuming a hypocaloric diet and performing modest levels of exercise. Our own experience with the famine response is consistent with that found in the literature. Treating to normalize thyroid hormone levels and eliminate hypothyroid symptoms results in the suppression of TSH. This is understood as a normal part of treatment once we accept that the thyroid set point has been lowered. This is not an argument to use thyroid hormones to increase metabolism above normal to achieve weight loss. Our goal is to correct the hypothyroid response in a weight loss patient and return him/her to normal metabolism so that the patient feels normal and is better able to lose weight and maintain that loss.*

**PROGNOSIS.** Severely hypothyroid conditions accompanied by pronounced atherosclerosis (resulting from abnormal lipid metabolism) may cause angina and other symptoms of CAD. Treatment of hypothyroidism-induced angina can be difficult because thyroid hormone replacement increases the heart's need for oxygen by increasing body metabolism. This increase in metabolism then precipitates angina and aggravates the anginal condition. In severe hypothyroidism, psychiatric abnormalities can occur and are described as "myxedema madness" in the older literature.

Rarely, severe or prolonged hypothyroidism may progress to myxedema coma when aggravated by stress such as surgery, infection, or noncompliance with thyroid treatment. Myxedema coma can be fatal because of the extreme decrease in the metabolic rate, hypoventilation leading to respiratory acidosis, hypothermia, and hypotension.

**SPECIAL IMPLICATIONS FOR THE THERAPIST 11.7**

### *Hypothyroidism*

In the case of myxedematous hypothyroidism, distinctive changes in the synovium can occur, resulting in a viscous noninflammatory joint effusion. Often the fluid contains calcium pyrophosphate dihydrate (CPPD) crystal deposits that may be associated with chondrocalcinosis (i.e., calcium salts in the synovium). When these hypothyroid clients have been treated with thyroid replacement, some have experienced attacks of acute pseudogout caused by the crystals in the periarticular joint structures (found in both the hyaline cartilage and fibrocartilage). Without medical treatment, this condition can lead to permanent joint damage.

Calcium pyrophosphate dihydrate crystal deposition disease (pseudogout) usually affects larger joints, but symptomatic involvement of the spine with deposition of crystals in the ligamentum flavum and atlantooccipital ligament can result in spinal stenosis and subsequent neurologic syndromes.[376] Effective treatment of pseudogout may include joint aspiration to relieve fluid pressure, steroid injection, and nonsteroidal antiinflammatories.[211,408] Although the synovium contains noninflammatory joint effusion, crystals may loosen, resulting in crystal shedding into the joint fluid, thereby causing an inflammatory response.

The role of the therapist is similar to that in the treatment of rheumatoid arthritis (see Chapter 27). Muscular complaints (aches, pain, and stiffness) associated with hypothyroidism are likely to develop into persistent myofascial trigger points. Clinically, any compromise of the energy metabolism of muscle aggravates and perpetuates trigger points. These do not resolve just with specific intervention by a therapist (e.g., trigger point therapy or myofascial release); they also require thyroid replacement.[402,221]

#### Hypothyroidism and Fibromyalgia

The correlation between hypothyroidism and fibromyalgia syndrome continues to be investigated.[39,40,278] Despite the correlation between hypothyroidism and fibromyalgia syndrome, thyroid dysfunction is seen at least three times more often in women with rheumatoid arthritis than in women with similar demographic features with noninflammatory rheumatic diseases such as osteoarthritis and fibromyalgia.[57,295] Studies have shown an association between hypothyroidism and fibromyalgia. Persons with fibromyalgia syndrome may have a blunted response to a hypothalamic-releasing hormone (thyrotropin) that stimulates the anterior pituitary to secrete TSH, or, in some cases, a possible tissue-specific resistance may exist to thyroid hormone.[268]

Reduced high-energy phosphate in muscle, related to impairment of carbohydrate metabolism (glycolysis abnormalities), may explain the chronic fatigue that can approach lethargy; it is noticeable on arising in the morning and is usually worse during midafternoon. These clients are particularly weather conscious and have muscular pain that increases with the onset of cold, rainy weather.[408]

#### Acute Care Setting

Dry, edematous tissues associated with hypothyroidism are more prone to skin tears and breakdown. Prevention of pressure injury requires careful monitoring of the usual pressure points (e.g., sacrum, coccyx, scapulae, elbows, greater trochanter, heels, and malleoli).

#### Hypothyroidism and Medication

Clients with cardiac complications are started on small doses of thyroid hormone because large doses can precipitate heart failure or myocardial infarction by increasing body metabolism, myocardial oxygen requirements, and consequently, the workload of the heart. Carefully observe for any signs of aggravated CVD, such as chest pain and tachycardia. Report any signs of hypertension or congestive heart failure in the older adult. After thyroid replacement therapy begins, watch for symptoms of hyperthyroidism (e.g., restlessness, tremor, sweating, dyspnea, and excessive weight gain; see also Table 11.4).

All pharmaceuticals taken to replace thyroid hormone use the same synthetic $T_4$ but the inactive ingredients can vary. Altered absorption (increased or decreased) can occur, resulting in additional symptoms. If a client begins to report a change in thyroid symptoms, ask about a recent change in drug brand or name. Changes in symptoms, especially if occurring shortly after a switch to a generic form of the medication, should be reported to the treating physician.

Older adults (aged 70 or older, especially those who have been treated long-term with levothyroxine for hypothyroidism) are at increased risk of bone fractures. Older adults with hypothyroidism have lower requirements for levothyroxine replacement; if dosage is not changed and lowered appropriately, overtreatment can lead to iatrogenic hyperthyroidism.[443] The resulting chronic hyperthyroidism is associated with a higher risk of osteoporosis and an increase in bone fractures. An excess of thyroid hormone can also affect neuromuscular function and muscle strength, increasing the risk of arrhythmias and falls.[33,60,340,381] The physical therapist can be instrumental in making sure older adults are screened for aberrant vital signs, history of falls or falls risk, and osteoporosis and evaluated routinely for correct medication dosage.

#### Hypothyroidism and Exercise

Activity intolerance, weakness, and apathy secondary to decreased metabolic rate may require developing increased tolerance to activity and exercise once thyroid replacement has been initiated. Increased activity and exercise are especially helpful for the client who is constipated secondary to slowed metabolic rate and decreased peristalsis. Exercise-induced myalgia leading to rhabdomyolysis (disintegration of striated or skeletal muscle fibers with acute edema and excretion of myoglobin in the urine) has been reported in undiagnosed[141] or untreated hypothyroidism or in individuals who are noncompliant with treatment.[97] Rhabdomyolysis also could occur possibly as a result of poor drug compliance in combination with other aggravating factors such as exercise.[97,273,393]

Although they occur infrequently, the therapist should remain alert to any signs or symptoms of rhabdomyolysis (e.g., unexplained muscle pain and weakness) in exercising clients with hypothyroidism. Rhabdomyolysis can progress to renal failure. Reduction in stroke volume and heart rate associated with hypothyroidism causes lowered cardiac output, increased peripheral vascular resistance to maintain systolic blood pressure, and a variety of electrocardiogram (ECG) changes (e.g., sinus bradycardia, prolonged PR interval, and depressed P waves).

In animal models, exercise can affect skeletal and cardiac muscle systems independent of thyroid hormone replacement, which supports the role of exercise in improving muscle and cardiovascular function for the person with hypothyroidism.[113,230] Because changes in lipid and lipoprotein levels occur with exercise, an exercise program can improve the lipid profile. This is especially important for the person with altered lipid metabolism and associated cardiovascular complications. However, if the client is hypothyroid with lipid abnormalities, the thyroid deficit should be corrected first. After treatment, if any lipid abnormality remains, exercise should be instituted to treat it.

### Goiter

Goiter, an enlargement of the thyroid gland, may be a result of lack of iodine, inflammation, or tumors (benign or malignant). Enlargement also may appear in hyperthyroidism, especially Graves disease. Goiter occurs most often in areas of the world in which iodine, which is necessary for the production of thyroid hormone, is deficient in the diet (Fig. 11.5). Factors that inhibit normal thyroid hormone production result in a negative feedback loop, with hypersecretion of TSH. The TSH increase results in the production and secretion of huge amounts of thyroglobulin (colloid) into the glandular follicles and the gland grows in size.

Thyroglobulin is the large glycoprotein molecule in which thyroid hormones ($T_3$ and $T_4$) are produced in the presence of iodine. When iodine is absent, only the thyroglobulin is made by the gland in response to repeated TSH stimulation. Because the thyroglobulin molecule is large, its increased production causes rapid glandular growth, and a marked increase in overall glandular mass occurs called a *colloid goiter*.[184] With the use of iodized salt and iodine-containing binders in commercial foods, this problem almost has been eliminated in the United States and Canada. Although the younger population in the United States may be goiter-free, aging adults may have developed

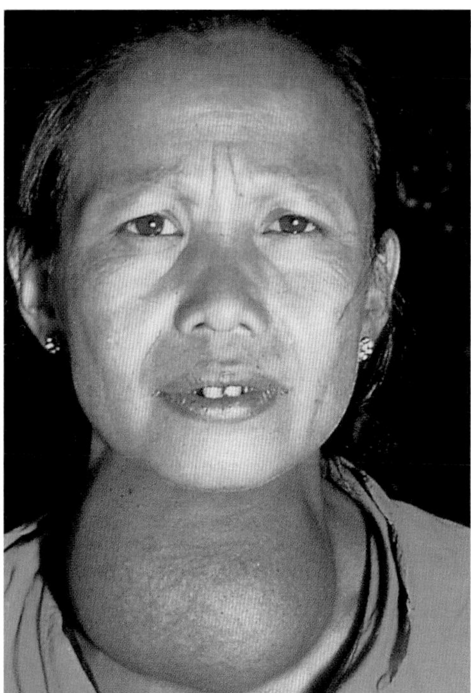

**Figure 11.5**

**Goiter.** The enlarged thyroid gland appears as a swelling of the anterior neck. This condition results from a low dietary intake of iodine and is rare in Canada and the United States but may be seen in other parts of the world. (From Thibodeau GA, Patton KT: *The human body in health & disease*, ed 4, St Louis, 2005, Mosby.)

goiter during their childhood or adolescent years and may still have clinical manifestations of this disorder.

Increased neck size may be observed, and when the thyroid increases to a certain point, pressure on the trachea and esophagus may cause difficulty breathing, dysphagia (difficulty swallowing), and hoarseness. Compression of the upper airway can be a fatal complication. Surgical intervention is essential when the trachea is compromised.

## Thyroiditis

Thyroiditis, inflammation of the thyroid, may be classified as *acute suppurative* (pus forming and very rare), *subacute granulomatous* (uncommon), and *lymphocytic* or *chronic* (Hashimoto disease). Acute and subacute thyroiditis are uncommon conditions caused by bacterial (*Streptococcus pyogenes*, *Staphylococcus aureus*, and *Pneumococcus pneumoniae*) and viral agents, respectively. Infected glands are painful and associated with systemic symptoms of fever and hyperthyroidism. Several varieties of related autoimmune causes of thyroiditis exist, such as Hashimoto (lymphocytic) thyroiditis and postpartum thyroiditis. These types of thyroiditis are generally painless, with only a rare case of Hashimoto causing pain. Only the most common form of Hashimoto thyroiditis is discussed further.

Hashimoto (chronic) thyroiditis affects women more frequently than it does men (10:1) and is most often seen in the 30- to 50-year-old age group. The disorder has an autoimmune basis, and genetic predisposition appears to play a role in the etiology. It is associated with HLA-DR3, which is also present in other autoimmune conditions (e.g., Graves disease, systemic lupus erythematosus, type 1 DM, pernicious anemia, myasthenia gravis, and rheumatoid arthritis).[295] Hashimoto thyroiditis causes destruction of the thyroid gland because of the infiltration of the gland by lymphocytes and antithyroid antibodies. This infiltration results in decreased serum levels of $T_3$ and $T_4$, thus stimulating the pituitary gland to increase the production of TSH.

The increased TSH causes hyperfunction of the tissue, and goiter formation (enlargement of the gland) results. In some cases, this increase in function helps maintain a normal hormonal level, but eventually, when enough of the gland is destroyed, hypothyroidism develops. Hashimoto thyroiditis is one of the most common causes of hypothyroidism in women older than age 50 years.

Signs of chronic thyroiditis usually include painless symmetric or asymmetric enlargement of the gland and an irregular surface, which occasionally causes pressure on the surrounding structures. This pressure may subsequently cause dysphagia or a more subtle "tight" sensation when swallowing, and respiratory distress.

Most clients are euthyroid (have a normally functioning thyroid), about 20% are hypothyroid, and fewer than 5% are hyperthyroid, with these people having combined Hashimoto and Graves disease caused by a genetic component.[207] The course of Hashimoto thyroiditis varies. Most people see a decrease in the size of the goiter and remain stable for years with treatment.

Treatment is directed toward suppressing the TSH to the lower end of the normal range to decrease TSH stimulation of the gland and to correct hypothyroidism if present. Tablets containing thyroxine ($T_4$) can help regulate and maintain adequate levels of circulating hormones. Generally, long-term or permanent therapy is advised.

SPECIAL IMPLICATIONS FOR THE THERAPIST 11.8

### *Thyroiditis*

Because the symptoms of thyroiditis are related to glandular function, and because the condition may be associated with hypothyroidism or hyperthyroidism, the therapist is referred to the sections relevant to client presentation.

## Thyroid Cancer

**Overview.** The thyroid gland contains two types of cells: follicular cells, which are responsible for the production of thyroid hormone, and C cells, which make calcitonin, a hormone that participates in calcium metabolism. There are four main types of thyroid cancer: papillary, follicular, medullary, and anaplastic thyroid cancer.[23]

**Papillary thyroid cancer** is the most common type of thyroid cancer. It develops from the follicular cells and grows slowly and is usually found in only one lobe; only 10% to 20% of papillary thyroid cancers appear in both lobes. **Follicular thyroid cancer** also develops from the follicular cells and is usually slow growing. It is less common than papillary thyroid cancer; both are curable when found early and in people younger than 45. Together, papillary and follicular thyroid cancers make up about 90% of thyroid cancers.

**Medullary thyroid cancer (MTC)** accounts for 5% of thyroid cancers and develops in the C cells. It can be the result of a genetic syndrome called multiple endocrine neoplasia type 2 (MEN2). MTC accounts for about 5% of thyroid cancers. **Anaplastic thyroid cancer** is a rare, fast-growing, poorly differentiated thyroid cancer that accounts for only 2% of thyroid cancers.

**Incidence and Etiology.** Although malignant tumors of the thyroid are rare (less than 1% of Americans will be diagnosed in their lifetime), thyroid cancer makes up more than 90% of all endocrine cancers and accounts for 63% of deaths from endocrine cancer, with an increasing incidence worldwide.[53] In the United States, 60,220 new cases of thyroid cancer were diagnosed in 2013 with 1850 deaths reported the same year,[397] with a slight decrease to 55,870 new cases in 2017 and 2010 deaths.[398]

Thyroid cancer affects women more than men (2:1 ratio), mainly between the ages of 40 and 60 years. However, the presence of a thyroid nodule in a man is regarded with greater suspicion for cancer. A past medical history of radiation to the head, neck, or chest (e.g., for an enlarged thymus or tonsils, acne, or Hodgkin disease) or cumulative exposure over a lifetime is the most obvious risk factor. In other countries iodine deficiency and excess iodine have been linked with thyroid cancer.

**Clinical Manifestations.** The usual presentation of thyroid cancer is the appearance of a hard, painless nodule on the thyroid gland or a gland that is multinodular. Most palpable nodules of the thyroid are benign adenomas and rarely become malignant or grow to a significant size to cause pressure against the trachea. Red-flag symptoms include vocal cord paralysis, ipsilateral cervical lymphadenopathy, and fixation of the nodule to surrounding tissues.[98,202,344]

## MEDICAL MANAGEMENT

**DIAGNOSIS, TREATMENT, AND PROGNOSIS.** Thyroid cancer is diagnosed by fine-needle aspiration (FNA) biopsy. More advanced molecular techniques for the diagnosis of thyroid nodules are being developed.[224,302] Molecular diagnostic assays using tumor-specific markers may improve the sensitivity and accuracy of FNA, possibly reducing the number of surgical procedures to remove lesions that later prove to be benign.[369]

Treatment usually involves removal of all or part of the thyroid. Neck resection of involved lymph nodes may be done for metastases to the neck. Radioactive ablation of remaining thyroid tissue is standard practice for most thyroid cancers. External radiation may be used in some situations. Major postoperative complications may involve damage to the laryngeal nerve, hemorrhage, and hypoparathyroidism.[333] Individuals treated for thyroid cancer require long-term follow-up to detect recurrent disease, which can present years after initial therapy.[254]

Most thyroid cancers are treatable; only about 5% of palpable nodules are malignant. Of the malignant nodules, most are a variety that seldom metastasize beyond regional lymph nodes of the neck, resulting in a good prognosis for most people. However, disease recurrence and metastasis may occur in as many as 20% of affected individuals.[53] Papillary and follicular thyroid cancers are very often curable, especially when diagnosed and treated early in adults younger than 45. Medullary thyroid cancer can be controlled if it is diagnosed and treated before it spreads. Anaplastic thyroid cancer grows very quickly, making it more difficult to treat successfully.[23]

**SPECIAL IMPLICATIONS FOR THE THERAPIST 11.9**

### *Thyroid Cancer*

A thyroid neoplasm can be the incidental finding in persons being treated for a musculoskeletal condition involving the head and neck. Most thyroid nodules are benign, but as mentioned previously, any time a therapist examines a client's neck and finds an asymptomatic nodule or unusual swelling or enlargement (with or without symptoms of pain), hoarseness, dyspnea, or dysphagia (difficulty swallowing), a medical referral is required.

The therapist may become involved with clients who have developed radiation therapy–induced fibrosis contractures. Early intervention to prevent loss of motion, fibrosis, and lymphedema (e.g., self-manual lymphatic drainage techniques, see Chapter 13) is advised, but studies have not been done to support this recommendation.

Individuals treated for head and neck cancers can present with complex, difficult-to-treat problems secondary to cancer treatment. Proper stretching to prevent loss of motion of the head, neck, and jaw is important, especially if fibrosis has impaired eating and swallowing. For clients with involvement of the head, neck, and jaw, baseline measurements should be taken to help document improvement. This can include mouth opening and tongue protrusion, as well as shoulder and neck active range of motion. Some clinicians advocate taking girth measurements circumferentially around the neck, as well as circumferentially around the head from the submandibular region to the hair line.[183,276]

## Parathyroid Glands

Two parathyroid glands are located on the posterior surface of each lobe of the thyroid gland. These glands secrete PTH, which regulates calcium and phosphorus metabolism.

PTH exerts its effect by the following:

1. Increasing the release of calcium and phosphate from the bone (bone demineralization).
2. Increasing the absorption of calcium and excretion of phosphate by the kidneys.
3. Promoting calcium absorption in the GI tract.[207]

Disorders of the parathyroid glands may come to the therapist's attention because these conditions can cause periarthritis and tendinitis. Both types of inflammation may be crystal induced, with formation of periarticular or tendinous calcification. Rarely, ruptured tendons resulting from bone resorption at the insertions occur in cases of primary hyperparathyroidism. These complications and problems are seen infrequently because most cases are diagnosed earlier with the advent of blood screening for identification of asymptomatic hypercalcemia.

### Hyperparathyroidism

**Definition and Incidence.** Hyperparathyroidism is a disorder caused by overactivity of one or more of the four parathyroid glands that disrupts calcium, phosphate, and bone metabolism. Women are affected more than men (2:1), usually after age 60 years (postmenopausal). Hyperparathyroidism is frequently overlooked in the over-60 population. Symptoms in the early stages for this group are subtle and easily attributed to the aging process, depression, or anxiety. Eventually the symptoms intensify as the level of serum calcium rises, but this situation is accompanied by increased bone damage and other complications.

**Etiologic and Risk Factors.** Hyperparathyroidism is classified as primary, secondary, or tertiary. *Primary hyperparathyroidism* develops when the normal regulatory relationship between serum calcium levels and PTH secretion is interrupted. This occurs when one or more of the parathyroid glands enlarge, increasing PTH secretion and elevating serum calcium levels. The most common cause is a single adenoma of the parathyroid gland. Hyperplasia of the gland without an identifying injury and multiple adenomas are less common causes. Medications, such as thiazide diuretics for hypertension and lithium carbonate for psychiatric disorders, have also been implicated as a cause or factor that exacerbates hyperparathyroidism.

*Secondary hyperparathyroidism* occurs when the glands are hyperplastic from malfunction of another organ system. A hypocalcemia-producing abnormality outside the parathyroid gland results in a compensatory response of the parathyroid glands to chronic hypocalcemia. This is usually the result of renal failure (decreased renal activation of vitamin D), but it also may occur with osteogenesis imperfecta, Paget disease, multiple myeloma, carcinoma with bone metastasis, laxative abuse, and vitamin D deficiency.

*Tertiary hyperparathyroidism* is seen almost exclusively in dialysis clients who have long-standing secondary hyperparathyroidism. Hyperplasia occurs, and the parathyroid glands ultimately become autonomous in function and unresponsive to serum calcium levels. Parathyroidectomy is required even after successful renal transplantation has resolved the cause of the secondary hyperparathyroidism.[149]

**Pathogenesis and Clinical Manifestations.** The primary function of PTH is to maintain a proper balance of calcium and phosphorus ions within the blood. PTH is not regulated by the pituitary or the hypothalamus and maintains normal blood calcium levels by increasing bone resorption and GI absorption of calcium. It also maintains an inverse relationship between serum calcium and phosphate levels by inhibiting phosphate reabsorption in the renal tubules.

Abnormal PTH production disrupts this balance; symptoms of hyperparathyroidism are related to this release of bone calcium into the bloodstream. Excessive circulating PTH leads to bone damage, hypercalcemia, and kidney damage (Table 11.7). In fact, hyperparathyroidism is the most common cause of hypercalcemia, which can lead to nervous system, musculoskeletal, metabolic, and cardiovascular problems. See Chapter 5 for further discussion of hypercalcemia.

***Bone Damage.*** Oversecretion of PTH causes excessive osteoclast growth and activity within the bones. Osteoclasts are active in promoting resorption of bone, which then releases calcium into the blood, causing hypercalcemia. This calcium loss leads to bone demineralization, and in time, the bones may become so fragile that pathologic fractures, deformity (e.g., kyphosis of the thoracic spine), and compression fractures of the vertebral bodies occur. If uncontrolled, osteoclast proliferation may cause lytic bone lesions (bone disintegrates, leaving holes).

Surgical treatment of hyperparathyroidism (parathyroidectomy) can be expected to result in biochemical cure and increased bone mineral density of the lumbar spine and femoral neck (areas rich in cancellous bone), in both symptomatic and asymptomatic clients. Cortical bone loss, however, is not as readily reversible in either group.[399] Early surgical treatment of hyperparathyroidism may assist in the prevention of spine and hip fractures in this population.

**Table 11.7** Systemic Manifestations of Hyperparathyroidism

| Early CNS Symptoms | Musculoskeletal Effects | Gastrointestinal Effects | Genitourinary Effects |
|---|---|---|---|
| Lethargy, drowsiness, paresthesias<br>Slow mentation, poor memory<br>Depression, personality changes<br>Easily fatigued<br>Hyperactive deep tendon reflexes<br>Occasionally glove-and-stocking distribution sensory loss | Mild to severe proximal muscle weakness of the extremities<br>Muscle atrophy<br>Bone decalcification (bone pain, especially spine; pathologic fractures; bone cysts)<br>Gout and pseudogout<br>Arthralgias involving the hands<br>Myalgia and sensation of heaviness in the lower extremities<br>Joint hypermobility | Peptic ulcers<br>Pancreatitis<br>Nausea, vomiting, anorexia<br>Constipation<br>Abdominal pain | Renal colic associated with stones<br>Hypercalcemia (polyuria, polydipsia, constipation)<br>Kidney infections<br>Renal hypertension |

Modified from Goodman CC, Heick J, Lazaro R: *Differential diagnosis for therapists: screening for referral*, ed 6, Philadelphia, 2017, Saunders.

***Hypercalcemia.*** As excessive PTH secretion results in bone resorption and hypercalcemia as just described, hypercalciuria (excessive calcium in the urine) eventually develops because the excessive filtration of calcium overwhelms this renal mechanism. High serum calcium levels also stimulate hypergastrinemia (excess gastrin, a hormone that stimulates secretion of gastric acid and pepsin in the blood), abdominal pain, peptic ulcer disease, and pancreatitis.

***Kidney Damage.*** As serum calcium levels rise in response to excessive PTH levels, large amounts of phosphorus and calcium are excreted and lost from the body. Excretion of these compounds occurs through the renal system, leaving deposits of calcium phosphate within the renal tubules. This produces a kidney condition called *nephrocalcinosis.* Because calcium salts are insoluble in urine, kidney stones composed of calcium phosphate develop. Serious renal damage may not be reversible with parathyroidectomy.

Some people with hyperparathyroidism may be completely asymptomatic, but even seemingly asymptomatic clients with elevated serum and PTH levels have been found to have paresthesias, muscle cramps, and loss of pain and vibratory sensation in a stocking-glove distribution. Others suffer from a wide range of symptoms as a result of skeletal disease, renal involvement, GI tract disorders, and neurologic abnormalities.

## MEDICAL MANAGEMENT

**DIAGNOSIS.** The diagnosis of hyperparathyroidism depends on measurement of PTH levels in persons found to be hypercalcemic (high serum levels of calcium). Serum calcium and PTH levels are elevated, serum phosphorus may be low normal or depressed, and urine calcium can range from low to high. Radiographic evidence of skeletal damage is important to measure in asymptomatic clients with mild hyperparathyroidism. Skeletal damage can be seen on x-ray as diffuse demineralization of bones, bone cysts, subperiosteal bone resorption, and loss of the laminae durae surrounding the teeth.

**TREATMENT AND PROGNOSIS.** Treatment for primary hyperparathyroidism is surgical removal (parathyroidectomy). Minimally invasive parathyroidectomy is advised even for individuals with mild elevation in calcium because of the risk for more serious complications of hyperparathyroidism such as renal failure, osteoporosis, and early death from CVD. Preoperative localization of the adenoma by scanning with technetium Tc 99m–labeled sestamibi allows for limited resection whenever possible.

The prognosis is good if the condition is identified and treated early. Untreated, hyperparathyroidism exacerbates many conditions among older adults such as osteoporosis and CAD. Emergency medical management of severe hypercalcemia includes use of drugs to lower serum calcium, such as hydration and loop diuretics, which promote calcium loss through the kidneys, and antiresorption agents, which inhibit calcium release from bone.

Long-term medical management of hypercalcemia with drugs is not as effective as parathyroid surgery, but if needed for short-term treatment, drugs, such as calcimimetics, bisphosphonates, estrogen, and calcitonin, can prevent progressive bone demineralization.[408]

SPECIAL IMPLICATIONS FOR THE THERAPIST 11.10

### *Hyperparathyroidism*

The therapist is likely to see skeletal, articular, and neuromuscular manifestations associated with hyperparathyroidism. Chronic low back pain and easy fracturing resulting from bone demineralization may be compounded by marked muscle weakness and atrophy, especially in the legs.[207]

Inflammatory erosive polyarthritis may be associated with chondrocalcinosis and calcium pyrophosphate dihydrate crystal deposits in the synovial fluid in some cases of hyperparathyroidism. This erosion, described as *osteogenic synovitis,* occurs as part of the bone destruction that can occur with hyperparathyroidism. When this complication develops, the Achilles, triceps, and obturator tendons are most commonly affected; other affected areas may include hands and wrists (CTS), shoulders, knees, clavicle, and axial skeleton. Because of better and earlier diagnosis, inflammatory erosive polyarthritis and chondrocalcinosis are much less common today than they were several decades ago. However, some older adults still experience these complications and may present with these problems. Concurrent illness and surgery (e.g., parathyroidectomy) are recognized inducers of acute arthritic episodes.

The therapist may be involved in treating the arthritis associated with this (or any other endocrine) condition, but unless the underlying cause is treated first, intervention for the arthritis will be frustrating and poorly effective. After medical treatment, the therapist's treatment of the residual arthritis is the same as for arthritis, regardless of the cause.

#### Acute Care

In the acute care setting, auscultate for lung sounds and listen for signs of pulmonary edema in the person receiving large amounts of intravenous (IV) saline solution, especially in the presence of pulmonary or cardiac disease. Monitor the person on digitalis carefully for any toxic effects produced by elevated calcium levels, because clients with hypercalcemia are hypersensitive to digitalis and may quickly develop toxic symptoms (e.g., arrhythmias, nausea, fatigue, or visual changes).

Clients with osteopenia are predisposed to pathologic fractures and must be treated with caution to minimize the risk of injury. Take every safety precaution, assisting carefully with walking, keeping the bed at its lowest position, raising the side rails, and lifting the immobilized person carefully to minimize bone stress. Schedule care to allow the person with muscle weakness recovery time and rest between all activities.

#### Postoperative Care

Postoperatively, after parathyroidectomy, the person should use a semi-Fowler position with support for the head and neck to decrease edema, which can cause pressure on the trachea. Observe for any signs of mild tetany, such as reports of tingling in the hands and around the mouth. These symptoms should subside quickly but may be prodromal signs of tetany resulting from hypocalcemia. Watch for increased neuromuscular irritability and other signs of severe tetany and report them immediately. Acute postoperative arthritis may occur secondary to gout or pseudogout.

Early ambulation (although uncomfortable) is essential, because weight bearing and pressure on bones speed up recalcification. The use of light ankle weights or light weight-resistive elastic for the lower extremities provides tension at the musculotendinous/bone interface, accomplishing the same response. The physician first must approve the same type of exercise program for the upper extremities because care must be taken not to disturb the surgical site.

### Home Health Care

For the person at home, fluids are important, and the use of cranberry or prune juice to increase urine acidity and help prevent stone formation may be recommended. Evaluate the living environment for any potential safety hazards that may predispose the client to injury, such as throw rugs, tub or shower stall without a rubber mat or decals to prevent slipping, missing hand and guard rails wherever necessary, and improper lighting. Encourage the use of a night-light in dark areas at all times.

Box 11.4

**CHARACTERISTICS OF HYPERPARATHYROIDISM AND HYPOPARATHYROIDISM**

*Hyperparathyroidism*

- Increased bone resorption
- Elevated serum calcium levels
- Depressed serum phosphate levels
- Hypercalciuria and hyperphosphaturia
- Decreased neuromuscular irritability

*Hypoparathyroidism*

- Decreased bone resorption
- Depressed serum calcium levels
- Elevated serum phosphate levels
- Hypocalciuria and hypophosphaturia
- Increased neuromuscular activity, which may progress to tetany

## Hypoparathyroidism

**Definition.** Hyposecretion, hypofunction, or insufficient secretion of PTH are ways to describe hypoparathyroidism.[47] Because the parathyroid glands primarily regulate calcium balance, hypoparathyroidism causes hypocalcemia and produces a syndrome opposite that of hyperparathyroidism with abnormally low serum calcium levels, high serum phosphate levels, and possible neuromuscular irritability (tetany) (Box 11.4).

**Etiologic Factors and Incidence.** Hypoparathyroidism is either iatrogenic, which is most common, or idiopathic. *Iatrogenic* (acquired) causes include accidental removal of the parathyroid glands during thyroidectomy or anterior neck surgery. Variations in location and color in addition to the minute size of parathyroid glands make identification difficult and may result in glandular damage or accidental removal during thyroid removal or anterior neck surgery. Other iatrogenic causes can include infarction of the parathyroid glands as a result of an inadequate blood supply to the glands during surgery, strangulation of one or more of the glands by postoperative scar tissue, and rarely, massive thyroid irradiation. Other secondary causes of hypoparathyroidism may include hemochromatosis, sarcoidosis, amyloidosis, tuberculosis, neoplasms, or trauma. Idiopathic causes affect children nine times as often as adults and affect twice as many women as men. Like Graves disease and Hashimoto thyroiditis, idiopathic hypoparathyroidism may be an autoimmune disorder with a genetic basis.

**Pathogenesis.** PTH normally functions to increase bone resorption to maintain a proper balance between serum calcium and phosphate. When parathyroid secretion of PTH is reduced, bone resorption and GI tract absorption slow, serum calcium levels fall, and severe neuromuscular irritability develops. Calcifications may form in various organs such as the eyes and basal ganglia. Serum phosphate levels rise without sufficient PTH because fewer phosphorus ions are secreted by the distal tubules of the kidneys with decreased renal excretion of phosphorus.

**Clinical Manifestations.** Mild hypoparathyroidism may be asymptomatic, but it usually produces hypocalcemia and high serum phosphate levels that affect the CNS and other body systems (Table 11.8). The most significant clinical consequence of hypocalcemia associated

**Table 11.8** Systemic Manifestations of Hypoparathyroidism

| CNS Effects | Musculoskeletal Effects[a] | Cardiovascular Effects[a] | Integumentary Effects | Gastrointestinal Effects |
|---|---|---|---|---|
| Personality changes (irritability, agitation, anxiety, depression)<br>Seizures | Hypocalcemia (neuromuscular excitability and muscular tetany, especially involving flexion of the upper extremity)<br>Spasm of intercostal muscles and diaphragm compromising breathing<br>Positive Chvostek sign | Cardiac arrhythmias<br>Eventual heart failure | Dry, scaly, coarse, pigmented skin<br>Tendency to have skin infections<br>Thinning of hair, including eyebrows and eyelashes<br>Fingernails and toenails become brittle and form ridges | Nausea and vomiting<br>Constipation or diarrhea<br>Neuromuscular stimulation of the intestine (abdominal pain) |

[a]The therapist should be aware of musculoskeletal and cardiovascular effects, which are the most common and important.

Modified from Goodman CC, Heick J, Lazaro R: *Differential diagnosis for therapists: screening for referral*, ed 6, Philadelphia, 2017, Saunders.

with hypoparathyroidism is neuromuscular irritability. In people with chronic hypoparathyroidism, this neuromuscular irritability may result in tetany. Hypocalcemia resistant to PTH, called *pseudohypoparathyroidism*, is determined genetically and is associated with shortened metacarpals and metatarsals.[241]

Acute (overt) tetany begins with a tingling in the fingertips, around the mouth, and occasionally, the feet. This tingling spreads and becomes more severe, producing painful muscle tension, spasms, grimacing, laryngospasm, and arrhythmias. Trousseau sign (carpal spasm) and Chvostek sign (hyperirritability of the facial nerve, producing a characteristic spasm when tapped) are apparent on examination. In severe cases, a tracheostomy may be required to correct acute respiratory obstruction secondary to laryngospasm.

### MEDICAL MANAGEMENT

**DIAGNOSIS.** Diagnosis of this condition is based on history, clinical presentation, examination, and laboratory values (low serum calcium, high serum phosphate, or low or absent urinary calcium). Radioimmunoassay for PTH demonstrates decreased PTH concentration.

**TREATMENT.** Acute hypoparathyroidism, with its major manifestation of acute tetany, is a life-threatening disorder. Treatment is directed toward elevation of serum calcium levels as rapidly as possible with intravenous calcium, prevention or treatment of convulsions, and control of laryngeal spasm and subsequent respiratory obstruction. Treatment of chronic hypoparathyroidism with pharmacologic management is accomplished more gradually than treatment for an acute situation. Surgical intervention is not appropriate and, in fact, is often the cause of this condition.

**PROGNOSIS.** Full recovery from the effects of hypoparathyroidism is possible when the condition is diagnosed early, before the development of serious complications. Unfortunately, once formed, cataracts and brain (basal ganglion) calcifications are irreversible. Death can occur from respiratory obstruction secondary to tetany and laryngospasms if treatment is not initiated early in acute hypoparathyroidism.

SPECIAL IMPLICATIONS FOR THE THERAPIST 11.11

### *Hypoparathyroidism*

Anyone experiencing acute tetany will be receiving acute medical care and will not be a likely candidate for therapy until the condition has resolved with treatment.

#### Chronic Hypoparathyroidism

For the person with chronic hypoparathyroidism, observe carefully for any minor muscle twitching or signs of laryngospasm because these may signal the onset of acute tetany. Chronic tetany is less severe, usually affects one side only, and may cause difficulty with gait and balance. Gait training and prevention of falls are key components of a therapy program. Hyperventilation may worsen tetany; focus on breathing during exercise is important.

Chronic hypoparathyroidism can lead to cardiac complications (e.g., arrhythmia, heart block, and decreasing cardiac output) that necessitate careful monitoring. Calcium in vitamin D preparations prescribed for this condition may result in hypercalcemia, which potentiates the effect of digitalis, thus requiring close monitoring for signs of digitalis toxicity and mild hypercalcemia. When one agent potentiates the effects of another agent, the enhancement is such that the combined effect is greater than the sum of the effects of the individual agents.

#### Home Health Care

Lifelong medication, dietary modifications, and medical care are required for the person with chronic hypoparathyroidism. Serum calcium levels must be checked by a physician at least three times a year to maintain normal serum calcium levels. If hypophosphatemia persists, cheese and milk should be omitted from the diet because they have a high calcium content. Other foods high in calcium but low in phosphorus are encouraged.

## Adrenal Glands

The adrenals are two small glands located on the upper part of each kidney (see Fig. 11.1). Each adrenal gland consists of two relatively discrete parts: an outer cortex and an inner medulla. The outer cortex is responsible for the secretion of mineralocorticoids (steroid hormones that regulate fluid and mineral balance), glucocorticoids (steroid hormones responsible for controlling the metabolism of glucose), and androgens (sex hormones).

The centrally located adrenal medulla is derived from neural tissue and secretes epinephrine and norepinephrine, which exert widespread effects on vascular tone, the heart, and the nervous system, and affects glucose metabolism. Together, the adrenal cortex and medulla are major factors in the body's response to stress.

Glandular hypofunction and hyperfunction characterize the major disorders of the adrenal cortex. Underactivity of the adrenal cortex results in a deficiency of glucocorticoids, mineralocorticoids, and adrenal androgens. Overactivity results in excessive production of these same hormones.

### Adrenal Insufficiency

Hypofunction of the adrenal cortex can originate from a disorder within the adrenal gland itself (primary adrenal insufficiency), or it may be due to hypofunction of the pituitary–hypothalamic unit (secondary adrenal insufficiency).[408] Adrenocortical insufficiency, whether primary or secondary, can be either acute or chronic.

**Primary Adrenal Insufficiency (Addison Disease)**

*Definition and Overview.* Addison disease is a condition that occurs as a result of a disorder within the adrenal gland itself, with insufficient cortisol release from the adrenal glands causing a wide range of problems. Addison disease was named for the physician who first studied and described the associated symptoms. Adrenal insufficiency affects about 4 adults in 100,000 each year in the

United States. Both sexes are affected, but the incidence is slightly higher in women than men. Addison disease can occur anytime across the life span with a preponderance of cases during middle age (40–60 years).

Primary forms of adrenal insufficiency are uncommon; the therapist is most likely to see secondary adrenal insufficiency as a result of suppression of ACTH by steroid therapy or secondary to opportunistic infections related to human immunodeficiency virus (HIV).

***Etiologic Factors.*** At one time, most causes of Addison disease occurred as a complication of tuberculosis, but now most cases are considered idiopathic or autoimmune. Because more than half of all people with idiopathic Addison disease have circulating autoantibodies that react specifically against adrenal tissue, this condition is considered to have an autoimmune basis.

Less frequent causes of primary insufficiency include bilateral adrenalectomy, adrenal hemorrhage or infarction, radiation to the adrenal glands, malignant adrenal neoplasm, and infections (e.g., histoplasmosis or cytomegalovirus). Destruction of the adrenal glands by chemical agents has been reported.[333] Medications, such as antifungals, adrenolytic agents, etomidate, rifampin, phenytoin, and phenobarbital, can also trigger Addison disease.

***Risk Factors.*** Surgery (including dental procedures); pregnancy (especially with postpartum hemorrhage); accident, injury, or trauma; infection; salt loss resulting from profuse diaphoresis (hot weather or with strenuous physical exertion); or failure to take steroid therapy in persons who have chronic adrenal insufficiency can cause acute adrenal insufficiency.

***Pathogenesis and Clinical Manifestations.*** This adrenal gland disorder results in decreased production of cortisol (a glucocorticoid) and aldosterone (a mineralocorticoid), two of the primary adrenocortical hormones. Glucocorticoid deficiency causes widespread metabolic disturbances. Consequently, when glucocorticoids become deficient, gluconeogenesis decreases, with resultant hypoglycemia and liver glycogen deficiency. The person grows weak, exhausted, hypotensive, and suffers from anorexia, weight loss, nausea, and vomiting. Emotional disturbances can develop, ranging from mild neurotic symptoms to severe depression. Glucocorticoid deficiency also diminishes resistance to stress.

In anyone who has previously been diagnosed with Addison disease, acute symptoms such as severe abdominal pain, low back or leg pain, severe vomiting, diarrhea, and hypotension may develop quickly in response to triggers such as trauma, infarction, or infection. The resulting condition, called *addisonian crisis*, can progress quickly to hypovolemic shock (e.g., hypotension, tachycardia, and loss of consciousness) from rapid fluid loss.

Chronic adrenal insufficiency with chronic cortisol deficiency results in a failure to inhibit anterior pituitary secretion of ACTH. The result is a simultaneous increase in ACTH secretion and melanocyte-stimulating hormone (MSH); excessive MSH increases skin and mucous membrane pigmentation. Persons with Addison disease may have a bronzed or tanned appearance, which is the most striking physical finding with primary adrenal insufficiency (not present in all people with this disorder). This change in pigmentation may vary in the white population from a slight tan or a few black freckles to an intense generalized pigmentation. The change in pigmentation is most commonly observed over extensor surfaces such as the backs of the hands (metacarpophalangeal joints), elbows, knees, creases of the hands, lips, and mouth. Increased pigmentation of scars formed after the onset of the disease is common. Members of darker-skinned races may develop a slate-gray color that is obvious only to family members.

Aldosterone deficiency causes numerous fluid and electrolyte imbalances. Aldosterone normally promotes conservation of sodium and therefore conserves water and excretion of potassium. A deficiency of aldosterone causes increased sodium excretion, dehydration, hypotension (low blood pressure causing orthostatic symptoms), and decreased cardiac output affecting heart size (decrease in size). Eventually, hypotension becomes severe and cardiovascular activity weakens, leading to circulatory collapse, shock, and death. Excess potassium retention (greater than 7 mEq/L) can result in arrhythmias and possible cardiac arrest.

Other clinical effects include decreased tolerance for even minor stress, poor coordination, fasting hypoglycemia (resulting from decreased gluconeogenesis), and a craving for salty food. Addison disease may also retard axillary and pubic hair growth in females, decrease the libido (from decreased androgen production), and in severe cases, cause amenorrhea (absence of menstruation).[483]

## MEDICAL MANAGEMENT

**DIAGNOSIS AND PROGNOSIS.** Diagnosis of Addison disease depends primarily on blood and urine hormonal assays and cortisol response to synthetic ACTH administration. Decreased serum cortisol levels are the hallmark of Addison disease. An ACTH stimulation test can help identify the presence of Addison disease and the type. In an ACTH stimulation test, baseline measurements of blood and urine cortisol levels are measured. The individual receives an intramuscular injection or intravenous infusion of ACTH to stimulate cortisol secretion. Blood cortisol and aldosterone measurements are repeated 30 to 60 minutes later. These levels should be greater than baseline levels; with adrenal insufficiency, the levels do not rise or rise only slightly.[368]

If the ACTH stimulation test is positive, a CRH stimulation test is conducted to determine if the adrenal insufficiency is primary or secondary. After injection of synthetic CRH, blood cortisol measurements are taken. A high ACTH level without increased cortisol signals primary adrenal insufficiency. An absent or delayed ACTH response without deficient cortisol level indicates secondary adrenal insufficiency.[199]

Complications from Addison disease such as hyponatremia, hypoglycemia, hyperkalemia, hypercalcemia, and metabolic acidosis will be apparent in the blood chemistry values obtained.

**TREATMENT.** Acute adrenal insufficiency is treated by replacing fluids, electrolytes, glucose, and cortisol while identifying the underlying cause of the problem. Medical management for chronic adrenal insufficiency is primarily pharmacologic, consisting of lifelong administration of synthetically manufactured corticosteroids and mineralocorticoids (fludrocortisone). If untreated, Addison disease is ultimately fatal. Adrenal crisis requires immediate hospitalization and treatment.

SPECIAL IMPLICATIONS FOR THE THERAPIST 11.12

### *Primary Adrenal Insufficiency (Addison Disease)*

With pharmacologic therapy, listlessness and exhaustion should gradually lessen and disappear, making exercise possible. Stress (including physical stress) should be minimized, with physical activity and exercise progressed very gradually per individual tolerance. Too much stress of any kind can put the client into an "addisonian crisis" as the body is unable to meet the cortisol demand caused by the extra "stress" of exercise.

Aquatic physical therapy may be contraindicated for anyone with Addison disease. The heat and humidity of the pool environment cause the body to require more cortisol so that blood vessels can respond in order to increase blood pressure and cool the body down. With adrenal insufficiency, the adrenal gland cannot produce enough cortisol for the demands on the individual.

The therapist should monitor vital signs in anyone with Addison disease, especially when initiating and progressing an exercise program. Even small changes in medication dose can create a medical emergency in people with Addison disease. Watch for any signs of an impending crisis such as dizziness, nausea, profuse sweating, elevated heart rate, and tremors or shaking.

Any signs of infection, such as sore throat or burning on urination, should be reported to the physician. The client may be directed by the physician to increase medication dosage during times of stress and self-limiting illnesses (e.g., colds and flu). The therapist may need to advise the person to check with the physician if illness or any of the listed risk factors develop at home or during outpatient care.

Individuals with known Addison disease who enter the hospital for orthopedic surgery are often administered increased doses of cortisol to adjust for the increased needs in stress situations. Clients with Addison disease should be assessed carefully for signs of hypercortisolism, which can result from excessive long-term cortisol therapy. Assess for signs of sodium and potassium imbalance as well.

Steroid-induced psychosis can occur but often has some of the same symptoms as addisonian crisis. There can be personality changes as the affected individual becomes suspicious, confused, and irritable. Slurred speech and difficulty moving with poor motor planning and motor incoordination may be compounded by severe exhaustion. The therapist is encouraged to be sensitive to clients experiencing medication-induced psychosis; what may appear as a lack of motivation or poor/noncompliance may require compassion, understanding, and patience until the medical condition is under control and the client can begin to make progress. The therapist must monitor and help the client monitor fatigue or periods of adrenal insufficiency to avoid the return of psychotic symptoms. Working closely with the orthopedic surgeon and endocrinologist is very important for these individuals.[368]

If steroid replacement therapy is inadequate or too high, changes in amounts of sodium and water are observed. Persons receiving glucocorticoid alone may need mineralocorticoid therapy if signs of orthostatic hypotension or electrolyte abnormalities develop. Older adults may be more sensitive to the side effects of steroid therapy, such as osteoporosis, hypertension, and diabetes, when these conditions already exist. The therapist must not overlook the presence of these other conditions when providing treatment intervention.

Anyone with identified Addison disease should wear an identification bracelet and carry an emergency kit containing dexamethasone or hydrocortisone. Steroids administered in the late afternoon or evening may cause stimulation of the CNS and insomnia in some people. Anyone reporting sleep disturbances should be encouraged to discuss this with the physician.

## Secondary Adrenal Insufficiency

Secondary adrenal insufficiency is caused by other conditions outside the adrenals, such as hypothalamic or pituitary tumors, removal of the pituitary or other causes of hypopituitarism, or too-rapid withdrawal of corticosteroid drugs. Long-term exogenous corticosteroid stimulation suppresses pituitary ACTH secretion and results in adrenal gland atrophy. Untimely discontinuation of adrenocorticosteroid therapy results in acute adrenal insufficiency and can become a life-threatening emergency. Anyone receiving adrenocorticosteroid therapy should be identified through the use of a bracelet or necklace. Steroid therapy must be discontinued gradually so that pituitary and adrenal function can normalize.

Clinical manifestations of secondary disease are somewhat different from symptoms of primary adrenal insufficiency. Whereas most symptoms of primary adrenal insufficiency arise from cortisol and aldosterone deficiency, symptoms of secondary disease are related to cortisol deficiency only. Because the gland is still intact, aldosterone is secreted normally, but the lack of stimulation from ACTH results in deficient cortisol secretion. Arthralgias, myalgias, and tendon calcification can occur, which resolve with treatment of the underlying condition.

Hyperpigmentation is not part of the clinical presentation because ACTH and MSH levels are low. Additionally, because aldosterone secretion may continue at fairly normal levels in secondary adrenal hypofunction, this condition does not necessarily cause accompanying hypotension and electrolyte abnormalities.[292]

As with primary adrenal insufficiency, treatment involves replacement of ACTH and monitoring for fluid and electrolyte imbalances. Too much cortisol replacement can result in the development of Cushing syndrome (see next section).

## Adrenocortical Hyperfunction

Hyperfunction of the adrenal cortex can result in excessive production of glucocorticoids, mineralocorticoids, and androgens. The three major conditions of adrenocortical hyperfunction are Cushing syndrome (glucocorticoid excess), Conn syndrome or aldosteronism (aldosterone excess), and adrenal hyperplasia (adrenogenital syndrome). This last condition is rare and congenital and is not discussed further in this text.

**Table 11.9** Pathophysiology of Cushing Syndrome

| Physiologic Effect | Clinical Result |
|---|---|
| Persistent hyperglycemia | "Steroid diabetes" |
| Protein tissue wasting | Weakness as a result of muscle wasting; capillary fragility resulting in ecchymoses; osteoporosis as a result of bone matrix wasting |
| Potassium depletion | Hypokalemia, cardiac arrhythmias, muscle weakness, renal disorders |
| Sodium and water retention | Edema and hypertension |
| Hypertension | Predisposes to left ventricular hypertrophy, congestive heart failure, cerebrovascular accidents |
| Abnormal fat distribution | Moon-shaped face; dorsocervical fat pad; truncal obesity, slender limbs, thinning of the skin with striae on the breasts, axillary areas, abdomen, and legs |
| Increased susceptibility to infection; lowered resistance to stress | Absence of signs of infection; poor wound healing |
| Increased production of androgens | Virilism in women (e.g., acne, thinning of scalp hair, hirsutism or abnormal growth and distribution of hair) |
| Mental changes | Memory loss, poor concentration and thought processes, euphoria, depression ("steroid psychosis") |

### Cushing Syndrome

***Definition and Overview.*** Hypercortisolism is a general term for an excess of cortisol in the body. This condition can occur as a result of hyperfunction of the adrenal gland (usually benign or malignant adenomas, rarely a carcinoma), an excess of corticosteroid medication, or an excess of ACTH stimulation from the pituitary gland (or other sites). ACTH secreted by the pituitary has a key role in cortisol release. When the hypothalamus senses low ACTH levels in the blood, it sends CRH to the pituitary to stimulate ACTH secretion, which in turn stimulates the adrenal glands to release cortisol. When blood cortisol levels are adequate or elevated, the hypothalamus and pituitary release less CRH and ACTH.[6,25]

Hypercortisolism resulting from adrenal gland oversecretion or from hyperphysiologic doses of corticosteroid medications is called *Cushing syndrome.* When the hypercortisolism results from oversecretion of ACTH from the pituitary, the condition is called *Cushing disease.* The clinical presentation is the same for both conditions.[298]

A separate condition called *pseudo-Cushing syndrome* occurs when conditions such as depression, alcoholism, estrogen therapy, or eating disorders cause changes like those of Cushing syndrome. In pseudo-Cushing syndrome, the symptoms will go away when the cause is eliminated.

***Etiologic Factors and Incidence.*** The primary causes of Cushing syndrome are hyperphysiologic doses of adrenocorticosteroids (exogenous cause) and adrenocortical tumors (endogenous cause). Cushing disease results from pituitary adenomas, which secrete an excess of ACTH, causing overstimulation of a normal adrenal gland (70% of all cases are Cushing disease caused by pituitary tumor).[6]

Therapists are more likely to treat people who have developed medication-induced Cushing syndrome (exogenous steroid administration). This condition occurs after these individuals have received large doses of cortisol (also known as hydrocortisone) or cortisol derivatives. Exogenous steroids are administered in individuals who have received organ transplants and for a number of rheumatologic, pulmonary, neurologic, and nephrologic diseases. Noniatrogenic Cushing syndrome occurs mainly in women (5:1 ratio of women to men), with an average age at onset of 25 to 40 years, although it can be seen in people up to age 60 years.

***Pathogenesis and Clinical Manifestations.*** Cushing syndrome occurs as a result of excess cortisol release from the adrenal glands or exogenously administered glucocorticoids. Cushing disease is usually due to an anterior pituitary tumor. When the normal function of the glucocorticoids becomes exaggerated, a wide range of physiologic responses can be triggered, including hyperglycemia, hypertension, proximal muscle wasting, and osteoporosis (Table 11.9).

Cortisol has a key role in glucose metabolism and a lesser part in protein, carbohydrate, and fat metabolism. Cortisol also helps maintain blood pressure and cardiovascular function while reducing the body's inflammatory responses. Overproduction of cortisol causes liberation of amino acids from muscle tissue with resultant weakening of protein structures (specifically muscle and elastic tissue). The end result may include a protuberant abdomen (Fig. 11.6) with purple striae (stretch marks), poor wound healing, thinning of the skin, generalized (progressive) muscle weakness, and marked osteoporosis that is made worse by an excessive loss of calcium in the urine. In severe cases of prolonged Cushing syndrome, muscle weakness and demineralization of bone may lead to pathologic fractures and wedging of the vertebrae, kyphosis (Fig. 11.7), osteonecrosis (especially of the femoral head), bone pain, and back pain.

The effect of increased circulating levels of cortisol on the muscles varies from slight to marked. Muscle wasting can be so extensive that the condition simulates muscular dystrophy. Marked weakness of the quadriceps muscle often prevents affected people from rising out of a chair unassisted.

Whenever corticosteroids are administered, the increase in serum cortisol levels triggers a negative feedback signal to the anterior pituitary gland to stop its secretion of ACTH. This decrease in ACTH stimulation of the adrenal cortex results in adrenocortical atrophy during the period of exogenous corticosteroid administration. If these medications are stopped suddenly rather than reduced gradually, the atrophied adrenal gland will not be able to provide the cortisol necessary for physiologic needs. A life-threatening situation known as *acute adrenal insufficiency* can develop, requiring emergency cortisol replacement.[459]

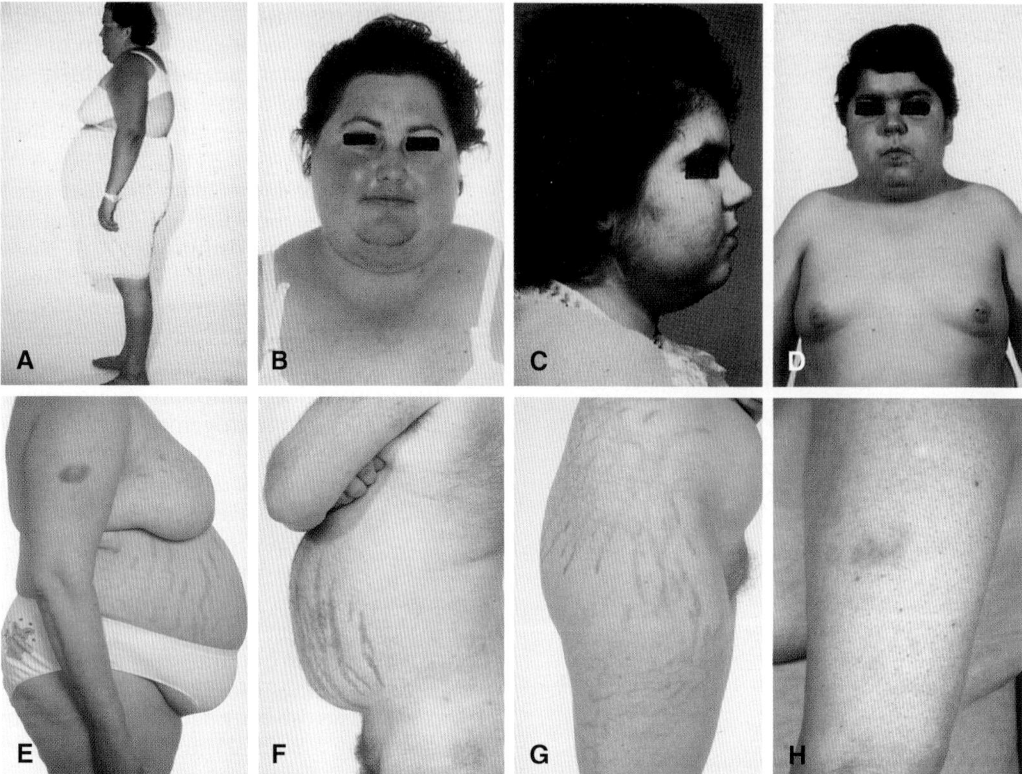


**Figure 11.6**

**Clinical features of Cushing syndrome.** (A) Central and some generalized obesity and dorsal kyphosis in a 30-year-old woman with Cushing disease. (B) Same woman as in A, showing moon facies (round face), hirsutism (hair growth), and enlarged supraclavicular fat pads. (C) Facial rounding, hirsutism, and acne in a 14-year-old girl with Cushing syndrome. (D) Central and generalized obesity and moon facies in a 14-year-old boy with Cushing syndrome. (E and F) Typical central obesity with visible abdominal striae ("stretch marks") seen in a 41-year-old woman and 40-year-old-man with Cushing syndrome. (G) Striae in a 24-year-old woman with congenital adrenal hyperplasia treated with excessive doses of dexamethasone as replacement therapy. (H) Typical bruising and thin skin of Cushing syndrome. In this case, the bruising has occurred without obvious injury. (From Larsen RP: *Williams textbook of endocrinology*, ed 10, Philadelphia, 2003, WB Saunders.)

## MEDICAL MANAGEMENT

**DIAGNOSIS.** Although there is a classic cushingoid appearance in persons with hypercortisolism (see Fig. 11.6), diagnostic laboratory studies, including measurement of urine and serum cortisol, are used to confirm the diagnosis. If the initial laboratory tests are positive (elevated cortisol levels), then confirmatory tests (e.g., 2-day low-dose dexamethasone, low-dose DST-CRH testing, or late-night salivary cortisol) can be ordered.[231]

Serum ACTH levels help determine whether Cushing syndrome is ACTH-dependent (e.g., pituitary tumor, which technically makes it Cushing disease). Adrenal imaging can be used to assess for Cushing that is ACTH-independent (adrenal tumor). Further testing (pituitary contrast-enhanced magnetic resonance imaging [MRI] and abdominal computed tomographic [CT] scan) is determined on the basis of these results. X-rays or dual-energy x-ray absorptiometry scans may be needed to assess for fractures or to rule out osteopenia or osteoporosis, respectively. These tests may be conducted to obtain a baseline measurement of bone density, or they may be obtained in response to an individual's report of musculoskeletal symptoms such as bone pain or backache.[324]

**TREATMENT AND PROGNOSIS.** Treatment to restore hormone balance and reverse Cushing syndrome or disease may require pituitary irradiation, drug therapy, or surgery (e.g., adrenalectomy, resection of tumors) depending on the underlying cause.[281] For individuals with muscle wasting or at risk for muscle atrophy, a high-protein diet may be prescribed. Lifelong glucocorticoid replacement is necessary when the pituitary is removed or destroyed and for individuals who undergo bilateral adrenalectomy.[6,345]

Prognosis depends on the underlying cause and the ability to control the cortisol excess. Surgical cure rates are approximately 80%, with a 25% recurrence rate by 5 years. Prognostic factors include experience of surgeon, degree of postoperative hypocortisolism, and finding of a tumor at surgery.[46] The more rare adrenocortical carcinomas are associated with a 5-year survival rate of 30% or less.[6]

**SPECIAL IMPLICATIONS FOR THE THERAPIST 11.13**

### *Cushing Syndrome*

See "Adverse Effects of Corticosteroids" in Chapter 5.

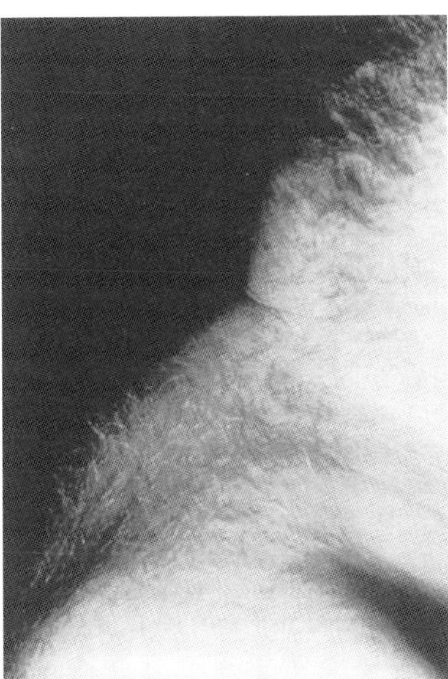

**Figure 11.7**

**Buffalo hump and hypertrichosis (excessive hairiness; hirsutism) in a male with Cushing syndrome.** This hump is a painless accumulation of fat that also may occur idiopathically in (usually) women. A familial pattern may exist (i.e., affected women report a similar anatomic change in their mothers). In the case of steroid-induced changes, this condition resolves when the individual stops taking the medication; in such cases, therapeutic intervention by the therapist has no permanent effect. Idiopathic fat deposits and underlying postural changes can be altered with postural correction and soft tissue and joint mobilization techniques. No studies have substantiated whether these changes are long-term. (From Callen JP, Jorizzo J: *Dermatological signs of internal disease*, ed 2, Philadelphia, 1995, WB Saunders.)

### Conn Syndrome

***Definition and Overview.*** Conn syndrome, or primary aldosteronism, occurs when an adrenal lesion results in hypersecretion of aldosterone, the most powerful of the mineralocorticoids. Its primary role is to conserve sodium, and it also promotes potassium excretion. The major cause of primary aldosteronism (an uncommon condition present most often in women aged 30 to 50 years) is a benign, aldosterone-secreting tumor called *aldosteronoma.*[161] Rarely, Conn syndrome develops as a consequence of adrenocortical carcinoma.

Secondary hyperaldosteronism also can occur as a consequence of pathologic lesions that stimulate the adrenal gland to increase production of aldosterone. For example, conditions that reduce renal blood flow (e.g., renal artery stenosis) or induce renal hypertension (e.g., nephrotic syndrome or ingestion of oral contraceptives) and edematous disorders (e.g., cardiac failure or cirrhosis of the liver with ascites) can cause secondary hyperaldosteronism.

***Pathogenesis and Clinical Manifestations.*** Aldosterone affects the tubular reabsorption of sodium and water and the excretion of potassium and hydrogen ions in the renal tubular epithelial cells; an excess of aldosterone enhances sodium reabsorption by the kidneys. This leads to the development of hypernatremia (excess sodium in blood, indicating water loss exceeding sodium loss), hypervolemia (fluid volume excess, increase in the volume of circulating fluid or plasma in the body), hypokalemia (low blood levels of potassium), and metabolic alkalosis. With the hypervolemia and hypernatremia, the blood pressure increases, often to very high levels, and renin production is suppressed. This hypertension can lead to cerebral infarctions and renal damage.

Without intervention, complications of chronic hypertension develop in the presence of hypertension, hypernatremia, and hypokalemia, heart failure, renal damage, and cerebrovascular accident. Hypokalemia results from excessive urinary excretion of potassium, causing muscle weakness; intermittent, flaccid paralysis; paresthesias; or cardiac arrhythmias.

This excessive urinary excretion of potassium (hypokalemia) leads to polyuria and resulting polydipsia (excessive thirst). DM is common because hypokalemia interferes with normal insulin transport. Finally, hypokalemia leads to metabolic alkalosis, which can cause a decrease in ionized calcium levels, resulting in tetany and respiratory suppression. However, low serum potassium and alkalosis are not always present at the time of diagnosis.

## MEDICAL MANAGEMENT

**DIAGNOSIS, TREATMENT, AND PROGNOSIS.** Diagnosis of primary hyperaldosteronism is based on elevations in serum and urine aldosterone studies and CT scanning of the abdomen for evidence of unilateral and sometimes bilateral adenomas of the adrenal gland.[161] Radiographic studies can reveal cardiac hypertrophy resulting from chronic hypertension. Radionuclide scanning techniques using radiolabeled substances allow visualization of any tumors present.

The goals of treatment are to reverse hypertension, correct hypokalemia, and prevent kidney damage. Surgical removal of the aldosterone-secreting tumor may also require adrenalectomy, which completely resolves the hypertension within 1 to 3 months. However, without early diagnosis and treatment, renal complications from long-term hypertension may be progressive. Pharmacologic treatment to increase sodium excretion and treat the hypertension and hypokalemia is a nonsurgical alternative.

**SPECIAL IMPLICATIONS FOR THE THERAPIST 11.14**

*Conn Syndrome*

The therapist treating someone with hyperaldosteronism, primary or secondary, may observe signs of tetany (muscle twitching and Chvostek sign) and hypokalemia-induced cardiac dysrhythmias, paresthesias, or muscle weakness. If these are encountered in an acute care setting, the medical team is usually well aware of such symptoms and is working to establish a fluid–electrolyte balance. When such signs and symptoms are observed in the outpatient setting, the client must seek medical attention.

## Adipose Tissue

Fat is most often viewed as a storage site for energy, with little other function. However, adipose tissue can also be classified as the largest endocrine organ in the body. Neurotransmitters and glucose (along with other molecules) directly act on adipocytes to induce the release of a number of different proteins collectively termed *adipokines* (or adipocytokines) that can act locally as autocrine hormones or through the bloodstream as endocrine hormones.[178] A large number of these mediators (adipokines) have been identified and studied (e.g., tumor necrosis factor alpha [TNF-α], leptin, adiponectin, resistin, chemerin, interleukin-6 [IL-6], visfatin).[73] Adipokines released by adipocytes function to maintain the balance of energy by regulating appetite, energy expenditure, insulin sensitivity, and lipid uptake. Other roles of adipokines that are beyond the conservation of energy include the induction of vasoconstriction (angiotensin), inflammation (leptin; see further discussion of inflammation below), or angiogenesis (vascular endothelial growth factor). Important advances related to these proteins are shedding new insights into the pathophysiologic mechanisms of many complicated diseases, such as obesity, diabetes, arthritis, and cardiovascular disease.

One reason that the role of adipose tissue in health and disease has been difficult to describe is due to the fact that fat from different parts of the body functions in various ways. In mammals, adipose tissue is divided into two categories: brown and white. Brown fat is a very specialized tissue that is important in thermoregulation, converting energy from food into heat.[71] Infants have more brown fat; thus, they are more sensitive to temperature changes, especially the cold. The amount of brown fat decreases into adulthood, but some does remain in specific locations through the life span. The activity of the adipocytes in brown fat is closely regulated by the sympathetic nervous system. White adipose tissue (white fat) is the classic adipose tissue responsible for storage of triglycerols to provide a long-term reservoir of energy for the body.[439] White adipose tissue is an important endocrine and secretory organ. Releasing a series of multiple-function mediators, white fat is involved in a wide spectrum of diseases, including not only cardiovascular and metabolic complications, such as atherosclerosis and type 2 diabetes, but also inflammatory- and immune-related disorders, such as rheumatoid arthritis and osteoarthritis.[73] Another consideration is the association between obesity and accumulation of *ectopic fat*, defined as abnormal lipid droplets in nonfat cells such as the heart, pancreas, liver, and skeletal muscle. In obesity, fat cells themselves become insulin resistant and cannot uptake and store excess calories. As a consequence, ectopic fat accumulates in organs and skeletal muscle. Ectopic fat may cause skeletal muscle cell death and a decrease in lean body mass.[418] Excess adipose tissue has been found in skeletal muscles of individuals with obesity and diabetes, and this has been associated with low muscle strength and impaired physical function.[4,198,288]

**SPECIAL IMPLICATIONS FOR THE THERAPIST 11.15**

### *Adipose Tissue*

Fat accumulated in the lower body (subcutaneous fat) results in a pear-shaped figure, whereas fat in the abdominal area (visceral fat) produces more of an apple shape. Specific genes have been identified that help dictate the number of fat cells and where they are located. This process is also influenced by hormonal production (decreased estrogen at menopause with increased ratio of androgens to estrogens).

Visceral fat produces cytokines (e.g., TNF or IL-6) that increase the risk of CVD by promoting insulin resistance and low-level chronic inflammation. Excess abdominal fat is considered a greater risk factor than overall obesity for cardiovascular disease and type 2 diabetes; it has also been linked to colorectal cancer, hypertension, and memory loss.[418] But the good news is that visceral fat can be reduced with diet and exercise. The therapist can offer education and guidance in this area of prevention and management.

Increasing physical activity and exercise to 1 hour daily may be ideal, but benefits have been observed with even 30 minutes of daily, moderate activity. Twice-weekly strength training has also been shown to prevent increases in body fat percentage and attenuate increases in abdominal fat in at least one study of overweight or obese women.[390]

The therapist can help individual clients assess BMI and waist circumference. BMI helps identify people whose weight increases their risk for several conditions such as heart disease, stroke, and diabetes. BMI can be misleading in individuals who are very muscular or very tall.

Waist circumference is used to measure abdominal adiposity. A tape measure is placed around the waist at about the level of the navel. Waist measurement greater than 35 inches for women and 40 inches for men indicates rising risk. A large waist correlates with diabetes risk (even when the BMI is within a normal range).

Relationships between BMI, waist circumference, and health risk may vary by ethnic group.[265,375,489] For example, a waist circumference above 31.5 inches in Asian women is considered a health risk.[188,303] The WHO consensus statement notes that although health risks do appear to occur at lower BMIs for Asian populations, the cut-off points for overweight and obesity vary by Asian countries. The range of cut-off points is 22 to 25 for overweight, so the consensus is to retain 25 as the cut-off point for overweight for all populations.

Waist-to-height ratio has been shown to be a good predictor of risk for diabetes and CVD from studies conducted in 14 different countries. Both waist circumference and waist-to-height ratios are stronger predictors than BMI. It has been suggested that "keep your waist circumference to less than half your height" may be a useful screening tool across cultures.

## Obesity

Because obesity is a multifactorial disease with complex interactions between lifestyle, environment, and genetics, it is important to understand how genetic expression through environmental influence causes an individual to be susceptible to obesity to develop effective prevention and treatment strategies. Physical therapists are in a unique position to positively affect the present obesity epidemic, through increasing physical activity, diet management, and education.

Rates of obesity have increased in adults during the last 30 years but have also increased dramatically in children, especially in the United States, which is of grave concern. In fact, some authors feel the current worldwide pandemic of obesity should be considered a communicable versus a noncommunicable disease because it is a "socially contagious feature of globalization." [55,233] The dramatic increase in obesity rates in the high-income world and across the United States affecting individuals of all ages and ethnic groups in the last half of the 20th century has raised questions of how a genome can change in a short period of time to predispose an entire world to obesity, if indeed these are heritable changes.

Recent and increasing evidence in animal and human studies support the involvement of epigenetic status of our genes in the obesity epidemic. Much evidence supports that environmental factors, lifestyle, and nutrition affect the epigenetic programming of parental gametes, the fetus, and the early postnatal development, so that the epigenetic marks induced in utero and in early life could determine a significant increase of obesity (and of other complex diseases, such as type 2 diabetes [T2D] and cardiovascular disease) and could be transmitted transgenerationally. [42,148]

Obesity is of great concern because of the direct effects on mortality and morbidity and the impact on health care costs as a high disease burden. It is also linked to other costly chronic diseases such as insulin resistance, T2D, fatty liver disease, endocrine and immune disorders, and cardiovascular disease.[42,148] Measures of obesity including BMI, waist circumference, and the waist–hip ratio (WHR) show an estimate of heritability between 40% to 70%.[148] Early hypotheses of a mechanism in an evolutionary perspective for obesity centered on the complimentary thrifty genotype and thrifty phenotype theories leading to (and further explaining) the present *fetal programing hypothesis*.[148] While these theories were considered simple explanations at the time, they do allow scholars, researchers, and clinicians to understand the role the environment and behavior choices play in the present obesity epidemic and the role epigenetics plays in this short generational change that has been observed.

**Definition and Measurement.** Obesity is defined as an excessive accumulation of fat in the body that contributes to numerous chronic diseases as well as early mortality and morbidity. *Bariatrics* is the branch of medicine concerned with the management of obesity.[416]

Prior to the development of the *Clinical Guidelines on the Identification, Evaluation and Treatment of Overweight and Obesity in Adults: The Evidence Report*,[319] measures used to determine weight status varied (e.g., weight–height tables, skinfold measurements, 20% higher than normal weight).

Currently, most research studies and clinical practice use one of three commonly accepted "field measures" to define obesity in adults: BMI, waist circumference, and waist-to-hip ratio. All of these measures are clinically simple and practical to administer and have been shown to relate to health risk. Ranges of BMI, calculated as a ratio of height to weight, are used to categorize body weight status and health risk. BMI has been empirically validated as the best simple tool for correctly identifying obesity.[401] Recently, research studies have begun to use more sophisticated methods, such as magnetic resonance imaging or dual energy x-ray absorptiometry (DEXA), which are so-called "reference measurements"—techniques that are typically used only in large research studies to confirm the accuracy of other body measurement techniques.[203] Air-displacement plethysmography with a popular commercial product called the Bod Pod is now used in many clinical research projects at universities and has replaced previously used underwater weighing densitometry. Bioelectric impedance analysis (BIA) measures impedance of the body to a small electric current. Multicompartment models are considered to be the most accurate method of measuring body composition because each of the abovementioned techniques actually measures different parts of body mass or body composition.[473]

The National Institutes of Health clinical guidelines and the WHO[490] define overweight in adults as a BMI equal to or greater than 25 kg/m$^2$. Obesity, defined as a BMI equal to or greater than 30 kg/m$^2$, is further divided into three classes. A BMI greater than or equal to 25 kg/m$^2$ is associated with increased risk for premature death and disability. As one progresses to a higher class of obesity, health risk and morbidity increase.[154] The term *morbid obesity* has been used by some authors to refer to a BMI greater than 40 kg/m$^2$.[210] BMI varies with age and sex in children and adolescents, necessitating the CDC to develop BMI guidelines that uniquely account for growth using weight and height. Among adults, there is a set cut point based on health risk, while among children, the definition is statistical and is based on a comparison to a reference population. BMIs[329] greater than or equal to the 85th and less than or equal to the 95th percentile signify a risk for being overweight; BMI greater than or equal to the 95th percentile signifies risk for being obese.[478] Regardless of the person's age, gender, or socioeconomic status, all medical practitioners should track weight and height regularly and address any concerns or weight-related risks with their patients/clients.

New strategies for measurement are being considered as researchers and practitioners seek the best measures for describing the extent of the obese condition and its relationship to health risk. For example, the Body Adiposity Index (BAI), a relationship between hip circumference and height, has been proposed as a clinically feasible strategy for measuring percentage of body fat. Thus far, however, the BAI measure is still being studied for its accuracy and ability to predict health risk.[44] Although BMI may not accurately reflect individual variations in fat-free mass, this measure is currently the most common measure of obesity and is an internationally accepted and understood definition of the condition. Regardless of the measure used, obesity is a condition that is inherently risky for health and longevity, especially if the distribution of such fat is in and around the abdomen (see Fig. 11.8).[498]

See further discussion of the diagnostic relevance of measures of obesity under "Diagnosis" later in this topic.

**Incidence and Prevalence.** Obesity is now regarded as a pandemic (affecting all people globally),[372] with implications for 300 million people across the world.[245] Obesity has begun to replace other known causes of mortality (e.g., undernutrition and infectious diseases) as the most significant contributor to ill health. It is second only to cigarette smoking as a leading cause of preventable

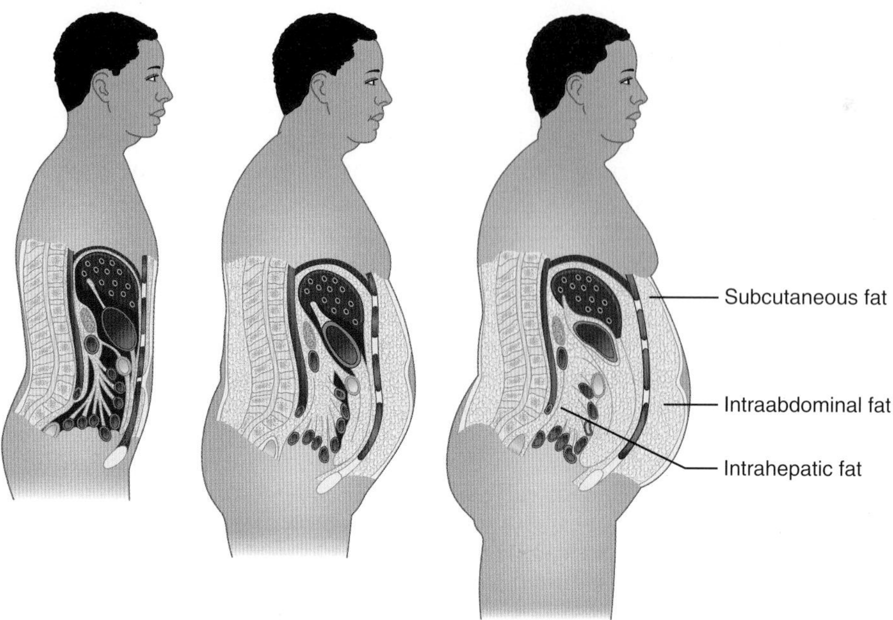


**Figure 11.8**

**Abdominal adipose tissue (fat) can accumulate as subcutaneous, intraabdominal, or intrahepatic (fatty lobules throughout the liver).** The body has an almost unlimited capacity to store fat. Central obesity has been linked with serious health consequences (e.g., cardiovascular disease, insulin resistance, diabetes mellitus).

death in the United States and contributes to 500,000 deaths annually; out of these deaths, the CDC reports that 30,000 are premature deaths. In the United States, it is estimated that 65% of adults can be categorized as overweight or obese.[234]

The prevalence of obesity among adults continues to increase[51,76]; from 1980 to 2002, obesity doubled in adults and overweight prevalence tripled in children and adolescents.[76] The prevalence of obesity was 39.8% and affected about 93.3 million U.S. adults in 2015 to 2016.[185] The adult obesity rate was at or above 35% in seven states and at least 30% in 29 states. West Virginia has the highest adult obesity rate at 38.1%, and Colorado has the lowest at 22.6%. Among both men and women, the prevalence of obesity followed a similar pattern by age. Men aged 40 to 59 (40.8%) had a higher prevalence of obesity than men aged 20 to 39 (34.8%). Women aged 40 to 59 (44.7%) had a higher prevalence of obesity than women aged 20 to 39 (36.5%). For both men and women, the prevalence of obesity among those aged 60 and over was not significantly different from the prevalence among those aged 20 to 39 or 40 to 59.[185]

This growth in the percentage of people who are overweight or obese is occurring across all age groups and is of significant concern in both pediatric and geriatric populations. The disease burden created by obesity is not felt equally across all populations; disparity exists across race, gender, age, socioeconomic status, and education level.[147,487] Also of concern is the medical cost associated with obesity in the United States, estimated to be at least $147 billion.[80]

Identifying childhood obesity is critical in the prevention of future modifiable mortality and spending, since those who are obese consume 42% more in health care dollars than healthy weight individuals.[75,330] As with obesity among adults, the financial burden of childhood obesity is high.[146,320,420] The direct annual health care costs of childhood obesity, including prescription drugs, emergency department visits, and outpatient medical care is $14.1 billion in the United States.[75] The American Heart Association confirms that obese children have worse lipid profiles, higher blood pressures, and higher glucose and insulin concentrations than their nonobese peers. These early risk factors are predictive of early atherosclerosis, cardiac pathology, additional morbidities, and mortality in adulthood.[419]

Race and ethnicity also play a role in childhood obesity, with Hispanic boys significantly more likely than non-Hispanic Caucasian boys to have high BMI. Furthermore, adolescent non-Hispanic black females were significantly more likely to have high BMI at all three cut points compared to non-Hispanic white females. However, there was no significant difference when comparing Hispanic girls to non-Hispanic white girls.[308]

It is estimated that 80% of adolescents who are overweight become obese as adults,[477] with about half of school-aged children who are obese remaining obese as adults.[153] Additionally, obese children under the age of 10 who had at least one obese parent had nearly double the chance of becoming obese as adults compared with children who did not have obese parents. Thus, it is apparent that parental obesity and obesity age of onset are important factors that impact whether or not a child remains obese as an adult. It is unclear if these traits are lifestyle choices or epigenetic changes as recent evidence seems to demonstrate.

Box 11.5

**RISK FACTORS FOR OBESITY**

- Sedentary lifestyle
- High-glycemic diet
- Underlying illness (e.g., hypothyroidism, polycystic ovary syndrome)
- Genetic disorder (Prader-Willi syndrome)
- Genetic, familial, or biologic factors
  - Medications (e.g., increased appetite or food cravings associated with prescription medications)
  - Corticosteroids (see Box 5.5)
  - Antidepressants
  - Antihypertensives
  - Anticonvulsants
  - Diabetes medications (short-acting insulin)
- Environmental or psychosocial/behavioral factors (e.g., history of sexual abuse, socioeconomic status, eating disorders, lack of sleep, stressful lifestyle, smoking cessation)

Existing evidence indicates that physical inactivity is strongly associated with body weight gain and that participation in purposeful and regular exercise and maintenance of a physically active lifestyle can be effective in maintaining a healthy body weight.[62,86,99,155,328,484] Although sedentary lifestyles have not been shown to be the cause of obesity, sedentary behavior (i.e., muscular inactivity) has been linked to metabolic risks,[123] and the risk of becoming sedentary increases with BMI.[310] Research has confirmed the importance of physical activity to maintain weight loss, especially if exercise commitment reached or exceeded 200 minutes per week.[252,262] Prescribing safe and specific regimens to meet this criterion is definitely in the scope of practice for physical therapists and the move to more precision-based physical therapy prescribed based on a person's genetic or epigenetic profile.[100,132]

**Etiologic and Risk Factors.** The development of obesity depends on an imbalance between energy intake and energy expenditure, with more energy consumed than is expended. Inactivity and an energy-dense diet (i.e., highly processed and refined foods without fiber) are known contributors to weight gain. Environmental factors (including lack of access to full-service grocery stores, increasing costs of healthy foods and the lower cost of unhealthy foods, and lack of access to safe places to play and exercise) all contribute to the increase in obesity rates by inhibiting or preventing healthy eating and active living behaviors.[234]

Absolute reasons why energy imbalance leads to obesity remain to be determined. However, several factors associated with the development of the energy imbalance and that may lead to excessive fat deposition and obesity are listed in Box 11.5. In addition, the failure of aging people to adjust food intake in response to lowered metabolism and diminished activity and weight cycling with fluctuations of body weight produced by repeated cycles of weight loss and gain appear to contribute to the inability to lose weight on a long-term basis.

Medication-induced weight gain also may occur as a result of increased appetite, episodes of hypoglycemia, or water retention. Other drugs, such as corticosteroids, make the body less able to absorb blood glucose, leading to increased fat deposits in the trunk. Antihypertensive medications, such as beta-blockers, may produce fatigue or shortness of breath, leading to reduced activity levels and increased weight gain.

A growing body of evidence suggests that some forms of obesity may result from biochemical defects rather than just consumption of excess calories.[227,482] After a 40-year search, scientists originally found three genes linked to obesity (ob, neuropeptide Y [Npy], and the Beacon gene). Npy and the Beacon gene produce a protein that stimulates the appetite, whereas the ob gene produces a protein (leptin) that switches off the appetite. In some obese people, the body does not respond to leptin; in others, the Beacon gene is working in overdrive, producing too much appetite-stimulating protein.[95]

Despite the new discoveries of single-gene mutations resulting in obesity, most cases of obesity are more likely the result of subtle interactions of several related genes with environmental factors that favor the net deposition of calories as fat. The increasing rates of obesity cannot be exclusively explained by changes in the gene pool, although genetic variants that were previously silent may now be triggered by the high availability of energy- and fat-dense foods and by the increasingly sedentary lifestyle of modern societies.[293,305]

The scientific community worldwide has been inspired to identify the contextual factors and behaviors (stand-alone as well as combined) correlated with childhood obesity. Previous exploratory studies have indicated there may be a relationship between BMI in children and factors including, but not limited to, screen time, socioeconomic status, sleep behaviors, religious practices, nutrition, and physical activity. Researchers in Canada used recursive partitioning to produce a classification tree predictive of elementary-age obesity associated with exposure to a combined series of variables. Their[452] results yielded seven definitive subgroups of combined variables that could be used to rank risk of obesity at baseline, though the same combination of variables did not predict subjects' BMI at the two-year conclusion of the study. Similar but separate research conducted with groups of children in Spain and in Britain looked to find predictive variables for obesity, but a similar study was not found for American children for whom culture, geography, and socioeconomic systems differ and, therefore, have presumably unique consequences.[326,479]

Research on childhood obesity in the United States, exploring the implications of socioeconomic and minority statuses, has consistently confirmed the beneficial effect of affluence on fitness, but the consequences of the intersection of race/ethnicity and household income requires further investigation.[35,309,327] Recently, a global research focus on the fitness ramifications of a modern construct, screen time, has dominated a number of studies.[143,495] In 2015, from a robust international sample of 5800 subjects, LeBlanc et al reported[264] common correlates of sedentary behavior and screen time: poor weight status, reduced physical activity, and having a

TV or computer in the child's bedroom. Published the same year, Ferrari et al[143] corroborated that children with electronic equipment in their bedroom are less likely to perform moderate to vigorous physical activity. Taking a unique tack, Xu and associates[495] established the influence of parental modeling in relation to children's physical activity and screen time behaviors.

**Pathogenesis.** The mechanisms proposed to explain the development or effects of obesity on the human body target neurologic, metabolic, and energy regulation systems.

Accumulating evidence indicates that obesity is a central nervous system–mediated *neuroendocrine dysfunction*. Because the central nervous system plays a key role in the regulation of food intake and energy balance, one explanation may be that either spontaneous genetic mutations or targeted gene deletions that impair central nervous system signaling cause disrupted food intake and body-weight control.[143] Researchers are studying the highly complex process of signaling molecules involved in the regulation of food intake and how inherited or acquired defects in the function of these hormonal and neuropeptide signaling pathways contribute to obesity.[391,488]

Another explanation involves the neuroendocrine system and suggests that *hormonal dysfunction* affecting the hypothalamic–pituitary–adrenal (HPA) axis results in a complex series of events. Stress stimulates daily, periodic elevations of cortisol secretion and results in impaired cortisol secretion, prolonged stimulation of the sympathetic nervous system, and subsequent hypothalamic arousal. The net effects of this neuroendocrine–endocrine cascade are poorly regulated cortisol secretion, insulin resistance, elevated blood pressure, and visceral accumulation of body fat (central obesity).[50] The result can be a collection of metabolic risk factors, referred to as the *metabolic syndrome*, which includes abdominal obesity, atherogenic dyslipidemia, elevated blood pressure, insulin resistance, and prothrombotic and proinflammatory state of the blood.

*Energy regulation* also has been a target for explaining the mechanism(s) of obesity. In this case, the sodium ($Na^+$)/potassium ($K^+$)/adenosine triphosphatase (ATPase) pump is thought to play a major role in the development of obesity. This enzyme pump transports sodium out of the cell and potassium into the cell at the expense of cellular energy in the form of adenosine triphosphate (ATP). Obese people are thought to have fewer ATPase pumps than the nonobese; the obese person uses less energy and expends fewer calories, keeping a state of equilibrium within the body.

The *adipose cell* theory postulates that some people inherently have an excessive number of fat cells (adipocytes), and the size of the fat cells is increased. Similarly, the *lipoprotein lipase* theory suggests that the enzyme lipoprotein lipase, which helps fat to be deposited in adipocytes, is elevated in obese persons, and weight reduction stimulates even more production of the enzyme, causing fat cells to return to their hypertrophic size.

More recently, researchers have proposed the theory that for some people, obesity is the result of intestinal microorganisms. The *microbial* theory of obesity suggests a biologic cause of weight gain from an altered level of bacterial intestinal microbes called *gut microflora*.[33,223,434] Gut microbes contribute to body weight regulation through an effect on the metabolic and immune system of each individual, resulting in an improved ability to extract and store energy from ingested food.[297,371,403,465]

In recent years, *viral infections* have been recognized as a possible cause of obesity, along with the traditionally recognized causes. A human virus, *adenovirus-36* (Ad-36), has been recognized as a potential cause of obesity (referred to as *infectoobesity*). This virus is known to increase the replication, differentiation, lipid accumulation, and insulin sensitivity in fat cells and reduce those cells' leptin secretion and expression (gene that switches off appetite).[159,457]

Linked to the regulation of leptin, there is some evidence that people who sleep less weigh more. Chronic sleep deprivation, defined as sleeping only 4 to 5 hours per 24-hour cycle, alters levels of the appetite-regulating hormones leptin and ghrelin, leading to increased appetite. Weight gain may occur as a result of increased wake time, altered appetite, and the resultant fatigue, which makes exercise more difficult.[338]

**Clinical Manifestations.** Regardless of the mechanisms of the condition, the outward signs and symptoms of obesity are readily observable (excess body fat). However, the effects and complications of obesity are less easily identified at onset.

Obesity is associated with significant increases in both morbidity and mortality from many conditions (Box 11.6) and is associated with three leading causes of death: cardiovascular disease, cancer, and diabetes mellitus.

***Diabetes Mellitus.*** Type 2 diabetes mellitus is often associated with obesity. Excessive food intake, with or without physical inactivity, stimulates hyperinsulinemia. Through a negative-feedback mechanism, excessive insulin levels decrease the number of insulin receptor sites on adipose cells. The decrease in insulin receptor sites decreases the amount of glucose that can enter the cells. This promotes

**Box 11.6**

**COMPLICATIONS ASSOCIATED WITH OBESITY**

- Metabolic syndrome
- Type 2 diabetes mellitus
- Liver diseases
- Osteoarthritis
- Sleep apnea
- Atherosclerosis, hypertension, cardiovascular diseases
- Stroke
- Asthma
- Cancer
- Menstrual disorders and infertility
- Lymphedema
- Impaired mobility
- Gallbladder disease
- Psychologic disturbances such as irritability, loneliness, depression, binge eating, and tension
- Premature death

Data from Deusinger SS et al: The obesity epidemic: health consequences and implications for physical therapy. *PT Magazine* 12(6):82–104, 2004.

high blood levels of glucose. The excess glucose is stored as glycogen in the liver or as triglycerides in adipose cells, thereby enhancing hypertrophy and hyperplasia of fat cells in the already obese person. Weight reduction can reverse this process.

***Asthma.*** Rising asthma rates and poor management of the disease are increasingly linked to obesity.[56,72] The mechanism for the causality is thought to be related to an inability of the person to take deep breaths, which leads to more reactive airways and, if severe enough, asthma. Research is mixed as to whether the link between obesity and asthma is the same for women and men.

***Functional Impairments.*** Obesity also is associated with significant functional deficits or problems that lead to functional impairments. Shortness of breath; fatigue; ADL limitations[403]; increased risk for falls[138]; and an increased incidence of hip, knee, and back pain in those who are obese[30] are potential problems. Given a strong association between obesity and osteoarthritis (OA) of the knee, the risk for dysfunction in functional activities, such as walking and stair climbing, has been investigated.[133,318] Weight loss has been shown both to reduce the risk of OA and to improve function in the face of this condition.[318]

Both perceptions and observed measures of functional limitations have been tested and found to be associated with difficulty of accomplishing daily tasks related to housework and self-care.[259,260] Thus the clinical manifestations of obesity have broad implications for numerous body systems and health dimensions.

***Lower Extremity Lymphedema.*** Obesity may be a cause of lower extremity lymphedema. Individuals with a BMI greater than 59 have been documented with lymphedema. It has been hypothesized that this may be the threshold above which lymphatic flow becomes impaired.[179] The mechanism for this relationship between BMI and lymphedema has not been established. Lymphatic vessels may be compressed or inflamed, resulting in impaired lymph flow, or alternatively, elevated production of lymph from the enlarged limb may overwhelm the lymph system's capacity to move/remove fluid.[179]

***Complications with Pregnancy.*** Obesity in pregnancy is of concern and affects maternal–fetal outcomes. Women who are obese face high risk of developing health problems during their prenatal and postnatal periods, increased risk of spontaneous abortions and still births,[107] gestational diabetes mellitus,[160] pregnancy-induced hypertension,[1,160] development of deep venous thrombosis,[107] and prolonged pregnancy and labor.[492] Risks to the fetus include birth defects,[212] macrosomia (birthweight more than 4000 g [9 lb]),[107] and shoulder dystocia[191] during birth; in addition, there is a higher risk of developing childhood obesity and glucose intolerance in adulthood.[191]

***Other Complications.*** Other complications may include nephrotic syndrome and renal vein thrombosis; other thromboembolic disorders; digestive tract diseases, such as gallstones and reflux esophagitis; asthma; obstructive sleep apnea; carpal tunnel syndrome; subfertility- and pregnancy-related issues in women; and subsequent pulmonary compromise with decreased gas exchange, vital capacity, and expiratory volume. As discussed, dietary patterns, portion control, and energy-dense choices in combination with physical inactivity contribute to obesity and metabolic consequences.

## MEDICAL MANAGEMENT

**PREVENTION.** The importance of physical activity in preventing obesity has long been established, yet there may be other barriers that contribute to this national epidemic, such as reduced access to parks, trails, recreation centers, and other forms of recreational activity.[41] However, the role these barriers play in the prevention of obesity has not been thoroughly researched nor understood. Moreover, in defiance of the association between physical activity and reduced rates of obesity and diabetes, in 2001, 25% of U.S. adults did not participate in any physical activities outside of their job requirements. Furthermore, less than 20% of adults attempted to meet the minimum guidelines of exercising more than 150 minutes a week or eating a healthy diet. For these reasons, developing educational programs that encourage awareness and healthy behaviors and identifying barriers to physical activity and fitness should be a priority for the United States.[445]

Insufficient amounts of physical activity (PA), increased screen time, and inadequate dietary intake are considered to be some of the modifiable risk factors for obesity in children.[24] The complexity of these health behaviors is influenced by a range of child, parent, and household factors and broader neighborhood factors, such as the physical and social environment.[124,152,237] Other proposed influential factors include the continual availability of healthy food, targeted unhealthy advertising, time and financial constraints, and cultural norms with respect to dietary and activity habits.[87]

In a review by Davison and Birch in 2001,[109] the Ecological Systems Theory (EST) model was used to examine the relationship between a child's personal environment and specific characteristics and the occurrence of that child being overweight. Research was reviewed on children's dietary patterns, and links were found correlating high amounts of fat intake and the child's preference for fat with a higher percent of body fat, fat mass, and skinfold thickness. The authors found that family characteristics can greatly influence a child's weight status.

One study indicated that children who are predisposed to obesity are at higher risk to gain weight from high-energy, high-fat foods than children with no family history of obesity.[109] Cunningham et al[104] found similar findings supporting the notion that eating patterns early in life have a strong correlation with risk of obesity.[104] It was also determined that the parents' education on nutrition influenced the types of foods they fed their children as well as their time available for food preparation. In a family where the adults were more physically active, the children tended to be more physically active as well. Higher levels of activity can compensate for high caloric intake, making it easier to maintain a healthy weight, whereas a sedentary lifestyle places a child at a higher risk for being overweight.[37] Likewise, increased screen time may limit physical activity and lead the child to a higher risk of being overweight.

Although previous research has explored the psychological, dietary, parental, physical activity, and home environment factors, the relationship between social and physical environments to adolescent physical activity and obesity needs to be further explored. Recent research indicates that the social environment may be a significantly influential factor in determining the physical activity levels of adolescents. Some experts attribute reduced activity levels to changes in childhood environments that resulted in decreased safe and suitable opportunities and spaces for activity. In a 2009 study by Franzini et al,[152] the association between physical activity, obesity, and physical and social environments was explored by analyzing data collected as part of the "Healthy Passages" community-based study in Alabama, California, and Texas. Social environment included well-studied factors such as perceived safety, collective efficacy (social cohesion and social control), collective socialization, neighborhood exchange, and social ties. Physical environment included traffic, disorder (graffiti and litter), and residential density. Physical environment is dependent on where you are (vicinity to parks and play), and social environment is dependent on who you are with (people who enjoy playing outdoors vs. video games).

As hypothesized by these authors, social environment was significantly and positively correlated with adolescent physical activity, higher intensity exercise, school-based physical activity, as well as active free-time activities of choice ($P < 0.05$), and was negatively correlated with child obesity when controlling for socio-demographic variables. Surprisingly, this was not the case for physical environment. As concluded by Franzini et al, social environment is substantially related to both physical activity and child obesity, and may therefore also be a potentially significant (albeit difficult) means for influencing childhood obesity in combination with other efforts.

It should be recognized that the social environment is also only one variable among many that impact health behaviors and status in adolescent populations. As previously discussed, many other factors may also place a child at high risk to become overweight, such as dietary preference and intake, activity level, television and computer habits, ethnicity, gender, community recreation opportunities, community planning, and parental modeling and education.[87] Thus, an ecological systems model, which conceptualizes the child as nested within a broader and multi-influence contextual system, is a useful guide for understanding the complex multilevel scales of influence on a child's behavior, which in turn affect the child's weight status.

In a recent study looking at children that were 5 years old, on average, they played outside approximately 2 hours a day and watched television more than two and a half hours a day. This same study showed that each hour of outdoor play lowered the child's percentile on BMI about a half point. For each additional hour a child had playing outdoors compared to watching television, their BMI percentile was on average 1.5 points lower. In addition, this study showed that children whose families were of higher socioeconomic status watched less television.[237] A longitudinal study in 2014 following a cohort of children from kindergarten to eighth grade found that in kindergarten, the difference between low- and high-income children's BMIs were not significant. When those same children reached eighth grade, a significantly higher proportion of the low-income group were obese compared to the high-income group.[219]

Preventing obesity from occurring or worsening is an important part of achieving a healthier population. Prevention includes maintenance of healthy weight, maintenance of weight loss, and prevention of weight gain. Identifying risk factors that can lead to obesity or cause related health problems and learning strategies toward achieving a healthy weight are the keys to successful prevention.[21] The CDC has recommended 24 strategies and appropriate measurements to help communities create environments that promote good nutrition and physical activity (available at http://www.cdc.gov/mmwr/preview/mmwrhtml/rr5807a1.htm?s_cid=rr5807a1_e). These strategies confirm the importance of a multidimensional approach to the causes and solutions for the obesity epidemic.

Physical therapists' scope of practice includes an imperative for involvement in all levels of prevention (primary, secondary, tertiary) of this important health risk. Physical therapists have been traditionally comfortable with tertiary prevention, which aims to limit the sequelae of chronic health conditions, and actively involved with secondary prevention, which focuses on reducing the severity or duration of existing conditions. Providing primary prevention services is a contemporary expectation that involves vigilance about health risk and promotion of lifestyle strategies that reduce risk and impart health. With regard to obesity, primary prevention would be aimed at achieving appropriate energy balance to avoid weight gain in the first place—especially during biologic or personal stages of life (e.g., puberty) shown to be related to potentially unhealthy weight gain.

**DIAGNOSIS.** Measurement of body composition should be an essential component of the physical therapy examination. This should be directed at determining the presence and distribution of body fat by measuring height, weight, body circumference (extremity and waist), and nutritional status. In addition, the presence of associated causes of obesity should be investigated.

Abdominal (visceral) fat is metabolically active. Measurement of abdominal circumference is needed to identify the distribution of body fat and to determine the risks associated with increased waist circumference. Waist circumferences that are higher than 40 inches for men and 35 inches for women increase the risk for premature death and disability as a consequence of overweight or obesity. Waist circumference is the best predictor of visceral (intraabdominal) fat and total fat. The most clinically telling physical sign of serious underlying disease is increased waist circumference, which is linked to insulin resistance, hypertension, dyslipidemia, type 2 diabetes, coronary heart disease, sleep apnea, and gallbladder disease.[190]

**TREATMENT.** Both physical activity and nutrition are important in addressing obesity. Physical activity and nutrition are modifiable factors that respond similarly to the same interventions. To maintain a healthy weight, it is important to keep energy expenditure at or above energy intake. This can be accomplished by decreasing caloric intake, increasing exercise energy expenditure, or both.

***Weight Loss.*** Weight loss is regarded as a major aspect of treatment for the person who is obese. Although the amount of weight loss necessary may be individual, 10% loss in body weight is regarded as a standard that improves health. The National Weight Control Registry (www.nwcr.ws/) reports that weight loss and maintenance of the weight loss are best accomplished if individuals participate in regular intensive exercise, attend support groups, restrict the amount and kinds of food eaten, and weigh themselves often.

A multidisciplinary approach with emphasis on weight loss and maintenance of that loss is appropriate for anyone with a BMI of 30 and above and for those people with a BMI in the 25 to 29 range who have associated health problems. Such a treatment program includes moderate calorie intake, behavior modification, exercise, and social support. The same recommendations are appropriate for individuals who have not yet become overweight but are at risk for the condition because of genetics, personal habits, or environment.

***Medications.*** Medications for obesity are widely available over the counter and by prescription. The use of pharmacologic agents to calm cravings, inhibit appetite, reduce fat absorption, and increase metabolic rate is highly controversial and provides at best only a short-term benefit. Drug therapy is thought to work best when it is part of an overall program aimed at lifestyle change involving dietary changes, exercise, and behavior modification.[463,472] To be effective, drug treatment for obesity should be continued indefinitely, much like treatment for any chronic condition.[20,137,472] Researchers continue to look for drugs that can prevent or alter the physiology of obesity.

***Surgery.*** Surgical treatment, referred to as *bariatric surgery*, may be considered for some obese people if serious attempts to lose weight have failed, if BMI is greater than 40 kg/m$^2$ with or without comorbidities, or if there is a BMI of 35 kg/m$^2$ with significant health-related comorbidities[20,137,322,425,472] and complications of obesity that are life-threatening. Surgical approaches rely on reconfiguring or redirecting the gastrointestinal system through bariatric weight loss surgery (e.g., Roux-en-Y gastric bypass, laparoscopic adjustable gastric banding, vertical banded gastroplasty). Bariatric surgery has been shown to provide the greatest degree of sustained weight loss in people with morbid obesity.[272]

Laparoscopic Roux-en-Y gastric bypass has been referred to as the "gold standard" operation for surgical control of obesity. It is effective in achieving weight loss, improving comorbidities and quality of life, and reducing recovery time and perioperative complications.[386] This procedure is safe and effective and decreases overall costs.[322]

Evidence supports this shift in surgical approach for individuals having laparoscopic surgery based on studies demonstrating improved SF-36 scores,[7,163,323,425] decreased recovery times,[7,323] earlier return to work,[323] less postoperative pain,[323,386] and comparable amounts of weight loss.[114,386]

***Behavioral and Lifestyle Changes.*** The relationship(s) between biologic and behavioral factors influencing obesity is not yet completely understood. However, regardless of the medical and surgical treatments available to treat obesity, behavioral change in the frequency and type of eating and exercise habits remains the foundation of both prevention and intervention.[461]

Behavior in both prevention and treatment is influenced by what options are available (e.g., vending machines, safe parks in which to walk), how and to whom health information is portrayed (e.g., media vs. health practitioner), and what type of support is given to individuals who seek and/or need to make a change.[214]

Practitioners require knowledge of various behavior change theories including what motivates change, how behavioral change occurs, what resources are needed to make change, and strategies useful for promoting and maintaining change. Across the theoretic foundations guiding this knowledge, the combined merits of providing accurate information, understanding barriers preventing change, anticipating personal readiness for change, and providing structure and support over extended periods to enable sustained new behaviors have been recognized as helpful.[36]

Although lifestyle programs have been shown to be the most successful in creating durable change, regulation of body weight (to either prevent gain or maintain loss) is still affected by a myriad of intrapersonal and environmental factors that interact to make obesity control difficult. Tailoring all interventions to the "personal environment" of each individual is critical in overcoming the intrinsic and extrinsic pressures in the American culture that affect the current epidemic of obesity.[279]

**PROGNOSIS.** The management of obesity continues to be challenging, particularly because its effect on the whole person is so broad and the causes/influences are so numerous that prognosis relies on significant and sustained lifestyle changes that must last a lifetime. When therapy is confined to dietary measures alone, treatment of obesity is less likely to be successful. Because the risk of mortality and morbidity from obesity rises in proportion to the degree of obesity and the presence of complications, treatment is essential. For example, among the cardiovascular problems associated with obesity, hypertension in combination with obesity increases the risk for development of cerebrovascular disease, specifically cerebral thrombosis.

Weight loss alters conditions associated with obesity, and even moderate weight loss in an obese person (i.e., 10 to 20 lb) provides substantial changes in risk factors. Following weight loss in individuals who are obese, a decrease in blood pressure usually occurs with a regression of left ventricular hypertrophy, total and high-density lipoprotein cholesterol are favorably changed, and glucose tolerance improves in those people with type 2 diabetes mellitus.

The addition of exercise to a comprehensive program of caloric reduction and behavior modification can improve results. Regular exercise can maximize body composition change and increase the probability of maintaining weight loss.

Patterns of fat distribution are important in determining the risks associated with obesity. Visceral fat within the abdominal cavity is more hazardous to health than subcutaneous fat around the abdomen. Upper body obesity around the waist and flank is a greater health hazard than lower body obesity marked by fat in the thighs and buttocks.

Although the connection between obesity (BMI greater than 30) and coronary heart disease is well established, it remains unknown whether a similar link exists for those who are mildly overweight. Research has shown that people whose BMI at midlife (30 to 55 years of age) was between 23 and 24.9 had a 50% higher risk of heart attack compared with those whose BMI was under 20. Women whose BMI was greater than 29 had a 3.6 times greater risk of heart attack compared with the leanest group.[480] Moderately higher adiposity at younger ages (18 years) is associated with increased premature death in younger and middle-aged women.[449]

**SPECIAL IMPLICATIONS FOR THE THERAPIST 11.16**

### *Obesity*

Obesity has negative effects on overall health; emerging evidence indicates that obesity has effects beyond those associated with chronic disease and may indeed be responsible for epigenetic changes that can lead to generational changes over time. For example, obesity has negative effects on overall physical function and mobility, although the contributions of obesity to overall musculoskeletal function are not well understood. For every day someone lies in bed or remains immobile, it takes even more time to regain the strength from that day of bed rest. Also, presumably the person was not losing weight at the same rate he or she was losing strength. Because sedentary habits have increased the disparity between body mass and strength over the last 5 years, those conditions create an even greater challenge when treating someone who is obese and who is chair or bed bound.

Problems associated with obesity commonly seen in a therapy program include back pain; arthritis; biomechanical dysfunction affecting the hips, knees, and ankle/foot; skin breakdown; and cardiopulmonary compromise. Obesity is a known risk factor in the development of type 2 diabetes mellitus, often accompanied by diabetic neuropathy, foot ulcerations, and neuropathic fractures (see "Diabetes Mellitus" in Chapter 11).

For the physical therapist, working with the individual who is obese poses a definite risk to personal safety and health. Using proper body mechanics, careful planning for transfers, and obtaining adequate help are essential during any lifting, transfers, and hands-on therapy. A screening tool, developed by Michael Dionne (Dionne's Egress Test, or DET) can be used to predict the safety of bariatric patient transfers. It provides a three-step process to evaluate a person's mobility to go from sit-to-stand, march in place, and step forward and back. The DET takes into account neurologic deficits that may be linked to balance, not muscle weakness, and may assist health care clinicians to determine whether someone with extreme obesity can safely mobilize out of bed or whether mechanical conveyance is indicated. The DET has been shown to be moderately reliable in a pilot study; validity has not been established.[410,411,417]

#### Obesity and Body Composition

Body composition (i.e., the relationship of fat mass to lean body mass) is an important variable in judging health risk and one that many people may seek to understand. The public has become aware that BMI is not a sufficient measure of body composition and is flawed when used (for example) in reference to professional athletes, who have a high ratio of lean body mass, or the elderly, who have less lean body mass.[135,453] Standard expectations for percent body fat are 10% to 22% for men and 20% to 32% for women.[10] Clearly, it is important to provide education about health risk from adiposity, not from accumulation of muscle from resistance training or other exercise strategies.

#### Obesity and Back Pain[70]

It is also now well-recognized that adipose tissue is an active endocrine organ that secretes many active cytokines and hormones,[232] some of which may be related to the development of musculoskeletal pain. Leptin, a proinflammatory adipokine, has been associated with pain and osteoarthritis in women.[497] Recent cross-sectional and longitudinal studies are beginning to highlight the important role of body composition in the development and worsening of joint pain, including the low back.[58] A recent systematic review and meta-analysis demonstrated that body fat is positively associated with joint pain in the low back, knee, and foot.[464] There is a suggestion that specifically elevated fat mass led to this association rather than just being overweight. Additional high-quality longitudinal studies are needed to further demonstrate this.

#### Obesity and Joint Pain

Obesity contributes to increases in musculoskeletal pain, demonstrated by increased odds ratios of 1.7 to 9.9 of work-restricting pain in obese subjects as compared to the general population.[341] There is an association between obesity and knee and hand OA but not hip OA or general OA.[180,426]

There is also some relationship between BMI and the frequency of hip and knee replacement surgery[474] and poorer outcomes after total knee arthroplasty,[150] but no association is demonstrated between BMI and the need for total hip or knee revision surgery.

Obese individuals should have greater joint loading forces; however, at least one study demonstrated that obese individuals could have gait loading forces in the knee that are less than normal-weight individuals, if they adjust their gait by adopting a slower self-preferred speed.[117]

There is also evidence that there is an association between BMI and pain in non–weight-bearing joints; therefore the relationship may not be due to strictly mechanical loading.[216]

#### Obesity and Mobility/Balance

Individuals with moderate and severe obesity have been found to report that their mobility is less than very good or excellent. They also demonstrate low levels of mobility on performance-based measures. Higher BMI categories are not associated with statistical differences in self-reported or physical measures of balance; however, a trend was observed, with a greater percentage of subjects with higher BMIs being unable to complete tests of unilateral stance.[193]

### Obesity and Physical Activity

Obesity might have a negative effect on performance of activities that require muscular strength or power, because the muscle would have to apply a greater force to move a larger mass. This was demonstrated in one study of children where obesity limited the ability to perform lower extremity activities such as vertical jump and standing long jump.[197]

In addition, walking requires a training level of moderate to high intensity in most obese women, 56% $VO_2$max in obese women versus 35% in normal-weight women.[296] Therefore, long and brisk walks should not be regarded as low intensity and fat-burning for obese women. Because walking in obese adults also has been shown to require more energy than in nonobese counterparts, pursuing greater participation in physical activity may not be motivating.[63]

Compliance may be improved with exercise and activity programs that require a lower $VO_2$max level, for example, bicycling, water activity, and simple calisthenics and weight resistance training. Another ADL that requires significant lower extremity strength is rising from a chair. One study demonstrated that in 8- and 9-year-old obese children, 69% needed assistance in rising from a chair.[239,468] This difficulty may accelerate the cycle of obesity and encourage sedentary behavior as a result of the difficulty in getting up to perform physical activity.

### Obesity and Operative Complications

There are technical challenges in preparing and operating on an obese individual. Imaging equipment may not be large enough to accommodate the very obese individual, and the quality of the image may be poor. Motion studies using flexion and extension radiographs may not assess range of motion adequately. Additional considerations include maintaining an open airway and accessing venous or arterial blood vessels because of adipose tissue getting in the way.[337]

There is no strong correlation between obesity and perioperative complications,[217,312] but there are many reports of operative complications in obese individuals after many different kinds of procedures (e.g., gynecologic, orthopedic, cardiovascular, transplantation, urologic). There are reports of positional neuropathies after surgery in morbidly obese individuals (BMI greater than 40). Positional palsies are attributed to increased weight causing traction or compression on peripheral neurovascular bundles, especially when the individual is placed in the prone position without adequate support and padding.[337]

Increased body mass also increases blood volume, placing added strain on the cardiovascular and respiratory systems. Over time, this can lead to decreased lung compliance and hypoxia. Preventing respiratory complications must be a team priority.[106] Early mobility to help prevent both respiratory complications and venous thromboembolism is advised. The American Society for Metabolic and Bariatric Surgery recommends early postoperative ambulation, perioperative use of lower extremity sequential compression devices, and chemoprophylaxis (anticoagulation regimen) unless contraindicated.[22]

### Bariatric Weight Loss Surgery

After bariatric surgery, vitamin and mineral deficiencies can occur; the physical therapist should watch for signs and symptoms such as brittle nails, poor wound healing, easy bruising, paresthesias of the hand and feet, and bone pain. Dumping syndrome, a problem associated with Roux-en-Y gastric bypass procedure, is characterized by nausea, weakness, perspiration, and diarrhea.

Changes in physical function and mobility following gastric bypass surgery (e.g., increased distance during the 6-minute walk test) and quality of life have been reported.[438] Additional research is needed to examine individual-specific interventions that can further enhance improvements in functional mobility and further define the role of the physical therapist with this patient population.

Postoperative complications can include chronic inflammation of the lower extremities; increased pendulous tissue in the abdomen, trunk, and extremities; and lymphedema of the head, neck, trunk, genitals, and extremities. Individuals with diabetes and/or vascular problems may have lower extremity lymphedema complicated by slow- or nonhealing wounds.

Techniques of lymphatic massage and compression strategies may be needed. Care must be taken to address postural and breathing issues (e.g., forward head, rounded shoulders, deep breathing in the upright position). The plan of care should also emphasize cardiopulmonary endurance, muscle strengthening, and adaptive techniques for hygiene and self-care.

### Prevention

Prevention and screening programs for adults and children are advocated in *Healthy People 2020* toward the goal of promoting health and reducing chronic disease associated with diet and weight because no state achieved the intended reduction in prevalence of adult obesity to 15%.[78] The physical therapist's role in prevention and wellness, including screening programs and health promotion, is discussed in Chapter 1 as presented by the APTA.

In the face of a true epidemic of obesity, our roles will undoubtedly be focused on secondary prevention (e.g., adapting exercise regimens to avoid high-impact activity for people carrying excess weight) or tertiary prevention (e.g., prescribing support stockings to potentially prevent vascular insufficiency). However, primary prevention of weight gain is a must for individuals still at low risk for obesity and could include prescription of multiple exercise strategies that sustain long-term participation and referral to literature or professionals dealing with proper (not fad) nutrition habits. There is a role for physical therapists to work with primary care physicians and pediatricians to establish safe and effective exercise programs for patients in order to prevent obesity in high- and low-risk individuals. Physical therapists should perform body composition measurements as a part of the routine physical therapist examination. See also previous discussions of physical activity and nutrition in this chapter.

Box 11.7

**STRATEGIES TO FACILITATE SUCCESSFUL EXERCISE PROGRAMS**

- Ask the client if he or she is currently exercising regularly (or was before illness or injury). Provide a brief description of benefits that the person could achieve from such a program.
- Stress exercise benefits of improving health rather than achieving weight loss.
- Allow the person to respond to the recommendation for an exercise program. Encourage the person to verbalize any thoughts or reactions to your suggestions.
- Determine whether the person believes that an exercise program will benefit him or her personally. Help the individual to set personal goals for exercise.
- Establish a patient/client self-charge contract and plan to monitor one's own success.
- Be aware of any cultural or philosophical beliefs the person may have regarding exercise.
- If resistance to the idea of an exercise program is encountered, give the person an opportunity to list potential barriers to exercise. Ask the person to suggest ways to overcome potential barriers.
- Whenever possible, provide a written copy (preferably just pictures because of the potential of undisclosed illiteracy) of the proposed exercise program. Review progress and reward attempts, successes, and progression of the exercise program.
- Make it fun to foster a lifestyle approach characterized by long-term adherence.

Physical therapists must be involved in screening for obesity and its comorbidities as suggested by the surgeon general to reinforce how important regular exercise is in enhancing physical and mental well-being and prevention of the comorbidities associated with obesity. Since obesity is often associated with an increased prevalence of cardiovascular risk factors, graded exercise testing may be indicated before prescribing an exercise program. Even morbidly obese people can be evaluated on the treadmill with some modification in the testing protocol such as beginning with slow walking without treadmill elevation, followed by gradual increases in speed to achieve maximal exertion. Submaximal exercise testing overcomes many of the limitations of maximal exercise testing and may be applicable to this population.[12,125]

## Exercise

The effects of overconsumption in adults can be addressed with just 3 minutes more walking per day. This means that closing the gap between energy intake (i.e., eating) and energy expenditure (e.g., moving) may require minimal additional energy expenditure.[454] Physical therapists recognize the challenges of encouraging lifestyle change in their patients/clients and must seek creative and individualized ways to promote healthy approaches to balancing the energy equation associated with the epidemic of obesity through individual behavior change but also an ecological approach that modifies the social and physical environment, allowing physical therapists to be involved in true primary prevention activities.

Box 11.8

**POTENTIAL COMPLICATIONS OF OBESITY DURING EXERCISE**

- Precipitation of angina pectoris or myocardial infarction
- Excessive rise in blood pressure
- Aggravation of degenerative arthritis and other joint problems
- Ligamentous injuries
- Injury from falling
- Excessive sweating
- Skin disorders, chafing
- Hypohydration and reduced circulating blood volume
- Heat stroke or heat exhaustion

From Skinner JS: *Exercise testing and exercise prescription for special cases: theoretical basis and clinical application*, ed 3, Philadelphia, 2005, Lea & Febiger.

Hill and colleagues,[196,238] using National Health and Nutrition Examination Survey[196,317] data over an 8-year period, have determined that the median energy accumulation is 15 kcal/day and that 90% of the population accumulates an excess of less than 50 kcal/day. On the basis of this information, much of the weight gain seen in the population could be eliminated by some combination of increasing energy expenditure and reducing energy intake, thus closing the energy gap.[116] For example, this can be accomplished for many people simply by walking an extra mile per day or for 15 to 20 minutes, or by reducing intake with smaller portions of food.

Prescribing exercise for obese people follows the principles used with healthy people (see Box 11.7), including modifications for mechanical limitations, awareness of potential hazards during exercise (Box 11.8), and awareness of the greater heat intolerance of the obese. Some equipment modifications may be necessary if the client is too large to use a stationary bicycle or exceeds the manufacturer's recommended weight capacity. For example, the client can pedal some stationary bikes while seated in a chair behind the bike.

A higher incidence of exercise-related injury exists among the obese that requires extra caution in the first few weeks of exercise participation. Recommendations include adequate warm-up and stretching and progressive increases in intensity, frequency, and duration. Severe obesity contributes to back pain and back injury and affects foot mechanics, which can lead to foot and ankle problems. Selection of appropriate footwear with possible orthotic devices that provide heel support or compensatory foot pronation is recommended to make exercise safer and more comfortable.

The American College of Sports Medicine[13,14] presents the benefits of low-intensity, short-duration regular exercise. Exercise regimens, paired with appropriate nutritional change, have healthful effects and may produce significant weight loss. Long-term continuation of this dual lifestyle change is required for both weight loss and maintenance. Accumulation of 60 minutes of formal exercise and daily physical activity is recommended. Performance at an appropriate frequency and intensity are the early goals toward achieving a habit of regular exercise rather than weight loss.

**Table 11.10** Regulation of Glucose Metabolism

| Gland | Regulating Function |
|---|---|
| **Pancreas** | |
| Alpha cells (islets of Langerhans) | Secrete glucagon; increase blood glucose level |
| Beta cells (islets of Langerhans) | Secrete insulin (glucose-regulating hormone); decrease blood glucose level; release connecting or C-peptide in equal amounts to insulin |
| Delta cells (islets of Langerhans) | Secrete somatostatin (regulates endocrine system and affects neurotransmission and cell proliferation); regulate the release of insulin and glucagon |
| Gamma cells (islets of Langerhans) | Secrete pancreatic polypeptide (self-regulate exocrine and endocrine pancreatic secretion activities) |
| **Adrenal Gland** | |
| Medulla: Epinephrine | Responds to stress; epinephrine stimulates liver and muscle glycogenolysis to increase the blood glucose level |
| Cortex: Glucocorticoids | Increase blood glucose levels by promoting the flow of amino acids to the liver, where they are synthesized into glucose |
| **Anterior Pituitary** | |
| Adrenocorticotropic hormone (ACTH) | Increases blood glucose levels |
| Human growth hormone (GH) | Limits storage of fat; favors fat catabolism; inhibits carbohydrate catabolism, raising blood glucose levels |
| **Thyroid** | |
| $T_3$ and $T_4$ | May raise or lower blood glucose levels |

Developing an exercise program the person likes and can complete over time is the initial focus. Finding the right match may take some time and several unsuccessful attempts. Moreover, studies indicate that improved fitness through regular physical activity reduces cardiovascular morbidity and mortality for overweight individuals even if they remain overweight. The ultimate goal for the exercising obese person is to make a lifelong commitment to achieving reasonable energy expenditure through routine physical activity.[405]

The influence of body weight on exertion and lower-extremity trauma may support an initial program of stationary cycling. Aquatic exercise programs can be an important part of reducing strain on joints by providing non–weight-bearing exercise for the obese person. Resistive exercises and weightlifting can be structured to produce aerobic gains by using a circuit style with low resistance, multiple repetitions, and short rests between sets. For most individuals, caloric expenditure with traditional strength-training techniques is not as great as with circuit lifting or aerobic conditioning, but strength training does use calories and can increase lean body mass.

Behavior modification focusing on routine daily activities that require no special equipment and involve only simple lifestyle changes may be the only type of physical activity that is continued for any length of time. For example, less reliance on vehicular transportation, parking a distance from the destination, avoiding elevators and using stairs, delivering messages within the work structure rather than telephoning, and walking 10 minutes during lunch are useful and easily accommodated suggestions for increasing energy expenditure.

## Pancreas (Islets of Langerhans)

The pancreas lies behind the stomach, with the head and neck of the pancreas located in the curve of the duodenum and the body extending horizontally across the posterior abdominal wall (see Fig. 11.1). It has two functions, acting as both an endocrine gland (secreting the hormones insulin and glucagon) and an exocrine gland (producing digestive enzymes). The cells of the pancreas that function in the endocrine capacity are the islets of Langerhans.

The islets of Langerhans have three major functioning cells: (1) the alpha cells produce glucagon, which increases the blood glucose levels by stimulating the liver and other cells to release stored glucose (glycogenolysis); (2) the beta cells produce insulin, which lowers blood glucose levels by facilitating the entrance of glucose into the cells for metabolism; and (3) the delta cells produce somatostatin, which is thought to regulate the release of insulin and glucagon (Table 11.10).[207]

### Diabetes Mellitus

**Definition and Overview.** DM is a chronic, systemic disorder characterized by hyperglycemia (excess glucose in the blood) and disruption of the metabolism of carbohydrates, fats, and proteins. Insulin, produced in the pancreas, normally maintains a balanced blood glucose level. DM is characterized as a group of metabolic diseases resulting from defects in the secretion of insulin, action of insulin, or both. The chronic hyperglycemia of DM is associated with long-term damage and dysfunction and impairment of tissues and organs, especially the eyes, kidneys, nerves, heart, and blood vessels.

The majority of cases of DM fall into two large categories: type 1 DM and type 2 DM, related to differences in etiology and pathogenesis of the disease. In type 1 DM (previously called *insulin-dependent DM [IDDM]* or *juvenile-onset DM*), the cause of hyperglycemia is an absolute deficiency of insulin production and secretion.

Most individuals with type 1 DM can be identified by serologic evidence showing an autoimmune process occurring in the islet cells of the pancreas along with specific genetic markers. People with type 1 DM are prone to ketoacidosis and specific metabolic derangements associated with hyperglycemia; they require exogenous insulin to maintain life.

Type 2 DM (previously called *non–insulin-dependent DM [NIDDM]* or *adult-onset DM*) is a much more prevalent form of diabetes, and the cause is a combination of cellular resistance to insulin action and an inadequate compensatory insulin secretory response. Individuals

**Table 11.11** Differences Between Types of Diabetes Mellitus

| Features | Type 1 (Ketosis-Prone) | Type 2 (Not Ketosis-Prone) |
|---|---|---|
| Age at onset | Usually <20 y | Usually >40 y; increasing number of cases in all ages, including children |
| Proportion of all cases | <10% | >90% |
| Type of onset | Abrupt (acute or subacute) | Gradual |
| Etiologic factors | Possible viral/autoimmune, resulting in destruction of islet cells | Obesity-associated insulin resistance |
| HLA association | Yes | No |
| Insulin antibodies | Yes | No |
| Body weight at onset | Normal or thin, obesity uncommon | Majority are obese (80%) |
| Endogenous insulin production | Decreased (little or none) | Variable (above or below normal) |
| Ketoacidosis | May occur | Rare |
| Treatment | Insulin, diet, and exercise | Diet, oral hypoglycemic agents, exercise, insulin, and weight control |

Modified from Goodman CC, Snyder TE: *Differential diagnosis for physical therapists*, ed 5, Philadelphia, 2013, Saunders.

**Table 11.12** Blood Glucose Levels

| Fasting Plasma Glucose Test | Two-Hour Oral Glucose Tolerance Test |
|---|---|
| Normal: <100 mg/dL | Normal: <140 mg/dL |
| Prediabetes: 100-125 mg/dL | Prediabetes: 140-199 mg/dL |
| Diabetes: >125 mg/dL | Diabetes: ≥200 mg/dL |

with type 2 DM are not as likely to exhibit the metabolic derangements common to the person with type 1 DM, and type 2 DM usually can be controlled with diet, exercise, and oral hypoglycemic agents. In some cases, however, people with type 2 DM do require insulin replacement.[91] A comparison of the primary differences between the two types of diabetes is shown in Table 11.11.

In recent years, the lines between type 1 and 2 DM have begun to blur. In addition, with increased obesity, type 2 DM is being diagnosed in younger and younger children which some have termed *maturity-onset diabetes of the young* (MODY).[8,357] An autoimmune type of diabetes that begins in middle to late adulthood, referred to as latent autoimmune diabetes in adults (LADA) or Type 1.5 diabetes has been identified. In addition, it has been suggested that obesity-related insulin resistance and type 2 DM may also have an autoimmune component.[441] It is important to understand that the characteristics of type 1 and 2 diabetes are not mutually exclusive and should be considered along a spectrum of attributes of the disease.

**Prediabetes.** Prediabetes occurs when the body cannot utilize glucose the way it should. After ingesting food, carbohydrates are converted into glucose. The pancreas releases insulin to help move the glucose into the cells to be used for energy. In someone with prediabetes, this process is not completed because either the body cells do not recognize all of the insulin (decreased insulin sensitivity) or the cells stop responding to the action of insulin (increased insulin resistance).

With less glucose moving into the cells, the blood glucose levels start to rise. This is the beginning of a condition referred to as *prediabetes*. In prediabetes, the blood glucose levels are higher than normal but not quite high enough to be considered diabetes (Table 11.12). Many people with prediabetes have hypertension and dyslipidemia. The trio of comorbidities increases the risk of developing type 2 diabetes and heart disease. Most people diagnosed with prediabetes do, in fact, go on to develop diabetes. More than half have diabetes within 10 years.

According to the American Diabetes Association,[91] two categories of hyperglycemia classifications fall between normal and a true diagnosis of diabetes. *Impaired glucose tolerance* and *impaired fasting glucose* refer to intermediate metabolic stages that fall between normal glucose metabolism and diabetes. Elevated glucose levels on either test is defined as prediabetes.

Individuals with impaired glucose tolerance often manifest hyperglycemia only when challenged with the oral glucose load used in the oral glucose tolerance test, which is a measure of how well insulin clears glucose from the bloodstream. Impaired fasting glucose is diagnosed in people whose fasting plasma glucose levels are equal to or greater than 100 mg/dL but less than or equal to 125 mg/dL. (Normal plasma glucose as defined by the American Diabetes Association is less than 100 mg/dL.)[91] A third test that may be used to define prediabetes and diabetes is glycated hemoglobin (A1C), which is a measure of the percentage of blood sugar attached to hemoglobin and is indicative of a person's average blood sugar level for the previous 3 months. Prediabetes is diagnosed in people with an A1C greater than or equal to 5.7% but less than or equal to 6.4%.

The terms *prediabetes*, *borderline diabetes*, and *insulin resistance syndrome* are sometimes used interchangeably, and sometimes the terms *insulin resistance syndrome* and *metabolic syndrome* are used to describe the same condition. There are slight differences in these terms, with some overlap. For example, because prediabetes represents both a state of decreased insulin sensitivity and increased insulin resistance, it is not strictly the same thing as just insulin resistance syndrome. The test for insulin resistance syndrome, called the euglycemic clamp, is complicated and costly and therefore not used in most doctors' offices. If blood tests are indicative of prediabetes, insulin resistance syndrome is likely present. Although prediabetes can develop without metabolic syndrome, many people with prediabetes also have metabolic syndrome. Metabolic syndrome includes central obesity, insulin resistance (the "prediabetes component"), and dyslipidemia.

Borderline diabetes is not a label accepted by everyone; the issue can be explained as one of difficulty metabolizing sugar because of overloading the body with excess food. Labeling the condition as borderline diabetes can have a negative effect on employment and insurance.

Most people with prediabetes do not exercise adequately, do not control their weight or restrict fat and calories. The Diabetes Prevention Program Intervention Trial showed that diet and exercise can lower the incidence of type 2 diabetes by 58% over 3 years among those at high risk.[119] The American Diabetes Association recommends people with prediabetes lose 5% to 7% of body weight and increase physical activity to at least 150 minutes of moderate exercise each week to prevent or delay the onset of type 2 DM.[92]

### Other Types and Categories of Diabetes Mellitus

In addition to the main categories of type 1 and type 2 DM, other rare specific types of DM exist, which are associated with a variety of etiologies, including the following:

- Genetic beta-cell defects
- Genetic defects in insulin action
- Disorders of the exocrine pancreas such as injury, neoplasm, cystic fibrosis, or infection
- Other endocrinopathies that antagonize insulin secretion or action (e.g., increased growth hormone, cortisol, glucagons, or epinephrine)
- Drug or chemically induced DM (e.g., glucocorticoids, thiazides, thyroid hormone)
- Uncommon forms of immune or genetically associated syndromes (e.g., stiff-man syndrome, Down syndrome, Klinefelter syndrome, Turner syndrome, and Wolfram syndrome)
- Infections (certain viruses, including rubella, coxsackievirus B, cytomegalovirus, adenovirus, and mumps, have been associated with beta-cell destruction in people with existing genetic markers)
- Gestational DM

The final category, gestational DM, is defined as any degree of glucose intolerance recognized with the onset of pregnancy. Approximately 6 weeks or more after pregnancy ends, the woman should be reclassified into one of the other categories, depending on whether or not her glucose tolerance resolves. She could be reclassified as normal if no glucose intolerance remains after the pregnancy is completed. Gestational DM accompanies approximately 8% of all pregnancies[501] and is most evident among women who are overweight and sedentary.

Most women who have gestational DM return to normal glucose metabolism after pregnancy.[91] However, with time, these women will likely be diagnosed with type 2 DM.[423] In addition, children born to women with gestational DM generally have delayed fine and gross motor skills and a higher prevalence of inattention or hyperactivity compared to children born of women without gestational DM.[331]

**Incidence and Prevalence.** According to the World Health Organization, more than 400 million people worldwide (about 1 in 11 persons) have been diagnosed with diabetes. In the United States, over 30 million people (about 1 in 10 persons) have been diagnosed with diabetes.[19,79,491] In addition, one third of U.S. adults are known to have prediabetes and are therefore at risk for developing type 2 diabetes, heart disease, and stroke.

**Box 11.9**

**RISK FACTORS FOR TYPE 1 AND TYPE 2 DIABETES MELLITUS**

***Type 1 DM Risk Factors***

- Presence of type 1 diabetes in a first-degree relative (sibling or parent)

***Type 2 DM Risk Factors***

- Positive family history (first-degree relative with diabetes mellitus)
- Ethnic origin: Black, Native American, Hispanic, Asian American, Pacific Islander
- Obesity (BMI >25)
- Increasing age (≥45 y)
- Habitual physical inactivity; sedentary lifestyle
- Previous history of gestational diabetes (GDM) or delivery of babies weighing more than 9 lb
- Presence of other clinical conditions associated with insulin resistance (e.g., polycystic ovary syndrome)
- History of vascular disease
- Previously identified impaired fasting glucose or impaired glucose tolerance
- Hypertension (≥140/90 mmHg in adults or on therapy for hypertension)
- HDL cholesterol level <35 mg/dL and/or triglyceride level ≥250 mg/dL
- Cigarette smoking

*DM*, Diabetes mellitus.

Diabetes, with its severe complications of heart disease, stroke, kidney disease, blindness, and loss of limbs, is the most common endocrine disorder, ranked as the seventh leading cause of death from disease in the United States (mostly because of increased rates of CAD). It is the leading cause of blindness and renal failure in adults.

Black, Native, Hispanic, Mexican, and Asian Americans are 1.5 to 2 times more likely to develop DM than are white Americans, with increasing incidence associated with advancing age. Nearly one half of all Americans with DM are older than 60 years and nearly one fourth of the U.S. population older than age 65 have diabetes[101]; males and females are affected equally.

Approximately 90% of all cases of DM are type 2. Type 1 DM and secondary causes (e.g., medications, genetic disease, or hormonal changes) account for the remaining 10%. Since the mid-1970s, the incidence of diabetes has steadily increased as a result of prolonged life expectancy; increased incidence of obesity; and reduced mortality resulting in increased live births to people with type 1 DM, whose children are predisposed to future development of type 1 DM.

**Etiologic and Risk Factors.** Risk factors for type 1 and type 2 DM have been identified (Box 11.9). Additionally, lifestyle factors, such as watching 2 or more hours of television daily, skipping breakfast, drinking a daily carbonated beverage, and having a waist measurement larger than 35 inches for women and 40 inches (a sign of abdominal fat) for men, may be linked with type 2 diabetes.

More television (sedentary lifestyle) is often linked with less activity, which can lead to weight gain. Eating nonnutritious snacks while watching television and/or drinking soda pop adds extra empty calories, which can also result in weight gain. Eating fast food more than twice a week raises the risk of obesity and the likelihood of becoming resistant to insulin.

High stress can interfere with the body's ability to make insulin and process glucose; cortisol is a key factor in glucose metabolism, and stress is linked with elevated cortisol levels. Stress can also interrupt sleep, and sleep disturbances may be linked with an increased risk of developing insulin resistance. Other lifestyle and risk factors under investigation for diabetes include consuming processed meat (e.g., bacon, hot dogs, and lunch meat[144]) and major depressive disorders.[429,451]

### Type 1 Diabetes Mellitus

Type 1 DM results from cell-mediated autoimmune destruction of the beta cells of the pancreas and is a condition of absolute insulin deficiency. This autoimmune process is detectable because markers of cellular destruction called *autoantibodies* are specific to pancreatic beta cells. One and sometimes more of these autoantibodies are present and detectable in 85% to 90% of individuals with type 1 DM when the disease initially is diagnosed. People with autoimmune destruction of beta cells are also prone to other autoimmune disorders such as Graves disease, Hashimoto thyroiditis, Addison disease, vitiligo, autoimmune gastritis, and pernicious anemia.[256]

In type 1 DM the rate of beta-cell destruction is rapid in some people (mainly infants and children) and slow in others (mainly adults). Even though immune-mediated diabetes commonly occurs in childhood and adolescence, it can occur at any age, even late in life. In about 10% of cases of type 1 DM, no definable autoimmune etiology exists. Some individuals in this category (usually of African or Asian origin) have permanent hypoinsulinemia and are prone to ketoacidosis but have no evidence of autoimmunity. Their need for insulin replacement is usually inconsistent.

Globally, the incidence of type 1 diabetes is rising about 2% to 3% per year. Interactions between genetic, environmental, and behavioral factors are implicated in this increase. Certain human leukocyte antigens (HLA-DR3 and HLA-DR4) on specific chromosomes appear to predispose persons to the development of type 1 DM. For example, there is a fourfold increased prevalence of Down syndrome among people with type 1 diabetes, supporting the theory that genes on chromosome 21 may confer risk for type 1 diabetes.[43] In addition to the two HLA genetic loci, over 60 non-HLA genetic loci have been associated with risk of type 1 DM. Environmental and behavioral factors that have been associated with type 1 DM include infant and adult diets, early vitamin D insufficiency, early viruses associated with islet inflammation, and decreased gut-microbiome diversity. In the future, a combination of familial, HLA and non-HLA, environmental, and behavioral risk factors could help improve the prediction of risk or development of type 1 DM and discrimination between type 1 and type 2.[120]

Up to 20% of women with type 1 DM have some kind of eating disorder that predisposes them to further complications with glucose control. Binge eating and use of intense, excessive exercise are common in preteen, teenage, and young women with type 1 DM.[96,170] The emphasis on weight control, dietary habits, and food at a time when poor self-esteem, stress, and altered image occur in young women with type 1 DM may contribute to an increased risk for eating disorders.[287]

Individuals with type 1 DM and eating disorders are more likely to practice insulin omission and reduction, symptoms that are unique to DM and increase the risk of DKA and microvascular complications, such as retinopathy, in this population group.[170]

### Type 2 Diabetes Mellitus

Type 2 DM is a form of diabetes in which individuals have endogenous insulin production but have difficulty with effective insulin action at the cellular level. People with type 2 DM may not need insulin treatment to survive but need other forms of therapy to prevent hyperglycemia and its resulting complications. However, over time, an imbalance in pancreatic beta cell production and apoptosis may also occur, resulting in a reduction in beta cell mass, progression in disease severity, and necessitating the use of insulin.[280]

Type 2 DM is associated with obesity. In fact, obesity-dependent diabetes in childhood is now referred to as *diabesity* and is considered an inflammatory metabolic condition. Both insulin resistance and defective insulin secretion appear very prematurely in obese individuals, and both worsen similarly toward diabetes.[289,389]

Most people with type 2 DM are obese and sedentary; these two risk factors cause some degree of insulin resistance. At least 80% of all persons with type 2 DM are obese, and the remaining 20%, who are not obese by traditional weight criteria, may have an increased percentage of body fat distribution, particularly in the abdominal area.[91]

Type 2 diabetes was originally called *late-* or *adult-onset diabetes* because it primarily occurred in people aged 60 years or older. Starting in the early 1990s, a trend toward the development of type 2 DM in children and adolescents was observed. Excess body fat and sedentary lifestyle are the key risk factors contributing to the development of type 2 DM in younger population groups. Type 2 DM susceptibility genes that lead to insulin resistance in humans have been identified.[282,382]

Cigarette smoking may also be a risk factor for developing type 2 DM. Smokers exhibit a significantly increased incidence of diabetes compared to people who have never smoked.[151]

People with this form of diabetes may have normal or elevated insulin levels, but the insulin produced is ineffective because the cells are resistant to attachment to their cellular receptors and subsequent action. Insulin secretion also is impaired, and the beta cells are unable to secrete increased amounts of insulin when needed. Ketoacidosis seldom occurs in this type of diabetes, but people with type 2 DM are at increased risk for developing macrovascular and microvascular complications. The risk of developing this form of diabetes increases with

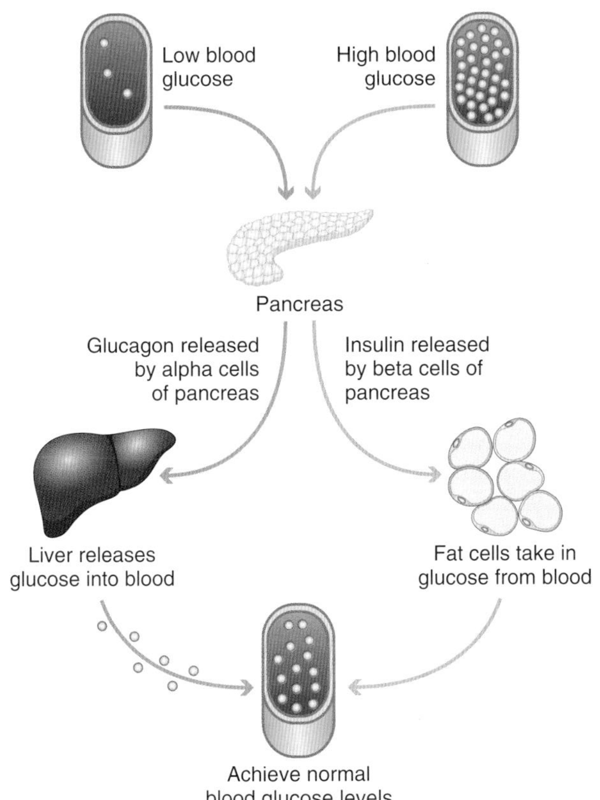


**Figure 11.9**

**Endocrine function of the pancreas.** Type 2 diabetes can promote excess sugar release from the liver, render the pancreas incapable of producing sufficient insulin, and dampen the effects of insulin on muscle and fat. Normally after intake of food, the stomach transforms food into glucose, which then enters the bloodstream. Rising blood glucose levels signal beta cells in the pancreas to release insulin. The insulin transports glucose into the cell and sets up a cascade of events (e.g., increased rate of glucose utilization and adenosine triphosphate [ATP] generation, conversion of glucose to glycogen, increase in protein and fat synthesis) that eventually results in a decline in blood glucose concentration and restoration of homeostasis. When the blood glucose levels drop (such as occurs in a hypoglycemic state or when fasting), alpha cells in the pancreas produce glucagon, which increases the blood glucose levels by stimulating the liver and other cells to release stored glucose (a process called *glycogenolysis*). The blood glucose concentration rises, thus restoring the proper balance and returning the body to a state of homeostasis. Either beta-cell dysfunction or insulin resistance can disrupt this process, resulting in decreased plasma insulin and ultimately hyperglycemia.

age, obesity, low cardiorespiratory fitness, and lack of exercise.[470] Type 2 DM occurs more frequently in women with prior gestational DM and in individuals with hypertension or dyslipidemia. Its frequency varies in different racial/ethnic groups (see Box 11.3).

**Pathogenesis.** Insulin is a hormone secreted by the beta cells of the pancreas that transports glucose into the cell for use as energy and storage as glycogen: it turns food into energy. It also stimulates protein synthesis and free fatty acid storage in the fat deposits. In DM, insulin is either insufficient in amount (type 1) or ineffective in action (type 2).

Insulin deficiency compromises the body tissues' access to essential nutrients for fuel and storage.[408] When glucose levels are elevated normally (e.g., after eating a meal), beta cells increase secretion of insulin to transport and dispose of the glucose into peripheral tissues, thereby lowering blood glucose levels and reestablishing blood glucose homeostasis. Defects in the pancreas, liver, or skeletal muscle, singularly or collectively, can contribute to abnormal glucose homeostasis when cells in each of these areas do not respond to insulin.

Normally, after a meal, the blood glucose level rises. The liver takes up a large amount of this glucose for storage or for use by other tissues such as skeletal muscle and fat. When insulin is deficient or its function is impaired, the glucose in the general circulation is not taken up or removed by these tissues; thus, it continues to accumulate in the blood, a condition called *hyperglycemia*. Because new glucose has not been deposited in the liver, the liver produces more glucose and releases it into the general circulation, which increases the already elevated blood glucose level (Fig. 11.9).[408]

When a true deficiency of insulin exists, such as that which occurs in type 1 DM diabetes, the following three major metabolic problems exist: (1) decreased utilization of glucose (as described), (2) increased fat mobilization, and (3) impaired protein utilization. Cells that require insulin for transporting glucose inside the cell, such as in skeletal and cardiac muscle and adipose tissue, are affected most, whereas nerve tissue, erythrocytes, and the cells of the intestines, liver, and kidney tubules, which do not require insulin for glucose transport, are affected the least.

In an attempt to restore balance and normal levels of glucose, the kidney excretes the excess glucose, resulting in glucosuria (sugar in the urine). Glucose excreted in the urine acts as an osmotic diuretic and causes excretion of increased amounts of water. This process results in fluid volume deficit (see Chapter 5). The conscious person becomes extremely thirsty and drinks large amounts of water (polydipsia).

Increased fat mobilization occurs because the body can rely on fat stores for energy when glucose is not available. The process of fat metabolism leads to the formation of breakdown products called *ketones*, which accumulate in the blood and are excreted through the kidneys and lungs. Ketones can be measured in the blood and the urine to indicate the presence of diabetes. Ketones interfere with the acid–base balance by producing hydrogen ions. The pH can fall, and the affected person can develop metabolic acidosis (see Chapter 5).

After the renal threshold for ketones is exceeded, the ketones appear in the urine as acetone (ketonuria). When large amounts of glucose and ketones are excreted, osmotic diuresis becomes more severe and fluid and electrolyte loss through the kidneys increases. Sodium, potassium, and other critical electrolytes are lost in the urine, resulting in severe dehydration and electrolyte deficiency and worsening acidosis. When fats are used for a primary source of energy, the body lipid level can rise to five times the normal amount. This elevated level can lead to atherosclerosis and its subsequent cardiovascular complications (see Chapter 12).

Impaired protein utilization occurs because the transport of amino acids (the chief constituent of proteins)

**Table 11.13** Cardinal Signs of Diabetes at Diagnosis

| Clinical Manifestations | Pathophysiologic Bases |
|---|---|
| Polyuria (excessive urination, types 1 and 2) | Water is not reabsorbed from renal tubules because of osmotic activity of glucose in the tubules |
| Polydipsia (excessive thirst, types 1 and 2) | Polyuria causes dehydration, which causes thirst |
| Polyphagia (excessive hunger, type 1) | Starvation secondary to tissue breakdown causes hunger |
| Weight loss (type 1) | Glucose is not available to the cells; body breaks down fat and protein stores for energy; dehydration |
| Recurrent blurred vision (types 1 and 2) | Chronic exposure of the lenses and retina to hyperosmolar fluids causes blurring of vision |
| Ketonuria (type 1) | Fatty acids are broken down so ketones are present in urine |
| Weakness, fatigue, and dizziness (types 1 and 2) | Dehydration leads to postural hypotension; energy deficiency and protein catabolism contribute to fatigue and weakness |
| Often asymptomatic (type 2) | Physical adaptation often occurs because rise in blood glucose is gradual |

into cells requires insulin. Normally, proteins are constantly being broken down and rebuilt. Without insulin to transport amino acids, thereby contributing to protein synthesis, the balance is altered and protein catabolism increases. Catabolism of body proteins and resultant protein loss hamper the inflammatory process and diminish the tissue's ability to repair itself.

Because the person with type 2 DM continues to produce and use some amount of endogenous insulin, the metabolic problems associated with inappropriate use of fat and protein for energy do not occur as severely. People with type 2 DM are not prone to ketoacidosis and the metabolic derangements associated with type 1 DM. They are, however, still at great risk for hyperglycemic osmotic diuresis, dehydration, shock, and loss of electrolytes.[408]

**Clinical Manifestations**

***Pathophysiology of Diabetic Complications.*** The long-term presence of DM affects the large blood vessels (macrovascular), small blood vessels (microvascular), and nerves throughout the body. The chronic hyperglycemia of diabetes results in the accelerated atherosclerosis that leads to macrovascular disease, affecting arteries that supply the heart, brain, and lower extremities. Insulin resistance syndrome has also been implicated in the macrovascular changes in diabetes.[59,168]

Diabetes is also associated with the development of diabetes-specific microvascular pathology in the retina, renal glomerulus, and peripheral nerve. As a result, diabetes is a leading cause of blindness, kidney failure, and a variety of debilitating neuropathies. The microvascular disease in the retina, glomerulus, and vasa nervorum has similar underlying pathophysiology.

Hyperglycemia causes abnormalities in blood flow and increased vascular permeability (caused by decreased activity of vasodilators, increased activity of vasoconstrictors, and abnormal production of extracellular matrix), and with time, microvascular cell loss and progressive capillary occlusion occur. In addition, hyperglycemia may also decrease production of trophic factors, which are required to maintain healthy endothelial and neuronal cells.

How does hyperglycemia cause these macrovascular and microvascular damages? Four main molecular mechanisms have been proposed: increased polyol pathway flux; increased advanced glycation end-product formation; activation of protein kinase C isoforms; and increased hexosamine pathway flux.[64,68] All four mechanisms seem to reflect a single hyperglycemia-induced process of overproduction of superoxide by the mitochondrial electron-transport chain. As an example, neuropathy in diabetes presumably results from the increased polyol pathway flux and is related to the accumulation in the nerve cells of sorbitol, a by-product of improper glucose metabolism. This accumulation then results in abnormal fluid and electrolyte shifts and nerve-cell dysfunction. The combination of this metabolic derangement and the diminished vascular perfusion to nerve tissues contributes to the severe problem of diabetic neuropathy.

***Cardinal Signs and Symptoms.*** In type 1 diabetes, symptoms of marked hyperglycemia include polyuria, polydipsia, weight loss with polyphagia, and blurred vision (Table 11.13). These symptoms occur as a result of the inability of the body to use glucose appropriately and the resulting osmotic diuresis, dehydration, and starvation of body tissues. In type 1 DM, the utilization of fats and proteins for energy causes severe hunger, fatigue, and weight loss. The person with this type of diabetes may present initially in DKA.

People with type 2 diabetes also may have some of these cardinal signs and symptoms, but the aging population may not recognize the abnormal thirst or frequent urination as abnormal for their age. The person with type 2 diabetes frequently goes undiagnosed for many years because onset of type 2 DM is often gradual enough that the classic signs of hyperglycemia are not noticed. More commonly, they may experience visual blurring, neuropathic complications (e.g., foot pain), infections, and significant blood lipid abnormalities. Type 2 DM is commonly diagnosed while the client is hospitalized or receiving medical care for another problem. Frequently, the person presents with one of the long-term complications of DM such as CVD, neuropathy, retinopathy, or nephropathy.

***Atherosclerosis.*** Because of the hyperglycemia and increased fat metabolism associated with type 1 DM, atherosclerosis begins earlier and is more extensive among people with diabetes than in the general population. Atherosclerotic changes in large blood vessels, caused by lipid accumulation and thickening of vessel walls, result in decreased vessel lumen size, compromised blood flow, and ischemia to adjacent tissues. As a consequence, people with diabetes have a much higher risk of myocardial infarction, stroke, and limb amputation.

Atherosclerosis and the accompanying large-vessel changes result in cardiovascular and cerebrovascular changes, skin and nail changes, poor tissue perfusion,

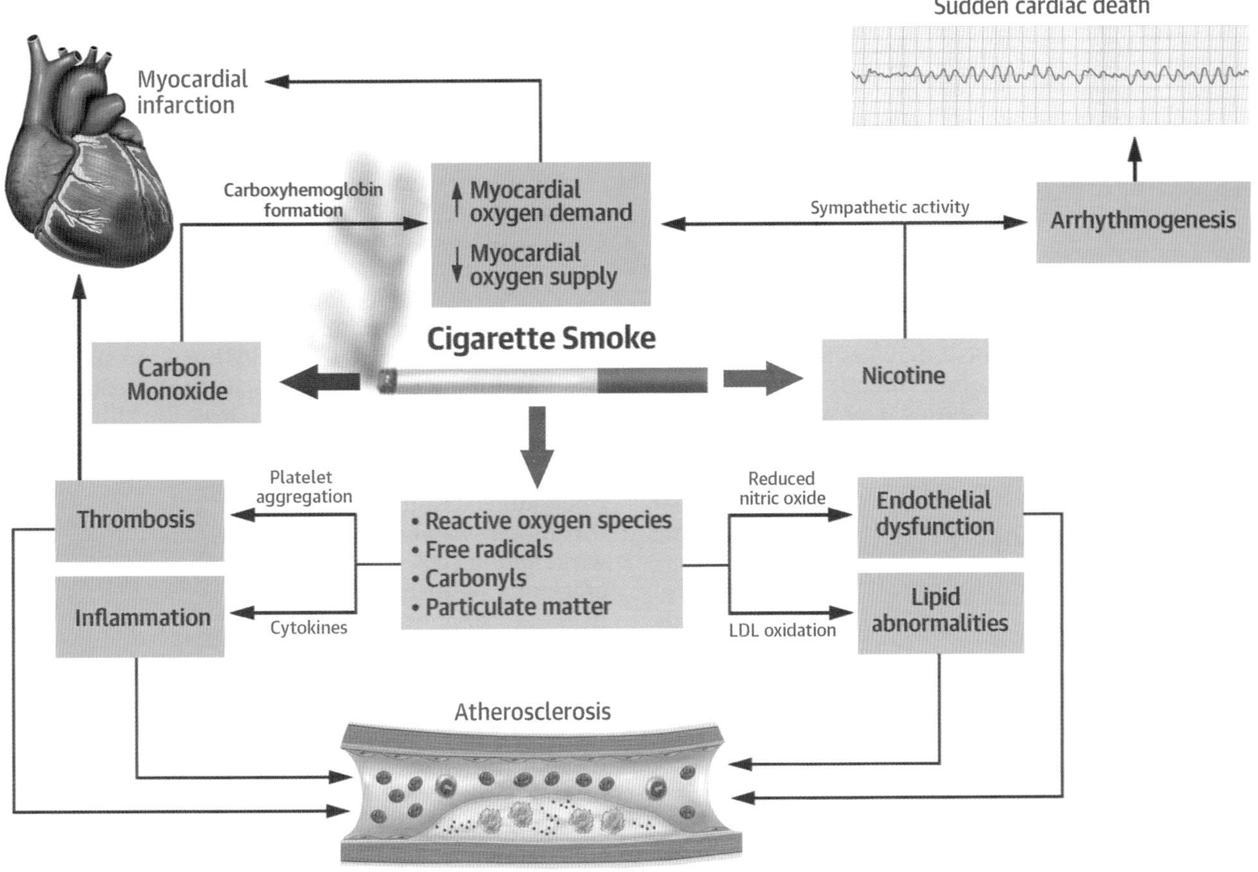


**Figure 11.10**

**Schematic showing the contribution smoking to the development of cardiovascular disease.** (From Kalkhoran S, Benowitz NL, Rigotti NA: Prevention and treatment of tobacco use. *J Am Coll Cardiol* 72(9):1030–1045, 2018. https://doi.org/10.1016/j.jacc.2018.06.036.)

decreased or absent pedal pulses, and impaired wound healing. Atherosclerosis combined with peripheral neuropathy and the subsequent foot deformities increases the risk for pressure injury of skin and underlying tissues and limb amputation.

Individuals with undiagnosed type 2 DM are at significantly higher risk for CAD, stroke, and peripheral vascular disease than the population without diabetes. Screening of the type 2 at-risk population is essential in the prevention and treatment of diabetes-related complications. In addition, all individuals with diabetes should be aware of the strong and consistent data regarding the risks of smoking and the exacerbation of atherosclerosis-related diabetic complications.

Clients and families should be consistently and continuously counseled and encouraged in smoking cessation. Smoking has been implicated in the progression from impaired glucose tolerance to development of type 2 DM. The combination of smoking and diabetes dramatically increases the risks related to atherosclerotic vessel disease, impaired wound healing, and the associated morbidity and mortality rates. Smoking is also associated with premature development of microvascular diabetes-related complications (Fig. 11.10).[15,400]

***Cardiovascular Complications.*** CVD is the leading cause of mortality and morbidity in diabetes and accounts for approximately two-thirds of all deaths among the diabetic population.[91] People with diabetes have 1.5- to 4-fold increased risk of having CAD, stroke, and myocardial infarction.[91] Although diabetes has long been recognized as a potent and prevalent risk factor of ischemic heart disease caused by coronary atherosclerosis, diabetes has also become associated with left ventricular dysfunction independent of hypertension and CAD. This is a disease of a cardiac muscle itself and is called *diabetic cardiomyopathy*.[3,140,210]

Individuals with diabetic cardiomyopathy initially exhibit frequent left ventricular diastolic filling and relaxation abnormalities, later followed by systolic dysfunction, left ventricular hypertrophy, and left heart failure.[311] Diabetic cardiomyopathy is not fully explained by the cellular effects of hyperglycemia alone; the important mechanisms include metabolic disturbances, myocardial fibrosis, small vessel disease, cardiac autonomic neuropathy, and insulin resistance.[140,181,311] Because of the presence of autonomic neuropathy, people with diabetes may have what is called "silent ischemia" or silent heart attack. They do not experience typical pain because of the damage to nerves that occurs in diabetes.

The cardiovascular and renal systems are intricately connected and affected by diabetes. Low blood flow to the kidney causes a release of renin, which in turn triggers a cascade of events as angiotensin is converted to angiotensin I and then to angiotensin II, resulting in large increases in blood pressure. The risk of myocardial infarction and stroke increases as well.

***Retinopathy and Nephropathy.*** Diabetic retinopathy is a highly specific vascular complication in persons with both type 1 and type 2 DM, and its prevalence is correlated closely with duration and control of high blood glucose levels. After 20 years with DM, nearly all individuals with type 1 DM and more than 60% of type 2 DM have some degree of retinopathy.

Diabetic retinopathy poses a serious threat to vision. People with type 1 and type 2 diabetes should undergo yearly comprehensive eye exams. Underlying microvascular occlusion of the retina resulting in progressive areas of retinal ischemia and tissue death causes diabetic retinopathy. Studies have established that intensive management of blood glucose level control to consistent near-normal levels can prevent and delay the progression of diabetic retinopathy.[118]

Exercise may be protective against the development of macular degeneration, and individuals with diabetic retinopathy may benefit from low- to moderate-intensity aerobic and resistance exercise.[274] However, individuals with proliferative or preproliferative retinopathy should be screened by a physician prior to beginning an exercise program. High-intensity exercise and high-impact activities and head-down activities can greatly increase eye pressure and should be avoided.[91,244]

Diabetes is now the leading cause of end-stage renal disease, which is kidney failure requiring dialysis or transplantation, in the United States and Europe.[77,270] Hardening and thickening of the glomerular basement membrane, which result in eventual destruction of critical renal filtration structures, cause diabetic nephropathy. The presence of small amounts of albumin in the urine, called microalbuminuria, is the earliest clinical evidence of nephropathy. Approximately one of four people with type 2 diabetes have microalbuminuria that, if untreated, gradually worsens. Eventual destruction of the filtering ability of the kidney causes chronic renal failure and the need for permanent dialysis or renal transplantation.

Renal destruction, as with retinopathy, can be slowed significantly with early detection and monitoring, tight glucose control, early treatment of hypertension (particularly with angiotensin-converting enzyme [ACE] inhibitors), careful monitoring of dietary protein, and strong encouragement of cessation of smoking.[118,127,194] Hypertension is managed with ACE inhibitors initially, and if blood pressure is not less than 130/85 mm Hg, a β-blocker may be added. However, combining a β-blocker with a diuretic can blunt awareness and symptoms of low glucose, so this combination usually is not recommended.

Even though protein excretion increases after exercise, exercise does not accelerate progression of diabetes-related chronic kidney disease (DM/CKD). Furthermore, greater participation in physical activity lowers the odds of developing DM/CKD and lowers risk or mortality in patients with the condition.[466] People with CKD/DM can safely engage in aerobic and resistance exercise from low to vigorous intensities commensurate with their level of physical fitness. Vigorous exercise should be avoided the day before urine protein tests are done to prevent false-positive readings. Low- to moderate-intensity exercise programs, supervised by a qualified health care professional, are recommended for patients with end-stage renal disease to support cardiovascular endurance and muscle strength. Supervised exercise can be performed during dialysis sessions or on alternate days.[91]

***Infection.*** Chronic, poorly controlled diabetes mellitus can lead to a variety of blood vessel and tissue changes that result in impaired wound healing and markedly increased risk for infections. Impaired vision and peripheral neuropathy contribute to the decreased ability of the person with diabetes to feel or see breaks in skin integrity and developing wounds. Vascular disease contributes to tissue hypoxia, which further decreases healing ability.

In addition, once pathogens are inside the body, they multiply rapidly because the increased glucose content in body fluids and tissues fosters bacterial growth. Because the blood supply to tissues is already compromised, white blood cells are not mobilized to the affected areas efficiently or adequately. Diabetes results in higher incidences of skin, urinary tract, vaginal, and other types of tissue infections.[207]

***Musculoskeletal Problems.*** Musculoskeletal complications are common, often involving the hands, shoulders, spine, and feet. Carpal tunnel syndrome, Dupuytren contracture, trigger finger (tenosynovitis), and adhesive capsulitis occur significantly more often in people with diabetes compared with those who do not have diabetes.[360] Available data show that more than 30% of people with type 1 or type 2 DM have some kind of hand or shoulder disease. More people with type 1 DM have musculoskeletal disorders than those with type 2 DM, and the degree of stiffness is greater with this type of diabetes. The exact mechanism by which the specific metabolic abnormalities of diabetes are linked to rheumatic manifestations remains unclear but appears to be linked to significantly higher A1c levels.[11,360]

Although these disorders are not life-threatening, they can add significant functional impairment to a person's life. See also the discussion of orthopedic problems that can develop secondary to sensory and motor neuropathy in "Sensory, Motor, and Autonomic Neuropathy" below.

Upper Extremity. In the hand, the syndrome of limited joint mobility (SLJM or LJM) and the stiff hand syndrome are unique to diabetes. SLJM is characterized by painless stiffness and limitation of the finger joints (Fig. 11.11). Flexion contractures typically progress to result in loss of dexterity and grip strength. The SLJM is an underdiagnosed complication of diabetes, largely because this type of loss of hand range of motion is considered a common normal sign of aging.[172] The severity of this syndrome in diabetes is correlated with the duration of disease, duration and quantity of insulin therapy, and smoking. Joint contractures also may develop in larger joints, such as the elbows, shoulders, knees, and spine.

The stiff hand syndrome often is confused with or included in SLJM, but it has a distinct pathogenesis and clinical presentation. The stiff hand syndrome occurs uniquely with diabetes and is seen more frequently with type 1 DM and poor blood glucose control. Paresthesias, which eventually become painful, are accompanied by subcutaneous tissue changes such as stiffness and

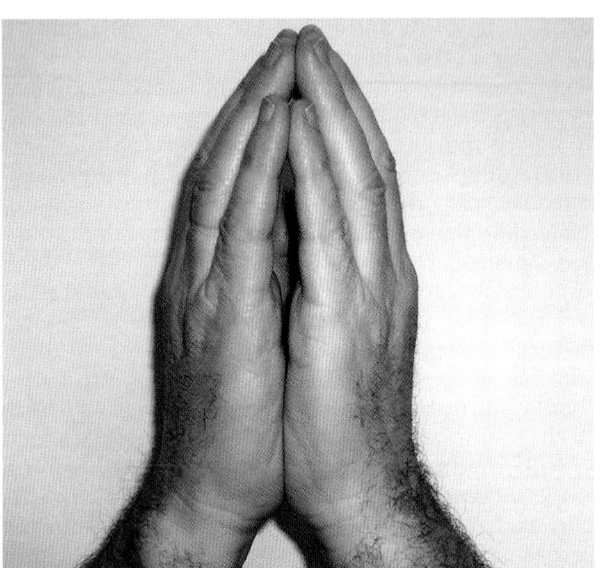

**Figure 11.11**

**The prayer sign.** The individual is unable to press the palms flat against each other, a diagnostic sign for the syndrome of limited joint mobility in diabetic persons. Other conditions also may result in loss of extension with a positive prayer sign. (From Drake WM, Glynn M: *Hutchison's clinical methods: An integrated approach to clinical practice,* ed 24, St. Louis, 2018, Elsevier Ltd.)

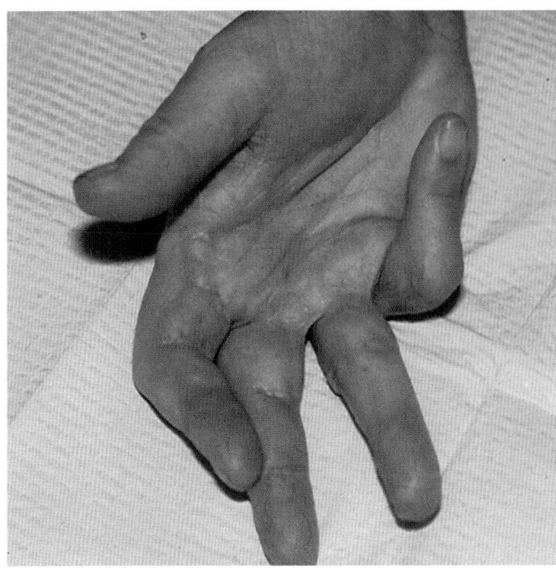

**Figure 11.12**

**Dupuytren contracture.** The contracture may be symptomatic (painful), but with or without pain it results in impaired hand function. (From Skirven TM, et al: *Rehabilitation of the hand and upper extremity,* ed 7, St. Louis, 2021, Elsevier.)

hardness. Vascular insufficiency may be the underlying cause or may be secondary to neuropathy, nodular tenosynovitis, and osteoarthritis.

Dupuytren contracture is characterized by the formation of a flexion contracture, palmar nodules, and thickening band or cord of palmar fascia (Fig. 11.12), usually involving the third and fourth digits in the population with diabetes (rather than the fourth and fifth digits in the population without diabetes). Pain and decreased range of motion are the primary presentation. Painless nodules develop in the distal palmar crease, often in line with the ring finger, which slowly mature into a longitudinal cord that is readily distinguishable from a tendon. The skin overlying the nodules is usually puckered.

In some cases, regression of symptoms does occur without intervention, although the underlying mechanism for this phenomenon remains unknown. Surgical excision has not been shown to be a reliable cure for the disease and is not recommended unless there is a contracture that is bothersome. It has been reported that if the disease recurs after surgical excision, the rate of progression may be faster.[364]

Flexor tenosynovitis (also called *chronic stenosing tenosynovitis*) is another rheumatologic condition seen more commonly in persons with diabetes. Tenosynovitis is caused by accumulation of fibrous tissue in the tendon sheath and can cause aching, nodularity along the flexor tendons, and contracture. Locking of the digit, called *trigger finger*, can occur in flexion or extension and may be associated with crepitus or pain. In the population with diabetes, tenosynovitis is found predominantly in women and affects the thumb, middle, and ring fingers most often.

Diabetes is the systemic disease most often seen in connection with peripheral neuropathy of the hand, including CTS. The clinical presentation of CTS is the same for the person with diabetes as for the person without diabetes, although in diabetes CTS can be either a neuropathic process or an entrapment problem. Both neuropathy and compression within the carpal tunnel may exist together.

Adhesive capsulitis (also known as *periarthritis* or *frozen shoulder*) is characterized by diffuse shoulder pain and loss of motion in all directions, often with a positive painful arc test and limited joint accessory motions. The pattern is slightly different from that of typical adhesive capsulitis, in which regional tightness in the anteroinferior joint capsule primarily compromises external rotation, followed by loss of abduction and, less often, internal rotation and flexion.

The pattern in diabetes is one of significant global tightness with external and internal rotation equally limited in the dominant shoulder, followed by limitations in abduction and hyperextension. External rotation and hyperextension are most limited in the nondominant shoulder, followed by internal rotation and abduction. The pathogenesis of the capsular thickening and adherence to the humeral head remains unknown. The long head of the biceps tendon may become glued down in its tendon sheath on the anterior humeral head.[427]

Adhesive capsulitis may be accompanied by vasomotor instability of the hand previously referred to as reflex sympathetic dystrophy but now classified as the complex regional pain syndrome. This condition is characterized by severe pain, swelling, and trophic skin changes of the hand (e.g., thinning and shininess of the skin with loss of wrinkling, sometimes with increased hair growth).

Skin changes in diabetic hand arthropathy, in addition to changes caused by complex regional pain syndrome, may occur in association with adhesive capsulitis. Other skin changes associated with diabetes include scleroderma

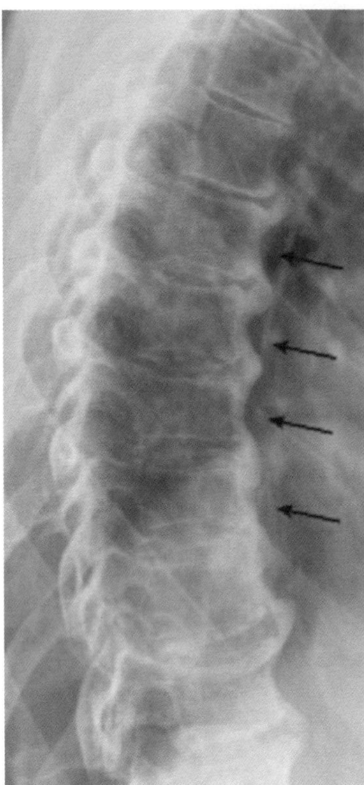

**Figure 11.13**

**Diffuse idiopathic skeletal hyperostosis (DISH), or ankylosing hyperostosis, associated with type 2 diabetes mellitus (DM).** DISH can occur with other conditions, such as ankylosing spondylitis. The thoracic spine is most commonly involved in diabetes. This type of DISH can be distinguished from ankylosing spondylitis by the preservation of sacroiliac joints, a site of typical involvement in ankylosing spondylitis. (From Devlin VJ: *Spine secrets*, ed 3, St. Louis, 2021, Elsevier.)

diabeticorum, an asymptomatic thickening of the skin that may lead to a peau d'orange appearance, which usually involves the posterior neck, upper back, and shoulders.[65] Skin and subcutaneous tissue atrophy and tendon flexion contractures develop. The natural history of this condition ranges from spontaneous remission to permanent loss of function.

Tendinopathy with thickening of the plantar fascia and Achilles tendon and tendo-Achilles tightening occurs as glucose deposits in tendons and ligaments result in loss of flexibility and rigid foot. In the diabetic population, loss of Achilles tendon flexibility, especially when combined with a flatfoot, increases pressure under the foot, adding to the compressive forces that contribute to pressure injury formation.[165]

Spine. Diffuse idiopathic skeletal hyperostosis (DISH; also known as *ankylosing hyperostosis* or *Forestier disease*) is a condition of the spine seen most often in people with type 2 DM, although it can occur in a person who does not have diabetes. In DISH, osteophytes develop into bony spurs, typically right-sided syndesmophytes that may join to form bridges (Fig. 11.13). The thoracic spine most commonly is involved. In contrast to ankylosing spondylitis, the sacroiliac joints are spared, and vertebral body osteoporosis is absent. Calcaneal and olecranon spurs may develop, and new bone may form around the hips, knees, and wrists.

People with DISH may be asymptomatic, or they may experience back pain and stiffness without limitations in range of motion. Dysphagia may develop if extensive cervical spine involvement occurs. The pathogenesis of DISH is unknown, and apparently no correlation exists between the degree of diabetic control and the extent of hyperostosis.

Arthritis. Nearly half of people with diabetes also have arthritis. Moreover, the prevalence of arthritis-attributable activity limitations is significantly higher in adults with both diseases compared to adults with arthritis but not diabetes.[84] The prevalence of arthritis is higher with increased age, BMI, and physical inactivity. Both rheumatoid arthritis and osteoarthritis have been associated with diabetes, in different ways. Type 1 DM and rheumatoid arthritis are both autoimmune diseases. Levels of inflammatory markers, including C-reactive protein, IL-6, and TNF-$\alpha$, high in people with rheumatoid arthritis, have also been found to be elevated in people with type 1 DM for longer than five years. The common connection between osteoarthritis and type 2 DM is obesity and related chronic inflammation.[84,481] This connection has important implications for exercise prescription. Thirty to 60 minutes of continuous walking per day is often recommended for weight management and blood sugar control. However, in people with knee osteoarthritis, continuous walking for greater than 30 minutes has been associated with high joint loads, elevation of a biomarker indicative of cartilage turnover, and increased joint pain. Interval walking regimens, incorporating rest breaks, may potentiate negative effects longer continuous bouts may have on the knee joint and also limit pain during exercise.[213]

Osteoporosis. Generalized osteoporosis usually develops within the first 5 years after the onset of DM and is more severe in persons with type 1 DM. It is hypothesized that bone matrix formation may be inadequate in the absence of normal circulating insulin levels. Results of bone density studies in persons with type 2 DM are conflicting, with some studies demonstrating decreased bone density and others indicating increased bone density. While bone mass may remain normal in people with type 2 DM, bone quality may be impaired.

As in any case of osteoporosis, regardless of the underlying cause, this condition places the person at greater risk for fractures. With the additional loss of sensation associated with diabetes, minor trauma easily produces injury. Microfractures can occur in already weakened bone and cartilage and may remain unrecognized because of the lack of pain appreciation. A vicious circle is started, leading to further damage.

A class of oral diabetes medication called glitazones and a medication called canagliflozin may promote bone loss and osteoporotic fractures in postmenopausal women.[186,336] Good blood sugar control, supported by a healthy diet and regular exercise, is important for bone health and prevention of fractures.

***Sensory, Motor, and Autonomic Neuropathy.*** Sensory, motor, and autonomic neuropathy associated with DM is a common phenomenon with known risk factors (e.g., duration of diabetes, current A1c [glycated hemoglobin value], BMI, smoking, hypertension, and high triglycerides). The presence of CVD doubles the risk of neuropathy.[432]

Neuropathy may affect the CNS, peripheral nervous system, or autonomic nervous system. The most common form of diabetic neuropathy is a sensory polyneuropathy, usually affecting the hands and feet and causing symptoms that range from mild tingling, burning, numbness, or pain to a complete loss of sensation (usually feet) and foot drop.

Sensory Neuropathy. Many people with diabetes suffer from *diabetic peripheral neuropathic pain* (DPNP) associated with nerve damage. Spontaneous pain, allodynia (painful response to benign stimuli), hyperalgesia, and other unpleasant symptoms are common with DPNP. Neuropathic pain often progressively increases in intensity throughout the day and is worse at night, significantly impairing sleep. Some individuals experience painful neuropathy called *insulin neuritis syndrome* at the beginning of therapy for diabetes; the feet are affected more often than the hands, and it is usually self-limiting.[458]

The loss of sensation in diabetic neuropathy predisposes joints to repeated microtrauma and progressive, noninfectious joint destruction. Chronic progressive degeneration of the stress-bearing portion of a joint associated with loss of proprioceptive sensation in the joint produces a condition called *Charcot disease, Charcot arthropathy, neuroarthropathy,* or *neuropathic arthropathy.* Diabetes is the most common cause of neuropathic joints. Charcot neuroarthropathy presents in people with type 1 diabetes after an average duration of 20 to 24 years and in individuals with type 2 diabetes after only 5 to 9 years.[351]

Several stages of neuropathic arthropathy (Charcot foot) occur involving autonomic dysfunction of blood flow leading to bone destruction and absorption resulting in dislocation, deformity, and an unstable joint. Bone fragments and debris are deposited in the affected joint. Subluxation of the tarsal and metatarsal joints commonly results in a rocker-bottom foot deformity and a redistribution of pressure on the plantar surface of the foot with progressive pressure injury (ulceration) and possible infection. An acute neuropathic joint is swollen, warm, and edematous with bounding distal pulses. Pain may be minimal because of the underlying altered sensation, but up to half of all affected individuals report some degree of pain.[61]

Left untreated, neuropathic changes can progress to complete destruction of the joint. The presence of autonomic neuropathy may hasten this process because the blood vessels are unable to respond appropriately (e.g., vasoconstrict) to even minor trauma. Prolonged and unregulated hyperemia in the foot may lead to excessive bone resorption, resulting in decreased bone mineral density, further increasing the risk of bone and joint destruction.[450]

Joints with less movement transmit abnormal forces through the foot to injure already damaged joints. This is especially true during walking, when large forces are placed on the midtarsal and tarsometatarsal joints. Obesity further increases these forces, and in the presence of any preexisting gait abnormalities or deformities, both create additional stress that compounds the condition.

Assessment of the underlying problem is important in planning the appropriate treatment intervention. For example, improving circulation may be a goal with macrovascular or peripheral vascular disease, whereas foot care and orthoses are more appropriate treatments for microvascular-caused neuropathy. The underlying neurologic disorder should be treated, but this has no effect on the existing arthropathy. Reduction of weight bearing, joint immobilization, and joint protection are important conservative treatment tools. Surgical fusion can be performed if all else fails, but joint replacement is contraindicated in this condition.[81,379]

Medications aimed at chronic neuropathic pain have included tricyclic antidepressants (e.g., amitriptyline, nortriptyline, or imipramine), but anticholinergic effects, such as dry mouth, blurred vision, constipation, cardiac arrhythmias, and orthostatic hypotension, often limit their use.

Anticonvulsants, such as gabapentin (Neurontin) and pregabalin (Lyrica), have met with greater success. Selective serotonin reuptake inhibitors (SSRIs), such as duloxetine (Cymbalta), can be used by some individuals to treat painful DPNP. By inhibiting the reuptake of these neurotransmitters, descending inhibitory pathways in the spinal cord are activated and block ascending pain signals to the brain.[456] For individuals who fail to respond to nonnarcotic medications, narcotic analgesics, such as tramadol and oxycodone, may be considered as a second medication. In a large multicenter clinical trial, alpha-lipoic acid (an antioxidant) was found to decrease neuropathic pain and improve nerve conduction. Modest decreases in pain have also been reported with acetyl-L-carnitine, which may be deficient in neural fibers of people with type 2 DM.[252]

Exercise is known to improve metabolic and micro- and macrovascular health factors that affect nerve health.[422] A growing body of evidence suggests that exercise as part of a healthy lifestyle intervention may have a protective effect, preventing DPN in people with diabetes. Furthermore, in people with DPN, exercise may preserve or facilitate growth in sensory nerve fibers and thereby mediate neuropathic pain.[242] With appropriate monitoring, weight-bearing exercise that meets U.S. Department of Health and Human Services guidelines[446] for physical activity has been shown to be safe and effective in improving physical function and metabolic health in people with diabetes and DPN.[267] However, the specific mechanism of exercise-induced nerve protection and regeneration and the dosage of exercise needed for prevention and management of DPN are not yet well understood.

Motor Neuropathy. Motor neuropathy is more common with long-standing disease and produces weakness and atrophy; bilateral but asymmetric proximal muscle weakness is called *diabetic amyotrophy*. Diabetic amyotrophy leads to bony deformities (e.g., claw toes, severe flatfoot with valgus of the midfoot, or collapse of the longitudinal arch) that contribute to biomechanical changes in foot function, resulting in abnormal patterns of loading. Pain and erythema of the forefoot may constitute forefoot osteolysis, which is sometimes considered another form of neuropathy distinguished from cellulitis or osteomyelitis by laboratory values (leukocyte count) and roentgenographic appearance.

Autonomic Neuropathy. Autonomic neuropathy is sometimes referred to as *diabetic autonomic neuropathy* and affects nerves that innervate heart, lung, stomach, intestines, bladder, and reproductive organs. It may manifest itself through the loss of control of blood pressure, blood glucose levels, temperature, regulation of sweating (skin becomes dry and cracked with buildup of callus), and blood flow in the limbs. Skin changes such as these can create more openings for bacteria to enter. The combination of all three types of neuropathy can ultimately lead to gangrene and possible amputation, largely preventable with proper care.

Cardiovascular autonomic neuropathy is manifested by the lack of heart rate variability in response to deep breathing and exercise, exercise intolerance, persistent sinus tachycardia, bradycardia, and postural hypotension. Stress testing should be considered before starting an exercise program, especially in the older adult.[26,27,92,201] Cardiovascular autonomic neuropathy may also result in reduced perception of ischemic pain, making a person with diabetes unaware of having a heart attack. This may delay appropriate medical treatment and lead to death.[457]

Diabetic autonomic neuropathy may lead to hypoglycemia without awareness because of loss of the warning signs of hypoglycemia such as sweating and palpitations. Being unaware of hypoglycemia and unresponsive to it are troublesome metabolic complications because they impair the person's ability to manage the disease and may result in death. Other forms of autonomic neuropathy include gastroparesis (decreased gastrointestinal motility accompanied by diarrhea and fecal incontinence), constipation, urinary tract infections (nerve damage can prevent the bladder from emptying completely, allowing bacteria to grow in the bladder and kidneys), urinary incontinence, and sexual (erectile) dysfunction.

Pressure Injury (Ulceration). Sensory neuropathy, occurring as a result of improper glucose metabolism and diminished vascular perfusion to nerve tissues, places the diabetic person at risk for the development of ulcers. Diabetic foot ulcers are caused primarily by repetitive stress on the insensitive skin with increased pressure and/or horizontal (shear) stress. Body weight and activity level increase the force that the foot must transmit, and this also may increase pressure and shear force, especially in the presence of an underlying bony prominence or foot imbalance. In addition, previously healed ulcers leave scars that transmit force to underlying tissues in a more concentrated manner and hold the fat pad locally so that it cannot function physiologically. As a result, it cannot transmit shear forces, and it becomes damaged easily.

The loss of autonomic nerve function eliminates the production of sweat, leaving the skin dry and inelastic. Changes in pressure and gait, fat atrophy, and muscle weakness are mechanical factors that, along with sensory neuropathy, influence the development of plantar skin abnormalities, especially ulceration.[49,407] Diabetes-induced changes in the skin are likely to contribute to ulceration because the collagen and keratin (a protein that is the principal constituent of epidermis, hair, and nails) may be glycosylated (saturated with glucose) with increased cross-linking, which makes the skin stiff. Keratin builds up in response to the increased pressure, covering the openings of unhealed ulcers, and cannot be removed as readily as normal keratin.

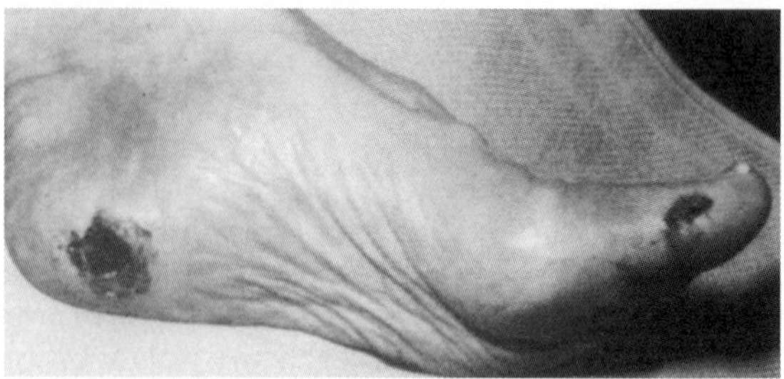

**Figure 11.14**

**Neurotrophic ulcers associated with diabetic neuropathy.** (From Callen JP, Jorizzo JL: *Dermatological signs of internal disease*, Philadelphia, 1995, WB Saunders.)

The areas most commonly affected by foot ulcers are the plantar areas of the metatarsal heads, the toes, and the plantar area of the hallux (Fig. 11.14). In the Charcot foot, the incidence of ulceration beneath the talus and navicular bones becomes more common because of the rigid rocker-bottom deformity.

Cognitive Function. Clearly, diabetes has deleterious effects on cardiovascular, renal, eye, peripheral nerve, and musculoskeletal function. The effects of diabetes on cognitive function are less well known. There is evidence that, in comparison to older adults without DM, older adults with DM may exhibit greater deficits in high-level cognitive processes responsible for planning, coordinating, and sequencing of cognitive operations. Impairments in these processes, collectively known as executive function, may contribute to balance and gait abnormalities, difficulty with activities of daily living, and increased risk of falls associated with diabetes.[374]

## MEDICAL MANAGEMENT

**PREVENTION.** Prevention of obesity-related health problems, including prediabetes and subsequent type 2 diabetes, is a key focus of the medical community. Therapists play an important role in providing education on the beneficial effects of exercise combined with proper nutrition. Studies have clearly shown that people who incorporate physical activity and exercise into their daily lives are less likely to develop type 2 diabetes no matter what their initial weight.[248-250]

A meta-analysis revealed a dose-response relationship for prevention of type 2 diabetes. People who adopted an activity program of 150 minutes weekly of moderate-intensity activity (e.g., brisk walking) similar to what the surgeon general advises had a 26% lower risk of developing type 2 DM compared to people who were sedentary. Achieving 300 and up to 600 minutes of moderate-intensity activity per week were associated with 36% and 53% reductions in risk, respectively.[409]

Studies using liposuction and studies using bariatric gastric bypass surgery in the overall treatment of obesity point to the efficacy of this treatment option to disrupt the pathway that brings about insulin insensitivity in the obese individual to prevent or put in remission type 2 diabetes. Fat removal by liposuction and by bariatric surgery has been linked with modification of cardiovascular risk and vascular inflammatory markers in the obese individual, with beneficial effects on insulin resistance as well.[134,342,385] New guidelines advocate for the consideration of bariatric surgery, along with medical and lifestyle management, to treat type 2 DM in patients with a BMI as low as 30 kg/m$^2$ or 27.5 kg/m$^2$ in Asian populations.[103]

**SCREENING.** The American Diabetes Association recommends universal screening for type 2 diabetes at age 45 and, if normal, repeat testing every three years. Testing should be considered in adults of any age who are overweight or obese (BMI >25) and who have one or more additional risk factors (see Box 11.9). Anyone who has been diagnosed with prediabetes should have their glucose monitored once a year.[19]

**DIAGNOSIS.** Diagnostic assessment may include a variety of testing procedures: fasting plasma glucose, oral glucose tolerance test, and A1c. A diagnosis of diabetes is confirmed by symptoms of hyperglycemia and blood and urine glucose and ketone abnormalities. Current defined criteria for definitive diagnosis of diabetes mellitus are the following:[19]

- Classic symptoms of diabetes (polyuria, polydipsia, and unexplained weight loss) plus a casual plasma glucose concentration ≥200 mg/dL. (*Casual* is defined as any time of day without regard to time since last meal.)

or

- Fasting plasma glucose (FPG) ≥126 mg/dL after no caloric intake for at least 8 hours.

or

- 2-hour postload glucose ≥200 mg/dL during an oral glucose tolerance test

or

- A1c ≥6.5%.

Obesity and type 2 diabetes are on the rise in children and adolescents. The American Diabetes Association recommends that children with body mass index at or over the 85th percentile for gender and age and two risk factors for DM (family history, race/ethnicity, signs/symptoms) be assessed for diabetes.[19]

**GLUCOSE MONITORING.** Individuals using multiple daily insulin injections or an insulin pump should perform self-monitoring of blood glucose (SMBG) three or more times a day. SMBG may also be useful for individuals using insulin injections that are less frequent, oral antidiabetes medications, or medical nutrition therapy. SMBG is also recommended when a new physical activity is introduced, such as occurs in an exercise or rehabilitation program, and should be continued until the individual's response to the change is known and predictable in maintaining stable blood glucose levels.

New insulins and easier blood glucose monitoring have improved the ability to obtain much tighter control of blood glucose levels with fewer fluctuations and reduced risk of hypoglycemia. There are two methods used to monitor glucose immediately and over time: direct blood sampling (fingersticks) and continuous glucose monitoring (CGM). CGM involves placement of a glucose sensor under the skin. The sensor measures glucose levels in the interstitial fluid and transmits this information to an electronic receiver (either an insulin pump or a pager-like device). CGM is considered to be useful for children and adults with type 1 diabetes and people with frequent hypoglycemia. In the past, CGM equipment required regular fingersticks for calibration; newer systems do not. Noninvasive technologies for SMBG such as near-infrared spectroscopy are under development. SMBG is an important management tool in the long-term treatment of this disease. Early screening and assessment of people at risk for diabetes are critical so that prevention and treatment of complications can be initiated before the onset of significant microvascular and macrovasular damage.

**Table 11.14** Correlating A1c to Mean Plasma Glucose Levels

| A1c (%) | Mean Plasma Glucose (mg/dL) |
|---|---|
| 6 | 135 |
| 7 | 170 |
| 8 | 205 |
| 9 | 240 |
| 10 | 275 |
| 11 | 310 |
| 12 | 345 |

Normal reference range for A1c is 4% to 6%. The goal for clients with diabetes is below 7% (target level is 6.5), but not everyone has the same target; it does depend on comorbidities, age, and duration of disease.[346] In general, higher levels are linked with greater risk of diabetes-related complications. A1c level of 7% correlates to an average daily plasma glucose level below 170 mg/dL. It is not used to diagnose diabetes and should not be measured too often in those who are using it to measure glucose control. Two measurements a year are sufficient in anyone who is meeting goals of treatment and who has stable control, and a maximum of 4 to 6 a year in people whose treatment has changed, or who are not meeting treatment goals.[283]
Data from American Diabetes Association, 2012.

In addition to being a diagnostic tool, A1c level is used to monitor blood glucose control over time (Table 11.14). The A1c test should be performed at least two times per year in individuals with controlled diabetes and four times per year for those whose blood sugar levels are not well controlled or who are on a new diabetes medication regimen. The American Diabetes Association recommends a target A1c level as 7% or less. A higher A1c target may be recommended for individuals who are older, have a history of severe hypoglycemic episodes, or diabetes-related health complications.[17,428] According to the U.K. Prospective Diabetes Study, a 1% reduction of the A1c level reduces the risk of microvascular complications such as retinopathy and nephropathy by 25% and heart attack by 14% or more. People with A1c concentrations less than 5% had the lowest rates of CVD and mortality.[235]

**TREATMENT.** There is no widely available cure for diabetes. The goal of overall care for persons with diabetes is control or regulation of blood glucose. Many large-scale studies have shown that tight glucose control reduces the risk of vascular complications in both type 1 and type 2 diabetes. Tight control of blood pressure lowers the risk of strokes, heart attacks, and heart failure and slows the progression of diabetic kidney disease.[424] Early identification and intervention are strongly linked with risk reduction of late complications.[268] Three key standards and goals in the treatment and self-management of DM include the following:[17,208]

- A1c less than 7%
- Blood pressure less than 130/80 mm Hg
- Low-density lipoprotein (LDL) <100 mg/dL, high-density lipoprotein (HDL) cholesterol >50 mg/dL, and triglycerides <150 mg/dL.

Data from the National Center of Health Statistics show that only 7.3% of adults with diabetes have achieved all three targets.[383] To help people with diabetes reach these goals, the National Diabetes Education Program has started an education program called *Control the ABCs*, in which *A* is A1c, *B* is blood pressure, and *C* is cholesterol). Education materials are available in English and Spanish and for Asian Americans and Pacific Islanders.[318] A new position statement from the European Association for the Study of Diabetes and the American Diabetes Association have also published new recommendations (rather than guidelines) designed to approach each person with type 2 diabetes as an individual rather than prescribing to the singular idea of "one number fits all" (referring to the A1c target).[108] The position statement lists seven key points related to glycemic targets; diet, exercise, and education; use of pharmaceuticals; consideration of individual preferences, needs, and values; and a clear focus on cardiovascular risk reduction.[6] Therapists are encouraged to read this document and help reinforce all of the concepts presented as part of their client education programs.

Data suggest that atherogenic and inflammatory mediators contributing to microvascular and macrovascular complications are elevated even before the onset of diabetes. There may even be a "metabolic memory" associated with these early changes. Comprehensive metabolic control instituted early may alter the natural history of diabetic complications by affecting this metabolic memory.[268,307]

Researchers continue to investigate drugs that would prevent the formation of fat cells, thereby reducing the problem of obesity before type 2 DM can develop. Studies of the use of gene therapy as a treatment for both types of diabetes are ongoing, utilizing a variety of approaches, such as direct delivery of the insulin gene to non–beta cells, improving insulin secretion from existing beta cells, and implanting genetically modified cells.[166,167,225,496] Experimental research is under way in the development of a vaccine for type 1 DM that may help stop the immune system attack of the insulin-producing beta cells of the pancreas.[460,475] Pancreatic islet cell and whole-pancreas transplants for treatment of diabetes is ongoing; the potential for immune rejection of the tissue remains problematic.[396,476]

**Type 1 Diabetes Mellitus.** Type 1 DM requires exogenous insulin administration and dietary management to achieve tight (near normal) blood glucose control. With no circulating endogenous insulin, the effect of aerobic exercise in providing increased glycemic control for the person with type 1 DM may be limited. To date, studies of the effect of aerobic exercise in type 1 DM have shown mixed results. Regardless, exercise should be taken into account as part of the total picture in order to minimize the complications associated with diabetes.

The insulin dosage schedule varies depending on the individual's age, level of compliance, and severity of diabetes (Table 11.15). Control over blood glucose levels dictates how "brittle" the diabetes is. *Brittle diabetes* (also known as *labile* or *unstable diabetes*) is a term used when a person's blood glucose level often swings quickly from high to low and from low to high. The individual with wide glucose excursions is considered very brittle.

Poorly controlled diabetes is ideally treated with more frequent administration of insulin (e.g., four times per day), whereas other individuals may receive insulin once or twice daily, sometimes mixing different types of

**Table 11.15** Types of Insulin and Insulin Action

| Type | Name | Onset of Action | Peak Response | Duration of Action |
|---|---|---|---|---|
| Rapid-acting insulin | Insulin lispro (Humalog) | 5 min | 30–90 min | 3–4 h |
| | Insulin aspart (NovoLog) | 15 min | 45–90 min | 3–5 h |
| | Insulin glulisine (Apidra) | 15 min | 3–5 h | 3–8 h |
| Short-acting or regular insulin | Insulin human regular (Humulin-R, Novolin-R) | 30 min | 2–3 h | 3–8 h |
| Intermediate-acting insulin | NPH insulin (Humulin N, Novolin N) | 1.5 h | 4–12 h | Up to 18 h |
| Long-acting insulin | Insulin glargine (Lantus) | 1.5-4 h | No peak | Up to 24 h |
| | Insulin detemir (Levemir) | | | |
| Premixed insulins (combination of two types of insulin) | 70/30 (%) (Humulin mix, Novolin mix)<br>50/50 (%) (Humalog mix)<br>75/25 (%) (Humalog mix)<br>70/30 (%) (NovoLog mix) | Depends on mixture; 5-30 min | Depends on mixture; 1–12 h | Up to 18 h |

**Onset of action** is how long it takes before the insulin reaches the bloodstream and starts to lower glucose levels.
**Peak response** is the time at which the insulin exhibits maximum effectiveness.
**Duration of action** is how long the insulin continues to lower blood glucose.
Data from Micromedex Healthcare Series [Internet database]. Greenwood Village, CO, Thomson Reuters Healthcare Inc. Updated periodically. Compiled by Tanner Higginbotham, PharmD, University of Montana Drug Information Service, 2012.

insulin (e.g., rapid-acting [human analog; Humalog]; short-acting [regular] with intermediate-acting [NPH] insulin). Humalog (Lispro) is a type of insulin that has rapid action. It works faster than short-acting insulin and must be taken with a meal to prevent hypoglycemia.[222] From a therapist's point of view, the client receiving more frequent dosages is less likely to develop hypoglycemia, especially when beginning an exercise program.

***Insulin Delivery System.*** A hybrid closed-loop insulin delivery system, sometimes called an artificial pancreas, that combines an insulin pump with a continuous glucose monitoring device is now available for children and adults. Information received from the continuous glucose monitor (CGM) is analyzed by the insulin pump, where a predictive algorithm is used to adjust the dose of insulin delivered accordingly throughout the day and night. The insulin pump is a lightweight, pager-sized device worn conveniently in a pocket or on a belt clip. The CGM is a lightweight disc (approximately 1 inch in diameter) that houses a small wire sensor inserted under the skin; it measures glucose readings in interstitial fluid. An adhesive patch holds the CGM on the skin (Fig. 11.15). This insulin delivery system is water resistant and can be modified to make swimming possible.

Individuals who have hybrid closed-loop systems that detect and respond to changes in the blood glucose level must do fingersticks only occasionally to monitor glucose levels and ascertain the system is working. The hybrid system may yield better glucose control and reduced risk of hypoglycemia in comparison to the traditional approaches using just an insulin pump or pen and fingersticks to determine insulin dosage needed. This new technology is more complex than traditional insulin delivery methods; for optimal efficacy, and safety, the wearer must understand and be confident in using a hybrid system.[431] Implantable pump options that can dispense insulin in constant, steady pulses throughout the day are still being tested. This type of pump would eliminate the need for an open needle site in the skin. Other methods for insulin delivery under investigation include nasal spray, suppositories, and iontophoresis.

**Type 2 Diabetes Mellitus.** Type 2 DM is most often treated with diet and exercise, sometimes in conjunction with oral hypoglycemic drugs (OHDs); insulin may also be required. *Exercise* is a recognized therapy for the prevention of complications in type 2 DM. Numerous studies have shown a consistent positive effect of regular exercise training on carbohydrate metabolism and insulin sensitivity. Some of the beneficial effects include decreased need for insulin, prevention of CVD and obesity, management of hypertension, reduction in very-low-density lipoprotein cholesterol, and improved mobility.[91,228,433]

A plant-based *diet* is becoming more widely known for its potential effects and benefits in the prevention and treatment of type 2 DM. The use of whole-grain or traditionally processed cereals and legumes has been associated with improved glycemic control in individuals with diabetes and in individuals who are insulin-resistant. Long-term studies have shown that whole-grain consumption reduces the risk of both type 2 diabetes and CVD.[215]

The combination of diet and exercise is more powerful than either one alone and may be even more effective than drugs for preventing type 2 DM. A low-fat, low-calorie diet with moderate exercise (30 minutes 5 times a week) has been shown to reduce new diabetes cases by 58% over a 3-year period. By contrast, the drug metformin, which lowers blood sugar levels and boosts insulin sensitivity, reduced new cases by 31%.[243] The LookAHEAD Clinical Trial involving over 5000 people with type 2 diabetes who were overweight or obese further demonstrated the additive positive effects of diet and exercise on glycemic control, body weight, and biomarkers for cardiovascular disease.

Another new class of drug for type 2 DM, incretin mimetics, is injected. Incretin mimetics, which include exanatide (Byetta), liraglutide (Victoza) and pramlintide (Symlin), mimic the action of GI hormones that increase

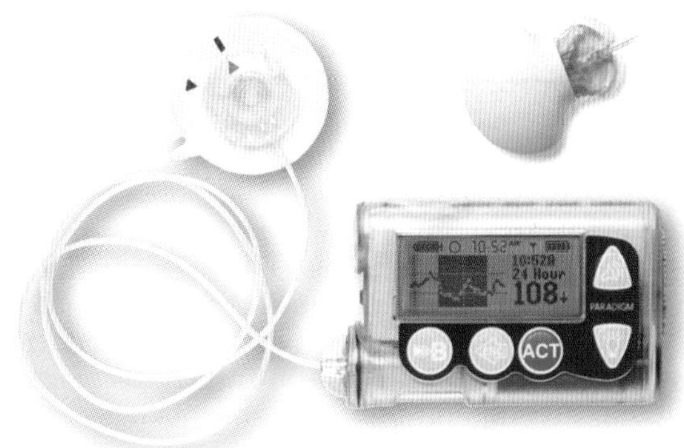


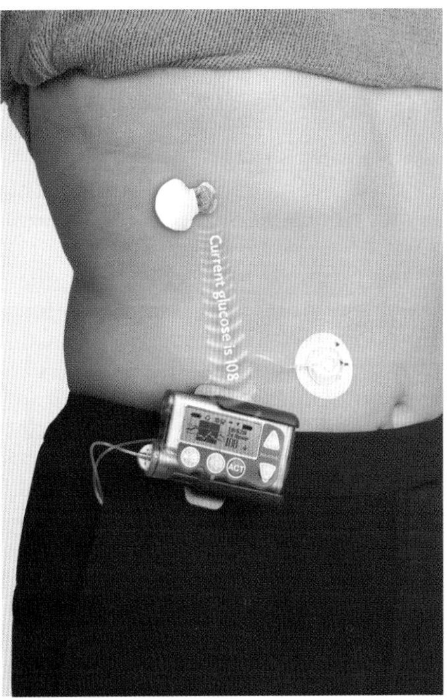


**Figure 11.15**

**The programmable insulin pump delivery system.** Compact and worn like a pager, the programmable insulin pump delivers fixed amounts of insulin continuously, based on continuous blood glucose levels determined by skin sensor. The device includes the pump itself (including controls, processing module, and batteries), a disposable reservoir for insulin (inside the pump), and a disposable infusion set, including a cannula for subcutaneous insertion (under the skin) and a tubing system to interface the insulin reservoir to the cannula. (Courtesy Medtronic MiniMed Paradign Revel Insulin Pump, Medtronic, Northridge, CA, 2013; see YouTube demonstration available online at http://www.youtube.com/watch?v=AU78ETXSLjQ.)

secretion of insulin, like GLP-1, and slow the rate of digestion. This class of drug does not lead to weight gain and has been associated with weight loss in some people. Possible adverse effects include pancreatitis and pancreatic cancer. See eBox 11.1 on the Evolve website for more information on OHDs.

**Treatment of Long-Term Complications.** Prevention of long-term complications is the goal for all clients with DM. Risk of complications is associated independently and additively with hyperglycemia and hypertension. Intensive treatment of both these risk factors is required to prevent and minimize the incidence of most complications.[421]

Medical treatment of long-term diabetic complications may include dialysis or kidney transplantation for renal failure and vascular surgery for large vessel disease. Currently, the American Diabetes Association advises that people with diabetes and increased cardiovascular risk take low-dose aspirin (75–162 mg) daily to help minimize risks such as heart attacks and strokes. This includes most men older than 50 years of age or women older than 60 years of age who have at least one additional major CVD risk factor. Prophylactic aspirin therapy is not recommended for adults with diabetes at low CVD risk because the potential adverse effects of gastrointestinal bleeding outweigh the potential benefits.[17]

Treatment guidelines from the American Diabetes Association recommend lifestyle modifications focusing on diet, weight loss, and physical activity to help people with diabetes achieve and maintain a normal lipid profile. The use of statins (cholesterol-lowering drugs such as Crestor, Lipitor, Zocor, Mevacor, or Pravachol), regardless of baseline lipid levels, is recommended for adults with diabetes and CVD and adults without CVD who have one or more CVD risk factors.[18] If lipid level targets (LDL < 100 mg/dL) are not reached with lifestyle modifications and statin therapy, other lipid-lowering medication may be considered.

Review of available data shows that statins reduced heart attacks and strokes by 22% to 44% in people with diabetes.[411] There is now evidence that statins are associated with increased risk of developing type 2 DM in some people. Likewise, there is controversy about the use of prophylactic statin therapy in adults without diabetes who are at moderate risk for developing CVD.[69,358]

***Diabetic Ulcers.*** The therapist often is involved in prevention and wound care for diabetic ulcers, which may help prevent amputation. Early recognition and prompt management of wounds, ulceration, and Charcot foot can facilitate healing. For example, a CDC study showed that people with diabetes who wore proper shoe protection had only a 20% recurrence rate of ulceration compared with an 80% rate for those without offloading.[412]

A handheld, noninvasive, infrared thermometer can be used to measure and compare skin surface temperature for the purpose of identifying increased skin temperatures, intended as an early warning of inflammation, impending infection, and possible foot ulceration. Temperature difference of four or more degrees between the right and left foot is a predictive risk factor for foot ulcers; self-monitoring has been shown to reduce the risk of ulceration in high-risk individuals.[30,31,262,426]

Offloading or pressure reduction is a key component for healing ulcers and preventing recurrence. The normal response to damaged areas is to spare them from pressure because they are painful. However, in the insensitive foot of a person with diabetes, this normal alteration of weight-bearing surface, pressure, and duration does not take place, resulting in repetitive stress and injury with subcutaneous and cutaneous necrosis and skin breakdown.

A marked improvement in the rate of healing for plantar ulcers has been reported using a combination of total-contact cast and tendo-Achilles lengthening (percutaneous heel cord lengthening), as opposed to total-contact cast alone.[30,271,313,378]

The results of at least one study show tendo-Achilles lengthening should not be done in anyone with complete anesthesia of the heel pad; increased dorsiflexion can increase the risk of heel ulceration. This procedure is advised only in a multidisciplinary setting able to provide adequate nutrition, wound care, surveillance, treatment of complications and other biomechanical abnormalities, and intervene early in any developing ulcerations.[200]

Other interventions include débridement, infection control, protective dressings, revascularization, proper nutrition, and client education. Active dressings, such as growth factors and living skin, are also in use. Topical application of growth factors on wounds without infection and with at least a minimal level of vascularization was introduced in the early 1990s and has progressed to include new techniques in skin transplantation.

Several different modalities have been applied as adjunctive interventions for diabetic peripheral neuropathy symptoms and diabetic foot wounds. Infrared light therapy, such as monochromatic near-infrared photo energy, has been applied to improve sensory impairment, reduce pain, and prevent and heal ulcers. Light absorbed by hemoglobin in the blood causes the release of nitric oxide, resulting in vasodilation and improved collateral circulation and, in theory, this will reverse loss of protective sensation. Laser therapy, delivered with devices emitting from one to four wavelengths (low- to high-level laser therapy) has been reported as an adjunctive procedure that promotes healing of chronic diabetic foot wounds by increasing blood flow and release of growth factors, and by reducing inflammation.[284] Cool laser therapy has been used as a revascularization therapy. Cool laser revascularization for peripheral artery therapy (CliRpath) uses a cool excimer laser and catheter system to vaporize arterial blockages, restoring blood flow and promoting wound healing. Acupuncture has been reported to reduce diabetic neuropathic pain.[494] Systematic reviews reveal a paucity of high-quality investigations on the effectiveness of modalities and conclude that existing clinical trials demonstrating positive results should be interpreted with caution because of small sample sizes and high risk of bias.[321]

***Transplantation.*** Research is being conducted on the use of transplanted pancreatic islet cells rather than the entire pancreas. The transplant recipient receives one or more infusions of pancreatic islet cells that include insulin-producing beta cells. High rates of insulin independence have been reported at 1 year in the leading islet transplant centers. Loss of insulin independence by 5 years occurs in the majority of recipients. Lifelong immunosuppression and its complications limit this treatment to candidates who have the most severely unstable glycemic control despite optimal insulin therapy.[395,396]

Stem cell research may find a way for people to use their own stem cells to develop them into islet cells and allow infusions without cell-rejection complications and the need for lifelong immunosuppression.[45]

**PROGNOSIS.** Diabetes control depends on the proper interaction between the following three factors: (1) food, (2) insulin or oral medication to lower blood glucose, and (3) activity (e.g., sedentary or exertional) or exercise. When diabetes is regulated successfully, complications of hyperglycemia and hypoglycemia can be avoided with minimal disruption to a normal lifestyle. However, diabetes can be fatal even with medical treatment, or it can cause major permanent disabilities and seriously impair functional abilities.

Studies have shown that type 2 DM raises a person's risk of dying from heart disease by 2 to 3 times.[414] In fact, about 50% of myocardial infarctions and 75% of strokes are attributable to diabetes. Diabetes is the leading cause of new blindness and is a contributory cause to renal failure and peripheral vascular disease.

Regardless of the modality of treatment used for the person with type 1 or type 2 DM, studies have shown clearly that tight glucose control (plasma glucose levels consistently within normal limits, approximately 100 mg/dL) delays onset and progression of diabetic complications. The only apparent danger in maintenance of tight control is the greater possibility of hypoglycemia, particularly in those people with type 1 DM who

**SPECIAL IMPLICATIONS FOR THE THERAPIST 11.17**

## *Diabetes Mellitus*

Client education is the key to therapeutic, nonsurgical treatment of the neuromusculoskeletal complications associated with diabetes. Extensive self-management is the focus of the educational program. *Diabetes Self-Management* is an invaluable tool for anyone with diabetes, available online at http://www.diabetesselfmanagement.com. Physical therapists should consider referring patients with risk factors for diabetes to the National Diabetes Prevention Program, a 16-week self-management training program developed by the Center for Disease Control that is held at local YMCAs, hospitals, and public health centers (https://www.cdc.gov/diabetes/prevention/).

Exercise is a key component of the overall intervention plan.[91] The client must be taught the importance of assessing glucose levels before and after exercise and judging what carbohydrate and insulin requirements are suitable for the activity or workout. People with diabetes and peripheral neuropathy have a high incidence of injuries (e.g., falls, fractures, sprains, cuts, and bruises) during walking or standing and a low level of perceived safety. Suggested strategies for appropriate clinical intervention to reduce these complications are available.[91]

### Complications of Insulin Therapy

#### *Hypoglycemia*

Insulin therapy can result in hypoglycemia (low blood glucose, also called an *insulin reaction*);[102] tissue hypertrophy, atrophy, or both, at the site of injection; insulin allergy; erratic insulin action; and insulin resistance. Symptoms of hypoglycemia are related to two body responses: increased sympathetic activity and deprivation of CNS glucose supply (Table 11.16). The clinical picture may be varied, from a report of headache and weakness to irritability and lack of muscular coordination (much like drunkenness) to apprehension, inability to respond to verbal commands, and psychosis.

Symptoms can occur when the blood glucose level drops to 70 mg/dL or less, although this value varies among those with diabetes and can be lower than 70 mg/dL before symptoms are elicited. In diabetes, an overdose of insulin, late or skipped meals, or overexertion in exercise may cause hypoglycemic reactions. Immediately provide carbohydrates in some form (e.g., fruit juice, honey, hard candy, or commercially available glucose tablets or gel); a blood glucose test should be performed as soon as the symptoms are recognized. The unconscious person needs immediate medical attention; to prevent aspiration, fluids should not be forced. Hospitalization is recommended when the following occur:

- The blood glucose is less than 50 mg/dL and/or the treatment of hypoglycemia has not resulted in prompt recovery of altered mental status.
- The individual has had seizures or is unconsciousness.
- A responsible adult cannot be with the person for the next 12 hours.
- A sulfonylurea drug causes the hypoglycemia; this type of drug reduces liver conversion of glycogen to glucose and prolongs the period of hypoglycemia.

It is important to note that clients can exhibit signs and symptoms of hypoglycemia when their elevated blood glucose level drops rapidly to a level that is still elevated (e.g., 400-200 mg/dL). The rapidity of the drop is the stimulus for sympathetic activity–based symptoms; even though a blood glucose level appears elevated, affected individuals may still have symptoms of hypoglycemia.

**Table 11.16** Clinical Signs and Symptoms of Hypoglycemia

| Sympathetic Activity (Increased Epinephrine) | CNS Activity (Decreased Glucose to Brain) |
|---|---|
| Pallor | Headache |
| Perspiration* | Blurred vision |
| Piloerection (erection of the hair) | Thickened speech |
| Increased heart rate (tachycardia) | Numbness of the lips and tongue |
| Heart palpitation | Confusion |
| Nervousness[a] and irritability | Emotional lability |
| Weakness[a] | Convulsion[a] |
| Shakiness/trembling | Coma |
| Hunger | |

[a]Signs most often reported by clients.

When a person with diabetes mentions the presence of nightmares, unexplained sweating, and/or headache causing sleep disturbances, hypoglycemia may be indicated during nighttime sleep (most often related to the use of intermediate and long-acting insulins given more than once a day). These symptoms should be reported to the physician.

Erratic insulin action (i.e., low blood glucose followed by high blood glucose) can occur as a result of a variety of factors such as overeating, irregular meals, irregular exercise, irregular rest periods, chronic overdosage of insulin (Somogyi effect), emotional or psychologic stress, failure to administer insulin, or intermittent use of hyperglycemic or hypoglycemic drugs (e.g., aspirin, phenylbutazone, steroids, birth control pills, or alcohol).

The Somogyi effect occurs when the blood glucose level decreases to the point at which stress hormones (epinephrine, growth hormone, and corticosteroids) are released, causing a rebound hyperglycemia. Treatment consists of increasing the amount of food eaten and/or decreasing the insulin. The therapist may be a helpful source of education to help clients remember the many factors affecting their condition.

### Lipogenic Effect of Insulin

Frequent injections of insulin at the same site can cause thickening of the subcutaneous tissues (hypertrophy or lipohypertrophy) and a loss of subcutaneous fat (atrophy or lipoatrophy), resulting in a dimpling of the skin that is lumpy and hard or spongy and soft. These abnormal tissue changes may cause decreased absorption of the injected insulin and poor glucose control.

The client usually is instructed to choose an injection site that is easily accessible (e.g., thighs, upper arms, abdomen, or lower back) and relatively insensitive to pain (away from the midline of the body). Sites of injection should be rotated, and rotation within each area is recommended. An individual can rotate within an area using 1 inch of the surrounding tissue at a time. The client who is going to exercise should avoid injecting sites or muscles that will be exercised heavily that day because exercise increases the rate of absorption. Following a definite injection plan can help avoid tissue damage.

Even with an insulin pump, the infusion site should be changed every 2 or 3 days or whenever the client's blood glucose is above 240 mg/dL for two tests in a row. Rotating insertion sites will help prevent infection and tissue damage.

### Diabetic Ketoacidosis

The therapist must always be alert for signs of ketoacidosis (e.g., acetone breath, dehydration, weak and rapid pulse, and Kussmaul respirations) progressing to hyperosmolar coma (polyuria, thirst, neurologic abnormalities, and stupor). Immediate medical care is essential. If it is not clear whether the symptoms are the result of hypoglycemia or hyperglycemia (Table 11.17), the health care worker is advised to administer fruit juice or honey. This procedure does not harm the hyperglycemic person but could potentially save the hypoglycemic person. Everyone with diabetes should wear a medical alert identification tag.

### Vitamin B Deficiency

Some individuals using metformin can develop vitamin $B_{12}$ deficiency, resulting in serious damage to the nervous system. Complications can be minimized with early detection and intervention. Anyone on metformin, especially high doses or a prolonged course of therapy, should be screened for the deficiency. The therapist can help monitor this with the client and recognize any early neurologic signs and symptoms.[435]

**Table 11.17** Comparison of Manifestations of Hypoglycemia and Hyperglycemia

| Variable | Hypoglycemia | Hyperglycemia |
|---|---|---|
| Onset | Rapid (minutes) | Gradual (days) |
| Mood | Labile, irritable, nervous, weepy | Lethargic |
| Mental status | Difficulty concentrating, speaking, focusing, coordinating | Dulled sensorium, confused |
| Inward feeling | Shaky, hungry, headache, dizziness | Thirst, weakness, nausea/vomiting, abdominal pain |
| Skin | Pallor, sweating | Flushed, signs of dehydration |
| Mucous membranes | Normal | Dry, crusty |
| Respirations | Shallow | Deep, rapid (Kussmaul respirations) |
| Pulse | Tachycardia | Less rapid, weak |
| Breath odor | Normal | Fruity, acetone |
| Neurologic | Tremors; late: dilated pupils, convulsion | Diminished reflexes, paresthesias |
| **Blood Values** | | |
| Glucose | Low: <50 mg/dL | High: ≥250 mg/dL |
| Ketones | Negative | High/large |
| pH | Normal | Low: ≤7.25 |
| Hematocrit | Normal | High |
| **Urine Values** | | |
| Output | Normal | Polyuria (early) to oliguria (late) |
| Glucose | Negative | High |
| Ketones | Negative/trace | High |

From Ignatavicius D, Workman M: *Medical-Surgical Nursing: Patient Centered Collaborative care*, ed 6, Saunders, 2010, Philadelphia.

Box 11.10

**DIABETES MELLITUS: KEY POINTS TO REMEMBER**

***General Guidelines***

- Although "safe" blood glucose levels are between 100 and 250 mg/dL (i.e., the person is not likely to experience diabetic ketoacidosis), the goal of therapy may be toward tighter control (e.g., in a young person with type 1 DM, 90 to 130 mg/dL) or moderate control (e.g., in an adult with type 2 DM, up to 150 mg/dL). A measurement more than 120 mg/dL should still be monitored closely in any age group. Blood glucose levels between 250 and 300 mg/dL are considered in the "caution zone"; test urine for ketones and wait to exercise if there is a high level until blood sugar drops to a safe preexercise range.
- If the blood glucose level is ≤100 mg/dL, a carbohydrate snack should be given and the glucose retested in 15 minutes to ensure an appropriate level. Food eaten in response to blood glucose levels between 70 and 100 mg/dL is symptom dependent (i.e., if a person's blood glucose is 80 mg/dL but no signs or symptoms of hypoglycemia are present, no snack is necessary).
- Observe carefully for signs or symptoms of diabetic ketoacidosis: acetone breath, dehydration, weak and rapid pulse, Kussmaul respirations.
- *Avoid exercise* if blood glucose is >250 mg/dL with evidence of ketosis; exercise is potentially permitted if blood glucose is up to 300 mg/dL without evidence of ketones in the urine.
- Administer fruit juice or honey to anyone with diabetes who is in a hypoglycemic state. If uncertain whether the person is hypoglycemic or hyperglycemic, provide juice or honey anyway.
- Exercise must be carefully planned in conjunction with food intake and administration of insulin or oral hyperglycemic agents.
- Do *not* exercise during peak insulin times. The peak activity of insulin occurs at different times depending on the type, dose, and time of the insulin injection (see explanation in text).
- When under stress, the person with diabetes has increased insulin requirements and may become symptomatic even though the disease is usually well controlled in normal circumstances.
- Avoid exercising late at night if this has not been gradually and consistently incorporated into the overall lifestyle. Delayed hypoglycemic reactions can occur during sleep hours after heavy, unaccustomed exercise late in the evening.

***Before Exercise***

- Take at least 16 ounces of fluid before exercise (approximately two 8-oz glasses).
- Glucose levels must be monitored immediately before exercise.
- Do not exercise when blood glucose levels are at or near 250 mg/dL with urinary ketones and use caution if glucose level is >300 mg/dL and no ketosis is present.[502]
- Do *not* exercise without eating at least 2 h before exercise (exercise about 1 h *after* a meal is best, but individual variations must be determined).
- Do *not* inject short-acting insulin in muscles or sites close to areas involved in exercise within 1 h of exercise because insulin is absorbed much more quickly in an active extremity.
- Clients with type 1 DM may have to reduce the insulin dose or increase food intake when initiating an exercise program.
- Ketosis can be checked by means of a urine test before exercise (e.g., if the blood glucose is close to 250 mg/dL). If the test is positive (i.e., showing large numbers of ketones in the urine), exercise should be delayed until the urine test shows negative or low numbers of ketones. The person should administer insulin. Delay exercise until glucose and ketones are under control.
- Do not use drugs that may contribute to exercise-induced hypoglycemia (e.g., beta blockers, alcoholic beverages, diuretics, estrogens, phenytoin).
- Menstruating women need to increase their insulin during menses, especially those who are inactive or who do not exercise on a regular basis.

***During Exercise***

- It is best to exercise regularly (5 times/wk or at least every other day) and consistently at the same time each day.
- Duration of exercise is optimal at 40 to 60 min, although as little as 20 to 30 min of continuous aerobic exercise is beneficial in improving glucose homeostasis.
- During prolonged activities, a readily absorbable carbohydrate snack (e.g., fruit) is recommended for each 30 minutes of activity. After exercise, a more slowly absorbed carbohydrate snack (e.g., bread, pasta, crackers) helps prevent delayed-onset hypoglycemia. Activities should be stopped with the development of any symptoms of hypoglycemia and blood glucose tested.
- Replace fluid losses adequately.
- Monitor blood glucose every 30 min during prolonged exercise.
- Anyone with diabetes should not exercise alone. Health care workers, partners, teammates, and coaches must understand the possibility of hypoglycemia and how to manage it.

***After Exercise***

- Glucose levels must be monitored 15 min after exercise, especially if exercise is not consistent.
- Increase caloric intake for 12 to 24 h after activity, according to intensity and duration of exercise.
- Reduce insulin, which peaks in the evening or night, according to intensity and duration of exercise.

*DKA*, Diabetic ketoacidosis; *DM*, diabetes mellitus.

### Diabetes and Exercise

An overwhelming body of evidence now exists that acute muscle contractile activity and chronic exercise improve skeletal muscle glucose transport and whole-body glucose homeostasis in the person with type 2 DM (Box 11.10).[83,92] High-intensity progressive resistance exercise has been shown to improve body composition, leading to better glucose control and less insulin resistance among older adults with type 2 diabetes.[297]

Exercise helps to increase insulin sensitivity, thus lowering blood glucose levels. Increased insulin sensitivity allows the body to utilize the available blood glucose for the person with type 2 diabetes; an increase in insulin sensitivity can last 12 to 72 hours after exercise. A combination

**Table 11.18 Benefits and Potential Risks of Exercise in People with Diabetes Mellitus**

| Benefits | Potential Risks[a] |
|---|---|
| Improves cardiovascular function | Hypoglycemia in people taking oral hypoglycemics or insulin |
| Improves maximum oxygen uptake | Worsening of hyperglycemia |
| Improves insulin binding and sensitivity | Cardiovascular disease, such as myocardial infarction, arrhythmias, excessive increases in blood pressure during exercise, postexercise orthostatic hypotension, or sudden death |
| Lowers insulin requirements (type 2 DM) | Microvascular disease, such as retinal hemorrhage or increased proteinuria |
| Improves sense of well-being and quality of life | Degenerative joint disease |
| Promotes other healthy lifestyle activities | Orthopedic injury related to neuropathy |
| Increases carbohydrate metabolism | |
| Improves blood glucose control[b] | |
| Reduces hypertension | |
| May help with weight reduction | |
| Improves lipid profile | |
| Reduces stress | |

[a]These are potential risks over the long term. In general, the benefits of regular exercise outweigh the risks.

[b]Not confirmed for insulin-dependent diabetes mellitus (type 1 DM).

Data from the following: Hordern MD, Dunstan DW, Prins JB, Baker MK, Singh MA, Coombes JS: Exercise prescription for patients with type 2 diabetes and pre-diabetes: a position statement from Exercise and Sport Science Australia. *J Sci Med Sport* 15(1):25–31, 2012, and Colberg SR, Sigal RJ, Fernhall B, Regensteiner JG, Blissmer BJ, Rubin RR, Chasan-Taber L, Albright AL, Braun B, American College of Sports Medicine, American Diabetes Association: Exercise and type 2 diabetes: the American College of Sports Medicine and the American Diabetes Association: joint position statement executive summary. *Diabetes Care* 33(12):2692–2696, 2010.

of both aerobic and resistance training (but not either one alone) has been shown to improve HbA1c levels[88,415] as well as produce greater benefit in some aspects of quality of life (e.g., bodily pain, mental health, vitality).[316]

There is a high prevalence of people with underlying skeletal muscle insulin resistance or impaired skeletal muscle glucose disposal such as occurs with inactivity, bed rest, limb immobilization, or denervation. Therapists must recognize, understand, and use the role of skeletal muscle in glucose homeostasis to address the needs of clients with any of these risk factors. For excellent, detailed reviews of the pathways of glucose transport into skeletal muscle and the pathophysiology of insulin action in skeletal muscle as it contributes to disturbances of whole-body glucose metabolism, refer to Turcotte and Fisher[442] and Sinacore and Gulve.[403]

A program of planned exercise, including all the elements of fitness (flexibility, muscle strength, and cardiovascular endurance) can benefit persons with diabetes, especially those with type 2 DM. Exercise increases carbohydrate metabolism (which lowers the blood glucose level); aids in maintaining optimal body weight; increases high-density lipoproteins (HDLs); and decreases triglycerides, blood pressure, and stress and tension (Table 11.18).

Exercise and physical activity (even leisure-time physical activity and activity on the job) have been shown to independently reduce the risk of total and cardiovascular mortality of adults with type 2 diabetes. Exercise capacity is reduced by diabetes-related CVD, but exercise training is an excellent therapeutic adjunct in the treatment of diabetic CVD.[228]

The favorable association of physical activity with longevity occurs regardless of BMI, blood pressure, smoking habits, and total cholesterol levels.[204,205] Once again, the therapist can be very instrumental in client education on the importance of exercise for a wide range of reasons and benefits to the individual with diabetes.

### General Exercise and Daily Movement Considerations

For anyone with diabetes, type 1 or type 2, the exercise prescription must take into account any of the complications present, especially cardiovascular changes, autonomic and sensory neuropathy, and retinopathy.[502] Muscle damage, with accompanying insulin resistance and impaired glucose uptake and disposal, can occur when untrained individuals begin to exercise.[403] For this reason, clients with diabetes must start any new activity at a well-tolerated intensity level and duration, gradually increasing over a period of weeks or even months.[502]

Some thought should be given to the specific type of exercise selected. The young individual, in good metabolic control, can safely participate in most activities. The therapist should always be aware of and screen for clients who may have eating disorders, especially those who engage in excessive, intense exercise as a means of controlling their weight. Specific screening methods and questions are available for the therapist.[173]

The middle-aged and older person with diabetes should be encouraged to be physically active, with consideration given to activity prescription, comorbidities, and age-related musculoskeletal changes.[92] These considerations are discussed in following sections. Specific recommendations for athletes and for adventure sports such as scuba diving are also described.

In people with or with risk factors for type 2 diabetes, higher amounts of sedentary time are associated with poorer glycemic control and increased morbidity and mortality. To reduce postprandial hyperglycemia and improve glycemic control people with diabetes should: (a) walk for 15 minutes after eating meals and (b) reduce total sitting time, interrupting sitting time every 30 minutes with 3 minutes of standing, walking or body-weight resistance exercise. Increasing daily movement may be a starting point for sedentary people with diabetes who have difficulty adhering to more structured exercise prescriptions.[92]

### Exercise and Diabetic Nephropathy

Although increases in blood pressure during a single bout of physical activity may temporarily increase levels of microalbumin in urine, exercise does not accelerate progression of kidney disease. Over the long run, the positive effects of exercise training on blood pressure and glycemic control may help slow progression of diabetic nephropathy.[17] Before initiating an exercise program individuals, with nephropathy should be screened for CVD and possible abnormal vital sign responses to exercise. Exercise should be initiated at low intensity and volume and progressed to moderate intensity and volume per the person's capabilities. High-intensity exercise and the Valsalva maneuver should be avoided to prevent large increases in blood pressure.[91] Aerobic capacity, muscle strength, and physical function may be poor in people with diabetic nephropathy. Both supervised exercise programs during dialysis and home-based exercise programs have been shown to improve quality of life and physical function in people with kidney disease.[220]

### Exercise Screening

As positive as exercise is in the prevention and control of diabetes, the therapist must keep in mind that diabetes is a metabolic disorder with cardiovascular and circulatory implications. Reduced blood flow to the skin and skeletal muscle can be further compromised by intense exercise, and recovery time is longer. All possible effects of exercise must be kept in mind when designing an exercise program to suit the individual's needs. Strenuous exercise can have some serious side effects for people with poorly controlled diabetes and related health complications.[266] However, with proper management of blood glucose and individualized evidence-based exercise plans, most people with diabetes can exercise in a safe and effective manner. Per current guidelines, a preexercise physical examination by a physician may not be necessary for people with controlled diabetes at low risk of coronary artery disease. However, a preexercise examination, conducted by a physician, and possible exercise stress test is recommended for sedentary and older people prior to beginning exercise more vigorous than a brisk walk, and people with diabetes-related health comorbidities.[91] Preexercise evaluations should include screening for the presence of macrovascular and microvascular complications and musculoskeletal conditions that may be worsened by the exercise program.[92]

### Exercise in Type 1 Diabetes Mellitus

The person with type 1 DM tends to be thin, may be poorly nourished, and, because of the islet cell deficiency, always needs exogenous insulin for adequate control of blood glucose. Exercise can increase strength and facilitate maintenance of weight and provide other important benefits (see Table 11.18), but unfortunately, exercise has not been proven to provide increased glycemic control for the person with type 1 DM.

### Glycemic Response to Exercise

In individuals without diabetes, plasma insulin levels decrease during exercise, and insulin counterregulatory hormones (glucagon and epinephrine) promote increased hepatic glucose production, which matches the amount of glucose used during exercise. As a result, during exercise in individuals without diabetes, blood glucose levels remain normal.

The glycemic response to exercise in people with type 1 DM as well as people with type 2 DM who require insulin therapy, insulin secretagogue therapy, or both is variable and is influenced by several factors including the type and timing of exercise. In general, aerobic exercise tends to decrease blood sugar levels. Hypoglycemia may occur when prolonged aerobic exercise is performed after a meal and the usual insulin dose was taken at mealtime. Aerobic exercise while fasted, such as before breakfast, may result in a lesser decrease in blood sugar levels. During anerobic exercise, such as resistance training or interval training, blood sugar may remain stable or rise if the intensity is high. Mixed aerobic and anaerobic sports activities, like tennis or soccer, are associated with better glucose stability than predominately aerobic activities.[365] Variability in glycemic responses to exercise in people with Type 1 diabetes make recommendations for management of insulin dosing and food intake complex. Blood glucose should be checked prior to exercise. Another approach to preventing exercise-induced hypoglycemia is to reduce insulin dose instead of or in conjunction with increasing carbohydrate intake.[91]

### Hypoglycemia During Exercise

Moderate periods (30–45 minutes) of moderate-intensity exercise provide beneficial effects, but longer periods may result in hypoglycemia. Lack of adequate glycogen stores (i.e., decreased glycogen stores in the liver and, to a lesser extent, in skeletal muscle) leads to impaired aerobic exercise endurance when compared with the nondiabetic person. Watch for symptoms of hypoglycemia such as sweating, shakiness, nausea, headache, and difficulty concentrating. The greatest risk of severe hypoglycemia occurs 6 to 14 hours after strenuous exercise. Strategies for avoiding hypoglycemia following exercise include (a) reducing insulin dose taken prior to exercise, (b) ingesting carbohydrate before and/or during exercise. Additional strategies include performing high-intensity bouts intermittently during moderate-intensity aerobic exercise or performing resistance exercise prior to aerobic exercise.[91] People who have a tendency for hypoglycemia should consult with their physician to develop a diabetes and exercise plan of action. It is also important that muscle and hepatic glycogen be restored during periods of rest. Insulin and caloric intake must be adjusted after strenuous exercise to avoid severe nocturnal hypoglycemia.

### Hyperglycemia

Hyperglycemia may result from high-intensity aerobic exercise in persons with and without diabetes. This can be challenging, particularly for people requiring insulin or insulin secretagogues. During high-intensity exercise, catecholamine (epinephrine and norepinephrine) levels increase significantly more than in moderate-intensity exercise. The change in catecholamines increases liver glucose production to levels exceeding muscle glucose uptake, resulting in hyperglycemia.

After high-intensity exercise, in people without diabetes and people with diabetes not requiring insulin, liver glucose production declines at a faster rate than declines in muscle glucose uptake, with blood glucose levels returning to normal within 1 to 2 hours. Postexercise hyperglycemia may persist and become problematic in people who use insulin and decrease their exercise insulin dose prior to exercise. Lower levels of insulin during recovery (attributed to reduction in dosing) slows the decline in hepatic glucose production and muscle glucose uptake.

When too little insulin is available, the cells are sensing starvation, so increased release of glucagon and catecholamines persists. These hormones further increase glucose mobilization into the bloodstream and significantly increase an already high level of glucose and ketones. If the hyperglycemia and ketosis is high enough and/or if the person is dehydrated, DKA can be precipitated.[91,182] Alternating bouts of high-intensity with low-intensity activity (interval training) does not appear to lead to less of a tendency for both hypoglycemia and hyperglycemia and therefore may be a good strategy for exercise prescription for people requiring insulin to control diabetes.[91,182]

### Sports Participation

Managing diabetes is very challenging for competitive athletes. The National Athletic Trainers' Association Position Statement on this topic and the Diabetes Exercise and Sports Association are helpful resources for therapists, trainers, and athletes.[218] In the past, people with diabetes, dependent on insulin, were discouraged from participating in adventure sports such as scuba diving and rock climbing. However, guidelines now exist that, if followed, may allow for safe participation in adventure sport activities.[354]

### Exercise in Type 2 Diabetes Mellitus

In contrast to Type 1 DM (discussed in previous section), people with type 2 DM are often obese, and exercise is a major contributor in controlling hyperglycemia. Exercise can improve short-term insulin sensitivity and reduce insulin resistance, making it possible to prevent type 2 DM in those persons at risk and to improve glycemic control in those with diabetes. These effects disappear a few days after exercise is discontinued.

Consequently, for exercise to be an effective means of controlling diabetes, there should be no more than 2 days between exercise bouts. Regular physical activity, a healthy diet, and weight loss of at least 7% to 10% in people who are overweight are cornerstones to management of type 2 DM.[92,201]

Hypoglycemia is not as common a problem for the persons with type 2 DM who do not require insulin or insulin secretagogues because endogenous insulin levels usually can be maintained. However, individuals with type 2 DM who receive insulin or sulfonylureas may have a risk for hypoglycemia similar to that of people with type 1 DM.[91,182] Many people with type 2 DM are obese, sedentary, and have additional health comorbidities that need to be considered in exercise prescription. Box 11.10 includes key considerations for exercise and blood glucose control for people with type 1 and type 2 DM. Another helpful resource is American Physical Therapy Association's (APTA's) Physical Fitness and Type 2 Diabetes Pocket Guide (http://www.apta.org/PFSP/). General guidelines for exercise prescription follow, and considerations for exercising with diabetes and health comorbidities, such as peripheral neuropathy and retinopathy, are discussed in subsequent sections.

### General Guidelines for Exercise Prescription

For blood glucose control, adults with type 2 DM should perform at least 150 minutes of moderate- to vigorous-intensity aerobic exercise spread out over at least 3 days, with not more than 2 consecutive days between bouts of exercise. Seventy-five minutes of vigorous activity may be sufficient for more physically fit individuals. Youth with type 2 DM should participate in 60 minutes of moderate to vigorous aerobic activity per day. In addition to aerobic exercise, youth and adults should engage in muscle strengthening activities 2 to 3 days per week. For adults, moderate to vigorous resistance training (50%–80% of 1 repetition maximum) 2 to 3 days per week is advised.[91] Each resistance training session should include 5 to 10 exercises covering all major muscle groups and one to three sets of 10 to 15 repetitions per exercise. Resistance exercise improves bone health, increases muscle mass, and benefits blood glucose control.[289]

Low-intensity exercise and interval training, alternating low–moderate aerobic exercise with resistance exercise may also reduce hyperglycemia. These types of exercise are better tolerated by people with poor exercise capacity, increasing the likelihood that they will regularly achieve the recommended amount of physical activity.[286]

Exercise should not be initiated if the blood glucose is 70 mg/dL or less in people with type 2 DM and 90 mg/dl or less in people with type 1 DM. In addition, anyone with blood glucose levels at or near 250 to 300 mg/dL and with positive ketone levels should *NOT* exercise, because vigorous activity also can raise the blood glucose level by releasing stored glycogen. Vigorous exercise should not be undertaken within 2 hours before going to sleep at night because this is when exercise-induced hypoglycemia can occur, with potentially fatal consequences.

Exercise in the morning is recommended to avoid hypoglycemia resulting from fluctuations in insulin sensitivity caused by factors such as diurnal variations in growth hormone. Growth hormone levels remain low in the afternoon, and less gluconeogenesis occurs. Vigorous or intense exercise late in the day or evening can lead to delayed hypoglycemia during sleep, which is dangerous.

### Balancing Insulin, Food, and Exercise

Because glucose can enter the cells without insulin during exercise, food should be eaten if the person is exercising more than usual. Conversely, when exercising less often, a lighter diet or more insulin is required.

Glucose levels should be monitored before and after exercise (or therapy activities), remembering that the effect of exercise can be felt up to 12 to 24 hours later. Those clients taking insulin should have their own glucose-monitoring devices (fingerstick or laser punctures).

After exercise, available glucose is important for the replenishment of muscle glycogen stores. Bouts of hypoglycemia can be delayed until hours after completion of exercise. The insulin-dependent person must regulate activity so that the rate of energy expenditure balances the amount and type of insulin and food intake (Table 11.19). Women who are menstruating may need to increase their insulin during menses.

### Exercise and the Insulin Pump and Continuous Glucose Monitoring

CSII therapy brings the exercising individual with diabetes a response as close to normal as possible. But anyone with diabetes who uses an insulin pump must make frequent insulin adjustments to mimic the normal metabolic response, thereby maintaining a more normal glycemic control, especially during periods of higher-intensity or longer-duration exercise.[93] Most people using an insulin pump have type 1 (insulin-dependent) DM, although anyone with type 2 DM who uses insulin can also wear a pump.

One of the disadvantages of an insulin pump is that it can malfunction or become displaced without the person knowing it. Exercise can exacerbate the situation when insulin delivery has been unknowingly disrupted and hypoinsulinemia is developing. The therapist should always be alert to any signs of DKA in clients using an insulin pump. Teach the client to be vigilant during exercise to maintain the integrity of the infusion site and to pay attention to any symptoms of impending DKA (e.g., thirst, nausea, weakness, or excessive urination). Continuous glucose monitoring may decrease the risk of exercise-induced hypoglycemia. However, the user must be aware of the potential for inaccurate blood glucose measurements and sensor breakage.

### Diabetic Autonomic Neuropathy

Many people with diabetes may not be able to exercise intensely to a calculated heart rate because of preexisting heart conditions, deconditioning, age, neuropathies, arthritis, or other joint problems. Exercise may be contraindicated in anyone with a severe form of autonomic neuropathy (Box 11.11), especially anyone with vasomotor instability, angina, and a history of myocardial infarction.[91] The therapist is advised to communicate and collaborate with the client and physician when considering an exercise program for anyone with this problem.

Generally, individuals with autonomic neuropathy have a poor ability to perform aerobic exercise because of decreased maximal heart rate and increased resting heart rate. Postexercise heart-rate recovery is lower and may even be a sensitive enough screening test for individuals needing a clinical autonomic evaluation.[377] Persons with a generalized form of autonomic neuropathy may have hypotensive episodes after exercising, especially those who are deconditioned. They also demonstrate a predisposition toward dehydration in the heat and poor exercise tolerance in cold environments.

People with diabetic autonomic neuropathy may have a higher resting heart rate but lower maximal heart rate, making exercise at safe levels more difficult. It may be better to use the percentage of heart rate reserve (% HRR), which is the difference between resting heart rate and maximum heart rate, as a valid measure in prescribing exercise intensity instead of the rating of perceived exertion (RPE) scale, which relies on self-assessment of exertion.[94]

When using % HRR to determine an appropriate exercise intensity, maximal HR should be directly measured using an exercise stress test rather than estimated from age for better accuracy. The American College of Sports Medicine (ACSM) recommends that individuals with diabetic autonomic neuropathy be screened and receive physician approval before initiating exercise and that exercise intensity levels for clients with diabetic autonomic neuropathy should remain in the 40% to 75% HRR span.[11,92,201]

Some people with autonomic neuropathy may have silent myocardial infarctions without angina. The first symptom may be shortness of breath resulting from congestive heart failure. Decrease in nerve innervation to the heart associated with this type of neuropathy may prevent a normal increase in heart rate with stress or exercise, requiring careful observation and monitoring of vital signs during exercise. Blood pressure regulation is altered with autonomic neuropathy; exercise can further stress the impaired system. Clients with autonomic neuropathy are prone to hypothermia, dehydration, and hypotension or hypertension.

Diabetes is associated with reduced tolerance to heat. Autonomic neuropathy may also include changes in thermoregulation with a decreased or altered ability to perspire. Exercise with a concomitant increase in core body temperature can lead to heat stroke.[349] Impairment of sweating has been demonstrated even with isometric exercise.[350] Proper hydration is essential, and precautions should be taken to avoid heat stroke. The Valsalva maneuver should be avoided.

### Diabetes and Neuromusculoskeletal Complications

The treatment of musculoskeletal problems does not differ from treatment for these same conditions in the nondiabetic population. Early aggressive therapy for adhesive capsulitis usually results in restoration of functional motion, even though full range of motion may not be achieved.

Hand function can be maintained and disease progression delayed with hand therapy, especially for the stiff hand syndrome. SLJM does not always benefit from therapy, but treatment intervention should be tried. For all neuromusculoskeletal conditions, the therapist must pay attention to elevated A1c levels because these have been linked with the presence of neuropathy and upper limb impairments.[360] The client must understand the importance of monitoring and maintaining control of the A1c levels. A self-directed exercise program established by the therapist can help prevent recurrence of symptoms and maintain functional outcomes.

Intervention for CTS must take into account the neuropathic and entrapment components in the person with diabetes; surgical decompression may not be beneficial because of the neuropathic component. Nonsurgical efforts should be the focus of treatment. In conditions such as adhesive capsulitis and complex regional pain syndrome, a successful outcome is more likely with early medical and therapeutic intervention.

### Diabetes and Foot Care

Disorders of the feet constitute a source of increasing

**Table 11.19** Making Food Adjustments for Exercise: General Guidelines

| Type of Exercise and Examples | If Blood Glucose Is[a] | Increase Food Intake By | Suggestions of Food to Use |
|---|---|---|---|
| Exercise of short duration and low moderate intensity (walking half mile or leisurely bicycling for <30 min) | <100 mg/dL<br>≥100 mg/dL | 10–15 g of carbohydrate per hour of exercise not necessary to increase food | 1 fruit or 1 starch/bread exchange |
| Exercise of moderate intensity (1 h of tennis, swimming, jogging, leisurely bicycling, golfing) | <100 mg/dL | 25–50 g of carbohydrate before exercise, then 10–15 g per hour of exercise | ½ meat sandwich with a milk or fruit exchange |
| | 100–179 mg/dL | 10–15 g per hour of exercise | 1 fruit or 1 starch/bread exchange |
| | 180–300 mg/dL<br>≥300 mg/dL | Not necessary to increase food<br>Do not begin exercise until blood glucose is under better control | |
| Strenuous activity or exercise (about 1–2 h of football, hockey, racquetball, or baseball games; strenuous bicycling or swimming; shoveling heavy snow) | <100 mg/dL | 50 g carbohydrate; monitor blood glucose carefully | 1 meat sandwich (2 slices of bread) with a milk and fruit exchange |
| | 100–179 mg/dL | 25–50 g carbohydrate, depending on intensity and duration | ½ meat sandwich with a milk or fruit exchange |
| | 180–300 mg/dL | 10–15 g carbohydrate | 1 fruit or starch/bread exchange |
| | ≥300 mg/dL | Do not begin exercise until blood glucose is under control | |

[a]100 mg/dL = 100 mL. The 100 mg/dL is a general guideline. Wide individual variations occur in this area. The timing of food intake may be symptom dependent. Some individuals may experience symptoms of hypoglycemia when the blood glucose is 150 mg/dL, others not until the level is below 80 mg/dL. and so on.

**Box 11.11**

**CONTRAINDICATIONS TO EXERCISE IN DIABETES MELLITUS**

- Poor control of blood glucose levels
- Unevaluated or poorly controlled associated conditions:
  - Retinopathy
  - Hypertension
  - Neuropathy (autonomic or peripheral)
  - Nephropathy
- Recent photocoagulation or surgery for retinopathy
- Dehydration
- Extreme environmental temperatures (hot or cold)

Data from Hordern MD, Dunstan DW, Prins JB, Baker MK, Singh MA, Coombes JS: Exercise prescription for patients with type 2 diabetes and pre-diabetes: a position statement from Exercise and Sport Science Australia, *J Sci Med Sport* 15(1):25–31, 2012; Colberg SR, Sigal RJ, Fernhall B, Regensteiner JG, Blissmer BJ, Rubin RR, Chasan-Taber L, Albright AL, Braun B; American College of Sports Medicine; American Diabetes Association: Exercise and type 2 diabetes: the American College of Sports Medicine and the American Diabetes Association: joint position statement executive summary, *Diabetes Care* 33(12):2692–6, 2010.

morbidity associated with diabetes. Foot problems are a leading cause of hospital admission in people with diabetes, and diabetes is the most common reason for lower limb amputation. Half of those cases are preventable with proper foot care.[407,458] Treatment of the underlying diabetes has little effect on any joint disease already present. The most beneficial intervention includes stabilizing the joint, minimizing trauma, maintaining muscular strength, and performing daily foot care.

The therapist must teach each person with diabetes proper foot and skin care. Regular foot checks after exercise using a mirror to inspect all surface areas and between the toes is advised. Having the therapist demonstrate and consistently carry this out with the client is a helpful educational tool. Any areas of warmth, erythema, swelling, or skin changes must be evaluated carefully and immediately. The therapist is advised to reinforce client education at each and every session.

### Diabetic Peripheral Neuropathy

Assess for risk factors for amputation (e.g., previous ulcer or amputation) and for signs of diabetic neuropathy (e.g., numbness or pain in hands or feet or footdrop). Scarborough[384] includes an excellent summary of assessment (tests and measures) for the foot and lower extremity. Vinik and Mehrabyan also offer an excellent review of diabetic neuropathies that will be of interest to any clinician working with this problem.[458]

Keep in mind that ankle-brachial index (ABI) measurements used to assess arterial circulation may have limited value in anyone with diabetes because calcification of the tibial and peroneal arteries may render them noncompressible.[67]

Provide clients with a monofilament for self-testing (Fig. 11.16). For a description of an easy and reliable method to test for protective sensation using the Semmes-Weinstein monofilaments, see the reference section.[115,315] This test is an easily used clinical indicator for identifying people who are at risk for developing foot ulcers and requiring subsequent amputations. It can clearly demonstrate physiologic changes in peripheral nerve function. If the person cannot feel the monofilament when applied with slight pressure against the skin, there is an increased risk of ulceration. The results of this test provide a definitive idea of who can benefit most from preventive care, education, and prescription of appropriate therapeutic footwear.[315]

Decreased sensation in the feet associated with diabetic neuropathy can affect both the timing and quality of gait, requiring retraining of the somatosensory and vestibular systems to help compensate for the somatosensory deficit.[192,348] Gait and strength training are important in the management of large-fiber neuropathies when impaired vibration, depressed tendon reflexes, and shortening of the Achilles tendon occur.[458] Diabetes gait may occur independent of sensory impairment. Increased joint movement, wider stance, and slower pace demonstrated in some individuals with type 2 diabetes may be neurologic in origin and not related to muscle weakness or loss of sensation in the feet.[347]

Anyone with peripheral neuropathy is advised to avoid soaking the feet. There is a danger of burns, and prolonged exposure to warm water leaves the skin susceptible to fungal infections. Whirlpools are contraindicated and baths are not advised (showering may be best). Bathing and soaking remove the protective barrier from the skin and can lead to other infections, especially if there are fissures from dry skin caused by decreased circulation.

In a new position statement on diabetic peripheral neuropathy pain, the American Diabetes Association recommends that opioids should only be prescribed when all other pharmacologic and nonpharmacologic treatments fail. Moderate-intensity aerobic exercise may help prevent the onset of peripheral neuropathy.[355] Exercise guidelines for people with diabetes and peripheral neuropathy have been changed to allow moderate-intensity weight-bearing exercise for individuals with peripheral neuropathy but no foot ulcers. Recent studies indicate that walking at moderate intensity does not increase risk of foot ulcer, including reoccurrence of ulcers in people with peripheral neuropathy.[266,444]

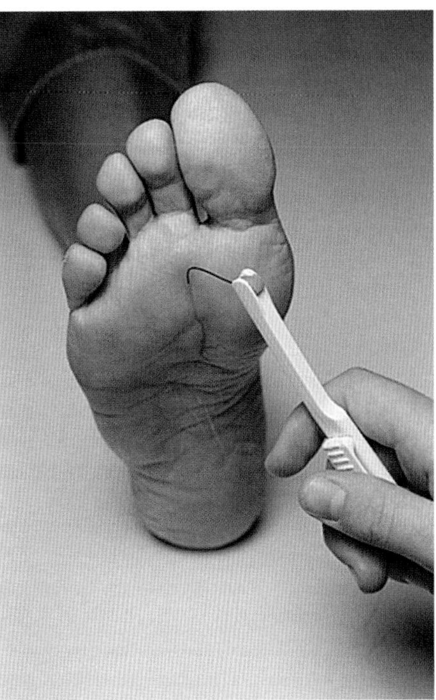

**Figure 11.16**

**Semmes-Weinstein monofilament testing for protective sensation.** Performed if the client is suspected of having peripheral neuropathy or known diabetes with possible peripheral neuropathy. The 5.07 monofilament (calibrated to apply 10 grams of force) has been adopted for screening in the diabetic population. The monofilament is applied perpendicular to the test site with enough pressure to bend the monofilament for 1 second. Abnormal response: client does not perceive the monofilament. Do not test over calloused areas. An initial foot screen should be performed on anyone with diabetes and at least annually thereafter. Anyone who is at risk should be seen at least four times a year to check their feet and shoes to help prevent foot problems from occurring. (From Seidel HM: *Mosby's physical examination handbook*, ed 6, St Louis, 2006, Mosby.)

### Neuropathic (Diabetic) Ulcers

All people with diabetes should have an annual comprehensive foot examination to identify risk factors predictive of neuropathic ulcers. The most common cause for neuropathic (diabetic) ulcers is excessive plantar pressure in the presence of sensory neuropathy and foot deformity. Neuropathic foot ulcers can occur at any areas where pressure or shear force is applied to the foot (top, sides, or bottom). Many occur beneath the metatarsal heads and are the result of painless trauma caused by excessive plantar pressures during walking.[314]

The presence of corns or calluses is an indication that footwear fits poorly and should be carefully evaluated by the therapist. Additionally, cartilage requires insulin for glucose uptake, metabolism of carbon dioxide, and collagen synthesis. Lacking an adequate supply, the articular cartilage in the person with diabetes does not tolerate repetitive trauma, compression, and motion, making proper footwear all the more important.[356]

Note the location of any foot ulcerations for possible causes that can be corrected. For example, ill-fitting shoes may cause ulcers on the medial or lateral borders of the feet, whereas ulcers on top of the foot may be caused by deformities such as hammer (claw) toes.

The risk of ulceration and poor wound healing in the diabetic population underscores the importance of therapists providing nonsurgical alternatives for these problems. Although the management of the diabetic foot (Charcot joint) sometimes requires surgery to restore osseous alignment, regain stability, and prevent ulceration,[255] most people can be treated with appropriate cast, shoe, orthotic devices, or other therapeutic footwear. When a neuropathic joint is detected early, offloading the joint and avoiding weight bearing for 8 weeks may prevent progression of disease.

The presence of a previous history of plantar ulceration may alert the therapist to the need to teach the client how to control activity levels to lessen shear forces on scars from previous ulcers.[65] Orthoses are often used to redistribute or move pressure away from a blister or other area of pressure. Soft, moldable orthoses are preferred to the rigid orthoses used by clients with other types of foot problems. An excellent review of various offloading techniques for the treatment of neuropathic ulcers is available.[394]

Total-contact cast is an effective intervention for neuropathic plantar ulcers. The cast encases the entire foot and ankle, with all major bony prominences padded with foam or felt, and reduces total loads on the foot by about one-third of the normal load. Frequent cast changes are made as the swelling goes down and to avoid ulceration in the cast. Monitoring of foot problems through the use of skin temperature changes using dermal thermography may provide valuable information to the clinician in the detection, treatment, and prevention of neuropathic foot problems.[29]

Total contact inserts and metatarsal pads can be used to reduce excessive plantar stresses, thereby preventing skin breakdown and ulceration. The total contact insert reduces excessive pressures at the metatarsal heads by increasing the contact area of weight-bearing forces. Metatarsal pads act by compressing the soft tissues proximal to the metatarsal heads and relieving compression at the metatarsal heads.[314]

The prevention of foot problems before they begin is always the most effective method in offsetting the development of foot ulceration and infection and their potentially devastating effects. The use of proper footwear, proper cleaning and lubrication of the feet, safe removal of corns or calluses, and removal of mechanical sources of foot pressure are critical components in the prevention of foot problems. Client education is a key component in the monitoring and detection of potential difficulties.[356]

### Delayed Wound Healing

Because wound healing (surgical and nonsurgical) is impaired in the diabetic foot, surgery can be accompanied by increased risks of poor healing and infection. Sympathectomy, arthrodesis, and joint immobilization have not been proved helpful. Organ transplantation in someone with diabetes is also a risk factor for delayed wound healing because of the long-term immunosuppression required.[404]

The detrimental effects of cigarette smoking on wound healing and peripheral circulation are well documented. Smoking increases insulin resistance, worsens diabetes complications, and has a negative effect on prognosis. People with diabetes who smoke have a higher all-cause mortality rate than those who do not smoke.[413]

Smoking cessation is one of the two most important ways to reduce macrovascular complications in adults with diabetes. Control of hypertension is the other. The American Diabetes Association recommends that all health care providers routinely identify the smoking (tobacco use) status of clients with diabetes and offer cessation support and education.[16]

Substance abuse of any kind can impair or slow the rehabilitation process, especially delaying wound healing. Client education in this area is an important aspect of treatment. Despite strong evidence that clinician support of smoking cessation is effective for smokers who have diabetes, only about half report that their physician ever advised them to stop or cut down on their smoking (or substance use).[282]

The U.S. Public Health Service Clinical Guideline[436] suggests health care providers use the 5 A's: ask, assess, advise, assist, and arrange. A brief nonconfrontational discussion of smoking cessation may help move the smoker to the next level of readiness. The clinician can help clients think about what will be better if they quit; moving the person to the contemplation stage (ready to quit in the next 6 months) doubles the chance of quitting during that time.[352,359]

### Diabetes and Physical Agents

Numerous studies from the 1980s and continued ongoing research have documented the large interindividual and intraindividual variability in subcutaneous insulin absorption, a major contributing factor in the variability of blood glucose. The therapist must be aware of these factors and plan intervention accordingly. Specifically, insulin absorption is impaired or altered by smoking, injection site, thickness of skinfold (adipose tissue), exercise, subcutaneous edema, local subcutaneous blood flow, ambient and skin temperature, and local massage.[28,195]

The application of heat causes local vasodilation and hyperemia (excess blood to an area), necessitating burn precautions in this population. In a therapy practice, heat application may take the form of hot packs, paraffin, hydrotherapy, fluidized therapy, infrared radiation, ultrasound, or aquatic (pool) physical therapy.

Heat from the use of hot baths, whirlpools, saunas, or sun beds has been shown to accelerate the absorption of subcutaneous injections of insulin by increasing skin blood flow. To reduce the risk of hypoglycemia, local application of heat to the site of a recent insulin injection should be avoided. The use of cryotherapy (cold) with its effects of vasoconstriction and decreased skin blood flow would be expected to slow or delay insulin absorption from the injection site.

### Diabetes and Menopause

As life expectancy increases, women are living a greater proportion of their lives in the postmenopausal phase, a time when the prevalence of type 2 diabetes also increases. The therapist should be aware that the consequences of CVD, osteoporosis, and cancer are more pronounced in women who have type 1 or type 2 diabetes, especially in women who have metabolic syndrome followed by the development of type 2 diabetes.

The transition from premenopause to postmenopause estrogen-deficient status is associated with the emergence of many features of the metabolic syndrome, such as central obesity (intraabdominal body fat), insulin resistance, and dyslipidemia, which are also known to be risk factors for CVD. The prevalence of the metabolic syndrome increases with menopause and may partially explain the apparent acceleration of heart disease after menopause.[71]

Women with type 1 diabetes frequently go through menopause at an earlier age than women who do not have diabetes. Premature or early menopause may be considered an unstudied complication of type 1 diabetes.[121] Risk factor assessment for any of these comorbidities throughout the life cycle is especially important for any woman who has diabetes.

As the woman with diabetes approaches menopause, changes in estrogen and progesterone affect how cells respond to insulin and therefore blood glucose levels. Menopause symptoms can mimic low blood glucose levels (e.g., moodiness or short-term memory loss).

Sleep disturbance and weight gain associated with menopause make it harder to control blood glucose levels. There is an increased risk of urinary tract infection, especially for the menopausal/postmenopausal woman on insulin and/or who has had diabetes for 10 or more years.[34] During the postmenopause years when female hormone levels remain low, insulin sensitivity may increase, with a drop in the expected blood glucose levels.[366]

There are conflicting reports on the role of hormone replacement therapy for postmenopausal women who have type 2 DM. Whether hormone replacement therapy improves glycemic control or worsens insulin sensitivity remains unproved. Results may vary according to the type of hormone replacement therapy, age of the woman, and route of administration.[174,235,239,300]

Polycystic ovary syndrome (PCOS) is an endocrine disorder characterized by multiple ovarian cysts and insulin resistance syndrome. Clinical signs include menstrual irregularities, infertility, acne, and obesity. PCOS affects about 10% of women. However, its prevalence may increase commensurate with current trends in increasing obesity, insulin resistance syndrome, and type 2 diabetes. Exercise and a healthy diet may be important components in treatment of PCOS.[438]

### Diabetes and Psychosocial Behavior

The therapist should keep in mind the psychologic and behavioral aspects of diabetes with regard to improving clinical outcomes. Most people with diabetes experience a high degree of emotional distress that continues throughout their lives but is rarely addressed by professionals.[406]

Common psychologic problems known to complicate diabetes management include depression, poor self-esteem, impact on the family dynamics, family and social support, compliance and motivation, eating disorders (particularly compulsive overeating), quality of life, and so on. Twenty percent to 40% of people with diabetes experience some level of depression, twice the rate of depression in people without diabetes.[131] Depression can negatively impact diabetes self-care. Exercise may help relieve depression.[263] It is also important to remember that symptoms of poor glycemic control, such as lethargy, look like symptoms of depression.

A team approach that includes close collaboration between diabetologists, psychologists, and physical therapists is important.[5] A good resource for information on depression and on eating disorders for both therapists and patients/clients is the Behavioral Diabetes Institute (http://behavioraldiabetesinstitute.org). Motivational interviewing and cognitive behavioral strategies including empowerment-based strategies have been proposed to improve metabolic and psychosocial outcomes. The therapist can be instrumental in helping the client formulate a personal self-management plan that incorporates experimentation and exploration to find what the stumbling blocks may be and what works best for achieving consistency in results and attaining goals.[157,177]

### Diabetes and Aquatic Physical Therapy

The Aquatics Section of the APTA has an annotated bibliography with relevant articles related to pool therapy, including the use of aquatics with medical conditions such as diabetes mellitus. This document is available through the Aquatics Section of the APTA.

Swimming may be a good choice to offer the individual with diabetes to improve exercise capacity and muscle function, especially those who have cardiovascular disease and peripheral complications that may hamper many types of conventional exercises.[32] The physical therapist can be very instrumental in providing education about providing meticulous foot care. Wearing boat shoes (specially designed shoes for water wear available in many local stores) can help prevent scraping the feet along the sides or bottom of the pool. Care must be taken to gently dry the feet, especially between the toes, after swimming to prevent infection. Anyone with abrasions or open sores should not enter a swimming pool environment.

A rise in ambient (surrounding) temperature such as a client might experience in an indoor, warm, and humid pool setting also causes an increase in insulin absorption from subcutaneous injection sites. The insulin disappearance rate may be as much as 50% to 60% greater with an increase of 15° in ambient temperature.[247]

Additionally, the ease of movement in the water allows increased activity without the same perceived intensity of exertion for the same amount of work performed outside the water. The combination of increased temperatures and increased activity can result in hypoglycemia. The therapist and client must work closely together to maintain a balance of activity, food intake, and insulin dosage.

When a client with diabetes begins aquatic physical therapy, both the time in the water and the intensity of exercise should be systematically progressed and monitored, with one of the parameters being increased with each session according to the client's tolerance. Before pool therapy, the client must not miss any meals or snacks and must measure blood glucose levels.

A snack or beverage, such as orange juice, should be readily available throughout the therapy session for anyone developing symptoms of hypoglycemia. Glucose testing should be performed after completion of the pool program. Exercise can have a positive effect in reducing blood glucose levels in persons with type 2 DM, but sudden drops in blood glucose levels after exercise should be avoided.

With careful management, the individual should be able to adjust food intake and exercise tolerance to avoid having to increase insulin dosage. Throughout the pool program, the therapist must closely monitor each individual with diabetes for any signs of hypoglycemia (see Table 11.16). The affected individuals must be cautioned to carry out self-monitoring and to respond to the earliest perceived symptoms.

### Insulin Resistance Syndrome

Insulin resistance refers to the phenomenon of having high levels of both circulating insulin and glucose in the bloodstream, but the insulin molecules cannot bind properly to the insulin receptor sites on the surface of the cell to allow glucose to enter the cells and be used for energy. A syndrome of insulin resistance has been proposed to explain the frequent association of hypertension, carbohydrate intolerance, abdominal obesity, dyslipidemia, and accelerated atherosclerosis associated with type 2 DM.

Although a primary insufficiency of insulin secretion is the pathology in the development of type 2 DM, obesity is a major risk factor for the development of this type of DM, caused in part by the associated insulin resistance. In 1988, the combination of hypertension, glucose intolerance, hyperinsulinemia, and dyslipidemia was called *syndrome X*, and later renamed *metabolic syndrome*, by Gerald Reaven, MD, a diabetes expert who predicted an increased incidence of coronary heart disease and type 2 diabetes.[362] In consideration of this, in 2009, a consensus definition was released by a group of professional organizations (e.g., American Heart Association, International Diabetes Federation, National Heart, Lung and Blood Institute) identifying specific criteria for the clinical diagnosis of metabolic syndrome. Criteria for metabolic syndrome in this consensus definition include the presence of three of these five measurements: abdominal obesity (waist circumference), elevated triglyceride levels, low HDLs, hypertension, and elevated fasting glucose.

Obesity is the single modifiable factor that sets off the metabolic syndrome. The syndrome is associated with alterations in the abdominal fat cells. With increased fat storage, these cells become distorted in shape, and the receptor site for insulin becomes "warped" or out of proper alignment, so the insulin molecule "key" no longer fits in the receptor. Insulin resistance makes it more difficult to lose weight, because the cells are not getting enough fuel and the individual perceives hunger when adequate amounts of circulating glucose exist. The affected individual may develop elevated blood pressure and problems with reactive hypoglycemia. When the excess insulin is suddenly used, glucose rushes into the cells and the blood glucose drops suddenly. This sequence creates intense sweet cravings, and the cycle repeats itself with increasing insulin resistance.[459]

The term *insulin resistance syndrome* (IRS) was suggested by the American College of Endocrinology and the American Association of Clinical Endocrinologists to more aptly describe the prediabetic state.[129] Although IRS has many of the same characteristics of metabolic syndrome, diagnosis is based on a fasting glucose level (100 mg/dL < IRS < 126 mg/dL). Insulin resistance, a generalized metabolic disorder in which the body cannot use insulin efficiently, appears to play a key role in metabolic syndrome. Although not everyone with insulin resistance has metabolic syndrome, most people with metabolic syndrome are also resistant to the action of insulin. At this prediabetic stage, changes in lifestyle will have the greatest impact on halting any disease progression. In fact, it may be the only time in the disease progression when changes in daily activity levels and nutritional status may have an impact.

**SPECIAL IMPLICATIONS FOR THE THERAPIST 11.18**

### *Insulin Resistance Syndrome/Metabolic Syndrome*

Physical therapists have a unique opportunity to address IRS/metabolic syndrome through reasonable dietary advice and carefully prescribed exercise counseling. After assessment, physical therapists should guide individuals toward an activity program that includes near-daily exercise that is progressive to a weekly expenditure exceeding 1200 kilocalories of aerobic activity.[206]

The therapist can provide education regarding the importance of weight loss, exercise, and dietary changes needed to help control dyslipidemia and hypertension. With appropriate lifestyle changes, people can reduce their risk of CVD, prediabetic states, and diabetes.

Studies have not yet determined the ideal exercise program for IRS/metabolic syndrome. Moderate aerobic exercise three times a week based on the ACSM guidelines was found to increase insulin activity in nonobese, nondiabetic subjects despite the fact that there were no changes in weight, BMI, waist-to-hip ratio, lipid profile, or oxygen consumption after 2 months of exercise.[92,189] Many studies indicate a dose response, with higher energy expenditures and higher exercise intensities, including high-intensity interval training, producing greater reductions in insulin resistance.[48] The mechanisms responsible for the improvement in insulin sensitivity after exercise training have been studied extensively but are not fully understood. Research focusing on insulin resistance in skeletal muscle and in particular its relation to changes in aerobic fitness in type 2 diabetes is ongoing.[332,387,442]

receive frequent exogenous insulin administration.[91] Less stringent glycemic control may be appropriate for patients with a history of frequent hypoglycemia. Current guidelines emphasize the importance of individualization of glycemic targets based on patient and disease factors.[17]

## Hyperglycemia

Two primary life-threatening metabolic conditions, DKA and hyperosmolar hyperglycemic state (HHS), can develop if uncontrolled or untreated DM progresses to a state of severe hyperglycemia (greater than 300 mg/dL).[240] Between DKA and HHS is a continuum of metabolic abnormalities.

### Diabetic Ketoacidosis

***Definition and Overview.*** DKA is most commonly seen in type 1 diabetes when complications develop from severe insulin deficiency. About one-half of the people who require hospitalization for DKA develop this hyperglycemic emergency secondary to an acute infection or failure to follow their prescribed dietary or insulin therapy.[462]

Most episodes of DKA occur in persons with previously diagnosed type 1 DM. However, the condition may occur in new cases of type 1 and in persons with type 2 DM (under stressful conditions in the latter such as during a myocardial infarction). It is characterized by the triad of hyperglycemia, acidosis, and ketosis.[408]

*Etiologic Factors.* Any condition that increases the insulin deficit in a person with diabetes can precipitate DKA. Causes of DKA commonly include taking too little insulin; omitting doses of insulin; failing to meet an increased need for insulin because of surgery, trauma, pregnancy, stress, puberty, or infection; and development of insulin resistance caused by insulin antibodies. Other precipitating causes are listed in Box 11.12.

The most common precipitating factor is infection, which occurs in up to half of all cases and may seem like a trivial condition such as mild cellulitis or upper respiratory tract infection. Omission of insulin, either because of noncompliance or because people mistakenly believe that insulin is not required on sick days when they are not eating well, is another important and preventable cause of DKA.

In young individuals with type 1 DM, psychologic problems complicated by eating disorders may be a contributing factor in 20% of recurrent ketoacidosis. Factors that may lead to insulin omission in younger people include fear of weight gain with improved metabolic control, fear of hypoglycemia, rebellion from authority, and stress of chronic disease. In approximately 15% to 30% of cases, no identifiable cause of DKA can be determined.[408]

*Pathogenesis.* The initiating metabolic defect in DKA is an insufficient or absent level of circulating insulin. Insulin may be present, but not in a sufficient amount for the increase in glucose resulting from the stressor (see Box 11.12). Inadequate insulin creates a biologic state of starvation, which triggers the excess secretion of counterregulatory hormones, particularly glucagon, in an attempt to get more glucose to the cells and tissues. The abnormal insulin-to-glucagon ratio, with excess circulating catecholamine, cortisol, and GH levels, initiates a host of complex metabolic reactions, leading to hyperglycemia, acidosis, and ketosis.

When the body lacks insulin and cannot use carbohydrates for energy, it resorts to fats and proteins. The process of catabolizing fats for fuel gives rise to incomplete lipid metabolism, dehydration, metabolic acidosis, and electrolyte and acid–base imbalances.

*Clinical Manifestations.* The signs and symptoms of DKA vary, ranging from mild nausea to frank coma (Table 11.20). Common symptoms are thirst, polyuria, nausea, and weakness that have progressed over several days. This condition also may develop quickly, with symptoms progressing to coma over the course of only a few hours. Other symptoms may include dry mouth; hot, dry skin; fruity (acetone) odor to the breath, indicating the presence of ketones; overall weakness, possible paralysis; confusion, lethargy, or coma; and deep, rapid respirations (Kussmaul respirations). Fever is seldom present even though infection is common, primarily a result of peripheral vasodilation. Severe abdominal pain, possibly accompanied by nausea and vomiting, easily mimics an acute abdominal disorder.

### Box 11.12

**PRECIPITATING CAUSES OF DIABETIC KETOACIDOSIS**

- Inadequate insulin under stressful conditions
- Infection
- Missed insulin doses
- Trauma
- Medications
  - Beta blockers
  - Calcium-channel blockers
  - Pentamidine (NebuPent, Pentam)
  - Steroids
  - Thiazides (diuretics)
- Alcohol abuse (inability to manage insulin because of mentation change; alcoholic ketoacidosis)
- Hypokalemia
- Myocardial ischemia
- Surgery
- Pregnancy
- Pancreatitis
- Renal failure
- Stroke

## MEDICAL MANAGEMENT

**DIAGNOSIS, TREATMENT, AND PROGNOSIS.** Prevention of DKA through client education is the key to avoiding this serious condition. Once DKA is suspected, the diagnosis must be established quickly, with immediate treatment after diagnostic confirmation (blood glucose level >300 mg/dL [>250 with serum ketones], pH <7.3, and bicarbonate level <18 mEq/L).

Treatment includes fluid administration, insulin therapy, and correction of metabolic abnormalities (potassium, bicarbonate, and phosphate), in addition to correction of any underlying illnesses (e.g., infection). Before the discovery of insulin in the 1920s, DKA was almost universally fatal. This complication is still potentially lethal, with an average mortality rate between 5% and 10%.

**Hyperosmolar Hyperglycemic State.** HHS is another acute complication of diabetes, a variation of DKA. HHS is characterized by extreme hyperglycemia (800–2000 mg/dL), mild or undetectable ketonuria, and the absence of acidosis. It is seen most commonly in older adults with type 2 DM.[240,268]

The precipitating factors of HHS may be similar to those for DKA, such as infections, inadequate fluid intake, medications (see Box 11.12), or stress. HHS may be the first indication of undiagnosed diabetes, and it may occur in the case of someone who is receiving total parenteral nutrition (hyperalimentation) or who is on renal dialysis and receiving solutions containing large amounts of glucose.

The major difference between HHS and DKA is the lack of ketosis with HHS. Because some residual ability exists to secrete insulin in type 2 DM, the mobilization of fats for energy is avoided. When adequate insulin is lacking, blood becomes concentrated with glucose. Because glucose molecules are too large to pass into cells, osmosis of water occurs from the interstitial spaces and cells to dilute the glucose in the blood. Osmotic diuresis occurs, and eventually the cells become dehydrated. If not treated promptly, the severe dehydration leads to vascular collapse and death.

Clinical manifestations of HHS are polyphagia, polydipsia, polyuria, glucosuria, dehydration, weakness, changes in sensorium, coma, hypotension, and shock. Lactic acidosis also can develop if tissue perfusion is compromised.

**Table 11.20** Clinical Symptoms of Life-Threatening Glycemic States

| | HYPERGLYCEMIA | HYPOGLYCEMIA |
|---|---|---|
| **Diabetic Ketoacidosis (DKA)** | **Hyperosmolar, Hyperglycemic Syndrome (HHS)** | **Insulin Shock** |
| Gradual onset[a]<br>Headache<br>Thirst (very dry mouth)<br>Hyperventilation<br>Fruity odor to breath<br>Lethargy/confusion/coma<br>Abdominal pain and distention<br>Dehydration<br>Polyuria, ketones in urine<br>Flushed face<br>Elevated temperature<br>Blood glucose level >300 mg/dL (250–300 is the "caution zone")<br>Arterial pH <7.30 | Gradual onset<br>Extreme thirst (may disappear over time)<br>Polyuria leading quickly to decreased urine output<br>Volume loss from polyuria leading quickly to renal insufficiency<br>Severe dehydration<br>Lethargy/confusion<br>Seizures<br>Hallucinations, coma<br>Blood glucose level >600 mg/dL<br>Arterial pH >7.30 | Sudden onset<br>Pallor<br>Perspiration<br>Piloerection<br>Increased heart rate<br>Palpitations<br>Irritability/nervousness<br>Weakness<br>Hunger<br>Shakiness<br>Headache<br>Double/blurred vision<br>Slurred speech<br>Fatigue<br>Numbness of lips/tongue<br>Confusion<br>Convulsion/coma<br>Blood glucose level <70 mg/dL |

[a]Less gradual than HHS.
Modified from Goodman CC, Snyder TE: *Differential diagnosis for physical therapists: screening for referral*, ed 5, Philadelphia, 2013, Saunders.

Treatment is with short-acting insulin, electrolyte replacement, and careful fluid replacement to avoid congestive heart failure and intercerebral swelling in older adults, who often have other cardiovascular or renal disorders.

## METABOLIC SYSTEM

As noted earlier, the endocrine system works with the nervous system to regulate and integrate the body's metabolic activities. Metabolism is the physical and chemical (physiologic) processes that allow cells to utilize food to continually rebuild body cells and transform food into energy. Metabolism is broken down into two phases: the anabolic (tissue-building) and catabolic (energy-producing) phases. The *anabolic phase* converts simple compounds derived from nutrients into substances the body cells can use, whereas the *catabolic phase* is a consumptive phase when these organized substances are reconverted into simple compounds with the release of energy necessary for the proper functioning of body cells.[184]

The body gets most of its energy by metabolizing carbohydrates, especially glucose. A complex interplay of hormonal and neural controls regulates the homeostasis of glucose metabolism. Hormone secretions of five endocrine glands dominate this regulatory function (see Table 11.10). The rate of metabolism can be increased by exercise, elevated body temperature (e.g., high fever or prolonged exertional exercise), hormonal activity (e.g., thyroxine, insulin, or epinephrine), and increased digestive action after the ingestion of food.

### SPECIAL IMPLICATIONS FOR THE THERAPIST 11.19

#### *Diabetic Ketoacidosis*

The therapist will be an active member of the health care team, emphasizing to anyone with type 1 DM the need for regular, daily self-monitoring of blood glucose, adherence to the diabetes management program, and early recognition of and intervention for mild ketosis. The therapist also must be able to recognize early signs and symptoms of DKA in addition to signs of infection, a major cause of DKA. The first sign of an infection in a foot or leg or an upper respiratory, urinary tract, or vaginal infection should be reported immediately to the physician.

DKA can cause major potassium shifts accompanied by muscular weakness that can progress to flaccid quadriparesis. The weakness is initially most prominent in the legs, especially the quadriceps, and then extends to the arms with involvement of the respiratory muscles.

### Fluid and Electrolyte Balance (see also discussion, Chapter 5)

Fluid and electrolyte balance is a key component of cellular metabolism. Homeostasis, maintaining the body's chemical and physical balance, involves the proper functioning of body fluids to preserve osmotic pressure, acid–base balance, and anion–cation balance. The goal of metabolism and homeostasis is to maintain the complex environment of body fluids that nourishes and supports every cell.

Body fluids, classified as intracellular and extracellular, contain two kinds of dissolved substances: those that dissociate (separate) in solution (electrolytes) and those that do not. For example, when dissolved in water, glucose does not break down into smaller particles, but sodium chloride dissociates into sodium cations (positively charged) and chloride anions (negatively charged).

The composition of these electrolytes in body fluids is electrically balanced, so the positively charged cations (sodium, potassium, calcium, and magnesium) equal the negatively charged anions (chloride, bicarbonate, sulfate, phosphate, and carbonic acid). Although these particles are present in relatively low concentrations, any deviation from their normal levels can have profound physiologic effects.

### SPECIAL IMPLICATIONS FOR THE THERAPIST 11.20

#### *Hyperosmolar Hyperglycemic State*

The therapist should be alert to any signs of HHS in the aging adult who may have a previous diagnosis of type 2 DM. Early recognition and treatment to restore fluid and electrolyte balance are important for a good prognosis in this condition.

Because many situations in the body cause both normal and abnormal fluid shifts, it is important to have a clear understanding of fluid compartments. The recognition of pathologic conditions, such as edema, dehydration, ketoacidosis, and various types of shock, can depend on the understanding of these concepts.

In the healthy body, fluids and electrolytes are constantly lost or exchanged between compartments. This balance must be maintained for the body to function properly. The amount used in these functions depends on such factors as humidity; body and environmental temperature; physical activity; metabolic rate; and fluid loss from the GI tract, skin, respiratory tract, and renal system. Normal balance is achieved through fluid intake and dietary consumption. Alterations in fluid and electrolyte balance are discussed more completely in Chapter 5.

## Acid–Base Balance

The proper balance of acids and bases in the body is essential to life. The body maintains the pH of extracellular fluid (fluid found outside cells) between 7.35 and 7.45 through a complex chemical regulation of carbonic acid by the lungs and base bicarbonate by the kidneys. The pH is essentially a measure of hydrogen ion concentration in body fluid. Nutritional deficiency or excess, disease, injury, or metabolic disturbance may interfere with normal homeostatic mechanisms and cause a lowering of pH called *acidosis* or a rise in pH called *alkalosis*.

Various bodily functions operate to keep the pH at a relatively constant level. Acid–base regulatory mechanisms include chemical buffer systems, the respiratory system, and the renal system. These systems interact to maintain a normal acid–base ratio of 20:1 bicarbonate to carbonic acid. The consequences of an acid–base metabolism disorder can result in many signs and symptoms encountered by the therapist. These conditions are discussed more completely in Chapter 5.

## Aging and the Metabolic System

Aging as measured by loss of physiologic function has not yet been defined precisely, so the distinction between usual, normal, and ideal metabolic changes remains undetermined. Studies of the aging population have shown that several physiologic parameters, such as body weight, basal metabolism, renal clearance, and cardiovascular function, decline with age. Protein-calorie nutritional status has pervasive effects on metabolic regulatory systems; nutritional status often declines with age, which contributes to metabolic dysfunction.[229]

Because the respiratory and renal systems are largely responsible for maintaining acid–base balance, changes in these systems associated with aging also have an impact on metabolic function. A common measure for metabolic loss in tissues is the decline in $VO_2max$, the maximum oxygen extraction capacity of the lungs.

Loss of muscle mass associated with aging can affect stroke volume capacity and oxidative metabolism.[339] The low-level metabolic acidosis that appears to occur in many people with advancing age may play a role in age-associated bone loss, a factor that has received little attention from those who study bone loss and aging.[294]

Oxidative stress has been implicated in the pathogenesis of a number of diseases and has been labeled the *free radical theory of aging* studies indicate that protection from the consequences of excess metabolic activity results in a slowing of the aging process, particularly in the postreproductive period of life.[74,156] Links between oxidative stress and aging focus on mitochondria in a theory called the *mitochondrial theory of aging*. Mitochondria, the principal site of adenosine triphosphate (ATP) synthesis (also containing DNA and RNA), is the cellular site of energy production from oxygen and the principal site of free radical damage.[110]

Free radical derivatives of oxygen are generated as a result of normal metabolic activity, producing destructive oxidation of membranes, proteins, and DNA. These free radicals (unstable oxygen molecules robbed of electrons) attempt to replace their missing electrons by scavenging the body and taking electrons from healthy cells, causing a chain reaction called *oxidation*.

The formation of free radicals can be triggered by many exogenous (outside) factors such as cigarette smoke, air pollution, anticancer drugs, ultraviolet lights, pesticides and other chemicals, uncontrolled diabetes, radiation, and emotional stress. The major defenses against these destructive by-products of normal metabolism are the protective enzymes, which remove the free radicals and remove, repair, and replace cell constituents.

Impairment of cellular function and metabolism occurs as proteins and DNA (which turn over slowly or not at all) are damaged over time.[128] The use of antioxidants found naturally in fruits and vegetables or ingested as a nutritional supplement to counteract this process is thought to increase longevity but remains under scientific investigation.[305,306]

## Signs and Symptoms of Metabolic Disease

Clinical manifestations of metabolic disorders vary, depending on the specific pathology present. Fluid and electrolyte disorders, disorders of acid–base metabolism leading to metabolic (nonrespiratory) alkalosis or acidosis, and their associated signs and symptoms are discussed in Chapter 5.

# SPECIFIC METABOLIC DISORDERS

*Metabolic bone disease* is discussed in Chapter 24, and *disorders of purine and pyrimidine metabolism* resulting in gout and pseudogout are discussed in Chapter 27.

## Metabolic Bone Disease

Metabolic disorders involving the connective tissue may result in pathologic loss of bone mineral density, such as occurs in osteomalacia or osteoporosis, or acceleration of both deposition and resorption of bone, as seen in Paget disease. These disorders differ in pathogenesis and treatment and are discussed in Chapter 24.

## Metabolic Neuronal Diseases

Metabolic neuronal diseases are rare and are not likely seen in a therapy practice. Phenylketonuria (PKU), Wilson disease, and porphyrias are the three most often encountered and are briefly discussed in this section.

### Phenylketonuria

PKU is an autosomal recessive disease resulting from a genetic defect in the metabolism of the amino acid phenylalanine (Phe). This condition is transmitted recessively through apparently healthy parents, who show signs of the disease only on testing. The lack of an enzyme (phenylalanine hydroxylase) necessary for the conversion of the amino acid Phe into tyrosine results in an accumulation of Phe in the blood with excretion of phenylpyruvic acid in the urine. If untreated, the condition results in mental retardation and other manifestations such as tremors, poor muscular coordination, excessive perspiration, mousy odor (resulting from skin and urinary excretion of phenylpyruvic acid), and seizures.

Although PKU cannot be cured, a simple screening test for PKU can be administered to newborns and is required by law in most states in the United States and in all provinces in Canada. Currently, between 160 and 400 of the 4 million babies born in the United States each year are affected. The practice of discharging newborns in 24 hours is resulting in an increase in the number of babies at risk of PKU.

Treatment is primarily through Phe restriction of the infant's diet to control the effects of PKU and is prescribed on an individual basis with the additional administration of a dietary protein substitute. The start of newborn screening for PKU during the early 1970s has given rise to an increasing number of people who have been identified and successfully treated for the disease in childhood. Initiation of nutritional therapy before conception for women assures a successful pregnancy outcome.[238] A need remains for maternal screening before pregnancy to identify undiagnosed maternal PKU and subsequent prophylactic treatment to prevent maternal PKU syndrome.[187]

The prognosis for people with PKU has improved greatly with early institution of treatment after birth. However, hyperphenylalaninemia can cause white matter abnormalities, psychiatric illness, and decreased performance on neuropsychologic tests for people with PKU compared with subjects without PKU. It has been shown that the diet necessary to reduce Phe levels cannot be terminated after adolescence without elevation of plasma levels, resulting in poor neuropsychologic performance.[111]

### Wilson Disease

Wilson disease, also known as *hepatolenticular degeneration*, is a progressive disease inherited as an autosomal recessive trait (both parents must carry the abnormal gene). This condition produces a defect in the metabolism of copper, with accumulation of copper in the liver, brain, kidney, cornea, and other tissues. Although the pathogenesis of Wilson disease is still uncertain, it seems likely that defective biliary excretion of copper is involved.

The disease is characterized by the presence of Kayser-Fleischer rings around the iris of the eye (from copper deposits), cirrhosis of the liver (see Chapter 17), and degenerative changes in the brain, particularly the basal ganglia. Liver disease is the most likely manifestation in the pediatric population, and neurologic disease is most common in young adults. Cerebellar intoxication from deposition of copper in the brain results in athetoid movements and an unsteady gait.

Other CNS symptoms may include pill-rolling tremors in the hands, facial and muscular rigidity, dysarthria, and emotional and behavioral changes. Musculoskeletal effects occur in severe disease and may include muscle atrophy and wasting, contractures, deformities, osteomalacia, and pathologic fractures.[408]

Treatment is pharmacologic (e.g., lifetime administration of vitamin $B_6$ and D-penicillamine) and is aimed at reducing the amount of copper in the tissues by promoting its urinary excretion. Managing hepatic disease is also important; if left untreated, Wilson disease progresses to fatal hepatic failure.

Neurologic abnormalities, acute abdominal pain, skin fragility, and photosensitivity and psychiatric problems are symptoms that characterize the porphyrias. Various drugs and chemicals can cause porphyria (e.g., large amounts of alcohol, hemodialysis, or other chemical toxins) or can trigger acute, potentially life-threatening attacks in susceptible individuals. Diagnosis is suspected when clinical symptoms are combined with substantial increases in porphyrins or porphyrin-precursors in the blood and urine.[85]

**SPECIAL IMPLICATIONS FOR THE THERAPIST 11.21**

*Wilson Disease*

For the person with Wilson disease, physical or vocational rehabilitation may be required. In the advanced stage of this disease, self-care is promoted to prevent further mental and physical deterioration. An exercise schedule is essential to encourage consistent focus on rehabilitation. Sensory deprivation or overload should be avoided, and prevention of integumentary and musculoskeletal injuries that could occur as a result of neurologic deficits is important.

**Porphyrias**

Porphyrias are a group of hereditary and sometimes acquired diseases characterized by enzymatic abnormalities in biosynthesis of the heme molecule. Normally, porphyrins and their precursors are necessary for the synthesis of the heme molecule. In porphyrias, because of enzyme deficiencies, an accumulation of excessive amounts of porphyrins and their precursors occurs. This accumulation results in generalized clinical symptoms.

### REFERENCES

To enhance this text and add value for the reader, all references are included in the enhanced ebook on Student Consult that accompanies this textbook. The reader can view the reference source and access it online whenever possible.

CHAPTER 12

# The Cardiovascular System

IRINA V. SMIRNOVA • PAMELA BARTLO

The cardiovascular system functions in coordination with the pulmonary system to circulate oxygenated blood through the arterial system to all cells in the body. The deoxygenated blood is then collected from the venous system and delivered to the lungs for reoxygenation (Fig. 12.1).

Pathologic conditions of the cardiovascular system are varied, multiple, and complex. This chapter presents cardiovascular diseases according to how they affect structure and function of individual components of the cardiovascular system, including diseases of the heart muscle and heart vessels, cardiac nervous system, heart valves, pericardium, and blood vessels.

Influence of aging on cardiovascular system components and function is discussed with emphasis on positive effects of physical exercise. Gender differences are described as they relate to the cardiovascular system and diseases. Whenever possible, ethnicity as it relates to cardiovascular diseases is included in each section. Although race itself may not cause cardiovascular diseases, ethnicity may cause or contribute to cardiovascular diseases, especially with regards to diet and seeking medical help.

Other factors, such as surgery, pregnancy, cardiogenic shock, and complications from other pathologic conditions (e.g., acquired immunodeficiency syndrome [AIDS], cancer treatment, diffuse connective tissue diseases) can also adversely affect the normal function of the cardiovascular system. Discussion of these additional factors is limited in this chapter (see specific chapters for each subject).

## PREVALENCE OF CARDIOVASCULAR DISEASE AND RISK FACTORS

Cardiovascular disease (CVD) causes one in three deaths reported each year in the United States.[50] The leading risk factors for CVD include hypertension, high serum cholesterol levels, physical inactivity, diabetes, suboptimal diet, overweight/obesity, and smoking.[50] Of these, at least one risk factor for CVD is present in nearly half (47%) of the adult population age 20 years and older.[50] Evaluation of family history is also important to improve cardiovascular risk assessment. This can lead to better and earlier prevention options.[50]

## CARDIOVASCULAR DISEASE PREVENTION STRATEGIES

With over 90 million U.S. adults affected by CVD,[50] its prevention is of utmost importance. *Primary prevention* is aimed at reducing chances of the first adverse cardiovascular event in persons with no clinically apparent CVD and is possible to achieve only through lifestyle and environmental changes. *Secondary prevention* encompasses approaches to decrease the recurrent cardiovascular events and reduce death resulting from CVD. Beyond primary and secondary prevention, *primordial prevention* is a more far-reaching idea. It includes "ensuring that the ideal levels of cardiovascular risk factors are observed in healthy children" and "are preserved into adulthood.[50]

## SIGNS AND SYMPTOMS OF CARDIOVASCULAR DISEASE

Cardinal symptoms of cardiac disease usually include chest, neck, or arm pain or discomfort; palpitations; dyspnea; syncope (fainting); fatigue; cough; and cyanosis. Edema and leg pain (claudication) are the most common symptoms of the vascular component of cardiovascular pathologic conditions. Symptoms of cardiovascular involvement should be reviewed by system as well (Table 12.1).

*Chest pain or discomfort* (e.g., tightness, pressure sensation) is a common presenting symptom of CVD and must be evaluated carefully. Chest pain of systemic origin may be cardiac or noncardiac and may radiate to the neck, jaw, upper trapezius, upper back, shoulder, or arms (most commonly the left arm). Radiating pain down the arm is in the pattern of ulnar nerve distribution. Noncardiac chest pain can be caused by an extensive list of disorders and is not covered in this text.

Cardiac-related chest pain may arise secondary to ischemia, myocardial infarction (MI), pericarditis, endocarditis, mitral valve prolapse, or aortic dissection with or without aneurysm. Location and description (frequency, intensity, duration) vary according to the underlying pathologic condition (see each individual condition).

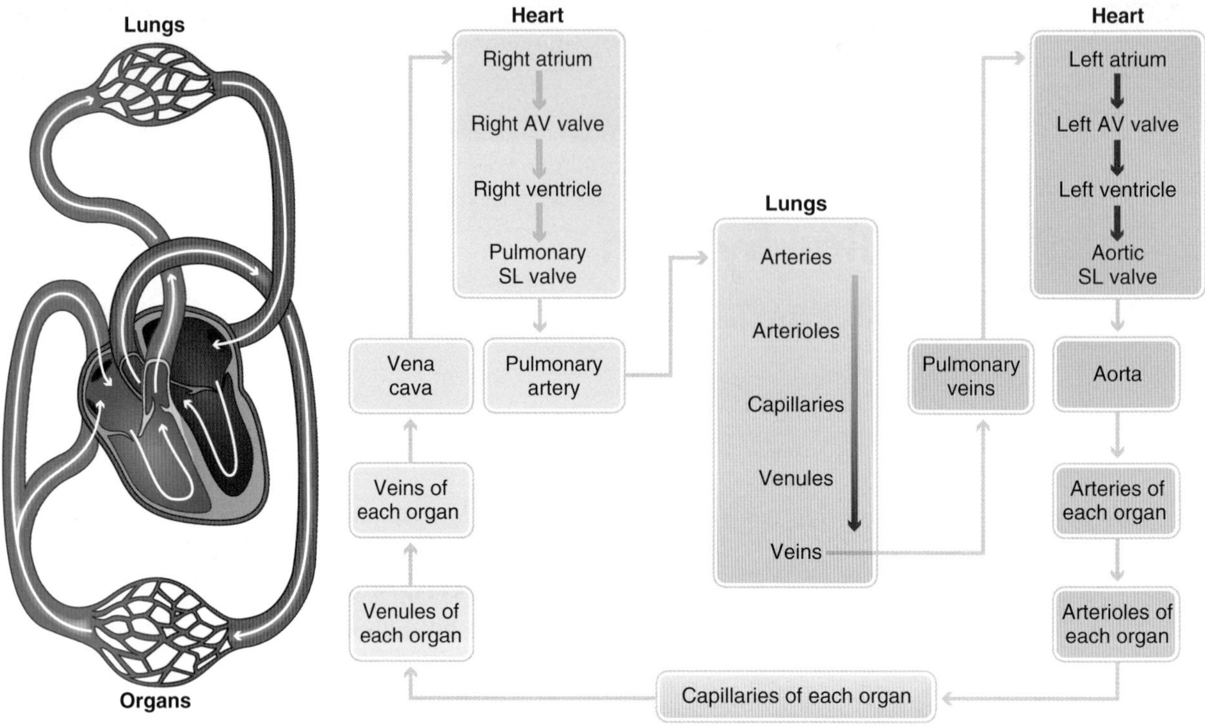


**Figure 12.1**

**Structure and circulation of the heart.** Blood flows from the superior and inferior venae cavae into the right atrium through the tricuspid valve to the right ventricle. The right ventricle ejects the blood through the pulmonic valve into the pulmonary artery during ventricular systole. Blood enters the pulmonary capillary system, where it exchanges the carbon dioxide for oxygen. The oxygenated blood then leaves the lungs via the pulmonary veins and returns to the left atrium. From the left atrium, blood flows through the mitral valve into the left ventricle. The left ventricle pumps blood into the systemic circulation through the aorta to supply all the tissues of the body with oxygen. From the systemic circulation, blood returns to the heart through the superior and inferior venae cavae to begin the cycle again. (From Thibodeau and Patton: *The human body in health and disease*, ed 6, St Louis, Mosby, 2014.)

*Angina* is a chest pain or discomfort occurring when a heart muscle does not get enough oxygen. It is a symptom of coronary artery disease (CAD). It usually starts behind the sternum, but it may radiate into either upper extremity, shoulder, neck, jaw, throat, and/or upper back. The pain is often described as pressure, squeezing, or tightness in the chest. Some people may mistake it for indigestion. Shortness of breath, weakness, light-headedness, and sweating may occur.

*Palpitations,* the presence of an irregular, fast, or "extra" heartbeat, may also be referred to as arrhythmias or dysrhythmias, which may be caused by a relatively benign condition (e.g., mitral valve prolapse, caffeine, anxiety, exercise) or a severe condition (e.g., CAD, cardiomyopathy, complete heart block, ventricular aneurysm, atrioventricular valve disease, mitral or aortic stenosis).

Palpitations may occur as a response to the bursts of adrenaline that occur with drops in estrogen levels, as a response to excess or erratic production of adrenaline-type compounds associated with panic disorder, or as a result of hyperthyroidism through other mechanisms.

Palpitations have been described as a bump, pound, jump, flop, flutter, butterfly, or racing sensation of the heart. Palpated pulse may feel rapid or irregular, as if the heart has skipped a beat. Some people report fluttering sensations in the neck rather than in the chest or thoracic area.

*Dyspnea,* also referred to as breathlessness or shortness of breath, can be cardiovascular in origin, but it may also occur secondary to pulmonary pathologic conditions, trauma, fever, certain medications, or obesity. Early onset of dyspnea may be described as a sensation of having to breathe too much or as an uncomfortable feeling during breathing after exercise or exertion. Shortness of breath with mild exertion (dyspnea on exertion) can be caused by an impaired left ventricle that is unable to contract completely. The result is an abnormal accumulation of blood in the pulmonary circulation. Pulmonary congestion and shortness of breath then ensue. With severe compromise of the cardiovascular or pulmonary system, dyspnea may occur at rest.

Dyspnea may be a predictor of death from cardiac or other causes.[287] The severity of dyspnea is determined by the extent of disease; the more severe the heart disease, the more readily episodes of dyspnea occur. More extreme dyspnea includes paroxysmal nocturnal dyspnea and orthopnea. *Paroxysmal nocturnal dyspnea* is sudden, unexplained episodes of shortness of breath that, at night awaken a person sleeping in a supine position. The person feels like they do not have enough air to breathe, and they have to sit upright. Moving to the upright position brings relief because the amount of blood returning to the heart and lungs from the lower extremities decreases in this position. This type of dyspnea frequently accompanies heart failure (HF) with congestive symptoms. *Orthopnea* is the term used to describe breathlessness that occurs during recumbency and is relieved by sitting upright, using pillows to prop the head and trunk. Orthopnea can occur anytime during the day or night.

**Table 12.1** Cardiovascular Signs and Symptoms by System

| System | Symptom |
|---|---|
| General | Weakness<br>Fatigue<br>Weight change<br>Poor exercise tolerance |
| Integumentary | Pressure ulcers<br>Loss of body hair<br>Cyanosis (lips, nail beds) |
| Central nervous system | Headaches<br>Impaired vision<br>Light-headedness or syncope (fainting) |
| Respiratory | Labored breathing, dyspnea (shortness of breath)<br>Productive cough<br>Orthopnea |
| Cardiovascular | Chest, shoulder, neck, jaw, or arm pain or discomfort (angina)<br>Palpitations<br>Peripheral edema<br>Intermittent claudication (leg pain) |
| Genitourinary | Frequent urination<br>Nocturia<br>Concentrated urine<br>Decreased urinary output |
| Musculoskeletal | Muscular fatigue<br>Myalgias<br>Chest, shoulder, neck, jaw, or arm pain or discomfort<br>Peripheral edema<br>Intermittent claudication (leg pain, cramping, or discomfort) |
| Gastrointestinal | Nausea and vomiting<br>Abdominal distention (caused by ascites)<br>Abdominal pain (abdominal angina) |

*Cardiovascular syncope* is a type of syncope. Syncope (loss of consciousness, or fainting; in a milder form, light-headedness) is caused by cerebral hypoperfusion (reduced oxygen supply to the brain). Cardiac syncope develops when the heart's pumping ability becomes compromised. When the heart does not pump as much blood, blood pressure drops low enough to cause fainting. Cardiac syncope can be caused by bradycardia (decreased heart rate), tachycardia (increased heart rate), or hypotension (low blood pressure).[331]

*Vasovagal syncope* is a term that is used for persons who have a very strong parasympathetic response that leads to vasodilation throughout the body. It can occur after a prolonged period of sitting or standing. Normally, in such a situation, blood tends to pool in the legs, requiring a sufficient heart rate and vasoconstriction to push the blood back to the heart. If this mechanism is not working, vasovagal syncope occurs, because the heart rate slows and vessels dilate, causing hypotension and cerebral hypoperfusion with subsequent fainting and/or falling.

The individual has a vagal response to the vascular system and passes out but regains consciousness right away (after being recumbent due to return of blood flow to the heart). This type of syncope is not as serious as cardiac syncope (except as a potential source of injury from falling). Vasovagal syncope is the most common cause of syncope in the general population.[331]

*Fatigue* after minimal exertion indicates a lack of energy that may be cardiac in origin (e.g., CAD, aortic valve dysfunction, cardiomyopathy, myocarditis), or it may occur secondary to neurologic, muscular, metabolic, or pulmonary pathologic conditions. Often fatigue of a cardiac nature is accompanied by associated symptoms, such as dyspnea, chest pain, palpitations, or headache.

*Cough* is primarily associated with pulmonary conditions but may occur as a pulmonary complication of a cardiovascular condition. Left ventricular dysfunction, including mitral valve dysfunction that results in pulmonary edema, may result in a cough when aggravated by exercise, metabolic stress, supine position, or paroxysmal nocturnal dyspnea. This type of cough is often hacking and dry. A cough caused by pulmonary edema may produce large amounts of frothy, blood-tinged sputum. In the case of HF with congestive symptoms, a cough develops because a large amount of fluid is trapped in the pulmonary tree, irritating the lung mucosa. Also, a persistent, dry cough can develop as a side effect of some cardiovascular medications (e.g., angiotensin-converting enzyme [ACE] inhibitors).

*Cyanosis* is a bluish discoloration of the lips and nail beds of the fingers and toes that accompanies inadequate blood oxygen levels (reduced amounts of bright-red oxygenated hemoglobin). While such discoloration is observed in the light-skin white population, gray color tones (instead of pink/red) along the gum line (buccal mucosa) are noted in the mouths of African Americans, Hispanics, or other dark-skinned individuals. Although cyanosis can accompany cardiac, pulmonary, hematologic, or central nervous system (CNS) disorders, visible cyanosis most often accompanies cardiovascular and pulmonary problems.

*Peripheral edema* is the hallmark of right ventricular failure; it is usually bilateral and dependent and may be accompanied by jugular venous distention, cyanosis (of lips, appendages), and abdominal distention from ascites. Right upper quadrant pain, described as constant, aching, or sharp, may occur secondary to an enlarged liver with this condition. Right-sided HF and subsequent edema can also occur as a result of cardiac surgery, venous valve incompetence or obstruction, or cardiac valve stenosis. Noncardiac causes of edema include pulmonary hypertension and lung dysfunction, resulting in right-sided HF, as well as kidney dysfunction, cirrhosis, burns, infection, lymphatic obstruction, and allergic reaction.

*Claudication,* sometimes described as cramping or burning in the lower extremities, is reported at a consistent amount of exercise or activity. The symptoms develop as a result of peripheral vascular disease (PVD), arterial or venous, often occurring simultaneously with CAD.[147] The symptoms are due to peripheral muscles reaching a point where oxygen demand is greater than oxygen delivery. Claudication can be more functionally debilitating than other associated symptoms, such as angina or dyspnea, and may occur in addition to these other symptoms. Other noncardiac causes of leg pain (e.g., sciatica, anterior compartment syndrome, gout, peripheral neuropathy, pseudoclaudication) must be differentiated from pain associated with PVD.[147] Low-back pain associated with *pseudoclaudication* often indicates spinal stenosis. The typical person affected is approximately 60 years old and bothered less by back pain than by a discomfort occurring in the buttock, thigh, or leg that (like true claudication) is brought on by walking but (unlike true claudication) can also be elicited by prolonged standing. The discomfort associated with pseudoclaudication is frequently bilateral and improves with rest or with flexion of the lumbar spine.

Biomarkers (biological markers), in a large sense, are "a broad subcategory of medical signs—that is, objective indications of medical state observed from outside the patient—which can be measured accurately and reproducibly."[345] As qualifiable characteristics of biologic processes, biomarkers serve as "an indicator of normal biological processes, pathogenic processes, or pharmacologic responses to a therapeutic intervention."[345] Examples of biomarkers for CVD include blood pressure, premature ventricular contraction, low-density lipoprotein cholesterol (LDL-C), C-reactive protein (CRP) and other circulating (in blood) molecular biomarkers.[7] Molecular biomarkers are substances released by cells under stress (i.e., inflammation of the tissue, stretching, injury, lack of oxygen to cells, free radical formation and oxidative stress) or as a result of cell rupture (death) and can point to an insult or damage to a specific organ or system. Biomarkers are used to predict the disease risk and monitor the disease progression and how the body responds to treatments. They allow tailoring treatment to individual differences and needs. Circulating biomarkers have been identified and characterized for specific CVDs and will be discussed below, when appropriately, in sections on specific CVD entities. They will be referred to as biomarkers.

SPECIAL IMPLICATIONS FOR THE THERAPIST 12.1

## *Signs and Symptoms of Cardiovascular Disease*

### Evaluation and Monitoring

As part of the evaluation, the physical therapist assesses cardiac signs and symptoms, the degree of risk of an adverse cardiac event, type and degree of impairment (dysfunction at the level of the tissue, organ or organ system, and circulation), and the level of disability (difficulty performing activities of daily life) and functional limitations (restrictions in the ability to perform specific actions).[126]

Individuals with cardiac impairment should be examined by a physician. Exercise testing to diagnose the specific level of pathology and impairment aids the therapist in prescribing an individual exercise program with specific parameters (mode, intensity, duration, frequency) determined based on the results of examination and testing.

In some cases, monitoring individuals closely and minimizing risk of an adverse event are a priority (e.g., the person awaiting further medical intervention). If the individual is symptomatic, recommendations are given to minimize life-threatening risks; interventions are directed at the underlying impairments whenever possible.

As a general guideline, the therapist monitors the unstable cardiac client (whether or not an initial electrocardiogram (ECG) readout is available) during initial exercise to keep intensity lower than the threshold at which cardiac symptoms appear. In other cases, when the degree of risk is low, the need for monitoring may be reduced accordingly, and treatment can be less conservative.

The evaluation and intervention strategies for clients with the cardiac symptoms described go beyond the scope of this text, and the physical therapist is referred to any of the specific cardiopulmonary texts available. Special implications included in this chapter should be supplemented by other such materials.

### Signs and Symptoms

Cervical disk disease, arthritic changes, and other musculoskeletal issues can mimic atypical *chest pain* requiring screening for medical disease. Pain of cardiac origin can be experienced in the shoulder because the heart (and diaphragm) are supplied by the C5 to C6 spinal segment, which refers visceral pain to the corresponding somatic area. Chest pain attributed to trigger points and other noncardiac causes is discussed in detail elsewhere.[153]

*Palpitations* lasting for hours or occurring in association with pain, shortness of breath, fainting, or severe light-headedness or dizziness require medical evaluation. Palpitations in any person with a personal history of cardiac disease or a family history of unexplained sudden death require urgent medical referral. Clients describing palpitations or similar phenomena may not be experiencing symptoms of heart disease.

Palpitations can be considered physiologic (i.e., fewer than six occurring per minute may be considered within the normal function of the heart), or they may occur as a result of an overactive thyroid, secondary to caffeine sensitivity, as a side effect of some medications, during menopause when estrogen levels decline, and through the use of stimulant drugs.

Encourage the client to report any such symptoms to the physician if this has not already been brought to the physician's attention. ECG monitoring of the heart's electrical impulses along with a diary of symptoms while wearing the monitor is most often used to identify the underlying condition.

Before referring the client to the physician, the therapist can help the client characterize the symptom or symptoms by asking a series of questions: Is the sensation long-lasting or transient? Palpitations that begin and end abruptly are more often true sustained arrhythmias. Episodes that gradually appear and disappear tend to be normal alterations in heart rhythm or related to caffeine or another stimulant.

Does anything precipitate the symptom or symptoms? Eliminating possible triggers (e.g., caffeine) one at a time may reduce or eliminate palpitations. Is there an association between hormonal status and palpitations (e.g., onset or change in frequency associated with ovulation or start or stop of menstruation)? If exercise brings on the palpitations, ventricular tachycardia may be the underlying cause.

On the other hand, sometimes starting an exercise program reduces the frequency of palpitations. Some people find that deep breathing, coughing, or relaxation can stop the symptom when it begins. If fainting occurs with the palpitations and there is a family history of sudden death, there may be an inherited cardiomyopathy or primary arrhythmia. For the experienced clinician, auscultation may provide additional useful information. Gathering this type of information for the physician's consideration can be very helpful in making the medical diagnosis.

*Dyspnea* may be a sign of poor physical conditioning, cardiac pump insufficiency, obesity, or pulmonary pathology. Anyone who cannot climb a single flight of stairs without feeling moderately to severely winded or who awakens at night or experiences shortness of breath when lying down should be evaluated by a physician. Anyone with known cardiac involvement in whom progressively worse dyspnea develops must also notify the physician of these findings.

Dyspnea relieved by specific breathing patterns (e.g., pursed-lip breathing) or by specific body positions (e.g., leaning forward on arms to lock the shoulder girdle) is more likely to be pulmonary than cardiac in origin. Because breathlessness can be a terrifying experience, the patient will avoid activity that provokes the sensation, which quickly reduces functional activities. Physical therapy intervention via pulmonary rehabilitation can favorably influence both exertional and clinically assessed dyspnea. The therapist is a key in preventing this vicious circle and in delaying decline of function in the cardiopulmonary population. There are various tools to measure dyspnea, so the therapist should pick the one correct for their patient population.[276]

*Syncope* without any warning period of light-headedness, dizziness, or nausea may be a sign of heart valve or arrhythmia problem. Dizziness or syncope can occur shortly after stopping exercise as a result of decreased venous return to the heart in a normal, healthy adult but should always be evaluated in light of the whole person and context of the situation. Syncope under any circumstance should not be ignored, as sudden death can occur; therefore medical referral is recommended for any unexplained syncope.

Athletes may experience neurocardiogenic syncope (neurally mediated hypotension; also known as vasodepressor syncope, vasovagal attack), a benign noncardiac cause of fainting in athletes. This disorder of autonomic cardiovascular regulation (i.e., blood pressure control system) is precipitated by prolonged standing after exertion, a warm environment, or stress, or it may occur during or after exercise, and is not life-threatening. Fainting during exertion, however, should always be evaluated by medical personnel.

*Fatigue* beyond expectations during or after exercise, especially in a client with a known cardiac condition, must be closely monitored. It should be remembered that β-blockers prescribed for cardiac problems can also cause unusual fatigue symptoms. For the client experiencing fatigue without a prior diagnosis of heart disease, monitoring vital signs may indicate a failure of the blood pressure to rise with increasing workloads.

Such a situation may indicate inadequate cardiac output to meet the demands of exercise. However, poor exercise tolerance is often the result of deconditioning, especially in the older adult population. Further testing (e.g., exercise treadmill test) may be helpful in determining whether fatigue is related to cardiac problems.

*Peripheral edema* in the form of a 3-lb or greater weight gain in 24 hours or gradual, continuous gain over several days with swelling of the ankles, abdomen, and hands, and shortness of breath, fatigue, and dizziness may be a red flag symptom of HF. When such symptoms persist despite rest, medical referral is required. Edema related to HF may necessitate ECG monitoring during exercise or activity, whereas edema of peripheral origin requires medical treatment of the underlying cause.

*Claudication* is always accompanied by diminished peripheral pulses in the presence of vascular disease, usually accompanied by skin discoloration and trophic changes (e.g., thin, dry, hairless skin). Core temperature, peripheral pulses, and skin temperature should be assessed. Cool skin is more indicative of vascular obstruction; warm to hot skin may indicate inflammation or infection. Sudden worsening of intermittent claudication may be a result of thromboembolism and must be reported to the physician immediately.

If persons with intermittent claudication have normal-appearing skin at rest, exercising the extremity to the point of claudication usually produces marked pallor of the skin over the distal one third of the extremity. This postexercise cutaneous ischemia occurs in both upper and lower extremities and is caused by selective shunting of the available blood to the exercised muscle and away from the more distal parts of the extremity.

## AGING AND THE CARDIOVASCULAR SYSTEM

CVD is the most common cause of hospitalization and death in the older population in the United States.[306] With the aging of America, by the year 2050, the number of people 65 years and older will more than double, reaching 25% of the population, and the number of people 85 years and older will triple, reaching 4.5% of the population.[78,135] With this increase in the number of older persons, CVD is likely to be even more of a major health problem in the future, as it accounts for greater than 30% of deaths in people age 65 years and above.[78] CVD is endemic in the US population surviving into old age.[135] In fact, more than half of adult Americans will have some form of CVD by 2030.[78]

### Specific Effects of Aging

The hearts of older persons, even fit, healthy, and active adults, pump less blood to peripheral organs; and the heart of the older person has to work much harder under the same circumstances (e.g., exercise in warm environments) than that of a younger person.

Aging of the heart is associated with a variety of molecular mechanisms and cellular pathways leading to changes in cardiac structure and function.[109,270] Disease-independent changes in the aging heart include reduced autophagy (intracellular degradation of unneeded proteins and cellular breakdown products), increased oxidative stress, development of cardiac fibrosis, reduction in the number of myocytes within the conduction tissue, reduction in calcium transport across myocyte membranes, lower capillary density, decreases in the intracellular response to β-adrenergic stimulation (sometimes referred to as blunted β-adrenoceptor responsiveness), and impaired autonomic reflex control of heart rate. Vascular aging involves endothelial dysfunction and increase in arterial wall thickness and stiffness. Other age-related events include atrial and ventricular remodeling (leading to atrial and ventricular dysfunction), degenerative valvular disease (including aortic stenosis), and changes in the structure of the sinus node (resulting in impaired conduction).

Although the specific organ changes associated with aging are discussed here, disease and lifestyle may have a greater impact on cardiovascular function than aging. Research now shows that even children need to control their modifiable risk factors for heart disease.

Postmortem heart studies of adolescents and young adults demonstrate that heart disease begins earlier than formerly expected. Atherosclerotic deposits and blood vessel changes have been demonstrated in early adolescence with substantial changes observed by age 30 years in some people. More recent studies of overweight and obese children and teens have confirmed their arteries are as stiff and thick as those of middle-aged adults.[203]

As the arteries age, increased collagen and calcium content and progressive deterioration of the arterial media combined with atherosclerotic plaque formation result in stiff and thickened arterial walls and narrowed lumen. A combination of increased systolic blood pressure and increased fatigue of arterial walls accelerates arterial damage. Age-related changes in aorta vary by anatomic region rather than occurring uniformly along its length. With aging, the greatest difference in aortic stiffness is found in the abdominal region, followed by the thoracic-descending region, the mid-descending region, and aortic arch,[175] and coinciding with the greatest degree of calcium deposition in the abdominal region.[243] Comprehensive explanation of the effects of aging on aorta and microvessels is provided by the Vascular Aging Continuum.[274]

## Effects of Aging on Function

Aerobic capacity, measured as peak oxygen uptake ($VO_2$), is reduced in aging. In healthy adults, peak $VO_2$ declines by 10% per decade, resulting in an 80-year-old having half of the peak $VO_2$ of a 30-year-old person. The reduction in peak $VO_2$ is partially mediated by a decline in maximal heart rate, due to impaired β-adrenergic receptor response.[135]

The changes described earlier have considerable consequences during cardiovascular stress, such as occurs with increased flow demand (e.g., exercise, postoperative), demand for acute autonomic reflex control (e.g., change in posture), or severe disease (e.g., uncontrolled hypertension, tachyarrhythmias, myocardial ischemia). Physiologic aging is accompanied by a progressive decline in resting organ function. Consequently, the reserve capacity to compensate for impaired organ function, heat elevation, drug metabolism, and added physiologic demands is impaired, and functional disability will occur more quickly and take longer to resolve.[109]

The heart undergoes some changes associated with advanced age in individuals who do not exercise and who have risk factors for cardiac disease.[212] Moderate thickening of the left ventricular wall (exaggerated in hypertensive clients) and increased left atrial size occur as a result of myocyte enlargement (hypertrophy) or replacement by fibrous tissue. Decreased ventricular filling compensated by increased systolic blood pressure occurs as a result of the changes in the ventricular wall. Left ventricular functioning is compromised in the presence of stress such as vigorous exercise or disease. Arrhythmia or hypertension may occur as a result.

Changes at the peripheral vessels, most often larger and medium-sized vessels, include calcium deposition and changes in the amount of elastin and collagen leading to loss of elasticity.

There is some evidence that age-related decline in steroid hormones, particularly the sex hormones (estrogen, progesterone, testosterone, dehydroepiandrosterone, pregnenolone) triggers a feedback loop to elevate cholesterol concentrations. This mechanism allows the body to maintain levels of vital hormones needed for tissue repair, maintenance, and response to physiologic stresses. But age-impaired hormone synthesis does not allow the elevated cholesterol to actually restore hormones to the optimum levels, thus resulting in damaging, elevated cholesterol levels, leading to coronary heart disease and stroke. Resting cardiac function (e.g., cardiac output, heart rate) shows minimal age-related changes, with changes in functional capacity being more apparent during exercise. The maximal heart rate, or the highest heart rate during exercise, does decline with age, possibly because of a decreased secretion of catecholamines and diminished cardiovascular response to them. This decline in maximal heart rate is reflected in the target zone heart rates for exercising senior citizens. Appendix B explains the standard calculation of target heart rates for sedentary and physically fit older adults. However, caution should be used with older adults as this calculation isn't always accurate for older ages. Exercise testing will provide the physical therapist with a more accurate measure of the patient's exercising ability. The effect of the Frank-Starling mechanism remains unaltered with age and is used effectively during exercise to maintain cardiac output through a higher stroke volume.

The Frank-Starling law states that the greater the myocardial fiber length (or stretch), the greater its force of contraction. The more the left ventricle fills with blood, the greater the quantity of blood ejected into the aorta. One can use an analogy with a rubber band: the more it is stretched, the more strongly it recoils or snaps back. Thus a direct relationship exists between the volume of blood in the heart at the end of diastole and the force of contraction during the next systole.

## Exercise and Age-Associated Changes in the Heart

It is commonly accepted that a decline in maximal oxygen uptake, maximal heart rate, and maximal cardiac output with aging occurs during exercise, even in older athletes. These cardiovascular alterations parallel changes that occur with deconditioning or disuse and may improve with increased activity. Exercise can reverse some of the age-associated changes in the heart at least partially,[212,270] supporting the hypothesis that age-related cardiovascular changes are mostly the result of inactivity or deconditioning.

In older people, aerobic exercise training lowers heart rate at rest, reduces heart rate and levels of plasma catecholamine, $VO_{2max}$ and improves quality of life.[135,179] Finally, exercise stress testing and exercise prescription for older people should be more conservative at first and monitored closely.[135] Recommendations and precautions to minimize the risk of adverse cardiac events among previously sedentary older adults who do not have symptomatic CVD and are interested in starting an exercise program are available.[17,360] The therapist is instrumental in conducting an examination and performing exercise testing to identify the specific level of pathology, impairment, disability, and/or functional limitations.[324] An individual exercise prescription is made (mode, intensity, duration, frequency) based on the results of the examination and testing.[17,132,155]

## GENDER DIFFERENCES AND THE CARDIOVASCULAR SYSTEM

There are some differences in the cardiovascular system between genders. This text can't cover all differences, so the reader is referred to other, more complete sources.[63,181,217,231,245,259] While men and women have, in general, similar traditional risk factors for CVD women have additional risk factors including disorders of pregnancy, adverse pregnancy outcomes, and menopause.[50]

Female hearts are not only smaller than male hearts, but also are constructed differently and respond to age and hypertrophic stimuli differently. For instance, structural differences in the mitral valve may explain why women are more prone to mitral valve prolapse than men. At puberty, a young woman's QT interval lengthens, and the woman with a long QT interval is at greater risk for a serious form of ventricular arrhythmia (known as *torsades de pointes*) and sudden cardiac death, especially when taking drugs that prolong the QT interval.[365]

Left ventricular mass increases with age in healthy women but remains constant in men. Under increased cardiac loading conditions (e.g., hypertension, aortic stenosis), this disparity between genders is even more obvious. The risk for drugs other than cardiac and psychotropic ones to cause prolongation of the QT interval has been recognized. Women also have a three times greater risk of potentially fatal arrhythmias from some cardiac and psychotropic medications. Complications from antiarrhythmic drug use are most common during the first 3 days or after a dosage increase.

Women metabolize many medications differently from men. Differences in body size and levels and repertoire of sex hormones are some of the causes.[218]

Women tend to have a higher incidence of bleeding episodes from thrombolytic agents. Women also have different outcomes with surgery and percutaneous coronary intervention (PCI; previously referred to as percutaneous transluminal coronary angioplasty, or PTCA), a procedure aimed at widening of a narrowed vessel lumen with either an inflated balloon (angioplasty) or an inserted stent. More repeat procedures of PCI are done in women, possibly because of smaller arteries, more advanced disease compared to men, or different tolerance to medications.[10] Women, in contrast to men, with premature coronary disease are at higher risk of developing vascular and ischemic complications after PCI.[10] Women with stable angina and acute coronary syndrome have higher in-hospital mortality rates.[245]

Women receive less-aggressive therapy than men for acute ischemic heart disease[181] or hypertension[245] and have a poorer outcome when treatment is received. Until recently, women in all age groups have been less likely to undergo diagnostic catheterization than men, and this difference was especially pronounced among older women (older than age 85 years). Women have been less likely than men to receive preventive care (drug treatment for lipid management; risk factor management through exercise, nutrition, and weight reduction), and timely thrombolytic therapy for heart attack (or stroke).[67,141] Women were less likely to undergo PCI and coronary artery bypass graft (CABG) when compared to men.[246] Now that these facts are recognized,[63,181,218,231,245,246,259] there is hope that this equal-opportunity disease will become an equally treated disease. A new generation of physicians trained to recognize differences between men and women will help.

Women also tend to delay longer than men before seeking help for symptoms of acute MI, referred to as *decision delay*, further compromising effective treatment and improved outcomes.[162,246] This is especially true given the evidence that first heart attacks in women may be more severe and that women are more likely to die in the first weeks and months after a heart attack. Increased rate of mortality is reported in middle-aged women with new-onset atrial fibrillation.[94] The increased risk of death is attributed to increased HF, stroke, and MI. Aggressive treatments are suggested, including anticoagulants and hypertension medications, in order to reduce the incidence of stroke and mortality risk.

For many years, women and minorities were underrepresented in studies conducted on heart disease and stroke, but this has changed over the last decade along with concomitant expansion of prevention and educational outreach programs for heart attack, stroke, and other CVDs in women.[63,181,218,259] Large observational studies report marked improvements in the accuracy of results for women undergoing exercise treadmill, echocardiography, and nuclear testing as a result of expanding risk parameters in the test interpretations and improved diagnostic accuracy of such tests.[249] As with older adults, the typical heart rate maximum equation may not be accurate for women either. Heart rate estimates for women should be based on a modified formula: peak heart rate = 206 − [age × 0.88].[158] Because of technological advances, improved surgical techniques, greater awareness of gender differences in heart disease, and increased funding for gender-based research, these trends are improving, and women now seem to do as well as men after surgical (revascularization) procedures to restore blood flow to the heart.

Although the American Heart Association (AHA) reports a decline in death rates in women for CAD and stroke,[67] women are still twice as likely as men to die within 1 year of having a heart attack, and women are at greater risk for second heart attacks and for disability because of HF. In 2007 in the United States, CVD was responsible for approximately one death per minute in women.[50] The death rate among African American women is 33.7% higher for stroke and 69% higher for heart disease than that of white women.[259] At the same time, African American women have significantly lower awareness of heart disease and stroke compared to white women.[259] Not surprisingly, almost half of all women do not realize the necessity of clinical care in case of acute cardiovascular event. Only 53% of women would call 911 if they suspected they were having the event.[259] The need for education and increasing awareness of CVD risk factors of women and their families is obvious.

In 2011, the AHA updated its guidelines on prevention of CVD in women, transforming them from evidence-based into effectiveness-based, stressing the effectiveness (benefits and risks derived from clinical practice) of preventive therapies versus efficacy (benefits derived from clinical research).[259]

## Coronary Artery Disease in Women

It was long believed that CAD was a more benign process in females, but this has been soundly disproved. A woman presenting with angina postmenopausally has the exact same mortality as a man presenting with angina in his sixties. CAD is the single leading cause of death and a significant cause of morbidity among women in the United States.[63,259]

Certain characteristics and clinical conditions may place women at higher risk of CAD development or progression, such as depression, being black, menopausal status, age, type 2 diabetes mellitus, and thyroid dysfunction. In addition, female gender may adversely influence the relative benefits of some risk modification interventions in older adults (e.g., cholesterol lowering, sedentary behavior, smoking cessation).[249] Many women die of CAD without any warning signs, and by age 65 years, one in four women has heart disease (the same proportion as in men). CAD claims the lives of nearly 240,000 women annually in the United States.[249] Women with type 2 diabetes die of CAD three times as often as men with this condition.[300] Despite these statistics, misperceptions still exist that CVD is not a real problem for women and that, despite the fact that some risk factors for CAD can be prevented, CAD is not curable. For these reasons, education and prevention are vitally important to reduce risk of heart disease. [236]

A new predictive model for women that combines newer risk markers with traditional risk factors and family history is being investigated. A family history of heart attack prior to age 60 years has been added to the list of risk factors of which women should be aware. The Reynolds Risk Score could help target women who could benefit from more aggressive preventive treatment, including diet, exercise, hormone therapy, nutriceuticals, and possibly a statin or other cholesterol-lowering medication.[98,298]

## Coronary Artery Surgery and Women

The number of women undergoing CABG continues to increase. Women may experience more chest wall discomfort as a common side effect of CABG than men; it is most often reported in those women who had an internal mammary artery graft.

Women undergoing bypass surgery have a death rate about twice as high as that of men; the difference is more evident in younger women (younger than 50 years old).[349] This has been attributed to the fact that women generally have smaller bodies, meaning smaller coronary arteries on which it may be technically more difficult to operate. As a result, a variation of CABG surgery has been developed, known as off-pump coronary artery bypass, which has reduced the death rate among women and brought about greater equalization in outcomes between men and women. Off-pump coronary artery bypass is less invasive because the procedure does not require a cardiopulmonary bypass, which stops the heart during surgery and directs the blood outside the body. However, even with this procedure, gender differences remain, as women still experience more postoperative complications.

## Coronary Microvascular Dysfunction

A "stealth" form of heart disease called *coronary microvascular dysfunction* or *disease* has been identified in women.[181] This phenotype does not show up on angiograms, and positron emission tomography (PET) is used to diagnose it. Classic signs of reduced blood flow to the heart (ischemia) are not present. Instead there are false-positive stress test results (significantly abnormal results on the stress test but clear arteries on an angiogram). It may be that the tiny blood vessels to the heart become constricted, reducing blood flow.

Scientists suspect ischemia may have different effects on women compared to CAD (Table 12.2). It was previously thought that women with chest pain but clear arteries had an aggravating case of coronary microvascular syndrome, but it was not considered harmful.

Research in the WISE study, a federally funded investigation into ischemic heart disease in women, was undertaken to investigate this phenomenon.[37,297,328] Autopsy comparisons of women and men have shown that women who die of heart attacks are more likely to have plaque buildup uniformly around the inside of the blood vessel, possibly as a result of chronic inflammation. Inflammation may not be the only cause of coronary microvascular dysfunction. Endothelial dysfunction, autonomic dysregulation, hormonal deficiency, and hyperinsulinemia have been shown to play a role.[181] Women with this type of heart disease are at increased risk for heart attack, stroke, and reduced quality of life.

## Hormonal Status

### Influence of Hormones on Coronary Artery Disease

Estrogen has been considered to have a cardioprotective benefit for women via a variety of mechanisms. It stimulates the formation of high-density lipoprotein cholesterol (HDL-C), the good cholesterol, which carries fat away from the artery wall and back to the liver to be

**Table 12.2** Ischemic Heart Disease

| | Coronary Artery Disease | Coronary Microvascular Disease |
|---|---|---|
| Clinical presentation | Chest pain often described as "crushing" radiating to the left arm, jaw, upper back; can present differently in women<br>Cold sweat, nausea | Diffuse discomfort<br>Extreme fatigue<br>Depression<br>Dyspnea<br>Older adult: confusion or increased confusion |
| Pathology | Plaque buildup extending in toward the blood vessel lumen | Microvascular constriction (narrowing of smaller coronary arteries) *plaque deposited uniformly around inside of the artery walls* |
| Diagnosis | Stress test, coronary angiography | Stress test[a], functional vascular imaging (e.g., multidirectional CT scan of the heart, stress echocardiography, SPECT) |
| Treatment | Surgery (angioplasty, CABG)<br>Medication (statins) | Medication (antihypertensives, anti-inflammatories, statins) |

[a]Stress echocardiography uses ultrasound to produce images of the heart after an exercise stress test.

*CABG*, Coronary artery bypass graft; *CT*, computed tomography (serves as a noninvasive angiogram; moves around the heart generating a three-dimensional image of the heart and coronary arteries); *SPECT*, single-photon emission computed tomography (injects a radioactive tracer into bloodstream to chart the flow of blood in the heart and coronary vessels).

Data from Bonow RO: *Braunwald's heart disease—a textbook of cardiovascular medicine*, ed 9, Philadelphia, 2011, WB Saunders.

broken down and excreted. Estrogen will also stimulate LDL-C receptors in the liver and possibly the blood vessel walls. These receptors bind the LDL-C, the bad cholesterol, and remove it from the circulation, preventing its deposit in atherosclerotic plaques.

Estradiol acts as a calcium channel blocker to relax artery walls, which helps dilate the arteries, improves blood flow throughout the brain and the rest of the body, and helps to lower blood pressure. Estrogen maintains the normal balance of prostacyclin and thromboxane, two chemicals that regulate clot formation. Estrogen increases arterial wall production of prostacyclin, which improves blood flow and decreases platelet aggregation. Estrogen exerts its action on cells and tissues through binding to a receptor. In addition to a classical estrogen receptor (ER) that mediates reproductive effects of estrogen, recently, a new G-protein coupled receptor (GPER) has been identified.[129] In the cardiovascular system GPER stimulates vasorelaxation, leading to lowering blood pressure, and regulates cholesterol metabolism in the liver, promoting clearance of LDL-C particles.

Another possible mechanism by which estrogen protects against heart disease before menopause is the release of nitric oxide (formerly referred to as endothelium-derived relaxing factor), a chemical stimulated by estrogen and responsible for dilating blood vessels to maintain normal blood pressure and flow. As women lose the biologically active estradiol, their incidence of CVD increases dramatically, matching the incidence among men within 10 years of menopause without hormone replacement therapy.

Myocardial ischemia may be more easily induced when estrogen concentrations are low, a finding that may be important for timing assessment and evaluating treatment in women with CAD.

### Hormone Replacement for Postmenopausal Women

The use of hormones for cardioprotection has been under investigation for many years. Because heart attacks tend to occur 10 years later in women than in men, it was assumed that the protective effect of estrogen was responsible. Exogenous (externally administered) estrogen has been reported to improve serum lipid profiles, carbohydrate metabolism, and vascular reactivity, but surprisingly, hormonal therapy did not produce overall cardiovascular benefit.[181] There is no concrete evidence showing that hormone replacement in postmenopausal women creates an improvement in cardiac autonomic modulation.[285]

### Oral Contraceptives

Studies show that women smokers older than age 35 years who use oral contraceptives are much more likely to have a heart attack or stroke than nonsmokers who use birth control pills. In the last 20 years, cardiovascular complications in all women taking oral contraceptives have become less common because current contraceptives contain the lowest dose of estrogen possible without breakthrough bleeding.

At this dose, the risk of thromboembolic disease is reduced to about 40 events per 100,000 women per year, approximately the same risk as in the general population.[66] There is much debate about the safety of newer formulations of oral contraceptives. There is still a risk of ischemic stroke and venous thromboembolic events, so these should be monitored in premenopausal women.[211]

## Hypertension in Women

More women than men eventually develop hypertension in the United States because of their higher numbers and greater longevity. White coat hypertension (rise in blood pressure when being evaluated by a physician or other health care worker) is more prevalent among women, and black women are more likely to have white coat hypertension than black men. Alcohol, obesity, and oral contraceptives are important causes of rise in blood pressure among women. It has been shown for quite some time that alcohol increases risks of cardiomyopathy, atrial fibrillation, systemic hypertension, and stroke.[204] Women, like men, may have excessive alcohol consumption; yet they are less likely than men to be identified as alcohol abusers at early stages of the illness. Thus, their rates of hypertension may be even higher than those of men. ACE inhibitors and angiotensin II receptor blockers are contraindicated in pregnancy and should be avoided in women with childbearing potential.[13] Infants who were exposed to ACE inhibitors in utero were found to be at increased risk of major congenital malformations that affected the cardiovascular and nervous systems.[99]

In the WISE study, early onset of high systolic blood pressure or pulse pressure (the difference between systolic and diastolic blood pressures) has been linked with a higher risk of having significant CAD.[36]

### Cholesterol Concerns for Women

Serum cholesterol is transported in serum with the help of lipoproteins. Lipoproteins are complexes of fat and proteins that help dissolve, transport, and utilize the cholesterol molecule. Depending on the nature of the lipoprotein carrier, cholesterol can be atherogenic (bad) or nonatherogenic (good). Atherogenic cholesterol LDL-C is a primary cause of atherosclerosis. Very-low-density lipoprotein (VLDL) is a carrier of triglycerides, and VLDL-C is atherogenic. HDL-C is a nonatherogenic cholesterol, which carries cholesterol away from the cells to be cleared in the liver. Elevated LDL-C levels are linked to increased risk of stroke and large-artery atherosclerosis in women.[50] Higher HDL-C levels reduced risks of ischemic stroke in men but not women.[50] Premature menopause (age <40 years) is associated with increased CVD risk in women.[157] After menopause, women have higher concentrations of total cholesterol than men do, but the significance of this finding remains unknown. Low levels of HDL-C cholesterol are predictive of CAD in women and appear to be a stronger risk factor for women older than 65 years than for men of the same age.[264]

The current guidelines for the treatment of elevated cholesterol have been addressed with regards to white women and women of color.[157] The guidelines do not use specific target cholesterol levels but rather rely on an individual's total risk for cardiovascular disease and setting an upper limit for their LDL-C levels.

## DISEASES AFFECTING THE HEART MUSCLE

### Ischemic Heart Disease, Coronary Heart Disease, Coronary Artery Disease

Coronary arteries carry oxygenated blood to the myocardium. When these arteries become narrowed or blocked, the areas of the heart muscle supplied by that artery do not receive a sufficient amount of oxygen and become ischemic and injured. If the ischemia continues for a prolonged period of time, infarction may result. The disorder of the myocardium owing to insufficient blood supply is known as ischemic heart disease, also referred to as CAD or coronary heart disease (CHD).

Despite improved clinical care, heightened public awareness, and widespread use of health innovations, atherosclerotic disease (resulting in narrowing of arteries) remains the number one cause of mortality and morbidity in the United States.

**Box 12.1**

**NONATHEROSCLEROTIC CAUSES OF CORONARY ARTERY OBSTRUCTION**

- Kawasaki disease
- Coronary embolism
  - Infective endocarditis
  - Prosthetic valves
  - Cardiac myxomas
  - Cardiopulmonary bypass
  - Coronary arteriography
- Metabolic syndrome
- Insulin resistance (hyperinsulinemia)
- Trauma to coronary arteries
  - Penetrating
  - Nonpenetrating
- Arteritis
  - Syphilis
  - Polyarteritis nodosa
  - Lupus erythematosus
  - Rheumatoid arthritis
- Connective tissue diseases
- Radiotherapy

An estimated 16.5 million persons in the United States have CHD. In 2018, approximately 750,000 people had first-time cardiac events and 335,000 had a recurrent event. Approximately 34.4% of those events were fatal. Eleven million Americans who are alive today have a history of angina pectoris, MI, or both, and an estimated 2 million middle-aged and older adults (more than 75 years) have silent myocardial ischemia.[50]

Although CAD death rates in the United States have decreased since reaching a peak during the late 1960s (146.2 cases per 100,000 in 1948 with a peak of 220.3 in 1963 to 87 cases per 100,000 in 1996), a decline in the incidence of CAD has not been achieved. In 1940, the rate of CAD was 26.4 per 100,000 people compared to 196.6 in 2016.[79]

The declining mortality rate does not apply to those adults with diabetes and has been attributed to improvements in lifestyle (e.g., reduced smoking, improved treatment for lipid lowering, improved coronary care), whereas the increased incidence may be related to the increasing number of people who are surviving past age 65 years.

Nonatherosclerotic causes of coronary artery obstruction and subsequent ischemic heart disease are uncommon (Box 12.1). For example, mediastinal radiotherapy for left-sided breast cancer, Hodgkin lymphoma, or non–Hodgkin lymphoma may be an independent risk factor in the development of ischemic heart disease.

Radiotherapy causes cardiac perfusion defects 6 months after treatment in most people, but it remains unknown if these changes are transient or permanent. Improvements in radiation technique have reduced complications, especially late cardiac deaths.

#### Arteriosclerosis

Arteriosclerosis represents a group of diseases characterized by thickening and loss of elasticity of the arterial walls, often referred to as hardening of the arteries. Arteriosclerosis can be divided into three types: (1) *atherosclerosis,* in which athero mas (plaques of fatty deposits) form in the

**Table 12.3** Coronary Artery Disease Risk Factors

| MODIFIABLE RISK FACTORS | | | NONMODIFIABLE RISK FACTORS | NEWER PREDICTORS OF RISK FACTORS |
|---|---|---|---|---|
| **Risk Factors for Which Intervention Has Been Shown to Reduce Incidence of CAD** | **Risk Factors for Which Intervention Is Likely to Reduce Incidence of CAD** | **Risk Factors for Which Intervention Might Reduce Incidence of CAD** | | **Risk Factors Under Investigation** |
| Cigarette smoking<br>Elevated total serum cholesterol level<br>Elevated LDL-C level >100 mg/dl<br>Hypertension | Obesity<br>Physical inactivity<br>Diabetes or impaired glucose tolerance; insulin resistance<br>Low HDL-C level<br>• Men <40 mg/dL<br>• Women <50 mg/dL<br>Hormonal status; oral contraceptives; hysterectomy or oophorectomy; menopause without hormone replacement (especially before age 40 yr)<br>Thrombogenic factors | Psychologic factors and emotional response to stress<br>Discriminatory medicine[a]<br>Oxidative stress<br>Excessive alcohol consumption or complete abstinence<br>Elevated triglycerides<br>Sleep-disordered breathing<br>Poor nutrition | Age<br>• Women >55 yr<br>• Men >45 yr<br>Male gender<br>Family history; genetic determinants<br>Ethnicity<br>Infection (viral, bacterial) | Elevated homocysteine (>15 μmol/L)<br>C-reactive protein (CRP)<br>• Below 1 mg/dL: low risk<br>• 1–3 mg/dL: moderate risk<br>• Above 3 mg/dL: high risk<br>Lipoprotein (a) or Lp(a) (>30 mg/dL)[b]<br>Troponin T<br>Plasminogen activator inhibitor (marker for recurrence of MI)<br>D-dimer (fibrin)<br>Male erectile dysfunction (impotence)<br>Ankle/brachial blood pressure index |

[a]Discriminatory medicine is not technically a risk factor for CAD but rather results in a different natural history for some individuals.
[b]Applies to whites and Asians but not to blacks.
*CAD*, Coronary artery disease; *LDL-C*, low-density lipoprotein cholesterol; *HDL-C*, high-density lipoprotein cholesterol; *MI*, myocardial infarction.

inner layer (intima) of the arteries; (2) *Mönckeberg arteriosclerosis*, involving the middle layer of the arteries with destruction of muscle and elastic fibers and formation of calcium deposits; and (3) *arteriolosclerosis* or *arteriolar sclerosis*, characterized by thickening of the walls of small arteries (arterioles). All three forms of arteriosclerosis may be present in the same person but in different blood vessels. Frequently, the terms *arteriosclerosis* and *atherosclerosis* are used interchangeably, although technically atherosclerosis is a most common form of arteriosclerosis.

### Atherosclerosis

Atherosclerosis can affect any of the arteries, and this pathologic process is referred to as atherosclerotic cardiovascular disease (often shortened to CVD).

When the arteries of the heart are affected it is referred to as CAD or CHD; when the arteries to the brain are affected, cerebrovascular disease is the term. Atherosclerosis of blood vessels supplying other parts of the body can result in PVD, aneurysm, and intestinal infarction. Atherosclerosis as it affects the heart vessels is discussed in this section. The effects of atherosclerosis on other blood vessels are discussed individually elsewhere.

### Etiologic and Risk Factors

The Framingham Heart Study, initiated in 1948 and now continuing with its third generation of participants, was the original research regarding CAD risk factors.[107] Results from that study and ongoing research have identified important modifiable and nonmodifiable risk factors associated with death caused by CAD.

Modifiable risk factors that can be *controlled* are referred to now as "risk factors for which intervention has been shown to *reduce* incidence of CAD"; other risk factors that can be *managed* are now referred to as "risk factors for which intervention is *likely to reduce* incidence of CAD" or "risk factors for which intervention *might reduce* incidence of CAD." Some risk factors cannot be altered (nonmodifiable), such as age, gender, family history of heart disease, ethnicity, and exposure to infectious agents (Table 12.3).

As the Framingham study continues to gather and analyze new data, results are reported that help modify existing health risk appraisal models relating risk factors to the probability of developing CAD. With these new models, blood lipid levels, diabetes, systolic blood pressure, and cigarette smoking are emphasized once again as independent predictors of risk.

It has been well documented that African American and Mexican American women and African American men have greater risk for CVD.[50] Differences in socioeconomic status (as measured by educational level and family income) do not explain the higher prevalence of CVD risk factors in these ethnic minority groups.

Higher prevalence of certain risk factors in African American women, particularly diabetes and obesity, may explain their increased risk of CAD. Dyslipidemia, diabetes, and smoking have been shown to have the greatest impact on CAD rates for African American men. Hispanic men had the greatest impact from dyslipidemia and family history.[23] Further research regarding the impact of ethnicities on CAD rates is still needed.

**Modification of Risk Factors That Reduce Incidence of Coronary Artery Disease.** *Cigarette smoking* remains the leading preventable cause of CAD. Products of tobacco burning, of which there are more than 4,000,[97] increase heart rate and blood pressure. They also decrease the oxygen-carrying capacity of blood; lead to accumulation of such poisonous compounds as carbon monoxide, cyanide, formaldehyde, and carbon dioxide; cause narrowing of blood vessels; and increase the work of the heart. By-products of tobacco smoking in the blood act as potent oxidizing agents. This oxidation damages the intimal lining of the arterial walls, exposes collagen, and accelerates platelet aggregation.

Nicotine itself enhances the process of atherosclerosis[97] by a direct effect on the blood vessel wall. It increases proliferation of vascular smooth muscle cells and aggregability of platelets, both contributing to atherosclerotic plaque formation in the coronary arteries. Nicotine elevates LDL-C levels in blood and increases the expression of LDL receptors on smooth muscle cells lining the plaque, priming the cells for the entry of LDL-C particles. Nicotine induces release of catecholamines, causing increase in blood pressure and heart rate.

People who smoke have 2 to 4 times higher risk of stroke compared to those who do not smoke or quit more than 10 years ago.[50] Quitting smoking at the age of 25 to 34 extends life for 10 years, at age 35 to 44 for 9 years, and at age 45 to 54 for 6 years.[50]

*Elevated total serum cholesterol levels* (>150 mg/dL) place a person at greater risk for heart disease (Table 12.4). Therapy to lower LDL-C levels can stabilize, reduce, or even reverse the progression of atherosclerotic plaques and coronary stenosis and reduce recurrent cardiac episodes. Cholesterol levels are influenced by a variety of factors including heredity, diet, exercise, alcohol consumption, obesity, medications, menopausal status, thyroid function, and smoking. Impaired thyroid function is a cause of elevated cholesterol and arterial stiffness.[311]

*Hypertension*, or high blood pressure, causes the heart to work harder and may injure the arterial walls, making them prone to atherosclerosis. Epidemiologic studies document a strong association between high levels of both systolic and diastolic blood pressure and risk of CAD (and stroke) in both men and women.

Hypertension is aggravated by obesity and a diet high in salt. It is also associated with diabetes and excessive alcohol use. It can be initiated or aggravated by the use of oral contraceptives, especially in women who smoke. Women who have undetected or uncontrolled hypertension are five times more likely to experience angina, heart attack, or sudden death than women with normal blood pressure. Weight reduction, dietary interventions, and pharmacologic intervention have important roles in the prevention and treatment of hypertension.

**Modification of Risk Factors That Are *Likely* to Reduce Incidence of Coronary Artery Disease.** Physical inactivity,[207] sedentary lifestyle,[379] and obesity[145] are parallel, interrelated epidemics in the United States that contribute to increased risk of CAD.

*Obesity* alone can lead to CAD, because the excess weight makes the heart work harder to pump blood throughout the body, as well as causing inflammation in the arteries,

**Table 12.4** Heart Disease Prevention Target Measurements[a]

| Risk Factors | Targets |
|---|---|
| **Body Measurements** | |
| • Body mass index (BMI): multiply your weight in pounds by 703, then divide that number by the square of your height in inches | 18.5–24.0 |
| • Waist-to-hip ratio (WHR): divide your waist measurement in inches by your hip measurement in inches | ≤0.8 |
| **Lipids, Lipoproteins** | |
| • Total cholesterol | <200 mg/dL |
| • HDL cholesterol | ≥40 mg/dL (men) ≥50 mg/dL (women) |
| • LDL cholesterol | ≤100 mg/dL |
| • Triglycerides | ≤200 mg/dL (<150 mg/dL)[b] |
| • Total cholesterol/HDL ratio | <4.5 |
| **Blood Pressure** | See Table 12.8 |

[a]These target measures are for healthy adults without evidence of heart disease.

[b]Grundy SM, Stone NJ, Bailey AL, et al. AHA/ACC/AACVPR/AAPA/ABC/ACPM/ADA/AGS/APhA/ ASPC/NLA/PCNA Guideline on the Management of Blood Cholesterol, *Journal of the American College of Cardiology*, 2018, doi: https://doi.org/10.1016/j.jacc.2018.11.003

leading to atherosclerosis.[189] Obesity is commonly associated with diabetes mellitus, high blood pressure, and high serum lipid (triglycerides and cholesterol) levels.[78] The prevalence of overweight and obesity has increased among both men (75% of all) and women (68% of all) in the United States in the past decade.[78] One of every five children and adolescents aged 2 to 19 is obese.[78] Table 12.4 lists target body measurements (adults) for the prevention of heart disease. Increasing research and knowledge related to nutrition have led to identification of several dietary factors that influence CAD risk. The epidemiologic evidence confirms that diets low in saturated fat and high in fruits, vegetables, whole grains, and fiber are associated with a reduced risk of CAD.

*Physical inactivity* is a major risk factor equal to increased cholesterol levels, cigarette smoking, and high blood pressure. Replacing 10 minutes of sedentary time with 10 minutes of light-intensity activity reduces mortality risk by 9%.[50] Physical inactivity increases risks of stroke (by 60%), CAD (by 45%), and high blood pressure (by 30%).[207] Eliminating physical inactivity worldwide would lead to 6% decrease in CAD and prolong life expectancy by 0.68 years.[121] AHA underscores the role of physical therapists in promoting physical activity and prescribing exercise to their clients.[229] Physical therapists are urged to be proactive in addressing assessment and promotion of physical activity, including educating the public on the role of the physical therapist in the management of CVD through exercise. Exercise has been recognized as "one of the most important and effective interventions physical therapists can incorporate into every patient plan of care to promote health and wellness."[229]

Physical activity is linked to lower rates of many chronic diseases including CVD. Regular aerobic exercise reduces CVD risk in part by lowering resting pulse rate and blood pressure, improving lipid profile and managing body weight.[121]

*Impaired glucose metabolism* (e.g., insulin resistance, hyperinsulinemia, glucose intolerance) is reported to be atherogenic. Impaired glucose tolerance and increased levels of glycated hemoglobin are powerful contributors to atherosclerotic cardiovascular events.[164]

Diabetes mellitus is a major risk factor for CVD, causing a two- to fourfold increase in the CVD risk. Moreover, the poorer the glycemic control, the higher the risk.[50,137] The risk for ischemic heart disease was 2.4-fold higher in men and 3.5-fold higher in women with diabetes compared with their nondiabetic counterparts.[300] Individuals with type 2 diabetes mellitus have a risk of MI equivalent to that of someone without diabetes who has had a previous MI. Kidney disease accompanied by hypertension is a serious complication affecting the cardiovascular system among people with diabetes.[137] Diabetes confers the same risk of CVD as aging 15 years.[56] More than 50% of persons who have diabetes die of CVD.[300] Among them, almost 70% of people older than 65 years die of some form of heart disease.[50] People with diabetes die of heart disease 2 to 4 times more often than people without diabetes.[50]

*Low levels of HDL-C* (and high levels of triglycerides) produce twice as many cases of CAD as any other lipid abnormality; this effect is exaggerated in women (see Table 12.4).

*Hormonal status* in the menopausal or postmenopausal woman is now known to be a likely contributing risk factor in the development of CAD.[245] The mechanism through which a protective effect is mediated by estrogen has not been explained completely.

**Modification of Risk Factors That *Might* Reduce Incidence of Coronary Artery Disease.** *Psychological factors and emotional stress* (e.g., depression, anxiety, anger, personality factors and character traits, social isolation, hostile environment, emotional disturbances, chronic life stress including job stress) contribute significantly to the pathogenesis and expression of CAD, especially in women.[8,83,245,291] Persons with depression have double risk of an MI.[83]

People who are negative, insecure, and distressed (type D personality) are three times more likely to experience a second heart attack than non–D types.[226] Inflammation elicited by type D stress is linked to increased risk of CAD in this population.[83]

Although in type A personality, increased risk of cardiovascular mortality was linked to cognitive hostility (hostile thoughts rather than hostile behavior) this population had better survival in CAD, perhaps due to better adherence to medical treatment.[83] People who have antagonistic personality have higher risk of MI or stroke. Studies showed that they have thicker carotid artery walls than people who are more agreeable.[348]

The long-held belief that anger can increase the risk of acute MI and can be an immediate trigger of heart attacks has been verified.[375] Negative emotions (anger, hostility) displayed in Twitter messages were found linked to increased risk of cardiovascular death.[83]

About one in four people experience symptoms of anxiety or depression after a heart attack or coronary bypass surgery. Moderate to severe depression is associated with altered cardiac autonomic modulation, including elevated heart rate, elevated norepinephrine, and reduced heart rate variability, known risk factors for cardiac morbidity and mortality. People with depression have lower levels of HDL-C.[83] Thus, treating anxiety and depression is an important step in preventing disability and premature death in people with CAD.

Whereas negative emotions trigger the stress response, increasing blood pressure and heart rate and altering platelet function, positive emotions and laughter can lower the risk of cardiovascular events.[245] One of the mechanisms involves changes in endothelial function and improved blood flow. In one study, people who watched movies that elicited laughter had their blood flow increased 22% compared to the baseline values. In contrast, those who watched stressful movies had blood flow reduced by 35%.[250] Cognitive behavioral therapy was able to increase HDL-C levels in acute-MI patients who previously had undergone CABG surgery or PCI. In addition, as these individuals' depression level was reduced, they were better at managing their anger and anxiety and showed significant improvements in self-rated health. Increasing evidence suggests that cognitive behavioral therapy and anger management may benefit cardiac clients by improving medical outcome.[83]

*Oxidative stress,* or the oxidation of LDL-C particles as part of the atherosclerotic plaque formation, is under active investigation. Oxidative stress is considered a significant risk factor for CVD. However, there isn't good evidence that antioxidant nutrients provide benefits for CVD.

This apparent paradox between the role of antioxidants in reducing oxidative stress and the failure of many antioxidant supplementations warrants further research. Meanwhile, according to the current AHA scientific statement, antioxidant vitamin supplements to prevent CVD are not listed as recommended.[33]

*Moderate alcohol consumption* decreases the risk of heart disease in some people.[260] This is attributed to alcohol's beneficial effects on hemostasis, including platelet aggregation, coagulation factors, and fibrinolytic system.[319] Specifically, alcohol intake increases activity of an enzyme called *tissue-type plasminogen activator (tPA)* that helps to keep blood flowing smoothly by initiating dissolving of clots (fibrinolysis).

Although a small amount of alcohol taken daily with meals may elevate levels of HDL-C and the bioflavonoids in red wine reduce atherosclerosis, most researchers oppose recommending drinking as a public health measure to fight heart disease and stress that no one, particularly people with a personal or family history of alcohol abuse, should drink alcohol to improve cholesterol. Dietary supplements containing flavonoids and antioxidants are now available without the sugar in grape juice or the alcohol in wine. It should always be remembered that heavy alcohol consumption and binge drinking increase risk of blood clot formation, cardiac arrhythmia, elevated blood pressure, and CVD. In fact, alcohol use is listed among 10 leading risk factors related to death.[50] Control of alcohol consumption is especially important for women as they have a higher risk of cardiovascular mortality.[383]

Greater concentrations of alcohol can contribute to CVD, and even light drinking has not been shown to reduce CVD risk more than abstaining from drinking all together.[130]

**Nonmodifiable Risk Factors.** The risk of CVD or CAD increases with *increasing age,* and the person older than 40 years is more likely to become symptomatic. *Gender* as a nonmodifiable risk factor is reflected in the fact that heart disease is more prevalent among men. Women generally experience heart attacks 10 years later than men, possibly because of the biologic protection factor provided premenopausally by estrogen, although hormone replacement therapy (HRT) did not prove beneficial for CAD.[245] Substantial disparity exists between men and women: one year after MI at the age of more than 45 years, 26% of women versus 19% of men die, and within five years after a first MI 47% of women versus 36% of men die.[245]

A *family history* of CVD (i.e., one or more members of the immediate family with the disease) is associated with increased incidence of heart disease. It is proposed that a mix of environmental and genetic factors leads to atherosclerosis of the coronary arteries in a complex, unpredictable, and unknown series of interactions. For selected individuals, genetic predisposition, especially abnormalities in lipoprotein metabolism, can play a very important role in their risk of developing atherosclerosis.

Current research is exploring the possibility of "candidate genes" that may be associated with an increased risk of CAD. One example is familial hypercholesterolemia affecting, 1 in 300 to 500 individuals in some populations. A majority of this population (80%–85%) has a mutation in the gene for the LDL receptor. Approximately 5% to 10% of people with the condition have mutations in the apolipoprotein B gene that results in an abnormality that prevents interaction of cholesterol particles with the LDL receptor. In familial hypercholesterolemia, serum LDL-C levels are double what are considered normal levels, predisposing a person to CAD from a young age. With this condition, a person under the age of 40 has a 100-fold increased risk of CAD.[258] Clinical guidelines from national professional organizations and societies, including the National Lipid Association and American Heart Association (AHA), call for universal screening for cholesterol levels in all individuals before 20 years of age, and beginning at age 2 with a family history of premature CVD and elevated cholesterol levels.[368]

Modern technology and information from the Human Genome Project, completed in 2003, now allow linkage in family studies to be supplemented with accurate localization of disease-causing or susceptibility (candidate) genes in the whole genome (our entire set of genes). In order to identify genomic changes leading to development of different diseases, genome-wide association studies (GWAS) are conducted. Complete genomes of many people are scanned in search of small genetic variations (known as SNPs, single nucleotide polymorphisms) associated with a particular disease. This approach proved to bring considerable success. Several thousands of GWAS have been performed that revealed association in more than 3,500 unique human diseases/traits,[252] including CVD.[200] Genetic variances in about 160 chromosomal loci have been identified as associated with the risk of CAD.[49] These variances affect gene products (proteins) involved in the cholesterol and triglyceride metabolism, vascular remodeling, inflammation, and blood pressure. Investigating genetic basis of diseases and conditions allows development of novel approaches for prevention and treatment.

Although a person's genetic makeup was always considered a nonmodifiable risk factor of CVD, evidence suggests that variations in genes associated with triglyceride levels may determine the beneficial level of physical activity. While exercise has been known for decreasing triglyceride levels, levels with exercise training will affect how much a person needs to exercise to achieve a desired decrease in triglyceride levels.[322]

A person's race has not been shown to be a specific risk factor for CAD, but a person's *ethnicity* is a risk factor. Certain ethnic groups have been shown to have a higher rate of heart disease.[50] The risk of heart disease is highest among African Americans, who are three times more likely to have extremely high blood pressure, a major risk factor for CAD, and who have a higher prevalence of other risk factors, such as diabetes mellitus, obesity, and cigarette smoking.[74]

Native Americans have an unusually high rate of obesity and diabetes. Their heart disease death rate is 20% higher than among other racial and ethnic groups in the United States. Native Americans die from heart disease at younger age.[21] Hispanics, in general, have a higher risk of CVD, due to high prevalence of dyslipidemia, obesity, diabetes mellitus, and high blood pressure.[312,329] High heterogeneity of the Hispanic population presents challenges in collecting comprehensive research data on cardiovascular risks.[312] The Hispanic paradox exists, presenting with lower mortality in the presence of higher cardiovascular risk factors, which may partially be explained by challenges in documenting cause of death in this diverse population.[329]

*Infections* (bacterial and viral) as a cause of atherosclerosis and thereby CAD in some people have been supported by experimental and clinical data. This discovery came about as researchers identified the presence of a common virus (cytomegalovirus) in arterial plaque as a contributing factor to angioplasty failure. Atherosclerosis, now recognized as an inflammatory process, and injury to the inner layer of the artery may be triggered by acute or chronic infection, particularly in more susceptible disease states such as diabetes. There is much research examining specific infections and CAD risk, but very few studies have shown direct links so far. However, human papillomavirus was added to the list of infectious agents associated with MI or stroke in women.[208]

**Newer Predictors.** Investigators may have identified markers for heart disease present in apparently healthy people, that is, components of blood or other factors that can help identify risk of CAD before symptoms develop (see Table 12.3). Serum cholesterol has been used for a long time, but many more potential predictors of risk are being examined.

*Homocysteine,* an amino acid that is generated as the body metabolizes another amino acid, methionine (found in animal-derived foods), occurs naturally in blood and tissues; it is not one of the 20 protein-building amino acids. Elevated levels of homocysteine are more common in people with CAD; it may be as much of a risk factor as high cholesterol or smoking.

*C-reactive protein (CRP)*, an acute-phase reactant that reflects low-grade systemic inflammation, is produced by the liver in response to trauma, tissue inflammation, and infection, and seems to predict hypertension, diabetes, heart attacks, and strokes before they occur.[380] People with even slightly elevated blood levels of CRP appear to be at increased risk for CAD and its complications regardless of age, gender, general health, or the presence of other CAD risk factors (see Table 12.3). Cigarette smokers have elevated levels of CRP, and individuals experiencing a heart attack who have high levels of CRP have a slower-than-normal response to antithrombotic medication. Preliminary data suggest that the relative effectiveness of secondary preventive therapies, such as cholesterol-lowering drugs and aspirin, may depend on an individual's baseline CRP level.[380]

Lipoprotein (a) (*Lp*(*a*)), an LDL-C particle with an additional protein attached, slows the breakdown of blood clots. People with high levels of Lp(a) are at greater risk for MI than those with lower levels of Lp(a).

*Pulse pressure* (<60 mm Hg), a measure of arterial stiffness *(systolic blood pressure minus diastolic blood pressure)*, has been investigated as an independent predictor of CAD risk. This has been especially noted in people with hypertension or diabetes.[264]

*Erectile dysfunction* (impotence) is of vascular etiology with underlying endothelial dysfunction. In younger men with no cardiac symptoms, erectile dysfunction is proposed as a marker of increased risk of CVD.[190]

*Metabolic syndrome* is an aggregation of multiple cardiovascular risk factors of metabolic origin in one individual that are linked to the development of atherosclerotic disease. Several definitions of metabolic syndrome were proposed by various organizations. AHA interprets metabolic syndrome as a group of the following five risk factors: elevated glucose level, hypertension, central obesity, and dyslipidemias (specifically, high levels of triglycerides and low levels of HDL-C).[58] Insulin resistance and central obesity are key underlying causes of the metabolic syndrome. Several related conditions including chronic inflammation, increased thrombosis (thrombosis is the formation of a clot; thrombus is the clot), nonalcoholic fatty liver disease, cholesterol gallstones, and sleep apnea are associated with metabolic syndrome.[50,58] Metabolic syndrome is diagnosed when any three of the five risk factors are present (Box 12.2).

In the United States, every third adult has metabolic syndrome.[379] The rising prevalence worldwide of this problem is largely due to increasing obesity and sedentary lifestyles. Metabolic syndrome is considered a disease of unhealthy lifestyle.[50] Individuals with metabolic syndrome are twice as likely to develop CVD over the next 5 to 10 years as individuals without the syndrome and five times more likely to develop type 2 diabetes mellitus.[9]

The primary goal of clinical management of metabolic syndrome is to reduce the risk for atherosclerotic CVD. When encountering clients presenting with abdominal obesity, physical therapists should appreciate that waist circumference may be associated with lipid abnormalities.[180]

Box 12.2

**CRITERIA FOR CLINICAL DIAGNOSIS OF METABOLIC SYNDROME**

Any three of these five components constitute a diagnosis of metabolic syndrome:

- Elevated waist circumference (in the United States: waist size of more than 40 inches [102 cm] in men and 35 inches (88 cm) in women; lower values are recommended for Asian, Middle Eastern, South American, and African groups)
- Reduced levels of HDL (good or "healthy" cholesterol): less than 40 mg/dL in men and 50 mg/dL in women
- Increased blood pressure of 130/85 mm Hg or greater
- Elevated fasting blood glucose level of 100 mg/dL or greater
- Elevated serum triglyceride levels of 150 mg/dL or greater

Data from Alberti KG, Eckel RH, Grundy SM, et al: *Harmonizing the metabolic syndrome.* Joint Interim Statement of the International Diabetes Federation Task Force on Epidemiology and Prevention; National Heart, Lung, and Blood Institute; American Heart Association; World Heart Federation; International Atherosclerosis Society; and International Association for the Study of Obesity, *Circulation* 120:1640–1645, 2009.

## Pathogenesis

The mechanism by which CAD develops is complex. Atherosclerosis plays a key role in the restriction of blood flow through coronary circulation, leading to CAD. It is commonly accepted now that atherosclerosis is a chronic inflammatory condition triggered by LDL-C depositions and immune activation in the arterial wall.[34] In some cases, the initial damage comes from LDL-C cholesterol that has been modified by free radicals. Free radicals are abundant in people who smoke and who have high blood pressure or diabetes. In other cases, high levels of homocysteine or bacteria may contribute to early damage of arterial linings.

Endothelial cells forming the inner lining of an arterial wall perform many regulatory functions, including production of smooth muscle relaxing and contracting factors, and procoagulant and anticoagulant mediators. Unfavorable conditions (such as hypertension, dyslipidemia, insulin resistance) cause endothelial cell dysfunction. This endothelial dysfunction leads to several detrimental factors for vascular wall events including inflammation, thrombogenesis, vasoconstriction, and oxidative stress (Fig. 12.2).

Proinflammatory mediators are then produced, triggering inflammation that damages the vessel wall. As a result, LDL-C particles circulating in blood flow into the arterial wall and start to build up an atherosclerotic plaque (or lesion) within the intima. The deposited LDL-C undergoes oxidation and further stimulates inflammation and production of cell adhesion molecules. Inflammatory and immune cells adhere to the lesion and amplify the inflammatory response by producing more mediators, leading to more wall damage and LDL-C and cell recruitment. Among immune cells, monocytes deposited into the lesions differentiate into tissue macrophages. The macrophages, through their cell surface receptors, uptake large amounts of LDL-C particles and convert into foam cells (lipid-laden macrophages), a hallmark of atherosclerotic

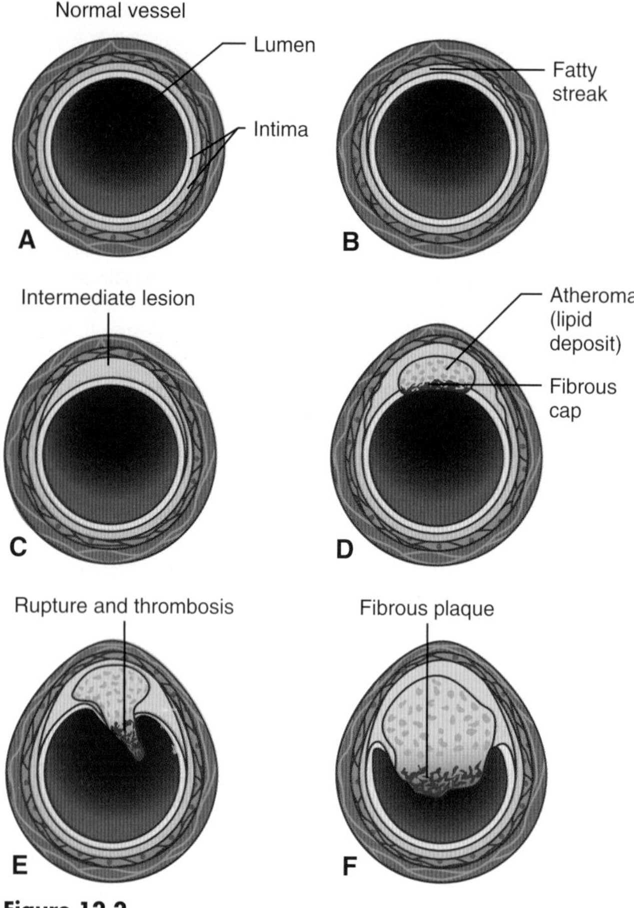


**Figure 12.2**

**Atherosclerosis model.** Atherosclerosis begins with an injury to the endothelial lining of the artery (intimal layer) that makes the vessel permeable to circulating lipoproteins. New technology using intravascular ultrasound shows the entire atherosclerotic plaque and has changed the way we view things. The traditional model held that an atherosclerotic plaque in the blood vessel, particularly a coronary blood vessel, kept growing inward and obstructing flow until it closed off and caused a heart attack. This is not entirely correct. It is more accurate to say that in the normal vessel (A), penetration of lipoproteins into the smooth muscle cells of the intima produces fatty streaks (B) and the start of a coronary lesion forms. (C and D) The coronary lesion grows outward first in a compensatory manner to maintain the open lumen. This is called *positive remodeling*. The blood vessel tries to maintain an open lumen until it can do so no longer. A little roof or "fibrous cap" separates the plaque from the inside of the lumen. A blood clot called an *intraplaque thrombosis* can form inside the plaque; the clot may never leave the plaque. (E) The plaque (atheroma) begins to build up, gradually pressing inward into the lumen with obstruction of blood flow and possible rupture and thrombus, potentially leading to myocardial infarction or stroke. Capped plaques are not as likely to rupture as the softer type packed with viscous cholesterol and white blood cells but only capped with a thin layer of collagen. (F) Vascular disease today is considered a disease of the wall. Some researchers like to say the disease is in the donut, not the hole of a donut, and that is a new concept. (From Goodman CC, Heick J, Lazaro RT: *Differential diagnosis for physical therapists: screening for referral,* ed 6, St Louis, 2018, Elsevier. Data from Horn HR: Insulin resistance, diabetes, and vascular disease: the rationale for prevention. Available online at http://www.medscape.com/viewarticle/466799_2. Accessed May 2019.)

lesions. T lymphocytes are recruited to the lesions, with LDL-C thought to be an autoantigen. A T lymphocyte subtype promotes formation of the fibrous cap, made of collagen, that covers the lesion, thus stabilizing the atherosclerotic plaque. Many cytokines and chemokines participate in the lesion formation process, including proinflammatory interleukin-1β (IL-1β), IL-6, interferon-γ and tumor necrosis factor-α (TNFα), anti-inflammatory IL-10, and transforming growth factor-β (TGFβ).[34]

In addition to inflammation and lipid accumulation, punctate calcium deposits are found in the atherosclerotic plaques. Pathologic deposition of calcium occurs in the arterial wall intima and media.[26] While calcium deposits within the atherosclerotic plaques destabilize them, wall deposits make the artery stiffer.[34] Calcium accumulations can be detected using imaging techniques.

As the atherosclerotic plaque develops, it becomes covered by a fibrous cap made of collagen, with contributions from smooth muscle cells. This fibrous cap is covered by a layer of endothelial cells, which stays intact until the later stages of atherosclerosis. The fibrous cap serves to protect the plaque content from contacting blood, thus preventing clotting. When this fibrous cap breaks down, the atherosclerotic plaque ruptures, exposing its thrombogenic surface. When endothelial cells that cover the plaque dislodge, they expose the subendothelial matrix leading to plaque erosion. The exposed matrix becomes thrombogenic. In either case, thrombus is formed, and it obstructs the lumen.[34]

In fact, the major clinical effect of atherosclerosis (the obstruction of the blood flow) develops not due to gradual narrowing of the vessel lumen but to rupture or erosion of the atherosclerotic plaque, precipitating thrombus formation that obstructs the lumen leading to MI.[51]

Although platelet activation is a normal response to injury, in atherosclerosis, once the platelets adhere, they also release chemicals that alter the structure of the blood vessel wall, so that what starts out as a small erosion in the wall can end up a swollen mound of platelets, muscle cells, and fibrin clots, an accumulation that obstructs the flow of blood through the vessel.

After a thrombus forms and causes static or reduced blood flow in the vessel, the fibrin clot is stabilized by crosslinking. This is commonly referred to as a *red thrombus* because of the presence of entrapped red blood cells. Within the thrombus is thrombin, which remains active and can activate platelets. Platelets also release plasminogen activator inhibitor-1 (PAI-1), a potent natural inhibitor of fibrinolysis, and vasoactive amines that can lead to vessel spasm, further platelet aggregation, and thrombus formation or reocclusion. This cycle of injury, platelet activation, and lipid deposition can lead to complete blockage of a vessel and result in ischemia and necrosis of tissue supplied by the obstructed blood vessel.

Evidence shows that even small atherosclerotic plaques can rupture and cause problems. These vulnerable plaques are covered by a thin cap rather than the thick, fibrous one shown in Figure 12.2. Inflammation and cellular changes weaken and degrade the thin cap until it ruptures, exposing its fat-rich thrombogenic core.

Several studies emphasize the fact that cholesterol deposits are only one of many mechanisms through which acute CAD develops. Information points to the endothelium as a modulating factor in the pathogenesis of CAD through the production of nitric oxide and angiotensin II, which maintain the homeostatic environment, influencing the progression of CAD. This imbalance tends to promote CAD in individuals who have multiple risk factors.

Endothelium-derived nitric oxide is an important mediator of exercise-induced changes in skeletal muscle blood flow. This molecule is responsible for the natural dilation of blood vessels.

Nitric oxide is an antilipid that provides a nonstick coating to the lining of blood vessels, much like Teflon. These two effects have helped explain how nitric oxide might prevent heart attacks and strokes and why nitroglycerin works—nitroglycerin is converted to nitric oxide inside vascular tissue, where it relaxes smooth muscle in arteries and causes blood vessels to dilate.

### Clinical Manifestations

Atherosclerosis by itself does not necessarily produce symptoms. For manifestations to develop, there must be a critical deficit in blood supply, and thus oxygen, to the heart or other structures supplied by affected blood vessels. For example, symptoms of CAD may not appear until the lumen of the coronary artery narrows by 75%. Then, pain and dysfunction may occur in the region supplied by the occluded artery.

When atherosclerosis develops slowly, collateral circulation develops to meet the heart's needs. Complications from atherosclerosis occur because it is a progressive disorder that results in more severe cardiac disease if it is not prevented or left untreated. Common sequelae of atherosclerosis affecting coronary arteries include angina pectoris, MI or heart attack, and sudden death.

Men experience angina as the first symptom of CAD in one third of all cases and heart attack or sudden death in the majority of cases. Half of all women experience angina, while the other half remain asymptomatic or present with atypical symptoms (see "Angina Pectoris" below).

## MEDICAL MANAGEMENT

**PREVENTION.** Overwhelming evidence indicates that CVD and CAD are largely preventable; therefore whenever possible, prevention of CVD and CAD is the goal for everyone. And atherosclerosis is not a disease of middle to old age; it begins in adolescence and young adulthood and develops slowly but progressively throughout the body.

Preventing heart disease means controlling LDL-C before atherosclerosis gets a chance to do much damage. Reduction in the serum level of LDL-C (at or below 100 mg/dL) throughout the life span through the use of diet, exercise, and statins or other cholesterol-lowering drugs is one way experts propose to do this. Healthy People 2020,[170] a U.S. federal initiative based on scientific data, has identified the following goals for heart disease and stroke: improvement of cardiovascular health and quality of life through the prevention, detection, and treatment of risk factors; early identification and treatment of heart attacks and strokes; and prevention of recurrent cardiovascular events. Aligned with the federal initiative, the AHA's 2020 Impact Goals include improvement of cardiovascular health of all by 20% and reduction of deaths from CVD and stroke by 20%.[19] An excellent guide to evidence-based primary prevention of CVD and similar recommendations for prevention of cerebrovascular disease (i.e., stroke) are available.[69,137,245,259,332,337]

Health perceptions, seeking medical health care, and willingness to participate in long-term preventive therapies are significantly influenced by age and cultural and socioeconomic factors.[32,207,350] Older individuals are less likely to be referred to cardiac rehabilitation and exercise-training programs and are less likely to attend than younger adults. Therefore, preventive cardiology, including primary and secondary preventive efforts such as cardiac rehabilitations should be directed at the older adult.[135,166]

Primary and secondary prevention programs are needed that are modified for the language, cultural, and medical needs of people of all age groups and ethnic backgrounds but especially for older ethnic minorities who are at increased risk for CVD.[332] Ethnic comparisons of health behaviors and prevalence of risk factors among teenagers support the need for health promotion intervention among ethnic teenagers.[40,312]

Women are less likely than men to receive health care advice on risk reduction while they are still healthy (i.e., before a significant cardiac event), even though they are more likely to die with the first heart attack. Because of the differences in MI symptoms between women and men, and that women's symptoms are not taken seriously or downplayed, women often experience delay with diagnosis and treatment that results in reduced outcomes.[259] For this reason, guidelines for prevention of CVD in women were published by AHA in 2007 and updated in 2011.[259] Specific guidelines for prevention of ischemic heart disease[245] and stroke[67] in women are available as well.

The bottom line is that even for people with a strong genetic component, modifying risk factors can slow the growth and spread of atherosclerotic plaque and reduce the risk of heart attack or stroke. The goal is to prevent cholesterol-filled plaque from rupturing or eroding, a key event that leads to the formation of blood clots that can block a coronary or carotid artery. Many people with significant nonmodifiable risk factors for heart disease but who follow a heart-healthy lifestyle live longer and in better health with better quality of life compared with those individuals who do not follow a heart-healthy plan.

**DIAGNOSIS.** Current national guidelines advise everyone older than age 20 years to have his or her cholesterol checked to establish a baseline, with follow-up once every 5 years (more often for those with risk factors for heart disease).[367]

Advances in technology are rapidly changing the diagnostic tools available to physicians for diagnosing and evaluating CAD. Coronary angiography (angiogram or arteriogram; x-ray examination of the arteries with dye injection) has been the most widely used anatomic test to assess the degree of atherosclerotic coronary disease and left ventricular contractility.

Angiograms are limited, though, by their inability to detect which plaques represent vulnerable sites for rupture. Overall, results of angiogram are similar between men and women, but clinicians do have increased difficulty specifying individual vessel occlusion for women compared with men.[114] Tests using ultrasound or nuclear agents are less reliable in women because signals are blocked by breast tissue. Angiography is much more accurate than echocardiography, although echocardiography improves the diagnostic accuracy of stress tests.

Echocardiography is a group of interrelated applications of ultrasound imaging (including Doppler, contrast, stress, and real-time three-dimensional [RT3D] echocardiography). Advances in echocardiography have expanded its use in assessment of regional myocardial function, analysis of diastolic function, and quantification of regional myocardial function in different pathologic conditions, including ischemic heart disease.

Echocardiography has the potential to image myocardial perfusion along with wall motion and wall thickening. Stress echocardiography showing responses of the heart can be performed during or after a number of different physical stressors. This is important, because responses of the heart to stressors are probably even more important in evaluating cardiac health than how the heart functions at rest.

Exercise treadmill testing to record symptoms and the electrical activity of the heart under stress continues to offer a means of assessing risk of future cardiac events in most groups (obese, sedentary, middle-aged or older men and women; studies among ethnic groups are underway).[93]

Other diagnostic test procedures available include ultrafast computed tomography (fast CT; "heart scan"), which allows for a computer image accommodating for the heart's pumping cycle. Multidirectional or multidetector CT (also referred to as the "new angiogram") generates up to 64 slice-like images of the heart. A computer then reconstructs these slices to create a detailed 3D image of the heart and coronary arteries. Although less expensive, this new technology is not yet considered a replacement for angiography as it exposes people to increased doses of radiation compared to a traditional coronary angiogram.

Magnetic resonance angiography (MRA) uses a powerful cylinder-shaped magnet that is able to vibrate in distinctive ways to create a signal that is translated into a picture. This technique is also synchronized to the heart cycle and is able to detect plaques. High-speed rotational angiography may be the next technologic diagnostic technique. MRA gives a dynamic multiple-angle perspective of the coronary tree during a single contrast injection.[235]

With a standard angiogram, the camera is placed at different angles and takes a series of pictures of the heart. Dye is injected with each angle photographed. High-speed rotational angiography allows the camera to sweep across the heart in an arc, taking all the (digital) pictures with one injection. The digital component allows the cardiovascular surgeon to stop and look at each frame.

In the future, advanced technology may be able to determine which plaques are most likely to rupture. Thermography using probes to check the temperature of arteries may also reveal vulnerable plaques that are at risk for rupture, because these will be inflamed with elevated temperatures. The routine measurement of newer predictors, such as Lp(a) and CRP, is not recommended at this time for prognostic use and will be delayed until the clinical benefits of altering their concentrations are made available.

***Modification of Risk Factors.*** Modifying risk factors whenever possible can decrease the risk of CVD/CAD. This includes cessation of cigarette smoking, management of diabetes and hypertension, body weight reduction, lipid management, preventing excessive blood clotting, and annual influenza vaccination.[340]

Changing dietary habits by reducing fat intake can result in regression and disappearance of fatty streaks consisting of lipid-laden macrophages, T lymphocytes, and smooth muscle cells before these components progress to form an atherosclerotic plaque.

Dietary changes are recommended for everyone, including children and adults, as it is now recognized that blood vessel changes associated with heart disease begin as early as 15 years of age[318] and the progression of the lesions is strongly influenced by the same risk factors that predict risk of clinically manifest coronary disease in middle-aged adults.[150] In addition, at least one third of all Americans younger than age 19 years are overweight or obese.[165] There are guidelines to help the therapist outline some of the major dietary and lifestyle recommendations for risk reduction throughout the lifespan.[20,33,121,272] The use of a health risk appraisal form may be beneficial as well.[113]

***Exercise and Physical Activity.*** Exercise and physical activity have been shown to reduce the risk for coronary events,[340] diabetes, and other vascular diseases or complications.[173,356]

The American College of Sports Medicine's position on the quantity and quality of exercise for developing and maintaining cardiorespiratory and muscular fitness and flexibility in healthy adults recommends aerobic endurance training at least 3 days/wk for at least 150 to 300 minutes/wk at a moderate intensity, or 75 to 150 minutes/wk of vigorous-intensity aerobic physical activity, or an equivalent combination of moderate- and vigorous-intensity aerobic activity. It is also recommended that adults perform resistance exercise involving large muscle groups at least 2 days per week at a moderate intensity level.[360] Aerobic exercise does not need to be a vigorous level for cardiovascular protection.[360] Substantial evidence supports the benefit of continued regular physical activity that does not need to be strenuous or prolonged and includes daily leisure activities, such as walking or gardening. Evidence shows that exercise helps keep the inner lining of the arteries healthy and less prone to injuries that lead to plaque formation. Regular expansion and contraction of arteries during exercise is thought to keep the vessels "in shape," maintaining endothelial function and limiting development of atherosclerotic plaques in the arterial walls. For individuals with CAD, moderate exercise (3 hr/wk), in combination with low-fat diet and stress management, improved endothelial function and reduced inflammatory markers associated with atherosclerosis.[117] In terms of exercise effects on platelet aggregation in CAD and other CVDs, the findings are contradictory.[184]

Heart rate recovery, a prognostic indicator and predictor of mortality, can be improved by exercise. Individuals with abnormal (slowed) heart rate recovery after 12 weeks of aerobic exercise performed 3 times per week for 30 to 50 minutes per session were able to normalize it and had mortality levels similar to persons with normal heart recovery rate.[223] Heart rate recovery is defined as a delayed decrease in heart rate during recovery after exercise to less than or equal to 12 beats per minute after the first minute while walking in recovery.[17]

The effect of exercise on cholesterol has been documented, but it remains unclear which component of exercise is the underlying beneficial mechanism. Exercise frequency may be more important than intensity in improving triglyceride and HDL-C levels and both aerobic and resistive exercise training have been reported effective with an additive effect when both exercises were combined.[145] Even so, many health benefits from physical activity can be achieved in shorter bouts at less intensity.[143] More studies are required to identify the ideal prescriptive exercise.

The benefits of strength training for people with heart disease have generated debate on both sides. In the past, there was some concern that abrupt surges of blood pressure could increase the risk of plaque disruption. But recommendations from the AHA show that resistance training can be safe and beneficial for individuals with heart disease at low risk.[132] This would include people who do not have HF, symptoms of exercise-induced angina, or severe heart arrhythmias.

Exercise alone independent of weight loss or diet changes can have significant beneficial effects on cardiovascular risk factors in overweight people with elevated cholesterol levels.[145] Exercise is the one single intervention with the ability to influence the greatest number of risk factors (e.g., aids in smoking cessation, alters cholesterol levels, reduces blood pressure, helps control blood glucose levels, reverses the effects of a sedentary lifestyle, contributes to weight loss, helps in managing stress-induced increases in heart rate and blood pressure).

***Pharmacotherapy.*** Clinical trials have proven conclusively that both fatal and nonfatal coronary events and strokes can be prevented. Pharmacologic management is used to reduce the risk of clotting, treat hypertension, reverse dyslipidemia, and reduce inflammation associated with atherosclerosis.[282]

Medications such as 3-hydroxy-3-methylglutaryl coenzyme A (HMG-CoA) reductase inhibitors (better known as "statins") are targeting the key enzyme of the cholesterol synthesis pathway. Statins are proven effective not only in lowering LDL-C levels and raising HDL-C levels (primary prevention) but also in reducing cardiovascular events (secondary prevention) in specific populations, for instance, in people with ischemic heart disease. An observational study of MI patients who already had low LDL-C levels (below 50 mg/dL) at the time of MI showed that these patients had reduced cardiac death and improved cardiac revascularization a year after the discharge on statins versus those patients who were not taking statins.[289] The use of statin medications has also been shown to be effective in patients with HF, especially if they have preserved ejection fraction.[273] Unfortunately, adherence to statin therapy needs to be better. Study showed that less than 40% of people, in the year after MI, were taking statins, even when the medications were provided free of charge.[89]

When statins alone are not effective or not tolerated well, another approach to lower the LDL-C is used, through inhibiting another protein in cholesterol metabolism, PCSK9. PCSK9 functions by binding to LDL receptors and not allowing the receptor to catch LDL-C in the bloodstream and remove it from circulation. Thus, if PCSK9 is inhibited LDL-C level in blood will decrease. PCSK9 inhibitors, in the form of monoclonal antibodies, have been developed and used, being especially effective in high-risk cardiovascular patients.[314]

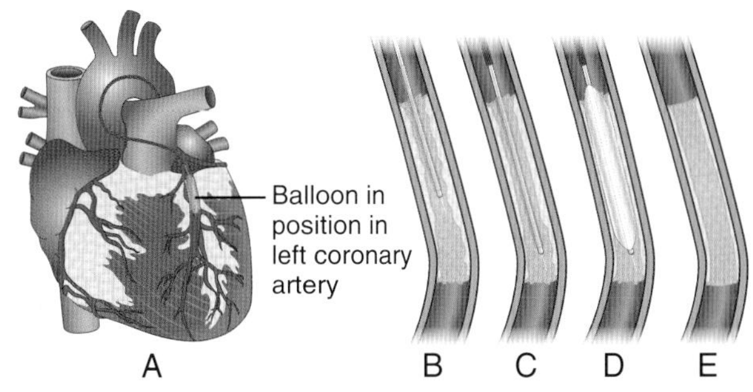


**Figure 12.3**

**Percutaneous coronary intervention (PCI) can open an occluded coronary artery without opening the chest, an important advantage over bypass surgery.** (A) Once coronary angiography has been performed to determine the presence and location of an arterial occlusion, a guide catheter is threaded through the femoral artery (groin) or the radial artery (wrist) into the left coronary artery. (B) When the angiography shows the guide catheter positioned at the site of occlusion, the uninflated balloon is centered in the obstruction. (C) A smaller double-lumen balloon catheter is inserted through the guide catheter. (D) The balloon is inflated, compressing the plaque against the arterial wall, and deflated until the angiogram confirms a reduced pressure gradient in the vessel. (E) The balloon is removed, and the artery is left unoccluded.

Table 12.4 lists target measurements to reduce risk factors developed by the American College of Cardiology and the AHA. The routine use of low-dose aspirin (75-162 mg/day) is recommended in everyone with CAD unless there are contraindications.[340] The AHA now recommends low-dose aspirin therapy of 81 mg/day or 100 mg every other day for all women age 65 years or older. Studies show that aspirin will not prevent heart attacks in individuals with diabetes who have no evidence of CVD, and routine use of low-dose aspirin is not recommended for healthy women younger than age 65 years, but it may still be considered for all women at risk for stroke who are not at increased risk of bleeding and whose blood pressure is controlled.[259]

**Treatment.** Medical management is directed toward the specific blood vessel occlusion and depends on complications, for example, occlusive disease of the peripheral vasculature, arterial disease in diabetic clients, occlusive cerebrovascular disease, or visceral artery insufficiency (intestinal ischemia) (see discussion of each individual complication).

***Surgery.*** Surgical management of atherosclerosis of the coronary arteries may include PCI (Fig. 12.3), CABG (Fig. 12.4), and/or coronary stents (Fig. 12.5). The current generation of drug-coated and drug-eluting stents are bare metal covered with a polymer (plastic) coating that holds and releases a drug to inhibit the growth of endothelial cells. Several companies are working on polymers that are more compatible with the body and less likely to trigger clots. Others are testing polymers that dissolve and disappear after some time.

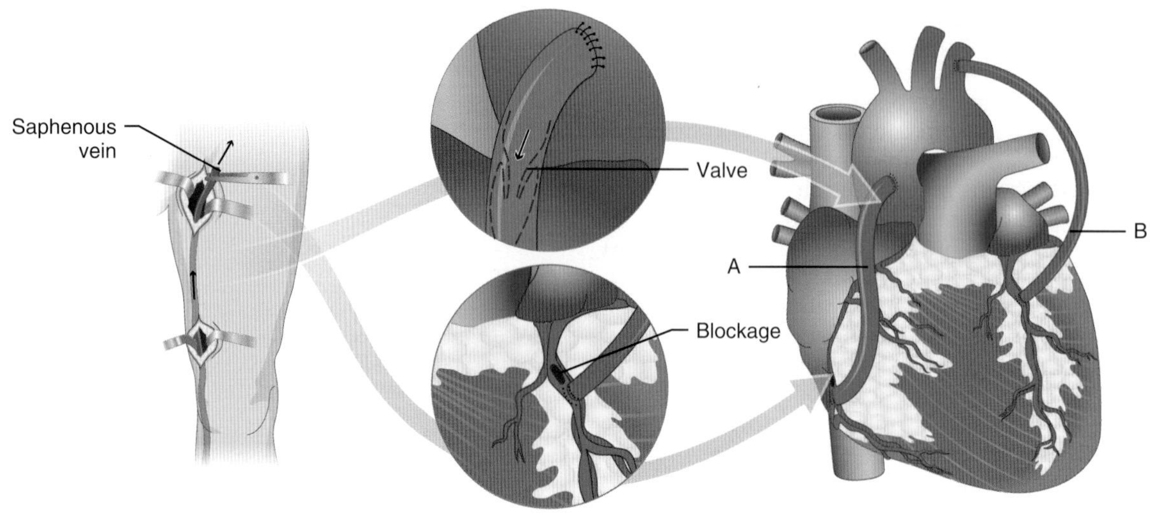


**Figure 12.4**

**Coronary artery bypass graft (CABG).** This procedure involves taking a portion of a vein or artery from the leg, chest, or arm and grafting it onto the coronary artery. In this illustration, a section of the saphenous vein (A) is used as a graft to route blood around areas of blockage. Bypassing the clogged vessel provides an alternative route (B) for blood to reach the heart muscle. The internal mammary artery and, more recently, radial or brachial arteries can be used as an alternate graft site. CABG has been a major surgery requiring a sternotomy but is being refined to possibly become an off-pump bypass grafting through a partial sternotomy. It is considered most effective in individuals who have several severely blocked coronary arteries and a previously damaged heart muscle or when repeated revascularization has failed. (From Black JM, Hawks JH, Keene AM: *Medical-surgical nursing: clinical management for positive outcomes,* ed 6, Philadelphia, 2001, WB Saunders.)

Angioplasty is performed more often than bypass surgery. However, the surgeon and patient should decide together which is the better surgical option. Angioplasty combined with a stent reduces the incidence of restenosis, especially for people with diabetes who have a high restenosis rate when treated by standard balloon angioplasty.[362] Antiplatelet treatment with aspirin (Table 12.5) is a standard pharmacologic regimen after coronary artery stenting for the prevention of thrombosis.

For the person with significant coronary and carotid artery disease, the importance of treating symptomatic stenosis of the carotid artery as a means of stroke prevention is now widely accepted. Carotid artery angioplasty and stenting constitute a procedure that is an alternative to carotid endarterectomy, especially for people considered at high risk for postoperative complications.

Blockages that are heavily calcified and that involve long stretches of coronary artery are difficult to treat successfully with angioplasty or stenting. In such cases, rotational atherectomy can be accomplished using a device called a *rotoblator* (catheter tipped with a tiny rotary blade). This procedure makes sharp cuts in plaque, shaving away the blockage and producing a relatively smooth luminal surface.

Other surgical techniques, such as mechanical thrombectomy using a device (AngioJet System) that removes blood clots in the coronary (or carotid) arteries before angioplasty are viable options in some cases but carry a higher rate of major complications, especially for women.

Intravascular ultrasound, a technology that combines echo with catheterization, may eventually allow diagnosis and therapy to be combined as the cardiologist uses a camera on the tip of a catheter to precisely target atherosclerotic blockage.

Although surgical intervention has been a mainstay for the treatment of CAD, researchers are questioning the necessity of heart surgery and studying the benefits of pharmacologic intervention combined with exercise and lifestyle changes. The role of exercise in the prevention of atherosclerosis has been discussed, but the role of exercise as a treatment modality is equally important.

***Cardiac Rehabilitation.*** The Science Advisory and Coordinating Committee of the AHA has recommended that health care providers implement a coordinated effort

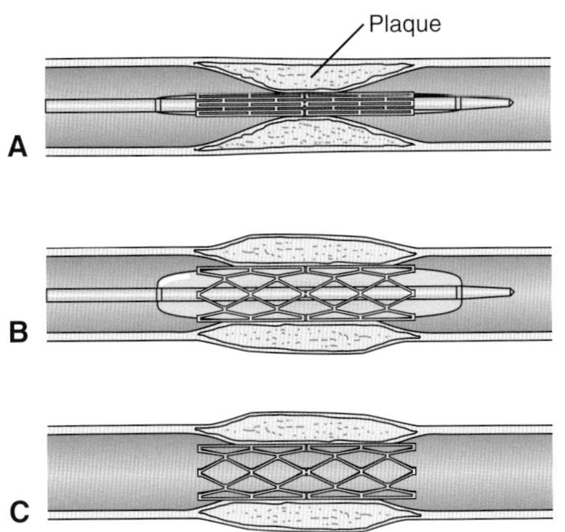


**Figure 12.5**

**Application of the coronary stent.** (A) Cross-section of a severely occluded coronary artery. (B) Blocked coronary artery can be held open using a balloon-expandable device called a *coronary stent.* (C) Stent shown here is in place to maintain opened vessel, allowing blood to pass through freely. Biodegradable stents are under development to reduce or eliminate problems associated with metal stents. Delivery of drugs or gene therapy to inhibit intimal hyperplasia and prevent post-angioplasty restenosis is under investigation.[293] (From Lewis SL et al: *Medical-surgical nursing: assessment and management of clinical problems,* ed 10, St. Louis, 2017, Elsevier.)

to promote outpatient cardiac rehabilitation to eligible individuals. Home health nurses and physical therapists are specifically highlighted as valuable agents in facilitating referral and enrollment and bridging the gap between acute care and outpatient status.[73] The AHA's report on clinical performance and quality measures for cardiac rehabilitation[354] has been endorsed by the American Physical Therapy Association.

Cardiac rehabilitation exercise training consistently improves objective measures of exercise tolerance, without significant cardiovascular complications or other adverse outcomes. Appropriately prescribed and conducted exercise training is recommended as an integral component of the treatment of atherosclerosis and CAD.[14]

Cardiac rehabilitation programs incorporate exercise training as well as education[236] on risk factors for CAD. A comprehensive cardiac rehabilitation program seeks to formulate an individual plan for each patient to address their specific lifestyle behaviors and monitor their own progression of physical activity. Exercise-based cardiac rehabilitation is effective in improving functional capacity and mortality.[354]

***Gene Therapy and Gene Editing.*** Gene therapy (i.e., gene transfer) is one strategy with the potential to prevent some of the sequelae after arterial injury, induce growth of new vessels ("therapeutic angiogenesis"), or remodel preexisting vessels.[293] Cardiac angiogenesis was viewed as the most promising approach, with delivery of genes for angiogenic growth factors, specifically vascular endothelial growth factor. When injected directly into the heart, this gene prompts the heart to sprout tiny new blood vessels to bypass the blocked vessels, restoring blood supply. While preclinical studies produced a lot of enthusiasm, the latest trials did not show expected efficacy.[160] More research is needed to optimize this promising therapy, including improve forms and routes of gene delivery.[160,293]

A novel approach for gene editing became available with the discovery of an advanced scientific tool, the CRISPR RNA-guided endonuclease system.[201] With this approach, a "defective" portion of a gene can be removed and a "correct" portion can be inserted, or a gene can be modified in part to produce a less active protein. One example when a less active protein would be desirable is PCSK9, a protein that prevents removal of cholesterol from the bloodstream. In fact, people with a loss-of-function variant of PCSK9 have lower risk of atherosclerotic CVD.[314] In an animal study, using CRISPR technology, a mutation of PCSK9 gene in a liver with a specific viral vector led to 40% decrease in cholesterol in blood.[201] This strategy could be used to decrease circulating triglycerides or other risk factors for CAD.

Genetic approaches will continue to identify genes and pathways involved in the predisposition to and pathophysiology of atherosclerosis. Targets for therapeutic intervention based on gene profiling continue to be the focus of research at this time.[49,201]

***Complementary and Integrative Medicine.*** The role of complementary and alternative or integrative medicine, sometimes referred to as mind–body therapies, is increasing as more people seek out self-management techniques.[376] At the same time, there is more evidence now, including from the AHA, to support the effects of these therapies on heart disease, blood pressure, lipid levels, morbidity, and mortality.[62,222]

Examples of these techniques include prayer or meditation[62,222] and/or religious attendance at church, synagogue, or other services[47,85]; yoga, Tai Chi, and other forms of martial arts;[62] BodyTalk, reiki, and acupuncture;[62] social support and/or support groups; cognitive-behavioral therapy; imagery; hypnosis; physiologic quieting; relaxation techniques; music therapy; and others (Table 12.6).

**Prognosis.** The AHA reports compelling scientific evidence that comprehensive risk factor interventions in people with cardiovascular heart disease extend overall survival, improve quality of life, decrease the need for interventional procedures, and reduce the incidence of subsequent MI. Even so, despite the well-documented benefit of preventive measures and cardiac rehabilitation, compliance with recommendations for reducing risk factors and utilization rates of rehabilitation programs remain low, especially among women.[259]

Prognosis depends on the site of the myocardial damage and the extent of myocardial necrosis. Fatality rates for CAD remain low before age 35 years, but these figures increase exponentially until age 75 years, with men generally experiencing mortality at approximately twice the rate of women until age 65 years. Total CAD mortality in women after age 65 years now exceeds that of men. Of the nearly 20,000 persons eligible for heart transplants, only 10% receive a new heart each year. Advanced atherosclerosis is usually fatal if vessels to the brain or heart are

**Table 12.5** Common Cardiovascular Medications

| Medications: Trade Names (Generic Names) | Indications and Side Effects[a] |
|---|---|
| **α-Adrenergic Receptor Agonists** | |
| Aldomet (methyldopa)<br>Catapres (clonidine)<br>Proamatine (midodrine)<br>Tenex (guanfacine)<br>Wytensin (guanabenz) | **Indication:** midodrine treats symptomatic orthostatic hypotension; clonidine, guanabenz, methyldopa, and guanfacine treat hypertension<br>**Side effects:**<br>Midodrine: supine hypertension, piloerection, dysuria, severe hypertension†;<br>Clonidine: contact dermatitis, erythema, xerostomia, dizziness, headache, sedation, somnolence, fatigue;<br>Guanabenz: xerostomia, asthenia, sedation, somnolence;<br>Methyldopa: asthenia, dizziness, headache, sedation, erectile dysfunction (impotence), reduced libido;<br>Guanfacine: orthostatic hypotension, abdominal pain, constipation, xerostomia, dizziness, headache, somnolence, hypotension,[b] syncope[b] |
| **α-Adrenergic Receptor Antagonists** | |
| Cardura (doxazosin)<br>Hytrin (terazosin)<br>Minipress (prazosin) | **Indication:** hypertension<br>**Side effects:** edema, orthostatic hypotension, nausea, dizziness, headache, somnolence, vertigo, fatigue, palpitations, asthenia, syncope[b] |
| **Angiotensin-Converting Enzyme (ACE) Inhibitors** | |
| Accupril (quinapril)<br>Altace (ramipril)<br>Capoten (captopril)<br>Lotensin (benazepril)<br>Prinivil (lisinopril)<br>Vasotec (enalapril)<br>Zestril (lisinopril) | **Indications:** heart failure, hypertension, ventricular dysfunction post-MI<br>**Side effects:** dry and persistent cough, fatigue, headaches, dizziness, syncope,[b] swelling of the throat, face or lips or swelling of feet or abdomen† |
| **Angiotensin II Receptor Blockers (ARBs)** | |
| Atacand (candesartan)<br>Avapro (irbesartan)<br>Benicar (olmesartan)<br>Cozaar (losartan)<br>Diovan (valsartan)<br>Edarbi (azilsartan)<br>Micardis (telmisartan) | **Indications:** heart failure, hypertension, ventricular dysfunction post-MI<br>**Side effects:** diarrhea, heartburn, headache, upper respiratory infection, fatigue, dizziness, cough, swelling of the throat, face, or lips,[b] muscle pain or tenderness[b] |
| **β-Adrenergic Receptor Antagonists (β Blockers)** | |
| Blocadren (timolol)<br>Bystolic (nebivolol)<br>Coreg (carvedilol)<br>Corgard (nadolol)<br>Inderal (propranolol)<br>Lopressor (metoprolol tartrate)<br>Sectral (acebutolol)<br>Tenormin (atenolol)<br>Toprol XL (metoprolol succinate)<br>Trandate (labetalol)<br>Visken (pindolol)<br>Zebeta (bisoprolol) | **Indications:** angina, cardiac arrhythmias, hypertension, heart failure, ventricular dysfunction post-MI<br>**Side effects:** bradycardia, dizziness, fatigue, bradyarrhythmia, headache, depression, peripheral edema, erectile dysfunction, somnolence, diarrhea, asthma,[b] bronchospasm,[b] heart failure,[b] arrhythmias[b] |
| **Antiarrhythmics** | |
| Cordarone (amiodarone)<br>Lanoxin (digoxin)<br>Multaq (dronedarone)<br>Quinaglute (quinidine)<br>Rythmol (propafenone)<br>Tambocor (flecainide)<br>Tikosyn (dofetilide) | **Indications:** cardiac arrhythmias, heart failure<br>**Side effects:** chest pain, diarrhea, headache, hypotension, photosensitivity, visual disturbances, dyspnea, taste disturbances, nausea, vomiting, abnormal gait, dizziness, fatigue, arrhythmias[b] |
| **Direct Renin Inhibitors** | |
| Tekturna (aliskiren) | **Indication:** hypertension<br>**Side effects:** diarrhea, dizziness, headache, cough, swelling of the throat, face, and lips[b] |

**Table 12.5** Common Cardiovascular Medications—cont'd

| Medications: Trade Names (Generic Names) | Indications and Side Effects[a] |
|---|---|
| **Calcium Channel Blockers** | |
| Adalat (nifedipine)<br>Calan (verapamil)<br>Cardene (nicardipine)<br>Cardizem (diltiazem)<br>Isoptin (verapamil)<br>Norvasc (amlodipine)<br>Plendil (felodipine)<br>Procardia (nifedipine)<br>Tiazac (diltiazem)<br>Verelan (verapamil) | **Indications:** angina, hypertension, cardiac arrhythmias<br>**Side effects:** bradycardia, palpitations, peripheral edema, flushing, nausea, vomiting, dizziness, headache, cough, bradyarrhythmia, fatigue, somnolence, constipation, gastroesophageal reflux, angina[b] |
| **Anticoagulants** | |
| Argatroban<br>Arixtra (fondaparinux)<br>Coumadin (warfarin)<br>Eliquis (apixaban)<br>Heparin, unfractionated<br>Low-molecular-weight heparins (LMWHs)<br>• Fragmin (dalteparin)<br>• Lovenox (enoxaparin)<br>Pradaxa (dabigatran)<br>Xarelto (rivaroxaban) | **Indications:** treatment and prevention of clot formation and emboli in the deep veins, heart, lungs, and extremities<br>**Side effects:** fever, diarrhea, nausea, hematoma, gastritis (dabigatran), gastroesophageal reflux disease (dabigatran), major bleeding/hemorrhage,[b] anemia,[b] syncope (rivaroxaban)[b] |
| **Antiplatelets** | |
| Brilinta (ticagrelor)<br>Ecotrin (aspirin)<br>Effient (prasugrel)<br>Kangreal (cangrelor)<br>Persantine (dipyridamole)<br>Plavix (clopidogrel)<br>Ticlid (ticlopidine) | **Indication:** prevention of clot formation and emboli in the deep veins, heart, and brain<br>**Side effects:** abdominal discomfort, diarrhea, nausea, dizziness, headache, hypertension (prasugrel), backache (prasugrel), cough (prasugrel), dyspnea (ticagrelor), severe bleeding/hemorrhage,[b] angina,[b] syncope,[b] arrhythmias (prasugrel),[b] swelling of the throat, face, and lips (prasugrel, ticagrelor)[b] |
| **Hemostatics** | |
| Amicar (aminocaproic acid)<br>Cyklokapron (tranexamic acid) | **Indications:** excessive bleeding, hemorrhage<br>**Side effects:** aminocaproic acid: nausea, vomiting, dizziness, headache, bradycardia, myopathy[b]; tranexamic acid: abdominal pain, arthralgia, backache, muscle cramp, musculoskeletal pain, headache, nasal sinus problems, anemia,[b] visual disturbance[b] |
| **Cholesterol-Modifying Agents** | |
| Crestor (rosuvastatin)<br>Lipitor (atorvastatin)<br>Livalo (pitavastatin)<br>Lescol (fluvastatin)<br>Lopid (gemfibrozil)<br>Mevacor (lovastatin)<br>Nia-Bid (niacin)<br>Niacor (niacin)<br>Nicobid (niacin)<br>Pravachol (pravastatin)<br>Questran (cholestyramine)<br>Zetia (ezetimibe)<br>Zocor (simvastatin) | **Indications:** prevention and treatment of coronary heart disease, dyslipidemias, hypercholesterolemia, hypertriglyceridemia, atherosclerosis<br>**Side effects:** diarrhea, abdominal pain, nausea, indigestion, arthralgia, pain in extremities (except cholestyramine), headache, flushing (niacin), myalgia (except cholestyramine),[b] rhabdomyolysis (except cholestyramine),[b] increased risk of myopathy (80 mg simvastatin) |
| **Antidiuretics** | |
| DDAVP (desmopressin) | **Indication:** central diabetes insipidus<br>**Side effects:** headache, rhinitis |

*Continued*

**Table 12.5** Common Cardiovascular Medications—cont'd

| Medications: Trade Names (Generic Names) | Indications and Side Effects[a] |
|---|---|
| **Diuretics** | |
| Aldosterone antagonists<br>• Aldactone (spironolactone)<br>• Inspra (eplerenone)<br>Carbonic anhydrase inhibitors<br>• Diamox (acetazolamide)<br>Loop diuretics<br>• Bumex (bumetanide)<br>• Demadex (torsemide)<br>• Lasix (furosemide)<br>Potassium-sparing diuretics<br>• Dyrenium (triamterene)<br>• Midamor (amiloride)<br>Thiazide/thiazide-like diuretics<br>• Diuril (chlorothiazide)<br>• Hydrodiuril (hydrochlorothiazide)<br>• Hygroton (chlorthalidone)<br>• Lozol (indapamide)<br>• Zaroxolyn (metolazone) | **Indications:** heart failure, hypertension, edema<br>**Side effects:** diarrhea, nausea, vomiting, headache, lethargy, fatigue, erectile dysfunction (impotence), increased urination, cough (eplerenone), gynecomastia (spironolactone), increased hair growth (spironolactone), electrolyte abnormalities,[b] orthostatic hypotension[b] |
| **Phosphodiesterase Inhibitors** | |
| Revatio (sildenafil)<br>Adcirca (tadalafil) | **Indication:** pulmonary arterial hypertension<br>**Side effects:** hypotension, flushing, indigestion, headache, visual disturbance, nasal congestion and bleeding, rhinitis, priapism[b] |
| **Vasodilators** | |
| Apresoline (hydralazine)<br>Imdur (isosorbide mononitrate)<br>Isordil (isosorbide dinitrate)<br>Loniten (minoxidil)<br>Nitro-Bid (nitroglycerin)<br>Nitrostat (nitroglycerin)<br>Sorbitrate (isosorbide dinitrate) | **Indications:** angina; hydralazine and minoxidil are used for hypertension<br>**Side effects:** nitroglycerin: dizziness, headache, flushing, severe hypotension[b]; isosorbide mononitrate and dinitrate: dizziness, headache, bradycardia; hydralazine: headache, palpitations, diarrhea, nausea, vomiting, chest pain[b]; minoxidil: hirsutism, edema, cardiac conduction abnormalities[b] |

[a]The therapist is more likely to see potential side effects that develop when the person is physically challenged and that are not otherwise present. Any unusual signs or symptoms and potential side effects should be documented and reported to the prescribing physician.
[b]Document and contact physician.
*MI*, Myocardial infarction.
Information in this table was reviewed and updated by the University of Montana College of Health Professions and Biomedical Sciences Drug Information Service (Sherrill J. Brown, DVM, PharmD, BCPS).
Data from: DiPiro JT, Talbert RL, Yee GC, et al, editors: *Pharmacotherapy: a pathophysiologic approach*, ed 10, New York, 2017, McGraw-Hill Education; Brunton LL, Hilal-Dandan R, Knollmann BC, editors: *Goodman & Gilman's the pharmacological basis of therapeutics*, ed 13, New York, 2017, McGraw-Hill Education; *Micromedex Healthcare Series* [https://www.worldcat.org/title/micromedex-healthcare-series/oclc/44535138], Greenwood Village, CO: Thomson Reuters (Healthcare); DrugReference: *Facts & Comparisons eAnswers* [https://www.wolterskluwercdi.com/facts-comparisons-online/], available from Wolters Kluwer; Merck Manual Professional Version: Drug Info [https://www.merckmanuals.com/professional/resources/brand-names-of-some-commonly-used-drugs].

affected, but new technology and new surgical intervention may reduce mortality in the decade ahead.

Surgical procedures are considered safe, and although complications can occur, the rates of complications (e.g., reintervention or repeat procedures, reexploration for bleeding) following CABG surgery have declined substantially in the last 15 years despite higher client risks. In the case of angioplasty, the risks of failure and mortality are higher with advanced age, female gender, diabetes mellitus, multivessel CAD, and HF.[221]

PCIs are associated with greater rates of restenosis among women, who are at greater risk for complications and have a higher mortality rate. Most studies attribute the higher mortality rate to the fact that women more often undergo the surgery during an emergency; they are usually older at the time of diagnosis than men; they

**Table 12.6** Medical Management of Cardiovascular Conditions[a]

| Coronary Artery Disease/Myocardial Infarction | Angina Pectoris | Hypertension | Congestive Heart Failure | Arrhythmias |
|---|---|---|---|---|
| Lifestyle changes (see text)<br>Prescriptive exercise<br>Medications:<br>• Morphine<br>• β-Adrenergic blockers<br>• Angiotensin-converting enzyme (ACE) inhibitors<br>• Angiotensin II receptor blockers (ARBs)<br>• Statins<br>• Nitrates<br>• Calcium channel blockers<br>• Antiplatelets<br>• Anticoagulants<br>• Thrombolytics<br>• Aldosterone antagonists | Lifestyle changes<br>Prescriptive exercise<br>Medications:<br>• β-Adrenergic blockers<br>• ACE inhibitors<br>• Statins<br>• Nitrates<br>• Calcium channel blockers<br>• Antiplatelets<br>• Anticoagulants | Lifestyle changes<br>Prescriptive exercise<br>Medications (frequent combination therapy):<br>• ACE inhibitors<br>• ARBs<br>• Diuretics<br>• β-Adrenergic blockers<br>• Calcium channel blockers<br>• $\alpha_1$-Adrenergic blockers<br>• Central $\alpha_2$-adrenergic agonists<br>• Peripheral adrenergic blockers<br>• Vasodilators<br>• Aldosterone antagonists<br>• Direct renin inhibitors | Lifestyle changes<br>Prescriptive exercise<br>Medications (frequent combination therapy):<br>• Hydralazine<br>• ACE inhibitors<br>• ARBs<br>• β-Adrenergic blockers<br>• Diuretics<br>• Calcium channel blockers<br>• Nitrates<br>• Aldosterone antagonists | Cardioversion (electrical or pharmacologic)<br>Medications:<br>• Aspirin<br>• Anticoagulants<br>• Antiarrhythmics:<br>  • Class I: Block sodium and potassium channels<br>  • Class II: β-Adrenergic blockers (used as antiarrhythmics drugs)<br>  • Class III: Block potassium channels<br>  • Class IV: Calcium channel blockers (used as antiarrhythmic drugs) |
| Surgery:<br>• Percutaneous coronary intervention(PCI)<br>• Coronary bypass graft (CABG)<br>• Coronary stent<br>• Implantation<br>• Atherectomy<br>• Mechanical thrombectomy<br>• Transmyocardial revascularization (TMR)<br>• Photo angioplasty<br>• Intraaortic balloon pump (IABP)<br>• Transplantation | Surgery:<br>• Revascularization procedures for unstable angina; see CAD/MI, this table<br>• TMR | Surgery:<br>• Transplantation | Surgery:<br>• Revascularization procedures (see CAD/MI, this table)<br>• IABP<br>• Left ventricular assistive device (see Chapter 21)<br>• Cardiac resynchronization therapy (CRT)<br>• Implantable cardioverter defibrillator (ICD)<br>• Transplantation | Surgery:<br>• Maze procedure (surgical or catheter)<br>• Pacemaker<br>• ICD<br>• Ventricular resynchronization therapy |

[a] The use of complementary-integrative therapies in the adjunctive treatment of each of these conditions is under investigation at this time (see text discussion in "Atherosclerosis: Treatment"). Research centered on pharmacologic and surgical approaches to these conditions is changing rapidly. This information represents a broad overview and may not include every option available.

The term *blocker* is synonymous with *antagonist.*

Combination medication therapy is frequently used in all of these cardiovascular conditions.

Antiplatelets, anticoagulants, and thrombolytics are used to treat overactive clotting but have distinct uses and mechanisms of action. Antiplatelets block platelet aggregation and platelet-induced clotting, anticoagulants inhibit the synthesis and action of clotting factors, and thrombolytics facilitate clot breakdown (fibrinolysis) after the formation of a clot.

Information in this table was reviewed and updated by the University of Montana College of Health Professions and Biomedical Sciences Drug Information Service (Sherrill J. Brown, DVM, PharmD, BCPS).

Data from: Susan Queen, PT, PhD, University of New Mexico, Albuquerque, NM (with permission); DiPiro JT, Talbert RL, Yee GC, et al, editors: *Pharmacotherapy: a pathophysiologic approach*, ed 10, New York, 2017, McGraw-Hill Education.

are more likely to have other complicating conditions (e.g., hypertension, diabetes); their coronary arteries are more calcified, prone to dissection, with atherosclerosis diffused and hard to localize, and are generally smaller, making surgery more difficult.[156]

The higher rates of morbidity and mortality associated with angioplasty have resulted in the use of the balloon-expandable stent, which is associated with a low restenosis rate and a favorable clinical outcome with event-free survival rate at 1 year. The need for repeat revascularization has also been significantly reduced.

SPECIAL IMPLICATIONS FOR THE THERAPIST 12.2

### *Ischemic Heart Disease, Coronary Heart Disease, Coronary Artery Disease*

Physical therapists can be instrumental in guiding individuals through a preoperative wellness program, including client education, risk factor reduction, and exercise program. The physical therapist is one of the health care professionals whose clinical judgment should assist a physician in selecting the most beneficial therapeutic approach for individuals with CVD.[30,354]

In the inpatient setting, physical therapists assessing patients' functional capacity and determining discharge placement may dramatically improve referral to outpatient cardiac rehabilitation.[30,354] This approach, referred to as a "paradigm shift,"[34] may be especially beneficial for people with CVD who demonstrate severe disability at discharge. Individuals with CAD who completed cardiac rehabilitation had reduced risk of morbidity and mortality, but only less than a third of eligible patients are undergoing cardiac rehabilitation.[354]

#### Prescriptive Exercise

The known benefits of regular physical activity and exercise in both primary and secondary prevention of CVD have been thoroughly documented (and discussed in this section; see "Prevention"). Exercise training increases cardiovascular aerobic capacity and decreases myocardial oxygen demand at any level of physical activity in apparently healthy people, as well as in most people with CVD.

Regular dynamic exercise is considered adjunctive therapy for lipid management along with dietary management and reduction of excess weight but must be maintained in order to sustain the training effects. Both short- and long-term endurance exercise can contribute to an improvement in blood lipid abnormalities.[316]

Although exercise and physical training have been shown to improve exercise capacity and recovery of the autonomic nervous activity,[53] there is an increased risk that exercise may precipitate cardiovascular complications and silent symptoms of ischemia, arrhythmias, or abnormal blood pressure. Heart responses to exercise and fatigue necessitate special considerations for the formulation and execution of physical conditioning programs. Determining how heart rate and blood pressure respond to exercise (e.g., at what point symptoms of oxygen deprivation occur) forms the basis for an exercise prescription.

Frequent premature ventricular contractions are considered a contraindication to exercise unless approved by the physician (e.g., as in the case of automatic implantable cardioverter-defibrillators). Indications for stopping an exercise test can be used as precautions during therapy or exercise. Therapists in all settings are encouraged to read the complete Scientific Statement on Exercise Standards for Testing and Training by the AHA[132] and the Guidelines for Cardiac Rehabilitation and Secondary Prevention Programs developed by the American Association of Cardiovascular and Pulmonary Rehabilitation.[14] Description of risks associated with resistance exercise in older adults and recommended guidelines for resistance exercise prescription in this population of cardiac rehabilitation clients are also available.[14]

#### Monitoring During Exercise

More than half of all ischemic episodes are not accompanied by angina. Patients with identified CAD risk factors or diagnosed CAD should inform the therapist of all unusual sensations, not just episodes of chest pain or discomfort. Exercise testing should be performed before beginning an exercise program, but sometimes this isn't feasible or available. In that case, the therapist should monitor the patient's heart rate and rhythm, respiratory rate, blood pressure, and pulse oximetry. It is important for the therapist to note any accompanying symptoms before, during, and after exercise. This type of monitoring can be modified for each individual and is recommended throughout therapy intervention. Documentation of vital signs can be an excellent way to demonstrate evidence-based outcomes of intervention.

Side effects of cardiovascular medications may not appear until the cardiovascular system is challenged, such as occurs during therapy intervention. Monitoring for drug-related problems is essential, and a basic understanding of how these medications work is helpful (see Table 12.5). Striking a balance between the benefits of cardiovascular medications and acceptable or tolerable side effects can be a challenge, and the therapist must keep this in mind when documenting and reporting drug-related effects that these medications often produce physiologic responses that increase the effectiveness of physical therapy. A more comprehensive discussion of this topic is available.[91]

Several drugs used in the treatment of CAD are known to alter the heart rate. For example, β-adrenergic blocking agents used in the treatment of angina and hypertension cause a reduction in resting and exercise heart rate. Anyone taking these medications may not be able to achieve a target heart rate above 90 beats/min; therefore, using symptoms (e.g., angina, diaphoresis, shortness of breath, dizziness, pallor, isolated [arm or leg] or overall fatigue) and rating perceived exertion may be a more appropriate means of monitoring. Avoid increases of more than 20 beats/min over the resting rate for individuals taking these medications.

Conservative limits postoperatively include a maximal heart rate of 130 beats/min, 120 beats/min for medically managed cases or an increase of 30 beats/min for surgical cases and 20 beats/min for medical cases. A safe rate of exercise will allow the heart rate to return to the resting level within 5 minutes after stopping exercise.

Almost all antihypertensive agents, including diuretics that may have a dual action of peripheral dilation and volume depletion, can have a profound effect on postexercise blood pressure. In some healthy people, when exercise is terminated abruptly, precipitous drops in systolic blood pressure can occur owing to venous pooling. Some people with CAD have higher levels of systolic blood pressure that exceed peak exercise values; a proper cool-down after vigorous exercise is important to prevent such an occurrence.

More detailed information on the effects of various drugs on the exercise response during training in clients with CAD can be found in *Guidelines for Exercise Testing and Prescription* by the American College of Sports Medicine.[17]

### Postoperative Considerations

Cardiac rehabilitation (phases I to III) is an important component of intervention for anyone treated medically for HF, arrhythmias, unstable angina, CAD, MI, valvular disease, or heart transplantation. This multidisciplinary program of education and exercise is designed to promote the development and maintenance of a desirable level of physical, social, and psychologic function in those individuals with an acute cardiovascular illness.

Specific goals of cardiac rehabilitation include stratifying risk, improving emotional well-being and psychologic factors, reducing CAD risk factors, and decreasing symptoms. In addition, older adults often have reduced functional capacity and quality-of-life scores compared with younger CAD clients, making this an important goal for those individuals.[86,135,339]

Implementation of phase I cardiac rehabilitation can be carried out by nurses or physical therapists. However, in many facilities, consultation with a physical therapist may be requested only when there are postoperative complications or preexisting conditions that limit phase I (e.g., amputation, cerebrovascular accident, polio, spinal cord injury). Phase I begins 1 to 3 days following CABG (or other) surgery or an MI. Primary emphasis is on postsurgical mobilization and monitoring for adverse responses to activity. Education is essential given the presence of comorbidities and the need for individualized prescriptive exercise. The patients should also be educated to begin to monitor their own responses to activity in case of adverse response.

### Sternal Precautions

Many facilities still utilize sternal precautions after cardiac surgery. These may include restricting upper extremity motion overhead or to the side, lifting/pushing/pulling objects over 2 pounds, and using upper extremities for certain transfers and with assistive devices for 6 to 12 weeks.[124] The original intent was to help prevent sternal dehiscence (separation of the sternal bone) and/or sternal infection. However, research has shown that these restrictions are unnecessary.[70,124,357] Therapists should still screen their clients for potential sternal complications prior to mobilizing them. The Sternal Instability Scale has been shown to be a valid tool to assess the client's risk of sternal dehiscence postsurgery.[122,123] If a client is found to be more at risk for sternal complications, more conservative movements and support should be used.

For all clients with median sternotomy incisions, supported coughing ("splinting") should be used. The use of thoracic support devices may be warranted for external support and pain control, especially in women (i.e. Posthorax®, Qualibreath®).[125,154] For those not at high risk for sternal complications, movement can be initiated the first 1 to 3 days after surgery. This includes upper extremity activity and the use of assistive devices for mobility.[124]

This shift towards early motion and less restriction has led to the development of the "Move in the Tube" concept instead of traditional sternal precautions[3] (Fig. 12.6). The Move in the Tube concept allows the client to complete functional motions and early activity without putting unsafe stress across the sternum. Therapists should educate the client how to move as if they have a tube wrapped around their thoracic cage and pelvis. The reference by Adams et al. and the included graphics (Fig. 12.6) give more specific explanations of Move in the Tube.[3] If applicable, a set of patient-specific precautions, rather than restrictive ones, with a focus on function is likelier to facilitate the client's recovery.[70]

Airway clearance is important after surgery, but coughing does put moderate to severe stress across the sternum. Airway clearance should consist of the patient coughing, as needed, with splinting across the sternal incision. Home monitoring of symptoms for the first weeks after surgery is essential following the guidelines in Box 12.3. The physician should be notified if the client experiences one or more of the signs and symptoms outlined. Transfusion is no longer a standard part of open heart surgery, so hematocrit levels are usually low (25%–29%) following this procedure, requiring modification of exercise guidelines unless directed otherwise by the physician.

Discharge instructions for the cardiovascular surgical population may vary according to physician and institution, but some general guidelines apply (Box 12.4). The therapist can be helpful in teaching about unexpected symptoms and ways to manage them. One of the most important aspects of early care by the therapist is education about what the client should and shouldn't feel during recovery and what to do in the event of an abnormal response.

Reassurance and education are extremely important for clients who are emotionally distressed. Although these people are successful in improving their functional status and physical capacity, they are more likely to experience angina during activities of daily living and during exercise and to be less successful in returning to work.

### Postoperative Exercise

Exercise rehabilitation is an important part of the recovery process after cardiothoracic surgery. Easy fatigability related to muscular weakness lessens with increased physical activity. Exercise-induced symptoms of angina and light-headedness or syncope disappear immediately after surgery with a successful result.

Guidelines developed by the AHA and the American College of Cardiology Foundation emphasize the importance of participating in a cardiac rehabilitation program after a heart attack or bypass surgery.[340] The exercise capacity of clients soon after MI and bypass surgery is determined by the same parameters as in healthy individuals or for other cardiac problems, including time since MI, age, physical training status, and amount of myocardial dysfunction that occurs with exercise. CNS dysfunction is a common consequence of otherwise uncomplicated CABG surgery that may affect exercise capacity. The exact cause of this neurologic phenomenon remains unknown, but it may be the result of preoperative intracranial or extracranial carotid artery disease contributing to compromised hemodynamics and cerebral hypoperfusion.

The physical activity program after coronary surgery should incorporate aerobic and resistance exercise. It should be guided by the timeline since surgery, medical stability of the client, and specific individual comorbidities. Discussion of specific exercise program needs and parameters for phase I–III cardiac rehabilitation can be found in textbooks specific to cardiothoracic physical therapy care.

### *Side Effects of Medication*

As shown in Table 12.5, there is a wide range of commonly prescribed cardiovascular medications with an equally wide variety of potential side effects. The therapist must make note of medications used by each client and observe for any of the common adverse effects.

Statins are widely prescribed and are recommended for the treatment of hypercholesterolemia. However, the therapist should be aware of myopathies or myalgias that can be associated with the use of statins.[169] Myalgia as a result of taking a statin medication usually occurs within a few weeks of starting the drug. Any unexplained muscle pain, cramps, stiffness, spasm, or weakness in an adult taking a statin should be reported to the physician. This is especially true if there are any predictive risk factors. Risk factors for this particular effect include age older than 80 years, small body frame or frail health, presence of kidney disease, and polypharmacy. For anyone experiencing adverse muscular effects from statin therapy, alternative approaches are recommended such as using a different dose of the same statin or using another drug from the statin group and using vitamin D and coenzyme Q10 supplements.[303]

Individuals taking some forms of statins (e.g., Zocor [simvastatin], Lipitor [atorvastatin], and Pravachol [pravastatin]) are warned to avoid drinking grapefruit juice while taking statins because grapefruit juice contains inhibitors of the enzyme responsible for breaking down one of the statin metabolites (products of statin's conversion in the body). Inhibition of the enzyme may lead to accumulation of the metabolite in the body and resulting toxicity.

## Angina Pectoris

### Definition and Incidence

As blood vessels become obstructed by the formation of atherosclerotic plaque, the blood supply to tissues supplied by these vessels becomes restricted. When the cardiac workload exceeds the oxygen supply to myocardial tissue, ischemia occurs, causing temporary chest pain or discomfort, called *angina pectoris.* It may feel like squeezing or pressure in the center of the chest. Angina is not a disease but a symptom of an underlying problem, typically CAD. The exact incidence of angina is unknown, although it is considered common, especially in people age 65 years and older; it occurs more often in men. In the United States, 3.4% of adults older than 20 years of age experience angina.[50]

**Box 12.5**

**TYPES OF ANGINA PECTORIS**

- Stable angina; classic exertional angina
- Unstable or preinfarction angina
- New-onset (unstable) angina
- Nocturnal angina
- Postinfarction angina
- Preinfarction angina (unstable); progressive, crescendo angina
- Prinzmetal, vasospastic or variant angina
- Resting angina (decubitus)
- Microvascular angina

### Overview

There are several types of anginal pain (Box 12.5).

*Stable angina,* classified as classic, exertional angina, occurs at predictable levels of physical or emotional stress, over a period of 1 to 4 months, and resolves promptly with rest or nitroglycerin. No pain occurs at rest, and the location, duration, intensity, and frequency of chest pain are consistent over time.

*Unstable angina* or *preinfarction angina* is unpredictable and is characterized by an abrupt change (increase) in the intensity and frequency of symptoms or decreased threshold of stimulus. This angina lasts longer than 15 minutes and is a symptom of worsening cardiac ischemia. It may be caused by a blood clot blocking an artery.

*New-onset angina* describes angina that has developed for the first time within the last 2 weeks and is also considered unstable.

*Nocturnal angina* may awaken a person from sleep with the same sensation experienced during exertion and is usually caused by increased heart rate associated with dreams or in response to underlying HF.

*Postinfarction angina* occurs after MI when residual ischemia triggers an episode of angina.

*Prinzmetal, vasospastic,* or *variant angina* produces symptoms similar to those of typical angina, but it is caused by abnormal or involuntary coronary artery spasm rather than directly by buildup of atherosclerotic plaques. These spasms periodically squeeze arteries shut and keep the blood from perfusing the heart. About two thirds of people with variant angina have severe coronary atherosclerosis in at least one major vessel. The pattern of variant angina is typically characterized by early morning occurrence, frequently at the same time each day, and it occurs at rest (i.e., it is unrelated to exertion).

Variant angina is more common in women younger than 50 years; it is often associated with various types of arrhythmias or conduction defects. It is not a benign condition but is less likely to lead to a heart attack than angina caused by atherosclerosis, because most heart attacks are caused by the rupture of an atherosclerotic plaque.

*Decubitus* or *resting angina* is considered atypical; it occurs most often when at rest and frequently occurs at the same

Keep Your Move in the Tube®

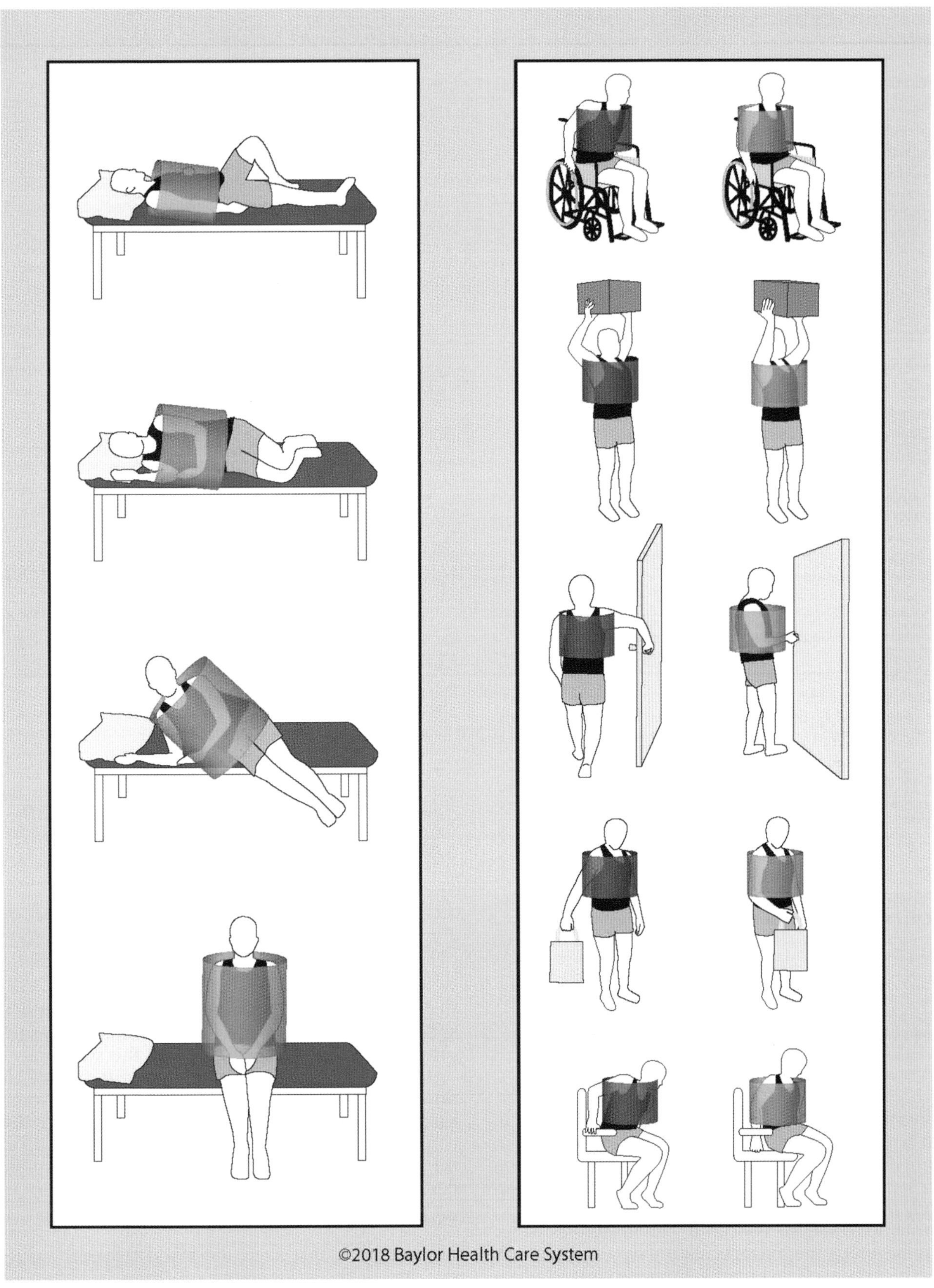


**Figure 12.6**

**Move in the Tube.** Clients that undergo thoracic surgery using a median sternotomy incision should follow the Move in the Tube guidelines for transfers, mobility, lifting, and limb movement for at least 4 weeks post-surgery. Clients should avoid lifting, pushing, or pulling movements that create force across the sternal area. However, lifting, pushing, and pulling that occur within the client's center of gravity of proximal sphere of movement are allowed and are safe when done correctly. (Copyright by Baylor Health Care System, 2018.)

Box 12.3

**INDICATIONS FOR DISCONTINUING OR MODIFYING EXERCISE[a]**

***Symptoms***

- New-onset or easily provoked anginal chest pain
- Increasing episodes, intensity, or duration of angina (unstable angina)
- Discomfort in the upper body, including chest, arm, neck, or jaw; chest pain unrelated to chest incision
- Fainting, light-headedness, dizziness
- Sudden, severe dyspnea
- Severe fatigue or muscle pain
- Nausea or vomiting
- Back pain during exercise
- Bone or joint pain or discomfort during or after exercise
- Severe leg claudication

***Clinical Signs***

- Pallor; peripheral cyanosis; cold, moist skin
- Staggering gait, ataxia
- Confusion or blank stare in response to inquiries
- Resting heart rate >130 beats/min or <40 beats/min
- >6 Arrhythmias (irregular heartbeats; palpitations) per hour
- Frequent premature ventricular contractions
- Uncontrolled diabetes mellitus (blood glucose level >250 mg/dL)
- Oxygen saturation <90% (98% is normal); some variability (individual and geographic)
- Acute infection or fever >37.8° C (100° F)
- Persistent drainage or change in drainage from any incision
- Increased swelling, tenderness, and redness around any incision site
- Inability to converse during activity
- Blood pressure (BP) abnormalities
  - Fall in systolic BP with increase in workload; specifically, a decrease of 10 mm Hg or more below any previously recorded BP accompanied by other signs or symptoms
  - Rise in systolic BP above 250 mm Hg or diastolic BP above 115 mm Hg
- Signs of CNS involvement (e.g., confusion or delirium, cognitive decline, encephalopathy, seizure, stroke)

***Other***

- Person indicates need or desire to stop
- Recent myocardial infarction (within 48 hours)

[a]Not all signs and symptoms require immediate cessation of exercise or intervention. The therapist is advised to document any clinical signs or symptoms observed or reported along with any modifications made in the intervention and notify the physician accordingly.

Adapted from Fletcher GF, Ades PA, Kligfield P, et al: Exercise standards for testing and training: a scientific statement from the American Heart Association, *Circulation* 128(8):873–934, 2013.

Box 12.4

**DISCHARGE INSTRUCTIONS AFTER CARDIOVASCULAR SURGERY**

- **Showers:** Permitted 2 days after surgery or hospitalization. Avoid tub baths or soaking in water until incisions are healed; avoid extremely hot water.
- **Incisions:** The incision should be kept dry but can be gently washed with mild soap and warm water (directly over the tapes); lotions, creams, oils, or powders are not permitted until the wound is completely healed unless prescribed by the physician.
- **Care of surgical leg** (for bypass graft involving the leg): Avoid crossing the legs, which impairs circulation; avoid sitting in one position or standing for prolonged periods. Elevate the involved leg when sitting or lying down. Swelling in the grafted leg is common until collateral circulation develops. Swelling should decrease after leg elevation but may recur when standing. Progressive edema must be reported to the physician.
- **Compression stockings:** Worn for at least 2 weeks after discharge during the daytime and removed at bedtime.
- **Rest:** A balance of rest and exercise is an essential part of the recovery process. Resting between activities and short naps are encouraged. Resting may include sitting quietly or reading for 20 to 30 minutes; loss of appetite is common for the first 2 weeks and may contribute to fatigue.
- **Walking:** Walking increases circulation throughout the body and to the heart muscle and is encouraged. Activity must be increased gradually, but frequent walks of short duration are recommended initially. Pacing of activities throughout the day, combined with energy conservation, is important.
- **Stairs:** Climbing stairs is permitted unless the physician indicates otherwise.
- **Sexual relations:** Sexual relations can be resumed when the client feels physically comfortable (usually 2–4 weeks after discharge; see also text discussion).
- **"Move in the tube" motions.**

***Stop any activity immediately if dyspnea, palpitations, chest pain or discomfort, or dizziness or fainting develops. Notify the physician if symptoms do not subside with rest within 20 minutes.***

Adapted from Fletcher GF, Ades PA, Kligfield P, et al. Exercise standards for testing and training: a scientific statement from the American Heart Association, *Circulation* 128(8):873–934, 2013.

time every day. This type of anginal chest pain is atypical in that it is paroxysmal in nature, not brought on by exercise, and not relieved by rest, but it is reduced when the person sits or stands up. It is more prevalent among women, particularly those who have undergone hysterectomy.

*Microvascular angina* associated with insulin resistance syndrome affects the microcirculatory system, a network of tiny blood vessels that branch from the large coronary vessels and that provide oxygen to each of the millions of myocardial cells. Why these vessels spasm and cause decreased blood flow remains undetermined; the cause may be a decrease in estrogen during menopause or a specific trigger from within the heart. Long-term survival rates are not reduced in women with this syndrome.

Microvascular angina is caused by reduction of blood flow through the smallest coronary arteries, coronary microvasculature. It develops when the arteries' walls are constricted. Chest pain usually lasts longer than 10 to 30 minutes. Microvascular angina is usually a symptom of coronary microvascular disease.

### Etiologic and Risk Factors

Any condition that alters the blood (oxygen) supply or demand of the myocardium can cause ischemia (Table 12.7). Increased oxygen needs of the heart, increased cardiac output, or reduced blood flow to the heart can cause angina. CAD accounts for 90% of all cases of angina,

**Table 12.7** Causes of Myocardial Ischemia

| Decreased Oxygen Supply | Increased Oxygen Demand |
|---|---|
| **Vessels** | |
| Atherosclerotic narrowing | Hyperthyroidism |
| Inadequate collateral circulation | Arteriovenous fistula |
| Spasm caused by smoking, emotion, or cold | Exercise or exertion |
| Coronary arteritis | Emotion or excitement |
| Hypertension | Digestion of large meal |
| Hypertrophic cardiomyopathy | |
| **Circulatory Factors** | |
| Arrhythmias (decreased blood pressure) | |
| Aortic stenosis | |
| Hypotension | |
| Bleeding | |
| **Blood Factors** | |
| Anemia | |
| Hypoxemia | |
| Polycythemia | |

Data from Bonow RO: *Braunwald's heart disease—a textbook of cardiovascular medicine*, ed 9, Philadelphia, 2011, WB Saunders; Goldman L, Schafer AI: *Goldman's Cecil medicine*, ed 24, Philadelphia, 2012, WB Saunders.

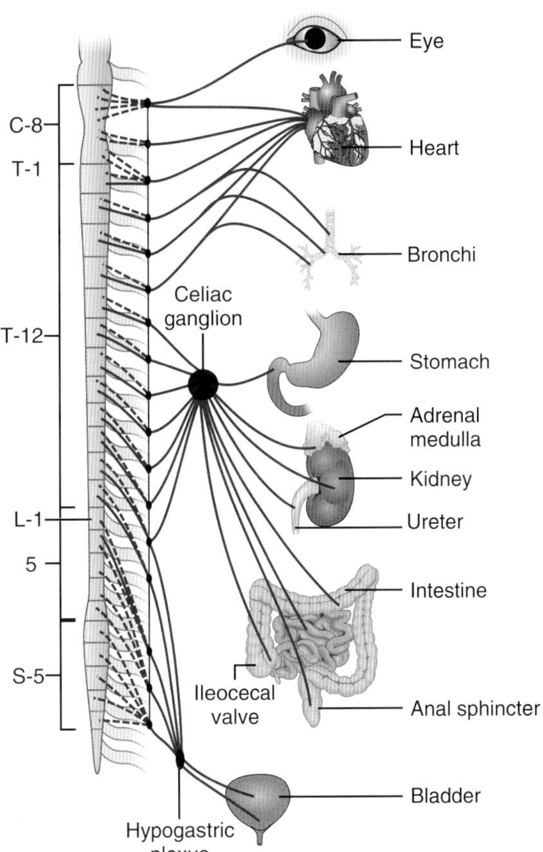


**Figure 12.7**

**Diagram of the autonomic nervous system.** The visceral afferent fibers mediating cardiac pain travel with the sympathetic nerves and enter the spinal cord at multiple levels (C3 to T4). This multisegmental innervation results in a variety of pain patterns associated with myocardial ischemia and infarction.

although other conditions affecting nonatherosclerotic vessels can also cause angina. Disorders of circulation, such as relative hypotension secondary to spinal anesthesia, antihypertensive drugs, or blood loss, can also result in decreased blood return to the heart and subsequent ischemic pain.

Onset of angina may be triggered by physical exertion or exercise, especially involving thoracic or upper extremity muscles or walking rapidly uphill. Increases in heart rate or blood pressure (e.g., psychologic or emotional stress) or vasoconstriction can also bring on anginal symptoms. Angina may also occur less commonly during sexual activity, at rest, or at night during sleep. In the case of variant angina, episodes can be triggered by cocaine, amphetamines, migraine medication, and herbal supplements such as ephedra or bitter orange.

## Pathogenesis

Angina is a symptom of ischemia usually brought on by an imbalance between cardiac workload and oxygen supply to myocardial tissue usually secondary to CAD (see previous discussion on pathogenesis of atherosclerosis). Disruption of a formed plaque with sudden total or near-total arterial occlusion may bring on unstable angina. Rupture leads to the activation, adhesion, and aggregation of platelets and the activation of the clotting cascade, resulting in the formation of an occlusive thrombus. If this process leads to complete occlusion of the artery, then MI occurs. If the process leads to severe stenosis but the artery remains open, then unstable angina occurs.

Chemical mediators within the ischemic segment of the myocardium (e.g., histamine, bradykinin, prostaglandins) and buildup of protons from lactic acid and reactive oxygen species irritate cardiac spinal afferent endings in the ventricles resulting in myocardial pain.[140] Afferent sympathetic fibers of the autonomic nervous system enter the spinal cord from levels C3 to T4 (Fig. 12.7), accounting for the varied locations and radiation patterns of anginal pain. The effects of temporary ischemia are reversible; if blood flow is restored, no permanent damage to or necrosis of the heart muscle occurs.

## Clinical Manifestations

Angina is characterized by temporary pain or, more often, discomfort that starts suddenly in the chest (substernal or retrosternal) and sometimes radiates to other parts of the body, most commonly to the left shoulder and down the ulnar border of the arm to the fingers. Pain or discomfort may also be referred to any dermatome from C3 to T4, presenting at the back of the neck, lower jaw, teeth, upper back, interscapular area, abdomen, and possibly down the right arm (Fig. 12.8). Location of anginal symptoms can vary between individuals and between genders.[209]

The sensation described is often referred to as squeezing, burning, pressing, heartburn, indigestion, or choking. It is usually mild to moderate (rarely reported as severe); it usually lasts 1 to 3 minutes, sometimes 3 to 5 minutes, but can persist up to 15 to 20 minutes. Symptoms are usually relieved by rest or nitroglycerin; in women with abdominal symptoms of angina, symptoms may be relieved by taking an antacid.

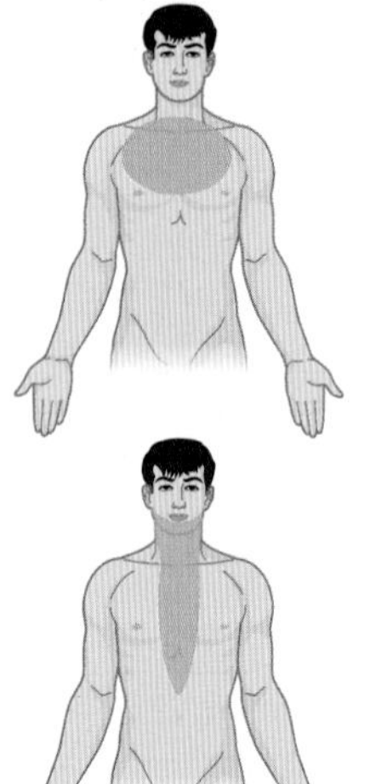
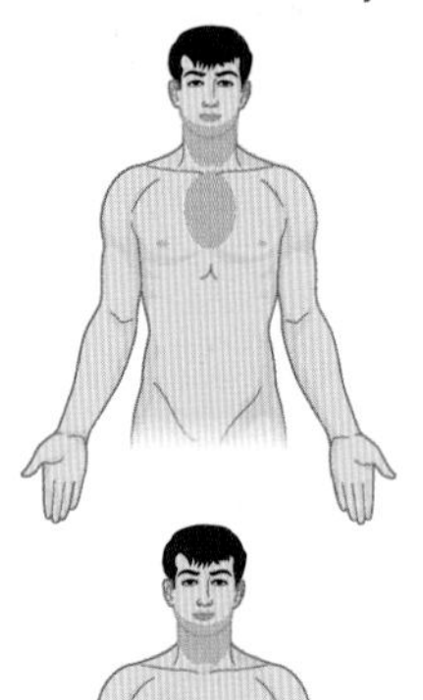
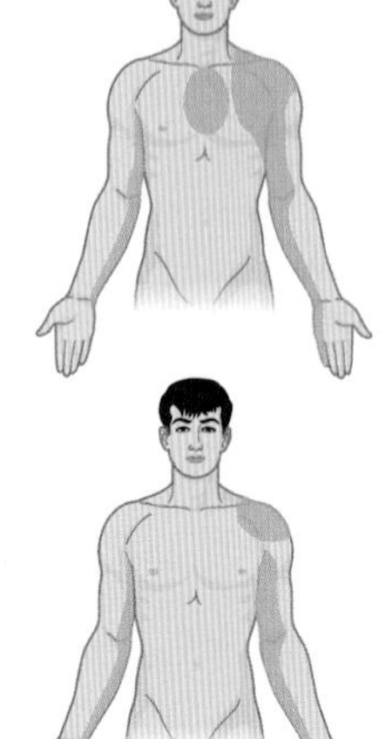
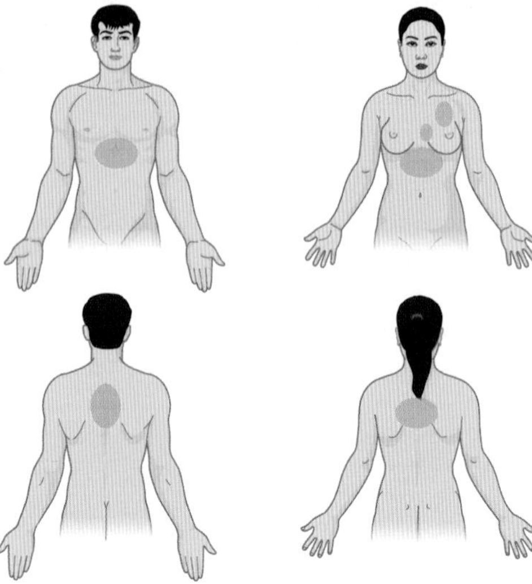


| Most common warning signs of heart attack | Atypical, less common warning signs (especially women) |
|---|---|
| • Uncomfortable pressure, fullness, squeezing, or pain in the center of the chest (prolonged)<br>• Pain that spreads to the throat, neck, back, jaw, shoulders, or arms<br>• Chest discomfort with llight-headedness, dizziness, sweating, pallor, nausea, or shortness of breath<br>• Prolonged symptoms unrelieved by antacids, nitroglycerin, or rest | • Unusual chest pain (quality, location, e.g., burning, heaviness; left chest), stomach or abdominal pain<br>• Continuous midthoracic or interscapular pain<br>• Continuous neck or shoulder pain<br>• Pain relieved by antacids; pain unrelieved by rest or nitroglycerin<br>• Nausea and vomiting; flu-like manifestation without chest pain/discomfort<br>• Unexplained intense anxiety, weakness, or fatigue<br>• Breathlessness, dizziness |

**Figure 12.8**

**Early warning signs of a heart attack.** Multiple segmental nerve innervation shown in Figure 12.6 accounts for the varied pain patterns possible. A woman can experience any of the various patterns described but is more likely to develop atypical symptoms of pain as depicted here. (Modified from Goodman CC, Heick J, Lazaro RT: *Differential diagnosis for physical therapists: screening for referral*, ed 6, St Louis, 2018, Elsevier.)

Recognizing symptoms of myocardial ischemia in women is more difficult, as the symptoms are atypical, less reliable, and do not follow the classic pattern described. Atypical symptoms of angina in women include breathlessness, pain in the left chest, upper abdominal pain, and back or arm pain (more rarely, isolated pain in the right biceps muscle) in the absence of substernal chest pain. The pain may be more diffuse and is described as sharp or fleeting, unrelated to exercise, unrelieved by rest or nitroglycerin, but relieved by antacids, and characterized by palpitations without chest pain. The pain may be repeated and prolonged. Chest pain in women with chronic stable angina is more likely to occur during rest, sleep, or periods of mental stress. Many women describe the pain in ways consistent with unstable angina, suggesting that they first become aware of their chest discomfort or have it diagnosed only after it reaches more advanced stages. Some experience a sensation similar to that of inhaling cold air rather than the more typical shortness of breath. Other women note only weakness and lethargy, and some have observed isolated pain in the midthoracic spine or throbbing and aching in the right biceps muscle.

## MEDICAL MANAGEMENT

**DIAGNOSIS.** The diagnosis of angina pectoris is strongly suspected if history is present and is supported if sublingual nitroglycerin shortens an attack and if prophylactic nitrates permit greater exertion or prevent angina entirely. Medical evaluation includes examination for signs of diseases that may produce angina or contribute to or accompany atherosclerotic disease.

Early and accurate triage to assess risk (low, intermediate, high) can help identify those people for whom medical therapy will probably fail and lead to better outcomes through a more appropriate management strategy. ECG is normal in approximately 25% to 30% of people with angina, so the exercise tolerance test is a more useful noninvasive procedure for evaluating the ischemic response to exercise in the client with angina. Diagnostic testing continues as for CAD (see "Atherosclerosis: Diagnosis" above and "Myocardial Infarction: Diagnosis" below).

**PREVENTION AND TREATMENT.** Prevention of attacks is the first step after the acute attack subsides. Treatment of underlying disorders such as hypertension is essential. The client is also encouraged to avoid situations and stressors that precipitate angina. This usually requires modifying all possible risk factors through changes in lifestyle and modifications of lifelong habits.

Short-acting sublingual nitroglycerin is the drug of choice for the acute attack, usually relieving symptoms within 1 to 2 minutes. Nitroglycerin oral spray is also available in a metered delivery system, which is especially useful for anyone having difficulty handling or swallowing pills. The spray is also easy to use in the dark and is more rapidly acting. Long-acting nitrates (e.g., oral sustained-release nitroglycerin, transdermal nitroglycerin patches, nitroglycerin ointment) are especially useful for people for whom sudden drop in blood pressure associated with taking nitroglycerin is not desirable (i.e., people with hypotension) or for those requiring more consistent treatment of anginal symptoms.

Pharmacologic therapy may include other vasodilators, such as β-blockers (i.e., β-adrenergic receptor blockers) and calcium channel blockers (see Table 12.5). Intravascular thrombosis is a key element in the pathophysiology of unstable angina and its progression to MI. Anticoagulation therapy using aspirin and/or heparin is an important part of treatment for unstable angina.[24]

Anticoagulants, such as aspirin and heparin, slow down or prevent clot formation, whereas thrombolytic agents, such as tPA, its modification Retavase (reteplase), urokinase, and streptokinase, facilitate breakdown of clots that have already formed. Both anticoagulants and thrombolytics are antithrombotics. Aspirin blocks platelet cyclooxygenase, preventing the formation of thromboxane $A_2$, thereby inhibiting platelet aggregation. Heparin binds to an enzyme inhibitor, antithrombin III, enabling it to inactivate clotting factors such as thrombin or factor Xa. tPA, retavase, urokinase, or streptokinase, all known as "clot busters," do not break clot themselves, but each can activate plasminogen to plasmin that lyses the clot.

Second-line alternatives to aspirin (sometimes referred to as "super aspirins"; (e.g., Ticlid [ticlopidine], Plavix [clopidogrel]) are more effective than aspirin in preventing platelet aggregation and thereby reducing the combined risk of ischemic stroke, MI, or death from vascular disease and may be useful in preventing coronary stent thrombosis.

Revascularization procedures are recommended for persons who do not become ischemia free on medical therapy, especially clients with progressive unstable angina. Surgical intervention, such as PCI, has been shown to relieve angina, but it does not halt the progress of atherosclerosis. It simply restores blood flow through the area that had been blocked. CABG can diminish the probability that ischemia will lead to necrosis and lethal infarction.

For people who are not good candidates for any of the proven procedures or whose angina persists despite angioplasty or bypass surgery, transmyocardial revascularization (TMR) may be recommended. In TMR, a computer-controlled laser drills tiny channels through the wall of the left ventricle while the chamber is filled with oxygenated blood. In theory, this allows blood to flow through the channels to the oxygen-deprived tissue, relieving angina. The openings on the heart's surface scar over quickly, but it is not known how long the channels stay open on the inside of the heart; long-term results remain unknown.

TMR is still not widely available in all centers, but studies have reported success in relieving severe angina that has been refractory to medical and surgical intervention.[206] This procedure is performed through a 4-inch incision between the ribs and does not require a bypass machine; efforts to develop noninvasive techniques for TMR using fiberoptic catheters are under investigation.

**PROGNOSIS.** Myocardial ischemia leaves the heart vulnerable to arrhythmias and MI, which can be fatal. About one third of all people who experience angina pectoris die suddenly from MI or arrhythmias. Prognosis depends primarily on left ventricular function (i.e., ejection fraction) but is influenced by type of angina, ability to prevent angina, and severity of underlying disease, such as hypertension or atherosclerosis.

**SPECIAL IMPLICATIONS FOR THE THERAPIST 12.3**

## *Angina Pectoris*

### Identifying Angina

Referred pain from the external oblique abdominal muscle and the pectoral major muscle can cause the sensation referred to as heartburn in the anterior chest wall, which mimics angina. When active trigger points are present in the left pectoralis major muscle, the referred pain is easily confused with that from coronary insufficiency. Physical therapy to eliminate the trigger points can aid in the diagnostic process.

Anterior chest wall syndrome with localized tenderness of intercostal muscles, Tietze syndrome with inflammation of the chondrocostal junctions, intercostal neuritis, and cervical or thoracic spine disease involving the dorsal nerve roots can all produce chest pain that mimics angina. Evaluation of range of motion, palpation of soft tissue structures, and analysis of relieving or aggravating factors usually differentiate these conditions from true angina.[153] Likewise, heartburn from indigestion, hiatal hernia, peptic ulcer, esophageal spasm, and gallbladder disease can also cause angina-like symptoms that require a medical evaluation for an accurate medical diagnosis. Occasionally the client may have radiating shoulder or scapular pain that must be differentiated from atypical anginal pain.

The development of unstable angina also requires immediate medical referral and may be reported as the onset of angina at rest, occurrence of typical angina at a significantly lower level of activity than usual, changes in the typical anginal pattern (e.g., symptoms occurring more frequently), or changes in blood pressure (decrease) or heart rate (increase) with levels of activity previously well tolerated. Educating the public about reducing delays and getting to an emergency department at the earliest signs of heart attack is essential.[236] Reperfusion therapy within the first 60 to 70 minutes of a heart attack can make a significant difference in outcome.

### Nitroglycerin

A person experiencing angina should reduce the intensity of or, if necessary, stop all activity and sit down for a few minutes until the symptoms disappear. Exercise can be resumed at a reduced intensity once symptoms dissipate. Interval-type training may be required (i.e., slow activity alternating with activity requiring more effort) to allow activity without anginal symptoms. Some experts suggest waiting several hours before resuming exercise. Anyone experiencing angina regularly with exercise or at a lower exertion than in the past may need a medical evaluation.

Nitroglycerin may be used prophylactically 5 minutes before activities likely to precipitate angina. This is especially true in the intervention or exercise setting for the person with chronic, stable, exertional angina. The use of nitroglycerin must be by physician order and cannot be decided solely by the therapist and client.

Clients must be reminded that they are not to alter their prescribed drug schedule without consulting their health care provider and that nitroglycerin should be taken as prescribed. For example, taking sublingual nitroglycerin orally markedly decreases its effectiveness. Clients should be seated when taking nitroglycerin to avoid syncope and falls. For anginal pain or discomfort that is not relieved by rest or relieved by up to three nitroglycerin doses in 10 to 15 minutes (i.e., the initial dose followed by a second dose 5 minutes later and a third dose 5 minutes after the second dose), the client should seek immediate medical care. Until the angina is controlled and coronary blood flow reestablished, the client is at risk of myocardial damage and possible infarction from myocardial ischemia.

Nitroglycerin tablets are inactivated by light, heat, air, and moisture, and they should be stored in the refrigerator in an amber container with a tight-fitting cover. Nitroglycerin has a short shelf life and needs to be replaced about every 3 months. A potent nitroglycerin tablet should produce a burning sensation under the tongue when taken sublingually (if it does not, the client should check the expiration date).

### Orthostatic Hypotension

Orthostatic hypotension (see more complete discussion of orthostatic [postural] hypotension later in this chapter) is one of the most common side effects of prophylactic medications for angina. Caution on the part of the therapist is required when exercising or ambulating with clients who take these medications. If the person becomes hypotensive, have the person assume a supine position with legs elevated to increase venous return and to ensure cerebral blood flow.

Extra caution must be taken when placing anyone with orthostatic hypotension and HF supine with legs elevated, because this may overload an already stressed ventricle. Keeping the head elevated and monitoring carefully are required in this circumstance. Vascular support hose may be recommended if the hypotension occurs regularly, and the person should be reminded to change positions slowly to minimize the effects of orthostatic hypotension. Headache, weakness, increasing pulse, or other unusual signs or symptoms should be reported to the physician. In a home health setting, the home should be evaluated for potentially hazardous conditions in case of a fall from hypotension. All clients should be encouraged to avoid hazardous activities until their condition is stabilized by medication, especially in the presence of dizziness.

### Monitoring Vital Signs

Exercise testing should be performed before a client begins an exercise program. However, sometimes the client has not undergone exercise testing or it is not appropriate for that particular client and therefore, baseline measurements are unavailable for use in planning exercise. In that case, the therapist should monitor the heart rate and blood pressure and note any accompanying symptoms during exercise. All factors and patient variables must be considered, including cognitive function, resting blood pressure, heart rate response to rest after physical activity and exercise, gait speed during ambulation, medications (especially antihypertensives), the presence of other co-morbidities that can affect vital signs, and so on.

Exercise and activity should be performed below the anginal threshold. The therapist must document heart rate and blood pressure when the ischemia began (as evidenced by symptoms of angina) to establish these parameters. Angina occurring after an MI is not considered normal and should be reported to the physician. Exercise testing is recommended before a client resumes an exercise program.

## Hypertensive Cardiovascular Disease

Hypertensive CVD includes hypertensive vascular disease and hypertensive heart disease. Other conditions affecting the heart caused by an underlying pulmonary pathologic condition (e.g., pulmonary hypertension, pulmonary heart disease) are discussed in Chapter 15.

### Hypertension (Hypertensive Vascular Disease)

**Definition and Overview.** Blood pressure is the force exerted against the walls of the arteries and arterioles; diastolic pressure (bottom number in the pressure measurement) is the pressure in these vessels when the heart is relaxed between beats, and systolic pressure (top number in the pressure measurement) is the pressure exerted in the arteries when the heart contracts. Between ages 55 and 60 years, diastolic blood pressure often begins to plateau and may even decline, whereas systolic blood pressure often starts to rise.

Hypertension, or high blood pressure, presents a serious threat to the health of the client's heart. Consistent elevated peripheral pressure puts added stress on vascular walls, as well as the myocardial muscle itself. Guidelines for prevention, evaluation, and treatment of hypertension define three categories for hypertension levels. Blood pressure between 120 and 129 mm Hg systolic AND less than 80 mm Hg diastolic is considered to be elevated. Hypertension stage 1 is labeled as values of systolic pressure between 130 and 139 mm Hg OR diastolic between 80 and 89 mm Hg. Systolic levels at least 140 mm Hg OR diastolic pressure levels at least 90 mm Hg are categorized as hypertension stage 2. There are also guidelines for hypertension levels in children and adolescents.[133] Therapists working with pediatric populations should become familiar with these values and incorporate them into their client care.

**Table 12.8** Categories of BP in Adults[a]

| BP Category | SBP | | DBP |
|---|---|---|---|
| **Normal** | <120 mm Hg | and | <80 mm Hg |
| **Elevated** | 120–129 mm Hg | and | <80 mm Hg |
| **Hypertension** | | | |
| **Stage 1** | 130–139 mm Hg | or | 80–89 mm Hg |
| **Stage 2** | ≥140 mm Hg | or | ≥90 mm Hg |

[a]Individuals with SBP and DBP in 2 categories should be designated to the higher BP category.
BP indicates blood pressure (based on an average of ≥2 careful readings obtained on ≥2 occasions, as detailed in diastolic blood pressure (DBP) and systolic blood pressure (SBP).
From Potter PA, et al: *Fundamentals of nursing*, ed 10, St. Louis, 2021, Elsevier.

Hypertension can be classified according to type (systolic or diastolic), cause, and degree of severity. Hypertension can also be classified based on risk according to the most recent guidelines (Table 12.8).[133,373]

*Primary* (or essential) *hypertension* is also known as idiopathic hypertension and accounts for 90% to 95% of all cases of hypertension. *Secondary hypertension* accounts for only 5% to 10% of cases and results from an identifiable cause. Intermittent elevation of blood pressure interspersed with normal readings is called *labile hypertension* or borderline hypertension. *Malignant hypertension* (also known as hypertensive crisis) is a syndrome of markedly elevated blood pressure (systolic pressure >180 mm Hg AND/OR diastolic blood pressure >120 mm Hg) with target organ damage (e.g., retinal hemorrhages, papilledema, HF, encephalopathy, renal insufficiency, stroke).[373] The elevation of systolic blood pressure independently of change in the diastolic blood pressure is now recognized as a medical condition referred to as *isolated systolic hypertension.*

**Incidence.** Worldwide, more than 31% of the adult population has hypertension.[50] The incidence of hypertension varies considerably among different groups in the American population, but it is estimated that one in three adult Americans older than 20 years of age (34%; 85+ million) has high blood pressure.[50] Two of every three adults older than age 60 years has high blood pressure.[50] Not surprisingly, hypertension contributes to every sixth death and more than half of all CVD-related deaths in the United States.[50] Sixteen percent of U.S. adults are not aware they have hypertension.[50] Hypertension is twice as prevalent and more severe among African Americans than whites.[50] This phenomenon has been attributed to heredity, greater environmental stress, and greater salt intake or salt sensitivity (i.e., responsiveness to changes in sodium balance and extracellular fluid and volume status), although the actual cause is not clear; reduced access to health care increases the prevalence of untreated hypertension.

The population that has the lowest prevalence of blood pressure control is adults 20 to 39 years of age.[50,79] Blood pressure control rates vary in minority populations and are lowest in Mexican Americans and Native Americans.[79] Socioeconomic factors and lifestyle may be important barriers to blood pressure control in some minority individuals.

Hypertension, except for smoking in men, is the highest risk factor for CVD mortality. If hypertension is eliminated, CVD mortality could decrease by 30% in men and 38% in women.[50]

**Etiologic and Risk Factors.** *Primary (essential) hypertension* has no established etiology but is probably related to genetics and other risk factors, such as smoking, obesity, and high cholesterol levels, and is more prevalent in people of color. It is estimated that 75% of occurrences of hypertension are related to obesity.[275] A familial association with hypertension has been documented, possibly attributable to common genetic background, shared environment, or lifestyle habits. In the recent past, advances in genomics studies led to uncovering genetics of hypertension and control of blood pressure.

A large-population GWAS identified over 1,000 genetic variants with more than 900 loci linked to hypertension.[268] As a complex trait, blood pressure is affected by many determinants, including vascular stiffness and endocrine and autonomic factors. While understanding of mechanisms for linking majority of genetic variants to hypertension is lacking, some of the discovered genetic variants are now linked to specific mechanisms that play a role in controlling blood pressure.[338] Among candidate genes, collagen 4, a component of vascular basement membrane, contributes to structural properties of the vascular wall. Variants in the genes responsible for synthesis and signaling of natriuretic peptides and nitric oxide affect sodium excretion and vessel dilation, respectively.

How the genetics of hypertension may affect environmental influences on the disease pathology is elucidated in the gene–environment interaction studies.[268] In this approach, genetic variants are viewed as predisposing people to be more or less vulnerable to a negative environment or be more or less responsive to positive environmental influences. Examples include genetic loci interacting with dietary salt intake ("saltsensitivity"), smoking, and alcohol consumption, all to influence blood pressure.[268]

With the abundance of antihypertensive medications, less than half of people with hypertension have it controlled.[50,268] While many factors contribute to this outcome, genetic variants may be partially responsible. Pharmacogenomics has the potential to predict the therapeutic effect and adverse response to classes of drugs based on the person's gene variants. Studies showed that blood pressure responses to β-blockers relate to the variants in the locus of the β1-adrenoceptor gene.[268]

Box 12.6

**CAUSES OF SECONDARY HYPERTENSION**

- Coarctation of the aorta
- Alcohol abuse
- Pregnancy induced
- Thyrotoxicosis
- Increased intracranial pressure from tumors or trauma
- Collagen disease
- Endocrine disease
  - Acromegaly
  - Cushing disease
  - Diabetes
  - Hypothyroidism
  - Hyperthyroidism
  - Pheochromocytoma (rare catecholamine-secreting tumor)
- Chronic kidney disease (most common cause in the general population: vascular renal disease)
- Drug induced or drug related (e.g., oral contraceptives, corticosteroids, cyclosporine, cocaine, anabolic steroids, amphetamines)
- Acute stress
  - Surgery
  - Psychogenic hyperventilation
  - Alcohol withdrawal
  - Burns
  - Pancreatitis
  - Sickle cell crisis
- Neurologic disorders
  - Brain tumor
  - Respiratory acidosis
  - Encephalitis
  - Sleep apnea
  - Guillain-Barré syndrome
  - Quadriplegia
  - Lead poisoning

Data from Whelton PK, Carey RM, Aronow WS, et al.: 2017 ACC/AHA/AAPA/ABC/ACPM/AGS/APhA/ASH/ASPC/NMA/PCNA Guideline for the Prevention, Detection, Evaluation, and Management of High Blood Pressure in Adults: A Report of the American College of Cardiology/American Heart Association Task Force on Clinical Practice Guidelines, *Circulation* 138(17):e484–e594, 2018.

Box 12.7

**RISK FACTORS OF PRIMARY (ESSENTIAL) HYPERTENSION**

***Modifiable***

- High sodium intake (causes water retention, increasing blood volume)
- Obesity (associated with increased intravascular volume)
- Insulin resistance and metabolic abnormalities
- Diabetes mellitus
- Hypercholesterolemia and increased serum triglyceride levels
- Smoking (nicotine restricts blood vessels)
- Long-term abuse of alcohol (increases plasma catecholamines)
- Continuous emotional stress (stimulates sympathetic nervous system)
- Personality traits (hostility, sense of hopelessness)
- Sedentary lifestyle
- White coat hypertension (see explanation in text)
- Hormonal status (menopause, especially before age 40 years and without HRT; hysterectomy/oophorectomy)

***Nonmodifiable***

- Positive family history of cardiovascular disease
- Age (>55 years)
- Gender (male <55 years; female >55 years)
- Ethnicity (African American,[a] Hispanic)

[a]From a pathogenetic point of view, recent research findings have suggested that β-adrenergic receptor downregulation is characteristic of hypertension in whites, whereas heightened vascular α-receptor sensitivity or early vascular hypertrophy may be a feature of hypertension in African Americans.[332a] African Americans demonstrate somewhat reduced blood pressure responses to monotherapy with β-bockers, ACE inhibitors, or angiotensin receptor blockers compared with diuretics or calcium channel blockers. These differential responses are largely eliminated by drug combinations.[27,373]

Adverse drug reactions associated with hypertension gene variants have been documented as well.[268]

Such findings are extremely important in providing new insights into the genetics and biology of blood pressure, and suggesting potential novel therapeutic pathways for the disease prevention and management.

Small arteries branching from the aorta, called arterioles, regulate blood pressure. Any condition that can narrow the opening of these arterioles can increase the blood pressure in the arteries. A variety of specific diseases or problems, such as chronic renal failure, renal artery stenosis, or endocrine disease, can cause *secondary hypertension* (Box 12.6). The risk for CVD in adults with hypertension is determined not only by the level of blood pressure, but also by the presence or absence of target organ damage or factors such as smoking, dyslipidemia, or diabetes. *Isolated systolic hypertension* has very distinct causes, often not directly vascular and often related to a specific organ or tissue, such as anemia, malfunctioning aortic valve, obstructive sleep apnea, kidney disease, or overactive thyroid.

Risk factors for hypertension may be modifiable or nonmodifiable (Box 12.7). The risk of hypertension increases with age as arteries lose elasticity and become less able to relax. Hypertension occurs slightly more often in men than in women and at an earlier age, but after age 64 years, hypertension begins to develop in more women than men.[50] In all groups the incidence of hypertension increases with age, with a poorer prognosis for people whose hypertension begins at a young age.

Similar to other anxiety-provoking situations that cause rises in blood pressure, white coat hypertension increases the risk of heart disease and CVD mortality.[50] The white coat effect is more pronounced in older adults. For every 10-year increase in age, there is an about 4 mm Hg increase in systolic blood pressure.[50] Personality traits such as hopelessness, hostility, anger, and stress are important factors in CVD, including hypertension.[50] Hypertension itself represents a significant risk factor for the development of CAD, stroke, HF, and renal failure, preceding HF in 90% of all cases and increasing in all other associated conditions. At 60 years of age, people with hypertension have a 60%

lifetime risk of CVD versus normotensive counterparts having a 45% risk.[50]

The use of nonsteroidal antiinflammatory drugs (NSAIDs) in hypertensive persons has been shown to increase blood pressure even more.[11,42] Given the high prevalence of NSAIDs use by older adults, especially for conditions such as arthritis, gout, and similar problems, the association between this drug use and blood pressure must be observed carefully.

Alcohol consumption at any dose increased a risk of hypertension in men. In women, higher consumption was associated with the risk of hypertension, while low doses (1–2 drinks/day) did not have an effect.[313]

Blood pressure is linked to sodium intake and modulated by the "salt gene" (angiotensinogen) in some people. Those who are salt sensitive (including those who do not yet have high blood pressure) may have an increased risk of death. Salt sensitivity is a measure of how blood pressure responds to sodium and is independent of other risk factors (including elevated blood pressure) for death from CVD.

Inadequate sleep has been identified as a risk factor for hypertension among adults in their fourth to sixth decades who sleep less than 5 hours each night.[111] Women have a stronger relationship between short sleep duration and hypertension.[142] Short sleep duration activates the hormones leptin and ghrelin, which affect appetite, making sleep deprivation a risk factor for obesity, as well as for diabetes, two conditions commonly linked with hypertension. Interventions to extend sleep and improve sleep quality have been proposed for hypertension.[142]

**Pathogenesis.** Blood pressure is regulated by two factors: blood flow and peripheral vascular resistance. Blood flow is determined by cardiac output (strength, rate, rhythm of heartbeat; blood volume). The resistance to flow is primarily determined by the diameter of blood vessels and, to a lesser degree, by the viscosity of blood.

Increased peripheral resistance as a result of the narrowing of the arterioles is the single most common characteristic of hypertension. Constriction of the peripheral arterioles may be controlled by two mechanisms, each with several components: (1) sympathetic nervous system activity (autonomic regulation) and (2) activation of the renin–angiotensin system.

In the case of the sympathetic nervous system, norepinephrine is released by the adrenal medulla in response to psychogenic stress or baroreceptor activity. The blood vessels constrict, causing an increase of peripheral resistance. At the same time, epinephrine is secreted by the adrenal medulla, resulting in increased force of cardiac contraction, increased cardiac output, and vasoconstriction.

With prolonged hypertension, the elastic tissue in the arteriole walls is replaced by fibrous collagen tissue. The thickened arteriole wall becomes less distensible, offering even greater resistance to the flow of blood. This process leads to decreased tissue perfusion, especially in the target organs of high blood pressure (i.e., heart, kidneys, brain). Atherosclerosis is also accelerated in persons with high blood pressure, contributing to the narrowing of the lumen and increase in blood pressure.

Within the renin–angiotensin system, vasoconstriction results in decreased blood flow to the kidney. Whenever blood flow to the kidney diminishes, renin is secreted, and it converts angiotensinogen to angiotensin I. Angiotensin I is converted, by ACE, to angiotensin II, causing vasoconstriction within the renal system and increased total peripheral resistance. Angiotensin II also stimulates the secretion of aldosterone, which promotes sodium and water retention by the kidney tubules, causing an increase in blood volume. All these factors increase blood pressure.

**Clinical Manifestations.** Hypertension is frequently asymptomatic, creating a significant health care risk for affected people. When symptoms do occur, they may include headache (usually occipital and present in the morning, worse on waking, and slowly improving with activity), vertigo, flushed face, spontaneous epistaxis, blurred vision, and nocturnal urinary frequency. Elevated blood pressure when measured, especially in the early stages, may be the only sign of hypertension.

Sleep-disordered breathing is also associated with systemic hypertension in middle-aged and older individuals of both genders and different ethnic backgrounds.[323] Progressive hypertension may be characterized by cardiovascular symptoms (dyspnea, orthopnea, chest pain, and leg edema) or cerebral symptoms (nausea, vomiting, drowsiness, confusion, and fleeting numbness or tingling in the limbs).

## MEDICAL MANAGEMENT

**PREVENTION.** The American Society of Hypertension recommends that everyone, regardless of age, know his or her blood pressure (the actual numbers). An annual blood pressure check is important for everyone; more frequent blood pressure measurements should be taken in anyone with risk factors or known hypertension. Elevated blood pressure in an adult younger than age 50 years can cause long-term accumulated damage that is irreversible by age 50 or 60 years; therefore, any elevation in blood pressure at any age must be addressed.

The most important prevention factor is physical activity and exercise; other key variables include weight control; limitations on salt, sugar, and alcohol intake; and modification of other risk factors present (see Box 12.7).

**DIAGNOSIS.** Blood pressure varies over the course of any single day depending on exertion, emotional state, ingestion of food, medications, and the presence of risk factors described previously. Thus it is important that blood pressure be measured at several different times and under consistent circumstances before a diagnosis of hypertension is made. Twenty-four-hour blood pressure monitoring using a portable device that automatically takes blood pressure readings at regular intervals is available and especially helpful in mapping out labile hypertension although it may not be clinically feasible. When available, the individual maintains a log of activities and emotions corresponding to the times when readings are taken; this information is compared with the computer-generated map of blood pressures generated from the data collected by the measurement device. No other tests are specific for essential hypertension.

Laboratory tests in the routine evaluation of hypertension include a complete blood count; urinalysis; serum electrolytes, lipid profile and creatinine; fasting blood glucose; thyroid-stimulating hormone; and ECG.[373] Other more specific tests may be needed for secondary hypertension, and more complete cardiac assessment may be required for selected individuals.

**TREATMENT.** Once diagnosed, hypertension requires ongoing management (see Table 12.6) despite the absence of symptoms. The goal is to achieve and maintain the lowest safe arterial blood pressure (without side effects); the intended target goal is to reduce blood pressure to less than 130/80 mm Hg as much as possible for each client depending on their age and other comorbidities.[373]

The decision to treat and the method and intensity of intervention are based on the concept of total risk, not just blood pressure measurements. This approach takes into account cardiovascular risk factors in people with hypertension (see Box 12.7) and the presence of target organ damage or clinical CVD (e.g., prior coronary revascularization, MI, stroke, peripheral artery disease, retinopathy).

Management of hypertension may begin with a "stepped care" approach including the increase of physical activity, dietary modification, smoking cessation, and other nonpharmacologic interventions as initial therapy for primary hypertension (including those with blood pressure on the high side of normal or a family history of hypertension). This approach has been shown effective in lowering blood pressure and can decrease other cardiovascular risk factors.

Even when lifestyle modifications alone are not adequate in controlling hypertension, they may reduce the dosage of medication needed to manage the condition.[232] This program may include weight reduction; smoking cessation; a regular program of aerobic exercise; moderation of alcohol, dietary fat, caffeine, and dietary sodium; administration of nutritional supplements (e.g., potassium, calcium, magnesium); and behavioral cognitive therapy for those with hypertension associated with certain personality traits. See "Atherosclerosis: Treatment" above.

If nonpharmacologic measures fail to produce the desired results or if the blood pressure is very high at the time of diagnosis, blood pressure–lowering medications are prescribed starting with the lowest effective dose (to avoid intolerable side effects) and modified accordingly. A large number of antihypertensive medications is currently available, and they can be classified by mode of action as listed in Table 12.6.

Only 30% of cases of hypertension can be controlled with one drug. Blood pressure control in more than two-thirds of individuals with hypertension cannot be done with one medication but requires a combination of two or more medications from different classes.[373] Combinations of drugs allow the achievement of greater blood pressure reduction at lower drug doses and thus with fewer side effects. Diuretics, alone or combined with drugs from other classes, are recommended as the first step in the pharmacologic management of uncomplicated hypertension. In high-risk conditions, medications from other classes, specifically ACE inhibitors, are recommended for use initially.[373] Because diuretics decrease plasma volume and cause potassium depletion and renal complications, the use of other classes of antihypertensive drugs is also important to consider.

African Americans tend to have a greater need for combination therapy to control blood pressure, as they are generally more responsive to calcium antagonists and diuretics than to β-blockers, ACE inhibitors, or angiotensin II receptor blockers. Older adults with hypertension are generally equally responsive to all classes of antihypertensive medications, but they have an increased likelihood of side effects. Pharmacologic therapy must be individualized, matching the individual's clinical presentation with medications available.

The use of home monitoring devices is an important part of the management program both to monitor the blood pressure and to evaluate the effect of antihypertensive medication. Home monitoring can also distinguish between sustained hypertension and white coat hypertension and improves program and medication compliance. In individuals with hypertension, the blood pressure readings taken in a clinic setting may be 5 to 10 mm Hg higher than measurements taken at home. Recommended frequency of readings is twice daily (morning and evening) on work and nonwork days for anyone newly diagnosed or in whom antihypertensive medication has recently been initiated or changed. Anyone with stable hypertension can take blood pressure reading several days per week.

More aggressive early treatment of people with diabetes and elevated blood pressure is recommended, while recommendations for treatment of people with metabolic syndrome have not been clearly defined.[373]

Obesity has long been associated with hypertension and is an independent risk factor for CVD and CAD. Regular exercise enhances weight loss and reduces blood pressure independent of weight loss.

It is also recommended that individuals with high blood pressure limit their intake of alcohol and refrain from binge-type drinking patterns.[373]

Older individuals, most African Americans, and hypertensive individuals are more sensitive to change in dietary sodium than are other individuals. A reduction of sodium intake alone may be enough to control blood pressure in persons with mild hypertension and may reduce the medication requirements in those who require drug therapy.

Dietary potassium deficiency may have a role in increasing blood pressure. Individuals may also become hypokalemic from increased urinary potassium excretion during diuretic therapy and require additional potassium. The diuretics may lead to magnesium losses in urine, and hypomagnesemia itself can lead to increased urinary potassium losses.

Magnesium and calcium influence vascular tone because magnesium acts to relax blood vessels and calcium assists in blood vessel contraction. A proper balance of these two ions is essential, as they compete for entry into the cell. When magnesium is low, an abnormally large amount of calcium enters the cells so that blood vessels begin to lose their ability to relax. Progressive vasoconstriction and subsequent spasms result in elevated blood pressure and eventual ischemia. Muscle weakness with depressed tendon reflexes may accompany this condition. A fall in serum potassium level also enhances the effects of cardiac glycoside digoxin, increasing the risk of digoxin toxicity (see Table 12.5). Although digoxin is an inhibitor of the sodium–potassium pump in heart muscle, it competes with potassium ions for binding to the pump.

**PROGNOSIS.** Hypertension is a leading cause of death in the world.[373] In the United States, hypertension is responsible for more deaths from CVD than any other modifiable risk factors.[373] More than 50% of people who died from CAD and stroke had high blood pressure. Hypertension is the second leading cause of end-stage renal disease, behind diabetes mellitus, causing 34% of cases. Hypertension accounts for 25% of such cardiovascular events as CAD, coronary revascularization, stroke, and HF. African Americans have the highest risk of developing hypertension when compared to whites, Hispanics, and Asians.[50,373]

When a person with hypertension achieves the target blood pressure, it must be emphasized that blood pressure control does not equal cure. Adherence to treatment and follow-up monitoring must be continued on an ongoing basis. Unfortunately, the cost of antihypertensives, side effects, and lack of symptoms sometimes lead to poor compliance with treatment. Treatment prolongs life, and antihypertensive medications have dramatically reduced the mortality rate associated with hypertension.

SPECIAL IMPLICATIONS FOR THE THERAPIST 12.4

## *Hypertension (Hypertensive Vascular Disease)*

It is estimated that hypertension remains undiagnosed in nearly half of the 85 million Americans who have it. It is possible that many patients in a therapy practice will be hypertensive without knowing it. Cardiac pathology may be unknown, requiring the therapist to remain alert for risk factors that require medical screening. For anyone with identified risk factors, a baseline blood pressure measurement should be taken on two or three separate occasions, and any unusual findings should be reported to the physician.

The role of the therapist in screening to identify conditions such as hypertension is important, as an essential early component of intervention for this condition includes exercise. The therapist has an important role in helping to identify people with undiagnosed hypertension and referring them for medical evaluation and treatment. Patient education includes emphasizing the importance of adherence to the medical treatment (i.e., taking medication as prescribed; not discontinuing medications without the medical doctor's approval) and follow-up, and teaching them how to identify signs and symptoms of stroke or MI that can occur as a result of a hypertensive crisis. The therapist is also instrumental in reviewing modifiable risk factors and encouraging clients to lose weight if necessary, stop smoking, and exercise appropriately.

Anyone with hypertension is at risk for a hypertensive crisis, especially anyone who discontinues prescribed hypertensive medications without physician approval or those individuals who have long-standing essential hypertension that has not been managed optimally. Elevated blood pressure with any symptoms of target organ damage (e.g., epistaxis, chest discomfort, back pain, headache, visual disturbances, shortness of breath, confusion, or other sign of altered mental state) is a red flag requiring immediate medical attention.[373]

The potential for osteoporosis and subsequent hip fractures in older adults (especially women) with hypertension points to the importance of osteoporosis screening and prevention in this population. The physical therapist has an important role in the primary prevention of impairments and functional limitations in people with hypertension. A sudden increase in blood pressure such as occurs with any increase in intraabdominal pressure during exercise or stabilization exercises can be dangerous for already hypertensive persons. The therapist must alert individuals with hypertension to this effect and teach proper breathing techniques during all activities.

### Medications

People with CAD taking NSAIDs for pain relief may also be at risk for a myocardial event during times of increased myocardial oxygen demand (e.g., exercise, fever). In addition, older adults taking NSAIDs and antihypertensive agents must be monitored carefully. Regardless of the NSAID chosen, it is important to check blood pressure within the first few weeks after therapy or exercise is initiated and periodically thereafter.

It has been shown that NSAIDs may cause an increased risk of serious cardiovascular thrombotic events, MI, stroke, HF, and hypertension.[105] Individuals with a prior history of CVD or with risk factors for CVD may be at greater risk.

It is important to follow up with the client to ensure that they are taking their medication as prescribed. The therapist should always review the client's medications list prior to the initial therapy session, and then as needed in subsequent sessions, to assess for potential side effects or implications for therapy. Any side effects noted may indicate that a medication adjustment is needed and should be brought to the physician's attention (see Table 12.5).

The following brief description of the impact of various drug classes (all of which dilate blood vessels) on exercise may assist the therapist in prescribing activities for those who require pharmacologic agents and provide insight into therapeutic decisions for active hypertensive individuals. Vasodilators such as nitroglycerin and other nitrates act as a prophylactic or rescue intervention for angina by dilating the coronary arteries and improving collateral cardiac circulation, increasing oxygen supply to the heart muscle, and decreasing the blood pressure, thereby decreasing symptoms of angina.

The β-adrenoreceptor antagonists (β-blockers) selectively inhibit an increase in heart rate. Clinically, this means that when the person increases his or her activity or exercise level, the normal physiologic response of increased heart rate is blunted. This requires a longer warm-up and cool-down period. Sudden changes in position (e.g., supine to standing) should be avoided to prevent dizziness and falls associated with the resulting orthostatic hypotension.

The β-blockers diminish catecholamine-induced elevations of heart rate, myocardial contractility, and blood pressure. These effects reduce myocardial oxygen requirements during exertion and stress, thereby preventing angina and allowing the person to exercise for longer periods before the onset of angina. The intended action of β-blockers may prevent normal blood pressure and heart rate responses to exercise; therefore, using heart rate as an index for monitoring response to exercise is not recommended. Although β-blockers are effective antihypertensives, most of them adversely alter aerobic capacity so that exercise capacity may be reduced.

An exercise prescription should be based on exercise stress test results using recommended guidelines.[17] Side effects of β-blockers include bronchospasm, which causes difficulty breathing, and chest tightness, which mimics angina; orthostatic hypotension; syncope; headache; and fatigue and weakness may also occur.

Diuretics are often the first-choice antihypertensive agents for many clients.[373] Diuretic use does not have a negative impact on exercise for those with angina or straight hypertension.[130] The use of loop diuretics may not be appropriate in clients with HF with congestive symptoms, and that will be discussed later in the chapter.[255,256]

Calcium plays a role in the electrical excitation of cardiac cells and in the mechanical contraction of the cardiac and vascular smooth muscle cells. Calcium channel antagonists inhibit calcium ion influx across the cell membrane during cardiac cell depolarization, relax coronary vascular smooth muscle, dilate coronary and peripheral arteries, and increase myocardial oxygen delivery in people with vasospastic angina. This class of vasodilators decreases peripheral vascular resistance at rest and during physical activity, thereby altering exercise tolerance by affecting heart rate and blood pressure during exercise.

During exercise, calcium channel antagonists have been observed to reduce systolic and diastolic pressure at submaximal loads, but higher systolic blood pressures measured during maximal exercise are not lowered. Side effects of calcium antagonists (e.g., drowsiness, dizziness, headache, peripheral edema, tachycardia, or bradycardia) may interfere with a client's ability to participate in an exercise program.

ACE inhibitors reduce blood pressure by lowering peripheral vascular resistance and are considered an initial treatment choice by many physicians. They are readily available as generic drugs (less expensive). One of the side effects of ACE inhibitors is chronic dry cough[115] that may vary in intensity, from tolerable to debilitating. Studies show that different doses of ACE inhibitors can have different effects on exercise capacity and cause possible renal issues.[96,112] Therefore, doses should be tailored to the individual to optimize functional benefits.

### Exercise and Blood Pressure

The benefits of resistive or dynamic exercise in people with and without CVD are well known and available for review.[301] A regular program of aerobic exercise, introduced gradually, facilitates cardiovascular conditioning, may assist in weight reduction, and may provide some benefit in reducing blood pressure. Postexercise hypotension (lowered blood pressure in response to exercise) in prehypertensive and hypertensive individuals has been observed for up to 10 and more hours after exercise.[61] Of relevance, reduction of resting arterial pressure by 3 mm Hg leads to decrease in risk of death from stroke by 8% and from CAD by 5%.[61] Overall, regular exercise will develop a protective response at the heart by decreasing hypertension levels.[216,261] On the other hand, blood pressure will return to its previous elevated level if training is discontinued.

Heavy isometric exercises and heavy weightlifting may be harmful, because the blood pressure often rises because of vasovagal reflexes that occur. Generally, antihypertensive drugs have not been found to affect the blood pressure response to isometric exertion.

### Exercise and Malignant Hypertension

There is always a concern for a stroke (cerebrovascular accident [CVA]) or recurrent stroke in anyone with uncontrolled, malignant hypertension. Therapists in the acute care setting must monitor vital signs closely in individuals with a history of hypertension-induced CVA. With malignant hypertension, the set point for cerebral autoregulation (i.e., ability of tissues/organs to remain evenly perfused with fluctuating blood/perfusion pressures) is higher, which means blood pressure must be higher to prevent hypoperfusion of the brain.

There are no evidence-based guidelines for an appropriate blood pressure level during exercise for people with CVA. It should be noted that facilities use different levels ranging from systolic levels of 160–180 or 210–220 mm Hg (depending on individual factors) and diastolic limits up to 110 mm Hg. Due to the lack of evidence outlining a specific blood pressure range, therapists should examine their facility's accepted values, speak with the physicians regarding their preferences in blood pressure values, and monitor the clients individually for stability with varying blood pressure levels.

### Exercise Training Guidelines

The intensity of exercise required to produce health benefits and decrease blood pressure has been confused with the level of exercise necessary to improve physical fitness. Health benefits can be achieved without large gains in fitness. Encouraging people to increase their level of total energy expenditure is the key to increasing activity levels rather than emphasizing physical fitness. The type, intensity, duration, and frequency of training, as well as progression, should be assessed regularly.

A preexercise evaluation and exercise testing may be prescribed by the physician. This information is helpful in establishing submaximal and maximal blood pressure responses. Monitoring vital signs before, during, and after exercise or activity is essential. Any person with an exaggerated systolic blood pressure response (higher than 250 mm Hg) or failure to reduce diastolic pressure (to less than 90 mm Hg) should be referred to the physician for reevaluation.

Training intensity does not need to be high, and it appears that low-intensity activity (65%–70% of maximal heart rate) three times per week is as effective as high-intensity activity in blood pressure reduction. Training intensity should be based on maximal heart rate using the calculated formulas or measured during a maximal exercise test. After 12 to 16 weeks, if the blood pressure is adequately controlled, the physician may reduce the antihypertensive medication slowly to determine the long-term effect of training on blood pressure. Several resources are available for determining the appropriate exercise program for the hypertensive client, whether symptomatic or asymptomatic.[16,359]

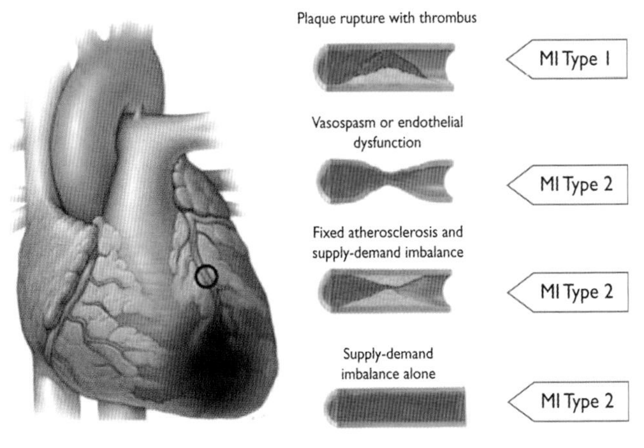


**Figure 12.9**

**Myocardial infarction type 1 and 2.** (From Mihatov N, Januzzi JL, Gaggin HK. Type 2 myocardial infarction due to supply-demand mismatch. *Trends in Cardiovascular Medicine* 2017;27(6):408–417.)

## Myocardial Infarction

### Definition and Incidence

MI, also known as a heart attack, is myocardial cell death due to prolonged ischemia,[355] with resultant necrosis of myocardial tissue. Any prolonged obstruction depriving the heart muscle of oxygen can cause an MI. Based on the type of obstruction, MI is classified into two major types.[355] MI type 1 is caused by CAD and is triggered by the atherosclerotic plaque disruption (rupture or erosion). MI type 2 develops due to a mismatch between oxygen supply and demand by myocardial tissue; no atherosclerotic plaque disruption occurs (Fig. 12.9).

MI occurs in over 800,000 persons in the United States each year, leading to 150,000 deaths. Every 40 seconds, an American has an MI. At first MI, the average age of a man is 65 years, and a woman is 72 years.[50]

### Etiologic and Risk Factors

Etiologic and risk factors are the same as for all forms of CVD, especially angina pectoris associated with CAD. The majority of MIs result from coronary thrombus at the site of a preexisting atherosclerotic stenosis. New cases of MI can occur in people with only a borderline risk profile or even lack of known risk factors, suggesting other unidentified risk factors.

Other causes may include cocaine use or other stimulant drugs (which cause vasoconstriction of the coronary arteries), vasculitis, aortic stenosis, or aortic root or coronary artery dissection. Smokers have more than twice as many heart attacks as nonsmokers, and sudden cardiac death occurs two to four times more frequently in smokers.[359] After an infarction, smokers have a poorer chance of recovery than nonsmokers.

It is a well-established fact that heart attacks occur more frequently in the early morning hours. This peak incidence is attributed to an increase in catecholamines with the resultant increased blood pressure, increased workload of the heart, as well as increased clotting factors in the early morning. Heart attacks also occur in a seasonal pattern with an increased incidence between Thanksgiving and New Year's Day across all ages, in both genders, and across geographic regions.[327] Whether this can be attributed to mood changes, weather, circadian rhythms, large quantities of food consumed, or some other mechanism remains unknown.

Acute respiratory tract infections, such as the common cold, influenza, and bronchitis, increase the risk of an MI by 17-fold within 1 week of the infection.[315] Early symptoms of heart attacks may, however, be mistaken for acute upper respiratory tract infection.

Every fifth MI is silent (or unrecognized).[50] Silent MI, while having objective signs of an infarct, presents with unrecognised, atypical symptoms or no symptoms.[361] Nonfatal silent MI significantly increases risk of mortality.[355,361] Silent myocardial ischemia (ischemia with no signs of angina) and silent MI are highly prevalent among people with diabetes,[361] presumably because of reduced sensitivity to pain due to autonomic neuropathy. Hypertension, prior CVD, and age are risk factors for silent MI.[361]

Obesity, with its effect on the cardiovascular system, increases risk of MI.[275] Fat tissue in the abdomen, epicardial and other areas, becomes an endocrine organ affecting other organs, such as skeletal muscles, liver, heart, brain, and vasculature. Fat promotes inflammation in coronary arteries, increasing heart attack risk. Free fatty acids accumulate in cardiomyocytes, as in other cells, causing lipotoxicity, leading to insulin resistance and atherogenicity.[275]

Waist circumference, the ratio of waist-to-hip measurements or the ratio of waist-to-height measurements may provide one of the best predictors of heart attack risk. Higher waist measurements relative to hip measurements increase heart attack risk even if BMI is within the acceptable range (85% or higher ratio for women and 90% or higher for men increases the risk). An improvement in waist-to-height ratio of 0.013 had a marked improvement in cardiovascular health.[330]

**Pathogenesis.** The myocardium receives its blood supply from the two large coronary arteries and their branches (Fig. 12.10; Table 12.9). One or more of these blood vessels may become occluded by a clot that forms suddenly when an atheromatous plaque ruptures through the sublayers of a blood vessel wall or undergoes erosion (MI type 1). In most MI cases, infarcts result from an occlusive thrombus superimposed on an atherosclerotic plaque. Plaque rupture is a more common cause of MI than plaque erosion. While 76% of men had fatal MI due to plaque rupture, only 55% of women had it as a cause of MI. Plaque erosion had higher prevalence in women, especially of younger age, when compared to men.[246] While MI type 1 is caused by CAD and resulting atherosclerotic plaque disruption (rupture or erosion), MI type 2 is unrelated to atherothrombosis and occurs due to insufficient perfusion of myocardium, resulting in unmet oxygen demand. The myocardial oxygen supply/demand imbalance may develop due to coronary atherosclerosis (no plaque disruption) narrowing the vessel lumen, coronary artery spasm, coronary microvascular dysfunction, coronary embolism, coronary artery dissection, or other mechanisms leading to reduced oxygen supply (respiratory failure, hypotension/shock) or increased oxygen demand (sustained tachyarrhythmia,

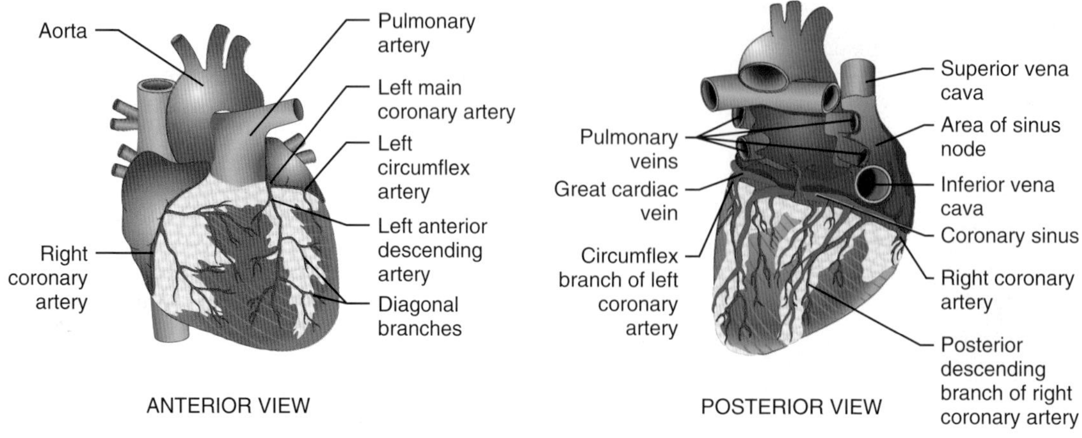


**Figure 12.10**

**Areas of myocardium affected by arterial insufficiency of specific coronary arteries.** The right and left coronary arteries branch off the aorta just above the aortic valve and normally supply the myocardium with oxygenated blood. Table 12.9 lists the most commonly affected arteries and the area of myocardium supplied.

**Table 12.9** Blood Supply to the Myocardium

| Area of Myocardium[a] | Supplied By |
|---|---|
| Anterior | Left coronary artery<br>Left anterior descending branch[b] |
| Posterior | Right coronary artery |
| Inferior | Right coronary artery |
| Anteroseptal | Left coronary artery<br>Left anterior descending branch |
| High Lateral | Circumflex artery<br>Left coronary artery<br>Diagonal branch |
| Apical | Usually left coronary artery<br>Left anterior branch<br>Sometimes right coronary artery<br>Posterior descending branch |

[a]Most commonly affected arteries and the area of myocardium supplied are listed in order of decreasing occurrence.

[b]Often referred to as the "widow maker," untreated blockage of the left anterior descending branch leads to permanent heart damage if the individual does not die first.

severe hypertension). Type 2 MI occurs more frequently in women.[355] Mortality rates for MI type 2 are generally higher than for MI type 1.[355]

The most common site of infarction is the left ventricle, the chamber of the heart with the greatest workload. Thrombosis of the anterior descending branch of the left coronary artery is the most common cause of infarction and affects the anterior left ventricle (Fig. 12.11).

Occlusion of the left circumflex artery produces anterolateral or posterolateral infarction. Right coronary artery thrombosis leads to infarction of the posteroinferior portion of the left ventricle and may involve the right ventricular myocardium and interventricular septum. The arteries supplying the atrioventricular node and the sinus node more commonly arise from the right coronary artery; thus atrioventricular block at the nodal level and sinus node dysfunction occur more frequently during inferior infarctions.

Ischemia of myocardium causes detrimental effects within a few minutes. Oxygen deprivation is accompanied by electrolyte disturbances, particularly cellular loss of potassium, calcium, and magnesium. Myocardial cells deprived of necessary oxygen and nutrients lose contractility, thereby diminishing the pumping ability of the heart. Sarcolemmal disruptions and mitochondrial abnormalities observed within 10 minutes after onset of ischemia[355] eventually lead to myocyte necrosis. In response to this necrosis, leukocytes aid in removing the dead cells, and cardiac fibroblasts produce fibrotic proteins, mostly collagens, and form a fibrous scar within the area of infarction (referred to as fibrosis). The remaining heart muscle cells enlarge to compensate for the loss in heart pump function. Usually the formation of fibrous scar tissue is complete within 6 to 8 weeks (Table 12.10). The infarcted myocardium presents with altered ECG (Fig. 12.12).

When blood flow is restored to ischemic myocardium, myocardial reperfusion injury develops. Paradoxically, restoration of blood flow in ischemic tissue makes cells generate massive amounts of reactive oxygen species (ROS) that damage intracellular components. Contributors to ROS production include mitochondria and enzymes such as xanthine oxidase, NADPH oxidase, and uncoupled nitric oxide synthase.[152] This phenomenon must be considered when revascularization approaches (PCI, CABG) are undertaken. Protection from reperfusion injury should be applied as early as possible in reperfusion, as cells die within the first minutes of blood reflow.

Despite our understanding of mechanisms of ischemia-reperfusion injury and promising animal model studies, translation of this knowledge into clinical settings has been unsatisfactory. Failure to develop effective cardioprotective strategies may be explained, at least partially, by the multifactorial nature of MI, with cardiomyocyte death occurring through multiple mechanisms, and nonmyocyte cells (cardiac fibroblasts, endothelial and smooth muscle cells, immune cells) being damaged. Successful cardioprotection may require a multitarget approach.[106] The multitarget cardioprotection may include protective modalities such as ischemic conditioning (controlled, brief application of ischemia and

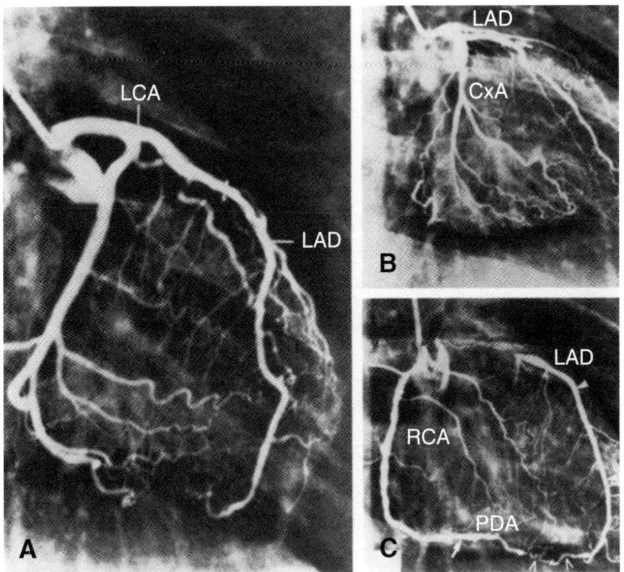


**Figure 12.11**

(A) Angiogram of a normal left coronary artery (LCA). (B) Angiogram of a totally obstructed left anterior descending (LAD) coronary artery. (C) Angiogram of the right coronary artery (RCA) and its major branch, the posterior descending artery (PDA) (same heart as in B). The LAD is seen because of collateral vessels connecting the LAD and the RCA system. (From Boucek R, Morales A, Romanelli R, et al: *Coronary artery disease: pathologic and clinical assessment,* Baltimore, 1984, Williams & Wilkins, pp. 4, 9.)

**Table 12.10** Tissue Changes After Myocardial Infarction

| Time After MI | Tissue Changes |
|---|---|
| 6–12 hr | No gross changes; healing process has not begun |
| 18–24 hr | Inflammatory response; intercellular enzyme release |
| 2–4 days | Visible necrosis; proteolytic enzymes remove debris; catecholamines, lipolysis, and glycogenolysis elevate blood glucose and increase free fatty acids to assist depleted myocardium recovery from anaerobic state |
| 4–10 days | Debris cleared; collagen matrix laid down |
| 10–14 days | Weak, fibrotic scar tissue with beginning revascularization; area vulnerable to stress |
| 6 wk | Scarring usually complete; tough, inelastic scar replaces necrotic myocardium; unable to contract and relax like healthy myocardial tissue |

Modified from McCance KL, Huether SE: *Pathophysiology: the biologic basis for disease in adults and children*, ed 7, St Louis, 2013, Mosby.

reperfusion), pharmacologic agents, and physical therapy interventions (hypothermia when applied before reperfusion, and electrical nerve stimulation). Timing of the application may be different (during ischemia, at reperfusion, or late into reperfusion). Different cellular targets (cardiomyocytes and nonmyocyte cells, including immune and inflammatory cells) and intracellular targets (inhibition of cell death pathways; stimulation of cell survival pathways) need to be considered. Ideally, when combined, the cardioprotective strategies would show additive or synergistic effect.[106]

Ischemic and injured myocardial tissues cause characteristic ECG changes. More profound shifts of ST segment or inversions of T wave with multiple leads are associated with a larger degree of myocardial ischemia and worse prognosis. Reperfusion is usually accompanied by a large and rapid reduction in ST segment elevation. As the myocardium heals, the ST segment and T waves gradually return to normal, but abnormal Q waves may persist. It is recommended that patients with suspected MI undergo ECG promptly (within 10 minutes) after first medical contact.[355]

**Clinical Manifestations.** The most notable symptom of MI is a sudden sensation of pressure, often described as prolonged crushing chest pain, occasionally radiating to the arms, throat, neck (as high as the occipital area), and back (Fig. 12.8). The pain is constant, lasting 30 minutes up to hours, and may be accompanied by pallor, shortness of breath, and profuse perspiration. Catecholamine release resulting in sympathetic stimulation may produce diaphoresis and peripheral vasoconstriction that cause the skin to become cool and clammy. Angina pectoris pain can be similar, but it is less severe, does not last for hours, and is relieved by cessation of activity, rest, or nitrates. Often, anginal symptoms will be a precursor to MI, but not always.

Symptoms do not always follow the classic pattern, especially in women. Two major symptoms in women are shortness of breath, sometimes occurring in the middle of the night, and chronic, unexplained fatigue. Atypical presentation may include continuous pain in the midthoracic spine or interscapular area, neck and shoulder pain, stomach or abdominal pain, nausea or indigestion as the only symptom, unexplained anxiety, or heartburn that is not altered by antacids. Women are more likely than men to have symptoms unrelated to chest pain such as aching, heaviness, or weakness in one or both arms, heat or flushing sensation, or racing heart.[246,384]

Nausea and vomiting may occur because of reflex stimulation of vomiting centers by pain fibers. Fever may develop in the first 24 hours and persist for a week because of inflammatory activity within the myocardium.

Postinfarction complications include arrhythmias, HF, cardiogenic shock, pericarditis, rupture of the heart, thromboembolism, recurrent infarction, and sudden death. Arrhythmias, affecting more than 90% of individuals, are the most common complication of acute MI and are caused by ischemia, hypoxia, autonomic nervous system imbalances, lactic acidosis, electrolyte imbalances, drug toxicity, or alterations of impulse conduction pathways or conduction defects.[384]

## MEDICAL MANAGEMENT

**PREVENTION.** See "Atherosclerosis: Prevention" and "Angina Pectoris: Prevention and Treatment" above.

**DIAGNOSIS.** Diagnosis of acute MI and determination of the site and extent of necrosis rely on the clinical history, interpretation of the ECG, and measurement of serum levels of cardiac enzymes. Further testing may determine if atherosclerosis was the cause of the MI and any need for surgical intervention (see also "Atherosclerosis: Medical Management"). Diagnostic uncertainty frequently arises because of a variety of factors.

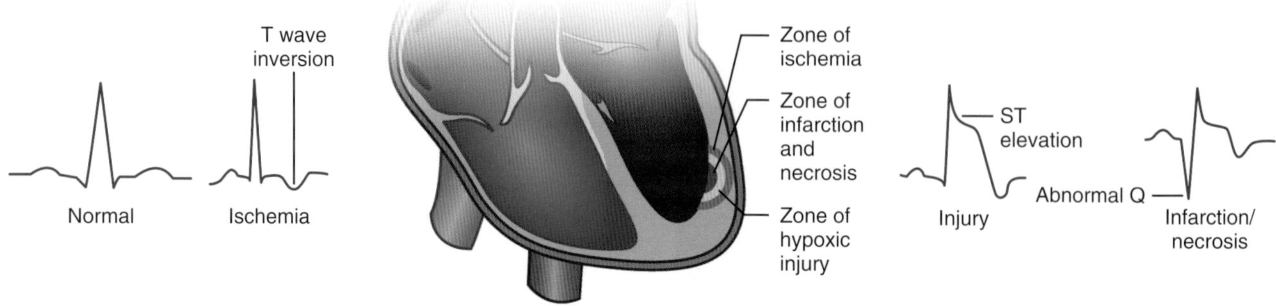


**Figure 12.12**

**Electrocardiographic (ECG) alterations associated with the three zones of myocardial infarction (MI).** When the myocardium has been completely deprived of oxygen, cells die, and the tissue becomes necrotic in an area called the *zone of infarction*. Immediately surrounding the area of infarction is a less-seriously damaged area of injury called the *zone of hypoxic injury*. This zone is able to return to normal, but it may also become necrotic if blood flow is not restored. With adequate collateral circulation, this area may regain its function within 2 to 3 weeks. Adjacent to the zone of hypoxic injury is another reversible zone called the *zone of ischemia*.

Many people with acute MI have atypical symptoms, and half of all people with typical symptoms do not have acute MI. Half of the people with acute MI have nondiagnostic ECGs, and some people are unable to provide a history of symptoms. Biochemical markers of cardiac injury are commonly relied on to diagnose or exclude acute MI. These laboratory tests dramatically reduce the cost of treating heart attacks by allowing physicians to quickly discharge people with noncardiac chest pain.

Biomarkers of myocardial injury are an essential component of a clinical picture of MI.[355] Abnormal cardiac biomarkers, on a background of acute myocardial ischemia, identify myocardial injury as MI. Cardiac troponin I (TnI) and cardiac troponin T (TnT) (regulatory proteins that help the heart muscle contract) are now being used as preferred biomarkers to evaluate myocardial injury.[355] TnI is very specific for myocardial ischemia and necrosis, while TnT may come from injured skeletal muscles. TnT begins to elevate 2 to 3 hours after an onset of acute MI, peaks at 3 to 4 days and remains elevated 5 to 7 days after an MI. Myocardial isoform of creatine kinase (CK-MB) is less specific and less sensitive. Myoglobin has also been found to be a marker of MI.[263]

Researchers are continuing to investigate other hemostatic markers based on the knowledge that coronary thrombosis involves both coagulation and fibrinolysis cascades. For example, increases of fibrinogen and D-dimer, a circulating marker of fibrin turnover, are significantly higher in people with acute ischemic events such as MI and unstable angina than in nonischemic individuals. Although D-dimer is still not a recommended marker of MI, there is some research indicating that it may be useful.[302] Other enzymes are emerging as possible markers of MI, but there is not enough evidence yet for their recommended use in diagnosing MI.[263]

Infarcted tissue is electrically silent and does not contribute to the ECG. Most clients with acute infarction have ECG changes, although this test provides only a crude estimate of the magnitude of infarction. When diagnosis by ECG and biomarkers is not possible (e.g., when people seek medical attention after MI), scintigraphic studies (radionuclide imaging) can show areas of necrotic myocardium and diminished perfusion. These tests, which use radiotracers, do not distinguish old damage from recent infarction, and false-positive results can occur.

Other test procedures may include echocardiography, which is useful in assessing the ability of the heart walls to contract and relax, and transesophageal echocardiography (TEE), an ultrasonic technique that provides a clearer image of the heart, including the posterior wall, valvular anatomy, and thoracic aortic structure, providing identification of structural heart diseases. Newer technology, such as RT3D imaging, has the potential to improve evaluation of heart function (especially ventricular) with TEE.

Magnetic resonance imaging (MRI) to evaluate structural defects of the heart and positron emission tomography (PET) to evaluate cardiac physiology and metabolism and assess tissue perfusion have contributed significantly to the understanding of the pathophysiology of the ischemic heart.

**TREATMENT.** The goal of treatment is reestablishing the flow of blood in blocked coronary arteries. Pharmacologic intervention is used to provide pain relief (essential because angina is evidence of ongoing ischemia), limit infarction size, reduce vasoconstriction, prevent thrombus formation, and augment repair. MI caused by intracoronary thrombi can be relieved by infusion of thrombolytic agents (e.g., tPA, its modification Retavase (reteplase), urokinase, streptokinase) that dissolve clots, promote vasodilation, and reduce infarct size.

PAI-1 is a naturally occurring substance that inhibits another natural substance, tPA. tPA is an enzyme released endogenously as part of the body's defense against thrombosis; it promotes degradation of fibrin, leading to dissolving of blood clots. tPA is now a genetically engineered drug used in thrombolytic therapy as well.

It has been established that initiation of tPA or other thrombolytic agent within the first 2 hours of symptom

Box 12.8

**CONTRAINDICATIONS TO EXERCISE AFTER MYOCARDIAL INFARCTION**

- Acute MI (<1 or 2 days after an MI without physician approval)
- Unstable angina; easily provoked angina

New ECG arrhythmias

- Signs and symptoms of MI (e.g., nausea, dyspnea, lightheadedness, chest pain)
- $PaO_2$ <60 mm Hg
- $O_2$ saturation <85%
- Hemoglobin <8 g/dL; hematocrit <26%
- Severe aortic outflow obstruction
- Suspected or known dissecting aneurysm
- Acute myocarditis or pericarditis
- Uncontrolled complex arrhythmias
- Active severe HF; resting respiratory rate >45 breaths/min
- Recent pulmonary embolism or thrombophlebitis
- Untreated third-degree heart block
- Severe systemic hypertension unresponsive to medication
- Uncontrolled diabetes
- Acute infections
- Digoxin toxicity

Modified from Bonow RO: *Braunwald's heart disease—a textbook of cardiovascular medicine*, ed 9, Philadelphia, 2011, WB Saunders.

onset is associated with improved survival.[271] After a thrombolytic agent is administered, intravenous (IV) heparin therapy is usually given with adjunctive drug therapy during and after MI, because platelet inhibitors and other cardiovascular medications are known to further reduce mortality when administered during the acute phase. Of note, women have higher bleeding than men with thrombolytic therapy after acute MI.[246] Recommendations for optimal care after acute MI emphasize reestablishment of coronary blood flow through PCI where available or thrombolytic therapy administration where PCI is not available or not appropriate.[271]

Exercise has been recommended as a means of increasing pain tolerance, increasing the threshold of the stimulus required to induce angina, alleviating depression, reducing anxiety, and inducing collateral circulation. Increasing evidence suggests that combining a low-fat diet and intensive exercise training can improve myocardial perfusion by regression of coronary atherosclerosis. Exercise training may be contraindicated for some people (Box 12.8; see also Box 12.3). Medical clearance must be obtained for entry into an exercise training program.

Exercise testing is the most useful tool to establish guidelines for exercise training in apparently healthy adults and is mandatory for people with known or suspected CVD.[17] Sub-maximal exercise testing can be done within 3 days of MI with a very low incidence of complications. Criteria for testing usually include clients who are off IV nitroglycerin with no angina at rest, uncontrolled cardiac failure, or arrhythmias. Early testing can lead to early triage and potential cost savings.

Other treatment interventions, including identification and modification of risk factors, angioplasty (PCI), atherectomy, gene therapy and gene editing, and cardiac rehabilitation utilizing exercise programs, have been previously discussed in detail (see "Ischemic Heart Disease: Medical Management" above).

**PROGNOSIS.** The size and anatomic location of the infarction, together with the amount of damage from previous infarctions, determine the acute clinical picture, the early complications, and the long-term prognosis. The first 24 hours after onset of symptoms is the time of highest risk for sudden death. The sooner someone reaches the hospital, the better the prognosis. Data indicate that African Americans had a 30% longer waiting time for chest pain at emergency departments than white patients.[50] Of those experiencing an acute MI, 80% survive the initial attack when transported to a coronary care unit. Patients with MI admitted on a weekend had significantly decreased odds of having early invasive intervention, with greater mortality.[50] After a first MI, the median survival time for men is 8.2 years and for women 5.5 years.[50] Substantial reductions in post-MI death have occurred over the last 5 decades because of improved intervention.

Factors negatively affecting prognosis include age (clients older than 80 years have a 60% mortality), evidence of other CVDs, respiratory diseases, uncontrolled diabetes mellitus, anterior location of MI (30% mortality rate), and hypotension (clients whose systolic blood pressure is less than 55 mm Hg have a 60% mortality rate). The risk of reinfarction is increased in women, people with elevated blood pressure, and people with elevated serum cholesterol.

Prognostic testing predictive of cardiac events includes standard exercise testing such as functional capacity and heart rate recovery[132] and imaging using single-photon emission computed tomography with contrast agents (e.g., thallium-201, technetium-99m sestamibi). In the imaging studies, a radioisotope is taken up by adequately perfused tissue, allowing detection of myocardial perfusion defects at rest and during exercise (areas of infarction appear as regions of diminished isotope activity or no activity, referred to as *cold spots*).

Study of the prognostic value of exercise testing in people after MI shows that workload (measured in metabolic equivalents) is predictive of future MIs and death.

SPECIAL IMPLICATIONS FOR THE THERAPIST 12.5

## *Myocardial Infarction*

### Early Postmyocardial Infarction Considerations

Although the myocardium must rest, bed rest puts the client at risk for development of hypovolemia (low blood volume), hypoxemia (hypoxia), muscle atrophy, pulmonary embolism, and general medical and integumentary risks. Developing a program of progressive physical activity with adequate pacing and rest periods begins within 24 hours after hospitalization for clients with uncomplicated MI. Evidence-based standards for mobility after administration of tPA remain lacking. Many institutions hold therapy until 24 hours after tPA infusion because of issues of perfusion, bleeding risks, or because of multiple other medical diagnostic procedures ordered (e.g., CT scans, echocardiograms).

Even if mobility is limited, therapeutic interventions are not. The therapist could perform certain evaluation and examination techniques, as well as have the patient perform certain range of motion or mobility. Therapists must use their clinical expertise and critical thinking skills to formulate an appropriate plan of care. For example, gentle movement exercises, deep breathing, and coughing can begin immediately as prophylactic measures. Transfers to the edge of the bed and possibly out of bed may be beneficial with low risk depending on the stability and tolerance of the client.

Early therapeutic exercise helps prevent cardiopulmonary complications, venous stasis, joint stiffness, and muscle weakness. Relaxation is often promoted with low-intensity activity. Activities that increase intrathoracic or intraabdominal pressure, such as breath holding and Valsalva maneuvers, can precipitate bradycardia followed by increased venous return to the heart, causing possible cardiac overload. For this reason, these actions are contraindicated and should not be performed in any stage of the rehabilitation program.[176]

During the first 6 weeks post-MI, the client is cautioned to avoid saunas, hot tubs, whirlpools, and excessively warm swimming pools. Early rehabilitation lasting 2 to 3 weeks is often followed by exercise testing, at which time water therapy may be permissible per physician approval. Specific aspects of cardiac rehabilitation and postoperative care are beyond the scope of this text. Other more specific texts are available to guide the therapist in this area.[139,176]

### Monitoring Vital Signs

The therapist must continually monitor for signs of further ischemia and possibly further infarction, including generalized or localized pain anywhere over the thorax, upper limbs, and neck; palpitations; dyspnea; light-headedness; syncope; sensation of indigestion; hiccups; and nausea (see Fig. 12.8). Pain medications, such as morphine, used to minimize discomfort initially may also depress the respiratory drive.

The coronary care unit therapist must monitor vital signs before, during, and after interventions. These should include heart rate, blood pressure, oxygen saturation, and ECG rhythm. The home health therapist must monitor pulse and blood pressure measurements for hypotension because of the side effects precipitated by antihypertensive medications, vasodilators, and other antianginal agents. Initial ambulation and activities at home should be roughly equivalent to levels achieved at the hospital at the time of discharge, depending on the client's physiologic response to the transition from hospital to home.

The client must increase activities gradually to avoid overtaxing the heart as it pumps oxygenated blood to the muscles. The metabolic equivalent system provides one way of measuring the amount of oxygen needed to perform an activity as a measure of the intensity of an activity. One metabolic equivalent of the task (MET) equals 3.5 mL of oxygen per kilogram of body weight per minute; 1 MET is approximately equivalent to the oxygen uptake a person requires when resting. At 2 METs, the individual is working at twice the individual's resting metabolic rate.

Very early mobilization activities after acute MI should not exceed 1 to 2 METs (e.g., brushing teeth, eating). By comparison, people who can exercise to 8 or more METs (oxygen uptake of 28 mL/kg/min or more) can perform vigorous-level physical activities. In general, 3 to 6 METs is considered the equivalent of moderate exercise. Activities with METs higher than 6 include singles tennis, cycling more than 10 mph, walking more than 4 mph, and cross-country skiing. A full compendium of the MET levels required to perform any activity is available.[5] Therapists can reference this list when assessing whether their client can perform a specific activity.

The MET system may not be as accurate for overweight, obese, or older adults. For example, because maximal aerobic capacity usually declines with age,[294] even when working at the same MET level as a younger person, the older individual's relative exercise intensity will usually be greater. In addition, research shows that using the MET system underestimates the energy used for an activity in overweight or obese individuals who may end up working at a level too high for them.[294] The therapist is advised to use the rate of perceived exertion (RPE; see Table 12.13) instead for these population groups.[136]

As activity level increases, the therapist must monitor heart rate, blood pressure, oxygen saturation (when able) and fatigue. Activities should be modified and adjusted as needed based on each client's individual hemodynamic response. During phase I cardiac rehabilitation (acute hospital), the heart rate should not rise more than 10 to 20 beats per minute above resting level, and blood pressure must not rise more than 25 mm Hg above resting level for the first 1 or 2 therapy sessions. After those sessions, if the therapist finds that the client's response to exercise has been stable, the vital signs can be pushed to slightly higher levels from resting using continued monitoring of symptoms and client response.

When systolic blood pressure falls or fails to increase as the intensity of exercise increases, exercise intensity should be immediately reduced. A drop in systolic blood pressure during exercise below the rest value as measured in the standing position is associated with increased risk of lethal arrhythmia in clients with a prior MI or myocardial ischemia.

Supplemental oxygen may be used to supply the myocardium with oxygen when the demand exceeds supply, thereby reducing myocardial stress and eliminating dyspnea. Caution must be exercised, as too much oxygen can be deleterious for clients with acute MI.[242] Even though supplemental oxygen can increase arterial oxygen level in MI, it reduces cardiac output, increases blood pressure, and increases resistance to blood flow. Only clients with low oxygen levels should be administered oxygen and only to the extent that it does not cause hyperoxia.[242] The therapist must monitor oxygen saturation levels during exercise or intervention, because these activities may increase myocardial oxygen demand.

The client who sustained an MI and also has chronic obstructive pulmonary disease (COPD) and receives oxygen therapy may develop hypercapnia (high levels of $CO_2$ in blood caused by hypoventilation) or experience its worsening and must be monitored very closely for symptoms of decreased ventilation, such as headache, giddiness, tinnitus (ringing in the ears), nausea, weakness, and vomiting. Elevated $CO_2$ levels in the COPD client eliminate the drive to breathe normally that is initiated by rising levels of $CO_2$. The only drive to breathe in the COPD client is hypoxia (reduced oxygen levels), and when the normoxic state is reached the hyperoxic drive becomes depressed. Appropriately prescribed oxygen is vital for the individual with COPD, whereas administration of excessive oxygen to a person with $CO_2$ retention can further depress the respiratory drive, resulting in death. Of importance, evidence shows that physical activity is a powerful drive that counteracts respiratory depression even in people with COPD who retain $CO_2$.

### Exercise after Myocardial Infarction

As little as 25 years ago, exercise was avoided following a heart attack, but research shows that a reasonable amount of regular exercise is the best way to strengthen the heart and control blood pressure, improve cholesterol status, manage diabetes, and control weight. Survivors who exercise usually require less medication, are less likely to need future invasive procedures (e.g., PCI, CABG), and are less likely to die of a second heart attack than those who remain sedentary.

It is recommended that individuals with a history of MI combine aerobic exercise (at least 3 days per week; 20–40 minutes each session; at 40%–80% of $VO_{2max}$; RPE of 11–15 on scale of 20), resistance training (2–3 days per week; 1–3 sets of 10–15 repetitions of 8–10 exercises; 40%–50% maximal voluntary contraction [avoid Valsalva maneuver]), and flexibility exercise aimed at static stretching of the upper and lower body (2–3 days per week; hold for 10–30 seconds).[16,299] For some people, the use of a cane or walker is an isometric use of muscles that can increase heart rate; therefore, careful monitoring of vital signs and indications of perceived exertion are required even with functional mobility. This is especially critical for high-risk cardiac clients. Special care for clients who receive antithrombotic or thrombolytic agents is necessitated to avoid tissue bleeding during exercise therapy.

In general, people that survive a heart attack are often people who have never exercised before and need sound advice and careful supervision by a physical therapist. Exercise may induce cardiac arrhythmias during diuretic and digoxin therapy, and recent ingestion of caffeine may exacerbate arrhythmias. Exercise-induced arrhythmias are generated by enhanced sympathetic tone, increased myocardial oxygen demand, or both. The immediate postexercise period is particularly dangerous because of high catecholamine levels associated with a generalized vasodilation. Sudden termination of muscular activity is accompanied by diminished venous return and may lead to a reduction in coronary perfusion while heart rate is elevated. A careful cool-down period is required with continued monitoring of vital signs after exercise.[24]

### Sexual Activity

People with cardiac disease, both men and women, are prone to sexual dysfunction. Often their concerns are voiced to the therapist. The link between CVD and erectile dysfunction in men has been the subject of recent studies. Erectile dysfunction is an early predictor of CAD and should be medically evaluated.[116,223]

Problems may be caused by medications, anxiety, depression, or limited physical capacity. Hypertensive medications are the most common drugs to cause sexual dysfunction (e.g., loss of sexual desire or ability to reach orgasm).

Fear of death during sexual intercourse, fear of another infarction caused by sexual activity, and diminished sexual ability caused by illness and aging may occur. The sexual partner may have many similar fears and may want to be included in any information provided about return to sexual function. The relative risk of triggering an MI by sexual activity is less than 1%.[223]

Sexual activity is considered a reasonable activity for most people with CVD. Before engaging in sexual activity, a comprehensive physical examination is recommended for anyone who has concerns or who is at risk for triggering an MI with sexual activity. A scientific statement from the AHA provides general recommendations for individuals with specific CVD conditions, following angioplasty and stenting, and after a heart attack.[223] A consensus document on sexual counseling for individuals with CVD and their partners is available from the AHA and the European Society of Cardiology Council on Cardiovascular Nursing and Allied Professions, guiding all members of the health care team including physical therapists on how to address sexual issues.[344]

Sexual intercourse with orgasm is physiologically equivalent to activities such as a brisk walk or climbing a flight of stairs. It has been equated to 5 METs of work on an exercise stress test; preorgasmic and postorgasmic phases require about 3.7 METs. It is important for the therapist to discuss with the client that sexual intercourse is an activity requiring moderate physical exertion and therefore, requires a certain level of aerobic capacity. Advice to clients should be based on consultation with the physician.

Some general guidelines include the following: (1) When the client can sustain a heart rate of 110 to 120 beats/min with no shortness of breath or anginal pain, the client can resume sexual activity; (2) sexual activity should be resumed gradually and only after activities such as walking moderate distances (equivalent to 3 or 4 miles on a level treadmill) or climbing stairs comfortably have been accomplished; (3) sexual activity causes the least amount of stress when it occurs in familiar surroundings with the usual partner in a comfortable environment; (4) gradual foreplay helps the heart prepare for coitus; less strenuous sexual activities, such as cuddling, kissing, touching, and hugging, can be engaged in without sexual intercourse; (5) positions requiring isometric contractions should be avoided; (6) eating a large meal or drinking alcohol 1 to 3 hours before sexual activity should be avoided; (7) anal penetration should be avoided, because it stimulates the vagus nerve and may cause chest pain and slows down the heart rate and rhythm, impulse conduction, and coronary blood flow; and (8) health professionals should advise clients who experience postcoital angina to use nitrates.[344]

Box 12.9

**NEW YORK HEART ASSOCIATION'S FUNCTIONAL CLASSIFICATION OF HEART DISEASE**

- **Class I:** Cardiac disease present but no limitation on physical activity. Ordinary physical activity does not cause undue fatigue, palpitation, dyspnea, or anginal pain.
- **Class II:** Slight limitation on physical activity. Comfortable at rest, but ordinary physical activity results in fatigue, palpitation, dyspnea, or anginal pain.
- **Class III:** Marked limitation of physical activity. Comfortable at rest, but less than ordinary physical activity causes fatigue, palpitation, dyspnea, or anginal pain.
- **Class IV:** Unable to carry on any physical activity without discomfort. Symptoms of cardiac insufficiency or of the anginal syndrome may be present even at rest. If any physical activity is undertaken, discomfort is increased.

Table 12.11 Etiologic and Risk Factors Associated with Heart Failure

| Etiologic Factors | Risk Factors[a] |
|---|---|
| Hypertension | Emotional stress |
| Coronary artery disease | Physical inactivity |
| Myocardial infarction | Obesity |
| Valvular heart disease | Diabetes mellitus |
| Congenital heart disease | Nutritional deficiency (vitamin C, thiamin) |
| Endocarditis | Fever |
| Pericarditis | Infection |
| Myocarditis | Anemia |
| Cardiomyopathy | Thyroid disorders |
| Chronic alcoholism | Pregnancy |
| Atrioventricular malformation | Paget disease |
| Thyrotoxicosis (arrhythmia) | Pulmonary disease |
| Chronic anemia | Medications (e.g., steroids, NSAIDs) |
| | Drug toxicity |
| | Renal disease |

[a]Risk factors for new onset or exacerbation of previous HF.
*NSAIDs,* Nonsteroidal antiinflammatory drugs.

## Heart Failure

### Definition and Overview

In the most recent, 2013, guidelines, the American College of Cardiology and AHA defined HF as "a complex clinical syndrome that results from any structural or functional impairment of ventricular filling or ejection of blood."[378] Previously, the term "congestive heart failure" was used for this condition; however, some patients present without signs or symptoms of volume overload; therefore, the term "heart failure" is preferred over "congestive heart failure."[378]

HF is a condition in which the heart is unable to pump sufficient blood to supply the body's needs. Pumping ability may be impaired due to disorders of pericardium, myocardium, epicardium, heart valves, or large vessels or some metabolic abnormalities. Failure typically develops on and predominantly affects one side of the heart (left-sided or right-sided) and may progress to the other side. Most patients develop HF due to impairment of the left ventricular myocardial function. HF is not the same as cardiomyopathy or left ventricular dysfunction, but each of them may cause HF. HF may be chronic over many years, requiring management by oral medications, or it may be acute and life-threatening, requiring more dramatic medical management to maintain an adequate cardiac output.

### Classifications

The American College of Cardiology and AHA classify HF into 4 stages, A–D; and the New York Heart Association (NYHA) divides HF into 4 functional classifications, I–IV (see Box 12.9).[378] While stages describe development and progression of HF, the NYHA classes focus on exercise capacity and symptoms of HF, both providing complementary information about the presence and severity of HF.

Based on the left ventricular ejection fraction, HF is classified into HF with reduced ejection fraction (HFrEF) and HF with preserved ejection fraction (HFpEF).

Left-sided HF occurs when the left ventricle can no longer maintain a normal cardiac output, and right-sided HF develops as a result of right ventricular dysfunction secondary to either left-sided HF or to pulmonary disease. Strictly classified, left ventricular failure is referred to as HF; acute right ventricular failure, seen almost exclusively in association with massive pulmonary embolism, is labeled cor pulmonale. Cor pulmonale is heart disease, but it arises from an underlying pulmonary pathologic condition. Right-sided heart dysfunction secondary to left-sided HF, vascular dysfunction, or congenital heart disease is excluded in the definition of cor pulmonale.

### Incidence

HF is a common complication of ischemic and hypertensive heart diseases. It is more common in the older adult but is also frequently seen in adults over the age of 45 after sustaining an MI. Because the heart muscle is damaged during a heart attack, many people who have a heart attack develop HF. In the United States, HF develops in 1 million individuals annually;[50] it is the most common cause for hospitalization in people older than 65 years, with an estimated 6.5 million men and women living with HF in the United States today.[50] This condition is on the increase as the population ages and more people survive heart attacks. The lifetime risk of HF in an adult at age 45 through 95 years is 20% to 45%.[50] African Americans have the highest risk of HF.[378]

### Etiologic and Risk Factors

About one in three adult Americans have at least one risk factor for HF.[50] Among the risk factors (Table 12.11), hypertension is one of the most prevalent and the single most important modifiable risk factor. The risk of HF increases with elevated blood pressure (especially systolic), duration of hypertension, and older age. Diabetes mellitus and metabolic syndrome are important risk factors in developing HF contributing through hyperglycemia, insulin resistance, obesity, and dyslipidemia. Atherosclerotic disease contributes to development of HF as well.

Many cardiac conditions predispose individuals to HF. People with preexisting heart disease are at greatest risk for the development of HF, because when the heart is stressed, compensatory mechanisms may be inadequate. For example, a faster redistribution of blood volume and increased demand for oxygen by the myocardium occur with increased activity, such as exercise, resulting in HF for those with already compromised heart function. Many different types of cardiomyopathies (diseases of the heart muscle) predispose a person to developing HF. Among them: dilated cardiomyopathy, both idiopathic and familial; cardiomyopathies due to endocrine and metabolic causes (obesity, diabetes, thyroid disease, acromegaly and growth hormone deficiency, iron overload); toxic cardiomyopathies (alcoholic, cocaine, related to cancer therapies); cardiomyopathies due to inflammation (myocarditis, rheumatologic disorders); cardiomyopathies due to infections (Chagas disease, AIDS); peripartum cardiomyopathy (develops in the last trimester of pregnancy); amyloidosis; and sarcoidosis.[378] After ischemic heart disease and dilated cardiomyopathy, valvular heart disease (mainly mitral and aortic valve disease) is the third leading cause of HF.

Pulse pressure appears to be the best single measure of blood pressure for predicting mortality in older people and helps explain apparently discrepant results for low diastolic blood pressure. Pulse pressure is more predictive than even systolic blood pressure alone. Each elevation of 10 mm Hg between systolic and diastolic blood pressure increases the risk of HF by 14%.[151,278,353] Although the literature supports the use of pulse pressure as a significant prognostic indicator, day-to-day clinical use is not common.

HF occurring during middle age as distinguished from HF at advanced age includes an increasing proportion of women.[50] In older adults, hypertension remains the most common etiology in women, while in men, CAD is the main contributor to HF.[196] Women with diabetes mellitus have a threefold increased risk of HF when compared to men.[378] Comparable treatment of women with HF produces better clinical outcomes.[181] Medications such as steroids or NSAIDs and drug toxicity are also risk factors for developing HF,[277] although not as common. For the person with chronic, stable HF, acute exacerbations may occur, caused by alterations in pharmacologic therapy, client noncompliance with medications, excessive salt and fluid intake, arrhythmias, pulmonary embolisms (PEs), infection, or progression of the underlying disease.

**Pathogenesis and Clinical Manifestations.** The main contributors to the pathogenesis of HF are changes in neurohormonal activation and left ventricular remodeling.[168] These processes are triggered by an "index event" (e.g., MI; hemodynamic pressure as in hypertension) and develop into a clinical syndrome characterized by impaired cardiac function, leading to decline in the heart pumping. The index event either causes damage to the cardiac muscle tissue or impairs its contracting ability. The neurohormonal changes and left ventricular remodeling are regulated by biologically active molecules that are overproduced in response to a triggering event. The body counteracts with compensatory mechanisms, including activation of the sympathetic nervous system and the renin–angiotensin–aldosterone system (to maintain cardiac output), peripheral arterial vasoconstriction and increased contractility, and release of inflammatory mediators (assisting with cardiac repair and remodeling). Continued activation of these systems leads to mediation by biomolecule structural changes, or remodeling, of the left ventricular myocardium. Left ventricular remodeling involves changes in cardiomyocyte structure and function, accumulation of fibrotic tissue (increased deposits of collagen in the extracellular matrix), changes in cardiac energetics and mitochondrial biology, and alteration in the architecture of the left ventricular chamber, all leading to deterioration of the left ventricular performance.

HF is a complex event involving one or both ventricles. This discussion is based on left ventricular failure. When the heart fails to propel blood forward normally (such as occurs with left ventricular failure), the body uses three neurohormonal compensatory mechanisms; these are effective for a short time but eventually become insufficient to meet the oxygen needs of the body.

First, the failing heart attempts to maintain a normal output of blood by enlarging its pumping chambers so that they can hold a greater volume of blood. This lengthening of the muscle fibers, called *ventricular dilation,* increases the amount of blood ejected from the heart. This compensatory mechanism has limits, because contractility of ventricular muscle fibers ceases to increase when they are stretched beyond a certain point.

During this *first compensatory phase,* the right ventricle continues to pump more blood into the lungs. Congestion occurs in the pulmonary circulation, with accumulation of blood in the lungs. The immediate result is shortness of breath (most common symptom), and if the process continues, actual flooding of the air spaces of the lungs occurs, with fluid seeping from the distended blood vessels; this is called *pulmonary congestion* or *pulmonary edema.* Congestion in the vascular system interferes with the movement of fluids in and out of the various fluid compartments, resulting in fluid accumulation in the tissue spaces and progressive edema. Resulting ventilation/perfusion mismatch occurs due to the fluid accumulation and this further deprives the heart, peripheral muscles, and body organs from oxygen-rich blood.

During the *second compensatory phase,* the sympathetic nervous system responds to increase the stimulation of the heart muscle, causing it to pump more often. In response to failing contractility of the myocardial cells, the sympathetic nervous system activates adaptive processes that increase the heart rate and increase its muscle mass to strengthen the force of its contractions. This results in ventricular hypertrophy and a need for more oxygen by the heart muscles themselves.

Eventually, the coronary arteries cannot meet the oxygen demands of the enlarged myocardium, and the person may experience angina pectoris owing to ischemia. Secondary compensatory mechanisms activate the sympathetic nervous system and release endothelin from vascular linings, vasopressin (antidiuretic hormone) from the pituitary gland, and atrial natriuretic hormone from the heart.

The *third compensatory phase* involves activation of the renin–angiotensin–aldosterone system. With less blood

**Table 12.12** Clinical Manifestations of Heart Failure

| Left Ventricular Failure | Right Ventricular Failure |
|---|---|
| Progressive dyspnea (exertional first) | Dependent edema (ankle or pretibial first) |
| Paroxysmal nocturnal dyspnea | Jugular vein distention |
| Orthopnea | Abdominal pain and distention |
| Productive spasmodic cough | Weight gain |
| Pulmonary edema | Right upper quadrant pain (liver congestion) |
| Extreme breathlessness | Cardiac cirrhosis |
| Anxiety (associated with breathlessness) | Ascites |
| Frothy pink sputum | Jaundice |
| Nasal flaring | Anorexia, nausea |
| Accessory muscle use | Cyanosis (nail beds) |
| Crackles (formerly called rales) | Psychologic disturbances |
| Tachypnea | |
| Diaphoresis | |
| Cerebral hypoxia | |
| Irritability | |
| Restlessness | |
| Confusion | |
| Impaired memory | |
| Sleep disturbances | |
| Fatigue, exercise intolerance | |
| Muscular weakness | |
| Renal changes | |

coming from the heart, less blood passes through the kidneys. The kidneys respond by retaining water and sodium in an effort to increase blood volume, which further exacerbates tissue edema. The expanded blood volume increases the load on an already compromised heart. These mechanisms are responsible for the symptoms of diaphoresis, cool skin, tachycardia, cardiac arrhythmias, and oliguria (reduced urine excretion).

When the combined efforts of these three compensatory mechanisms achieve a normal level of cardiac output, the client is said to have compensated HF. Ultimately, however, the body's efforts to compensate may backfire and produce higher blood volume, higher blood pressure, and more stress on the already weakened heart. The heart's ongoing failure to supply the body with blood compels the body to keep compensating in ways that further burden the heart, and the cycle perpetuates itself. At times, these mechanisms may not be enough to keep the heart/body dynamic stable, and the person will experience a "HF exacerbation." Reestablishing fluid levels in the body typically helps to stabilize the client again. This is usually accomplished through medications and close restriction and monitoring of fluid intake and output. When these mechanisms are no longer effective and the disease progresses to the final stage of impaired heart function, the client has decompensated HF.

Decompensated HF ranges from mild congestion with few symptoms to life-threatening fluid overload and total heart failure (Table 12.12). Symptoms usually develop very gradually so that many people do not recognize or report signals of serious disease. The older adult, in particular, may wrongly associate early symptoms with a lack of fitness or consider them a sign of normal aging.[306] Confusion and impaired thinking can characterize HF in older adults. Clients with HF often feel anxious, frightened, and depressed. Fears may be expressed as frightening nightmares, insomnia, acute anxiety states, depression, or withdrawal from reality.

***Left-Sided Heart Failure.*** Failure of the left ventricle (Fig. 12.13) prevents the heart from pumping enough blood through the arterial system to meet the body's metabolic needs and causes either pulmonary edema or a disturbance in the respiratory control mechanisms. The degree of respiratory distress varies with the client's position, activity, and level of emotional or physical stress, but any of the symptoms listed under "Pulmonary Edema" in Chapter 15 may occur.

*Dyspnea* is subjective and does not always correlate with the extent of heart failure; exertional dyspnea occurs in all clients to some degree. Time for dyspnea to subside is an indication of progress or deterioration in a client's status, and it can be measured for documentation. Paroxysmal nocturnal dyspnea resembles the frightening sensation of awakening with suffocation. Once the client is in the upright position, relief from the attack may not occur for 30 minutes or longer. The client often assumes a three-point position, sitting up with both hands on the knees and leaning forward. In severe HF, the client may resort to sleeping upright in a chair or recliner. Other sleep disturbances may occur from central sleep apnea, which is present in approximately 40% of all adults with HF.

*Fatigue* and *muscular weakness* are often associated with left ventricular failure because dyspnea develops along with weight gain and a faster resting heart rate, which decrease the person's ability to exercise. Inadequate cardiac output leads to decreased peripheral blood flow and blood flow to skeletal muscle. The resultant tissue hypoxia and slowed removal of metabolic wastes cause the person to tire easily. Disturbances in sleep and rest patterns may aggravate fatigue; muscle atrophy is common in advanced HF. As the client begins to feel more short of breath with any exertion, they restrict their physical activity, which further perpetuates the problems.

*Renal changes* can occur in both right- and left-sided HF, but they are more evident with left-sided failure. During the day, the client is upright, decreased cardiac output reduces blood flow to the kidneys, and the formation of urine is reduced (oliguria). Sodium and water not excreted in the urine are retained in the vascular system, adding to the blood volume.

Diminished blood supply to the renal system causes the kidney to secrete renin, stimulating production of angiotensin II, which causes vasoconstriction, thereby causing an increase in peripheral vascular resistance, increasing blood pressure and cardiac work, and resulting in worse HF. Renin secretion also indirectly stimulates the secretion of aldosterone from the adrenal gland. Aldosterone acts on the renal tubules, causing them to increase reabsorption of sodium and water, further increasing fluid volume. At night, urine formation (nocturia) increases with the recumbent position as blood flow to the kidney improves. *Nocturia* may interfere with effective sleep patterns, which contributes to fatigue, as mentioned.

***Right-Sided Heart Failure.*** Failure of the right ventricle (see Fig. 12.13) to adequately pump blood to the

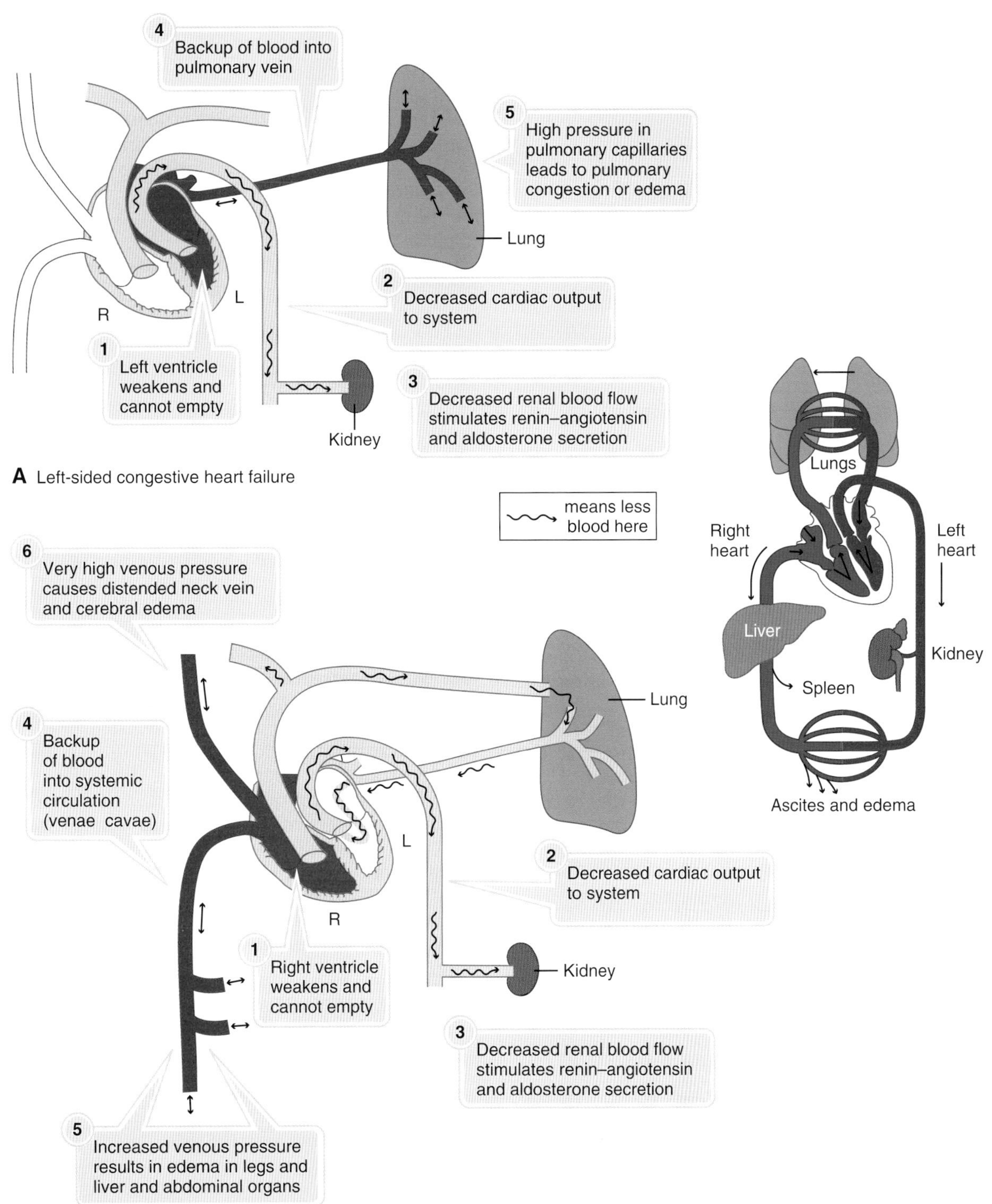


**Figure 12.13**

**Pathophysiologic mechanisms of heart failure.** (A) Left-sided heart failure leads to pulmonary edema (see text description). (B) Right ventricular failure causes peripheral edema that is most prominent in the lower extremities. *Inset,* Integration of the pulmonary and systemic circulation. When the heart contracts normally, it pumps blood simultaneously into both loops, but pump failure causes circulatory or pulmonary problems, depending on the underlying pathologic mechanism. (A and B from Gould B: *Pathophysiology for the health professions,* ed 2, Philadelphia, 2002, WB Saunders, p. 286; inset from Damjanov I: *Pathology for the health-related professions,* ed 3, Philadelphia, 2006, WB Saunders.)

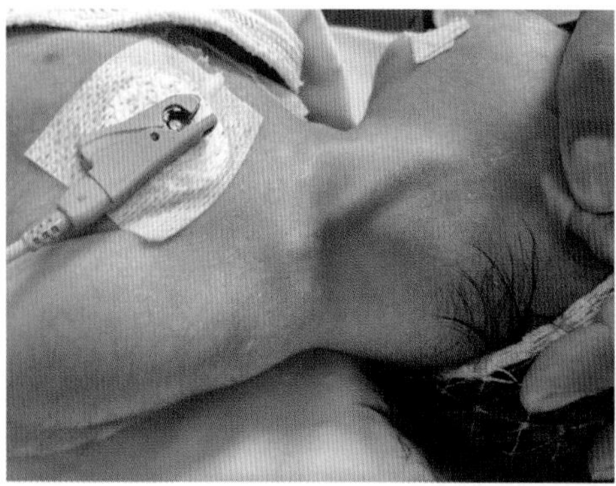

**Figure 12.14**

Jugular venous distention can be a sign of right-sided heart failure. (From Kanburoglue MK: Corrigan pulse and fullness of the neck vessels in a neonate, *The Journal of Pediatrics,* 187: 329, 2017.)

lungs results in peripheral edema and venous congestion of the organs. Symptoms result from congestion in the heart's right side and throughout the venous system.

*Dependent edema* is one of the early signs of right ventricular failure, although significant HF can be present in the absence of peripheral edema. In HF with congestive symptoms, fluid is retained because the baroreceptors of the body sense a decreased volume of blood as a result of the heart's inability to pump an adequate amount of blood. The receptors subsequently relay a message to the kidneys to retain fluid so that a greater volume of blood can be ejected from the heart to the peripheral tissues. Unfortunately, this compounds the problem and makes the heart work even harder, which further decreases its pumping ability, causing a sense of weakness and fatigue and resulting in peripheral edema.

The retained fluid commonly accumulates in the extracellular spaces of the periphery. The resultant edema is usually symmetric and occurs in the dependent parts of the body, where venous pressure is the highest. In ambulatory persons, edema begins in the feet and ankles and ascends up the lower legs (pretibial areas). It is most noticeable at the end of a day and often decreases after a night's rest. In the recumbent person, pitting edema may develop in the presacral area and, as it worsens, progress to the medial thighs and genital area.

*Jugular venous distention* also results from fluid overload. The jugular veins empty unoxygenated blood directly into the superior vena cava. Because no cardiac valve exists to separate the superior vena cava from the right atrium, the jugular veins give information about activity on the right side of the heart. As fluid is retained and the heart's ability to pump is further compromised, the retained fluid backs up into both the lungs and the venous system, and the jugular veins reveal this. Jugular venous pulsations are examined by inspecting the silhouette of the neck with the person reclining at a 45-degree angle (Fig. 12.14). The use of the right internal jugular vein is recommended because the left internal jugular may be falsely elevated in some people.

Although not as common as peripheral edema, fluid collection in and around the liver can also occur. As the liver becomes congested with venous blood, it becomes enlarged, and *abdominal pain* occurs. If this occurs rapidly, stretching of the capsule surrounding the liver causes severe discomfort, and the person may notice either a constant aching or a sharp *right upper quadrant pain.* In chronic HF, longstanding congestion of the liver with venous blood and anoxia can lead to ascites and jaundice, which are symptoms of liver damage. Anorexia, nausea, and bloating develop secondary to venous congestion of the gastrointestinal (GI) tract.

*Cyanosis* of the nail beds appears as venous congestion reduces peripheral blood flow.

***Heart Failure with Reduced Ejection Fraction.*** Symptoms of HF, with an ejection fraction of 40% or more, define HFrEF. About 50% of HF patients have HFrEF. About half of HFrEF patients have enlarged left ventricle. Systolic dysfunction is common (HFrEF is also known as systolic HF). The weakened left ventricle does not contract fully and expels less blood. Symptoms include dyspnea and fatigue. CAD and MI are common causes of HFrEF. Efficacious therapies are available for patients with HFrEF.

***Heart Failure with Preserved Ejection Fraction.*** Symptoms of HF, but with an ejection fraction of 50% or less, define HFpEF. HFpEF is characterized by a heart that is normal in size but with stiffness of the heart muscle both when relaxed and when contracting. These changes interfere with the diastole (filling) phase of heart function (HFpEF is also known as diastolic HF) and present with symptoms of dyspnea, coughing, wheezing, and fatigue. If left untreated, pulmonary and peripheral edema can develop suddenly. Triggers for the development of this type of "flash" pulmonary edema include sudden surges of emotion or activity, high-fat meals, sudden excessive exercise, or forgetting to take prescription cardiovascular medications. The major cause of HFpEF is hypertension. HFpEF is associated with aging. A typical patient is an older woman with a history of hypertension. Development of optional treatments for this type of HF is ongoing.

## MEDICAL MANAGEMENT

**DIAGNOSIS.** Diagnosis is based on the clinical picture and depends on where symptoms are on the continuum of mild to severe. Because the two sides of the heart serve different functions, distinguishing the symptoms of left-sided HF from those of right-sided HF is critical in both diagnosis and treatment in the early stages of HF. As HF develops, both sides of the heart become involved due to retrograde progression. So if the therapist is seeing a client well after HF has developed, it may be unclear which side of the heart the HF began with. Whether the client is being treated earlier or later in the disease progression, it is important to consider whether there is systolic and diastolic dysfunction, both of which indicate a functional or structural defect in the ventricles.

An echocardiogram is the main diagnostic tool. Noninvasive cardiac tests such as ECG and chest radiography are secondary tools that can determine left ventricular size and function well enough to confirm the diagnosis. Cardiac catheterization is not routinely performed, but it may be useful in certain cases (e.g., atherosclerotic heart disease, which is potentially correctable). Arterial blood gases are measured to evaluate oxygen saturation. Liver enzymes (e.g., aspartate transaminase, alkaline phosphatase) are often elevated; liver involvement with hyperbilirubinemia commonly occurs, resulting in jaundice.

Biomarkers became an important supplement for predicting HF, confirming the diagnosis, evaluating the prognosis, and directing therapies. Measuring B-type natriuretic peptide (BNP), a protein secreted from the cardiac atria in response to wall tension and pressure overload, can reliably predict the presence or absence of HF.[90] BNP is a stronger predictor of HF than its relative, atrial natriuretic peptide (ANP).[90] In addition to the natriuretic peptides, next-generation biomarkers are in development to use with application to HF. The candidate biomarkers may come from pathways of neurohormonal regulation, extracellular matrix remodeling, inflammation, oxidative stress, myocyte stress and injury, and other processes in the diseased heart.[90] A comprehensive review of biomarkers related to HF and their role in prevention, assessment, and management of HF has been published by the AHA.[90]

**PREVENTION AND TREATMENT.** Managing HF begins with treatment of the underlying cause whenever possible. Nonpharmacologic interventions such as diet and exercise that alter interactions between the heart and the periphery are now accepted therapeutic approaches.

Alterations in lifestyle reduce symptoms and the need for additional medication. There is an urgent need to develop more effective strategies for the prevention and treatment of this increasingly common disorder. Multiple comorbidities in older clients require a multidisciplinary approach to management. Persons with HF are placed on a sodium-restricted diet, sometimes with limited fluid intake. Emotional and physical rest during the initial phases of intervention is also important in diminishing the workload of the heart.

***Activity and Exercise.*** Exercise programs have proved to quantitatively achieve results similar to those attained with most effective drug therapies. These findings have shifted attention away from treating the heart toward exercising the muscles.

Whenever possible, physical activity and exercise are prescribed per client tolerance. Clients should perform a combination of aerobic and resistance exercise,[29] similar to those for people after MI (see "Exercise After Myocardial Infarction"). Physical training for clients with HF results in an improvement in skeletal and inspiratory muscle strength, endurance, aerobic characteristic of skeletal muscles, peripheral vascular function, and autonomic nervous system balance.[29] Improved blood flow to the muscles, uptake of oxygen by the muscles, and venous return away from the periphery are all improved in people with HF following regular exercise. Physical activity has been determined to be a safe therapy for individuals with HF.[378] Exercise training also improves exercise and functional capacities,[29,41] reduces symptoms, improves health and psychosocial status, improves overall quality of life,[41] and decreases mortality.[378] Clients with HF have shown lower physical activity tolerance if they have sleep disturbance too.[88] Therefore, it is important to discuss sleep patterns and disturbances with HF clients, as sleep issues often arise due to fluid accumulation in the lungs, causing shortness of breath at night in the supine position.

***Pharmacotherapy.*** Pharmacologic therapy for HF[377] is driven by our understanding of HF as a cascade of neurohormonal events centered on ventricular remodeling. Pharmacologic agents are used to reduce the heart's workload, increase muscle strength and contraction, and inhibit neuroendocrine responses to heart failure (see Tables 12.5 and 12.6).

ACE inhibitors have become standard therapy for HF because of their ability to block the renin–angiotensin–aldosterone system, increasing renal blood flow and decreasing renal vascular resistance, thereby enhancing diuresis. ACE inhibitors reduce left ventricular filling pressure and moderately increase cardiac output. Vasodilator therapy in combination with ACE inhibitors prolongs life in persons with moderate to severe HF.

Diuretics are also standard care for people with HF to control fluid buildup and prevent congestion. It is important for the client, therapist, and physician to monitor the diuretic's dose and the client's fluid balance. Too much diuresis can deplete potassium, which can cause life-threatening arrhythmias. Digoxin may be added to stimulate the heart's pumping action if symptoms persist despite treatment with ACE inhibitors and diuretics. Angiotensin II receptor blockers have been added to function as an antihypertensive and enhance the clearance of sodium and water. Aldosterone antagonists are used as potassium-sparing diuretics.

The β-blockers, once rarely considered in the treatment of HF, are effective in reducing symptoms, improving clinical status, reducing hospitalizations, and reducing the risk of death.[28] Combining β-blockers with ACE inhibitors can produce additive effects on two neurohormonal systems (renin–angiotensin–aldosterone system and sympathetic nervous system).

***Surgery.*** Surgical intervention may include CABG for underlying myocardial ischemia and infarction. If the HF is caused in full or in part due to heart valve abnormalities, reconstruction of the incompetent heart valve(s) may be performed. Internal counterpulsation (Fig. 12.15) or external counterpulsation, which uses an external pump or balloon to adjust the aortic blood pressure; temporary ventricular assistive devices for people unable to come off bypass; and use of an artificial heart or cardiac transplantation are all other possible surgical interventions.

Cardiac transplantation is now more common for treatment of HF. Transplantation is successful for selected individuals, usually those who are treated early in the course of HF, before advanced symptoms develop. Reform of the selection process is recommended to identify people who, although not critically ill, will not survive without early transplantation.

Cardiac resynchronization therapy (CRT) is when a pacemaker is inserted to stimulate both ventricles (biventricular pacing) in an effort to improve the heart's overall cardiac efficiency by coordinating the heart's contractions (both ventricles pump at the same time, making the heart pump more forcefully). CRT allows greater contractility of the ventricles, thus improving cardiac output and activity tolerance.[104,174] It has also been shown to improve longevity in people with HF.[104,174] There is also some limited data that shows that CRT may cause electrical remodeling at the heart.[6]

***Self-care.*** AHA has issued a scientific statement on promoting self-care for individuals with CVD, including heart

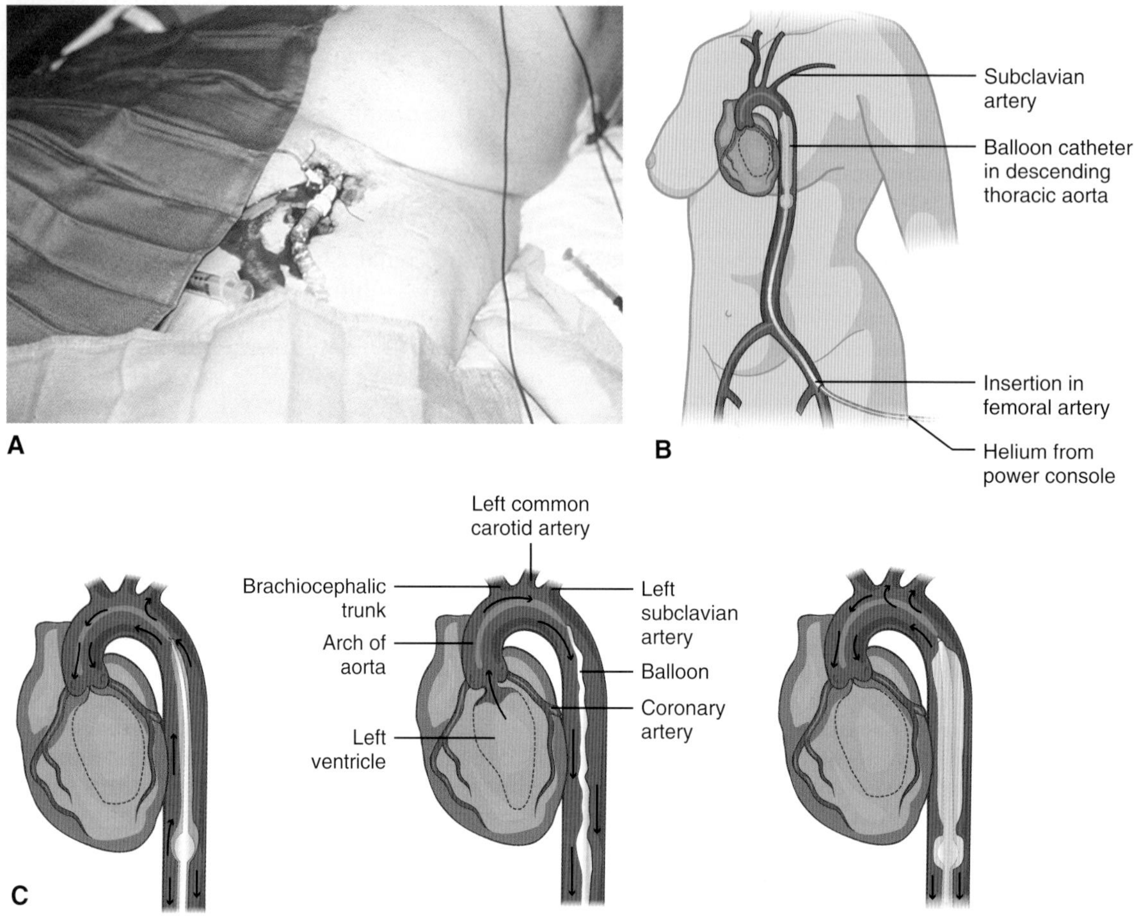


**Figure 12.15**

The intraaortic balloon pump is a common type of cardiac assist device that is used to improve myocardial oxygen supply–demand for individuals with deteriorating hemodynamics or ongoing ischemia, as evidenced by rest pain or electrocardiographic changes in the region of the infarct. The primary functions of balloon counterpulsation are to reperfuse the coronary arteries at the end of systole and reduce the left ventricular afterload (the amount of work the ventricle must do), thereby decreasing myocardial oxygen consumption and improving cardiac output. These intravascular catheter-mounted counterpulsation devices are traditionally used for cases of cardiogenic shock following cardiac surgery or an acute myocardial infarction as well as for people who have chronic end-stage heart failure and who are not candidates for long-term ventricular assistive device support. The rationale for intraaortic balloon pump counterpulsation in this latter situation is to maintain systemic perfusion and preserve end-organ function until cardiac transplantation occurs. (A) The catheter is usually placed through the femoral artery, and the balloon is moved up the iliac artery to the descending aorta, where it is then placed, (B) above the renal arteries and below the subclavian artery. This position is critical in order to prevent ischemia to the upper extremities or kidneys. (C) When the heart contracts (systole), the balloon is deflated, creating a decline in aortic pressure. After the heart contracts (during diastole), the balloon is filled with air, causing the blood to regurgitate back toward the root of the aorta, thereby perfusing the coronary arteries. When the left ventricle is ready to pump, the balloon is deflated (cardiac systole again), reducing ventricular afterload. (A, courtesy Chris Wells, PT, MS, PhD, University of Pittsburgh Medical Center, 2001. B, from Black JM, Hawks JH, Keene AM: *Medical-surgical nursing: clinical management for positive outcomes,* ed 7, Philadelphia, 2005, WB Saunders. C, from Lewis SL, Heitkemper MM, Dirksen SR: *Medical surgical nursing: assessment and management of surgical problems,* ed 7, St Louis, 2007, Mosby.)

failure, and stroke[308] advocating for self-care as a method of prevention, management, and improving outcomes. Self-care is defined as a "naturalistic decision-making process addressing both the prevention and management of chronic illness, with core elements of self–care maintenance, self–care monitoring, and self–care management."[308]

Specific self-care behaviors include medication adherence, understanding of health status and risk awareness ("know your numbers"), symptom monitoring, dietary adherence, controlled alcohol use, weight control, exercise, smoking cessation, preventive behaviors (personal hygiene, dental health, immunizations, etc.), and nonprescription medication taking (physician-approved vitamins). There is a variety of factors that make self-care difficult, including comorbid conditions, depression, anxiety, age-related issues, impaired cognition, sleep disturbances, poor health literacy,[236] and problems with the health care system. Skill development, behavioral changes, and family support are recognized interventions that promote self-care. Poor quality of life and early mortality in individuals with heart failure may be reduced if the people are actively engaged in consistent self-care.[308]

**Prognosis.** Treatment of HF remains difficult; although declines in mortality have been observed recently, associated with treatments of HF risk factors, advances in pharmacologic therapy, cardiac revascularization approaches, and CRT.[50] Annual mortality rates range from 10% in stable clients with mild symptoms to greater than 50% in people with advanced, progressive symptoms. Approximately 40% to 50% of clients with HF die suddenly, probably owing to ventricular arrhythmias. Half of those who have HF will die within 5 years of diagnosis.[378] HF accounts for 7% of all deaths from CVD.[378]

To achieve the maximal benefit from drug therapy, symptoms must be recognized as early as possible and intervention initiated. Because this condition often develops gradually, intervention is delayed, full resolution is not usually possible, and HF becomes a chronic disorder.

NYHA class is the greatest predictor of mortality in people with HF.[39] The NYHA classes are based on a client's physical activity abilities,[103] so the therapist should use the client's NYHA class to perform risk stratification (see Box 12.9). Older age and lower glomerular filtration rate were the other two major predictors of mortality for people with HF.[39]

Other signs of poor prognosis include severe left ventricular dysfunction, severe symptoms and limitation of exercise capacity, secondary renal insufficiency, and elevated plasma catecholamine levels.

## SPECIAL IMPLICATIONS FOR THE THERAPIST 12.6

### *Heart Failure*

Therapists have a unique role in the prevention, medical management, and rehabilitation of people with HF. Physical therapists can provide programs that profoundly improve the exercise tolerance and functional status of individuals with HF.

Medical intervention can be more objectively implemented by using information obtained during physical therapy assessments and interventions. Tests such as the 6-minute walk test may be helpful in predicting peak oxygen consumption and early survival, as well as in implementing a proper exercise conditioning program for people with advanced HF.[292]

Education of physicians and other health care professionals about the role of the physical therapist in defining prescriptive exercise is important.[30] Consideration for the complex pathologic conditions and comorbidities of people in this population is an important contribution to cardiac rehabilitation from the physical therapist's training. Clients should be referred to rehabilitation before the $\dot{V}O_{2max}$ drops below 14 mL/kg/min and when the wedge pressure is still greater than 16 mm Hg (i.e., before clients progress in a downward spiral requiring transplantation).

#### Early Considerations

Clients hospitalized with severe HF require a therapy program to maintain pulmonary function and prevent complications of bed rest (e.g., skin breakdown, venous stasis, venous thrombus, PEs). An important aspect of intervention is functional assessment (Box 12.9) and physical exercise within the limitations set by the physician and as determined appropriate by the therapist. See also established guidelines for exercise training in HF.[69,281] Physical therapy assessment of cardiopulmonary status is beyond the scope of this text. The clinician is referred to any of the specific examination and assessment texts available.[139,176]

The therapist should be aware of other factors that impact the progression and management of HF. These include psychosocial considerations, especially in older adults with HF. Neuropsychiatric conditions such as Alzheimer dementia and complications such as delirium are common in older adults with HF. Persistent alcohol abuse and cigarette smoking often contribute to the onset and progression of HF. Major depression, other depressive disorders, anxiety, and social isolation are also factors that can have adverse effects on functional status, quality of life, and prognosis. Working as a team with psychologists, nurses, and social workers can address these issues effectively.

#### Monitoring Vital Signs

Aerobic capacity is likely impaired with HF and even more so if the client is deconditioned. Adaptive responses to activity may be attenuated or inadequate; activity may exacerbate cardiovascular pump dysfunction; and signs of fatigue and shortness of breath are common. The downward cycle of disease, deconditioning, decreased activity, and disability necessitates the monitoring of vital signs.[139] During acute exacerbations of HF, the therapist should monitor vital signs at rest, during activity, and after a 2- to 3-minute recovery period. For the patient with chronic HF, the therapist should monitor vital signs intermittently or as needed with exercise. Oxygen can be assessed through pulse oximetry. The amount needed can be determined by the therapist's consultation with the client's physician. Oxygen may be administered by mask or cannula. The therapist should monitor the need to increase oxygen delivery values during exercise and discuss with the physician as needed.

Monitor the client for signs of increasing peripheral edema by assessing jugular neck vein distention, peripheral edema in the legs or sacrum, and any report of right upper quadrant pain. In the outpatient or home health setting, the client is advised to call the nurse or physician if shoes, belt, or pants become too tight to fasten, usual activities of daily living or tasks become difficult, extra sleep is needed, or urination at night becomes more frequent. It is important for the client to check their weight daily. If they gain 2 or more pounds in a day or 5 or more pounds in a week, they should contact their physician immediately, as this could be a sign of fluid retention due to their HF.[15]

Monitoring blood pressure is essential to detect HF; observe for decreasing blood pressure and report any change in status to the nurse or physician immediately. Exaggerated increases in heart rate may be observed as the heart attempts to maintain adequate cardiac output. The therapist should observe for dyspnea at rest and/or with activity and auscultate for changes from baseline during activity.[139]

Continuous supervision and frequent monitoring of blood pressure are necessary when starting an exercise program for someone with HF. RPE should range from 11 to 14 (light to somewhat hard; Table 12.13). Anginal symptoms should not exceed 2 on the 0 to 4 angina scale (moderate to bothersome), and exertional dyspnea should not exceed a rating of mild, some difficulty with activity. Initially, full resuscitation equipment should be available.[14]

#### Positioning

Positioning is important, and the client is taught to use a high Fowler position (head of the bed elevated at least 20 inches above the level position or roughly 45 degrees) or chair to reduce pulmonary congestion, facilitate diaphragmatic expansion and ventilation, and ease dyspnea.

The legs are maintained in a dependent position as much as possible to normalize venous return. Range of motion to decrease venous pooling and monitoring for the development of thrombophlebitis (e.g., unilateral swelling, calf pain, pallor) are required.

Activity in the upright position is preferred (again because of increased venous return in the supine position). This guideline should apply during aquatic activities as well. Monitoring vital signs is important, as these individuals can deteriorate at any time. Extra caution is advised if the systolic blood pressure is less than 80 mm Hg and resting heart rate is less than 50 beats/min or more than 100 beats/min. Worsening orthopnea may be suspected if the individual requires more and more pillows in the upright position.

### Exercise and Heart Failure

The best guideline is to customize initial exercise intensity for each individual,[281] keeping in mind the individual's goals and expected outcomes (e.g., preparation for transplantation, improved functional daily living, perceived quality of life). Using an interval training approach is helpful with those individuals who demonstrate marked exercise intolerance.

The American College of Sports Medicine's guidelines[18] suggest that HF clients entering an exercise program should start with moderate-intensity exercise (40%-60% $VO_{2max}$) for a duration of 2 to 6 minutes, followed by 2 minutes of rest. Blood pressure and heart rhythm should be routinely monitored at rest, intermittently during exercise, and after cool-down. The goal is to gradually increase the intensity and duration of exercise.

Others advocate starting HF clients at a low to moderate exercise intensity (less than 40% $VO_{2max}$) with a shorter duration of exercise initially and a shorter rest period of less than 2 minutes). Recommendations for interval exercise training have also been reported.[185] There is some research regarding high intensity interval training (HIIT) with clients with HF that has been positive.[149,342] However, these data are limited and are not generalizable to all people with HF. Most studies were with clients with good NYHA class who were already performing some interval training. The therapist should use current research and clinical judgement before deciding to prescribe a HITT for their client with HF.

Symptoms and general fatigue level serve as a guideline to determine exercise frequency, and warm-up/cool-down periods should be longer than normal for observation of possible arrhythmias. This is especially important for anyone with HFpEF as they are prone to atrial fibrillation and subsequent risk of blood clots and stroke. These individuals are also prone to a condition called *chronotropic incompetence*, which is difficulty getting the heart rate to increase during exercise.[326]

For anyone with HF, determination of appropriate exercise intensity based on 40% to 60% $VO_{2max}$ is recommended (rather than based on heart rate peak) because the response to exercise is frequently abnormal. Alternatively, the initial exercise intensity should be 10 beats below any significant symptoms, including angina, exertional hypotension, arrhythmias, and dyspnea.

Rehabilitation personnel must observe the client for symptoms of cardiac decompensation during exercise, including cough or dyspnea, hypotension, light-headedness, cyanosis, angina, and arrhythmias. Exercise progression following these recommendations is available in detail.[14,18]

The therapist should keep in mind that some older HF clients are unable to increase their exercise intensity or duration despite starting very slowly. These people do not achieve the goal of increased endurance and often leave the program owing to increased symptoms and exercise intolerance. Maintaining or even improving functional activities and independence at home may be more appropriate goals for this group.

### Medications

Diuretics can produce mild to severe electrolyte imbalance, requiring special consideration. A small drop in the serum potassium level can precipitate digoxin poisoning (digoxin toxicity) and serious arrhythmias, as a consequence of digoxin competing with potassium ions for binding to its target sodium-potassium pump. This situation is a life-threatening condition and may present with systemic or cardiac manifestations. The occurrence of digoxin toxicity has decreased over the years because of less usage, lower doses, and better monitoring and today occurs in approximately 1% of patients.[44] Any sign or symptom of digoxin toxicity (see Table 12.5) should be reported to the physician.

Digoxin toxicity may occur for a variety of reasons. Most commonly, it is due to worsening renal function, inappropriate dosing, client taking the medication inappropriately, or due to a suicidal gesture. Recommendations for the dosing of digoxin are now between 0.125 mg/day and 0.25 mg/day. If the serum albumin level is low, digoxin may not be bound to albumin and will be circulating as "free" digoxin, producing toxic effects. It is possible, however, for the digoxin toxicity to occur when digoxin blood levels are in therapeutic range and albumin levels are normal. Albumin levels are not always abnormal when side effects occur.

Digoxin toxicity can cause a dip in the ST segment on ECG; whenever possible, the ECG should be monitored during exercise. Activity should not increase the magnitude of the altered ST segment. A physical therapist should watch for a low, irregular pulse (less than 60 beats/min); the heart rate normally increases to compensate for HF, but in the presence of digoxin, heart rate decreases.

NSAIDs, including nonprescription drugs such as ibuprofen, increase fluid retention independently and significantly blunt the action of diuretics and other cardiovascular drugs (especially ACE inhibitors), exacerbating preexisting HF and causing isolated lower extremity edema. The major consideration for exercise in clients taking ACE inhibitors is the possibility of hypotension and accompanying arrhythmias. These problems should be reported to the physician and can be addressed by maintaining proper hydration and by altering dosages and the simultaneous use of other medications.

## Orthostatic (Postural) Hypotension

### Definition and Overview

The term *orthostatic (postural) hypotension* signifies a decrease of 20 mm Hg or greater in systolic blood pressure or a drop of 10 mm Hg or more in both systolic and diastolic arterial blood pressure with a concomitant pulse increase of 15 beats/min or more on standing from a supine or sitting position.

Orthostatic hypotension may be acute and temporary or chronic. Orthostatic hypotension occurs frequently in older adults and occurs in more than one half of all frail older adults, contributing significantly to morbidity from syncope, falls, vital organ ischemia (e.g., MI, transient ischemic attacks), and mortality among older adults with diabetic hypertension. It is highly variable over time but most prevalent in the morning, when supine blood pressure is highest, and on first arising from a seated position.

### Etiologic Factors

Orthostatic hypotension is recognized in all groups as a cardinal feature of autonomic nervous dysfunction, as well as other nonneurogenic etiologies (Box 12.10).

Postural reflexes are slowed as part of the aging process for some, but not all, people. Normal aging is associated with various changes that may lead to postural hypotension. Cardiac output declines with age; in the older adult with hypertension, it is even lower. When subjects older than age 65 years are put under passive postural stress (60 degree upright tilt), their stroke volume decreases even further. These normal changes obviously predispose the aging adult to postural hypotension from any process that further reduces fluid volume or vascular integrity. For example, pooling of blood after eating may lead to profound hypotension, called *postprandial hypotension*.

In addition, as systolic pressure rises from atherosclerosis, baroreceptor sensitivity and vascular compliance are reduced further, increasing the likelihood of postural hypotension. In general, older adults with postural hypotension have higher rates of CVD, but there is no evidence of a direct cause of CAD by postural hypotension, just a positive relationship between the two.[75,227]

Most commonly, orthostatic hypotension develops due to dehydration and medications, specifically diuretics and vasodilators.[330] Drugs are a major cause of orthostatic hypotension, particularly in older adults. Many have effects on the autonomic nervous system, both centrally and peripherally, and on fluid balance. Diuretics, calcium channel blockers, nitrates, and L-dopa have hypotensive effects. Antidepressants are a common, overlooked cause of orthostasis, even though this is a known side effect of these medications. A general adverse result of treatment for hypertension may be excessive hypotension. In addition, many older adults with systolic hypertension have postural hypotension that may require management before the hypertension is addressed.

Chronic orthostatic hypotension may occur secondary to a specific disease, such as endocrine disorders, metabolic disorders, nephropathy, or neurogenic disorders affecting the autonomic or central nervous system. Alcohol and drugs such as vincristine used in the treatment of cancer can cause autonomic neuropathy, leading to the impairment of vasoconstrictive mechanisms, resulting in orthostatic hypotension.

**Table 12.13** Borg Scale of Perceived Exertion[58,a]

| Numerical Rating Scale | Verbal Rating |
|---|---|
| **6** | No exertion at all |
| 7 | Extremely light |
| 8 | |
| 9 | Very light |
| 10 | |
| 11 | Light |
| 12 | |
| 13 | Somewhat hard |
| 14 | |
| 15 | Hard |
| 16 | |
| 17 | Very hard |
| **18** | |
| 19 | Extremely hard |
| 20 | Maximal exertion |

[a]Using a perceived exertion scale is a useful approach to activity prescription. The individual is prescribed a desirable rating of perceived exertion and uses that level of intensity as a daily guideline for activity. A suggested rating of perceived exertion for most healthy individuals is 13 to 15 (somewhat hard to hard on the scale). For the compromised person, a more moderate level of perceived exertion may be recommended by the physician.

**Box 12.10**

**CAUSES OF ORTHOSTATIC HYPOTENSION**

- Volume depletion (e.g., burns, diabetes mellitus, or potassium depletion)
  - Side effects of alcohol and other drugs that cause volume depletion (e.g., antidepressants, antihypertensives, diuretics, ACE inhibitors, vasodilators)
- Venous pooling (e.g., pregnancy, varicosities of the legs)
- Prolonged immobility
- Starvation, malnutrition, alcoholism, eating disorders
- Performing Valsalva maneuver
- Sluggish normal regulatory mechanisms (e.g., anatomic variation, altered body chemistry)
- Autonomic nervous system dysregulation (e.g., diabetes mellitus, Parkinson disease, aging, fibromyalgia syndrome, chronic renal failure)

Modified from Bonow RO: *Braunwald's heart disease—a textbook of cardiovascular medicine*, ed 9, Philadelphia, 2011, WB Saunders.

### Pathogenesis

Orthostasis is a physiologic stress related to upright posture. When a normal individual stands up, the gravitational changes on the circulation are compensated for by several mechanisms, including the circulatory and autonomic nervous systems. On standing, the force of gravity in the vertical axis causes venous pooling in the lower limbs, a sharp decline in venous return, and reduction in filling pressure of the heart, which increase further on prolonged standing because of shifting of water to interstitial spaces and hemoconcentration.

These mechanical events can cause a marked reduction in cardiac output and consequent fall in arterial blood pressure. In healthy people, cardiac output and blood pressure regulation are maintained by powerful compensatory mechanisms involving a rise in heart rate. Blood pressure is maintained by a rise in peripheral resistance.

These compensatory mechanisms are initiated by the baroreceptors located in the aortic arch and carotid bifurcation. Orthostatic hypotension results from failure of the arterial baroreflex, most commonly because of disorders of the autonomic nervous system.[48]

In people with autonomic failure or dysreflexia (e.g., Parkinson disease, aging, diabetes, fibromyalgia), orthostatic hypotension results from an impaired capacity to increase vascular resistance during standing. This dysfunction leads to increased downward pooling of venous blood and a consequent reduction in stroke volume and cardiac output that exaggerates the orthostatic fall in blood pressure.

Approximately 80% of the blood pooled in the lower limb is contained in the upper leg (thighs, buttocks), with less pooling in the calf and foot. The location of the additional venous pooling has not been clearly identified, but present data suggest the abdominal compartment and perhaps leg skin vasculature. The pooled blood in the veins of the feet and calves is arterial in origin in that it arises as a result of decreased venous drainage of that region.

In contrast, the blood pooled in the thighs, buttocks, pelvis, and abdomen arises primarily from venous reflux. The pooled blood is not actually stagnant; its mean circulatory time through the dependent region is merely increased by changes in the pressure gradient across the vascular bed, increases in venous volume, and possibly decreases in venous tone. The identification of venous pooling may offer insights for intervention techniques in the future.

### Clinical Manifestations

Orthostatic hypotension is often accompanied by dizziness, blurring or loss of vision, and syncope or fainting. There are three main modes of presentation in the older adult: (1) falls or mobility problems, (2) acute or chronic mental confusion, and (3) cardiac symptoms.

A common clinical picture is the person whose legs give way when attempting to stand, usually after prolonged recumbency, after physical exertion, or in a warm environment. These episodes may be accompanied by confusion, pallor, tremor, and unsteadiness. Loss of consciousness may cause frequent falls and additional injuries that can be quite serious. Clients may also become light-headed and/or have syncopal episodes associated with quick position changes that lead directly into ambulation. The venous system does not have adequate time to increase venous return, so the client has additional pooling and orthostasis. Ischemic symptoms of orthostatic hypotension are nonspecific, including lethargy, weakness, low backache, calf claudication, and angina. Orthostatic hypotension may also be an early sign of some other illness or the effects of medication.

## MEDICAL MANAGEMENT

There are several general and specific approaches to the management of orthostatic hypotension[253] but no curative intervention for orthostatic hypotension of unknown cause. Prevention is important, and whenever the underlying disorder causing hypotension is corrected, symptoms cease. Nonneurogenic causes, such as diminished intravascular volume, are treated specifically. In orthostatic hypotension caused by autonomic failure, there are considerable difficulties in reestablishing sympathetic or parasympathetic efferent activity.

Tilt study or tilt-table testing may be used to assess hypotension by monitoring blood pressure and pulse while tilting a person from horizontal supine to 60 degrees upright. This test has proved very valuable in determining the cause of dizziness or syncope and can reveal irregularities in the vascular regulating system. A combination of general measures and pharmacologic measures is needed in the management of neurogenic postural hypotension.

## SPECIAL IMPLICATIONS FOR THE THERAPIST 12.7

### *Orthostatic Hypotension*

Many medications used to treat hypertension can result in hypotension, especially when combined with interventions or exercise that result in vasodilation. Of particular concern are heat modalities, such as the whirlpool or aquatic therapy in a warm pool. In addition, moderate to vigorous exercise of large muscle groups can produce significant vasodilation and can result in hypotension. This is particularly true following exercise, when venous return diminishes as exercise abruptly ceases. A cool-down period is essential, and safety measures must be employed.[176]

Stationary standing, as is performed in many activities of daily living, can produce hypotension, especially among those individuals with autonomic failure. With autonomic failure, symptoms of postural hypotension are also increased on standing after exercise. The therapist can instruct the individual in protective measures that reduce excessive orthostatic blood pooling, including avoidance of precipitating factors.

Anyone with orthostatic hypotension, especially persons taking antihypertensive agents, should be instructed to rise slowly from the bed or chair after a long period of recumbency or sitting to avoid loss of balance and prevent falls. Dorsiflexing the feet (ankle pumps), raising the arms overhead with diaphragmatic breathing, and abdominal compression before standing often promote venous return to the heart, accelerate the pulse, and increase blood pressure, thus lessening a hypotensive response to the change in position.

The use of abdominal binders and elastic stockings may also help with venous return.[253] Stockings should not be taken off at night to avoid falls when getting up to go to the bathroom or when getting out of bed in the morning. Elevating the head of the bed 5 to 20 degrees prevents the nocturnal diuresis and supine hypertension caused by nocturnal shifts of interstitial fluid from the legs to the rest of the circulation. Eating small meals may help to avoid postprandial (after eating) hypotension.

The person who becomes hypotensive should assume a supine position with legs elevated to increase venous return and to ensure cerebral blood flow. As previously mentioned, this position must be monitored carefully for anyone with orthostatic hypotension and HF, possibly requiring modifying the position to include slight head and upper body elevation. Crossing the legs, which involves contraction of the agonist and antagonist muscles, also has been shown to increase cardiac output, thereby increasing blood pressure.[363]

The physician should be notified if the person remains symptomatic after these measures have been taken. Anyone who is considered borderline hypotensive when tested in the supine position should have blood pressures measured and pulses counted in a sitting position with the legs dangling. If no change occurs when this is done, repeat the measurements with the person standing, if possible. A drop in systolic pressure of 10 to 20 mm Hg or more that is associated with an increase in pulse rate of more than 15 beats/min suggests depleted intravascular volume (Fig. 12.16). Some normovolemic persons with peripheral neuropathies or those taking antihypertensive medications may demonstrate an orthostatic fall in blood pressure but without an associated increase in pulse rate.

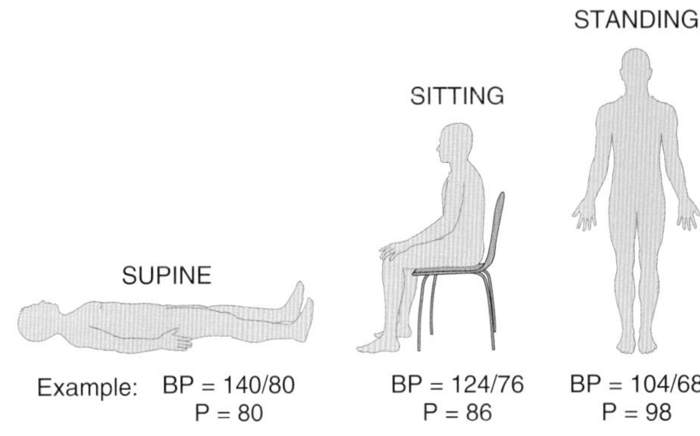


**Figure 12.16**

**Assessing postural hypotension.** After measuring the blood pressure (BP) and pulse (P) in the supine position, leave the blood pressure cuff in place and assist the person in sitting. Remeasure the blood pressure within 15 to 30 seconds. Assist the person in standing, and measure again. A drop of more than 20 mm Hg systolic and more than 10 mm Hg diastolic indicates postural hypotension. Sample measurements are given. (From Freeman R, Wieling W, Axelrod FB, et al. Consensus statement on the definition of orthostatic hypotension, neurally mediated syncope and the postural tachycardia syndrome. *Auton Neurosci.* 2011;161(1–2):46–48.)

## Myocardial Disease

### Myocarditis

Myocarditis is a relatively uncommon acute or chronic inflammatory condition of the muscular walls of the heart (myocardium). It has been classified by the AHA as a primary acquired (inflammatory) cardiomyopathy.[240]

It is most often a result of bacterial or viral infection, but it also includes those inflammatory processes related to infectious and noninfectious causes of ischemic heart disease. Other possible causes of myocarditis include chest radiation for treatment of malignancy, sarcoidosis, and drugs, such as lithium, IL-2, and cocaine.

The therapist is most likely to treat the person with systemic lupus erythematosus (SLE) who may have a type of myocarditis called *lupus carditis*. SLE is a multisystem autoimmune disease characterized by a release of autoantibodies into the circulation, with a subsequent inflammatory process that can target the heart and vasculature.

Myocarditis typically progresses through active, healing, and healed stages. Its pathobiology includes infiltration by inflammatory cells, leading to interstitial edema and focal myocyte necrosis, with replacement fibrosis developing over time. The heart electrical system changes, triggering the development of ventricular tachyarrhythmias. In some cases, myocarditis progresses to dilated cardiomyopathy with left ventricular dysfunction.[240]

Clinical evidence of cardiac involvement is found in up to 50% of all people with SLE. Clinical manifestations may include mild continuous chest pain or soreness in the epigastric region or under the sternum, palpitations, fatigue, and dyspnea; and onset may follow a viral upper respiratory tract illness in the population at large as well as in persons with SLE. Complications include HF, arrhythmias, dilated (congestive) cardiomyopathy (see next section), and sudden death.

Myocarditis usually resolves with treatment of the underlying condition or cause; specific antimicrobial therapy is prescribed if an infectious agent can be identified. Viral myocarditis is treated with medications that improve cardiac output and reduce arrhythmias, if present.

Management of myocarditis in SLE is usually with corticosteroids, but immunosuppressive agents may be required. Myocarditis that progresses to dilated cardiomyopathy with HF is frequently fatal without heart transplantation.

SPECIAL IMPLICATIONS FOR THE THERAPIST 12.8

*Myocarditis*

Active myocarditis is considered a contraindication for therapy, because this condition can progress very quickly and stress must be avoided. Each case should be evaluated by the physician. Athletes in whom myocarditis is suspected or diagnosed should discontinue all sports for 6 months after onset of symptoms. A follow-up with a cardiologist and exercise testing should be done before the athlete returns to sport.[284]

If an impairment of myocardial contractility is present, diastolic blood pressure may be elevated to maintain stroke volume. Disruptions leading to lethal cardiac arrhythmias cannot be predicted.

### Cardiomyopathy

**Definition and Overview.** Cardiomyopathy is part of a group of conditions affecting the heart muscle itself, so that contraction and relaxation of myocardial muscle fibers are impaired. The AHA uses the following definition for cardiomyopathy, reflecting the failure of myocardial performance due to mechanical (diastolic or systolic dysfunction) or electrical (arrhythmias) deficiency.

Cardiomyopathies are a heterogeneous group of diseases of the myocardium associated with mechanical and/or electrical dysfunction that usually (but not invariably) exhibit inappropriate ventricular hypertrophy or dilation and are the result of a variety of causes that frequently

**Table 12.14** American Heart Association (AHA) Classification of Cardiomyopathies

| Primary[a] | Secondary[b] |
|---|---|
| **Genetic**<br>• Hypertrophic cardiomyopathy<br>• Arrhythmogenic right ventricular cardiomyopathy/dysplasia (rare)<br>• Left ventricular noncompaction<br>• Conduction defects<br>• Ion channel disorders<br>**Mixed (genetic and nongenetic)**<br>• Dilated cardiomyopathy<br>• Restrictive (nonhypertrophied; rare)<br>**Acquired**<br>• Myocarditis (inflammatory cardiomyopathy)<br>• Stress-induced<br>• Peripartum/postpartum (rare)<br>• Infants of mothers with insulin-dependent diabetes mellitus | **Infiltrative**<br>Amyloidosis<br>Gaucher disease (genetic/familial)<br>Hurler disease (genetic/familial)<br>Hunter disease (genetic/familial)<br>**Storage**<br>Hemochromatosis<br>Glycogen storage disease<br>Niemann-Pick disease (genetic/familial)<br>Toxicity<br>Drugs, heavy metals, chemical agents<br>**Endomyocardial fibrosis**<br>**Inflammatory (sarcoidosis)**<br>**Endocrine**<br>Diabetes<br>Hyperthyroidism<br>Hypothyroidism<br>Hyperparathyroidism<br>Pheochromocytoma<br>Acromegaly<br>**Neuromuscular/neurologic**<br>Friedrich ataxia disease (genetic/familial)<br>Muscular dystrophy (genetic/familial)<br>Neurofibromatosis (genetic/familial)<br>Tuberous sclerosis<br>**Nutritional deficiencies**<br>Autoimmune<br>• Systemic lupus erythematosus<br>• Dermatomyositis<br>• Rheumatoid arthritis<br>• Scleroderma<br>• Polyarteritis nodosa<br>**Electrolyte imbalance**<br>**Cancer treatment (chemotherapy, radiation therapy)** |

[a]Predominantly involves the heart.
[b]Myocardial changes occur as part of a generalized systemic disorder affecting many organs. Only the most common diseases associated with cardiomyopathies are listed.
Data from Maron BJ, Towbin JA, Thiene G, et al: Contemporary definitions and classification of the cardiomyopathies: an American Heart Association Scientific Statement from the Council on Clinical Cardiology, Heart Failure and Transplantation Committee; Quality of Care and Outcomes Research and Functional Genomics and Translational Biology Interdisciplinary Working Groups; and Council on Epidemiology and Prevention, *Circulation* 113(14):1807–1816, 2006.

are genetic. Cardiomyopathies either are confined to the heart or are part of generalized systemic disorders, often leading to cardiovascular death or progressive heart failure–related disability.[240]

Cardiomyopathies are classified as *primary* and *secondary*, based on predominant organ involvement. Primary cardiomyopathies are confined to the heart muscle. Secondary cardiomyopathies include myocardial pathology that develops as part of a variety of generalized systemic disorders that affect the heart along with other organs at the same time.

Primary cardiomyopathies include genetic, mixed (genetic and nongenetic), and acquired (Table 12.14).

Genetic cardiomyopathies include hypertrophic and arrhythmogenic right ventricular cardiomyopathies, left ventricular noncompaction, conduction system disease, and ion channelopathies. In general, these congenital or familial types of cardiomyopathies are fairly uncommon individually, but a growing number of different types caused by mutations in genetic encoding have been identified. Mixed cardiomyopathies include dilated and primary restrictive nonhypertrophied cardiomyopathies. An example of an acquired cardiomyopathy is myocarditis. Considerable overlap can occur among the primary classifications within the same person, as sometimes cardiomyopathy progresses from one category to another during the natural history of the disease.

**Incidence and Risk Factors.** Cardiomyopathy can affect any age group and is often seen in young adults in the second and third decades. The actual incidence is unknown, but the disease may be more common than was previously realized.

This increase in incidence may be attributed to two important variables: (1) improved technology, which has allowed for more accurate evaluation of ventricular dimensions and ventricular wall movement; and (2) an increased incidence of myocarditis, an important precursor to cardiomyopathy, as a result of a wide variety of pathogens, toxins, and autoimmune reactions. There is a subset of patients that develop cardiomyopathy after an MI. In these patients, the higher incidence is attributable to advances in care for MI, so there is lower incidence of immediate mortality.

*Hypertrophic cardiomyopathy* is an autosomal dominant genetic trait. Over 2,000 mutations in 11 genes coding for sarcomeric proteins have been linked with hypertrophic cardiomyopathy.[239] It is the most frequently occurring cardiomyopathy (prevalence is 1 in 500; 1 in 200 if estimated using both clinical and genetic diagnoses) and the most common cause of sudden cardiac death in the young (including trained athletes).[239,240] Although the disease affects an estimated 750,000 people in the United States, only 100,000 have been diagnosed; women and African Americans have been especially underdiagnosed. This form of cardiomyopathy occurs more often in adolescents and young adults.

*Dilated cardiomyopathy* occurs most often in persons in their third or fourth decade.[59] With a prevalence of 1:2,500 it is the third most frequent cause of HF and most frequent cause of heart transplantation. About 20% to 35% of cases are linked to mutations in a diverse group of genes, and the remainder result from some known disease process (e.g., viral or bacterial infection toxins, rheumatic fever, myasthenia gravis, progressive muscular dystrophy, hemochromatosis, amyloidosis, sarcoidosis).[240] Risk factors for dilated cardiomyopathy include long-term alcohol abuse, myocarditis, drugs, toxins, endocrine disturbances, and inborn errors of metabolism (in children). African Americans have a threefold higher risk of developing dilated cardiomyopathy and a 1.5- to 2-fold risk of dying from it compared to white populations.[59]

*Restrictive cardiomyopathy* occurs as a result of myocardial fibrosis (e.g., amyloidosis, sarcoidosis, hemochromatosis), hypertrophy, infiltration, or defect in myocardial relaxation. Some cases have familial origin. It is the least common form of cardiomyopathy.

*Peripartum (postpartum) cardiomyopathy* is a rare but very serious disease that results in HF. It is a dilated form and may appear for no apparent reason during the last month of pregnancy or the first 5 months after delivery. In half of the cases, it resolves within 6 months. Incidence is higher among multiparous women older than 30 years, particularly those with malnutrition or preeclampsia. Estimates vary, but the occurrence may be 1 in every 1,300 to 4,000 deliveries.[159] Maternal death from HF, blood clots, infection, and stillbirth can occur. Symptoms of orthopnea, cough, palpitations, and high blood pressure may not occur until several weeks after delivery.

*Chemotherapy-induced cardiomyopathy* is one of the cardiovascular complications of cancer therapy. Risk factors for its development include increasing doses of chemotherapeutic agents and their nature.[82,167] Anthrocyclines are the major cause of this type of cardiomyopathy. Other cancer therapy agents such as trastuzumab and protease inhibitors can also cause cardiomyopathy.[81]

**Pathogenesis.** The exact pathogenesis of cardiomyopathy is unknown; the risk factors mentioned previously seem to lower the threshold for the development of cardiomyopathy. For example, heavy consumption of alcohol is thought to cause dilated cardiomyopathy through several mechanisms:

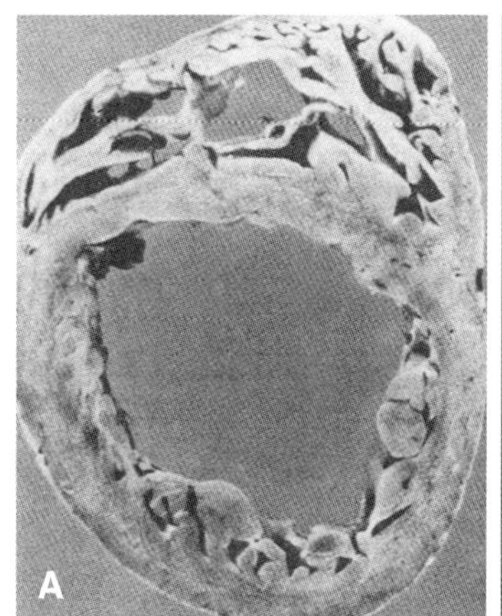


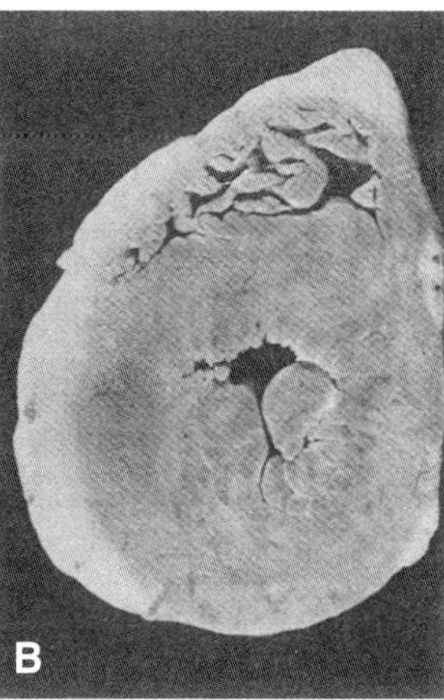


**Figure 12.17**

(A) Cross-sectional view of dilated cardiomyopathy. (B) Hypertrophied heart. (From Kinney M: *Comprehensive cardiac care,* ed 7, St Louis, 1991, Mosby, pp. 346, 349.)

direct toxic effect of alcohol or of its metabolites; effects of nutritional deficiencies, especially thiamine deficiency; and toxic effects of beverage additives, such as cobalt.

Obesity produces an increase in total blood volume and cardiac output because of the high metabolic activity of excessive fat. In moderate to severe cases of obesity, this may lead to left ventricular dilation, increased left ventricular wall stress, and left ventricular diastolic dysfunction.

Hypertrophic cardiomyopathy is distinguished by inappropriate and excessive left ventricular hypertrophy (thickening of the wall and interventricular septum) and normal or even enhanced cardiac muscle contractile function. Over time, the overgrowth of the wall leads to rigidity in the myocardium. The result is decreased diastolic functioning, because the rigid myocardium cannot relax during the diastolic phase, reducing the amount of blood flowing into the ventricles.

Regardless of the underlying cause, dilated cardiomyopathy results from extensively damaged myocardial muscle fibers and is characterized by cardiac enlargement. The heart ejects blood less efficiently than normal, so that a large volume of blood remains in the left ventricle after systole, which results in ventricular dilation with enlargement and dilation of all four chambers and eventually leads to HF (Figs. 12.17 and 12.18).

Restrictive cardiomyopathy is characterized by marked endocardial scarring (fibrosis) of the ventricles, and the resulting rigidity impairs diastolic filling due to lack of myocardial distension.

**Clinical Manifestations.** Generally, the symptoms of cardiomyopathy are the same as for HF (e.g., dyspnea, orthopnea, tachycardia, palpitations, peripheral edema, distended jugular vein).

Hypertrophic cardiomyopathy is frequently asymptomatic, sudden death being the presenting sign. In fact, hypertrophic cardiomyopathy is the most common cause of sudden death in young competitive athletes.[369] The most common symptom is dyspnea caused by high pulmonary pressures produced by the elevated left ventricular diastolic pressure; symptoms are often exacerbated during strenuous exercise.

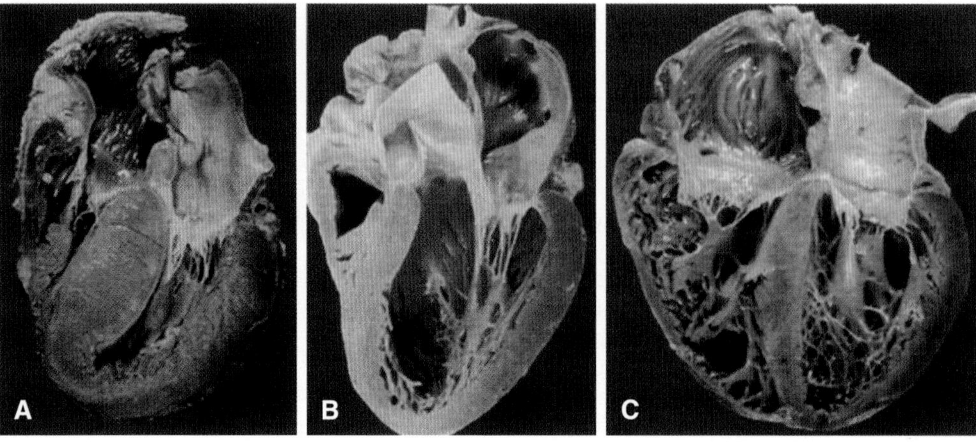


**Figure 12.18**

**Gross pathologic specimens of the cardiomyopathies.** (A) Hypertrophic cardiomyopathy, showing a marked increase in myocardial mass and preferential hypertrophy of the interventricular septum. (B) Normal heart, with normal left ventricular dimensions and thickness. (C) Dilated cardiomyopathy, showing marked increase in chamber size. Atrial enlargement is also evident in both cardiomyopathies (A and C). (From Seidman JG, Seidman C: The genetic basis for cardiomyopathy: from mutation identification to mechanistic paradigms, *Cell* 104:557, 2001.)

Dilated cardiomyopathy is characterized by fatigue and weakness; chest pain (unlike angina) may occur. Blood pressure is usually normal or low.

Restrictive cardiomyopathy causes clinical manifestations related to decreasing cardiac output. As cardiac output falls and intraventricular pressures rise, signs of HF appear. The earliest manifestations may include exercise intolerance, fatigue, and shortness of breath, followed by other symptoms such as peripheral edema and ascites.

## MEDICAL MANAGEMENT

**DIAGNOSIS AND TREATMENT.** Diagnosis requires exclusion of other causes of cardiac dysfunction, especially causes of HF and arrhythmias. Catheterization to assess arteries and valves, echocardiography, chest radiography, blood chemistries, genetic mutation analysis (for hypertrophic cardiomyopathy), and ECG are specific tests that are performed. Researchers continue to investigate ways to monitor people with cardiomyopathy and to devise noninvasive diagnostic techniques.

Comprehensive practice guidelines are available for the diagnosis and treatment of hypertrophic[148] and dilated[59] cardiomyopathies. Treatment of patients with established cardiomyopathy is directed at clinical symptoms of HF and arrhythmias. The specific treatment of cardiomyopathy is determined by the underlying cause and may include physical, dietary, or pharmacologic interventions; mechanical circulatory support; or surgical intervention, including transplantation. Cardiac resynchronization therapy has been shown to be effective in the treatment of cardiomyopathy.[244]

ACE inhibitors and β-blockers are used for some forms of hypertrophic[148]and dilated[59] and cardiomyopathies. Calcium channel blocking agents (see Table 12.5) may be used to relieve symptoms and reduce exercise intolerance. Restrictive cardiomyopathy has no specific treatment interventions. The goal is to control HF through the use of diuretics, vasodilators, and salt restriction.

**PROGNOSIS.** Seventy-five percent of persons diagnosed with idiopathic dilated cardiomyopathy die within 5 years after the onset of symptoms, because diagnosis does not usually occur until advanced stages. Persons with hypertrophic cardiomyopathy can lead long, relatively asymptomatic lives. Some people have a history of gradually progressive symptoms, but others experience sudden death, especially during exercise, as the initial diagnostic event. Restrictive cardiomyopathy may cause sudden death as a result of arrhythmia, or a more progressive course may occur, with eventual HF. Intervention rarely results in long-term improvement.

Many persons with various types of cardiomyopathy experience stabilization or even an improvement in symptoms, but the end result of cardiomyopathy is sudden death or a fatal progression toward HF. No cure exists, outside of cardiac transplantation. Heart transplantation shows a 1-year survival rate of greater than 80% and a 3-year survival rate of 70% for dilated cardiomyopathy. The 1-year survival rate without transplantation is 5%.

**SPECIAL IMPLICATIONS FOR THE THERAPIST 12.9**

### *Cardiomyopathy*

Sudden death can occur, but the incidence is rare. It occurs more often in younger people who have cardiomyopathy, and it may be avoided by eliminating strenuous exercise (e.g., running, competitive sports) when a diagnosis has been established. Rest improves cardiac function and reduces heart size.

During the early stages of the disease, many people find it difficult to accept activity restrictions and need encouragement to follow guidelines for activity restriction. Clients should avoid poorly tolerated activities; combine rest with activity; understand that physical stress and emotional stress exacerbate the disease; learn correct breathing techniques, avoid any Valsalva maneuver as it decreases the inflow of venous blood and impairs outflow; and understand that alcohol depresses myocardial contractility and should be eliminated.

The therapist can provide valuable information regarding energy conservation techniques to assist persons with continued independence in activities of daily living and possibly even with improvement of activity tolerance. This is especially true for the person awaiting a cardiac transplant. The therapist involved with athletes (of all ages) is advised to follow the AHA guidelines for preparticipation screening and identifying athletes at risk for sudden cardiac death.[241]

Cardiomyopathy associated with cardiotoxicity following chemotherapy is often clinically silent because of the clients' low levels of physical activity. An evaluation to screen for potential cardiopulmonary dysfunction is essential with these clients.

The evaluation should include an assessment of current physical activity levels and exercise tolerance and monitoring of heart rate and rhythm, blood pressure, respiratory responses, and any other signs and symptoms of exercise intolerance (e.g., dyspnea, fatigue, light-headedness or dizziness, pallor, palpitations, chest discomfort). A scale that rates perceived exertion (see Table 12.13) is often useful during the evaluation and for establishing initial exercise guidelines toward improving endurance.

For the person who has been hospitalized and has not ambulated yet, the therapist will need to assess tolerance to activities at the edge of the bed before ambulating. During activities, monitor pulse, oxygen saturation, respirations, blood pressure, and color. The heart rate, systolic blood pressure, and respiratory rate normally increase in proportion to the exercise (movement) intensity, whereas the diastolic blood pressure changes minimally (±10 mm Hg).

Improved activity tolerance may be demonstrated by minimal change in pulse or blood pressure during activities with minimal fatigue after the activity. Pulse, respirations, and blood pressure should return to a normal range within 3 minutes of the end of the activity. Discontinue any activity that results in chest pain, severe dyspnea, cyanosis, dizziness, hypotension, or sustained tachycardia. Abnormal responses include either blunted or excessive rises in heart rate or systolic blood pressure, excessive increases in diastolic blood pressure or respiratory rate, a fall in systolic blood pressure with increasing activity, or increasing irregularity of the pulse. These signs may be the result of cardiopulmonary toxicity or simply the result of deconditioning. Any signs of intolerance to activity should be documented, and cardiac changes outside of the normally expected changes should be discussed with the physician. If the person is receiving diuretics, monitor for signs of too-vigorous diuresis (e.g., muscle cramps, orthostatic hypotension). If the person becomes hypotensive, use a supine position with legs elevated to increase venous return and to ensure cerebral blood flow.

## Trauma

### Nonpenetrating

Any blunt chest trauma may produce myocardial contusion, resulting in myocardial hemorrhage with little if any myocardial scar once healing is complete. The most common blunt trauma to the chest occurs by the steering wheel impact from an automobile accident or striking the chest onto an object during a fall. Large contusions may lead to myocardial scars, cardiac rupture, HF, or formation of aneurysms. When a client sustains a chest trauma, it is important to watch for pericardial effusion. Fluid can build up in the pericardial space after the trauma and if left untreated it can lead to HF or death.

The chest pain of myocardial contusion is similar to that of MI and is often confused with musculoskeletal pain from soft tissue consequences of chest trauma. Myocardial contusion is usually treated similarly to MI, with initial monitoring and subsequent progressive ambulation and cardiac rehabilitation.

### Penetrating

Penetrating cardiac injuries are most often caused by external objects, such as bullets or knives, and sometimes from bony fragments secondary to chest injury. Iatrogenic causes of cardiac penetrating injury include perforation of the heart during catheterization and cardiac trauma from cardiopulmonary resuscitation. Complications include arrhythmias, aneurysm formation, death from infection (e.g., bacterial endocarditis or infection from a retained foreign body), a form of pericarditis associated with this type of injury, ventricular septal defects, and foreign body embolus.

## Myocardial Neoplasm

Primary cardiac tumors are rare, with an autopsy frequency of 0.001 to 0.030%.[102] Malignant cardiac tumors account for 9.5% of primary cardiac tumors, with 95% to 98% of these tumors being sarcomas arising from connective tissue (e.g., myxoma, rhabdomyoma, mesothelioma, fibroelastoma) and the remaining 2% to 5% being lymphomas.[102]

Some of these sarcomas are limited to the myocardium, replacing functional cardiac tissue with cancerous cells without any intracavity extension. These tumors may produce no cardiac symptoms or may present with arrhythmias and conduction disturbances.

Tumors projecting into a cardiac cavity may present with progressive HF, precordial pain, pericardial effusion tamponade, arrhythmias, conduction disturbances, and sudden death. Because these tumors occur more frequently in the right side of the heart, right-sided heart failure is more common (jugular venous distention, ascites, systemic edema). People with sarcomas face a rapid functional decline, with death occurring from a few weeks to 2 years after onset of symptoms. These tumors proliferate rapidly, invading and damaging not only the myocardium but contiguous structures such as the venae cavae and tricuspid valve as well.[68]

Benign primary cardiac tumors occur approximately three times more often than malignant primary tumors, with myxomas accounting for nearly 50% of these primary benign tumors.[102] Myxomas arise most often from the endothelial surface of the left atrium, causing mechanical interference with cardiac function including intracardiac obstruction. Tumors located in other cardiac chambers account for 10% of myxomas. Other benign cardiac tumors (also rare) include lipoma, papilloma, fibroelastoma, rhabdomyoma, and fibroma.

Signs of obstruction can include right-sided heart failure, pulmonary edema, orthopnea, and dyspnea. Constitutional symptoms include fatigue, fever, weight loss, arthralgia, and myalgia. Embolization caused by fragments from the tumor can also occur in these individuals. If the tumor is in the left side of the heart, the emboli result in infarction damage to the viscera, including the heart, limbs, kidneys, and CNS.[304] Because these tumors often lie in the atrial cavity they can (if large enough) cause damage to the mitral valve or even block the orifice of this valve, leading to sudden death. Tumors found in the right side of the heart infrequently lead to pulmonary hypertension and PEs.

Metastases to the heart and pericardium are much more common, occurring 100 to 1000 times more often than primary cardiac tumors.[68,309] Melanoma has the highest frequency of metastasis to the heart, with metastases also possible from carcinomas of the lung, breast, and esophagus and malignant leukemia and lymphoma.[305]

A tumor may involve the heart by one of four metastatic pathways: retrograde lymphatic extension, hematogenous spread, direct contiguous extension, or transvenous extension. Metastatic involvement of the heart and pericardium may go unrecognized until autopsy. Impairment of cardiac function occurs in approximately 30% of cases and is usually attributed to pericardial effusion. The clinical presentation includes shortness of breath, cough, anterior thoracic pain, pleuritic chest pain, or peripheral edema. Cardiac neoplasms come to the attention of a therapist when (1) progressive interference with mitral valve function results in exercise intolerance or exertional dyspnea; (2) embolus causes a stroke; or (3) systemic manifestations occur, including muscle atrophy, arthralgias, malaise, or Raynaud phenomenon.

Diagnosis of myxomas and other cardiac neoplasms is usually made by echocardiography followed by imaging studies, with MRI being of greater value in delineating cardiac tumors.[309] There are no specific physical or laboratory tests for metastatic heart disease, and diagnosis is difficult, as these tumors can masquerade as other cardiac defects. ECG is nonspecific, chest radiography may reveal an enlarged cardiac silhouette, and radionuclide angiography is helpful in diagnosing intracavity tumors. Two-dimensional echocardiography is the method of choice to detect cardiac metastases.[305]

Treatment of choice for myxomas is usually resection of the tumor, which in most cases is curative. Cardiac rehabilitation may be required according to the individual's postoperative cardiovascular condition and the amount of heart tissue removed. Recurrence is rare and appears to be the result of incomplete resection of the tumor or intraoperative dislocation of tumor material. The presence of cancer cells in more than one area of the myocardium (multifocal genesis) may also lead to recurrence despite treatment.[267]

In most cases, cardiac metastases are treated with palliative care because advanced disease is present at the time of diagnosis. Radiation is not typically used to treat cardiac neoplasms, which means that radiation heart disease occurs secondarily to radiation therapy for tumors in the area of the heart (e.g., mediastinum, breast, head and neck, and thyroid). A history of such tumors should alert the therapist to the possibility that cardiac defects may be present.

## Congenital Heart Disease

### Overview and Incidence

Congenital heart disease is an anatomic defect in the heart that develops in utero during the first trimester and is present at birth in approximately 1% of births in the United States.[50] Over the past 3 decades, major advances have been made in the diagnosis and treatment of congenital heart disease, resulting in many more children who have survived to adulthood with surgically corrected or uncorrected anomalies. Today, there are more than 2 million children and adults with congenital heart conditions. Congenital heart disease affects about 10 of every 1000 babies born in the United States, making this the most common category of congenital structural malformation.[237] Other than prematurity, it is the major cause of death in the first year of life. Children with congenital heart disease are also more likely to have extracardiac defects, such as tracheoesophageal fistula, diaphragmatic hernias, and renal abnormalities.

There are two categories of congenital heart disease: cyanotic and acyanotic (Table 12.15). In clinical practice, this system of classification is problematic, because children with acyanotic defects may develop cyanosis, and those with cyanotic defects may be pink and have more clinical signs of HF.

*Cyanotic* defects result from obstruction of blood flow to the lungs or mixing of oxygen desaturated blue venous blood with fully saturated red arterial blood within the chambers of the heart. Most *acyanotic* defects involve primarily left-to-right shunting through an abnormal opening.

### Etiologic Factors

Many congenital heart diseases have genetic causes with well-known chromosomal anomalies (e.g., trisomy 13, 18, 21; Turner syndrome). They account for 9% to 18% of all congenital heart defects. Single-point mutations, particularly in genes of cardiac transcription factors, are implicated in congenital cardiovascular defects. Approximately 10% of the defects are caused by de novo mutations, mostly in chromatin-regulating genes.[50] For the remainder, the causes are either unknown or involve multiple factors,[50] such as alcohol consumption, smoking[12] (including secondhand smoking), air pollutants, maternal rubella infection during the first trimester, preeclampsia, folate deficiency, altitude, maternal obesity,[286] and diabetes (both pregestational and gestational).[50,366]

### Pathogenesis

The heart begins to form from a tube-like structure during the fourth week after conception. As development progresses, the tube lengthens and forms chambers, septa, and valves. Anything that interferes with this developmental process during the first 8 to 10 weeks of pregnancy can result in a congenital defect (Fig. 12.19).

**Cyanotic.** In *transposition of the great vessels,* no communication exists between systemic and pulmonary circulations, so that the pulmonary artery leaves the left

**Table 12.15** Congenital Heart Disease

| Defect | Incidence | Clinical Manifestations | Prognosis |
|---|---|---|---|
| **Cyanotic** | | | |
| Transposition of the great vessels | 16%[a]; 3:1 male-to-female ratio | Depends on size and type of defects; cyanosis; HF (newborn) | Improved surgical treatment provides excellent long-term outcome |
| Tetralogy of Fallot | 10%–15% | *Infants:* acutely cyanotic at birth or progressive cyanosis first year<br>*Children:* hypoxic events with tachypnea, increasing cyanosis, digital clubbing; poor growth and development; seizures, loss of consciousness, death possible<br>*Adults:* dyspnea, limited exercise tolerance | At risk for sudden lethal arrhythmias; mild obstruction progresses with age; reduced life expectancy |
| Tricuspid atresia | <1%; relatively rare | Newborn cyanosis; tachycardia; dyspnea digital clubbing (older child) | Unreported; depends on success of treatment |
| **Acyanotic** | | | |
| Ventricular septal defect | 25%; single most common CHD; 25%–40% close spontaneously by age 2 yr; 90% close by age 10 yr | Asymptomatic with small defect; HF (age 1–6 mo); history of frequent respiratory infections; poor growth and development; dyspnea, fatigue and exercise intolerance (older child) | No physical restrictions |
| Atrial septal defect | 10% children; 2:1 female-to-male ratio<br>Accounts for 33% of all congenital heart disease cases surviving to adulthood | *Older child*: asymptomatic; growth failure; HF<br>*Adult*: fatigue or dyspnea on exertion | No physical restrictions if corrected; frequent complications in adults |
| Coarctation of the aorta | 6%; 3:1 male-to-female ratio | High systolic blood pressure and bounding pulses in arms; weak or absent femoral pulses; cool lower extremities with lower blood pressure<br>*Infants:* HF<br>*Children:* headaches, fainting, epistaxis (hypertension); exercise intolerance, easy fatigability<br>*Adults:* asymptomatic or signs of hypertension (headache, epistaxis, dizziness, palpitations) | No physical restrictions if corrected; frequent complications in adults |
| Patent ductus arteriosus | 12%; spontaneous closure in normal term infants by day 4; common in children born to mothers affected by rubella during first trimester; increased incidence in infants born at high altitudes (higher than 10,000 ft); present in 20%–60% of premature infants weighing <1500 g | *Children:* asymptomatic; HF<br>*Adult:* if symptomatic: fatigue, dyspnea, palpitations | Closure may occur up to age 2 yr; normal life expectancy with small defect; aneurysm and rupture can occur; poor prognosis for large defect without transplantation |
| Aortic stenosis | 5% of all congenital heart disease | Asymptomatic; exercise intolerance, dizziness, and chest pain with prolonged standing | Good with early detection and surgical treatment; exercise testing recommended before participation in athletics |

[a]Figures account for percentage of all congenital heart disease.
*CHD*, Congenital heart disease; *HF*, heart failure.

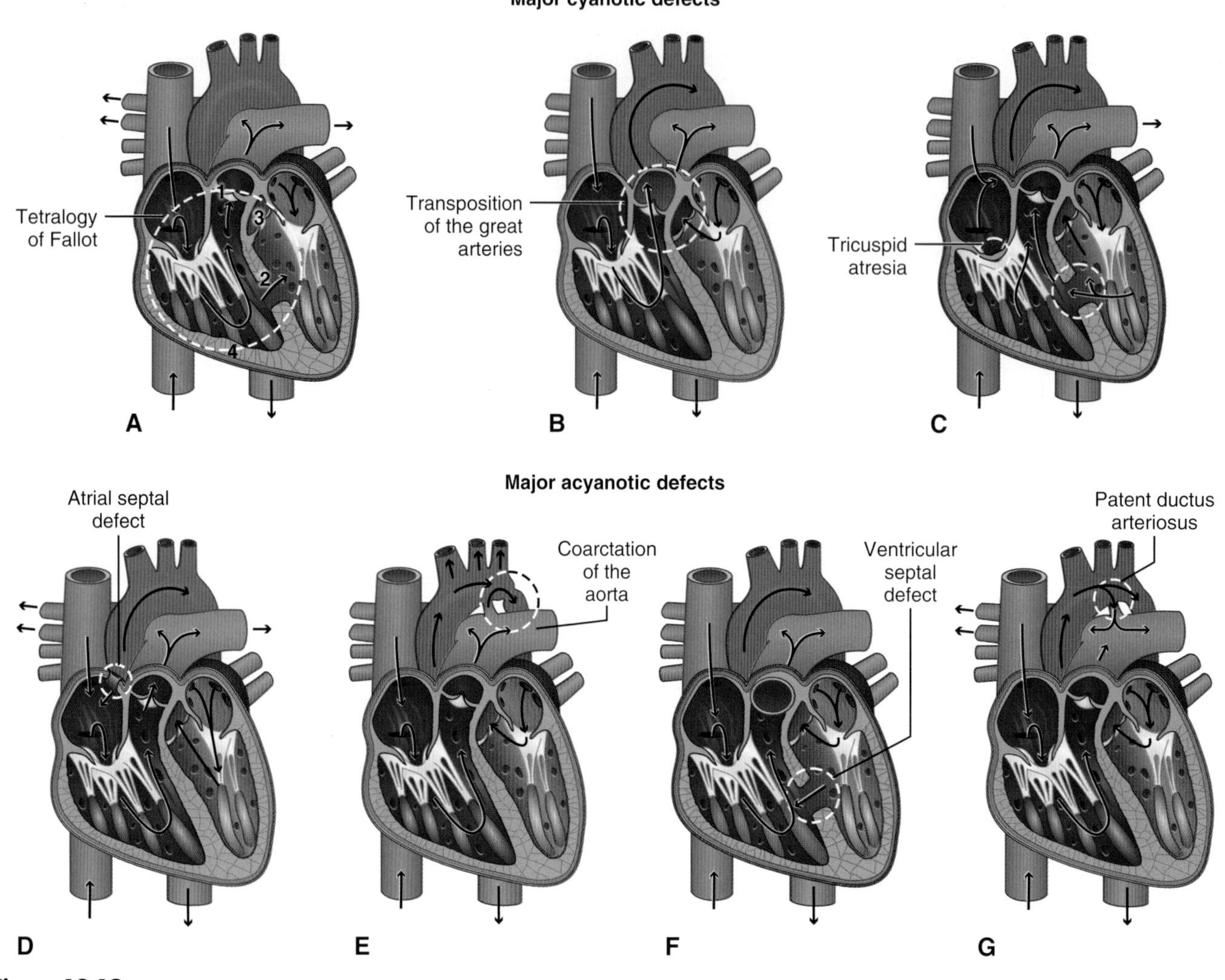


**Figure 12.19**

**Major cyanotic defects (see Fig. 12.1 for normal structure and circulation of the heart).** (A) *Tetralogy of Fallot* has four defects: (1) pulmonary stenosis: narrowing at or just below the pulmonary valve; (2) ventricular septal defect (VSD): hole between the two bottom chambers (ventricles) of the heart; (3) aorta is positioned over the ventricular septal defect instead of in the left ventricle; (4) right ventricle is more muscular than normal. (B) *Transposition of the great arteries:* systemic venous blood returns to the right atrium and then goes to the right ventricle and on to the aorta instead of going to the lung via the pulmonary artery. (C) *Tricuspid atresia:* failure of the tricuspid valve to develop with a lack of communication from the right atrium to the right ventricle. Major acyanotic defects: (D) *Atrial septal defect:* blood from the pulmonary vein enters the left atrium, and some blood crosses the atrial septal defect into the right atrium and ventricle. (E) *Coarctation of the aorta:* severe obstruction of blood flow in the descending thoracic aorta. (F) *Ventricular septal defect:* when the left ventricle contracts, it ejects some blood into the aorta and some across the ventricular septal defect into the right ventricle and pulmonary artery. (G) *Patent ductus arteriosus:* some of the blood from the aorta crosses the ductus arteriosus and flows into the pulmonary artery.

ventricle and the aorta exits from the right ventricle. For the infant with this condition to survive, there must be communication between the two circuits. In approximately one third of all cases, another associated defect occurs that permits intracardiac mixing (e.g., atrial septal defect, ventricular septal defect, patent ductus arteriosus), but two thirds of cases have no other defect present, and severe cyanosis develops.[60]

*Tetralogy of Fallot* consists of four classic defects: (1) pulmonary stenosis, (2) large ventricular septal defect, (3) aortic communication with both ventricles, and (4) right ventricular hypertrophy. This infant will need urgent reconstruction due to the complications from these four abnormalities. *Tricuspid atresia* is a failure of the tricuspid valve to develop, with a lack of communication from the right atrium to the right ventricle. Blood flows through an atrial septal defect or a ductus arteriosus to the left side of the heart and through a ventricular septal defect to the right ventricle and out to the lungs. There is complete mixing of unoxygenated and oxygenated blood in the left side of the heart, resulting in systemic desaturation and varying amounts of pulmonary obstruction.

**Acyanotic.** *Ventricular septal defect* is an abnormal opening between the right and left ventricles that may vary in size from a small pinhole to complete absence of the septum, resulting in a common ventricle. *Atrial septal defect* is an abnormal opening between the atria, allowing blood from the higher-pressure left atrium to flow into the lower-pressure right atrium.

*Coarctation of the aorta* is a localized narrowing near the insertion of the ductus arteriosus, resulting in increased pressure proximal to the defect (head, upper extremities) and decreased pressure distal to the obstruction (body, lower extremities).

*Patent ductus arteriosus* is a failure of the fetal ductus arteriosus (artery connecting the aorta and pulmonary artery) to close within the first weeks of life. The continued function of this vessel allows blood to flow from the high-pressure aorta to the low-pressure pulmonary artery, causing continuous flow from the aorta to the pulmonary artery (referred to as left-to-right shunting). A patent ductus arteriosus rarely closes spontaneously after infancy.

*Congenital aortic stenosis* is discussed later in this chapter in "Diseases Affecting the Heart Valves."

### Clinical Manifestations

The most common signs and symptoms include cyanosis and signs of HF (e.g., dyspnea, pulmonary edema, fatigue). See Table 12.15 for clinical manifestations of each particular defect. Complications may include HF, pulmonary edema, pneumonia, hypoxia, and sudden death. There is often a risk of bacterial endocarditis and pulmonary vascular obstructive disease later in life.

It is important to recognize the presence of neurodevelopmental delays or disabilities seen in those with congenital heart disease.[333] As these children reach school age, they have a two to three times higher incidence of neurodevelopmental disabilities and 10% to 15% incidence of behavioral disorders (anxiety, mood changes) than seen in the general population of children the same ages.[146] It is possible that both congenital heart disease and abnormal brain development may be influenced by genetic contributions, causing a developmental delay in both.

A decrease in the infant's ability to grow in weight, called failure to thrive, is also very common postsurgically in infants with congenital heart disease.[101] Up to 15% of the infants have been found to be malnourished and about 35% undernourished.[265] Weight loss postsurgery can lead to higher mortality rates,[171] as well as cognitive and/or behavioral issues as the child develops.[120] Therefore, it is important for the therapist to work with the dietician and the child's parents to ensure proper nutrition. Doing so will allow the child to have enough energy for physical activity and ability to reach physical developmental milestones.

### MEDICAL MANAGEMENT

**PREVENTION AND DIAGNOSIS.** With the whole genome sequenced and advances in genetic tools, identification of genetic mutations predisposing to congenital heart disease may allow preventive measures by modulation of secondary genetic or environmental factors. Until then, most forms of congenital heart disease can potentially be detected in utero with the routine use of ultrasonography.

The prenatal diagnosis of a major cardiac malformation requires further assessment for extracardiac and chromosomal disorders. Conversely, diagnosis of Down syndrome (prenatally or postnatally) requires early cardiologic assessment for cardiac anomalies, most commonly atrioventricular and ventricular septal defects. Prenatal knowledge of cardiac anomalies allows for optimal prenatal and postnatal management.

Prenatal screening for maternal rubella antibodies provides important information for further diagnostic testing. In cases where prenatal diagnosis does not occur and when there are no symptoms initially, cardiac anomalies can remain undetected for years and even decades. For example, a person with atrial septal defect may have normal sinus rhythm for the first three decades of life and then develop atrial fibrillation (AF) and supraventricular tachycardia (SVT).[60] Occasionally a diagnosis isn't made until late adolescence or adulthood, when the client's growing body puts too much stress on their compromised heart. Clinical diagnosis begins with detection of signs and symptoms, auscultation, and detection of heart murmur. TEE, Doppler color-flow echocardiography, and now RT3D echocardiography provide a definitive diagnosis without invasive cardiac catheterization and angiography.

**TREATMENT AND PROGNOSIS.** Remarkable innovations in medical and surgical approaches over the past several decades now allow for correction of major cardiac defects in children, even in early infancy.[367] In utero correction, called fetal cardiac intervention, is possible. This is only done in specific cases, and the physician weighs all the risks with the possible benefits.[1] Typically, fetal cardiac intervention is reserved for clients when the morbidity rates are very high. Postnatally, curative or palliative (providing relief of symptoms) surgical correction is available for more than 90% of persons with congenital heart disease.

There is a clear trend toward complete correction of malformations rather than staged procedures to obtain initial palliation and delayed correction. The risk for most surgical procedures is low (between 1% and 5%).

Considering the neurodevelopmental component in congenital heart disease, interdisciplinary neurocardiac care program (involving developmental pediatricians, neurologists, occupational and physical therapists, speech and language pathologists, social workers, nurses, and dietitians) should be beneficial at improving the outcomes for these children.

**SPECIAL IMPLICATIONS FOR THE THERAPIST 12.10**

### *Congenital Heart Disease*

Therapists need to be alert to signs of HF in children with congenital heart disease and in infants with suspected congenital heart disease. Signs of HF indicate a worsening clinical condition; the earlier these are detected, the sooner intervention can be initiated.

The surgical procedures associated with the repair of congenital heart disease (e.g., bypass, deep hypothermia) can cause other complications or conditions. Although they are not very common, neurodevelopmental deficits such as choreoathetosis, cerebral palsy, or hemiparesis can result from surgical repair of a cardiac defect.[54]

Gross motor development can be negatively impacted by prolonged hospitalization, deficiencies in cardiovascular status, surgical techniques used to minimize blood loss, or any combination of these factors. The more complex the defect or defects and the more numerous the open heart surgeries required, the greater the risk for neurologic impairment.

Most children with significant heart defects will have had heart surgery before they start school. In addition to a developmental assessment, the therapist should evaluate for soft tissue restriction at the site of the healed scar (either sternal or thoracic), which may affect breathing capacity.

Physiologic response to therapy intervention can be assessed by observing skin color, respiratory effort, and behavioral response. Oxygen saturation monitors may not be helpful, because these children have abnormally low readings as their baseline level.

In general, anyone who has had successful surgery is allowed unrestricted sports activity. Young children with unrepaired tetralogy of Fallot instinctively learn to squat, getting into the flat-footed baseball catcher's stance when they are fatigued. This posture increases the tension in the leg muscles, reduces blood flow to the leg muscles, and raises peripheral resistance and blood pressure.

Care of pregnant women with congenital heart disease requires understanding of the specific congenital defect, the nature of previous surgical correction, and the presence of any complications or sequelae.[334]

## DISEASES AFFECTING THE CARDIAC NERVOUS SYSTEM

### Arrhythmias: Disturbances of Rate or Rhythm

#### Definition and Overview

The heart rhythm and the number of times the heart beats (rate) are generated and regulated by the sinoatrial (SA) node, the internal pacemaker located in the upper right portion of the heart. The signal from the SA node travels through the cardiac conduction system, first through the walls of the atria and then through the walls of the ventricles, causing the atrial (supraventricular) and ventricular chambers of the heart to contract and relax at regular rates necessary to maintain circulation at different levels of activity. An arrhythmia (dysrhythmia) is a disturbance of heart rate or rhythm caused by an abnormal rate of electrical impulse generation by the SA node or the abnormal conduction of impulses.

Arrhythmias can be classified according to their origin as ventricular or supraventricular (atrial), according to the pattern (fibrillation or flutter), or according to the speed or rate at which they occur (tachycardia or bradycardia).

Several types of AF are now recognized, including first-detected-episode AF (may or may not be symptomatic; may self-resolve), recurrent paroxysmal AF (two or more episodes that resolve spontaneously), persistent AF, and permanent AF. Persistent AF is sustained for more than 7 days. It can occur after a first-detected-episode AF or after recurrent paroxysmal AF. Permanent AF, also known as chronic AF, occurs when sinus rhythm cannot be sustained after cardioversion (normal heart rhythm returns spontaneously) or when the decision has been made to let AF continue without efforts to restore normal sinus rhythm.[190]

Arrhythmias vary in severity from mild, asymptomatic disturbances that require no intervention (e.g., sinus arrhythmia, in which the heart rate increases and decreases with respiration) to catastrophic ventricular fibrillation, which requires immediate resuscitation. The clinical significance depends on the effect on cardiac output and blood pressure, which is partially influenced by the site of origin.

#### Etiologic and Risk Factors and Incidence

Arrhythmias may be congenital or may result from one of several factors, including hypertrophy of heart muscle fibers secondary to hypertension, previous MI, HF, valvular heart disease, irritability after surgery, or degeneration of conductive tissue that is necessary to maintain normal heart rhythm (called *sick sinus syndrome*). Among risk factors diabetes, obstructive sleep apnea, smoking, alcohol use, increased pulse pressure, family history, left ventricle enlargement, and left ventricular wall thickness are listed.[190]

Between 2.7 and 6.1 million people in the United States have AF.[50] The prevalence of AF doubles with each advancing decade of age beginning at age 50 to 59 years, with a statistically significant increase among men ages 65 to 84 years, although this gap closes with advancing age and remains unexplained.[228]

BMI appears to correlate strongly with the risk of AF.[129] With each unit increment of BMI, the risk of AF increases 3%. A person who is obese has approximately a 34% greater risk of AF when compared to a person with normal BMI. Moreover, people in the heaviest BMI category have 2.3 times the risk.[118] Improved cardiac care has increased the number of survivors of cardiac incidents who may experience subsequent complications, such as AR or another arrhythmia.

Cardiac arrhythmias are very common in the setting of HF, with atrial and ventricular arrhythmias often present in the same person. Arrhythmias can occur when a portion of the heart is temporarily deprived of oxygen, disturbing the normal pathway of the heartbeat. Toxic doses of cardioactive drugs (e.g., digoxin and other cardiac glycosides), exposure to phenylpropanolamine found in some decongestants, alcohol and caffeine consumption, high fever, and excessive production of thyroid hormone (hyperthyroidism) may also lead to arrhythmias. In many cases, particularly in younger people, there is no known or apparent cause.

#### Pathogenesis and Clinical Manifestations

Arrhythmias can be changes in either the heart's rate or its cardiac conduction pattern. Some arrhythmias will affect rate only, some rhythm only, and some will affect both rate and rhythm.

**Rate.** The adult heart beats an average of 60 to 100 beats/min; an arrhythmia is considered to be any significant deviation from the normal range. Whether change in heart rate (number of contractions of the cardiac ventricles per period of time) produces symptoms at rest or on exertion depends on the underlying state of the cardiac muscle and its ability to alter its stroke output to compensate.

Rate arrhythmias are of two basic types: tachycardia and bradycardia. Tachycardia occurs when the heart beats too fast (more than 110 beats/min in an adult). Tachycardia develops in the presence of increased sympathetic stimulation, such as occurs with fear, pain, emotional stress, exertion, or exercise; or with ingestion of artificial stimulants, such as caffeine, nicotine, and amphetamines. In these instances, the tachycardia may not be pathologic but just transient based on the patient's immediate physiologic state (i.e., during exercise).

Tachycardia is also found in situations in which the demands for oxygen are increased, such as fever, HF, infection, anemia, hemorrhage, myocardial injury, and hyperthyroidism. Usually the individual with tachycardia perceives no symptoms, and medical intervention is directed toward the underlying cause.

Bradycardia (less than 50 beats/min in an adult) is normal in well-trained athletes, but it is also common in individuals taking β-blockers, those who have had traumatic brain injuries or brain tumors, and those experiencing increased vagal stimulation (e.g., from suctioning or vomiting) to the physiologic pacemaker.

Organic disease of the sinus node, especially in older people and those with heart disease, can also cause sinus bradycardia that is pathologic in nature. Bradycardia is usually asymptomatic, but when it is caused by a pathologic condition, the person may experience fatigue, dyspnea, syncope, dizziness, angina, or diaphoresis (profuse perspiration). Medical intervention is not usually required unless symptoms interfere with function, cardiac output is too low to sustain the individual, or it is drug or angina induced. When symptoms or complications arise due to bradycardia, atropine or a mechanical pacemaker can be used to re-establish a more normal heart rate.

**Rhythm.** Arrhythmias as variations from the normal rhythm of the heart (especially the heartbeat) are detected when they become symptomatic or during monitoring for another cardiac condition. Abnormalities of cardiac rhythm and electrical conduction can be lethal (sudden cardiac death), symptomatic (syncope or near syncope, dizziness, chest pain, dyspnea, palpitations), or asymptomatic. They can be dangerous because they alter cardiac output so that perfusion of the brain or myocardium is impaired, or they tend to deteriorate into more serious arrhythmias with the same consequences.

The many different types of abnormal cardiac rhythms are usually classified according to their origin (atrial, ventricular), but only the most common ones are included here. Complete discussion of all other cardiac arrhythmias is available.[176]

*Sinus arrhythmia* is an irregularity in rhythm that may be a normal variation in athletes, children, and older people or may be caused by an alteration in vagal stimulation. Sinus arrhythmia may be respiratory (increases and decreases with respiration) or nonrespiratory and associated with infection, drug toxicity (e.g., digoxin, morphine), or fever. Treatment for the respiratory type of sinus arrhythmia is not necessary; all other sinus arrhythmias are treated by providing intervention for the underlying cause.

AF is the most common type of supraventricular tachycardia (SVT) or chronic arrhythmia. SVT is also called paroxysmal SVT or paroxysmal atrial tachycardia. It is characterized by rapid, involuntary, irregular muscular contractions of the atrial myocardium—quivering or fluttering instead of contracting normally. Consequently, blood remains in the atria after they contract, and the ventricles do not fill properly. As the heart rate increases, there is less time for passive ventricular filling from the atria. Since the atria don't contract fully to push blood into the ventricles and the heart rate is fast, blood flow may diminish, creating a drop in oxygen levels that results in symptoms of shortness of breath, palpitations, fatigue, and, more rarely, fainting. AF occurs most often as a secondary arrhythmia associated with rheumatic heart disease, dilated cardiomyopathy, atrial septal defect, hypertension, mitral valve prolapse, recurrent cardiac surgery, after acute MI, and hypertrophic cardiomyopathy (conditions that affect the atria).

Secondary AF can also occur in people without cardiac disease, but in the presence of a systemic abnormality that predisposes the individual to arrhythmia (e.g., hyperthyroidism, medications, diabetes, obesity, pneumonia, or alcohol intoxication or withdrawal). People with AF are prone to blood clots because blood components that remain in the atria aggregate and attract other components, triggering clot formation. The effect rarely occurs before 72 hours of the first abnormal contraction. AF can result in HF, cardiac ischemia, and arterial emboli that can result in an ischemic stroke.

*Ventricular fibrillation* is an electrical phenomenon that results in involuntary, uncoordinated muscular contractions of the ventricular muscle; it is a frequent cause of cardiac arrest. Treatment is directed toward depolarizing the muscle, thus ending the irregular contractions and allowing the heart to resume normal regular contractions.

*Heart block* is a disorder of the heartbeat caused by an interruption in the passage of impulses through the heart's electrical system. This may occur because the SA node misfires or the impulses it generates are not properly transmitted through the heart's conduction system. Heart blocks are differentiated into three types determined by ECG testing: first-degree, second-degree, and third-degree (complete) heart block. Causes include CAD, hypertension, myocarditis, acute MI, and overdose of cardiac medications (e.g., digoxin, calcium channel blockers, β-blockers). Depending on the degree of the heart block, it can cause fatigue, dizziness, or fainting. Heart block can affect people at any age, but this condition primarily affects older people. Mild cases do not require intervention. When treatment is necessary, medications and pacemakers are the two primary forms of management.

*Sick sinus syndrome,* or brady-tachy syndrome, is a complex cardiac arrhythmia and conduction disturbance that is associated with advanced age, CAD, HF, or drug therapy (e.g., digoxin, calcium channel blockers, β-blockers, antiarrhythmics). Sick sinus syndrome as a result of degeneration of conductive tissue necessary to maintain normal heart rhythm occurs most often among older people. A variety of other heart diseases and other conditions (e.g., cardiomyopathy, sarcoidosis, amyloidosis) also may result in sinus node dysfunction. Sick sinus syndrome is characterized by bradycardia alone, bradycardia alternating with tachycardia, or bradycardia with atrioventricular block, resulting in cerebral manifestations of light-headedness, dizziness, and near or true syncope.

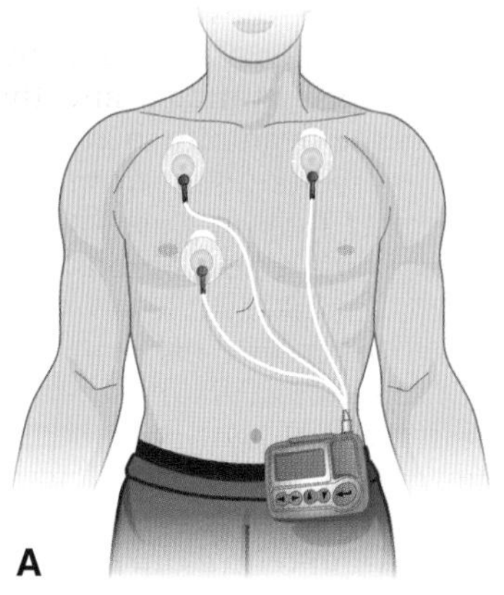


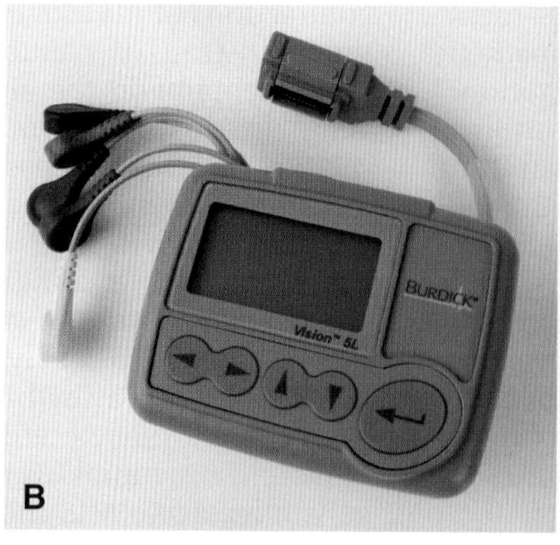


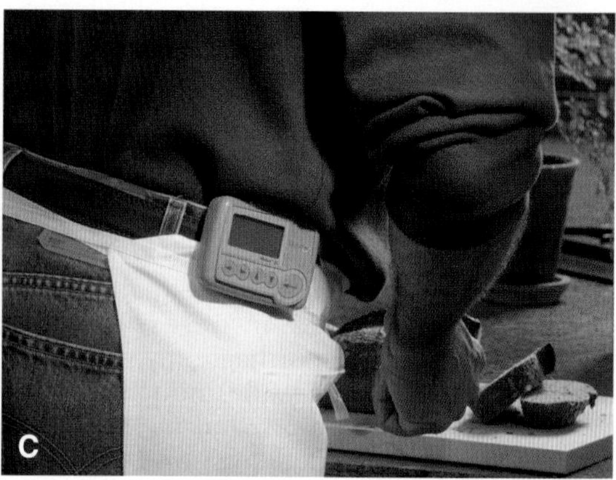


**Figure 12.20**

(A) External cardiac monitoring (a form of telemetry, also called ambulatory electrocardiography [ECG] or Holter monitoring) uses a tape recorder that is attached to the skin by ECG electrodes. It is able to record the heart rhythm over a 24-hour period. Any symptoms experienced while wearing the unit should be recorded by the individual wearing the device. The recording is then analyzed. It may detect changes in heart rhythm or changes in the ECG that might indicate a lack of blood supply to the heart. (B) Any number of electrodes up to 12 leads can be used. The standard three-electrode system in A consists of positive electrode, negative electrode, and ground electrode. (C) The unit is small and convenient and can be clipped to the belt or waistband or slipped into a pocket. (Courtesy Cardiac Science Corporation, Bothell, WA. Used with permission.)

Sinus node dysfunction is suspected in the older adult experiencing episodes of syncope or near syncope, especially in the presence of heart palpitations. An accurate diagnosis is made with ECG, often requiring a 24-hour Holter monitor to document the arrhythmias described.

Treatment for the symptomatic person varies according to the specific arrhythmia manifestations and may include antiarrhythmic agents alone or combined with a permanent-demand pacemaker or withdrawal of agents that may be responsible for the arrhythmia.

*Holiday heart syndrome* may occur when the heart responds to the increase in catecholamines (epinephrine, norepinephrine) brought on by excessive alcohol intake. Alcohol metabolites may also cause conduction delays. The toxic effects of alcohol can also cause a rise in the level of free fatty acids, contributing to the onset of this condition.[64]

## MEDICAL MANAGEMENT

**DIAGNOSIS.** ECG is the most common test procedure to document arrhythmias, but if the person is not experiencing symptoms, the heart rhythm may look normal. Recorded ambulatory ECG may be used to document arrhythmias. The individual may use continuous monitoring (external cardiac monitoring; Holter monitoring; Fig. 12.20) recording all cardiac cycles over a prescribed period of time (usually 24–48 hours) or cardiac event monitoring recording ECG just when symptoms are perceived.

Monitoring is especially helpful in recording sporadic arrhythmias that an office or stress test ECG might miss. Monitoring may also be used by persons recovering from MIs, receiving antiarrhythmic medications, or using pacemakers. Pocket-sized devices and devices that interface with smart phones or computers allow home monitoring when they are available. Readings on portable devices may be stored and then transmitted electronically, or the device can be hooked up to the physician's ECG or diagnostic computer. Monitoring units do not replace an ECG and should not be used without a physician's approval.

TEE imaging using an ultrasonic transducer mounted on the tip of a flexible instrument is used to detect cardiac emboli before medications are initiated to control heart rate and rhythm. If a serious arrhythmia is suspected, an electrophysiologic study can be performed. This test is an invasive study that uses wires placed via catheterization to electronically stimulate the heart in an attempt to reproduce the arrhythmia.

**TREATMENT.** The goal of treatment is to control ventricular rate, prevent thromboembolism, and restore normal sinus rhythm if possible. Normal heart rhythm returns spontaneously (called *cardioversion*) almost immediately in some cases, especially if there is no underlying heart disease. When conversion to normal rate and rhythm does not occur, there are two major approaches to cardioversion: electrical and pharmacologic.[190]

The electrical method employs the use of a device called a *defibrillator* and is usually most effective and may require several weeks (or longer) of anticoagulant therapy (warfarin) to reduce stroke risk. Anyone who has been in AF less than 48 hours but is hemodynamically unstable with serious signs and symptoms related to AF will need immediate electrical cardioversion. Low-voltage electric shocks interrupt the irritable foci of the heart, letting the SA node resume its role as a primary pacemaker.[310] One-time cardioversion may be performed externally. If the client is at risk for periodic ventricular arrhythmias, an internal defibrillator may be surgically placed.

Pharmacologic treatment may include agents prolonging depolarization and/or other cardiovascular medications[190] (see Table 12.5). If successful, cardioversion restores sinus rhythm, and drug therapy is used to maintain normal heart rate and rhythm. Even with successful electrical cardioversion, long-term antiarrhythmic and anticoagulation drug therapy is used to sustain normal sinus rhythm.

Some tachycardias can be treated with radiofrequency ablation, a nonsurgical but invasive technique that uses catheterization to thread wires into the heart through

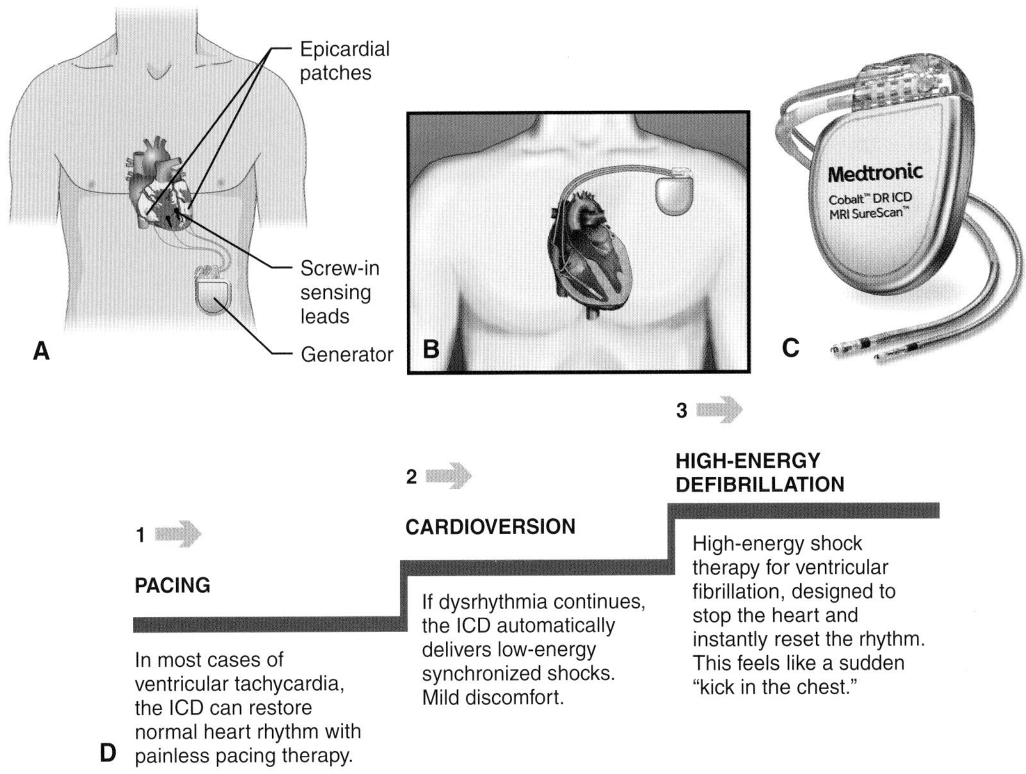


**Figure 12.21**

(A) Placement of an implantable cardioverter-defibrillator (ICD) and epicardial lead system. The generator is placed in a subcutaneous "pocket" created in the left upper abdominal quadrant. The epicardial screw-in sensing leads monitor the heart rhythm and connect to the generator. If a life-threatening dysrhythmia is sensed, the generator can pace-terminate the dysrhythmia or deliver electrical cardioversion or defibrillation through the epicardial patches. With this system, the leads/patches must be placed during open chest surgery. (B) Illustration of the implant position of Medtronic Colbalt™ XT DR ICD MRI SureScan™. Transvenous lead system. The pacing/cardioversion/defribilation functions are all contained a lead (or leads) inserted into the right atrium and ventricle. This generator is small enough to place in the pectoral region. (C) The Medtronic Colbalt™ XT DR ICD MRI SureScan™. [A and D] From Urden LD: *Thelan's critical care nuring: diagnosis and management,* ed 5, St Louis, 2006, Mosby; [B and C] From Medtronic, Inc. Reproduced with permission of Medtronic, Inc. Minneapolis, MN.

which radio waves can be aimed at the heart tissue where the arrhythmia originates. The catheter-delivered quick bursts of current destroy (or cauterize) the specific areas of heart muscle that are generating the abnormal electrical signals causing the arrhythmia. One complication of this technique is the potential destruction of the conducting system (the heart's own internal pacemaker), which necessitates surgical implantation of an artificial pacemaker for some people. Another complication is the failure of the ablation to correct the arrhythmia. Recurrence of arrhythmia, especially AF, is common, and more than one ablation procedure may be needed in order to permanently correct the arrhythmia, if at all possible.[364]

*Pacemakers,* implants designed to replace the heartbeat by delivering a battery-supplied electrical stimulus through leads attached to electrodes in contact with the heart, may be used in cases of bradycardia, heart block, or refractory tachycardia. Refractory tachycardia is a condition in which the heart is beating very quickly, but only a portion of those beats are functional. Many more beats just echo or make a beat but without contractile force behind the blood flow. Functionally, the heartbeat is actually very slow.

Pacemakers initiate the heartbeat when the heart's intrinsic conduction system fails or is unreliable. In the case of life-threatening arrhythmias (e.g., ventricular tachycardia, ventricular fibrillation) that do not respond to other types of intervention, a device called an implantable cardioverter-defibrillator (ICD) may be implanted (Fig. 12.21). The ICD monitors the heart rhythm, and if the heart starts beating abnormally, it generates an electric shock to restore the normal sinus (heart) rhythm.

For people whose arrhythmias are resistant to pharmacologic therapy, another surgical intervention is available called the *maze procedure.* This procedure is done with a scope, catheter, and robotics to make a series of maze-like cuts in the atria, which are then sewn back together. The scar tissue that forms during the healing process blocks faulty circuits, preventing AF. Many people may still need a pacemaker and drug therapy to maintain normal rate and rhythm even after the maze procedure. A more refined version of this procedure (catheter maze) takes a percutaneous, nonsurgical, noninvasive approach using radiofrequency ablation to destroy tissue.

*Ventricular resynchronization therapy* can also treat intraventricular conduction disturbances associated with HF. This specific type of pacemaker resynchronizes the right and left ventricles so they pump at the same time, making the heart pump more forcefully instead of pumping faster (as occurs with a typical pacemaker or in the case of HF, when the heart beats faster to compensate for a weak pumping mechanism).[104,174]

**PROGNOSIS.** About half of all individuals with AF will spontaneously convert to normal sinus rhythm within 24 to 48 hours; this is less likely to occur in people whose AF has lasted longer than 7 days.[374]

Sudden cardiac arrest (sudden death) is responsible for 22% of deaths from all causes of people with AF[50] and is often preceded by fatal heart dysrhythmias in people who have no prior history of heart disease. In fact, data from the Framingham Heart Study indicate that AF is independently associated with a substantially increased risk for death in both men and women, even after adjustment for age and associated factors, such as hypertension, HF, and stroke.[230]

Defibrillation within the first few minutes of cardiac arrest can save up to 50% of lives; by comparison, fewer than 5% of people who sustain sudden cardiac arrest outside of a hospital survive without defibrillation. Early defibrillation is the key to survival.[266] Therefore, most public and many private companies and facilities have defibrillators on site.

The most appropriate and effective drug or drug combination remains unknown, and side effects of long-term rate and rhythm control intervention (e.g., organ toxicity of the lung, liver, and thyroid; aggravation of a preexisting arrhythmia or development of a new arrhythmia instead of preventing it) may prevent long-term use of drug therapy.

## SPECIAL IMPLICATIONS FOR THE THERAPIST 12.11

### *Arrhythmias*

Any time a person's pulse is abnormally slow, rapid, or irregular, especially in the presence of known cardiac involvement, documentation and notification of the physician are necessary. Early detection and treatment of AF can be critical in reducing the client's risk of stroke and hemodynamic compromise.

Predisposing factors for arrhythmias include fluid and electrolyte imbalance and drug toxicity. To prevent postoperative cardiac arrhythmias, the therapist should determine the client's blood oxygen level using pulse oximetry and/or blood gas analysis and, in consultation with the physician, provide adequate oxygen during activities that increase the heart's workload. Physical activity workloads should be adjusted on an individual client basis, making sure to not overtax the client's aerobic capacity, as doing so could cause an arrhythmia.

Individuals experiencing exercise intolerance as a result of palpitations, fatigue, and shortness of breath should be assessed further. Keep in mind that people with arrhythmias can be completely asymptomatic. And it is possible that clients describing palpitations or similar phenomena may not be experiencing symptoms of arrhythmic heart disease at all.

Palpitations can occur as a result of an overactive thyroid, secondary to caffeine sensitivity, as a side effect of some medications, from decreased estrogen levels, and through the use of drugs such as cocaine. Encourage the client to report any such symptoms to the physician if this has not already been brought to the physician's attention.

It is the position of the American Physical Therapy Association that properly trained physical therapists should be authorized to perform advanced cardiac life support procedures, including cardiac monitoring for arrhythmia recognition and cardiac defibrillation.[22]

Physical therapists prescribe exercise for many people with a history of personal or family heart disease or known risk factors for cardiac disease potentially necessitating cardiopulmonary resuscitation. When treating clients with known arrhythmias, it is important to have advanced cardiac life support equipment available in case of emergency.

Performing an assessment of falls for individuals with cardiac disease, especially for anyone with a personal or family history of arrhythmias, is highly recommended. Screening for syncope, assessing balance and fall risk, and falling prevention programs are important components of a therapist's evaluation. If the individual is also on anticoagulation therapy, the individual should be monitored (and taught how to self-monitor) for signs and symptoms of bleeding; in the acute care setting, the therapist can monitor international normalized ratio. Evaluations of specific assessment and screening tests are available.

#### Exercise and Arrhythmias

Individuals with a history of atrial fibrillation should be encouraged to maintain as normal and active a lifestyle as possible. They should be informed that exercise can increase arrhythmias because of the increase in activity of the sympathetic nervous system and the increase in circulating catecholamines. Exercise may induce cardiac arrhythmias under several specific conditions, including diuretic and digoxin therapy or following recent ingestion of caffeine. Avoiding triggers such as caffeine, alcohol, or overeating can help mitigate risk of arrhythmias and should be encouraged. Good nutrition, smoking cessation for those who use tobacco, and regular physical activity and exercise are key components of the management of arrhythmias.

Exercise-induced arrhythmias are generated by enhanced sympathetic tone, increased myocardial oxygen demand, or both. The therapist can be involved in preparticipation screening of all athletes for conditions that put them at risk for sudden cardiac death.[385] At times, the arrhythmias may disappear with exercise and increased perfusion. Exercise recommendations for athletes with selected arrhythmias are available.[138,351]

Medications that are effective in controlling arrhythmias at rest may not be as effective during exertion or stress. In addition, side effects of antiarrhythmic agents may be more apparent during exercise. For example, decreases in either exercise performance or blood pressure during exercise may occur. Because of their effects on the electrophysiologic characteristics of cardiac cells, these medications have the potential to cause abnormal rhythms. The effect of slowing the impulse through the myocardium may manifest itself during exercise as a partial or complete heart block.

Individuals with known arrhythmias and clients who are taking antiarrhythmic medications may need to be evaluated under conditions of graded exercise to ensure that the arrhythmia remains under control during activity. Monitoring heart rate and blood pressure during activity and palpation of peripheral pulses are essential in the absence of ECG.

Continued monitoring and observation during the recovery period are also important, because arrhythmias often occur during recovery rather than during peak exercise. If the exercise is stopped abruptly and the individual remains upright, pooling of blood in the lower body occurs. The decreased venous return and subsequent decreased blood flow to the heart may facilitate an irregular rhythm. By adding a cool-down period to an exercise session, a sudden decrease in venous return is avoided.

For the client who is wearing or has worn a cardiac monitor (Holter, event, loop), the therapist must obtain the interpretation of the results to determine if modifications are needed in the person's activities. Anyone with life-threatening arrhythmias should not begin physical therapy activity until intervention for the arrhythmia is initiated and the condition is stabilized. Increasing frequency of arrhythmias developing with activity must be evaluated by the physician.[176]

### Pacemaker

For the client wearing a pacemaker, the first weeks after surgery may be characterized by fatigue, during which time activity restrictions apply. Most people can drive, but strenuous activities using the arms (e.g., housework, golf, tennis, hunting, lifting more than 10 lb) are not recommended and may be contraindicated. Once the incision is fully healed and the pacemaker is stable, scar mobilization is permissible. The usual precautions for scar mobilization apply, including mobilizing the tissue in the direction of the scar before using any cross-transverse techniques and mobilizing toward the scar rather than away from the scar to avoid overstretching the healing tissue.

Problems with pacemakers are uncommon, but any unusual deviation from the set heartbeat expected or the development of unusual symptoms, such as dyspnea, dizziness or light-headedness, and syncope or near syncope, must be reported immediately to the physician. If the client notices an increase in fatigue level, that may also be an indication of a complication or mechanical failure of the device. It is important that the therapist understands the underlying cardiac problem, as well as the type of pacemaker the client is using, before monitoring the client's response to an exercise program. More detailed information regarding types of pacemakers and pacemaker implantation is available;[199] see also information from pacemaker manufacturers.

It should be noted that MRIs and prolonged exposure to electromagnetic waves are contraindicated in anyone who is pacemaker dependent. Most exposures to electromagnetic interference are transient and pose no threat to people with pacemakers and ICDs. Electromagnetic interference between cellular phones and pacemakers or ICDs is possible but extremely rare. Clients with pacemakers who notice a change in the mechanical functioning should consult with their physician to see if it is related to their cellular phone or other mobile device.

Most pacemakers currently used contain a setting for heart rate modulation. This allows the heart rate to increase based on physical demand, although still to a set rate. It is important for the client to have a warm-up period of movement (5–10 min) before aerobic or resistance exercise begins. This allows the pacemaker time to increase the client's heart rate based on physiologic demand. Exercise intensity may be limited only by the underlying heart disease and left ventricular function. If the pacemaker recipient has undergone exercise testing safely, aerobic conditioning and endurance training can be initiated, although precaution is still advised regarding vigorous upper-body activities. In some individuals who have suffered cardiac arrest and now have a pacemaker (or other implantable device), the response to surviving cardiac arrest has been compared to posttraumatic stress disorder that can occur after a person experiences a traumatic event that is outside the realm of usual human experience. Depression, anxiety, difficulty concentrating, negative health beliefs, and increased somatic complaints may be present with or without persistent emotional disability and maladaptation to the event. The therapist should screen all clients with new pacemaker implantation for depression or anxiety and refer them to the physician or mental health professional when appropriate.

## DISEASES AFFECTING THE HEART VALVES

Heart problems that occur secondary to impairment of valves may be caused by infections such as endocarditis, congenital deformity, or disease (e.g., rheumatic fever, coronary thrombosis). Valve deformities are classified as functional (e.g., stenosis, insufficiency) or anatomic (e.g., prolapse; congenital deformities; and deformities caused by rheumatic fever, trauma, infection, ischemia) (Fig. 12.22).

*Stenosis* is a narrowing or constriction that prevents the valve from opening fully and may be caused by fibrosis, scarring, or abnormal calcium deposits on the leaflets. Valvular stenosis causes obstruction to blood flow, and the chamber behind the narrow valve must produce extra work to sustain cardiac output. Often the muscles of that chamber become hypertrophied due to the extra workload placed on them to get blood past the narrowed valve.

*Insufficiency* (also referred to as *regurgitation*) occurs when the valve does not close properly and causes blood to flow back into the heart chamber. The heart chamber behind the insufficient valve gradually dilates in response to the increased volume of blood. Severe degrees of incompetence are possible in the absence of symptoms. *Prolapse* affects the mitral or tricuspid valve and occurs when enlarged leaflets bulge backward into the atrium.

Valve conditions increase the workload of the heart and require the heart to pump harder to force blood through a stenosed valve or to maintain adequate flow if blood is seeping back. Initially the cardiovascular system compensates for the overload, and the person remains asymptomatic, but eventually as stenosis or insufficiency progresses, cardiac muscle dysfunction and accompanying symptoms of HF (breathlessness, dyspnea) develop.

The presence of CAD in clients with valve disease is similar to that of the general population. However, clients

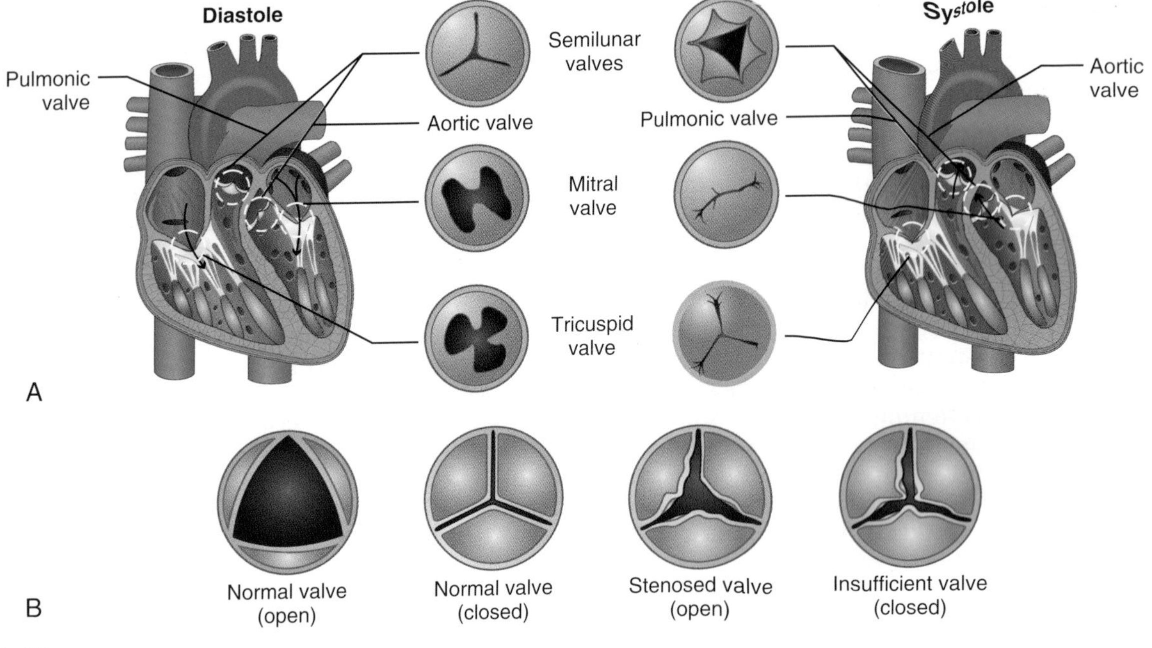


**Figure 12.22**

**Valves of the heart.** (A) The pulmonic, aortic, mitral, and tricuspid valves are shown here as they appear during diastole (ventricular filling) and systole (ventricular contraction). (B) Normal position of the valve leaflets, or cusps, when the valve is open and closed; fully open position of a stenosed valve; closed regurgitant valve showing abnormal opening into which blood can flow back.

with mitral or aortic valve disease especially, can have a higher risk of complications from CAD.[77]

## Mitral Stenosis

### Etiologic Factors and Pathogenesis

Mitral stenosis is most often a sequela of rheumatic heart disease and primarily affects women. Often a history of rheumatic fever is absent. Because the mitral valve is thickened, it opens in early diastole with a snap that is audible on auscultation and then closes slowly with a resultant murmur.

The anterior and posterior leaflets are fixed like a funnel with an opening in the center, and they move together rather than in opposite directions. When the valve has narrowed sufficiently, left atrial pressure rises to maintain normal flow across the valve and to maintain a normal cardiac output. This results in a pressure difference between the left atrium and the left ventricle during diastole.

### Clinical Manifestations

In mild cases, left atrial pressure and cardiac output remain normal, and the person is asymptomatic, perhaps until pregnancy or the development of AF, when dyspnea and orthopnea develop. In moderate stenosis, dyspnea and fatigue appear as the left atrial pressure rises and mechanical obstruction of filling of the left ventricle reduces cardiac output.

With severe stenosis, left atrial pressure is high enough to produce pulmonary venous congestion at rest and reduce cardiac output, with resulting dyspnea, fatigue, and right ventricular failure. Lying down at night further increases the pulmonary blood volume, causing orthopnea and paroxysmal nocturnal dyspnea.

### MEDICAL MANAGEMENT

**DIAGNOSIS, TREATMENT, AND PROGNOSIS.** Echocardiography is the most valuable technique for assessing mitral valve stenosis and providing information about the condition of the valve and left atrium size. If the left ventricular heart muscles hypertrophy, it can be seen and measured on the echocardiography. Doppler techniques (measuring blood flow using ultrasound) can be used to determine the severity of the valve problem.

Because mitral stenosis may be asymptomatic, intervention is delayed until symptoms develop. Mitral stenosis may be present for a lifetime with few or no symptoms, or it may become severe in a few years. The onset of AF accompanied by more severe symptoms may be treated pharmacologically (digoxin, antiarrhythmic agents, anticoagulants).

Surgery may be indicated in the presence of uncontrollable pulmonary edema, severe dyspnea limiting function, pulmonary hypertension, arrhythmia, or systemic emboli uncontrolled by anticoagulation treatment. Surgical procedures include valve repair (commissurotomy to break apart the adherent leaves) or replacement with an artificial valve.

Operative mortality rates are low. However, when there are complications, they are typically due to thrombosis, leaking, endocarditis, or degenerative changes in valve tissue.

## Mitral Regurgitation

### Incidence, Etiologic Factors, and Pathogenesis

Mitral regurgitation is found in 1.7% of adults in the United States, occurring at 0.5% at age 18 to 44 years and 9.3% at 75 years or older,[50] clearly indicating its association with aging. Mitral regurgitation has many possible causes, but involvement of the mitral valve from ischemic heart disease accounts for approximately half of all cases. Other secondary causes include infective endocarditis (valve perforation), dilated cardiomyopathy, rheumatic disease, collagen vascular disease, rupture of the chordae tendineae, and, rarely, cardiac tumors. It is independently associated with female gender, lower BMI, and older age. Valve issues in general are higher in clients that are obese.[216]

During left ventricular systole, the mitral leaflets do not close normally, and blood is ejected into the left atrium as well as through the aortic valve. In acute regurgitation, left atrial pressure rises abruptly, possibly leading to pulmonary edema. When regurgitation is a chronic condition, the left atrium enlarges progressively; the degree of enlargement usually reflects the severity of regurgitation.

### Clinical Manifestations

Unfortunately, people with mitral regurgitation lack early warning signs and may remain asymptomatic until severe and often irreversible left ventricular dysfunction occurs. For many years, the left ventricular end-diastolic pressure and the cardiac output may be normal at rest, even with considerable increase in left ventricular volume. Eventually, left ventricular overload may lead to left ventricular failure. People with mitral regurgitation experience exertional dyspnea (because of increased left atrial pressure) and exercise-induced fatigue (because of reduced cardiac output). AF may also develop.

## MEDICAL MANAGEMENT

**DIAGNOSIS, TREATMENT, AND PROGNOSIS.** The diagnosis is primarily clinical (auscultation), but it can be confirmed and quantified by echocardiography. Other testing procedures may include cardiac catheterization to assess the regurgitation, left ventricular function, and pulmonary artery pressure; coronary arteriography to determine the cause of the lesion and for preoperative evaluation; and nuclear medicine techniques to measure left ventricular function and estimate the severity of regurgitation.

Persons with chronic valve insufficiency/regurgitation who are asymptomatic require careful monitoring for left ventricular function and may require surgery even if no symptoms are present. Unlike stenosis, regurgitation may progress insidiously, causing left ventricular damage before symptoms have developed.

Surgical intervention may be recommended if left ventricular function is impaired or when activity becomes severely limited. Mitral valve repair has a lower operative mortality and a better late outcome than mitral valve replacement.[233] Acute mitral regurgitation secondary to MI often requires emergency surgery, but the surgical risk is high and the outcome poor. Acute non–MI-related mitral regurgitation has a much better prognosis with higher postoperative survival after well-timed mitral valve repair. Indicators of poorer prognosis include mitral valve replacement, age older than 75 years, and the presence of CAD.

## Mitral Valve Prolapse

### Incidence and Etiologic Factors

Mitral valve prolapse (MVP) has been described as a common disease with frequent complications. MVP occurs in approximately 2% to 3% of "normal" adults, especially young women, and is detected most often during pregnancy.[108] Men seem to have a higher incidence of complications.[50]

MVP is characterized by a slight variation in the shape or structure of the mitral (left atrioventricular) valve. This structural variation has many other names, including floppy valve syndrome, Barlow syndrome, myxomatous mitral valve syndrome, and click-murmur syndrome. Barlow syndrome is a controversial clinical syndrome that may have as its only manifestation MVP without regurgitation. MVP usually occurs in isolation; however, it can be associated with a number of other conditions, such as Marfan syndrome, rheumatic fever, endocarditis, myocarditis, atherosclerosis, SLE, muscular dystrophy, acromegaly, adult polycystic kidney disease, and cardiac sarcoidosis. Genetic variants for the rare X-linked valvular dystrophy and autosomal dominant inheritance genes (for filamin A and other proteins) have been linked to MVP.[50]

### Pathogenesis

MVP is a pathologic, anatomic, and physiologic abnormality of the mitral valve apparatus affecting mitral valve leaflet motion. Normally, when the lower part of the heart contracts, the mitral valve remains firm and prevents blood from leaking back into the left atrium. In MVP, the slight variation in shape of the mitral valve allows one part of the valve, the leaflet, to billow back into the left atrium during contraction of the ventricle. One or both of the valve leaflets may bulge into the left atrium during ventricular systole. Usually the amount of blood that leaks back into the left atrium is not significant, but in a small number of people, it develops into mitral regurgitation. MVP is the most common cause of isolated mitral regurgitation. The consistent regurgitation of blood into the left atrium will cause the atrium to dilate, thus altering the myocardial muscles' length-tension relationships and the dynamic of blood volume in the heart.

The presence of symptoms linked to neuroendocrine dysfunctions or to the autonomic nervous system has led to the recognition of a pathologic condition known as *mitral valve prolapse syndrome (MVPS)*. Usually diagnosed by chance in asymptomatic individuals during routine tests, MVPS (prolapse with or without mitral regurgitation) has a high clinical incidence of neuropsychiatric symptoms (e.g., anxiety disorder, panic attacks, depression), as well as symptoms of autonomic dysfunction (e.g., postural hypotension, palpitations, cold hands and feet, shortness of breath, chest pain).

As the autonomic nervous system is being formed in utero, the mitral valve is also being formed. If there is a slight variation in the structure of the heart valve, there is also a slight variation in the function or balance of the autonomic nervous system. The importance of recognizing that MVP may occur as an isolated disorder or with other coincident findings has led to the use of both terms.

### Clinical Manifestations

More than 50% of all people with MVP are asymptomatic, another 40% experience occasional symptoms that are mildly to moderately uncomfortable, and only

1% suffer severe symptoms and lifestyle restrictions. Although the malformation occurs during gestation, it usually remains unnoticed until young adulthood. In women, the valve disorder often doesn't become symptomatic until they become pregnant. MVP is the most common cardiac disorder in women who are pregnant.[382] Men and women with MVP usually become aware of symptoms suddenly, and there does not appear to be any correlation between the severity of symptoms and the severity of the prolapse.

The most common triad of symptoms associated with MVP is profound fatigue that cannot be correlated with exercise or stress, palpitations, and dyspnea. Fatigue may not be related to exertion, but deconditioning from prolonged inactivity may develop, further complicating the picture.

The therapist is more likely to see the individual with MVP associated with connective tissue disorders or the MVPS with autonomic dysfunction. Frequently occurring musculoskeletal findings in clients with MVPS include joint hypermobility, temporomandibular joint syndrome, pectus excavatum, mild scoliosis, straight thoracic spine, and myalgia.[210]

Other symptoms associated with MVPS may include tremors, swelling of the extremities, sleep disturbances, low-back pain, irritable bowel syndrome, excessive perspiration or inability to perspire, rashes, muscular fasciculations, visual changes or disturbances, difficulty in concentrating, memory lapses, and dizziness.

Chest pain or discomfort may occur as a result of autonomic nervous system dysfunction (dysautonomia). The autonomic nervous system imbalance results in inadequate relaxation between respirations and eventually causes the chest wall muscles to go into spasm. The chest pain is sharp, lasts several seconds, and is usually felt to the left of the sternum. It is intermittent pain that may occur frequently for a few weeks and then disappear completely, only to return again some weeks later.

### MEDICAL MANAGEMENT

**DIAGNOSIS, TREATMENT, AND PROGNOSIS.** MVP is often discovered during routine cardiac auscultation or when echocardiography is performed for another reason. It is characterized by a symptomatic clinical presentation and clicking noise on auscultation in late systole, with or without sounds of valvular leak (murmur).

The mitral valve begins to prolapse when the reduction of left ventricular volume during systole reaches a critical point at which the valve leaflets no longer coapt (edges approximate together); at that instant, the click occurs and the murmur begins. Complete diagnostic (major and minor) criteria have been outlined elsewhere.[384] Echocardiography may be used to confirm the diagnosis, and ECG, event, or Holter monitoring (see Fig. 12.20) to show arrhythmias associated with the prolapse may be used.

Management includes routine monitoring of stability or progression of MVP; β-blockers to control arrhythmias; an exercise program to improve overall cardiovascular function; counseling to eliminate caffeine, alcohol, and cigarette use; and administration of antibiotics before any invasive procedure (including dental work, sigmoidoscopy) as prophylaxis against endocarditis.

Surgical replacement of the valve is typically not recommended unless severe structural problems are present that contribute to reduced activity or deterioration of left ventricular function from progression of MVP to mitral regurgitation.

MVP or MVPS is a benign condition in the vast majority of people. It is not life-threatening, and only rarely does it result in complications or significantly alter a person's lifestyle. Progressive mitral regurgitation with gradual increase in left atrial and left ventricular size, AF, pulmonary hypertension, and the development of HF occur in 10% to 15% of people with both murmurs and clicks. Men older than 50 years are most often affected.[384]

## Aortic Stenosis

### Etiologic Factors and Pathogenesis

Aortic stenosis is a disease of aging that is likely to become more prevalent as the proportion of older people in our population increases. In the United States, the prevalence of aortic stenosis is 0.4%, with severe to moderate calcific aortic stenosis at the age of 75 years or older at 2.8%.[50] It is most commonly caused by progressive valvular calcification either superimposed on a congenitally bicuspid valve or, in the older adult, involving a previously normal valve following rheumatic fever. Aortic valve calcification is linked to LDL-C–related genetic variants.[50]

Risk factors for progression of aortic stenosis are the same as those for heart disease and include obesity, metabolic syndrome, diabetes, CAD, older age, smoking, high cholesterol, hypercalcemia, and renal insufficiency.[50] More than 80% of affected persons are men, and when women are affected, differences are noted (e.g., women with aortic stenosis have thicker ventricular walls, reducing wall stress and higher ejection fractions) that require different postoperative management (e.g., low cardiac output requiring volume expansion rather than the use of pressor agents).[321]

Ejection fraction is the amount of blood the ventricle ejects; the normal resting ejection fraction is approximately 55% to 60%. A decreased resting ejection fraction is a hallmark finding of ventricular failure. Due to the added stress on the left ventricular muscles, aortic stenosis often manifests as a decreased resting ejection fraction.

Although the deformed valve is not stenotic at birth, it is subjected to abnormal hemodynamic stress, which may lead to thickening and calcification of the leaflets with reduced mobility. The orifice of the aortic valve narrows, causing increased resistance to blood flow from the left ventricle into the aorta.

Outflow obstruction increases pressure within the left ventricle as it tries to eject blood through the narrow opening, causing decreased cardiac output, left ventricular hypertrophy, and pulmonary vascular congestion. Preschool and school-age children are more likely to have a bicuspid valve; teenagers and young adults present with three leaflets, but the three leaflets are partially fused.

### Clinical Manifestations

In adults, aortic stenosis is usually asymptomatic until the sixth (or later) decade. Characteristic sounds may be heard on auscultation, but cardiac output is maintained until the stenosis is severe and left ventricular failure, angina pectoris, or exertional syncope develops. The origin of exertional syncope in aortic stenosis remains controversial. It is perhaps caused by an exercise-induced decrease in total peripheral resistance, which is uncompensated because cardiac output is restricted by the stenotic valve. The most common sign of aortic stenosis is a systolic ejection murmur radiating to the neck (usually heard best in the aortic area). Aortic stenosis can lead to symptoms such as fatigue, chest pain, dizziness, and shortness of breath (breathlessness). Sudden death may occur, even in previously asymptomatic individuals.

#### MEDICAL MANAGEMENT

**DIAGNOSIS, TREATMENT, AND PROGNOSIS.** The clinical assessment of aortic stenosis can be difficult, especially in the older person. Echo Doppler (echocardiography with Doppler ultrasonography) is diagnostic in most cases. ECG may show left ventricular hypertrophy, and x-ray or fluoroscopy may show a calcified aortic valve. Coronary angiography and possible subsequent coronary intervention may be necessary in older adults at risk for CAD before valve replacement.

Pharmacologic therapy has limited use in this condition. Surgical intervention is usually required for the symptomatic person but also should be strongly considered for the asymptomatic person because of the risk of sudden death due to the added stress on the left ventricle.

Surgical procedures may include valve replacement with a mechanical prosthesis or bioprosthesis (made with biologic material) or use of the pulmonary valve in place of the aortic valve and replacement of the pulmonary valve with a homograft (Ross procedure). Homografts have been shown to have a superior durability compared to xenogenic biologic prostheses. They have a low rate of thromboembolic events and good outcomes of durability.[202]

The aortic valve may be replaced through sternotomy incision ("open heart" surgery) or without opening the thoracic cavity (transcatheter aortic valve replacement). In the transcatheter technique, the new valve is delivered to the heart through a catheter inserted through an artery in the groin. There are risks associated with the transcatheter procedure, so typically younger adults will undergo traditional sternotomy technique and older adults, at high risk for open heart technique, will undergo the transcatheter technique.[31]

Adults with aortic stenosis are at risk for infective endocarditis. It is important that they have routine monitoring by their physician and report any abnormal symptoms immediately.

## Aortic Regurgitation (Insufficiency)

### Etiologic Factors and Pathogenesis

In the past, aortic regurgitation occurred secondary to rheumatic fever, but antibiotics have reduced the number of rheumatic fever–related cases. Nonrheumatic causes account for most cases today, including congenitally bicuspid valves, infective endocarditis (valve destruction by bacteria), and hypertension. Aortic regurgitation may also occur secondary to aortic dissection with or without aortic aneurysm, ankylosing spondylitis, Reiter syndrome, collagen vascular disease, syphilis, or Marfan syndrome. Prevalence of aortic regurgitation is 0.5%, reaching 2% among people 75 years of age or older.[50]

When cardiac systole ends, the aortic valve should completely prevent the flow of aortic blood back into the left ventricle. A leakage during diastole is referred to as *aortic regurgitation* or *aortic insufficiency*. When aortic regurgitation develops gradually, the left ventricle compensates by both dilation and enough hypertrophy to maintain a normal wall thickness/cavity ratio, thereby preventing development of symptoms. Left ventricular wall characteristics from aortic insufficiency are similar to those of dilated cardiomyopathy. Eventually the left ventricle fails to stand up under the chronic overload, and symptoms develop.

### Clinical Manifestations

Longstanding aortic regurgitation may remain asymptomatic even as the deformity increases, causing enlargement of the left ventricle. The large total stroke volume in aortic regurgitation produces a wide pulse pressure and systolic hypertension, resulting in exertional dyspnea, fatigue, and excessive perspiration with exercise as the most frequent symptoms; paroxysmal nocturnal dyspnea and pulmonary edema may also occur. Angina pectoris or atypical chest pain may be present, but this is uncommon in the absence of CAD.

#### MEDICAL MANAGEMENT

**DIAGNOSIS, TREATMENT, AND PROGNOSIS.** Once aortic regurgitation is suspected on physical examination, echocardiography with Doppler examination of the aortic valve can help estimate its severity. Aortography during catheterization helps confirm the severity of the disease. Scintigraphic studies can quantify left ventricular function and functional reserve during exercise and provide a useful predictor of prognosis.

Acute aortic regurgitation may lead to left ventricular failure; surgical reconstruction or replacement of the valve (Ross procedure) is advisable before onset of permanent left ventricular damage (usually before ejection fraction falls below 55%), even in asymptomatic cases. Chronic regurgitation carries a poor prognosis without surgery when significant symptoms develop. Medical therapy may include vasodilators to reduce the severity of regurgitation and diuretics and digoxin to stabilize or improve symptoms.

## Tricuspid Stenosis and Regurgitation

Tricuspid stenosis may be congenital or rheumatic in origin and is less common than aortic or mitral. Exercise testing and rehabilitation do not occur until after valve surgery. Tricuspid regurgitation may occur secondary to carcinoid syndrome, SLE, or infective endocarditis among injection drug users and in the presence of mitral valve disease. Surgical repair is more common than valvular replacement for tricuspid valve disease.

## Pulmonary Valve Stenosis and Regurgitation

The pulmonary valve is the least common valve to have abnormalities. Pulmonary stenosis is usually a congenital malformation. It occurs in about 8% to 10% of congenital cardiac conditions.[317] The initial sign of pulmonary stenosis is usually hearing a murmur during heart auscultation. Echocardiography is then performed to diagnose the stenosis. Symptoms of pulmonary stenosis include abdominal distention, cyanosis, fatigue, failure to thrive in infants, and shortness of breath. Symptoms may get worse with activity or exercise.

Pulmonary regurgitation is also usually a congenital cardiac condition. It is most commonly a secondary complication from another cardiac condition such as tetralogy of Fallot. Clients are typically nonsymptomatic until the regurgitation becomes severe. Once symptomatic, the client will present with decreased activity tolerance, signs of HF, and possibly ventricular arrhythmias, or sudden death.[100] Surgical replacement or repair of the pulmonary artery is utilized when symptoms are moderate to severe and medications have not helped stabilize the client.

SPECIAL IMPLICATIONS FOR THE THERAPIST 12.12

## *Valvular Heart Disease*

People with mild valvular malfunction have few to no symptoms and can usually exercise vigorously and take part in intense sports activities without adverse effects. Although exercise will not improve the mechanical function of a valve, improvement in submaximal cardiac capacity can occur. Exercise is usually stopped for the same reason as it is in healthy adults (i.e., when respiratory distress occurs or when the person expresses a desire to stop). If the valvular disease is moderate or severe, the client will typically undergo surgical repair or replacement. Physical therapy after surgery is similar to that after other cardiac surgical procedures.

Involvement of more than one valve is not uncommon in people with rheumatic valvular disease and in people who develop valvular regurgitation as a result of ventricular dilation. Usually symptoms and clinical course are determined by the predominant pathologic condition. When two valves are affected equally, symptoms are determined by the most proximally located valve. The combination of aortic regurgitation with mitral valve regurgitation is the most common, but the combination of mitral valve disease (either regurgitation or stenosis) with aortic stenosis is the most problematic.[981,380]

### Exercise

*Exercise testing* for most people with valvular disease is of limited value. For example, there is poor correlation between the degree of mitral stenosis and the duration of symptom-limited treadmill exercise. However, exercise echocardiography performed while the individual is on a stationary cycle can be a valuable means for determining left ventricular function in people during exercise.

*Prescriptive exercise* must be individualized based on the underlying pathologic condition, medical intervention, and condition of the person. Both aerobic and resistance training can be performed. However, resistance training should be monitored more closely with specific instructions to the client to avoid overexertion and any isometric movements or the Valsalva maneuver.

A perceived exertion between light and somewhat hard (rate of perceived exertion of 11–14; see Table 12.13) is the goal, but the individual will usually begin with a much lighter workout and progress over time to this level. Tolerance to symptoms and current exercise habits are important determinants in progressing an exercise program.

Some people with valvular disease avoid physical activity as much as possible and never exercise to the point of developing any symptoms of dyspnea, fatigue, or muscular discomfort. This is counterproductive, as symptoms will then typically develop at lighter exertion loads due to the body being unaccustomed to any physical activity. Other people force themselves to ignore mild (or even moderate to severe) symptoms to stay on the job or finish a task started, which is also unadvisable.

Fatigue, weakness, and pallor are signs of an inadequate cardiac output for the demands of the exercise. These signs and symptoms are partly subjective, and it is a clinician's decision as to how far to allow these people to continue exercising. Chest pain may indicate myocardial ischemia or pulmonary hypertension, or it may be a noncardiac symptom arising from the chest wall.

Exercise prescription should follow precautions similar to those for angina pectoris. Exercise should be stopped immediately when any signs of reduced cerebral blood flow develop, such as severe facial pallor, confusion, dizziness, heart palpitations, or unsteady gait (see also Boxes 12.4 and 12.9).

Pulmonary edema can be produced by exercising beyond a certain point in people with valvular disease, especially those with mitral stenosis. Pulmonary congestion induced by exercise may cause coughing rather than dyspnea, and exercise should be stopped if coughing becomes significant. HF may occur secondary to chronic, progressive valvular disease. Peripheral edema, nocturia, mild nocturnal dyspnea, unexpected weight gain, or more than the usual amount of fatigue can be minor symptoms that are passed over unless specifically sought. Such symptoms must be reported to the physician.

The status of the myocardium is another important variable in exercise impairment relative to valvular heart disease. Severe aortic regurgitation is well tolerated for many years until myocardial weakness occurs. In all forms of heart disease, the healthy myocardium can compensate and maintain the systemic blood flow at or near normal levels for an extended period of time. For the client with valvular disease and myocardial disease or associated CAD, this compensation is not possible, and a lower exercise capacity results.

### Stenosis

Valvular stenosis develops or progresses gradually, and because the normal valve orifice is larger than is necessary, stenosis is usually severe before exercise symptoms occur (i.e., a normal valve is larger than is needed for normal functioning and therefore has excess capacity).

Stress testing may be performed before initiation of an exercise program; with or without those test results, clients should be monitored closely, possibly using the perceived exertion or dyspnea scales mentioned earlier in this chapter. Because of reduced cardiac output, muscle perfusion is reduced and lactate is produced at low workloads. Maximal heart rate may be reduced when dyspnea is the cause of premature termination of exercise. Exercise systolic blood pressure may reach only 130 mm Hg because of low output. Exercise capacity in clients with mitral stenosis can be improved by slowing heart rate and prolonging the diastolic filling period with the use of β-blocking agents.

In the case of symptomatic aortic stenosis, clients are not candidates for exercise programs because of the danger of sudden death. Persons who are asymptomatic must be carefully evaluated before increasing their physical activity, and for most, exercise intensity should be mild. Angina with exercise is a common symptom when the aortic stenosis is severe.

#### Regurgitation

Exercise capacity may be unaffected in cases of mild regurgitation. Mitral regurgitation increases when aortic blood pressure is increased, such as occurs during isometric contractions. Light to moderate rhythmic and repetitive exercise reduces peripheral resistance and is recommended in place of isotonic exercise, which increases the heart rate. Individuals with valvular regurgitation due to a genetic condition, such as Marfan syndrome or Ehlers-Danlos syndrome, should avoid competitive sports, physical activities that may involve collisions, or isometric physical activities.[87,336] If no evidence of regurgitation or aortic dilation is evident, greater physical activity can be performed by these individuals.

#### Prolapse

Most people with MVP can participate in all sports activities, including intense competitive sports. Exercise is a key component in the management of MVP in order to improve overall cardiovascular function. However, at times, symptoms of fatigue and dyspnea caused by the MVP may limit physical activity, leading to deconditioning and contributing to a cycle of even more fatigue and shortness of breath.

Caution is advised in the use of weight training for the client with MVP; gradual buildup using light weights and increased repetitions is recommended. Some people with MVPS are prone to exercise-induced arrhythmias, which can (rarely) result in sudden death. Any time tachycardia develops in someone with known MVP, immediate medical referral is necessary.

#### Postoperative Considerations

Postoperative considerations are the same as for people who have had other types of cardiothoracic surgery. After uncomplicated valve ballooning, a return to normal activities is possible within 5 to 7 days. Gradual walking programs can be initiated at home for most people within a few days after surgery, or the client may enroll in a structured cardiac rehabilitation program.

Cardiac rehabilitation postoperatively in people with valvular heart disease is similar to that in post-CABG clients. Care should be taken to avoid high-impact exercises or exercises with a risk of trauma in people who are receiving anticoagulation therapy to avoid hemarthrosis and bruising.

Exercise outcomes differ after aortic, mitral, and mitral/aortic valve surgery. The degree of improvement in exercise capacity depends on the degree of residual dysfunction, presence or absence of arrhythmia, age of the subject, and the effort made to improve exercise capacity.[335] Functional capacity is substantially increased following aortic valve surgery but remains limited following mitral and mitral/aortic surgery, possibly because of differences in oxygen uptake. As mentioned, for people with mitral stenosis, exercise provides an early warning system, because the onset of dyspnea with strenuous exercise signals the beginning of clinical deterioration.

People who receive valve replacements may not be able to achieve maximal levels of exertion, but they should be able to achieve moderate to high levels depending on their other physical abilities and overall health. Because stress testing results can be normal after valve replacement, exercise Doppler echocardiography has been used to help prescribe physical activity in clients with prosthetic valves.

## Infective Endocarditis

### Definition and Incidence

Infective, or bacterial, endocarditis is an infection of the endocardium, the lining inside the heart, including the heart valves. It most commonly damages the mitral valve, followed by the aortic, tricuspid, and pulmonary valves. Endocarditis is categorized as either acute or subacute, depending on the clinical course, organisms, and condition of the valves. It affects 15 out of 100,000 people in the United States.[50]

### Etiologic and Risk Factors

Endocarditis can occur at any age, but rarely occurs in children. Half of all clients diagnosed are older than 60 years. Older adults may be at greater risk of endocarditis because valvular endocardial disruption is more common, immunity is impaired, and nutrition is poor. Endocarditis is more prevalent among men than women. MVP and mitral regurgitations increase risk of endocarditis.

Bacterial endocarditis may involve normal valves, but more often affects valves that have been damaged by some other previous pathologic process (e.g., rheumatic disease, congenital defects, cardiac surgery). Endocarditis is frequently caused by bacteria (particularly streptococci or staphylococci) normally present in the mouth, respiratory system, or GI tract or as a result of abnormal growths on the closure lines of previously damaged valves. In addition, persons with prosthetic heart valves, injection drug users, immunocompromised clients (including individuals receiving treatment for cancer), women who have had a suction abortion or pelvic infection related to intrauterine contraceptive devices, and postcardiac surgical clients are at high risk for developing endocarditis. Congenital heart disease and degenerative heart disease, such as calcific aortic stenosis, may also cause endocarditis. Dental procedures were thought to contribute to incidences of

**Table 12.16** Clinical Manifestations of Infective Endocarditis

| Systemic Infection | Intravascular Involvement | Immunologic Reaction | Musculoskeletal | Neurologic |
|---|---|---|---|---|
| Fever<br>Chills<br>Sweats<br>Malaise<br>Weakness<br>Anorexia<br>Weight loss<br>Cough<br>Dyspnea<br>Hemoptysis | Chest pain<br>Congestive heart failure<br>Cold and painful extremities<br>Clubbing<br>Petechiae<br>Splinter hemorrhages<br>Osler nodes | Arthralgia<br>Proteinuria<br>Hematuria<br>Acidosis<br>Arthritis | Arthralgia<br>Myalgias<br>Low-back pain | Confusion<br>Abscess<br>Cerebritis<br>Meningitis<br>Stroke (embolic or hemorrhagic) |

infective endocarditis; however, it was estimated that the risk is as low as 1 case per 14 million dental procedures.[50]

Hospital-acquired infective endocarditis has become more common as a result of iatrogenic endocardial damage produced by surgery, intracardiac pressure-monitoring catheters, ventriculoatrial shunts, and hyperalimentation lines that reach the right atrium. Portals of entry for microorganisms are also provided by wounds, biopsy sites, pacemakers, IV and arterial catheters, indwelling urinary catheters, and intratracheal airways.

### Pathogenesis

As an infection, endocarditis causes inflammation of the cardiac endothelium with destruction of the connective tissue. As these bloodborne microorganisms adhere to the endocardial surface, destruction of the connective tissue occurs as a result of the action of bacterial lytic enzymes. The surface endocardium becomes covered with fibrin and platelet thrombi that attract even more thrombogenic material.

The result is the formation of wart-like growths called *vegetations*. These vegetations, consisting of fibrin and platelets, can break off from the valve, embolize, and cause septic infarction in the myocardium, kidney, brain, spleen, abdomen, or extremities. These thromboemboli contain bacteria that not only cause ischemic infarcts, but also form new sites of infection, transforming into microabscesses. Bacteria may further invade the valves, causing intravalvular inflammation, destroying portions of the valves, and causing valve deformities.

Infective endocarditis of the right-side heart valves occurs commonly in injection drug users. Although a variety of hypotheses have been put forward to explain this phenomenon, no single explanation has been proven.

### Clinical Manifestations

Endocarditis can develop insidiously, with symptoms remaining undetected for months, or it can cause symptoms immediately, as in the case of acute bacterial endocarditis. Clinical manifestations can be divided into many groups (Table 12.16). It causes varying degrees of valvular dysfunction and may be associated with manifestations involving any number of organ systems, including lungs, eyes, kidneys, bones, joints, and CNS. The mitral, aortic, tricuspid, and pulmonary valves can be affected (descending order). Also, more than one valve can be infected at the same time. Neurologic signs and symptoms are predominant in about one third of all cases in those people older than 60 years. The classic findings of fever, cardiac murmur, and petechial lesions of the skin, conjunctivae, and oral mucosa are not always present.

Up to 50% of people with infective endocarditis initially have musculoskeletal symptoms, including arthralgia (most common), arthritis, low-back pain, and myalgia. Half of these people will have only musculoskeletal symptoms without other manifestations of endocarditis. The early onset of joint pain and myalgia as the first sign of endocarditis is more likely if the person is older and has had a previously diagnosed heart murmur.

Proximal joints are most often affected, especially the shoulder, followed by the knee, hip, wrist, ankle, metatarsophalangeal and metacarpophalangeal joints, and acromioclavicular joints (order of declining incidence). Most often one or two joints are painful, and symptoms begin suddenly, accompanied by warmth, tenderness, and redness. Symmetric arthralgia in the knees or ankles may lead to a diagnosis of rheumatoid arthritis, but as a rule, morning stiffness is not as prevalent in clients with endocarditis as in those with rheumatoid arthritis or polymyalgia rheumatica.

Bone and joint infections are particularly common among injection drug users. The most common sites of osteoarticular infections are the vertebrae, wrist, and sternoclavicular and sacroiliac joints, often with multiple joint involvement.[262]

Almost one third of clients with endocarditis have low-back pain, which may be the primary symptom reported. Back pain is accompanied by decreased range of motion and spinal tenderness. Pain may affect only one side, and it may be limited to the paraspinal muscles. Endocarditis-induced back pain may be very similar to that associated with a herniated lumbar disk, as it radiates to the leg and may be accentuated by raising the leg or by sneezing, coughing, or laughing. However, neurologic deficits are usually absent in persons with endocarditis. Rarely, other musculoskeletal symptoms, such as osteomyelitis, tendinitis, hypertrophic osteoarthropathy, bone infarcts, and ischemic bone necrosis, may occur.

## MEDICAL MANAGEMENT

**DIAGNOSIS, TREATMENT, AND PROGNOSIS.** Infective endocarditis is often difficult to diagnose because it can present with a wide array of signs and symptoms, as well as a confusing clinical picture. Blood cultures to identify specific pathogens in the presence of septicemia are required to determine appropriate antibiotic therapy, which is the primary medical intervention.

Other laboratory test results indicative of infectious endocarditis include elevated erythrocyte sedimentation rate, proteinuria, and hematuria. Echocardiography may be used to confirm the diagnosis and is useful in showing underlying valvular lesions and quantifying their severity. This test is not as useful in older adults, because it is common to find echogenic areas around and on degenerative valves that are impossible to distinguish from the infective vegetations seen in infective endocarditis. Large masses on valves are much more diagnostic.

Although it is easily prevented (for the at-risk person) by taking antibiotics before and after procedures, genitourinary instrumentation, and open cardiovascular surgery, endocarditis is difficult to treat and can result in serious heart damage or death. Potential complications are many, including HF and arterial, systemic, or PEs. Therapy with antibiotics may be prolonged and, without complete treatment, relapse can occur up to 2 or more weeks after medical intervention. Surgical valve replacement may be necessary, depending on the response to treatment, sites of infection, recurrent infection, or infection of a prosthetic valve. Care is taken by the medical staff to prescribe antibiotics long enough to completely eradicate the infection but not prolong their use beyond that, putting the client at risk for antibiotic-resistant infections in the future.[35]

SPECIAL IMPLICATIONS FOR THE THERAPIST 12.13

### *Infective Endocarditis*

Physical exertion beyond normal activities of daily living is usually limited for the person receiving antibiotic therapy for endocarditis and during the first few weeks of recovery. The therapist treating a person with infective endocarditis during this acute phase should focus on functional movements and mobility only. Due to early manifestations of endocarditis being primarily peripheral (musculoskeletal or cutaneous) in nature, the therapist may be the first to recognize signs and symptoms of a systemic disorder and should refer the client back to the physician if endocarditis is suspected.

Splinter hemorrhages (dark red linear streaks resembling splinters under the nail bed), clubbing, petechiae, purplish red subcutaneous nodes on the finger and toe pads, and lesions on the thenar and hypothenar eminences of the palms, fingers, and sometimes the soles are very often present in individuals with infective endocarditis.

For any client with known risk factors or a recent history of endocarditis, the therapist must be alert for signs of endocarditis, indications of complications (easy fatigue associated with HF or peripheral emboli), lack of response to therapy intervention, or signs indicating relapse. Often, the client thinks the symptoms are recurrent bouts of the flu or other general illness.

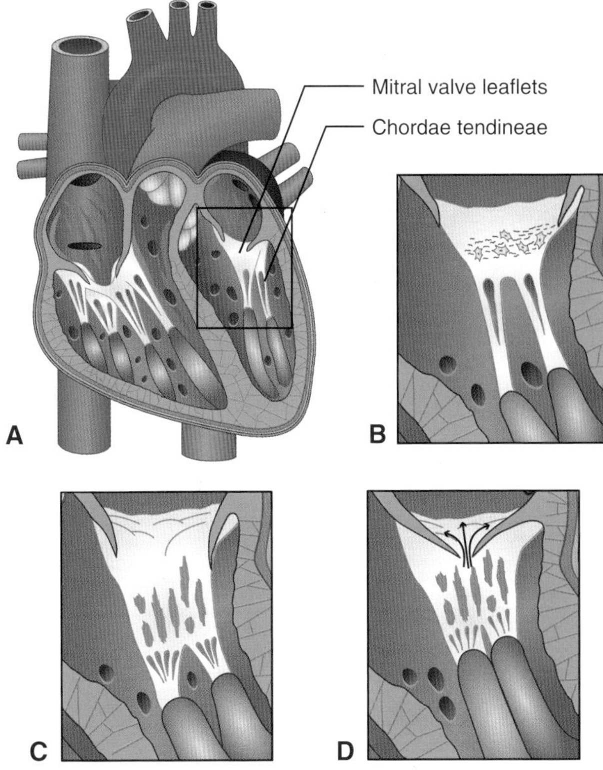


**Figure 12.23**

**Cardiac valvular disease caused by rheumatic fever.** (A) Inflammation of the membrane over the mitral (and aortic) valves may cause edema and accumulation of fibrin and platelets on the chordae tendineae. (B) This accumulation of inflammatory materials produces rheumatic vegetations that affect the support provided by the chordae tendineae to the atrioventricular valves. (C) In this view, the mitral valve leaflets have become thickened with scar tissue and calcified. The chordae tendineae often fuse. (D) As a result, the scarred valve fails to close tightly (mitral stenosis), and regurgitation or backflow of blood into the atrium develops. Prolonged, severe stenosis with mitral regurgitation leads to symptoms of congestive heart failure. (Modified from Goodman CC, Snyder TE: *Differential diagnosis in physical therapy*, ed 3, Philadelphia, 2000, WB Saunders, p. 110.)

## Rheumatic Fever and Heart Disease

### Overview, Incidence, and Etiologic Factors

Rheumatic fever is one form of endocarditis (infection), caused by streptococcal group A bacteria, that can be fatal or may lead to rheumatic heart disease (10% of cases), a chronic condition caused by scarring and deformity of the heart valves (Figs. 12.23 and 12.24). It is called rheumatic fever because two of the most common symptoms are fever and joint pain.

The infection generally starts with strep throat in children between ages 5 and 15 years and damages the heart in approximately 50% of cases. The aggressive use of specific antibiotics in the United States had effectively reduced the incidence of rheumatic fever to around 0.5 cases per 1,000 school-age children and removed it as the primary cause of valvular damage.[45] While incidence of rheumatic heart disease is very low in high-income countries, including the United States, it is endemic in some low- and middle-income countries.[50]

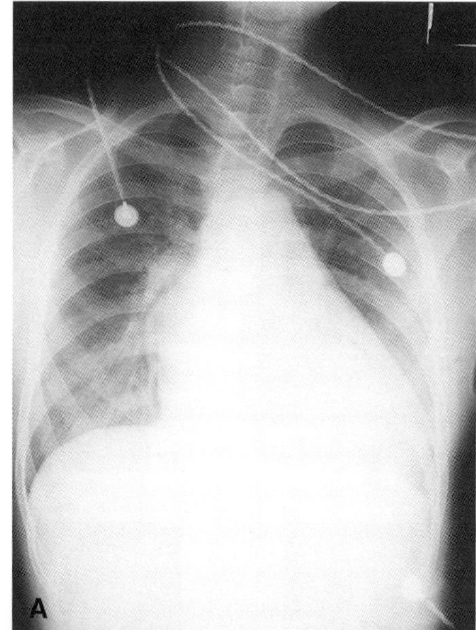


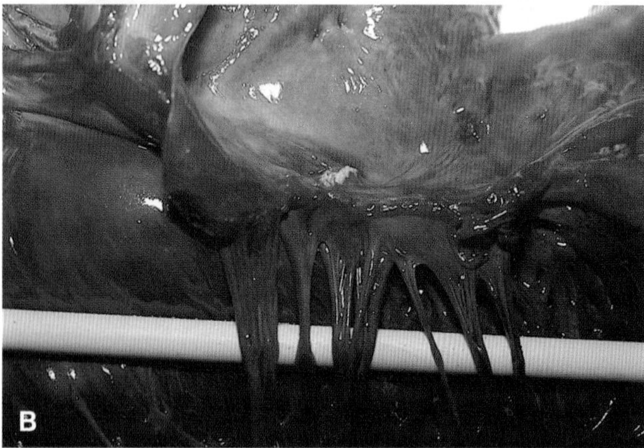


**Figure 12.24**

(A) Chest radiograph of a 15-year-old boy who had multiple occurrences of acute rheumatic fever, showing gross cardiac enlargement and failure. He had mitral regurgitation and stenosis and aortic regurgitation and stenosis. (B) Postmortem cardiac examination of the same boy, showing thickened, shortened mitral valve cusps with calcific vegetation and thickened chordae tendineae. Chordae are the tendinous cords connecting the two atrioventricular (AV) valves (the tricuspid valve between the right atrium and right ventricle and the mitral valve between the left atrium and left ventricle) to the appropriate papillary muscles in the heart ventricles; the chordae tendineae in effect anchor the valve leaflets. This support to the AV valves during ventricular systole helps prevent prolapse of the valve into the atrium. (Courtesy Professor Bart Currie, Menzies School of Health Research, Darwin, NT, Australia.)

## Pathogenesis

The exact pathogenesis is not well understood. In response to the streptococcal bacterial infection, the body's T cells are activated, and B cells produce antibodies against different components of the bacterium to fight the infection. As it happens, these streptococcal cell components have structural similarities with the host body proteins, and activated T cells start infiltrating tissues and the antibodies start binding to proteins on the heart, brain cells, muscles, and joints, beginning the autoimmune response. Infiltration of T cells and immune complex deposits trigger extensive inflammation in tissues. Thus rheumatic fever is classified as an autoimmune disease. In the case of the heart valves, the inflammation affects the valve tissue and myocardium. All layers of the heart (epicardium, endocardium, myocardium, pericardium) (Fig. 12.25) may be involved.

Endocardial inflammation causes swelling of the valve leaflets, with secondary erosion along the lines of leaflet contact. Small, bead-like clumps of vegetation containing platelets and fibrin are deposited on eroded valvular tissue and on the chordae tendineae. The mitral and aortic valves are those most commonly affected.

Over time, scarring and shortening of the involved structures occur, and the leaflets adhere to each other as the valves lose their elasticity. As many as 25% of clients will have mitral valvular disease 25 to 30 years after rheumatic fever, developing fibrosis and calcification of valves, fusion of commissures (union or junction between adjacent cusps of the heart valves) and chordae tendineae, and mitral stenosis with fish-mouth deformity (Fig. 12.26).

## Clinical Manifestations

Although strep throat is the most common manifestation of the streptococcal bacterial invasion, streptococcal infections can also affect the skin, kidneys, and, less commonly, the lungs. In some cases of strep throat, the initial triggering of sore throat or pharyngitis does not cause extreme illness, if any discomfort at all.

However, the major manifestations of acute rheumatic fever are usually carditis, acute migratory polyarthritis, and chorea, which may occur singly or in combination with other symptoms. In the acute, full-blown sequelae, shortness of breath and increasing nocturnal cough also occur. A ring- or crescent-shaped rash with clear centers on the skin of the limbs or trunk (erythema marginatum) is present in fewer than 2% of persons in an acute episode. Subcutaneous nodules may occur over bony prominences and along the extensor surfaces of the arms, heels, knees, or back of the head, but these do not interfere with joint function.

*Carditis* is most likely to occur in children and adolescents. Mitral or aortic valve dysfunction may result in a previously undetected murmur. Chest pain caused by pericardial inflammation and characteristic heart sounds may occur. *Polyarthritis* may develop in a child or young adult with acute rheumatic fever 2 to 3 weeks after an initial cold or sore throat. Sudden or gradual onset of painful migratory joint symptoms in knees, shoulders, feet, ankles, elbows, fingers, or neck; fever (37.2°–39.4° C [99°–103° F]); palpitations; and fatigue are present. Malaise, weakness, weight loss, and anorexia may accompany the fever.

The migratory arthralgias usually involve two or more joints simultaneously or in succession and may last only 24 hours, or they may persist for several weeks. However, in adults, only a single joint may be affected. Joints that are sore and hot and contain fluid completely resolve, followed by acute synovitis, heat, synovial space tenderness, swelling, and effusion present in a different area the next day. The persistence of swelling, heat, and synovitis in a single joint or joints for more than 2 to 3 weeks is extremely unusual in acute rheumatic fever.

Rheumatic *chorea* (also called Sydenham chorea or St. Vitus dance) occurs in 3% of cases 1 to 3 months

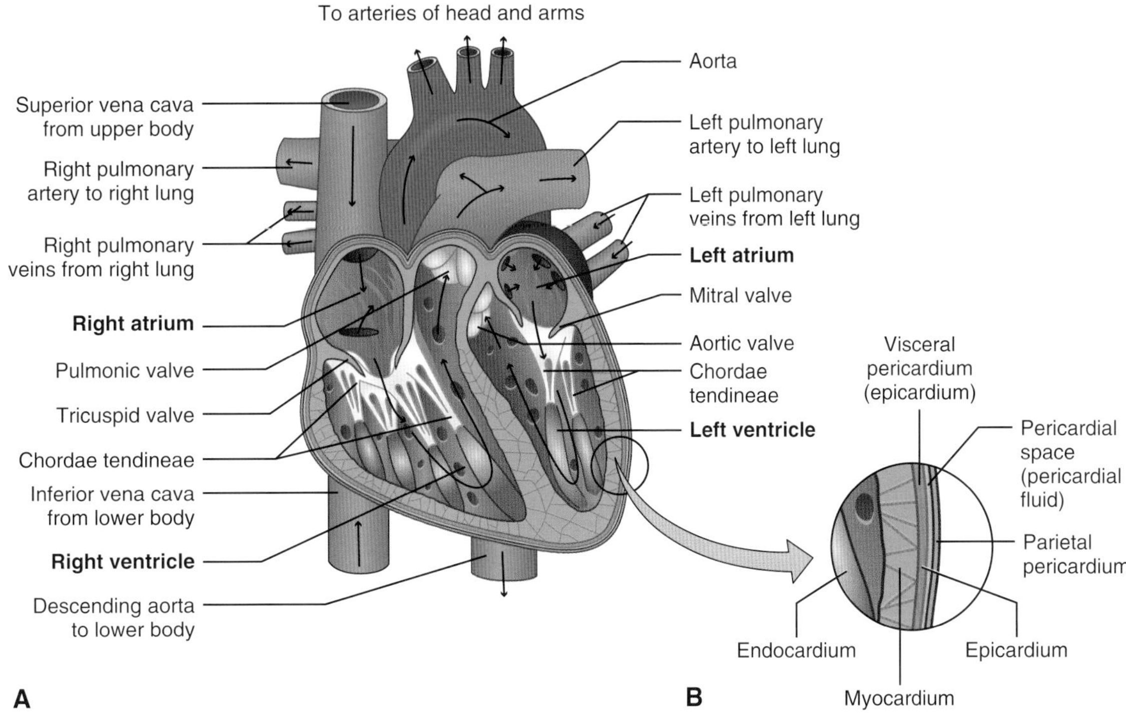


**Figure 12.25**

(A) Structure and circulation of the heart. Blood flows from the superior and inferior venae cavae into the right atrium through the tricuspid valve to the right ventricle. The right ventricle ejects the blood through the pulmonic valve into the pulmonary artery during ventricular systole. Blood enters the pulmonary capillary system, where it exchanges the carbon dioxide for oxygen. The oxygenated blood then leaves the lungs via the pulmonary veins and returns to the left atrium. From the left atrium, blood flows through the mitral valve into the left ventricle. The left ventricle pumps blood into the systemic circulation through the aorta to supply all the tissues of the body with oxygen. From the systemic circulation, blood returns to the heart through the superior and inferior venae cavae to begin the cycle again. (B) Sagittal view of the layers of the heart wall.

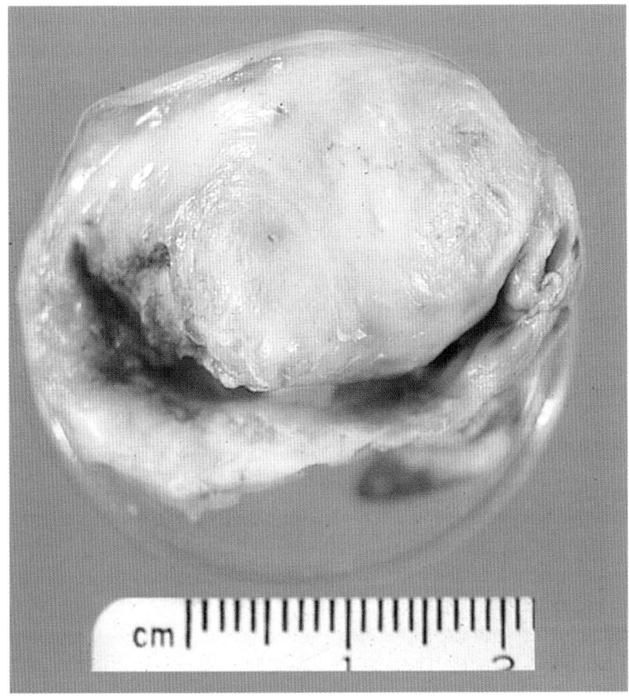


**Figure 12.26**

A severely stenotic mitral valve has a narrowed orifice that has the appearance of a classic "fish mouth" deformity. (From Aliya N, Husain MD: *High-yield thoracic pathology*, Philadelphia, 2012 Elsevier, pp 497–497.)

after the streptococcal infection and is always preceded by polyarthritis. Chorea in a child, teenager, or young adult is almost always a manifestation of acute rheumatic fever. Other causes of chorea are SLE, thyrotoxicosis, and cerebrovascular accident, but these are uncommon and unlikely in a child.

The chorea develops as rapid, purposeless, nonrepetitive movements that may involve all muscles except the eyes. This pattern of movement may last for 1 week, several months, or even several years without permanent impairment of the CNS.

## MEDICAL MANAGEMENT

**DIAGNOSIS AND TREATMENT.** Late diagnosis can have serious consequences requiring immediate antibiotic and antiinflammatory treatment. Jones criteria are used as the basis for diagnosis (Table 12.17), and results of throat culture for group A streptococci are usually positive. Echocardiography combined with Doppler technology provides reliable hemodynamic and anatomic data in the assessment of rheumatic heart disease.

Aspirin may be used to treat the joint manifestations and as a general antiinflammatory agent. Corticosteroids are used when there is clear evidence of rheumatic carditis. Children with acute chorea are generally treated with some form of CNS depressant, such as phenobarbital. Commissurotomy and prosthetic valve replacement may be necessary for valvular dysfunction associated with chronic rheumatic disease.

**Table 12.17** Jones Criteria for Diagnosis of Rheumatic Fever

| Major Manifestations | Minor Manifestations | Supporting Evidence of Streptococcal Infection |
|---|---|---|
| Carditis<br>Polyarthritis<br>Chorea<br>Erythema marginatum<br>Subcutaneous nodules | Previous rheumatic fever or rheumatic heart disease<br>Arthralgia<br>Fever<br>Elevated appearance of C-reactive protein<br>Leukocytosis<br>ECG changes | Recent scarlet fever<br>Positive throat culture for group A *Streptococcus*<br>Other positive laboratory tests |

*ECG*, Electrocardiogram.

Data from Dajani AS, Ayoub A, Burman FZ, et al: American Heart Association medical/scientific statement: guidelines for the diagnosis of rheumatic fever: Jones criteria, 1992 update, *Circulation* 87:302–307, 1993. Jones criteria have been reviewed and remains valid per the Jones Criteria Working Group. In Ferrieri P: Proceedings of the Jones Criteria Workshop, *Circulation* 106:2521–2423, 2002.

**PROGNOSIS.** Initial episodes of rheumatic fever last weeks to months, but 20% of children affected have recurrences within 5 years and may progress to severe disease, requiring valve surgery over 7.5 years.[50] Relapses increase the risk of heart damage that leads to rheumatic heart disease, with mitral or aortic stenosis or insufficiency caused by progressive valve scarring. Mortality for acute rheumatic fever is low (1%–2%), but persistent rheumatic activity with complications (enlarged heart, AF, arterial embolism, HF, pericarditis) is associated with long-term morbidity and mortality.

**SPECIAL IMPLICATIONS FOR THE THERAPIST 12.14**

### *Rheumatic Fever and Heart Disease*

The increased incidence of infection with streptococcal group A bacteria in the adult population may result in cases of sudden or gradual onset of painful migratory joint symptoms affecting the knees, shoulders, feet, ankles, elbows, fingers, or neck. Any time an adult presents with intermittent or migratory joint symptoms, their temperature must be taken.

The therapist should ask about recent exposure to someone with strep throat and a recent history or symptoms such as presence of rash anywhere on the body, sore throat, or cold. The sore throat or cold symptoms may be mild enough that the person does not seek medical care of any kind. The presence of fever accompanied by a clinical presentation of migratory arthralgias or a history of recent illness as described requires medical evaluation.

As many as 25% of people affected by rheumatic fever develop mitral valve dysfunction 25 to 30 years later. Adults who experience exercise intolerance or exertional dyspnea of unknown cause and who have a previous history of childhood rheumatic fever may be experiencing the effects of MVP. Dyspnea associated with MVP is most commonly accompanied by fatigue and palpitations. This history in combination with this triad of symptoms requires evaluation by a physician. In the case of a confirmed diagnosis of rheumatic fever–related mitral valve involvement, exercise will not improve the mechanical function of the valve, but improvement in cardiovascular function can occur.

## DISEASES AFFECTING THE PERICARDIUM

The pericardium consists of two layers: the inner visceral layer, which is attached to the epicardium, and an outer parietal layer (see Fig. 12.25).

The pericardium stabilizes the heart in its anatomic position despite changes in body position and reduces excess friction between the heart and surrounding structures. It is composed of fibrous tissue that is loose enough to permit moderate changes in cardiac size but that cannot stretch fast enough to accommodate rapid dilation or accumulation of fluid without increasing intracardiac pressure.

The pericardium may be a primary site of disease and is often involved by processes that affect the heart. It may also be affected by diseases of the adjacent tissues. Pericardial diseases are common and have multiple causes. Three conditions primarily affect the pericardium: acute pericarditis, constrictive pericarditis, and pericardial effusion. These three diseases are grouped together for ease of understanding in the following section.

### Pericarditis

#### Definition and Overview

Pericarditis or inflammation of the pericardium, the double-layer membrane surrounding the heart, may be a primary condition or may be secondary to a number of diseases and circumstances (Box 12.11). It may occur as a single acute event, or it may recur and become a chronic condition called *constrictive pericarditis* (uncommon).

#### Incidence and Etiologic Factors

The most common types of pericarditis encountered by the therapist will be drug induced, those present in association with autoimmune diseases (e.g., connective tissue disorders such as SLE, rheumatoid arthritis), after MI, in conjunction with renal failure, after open heart surgery, or after radiation therapy.

Other types encountered less often include viral pericarditis (e.g., Epstein-Barr, hepatitis, human immunodeficiency virus [HIV]) and neoplastic pericarditis (from spread to the pericardium of adjacent lung cancer or invasion by breast cancer, leukemia, Hodgkin lymphoma).

Box 12.11

**CAUSES OF PERICARDITIS**

- Idiopathic (85%)
- Infections
  - Viral (Coxsackie, influenza, Epstein-Barr, hepatitis B, HIV, cytomegalovirus, varicella zoster, herpes simplex)
  - Bacterial (tuberculosis, *Staphylococcus, Streptococcus,* meningococcus, pneumonia, *Salmonella, Neisseria gonorrhoeae, Pseudomonas*)
  - Parasitic
  - Fungal
- Myocardial injury
  - MI
  - Cardiac trauma: instrumentation; blunt or penetrating pericardium; rib fracture
  - Postcardiac surgery
- Hypersensitivity
  - Collagen diseases: rheumatic fever, scleroderma, SLE, rheumatoid arthritis
  - Drug reaction
  - Radiation or cobalt therapy
- Metabolic disorders
  - Uremia
  - Myxedema
- Chronic anemia
- Neoplasm
  - Lymphoma, leukemia, lung or breast cancer
- Aortic dissection
- Graft-versus-host disease

Data from Bonow RO: *Braunwald's heart disease—a textbook of cardiovascular medicine*, ed 9, Philadelphia, 2011, WB Saunders.

### Pathogenesis

Many causes of pericarditis affect both the pericardium and the myocardium (myopericarditis) with varying degrees of cardiac dysfunction. Constrictive pericarditis is characterized by a fibrotic, thickened, and adherent pericardium that is compressing the heart. The heart becomes restricted in movement and function. Diastolic filling of the heart is reduced, venous pressures are elevated, cardiac output is decreased, and eventual cardiac failure may result.

When fluid accumulates within the pericardial sac, it is referred to as *pericardial effusion.* Blunt chest trauma or any cause of acute pericarditis can lead to pericardial effusion. Rapid distention or excessive fluid accumulation from this condition can also compress the heart (cardiac tamponade) and reduce ventricular filling and cardiac output.

### Clinical Manifestations

The presentation and course of pericarditis are determined by the underlying etiology. For example, pericarditis may occur 2 to 5 days after infarction as a result of an inflammatory reaction to myocardial necrosis, or it may occur within the first year after radiation initiates a fibrotic process in the pericardium. Often there is pleuritic chest pain that is made worse by lying down, deep breathing, and coughing and is relieved by sitting upright or leaning forward. The pain is substernal and may radiate to the neck, shoulders, upper back, upper trapezius, left supraclavicular area, or epigastrium, or down the left arm.

Other symptoms may include fever, joint pain, dyspnea, or difficulty swallowing. Auscultation of the lower left sternal border where the pericardium lies close to the chest wall will produce a pericardial friction rub, a high-pitched scratchy sound that may be heard at end expiration. This sound is produced by the friction between the pericardial surfaces that results from inflammation and occurs during heart movement. Symptoms of constrictive pericarditis develop slowly and usually include progressive dyspnea, fatigue, weakness, peripheral edema, and ascites. Constrictive disease can lead to diastolic dysfunction and eventual HF.

## MEDICAL MANAGEMENT

**DIAGNOSIS.** Clinical examination, including clinical presentation, auscultation, and client history, may assist with the diagnosis. A classic sign of pericarditis is the pericardial friction rub heard on auscultation. Other diagnostic tools include chest x-ray (showing enlarged cardiac shadow), characteristic ECG changes (showing evidence of an underlying inflammatory process), and laboratory studies (e.g., elevated erythrocyte sedimentation rate or elevated white blood cell count [nonspecific indicators of inflammation] and elevated cardiac enzymes [post-MI]). CT, MRI, and echocardiography are modalities used for imaging the pericardium and pericardial disease.

**TREATMENT.** New treatments for pericardial diseases are being developed as a result of modern imaging, new understanding of molecular biology, and immunologic techniques. Comprehensive and systematic implementation of new techniques of pericardiocentesis, pericardial fluid analysis, pericardioscopy, and epicardial and pericardial biopsy, as well as the application of new techniques for pericardial fluid and biopsy analyses, have permitted early specific diagnosis, creating foundations for etiologic intervention in many cases.[186]

Conventional treatment remains twofold, directed toward prevention of long-term complications and treatment of the underlying cause. For example, while any underlying infection is treated when possible (antibiotics for bacterial pericarditis), symptomatic treatment is provided for idiopathic, viral, or radiation pericarditis. Anti-inflammatory drugs are given for severe, acute pericarditis or pericarditis associated with connective tissue disorders. Chemotherapy is given for neoplastic pericarditis; and dialysis is performed for uremic pericarditis. Analgesics may be prescribed for the pain and fever. Pericardiocentesis (surgical drainage with a needle catheter through a small subxiphoid incision) may be performed if cardiac compression from pericardial effusion (cardiac tamponade) does not resolve.

Treatment for constrictive pericarditis is both medical and surgical, including digoxin preparations, diuretics, sodium restriction, and pericardiectomy (surgical excision of the damaged pericardium).

**PROGNOSIS.** The prognosis in most cases of acute viral pericarditis is excellent when there is no (or only minimal) myocardial involvement, because this is frequently a self-limited disease. Without medical intervention, shock and death can occur from decreased cardiac output with cardiac involvement. Constrictive pericarditis is a progressive disease without spontaneous reversal of symptoms. Most people become progressively disabled over time. Surgical removal of the pericardium is associated with a high mortality rate when progressive calcification in the epicardium and dense adhesions or fibrosis between the pericardial layers are present.

SPECIAL IMPLICATIONS FOR THE THERAPIST 12.15

### *Pericarditis*

Pericardial pain can be mistaken as a musculoskeletal problem, presenting as just upper back, neck, or upper trapezius pain. In such cases, the pain may be diminished by holding the breath or aggravated by swallowing or neck or trunk movements, especially side bending or rotation.

Pain is also aggravated by respiratory movements, such as deep breathing, coughing, and laughing. The therapist must screen for medical disease by assessing aggravating and relieving factors and by asking the client about a history of fever, chills, upper respiratory tract infection (recent cold or flu), weakness, heart disease, or recent heart attack.

Special precautions depend on the underlying cause of the pericarditis. Mild cases have few precautions, and therapy intervention is guided by client tolerance, while the therapist also monitors for any symptoms of HF. A mild pericarditis can quickly progress to a severe condition that requires medical evaluation. The clinician is referred to each individual section in this text representing the etiology of pericarditis for precautions.

## DISEASES AFFECTING THE BLOOD VESSELS

Diseases of blood vessels observed in a therapy setting can include aneurysm, PVD, vascular neoplasm, and arteriovenous malformation.

### Aneurysm

Definition and Overview

An aneurysm is an abnormal stretching (dilation) in the wall of an artery, a vein, or the heart with a diameter that is at least 50% greater than normal. When the vessel wall becomes weakened from trauma, congenital vascular disease, infection, or atherosclerosis, a permanent sac-like formation develops. A false aneurysm (pseudoaneurysm) can occur when the wall of the blood vessel is ruptured and blood escapes into surrounding tissues, forming a clot (Fig. 12.27). Dissection is the disruption of the tunica media layer of the vessel wall with bleeding occurring within and along the wall that results in the separation of the wall layers.[178]

Aneurysms are of various types (either arterial or venous) and are named according to the specific site of

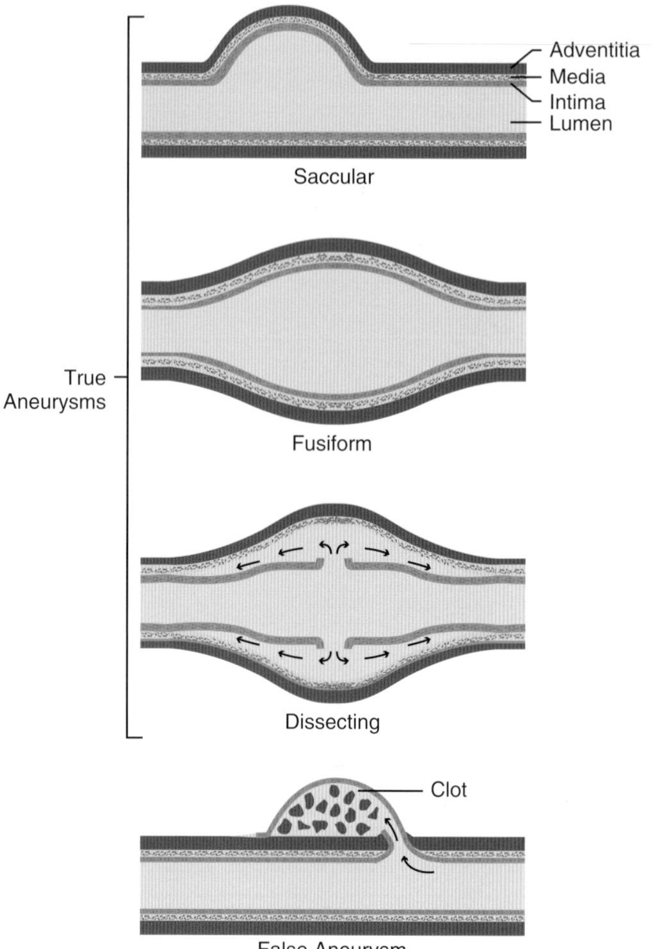


**Figure 12.27**

**Longitudinal sections showing types of aneurysms.** In a true aneurysm, layers of the vessel wall dilate in one of the following ways: saccular, a unilateral outpouching; fusiform, a diffuse dilation involving the entire circumference of the artery wall; or dissecting, a bilateral outpouching in which layers of the vessel wall separate, with creation of a cavity. In a false aneurysm, the wall ruptures, and a blood clot is retained in an outpouching of tissue.

formation (Fig. 12.28). The most common site for an arterial aneurysm is the aorta, forming a thoracic aortic aneurysm (which involves the ascending, transverse, or first part of the descending portion of the aorta) or an abdominal aortic aneurysm (commonly abbreviated as AAA and which generally involves the aorta between the renal arteries and iliac branches).

*Thoracic aortic aneurysms* located above the diaphragm occur less often than other types but tend to be more life-threatening.

*Abdominal aortic aneurysms* located below the diaphragmatic border occur about 4 times more often than thoracic aneurysms, most likely because the aorta is not supported by skeletal muscle at this location.

*Peripheral arterial aneurysms* affect the femoral and popliteal arteries and are not as common.

*Intracranial (cerebral) aneurysms* affect cerebral arteries or veins. Unruptured intracranial aneurysms occur in 0.2% to 10% of the general population. Fifty percent to

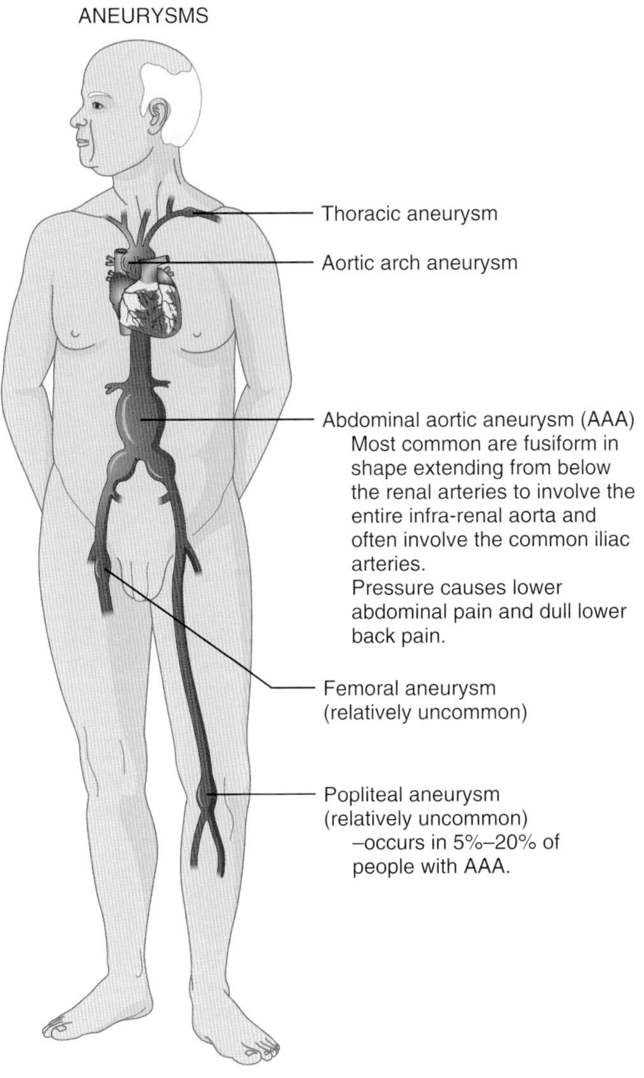


**Figure 12.28**

**Aneurysms are named according to the specific site of formation.** Abdominal aortic aneurysms are the most common type; more than 95% of abdominal aortic aneurysms are located below the renal arteries and extend to the umbilicus, causing low-back pain. (From Jarvis C: *Physical examination and health assessment,* ed 5, Philadelphia, 2008, WB Saunders.)

80% of all intracranial aneurysms do not rupture in the course of a person's lifetime.

## Incidence and Etiologic and Risk Factors

According to the Society for Vascular Surgery, approximately 200,000 people in the United States are diagnosed annually with abdominal aortic aneurysm, and 14,000 of those aneurysms are severe enough to rupture, causing death.[341]

Age is the most significant risk factor for AAA,[80] usually beginning after age 50 years, presumably as a result of chronic inflammatory vascular wall changes, resulting in atherosclerosis. Atherosclerosis or any injury to the middle or muscular layer of the arterial wall (tunica media) is responsible for most arterial aneurysms. However, someone without evidence of atherosclerosis/injury can develop an aneurysm, especially in the presence of congenital weakness of the blood vessel walls. The prevalence of AAA is 1.4% for people between 50 and 84 years of age,[80] and the incidence is increasing, probably due to the increasing number of older adults and the increasing number of people with peripheral hypertension.

Aneurysms occur much more often in men than in women, although women have a higher risk of aneurysm rupture.[80] AAA is less common for African Americans, Hispanics, Asian Americans, and in people with diabetes.[80] Cigarette smoking increases the risk of aneurysm sevenfold, and more than 90% of people with AAA smoked at some point in their life. Other risk factors include increased salt intake, hypertension, and presence of peripheral artery disease and cerebrovascular disease. The risk is decreased in those eating fruits and vegetables more than 3 times per week and exercising more than once a week.[80]

First-degree related family members (parent, adult child, or sibling) of anyone with an aneurysm have a 20% increased risk of AAA.[80] GWAS identified variants in genes for ACE, angiotensin II type 1 receptor, IL-10, matrix metalloproteinase 3, and transforming growth factor β receptor II are linked to AAA.[80] Moreover, specific allelic variations have been identified that may influence respiratory epithelium response to cigarette smoking, providing an insight on smoking as a significant risk factor.

Thoracic aortic aneurysms account for approximately 10% of all aortic aneurysms. The incidence is about 10 per 100,000 persons per year.[178] Risk factors include hypertension, smoking, chronic obstructive pulmonary disease, bicuspid aortic valve anomaly, and inflammatory disease.[178] Some genetic syndromes that affect connective tissue are associated with thoracic aortic aneurysms, including Marfan syndrome (caused by mutation in one of the connective tissue proteins, fibrillin 1) and Ehler-Danlos syndrome (mutation in another connective tissue protein, collagen, mostly type III). This knowledge is exciting, as it allows physicians to employ strategies used in individuals with Marfan syndrome, for instance, to prevent or treat aortic aneurysms and dissections. Turner syndrome (presence of only one X chromosome in females) is also linked to development of thoracic aortic aneurysm.[178]

## Pathogenesis

The vessel wall weakens as a result of the decrease or loss of elastic fibers that are replaced with nonstretchable proteoglycans, and loss of smooth muscle cells in the tunica media.[178] Increased levels of matrix metalloproteinases, which have elastolytic activity, detected in the media of aortic aneurysms are associated with degradation of elastin, the structural component of elastic fibers.[178] Most thoracic aneurysms are caused by these degenerative changes in the vessel wall, with atherosclerotic plaques and inflammatory processes probably contributing to thinning and weakening of the wall.[178]

Plaque formation erodes the vessel wall, predisposing the vessel to stretching of the inner and outer layers of the artery and formation of a sac. When a dissection occurs, the innermost layer of the aorta tears, creating a false channel that allows blood to flow into the middle layer. With each heartbeat, the dissection can extend, causing the aortic wall to further separate or dissect.

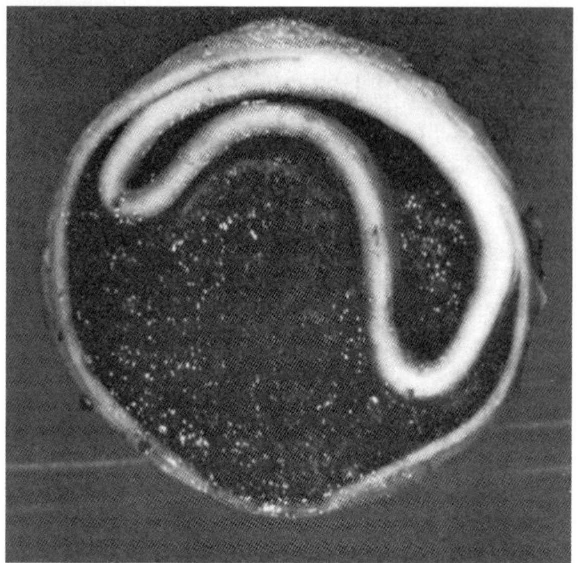

**Figure 12.29**

**Dissecting aneurysm.** Cross-section of the aorta with dissecting aneurysm showing true aortic lumen (*above* and *right*) compressed by dissecting column of blood that separates the media and creates a false lumen. (From Kissane JM, ed: *Anderson's pathology,* St Louis, 1990, Mosby.)

With time, the aneurysm becomes more fibrotic, but it continues to bulge with each systole, thus acting as a reservoir for some of the stroke volume. In the case of thoracic aortic aneurysms, the sheer force of elevated blood pressure causes a tear in the intima with rapid disruption and rupture of the aortic wall. Subsequent hemorrhage causes a lengthwise splitting of the arterial wall, creating a false vessel (Fig. 12.29), and a hematoma may form in either channel (i.e., the false or true lumen).

### Clinical Manifestations

Aneurysms may be asymptomatic. However, when they do occur, manifestations depend largely on the size and position of the aneurysm and its rate of growth. Persistent but vague substernal, back, neck, or jaw pain may occur as enlargement of the aneurysm impinges adjacent structures or interrupts blood flow to other areas.

Aortic dissection may be experienced as extreme, sharp pain felt at the base of the neck or along the back into the interscapular area. When pressure from a large volume of blood is placed on the trachea, esophagus, laryngeal nerve, lung, or superior vena cava, symptoms of dysphagia; hoarseness; edema of the neck, arms, or jaw and distended neck veins; and dyspnea and/or cough may occur, respectively.

Other signs and symptoms may be present in the case of *acute aortic dissection* as a result of compression of branches of the aorta. These include acute MI, reversible ischemic neurologic deficits, stroke, paraplegia, renal failure, intestinal ischemia, and ischemia of the arms and legs. Acute chest pain may also result from a nondissecting, intramural hematoma of the aorta or erosion of a penetrating atherosclerotic ulcer.[178]

In the case of an untreated AAA, expansion and rupture can occur in one of several places, including the peritoneal cavity, the mesentery, the retroperitoneum, into the inferior vena cava, or into the duodenum or rectum. Rupture refers to a tearing of all three tunicae (tunica adventitia, tunica media, tunica intima) with bleeding into the thoracic or abdominal cavity. The most common site for an AAA is just below the renal arteries, and it may involve the bifurcation of the aorta (see Fig. 12.28).

Most abdominal aortic aneurysms are asymptomatic, but intermittent or constant pain in the form of mild to severe mid-abdominal or lower back discomfort is present in some form in 25% to 30% of cases. Groin or flank pain may be experienced because of increasing pressure on other structures. Women may initially believe this pain related to menstruation, but pain from AAA is not cramping in nature; instead, it tends to be stronger and nagging.

Early warning signs of an impending rupture may include abdominal heartbeat when lying down or a dull ache (intermittent or constant) in the mid-abdominal left flank or lower back. Rupture is most likely to occur in aneurysms that are 5 cm or larger, causing intense flank pain with referred pain to the back at the level of the rupture. Pain may radiate to the lower abdomen, groin, or genitalia. Back pain may be the only presenting symptom before rupture occurs. Detection of an AAA is through physical exam and imaging. Physical exam should include history, auscultation of abdominal aorta listening for bruits, palpation of abdominal aorta margins, and general abdominal screening. It is important to note that physical exam alone is only reliable at diagnosing AAA about 20% of the time,[55] and therefore, imaging is a more reliable tool for diagnosing AAA. Imaging may be performed using CT, ultrasound, or MRI, with ultrasound considered to be the gold standard for diagnosis.[55]

The most common site for peripheral arterial aneurysm is the popliteal space in the lower extremities. Most are caused by atherosclerosis and occur bilaterally in men. Popliteal aneurysm presents as a pulsating mass, 2 cm or more in diameter, and causes ischemic symptoms in the lower limbs (e.g., intermittent claudication, rest pain, thrombosis, and embolization, resulting in gangrene). Femoral aneurysm presents as a pulsating mass in the femoral area on one or both sides.

## MEDICAL MANAGEMENT

**DIAGNOSIS.** Detection of abdominal and peripheral aneurysms often occurs when the physician palpates a pulsating mass during routine examination or when x-rays are taken for other purposes (although not all aortic aneurysms show abnormalities on chest radiography). Radiography, ultrasonography, echocardiography with color Doppler imaging, CT, MRI, arteriography, and aortography may be used for investigation.[178]

**PREVENTION AND TREATMENT.** Annual examination to ensure early identification is recommended for family members (parent, adult child, or sibling) of anyone who has previously been diagnosed with an aortic aneurysm. Anyone with a family risk or signs of diseased arteries should take preventive measures, including smoking cessation, regular exercise, blood pressure control, and cholesterol management.[178]

Treatment is determined based on the size of the bulge, how fast it is expanding, and the individual's clinical presentation. The goal in managing dissecting aneurysms is to prevent further dissection and minimize the damage to organs that may not have received enough blood flow.[178]

For small aneurysms of any type, watchful waiting is often advised. Watchful waiting and preventive pharmacology (e.g., statin to lower cholesterol; β-blocker or ACE inhibitor to control blood pressure and prevent the aneurysm from getting larger or bursting) may be advised depending on individual factors. As a less-invasive alternative to open surgery, an endovascular treatment is used for some types of thoracic aortic aneurysm and dissection.[178] It involves insertion of an endovascular stent graft, a fabric tube supported by a metal mesh. This supports the aorta externally to prevent further dissection during asystole.

For peripheral aneurysms, open or endovascular repair techniques are recommended.[25] Surgical intervention before rupture provides a good prognosis; at 5.5 cm distention in diameter (about 2 inches), the risk of rupture exceeds the risk of repair. A less invasive endovascular repair procedure known as endoluminal stent-graft may offer an alternative to traditional open abdominal surgery with better survival rates even for older, sicker adults. Guided by angiographic imaging, a catheter is inserted through the femoral or brachial artery to the aneurysm. A balloon within the catheter is then inflated, pushing open the stent graft, which attaches with tiny hooks to healthy arterial wall above and below the aneurysm. This creates a channel for blood flow that bypasses the aneurysm.[238]

**PROGNOSIS.** The mean growth rate of the AAA is 2.21 mm per year, and does not seem to depend on age or sex.[50] Aneurysm rupture rate and mortality associated with AAA is reduced by ultrasound screening. AAA patients with elective repair have better outcomes, at least for the first 3 years, if they have the endovascular procedure versus open repair. Data for thoracic aortic aneurysm repair is not as conclusive.[50]

The standard open surgical approach to replace the diseased aorta is steadily improving but is still associated with high morbidity and substantial mortality rates. MI, respiratory failure, renal failure, and stroke are the principal causes of death and morbidity after surgical procedures performed on the thoracic aorta.

At the same time, the endoluminal stent-graft comes with its own set of complications, including fever, breakdown or migration of the device, leaks, and unknown durability. Further studies to improve treatment are ongoing.

AAA rupture risk increases with the aneurysm diameter. A person with an aneurysm larger than 8 cm in diameter has a 30% to 50% rupture risk per year, while a person with an aneurysm smaller than 4 cm has close to 0% risk of rupture.[50] Aneurysm rupture is associated with a high mortality; frequently, aneurysms are discovered only at autopsy.

SPECIAL IMPLICATIONS FOR THE THERAPIST 12.16

### *Aneurysm*

Because the prevalence of all diseases of the aorta increases with age and because the population in the United States is aging, it is expected that aortic aneurysm at all levels will be encountered with increasing frequency. Knowledge of the natural history, familial history, and clinical features of this disorder may alert the therapist to the need for medical intervention.

For the person who has had a surgically repaired aneurysm (open or endovascular repair), activities are initially restricted and are then gradually reintroduced. The therapist may be involved in bedside exercises and early mobility, which are especially important to prevent thromboembolism as a result of venous stasis during prolonged bed rest and immobility, as well as to verify functional movements with safe cardiovascular responses.

Because of the invasiveness of open abdominal surgery, anyone undergoing this procedure is at high risk for pulmonary complications. In fact, anyone with complications associated with an aneurysm is also at risk for pulmonary complications. Even with less-invasive endovascular repair, traditional manual muscle testing (or other activities involving isometric contraction) can significantly increase arterial blood pressure and thus should be avoided in people with aortic aneurysm. The therapist must be careful in documenting deficits in strength, endurance, and balance without overtly increasing blood pressure, especially in the early stages of rehabilitation.[290]

Incisional pain and the use of abdominal musculature in coughing discourage the person from full inspirations as well as effective forceful huffing or coughing. The acute care therapist will utilize clinical techniques to assist with cough with pillows or towel rolls at the incisional site and forceful huffing.[176] It is important for the therapist to encourage the patient to perform deep breathing and coughing as much as possible to prevent pulmonary complications.

Proper lifting techniques should be reviewed before discharge, even though the client will not be able to provide a return demonstration. Activities that require pushing, pulling, straining, or lifting more than 10 lb are restricted for 6 to 10 weeks postoperatively.

Anterior or abdominal soft tissue mobilization for persons with back pain who have postoperative abdominal scars may require indirect techniques. This precaution is especially true for the person with a previous abdominal aneurysm, the person with a known nonoperative aneurysm (less than 5 cm), or the person with a family history of aneurysm or an undiagnosed aneurysm.

The therapist must always palpate the abdomen for a pulsating mass before performing anterior or abdominal therapy. It is possible to palpate the width of the pulse beginning at the abdominal midline and progressing laterally. The pulse should be characterized by a uniform width on either side of the abdominal midline until the umbilicus is reached, at which point the aortic bifurcation results in expansion of the pulse width. Throbbing pain that increases with exertion should alert the therapist to the need to monitor vital signs and palpate pulses.

**Box 12.12**
**PERIPHERAL VASCULAR DISEASES**

***Inflammatory Disorders***

- Vasculitis (see also Table 12.18)
- Polyarteritis nodosa
- Arteritis
- Allergic or hypersensitivity angiitis
- Kawasaki disease
- Thromboangiitis obliterans (Buerger disease)

***Arterial Occlusive Disorders***

- Arterial thrombosis/embolism
- Thromboangiitis obliterans
- Arteriosclerosis obliterans

***Venous Disorders***

- Thrombophlebitis
- Varicose veins
- Chronic venous insufficiency

***Vasomotor Disorders***

- Raynaud disease
- Complex regional pain syndrome (formerly reflex sympathetic dystrophy)

## Peripheral Vascular Disease (PVD)

Although PVD is usually thought to refer to diseases of the blood vessels supplying the extremities, in fact, PVD actually encompasses pathologic conditions of blood vessels supplying the extremities and the major abdominal organs, most often apparent in the intestines and kidneys.

PVD is organized based on the underlying pathologic finding (e.g., inflammatory, arterial occlusive, venous, or vasomotor disorders) (Box 12.12). Although the terms *peripheral artery disease* (PAD) and *peripheral vascular disease* (PVD) are often used interchangeably, PVD is a broader, more encompassing grouping of disorders of both the arterial and venous blood vessels, whereas PAD only refers to arterial blood vessels. PVD typically affects the legs more often than the arms, but upper extremity involvement is not uncommon.

Approximately 8.5 million Americans older than age 60 years are affected by PVD; and in this age group, 12% to 20% of people have it. It is a leading cause of disability in this age group and in people with diabetes. Like CAD and cerebrovascular disease, arterial occlusive forms of PVD are most common as a result of atherosclerosis. Intermittent claudication, or cramping/burning pain related to activity level, is the classic symptom of PAD. Like angina associated with CAD, intermittent claudication associated with PAD is predictable and nearly always develops after the same amount of exertion (e.g., walking a specific distance), generally occurs in the calves and less commonly in the thighs and buttocks,[76] and usually improves rapidly with rest.[147]

Intermittent claudication sharply increases in late middle age and is somewhat higher among men than women. However, in later decades, rates of women with PVD catch up to those of men.[84] It is believed that the true prevalence of PAD may be significantly higher than reported due to people not reporting intermittent claudication yet, and therefore, the PVD isn't diagnosed yet.[84] While 10% of people with PAD have classic symptoms of intermittent claudication, 50% have leg symptoms different from claudication, and 40% do not complain about leg pain.[50]

Specific symptoms of the various forms of PVD depend on the underlying pathologic condition, the blood vessels involved (arteries or veins), and the location of the affected blood vessels; each form is discussed individually in the following sections.

### Inflammatory Disorders

Inflammatory conditions of the blood vessels are often triggered by immunologic conditions, often an autoimmune disease. The resulting inflammation causes damage to various vessels, leading to end-stage organ damage. Vasculitis (e.g., polyarteritis nodosa, giant cell arteritis, Kawasaki disease) is the most commonly encountered inflammatory blood vessel disease in a therapy practice.

**Vasculitis.** Vasculitis is actually a group of disorders that share a common pathogenesis of inflammation of the blood vessels, involving arteries and veins, and resulting in narrowing or occlusion of the lumen or formation of aneurysms that can rupture. Nerves may be affected by vasculitis as well. Vascular inflammation is a central feature of many rheumatic autoimmune diseases, especially rheumatoid arthritis and scleroderma.

Vasculitis can involve blood vessels of any size, type, or location, and can affect any organ or system, including the nervous system. Neurologic manifestations of vasculitis can occur in conjunction with any of the vasculitides, affecting the peripheral nervous system or the CNS. Vasculitis may occur as an isolated peripheral nerve vasculitis (localized vasculitis). The primary target organ involvement is usually muscle, peripheral nerve, skin, testicle, or kidney, and, less often, the CNS.

Vasculitis is broadly divided into infectious vasculitis, when a vessel wall is invaded by a pathogen (hepatitis B or C, HIV, cytomegalovirus, rickettsia), and noninfectious vasculitis. The current nomenclature of noninfectious vasculitis was adopted at the 2012 International Chapel Hill Consensus Conference on the Nomenclature of Systemic Vasculitides.[193] The categorization of vasculitis types was based on the size of the predominant vessels involved (Table 12.18). Based on pathologic mechanisms, there is immune-complex mediated, antineutrophil cytoplasmic (ANCA)-mediated, or cell-mediated immune vasculitis.[194] Vasculitis may be acute or chronic, with varying degrees of involvement. The distribution of lesions may be irregular and segmental rather than continuous.

Immune (antibody–antigen) complexes can be formed between an antibody made against a foreign antigen or an autoantibody against a self antigen (autoimmune response). The immune complexes are deposited in the blood vessel walls, resulting in activation of the complement cascade that generates massive inflammatory response contributing to endothelial damage. The released inflammatory factors activate endothelial cells, smooth muscle cells, and fibroblasts leading to pathologic changes in the vessel wall, including its thickening. Vessel occlusion and tissue ischemia follows, affecting nerves, among other structures, with axonal degeneration and the resultant neuropathy.

**Table 12.18** Vasculitis

| Vessels Involved | Vasculitides | Organ Systems Involved |
|---|---|---|
| Small vessels (arterioles, capillaries, venules) | Inflammatory bowel disease vasculitis | Skin, viscera, heart, synovium, GI tract |
| | Hypersensitivity vasculitis; drug-induced vasculitis | According to underlying cause and involved structures |
| | Vasculitis associated with infections or other diseases | |
| | Immune-complex small vessel vasculitis associated with autoimmune conditions (paraneoplastic vasculitis) | |
| Medium-size and small vessels | Vasculitis associated with malignancy | Determined by site of malignancy |
| | Thromboangiitis obliterans (Buerger disease) | Arteries and veins of digits and limbs |
| | Kawasaki disease (muscular arteries, rarely veins) | Cardiac, iliac, renal, internal mammillary |
| | Polyarteritis nodosa | Aorta and its primary and secondary branches, renal and visceral arteries, muscle, testes, nerves |
| | Vasculitis in rheumatic disease and connective tissue disorders | Synovium, skin, nail beds |
| | Angiitis of the CNS | CNS |
| | Wegener granulomatosis (uncommon) | Local: nasal structures<br>Systemic: lungs (upper and lower respiratory tracts), renal (glomerulonephritis), any organ can be involved |
| Large and medium-size vessels | Takayasu arteritis (rare) | Aorta and its primary branches, renal and visceral arteries |
| | Giant cell (temporal) arteritis | Extracranial arteries of the head and neck; any other artery but less common |
| Peripheral nervous system | Localized vasculitis | Vasa nervosum at the level of the epineural arteries (i.e., blood vessels supplying the neural arch in the spinal axis) |

*GI*, Gastrointestinal; *CNS*, central nervous system.
Adopted from Jennette JC, Falk RJ, Bacon PA, et al: 2012 revised International Chapel Hill Consensus Conference Nomenclature of Vasculitides, *Arthritis Rheum* Jan;65(1):1–11, 2013.

**Polyarteritis Nodosa**

***Overview and Etiologic Factors.*** Polyarteritis nodosa refers to a condition consisting of multiple sites of inflammatory and destructive lesions in the arterial system, the lesions being small masses of tissue in the form of nodes or projections (nodosum). The cause of polyarteritis nodosa is unknown, and infections are suspected, at least partially. While a few dozen years ago, hepatitis B was present in 50% of cases, currently only 5% of people with polyarteritis nodosa have hepatitis B.[194] Polyarteritis occurs more commonly among IV drug abusers and other groups who have a high prevalence of hepatitis B, hepatitis C, and HIV infection. Any age can be affected, but it is more common among older adults.[194]

***Clinical Manifestations.*** Polyarteritis nodosa affects small and medium-sized blood vessels, resulting in a variety of clinical presentations depending on the specific site of the blood vessel involved. Some of the more likely symptoms include abrupt onset of fever, chills, tachycardia, arthralgia, and myositis with muscle tenderness.

Any organ of the body may be affected, but most often involved are the kidneys, heart, liver, GI tract, muscles, and testes. Abdominal pain, nausea, and vomiting are common with GI tract involvement, which is present in half of the cases.[194] Pericarditis, myocarditis, arrhythmias, and MI reflect cardiac involvement. Complications may include aneurysm, hemorrhage, thrombosis, and fibrosis, leading to occlusion of the vessel lumen. Multiple asymmetric neuropathies (motor and sensory distribution) can occur when vasculitis affects the arteries of the peripheral nerves (vasa nervorum). Paresthesias, pain, weakness, and sensory loss occur, involving several or many peripheral nerves simultaneously. Peripheral neuropathy is observed in 75% of patients with polyarteritis nodosa.[194]

## MEDICAL MANAGEMENT

**DIAGNOSIS, TREATMENT, AND PROGNOSIS.** Diagnosis is made by characteristic laboratory findings, biopsy of symptomatic sites (especially muscle or nerve), and, possibly, visceral angiography. When CNS vasculitis is suspected, angiography is necessary, because MRI and CT do not provide sufficient evidence to confirm the diagnosis.

Prolonged use of corticosteroids is necessary to control fever and constitutional symptoms while vascular lesions are healing. Immunosuppressants may be used in conjunction with steroids to improve survival. Withdrawal from drugs is often followed by relapse of the polyarteritis nodosa. Treatment of the polyarteritis nodosa associated with hepatitis B is more complicated, because cytotoxic drugs used to treat the vasculitis can exacerbate the hepatic disease. Prognosis is poor without intervention, with a 5-year survival rate of only 20%. Pharmacologic therapy with corticosteroids increases survival to 50%, and steroids combined with immunosuppressive drugs have improved 5-year survival to 90%.

**Giant Cell Arteritis**

***Overview and Incidence.*** Giant cell arteritis (GCA), or cranial or temporal arteritis, is a vasculitis primarily involving multiple sites of temporal and cranial arteries (i.e., arteries of the head and neck and sometimes the aortic arch).

It is the most common vasculitis in the United States and affects older people with the incidence increasing with age after 50 years. Women age 70 to 79 have the highest incidence, and women are typically affected 3 times more often than men.[288] The most common comorbidity is polymyalgia rheumatica (PMR), but others include hypertension, spine pain, and osteoporosis.

*Etiologic Factors and Pathogenesis.* Multiple human leukocyte antigen loci and loci that influence function of T helper and T regulatory cells were identified as risk factors for GCA.

Cell-mediated immune mechanisms are implicated in GCA. T cells and macrophages are recruited in the vessel walls triggering the release of cytokines (IL-6, 12, 17), activating endothelial cells, smooth muscle cells, and fibroblasts. The middle layer (tunica media) of the large and medium-size arteries, particularly those blood vessels supplying blood to the head, is inflamed, causing the artery walls to thicken (stenosis) and obstruct blood flow. Ischemic complications and secondary thrombosis may occur. Healing produces fibrosis of the arterial wall, and the affected blood vessel becomes cord-like, thickened, and nodular, which can be observed externally when the temporal artery is involved.

*Clinical Manifestations.* The onset of arteritis is usually sudden, with severe, continuous, unilateral, throbbing headache and temporal pain as the first symptoms, accompanied by flu-like symptoms or visual disturbances. The pain may radiate to the occipital area, face, or side of the neck. Visual disturbances range from blurring to diplopia to visual loss. Irreversible blindness may occur anywhere in the course of the disease secondary to involvement of the ophthalmic artery.

Other symptoms may include enlarged, tender temporal artery; scalp sensitivity; and jaw claudication (i.e., pain in response to chewing, talking, or swallowing) when involvement of the external carotid artery causes ischemia of the masseter muscles. In that case, the pain is relieved by rest. Left untreated, the condition may lead to blindness and occasionally to a stroke, heart attack, or aortic dissection.

## MEDICAL MANAGEMENT

**DIAGNOSIS.** Early diagnosis is important to prevent blindness caused by obstruction of the ophthalmic arteries. Diagnosis is made by recognition of the presenting symptoms, and in some cases, arteritis follows PMR, a similar condition. Although GCA and PMR may occur as separate entities, most epidemiologic surveys group these two conditions together as one disorder. These may be two forms of a common pathophysiologic process characterized by varying degrees of synovitis and arteritis. They may actually represent two points along a single disease continuum.

Biopsy of the temporal artery may be performed, but results are often negative given the focal (segmental) nature of the disease. Color ultrasonography of the temporal arteries detects characteristic signs of vasculitis with a high sensitivity and specificity even in the absence of clinical signs of vascular inflammation (helpful in diagnosing temporal arteritis in people with previously diagnosed PMR).

People with extracranial GCA present with occlusive arterial lesions that may be detected with multiple imaging modalities: arteriography, IV digital subtraction angiography, CT scanning, and MRA. However, inflammation of the arterial wall cannot be detected by these means.

PET, standard CT imaging with contrast enhancement and certain magnetic resonance sequences, as well as ultrasound, permit identification of the edema and inflammation of the vessel wall. This is an important marker for active disease. Laboratory findings include elevated erythrocyte sedimentation rate, reflective of the underlying inflammatory process.

**TREATMENT AND PROGNOSIS.** Treatment of arteritis to prevent blindness and other vascular complications is with oral antiinflammatory drugs (usually a corticosteroid such as prednisone), providing symptomatic relief in 3 to 5 days. Visual loss can be permanent if allowed to persist for several hours without adequate intervention. With proper intervention, arteritis is a self-limiting disease, usually resolving within 6 to 12 months. Approximately 30% of affected individuals relapse in the first year of treatment during dose tapering. Combined pharmacology with corticosteroids and immunosuppressants as well as methotrexate and cyclophosphamide may be used.[194]

**Hypersensitivity Angiitis.** Hypersensitivity angiitis, a form of vasculitis, can occur at any age, but it most commonly affects children and young adults. The etiology is unknown, but the disease often follows an upper respiratory tract infection, and allergy or drug sensitivity plays a role in some cases. It is usually localized to the small vessels of the skin, first appearing on the lower extremities in a variety of lesions.

A classic triad of symptoms occurs in 80% of cases that includes purpura (bruising and petechiae or round purplish red spots under the skin), arthritis, and abdominal pain. Inflammation and hemorrhage may occur in the synovium and CNS. Medical management (diagnosis, treatment, prognosis) is the same as for the other forms of vasculitis already discussed.

**Kawasaki Disease**

*Overview and Etiologic Factors.* Kawasaki disease, also known as mucocutaneous lymph node syndrome, is an acute febrile illness associated with systemic (multiorgan) vasculitis. It predominantly affects medium and small arteries. It can occur in any ethnic group but seems most prevalent in Asian populations (especially Japanese, with equal incidence in Japan and in the United States among Japanese or Japanese descendants).

Children younger than age 4 years comprise 80% of all cases, and 20% develop cardiac complications that can be fatal. The etiology is unknown, but because seasonal and geographic outbreaks appear to occur, an infectious cause is suspected. It is thought that most cases of Kawasaki syndrome are related to an immunologic response to an infectious, toxic, or antigenic substance.[358]

*Pathogenesis.* Substantial evidence suggests that immune activation has a role in the pathogenesis of Kawasaki syndrome. The principal area of pathologic findings is the cardiovascular system. Kawasaki disease progresses pathologically and clinically in stages. During the acute stage of the illness (first 2 weeks), vascular inflammation and immune activation within the arterioles, venules, and capillaries occur, which later progress to include the main coronary arteries, the heart, and the larger veins.

In the acute phase, transmural necrotizing inflammation develops, with infiltration of neutrophils and monocytes, leading to degeneration of vascular walls and aneurysm formation. In the chronic, sclerotic phase, the vessels develop scarring, intimal thickening, calcification, and formation of thrombi. If death occurs as a result of this disease (rare), it is usually the result of aneurysm, coronary thrombosis, or severe scar formation and stenosis of the main coronary artery.

*Clinical Manifestations.* Clinical manifestations present in three phases: acute phase, subacute phase, and convalescent phase. In the *acute phase,* a sudden high fever (lasting over 5 days) that is unresponsive to antibiotics and antipyretics is followed by extreme irritability.

During the *subacute phase* (lasting approximately 25 days), the fever resolves, but the irritability persists along with other symptoms, such as anorexia, rash (exanthema) of the trunk and extremities with reddened palms and soles of the hands and feet, and subsequent desquamation (skin scales off) of the tips of the toes and fingers, peripheral edema of the hands and feet, cervical lymphadenopathy (usually unilateral), bilateral conjunctival infection without exudate, and changes in the oral mucous membranes (e.g., erythema, dryness and cracks or fissures of the lips, reddening or strawberry tongue).

In one third of all cases, children develop arthralgias and GI tract symptoms, typically lasting about 2 weeks. Joint involvement may persist for as long as 3 months. During this subacute phase, the person is at risk for cardiac involvement, especially the development of myocarditis, pericarditis, and arteritis that predisposes to the formation of coronary artery aneurysm in nearly 25% of cases not treated within 10 days of fever onset.

The *convalescent phase* occurs 6 to 8 weeks after onset of Kawasaki disease and is characterized by a resolution of all clinical signs and symptoms. However, during this phase, the blood values have not returned to normal. At the end of the convalescent phase, all values return to normal, and the child has usually regained his or her usual temperament, energy, and appetite.

## MEDICAL MANAGEMENT

**DIAGNOSIS, TREATMENT, AND PROGNOSIS.** Early recognition and prompt management of the acute syndrome are critical. Diagnosis is made on the basis of clinical manifestations and associated laboratory tests. There are no specific laboratory tests for Kawasaki disease, but indicators of acute inflammation (elevated CRP and erythrocyte sedimentation rate) are looked at. Echocardiograms are useful in providing a baseline and for monitoring myocardial and coronary artery status, but echocardiograms cannot fully diagnose Kawasaki syndrome.

The introduction of high-dose IV gamma globulin in combination with aspirin therapy to reduce fever and control inflammation and aneurysm formation has significantly reduced the prevalence of coronary artery abnormalities.

Prognosis is good for recovery with intervention, although serious cardiovascular problems (e.g., coronary thrombosis, aneurysm) may occur later in persons with cardiac sequelae. In 10% to 20% of patients, coronary arteritis develops, and of these, 2% have MI.[194] Giant aneurysms (diameter exceeding 8 mm) have the worst prognosis, because these are unlikely to regress or resolve, with death common in this subgroup population. Occasionally, severe ischemic heart disease requires cardiac transplantation.[251]

**Thromboangiitis Obliterans (Buerger Disease)**

*Overview and Pathogenesis.* Thromboangiitis obliterans, also referred to as Buerger disease, is a vasculitis (inflammatory and thrombotic process) affecting the peripheral blood vessels (both arteries and veins), primarily in the extremities. The cause is not known, but it is most often found in men younger than 40 years who smoke heavily, although the incidence in women is increasing.

The pathogenesis of thromboangiitis obliterans is unknown, but general inflammatory concepts apply. The inflammatory lesions of the peripheral blood vessels are accompanied by thrombus formation and vasospasm, occluding and eventually obliterating (destroying) small and medium-size vessels of the feet and hands.

Studies have linked elevated levels of homocysteine to Buerger disease.[183,198] Homocysteine has many potential effects: it limits the bioavailability of nitric oxide, impairs endothelium-dependent vasorelaxation, increases oxidative stress, stimulates smooth muscle cell proliferation, alters the elastic properties of vessel walls, and generates a prethrombotic state through the activation of factor V.

*Clinical Manifestations.* Clinical manifestations of pain and tenderness of the affected part are caused by occlusion of the arteries, reduced blood flow, and subsequent reduced oxygenation of tissues. The symptoms are episodic and segmental, meaning that the symptoms come and go intermittently over time and appear in different asymmetric anatomic locations. The plantar, tibial, and digital vessels are most commonly affected in the lower leg and foot. Intermittent claudication centered in the arch of the foot or the palm of the hand is often the first symptom.

When the hands are affected, the digital, palmar, and ulnar arteries are most commonly involved. Pain at rest occurs, with persistent ischemia of one or more digits. Other symptoms include edema, cold sensitivity, rubor (redness of the skin from dilated capillaries under the skin), cyanosis, and thin, shiny, hairless skin (trophic changes) from chronic ischemia. Paresthesias, diminished or absent posterior tibial and dorsalis pedis pulses, painful ischemic ulceration, and eventual gangrene may develop. Inflammatory superficial thrombophlebitis is common.

## MEDICAL MANAGEMENT

**DIAGNOSIS, TREATMENT, AND PROGNOSIS.** Arteriography may be used in the diagnosis, but definitive diagnosis of thromboangiitis obliterans is determined by histologic examination of the blood vessels (microabscesses in the vessel wall) in a leg amputated for gangrene.

Intervention should begin with cessation of smoking and avoidance of any environmental or secondhand smoke inhalation. All other treatment techniques are aimed at improving circulation to the foot or hand, including pharmacologic intervention (e.g., vasodilators, pain relievers) and physical or occupational therapy (see also "Atherosclerosis: Medical Management" above).

Regional sympathetic ganglionectomy may produce vasodilation and increase blood flow. If ulcerations develop, wound care is needed, and amputation (sometimes multiple sites or levels) may be required when the individual is unable to quit smoking or when conservative care fails. With the findings of elevated levels of plasma prothrombotic factors associated with Buerger disease, screening and treatment for elevation of these factors is recommended, especially to assess which clients may eventually require amputation.

Thromboangiitis is not life-threatening, but it can result in progressive disability from pain and loss of function secondary to amputation. Cessation of smoking is the key determinant in prognosis.

**SPECIAL IMPLICATIONS FOR THE THERAPIST 12.17**

### *Inflammatory Disorders*

Peripheral neuropathy is a well-known and frequently early manifestation of many vasculitic syndromes. The pattern of neuropathic involvement depends on the extent and temporal progression of the vasculitic process that produces ischemia. A severe, burning dysesthetic pain in the involved area is present in 70% to 80% of all cases.

Other symptoms may include paresthesias and sensory deficit, as well as severe proximal muscle weakness and muscular atrophy that can occur secondary to the neuropathy. In the early phase, one nerve is affected and causes symptoms in one extremity (mononeuritis multiplex), but other nerves can become involved as the disorder progresses.

The therapist should watch for anyone with neuropathy who exhibits constitutional symptoms, such as fever, arthralgia, or skin involvement. This may herald a possible vasculitic syndrome and requires medical referral for accurate diagnosis. Early recognition of vasculitis can help prevent a poor outcome. With no treatment or with a poor outcome to intervention, CNS involvement (e.g., encephalopathy, ischemic and hemorrhagic stroke, cranial nerve palsy) can occur late in the course of vasculitis.

When corticosteroids (e.g., prednisone alone or sometimes in combination with other medications) are used (e.g., in the case of vasculitic neuropathy), the therapist must be aware of the need for osteoporosis prevention and attend to the other potential side effects from the chronic use of these medications.

Alternative methods of pain control may be offered in a rehabilitation setting, such as biofeedback, transcutaneous electrical nerve stimulation, and physiologic modulation (e.g., using a handheld temperature sensor to control autonomic nervous system function).

#### Vasculitis (Inflammatory Disease of Arteries and Veins)

The therapist's role in management of vasculitis may be primarily for relief of painful muscular and joint symptoms when present and in the prevention of functional loss in the case of neuropathies. For the client with thromboangiitis obliterans (Buerger disease), exercise must be graded to avoid claudication, and the client must be instructed in a home program for preventive skin care (see Box 12.13). Gangrene can occur as a result of prolonged ischemia from vessel obliteration; clients are typically treated for wound care and postoperatively after amputation.

Often a client with some other primary orthopedic or neurologic diagnosis has also been medically diagnosed with vasculitis.

#### Arteritis

Early recognition and referral can prevent the serious complications associated with arteritis. Older adults who experience sudden or unexplained headaches, lingering flu-like symptoms such as muscle aches (myalgia) and fatigue, persistent fever, unexplained weight loss, jaw pain when eating, or visual disturbances must be referred to their physicians. This is especially true for anyone with a previous diagnosis of PMR.

The long-term use of corticosteroids can result in side effects such as osteoporosis and bone fractures, weight gain, diabetes, and high blood pressure. The client must be advised regarding an osteoporosis prevention program and how to handle an increase in appetite. Remaining physically active and exercising are key components for both these issues.

### Arterial Occlusive Diseases

Occlusive diseases of the blood vessels are a common cause of disability and usually occur as a result of atherosclerosis. Other causes of arterial occlusion include trauma, thrombus or embolism, vasculitis, vasomotor disorders such as Raynaud disease or phenomenon and complex regional pain syndrome (formerly reflex sympathetic dystrophy), arterial punctures, polycythemia, and chronic mechanical irritation of the subclavian artery as a result of compression by a cervical rib. For each individual case, see the discussion of the underlying cause of the occlusion to understand etiologic and risk factors and pathogenesis.

Atherosclerotic occlusive disease can also affect vessels throughout the body other than the coronary vessels. For example, occlusive disease affecting the intestines results in acute intestinal ischemia or ischemic colitis, depending on the location of the occlusion.

Occlusive cerebrovascular disease as a result of atherosclerosis accounts for many episodes of weakness, dizziness, blurred vision, transient ischemic attack or cerebrovascular accident or stroke. Extracranial arterial ischemia (e.g., common carotid bifurcation, vertebral artery) accounts for more than half of these types of strokes.

**Arterial Thrombosis and Embolism.** Occlusive diseases may be complicated by arterial thrombosis and embolism (Fig. 12.30). Chronic, incomplete arterial obstruction usually results in the development of collateral vessels before complete occlusion threatens circulation to the extremity. Arterial embolism is generally a complication of ischemic or rheumatic heart disease, with or without MI.

Box 12.13

### GUIDELINES FOR TEMPERATURE PROTECTION AND SKIN CARE

#### *Temperature Protection*

- Nicotine causes vasoconstriction of the small vessels in the hands and feet; avoid all tobacco products.
- Recognize and avoid other triggers that cause vasoconstriction (e.g., emotional distress, caffeine, cold or cough remedies that contain a decongestant).
- Wear layers of clothing made of natural fibers, such as cotton, to draw moisture away from the skin; in cold weather, wear a hat and scarf because heat is lost through the scalp; silk is a good insulator, so consider it for socks and long underwear.
- Wear thick mittens, which are warmer than gloves, and socks purchased from an outdoor clothing or ski shop designed to wick moisture away while retaining body heat.
- Avoid air conditioning; wear warmer clothes, layer light clothing, or wear a sweater or jacket in air conditioning; be careful when going into an air-conditioned environment after being out in the heat or vice versa.
- Test water temperature before bathing or showering or have a member of the family test first; use other portion of the body to test if insensitivity exists in hand or foot.
- Use a heating pad, hot water bottle, or electric blanket to warm the sheets of your bed before getting into bed, but *do not* apply these directly to the skin, and do not sleep with any electric device left on; if necessary, wear light socks and mittens or gloves to bed. Do not soak hands or feet in hot water.
- Keep household temperatures at a constant, even, and comfortable level.
- Keep protective covering available at all times, even in the summer.
- Avoid contact with extremes of temperature, such as oven, dishwasher (hot dishes), refrigerator, or freezer; wear thick oven mitts whenever reaching into the oven. Keep mittens or warm gloves by the refrigerator and freezer to prevent symptoms when reaching into it.
- Wear rubber gloves whenever cleaning, washing dishes, or rinsing or peeling vegetables under water.
- Avoid holding ice, ice-cold fruit, hot or cold drinks, or frozen foods; wear protective gloves whenever making contact with any of these items.

#### *Skin Care*

- Take care of your skin, and give your hands and feet extra care and protection; examine hands and feet daily; at the first sign of bruising, skin changes (e.g., cracking, calluses, blisters, redness), swelling, infection, or ulcer, immediately contact a member of your health care team (e.g., nurse, physical therapist, physician). If vision is impaired, have a family member or health care professional inspect your hands and feet.
- Circulation problems tend to create dry skin and delay healing; keep your skin clean and well moisturized; wash with a mild, creamy, or moisturizing liquid soap or gel; clean carefully between fingers and toes; *do not* soak them.
- Avoid perfumed lotions, and do not put lotion on sores or between toes.
- Observe carefully for any activities that might put pressure on your fingertips, such as using a manual typewriter, playing a musical instrument (e.g., guitar, piano), and doing crafts or needlework.
- Do not go barefoot indoors or outdoors; this includes getting up at night; avoid wearing open-toed shoes, pointy-toed shoes, high heels, or sandals; always wear absorbent socks or socks that wick perspiration away from skin; avoid nylon material (including pantyhose material); avoid stockings with seams or with mends; change socks or stockings daily.
- Make sure shoes provide good support without being too tight, avoid shoes that cause excessive foot perspiration, and alternate shoes throughout the week (i.e., do not wear the same shoes every day). Do not wear shoes without socks or stockings.
- Avoid hot tubs and prolonged baths; dry carefully between toes; water temperature should be between 32.2° and 35° C (90° and 95° F).
- Use heel protectors, sheepskin, and other protective devices whenever recommended.

#### *Other Tips*

- For Raynaud disease or phenomenon, avoid situations that precipitate excitement, anxiety, or feelings of fear; teach yourself how to recognize early signs of these emotions and use relaxation techniques to reduce stress.
- For Raynaud disease or phenomenon, when you have an attack, gently rewarm fingers or toes as soon as possible; place your hands under your armpits, wiggle fingers or toes, or move or walk around to improve circulation; if possible, run warm (*not* hot) water over the affected body part until normal color returns.
- Do not use razor blades; use electric razors.
- Avoid medications and substances (e.g., nicotine; caffeine in chocolate, tea, coffee, and soft drinks) that can cause blood vessels to narrow; discuss all medications with your physician.
- Maintain good circulation; do not stay in one position for more than 30 minutes; use breathing and stretching exercises whenever confined to a desk, chair, car, or bed for more than 30 minutes.
- Do not wear constricting or tight clothing, especially tight socks; avoid elastic around wrists or ankles.
- Do not wear jewelry, such as watches or bracelets, to bed at night.
- Leave a night light on in dark areas; turn on lights in dark areas and hallways.
- Do not sit with legs crossed because this can cause pressure on the nerves and blood vessels.
- Avoid sunburn.
- Do not scratch insect bites; do not scratch areas of itchy skin.
- Do not do bathroom surgery on corns or calluses; do not use chemical agents for the removal of corns or calluses; see your physician.

#### *Care of Nails*

- Use clippers, not scissors; *do not* use razor blades; cut toenails straight across, but file fingernails in a rounded fashion to the tips of your fingers.
- Take care of your nails; use cuticle softener or moisturizing cream or lotion around cuticles; push the cuticles back very gently with a cotton swab soaked in cuticle remover; *do not* push cuticles back with a sharp object, and *do not* cut the cuticles with scissors or nail clippers.
- Use lamb's wool between overlapping toes.

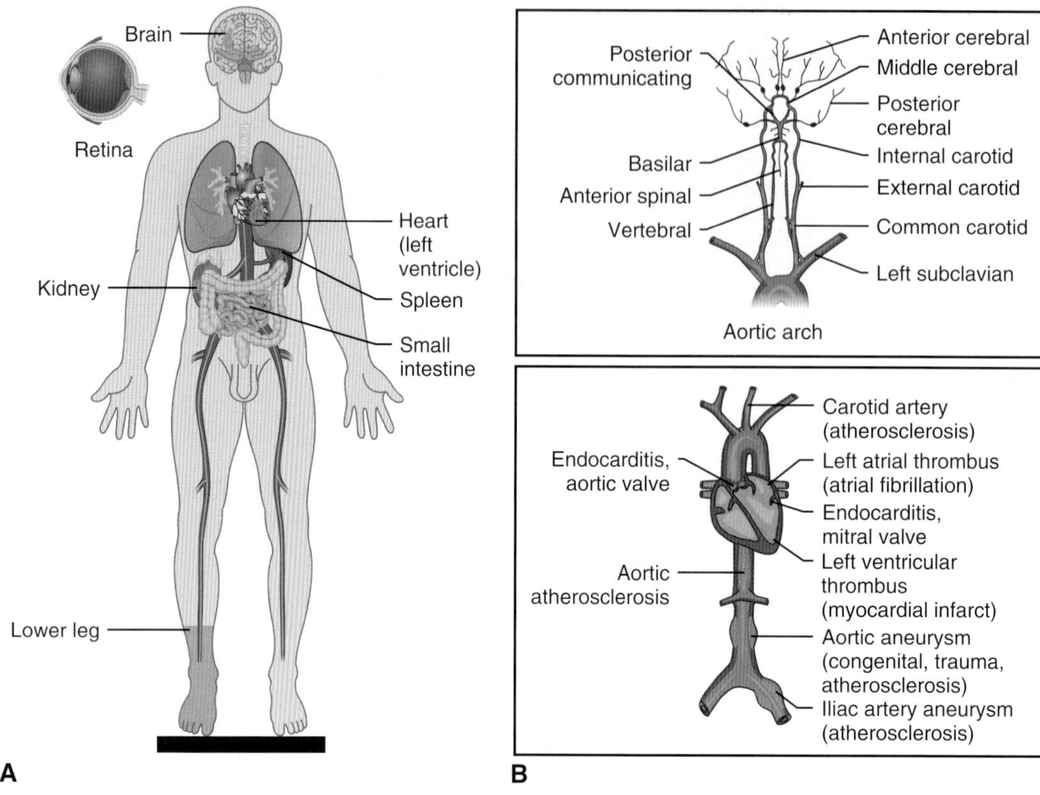


**Figure 12.30**

(A) Common sites of infarction from arterial emboli. (B) Sources of arterial emboli.

Signs and symptoms of pain, numbness, coldness, tingling or changes in sensation, skin changes (pallor, mottling), weakness, and muscle spasm occur in the extremity distal to the block (Fig. 12.31). Treatment may include immediate or delayed embolectomy, anticoagulation therapy (e.g., heparin), and protection of the limb.

**Thromboangiitis Obliterans (Buerger Disease).** Thromboangiitis obliterans is discussed as a vasculitis in an earlier section (see Inflammatory Disorders) but is mentioned here as an occlusive disorder because the inflammatory lesions of the peripheral blood vessels are accompanied by thrombus formation and vasospasm, occluding blood vessels.

**Arteriosclerosis Obliterans (Peripheral Artery Disease)**

***Definition and Overview.*** Arteriosclerosis obliterans, defined as arteriosclerosis in which proliferation of the intima has caused complete obliteration of the lumen of the artery, is also known as atherosclerotic occlusive disease, chronic occlusive arterial disease, obliterative arteriosclerosis, and PAD. It is the most common arterial occlusive disease and accounts for approximately 95% of cases. It is a progressive disease that causes ischemic ulcers of the legs and feet and is most often seen in older clients, associated with diabetes mellitus. Obesity may also contribute to the formation of arteriosclerosis obliterans.

***Etiologic and Risk Factors.*** PAD has risk factors that are similar but not identical to those for CAD. Smoking is a more potent risk factor for PAD than for CAD. Atherosclerosis as the underlying cause of occlusive disease, with its known etiologic and associated risk factors, is discussed earlier in this chapter. PAD also correlates strongly with diabetes and high cholesterol. In fact, smoking, diabetes, hypertension, and hypercholesterolemia together are responsible for 75% of risk of PAD.[50] Other risk factors include older age, sedentary lifestyle, family history of PAD, elevated inflammatory biomarkers, and increased homocysteine.[50,147]

It has been reported that PAD is more prevalent in women than generally appreciated, but estimates vary greatly according to the diagnostic criteria applied. Prevalence and incidence rates do not differ significantly by gender, although incidence rates in women lag behind those in men in a pattern similar to that for CAD.[259]

Individuals with PAD are more likely to have CAD and cerebrovascular disease than those without PAD.[50] In fact, the prevalence of atherosclerosis in other arterial beds (coronary, carotid, and renal arteries) in people with PAD is higher than in those without PAD.[147]

***Pathogenesis.*** See also "Atherosclerosis: Pathogenesis" above.

Because peripheral arterial disease is one expression of atherosclerosis, understanding the pathogenesis of atherosclerosis is important. The arterial narrowing or obstruction that occurs as a result of the atherosclerotic process reduces blood flow to the limbs during exercise, and as the atherosclerosis progresses, it occurs even at rest. Muscular reactivity is also adversely affected in PAD. Prostacyclin and nitric oxide usually activate vascular relaxation. In PAD, these relaxation factors are reduced, and constrictive factors such as endothelin are increased. This imbalance of vascular reactivity contributes to decreased blood flow.

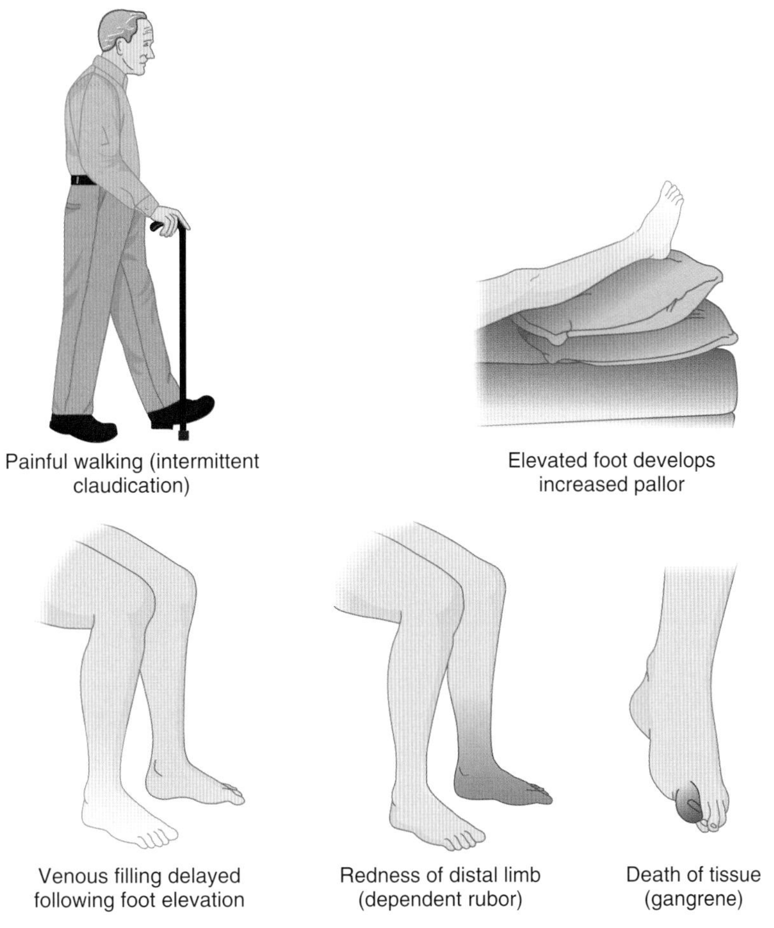


**Figure 12.31**

**Signs and symptoms of arterial insufficiency.**

*Clinical Manifestations.* In peripheral vessels, claudication symptoms appear when the diameter of the vessel narrows by 50% or more. PAD affecting the lower extremities is primarily one of large and medium-size arteries and most frequently involves branch points and bifurcations. Symptoms of arterial occlusive disease usually occur distal to the narrowing or obstruction. Acute ischemia may present with some or all of the classical symptoms, such as pain (typically cramping and/or burning in nature), pallor, paresthesia, paralysis, and pulselessness. However, arteries can become significantly blocked without symptoms developing, a phenomenon referred to as *silent ischemia.*

Even though silent ischemia is not associated with symptoms, it poses the same long-term sequelae and complications as overt ischemia and must be treated. It is strongly suspected when systolic blood pressure is lower at the ankle than at the arm (see further discussion of ankle/brachial index in this section).

Occlusive disease of the distal *aorta* and *iliac arteries* usually begins just proximal to the bifurcation of the common iliac arteries, causing changes in both lower extremities (Fig. 12.32; Table 12.19). Bilateral, progressive, intermittent claudication (pain, ache, or cramp in the muscles, causing limping) is almost always present in the calf muscles and is usually present in the gluteal and quadriceps muscles, presenting as buttock, thigh, and calf pain.

The distance a person can walk before the onset of pain indicates the degree of circulatory inadequacy. The primary symptom may only be a sense of weakness or tiredness in these same areas; both the pain and weakness or fatigue are relieved by rest.

Occlusive disease of the *femoral and popliteal arteries* usually occurs at the point at which the superficial femoral artery passes through the adductor magnus tendon into the popliteal space. Occlusion of these regions is also marked by intermittent claudication of the calf and foot that may radiate to the ipsilateral popliteal region and lower thigh. Although symptoms occur ipsilateral to the occlusion anywhere distal to the bifurcation of the aorta, most people have bilateral disease and therefore bilateral symptoms. There are definite changes of the affected lower leg and foot as listed in Table 12.19.

Occlusive disease of the *tibial* and *common peroneal arteries,* as well as the pedal vessels and small digital vessels, occurs slowly and progressively over months or years. The eventual outcome depends on the vessels that are occluded and the condition of the proximal and collateral vessels. Arterial ulcers may develop as a result of ischemia, usually located over a bony prominence on the toes or feet (e.g., metatarsal heads, heels, lateral malleoli).

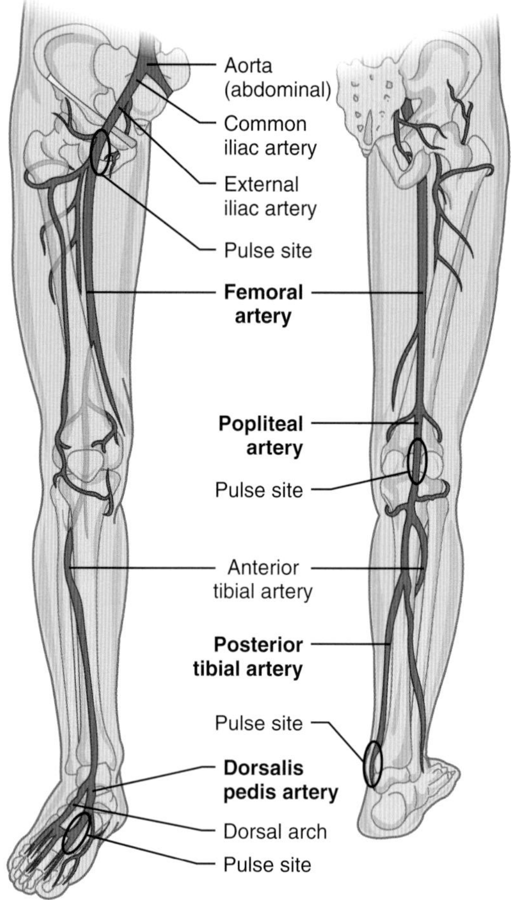


**Figure 12.32**

**Arteries in the leg.** The abdominal aorta branches (aortic bifurcation) into the right and left common iliac arteries. These arteries pass through the pelvic cavity and under the inguinal ligament to become the major arteries supplying the leg, called the femoral arteries. Each femoral artery travels down the thigh until, at the lower thigh, it courses posteriorly, where it becomes the popliteal artery. Below the knee, the popliteal artery divides into the anterior tibial artery and posterior tibial artery. The anterior tibial artery travels down the front of the leg onto the dorsum of the foot, where it becomes the dorsalis pedis artery. In the back of the leg, the posterior tibial artery travels down behind the malleolus and forms the plantar arteries in the foot. (From Jarvis C: *Physical examination and health assessment,* ed 5, Philadelphia, 2008, WB Saunders.)

The skin is shiny and atrophic, and fissures and cracks are common. Loss of hair on the feet and toes is also common.

Pain at rest indicates more severe involvement, which may mimic deep vein thrombosis (DVT), but relief from the occlusive disease can sometimes be obtained by dangling the uncovered leg over the edge of the bed. This dependent position would increase symptoms of DVT, which is usually treated by leg elevation. Exercise may cause pedal pulses to disappear in some people as the smaller artery is occluded during the time of muscle use. Prolonged occlusion of the arteries, usually at the level of one of these smaller branches, results in necrosis. The necrotic tissue may become gangrenous and infected, requiring surgical intervention.

**Table 12.19** Arterial Occlusive Disease

| Site of Occlusion | Signs and Symptoms |
|---|---|
| Aortic bifurcation | Sensory and motor deficits<br>• Muscle weakness<br>• Numbness (loss of sensation)<br>• Paresthesias (burning, pricking)<br>• Paralysis<br>Intermittent claudication (lower back, gluteal muscles, quadriceps, calves; relieved by rest)<br>Cold, pale legs with decreased or absent peripheral pulses |
| Iliac artery | Intermittent claudication (buttock, hip, thigh; relieved by rest)<br>Diminished or absent femoral or distal pulses<br>Erectile dysfunction in males |
| Femoral and popliteal artery | Intermittent claudication (calf, foot; may radiate)<br>Leg pallor and coolness<br>Dependent rubor<br>Blanching of feet on elevation<br>No palpable pulses in ankles and feet<br>Gangrene |
| Tibial and common peroneal artery | Intermittent claudication (calves; feet occasionally)<br>Pain at rest (severe disease); possibly relieved by dangling affected leg<br>Same skin and temperature changes in lower leg and foot as described above<br>Pedal pulses absent; popliteal pulses may be present |

Occlusive arterial disease for the person with diabetes mellitus is further complicated by very slow healing, and healed areas may break down easily. In the case of long-term diabetes, diabetic neuropathy with diminished or absent sensation of the toes or feet often occurs, predisposing the person to injury or pressure ulcers that may progress because of poor blood flow and subsequent loss of sensation (Table 12.20). Amputation rate in people with diabetes is markedly higher than for those individuals with PAD without diabetes.[50]

## MEDICAL MANAGEMENT

**DIAGNOSIS.** Diagnosis is based on client history and clinical examination. Diagnostic tools may include noninvasive vascular tests (e.g., ankle/brachial index, segmental limb pressures, pulse volume recordings, duplex ultrasonography, computed tomography angiography, magnetic resonance angiography) or, if invasive tests are required, arteriography with contrast or with MRI. An in-depth discussion of the diagnosis and intervention strategies for chronic arterial insufficiency of the lower extremities is available.[25,147]

**Prevention and Treatment.** Prevention is the key to reducing the incidence of PAD caused by atherosclerosis. The AHA and American College of Cardiology have recently updated their guideline for the management of people with PAD.[25,147]

Risk factor reduction and lifestyle measures are the first steps, with smoking cessation (or not ever starting)

**Table 12.20** Comparison of Arterial, Venous, and Neuropathic Ulcers

| | Arterial Ulcer | Venous Ulcer | Neuropathic (Diabetic) Ulcer |
|---|---|---|---|
| Etiology[a] | Arteriosclerosis obliterans<br>Atheroembolism<br>Large- or medium-vessel atherosclerosis<br>Raynaud disease<br>Diabetes mellitus<br>Collagen disease<br>Vasculitis | Valvular incompetence<br>History of DVT<br>Venous insufficiency accompanied by hypertension<br>Peripheral incompetence; varicose veins | Diabetes mellitus; combination of arterial disease and peripheral neuropathy<br>Repetitive unrecognized trauma |
| Location | Anywhere on leg or dorsum of foot or toes<br>Bone prominences (anterior tibial)<br>Lateral malleolus | Medial aspect of distal one third of lower extremity<br>Behind medial malleolus | Same areas in which arterial ulcers appear, especially toes<br>Areas where peripheral neuropathy occurs (pressure points on plantar aspect of foot, toes, heels) |
| Clinical Manifestations | Painful, especially with legs elevated<br>Pulses poor quality or absent Intermittent claudication (exertional calf pain)<br>Rest pain or nocturnal aching of foot or forefoot relieved by dependent dangling position<br>Integumentary (trophic) changes<br>Hair loss<br>Thin, shiny skin<br>Ischemia: pale, white skin color<br>Areas of sluggish blood flow: Red-purple mottling<br>Hypersensitivity to palpation<br>History of minor nonhealing trauma | Can be very painful; venous insufficiency can cause aching pain; more comfortable with legs elevated<br>Normal arterial pulses<br>Eczema or stasis dermatitis<br>Edema<br>Venous perimound (dark pigmentation) is called hemosiderin or staining; Leakage of hemosiderin is due to blood that cannot return because of vascular incompetence | Classic symmetric ascending stocking-glove distribution of sensory loss (begins in feet and ascends to knees, then symptoms begin in the hands)<br>May not be painful because of loss of sensation (e.g., neuropathic ulcers are painless or insensate when palpated)<br>Some people experience unpleasant sensations (tingling or hypersensitivity to normally painless stimuli)<br>Loss of vibratory sense and light touch<br>Pulses may be present or diminished (arteries become calcified)<br>Neuropathic foot is warm and dry<br>Loss of vascular tone increases arteriovenous shunting and impairs blood flow necessary for wound healing; sepsis common<br>Altered biomechanics and weight bearing |
| | 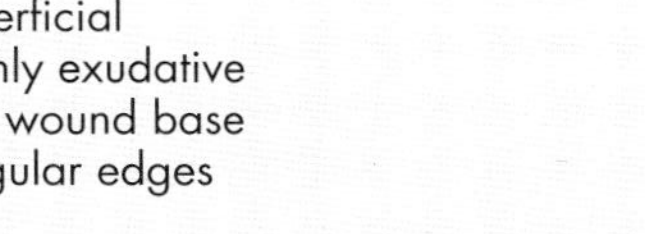 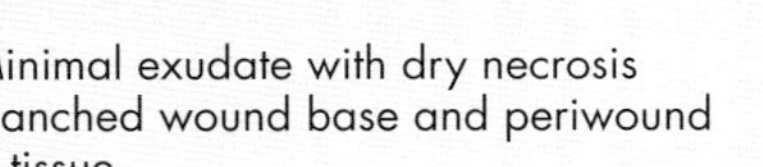 | 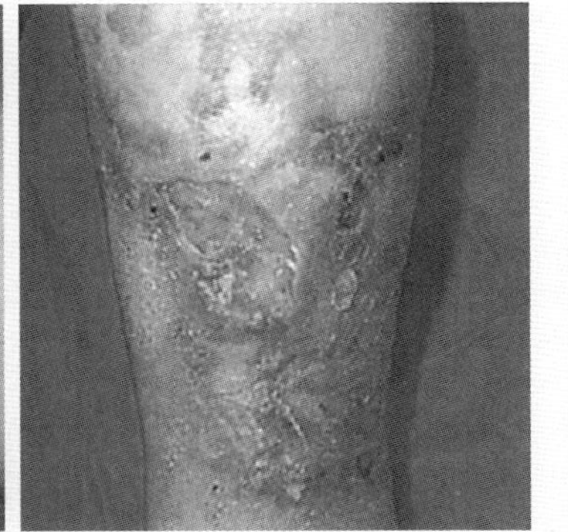 | |
| Wound Appearance | Minimal exudate with dry necrosis<br>Blanched wound base and periwound tissue | Superficial<br>Highly exudative<br>Red wound base<br>Irregular edges | Round, craterlike with elevated rim; diabetes hastens changes described in figure at left (arterial ulcer)<br>Minimal drainage<br>Frequently deep<br>High infection rate |

[a]Ulceration may also occur as a result of lymphatic disorders, skin cancer, metabolic abnormalities, and vasculitis.
*DVT*, Deep vein thrombosis.

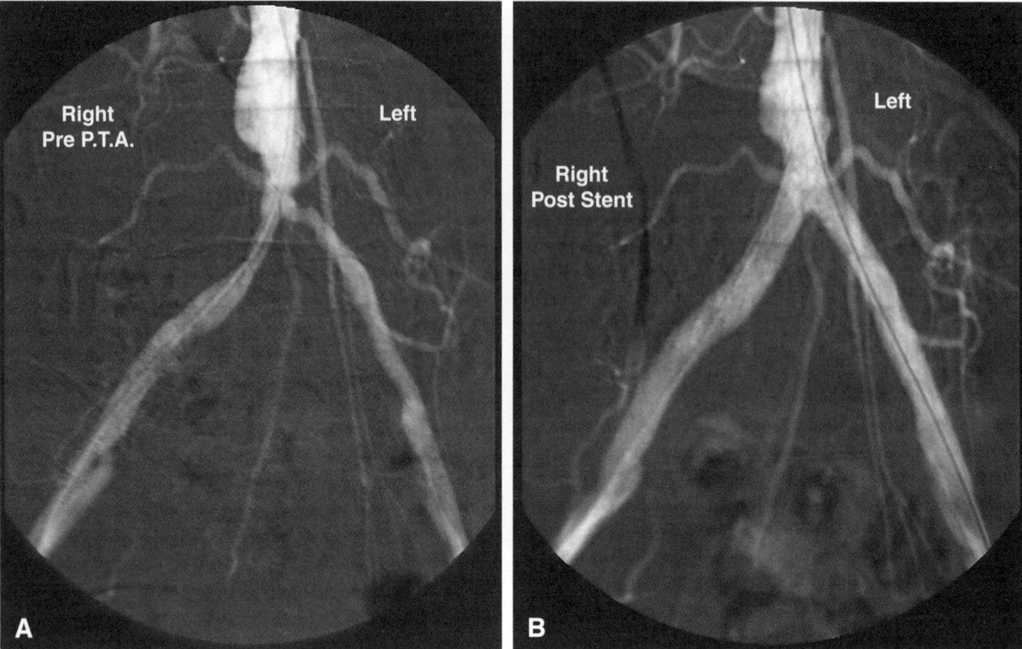


**Figure 12.33**

**Percutaneous transluminal angioplasty (PTA) may be used in peripheral vascular disease.** (A) Significant narrowing of the aortic bifurcation and both common iliac arteries. The narrowing in both iliac arteries was successfully treated by angioplasty, and bilateral stents were inserted to maintain patency. (B) The client had presented with bilateral calf claudication, which was relieved by this procedure. (From Forbes CD, Jackson WF: *Color atlas and text of clinical medicine,* ed 3, London, 2003, Mosby.)

as the single most effective prevention tool. A conservative approach to care that includes a program of dietary management to decrease cholesterol and other fats, pain control, and daily physical activity and exercise therapy to improve collateralization and function has been uniformly endorsed by experts in vascular disease.[25,147] Careful attention must be given to preventive skin care (Box 12.13) to avoid even minor injuries, infections, or ulcerations.

Recommendations for antiplatelet drugs[147] include administering of aspirin in a wide range of doses (75–325 mg per day) as an antiplatelet agent. As an alternative to aspirin therapy, clopidogrel can be given. Antiplatelet therapy reduces the risk of vascular events in people with PAD by 26%.[50] Combination antiplatelet therapy with aspirin and clopidogrel can be used for certain high-risk individuals with PAD who are not considered at increased risk of bleeding. Oral anticoagulation therapy (such as warfarin) in addition to antiplatelet therapy is not recommended for prevention of cardiovascular events among people with PAD.[147]

Statins are indicated for all patients with PAD.[147] They reduce the risk of adverse cardiovascular events and amputations and improve limb-related outcomes.[50,147]

Antihypertensive therapy is recommended for patients with PAD and high blood pressure to decrease risk of MI, stroke, HF, and death due to cardiovascular causes.

Smoking cessation should be advised to patients with PAD. Approaches may include pharmacotherapy (i.e., nicotine replacement therapy) and/or smoking cessation programs.

Revascularization is a component of a tailored patient care plan that includes medical therapy (see above), structured exercise therapy (see below), and care to minimize tissue loss.[147] The decision about revascularization intervention is usually made after exercise therapy combined with risk factor modification has been unsuccessful in preventing the impairment and subsequent disability. Revascularization for claudication is indicated if blood flow is compromised enough to produce symptoms of ischemic pain at rest, if tissue death has occurred (gangrene), or if claudication interferes with essential activities or work.[36,147] Revascularization can include endovascular revascularization, surgery, or both.

Endovascular techniques include percutaneous transluminal angioplasty (PTA; Fig. 12.33), stents and atherectomy.[147] PTA, performed with a balloon, can be done with or without stent insertion. Stents are generally used in larger arteries (iliac, renal) with high blood flow, while balloons are used in smaller arteries and long occlusions.

Surgical revascularization with a femoral-popliteal bypass is the most common surgical procedure for claudication, because the superficial femoral and proximal popliteal arteries are the most common sites for occlusion and stenosis.[147] Cessation of smoking may be required by the physician before surgery is considered.

Persons with localized occlusions of the aorta and iliac arteries less than 10 cm in length, with relatively normal vessels proximally and distally, are good candidates for angioplasty or stenting (see Figs. 12.3 and 12.5). Conversely, people with multisegmented arterial disease with more involved symptoms are at greater risk of amputation, and therefore, endovascular and open surgical treatment are recommended for limb salvage in these types of clients.

Prescriptive exercise is discussed in great detail later in the chapter, and a comprehensive review published by the AHA is available about optimal exercise programs for people with

PAD, including discussion of traditional and novel exercise modalities, selection of outcome measures, assessment of exercise efficacy, and comparison of exercise therapy outcomes with other therapeutic interventions.[356] Several mechanisms have been implicated in the benefits of physical activity for PAD. They include decrease in proinflammatory biomarkers,[110] increase in endothelium-dependent vasodilation,[192] increase in calf muscle blood flow and oxygen extraction,[38] increase in gastrocnemius capillary density,[119] and increase in endothelial stem and progenitor cells (cells that line the blood vessels capable of blood vessel repair).[316] Exercise can protect against atherothrombotic events by enhancing fibrinolysis[283] and favorably altering cardiovascular risk factor profile (e.g., improved lipid profile, reduced blood pressure),[191] an important element in the management of PAD.[214] Involvement of multiple mechanisms may explain the efficacy of exercise training over other treatments. In PAD, supervised exercise is superior to both iliac artery stenting and optimal medical care when treadmill walking distance is compared.[50] Patients with PAD who maintain higher physical activity levels in daily life have slower rates of functional decline, lower risk of CVD-related death, and better overall survival rate.[50]

**PROGNOSIS.** Arterial occlusive diseases are not life-threatening, but people with symptoms such as intermittent claudication often have a decreased quality of life because of mobility limitations. In fact, lower quality of life is reported regardless of the presence of leg symptoms.[50] People with PAD have reduced walking endurance, and claudication is associated with 50% decline in peak oxygen consumption.[356] These limitations, combined with avoidance of physical activity, especially walking, lead to further decline in functional status and cardiovascular health. The effects of occlusive diseases may also cause the need for amputation, which then increases the client's risk of mortality from complications at that time or in the future. Symptoms of chronic arterial insufficiency progress slowly over time, so that progressive disability from pain, ulceration, gangrene, and loss of function or limbs is more likely to occur than death as a result of peripheral occlusive diseases.

On the other hand, because people with either asymptomatic or symptomatic PAD have widespread arterial disease, they have a significantly increased risk of stroke, MI, and cardiovascular death. People with PAD who continue smoking have a much greater risk of death, MI, and amputation compared to those who quit smoking.[50]

**SPECIAL IMPLICATIONS FOR THE THERAPIST 12.18**

## *Arteriosclerosis Obliterans (Peripheral Artery Disease)*

### Arterial Tests and Measures

Graded treadmill protocols that give highly reproducible results have been developed to test people with PAD and are able to evaluate change in exercise performance. Two widely used graded protocols maintain a walking speed of 2 mph, one with grade increases of 3.5% every 3 minutes, the other with grade increases of 2% every 2 minutes. As the individual walks on the treadmill, time to pain and maximal walking time are recorded. All people limited by claudication are reproducibly brought to maximal levels of discomfort using either of these protocols.[18]

Claudication time is the measure of how far or how long a client can walk until their claudication symptoms present. This can be measured as part of the graded treadmill protocol or through ambulation on a level surface at the client's self-selected walking speed. The therapist documents that the client can walk "x" min (or "x" feet) at "x" gait speed before symptoms commence. Then the therapist reevaluates and re-documents claudication time after several weeks of therapy intervention.

The ankle-brachial index (ABI) (Box 12.14) is another measure of arterial perfusion at the level measured available to therapists for use in documenting the need for and benefit of a prescriptive exercise program. The ABI is a simple, inexpensive, and noninvasive tool that correlates well with angiographic disease severity and functional symptoms. It is well established as an independent predictor of cardiovascular morbidity and mortality.[2]

Blood pressures are measured, on the same side, in both the arm (brachial blood pressure) and the ankle with the client in a supine position for both measures. The ankle blood pressure may be auscultated using the dorsalis pedis pulse or posterior tibialis artery with the cuff placed above the ankle or using Doppler if available. The systolic ankle pressure is divided by the brachial systolic pressure.

With increasing degrees of arterial narrowing, there is a progressive fall in systolic blood pressure distal to the sites of involvement. If both pressures are measured with the person in the supine position and the vessels are unobstructed, the ratio of ankle to brachial pressures should be 1.0.[325]

If flow to the lower extremity is decreased, the ratio will be less than 1.0. The reference standard of ABI less than 0.90 at rest indicates PAD.[147] ABI measurements (>1.40) may be of limited value in anyone with diabetes, because calcification of the tibial and peroneal arteries may render them noncompressible. In such cases, the toe-brachial index (TBI) is used.[147] ABI below 0.9 (0.8 in some facilities) at rest may exclude individuals from early ambulation and compression in the acute care setting as part of a DVT protocol decision-making algorithm regarding ambulation and compression.

ABI can be measured before and after exercise to assess the dynamics of intermittent claudication. This can be accomplished by leaving the ankle pressure cuffs in place during the exercise. Once the walk is completed or pain develops, the person rapidly assumes a supine position and the ankle pressures are measured.

At modest workloads, the healthy adult can maintain ankle systolic pressures at normal levels. If the exercise is strenuous, there may be a transient fall in systolic pressure that rapidly returns to baseline levels. In people with intermittent claudication, a different response is seen, even at low workload. If the person walks to the point of claudication, ankle systolic pressure falls precipitously, often to unrecordable levels, and will not return to baseline levels for several minutes as blood flow is reestablished in the area.

It is not necessary (and may be misleading) to measure arm systolic pressure after exercise, because this will increase by an amount related to the workload, and the most important variable is the extent to which ankle pressure falls and the time it takes to recover (i.e., the period of postexercise ischemia). In general, if ankle pressure falls by more than 20% of the baseline value and requires more than 3 minutes to recover, the test result is considered abnormal.[279]

However, a difference of 10 to 15 (or more) points in systolic blood pressure between the arms may signify peripheral vascular disease and warrants further vascular assessment.[92]

### Prescriptive Exercise

Supervised exercise programs are more effective than unsupervised programs in improving treadmill walking distances for individuals with intermittent claudication.[65,163,356] In prescribing an exercise program for someone with claudication secondary to occlusive disease, exercise tolerance must be determined. A training heart rate should be based on the exercise tolerance test, because persons with PAD frequently have CAD as well. Frequently, symptoms of claudication occur before training heart rate is reached, but the heart rate should be monitored and should not exceed the training heart rate, even in the absence of symptoms. Anginal chest pain is a red flag to decrease exercise intensity.

A progressive conditioning program, including walking for fixed periods, is essential, even if the initial length of walking time is only 1 minute. The greatest improvement occurs with intermittent exercise to near-maximal pain, followed by rest, followed by exercise to near-maximal pain again. This is most commonly achieved via walking on a treadmill. This pattern is repeated starting with intervals as short as 1 to 5 minutes, alternating with rest periods of sufficient duration to eliminate pain (usually 2–10 minutes). Without complicating factors, the individual is usually able to complete at least a 30- to 45-minute walk without pain or rest breaks within 6 to 8 weeks.

Claudication is influenced by the speed, incline, and surface of the walk and should be modified whenever possible to improve exercise tolerance. Impairment measures, functional measures, quality-of-life assessment, and specific walking parameters are outlined in detail elsewhere.[325] Social support may also play an important role in the client's physical function and quality of life.

After exercise, numbness in the foot as well as pain in the calf may occur. The foot may be cold and pale, which is an indication that the circulation has been diverted to the arteriolar bed of the leg muscles. Many people with claudication are already receiving β-blockers for angina or hypertension.

The main factor limiting success of exercise therapy is lack of client motivation. For this reason, the most successful programs prescribe regular exercise sessions, either supervised or unsupervised, based on the client's abilities and preferences. There has been little to no difference shown in the effectiveness of supervised compared with unsupervised exercise programs.[163] It is more important to stress regularity of exercise than intensity.

Comorbid diseases, such as CAD or diabetes mellitus, and severity and location of arterial occlusive disease do not preclude successful response to prescriptive exercise. Unstable cardiopulmonary conditions require more careful consideration and collaboration with the health care team.[147]

### Precautions

When arterial thrombosis or embolism is suspected, the affected limb must be protected by proper positioning below the horizontal plane and protective skin care provided. Heat or cold application and massage are contraindicated, and family members must also be notified of these restrictions. The home health therapist must be alert to the possibility of hot water bottles, heating pads, electric blankets, and hot foot soaks being used by the client without physician approval. This precaution is especially true for people with diabetes-associated peripheral neuropathies and for people with paraplegia.

The therapist should encourage the person with vascular disease to prevent becoming chilled by keeping the thermostat at home set at 21.1° to 22.2° C (70°–72° F) and to avoid prolonged exposure to cold outdoors.

In addition, many people with PAD and diabetes mellitus have peripheral sensory neuropathy and are at greater risk for skin breakdown on the foot from weight-bearing activities such as walking or running (see Box 12.13). These individuals should participate in alternative forms of exercise (e.g., bicycling, swimming/aquatics) even though these exercises may not improve walking ability as much as a structured walking program.[134]

## VENOUS DISEASES

Venous disease can be acute or chronic; acute venous disease includes thrombophlebitis, and chronic venous disease includes varicose vein formation and chronic venous insufficiency.

**Thrombophlebitis.** Thrombophlebitis is swelling of a vein because of vein wall inflammation (phlebitis) occurring as a result of thrombus (blood clot) deposition in

**Box 12.14**

**ANKLE-BRACHIAL INDEX[a]**

- ≥1.1: Suspicious for arterial calcification; blood vessels do not compress (e.g., diabetes)
- 1.0: Adequate blood supply; compression acceptable
- <1.0: Inadequate blood supply; impaired wound healing; requires medical evaluation; prescriptive exercise beneficial
- 0.5–0.9: Indicates arterial occlusion; prescriptive exercise may be beneficial; delayed wound healing; light compression acceptable
- <0.5: Severe arterial occlusive disease; may require surgical revascularization procedure; wound healing unlikely; rarely compress; DVT protocol: excluded from early ambulation and compression

[a]Values vary slightly from institution to institution and geographically from one area of the United States to another. Consider these values a general guideline and check the standard used at your current facility/location.

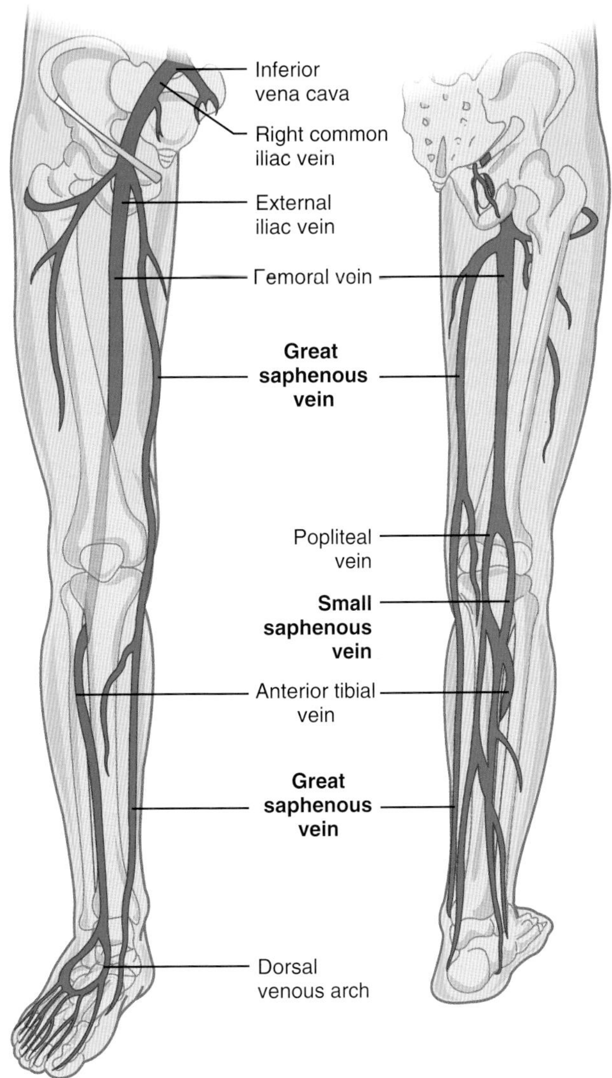


**Figure 12.34**

**Veins in the leg.** The legs have three types of veins: deep veins (femoral and popliteal) coursing alongside the deep arteries to conduct most of the venous return from the legs; superficial veins, the great and small saphenous veins; and perforators (not pictured), the connecting veins that join the two sets and route blood from the superficial into the deep veins. The great saphenous vein starts at the medial side of the dorsum of the foot and ascends in front of the medial malleolus, crossing the tibia obliquely and ascending along the medial side of the thigh. The small saphenous vein starts on the lateral side of the dorsum of the foot and ascends behind the lateral malleolus and up the back of the leg, where it joins the popliteal vein. (From Jarvis C: *Physical examination and health assessment*, ed 5, Philadelphia, 2008, WB Saunders.)

the vein. Depending on the depth location of the affected veins, there are two different types: DVT and superficial thrombophlebitis.

### Deep Vein Thrombosis and Pulmonary Embolism

*Definition and Overview.* Vein thrombosis is a partial occlusion (mural thrombus) or complete occlusion (occlusive thrombus) of a vein by a thrombus (clot) with secondary inflammatory reaction in the wall of the vein (thrombophlebitis). A venous thrombus is an intravascular collection of fibrin network, platelets, erythrocytes, and leukocytes, the end result of the activation of the clotting cascade with the potential to produce significant morbidity and mortality.[177]

Together, DVT and pulmonary embolism (PE) are referred to as venous thromboembolism (VTE). The presence of a VTE in the venous system is divided by depth and proximity. In the lower extremity, the superficial system is comprised of the great (long) and small (short) saphenous veins (Fig. 12.34). The deep veins are divided into distal and proximal. The distal deep veins include the anterior tibial, posterior tibial, and peroneal veins. The proximal deep veins include the popliteal, superficial femoral, deep femoral, common femoral, and external iliac veins.

A DVT is classified as distal if it is below the knee and proximal if it is located in the popliteal vein or above.[177] The most common superficial vein thrombosis occurs in the saphenous vein in the lower extremity (see Fig. 12.34); and the most common DVT occurs in the femoral or iliac veins.

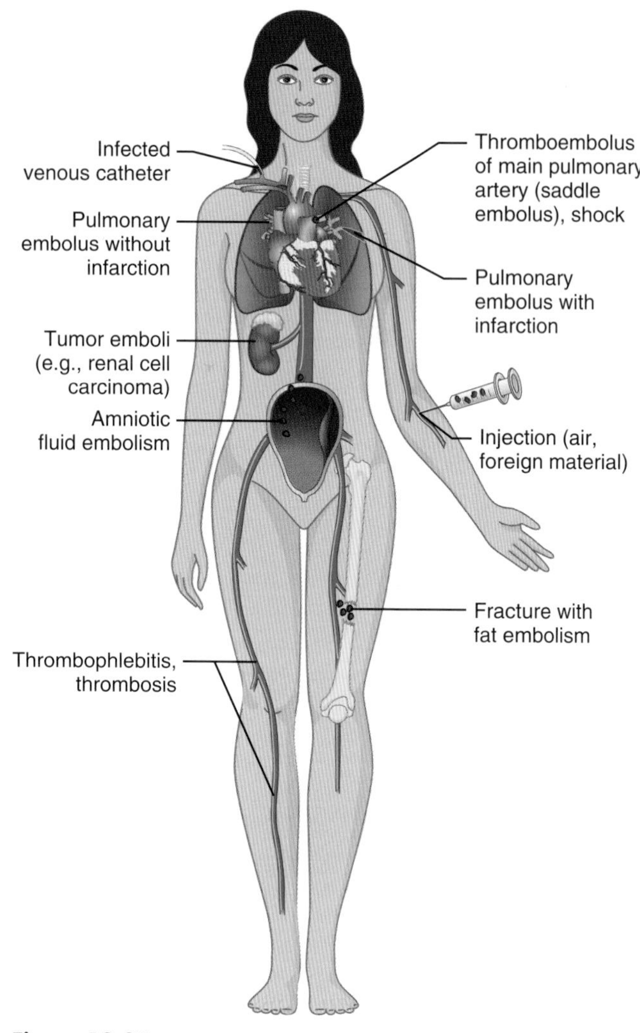


**Figure 12.35**

**Sources and effects of venous emboli.**

A PE can occur when part of a thrombus (embolus) in a DVT breaks loose and travels through the right side of the heart into the pulmonary artery. An embolus lodged in a pulmonary artery or one of its branches occludes blood flow to that part of the lung, damaging the lung and impairing gas exchange.

If a thrombus occludes a major vein (e.g., femoral, vena, axillary), the venous pressure and volume rise distally. However, if a thrombus occludes a deep small vein (e.g., tibial, popliteal), collateral vessels develop and relieve the increased venous pressure and volume. This is why the majority of PEs come from proximal DVTs.

***Incidence, Etiology, and Risk Factors.*** The number of people affected by VTE (DVT and PE combined) is unknown; estimates are wideranging because there is not an organized national surveillance system,[50] and variable presentations lead to diagnostic challenges. The annual incidence of VTE is estimated to be between 1.0 and 2.2 per 1,000 persons,[50,225] reaching between 300,000 and 600,000 people per year in the United States, with numbers likely being underestimated.[50] Within 10 years, the number of hospitalized patients with DVT has increased by 34% and with PE by 53%.[50]

Incidence of VTE increases significantly with age regardless of gender, with PE accounting for the larger proportion of all VTE. Lifetime risk of VTE at age 45 is 8%. Incidence of VTE is higher in African Americans and lower in Asian Americans and Native Americans when compared to the white population.[50]

VTE has become a significant health problem and is considered to be the most preventable cause of hospital-related death and is among the top causes of pregnancy-related death.[46]

Approximately 30% to 60% of all people (women more than men) undergoing major general surgical procedures or having common pathologies such as cerebrovascular accidents develop clinical manifestations of DVT up to 4 weeks after the operation or incident (Fig. 12.35).[127]

VTE is the most common reason for hospital readmission and death after total hip and total knee arthroplasty.[127] High-risk surgical candidates have a history of recent VTE or have undergone extensive pelvic or abdominal surgery for advanced malignancy, CABG, renal transplantation, splenectomy, or major orthopedic surgery to the lower limbs (e.g., hip or knee arthroplasty, surgery for fractured hip, tibial osteotomy).

Emboli can be formed of other substances besides a blood clot. Air bubbles, fat droplets, amniotic fluid, clumps of parasites, or tumor cells can lead to a VTE. Fat embolism syndrome from fat thromboembolic phenomenon is a well-known consequence of femoral total hip replacement arthroplasty. Intravasation of fat into the bloodstream during prosthetic implantation has been linked with postoperative confusion and cognitive decline. The risk of fat embolism syndrome is four times greater with simultaneous bilateral total knee or total hip replacements. Changes have been made in the arthroplasty surgical technique that may result in a reduced incidence of this complication.

Approximately 50% of VTE are triggered by immobility, surgery, trauma, or hospitalization; 20% are linked to cancer.[50] History of thrombosis, obesity, nursing home residence, central venous catheter, infection, kidney disease, long-distance travel, pregnancy, and postpartum periods in females are considered risk factors for VTE.[50]

Venous thrombus formation is usually attributed to the Virchow triad: venous stasis, hypercoagulability, or injury to the venous wall,[4] although other risk factors may be present (Box 12.15).[50,131] It is commonly held that at least two of these three conditions must be present for a thrombus to form. Fifty percent of all DVT cases are viewed as idiopathic.[46]

Genetics is highly implicated in VTE. The connection has been established with mutations for antithrombin III, protein S, protein C, factor V Leiden, prothrombin (mutation variant 20210A), and sickle cell disease trait.[50] Several genetic factors have been demonstrated to interact adversely with lifestyle influences, such as oral contraceptives and smoking.

***Pathogenesis.*** Any trauma to the endothelium of the vein wall exposes subendothelial tissues to platelets and clotting factors in the venous blood, initiating thrombosis. Platelets adhering to the vein wall attract the deposition of fibrin, leukocytes, and erythrocytes, forming a thrombus that may remain attached to the vessel wall.

Box 12.15

**RISK FACTORS FOR DEEP VENOUS[a] THROMBOSIS**

***Immobility (Venous Stasis)***

- Hospitalization
- Prolonged bed rest (e.g., burns, fracture)
- Prolonged air travel
- Neurologic disorder (e.g., spinal cord injury, stroke)
- Cardiac failure
- Absence of ankle muscle pump

***Trauma (Venous Damage)***

- Surgery
- Local trauma (e.g., direct injury)
- Indwelling venous access devices
- Intravenous injections
- Fracture or dislocation
- Childbirth and delivery
- Sclerosing agents

***Lifestyle***

- Hormonal status
  - Oral contraceptive use
  - Hormonal medications (e.g., tamoxifen, Adriamycin [doxorubicin])
  - Pregnancy and postpartum period
  - In vitro fertilization
- Smoking

***Hypercoagulation***

- Genetics (hereditary thrombotic disorders)
- Neoplasm (especially viscera, ovary)
- Increasing levels of coagulation factors (VIII, XI)
- Prothrombin mutation
- Increasing levels of homocysteine
- Activated protein C syndrome

***Other***

- Family history
- Diabetes mellitus and other chronic diseases
- Obesity
- Previous DVT
- Buerger disease
- Age >60 years
- Idiopathic (50% of all DVT cases)

[a]The terms *venous* and *vein* are used interchangeably in the literature and in this text.

***Clinical Manifestations.*** In the early stages, approximately half of the people with DVT are asymptomatic for any signs or symptoms in the affected extremity. The lower extremities appear to be affected most often (more than 90%), but upper extremity venous thrombi can also develop.

Lower-Extremity Vein Thrombosis. When symptoms occur in the lower extremity, the client may report a dull ache, a tight feeling, or pain in the calf, often misdiagnosed as some other cause of leg pain. In 80% of the cases with symptoms, the DVT is proximal, above the trifurcation of the popliteal vein.[177] It is important to realize that proximal DVTs more often lead to severe consequences of DVT and that at the time of diagnosis, more than 50% of the affected individuals already have PE.[307]

Signs are often absent; when present but taken alone, they may be variable and unreliable. Signs and symptoms include leg or calf swelling, pain or tenderness, dilation of superficial veins, and pitting edema. The skin of the leg and ankle on the affected side may be relatively warmer than on the unaffected side (the therapist should check for temperature changes with the backs of the fingers or a skin thermometer). If venous obstruction is severe, the skin may be cyanotic.

Any of these symptoms can occur without DVT, possibly associated with other vascular, inflammatory, musculoskeletal, or lymphatic conditions that produce signs and symptoms similar to those of DVT.

PEs, most often from the large, deep veins of the pelvis and legs, are the most devastating complication of DVT and can occur without apparent warning, ending in sudden death. Signs and symptoms of PE are dependent on the size and location of the PE[307] and may include the following: pleuritic chest pain; diffuse chest discomfort; tachypnea; tachycardia; hemoptysis; anxiety, restlessness, apprehension; dyspnea; and persistent cough.

Upper-Extremity Vein Thrombosis. Venous thrombosis of the upper extremity accounts for up to 10% of all cases of DVT, most often affecting the subclavian vein, axillary vein, or both, with occurrences less often affecting the internal jugular and brachial vein.[224] Primary upper-extremity DVT is either idiopathic or associated with strenuous physical activity (effort-induced thrombosis). Secondary upper-extremity DVT is usually associated with infection, a systemic illness (e.g., cancer), the use of indwelling peripherally inserted central catheter (PICC) lines or central venous catheters (CVCs) (e.g., used in the treatment of cancer, parenteral nutrition), or, less often, hemodialysis.[195,213,224]

In the case of upper-extremity superficial vein thrombosis, dull pain and local tenderness in the region of the involved vein may be accompanied by signs of superficial induration (firm or hard cord) and redness.

Upper-extremity *superficial* vein thrombosis is self-limiting and does not typically cause PE, because the blood flows to deeper veins through small perforating venous channels. Iatrogenic superficial vein thrombosis is often secondary to prolonged IV catheter use. Upper-extremity *deep* vein thrombosis is not as common as in the lower extremity, but, again, incidence may be on the rise as a consequence of the increasing use of PICC lines or CVCs.

Unfortunately, the first clinical manifestation of *deep* thrombosis may be PE, and as a consequence of upper extremity DVT, it can be fatal.[4] Symptoms (when present) are similar to those for the lower extremity. The therapist should be aware of the presence of any risk factors and watch for pain and pitting edema or swelling of the entire (usually upper) limb and/or an area of the limb that is 2 cm or more larger than the surrounding area, indicating swelling requiring further investigation.

Other symptoms include numbness, heaviness, redness or warmth of the arm, dilated veins, or low-grade fever possibly accompanied by chills and malaise. Bruising or discoloration of the area or proximal to the thrombosis has been observed in some cases.[213] Swelling can contribute to decreased neck or shoulder motion. In addition to any of the signs and symptoms listed here, the individual with a PICC line may also report pain or tenderness at or above the insertion site.

**Table 12.21** Wells Clinical Decision Rule for Deep Vein Thrombosis*

| Clinical Presentation | Score |
|---|---|
| Active cancer (within 6 months of diagnosis or receiving palliative care) | 1 |
| Paralysis, paresis, or recent immobilization of lower extremity | 1 |
| Bedridden for more than 3 days or major surgery in the last 4 weeks | 1 |
| Localized tenderness in the center of the posterior calf, the popliteal space, or along the femoral vein in the anterior thigh/groin | 1 |
| Entire lower-extremity swelling | 1 |
| Unilateral calf swelling (more than 3 mm larger than uninvolved side) | 1 |
| Unilateral pitting edema | 1 |
| Collateral superficial veins (nonvaricose) | 1 |
| An alternative diagnosis is as likely (or more likely) than DVT (e.g., cellulitis, postoperative swelling, calf strain) | −2 |
| **Total Points** | |

*DVT*, Deep vein thrombosis.
Key:
−2 to 0: Low probability of DVT (3%)
1 to 2: Moderate probability of DVT (17%)
≥3: High probability of DVT (75%)
Medical consultation is advised in the presence of low probability; medical referral is required with moderate or high score.
From Wells PS, Anderson DR, Bormanis J et al.: Value of assessment of pretest probability of deep-vein thrombosis in clinical management. *Lancet* 350:1795–1798, 1997. Used with permission.

Chronic venous insufficiency or postthrombotic syndrome are possible sequelae to upper extremity DVT.[213]

## MEDICAL MANAGEMENT

**PREVENTION.** Primary prevention of DVT/VTE through the use of early mobilization for low-risk individuals and prophylactic use of anticoagulants (see Table 12.5) in people considered at moderate to high risk for DVT is important. Mobilization and compression stockings following acute DVT reduce the risk of postthrombotic syndrome.[177] Although such interventions reduce the risk of DVT, it must be understood that even people receiving anticoagulant therapy can still develop DVT.

Routine use of knee elastic stockings in all postoperative clients has been adopted in most hospitals, and many facilities use pneumatic pressure devices with on/off cycles applied for the first few hours after major surgery to mimic the calf pump. There is strong evidence to advocate for the use of intermittent compression devices to prevent DVT.[177] Once the person is able, ankle pumping and mobility are added.

Evidence-based clinical practice guidelines have been published for the prevention of VTE in orthopedic surgery through preventing thrombosis with antithrombotic therapy, by the American Academy of Orthopedic Surgeons,[254] and by the American College of Chest Physicians;[127] for diagnosis of VTE, by the American Society of Hematology;[225] as well as the VTE Clinical Practice Guidelines published by the American Physical Therapy Association.[177]

**DIAGNOSIS.** The diagnosis of a DVT has been aided by the inclusion of Clinical Decision Rules (CDRs), or more currently named as Risk Assessment Tools.[72] One such tool is the use of the Wells Risk Assessment,[371,372] which has been shown to be a reliable and valid tool for clinical assessment for predicting the risk of DVT in the lower extremity.[177] A simple model to predict upper-extremity DVT has also been proposed but has not been routinely adopted since the initial study.[95] The best available test for the diagnosis of upper-extremity DVT is venous duplex ultrasonography.[224]

Use of the Wells Risk Assessment has been specifically shown to be valid with different populations and is recommended to help determine the likelihood of DVT.[177] Utilization of the Wells Risk Assessment in anyone with suspected DVT clusters signs, symptoms, and risk factors and classifies the person's likelihood of having DVT as low, moderate, or high (Table 12.21). There are several risk assessment models that may help the therapist in predicting who may be at risk for DVT.[177] These include the Padua score for assessing VTE risk in hospitalized patients, the IMPROVE VTE RAM, the Autar DVT Risk Assessment Scale, and the Geneva Risk Score. These can be used in conjunction with the Wells scale to assist the therapist in referring appropriate clients for further testing for DVT. It is important for the therapist to keep this in mind, as one study has shown that physical therapists often underestimate the likelihood of DVT in high-risk individuals and frequently do not refer to a physician when they should.[307] Moreover, survey of physical therapy clinical instructors uncovered that two-thirds of those surveyed not only were using outdated DVT/VTE screening tools but were unable to identify major risk factors for DVT/VTE.[172]

At-risk clients as assessed by history and clinical examination receive a D-dimer blood test (checking for fibrin breakdown products released from a thrombus) to determine the DVT risk level. Moderate- to high-risk individuals (D-dimer level above 500 ng/mL) receive Doppler duplex ultrasonography as a rapid screening procedure to detect thrombosis. Venous duplex ultrasonographic scanning has replaced contrast venography as the primary diagnostic test for DVT because it allows noninvasive real-time visualization of the vein while simultaneously providing information on venous flow.

It is recognized that often, other calf muscle strain or contusion may be difficult to differentiate from vein thrombosis. Further diagnostic testing may be required to determine the correct diagnosis. Occasionally, a ruptured Baker cyst may produce unilateral pain and swelling in the calf. A history of arthritis in the knee of the same leg and the disappearance of the popliteal cyst at the time symptoms develop are clues the physician can use to make the differentiation. Although the Homans sign was once used for differential diagnosis of acute DVT, it is no longer considered a sensitive or specific test for ruling in or out DVT. Its use is not recommended due to high rates of both false-positive and false-negative results in the diagnosis of DVT.

**TREATMENT.** The goals of DVT management are to prevent progression to PE, limit extension of the thrombus, limit damage to the vein, and prevent another clot from forming. Current therapy is to administer anticoagulants. The primary anticoagulants used are low-molecular-weight heparins (LMWHs). Other alternatives are Arixtra (fondaparinux), oral thrombin or factor Xa inhibitors, unfractionated heparin, or Coumadin (warfarin) (see Table 12.5).[43,177] Anticoagulation therapy for acute DVT prevents enlargement of the thrombus and allows for further attachment of the thrombus to the vessel wall, thereby reducing the likelihood of PE. Anticoagulants prevent or slow down the clot formation, whereas thrombolytics facilitate the dissolution of the clot. The rate of clot lysis in individuals treated only with anticoagulants is slower than in combination with thrombolytic therapy, and it can take up to several months in some cases for the clot to completely resolve.[370] Combined use of anticoagulants and thrombolytics increases the patency of the veins and decreases the frequency of postthrombotic syndromes by one third, compared to anticoagulation therapy alone.[370] However, the use of thrombolytics increases risk of bleeding incidence twofold.[370] This complication, together with the prohibitive cost and the need for strict selection of patients who will most likely benefit despite the possibility of bleeding, may delay or prevent wide use of thrombolytic therapy in DVT.[197]

Anticoagulants can be very effective in treating a thrombus. However, anticoagulation therapy does not effectively address the need to restore venous function in the thrombosed veins.[370]

Elastic stockings must be worn whenever the person is ambulating or in the upright position. Once anticoagulation has been initiated and the client has received the appropriate dose for that medication, then the therapist should begin mobilizing the person.[177] Clients are advised to remain active but avoid any straining maneuvers.

For cases of massive DVT, thrombolysis, thrombectomy, and embolectomy (often performed in an interventional angiography laboratory) can be performed.

**PROGNOSIS.** DVTs that are not diagnosed can lead to life-threatening consequences, such as PE. With appropriate intervention and in the absence of complications, a return to normal health and activity can be expected within 1 to 3 weeks for the person with an upper-extremity or calf DVT and within 6 weeks for the person with thigh or pelvic DVT.

Prognosis depends on the size of the vessel involved, the presence of collateral circulation, and the underlying cause of the thrombosis (e.g., spinal cord injury, stroke, or cancer may prevent return to former health).

A potential long-term complication of DVT is venous stasis or insufficiency (postthrombotic syndrome) when permanent damage to the vein has occurred. Approximately 30% of people who had proximal lower-extremity DVT will develop postthrombotic syndrome or venous stasis syndrome in the first 20 years following DVT, and 3.7% develop venous ulcer.[50]

## SPECIAL IMPLICATIONS FOR THE THERAPIST 12.19

### *Vein Thrombosis and Pulmonary Embolism*

(See also "Special Implications for the Therapist 15.23: Pulmonary Embolism and Infarction.") The APTA published specific Clinical Practice Guidelines for the physical therapist's role in the management and treatment of VTE from DVT. Most of those guidelines are reflected in this chapter, but the therapist is encouraged to go directly to the publication for complete discussion of recommended guidelines.[177]

#### Risk Assessment

Populations at risk (see Box 12.15), especially postoperative, postpartum, and immobilized clients, should be identified by the medical staff and observed carefully. Risk factor assessment models (e.g., Autar DVT scale, Wells Risk Assessment for DVT or PE, Padua score, the IMPROVE VTE RAM, and the Geneva Risk Score) for use in a therapy practice are available.[43,177] Using risk categories (i.e., increasing age, BMI, immobility, special DVT risk, trauma, surgery, high-risk disease), the therapist can accurately predict and categorize each person's risk for VTE disease as no risk (less than 10%), low risk (10%), moderate risk (11%-40%), or high risk (greater than 41%).

The person at risk for DVT secondary to fracture and subsequent immobility involving a lower-extremity cast should be carefully evaluated when the cast is removed. Normally, calf muscle atrophy is easily observed when the cast is removed. Normal calf size (less than 1 cm difference between left and right) without atrophy on cast removal may signal swelling associated with DVT.

For the client with diagnosed thrombophlebitis, the therapist should monitor and report any signs of PE, such as chest pain, hemoptysis, cough, diaphoresis, dyspnea, and apprehension. Clients with a history of DVT may develop chronic venous insufficiency even years later and therefore must be monitored periodically for life.

#### Precautions During Anticoagulation Therapy

Anyone receiving anticoagulant therapy that is not a LMWH (e.g., warfarin) must be monitored for manifestations of bleeding, as evidenced by blood in the urine, in the stool, or along the gums or teeth; subcutaneous bruising; or back, pelvic, or flank pain. The presence of any of these signs or symptoms must be reported to the physician immediately.

The risk for bleeding is increased with alcohol use, especially if there is concomitant liver disease, as alcohol also can potentiate warfarin. Many herbs have natural anticoagulant effects that can potentiate the effect of warfarin, and others can counteract its effect. Ginkgo biloba, garlic, dong quai, dan shen, and ginseng (herbs commonly ingested in supplemental form) should not be used or taken at the same time as warfarin. Anyone using these products should be encouraged to discuss medication dosage with the prescribing physician. Eating large quantities of vitamin K–rich foods can also interfere with the drug's anticoagulant effects, requiring careful monitoring of food intake while on warfarin.

Bleeding under the skin and easy bruising in response to the slightest trauma can occur when platelet production is altered. This condition necessitates extreme care in the therapy setting, especially any intervention requiring soft tissue mobilization, manual therapy, or the use of any equipment, including any modalities and weight-training devices. Rarely, skin necrosis associated with the use of warfarin occurs, presenting as large hemorrhagic blisters on the breasts, buttocks, thighs, and penis requiring wound management.

Most, if not all, of these complications do not occur in the person taking a LWMH, so less caution is needed for mobilization, and there are fewer dietary restrictions.

#### Prevention and Intervention

Prevention is the key to treatment of thrombophlebitis, both preventing thrombus formation and preventing thrombi from becoming emboli. Preventive therapy can be tailored to the individual's level of risk while focusing on physical activity, exercise, prophylactic use of anticoagulants, and compression. The activity and exercise protocol may include active and passive range-of-motion exercise, early ambulation for brief but regular periods whenever possible, coughing and deep-breathing exercises, and proper positioning.

After thrombosis of a deep calf vein, elastic support hose should be worn for at least 6 to 8 weeks or longer if risk assessment is moderate or high. Helping the client find easier ways to put the hose on and explaining the purpose may increase compliance in using the hose consistently and correctly.

The use of TED (antiembolism) hoses should be restricted to individuals who are nonambulatory for short periods of time. They do provide compression in the range of 13 to 18 mm Hg but are not intended for use while ambulating. A light gradient compression stocking of 20 to 30 mm Hg (available off the shelf) is advised to prevent blood clot formation when medically necessary in individuals who are upright, active, or ambulatory. (This would be a much better choice for orthopedic patients postoperatively once they are ambulatory.)

Support pantyhose may be an acceptable alternative for some people who have trouble putting on the compressive stockings or who live in very hot climates. The rationale for the use of compressive or elastic stockings is that the compressive force applied by the stocking causes the vessel wall to become applied to the thrombus, thereby keeping the thrombus in its location and preventing movement inside the blood vessel. Without the external compressive force of the stocking, once the person stands, increased hydrostatic pressure causes venous distention and permits the thrombus to become free floating inside the vessel.

The American College of Chest Physicians recommends that anyone flying or sitting in a motor vehicle for more than 8 hours avoid wearing constrictive clothing around the waist or legs, stay hydrated, and perform frequent ankle pumps or other foot and leg exercises.[182]

Regarding positioning, the person at risk must be taught the importance of avoiding one position for prolonged periods and avoiding pillows under the legs postoperatively to facilitate venous return. At the same time, elevation of the legs just above the level of the heart aids blood flow by gravitational force and prevents venous stasis as a contributing factor to the formation of new thrombi. Prolonged sitting in a chair in the early postoperative period should be avoided.

### DVT and Ambulation

Mobilization and ambulation is important for people with DVT after an adequate anticoagulant has been administered and if local symptoms and general client condition permit. The concern in an acute care or rehabilitation setting is the increased risk of PE in clients who are aggressively mobilized too soon after a diagnosis of a DVT and before adequate anticoagulation has been administered. The therapist should reference the APTA guidelines for VTE or the specific facility protocol for the appropriate length of bed rest needed prior to mobilization after each type of anticoagulant. These times can rage from 10 min to 24 hrs, so it is important to know the specific time at each health care facility or for each type of medication.

Due to the sequelae that can happen from bedrest, therapists are encouraged to mobilize clients as soon as appropriate.[177,182]

Knowledge of the evidence and current practice guidelines allows therapists to collaborate with physicians and make the most appropriate decisions for their clients, potentially avoiding unnecessary and detrimental bed rest/immobility. Compression along with anticoagulation when mobilizing remains the standard practice.[177,182]

### DVT and Laboratory Values

Therapists need to know what anticoagulant medication patients are taking and how to determine if the medication is therapeutic. Warfarin is monitored by the international normalized ratio (INR), and unfractionated heparin is monitored by partial thromboplastin time (PTT). LMWH is therapeutic almost immediately after given and, unlike the others, does not require a lab value to determine achievement of a therapeutic range.

The INR is a measure of coagulability and was developed to provide results that would not vary between laboratories. Individuals receiving anticoagulation therapy because of history of DVT, CAD, cerebrovascular disease, atrial fibrillation, and other reasons are usually anticoagulated to an INR of 2 to 3.[27]

As INR increases, however, the risk of bleeding with minor trauma increases, and excessive bleeding may occur during surgery, as well as spontaneous bleeding. Therapists must keep INR levels in mind when working with clients. An INR between 2 and 3 is considered "therapeutic" for anticoagulation. Guidelines have not been published for levels above which physical activity would be contraindicated.

As with any clinical decision, the individual being considered would be evaluated, taking factors such as medical history; symptoms related to activity; type of activity (bed exercises or out-of-bed activities); size, location, and number of thrombi; clinical presentation (e.g., obvious signs of severe swelling, redness, warmth, tenderness; evidence of PE); and cognitive function in following directions.

## Varicose Veins

***Definition and Incidence.*** Varicose veins are an abnormal dilation of veins, usually the saphenous veins of the lower extremities, leading to tortuosity (twisting and turning) of the vessel, incompetence of the valves, and a propensity to thrombosis.

Women are affected with leg varicosities more often than men (secondary to pregnancy) until age 70 years, when the gender difference disappears. The incidence of varicose veins is 2.6% in women and 1.9% in men.[50] This condition most often develops between the ages of 30 and 50 years for all persons.

A separate but similar condition called *spider veins* or *telangiectasia* (broken capillaries) results in fine-lined networks of red, blue, or purple veins, usually on the thighs, calves, and ankles. The veins may form patterns resembling a sunburst, a spider web, or a tree with branches but can also appear as short, unconnected, or parallel lines.

***Etiologic and Risk Factors.*** Family history is associated with the development of this condition, and several genes have been implicated.[50] While varicose veins may be an inherited trait, it is unclear whether the valvular incompetence is secondary to defective valves in the saphenous veins or to a fundamental weakness of the walls of the vein leading to dilation of the vessel.

Periods of high venous pressure associated with heavy lifting or prolonged sitting or standing are risk factors. Hormonal changes (e.g., pregnancy, menopause, hormonal therapy) often contribute to the development of this condition by relaxing the vein walls.

Other risk factors include pressure associated with pregnancy or obesity, HF, hemorrhoids, constipation, esophageal varices, and hepatic cirrhosis. Occurrence of a varicose vein in one location predisposes the client to varicosities in other veins as well. Risk factors for spider veins are similar to those for varicose veins (age, hormones, familial predisposition) but also include local injury (past or present).

***Pathogenesis.*** Blood returning to the heart from the legs must flow upward through the veins, against the pull of gravity. This blood is milked upward, principally by the massaging action of the muscles against the veins. To prevent the blood from flowing backward, the veins contain one-way valves located at intervals, which operate in pairs by closing to stop the reverse movement of the blood.

The vessels most commonly affected by varicosities are located just beneath the skin superficial to the deep fascia and function without the kind of support deep veins of the legs receive from surrounding muscles. As the one-way valves become incompetent or the veins become more elastic, the veins engorge with stagnant blood and become pooled.

Any condition accompanied by higher pressure changes places a strain on these veins, and the lack of pumping action of the lower leg muscles causes blood to pool. Other sites involved include the hemorrhoidal plexus of the rectum and anal canal (either inside or outside the anal sphincter), submucosal veins of the distal esophagus, and the scrotum (varicocele).

The weight of the blood continually pressing downward against the closed venous valves causes the veins to distend and eventually lose their elasticity. When several valves lose their ability to function properly, the blood collects in the veins, causing the veins to become swollen and distended. During pregnancy, the uterus may press against the veins coming from the lower extremities and prevent the free flow of returning blood. More force is required to push the blood through the veins, and the increased back-pressure can result in varicose veins.

***Clinical Manifestations.*** The clinical picture is not directly correlated with the severity of the varicosities. Extensive varicose veins may be asymptomatic, but minimal varicosities may result in multiple symptoms. The development of varicose veins is usually gradual, with the most common symptoms reported as a dull, aching

NORMAL VEINS
Functional valves aid in flow of venous blood back to heart

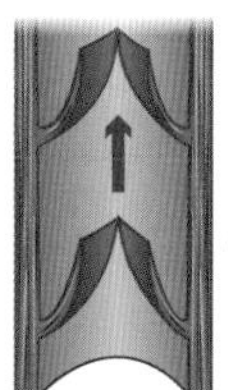

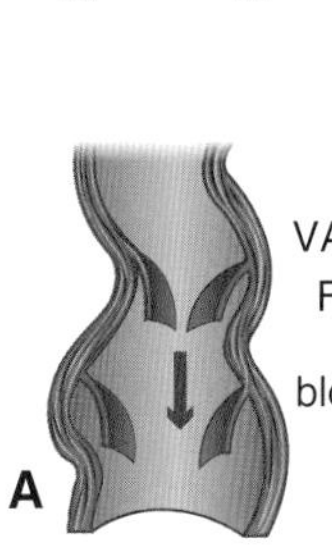


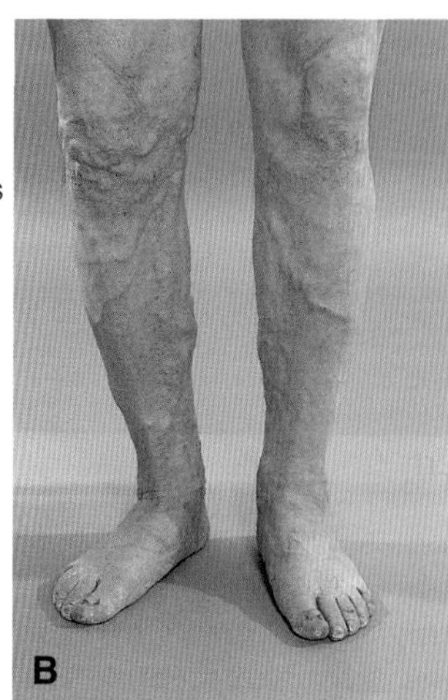


**Figure 12.36**

(A) Diagrams of normal *(top)* and varicose *(bottom)* veins. (B) Person with varicose veins. (A, from O'Toole M, ed: *Miller-Keane encyclopedia and dictionary of medicine, nursing, and allied health*, ed 6, Philadelphia, 1997, WB Saunders, p. 1702. B, from Forbes CD, Jackson WF: *Color atlas and text of clinical medicine*, ed 3, London, 2003, Mosby.)

heaviness, tension, or feeling of fatigue brought on by periods of standing. Cramps of the lower legs may occur, especially at night, and elevation of the legs often provides relief. Itching from an associated dermatitis may also occur above the ankle.

The most visible sign of varicosities is the dilated, tortuous, elongated veins beneath the skin, which are usually readily visible when the person is standing (Fig. 12.36). Varicosities of long duration may be accompanied by secondary tissue changes, such as a brownish pigmentation of the skin and a thinning of the skin above the ankle. Swelling may also occur around the ankles.

Untreated, the veins become thick and hard to the touch; impaired circulation and skin changes may lead to ulcers of the lower legs, especially around the ankles (see Table 12.20). One of the most important distinctions between varicose veins and spider veins is that, in some cases, varicose veins can result in thromboses (blood clots) and phlebitis (inflammation of the vein) or venous insufficiency ulcers, whereas spider veins are merely a cosmetic issue with no adverse effects.

## MEDICAL MANAGEMENT

DIAGNOSIS. The physician must distinguish between the symptoms of arteriosclerotic PVD, such as intermittent claudication and coldness of the feet, and symptoms of venous disease, because occlusive arterial disease usually contraindicates the operative management of varicosities below the knee. When the two conditions coexist, the reduced blood flow caused by the atherosclerosis may even improve the varicosities by reducing blood flow through the veins.

Patient history of symptoms should be used in conjunction with visual inspection and palpation to identify varicose veins of the legs. Doppler ultrasonography or the duplex scanner is useful in detecting the location of incompetent valves. Endoscopy or radiographic diagnosis identifies esophageal varices; rectal examination or proctoscopy is used to diagnose hemorrhoids; and palpation identifies varicocele (scrotal swelling).

**TREATMENT.** Treatment of mild varicose veins is conservative, consisting of periodic daily rest periods with feet elevated slightly above the heart. External massage directing fluid back towards the direction of the heart may help to relieve some symptoms. Client education as to the importance of promoting circulation is stressed, including instructions to make frequent changes in posture, a daily exercise program, and the appropriate use of properly fitting elastic stockings.

When varicosities have progressed past the stage at which conservative care is helpful, surgical intervention and compression sclerotherapy may be considered. In the past, surgical treatment of varicose veins consisted of removing the varicosities and the incompetent perforating veins (ligation and stripping), a procedure sometimes referred to as *stripping the veins* or *miniphlebectomy*. The conservative hemodynamic correction of venous insufficiency (CHIVA) procedure is another surgical option that has been found to be highly effective, even more so than vein stripping.[280]

However, newer techniques including the use of lasers have been found to be effective with less risk than the surgical procedures.[52] Other procedures for varicose veins have been developed too, including radiofrequency ablation (radio waves used to seal off the vein) and sclerotherapy (injections of a hardening, or sclerosing, solution; over several months' time, the injected veins atrophy, and blood is channeled into other veins).

Radiofrequency and laser treatments were found comparable with respect to the venous occlusion rates at 3 months after treatment with the former procedure accompanied with less pain, lower analgesia levels, and reduced bruising.[269]

Some individuals may try oral dietary supplementation as an addition to traditional management of varicose veins, but this is not a standard recommendation for treatment.

**PROGNOSIS.** Good results with relief of symptoms are usually possible in the majority of cases. Early conservative care for varicose veins during initial stages may help prevent the condition from worsening, but advanced disease may not be prevented from recurring, even with surgical intervention or sclerotherapy. Although surgery for varicose veins can improve appearance, it may not reduce the physical discomfort, suggesting that most lower limb symptoms may have a nonvenous cause. A high mortality is associated with ruptured, bleeding esophageal varices.

SPECIAL IMPLICATIONS FOR THE THERAPIST 12.20

### *Varicose Veins*

The therapist can be instrumental in developing prescriptive exercise and preventive measures for anyone at risk for, or already diagnosed with, varicose veins. Because excessive sitting or standing contributes to this condition, the therapist can individualize a program to help the person avoid static postures and utilize quick stretching or movement breaks coordinated with deep-breathing exercises.

Nonprescription pantyhose should be replaced with special compression garments that do not constrict behind the knee, upper leg, waist, or groin. These should be worn as much as possible during the daytime hours (including during exercise for some people) but may be removed at night. After exercise and at the end of the day, the therapist should instruct the individual to elevate the legs in a supported position above the level of the heart for 10 to 15 minutes.

The therapist should encourage the person to practice good breathing techniques during this time. Aerobic exercise, strength training, or resistive exercises are encouraged, but high-impact activities, such as jogging or step aerobics, should be avoided. Brisk walking, cycling, cross-country skiing or NordicTrack equipment, rowing, and swimming are all good alternatives to high-impact activities.

## Chronic Venous Insufficiency

**Definition and Incidence.** Chronic venous insufficiency (CVI), also known as postphlebitic syndrome and venous stasis, is defined as inadequate venous return over a long period of time. This condition follows most severe cases of DVT, although it is possible to develop CVI without prior episodes of DVT. CVI may also occur as a result of leg trauma, varicose veins, and neoplastic obstruction of the pelvic veins. The long-term sequelae of CVI may be chronic leg ulcers, accounting for the majority of vascular ulceration; incidence is expected to continue rising with the aging of America.[78] In the United States, 25 million people have varicose veins.[50]

**Etiologic Factors and Pathogenesis.** CVI occurs when damaged or destroyed valves in the veins result in decreased venous return, thereby increasing venous pressure and producing venous stasis. Without adequate valve function and in the absence of the calf muscle pump, blood flows in the veins bidirectionally, causing high ambulatory venous pressures in the calf veins (venous hypertension). Superficial veins and capillaries dilate in response to the venous hypertension. Red blood cells, proteins, and fluids leak out of the capillaries into interstitial spaces, producing edema and the reddish brown pigmentation characteristic of CVI. Hair loss in the lower extremity usually accompanies the change in skin color and edema. More severe venous disease is often accompanied by hyperpigmentation, venous eczema, and venous ulcers.[50]

Chronic pooling of blood in the veins of the lower extremities prevents adequate cellular oxygenation and removal of waste products. Any trauma, especially pressure, further lowers the oxygen supply by reducing blood flow into the area. Cell death occurs, and necrotic tissue develops into venous stasis ulcers. The cycle of reduced oxygenation, necrosis, and ulceration prevents damaged tissue from obtaining necessary nutrients, causing delayed healing and persistent ulceration. Poor circulation impairs immune and inflammatory responses, leaving venous stasis ulcers susceptible to infection.

Presence of flat feet and leg injury in women and smoking in men predispose to CVI.[50] Other contributing factors may include poor nutrition, immobility, diabetes, obesity, and local trauma (past or present). A previous history of burns requiring skin grafts predisposes the individual to venous insufficiency. The area of the graft usually lacks superficial veins, properly functioning capillaries, or both, resulting in blood pooling in these areas. As a result, previously burned areas and skin grafts in the lower extremity are susceptible to vascular ulceration.

**Clinical Manifestations.** CVI is characterized by progressive edema of the leg; thickening, coarsening, and brownish pigmentation of skin around the ankles; and venous stasis ulceration (see Table 12.20). Venous insufficiency ulcers constitute approximately 80% of all lower extremity ulcers, occurring most often above the medial malleolus, where venous hypertension is greatest.

These ulcers characteristically are shallow wounds with a white creamy to fibrous slough over a base of good granulation tissue. They can be very painful, with a moderate to large amount of drainage. The wounds typically have irregular borders and are partial to full thickness, often with signs of reepithelialization (e.g., pink or red granulation base). Frequently, moderate to severe edema is present in the limb. In longstanding cases, this edema becomes hardened to a dense, woody texture. The skin of the involved extremity is usually thin, shiny, dry, and cyanotic. Dermatitis and cellulitis may develop later in this condition.

## MEDICAL MANAGEMENT

The physician will differentiate between CVI and other causes of edema and ulceration of the lower extremities using client history, clinical examination, and diagnostic tests to rule out or confirm superimposed acute phlebitis. Arterial and venous insufficiency may coexist in the same person.

Treatment goals and techniques are as for varicose veins (increase in venous return, reduction of edema). Conventional methods of compression and rest and elevation (e.g., more frequent periods of leg elevation above the level of the heart are encouraged throughout the day with the foot of the bed elevated 6 inches at night) have been augmented by surgical intervention.

Rapid progress in endovascular procedures with angioplasty and stenting has made it possible for the development of techniques to relieve obstruction and repair reflux in the deep veins. Venous stasis ulcers require ongoing treatment, usually involving the therapist (e.g., primary intervention for edema reduction and topical ulcer and wound care). Graduated lower extremity compression wrapping or garments are a large part of wound care for venous stasis wounds.[295] More detailed information on wound care for venous stasis wounds is available.[346] Researchers are developing bioengineered skin, a living human dermal replacement, for the management of venous ulcers.

The prognosis is poor for resolution of CVI, with chronic venous stasis ulcers causing loss of function and progressive disability. Recurrent episodes of acute thrombophlebitis may occur, and noncompliance with the treatment program is common.

SPECIAL IMPLICATIONS FOR THE THERAPIST 12.21

### *Chronic Venous Insufficiency*

The therapist can be instrumental in providing clients with venous insufficiency with education and prevention to avoid complications that can occur with vascular ulceration and chronic wounds. Formulating an exercise prescription; collaborating with a nutritionist; and understanding the underlying etiology, hemodynamics, comorbidities, and principles of tissue repair are essential in developing a plan of care.

Compression therapy (e.g., bandages, gradient compression stockings, pumps) is the gold standard for treatment of venous insufficiency, especially when venous leg ulcers are present.[295] The goal is to promote venous return from peripheral veins to central circulation. The therapist may also use layered gradient compression wraps. Antiembolism TED hospital stockings are not an effective treatment for vein disease. They do offer mild equalized compression for individuals who are bedridden, but they cannot support the vein walls for individuals who are upright. They also do not provide graduated compression to ensure venous return toward the heart. The presence of HF is considered a precaution to the use of external compression and requires close collaboration between the physician and therapist.

Before initiating compression therapy, the ABI should be measured. ABI is determined using a noninvasive arterial Doppler study to assess the level of circulation. Compression may not be tolerated and/or may have to be modified if arterial circulation is compromised. Arterial obstruction in the presence of venous insufficiency may not be readily recognized.

The ABI is the result of a vascular diagnostic test comparing the systolic blood pressure between the ankle and brachial pulses. ABI results should be reported with noncompressible values defined as greater than 1.40, normal values 1.00 to 1.40, borderline 0.91 to 0.99, and abnormal 0.90 or less.[147]

An index result of 1.0 indicates an adequate arterial blood supply; an index less than 1.0 indicates insufficient blood flow to the distal regions for healing to occur (see Box 12.14, which includes acceptable values for compression therapy). ABIs can be higher than 1.0 in individuals with diabetes, as the vessels do not compress because of arterial calcification.[148]

Assessing ABI is also warranted if wounds associated with CVI do not demonstrate healing within 2 weeks of beginning wound care. An assessment of the legs should be performed frequently to observe for insufficiency (stasis) ulcers, skin changes (e.g., color, texture, loss of hair, temperature), impaired growth of nails, and discrepancy in size of extremities, including observations and measurements for edema.

In the home health setting, the client or family should be instructed to contact a member of the medical team if any edema or change in the condition of the extremity occurs. When a stasis ulcer of any size is detected, treatment is initiated. A wound care specialist (usually a physical therapist or a nurse) is a vital part of the health care team in the management of stasis ulcers. Information on specific wound care management is available elsewhere.[346]

Pulsatile débridement devices may be beneficial in the removal of loose debris. However, they should be used with caution due to suction pressure that could exacerbate venous pooling if too high or in one area for too long.

The client should be advised to avoid prolonged standing and sitting; crossing the legs; sitting too high or too deep for feet to touch the floor, causing pressure against the popliteal space; and wearing tight clothing (including girdles, elastic waistbands, or too-tight jeans) or support hose or stockings that extend above the knee, which act as a tourniquet at the popliteal fossa. Elastic stockings are recommended, but they must be worn properly to avoid bunching behind the knee or uneven compression in the popliteal fossa.

Box 12.16

**COLLAGEN VASCULAR DISEASES**

- Ankylosing spondylitis
- Dermatomyositis
- Localized (cutaneous) scleroderma
- Mixed connective tissue disease
- Polyarteritis nodosa
- Polymyalgia rheumatica
- Polymyositis
- Rheumatoid arthritis
- Sjögren syndrome
- SLE
- Systemic sclerosis (scleroderma)
- Temporal arteritis

## Vasomotor Disorders

### Raynaud Disease and Raynaud Phenomenon

***Definition and Overview.*** Intermittent episodes of small artery or arteriole constriction of the extremities causing temporary pallor and cyanosis of the digits (fingers more often than toes) and changes in skin temperature are called *Raynaud phenomenon.* These episodes occur in response to cold temperature or strong emotion, such as anxiety or excitement. When this condition is a primary vasospastic disorder, it is called (idiopathic) *Raynaud disease* or *primary Raynaud.* If the disorder is secondary to another disease or underlying cause, the term *Raynaud phenomenon* or *secondary Raynaud* is used.

*Incidence and Etiologic and Risk Factors*

Raynaud Disease. Eighty percent of persons with Raynaud disease are women between the ages of 20 and 49 years. The exact etiology of Raynaud disease remains unknown, but it appears to be caused by hypersensitivity of digital arteries to cold. Raynaud disease accounts for 65% of all people affected by this condition.[257] Risk factors include female gender, having family members with Raynaud disease, smoking, and manual occupation.[144] People with Raynaud disease experience migraine 4 times more often than people without it.[144] Raynaud disease is usually experienced as more annoying than medically serious.

Raynaud Phenomenon. Epidemiologists estimate that Raynaud phenomenon is a problem for 3% to 5% of the general population; it affects women 20 times more frequently than men, usually between the ages of 15 and 40 years.[257] Risk factors for Raynaud phenomenon are different between men and women. The Framingham Offspring Study reports that age and smoking are associated with Raynaud phenomenon in men only, whereas an association with marital status and alcohol use was observed in women only.[347] These findings suggest that different mechanisms influence the expression of Raynaud phenomenon in men and women.

Raynaud phenomenon as a condition secondary to another disease is often associated with Buerger disease or connective tissue disorders (collagen vascular diseases), such as Sjögren syndrome, scleroderma, polymyositis and dermatomyositis, mixed connective tissue disease, SLE, and rheumatoid arthritis[220] (see Box 12.16). Raynaud phenomenon can be a sign of occult (hidden) neoplasm, especially suspected when the presentation is unilateral.

Raynaud phenomenon may also occur with change in temperature, such as occurs when going from a warm outside environment to an air-conditioned room. In addition, Raynaud phenomenon may be associated with occlusive arterial diseases and neurogenic lesions, such as thoracic outlet syndrome, or with the effects of long-term exposure to cold (occupational or frostbite), trauma, or use of vibrating equipment such as jackhammers. Injuries to the small vessels of the hands may produce Raynaud phenomenon. Also, the trauma can be a result of repetitive stress that comes from using crutches for extended periods, typing on a computer keyboard, or even playing the piano.

Several medications (e.g., β-blockers, ergot alkaloids prescribed for migraine headaches, antineoplastics used in chemotherapy) have also been implicated.[220] Because nicotine causes small blood vessels to constrict, smoking can trigger attacks in persons who are predisposed to this phenomenon.

***Pathogenesis and Clinical Manifestations.*** The exact pathogenesis for Raynaud disease and Raynaud phenomenon is not known; a combination of vascular, neural, and humoral factors is implicated.[220] Although the causes differ for Raynaud disease and Raynaud phenomenon, the clinical manifestations are the same, based on a pathogenesis of arterial vasospasm in the skin.

It begins with the release of chemical messengers that cause blood vessels to constrict and remain constricted. The flow of oxygenated blood to these areas is reduced, and the skin becomes pale and cold. In the constricted vessels, the blood, which has released its oxygen to the tissues surrounding the vessels, pools in the tissues, producing a bluish or purplish color.

In the case of fibromyalgia-associated Raynaud phenomenon, symptoms may be the result of cold-induced spasms of the arteries caused by a problem in the autonomic nervous system control of the blood supply to the extremities. This could explain why the cold-induced pain is significant but without skin color changes in this population.

In most cases, the skin color progresses from blue to white to red. First, ischemia from vasospastic attacks causes cyanosis, numbness, and the sensation of cold in the digits (thumbs usually remain unaffected). The affected tissues become numb or painful, and skin temperature decreases. For unknown reasons, the flow of chemical that triggered the process eventually stops. The vessels relax, and blood flow is restored. The skin becomes white (characterized by

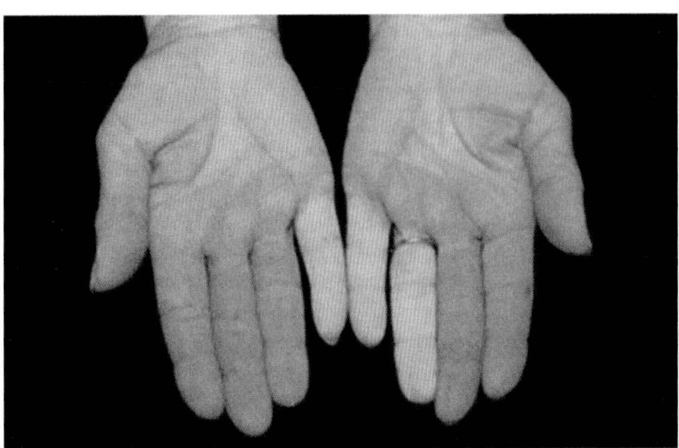

**Figure 12.37**

**Raynaud disease or phenomenon.** White color (pallor) from arteriospasm and resulting deficit in blood supply may initially involve only one or two fingers, as shown here. Cold and numbness or pain may accompany the pallor or cyanosis stage. Subsequent episodes may involve the entire finger and may include all the fingers. Toes are affected in 40% of cases. (From Jarvis C: *Physical examination and health assessment*, ed 4, Philadelphia, 2004, WB Saunders.)

pallor) and then red (characterized by rubor) as the vasospasm subsides and the capillaries become engorged with oxygenated blood. Oxygen-rich blood returns to the area, and as it does so, the skin becomes warm and flushed. The person may experience throbbing, paresthesia, and slight swelling as the blood flow is reestablished.

Sensory changes, such as numbness, stiffness, diminished sensation, and aching pain, often accompany vasomotor manifestations. Initially, no abnormal findings are present between attacks, but over time, frequent, prolonged episodes of vasospasm cause ischemia to interfere with cellular metabolism, causing the skin of the fingertips to thicken and the fingernails to become brittle.

In severe, chronic Raynaud phenomenon, the underlying condition may produce scars in the vessels, reducing the vessel diameter and therefore blood flow. When attacks occur, they are often more severe, resulting in prolonged loss of blood to fingers and toes, which can produce painful skin ulcers; and rarely, gangrene may develop. Episodes of Raynaud disease are often bilateral, progressing distally to proximally along the digits. Raynaud phenomenon may be unilateral, involving only one or two fingers, but this clinical presentation warrants a physician's differential diagnosis, as it can be associated with cancer (Fig. 12.37).

## MEDICAL MANAGEMENT

**DIAGNOSIS AND PROGNOSIS.** Diagnosis is usually made by clinical presentation and past medical history. If possible, evaluation during an attack can assist with diagnosis. Raynaud disease is diagnosed by a history of symptoms for at least 2 years with no progression and no evidence of underlying cause. Raynaud disease must be differentiated from the numerous possible disorders associated with Raynaud phenomenon. Untreated and uncontrolled Raynaud may damage or destroy the affected digits. Rarely, necrosis, ulceration, and gangrene result. Even with intervention, the person with Raynaud disease or phenomenon may experience disability and loss of function.

**PREVENTION AND TREATMENT.** Treatment for *Raynaud disease* is limited to prevention or alleviation of the vasospasm because no underlying cause or condition has bee n discovered. There continues to be research into pharmacologic agents, including topical gels and creams, for treatment of primary and secondary Raynaud, but nothing is routinely recommended at this time. Clients are encouraged to avoid stimuli that trigger attacks, such as cool or cold temperatures, changes in temperature, and emotional stress, and to eliminate use of nicotine, which has a constricting effect on blood vessels.

Physical or occupational therapy is often prescribed and should include client education about managing symptoms through protective skin care and protection from cold (see Box 12.13), stress management and relaxation techniques, whirlpool or other gentle heat modalities, and exercise. Large-movement arm circles in a windmill fashion can restore circulation in some people. The individual will have to experiment with the speed at which to move the arms. Some people benefit from slow, gentle movement, whereas others find greater success with fast rotations.

Pharmacologic intervention is pursued when conservative therapy fails. Its goal is to make attacks less frequent and severe, not to cure the underlying disease. Calcium channel blockers are an effective pharmacologic treatment of secondary Raynaud and remain first-line therapy for this condition.[220] Other medications used are alpha-adrenergic blockers, prostaglandins, and endothelin inhibitors.[220] The medications may improve circulation by dilating blood vessels and reducing blood cell clumping. Pharmacologic management may also include non-addictive analgesics for pain. Therapists can be instrumental in teaching physiologic modulation starting with hand warming.

When conservative care fails to relieve symptoms and the condition progresses clinically, sympathetic blocks followed by intensive therapy may also be helpful. Sympathectomy may be necessary for persons who only temporarily benefit from the sympathetic blocks.

Treatment for Raynaud phenomenon consists of appropriate treatment for the underlying condition or removing the stimulus causing vasospasm. The clinical care described for Raynaud disease may also be of benefit.

**SPECIAL IMPLICATIONS FOR THE THERAPIST 12.22**

### *Vasomotor Disorders*

**Raynaud Disease and Phenomenon**

Prevention of episodes of Raynaud is important. The affected individual must be encouraged to keep warm, avoid air conditioning, and dress warmly in the winter (e.g., protect the extremities as well as the head, chest, and back to maintain overall body temperature).

Aquatic therapy is often helpful in diminishing symptoms, but again, the individual must be careful when moving from place to place with extreme temperature changes (e.g., from outside winter temperatures into a warm pool area and back outside). The use of antihypertensives for Raynaud can result in postural hypotension; the physician should be notified of these findings to alter the dosage.

SPECIAL IMPLICATIONS FOR THE THERAPIST 12.23

### *Peripheral Vascular Disease*

Even though Special Implications for the Therapist boxes for each individual disease making up PVD have been presented, a brief overview or summary of PVD as a whole seems warranted and a reminder that because of the prevalence of atherosclerotic disease in anyone with PVD, heart rate and blood pressure should be monitored during the evaluative process and during initial interventions. This is especially important in those with diabetes mellitus and for anyone who has undergone an amputation, which implies severe disease.

Notably, people with PAD may exhibit precipitous rises in blood pressure during exercise owing to the atherosclerotic process present and the diminished vascular bed. Examination of the pedal pulses should be part of the physical examination for all clients older than 55 years, and measurement of the ABI is recommended for those who have diminished or nonpalpable pedal pulses but who do not have diabetes.[147]

For the client with back pain, buttock pain, or leg pain of unknown or previously undiagnosed cause, screening for medical disease, including assessment of risk factors, past medical history, and special tests and measures (e.g., bicycle test, palpation of pulses), is essential.[153]

PVD can be confusing, with the wide range of diseases affecting veins and arteries, the etiology of which is sometimes occlusive, sometimes inflammatory, and, occasionally, as in the case of Buerger disease, both occlusive and inflammatory. The basic point to keep in mind is how arterial disease differs (significantly) from venous disease in clinical presentation, pathogenesis, and management.

Focusing on the underlying etiologic factors is the key to choosing the most appropriate and effective intervention. For example, in the case of acute arterial disease, the tissues are not oxygenated, and ischemia can result in local necrosis; gangrene can develop quickly. The goal is to increase oxygen without increasing demand or need for oxygen. Claudication occurs when the activity causes increased oxygen demand in an already compromised area.

During the acute phase of arterial ischemia rehabilitation, intervention and movement are minimized, heat and massage are contraindicated, and the person is instructed in the use of positions that will increase blood flow to the tissues involved (e.g., head elevated with legs slightly lower than the heart).

Chronic arterial disease can be treated by the therapist by concentrating on improving collateral circulation and increasing vasodilation, most often through low-intensity aerobic exercise over a period of several weeks. The role of exercise in PAD (especially in reducing claudication) is well documented.[356]

In venous disorders, the tissues are oxygenated but the blood is not moving, and stasis occurs. With venous occlusion, the skin is discolored rather than pale (ranging from angry red to deep blue-purple), edema is prominent, and pain is most marked at the site of occlusion, although extreme edema can render all the skin of the limb quite tender.

The goal of therapy is to create compressive pumping forces to move fluid volume and reduce edema. For this reason, heat or cold, compression stockings, massage, and activity (e.g., ankle pumps, heel slides, quad sets, ambulation) are part of the treatment protocol.

Further guidelines for exercise in the management of PVD are outlined elsewhere.[18] Modifying cardiovascular risk factors, improving exercise duration and decreasing claudication, preventing joint contractures and muscle atrophy, preventing skin ulcerations, promoting healing of any pressure ulcers, and improving quality of life are part of the therapy plan of care.

For people with vascular ulcers, improving the arterial supply or venous return will lessen pain, increase mobility, and allow ulcers to heal. Whenever ulcers are present, understanding the type of ulcer and underlying etiology will point to the best intervention. The assessment of and therapeutic intervention for vascular wounds are beyond the scope of this text; the reader is referred to other, more appropriate texts.[346]

## Vascular Anomalies

Vascular (i.e., involving the blood vessels) anomalies include vascular tumors and vascular malformations.[187]

### Vascular Neoplasms

Vascular tumors are classified as benign, locally aggressive or borderline, or malignant.[187,248]

Benign tumors include different types of hemangiomas (infantile; congenital; spindle cell; epithelioid). Locally aggressive or borderline tumors include some hemangioendotheliomas (kaposiform; retiform; composite) and Kaposi sarcoma. Malignant tumors include angiosarcoma and epithelioid hemangioendothelioma.

Infantile hemangioma is the most common vascular lesion observed in children. It presents as a single cutaneous lobular "strawberry mark" and is visible in the first weeks of the child's life. White females have it more often than males, with the ratio 3:1. Typically, no intervention is needed and no complications develop.

Kaposiform hemangioendothelioma, in 90% of cases, is encountered in infancy. It is a locally invasive neoplasm that may be accompanied by an enlarging cutaneous/subcutaneous mass. This lesion can affect any organ or region but mainly the extremities. Treatments are directed toward the underlying lesion. Due to the infiltrative nature of the neoplasm, surgical excision of the entire lesion is rarely possible; otherwise it would be curative.

Kaposi sarcoma occurs in people with compromised immune system, including people with AIDS or transplant patients who are on immunosuppressants to avoid tissue/organ rejection. It is caused by the Kaposi sarcoma–associated herpesvirus. Some lesions resemble a simple hemangioma with tightly packed clusters of capillaries, most often visible on the skin. They are not usually a cause of death. However, if the lesions spread to other parts of the body (digestive tract, lungs), they may cause detrimental effects, such as bleeding and organ dysfunction.

Malignant vascular neoplasms are extremely rare and represent only 2% of all vascular neoplasms.[248] *Angiosarcoma* can occur in either gender and at any age, most commonly appearing as small, painless, red nodules on the skin, soft tissue, breast, bone, liver, and spleen. A quarter of patients present with tumor rupture, and more than half of people with angiosarcoma have metastases at diagnosis. Those with no metastases at diagnosis have 25% to 30% survival chance after 5 years.[248]

### Vascular Malformations

Vascular malformations are lesions arising during vascular development due to congenital errors.[248] The cells do not properly proliferate but undergo increased turnover. The lesion grows commensurate with the patient. The growth rate is stimulated by hormones (puberty, pregnancy), hemorrhage, or infection.

Vascular malformations are classified as simple, combined, those of major named vessels, and those associated with other anomalies.[187,248]

Simple vascular malformations are capillary, lymphatic, venous, and arteriovenous malformations (AVM), and arteriovenous fistula.

A combination of a few different simple malformations in one person constitutes a combined vascular malformations. Combinations of all types of simple malformations can also occur. The combined lesions typically extend throughout a limb and parts of the trunk and/or head/neck. Long-term pain and functional issues are present in patients with such lesions.

Major vessels can be affected in many aspects, including alternate origin, length, diameter (focal stenosis; aneurysm), valves, and communication. Examples of such abnormalities include partial or complete congenital absence of the portal vein, carotid artery anomalies, and sciatic vein persistence.

**Arteriovenous Malformations.** AVMs are congenital vascular malformations. They may occur in any blood vessel, but the most common sites include the brain, lungs, GI tract, and skin. AVMs are the result of localized maldevelopment of part of the primitive vascular plexus consisting of abnormal arteriovenous communications without intervening capillaries. There is a central tangled mass of fragile, abnormal blood vessels called the *nidus* that shunts blood from cerebral feeding arteries directly into cerebral veins. The loss of the normal capillary network between the high-pressure arterial system and the low-pressure venous system results in a faster flow and elevated pressure within the delicate vessels of the AVM. The lack of a gradient pressure system predisposes the lesion to rupture.

AVMs vary in size, ranging from massive lesions that are fed by multiple vessels to lesions too small to identify. Perfusion to adjacent brain tissue may be impaired because blood flow is diverted to the AVM, a phenomenon referred to as *vascular stealing*. Approximately 10% of cases present with aneurysms. Small AVMs are more likely to bleed than large ones, and once bleeding occurs, repeated episodes are likely.

Clinical presentation depends on the location of the malformation and may relate to hemorrhage from the malformation or an associated aneurysm or to cerebral ischemia caused by diversion or stasis of blood. Seizures, migraine-like headaches unresponsive to standard therapy, and progressive neurologic deficits may develop.

Diagnostic testing and planned intervention rely on cerebral angiography to show the AVM size, location, feeding vessels, nidus, and venous outflow vessels. Other tests may include MRI, x-rays, ultrasound, electroencephalography, and arteriography. The most common treatment for brain AVM is surgery. Surgical resection (removal), endovascular embolization (injection of a small particle—an embolizing agent—to block the artery and reduce blood flow into the AVM), and stereotactic radiosurgery (delivery of extremely precise doses of radiation to destroy abnormal blood vessels) are available options. Treatment options are individualized depending on the size and location of the lesion, as well as any other surgical risks present.

SPECIAL IMPLICATIONS FOR THE THERAPIST 12.24

*Arteriovenous Malformations*

Generally, the individual with a known AVM is advised to avoid activities and exercise that can increase intracranial or blood pressure (see Box 16.1). Weight training and contact sports are contraindicated, and some physicians advise against highly aerobic exercise, including running.

Postoperative complications can include hemorrhage, seizures, nausea, vomiting, or headache, and symptomatic perilesional edema can occur up to 1 year after the procedure. Neurologic deficits vary but are usually transient; radiation-induced brain injury is rare. The radiation's effect begins immediately, but complete obliteration of the lesion can take up to 3 years, during which time the affected individual must continue to maintain a normal blood pressure.

## OTHER CARDIAC CONSIDERATIONS

Despite the success of new immunosuppressive regimens and better results with transplantation, few people who are dying of HF will actually have the opportunity to receive a heart transplant. The mechanical technology may eventually allow selected persons to receive long-term (permanent) support as a substitute for cardiac transplantation (left ventricular assist devices [LVAD]). Use of LVAD can act as a bridge to transplant or as the permanent intervention. It can decrease mortality and improve quality of life for those with HF.[234]

Research is still exploring tissue engineering to replace transplantation, but tissue engineering is not available yet. Mechanical devices (e.g., artificial heart, implanted cardiac assistive devices or other bridges to transplantation) are used to help keep people alive while they await heart transplant or as a replacement intervention for transplantation.

### The Cardiac Client and Surgery

Postsurgical complications following cardiac surgery can include myocardial injury, blood loss, superficial incisional infections, AF, pneumonia, cognitive impairments, brachial plexus injuries, and subxiphoid incisional hernias. Complications associated with a cardiopulmonary bypass machine can include AF, altered cognition, and/or memory associated with systemic inflammation, cerebral hypoperfusion, atheromatous debris, and microemboli (e.g., platelet aggregates, red blood cell fragments, air bubbles).[70]

Persons with previously diagnosed cardiac disease undergoing general or orthopedic surgery are at risk for additional postoperative complications. Anesthesia and surgery are often associated with marked fluctuations of heart rate and blood pressure, changes in intravascular volume, myocardial ischemia or depression, arrhythmias, decreased oxygenation, and increased sympathetic nervous system activity. In addition, changes in medications, surgical trauma, wound healing, infection, hemorrhage, and pulmonary insufficiency may overwhelm the already compromised heart. All these factors place an additional stress on the cardiac client during the perioperative period regardless of the type of surgery being performed.

Cardiac surgery via traditional median sternotomy requires a longitudinal incision and disruption of the sternum. During the operative procedure, the bone is rewired with stainless steel wire.

Complications following a sternotomy include mediastinitis, sternal dehiscence (separation), poor wound healing, chronic pain, posttraumatic stress disorder, and, more rarely, brachial plexus injury. Risk factors for these complications may include obesity, osteoporosis, diabetes or other comorbidities, large breasts in women (the weight of both breasts puts additional traction on sutures), and client noncompliance or poor compliance.

Less invasive means of performing cardiac surgery are now possible with advances in technology, especially videoscopic visualization and the ability to provide myocardial protection. More and more surgeons are using minimally invasive techniques such as a partial upper sternotomy or small right thoracotomy instead of the traditional median sternotomy in hopes of reducing operative stress, postoperative pain, and postoperative recovery time.

A minithoracotomy or "keyhole" thoracotomy via a small incision allows surgeons to operate on a beating heart. These alternative surgical techniques involve passing instruments through small incisions in the skin and muscle and between the ribs. Surgeons can suture bypass vessels around blocked coronary arteries without shutting down the heart and rerouting the blood through a bypass machine.

**SPECIAL IMPLICATIONS FOR THE THERAPIST 12.25**

## *The Cardiac Client and Surgery*

### Noncardiac Surgery

Therapy for people with CVD undergoing noncardiac (orthopedic, neurologic) surgery is altered only by the need for more deliberate and careful monitoring of the person's response to activity and exercise. Comprehensive guidelines for perioperative and postoperative care for such patients are available.[13]

Postoperative rehabilitation may take longer because of the underlying cardiac condition and any complications that may arise as a result of cardiovascular compromise. Evaluation for postsurgical arrhythmias is an important part of the early postoperative care. Careful observation for DVT must be ongoing during the first 1 to 3 weeks postoperatively. Anyone with polycythemia or thrombocytopenia is at increased risk for hemorrhage, necessitating additional special precautions.

Physical therapy initiated in the intensive care unit focuses on restoring mobility, increasing strength, and improving balance and reflexes. Active motion exercises of upper and lower extremities; upright positioning and sitting tolerance; and bedside standing and ambulation (as able) are included in the early postoperative protocol. Airway clearance techniques (formerly, chest physical therapy, pulmonary physical therapy, pulmonary hygiene) and breathing exercises are essential to prevent atelectasis (particularly left lower lobe atelectasis) and improve ventilatory ability (especially for inspiratory volumes). Airway clearance techniques are very important in the case of implantation of an artificial heart, because of the location of the device. Frequent, slow, rhythmic reaching, turning, bending, and stretching of the trunk and all extremities many times throughout the day help alleviate the surgical pain-tension cycle and facilitate pulmonary function.

### Cardiac Surgery

Individuals undergoing cardiothoracic procedures have some unique challenges to overcome. The damaged heart is subjected to the stress of paralysis and reinitiation of function when cardiopulmonary bypass is part of the procedure. Trauma from the cardiac event, combined with trauma from the cardiac surgery, alters the heart's ability to resume a normal working load immediately after surgery. Physical activity must be titrated or applied in a dosing fashion to load the heart according to each individual's hemostatic status and tolerance. Exercise intensity and duration should be progressed over several weeks and months.

Progressive ambulation can be initiated as soon as the client can transfer out of bed. In the case of open heart surgery, sternal precautions should follow the Move in the Tube guidelines (see Fig. 12.15).

When the client can ambulate 1,000 feet, the treadmill (1 mile/hr) or exercise cycle (0.5 rate of perceived exertion) can be used (see Table 12.13), usually around the fourth postoperative day if there are no complications. Whether to use the treadmill or bicycle is generally an individual decision made by the client based on personal preference. Presence of orthopedic problems must be taken into consideration as well.

Chest (and in women, breast) discomfort, shortness of breath, upper quadrant myalgia (chest, arms, neck, upper back), palpitations, a pulling sensation in the upper chest, low activity tolerance, mood swings, and localized swelling in the case of grafts taken from the leg are all commonly reported in the early days and weeks after cardiac surgery. These clinical manifestations are minimized but not completely eliminated with the less invasive keyhole (minithoracotomy) surgery performed in some facilities.

### Exercise

The use of lower-extremity–derived aerobic exercise to improve hemodynamics, normalize heart rate, improve oxygen uptake and delivery, and decrease diastolic blood pressure has been well documented and was discussed earlier in this chapter. Many of the individuals undergoing surgery have not exercised in years and demonstrate balance deficits, deconditioning, significant endurance limits (fatigue), and/or are fearful of exercise. Those who walk into their scheduled surgery may not have endurance limits from longstanding disease, so exercise and physical activity recommendations are less limited.

The therapist must firmly encourage active participation in a program of physical activity and exercise for anyone who has given up and chosen to remain sedentary. Exercise tolerance must be monitored closely during the early weeks after surgery. This should be accomplished by measuring vital signs, ECG, and client perceived exertion. Regular exercise sessions at least three times per week for at least 40 to 60 min in total duration are advised until a moderate to somewhat hard level of exertion is reached (e.g., 12–14 on the Rate of Perceived Exertion scale or 4 out of 10 on the modified Borg scale). For all cardiac patients, the therapist is encouraged to use perceived exertion scales, such as the dyspnea index or Borg Scale (see Table 12.13), monitor changes in diastolic pressure, and rely on measurements of oxygen uptake to set exercise limits.

In the case of median sternotomy, altered pulmonary function and movement impairments of the chest and abdomen may be present. Posture is important, especially for anyone with a kyphotic posture for any reason. Optimizing capacity and increasing activity intensity depends on an upright posture to enhance rib mobility, chest movement, and lung expansion.

### Psychosocial Considerations

Psychologic and emotional recovery from cardiac surgery is not always addressed or discussed. Recent research has documented that cardiac surgery is often accompanied by significant cognitive decline, especially memory loss (verbal and visual) and decline in task planning ability (visuoconstruction) and psychomotor speed. This has been shown to be at least slightly greater in people who are "on" bypass pump during CABG surgery as opposed to those whose surgeries are performed "off" pump.[296]

There is no definitive answer as to whether the observed cognitive decline is related to the surgery itself (e.g., effects of anesthesia, hypoperfusion associated with use of the heart-lung bypass machine, disruption of atherosclerotic plaque-forming emboli), normal aging in a population with cardiovascular risk factors, or a combination of these and other factors.[321] However, there is evidence that people who are of older age, female, or with high postoperative creatinine levels are more at risk for developing cognitive impairments after cardiac surgery.[162]

Depression is commonly reported after CABG and after cardiac surgery in general. However, the majority of people who are depressed after cardiac surgery were most likely depressed before surgery. There does not appear to be any correlation between depressed mood and cognitive decline after cardiac surgery, which suggests that depression alone cannot account for the cognitive decline.

Because cardiac surgery is increasingly performed in older adults with more comorbidities, identifying people at risk for adverse neurocognitive outcomes is helpful in protecting them by modifying the surgical procedure or by more effective medical therapy.[321]

## Circulatory Shock

Circulatory shock (often referred to as shock) is acute, severe circulatory failure leading to underperfusion of peripheral tissues. Shock may develop due to a variety of precipitating conditions. Regardless of the cause, shock is associated with marked reduction of blood flow to vital organs, eventually leading to cell damage, due to lack of oxygen for energy production, and death. See Table 14.1 for categories and causes of shock.

The therapist may see a client in one of three stages of shock. *Stage 1*, compensated hypotension, is characterized by reduced cardiac output that stimulates compensatory mechanisms that alter myocardial function and peripheral resistance. During this stage, the body tries to maintain circulation to vital organs such as the brain and the heart, and clinical symptoms are minimal. Blood pressure may remain normotensive.

In *stage 2*, compensatory mechanisms for dealing with the low delivery of oxygen and nutrients to the body are overwhelmed, and tissue perfusion is decreased. Early signs of cerebral, renal, and myocardial insufficiency are present. Cardiogenic shock (a type of shock due to inadequate cardiac function) may result from disorders of the heart muscle, valves, or electrical pacing system. Shock associated with MI or other serious cardiac disease carries a high mortality rate.[219] The therapist is only likely to see this type of client in a coronary care unit setting.

*Stage 3* is characterized by severe ischemia with damage to organs. The kidneys, liver, and lungs are especially susceptible; ischemia of the GI tract allows ulcerations and invasion by bacteria with subsequent infection.

Clinical manifestations of shock may include (in *early* stages) tachycardia, increased respiratory rate, and distended neck veins. In early septic shock (vascular shock caused by infection), there is hyperdynamic change with increased circulation, so that the skin is warm and flushed and the pulse is bounding rather than weak.

In the second phase of shock (*late* shock), hypoperfusion (reduced blood flow) occurs, with cold skin and weak pulses, hypotension (systolic blood pressure of 90 mm Hg or less), mottled extremities, with weak or absent peripheral pulses, and collapsed neck veins. This phase is usually irreversible; the client is unresponsive, and cardiovascular collapse eventually occurs. The therapist should be aware that some healthy adults may have blood pressure levels this low without ill effects or with only minor symptoms of orthostatic hypotension when changing positions quickly.

Treatment is directed toward both the manifestations of shock and its cause.

**SPECIAL IMPLICATIONS FOR THE THERAPIST 12.26**

### *Circulatory Shock*

The therapist in an acute care or home health setting may be working with a client who is demonstrating signs and symptoms of impending shock. Careful monitoring of vital signs and clinical observations will alert the therapist to the need for medical intervention. The client in question may demonstrate normal mental status or may become restless, agitated, and confused. Medical care at the earliest possible sign of shock is the best chance for client survival.

For the acute care therapist, people hospitalized with shock are critically ill and are usually unresponsive. Cardiopulmonary and musculoskeletal function as well as prevention of further complications will be the focus of the therapist. Treatment for the immobile person in shock, which is directed toward positioning, skin care, and pulmonary function, must be short in duration but effective to avoid fatiguing the person.

## The Cardiac Client and Pregnancy

Normal physiologic changes during pregnancy can exacerbate symptoms of underlying cardiac disease, even in previously asymptomatic individuals. The most common cardiovascular complications of pregnancy are peripartum cardiomyopathy, valvular dysfunction, aortic dissection, and pregnancy-related hypertension.

Peripartum cardiomyopathy or cardiomyopathy of pregnancy is discussed briefly earlier in the chapter. Pregnancy predisposes to aortic dissection, possibly because of the accompanying connective tissue changes. Dissection usually occurs near term or shortly postpartum in the arteries (including coronary arteries) or the aorta, and special implications are the same as for aneurysm.

## The Heart in Collagen Vascular Diseases

Collagen vascular diseases, or connective tissue diseases (Box 12.16), is a group of disorders affecting connective tissue, of which collagen is an essential component. Some of these disorders are autoimmune diseases (when the body's immune system produces antibody against its own connective tissue components), and some are hereditary, with mutations occurring in genes coding for collagen or other connective tissue proteins. Collagen vascular diseases often involve the heart, although cardiac symptoms are usually less prominent than other manifestations of the disease.

### Systemic Lupus Erythematosus

SLE is a multisystem clinical illness characterized by an inflammatory process that can target all parts of the heart, including the coronary arteries, pericardium, myocardium, endocardium, conducting system, and valves. Lupus cardiac involvement (lupus carditis) may include pericarditis, myocarditis, endocarditis, or a combination of the three. Cardiac disease can occur as a direct result of the autoimmune process responsible for SLE or secondary to hypertension, renal failure, hypercholesterolemia (excess serum cholesterol), drug therapy for SLE, and, more rarely, infection (infective carditis).

*Pericarditis* is the most frequent cardiac lesion associated with SLE, presenting with the characteristic substernal chest pain that varies with posture, becoming worse in recumbency and improving with sitting or bending forward. In some people, pericarditis may be the first manifestation of SLE.

*Myocarditis* is a serious complication reported to occur in less than 10% of people with SLE; although the simultaneous involvement of cardiac and skeletal muscle may occur more commonly than previously suspected. More sensitive diagnostic techniques now make early detection of occult myocarditis possible. Myocarditis in association with SLE occurs most often as left ventricular dysfunction and conduction abnormalities with varying degrees of heart block.

Lupus *endocarditis* occurs in up to 30% of persons affected by SLE. Major lesions associated with lupus endocarditis include the formation of multiple noninfectious wart-like elevations (verrucae) around or on the surface of the cardiac valves, most commonly the mitral and tricuspid valves.

Other types of valvular disease associated with SLE include mitral and aortic regurgitation or stenosis.

### Rheumatoid Arthritis

On rare occasions, the heart is involved as a part of rheumatoid arthritis, a chronic, systemic, inflammatory disorder that can affect various organs but predominantly involves synovial tissues of joints. When the heart is affected, rheumatoid granulomatous inflammation with fibrinoid necrosis may occur in the pericardium, myocardium, or valves. Involvement of the heart in rheumatoid arthritis does not typically compromise cardiac function.

### Scleroderma

Scleroderma or systemic sclerosis is a rheumatic disease of the connective tissue characterized by hardening of the connective tissue. Involvement of the heart in persons with scleroderma is the third leading cause of death in this population behind renal disease and pulmonary complications.[343] The myocardium exhibits intimal sclerosis (hardening) of small arteries, which leads to small infarctions and patchy fibrosis. As a result, HF and arrhythmia are common. Cor pulmonale may occur secondary to interstitial fibrosis of the lungs, and hypertensive heart disease may occur as a result of renal involvement.

### Polyarteritis Nodosa

Polyarteritis refers to a condition of multiple sites of inflammatory and destructive lesions in the arterial system; the lesions consist of small masses of tissue in the form of nodes or projections (nodosum) (see previous discussion of polyarteritis nodosa in this chapter). The heart is involved in up to 75% of cases of polyarteritis nodosa. The necrotizing lesions of branches of the coronary arteries result in MI, arrhythmias, and heart block. Cardiac hypertrophy and failure secondary to renal vascular hypertension occur.

### Ankylosing Spondylitis

Ankylosing spondylitis is a chronic, progressive inflammatory disorder affecting fibrous tissue primarily in the sacroiliac joints, spine, and large peripheral joints. A characteristic aortic valve lesion develops in as many as 10% of persons with longstanding ankylosing spondylitis. The aortic valve ring is dilated, and the valve cusps are scarred and shortened. The functional consequence is aortic regurgitation (see "Aortic Regurgitation [Insufficiency]" above).

SPECIAL IMPLICATIONS FOR THE THERAPIST 12.27

### *Collagen Vascular Diseases*

Treatment of the collagen vascular diseases described must take into consideration the possibility of cardiac involvement. The physician has usually diagnosed concomitant cardiac disease, but complete health care records are not always available to the therapist. If the therapist identifies signs or symptoms of cardiac origin, the client may be able to confirm previous diagnosis of the condition. In such cases, careful monitoring may be all that is required. However, the alert therapist may be the first health care provider to identify signs or symptoms of underlying dysfunction during onset, necessitating medical referral. (See each collagen vascular disease for discussion of individual implications.)

## Cardiac Complications of Cancer and Cancer Treatment

People with cancer experience all the usual cardiac problems that occur in the general population in addition to complications of cancer and its therapy. Tumor masses can cause compression of the heart and great vessels, resulting in pericardial effusions and tamponade. Certain tumors can cause arrhythmias and may secrete mediators that are directly toxic to the heart. Pericardial effusions and tamponade can follow surgery, radiation, or chemotherapy.

Many treatments for cancer are known to be cardiotoxic. A new discipline, cardio-oncology, emerged in the field of cardiovascular medicine to provide the best cancer treatment while preserving cardiovascular health.[71,247]

Cardiac toxicity may occur following chest irradiation, especially when combined with the administration of many chemotherapeutic agents. Chest radiation for any type of cancer exposes the heart (and lungs) to varying degrees and doses of radiation. Previous mediastinal radiation and increasing cumulative doses of chemotherapy are known risk factors for the development of cardiotoxicity.[247]

Radiation exposure can cause considerable scarring within the subendocardial adipose tissue, endocardial thickening, and interstitial fibrosis.[309] Collectively, the latter three defects would make the heart less capable of expanding during systole. Pericardial effusion is the most common manifestation of radiation-induced heart disease, but other cardiac complications of radiation include coronary artery fibrosis or luminal narrowing, which can result in hypertension, angina, and MI.

Often, effects of chemotherapy are not seen until years or decades after treatment with the drug has been completed. Many other chemotherapeutic agents are cardiotoxic, but not to the extent that doxorubicin, an anthracycline antibiotic, was in the 1970s, and the effects of present chemotherapeutic agents tend to be more acute than chronic.

Cardiotoxic effects of cancer treatment are various, from left ventricular dysfunction to HF. The most common side effect of chemotherapy is left ventricular systolic dysfunction.[247] Chemotherapy agents may prompt acute and chronic HF or coronary spasm leading to angina, MI, arrhythmias, or sudden death. Other cardiac problems that may develop include acute or chronic pericarditis, blood pressure changes, ECG changes, myocardial fibrosis with a resultant restrictive cardiomyopathy, conduction disturbances, accelerated and radiation-induced CAD, and valvular dysfunction. These may occur during or shortly after treatment or within days or weeks after treatment; or they may not be apparent until months and sometimes years after completion of chemotherapy. Anthracycline effects on the heart reduce exercise tolerance.

While traditional radiation treatment and chemotherapy remain foundational therapies for many treatment protocols, targeted therapy and immunotherapy have been successfully used for many cancers. Targeted therapy is based on using drugs (small synthetic molecules) to affect specific molecules or pathways (both are targets) involved in cancer cell growth and spreading, leading to inhibiting or stopping cancer cell progression. Immunotherapy is a type of biologic therapy that helps the body's immune system to kill cancer cells directly (by equipping T cells against a specific tumor), or boosts the immune system (using biologic response modifiers, including interferons and interleukins) to fight cancer more efficiently in general. These newer therapies have fewer adverse cardiac effects, but they may affect other body systems (GI tract, liver, skin).

A number of risk factors may predispose someone to cardiotoxicity, including total daily dose, increasing cumulative dose, schedule of administration, concurrent administration of cardiotoxic agents, prior chemotherapy, mediastinal radiation, age (younger than 18 years or older than 70 years), female gender, history of preexisting cardiovascular disorders, or other comorbidities such as obesity and diabetes.[247]

Early detection of cardiotoxicity in cancer treatment is essential, as it allows the identification of individuals who need to be protected with heart medications in order to continue the cancer treatment or to seek alternative therapies.[247] Echocardiography is recommended to assess cardiotoxicity and left ventricular function in cancer patients after chemotherapy and radiation.[386] Although clinical guidelines are available for addressing cardiotoxicity in cancer survivors,[352] further work is needed to determine optimal cancer interventions for people with CVD risk factors.

Vascular and metabolic toxicity of cancer therapy have been recognized.[71] Vascular toxicity is associated with endothelial injury and cell death, increased platelet aggregation, and induction of vascular oxidative stress. Vascular complications include coronary vasospasm, capillary leak, hypertension, venous thromboembolic disease, myocardial ischemia, and cerebrovascular events. Dysregulation of metabolism after cancer therapy may lead to cardiac and vascular sequelae. One example of metabolic complications in cancer treatment is dysregulation of glucose metabolism.

Different strategies are used to lessen the adverse effects of cancer treatments on cardiovascular health. Newer radiation techniques are available that limit the overall radiation dose and the heart exposure to radiation. Cardioprotective agents, such as dexrazoxane for anthracycline chemotherapy, have been used to mitigate the cardiotoxic effects of cancer therapy.[247]

SPECIAL IMPLICATIONS FOR THE THERAPIST 12.28

### *Cardiac Complications of Cancer Treatment*

Any client referred to therapy who has completed oncologic treatment should be assessed for potential cardiac (and pulmonary) dysfunction, including questions about previous and current activity levels, evaluation of exercise tolerance or endurance, and monitoring of heart rate and rhythm, blood pressure, and respiratory responses.

Any symptoms of exercise intolerance (shortness of breath, light-headedness or dizziness, fatigue, pallor, palpitations, chest pain or discomfort) must be noted.

Clients may be asymptomatic, with the only manifestation being ECG changes. Ideally, the oncology and cardiac team will recommend continuous cardiac monitoring with baseline and regular ECG and echocardiographic studies and measurement of serum electrolytes and cardiac enzymes for those individuals with risk factors or a history of cardiotoxicity.

Specific exercise guidelines have also been outlined for the inclusion of gradual endurance training as a part of the treatment plan for anyone with cardiotoxicity secondary to oncologic treatment.

Cardiotoxicity can be prevented by screening and modifying risk factors, aggressively monitoring for signs and symptoms as chemotherapy is administered, and continuing follow-up after completion of a course or the entire treatment.

For those clients simultaneously involved in a cardiac rehabilitation program (or physical therapy care for another pathology) and receiving care for cancer, exercise prescription should be graded to the individual's abilities and fatigue levels. The therapist should work with the client to schedule therapy sessions and home exercise around chemotherapy or radiation treatments.

## REFERENCES

To enhance this text and add value for the reader, all references are included in the enhanced ebook on Student Consult that accompanies this textbook. The reader can view the reference source and access it online whenever possible.

CHAPTER 13

# The Lymphatic System

BONNIE B. LASINSKI • JOY COHN

The lymphatic system develops embryologically from the venous system. Two major theories of the embryologic origin of the lymphatic system exist: the *centrifugal*, or venous budding, theory and the *centripetal* theory. The centrifugal theory states that the lymphatic endothelium develops from the venous endothelium; the centripetal theory states that both systems (venous and lymphatic) develop from undifferentiated (stem type) mesenchymal cells. Advances in lymphangiogenesis research may clarify which theory is correct; this information will have a great impact on genetic research and the eventual molecular treatment of lymphangiodysplasias.[191]

The interstitial fluid that is created by ultrafiltration from the blood capillary beds is taken up by the initial lymphatic vessels into larger collecting vessels, into lymphatic trunks, and back into the right side of the heart via the lymphatic ducts that empty into the right and left subclavian veins in the neck.[59,101,185] This is a one-way regional system that moves fluid from the periphery to the central circulation. It is designed to absorb macromolecules (protein and fatty acids); help maintain fluid balance in the tissues; fight infection; and assist in the removal of cellular debris and waste products from the extracellular spaces. In many ways, it functions similarly to the sanitation system of a major city. It is largely ignored and goes unnoticed until it is disrupted and the "garbage" (in the form of lymphedema) piles up. This drainage system is separate from the general circulatory system but is the conduit for returning macromolecules and interstitial fluids to the circulatory system.[59,185]

The cardiovascular system is a closed system of vessels with a pump (the heart) to move the fluid (blood) through arteries and capillaries, providing nutrition to cells, and then back to the heart via the veins. Fluid leaves the capillary bed in processes called *diffusion* and *ultrafiltration* that nourish the tissues and cells. Diffusion is free movement of fluid in both directions through the capillary walls; ultrafiltration is a primarily one-way movement of some additional fluid and molecules through the semipermeable capillary wall into the interstitial space.

The lymphatic system is responsible for carrying this capillary ultrafiltrate fluid volume as well as the escaped plasma proteins back to the blood circulation. Most protein molecules are too large to be reabsorbed through the endothelium of the blood capillaries. A small amount of protein, if broken down into smaller molecules by macrophages, can pass through the open junctions in the endothelium. However, the majority of extracellular protein must be recycled via the lymphatic system. The lymphatic system, in addition, absorbs digested fatty acids from the gut so that they can be made available to the body for metabolism.[126]

The lymphatic system is a pressure-driven system based on the principles of osmotic diuresis. If the normal lymphatic transport mechanisms are disrupted (e.g., by scar tissue, removal/damage of nodes, or reduced muscle pumping), significant accumulations of water and protein can remain in the tissue spaces, resulting in latent, acute, or chronic lymphedema. The proteins are a result of cellular metabolism and are not related to protein ingested from food.

The dynamics of fluid exchange in the tissues are controlled by the microcirculation unit consisting of the arterial and venous capillaries, the tissue channels, the proteolytic cells (macrophages) in the tissues, and the initial lymphatics (see the description of initial lymphatics in Anatomy and Physiology of the Lymphatic System later).

## MICROCIRCULATION UNIT: PRINCIPLES OF FLUID DYNAMICS AND EXCHANGE

### Starling's Hypothesis

In 1897, Starling proposed the mechanism governing fluid flow out of the blood capillaries into the tissues and back into the capillaries again. There are four pressures that are important in Starling's law: (1) *plasma hydrostatic pressure*, the pressure inside the capillaries that decreases owing to peripheral resistance as fluid passes from the arterial to the venous side of the capillary loop; (2) *tissue hydrostatic pressure*, the pressure of fluid in the tissue channels (usually negative or less than atmospheric pressure) that tends to pull fluid from the capillaries into the tissues[a]; (3) *plasma colloidal osmotic pressure,* the pressure caused by plasma proteins that creates a siphon effect and pulls fluid into the capillaries; and (4) *tissue colloidal osmotic pressure,* the pressure caused by plasma proteins in the tissues that causes a net movement of fluid into the tissues. All of these pressure systems determine how much fluid moves and where it moves within the body.

### Fluid Dynamics

The laws of basic fluid dynamics dictate that fluid flows from an area of high pressure to an area of lower pressure until equilibrium is reached. Starling's law simplified means that fluid in the blood capillary will tend to flow into the tissue spaces because plasma (blood) hydrostatic pressure is higher than the tissue hydrostatic pressure.

When the blood reaches the venous side of the capillary, the plasma hydrostatic pressure will be lower owing to peripheral resistance, and ultrafiltration will reduce to almost nothing.

In Starling's view, there was significant reabsorption on the venous side of the capillary beds because when the blood reaches the venous side of the capillary, the plasma hydrostatic pressure will be lower than the plasma colloid (protein) osmotic pressure, and the fluid will be drawn back into the venous side of the capillary by the hydrophylic nature of the blood plasma. More precise modern measurements have demonstrated that there is a dwindling ultrafiltrate across the capillary beds and that there is no reabsorption into the venous capillaries. "Tissue fluid balance thus depends critically upon lymphatic function."[126] The initial lymphatic capillaries will take up interstitial fluid (where it becomes *lymph*) and drain it to the collecting lymphatics and larger lymphatic trunks, through regional lymph nodes, and eventually into the right lymphatic duct or the thoracic duct and back into the subclavian veins (Fig. 13.1).

Lymphatic flow measured at the ducts demonstrates a volume of 1 to 4 L/day; it was assumed that this was the entire volume absorbed by the lymphatics, but it has been demonstrated that as much as one-half of the water volume absorbed by the lymphatics is removed in the lymph nodes via close connection with blood capillaries in the cortex of the nodes. The actual normal lymphatic load per day is 8 L or more.[105] With excessive ultrafiltration, edema results. In the presence of lymphatic dysfunction, fluid volume *and proteins* will remain trapped in the tissue spaces and cause lymphedema. With lymphedema, the challenge for the therapist is to effectively move that fluid and protein back into functioning lymphatics and then into the central circulation. This model is a very gross simplification, but it can be helpful in understanding the basics of fluid dynamics in the capillary loop. Many other factors affect the tissues in addition to those mentioned previously.[33,106,190]

[a]However, in edema, it can become positive and tend to keep fluid out of the tissues. This is the one "safety factor" that controls lymphedema (i.e., the fibrous tissue actually helps to increase tissue hydrostatic pressure and control the size of the limb to some extent).

## ANATOMY AND PHYSIOLOGY OF THE LYMPHATIC SYSTEM

The lymphatic system is composed of superficial and deep lymph vessels and nodes. Other lymphatic organs and tissues include the thymus, bone marrow, spleen, tonsils, and Peyer patches of the small intestine. These perform important immune functions, which are discussed in Chapter 7. The central nervous system (CNS) was thought for centuries to be devoid of lymphatic vasculature.[105] It has been demonstrated more recently[112] that there are several drainage pathways in the CNS: functional lymphatic vessels in the meninges that line the dural sinuses and drain to the cervical lymph nodes via a pathway termed *glymphatic*.[148] The glymphatic pathway is thus named because it mimics the glial and lymphatic pathways in clearing waste from the brain, ultimately draining to the cervical lymph nodes. Of great interest is that this clearance has been demonstrated to double during sleep. As in normal soft tissue outside of the CNS, the abnormal accumulation of "waste" in the form of proteins causes dysfunction. These may play an important role in neurologic conditions such as Alzheimer disease, in which the abnormal deposition of a macromolecule, amyloid beta, in the brain is a hallmark of the condition.[111]

Superficial vessels rely on an interaction of oncotic and hydrostatic pressures, muscle contraction, arterial pulsation, and gentle movement of the skin to absorb and transport lymph fluid, whereas the deeper vessels, which generally parallel the venous system, contain smooth muscle and valves and help prevent backflow. Respiratory effort also enhances flow in the trunks and ducts.[32,101]

The anatomy of the lymphatic vessel system can be compared with the vein system on the leaves and stems of trees. The smallest vessels, or veins, are at the periphery of the tissues (leaves), and the diameter of these vessels gradually increases in the stem of the leaf as the system progresses into larger and larger vessels (corresponding to deeper tissues) and continues to progress to larger stems and branches of the tree until the trunk is reached.

### Initial Lymphatics

The smallest lymphatic vessels (diameter 20 to 40 μm), called *lymphatic capillaries,* begin as blind-ended sacs of subepidermal endothelium.[32,47,59] These are referred to as the *initial lymphatics* and are in close proximity to the blood capillary loops (Fig. 13.2).

The vessel walls of these initial lymphatics are one cell thick, formed by overlapping endothelial cells with many loose junctions between cells similar to pores (Fig. 13.3). These intermittently open pores allow for movement of water and proteins into the vessel and prevent the escape of protein into the interstitium as they close with filling of the vessel.

The capillaries are connected to the surrounding tissue matrix by anchoring filaments that act as guidewires to pull the cell junctions open when the tissue pressure rises as a result of increased extracellular fluid volume (Fig. 13.4).[22,101] These vessels are arranged in a meshlike

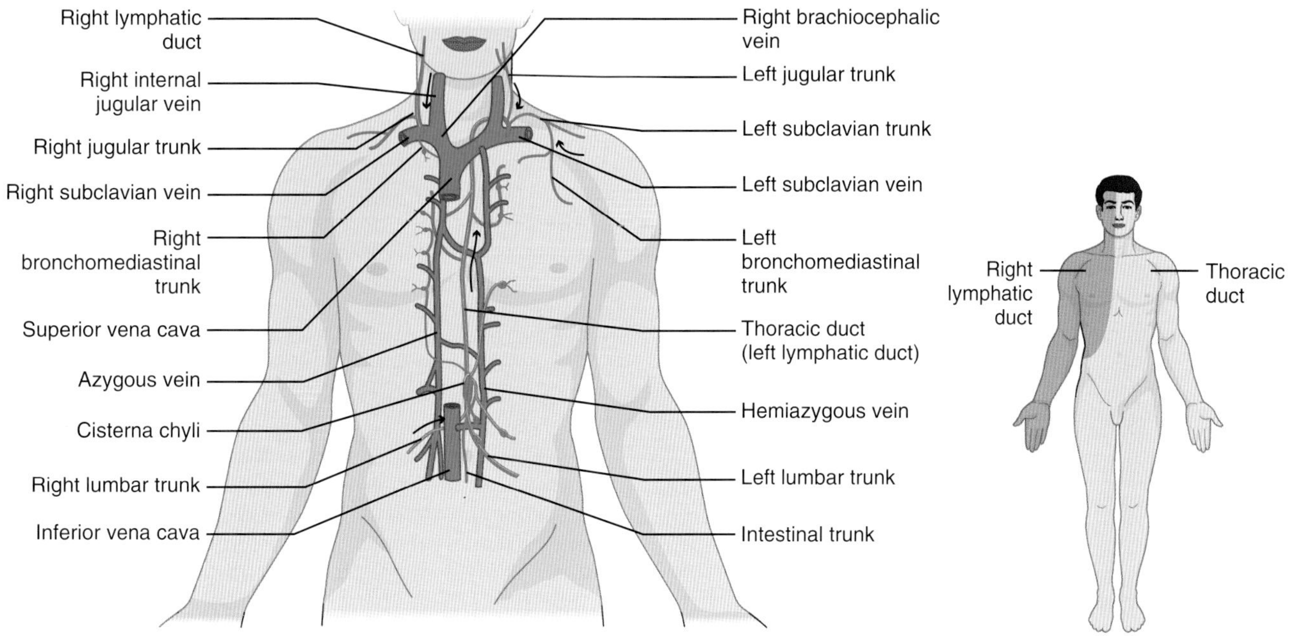


**FIGURE 13.1**

**Lymphatic ducts.** The thoracic duct *(green)* leading from the cisterna chyli to discharge into the left subclavian vein in the neck. (The blood vessels are shaded *blue*.) The right lymphatic duct is also shown (see figure on right). This carries far less lymph than the thoracic duct, draining mainly the right arm and head, the heart and lungs, and the anterior chest wall. These two main trunks sometimes are linked by large collateral lymphatics. (From Casley-Smith JR, Casley-Smith JR: *Modern treatment for lymphoedema*, ed 5, Adelaide, Australia, 1997, Lymphoedema Association of Australia. *Inset,* Jarvis C: *Physical examination and health assessment*, ed 6, Philadelphia, 2011, Saunders.)

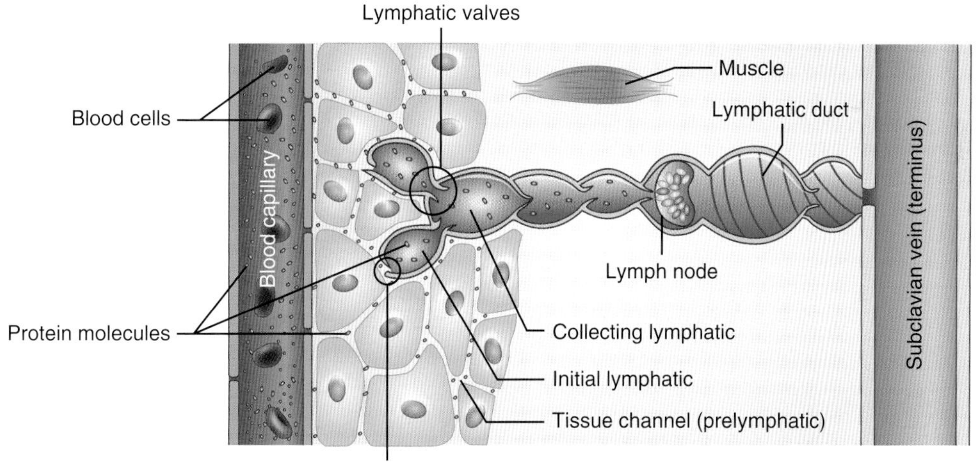


**FIGURE 13.2**

**Anatomy of the lymphatic vessel system (schematic).** This diagram shows the passage of protein *(dots)* in normal tissue from the blood capillary, through the tissue channels, into and through the lymphatic system, back to the venous system, and eventually emptying into the subclavian vein. Terminology has changed over the years; the reader should be aware that the terms *initial lymphatic* and *lymphatic capillary* refer to the same structure. Note that the protein molecules are not on the venous side of the diagram because for the most part, these molecules are too large to pass through the openings in the venous endothelium. Also note that this is a schematic diagram and not drawn to scale; the lymphatic duct depicted emptying into the venous system (subclavian vein) is much deeper (under the fascia) than this two-dimensional illustration can portray. Various malfunctions are illustrated in Fig. 13.15. (From Casley-Smith JR, Casley-Smith JR: *Modern treatment for lymphoedema*, ed 5, Adelaide, Australia, 1997, Lymphoedema Association of Australia.)

plexus; for every square millimeter of tissue, 7 mm of lymphatics are available to drain it.[32]

The initial lymphatics function as force pumps powered by variations in total tissue pressure caused by movement; muscular contraction; and variations in external pressure caused by stretch, gravity, change in position, and other similar factors. Without changes in total tissue pressure, these force pumps cannot function, and fluid will accumulate in the interstitium, leading to edema.

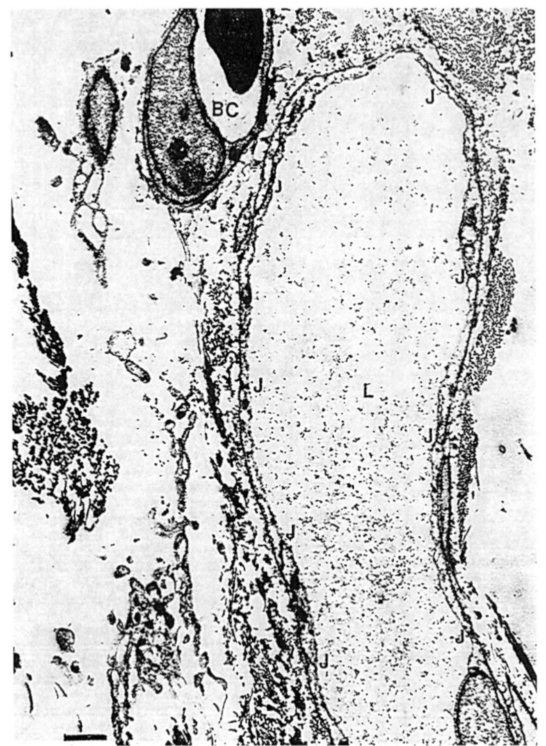


**FIGURE 13.3**

**An initial lymphatic *(L)* in a quiescent (at rest or inactive) tissue.** Many closed (narrow or tight) junctions *(J)* are evident. A blood capillary *(BC)* is shown for comparison of size, endothelial opacity, and other characteristics. The bar at the lower left (1 μm) is provided to give the viewer size perspective. (From Casley-Smith JR, Casley-Smith JR: *Modern treatment for lymphoedema*, ed 5, Adelaide, Australia, 1997, Lymphoedema Association of Australia. Modified from Casley-Smith JR: Endothelial permeability. II. The passage of particles through the lymphatic endothelium of normal and injured ears. *Br J Exp Pathol* 46:35–49, 1965.)

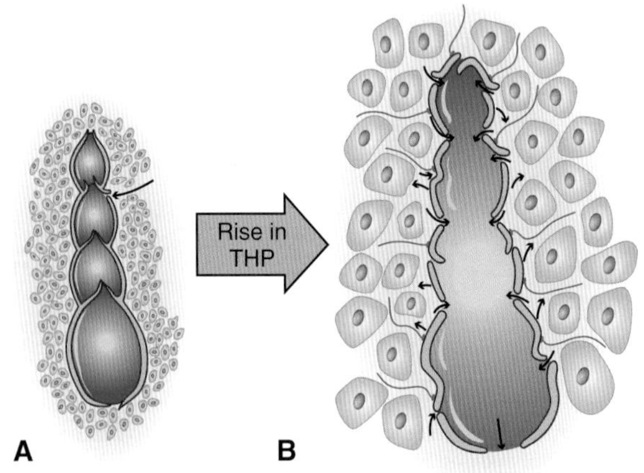


**FIGURE 13.4**

**Effects of elevated tissue hydrostatic pressure *(THP)* on initial lymphatic functioning.** (A) Normal lymphatic vessel at a fairly low THP and normal lymphatic drainage. (B) Tissue response to a tremendous increase in THP (represented by the *large arrow*). The swelling in the interstitial tissues pulls on the anchoring filaments, pulling and holding open the initial lymphatic endothelial junctions (*thin arrows* pointing outward), allowing fluid to pour into the initial lymphatic in an attempt to reduce edema. In this way, in place of a few widely open junctions, there are many slightly open ones through which fluid is forced (*thicker arrows* directed inward) down a hydrostatic pressure gradient. (From Casley-Smith JR, Casley-Smith JR: *Modern treatment for lymphoedema*, ed 5, Adelaide, Australia, 1997, Lymphoedema Association of Australia.)

## Lymph Vessel Network

Deeper in the dermis are *precollectors* (Fig. 13.5), which flow into *collecting lymphatics* located in the subcutaneous tissue (Fig. 13.6). The true collecting vessels have valves to prevent backflow and some muscle tissue in their walls to further enhance their pumping action.[32,190] Extrinsic muscle contraction, autonomic stimulation, or manual lymphatic drainage (MLD) also increases this pumping action.

Collecting lymphatics do not form a plexus, but there can be connections between them. Their diameter gradually increases in size to form the *lymph trunks,* which lie near the deep fascia. Each segment of collecting lymphatic vessel between two valves is called a *lymphangion* (Fig. 13.7). The muscle in the collecting lymphatic walls contracts rhythmically. Smooth muscle cells around the endothelial cell layer face the lumen of the vessel. These are innervated by the autonomic nervous system and contract at rest an average of 5 to 10 times per minute.[192] This lymphangiomotoricity combines with the contraction of the lymphangion itself, which is triggered by distention of the vessel wall. The greater the stretch, the greater the force of the contraction. If many lymphangions contract at once and outflow is obstructed (e.g., by scarred or irradiated lymph nodal areas), pressure inside the vessel can reach 100 mm Hg or more.

Sustained high intravascular pressure fatigues the muscle wall, leading to ineffective smooth muscle contraction and ultimately to vessel failure. The walls dilate, preventing closure of valve flaps, and a backflow of lymph distal to the site of obstruction occurs, causing lymphedema. This is one plausible explanation for the fact that many individuals with a limb at risk develop lymphedema months or even years after their original surgery. For a time, the remaining lymphatics function marginally without evidence of clinical lymphedema, but these units become overtaxed, eventually the walls fatigue, and latent lymphedema progresses to acute and then to chronic lymphedema.

The lymph trunks in the extremities join into the larger lymph vessels of the trunk, which join to form the *thoracic duct* and the *right lymphatic duct* that pump the lymph into the central circulation at the left and right subclavian veins in the root of the neck. The deep lymphatic vessels are embedded in fatty tissue and accompany the chains of lymph nodes along the blood vessels.[47] This explains why injury to blood vessels in an area also implies injury to lymphatic vessels in that area, regardless of whether it is unexpected or controlled trauma, as in surgery.

As lymph flows from the periphery to the root of the limbs and on to the central circulation, it passes through many *lymph nodes,* which act as filters to cleanse the lymph of waste products and cellular debris. Vessels distal to nodes are called *afferent lymph vessels.* Vessels leaving lymph nodes for more proximal points are called *efferent lymph vessels.*

Lymph nodes also adjust the fluid concentration[105]; produce lymphocytes and macrophages, which are critical for immune function; destroy foreign bacteria, harmful viruses, and cancer cells; and filter waste products. Lymph nodes offer 100 times the normal resistance to flow of lymph within the lymphatic vessels themselves,

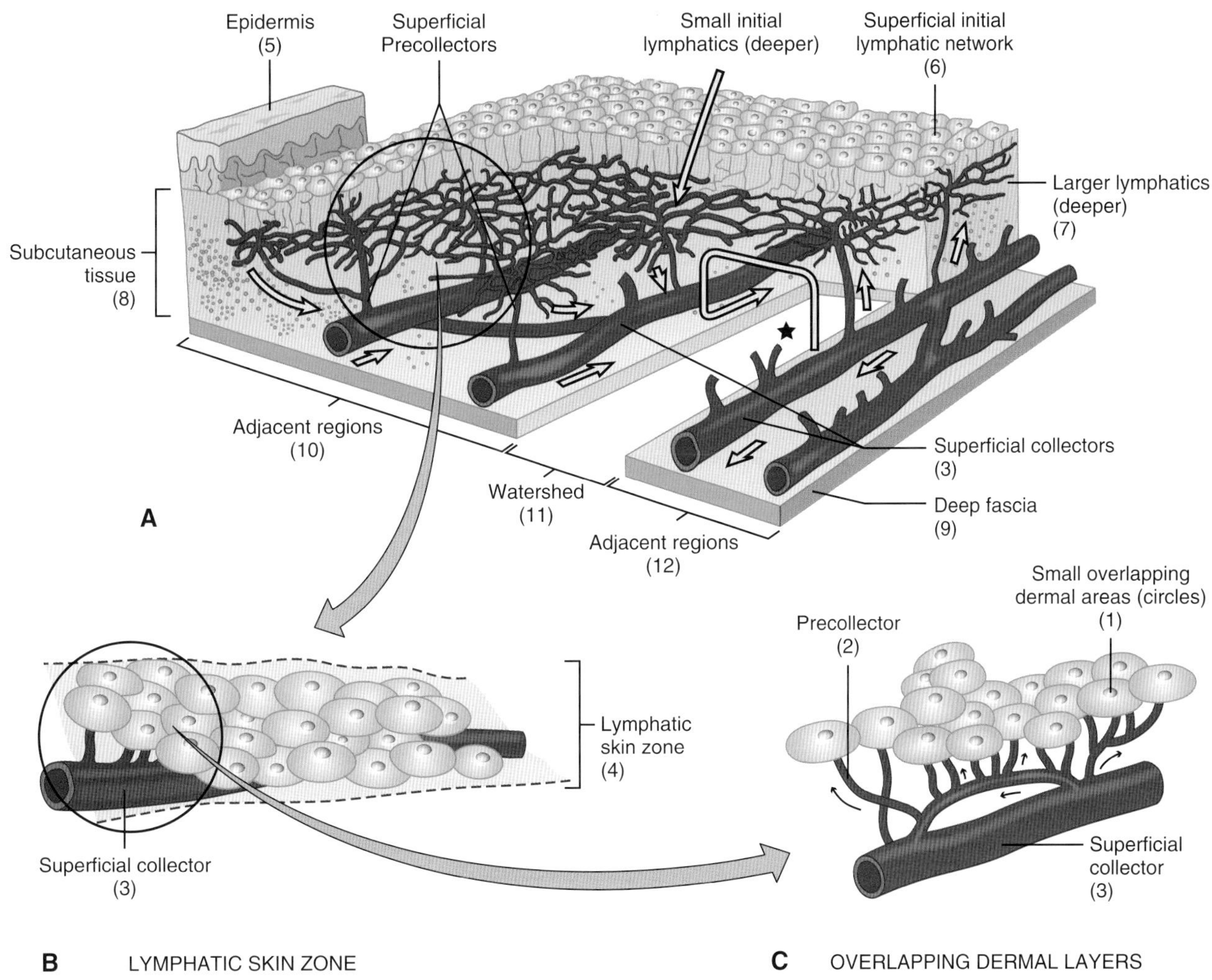


**FIGURE 13.5**

**Overview of the lymphatic drainage system.** (A) Overview of the lymphatic drainage paths from a skin region. The epidermis *(5)* is superficial to a superficial initial lymphatic network *(6)*, which sends blindly ending vessels into the dermis and which is linked to the deep dermal plexus of larger initial lymphatics *(7)* in the subcutaneous tissue *(8)* by many connections. The superficial collecting lymphatics *(3)*, which discharge into the larger ones (not shown), lie next to the deep fascia *(9)*. A watershed *(11)* lies between two adjacent regions (*10* and *12*), which drain in opposite directions *(medium arrows)*. One of these is obstructed *(red vessels)*. The deep and superficial initial lymphatic plexus overlap across this watershed. These groups of cross-connections provide collateral drainage and are enlarged by manual massage. The large *U-shaped arrow (star)* shows this path. (B) Lymphatic skin zone *(4)* that extends along the length of a superficial collector *(3)*. Certain areas of the skin drain into a specific superficial collector, which accounts for the clinical observation of lymphedema in portions of an extremity (e.g., pockets of extra swelling or asymmetric edema). When a specific superficial collector is blocked (or if the deep collector into which it drains is blocked), the result is edema at that site. (C) Small overlapping dermal areas *(1, circles)* drain into networks of initial lymphatics (not shown), which drain into small collecting lymphatics called precollectors *(2)* and then to larger superficial collectors *(3)*. (From Casley-Smith JR, Casley-Smith JR: *Modern treatment for lymphoedema*, ed 5, Adelaide, Australia, 1997, Lymphoedema Association of Australia. Modified from Földi M, Kubik S: *Lehrbuch der lymphologie fur mediziner und physiotherapeuter mit anhang: praktische linweise fur die physiotherape*, Stuttgart, Germany, 1989, Gustav Fischer Verlag.)

which explains why they are often the sites of obstruction in lymphatic dysfunction.[32,59,60,190]

## Lymphatic Territories and Watersheds

The anatomy of the lymphatic system is regional. The superficial body is divided into a series of lymph drainage areas called *territories*, which are bordered and separated by so-called watershed areas. Within a territory, smaller divisions called lymphotomes designate areas specific to certain of the regional nodes. The watershed boundaries are characterized by sparse collateral flow to adjacent territories,[14,59,101] but connections exist between these territories in the superficial and deep plexus and via collateral lymphatics between deep collectors in adjacent territories located just above the deep fascia. Under normal conditions, the lymph drains in opposite directions on either side of these watersheds to the adjacent regional nodes (Fig. 13.8).

### Trunk Quadrants

The trunk can be divided into four quadrants: the left and right axillary territories and the right and left inguinal territories. Each set of regional nodes (axillary or inguinal) drains the truncal quadrant (anterior and posterior portions) as well as the limb where the nodes are located.

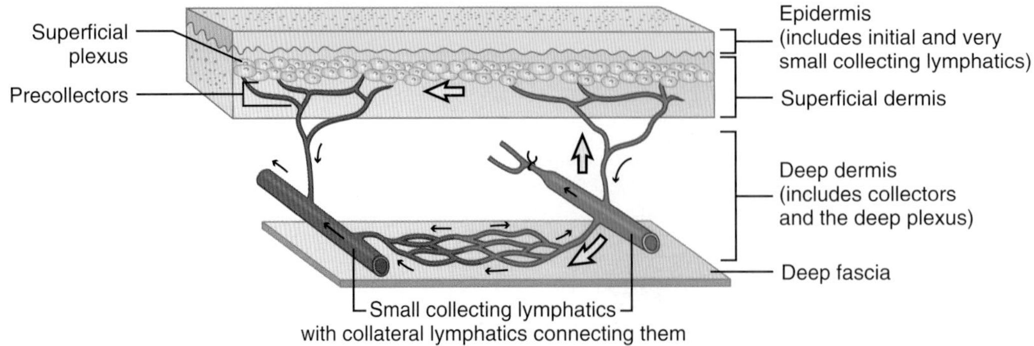


**FIGURE 13.6**

**Lymphatic vessel network.** Lymphatics traverse through the superficial dermal layer to the deeper dermis and deep fascia via lymphatic vessels that increase in size as they go deeper into the tissues. Two layers of lymphatic plexus are in the skin: superficial and deep. The dermis (layer just below the epidermis, formerly called the corium) contains blood and lymphatic vessels, nerves and nerve endings, glands, and hair follicles. Lymphatic vessels in the dermal layer can divert fluid from a blocked area and drain it into a normally functioning area or areas. In this illustration, one of the two larger collectors (right) is blocked; note the watershed between the blocked and the open collecting lymphatic. The lymph that would normally be transported along this blocked collector instead passes up into the superficial plexus and down into the deeper plexus formed by collaterals in the watershed area located just above the deep fascia. In these, the lymph passes to the nonblocked collector (left) and then drains into larger lymph vessels (not shown). When edema exists, the valve flaps in the collaterals are dilated and do not meet, thereby allowing lymph to move in either direction across these vessels (i.e., across the watershed). (From Casley-Smith JR, Casley-Smith JR: *Modern treatment for lymphoedema*, ed 5, Adelaide, Australia, 1997, Lymphoedema Association of Australia. Modified from Földi M, Kubik S: *Lehrbuch der lymphologie fur mediziner und physiotherapeuter mit anhang: praktische linweise fur die physiotherape*, Stuttgart, Germany, 1989, Gustav Fischer Verlag.)

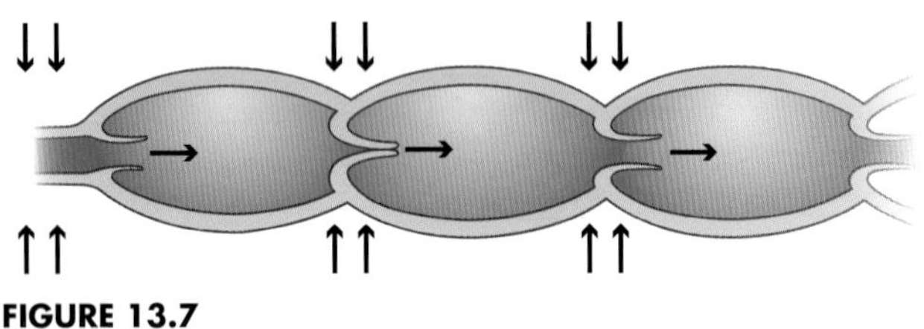

**FIGURE 13.7**

**The lymphangion.** Many lymphangions may contract at once, but sometimes only one lymphangion is triggered. The pressure exerted by each lymphangion is usually a few millimeters of mercury but can be greater than 100 mm Hg if outflow is obstructed and many units are contracting at once. Contraction is triggered by distention (i.e., greater filling creates greater force) but can be modified by humoral (including medications) and nervous factors. Pumping is greatly aided by varying total tissue pressure (e.g., from adjacent muscles, respiration, or manual lymphatic drainage), as previously mentioned in the text. (From Casley-Smith JR, Casley-Smith JR: *Modern treatment for lymphoedema*, ed 5, Adelaide, Australia, 1997, Lymphoedema Association of Australia.)

Some individuals possess an additional axillary drainage pathway from the lateral aspect of the upper arm called the *deltoid-pectoral* or *cephalic chain.* This pathway drains directly into the ipsilateral subclavian nodal area, bypassing the axilla entirely. If this pathway is present, an individual may be less likely to develop upper extremity lymphedema secondary to axillary disruption (surgical or by irradiation), as the pathway may provide sufficient residual lymph transport capacity for the upper extremity. This pathway can be disrupted by supraclavicular irradiation sometimes used to treat a wider region or for recurrent cancer of the chest wall.[102]

The left and right abdominal lymphotomes drain into the left and right superficial inguinal nodes, respectively. Each leg as well as corresponding half of the lumbar, gluteal, and genital region drains to the ipsilateral superficial inguinal nodes. From there, fluid drains into the deep inguinal, pelvic, and abdominal nodes, into the cisterna chyli, the thoracic duct, and to the left subclavian vein (see Fig. 13.1).[59] Most of the lower leg drains via the femoral trunks, which run on the anterior/medial thigh to the inguinal nodes, also draining the medial and lateral thigh lymphotomes. There is a small posterior lower leg lymphotome draining to the popliteal nodes by way of the dorsolateral trunks. Notably the collectors tend to coalesce on the medial surfaces of the arm and leg—this is most important in the lower leg, where almost all of the flow from the lower half of the leg, comes into and past the medial knee, and thus an injury to this region may have extensive consequences. A midline watershed divides the head, neck, and face areas. The right side drains to the right cervical nodes and then to the right supraclavicular nodes; the left side drains to the left cervical nodes and then to the left supraclavicular nodes. The posterior aspect of the head and neck drains into the vertebral lymphatics that drain into the supraclavicular nodes on the ipsilateral side.[32,59]

SPECIAL IMPLICATIONS FOR THE THERAPIST 13.1

## *Anatomy of the Lymphatic System*

It is important to realize that the right upper extremity and truncal quadrant drain into the right lymphatic duct and that the left upper extremity, left truncal quadrant and both lower extremities, external genital areas, and abdominal lymphotomes drain into the left subclavian vein via the thoracic duct. The superficial lymphatic drainage to regional nodes is very symmetric, but the deep lymphatic drainage is very asymmetric, with three-fourths of the total flow draining to the left subclavian vein. Lymphatic obstruction or impairment affects the trunk quadrants *and* extremities. In addition to extremity edema, individuals may develop

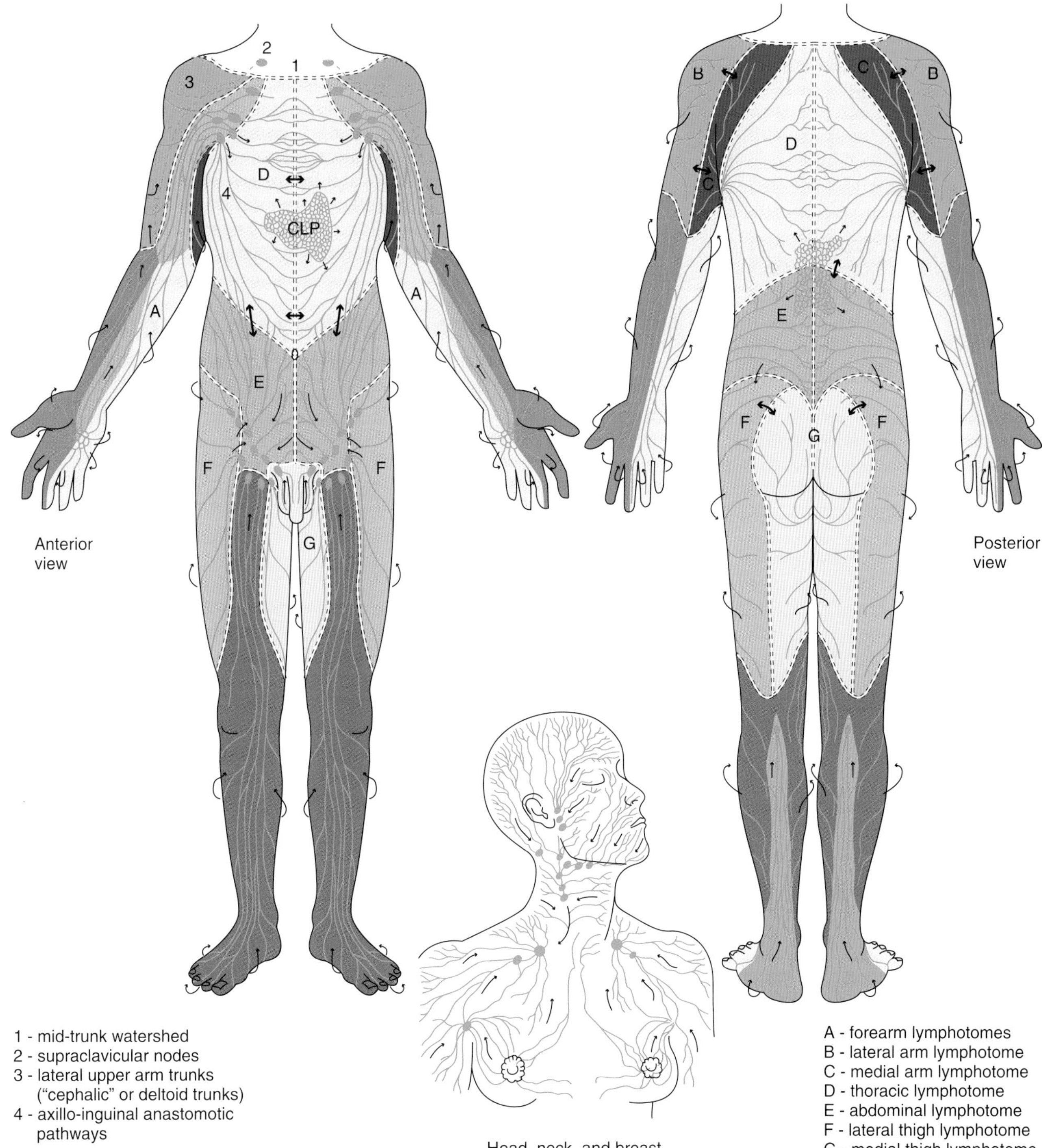


**FIGURE 13.8**

**Regional lymphatic system.** The dermal and subcutaneous lymph territories (lymphotomes are indicated by different shadings) of the lymphatic system are separated by watersheds (marked by = = = =). *Arrows* indicate the direction of the lymph flow. Normal drainage is away from the watershed, but collaterals cross the watershed *(thick double arrows)*. When the main drainage paths from each of these regions are blocked, lymph *(thick single arrows)* has to be carried across the watersheds via collaterals and plexus. The cutaneous lymphatic plexus *(CLP)* is shown in the center of the chest only. It is filled from the tissues and covers the entire body; this is not shown to avoid confusion. These initial lymphatics fill superficial collectors, which drain into deep ones and then into the lymphatic trunks *(small arrows)*. The lymphotome of the external genitals and perineum is shown but unlabeled. (From Casley-Smith JR, Casley-Smith JR: *Modern treatment for lymphoedema*, ed 5, Adelaide, Australia, 1997, Lymphoedema Association of Australia. Modified from Földi M, Kubik S: *Lehrbuch der lymphologie fur mediziner und physiotherapeuter mit anhang: praktische linweise fur die physiotherape*, Stuttgart, Germany, 1989, Gustav Fischer Verlag.)

lymphedema of the adjacent breast, lateral trunk, abdomen, genitals, suprapubic area, or buttocks depending on the affected regional nodes.

### Collateral Lymph Flow

Drainage can be redirected from one territory to another by redirecting lymph from an overloaded one toward a normal one, even across two or three intermediate overloaded areas (see Fig. 13.6). This change in flow occurs through the most superficial plexus, which then drains into the deeper (but still epifascial) collectors and deep trunks. The deep trunks also have collaterals crossing the watersheds to accomplish this flow. The dilation of the collectors and collaterals together with the superficial plexus accounts for the success of therapy, using MLD as part of the program.

Improper treatment of extremity edema without considering the impact of that treatment on the trunk quadrant adjacent to the limb or limbs involved can result in the development of truncal, breast, or genital edema, when none existed before intervention for the extremity edema.[16]

### Lymph Nodes

Normal, healthy lymph nodes are soft and nonpalpable. Palpable lymph nodes do not always indicate serious or ongoing disease, but this determination requires an evaluation by a physician. Therapists may identify suspicious palpable lumps in a client who has already been examined by a physician. However, the therapy profession offers greater opportunity for identification of suspicious nodes, given the specificity of palpatory skills and techniques practiced by a therapist. For this reason, the therapist should not hesitate to return a client to the referring or primary physician for further evaluation.

Past medical history is extremely helpful in determining the urgency of referral. A suspicious, palpable node in the presence of a previous history of cancer warrants immediate medical referral. Supraclavicular and inguinal nodes are common metastatic sites for cancer. Nodes involved with metastatic cancer are usually hard and fixed to the underlying tissue.

### Lymphadenopathy

In acute infections (lymphadenitis), nodes are tender asymmetrically, enlarged, and matted together, and the overlying skin may be red and warm (erythematous). Changes in size (>2 cm) of lymph nodes, immobile lymph nodes, and firm or hard lymph nodes in one or more areas or the presence of painless enlarged lymph nodes must be reported to the physician.[79]

In the case of recent pharyngeal or dental infections, minor, residual enlargement of cervical nodes may be observed. Intraoral infection may also cause an inflamed cervical node. The therapist may first be alerted to this condition by a spasm of the sternocleidomastoid muscle causing neck pain.

Palpation may appear to aggravate a primary spasm, as if the spasm were originating in the muscle, when in fact a lymph node under the muscle is the source of symptoms. In such cases, the past history is the key to quickly identifying the need for medical referral or follow-up care.

Lymphadenopathy in certain anatomic areas such as preauricular or postauricular (in front of or behind the ear) and especially supraclavicular or scalene regions is viewed by the medical community with greater suspicion because these areas are not usually enlarged as a result of local subclinical infections or trauma.[79] In very thin individuals, inguinal nodes may be palpable but normal, as they tend to be somewhat larger than other nodes and sit directly on the fascia at the inguinal ligament.

## INFLAMMATION AND INFECTION IN THE LYMPHATIC SYSTEM

Disorders of the lymphatic system may result from *lymphangitis* (inflammation of a lymphatic vessel), *lymphadenitis* (inflammation of one or more lymph nodes), *lymphedema* (an increased amount of lymph fluid in the soft tissues), or *lymphadenopathy* (enlargement of the lymph nodes). Lymph nodes act as defense barriers and are secondarily involved in virtually all systemic infections and in many neoplastic disorders arising in the body.

The specific node, or nodes, affected in an infectious disease depends on the location of the infection, the nature of the invading organism, and the severity of the disease. For example, infections involving the pharynx, salivary glands, and scalp often cause tender enlargement of the neck nodes, referred to as *reactive cervical lymphadenopathy. Generalized lymphadenopathy,* enlargement of two or three regionally separated lymph node groups, is usually a result of inflammation, neoplasm, or immunologic reactions.

These two types of lymphadenopathy are normal reactions to infection that result in large and tender lymph nodes, but the node is not necessarily infected (warm or reddened, as with lymphadenitis). The presence of lymphadenopathy is usually of greater significance in people older than 50 years; lymphadenopathy in people younger than age 30 is usually from benign causes, but this must be medically determined.

### Lymphedema

#### Definition

Lymphedema is a swelling of the soft tissues that results from the accumulation of protein-rich fluid in the extracellular spaces. It is often accompanied by tissue fibrosis secondary to chronic inflammation with prolonged swelling. It is caused by decreased lymphatic transport capacity and/or excessive lymphatic load and is most commonly seen in the extremities but can occur in the head, neck, abdomen, and genitalia.

#### Classification of Lymphedema

Lymphedema is divided into two broad categories: primary (idiopathic) and secondary (acquired) lymphedema. In the past, primary lymphedema was classified as connatal if it appeared at birth, praecox if it appeared at puberty, or tarda if it developed after age 35 years.

Box 13.1

**STAGES OF LYMPHEDEMA**

***Stage 0 (Latent Lymphedema)***

- Lymph transport capacity is reduced; no clinical edema is present
- Symptomatic complaints possible: achiness, heaviness, unusual sensations

***Stage I***

- Accumulation of protein-rich, pitting edema
- Reversible with elevation; area affected may be normal size on waking in the morning
- Increases with activity, heat, and humidity

***Stage II***

- Accumulation of protein-rich, nonpitting edema with connective scar tissue
- Irreversible; does not resolve overnight; increasingly more difficult to pit
- Clinical fibrosis is present
- Skin changes present in severe stage II

***Stage III (Lymphostatic Elephantiasis)***

- Accumulation of protein-rich edema with significant increase in connective and scar tissue
- Severe nonpitting fibrotic edema
- Atrophic changes (hardening of dermal tissue, skin folds, skin papillomas, hyperkeratosis)

The term *connatal* (present from birth) applies to most primary lymphedemas that are present at birth, rather than the term *congenital,* which implies a specific genetic abnormality. The severity of lymphedema is graded using the scale from the International Society of Lymphology: stage 0 (latent lymphedema), stage I, stage II, and lymphostatic elephantiasis (stage III) (Box 13.1).[10,84–86]

In *stage 0* (or *latent lymphedema*), lymph transport is impaired, but there is no clinical evidence of swelling. Interstitial fluid must increase more than 30% above the normal volume for swelling to be evident.[75] The interstitial tissue contains both collagen fibers and proteoglycan filaments. The amount of free fluid normally is negligible. When the tissue develops edema, small pockets and rivulets of fluid expand tremendously until one-half or more of the edema becomes free-flowing and at that point demonstrates clinical pitting.[76] Stage 0 may last months or years. Understanding the concept of latent lymphedema is critical in providing guidance to individuals at risk as well as in recognizing the early signs and symptoms of progression from stage 0 to stage I. These may include a sensation of heaviness, fatigue, achiness, or pain in the limb at risk.[5]

*Stage I lymphedema* is soft, pits on pressure, and reverses with elevation (as in sleep). In the early stages, there is a chronic inflammatory response to the excessive protein in the interstitium.[2,135] The subcutaneous tissues begin to fibrose, progressing the lymphedema from stage I to stage II. A lymphedematous limb may be stage II in the foot and ankle and stage I in the thigh.

*Stage II lymphedema* is nonpitting and does not resolve on elevation of the limb, and clinical fibrosis is present. Atrophic skin changes (such as loss of hair growth and dryness) and lymph fistulae are common in severe stage II lymphedema. Chronic inflammation and poor skin integrity with a compromised immune response can lead to recurrent bacterial and fungal infections.

The most severe, *stage III lymphedema,* is referred to as lymphostatic elephantiasis. This is characterized by severe nonpitting, fibrotic edema with hyperkeratosis, papillomas, skin folds with tissue flaps, and leaking lymph fistulae. Lymphangiomas (a form of lymphangiectasia) may also be present.

### Incidence and Risk Factors

The exact prevalence of lymphedema is unknown because many people remain undiagnosed; there is no agreement on the exact method for diagnosis or, if diagnosed, treatment or follow-up care does not occur, and the condition remains unreported.[103] Ascertaining prevalence is difficult, but it is estimated to be present in 1.33 to 1.44 persons/1000.[152]

**Primary Lymphedema.** Estimations of the prevalence of any type of primary lymphedema are that in people younger than 20 years old, 1.15/100,000 are affected.[152] Approximately 15% of primary lymphedemas are present at birth. The most common form of primary lymphedema (with onset from adolescence to midlife) accounts for 75% of primary lymphedema in a 4:1 ratio of females to males (formerly called *lymphedema praecox* or *Meige disease*). Of all primary lymphedemas, 10% to 20% appear abruptly after age 35 years (formerly called *lymphedema tarda*).[29] A small percentage of primary lymphedemas occur in association with rare genetic syndromes such as Milroy disease (appears at birth) or lymphedema-distachiasis syndrome, accounting for approximately 2% of primary lymphedemas.

**Secondary Lymphedema.** The incidence of secondary lymphedema also remains an approximate figure. Lymphatic filariasis is the number one cause of secondary lymphedema worldwide. It is a parasitic infection spread via mosquitoes and affects more than 120 million people in 80 countries throughout the tropics and subtropics of Asia, Africa, the Western Pacific, and parts of the Caribbean and South America. Currently, more than 1.3 billion people in 72 countries are at risk. Approximately 65% of persons infected live in the World Health Organization (WHO) South-East Asian Region, 30% live in the WHO African Region, and the remainder live in other tropical areas.[193] At the present time, no detailed maps are available of the geographic distribution of secondary lymphedema caused by filariasis, but distribution may be governed by climate, with an estimated 420 million people exposed to this infection in Africa in 2013.[108] The WHO estimates 700,000 people in the Americas are affected today (including 400,000 in Haiti and 100,000 in the Dominican Republic). In First World countries, the systematic eradication of mosquitoes has reduced the incidence to a negligible number.[49]

Clinical reports on the incidence of secondary lymphedema from other causes vary depending on the criteria used to define lymphedema, the measurement tool used, and the length of time individuals are followed after treatment, with an estimated 3 million new cases in the United States each year.[49]

### Incidence Associated With Cause

**Medical Procedures—Upper Extremity.** Reported incidence of lymphedema is 0% to 5% after sentinel lymph node biopsy (SLNB), 13% after axillary lymph node dissection (ALND), and 22% after surgery with irradiation.[152] In one large registry review, 75% of breast cancer–related lymphedema (BCRL) cases occurred within 1 year of surgery, with 90% of BCRL cases developing within 3 years of treatment.[134] However, the risk persists even years later. The risk of BCRL was not substantially different comparing patients with surgery alone—SLNB versus ALND (4.1% versus 3.5%) rates were similar, but the addition of radiation or radiation plus chemotherapy created a much higher risk. The BCRL rate in patients with ALND plus radiation was 9.5% at 5 years compared with 3.5% without radiation. The patients at greatest risk had multiple therapies for their cancer (>25% incidence).[134] This increase in incidence with multimodal treatment when surgery, radiation, and chemotherapy are combined has been demonstrated frequently.[28,38,128] This risk profile is linked to higher-stage disease at diagnosis, as these patients require more intensive treatment. Individuals at risk have a 50% risk of developing any stage of lymphedema by 20 years after treatment, though it should be noted that this study is based on older treatment protocols.[143]

Individuals who undergo lumpectomy receive either ALND or SLNB and radiation therapy. As mentioned previously, these treatments increase an individual's risk of developing lymphedema.

A 2017 report on considerations for clinicians managing breast cancer reported the risk of lymphedema as 3% to 8% after SLNB and 13% to 14% after ALND.[117] The risk increases to 25% to 40% with axillary surgery plus radiation. A 2015 study on the treatment of melanoma reported secondary lymphedema in 10.9% of cases that received ALND.[67]

Bevilacqua and colleagues[11] created validated nomograms to assist in predicting risk of BCRL after ALND for breast cancer. The authors collected data from a prospective cohort of 1054 women with unilateral breast cancer, defining lymphedema as a 200-mL difference between arms at 6 months or more after surgery. Risk factors included age, body mass index (BMI), ipsilateral arm chemotherapy infusions, level of ALND, location of radiation field, development of postoperative seroma, infection, and early edema.

A Cochrane review concluded that overall survival rates were similar when comparing SLNB with ALND and that lymphedema was less likely after SLNB.[19] Researchers are looking at evidence comparing long-term outcomes after SLNB versus ALND, debating whether there may be a subset of women who may not need axillary surgery if treated with systemic therapy (chemotherapy or radiation).

Prospective surveillance for lymphedema, most commonly advocated for patients with breast cancer, has become a paradigm shift in the management and detection of lymphedema.[117] Investigations into predictive factors for lymphedema after breast cancer surgery have identified the following: individuals with lymphedema are more likely to be overweight (BMI ≥25) and to have had axillary radiation, mastectomy versus lumpectomy, more positive lymph nodes, chemotherapy, fluid aspirations after surgery, and active cancer.[117,177] Controlling the predisposing controllable risk factors has a significant effect on the probability of developing lymphedema. See the discussion later in this chapter regarding appropriate strengthening of an at-risk arm to reduce the risk of lymphedema.

The effect of weight reduction on lymphedema has been studied in a small number of women with BCRL. Weight reduction with a corresponding decrease in BMI reduced the volume of affected limbs more than twice that of the unaffected limb. Several possible explanations for the greater volume loss in the affected limbs include improvement in lymph drainage because of fat loss, the actual change in composition of the tissues in the limb with reduced fat, and loss of fat, allowing improved function of elastic compression garments.[166] Body weight is one significant risk factor that the person can be empowered to impact by exercise and dietary modification.[9] Studies looking at the potential of weight reduction strategies to reduce BCRL are promising but not definitive.[77]

**Medical Procedures—Lower Extremity.** The incidence of lower extremity lymphedema after inguinal lymph node dissection to treat melanoma has been reported to be 32.1% in patients who underwent inguinal lymph node dissection.[67] The average reported incidence of lower extremity lymphedema after treatment for prostate cancer has been reported to be 4% (range, 1% to 18%). The overall risk of lymphedema in individuals with prostate cancer after pelvic node dissection has been reported to be 8%, increasing to 16% after radiation treatment.[41] In a review of gynecologic cancer treatment, the risk of lymphedema ranged from 0% to 70% but differed with various cancer types.[12] In endometrial cancer the risk is 1.2% to 47% depending on the assessment method used, with prominent risk factors reported as pelvic/paraaortic lymphadenectomy, postoperative radiation, and obesity. In cervical cancer, the standard treatment (radical hysterectomy with pelvic lymph node dissection) led to a reported range of 0% to 55.9%. Risk factors included postoperative radiation, larger number of dissected nodes, and suprafemoral node dissection. In ovarian cancer, the reported incidence is 4.7% to 40.8%. In the majority of cases (86.2%), lymphedema developed in the first year after surgery. In vulvar cancer, the incidence is reported to be 30% to 70%. SLNB may reduce the risk of lymphedema in this population, though this remains controversial[12] regarding oncologic management.

### Etiologic Factors

**Primary Lymphedema.** The exact cause of *primary lymphedema* is unknown and cannot be linked to any significant traumatic event (Table 13.1). Primary lymphedema is most likely the result of lymphangiodysplasias or malformations of the lymphatic vessels present at birth (Fig. 13.9) but sometimes delayed in symptomatic presentation. Although a small percentage of primary lymphedemas are linked to genetic causes (e.g., Milroy disease), most cases are not genetically linked and are more likely the result of some developmental abnormality in the fetus. A family history of lymphedema is present in only 10% to 20% of all people with primary lymphedema.[29]

**Table 13.1** Etiology and Risk Factors for Lymphedema

| Primary | Secondary[a] |
|---|---|
| Unknown | Filariasis |
| Hereditary | Primary or metastatic neoplasm (benign or malignant) |
| Developmental abnormality | Surgery (lymph node dissection or removal; other surgery: see text) |
| Aplasia | Radiation treatment |
| Hypoplasia | Chemotherapy |
| Hyperplasia | Severe infection |
| | Lipedema |
| | Chronic venous insufficiency |
| | Liposuction |
| | Crush injury |
| | Compound fracture |
| | Severe laceration |
| | Degloving skin injury |
| | Burns |
| | Obesity |
| | Multiparity |
| | Paralysis |
| | Medications |
| | Prolonged systemic use of cortisone (cortisone skin) |
| | Tamoxifen/Adriamycin |
| | HIV/AIDS |

[a]Listed in approximate descending order of frequency.

*Note:* For additional resources, see Box 13.2. For more detailed information for individuals diagnosed with lymphedema, go to www.lymphnet.org.

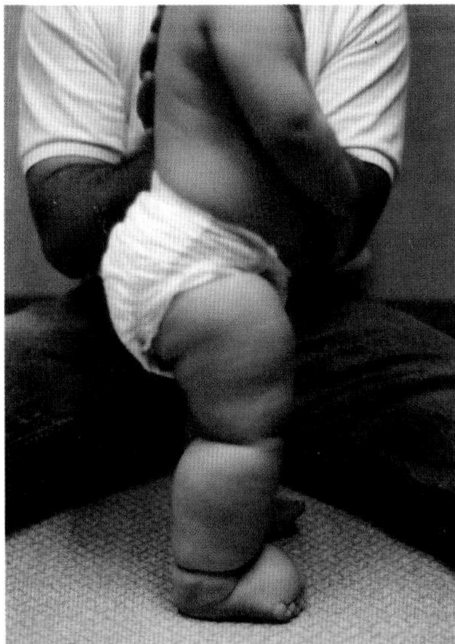

**FIGURE 13.9**

**A 13-month-old child with primary lymphedema of the right lower extremity, right buttock, and genital area since birth.** (Courtesy Lymphedema Therapy, Woodbury, NY.)

Klippel-Trénaunay syndrome is a rare occurrence in embryonic development and is associated with numerous anomalies. These can include varicose veins, cavernous hemangioma of the skin, and hypertrophy of bones and soft tissues in one or several extremities. In

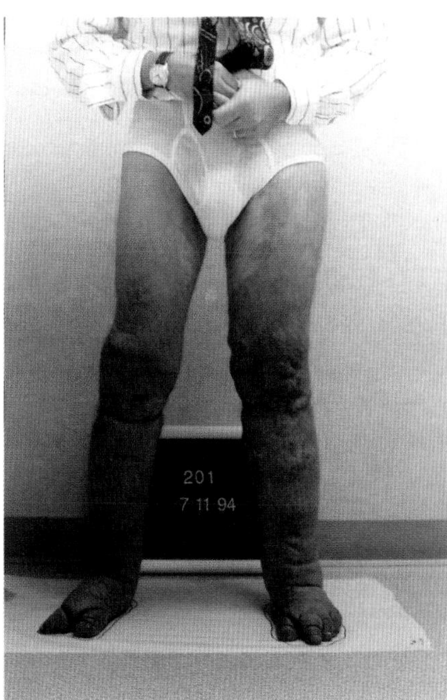


**FIGURE 13.10**

**A 50-year-old man with Klippel-Trénaunay-Weber syndrome, a lymphangiodysplasia that caused lymphedema in both lower extremities.** Note the skeletal abnormalities of the toes, the large hemangioma on the left thigh, and the venous varicosities in the lower legs. (Courtesy Lymphedema Therapy, Woodbury, NY.)

addition, dysplasia of the lymphatic system and neurogenic and visceral vascular malformations can occur. Dysplasia of the lymphatics can result in lymphedema in the involved extremities (Fig. 13.10).[22]

Malformations of the lymphatic vessels associated with primary lymphedema can be divided into three types: aplastic, hypoplastic, and hyperplastic. *Aplasia* occurs when the lymphatic collectors are so few that they are considered absent. Aplasia may also involve the absence of lymph capillaries that render the adequate collectors less functional. Aplasia is most often combined with hypoplasia; complete aplasia would result in tissues unable to support life.

*Hypoplasia* refers to less than the normal expected number of lymph collectors in the affected region and may also occur when collectors present are unable to function as transport vessels. Hypoplasia represents the most common cause of primary lymphedema, occurring in 75% of cases. *Hyperplasia* accounts for 15% of primary cases and is characterized by grossly dilated and enlarged lymphatics that can become varicose. Hyperplasia can occur in the lymphatics of the superficial plexus of the skin or in the main lymph trunks. As a result of the overdilation of the vessels, the intralymphatic valve flaps do not seal, and a reflux of lymph occurs.

When this occurs in the mesenteric and intestinal lymphatics, a reflux of chyle to distal areas also takes place—that is, to the skin of the genitals, buttocks, and thighs or to the knee joint (Fig. 13.11). Chyle is the protein-rich, milky fluid taken up by the intestinal lymphatics during digestion, consisting of lymph and triglycerides in a stable

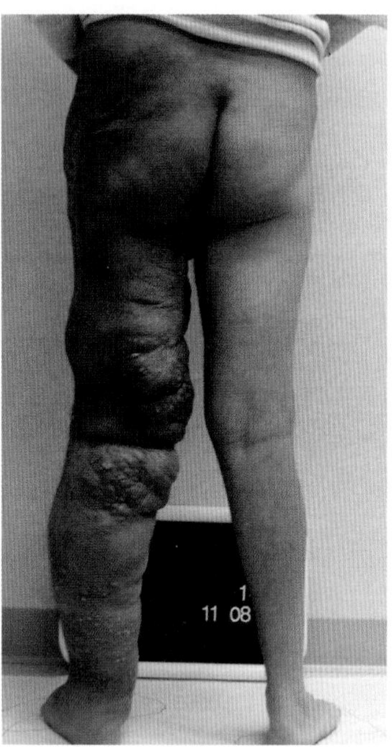


**FIGURE 13.11**

**A 19-year-old man with primary lymphedema of the left lower extremity (onset at age 8 years).** Lymphedema progressed to involve the buttocks and genitalia after prolonged pneumatic compression pump usage. This young man had three microsurgical procedures (lymphovenous and lympholymphatic anastomoses) in an attempt to reduce the genital and extremity edema. In addition, he had two debulking surgeries, which also were unsuccessful in reducing the lymphedema. He developed chylous reflux and eventually had sclerotherapy to his leaking abdominal lymphatics, which was very successful in stopping the severe leakage of chyle from his scrotum, medial thigh, and buttock. The chyle-filled papules are visible on the posterior aspect of the thigh and calf. Notice the abnormal bulges and skin folds on the posterior thigh, which result when the debulked areas fill in with edema fluid. (Courtesy Lymphedema Therapy, Woodbury, NY.)

emulsion, and transported with the other lymphatic volume by the thoracic duct to the venous system.

*Lymphangiectasia* refers to lymphatic hyperplasia in a deeper organ or localized area of a limb. Lymphangiomas and lymph cysts are forms of lymphangiectasia.[29,59]

**Secondary Lymphedema.** Secondary lymphedema occurs as the result of known damage to otherwise normal lymphatic vessels or nodes in one or more regions. The most common cause of secondary lymphedema worldwide is *filariasis*. This is a parasitic worm, introduced to the body by a mosquito bite in endemic regions. The larvae of the worm are injected into the dermis with the bite. They pass into the initial lymphatics and larger collecting lymphatics and can grow to 20 cm in length and 1 to 2 cm in diameter as they mature into the adult worm forms. The greatest damage, however, is done after the worm dies, often 5 to 10 years after the initial infection. At that time, foreign proteins from the worm body cause severe local inflammatory reactions that lead to severe fibrosis and scarring of the tissues, totally blocking the larger lymph collectors. This total blockage results in massive swelling distal to that locale.[65,154,190]

In the United States and other regions of the world where the filaria parasite does not exist or has been eradicated, the most common cause of secondary lymphedema is invasive procedures used in the diagnosis and treatment of cancer. *Regional lymph node dissection* for diagnostic staging and eradication of tumor sites disrupts the lymphatic system. Radiation therapy, reconstructive or other surgical procedures, and the combination of these procedures are well-known contributing factors to the development of lymphedema.

*Local radiation treatment* after surgery for cancer increases the incidence of secondary lymphedema three times that of surgery alone, probably a result of the increase in local tissue fibrosis that further impairs lymph flow through the remaining functioning lymphatic vessels and nodes.[32,101] If there is significant burning and blistering of the skin during radiation treatment, the risk of lymphedema is increased owing to fibrosis of the skin and subcutaneous tissues.[156]

*Other causes* of secondary lymphedema include bacterial or viral infection; multiple abdominal surgeries, particularly in obese individuals; any trauma or surgery that impairs the lymphatics; or repeated pregnancies (see Table 13.1). Liposuction done for cosmetic reasons to enhance appearance, when performed on an individual with an asymptomatic but marginal lymphatic system, can trigger lymphedema in the at-risk limb.

Crush injuries, severe burns, compound fractures, or severe lacerations or degloving injuries to the skin can significantly impair lymph flow. These traumatic injuries are also usually associated with damage to blood vessels. The damaged blood vessels leak fibrinogen, blocking the tissue channels and initial lymphatics and thus contributing to the development of lymphedema. Other known causes that have been reported to be associated with secondary lymphedema include paralysis; lipedema; chronic venous insufficiency; obesity[121]; skin thinned by cortisone (sometimes referred to as *cortisone* or *steroid skin*); and AIDS, particularly if Kaposi sarcoma is present.[33]

Deep vein thromboses (DVT) are a higher risk in individuals with active cancer diagnoses. Lower extremity or pelvic surgeries or a history of 3 or more days of bed rest are also risk factors.[149] Certain medications used in cancer care are known to increase the risk of DVT, for example, tamoxifen. This can lead to an increase in lymphatic load owing to venous obstruction and lead to lymphedema in an at-risk limb.

*Surgery* is controlled trauma, but it is trauma nevertheless; the more extensive the procedure, the more extensive is the trauma. Surgery in individuals with a marginal lymphatic system (where the lymph transport capacity equals the normal lymph load) can cause enough of an overload to trigger lymphedema. For example, an individual undergoing a joint replacement may develop chronic leg edema that is often misdiagnosed as venous insufficiency or cardiac related. This is particularly true in an older, obese individual who has poor functional mobility. If the diagnosis of lymphedema is delayed or never made and is not addressed, the individual may not be able to succeed in postoperative rehabilitation (Fig. 13.12).

In the past, most health care professionals knew about upper limb lymphedema secondary to axillary dissection for breast cancer, but many were not aware that an individual who had a previous DVT and inguinal node

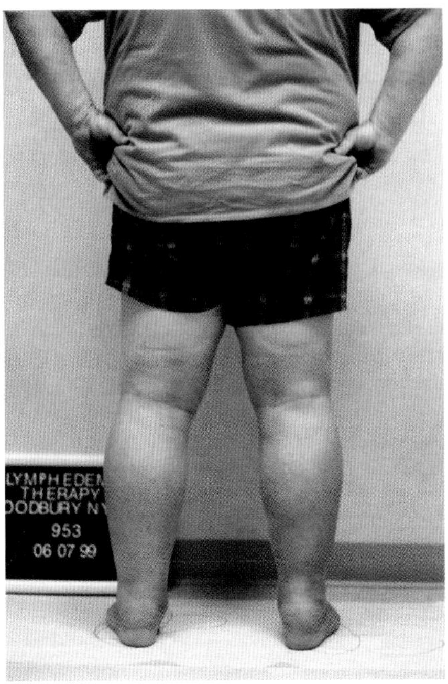


**FIGURE 13.12**

**A 63-year-old man with lymphedema of both lower extremities, left greater than right.** The swelling developed in the left leg 1 year after a coronary artery bypass graft procedure in which veins were harvested from the left leg. The swelling began in the right leg, worsened in the left leg, and progressed into the abdomen after radium seed implantation for prostate cancer. This man's marginal lymphatic system was overwhelmed by the trauma caused by the coronary artery bypass graft procedure and the radium seed implantation procedure. (Courtesy Lymphedema Therapy, Woodbury, NY.)

dissection for melanoma in the leg or any cancer in the pelvic region was at risk for lymphedema of the leg and possibly the genitals, buttocks, or abdomen.

A person with chronic postoperative edema after a fracture or total hip or knee replacement is often not routinely evaluated for lymphedema. The combination of venous edema and lymphedema is often overlooked in the management of edema secondary to trauma. Many cases of chronic edema with recurrent infection and skin ulcerations are treated as pure venous edemas with poor results because the lymphatic component of the edema is not addressed.

*Obesity* may be a cause of lower extremity lymphedema.[74] There is a threshold defined by BMI beyond which lymphatic dysfunction can be demonstrated. Individuals who are obese but below that threshold (while they may have a normally functioning lymphatic system) can have significant venous edema. The threshold appears to be a BMI of 30 for an increased risk of BCRL and between 53 and 59 for the lower extremity in obese individuals without any other risk factors.[121] Proximal transport of lymphatic fluid from the extremity depends on normal clearance function of the lymphatic vasculature. Anything that can increase the volume of lymph produced by the tissues increases the load. With increased adipose tissue, there can be increased compression on the lymphatic vessels, reducing lymphatic flow. At the same time, increased lymph production from the enlarging limb may overwhelm the capacity of a normal functioning lymphatic system to move and remove the fluid from the extremity.[74] Another phenomenon seen in morbidly obese patients is called massive localized lymphedema. This is characterized by a very local lymphatic dysfunction seen in the most dependent part of an enlarged abdominal pannus or fatty lobule—usually in the medial distal thigh. A differentiation from fatty tissue can be made by the most dependent skin having a peau d'orange texture.[95]

**A THERAPIST'S THOUGHTS[a]**

***A Helpful Analogy to Understand Pathogenesis***

Simply stated, you can think of the lymphatic vessels as the lanes on a highway, the lymph nodes as the toll booths, and lymph as the cars to be transported on that highway. As long as the number of cars (lymph load) is equal to or less than the number of lanes open (lymph vessels), there is homeostasis. If there is a sudden increase in cars entering the highway (acute injury, infection, inflammation), there may be a temporary traffic jam (edema) that can resolve in a short time (days or weeks). However, if a number of lanes or toll booths are closed (lymph vessels or nodes excised or lymph nodes are irradiated), the transport capacity is reduced, and even though the number of cars on the highway has not increased (lymph load is stable), traffic (lymph) builds up and lymphedema develops.

[a]Bonnie Lasinski

### Pathogenesis

Lymphedema by definition is a low-flow, high-protein edema that occurs when the lymph transport capacity is inadequate to recycle proteins and transport the normal volume of lymph. It is a failure of the safety valve mechanisms (Fig. 13.13). This can occur when the lymph load is normal, but the lymph transport capacity is inadequate *(decreased absorption of lymph in lymph nodes)*, or when there is an increase in the lymphatic load (e.g., protein/fluid entering the tissues), and the transport capacity is inadequate *(subtotal lymphatic blockage)*.

In reality the body adjusts the flow if the capacity alters in response to changes in tissue hydrostatic pressure and other changes in homeostasis *(remaining lymphatics increase their pumping activity)*, and conversely, the capacity can be adjusted if the load alters *(intralymphatic pressure increases)*. When the safety valve mechanisms are no longer effective or become overwhelmed, the body's normal compensation is not enough, and lymphedema develops.

Why some individuals develop lymphedema after lymph node dissection and others do not remains a puzzle. It has been found that muscle lymph flow is higher in both arms of women who ultimately develop lymphedema compared with women who do not. Higher fluid filtration in the upper extremity may be a predisposing factor for lymphatic failure after lymphatic obstruction occurs.[172]

Higher arterial blood flow and lower amplitude venous blood flow pulse have been observed in women with lymphedema.[125] Stout and colleagues[175,176] studied

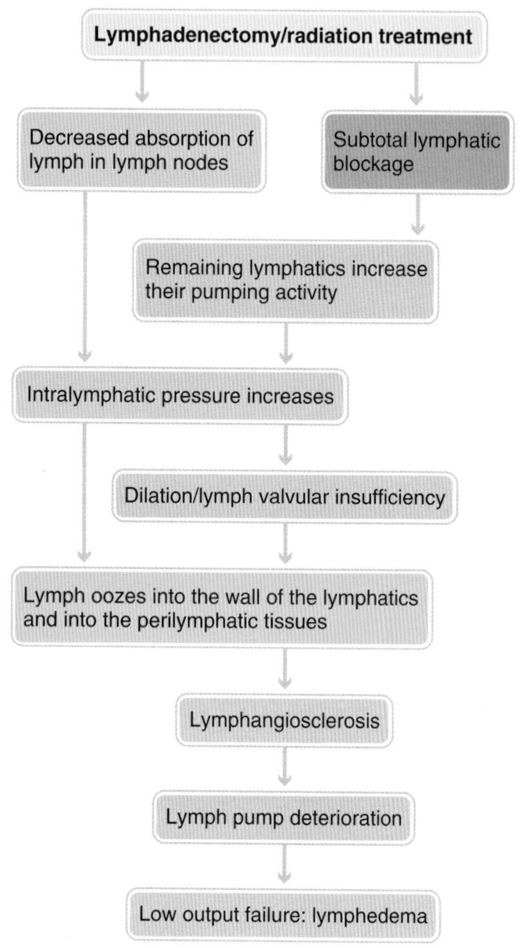


**FIGURE 13.13**

**Pathogenesis of lymphedema.** This flow chart follows the progression from an at-risk or latent phase of lymphedema to acute lymphedema after lymphadenectomy and/or radiation treatment to the nodal area. (Courtesy Dr. Michael Földi, June 1999.)

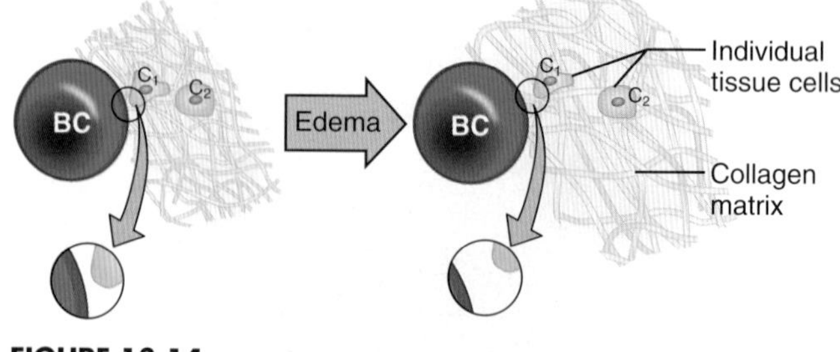


**FIGURE 13.14**

**Reduction of gas (oxygen) exchange.** Even a relatively minor amount of edema, which moves the fibers and individual tissue cells *(C1, C2)* apart by only a small amount, can cause a great increase in the resistance to diffusion of gases (and other small lipid-soluble molecules) between the cells and the blood capillaries *(BC)*. The magnified view of the distance between the BC and the tissue cell (representing the cell's oxygen supply) is greatly increased in the edematous state. The greater distance for oxygen to diffuse to nourish the cells will eventually lead to a hypoxic state. (From Casley-Smith JR, Casley-Smith JR: *Modern treatment for lymphoedema*, ed 5, Adelaide, Australia, 1997, Lymphoedema Association of Australia.)

segmental limb volume changes over time from before surgery to 12 months after surgery in 46 women who were at risk for BCRL. Increases in segmental volume were found in two segments in the affected forearm before the onset of lymphedema. This study highlights the importance of prospective surveillance in individuals at risk to develop lymphedema.[175,176] Lymphedema causes the lymphatic vessels to dilate; the valve flaps become incompetent *(dilation/lymph valvular insufficiency)*, and the protein-rich lymphatic fluid refluxes to the tissue spaces *(perilymphatic tissues)*. At first, a proliferation of initial lymphatic vessels occurs as the system tries to cope with the accumulation of lymphatic load. Lymph vessels can reconnect, or collateral lymphatics can develop to bypass the damaged area.

**Chronic Inflammation.** A state of chronic inflammation exists in lymphedematous tissue.[137] This chronic inflammation leads to progressive tissue fibrosis, resulting in a state of relative hypoxia in the tissues, further impeding tissue oxygenation and contributing to a cycle of chronic inflammation and increased risk of infection.

**Infection or Delayed Wound Healing.** In either primary or secondary lymphedema, infection or delayed wound healing (the latter can be directly related to the low oxygen state caused by edema) will add to the high-protein edema. Infection in the tissues (cellulitis) or infection in the lymph vessels (lymphangitis) can cause progressive tissue fibrosis and/or scarring in the lymph vessels *(lymphangiosclerosis)*. Although some recanalization and collateralization of lymph vessels occur, lymphatic function remains compromised. An increase in the size of the tissue channels occurs with an increase in the distance for the oxygen to diffuse from the capillaries to the cells (Fig. 13.14). Gas exchange and metabolism of cellular waste products are impaired.

**Lymph Pump Deterioration.** Although the number of macrophages increases, their activity is decreased in the lymphedema fluid for reasons not clearly understood. Some theories suggest that the chronic lack of essential nutrients (e.g., oxygen) or perhaps a toxic factor produced by the stagnant proteins or the damaged tissues contribute to the deterioration of macrophages.[28,30] In chronic lymphedema, the muscle wall of the collecting lymphatics hypertrophies and eventually scleroses, reducing the effective pumping power of these vessels *(lymph pump deterioration)*.

**Impaired Transport Mechanism.** The effect of lymphedema on the blood vessels causes a proliferation of new small blood vessels and the development of arteriovenous anastomoses. These new small vessels may leak as a result of abnormal changes in total tissue pressure in the lymphedematous region, further overloading the area. Proteins, fats, cellular waste products, and the interstitial fluid have no alternative transport pathway from the soft tissue to the venous system except via the lymphatic system. When this transport mechanism is impaired, lymphedema develops (Fig. 13.15A). The impairment can be structural or functional.

***Structural Impairment.*** Aging and damaged blood vessels are associated with structural impairment as fibrin physically narrows or blocks tissue channels (Fig. 13.15B). Hypoplasia of the collecting lymphatics is also associated with the pathogenesis of structural lymphedema (Fig. 13.15C).

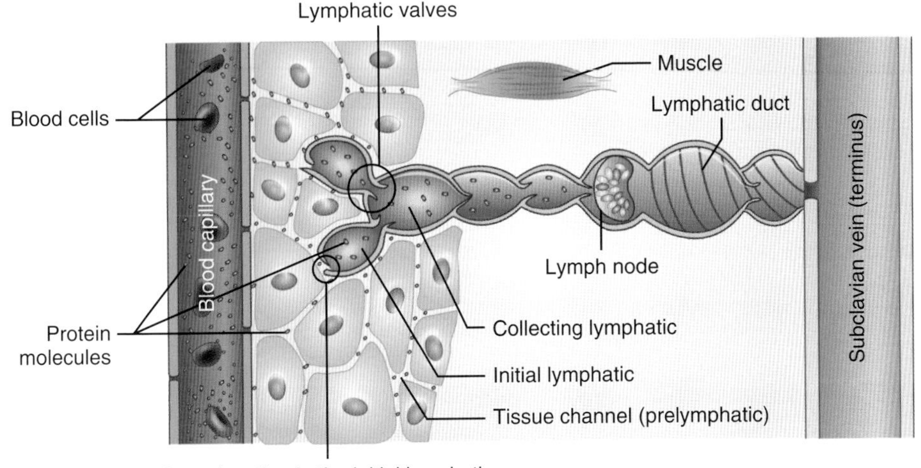


B

C

**FIGURE 13.15**

**Low-flow, high-protein lymphedema caused by structural impairment.** (A) Normal tissue for comparison showing the passage of protein *(dots)* in normal tissue from the blood capillary through the tissue channels, into and through the lymphatic system, and back to a vein. (B) Altered interstitial tissue (e.g., too few or too narrow tissue channels). Notice that the prelymphatic channels are much narrower than in the normal tissue, and the protein molecules are stacked up on the arterial side, unable to move easily through the narrow tissue channels, causing impaired lymph flow (and eventual tissue fibrosis). Inlet valves are closed because the endothelial cell junctions cannot open properly in fibrosed tissues, contributing to poor lymph drainage. (C) Abnormally few initial lymphatics. This may occur developmentally or because some of the vessels become blocked (e.g., by fibrin). In this case, too few initial lymphatics are evident. Notice the dilation of the prelymphatic channels, the greater concentration of protein molecules in the tissue channels, and the malformed inlet valve. Low-flow, high-protein lymphedema caused by structural impairment.

Primary lymphedema with onset at puberty can be explained by a growth spurt and increase in tissue mass, causing the body to outgrow or outstrip the capacity of the lymphatic system. The functioning vessels become overwhelmed, and the walls fail, dilate, and result in valvular incompetence, causing increased peripheral intralymphatic pressures and peripheral lymphedema.

Structural lymphedema may also occur when the flaps of incompetent valves of the collecting lymphatics (Fig. 13.15D) no longer meet, allowing reflux of lymph to regions distal to the blockage. The initial lymphatics eventually dilate as well, their endothelial junctions remain open, and lymph refluxes to the tissues.

Other causes of structural lymphedema include gaps and tears in the initial lymphatic walls associated with trauma and inflammation (Fig. 13.15E); physical obstruction of collecting lymphatics (Fig. 13.15F) associated with fibrosis, radiation therapy, tumor growth, and surgical excision of lymphatics during tumor removal; and torn anchoring filaments (Fig. 13.15G) associated with sudden acute edema. Sudden acute edema may occur secondary to massive trauma or infection and can tear the microfilaments that connect the initial lymphatics to the interstitial tissues, resulting in the collapse of the initial lymphatics because of the high total tissue pressure.[29]

***Functional Impairment.*** Anything that causes a lack of variation in total tissue pressure may cause lymphedema. Bed rest, paralysis, or prolonged immobility combined with dependency of the limb can severely limit changes in total tissue pressure. This variation contributes to a pressure gradient between the interstitial tissues and the intralymphatic pressure. Normally, this pressure gradient stimulates the lymphangions to contract, which enhances the flow of lymph from the periphery to the center of the

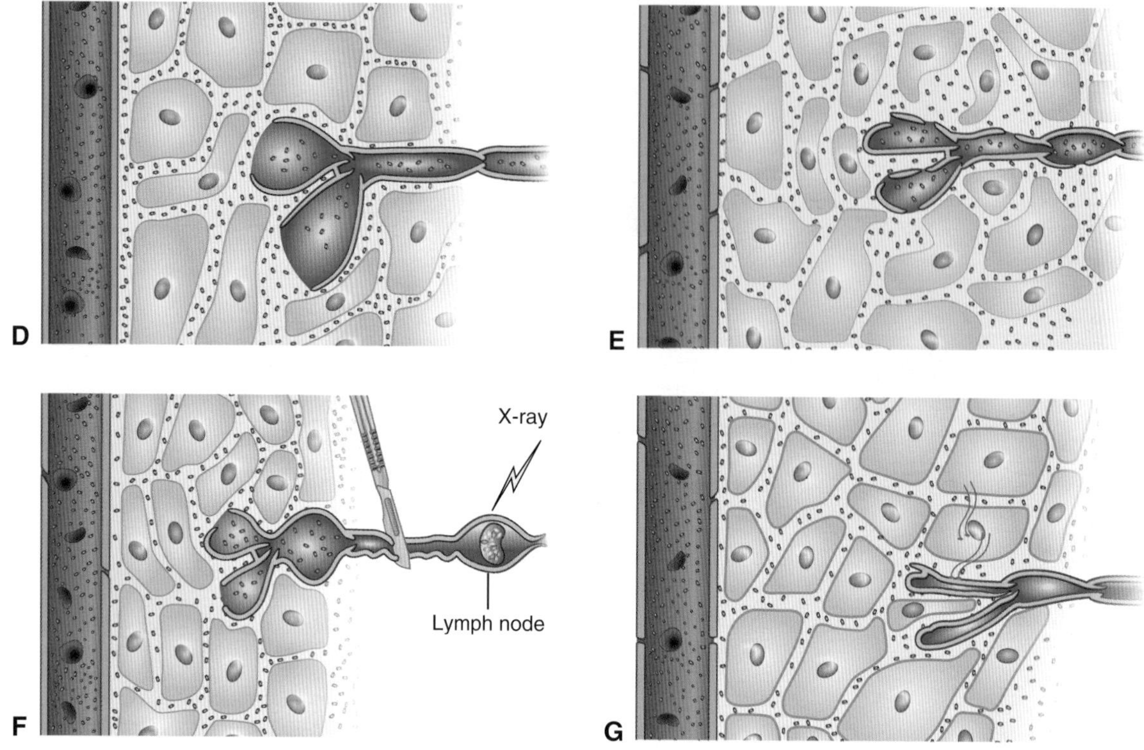


**FIGURE 13.15 cont'd**

**Low-flow, high-protein lymphedema caused by structural impairment.** (D) Malformations of the initial lymphatics preventing their inlet valves from sealing; the prelymphatic tissue channels are dilated, a high-protein concentration exists there, and the tissue channels become dilated and stretched. This can happen in both primary and secondary lymphedema; in secondary lymphedema, it occurs after prolonged lymphostasis from a more proximal blockage. (E) Injuries to the walls of the very fragile initial lymphatics. Lymph refluxes into the tissue channels, causing them to dilate. The high concentration of protein in the extracellular tissues causes a chronic inflammatory response and greater risk of infection. Note the larger spaces between the tissues. This results in a larger distance for oxygen to diffuse and leads to tissue hypoxia. (F) Iatrogenic factors (e.g., surgery, irradiation, tumor growth) that damage the lymphatic ducts or larger vessels impair lymph flow from the periphery. When movement of lymph from the tissue channels into the initial lymphatics is impaired, the tissue channels dilate, lymph stasis occurs, and there is a high-protein concentration in the tissues with subsequent chronic inflammation, increased risk of infection, and progressive swelling of the limb. (G) Anchoring filaments tearing away from the interstitial tissue. This occurs in severe edema from other causes (e.g., rapid swelling from acute lymphedema as a result of trauma can tear the anchoring filaments from the surrounding tissues). The initial lymphatics can no longer function as conduits, as they would normally. The lymphostasis this produces worsens the existing edema. (From Casley-Smith JR, Casley-Smith JR: *Modern treatment for lymphoedema*, ed 5, Adelaide, Australia, 1997, Lymphoedema Association of Australia.)

body. When the tissue pressure does not change or vary, the force pumps remain inactive.

Other factors contributing to functional impairment of the lymphatic system may include spasm of collecting lymphatics (e.g., lymphangiospasm caused by inflammation stimulating sympathetic nerves), paralysis of the collecting lymphatics (e.g., prolonged distention leading to fatigue and ultimately failure), and impaired contraction of the collecting lymphatics caused by physical obstruction of fibrotic tissue surrounding lymphatic vessels. This type of functional impairment is common in severe stage II lymphedema and stage III lymphostatic elephantiasis. If collectors cannot pump, lymph refluxes peripherally, causing overdilation of the collecting lymphatics, valvular incompetence, lymphatic failure, and ultimately lymphedema.[29,59,190]

**Clinical Manifestations.** Primary or secondary lymphedema is characterized by clinical signs and symptoms caused by the effects of lymphedema on the lymphatics, body tissues, and blood vessels. Lymphedema resulting from filariasis is reversible in its early stages; secondary lymphedema can be transient if damage is minor. Secondary lymphedema can develop immediately postoperatively or weeks, months, or years after surgery.[5]

Lymphedema can develop in any part of the body or limbs. Signs or symptoms of lymphedema include a full, heavy, or tight sensation in the affected body part; numbness, burning, aching, pain; decreased flexibility in the hand, wrist, or ankle; difficulty fitting into shoes or clothing in one specific area; or jewelry tightness. Increased girth and weight of the limbs along with postural changes and limitation in joint motion leads to functional deficits. In advanced cases, loss of skin integrity allows portals of entry for bacteria to invade the skin and cause recurrent infection. Significant edema of the head and neck can cause severe functional impairments in speech, swallowing, and respiration, in addition to the pain and psychologic trauma from cosmetic disfigurement.

These physical impairments can lead to functional limitations and disability along with the potential for psychosocial morbidity (e.g., social isolation, depression, or suicide).[6,90] Healing time is increased, and all of this is occurring in a heavy, painful, and clumsy limb that is more prone to injury because of its abnormally large size and decreased functional mobility. Risk of injury is increased when oxygenation and metabolism of waste and cellular debris are decreased. This is an extremely dangerous environment.

**Complications of Lymphedema.** As lymphedema progresses, atrophic skin changes can occur as a result of the low oxygen state, including loss of hair and sweat glands, formation of keratotic patches on the skin, and development of papillomas (mushroom-like outgrowths of the skin) that sometimes leak lymphatic fluid. Lymphangiosarcoma (Stewart-Treves syndrome) is a rare, highly malignant secondary cancer that can develop into an advanced, chronic lymphedema when left untreated.[190]

Primary lymphedema can be present in many parts of the body, and if it is present from birth, the deep internal organs often are affected. Clinical cases of primary lymphedema of the lower extremities may involve the buttocks, genitals, and intestines with reflux of intestinal chyle (chylous reflux/protein-losing enteropathy) through fistulae on the genitals, buttocks, and legs or the leakage of protein-rich chyle from the intestinal lymphatics into the abdomen or thoracic cavity (see Fig. 13.23). This protein-losing enteropathy is a medical emergency. Individuals who complain of abdominal bloating, chronic diarrhea, or intolerance of fatty foods may also experience fluid accumulation in the abdomen and genitals from the pressure of the fluid leaking from the intestinal lymphatics. In some cases, these clients are treated medically or surgically with sclerotherapy to seal off these leaking lymphatics in an attempt to halt the reflux of this fluid.

As lymphedema progresses, the dermal layer of the skin thickens, the skin itself dries and cracks, and ulcerations often develop. These ulcers may not heal because of the tension on the tissues from the edema and the decreased oxygenation state, coupled with the subcutaneous fibrosis and chronic inflammation. As the skin and tissues stretch and fill, skin folds and lobules can develop. These folds and lobules become breeding grounds for fungal and bacterial infections that further damage skin integrity, creating new portals of entry for the bacteria as the skin macerates and cracks.

Chronic fungus (tinea) is common on the foot and toes of anyone with lymphedema of the legs as well as in the groin and under the breast. This fungus can be difficult, if not impossible, to treat topically. If tinea is not addressed during treatment, a successful outcome is not possible (Fig. 13.16).[29]

The progressive increase in girth and weight of the affected areas contributes to pathologic alterations in the gait pattern and decreases in functional range of motion and strength caused by fatigue and inactivity. Coupling this with impairments in shoulder mobility caused by tightness of the trunk and pectoralis major and minor muscles secondary to radiation treatment for breast cancer, there is a risk for development or worsening of shoulder impingement or rotator cuff problems.[104,164] With increasing edema and subcutaneous fibrosis, tactile sensation and kinesthetic awareness are impaired, increasing the risk of injury to the affected areas.

If the edema progresses into the trunk quadrant adjacent to the lymphedematous limb, a further loss of trunk strength and function can occur. Some individuals, for example, must sleep in a recliner chair to prevent losing their independence, as they can no longer mobilize themselves and their heavy limbs in bed. A vicious cycle develops with decreasing mobility, unrelieved dependency of the limbs, and loss of strength, leading to joint contractures, further increasing the risk to the already impaired skin. Balance may be impaired, and the individual may no longer be able to shower or bathe independently, as a result of the fear of falling or inability to move the heavy limbs over the bath or shower ledge. Hygiene becomes a problem, further increasing the risk for fungal and bacterial infections.[118,130]

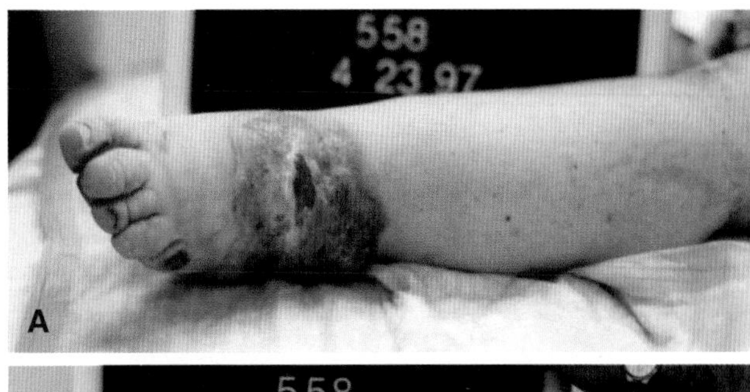


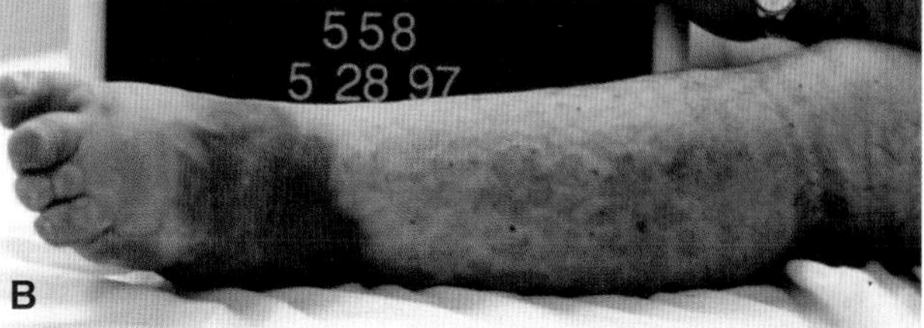


**FIGURE 13.16**

**A 30-year-old man with spina bifida and lymphedema secondary to paralysis and unsuccessful plastic surgery with skin graft for a chronically itchy, 2-cm keratotic lesion on the left anterior ankle crease.** (A) Chronic ulceration complicated by fungal infection of the ulcer itself and the foot or toes. Note the hypertrophic fibrotic skin at the ankle and warty changes on the toes. (B) After 4 weeks of complex lymphedema therapy (débridement of the ulcer was done daily in addition to lymphatic drainage, compression bandaging, and other skin care). Exercise was not possible because of paralysis; deep abdominal breathing exercises and modified self–lymphatic drainage were taught and then practiced daily. Note that the wound healed completely and the infection resolved. (Courtesy Lymphedema Therapy, Woodbury, NY.)

## MEDICAL MANAGEMENT

Remarkable progress has occurred in diagnosis and management of lymphedema in the United States since 1990. Ironically, this has occurred despite the incorrect prediction for people with breast cancer that the advent of breast-conserving lumpectomy would eliminate upper extremity lymphedema so commonly seen in individuals following mastectomy.

### Diagnosis

***Primary Lymphedema.*** An easy-to-perform clinical test for determining primary lower extremity lymphedema is observation of the Stemmer sign, a thickened cutaneous fold of skin over the second toe, typically present in the early stages. This allows for differential diagnosis of a primary ascending lymphedema without false-positive findings. The Stemmer sign appears in the late stages of descending lymphedema (Fig. 13.17).[173] It is possible

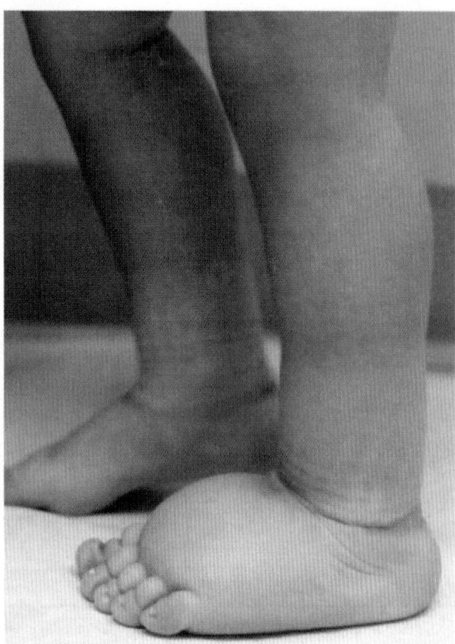

**FIGURE 13.17**

Stemmer sign is clearly visible as a thickening of the skin folds of the toes of this 22-month-old child with a history of primary lymphedema of the left lower extremity diagnosed at birth. (Courtesy Lymphedema Therapy, Woodbury, NY.)

to have primary lymphedema without a Stemmer sign present.

***Secondary Lymphedema.*** The clinical diagnosis of secondary lymphedema is fairly straightforward in a limb at risk when there is known disruption to the regional lymphatics (e.g., after axillary dissection/radiation or after inguinal or pelvic node dissection/radiation). A detailed medical history, including *all* surgical procedures and their chronology relative to the onset or worsening of the edema, is the cornerstone of a successful lymphologic evaluation. In secondary lymphedema, other diagnostic tests are rarely needed to confirm the diagnosis in the majority of cases.

Of concern to a therapist should be a client who presents with unilateral limb swelling with no obvious cause by history; venous obstruction via a DVT or occult tumor should always be considered before treatment in this instance. A venous Doppler study of the edematous limb is often done to rule out a DVT as the cause of the swelling, but computed tomography (CT) or magnetic resonance imaging (MRI) of the upper or lower body may also be necessary if the Doppler study is negative. Lymphedema may also be the first sign of cancer recurrence even years after cancer treatment. The prospect of recurrent disease is a frightening one, but it must be ruled out. Malignant lymphedema (i.e., directly resulting from neoplasm blocking a major nodal region or lymph vessel) is typically worse and progresses more rapidly than nonmalignant secondary lymphedema. Malignant lymphedema begins usually in the proximal portion of the limb, and alterations in skin color and texture are common (Fig. 13.18). It is also associated with severe neurogenic pain and/or sensorimotor deficits, particularly in the upper extremity when the brachial plexus is involved. These symptoms must be differentiated from the pain and weakness of radiation plexopathy, which sometimes progresses more slowly but causes the same type of functional deficits without such rapid onset.

***Diagnostic Tests.*** In cases of unexplained swelling, particularly in the lower extremities when no known trauma or surgery is evident, the clinical examination and history may not provide a definitive medical diagnosis. Standard MRI or CT scan of the chest or pelvis may reveal a previously unsuspected tumor and will clearly show edema fluid in a limb or region, but these tests do not provide a description of lymphatic function. Several tests are available to assess lymphatic function, including lymphoscintigraphy, fluorescence lymphography, and magnetic resonance lymphangiography.[34,187] Lymphoscintigraphy assesses clearance of a radioactive tracer injected into subepidermal tissue and can describe the flow pattern, timing of clearance, or pooling in the limb. Fluorescence lymphography allows visual assessment of flow through lymphatic collectors superficially via visualization with specialized goggles of the fluorescence of indocyanine green as it is cleared after injection into the skin. Magnetic resonance lymphangiography does not require contrast enhancement and is best for visualizing congested proximal vessels. These specialized tests rarely give additional information when treating uncomplicated lymphedemas.[34,187]

**Treatment.** The primary focus in a case of lymphedema triggered by a new or metastatic cancer is to treat the cancer first and then manage the lymphedema. Input on how to minimize exacerbation of the lymphedema during the cancer treatment is often well received if given with the intent to provide comfort and function.

On one hand, individuals are encouraged to undergo the cancer treatment that they wish to pursue, without guilt or fear that it will worsen the lymphedema. They need to know the possibilities and risks, but they should not be frightened away from necessary treatment for the cancer by a well-meaning health care professional.

On the other hand, the lymphedema should not be ignored. Management of the lymphedema must be coordinated with the medical team (e.g., medical oncologist, surgeon, and radiation oncologist) and the client. This communication can avoid further overloading the person with additional appointments and adding more to their daily activities than they can handle. Adjustable low-stretch Velcro-style garments are useful, as they are more comfortable, easier to put on, and able to adjust to limb fluctuations in this setting.

**Medications.** No clear-cut pharmaceutical drug is available to treat lymphedema. A class of drugs called benzopyrones was investigated in Australia but were found to cause severe liver problems in some people. They have never been approved for use in the United States by the Food and Drug Administration. These drugs increased proteolysis, helping to reduce the interstitial protein concentration, signaling the body to reabsorb more extracellular fluid, thereby reducing the lymphedema. These substances have been shown to soften fibrotic tissue and increase the healing of chronic ulcerations and bacterial infections in stage III lymphedema, probably a result of the activity of the macrophages, stimulating the immune

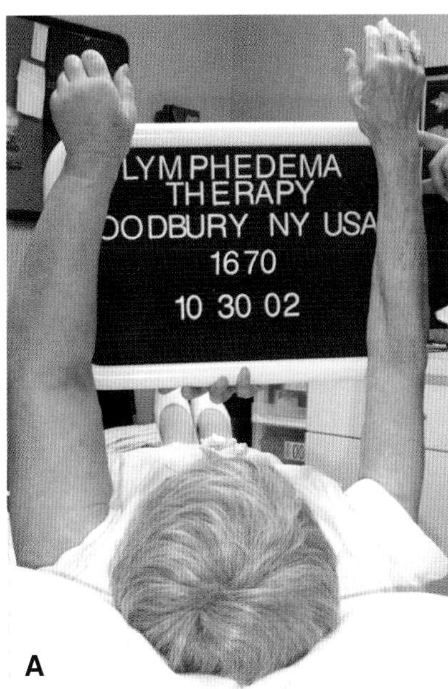


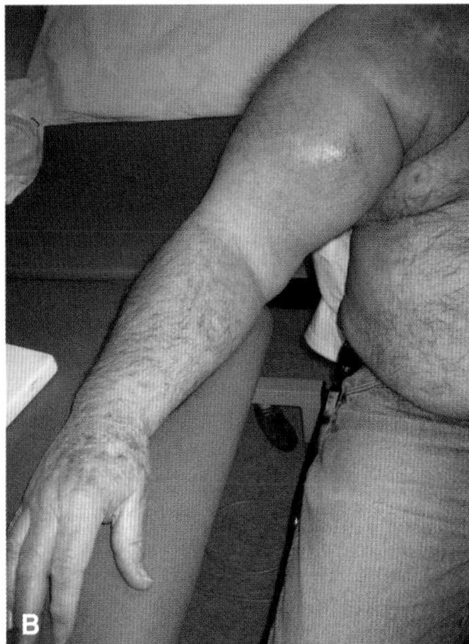

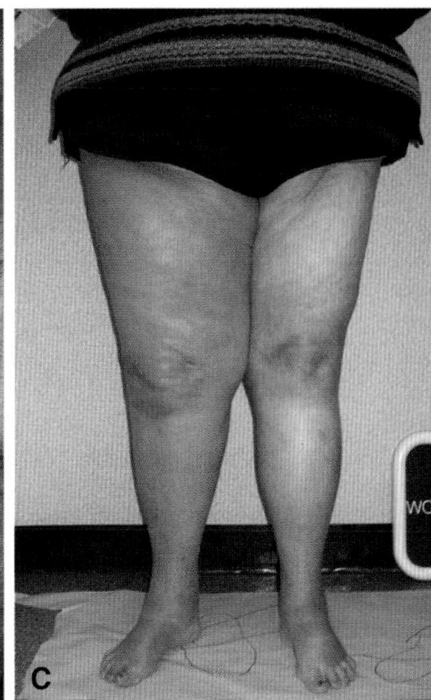

**FIGURE 13.18**

(A) Malignant lymphedema left upper extremity; edema is more marked in the upper arm. Note dusky color and shiny quality of the skin. Note obvious weakness in the left shoulder—the patient is unable to elevate the left arm as far as the right. She is status postlumpectomy and radiation treatment for breast cancer 2 years before sudden onset of painful proximal limb swelling with progressive weakness of the left shoulder. Recurrence of cancer in the axilla was diagnosed, and she was treated with chemotherapy. Lymphedema treatment was recommended in consultation with her oncologist and primary care provider to reduce pain and improve quality of life. (B) Malignant lymphedema right upper extremity secondary to recurrent melanoma of the right axilla. Note varices in the right upper arm and extension of the swelling into the right anterior axillary line and into the right chest wall. (C) Malignant lymphedema both lower extremities, right greater than left. Edema is more marked in the thigh than in the lower leg. Note dusky color and shiny quality of the skin of the right leg. This woman had recurrence of ovarian cancer with severe pain in the right hip, groin, and genital areas with marked genital edema. Not shown in this photo are the proximal varices that were present in the right proximal thigh extending over the inguinal crease—a sign that is frequently seen with recurrent cancer in the pelvis/abdomen. (In the case of malignant lymphedema of the upper extremity, varices are often seen in the proximal aspect of the upper arm extending into the chest wall.) (Courtesy Lymphedema Therapy, Woodbury, NY.)

response.[a] Current literature on the treatment of lymphedema does not recommend the use of pharmaceuticals.[36]

***Diuretics.*** Diuretics work well on sodium retention edemas but do not help lymphedema, yet they continue to be prescribed. Although it is true that taking large doses of diuretics will reduce total body fluid volume, these medications do not address the cause of the lymphedema (i.e., that the lymph load is exceeding the reduced lymph transport capacity). Furthermore, diuretics may remove the "water" component of the lymphatic fluid, further concentrating the extracellular protein in the tissues increasing fibrosis, and may lead to a rebound swelling. Moreover, long-term use of high-dose diuretics leaves the individual at great risk for developing electrolyte disturbances and renal impairments.

Experts agree that diuretics may be indicated in cases of malignant lymphedema. Individuals with comorbid conditions that require the use of diuretics, such as arterial hypertension, nephritic syndrome, or congestive heart disease, must be strongly advised to continue their medication and to consult with their primary physician/specialist with questions regarding their prescription.[22,59] If the treating therapist feels that a client is taking a diuretic inappropriately, this must be discussed with the referring physician only.

[a] References 22, 33, 29, 31, 59, 60, 110, 127, 141, and 182.

***Medications That Can Cause or Worsen Edema.*** Some nonsteroidal antiinflammatory drugs that are cyclooxygenase-2 inhibitors such as celecoxib (Celebrex) have a warning in the package insert about leg edema being a possible side effect. This has been clinically reported in several cases with lymphedema and arthritis; the individual with arthritis may experience an increase in edema when taking these drugs.[17]

Other commonly prescribed drugs such as amlodipine (Norvasc; used to treat hypertension) and rosiglitazone (Avandia; used to treat diabetes) can cause leg edema. Pregabalin (Lyrica) and ropinirole (Requip), drugs prescribed for neuropathy (used with diabetic neuropathy and shingles) and restless legs syndrome, may cause heart failure and limb edema. Many people do have neuropathy from chemotherapy (e.g., docetaxel [Taxotere] or platinum drugs) that is permanent and take these medications to manage the symptoms of neuropathy. Paclitaxel and docetaxel chemotherapy as well as some immunotherapies can cause edema in both lower extremities in patients with breast cancer and other cancers. This is not a true lymphedema, as lymphatic damage to the nodes of the inguinal region/pelvis rarely occurs, but the drugs can cause a capillary leak syndrome with severe ultrafiltration and edema.[7,20] Therapists[71] must be aware of this possible side effect with any of these medications and not assume that increased edema is a result of, for example, behavioral nonadherence or a problem with fit of a compression garment.

Clients may experience similar problems as new drugs for other conditions are introduced into the market. Even if the package does not warn of edema as a possible side effect, the therapist and client must observe carefully for any early signs or symptoms associated with the use of a new prescription. A useful resource for cancer drugs is www.oncolink.org.

**Surgery.** Surgery has been used to treat severe lymphedema in the past with limited success. It is still done today if an individual receives no benefit from conservative treatments or does not have access to these treatments. Numerous surgical approaches have been proposed to treat chronic lymphedema of the extremity.

***Microsurgery.*** Microsurgical procedures attempt to anastomose a lymph vessel or node with a vein or with another functioning lymph vessel or lymph node. The morbidity and mortality from these procedures can be significant. These procedures may fail soon after the surgery, leaving the individual with more superficial scarring that further blocks collateral lymph flow from the obstructed limb. Animal and cadaver studies continue investigating surgical techniques to resect tumors, reconstruct breast tissue, or perform liposuction[66,70] that will prevent venous occlusion and subsequent lymphatic dysfunction.

Vascularized lymph node transfer procedures involve transplanting lymph nodes or lymphatic tissue from a distant site to an affected limb. The indications include lymphedema that does not respond well to conservative treatment and chronic infections. Studies have also demonstrated beneficial effects for select individuals.[8,36,158] Most of the published reports, however, are based on small numbers of people, use different tools to measure lymphedema, and lack long-term follow-up. The risk of developing lymphedema at the sites distal to the harvest site is not reported.

***Debulking.*** Debulking procedures (e.g., the Charles operation) seek to physically remove the excess fibrosclerotic connective tissue. (These procedures are done rarely in the United States except in extreme cases; debulking is still done in other countries.) These operations create extensive longitudinal scars on the involved extremities or involve complete removal of all soft tissue down to the muscle fascia with split-thickness skin grafts to cover. Although these procedures attempt to address the size of the limb, they leave a poor cosmetic appearance, and they do not address the cause of the impairment, which is decreased lymph transport capacity. This problem is unchanged or exacerbated by these procedures; over time, without maintaining continuous compression on the limbs with compression bandages or garments, the limbs begin to swell again, often with disfiguring asymmetric lobules and severe skin changes (see Fig. 13.11).[29,59]

Brorson and colleagues,[21] working in Sweden, reported successful maintenance of limb volume reduction following liposuction to reduce chronic, fibrotic lymphedema. The majority of their cases were individuals with BCRL; they emphasized that these individuals must commit to wearing compression garments 24 hours daily to avoid recurrence of swelling.[21] In the United States, it has been reported that affected individuals were able to reduce or stop use of compression garments when a combination of suction lipectomy and vascularized lymph node transfers were used.[73]

***Reconstructive Breast Surgery.*** Lymphedema can develop as a complication of breast reconstructive surgery, though a recent review stated a lower association than with mastectomy alone or lumpectomy.[168] Many different procedures are available, ranging from the insertion of a tissue expander followed later by the insertion of a permanent saline implant to more extensive myocutaneous or free flap procedures (i.e., transverse rectus abdominal muscle flap, latissimus flap, deep inferior epigastric artery perforator flap, gluteal artery perforator flap, transverse upper gracilis flap) involving transplanting flaps of muscle and skin or tissue and skin with blood vessels to the breast area to form a more "natural" breast.[169] See complete discussion in Chapter 20.

The transverse rectus abdominal muscle flap, a pedicled flap, uses the contralateral rectus abdominis muscle and skin by tunneling it across the abdomen and up to the breast area while remaining attached to its blood supply in the abdomen. The deep inferior epigastric artery perforator flap, a free flap, moves soft tissue and skin to the breast area, where it is reconnected to a blood supply microsurgically, leaving the abdominal muscles intact. Lower abdominal free flap reconstruction can include transfer of nodes, and this has been reported to improve postoperative lymphatic function in the associated arm in limited series.[36] These procedures usually consist of two other minor procedures performed separately to tattoo a new areola and create a nipple.

These procedures involve extensive scarring in the lower abdomen extending from hip to hip, in addition to the individual scars on the breast area. The horizontal hip-to-hip scar effectively blocks a large area of collateral lymph flow from the ipsilateral axillary region through the lower abdomen to the superficial inguinal nodes and sometimes leads to abdominal edema above the scar. This area of collateral lymph drainage is then compromised for the treatment of ipsilateral upper extremity lymphedema that can develop after axillary dissection and mastectomy.

The latissimus flap procedure also creates a long transverse scar on the ipsilateral posterolateral thorax, effectively blocking a large area of collateral lymph drainage from the upper extremity to the ipsilateral inguinal nodes. This lymphatic pathway may be needed to treat a secondary upper extremity lymphedema with MLD. These procedures may lead to truncal lymphedema, which is often not recognized and sometimes discounted as psychosomatic and can cause considerable disability, impairment of function, and psychosocial distress.[52]

The scar from the gluteal artery perforator flap, which transfers tissue and skin from the buttock, is concealed in the gluteal fold and does not obstruct any lymphatic pathways for the upper extremity. The transverse upper gracilis flap transfers the small adductor gracilis muscle and skin, leaving a scar on the medial aspect of the proximal thigh. Although the scars from these procedures do not obstruct collateral lymphatic pathways, these procedures remove tissue/muscle from one side of the body (buttock and the medial thigh) that may require tissue reduction on the contralateral side to obtain acceptable cosmetic symmetry.169 It should be noted that with transfer of muscles in any of these procedures, weakness and muscle imbalances are common and are amenable to rehabilitation.[124,119]

**Prognosis.** Thanks to advances in surgery and chemotherapy and the emphasis on early detection, many more individuals are surviving cancer for many years, living and functioning well with limbs at risk for lymphedema. It is hoped that refinement in measurement tools as well as the inclusion of self-reported symptoms, which may be present well before a 2-cm difference between measurement sites can be recorded, will lead to earlier diagnosis and management of lymphedema. Prospective surveillance is strongly recommended for individuals at risk.[78]

Left untreated, lymphedema is a progressive disease; current surgical and pharmacologic approaches do not bring about a cure. Lymphedema is a lifelong, chronic condition but one that can be managed effectively or reversed to a large degree with proper intervention, client education, and regular follow-up care.

When scarring and lymphatic dysfunction are severe, treatment, such as MLD, cannot always restore normal cosmesis; however, it can successfully reduce some of the edema, leading to improved function and reduced risk for cellulitis.[94] It has been suggested that recurrent cellulitis may also be reduced by several of the surgical procedures described to address lymphedema, including vascularized lymph node transfer and lymphovenous anastomosis.[165]

In an example of improved function, in individuals with severe edema of the throat and neck after surgery and radiation for tongue cancer, lymphatic drainage can reduce the swelling enough to allow the person to discontinue use of a tracheotomy tube previously considered permanent. Some clients are able to eat solid foods again; others with severe periorbital and lower facial edema may be able to open their eyes and read and watch television again. Although these are not cures, they are great improvements in function that are important to individual quality of life.

## SPECIAL IMPLICATIONS FOR THE THERAPIST 13.2

### *Lymphedema*

It is critical to advise individuals who are at risk for lymphedema of the signs and symptoms of lymphedema and to educate them on risk-reduction strategies (https://lymphnet.org) to minimize stress on their marginal lymphatic systems (Fig. 13.19). Great care must be taken to avoid further overloading an already compromised area by the application of various modalities or ill-advised therapeutic exercises.

Stout and colleagues[176] proposed a prospective surveillance model to monitor and screen clients at risk for BCRL. They followed two groups of women. The prospective surveillance model (PSM) group was assessed preoperatively, including range of motion, muscle strength, limb volume, BMI, functional status, and level of physical activity. Subjects received education in lymphedema risk reduction and advice on postoperative activity. They returned for follow-up assessment of the above-mentioned parameters at 3-month intervals postoperatively for 1 year. Lymphedema onset would be identified at an early stage, potentially requiring less intensive treatment to manage it at the earlier stage.

The other group, the traditional model of care, assumed that the physician would identify women with lymphedema at the same average incidence rate (one-third of women over a 1-year period) and refer those women for treatment. Costs for treatment for each model were estimated, and the savings in the PSM group were considerable: the treatment cost was $636.19 in the PSM group compared with $3124.92 in the traditional-model-of-care group. Early identification and treatment minimize progression of lymphedema to a more advanced stage, potentially necessitating fewer treatment visits at a considerable cost savings.[167,176]

For clients who are free of lymphedema but receiving radiation therapy, the irradiated area may show signs such as blistering, discoloration, erythema (redness), or increased skin temperature changes. These are common acute skin changes associated with radiation that normally resolve within 2 to 3 weeks after radiation. If these skin changes do not resolve, they are of concern. The limb should be assessed for girth increases in the ipsilateral limb *during* radiation, and light compression (though not over tissue being irradiated) can be used if noted. Once radiation treatment is completed, any residual swelling can be addressed effectively.

Many people do not report edema during the interview and history-taking portions patient/client consultations unless it is severe. The client's leg may be four times the size of the normal leg, yet the individual will say the swelling "just started" or "only just started to bother me" or "never swelled like this." When clients are asked if they ever noticed even a little swelling in the foot or ankle, a mark when they removed socks or shoes, or swelling when it was hot or when they stood for a long time, they often report all of these events have occurred for years, "but it never bothered me" or "it was not really bad," and so on. This behavior is particularly common in heavier clients who do not have a perception of how overweight they are or really cannot see or reach their feet.

Lymphodynamic insufficiency is a concern when treating lymphedema. Clients, particularly those with primary lymphedema of the lower extremities, should be evaluated for abdominal and genital edema before undergoing any treatment to reduce the extremity lymphedema to avoid the complication of moving more fluid into an already overloaded abdominal area.

Throughout the episode of care, observe and/or lightly compress the areas adjacent to the lymphedematous limb or region (the ipsilateral buttock, suprapubic/genital areas, ipsilateral breast/lateral trunk, or contralateral lower extremity in a case with pelvic/abdominal node obstruction) to ensure that treatment of the peripheral lymphedema does not create lymphedema in adjacent lymph drainage areas.

An increased risk of this fluid movement may occur when using gradient compression pump therapy

# Healthy Habits for Patients at Risk for Lymphedema

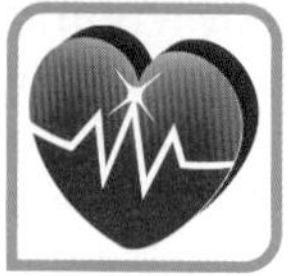

### Healthy Lifestyle:

*A healthy diet and exercise are important for overall good health.*

- Maintain optimal weight through a healthy diet and exercise to significantly lower risk of lymphedema.
- Gradually build up the duration and intensity of any activity or exercise. Review the Exercise Position Paper.*
- Take frequent rest periods during activity to allow for recovery.
- Monitor the at-risk area during and after activity for change in size, shape, tissue, texture, soreness, heaviness, or firmness.

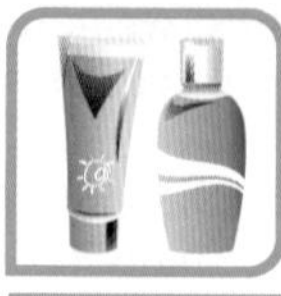

### Skin Care:

*Make sure that your skin is in good condition.*

- Keep your at-risk body part clean and dry.
- Apply moisturizer daily to prevent chapping/chafing of skin.
- Pay attention to nail care and do not cut cuticles.
- Protect exposed skin with sunscreen and insect repellent.
- Use care with razors to avoid nicks and skin irritation.

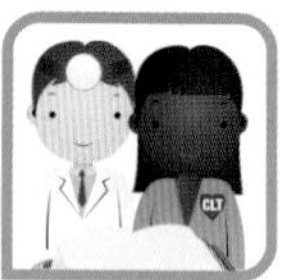


### Medical Check-ups:

*Find a certified lymphedema therapist (CLT).**

- Review your individual situation, get screened for lymphedema, and discuss risk factors with your CLT.
- Ask your CLT or healthcare professional if compression garments for air travel and strenuous activity are appropriate for you.
- If a compression garment is recommended, make sure it is properly fitted and you understand the wear, care, and replacement guidelines.
- Set a follow-up schedule based on your needs with your CLT.
- Report any changes in your at-risk body part to your CLT.

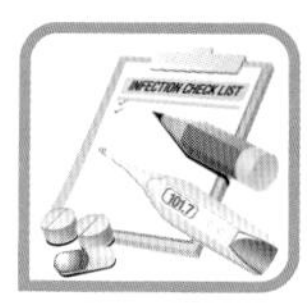


### Infection Education:

*Know the signs of infection and what to do if you suspect you have one.*

- Signs of infection: rash, itching, redness, pain, increased skin temperature, increased swelling, fever, or flu-like symptoms.
- If any of these symptoms occur, contact your healthcare professional immediately for early treatment of possible infection.
- If a scratch or puncture to your skin occurs, wash it with soap and water, apply topical antibiotics, and observe for signs of infection.
- Keep a small first aid kit with you when traveling.

## TRY TO AVOID POSSIBLE TRIGGERS

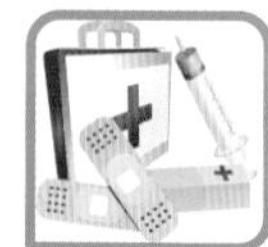

**Injury or Trauma**

- Wear gloves while doing activities that may cause skin injury (e.g., washing dishes, gardening, using chemicals like detergent).
- Try to avoid punctures (e.g., injections and blood draws).

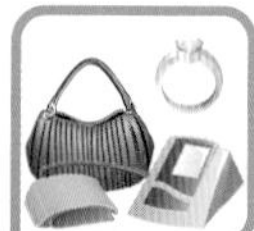

**Limb Constriction**

- Wear loose jewelry and clothing.
- Avoid carrying a heavy bag or purse over the at-risk limb.
- Try to avoid blood pressure cuffs on the at-risk limb.

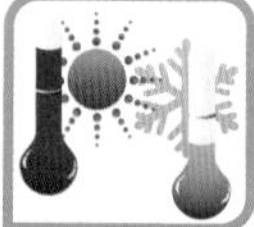

**Extreme Temperatures**

- Avoid exposure to extreme cold, which can cause rebound swelling or chapping of skin.
- Avoid prolonged (> 15 min.) exposure to heat, particularly hot tubs and saunas.

**Prolonged Inactivity**

At-risk for leg lymphedema?

- Avoid prolonged standing or sitting by moving and changing position throughout the day.
- Wear properly fitted footwear and hosiery.

*Please Note:* These guidelines are meant to help reduce your risk of developing lymphedema and are NOT prevention guidelines. Because there is little research about risk reduction, many of these use a common-sense approach based on the body's anatomy and knowledge gained from decades of clinical experience by experts in the field. Risk reduction should always be individualized by a certified lymphedema therapist and healthcare professional.

*To review the NLN's other position papers, visit www.lymphnet.org.

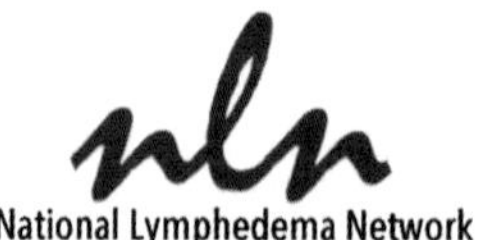


**FIGURE 13.19**

**Healthy habits for patients at risk for lymphedema.** (From the National Lymphedema Network.)

(intermittent pneumatic compression [IPC]) to treat extremity lymphedema. See Compression Pumps: Intermittent Pneumatic Compression and A Therapist's Thoughts: Intermittent Pneumatic Compression below.

### Orthopedic Lymphedema

Postsurgical lymphedema may occur after, for example, total knee or total hip replacement.[39] If the individual is poorly mobile and had some degree of edema in the legs preoperatively (often attributed to arthritis but may represent chronic venous insufficiency or a true lymphedema), the increase in edema postoperatively is often considered the normal sequelae for the procedure. Important loss of time in rehabilitation occurs for these people who are in pain and experience decreased range of motion and strength because of the increasing edema.

When the edema is properly reduced and maintained, rehabilitation can progress quite well, provided that the therapist remembers the concept of limiting lymph load so as not to exceed the individual lymph transport capacity.

This clinical skill comes with experience and constant monitoring in the early stages of activity to assess which activities increase the person's subjective feeling of congestion and fullness in the affected areas. Heat modalities will increase superficial vasodilation and ultrafiltration, increasing edema, and therefore should be used with great caution. A past history of multiple abdominal or thoracic surgeries, vein stripping or sclerotherapy, and liposuction in the legs should remind the evaluating therapist to carefully assess signs and symptoms of lymphedema. A limb that was perceived as "less than perfect" can become a severely swollen, distorted limb, psychologically devastating to the individual whose appearance was of paramount importance.

### Evaluation

When evaluating an individual with suspected lymphedema (or an individual with unexplained edema of an extremity or extremities, trunk, or head and neck), cardiac, renal, hepatic, thyroid, and arteriovenous disease must be ruled out medically. The results of specific tests used to diagnose the edema should be reviewed.

Functional scans for lymphatics that are useful to differentiate between venous edema, lipedema, and lymphedema have already been discussed. Remember that a combination of these conditions can coexist. The intervention of an experienced lymphologist is needed in cases complicated by genetic lymphangiodysplasias.[22,59,60,110]

### Importance of Past Medical History

A detailed and complete medical history and clinical examination are almost always the only information needed to diagnose uncomplicated lymphedema.[61] A detailed history must be taken, including past medical history, especially cancer, and all surgeries; information about swelling including onset and progression; tests conducted to evaluate and diagnose the condition; vein stripping; bypass stents; insertion or removal of central lines and ports; and all medications. An accurate history of infections in the affected areas, how these were treated, and how they responded to treatment is also critical. A chronologic review of the person's previous treatments and/or interventions for lymphedema and the response to treatment is important.

It is essential to keep in mind that secondary lymphedema can be the result of an orthopedic surgery or trauma that further disrupted marginal lymphatics. Individuals with extensive acute or chronic edema after trauma or surgery should be evaluated for lymphedema. Early intervention and management of this type of lymphedema can significantly minimize the complications of advanced, untreated lymphedema mentioned earlier.

In the case of a known history of cancer, lymphedema that does not respond to proper treatment may be caused by metastases blocking lymphatic flow. In such a case, treatment may result in a reduced response compared with what is expected when treating a nonmalignant lymphedema. The therapist must remain alert to the difference in clinical presentation at the outset of treatment as discussed earlier and be alert to a change in response during treatment.

### Clinical Assessment

Clinical evaluation includes a detailed description of skin integrity. This description should include the presence of edema or fibrosis on the trunk quadrants, the head and neck, and the limbs; location and condition of scars, fibrotic areas, and open wounds; evidence of healed ulcerations; and location of papilloma, warts, leaking edema, and/or subcutaneous fibrosis; presence of folliculitis; location of a previous radiation field; and presence of palpable nodes in the axillary or inguinal areas. The presence of a fungal infection, presence or absence of pitting and subcutaneous fibrosis, presence or history of folliculitis, and palpable nodes in the axilla or inguinal areas should also be noted.

Signs and symptoms of cording or axillary web syndrome may be present in individuals after axillary dissection. The therapist may palpate a firm cordlike structure extending from the axilla to the forearm through the antecubital fossa or even to the wrist. The affected individual reports a pulling sensation/pain when attempting to elevate the arm. These cords limit mobility of the shoulder and can significantly impair activities of daily living.[62,135,163,184] Experts debate whether these are venous or lymphatic in origin or a combination of both structures, possibly caused by contracture of these vessels after being resected during axillary dissection.[194] ALND and younger age were reported as risk factors in one study.[135] There was no association with BMI, but BMI may be associated with a higher risk of lymphedema.

The presence or absence of pain, paresthesias, or other sensory impairments is documented. Using a visual analog scale of 0 to 10 is the easiest documentation for this assessment.

### Role of Photography in Documentation

Photographs are helpful to detail changes in skin color, appearance, and size of the limb. A digital camera is very helpful to document progress. A photo release should be obtained from the client, and images should be stored securely; it is important to avoid identification of the client per Health Insurance Portability and Accountability Act guidelines. Subsequent photos can document improvement and encourage patients/clients greatly, as it is easy to forget how involved a limb was when it is treated and improving. These images are also helpful to assist in obtaining additional insurance coverage if required. Volumetric measurements calculated from circumferential measurements taken at set intervals on the limbs have become the standard in clinical settings. Water displacement for volumetric assessment is the gold standard but is impractical in clinical settings.[40,142] In some research and clinical settings, perometry, a computer-generated limb volume, is used. The perometer, an optoelectric device, calculates limb volume with infrared light that transects the limb every 3 mm. The perometer, while accurate and a valid measure, is very expensive (>$20,000) and not practical in the typical clinic setting. There are no standardized measurement tools for truncal or head and neck lymphedema.

Photographs taken in fixed positions from a standardized height and distance are helpful to detail asymmetry and changes. Hemicircumferences of the trunk taken at intervals measured from the floor to specific heights can give a relative difference in volume if the swelling is unilateral. There are some reports of individual measurement strategies used to document head and neck edema.[48]

### Documenting Functional Impairments

Careful documentation of the individual's functional impairments related to the lymphedema is key to evaluating the outcome of any treatment that is recommended.[50] Many individuals with chronic lymphedema have "learned to live with it" and often do not consider lymphedema as a "limitation." Tactful questioning can uncover the many compensating mechanisms employed to get through the day.[69] Outcome measures to screen and assess for the functional limitations associated with lymphedema have been described.[122,189] Other commonly used outcome measures include the Disabilities of Arm, Shoulder and Hand (DASH) score, Quick DASH score, and Penn Shoulder Score for upper extremity function in breast cancer. A recently validated outcome specific to lymphedema of both upper and lower extremities is the Lymphedema Life Impact Scale (LLIS). Lymphedema and lymphedema treatment impact quality of life in many domains other than functional, including psychologic, economic, and social. The therapist and client need to collaborate as a team to develop a strategy that affords the client the best outcome in all domains.[4,99,150,151]

### Early Recognition of Lymphedema

A preoperative screening evaluation should record baseline measurements of both operative and nonoperative extremities. Circumferential measurements taken with a flexible tape measure are the easiest, most economical measurements to take. These measurements assess the shape and contour of a limb more accurately than a volumetric measure; however, volumetric measures are a more precise measure of total volume of a limb.

Volumes from circumferential measurements have a high validity compared with volumes from water displacement, but they are slightly larger.[183] Tissue texture, unusual limb asymmetries or contours, skin color, strength, and functional range of motion are recorded.

Perometry, tonometry, and bioimpedance also have been used to quantify lymphedema.[81] A tonometer measures tissue compliance, and the degree of compression provides an assessment of tissue fibrosis.[23] There is minimal evidence that tonometry is reliable for use in lymphedema.[81]

Bioimpedance is another noninvasive technique that measures total body fluid and extracellular fluid in extremities by measuring the resistance of various tissues to the flow of an electrical current. It detects very small differences in the extracellular volumes of arms and legs, suggesting that this technique may be able to diagnose lymphedema in its first stage, before the onset of visible swelling and discomfort.[43,45,170] It is not a useful technique in individuals with bilateral limb involvement.[40]

There is still no consensus on what amount of limb volume change defines lymphedema. However, lymphedema is not defined only by a change in limb volume. Sensations of limb heaviness, tightness, soreness, fatigue, and pain accompany subtle changes in limb volume that may or may not be readily detectable in the early stages of lymph stasis that occur on the continuum from latent lymphedema (stage 0) to where obvious pitting edema is present in stage I.

Further study is needed to examine these factors and their relationship to the progression of lymphedema.[3,69,151] Any sensory abnormalities or neurologic impairments should be noted. Risk-reduction strategies with emphasis on proper skin hygiene and recognition of the early signs of lymphedema and secondary infection are reviewed with the individual.

A list of resources including whom to contact should a problem arise (and when available) is provided to the individual. Discussion of individual activities of daily living and brief task analysis of job and home can point to possible problem areas that may need to be modified to reduce the risk of triggering lymphedema from overuse of the postoperative extremity or reduce potential exposure to trauma, chemicals, excessive heat, or repetitive tasks.

### Physical Therapist's Intervention

Regardless of the treatment approach or training of the therapist, several overall components of the following interventions may be modified, according to each individual client:

- MLD
- Multilayer short-stretch compression bandaging
- Exercise
- Compression garments
- Compression pumps (IPC)
- Education (e.g., basic anatomy, skin and nail care, self-MLD, self-bandaging, garment care, infection management)
- Psychologic and emotional support

These components make up a multifactorial treatment approach referred to as *comprehensive lymphedema management* that is similar in concept, though may vary slightly in detail, for all the combined lymphedema therapy approaches and is carried out in two distinct phases: the initial intensive intervention phase and the optimization (maintenance) phase. Different countries use different acronyms for this treatment approach; comprehensive lymphedema management is sometimes referred to as *complete decongestive therapy (CDT)*, *combined decongestive physiotherapy (CDP)*, *complex lymphedema/lymphatic therapy (CLT)*, *decongestive lymphatic therapy (DLT)*, or *complex physical therapy (CPT)*. In the United States, the more common usage is CDT or CLT.

### Initial Intensive Intervention Phase

During this phase of treatment, daily intervention requiring maximum adherence is often necessary to disperse lymph fluids through the superficial lymphatic vessel network and to prevent congestion of fluid in areas proximal to the compression bandages. Components of treatment include the following:

1. Meticulous skin care and treatment of any infections: This may also include careful moisturizing, débridement of ulcers, and wound care.
2. Manual lymphatic drainage (MLD): Variations exist in specific stroke and pressure techniques such as Vodder, Leduc, Földi, and Casley-Smith; however, all schools of thought work to decongest the trunk quadrants first before addressing the lymphedematous extremity/areas, decongesting the proximal portions of the limb first and progressively working distally to the end of the limb with the direction of flow always toward the trunk. Special strokes are available for fibrotic areas.
3. The affected limb or limbs are then bandaged with multilayer short-stretch compression bandages during the initial treatment phase and fitted with a compression garment/bandage alternative with a reduced, plateaued volume.
4. Each individual is instructed in specific self-care, self-MLD techniques, and exercises that are modified for the individual. The basic principle is to enhance the lymphatic pumping and collateral lymph flow from the involved or impaired areas into adjacent, normally functioning areas in the trunk with return to the central circulation via the right lymphatic duct and the thoracic duct.[14,15,62,101]

### Optimization (Maintenance) Phase

During this second phase, the individual home program is finalized, continuing with the components of comprehensive lymphedema management from the initial intervention phase now modified for each person according to the clinical presentation and individual needs. During this phase, customized pressure gradient elastic support garments may replace compression bandaging when the limb is normal or close to normal. Inelastic compression garments with Velcro closures are an option for night compression or for individuals who cannot manage elastic compression garments or prefer the ease of Velcro for donning and doffing.[99]

### Components of Comprehensive Lymphedema Therapy

Considerable advances were made in the treatment of lymphedema after Kubik's detailed description of the regional anatomy of the lymphatic system published in 1985 (see Fig. 13.8). Földi and Földi reported the successful results of their techniques, referred to as *CDP*, documenting 50% reductions in lymphedema in individuals after a 4-week course of daily CDP. Of those individuals, 50% maintained that reduction by adhering to a home program of self-MLD, exercises, and continuous compression on the affected limb using compression garments or bandages.[56,58]

Casley-Smith and Casley-Smith[29] presented results of another conservative treatment, referred to as *CPT*, reporting reductions of more than 60% in 618 lymphedematous limbs.

### Manual Lymph Drainage

Von Winiwarter first introduced the concepts of MLD in 1882. These techniques were improved by Vodder in the 1930s, but were originally applied to improve the functioning of normal lymphatics.[192] Moreover, the reductions in edema obtained with MLD in those early years could not be maintained because of a lack of adequate compression bandages and garments. The Vodder techniques were modified by Asdonk and Leduc and later by Földi and Casley-Smith.[27] MLD, a gentle, manual treatment technique consisting of several basic strokes, is designed to improve the absorption of interstitial protein and fluid and transport activity of intact lymph vessels by providing mild mechanical stretches on the wall of the lymph capillaries and collectors. Some proponents of MLD advise against the use of the word massage (e.g., manual lymphatic massage or lymphatic drainage massage) because the term massage means "to knead." MLD does not have kneading elements and is generally applied suprafascially and with gentle stretch, whereas massage is usually applied to subfascial tissues with deep kneading.[59]

The major contributors to the management techniques have developed training programs to teach their methods. The Lymphology Association of North America (LANA) (www.clt-lana.org), a nonprofit organization composed of physicians, nurses, physical and occupational therapists, massage therapists, and researchers who specialize in lymphedema management, has developed standards for lymphedema therapists in the United States to educate the American medical community to the training and treatment considered to be adequate to effectively treat lymphedema. This will help ensure access to adequate treatment for all individuals living with lymphedema. The Education Committee of the International Lymphoedema Framework Project (www.lympho.org) continues to work with partner countries to determine core concepts in lymphology critical in health professional education at both the basic and the advanced levels. The United States has representation on this committee by members of the American Lymphedema Framework Project (www.alfp.org). The American Physical Therapy Association (APTA) (www.apta.org) through the Academy of Oncologic Physical Therapy also offers training in the management of peripheral edema.

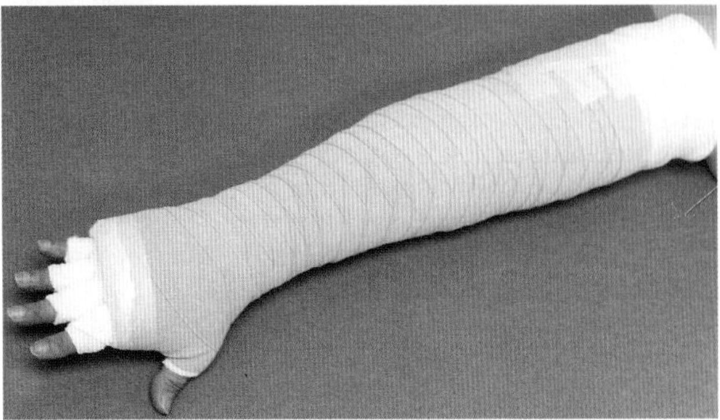

**FIGURE 13.20**

**Example of multilayer short-stretch compression bandaging of the upper extremity.** (Courtesy Lymphedema Therapy, Woodbury, NY.)

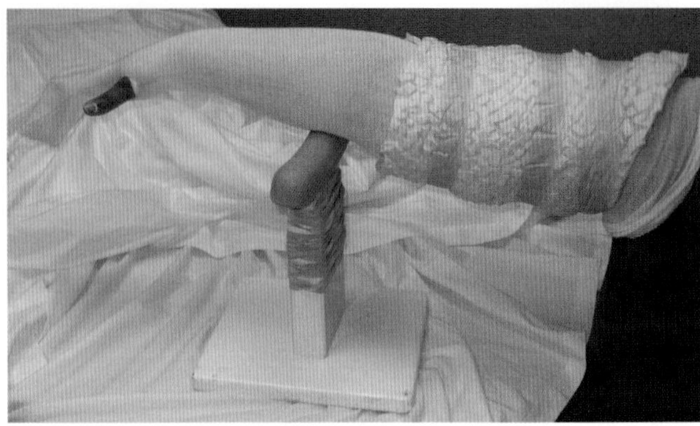

**FIGURE 13.21**

**Example of therapist-made custom foam chip pads that are placed under the compression layer to soften fibrosis and reshape the limb.** (Courtesy Lymphedema Therapy, Woodbury, NY.)

## Compression Bandaging

### Short-Stretch Compression Bandages

Short-stretch compression bandages applied to the lymphedematous extremity after lymphatic drainage help maintain the edema reduction achieved through lymph drainage (Fig. 13.20). Short-stretch bandages have minimal recoil because they do not contain elastic fibers and stretch only 30% to 40% of their unstretched length. They have a low resting pressure (i.e., when the bandaged limb is at rest, they exert minimal pressure on the skin), avoiding any skin ischemia or breakdown. Conversely, they have a high working pressure. When the muscles in the bandaged limb contract against the short-stretch bandage, the bandage provides a semirigid container, creating an increase in interstitial tissue fluid pressure, an increase in lymph uptake, and increased pumping of the collecting lymphatics. Consequently, these bandages are comfortable when the limb is at rest and greatly increase the transport of lymph when the limb is in motion.[46]

The effects of low-stretch compression bandaging alone and in combination with MLD can create an additional 11% reduction in arm lymphedema when MLD is added to compression bandaging.[87] An additional 20% limb volume reduction was demonstrated in a group of women with BCRL when MLD was added to compression bandaging.[89] The same benefit was reported in a randomized controlled trial of 50 women with BCRL.[120] In a trial of patients with BCRL comparing low-stretch compression bandaging with an adjustable low-stretch bandage alternative garment in two groups who both received MLD before application, the volume reduction achieved was significant and similar in both groups immediately and at 3 months after treatment ended.[145]

### Long-Stretch Compression Bandages

Long-stretch compression bandages, with elastic fibers, have a low working pressure and a high resting pressure; that is, they are not very effective in increasing the transport of lymph when the bandaged limb is moving, and they can become dangerously tight when the limb is at rest, creating a tourniquet effect on the limb at rest. These are not the bandages of choice for individuals with lymphedema.

Proper bandaging techniques use sufficient padding materials including cotton padding and foams of varying thicknesses over bony prominences and to even out unusual limb contours to ensure that a gradient of pressure is achieved. This gradient must be greatest at the most distal point of the involved limb, gradually decreasing as the bandage layers reach the proximal portion of the limb. This gradient is particularly critical in limbs where lobules, large balloon-like areas separated by a deep skinfold or ridge, occur, often in the vicinity of a joint (usually on the medial side of the limb).

### Maintaining a Proper Compression Gradient

According to the Laplace law, the pressure applied by the bandage is inversely proportional to the radius of the limb segment bandaged; that is, the smaller the radius of the limb segment, the greater is the pressure applied by the bandage. For example, when bandaging an upper extremity with significant edema in the dorsum of the hand but a narrow wrist relative to the hand and forearm, the wrist area must be sufficiently padded to increase the radius (of the wrist limb segment) to be larger than the radius of the hand. If this is not done, the bandaging may act as a tourniquet to the hand.[26]

A proper compression gradient achieved with short-stretch bandages can increase tissue pressure, improve the activity of the lymphangion, and increase the efficiency of the muscle pump in the involved limb. It not only maintains the reduction in the involved limb that was achieved through lymph drainage, but it also can increase that reduction by enhancing the muscle pump during activity.[116]

In addition, a layer of crafted foam pieces and/or the application of varying densities of foam pieces or "chips" encased in adhesive gauze, stockinette, or fabric may be applied under the compression bandages (Fig. 13.21). Foam helps to improve comfort, recontour the limb, and soften fibrotic tissue.

Compression bandaging is usually worn 23/24 hours 7 days/week during the initial intensive phase of treatment, removed only for bathing, skin care, and lymph drainage and immediately reapplied. After the initial treatment phase, the individual is able to maintain adequate compression during the day with a compression garment (elastic or low-stretch with Velcro closures). Getting the individual to understand that they must also maintain some form of nighttime compression is the key to success in the optimization phase of the program, as blood circulation and the tendency to swell are constant.[30,93,94,99]

Short-stretch bandages, because of their low resting pressure and customized fit, provide the optimal nighttime compression. The drawback to these bandages is that self-bandaging is time-consuming and difficult for individuals with limited mobility, obese individuals, and individuals with a very large, heavy limb. Many bandage alternatives are now available for this purpose that use various fabric sleeves/leggings with foam padding and Velcro closures for easier application and rely on the LaPlace law for their effect as well. Results of one clinical study reported that individuals who wore their compression garments day and night maintained their reductions during the optimization phase.[15]

No skin problems or tissue breakdown have resulted from wearing the garments to bed. It should be noted, however, that most of the involved individuals had custom-made, low-elasticity, or inelastic garments that were not measured and fitted until the involved limbs were fully reduced (plateaued in reduction).[15]

### Exercise Guidelines

Lymph transport capacity can be impaired in 27% to 49% of individuals after breast cancer treatment.[97] The exact pathology and etiology of BCRL is thought to be multifactorial and not as simple as a "stop-cock" effect. The stop-cock effect is like putting a cork in a bottle. Various factors such as cutting lymph vessels and nodes have the stopcock effect of impairing flow of lymph fluid. Venous impairment/impingement, the action of inflammatory mediators, and tissue changes related to late effects of radiation are other factors that may contribute to the development of BCRL because of this effect. Exercise helps mediate this effect.

Impairment in venous circulation from chronic venous insufficiency or surgery and/or radiation treatment may contribute significantly to impaired fluid transport in the at-risk or affected limb.[97,172] In a cohort of 365 subjects with lymphedema and suspected presence of mixed lymphatic and venous edema, Szuba and colleagues[180] found clinically relevant venous stasis (on evaluation of 35 radiocontrast venograms) in 5 of 7 subjects with edema of the upper extremity and venous occlusion in 2 of 7 subjects with upper extremity edema. This situation of a mixed edema with lymphatic and venous components is common in morbidly obese people as discussed earlier. Again, exercise can be beneficial in facilitating decompression.

Exercise activates muscle groups and joints in the affected extremity. Combining a specific exercise program for each client with the use of sufficient compression facilitates the process of decongestion by using the natural pumping effect of the muscles to increase lymph flow while preventing limb refilling.[37]

Most clinicians experienced in lymphedema treatment agree on basic guidelines for remedial exercise. These exercises are specifically designed to encourage lymphatic flow following the same concepts used for MLD: encourage proximal flow first—that is, work the trunk/neck muscles first, followed by the limb girdle muscles, working from proximal to distal on the limb and finishing with trunk exercises and deep abdominal breathing to enhance flow through the thoracic duct.[24,59]

It is prudent to exercise with a compression garment or compression bandages on the involved limbs to enhance the variation in total tissue pressure to facilitate increased lymph flow. In addition, therapists must remember that lymph load must not exceed lymph transport capacity, or the exercise or activity will increase the lymphedema or possibly trigger lymphedema in a client with limbs at risk for lymphedema.[159-161]

Activities such as brisk walking, cycling, swimming, cross country skiing, and Tai chi are thought to be lower-risk activities.[59] Many activities or sports can be resumed after developing lymphedema, but the key to return to activity is gradual resumption while wearing effective compression. The mantra of the Physical Activity and Lymphedema Trial (PAL) trial was "start low, progress slow."[159-161]

### Weight Training

There is substantial current research evidence that exercise is safe in clients with breast cancer.[96,159-161] There is minimal evidence in other lymphedema populations.[96,91]

Schmitz and colleagues[159] followed 141 breast cancer survivors (previously diagnosed with lymphedema) who participated in a supervised, twice-weekly weight-lifting program for 1 year (PAL trial). Participants all wore compression garments on their affected arm and hand during the trial. Participants received proper instruction in small groups to ensure that they performed proper warm-up, weight-training, cooldown, and stretching exercises. Throughout the course of the study, participants exercised with constant access to fitness trainers when needed. The importance of individualized instruction and proper progression of any exercise program cannot be overemphasized. Lymphedema did not worsen with exercise, and participants reported improvement in arm and hand symptoms, reduction in exacerbations of lymphedema, and improved upper extremity strength.[159,161,171]

A contemporaneous study was published in 2010, following 154 breast cancer survivors (from 1 to 5 years postoperatively) *at risk* for lymphedema who participated in a similar supervised weight-lifting exercise program.[160] The reported incidence of lymphedema during the trial period was no greater for the exercise group than for the control group (11% exercise group versus 17% control group and in women with five or more lymph nodes removed 7% exercise group versus 22% control group). This suggests that weight lifting does not increase the risk for breast cancer–related lymphedema.[160]

Turner and colleagues[186] followed 10 women after breast cancer treatment for 3 months after they participated in a moderate-intensity exercise program consisting of mild strengthening exercises and cardiovascular exercises. Participants reported a decrease in fatigue and improved quality of life with no precipitation or exacerbation of lymphedema.[186] Courneya and associates[44] conducted a multisite randomized controlled trial in Canada including 242 individuals treated for breast cancer who were beginning adjuvant chemotherapy. One group ($n$ = 82) received standard care, another group ($n$ = 82) participated in supervised resistance exercises, and a third group ($n$ = 78) participated in supervised aerobic exercise for the 17 weeks that they were undergoing the chemotherapy. Cancer-related fatigue, quality of life, and lymphedema were measured. Neither aerobic nor resistance exercise was shown to trigger lymphedema in the study groups.[44] Further studies are needed in this area.[96]

### Compression Garments

Elastic compression garments were never designed to treat and reduce lymphedema but rather were meant to maintain a limb that had already been reduced. Because lymphedema damages the elastic fibers of the skin, compression of the affected area is necessary to prevent reaccumulation of the lymphatic fluid.

Originally, compression garments were engineered to treat venous edema and were meant to be applied to the edema-free extremity before the individual got out of bed after a night of limb elevation. The same premise should apply to the lymphedematous extremity—that is, the edema must be reduced through treatment for the garment to work effectively because gravity does not have the same overnight effect on most stages of lymphedema.

Care must be given to the fit and function of the myriad fabrics, compression grades, and styles available, with proper instruction in donning and doffing. In addition, realistic expectations concerning these garments are a must to achieve client success and comfort.[15,33,52,60,113]

Clients need to understand that blood moves into the affected extremity with each beat of the heart, approximately 60 to 70 times/min, 60 min/h, 24 h/day. When there is obstruction to lymph flow back to the central circulation at a regional lymph node basin, the only way to assist that flow is to apply external pressure over the skin of the affected extremity on a continuous (day and night) basis.

Elastic compression garments are a means to achieve this, but they are only one component of a total self-care program meant for daytime usage. However, they are an essential component. For example, a client with lymphedema in the fingers, hand, and arm will not achieve good control of the lymphedema by wearing a wrist-to-axilla compression sleeve without a glove or gauntlet. In fact, wearing a compression sleeve without a glove may actually cause edema in the hand or worsen edema if present. Removing the compression sleeve may allow some of the hand swelling to shift into the forearm and make the hand appear better, but that is not a solution to the problem—a well-fitting compression glove designed to be worn with the compression sleeve is a more effective solution.

Designing, measuring, and fitting compression garments is as much art as it is science. What works for one client may be inappropriate for another. Experience, knowledge of the variety of garments available, and honest client/therapist communication lead to the best outcomes. Regular follow-up to evaluate the efficacy of the compression garments is important to determine when modifications in style or compression are needed to optimize client adherence.

### Education and Home Program

Education begins on the first day of therapy intervention and is an essential part of both phases of the program. Lymphedema is a chronic condition, and the affected individual must "own" it and understand how to self-manage it. Simple analogies such as the traffic jam analogy presented earlier can help clients gain an understanding of the physiologic reasons why they are doing what they are doing for each component of therapy. It is this understanding that helps them carry through on discharge into their home program. The success of any combined lymphedema treatment program hinges on adherence with the home maintenance program.[150]

Client education includes instruction in the basic anatomy and physiology of the lymphatic system, pathophysiology of the individual's particular lymphedema, individual self-drainage pathways to follow during the self-care program, basic principles of the individual exercise program, risk of infection and how to reduce that risk, wear and care for compression bandages or garments, and individual skin care regimens.

Hands-on instruction in self-bandaging techniques requires practice and patience but is essential for the individual (or those able to assist them) to master. In the home maintenance phase after initial intensive treatment, consistent use of compression, skin care, and risk reduction are three of the most important components of the home program. Psychologic support, including support groups, is another critical component of a comprehensive lymphedema management program.

### Importance of Adherence

Maintaining reductions of lymphedema has been documented with adherence to a home program of skin care, exercise with self–lymphatic drainage, and compression garment wear. Significant decreases in microlymphatic hypertension (measured by fluorescence microlymphography and lymph capillary pressure measurement), decreases in extremity lymphedema, and improvements in lymphoscintigraphic findings have been reported after a course of CDT.[64,82] Individuals with less than 100% adherence to their home program lose a portion of their reductions (Figs. 13.22, 13.23, and 13.24).[15,94,98]

### Compression Pumps: Intermittent Pneumatic Compression

Historically in the United States a person with lymphedema was given a prescription for a compression garment and range-of-motion exercises. In some cases, treatment with a pneumatic compression pump (also known as an IPC) was prescribed as the edema progressed. The degree and intensity of this treatment varied greatly because of the lack of verified, long-term

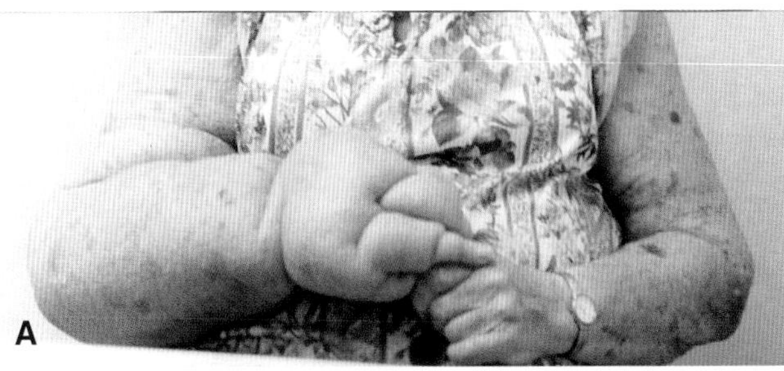


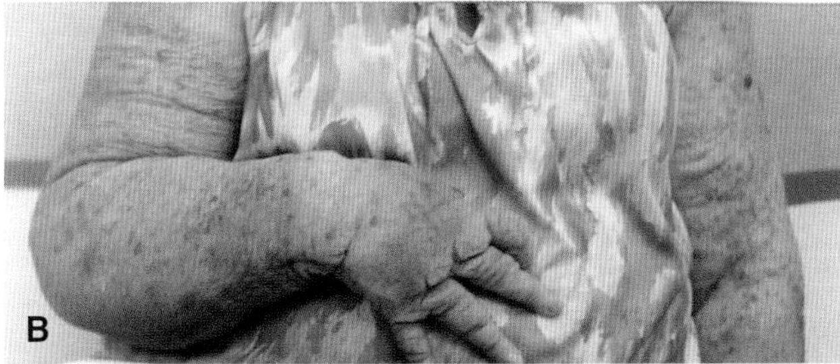


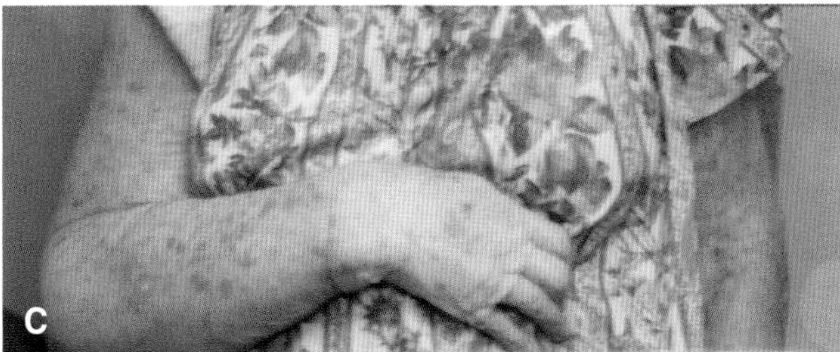


**FIGURE 13.22**

(A) Before treatment, an 84-year-old woman with severe, elephantitic lymphedema of her right upper extremity for 20 years secondary to surgery and radiation treatment for breast cancer 30 years ago. Her right hand was essentially nonfunctional. She needed assistance in all areas of activities of daily living. (B), After 20 complete decongestive therapy (CDT) treatments, she achieved a 77% reduction in lymphedema in her right upper extremity and began to use her right hand functionally again. (C) Four years after CDT treatment. She follows through with a home exercise program, skin care, and compression garment wear. She has not had any additional treatments other than the initial 20 CDT treatments, and she has improved her reduction to almost 100% in the years after treatment. She is more independent in activities of daily living and can even don her compression glove and sleeve with minimal assistance. (Courtesy Lymphedema Therapy, Woodbury, NY.)

scientific studies proving the efficacy of one treatment over another.

Treatment with pneumatic compression consisted of placing the involved limb into a rubber sleeve that inflated with air from the pump, squeezing the limb, and moving fluid proximally toward the trunk. Over time, the pumps became more technologically sophisticated, allowing for a gradient pressure from distal to proximal and allowing for intermittent application of pressure.[53] Olszewski and colleagues[136] studied the effect of applying IPC on the movement of lymph in 15 individuals with lower extremity lymphedema caused by obstruction. They found that IPC moved an isotope in lymph that remained in functioning lymphatics and in tissue fluid in the interstitial spaces toward the inguinal region, but lymph did not cross the inguinal crease into the pelvis/abdomen. It collected at the proximal thigh.[137] Pumps available in single or multichamber models can apply pressures from 10 to 100 mm Hg; the walls of the superficial lymphatics may collapse with greater than 60 mm Hg pressure.[16,25,51,57] A consensus document stated that a wide range of compression from 5 to 10 mm Hg up to greater than 120 mm Hg may be effective in venous and lymphatic diseases.[139] However, other research states that it is prudent to use IPC at lower pressures to reduce the risk of the collapse of superficial lymphatic vessels when done as part of CDT. The recommended pressure in this study was 50 mm Hg.[178]

Significant discrepancies have been found between target pressures set on the compression device control dial (30, 60, 80, or 100 mm Hg) and the actual pressures measured inside the cuff chamber (54, 98, 121, or 141 mm Hg). It has been recommended that the devices be set at much lower target pressures (<30 mm Hg) than those typically applied in clinical practice.[162]

Newer devices have added a truncal appliance and many additional chambers that provide programmable compression to the trunk and lymph node basins at the root of the treated limb to prepare the trunk to receive fluid from the treated limb. There is a small body of research evidence that these pumps improve quality of life and function and can reduce cellulitic episodes.[88,131] However, there is minimal evidence that they facilitate movement of proteins from the interstitium.[53] More studies are required to prove positive effects on lymphatic flow. In the case of a patient with a chronic disease requiring lifelong care, the prescription of a pump alone is a disservice to the patient. A systematic review of IPC stated that it was an "acceptable home based treatment modality in addition to wearing compression garments."[53] In addition, most studies of IPC use report a follow-up of usually 30 to 60 days or up to 1 year. Overall, studies conclude that there is minimal guidance on the appropriate dosage for treatment: amount of pressure, number of cycles, and frequency/duration of use.[53,63]

### Skin Care

Generally, for most people an hour a day spent on exercise and garment care is reasonable for this condition. It is reasonable to spend 20 minutes twice daily on exercise and self-massage and another 20 minutes on skin care and washing or caring for compression garments. The better the individual understands the pathophysiology of the lymphedema, the greater the adherence.

Instruction in skin care includes the use of low-pH or neutral-pH soaps, cleansers, and moisturizers; the proper care of fingernails and toenails (see Fig. 13.19); use of topical antibiotic or antifungal preparations; and instruction in skin hygiene and compression garment/bandage washing for good hygiene.

The normal pH of healthy skin is acidic (<7.0) and accounts for the waterproof barrier of the skin surface and reduced microflora.[109] Repeated use of alkaline soaps and cleansers on the skin will result in the loss of this waterproof property, drying the skin and causing microscopic cracks in the skin surface, increasing the likelihood of bacterial invasion.

The elements of a personal first aid kit including basic wound care supplies can be discussed. The client is

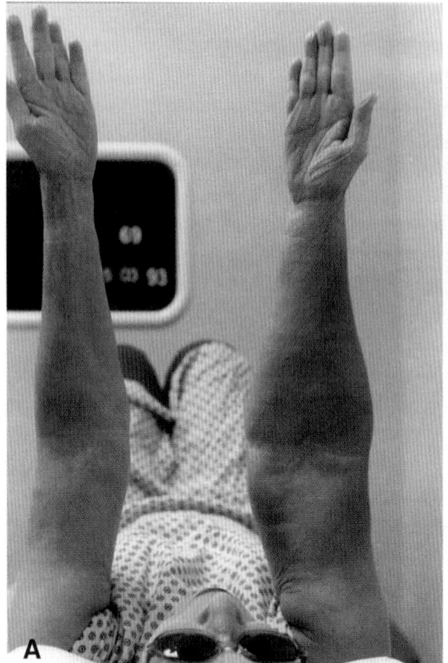

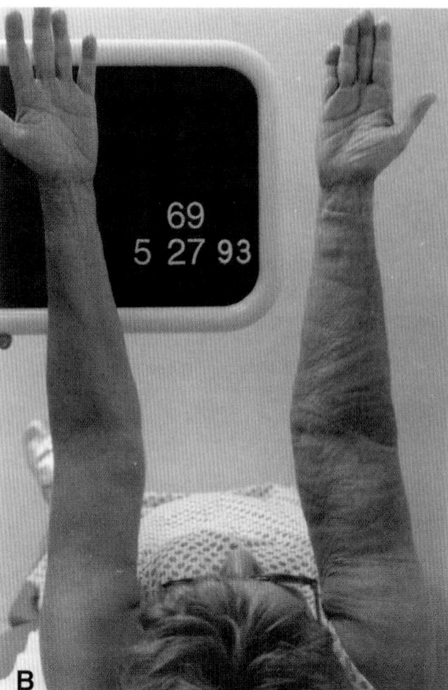


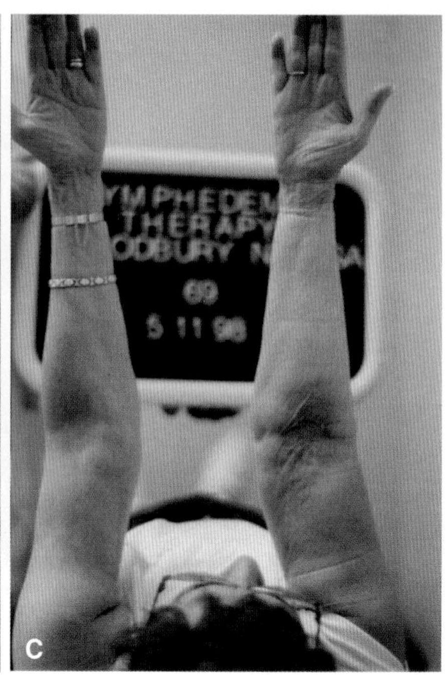

**FIGURE 13.23**

(A) Before treatment, a 69-year-old woman with stage II lymphedema of the right upper extremity of 20 years' duration secondary to breast cancer surgery and treatment. For the past few years, she has had recurrent cellulitis infections in the right arm, with hospitalization several times per year to receive intravenous antibiotics. (B) After 18 complete decongestive therapy (CDT) treatments, she achieved a 57% reduction in lymphedema in the right upper extremity. The wrinkling in her forearm and upper arm is from the compression bandaging, which was removed shortly before taking this photograph. These wrinkles were only temporary. Note the significant reduction in lymphedema. (C) Five years after CDT treatment. She has improved the reduction in the lymphedema of her right upper extremity to 64%. She has had no additional treatment for lymphedema, but she follows her home program of self-massage, exercise, skin care, and compression garment wear. She has had only two cellulitis infections in the past 5 years, which were treated successfully with oral antibiotics. Note the reshaping of the forearm and upper arm since previous photos were taken. (Courtesy Lymphedema Therapy, Woodbury, NY.)

instructed to carry this kit whenever traveling. For individuals with recurrent cellulitis, a prescribed antibiotic for use if needed is recommended. For older adults, individuals with limited mobility, or visually impaired persons, a caregiver can be instructed in how to inspect the lymphedematous limb or area daily for signs of skin irritation or infection. A large magnifying mirror on a long handle or a full-length wall mirror can assist clients to inspect the back of their limbs, torso, and side of body for signs of reduced skin integrity.

Although consistency in using these techniques is very important, many people experience exacerbation of the lymphedema from an infection or skin problem, necessitating removal of the compression garment to avoid spread of the infection until treated. These incidents can be minimized if individuals know what to look for and how to proceed when an infection occurs. Knowing the procedure for an emergency visit, whom to contact, and how to advocate for their own care within the medical system should be discussed and reviewed at the time of discharge and at subsequent follow-up visits.[100]

If an infection develops, treatment must be discontinued owing to the risk of spread until symptoms are reduced. Treatment can resume once an effective antibiotic is part of the care regimen.[114,147] Any sign or symptom of infection always requires immediate medical attention.

### Guidelines for Job and Lifestyle Modifications

The same principles for exercise also apply to pacing and modifying work activities and ADLs to avoid overload. Affected individuals do not necessarily have to give up a job just because lymphedema has been diagnosed. Cooperative discussion may be helpful between the therapist, the client, and the client's employer to implement simple task modifications ensuring client safety and comfort at work.

Some work requirements may have to be reduced, modified, or eliminated, and the employer should be aware of any special needs the employee may have (e.g., the need to wear compression garments and to protect them with constant changes of vinyl gloves throughout the day in a food service job or the need for a hair stylist to rest with arm or arms elevated in between customers).

Successful management of lymphedema should mean greater "ability" for the individual, not "disability." It may be necessary to modify a workstation to provide more comfort for an individual with leg edema. Interactive education is the key to success. If the employer understands the problem of lymphedema and is assisted in providing a simple solution, everyone wins. For example, an individual with lower extremity lymphedema may need to get up from the workstation every hour and walk around for 5 minutes. A place to elevate the affected leg under the desk may be needed.

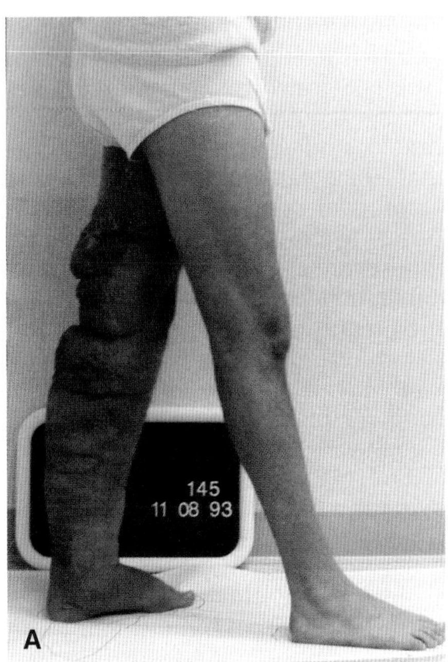

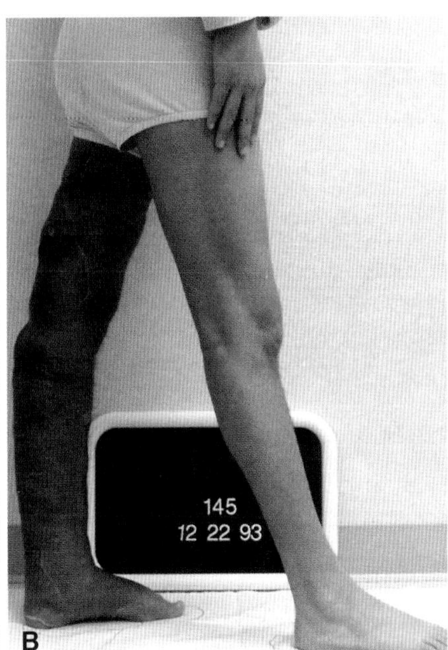

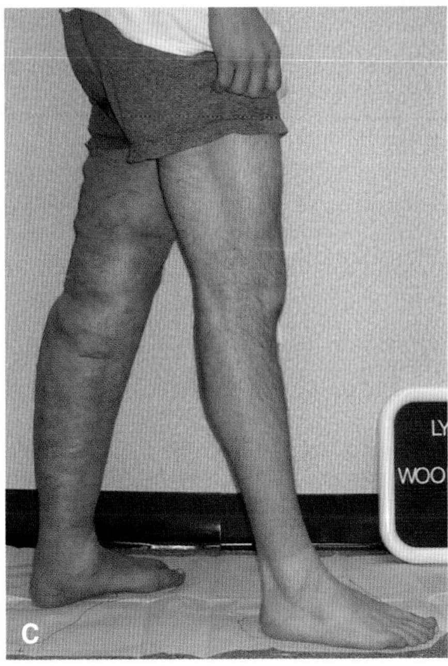


**FIGURE 13.24**

(A) Before treatment, a 19-year-old man with severe stage II primary lymphedema of the left lower extremity progressing to the left buttock and genitals with chylous reflux to the scrotum, buttock, and thigh. The onset of the edema was at age 8 years (see Fig. 13.11). He spent most of his high school years in and out of the hospital. In the 24 months before treatment, he was hospitalized 22 times for cellulitis in the left lower extremity and placed in the intensive care unit with septic shock three times. (B) After one course of complete decongestive therapy (CDT) of 30 treatments interrupted by a 2-week hospitalization (1 week in intensive care unit) for cellulitis of the left leg and buttock with severe chylous leakage from the scrotum, buttock, and thigh. He went into septic shock and needed hyperalimentation to treat the hypoproteinemia (that resulted from the chylous leakage) via a central venous line. Despite the massive increase in swelling and open areas on the posterior left thigh and buttock resulting from the cellulitis, he achieved a 67% reduction in lymphedema of his left lower extremity with reductions in the abdominal, suprapubic, and genital swelling as well. (C) Twelve-and-a-half years after CDT. Note that some increase in the girth of the left lower extremity has occurred, particularly in the areas just proximal and distal to the knee, where the tissues are lax from the original debulking surgery. These areas fill in quickly without compression. Some of the girth increase is due to weight gain now that he no longer has recurrent cellulitis and the chylous reflux is under control. This young man, having spent his high school years in and out of the hospital, was able to complete his college degree and is now a registered nurse working in an emergency department. Since his CDT treatment, he has made his lymphedema management home program a priority in his life and continues to maintain a 60% reduction in lymphedema in his left lower extremity. (Courtesy Lymphedema Therapy, Woodbury, NY.)

Requesting reasonable accommodations is an important goal, but sometimes certain job tasks cannot be modified. For example, a nurse with significant upper extremity lymphedema may have difficulty getting assistance every time it is necessary to move and lift a patient or resident. Constant lifting and positioning heavy patients or residents can worsen upper extremity lymphedema. Working as an obstetric or operating room nurse where handwashing and constant changing of gloves is necessary may preclude use of a compression glove to manage swelling and require a change to a different environment of care. In such cases the decision rests with the individual and employer whether a job change is needed or whether it will be necessary to stay and make the best of things.

### Psychosocial Considerations and Quality of Life

Great emphasis has been given to the myriad physical symptoms and resulting impairments associated with lymphedema. Little is reported on the psychologic distress these individuals experience on a daily basis. People are curious about the change in size and shape of the affected limb. Individuals are faced with tremendous alterations in body image and often deal with chronic pain and impaired mobility/function, and many feel embarrassed. Some experience the scorn of a public perception that they are deformed or distorted. Some feel that their job security may be threatened because of their appearance or the perception that they "cannot do the job."[42,69] Individuals with severe leg lymphedema with chronic infections and ulcerations may leak lymphatic fluid from their limbs and experience public humiliation when people turn away from them in fear and ignorance. Affected individuals become prisoners in their own homes, too embarrassed or afraid to go out in public. Many are judged by others who do not understand "how this could happen" and why it was not "taken care of." Individuals living with lymphedema can experience tremendous guilt and self-doubt. Many clients have been told by numerous medical professionals, "There is nothing to be done; just learn to live with it." Even today, some physicians and therapists in the United States still tell individuals with lymphedema that not much can be done except to "elevate the limb and wear loose long sleeves or long pants."

Individuals with lymphedema need tremendous psychologic support to cope with the problems associated with living with such a chronic condition.[120,133]

Box 13.2

**IMPORTANT RESOURCES IN THE TREATMENT OF LYMPHEDEMA[a]**

- American Cancer Society
  The American Cancer Society sponsored an international meeting on breast cancer–related lymphedema 1998 and sponsored a symposium in 2012. Both of these meetings brought together international experts on breast cancer and lymphedema. The symposium findings were published in the journal *Cancer* (*Cancer* 83:2775–2890, 1998, and *Cancer* 118(S8), 2012). Available from the American Cancer Society: (800) 227–2345.
  www.cancer.org
- American Lymphedema Framework Project (ALFP)
  www.alfp.org
- American Physical Therapy Association (APTA): Academy of Oncologic Physical Therapy—Lymphedema Special Interest Group (SIG)
  www.oncologypt.org
- Casley-Smith International (CSI)
  www.casleysmithinternational.org
- International Lymphoedema Framework Project (ILF)
  There are many downloadable monographs on this website.
  www.lympho.org
- International Society of Lymphology (ISL)
  The University of Arizona College of Medicine
  University Medical Center
  1510 North Campbell Avenue
  Tucson, AZ 85724
  (520) 626-6360
  FAX: (520) 626-0822
  A quarterly journal is available on international research on lymphedema.
  www.internationalsocietyoflymphology.org
- Step Up–Speak Out (SU-SO)
  www.stepup-speakout.org
- Australasian Lymphology Association
  www.lymphoedema.org.au.
- Lymphology Association of North America (LANA)
  www.clt-lana.org
- The Lymphatic Education & Research Network
  261 Madison Avenue 9th Floor
  New York, NY 10016
  (516) 625-9675
  Fax (516) 625-9410
  www.lymphaticnetwork.org
  e-mail contact: lern@lymhaticnetwork.org
- Canadian Lymphedema Framework
  www.canadalymph.ca
- National Lymphedema Network
  The newsletter was discontinued.
  www.lymphnet.org.
- Lipedema Foundation
  39 Lewis Street 4th Floor
  Greenwich, CT 06830
  www.lipedema.org

[a]The listing of any particular program or the omission of others does not denote support or preference for one method of lymphedema intervention over another. This list of resources is meant to guide the interested therapist to further information. These resources were current as of December 2018.

Innovative lymphedema treatment programs offer support groups (Box 13.2). The National Lymphedema Network, an advocacy organization, is one source of information in the United States. Patient advocates supported by lymphedema specialists offer online education and outreach to individuals who may not have access to specialty care in their communities (http://www.stepup-speakout.org).

Radina and Armer[146] studied women's coping strategies and found that "the potential 'pile up' of stressors leading to vulnerability after breast cancer treatment lymphedema reported by participants included modification of daily household and work-related tasks, living with a constant reminder of the cancer, and feelings of abandonment by medicine." They state that "resiliency … is characterized as adjustment, adaptation, or crisis" and suggest that practitioners "need to serve the patient and the family." A more recent review of the impact of BCRL on quality of life concluded that "While improvements in breast cancer therapy have contributed to a decrease in the incidence of lymphedema, the overall negative impact the condition has on patients and survivors has remained unchanged."[181] This is particularly true for older cancer survivors. Older adults may have multiple medical comorbidities that cause chronic impairments in mobility and function that affect their ability to undergo an intensive treatment program as well as to adhere to an ongoing self-care program for lymphedema.[4]

Great strides are being made in recognizing lymphedema as a condition that deserves to be acknowledged and treated early and aggressively. Theoretically, all clinicians know that psychologic support is crucial to success in managing a chronic illness or condition. However, having the practical applications in place to help the individual takes a tremendous commitment in personal time and financial resources. Nevertheless, a successful lymphedema treatment program must offer ongoing support and follow-up care.

## A THERAPIST'S THOUGHTS[a]

### *Risk Reduction Strategies*

Although no double-blind studies have been published that prove that these strategies are effective in reducing risk of developing lymphedema, the guidelines available from the National Lymphedema Network (see Box 13.2) follow the commonsense application of the anatomic and physiologic principles of lymphatic function and are fully referenced from the literature in the document titled *Risk Reduction*. This document addresses both individuals at risk for lymphedema and individuals who have lymphedema. A few areas are often questioned by our clients.

**Blood Pressure Assessment as a Potential Trigger**

Although there is no proof that taking blood pressure (BP) measurements on the limb at risk will trigger lymphedema, it is logical to consider that applying the BP cuff and inflating it to 200 mm Hg will compress veins and lymphatics under the area of the cuff, abruptly increasing the lymphatic load distal to the cuff.[35,54] If the limb at risk must be used, it is helpful to avoid inflating the cuff to more than the person's average systolic pressures using a manual cuff rather than an automatic BP device. This would limit the compression of the local lymphatics as much as possible and is not especially onerous to medical professionals. Clients should be educated to request this.[138]

Individuals who are obese are more likely to be hypertensive, requiring inflation of the BP cuff to higher pressure to get the baseline measure. Because obesity and weight gain during treatment are primary risk factors for lymphedema, this subset of clients with breast cancer may warrant more caution; again, no data support clinical practice guidelines at this time.[35,144]

It is recommended that clients who have undergone ALND, SLNB, or radiation therapy avoid having BP measurements taken on the affected side if possible. Although it has been suggested that a client who has had bilateral ALND or SLNB should have BP measurements taken in the leg, this is not standard clinical practice in the United States. Some oncology staff advise taking BP measurements in the arm with the least amount of nodal dissection. For clients who have had a mastectomy without ALND (i.e., prophylactic mastectomy), BP can be obtained in either arm.[107]

**Venipuncture or Surgery as a Potential Trigger**

There is a small risk of introducing bacteria with the needlestick as well as potential damage to the local veins and lymphatics depending on the degree of compression under the tourniquet and how many times the person has to be punctured to get a full sample. Surgery causes trauma, and there is a known risk of infection from any surgery. Again, it makes sense to err on the side of caution and to avoid using the limb at risk for venipuncture unless there is no other option. For people who have had bilateral ALND, this poses a problem. Many laboratories do not have personnel who are competent in venipuncture on the leg or foot. Some physicians believe that the risk of DVT in the leg is too great and will not recommend using the leg or foot to draw blood. It has been suggested to try to minimize tourniquet time or to eliminate the use of the tourniquet during venipuncture to reduce the risk of damaging lymphatics. When elective upper extremity surgery is necessary in an at-risk or lymphedematous limb, surgery should not be avoided simply because of lymphedema, as there is minimal risk described and preoperative and postoperative conservative care of the lymphedema can ameliorate any long-term consequences.[80]

**Air Travel**

The reduced atmospheric pressure while flying combined with inactivity with dependent limbs is thought to be a trigger for lymphedema. There is minimal evidence to demonstrate this risk.[35,54] In one study, individuals without lymphedema who wore precautionary compression were more likely to develop swelling. Individuals with a diagnosed lymphedema can be advised to wear their regular compression during flight and to get up and move frequently during long flights to reduce blood pooling by musculoskeletal activation and remain hydrated. This is the same advice given to people at risk for DVT.[72]

There are no absolutes, and the guidelines are just that—guidelines for clients to discuss with their physicians. Many of the other precautions are commonsense recommendations. In an individual with known immunocompromise, maintaining and protecting the skin is paramount—moisturize well with nonfragranced moisturizers (fragrances are usually the culprit in allergic reactions), protect the skin from sunburn and irritations by harsh chemicals, and protect the skin from injury (e.g., by wearing gardening gloves).

Exercise has in the past been considered dangerous to at-risk and lymphedematous limbs. Affected individuals will often report they no longer use the at-risk limb for any activities. This is incorrect. The evidence is strong that exercise is beneficial for both groups and does not increase the risk of lymphedema when appropriately introduced to the client's self-care regimen. The Physical Activity and Lymphedema (PAL) trial, a large randomized controlled trial, instructed women with or at risk for unilateral BCRL in a progressive resistance exercise program for the upper extremities as part of a whole-body flexibility and strength program that was performed for 1 hour twice/week for a year. The women demonstrated notable strength gains, improved quality of life and self-esteem, and no increased risk of development or exacerbation of lymphedema.[159–161]

Currently there is no cure for lymphedema. Any strategy that might delay the onset of this condition is worth pursuing. Individuals with a limb at risk should be educated about these risk-reduction strategies so that they can "live smart" by incorporating some or all of them into their daily activities if they choose. It is the client's right to choose, but he or she needs to have appropriate information to make an informed choice.[68,132]

[a]Bonnie Lasinski and Joy C. Cohn.

## A THERAPIST'S THOUGHTS[a]

### *On Infection*

Understanding the risk for infection is critical when evaluating and educating individuals with or at risk for lymphedema. These individuals are extremely prone to local infection from minor trauma, abrasion, or insect bite or without any obvious trigger and must be educated in risk reduction and proper skin care to minimize their risk for recurrent infections. Ryan[155] eloquently explained the rationale behind meticulous skin care: "The epidermis and adipose tissues ... are likely factories of growth factors and mediators of inflammation. ... [C]ytokines manufactured by the epidermis ... are perhaps also responsible for recurrent inflammatory episodes. ... [A]pplication of external emollients that are antiinflammatory ... should be looked upon as being proactive in the management of lymphedema."

Minor irritations, local areas of redness of the skin, and minor dermatitis reactions must be observed and treated aggressively to avoid progression to a major infection. In a therapy department, the treatment environment and all equipment must be meticulously cleaned, including the tape measure used for circumferential measurements between clients. The tape measure can be cleaned with an alcohol wipe and then air drying, or single-use measurement tapes can be used. Universal precautions must be applied. Gloves are not necessary unless there is an actual concern for cross contamination such as in a region with a fungal infection or open wound. (See Infectious Diseases in Chapter 8 and Standard Precautions in Appendix A.)

Many people with lymphedema are unaware of the increased risk of infection or are lulled into complacency by health care professionals who tell them "not to worry" because antibiotics are available if an infection develops. Any infection further stresses the already overloaded regional lymphatic system, sometimes irreversibly causing damage to the cutaneous lymphatics owing to the intense inflammatory response that accompanies a cellulitis.

Any infection in a lymphedematous limb, even a local infection, must be medically treated immediately without delay. Patients/clients must be educated as to the signs and symptoms of a cellulitic infection so that they will react immediately if suspected. Those symptoms may include pain, increased warmth, swelling, and redness of the skin often accompanied by a fever.[147] Early recognition can save precious time, eliminating severe inflammation with timely administration of an appropriate antibiotic. Cellulitis can rarely be cultured, but reevaluation 24 to 72 hours after starting antibiotics should demonstrate reduced symptoms to allow for treatment to be reinitiated with the physician's approval. Courses of antibiotics are prescribed for 5 to 14 days. Treatment for recurrent cellulitic infections should include an infectious disease specialist. Excellent guidelines for this treatment have been published by the International Lymphoedema Framework Project[83,92] and British Lymphology Society.

[a]Bonnie Lasinski and Joy C. Cohn.

## A THERAPIST'S THOUGHTS[a]

### *Exercise and Activity*

Simply stated, the greater the intensity of the exercise, the greater the oxygen demand. With increased oxygen demand comes increased blood flow to the muscles, which provides the oxygen to do the work. Signs of limb "overload" are aching; congested, full feeling; discomfort in the proximal lymph nodal area (axilla or inguinal areas); pain; throbbing; or change in skin color. If any of these signs or symptoms occurs, the activity should be discontinued, and the limb should be elevated. Deep breathing exercises and some self–lymphatic drainage may help decongest the trunk and limbs and reduce the discomfort.[129] The individual must learn to listen to his or her body and grade future activity accordingly to avoid overloading the system.[157]

[a]Bonnie Lasinski.

## A THERAPIST'S THOUGHTS[a]

### *Commonsense Explanations to Facilitate Adherence to Compression Garments and Exercise/Self-MLD*

Lymphedema results when lymph load (amount of lymph fluid to be moved) exceeds the ability of the system to move that fluid (lymph transport capacity). Lymph transport capacity can be impaired by damage or removal of lymph vessels and/or nodes (as in secondary lymphedema) or by maldevelopment of lymph vessels or nodes (as in primary lymphedema).

To expand on the analogy of lymph fluid being like cars on a highway where the lanes/tollbooths are the lymph vessels/nodes mentioned earlier in the chapter, consider this next idea. If the client imagines that three of six tollbooths are suddenly shut down, the same number of cars have to pass through, so traffic (lymph) backs up. Once the initial backlog is cleared, traffic may start to move again, but very slowly, inching along (lymphedema is decreased by treatment and compression garment wear). Now someone jams on their brakes (compression garment is removed), and traffic (lymph) backs up again. The only way to keep traffic moving is to keep that slow flow going consistently (wear compression garment and perform self-MLD daily) so that lymph load does not exceed lymph transport capacity.

Once traffic backs up, it takes a long time to get it going again, and sometimes it never gets back to normal (an exacerbation of lymphedema related to infection, injury, recurrent malignant disease, or nonadherence to self-care may not resolve). Modi and colleagues[123] showed this in individuals who had BCRL. They applied a BP cuff to the affected arms and showed that when they decreased the pressure in the cuff, the lymph did not begin to flow in the affected arm until much later and at a lower pressure than their unaffected arm. When the affected arm is constricted and flow is stopped, it takes a lot longer for the flow to begin again once the constriction is removed. Lymphedema not only worsens but when the constriction is removed, resumption of flow is slow so that more interstitial fluid is building up and not moving out of the tissues, again because the resumed flow is so slow.

So, even if some of the tollbooths open again (collateral lymph flow; person does self-MLD and puts compression bandages or garment back on), the signal person does not let the cars start to drive through again for another few minutes, so more cars (lymph) back up even though some lanes have reopened—so more of a back-up than before and longer for the traffic (lymph flow) to get back to its "normal" flow, which, in the case of a limb with lymphedema, is slow to begin with. Clients who understand this concept have an easier time adhering to their self-care program of exercise and compression garment wear because they know how it affects their lymphedema.

[a]Bonnie Lasinski.

## A THERAPIST'S THOUGHTS[a]

### *Intermittent Pneumatic Compression*

Not all IPC devices are the same. It is important for the clinician to be familiar with the specific parameters and pressures provided by each unit to determine what unit best fits the individual goals of a client's treatment plan.[115,116]

In the presence of soft tissue injury, vigorous massage or the use of compression pumps at pressures higher than 60 mm Hg can cause severe damage to the walls of the initial lymphatic vessels (possibly by tearing the anchoring microfilaments mentioned earlier). This collapse of the initial lymphatic walls impairs lymphatic transport capacity and results in lymphedema and extravasation of lymphedema into an adjacent trunk quadrant.[16]

Atrophy or hypertrophy of the skin can further compromise lymphatic function as a result of the loss of elasticity. A network of collagen and elastin fibers surrounding the lymphatic system helps the skin respond to movement, so any variable that can damage the lymph system of the skin (e.g., aging, chronic sun exposure, or prolonged use of systemic steroids) compromises the response of the tissues to movement caused by massage or pneumatic compression.

The resultant injury to the blood vessels and lymphatics causes fluid and protein to leak from the damaged vessels, setting up a chronic inflammatory response, potentially leading to permanent fibrosclerotic changes.[156] These fibrosclerotic changes further compromise oxygen perfusion in the tissues, resulting in a repetitive cycle of hypoxia and chronic inflammation,[2,135] which is the perfect environment for bacterial and fungal infections to flourish. In addition, IPC treatment protocols require daily use for hours per day, physically and psychologically restricting the person who is "tied to the machine" for hours at a time.

Although IPC can be helpful in early-stage I lymphedema, when simple elevation overnight usually reduces the edema, it may be less helpful in stage II fibrotic lymphedema. Although the pumps increase the reabsorption of water into venous capillaries, they do not move the extracellular protein because these molecules are too large to enter the venous fenestrae. Proteins must be transported via the lymphatics and are the key to good control.

This is a situation that may trigger a rebound edema by diluting the concentrated protein in the soft tissue space. The higher protein concentration remaining in the tissues also causes the chronic inflammatory response discussed earlier, triggering the development of more subcutaneous fibrosis. The vicious cycle of lymphedema repeats itself. The chronic inflammatory response increases the individual's risk of developing secondary infections (cellulitis/lymphangitis).

Therapists should monitor truncal measurements in addition to full limb measurements when treating individuals with IPC. IPC used at lower pressures may be effective for immobile individuals who sit for prolonged periods with their legs in the dependent position, provided that they do not have comorbid conditions that contraindicate the use of IPC such as congestive heart failure, active infection, malignant disease in the limb to be treated, or acute DVTs.[140] IPC can be very helpful for a patient who is less mobile and has limited access to expert lymphedema management. It also may be a good replacement for self-MLD for a patient who cannot adequately perform it, but it is never a substitute for consistently worn compression garments during the day.

[a]Bonnie Lasinski.

## A THERAPIST'S THOUGHTS

### *Low Level Laser Therapy*[a]

Low Level Laser Therapy (LLLT) or Photobiomodulation is an intervention that was approved by the FDA in 2007 for use in the breast cancer population.[7a] It is an intervention that has non-thermal effects on soft tissue and may be helpful by "increasing lymphatic flow through lymghangiogenesis, stimulation of lymphatic motoricity and prevention of tissue fibrosis that could potentially disrupt lymphatic function."[168a] In a pooled analysis,[168a] moderate strength evidence supported LLLT in the reduction of volume in BCRL. In a systematic review[7a] strong evidence showed LLLT to be more effective at reducing volume than a sham treatment, but conflicting evidence led to the conclusion that LLLT was not more effective than other conventional interventions for BCRL. The specific parameters for the use of LLLT are not clear from the literature but 904 nm wavelength with 1.5 J/cm$^2$ to 2.4 J/cm$^2$ dosage were commonly used. Treatment frequency was often 3 times per week with a minimum of 3 to 4 weeks up to 12 weeks duration in the studies reviewed in these two analyses.[7a,168a] The axilla is the most commonly treated region in BCRL.

[a]Joy Cohn.

## Lymphadenitis

Infections elsewhere in the body can lead to lymphadenopathy as described previously. When the lymph node becomes overwhelmed by the infection, the lymph node itself can become infected; this is called *lymphadenitis*. Lymphadenitis can be classified as acute or chronic; acutely inflamed lymph nodes are most common locally in the cervical region in association with infections of the teeth or tonsils or in the axillary or inguinal regions secondary to infection of the extremities.

In acute lymphadenitis, the lymph nodes are enlarged, tender, warm, and reddened. In the case of chronic lymphadenitis, long-standing infection from a variety of sources results in scarred lymph nodes with fibrous connective tissue replacement. The nodes are enlarged and firm to palpation but not warm or tender. The management of lymphadenitis is treatment of the underlying disorder.

## Lymphangitis and Cellulitis

Lymphangitis, an acute inflammation of the subcutaneous lymphatic channels, usually occurs as a result of hemolytic streptococci or staphylococci (or both) entering the lymphatic channels from an abrasion or local trauma, wound, or infection (usually cellulitis; see further discussion of cellulitis in Chapter 10). The involvement of the lymphatics is often first observed as a red streak under the skin (referred to in layperson terms as *blood poisoning*), radiating from the infection site in the direction of the regional lymph nodes.

The red streak may be very obvious, or it may be very faint and easily overlooked, especially in dark-skinned people. The nodes most commonly affected are submandibular, cervical, inguinal, and axillary, in that order. Involved nodes are usually tender and enlarged (>3 cm).

Systemic manifestations include fever, chills, malaise, and anorexia. Other symptoms may occur in association with the underlying infection located elsewhere in the body. Bacteremia from any cause can result in suppurative arthritis (inflammatory with pus formation), osteomyelitis, peritonitis, meningitis, or visceral abscesses.

When cellulitis results in lymphangitis, throbbing pain occurs at the site of bacterial invasion, and the client presents with a warm, edematous extremity (or possible scrotal lymphedema in male clients and occasionally vulvar lymphedema in female clients).

### MEDICAL MANAGEMENT: INTACT LYMPHATIC SYSTEM

DIAGNOSIS. Lymphangitis may be confused with superficial thrombophlebitis, but the erythema associated with lymphangitis is first seen as a red streak under the skin radiating toward the regional lymph nodes (usually ascending proximally), whereas the erythema associated with thrombosis is usually over the thrombosed vein with local induration and inflammation.

However, suppurative thrombophlebitis may develop if bacteria are introduced during intravenous therapy, especially when the needle or catheter is left in place for more than 48 hours. The physician also needs to differentiate cellulitis from soft tissue infections (e.g., gangrene or necrotizing fasciitis) that may require early and aggressive incision and resection of necrotic infected tissue.

A person with a history of vascular disease taking anticoagulant medication should have a Doppler ultrasound to rule out DVT before being treated. Laboratory tests are often not required but may include blood culture (often positive for staphylococcal or streptococcal species) and culture and sensitivity studies on the wound exudate or pus.

**Treatment and Prognosis.** Prompt parenteral antibiotic therapy is mandatory, because bacteremia and

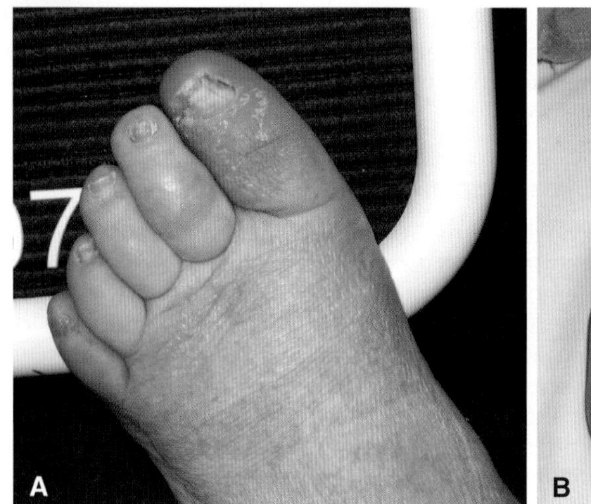

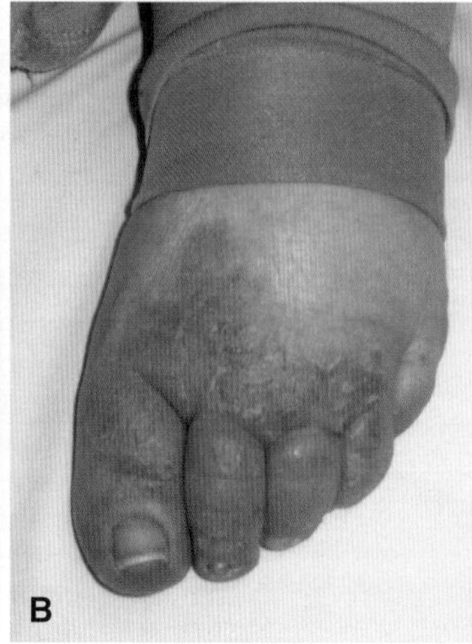

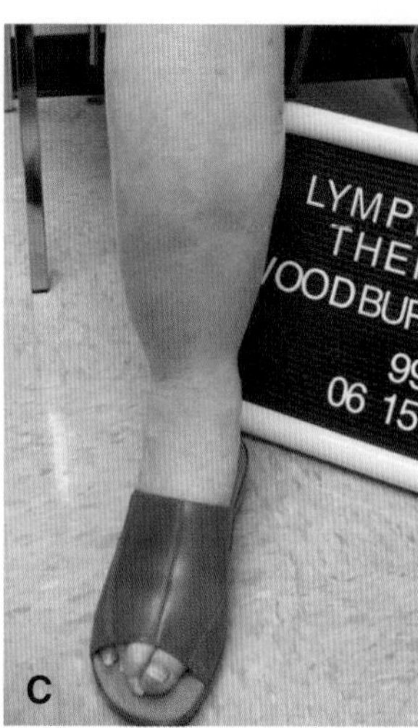

**FIGURE 13.25**

(A) Cellulitis of the left great toe/forefoot owing to an ingrown toenail in a man with diabetes and lymphedema in the lower extremities secondary to chronic venous insufficiency. (B) Cellulitis of the left toes/foot in a woman with primary lymphedema of the left lower extremity. This young woman often worked double shifts as a waitress. Her foot would swell and the skin would become irritated/blistered in her shoe, causing recurrent infections of the left foot/leg accompanied by fever, chills, malaise, and pain. A change in footwear resulted in a marked reduction in frequency of the infections. (C) Cellulitis of the right lower leg owing to an insect bite in a woman with lymphedema secondary to pelvic lymph node dissection and radiation to treat cervical cancer. (Courtesy Lymphedema Therapy, Woodbury, NY.)

systemic toxicity develop rapidly once organisms reach the bloodstream via the thoracic duct. Antibiotic treatment may be accompanied by general measures such as heat, elevation, immobilization of the infected area, and analgesics for pain.

Appropriate wound care may include drainage of the pus from an infected wound when it is clear that an abscess is associated with the site of initial infection. An area of cellulitis should not be excised, because the infection may be spread by attempted drainage when pus is not present. Treatment as described should be effective against invading bacteria within a few days.

## MEDICAL MANAGEMENT: INFECTIONS WITH IMPAIRED AND AT-RISK LYMPHATIC SYSTEM AND LYMPHEDEMA

**DIAGNOSIS.** Confusion of cellulitis or lymphangitis with thrombophlebitis in an individual with lymphedema or at risk for lymphedema is common and has a disastrous impact on the severity of the lymphedema. An episode of cellulitis or lymphangitis often triggers the development of lymphedema in an individual who is at risk but has no clinical signs of edema. Improper, inadequate treatment of these infections can lead to chronic infection or inflammation and progression of the lymphedema.

The individual who has had regional lymph node dissection and/or radiation has an impaired immune response in the areas that drain to that regional nodal area. Consequently, infection can spread rapidly in those regions, and any delay in treatment while awaiting blood cultures and vascular tests can cause progression of the infection.

The combination of the impaired nodal area and the inactivity of the macrophages in the lymphedematous region allows the bacteria to multiply rapidly, feeding on the high-protein lymphedema fluid. It is not uncommon for a person to develop a high fever with shaking chills (40.5 °C [105 °F]) within 30 minutes of feeling ill or feeling an ache or pain in the lymphedematous region. It is

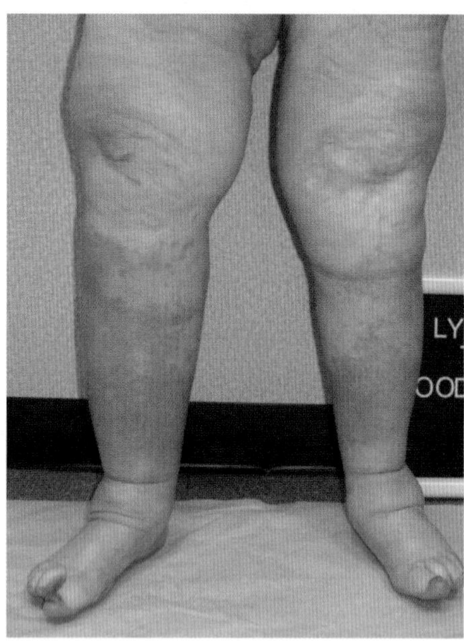

**FIGURE 13.26**

**This woman had experienced pain, increased swelling, and itching of the skin on both legs for months.** She had swollen ankles and feet as a teen, and the swelling worsened as she aged. She saw a vascular surgeon who performed Doppler studies and ruled out deep vein thrombosis but had no diagnosis for her problem. She saw a dermatologist who diagnosed a contact dermatitis and prescribed topical cortisone cream. Her podiatrist referred her to a lymphedema specialist, who promptly diagnosed primary lymphedema of both legs, complicated by cellulitis. (Courtesy Lymphedema Therapy, Woodbury, NY.)

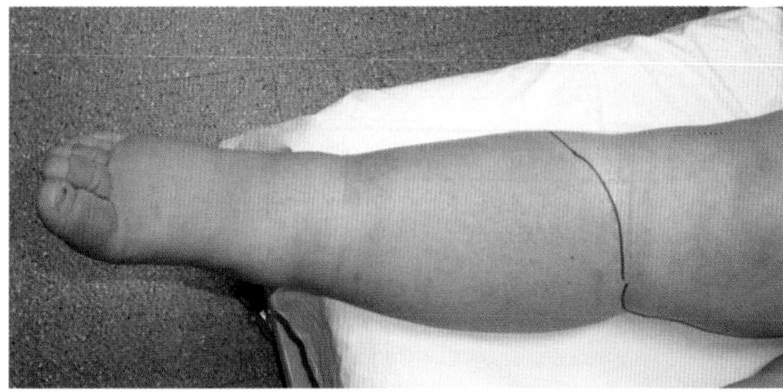

**FIGURE 13.27**

**A woman with primary lymphedema in the lower extremities with cellulitis in the lower leg.** Note the black line drawn by the therapist to mark the extent of the infection. This is important to monitor the course of the infection. The person was prescribed an oral antibiotic and advised by the physician that if the redness progressed proximal to the black line, she must go to the emergency department and be assessed for intravenous antibiotics. Note the severity of the swelling and fibrosis of the toes. Examination of the skin between her toes revealed that she had a fungal infection that caused the skin to macerate and crack. Bacteria can then enter the broken skin and cause a secondary bacterial infection. This is a common problem in people with lymphedema of the lower extremities. (Courtesy Lymphedema Therapy, Woodbury, NY.)

not acceptable for these people to "wait and see" and call their physician in a day or two. They must be seen and evaluated by a physician immediately to rule out thrombosis versus cellulitis or lymphangitis and initiate appropriate treatment immediately.

The more insidious onset of local infection (cellulitis) may manifest with an area of redness on the skin that looks like a rash or sunburn. The area may be warm to touch but not initially painful, and the individual may not develop any pain or fever. In fact, cellulitis is often mistaken for an allergic reaction, thought to be a reaction to an insect bite, or a local reaction to a sprain or strain, even when these triggers were not present (Fig. 13.25).

Individuals with advanced stage II and stage III lymphedema may develop recurrent cellulitis that is mistaken for "normal" skin changes associated with chronic lymphedema (Fig. 13.26).

**TREATMENT AND PROGNOSIS.** Treatment of cellulitis or lymphangitis in an individual with lymphedema or at risk for lymphedema differs from treatment of these conditions in an individual with an intact lymphatic system. In a healthy individual, cellulitis and lymphangitis are relatively rare. Many cases of primary lymphedema are missed in young individuals who present with unexplained recurrent cellulitis in the absence of injury or trauma. Recurring cellulitis does not develop unless some underlying pathology is causing it (usually primary lymphedema).

In a healthy individual, heat is often prescribed as an adjunct to relieve pain in the inflamed area, whereas heat should *never* be applied to individuals with lymphedema or those at risk for developing lymphedema. This contraindication includes individuals who have developed lymphedema after orthopedic surgeries.

Local heating will increase vasodilation and ultrafiltration of more fluid into the interstitial spaces, further overloading the decompensated lymphatic transport capacity, exacerbating the existing lymphedema, or possibly triggering lymphedema in the limb at risk, where no clinical lymphedema existed before the onset of the infection. Rest and immobilization of the involved areas are recommended measures. Cold can be applied to relieve pain.

Experienced lymphologists initiate immediate oral antibiotic therapy, usually with high doses of broad-spectrum antibiotics and periodic medical monitoring in the first 48 to 72 hours to observe the area for spread of the infection. It is imperative that the original area of redness be outlined with indelible marker to check on the progress or regression of the infection (Fig. 13.27).

If a poor response to the oral antibiotics is evident, hospitalization for intravenous antibiotic therapy may be necessary. A local infection can progress to septic shock if not treated effectively. A common cause of recurrent cellulitis or lymphangitis is poor, inadequate treatment of a previous infection. A common manifestation is recurrent infection in the same area of the same limb every 2 to 3 weeks. In fact, this is more likely the same infection that was never eradicated the first time. Cases such as this often have a common history of administration of too short (3 to 5 days) or inadequate doses of oral antibiotics to treat the cellulitis or lymphangitis associated with lymphedema.

**SPECIAL IMPLICATIONS FOR THE THERAPIST 13.3[a]**

### *Lymphangitis and Cellulitis*

Clinicians must remember the pathophysiology of lymphedema to understand the seriousness of these infections. Obviously, not every local infection will progress to septicemia. However, the risk is there, given the low oxygen state in the lymphedematous area; the limited response of the macrophages; and the diminished immune response in the individual with nodal dissection or irradiation or, in the case of primary lymphedema, too few, fibrosed, or poorly developed nodes. In addition, a soft tissue infection can make lymphatic dysfunction worse, sometimes leading to an overall poorer long-term condition.

At the first sign of infection, the affected individual must seek medical consultation immediately and discontinue all current lymphedema treatment modalities, including MLD, pumps, bandaging, and garments, until the physician determines it is safe to resume.

If the infection is treated early, some physicians may allow resumption of bandaging or garments as tolerated to avoid the limb ballooning out of control as the infection is resolving. This is determined on a case-by-case basis by the physician who is familiar with the individual, follows the individual's care closely, and provides emergency treatment as needed for that person.

[a] Bonnie Lasinski.

## Lipedema

### Overview and Etiologic Factors

The term *lipedema* was first used by Allen and Hines[1] to describe a symmetric "swelling" of both legs, extending

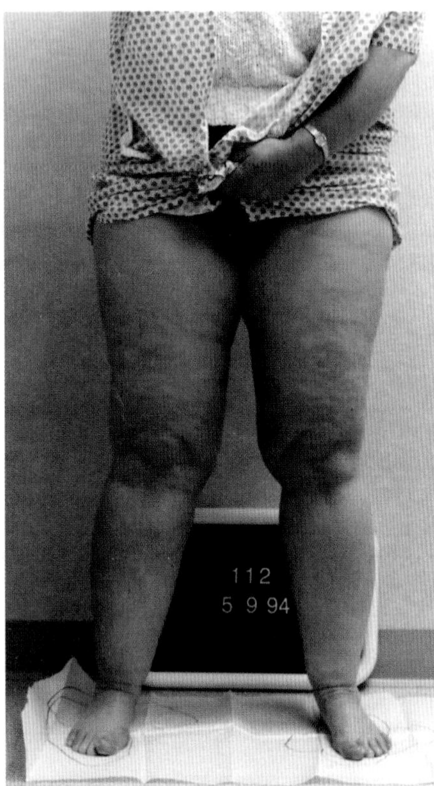


**FIGURE 13.28**

**Stage I lipedema.** Note that the feet are free of edema and the ankles and lower legs have pitting edema. Fatty nodules are beginning to appear on the distal thighs. (Courtesy Lymphedema Therapy, Woodbury, NY.)

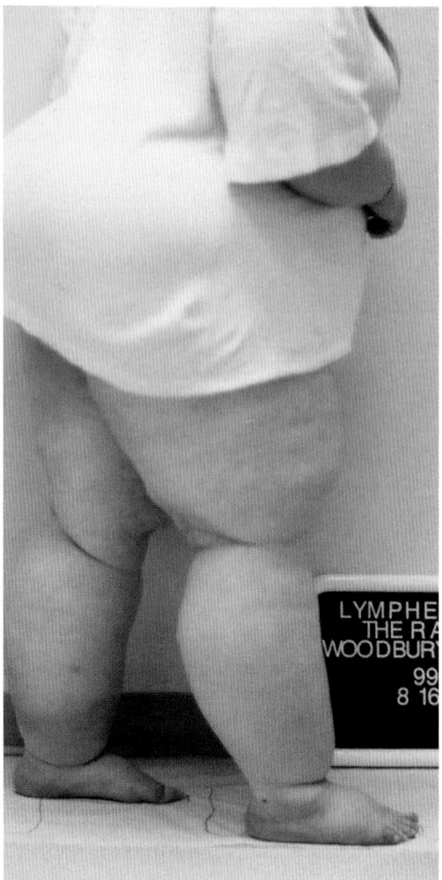

**FIGURE 13.29**

**Stage II lipedema.** Obvious pitting edema on the dorsum of the feet is evident, and the tissues are beginning to hang over the medial and lateral ankles and above the knees. The discoloration at the anterodistal left lower leg is due to a resolving cellulitis owing to the lymphedema that developed secondary to the lipedema. (Courtesy Lymphedema Therapy, Woodbury, NY.)

from the hips to the ankles, caused by deposits of subcutaneous adipose tissue. The underlying etiologic factors of these fat deposits remain unknown. Although lipedema is not a disorder of the lymphatic system per se, it is often confused with bilateral lower extremity lymphedema and may be a secondary cause for long-term lymphedema. It occurs almost exclusively in women, may have an associated family history (20% of cases), and is usually accompanied by hormonal disorders.[55] If present in a man, it is accompanied by massive hormonal disorder, often of the pituitary.

Fat deposition in the lower extremities extends from the malleoli to the pelvic brim, often with lobules hanging over the feet. The feet are not affected. Occasionally, lipedema is found in the arms. Typically, fatty bulges are in the lateral proximal thigh and the medial distal thigh, just above the knee. Clinically affected individuals present with easy bruisability, pain to palpation, and orthostatic edema as the day progresses; the edema is relieved by prolonged elevation of the leg or legs overnight.[33,153] The fatty depositions are not reduced substantially by dieting or even by bariatric surgery and so are called "diet resistant." However, many individuals with lipedema are clinically obese, which is amenable to nutritional and dietary changes.

## Stages of Lipedema

In stage I the skin is still soft and regular, but nodular changes can be felt on palpation (Fig. 13.28). No color changes occur in the skin, and the subcutaneous tissues have a spongy feel, similar to a soft rubber doll. In stage II the subcutaneous tissue becomes more nodular and tough. Large fatty lobules begin to form on the medial distal and proximal thighs and medial and lateral ankles just above the malleoli (Fig. 13.29). Pitting edema is common, increasing as the day progresses. The individual may report hypersensitivity over the anterior tibial area. Skin color changes occur in the lower leg, indicative of venous insufficiency, which can progress to a true lymphedema Stage III lipedema involves massive fat deposition, generally between hips and knees.[55] Progression to lipolymphedema is not indicated by the stage of lipedema but is diagnosed when Stemmer's sign becomes positive.

## Pathophysiology of Lipedema

There has been no definite genetic link demonstrated.[55] Many histologic and physiologic changes occur in lipedema. A decrease in the elasticity of the epidermis and subcutis also occurs. The basement membrane of vessels is thickened, and disturbances in vasomotion take place. The venoarterial reflex is disturbed, causing decreased vascular resistance, increased skin perfusion, and increased capillary filtration. Under normal circumstances, the venoarterial reflex is an important mechanism for the regulation of microcirculation and interstitial fluid exchange. It is measured as a ratio between skin perfusion in the supine versus the standing position using a laser Doppler flowmeter.

Increased venous or blood capillary pressure causes increased ultrafiltration. These changes, combined with the decreased efficiency of the calf muscle pump, result in both the dependent pitting edema seen in stage I and the secondary lymphedema (that is due to long-standing lymphatic overload) that often complicates lipedema in its later stages.[59] Histologic changes seen in lipedema include a thinning of the epidermal layer, thickening of the subcutaneous tissue layer, fibrosis of arterioles, tearing of elastic fibers, dilated venules and capillaries with increased permeability, and hypertrophy and hyperplasia of fat cells. Clinical studies show enlargement of the prelymphatic channels[174] and defects in capillary perfusion.[188] Some authors have reported no alteration in lymphatic transport,[18] whereas others[13] have reported decreased lymph outflow in individuals with lipedema. Földi and Földi[60] reported an increase in fat cell growth during lymphostasis. Overall the condition is characterized by fatty tissue, abnormally deposited with a slow onset at the time of puberty, which may be due to abnormal fat metabolism and/or hormonal changes associated with puberty and/or endocrine dysfunction.[55]

## MEDICAL MANAGEMENT

**DIAGNOSIS.** The diagnosis of lipedema is difficult if the clinician is unfamiliar with this condition. Often, affected individuals are told that they are "fat" and should just lose weight to resolve the problem. For reasons still unknown, the fatty tissue accompanying this condition cannot be significantly decreased by diet. It is not uncommon for a diagnosis of primary lymphedema to be made. This results in frustration for the person who then seeks out lymphedema therapy, with poor results.

Several significant clinical differences exist between lipedema and bilateral primary lymphedema. The feet are not involved in lipedema; although they are edematous with a positive Stemmer's sign in lymphedema, Stemmer's sign is absent in lipedema (see Fig. 13.17). The "swelling" in lipedema is symmetric, whereas in primary lymphedema, one limb may be more involved than the other. The subcutaneous tissues feel rubbery in lipedema. In advanced stage II lymphedema, significant subcutaneous fibrosis occurs, which feels firmer than lipedema.

Although incidences of cellulitis in stage II lipedema, usually with a component of lymphedema as well, have been reported, the frequency of cellulitis in stage II lymphedema is much higher. The time of onset of the "swelling" in lipedema is usually around puberty, and 90% of these cases have accompanying diagnoses of hormonal disturbance (thyroid, pituitary, or ovarian). This is usually not the case with primary lymphedema.

A lymphoscintigram may be helpful to differentiate between lymphedema and lipedema; however, results can be conflicting because lymphedema often occurs to some degree in the later stages of lipedema, probably a result of impairment of lymph flow caused by the pressure of fatty tissue.

Obesity is common in conjunction with lipedema, as this diagnosis causes great psychologic distress owing to poor recognition of the disorder and futile attempts to "diet away" the condition. Obesity does not cause lipedema but often accompanies it. The cause of lipedema is not entirely clear but results in excessive deposition of adipose tissue, most often in the lower extremities (see Figs. 13.28 and 13.29), although it can occur in the upper extremities, too.

**TREATMENT AND PROGNOSIS.** No effective medical treatment for lipedema is available, and the prognosis is guarded; however, significant functional improvements and pain relief are possible with CDT with shorter duration of treatment and good program adherence. Following decongestion and rehabilitation, good results may be further improved by use of tumescent liposuction. This is a specialized form of liposuction that preserves the connective tissue and lymphatic vessels by use of localized fluid infiltration of the tissues and then removal selectively of the fat lobules with microcannules that vibrate.[55] Medical management involves treating the hormonal disturbance as effectively as possible and providing nutritional guidance to avoid additional weight gain. Many of these individuals have endured years of ridicule because of their physical appearance and become recluses in their homes, further limiting their activity level.

As lipedema progresses and the hypersensitivity increases, individuals feel less inclined to walk or exercise because of the pain. They inevitably gain more weight as a result of the inactivity and depression, often finding food their only comfort.

### SPECIAL IMPLICATIONS FOR THE THERAPIST 13.4[a]

#### *Lipedema*

The primary goal of therapy intervention in a person with lipedema is symptomatic relief and realistic improvement of trunk and lower extremity function. Application of the combined lymphedema treatments has shown some success in relieving the pain and hypersensitivity in the lower legs and improving general mobility.[179] Usually, a lower level of compression is needed to support a lipedematous limb compared with a lymphedematous limb of the same size and girth. This guideline applies to the compression garments, too.

These individuals often require more padding under the compression bandages, particularly in the anterior tibial area. They do not tolerate circular knit garments, as they tend to cut into the soft tissues or at the ankle, and usually require a lower class of compression garment than someone with uncomplicated lymphedema. The therapist must remember, however, that later-stage lipedema is often accompanied by lymphedema, too, and that treatment includes compression garments, often of a higher compression class, though still flat knit.

The main goals of intervention are to decrease pain and hypersensitivity, decrease the lymphedematous component of the disease, and assist the individual in maintaining and/or reducing adipose tissue through exercise and nutritional guidance. The compression garments can help support the adipose tissue for exercise to assist weight loss. The most difficult task is fitting the compression garments. Flat knit garments are more comfortable, as circular knit fabrics tend to cut into the very soft fatty tissue or at the ankles. They must be custom-made because of the large size of the individual and can be uncomfortable at the waist if not carefully measured, particularly when sitting.

It may be more functional to compromise with compression ending just below the knee if that is all that the individual can tolerate. Compression garments can be designed in two pieces, one from the toes to just below the knee and a second layer from below the knee to the waist in a lighter fabric that can be removed if needed, leaving the lower leg garment intact.

Making the radical change in daily activity level is most challenging for these individuals. Providing continued support and encouragement is important. Networking is helpful and is facilitated by offering a support group, which can be held on an irregular, informal basis. An hour-long educational meeting, even if only offered three or four times per year, can provide a neutral meeting place for people to begin networking.

Nothing can compare with the encouragement and hope that an individual with lipedema or lymphedema can derive from seeing and talking with someone else living with the same problem and hearing how others cope on a day-to-day basis. Therapists can receive some of the best guidance on exercise and coping with compression garments in a group like this.

[a]Bonnie Lasinski and Joy C. Cohn.

## REFERENCES

To enhance this text and add value for the reader, all references are included in the enhanced ebook on Student Consult that accompanies this textbook. The reader can view the reference source and access it online whenever possible.

CHAPTER 14

# The Hematologic System

CELESTE KNIGHT PETERSON

Hematology is the branch of science that studies the form, structure, and function of blood and blood-forming tissues. Two major components of blood are examined: plasma and formed elements (erythrocytes, or red blood cells [RBCs]; leukocytes, or white blood cells [WBCs]; and platelets, or thrombocytes).

Delivery of these formed elements throughout the body tissues is necessary for cellular metabolism, defense against injury and invading microorganisms, and acid–base balance. The formation and development of blood cells, which usually take place in the bone marrow, are controlled by hormones (specifically erythropoietin) and feedback mechanisms that maintain an ideal number of cells.

The hematologic system is integrated with the lymphatic and immune systems; for a complete understanding of these systems, see Chapters 7 and 13. The lymph nodes are part of the lymphatic system but also part of the hematopoietic (blood-forming) system and the lymphoid system, which consists of organs and tissues of the immune system.

Lymph fluid passes through these nodes, or valves, which are located in the lymph channels at 1- to 2-cm intervals. As the fluid passes through the nodes, it is purified of harmful bacteria and viruses. Networks of the lymphatic system are situated in several areas of the body and may be considered primary (thymus and bone marrow) or secondary (spleen, lymph nodes, tonsils, and the Peyer patches of the small intestine).

All the lymphoid organs link the hematologic and immune systems in that they are sites of residence, proliferation, differentiation, or function of lymphocytes and mononuclear phagocytes (mononuclear phagocyte system: macrophage and monocyte cells capable of ingesting microorganisms and other antigens).

Lymphocytes are any of the nonphagocytic leukocytes (WBCs) found in the blood, lymph, and lymphoid tissues that make up the body's immunologically competent cells. They are divided into two classes: B and T lymphocytes. For example, in the hematologic system, the lymphocytes of the spleen produce approximately one-third of the antibody available to the immune system.

## SIGNS AND SYMPTOMS OF HEMATOLOGIC DISORDERS

Disruption of the hematologic system results in circulatory disorders, as well as signs and symptoms noted in the hematologic tissues themselves. The circulatory disorders can be characterized by edema and congestion, infarction, thrombosis and embolism, lymphedema, bleeding and bruising, and hypotension and shock (Box 14.1).

*Edema* is the accumulation of excessive fluid within the interstitial tissues or within body cavities. *Congestion* is the accumulation of excessive blood within the blood vessels of an organ or tissue. The forms of lymphedema include cerebral edema, inflammatory edema, peripheral dependent edema, and pulmonary edema. Congestion may be localized, as with a venous thrombosis, or generalized, as with heart failure, which results in congestion in the lungs, lower extremities, and abdominal viscera.

*Infarction* is a localized region of necrosis caused by reduction of arterial perfusion below a level required for cell viability. Such a situation occurs as a result of arterial obstruction caused by atherosclerosis, arterial thrombosis, or embolism, when oxygen supply fails to meet the oxygen requirements of organs with end arteries, such as the gastrointestinal (GI) tract, the heart, and, less often, the kidneys and spleen. Cerebral cortical neurons (cerebral infarction) and myocardial cells (myocardial infarction) are most vulnerable to ischemia, although protective collateral blood flow develops in the heart through anastomoses.

A *thrombus* is a solid mass of clotted blood within an intact blood vessel or chamber of the heart. An *embolus* is a mass of solid, liquid, or gas that moves within a blood vessel to lodge at a site distant from its place of origin. Most emboli are thromboemboli. Thrombosis (development of a thrombus or clot) results from pathologic activation of the hemostatic mechanisms involving platelets, coagulation factors, and blood vessel walls. Endothelial injury, alteration in blood flow (stasis and turbulence), and hypercoagulability of the blood (e.g., protein abnormalities either primary or associated with cancers) promote thrombosis and thromboembolism.

**Box 14.1**

**MOST COMMON SIGNS AND SYMPTOMS OF HEMATOLOGIC DISORDERS**

- Edema
  - Lymphedema
  - Cerebral edema
  - Inflammatory edema
  - Peripheral dependent edema
  - Pulmonary edema
- Lymphadenopathy
- Congestion
- Infarction (brain, heart, GI tract, kidney, spleen)
- Thrombosis
- Splenomegaly
- Embolism
- Bleeding and bruising
- Shock
  - Rapid, weak pulse (late phase)
  - Hypotension (systolic blood pressure <90 mm Hg)
  - Cool, moist skin (late phase)
  - Pallor
  - Weak/absent peripheral pulses

*Lymphedema*, or chronic swelling of an area from accumulation of interstitial fluid (edema), occurs in hemolymphatic disorders secondary to obstruction of lymphatic vessels or lymph nodes. Obstruction may be of an inflammatory or mechanical nature from trauma, regional lymph node resection or irradiation, or extensive involvement of regional nodes by malignant disease.

Women who have been treated surgically for breast cancer with lymph node dissection, mastectomy, and/or radiation therapy are at double the risk of developing lymphedema of the arm and/or chest wall. When the obstruction that slows the lymph fluid exceeds the pumping capacity of the system, the fluid accumulates in the tissues in the extremity, causing edema in one or more limbs. This accumulation of fluid may become a source for bacterial growth, leading to infection, fibrosis, and possible loss of functional limb use.

*Bleeding and bruising* can occur from trauma of various types and are normal consequences of injury. However, when bleeding and bruising are elicited with minor trauma (e.g., brushing teeth) or bleeding continues longer than normal, there is more concern for a disorder of the blood. These symptoms are often a result of platelet abnormalities (function or quantity) such as idiopathic thrombocytopenic purpura, thrombotic thrombocytopenic purpura, or von Willebrand disease.

Purpura is a hemorrhagic condition that occurs when not enough normal platelets are available to plug damaged vessels or prevent leakage from even minor injury to normal capillaries. Purpura is characterized by movement of blood into the surrounding tissue (extravasation), under the skin, and through the mucous membranes, producing spontaneous ecchymoses (bruises) and petechiae (small, red patches) on the skin. When accompanied by a decrease in the circulating platelets, it is called *thrombocytopenic purpura*. In the acute form, bleeding can occur from any of the body orifices, such as hematuria, nosebleed, vaginal bleeding, and bleeding gums.

**Table 14.1** Etiologic Factors of Shock

| Category of Shock | Causes |
|---|---|
| Hypovolemic | Hemorrhage (loss of blood, shock)<br>Vomiting<br>Diarrhea<br>Dehydration secondary to:<br>• Decreased fluid intake<br>• Diabetes mellitus (diuresis during diabetic ketoacidosis or severe hyperglycemia)<br>• Diabetes insipidus<br>• Inadequate rehydration of long-distance runner<br>Addison disease<br>Burns |
| Cardiogenic | Arrhythmias<br>Acute valvular dysfunction<br>Acute myocardial infarction<br>Severe congestive heart failure<br>Cardiomyopathy<br>Obstructive<br>Septic<br>Neurogenic<br>Obstructive valvular disease (aortic or mitral stenosis)<br>Cardiac tumor (atrial myxoma) |
| Reduced system vascular resistance | Bacteremia; overwhelming infections<br>Spinal cord injury<br>Pain<br>Trauma<br>Vasodilator drugs<br>Burns<br>Thyrotoxicosis<br>Pancreatitis<br>Anaphylaxis<br>Liver failure |

*Shock* occurs when the circulatory system (heart as well as arteries) is unable to maintain adequate pressure in order to perfuse organs. Common clinical signs include tachycardia, tachypnea, cool extremities, decreased pulses, decreased urine output, and an altered mental status. Hypotension is typically present but may be initially absent. The end result is hypoxia to end-organ tissues, particularly the kidneys, brain, and heart.

Diagnosis as to the cause of shock should include an evaluation of the heart, a search for infection, or source of bleeding. Myocardial infarction and heart failure are problems that make it difficult for the heart to pump an adequate amount of blood to the body. Decreased blood volume (hypovolemia) from hemorrhaging or severe volume depletion (e.g., nausea, vomiting, and diarrhea) also reduces the body's ability to perfuse tissue.

Disorders that cause a decrease in the arterial pressure include sepsis (infection from any source), liver failure, severe pancreatitis, anaphylaxis, and thyrotoxicosis. The three most common classes of shock therefore are cardiogenic (heart related), hypovolemic, and causes related to reduced systemic vascular resistance, although many overlap (Table 14.1).

*Lymphadenopathy* is the abnormal enlargement of a lymph node(s). Lymph nodes filter lymph as it returns to the heart. Infectious organisms (e.g., Epstein-Barr virus [EBV] and tuberculosis) and autoimmune disorders (e.g., rheumatoid arthritis [RA] and systemic lupus erythematosus [SLE]) can cause an inflammatory expansion and enlargement of lymph nodes. Malignant diseases, such as lymphoma, chronic lymphocytic leukemia, and Hodgkin lymphoma, can also cause enlarged lymph nodes.

Lymph nodes are typically "rubbery" in feel, unattached to surrounding tissue (mobile), and small (usually less than 1 cm). Inflammatory nodes may be tender to the touch, warm, and enlarged but usually remain mobile and soft. Malignant nodes are often not tender or mobile; they are firm and enlarged. Most cases of lymphadenopathy are not malignancy related, although all instances of abnormal adenopathy should be investigated.

Enlargement of the spleen, or *splenomegaly*, is present in many hematologic diseases. The spleen is normally involved in removing old or deformed erythrocytes, producing antibodies, and removing antibody-laden bacteria or cells. When the spleen exceeds normal function in one of these areas, it becomes enlarged. For example, if a client has hereditary spherocytosis and forms abnormally shaped erythrocytes, the spleen attempts to remove all these cells, thereby increasing in size to accomplish this task.

Splenomegaly is often noted in people with infectious mononucleosis or malignancies such as Hodgkin lymphoma (where the spleen is infiltrated by disease). If the bone marrow is unable to produce cells (because of an infiltrative process), the spleen often assumes that role and becomes enlarged (extramedullary hematopoiesis).

SPECIAL IMPLICATIONS FOR THE THERAPIST 14.1

## *Hematologic Disorders*

Hematologic conditions alter the oxygen-carrying capacity of the blood and the constituents, structure, consistency, and flow of the blood. These changes can contribute to hypocoagulopathy or hypercoagulopathy, increased work of the heart and breathing, impaired tissue perfusion, and increased risk of thrombus.

Hematologic abnormalities require that the results of the client's blood analysis and clotting factors be monitored so that therapy intervention can be modified to minimize risk.[84] Precautions and interventions for the client with lymphedema are discussed in Chapter 13.

Platelet disorders require special consideration by the therapist during exercise. Decreased platelets are associated with the risk of life-threatening hemorrhage; physical therapy intervention must be tailored to the individual's platelet levels. For example, platelet levels between 40,000 and 60,000 μL face an increased risk of postsurgical or traumatic bleed. Low-load resistance exercise is permitted with 1- to 2-lb weights. Safe exercise includes walking, stationary bicycling with light resistance, and minimal activities of daily living.

For clients with platelet levels in the 20,000 to 40,000 range, low-intensity exercise with no weights or resistance up to 2 lb is permitted but with no resistance during stationary biking. Activity and exercise restriction is even more stringent when platelet levels are below 20,000. Below 10,000, spontaneous central nervous system, GI, and/or respiratory tract bleeding may occur.[484] In all cases, clients are monitored carefully for any signs of bleeding. Guidelines vary from one geographic region to another and even from center to center within a single geographic location.

### Splenomegaly

Because splenomegaly is often associated with conditions characterized by rapid destruction of blood cells, it is important to follow the usual precautions for anyone with poor clotting abilities.

The client must be taught proper breathing techniques in conjunction with ways to avoid activities or positions that could traumatize the abdominal region or increase intracranial, intrathoracic, or intraabdominal pressure.

The person with a small or absent spleen is more susceptible to streptococcal infection, which calls for prevention techniques such as good handwashing.

### Exercise and Sports

Exercise training can induce blood volume expansion immediately (plasma volume) and over a period (erythrocyte volume) and is associated with healing, improved quality of life, and improved exercise capabilities in cases of anemia from hemorrhage, trauma, renal disease, and chronic diseases. The reestablishment of erythropoiesis through exercise and effects of exercise on blood volume in other groups remain unknown but are a potential area for further investigation and consideration in the clinical setting.[106,378]

Improvements in athletic performance with exogenous erythropoietin (referred to as "blood doping") have been documented as improvements in running time and maximal oxygen uptake. However, these effects are not without risk for increased blood viscosity and thrombosis, with potentially fatal results. Until a definitive test is developed for detection of exogenous erythropoietin, the therapist must remain aware of this potential problem.[397,398]

### Monitoring Vital Signs

Clients in whom shock develops may exhibit orthostatic changes in vital signs. A drop in systolic blood pressure of 10 to 20 mm Hg or more, associated with an increase in pulse rate of more than 15 beats/min, may indicate a depleted intravascular volume.

The therapist is unlikely to see a client with acute hypovolemia; hypovolemia is more likely the result of dehydration, as in the case of the long-distance runner or the client with severe diarrhea or slow GI tract bleeding. The aging population is especially vulnerable to development of unknown slow intestinal bleeding, especially with the use of aspirin or nonsteroidal antiinflammatory drugs.

Clients with peripheral neuropathies or clients taking medications such as certain antihypertensive drugs may be normovolemic and experience an orthostatic fall in blood pressure but without associated increase in pulse rate. If any doubt exists, the client should be placed in the supine position with legs elevated to maximize cerebral blood flow. The Trendelenburg position, in which the head is lower than the rest of the body, is no longer used because of the increased difficulty of breathing in this position.

## AGING AND THE HEMATOPOIETIC SYSTEM

As a person ages, there are associated changes in the bone marrow. Generally, there is a decrease in the production of RBCs and lymphocytes with a comparative increase in the production of myeloid cells. Hematopoietic stem cells (HSC) lose their ability to self-renew and differentiate into various mature cells. This process is driven by selective pressures that may be due to exposure to infective agents or other stresses. Changes in chemokines and cytokines most likely direct the selection of specific types of HSCs. HSCs, then, become clonal, and destined for only specific cell types. This results in more myeloid cells with a bias for the innate immune system over the production of lymphocytes (T and B cells) with a reduced ability for adaptive immune response. It also reduces the variation and diversity of the lymphocyte pool. HSCs exhibit changes in methylation regulation of the DNA and telomere shortening (although this varies between older people and may account for individual variation in aging). Aging HSCs demonstrate changes in cell cycle distribution as well as acquire DNA damage with the inability to make repairs.[62,81]

Bone marrow also has mesenchymal derived stem cells (MSCs) that differentiate into osteoblasts, adipocytes, myocytes, and chondrocytes. These cells aid in the structural formation of the bone marrow and provide the microenvironment and various "niches" for the maturation of cells. With aging, the cells of the microenvironment may alter production of cytokines/chemokines and influence changes in HSCs.[222]

Platelets signal WBCs in regards to inflammation and thrombosis. As people age, platelet products change, inducing monocytes to secrete cytokines that are proinflammatory, which may contribute to chronic inflammation often seen in the elderly.[43]

Age-related changes in the peripheral blood include slightly decreased hemoglobin and hematocrit, although levels remain within the normal adult range. Diseases or vitamin deficiencies can cause low hemoglobin levels noted in aging adults. Iron deficiency (usually via blood loss such as ulcer, colon polyps, or cancer) can be associated with a longstanding condition such as rheumatologic conditions often seen in a therapy practice (referred to as *anemia of chronic disease*). Vitamin $B_{12}$, which is required to produce blood cells, and the subsequent development of anemia (resulting from a $B_{12}$ deficiency) with its hematologic, neurologic, and GI manifestations, are discussed later in this chapter.

## BLOOD TRANSFUSIONS

Advances in treating hematologic/immunologic disorders through blood transfusions and hematopoietic cell transplantation (HCT) have provided new success in long-term treatment and a cure for some previously fatal disorders. Modern blood banking and transfusion medicine have developed techniques to administer only the blood component needed by the client, such as packed RBCs for anemia, specific factors for people with coagulation deficiencies (such as factor VIII deficiency or hemophilia), or platelets for people with active bleeding or leukemias.

Clients in a therapy setting who have undergone numerous surgical procedures (e.g., traumatic injuries) or elective orthopedic or cardiac procedures may also receive autologous blood transfusions (i.e., reinfusion of a person's own blood) when significant blood loss may be a complication and a transfusion may be anticipated.

The development of recombinant human erythropoietin, with its ability to stimulate erythropoiesis (bone marrow production of red cells) and elevate RBCs, has reduced the need for blood transfusion in a variety of clinical situations (e.g., chronic renal disease, anemia following chemotherapy and hematopoietic cell transplantation, and surgical procedures, especially joint arthroplasty and cardiac procedures).

### Reaction to Blood and Blood Products

#### Febrile Nonhemolytic Reaction

Because blood products are most often donated from another person, reactions may occur. The most common transfusion-related reaction is a febrile, nonhemolytic reaction (occurring in 0.5%-1% of erythrocyte transfusions). The condition is characterized by an increase in temperature by more than 1.0° C (1.8° F) or higher than 38° C (100.4° F) during or within 4 hours after the transfusion. These reactions are usually a result of donor-derived cytokines during storage.

Treatment includes stopping the transfusion, checking the blood for a direct hemolytic process (in the laboratory), and administering antipyretics. Symptoms are usually transient, and the removal of donor leukocytes from the blood (leukocyte reduction) can reduce the risk of another similar reaction (Box 14.2).

#### Transfusion-Associated Circulatory Overload

Transfusion-associated circulatory overload (TACO) is a relatively common type of transfusion reaction but is often underrecognized. Historically it has been

Box 14.2

**SIGNS AND SYMPTOMS OF REACTIONS TO BLOOD AND BLOOD PRODUCTS**

***Febrile, Nonhemolytic Transfusion Reaction***

- Fever/chills
- Headache
- Nausea/vomiting
- Hypertension
- Tachycardia

***Transfusion-Related Acute Lung Injury***

- Pulmonary edema
- Acute respiratory distress
- Severe hypoxia

***Acute Hemolytic Transfusion Reaction***

- Fever/chills
- Nausea/vomiting
- Flank, abdominal pain
- Headache
- Dyspnea
- Hypotension
- Tachycardia
- Red urine

***Delayed Hemolytic Transfusion Reaction***

- Unexplained drop in hemoglobin—anemia
- Increased bilirubin level—jaundice
- Increased lactate dehydrogenase level

***Allergic Reactions***

- Hives/rash
- Wheezing
- Mucosal edema

***Anaphylaxis***

- Abrupt hypotension
- Edema of the larynx
- Difficulty breathing
- Nausea
- Abdominal pain
- Diarrhea
- Shock
- Respiratory arrest

***Septic Reactions***

- Fever/chills
- Hypotension
- Headache
- Back, chest, abdominal pain
- Shortness of breath

***Circulatory Overload***

- Red face
- Shortness of breath
- Tachycardia
- Orthopnea
- Hypertension
- Headache
- Seizures

reported in less than 1% of transfusions, but this is probably low and may be more likely 1% to 8% of transfusions. TACO is due to volume overload from a rapidly infused transfusion. It is most often noted in clients who are older, with comorbidities such as heart or kidney disease. Shortness of breath typically begins within 6 hours of transfusion associated with elevated central venous pressure, chest radiograph consistent with pulmonary edema, and elevated B-type natriuretic peptide. Treatment is the use of diuretics and respiratory support.

### Transfusion-Related Acute Lung Injury

Transfusion-related acute lung injury (TRALI) occurs in as many as 1 in every 5000 transfusions, although actual rates are unknown due to poor recognition of the syndrome.[356,402] However, since the implementation of strategies to reduce the risk of TRALI in the mid 2000s, the incidence has significantly decreased.[97,310] Yet TRALI remains the most common cause of transfusion-related death (mortality rate historically of 5% but studies demonstrate more recent rates of 13% to 21%).[460] Higher rates of mortality are seen in people who are critically ill and then develop TRALI. Transfusion-related acute lung injury occurs as a consequence of HLA or neutrophil-specific antibodies in donor plasma directed against recipient leukocytes in the pulmonary vasculature. This reaction typically presents within 6 hours of the transfusion. Common findings include fever, hypotension, and pulmonary edema. Unlike adult respiratory distress syndrome, improvement can sometimes be seen within days. With appropriate respiratory intervention (people often require intubation and ventilation), most individuals recover without permanent pulmonary damage.

### Acute Hemolytic Transfusion Reaction

Less common than other types of transfusion reactions (only 1 in every 70,000 transfusions),[155] acute hemolytic transfusion reaction, an ABO incompatibility, is the most feared complication. Typically, a mistake is made by giving a person the wrong blood or blood is mislabeled. Symptoms begin soon after the transfusion is begun (within 24 hours), including fever and flank pain; if this progresses to disseminated intravascular coagulation (DIC), clients may manifest hypotension and bleeding (see Box 14.2). Erythrocytes are destroyed intravascularly with resultant red plasma and red urine.

The mortality rate is high, ranging from 17% to 60%. The transfusion is immediately terminated and the client given cardiovascular support. Renal failure, disseminated intravascular coagulation, and severe hypotension may occur.

### Delayed Hemolytic Transfusion Reaction

Delayed hemolytic transfusion reactions typically occur 7 to 14 days after a transfusion. This reaction is a consequence of an amnestic response from antibodies to minor or non-ABO proteins that were produced in a previous transfusion, but are not immediately detectable during a subsequent pretransfusion testing. These reactions are often asymptomatic and are noted only because the hemoglobin does not rise as predicted following the transfusion.

### Allergic Reaction/Anaphylaxis

Mild allergic reactions (such as pruritus and urticaria) are common (1%-3% of transfusions), particularly in clients who have received multiple transfusions. The allergy is usually caused by donor plasma proteins and often does not recur.

More severe respiratory symptoms may occur, such as wheezing, shortness of breath, abdominal symptoms, hypotension, and mucosal edema and are classified as anaphylaxis or anaphylactoid reactions. Anaphylactic or anaphylactoid reactions are rare (approximately 1 in 20,000-50,000 transfusions) and may occur with or without allergic reactions. It is usually seen in people who are immunoglobulin (Ig) A deficient and make anti-IgA antibodies that react to a donor's IgA. These reactions are also noted in clients who are allergic to a protein in the donor blood product. This reaction can be severe and fatal and is associated with shock, respiratory failure, and vascular collapse. Treatment consists of immediately discontinuing the transfusion, administering antihistamines and/or epinephrine, and providing cardiovascular and respiratory support. All subsequent transfusions require washing of all blood products. Plasma products must be obtained from IgA-deficient donors if the person is IgA deficient.

### Septic Reactions

Rarely, septic reactions can occur secondary to bacterial contamination of blood products, principally platelets (they are not stored at cold temperatures). Sepsis is seen in approximately 1:50,000 platelet transfusions and only 1:5,000,000 RBC transfusions. In March 2004, all blood banks began to routinely screen platelets for bacterial contamination, with a subsequent reduction in septic reactions. Symptoms of such reactions include fever/chills; hypotension; headache; back, chest, and abdominal pain; and shortness of breath. Culture of the product and appropriate antibiotics and cardiovascular support are the mainstays of treatment.

Transfusion as a source for hepatitis (B and C) has been reduced since the initiation of donor screening for hepatitis antibodies. Newer testing techniques, such as nucleic acid testing (NAT), have reduced the risk even further. Current risk of contracting hepatitis C from a blood transfusion is less than 1:1,000,000 transfusions. People with hemophilia can receive various medications and products to treat their disease. One option is plasma-derived factor concentrates, which have been free of hepatitis B, hepatitis C, and HIV viruses since 1993, or recombinant products (nonhuman plasma factors made in the lab), which are now considered the standard of care and avoid the risk of contracting an infectious disease.

The risk of HIV infection by transfusion is low overall, calculated at 1:1.5 to 2 million transfusions.[487] The risk of HIV transmission by blood transfusion has been continually reduced through the elimination of high-risk individuals from blood donor pools and the use of more sensitive screening (e.g., NAT). The transmission of HIV is possible if the donor has contracted the virus but has not developed any detectable laboratory markers. Effort has also been directed at inactivating HIV even in products that have tested negative for HIV through inactivation/purification processes.

**SPECIAL IMPLICATIONS FOR THE THERAPIST 14.2**

### *Blood Transfusions*

As a general rule, people are not usually exercising or being treated by the physical therapist during a blood transfusion. There are no published guidelines for this protocol and it is not a hard and fast rule. Each case can be evaluated on its own merits person by person.

The therapist must consider why a person is receiving a blood product, what is the underlying medical condition and the goals of therapy for that day/week. Consideration should be given for what is in the best interest of the individual's health and safety. In other words, will mobilizing the person during a blood transfusion be beneficial or detrimental? Can treatment be held (postponed) until a later time either later in the transfusion process or later in the day or the next day?

In some facilities, cautious therapy can be carried out during blood transfusions for those individuals who can tolerate it. Movement and gentle exercise or range-of-motion is not advised until the nursing staff approves it.

The reasons for holding physical therapy during blood transfusion are not always physiologic. Sometimes it is more a matter of logistics. For example, during the transfusion procedure, nothing the therapist does should compromise (dislodge) the intravenous line. The policy of physical therapists working with individuals receiving blood transfusions varies from region to region and even within the same facility. Perhaps it is more a matter of how routine the procedure is for the health care staff. For example, nurses in intensive care units are often more comfortable getting people mobilized with multiple lines and while watching unstable hemodynamics. On orthopedic floors, where multiple lines are not standard, nurses may wait for very stable hemodynamics before mobilizing postoperative patients.

On the orthopedic floor, therapists may only do supine therapeutic exercise with individuals receiving transfusion, when in fact there is no reason to withhold treatment. In reality, blood transfusions through an intravenous line are no different than any other fluid administered in the same way. Monitor vital signs, observe for tolerance to treatment, and carry on as usual.

Most blood transfusion reactions occur during the actual transfusion and are not of consequence to the therapist unless working with the individual during the actual transfusion. Exercise or therapy of any kind is not advised during the first 30 minutes (possibly up to 60 minutes) of the transfusion. This allows the nurses to evaluate how the patients are responding to the blood while monitoring for any adverse reactions. Most adverse reactions occur during the first 15 minutes (e.g., fever, chills, urticaria, acute respiratory distress, transfusion-related acute lung injury). Once the therapist begins working with the individual being transfused, then it is important to monitor for signs of adverse reactions to the transfusion and signs of orthostatic hypotension.

There may be some question as to the appropriateness of physical therapy treatment for individuals receiving a blood transfusion for anemia. If the person is anemic enough to need a blood transfusion, is the person able to tolerate therapeutic exercise?

If the person is asymptomatic, the IV site is stable, and activity or movement is tolerated, then therapeutic exercise may be prescribed. When autologous transfusion is unavailable or inappropriate, the therapist must be alert for any signs of adverse reaction. Among the most common transfusion reactions are febrile, nonhemolytic transfusion reactions and delayed hemolytic transfusion reactions. Clinical symptoms from these reactions are typically mild and can usually be prevented on subsequent transfusions.

One of the most severe, but uncommon, reactions is the acute hemolytic transfusion reaction. This is a result of antigen–antibody reactions resulting from blood type incompatibility, with clumping of cells, hemolysis, and release of cellular elements into the serum. Box 14.2 lists the signs and symptoms indicating such a reaction.

Occasionally, a client may develop an allergic reaction observed as dyspnea or hives; the latter may be brought to the therapist's attention after local modality intervention. The therapist may also be the first to recognize early signs of hepatitis (jaundice), especially changes in sclerae or skin color or reported changes in urine (dark or tea colored) and stools (light colored or white).

## Bloodless Medicine and Surgery

Karen Wilk, PT, DPT

Bloodless medicine and surgery, the use of technological and pharmaceutical techniques to minimize blood loss and avoid the use of allogeneic blood transfusions, has advanced in recent years into the concept of patient blood management.[392] Patient blood management uses evidence-based medicine to develop an individualized plan for each person to minimize or eliminate the need for transfusions. This is based on three main principles applied to medical and surgical patients: manage anemia, minimize blood loss, and optimize hemostasis.[391,445]

Why has there been a movement away from transfusions? For generations blood transfusions have been viewed by the medical community and recipients as a lifesaving treatment. A number of factors are moving the medical community in this direction. One is the community of Jehovah's Witnesses, who seek medical care but decline the use of most forms of transfusions. Rather than refuse to treat these individuals without the use of transfusions, some physicians worked to find techniques that were compatible with the religious beliefs of this group.[391]

Second, although the blood supply can be considered safer than ever as a result of donor prescreening and postdonation testing, new infectious agents are possible and donor history of HIV and/or hepatitis have made some people caution in accepting blood transfusions.[390,393]

Finally, there is a growing body of evidence that there are risks to receiving a transfusion. Risks of receiving transfusions include infections, increased length of stay in ICU and hospital, increased renal and cardiac events, acute respiratory distress syndrome, cancer recurrence, and death.[390,393,445] Despite safeguards in place, human error cannot be eliminated from the transfusion process, and currently mistransfusion is the greatest risk of mortality from transfusion.[393,445] For these reasons, individuals whose religious beliefs are incompatible with transfusions are seeking bloodless alternatives.

### Objectives

The first objective of patient blood management is the control of anemia. Anemia is related to the decreased production or increased destruction of blood cells or a combination of both. In trauma patients, the rapid loss of blood may require the use of transfusions. For the nontrauma patient the identification and treatment of anemia is critical.

For surgical patients adequate timely screening is needed. It is important to review personal or family history of anemia prior to surgery. The presence of undetected anemia must be discovered and treated prior to surgical intervention. Treatment of preoperative anemia can include iron, recombinant human erythropoietin and folic acid, with the goal of normal range hemoglobin by the time of surgery.[390,391,393,445]

Some patients consider the predonation of their own blood preoperatively. Blood donated in this way must be timed well with the surgical date and is therefore subject to the same changes all blood undergoes during cold storage, including changes to the RBCs. Also, some people who predonate their own blood face issues of anemia in the preoperative phase and may need treatment for anemia.[391,393]

### Minimizing Blood Loss

During surgery, steps can be taken to minimize blood loss. These measures can include positioning the individual to elevate the area of blood loss, use of a tourniquet, and gentle handling of tissues.[391,393] Instruments that minimize blood loss include the harmonic scalpel, argon beam, and radiofrequency assisted thermal ablation.[393] There are also topical and systemic agents that contain collagen, thrombin, and fibrinogen to promote coagulation.[391]

Acute normovolemic hemodilution can be used when blood loss is expected. Just before surgery several units of blood are removed and replaced with crystalloid or colloid solutions so blood volume is maintained. Any fluid lost during surgery contains fewer RBCs and clotting factors are preserved. At the conclusion of the surgery the blood is reinfused to the patient. The entire process is completed through a closed circuit.[389,393]

Another way to impact blood loss in the operating room is to avoid hypothermia. Hypothermia can impede platelet function, resulting in increased blood loss.[391,417] During surgery blood that is lost can be suctioned and saved. It is collected, mixed with anticoagulants, filtered, and reinfused to the patient. The use of cell salvage can continue into the postoperative phase through the use of drains.[391,393] Anyone diagnosed with cancer cannot use this technique because of concerns about cancer spread.

### Postoperative Concerns

Postoperatively, continuing steps to minimize blood loss should be taken. If there is postoperative bleeding, the patient may need to return to the operating room. Postoperative phlebotomy should be minimized and microsampling techniques used, because routine blood draws can cause anemia.[456]

Clinician acceptance of lower hemoglobin levels is essential. It is not uncommon for surgical patients to experience a drop in postoperative hemoglobin levels. Monitoring to ensure it is in the range of acceptability is prudent.[417] Research shows there is a hemoglobin reserve that allows individuals to tolerate lower hemoglobin levels than previously thought if tissue perfusion is maintained. Hemoglobin levels alone should not be a trigger for transfusion, rather the individual should be looked at as a whole.

The number of bloodless medicine and surgery programs is growing, allowing an increasing number of patients access to these techniques for surgeries, including Whipple procedure for pancreatic cancer, joint replacements, and coronary artery bypass.

SPECIAL IMPLICATIONS FOR THE THERAPIST 14.3

### *Bloodless Medicine and Surgery*

Therapists who work in acute care, surgical, and postoperative settings need to have an awareness of the impact of lower hemoglobin levels on the patient's ability to participate in therapy. The therapist should review blood work results prior to each therapy session, looking specifically at hemoglobin levels. Routine vital signs, including pulse oximetry, must be monitored throughout the session. Watch and talk to the patient and monitor how the patient is tolerating the activity level. There are no studies looking at hemoglobin levels and safe activity levels, but individuals participating in bloodless medicine programs tolerate therapy sessions well with hemoglobin levels in the 6.5 to 9.0 range. Practice guidelines for blood management are published by the Society of Thoracic Surgeons (STS) and updated every 3 years. The most recent update may be of interest to therapists working in settings where blood conservation is employed. For the full text of this and other STS Practice Guidelines, visit http://www.sts.org/resources-publications at the official STS website (www.sts.org).[112]

# DISORDERS OF IRON ABSORPTION

## Hereditary Hemochromatosis

Hereditary hemochromatosis (HH) is an autosomal recessive hereditary disorder characterized by excessive iron absorption by the small intestine. Most people with HH have the C282Y mutation in the *HFE* gene, but a small percentage have both the C282Y mutation and the H63D mutation. The genetic susceptibility is seen in 1 in 250 people[330] of Northern European descent; however, only 70% that are homozygous for the C282Y mutation with demonstrate evidence of the disease and only 10% of people homozygous for C282Y will develop the full expression of the disease with organ damage.[19,146] Hemochromatosis is present at birth but remains asymptomatic until the development of iron overloading and onset of symptoms between ages 40 and 60 years (sometimes as early as age 30 years). The prevalence is equal among men and women, but men experience symptoms 5 to 10 times more often than do women (menstruation and pregnancy help to slow progression of the disorder).

### Pathogenesis

Hemochromatosis can be caused by mutations in the genes of any of the proteins that regulate the entry of iron into the blood, including alterations in the hepcidin and ferroportin genes, and iron regulatory proteins, such as human hemochromatosis protein (HFE), hemojuvelin, and transferrin receptor 2.[125,197,333]

The most common inherited form of the disease is caused by abnormalities of the *HFE* gene (type I) located on chromosome 6.[20] The product of the *HFE* gene interacts with other receptors and proteins to regulate hepcidin production. Hepcidin is the main iron-regulatory protein produced by the liver and, when present in the circulation, decreases iron absorption from the gut and inhibits the release of iron from macrophages.[294] Mutations in the *HFE* gene lead to a decreased production of hepcidin, resulting in increased absorption of iron by intestinal enterocytes and release of iron by macrophages.

The severity of the disease depends on several factors, including how many and which genes are affected. For example, 85% of people with clinical hemochromatosis have homozygous mutations for C282Y[19]; yet even among people with this type of mutation, they are only predisposed for the disease, and there is significant variability in the clinical manifestation. Those with mild iron overload may be homozygous for H63D but heterozygous for C282Y and H63D (one gene of each affected). But people who are heterozygotes for C282Y rarely develop the disease. Environmental factors are also thought to play a role in the clinical manifestations of the disease, such as blood loss, alcohol intake, coexistence of chronic hepatitides B and C, and nonalcoholic fatty liver disease.[328,334]

### Clinical Manifestations

The body typically absorbs iron at a rate equal to body requirements. But in hemochromatosis, there is an uncoupling between absorption and body needs. Excess iron is slowly deposited in cells, particularly in the liver, heart, pancreas, and, to a lesser extent, other endocrine glands (e.g., the pituitary gland).

Signs and symptoms can include weakness, chronic fatigue, myalgias, joint pain (particularly the second and third metacarpophalangeal joints [MCPs]),[449] abdominal pain, hepatomegaly, elevated hemoglobin, and elevated liver enzymes. Continued iron overload leads to tissue damage. The liver is the most commonly affected organ, and clients may present with hepatomegaly without liver enzyme abnormalities. If the disease progresses without treatment, cirrhosis and liver cancer may ensue.

Other complications of untreated hemochromatosis include diabetes mellitus, cardiac myopathy (with associated HF) and arrhythmias, hyperpigmentation or "bronzing" of the skin, destructive arthritis, and impotence (men) or decreased libido (women) and sterility.

Clients have noted that symptoms often began up to 10 years before a diagnosis was made.[253] Due to routine laboratory testing, elevations in liver enzymes and serum iron markers (ferritin and transferrin saturation) often prompt an evaluation for asymptomatic HH, prior to irreversible tissue damage.

### MEDICAL MANAGEMENT

**DIAGNOSIS.** Diagnosis can best be made through blood tests. The most sensitive screening test is the measurement of transferrin saturation. Levels higher than 45% are suggestive of the disease.[19] A ferritin greater than

200 ng/mL in men and 150 ng/mL in women with iron overload is also indicative of the disease. Individuals who have screening tests compatible with HH should undergo genetic testing for the C282Y mutation.

In the past, a liver biopsy was required to confirm the diagnosis. However, with current available genetic tests, liver biopsies are only required in situations such as determining the severity of the disease or when alternative diagnoses are in question. MRI is able to estimate hepatic and cardiac iron overload, whereas ultrasound-based elastography aids in recognizing hepatic fibrosis.[450] In families where hemochromatosis has been previously diagnosed, all first-degree blood relatives should be genetically screened for hemochromatosis. Careful monitoring of affected family members can be done through blood tests.

TREATMENT. Treatment should begin as early in the disease process as possible. Individuals who are symptomatic or demonstrate end-organ damage need immediate treatment. People with iron levels that progressively exceed normal values benefit from treatment prior to the deposition of iron in tissue.[298] Clients with ferritin levels below 500 ng/mL can safely be monitored. Medical intervention consists of weekly to twice-weekly therapeutic phlebotomy. This is performed until iron stores are at normal levels, with ferritin between 50 and 100 ng/mL (for some clients this may take 2-3 years), after which maintenance therapy is done as needed to maintain appropriate levels (typically every 2-4 months). Ferritin levels should be monitored every 3 months.[373]

Chelating agents (i.e., agents that bind iron) may be given parenterally in cases where anemia or protein loss is severe and the client cannot tolerate phlebotomy.[283] Phlebotomy, however, is less expensive and safer. Affected individuals are instructed to avoid ingesting alcohol because it increases the risk of developing cirrhosis.

### PROGNOSIS

The prognosis is good, with improved or normal life expectancy as long as the iron levels remain in the normal range and the disease has not caused organ damage. With treatment, malaise, fatigue, abdominal pain, liver function, and cardiac function improve, skin color lightens, and approximately 40% of clients with diabetes mellitus have improved glycemic control. Cirrhosis does not improve with therapy and 30% of clients go on to develop hepatocellular carcinoma. Hypogonadism and arthropathy typically do not improve with treatment, and joint symptoms may actually progress despite therapy.[19]

#### SPECIAL IMPLICATIONS FOR THE THERAPIST 14.4

*Hemochromatosis*

Arthropathy occurs in 40% to 60% of individuals with hemochromatosis and can be the first manifestation of the disease.[182] The arthropathy associated with hemochromatosis is not reversible and often continues to progress even with effective medical intervention.

Osteoarthritic manifestations are diverse, with minimal joint inflammation at first. The affected individual may report twinges of pain on flexing the small joints of the hand, especially the second and third metacarpophalangeal joints. Involvement of these joints often helps to distinguish hemochromatosis-related arthropathy from osteoarthritis.

Acute joint presentation can occur with progression that involves the large joints, including the hips, knees, and shoulders, accompanied by destruction to the joint, severe impairment, and resulting disability. Hemochromatosis may be associated with calcium pyrophosphate dihydrate deposition disease. This presents as an acute inflammatory arthritis.[409]

Therapeutic intervention is essential in providing flexibility, strength, and proper alignment to promote function, prevent falls, and prevent the loss of independence in activities of daily living. The therapist can be very helpful in evaluating the need for assistive devices, orthotics, and splints toward these goals.

## DISORDERS OF ERYTHROCYTES

### The Anemias

#### Definition

Anemia is a pathologic state resulting in a reduction of the oxygen-carrying capacity of the blood from an abnormality in the quantity or quality of RBCs. The World Health Organization (WHO) has defined anemia in terms of the level of hemoglobin: less than 13 g/dL for men and less than 12 g/dL for women. Different ranges exist for men and women, infants and growing children, and different metabolic and physiologic states.[47]

These normal values must be evaluated on an individual basis; normal levels may be inadequate if tissue oxygen delivery is impaired by pulmonary insufficiency, cardiac disorders, or an increase in hemoglobin oxygen affinity.

#### Overview

Anemia is not a disease entity in itself; rather, it is a symptom of many other diseases, such as dietary deficiency (anemia caused by folate or vitamin $B_{12}$ deficiency); acute or chronic blood loss (iron deficiency); congenital defects of hemoglobin (sickle cell diseases); exposure to industrial poisons; diseases of the bone marrow; chronic inflammatory, infectious, or neoplastic disease; or any other disorder that upsets the balance between blood loss through bleeding or destruction of blood cells and production of blood cells. Anemia may be classified into three main pathophysiologic states and results from either (1) blood loss, (2) decreased production of erythrocytes, or (3) peripheral destruction of erythrocytes (Box 14.3). Anemias are also described according to cellular morphology (form/structure) (Box 14.4). Descriptions of anemias based on erythrocyte morphology refer to the size and hemoglobin content of the RBC. In some anemias, variations occur in size (e.g., anisocytosis) or shape (e.g., poikilocytosis) of erythrocytes.

#### Etiologic Factors and Pathogenesis

Anemia results from (1) excessive blood loss, (2) increased destruction of erythrocytes, or (3) decreased production of erythrocytes. Anemia is the most common hematologic abnormality; only the anemias most commonly observed in rehabilitation or therapy settings are

Box 14.3

**CAUSES OF ANEMIA**

***Excessive Blood Loss (Hemorrhage)***

- Trauma, wound
- GI cancers
- Angiectasia
- Bleeding peptic ulcer
- Excessive menstruation
- Bleeding hemorrhoids
- Varices, diverticulosis

***Destruction of Erythrocytes (Hemolytic)***

- Mechanical (e.g., microangiopathic hemolytic anemia; damage by a mechanical heart valve)
- Autoimmune hemolytic anemia
- Hemoglobinopathies (e.g., sickle cell diseases)
- Enzyme defects (e.g., glucose-6-phosphate dehydrogenase deficiency)
- Parasites (e.g., malaria)
- Hypersplenism
- Cell membrane abnormalities (e.g., hereditary spherocytosis)
- Thalassemias

***Decreased Production of Erythrocytes***

- Chronic diseases (e.g., rheumatoid arthritis, tuberculosis, cancer)
- Nutritional deficiency (e.g., iron, vitamin $B_{12}$, alcohol abuse, folic acid deficiency)
- Cellular maturational defects (e.g., thalassemias, cytotoxic or antineoplastic drugs)
- ↓ Bone marrow stimulation (e.g., hypothyroidism, decreased erythropoietin production)
- Bone marrow failure (e.g., leukemia, aplasia)
- Bone marrow replacement (myelophthisis; neoplasm)
- Myelodysplastic syndromes (sideroblastic anemia)

Box 14.4

**ANEMIA CLASSIFIED BY MORPHOLOGY**

- Normocytic (normal size)
- Macrocytic (abnormally large)
- Microcytic (abnormally small)
- Normochromic (normal amounts of hemoglobin)
- Hyperchromic (high concentration of hemoglobin)
- Hypochromic (low concentration of hemoglobin)
- Anisocytosis (various sizes)
- Poikilocytosis (various shapes)

discussed here, using the three etiologic categories from Box 14.3 as a guideline.

The underlying pathogenesis can be multifactorial and depends on the condition causing the anemia. A number of physiologic compensatory responses to anemia occur, depending on the rapidity of onset and duration of anemia and the condition of the individual.

The production of erythrocytes is controlled by the hormone erythropoietin. When the kidneys detect hypoxia or anemia, erythropoietin is released, which results in the activation of transcription factors. These factors begin the process of erythropoiesis on the level of hematopoietic stem cells. Erythropoietin, a growth factor, along with other growth factors (such as IL-3 and GM-CSF), regulates and controls the proliferation and maturation of erythroid progenitor cells. Erythropoietin is required for the final maturation of erythroid cells and stimulates the release of RBCs from the bone marrow, and, depending on the severity of the anemia, the spleen and liver.[324] Other factors are also required for making an RBC, including iron, cobalamin, folate, and healthy bone marrow.

In acute-onset anemia with severe loss of intravascular volume, peripheral vasoconstriction and central vasodilation occur to preserve blood flow to the vital organs.

If the anemia persists, small-vessel vasodilation will provide increased blood flow to ensure better tissue oxygenation. These vascular compensations result in decreased systemic vascular resistance, increased cardiac output, and tachycardia, resulting in a higher rate of delivery of oxygen-bearing erythrocytes to the tissues. Other compensatory mechanisms include an increase in plasma volume to maintain total blood volume and enhance tissue perfusion and stimulation of erythropoietin production to increase new erythrocyte production.

**Excessive Blood Loss.** Excessive blood loss, such as occurs with GI bleeding, is a cause of anemia seen in a therapy practice. Slow, chronic GI blood loss from medication (aspirin or NSAIDs) or any GI disorder (e.g., peptic and duodenal ulcers, GI cancers, hemorrhoids, diverticulitis, ulcerative colitis, and colon polyps) can result in iron-deficiency anemia.

**Destruction of Erythrocytes.** Destruction of erythrocytes (hemolysis) can occur as a result of congenital or acquired disorders caused by congenital RBC membrane abnormalities, lack of necessary enzymes needed for normal metabolism, autoimmune processes, or infection. All but the autoimmune processes are discussed elsewhere in this chapter.

Autoimmune hemolytic anemia (AIHA) is caused by an autoantibody that attaches to the RBC, leading to its destruction. AIHA is classified according to the temperature at which the antibodies optimally bind to the RBC. The most common form of AIHA is warm antibody-mediated, an IgG autoantibody that binds to erythrocyte Rh antigens at body temperature (warm autoimmune hemolytic anemia [WAIHA]). Phagocytic or cytotoxic cells are attracted to the attached autoantibody and are able to phagocytize the RBC completely or partially. Partially phagocytized cells become spherical and are removed by the spleen. Some of these IgG autoantibodies also bind and activate complement, although this mechanism is less effective at causing cell lysis. WAIHA can be a primary disorder or secondary to medications, such as penicillins and cephalosporins; lymphoproliferative disorders (chronic lymphocytic leukemia); or autoimmune disorders, such as systemic lupus erythematosus (SLE).

Cold agglutinin disease is another autoimmune hemolytic process caused by IgM autoantibodies that bind to erythrocytes (glycoprotein antigens I or i) at temperatures less than 37° C (98.6° F) and trigger complement fixation and clumping of erythrocytes. These complement-laden erythrocytes may be destroyed intravascularly or removed by the liver. Cold agglutinin hemolytic anemia can be seen in clients with a lymphoproliferative disorder or in people with *Mycoplasma* and Epstein-Barr virus infections.

**Decreased Production of Erythrocytes.** Anemias resulting in the underproduction of RBCs usually stem from either a lack of erythropoietin, a hormone produced in the kidney that stimulates production and maturation of RBCs (as seen in chronic kidney disease), or an inability of the bone marrow to respond to erythropoietin and make RBCs. Hyporesponsiveness of the bone marrow may be a result of a nutrient deficiency or a chronic disease such as RA, SLE, tuberculosis, or cancer.

Nutritional deficiency as a cause of anemia can occur at any age. Iron, vitamin $B_{12}$, and folate are among the most important vitamins and minerals in the production of hemoglobin and the formation of erythrocytes. Iron is necessary for DNA synthesis and repair and is required for hemoglobin to transport oxygen.[347] Iron deficiency can occur secondary to blood loss (RBCs are the principal site of iron storage), malabsorption, and pregnancy. Menstruating women, pregnant women, growing children, lower socioeconomic groups, and older adults (as a result of economic constraints, lack of interest in food preparation, and poor dentition) are the most common groups to develop iron-deficiency anemia.

Vitamin $B_{12}$ (cobalamin) is required for DNA synthesis and methylation, as well as RNA synthesis. $B_{12}$ also is involved with neuronal myelination and deficiency can be serious, resulting in neurologic disorders. $B_{12}$ is only found in animal products, so deficiency of the vitamin may occur because of a lack in the diets of strict vegetarians or vegans. People (especially the elderly)[12] may also become deficient due to conditions that block or interfere with the absorption of vitamin $B_{12}$, such as bariatric surgery, intestinal bacterial overgrowth, achlorhydria (acid production reduced) from antacids, and/or excessive alcohol intake.[140] Other causes include pancreatic insufficiency, medications (e.g., metformin) and severe Crohn disease (Crohn disease can cause sufficient destruction of the ileum to retard vitamin $B_{12}$ absorption). However, vitamin $B_{12}$ deficiency most often develops because of an absence of intrinsic factor (IF) and results in pernicious anemia (PA). Vitamin $B_{12}$ in food is typically bound to proteins, but once chewed and swallowed, is released due to the acidity and the enzyme pepsin in the stomach. The saliva contains R-binders that bind to vitamin $B_{12}$ in the stomach. These R-binders are cleaved by pancreatic enzymes on entering the duodenum. Gastric parietal cells of the stomach secrete intrinsic factor that, once passed into the duodenum, binds newly released vitamin $B_{12}$. Mucosal cells in the ileum absorb this $B_{12}$-IF complex; vitamin $B_{12}$ is not absorbed without IF.

Pernicious anemia is caused by autoantibodies that block the formation of the $B_{12}$-IF complex. Autoantibodies develop against either IF or gastric parietal cells. Parietal cells become atrophic, resulting in a lack of IF production (may be related to chronic *H. pylori* infection).[26,372] Autoantibodies toward gastric parietal cells are seen in other autoimmune diseases, so are not specific for PA, whereas autoantibodies against IF are more specific but not as sensitive. Destruction of IF production sites may also occur with partial gastrectomy.

Folate, similar to $B_{12}$, is required for DNA synthesis and methylation. Folic acid deficiency has become rare in the United States due to food supplementation. Folic acid deficiency has many causes, but it can result from inadequate dietary intake, chronic alcoholism, malabsorption syndromes (e.g., surgery or celiac disease), medications (trimethoprim or phenytoin), anorexia, and disorders associated with increased cell turnover (e.g., pregnancy, hemolytic anemias). Pregnant women need twice the normal amount of folic acid to meet the needs of the developing fetus.

Anemia of chronic disease (ACD), also known as anemia of inflammation, is very common in the therapy setting. It is characterized by a modest reduction in hemoglobin (9-11 g/dL), the presence of inflammation, and decreased responsiveness of the bone marrow to erythropoietin. Conditions associated with this type of anemia are diverse and broad. Such causes include: infections (i.e., tuberculosis, osteomyelitis), malignancies, inflammation, chronic kidney disease, and diabetes mellitus. Many diseases associated with inflammation have accompanying elevated levels of cytokines (including interleukin [IL]-1 and IL-6, TNFα), which lead to altered erythropoietin responsiveness. Erythropoietin production is downregulated in the kidney and the erythroid precursor's response to erythropoietin is blunted. IL-6 induces the production of hepcidin, a protein synthesized by the liver, which regulates iron absorption.[83] Hepcidin both inhibits the absorption of iron from the gut and the release of iron from macrophages for bone marrow use. Clients with an underlying chronic illness usually have adequate iron stores, so anemia of chronic disease does not respond to supplemental iron. Increased macrophage activity may result in a modest reduction in RBC life span.

Anemia also results from chronic kidney disease with subsequent decreased erythropoietin production. Most dialysis clients respond to erythropoiesis-stimulating agents.

Bone marrow disorders constitute another source of anemia caused by decreased production of erythrocytes in a therapy practice. Aplastic anemia, marrow replacement with fibrotic tissue or tumor, acute leukemia, and infiltrative disease (e.g., lymphoma, myeloma, and carcinoma) fall into this etiologic category.

Anemias of radiation-induced bone marrow failure occur because the bone marrow stem cells are destroyed and mitosis (cell division) is inhibited, preventing the synthesis of RBCs. Antimetabolites used in cancer therapy also cause bone marrow failure by blocking the synthesis of purines or nucleic acids required for synthesis of DNA within the cell. Aplastic anemia may result from either damage to the stem cells or immune-mediated destruction of the stem cells.

### Clinical Manifestations

Signs and symptoms associated with anemia are related to the severity of anemia and the amount of time over which the erythrocytes were lost. Mild anemia often causes only minimal and usually vague symptoms, such as fatigue, until hemoglobin concentration is significantly reduced. As the anemia progresses, general signs and symptoms caused by the inability of anemic blood to

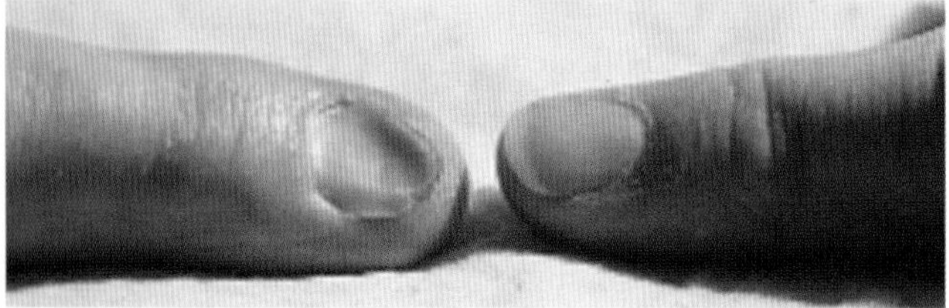

**Figure 14.1**

Normal nail *(right)* compared with nail referred to as koilonychia and sometimes called spoon-shaped nails or spoon nails *(left)*. They are thin, depressed nails with lateral edges turned up and are concave from side to side. They may be idiopathic, congenital, or a hereditary trait and are occasionally caused by iron-deficiency anemia. (Reprinted from Swartz MH: *Textbook of physical diagnosis*, ed 5, Philadelphia, 2006, WB Saunders.)

supply the body tissues with enough oxygen may include weakness, dyspnea on exertion, easy fatigue, pallor, tachycardia, increased angina in people with preexisting heart disease, and, occasionally, koilonychia (Fig. 14.1). Signs and symptoms indicative of hemolysis include jaundice (secondary to hemolysis of hemoglobin), splenomegaly, and gallstones.

Pallor in dark-skinned people may be observed by the absence of the underlying red tones that normally give brown or black skin its luster. The brown-skinned individual demonstrates pallor with a more yellowish-brown color, and the black-skinned person appears ashen or gray.

Mild iron deficiency may produce symptoms of irritability, lack of exercise tolerance, and headaches. Rarely, more substantial iron deficiency can lead to the tendency to eat ice, clay, starch, and crunchy materials (pica).

Neuropsychiatric complications such as dementia, ataxia, psychosis, and peripheral neuropathies can develop in cases of $B_{12}$ deficiency. These abnormalities are caused by lesions in the spinal column, the cerebrum, and peripheral nerves. The lack of cobalamin initially leads to demyelination of the nerves followed by axonal degeneration. Axonal death may result if cobalamin deficiency persists.

Reversal of symptoms may be possible if treatment is initiated before permanent damage to the nerves. The findings typically consist of a symmetric sensory neuropathy that begins in the feet and lower legs, although rarely it may involve the upper extremities, especially fine motor coordination of the hands. This upper-extremity neuropathy may clinically manifest as problems with deteriorating handwriting.

Affected individuals may also describe moderate pain or paresthesias of the extremities, especially the feet. Individuals may interpret the neuropathy as difficulty with locomotion when, in fact, they are experiencing the loss of proprioception. The affected individual may need to hold on to the wall, countertops, or furniture at home due to difficulties maintaining balance. An associated positive Romberg sign may be present. Loss of motor function is a late manifestation of $B_{12}$ deficiency.

Although a symmetrical neuropathy is the usual pattern, $B_{12}$ deficiency occasionally presents as a unilateral neuropathy and/or bilateral but asymmetrical neuropathy.

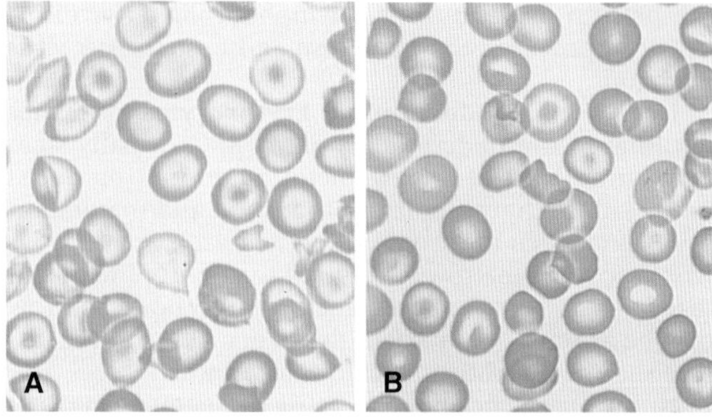


**Figure 14.2**

Thalassemia is a hemolytic hemoglobinopathy anemia characterized by microcytic, short-lived RBCs caused by deficient synthesis of hemoglobin polypeptide chains. Classification of type depends on the chain involved ($\alpha$-thalassemia, $\beta$-thalassemia). $\beta$-Thalassemia occurs in two forms: (A) thalassemia major and (B) thalassemia minor. Characteristic bull's-eye or target cells are shown here in both forms. (Reprinted from Damjanov I, Linder J: *Pathology: a color atlas*, St Louis, 2000, Mosby.)

Central nervous system (CNS) manifestations range from mild cognitive changes to dementia to frank psychosis. Clients may present with personality changes and/or inappropriate behavior.

Complications depend on the specific type of anemia; severe anemia can cause heart failure and hypoxic damage to the liver and kidney, with all the signs and symptoms associated with either of those conditions. Anemia in the presence of a coronary obstruction precipitates cardiac ischemia and is a risk factor for heart attack.

## MEDICAL MANAGEMENT

**DIAGNOSIS.** Anemia in the early stages often goes unnoticed because symptoms may not be recognized until hemoglobin concentration is reduced. Once symptoms become pronounced or noted on routine laboratory tests, the diagnosis is most often made by blood tests.

A complete blood count (CBC) gives the percentage of blood volume composed of erythrocytes, the concentration of hemoglobin, the erythrocyte count, and RBC indices. Included in the RBC indices is the size (reported as mean corpuscular volume), shape, and size distribution (RBC distribution width). Although normal levels of hemoglobin may vary according to laboratories, normal hemoglobin can be considered 13.5 to 17.5 g/dL for men (androgen effect), whereas for women it is 12 to 16 g/dL (depending on menses).

The RBC indices indicate if the RBCs are normal (normocytic), larger than normal (macrocytic, as seen with $B_{12}$ and folate deficiency), or smaller than normal (microcytic, as seen with thalassemias and iron deficiency). The peripheral smear may reveal structural characteristics, which give clues to the underlying cause of the anemia. For example, target cells (bull's-eye erythrocytes) are often associated with thalassemia (Fig. 14.2) and microspherocytes can be seen in warm antibody-induced hemolysis, whereas sickled erythrocytes are noted with sickle cell disease (Fig. 14.3). Tear-drop cells suggest bone marrow fibrosis, whereas schistocytes

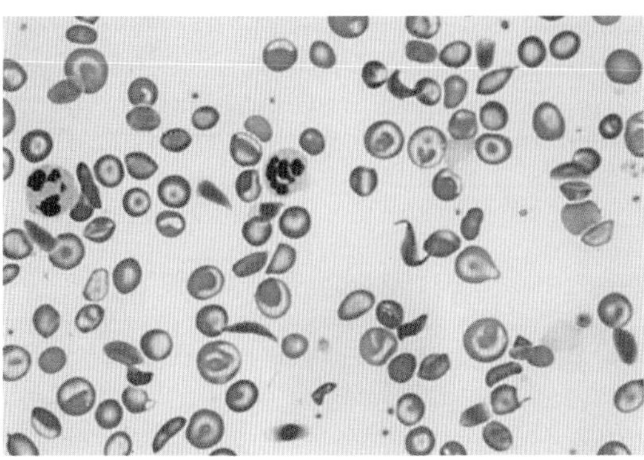

**Figure 14.3**

**Target and sickle cells typical of sickle cell anemia (×200).** (Reprinted from Goldman L: *Cecil textbook of medicine*, ed 22, Philadelphia, 2004, WB Saunders. Courtesy Jean Shafer.)

(pieces of RBCs) are indicative of a microangiopathy (thrombotic thrombocytopenic purpura, hemolytic uremic syndrome, and disseminated intravascular coagulation [DIC]) or hemolysis.

A reticulocyte count (the amount of new RBCs) is often very telling; underproduction anemias tend to have low reticulocyte counts (the bone marrow is unable to compensate), whereas anemias resulting from blood loss or peripheral destruction have a high reticulocyte count (the bone marrow is able to compensate). Laboratory values indicative of hemolysis include an elevated indirect bilirubin (product of RBC breakdown) and lactate dehydrogenase (LDH) (released with cell damage), decreased haptoglobin (protein that clears free hemoglobin), and a positive direct Coombs test (immune complexes attached to RBCs).

Personal and family history may point to congenital anemia, and a physical examination may elicit signs of primary hematologic diseases, such as lymphadenopathy, hepatosplenomegaly, skin and mucosal changes, stool positive for blood, or bone tenderness.

Following these initial tests, more specific laboratory tests can be done to verify the diagnosis. These may include an iron profile, serum ferritin (low in iron deficiency), haptoglobin, $B_{12}$ level, methylmalonic acid and homocysteine (both are elevated in cobalamin deficiency but only homocysteine is elevated in folate deficiency), folate level, antibodies to intrinsic factor, and LDH (high in hemolysis).

**TREATMENT.** Treatment of anemia is directed toward alleviating or controlling the causes, relieving the symptoms, and preventing complications. It is critical that the underlying cause of anemia is determined so that appropriate treatment can be given. For example, endoscopy to identify the source of GI blood loss for a client with a long-term history of NSAID use would indicate the need to stop taking the medication and prescribe the use of proton pump inhibitors.

Treating the underlying cause can include the replacement of deficient vitamins and minerals (e.g., vitamin $B_{12}$, folate, or iron) or corticosteroids for warm AIHA. The anemia of cold agglutinin disease is typically mild, requiring only a warm environment, whereas chemotherapy may be required for malignancies.

**PROGNOSIS.** The prognosis for anemia depends on the etiologic factors and potential treatment for the underlying cause. For example, the prognosis is good for anemia related to nutritional deficiency but worse for lymphoproliferative diseases. Likewise, treatment is aimed at correcting the underlying pathogenesis.

Untreated or misdiagnosed $B_{12}$ deficiency can be progressive, resulting in irreversible neurologic damage. Anemia in the older adult (age 85 years or older) is associated with an increased risk of death. Although anemia was once considered a normal consequence of aging, it is now recognized as a sign of other disease in the older adult (e.g., hip fracture, RA, erosive gastritis, peptic ulcer, malnutrition, cirrhosis, ulcerative colitis) requiring further assessment.[419]

## SPECIAL IMPLICATIONS FOR THE THERAPIST 14.5

### *The Anemias*

Anemia of chronic disease (also known as *anemia of inflammation*) is very common in the therapy setting.[123] It is characterized by a modest reduction in hemoglobin (9-12 g/dL), the presence of inflammation (secondary to inflammation, infection, and some malignancies), and decreased responsiveness of the bone marrow to erythropoietin. Chronic illness or inflammation signals the immune system to release a steady supply of inflammatory proteins that interfere with the production of red blood cells.

Bone marrow disorders constitute another source of anemia caused by decreased production of erythrocytes in a therapy practice. Aplastic anemia, marrow replacement with fibrotic tissue or tumor, acute leukemia, and infiltrative disease (e.g., lymphoma, myeloma, and carcinoma) fall into this etiologic category.

#### Exercise and Anemia

The impact of anemia on functional recovery in the acute care or rehabilitation setting and the theoretical risk of increased morbidity and mortality during prescribed therapeutic exercise have not been thoroughly investigated. Further study is indicated to examine the implications for anemia on functional recovery and cardiopulmonary complications during rehabilitation.[89]

The following guidelines should be used until proven protocols are developed. Exercise prescription for any anemic person should be reviewed with the physician.

Diminished exercise tolerance may be expected in anyone with anemia along with easy fatigability, depending on the cause of the anemia. Increased physical activity increases the demand for oxygen, which may not be adequately available in the circulating blood. Pacing and training that distribute the intensity of the workload over time can be used to promote physiologic recovery.[84]

Progress slowly for anyone with decreased exercise tolerance and monitor vital signs closely. For the sedentary aging adult, decreased activity can mask exercise intolerance; observe carefully for any changes in mental status.

The prevalence of iron-deficiency anemia is likely to be higher in athletic populations and groups, especially in younger female athletes, than in sedentary individuals. In anemic individuals, iron deficiency decreases athletic performance and impairs immune function, leading to other physiologic dysfunction.

Although it is likely that blood losses secondary to exercise, such as foot-strike hemolysis or iron loss through sweat, may contribute to anemia, nonathletic causes must also be considered. Dietary choices explain much of a negative iron balance, but the GI and genitourinary systems must be evaluated for blood loss.[398]

Evidence also exists for increased rates of RBC iron and whole-body iron turnover. The young female athlete may want to consult with medical or dietary consultants about the use of low-dose iron supplements during training.[24,486]

Research shows that people with chronic renal failure who have severe anemia are able to exercise but must do so at a lower intensity than the normal population. The maximum oxygen consumption ($VO_2max$) for the anemic client is at least 20% less than that for the normal population. Exercise testing and prescribed exercise(s) in anemic clients must be initiated with extreme caution and should proceed gradually to tolerance and/or perceived exertion levels.[95,312]

### Precautions

Knowing the underlying cause of the anemia may be helpful in identifying red flag symptoms indicating the need for alteration of the program or medical referral. For example, GI blood loss associated with NSAID use may worsen suddenly, precipitating a crisis in a therapy setting. After major noncardiac surgery (e.g., orthopedic procedures), even mild anemia is associated with increased morbidity and mortality. Rates of postoperative conditions, such as sepsis and venous thromboembolism, can be much higher associated with anemia.[280]

It is not uncommon for clients to present with both anemia and cardiovascular disease, precipitating angina. Studies show that the amount of oxygen-carrying hemoglobin (Hb) circulating in the blood of older women is an independent risk factor for mobility problems. Hb perceived as mildly low and even low-normal (12 g/dL) in women at least 70 years old increases the likelihood of difficulty performing daily tasks by 1.5 times.[58,59]

The therapist may identify older adults who have a difficult time with general mobility, such as walking more than one block, climbing a flight of stairs, or doing housework. When they have difficulty, they become more sedentary, resulting in a decline in independence. The condition of mildly low Hb is no longer considered clinically benign because mortality risk has been shown to be lower with higher Hb levels.[60] It may be appropriate to request assessment of Hb levels and/or communicate with the physician about the potential harm of low-normal Hb levels.

Bleeding under the skin and easy bruising in response to the slightest trauma often occur when platelet production is altered (thrombocytopenia) secondary to hypoplastic or aplastic anemia. This condition necessitates extreme care in the therapy setting, especially any intervention requiring manual therapy or the use of any equipment, including modalities and weight-training devices. Splenomegaly associated with some types of anemia requires precautions in performing soft tissue techniques in the left upper quadrant, especially up and under the rib cage; indirect techniques away from the spleen are indicated.

Decreased oxygen delivery to the skin results in impaired healing and loss of elasticity, as well as delayed wound healing and healing of other musculoskeletal injuries. If the anemia is caused by vitamin $B_{12}$ deficiency (e.g., pernicious anemia, pregnancy, hyperthyroidism), the nervous system is affected.

Alteration of the structure and function of the peripheral nerves, spinal cord (myelin degeneration), and brain may occur. Paresthesias, especially numbness mimicking carpal tunnel syndrome; gait disturbances; extreme weakness; spasticity; and abnormal reflexes can result. Permanent neurologic damage unresponsive to vitamin $B_{12}$ therapy can occur in extreme cases when intervention has been delayed.

### Monitoring Vital Signs

Many individuals who are anemic are asymptomatic. Careful monitoring is required. Tachycardia may be the first change observed when monitoring vital signs, usually accompanied by a sense of fatigue, generalized weakness, loss of stamina, and exertional dyspnea. Systolic blood pressure may not be affected, but diastolic pressure may be lower than normal, with an associated increase in the resting pulse rate.

Resting cardiac output is usually normal in people with anemia, but cardiac output increases with exercise more than in nonanemic people. As the anemia becomes more severe, resting cardiac output increases and exercise tolerance progressively decreases until dyspnea, tachycardia, and palpitations occur at rest.

### A THERAPIST'S THOUGHTS

***Anemia***

Anemia may be defined differently from region to region, hospital to hospital, and even physician to physician. Hemoglobin less than 8 g/dL is no longer a complete contraindication to physical therapy intervention.

A general guideline is to review and possibly modify or restrict activity and exercise when hemoglobin is less than 8 with a hematocrit level less than 25. This is especially applicable to individuals who are not critically ill or who are in the intensive care unit with acute coronary syndromes. Some institutions use less than 7 as a guideline for individuals in intensive care who have stable cardiac disease.

Low-impact and low-intensity aerobics (e.g., stationary bicycle) may be tolerated by individuals with anemia and hemoglobin levels between 10 and 12 g/dL. Isometrics and resistive exercise can also be incorporated slowly and carefully in this population group. Hemoglobin levels between 8 and 10 g/dL may be a contraindication to aggressive therapeutic strengthening and endurance training. Use the guidelines offered here to guide your thinking for each individual.

Remember to look at the *trend* an individual's hemoglobin levels over the last few days and try to understand what is going on with that particular person. Consider the past medical history, as well as the current medical and physical (conditioning) status.

Look for acute blood loss (even with normal or near-normal hemoglobin levels) versus chronic anemia. Engage in discussion with the medical staff to more fully understand the person's physiologic status. A person who is chronically anemic (e.g., chronic kidney disease) will probably be better able to withstand exercise at a lower hemoglobin level compared with an individual who is at the same level but has had an acute drop in hemoglobin.

*Eva Gold, PT

Box 14.5

**CAUSES OF LEUKOCYTOSIS**

- Acute hemorrhage
- Infection (viral, bacterial, or fungal)
- Malignancies (leukemia, lymphoma, non–small cell lung cancer, multiple myeloma)
- Myeloproliferative disorders
- Glucocorticosteroid therapy
- Trauma (burns)
- Tissue necrosis (infarction)
- Inflammation (autoimmune-mediated such as myositis or vasculitis)

## DISORDERS OF LEUKOCYTES

Alterations in blood leukocyte (WBC) concentration and in the relative proportions of the several leukocyte types are recognized as measures of the reaction of the body to infection, inflammation, tissue damage, or degeneration. In many instances, these alterations give useful indications of the nature of the pathologic process and may be seen in association not only with acute infections but also with many chronic ailments treated by the therapist.

Leukocytes may be classified in three main groups: granulocytes (basophils, eosinophils, neutrophils, mast cells), monocytes, and lymphocytes. *Granulocytes* contain proteins (histamine, cytokines, chemokines, enzymes or growth factors) that are helpful in the body's immune response. The main type of granulocyte is the neutrophil, also called the *polymorphonuclear leukocyte (PMN)*; these are usually not found in normal "healthy" tissue and are referred to as the first line of hematologic defense against invading pathogens.

Granulocytes are also involved in the pathophysiology of organ damage in ischemia/reperfusion, trauma, sepsis, or organ transplantation. Eosinophils are involved with allergic reactions and respond to parasitic and fungal infections. Basophils aid in antigen presentation and differentiation of specific T cells. Mast cells are found in connective tissue and mediate allergic reactions and tissue-related response to pathogens.

*Monocytes* are the largest circulating blood cells and represent an immature cell until it leaves the blood and travels to the tissues. Once migrated, monocytes form macrophages when activated by foreign substances, such as bacteria. Monocytes/macrophages participate in inflammation by synthesizing numerous mediators and eliminating various pathogens.

*Lymphocytes* are further divided into B and T cells. B lymphocytes are responsible for the humoral portion of the immune system and once differentiated into plasma cells, secrete antibodies that react with antigens and initiate complement-mediated destruction or phagocytosis of foreign pathogens, particularly bacteria. Other B cells become memory B cells, ready to recognize the same antigen if re-presented. T lymphocytes are in control of cell-mediated immunity and differentiate into helper, regulatory, cytotoxic or memory cells. Helper T cells secrete cytokines that stimulate B cells to differentiate into plasma cells. Regulatory T cells regulate the immune response, while cytotoxic T cells (once activated by cytokines) are able to recognize, bind to, and destroy cells altered by viruses or cancer cells. Memory T cells, like memory B cells, have an extended life and are ready to react to the same antigen.

These cells are also responsible for coordinating the immune response through the release of lymphokines and inflammatory modulators, creating a cell-to-cell communication with B cells and monocytes. The exact role or function of leukocytes during inflammatory processes remains the subject of considerable investigation.

### Leukocytosis

#### Definition and Etiology

Leukocytosis, defined as an increase in the number of leukocytes in the blood, may occur as a result of a variety of causes (Box 14.5), particularly infection and most ominously as leukemia. It may also occur as a normal protective response (demargination of neutrophils) to physiologic stressors such as strenuous exercise, emotional changes, temperature changes, anesthesia, surgery, pregnancy, some drugs, toxins, and hormones.[54,362]

Leukocytosis develops within 1 or 2 hours after the onset of acute hemorrhage and is greater when the bleeding occurs internally (e.g., into the peritoneal cavity, pleural space, or joint cavity, GI bleeding, or as a result of a skull fracture with associated intracranial bleed or subarachnoid hemorrhage) than when the bleeding is external.[25,55]

Leukocytosis is a common finding in and characterizes many infectious diseases recognized by a count of more than 10,000 WBCs/mm$^3$. An elevated WBC count (greater than 50,000/mm$^3$, with the majority of cells being neutrophils and neutrophil precursors) in response to a serious underlying process is referred to as a leukemoid reaction (see Box 14.5). It carries a grave prognosis in the elderly and in children, putting them at higher risk for the development of leukemia and pneumonia.[176,343]

Leukocytosis frequently results from an increase in circulating neutrophils (neutrophilia), recruited in large numbers in the course of infections and in the presence of some rapidly growing neoplasms (e.g., leukemia, non–small cell lung cancer, renal cell carcinoma, and gastric carcinoma).[451] The counts may be especially high in tumors with significant necrosis. Some tumors can also release hormone-like substances that cause leukocytosis.

### Clinical Manifestations

Clinical signs and symptoms of leukocytosis are usually associated with symptoms of the conditions listed in Box 14.5 and may include fever, headache, shortness of breath, symptoms of localized or systemic infection, and symptoms of inflammation or trauma to tissue.

## MEDICAL MANAGEMENT

**DIAGNOSIS, TREATMENT, AND PROGNOSIS.** Major leukocyte functions are accomplished in the tissues so that the leukocytes in the blood are in transit from the site of production or storage to the tissues. Variations in the blood concentrations of each leukocyte type may be of brief duration and easily missed or may persist for days or weeks. Laboratory tests for detecting leukocyte abnormalities include total leukocyte count, leukocyte differential cell count (see Chapter 40), peripheral blood morphology, and bone marrow morphology.

Treatment is directed toward the underlying cause of the change in leukocytes and control of any infections. Prognosis depends on the etiology of the leukocytosis.

### Basophilia

Basophilia refers to a condition where the number or proportion of basophils to other leukocytes in the blood or tissue is increased. Basophilia is primarily associated with myeloproliferative disorders, particularly chronic myeloid leukemia. It is also seen in allergic and chronic inflammatory reactions or infections (such as tuberculosis), as well as in autoimmune disorders and drug exposure.[375,431] Basophils are the least common subtype of leukocytes, accounting for 0.5% of all leukocytes. Basophils express multiple types of receptors (cytokine, chemokine, complement, immunoglobulin, and prostaglandin). Basophils mature in the bone marrow and circulate in the periphery. They have a half-life of only a few days. Although basophils are typically not found in tissue, they are able to infiltrate to inflamed tissue such as seen in asthma and atopic dermatitis.[193,428]

Aggregation of immunoglobulin Fc receptor (expressed by the surface of the basophil) bound by antigen to IgE results in basophil activation and granule and mediator release (Type-2 immunity).[408] Other cytokines and chemokines activate basophils or prime basophils for activation. Mediators that are released include histamine, heparin (less than mast cells contain), cytokines (such as IL-4), and leukotrienes (potent bronchorestrictors that can increase vascular permeability).

### Eosinophilia

Eosinophilia is the increased number of eosinophils in tissue or blood. Eosinophils are a prominent feature of helminthic infections, allergy, asthma, and pulmonary and vascular disorders. Eosinophils mature in the bone marrow and are stimulated to differentiate and develop by IL-5, IL-3 and GM-CSF.[1a] Once mature, they are released into the circulation and migrate into tissue. These tissues are often in areas that have contact with the external environment, such as the skin, GI tract, and lungs. Eosinophils may also be seen in the vasculature, heart, kidney, and brain. Eosinophils express a wide variety of cell surface receptors (immunoglobulin IgG and IgA, chemokines, cytokines, complement, and adhesion molecules) and can be activated by various antibodies and interleukins and stimulated to release proinflammatory mediators (such as chemokines, growth factors, cytokines, peroxidase, and other modulating proteins).[408]

An elevation in the number of eosinophils in the blood, eosinophilia (eosinophil count greater than 500/mm$^3$) is seen most often in mild atopic asthma, allergic reactions to drugs (ibuprofen, aspirin, sulfonamides, penicillins, anticonvulsants), helminthic reactions, malignancies, connective tissue disorders and hypereosinophilic syndromes.[208] Hypereosinophilia syndromes (typically with elevated peripheral blood eosinophils >1500/mm$^3$) are associated with marked, persistent eosinophilia with or without end-organ damage and exclusion of other known causes of eosinophilia. Allergic diseases such as allergic rhinitis, atopic asthma, and atopic dermatitis, may have a mild eosinophilia, but the number of eosinophils in tissues is typically more significantly elevated than in the blood.[428] If the peripheral blood eosinophilia is significantly elevated, a cause other than an allergic disorder should be sought.

### Neutrophilia

Neutrophils, or polymorphonuclear neutrophils (PMN), constitute approximately 60% to 70% of leukocytes in the peripheral blood and are, therefore, the most common leukocyte. Neutrophilia refers to an elevation in the amount of neutrophils in the blood (usually defined as two standard deviations above normal or an absolute neutrophil count of around 7,700/microL). Neutrophilia can occur through either an increase in the number of PMNs produced by the bone marrow or demargination of PMNs (about half of circulating PMNs reversibly adhere to the endothelium and are released when stimulated or demarginate). Neutrophils are the first cells to reach an infected or inflamed area. They release cytokines that then signal and recruit other cells, thereby amplifying the inflammatory response. Neutrophils are able to recognize foreign antigens and begin the process of phagocytizing and killing them.[249]

The many potential causes of neutrophilia include inflammation or tissue necrosis (e.g., after surgery from tissue damage, severe burns, myocardial infarction, pneumonitis, RA); acute infection (e.g., *Staphylococcus, Streptococcus, Pneumococcus*); drug- or chemical-induced causes (e.g., epinephrine, steroids, heparin, histamine); metabolic causes (e.g., acidosis associated with diabetes, gout, thyroid storm, eclampsia); and myeloproliferative malignancies, or metastatic neoplasms.[138] Physiologic neutrophilia may also occur as a result of exercise, extreme heat/cold, third-trimester pregnancy, and emotional distress. Cigarette smoking may also mildly increase the neutrophil count.

### Monocytosis

Monocytes are the circulating blood cells that give rise to macrophages and dendritic cells. Monocytes may be part of the initial immune response with beneficial results or part of acute and chronic inflammation.[96] Monocytosis, an increase in monocytes, is most often seen in chronic infections, such as tuberculosis, syphilis, and subacute endocarditis, and other inflammatory processes, such as SLE and RA, hemolytic anemias, and both hematologic and nonhematologic neoplasms. Monocytosis is present in up to 50% of people with collagen vascular disease.

Clients with sarcoidosis or other granulomatous processes may also have elevated monocytes. Monocytosis also exists as a normal physiologic response in newborns (first 2 weeks of life). Although not common, monocytes can go through a transformation, becoming leukemia, or an elevation of normal monocytes can be seen in malignancies such as Hodgkin and non-Hodgkin lymphoma. Monocytosis can be indicative of bone marrow recovery following a drug-induced loss of granulocytes.

**SPECIAL IMPLICATIONS FOR THE THERAPIST 14.6**

*Leukocytes*

It is important for the therapist to be aware of the client's most recent leukocyte (WBC) count before and during episodes of care if that person is immunosuppressed. At that time, the client is extremely susceptible to opportunistic infections and severe complications.

The importance of good handwashing and hygiene practices cannot be overemphasized when treating immunocompromised clients. Some centers recommend that people with a WBC count of less than $1000/mm^3$ or a neutrophil count of less than $500/mm^3$ wear a protective mask. Therapists should ensure that these people are provided with equipment that has been disinfected according to standard precautions.

## Leukopenia

### Definition and Etiology

White blood cells are classified as lymphocytes, granulocytes, or monocytes. A decrease in any or all of these cell types leads to leukopenia; however, the reduction in neutrophils (a type of granulocyte) is the most common cause of low WBC. Leukopenia can be caused by a variety of factors, such as HIV (or other viral infection, such as hepatitis), alcohol and nutritional deficiencies, infectious diseases (e.g., tuberculosis), overwhelming infections, medications, and autoimmune disorders (e.g., SLE, rheumatoid arthritis). It can occur in many forms of bone marrow failure, such as that following antineoplastic chemotherapy or radiation therapy or in myelodysplastic syndromes.

People with leukemia, lymphoma, and myeloma have serious underlying WBC abnormalities that reduce the amount of normally functioning WBCs, contributing to the risk of infection associated with leukopenia. Unlike leukocytosis, leukopenia is never beneficial. As the leukocyte count decreases, the risk for various infections increases.

### Clinical Manifestations

Leukopenia may be asymptomatic (and detected by routine tests) or associated with clinical signs and symptoms consistent with infection, such as sore throat, cough, high fever, chills, sweating, ulcerations of mucous membranes (e.g., mouth, rectum, vagina), frequent or painful urination, or persistent infections.

### MEDICAL MANAGEMENT

**DIAGNOSIS AND TREATMENT.** As with leukocytosis, diagnosis is by laboratory testing for leukocyte abnormalities. Treatment is directed toward elimination of the cause of the reduced leukocytes and control of any infections. Pharmacologic therapy includes the use of antibiotics, antifungal agents, and colony-stimulating factor drugs such as filgrastim. This, and similar drugs, markedly assist in decreasing the incidence of infection in people who have received bone marrow–depressing antineoplastic agents.

## NEUTROPENIA

Neutropenia is the condition associated with a reduction in circulating neutrophils. Neutrophils are often the first-line defense against infectious organisms, so a significant decrease in the number can have serious complications. Risk for infection is determined by the absolute neutrophil count (ANC), which is calculated by the WBC × (percent of polymorphonuclear cells [PMNs] + bands) ÷ 100. Neutropenia is defined as an ANC of less than 1500/microL (although this may vary from institution to institution). When the ANC falls below 1000/microL, the risk for infection rises; the highest risk occurs when the ANC is less than 500 micro/L. Persons at highest risk for infection and severe complications are those with an ANC of less than 100/microL (profound neutropenia) for greater than 7 days.[118] A fever that occurs in the setting of neutropenia is called a *neutropenic fever*, and can be a medical emergency. Causes are either acquired or congenital. Acquired neutropenias are typically a result of toxicity to neutrophil precursors in the bone marrow. This may be from drugs (e.g., chemotherapy agents, immunosuppressive agents, sulfonamides, macrolides, anticonvulsants) or infectious agents (e.g., hepatitis B, cytomegalovirus, EBV, HIV). Other drugs can cause an autoimmune-related peripheral destruction of neutrophils, leading to neutropenia.

Other causes of neutropenia include carcinoma of the lung, breast, prostate, and stomach and malignant hematopoietic disorders that can occupy enough of the bone marrow to cause global marrow failure, with resultant pancytopenias (all cell lines are decreased in number). Congenital causes usually come to attention early in life and are much less common than acquired causes.

The longer an individual exists without neutrophils, the higher the risk for significant infection. Administration of myeloid growth factors, such as granulocyte colony-stimulating factor (G-CSF) and granulocyte-macrophage colony-stimulating factor (GM-CSF) are utilized prophylactically in people who will receive chemotherapy that will cause neutropenia (primary prophylaxis of neutropenic complications); in clients who have had previous chemotherapy and a neutropenic fever and will receive another round of chemotherapy (secondary prophylaxis); and to reduce the duration of severe chemotherapy-induced neutropenia. Most guidelines suggest the prophylactic use of myeloid growth factors in the setting of chemotherapy when the anticipated level of neutropenia carries a 20% or higher risk of neutropenic fever.[407] Exceptions to using these factors include individuals with acute leukemia, myelodysplastic syndromes, and hematopoietic cell transplantation. Drug-induced neutropenia generally resolves in one to three weeks, once the offending drug is discontinued; in people exhibiting an infection, the use of G-CSF can be considered in order to shorten the duration of neutropenia.[442]

### Lymphocytosis/Lymphocytopenia

*Lymphocytosis* occurs most commonly in acute viral infections, especially those caused by EBV. Other causes include endocrine disorders (e.g., thyrotoxicosis, adrenal insufficiency) and malignancies (e.g., acute and chronic lymphocytic leukemia).

Lymphocytopenia may be acquired or congenital. Acquired lymphocytopenias can be attributed to abnormalities of lymphocyte production associated with neoplasms and immune deficiencies and destruction of lymphocytes by drugs, viruses, or radiation.

Other causes include corticosteroid therapy, severe systemic illnesses (e.g., miliary tuberculosis), SLE, sarcoidosis, viral hepatitis, or severe right-sided heart failure. For individuals with HIV, lymphocytopenia can be a major problem, increasing their susceptibility to viral illnesses, malignancies, and fungal infections.

## NEOPLASTIC DISEASES OF THE BLOOD AND LYMPH SYSTEMS

Hematologic malignancies include diseases in any hematologic tissue (e.g., bone marrow, spleen, thymus, lymphoid tissue) that arise from changes in stem cells or clonal (genetically identical cells) proliferation of abnormal cells. The primary hematologic disorders that result from stem cell abnormalities include the myeloproliferative neoplasms (e.g., polycythemia vera, essential thrombocythemia, chronic myeloid leukemia, and myelofibrosis with myeloid metaplasia) and acute myeloid leukemia. Myelofibrosis is the replacement of hematopoietic bone marrow with fibrous tissue, such as fibroblasts and collagen.

Multiple myeloma and plasma cell diseases arise from clonal proliferation of abnormal plasma cells. Lymphoid malignancies are also a clonal proliferation of malignant cells and can be categorized according to the malignant cell type: B-cell, T-cell/natural killer cell, and Hodgkin lymphoma. For ease of discussion, the leukemias are presented together.

### Hematopoietic Cell Transplantation

Hematopoietic cell transplantation (HCT) is often a treatment choice for many of the neoplastic diseases of the blood and lymph systems. Technical explanations of HCT are found in Chapter 21.

### The Leukemias

Leukemia is a malignant neoplasm of the blood-forming cells that replaces the normal bone marrow with a malignant clone (genetically identical cell) of lymphocytic or myelogenous cells.

The disease may be acute or chronic based on its natural course; acute leukemias have a rapid clinical course, resulting in death in a few months without treatment, whereas chronic leukemias have a more prolonged course. The four major types of leukemia are acute or chronic lymphocytic and acute or chronic myeloid leukemia (Table 14.2).

When leukemia is classified according to its morphology (i.e., the predominant cell type and level of maturity), the following descriptors are used: *lympho-*, for leukemias involving the lymphoid or lymphatic system; *myelo-*, for leukemias of myeloid or bone marrow origin involving hematopoietic stem cells ; *-blastic*, for leukemia involving large, immature (functionless) cells; and *-cytic*, for leukemia involving mature, smaller cells. If classified immunologically, T-cell/natural killer cell and B-cell leukemias are described.

*Acute leukemia* is an accumulation of neoplastic, immature lymphoid or myeloid cells in the bone marrow and peripheral blood. It is defined, using the WHO classification, as more than 20% blasts in the bone marrow.[15]

*Chronic leukemia* is a neoplastic accumulation of mature lymphoid or myeloid elements of the blood that usually progresses more slowly than an acute leukemic process and permits the production of greater numbers of more mature, functional cells. With rapid proliferation of leukemic cells, the bone marrow becomes overcrowded with abnormal cells, which then spill over into the peripheral circulation. Crowding of the bone marrow by leukemic cells inhibits normal blood cell production.

The three main symptoms that occur as a consequence of this infiltration and replacement process are (1) *anemia* and reduced tissue oxygenation from decreased erythrocytes, (2) *infection* from neutropenia as leukemic cells are functionally unable to defend the body against pathogens, and (3) *bleeding tendencies* from decreased platelet production (thrombocytopenia) (Fig. 14.4).

Leukemia is not limited to the bone marrow and peripheral blood. Abnormalities in the CNS or other organ systems can result from the infiltration and replacement of any tissue of the body with nonfunctional leukemic cells or metabolic complications related to leukemia.

Leukemia is a complex disease that requires careful identification of the subtype for appropriate treatment. Molecular probes can be used to establish a morphologic diagnosis of the type of leukemia, which then aids in treatment and prognosis. Molecular markers have generally been used to determine the presence or absence of leukemic cells remaining after intensive therapy, so-called residual disease, although no test has perfect sensitivity.[179,463,479]

Over the last 30 years, death rates for leukemia have been falling significantly (57% decline) for children and more modestly for adults younger than age 65 years. These declines in mortality reflect the advances made in the biologic and pathologic understanding of leukemia, technologic advances in medical care, and subsequent treatment that is more specifically targeted at the molecular level.

The aim of treatment is to bring about complete remission, or no evidence of the disease, with return to normal

**Table 14.2** Overview of Leukemia

| | Acute Lymphocytic Leukemia (ALL) | Chronic Lymphocytic Leukemia (CLL) | Acute Myelogenous Leukemia (AML) | Chronic Myelogenous Leukemia (CML) |
|---|---|---|---|---|
| Incidence (% of all leukemias) | 20% | 25% | 40% | 15% |
| Adults | 45% | 100% (common) | 80% (most common) | 95%–100% |
| Children | 55% (most common | NA | 20% | 2% |
| Age (yr) | Peak: 3–7 | Median age: 70 years | Mean age: 68; incidence increases with age from 45–80+ | Average age 65 (mostly adults) |
| Etiologic factors | ? Unknown; chromosomal abnormalities; Down syndrome (high incidence) | Chromosomal abnormalities; environmental factors | Benzene; alkylating agents; radiation; myeloproliferative disorders; chromosome abnormalities | Philadelphia chromosome; radiation exposure |
| Prognosis | Children: 90% survival<br>5-year overall survival: 71.6% | 5-year survival: 86.8% | Adults:<br>Disease-free survival: > 60 years: 5–10%<br>< 60 years: 30% | 5-year overall survival: 68.7% |

blood and marrow cells without relapse. For leukemia, a complete remission that lasts 5 years after treatment often indicates a cure. Future clinical and laboratory investigation will likely lead to the development of new, even more effective treatments, specifically for different subsets of leukemia. The development of new chemotherapeutic and biologic agents, combined with refined dose and schedule and hematopoietic cell transplantation, has already contributed to the clinical success of treatment.

## Acute Leukemia

Acute leukemia is a rapidly progressive malignant disease that results in the accumulation of immature, functionless cells called *blast cells* in the bone marrow and blood that block the development of normal cell development.

The two major forms of acute leukemia are *acute lymphoblastic leukemia* (ALL) and *acute myeloid leukemia* (AML). Lymphocytic leukemia involves the lymphocytes (B or T lymphoblasts) and lymphoid organs, and myeloid leukemia involves hematopoietic stem cells that are committed to differentiate into myeloid cells (monocytes, granulocytes, erythrocytes, and platelets).

### Acute Myeloid Leukemia

**Incidence and Risk Factors.** AML is an uncommon disease, only 1% of cancers, with an estimated 19,250 cases in 2018.[45] It is the most common leukemia in adults, constituting 80% of adult acute leukemias[401]; only 6% of individuals with AML are children. AML is more common in men than women with a ratio of 5:3 respectively.

The incidence of AML increases with each decade of life, with the median age at onset of 68 years.[45] It is uncommon in people under the age of 45. Most cases of AML develop for unknown reasons, whereas some cases occur following treatment for another cancer (chemotherapy or radiation induced), from a preexisting myelodysplastic syndrome, or a bone marrow failure syndrome (such as aplastic anemia).[468]

Two predominant types of treatment-related AML (t-AML) are described. The first typically occurs 5 to 7 years following exposure to an alkylating agent (i.e., cyclophosphamide, cisplatin) and/or radiation and is often heralded by a dysplastic phase. The other appears shortly after exposure to a topoisomerase II inhibitor (approximately 1 to 3 years) and lacks a dysplastic phase. Abnormalities in chromosome 5 and/or 7 are often seen in treatment-related AML and carry a worse prognosis than those cases that are idiopathic.[15,131,370]

Other risk factors for AML include previous radiation exposure and chemical/occupational exposure (e.g., benzene, herbicides, pesticides, cigarette smoking). Persons with uncommon genetic disorders, such as Down syndrome or Fanconi syndrome, also have a higher incidence of developing acute leukemia than the general population.

**Pathogenesis.** AML is a heterogeneous group (not all the same) of neoplastic myeloid cells. Myeloid stem cells have the capability of differentiating into granulocytes, monocytes, erythrocytes, and platelets; neoplastic changes can occur along any line, resulting in many subtypes of AML. These clonal cells (meaning they originate from the same stem cell or progenitor cell) are able to quickly divide, but unable to mature and differentiate into normal, functioning cells.

Current techniques allow for cytogenetic analyses that can reveal specific chromosomal abnormalities. These aberrant changes include gain or loss of part or all of a chromosome; or portions of a chromosome translocate (move) and fuse with another gene, creating a fusion gene. Some of the genes that are altered in AML include genes for protein transcription factors (e.g., RARA), proteins that act as tumor suppressors (e.g., TP53), and proteins involved in intracellular signaling (e.g., FLT3).[78,323] It is these successive abnormalities that lead to the development of leukemia, either allowing the cell to divide without regulation or failing to undergo programmed cell death (apoptosis).[132]

**Clinical Manifestations.** Initial clinical indications of AML are related to pancytopenia (reduction in all cell lines), reflecting leukemic cell replacement of bone marrow. Clients often have infections because of a lack of neutrophils or bleeding secondary to platelet deficiency (thrombocytopenia).

Anemia accompanied by pallor, fatigue, malaise, hypoxia, and bleeding (gum bleeding, epistaxis, ecchymoses, petechiae, retinal hemorrhage)

**Cause:** Rapidly proliferating development of leukocytes inhibiting erythrocytes and thrombocytes.

Severe infections (pneumonia, septicemia), ulcerations of the mouth and throat

**Cause:** High numbers of immature or abnormal leukocytes unable to fight and destroy microorganisms.

Increased metabolic rate accompanied by weakness, pallor, and weight loss

**Cause:** Increased leukocyte production requiring large amounts of nutrients; cell destruction increases the amount of metabolic wastes.

Headache, disorientation

**Cause:** Abnormal white cells infiltrating the central nervous system.

Hyperuricemia causing renal pain, obstruction (from stone formation), and infection; a late development is renal insufficiency with uremia

**Cause:** Large amounts of uric acid released as a result of destruction of great numbers of leukocytes; in late stages, abnormal leukocytes infiltrate the kidneys.

Enlarged organs (splenomegaly, hepatomegaly) exerting pressure on adjacent organs

**Cause:** High numbers of white cells accumulating within the liver and spleen, causing distention of tissues.

Lymphadenopathy and bone pain

**Cause:** Excessive numbers of white cells accumulating in lymph nodes and bone marrow.

**Figure 14.4**

**Pathologic basis for the clinical manifestations of leukemia.** (Modified from Black JM, Matassarin-Jacobs E, editors: *Luckmann and Sorensen's medical-surgical nursing*, ed 4, Philadelphia, 1993, WB Saunders.)

Spontaneous bleeding or bleeding with minor trauma often occurs in the skin and mucosal surfaces, manifested as gingival bleeding, epistaxis, midcycle menstrual bleeding, or heavy bleeding associated with menstruation (see Fig. 14.4). Petechiae (small, purplish spots caused by intradermal bleeding) are common clinical manifestations of thrombocytopenia particularly noted on the extremities after prolonged standing or minor trauma.

Fatigue, loss of energy, and shortness of breath with physical exertion are common because of anemia. Leukemia cells may infiltrate the skin (known as leukemia cutis), seen most often in the acute monocytic or myelomonocytic subtypes of AML. Leukemia cutis may present as multiple purplish papules or as a diffuse rash (Fig. 14.5). Uncommonly, AML cells may also form masses in the skin, tissue, or bone [21]

Modest splenomegaly is seen in 10% of clients with AML, whereas lymphadenopathy is uncommon. Discomfort in the bones, especially of the sternum, ribs, and tibia, caused by expanded leukemic marrow may occur. In the older adult, the disease can present insidiously

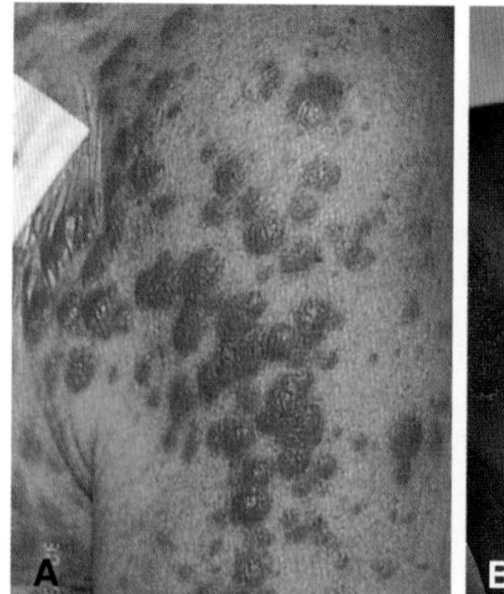


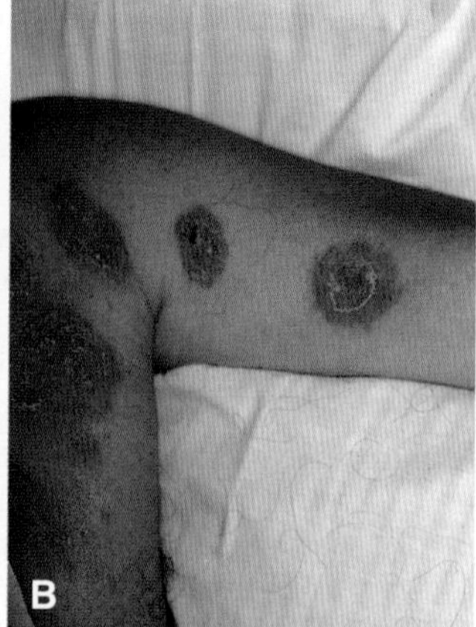


**Figure 14.5**

(A) Leukemia cutis in an individual with monoblastic leukemia. (B) Another example of leukemia cutis in the form of erythematous nodular tumors. (A, Reprinted from Hoffman R: *Hematology: basic principles and practice*, ed 4, Philadelphia, 2005, Churchill Livingstone. B, Reprinted from Noble J: *Textbook of primary care medicine*, ed 3, St Louis, 2001, Mosby.)

with progressive weakness, pallor, a change in sense of well-being, and delirium.

CNS involvement is uncommon, occurring in only 1% to 2% of adults presenting with AML.[22] These people present with symptoms similar to meningitis (e.g., headache, stiff neck, and fever). Some clients may develop cerebral bleeding or meningitis because of pancytopenia. In a small number of cases, AML may be more subtle, presenting at first with progressive fatigue and normal blood counts.

## MEDICAL MANAGEMENT

**DIAGNOSIS.** Initial blood tests often reveal an elevated leukocyte count with an excessive amount of immature cells although low counts may be seen, especially in the elderly. Uncommonly, initial counts may be normal. Sometimes Auer rods (linear groupings of primary granules) are seen on peripheral blood smear, which are indicative of AML, rather than ALL. Diagnosis usually requires a bone marrow biopsy and aspiration in order to view bone marrow architecture and perform further tests, such as cytogenetics, immunophenotyping, and flow cytometry. The diagnosis of AML is made when more than 20% of blasts are detected in the bone marrow.

Because most AML does not involve the CNS, lumbar punctures are not needed unless clinically indicated. Treatment is determined by lineage, and AML treatment differs from ALL treatment. AML can be subdivided into various subtypes or classifications, and each subtype may receive varying initial therapy

The WHO has provided a revised classification of AML, using cytogenetic information (chromosomal abnormalities) and clinical information. The categories include AML with recurrent genetic abnormalities, AML with myelodysplasia-related changes, therapy-related AML, and AML not otherwise specified (NOS), with other provisional diagnoses.[15] AML NOS is similar to the older French-American-British (FAB) system of classification.

Some of the more common genetic abnormalities include a translocation between chromosomes 8 and 21 (which is a favorable mutation); a translocation or inversion in chromosome 16 (more favorable mutation); rearrangements in chromosome 11 and translocation of parts of chromosomes 9 and 11; and a translocation between chromosomes 15 and 17 (favorable fusion mutation called PML-RARA). The latter translocation, known as acute promyelocytic leukemia (APL), is important to identify, because it is treated differently from other AML subtypes and carries a better prognosis.

Other abnormalities that have been identified include mutations of the fms-like tyrosine kinase 3 gene (*FLT3*), associated with a poor prognosis, and nucleophosmin gene (*NPM1*) mutation, which is associated with a better prognosis.[299] Pretreatment cytogenetics often prognosticate outcomes (favorable, intermediate, and high risk for recurrence) and influence therapy.[225]

**TREATMENT.** The treatment of acute leukemia can be a medical emergency, especially if the WBC count is high (about 20% of people with AML have a WBC greater than 100,000/mL), placing the person at risk for cerebral hemorrhage caused by leukostasis (obstruction of and damage to blood vessels plugged with rigid, large blasts). Clients with a high WBC prior to receiving chemotherapy are at risk for tumor lysis syndrome (see "Acute Lymphoblastic Leukemia [Acute Lymphocytic Leukemia]" below). Clients diagnosed with the subtype acute promyelocytic leukemia (APL) require emergent treatment with all-*trans* retinoic acid (ATRA) because this type of AML is associated with disseminated intravascular coagulation (DIC). ATRA promotes differentiation of immature, malignant promyelocytes to mature neutrophil cells.

Treatment decisions are based on the subtype of AML and cytogenetics. Most induction (initial) treatment protocols utilize aggressive combination chemotherapy (typically cytarabine and an anthracycline) in order to eradicate the neoplastic cells and restore normal hematopoiesis. Supportive care, including fluids, blood product replacement, and prompt treatment of infection with broad-spectrum antibiotics, is frequently needed during the 3- to 4-week hospitalization required for bone marrow recovery. Significant complications occur during this period, with a treatment mortality death rate of 3% to 10%.[309] People over the age of 60 often receive a low-intensity combination therapy induction that results in lower toxicities but with poorer outcomes.[309,342,471]

Induction chemotherapy is followed by consolidation chemotherapy, which is intended to maintain a complete remission and eradicate residual disease. Consolidation treatment is administered in 3 to 4 courses.

People who are young, with cytogenetics consistent with a good prognosis, can undergo consolidation therapy. Individuals at high risk for recurrent disease should consider allogeneic HCT after induction chemotherapy. Older people with favorable-to-intermediate cytogenetics typically receive an abbreviated consolidation treatment. Elderly clients with high-risk disease and comorbidities may not be able to tolerate aggressive therapy, in which case they are offered supportive care. This usually consists of transfusions, antibiotics, and low-dose chemotherapy (such as hydroxyurea) to control leukocytosis. Medically fit older adults with unfavorable cytogenetics may opt for a nonmyeloablative allogeneic HCT associated with a clinical trial.[108,252]

The discovery of mutations and translocations that may be causing leukemia has led to the development of targeted therapeutic agents. One example is all-*trans*-retinoic acid (ATRA). It is used against acute promyelocytic leukemia along with chemotherapy and targets the promyelocytic leukemia–retinoic acid receptor-α fusion transcript of the t(15,17) translocation.

**PROGNOSIS.** If left untreated, all leukemias are fatal. Adverse prognostic features include older age (often have more chromosome abnormalities and comorbidities), history of previous myelodysplastic syndrome or myeloproliferative disorder, previous exposure to chemotherapy and/or radiation, or chromosome abnormalities associated with a poor prognosis. With induction treatment, approximately 60% to 70% of clients younger than 60 years achieve a remission. The rate of remission decreases as age increases over 60 years.

On average, clients older than 60 years of age have a 5-year disease-free survival of 5% to 10%,[134] whereas those younger than 60 years have a 5-year disease-free survival of 30%. The overall 5-year survival rate is 27%.[45]

Current research is focused on cytogenetics and targeted therapies in hopes of improving long-term survival.

### Acute Lymphoblastic Leukemia (Acute Lymphocytic Leukemia)

**Incidence and Risk Factors.** In contrast to AML, ALL is diagnosed more frequently in children, with approximately 5900 cases per year and a median age of diagnosis of 15 years. Between the years 2011 and 2015, over 55% of the cases occurred in individuals under the age of 20, whereas the remaining cases were diagnosed in adults. Yet of the approximately 1500 annual deaths, about 85% occurred in adults, with a median age of 56. Unfortunately, the incidence of ALL has slowly increased over the past 25 years; however, the death rate has slightly improved.[45,406]

Like AML, most ALL cases develop for unknown reasons. A few risk factors have been identified, including previous exposure to chemotherapy and/or radiation. Persons with genetic disorders such as Down syndrome also have an increased risk. Questions have arisen as to whether other environmental factors, such as exposure to infectious agents or electromagnetic fields, such as those generated in high-voltage power lines, increase the risk of developing ALL. Studies are ongoing, however, evidence is lacking.[386]

**Pathogenesis.** Acute lymphoblastic leukemia is characterized by the inability of lymphocytic progenitor cells, lymphoblasts, to mature into normal T and B cells. About 85% of ALLs have a B-cell lineage, 10% to 15% a T-cell lineage, while a natural killer (NK) cell linage is rare and comprises less than 1% of ALL cases. Abnormal cytogenetics or translocations and mutations are frequently seen in ALL cases. These abnormalities are noted in varying rates among children versus adults and may herald a poor versus good prognosis. The *BCR-ABL1* fusion gene (Philadelphia chromosome) t(9;22) is more often associated in adults with ALL than in children, while children demonstrate the t(12;21) mutation more frequently than adults. Children under the age of 12 months frequently exhibit the t(4;11) abnormality, although it is rarely seen in adults. The t(4;11) and t(9;22) have a poor prognosis, whereas cases involving the t(12;21) or hyperdiploidy (50-60 chromosomes in the leukemic cells) have better treatment results.[270] Genetic abnormalities found in children with T-cell ALL currently do not appear to influence prognosis.

**Clinical Manifestations.** Individuals with ALL most commonly present with hepatomegaly/splenomegaly, fever, lymphadenopathy, abnormal blood counts, and musculoskeletal pain.[65] Many of these signs/symptoms are due to an abnormal bone marrow that is unable to engage in normal hematopoiesis. Hepatosplenomegaly and lymphadenopathy (particularly in the mediastinum) are frequently encountered, as abnormal cells infiltrate the liver, spleen, and lymph nodes. A mediastinal mass may be present, which if large enough, may lead to difficulty breathing or upper extremity swelling due to increased pressure on the bronchus or superior vena cava (SVC syndrome). Stridor and SVC syndrome require immediate attention. Fever may be due to infection (secondary to a lack of neutrophils) or the body's response to the leukemia itself. Easy bleeding and bruising are indicative of thrombocytopenia, and clients are often tired as a result of anemia.

ALL is more likely than AML to have leukemic cells spread to extramedullary sites. Although symptoms are not typically present at diagnosis, the CNS is frequently involved, and can cause headache, weakness, seizures, vomiting, difficulty with balance, radiculopathy, cranial nerve palsy, and blurred vision.[85,276] Testicles in males and ovaries in females may harbor leukemic cells and are difficult to reach with chemotherapy agents.

Bone and joint pain from leukemic infiltration or hemorrhage into a joint may be the initial symptoms (more common finding in children than adults). Involvement of the synovium may lead to symptoms suggestive of a rheumatic disease, especially in children.

Tumor lysis syndrome is common at diagnosis or shortly after the instigation of chemotherapy. This life-threatening condition occurs when there is a high turnover rate of cells (seen in acute leukemias) or chemotherapy agents lyse significant numbers of cells, resulting in high levels of potassium, phosphate, and uric acid accompanied by low levels of calcium. Complications such as acute renal failure, cardiac arrhythmias, seizures, and multiorgan failure may also occur.[180] Prevention of tumor lysis syndrome is accomplished with hydration and the use of allopurinol or rasburicase. For serious cases, dialysis may be required. See also discussion of tumor lysis syndrome in Chapter 9.

## MEDICAL MANAGEMENT

**DIAGNOSIS.** The diagnosis of ALL is similar to that of AML (see "Diagnosis" in "Acute Myelogenous Leukemia" above). The peripheral blood smear is examined, and additional special tests are performed using peripheral blood and bone marrow. A bone marrow biopsy and aspirate are needed for many of these tests. Diagnosis requires at least 25% of lymphoblasts on bone marrow examination.

Bone marrow is used to perform flow cytometry/immunophenotyping to determine if the leukemic cells are myeloid or lymphoid in origin (rarely there are cells that express features of both). Flow cytometry immunohistochemistry studies are also able to identify if the cells are from B- or T-cell lineage, which determines treatment. Cytogenetic studies are performed to aid in WHO classification, prognosis, and determining subsequent treatment.[432]

Because ALL commonly involves the CNS, a lumbar puncture is done to collect cerebral spinal fluid for analysis. As with AML, ALL is a heterogeneous group of lymphoid leukemias with varying prognoses.

The FAB classification of ALL is no longer used because it lacked prognostic significance. The WHO classifies ALL as either B-ALL, not otherwise specified (NOS); B-ALL with recurrent genetic abnormalities; T-ALL; and early T cell precursor lymphoblastic leukemia.[432]

**TREATMENT.** ALL treatment protocols vary depending on age (adult or child), subtype of ALL, and genetic abnormalities associated with risk of recurrence. Most centers treat ALL on a risk-based assessment (i.e., age, morphology, cytogenetics).[385] All therapy is given in phases: induction, consolidation, and maintenance. Initial treatment is called remission-induction therapy and consists of aggressive chemotherapy typically utilizing vincristine, L-asparaginase, and a corticosteroid. An anthracycline, such as doxorubicin or daunorubicin, is often added to regimens for clients at high risk for recurrence. Bone marrow is examined during induction treatment to assess therapy. Flow cytometry or quantitative PCR testing of bone marrow at the end of induction can determine if residual disease is present, termed measurable residual disease (MRD). Bone marrow without MRD indicates a complete remission and signals a better outcome.

Although only 5% of clients present with CNS involvement, prior to prophylactic CNS treatment up to 80% of individuals who were in remission relapsed with ALL-related meningitis. Currently, prophylactic intrathecal chemotherapy is periodically administered throughout treatment,[228] and those at high risk for CNS relapse may receive reduced doses of cranial radiation. Intensification or consolidation therapy is administered following successful induction treatment (no MRD) and lasts for 4 to 8 months. This consists of the administration of agents with mechanisms of action different from those used in induction therapy in an attempt to destroy cancer cells that may already be resistant to drugs used in induction. Consolidation may be followed with an intensification phase, where agents originally used in induction are given over 5 to 8 weeks, termed "delayed intensification." The last phase of treatment is the maintenance therapy, consisting of cyclic use of other chemotherapy agents over a period of 2 years or longer.

Selection of these agents is based on risk of recurrence, age, and subtype. Drugs, dosages, and scheduling can be individualized, although most are treated through clinical trial protocols. For ALL subtypes at high risk of recurrence, allogeneic HCT is offered. Adults frequently require transplantation and can achieve long-term survival rates of approximately 26% to 49%.[447]

Tyrosine kinase inhibitors (TKI), such as imatinib, dasatinib, nilotinib, and bosutinib, in combination with intensive chemotherapy, are available for the treatment of ALL with the Philadelphia chromosome t(9;22) translocation, providing significantly improved outcomes.[384] Studies are underway to determine if chemotherapy with a TKI or HCT after first remission offers the best long-term survival.

Although therapy is very successful in inducing remission and cure, a small percentage of people still die due to toxicities from aggressive chemotherapy, referred to as treatment-related death. Infants and older children had higher rates of treatment-related death, occurring in about 1% to 3% of ALL cases.[369,388]

Ninety-eight percent of children and 85% of adults achieve a complete remission following remission-induction therapy. With such favorable results, efforts are being made to reduce toxicities associated with aggressive combination chemotherapy, especially in children with standard-risk ALL with favorable cytogenetics.

Studies show that children who survive cancer go on to develop significant long-term medical problems, including other cancers, heart disease, learning disabilities, cognitive dysfunction, joint replacement, short stature, and hearing/vision loss.[305,346] Some of the strategies being implemented in protocols include a dose reduction of vincristine in infants, the omission of cranial irradiation, and a dose reduction of methotrexate in clients with Down syndrome.[377]

**PROGNOSIS.** Children with ALL do better than adults (the older the client, typically the worse the prognosis) and the survival rate has been improving; for children and adolescents, the 5-year survival rate is approximately 90%[183,331] with a cure rate of greater than 80%. Infants (younger than 1 year) have a poor prognosis and often die as a consequence of complications of therapy.[332] Although 80% to 90% of adults achieve a remission following induction therapy, about half will relapse, resulting in a 30% to 40% cure rate. The overall 5-year survival rate is approximately 68%.[44]

## Chronic Leukemia

Chronic leukemia is a malignant disease of the bone marrow and blood that progresses slowly and permits numbers of more mature, functional cells to be made. Chronic leukemia has two major groups: chronic myeloid leukemia (CML) and chronic lymphocytic leukemia (CLL), each with several subtypes.

These are entirely different diseases and are presented separately. CML is also known as chronic myelogenous leukemia or chronic myelocytic leukemia and is one of the myeloproliferative diseases. Other less-common forms include prolymphocytic leukemia (terminal transformation of CLL) and hairy cell leukemia (accounting for only 1%-2% of adult leukemias).

### Chronic Myeloid Leukemia

**Incidence and Etiologic Factors.** CML is a neoplasm of the hematopoietic stem cell committed to the myeloid lineage. The genetic abnormalities created in the stem cell are the result of acquired injury to the DNA and passed on to all related cell lines, resulting in increases in myeloid cells and clonal anomalies in erythroid cells and platelets. This leads to abnormal cells in peripheral blood and marked hyperplasia in the bone marrow.

CML accounts for 15% of all leukemias,[401] with approximately 8400 cases diagnosed per year. The median age at diagnosis is 65 years, with an incidence of 1.8 cases per 100,000 people.[46] This type of leukemia occurs mostly in adults, with only 2% developing in children. Although the exact etiologic factors are unknown, the incidence of CML is increased in people with severe radiation exposure. No chemical or other environmental risk factors are known to cause CML.

**Pathogenesis.** CML originates in the hematopoietic stem cell that is committed to the myeloid line (i.e., this cell has the ability to develop into any one of several blood cells along the myeloid lineage) and involves overproduction of myeloid cells. The genetic defect detected in CML cells is called the Philadelphia chromosome. This translocation, t(9,22), was the first consistent chromosomal anomaly identified in a cancer and is now detected in all cases of CML and known to be the cause of CML.

The abnormal chromosome develops from the accidental translocation and fusion of the *BCR* gene on chromosome 22 and the *ABL* gene on chromosome 9, creating a unique gene *(BCR-ABL1)*. The *BCR-ABL1* gene encodes for an abnormal protein product that acts as a tyrosine kinase, resulting in a dysregulated proliferation signal.

Tyrosine kinase is an enzyme that is necessary for intracellular signaling and cell growth. In normal cells the enzyme turns on and off as it should, but in people with CML this enzyme appears to be in the perpetual "switched on" state, eliminating the normal checks and balances on proliferation and allowing cells to escape from apoptosis (programmed cell death). CML has a chronic phase and an accelerated phase or blast crisis. In order for CML to progress from chronic to accelerated phase, several events appear necessary: increased levels of BCR-ABL1 protein, inactivation of tumor suppressor genes (such as the p53 tumor suppressor gene), additional chromosomal abnormalities (trisomy of chromosomes 8 and 19 or duplication of the Philadelphia chromosome), and differentiation arrest (cells become more immature in their development).

Unlike AML, CML initially permits the development of mature WBCs that generally function normally. This important distinction from acute leukemia accounts for the less-severe early course of the disease.

**Clinical Manifestations.** The majority of people with CML present in the chronic phase (85%), and presenting signs and symptoms are often quite nonspecific. The most typical symptoms at presentation are fatigue, anorexia, and weight loss, although approximately 40% of affected individuals are asymptomatic. Sweats, malaise, and shortness of breath during physical activity are also reported.

Splenomegaly is present in 50% of all cases, with corresponding complaints of left upper quadrant pain and early satiety. Thrombocytosis is also very common. The natural history of CML is a progression (over years) from a proliferative phase (chronic phase), into an accelerated phase (more symptoms and an increase in the number of immature cells, but not acute leukemia), to an aggressive acute leukemia (blast crisis) that can be rapidly fatal without treatment. In a minority of cases, the clinical progression may be biphasic from chronic phase directly to blast crisis.

## MEDICAL MANAGEMENT

**DIAGNOSIS.** Early in the disease process, only vague symptoms or routine blood analysis may herald the disease. Peripheral blood counts and smears often demonstrate an abnormal leukocytosis, which leads to further testing. The peripheral blood smear will often reveal a wide range of cells in a variety of stages, with the majority along the neutrophil line. Basophilia is often seen and associated with CML. The appearance of both mature and immature cells in the peripheral blood is suggestive of CML but must be differentiated from other myeloproliferative diseases. WBC counts are often over 100,000/microL (50%-70%) and platelet counts between 600,000 and 700,000/microL (15%-30%).[475] Although these cells may appear morphologically normal, they have cytochemical abnormalities and do not function appropriately, resulting in infection and bleeding.

The diagnosis is made by detecting the BCR-ABL1 fusion gene by routine cytogenetics or fluorescence in situ hybridization (FISH) or by reverse transcription–polymerase chain reaction (RT-PCR). Cytogenetic testing and bone marrow evaluation determine the phase of the disease.

**TREATMENT AND PROGNOSIS.** All people diagnosed with CML require treatment, even those who are asymptomatic. Recent research has significantly changed the treatment and prognosis of CML. Knowledge that the cause of the disease was an abnormal *BCR-ABL1* gene led to the development of the drug imatinib mesylate, designed to target and inhibit tyrosine kinase. In clients with chronic-phase disease, treatment with imatinib led to an overall survival of 89% at 5 years. However, with time most people develop resistance to imatinib, requiring further treatment. Nilotinib and dasatinib, more potent tyrosine kinase inhibitors, are second-line therapies with similar results to imatinib.[319,367] As long as the individual is responding and able to tolerate the drug, TKIs are given indefinitely; although some clients are able to stop treatment for a time once they obtain a molecular remission, a so-called "treatment-free remission." Guidelines are being established for the safe discontinuance of treatment, as well as monitoring to determine when therapy should be resumed.[376]

The overall 5-year survival rate is approximately 68% but is improving for some individuals treated with new treatment options.[46] For most people who present in chronic phase and are treated with TKIs, their life expectancy approaches that of the general population (age matched).[29] Overall survival decreases with age and comorbidities.[34] For those individuals with CML who are not responsive to TKIs (or for those who are unable to tolerate TKIs), chemotherapy can control the symptoms for a time. HCT continues to be an option that may provide a cure. This procedure is for select people with resistant disease (regardless of phase) or with accelerated or blast-phase disease.

### Chronic Lymphocytic Leukemia

**Incidence, Etiologic Factors, and Risk Factors.** CLL is the most common type of leukemia in adults, accounting for 25% to 30% of all leukemias, with over 20,000 cases per year.[387,401] The incidence of CLL increases with advancing age, with the median age of presentation being 70 years; 90% are older than 50 years, and men are affected more often than women.[387] CLL and small lymphocytic lymphoma are the same disease but the distinction is based on presence of the disease principally in the blood stream and bone marrow (termed leukemia) or in lymph nodes (called lymphoma). Both receive the same treatment. For this reason, CLL is often grouped with lymphomas in treatment centers.

The cause of CLL is also unknown but a few environmental factors are implicated, such as farming pesticides and the chemical warfare herbicide Agent Orange, although conclusive evidence is lacking. Some groups of people may have a genetic predisposition, including persons with a first-degree family member with CLL.[482]

**Pathogenesis.** The cell type responsible for more than 95% of the cases of CLL is the B cell (T cell CLL is uncommon). When a normal B cell is stimulated by an antigen, it enters a proliferative phase, creating clones able to fight infection. It is during this proliferative stage that a cell may develop mutations and predispose it to becoming cancerous, called monoclonal B-cell lymphocytosis (MLB).[120] Once MLB is established, it is presumed that further mutations or changes in the environment then allow for the progression to CLL. Most cases of MLB do not progress to CLL. Despite the uniform name for this type of leukemia, the disease is heterogeneous, with many types of genetic changes and expressions of the disease.[478] Each individual with CLL may demonstrate several different malignant clone populations.[220,282] The pathway to becoming malignant consists of multiple steps; some of the mutations and stages are known and others require more research. These cancerous cells are able to proliferate independent of antigen stimulation and lack the ability to undergo apoptosis (programmed cell death).

Fluorescence in situ hybridization is performed on the peripheral blood, looking at specific chromosomal abnormalities such as del(17p), del(13q), del(11q) and trisomy 12. The tumor-suppressor gene, TP53, is located on chromosome 17. For individuals with the 17p deletion, this gene is no longer able to function. At diagnosis of CLL, only about 10% of people have this mutation but, with time and evolution of genetic mutations, the presence of del(17p) becomes much higher, particularly in people with refractory or relapse of disease.[148]

Del(11q) occurs in about 20% of people with CLL. In the past, clients with this abnormality either did not respond to treatment or relapsed soon after achieving remission; however, newer treatments with fludarabine, cyclophosphamide, and rituximab have improved outcomes. The most common mutation is the deletion of 13q, seen in up to 50% of clients with CLL.[91] This genetic abnormality carries a more benign prognosis, with slowly progressive disease. Another abnormality, noted in 15% of people with CLL, is trisomy 12 which may be associated with progressive disease, although if it is the only abnormality noted, it often is indicative of low-risk disease.[368]

**Clinical Manifestations.** In the early stages of the disease, most clients remain asymptomatic or complain of vague, nonspecific symptoms such as fatigue or enlarged lymph nodes. Lymphadenopathy is the most common sign in people with CLL, noted in 50% to 90%. Splenomegaly is also a common finding, present in 25% to 50% of cases. Between 5% to 10% of individuals may also describe what are termed "B" symptoms, such as fever, night sweats, and unintentional weight loss. Malignant lymphocytes may also uncommonly infiltrate the skin (leukemia cutis) manifesting as macules, papules, plaques, nodules or exfoliative erythroderma in the head and neck area.[5,231] Depending on the mutations present in the abnormal clone, clients may experience a prolonged, indolent course with few symptoms.

Those people with more aggressive CLL develop pancytopenia (with accompanying symptoms of infections, hemorrhage, and significant fatigue) and decreased immunoglobulin levels. The most common opportunistic infections include encapsulated bacteria (*Streptococcus pneumoniae, Haemophilus influenzae*) while herpes simplex virus and herpes zoster are the most common viruses encountered. Approximately 10% of clients develop the complication of autoimmune hemolytic anemia (AIHA),[321] and immune thrombocytopenia occurs in 2% of cases.[36] Approximately 2% to 9% of people with CLL develop a rapidly progressive large-cell lymphoma called Richter transformation, requiring more aggressive therapy.[318]

## MEDICAL MANAGEMENT

**DIAGNOSIS AND STAGING.** Examination of the peripheral blood smear, CBC, and flow cytometry are performed to make a diagnosis. The peripheral blood smear may demonstrate "smudge cells"; although these cells appear mature, they are often fragile and break easily. Bone marrow examination is not required but may be helpful. Staging is established according to the Rai and Binet systems.

The Rai system recognizes stages conferring a low (stage 0), intermediate (I, II), and high (III, IV) risk of progression. This staging determines which clients should receive treatment and when, but this staging system does not provide reliable prognostic information. The Binet system uses hemoglobin, platelet count, and number of involved lymph node groups, classifying the disease into stages A, B, and C.

**Treatment.** There has been significant advancement in the number of agents able to treat CLL. Although they do not provide a cure, these drugs can offer durable remissions. Many people are diagnosed early, prior to symptoms, due to an elevated lymphocyte count.

Clients who are found to be at low risk for progression require careful monitoring and frequent examinations, with treatment initiated when symptoms worsen or if there is evidence of rapidly progressive leukemia. Treatment prior to the presence of symptoms has not been shown to be of benefit.[28,38] Clients with symptoms or rapidly progressive disease can be treated with traditional chemotherapy agents, such as alkylating agents (cyclophosphamide, chlorambucil) and purine nucleoside analogues (fludarabine, cladribine). However, monoclonal antibodies (rituximab, alemtuzumab, and ofatumumab), the phosphoinositide-3 kinase inhibitor idelalisib, and the Bruton kinase inhibitor ibrutinib,[272,476] have been approved for treatment of CLL and are now often used prior to traditional chemotherapy agents (particularly ibrutinib) due to efficacy and improved side-effect profiles. Choice of agent is often determined by age and the individual's comorbidities.

Lenalidomide, an immunomodulating agent used in treating multiple myeloma and myelodysplastic syndromes, is also approved for treatment of CLL.[57,267] The use of HCT for the treatment of CLL is not often utilized, but remains a successful option in a limited number of refractory cases.[262]

## PROGNOSIS

CLL continues to be a fatal disease with a significant impact on life expectancy, but in the last few years a trend toward an improvement in overall survival has taken place (overall 5-year survival rate of 84%).[209,287]

Because CLL is a heterogenic disease, prognosis varies greatly at diagnosis. Prognostic information includes stage of disease at diagnosis and the presence or absence of prognostic chromosomal or gene markers.

Clients who present in Rai stages III–IV have an average life expectancy of 5 years, whereas those with less aggressive leukemia may never require treatment (depending on the age at diagnosis). Approximately 70% of people with CLL eventually require treatment.[198]

Chromosomal abnormalities and measurement of beta-2 microglobulin (higher levels have a worse prognosis) also aid in prognosis. Specific chromosomal abnormalities are prognostic indicators, such as del(17p), del(13q), del(11q) and trisomy 12. Newer markers include ZAP-70, CD38, and the gene mutations TP53 (seen with del(17p)) and SF3B1. Del(13q) and trisomy 12 are associated with a better prognosis, with a median survival of 133 and 114 months respectively; cases involving del(17p), TP53, ZAP-70 and CD38 are known to be progressive, resistant to therapy or relapse early.[91,426] People with del(17p) have a 32-month median survival. Mutations in the immunoglobulin heavy chain variable region carry a better prognosis. The chromosomal abnormalities may be used predictively, but the prognostic use of newer markers is still to be determined in clinical trials.

## SPECIAL IMPLICATIONS FOR THE THERAPIST 14.7

Like all cancers, medical innovations in the treatment of leukemia are increasing the affected individual's life span while increasing the likelihood of treatment side effects. Strengthening and energy-enhancing programs during cancer treatment can significantly improve symptoms of fatigue and depression, increase cardiovascular endurance, and maintain quality of life.[101]

Many more research studies are available now on the role of exercise specifically during the medical management of pediatric and adult leukemias. Significant improvement in health-related quality of life, fitness, mental health, and reduced symptom interference on daily life activities have been reported.[8,133,189] Observational studies also report low physical activity levels among survivors of leukemias, with the potential for adverse health effects as a result.

There is a growing body of literature with evidence to support the idea that regular physical activity is safe and has potential benefits for both adult and pediatric hematologic cancer survivors.[473] The physical therapist working with this group of individuals can be very instrumental in client education and supervised exercise programs to potentially improve muscle strength, physical function, and cardiorespiratory fitness, while reducing fatigue and improving overall quality of life.[473]

### Precautions

The period after chemically induced remission is critical for each client, who is now highly susceptible to spontaneous hemorrhage and defenseless against invading organisms. The usual precautions for thrombocytopenia, neutropenia, and infection control must be adhered to strictly. The importance of strict handwashing technique cannot be overemphasized. The therapist should be alert to any sign of infection and report any potential site of infection, such as mucosal ulceration, skin abrasion, or a tear (even a hangnail). Precautions are as for anemia, outlined earlier in this chapter (see "The Anemias.").

Anticipating potential side effects of medications used in the treatment of leukemia can help the therapist better understand client reactions during the episode of care. Drug-induced mood changes, ranging from feelings of well-being and euphoria to depression and irritability, may occur; depression and irritability may also be associated with the cancer. Exercise intensity and duration and activity modifications are necessary for clients with anemia.

Clients with a history of prolonged corticosteroid use should be assessed for muscle weakness and avascular necrosis of the hips and shoulders.

### Joint Involvement

Arthralgia or arthritis occurs in approximately 12% of adults with chronic leukemia, 13% of adults with acute leukemia, and up to 60% of children with ALL. Articular symptoms are the result of leukemic infiltrates of the synovium, periosteum, or periarticular bone or of secondary gout or hemarthrosis. Asymmetrical involvement of the large joints is most commonly observed. Pain that is disproportionate to the physical findings may occur, and joint symptoms are often transient.

### Children with Leukemia

Because of increasing survival rates for children with ALL and the extensive side effects of the treatments, the therapist must pay attention to specific measures of cognition, function, activity, and participation when planning an appropriate intervention program. All components are needed in a comprehensive program.[243]

Short- and long-term impairments can affect any or all of these components. Decreased hemoglobin levels, osteonecrosis, joint range of motion, strength, gross and fine motor performance, fitness, and attendance or absence from school are all factors to consider.[243]

Long-term effects of treatment and CNS prophylaxis can include peripheral neuropathies, neuropsychologic disorders, problems with balance, decreased muscle strength, and obesity. CNS prophylaxis includes intrathecal chemotherapy (injection of drugs into the spinal fluid) and cranial irradiation. Cranial irradiation and obesity are significant predictors of impaired balance.[477]

Preschool children with immature nervous systems may be more sensitive to the neurotoxicity of radiation and chemotherapy, placing them at a greater risk for CNS damage than children with fully developed neurologic systems.[269] Learning difficulties, cognitive deficits, attention problems, and lack of participation in physical activities can be sequelae of medical treatment.[477]

Personal factors such as a family's cultural belief system may influence how children and their parents perceive rehabilitation and specific interventions. Health-related quality of life and goals may be driven by family and cultural values that are not necessarily what the therapist perceives as in the best interest of the child's function and fitness.

The therapist should try to match the program with the family's cultural expectations, ability to participate, and emotional and financial resources. Expecting from the family only what they can succeed at and providing support and education where they are needed to help the family grow and care for their child with medical needs will create the best therapeutic environment for the child to thrive in.

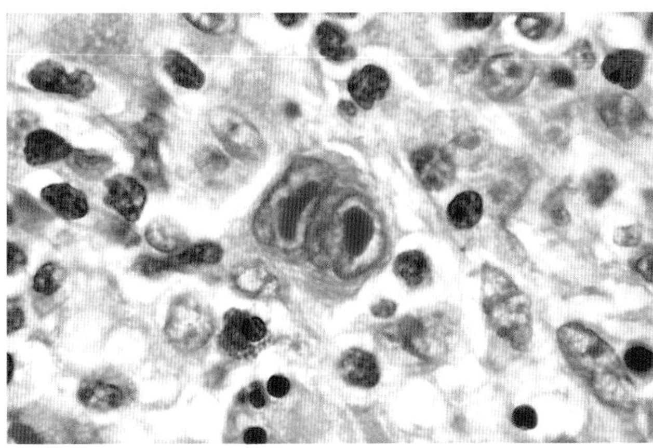

**Figure 14.6**

**Reed-Sternberg cell.** Named for Dorothy M. Reed, American pathologist (1874–1964), and Karl Sternberg, Austrian pathologist (1872–1935). This is one example of the large, abnormal, multinucleated reticuloendothelial cells in the lymphatic system found in Hodgkin lymphoma. The number and proportion of Reed-Sternberg cells identified are the basis for the histopathologic classification of Hodgkin lymphoma. (Reprinted from Kumar V, Cotran RS, Robbins SL: *Basic pathology*, ed 6, Philadelphia, 1997, WB Saunders. Courtesy Dr. Robert W. McKenna, University of Texas Southwestern Medical School, Dallas.)

## Malignant Lymphomas

*Lymphoma* is a general term for cancers that develop in the lymphatic system. Lymphomas are divided into two groups: Hodgkin lymphoma (HL; also known as Hodgkin disease) and non-Hodgkin lymphoma (NHL).

It is becoming more useful to categorize lymphomas according to their clinical behavior—indolent or aggressive—and their chromosome features. Currently HL is distinguished from other lymphomas by the presence of a characteristic type of cell known as the Reed-Sternberg cell. All other types of lymphoma are called NHL and have multiple subsets.

### Hodgkin Lymphoma

**Definition and Overview.** HL is a lymphoid neoplasm with the primary histologic finding of giant Reed-Sternberg cells in the lymph nodes. These cells are of B-cell lineage and have twin nuclei and nucleoli that give them the appearance of owl eyes (Fig. 14.6).

Although this malignancy originates in the lymphoid system and primarily involves the lymph nodes, it can spread to other sites, such as the spleen, liver, and bone marrow. There are two groups of HL: classic HL (further divided into four categories) and nodular lymphocyte-predominant HL (NLPHL). NLPHL is uncommon and represents only 10% of HL cases.

**Incidence and Risk Factors.** Classic HL can occur in both children and adults but peaks at two different ages: about the age of 20 and 65 years, with a median age of 39 at diagnosis. Children younger than 5 years rarely develop this disease, and only 10% of HL cases occur in children 16 years old and younger. LPHL typically has only one peak incidence around the fourth decade. It is estimated that 8500 new cases of HL were diagnosed in 2018, with 1050 deaths.[301]

Although the exact cause of HL remains under investigation, certain risk factors have been identified. One factor that has been related to HL is previous infection with EBV.[164] The DNA of this virus has been found in the Reed-Sternberg cells of approximately 30% to 50% of clients with classic HL.[246] People with HIV or other types of immunosuppression (post-transplantation) are also at increased risk for developing HL,[322] as are individuals with an autoimmune disorder.[172]

**Pathogenesis.** The pathologic cell of classic HL is the Reed-Sternberg cell, which is a clonal lymphoid cell, and usually is of B lineage.[215] Other malignant cells seen in HL include "mummified cells," "lacunar cells," "Hodgkin cells," and "popcorn cells." Depending on the subtype of HL, the presence and composition of cells varies. These neoplastic cells are surrounded by inflammatory cells—granulocytes, lymphocytes, plasma cells, and fibroblasts. The reason for the transformation from a normal B cell to a malignant cell is still under investigation, but significant progress has been made. The Reed-Sternberg cells are missing many of the specific B cell transcription factors (such as those that aid in immunoglobulin formation) and B cell markers (markers that define B cells), yet may demonstrate markers more specific for T cells.[382] They also overexpress programmed death 1 and/or 2 ligands (PD-L1 or L2) that bind to PD-1 receptors on T cells, leading to an "exhaustion" of the T cell and eventual inactivation. This inactivation creates an area of local immunosuppression and allows the Reed-Sternberg cell to evade detection and destruction by T cells.[48] Other molecules and factors are expressed by the Reed-Sternberg cells that promote B cell activation and longevity. For example, nuclear factor kappa B (NF-κB) is involved in signaling pathways for B cell DNA transcription, cytokine production, and longevity. HL cells have mutations that promote the production of NF-κB while simultaneously reducing negative regulation, thereby evading apoptosis and making the cell immortal.[201,472]

Most likely there are various causes that account for the bimodal distribution of the disease (i.e., younger people may develop HL caused by a different etiology than older people). Recent evidence suggests that an infection or inflammation may be involved. As just discussed, genes from EBV are found in one-third to one-half of all HL cases in the industrialized world. Yet, other factors in concert with EBV infection, such as an abnormal antibody response to EBV,[226,274] are likely required for malignant transformation.[163]

Many cytokines, particularly interleukins, are involved in producing an environment where the Reed-Sternberg cells thrive. For example, some interleukins attract inflammatory cells (eosinophils, monocytes, and mast cells), which aid in the survival of the cell.[7,165] In the laboratory, if these inflammatory cells are not surrounding the Reed-Sternberg cells, they do not survive.

**Clinical Manifestations.** See Fig 14.7.

Classic HL and NLPHL present with different clinical manifestations and progression of disease. Because of these distinctions, these two subgroups are discussed separately.

***Classic Hodgkin Lymphoma.*** Classic HL begins in a lymph node and spreads contiguously to other lymph

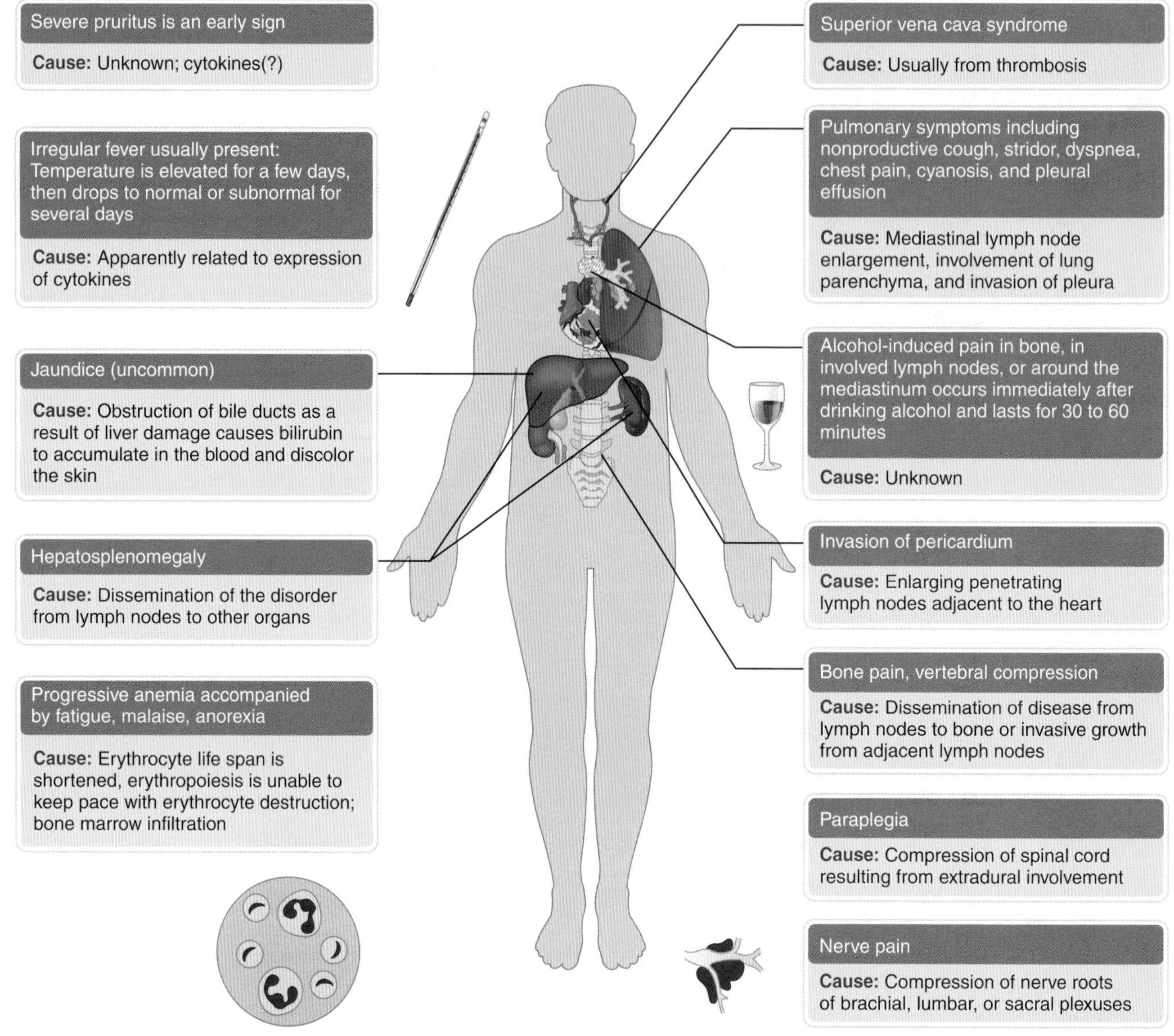


**Figure 14.7**

Pathologic basis for the clinical manifestations of HL.

node chains. The cervical, supraclavicular, and mediastinal lymph nodes are the most common initial locations for involvement (Fig. 14.8). These lymph nodes are typically nontender and firm.

Nodular sclerosing HL typically presents with supradiaphragmatic lymph node involvement, whereas mixed cellularity classic HL (MCHL) often exhibits smaller involved lymph nodes in a subdiaphragmatic location or involves organs. Clients who have disease below the diaphragm, MCHL, or "B" symptoms (fever, night sweats, weight loss) are more likely to develop splenic involvement. Splenic involvement is seen in 25% to 50% of people with HL, but detection is often difficult. An enlarged spleen does not necessarily indicate involvement, and a normal-size spleen does not rule out involvement. HL in the liver is uncommon and may be associated with splenic involvement and "B" symptoms.

Bone marrow involvement occurs in less than 10% of newly diagnosed cases. If lymph nodes become large and bulky, they can lead to further symptoms, such as tracheal or bronchial compression with accompanying shortness of breath, chest pain, or cough. Uncommonly it may cause superior vena cava syndrome. Lymph node masses in the abdomen can obstruct the GI tract. Lymph nodes may grow and enlarge and finally perforate the lymph node capsule, continuing to grow and invade into adjacent tissue or organs. This can occur in the lung, pericardium, pleura, chest wall, gut, or bone.

Pruritus is an early manifestation of HL occurring in 10% to 15% of clients with HL; many people develop pruritus at some point in the course of their disease. Those with severe pruritus have a poorer prognosis.

One uncommon but specific clinical sign for HL is the development of pain with the consumption of alcohol. When present, pain is typically noted in areas with HL or bony involvement.

Effusions (collections of fluid) may also develop in the lung, heart, or abdominal cavity. Tumor can spread not

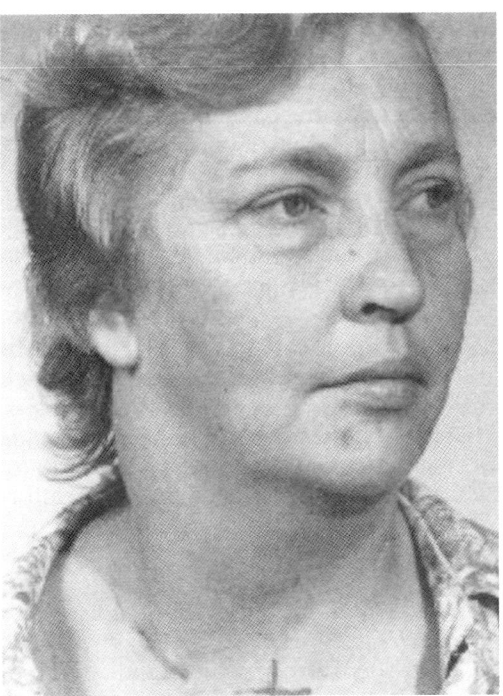

**Figure 14.8**

**Enlarged cervical lymph node associated with HL.** (Reprinted from del Regato J, Spjut HJ, Cox JD: *Cancer: diagnosis, treatment, and prognosis*, ed 6, St Louis, 1985, Mosby–Year Book.)

only from lymph node to adjacent lymph node, but via the bloodstream to lung, liver, bone marrow, and bone, particularly in disease relapse. Involvement in these areas is often indicative of extensive disease. As bone marrow is replaced, infections, anemia, and thrombocytopenia result.

HL involvement of the CNS is very rare and may include cranial nerve palsies, motor/sensory deficits and seizures.[359] Occasionally spinal cord involvement may occur in the dorsal and lumbar regions, and compression of nerve roots of the brachial, lumbar, or sacral plexus can cause nerve root pain. Epidural involvement (also uncommon) causes back and neck pain with hyperreflexia.[126]

***Nodular Lymphocyte-Predominant Hodgkin Lymphoma.*** NLPHL typically presents with involvement of peripheral rather than central lymph nodes, such as the cervical, axillary, or inguinal lymph node chains. Unlike classic HL, NLPHL does not follow an orderly pattern of spread, but can be found in lymph nodes distant from the original node of disease. NLPHL infrequently involves the bone marrow, spleen, or lung. "B" symptoms rarely occur. NLPHL has an indolent clinical course with long disease-free intervals. Relapse is common but responds well to treatment.

### Special Considerations

***Pregnancy and Hodgkin Lymphoma.*** Because the mean age at diagnosis of HL is 39 years, it is not uncommon for women to develop HL while pregnant. The management of HL during pregnancy must be individualized. Initial diagnostic staging can be accomplished safely with ultrasound or magnetic resonance imaging (MRI).[192,297] Many women have been successfully treated while pregnant without adverse effects on the fetus.[110,187] Chemotherapy agents are known teratogens and treatment during the first trimester should be avoided if the option is available to delay therapy. Treatment during the second and third trimesters can lead to low birth weight, intrauterine growth restriction, and cognitive disabilities. However, many women have received ABVD treatment while pregnant in the second and third trimesters, with normal outcomes.[18,102] Women presenting in later pregnancy are often able to have therapy delayed until after delivery or can undergo modified or standard combination chemotherapy and radiation therapy.[363]

With the increased use of ABVD therapy (Adriamycin [doxorubicin], bleomycin, vinblastine, and dacarbazine) and reduced reliance on radiation therapy, the use of radiation can be avoided. However, with appropriate shielding, the estimated fetal dose of radiation can be reduced by 50% or more in most cases if emergently required.[143] In nonpregnant women, to further reduce any risk, it is advisable to delay pregnancy for 12 months after completion of radiation therapy.[110] Ovarian function and ability to become pregnant following therapy is similar to the general population, if treatment did not include an alkylating agent or pelvic radiation.[205]

Although men who survive HL have a good chance of preserving fertility,[423] long-term semen banking is available for men whose future fertility may be compromised by aggressive treatment.[177]

## MEDICAL MANAGEMENT

**DIAGNOSIS AND STAGING.** The diagnosis of HL is made through the evaluation of an affected lymph node. This requires an excisional biopsy of involved tissue (usually an accessible lymph node). Needle biopsy usually does not provide enough cells for diagnosis because only 2% to 3% of the cells in a lymph node may be malignant. Biopsied tissue is sent for molecular testing (cytogenetics, gene expression, FISH), immunophenotyping, and histopathologic studies in order to make the diagnosis. Identification of EBV may also aid in the differential diagnosis. The presence of the Reed-Sternberg cells is required for the diagnosis; however, Reed-Sternberg cells are seen in other disorders.

Currently there are two systems to classify and stage HL: the WHO/Revised European-American Lymphoma classification and the Lugano classification (Box 14.6). The WHO/Revised European-American Lymphoma classifies HL into two groups: nodular lymphocytic-predominant HL and classic HL which has four subgroups: nodular sclerosis classic HL, lymphocyte-rich classic HL, MCHL, and lymphocyte-depleted classic HL.

The Lugano classification was published in 2014 and updated the Cotswold modification of the Ann Arbor staging system.[61] Staging of HL is divided into stages I through IV and adds prognostic information concerning bulky disease (worse prognosis if more than 10 cm), regions of lymph node involvement (local vs. extranodal extension), and the presence of "B" symptoms (fever, night sweats, weight loss). Complete physical, blood tests, and positron emission tomography with computed tomography (PET-CT) scans of the chest, abdomen, and pelvis (Fig. 14.9) aid in staging. PET-CT scans can be helpful in assessing the stage, response to treatment, and prognosis. Treatment of HL is dictated by

Box 14.6

**LUGANO STAGING CLASSIFICATION FOR HODGKIN LYMPHOMA[a]**

| | |
|---|---|
| Stage I | Involvement of a single lymph node or group of adjacent nodes, or a single extralymphatic site without lymph node involvement IE (e.g., spleen, thymus, Waldeyer ring) except liver and bone marrow |
| Stage II | Involvement of two or more lymph node regions on the same side of the diaphragm or limited contiguous extranodal involvement (the number of regions involved is noted after the stage, i.e., stage II-3) |
| Stage III | Involvement of lymph node regions or structures on both sides of the diaphragm; may include spleen |
| Stage IV | Noncontiguous extralymphatic involvement (including lung, bone marrow, liver) |
| Bulky disease | A single node mass measuring >10 cm or > 1/3 of the transthoracic diameter determined by CT |
| E | Extranodal contiguous extension that can be included in a radiation field. |
| A/B | B symptoms: weight loss >10%, fever, night sweats |

[a]For all stages: A, asymptomatic; B, constitutional or systemic symptoms.

Staging of disease determined by PET-CT or CT adapted from the Cotswold Modification of the Ann Arbor Staging Classification. Cheson BD, Fisher RI, Barrington SF, et al: Recommendations for initial evaluation, staging, and response assessment of Hodgkin and non-Hodgkin lymphoma: the Lugano classification, *J Clin Oncol* 32(27):3059-3068, 2014.

staging, classified as limited or early (stages I and II, non-bulky) or advanced (stages III and IV). Those with early disease are often then classified as favorable or unfavorable. Advanced disease is further stratified according to the presence of 11 risk factors (International Prognostic Score). Some factors denoting a worse prognosis include a low serum albumin, low hemoglobin, age older than 45 years, and male gender (despite stage). Other factors that carry a poorer prognosis include "B" symptoms, stage IV disease, too high or too low lymphocyte count, or high WBC count. These factors are often considered in subsequent treatment options.

Bone marrow biopsy or aspirate is typically not needed unless abnormal blood counts are seen and there is a suspicion for bone marrow involvement. Because systemic chemotherapy is utilized, extensive staging is no longer required, including exploratory laparotomy or splenectomy (which can be more dangerous than helpful).

**TREATMENT.** HL is a highly curable disease. People with classic HL are treated with chemotherapy, despite the stage at presentation (early disease benefits from chemotherapy). Clients with localized disease and favorable disease characteristics are usually treated with radiation to diseased tissue (involved field radiation only)[16,99] and two courses of chemotherapy consisting of ABVD (doxorubicin, bleomycin, vinblastine, and dacarbazine). If radiation is not desired due to long-term side effects, another option is to receive four to six cycles of chemotherapy. Chemotherapy alone is utilized for clients with more advanced disease. A PET scan is obtained after two to three courses of chemotherapy to determine response to treatment. Individuals with early disease and a good response by PET may be able to avoid radiation.

Standard treatment involves combination chemotherapy consisting of six cycles of ABVD with or without radiation.[260] Unlike NHL, HL subtypes are treated in a similar manner, with the exception of NLPHL. NLPHL is typically discovered in early stages; however, there is a higher risk for late relapse in distant locations from the original cancer. People with this type of HL can receive radiation alone for localized disease or, for more advanced disease, treatment may include rituximab alone or accompanied

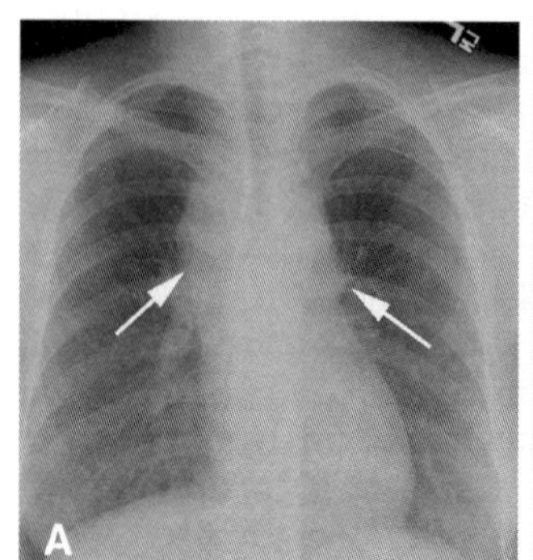

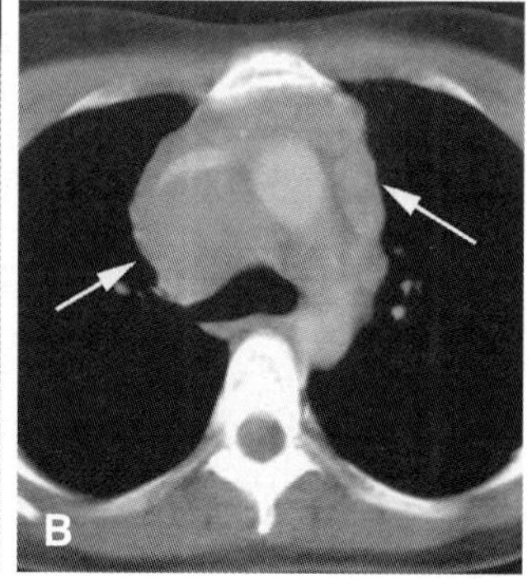

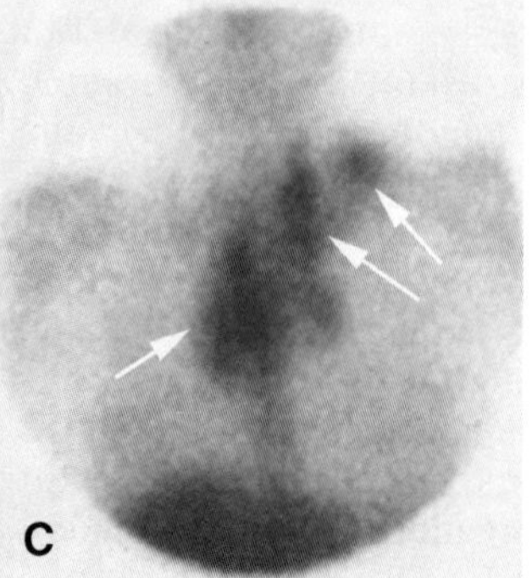

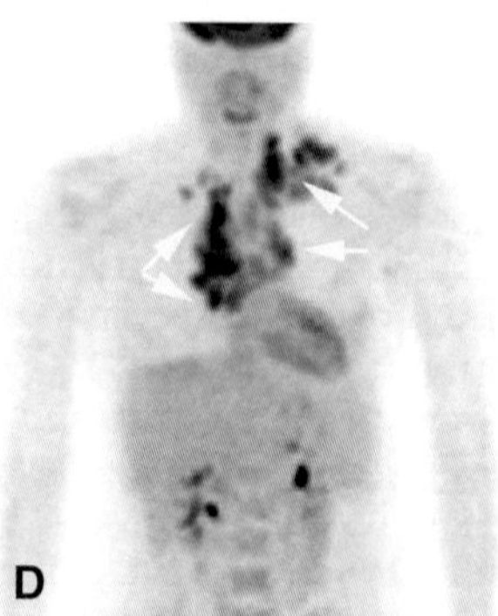


**Figure 14.9**

HL as seen on chest radiograph (A); CT scan of the chest (B); gallium scan of the head, neck, and chest (C); and positron emission tomography (PET) scan (D). The *arrows* indicate sites of diseases. Note that PET and CT scans provide more detailed information compared with chest radiograph and gallium scan. (Reprinted from Goldman L: *Cecil textbook of medicine*, ed 22, Philadelphia, 2004, WB Saunders.)

with chemotherapy. Clients with relapsed disease often respond well to repeat therapy.[153]

Salvage chemotherapy and autologous or allogeneic HCT is offered to people who do not respond to therapy or have relapsed disease. Autologous HCT is the procedure of choice because of the more-severe complications of allogeneic HCT. If an autologous HSCT fails, allogeneic HSCT remains an option. The monoclonal antibody brentuximab vedotin and the programmed death-1 antibodies (pembrolizumab, nivolumab) are also utilized in treating relapsed and refractory disease.

Survivors of HL are at high risk for developing a secondary malignancy, even as long as 40 years following treatment.[379] The incidence of developing thyroid cancer, soft tissue sarcoma, mesothelioma, and non-Hodgkin lymphoma is ten times higher compared to the general population. Leukemia, esophageal, stomach, pancreatic, and lung cancer was seen five to ten times more often.[379] Cardiac disease is the most common nonmalignant cause of death in HL survivors.[295] Clients who were treated with chemotherapy (particularly with doxorubicin) have a higher risk of heart failure,[453] and people that received radiation to the chest were more likely to have a fatal myocardial infarction (presumed to be caused by damage to the intimal lining of the coronary arteries).

The risk of stroke or transient ischemic attack also increases in survivors of HL (two to three times greater than the general population). This is most likely related to radiation to the neck and chest.[80]

The chemotherapy drug bleomycin can cause delayed (6 months following completion of treatment) lung injury in approximately 25% of people, which can be sustained. The most severe lung injury is pulmonary fibrosis, seen more commonly in the elderly who receive high doses. Neuropathies and muscular weakness are also seen due to treatment with the drugs vinblastine and brentuximab vedotin. The peripheral neuropathy often improves over time. Radiation has been known to cause severe atrophy and weakness of the head and upper chest muscles,[452] often referred to as "dropped-head syndrome" because of the difficulty of keeping the head upright. This may occur many years following treatment.

ABVD has not been shown to cause subfertility in men or women, as do the older alkylating agents previously used.[167] Because of the increased long-term complications, the use of radiation has been limited to only areas in field, and lower doses are being used, particularly in children. The combination therapy of ABVD appears to be a better long-term choice for treatment.[92] Treatment options have attempted to balance toxicities with high cure rates.[199,203]

**PROGNOSIS.** HL is considered one of the most curable forms of cancer, and death rates have decreased 60% since the early 1970s. Prognosis depends on the staging and presence of risk factors at presentation including: age older than 45 years, male sex, leukocyte count greater than 15,000/μL, serum albumin level less than 4 g/dL, and hemoglobin level less than 10.5 g/dL. For clients without risk factors and localized disease, the 5-year survival rate is over 90%.[98,300,301] Those diagnosed with stage IV disease have a 73% 5-year survival rate and the 5-year overall survival rate is 86.6%.[301]

The cause of death in the majority of cases prior to 15 years is recurrent disease. After 15 years, most die of other causes, including secondary neoplasms derived from HL therapy.

**SPECIAL IMPLICATIONS FOR THE THERAPIST 14.8**

### *Hodgkin Lymphoma*

The therapist may palpate enlarged, painless lymph nodes during a cervical, spine, shoulder, or hip examination. Lymph nodes are evaluated on the basis of size, consistency, mobility, and tenderness. Lymph nodes up to 2 cm in diameter, soft consistency, freely and easily moveable, tender to palpation, and transient are considered within normal limits but must be followed carefully.

Lymph nodes greater than 2 cm in diameter that are firm in consistency, nontender to palpation, fixed, and hard are considered suspicious and require evaluation. Enlarged lymph nodes associated with infection are more likely to be tender than slow-growing nodes associated with cancer.

*Changes* in size, shape, tenderness, and consistency should raise a red flag. The physician should be notified of these findings and the client advised to have the lymph nodes evaluated by the physician; in someone with a history of cancer, immediate medical referral is necessary.

The therapist's role in lymphoma includes, but is not limited to, assessing and/or addressing (1) quality-of-life issues, including emotional and spiritual needs; (2) impairments, functional limitations, and disabilities; and (3) physical conditioning and deconditioning.

Generalized weakness, decreased endurance, impaired mobility, altered kinesthetic awareness and balance, including unstable gait; respiratory impairment; involvement of the lymphatic system (lymphedema); and pain are only a few of the identified signs and symptoms of impairment common with this group of people.

Requirements for infection control and treatment subsequent to the cytotoxic effects on the CNS are outlined previously in the section on the leukemias. Additionally, side effects of radiation and/or chemotherapy must be considered.

Depending on the results of the therapist's examination and evaluation, intervention strategies may include client and family education, pain management, mobility and gait training, therapeutic exercise, balance training, aerobic conditioning, respiratory rehabilitation, and lymphedema management.

Monitoring vital signs is important, as is daily evaluation of laboratory values (e.g., hemoglobin, platelets, WBC, hematocrit

## Non-Hodgkin Lymphomas

**Overview and Incidence.** NHL comprises a large group (about 30 specific types described) of lymphoid malignancies that present as solid tumors arising from cells of the lymphatic system. More than 70,000 people develop NHL per year,[300] making it the most common hematologic malignancy and the seventh most common cancer in the United States. NHL is about nine times more common than HL.

Ninety-eight percent of NHL occurs in adults and less than 2% develops in children; yet the types of NHL seen in adults are different than those seen in children. The average age of onset in adults is about 67 years, with the majority developing NHL being older than 55 years of age.[300]

The lymph nodes are usually involved first, although extranodal lymphoid tissue, particularly the spleen, thymus, and GI tract, may also be involved. The bone marrow is commonly infiltrated by lymphoma cells, but this is rarely the primary site of a lymphoma.

The most commonly used classification system is the Revised European-American Lymphoma/WHO system, which relies on the histochemical, genetic, and cytologic features of the lymphoma. Approximately 85% of NHLs are B cell lymphomas, whereas only 15% are of T cell origin (uncommonly NK-cell). The clinical course for each of the NHLs, even subtypes, is variable.

The most common lymphoma is diffuse large B cell lymphoma (DLBCL), which comprises 30% of all NHLs. It is an aggressive, fast-growing tumor. The second most common is follicular lymphoma, constituting 30% of NHL cases. It is an indolent, slow growing tumor that responds to therapy but often relapses.

**Etiologic and Risk Factors.** Some studies have linked benzene (found in cigarette smoke, gasoline, and industrial pollution) and polychlorinated biphenyls to the development of NHL. More research is needed to solidify this causal association. People that have been previously exposed to chemotherapy and/or radiation, received organ transplantation, or been treated with immunosuppressive agents also have a higher risk of developing NHL.[64]

A wide variety of autoimmune diseases (RA and SLE) and immunodeficiency disorders are associated with an increased incidence of lymphomas. This phenomenon may reflect a decrease in the host's surveillance mechanism against transformed cells or be from prolonged exposure to oncogenic agents, such as EBV, as a consequence of failure to mount an adequate immune response.

In people with HIV, the risk of developing NHL is significantly elevated compared with noninfected people. Hepatitis C is also associated with certain subtypes of NHL, including lymphoplasmacytic lymphoma. The presence of *Helicobacter pylori* (bacteria) in the stomach lining is associated with the development of gastric mucosa-associated lymphoid tissue lymphomas (gastric MALT), but this comprises a very small proportion of cases.

**Pathogenesis.** NHL subtypes may develop at various stages of maturation, particularly during those processes that require gene rearrangements and alterations. Normally a B cell begins to develop in the bone marrow and once mature expresses IgM on its surface (antigen-naïve). The B cell then migrates to a secondary lymphoid site (lymph node or spleen) to complete maturation. On arrival at the lymph node, some B cells stay in the follicle mantle zone, while others are exposed to antigens and move to the germinal center. Here the cell begins two main processes: class-switch recombination and somatic hypermutation. A germinal center is composed of other cells, such as dendritic and T cells,[355] that aid in the proliferation and maturation of the B cells. These B cells, termed centroblasts, proliferate and mature into centrocytes. They then migrate to the light zone of the germinal center after undergoing somatic hypermutation of the immunoglobulin variable region. Somatic hypermutation, occurring during the centroblast phase, introduces point mutations and small insertions/deletions in order to increase the affinity of the produced antibody for its antigen. Somatic hypermutation may also produce antibodies that have less affinity for their own antigen, and only the antibodies with high affinity for an antigen are selected out in the light zone. It is also during this time that the B cells switch from expressing IgM to the more antigen-specific IgG or IgA. From this point B cells may become memory cells or terminally differentiated plasma cells.

For most subtypes of NHL, a progenitor cell has been identified along the development pathway where mutations have occurred, causing the disease.[154] B cells that undergo malignant changes in the mantle zone are thought to give rise to mantle cell lymphoma. Centroblasts are felt to be the progenitor cells for Burkitt and diffuse large B cell lymphomas. Follicular lymphoma may be derived from centrocytes, whereas marginal cell lymphoma arises from cells in the marginal zone.

T cell maturation is similar in that they begin maturation in the bone marrow and then migrate to the thymus. Here they remain antigen-naïve but continue to mature. During this process the DNA for the receptor expressed on the T cell surface is rearranged. Those with the alpha and beta receptors leave the thymus as CD4 or CD8 positive T cells; once they are presented with an antigen, they are stimulated into lymphoblasts, which mature into cytotoxic T cells, helper T cells, and memory cells. Natural killer cells (NK) mature in the bone marrow and are then released to migrate to the spleen, mucosal tissue, and blood. The T cells in the thymus are presumed to be the progenitor cells for lymphoblastic T cell NHL.

Although the exact causes of NHL are unknown, studies using techniques of molecular biology have provided clues to the pathogenesis. Malignant lymphomas can develop from the accumulation of genetic mutations affecting protooncogenes or tumor suppressor genes, leading to the clonal expansion of a neoplastic lymphocyte that is arrested at a specific stage of B- or T/NK-lymphoid cell differentiation. This occurs most often when the genes are undergoing rearrangement or insertions/deletions. Oncogenes can be activated by chromosomal translocations. The most common translocation is the t(14;18)(q32;q21) translocation, seen in 85% of follicular lymphomas.[350] The 8q24 translocation leads to dysregulation of the *c-Myc* gene and is noted in Burkitt and non-Burkitt small noncleaved lymphoma.[259] Tumor suppressor genes (TP53) can be inactivated by genetic deletions or mutations. DLBCL demonstrates multiple changes involving epigenetic remodeling (not involving DNA), interruption of cell differentiation, and changes in signaling pathways.[320] Eventually these malignant cells crowd out healthy cells, creating tumors and enlarging lymph nodes.

**Clinical Manifestations.** The NHLs are variable in clinical presentation and course, varying from indolent disease to rapidly progressive disease. The most common finding is lymphadenopathy (palpable or noted on CT or other scans). About 50% of people with NHL will develop extranodal disease. Other general but uncommon symptoms include fatigue, pruritus, hypersensitity reaction to insect bites, and effusions. Depending on the location and size of lymph node masses, some presenting symptoms may be oncologic medical emergencies, such as spinal cord compression, pericardial tamponade, superior vena cava compression, lymphomatous meningitis, intestinal obstruction, or thromboembolic disease.

Indolent lymphomas, such as follicular lymphoma, are often asymptomatic and even after diagnosis may not require therapy for several years. When symptoms are present they include painless, slow growing, peripheral lymphadenopathy (may be bulky, causing compression), hepatomegaly and splenomegaly. Occasionally there is spontaneous regression of disease, although relapse is the norm. Extranodal disease and "B" symptoms (fever, weight loss, and night sweats) are not usually seen at diagnosis, unless the disease is advanced. The bone marrow is frequently involved, resulting in cytopenias.[485] Follicular lymphoma may undergo a transformation to a more aggressive lymphoma with associated symptoms.

The aggressive lymphomas vary in presentation and progression, yet most display rapidly progressive lymphadenopathy. About 10% to 35% of people exhibit extranodal disease at diagnosis; the most common sites being the GI tract followed by the skin. Other extranodal sites include bone marrow, thyroid, CNS, genitourinary tracts, testis, bone, and kidney. "B" symptoms are common and noted in 30% to 40% of clients, particularly in people with liver or extranodal disease. Splenomegaly is seen in approximately 40% of people with NHL.

Lymphoblastic lymphoma, a high-grade lymphoma, can present with lymph node enlargement in the chest, leading to compression of the trachea or bronchus, causing shortness of breath and coughing. Development of the superior vena cava syndrome can occur secondary to compression of the superior vena cava by enlarged nodes; this causes edema of the upper extremities and face; superior vena cava syndrome is life-threatening and requires immediate attention. This type of lymphoma may also cause cranial nerve palsies as a result of leptomeningeal involvement.

Clients with Burkitt lymphoma may present with bowel obstruction caused by large abdominal masses or obstructive hydronephrosis from bulky lymph nodes obstructing the ureters.

Primary CNS lymphomas are restricted to the nervous system at diagnosis and are seen more frequently in clients with immunodeficiencies (HIV, genetic immunodeficiencies, posttransplantation).[111] Epstein-Barr virus is related to primary CNS lymphomas, with genomic DNA found in the malignant cells. Presenting symptoms may include headache, confusion, seizures, extremity weakness/numbness, personality changes, difficulty speaking, and lethargy. Prior to the spread of HIV, this type of lymphoma was rare.

*HIV and Non-Hodgkin Lymphoma.* NHL is more common in clients with HIV than is HL and is an AIDS-defining illness. Typically, lymphomas that occur in clients with HIV are aggressive, fast-growing tumors. The two major subtypes of lymphomas are CNS and systemic lymphomas (with or without CNS involvement).

Two rare lymphomas seen more frequently in people with HIV are primary effusion lymphoma and plasmablastic lymphoma of the oral cavity, but the most common types are DLBCL and Burkitt lymphoma. Tumor is frequently diffusely spread at the time of diagnosis, with extranodal involvement common.

As discussed above, many illnesses that are accompanied by a reduced immune system demonstrate an increased incidence of NHL. Prior to aggressive HIV therapy (i.e., ART), lymphomas in persons with HIV were associated with a very poor prognosis. Currently the use of ART has significantly reduced the risk of developing NHL and also improved tolerance for chemotherapy once diagnosed with NHL.[145] This reduction is based on higher CD4 counts and improving the immune system. It appears that if ART therapy is not effective, people with AIDS still have the same increased risk of developing NHL. The improved immune status derived from ART has increased treatment options for HIV-related lymphoma. Clients are now treated with the intent to cure, receiving chemotherapy, immune modulators, and HCT.

## MEDICAL MANAGEMENT

**STAGING/DIAGNOSIS.** Clinical staging of NHL is according to the Lugano classification system (based on the Ann Arbor staging system), ranging from stage I to stage IV. Unlike staging for HL, NHL does not utilize "B" symptom findings into staging. Compared with HL, NHLs are more likely to present in an extranodal site, and the progression of the NHL does not follow the orderly anatomic progression from one lymph node to the next but rather disseminates hematogenously. About 40% of NHLs present in stage I and II, while 50% are diagnosed in stage III and IV; about 10% are of an unknown stage at diagnosis.[301]

Accurate diagnosis is important because other clinical conditions can mimic malignant lymphomas (e.g., infection, tuberculosis, SLE, lung and bone cancer) and a biopsy is required to establish a definitive diagnosis. Molecular genetic techniques that take advantage of the clonal nature of this malignancy are now being applied to better characterize and diagnose lymphomas.

The type of imaging employed in staging is determined by the avidity of the tumor for fluorodeoxyglucose (FDG). Those tumors that are FDG-avid are best evaluated by PET-CT. Tumors that are not FDG-avid utilize CT alone. Imaging of the chest, abdomen, and pelvis are performed. Bone marrow is examined for staging and peripheral blood should be tested for hepatitis B and C serology and HIV. If clinical symptoms warrant, a lumbar puncture for spinal fluid may be performed. Immunohistochemistry, flow cytometry, or cytogenetic testing is done to distinguish one type of NHL from another.

PET-CT imaging is becoming more widespread and can be performed to aid in the initial diagnosis and help ascertain if a lymph node is malignant or benign. PET is also used following chemotherapy (frequently along with

CT) to determine if the lymphoma is reduced in size and the treatment is effective.[61]

The chemokine CXCL-13 was found to be elevated years prior to diagnosis of HIV-associated NHL. This may, in the future, serve as a biomarker for early detection.[184]

**TREATMENT.** Treatment varies for NHL depending on the stage, bulkiness of disease, phenotype (B or T/NK type), tumor grade (low, intermediate, high), age, and presence of comorbidities. NHL is often clinically separated into two general prognostic groups: indolent and aggressive.

In general, fast-growing tumors can be cured but require aggressive treatment. Slow-growing tumors often cannot be cured, particularly in advanced stages, but the clinical course is chronic and therapy is often reserved until symptoms develop, such as for follicular lymphoma. Localized disease (stage I or II) may be treated with radiation, whereas disseminated disease requires chemotherapy. The most common chemotherapy combination is CHOP (cyclophosphamide, doxorubicin, vincristine, and prednisone), but multiple regimens are used.

Because many risk factors for NHL are associated with a reduced immune system, immune modulators, such as monoclonal antibodies, have been employed to combat NHL. Combining the monoclonal antibody rituximab with an alkylating agent, such as bendamustine, has produced high rates of remission (up to 90%) in clients with follicular lymphoma. Rituximab is often used as a single agent following successful induction and frequently provides a durable remission. Rituximab is often given as part of CHOP therapy (R-CHOP) and is the treatment of choice for DLBCL.[74,200] Clinical studies suggest that the immune modulator rituximab may alter the sensitivity of B cell lymphoma to chemotherapy, as well as induce apoptosis and cause the lysis of B cells. Radiation may be used to treat bulky disease. Following treatment, residual masses often remain. Most are not cancerous, however PET scans are often able to distinguish active cancer from benign masses that represent scarring from therapy.

HCT may be used for individuals who relapse or do not completely respond to treatment (which often occurs with aggressive lymphomas or with refractory follicular lymphoma). Combined with intensive chemotherapy, HCT (autologous or allogeneic) can be curative.[100] Nonmyeloablative (i.e., the doses of chemotherapy are not high enough to ablate the bone marrow) transplants can be performed for older clients who normally cannot tolerate high-dose chemotherapy, but graft-versus-host complications are problematic.

Radioimmunotherapy, radioactive labeling of a monoclonal antibody, is also under investigation to provide targeted therapy and provide tumor-free grafts for transplant.[40,139]

The optimal management of women with NHL who are pregnant requires special considerations because of the poor prognosis without treatment. Treatment during the first trimester is associated with significant risk to the developing fetus and should be avoided. Treatment during the second or third trimester appears safe and should include standard chemotherapy, despite the potential risk to the developing fetus.[335]

**PROGNOSIS.** Good prognostic features include age younger than 60 years, limited disease at diagnosis (stage I or II), lack of extranodal disease, and a normal LDH level. Individuals with NHL survive for long periods when involvement is only regional. The presence of diffuse disease reduces survival time.

In general the 5-year survival rate of NHL is 70%,[300] with a 30% cure rate for aggressive lymphomas. The indolent lymphomas are usually systemic and widespread and cure cannot be achieved, whereas intermediate- and fast-growing lymphomas are more likely to present as treatable and even curable localized disorders but require aggressive therapy. The 5-year overall survival rate for aggressive lymphomas in low-risk clients is 73%, whereas the rate significantly decreases for high-risk clients to 26%.

Traditionally, high-grade NHL associated with AIDS was associated with an extremely poor prognosis. But with the advent of antiretroviral therapy for HIV and a multidisciplinary approach to complex AIDS cases involving malignancy, return to functional health has become possible for many individuals. Although survival rates have improved, clients with HIV still experience a higher mortality rate compared to those without HIV.[63,87,88,365]

Survivors of NHL are approximately 15% more likely to develop secondary malignancies as a result of treatment, particularly those who were diagnosed at younger ages. The risk continues for up to 30 years following completion of therapy. Survivors are also at higher risk for cardiovascular disease, infertility, endocrine dysfunction (such as hypothyroidism), and cognitive dysfunction (especially if treated for CNS involvement).

SPECIAL IMPLICATIONS FOR THE THERAPIST 14.9

### *Non-Hodgkin Lymphoma*

See "Special Implications for the Therapist 14.8: Hodgkin Lymphoma" above.

Although uncommon, the association between the use of methotrexate in RA and the development of lymphoma has been reported.[31,79] Any time an individual receiving methotrexate for RA complains of back pain accompanied by constitutional symptoms and/or GI symptoms and/or the therapist palpates enlarged lymph nodes at any of the nodal sites, a medical referral is warranted.

## Multiple Myeloma

**Definition and Overview.** Multiple myeloma (MM) is a primary malignant neoplasm of plasma cells arising in the bone marrow. This tumor initially affects the bones and bone marrow of the vertebrae, ribs, skull, pelvis, and femur. Progression of the disease causes damage to the kidney, leads to recurrent infections, and damages bone and nerves. The extent, clinical course, complications, and sensitivity to treatment vary widely among affected people, depending upon specific genetic alterations.

Several disorders and malignancies develop from the proliferation of monoclonal plasma cells and should be distinguished from MM, such as monoclonal gammopathy of undetermined significance (MGUS) (which frequently leads to MM), AL amyloidosis (a disease involving the precipitation of proteins that results in end-organ damage), and Waldenström macroglobulinemia (a lymphoplasmacytic malignancy). MGUS arises prior to the development of MM, although not all people with MGUS will go on to convert to MM. A certain subset of people demonstrates an intermediate clinical picture between MGUS and MM called "smoldering multiple myeloma." These individuals have a higher cellular burden but do not have end-organ damage.

MM cells secrete monoclonal proteins (called M-proteins). They may be intact immunoglobulins with a heavy chain (IgA, IgG, IgD) and light chain (κ or λ), or free light chains (16% of cases), or, uncommonly, may not secrete proteins.

**Incidence and Etiologic Factors.** Approximately 32,000 new cases of MM are diagnosed each year and the number continues to rise. The incidence, based on data between 2012 and 2016, is 6.9 cases per 100,000 men and women. MM occurs less often than the most common cancers (e.g., breast, lung, or colon), accounting for 1% of cancers, but is the second most common cause of hematologic cancers (10%).[313] This disease can develop at any age, but is most commonly seen in older people. The median age of diagnosis is 69 years of age; only 4% of people diagnosed with MM are younger than 44 years, whereas almost 10% are older than age 85.[181]

Black men are affected twice as often as white men, and MM is slightly more common in men than in women.[181] Risk factors and causes of MM are not clearly identifiable, but exposure to ionizing radiation may be linked. Certain occupational hazards found in the petroleum, leather, lumber, and agricultural industries may also increase the risk for developing MM. Each year, approximately 1% of people with MGUS go on to develop MM; those with smoldering multiple myeloma are at higher risk for developing MM and have a 10% progression rate per year.[216,218]

**Pathogenesis.** MM is caused by multiple genetic abnormalities and microenvironmental changes that lead to the transformation of plasma cells to cancerous cells.

The normal maturation process of plasma cells is tightly controlled and begins with the differentiation of a hematopoietic stem cell in the bone marrow that becomes committed to the B-cell lineage through transcription factors. Upon leaving the bone marrow, they migrate to the spleen or lymph nodes. Transcription factors, T cells, and dendritic cells aid in the maturation of the B cell. It is here that the B cell may be exposed to an antigen and move to the germinal center. Two principal processes then occur: class-switch recombination and somatic hypermutation. Class-switch recombination is the rearrangement of the immunoglobulin heavy chain (IgH) genes of pro-B cells to form IgG or IgA antibodies. Somatic hypermutation is the process of genetic alterations consisting of insertions/deletions and point mutations in order to significantly increase the affinity of the antibody for the antigen. B cells then migrate to the light zone of the germinal center and may become memory cells (ready to fight a future infection) or plasma cells (ready to fight a current infection). Somatic hypermutation also produces antibodies with poor affinity for antigen, and only the B cells with high affinity for antigen are selected in the light zone of the germinal center. Plasma cells are the mature B cells that have undergone terminal differentiation.

MM develops from a premalignant plasma cell dyscrasia called monoclonal gammopathy of undetermined significance (MGUS).[221] These cells are thought to have mutations (most likely during antigenic stimulation) that allow for clonal proliferation and production of a monoclonal immunoglobulin but do not cause end-organ tissue damage. About 3% of the population over the age of 50 has MGUS, but only 1% per year goes on to develop MM. Research is still being done in order to understand the progression from MGUS to MM, but it is believed that the MGUS cells either sustain further genetic abnormalities and/or the microenvironment of the bone marrow contributes to this conversion.[104]

Plasma cells normally express a transcription repressor (among other factors) termed BLIMP1, which results in the inability to divide or form germinal centers while inducing immunoglobulin secretion.[395] Whereas plasma cells undergo apoptosis (controlled cell death) in the spleen after a few weeks, plasma cells in the bone marrow may continue to secrete antibodies for up to a year.

It has been proposed that MM develops when abnormal B cells return to the bone marrow and, under the influence of surrounding cells in the microenvironment, lose this repression and begin to proliferate. Early, initial genetic changes in the IgH chain or the formation of trisomies can lead to both MGUS and MM. Furthermore, secondary chromosomal abnormalities are seen in MM, but rarely in MGUS (such as MYC [8q24], MAFB [20q12], and IRF [6p25]), whereas additional mutations are specific to MM but not MGUS, including MYC dysregulation and deletion in 17p13 with p53 mutations.[360]

Genetic changes determine the characteristics of the disease, which result in a heterogeneity of tumor growth, progression of disease, and resistance to therapy.[313] Myeloma cells, caused by genetic mutations, alter the expression of adhesion molecules that change the interaction between the malignant myeloma cells and the surrounding stromal cells and extracellular matrix proteins. When myeloma cells adhere to hematopoietic and stromal cells, there is a resultant release of cytokines and growth factors (principally IL-6, vascular endothelial growth factor, IL-10, insulin-like growth factor 1, members of the tumor necrosis factor family, and transforming growth factor β1). Response to growth stimuli is also altered, leading to the production of apoptotic proteins; other abnormalities include the induction of blood vessel formation (angiogenesis).[313] It is also these adhesion molecules that attract malignant plasma cells together, forming plasmacytomas or masses of plasma cells.

An imbalance in the function of bone cells, osteoclasts (break down bone), and osteoblasts (bone building), results in the characteristic lytic bone lesions. One pathway, the Wnt pathway, is inhibited, thereby suppressing osteoblasts. Stromal cells are induced to increase production of the RANK (receptor activator of nuclear factor-kappa B) ligand that binds to osteoclasts, thereby stimulating bone destruction. RANK ligand also leads to the inhibition of osteoclastic apoptosis (programmed cell death).[239]

**Clinical Manifestations.** MM is categorized as either asymptomatic (smoldering) or symptomatic, depending on the presence of signs and/or symptoms of organ or tissue dysfunction. The onset of MM is usually gradual and insidious. Common presenting features include fatigue, bone pain, neurologic symptoms, renal insufficiency, hypercalcemia, and recurrent infections. Fatigue is a frequent problem that is caused by anemia and elevated levels of cytokines. Anemia, caused by bone marrow infiltration and/or renal insufficiency, is present in 73% of people presenting with MM. Bony lesions were noted in 80% of newly diagnosed MM clients, whereas 58% reported bone pain.[313] Renal insufficiency is seen in approximately 20% to 40% of clients at presentation. Hypercalcemia is present in 13%,[217] whereas elevated creatinine levels are noted in 48% of newly diagnosed individuals.

The risk for infections is increased prior to treatment and with refractory disease, particularly with gram-negative organisms (60% of infections).[303] However, this risk decreases with response to therapy. Sinopulmonary infections are the most common. MM in older adults (older than 75 years) is the same as that reported in younger people except for a higher rate of infection in the older population.[364] These malignant plasma cells can also form large masses known as plasmacytomas, which can grow in bones and soft tissues.

***Musculoskeletal.*** Most people with MM develop bone pain and other bone-related problems as bone marrow expands and bone is destroyed. Bone pain is seen particularly in the ribs, pelvis, spine, clavicles, skull, and humeri. Bone loss, the major clinical manifestation of MM, often leads to pathologic fractures, spinal cord compression, and bone pain.

Initially, the bone pain may be mild and intermittent, or may occur acutely as severe pain in the back, rib, leg, or arm, often the result of an abrupt movement or minor effort that results in a spontaneous (pathologic) bone fracture. The pain is often radicular and sharp to one or both sides and is aggravated by movement. Symptoms associated with bone pain usually subside within days to weeks after initiation of systemic chemotherapy, but if the disease progresses there is associated progression of bone destruction. Bone destruction can lead to hypercalcemia, seen in 30% to 40% of people with MM, which can be life-threatening. Symptoms of hypercalcemia may include confusion, increased urination, loss of appetite, abdominal pain, constipation, and vomiting.

Muscular weakness and wasting affect nearly half of all individuals with cancer and contribute to the cause of cancer-related fatigue. Muscle wasting occurs as a result of disuse, pathology, anemia, nutritional imbalances, or decreased rates of muscle protein synthesis.

***Neurologic.*** Neurologic complications of MM stem from bone loss or tumor invasion or are protein related. As bone is destroyed in the vertebrae, collapse of the bone with subsequent compression of the nerves can occur. Clients may complain of back pain, numbness, tingling, or loss of strength.

Large plasmacytomas (particularly in the spinal canal or skull) can compress nerves, leading to spinal cord or cranial nerve compressions. Spinal cord compression is usually observed early or in the late relapse phase of the disease. Presenting symptoms include back pain with radiating numbness/tingling, muscle weakness or paralysis of the lower extremities, and loss of bowel or bladder control. Spinal cord compression is a medical emergency requiring immediate attention.

High concentrations of protein are also neuropathic. Amyloidosis (deposits of insoluble fragments of a protein) develops in approximately 10% of people with MM. These deposits cause tissues to become waxy and immobile and may affect nerves, muscles, and ligaments, especially the carpal tunnel area of the wrist. Carpal tunnel syndrome with pain, numbness, or tingling of the hands and fingers may develop.

***Renal.*** Renal impairment is a common complication of MM.[185] The pathogenesis is multifactorial, including toxic effect of the excess proteins on the renal tubules, dehydration, nephrotoxic drugs, and hypercalcemia. The large amount of monoclonal light chains secreted by the malignant plasma cells can form large casts in the tubules of the kidneys, causing dilation and atrophy, which leads to the inability of the nephron to function and interstitial nephritis.

Hypercalcemia occurs from increased bone destruction and absorption of calcium into the blood. In an effort to rid the body of the excess calcium, the kidneys increase the output of urine, which can lead to serious dehydration and result in further kidney damage if intake of fluids is inadequate.

Calcium can also be deposited in the kidney, creating another source of interstitial nephritis. Hypercalcemia is a common presenting feature but is less common after adequate chemotherapy. Recurrent urinary tract infections are also common and detrimental to the kidneys.

Many medications are nephrotoxic, including some antibiotics, radiographic dyes, and chemotherapy agents. NSAIDs can reduce blood flow to the kidneys, causing further damage. Because of the many factors that can cause injury to the kidneys, nephrotoxic medications should be avoided or used with caution in clients with MM because renal dysfunction and renal failure can occur.

## MEDICAL MANAGEMENT

**DIAGNOSIS.** The diagnosis of MM is determined by clinical and laboratory factors as well as bone marrow examination. Because other diseases also present with an elevated monoclonal gammopathy (i.e., MGUS and AL amyloidosis), criteria have been developed by the revised International Myeloma Working Group to aid in the diagnosis and distinction of these plasma cell dyscrasias so as to provide appropriate treatment (Table 14.3).[351,354] The principal difference is the involvement of tissue and organs in persons with MM, which may include hypercalcemia, renal failure, anemia, and osteolytic bone lesions (CRAB features). The new guidelines utilize biomarkers and more modern imaging techniques as part of diagnosis and staging.

Clients with a serum M-protein less than 3 g/dL, a clonal plasmacytosis in the bone marrow of less than 10%, and no evidence of organ or tissue involvement are categorized as having MGUS. Those with serum M-protein levels greater than 3 g/dL or urinary monoclonal

**Table 14.3** International Myeloma Working Group Diagnostic Criteria

| Diagnosis | M Protein (g/dL) | Bone Marrow Plasma Cell Percentage by Biopsy | Tissue or Organ Dysfunction Caused by MM–CRAB features (increased calcium level, renal insufficiency, anemia [Hgb<10 g/dL], and bone lesions) | Presence of a Biomarker |
|---|---|---|---|---|
| MGUS | <3 g/dL | <10% | No | Absent |
| Asymptomatic, smoldering MM | ≥3 g/dL | ≥10% | No | 10–60% bone marrow plasma cells<br>No end-organ damage |
| Symptomatic MM | present | ≥10% | Yes | >60% clonal plasma cells in the bone marrow; involved/uninvolved FLC ratio of 100 or more; MRI showing more than one focal lesion (bone or bone marrow) |

*MGUS*, Monoclonal gammopathy of undetermined significance; *MM*, multiple myeloma; *FLC*, free light chain.
Rajkumar SV, Dimopoulos MA, Palumbo A, Blade J, et al: International Myeloma Working Group updated criteria for the diagnosis of multiple myeloma, *Lancet Oncol* 15(12):e538, 2014.

protein of 500 mg/24 hr or more, a clonal plasmacytosis greater than 10% in the bone marrow, and no evidence of organ or tissue involvement are considered as having smoldering MM. MM is diagnosed if M-protein is present, the bone marrow exhibits a monoclonal gammopathy of greater than 10% or documented extramedullary plasmacytoma, and there is evidence of organ or tissue involvement referred to as a myeloma defining event (CRAB features). Osteolytic lesions may be documented by skeletal radiography, CT or PET-CT. Other myeloma defining events include biomarkers of malignancy, such as bone marrow clonal plasma cells of 60% or greater, serum free light chain (FLC) ratio of 100 or higher, or more than one focal lesion on MRI that is larger than 5 mm. Approximately 40% of people with MM display less than 3 g/dL of M-protein and 5% have less than 10% bone marrow plasmacytosis. In a small percentage of cases the MM cells do not express M-protein.

Persons diagnosed with smoldering MM are placed in risk categories for progression to MM, depending on the presence or absence of biomarkers. Myelomas that display del(17p), t(14;16), and t(14;20) are considered high risk for progressing to MM. The translocation t(4;14) and gain(1,q) are both considered intermediate risk. Other genetic abnormalities are thought to confer normal risk.[352]

The revised International Staging System was developed for MM[314] to establish prognosis. It defines three risk groups based on the serum $\beta_2$-microglobulin albumin levels: Stage 1 includes serum $\beta_2$-microglobulin of less than 3.5 mg/L and serum albumin greater than or equal to 3.5 g/dL while LDH is normal and cells without high risk cytogenetics; Stage 2 demonstrates values between stages 1 and 2; Stage 3 has a serum $\beta_2$-microglobulin greater than 5.5 mg/L. The mSMART risk stratification adds more criteria for staging that can be more helpful in guiding therapy.[264]

Tests performed to determine if criteria are met for the diagnosis of MM include a bone marrow biopsy and aspiration, measurement of M-protein in the blood (serum protein electrophoresis), serum immunofixation, serum free light chain (FLC) assay, and biopsy of any suspect mass. Cells from the bone marrow should be evaluated by FISH probes to detect genetic abnormalities such as t(14;16) and del(17p) to aid in risk stratification.[213]

A radiographic skeletal survey, CT or PET-CT can help to determine bone involvement. MRI is recommended if plain radiographs suggest a plasmacytoma[90]; if spinal cord compression is suspected, an emergent MRI or CT should be performed. PET scans are being used more frequently, particularly to determine the extent of the disease at the time of diagnosis, and contributing to more accurate staging.[32]

**TREATMENT.** MM is not curable but most people with MM are able to live almost 10 years after diagnosis. Treatments that have become available over the past few years have significantly improved survival.[352] Unlike other diseases, individuals with MM that are deemed eligible initially undergo autologous hematopoietic cell transplantation (HCT) after receiving induction chemotherapy with multiple agents. These agents consist of immunomodulatory drugs (lenalidomide or thalidomide), glucocorticoids, an alkylating agent (melphalan or cyclophosphamide), and a proteasome inhibitor (bortezomib). Although autologous HCT is not curative of MM, it does provide improvement in survival.

Eventually clients will relapse. There are several new drugs for the treatment of refractory or relapsed disease: proteasome inhibitors (carfilzomib and ixazomib), histone deacetylase inhibitors (panobinostat), immunomodulatory drugs (pomalidomide), and monoclonal antibodies (daratumumab and elotuzumab).

Use of these medications requires monitoring for their unique side effects. Bortezomib and thalidomide can cause peripheral nephropathy, while lenalidomide and pomalidomide increase the risk for thromboembolic events (VTE), and prophylaxis should be considered. Bortezomib may also lead to thrombocytopenia and herpes zoster reactivation and the prophylactic use of acyclovir is recommended. Thalidomide and lenalidomide are known teratogenic agents.

Conventional therapy combined with thalidomide, lenalidomide, or bortezomib can be offered to older people who cannot tolerate stem-cell transplantation.[313] Biologic age, however, should be the main consideration over chronologic age when a therapy and drug dose are selected. Consolidation and maintenance therapy is given following stem-cell transplantation.

Treatment of people with high-risk smoldering MM may improve the survival;[247] however, specific criteria are being evaluated, and currently this is not standard of care. Treatment typically is not instituted until criteria are met for MM with associated evidence of tissue/organ dysfunction.[217] Clients should be carefully followed in order to receive treatment once disease does progress from smoldering MM to MM.

Advances have also been made in correcting symptoms caused by the myeloma and surrounding cells. Bone pain is one of the most significant problems faced by clients with MM. Pathologic fractures are treated with surgery and pain control. Kyphoplasty can improve pain from vertebral-body compression fractures. Lytic lesions often require radiation for pain relief, along with opioids. Radiation may be all that is needed to decrease pain and stabilize the cervical spine when metastases occur. In some cases radiation has been shown to stop and even reverse bone destruction.[122]

The bisphosphonates pamidronate and zoledronic acid reduce vertebral fractures, skeletal related events, and pain.[261] Clients should be monitored for hypocalcemia and jaw osteonecrosis.

Hypercalcemia is treated with hydration, corticosteroids, and bisphosphonates. Anemia improves with myeloma treatment, but the use of erythropoietin can speed up recovery of erythrocyte production following chemotherapy.

Oncologists are looking toward individualizing treatment, depending on the types of mutations present in the myeloma cells that are indicative of high or low risk progression or aggressive disease. Treatments attempt to disrupt the abnormal signaling pathways that support the uncontrolled growth and migration of malignant plasma cells. They also endeavor to stimulate apoptotic pathways and disrupt abnormal cell adhesion and angiogenesis.

**PROGNOSIS.** Current medications for MM have extended overall survival but it remains an incurable disease. The median overall survival for people with standard risk MM is greater than 7 years, while those with high-risk biomarkers have a median overall survival of 3 years.[353] The 5-year survival rate is approximately 67% in cases that were diagnosed with local disease. For those with distant disease, the 5-year survival is reduced to 40% with an overall 5-year survival rate of 52.2%.[181]

The risk of smoldering MM progressing to MM or a related disorder during the first 5 years after diagnosis is 10% per year. Over the next 5 years the risk is 3% per year, whereas over the next 10 years the risk decreases to 1% to 2% per year.[216]

A poorer prognosis is seen in persons with any chromosomal abnormality. Specific translocations in the IgH chain (such as t(4;14), deletion 17p13, and chromosome 1 abnormalities) are also associated with a poor prognosis. Much research has been done and continues in order to profile each client's genetic mutations to determine prognosis and best treatment.[313]

If untreated, unstable MM can result in skeletal deformities, particularly of the ribs, sternum, and spine. Diffuse osteoporosis develops, accompanied by a negative calcium balance. Prognosis is affected by the presence of renal failure (poorer prognosis if present at the time of diagnosis), hypercalcemia, or extensive bony disease; infection and renal failure are the most common causes of death.

SPECIAL IMPLICATIONS FOR THE THERAPIST 14.10

## *Multiple Myeloma*

MM can have severe and devastating effects on the musculoskeletal system. Fatigue and skeletal muscle wasting can result in a weak and debilitated individual who is at risk for falls and subsequent musculoskeletal injuries. Bone pathology with fracture can also be very painful and disabling, affecting function and quality of life. The therapist may be instrumental in early detection and referral to minimize detrimental secondary effects.[194]

### Multiple Myeloma and Exercise

Therapists can assist individuals with MM to manage both the disease and treatment-related symptoms, improve overall quality of life, and prevent further complications associated with decreased activity and exercise.

The therapist may play an important role in various stages of the progression of this disease, including prevention and management of skeletal muscle wasting, cancer-related fatigue, and pathologic fractures.[194] Individualized exercise programs for individuals receiving aggressive treatment for MM may be effective for decreasing fatigue and mood disturbance and for improving sleep.[69]

Symptoms such as fatigue can be so overwhelming at times that some people have even said that they would rather just die than continue suffering the extremes of fatigue and malaise.[73] The National Comprehensive Cancer Network continues to recommend exercise in their updated clinical practice guidelines for the management of cancer-related fatigue.[285,286]

The guidelines suggest referral to physical therapy for fitness assessment and exercise recommendations, with emphasis on getting clients to gradually increase their activity level to avoid sustaining an injury or becoming discouraged. Short, low-intensity exercise programs may be helpful at first. The key is to get the individual to implement and maintain the program.

Individuals with MM have a number of intrinsic and extrinsic factors that can challenge their ability to engage in an exercise program. Intrinsic factors include a belief that exercise will help, a commitment to one's health, creation of personal goals, and a plan to reach them. Extrinsic factors include a good support system and adequate medical care (e.g., prophylactic epoetin alfa used to treat anemia).[71]

The therapist's ability to implement falls assessment and prevention programs can be a life-saving intervention for the individual at risk for pathologic fractures. Exercise interventions to improve function and decrease muscle wasting and cancer-related fatigue during and after cancer treatment for MM have been shown effective. Suggested exercise protocols for MM are available.[429]

### Complications

Specific examination and evaluation can provide early recognition of complications such as hypercalcemia and spinal cord compression. Any symptoms of hypercalcemia must be reported to the physician; the client should seek immediate medical care, as this condition can be life-threatening. Adequate hydration and mobility help minimize the development of hypercalcemia.

The client with MM who develops signs of cord compression must be referred to the physician. Emergency MRI is required to locate the area of cord compression. A laminectomy may be required when spinal cord compression occurs, but immediate radiation and high-dose glucocorticoid therapy usually relieve the compression, avoiding the need for surgical intervention.

Spinal instability may be a problem. Orthopedic back braces may help with pain management and reduce the risk of further trauma but are often poorly tolerated; newer lightweight supports with hook-and-loop fasteners may be more useful. Vertebroplasty and kyphoplasty procedures may help improve spinal stability; cement injected into the collapsed vertebrae reinforces the bone. In the case of kyphoplasty, vertebral height is restored.[117]

### Weight Bearing

There is little clinical evidence to guide the therapist in choosing a safe amount of weight bearing through cancer-lysed metastatic bone during exercise, transfers, ambulation, or other activities of daily living skills.[72] Some general guidelines based on radiographic findings have been suggested for individuals with bone metastases[124]:

| | |
|---|---|
| >50% (cortical metastatic involvement) | Non–weight bearing with crutches or walking; touch down permitted |
| 25%-50% | Partial weight bearing; avoid twisting or stretching |
| 0%-25% | Full weight bearing; avoid lifting or straining |

These recommendations must be used with caution, taking into consideration the client's age, general health, overall level of fitness, and level of pain. Through careful assessment, the therapist guides the client in maintaining mobility as much as possible while preventing fracture. Continual monitoring of symptoms to detect developing or new fracture is imperative. The affected individual must be taught what to look for and when to seek medical attention if signs and symptoms of new fracture appear.

### Supportive and Palliative Care

In preterminal and terminal stages, attention to supportive therapy and palliation are integral and can have a great impact on the individual and family's quality of life. The role of the therapist increases in late stages when immobility and renal failure complicate the clinical picture.[344]

## Myeloproliferative Neoplasms (Myeloproliferative Disorders)

Myeloproliferative neoplasms are a group of diseases of the bone marrow in which excess cells are produced. There is a transformation of hematopoietic stem cells that allows the cells to mature and function, yet there is uncontrolled production. Myeloproliferative neoplasms also share other characteristics, including a hypercellular bone marrow, tendency toward thrombosis and hemorrhage, and an increased risk of evolving into acute leukemia over time.[42] Myeloproliferative neoplasms are related to (and may transform into) myelodysplastic syndrome, a common blood cancer of the elderly that can progress to AML.

The four classic myeloproliferative neoplasms include CML, polycythemia vera (PV), essential thrombocythemia, and primary myelofibrosis. Even though all of these disorders can exhibit elevations in all cell lines, each disease has a particular cell line that is affected. As a result of specific molecular abnormalities being discovered in association with these disorders, the WHO revised the diagnostic criteria for these conditions and the term chronic myeloproliferative disorders was changed to myeloproliferative neoplasms.[441]

Polycythemia vera is an uncontrolled production of erythrocytes. Essential thrombocythemia is characterized by an elevated platelet count. Excessive fibrosis of the marrow is a dominant feature of primary myelofibrosis. Myelofibrosis and other more rare diseases are not covered in this text. CML is discussed with the leukemias.

### Polycythemia Vera

**Definition, Overview, and Etiologic Factors.** PV is a myeloproliferative neoplasm of bone marrow stem cells affecting the production of erythrocytes. The term *polycythemia* means an elevated RBC mass that may be primary or secondary.

Secondary polycythemia is typically acquired as a result of decreased oxygen availability to the tissues; the body attempts to compensate for the reduced oxygen by producing more erythrocytes (e.g., smoking, high altitudes, sleep apnea, and chronic heart and lung disorders). However, PV is a primary cause of polycythemia and results from a genetic abnormality that allows for the uncontrolled production of erythrocytes from a neoplastic hematopoietic stem cell.

The prevalence of PV is approximately 22 cases per 100,000.[235] It typically occurs in older people between the ages of 50 and 75 years, with approximately 5% to 10% diagnosed younger than the age of 40. The etiologic factors of PV are attributed to benzene and other occupational exposures, including radiation, although the majority of people diagnosed with PV do not have a history of these exposures.

**Pathogenesis.** PV results from mutations occurring in a hematopoietic stem cell, resulting in a proliferation of clonal cells. Not only does this cell produce RBCs, but often develops into leukocytes and platelets. Nearly all people with PV (more than 95%) have a mutation in the Janus kinase 2 *(JAK2)* gene, where valine is replaced for phenylalanine at position 617 (JAK2 V617F). Normally, once induced by erythropoietin, the *JAK2* gene produces a kinase that is responsible for intracellular communication and ultimately leads to cell production.

This gene normally exerts a negative effect in that it controls signals and the production of cells. But with this mutation, cellular production occurs despite the lack of binding erythropoietin and cytokines (cells become cytokine independent), leading to many of the problems seen in myeloproliferative neoplasms, including PV.

Other genetic abnormalities are also described, and several genetic modifications are most likely required for cellular transformation, with the *JAK2* mutation seen as a later, secondary mutation.[10] There is also an increased risk of PV evolving into AML over time. Although the mechanisms are not understood, people without the *JAK2* mutation can develop AML, demonstrating that other mutations may be the initial source of PV.

**Clinical Manifestations.** The symptoms of PV are often insidious in onset and characterized by vague complaints such as general malaise and fatigue, headache, and gastrointestinal disturbances. Although most cases are detected due to abnormal laboratory values, diagnosis may not be made until a secondary complication, such as stroke or thrombosis, occurs.

Symptoms are related to hyperviscosity, hypervolemia, and hypermetabolism. The increased concentration of erythrocytes frequently causes hypertension or neurologic symptoms, such as headache, blurred vision, feeling of fullness in the head, acral paresthesias and erythromelalgia (burning sensation in the hands and feet), dizziness, ringing in the ears, or vertigo. Bone pain may develop from increased production of cells. Abnormal interactions among erythrocytes, leukocytes, platelets, and the endothelium lead to thrombosis (e.g., cerebrovascular event, myocardial infarction, pulmonary embolus). Unusual thrombotic events, such as splenic infarctions and Budd-Chiari syndrome,[405] (thrombosis of the hepatic vein) should suggest the diagnosis of PV. Bleeding is seen in cases of platelet counts over 1 million (acquired von Willebrand syndrome) or with bone marrow that is fibrotic. On physical exam splenomegaly is common. Dyspnea may develop secondary to hypervolemia.

Gout and uric acid stones may develop because of hypermetabolism or increased turnover of RBCs. Intolerable pruritus (itching), especially after bathing in warm water, may be prominent and is characteristic of PV.

End-stage disease may manifest as progressive hepatosplenomegaly and associated cytopenias. As the bone marrow fills with fibroblasts, hematopoiesis is transferred to the liver and spleen. Clients may require transfusions.

## MEDICAL MANAGEMENT

**DIAGNOSIS.** PV is frequently asymptomatic and is often detected from a laboratory value obtained for another reason. Diagnosis is established by history, examination, and laboratory analysis and should be distinguished from secondary causes of polycythemia. In 2016 the WHO redefined criteria for the diagnosis of PV.[432] Previously, the arbitrary hemoglobin value of 18.5 for men and 16.5 for women was utilized; however a subgroup of people demonstrated the *JAK2* mutation and bone marrow changes consistent with PV, but did not meet defined hemoglobin levels. These people were more likely to have thrombosis than those individuals who met all diagnostic criteria, most likely due to lack of treatment.[266] New major diagnostic criteria include: an elevated hemoglobin of 16.5 for men and 16 for women; bone marrow biopsy demonstrating hypercellularity of all three lineages; and the presence of *JAK2* mutation.[23] WBC and platelet counts are often elevated in people with PV and are normal in most people with secondary polycythemia.

The presence of the *JAK2* mutation can be identified by FISH and other sensitive tests of molecular markers. A positive *JAK2* mutation (seen in 95% of people with PV), low erythropoietin level, and appropriate clinical factors may be enough information to make the diagnosis.

**TREATMENT.** Treatment goals are to reduce erythrocytosis and blood volume, control symptoms, and prevent thrombosis. Repeated phlebotomy is the most common treatment that is used to maintain a stable hemoglobin of less than 45%, causing iron deficiency and reducing the ability of the bone marrow to overproduce RBCs.[244]

Low-dose aspirin, if no contraindications exist, has been found to be beneficial to all people with PV in reducing the risk of thrombotic events.

For clients who do not respond to aspirin and phlebotomy, alternative medications include the antimetabolite hydroxyurea (particularly helpful for people at high risk for thrombosis, comprising people who have had a previous thrombotic event and/or are over the age of 60 years), and ruxolitinib, a *JAK1/2* inhibitor.[35]

**PROGNOSIS.** The life expectancy for people with PV is somewhat reduced, particularly for those with leukocytosis, thrombosis, or age over 60 years. The median survival is 14 years (people under the age of 60 have a median survival of 24 years);[440] however, those individuals who experience a transformation to MF or AML have severely reduced survival rates and poor outcomes. Approximately 5% to 6% of people will transform to MF after 10 years, and 2% to 14% transform to AML after 10 years.[53] The risk for stroke, myocardial infarction, and thromboembolism is high for people with this condition (27%-31%); thrombosis or hemorrhage is the major cause of death. Mortality rate increases with age starting at age 50 years.[421] Late in the course of this disease, bone marrow may be replaced with fibrous tissue (myelofibrosis) or be transformed into AML (10%-15%),[53] which are the most serious complications of PV and account for many dea ths.[214,236]

**SPECIAL IMPLICATIONS FOR THE THERAPIST 14.11**

### *Polycythemia Vera*

Thrombosis occurs more often in clients with PV, which requires the therapist to be alert to any possible signs of Budd-Chiari syndrome (abdominal pain, ascites, and liver function abnormalities) and deep vein thrombosis or stroke (e.g., weakness, numbness, inability to speak, visual changes, headache). Older age (greater than 60 years) and a previous history of thrombosis are standard risk factors for thrombosis. Risk may increase for those who are hypertensive, smoke or use other tobacco products, or have diabetes or hyperlipidemia.

GI bleeding, bruising, and epistaxis are also common. Watch for other complications, such as dyspnea and splenomegaly. If the person has symptomatic splenomegaly, follow precautions for soft tissue techniques required in the left upper quadrant, especially up and under the rib cage. These procedures must be secondary or indirect techniques away from the spleen.

### Essential Thrombocythemia

**Overview and Etiology.** Essential thrombocythemia (ET) is categorized as one of the myeloproliferative neoplasms. It is defined as a sustained and elevated platelet count greater than 450,000/µL without secondary causes.

ET is a primary thrombocytosis disorder resulting from a transformation of a hematopoietic stem cell and occurs most frequently in middle-aged to older adults (average age of onset is between 50 and 60 years). The incidence has significantly increased over the last decade due to the use of *JAK2* gene testing and the ability to diagnose the disease earlier.[129] Approximately 6000 cases are diagnosed in the United States each year.

Secondary causes of thrombocytosis occur as a result of conditions such as acute bleeding, iron deficiency, infection (e.g., tuberculosis), chronic inflammatory disease (e.g., RA), and malignancy, and resolve with treatment of the underlying pathology.[380] Secondary thrombocytosis may also be seen following splenectomy because platelets that normally would be stored in the spleen return to the circulating blood.

**Pathogenesis.** Approximately 50% of clients with ET demonstrate the *JAK2* mutation, linking it with other myeloproliferative neoplasms (see "Polycythemia Vera" above). The *JAK2* mutation is known to significantly increase the activity of the *JAK2* gene, induce cytokine-independent signaling, and activate downstream communications.[448] Thrombosis, a serious problem seen in ET, may develop as a result of an abnormal interaction among leukocytes, platelets, and vascular endothelium; although leukocytosis may be a better indicator of thrombosis risk than absolute platelet count.[105] Other genetic abnormalities are most likely responsible for the remaining cases that do not exhibit the *JAK2* mutation.

**Clinical Manifestations.** The most prominent feature is a platelet count elevation above 450,000/µL. Many people with ET also exhibit splenomegaly (50%) and episodes of bleeding and/or thrombosis, such as microvascular thrombi causing digital ischemia. The risk of thrombosis or hemorrhage at 15 years is 10% to 15% and 7%, respectively.

Visual disturbances, headache, burning sensation of the feet and hands accompanied by redness (erythromelalgia), and skin changes (livedo reticularis; Fig. 14.10) develop with increasing platelet counts. The most serious complications of bleeding and thrombosis occur secondary to a qualitative platelet dysfunction. Platelet counts above 1,000,000/µL can lead to acquired von Willebrand syndrome with associated bleeding episodes. Although major bleeding is uncommon, the likelihood increases as platelet counts exceed.

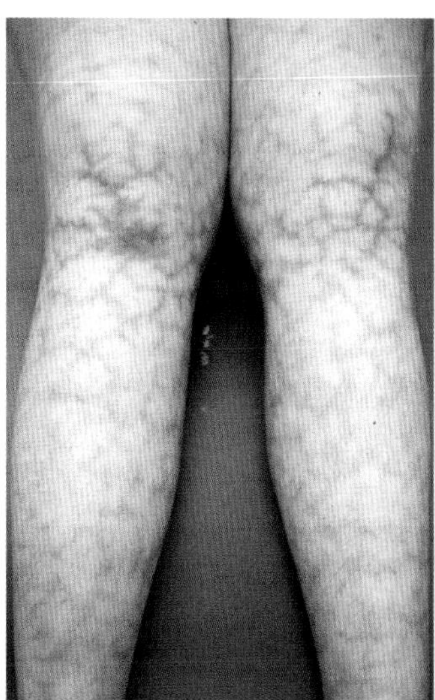

**Figure 14.10**

**Livedo reticularis associated with thrombocythemia (elevated platelet count).** The classic fishnet pattern is shown. (Reprinted from Piccini JP, Nilsson KR: *The Osler medical handbook*, ed 2, Baltimore, 2006, Johns Hopkins University.)

#### MEDICAL MANAGEMENT

DIAGNOSIS. Because most people are asymptomatic at diagnosis, the disease is usually identified from incidental laboratory tests. Causes of secondary thrombocytosis need to be eliminated in order to diagnose ET. Approximately 50% of people with ET exhibit a mutation in the *JAK2* gene. The presence of this mutation may portend a more aggressive course of disease. Other mutations related to ET include alterations of the *MPL* and *CALR* genes. A sustained, elevated platelet count; the *JAK2* mutation or other associated mutations; splenomegaly; and abnormal bone marrow are features indicative of ET.

TREATMENT. The treatment of ET is not curative and is designed to reduce symptoms and complications. Therapy depends on the age and symptoms of the person. Asymptomatic, young clients (age younger than 65 years) with a platelet count less than 1,000,000/µL may not require treatment. People experiencing vasomotor symptoms or are at high risk for thrombosis, such as those over the age of 60 years and/or have a history of thrombosis, should be treated with low dose aspirin. Hydroxyurea is utilized to reduce the platelet count to less than 400,000/µL for clients at high risk for thrombosis. This therapy significantly reduces the risk of bleeding or another thrombotic event.

Anagrelide reduces platelet counts in persons who are able to tolerate it. Side effects include arrhythmias, palpitations, hypotension, fluid retention, and heart failure. It should not be used in elderly persons with heart problems. Interferon-α, low-dose, may also be beneficial.[404]

Persons who develop acute ischemic events and have a platelet count greater than 1,000,000/µL can receive immediate plateletpheresis. If surgery is required, the platelet count should be brought to near-normal levels to reduce the risk of bleeding and thrombosis perioperatively.

**PROGNOSIS.** Most people with ET have near-normal life expectancies, with a median survival of 20 years. For people under the age of 60, life expectancies approach 30 years after diagnosis.[440] ET carries a small (less than 3% at 10 years) risk of transforming into acute leukemia, and has a 1% to 5% risk of developing into myelofibrosis at 10 years.[53] Bleeding and thrombotic events are the most serious complications and can be life-threatening.

SPECIAL IMPLICATIONS FOR THE THERAPIST 14.12

*Thrombocythemia*

The therapist may recognize this condition when the client presents with livedo reticularis accompanied by reports of headache, burning sensation in the hands and feet, and visual disturbances. Medical referral is required if the person has not been previously evaluated.

In cases of known thrombocythemia, the therapist must maintain surveillance for arterial and venous thrombotic episodes and educate the client about what to watch for and when to seek medical assistance immediately. Signs and symptoms of arterial emboli include pain, numbness, coldness, tingling or changes in sensation, skin changes (pallor, mottling), weakness, and muscle spasm occurring in the extremity distal to the block.

With venous occlusion, the tissues are oxygenated, but the blood is not moving, and stasis occurs. The skin is discolored rather than pale (ranging from angry red to deep blue-purple), edema is present, and pain is most marked at the site of occlusion, although extreme edema can render all the skin of the limb quite tender.

### Myelodysplastic Syndrome

**Overview.** Myelodysplastic syndrome (MDS) is a heterogeneous group of disorders resulting from the clonal expansion of a malignant hematopoietic stem cell. In comparison to myeloproliferative disorders, MDS typically presents with anemia and cytopenias. MDS can have a significant impact on quality of life and survival[116]; it also progresses at a variable rate to AML.

MDS has been underdiagnosed and underrecognized in the past. In 1995, only 1500 cases were reported, whereas between 2001 and 2004 there were about 10,000 new cases per year. MDS is more common in older people, with an incidence rate of about 75 to 162 per 100,000 in people 65 years of age and older.[67,68] Approximately 86% of people with MDS were 60 years of age or older, whereas only 6% were younger than age 50.[233] White men have the highest incidence of MDS.

**Etiology.** Most cases of MDS do not have an etiology. However, some established risk factors associated with secondary MDS include ionizing radiation and chemotherapy from a previous malignancy treatment; exposure to benzene (such as cigarette smoking)[325]; genetic disorders (i.e., Down syndrome); and the congenital diseases (i.e., Fanconi anemia). MDS that results from previous cancer treatment carries a poorer prognosis. The number of secondary cases has significantly increased, most likely because of the increase in people who have survived previous malignancies. Other factors that may be related include pesticides, alcohol consumption, and increased body mass index.[234]

**Pathogenesis.**[107,227]**.** A variety of genetic abnormalities are associated with MDS. These mutations have been noted to impair important cellular functions, such as DNA repair, mRNA splicing, and gene regulation.[483] The final common pathway of these abnormalities is a hematopoietic stem cell that is unable to effectively mature and develop, leading to the formation of dysplastic cells. Bone marrow microenvironment, cellular communication and signaling, as well as genetic mutations may all play a role in the development of MDS.

**Clinical Manifestations.** Because the cells are unable to effectively differentiate or function, they eventually undergo apoptosis. This results in ineffective hematopoiesis in the bone marrow, leading to various cytopenias. Clinical manifestations of MDS vary depending on the presence and severity of the cytopenias. Many people remain asymptomatic, and MDS is only suspected by laboratory values obtained for other clinical symptoms. Anemia (usually macrocytic) is the most common laboratory manifestation, noted in 80% to 85% of people presenting with MDS. Clients typically exhibit fatigue or exacerbation of underlying comorbidities, such as CHF or chronic obstructive pulmonary disease. Neutropenia is seen in 40% to 50% of newly diagnosed individuals, whereas thrombocytopenia is noted in 25% of clients.[116] People with MDS may be more prone to infections (particularly bacterial) or bleeding. MDS should be suspected in any elderly client with unexplained anemia and progressive cytopenias.

#### MEDICAL MANAGEMENT

**DIAGNOSIS.** Because MDS previously was thought to be rare, a primary care provider should have a high suspicion for MDS when evaluating older persons with anemia. Although anemia is common in the elderly, it is not an expected result of normal aging.[149] When taking a history, particular attention should be given to past cancer treatment, occupational exposures, tobacco use, or congenital/genetic disorders. Symptoms of fatigue, infection, and bleeding should be addressed.

For clients with one or more cytopenias and suspected MDS, the National Comprehensive Cancer Network guidelines[141] recommend a thorough history and exam; a bone marrow biopsy and aspiration with iron staining and cytogenetics; a serum erythropoietin level; RBC folate and vitamin $B_{12}$ levels; a CBC with reticulocyte count; a peripheral blood smear; HLA typing; HIV serology; and a total iron binding capacity and serum ferritin level. The peripheral blood smear may demonstrate hypolobulated, hypogranulated neutrophils and nucleated erythrocytes.

MDS is difficult to diagnose. Often other entities that present with anemia and dysplasia of blood cells must be excluded. This is particularly true in people who have early disease or mild dysplasia. The three main diagnostic features of MDS include: the presence of a cytopenia (hemoglobin less than 10 g/dL, absolute neutrophil count less than 1.8/microL, or platelets less than 100,000/microL);

peripheral blood smear or bone marrow aspirate/biopsy significant for cellular dysplasia; blast count in the bone marrow of less than 20%.

Several classification systems and prognostic models are used to aid in the diagnosis and stratification of clients according to determining risk for progression to AML. The FAB classification is based on cell morphology and bone marrow blast count. The WHO classification recognizes six variants of MDS, taking into account cytogenetics and immunophenotypic characteristics in addition to the FAB classification.[15,268,454] The Revised International Prognostic Scoring System (IPSS-R) utilizes bone marrow blast percentage, absolute neutrophil count, platelet count, hemoglobin, and cytogenetics as features that tend to determine outcome.

**TREATMENT.** Treatment of MDS is often determined by IPSS-R classification, whether high or low risk for progression to AML, life expectancy, or ability to tolerate medications or hematopoietic cell transplantation (HCT). Therapies are directed toward relieving symptoms and reducing the risk for progression to AML. People at low risk for developing AML can use the "watch and wait" approach, because there is currently no evidence that treating people who are asymptomatic improves outcomes.

Symptomatic anemia requires treatment, and therapy usually consists of transfusions, although this leads to iron overload and must be carefully monitored. Iron chelation therapy may be considered for those clients who have received 20 to 30 transfusions or have an elevated ferritin level of 2,5000 ng/mL. Bleeding may require platelet transfusions, and infections are treated with appropriate antibiotics. Attempts at avoiding chronic transfusion dependence are essential and may include the use of erythrocyte-stimulating agents, epoetin and darbepoetin alfa, granulocyte colony-stimulating factor, or granulocyte-macrophage colony-stimulating factor.

Medications that have improved MDS treatment include lenalidomide (an immunomodulating agent), azacitidine and decitabine (hypomethylating agents), and combination chemotherapy (for people at high risk for developing AML).

Those at high risk for progression to AML should receive treatment immediately. Because allogeneic HCT is potentially the only cure for MDS, treatment decisions must be made with this in mind. Good candidates for HCT include age younger than 55 (although performance status is more important), good performance status, high-risk MDS, and suitable donor.

**PROGNOSIS.** Because MDS is a heterogenic group of related disorders, the progression and prognosis vary substantially between variants. Data from the IPSS-R demonstrates an 8.8-year median overall survival for people at very low risk and 1.6 years for those at high risk.[142] Twenty-five percent of individuals with high-risk disease go on to develop AML within 1.4 years (median time).

## DISORDERS OF HEMOSTASIS

*Hemostasis* is the arrest of bleeding after blood vessel injury and involves the interaction among platelets, blood vessel wall, and the plasma coagulation proteins. Normal hemostasis is divided into two separate and independent processes (although they intersect): primary and secondary.[121]

*Primary hemostasis* involves the formation of a platelet plug at the site of vascular injury. When a vessel is disrupted, platelets become exposed to subendothelial matrix, which, with the aid of von Willebrand factor (VWB) and other adhesive proteins, leads to the adhesion and activation of platelets. VWF, which is usually coiled when inactive, upon activation becomes uncoiled and binds the collagen fibrils to the platelets via special receptors on the platelets. This ultimately leads to the formation of a platelet plug.

*Secondary hemostasis* (extrinsic pathway) is triggered when vascular damage exposes tissue factor. Tissue factor is found in places not normally exposed to blood flow, where the presence of blood is pathologic.

Tissue factor then binds clotting factor VII, which, in turn, activates factors X and IX. Activated factors IX and VIII also activate factor X. Activated factor X, along with activated factor V, form the prothrombinase complex, which is able to catalyze the conversion of prothrombin into thrombin. Thrombin cleaves soluble fibrinogen into insoluble fiber monomers that polymerize, creating a fibrin clot at the site of injury.

Normal primary hemostasis requires normal number and function of platelets and VWF. Persons who have abnormalities in primary hemostasis have defects in either the number or function of platelets or a deficiency or dysfunction of VWF.

A decrease in the number of platelets, called *thrombocytopenia*, can prevent hemostasis. An exceptionally high number of platelets, called thrombocytosis, may cause bleeding, thrombosis, or both. Persons with a deficiency or dysfunction in VWF have von Willebrand disease (VWD).

Bleeding caused by platelet disorders or VWD is characterized by easy bruising or mucosal bleeding. Normal secondary hemostasis necessitates the presence of clotting factors. Defects in secondary hemostasis result from clotting factor deficiencies or dysfunction, such as those seen in hemophilias A and B. Persons with abnormalities in secondary hemostasis tend to have more serious bleeding, such as deep muscle hematomas and spontaneous hemarthrosis.

### von Willebrand Disease (VWD)

#### Definition and Overview

VWD is the most common inherited bleeding disorder. It affects both genders and is caused by a lack (deficiency) or dysfunction of von Willebrand factor (VWF). The prevalence of this illness may be 1% of the population (based on population screening studies) although many Americans do not know they have it due to the mildness of their VWF deficiency.

VWF is a plasma protein that mediates the initial adhesion of platelets at sites of bleeding injuries; it binds and stabilizes blood clotting factor VIII in the circulation. Defects in VWF can cause bleeding by impairing platelet adhesion or by reducing the concentration of factor VIII. VWF binds collagen fibrils and platelets in areas of vascular injury to create a platelet plug. It also stabilizes factor

VIII and prevents it from being inactivated and cleared from the plasma during times of bleeding.

VWD represents a range of genetic diseases with the clinical manifestation of mucocutaneous bleeding, generally milder than hemophilia. VWD is classified into three main subtypes: types 1, 2, and 3. Type 1 is the most common subtype and accounts for 75% of clients with VWD. Persons with this subtype have 5% to 30% of the normal amount of VWF, leading to mild to moderate symptoms. Type 1 is inherited in an autosomal dominant fashion.

Type 2 is less common and seen in only 10% to 30% of VWD cases. It is caused by a dysfunction in VWF rather than a reduction in quantity of VWF.[434] This subtype is further divided into types 2A, 2B, 2M, and 2N, depending on the adhesion/binding protein abnormalities or multimerization defects. This subtype is also inherited in an autosomal dominant manner, except 2N is transmitted as an autosomal recessive trait.

The rarest (and most severe) form of VWD subtypes is type 3, which makes up only 1% to 5% of cases. Persons affected with this form have less than 1% of the normal plasma levels of VWF (levels may be undetectable) and very low levels of functional clotting factor VIII. Because these clients are lacking both VWF and factor VIII, their symptoms are more severe and resemble hemophilia A. Inheritance is autosomal recessive.

### Pathogenesis

VWF plays a vital role in primary hemostasis by aiding in platelet-to-platelet adhesion, linking platelets to vascular subendothelial collagen, and factor VIII protection. Endothelial and megakaryocytes produce VWF, which circulates in the blood as a multimer. Initially these newly secreted multimers are unusually large with a prothrombotic tendency, but then undergo processing into smaller multimers. People with low levels of VWF may have bleeding, while those individuals with high levels are prone to thrombosis.

Mutations in the VWF gene, located on chromosome 12, are responsible for VWD, although the specific type of mutation determines the clinical manifestations and type of disease (i.e., type 1, 2A, etc). Abnormalities in other non-VWD genes, such as those involved in ABO blood groups, may also contribute to disease expression. For example, people with type O blood have VWF levels that are reduced by 25%. Thus, often only one mutation leads to multiple deficits, such as problems with formation of multimers, secretion, or premature clearance of VWF.[435]

VWD occurs because of a qualitative lack of VWF or due to an abnormally functioning VWF (although VWF is produced, a mutation causes a malformation in the function of the proteins). Significant investigation has been placed into the discovery of the genetic abnormalities and how they correlate with VWD phenotypes.[114] More than 750 mutations of multiple types have been documented.[82]

### Clinical Manifestations

Symptoms experienced by clients with VWD vary depending on the subtype and severity of the abnormality. Many people with VWD do not realize they have the disease, often due to the mild nature of the defect and lack of a bleeding challenge. Clients with type 1 experience bleeding consistent with a primary hemostasis defect. This most frequently involves easy bruising and mucocutaneous bleeding, such as nosebleeds, gum bleeding, and/or prolonged oozing of blood after minor trauma, dental extraction or surgery. Symptoms associated with type 2 depend on the severity of the mutation and the quantity of functional VWF.

It is estimated that 10% to 15% of women with menorrhagia (excessive menstruation) have VWD.[394] Menorrhagia is a common presenting symptom yet is frequently overlooked and undiagnosed because gynecologists infrequently perform tests to confirm or exclude a bleeding disorder. Women also experience significant postpartum hemorrhaging and endometriosis.[223]

Type 2N and 3 clients present not only with symptoms of mucocutaneous and gastrointestinal bleeding but also more frequent and severe symptoms, including hemarthrosis and muscular hematomas (similar to hemophilia A). Women with type 3 VWD are particularly vulnerable to bleeding problems associated with their menstrual cycle, resulting in anemia and fatigue. Pregnancy places these women at risk for early trimester miscarriage or prolonged bleeding during delivery and postpartum. Type 3 VWD often presents in childhood due to the severe nature of the defect.

## MEDICAL MANAGEMENT

**DIAGNOSIS.** Diagnosis relies on the triad of a personal history of excessive mucocutaneous bleeding, laboratory tests consistent with VWF, and a positive family history of the condition. The most common screening laboratory tests used to assess coagulation are the activated partial thromboplastin time (aPTT is usually normal or slightly prolonged in VWD) and the prothrombin time (PT is typically normal). The Platelet Function Analyzer-100 (PFA-100) evaluates platelet function and in VWD the results are usually prolonged. CBC and platelet counts are also assessed. In the laboratory, measurement of VWF antigen (VWF protein levels) and activity, as well as Factor VIII activity levels, continue to be the most important diagnostic studies. VWF activity refers to testing the ability of a client's VWF to bind to platelets, collagen, and factor VIII. In order to standardize and reduce false-positive results, the National Heart, Lung, and Blood Institute have set guidelines and cutoff values for VWF activity and antigen levels. Clients with less than 30 international units/dL (<30%) with associated bleeding and positive family history for bleeding, are considered to have VWD. Clinical correlation must be made for individuals with 30 to 50 international units/dL (levels may be elevated due to inflammation, stress or other factors) and are labeled as having low VWF.[224] Once the diagnosis is established, testing for the type of disease is accomplished through tests such as the ratio of VWF activity to VWF antigen, ratio of factor VIII activity to VWF antigen, VWF multimer analysis, and ristocetin-induced platelet aggregation (RIPA).

Despite available tests, many clinicians find making the diagnosis very difficult—particularly for clients with mild disease. Because of the fluctuation of VWF from stress, exercise, estrogen, inflammation, and bleeding, testing may need to be repeated. Genetic analysis is also available to determine defects that are not otherwise detectable using standard testing.[135]

**TREATMENT AND PROGNOSIS.** The treatment of VWD centers on increasing VWF levels, or as needed, factor VIII activity. VWF and factor VIII concentrates are used for severe bleeding episodes, particularly for clients with type 3 VWD. They may also be utilized in prophylactic administration during pregnancy, prior to an invasive procedure or in people with recurrent hemarthrosis or frequent GI bleeding. Long-term prophylaxis is not done as routinely as in hemophilia, although some subgroups with severe disease appear to benefit.[174] Various VWF concentrates are available, including a plasma-derived concentrate (containing both VWF and factor VIII). In 2015 a recombinant VWF concentrate was approved for adults.[128,396] If synthetic concentrates are not available, other plasma replacements can be used. Fresh-frozen plasma contains both VWF and factor VIII but is accompanied by a large volume, and multiple bags can cause volume overload. Cryoprecipitate contains both proteins in a smaller, concentrated volume but has the potential of viral transmission, so is not currently recommended.

Most clients with VWD (especially type 1) do not require treatment except during times of surgery or trauma or after delivery of a baby. Women with mild disease and heavy menstrual bleeding may benefit from estrogen-containing oral contraceptives, which can increase the levels of VWF. Desmopressin (DDAVP) is the principal drug of choice for treating most cases of VWD (except type 3). It is a synthetic antidiuretic-hormone derivative that induces the secretion of VWF and factor VIII from cellular storage. This medication can be given intravenously, subcutaneously (not available in the United States), or intranasally. Other available medications, which are used for dental, menses or minor mucosal bleeding, include antifibrinolytic agents, such as tranexamic acid or ε-aminocaproic acid.[296] Along mucosal linings of the body there is fibrinolytic activity, which prevents fibrin from forming a clot. Antifibrinolytic amino acids can be given to inhibit this activity. Frequently, they are used as adjuvant medications along with concentrates and desmopressin during major and minor surgery.

Despite advancement in treatment, clients with type 3 VWD still face the challenge of developing inhibitors to available treatment. These inhibitors are typically antibodies that clear VWF from the plasma. Further use of concentrates with VWF can lead to anaphylaxis. Recombinant activated factor VII is a concentrate that can be used for clients with VWD (typically type 3) who have developed inhibitors to concentrates. Due to the increased risk of thrombosis, this agent should be used with caution in people who have a history of ischemic heart disease.

Pregnancy increases levels of VWF and factor VIII so that by term, many women with mild disease have normal levels. However, pregnant women with more severe disease or functional abnormalities (some type 2) must be followed very carefully throughout their pregnancy. Concentrates and antifibrinolytics are drugs of choice for prophylaxis or treating bleeding episodes. DDAVP may cause uterine contractions and is typically avoided prior to delivery. At delivery, most women require treatment. Concentrates and desmopressin are routinely used at birth and during the immediate postpartum period.[361] Care must also be taken when treating the newborn because the baby may have VWD as well. Intramuscular injections, surgery, and circumcision should be avoided in babies with a high risk of a bleeding disorder until an adequate diagnosis is made.

Orthopedic surgery is possible for individuals with VWD but requires a multidisciplinary approach with careful planning and communication among all concerned.[242]

## Hemophilia

### Overview

Hemophilia is a bleeding disorder inherited as an X-linked autosomal recessive trait. The two primary types of hemophilia are *hemophilia A* and *hemophilia B*. Hemophilia A results from a lack of clotting factor VIII and constitutes 80% of all cases of hemophilia. Hemophilia B is less common, affecting approximately 15% of all people with hemophilia, and is caused by a deficiency of factor IX. Other, less-common deficiencies, such as deficiencies of clotting factors I, II, V, VII, X, or XIII, are rare and are not fully discussed in this text. Unless otherwise noted, *hemophilia* refers to both hemophilia A and hemophilia B in this text.

Factors VIII and IX are required in secondary hemostasis (in contrast to VWF, which is needed in primary hemostasis). These clotting factors are activated and result in the production of thrombin, which cleaves fibrinogen to fibrin, creating a stable clot.

The level of severity of the disease depends on the defect in the clotting factor gene and is classified according to the percentage of clotting factor present in plasma (determined through blood tests): mild (6%-30%), moderate (1%-5%), and severe (less than 1%). Normal concentrations of coagulation factors are between 50% and 150%.

For people with *mild* hemophilia (25% of all cases), spontaneous hemorrhages (bleeding that occurs with no apparent cause) are rare, and joint and deep muscle bleeding are uncommon. Surgical, dental, or other injury or trauma precipitates symptoms that must be treated the same as for severe hemophilia.

For those people with *moderate* hemophilia (15% of all people with hemophilia), spontaneous hemorrhage is not usually a problem, but major bleeding episodes can occur after minor trauma.

People with *severe* hemophilia make up 60% of people with hemophilia and may bleed spontaneously or with only slight trauma, particularly into the joints and deep muscle.

### Incidence

Hemophilia A is relatively rare. It affects approximately 1 in 5000 male births and each year about 400 babies are born with the disease. Although it is not known how many individuals live with the disorder, a Centers for Disease Control and Prevention study done in 1994 estimated that about 17,000 people had hemophilia at that time. Based on those numbers, it is estimated that 20,000 people now live with hemophilia.[51,415] Hemophilia primarily affects males, without bias for race or

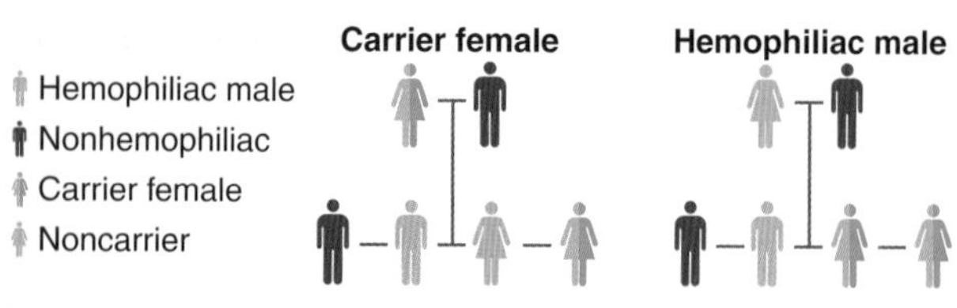


**Figure 14.11**

**Inheritance patterns in hemophilia for all family members.** A woman is definitely a carrier if she is (1) the biologic daughter of a man with hemophilia; (2) the biologic mother of more than one son with hemophilia; or (3) the biologic mother of one hemophilic son with at least one other blood relative with hemophilia. A woman may or may not be a carrier if she is (1) the biologic mother of one son with hemophilia; (2) the sister of a male with hemophilia; (3) an aunt, cousin, or niece of an affected male related through maternal ties; or (4) the biologic grandmother of one grandson with hemophilia. (Reprinted from Beare PG, Myers JL: *Adult health nursing*, ed 3, St Louis, 1998, Mosby.)

socioeconomic group. Hemophilia B is seen in 1 in every 30,000 male births and is more rare than hemophilia A.

## Etiologic Factors

The gene responsible for factors VIII and IX is located on the X chromosome, making hemophilia a gender-linked recessive disorder. Because females normally carry two X chromosomes, they only develop hemophilia if both genes are affected, if the normal X gene is inactivated, or if they only have one X chromosome (i.e., Turner syndrome), making hemophilia rare in females.

Males, on the other hand, only inherit one X chromosome and therefore develop hemophilia because they lack another normal X chromosome to provide these clotting factors (as most females do). Thus females are the carriers of the abnormality, whereas males present with the disease (Fig. 14.11).

Every carrier has a one in four chance of having a child with hemophilia. Men with the mutation will pass this on to their daughters (making them carriers), yet their sons will only inherit a normal Y chromosome and not develop hemophilia. Although in two-thirds of cases of hemophilia a known family history is evident, this disorder can occur in families (approximately one-third) without a previous history of blood-clotting disorders because of spontaneous genetic mutation. The remaining rare clotting factor deficiencies are inherited in an autosomal recessive manner.

## Pathogenesis

At least 10 proteins called *clotting factors* in the blood must work in a precise order to make a blood clot. Hemophilia A is caused by a deficiency of the protein clotting factor VIII, whereas hemophilia B is caused by a lack of factor IX. These clotting factors are produced by the liver (factor VIII by endothelial cells and factor IX by hepatocytes) and released into the blood. Factor VIII, once in the plasma, combines with VWF as part of this hemostasis cascade (as previously discussed). Factors VIII and IX are necessary for the formation of thrombin, which converts fibrinogen into fibrin, generating a clot. Clients with these factor deficiencies are unable to produce thrombin or a stable clot.

The genetic pattern of hemophilia is quite different from that of disorders such as sickle cell disease, in which every affected individual has the identical genetic defect. The presence of such variable defects in the same gene accounts for the differences in severity of hemophilia.

Many different genetic mutations cause factor VIII deficiency, such as gene deletions, duplications, insertions, inversions, and substitutions, which cause the clotting factor to be made incorrectly or not at all. Not all mutations are inherited; 25% to 30% of cases are caused by new mutations. To date, the CDC has created a list with over 2,000 known genetic mutations causing hemophilia A (F8 mutations) and 1,000 causing hemophilia B.[326] Most of these mutations are nucleotide substitutions (missense) or small deletions; however, one common mutation noted in more than 40% of people with severe hemophilia A is a partial inversion.[265]

## Clinical Manifestations

Clinically, hemophilia A and hemophilia B present with the same symptoms and can only be distinguished by specific factor assay tests. Unlike most clients with VWD, those with hemophilia manifest joint and deep muscle bleeding as well as excessive or delayed bleeding after trauma/surgery. Although people with hemophilia display mucocutaneous bleeding, small cuts typically do not bleed excessively. Disease severity is classified according to factor levels: mild disease has 6% to 30%, moderate expresses 1% to 5%, while severe disease has less than 1% of normal levels. There is some evidence that hemophilia B is less severe than hemophilia A based on patient registries and data from various sources.[258] Much of the clinical difference noted between hemophilia A and B is determined by the severity of the genetic mutation.[400] Regular prophylaxis is used less often for individuals with hemophilia B, and there is less need for orthopedic surgery among adults with hemophilia B with fewer joint replacements.[240]

Occurrences of bleeding are noted during the newborn period in infants who have severe hemophilia. The most common instances include immunizations, heel sticks, blood draws, and circumcision. If a child is born to a known carrier, circumcision should not be performed until appropriate tests are completed. As the child grows, bleeding problems will continue to be manifested.

Hematoma formation may result from injections or after firm holding (such as occurs when a child is held under the arms or by the elbow and lifted), excessive bruising from minor trauma, delayed hemorrhage (hours to days after injury) after a minor injury, persistent bleeding after tooth loss, and recurrent bleeding into muscles and joints.

Bruising, bleeding from the mouth or frenulum, intracranial bleeding, hematomas of the head, and hemarthrosis (bleeding into the joints) can occur during early ambulation. By age 3 to 4 years, 90% of children with severe hemophilia have had an episode of persistent bleeding not seen in mild cases.

Clients with severe hemophilia often display episodes of spontaneous bleeding (into the joints, muscles, and internal organs) along with severe bleeding with trauma or surgery. Those persons affected with mild to moderate hemophilia do not commonly have spontaneous bleeding but exhibit excessive bleeding with trauma and surgery.

**Women with Hemophilia.** Women with hemophilia experience excessive uterine bleeding during their menstrual cycle, with possible oozing from the ovary after ovulation mid-cycle. Heavy menstrual flow is often the symptom that initiates a coagulation evaluation or more often is reported but not adequately diagnosed.

Female carriers of a factor VIII mutation may have abnormal bleeding.[400] Although expected to have 50% of normal factor VIII levels, uncommonly, a woman who is a carrier of hemophilia can have very low levels of factors VIII or IX. This is because in every cell of the body either the normal X chromosome or the affected X chromosome is randomly inactivated (turned off) in a process called *lyonization*. If the majority of the inactivated chromosomes are the normal X, then the levels of clotting factors may be very low, and such carriers may experience excessive bleeding. Women may also have only one X chromosome (as seen in Turner syndrome), or inherited abnormal factor VIII genes from both the father and mother (carrier).

These women may experience mild abnormal bleeding from dental extractions, abortion or miscarriage, complications of pregnancy (e.g., placenta not delivered completely, episiotomy or tearing, prolonged postpartum hemorrhage), nosebleeds, and minor trauma (such as cuts with prolonged oozing).[340] The bleeding may be overlooked due to the misconception that hemophilia does not occur in women.

**Joint.** Spontaneous bleeding into the joint spaces (hemarthrosis) is one of the most common clinical manifestations of severe hemophilia (occurring during the first year after birth), occurring in 75% to 90% of clients. The knee is the most frequently affected joint, followed by the ankle, elbow, hip, shoulder, and wrist. Bleeding in the synovial joints of the feet, hands, temporomandibular joint, and spine is less common. Prophylaxis therapy begun early in childhood has been shown to prevent joint disease.[237] Most children with severe hemophilia and those with more than one bleeding episode receive prophylactic treatment. Children who are obese have also been found to be more likely to develop decreased joint movement, and programs are in place to help children with hemophilia maintain an optimal, healthy weight.[414]

If prophylaxis is not pursued or effective, joints can become significantly affected. Joints with 3 or more spontaneous bleeds in 6 months are called target joints (meaning they are more susceptible to another bleed), and in children with severe hemophilia, this can occur as a toddler. When blood is introduced into the joint, the joint becomes distended, causing swelling, pain, warmth, and stiffness. The synovial membrane responds by producing an increased number of synovial villi and undergoing vascular hyperplasia in an attempt to reabsorb the blood. Blood is an irritant to the synovium, which releases enzymes that break down RBCs and the cell by-products (e.g., iron). This process causes the synovium to become hypertrophied, with formation of fingerlike projections of tissue extending onto the articular surface.

The mechanical trauma of normal weight-bearing motion may then impinge and further injure the inflamed synovium. Iron in the form of hemosiderin is deposited in the synovium, which impairs the production of synovial fluid. A vicious cycle is established as the synovium

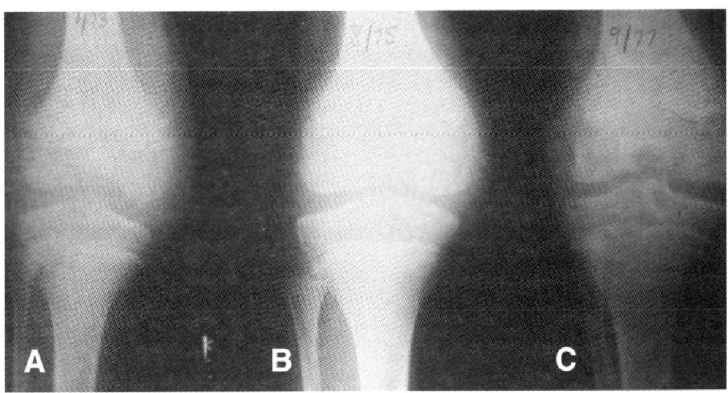


**Figure 14.12**

**Stages of hemophilic arthropathy according to the Arnold-Hilgartner scale.** (A) Stage I (1973). (B) Stage III (1975). (C) Stage IV (1977). (Courtesy Mountain States Regional Hemophilia Center, Colorado State Treatment Program, Denver, 1995.)

attempts to cleanse the joint of blood and debris, becoming more hypertrophic and susceptible to still further bleeding. Erosive damage of the cartilage follows these changes in the synovium with narrowing of the joint space (Fig. 14.12), erosions at the joint margins, and subchondral cyst formation. Collapse of the joint, joint sclerosis, and eventual spontaneous ankylosis may occur.[188]

In later stages of joint degeneration, chronic pain, severe loss of motion, muscle atrophy, crepitus, and joint deformities occur. Despite advances in medical management, target joints can progress to advanced arthropathy. This is most commonly seen in people with severe hemophilia. The articular cartilage softens, turns brown (from hemosiderin), and becomes pitted and fragmented. The inflamed synovium is thick and highly vascularized and can grow over the joint surfaces, becoming pannus.

Eventually, lesions in the deeper layers of cartilage result in subchondral bone breakdown and the formation of subchondral cysts. Osteophyte formation occurs along the edges of the joint (Box 14.7 and Table 14.4). With the destruction of the cartilage, little to no joint space is left. This bone-on-bone contact can lead to significant pain, limitation of motion, joint malalignment, muscle atrophy, functional impairment, and disability.

At this point joint bleeds are rare. For the child, recurrent bleeds into the same joint can lead to growth abnormalities. The epiphyses, where bone growth takes place, are stimulated to grow in the presence of hyperemia caused by bleeding. Postural asymmetries may develop (e.g., leg length differences, angulatory deformities, bony enlargement at the affected joint).

***Classification of Hemophilic Arthropathy.*** Several different classification scales are used to identify progression of hemophilic arthropathy. The Arnold-Hilgartner and Pettersson score classification scales have been in use for many years. With the Arnold-Hilgartner scale, the arthropathy is divided into stages that are assumed to be progressive. With the Pettersson score, a number of specific findings are evaluated and the additive sum of the assigned points is calculated.

In addition, there is now MRI information being used for classification as well. With improvements in hemophilia care, evaluation of subtle joint changes not readily apparent with conventional radiography has become

Box 14.7

**ARNOLD-HILGARTNER HEMOPHILIC ARTHROPATHY STAGES**

Staging scheme to classify joint changes seen on x-ray:

| | |
|---|---|
| 0 | Normal joint |
| I | No skeletal abnormalities; soft tissue swelling |
| II | Osteoporosis and overgrowth of epiphysis; no erosions; no narrowing of cartilage space |
| III | Early subchondral bone cysts, squaring of the patella; intercondylar notch of distal femur and humerus widened; cartilage space remains preserved |
| IV | Finding of stage III more advanced; cartilage space narrowed significantly; cartilage destruction |
| V | End stage; fibrous joint contracture, loss of joint cartilage space, marked enlargement of the epiphyses, and substantial disorganization of the joints |

Data from Arnold WD, Hilgartner MW: Hemophilic arthropathy, *J Bone Joint Surg Am* 59:287–305, 1977.

**Table 14.4** Pettersson Radiologic Classification of Hemophilic Arthropathy

| Type of Change | Finding | Score[a] |
|---|---|---|
| Osteoporosis | Absent | 0 |
| | Present | 1 |
| Enlarged epiphysis | Absent | 0 |
| | Present | 1 |
| Irregular subchondral surface | Absent | 0 |
| | Slight | 1 |
| | Pronounced | 2 |
| Narrowing of joint space | Absent | 0 |
| | <50% | 1 |
| | >50% | 2 |
| Subchondral cyst formation | Absent | 0 |
| | 1 Cyst | 1 |
| | >1 Cyst | 2 |
| Erosions at joint margins | Absent | 0 |
| | Present | 1 |
| Incongruence between joint surfaces | Absent | 0 |
| | Slight | 1 |
| | Pronounced | 2 |
| Joint deformity (angulation and/or displacement between articulating bones) | Absent | 0 |
| | Slight | 1 |
| | Pronounced | 2 |

A joint scoring system based on radiographic findings used to classify and monitor joint changes and damage.

[a]Note: Possible total joint score is 0 to 13 points.

From Anderson A, Holtzman TS, Masley J: *Physical therapy in bleeding disorders,* New York, 2000, National Hemophilia Foundation.

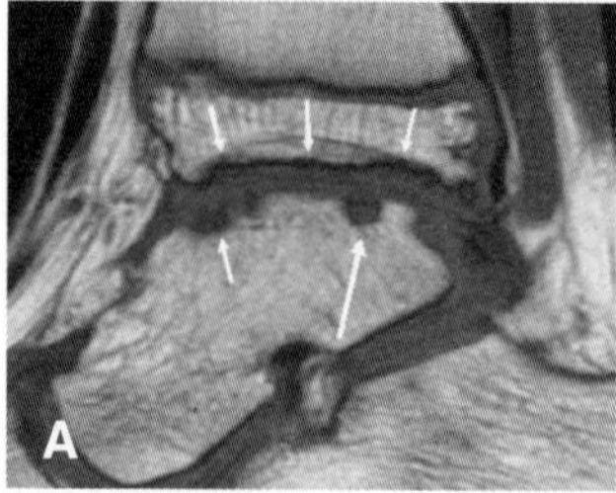

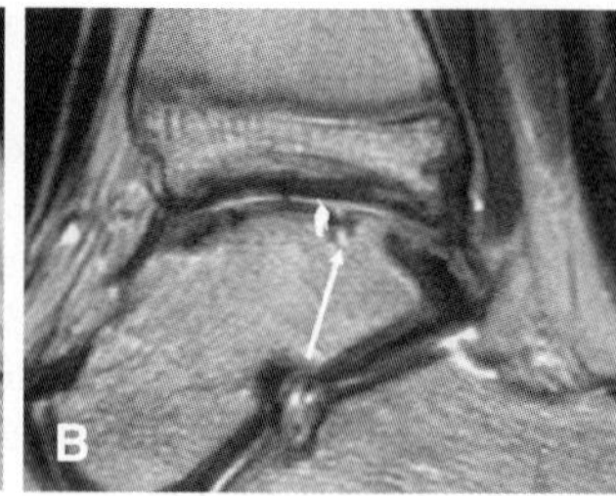


**Figure 14.13**

**MRI of hemophilic arthropathy.** (A) Left ankle of a 9-year-old boy with moderate hemophilia. Sagittal spin echo (SE) T1-weighted sequence. (B) Sagittal turbo spin echo (TSE) T2-weighted sequence. Cortical irregularity (best seen on T1-weighted image, *small arrows*) is the hallmark of surface erosions. Different types of subchondral cysts have different signal characteristics. In this joint a cyst is discerned in the dorsal part of the talar dome (intermediate signal on T1-weighted image and bright signal on T2-weighted image, *large arrows*), and a focal defect in the overlying cartilage is revealed (joint fluid in defect is bright on T2-weighted image). (Courtesy Bjorn Lundin, MD, University Hospital of Lund, Sweden.)

increasingly important. MRI can visualize effusion, hemarthrosis, synovial hypertrophy and/or hemosiderin deposition, subchondral cysts and/or surface erosions, and loss of cartilage (Fig. 14.13).

Different MRI methods for joint scoring use either a progressive or additive scoring strategy. Using proposed MRI scoring methods, imaging specialists can detect and monitor early joint changes, assess therapeutic outcomes, and further define the pathophysiology of hemophilic joint disease. An in-depth discussion of these techniques is available for readers interested in the specifics.[119,232,284]

The World Haemophilia Federation published a Hemophilia Joint Health Score (HJHS) tool to aid in identifying and quantifying the early changes seen in hemophilia joint disease. It is an 11-item scoring tool for assessing joint impairment in boys with hemophilia. It has been validated and is highly sensitive.[109,113,115,162] Drawbacks to the HJHS may include that while it is sensitive, it is not specific and may not correlate with need for referral or imaging.[50]

**Muscle.** Muscle hemorrhages can be more insidious and massive than joint bleeding, and although they can occur anywhere, muscle hemorrhages most often involve leg muscles (e.g., iliopsoas, quadriceps, gastrocnemius) and the arm (forearm flexors). Intramuscular hemorrhage may be visible in superficial areas such as the calf or forearm and may be accompanied with pain and limitation of motion of the affected part. Intramuscular hemorrhage that occurs in large muscles, such as the iliopsoas, may be less obvious without noticeable bruising or a palpable hematoma. Clients may demonstrate groin pain, pain on extension of the hip, and reflexive flexion of the hip and thigh. Presentation may include compression of the femoral nerve with subsequent weakness; decreased sensation over the thigh and knee in the L2, L3, and L4 distribution; decreased or absent knee reflexes; temperature changes; and even permanent impairment. Iliopsoas bleeds are considered a medical emergency requiring immediate referral to a physician.

A large hemorrhage can cause a compartment syndrome (particularly in leg and forearm) with pain (greater than expected), tightness of the skin, swelling, and neurologic changes secondary to compression of the neurovascular bundle. This may include numbness, tingling, and muscle weakness.

**Nervous System.** Intracranial hemorrhage (ICH) is not the most common site of bleeding in a person with hemophilia; however, it is the most serious and deadly complication. It occurs more frequently in newborns than older children and adults, with a prevalence rate of approximately 4%/year.[211,229] ICH may occur spontaneously or be trauma induced, leading to long-term consequences such as paralysis, seizures, cerebral palsy, and other neurologic deficits.

Although signs and symptoms of ICH may be dramatic (e.g., seizures, paralysis, apnea, unequal pupils, excessive vomiting, or tense and bulging fontanelles), they are often vague (e.g., crankiness or irritability, lethargy, feeding difficulty), leading to a delay in diagnosis. Many are asymptomatic and unreported. ICH in clients with hemophilia carries a mortality of about 20% when it occurs.

**Inhibitors.** With the production of safer factor concentrates, the development of antibody inhibitors (antibodies that remove or inhibit the function of the infused factor) poses a serious complication to hemophilia treatment, including death.[467] Often the development of inhibitors is clinically silent until a bleeding episode occurs and treatment is ineffective.[413] Individuals with hemophilia A develop inhibitors more frequently than those with hemophilia B. Racial differences are also noted with inhibitors more commonly seen in blacks (up to 50%) than whites (20%-30%). Clients affected most often are people who have severe hemophilia A, although people with mild to moderate disease may also develop inhibitors. Anaphylaxis may occur, particularly in people receiving factor IX concentrates who develop factor IX inhibitors. Routine screening is performed to monitor for inhibitors and people receiving factor IX infusions should receive the first 20 doses in a setting able to treat anaphylaxis.

The risk of developing an inhibitor does not remain the same during the lifetime of a person with hemophilia, and the appearance of antibodies can be transient or in low titers. Factors that increase the risk for developing inhibitors include timing, dose, and choice of replacement factor; specific genetic mutations; immune response mediators; and presence of "danger signals" received by the immune system from stressed cells. Clients with high-responding inhibitors (may be present in low titers but quickly increase in number upon exposure) may receive bypassing products (rFVIIa or an activated prothrombin complex concentrate) for acute bleeding or undergo immune tolerance therapy (ITI) (frequent infusions of factor) during periods without bleeding. All treatment decisions should be made in conjunction and consultation with a comprehensive hemophilia treatment center.[413]

**Transmissible Diseases.** Individuals, primarily those with severe hemophilia, who were treated before current purification techniques for factor concentrates (before 1986) may have been exposed to hepatitis B or C and/or HIV. Approximately 50% of people with hemophilia during this period became infected with HIV.[210] No other at-risk group had such a high prevalence; however, since 1986 no further HIV transmission has occurred.

Transmission of hepatitis is equally serious, and approximately 70% to 90% of people with hemophilia who received clotting factor before the mid-1980s test positive for hepatitis C.[212,273] This high rate of infection signifies that many people became coinfected with both HIV and hepatitis C. Coinfection can lead to an acceleration of liver disease, which may not respond to treatment, and the development of hepatocellular carcinoma.[103] Current improved methods of viral inactivation of factor concentrates through pasteurization and solvent treatment and monoclonal and recombinant technology have resulted in safer products.

Improved screening methods to identify donors with hepatitis have also reduced the risk of hepatitis transmission. As of 1998, there have been no reports of hepatitis or HIV transmission through clotting factor treated with these improved processes.[173,178]

The transmission of hepatitis A and parvovirus B19 has also been reduced in plasma-derived products (but not eradicated), but hepatitis A can now be prevented by immunization with a vaccine. All newborns with hemophilia now receive the hepatitis B vaccination series, but older clients often have hepatitis B along with its long-term sequelae. Transmission of parvovirus B19 in plasma-derived factors continues to be problematic.[411]

## MEDICAL MANAGEMENT

**DIAGNOSIS.** Effective treatment of hemophilia is based on an accurate diagnosis of the deficient clotting factor and its level in the blood. Diagnosis is not always straightforward, because a variety of factors can confound the test results (e.g., blood type; factor levels can be elevated by stress, hyperthyroidism, and pregnancy, yet decreased in hypothyroidism). Additionally, cord blood sample at birth may have physiologically low levels of factor IX that only reach adult values by 3 to 6 months of age. Initial blood tests include CBC, platelets, prothrombin time (PT), and activated partial thromboplastin time (aPTT). Most people with hemophilia will have a normal platelet count and PT; however, the aPTT is often prolonged, depending on the severity of the disease. Individuals with mild hemophilia may have enough factor VIII or IX for aPTT results to test normal, so if hemophilia is suspected, specific factor analysis should be pursued. Mixing studies are performed in people who have a prolonged aPTT. Normal plasma is added to the client's plasma and when retested, aPTT is normal due to factors present in the donor's plasma. If the mixing studies demonstrate correction of the aPTT, then assays for specific clotting factor activity are performed. Type 3 VWD may present similarly and VWF levels should be evaluated. Genetic testing is completed in order to identify the specific mutation as well as the risk for the development of an inhibitor. Other tests may be added depending on individual variables. It is also important for female relatives of those with hemophilia to identify their carrier status through DNA testing. Factor level analysis is important to aid in management.

**TREATMENT.** Currently no known cure or prenatal treatment for hemophilia exists. Until a medical cure is developed, primary goals for intervention in the case of bleeding episodes are to stop any bleeding that is occurring as quickly as possible and to infuse the missing factors until the bleeding stops (of note, if factor replacement is not effective, the person may have an inhibitor).

Treatment for severe forms of hemophilia is recommended to take place in comprehensive hemophilia treatment centers. In these centers the specialized care required can be provided through a multidisciplinary team approach with appropriately trained and experienced health care providers. Treatment at a hemophilia treatment center has been shown to minimize disability, morbidity, and mortality rates.[412]

Factor replacement therapy, given intravenously, is currently the mainstay of hemophilia treatment.[241] Most factor VIII concentrates are produced using recombinant techniques to provide virus-free products. Current fourth-generation products do not contain animal or added human plasma proteins. Methods used prior to the availability of recombinant technology to manufacture factor VIII concentrates utilized plasma pooled from thousands of donors that was then purified for factor VIII. This purified concentrate was treated to deplete viruses (heating in an aqueous solution, treated by a solvent detergent, or immunoaffinity purification). Although this type of product is still available and there have been no reports of clients being infected with hepatitis B or C or HIV, the risk remains that these pooled-plasma products could possibly lead to viral transmission. This possible increased risk of transmitting a virus makes recombinant concentrates the recommended treatment of choice. Recombinant concentrates are also available with modifications that increase the half-life of the drug. Although these products are more expensive, they have the advantage of less frequent administration, making the requirement for a central line less stringent. This has led to improved compliance, fewer bleeding episodes, and improved quality of life, which often offset the cost of the drug.[159]

Clients may receive either concentrate on-demand (due to bleeding) or prophylactically on an intermittent or regularly scheduled basis. Choice of therapy should be individualized and take into consideration the severity of the disease, age, bleeding pattern, joint health, comorbidities, and personal preferences.[14] Prophylaxis of recombinant factors is often instituted for severe hemophilia or individuals with more than one bleeding episode in order to maintain blood factor levels in the moderate range. Prophylaxis has been shown to reduce long-term complications, such as chronic arthropathy, as well as decrease the incidence of cerebral hemorrhage.[11,308] Prophylaxis therapy is very expensive (concentrates, need for catheters, etc.), but treatment improves quality of life, pain control, activity, and joint health.[238] Intermittent prophylaxis consists of receiving concentrates for weeks to months for specific activities, such as physical activity or surgical procedures. On-demand or episodic therapy may be better suited for individuals with mild or moderate factor deficiencies.

Emicizumab is approved as prophylaxis for people with hemophilia A, with and without inhibitors, to bypass the need for factor VIII. It is a monoclonal antibody that binds both factors IX and X together, activating factor X. This drug is not approved for acute bleeding, because a loading dose is required. Maintenance dosing frequency is every few weeks (depending on the dose) and is given subcutaneously. Complications include thrombotic events including thrombotic microangiopathy.

Persons with mild hemophilia A can use the drug desmopressin when possible. If this medication does not provide adequate hemostasis or the client is pregnant or younger than 2 years, factor VIII concentrates should be utilized. Antifibrinolytics, including tranexamic acid and ε-aminocaproic acid may also be of benefit for controlling bleeding associated with dental procedures.

Most babies that are born with hemophilia have a known family history of bleeding and hemophilia (although one-third of cases are spontaneous). Women who are known carriers undergo noninvasive ultrasound to determine the gender of the child. If the baby is male, a multidisciplinary approach is best to plan the mode of delivery and anesthesia. Procedures and monitoring methods should be noninvasive; avoiding forceps or vacuum delivery as well as fetal scalp electrodes, fetal venous sampling, and circumcision until laboratory confirmation is verified. Blood is typically obtained from the cord.

About 25% of people with hemophilia A develop inhibitors to factor VIII concentrates, while this occurs in only 3% to 5% of clients with hemophilia B. Inhibitors are typically antibodies that bind and remove the factor from the blood. Clients undergo routine testing for inhibitors or they may be noted when factor concentrates are not effective. If inhibitors are detected, individuals may receive bypassing products (rFVIIa or an activated prothrombin complex concentrate) for an episode of acute bleeding, or undergo immune tolerance therapy (ITI) (frequent infusions of factor) during times when there is no bleeding. (See previous section on inhibitors.)

***Hemophilia B.*** Treatment for clients with hemophilia B consists of factor IX concentrates. Recombinant factor IX concentrates do not use animal or human plasma proteins in the purification process, making the product safe from viruses. Pooled plasma–derived factor IX products are available, and like the factor VIII concentrates from pooled plasma, undergo a viral-depletion step. However, because of the safety factor of recombinant technology, recombinant factor IX concentrate is the medication of choice. Factor IX preparations are also available with an extended half-life.

***Pain Control.*** Comprehensive medical management of hemophilia may involve the use of drugs to control pain in acute bleeding and chronic arthropathies. People with hemophilia cannot use the common pain relievers aspirin or ibuprofen because these agents inhibit platelet function. More precisely, platelets do form an initial clot, but factor VIII or IX is unavailable to stabilize the clot. Some medications contain derivatives of aspirin and must be used cautiously. Corticosteroids or cyclooxygenase inhibitors are used occasionally and for a short duration for the treatment of chronic synovitis. Acetaminophen is a suitable aspirin substitute for pain control, especially in children. Most centers use opioid medications, such as codeine, to treat chronic pain for select individuals. For clients with cardiovascular disease, decisions regarding anticoagulation should be made in consultation with a hemophilia treatment center. Currently, there are no clinical practice guidelines on pain management in people with hemophilia who experience acute, disabling pain from hemarthroses and chronic arthropathy.[17,136,175]

***Gene Therapy.*** Gene therapy is still in experimental stages but appears very promising. When successful, gene therapy will deliver a normal (unaffected) copy of a gene into a target cell that contains a defective gene. Human trials are underway for hemophilias A and B using a variety of different delivery techniques. In fact, hemophilia is considered a model disease for treatment with gene therapy because it is caused by a single malfunctioning gene, and only a small increase in clotting factor could provide a great benefit.[358]

**Prognosis.** Years ago most males with hemophilia died in their youth. For the past 50 years, the care for individuals with hemophilia has improved significantly to the point that a newborn with hemophilia living in a developed nation can expect to have a normal life span and a high quality of life.[77] Currently, the majority of deaths in persons with hemophilia are due to liver failure (typically related to hepatitis B and C).[250]

Tremendous improvement has been made in carrier detection and prenatal diagnosis to provide early treatment and prevent complications. Gene therapy for hemophilias A and B holds promise of a cure, but whether gene therapy will be sufficiently safe and cost-effective to eventually replace factor-replacement therapy remains to be seen.[161,357,466] Additionally, home infusion therapy provides immediate treatment with clotting factor for joint and muscle bleeds recognized early. Early treatment has significantly reduced the morbidity formerly associated with hemophilia.

Medical treatment prolongs life and improves quality of life associated with improved joint function; however, people with severe hemophilia continue to have a significant number of bleeding episodes (one-third of people reported >5 bleeds/6 months) and 1 in 4 individuals continue to form target joints with associated disability and pain.[250]

Fortunately, improvements in blood screening tests, more stringent donor exclusion criteria, improved viral inactivation methods, and the introduction of recombinant hemophilia therapies have combined to dramatically reduce the rate of new bloodborne viral infections among people with hemophilia, especially those children born in the last 20 years.

ICH still remains a deadly complication of hemophilia, but prophylaxis treatment and improved understanding of the signs and symptoms associated with ICH may help to improve outcomes. Long-term effects of prophylaxis may present additional challenges in terms of safety, efficacy, and pharmacokinetics and remain the focus of research efforts. And with the normalization of lives as a result of improved treatment, new comorbidities are developing, including obesity, diabetes, cancer, and osteoporosis.[481] Clients with hemophilia continue to have significant quality of life issues, including social avoidance, occupational disability, chronic pain, and long-term sequelae from bleeding.[341]

SPECIAL IMPLICATIONS FOR THE THERAPIST 14.13

## *Hemophilia*

> **Note to Reader:**
> Only a brief discussion of treatment for the adult or child with hemophilia can be included in this text. For a more detailed examination, evaluation, and interventions, the reader is referred to other more specific publications by the National Hemophilia Foundation endorsed by the Medical and Scientific Advisory Committee (MASAC).[37,160,255,255,275,287-291]

Physical therapy intervention has been effective in reducing the number of bleeding episodes through protective strengthening of the musculature surrounding affected joints, muscle reeducation, gait training, and client education. Physical therapy is used during episodes of acute hemorrhage to control pain and additional bleeding and to maintain positioning and prevent further deformity.

Physical therapy intervention for individuals with hemophilia has undergone a drastic change. Two decades ago, everyone in the hemophilia community had joint disease in varying degrees of severity. Today treatment protocols are more aggressive, with more frequent infusions given at younger ages, resulting in less joint damage.[66] Many children with hemophilia are growing up without having a single joint bleed. The focus has shifted from rehabilitation to prevention; therapists are important health care professionals in helping these individuals lead normal, active lives.[66]

### Hemophilia, Physical Activity, and Exercise

A regular exercise program, including appropriate sports activities, resistance training, cardiovascular/aerobic training, and therapeutic strengthening and stretching exercises for affected extremities, is an important part of the comprehensive care of the individual with hemophilia.[416] In fact, regular physical activity and exercise can be considered a nonpharmacologic treatment used in conjunction with conventional treatment.[416]

The therapist can help individuals with hemophilia identify, seek out, and enjoy physical activity, exercise, and sport participation that provides benefits that outweigh the risks.[160] Patient/client education is key here because many people with bleeding disorders participate minimally in exercise[292] and have even expressed fear of exercise-induced bleeding, pain, or physical impairment.[275] But as Mulvany et al. demonstrated, with an individualized and supervised exercise program, benefits gained are measurable and significant, especially for those individuals with the most severe joint damage and coexisting illness.[275] The therapist can present the individual with evidence that refraining from exercise results in decreased strength, range of motion, function, and quality of life (see Mulvany et al.[275] for details).

Specific protocols for prescriptive exercise based on evidence are not yet available, leaving the physical therapist to design a program for each individual, relying on an understanding of tissue healing, best practice, expert opinions, and clinical judgment. Physical therapists may find a review of reference-based global recommendations and suggestions from clinicians with specialized training in the management of hemophilia valuable as provided by the Adult Bleeding Disorders Clinic in Canada.[27]

Vigorous physical activity may be transiently associated with a moderate relative risk of bleeding, but the absolute risk of bleeds is small.[33] Physical activity and exercise not only promote physical wellness in the form of improved work capacity, it also protects joints, enhances joint function, and is beneficial for decreasing the frequency of bleeds and has been shown to temporarily increase the levels of circulating clotting factor in individuals with a factor VIII deficiency.[293] Immobilization of joints can lead to deterioration of muscles, which, in turn, leads to joint instability and repeated bleeding and premature development of arthropathy.[271,427]

Growing evidence suggests that exercise, coupled with a healthy diet, may boost the immune system of people with hemophilia who also have HIV and/or are living with hepatitis C.[469] The therapist can be instrumental in helping the person with hemophilia to individualize an exercise or sports activity plan with specific but realistic goals and a schedule with alternating exercises (cross-training).

Although many factors related to joint bleeding are fixed, one risk factor that can be modified by the therapist is the body mass index. Clients with more severe disease develop joint problems earlier with accompanying range-of-motion problems. An increased body mass index also increases the risk of limited joint range-of-motion and may be a modifiable risk factor in clients with hemophilia.[410]

An overall therapy program includes client education early on for family, client, school personnel, and coaches for prevention, conditioning, and wellness. Specific guidelines are available, including all age levels from infants, toddlers, and preschoolers to adults, including sports safety information and the categorization of sports and activities by risk.[287]

For older children and adolescents, selecting a sport with a good chance of success and adequate preparation (e.g., stretching and flexibility, conditioning including strength and weight training, endurance including an aerobic component, and possibly infusion before participation) for the sport are crucial. There is some early evidence that high-intensity exercise can increase endogenous factor VIII in individuals with mild to moderately severe hemophilia, A. Further evidence is needed before promoting high-intensity activity to reduce bleeding risk prior to participation in sports.[144]

The National Hemophilia Foundation has mapped out categories of activity that are safe to participate in for anyone with hemophilia, along with precautions for some forms of exercise and contraindications to others (Table 14.5).

**Table 14.5** Categories of Activities Based on Risk

| Category 1 (Safest) | Category 2 (Moderately safe) | Category 3 (Potentially dangerous) |
|---|---|---|
| Archery | Baseball | All-terrain vehicle |
| Badminton | Basketball | Boxing |
| Bicycling | Bowling | High diving (competitive) |
| Dancing | Cross-country skiing | Football |
| Fishing | Diving (recreational) | Hockey |
| Frisbee | Dog sledding | Lacrosse |
| Golfing | Gymnastics | Motorcycling |
| Hiking | Horseback riding | Racquetball/handball |
| Ping pong | Ice skating | Rock climbing/rappelling |
| Snowshoeing | Jogging | Rugby |
| Swimming | Martial arts | Wrestling |
| Tai Chi/yoga/qi gong | Mountain biking | Power lifting; competitive weight lifting |
| Walking | River rafting | |
| Low-impact workout machines | Roller skating/blading | |
| | Rowing/crew | |
| | Running | |
| | Skiing (downhill or cross-country) | |
| | Snowboarding | |
| | Snowmobiling | |
| | Soccer | |
| | Tennis | |
| | Track and field | |
| | Volleyball | |
| | Water skiing | |
| | Weight lifting | |

This is not an exhaustive list of possible activities but provides a guideline to use when assessing activities for safety.
Data from Anderson, A, Forsyth, A: *Playing it safe: bleeding disorders, sports, and exercise*, National Hemophilia Foundation, 2012.

Category 1 involves primarily aerobic activities that are considered "safe" for most individuals with hemophilia. Category 1 activities build muscles to protect joints and help decrease the frequency of bleeds. Gaining flexibility and core strength through category 1 activities is a prerequisite for anyone with hemophilia before participating in category 2 activities.

Category 2 activities include sports and recreational activities in which the physical, social, and psychologic benefits of participation outweigh the risks. Individuals with severe hemophilia may have to avoid category 2 activities. Category 3 activities should be avoided by anyone with hemophilia; they are dangerous even for people without hemophilia. The risks outweigh the benefits.

Although it is obvious that some bleeding may result from participation in a sport, fewer bleeding episodes occur when children engage in physical activities on a regular basis than when they are sedentary. When a particular sport or activity is often followed by bleeding, then that activity should be reevaluated. A joint that requires multiple infusions to stop bleeding, remains symptomatic, or has persistent synovitis is not likely to withstand the stresses of a sport that relies on that joint.[287] Breakthrough bleeding despite prophylaxis occurs more often than previously recognized and should be part of a daily surveillance program.

As orthopedic problems occur, a problem-oriented program is developed specific to the pathology. Generally, a therapy program includes exercises to strengthen muscles and improve coordination; methods to prevent and reduce deformity; methods to influence abnormal muscle tone and pathologic patterns of movement; techniques to decrease pain; functional training related to everyday activities; special techniques such as manual traction and mobilization; massage; and physiotechnical modalities such as cold, heat (including ultrasound), and electric modalities. Orthotics may improve participation in activities and have been shown to reduce joint pain.[230,345]

Aquatic therapy is an excellent modality, especially for chronic arthropathy to improve physical functioning and quality of life.[195,461] The buoyancy of the water allows for ease of active movements across joints without the compressive force induced by gravity, thus decreasing pain. Water's density creates a resistive force to allow muscle strengthening, and the hydrostatic pressure can help reduce swelling.[195]

### *Guidelines to Strength Training*

In the past people with bleeding disorders were told to avoid strenuous exercise and any kind of weight training to avoid the risk of bleeding episodes. Today we know that a well-planned, supervised exercise program (Box 14.8) can be extremely beneficial to all

**Box 14.8**

**SUPERVISED EXERCISE PROGRAM FOR PEOPLE WITH BLEEDING DISORDERS AND HEMOPHILIC ARTHRITIS**

***Strength Training Protocol and Progression***

1. Progression to next level only if no adverse reaction to previous week of exercise.
2. Prophylaxis: Factor infusion recommended for people with severe hemophilia; people with mild and moderate hemophilia to have medications available, if needed.
3. Intensity: percent of isometric Nicholas dynamometry muscle test to assess pounds of weight to use or color of Thera-Band exercise band. The Hygenic Corporation[a] reports correspondence of colors to weight resistance as the following: yellow = 2.5 lb, red = 4.5 lb, green = 5.0 lb, blue = 7.5 lb, black = 9.0 lb, and silver = 15 lb.
4. Repetitions: to be done only in pain-free range.
5. Rate: 5-10 seconds concentric with exhale; 5-10 seconds eccentric with inhale.

**Level 1:** Prescribed for the most fragile joints, target joints, previously injured muscle, and joints with painful active range of motion, passive range of motion, or weight bearing. No acute swelling or bleeding within past 2 weeks.

| | Progression Intensity | No. of Repetitions | No. of Sets |
|---|---|---|---|
| Week 1 | 40% | 10 | 1 |
| Week 2 | 45%–50% | 10–20 | 2 |
| Week 3 | 50%–60% | 10–20 | 3 |
| Week 4 | 55%–65% | 10–20 | 3 |
| Week 5 | 60%–70% | 10–20 | 3 |
| Week 6 | 65%–75% | 10–20 | 3 |

**Level 2:** Prescribed for joints and muscles with history of bleeding and chronic, mild-to-moderate impairment. No bleeding in past 6 months.

| | Progression Intensity | No. of Repetitions | No. of Sets |
|---|---|---|---|
| Week 1 | 50% | 10 | 1 |
| Week 2 | 55%–60% | 10–20 | 2 |
| Week 3 | 60%–70% | 10–20 | 3 |
| Week 4 | 65%–75% | 10–20 | 3 |
| Week 5 | 70%–75% | 10–20 | 3 |
| Week 6 | 75% | 10–20 | 3 |

**Level 3:** Prescribed for joints and muscles with minimal history ofbleeding and no signs of impairment.

| | Progression Intensity | No. of Repetitions | No. of Sets |
|---|---|---|---|
| Week 1 | 60% | 10–20 | 1 |
| Week 2 | 65%–70% | 10–20 | 2 |
| Week 3 | 70%–75% | 10–20 | 3 |
| Week 4 | 75% | 10–20 | 3 |
| Week 5 | 75% | 10–20 | 3 |
| Week 6 | 75% | 10–20 | 3 |

***Example***

Participant 4, a 23-year-old man with severe hemophilia.

Right elbow = level 1: Target joint; had six episodes of bleeding over past 2 months. Active and passive range of motion painful at end range of flexion and extension. No acute swelling, no bleeding within past 2 weeks. Right biceps: isometric Nicholas dynamometry muscle test = 5 lb.

Left elbow = level 3: Only two episodes of bleeding in past. Last episode of bleeding was 2 years previously. Pain-free motion, no swelling or crepitus. Normal end-feel.

Left biceps: isometric Nicholas dynamometry muscle test = 30 lb.

Week 1:

Right elbow flexion: 40% of 5 lb = 2 lb or use yellow Thera-Band for 1 set of 10 repetitions in pain-free range.

Left elbow flexion: 60% of 30 lb = 18 lb or double thickness of black Thera-Band for 1 set of 10-20 repetitions in pain-free range.

[a] The Hygenic Corporation, 1245 Home Ave, Akron, OH 44310.

From Mulvany R, Zucker-Levin AR, Jeng M, et al: Effects of a 6-week, individualized, supervised exercise program for people with bleeding disorders and hemophilic arthritis, *Phys Ther* 90:509-526, 2010. Used with permission American Physical Therapy Association.

individuals with a bleeding disorder.[275] Weight training is still approached with caution as overly strenuous free-weight lifting can cause microtears in the muscles and intramuscular bleeds.[6,254]

Strength training, also known as resistance training, builds muscle, increases strength, stabilizes joints, improves circulation, and potentially reduces the risk of injury and spontaneous bleeding episodes. It is not body building, power lifting, or competitive weightlifting; these activities should be avoided.

The importance of warm-up and cool-down periods should be emphasized. Little or no weight is used until the individual can complete 10 to 15 repetitions with proper form. Weight or resistance can be gradually increased by 5% to 10% when the first phase of 10 to 15 repetitions is easy. The client should be reminded never to attempt to lift maximal weight.[6,9]

As with all strength training, it is best to utilize full pain-free range of motion slowly and with good breathing throughout the cycle of contraction and relaxation. Maintain adequate hydration at all times. Adolescents must especially be reminded that pain is a red flag to stop and seek help. Most injuries result from improper form and performing the exercise too fast. Any time an individual of any age with hemophilia experiences joint trauma or injury, strength training may have to be discontinued and gradually reintroduced after healing occurs.[6]

### Maintaining Joint Range of Motion

The therapist and client must be alert to recognize any signs of early (first 24-48 hours) bleeding episodes (Table 14.6). Providing immediate factor replacement to stop the bleeding and following the RICE (rest, ice, compression, and elevation) principle (Table 14.7) to promote comfort and healing are two goals for treating an acute joint (hemarthrosis) or muscle bleed (intramuscular hemorrhage).

The joint range of motion can be measured during this acute episode in the pain-free range but should not be strength tested. Elastic wraps, splints, slings, and/or assistive devices may be necessary and a tolerance and/or weaning schedule established. Static or dynamic night splints may be used to apply a low-load stretch to a muscle shortened because of an underlying condition such as synovitis or articular contracture.

A static splint made of plaster, synthetic casting materials, or thermoplastic splinting materials holds the joint in a single position. The material is molded to the extremity, then hardens, and straps are applied to keep it in place on the extremity. A static splint does not bend or straighten the joint. It must be remolded or remade as the individual gains range of motion.[191]

A dynamic splint applies a small amount of pressure (1-2 lb) to stretch a joint over a long period. The individual can still bend and straighten the joint and the therapist can adjust the amount of load applied as needed. There is less irritation and fewer bleeds with the dynamic splint.

**Table 14.7** Management of Joint and Muscle Bleeds

| Joint: Acute Stage | Joint: Subacute Stage | Muscle |
|---|---|---|
| Factor replacement<br>RICE<br>Pain-free movement; non (or minimal) weight-bearing<br>Pain medication; splinting and support as appropriate | Factor replacement (if indicated)<br>Progressive weight-bearing, movement, and exercises<br>Wean from splints and slings | Factor replacement<br>RICE<br>Progressive movement; appropriate weight-bearing status<br>Bed rest for iliopsoas bleed |

*RICE*, Rest, ice, compression (applying pressure to the area for at least 10-15 minutes), and elevation (immobilization and elevating the body part above the heart level while applying the ice).

Modified from Anderson A, Holtzman TS, Masley J: *Physical therapy in bleeding disorders,* New York, 2000, National Hemophilia Foundation. See also *Physical Therapy Practice Guidelines for Persons with Bleeding Disorders: Joint Bleeds.* Available online at http://www.hemophilia.org/sites/default/files/document/files/ptJointBleedGuidelines.pdf. Accessed July 11, 2014.

**Table 14.6** Clinical Signs and Symptoms of Hemophilia Bleeding Episodes

| Acute Hemarthrosis | Muscle Hemorrhage | Gastrointestinal Involvement | Central Nervous System Involvement |
|---|---|---|---|
| Aura, tingling, or prickling sensation<br>Stiffening into the position of comfort (usually flexion)<br>Decreased range of motion<br>Pain/tenderness<br>Swelling<br>Protective muscle spasm<br>Increased warmth around joint | Gradually intensifying pain<br>Protective spasm of muscle<br>Limitation of movement at the surrounding joints<br>Muscle assumes a position of comfort (usually shortened)<br>Loss of sensation | Abdominal pain and distention<br>Melena (blood in stool)<br>Hematemesis (vomiting blood)<br>Fever<br>Low abdominal/groin pain from bleeding into wall of large intestine or iliopsoas muscle<br>Hip flexion contracture due to spasm of the iliopsoas muscle secondary to retroperitoneal hemorrhage | Impaired judgment<br>Decreased visual and spatial awareness<br>Short-term memory deficits<br>Inappropriate behavior<br>Motor deficits: spasticity, ataxia, abnormal gait, apraxia, decreased balance, loss of coordination |

Modified from Goodman CC, Snyder TE: *Differential diagnosis for the physical therapist: screening for referral,* ed 5, Philadelphia, 2013, WB Saunders.

Repeated bleeds in the same area can cause a muscle to shorten, limiting joint range of motion. Individuals with inhibitors or limited access to treatment are at increased risk for this type of problem. Night splints may be a good option for people who have muscle contractures that are not responding to other treatment interventions. The desired effect can be obtained in 6 to 8 weeks for individuals who do not have an inhibitor. For those clients with inhibitors, night splinting can take much longer (6 months to 1 year).[191] Serial casting may be a better choice for clients with long-standing problems; either splinting or casting should be used before resorting to surgery.[127,366]

The therapist must watch for leg length discrepancy as a long-term result of joint arthropathy. Even minor discrepancies can affect standing posture and gait mechanics and contribute to low back pain and other lower quadrant impairments. Shoe lifts in conjunction with appropriate prophylactic therapy and exercise can be effective.[150,190]

### Specific Exercise Guidelines

Initiation of exercise after a bleed must be delayed, and rehabilitation progress is typically slower for individuals with factor VIII and factor IX deficiency who develop factor inhibitors. Prognosis for full return of function is diminished in such cases. In all cases of joint bleed, the use of heat is contraindicated; if used, hydrotherapy or aquatic intervention must be performed in comfortable but not hot temperatures to avoid blood vessel dilation.

When active bleeding stops, isometric muscle exercise should be initiated to prevent muscular atrophy. This exercise is especially critical with recurrent knee hemarthroses to prevent the visible atrophy of the quadriceps femoris muscle. As pain and edema diminish, the client should begin gentle active range-of-motion exercises, followed by slowly progressing strengthening exercises when the joint is pain free through its full range. In the case of an iliopsoas bleed, when ambulation is resumed, crutches and toe-touch weight bearing are initiated. Active movement should be performed in a pain-free range and progressed very slowly.

For all muscles, as the strengthening program is progressed, strengthening aids such as elastic bands or tubing and cuff weights can be used before transitioning to weight equipment. Preadolescents should avoid using high–weight lifting machines.

Postbleed exercise should also take into consideration any damage that may have occurred to the joint, such as ligamentous or capsular stretching. Closed chain and other exercises to restore proprioception should be incorporated into the rehabilitation program.

As a prophylactic measure, clients with severe hemophilia generally need to infuse with clotting factor when participating in a strengthening program. With careful supervision and progression of the exercise program, the individual can progress to aerobic activities.

In some individuals, increased stress levels result in increased frequency of spontaneous bleeding. Biofeedback may be considered especially helpful for these clients who experience spontaneous bleeding during emotional upsets and periods of depression. Biofeedback can also be used for muscle retraining or relaxation techniques to control muscle spasm and allow range of motion.

### Psychosocial Aspects of Hemophilia

Psychosocial factors have a significant impact on quality of life for individuals with chronic diseases such as hemophilia. Physical therapists have an important role in supporting the psychosocial needs of affected individuals as well as their families. Providing information and assistance, answering questions, and teaching coping strategies to minimize the impact of disabilities may help to maximize functional outcomes and improve quality of life for the individual and their families.[49]

The physical therapist can be helpful in encouraging consistent adherence to prophylaxis, an essential part of the treatment program to prevent and control bleeding episodes and their debilitating complications.[374,383] Technology such as web-based and mobile tools can help track bleeding episodes and infusions to assist individuals in managing this disease. The first tool available for this purpose (called ATHNadvoy) was developed in 2001 and donated to the American Thrombosis & Hemostasis Network in 2010.

A recent review of the literature[49] in this area showed that quality of life is reduced in persons with hemophilia, with a potential impact on education, employment and career, interpersonal relationships, family dynamics, and lifestyle decisions.[147,304] These findings were especially true when prophylactic treatment was not available. Carrier status in women may have a psychosocial impact and affect reproductive choices. There is a need for more international, multifaceted research to explore and quantify the social and psychological aspects of life with hemophilia.[49]

Depression is known to increase in individuals of all ages with chronic illnesses and early childhood trauma. Adults with hemophilia who also have life-threatening comorbidities associated with hemophilia (e.g., hepatitis C and/or HIV) are especially at risk for depression. The physical therapist may need to screen for depression (or suggest screening to the multidisciplinary team); a comprehensive treatment program that includes treatment for depression may improve overall health outcomes.[186]

### The Older Adult with Hemophilia

Life expectancy has increased dramatically with modern treatment for hemophilia extending life expectancy to nearly that of the general population.[202,424] Adults with hemophilia are reaching older age and experiencing various age-related health conditions never before seen in this population.[202] Consequently, they are not spared from other health care concerns, such as diabetes, heart disease, stroke, or cancer. The management of comorbidities may be complicated even more by the bleeding disorder. Age-related orthopedic comorbidities include degenerative joint changes, osteoporosis, muscle atrophy or sarcopenia, muscle weakness, and disturbance of gait and balance. Increased pain, muscle weakness and atrophy, along with an increased risk of falling are key features of advanced hemophilic arthropathy and aging.[424]

Although today's treatments have reduced the number and severity of joint bleeds, middle-aged and older adults with hemophilia did not have the benefit of powdered concentrates and prompt home care earlier on in their lives.

As children they were hospitalized and/or bed bound with casts, packed in ice while whole blood was administered slowly by intravenous drip. It took days for their levels to go up. Before factor replacement, it could take weeks to get a joint bleed under control. The consequence of this type of treatment was contracted joints and severe arthritis.[41]

Today's older adult still may not have quick and easy access to factor replacement. Mobility impairments can make it difficult, if not impossible, to get to a hemophilia treatment center. Loss of fine motor control or the onset of tremors makes self-care at home equally problematic.

The therapist can begin education about long-term planning with middle-aged clients. Introducing the idea of home modifications to improve accessibility should begin early. The importance of staying active cannot be overemphasized. All older adults find that recovery time and rehabilitation take longer as they advance through the decades. Resuming normal activities after injury, surgery, or health conditions that set them back is extremely important.[41]

It is also important to keep educating young clients who are noncompliant with their treatment and ignore recommendations. These individuals likely will have problems in the future similar to those experienced by today's older adult population, who did not have the benefit of modern treatment interventions.

The same is true for young adults during the college years or transitioning from living at home with adult supervision during high school to living on their own independently. For many people with bleeding disorders, this is the first time they will assume "ownership" of their disease.[254] Maintaining physical fitness at every stage of life is a key part of management for hemophilia.

### Orthopedic, Surgical, and Medical Interventions

Whereas factor replacement can be used to control bleeding associated with surgery, any operative or invasive medical procedure can create complications for individuals with hemophilia, especially those who develop inhibitors. For example, deep venous thromboses are a concern for individuals with bleeding disorders who require central venous catheters. According to one study,[72] central venous catheter–related deep venous thrombosis is common in children with inherited bleeding disorders and likely occurs earlier than previously thought.

Sometimes, even with optimal infusion therapy and aggressive hemophilia care, a joint becomes a chronic problem. In such cases orthopedic or surgical intervention may be indicated to alleviate pain and deformity and to restore the joint to a more functional state. This may include prescription for an orthosis or a splint or serial casting to increase range of motion. Joint replacement (arthroplasty) is now a treatment option as well.

*Synovectomy* (removal of the joint synovium) is recommended to stop a target joint from its cycle of bleeding. This procedure is not usually done to improve range of motion or to decrease pain, but rather to reduce the rate of destruction and prevent further damage to the joint caused by bleeding. Arthroscopic synovectomy is best performed before joint degeneration has progressed beyond stage II on the Arnold-Hilgartner scale (see Box 14.7).

Injection of a radioactive isotope (referred to as *isotopic synovectomy* or *synoviorthesis*, usually phosphorus-32 in the United States), which causes scarring to the synovium to arrest bleeding, is an option. This procedure has unique advantages and disadvantages and may be more appropriate for one type of client than another.[93,94]

*Arthroplasty* (joint replacement) is indicated when a joint shows end-stage damage and has become extremely painful. Client age, range of motion, and level of pain and function are determinants as to the timing of this procedure. Knees, hips, and shoulders are most commonly helped through arthroplasty, with restoration of pain-free joint movement.

The benefits of a 6-week preoperative physical therapy program (prehabilitation) combined with 6 weeks of postoperative rehabilitation have been demonstrated. An individually tailored and supervised program to increase range of motion and muscle strength enables rapid mobilization and recovery of function while minimizing the risk of bleeding.[425]

Long-term results of joint replacement are still under investigation. Mechanical survival of the implant is reported as good or excellent for 80% of knees, but complication rates are higher than in the nonhemophilic population and the incidence of late infection (months to years later) resulting in implant failure remains high (16%).[302,403,470]

With anyone with a bleeding disorder, the question of thromboembolic prophylaxis comes up. Although the American College of Chest Physicians and the American Academy of Orthopaedic Surgeons have set guidelines for thromboembolic prophylaxis in the general population, no such standard of care is in place for individuals with hemophilia. The risk of thrombosis in people with hemophilia following joint replacement (hip and knee) is thought to be lower, but cases have been reported of pulmonary embolism and deep vein thrombosis in these individuals.[422]

*Arthrodesis* (joint fusion) may be performed in a joint with advanced, painful arthropathy untreatable by arthroplasty. Joint fusion can relieve or eliminate pain to provide improved quality of life, but it also causes permanent loss of joint motion. Arthrodesis can be a very effective way to provide the individual a more stable base for weight-bearing activities.

*Osteotomy* (removal of a section of bone) may be done to correct angular deformities in a joint and may be considered before arthroplasty to reduce the stresses placed on a joint caused by poor alignment. Other, less-common interventions may include excision of a hemophilia pseudotumor or removal of cysts or exostoses.

### The Person with Hemophilia and HIV

It is important for anyone with both hemophilia and HIV to maintain optimal care of their musculoskeletal systems during and between bleeding episodes. It is especially important in the presence of chronic arthropathy and HIV or AIDS to maintain joint function through nonsurgical means, especially exercise.

Surgery may be contraindicated if the risk of infection is too great (e.g., when the CD4 cell count is less than 200). Activities such as tai chi and yoga provide stretching, strengthening (including weight bearing), and a mild aerobic component. Aquatics or swimming must be approached with caution because of the potential for transmission of *Cryptosporidium* oocysts, which cause infection in immunocompromised individuals.

## Thrombocytopenia

Thrombocytopenia, a decrease in the platelet count below 150,000/microL of blood, is caused by inadequate platelet production from the bone marrow, increased platelet destruction outside the bone marrow, or splenic sequestration (entrapment of blood and enlargement in the spleen). Thrombocytopenia can be further divided into mild (100,00 to 150,000/microL), moderate (50,000 to 99,000/microL), and severe (less than 50,000/microL).

Medications and supplements are a common cause of thrombocytopenia and should be reviewed with the client, including those taken over-the-counter. Alcohol and drug use, including quantity and frequency, should also be noted. Viral infections, such as hepatitis C and HIV, can lead to thrombocytopenia as well as thyroid disorders. Thrombocytopenia is a common complication of leukemia or metastatic cancer (bone marrow infiltration) and aggressive cancer chemotherapy (cytotoxic agents). Thrombotic thrombocytopenic purpura (TTP) (typically due to an antibody against ADAMTS13) and immune thrombocytopenic purpura (ITP)(antibodies against platelet proteins) are uncommon causes of thrombocytopenia with serious complications requiring immediate medical attention. Box 14.9 lists other causes.

Mucosal bleeding is the most common event and occurs by simply blowing the nose or brushing the teeth. Other sites of mucosal bleeding may include the uterus, GI tract, urinary tract, respiratory tract, and brain (ICH). Symptoms include epistaxis (frequent and difficult to stop), petechiae and/or purpura in the skin (especially the legs) and oropharynx, easy bruising, melena, hematuria, excessive menstrual bleeding, and gingival bleeding. Spontaneous bleeding may be seen with platelet counts less than 10,000/microL. For clients undergoing surgery, there is an increased risk of bleeding with platelet counts less than 50,000/microL and a platelet count of over 100,000/microL is preferred for neurosurgical procedures.

Box 14.9

**CAUSES OF THROMBOCYTOPENIA**

***Increased Platelet Destruction***

- Immune thrombocytopenic purpura (ITP)
- Drug-induced (immune-related) (heparin, penicillins, sulfonamides)
- Thrombotic thrombocytopenic purpura (TTP)
- Disseminated intravascular coagulation (DIC)
- Hemolytic uremic syndrome (HUS)
- Antiphospholipid syndrome (APS)
- Bypass during heart surgery
- Mechanical heart valve

***Decreased Platelet Production***

- Bone marrow infiltration (metastatic neoplasms, myelofibrosis, granulomatous disease)
- Bacterial infections
- Viral infections (HIV, cytomegalovirus, hepatitis C)
- Nutritional deficiencies (folate, vitamin $B_{12}$)
- Myelodysplasia
- Aplastic anemia
- Drug-induced (non–immune-related) (alcohol, chemotherapy agents, valproic acid)

***Platelet Sequestration in the Spleen***

- Splenomegaly

Diagnosis requires laboratory examination of blood and perhaps bone marrow (if clinically indicated) to confirm the diagnosis. Examination of the peripheral smear can distinguish between pseudothrombocytopenia and true thrombocytopenia. Pseudothrombocytopenia occurs when platelets clump together due to antibodies the person has to EDTA (which is in the collection tube), and a true count is not possible. If clumps are seen on the peripheral smear, blood can be drawn in a tube containing heparin or citrate to bypass this complication. In cases of confirmed thrombocytopenia the peripheral smear lacks a significant amount of platelets, which is verified by machine count.

Treatment depends on the precipitating cause. Cessation of offending medications, supplements, drugs or alcohol can resolve many cases. Transfusions are frequently used as a part of cancer therapy. TTP is treated with immediate plasma exchange, removing high-molecular-weight VWF multimers and replacing the deficient ADAMTS13. Glucocorticoids are also utilized to decrease antibody production. ITP is treated once a person is symptomatic (i.e., bleeding) or the platelet count is below 30,000/microL. First-line treatment consists of glucocorticoids or intravenous immune globulin (IVIG).

The prognosis is variable depending on the underlying cause; it is poor when associated with leukemia or aplastic anemia but good with conditions amenable to treatment.

SPECIAL IMPLICATIONS FOR THE THERAPIST 14.14

### *Thrombocytopenia*

Thrombocytopenia can cause bleeding into the muscles or joints, and the therapist may encounter the severe consequences of this condition. The therapist must be alert for obvious skin or mucous membrane symptoms of thrombocytopenia, such as severe bruising, external hematomas, and the presence of petechiae.

Such signs usually indicate a platelet level below 150,000/mm$^3$. Instruct the client to watch for signs of thrombocytopenia and when noted to immediately apply ice and pressure to any external bleeding site. They should avoid aspirin and aspirin-containing compounds without a physician's approval because of the risk of increased bleeding.

Strenuous exercise or any exercise that involves straining or bearing down could precipitate a hemorrhage, particularly of the eyes or brain. Exercise prescription is highly individualized and should take into account intensity, duration, and frequency appropriate for the individual's condition, age, and previous activity level.

Blood pressure cuffs and similar devices must be used with caution. When used, elastic support stockings must be thigh high, never knee high. Mechanical compression with a pneumatic pump and soft tissue mobilization are contraindicated unless approved by the physician. Practice good handwashing and observe carefully for any signs of infection.

## Effects of Aspirin and Other Nonsteroidal Antiinflammatory Drugs on Platelet Function

Acquired disorders of platelet function can occur through the use of aspirin and other NSAIDs that inactivate platelet cyclooxygenase. This key enzyme is required for the production of thromboxane $A_2$, a potent inducer of platelet aggregation and constrictor of arterial smooth muscle.

A single dose of aspirin can suppress normal platelet aggregation for 48 hours or longer (up to 1 week) until newly formed platelets have been released. Platelets are anucleated, and once aspirin irreversibly inhibits cyclooxygenase, the platelet is unable to synthesize new enzyme and remains inactive for the rest of its life span.

NSAIDs have less-potent antiplatelet effects than aspirin because they reversibly inhibit cyclooxygenase-1 (COX-1). Symptoms from this phenomenon are mild and may consist of easy bruising and bleeding, usually confined to the skin. NSAIDS that bind COX-2 have no effect on platelet function. The use of aspirin or NSAIDs is usually contraindicated before any surgical procedure. Prolonged oozing following dental procedures or surgery may occur.

## Disseminated Intravascular Coagulation

### Definition and Overview

Disseminated intravascular coagulation (DIC), sometimes referred to as *consumption coagulopathy*, is a process of uncontrolled activation of both coagulation and fibrinolysis. DIC may be acute (uncompensated and life-threatening) or chronic (compensated and subclinical).

It is an acquired disorder with diffuse or widespread coagulation occurring within blood vessels all over the body. DIC is actually a paradoxic condition in which clotting and hemorrhage occur simultaneously within the vascular system. Hemorrhage may occur in the kidneys, brain, liver, adrenals, heart, and other organs.

### Incidence and Etiologic Factors

DIC is common and in a study performed at tertiary care hospitals, was diagnosed in 1% of admissions.[248] It is particularly associated with sepsis, obstetric/gynecologic complications, cancer, intravascular hemolysis, and massive trauma. People with acute promyelocytic leukemia may present with acute DIC at high risk for serious hemorrhaging. Pancreatic cancer and other mucinous cancers, such as colon, gastric, breast, prostate, and ovarian cancer, also increase the risk of developing DIC.

### Pathogenesis

In the normal steady state there is a balance between the procoagulant and the anticoagulant factors, which keeps blood flowing. If an injury occurs, the coagulation process is initiated, with the resultant formation of a clot only where the vessel is damaged. Once the clot is stabilized, there is gradual breakdown of the clot as the tissue is repaired. There are also feedback systems that balance the timing and scale of responses. When DIC occurs there is serious disruption of this system. Several procoagulant factors can instigate DIC. The most common include tissue factor (TF), which becomes exposed after disruption of a vessel; bacterial components; DNA, histones, and DNA-binding proteins (extracellular); proteolytic enzymes produced by mucinous cancers; and microparticles that may contain TF. Once a procoagulant initiates coagulation, a cascade of events follows, resulting in the production of thrombi in small and large vessels. Thrombi consist of fibrin and platelets. Fibrinolysis (the breakdown of fibrin) then begins, creating fibrin degradation products (FDP). If FDPs are present in large amounts, they can interfere with both fibrin clot formation and platelet aggregation (acting as an anticoagulant).

Acute DIC may occur when large amounts of a procoagulant are exposed to blood (such as TF) or are present in the blood. This large exposure leads to a broad activation of the coagulation system, using clotting factors faster than they are produced and released, and forming thrombi throughout the vasculature. Once fibrinolysis is initiated, the FDPs produced interfere with further formation of clots. The loss of coagulation factors paired with the inability to form a clot promotes bleeding. Acute DIC is seen in people with sepsis, trauma, malignancy, or ABO-incompatible blood transfusions.

If the blood is exposed to small amounts of a procoagulant, chronic DIC may develop. Chronic DIC progresses at a slower rate than acute DIC, with the liver able to compensate by adequately producing coagulation factors and clearing FDPs. Due to this compensation, individuals with chronic DIC may experience thrombosis more frequently than hemorrhaging. Chronic DIC is more common in people with malignancy (mucinous cancers).

In DIC, the formation of thrombi, with complete occlusion or reduced perfusion of blood, along with bleeding leads to tissue and organ damage.

### Clinical Manifestations

Both acute and chronic DIC may present with thrombosis, bleeding or both, although chronic DIC typically presents with thrombosis instead of bleeding. Clients with acute DIC may demonstrate oozing from venipuncture sites, catheters, or areas of trauma. Nosebleeds or petechiae may be noted. More serious hemorrhaging can occur in the CNS, the gastrointestinal tract, or the lungs. Clients may experience delirium or focal neurologic deficits; hematochezia or melena; while hemorrhaging in the lungs causes difficulty breathing and hypoxia. Both venous thromboembolism and arterial thrombosis occur, causing ischemia to tissues and organs. This may manifest as acute renal failure or liver dysfunction. Jaundice may develop with hepatic dysfunction.

### MEDICAL MANAGEMENT

**DIAGNOSIS, TREATMENT, AND PROGNOSIS.** Diagnosis is made based on clinical presentation in combination with client history and laboratory testing. Laboratory findings suggestive of DIC include elevated D-dimer levels, prolonged PT and aPTT, thrombocytopenia, low fibrinogen, and presence of schistocytes (red cell fragments) on peripheral blood smear.

Treatment is always directed toward the underlying cause and must be highly individualized according to the person's age, nature and origin of DIC, site and severity of hemorrhage or thrombosis, and other clinical parameters. The hemorrhagic or thrombotic symptoms may be alleviated by appropriate blood product replacement, but the coagulopathy will continue until the causative process is reversed. Supportive methods include platelet and RBC transfusions, fresh frozen plasma, and cryoprecipitate for people who are hemorrhaging.[464,465] Heparin may be considered in cases where thrombotic features are dominant and the client is nonsymptomatic (such as chronic DIC).[464,465] Synthetic protease inhibitors and antifibrinolytic therapy (such as tranexamic acid) may be appropriate for people with significant bleeding due to a hyperfibrinolytic state, while natural protease inhibitors may be utilized to treat organ failure.

Morbidity and mortality are dependent on the extent of thrombosis, degree of hemorrhaging, and ability to correct the underlying disorder. Morbidity and mortality can be high for those whose underlying disease process is difficult to treat, such as sepsis and trauma.[464,465]

**SPECIAL IMPLICATIONS FOR THE THERAPIST 14.15**

#### *Disseminated Intravascular Coagulation*

Clients with DIC are treated by the therapist in oncology or intensive care units. DIC is either the consequence of malignancy or the end result of multisystem organ failure after trauma affecting multiple systems (e.g., severe trauma or burns).

Clients are in critical condition and require bedside care. Care must be taken to avoid dislodging clots and causing new onset of bleeding. Monitor the results of serial blood studies, particularly hematocrit, hemoglobin, and coagulation times prior to any intervention. To prevent injury, bed rest during bleeding episodes is required.

When monitoring vital signs, watch for hypotension and tachycardia. Regularly assess for signs and symptoms of bleeding, such as bleeding gums, bruising, petechiae, nosebleeds, reports of melena or hematuria, headaches, or changes in mental status. Assess the skin for necrosis and hematomas.

## Hemoglobinopathies

Several diseases result from an abnormality in the formation of hemoglobin (Hb). Because Hb is essential for life, anomalies in the shape, size, content, or oxygen-carrying capacity can lead to severe problems. Sickle cell disease and thalassemia are two hemoglobinopathies with potential for serious complications and are discussed further.

Hereditary spherocytosis, hereditary elliptocytosis, hereditary stomatocytosis, and pyropoikilocytosis are rare diseases that occur because of defects in the erythrocyte membrane that cause premature clearance of RBCs (hemolysis). Glucose-6-phosphate dehydrogenase deficiency also leads to hemolysis. Discussions of these diseases can be found elsewhere.

### Sickle Cell Disease

**Overview and Incidence.** *Sickle cell disease* (SCD) is an autosomal recessive disorder characterized by the presence of an abnormal form of Hb, called hemoglobin S (Hb S), within the erythrocytes. This irregular form of Hb is the result of a single mutation in the β-Hb chain where the amino acid glutamic acid at position 6 is substituted with valine.

The presence of Hb S can cause RBCs to change from their usual biconcave disk shape to a crescent or sickle shape once the oxygen is released (deoxygenated) or under hypoxic conditions. SCD occurs when two sickle cell genes are inherited (one from each parent) or one sickle cell gene and another abnormal Hb is inherited, so that almost all of the Hb is abnormal.

*Homozygous Hb SS* occurs when an individual inherits two sickle cell genes. *Heterozygous Hb SC* is the result of inheriting one sickle cell gene and one gene for another abnormal type of Hb called C. Persons with this type of abnormality have fewer complications than those with homozygous Hb S, but they exhibit more ophthalmologic and orthopedic complications, due to increased blood viscosity.

Heterozygous *Hb S β-thalassemia* is the result of inheriting one sickle cell gene and one gene for a type of thalassemia, another inherited anemia. β-Thalassemias are caused by genetic mutations that abolish or reduce production of the β-globin subunit of Hb.

The sickle cell trait refers to people who carry only one *Hb S* gene and is discussed at the end of this section. Hb F, or fetal Hb, is found in infants. Although most infants switch to making α- and β-Hb, some continue to make Hb F, termed hereditary persistence of Hb F. Those people who inherit one sickle gene and the hereditary persistence of Hb F abnormalities make $\alpha_2\gamma_2$ Hb and do not develop the severe symptoms of SCD.

Although exact numbers are not available, the Centers for Disease Control and Prevention estimates that 1 of every 365 African American newborns and 1 of every 16,300 Hispanic Americans has SCD. It is further estimated that 100,000 Americans have SCD and 1 in 13 African American babies has sickle cell trait.[52] It is a worldwide health problem, affecting many races, countries, and ethnic groups, and is the most common inherited hematologic disorder. The WHO estimates that each year more than 300,000 babies are born worldwide with severe Hb disorders.[443] The disease is particularly common among people whose ancestors come from sub-Saharan Africa, India, Saudi Arabia, and Mediterranean countries.

Sickle cell disease carries significant morbidity and mortality, as well as economic costs. From 1989 to 1993, over $475 million was spent on hospitalizations alone.[52]

The two primary pathophysiologic features of sickle cell disorders are chronic hemolytic anemia and vasoocclusion resulting in ischemic injury. Children with SCD are at increased risk for severe morbidity and mortality, especially during the first 3 years of life.

When a sickled cell reoxygenates, the cell resumes a normal shape, but after repeated cycles of sickling and unsickling the erythrocyte is permanently damaged and hemolyzes. This hemolysis is responsible for the anemia that is a hallmark of SCD. A brief discussion of the related sickle cell syndromes is presented, but only the most severe disorder, sickle cell anemia, is fully discussed in this text.

**Etiologic Factors.** The cause of SCD and its worldwide incidence is the result of several factors. The sickle cell trait may have developed as a single genetic mutation that provided a selective advantage against severe forms of falciparum malaria.

Anyone who carries the inherited trait for SCD but does not have the actual illness is more resistant against this form of malaria. In countries with malaria, children born with sickle cell trait survived and then passed the gene for SCD to their offspring. As populations migrated (including the slave trade), the sickle cell trait and SCD moved throughout the world.

Several theories purport to explain the origination of SCD, but its actual origin is unknown. Four separate haplotypes are known; each is related to the severity of illness and each is associated with a different geographic location, including different locations in Africa, eastern Saudi Arabia, and India.

**Risk Factors.** Because SCD is inherited as an autosomal recessive trait, both parents of an offspring must have the Hb S gene. When both parents have sickle cell trait, they have a 25% chance with each pregnancy of having a child with sickle cell anemia. If one parent has sickle cell trait and the other has a β-thalassemic disorder, they are at the same risk for having a child with a sickle β-thalassemia syndrome.

In couples in which one individual has sickle cell trait and one has Hb C trait, the chance of having a child with Hb SC disease is also 25% with each pregnancy. If one parent has SCD and the other has the sickle cell trait, the risk of having a child with SCD is 50% (Fig. 14.14).

Individuals with sickle cell trait can receive nondirective genetic counseling (given objective information without personal bias and without provision of specific recommendations) after Hb electrophoresis and other measurements have been performed on each prospective parent.

Risk factors likely to induce symptoms or episodes, previously called crises, are factors that cause physiologic stress, resulting in sickling of the erythrocytes. Stress from viral or bacterial infection, hypoxia, dehydration, extreme temperatures (hot or cold), alcohol consumption, or fatigue may precipitate an episode.

Additionally, episodes may be precipitated by the presence of acidosis; exposure to low oxygen tensions as a result of strenuous physical exertion, climbing to high altitudes, flying in nonpressurized planes, or undergoing anesthesia without receiving adequate oxygenation; pregnancy; trauma; and fever. Any of these factors may increase the body's need for oxygen, increasing the percentage of erythrocytes that deoxygenate, thereby precipitating an episode.

**Pathogenesis.** The sickle cell defect occurs in Hb, the oxygen-carrying constituent of erythrocytes. Hb contains four chains of amino acids. Two of the amino acid chains are known as *α-globin chains*, and two are called *β-globin chains*.

In normal Hb, the amino acid in the sixth position on the β-globin chains is glutamic acid. In people with SCD, the sixth position is occupied by another amino acid, valine (Fig. 14.15). This single-point mutation of valine for glutamic acid results in a loss of two negative charges that causes surface abnormalities. The sickle Hb transports oxygen normally, but after releasing oxygen, those Hb molecules that contain the β-globin chain defect stick to one another instead of remaining separate. The Hb then polymerizes (change molecular arrangement), forming long, rigid rods or tubules inside RBCs.

The higher the concentration of deoxygenated sickle Hb molecules and the lower the blood pH, the faster the polymerization occurs.[339] The rods cause the normally smooth, doughnut-shaped RBCs to take on a sickle or curved shape and to lose their vital ability to deform and squeeze through tiny blood vessels (Fig. 14.16).

For a time, this sickling is reversible because the cells are reoxygenated in the lungs; however, eventually the change becomes irreversible. In the process of sickling and unsickling, the erythrocyte membrane becomes damaged and the cells are removed (hemolyzed).

The sickled cells can adhere to the endothelium of blood vessels, which in small vessels can become occluded, depriving tissue from receiving an adequate blood supply. Under stress, tissues experience increased oxygen requirements, which causes more Hb to release its oxygen, leading to increased numbers of deoxygenated and polymerized cells.

Deoxygenation of sickle cells induces potassium (followed by water) efflux, which increases cell density and the tendency of Hb S to polymerize. The sickle cell also has a chemical on the cell surface that binds to blood vessel walls, leading to endothelial cell activation. As a result, these sickle-shaped, rigid, sticky blood cells cannot pass through the capillaries, blocking the flow of blood.

Occlusion of the microcirculation increases hypoxia, which causes more erythrocytes to sickle; thus a vicious cycle is precipitated. This accumulation of sickled erythrocytes obstructing blood vessels produces tissue injury.

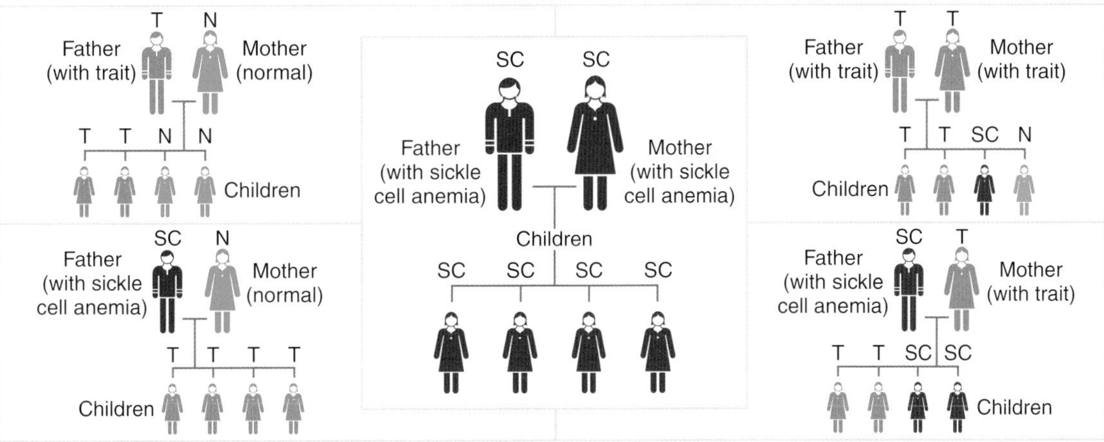


**Figure 14.14**

**Statistical probabilities of inheriting sickle cell anemia.** (Reprinted from O'Toole MT: *Miller-Keane encyclopedia and dictionary of medicine, nursing, and allied health,* rev ed, Philadelphia, 2005, WB Saunders.)

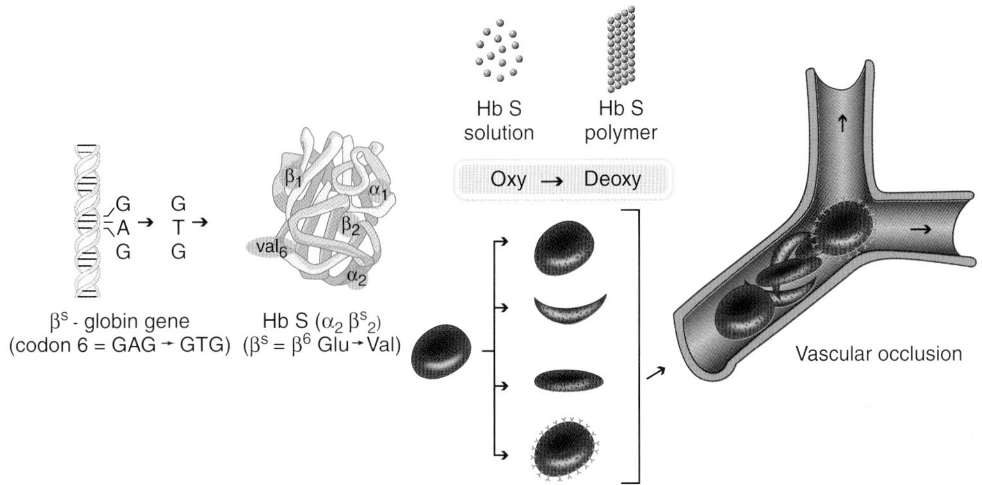


**Figure 14.15**

**Schematic view of the pathophysiologic characteristics of SCD.** The double-stranded DNA molecule on the *left* represents a β-globin gene in which a GAG→GTG substitution in the sixth codon has created the sickle cell gene. Valine is substituted for glutamic acid as the sixth amino acid, creating a mutant Hb tetramer (Hb S). A tetramer is a protein with four subunits (tetrameric). Hb S loses solubility and polymerizes when deprived of oxygen. Upon deoxygenation, most sickle cells lose deformability. Some cells sickle; a fraction becomes dehydrated, irreversibly sickled, and poorly deformable; a few become highly adherent. Vasoocclusion *(right)* is initiated by adherent cells sticking to the vascular endothelium, thereby creating a nidus that traps rigid cells and facilitates linking together in a chain formation, a process called polymerization. (Reprinted from Goldman L: *Cecil textbook of medicine,* ed 22, Philadelphia, 2004, WB Saunders.)

The organs at greatest risk are those with sluggish circulation, low pH, and a high level of oxygen extraction (spleen and bone marrow) or those with a limited terminal arterial supply (eye, head of the femur). No tissue or organ is spared from this injury. The higher the concentration of deoxygenated cells, the more severe (clinically) the complications.

Average sickle RBCs last only 10 to 20 days (normal is 120 days). The RBCs cannot be replaced fast enough, and anemia is the result. Although significant injury occurs in the microvasculature as a result of sickling, the most severe complication of SCD is a cerebral infarct, which occurs in the large blood vessels, where blood is moving rapidly and the diameter is wide.

Research has shown that not only are the Hb cells abnormal, but so are the blood vessel walls. This is likely a product of sickle cells adhering to and damaging endothelium, which leads to an inflammatory response of WBCs, cytokines, chemoattractants, and procoagulants. Over time, smooth muscle cells migrate into the wall, where they proliferate and narrow the lumen of the vessel.[338]

Significantly narrowed or stenotic arteries can further collect sickled cells, thereby occluding the lumen, resulting in stroke. Further complicating stroke and pulmonary hypertension is the lack of nitric oxide production. Normally, when hypoxia is present, nitric oxide is produced to cause local vasodilation, inhibit endothelial damage, and prevent proliferation of vascular smooth muscle.[458] However, free hemoglobin, released due to hemolysis, scavenges nitric oxide, thus blocking the normal beneficial effects of nitric oxide.[196] Hemolyzed erythrocytes also

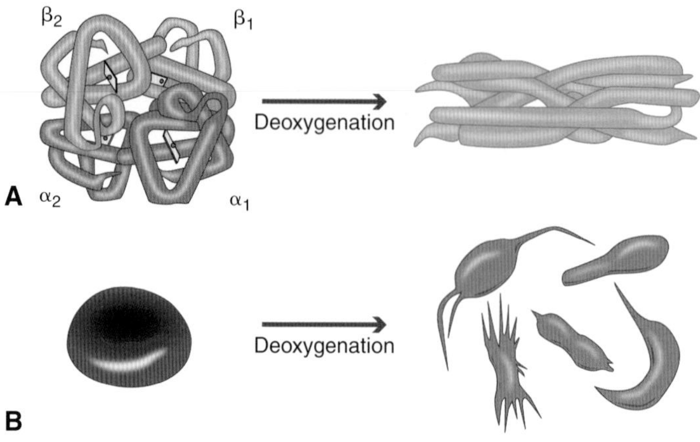


**Figure 14.16**

(A) The molecular structure of Hb contains a pair of α polypeptide chains and a pair of α chains, each wrapped around a heme group (an iron atom in a porphyrin ring). The quaternary structure of the Hb molecule enables it to carry up to four molecules of oxygen. In the folded β-globin chain molecule, the sixth position contacts the α-globin chain. The amino acid substitution at the sixth position of the β-globin chain occurring in sickle cell anemia causes the Hb to aggregate into long chains, altering the shape of the cell (Hb S). (B) The change of the RBC from a biconcave disk to an elongated or crescent (sickle) shape occurs with deoxygenation.

release arginase, an enzyme that breaks down arginine, a precursor for nitric oxide.

**Clinical Manifestations.** Sickled erythrocytes lead to hemolytic anemia and tend to occlude the microvasculature, resulting in both acute and chronic tissue injury. Intravascular sickling and hemolysis can begin by 6 to 8 weeks of age, but clinical manifestations do not usually appear until the infant is at least 6 months old, at which time the postnatal decrease in Hb F, which inhibits sickling, and increased production of Hb S lead to the increased concentration of Hb S.

Acute clinical manifestations of sickling, called *episodes*, usually fall into one of four categories: vasoocclusive or thrombotic, aplastic, sequestration or, rarely, hyperhemolytic (Fig. 14.17).

Pain caused by the blockage of sickled RBCs (thrombosis) is the most common symptom of SCD, occurring unpredictably in any organ, bone, or joint of the body, wherever and whenever an occlusion develops. The symptoms and frequency, duration, and intensity of the painful episodes vary widely (Box 14.10). Some people experience painful episodes only once a year; others may have as many as 15 to 20 episodes annually. The vasoocclusive episodes causing ischemic tissue damage may last 5 or 6 days, requiring hospitalization and subsiding gradually. Older clients more often report extremity and back pain during vascular episodes.

***Chest Syndrome.*** Two life-threatening thrombotic complications associated with SCD include acute chest syndrome and stroke. Acute chest syndrome results from the inability of sickled cells to become reoxygenated in the lungs. Sickled cells then adhere to lung endothelium cells, resulting in further inflammation, occluding vessels, and resulting in infarction. The most common precipitants are infection, fat emboli (from infarcted bone marrow), and infarction.

Symptoms include chest pain, shortness of breath, fever, wheezing, and cough (Box 14.11). Chest radiographs typically demonstrate an infiltrate, sometimes days after the symptoms began. Prognosis for this complication is poor and is one of the most common causes of death.[339]

Pulmonary hypertension can be a severe consequence of repeated microthrombotic events in the lung, even without a history of acute chest syndrome, seen in 6% to 10% of people with SCD.[257,317] Many factors may lead to pulmonary hypertension, with full understanding of the pathogenesis still lacking. Chronic hemolysis from sickled cells contributes to a reduction in nitric oxide (a potent vasodilator), which allows for continual vasoconstriction.[158] Chronic intravascular damage leads to acute and chronic inflammation of small vessels, which become thickened and blocked by thrombin and fibrous tissue, with the loss of the vascular bed. This process often proceeds without clinical symptoms until the person is short of breath, at which time the damage is irreversible. Affected persons exhibit symptoms of right heart failure, such as lower extremity edema, shortness of breath, fatigue, dyspnea on exertion, syncope/near syncope and chest pain. Pulmonary hypertension increases the risk of sudden death and is a significant cause of death in people with SCD.

***Stroke.*** Stroke, both hemorrhagic and ischemic, is another serious complication of SCD. By the age of 45 years, 24% of people with SCD will have experienced a stroke.[455] Stroke occurs in 11% of SCD clients younger than age 20 years, causing death or severe disability.[306] Stoke is usually caused by occlusion of large arterial blood vessels rather than a venous thromboembolism.[70] Abnormal proliferation of the endothelium results from chronic endothelial damage and interactions between platelets, WBCs, and abnormal RBCs. Progressive stenosis occurs secondary to decreased nitric oxide and other signaling proteins that alter regulation of vasoconstriction and vasodilation. Once the diameter of an affected artery is significantly narrowed, acute occluding of the vessel by a clot made of sickle and normal cells, WBCs, platelets, and thrombin, may happen, resulting in a cerebral infarct.[338]

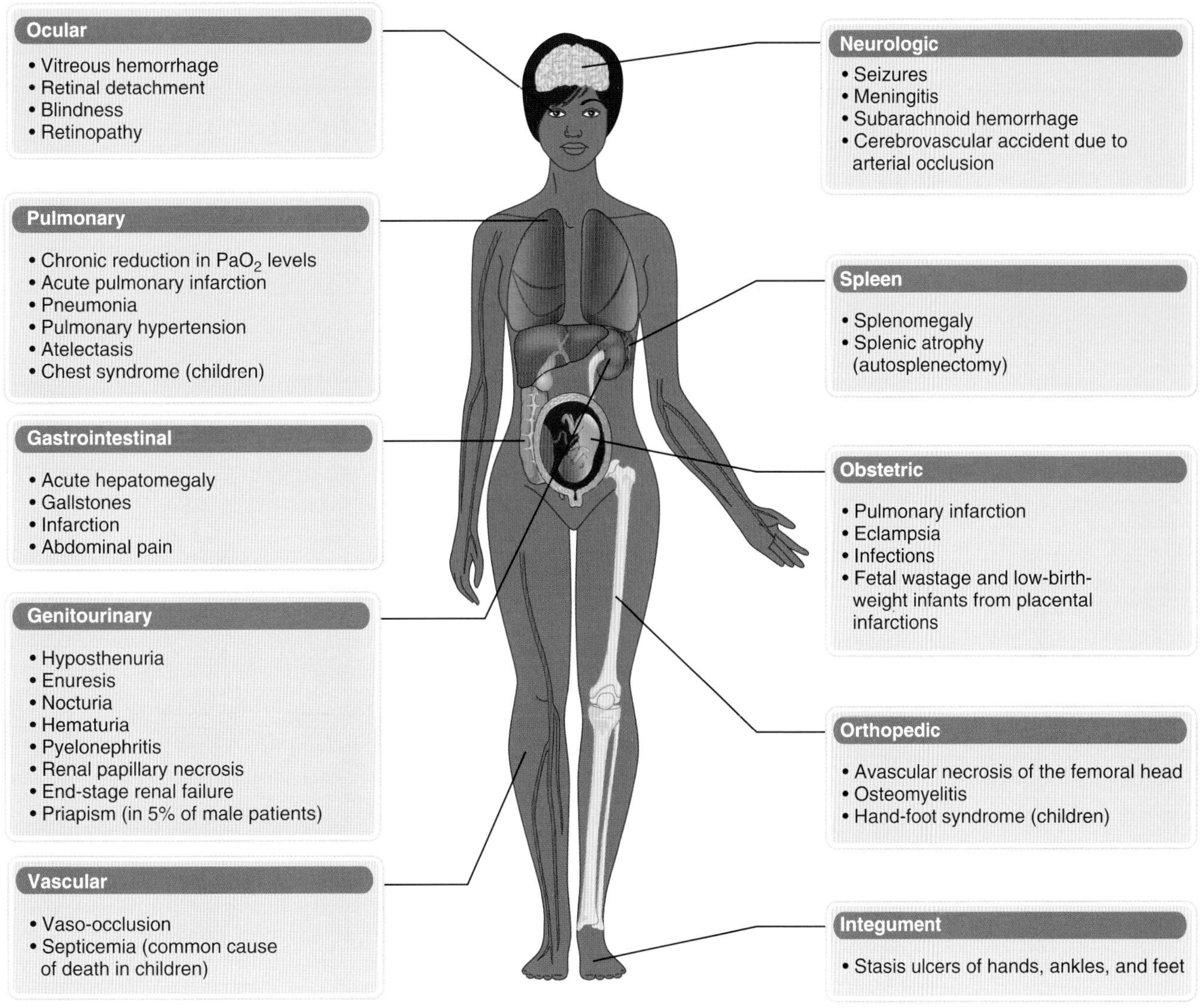


**Figure 14.17**

**Clinical manifestations and possible complications associated with SCD.** These findings are a consequence of infarctions, anemia, hemolysis, and recurrent infections.

Hemorrhagic stroke is less well understood but may be related to weakened vessels due to chronic injury and aneurysms.[281,433]

Ischemic reperfusion type injury may occur (similar to myocardial infarction followed by reperfusion) caused by endothelial cell damage, platelet clumping, release of cytokines, and the attraction of granulocytes, macrophages, T cells, and NK T cells to the site.[30] The acute obstruction and resulting inflammation lead to further hypoxia and acidosis and a cycle of continued sickling.[455]

Symptoms are similar to strokes in people without SCD, including paralysis, weakness, speech difficulties, seizures, and tingling/numbness of extremities. Infarcts can occur in the microvasculature as well. MRI and magnetic resonance angiography of the head and neck may show more extensive changes than are seen clinically, suggesting that silent strokes are not uncommon.

Additionally, many cognitive effects from these microvasculature strokes result in learning problems. Children demonstrate problems with memory, attention, visual–motor performance, and academic or social skills; neuromotor delays; mild hearing loss and auditory processing disorders; and failed speech and language screening.[4,170,204,420]

***Other Complications.*** For most people with SCD, the incidence of complications can be reduced by simple protective measures, such as prophylactic penicillin in children (until about age 5 years),[251] maintaining current vaccinations (to pneumococcus, meningococcus, *Haemophilus influenzae* type b, hepatitis B virus, and an annual vaccination against influenza virus), avoidance of excessive heat or cold and dehydration, and contact as early as possible with a specialist center. These precautions are most effective if susceptible infants are identified at birth.

Other thrombotic complications include *hand-and-foot syndrome* (dactylitis), which occurs when a microinfarction (clot) occludes the blood vessels that supply the metacarpal and metatarsal bones, causing ischemia; it may be an infant's first problem caused by SCD. It presents with low-grade fever and symmetric, painful, diffuse,

**Box 14.10**

**CLINICAL MANIFESTATIONS OF SICKLE CELL ANEMIA**

***Pain***

- Abdominal
- Chest
- Headaches

***Bone and Joint Episodes***

- Low-grade fever
- Extremity pain
- Back pain
- Periosteal pain
- Joint pain, especially shoulder and hip

***Vascular Complications***

- Cerebrovascular accidents
- Chronic leg ulcers
- Avascular necrosis of the femoral head
- Bone infarcts

***Pulmonary Episodes***

- Hypoxia
- Chest pain
- Dyspnea
- Tachypnea

***Neurologic Manifestations***

- Seizures
- Hemiplegia
- Dizziness
- Drowsiness
- Coma
- Stiff neck
- Paresthesias
- Cranial nerve palsies
- Blindness
- Nystagmus
- Transient ischemic attacks

***Hand-Foot Syndrome***

- Fever
- Pain
- Dactylitis

***Splenic Sequestration Episodes***

- Liver and spleen enlargement, tenderness
- Hypovolemia

***Renal Complications***

- Enuresis
- Nocturia
- Hematuria
- Pyelonephritis
- Renal papillary necrosis
- End-stage renal failure (older adult population)

Modified from Goodman CC, Snyder TE: *Differential diagnosis for the physical therapists: screening for referral*, ed 5, Philadelphia, 2013, WB Saunders.

**Box 14.11**

**COMPLICATIONS ASSOCIATED WITH PEDIATRIC SICKLE CELL ANEMIA**

***Chest Syndrome***

- Severe chest pain
- Fever of ≥38.8° C (≥102° F)
- Very congested
- Cough
- Dyspnea
- Tachypnea
- Sternal or costal retractions
- Wheezing

***Stroke***

- Seizures
- Unusual or strange behavior
- Inability to move an arm and/or a leg
- Ataxia or unsteady gait (do not assume these are guarding responses to pain)
- Stutter or slurred speech
- Distal muscular weakness in the hands, feet, or legs
- Changes in vision
- Severe, unrelieved headaches
- Severe vomiting

nonpitting edema in the hands and feet, extending to the fingers and toes (Fig. 14.18). The pain may be severe. This is a fairly common phenomenon seen almost exclusively in the young infant and child until the age of 4 years. The syndrome is typically self-limiting, and bones usually heal without permanent deformity (Fig. 14.19).

*Priapism* is also a thrombotic complication and requires immediate medical attention. Repeated and prolonged episodes can lead to impotence. SCD also affects the kidneys, demonstrating thrombotic complications and slowly losing function. End-stage renal disease can occur.

*Jaundice* is another common manifestation of SCD. Sickled cells do not live as long as normal cells and therefore die more rapidly than the liver can filter them. Bilirubin from these broken down cells builds up in the system, causing jaundice.

*Anemia* is a constant feature of SCD, with an Hb concentration of around 8 g/dL; acute, severe anemia, termed an aplastic crisis or episode, can occur when erythropoiesis abruptly stops. Clinical manifestations are pallor, fatigue, and jaundice. This is typically a result of parvovirus B19 infection.

Folate deficiency is another cause of severe anemia (often because of noncompliance in taking folate supplements). Anemia can also be worsened by renal insufficiency (decreased levels of erythropoietin) secondary to thrombosis.

Some of the complications associated with SCD are treated with transfusions, resulting in iron overload.

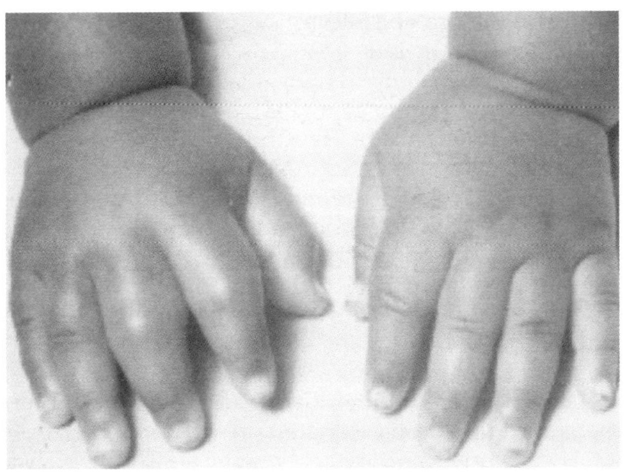

**Figure 14.18**

**Dactylitis.** Painful swelling of the hands or feet can occur when a clot forms in the hands or feet. This problem, known as hand-and-foot syndrome, occurs most often in children affected by SCD. (Reprinted from Gaston M: *Sickle cell anemia*, NIH Pub No 90-3058, Bethesda, MD, 1990, National Institutes of Health.)

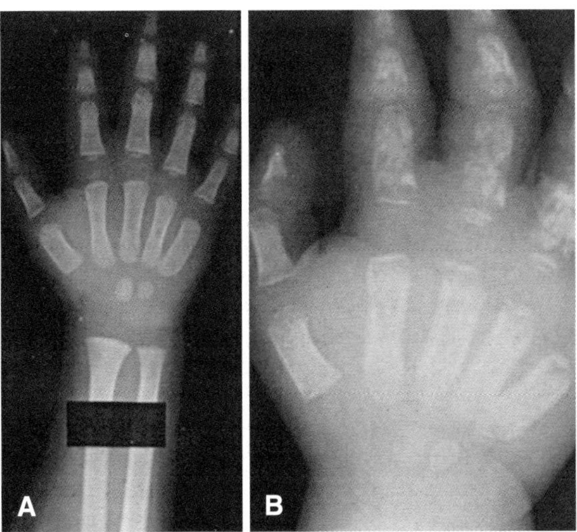


**Figure 14.19**

**Radiographs of an infant with sickle cell anemia and acute dactylitis.** (A) The bones appear normal at the onset of the episode. (B) Destructive changes and periosteal reaction are evident 2 weeks later. (Reprinted from Behrman RE: *Nelson textbook of pediatrics*, ed 17, Philadelphia, 2004, WB Saunders.)

*Hyperhemolysis* develops in some clients as a consequence of the formation of alloimmune responses to erythrocyte antigens, resulting in a delayed transfusion reaction with significant acute hemolysis of erythrocytes.

The spleen is an organ that is very susceptible to thrombotic occlusions (i.e., low blood flow, low oxygen tension, and low pH). Sickle-shaped RBCs frequently become trapped or sequestered in the spleen, often precipitated by infection. In sequestration episodes, large numbers of cells undergo sickling in the spleen, leading to ischemia, acute hemolysis, and necrosis of the spleen. Over time the spleen is destroyed in most children with SCD, becoming completely fibrotic, termed *autosplenectomy*. Children without a functioning spleen are at significant risk for overwhelming bacterial infections. *Hypovolemic shock* can occur, particularly in children, accompanied by a tender spleen and splenomegaly, leading to a serious risk of death before the age of 7 years from a sudden, profound anemia associated with rapid splenic enlargement.

Sequestration can occur in the liver but less frequently than splenic sequestration. Children with severe manifestations of sickle cell anemia have low bone mineral density and possess significant deficits in dietary calcium and circulating vitamin D, which complicates growth. Most children have growth retardation by the age of 2 years (weight more than height), which leads to osteoporosis and other bone abnormalities.[219]

## MEDICAL MANAGEMENT

**PREVENTION.** SCD can be prevented. Couples at risk of having affected children can be identified by inexpensive and reliable blood tests; chorionic villus sampling from 8 weeks' gestation can be performed for prenatal diagnosis.

Adoption of such measures goes hand in hand with health education. However, prenatal diagnosis can raise ethical questions that differ from one culture to another. Experience has clearly shown that genetic counseling, coupled with the offer of prenatal diagnosis, can lead to a large-scale reduction in births of affected children.

The risk of having affected children can be detected before marriage or pregnancy; however, to do so requires a carrier screening program. There is extensive experience with such programs in low- and high-income countries.

The WHO recommends these approaches be practiced in conformity with the three core principles of medical genetics: the autonomy of the individual or the couple, their right to adequate and complete information, and the highest standards of confidentiality.[443]

**DIAGNOSIS.** It is required in every state that all infants be screened for SCD regardless of race or ethnic background (universal screening). This recommendation is based on the following factors: (1) although SCD is more prevalent in certain racial and ethnic groups, it is not possible to define accurately an individual's heritage by physical appearance or surname; and (2) prophylactic penicillin and pneumococcal vaccination reduce both morbidity and mortality from pneumococcal infections in infants with sickle cell anemia and sickle thalassemia.

Screening targeted to specific racial and ethnic groups will therefore miss some affected infants, subjecting them to an increased risk of early mortality. Universal screening is the best, most reliable, and most cost-effective screening method to identify affected infants.[315] For newborns in the United States, blood for screening is obtained from the cord or a heel stick.

Screening of newborns for sickle cell disease or any of the other hemoglobinopathy can be made using high-performance liquid chromatography (HPLC), gel electrophoresis, or thin-layer isoelectric focusing. If test results are questionable, repeat testing should be done between the age of 3 and 6 months, when the beta hemoglobin chain is fully produced. DNA testing may be necessary to confirm the diagnosis, particularly if the infant has persistently elevated levels of hemoglobin F.

Diagnostic testing for children and adults is preferably made by HPLC, which is highly sensitive and specific.[263]

Alternative tests include isoelectric focusing and gel electrophoresis, although these are not as sensitive as HPLC.

Test results for sickle cell hemoglobinopathies using HPLC and isoelectric focusing are as follows: sickle cell anemia demonstrates 0% HbA, less than 2% HbF with the remainder HbS; sickle cell trait pattern shows greater than 50% as HbA, 35% to 45% HbS, and less than 2% HbF; hemoglobin SC disease expresses both HbS and HbC.

Prenatal diagnosis for SCD is possible as early as 8 to 10 weeks' gestation. Fetal cells are obtained by chorionic villus sampling and then the DNA is extracted, amplified using PCR, and analyzed for hemoglobinopathies. Preimplantation testing protocols are currently being developed in which DNA is evaluated from single cells prior to the embryo being implanted in the uterus.[245]

**TREATMENT.** Supportive care is essential for all pain crises and complications, including rest, pain medication (opioid and nonopioid), oxygen, administration of intravenous fluids, electrolytes, antibiotics, and physical and occupational therapy for joint and bone involvement. Routine health maintenance is required, including updating vaccinations, regular ophthalmologic care, screening for proteinuria, and pulmonary hypertension.

The medication hydroxyurea has been shown to reduce the number of painful episodes, hospitalizations, and acute chest syndrome.[430,462,474] It has multiple mechanisms of action and requires weeks before becoming effective, acting to prevent episodes rather than treat acute complications. Hydroxyurea is recommended for clients younger than 9 months with symptomatic disease, all children and adolescents over the age of 9 months, and symptomatic adults.[337,474]

Because all people with SCD are at risk for stroke, annual transcranial Doppler ultrasound should be initiated at the age of 2 years and continue until the age of 16 years to evaluate blood flow in the brain. All children with developmental delays or cognitive problems should undergo MRI to screen for silent infarcts. Acute stroke is managed with exchange transfusions to reduce the amount of Hb S to less than 30% while keeping the total Hb (through transfusions) at 10 g/dL. Because sickle cells function best at lower viscosities, blood is exchanged rather than just transfused.

The likelihood of a second stroke is increased, and prophylactic transfusions (this inhibits their own erythropoiesis of Hb S) have been shown to help decrease the risk of stroke and reduce the stenosis of arteries.[2,3] Complications with iron overload are common and can have significant long-term problems as well as alloimmunization (creating antibodies against "foreign" transfused cells). Chelating therapy is available but is often difficult for children to tolerate.

Acute chest syndrome (ACS) is treated with oxygen, antibiotics, pain medication, and avoidance of overhydration. Incentive spirometry may improve atelectasis, whereas bronchodilators aid in reactive airway symptoms. Simple transfusion of RBCs is helpful for mild cases of ACS, while exchange transfusion may be required if hypoxia continues despite supplemental oxygen. Clients also receive prophylaxis for thromboembolisms. Prophylactic exchange transfusions may be indicated for people with two or more episodes of ACS (moderate to severe despite maximal hydroxyurea therapy).

Some complications require diagnostic testing, such as pulmonary hypertension (PH). Because symptoms of pulmonary hypertension are subtle and may be equated with anemia or deconditioning, children 8 years and older should receive a baseline Doppler echocardiogram. Adults should have an echocardiogram every one to three years, depending on the tricuspid regurgitant jet velocity (TRV) and symptoms. TRV of 2.5 m/sec or greater is indicative of increased morbidity and mortality. All clients with symptoms suggestive of PH, along with an elevated TRV and N-terminal-pro-brain natriuretic peptide 160 pg/ml or greater, should undergo right heart catheterization. A resting mean pulmonary arterial pressure greater than 20 mm Hg diagnoses pulmonary hypertension. Other causes of PH should be excluded and/or treated, such as obstructive sleep apnea, chronic venous thromboembolism, portal hypertension, or HIV infection.[206]

First-line treatment for pulmonary hypertension includes hydroxyurea, with chronic transfusions as an alternative therapy for people who do not tolerate hydroxyurea or demonstrate no benefit.[206] Pulmonary hypertension specific medications are best suited for select individuals with verified PH with an elevated pulmonary vascular resistance (the resistance that needs to be overcome to push blood from the right ventricle to the lungs)[56] and a normal pulmonary capillary wedge pressure (an estimate of left atrial pressure). Although phosphodiesterase-5 inhibitors are contraindicated (increase vaso-occlusive episodes), prostacyclin agonists (e.g., epoprostenol) or endothelin receptor therapies (e.g., bosentan) can be used.[206]

Acute aplastic episodes can be treated with a transfusion if the anemia is severe and the reticulocyte count is low. Most often this is self-limiting and erythropoiesis resumes in a few days.

Simple transfusions are used in specific situations, including symptomatic anemia and surgical interventions.[349] Prophylactic transfusions (manually done by transfusing and alternately phlebotomizing or using an apheresis machine) are given preoperatively or to reduce SCD complications. Exchange transfusions are indicated for acute stroke and secondary stroke prevention; acute chest syndrome with significant hypoxia and secondary prevention of acute chest syndrome; prevention of recurrent priapism; progressive pulmonary hypertension; and multiorgan failure/hepatopathy. Transfusions have not been found to be beneficial for clients admitted to the hospital for a pain episode without symptomatic anemia.

Splenic sequestration can be a life-threatening event in infants and children. Treatments include maintenance of euvolemia, realizing that if a transfusion is given, the blood in the spleen is still available to later return to the circulatory system. Transfusing half the typical amount of blood may be considered.

Prenatal and neonatal screening can identify this disorder and significantly reduce morbidity and mortality through the use of prophylactic antibiotics. Infants with documented SCD (sickle cell anemia or Hb S β-thalassemia) should be started on oral prophylactic penicillin as soon as possible but no later than 3 months of age and continue at least until the age of 5.[480] Children who have experienced pneumococcal sepsis may remain on prophylactic penicillin indefinitely.

Most people with SCD should take supplemental folic acid and may need replacement of HCT, which has been shown to help, and possibly cure, individuals with SCD.[75] Matched related donors are best, providing an overall survival of over 90%.[130] HCT is best utilized in children under the age of 16[130] and often is considered for individuals with early complications at high risk for early death.[399] Individuals that should consider HCT include those who have significant complications that are not managed with hydroxyurea, such as frequent acute chest pain syndrome, stroke, or pain episodes. Due to the risks associated with HCT, the decision must be tailored to the person, depending on donor availability, comorbidities, and risk for death due to SCD complications.

**PROGNOSIS.** Historically, SCD has been associated with high mortality in early childhood from overwhelming bacterial infections, acute chest syndrome, and stroke. In the mid-1970s the average life expectancy was only 14.3 years. By 1994 the life expectancy had increased to 42 years for men and 48 years for women with sickle cell anemia.[336] Between 1999 and 2002, the mortality rate for blacks and African Americans younger than age 4 years fell by 42%. This dramatic drop is thought to be secondary to the introduction of the pneumococcal vaccine.[52]

Overall survival for people with SCD continues to improve with the delivery of health care at comprehensive sickle cell centers.[76] More people affected with SCD are now living longer but with significant end-organ damage.[348] SCD remains a devastating condition with recurrent episodes leading to early death. The complications of SCD can be life-threatening depending on their location. Recovery may be complete in some cases, but serious neurologic damage is more likely to occur, and repeated cerebrovascular accidents may lead to increased neurologic involvement, permanent paralysis, or death. Permanent damage from blood clots to the heart, kidney, lungs, liver, or eyes (blindness) can occur.

**SPECIAL IMPLICATIONS FOR THE THERAPIST 14.16**

*Sickle Cell Disease*

It is important for the therapist to recognize signs of complications, especially signs of acute chest syndrome, stroke, and neurodevelopmental impairment (see Box 14.11). Providing client education is also an important role. Clients should be taught about risks and risk prevention, including the importance of physical activity and/or mobility, prevention of pulmonary complications using breathing and incentive spirometry, and the importance of remaining well hydrated. Screening for referral to other rehabilitation or behavioral services is also part of the therapist's intervention. Be aware, too that A1C lab values can be altered in individuals with sickle hemoglobin, an important finding in the long-term management of diabetes.[157]

Stroke is a relatively infrequent complication in the young infant; the median age for occurrence of stroke in children is 7 years. Splenic sequestration (entrapment of blood and enlargement in the spleen) can occur in children younger than 6 years with homozygous Hb S and at any age with other types of SCD. Circulatory collapse and death can occur in less than 30 minutes.

Any signs of weakness, abdominal pain, fatigue, dyspnea, tachycardia accompanied by pallor, and hypotension require emergency medical attention. Client and family education should emphasize the importance of regularly scheduled medical evaluations for anyone receiving hydroxyurea. The risk of developing an undetected toxicity that can result in severe bone marrow depression must be explained. Outward signs of drug complications are rarely evident.

**Neurodevelopment**

SCD is a blood disorder; however, the CNS is one of the organs frequently affected by the disease.[171,381] Brain disease can begin early in life and often leads to neurocognitive dysfunction.

Approximately one-fourth to one-third of children with SCD have some form of CNS effects from the disease, which typically manifest as deficits in specific cognitive domains and academic difficulties.

The impact of the disease on families shares many features similar to other neurodevelopmental disorders; however, social-environmental factors related to low socioeconomic status, worry and concerns about social stigma, and recurrent, unpredictable medical complications can be sources of relatively higher stress in SCD.

Greater public awareness of the neurocognitive effects of SCD and their impact on child outcomes is a critical step toward improved treatment, adaptation to illness, and quality of life.

**Exercise**

Multiple factors contribute to exercise intolerance in individuals with sickle cell anemia, but little information exists regarding the safety of maximal cardiopulmonary exercise testing or the mechanisms of exercise limitation in these clients.

For example, low peak $VO_2$, low anaerobic threshold, gas exchange abnormalities, and high ventilatory reserve comprise a pattern consistent with exercise limitation due to pulmonary vascular disease in this population group. Low peak $VO_2$, low anaerobic threshold, no gas exchange abnormalities, and a high heart rate reserve reflect peripheral vascular disease and/or myopathy. Low peak $VO_2$, low anaerobic threshold, no gas exchange abnormalities, and a low heart rate reserve are best explained by anemia.[39] These kinds of cardiopulmonary factors must be considered when prescribing exercise for this population.[311]

During a sickle cell episode, the therapist may be involved in nonpharmacologic pain control or management. Precautions include avoiding stressors that can precipitate an episode, such as overexertion, dehydration, smoking, and exposure to cold or the use of cryotherapy for painful, swollen joints. (See "Special Implications for the Therapist 14.1: Hematologic Disorders" above.)

Fear of movement (kinesophobia) has been reported among individuals with sickle cell disease; greater kinesophobia is associated with greater pain and psychologic distress.[327] Addressing anxiety and fear and the effects of these emotions on pain, movement, and disability may help the individual remain active and able to participate in physical activity and exercise. Should a person with SCD experience an isolated musculoskeletal injury (e.g., sprained ankle) in the absence of any sickle cell episodes, careful application of ice can be undertaken.

### Pain Management

People with SCD suffer both physically and psychosocially. They may describe feelings of helplessness against the disease and fear a premature death. Frequent hospitalizations and consequent job absences often result in stressful financial constraints.

Depression is a common finding in this group of people. A program offering holistic treatment focuses on pharmacologic and nonpharmacologic strategies, offering the client multiple self-management options. The sickle cell pain can be successfully managed using whirlpool therapy at a slightly warmer temperature (38.9°-40° C [102°-104° F]), facilitating muscle relaxation through active movement in the water.

The therapist should teach the client alternative methods of pain control, such as the appropriate application of mild heat to painful areas or the use of visualization or relaxation techniques. Combined use of medications, psychologic support, relaxation techniques, biofeedback, and imagery is a useful intervention to lessen the effects of painful episodes.[166] Cognitive-behavioral therapy can be helpful in the management of sickle pain because of the high level of psychologic stress people with SCD experience.[444]

Joint effusions in SCD can occur secondary to long bone infarctions with extension of swelling and septic arthritis. Clients with SCD may also have coexistent rheumatic or collagen vascular disease or osteoarthritis, necessitating careful evaluation to determine the presence of marked inflammation or fever before initiating intervention procedures.

Teaching joint protection is important and may include assistive devices, equipment, and technology and pain-free strengthening exercises. Persistent thigh, buttock, or groin pain in anyone with known SCD may be an indication of aseptic necrosis of the femoral head. Blood supply to the hip is only adequate, even in healthy people, so the associated microvascular obstruction can leave the hip especially vulnerable to ischemia and necrosis. Up to 50% of sickle cell cases develop this condition.

Total hip replacement may be indicated in cases in which severe structural damage occurs; sickle cell–related surgical complications most commonly include excessive intraoperative blood loss, postoperative hemorrhage, wound abscess, pulmonary complications, and transfusion reactions.[457]

### Tolerance, Dependence, and Addiction

It is helpful if the client, family, and clinician understand the differences among tolerance, dependence, and addiction as they relate to the individual with SCD receiving or needing narcotic medications. Tolerance and dependence are both involuntary and predictable physiologic changes that develop with repeated administration of narcotics; these terms do not indicate the person is addicted.

*Tolerance* occurs when, after repeated administration of a narcotic, larger doses are needed to obtain the same effect. *Dependence* has occurred if withdrawal symptoms emerge when the narcotic is stopped abruptly. In either case, this means that once the medication is no longer needed, the dosage will have to be tapered down to avoid withdrawal symptoms.

Addiction, although also based on physiologic changes associated with drug use, has a psychologic and behavioral component characterized by continuous craving for the substance. Addicted people will use a drug to relieve psychologic symptoms even after the physical pain is gone.

The chronic use of narcotics for pain relief may lead to addictive use in vulnerable individuals, but even if someone is addicted, the pain should still be treated and narcotics should not be withheld if they are the drugs of choice for the pain condition. Ironically, undertreating the pain because of fear of fostering addiction actually encourages a pattern of drug-seeking and drug-hoarding behaviors.[137]

## Sickle Cell Trait

Sickle cell trait is not a disease but rather a heterozygous condition in which the individual has the mutant gene from only one parent ($\beta^s$ gene), and the normal gene ($\beta^A$ globin gene), resulting in the production of both Hb S and Hb A, with a predominance of Hb A (60%) over Hb S (40%). One in 12 African Americans has the sickle cell trait, and many other races and nationalities also carry the genetic defect.

Under normal circumstances, sickle cell trait is rarely symptomatic; symptoms may occur with conditions associated with marked hypoxia and at high altitudes. No increased risk is evident for individuals with sickle cell trait who undergo general anesthesia, and a normal life expectancy is predicted. It was previously reported that no increased risk of sudden death was evident for those who participate in athletics, but a small number of cases have now been reported.[13] However, it remains controversial whether the pathogenesis of these exercise-related deaths involved microvascular obstruction by sickled erythrocytes, because sickling can occur postmortem. The recommendations are that athletes with sickle cell trait adhere to compliance with general guidelines for fluid replacement and acclimatization to hot conditions and altitude.[398]

In 2010, the National Collegiate Athletic Association (NCAA) recommended all players be screened for sickle cell trait as a prerequisite prior to participation in athletics.[439] The American Society of Hematology, however, does not support this recommendation, commenting that it could harm the student athletes and the sickle cell community because all athletes should adhere to rules for hydration and avoiding adverse conditions, like any other athlete.[1,207] More research needs to be completed to substantiate this policy.[156]

### The Thalassemias

**Definition.** The thalassemias are a group of inherited disorders of Hb synthesis with abnormalities in one or more of the four globin genes. Hb is composed of four protein chains: two α-globin chains and two β-globin chains (see Fig. 14.16). These four proteins are attached to heme (iron and protoporphyrin), which allows a molecule of oxygen to reversibly bind to this complex molecule.

Depending on which globin chain is affected, people may have β-thalassemia or α-thalassemia. α-Thalassemia is common among people from Africa, the Mediterranean (*thalassa* is Greek for "sea," referring to early cases of SCD reported around the Mediterranean), the Middle East, and Asia. β-Thalassemia is most prevalent in the Mediterranean, Southeast Asia, India, and Pakistan.

**Overview and Pathogenesis.** The thalassemias are characterized by abnormalities in the globin genes, leading to incomplete or abnormal formation of Hb. This results in ineffective erythropoiesis and chronic hemolysis. Because there are four α-globin genes, several diseases can occur.

Clients who lack only one α gene (–α/αα) manifest no clinical symptoms and are carriers of the disorder. If two α genes are deleted (–,α or –α/–α), this condition is termed α-thalassemia trait and results in mild anemia. Hb H disease is characterized by three α gene deletions (–,–α) and results in severe anemia, CHF, and death. Fetal death occurs when all four of the α genes are deleted (hydrops fetalis).

Whereas α-thalassemia occurs with gene deletions, β-thalassemia is a heterogenous group of disorders caused by various genetic anomalies (usually point mutations), resulting in defects in the production of β-globin chains.

Thalassemia major (β°, also called Cooley anemia) results from significant genetic defects in both β-globin genes, leading to a lack of β-globin chain synthesis. β-Thalassemia intermedia is caused by a mutation in each of the β-globin genes, with one mutation being mild, allowing for more β-globin chains to be produced with improved function compared with β-thalassemia major.

β-Thalassemia trait ($\beta^+$) is characterized by only one gene having a mutation. Normally, the α- and β-globin chains are produced in an even ratio. When thalassemia occurs, there is a mismatch of globin chains produced. In persons affected with severe mutations, there are five to six times the number of normal precursor erythrocytes and 15 times the number of cells in apoptosis (programmed cell death) in the bone marrow as the body attempts to compensate for anemia. The cells that are released from the bone marrow may be rigid and unable to adapt to the size of the small capillaries or cleared by the immune system, resulting in hemolysis.[371]

**Clinical Manifestations.** α-Thalassemia is not as common as β-thalassemia. The clinical manifestations of β-thalassemia vary depending on the severity and number of mutations. The clinical manifestations of thalassemia are primarily attributable to (1) defective synthesis of Hb (ineffective erythropoiesis), (2) structurally impaired RBCs, and (3) hemolysis or destruction of the erythrocytes.

β-Thalassemia major exhibits the most severe complications of the β-thalassemias as a result of significant genetic mutations. Most of these complications are a result of severe anemia and iron overload (from blood transfusions and increased absorption from the gut).

Clients with β-thalassemia major require frequent and regular transfusions beginning in infancy. Anemia and iron overload lead to endocrinopathies, cardiomyopathy, and cirrhosis of the liver.[277,278] The endocrinopathies can be severe, including diabetes mellitus, hypoparathyroidism, hypopituitarism, delayed puberty, testicular and ovarian failure, and hypothyroidism.

These endocrine problems along with the anemia result in decreased bone mineral density, bone deformities, and osteoporosis (increasing the risk for pathologic fractures).[152] Even with appropriate management (i.e., well-transfused and iron-chelated individuals with thalassemia major), osteoporosis affects 40% to 50% of all affected children and adults (the most common complication of thalassemia intermedia).[152,437] Some of the bone deformities that occur due to extramedullary hematopoiesis include the face (enlarged maxillary bones, saddle nose, depressed cranium), pelvis, and spine.

As a reaction to the anemia, the body attempts to compensate by making erythrocytes in extramedullary locations, including the spleen and liver (causing hepatosplenomegaly). Because the bone marrow is filled with more cells than normal, there is bone expansion (often noted on the skull).

Multiple and frequent transfusions (usually for individuals with thalassemia major and many with thalassemia intermedia) place the client at risk for all complications related to transfusions, although cardiomyopathy is the most common cause of death.[329,371] Clients with thalassemia intermedia exhibit mild to moderate anemia but can become transfusion dependent during adulthood. Transfusion requirements are less than that received by clients with thalassemia major, but depending on the severity of the mutations, clients may still develop splenomegaly, iron overload, and bone deformities. Persons with the thalassemia trait typically have mild or no anemia. Their erythrocytes may be very small (microcytic anemia often incorrectly assumed to be iron deficiency), but splenomegaly and bone deformities do not develop. Due to the continued hemolysis and ineffective erythropoiesis, people with thalassemias (particularly β-thalassemia major) often exhibit cholelithiasis. Thrombosis and leg ulcers are also noted complications.

## MEDICAL MANAGEMENT

**DIAGNOSIS.** Once history and clinical exam are suspicious for the disease, diagnosis is by laboratory testing. The peripheral blood smear may demonstrate target cells (RBCs that appear like a target), fragments of erythrocytes (due to hemolysis), and very small RBCs (see Fig. 14.2). CBC reveals microcytic RBCs and anemia (depending on the mutations/deletions). The serum bilirubin and fecal and urinary urobilinogen levels may be elevated due to the severe hemolysis of abnormal cells. Iron studies should be obtained to evaluate for iron overload. High-performance liquid chromatography and electrophoresis are utilized most often to diagnose hemoglobinopathies.

Genetic testing can be done to confirm the diagnosis, carrier status and mutations. Because children under the age of 6 months do not express β-globin, they are most likely to have α-thalassemia.

**Treatment.** The anemia associated with thalassemia intermedia may range from mild (not requiring transfusions) to more moderate, requiring occasional transfusions. The goal is to maintain an Hb level of 9 to 10 g/dL, which allows for more normal development and growth and reduces the incidence of hepatosplenomegaly and bone deformities. Clients requiring more frequent transfusions can develop clinical manifestations as described above and should be closely monitored for iron overload and treated when present. Individuals with α-thalassemia require supplemental folate and care should be taken to avoid supplemental iron in multivitamins.

Treatment for thalassemia major consists of optimizing transfusions, providing chelation therapy for iron overload, and implementing hormone replacement as needed. Splenectomy can decrease transfusion requirements for selected people, although due to increased risk of overwhelming infections and thromboembolism, it is avoided. Thalassemia major requires lifelong transfusion, which places these persons at risk for transfusion-related infectious diseases.

The blood supply in the United States is rigorously tested, resulting in a significantly decreased incidence of hepatitides B and C and HIV.

MRI of the heart and liver are performed at baseline and to determine iron concentration in these organs. Ferritin is followed carefully and MRI can be performed if the ferritin is elevated or the client exhibits symptoms of organ involvement (e.g., heart failure, endocrinopathies). Chelation therapy should be initiated when ferritin is greater than 1000microL, liver iron concentration is 3 mg Fe/g dry weight, and/or if 20 to 25 units of RBCs have been transfused. Chelators remove iron from the bloodstream, and routine use in these clients has led to a doubling of life expectancy.[168] Deferasirox is commonly given due to the ease of oral administration.[169] Serious events associated with deferasirox use include severe gastrointestinal bleeding, renal and hepatic toxicity. Deferiprone, also given orally, is effective but only available in a few countries. Deferoxamine is commonly used as an initial treatment, although its parenteral administration makes it a less desirable agent.[436] Major side effects include changes in vision and hearing (often reversible upon discontinuation); renal and hepatic toxicities; and growth impairment. Some countries use a combination of deferiprone and deferoxamine, which has been shown to be highly effective in treating iron overload of the heart.[438] Progressive disease (or in clients who do not respond to chelation therapy) often requires hormone replacement. Clients can receive growth hormone, hormone replacement for testicular and ovarian failure, insulin for diabetes, levothyroxine for hypothyroidism, and calcium and vitamin D (and perhaps bisphosphonates) for osteoporosis.

HCT is a possible curative treatment option for those with severe disease, although long-term complications can be significant and donor availability and cost may be prohibitive.[418] Gene therapy appears promising and has been successful in humans, but remains challenging.[418,446]

Other experimental treatments include agents that increase fetal Hb production, such as histone deacetylase inhibitors and hypomethylating agents, although transfusion decreases the responsiveness of the bone marrow to these agents.[279,307]

**Prognosis.** Thalassemia trait does not affect life expectancy, but clients who carry the mutation need genetic counseling. People with α-thalassemia and β-thalassemia intermedia have varying symptoms and need for transfusions. Until recently the outlook for clients with thalassemia major has been poor, with lethal, severe hemolytic anemia and subsequent iron overload and dysfunction of almost all organ systems. Presently, due to aggressive chelation therapy beginning in childhood, there is a significant improvement in overall survival of individuals with transfusion-dependent thalassemia. Life expectancy has improved from early puberty into the fifth or sixth decades of adulthood.[459] Cardiac complications continue to be the principle cause of death, most often due to iron overload. Death from *hydrops fetalis* occurs in homozygous α-thalassemia and consistently results in stillbirth or death in utero.

SPECIAL IMPLICATIONS FOR THE THERAPIST 14.17

### β-*Thalassemia Syndromes*

Intervertebral disc degeneration is also possible, caused by transfusional iron overload or the use of deferoxamine.[152] Back pain is common secondary to osteoporosis, compression fractures, and disc degeneration.[86] Spinal asymmetry and scoliosis are also common in this group of individuals. Progression of deformity is less than reported in individuals with idiopathic scoliosis and is mainly attributed to anemia, hemosiderosis, iron chelation therapy, and associated endocrinologic disorders. In some cases (smaller curves), the curve resolves spontaneously. Optimal treatment for any of the musculoskeletal effects (osteoporosis, degenerative disc disease, scoliosis) remains an area for future investigation.[316]

Individuals with β-thalassemia syndromes may develop soft tissue masses in many areas, but especially along the paraspinal region. Neural compression can result in back pain, lower extremity pain, paresthesia, abnormal proprioception, exaggerated or brisk deep tendon reflexes, Babinski response, Lasègue sign, ankle clonus, urgency of urination, and bowel incontinence.[151] For an excellent review of spine involvement in individuals with this condition, the reader is referred to Haidar.[152]

## REFERENCES

To enhance this text and add value for the reader, all references are included in the enhanced eBook on Student Consult that accompanies this textbook. The reader can view the reference source and access it online whenever possible.

# CHAPTER 15

# The Respiratory System

LORA PACKEL • JOHN D. HEICK (PULMONARY EMBOLISM AND INFARCTION) • KAREN VON BERG (CYSTIC FIBROSIS)

The authors acknowledge the contributions of John Heick and Karen von Berg in the fourth edition of this text.

## OVERVIEW

Anatomically, the respiratory system can be divided into three main portions: the upper airway, the lower airway, and the terminal alveoli (Fig. 15.1). The upper airway consists of the nasal cavities, sinuses, pharynx, tonsils, and larynx. The lower airway consists of the conducting airways, including the trachea, bronchi, and bronchioles (Fig. 15.2). The alveoli, or air sacs, at the end of the conducting airways in the lower respiratory tract are the primary lobules, sometimes called the *acini*, of the lung.

Physiologically, lung function is comprised of ventilation and respiration. *Ventilation* is the ability to move the air in and out of the lungs via a pressure gradient. It can be thought of as moving air through tubes. *Respiration* refers to the gas exchange that moves oxygen into the blood stream to supply the body and removes carbon dioxide from the blood stream. Pathology of the airways, lungs, chest wall, or diaphragm will affect ventilation. Pathology of the gas exchange tissues or the cardiovascular system will affect respiration.

### Major Sequelae of Pulmonary Disease or Injury

Hypoxemia is the most common condition caused by pulmonary disease or injury. *Hypoxemia*, deficient oxygenation of arterial blood, may lead to *hypoxia*, a broad term meaning diminished availability of oxygen to the body tissues. Prolonged hypoxia will cause tissue damage or death. Hypoxemia is caused by respiratory alterations (Table 15.1) or cardiovascular compromise, whereas hypoxia may occur anywhere in the body caused by alterations of other systems and may not be related to changes in the pulmonary system.

Signs and symptoms of hypoxemia vary, depending on the level of oxygenation in the blood (Table 15.2). Sampling of arterial blood is an invasive measure of oxygenation, whereas pulse oximetry is a noninvasive measurement of arterial oxyhemoglobin saturation. These measurements can be taken at rest or during a standardized exercise test.

### Oxygen Transport Deficits in Systemic Disease

Although this chapter focuses on primary pulmonary impairment, pathologic conditions of every major organ system can have secondary effects on pulmonary function and on the oxygen transport pathway (which includes the cardiovascular system). These effects can include a variety of impairments, such as altered ventilation and/or perfusion, reduced static and dynamic lung volumes and flow rates, atelectasis; reduced surfactant production and distribution; impaired mucociliary transport; secretion retention; pulmonary aspiration; impaired lymphatic drainage; pulmonary edema; impaired coughing; and respiratory muscle weakness or fatigue.[136]

When assessing signs and symptoms of pulmonary disease, the therapist must consider the underlying cause of these symptoms and determine which therapy interventions can alleviate symptoms and improve functional capacity. Therapists must also recognize medical instability and determine the need for urgent or nonurgent referrals to the medical team.

### Signs and Symptoms of Pulmonary Disease

Pulmonary disease can be classified as acute or chronic, obstructive or restrictive, infectious, or oncologic, and is associated with many common signs and symptoms. The most common of these are cough and dyspnea. Other manifestations include chest pain, abnormal sputum, hemoptysis, cyanosis, digital clubbing, wheezing, and altered breathing patterns (Box 15.1 and Table 15.3).

#### Cough

Cough is considered a reflex that protects the pulmonary system. Sensory nerves are located throughout the pulmonary system and respond to both mechanical and chemical triggers.[333,383] Sensory information is carried by the vagus nerve to the medulla. Impulses are carried by the vagus nerve, phrenic nerve, and motor nerves to the expiratory muscles and by the superior laryngeal and recurrent laryngeal branches of the vagus to the larynx, trachea, and bronchi. These signals result in bronchoconstriction and contraction of expiratory muscles, resulting in a cough.[333,383] An acute cough is one that lasts less than 3 weeks, subacute cough lasts 3 to 8 weeks, and a chronic cough lasts 8 or more weeks.[333] As a physiologic response, cough occurs frequently in healthy people, but a persistent dry cough may be caused by a tumor, congestion, or hypersensitive airways (allergies). A productive cough with purulent sputum (yellow or green) may indicate infection, whereas a productive cough with nonpurulent sputum (clear or white) is nonspecific and indicates airway irritation. Hemoptysis (coughing and spitting blood) indicates a pathologic condition—infection, inflammation, abscess, tumor, or infarction. Rust-colored sputum can be a sign of pneumonia. Therapists should include the following in a cough history: duration, characteristics, production and

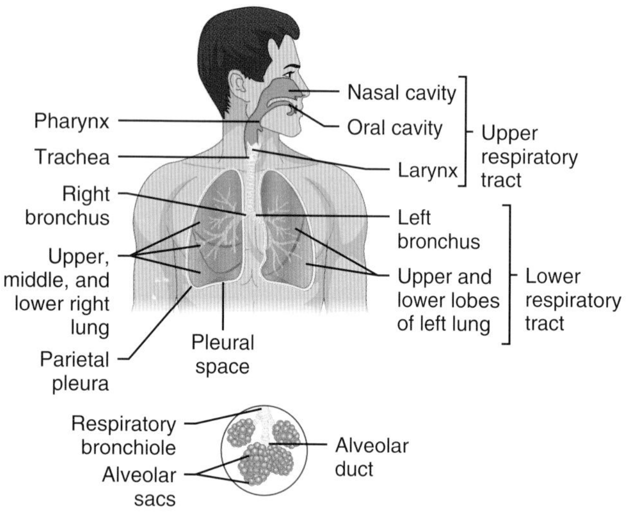

**Figure 15.1**

**Structures of the upper and lower respiratory tracts.** The upper respiratory tract consists of the nasal cavity, pharynx, and larynx; the lower respiratory tract includes the trachea, bronchi, and lungs. The circle shows the acinus, the terminal respiratory unit, which consists of the respiratory bronchioles, alveolar ducts, and alveolar sacs. This is the portion of the lungs where oxygen and carbon dioxide are exchanged.

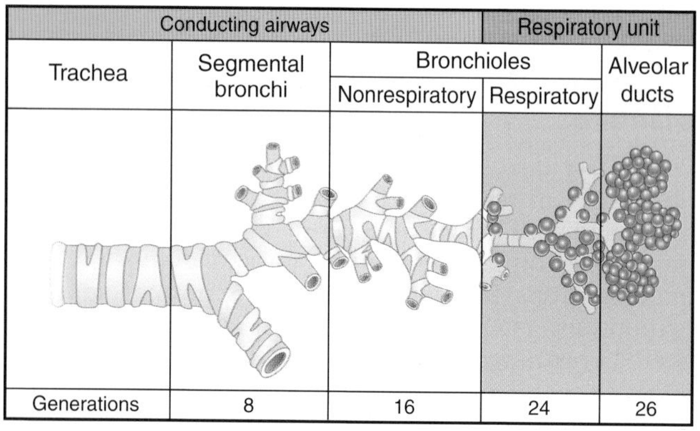

**Figure 15.2**

**Structures of the lower airway.** The first 16 generations of the airways branching in human lungs are purely conducting; transitional airways lead into the final respiratory zone, consisting of alveoli where gas exchange takes place.

**Table 15.1** Causes of Hypoxemia

| Mechanism | Common Clinical Cause |
|---|---|
| Ventilation–perfusion mismatch | Asthma<br>Chronic bronchitis<br>Pneumonia |
| Decreased oxygen content | High altitude<br>Low oxygen content<br>Enclosed breathing space (suffocation) |
| Hypoventilation | Lack of neurologic stimulation of the respiratory center<br>• Oversedation<br>• Drug overdose<br>• Neurologic damage<br>Chronic obstructive pulmonary disease |
| Alveolocapillary diffusion abnormality | Emphysema<br>Fibrosis<br>Edema |
| Pulmonary shunting | Acute respiratory distress syndrome (ARDS)<br>Hyaline membrane disease (ARDS in newborn)<br>Atelectasis |

Modified from McCance KL, Huether SE, editors: *Pathophysiology: the biologic basis for disease in adults and children*, ed 3, St Louis, 1998, Mosby-Year Book.

**Table 15.2** Signs and Symptoms of Hypoxemia

| $PaO_2$ (mm Hg) | Signs and Symptoms |
|---|---|
| 80–100 | Normal |
| 60–80 | Moderate tachycardia, possible onset of respiratory distress, dyspnea on exertion |
| 50–60 | Malaise<br>Light-headedness<br>Nausea<br>Vertigo<br>Impaired judgment<br>Incoordination<br>Restlessness |
| 35–50 | Marked confusion<br>Cardiac arrhythmias<br>Labored respiration |
| 25–35 | Cardiac arrest<br>Decreased renal blood flow<br>Decreased urine output<br>Lactic acidosis<br>Lethargy<br>Loss of consciousness |
| <25 | Decreased minute ventilation[a] secondary to depression of the respiratory center |

*$PaO_2$*, Partial pressure of arterial oxygen.
[a]The total expired volume of air per minute.
Modified from Frownfelter DL, Dean E: *Principles and practice of cardiopulmonary physical therapy*, ed 4, St Louis, 2006, Mosby-Year Book, p. 234.

description of sputum, associated symptoms such as fever, triggers if known, and treatments and their effectiveness.[333]

### Dyspnea

Dyspnea, or shortness of breath, is defined by the American Thoracic Society as, "a subjective experience of breathing discomfort that consists of qualitatively distinct sensations that vary in intensity.…[It] derives from interactions among multiple physiological, psychological, social, and environmental factors, and may induce secondary physiological and behavioral responses."[318] Dyspnea is a common symptom and can be associated with a variety of causes, including anxiety, heart failure, acute coronary syndrome, pulmonary embolus, COPD, upper respiratory infection, asthma, pneumonia, and lung cancer.[46] Factors contributing to the sensation of dyspnea include increased work of breathing (WOB), respiratory muscle fatigue, increased systemic metabolic demands, and decreased respiratory reserve capacity. Dyspnea when the person is lying down is called *orthopnea* and is caused by redistribution of body water. Fluid shift leads to increased fluid in the lung, which interferes with gas exchange and leads to orthopnea. In supine and prone, the abdominal contents also exert pressure on the diaphragm, increasing the WOB and often limiting vital capacity.

**Box 15.1**

**MOST COMMON SIGNS AND SYMPTOMS OF PULMONARY DISEASE**

- Cough
- Dyspnea
- Abnormal sputum
- Chest pain
- Hemoptysis
- Cyanosis
- Digital clubbing
- Altered breathing patterns

### Chest Pain

Pulmonary pain patterns are usually localized in the substernal or chest region over involved lung fields. However, pulmonary pain can radiate to the neck, upper trapezius, costal margins, thoracic area of the back, scapulae, or shoulder. Shoulder pain caused by pulmonary involvement may radiate along the medial aspect of the arm, mimicking other neuromuscular causes of neck or shoulder pain. Musculoskeletal causes of chest (wall) pain must be differentiated from pain of cardiac, pulmonary, epigastric, and breast origins.

Extensive disease may occur in the lung without occurrence of pain until the process extends to the parietal pleura (Fig. 15.3). Pleural irritation then results in sharp, localized pain that is aggravated by any respiratory movement. Clients usually note that the pain is alleviated by lying on the affected side, which diminishes the movement of that side of the chest.[414,440]

### Cyanosis

The presence of cyanosis, a bluish color of the skin and mucous membranes, depends on the oxygen saturation of arterial blood and the total amount of circulating hemoglobin. It is further differentiated as central or peripheral. Central cyanosis is best observed as a bluish discoloration in the oral mucous membranes, lips, and conjunctivae (i.e., the warmer, more central areas) and is most often associated with cardiac right-to-left shunts

**Table 15.3** Descriptions of Altered Breathing Patterns and Sounds

| Breathing Pattern or Sound | Description |
|---|---|
| Apneustic | Gasping inspiration followed by short expiration |
| Biot respiration (ataxia) | An irregular pattern of deep and shallow breaths; fast, deep breaths interspersed with abrupt pauses in breathing |
| Cheyne-Stokes respiration | Repeated cycle of deep breathing followed by shallow breaths or cessation of breathing |
| Crackles/rales | Discontinuous, low pitched sounds, predominantly heard during inspiration and indicate secretions in the peripheral airways[132] |
| Hyperventilation | Abnormally prolonged and deep breathing |
| Hypoventilation | Reduction in the amount of air entering the pulmonary alveoli, which causes an increase in the arterial $CO_2$ level |
| Kussmaul respiration | A distressing dyspnea characterized by increased respiratory rate (>20/min), increased depth of respiration, panting, and labored respiration typical of air hunger |
| Lateral-costal breathing | Chest becomes flattened anteriorly with excessive flaring of the lower ribs (supine position); minimal to no upper chest expansion or accessory muscle involvement with outward flaring of the lower rib cage instead; the person breathes into the lateral plane of respiration (gravity eliminated) because the weakened diaphragm and intercostal muscles cannot effectively oppose the force of gravity in the anterior plane; used to focus expansion in areas of the chest wall that have decreased expansion (e.g., spinal cord injury with atelectasis or pneumonia, asymmetric chest expansion with scoliosis)[a] |
| Paradoxical breathing (sometimes referred to as reverse breathing) | All or part of the chest wall falls in during inspiration; may be abdominal expansion during exhalation, can lead to a flattened anterior chest wall or pectus excavatum |
| Stridor | A shrill, harsh sound heard during inspiration in the presence of laryngeal obstruction |
| Wheezing | High pitched, continuous whistling sound, usually with expiration and related to bronchospasm or other constriction of the airways |

[a]From Massery M: Personal communication.

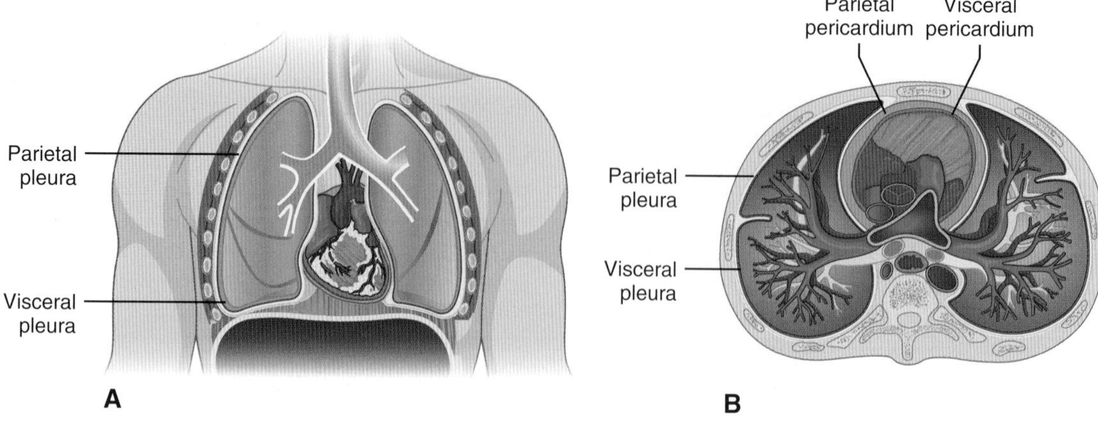


**Figure 15.3**

Chest cavity and associated structural linings shown in anterior (A) and cross-sectional (B) views. For instructional purposes the layers are depicted larger than actually found in the human body.

and pulmonary disease. Peripheral cyanosis is associated with decreased perfusion to the extremities, nail beds, and nose (i.e., the cooler, exposed areas) and is commonly caused by cold external temperature, anxiety, heart failure, or shock.

Clinically detectable cyanosis depends not only on oxygen saturation but also on the total amount of circulating hemoglobin that is bound to oxygen. For example, someone with severe anemia may not be cyanotic because all available hemoglobin is fully saturated with oxygen. However, someone with polycythemia may demonstrate signs of cyanosis because the overproduction of red blood cells results in increased amounts of hemoglobin that are not fully saturated with oxygen. In some instances, however, such as in carbon monoxide poisoning, hemoglobin is bound with a substance other than oxygen. There is no cyanosis, as the hemoglobin binding sites are fully occupied, however there is hypoxia due to lack of oxygen availability.

## Clubbing

Thickening and widening of the terminal phalanges of the fingers and toes result in a painless club-like appearance recognized by the loss of the angle between the nail and the nail bed (Fig. 15.4). Conditions that chronically interfere with tissue perfusion and nutrition may cause clubbing, including cystic fibrosis (CF), chronic obstructive pulmonary disease (COPD), lung cancer, bronchiectasis, pulmonary fibrosis, congenital heart disease, and lung abscess. Although 75% to 85% of clubbing is caused by pulmonary disease and resultant hypoxia (diminished availability of blood to the body tissues), clubbing does not always indicate lung disease. It is sometimes present in heart disease, peripheral vascular disease, and disorders of the liver and gastrointestinal tract.

## Altered Breathing Patterns

Changes in the rate, depth, regularity, and effort of breathing occur in response to any condition affecting the pulmonary system (see Table 15.3). Breathing patterns can vary, depending on the neuromuscular or neurologic disease or trauma (Box 15.2).

In a large cross-section of people and clinical disorders, hypoventilation is one of the most common changes in breathing patterns observed. Anything that can cause hypoxemia (e.g., fever, malnutrition, metabolic disturbance, loss of blood or blood flow, or availability of oxygen) reduces energy supplies and results in respiratory muscle dysfunction and altered breathing patterns. When hypoxemia is accompanied by skeletal muscle atonia associated with any neuromuscular cause, hypoventilation may further jeopardize the ventilatory pump.

Breathing pattern abnormalities seen with head trauma, brain abscess, diaphragmatic paralysis of chest wall muscles and thorax (e.g., generalized myopathy or neuropathy), heat stroke, spinal meningitis, and encephalitis can include *apneustic breathing, ataxic breathing,* or *Cheyne-Stokes respiration.*

Apneustic breathing localizes damage to the mid pons and is most commonly a result of a basilar artery infarct. Ataxic, or Biot, breathing is caused by disruption of the respiratory rhythm generator in the medulla. Cheyne-Stokes respiration is characterized by a crescendo and decrescendo pattern in respiratory rate followed by a brief period of apnea.[399] The most common cause of Cheyne-Stokes respiration is severe congestive heart failure, but it can also occur with renal failure, meningitis, drug overdose, and increased intracranial pressure. A similar pattern exists in infants younger than 6 months of age and is called "periodic" breathing. This pattern in infants is normal and changes to a regular pattern between 6 months and 1 year.

Spinal cord injuries above C3 result in loss of phrenic nerve innervation, necessitating a tracheostomy and ventilatory support. Upper thoracic injuries may also require ventilatory support, depending on the remaining respiratory muscles' ability to generate adequate negative pressure for inhalation. *Ventilatory support* is used to refer to a variety of interventions, including mechanical ventilation via endotracheal intubation, noninvasive ventilatory support with continuous positive airway pressure (CPAP),

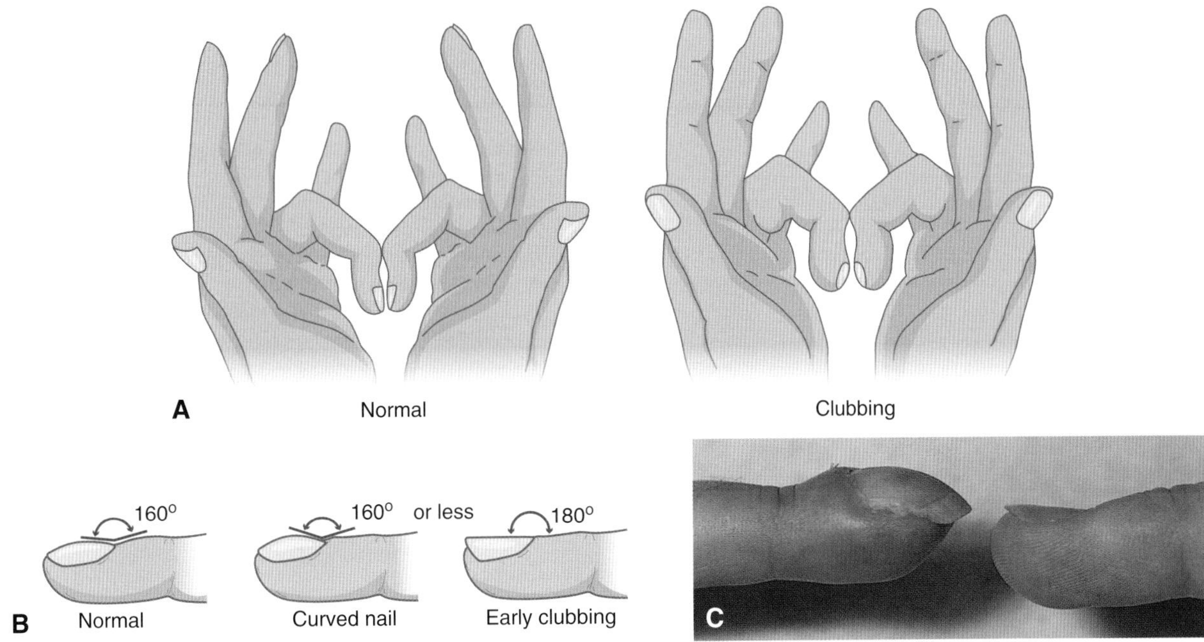


**Figure 15.4**

(A) Assessment of clubbing by the Schamroth method. The client places the fingernails of opposite fingers together and holds them up to a light. If a diamond shape can be seen between the nails, there is no clubbing. (B) The profile of the index finger is examined, and the angle of the nail base is noted; it should be approximately 160 degrees. The nail base is firm to palpation. Curved nails are a variation of normal with a convex profile and may look like clubbed nails, but the angle between the nail base and the nail is 160 degrees or less. In early clubbing, the angle straightens out to 180 degrees and the nail base feels spongy to palpation. (C) Photograph of advanced clubbing of the finger *(left)* compared with normal finger *(right)*. (A and B, from Swartz MH: *Textbook of physical diagnosis: history and examination*, Philadelphia, 1989, WB Saunders; C, from Swartz MH: *Textbook of physical diagnosis: history and examination*, ed 6, Philadelphia, 2009, WB Saunders.)

positive end-expiratory pressure (PEEP), and bilevel positive airway pressure. Those with lower thoracic injuries or incomplete injuries may also have altered breathing mechanics. These altered mechanics may place the person with spinal cord injury at risk for pulmonary infections, including pneumonia. Physical therapy interventions can improve breathing patterns and airway clearance, promoting good pulmonary hygiene.[420]

Clients with generalized weakness, as in the Guillain-Barré syndrome, some myopathies or neuropathies, or incomplete spinal cord injuries, may show a tendency toward a specific breathing pattern called *lateral-costal breathing* (see Table 15.3). Others who are experiencing failure of the ventilator system may demonstrate a paradoxical breathing pattern where the abdomen moves "inward" during inspiration instead of expanding.

## SPECIAL IMPLICATIONS FOR THE THERAPIST 15.1

### *Signs and Symptoms of Pulmonary Disease*

Many people with neuromusculoskeletal conditions, as well as people with primary or secondary pulmonary pathology, have the potential for oxygen transport deficits, impaired ventilation, and altered breathing patterns. For each type of condition, the therapist must identify those steps in the oxygen transport pathway that are affected, so that intervention targets the specific underlying problem.

Monitoring the cardiopulmonary status is important because many of the interventions provided by a therapist elicit an exercise stimulus and stress the oxygen transport system. Because impairment can result from diseases other than cardiopulmonary conditions, therapists in all settings need expertise in anticipating and detecting pulmonary dysfunction in the absence of primary pulmonary disease.[136,173]

Recognizing abnormal responses to interventions is important in identifying the client who needs additional intervention or who needs to be referred to another health care professional. Clinical observation of the client as the client breathes is important (Box 15.3) and can alert the therapist to respiratory pathologic conditions. Therapists should assess the muscle groups (abdominal and intercostal muscles, accessory muscles, and the diaphragm) involved in normal ventilatory function. Techniques to improve ventilation can enhance motor performance and improve a client's functional level.

High pressure in the pulmonary circulation (pulmonary hypertension) can cause pain during exercise that is often mistaken for cardiac pain (angina pectoris). For the therapist, musculoskeletal causes of chest pain must be differentiated from pain of cardiac, pulmonary, epigastric, and breast origins before treatment intervention begins.[197] The therapist involved in performing airway clearance techniques and pulmonary rehabilitation must recognize precautions for and contraindications to therapy interventions in the medical client (Table 15.4).

Box 15.2

**BREATHING PATTERNS AND ASSOCIATED CONDITIONS**

***Hyperventilation***

- Anxiety
- Acute head injury
- Hypoxemia
- Fever

*Kussmaul*

- Strenuous exercise
- Metabolic acidosis

*Cheyne-Stokes*

- Congestive heart failure
- Renal failure
- Meningitis
- Drug overdose
- Increased intracranial pressure
- Infants (normal)
- Older people during sleep (normal)

***Hypoventilation***

- Fibromyalgia syndrome
- Chronic fatigue syndrome
- Sleep disorder
- Muscle fatigue
- Muscle weakness
- Malnutrition
- Neuromuscular disease
  - Guillain-Barré
  - Myasthenia gravis
  - Poliomyelitis
  - Amyotrophic lateral sclerosis
- Pickwickian or obesity hypoventilation syndrome
- Severe kyphoscoliosis
  - Apneustic
  - Mid pons lesion
  - Basilar artery infarct

***Biot (Ataxia)***

- Exercise
- Shock
- Cerebral hypoxia
- Heat stroke
- Spinal meningitis
- Head injury
- Brain abscess
- Encephalitis

Box 15.3

**CLINICAL INSPECTION OF THE RESPIRATORY SYSTEM**

- Respiratory rate, depth, and effort of breathing
  - Tachypnea
  - Dyspnea
  - Gasping respirations
- Breathing pattern or sounds (see also Table 15.3)
  - Cheyne-Stokes respiration
  - Hyperventilation or hypoventilation
  - Kussmaul respiration
  - Upper chest breathing
  - Diaphragmatic breathing
  - Lateral-costal breathing
  - Paradoxical breathing
  - Prolonged expiration
  - Pursed-lip breathing
  - Wheezing/rhonchi
  - Crackles (formerly called rales)
- Cyanosis
- Pallor or redness of skin during activity
- Clubbing (toes, fingers)
- Nicotine stains on fingers and hands
- Retraction of intercostal, supraclavicular, or suprasternal spaces
- Use of accessory muscles
- Nasal flaring
- Tracheal tug
- Chest wall shape and deformity
  - Barrel chest
  - Pectus excavatum
  - Pectus carinatum
  - Kyphosis
  - Scoliosis
- Cough
- Sputum: clear or white (normal) frothy; red-tinged, green, or yellow (pathologic)

## AGING AND THE RESPIRATORY SYSTEM

Aging affects not only the physiologic functions of the lungs (ventilation and respiration) but also the ability of the respiratory system to defend itself. More than any other organ, the lung is susceptible to infectious processes and environmental and occupational pollutants (see "Environmental and Occupational Diseases" below). These factors, combined with the normal aging process, contribute to the decline of lung function.

Age-related alterations in the respiratory system are based on structural changes that result from repeated episodes of damage, lifelong exposure to the environment, and shortening of telomeres that ultimately result in cell death.[60] These changes over time lead to functional impairment of gas exchange.[449,517] Chest wall compliance decreases with aging due to calcification of costal cartilage and changes in the joints of the ribs and spine, as well as alterations in collagen. This increased stiffness affects the volume of air moved and the WOB. Elastic recoil also is decreased, with lower levels of elastin and higher levels of collagen.[60] Alveolar walls flatten, surface area is reduced, and the small airways more readily collapse and trap air, reducing the capacity for gas exchange.[173,244] Moreover, there is an increase in pulmonary arterial pressure, diminished vasodilation, and lower levels of nitric oxide that reduce the efficiency of alveolar capillary exchange.[60,410] Dead space increases with age, contributing to pulmonary limitations to exercise.[410]

Many changes that occur with aging affect the lower airway, but in the upper airway the movement of the cilia slows and becomes less effective in sweeping away mucus and debris. This reduced ciliary action, combined with the other changes noted, predisposes the older client to increased respiratory infections.

Reduction in respiratory muscle strength and endurance and subsequent increase in the WOB requiring greater muscle oxygen consumption at any workload are observed with increasing age.[54,173] The respiratory

**Table 15.4** Considerations for and Contraindications to Airway Clearance Techniques in the Medical Client

| Considerations | Contraindications |
|---|---|
| Hemoptysis | Untreated tension |
| Fragile ribs (e.g., metastatic bone cancer, osteoporosis, flail chest, rib fractures, osteomyelitis of the ribs) | Pneumothorax; treat when chest tube has been inserted and client is stable |
| Burns, open wounds, skin infections in thoracic area | Unstable |
| Pulmonary edema, congestive heart failure | Cardiovascular system |
| Large pleural effusion | Hypotension |
| Pulmonary embolism (controversial) | Uncontrolled hypertension |
| Symptomatic aneurysm or decrease in circulation of the main blood vessels | Acute myocardial infarction |
| Platelet count between 20,000 and 50,000/$mm^3$ | Arrhythmias |
| Postoperatively | Conditions prone to hemorrhages (platelet count <20,000/$mm^3$ must have physician approval) |
| Neurosurgery (positioning may cause increased intracranial pressure; can begin gentle breathing exercises) | Unstabilized head and neck injury |
| Esophageal anastomosis (gastric juices may affect suture line) | Intracranial pressure >20 mm Hg |
| Orthopedic clients who are limited in positioning | |
| Recent spinal fusion | |
| Surgical complications (e.g., pericardial sac tear) | |
| Recent skin grafts or flaps | |
| Resected tumors (avoid tumor area) | |
| Recently placed pacemaker | |
| Older or nervous clients who become agitated or upset with therapy | |
| Acute spinal injury or recent spinal surgery such as laminectomy (precaution: log-roll and position with care to maintain vertebral alignment) | |

muscles, including the diaphragm, become stiffer with age due to increased collagen. Moreover, the diaphragm's length tension is altered due to the increase in anterior-posterior diameter of the chest wall.[368,410] Loss of respiratory muscle strength can lead to dyspnea and, ultimately, to ventilatory pump failure.

Normal minute ventilation of older adults is comparable to that of younger people, although tidal volumes are smaller and rate is higher. There is a significant blunting of response to hypoxia and hypercapnia from both the respiratory and cardiovascular systems, particularly at rest. The hypercapnia response during exercise is greater in older adults, contributing to more dyspnea for a given workload even in the absence of oxygen desaturation or metabolic acidosis.

Most adults attain maximal lung function (as measured by forced expiratory volume [FEV]) during their early 20s, but with increasing age, especially after age 55 years, there is an overall decrease in the functional ability of the lungs to move air in and out. This decline peaks by age 75 years, falling to approximately 70% of our maximum. Aging reduces the reserve capacity of virtually all pulmonary functions regardless of lifestyle, although a sedentary lifestyle accelerates the decline.[279] With age, there are decrements in inspiratory capacity and vital capacity, and increases in functional residual capacity and residual volume. Total lung capacity stays about the same if changes in height that occur with aging are considered.[368]

All of these changes contribute to the increased WOB, resulting in a higher effort for the same activity compared to a younger person. These changes are amplified in the person who smokes or who is inactive.

Pulmonary complications during anesthesia and the postoperative period are significantly increased in older adults with preexisting diseases. Loss of an effective cough reflex contributes to an increased susceptibility to pneumonia and postoperative atelectasis in the older population. Other contributing factors to the loss of an effective cough reflex include conditions more common in older age, such as reduced consciousness, use of sedatives, impaired esophageal motility, dysphagia, and neurologic diseases.

**SPECIAL IMPLICATIONS FOR THE THERAPIST 15.2**

### *The Aging Respiratory System and Exercise*

The therapist working with older adults needs to understand the limitations to exercise to determine appropriate interventions. Various systems that are impacted by aging affect exercise tolerance, including the pulmonary system, cardiovascular system, and muscular system.

$VO_{2max}$declines with age, however this is largely attributed to inactivity, $VO_{2max}$ lower maximal heart rates, and changes to oxygen delivery at the muscle level that occur with aging.[410]

In order to "power" exercise, the body must get oxygen into the system (and carbon dioxide out), deliver it to the left side of the heart and the system, and extract oxygen at the muscle level to power the mitochondrial machinery. Aging-related changes to the lung tissue, the vasculature, and the thoracic cage decrease the ability of the lungs to power exercise over time. Again, this can be mediated by lifelong physical activity.

Ventilation of the airways involves moving air through "tubes." With age, the bronchi narrow and produce more mucus, impeding airflow. Moreover, the body has increased difficulty generating the muscular forces needed to change intrathoracic pressures. Changes to the thoracic cage with aging increase the anterior-posterior diameter of the chest wall, which diminishes the power output of the intercostals and diaphragm. The workload and efficiency of breathing is also hampered by stiffness in the costovertebral and costochondral joints. Respiration, which involves gas exchange, is also diminished due to the increased vascular resistance in the lungs, increased surface tension in the alveoli, and reduced diffusion capacity across the alveolar-capillary membrane.[410]

With age, there is a decline in muscle size and decrements in the neuromuscular junction that contribute to exercise intolerance. There is also a decrease in oxygen delivery to the muscle due to age-related impaired vasodilation.[410]

The above cardiac, vascular, and pulmonary changes that occur with aging result in fatigue with exercise, dyspnea on exertion, and increased work of breathing. An important message that physical therapists can and should convey to the older client is the power of physical activity to mediate these losses.

## INFECTIOUS AND INFLAMMATORY DISEASES

### Pneumonia

#### Overview and Etiologic Factors

Pneumonia is considered an acute lung injury (ALI) where an inflammatory process affects the parenchyma of the lungs. Pneumonia can be caused by (1) a bacterial, viral, fungal, or mycoplasmal infection (organisms that have both viral and bacterial characteristics); (2) inhalation of toxic or caustic chemicals, smoke, dusts, or gases; or (3) aspiration of food, fluids, or vomitus. It may be primary or secondary, and it often follows influenza. The common feature of all types of pneumonia is an inflammatory pulmonary response to the offending organism or agent. This response may involve one or both lungs at the level of the lobe (lobar pneumonia) or more distally at the bronchioles and alveoli (bronchopneumonia).

#### Routes of Infection

The major routes of infection are airborne pathogens, circulation, sinus infection, and aspiration. Hospital-acquired pneumonia and ventilator associated pneumonia are the most common infections in hospitalized patients and carry significant mortality and morbidity.[285]

#### Incidence

Pneumonia is a commonly encountered disease with an incidence rate of approximately 248 per 10,000 U.S. adults.[509] Approximately 30% of pneumonias are bacterial and are especially prevalent in the older adult. Viral pneumonia, accounting for nearly half of all cases, is not usually life-threatening, except in the immunocompromised person. The remaining 20% of all cases are caused by *Mycoplasma*.

#### Risk Factors

Infectious agents responsible for pneumonia are typically present in the upper respiratory tract and cause no harm unless resistance is lowered by some other factor or if something disrupts the flora typically present in the respiratory system. Risk factors for pneumonia in adults include older age, smoking, poor nutrition, previous pneumonia, COPD, asthma, reduced function, poor oral hygiene, environmental exposures such as dust and metals, immunosuppressive status, use of oral steroids, and use of acid reducing medications.[345, 11] Older adults, especially those who are bedridden or who have multiple comorbidities and those with altered consciousness (e.g., caused by alcoholic stupor, head injury, seizure disorder, drug overdose, or general anesthesia) are most vulnerable. Inactivity and immobility cause pooling of normal secretions in the airways that creates an environment promoting bacterial growth. In addition, hospitalization, confinement to an extended care facility or intensive care unit, surgery, mechanical ventilation, and urinary incontinence promotes rapid colonization of pathogenic organisms. People who have difficulty swallowing, those who have an inability to take oral medications, or those whose cough reflexes are impaired by drugs, alcohol, or neuromuscular disease are at increased risk for the development of aspiration pneumonia. Children younger than two, those born prematurely, and those with neurodevelopmental disorders are at a higher risk.[207,346]

#### Pathogenesis

Newer theories of pneumonia pathogenesis include disruption of the normal biome of the respiratory system that causes overgrowth of flora that is already present.[509] Although a common disease, pneumonia is relatively rare in healthy people because of the effectiveness of the respiratory host defense system and the fact that healthy lungs are generally kept sterile below the first major bronchial divisions. In the compromised person, the normal release of biochemical mediators by alveolar macrophages as part of the inflammatory response does not eliminate invading pathogens. The multiplying microorganisms release damaging toxins, stimulating full-scale inflammatory and immune responses with damaging side effects.

Once a pathogen enters the pulmonary system, macrophages are activated and release cytokines (TNFα, IL-1, IL-8) which beckon inflammatory cells to the site of infection. Macrophages also help to activate cell-mediated immunity (e.g., T cells), amping up the immunologic response. The result of immune activation is flooding of the lung parenchyma with inflammatory cells and leakage of the pulmonary vasculature.[243]

Endotoxins released by some microorganisms damage bronchial mucous and alveolar-capillary membranes as well as damage type II cells, which produce surfactant.[388] Inflammation and edema cause the respiratory exchange units to fill with infectious debris and exudate so that air cannot efficiently enter the alveoli and gas exchange is impaired, leading to ventilation–perfusion abnormalities and dyspnea. Production of interleukin (IL)-1 and tumor necrosis factor by alveolar macrophages can contribute to many of the systemic effects of pneumonia, such as fever, chills, malaise, and myalgia.

Resolution of the infection with eventual healing occurs with successful containment of the pathogenic microorganisms. When there is only mild or moderate damage to the epithelium, types I and II cells grow and restore the alveolar capillary membrane. In some with severe injury or with a history of smoking, inflammation is followed by laying down of fibroblasts and leads to pulmonary fibrosis and gas exchange abnormalities.[388]

**Aspiration Pneumonia.** Aspiration pneumonia (AP) refers to pneumonia that occurs due to fluids or other material from the oral cavity or GI tract is aspirated into the lower respiratory tract. Risk factors for AP include increasing age, dysphagia, depressed central nervous system impacting the cough reflex, reflux, anatomic abnormalities (laryngeal cleft or tracheoesophageal fistula), and debilitating illnesses. Although any region may be affected, the right side, especially the right upper lobe in the supine person, is commonly affected because of the anatomic configuration of the right main-stem bronchus. In addition to the typical symptoms and signs associated with pneumonia, AP should be suspected if patients are coughing at or shortly after meals.

**Fungal Pneumonia.** Pneumonia caused by fungi may present with mild symptoms, though some people become very ill. The three most common types, *histoplasmosis*, *coccidioidomycosis*, and *blastomycosis*, are generally specific to a limited geographic area. Other fungal lung infections primarily affect people with compromised immune systems. Diagnosis is made by culturing sputum samples.

**Viral Pneumonia.** Viral pneumonia is usually mild and self-limiting, often bilateral and panlobular but confined to the septa rather than the intraalveolar spaces as is more likely with bacterial pneumonia. Viral pneumonia can be a primary infection creating an ideal environment for a secondary bacterial infection, or it can be a complication of another viral illness. The virus destroys ciliated epithelial cells and invades goblet cells and bronchial mucous glands. Bronchial walls become edematous and infiltrated with leukocytes. The destroyed bronchial epithelium sloughs throughout the respiratory tract, preventing mucociliary clearance.

**Bacterial Pneumonia.** Destruction of the respiratory epithelium by infection with the influenza virus may be one mechanism whereby influenza predisposes people to bacterial pneumonia. The lung parenchyma, especially the alveoli in the lower lobes, is the most common site of bacterial pneumonia. When bacteria reach the alveolar surfaces, most are rapidly ingested by phagocytes.

Once phagocytosis has occurred, intracellular lysis proceeds but at a slower rate for bacteria than for other particles. As the condition resolves, neutrophils degenerate and macrophages appear in the alveolar spaces, which ingest the fibrin threads, and the remaining bacteria in the respiratory bronchioles are then transported by lung lymphatics to regional lymph nodes. The infection is usually limited to one or two lobes.

### Clinical Manifestations

Most cases of pneumonia are preceded by an upper respiratory infection. Signs and symptoms include pleuritic chest pain aggravated by chest movement, and a productive cough (with rust-colored sputum in bacterial pneumonia and watery sputum in viral). Other symptoms include dyspnea, tachypnea, crackles or adventitious breath sounds, fatigue, fever, chills, and generalized myalgias.

Older adults with pneumonia have fewer symptoms than younger people, and may present with vague symptoms, such as loss of appetite, fatigue, and decreased cognition/attention.[468] Associated changes in gas exchange (hypoxia and hypercapnia) may result in altered mental status (e.g., confusion) and may lead to falls.

Most cases of pneumonia are relatively mild and resolve within 1 to 3 weeks, although symptoms may linger for 1 or 2 more weeks (more typical of viral or *Mycoplasma* pneumonia). If the infection develops slowly with a fever so low as to be unnoticeable, the person may have what is referred to as "double pneumonia" (both lungs involved) or "walking pneumonia." This form tends to last longer than any other form of pneumonia. Complications of pneumonia can include pleural effusion (fluid around the lung), empyema (pus in the pleural cavity), and, rarely, lung abscess.

## MEDICAL MANAGEMENT

**DIAGNOSIS.** Community-acquired pneumonia typically presents with a productive cough, fever, and pleuritic chest pain, with a recent upper respiratory infection. Diagnosis is further supported by a new infiltrate on chest radiograph, lung auscultation, and microscopic examination of respiratory secretions.[316,509] For aspiration pneumonia, diagnosis may include a swallowing study. Gram stain, color, odor, and cultures are part of the sputum analysis. A blood culture may help identify the bacteria, but bacterial counts are only positive in approximately 10% of bacterial pneumonias; 90% of bacterial pneumonias do not show a positive bacterial count. The most common pathogens after the widespread delivery of the pneumococcal vaccine are rhinovirus, influenza, and *Streptococcus pneumoniae*. New pathogens continue to emerge with varying virulence, resulting in mild cases of pneumonia to pandemics. Viruses such as respiratory syncytial virus (RSV) are common in infants along with influenza, with *Streptococcus pneumoniae* the most prevalent bacterial pathogen.[207]

Urine antigen testing may also be used and provides a quick diagnosis, providing results for detecting *Streptococcus pneumoniae* in 15 minutes. Due to moderate sensitivity and the risk for false positives, this test is used in conjunction with other methods.[107]

Other diagnostic procedures may include chest radiographs that may reveal infiltrates involving a single lobe (lobar pneumonia from staphylococci) or multiple lobes. Radiographs have poor sensitivity, resulting in an upsurge in the use of CT scans for diagnosis.[509] In infants and children, pathogens are identified via nasopharyngeal secretions which are analyzed with polymerase chain reaction (PCR) techniques.[207] Physical examination, including percussion and auscultation of the chest, may reveal signs of lung consolidation such as dullness, or adventitious breath sounds.

**TREATMENT.** The primary treatment for bacterial and mycoplasmic forms of pneumonia is antibiotic therapy along with fluids. Treatment with specific antibiotics is based on the history; whether the pneumonia was community-acquired, hospital-acquired, or extended-care facility–acquired; and on the medical status and overall condition of the client (e.g., otherwise healthy or debilitated). Patients are typically started on empiric antibiotic therapy until a pathogen is determined. Airway clearance techniques and early mobility may aid in clearing purulent sputum.

Fungal pneumonia is treated with antifungal drugs. Viral pneumonia is treated symptomatically unless secondary bacterial pneumonia develops. Hospitalization may be required for the immunocompromised or frail client.

The U.S. Centers for Disease Control and Prevention (CDC) recommends two pneumonia vaccines and the influenza vaccine for those aged 65 and older; for people with chronic disorders; for individuals with poorly controlled diabetes mellitus; and for those with a compromised immune system or confined to a long-term care facility. Unfortunately, only 69% of those eligible get vaccinated.[90]

Infants and children in the United States are vaccinated against *Haemophilus influenzae* type b (Hib), and the influenza vaccine is recommended annually for children 6 months and older (NHLBI, pneumonia). A pneumococcal conjugate vaccine is recommended for all children younger than 2 years of age (series of four doses).[108]

For aspiration pneumonia, treatment should include swallowing rehabilitation, oral care, positioning to improve swallowing, and vaccines. Physical therapy and early mobility may reduce mortality rates in the elderly admitted with AP.[468]

**PROGNOSIS.** Community-acquired pneumonia (CAP) remains a common and serious clinical problem despite the availability of potent antibiotics and aggressive supportive measures. It is the eighth leading cause of death in the United States, claiming the lives of approximately 51,000 Americans annually.[215] Those admitted to the hospital with CAP are at a higher risk for myocardial infarction, rhythm disturbances, and heart failure. Moreover, patients who recover from CAP have a 30% higher mortality rate in the following 2 to 5 years.[509] In children, pneumonia accounts for approximately 16% of all deaths in children under 5 years of age.[386] Highly effective prevention and treatment methods can improve survival and reduce the likelihood of developing pneumonia, especially if vaccination rates were higher. The *Healthy People 2020* Objective 1-9c is to reduce hospitalization for immunization-preventable pneumonia to 8 per 10,000 in persons age 65 years or older.

SPECIAL IMPLICATIONS FOR THE THERAPIST 15.3

### *Pneumonia*

The CDC recommends different precautions depending on the pathogen causing pneumonia. For example, for viral pneumonia in adults, standard precautions are recommended, whereas standard and droplet precautions are used for those with *Streptococcus* Type A for 24 hours after treatment is initiated.[88] Interventions that should be considered in the person with pneumonia are: elevation of the head of the bed to 30 to 45 degrees, early mobilization, minimizing use of sedatives, and judicious fluid management. Prone positioning and chest physical therapy are no longer recommended for first-line interventions, but may be considered given to patients with other comorbidities and presentation.[274] Proper positioning to prevent aspiration during the postoperative period and for all people who are immobilized or who have a poor gag reflex is important.

Occasionally, a lower-lobe infection can irritate the diaphragmatic surface so that pain referred to the shoulder is the presenting symptom. For the client with a known diagnosis of pneumonia, the breathing pattern and the position assumed in bed can indicate the client's discomfort, reveal tachypnea, and demonstrate splinting of the chest to minimize pleuritic pain (i.e., lying on the affected side reduces the pleural rubbing that often causes discomfort).

Lobes affected by pneumonia will remain vulnerable to further infection for some time, especially in the bedridden, debilitated, or in those with neuromuscular compromise. However, the client, family, or caretakers should be instructed in breathing exercises and a positional rotation program with frequent positional changes to prevent secretions from accumulating in dependent positions and to optimize ventilation–perfusion matching.

## Pneumocystis carinii Pneumonia

### Definition, Etiology, and Risk Factors

*Pneumocystis carinii* pneumonia (PCP) is a fungal pneumonia that affects people with altered immunity. It has recently been renamed *Pneumocystis jirovecii*, after the fungus that initiates this disease. This pathogen is now thought to be a normal part of the pulmonary biome, but is reactivated or introduced in those who are immunocompromised.[133] Risk factors for PCP pneumonia include: low CD4 counts, graft-versus-host disease, immunosuppression, low serum albumin, and coinfection with a bacteria, cytomegalovirus, or aspirgillious.[502]

### Pathogenesis and Clinical Manifestations

PCP is thought to be transmitted as aerosolized particles.[422] The mechanism of spread is not fully known, but recently attention has been given to theories that point toward an infection in early childhood that either resurfaces in adulthood in immunosuppressed states or primes the host to reacquire the infection in adulthood.[422]

PCP is mostly a disease that affects the lungs, but can occasionally spread to other organs. Infection begins with the attachment of the *Pneumocystis* trophozoite (the feeding stage of a sporozoan parasite) to the alveolar lining cell. The trophozoite feeds on the host cell, enlarges, and transforms into the cyst form that ruptures (excystment) to release new trophozoites, repeating the cycle. The cell wall of PCP also elicits a brisk inflammatory response in the host and can contribute to respiratory failure in those with a significant pneumonia.[422] If the process is uninterrupted by the immune system or antibiotic therapy, the affected alveoli progressively fill with organisms and proteinaceous fluid until consolidation disrupts gas exchange, slowly causing hypoxia and death.

The physiologic response to PCP includes fever, impaired gas exchange, and altered respiratory function. Symptoms of PCP develop slowly in those with HIV and present as fever and progressive dyspnea, accompanied by a nonproductive cough. Fatigue, tachypnea, weight loss, and other manifestations of underlying immunosuppressive disease may be present and worsened as a result of the increased metabolic demands. In those who are immunocompromised without HIV, the presentation is more rapid, with significant shortness of breath (SOB) and fever.[422,502]

### MEDICAL MANAGEMENT

**DIAGNOSIS, TREATMENT, AND PROGNOSIS.** PCP must be considered in the differential diagnosis in individuals with immune dysfunction or suppression. Diagnosis is made based upon clinical symptoms, chest radiographs, CTs, and PCR evaluation of the pathogen. Combination of tests may also improve early detection. Specimens are acquired through bronchioalveolar lavage, tissue sampling, or sputum cultures.[422]

PCP is primarily treated with combination antibiotics (trimethoprim-sulfamethoxazole), although some people with HIV also receive corticosteroids. Prophylaxis with antibiotics is now recommended for those who are immunosuppressed, including those on steroids, certain people undergoing treatment for cancer, and those who are undergoing solid or liquid transplantation.

The mortality rates have decreased over the past 10 years, with rates reported between 10% and 53%.[133,303] In one retrospective study across 17 years, mortality rates were higher in those with non-HIV PCP.[422] Risk factors associated with higher mortality rates in those without HIV include older age, delay in diagnosis, solid tumors, female sex, and low albumin.[502]

## Pulmonary Tuberculosis

### Definition

Tuberculosis (TB), formerly known as consumption, is an infectious, inflammatory systemic disease that affects the lungs and may disseminate to involve other organs. TB is caused by infection with *Mycobacterium tuberculosis* (MT) and is characterized by granulomas, caseous (resembling cheese) necrosis, and subsequent cavity formation. Latent infection is defined as harboring MT without evidence of active infection; active infection is based on the presence of clinical and laboratory findings.

### Overview

MT is spread through droplets in the air and can be completely eradicated through normal immune defenses, cause a primary TB infection, or get walled off by the body's immune system, temporarily controlling the disease. This is referred to as a latent infection that can become reactivated later in life in approximately 5% to 10% of people.[421]

TB may be primary or secondary. The first or primary infection with MT is usually asymptomatic and almost always remains quiet after the development of a hypersensitivity to the microorganism. The primary infection usually involves the middle or lower lung area, with lesions consisting of exudation in the lung parenchyma. These lesions quickly become caseous and spread to the hilum, where they gain access to the bloodstream and predispose the person to the subsequent development of chronic pulmonary and extrapulmonary TB at a later time.

Secondary TB develops as a result of either endogenous or exogenous reinfection by MT. This is the most common form of clinical TB. Reactivated TB usually causes abnormalities in the upper lobes of one or both lungs. In the United States, development of secondary TB is almost always the result of endogenous reinfection that occurs when the primary lesion becomes active as a result of debilitation or lowered resistance.

### Incidence

Despite improved methods of detection and treatment, TB remains a global health problem, with an estimated 10 million people around the world with TB and 1.3 million deaths annually from active TB.[97] The highest rates of new TB cases are from 30 "high risk" countries, with the following eight countries accounting for most of the new cases: India, China, Indonesia, Philippines, Pakistan, Nigeria, Bangladesh, and South Africa.[505]

In 2017, there were 9,105 cases of TB in the United States, which is a 2.3% decrease from the prior year.[97] Incidence rates have decreased in the United States for all racial and ethnic groups.[96]

Foreign-born persons and racial/ethnic minorities continue to bear a disproportionate burden of TB disease in the United States. Seventy percent of reported TB cases in the United States occurred in foreign-born people and is 15 times higher than in U.S.-born individuals.[96] Immigrants to the United States undergo testing for TB as part of the immigration process. Limited access to health care because of socioeconomic status or illegal alien status, language barriers, sociocultural differences, and other social determinants of health contribute to higher rates of TB among minorities.

Multidrug-resistant TB has emerged as a major infectious disease problem throughout the world. The percentage of TB cases that are drug resistant has remained stable for the last 20 years, indicating an ineffective strategy to address this issue.[96]

The infected individual begins taking the prescribed medication, feels better, and discontinues taking the drugs, which are normally required to be taken for 6 to 9 months. The disease flares up months later and is now resistant to the medications, and the infected person passes it along as a new drug-resistant strain characterized by mutations in existing genes.[172]

### Risk Factors

Although TB can affect anyone, certain segments of the population have an increased risk of contracting the disease, particularly those with HIV infection, people age 65 years and older, and those who are immunocompromised. Other groups at risk include (1) people with diabetes,[209](2) IV drug users and those dependent on alcohol, (3) economically disadvantaged or homeless people living in overcrowded areas, (4) infants and children younger than age 5 years, (5) current or past prison inmates, (6) family and friends of a person with infectious TB, (7) people with end-stage renal disease, (8) others who are immunocompromised (those who are malnourished, organ transplant recipients, anyone receiving cancer chemotherapy or prolonged corticosteroid therapy, those on immune modulating drugs for autoimmune diseases), (9) women who are pregnant, (10) people from areas with high rates of TB, and (11) people who work in facilities that house high-risk people (hospitals, nursing homes, homeless shelters, prisons).[507]

Environmental factors that enhance transmission include contact between susceptible persons and an infectious person in relatively small, enclosed spaces (e.g., inadequate ventilation that results in insufficient dilution or removal of infectious droplet nuclei (e.g., older buildings such as hospitals, prisons, government buildings, universities); and recirculation of air containing infectious droplet nuclei. Adequate ventilation is the most important measure to reduce the infectiousness of the environment. Mycobacteria are susceptible to ultraviolet irradiation (i.e., sunshine), so outdoor transmission of infection rarely occurs.

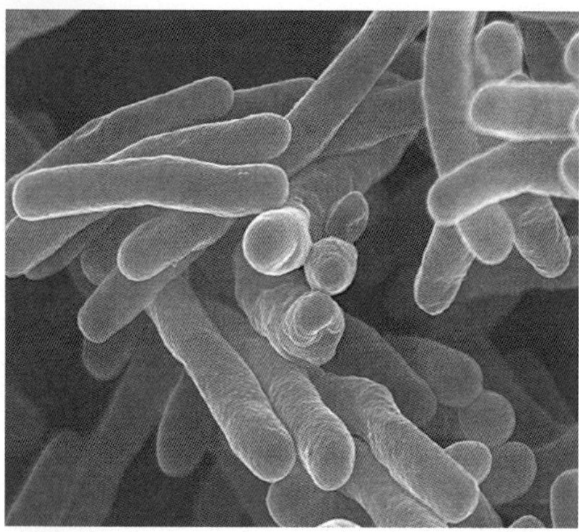

**Figure 15.5**

**Tuberculosis bacteria.** (Courtesy National Institute of Allergy and Infectious Diseases, National Institutes of Health, Bethesda, MD, 2001.)

## Etiologic Factors

The causative agent is the tubercle bacillus (Fig. 15.5), commonly transmitted in the United States by inhalation of infected airborne particles, known as droplet nuclei, which are produced when the infected persons sneeze, laugh, speak, sing, or cough. The mycobacterium that infect humans are *M. tuberculosis*, *M. bovis*, and *M. africanum*.[198]

Casual contact or brief exposure to a few bacilli will not result in transmission of sufficient bacilli to infect a person. Rather, longer duration and closer proximity to the infected individual contribute to transmission rates. In other parts of the world, bovine TB carried by unpasteurized milk and other dairy products from tuberculous cattle is more prevalent.

The tubercle bacillus is capable of surviving for months in sputum that is not exposed to sunlight. Within the body it becomes encapsulated and can lie dormant for decades and then become reactivated years after an initial infection. This secondary TB infection (endogenous reinfection) can occur at any time the person's resistance is lowered (e.g., alcoholism, immunosuppression, advancing age, comorbid conditions, or cancer).

## Pathogenesis

There are three primary stages of TB: primary infection, latent infection, and active disease. Primary infection occurs when a person inhales droplet nuclei containing *M. tuberculosis* (MT) and bacilli are ingested by macrophages. If the macrophage doesn't kill the MT, the bacilli replicate inside of the macrophage. A proliferation of epithelial cells surrounds and encapsulates the multiplying bacilli in an attempt to wall off the invading organisms, thus forming a granuloma. Granulomas have a necrotic center filed with alveolar macrophages infected with MT, surrounded by a variety of immune cells.[401] Caseous refers to the granulomas' gross appearance, which is similar to curdled cheese. In some people, infected macrophages can move to regional lymph nodes and spread to the system via the bloodstream (extrapulmonary TB). Bacilli enter the circulatory system and are carried to all areas of the body and may lodge in any organ, especially the lymph system, spine and weight-bearing joints, urogenital system, and meninges. Similar pharmacologic treatment is used for extrapulmonary and pulmonary TB.

Two to 10 weeks after initial human infection with the bacilli, acquired cell-mediated immunity usually limits further multiplication and spread of the TB bacilli, enabling the pathogen to survive symbiotically with its human host. Although the TB bacilli are walled off, the bacilli are not necessarily destroyed; they can remain alive but dormant inside the structure. In persons with intact cell-mediated immunity, collections of activated T cells and macrophages form granulomas that limit multiplication and spread of the organism, rendering the infection inactive, or *latent*. The tubercles stay intact as long as the immune system is maintained.

For the majority of individuals with an intact immune system, latent infection is clinically and radiographically undetected; a positive tuberculin (purified protein derivative) skin test result or a blood test is the only indication that infection has taken place. Individuals with latent TB infection but not active disease are not infectious and cannot transmit the organism. When residual lesions are visible on chest radiograph, these sites remain potential lesions for reactivation.

If, however, the infection is not controlled by the immune defenses, the person develops symptoms of active TB. In some people, active TB occurs due to reinfection by TB as opposed to activation of latent TB. Recent theories of TB include development of lipid pneumonia that causes liquefactive necrosis, resulting in cavity formation.[401] The inflammatory response and resultant lung damage are likely influenced by host characteristics such as comorbidities, immune system defenses, and genetic influence on immune responses. The cavities contain larger numbers of MT that can be spread through coughing, sneezing, and singing.

TB in the lungs can cause both restrictive and obstructive patterns and gas exchange abnormalities identified by pulmonary function testing and diffusion capacity for carbon monoxide.[401]

## Clinical Manifestations

Most symptoms associated with TB do not appear in the early, most curable stage of the disease, although TB could be detected via a skin or blood test. At this stage, chest radiographs are often normal, as are sputum tests.[98]

Signs and symptoms of active TB include the following:[98]

- Productive cough for 3 or more weeks
- Unexplained weight loss
- Night sweats
- Fever
- Fatigue
- Chest pain
- Adventitious breath sounds
- Symptoms associated with other organs affected by TB

Pulmonary complications associated with TB can include bronchopleural fistulae, esophagopleural fistulae, pleurisy with effusion, tuberculous pneumonia or laryngitis, and sudden lung atelectasis, indicating that a deep tuberculous cavity in the lung has perforated or created an opening into the pleural cavity, allowing air and infected material to flow to it (Fig. 15.6).

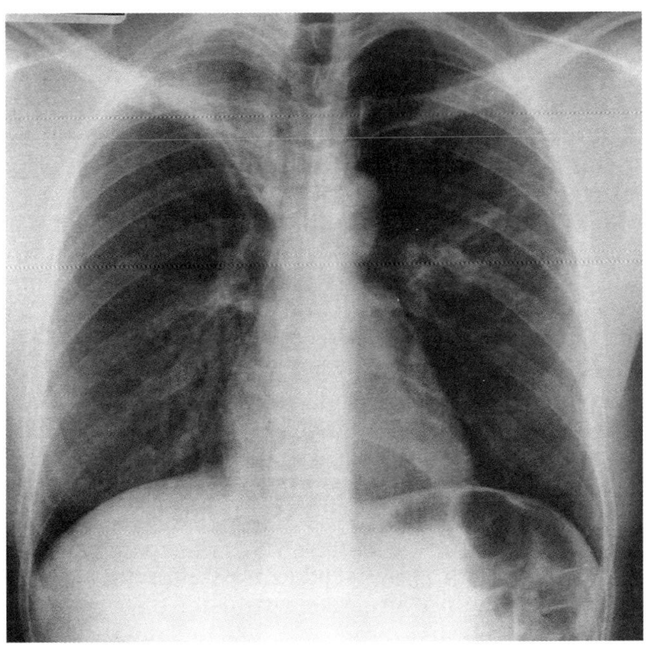

**Figure 15.6**

**Segmental consolidation in tuberculous bronchopneumonia.** The right upper lobe is grossly collapsed, scarred, and bronchiectatic. It had remained stable for many years until segmental nodular and linear consolidation appeared in the left mid zone, signaling reactivation. The segmental lesion was thought to be secondary to aspiration of bacteria from the right upper lobe. (From Grainger RG, Allison D: *Grainger and Allison's diagnostic radiology: a textbook of medical imaging*, ed 4, Philadelphia, 2001, Churchill Livingstone. Used with permission.)

TB can develop solely outside of the lungs or spread from the lungs to other areas in the body, which is termed extrapulmonary TB (EPTB). The most common sites for EPTB are lymph nodes, pleura, genitourinary system, gastrointestinal tract, bones, and the central nervous system. The pathophysiology of EPTB is not fully elucidated.[392] Extrapulmonary TB is higher in females, those with HIV, in immunosuppressed patients, in those with end-stage renal disease, those who had heavy alcohol use in the last year, and in younger people and those of African or Asian origin.[254,392]

## MEDICAL MANAGEMENT

**PREVENTION.** The World Health Organization has implemented an "End TB Strategy" that sets a vision of a "world free of tuberculosis." Milestones for 2025 include 75% reduction in TB deaths, 50% reduction in TB incidence, and no families facing catastrophic medical costs as a result of TB. The targets are advanced for the next milestone set for 2035. The three strategic pillars used to reach this goal are: (1) integrated, patient-centered care and prevention, (2) bold policies and supportive systems, and (3) intensified research and innovation. Key components of these pillars include early diagnosis of TB with appropriate drug-susceptibility testing, systematic screening of high risk-groups, vaccination against TB, and collaborative efforts with the HIV community. Other strategies include universal health coverage, addressing health disparities, and enacting policies to promote resource allocation for identification, treatment, and research.[508]

Testing for TB is a main strategy for early detection and prevention of spread. High-risk groups should be tested for TB, such as those exposed to TB, those from countries where TB disease rates are high; people who work in settings that increase risk, such as long-term care facilities, homes, and prisons; health care workers; those with HIV; and those who are immunosuppressed. Those who have latent TB should be treated to prevent active TB and further dissemination of the disease to others (see following section on treatment).

Preventing the transmission of TB is essential and can be done by using such simple measures as covering the mouth and nose with a tissue when coughing and sneezing, reducing the number of organisms excreted into the air. However, preventive and therapeutic interventions must address not only the bacillus but also the financial, nutritional, and employment status of those people at risk.

Adequate room ventilation and preventing overcrowding such as in homeless shelters and prisons are well-known preventive measures, but preventing this infection in many high-risk groups is complicated. Adherence to medication regimens is another area of focus to prevent drug-resistant TB.

**DIAGNOSIS.** Diagnostic measures for identifying TB currently include history, physical examination, chest radiograph, and more definitive testing via tuberculin skin test (TST), Xpert MTB/RIF© assay, blood tests (QuantiFERON®-TB Gold In-Tube test or T-SPOT® TB test) and microscopic examination of sputum. The two-step tuberculin skin test (TST) is typically used for health care workers and involves injecting inactive tuberculin into the skin. The person returns 48 to 72 hours later to determine results and then has a second administration of the skin test 1 to 3 weeks later. The skin and other tissue become sensitized to the protein part of the tubercle bacilli. A positive reaction causes a swelling or hardness at the site of infection and develops 3 to 10 weeks after the initial infection. A positive skin test reaction indicates the presence of a TB infection but does not indicate whether the infection is dormant or is causing a clinical illness.[85] The QuantiFERON-TB Gold test uses an enzyme-linked immunoassay (ELISA) to detect IF-$\gamma$ in blood when it interacts with two proteins that mimic TB. These proteins are different from those seen in people who get the BCG vaccine and therefore this test is more specific than the TST for this population. QantiFERON Gold test results are available in 48-72 hours.[75] The newest test is the Xpert MTB/RIF assay that can detect TB and multidrug-resistant TB.[76] This test analyzes a sputum sample, with results available in less than two hours.

People who are born outside of the United States may have been vaccinated with bacilli Calmette-Guerin (BCG). BCG is not routinely utilized in the United States because the strain of TB that is common in the United States is different from those found abroad, and due to its inconsistent effectiveness in preventing pulmonary TB. The BCG vaccine may cause false positives to the TST, and is often followed up with radiographs, blood tests, and physical examinations to assist in ruling out latent or active infection [79]

Because of the dormant properties of the tubercle bacillus, anyone infected with TB should have periodic TB testing performed. In the case of someone with known TB, the skin test will always be positive, requiring periodic screening with chest radiographs.

Treatment may be initiated with only a positive skin test even if chest film and sputum analyses show no evidence of the disease. In this way, the disease is less likely to reactivate later in life when the immune system performance declines with age.

**TREATMENT.** Treatment for latent TB prevents active TB. According to the CDC, more than 80% of cases of active TB result from untreated latent TB. Pharmacologic treatment through medication is the primary treatment of choice and renders the infection noncontagious and nonsymptomatic. These agents work by inhibiting cell wall biosynthesis, but the intracellular response that occurs is complex and poorly understood at this time.

The common drug regimens used to treat latent TB are isoniazid (INH) and rifapentine (RPT); rifampin (RIF); and isoniazid. The duration of treatment is dependent on the medical regimen and ranges from 3 to 9 months. Some of the medications are taken daily while others are taken 1 to 2 times per week.[80] The CDC recommends using the shortest duration medical regimen to encourage completion of the treatment. This regimen is referred to as 3HP, three refers to the length of treatment in months, H refers to the medication INH, and the P refers to the medication RPT.

Treatment for active TB includes taking medications for 6 to 9 months. As of this writing there are ten medications approved for treating active TB, the most common of which are isoniazid, rifampin, ethambutol (EMB), and pyrazinamide (PZA).[86]

**PROGNOSIS.** Pulmonary TB is a major cause of morbidity and mortality worldwide, resulting in the greatest number of deaths from any one single infectious agent. Predictive equations are published, but not used consistently. In a recent model, the following variables were associated with higher mortality rates: age over 65 years, TB meningitis, chronic kidney disease, coinfection with HIV, and pulmonary abnormalities identified on radiographs.[351]

Untreated, TB is 50% to 80% fatal, and the median time to death is 2.5 years.

## Lung Abscess

### Definition

Lung abscesses are thick-walled cavities with purulent exudate within the lung. An abscess usually develops as a complication of pneumonia, especially aspiration and staphylococcal pneumonia. This can occur when bacteria are aspirated from the oropharynx along with foreign material or vomitus, or it can occur from septic embolus from a heart valve.

### Risk Factors

There are systemic and focal risk factors for absesses.[154] Systemic factors include age greater than 65 years, corticosteroid use, immunosuppression, sepsis, malnutrition, diabetes, alcoholism, altered mental status, recumbent positioning, and cystic fibrosis.[154] Focal risk factors include seizures, neuromuscular disorders, oropharyngeal dysfunction, endotracheal intubation, reflux, periodontal infections, bronchial obstruction, pneumonia, and tube feeding.[154]

SPECIAL IMPLICATIONS FOR THE THERAPIST 15.4

### *Pulmonary Tuberculosis*

Health care workers should be alert at all times to the need for preventing TB transmission when cough-inducing procedures are being performed, but especially in cases of known TB or HIV infection. Isolation measures for anyone who may be dispersing *M. tuberculosis* must be taken both in the acute care setting and in outpatient areas. Inpatient rooms must be posted with airborne/droplet precautions.

If there is a high degree of suspicion or proved TB, clients should be cared for in negative-pressure isolation rooms while undergoing assessment and/or treatment. Procedures that may generate infectious aerosols should be carried out in similarly ventilated rooms. Precautions must be followed by all health care personnel having contact with clients diagnosed with TB (Box 15.4).

Therapists may be asked to assist individuals with a weak cough to generate a stronger one, either to improve ventilation or sometimes to obtain a sputum sample without undergoing the more invasive bronchoscopy. In such cases, the therapist should always check to see if the person has ever been diagnosed with pulmonary TB or had a recent TB test. When in doubt, the therapist should practice self-protective measures such as wearing a high-efficiency particulate air (HEPA) respirator or a protective mask. Training in the use of the mask and the proper sizing for the therapist are important when using these devices.

For the therapist evaluating a client with pulmonary TB, a thorough chest assessment and musculoskeletal evaluation should be performed. Chest expansion may be decreased because of diffuse fibrotic changes in progressive disease. Tracheal deviation may be present if there is a significant loss of volume in the upper lobes. Postural adaptations may have developed in late stages of the disease because of poor breathing patterns.[178] Other areas of assessment should include overall posture, gait, muscle strength, balance, and functional mobility.

People with TB typically have a poor nutritional status and progressive weight loss that may have secondary effects on the musculoskeletal system, such as postural defects and trigger point irritability. The effects of isolation result in disuse atrophy and cardiopulmonary and physical deconditioning, including progressive dyspnea.

Finding the balance between exercise and clinical limitations is challenging and there is little evidence that exercise is effective in people with active TB. There are limited studies looking at exercise and/or pulmonary rehabilitation post-TB; however, the studies indicate a positive outcome related to quality of life, and exercise capacity.[253]

Side effects of the medication can lead to peripheral neuritis that may be brought to the attention of the therapist. This and any other complication, such as hepatitis, hemoptysis, optic neuritis, or purpura, should be reported to the physician. Isoniazid-induced liver injury may present, with excess fatigue, nausea,

Box 15.4

**GUIDELINES FOR THERAPISTS FOR PREVENTING TRANSMISSION OF TUBERCULOSIS**

All TB control recommendations for inpatient facilities apply to hospices and home health services and outpatient settings.
All facilities should have a supervisor in charge of infection control compliance.
All new employees (and student therapists) should be screened with the two-step tuberculin skin test or Blood Assay *M. tuberculosis* test (BAMT).
Doors to airborne infection isolation rooms must be kept closed.
Clients infected with TB must cover mouth and nose with tissues when coughing, sneezing, or laughing.
Cough-inducing procedures should not be performed on TB clients unless absolutely necessary; such procedures should be performed using local exhaust, in a high-efficiency particulate air (HEPA)–filtered booth or individual TB isolation room. After completion of treatment, such persons should remain in the booth or enclosure until the cough subsides.
Clients must wear a mask when leaving the room.
Anyone entering the room must wear a gown and protective mask, called a HEPA respirator, properly.
Therapists must be adequately trained in the use and disposal of masks and should use a particulate respirator (PR; a special mask)[a] whenever the client is undergoing cough-inducement or aerosol-generating procedures.

- The therapist must check the condition of both the face piece and face seal each time the PR or HEPA respirator is worn.
- Gloves are used for Standard Precautions
- Disinfect the stethoscope between treatment sessions.
- Staff and employees are screened for TB yearly or more if working with high-risk populations.
- Hand washing is required before and after contact with the client.
- Isolation precautions must be continued until a clinical and bacteriologic response to medical treatment has been demonstrated.
- Environmental surfaces (e.g., walls, crutches, bed rails, walkers) are not associated with transmission of infections; only routine cleaning of such items is required.
- Therapists with current pulmonary or laryngeal TB should be excluded from work until adequate treatment is instituted, cough is resolved, and sputum is free of bacilli on three consecutive smears.
- Home health personnel can reinforce client education about the importance of taking medications as prescribed.

[a]There are several types of face masks designated as particulate respirators; all National Institute for Occupational Safety and Health (NIOSH)–certified respirators are acceptable protection for health care workers against *Mycobacterium tuberculosis*. The respiratory protection standard set by the Occupational Safety and Health Administration (OSHA) requires a NIOSH-certified respirator; when such a respirator is used, the law requires that a training and fit-test program be present.

vomiting, and abdominal pain mimicking the flu. All health care workers should be alert to these symptoms in anyone taking this medication. Early diagnosis and treatment can affect outcomes considerably.[95]

Extrapulmonary TB is much less common than pulmonary TB but occurs in 50% of individuals with concurrent HIV. Musculoskeletal and nervous system lesions are prevalent in extrapulmonary TB cases. Treatment of Pott disease follows the same chemotherapy regimen, with prompt response. Immobilization and avoidance of weight bearing may be required to relieve pain, with attention to maintaining strength and range of motion.

### For the Health Care Worker

Health care workers now take a two-step purified protein derivative test to screen for TB. The skin test is given on two separate occasions to reduce the likelihood of a false reading. For the health care worker who is exposed to TB and develops active disease, treatment will yield a "cure" if the appropriate pharmacologic intervention is followed for the full course prescribed, usually a minimum of 6 months. A cure simply means the active TB will not likely recur, but the person can be reexposed and reinfected. Treatment failure (not taking enough medication or for long enough duration) is a more likely outcome than reinfection because treatment compliance (i.e., noncompliance) is a much bigger problem. After 2 weeks on effective medication, more than 85% of people with positive sputum cultures convert to a noninfectious status. Although the individual is no longer considered infectious, a minimum of 6 months is required before the disease is considered cured.

If the health care worker is exposed and infected but does not develop active disease (approximately 90% of all cases), there is a 10% lifetime risk that active disease can develop; half of that risk takes place in the first 2 years. That 10% risk can be reduced to approximately a 1% risk if a single prophylactic medication is taken properly for 6 months.

In such cases, the individual is considered a "TB reactor" and will always skin test positive for TB. These individuals will require TB clearance in order to work in health care settings, schools, or other similar settings. Clearance is provided via medical documentation of treatment and with a letter from the attending physician. The TB bacterium must be inhaled and cannot be transmitted by physical contact with extrapulmonary sites unless the organism is expelled, aerosolized, and then inhaled. Although unusual, this type of situation may be encountered during wound care involving the integument and should be approached with appropriate standard precautions.

## Pathogenesis and Clinical Manifestations

As with all abscesses, a lung abscess is a natural defense mechanism in which the body attempts to localize an infection and wall off the microorganisms so they cannot spread throughout the body. As the microorganisms destroy the local parenchymal tissue (including alveoli, airways, and blood vessels), an inflammatory process causes alveoli to fill with fluid, pus, and microorganisms (consolidation). Death and decay of consolidated tissue may progress proximally until the abscess drains into the bronchus, spreading the infection to other parts of the lung and forming cavities (cavitation).

Clinical signs and symptoms of abscess include cough, fever, night sweats, purulent sputum, and pleuritic chest wall pain.[154] Affected individuals may present acutely or have a history of these symptoms for 2 to 3 weeks before presenting to the physician.

### MEDICAL MANAGEMENT

**DIAGNOSIS.** The radiographic appearance of a thick-walled solitary cavity surrounded by consolidation suggests lung abscess but must be differentiated from other possible lesions. Cavitary lesions in the apex of the upper lobes are frequently caused by TB rather than bacterial abscess. CT may also be used to rule out malignancy or pleural effusion.[154,512] Sputum cultures may be used to determine the exact microbes in the abscess.

**TREATMENT AND PROGNOSIS.** Treatment includes a course of antibiotics and good nutrition. If antibiotics are unsuccessful, surgical drainage will be considered. Risk factors for surgical intervention include abscess larger than 6cm at diagnosis and unresponsiveness to antibiotics.

Prognosis is good if antibiotics can treat the underlying cause, leaving only a residual lung scar. However, mortality remains in the range of 10% to 20% and is influenced by the severity of the primary disease that initially caused consolidation, low albumin levels, anemia, and infection by particular microbes.[342,512]

## Pneumonitis

Pneumonitis, an acute inflammation of lung tissue usually caused by infections, is discussed in this chapter (see "Environmental and Occupational Diseases" below) under its most common presentation as hypersensitivity pneumonitis. Other causes of pneumonitis include lupus pneumonitis associated with systemic lupus erythematosus (SLE), aspiration pneumonitis associated with inspiration of acidic gastric fluid, obstructive pneumonitis associated with lung cancer, and interstitial pneumonitis associated with AIDS. Consolidation with impaired gas exchange may occur in the involved lung tissue, but with successful inactivation of the infecting agent, resolution occurs with restoration of normal lung structure.

## Acute Bronchitis

Acute bronchitis is an inflammation of the trachea and bronchi (tracheobronchial tree) that is of short duration (2-3 weeks), is self-limiting, and typically is caused by a viral infection.[272] It may also result from chemical irritation such as smoke, fumes, or gas, or it may occur with viral infections such as influenza, measles, chickenpox, or whooping cough.

Symptoms of acute bronchitis include the early symptoms of an upper respiratory infection or a common cold, which progress to fever after a few days; a dry, irritating cough caused by transient hyperresponsiveness; sore throat; possible laryngitis; nasal congestion, and chest pain from the effort of coughing. Later, the cough becomes more productive of purulent sputum, followed by wheezing. Cough can last weeks and may be the issue that brings patients to their care team. There may be constitutional symptoms, including moderate fever with accompanying chills, back pain, muscle pain and soreness, and headache.

Clients with viral bronchitis present with a nonproductive cough that frequently occurs in paroxysms and is aggravated by cold, dry, or dusty air. Bacterial bronchitis (common in clients with COPD) causes retrosternal (behind the sternum) pain that is aggravated by coughing. Diagnostic testing is usually limited unless there is high suspicion for influenza or pertussis that could be treated with antibiotics.

Acute bronchitis should be differentiated from chronic bronchitis, pneumonia, whooping cough, rhinosinus conditions, and gastrointestinal reflux disease before treatment begins.[58] Treatment is conservative and symptomatic with rest, humidity, and nutrition and hydration.

Prognosis is usually good with treatment, and although acute bronchitis is typically mild, it can become complicated in people with chronic lung or heart disease and in older adults because they are more susceptible to secondary infections.

The use of chest physical therapy in children and adults with bronchitis is controversial, with limited large-scale studies to determine its effectiveness.[195,455] It is generally not recommended as a first line treatment for hospitalized adults.

# OBSTRUCTIVE DISEASES

## Chronic Obstructive Pulmonary Disease

### Definition

COPD is, "a common, preventable and treatable disease that is characterized by persistent respiratory symptoms and airflow limitation that is due to airway and/or alveolar abnormalities usually caused by significant exposure to noxious particles or gases."[3]

### Incidence and Risk Factors

Chronic lower respiratory disease is the third leading cause of death in the United States.[99] Fifteen million people reported that they had COPD in 2013.[99] Worldwide, it's expected to be the third leading cause of death by 2020.[3] Mortality rates have declined for men, but not for women, with the highest mortality seen along the Ohio and Mississippi rivers.[100] The burden from COPD is expected to increase over the next few decades as a consequence of the aging population and chronic exposure to risk factors.[189]

COPD is almost always caused by exposure to environmental irritants, especially smoking, which is the most common cause of COPD. Other risk factors for COPD are genetic predisposition (alpha-1 antitrypsin deficiency) as well as other genes currently under investigation.[3] As with all chronic diseases, the prevalence of COPD is strongly associated with age and usually presents at age 55 to 60 years. It is unclear if this is normal aging or if this represents cumulative exposure to particles. Due to changes in smoking patterns, there is an approximately equal incidence between genders. Other risk factors include infections and other factors that may impair lung development in childhood, exposure to particles such as cigarettes, pipes, cigars, marijuana, environmental smoke, occupational exposures, and particulates from burned wood or crops. People with a lower socioeconomic status are more likely to develop COPD, as are those with asthma. Air pollution is a potential risk factor, with an impact on lung development in children.[3]

## Pathogenesis and Clinical Manifestations

In those with COPD there is an abnormal chronic inflammatory cycle that results in structural changes to the airways and vasculature. Common characteristics are airway obstruction, air trapping, gas exchange abnormalities, mucus secretion, static and dynamic hyperinflation, pulmonary hypertension, exercise intolerance, and systemic features.[189,395] Clients will present with varying degrees of these pathophysiologic changes, depending on the severity and location of their disease.

In COPD a protease-antiprotease imbalance is seen, resulting in decreased elastin.[3] There is also upregulation of inflammatory cells and cellular signaling that perpetuates the inflammatory cycle. Functionally, these cellular changes result in reduction of expiratory flow with gas trapping that results in static and dynamic hyperinflation.[3] Narrowing in the airways prevents full emptying during expiration, causing trapping of air and increased functional residual capacity. The trapped air causes two main issues: decrements in inhalation volume and decreases in respiratory muscle function. The trapped air and hyperinflation decrease the volume of air that can enter the lungs on inhalation. This is worsened with elevations in respiratory rate as one would see with exercise and is termed dynamic hyperinflation, a significant limiter to exercise. The hyperinflation also changes the length–tension relationship and contractile properties of the respiratory musculature, lowering their efficiency and contributing to shortness of breath. Gas exchange abnormalities also occur due to structural changes in the alveoli, poor ventilation, and retention of $CO_2$ due to incomplete emptying of the lungs during exhalation.[3] Those with COPD also have muscle cachexia and shifting of muscle type, resulting in a reduction of aerobic type I fibers.

Common presenting signs of COPD include some or all of the following: dyspnea, sputum production, activity intolerance, and chronic cough. Dyspnea is often described as having difficulty breathing, heaviness, and having "air hunger."[189] People with COPD may also experience neurocognitive dysfunction as a result of chronic hypoxia and systemic inflammation.[267] There is no correlation between Global Initiative Chronic Obstructive Lung Disease (GOLD) stage of COPD and quality of life or exercise tolerance, indicating that there is a varied experience of COPD within each disease category.[490]

The pathogenesis and clinical manifestations of each component of COPD are discussed separately in their respective sections. Figure 15.7 provides a broad overview

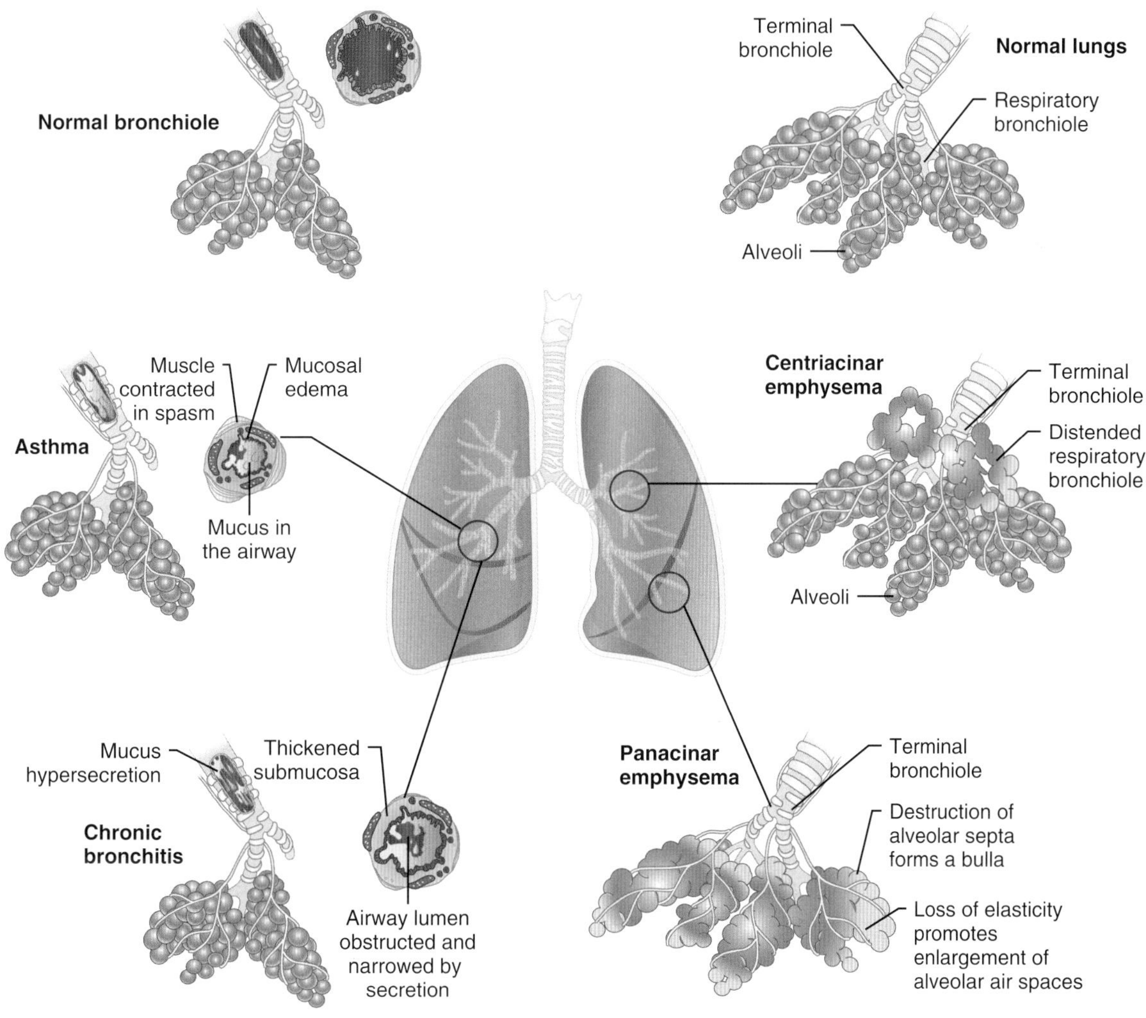


**Figure 15.7**

What happens in chronic obstructive lung disease/chronic airflow limitation.

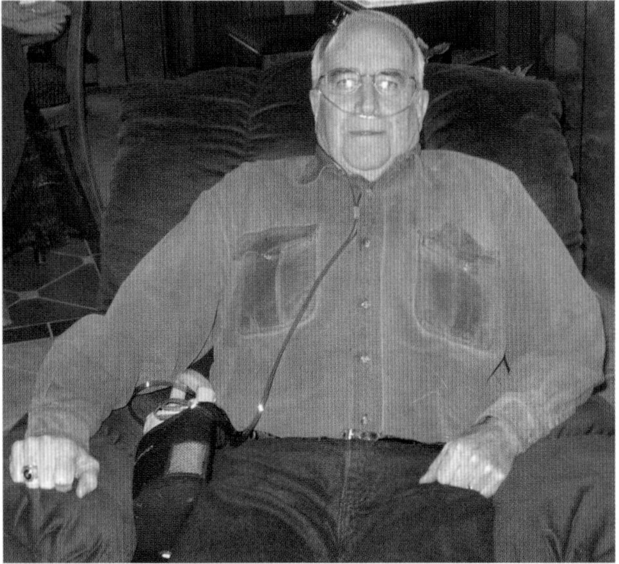

**Figure 15.8**

Characteristic look of chronic obstructive pulmonary disease (COPD) with shoulders raised and muscles tensed from shortness of breath (SOB) and the increased work of breathing (WOB). This man had a 30-year history of smoking 1.5 packs/day combined with asthma, eventually leading to stage IV emphysema and COPD. The effects of asthma and emphysema weakened the heart, resulting in congestive heart failure. Symptoms of SOB, productive cough, fatigue, dizziness, and muscular pain (caused by lack of oxygen) result in disability and reduced quality of life. Use of portable oxygen is required at all times. (Courtesy William T. Cannon, Missoula, MT. Used with permission.)

of COPD. The person with COPD often develops a characteristic look with shoulders raised and muscles tensed from SOB and the increased WOB (Fig. 15.8).

## MEDICAL MANAGEMENT

**DIAGNOSIS.** Physical examination, risk factor assessment, and airflow limitation as measured by pulmonary function tests (PFTs) are used to determine the presence and extent of COPD. COPD should be considered in anyone age 40 years or older with any of the following symptoms; progressive dyspnea that is worse with exercise, chronic cough, intermittent or persistent sputum production, exposure to risk factors, or a family history of COPD.[189]

Spirometry is the most basic and frequently performed test of pulmonary (lung) function. The spirometer measures how much air the lungs can hold and how well the respiratory system is able to move air into and out of the lungs. A postbronchodilator ratio of $FVC/FEV_1$ of less than 0.70 is diagnostic for COPD. If the ratio is between 0.6 and 0.8, the postbronchodilator test should be repeated.[438] After $FVC/FEV_1$ ratio of less than 0.7 is determined, the $FEV_1$ value is then utilized to categorize the severity as GOLD 1 (mild, $FEV_1$ >80% predicted); GOLD 2 (moderate, $FEV_1$ 50-80% predicted); GOLD 3 (severe, $FEV_1$ 30-49% predicted) or GOLD 4 (very severe, FEV1 <30% predicted). In conjunction with spirometry, symptom assessment using validated measures such as the COPD Assessment Test (CATTM) is strongly recommended.[438] The third component of medical diagnosis includes a history of exacerbations. These three components are combined to categorize patients into A, B, C, or D with associated recommendations for medical interventions.[438]

History, clinical examination, x-ray studies, and laboratory findings usually enable the physician to distinguish COPD from other obstructive pulmonary disorders, such as bronchiectasis, adult CF, and central airway obstruction. High-resolution computed tomography (CT) scan is used to diagnose and quantify emphysema. Laboratory analysis may include blood gas measurements and blood pH to indicate the presence of hypoxemia or hypercapnia (excess carbon dioxide in blood) and acid–base balance, and sputum culture to identify the presence of immunoglobulin E (IgE) antibodies against specific allergens. Skin testing for allergens that trigger attacks is most useful in young clients with extrinsic allergic asthma.

**TREATMENT.** The successful management of COPD requires a multifaceted approach that includes smoking cessation, pharmacologic management, airway clearance as needed, exercise (aerobic, strength, flexibility, posture, and breathing), control of comorbidities, avoidance of irritants, psychologic support, and dietary management.

The main goals for the client with COPD are to improve oxygenation, decrease carbon dioxide retention, and maximize quality of life. These are accomplished by (1) reducing airway edema secondary to inflammation and bronchospasm (asthma) through the use of bronchodilator medication, (2) facilitating the elimination of bronchial secretions, (3) preventing and treating respiratory infection, (4) increasing exercise tolerance, (5) managing comorbidities, (6) avoiding airway irritants and allergens, (7) relieving anxiety and treating depression, and (8) exercising to improve muscle oxidative capacity.

Decreasing and eliminating smoking is a top priority for the prevention and management of COPD. Comprehensive programs that include behavioral counseling combined with pharmacologic agents or nicotine replacement therapy can be effective.[438] Pneumococcal vaccination for the person with COPD decreases mortality rates and hospitalizations and is recommended for former smokers, current smokers, and all people with COPD.[284] Annual prophylactic vaccination against influenza is also recommended.

Medications are used to manage symptoms and prevent exacerbations to improve function and overall quality of life. Common classifications of medications used in the treatment of COPD include long-acting or short-acting $\beta_2$ agonists (LABA or SABAs), anticholinergics, combination devices (SABA with anticholinergic), antimuscarinics, methylxanthines, combination of LABA and corticosteroids, mucolytics, and phosphodiesterase-4 inhibitors. Systemic corticosteroids are of some help in acute exacerbations of COPD but have some immediate side effects, such as hyperglycemia, hypertension,[504] osteoporosis, and proximal muscle weakness (steroid myopathy), without producing any long-term benefits (Table 15.5).[354]

Long-term oxygen treatment, defined as longer than 15 hours per day,[189] reduces morbidity and extends life in clients with significant daytime hypoxemia.[127] People with $PaO_2$ of 55 or less, or a resting oxygen saturation of 88% or less, measured at two time periods 3 weeks apart (see Table 15.2), are considered for long-term oxygen therapy.[190] Oxygen therapy is also considered for those

**Table 15.5** Pharmacotherapy for Chronic Obstructive Pulmonary Disease and Asthma

| | COPD | Asthma |
|---|---|---|
| Maintenance | **Inhaled Bronchodilators**<br>$\beta_2$-Adrenergic agonists<br>• Short-acting<br>  • Albuterol<br>  • Levalbuterol<br>• Long-acting<br>  • Salmeterol<br>  • Formoterol<br>  • Arformoterol<br>Anticholinergics<br>• Short-acting<br>  • Ipratropium<br>• Long-acting<br>• Tiotropium<br>**Oral Bronchodilators**<br>• Methylxanthines<br>  • Theophylline<br>  • Aminophylline<br>**Inhaled Corticosteroids**<br>• Fluticasone<br>• Budesonide | **Inhaled Bronchodilators**<br>$\beta_2$-Adrenergic agonists<br>• Short-acting<br>  • Albuterol<br>  • Levalbuterol<br>• Long-acting<br>  • Salmeterol<br>  • Formoterol<br>**Oral Bronchodilators**<br>• Methylxanthines<br>  • Theophylline<br>  • Aminophylline<br>**Inhaled Corticosteroids**<br>• Fluticasone<br>• Budesonide<br>• Mometasone<br>**Oral Corticosteroids**<br>• Methylprednisolone<br>• Prednisone<br>• Prednisolone<br>**Leukotriene Modifiers**<br>• Montelukast<br>• Zafirlukast<br>• Zileuton<br>**Mast Cell Stabilizers**<br>• Cromolyn<br>**Anti-IgE Antibodies**<br>• Omalizumab |
| • Acute exacerbations | **Inhaled Bronchodilators**<br>$\beta_2$-Adrenergic agonists<br>• Short-acting<br>  • Albuterol<br>  • Levalbuterol<br>Anticholinergics<br>• Short-acting<br>• Ipratropium<br>**Oral and Intravenous Corticosteroids**<br>• Methylprednisolone<br>• Prednisone<br>• Prednisolone<br>**Antibiotics**<br>• Macrolides<br>• Cephalosporins<br>• Fluoroquinolones<br>• Doxycycline | **Inhaled Bronchodilators**<br>$\beta_2$-Adrenergic agonists<br>• Short-acting<br>  • Albuterol<br>  • Levalbuterol<br>Anticholinergics<br>• Short-acting<br>• Ipratropium<br>**Oral and Intravenous Corticosteroids**<br>• Methylprednisolone<br>• Prednisone<br>• Prednisolone |

Sources for pharmacotherapy updates: Global Initiative for Chronic Obstructive Lung Disease, Inc. Global initiative for chronic obstructive lung disease. *Global strategy for the diagnosis, management, and prevention of chronic obstructive pulmonary disease* (12/2011). Available at: http://www.goldcopd.org/uploads/users/files/GOLD_Report_2011_Feb21.pdf. Accessed July 17, 2012; and National Heart, Lung, and Blood Institute. *National asthma education and prevention program. Expert panel report 3: guidelines for the diagnosis and management of asthma. Full report 2007* (8/28/2007). Available at: http://www.nhlbi.nih.gov/guidelines/asthma/asthgdln.pdf. Accessed July 18, 2012.

who desaturate during sleep or exercise, although the present research does not show a survival advantage for oxygen therapy in those with mild daytime hypoxia or nocturnal hypoxia.[267,438]

Surgical treatment for COPD may include lung-volume reduction surgery (LVRS) for appropriate individuals. In surgical LVRS, large bullae or overdistended nonfunctional alveoli are removed, enabling compressed lung tissue to reexpand, thereby reducing overall dead space. LVRS is most successful in those with upper lobe disease who have a post rehabilitation low exercise capacity, and has been shown to reduce hyperinflation, improve respiratory mechanics, and reduce morbidity.[87,189,220] Lung transplantation may also be considered to improve quality of life, with a median survival of 5.5 years.[438]

Endobronchial valve procedures place stents designed to block air from entering diseased lung tissue during inhalation but allowing air to exit during exhalation. This type of device is intended to provide one-way airflow in segmental or subsegmental bronchi in individuals with pulmonary conditions complicated by air leaks or hyperinflation.[477]

Pulmonary rehabilitation is a multidimensional program that utilizes exercise, group education, smoking cessation, and nutritional guidance to improve symptoms and function in those with respiratory diseases. Pulmonary rehabilitation improves exercise performance, quality of life, dyspnea, and reduces the number of hospitalizations.[12,189,281,438]

**PROGNOSIS.** The prognosis for chronic bronchitis and emphysema is poor because these are chronic, progressive, and debilitating diseases. COPD mortality is steadily declining in men, but still rising in women.[103,171]

COPD is largely preventable, and many believe that early recognition of small airway obstruction with appropriate treatment and cessation of smoking may prevent disease progression. Early treatment of airway infections and vaccination against influenza and pneumococcal disease have an effect on morbidity and mortality of individuals with COPD, as do public health campaigns that address environmental toxins.

There is no cure for COPD, but smoking cessation increases the survival rate. Pulmonary rehabilitation also increases survival,[23] improves quality of life, decreases hospitalizations, and decreases incidence of COPD exacerbations.[23,55,430]

SPECIAL IMPLICATIONS FOR THE THERAPIST 15.5

## *Chronic Obstructive Pulmonary Disease*

### Pulmonary Rehabilitation

Pulmonary rehabilitation (PR) is a multidimensional and comprehensive approach to improving quality of life. It includes patient-specific exercise training, education in self-management, psychosocial support, smoking cessation, medication adherence, and nutrition.

Pulmonary rehabilitation is effective in reducing the risk of hospitalization, reducing mortality, improving health-related quality of life, and increasing exercise capacity.[390,438] Patients at all levels of GOLD classification can benefit from PR. Despite its benefits in improving dyspnea, quality of life, readmissions, and mortality, there are low referral rates to PR and limited access. Newer studies are identifying similar gains in many areas with home rehabilitation.[438]

Treatment of COPD includes breathing exercises, airway clearance techniques, physical training, a program to improve posture, and conditioning of respiratory musculature. For the motivated child with asthma, breathing exercises and controlled breathing are of value in preventing overinflation, improving the strength of respiratory muscles and the efficiency of the cough, and reducing the WOB.

People with COPD often adopt a sedentary lifestyle, which leads to progressive deconditioning.[438] Deconditioning will lead to progressive deterioration in limb and respiratory muscle function that could adversely affect exercise capacity. A focus on education is key in helping clients with COPD make important lifestyle changes (e.g., increasing physical activity, reducing smoking), taking medications as prescribed, and seeking care early on for any signs of new onset upper respiratory infection.[251]

### Exercise

Exercise limitation is a common manifestation of COPD. The skeletal muscle dysfunction seen in COPD is associated with increased mortality, reduced exercise capacity, and increased use of health care resources.[267] Muscle weakness is caused by a combination of factors, including deconditioning, chronic hypoxia, and systemic inflammation.[267] Hypoxia is implicated as the initiating factor for systemic inflammation as well as for an increase in oxidative stress, which causes muscle weakness and decreased aerobic capacity. Exercise tolerance can be improved despite the presence of fixed structural abnormalities in the lung. This suggests that factors other than lung function impairment (e.g., deconditioning and peripheral muscle dysfunction) play a predominant role in limiting exercise capacity in people with COPD.

Muscle weakness in stable COPD does not affect all muscles the same. For example, proximal upper limb muscle strength may be impaired more than distal upper limb muscle strength, peripheral muscle may be limited mainly by endurance capacity, and the diaphragm muscle may be altered structurally (e.g., changes in muscle length and configuration affecting the mechanical force and action)[72] and limited in strength capacity.

Clients with COPD must be encouraged to remain active, with specific attention directed toward activities they enjoy. Training in pacing and energy conservation allows even those with limited exercise tolerance to increase their daily activities. Exercise testing with gas exchange and/or functional walk tests, individualized to the specific client's needs and goals, are used to determine the person's baseline and for prescribing a training regimen. A combination of aerobic and strength training is recommend at 60% to 80% of the symptom-limited maximum heart rate achieved on a peak test or a RPE of 4 to 6 out of 10.[438] Strength training is not associated with improvements in exercise tolerance, however it can increase upper extremity (UE) endurance that can translate into improved functional capacity.[438] Simple arm elevation results in significant increases in metabolic and ventilatory requirements in clients with long-term airflow limitations. Pulmonary rehabilitation (PR) that includes upper extremity training (progressive resistance exercises) reduces metabolic and ventilatory requirements for arm elevation. This type of program may allow clients with COPD to perform sustained upper extremity activities with less dyspnea.[186] People with chronic airflow obstruction report disabling dyspnea when performing seemingly trivial tasks (e.g., activity with unsupported arms). Some muscles of the upper torso and shoulder girdle share both a respiratory and a positional function for the arms, resulting in functional limitations in many clients with lung disease during unsupported upper extremity activities.

Therapists can also consider inspiratory muscle training as part of a comprehensive program. Most studies show benefits in exercise performance and quality of life with 6 to 8 weeks of PR, with no additional gains at 12 weeks or beyond.[438] Finally, a recent meta-analysis revealed improvements in lower extremity (LE) strength and exercise capacity with the addition of neuromuscular electrical stimulation (NMES).[113]

Continuous walking is the most common form of exercise for COPD, although more recent evidence supports the use of high-intensity interval training. This type of training utilizes the overload principle, but because of the rest breaks, elicits a lower lactate response and lower ratings of perceived exertion.[281] Swimming is a preferred exercise option for clients with bronchial asthma (see next discussion).

When tolerated, high-intensity (continuous or interval), short-term training may lead to greater improvements in quality of life and aerobic fitness than low-intensity training of longer duration, but it is not absolutely necessary to achieve gains in exercise endurance.[55,175] Therapists working with these clients should encourage them to maintain hydration by drinking fluids (including before, during, and after exercise) to prevent mucous plugs from hardening and to take medications as prescribed.

Exercise tolerance may improve after exercise training (including weight training)[91] because of gains in aerobic fitness or peripheral muscle strength,[118,314] enhanced mechanical skill and efficiency of exercise, and improvements in respiratory muscle function, breathing pattern, or lung hyperinflation. Exercise improves muscle oxidative capacity and recovery in individuals with COPD.[389]

Exercise training can also reduce anxiety, fear, and dyspnea previously associated with exercise in the deconditioned person. Exercises for flexibility, posture, and motor control can improve mechanical and kinetic efficiency and thus can reduce oxygen demand during daily activities and exercise.

### Monitoring Vital Signs

Using a pulse oximeter can help the therapist and client observe for a decrease in oxygen saturation before hypoxemia occurs. Oxygen saturation is generally kept at 90% or above by titrating oxygen when a medical order to do so has been received. Altering physiologic responses using principles of self-induced biofeedback and breathing techniques may be able to help some clients self-regulate oxygen saturation levels (see reference 318 for a description of these techniques).

Some people with COPD retain carbon dioxide and have a depressed hypoxic drive, requiring low oxygen levels to stimulate the respiratory drive. In such cases the upward adjustment of supplemental oxygen levels must be monitored very carefully; increasing total oxygen administered via nasal canula requires careful monitoring of respiratory rate and breathing pattern, documentation, and consultation with other members of the PR team.

Blood pressure and pulse should be observed at rest and in response to exercise, especially in anyone with COPD and cardiac arrhythmias. Most people with COPD who have mild arrhythmias at rest do not tend to have increased arrhythmias during exercise.

In people with expanded lung volumes because of air trapping,[119] such as occurs in COPD (especially emphysema), the first heart sound is best heard under the sternal area (put the scope in the client's left epigastric area) rather than the apical or mitral area. The hyperinflation of the lungs causes the heart to elongate, displacing the left ventricle downward and medially.

**Box 15.5**

**IMPORTANT CONCEPTS IN THE USE OF A METERED-DOSE INHALER**

The therapist should observe the client self-administer the medication at least one time. Schedule the use of the metered-dose inhaler (MDI) for 15-20 minutes before exercise so as to maximize ventilation.

- MDIs are used to deliver medication to the lungs, avoiding deposition of the medication on the tongue and back of the throat. For this to occur, users must take in a slow deep breath over the course of 10 seconds while maintaining a good seal on the device.
- Each manufacturer has specific use instructions as well as cleaning instructions. Refer to the user manual for the specifics of each device.
  - Be sure to note directions for use, including cleaning and the need for priming the MDI.
- A therapist should evaluate the ability of the child or adult to adequately press on the device to release medication and to coordinate this with inhalation.
- A spacer may be used in conjunction with the MDI. With a spacer, the medication is released into the chamber and the user can slowly take a deep breath in without having to focus on coordinating the pressing of the device with inhalation.

Instructions for the use of different inhalers and video demonstrations are available online. When appropriate, the therapist should review proper administration with each individual based on the type of inhaler used.

Lung sounds are also changed because the loss of interstitial elasticity and the presence of interalveolar septa lead to air trapping, with increased volume of air in the lungs. Air pockets are poor transmitters of vibrations; thus vocal fremitus (the client whispers "99, 99, 99"), breath sounds, and the whispered and spoken voice are impaired or absent on auscultation. When there is fluid in the lung or lungs, consolidation, or collapse (e.g., atelectasis), whispered words are heard perfectly and clearly. This is the earliest sign of atelectasis.

A peak flowmeter, a home monitoring device to measure fast expiratory flow (a reflection of bronchorestriction), can be used to determine how compromised a client with asthma or reactive airways may be, compared to the normal values for that person. This may be a useful measure in determining response to therapy intervention and documenting measurable outcomes.

### Exercise and Medication

The majority of pulmonary medications are used to promote bronchodilation and improve alveolar ventilation and oxygenation and are delivered as an aerosol spray through a device called a *metered-dose inhaler* or in powder form with a dry powder inhaler.

Proper technique is important to ensure delivery of the medication to the desired location (Box 15.5).[56] When medications are properly used, their effects should improve an individual's ability to exercise and more effectively obtain the benefits of training.

## Chronic Bronchitis

### Definition and Overview

Chronic bronchitis (CB) is clinically defined as a condition of productive cough lasting for at least 3 months (usually the winter months) per year for 2 consecutive years. Chronic bronchitis can exist alone in people with normal spirometry, or in combination with airway obstruction.[8,189] Having chronic bronchitis increases one's risk of developing COPD.[164] People with CB have a rapid decline in $FEV_1$, frequent exacerbations, and poor quality of life.[329]

### Risk Factors and Pathogenesis

Chronic bronchitis is characterized by inflammation and scarring of the bronchial lining. This inflammation may obstruct airflow to and from the lungs and increases mucus production. Irritants, such as cigarette smoke, long-term dust inhalation, or air pollution, cause mucus hypersecretion and hypertrophy (increased number and size) of mucus-producing glands in the large bronchi. Epithelial atrophy, changes in squamous cells, and hypertrophy of smooth muscle cells occur.[460]

The swollen mucous membrane and thick sputum obstruct the airways, causing wheezing and a subsequent cough as the person tries to clear the airways. In addition, impaired ciliary function reduces mucus clearance and increases client susceptibility to infection. Infection results in even more mucus production, with bronchial wall inflammation and thickening. If airway collapse is present, air is trapped in the distal portion of the lung, causing reduced alveolar ventilation, hypoxia, and acidosis. This downward spiral continues because the client now has an abnormal ventilation/perfusion ($\dot{V}/\dot{Q}$) ratio and resultant decreased $PaO_2$.

As compensation for the hypoxemia, polycythemia (overproduction of erythrocytes) occurs. Cyanosis results from insufficient arterial oxygenation and peripheral edema from right ventricular failure. Pulmonary vascular resistance caused by inflammation and loss of capillary beds will contribute to cor pulmonale (right-sided congestive heart failure).

### Clinical Manifestations

The symptoms of chronic bronchitis are persistent cough and sputum production (worse in the morning and evening than at midday). The increased secretions from the bronchial mucosa and obstruction of the respiratory passages interfere with the flow of air to and from the lungs. The result is SOB, prolonged expiration, persistent coughing with expectoration, and recurrent infection. Infection may be accompanied by fever and malaise.

If the person goes on to develop COPD, reduced chest expansion, wheezing, cyanosis, and decreased exercise tolerance may occur. In addition, the obstruction present results in decreased alveolar ventilation and increased $PaCO_2$. Hypoxemia leads to polycythemia and cyanosis. If not reversed, pulmonary hypertension leads to cor pulmonale. Severe disability or death is the final clinical picture.

#### MEDICAL MANAGEMENT

In stable conditions, reducing irritants and using a combination of bronchodilators is effective. There is no evidence for use of antibiotics, oral corticosteroids, expectorants, or postural drainage. In significant acute exacerbations of chronic bronchitis, antibiotics and oral or IV corticosteroids can be effective.[59]

## Emphysema

### Definition and Overview

Emphysema is defined as an enlargement of the air spaces beyond the terminal bronchiole, and is associated with a loss of elasticity in the distal airways, airway collapse, and gas trapping.[266] There are three types of emphysema (see Fig. 15.7). Centrilobular emphysema, the most common type, produces destruction in the bronchioles of the upper lung regions. Inflammation develops in the bronchioles, but usually the alveolar sac (distal to respiratory bronchioles) remains intact. Centrilobular emphysema is the most common type in smokers.[266]

Panlobular emphysema destroys the air spaces of the entire acinus and most commonly involves the lower lung. Panlobular is common in those with $\alpha_1$-antitrypsin deficiency. Paraseptal (panacinar) emphysema destroys the alveoli in the lower lobes of the lungs, resulting in isolated blebs along the lung periphery. Paraseptal emphysema often occurs alongside of centrilobular in chronic smokers. Paraseptal emphysema is believed to be the likely cause of spontaneous pneumothorax. Those with emphysema have less hypoxia than those with CB, more breathlessness, and typically have a lower incidence of cor pulmonale.

### Etiologic Factors

Cigarette smoking is the major etiologic factor in the development of emphysema and has been shown to increase the numbers of alveolar macrophages and neutrophils in the lung[a], enhance protease release[b], and impair the activity of antiproteases. However, other factors, such as heredity, must determine susceptibility to emphysema because less than 10% to 15% of people who smoke develop clinical evidence of airway obstruction.

In many cases, emphysema occurs as a result of prolonged respiratory difficulties, such as chronic bronchitis that has caused partial obstruction of the smaller divisions of the bronchi. Emphysema can also occur without serious preceding respiratory problems as in the case of a defect in the elastic tissue of the lungs or in older persons whose lungs have lost their natural elasticity.

---

[a]Neutrophils, the most numerous type of leukocytes (white blood cells), increase dramatically in number in response to infection and inflammation. However, neutrophils not only kill invading organisms but also may damage host tissues when there are too many.

[b]Proteases, or proteolytic enzymes, are enzymes that destroy cells and proteins. The airway goblet cells and serous cells of bronchial glands normally secrete a protein called secretory leukoprotease inhibitor, which is capable of inhibiting neutrophils. The cellular interactions associated with smoking result in inactivation of protease inhibitors. This results in an imbalance between proteases and antiproteases (in favor of proteases), allowing even more cellular destruction than warranted by the inflammatory process already present.

Approximately 1% to 5% of people with early onset of COPD have an inherited deficiency of (low levels or absent) $\alpha_1$-antitrypsin, a protective protein.[151,476] $\alpha_1$-Antitrypsin is made primarily in the liver, but also in lung cells, monocytes, and intestinal epithelial cells.[476] The role of this protein is to dampen inflammation, control protease activity, and to inhibit cell apoptosis. When absent or in low quantities, people with this inherited mutation are at risk for developing COPD in the third to fifth decade of life.[476]

Those with $\alpha_1$-antitrypsin who are also smokers have accelerated COPD and die approximately 10 to 20 years earlier than nonsmokers. Systemic effects of $\alpha_1$-antitrypsin include low bone mineral density, increased aortic stiffness, and low lean muscle mass.[151] These effects may be amenable to the risk reduction provided by pulmonary rehabilitation.

### Pathogenesis

Inhaled particles impair the mucociliary escalator and induce inflammation and damage of the airways. This can lead to increased compliance of the airways, chronic inflammation, airway trapping, and chronic sputum production. In emphysema, there is destruction of elastin protein in the lung that normally maintains the strength of the alveolar walls, which leads to permanent enlargement of the acini. It is suspected that an interaction of accelerated cellular apoptosis, inflammation, and proteolysis causes the tissue destruction associated with emphysema.[460]

Eventually the loss of elasticity in the lung tissue causes narrowing or collapse of the bronchioles so that inspired air becomes trapped in the lungs. The alveoli lose their connections to each other, contributing to changes in compliance in the airways and air trapping. During exercise, air trapping is worsened, with inhalation occurring before full expiration, resulting in stacking of breaths and dynamic hyperinflation of the lungs.[266] Obstruction results from changes in lung tissues, rather than from mucus production and swelling as in chronic bronchitis.

The permanent overdistention of the air spaces with destruction of the walls (septa) between the alveoli is accompanied by partial airway collapse and loss of elastic recoil. Pockets of air form between the alveolar spaces (blebs) and within the lung parenchyma (bullae). This process leads to increased ventilatory dead space, or areas that do not participate in gas exchange, diminishing $\dot{V}/\dot{Q}$ matching (Fig. 15.9).[267] There are also abnormalities in the vasculature, with increased smooth muscle proliferation and changes to the intima that further worsen gas exchange.[45] Moreover, the microbiome of those with emphysema is different from those without this condition, which is an area under active investigation.[45]

The WOB is increased as a result of ventilatory drive from hypoxemia and hypercapnia, increased effort during exhalation (normally passive recoil), and flattening of the diaphragm caused by hyperinflation. As the disease progresses, there is increasing dyspnea and risk of pulmonary infection. Pulmonary hypertension develops from capillary loss and vessel intimal thickening, and this eventually leads to cor pulmonale (right-sided heart failure).

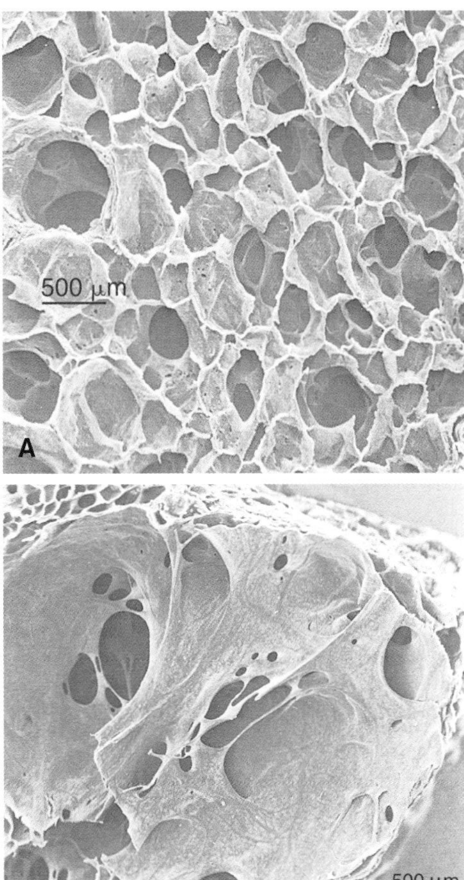


**Figure 15.9**

**Effects of emphysema seen in these scanning electron micrographs of lung tissue.** (A) Normal lung with many small alveoli. (B) Lung tissue affected by emphysema. Notice that the alveoli have merged into larger air spaces, reducing the surface area for gas exchange. (From Thibodeau GA, Patton KT: *Structure and function of the body*, ed 14, St Louis, 2012, Mosby. Used with permission.)

In centrilobular emphysema the destruction of the lung is uneven and originates around the airways. The membranous bronchioles are thicker, narrower, and more reactive than in panlobular emphysema. Lung compliance is low or normal and does not relate to the extent of the emphysema (i.e., not to the losses of elastic recoil), but rather the decrease in airflow is related mainly to the degree of airway abnormality.

In contrast, panlobular emphysema is characterized by even destruction of the lung and the small airways appear less narrowed and less inflamed than in centrilobular emphysema. Lung compliance is increased and is related to the extent of the emphysema; the decrease in airflow is primarily associated with the loss of elastic recoil rather than with the abnormalities in the airways.[122]

At the molecular and microvascular levels, protease–antiprotease (associated with $\alpha_1$-antitrypsin disease [AATD] emphysema) and oxidant–antioxidant theories continue under investigation as theories related to impaired reparative mechanisms in the causation of emphysema. Oxidative damage by free radicals, which

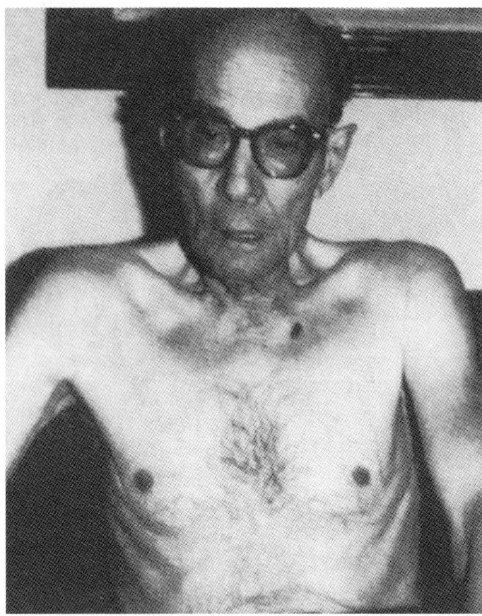

**Figure 15.10**

**The person with emphysema presents with classic findings.** Use of respiratory accessory (intercostal, neck, shoulder) muscles and cachectic appearance (wasting caused by ill health) reflect two factors: (1) shortness of breath, the most disturbing symptom, and (2) the tremendous increased work of breathing necessary to increase ventilation and maintain normal arterial blood gases. (From Kersten LD: *Comprehensive respiratory nursing*, Philadelphia, 1989, WB Saunders.)

is the basis for the free radical theory of aging (see discussion in Chapter 6), identifies cigarette smoke as the main source of oxidants contributing to epithelial damage associated with smoking-induced emphysema. Determining the mechanisms regulating the antioxidant responses is critical to understanding the role of oxidants in the pathogenesis of smoking-induced lung disease and to developing future strategies for antioxidant therapy.[430]

Muscle wasting in emphysema and COPD is linked to increased tumor necrosis factor-α production. Respiratory muscle atrophy can lead to deterioration of lung function and increased WOB.[460]

## Clinical Manifestations

At first, symptoms may be apparent only during physical exertion, but eventually marked exertional dyspnea progresses to dyspnea at rest. This occurs as a result of the irreversible destruction reducing elasticity of the lungs and increasing the effort to exhale trapped air. Cough is uncommon, with little sputum production. The client is often thin, has tachypnea with prolonged expiration, and must use accessory muscles for ventilation. To increase lung capacity and use of accessory muscles, the client often leans forward with arms braced on the knees, supporting the shoulders and chest. The combined effects of trapped air and alveolar distention change the size and shape of the client's chest, causing a barrel chest and increased expiratory effort appearance (Fig. 15.10).

Nocturnal hypoxemia is another clinical manifestation of emphysema. During sleep (especially rapid eye movement stage) there is a decrease in the sensitivity of chemoreceptors, decreased firing of the intercostal muscles, and increased airway resistance. These changes can be significant for the person with emphysema and worsen V/Q matching, leading to nocturnal hypoxia.[267] This may be worsened in people who also have obstructive sleep apnea. Persons with emphysema have three times the rate of anxiety as the general public. This anxiety is associated with dyspnea or fear of dyspnea. Antianxiety medications, particularly selective serotonin reuptake inhibitors, and cognitive behavioral therapy have been shown to be helpful, although more research is needed.[61]

The most common signs and symptoms of AATD include dyspnea, wheezing, cough, chronic allergies (year round), asthma that does not respond to treatment, and liver problems. A high prevalence of wheezing to allergen and irritant exposures with symptoms of atopy suggests that asthma is common in AATD but is usually associated with COPD. Individuals with AATD who are susceptible to asthma require allergy evaluation and aggressive anti-inflammatory management.[153]

## MEDICAL MANAGEMENT

DIAGNOSIS AND TREATMENT. Diagnosis is made on the basis of history (usually cigarette smoking), physical examination, chest film, chest CT, and pulmonary function tests. The most important factor in the treatment of emphysema is cessation of smoking. Human lungs benefit no matter when someone quits smoking; quitting smoking is the most effective way of preventing lung function decline caused by emphysema (and chronic bronchitis).

Pursed-lip breathing causes resistance to outflow at the lips, which in turn maintains intrabronchial pressure and improves the mixture of gases in the lungs. This type of breathing should be encouraged to help the client get rid of the air trapped in the lungs. Diaphragmatic breathing may benefit some clients in the early stages of emphysema. Methods to examine diaphragmatic movement and the potential for success with diaphragmatic breathing are available.[67] Pulmonary rehabilitation and supplemental oxygen are critical aspects of management of COPD.[87]

Lung transplantation is an established treatment for individuals with advanced emphysema. Double-lung transplantation may help avoid complications following single-lung transplantation, including native lung hyperinflation. However, single-lung transplantation is done more often because of limited donor organ availability.[503]

LVRS (surgically removing damaged areas of the lung) may help improve breathing, ventilation, and survival.[7] Those with upper lobe dysfunction and low exercise tolerance benefit the most from LVRS.[445] Endobronchial valves are one-way valves that are placed in the bronchi of affected lobes, which prevent air from entering but enable air to leave the segment. The collapse of the lobe decreases dead space in the lung. There are other techniques similar to valves under investigation that show early promise; however, long-term benefits are still unknown at the time of this writing.[247]

In the case of AATD, serum testing to measure the levels of $\alpha_1$-antitrypsin is required to identify this problem. Underrecognition of AATD is common, with diagnostic and treatment delays documented.[451] AATD is treated with weekly intravenous augmentation therapy to slow down or halt the destruction of lung tissue. Home infusion is available for some people.

Infusion of purified $\alpha_1$-antitrypsin from pooled human plasma raises the concentration in serum and epithelial-lining fluid above the protective threshold. Although evidence suggests this treatment slows the decline of lung function and may reduce infection rates while enhancing survival, the cost-effectiveness has been questioned.[450] Only nonsmokers can benefit from this treatment regimen; smoking increases neutrophils, which, in turn, inhibit $\alpha_1$-antitrypsin.

**PROGNOSIS.** Prognosis for individuals with symptomatic AATD is poor, with a high incidence of transplantation for liver and lung disease and even more on a transplant waiting list.[453]

## Asthma

### Definition and Overview

Asthma is defined as a reversible obstructive lung disease characterized by inflammation and increased reactivity of smooth muscle of the airways to various stimuli, causing bronchoconstriction and airflow resistance. It is a chronic condition with acute exacerbations and characterized as a complex disorder involving biochemical, autonomic, immunologic, infectious, endocrine, and psychologic factors. This condition can be divided into two main types according to causative factors: extrinsic (allergic) and intrinsic (nonallergic), but other recognized categories include adult-onset, exercise-induced, aspirin-sensitive, *Aspergillus*-hypersensitive, and occupational asthma (Table 15.6).

**Table 15.6** Types of Asthma

| Classification | Triggers |
|---|---|
| Extrinsic | Immunoglobulin E–mediated external allergens<br>• Foods; sulfite additives (wines)<br>• Indoor and outdoor pollutants, including ozone, smoke, exhaust<br>• Pollen, dust, molds<br>• Animal dander, feathers |
| Intrinsic | Unknown; secondary to respiratory infections |
| Adult-onset | Unknown |
| Exercise-induced | Alteration in airway temperature and humidity; mediator release |
| Aspirin-sensitive (associated with nasal polyps) | Aspirin and other nonsteroidal antiinflammatory drugs |
| Allergic bronchopulmonary aspergillosis | Hypersensitivity to *Aspergillus* species |
| Occupational | Metal salts (platinum, chrome, nickel)<br>Antibiotic powder (penicillin, sulfathiazole, tetracycline)<br>Toluene diisocyanate<br>Flour<br>Wood dusts<br>Cotton dust (byssinosis)<br>Animal proteins<br>Smoke inhalation (firefighters)<br>Latex-induced<br>Emotional stress |

### Incidence and Prevalence

In 2015, there were over 11 million visits to physicians for the management of asthma.[78] More than 20.4 million adults and 6.1 million children in the United States have been diagnosed with asthma.[77] Over 400,000 children and adults were discharged from the hospital in 2010 with issues related to asthma, with the highest rates seen in African American children and adults.[81] Asthma is most prevalent in African Americans, American Indians or Alaska Natives, and in those reporting two or more races.[84] Asthma prevalence in children decreased from 2010 to 2016 except in Mexican Americans.[14]

### Risk Factors

Risk factors for asthma include age, with asthma diagnosed more frequently in children although it can be diagnosed at any age. Other risk factors include heredity, exposure to smoke, maternal use of antibiotics in the third trimester, low birth weight, viral infections before age 3, low socioeconomic status, and cockroach/rodent infestations in the primary living areas.[52,326]

The environment, including air pollution and exposure to other environmental toxins (including pesticides),[186,230] homes that are airtight, exposure to pets, and windowless offices may also be risk factors contributing to the significant rise in incidence.

Large families, early exposure to pets, early infections, having older siblings, and attending daycare may protect against allergic sensitization.[478] Asthma can occur at any age, although it is more likely to occur for the first time before the age of 5 years. Antibiotic exposure during infancy appears to be a risk factor for developing childhood asthma. In childhood, it is three times more common and more severe in boys; however, after puberty, girls are more likely to be diagnosed.[161]

Asthma is found most often in urban, industrialized settings; in colder climates; and among the urban disadvantaged population (areas of poverty). Asthma is more prevalent and more severe among black children, but this may not be a result of race or low income per se but rather of demographic location because all children living in an urban setting are at increased risk for asthma.[9]

Overcrowded living conditions with repeated exposure to cigarette smoke, dust, cockroaches, and mold and where the use of a gas stove or oven is used for heat may be contributing factors.[292]

There is a relationship between weight and asthma, with a "U" shaped association.[70] There is a higher risk of asthma in those who are underweight and in those who are overweight.[70] There are suggestions that physical activity may be the modifying variable effecting the U-shaped curve; however it is difficult to draw strong conclusions because those without asthma may be more active and therefore have a lower body mass index. Obesity is linked to elevations in inflammatory markers. Adipocytes contain proinflammatory mediators such as leptin, tumor necrosis factor, and interleukin-6.[70] Some evidence indicates that these inflammatory markers influence T helper cells that are associated with airway inflammation. Obesity related asthma demonstrates different airway inflammation compared to other types of asthma, with increased neutrophils in sputum and lower levels of eosinophils. Obesity related asthma tends to be less responsive to medications, however asthma control can improve with a weight loss of 5% to 10%.[70]

## Etiologic Factors

Asthma occurs in families, which indicates that it is an inherited disorder. Asthma is influenced by two genetic tendencies: one associated with the capacity to develop allergies (atopy) and the other with the tendency to develop hyperresponsiveness of the airways independent of atopy. Environmental factors interact with inherited factors to cause attacks of bronchospasm. Asthma can develop when predisposed persons are infected by viruses or exposed to allergens or pollutants.

*Extrinsic asthma,* also known as atopic or allergic asthma, is the result of an allergy to specific triggers; usually the offending allergens are environmental antigens suspended in the air in the form of pollen, dust, molds, smoke, automobile exhaust, or animal dander. In this type of asthma, mast cells, sensitized by IgE antibodies, degranulate and release bronchoactive mediators after exposure to a specific antigen. More than half of the cases of asthma in children and young adults are of this type.

*Intrinsic asthma,* or nonallergic asthma, has no known allergic cause or trigger, has an adult onset (usually older than 40 years of age), and occurs more frequently in women.[376] Comorbidities that are associated with intrinsic asthma include nasal polyps, rhinosinusitis, and gastroesophageal reflux.[376] This type of asthma may develop from a hypersensitivity to the bacteria, or more commonly, viruses causing the infection. Other factors precipitating intrinsic asthma include drugs (aspirin and β-adrenergic antagonists), environmental irritants (occupational chemicals and air pollution), cold dry air, and exercise.

*Occupational asthma* or work exacerbated asthma is defined as variable narrowing of airways, causally related to exposure in the working environment to specific airborne dusts, gases, acids, molds, dyes, vapors, or fumes. Many of these substances are very common and not ordinarily considered hazardous. It is estimated that 15% of adult asthma is work related.[314]

High-risk occupations for asthma include farmers, animal handlers, and agricultural workers; painters; plastics and rubber workers; cleaners and homemakers (especially if cooking is done with a gas stove); textile workers; metal workers; and bakers, millers, and other food processors.

## Pathogenesis

Asthma is characterized by chronic airway inflammation and intermittent bronchospasm and bronchorestriction, as well as increased secretion production in response to allergens or irritants. The airways are the site of an acute inflammatory response consisting of cellular infiltration, epithelial disruption, mucosal edema, and mucous plugging (Fig. 15.11). The release of inflammatory mediators produces bronchial smooth muscle spasm; vascular congestion; increased vascular permeability; edema formation; production of thick, tenacious mucus; and impaired mucociliary function. Investigations are underway to examine the influence of the biome in the lung, which may predispose people to asthma as well as the gut–lung axis which proposes a connection between the gut microbiome and lung health.[487]

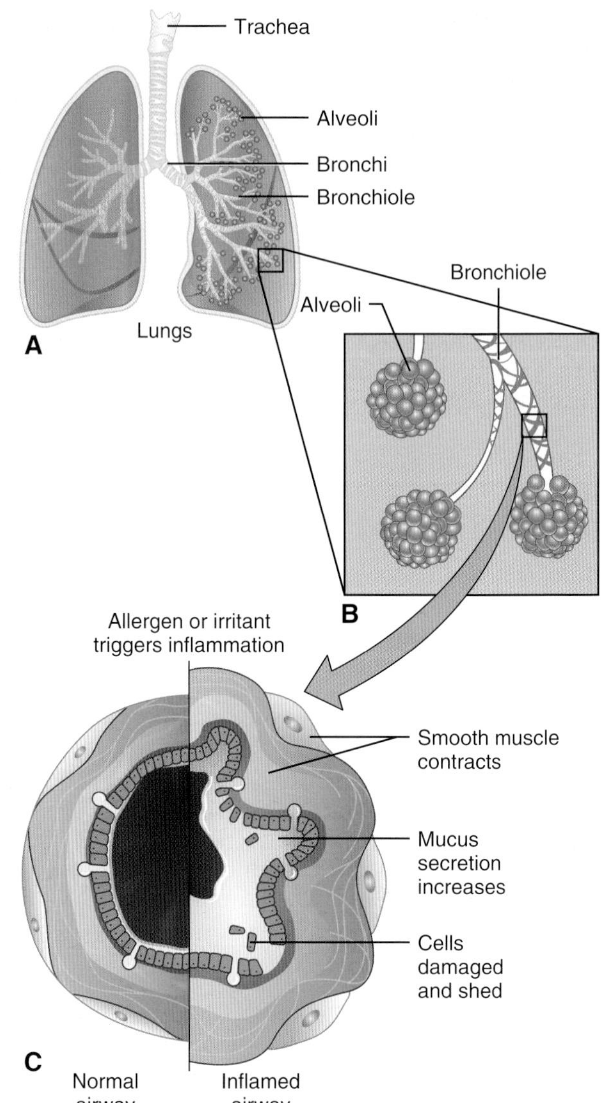


**Figure 15.11**

**Bronchiole response in asthma.** (A) Air is distributed throughout the lungs via small airways called *bronchioles.* (B) Healthy bronchioles accommodate a constant flow of air when open and relaxed. (C) In asthma, exposure to an allergen or irritant triggers inflammation, causing constriction of the smooth muscle surrounding the bronchus (bronchospasm). The airway tissue swells; this edema of the mucous membrane further narrows airways, with production of excess mucus also interfering with breathing.

Chronic inflammation can lead to airway remodeling, with permanent structural changes in the airways associated with progressive loss of lung function. Several mediators cause thickening of airway walls, goblet cell hyperplasia, and increased contractile response of bronchial smooth muscles. These changes in the bronchial musculature, combined with the epithelial cell damage caused by eosinophil infiltration, result in the airway hyperresponsiveness characteristic of asthma.

Once the airway is in spasm and airways are swollen, mucous plugs the airway, trapping distal air. $\dot{V}/\dot{Q}$ mismatch, hypoxemia, obstructed expiratory flow, and increased workload of breathing follow. Most attacks of asthmatic bronchospasm are short-lived, with relief from symptoms between episodes, although airway inflammation is present, even in people who are asymptomatic.

Although definitive causes of asthma have not been determined, there is much known about the immune system mechanisms that lead to allergic airway obstruction. T helper cells secrete cytokines, which contribute to inflammation that is mediated by IgE. IgE is present on mast cells and other airway cells. After repeated contact with antigens, these cells break down and release toxins, particularly leukotrienes, which cause bronchospasm and hypersecretions.[34]

## Clinical Manifestations

Clinical signs and symptoms of asthma differ in presentation (Box 15.6), degree (Table 15.7), and frequency among clients. Although current symptoms are the most important concern of affected people, they reflect the present level of asthma control more than underlying disease severity.[241]

During full remission, clients are asymptomatic and pulmonary function tests are normal. Over time, repeated attacks cause airway remodeling, chronic air trapping, proliferation of submucosal glands, and hypertrophied smooth muscle. This may progress to irreversible changes and COPD.

At the beginning of an attack, there is a sensation of chest constriction described as "chest tightness" or a sense of suffocation caused by the constriction of the smooth muscle in the respiratory tract and the inflammatory response in the lungs. Inspiratory and expiratory wheezing occurs when the airways narrow; prolonged expiration is seen in a 1:3 or 1:4 ratio (instead of the normal inspiratory-to-expiratory ratio of 1:2).

Nonproductive coughing fails to mobilize secretions and can intensify an attack as well as interfere with sleep. Production of yellow or green sputum requires medical evaluation for infection. Other symptoms may include tachycardia, tachypnea, fatigue, a tickle in the back of the throat accompanied by a cough in an attempt to clear the airways, and nostril flaring (advanced). Decreased oxygen saturation (hypoxemia; less than 90%) can occur quickly. Oxygen saturation level can be measured and monitored in order to respond quickly to changes in $SpO_2$. The individual may become agitated, restless, anxious, and hypertensive, with tachycardia, tachypnea, and diaphoresis.

The person usually assumes a classic sitting or squatting position to reduce venous return, leaning forward to use the accessory muscles of respiration. The skin is usually pale and moist with perspiration, and in a severe attack there may be cyanosis of the lips and nail beds. In the early stages of the attack coughing may be dry, but as the attack progresses, the cough becomes more productive of a thick, tenacious mucoid sputum. The nocturnal worsening of asthma is a common feature of this disease and may affect daytime alertness, even in children.[140] Rhinitis, chronic cough, snoring, and apnea may be responsible for sleep disturbance.

An acute attack that is not responsive to medical therapy is called *status asthmaticus*. This is a medical emergency requiring more vigorous pharmacologic and support measures, possibly including mechanical ventilation. Despite appropriate treatment, this condition can be fatal. With severe bronchospasm, the workload of breathing increases by 5 to 10 times, which can lead to acute cor pulmonale. When air is trapped, a severe paradoxical pulse develops as venous return is obstructed; blood pressure drops over 10 mm Hg during inspiration. Pneumothorax occasionally develops. If status asthmaticus continues, hypoxemia worsens and acidosis begins. If

Box 15.6

### CLINICAL MANIFESTATIONS OF BRONCHIAL ASTHMA

**Cough**

- Hacking, paroxysmal, exhausting, irritative, involuntary, nonproductive
- Becomes rattling and productive of frothy, clear, gelatinous sputum
- Main or only symptom
- Tickle in the back of the throat accompanied by a cough

**Respiratory-Related Signs**

- Shortness of breath; may occur at rest
- Prolonged expiratory phase
- Audible wheeze on inspiration and expiration or on expiration only; never on inspiration only
- Often appears pale
- May have a malar flush and red ears
- Lips deep dark red color
- May progress to cyanosis of nail beds, mouth, and lips
- Restlessness
- Apprehension
- Anxious facial expression
- Itching around nose, eyes, throat, chin, scalp
- Sweating may be prominent as attack progresses
- May sit upright with shoulders in a hunched-over position, hands on the bed or chair, and arms braced (older children)
- Speaks with short, panting broken phrases

**Chest**

- Coarse, loud breath sounds (may become quiet or silent if severe)
- Prolonged expiration
- Generalized inspiratory and expiratory wheezing; increasingly high-pitched
- Loss of breath sounds with severe cases

**With Repeated Episodes**

- Barrel chest
- Elevated shoulders
- Use of accessory muscles of respiration
- Skin retraction (clavicles, ribs, sternum)
- Facial appearance: flattened malar bones, circles beneath the eyes, narrow nose, prominent upper teeth, nostrils flaring

Modified from Wong DL: *Whaley and Wong's essentials of pediatric nursing*, ed 5, St Louis, 1997, Mosby-Year Book.

**Table 15.7 Stages of Asthma**

| Stage | Symptoms |
|---|---|
| Mild | Symptoms reverse with cessation of activity; daytime symptoms ≤2 times/wk; nighttime symptoms ≤2 times/mo; inhaled medication as needed (not usually daily) |
| Moderate | Audible wheezing<br>Use of accessory muscles of respiration<br>Leaning forward to catch breath<br>Daily (but not continual) daytime symptoms requiring short-acting inhalant and long-term treatment<br>Episodes ≥2 times/wk; nighttime symptoms ≥4 times/mo |
| Severe | Blue lips and fingernails<br>Tachypnea (30-40 breaths/min) despite cessation of activity<br>Cyanosis-induced seizures<br>Skin and rib retraction<br>Activity limited; frequent daytime and nighttime episodes, sometimes continual |

the condition is untreated or not reversed, respiratory or cardiac arrest will occur.

## MEDICAL MANAGEMENT

**PREVENTION.** Heavier emphasis on teaching self-management and especially prevention for anyone with asthma is recommended by the American Academy of Allergy, Asthma, and Immunology. *Healthy People 2020* has identified 11 objectives specifically related to this condition, including increasing the proportion of people with asthma who receive formal education as part of their management program (see *Healthy People 2020*: http://health.gov/healthypeople/). People with asthma must take an active role in preventing an asthma attack and treating it appropriately when one occurs. Each child and adult with asthma should utilize a peak flow meter to monitor their flow rates. This peak flow reading should be a part of their asthma action plan (Fig. 15.12) and this should be given to school nurses and any health care professional caring for a person with asthma.[13]

## DIAGNOSIS

Asthma is diagnosed through clinical assessment and spirometry. Patient history suggestive of asthma includes complaints of wheezing, coughing, chest tightness, seasonal allergies, nocturnal cough, and family history. Blood tests may reveal eosinophilia and elevated IgE. Skin prick testing may show specific allergens that can trigger an asthma episode.[325] In those with normal spirometry, a methacholine challenge may be used to diagnose asthma. Asthma diagnosis is considered when the $FEV_1$/FVC ratio is less than 70% and there is improvement of 12% or more in $FEV_1$ after a bronchodilator reversibility test. Diagnosis of asthma, according to the U.S. National Asthma and Education Prevention Program, is comprised of two components: impairment and risk. Impairment measures include airway obstruction as measured by spirometry, the frequency and intensity of daytime and nocturnal symptoms, frequency of a patient's use of short-acting β2 agonists, and activity limitations due to symptoms. The risk measure assesses the frequency of exacerbations. The combination of impairment and risk places the patient older than 12 years into two main categories: intermittent asthma and persistent asthma. Persistent asthma is further subdivided into mild, moderate, and severe. Once categorized, there is a stepwise progression of interventions, described below in the treatment section. Because asthma symptoms are not highly correlated to pulmonary function, standardized and validated questionnaires such as the Asthma Quality of Life Questionnaire should be used to inform treatment decisions.[325]

Diagnosis may be delayed in older clients who have other illnesses that cause similar symptoms or who attribute their breathlessness to the effects of aging and respond to the onset of asthma by limiting their activities to avoid eliciting symptoms. The diagnosis of occupational asthma is usually based on history of a temporal association between exposure and the onset of symptoms and objective evidence that these symptoms are related to airflow limitation.

**TREATMENT.** Treatment goals for asthma include improving quality of life, reducing symptoms, stabilizing/improving pulmonary function, and reducing the number and severity of exacerbations.[325] Patients should receive an Asthma Action Plan that can help identify early symptoms that warrant intervention, thereby preventing asthma attacks and exacerbations.

Identifying specific allergens for each individual, avoidance of asthma triggers, and a stepwise approach to pharmacologic management are recommended for the management of asthma. As discussed previously, there is a stepwise approach to pharmacologic therapy, depending on whether the person has intermittent or persistent asthma. For intermittent and persistent asthma, each treatment stage includes patient education, control of the environmental triggers, and management of comorbidities. For intermittent asthma, patients are typically prescribed a short-acting β-agonist (SABA), which relaxes the smooth muscles in the respiratory tracts resulting in bronchodilation. If a patient uses the SABA, more than 2 days per week, they should be reevaluated to improve symptom control (see Box 15.5 and Table 15.5). For those with persistent asthma, a long-acting β-agonist is prescribed along with a SABA, which is used as a "rescue" inhaler for acute symptoms. If symptoms are not controlled, inhaled corticosteroids are typically added to the regimen.[325] Antiinflammatory drugs have a preventive action by interrupting the development of bronchial inflammation. It is now clear that asthma attacks are actually episodic flare-ups of chronic inflammation in the lining of the airways, necessitating the use of inhaled antiinflammatories to suppress the underlying inflammation and allow the airways to heal.

It is important that people with asthma know the difference between medications that must be taken daily to prevent asthma symptoms and medications that relieve symptoms once they begin. Low-dose corticosteroid inhalants are recommended to reduce the risk of side effects (e.g., psychiatric problems, reduced growth

## Asthma Action Plan

For: ______ Doctor: ______ Date: ______

Doctor's Phone Number ______ Hospital/Emergency Department Phone Number ______

**GREEN ZONE**

### Doing Well

- No cough, wheeze, chest tightness, or shortness of breath during the day or night
- Can do usual activities

**And, if a peak flow meter is used,**

**Peak flow:** more than ______ (80 percent or more of my best peak flow)

My best peak flow is: ______

**Take these long-term control medicines each day (include an anti-inflammatory).**

| Medicine | How much to take | When to take it |
|---|---|---|
| | | |
| Before exercise ❒ ______ | ❒ 2 or ❒ 4 puffs ______ | 5 minutes before exercise |

**YELLOW ZONE**

### Asthma Is Getting Worse

- Cough, wheeze, chest tightness, or shortness of breath, or
- Waking at night due to asthma, or
- Can do some, but not all, usual activities

**-Or-**

**Peak flow:** ______ to ______ (50 to 79 percent of my best peak flow)

**Add: quick-relief medicine—and keep taking your GREEN ZONE medicine.**

**First** ______ (short-acting beta$_2$-agonist) ❒ 2 or ❒ 4 puffs, every 20 minutes for up to 1 hour ❒ Nebulizer, once

**Second**

**If your symptoms (and peak flow, if used) return to GREEN ZONE after 1 hour of above treatment:**
❒ Continue monitoring to be sure you stay in the green zone.

**-Or-**

**If your symptoms (and peak flow, if used) do not return to GREEN ZONE after 1 hour of above treatment:**
❒ Take: ______ (short-acting beta$_2$-agonist) ❒ 2 or ❒ 4 puffs or ❒ Nebulizer
❒ Add: ______ (oral steroid) mg per day For ______ (3–10) days
❒ Call the doctor ❒ before/ ❒ within ______ hours after taking the oral steroid.

**RED ZONE**

### Medical Alert!

- Very short of breath, or
- Quick-relief medicines have not helped, or
- Cannot do usual activities, or
- Symptoms are same or get worse after 24 hours in Yellow Zone

**-Or-**

**Peak flow:** less than ______ (50 percent of my best peak flow)

**Take this medicine:**

❒ ______ (short-acting beta$_2$-agonist) ❒ 4 or ❒ 6 puffs or ❒ Nebulizer
❒ ______ (oral steroid) mg

**Then call your doctor NOW.** Go to the hospital or call an ambulance if:
- You are still in the red zone after 15 minutes AND
- You have not reached your doctor.

**DANGER SIGNS**
- **Trouble walking and talking due to shortness of breath**
- **Lips or fingernails are blue**

- **Take ❒ 4 or ❒ 6 puffs of your quick-relief medicine AND**
- **Go to the hospital or call for an ambulance ______ (phone) NOW!**

See the reverse side for things you can do to avoid your asthma triggers.

**Figure 15.12**

**Asthma Action Plan.** (From National Heart, Lung, and Blood Institute. NIH Publication No. 07-5251, April 2007. Available online at: http://www.nhlbi.nih.gov/health/public/lung/asthma/asthma_actplan.pdf.)

in children, ocular effects, death, osteoporosis, or alopecia and hirsutism) from prolonged use.[135,456] Leukotriene-receptor antagonists inhibit inflammation and have been shown to be safe and effective in adults with asthma and allergic rhinitis.[488] Newer treatment interventions on the horizon include the use of immunotherapy and monocolonal antibodies to target specific pathways in asthma.

In those with asthma, there is some evidence that low vitamin D levels are associated with an increased risk of exacerbation.[204] There is some evidence that fresh fruits, a Mediterranean diet, and antioxidants may be protective.[179]

Many complementary treatments have been used to ameliorate asthma symptoms though there has been minimal research to validate most of these claims. Much of the research has been conducted in small samples or in single trials.[278] There is minimal but growing evidence to support the use of acupuncture.[63,307] Complementary treatments are still being studied for benefits and adverse effects.[48]

**PROGNOSIS.** The outlook for clients with *bronchial asthma* is excellent despite the recent increase in the death rate. Childhood asthma may disappear, but only about one-quarter of the children with asthma become symptom-free when their airways reach adult size. Factors that predict adult asthma include gender (males are more likely to outgrow asthma), smoking, allergy to dust mites, degree of airway hyperresponsiveness, and early age of onset.[426,467]

There is presently controversy regarding the term *asthma-COPD overlap syndrome*, with the suggestion that this is a distinct phenotype that has features of both asthma and COPD.[298] The risk of lung cancer, however, is greater in people with asthma compared with those who do not have a history of asthma.[4,393]

Attention to general health measures and use of pharmacologic agents permit control of symptoms in nearly all cases. In some people, chronic inflammation can lead to airway remodeling, with permanent structural changes in the airways associated with progressive loss of function. For these individuals, remodeling is not fully reversed by current therapy.

*Status asthmaticus* is acute, severe asthma exacerbation that is unresponsive to medications and can result in respiratory or cardiac arrest and possible death (see previous discussion). If ventilation becomes necessary, prognosis for recovery is poor.

## Exercise-Induced Bronchospasm or Bronchoconstriction

Exercise-induced bronchoconstriction (EIB), formerly called exercise-induced asthma, is an acute, reversible, usually self-terminating airway obstruction that develops 5 to 15 minutes after vigorous intensity exercise. During exercise, a person increases their respiratory rate and humidification is lost. This results in mast cell degranulation and release of leukotrienes, histamine, tryptase, prostaglandins, and eosinophils, causing bronchoconstriction and inflammation. The air humidity and the respiratory rate both influence EIB.[498]

### Prevalence

EIB occurs in 10% to 20% of children and adults, however this prevalence estimate depends on the diagnostic criteria used. Prevalence estimates in elite athletes vary widely depending on diagnostic criteria and the sport. EIB prevalence is higher in ice skaters, cross-country skiers, and in endurance sports such as distance running and mountain biking. There is preliminary evidence that there are racial differences as well, with African Americans and Asians demonstrating higher rates of EIB compared to Caucasians.[498]

### Risk Factors

EIB can occur without a diagnosis of underlying asthma. If EIB occurs in a person with diagnosed asthma, it may indicate the need for tighter control of symptoms. Other risk factors include female athletes, winter sport, exercise in dry air, presence of chloramines in water, exposure to emissions from ice-cleaning equipment, playgrounds/fields close to traffic or with high air particulate matter, and participation in endurance sports.[124,498] Low-risk sports include sports requiring less than a 5- to 8-minute effort, such as sprinting, hurdles, tennis, gymnastics, and weight-lifting. Moderate-risk sports are those requiring a continuous effort for 5 to 8 minutes, such as soccer, football, basketball, and field hockey. High-risk sports are those requiring more than a 5- to 8-minute effort in dry/cold air or in an environment with pollutants, such as swimming, endurance running, ice hockey, cross-country skiing, and high altitude sports.[124]

### Pathophysiology

There are two main theories of EIB: osmotic and thermal, with more evidence supporting the osmotic theory. The thermal theory states that airways exposed to cool air cause vasoconstriction of bronchial vasculature. When exercise is terminated, the airways rewarm, causing a reactive hyperemia and edema of the airways. The osmotic theory focuses on dehydration of airways as the trigger for bronchoconstriction.[498] When ventilation increases with exercise, the airways become dehydrated, changing the osmolarity of the airway surface liquid, which decreases mucociliary clearance and activation of leukocytes, mast cells, and eosinophils.[498] This triggers bronchoconstriction, inflammation, and the classic symptoms of asthma.

### Symptoms and Diagnosis

Symptoms of EIB include wheezing, dyspnea, cough, chest tightness, and mucus production during or after an exercise bout. Patients with EIB may have normal $FEV_1$. This parameter may improve after a bronchodilator is given, however this does not occur in all patients. The person with EIB demonstrates a 10% to 15% or greater drop in $FEV_1$[c] when they reach at least 80% of maximum heart rate for at least 4 minutes.[451,497] If spirometry is normal but EIB is suspected, patients should undergo an exercise test to note changes in $FEV_1$ before and after exercise, or hyperosmolar challenge with eucapnic voluntary hyperpnea (EVH) or mannitol. The EVH test involves hyperpnea with a dry gas inhalant to dry the airways, similar to what occurs with exercise.[235] There are two main protocols for EVH that involve breathing at a percentage of maximal voluntary ventilation for a period of time with spirometry at staged intervals.[235] EIB is diagnosed when there is a drop in $FEV_1$ of 10% or more compared to baseline.

### Treatment

The recommended treatment for EIB focuses on prophylaxis, with the affected individual taking a short-acting β-agonist prior to exercise less than 4 times per week to avoid building of tolerance to the medication. Leukotriene inhibitors can be used daily in those with EIB, but are not effective in all patients. Inhaled corticosteroids may also be used to decrease the frequency of EIB[498], as well as having an adequate warm-up period. Nonpharmacologic interventions include a prolonged warm-up to reduce the severity of EIB.[498] Warm-up should be continuous exercise at 60% to 80% of HRmax with increased efficacy when combined with medications.[498] Other preventative measures include breathing through a mask or scarf to maintain airway humidity and reducing exposure to environmental pollutants.[1] There are small studies that support the use of a low salt diet to attenuate symptoms, however larger trials are needed. There may also be a role for noninvasive ventilation and respiratory muscle training to reduce the hyperresponsiveness of airways.

---

[c]FEV1 is the forced expiratory volume, a measure of the greatest volume of air a person can exhale during forced expiration; the subscript is added to indicate the percentage of the vital capacity that can be expired in 1 second. FVC is forced vital capacity, a measure of the greatest volume of air that can be expelled when a person performs a rapid, forced expiratory maneuver. This usually takes about 5 seconds.

SPECIAL IMPLICATIONS FOR THE THERAPIST 15.6

## Asthma

Because physical therapists prescribe and observe exercise, they may be the first to recognize symptoms of undiagnosed asthma. Coughing is the most common symptom of EIB, but other symptoms include chest tightness, wheezing, and SOB. The affected (but undiagnosed) individual may comment, "I am more out of shape than I thought." This should be a red flag for the therapist to consider the possibility of asthma and need for medical diagnosis and intervention.

If an asthma attack should occur during therapy, first assess the severity of the attack. Place the person in the high Fowler position and encourage diaphragmatic and pursed-lip breathing. If the client has an inhaler available, provide whatever assistance is necessary for that person to self-administer the medication. Typically, the patient takes 4 puffs of their reliever medication and waits 4 minutes unless instructed differently in their asthma action plan. If the patient still exhibits signs of respiratory distress, often they are instructed to take 4 more puffs of the reliever. If the patient continues to demonstrate respiratory distress, call an ambulance. Other signs and symptoms that warrant an emergency response are: inability to speak due to dyspnea, perioral cyanosis or fingernail cyanosis, or chest pain.[21]

### Effect of Exercise

There are many barriers to exercise for people with asthma, including lack of motivation, time constraints, weather conditions, poor communication with their health care team, misunderstanding about medication regimen, lack of understanding about asthma, and belief that exercise is not good for this condition.[315,334] To prevent secondary complications of a sedentary lifestyle and because obesity can contribute to the inflammatory process associated with asthma, exercise and education about exercise should be part of any treatment program.

There is strong evidence to support physical training for cardiovascular training in this population.[396] There is inadequate evidence for a positive effect of breathing exercises and inspiratory muscle training in individuals who have asthma.[227,397] In children, a program of training 2 times/week for 6 to 8 weeks improved nocturnal symptoms of asthma, and there is some evidence of reduced inflammation. In nonobese adults, supervised exercise for 12 weeks was found to improve sleep quality, however there were insignificant results for unsupervised programs.[134] In a recent systematic review, exercise training in those with asthma improved fitness as measured by $VO_2$ peak and quality of life. There were mixed results for improvements in lung function and inflammation, possibly due to the varied exercise protocols and doses.[255]

### Exercise and Medication

Bronchospasm can occur during exercise (especially in EIB) if the person with asthma has a low blood oxygen level before exercise. For this reason, it is helpful to take bronchodilators by metered-dose inhaler before exercise, performing mild stretching and warm-up exercises during that time period to avoid bronchospasm with higher workload exercise. Increased exercise should be accompanied by good bronchodilator coverage to promote bronchodilation and improve alveolar ventilation and oxygenation. Exercise guidelines for adults with asthma can be modified from recommendations for children with asthma (Table 15.8).

**Table 15.8** Exercise Guidelines for Children With Asthma

| Recommendation | Benefit |
|---|---|
| General exercise, school-based physical education | Maintains motor control, flexibility, strength, cardiovascular fitness, and prevents or reverses side effects of medication (e.g., corticosteroids)<br>Raises threshold for strenuous exercise before mouth breathing and EIB occur |
| Low-impact exercise (aerobics, weight training, stationary bike) | Permits exercise without increased bronchospasm |
| Warm-up before aerobic activity | Helps control airway reactivity; gradually desensitizes mast cells, reducing release of bronchoconstrictive mediators |
| Exercise in a trigger-free environment (i.e., avoid cold, pollution, or increased pollen outdoors; exercise indoors; avoid tobacco smoke; swimming program is ideal) | Prevents bronchospasm; controls symptoms |
| Take prescribed medication properly before exercise or activity producing bronchospasm | Prevents bronchospasm |
| Monitor $FEV_1/FVC$ ratio before, during, and after physical activity[a]<br>Decrease of 10% requires slowing activity<br>Drop of 15%-20% from initial measurement requires cessation of exercise | Determines whether shortness of breath is caused by intensity of exercise or by diminished airflow as a result of bronchospasm |

*EIB*, Exercise-induced bronchospasm; *$FEV_1/FVC$*, ratio of forced expiratory volume in 1 second to forced vital capacity.

[a]Peak flowmeters can be used to obtain this information. Determine the child's normal range of lung function by having the child blow in the meter in the morning and evening for 1 week. The average level measured varies from person to person and is influenced by gender and height. Testing should establish a peak flow protocol against which lung function can be compared to determine if deterioration has occurred.

Many clients have found that using their inhalers in this way before exercise permits them to exercise without onset of symptoms. Proper administration of a metered-dose inhaler is essential (see Box 15.5). The first dose induces dilation of the larger, central bronchial tubes, relaxing smooth muscles in the airways; the second dose dilates the bronchioles (smaller airways).

Some athletes do not achieve the control needed for the performance demands of competition. The effectiveness of short-acting medications and medications in general for asthma varies widely among people with asthma while exercising. The preventive benefits of each medication dose may wane after taking a new drug for several weeks. Any athlete with asthma who cannot perform at the levels desired or expected because of asthma symptoms should be advised to review medications and medication use with the physician.

### Monitoring Vital Signs

Monitoring vital signs can alert the therapist to important changes in cardiorespiratory function. Lungs should be auscultated before, during, and after activity to monitor changes in lung sounds and quality of air movement. This should be paired with assessment of pulse rate, rhythm, and strength, blood pressure, rating of perceived exertion, and pulse oximetry. Therapists should also observe breathing pattern, looking for signs of intolerance such as use of accessory muscles and sternal retractions.

Status asthmaticus is severe, acute asthma that is unresponsive to bronchodilators and corticosteroids. Therapy can augment the medical management of the client with status asthmaticus. In coordination with the individual's medications, the therapist helps to remove secretions; promotes relaxed, more efficient breathing; enhances V/Q matching; reduces hypoxemia; and teaches the client to coordinate relaxed breathing with general body movement.

Caution needs to be observed to avoid stimuli that bring on bronchospasm and deterioration (e.g., aggressive percussion, forced expiration maneuvers, aggressive bag ventilation, or manual hyperinflation with an intubated individual). Certain body positions may have to be avoided because of client intolerance or exacerbation of symptoms in those positions.[136] Immediate medical care is recommended for anyone with asthma who fails to have a response to 4 doses of a short-acting $\beta_2$-agonist, subcostal retractions, cyanosis, inability to drink or speak because of SOB, or oxygen saturation on room air below 92%.[513] If present, therapists should reference the patient's asthma action plan.

## Asthma-COPD Overlap Syndrome

### Definition

Asthma-COPD Overlap Syndrome (ACOS) refers to asthma and COPD diagnoses in the same patient.[409] There is controversy over this diagnosis with no agreed-upon diagnostic criteria. Broadly, people present with persistent airflow limitation similar to COPD, a history of asthma with airflow reversibility with bronchodilation of 400 mL and improvement in $FEV_1$ of 15% or more.[466] Due to ambiguity about diagnosis, there are wide variations in incidence, prevalence, and treatment approaches at the time of this writing.

## Bronchiectasis

### Definition

Bronchiectasis is a progressive condition with irreversible destruction and dilation of airways. Abnormal and permanent dilation of the bronchi and bronchioles develops when the supporting structures (bronchial walls) are weakened by chronic inflammatory changes associated with secondary infection. This results in chronic productive cough, frequent respiratory infections, and chronic inflammation.[349]

### Incidence and Etiologic and Risk Factors

The incidence of bronchiectasis is rising, possibly as a consequence of the use of high-resolution chest CT, which is helping physicians to identify cases in their early stages.[192,212] Risk factors for bronchiectasis include infection with *H. influenza, S. pneumonia, Moraxella catarrhalis, Staphylococcus aureus, P. aeruginosa*, TB, non-TB mycobacteria, *Mycoplasma pneumoniae*, and adenovirus.[359]Other risk factors include older age (>60), older females, rheumatoid arthritis, Marfan syndrome, HIV, inflammatory bowel disease, COPD, cystic fibrosis (CF), and primary ciliary dyskinesia.[359] The most common cause of bronchiectasis is chronic inflammation that occurs after a pulmonary infection. The most common congenital issue associated with bronchiectasis is primary ciliary dyskinesia. In primary ciliary dyskinesia, ineffective clearance of secretions increases the risk of chronic or recurrent respiratory infections that precipitate bronchiectasis. Bronchiectasis also develops in people with immunodeficiencies involving humoral immunity, and recurrent aspiration.

CF causes about half of all cases of bronchiectasis. Rheumatoid arthritis, sinusitis, dextrocardia (heart located on right side of chest), Kartagener syndrome (alterations in ciliary activity), defective development of bronchial cartilage (Williams-Campbell syndrome), and endobronchial tumor predispose a person to bronchiectasis. Bronchiectasis may also affect those with COPD, worsening the dyspnea and lung function as compared to those without bronchiectasis.[192]

### Pathogenesis

Although bronchiectasis has been viewed as a progressive disease of destruction and dilation of the medium and large airways, there is now evidence of the importance of the small airways in the pathogenesis of this condition. Cole's hypothesis states there are four phases of bronchiectasis: (1) chronic infection, (2) chronic inflammatory response, (3) impaired defense of microorganisms and reduced mucociliary function, and (4) dilation of airways.[222]

Chronic inflammation of the bronchial wall by mononuclear cells is common to all types of bronchiectasis, with the inflammatory process often continuing after the infection has been cleared.[192] Abnormal

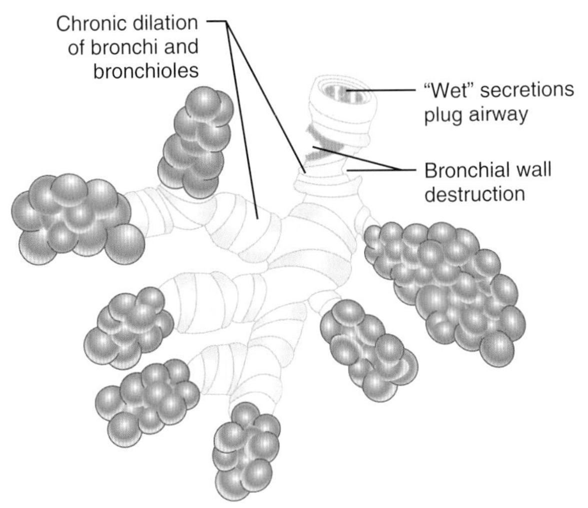


**Figure 15.13**

**Airway pathology in bronchiectasis.**

bronchial dilation is the result of enzymatic degradation of the airway's connective tissue. Infection, inflammation of the airways and dilation cause an increase in mucus production, airway plugging, and bronchospasm (Fig. 15.13).[475] People with bronchiectasis demonstrate a decline in $FEV_1$, with more significant decreases in those with systemic inflammation and more frequent and severe exacerbations.[192]

In response to these changes, large anastomoses develop between the bronchial and pulmonary blood vessels to increase the blood flow through the bronchial circulation. V/Q mismatch causes hypoxia and hypercapnia. Damage to these anastomoses is responsible for the hemoptysis present in persons with bronchiectasis.

## Clinical Manifestations

There is a varied presentation and symptom experience in those with bronchiectasis. The most common symptoms of bronchiectasis include persistent coughing, with large amounts of purulent sputum production (worse in the morning). Dyspnea is quite common in adults, along with chest pain, rhinosinusitis, fatigue, weight loss, and exercise intolerance. Children will also experience shortness of breath, a productive cough, and may also exhibit poor growth.[349] Clubbing may also occur, as well as cardiac issues such as pulmonary hypertension. Exacerbations in adults are defined as a person with documented bronchiectasis who has three or more of the following symptoms for 48 hours or more: cough, sputum volume and/or consistency, sputum purulence, breathlessness and/or exercise intolerance, fatigue and/or malaise, hemoptysis, and a clinician determines that a change in treatment is necessary.[218] There is a known correlation between bronchiectasis and rheumatoid arthritis, but the exact mechanism remains unknown.

## MEDICAL MANAGEMENT

**DIAGNOSIS.** Bronchiectasis is diagnosed through a combination of sputum culture, high-resolution CT imaging, and pulmonary function testing.[349,358] Underlying conditions that may contribute to the development of bronchiectasis are also evaluated, including tests for CF, inflammatory bowel disease, and ciliary dysfunction.[192] Serial CT scans increase radiation dose, limiting its utility. MRI is being evaluated as a possible diagnostic tool for monitoring. It is also recommended that patients undergo pulmonary function testing at diagnosis and annually, with obstructive and mixed patterns as well as normal PFTs as common findings.[349]

Bronchiectasis is diagnosed by CT if the airway diameter is greater than the adjacent blood vessel and there is wall thickening. The degree of bronchiectasis is determined by the extent of the dilation, the severity of mucous plugging, and the extent of airway dysfunction.

**TREATMENT.** Treatment interventions differ for those with CF-related bronchiectasis versus non-CF bronchiectasis. In those with CF, airway clearance techniques (chest physical therapy, autogenic drainage, high-frequency chest wall oscillation, active cycle of breathing) are recommended to aid secretion removal. The evidence to support the role of airway clearance in non-CF bronchiectasis is sparse, however it is still a recommended treatment. Bronchiectasis exacerbations are treated with antibiotics and bronchodilators. Other strategies include education about smoking cessation and vaccination for influenza virus and pneumococcal infection, and good nutrition.[358] Hydration is important, and oxygen may be administered. Mucolytic agents, inhaled corticosteroids, bronchodilators, and antibiotics are used to manage bronchiectasis.[358] Surgical resection is reserved for the few clients with localized bronchiectasis and adequate pulmonary function who fail to respond to conservative management or for the person with massive hemoptysis.

Other techniques that may be of use to facilitate sputum production include vibratory PEP devices, active cycle of breathing, and exercise.[295] The airway clearance interventions are similar to those used in CF, so the reader is encouraged to reference those sections of the book and refer to the excellent review by Lee et al.[295]

**PROGNOSIS.** The morbidity and mortality associated with bronchiectasis have declined markedly. Prognosis typically is good, depending on the patient's comorbidities and self-care. Mortality rates for bronchiectasis are in line with those for COPD and asthma.[157] Lower life expectancy was associated with increased age, lower activity scores as measured by the St. George Respiratory Questionnaire, infection by *Pseudomonas aeruginosa*, CF diagnosis, and reduced lung function.[303] The Bronchiectasis Severity Index is comprised of nine variables that predict mortality, hospitalization, exacerbations, and quality of life. Predictors of mortality are older age, low $FEV_1$, low BMI, and three or more exacerbations in the previous year.[328] Complications of bronchiectasis include recurrent pneumonia, lung abscesses, metastatic infections in other organs (e.g., brain abscess), and cardiac and respiratory failure.

# Bronchiolitis

## Definition and Overview

Bronchiolitis refers to several morphologically distinct pathologic conditions that involve the small airways.

Acute bronchiolitis is a commonly occurring, diffuse, and often severe inflammation of the lower airways (bronchioles) in children younger than age 2 years that is caused by a viral infection. Bronchiolitis in adults is typically due to other treatments, such as bone marrow transplantation, organ transplantation, and chest radiation.[131]

Bronchiolitis was once classified as a type of chronic interstitial pneumonia and referred to as *small airways disease*. Progress in pathology has provided more specific etiology-directed diagnoses that reflect the individual reaction patterns observed.

Bronchiolitis in the adult is classified as acute or chronic, with identification of these special forms (e.g., obliterative, eosinophilic bronchiolitis in asthma, necrotizing bronchiolitis in viral infection, or toxic fume bronchiolitis after exposure to noxious gases and the development of chemical pneumonitis).[261,489] Bronchiolitis obliterans (BO) is the most important clinical complication in transplant recipients, may represent a form of allograft rejection, and is associated with a 3- to 5-year median survival.[131]

### Incidence and Etiologic Factors

Bronchiolitis is the leading cause of hospitalization in infants less than 1 year old.[74] Constrictive bronchiolitis in adults usually occurs with chronic bronchitis; bronchiolitis in children is associated with pulmonary infections, such as respiratory syncytial virus (RSV) which accounts for 80% of cases, rhinovirus, adenovirus, coronavirus, human metapneumovirus, influenza and parainfluenza.[74,283] Primarily present in winter and spring, it is easily spread by hand-to-nose or nose-to-eye transmission. Exudative bronchiolitis, which is inflammation of the bronchioles with exudation of gray tenacious sputum, is often associated with asthma.

### Pathogenesis and Clinical Manifestations

Variable degrees of obstruction occur in response to infection as the bronchiolar mucosa swells and the lumina fill with mucus and exudate. Depending on the type, these changes occur as the walls of the bronchi and bronchioles are infiltrated with inflammatory cells, increased goblet cells, and fibroblasts.

Bronchiolitis in the adult is characterized by fibrosis of the submucosa and peribronchial tissues. The bronchial epithelium becomes damaged, and the resulting inflammatory process triggers a fibrotic repair process that obliterates the airways. Airways distal to the area impacted by BO can be normal.[131] Hyperinflation, obstructive emphysema from partial obstruction, and patchy areas of atelectasis may occur distal to the inflammatory lesion as the disease progresses.

Cough, respiratory distress, and cyanosis occur initially, followed by a brief period of improvement. Dyspnea, paroxysmal cough, sputum production, and wheezing with marked use of accessory muscles follow as the disease progresses. Apnea may be the first indicator of RSV infection in very young infants. Severe disease may be followed by a rise in $PaCO_2$ (hypercapnia), leading to respiratory acidosis and hypoxemia.

## MEDICAL MANAGEMENT

**PREVENTION.** Currently there is no vaccine for RSV. High-risk infants (premature or those with other health conditions) may receive palivizumab, which is a monoclonal antibody that can modulate the severity of RSV.[105] Understanding RSV disease mechanisms in order to develop a vaccine is difficult because there is a wide range of RSV disease phenotypes in humans and disparities in RSV disease phenotypes among the animal models used in research.[338]

Frequent handwashing and not sharing items, such as cups, glasses, and utensils, with persons who have RSV illness can decrease the spread of virus to others. Excluding children with colds or other respiratory illnesses (without fever) who are well enough to attend childcare or school settings may not decrease the transmission of RSV, because it is often spread in the early stages of illness. In a hospital setting, RSV transmission can and should be prevented by strict attention to contact precautions such as meticulous hand hygiene and wearing gowns and gloves.

**DIAGNOSIS AND TREATMENT.** Diagnosis is made on the basis of clinical findings, age, the season, and the epidemiology of the community. Infants present with rhinorrhea, cough, and low-grade fever. Children may also present with tachypnea, inspiratory crackles, expiratory wheezes, and apnea. Chest radiographs, blood testing, urine testing or virology are not recommended by national guidelines.[74]

There is no specific treatment for bronchiolitis, and medical therapy is controversial. National guidelines do not recommend use of β2-agonists, steroids, or antibiotics nor do they recommend nebulized hypertonic saline or chest physical therapy.[74] Oxygen may be indicated if saturations are less than 92%, and CPAP may be considered if in respiratory failure.[74] Antibiotics may be used initially when a bacterial cause of illness has not been ruled out or for secondary infections, but are not indicated if the pathogen is viral.[347] Complementary and alternative medicine has not been shown to be effective.[283] Prevention should include proper hand hygiene and possibly the use of palivizumab, a monoclonal antibody used to prevent RSV in high-risk populations.[74]

**PROGNOSIS.** The acute disease lasts about 3 to 10 days, and the majority of cases can be managed at home with a good prognosis. Hospitalization may be necessary for anyone with complicating conditions, such as underlying lung or heart disease, associated debilitated states, poor hydration, or questionable care at home. Some children deteriorate rapidly and die within weeks; others may follow a more long-term course. In the adult, the acute form usually has a good prognosis, but the prognosis for bronchiolitis obliterans is poor.

**SPECIAL IMPLICATIONS FOR THE THERAPIST 15.7**

### *Bronchiolitis*

RSV is the most common cause of pediatric acute bronchiolitis and pneumonia (see the section on RSV in Chapter 8). For this reason, any staff member with evidence of upper respiratory infection serves as a potential reservoir of RSV and should be excluded from direct contact with high-risk infants. All persons who come within 3 feet of an RSV client must wear a gown and mask with an eye shield and keep hands away from the face, especially the eyes, nose, and mouth. Hands must be washed before and after caring for any client and after handling potentially contaminated client care equipment. Standard precautions must be strictly carried out.

Because RSV is readily transmitted by close contact with personnel, families, and other children both by direct contact (especially lifting or holding) and through contact with objects handled by the child, precautions against cross-infection are important. The primary routes of inoculation for the organisms are large-droplet inhalation through the nose and eyes. When contact is made with mucous discharge or drainage from the eye, nose, or mouth, the therapist is reminded to wear an exterior hospital gown and to discard the gown (or change clothing) when leaving.

Pregnant female personnel or visitors should be advised of the risk of potential physical defects in the developing embryo from contact with RSV. Immunoprophylaxis to prevent RSV in high-risk infants is effective, and prevention of RSV may be possible in the future, with active maternal immunization during pregnancy providing passive immunity of infants.[188,486]

## Sleep-Disordered Breathing

### Definition

Sleep-disordered breathing comprises a collection of syndromes characterized by breathing abnormalities during sleep that result in intermittently disrupted gas exchange and sleep interruption. Sleep-disordered breathing includes Cheyne-Stokes respiration, hypoventilation syndromes with and without chronic lung disease, heavy snoring with daytime sleepiness (upper airway resistance syndrome), and sleep apnea. The most common sleep apnea syndrome, and the only one discussed here, is obstructive sleep apnea, defined as significant daytime symptoms (e.g., sleepiness) in conjunction with evidence of sleep-related upper airway obstruction and sleep disturbance.[44,372]

There are three types of sleep apnea: central, obstructive, and mixed. *Central sleep apnea* is caused by altered chemosensitivity and cerebral respiratory control. In this type of apnea, the brain misconstrues small rises in $PaCO_2$ and causes hyperventilation, resulting in the lowering of $PaCO_2$. This signals the brain to reduce or stop inspiration in order to assist in raising $PaCO_2$ to normal levels, causing apnea or hypopnea. $PaCO_2$ rises and then the cycle repeats, causing multiple episodes of hypopnea or apnea during sleep.[125] Brief (<10 second) periods of apnea in the newborn is considered normal and is termed periodic breathing. This pattern typically disappears a few weeks or months after birth. *Mixed sleep apnea* is a central apnea that is immediately followed by an obstructive event. At the time of this writing, a new condition called overlap syndrome (OVS) has been defined by the American Thoracic society. OVS refers to the co-occurance of obstructive sleep apnea and chronic obstructive pulmonary disease. Outcomes for those with OVS are worse than with sleep apnea or COPD alone, however research in this area is still limited.[311]

### Incidence and Prevalence

Prevalence estimates for obstructive sleep apnea are 2% to 4%, rising to 30% to 60% in men 60 years old or above and approximately 9% in middle-aged people. Sleep apnea also occurs in children, with an estimated prevalence of 1% to 5%.[187,348]

Forty percent of obese people have OSA, and 70% of people with sleep apnea are obese. OSA in children without neurologic impairment is most commonly caused by adenotonsillar hypertrophy, although obesity is positively correlated with this disorder in children as well.[25] Children with Down syndrome are particularly vulnerable to OSA and should be tested at age 3 to 4 years.[436]

### Etiologic and Risk Factors

OSA is caused by partial or complete pharyngeal collapse during sleep, leading to either reduction (hypopnea) or cessation (apnea) of breathing. Relaxation of the musculature of the pharynx and tongue during sleep obstruct ventilation. Obesity accounts for the majority of cases of OSA.[125] A neck circumference greater than 16 inches for a woman or greater than 17 inches in a man correlates with an increased risk for this disorder.[241]

People with craniofacial abnormalities (e.g., anatomically narrowed upper airways, such as occur in micrognathia; macroglossia (large tongue); and adenoid, uvula, elongated soft palate, or tonsillar hypertrophy), are predisposed to the development of OSA. Fat deposits or swelling in any or all of these tissues causes further obstruction.

Medical conditions that are associated with OSA include cardiovascular disease (hypertension, coronary artery disease, heart failure, dysrhythmias), cerebrovascular disorders (stroke, dementia, transient ischemic attacks), hypothyroidism,[405] depression, and erectile dysfunction.[372]

Other risk factors include older age, male gender (prior to menopause, then prevalence is about equal), and African American or Asian descent.[125] The evidence to support smoking is equivocal, however alcohol may aggravate OSA as a result of lowered airway tone and a lowered central respiratory drive.[125]

In children, risk factors include adenoid and tonsillar hypertrophy, craniofacial abnormalities, obesity, midface deficiency, mandibular hypoplasia, prematurity, allergic rhinitis, and neurologic disorders such as Down syndrome, cerebral palsy, and myotonias.[10,258]

### Pathogenesis and Clinical Manifestations

There are several hypotheses as to the pathogenesis of OSA syndrome. Collapse or obstruction of the airway may occur with the inhibition of muscle tone that characterizes some phases of non–rapid eye movement sleep, and rapid eye movement sleep.[299] During inspiration, the negative pressure generated by the respiratory muscles triggers a reflex in pharyngeal muscles that causes upper airway dilation. This reflex is dampened during sleep, causing those with OSA syndrome to have partial or complete collapse of the upper airway. When the airway is obstructed, there is a drop in oxygenation and a concomitant increase in carbon dioxide. In addition to a decrease in upper airway tone during sleep, there is also a drop in the sensitivity of chemoreceptors, further exacerbating loss of upper airway tone.[299]

By definition, apnea is a complete cessation of ventilation and therefore is precipitated by complete pharyngeal collapse, whereas hypopnea results from partial pharyngeal closure and is manifested by a substantial reduction in, but not a cessation of, breathing.

The cycle of recurrent pharyngeal collapse with subsequent arousal from sleep as the brain signals the person to wake up in order to breathe leads to the primary symptoms of daytime somnolence and an increase in the sympathetic drive.[169,299] Heart rate and blood pressure are elevated acutely after the apneic episode ends and there are chronic elevations as well. There are a number of physiologic consequences to OSA that are of particular import to the physical therapist. Intermittent apnea or hypopnea triggers inflammatory markers and genes that impact oxygen delivery, and the sympathetic nervous system is upregulated.[125] Activation of the sympathetic nervous system fight-or-flight response increases heart rate, blood pressure, respiratory rate, and glucose levels. Over time, the loss of deep or restful sleep from repeated apneic episodes results in hypertension,[225] daytime sleepiness, higher metabolic demands, impairments in myocardial relaxation, and lower cardiac output, fatigue, and difficulty concentrating.[288]

In OVS, the cyclical process described above is worsened by the airway resistance and hyperinflation associated with COPD. To compensate for these changes, respiratory rate increases, shortening time in expiration which, in the person with COPD, contributes to dynamic hyperinflation, further disrupting the sleep cycle.[311]

Neurocognitive effects may include personality changes; irritability, hyperactivity, judgment impairment, difficulty concentrating, poor school or work performance, automobile accidents, and memory loss.[117,219] Neurocognitive effects of apnea may also cause a mood disorder leading to an erroneous diagnosis of dysthymia (depressive mood disorder); treatment with standard antidepressant medications may exacerbate the condition.[261]

Fragmented sleep with its repetitive cycles of snoring, airway collapse, and arousal contributes to the development of hypertension and dysrhythmias such as bradycardia, atrioventricular blocks, atrial fibrillation, and nonsustained ventricular tachycardia.[125] People with sleep apnea are also at a higher risk for developing myocardial ischemia and ischemic stroke.[125,224]

The primary symptom in children is hyperactivity, not daytime somnolence. OSA syndrome in children is associated with impaired growth, inattention, depression, and an increased risk for cardiovascular conditions.[10]

## MEDICAL MANAGEMENT

**DIAGNOSIS.** Bed partners usually report loud cyclic snoring with periods of silence (breath cessation), restlessness, frequent episodes of waking up gasping, and often thrashing movements of the extremities during sleep. Other signs and symptoms include daytime sleepiness (not as common in those with heart failure), erectile dysfunction, morning headaches, memory issues, nocturia, and depression.[125]

Diagnosis may be made using sleep monitoring devices, overnight pulse oximetry, radiologic imaging, laboratory assays, questionnaires, and clinical signs and symptoms. An in-home system for diagnosing OSA is available, but the most reliable test to confirm the diagnosis is overnight polysomnography in both children and adults (i.e., monitoring the subject during sleep for periods of apnea and lowered blood oxygen saturation).[258] Disease severity is determined by the apnea-hypopnea index or AHI. Apnea is defined as a lowering of airflow to 90% or less of baseline for 10 or more seconds. Hypopnea is a reduction of airflow to 30% or less of baseline for 10 or more seconds with a drop in $PaO_2$ of 3% or more.[125] Severity is classified as mild (5-14 episodes of apnea/hypopnea per hour), moderate (15-30 episodes), or severe (more than 30 episodes).[372] Some physicians will use overnight pulse oximetry as the first step in diagnosis in people with heart failure. Sleep apnea can be diagnosed with 12.5 desaturations of greater than 3% per hour.[125] In children, the AHI of greater than 1 episode per hour along with symptoms of sleep apnea is used to make a diagnosis.[258]

The physician must differentiate sleep apnea syndrome from seizure disorder, narcolepsy, or psychiatric depression. A hemoglobin level is obtained, and thyroid function tests are performed. Several clinical diagnostic predictive formulas are being studied.[369]

**TREATMENT.** New clinical practice guidelines recommend weight loss for patients who are overweight or obese, with a body mass index of 25 $kg/m^2$ or above. For those who have a BMI of 27 $kg/m^2$ or greater who have not been able to achieve weight loss with a comprehensive program, pharmacotherapy and/or bariatric surgery should be considered. The recommendations include a comprehensive approach to weight loss, including reduced caloric intake, exercise/increased physical activity, and behavioral counseling.[233]

Obstructive and mixed types of sleep apnea syndrome can be treated. Because many clients with sleep apnea are overweight, weight loss is recommended. Mandibular advancement devices (MAD) may help in those with mild disease or those that have poor jaw occlusion. These devices position the mandible to increase the size of the upper airway and reduce collapse.[275] MADs are inferior to treatment with CPAP, but are indicated in those with mild OSA and in those intolerant or nonadherent to CPAP.[275] Compared to CPAP, MADs have lower success rates (as measured by the AHI), however higher adherence rates with MADs make them an attractive treatment option.[275]

The most common treatment for OSA is positive airway pressure (continuous, bilevel, or autopositive) used during sleep. The positive pressure from the pump's stents opens the airway, preventing or minimizing obstruction. Patients may undergo an overnight trial with a system to determine the ideal pressure settings to reduce episodes of apnea; newer devices can autocorrect. Currently, phrenic nerve stimulators and hypoglossal nerve stimulators are under investigation. These devices can sense periods of apnea and stimulate the phrenic nerve to initiate inhalation or the hypoglossal nerve to increase airway tone.[125]

In adults, positive airway pressure is more effective than no treatment and treatment with oral appliances in reducing apnea, decreasing blood pressure, and improving quality of life.[185] Surgery is recommended if an airway obstruction can be determined as the cause of the sleep apnea. Maxillomandibular surgery to correct anatomic factors is invasive with potential complications but can be very successful in alleviating OSA for carefully selected individuals.[332]

Neurogenic causes of sleep apnea are more difficult to control. There is insufficient evidence to draw any conclusions about the effectiveness of medication. Medication has been directed at improving tone in the upper airway, increasing ventilatory drive, reducing rapid eye movement sleep, and reducing airway resistance or surface tension. Alcohol and hypnotic medications should be avoided. In children, tonsillectomy/adenoidectomy is effective in a majority of cases.[403,434]

In children, treatment may be initiated for those with an AHI of 5 or more episodes per hour or in those with lower AHI if they also present with cardiovascular morbidity, growth delay/failure, or decreased quality of life.[258] Treatment for children may include weight loss, nasal corticosteroids, adenotonsillectomy, mandibular devices, craniofacial surgery for those with deformities, and CPAP/NPPV.[258]

**PROGNOSIS.** Evidence indicates that OSA may be associated with increased long-term cardiovascular and neurophysiologic morbidity. Cardiac and vascular morbidity may include systemic hypertension, cardiac arrhythmias, pulmonary hypertension, cor pulmonale, left ventricular dysfunction, stroke, and sudden death. In fact, the death rate for people with untreated sleep apnea is three times higher than for those who do not have this problem.[514] Recognition and appropriate treatment of OSA and related disorders will often significantly enhance the client's quality of life, overall health, productivity, and safety on the highway and job.

**SPECIAL IMPLICATIONS FOR THE THERAPIST 15.8**

### *Sleep-Disordered Breathing: Apnea*

Therapists should be aware that OSA increases with age and know the risk factors. Individuals with risk factors should be referred to a sleep center. Sleep position can affect the tongue's position. Individuals with sleep-aid devices, such as continuous positive airway pressure, often report noncompliance with use when asked; the therapist can encourage individuals to use these pumps routinely to improve function and to prevent cardiovascular morbidity. Any devices placed inside the mouth that are designed to hold the lower jaw in a forward position can put strain on the temporomandibular joint and affect jaw movements. The therapist should evaluate and monitor these potential adverse effects of these appliances.

Therapists can also work with individuals to find comfortable sleep positions that minimize the anatomic effects contributing to this problem. For example, raising the head of the bed with a wedge, or using a hospital bed can help bring the tongue forward and reduce symptoms of reflux at the same time. Using pillows to elevate the head should be discouraged if it causes increased cervical flexion and/or increased intraabdominal pressure.

Exercise is beneficial for those with OSA. A recent meta-analysis demonstrated that exercise can reduce AHI and improve subjective complaints as measured by sleep scales. This finding held no matter the type, duration, or frequency of exercise, with exercise showing benefits in AHI even if no there were no changes in BMI.[5]

Exercise is also beneficial for weight loss, with a recommended dose of 150 minutes/week of moderate intensity exercise. Increasing to 200 to 300 minutes per week will help to prevent weight gain.[233]

Pulmonary rehabilitation may be an effective adjunct intervention to improve quality of life and cardiovascular fitness and to assist with weight loss. Because of the possible cardiovascular complications associated with clients who have OSA, vital signs should be monitored before, during, and after submaximal or maximal exercise. The client should not be left in the supine position for prolonged periods of time, even while awake.

There are some reports of sleep apnea in association with cervical lesions (e.g., osteophytes caused by diffuse idiopathic skeletal hyperostosis),[310] as well as after anterior cervical spine fusion.[200] Individuals with rheumatoid arthritis complicated with temporomandibular joint destruction and cervical involvement can also develop OSA.[367] Physical therapy may be explored in developing treatment protocols when the musculoskeletal structures of the mandible contribute to the problem.

## Restrictive Lung Disease

### Overview

Restrictive lung disorders are a major category of pulmonary problems, including any condition that reduces chest wall movement and lung volume. Pulmonary function tests are characterized by a decrease in total lung capacity. There are many causes of restrictive lung disease that are covered in other sections of this chapter or book. More than 100 identified interstitial lung diseases can cause restrictive lung disease.

Extrapulmonary causes may include neurologic or neuromuscular disorders (e.g., head or spinal cord injury, amyotrophic lateral sclerosis, myasthenia gravis, Guillain-Barré syndrome, muscular dystrophy, or poliomyelitis), musculoskeletal disorders (e.g., ankylosing spondylitis, kyphosis or scoliosis, or chest wall injury or deformity), postsurgical conditions, particularly involving the abdomen or thorax, obesity, and collagen vascular diseases (scleroderma, systemic lupus, rheumatoid arthritis).

### Clinical Manifestations

Clinical presentation varies according to the cause of the restrictive disorder. Generally, clients exhibit a rapid, shallow respiratory pattern. Chronic tachypnea (fast rate) occurs in an effort to overcome the effects of reduced lung volume and compliance.

Exertional dyspnea progresses to dyspnea at rest because of the loss of inspiratory reserves. As the disease progresses, respiratory muscle fatigue may occur, leading to inadequate alveolar ventilation and carbon dioxide retention. Decreased chest wall movement and increased use of accessory muscles of ventilation are accompanied by the characteristic rapid, shallow breathing. Hypoxemia with digital clubbing is a common finding, especially in the later stages of restrictive disease.

### MEDICAL MANAGEMENT

**TREATMENT AND PROGNOSIS.** The management of restrictive lung disease is based in part on the underlying cause, but is also guided by the severity of the disease. Treatment goals are oriented toward adequate oxygenation, maintaining an airway, and obtaining maximal function. For example, persons with spinal deformities may be helped with corrective surgery and obese persons may experience improved breathing after weight loss.

Corticosteroids may help control inflammation and reduce further impairment, but previously damaged alveolocapillary units cannot be regenerated or replaced. Some clients with end-stage disease may be candidates for heart/lung transplantation. Most restrictive lung diseases are not reversible, and the disease progresses to include pulmonary hypertension, cor pulmonale, severe hypoxia, and eventual ventilatory or cardiac failure.

**SPECIAL IMPLICATIONS FOR THE THERAPIST 15.9**

### *Restrictive Lung Disease*

Restrictive lung disease is less prevalent than many of the other conditions discussed in this chapter. Most of the guidelines offered in other sections apply here as well. Exercise testing (6-Minute Walk Test or other submaximal exercise evaluation) plays an important role in determining the extent of the disease and assessing outcomes. Many residual effects of pulmonary pathology are neuromuscular in nature and can be addressed by appropriate physical therapy.[319]

A primary problem for clients with restrictive lung disease secondary to generalized weakness and neuromuscular disease is ineffective cough. Airway clearance techniques to facilitate cough and effective dislodging of secretions to the central airways may be exhausting for the client. Rest periods must be incorporated in the treatment. A person with restrictive lung disease will be more adversely affected by the restriction of lung function in the recumbent position, emphasizing the importance of routine positioning for immobile clients and active or active-assisted movements whenever possible. Extrapulmonary causes of restriction are most amenable to physical therapy intervention. Consider manual therapy for improving chest wall compliance with injury or after surgery, as well as flexibility exercises. Assess and address muscle weakness, impaired mobility, and difficulty with self-care. Educate the client to watch for and report adverse effects of medications.

## Pulmonary Fibrosis

### Definition and Overview

Pulmonary fibrosis is a type of interstitial lung disease in which ongoing epithelial damage leads to an inflammatory process and progressive scarring (fibrosis) of the lungs, predominantly fibroblasts and small blood vessels that progressively remove and replace normal tissue.[356] Affected individuals commonly present with progressive dyspnea and a nonproductive cough. Pulmonary function tests show a decreased total lung capacity, forced vital capacity, and $FEV_1$.[232] Incidence appears to be increasing, though in many cases, the etiology remains uncertain.[167]

### Etiologic and Risk Factors

Two-thirds of cases of pulmonary fibrosis are idiopathic pulmonary fibrosis (IPF), in which the cause is unknown. In the remaining one-third, fibrosis in the lung is caused by healing scar tissue after active disease, such as TB, systemic sclerosis, CF, or adult respiratory distress syndrome (ARDS). IPF is often diagnosed between 50 and 70 years of age, with a median age at diagnosis of 66.[232,271]

Other risk factors include smoking, male gender, genetic susceptibility, gastroesophageal reflux disease, and exposure to metal dust or livestock.[261,433] Additionally, some infections and connective tissue diseases, such as rheumatoid arthritis or SLE, certain drugs (particularly some chemotherapy agents), and, in rare cases, genetic or familial predisposition, increase the risk for developing pulmonary fibrosis. More recently mutations in genes that code for telomere length and others that impact cell adhesion and integrity have been implicated as etiologic factors.[420]

Thoracic radiation (e.g., postmastectomy radiation of the chest wall and regional lymphatics in clients with breast cancer) may result in pericarditis and pneumonitis, which can progress to pulmonary fibrosis weeks, or even months, after radiation treatments have ended. In addition, some chemotherapies can cause pulmonary fibrosis.[364]

### Pathogenesis and Clinical Manifestations

Fibroblast proliferation (fibrosis) irreversibly distorts and shrinks the lung lobe at the alveolar level and causes a marked loss of lung compliance. The lung becomes stiff and difficult to ventilate, with decreased diffusing capacity of the alveolocapillary membrane, causing hypoxemia. There does not appear to be an inflammatory process but rather abnormal wound healing in response to multiple, microscopic sites of ongoing alveolar epithelial injury and fibrosis.[256,429] Apoptosis of the alveolar epithelial cells, imbalance of oxidants and antioxidants in the lung, and alterations in telomerase activity have all been implicated in the etiology of IPF.[232] The course of pulmonary fibrosis varies, with early nonspecific symptoms such as SOB, fatigue, and a dry cough.

### MEDICAL MANAGEMENT

**DIAGNOSIS.** Diagnosis of IPF is made by high-resolution CT combined with clinical presentation and the exclusion of other possible lung disorders or autoimmune diseases. If the CT is borderline, a lung biopsy may be performed.[361]

Clinical assessment, pulmonary function tests showing a restrictive pattern, and radiographic studies support the pathologic findings.

**TREATMENT AND PROGNOSIS.** Two medications have been approved for IPF: pirfenidone (antifibrotic) and nintedanib (kinase inhibitor).[433] Patients may also be referred to pulmonary rehabilitation to improve peripheral muscle function and to learn to improve breathing efficiency. Pulmonary rehabilitation improves exercise capacity and health related quality of life.[130,419] Oxygen with activity and nocturnal oxygen may also be prescribed.

Lung transplantation may be indicated for those with severe IPF, with a 5-year survival rate of approximately 44%.[271] The clinical course of people with pulmonary fibrosis and rheumatoid arthritis is chronic and progressive. Response to treatment is unpredictable, and the overall prognosis is poor, with median survival time of less than 2 to 3 years. Older age is associated with a lower median survival. Some physicians will use the GAP index to predict the clinical course, which includes PFTs, gender, and age.[433]

## Systemic Sclerosis Lung Disease

### Definition

Systemic sclerosis (SSc), or scleroderma, is a chronic and progressive autoimmune disease of connective tissue characterized by excessive collagen deposition in the skin and internal organs, particularly the kidneys and lungs, and destruction of small arteries in the skin and organs. This condition is discussed in detail in Chapter 10.

### Incidence

Idiopathic lung disease accounts for 30% of the mortality in scleroderma, with a median survival of 5 to 8 years.[182] The lungs, as a result of a rich vascular supply and abundant connective tissue, are a frequent target organ (second to the esophagus in visceral involvement). Skin changes generally precede visceral alterations, and lung involvement rarely presents symptoms at first, but pulmonary symptoms develop after an average of 7 years.[43] Poor prognostic factors in those with lung involvement include greater than 20% involvement of total lung involvement, decrease in diffusion capacity of carbon monoxide, elevated CRP levels, presence of reflux, pulmonary artery hypertension, older age, and male gender.[116]

### Pathogenesis and Clinical Manifestations

Three pathways produce organ damage. First, inflammation is caused by T cells and cytokines, resulting in alveolitis before fibrosis. Second, severe thickening and obstruction of vessels occurs, resulting in pulmonary hypertension and renal failure. Third, cutaneous fibrosis occurs.[447] Immunosuppressive therapy may delay onset of symptoms by up to 4 years.[43]

Oxidative stress contributes to disease progression by a rapid degeneration of endothelial cell function in SSc. Daily episodes of hypoxia-reperfusion injury produce free radicals that cause endothelial damage, intimal thickening, and fibrosis along with inactivation of antioxidant enzymes.[176]

Studies have determined that the balance between fibrotic and inflammatory mediators may be important to developing pathology.[216] Lung biopsy of early lesions shows capillary congestion, hypercellularity of alveolar walls, increased fibrous tissue in the alveolar septa, and interstitial edema with fibrosis. As a result, initial symptoms of dyspnea on exertion and nonproductive cough develop. As fibroblast proliferation and collagen deposition progress, fibrosis of the alveolar wall occurs and the capillaries are obliterated. Clinically, the client demonstrates more severe dyspnea and has a greater risk of deterioration in pulmonary function.

### MEDICAL MANAGEMENT

**DIAGNOSIS.** Traditional tests, such as pulmonary function tests and chest radiographs, are insensitive and not predictive of outcome. High-resolution CT is very sensitive for early diagnosis of SSc lung involvement. Lung ultrasound is a new modality that may improve early diagnosis of lung disease in those with SSc.[116]

**TREATMENT.** Pharmacologic treatments include corticosteroids and immunosuppressive agents.[182] Lung transplantation is a viable option for carefully selected individuals with scleroderma-related lung disease.[431] Single-lung transplantation may be indicated in those without significant visceral dysfunction. Survival rates are equivalent to lung transplant recipients with other disorders, with a 2-year survival rate of 64%.[176,321,431]

**PROGNOSIS.** SSc lung disease is unpredictable and may be a mild, prolonged course, but as the pulmonary fibrosis advances and causes pulmonary hypertension, cor pulmonale characterized by peripheral edema may develop, progressing rapidly to respiratory failure and death. Lung disease is the most frequent cause of death from SSc.

## Chest Wall Trauma or Lung Injury

### Blunt Chest Trauma

Chest or thoracic trauma ranges from superficial wounds such as contusions and abrasions to life-threatening tension pneumothorax. Rib fractures account for 50% of blunt thoracic injuries.[259] Flail chest consists of fractures of three or more adjacent ribs on the same side, and possibly the sternum, with each bone fractured into two or more segments.[355] The fractured rib segments are detached (free-floating) from the rest of the chest wall and move paradoxically with respiration as the inspiratory force of the diaphragm causes inward movement of the fractured ribs. Forty percent of those with flail chest acquire pneumonia.[424] Flail chest has an associated mortality of 5% to 36%, with higher mortality rates when there are other pulmonary complications such as pneumonia and sepsis.[259] Trauma to ribs 1 to 4 typically results from high-energy trauma and may result in vascular injuries.[259] Middle zone fractures (ribs 5-9) are most likely to have pulmonary complications, while ribs 10 and below may result in liver, splenic or renal injuries.[259] Pulmonary complications include pneumothorax, pneumonia, pulmonary contusion, and pulmonary laceration.[463]

**Clinical Manifestations.** The primary complaint for a rib fracture is pain. If there is pulmonary involvement, patients may present with severe dyspnea,

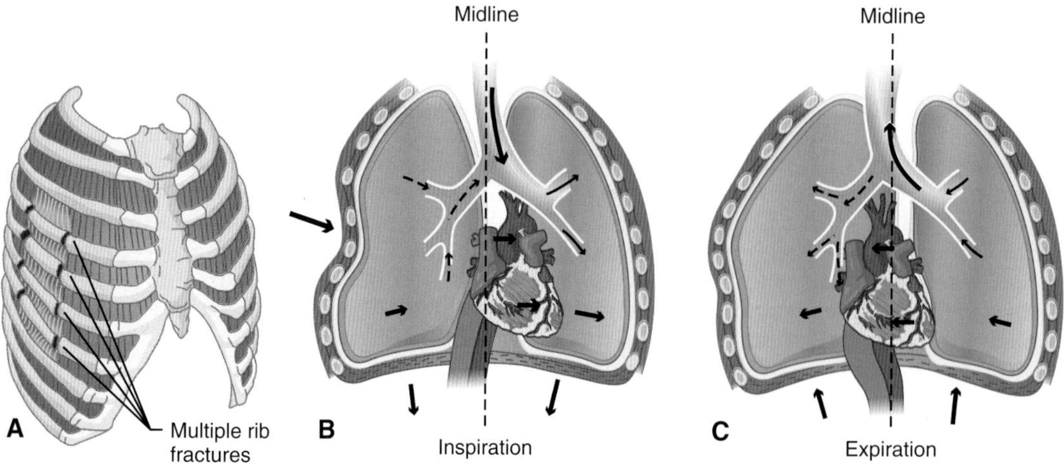


**Figure 15.14**

**Flail chest.** *Arrows* indicate air movement or structural movement. (A) Flail chest consists of fractured rib segments that are detached (free-floating) from the rest of the chest wall. (B) On inspiration, the flail segment of ribs is sucked inward. The affected lung and mediastinal structures shift to the unaffected side. This compromises the amount of inspired air in the unaffected lung. (C) On expiration, the flail segment of ribs bellows outward. The affected lung and mediastinal structures shift to the affected side with the diaphragm elevated on that side (not shown). Some air within the lungs is shunted back and forth between the lungs instead of passing through the upper airway.

hypoventilation, cyanosis, and hypoxemia. Fractured ribs can tear the pleura and lung surface, thereby producing hemopneumothorax. This causes the lung to collapse from the loss of negative pressure. Fractured ribs can also lacerate abdominal organs, the brachial plexus, and blood vessels.[463] In flail chest, the paradoxical chest motion impairs movement of gas in and out of the lungs (Fig. 15.14), promotes atelectasis, and impairs pulmonary drainage. Pulmonary contusions cause bleeding into the gas exchange areas, causing dyspnea and hypoxia if extensive.[463]

## MEDICAL MANAGEMENT

DIAGNOSIS. Rib fractures and/or flail chest are diagnosed by clinical examination and radiograph. If the impact is high energy, then imaging with chest CT and CT angiography is indicated.[259,463]

TREATMENT. Treatment for uncomplicated rib fractures includes pain management with over-the-counter medications, nonsteroidal antiinflammatory medications or, if more extensive, with epidurals, intercostal rib blocks or opioids.[463] If there is pulmonary involvement, the ABCs (airway, breathing, and circulation) of emergency management are followed. A chest tube removes both air and blood in the pleural cavity after chest trauma, which helps restore the negative pressure in the pleural space so that the lungs can remain inflated. The tube is usually positioned in the sixth intercostal space in the posterior axillary line. In those with flail chest, treatment involves pain management, chest physical therapy, noninvasive mechanical ventilation as needed, and the consideration for surgical stabilization.[152,355,424] Surgical fixation may be considered for flail chest, in ventilated patients, and in those with nonunion.[259] Whenever pulmonary function is adequate, intubation is avoided to help reduce infection, the most common complication associated with morbidity and mortality in clients with flail chest.

SPECIAL IMPLICATIONS FOR THE THERAPIST 15.10

### *Chest Wall or Lung Injury*

The emergency room therapist is the most likely therapist to evaluate and treat someone with a flail chest, although this varies by geographic region. Transcutaneous electrical nerve stimulators may aid in pain management although there is limited evidence to support this intervention in rib fracture.

Once the person has been stabilized and moved to the acute care setting, therapists may come into contact with patients who experience chest wall injuries. Manual techniques for secretion removal may be used, but the presence of a lung contusion directs medical intervention more toward drainage or aspiration of any blood pooled in the area.

Airway clearance techniques may have a role in facilitating chest tube drainage, but must be used carefully in the presence of any rib fractures. Percussion and vibration techniques are contraindicated directly over fractures, but can be used over other lung segments. Rib or chest taping and ultrasound over the site of the fracture should not be used. Once the fractures have healed, rib mobilization and soft tissue mobilization for the intercostals may be necessary to restore normal respiratory movements.

It should be noted that airway clearance techniques can cause rib fractures and that infants are particularly vulnerable to rib fractures.[109] Frequent turning and position changes, as well as deep-breathing and coughing exercises, are important. A semi-Fowler position may help with lung reexpansion necessary to prevent atelectasis.

In the case of flail chest from injury, simultaneous cardiac damage (myocardial contusion) may have occurred, necessitating the same care as for a person who has suffered a myocardial infarction.

Scapular fractures are often overlooked when only supine chest radiographs are performed. The therapist may recognize a suspicious clinical presentation (e.g., loss of scapular–humeral motion, symptoms disproportionate to the injury, or development of previously undocumented large hematomas) suggesting the need for more definitive medical diagnosis. In the case of all fractures, once the fracture is healed the therapist may become involved in restoration of movement and strength.

## ENVIRONMENTAL AND OCCUPATIONAL DISEASES

The relationship between occupations and disease has been observed, studied, and documented for many years. An in-depth discussion of this broad topic is included in Chapter 4. This chapter discusses only environmental and occupational diseases related to the lung. Occupational diseases can be divided into three major categories: (1) inorganic dusts (pneumoconioses); (2) organic dusts (hypersensitivity pneumonitis); and (3) fumes, gases, and smoke inhalation. These three categories have pathologic characteristics in common, including involvement of the pulmonary parenchyma with a fibrotic response.

### Pneumoconiosis

#### Overview

Any group of lung diseases resulting from inhalation of particles of industrial substances, particularly inorganic dusts (e.g., iron ore or coal), with permanent deposition of substantial amounts of such particles in the lung, is included in the generic term *pneumoconiosis* (dusty lungs). Clinically, common pneumoconioses include coal workers' pneumoconiosis, silicosis, and asbestosis. Other types of pneumoconiosis include talc, beryllium lung disease (berylliosis), aluminum pneumoconiosis, cadmium workers' disease, and siderosis (inhalation of iron or other metallic particles). Farmers in dry climate regions exposed to respirable dust (inorganic agricultural dusts) during farming activities (e.g., plowing and tilling) and toxic gases (e.g., from animal confinement) may develop chronic bronchitis, hypersensitivity pneumonitis, and pulmonary fibrosis.

#### Incidence, Prevalence, and Etiologic Factors

Pneumoconiosis is most common among miners, sandblasters, stonecutters, asbestos workers, insulators, and agriculture workers. Incidence increases with age due to the cumulative effects of exposure. Occupational asthma (new onset asthma caused by occupational environment) and work-exacerbated asthma (previously diagnosed asthma that is worsened by work environment) account for 17% of all asthma cases in adults.[102] The prevalence of coal workers pneumoconiosis (CWP) is estimated to be 10%, with a higher prevalence in central Appalachia, estimated to be 20.6%.[50]

*Silicosis,* formerly called *potters' asthma, stonecutters' cough, miners' mold,* and *grinders' rot,* is most likely to be contracted in today's industrial jobs involving sandblasting in tunnels, hard-rock mining (extraction and processing of ores), and preparation and use of sand. It can occur in anyone habitually exposed (usually over a period of 10 years) to the dust contained in silica, and any miner is subject to it. Usually, silicosis is associated with extensive or prolonged inhalation of free silica (silicon dioxide) particles in the crystalline form of quartz.

#### Risk Factors

Higher-risk workplaces are those with obvious dust, smoke, or vapor or those in which there is spraying, painting, or drying of coated surfaces. Heavier exposure occurs when there is friction, grinding, heat, or blasting; when very small particles are generated; and in enclosed spaces.

Not all clients exposed to occupational inhalants will develop lung disease. Harmful effects depend on the (1) type of exposure, (2) duration and intensity of exposure, (3) presence of underlying pulmonary disease, (4) smoking history, (5) particle size and water solubility of the inhalant, (6) and possibly genetic predisposition.[40] The larger the particle, the lower the probability of its reaching the lower respiratory tract; highly water-soluble inhalants tend to dissolve and react in the upper respiratory tract, whereas poorly soluble substances may travel as far as the alveoli.

The risk of lung cancer in those who both smoke and are exposed to asbestos is increased in a multiplicative way.[49] Exposure to significant amounts of asbestos is most common when asbestos materials are disturbed during renovation, repair, or demolition of older buildings containing asbestos materials.

Exposure while washing clothes soiled with these toxic substances has caused mesothelioma (malignancy associated with asbestos exposure) and berylliosis (beryllium lung disease associated with exposure to beryllium used in the manufacture of fluorescent lamps before 1950). Beryllium is used today as a metal in structural materials employed in aerospace industries, in the manufacture of industrial ceramics, and in atomic reactors, so exposure is still possible.

#### Pathogenesis

Dust particles (indestructible mineral fibers) that are not filtered out by the nasociliary mechanism or mucociliary escalator may be deposited anywhere in the respiratory tract and lungs, especially the small airways and alveoli. Each disease has its own pathogenesis, but in general the most dangerous dust particles measure 2 μm or less and are deposited in the smallest bronchioles and the acini (see Fig. 15.2).

The particles are ingested by alveolar macrophages, and most of the phagocytosed particles ascend to the mucociliary lining and are expectorated or swallowed. Some migrate into the interstitium of the lung and then into the lymphatics. These indestructible mineral fibers can actually pierce the lung cells. In response to the continued presence of these fibers, alveolitis may occur with an altered immune response that triggers activated macrophages to secrete fibroblast-stimulating factor, which in turn mediates excessive fibrosis (i.e., the thickening and scarring of lung tissue that occur around the mineral fiber).[28]

In *coal workers' pneumoconiosis*, ingestion of inhaled coal dust by alveolar macrophages leads to the formation of coal macules, which appear on the radiograph as diffuse small opacities (or white areas) in the upper lung.[375]

In work-related asthma, substances such as cereals, coffee beans, flour, plant proteins, dyes, animal dander, cleaning products, mold, and formaldehyde trigger an inflammatory process that results in inflammation, edema, and bronchoconstriction.[102]

Silica particles under 10 micrometers can penetrate deep into the lungs. These particles cause direct cytotoxicity to the lungs, produce reactive oxygen species, and secrete inflammatory and fibrotic messengers, resulting in fibrosis and cell death. Direct damage is caused by damage to lipids in the membrane of bronchoalveolar cells. Reactive oxygen species damage mitochondria and DNA. Activated macrophages play a role in secreting cytokines that activate fibroblasts and collagen deposition.[304] Between 10 and 40 years after initial exposure to silica, small rounded opacities called *silicotic nodules* form throughout the lung. These fibrotic nodules scar the lungs and make them receptive to further complications (e.g., TB, bronchitis, or emphysema).

*Asbestosis* is characterized by inhalation of asbestos fibers, a fibrous magnesium and calcium silicate nonburning compound used in roofing materials, insulation for electric circuits, brake linings, and many other products that must be fire resistant. As with the other pneumoconioses, asbestos particles are engulfed by macrophages. Once activated, macrophages then release inflammatory mediators, resulting in nodular interstitial fibrosis that can be seen on radiographs along with thickened pleura.

After an interval of 10 to 20 years between exposure and further complications, calcified pleural plaques on the dome of the diaphragm or lateral chest wall develop. The lower portions of the lungs are more often involved than the upper portions in asbestosis.

How asbestos causes mesothelioma is unclear; the formation of oxygen free radicals by macrophages can be a cause of chromosomal damage, or there may be a growth factor that governs individual susceptibility to mineral fiber–induced mesothelioma.

### Clinical Manifestations

Symptoms of pneumoconioses from dust exposure may be initially difficult to separate from common conditions such as chronic bronchitis and COPD.[375] Symptoms include progressive dyspnea, chest pain, chronic cough, and expectoration of mucus containing the causative particles. In rare cases, rheumatoid arthritis coexisting primarily with coal workers' pneumoconiosis but also with silicosis and asbestosis causes Caplan syndrome, a condition characterized by the presence of rheumatoid nodules in the periphery of the lung. Long-term exposure to acid and other substances produces ulceration and perforation of the septum, whereas nickel and certain wood dusts cause nasal carcinoma.

Silicosis is usually asymptomatic and has no effect on routine pulmonary function tests. As the disease progresses, mucus tinged with blood, loss of appetite, chest pain, and general weakness may occur. In complicated silicosis, dyspnea and obstructive and restrictive lung dysfunction occur.

Asbestosis is characterized by dyspnea, inspiratory crackles (on auscultation), and sometimes clubbing and cyanosis. As in the case of the other pneumoconioses, the simple or uncomplicated form of coal workers' pneumoconiosis is uncommon, but the chronic form is often associated with chronic bronchitis and infections.

## MEDICAL MANAGEMENT

**PREVENTION.** Prevention is the first line of defense against occupational diseases. Workplace-based education, preemployment screening, yearly physical examinations, surveillance and exposure reduction, and elimination of the pathogen are essential components of a strategy to prevent occupational lung disorders. Yearly monitoring of lung function with pulmonary function testing and chest radiographs is recommended.[375] Precautions such as the use of face masks, protective clothing, and proper ventilation, and periodic monitoring of particulate levels in the air are essential.

In 1971, asbestos became the first material to be regulated by the U.S. Occupational Safety and Health Administration. The Environmental Protection Agency (EPA) has classified asbestos as a Group A human carcinogen, causing both lung cancer and mesothelioma. Approximately 55 countries have banned asbestos, however it continues to be used in the United States.[396]

**DIAGNOSIS.** Identifying a workplace-related cause of disease is important because it can lead to prevention for others. The recognition of occupational causes can be difficult because of the latency period, delayed responses that occur at home either after work or years after exposure. Diagnosis is by history of exposure (which may be minimal with asbestosis and far removed in time from the onset of disease; the person may even be unaware of the exposure), sputum cytology, lung biopsy, chest film showing nodular or interstitial fibrosis, and pulmonary function studies.

Other pulmonary imaging techniques used in conjunction with the initial chest radiograph include conventional CT, high-resolution CT, and gallium scintigraphy. High-resolution CT scanning is the best imaging method to differentiate different origins of pneumoconiosis because presentation varies with the stimulus (silica, coal dust, iron dust, or asbestos). Magnetic resonance imaging (MRI) is helpful to distinguish progressive fibrosis from lung cancer.[115,317] Imaging alone is inadequate to make most diagnoses; clinical presentation of symptoms and lung function are also important.[412] Genetic susceptibility may be associated with beryllium-induced disease and may play a role in mediating other types of pneumoconiosis.[170]

**TREATMENT.** There is no standard treatment for these diseases. The dust deposits are permanent so treatment is directed toward relief of symptoms. Many of the pharmacologic interventions used for other pulmonary disease may be utilized (corticosteroids, bronchodilators, etc.). When lung neoplasm occurs, surgical removal and therapeutic modalities, such as radiotherapy or chemotherapy, may be employed. Lung transplantation has been increasingly used in pneumoconiosis.[51]

**PROGNOSIS.** The devastating feature of pneumoconioses is that there may be no obvious symptoms until the disease is in an advanced state. Once fully developed, prognosis is poor for most occupational lung diseases, with progressive and disabling results.

Although now uncommon, acute silicosis resulting from heavy exposure to silica rarely responds to treatment and progresses rapidly over a few years when it occurs. The increased incidence of TB among people with silicosis presents an additional negative factor to the prognosis.

Exposure to asbestos, radon, silica, chromium, cadmium, nickel, arsenic, and beryllium may result in neoplasm. Crystalline silica is a known human carcinogen, but this link is not defined and may be overestimated.[287,374] Both bronchogenic carcinoma and mesotheliomas of the pleura and peritoneum have been linked to asbestos. The exposure typically occurs 20 years before the development of bronchogenic carcinoma and approximately 30 to 40 years before the appearance of mesothelioma. The disease culminates in the sixth decade, with few cases occurring before age 40 years. Although progress has been made, median survival is approximately 1 year after diagnosis.[324]

## Hypersensitivity Pneumonitis

Hypersensitivity pneumonitis is a relatively rare disease that results from exposure to organic dusts. The alveoli and distal airways are most often involved as a result of inhalation of organic dusts and active chemicals. Most of the diseases are named according to the specific antigen or occupation and involve organic materials such as molds (e.g., mushroom compost, moldy hay, sugar cane, or logs left unprotected from moisture), fungal spores (e.g., stagnant water in air conditioners and central heating units), plant fibers or wood dust (particularly redwood, maple, and cotton), cork dust, coffee beans, bird feathers, and hydroxyurea (cytotoxic agent). Gram-bacterial endotoxins may be more to blame than dust in causing pneumonitis in cotton textile workers.[491] Mycobacteria have also been shown to be responsible for hypersensitivity pneumonitis in industrial metal grinding and in "hot tub lung."[6,206]

Regardless of the specific antigen involved in the pathogenesis of hypersensitivity pneumonitis, the pathologic alterations in the lung are similar. A combination of immune complex–mediated and T cell–mediated hypersensitivity reactions occurs, although the exact mechanism of these processes is still unknown. There is granulomatous inflammation of the airways initiated by an allergic reaction to an occupational or environmental molecule.[394]

Symptoms may develop 2 to 9 hours after exposure, with symptoms occurring days to weeks after the exposure (acute hypersensitivity pneumonitis) or have an insidious onset of weeks to months.[394] Common symptoms are vague and include fever, dyspnea, coughing, and systemic symptoms such as chills and body aches.[222,394] Diagnosis is made through clinical history and occupational exposures, radiograph, pulmonary function tests, bronchoalveolar lavage, and high-resolution chest CT. Lab tests may show antigen-specific IgG antibodies, while a bronchioalveolar lavage may show elevated levels of CD8+T cells, lowering the CD4:CD8 ratio.[394] On chest CT, there is the presence of bilateral ground glass opacities, centrilobular nodular opacities, thin-walled cysts, and air trapping.[222]

Initially, symptoms may be reversed by removing the worker from the exposure (the only adequate treatment), modifying the materials-handling process, or using protective clothing and masks. The symptoms typically remit within 24 to 48 hours but return on reexposure and, with time and in some people, may become chronic. If severe, treatment may include corticosteroids or oxygen to dampen inflammation.[222]

Hypersensitivity pneumonitis may present as acute, subacute, or chronic pulmonary disease, depending on the frequency and intensity of exposure to the antigen. Chronic pulmonary impairments differ depending on the offending agent; however, many people will only have mild airflow obstruction or have complete resolution with avoidance of the offending antigen.

## Noxious Gases, Fumes, and Smoke Inhalation

Exposure to toxic gases and fumes is an increasing problem in modern industrial society. Any time oxygen in the air is replaced by another toxic or nontoxic agent, asphyxia (deficient blood oxygen and increased carbon dioxide in blood and tissues) occurs. Such is the case when products manufactured from synthetic compounds are heated at high temperatures, releasing fumes. For example, workers who use heating elements to seal meat in plastic wrappers and workers involved in the manufacture of plastics and packaging materials made of polyvinyl chlorides are exposed to these fumes. Workers exposed to the artificial butter flavoring for popcorn, diacetyl, have developed significant respiratory obstruction.[282]

The most common mechanism of injury is local irritation, the specific type and extent depending on the type and concentration of gas and the duration of exposure. For example, highly soluble gases, such as ammonia, rapidly injure the mucous membranes of the eye and upper airway, causing an intense burning pain in the eyes, nose, and throat. Insoluble gases, such as nitrogen dioxide, encountered by farmers cause diffuse lung injury.

*Metal fume fever* is a systemic response to inhalation of certain metal dusts and fumes such as zinc oxide used in galvanizing iron, the manufacture of brass, and chrome and copper plating. Symptoms include fever and chills, cough, dyspnea, thirst, metallic taste, salivation, myalgias, headache, and malaise. Welding fumes create exposure to multiple hazardous agents and cause varied respiratory and systemic pathology.[331] *Polymer fume fever*, associated with heating of polymers, may cause similar symptoms. With brief exposures, the symptoms associated with these two syndromes are self-limiting, but prolonged exposure results in chronic cough, hemoptysis, and impairment of pulmonary function associated with a wide range of lung pathologic conditions.

*Chemical pneumonitis* can result from exposure to toxic fumes. The acute reaction may produce diffuse lung injury characterized by air space disease typical of pulmonary edema. In its chronic form, constrictive bronchiolitis develops.

*Smoke inhalation injury* produces direct mucosal injury secondary to hot gases, tissue anoxia caused by combustion products, and asphyxia as oxygen is consumed by fire. Thermal injury seen in the upper airway is characterized by edema and obstruction. Incomplete combustion of industrial compounds produces ammonia, acrolein, sulfur dioxide, and other substances in today's fires.

*Environmental tobacco smoke* (ETS), or exposure to secondhand smoke among nonsmokers, is widespread. In middle and high school students, their exposure to second hand smoke occurs in public areas (35%), at work (27.1%), at school (16.8%), at home (15.5%), or in a vehicle[377] (14.7%). In 2013 to 2014, 37.9% of children 3 to 11 years of age were exposed to ETS, 50.3% of non-Hispanic blacks, and 47.9% of those living in poverty.[474] ETS is composed of 85% sidestream smoke (SS) and 15% mainstream smoke (MS).[145] Some compounds, such as volatile amines, ammonia, and nicotine decomposition products have higher concentrations in SS compared to MS and if smaller than 2.5 μm, can easily enter the respiratory system.[145] ETS increases the risk of heart disease, respiratory infections, asthma, otitis media, and is a major risk factor for sudden infant death syndrome.[300,377] ETS also increases the risk for neurobehavioral problems such as attention-deficit hyperactivity disorder and decreased school performance.[237]

Infants born to women exposed to ETS during pregnancy have an increased chance of decreased birth weight and intrauterine growth retardation.[215] Nicotine may contribute to abnormal lung branching and changes to the structure of conducting airways.[377] Prenatal exposure also promotes airway hyperresponsiveness and early development of asthma and allergy, and double the odds of future attention-deficit hyperactivity disorder.[242,290] The effects of prenatal ETS can last through adolescence and beyond, with new evidence that female children exposed to ETS are twice as likely to develop COPD as adults.[237,377] Children are highly susceptible to ETS because of their proximity to parents while the parents are smoking, surface-area-to-body-weight ratio, and immaturity of their systems to metabolize ETS.[237]

Adults are also exposed to ETS; however, this exposure is declining as a consequence of new laws regarding smoking in public places. Approximately 58 million nonsmokers in the United States were exposed to ETS in 2011 to 2012, whereas 2 out of every 5 children ages 3 to 11 and 7 out of every 10 black children were exposed to SHS.[82] Nonsmoking adults who are exposed to ETS increase cardiovascular risk by up to 40% and have an elevated risk for lung cancer. Cardiovascular effects of ETS include endothelial dysfunction, increased arterial stiffness, increased LDL, and increased platelet activation, all of which contribute to the development of atherosclerosis.[145]

Third-hand smoke (THS) is also emerging as a risk factor for disease. THS refers to the constituents of tobacco smoke that are left on surfaces such as carpets and drapes or in the air after the THS has moved into the gas phase.[323] THS may remain on surfaces for weeks to months after smoking.[323] Research on the acute and long-term effects of THS is in its infancy at the time of this writing. E-cigarette use is on the rise in the United States. While e-cigarettes don't contain tobacco, they do contain nicotine and other toxins.[377] E-cigarette vapors also contain a variety of chemicals and small particles that in some cases are in higher concentrations than regular cigarettes.[145] Research on THS stemming from e-cigarettes is limited at this time.

## DROWNING

### Definition

Near drowning was a term previously used to describe an episode of drowning with survival, but the term "drowning" is now preferred. Drowning is defined by the World Health Organization as, "...the process of experiencing respiratory impairment from submersion/immersion in liquid."[340] Drowning occurs in three forms: (1) dry drowning, inhalation of little or no fluid with minimal lung injury because of laryngeal spasm (10%-15% of cases); (2) wet drowning, aspiration of fluid with asphyxia or secondary changes caused by aspiration (85%); and (3) recurrence of respiratory distress secondary to pneumonia or pulmonary edema within 1 to 2 days after a drowning incident. Recovery is rapid if respiration and circulation are restored before permanent neurologic damage occurs. Death may occur from asphyxia secondary to reflex laryngospasm and glottic closure.

### Incidence and Risk Factors

Drowning is highest in children under 5 and young adults aged 15 to 24.[104] Eighty percent of those who die by drowning are male, which is generally attributed to their choice of higher-risk activities, overestimation of swimming ability, and use of alcohol.[92,104] There are also racial disparities, with African American children (5-14 years) drowning at a rate three times that of Caucasian children.[104] Alcohol consumption while swimming or boating is involved in approximately 70% of drowning deaths in adolescents and adults.[104] Other risk factors include epilepsy, intellectual developmental disorder, heart attack, head or spinal cord injury at the time of the accident, failure to use personal flotation devices, increased use of hot tubs and spas, and lack of proper swimming training or overestimation of endurance by those who can swim, and low socioeconomic status.[92,506]

### Pathogenesis

The complications of drowning fall into two categories: the effects of prolonged anoxia on the brain and kidney, which as end organs may experience complications that are irreversible (determining the final prognosis), and ALI from aspiration of fluids. When aspiration accompanies drowning, severe pulmonary injury often occurs, resulting in persistent arterial hypoxia and metabolic acidosis, even after ventilation has been restored.

In the past, a distinction was made between the effects of saltwater and freshwater drowning (e.g., cardiovascular function and changes in blood volume and serum electrolyte concentrations), but it is now known that hypoxia is the most important determinant of survival in human drowning, regardless of the type of water involved.

The duration of submersion and the water temperature determine the pathologic events. Hypoxia results in global cell damage; different cells tolerate variable lengths

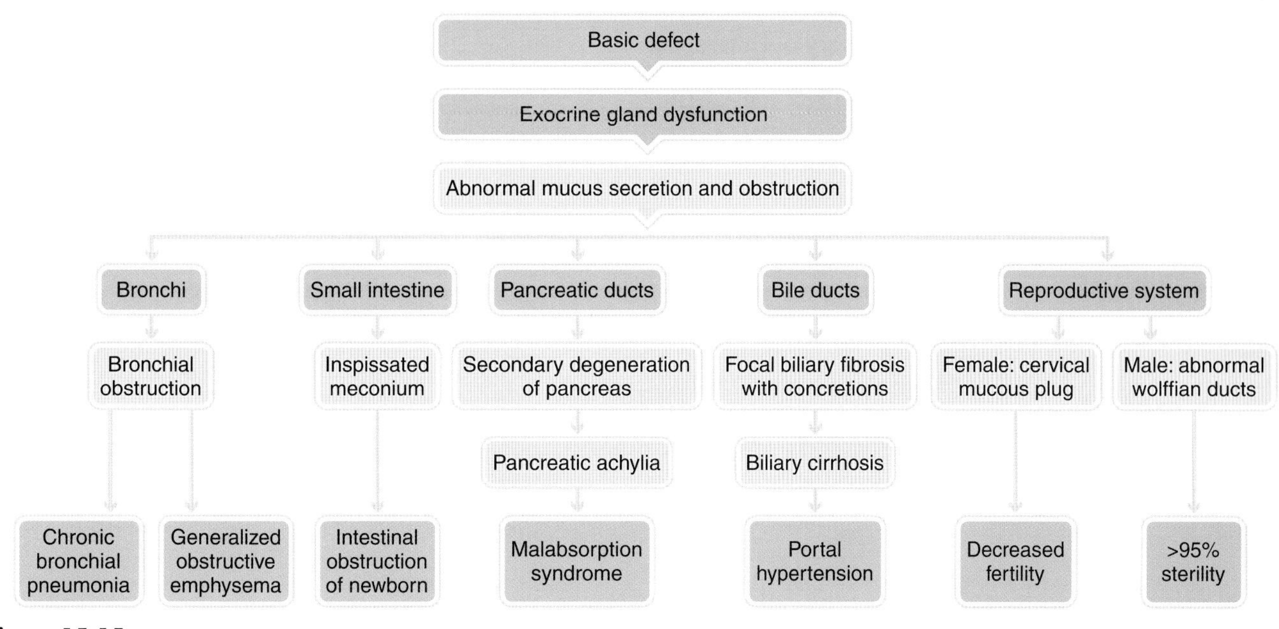


**Figure 15.15**

**Various effects of exocrine gland dysfunction in cystic fibrosis.** (From Wong DL: *Whaley and Wong's essentials of pediatric nursing*, ed 4, St Louis, 1993, Mosby.)

of anoxia. Neurons, especially cerebral cells, sustain irreversible damage after 4 to 6 minutes of submersion. The heart and lungs can survive up to 30 minutes.

The extent of CNS injury tends to correlate with the duration of hypoxia, but hypothermia accompanying the incident is associated with changes in neurotransmitter release (glutamate, dopamine) and may reduce the cerebral oxygen requirements and help reduce CNS injury.

## Clinical Manifestations

The clinical features in drowning are variable, and the person may be unconscious, semiconscious, or awake but apprehensive. Pulmonary and neurologic symptoms predominate, with cough, tachypnea, and possible development of ARDS with progressive respiratory failure.

Other pulmonary complications include pulmonary edema, bacterial pneumonia, pneumothorax, or pneumomediastinum secondary to resuscitation efforts. Fever occurs in the presence of aspiration during the first 24 hours, but can occur later in the presence of infection.

Early neurologic manifestations include seizures, especially during resuscitative measures, and altered mental status, including agitation, combativeness, and coma. Speech, motor, or visual abnormalities may occur, improve gradually, and resolve over several months.

### MEDICAL MANAGEMENT

**TREATMENT.** Restoration of ventilation and circulation by means of resuscitation at the scene of the accident is the primary goal of treatment to restore oxygen delivery and prevent further hypoxic damage. Other treatment is largely supportive, with antibiotics for pulmonary infection, maintenance of fluid and electrolyte balance, possible transfusion for significant anemia, and management of acute renal failure.

Comatose drowning victims frequently have elevated intracranial pressure caused by cerebral edema and loss of cerebrovascular autoregulation. Reduction of cerebral blood flow adds ischemic injury to already damaged brain tissue. To reserve cerebral function in such cases, cerebral resuscitation (controlled hyperventilation, deliberate hypothermia, or use of barbiturates, glucocorticoids, and diuretics) may be utilized.

**PROGNOSIS.** The prognosis depends in large part on the extent and duration of the hypoxic episode and is not related to type of water.[340] Submersion for six minutes or longer has poorer outcomes, whereas providing rescue breaths while still in the water is associated with better outcomes.[340] If laryngospasm is finally overcome and the person aspirates water or if aspiration of vomitus occurs during resuscitative measures, prognosis is worse than without these complications.

Coincident head trauma or subdural hematoma presents an additional prognostic complication. Neurologic injury is the most serious and least reversible complication in those persons successfully resuscitated. Little, if anything, has been shown to help, and it carries a grave prognosis.

# CONGENITAL DISORDERS

## Cystic Fibrosis

### Definition and Overview

Cystic fibrosis (CF) is an inherited disorder of ion transport (sodium and chloride) in the exocrine glands affecting the hepatic, digestive, reproductive (the vas deferens is functionally disrupted in nearly all cases; decreased fertility in both sexes), and respiratory systems (Fig. 15.15). The basic genetic defect predisposes people with CF to

**Table 15.9** Respiratory Disease: Summary of Differences

| Disease | Primary Area Affected | Result |
|---|---|---|
| Acute bronchitis | Membrane lining bronchial tubes | Inflammation of lining |
| Bronchiectasis | Bronchial tubes (bronchi or air passages) | Bronchial dilation with inflammation |
| Pneumonia | Alveoli (air sacs) | Causative agent invades alveoli with resultant outpouring from lung capillaries into air spaces and continued healing process |
| Chronic bronchitis | Larger bronchi initially; all airways eventually | Increased mucous production (number and size) causing airway obstruction |
| Emphysema | Air spaces beyond terminal bronchioles (alveoli) | Breakdown of alveolar walls; spaces enlarged |
| Asthma | Bronchioles (small airways) | Bronchioles obstructed by muscle spasm, swelling of mucosa, thick secretions |
| Cystic fibrosis | Bronchioles | Bronchioles become obstructed and obliterated; later larger airways become involved<br>Mucous plugs cling to airway walls, leading to bronchitis, bronchiectasis, atelectasis, pneumonia, or pulmonary abscess |

From Goodman CC, Snyder TE: *Differential diagnosis for the physical therapist*, ed 4, Philadelphia, 2007, Saunders.

chronic bacterial airway infections, and almost all persons develop obstructive lung disease associated with chronic infection that leads to progressive loss of pulmonary function.

CF was previously thought to be a multisystem disease that manifests either at birth (with intestinal obstruction) or in infancy/early childhood (with growth failure and recurrent sinopulmonary symptoms). It is now recognized that CF is a genetic disease; a broad spectrum of conditions are associated with mutations in the CF transmembrane conductance regulator (CFTR) gene. This also includes older children and adults presenting with manifestations in one organ, including sinopulmonary diseases, pancreatitis, or obstructive azoospermia. In many of these individuals, a diagnosis of CF is difficult to establish or exclude.[362]

### Incidence

CF is the most common inherited genetic disease in the white population, affecting approximately 30,000 children and young adults (equal gender distribution) in the United States. Approximately 1,000 new cases are diagnosed each year; nearly 70% of these diagnoses occur in the first year of life. When diagnosed prior to onset of symptoms, there is evidence to suggest nutritional and pulmonary outcomes are better later in life.

The disease is inherited as an autosomal recessive trait, meaning that both parents must be carriers so that the child inherits a defective gene from each one. In the United States, 5% of the population, or 12 million people, carry a single copy of the defective (CF) gene. Each time two carriers conceive a child, there is a 25% chance (1:4) that the child will have CF, a 50% (1:2) chance that the child will be a carrier, and a 25% chance (1:4) that the child will be a noncarrier.

### Etiologic Factors

In the last few decades, there have been major advances in understanding the underlying genetic factors related to this disease. In 1985, the CF gene was located on the long arm of chromosome 7. In 1989, the gene for CF was cloned and abnormalities in the CFTR protein were attributed to CF.

In healthy people, this CFTR protein provides a channel by which chloride (a component of salt) can pass in and out of the plasma membrane of many epithelial cells, including those of the kidney, gut, and conducting airways. People with CF have a defective gene that produces a mutant protein that interferes with cells' ability to manage chloride. More than 1,800 mutations in the CFTR gene have been identified; these mutations can be divided into several classes. In some mutations, the CFTR protein is synthesized to a lesser degree or not synthesized at all. In others, CFTR is made, but is not activated normally or not processed normally due to abnormal chloride channels. At least one copy of F508del, the most common CFTR mutation, is found in 90% of people with CF. This mutation results in production of a misfolded protein that does not reach the cell surface.

### Pathogenesis

The impermeability of epithelial cells to chloride results in (1) dehydrated and increased thickening of mucous gland secretions, primarily in the lungs, pancreas, intestine, and sweat glands; (2) elevation of sweat electrolytes (sodium chloride); and (3) pancreatic enzyme insufficiency. The dehydration results in thickened dry and gooey secretions that cause the mechanical obstruction responsible for multiple clinical manifestations of CF.

In the pancreatic ducts, the flow of digestive enzymes is blocked. As a result, absorption of food becomes increasingly difficult, particularly fat. Because of this effect, without supplemental enzymes, children with CF fall below norms for weight and height. In the airways, bronchial and bronchiolar obstruction by the abnormal mucus predisposes the lung to infection and causes patchy atelectasis with hyperinflation. The disease progresses from mucus plugging and inflammation of small airways (bronchiolitis) to bronchitis, followed by bronchiectasis, pneumonia, fibrosis, and the formation of large cystic dilations that involve all bronchi. Table 15.9 summarizes the differences among these various respiratory diseases.

Box 15.7

**CLINICAL MANIFESTATIONS OF CYSTIC FIBROSIS**

***Early Stages***

- Persistent coughing
- Sputum production
- Persistent wheezing
- Recurrent pulmonary infection
- Excessive appetite, poor weight gain
- Salty skin and sweat
- Bulky, foul-smelling stools

*Pulmonary Initial*

- Wheezy respirations
- Dry, nonproductive cough

*Progressive Involvement*

- Increased dyspnea
- Decreased exercise tolerance
- Paroxysmal cough
- Tachypnea
- Obstructive emphysema
- Patchy areas of atelectasis
- Nasal polyps, chronic sinusitis

***Advanced Stage***

- Barrel chest
- Kyphosis
- Pectus carinatum
- Cyanosis
- Clubbing (fingers and toes)
- Recurrent bronchitis
- Recurrent bronchopneumonia
- Pneumothorax
- Hemoptysis
- Right-sided heart failure secondary to pulmonary hypertension

*Gastrointestinal*

- Voracious appetite (early)
- Anorexia (late)
- Weight loss
- Failure to thrive or grow; protein-calorie malnutrition
- Distended abdomen
- Thin extremities
- Sallow (yellowish) skin
- Acute gastroesophageal reflux
- Intussusception

*Distal Intestinal Obstruction Syndrome (Meconium Ileus)*

- Abdominal distention
- Colicky, abdominal pain
- Vomiting
- Failure to pass stools (constipation)
- Rapid development of dehydration
- Anemia

*Liver*

- Cirrhosis
- Portal hypertension

*Pancreatic*

- Large, bulky, loose, frothy, foul-smelling stools (pancreatic enzyme insufficiency)
- Fat-soluble vitamin deficiency (vitamins A, D, E, K)
- Recurrent pancreatitis
- Iron-deficiency anemia
- Malnutrition
- Diabetes mellitus

*Genitourinary*

- Male urogenital abnormalities
- Delay in sexual development
- Sterility (most males); infertility (some females)

*Musculoskeletal*

- Marked tissue wasting, muscle atrophy
- Myalgia
- Osteoarthropathy (adult)
- Rheumatoid arthritis (adult)
- Osteopenia/osteoporosis (adult)

### Clinical Manifestations

The consistent finding of abnormally high sodium and chloride concentrations in the sweat is a unique characteristic of CF. Parents frequently observe that their infants taste salty when they kiss them. Almost all clinical manifestations of CF are a result of overproduction of extremely viscous mucus and deficiency of pancreatic enzymes. Box 15.7 gives a complete list of clinical manifestations by organ and in order of progression. Recurrent pneumothorax, hemoptysis, pulmonary hypertension, and cor pulmonale are serious and life-threatening complications of severe and diffuse CF pulmonary disease.

**Pancreas.** Approximately 90% of people with CF have pancreatic insufficiency, with thick secretions blocking the pancreatic ducts and causing dilation of the small lobes of the pancreas, degeneration, and eventual progressive fibrosis throughout. The blockage also prevents essential pancreatic enzymes from reaching the duodenum, thus impairing digestion and absorption of nutrients. Clinically, this process results in greasy, bulky, frothy (undigested fats because of a lack of amylase and tryptase enzymes), and foul-smelling stools (decomposition of proteins producing compounds such as hydrogen sulfide and ammonia).

As the life expectancy for people with CF has improved, the incidence of glucose intolerance and CF-related diabetes has increased because pancreatic damage can eventually affect the β cells. Approximately 30% of adults with CF have CF-related diabetes. Hyperglycemia may adversely influence nutritional status and weight, pulmonary function, and development of late microvascular complications.

**Gastrointestinal.** The earliest manifestation of CF, *meconium ileus* (sometimes referred to as distal intestinal obstruction syndrome (DIOS)), is present in approximately 20% of newborns with CF; the small intestine is blocked with thick, putty-like tenacious meconium.

Prolapse of the rectum is the most common gastrointestinal complication associated with CF, occurring most often in infancy and childhood.

People of all ages with CF are susceptible to intestinal obstruction from thickened, dried, or impacted stools (inspissated meconium). Advances in investigative techniques have led to increasing reports of Crohn disease and ischemic bowel disease in persons with CF. Prolonged administration of excessive doses of pancreatic enzymes is associated with the development of fibrosing colonopathy. To avoid this complication, people with CF should work closely with a dietitian to determine appropriate dosage of enzymes based on their individual diet. Correct dosage promotes digestion of carbohydrates, proteins, and fats, absorption of essential nutrients, and maintenance of a healthy weight. Higher BMI in people with CF correlates with better lung function.[443] Although these data do not demonstrate a causal relationship, they reinforce the importance of maintaining adequate nutrition and striving to maintain a normal BMI.

**Pulmonary.** Chronic cough and purulent sputum production are symptomatic of lung involvement. It can be difficult to expectorate the mucus because of its increased viscosity. This retained mucus provides an excellent medium for bacterial growth, placing the individual at increased risk for infection. Common bacteria are *Staphylococcus aureus* and *P. aeruginosa*, infecting 70% and 45%, respectively. Reduced oxygen–carbon dioxide exchange causes variable degrees of hypoxia, clubbing (see Fig. 15.4), cyanosis, hypercapnia, and resultant acidosis. Chronic pulmonary infection and hyperinflation lead to secondary manifestations of barrel chest, pectus carinatum, and kyphosis.

The most common complication of CF is progressive decline of lung function, with episodes of acute worsening of respiratory symptoms, often referred to as "pulmonary exacerbations." Although a generally applicable definition of a pulmonary exacerbation has not been developed, clinical features of an exacerbation have been described (Box 15.8). Pulmonary exacerbations require medical and physical therapy intervention but can still have an adverse impact on the individual's quality of life and a major impact on the overall cost of care.[168] Respiratory failure is a frequent complication of severe pulmonary disease in persons with CF and is the most common cause of CF-related deaths.

Liver involvement in CF is much less frequent than both pulmonary and pancreatic diseases, which are present in 80% to 90% of individuals with CF. Liver disease affects only 10% of the CF population; however, because of the decreasing mortality from extrahepatic causes, its recognition and management are a relevant clinical issue.

Recent observations suggest that clinical expression of liver disease in CF may be influenced by genetic modifiers; their identification is an important issue because it may allow recognition of people at risk for the development of liver disease at the time of diagnosis of CF and early institution of prophylactic strategies.[120]

**Genitourinary.** Genitourinary manifestations are primarily related to reproduction; infertility once thought to be universal in men and common in women can be treated successfully with in vitro fertilization. The vas deferens may be absent bilaterally, or if present, it is obstructed so that although sperm production is normal, blockage or fibrosis of the vas deferens prevents release of the sperm into the semen (azoospermia). Delayed puberty and amenorrhea due to malnutrition are common in females with CF. Women experience decreased fertility because thick mucus in the cervical canal can make conception more difficult.

**Box 15.8**

**SIGNS AND SYMPTOMS OF PULMONARY EXACERBATION IN CYSTIC FIBROSIS**

- Increased cough
- Increased sputum production and/or a change in appearance of sputum
- Fever
- Weight loss
- School or work absenteeism (because of illness)
- Increased respiratory rate and/or work of breathing
- New findings on chest examination (e.g., wheezing, crackles)
- Decreased exercise tolerance
- Decrease in $FEV_1$ of 10% or more from baseline value within past 3 months
- Decrease in hemoglobin saturation of 10% or more from baseline value within past 3 months
- New finding(s) on chest x-ray

*$FEV_1$*, Forced expiratory volume in 1 second.

For further information, see Flume PA: Cystic fibrosis pulmonary guidelines: treatment of pulmonary exacerbations, *Am J Respir Crit Care Med* 180(9):802–808, 2009. Available online at http://www.cff.org/UploadedFiles/treatments/CFCareGuidelines/Respiratory/CF-Care-Guidelines-Pulmonary-Exacerbations.pdf.

**Musculoskeletal.** By the 1990s, the majority of children with CF were living long enough to reach skeletal maturity.[205] Musculoskeletal dysfunctions can impair the person's ability to support the function of the lungs, thus contributing to the overall morbidity and mortality of the disease.[190] The muscles of respiration and posture are one and the same. As the WOB increases, the postural role of the trunk muscles is compromised.[321] Clinically, this is seen as altered spinal alignment (scoliosis, kyphosis) and abdominal muscle and pelvic floor muscle dysfunction (e.g., low back pain, stress urinary incontinence).

Decreased bone mineral density and bone mineral content are common at all ages in CF and attributed to multifactorial causes (e.g., nutrition, exposure to glucocorticoid therapy, gonadal dysfunction, age, body mass, or activity). Osteopenia and osteoporosis are common; consequences of bone loss include excessive kyphosis, neck and back pain, and an increased incidence of fractures.

Hypertrophic pulmonary osteoarthropathy occurs more frequently with increasing age and severity of disease in greater than 6% of individuals. This condition is accompanied by clubbing of the fingers and toes; arthritis; painful periosteal new bone formation (especially over the tibia); and swelling of the wrists, elbows, knees, or ankles. The periostitis is observed radiographically in the diaphysis of the tubular bones and may be a single layer or a solid cloaking of the bone.

Separately and usually without association with other manifestations of CF, attacks of episodic arthritis accompanied by severe joint pain, stiffness, rash, and fever may occur intermittently but repeatedly. Also related to CF are rheumatoid arthritis, spondyloarthropathies, sarcoidosis, and amyloidosis, which are caused by coexistent conditions and drug reactions.[53] Muscle pain is reported and may be alleviated with proper nutrition and exercise, although this is based on anecdotal information and has not been verified in studies.

## MEDICAL MANAGEMENT

**DIAGNOSIS.** Now that the gene responsible for CF has been identified, prenatal diagnosis and screening of carriers are possible as part of genetic counseling. The test is more than 99% accurate when positive. A negative genetic screening test is not as accurate because this only screens for a limited number of mutations. Prepregnancy genetic testing that involves DNA analysis of oocytes is available for couples at risk for having children with CF.

In 2004, the CDC issued a recommendation that all newborns be screened for CF and currently all 50 states and the District of Columbia do routine screening. A blood test from the newborn will check levels of immunoreactive trypsinogen (IRT), a chemical made by the pancreas. An elevated IRT is considered a positive screen; this is not a diagnostic test but will lead to other tests that can confirm or rule out CF: sweat test, genotype analysis, and nasal potential difference.

CF is traditionally diagnosed using pilocarpine iontophoresis, also known as the sweat test; a positive test occurs when the sodium chloride concentration is greater than 60 mEq/L for anyone younger than 20 years (reference value: 40 mEq/L) and above 80 mEq/L for those older than 20 years.[446]

Although elevated sweat electrolytes are associated with other conditions, a positive sweat test coupled with the clinical picture usually confirms the diagnosis. The test should be performed at an accredited CF center and repeated a second time. Alternatively, CF can be diagnosed by genotype analysis (performed prenatally or postnatally). Testing of the most common 23 mutations in the United States will detect greater than 90% of whites with CF. CF can be diagnosed on DNA alone. Nasal potential difference measures salt transport in the nasal epithelial cells. Nasal potential difference is very sensitive at detecting abnormalities and can be used to diagnose CF but is only available at a limited number of CF research centers.[337]

The age at presentation can vary, and some people are not diagnosed until adulthood. However, now that CF is included in newborn screening, in future years fewer cases will be diagnosed later in life. Diagnosis of CF in adulthood is generally attributable to a milder presentation of the disease and has a more favorable prognosis. Adults with unexplained chronic respiratory infections, bronchiectasis, pancreatitis, or absence of vas deferens should be screened for CF.[353,446]

***Clinical Screening Tests.*** Pancreatic elastase-1 (EL-1), a marker of exocrine pancreatic insufficiency in CF, can be measured in feces. EL-1 is a specific human protease synthesized by the acinar cells of the pancreas and is a reliable test of pancreatic sufficiency in newborns older than age 2 weeks. Fecal elastase has good sensitivity and specificity and predictive values for severe cases of pancreatic insufficiency. This test can be used to confirm the need for pancreatic enzymes and for annual monitoring of pancreatic-sufficient individuals to detect the onset of pancreatic insufficiency. Pulmonary function tests are performed in affected individuals from the age of 5 years and up to measure and monitor lung function over time. These tests are used to classify the severity of baseline lung disease. Almost all measures are based on the flow of air into and out of the lungs in a given period of time.

The two most common lung function measures are $FEV_1$ and FVC (forced vital capacity). These tests should be performed at least four times each year to assess the effectiveness of treatment; pulmonary function declines with progressive lung disease.

Several scoring systems have been developed to assess disease severity, measure acute changes, and evaluate appropriateness for lung transplantation. The most reliable and useful are the modified Shwachman and modified Huang scores. There is a need for a longitudinal assessment tool to follow individuals with milder CF.[201] High-resolution CT scans are more sensitive than $FEV_1$ at detecting changes in people with mild disease but introduce a risk of radiation exposure. Lung clearance index, obtained via a breath test, may be sensitive (and safer than high-resolution CT)[30] at detecting mild disease, in the presence of normal $FEV_1$.

A formal cardiopulmonary exercise test (CPET) with pulse oximetry and ventilatory gas analysis will provide the clinician with information on the status of the pulmonary system, as well as multiple other systems. Although maximal oxygen consumption ($VO_{2max}$) has been shown to be a better predictor of mortality in CF than $FEV_1$, it is not yet widely used in the assessment of people with CF. The recommended CPET for people with CF is cycle ergometry, using the Godfrey protocol.

Annual screening for CF-related diabetes mellitus (CFRD) with a glucose tolerance test should begin at the age of 10 years and is treated with insulin, dietary management, and exercise from the time of diagnosis. Symptoms of CFRD are often confused with pulmonary infection. Diabetes significantly impacts the course of CF, leading to worse nutrition, lower lung function, more hospitalizations, and worse mortality.[445]

Bone mineral density should be monitored routinely in people with CF. By the age of 18 years all people with CF should have a dual-energy x-ray absorptiometry (DEXA) scan to detect osteopenia or osteoporosis. A repeat scan is recommended every 1 to 5 years, based on the DEXA results, as well as other factors, such as $FEV_1$ and BMI.

**TREATMENT.** A multidisciplinary approach must be taken to work toward the goal of promoting a normal life for individuals with CF. Everyone should be followed at an accredited CF center where all disciplines are present and work together. The treatment of CF depends on the stage of the disease and which organs are involved. Some care teams take an aggressive approach from a young age, prior to onset of clinical symptoms. Medical management is oriented toward managing and preserving lung function and includes the use of antibiotics, antiinflammatories,

**Table 15.10** Inhaled Pharmacotherapy for Cystic Fibrosis

| Type of Therapy | Medication |
|---|---|
| Bronchodilator therapy | AccuNeb (albuterol)<br>ProAir HFA (albuterol)<br>Proventil HFA (albuterol)<br>Ventolin HFA (albuterol) |
| Mucus clearance therapies | HyperSal (sodium chloride solution)<br>Pulmozyme (dornase alfa) |
| Antibiotic therapies | Tobi (tobramycin)<br>Coly-Mycin M (colistimethate)[a]<br>Cayston (aztreonam) |

[a]Colistimethate is available as a solution for injection and must be diluted appropriately for nebulization.

Courtesy Tanner Higginbotham, PharmD, Drug Information Specialist, Skaggs School of Pharmacy, Department of Pharmacy Practice, University of Montana, Missoula, Montana.

aggressive pulmonary therapy with drugs (mucolytics) to thin mucous secretions, airway clearance techniques, exercise, and supplemental oxygen. Adequate hydration, caloric intake, and pancreatic enzymes administered with meals will enhance nutritional outcomes.

***Pharmacotherapy.*** Drug therapy for CF is primarily directed at preventing accumulation of thick, sticky mucus, managing infection, and preserving lung function. Discussion here is in the order in which medications are typically administered (e.g., bronchodilator, saline, dornase alfa, antibiotic, steroid).

Pharmacologic treatment may include sympathomimetics to control bronchospasm, parasympatholytics to offset smooth muscle constriction and bronchodilation, mucolytics to thin mucous secretions, aerosolized antibiotics (e.g., tobramycin), and inhaled antiinflammatory agents to decrease the amount of inflammation in the airways (Table 15.10).

A combination of treatments can result in fewer flare-ups and faster recovery.[156] First, a bronchodilator is administered to open the airways and improve mucociliary clearance. Inhaled bronchodilators are effective in individuals who have bronchial hyperresponsiveness.[203] Next, hypertonic saline, an inexpensive "low-tech" intervention, is inhaled. Saline, with a high concentration of salt (typically 7%), rehydrates the airway secretions, replenishes the airway surface liquid, and often induces a cough. Recombinant human deoxyribonuclease (rhDNase), known as dornase alfa (Pulmozyme®), a mucolytic, is effectively used to reduce sputum viscosity and increase mucociliary clearance.[457]

Hypertonic saline improves airway clearance but is not as effective as DNase in longer-term lung improvement.[494] Historically, it has been recommended to administer DNase 30 minutes prior to performing airway clearance techniques. However, a 2011 systematic review[139] suggests the timing of DNase in relation to airway clearance should be based largely on the individual's preference.

Tobramycin (Tobi) is an aminoglycoside antibiotic that works by stopping the growth of *P. aeruginosa*. It can be given intravenously or via nebulizer. Less than 50% of people with CF are infected with *P. aeruginosa*. The prevalence of *P. aeruginosa* is declining, likely due to widespread effort to eradicate initial acquisition. Another common antibiotic in CF care is aztreonam (Cayston®), a monobactam. When inhaled, antibiotics should be administered after the person performs airway clearance techniques. Additional antimicrobials are available to patients and more are in development. Many individuals who require frequent courses of intravenous antibiotics may have an implantable intravenous access device put in place. The risks of mechanical failure, sepsis, and thrombosis have made this device more successful when inserted and cared for at a CF center.[24,159,261]

High-dose ibuprofen may be used to slow the deterioration of the lungs by reducing inflammation and breaking the cycle of mucus buildup, infection, and inflammatory destruction. Neutrophils are responsible for much of the inflammatory response and are unresponsive to traditional chemotherapeutic treatment.

Pharmacologic intervention with microencapsulated pancreatic enzymes is critical when pancreatic involvement is severe. Aggressive nutritional management is needed to ameliorate the effects of malabsorption and the side effects of therapeutic intervention. Calcium supplements are warranted because of the high incidence of osteopenia and fractures.[26] Deficiency of vitamin D is common in individuals with CF and is associated with decreased bone mass in children and osteoporosis in adults and may impact other comorbidities common in CF. Vitamin $D_3$ (cholecalciferol) is recommended for all individuals with CF to achieve and maintain serum 25-hydroxyvitamin D levels of at least 30 ng/mL.[464]

***Gene Therapy.*** The identification of the mutated CF gene in 1989 was followed by the first phase of gene therapy in 1993 to correct the basic defect in CF cells, rather than relying on treatment of the symptoms. Finding a way to deliver the normal copy of the gene into the lung or intrahepatic biliary epithelial cells with adequate gene expression remains a challenge. Obstacles include vector toxicity and ineffective transgene expression.[155] The expectation is that the normal CFTR will reverse the physiologic defect in CF cells.

The FDA has approved a few drugs that target restoring function of the CFTR protein: ivacaftor, lumacaftor/ivacaftor, and tezacaftor/ivacaftor. Most recently, a triple-combination modulator therapy was approved—elexacaftor/tezacaftor/ivacaftor—for those with at least one F508del mutation; this includes nearly 90% of all people with CF. As of this writing, this triple-combination therapy is only available for people at least 12 years of age. In addition to restoring CFTR function, multiple key symptoms have improved for people taking these medications, including a greater than 10% increase in lung function. Several other drugs designed to treat more CFTR mutations are in clinical trials. These drugs will only help people who have some function of the CFTR protein. Research is ongoing to develop treatments for those with rare and nonsense mutations that do not produce any CFTR protein.

***Transplantation.*** Double-lung transplantation becomes a reality for many people with CF. Transplantation is not a cure for CF, but a bridge to allow people to live longer with a better quality of life. In the United States, the United Network for Organ Sharing has addressed perceived inequities in organ distribution by allocating organs by illness severity rather than time on the waiting list. A lung allocation score ranks severity for potential recipients 12 years of age and older for transplantation based on variables including lung function, oxygen and ventilatory needs, diabetes, weight, and physical performance via the Six-Minute Walk Test.[301]

Long-term survival has yet to be determined, but improved quality of life has been achieved. The new lungs do not acquire the CF ion-transport abnormalities but are subject to the usual posttransplantation complications. CF problems in other organ systems persist and may be worsened by some of the immunosuppressive regimens.[511]

CNS complications occur more frequently in CF transplant recipients than in other lung transplant recipients.[194] Criteria for lung transplantation are published, and early referral, when candidates have a greater than 50% risk of death within 2 years without transplant, is recommended.

Liver transplantation should be offered to anyone with CF and progressive liver failure and/or with life-threatening sequelae of portal hypertension, who also have mild pulmonary involvement that is expected to support long-term survival.[120,238]

**PROGNOSIS.** Using its innovative CF patient registry, which tracks information on nearly 30,000 people who receive care through the CF Foundation's Care Center Network, researchers have analyzed the numbers and continue to assess trends in the health status of registered individuals. When first distinguished from celiac disease in 1938, life expectancy with CF was approximately 6 months.[132]

The natural history of CF lung disease has been one of chronic progression with intermittent episodes of acute worsening of symptoms frequently called acute pulmonary exacerbations. These exacerbations typically warrant medical intervention.[168] But data show that the prognosis has steadily improved over the past 30 years, with a gradual increase in longevity; at the time of this publication the median survival for babies born in 2018 is 47 years, with more than 50% of children with CF living into adulthood.

Improvement in both the length and quality of life for adults with CF is primarily the result of newborn screening to identify and treat affected individuals before pulmonary or nutritional problems arise, as well as the development of new therapies (e.g., antimicrobials, CFTR modulators). Standardization of care, implementation of best practices, and continuous multidisciplinary care provided by specialists in CF centers also lead to improved nutrition and pulmonary function.

Lung disease is the primary cause of death for 80% for individuals with CF. Lung transplantation is an important therapeutic option for this group; CF accounts for 17% of pretransplant diagnoses. The primary goal of transplantation has always been to treat individuals with end-stage CF lung disease for whom medical therapies have failed. The secondary goal has been to improve quality of life.[301]

Since the first lung transplant for CF in 1983, survival rates have improved. Refinements in surgical technique, medications, and improved selection criteria have gradually improved postsurgical survival.[301] Individuals with CF who are listed for lung transplantation may require mechanical ventilatory support before transplantation. Negative predictive factors for prognosis after transplantation include *Burkholderia cepacia* and *S. aureus* infection, young age, and arthropathy.

Patients with CF who survive beyond the first year posttransplant have a median survival of 10.5 years. Approximately 35% of deaths within the first year following transplantation are due to acute infections. Rehabilitation plays an important role both pre- and posttransplant to improve limb strength, exercise capacity, and quality of life.

## SPECIAL IMPLICATIONS FOR THE THERAPIST 15.11

### *Cystic Fibrosis*

> **Note to Reader:** There is a document written by physical therapists that presents the scope of physical therapy practice for cystic fibrosis in the United States, available through the Cystic Fibrosis Foundation.[458]

#### Airway Clearance Techniques

The therapist will be involved with airway clearance techniques (ACTs) carried out several times per day or as often as the person is able to tolerate it without undue fatigue. It is generally recommended for individuals to perform ACTs twice daily, for maintenance, when healthy and increase frequency to at least three to four times per day during a pulmonary exacerbation. ACTs should not be performed before or immediately after meals, so treatment must be scheduled to avoid mealtimes for those who experience nausea, vomiting, or any other type of discomfort during treatment.

The therapist must always be aware that anyone with CF is susceptible to infections, in particular *Burkholderia cepacia*. Care must be taken to avoid transmission via equipment, other people, or oneself. Hand hygiene is essential, and high-alcohol hand rubs may be more effective.[191]

Aerosol therapy to deliver medication to the lower respiratory tract should be administered just before airway clearance techniques to maximize the effectiveness of both treatments. Breathing exercises, improving postural alignment, mobilizing the thorax through active exercise, and manual therapy are part of promoting good breathing patterns and improving inspiratory muscle endurance.

Although routine airway clearance is recommended for all individuals with CF, there is not one airway clearance technique proven to be more beneficial than the others. The prescribed ACTs should be individually tailored based on the individual's age, availability of a caregiver, ability of the individual to learn a technique, and the specifics of the lung disease. The many difficulties surrounding percussion and postural drainage (e.g., gastroesophageal reflux, decrease in oxygen saturation, poor compliance, time required, and the requirement for assistance of a trained individual) have resulted in the development of alternative airway clearance techniques that can be accomplished without the assistance of another caregiver and without adverse side effects. Some of these techniques include breathing exercises (active cycle of breathing and autogenic drainage), positive expiratory pressure (PEP) devices, and high-frequency chest wall oscillation (HFCWO) (Fig 15.16 and 15.17). Further specifics of ACTs for this population are beyond the scope of this text; the reader is referred to the more detailed materials available.[325a, 335]

## A THERAPIST'S THOUGHTS*

### *Tipping*

Postural drainage using traditional head-down positions can have detrimental effects, as mentioned above. This has been well documented in infants and the current standard of practice is to perform modified postural drainage (no head down; positions angled up to 30 degrees) when treating infants.[66,291] However, there is limited evidence for the older child and adult populations. Some therapists feel strongly and avoid Trendelenburg positioning in treatment of all ages. Other therapists argue that the benefits (improved ventilation and perfusion as well as secretion clearance) outweigh the risks. Therapists should consider that many adults with CF have diagnosed reflux, while others may have undiagnosed or silent reflux and aspiration. Each person should be assessed individually, and alternative treatments or modified positions should always be considered, even in an ICU setting.

## A THERAPIST'S THOUGHTS*

### *Airway Clearance*

Traditionally, ACT was the main role of physical therapists involved in CF care. At many hospitals today, ACT is performed by respiratory therapists. However, the physical therapist should still be involved in the care of all individuals with CF. Early intervention will detect musculoskeletal changes and improve outcomes. Many people with CF have spine and rib mobility restrictions as well as postural impairments. When the rib cage is aligned over the pelvis, the relationship of the diaphragm and pelvic floor muscles is optimized; this can improve breathing mechanics, secretion clearance, pain and quality of life, as well as decrease the incidence of stress urinary incontinence. Physical therapy goals also include improving strength, flexibility, and exercise capacity. Combining breathing exercises (active cycle of breathing technique, forced expiration technique) with stretches and manual therapy can enhance ventilation, airway clearance and general mobility. Individuals with cystic fibrosis often feel much better after these sessions than they do after ACT or exercise alone.

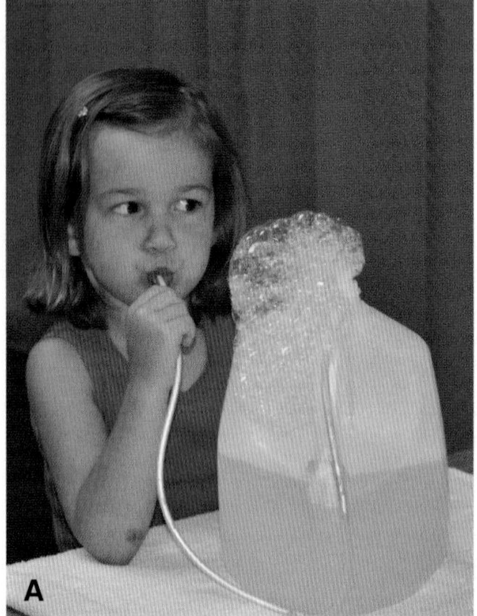


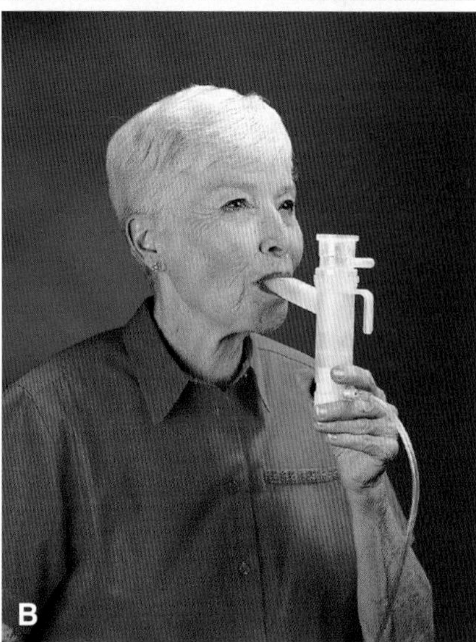


**Figure 15.16**

**PARI PEP.** The positive expiratory pressure (PEP) device maintains pressure in the lungs, keeping the airways open and allowing air to get behind the mucus to improve airway clearance, lung volume capacity, and oxygenation. The device can be used by children (A) and adults (B). Bubble PEP as seen in (A) can make breathing treatments fun for young children. They can begin to learn breathing control while getting the benefits of PEP therapy. Amount of expiratory resistance can be adjusted as needed for individuals by changing the amount of water and diameter of the tubing. ([A] Courtesy Karen von Berg. [B] From PARI, GmbH. PARI PEP is a registered trademark of PARI GmbH. Used with permission.)

### Musculoskeletal and Neuromuscular Complications

As people with CF are living longer, the role of the physical therapist in CF care is evolving. Musculoskeletal and neuromuscular complications are becoming more prevalent. Changes in postural alignment and decreases in bone mineral density are seen in grade-school-age children. It is much easier to prevent, rather than correct, musculoskeletal and neuromuscular impairments. Therefore, the physical therapist should be a part of the interdisciplinary care team throughout the life span.

Annual screening for posture, range of motion, and strength is recommended. Because stress urinary incontinence is present in up to 49%[147] of girls and 73% of women[485] with CF, screening should include pelvic floor muscle health. Any impairments noted on screening should be followed up with a more detailed examination with appropriate interventions recommended. Interventions should include, but are not limited to neuromuscular reeducation, manual therapy (i.e., spine and rib mobilizations, myofascial release), and therapeutic exercise for trunk, extremities, and pelvic floor musculature. For further assessment

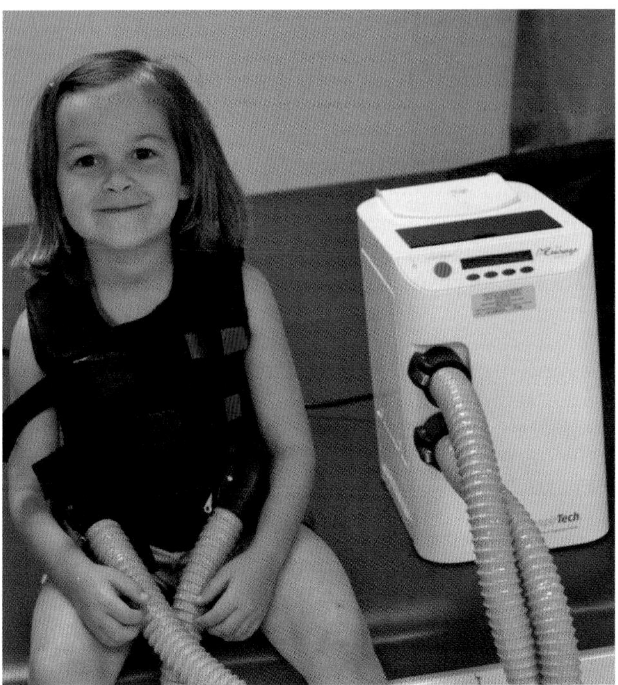

**Figure 15.17**

**High-frequency chest wall oscillation (HFCWO) vest.** A 5-year-old using the RespirTech inCourage system to assist with airway clearance therapy. During a hospital stay, some form of airway clearance is performed at least three times per day. HFCWO settings (frequency, pressure, and time) should be monitored and adjusted as needed to increase treatment effectiveness. Huffs are performed at regular intervals. The home program is adjusted accordingly. Any changes are documented and communicated with the outpatient CF team. (Courtesy Karen von Berg. Used with permission.)

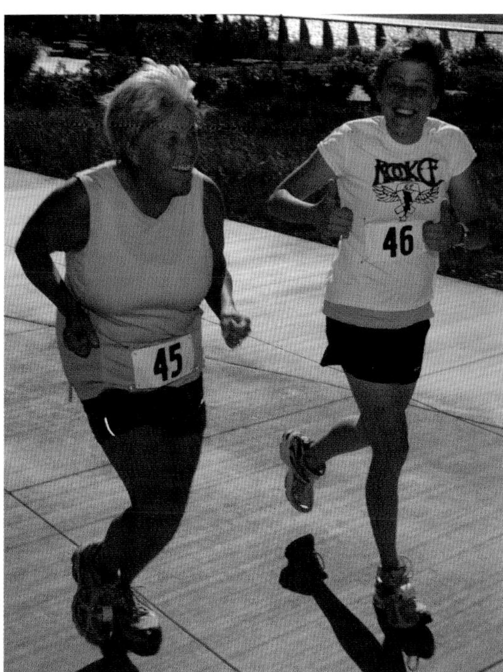


**Figure 15.18**

**Value of exercise for individuals with cystic fibrosis.** The 30-year-old woman on the right reports this photo was taken during her sixth half marathon. She reports that within 3 months of starting to run and train for a 5-km road race she noticed that her lung function improved measurably. This motivated her to keep gradually increasing her level of exercise. She says, "To me exercise is now just as important as the other treatments that I do each day. Everyone is different so starting slow and setting real goals is very important. I couldn't run a block 5 years ago when I started, so it does take time to build up and reach your goals." (Courtesy Emily Schaller. Used with permission.)

and treatment options, the reader is referred to a case study by Mary Massery.[321]

### Nutrition

Malnutrition and deterioration of lung function are closely interrelated and interdependent in the person with CF. Each affects the other, leading to a spiral decline in both. The occurrence of malnutrition during childhood seems to be associated with impaired growth and repair of the airway walls. In children, when growth in body length occurs, good nutrition is associated with better lung function. When adequate nutrition is combined with physical training and aerobic exercise, improved body weight, respiratory muscle function, lung function, and exercise tolerance occur with increases in both respiratory and other muscle mass.[210] Current guidelines recommend children with CF maintain a BMI greater than 50%. In those older than age 18 years, greater than 23% is ideal for males, and at least 22% for females.

### Exercise

Increasingly, exercise and sport are being advanced as core components of treatment for individuals with CF of all ages. A large portfolio of exercise literature has already established that supervised exercise programs enhance fitness (and thereby improve survival), increase sputum clearance, delay the onset of dyspnea, delay declines in pulmonary function, prevent decrease in bone density, enhance cellular immune response, decrease pulmonary exacerbations and hospitalizations, and increase feelings of well-being, thereby potentially improving self-image,[371] self-confidence, and quality of life for the person with CF. Both short- and long-term aerobic and anaerobic training have positive effects on exercise capacity, strength, and lung function[57] (Fig. 15.18).

Reduced systemic oxygen extraction is an important factor limiting exercise in many individuals with CF, but the specific parameters of this limitation remain unknown and probably vary from person to person.[339,360] Even unsupervised programs produce a training effect and pulmonary benefits.[337] Inspiratory muscle training alone in individuals with CF has shown improved lung function and increased work capacity, as well as improved psychosocial status.[137,158]

Exercise is an important adjunct to airway clearance. Although physical activity can increase expiratory airflow (shears mucus from the airway walls) and minute ventilation (opens previously collapsed airways), there is limited evidence to support exercise as a sole form of airway clearance. The therapist helps each individual develop an exercise routine that includes strengthening, stretching, aerobic, and endurance components, with special attention to breathing exercises to aerate all areas of the lungs. Exercise testing is recommended for activity counseling and recommendations as well as for routine monitoring and assessment of exercise-related symptoms, interim functional assessments, and pretransplant assessments. Cycle ergometry using the Godfrey protocol with pulse oximetry and gas exchange measures is the preferred test for all of the above except interim functional assessments. Treadmill tests (Bruce protocol with or without gas exchange measures) and maximal incremental field tests are second best options. A 6-minute walk test is required as part of the pretransplant listing process. For interim assessment of function, maximal incremental tests, submaximal tests, and task-specific tests are preferred. The reader is referred to a consensus statement for further rationale of the importance of exercise testing in CF as well as descriptions of the recommended tests.

Weight loss with exercise is of special concern in this population. The therapist can be very instrumental in providing client and family education about the importance of combining good nutrition and exercise/activity.

Energy expenditure is higher than usual for individuals with CF because of increased WOB consistent with higher ventilatory requirements.[493] This requires careful collaboration among patient/family, therapist, and nutritionist/dietician. In addition, systemic inflammatory response to exercise may be greater for individuals with CF, potentially exacerbating the disease.[251]

Individuals with CF awaiting a transplant must remain as active as possible; whenever possible, the therapist can design a safe but effective exercise program. If significant oxygen desaturation or severe breathlessness limits activity, then exercise on a treadmill, stationary bike, or even a stationary device for seated pedaling is recommended, with supplemental oxygen supplied at sufficient flow to match minute ventilatory requirements.[495] Exercise programs should also address any impairments in musculoskeletal strength and range of motion, especially trunk mobility.

Studies of exercise performance in lung transplant recipients with end-stage CF report that exercise performance improves after transplantation but remains well below normal.[360] In a study of 12 individuals 8 to 95 months after lung transplant, the diaphragm and abdominal muscle strength was preserved relative to healthy controls, but quadriceps strength was significantly diminished and affected exercise performance. Corticosteroid and antirejection medications have been shown to negatively impact muscle size and strength.[380]

The reader is referred to an evidence-based guide for appropriate physical activity and exercise prescription for people with CF.

### Athletes with Cystic Fibrosis

All people with CF are encouraged to exercise and participate in enjoyable physical activities, but some activities should be avoided. Scuba diving and high-altitude mountaineering pose risks (e.g., pneumothorax, high-altitude pulmonary edema) due to changes in air pressure and ambient pressure of oxygen, respectively. Contact sports and activities with increased potential for trauma (e.g., bungee jumping, horse jumping) should be avoided in any patients with impaired clotting function.

Therapists and dietitians should work with patients/families to ensure appropriate calorie intake to avoid weight loss as well as consumption of salty snacks and sports drinks to maintain electrolyte levels and avoid hyponatremia (deficiency of sodium in the blood, see Chapter 5) that can occur with excessive sweating. Many people with CF will expectorate more secretions during exercise; coaches and physical education teachers may need to be educated that coughing during exercise is acceptable and should not be feared.

### Adults with Cystic Fibrosis

As people with CF are living longer lives, there comes a time when they need to transition from pediatric to adult CF care centers (Fig 15.19). To minimize stress, pediatric centers should start the transition process early, allowing parents/caregivers and young patients time to gradually adjust to patients having more autonomy. Physical therapists can and should have an integral role in preparing patients for a more independent role as they become adolescents and young adults. Transition programs should be flexible enough to meet the needs of a wide range of young people, health conditions, and circumstances. The actual transfer of care should be individualized to meet the specific needs of young people and their families.[411] Family involvement, including parents, guardians, and the patient, is essential to the success of any transition phase. The omission of any key people from the transition team can result in frustration, feelings of abandonment, and miscommunication, which could ultimately lead to compromised care for the individual with CF. The CF R.I.S.E. program is a resource intended to guide centers in the transition process; centers can implement these tools as needed for each individual patient/family.

As individuals with CF survive longer into adulthood, the unique needs of this population need to be considered. In addition to progressive lung disease, some of the challenges facing adults with CF include health care insurance, pregnancy and family planning, male infertility, menopause, colorectal cancer, bone health, transplant, and end-of-life care. Individuals with CF and parent caregivers are at risk for anxiety, depression, and other psychological symptoms; routine mental health screening is recommended and guidelines for care are available. Life events such as going away to college and starting a career are also important considerations when caring for adults with CF. The physical therapy plan of care should be adapted to each individual patient's unique needs. Adult care resources are available for patients as well as clinicians.

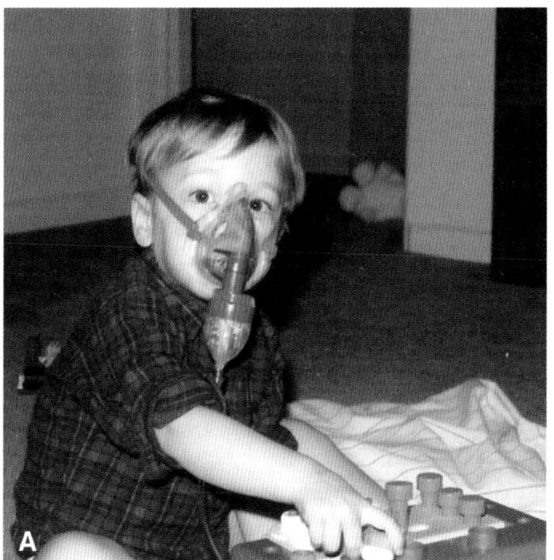
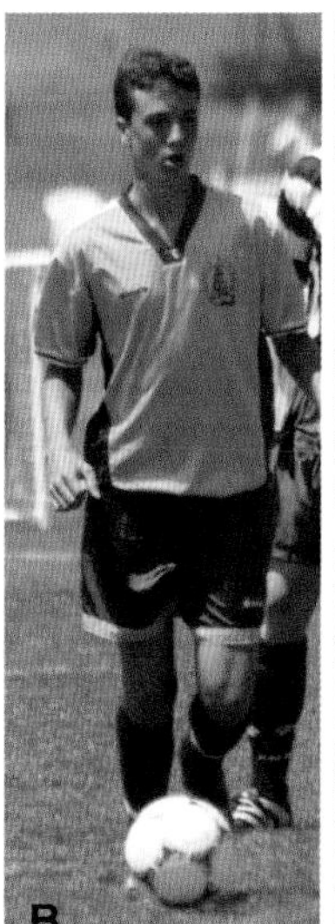
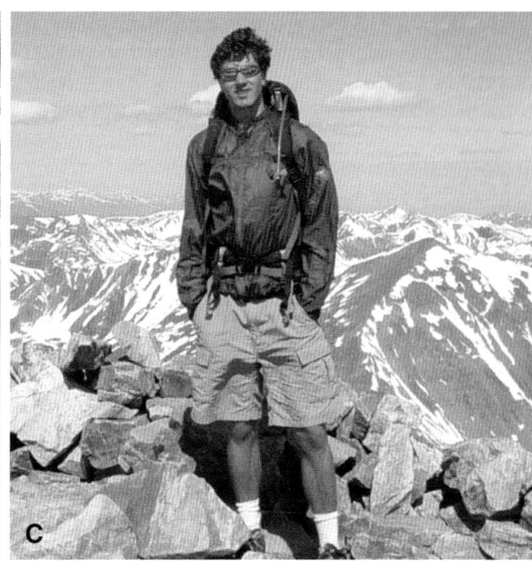

**Figure 15.19**

(A) An 18-month-old boy shortly after diagnosis; the face mask is a nebulizer (device designed to create and throw an aerosol) that is delivering albuterol (bronchodilator). (B) This same individual in 1999 at age 15 years (6 feet tall; 145 lb) competing in a regional soccer tournament. (C) Same young man at 23 years (6 feet 2 inches, 175 lb), still actively hiking, cycling, running, and playing intramural sports, while enrolled in graduate school. (Courtesy Kevin Hanson, Helena, MT, 2007. Used with permission.)

## PARENCHYMAL DISORDERS

### Atelectasis

#### Definition

Atelectasis is the collapse of normally expanded and aerated lung tissue at any structural level (e.g., lung parenchyma, alveoli, pleura, chest wall, bronchi) involving all or part of the lung. Atelectasis can impair gas exchange and is a risk factor for pneumonia, so prevention and early intervention are important to prevent untoward sequela.

#### Risk Factors, Etiologic Factors, and Pathogenesis

Risk factors for atelectasis include anesthesia, comorbid lung disease, neuromuscular disease, chronic disease, obesity, mucus plugging, prolonged bed rest, older age, and shallow breathing commonly due to pain.[413] Atelectasis after anesthesia can occur as a result of relaxation of the diaphragm, causing it to move cephalad and compress lung tissue.[413] Atelectasis may also occur due to the increased partial pressure of oxygen associated with the use of supplemental oxygen during surgery. This drives oxygen out of the alveoli and into the capillaries, decreasing alveolar volume and facilitating collapse and underventilation.[413] Finally, anesthesia-related atelectasis may also result from damage to surfactant from abnormal alveolar expansion and deflation that occurs with mechanical ventilation. Another cause of atelectasis includes obstruction of the bronchus (e.g., by tumors, mucus, or foreign material). With obstruction, atelectasis occurs as air in the alveoli is slowly absorbed into the bloodstream with subsequent collapse of the alveoli. Atelectasis can also develop when there is interference with the natural forces that promote lung expansion (e.g., hypoventilation due to paralysis, pleural disease, diaphragmatic disease, severe scoliosis, or masses in the thorax). Shallow breathing postoperatively due to sedation, immobility, pain, or splinting also reduces ventilation, resulting in atelectasis.

Insufficient pulmonary surfactant can also interfere with alveolar expansion. Reductions in surfactant can be found in such conditions as respiratory distress syndrome in infants, anesthesia, high concentrations of oxygen, lung contusion, aspiration of gastric contents, smoke inhalation, or with pneumoconiosis.

Finally, atelectasis can also be caused by compression resulting from pneumothorax, hemothorax, hydrothorax or abdominal distension.

#### Clinical Manifestations

Patients may present with dyspnea, cough, intercostal retractions, tachypnea, crackles, low oxygen saturation or decreased breath sounds.[413] When sudden obstruction of the bronchus occurs, there may be dyspnea, tachypnea, cyanosis, elevation of temperature, drop in blood pressure, substernal retractions, or shock. Physical therapists may hear crackles or decreased breath sounds in dependent lung bases in the postsurgical or immobile patient.

#### MEDICAL MANAGEMENT

DIAGNOSIS. Chest radiographs and clinical presentation are used to diagnosis atelectasis. Radiographs may show a shadow in the area of collapse or, if an entire lobe is collapsed, the radiograph will show the trachea, heart, and mediastinum deviated toward the collapsed area, with the diaphragm elevated on that side (see Fig. 15.14). Chest auscultation demonstrating absent breath sounds, diminished breath sounds, or crackles, adds to the clinical diagnostic picture. Blood gas measurements and pulse oximetry may show decreased oxygen saturation.

**PREVENTION, TREATMENT, AND PROGNOSIS.** To prevent atelectasis, smokers should refrain for 6 to 8 weeks prior to surgery.[413] Those that have underlying lung disease may be directed to increase bronchodilators and increase any airway clearance techniques they utilize.[413] Managing pain and early mobilization enable patients to breathe deeply and ventilate dependent airways.[413] Once atelectasis occurs, treatment is directed toward removing the cause whenever possible. Suctioning or bronchoscopy may be employed to remove airway obstruction. Airway clearance techniques may be helpful to remove secretions and promote segmental inflation after the obstruction has been removed. Breathing techniques that employ a breath hold to allow for cross-ventilation between alveoli are also used to improve alveolar expansion.

Surfactant has been used to resolve atelectasis in infants with respiratory distress syndrome, meconium aspiration, and other pathologies.[166] Antibiotics are used to combat infection accompanying secondary atelectasis. Reexpansion of the lung is often possible, but the final prognosis depends on the underlying disease.

SPECIAL IMPLICATIONS FOR THE THERAPIST 15.12

### *Atelectasis*

Atelectasis is a postoperative complication of thoracic or high abdominal surgery, with approximately 90% of patients experiencing atelectasis after anesthesia.[413]

Diminished respiratory movement as a result of postoperative pain is often addressed by the therapist. Early mobility, deep breathing, segmental reexpansion techniques, and cough training may help promote good pulmonary hygiene. Deep breathing with an inspiratory hold and effective coughing enhance lung expansion and may prevent atelectasis. Deep breathing is beneficial because it promotes the ciliary clearance of secretions, stabilizes the alveoli by redistributing surfactant, and permits collateral ventilation of the alveoli, through the Kohn pores in the alveolar septa.

The Kohn pores, which open only during deep breathing, allow air to pass from well-ventilated alveoli to underventilated alveoli, minimizing their tendency to collapse. To minimize postoperative pain during deep-breathing and coughing exercises, teach the client to hold a pillow firmly over the incision.

Early evidence supports early mobilization combined with respiratory interventions to prevent postoperative pulmonary complications, including atelectasis.[408]

## Pulmonary Edema

### Definition and Incidence

Pulmonary edema or pulmonary congestion is an excessive fluid accumulation in the lungs that develops in the interstitial tissue, air spaces (alveoli), or both. The fluid interrupts normal gas exchange and can lead to respiratory distress. Pulmonary edema is a common complication of many disease processes that occur at any age, but is more commonly experienced by older adults with left-sided heart failure.

### Etiologic and Risk Factors

Most cases of pulmonary edema are caused by left ventricular failure, acute hypertension, mitral valve disease, or fluid overload, but noncardiac conditions, especially kidney or liver disorders that cause sodium and water retention, can also produce pulmonary edema. These causes of pulmonary edema include intravenous narcotics, increased intracerebral pressure, brain injury, high altitude, diving and submersion, sepsis, medications, inhalation of smoke or toxins (e.g., ammonia), blood transfusion reactions, shock, and disseminated intravascular coagulation.[37,119,177]

Other risk factors include hyperaldosteronism, Cushing syndrome, use of glucocorticoids, and use of hypotonic fluids to irrigate nasogastric tubes. Pulmonary edema itself is a major predisposing factor in the development of pneumonia that complicates heart failure and ARDS.

### Pathogenesis

Pulmonary edema occurs when the pulmonary vasculature fills with fluid that leaks into the alveolar spaces, decreasing the space available for gas exchange. Normally the lung is kept dry by lymphatic drainage and a balance among capillary hydrostatic pressure, capillary oncotic pressure, and capillary permeability. A newer pathogenesis model has emerged which partially challenges previous mechanisms. A newer theory purports that the endothelial lining plays a critical role in balance of fluids.[29] The endothelium contains endothelial glycocalyx (EG), which provides an oncotic force to keep fluids within the vasculature. When this layer is damaged, as with surgery, the ability to control the movement of fluids into the interstitium is disturbed. Moreover, the EG is sensitive to hydrostatic pressure and when elevated, fluid may leak into the interstitium.[29]

Pulmonary edema develops as a result of (1) fluid overload, (2) decreased serum and albumin, (3) lymphatic obstruction, and (4) disruption of capillary permeability (tissue injury or immunoresponse) (Fig. 15.20).

**Fluid Overload.** When the filling pressures on the left side of the heart increase, the increased pressure is transmitted "upstream" to the left atrium and then the pulmonary vasculature. If it surpasses the oncotic pressure that holds fluid in the capillaries, fluid is drawn from capillaries in the interstitial space and then into the alveoli.[370] Normally, the lymphatic system removes this fluid from the lungs, but if the flow of fluid into the interstitium exceeds the ability of the lymphatic system to remove it, fluid overload and consequently pulmonary edema develops.

Pulmonary edema is commonly seen when the left side of the heart fails to pump adequately (e.g., myocardial ischemia or infarction, heart failure, or mitral or aortic valve damage). Increased left atrial pressure may also result from inadequate emptying of the atria, as occurs with atrial fibrillation. This increased left atrial pressure is transmitted to the pulmonary vasculature, eventually disrupting fluid homeostasis and causing the alveoli to flood.

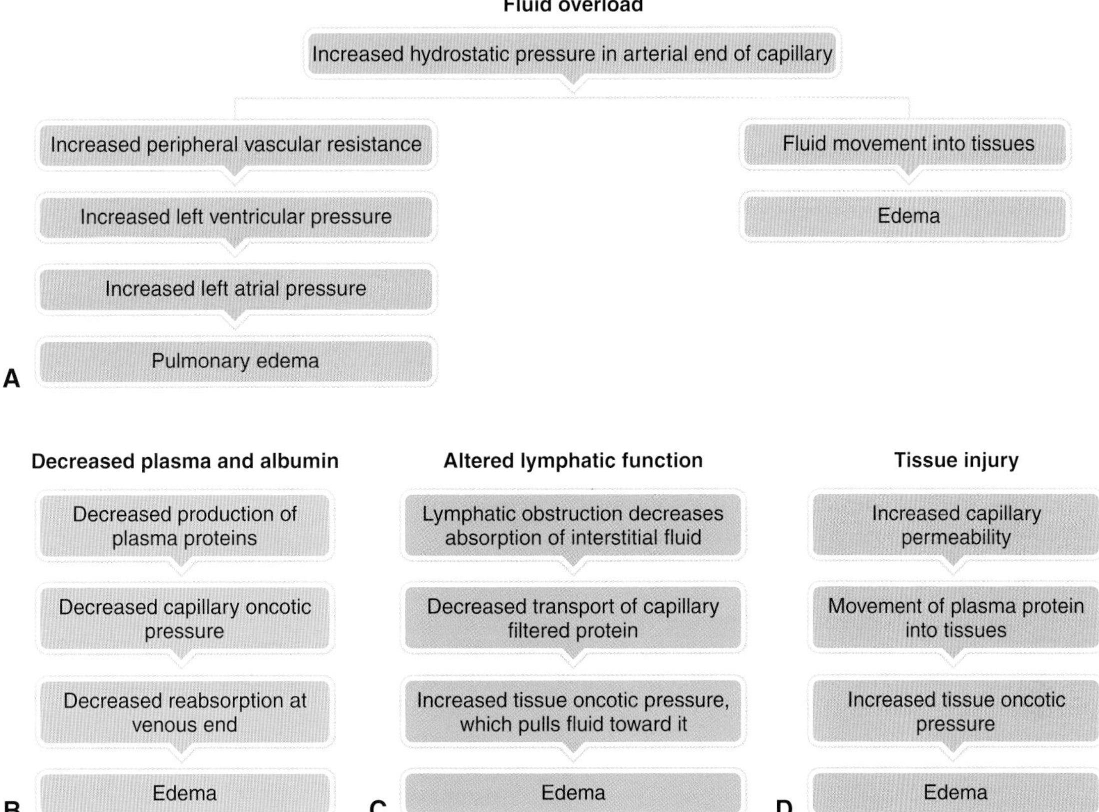


**Figure 15.20**

**Mechanisms of pulmonary edema formation.** (A) Fluid overload. (B) Decreased serum and albumin. (C) Lymphatic obstruction. (D) Tissue injury. (From Black JM, Hawks JH, eds: *Medical-surgical nursing*, ed 7, St Louis, 2005, WB Saunders.)

**Decreased Serum and Albumin.** In the case of liver cirrhosis, the serum protein and albumin levels are reduced in the vascular fluids. Thus less fluid reabsorption from the tissue spaces occurs, which results in pulmonary and peripheral edema and ascites.

**Lymphatic Obstruction.** When lymphatic channels are obstructed, have reduced function, or their functional capacity is exceeded, tissue oncotic pressure rises and results in edema. This obstruction can occur as a result of tumor seeding, but most often occurs in association with cardiogenic causes of pulmonary edema. When hemodynamic alterations (changes in the movement of blood and the forces involved) in the heart increase the perfusion pressure in the pulmonary capillaries, lymphatics cannot sufficiently remove excess fluid.

**Tissue Injury.** Disruption of capillary permeability is the cause of pulmonary edema in ALI associated with ARDS, inhalation of toxic gases, aspiration of gastric contents, viral infections, and uremia. In these conditions, destruction of endothelial cells or disruption of the tight junctions between them alters capillary permeability. Transfusion reactions are caused by leukocyte antibodies and result in increased capillary permeability.[128]

### Clinical Manifestations

Clinical manifestations of pulmonary edema occur in stages. During the initial stage, clients may be asymptomatic or they may complain of restlessness and anxiety and the feeling that they are developing a common cold. Other clinical symptoms and signs include dyspnea on exertion, decreases in physical activity, cough, crackles, and orthopnea.[143] If the pulmonary edema worsens or occurs rapidly, respiratory rate increases, and there may be audible wheezing. If the edema is severe, the cough becomes productive of frothy sputum tinged with blood, giving it a pinkish hue. If the condition persists, the person becomes hypoxic, less responsive, and may require mechanical ventilation.

## MEDICAL MANAGEMENT

PREVENTION. Prevention is a key component with persons at increased risk for the development of pulmonary edema. Preventive measures may include lowering salt intake and managing fluids in those with heart failure or pharmacologic interventions to manage ischemia/infarction and heart failure.

DIAGNOSIS. Pulmonary edema is usually recognized by its characteristic clinical presentation. Cardiogenic pulmonary edema is differentiated from noncardiac causes by the history and physical examination. An underlying cardiac abnormality can usually be detected clinically or by the electrocardiogram (ECG), chest film, cardiac CT, or echocardiogram. A chest radiograph may show Kerley lines (thin horizontal lines), ground glass appearance, lung consolidation, or indistinct pulmonary vessels.[29] Lung ultrasound is emerging as a quick modality to help identify pulmonary edema, however its use is not yet widespread.

There are no specific laboratory tests diagnostic of pulmonary edema; when the condition progresses enough to cause liver involvement, the physician may observe the hepatojugular reflex (positional or palpatory pressure on the liver results in distention of the jugular vein). Auscultation reveals crackles or discontinuous, explosive breath sounds typically heard on inhalation.[29] Blood gas measurements indicate the degree of functional impairment, and sputum cultures may indicate accompanying infection.

**TREATMENT.** Once pulmonary edema has been diagnosed, treatment is aimed at enhancing gas exchange, reducing fluid overload, and addressing the underlying cause. Supplemental oxygen, noninvasive ventilator support, or mechanical ventilation may be used along with medications to address the underlying cause or to improve ventilation. Morphine to relieve anxiety and reduce the effort of breathing may be used for people who do not have narcotic-induced pulmonary edema.

**PROGNOSIS.** The prognosis depends on the underlying condition. The presence of pulmonary edema is a medical emergency requiring immediate intervention to prevent further respiratory distress and death. It is often reversible with clinical management.

**SPECIAL IMPLICATIONS FOR THE THERAPIST 15.13**

*Pulmonary Edema*

Signs and symptoms of pulmonary edema that may come to the therapist's attention include engorged neck and hand veins (because of peripheral vascular fluid overload), pitting edema of the extremities, adventitious breath sounds, and paroxysmal nocturnal dyspnea so common with this condition. One of the first signs of dyspnea may be increased difficulty in breathing when lying down, relieved by sitting up (orthopnea). Pulmonary edema can become life-threatening within minutes, requiring immediate action by the therapist to get medical assistance for this person.

Jugular vein distention may occur with liver involvement. Positional or palpatory pressure on the liver may result in right upper quadrant or right shoulder pain, as well as jugular vein distention. The distention may be best observed with the person positioned sitting 30 to 45 degrees up from a fully supine position.

Liver involvement requires precautions when performing any soft tissue mobilization techniques to the anterior part of the abdomen, including the diaphragm. Indirect techniques or mobilization away from the liver is recommended.

When working with a client already diagnosed with pulmonary edema, the high Fowler position is preferred, with legs dangling over the side of the bed or plinth. This facilitates respiration and reduces venous return. If oxygen is being administered, the therapist monitors the oxyhemoglobin saturation levels and titrates oxygen accordingly with physician orders. It may be necessary to increase oxygen levels before exercise, but respiratory rate and breathing pattern must be monitored. Monitor for decreased respiratory drive (fewer than 12 breaths per minute is significant), which should be documented and reported immediately. Therapists should consider use of breathing facilitation techniques to enhance ventilation of the lower airways. Early mobilization and progressive activity is indicated as long as the therapist monitors the patient closely through pulse oximetry, lung auscultation, heart rate and rhythm, blood pressure, and telemetry.

## Acute Lung Injury and Acute Respiratory Distress Syndrome

### Definition

ALI/ARDS is a form of acute respiratory failure after a systemic or pulmonary insult. It is a syndrome and not a specific diagnosis, often a fatal complication of serious illness (e.g., sepsis), trauma, or major surgery. The Berlin definition of ARDS is:[471]

- Onset within 7 days after a known clinical insult or new/worsening pulmonary symptoms
- Bilateral opacities on chest radiograph or chest CI consistent with pulmonary edema
- Minimum of 5 cm $H_2O$ PEEP
- Respiratory failure not explained by heart failure or fluid overload

ARDS severity is categorized as:

- Mild: $PaO_2$:$FiO_2$ 201 to 300 mm Hg
- Moderate: $PaO_2$:$FiO_2$ 101 to 200 mm Hg
- Severe: $PaO_2$:$FiO_2$ 100 mm Hg or less

### Incidence

Worldwide estimates of ARDS are 10 to 86 cases per 100,000,[472] and ARDS accounts for about 10% of ICU admissions.[42] ALI/ARDS mortality rates have declined since the mid-1990s but still carries a relatively high mortality rate of 31% to 46%, depending on comorbidities and risk factors.[42,252]

### Risk Factors

ALI/ARDS can affect anyone at any time regardless of gender, age, or health status. Factors that increase the risk of ALI/ARDS include increasing age, sepsis, pneumonia, aspiration of gastric contents, pulmonary contusion, trauma, and near drowning (Box 15.9).[252,471] Indirect risk factors include sepsis originating outside of the lungs, hemorrhagic shock, pancreatitis, significant burns, drug overdose, receipt of blood products, cardiopulmonary bypass, and reperfusion after lung transplantation.[471] ARDS does not develop in the majority of people who have these risk factors, and it remains unclear why some develop it and others do not.

### Pathogenesis

There are three phases in the development and resolution of ARDS, although some patients only experience phases 1 and 2. Phase 1 is termed the exudative phase and

Box 15.9

**CAUSES OF ACUTE (ADULT) RESPIRATORY DISTRESS SYNDROME***

- Severe trauma (e.g., multiple bone fractures)
- Septic shock
- Pancreatitis
- Cardiopulmonary bypass surgery
- Diffuse pulmonary infection
- Burns
- High concentrations of supplemental oxygen
- Aspiration of gastric contents
- Massive blood transfusions
- Embolism: fat, thrombus, amniotic fluid, venous air
- Drowning
- Radiation therapy
- Inhalation of smoke or toxic fumes
- Thrombotic thrombocytopenic purpura
- Indirect: chemical mediators released in response to systemic disorders (e.g., viral infections, pneumonia)
- Drugs (e.g., aspirin, narcotics, lidocaine, phenylbutazone, hydrochlorothiazide, most chemotherapeutic and cytotoxic agents)

*Listed in order of decreasing frequency.

involves damage of the alveolar-capillary membranes. This causes protein-rich fluid to accumulate in the alveoli and interstitium, disrupting gas exchange and reducing lung compliance.[129,471] Inflammation and injury to these areas are heightened through activation of macrophages and proinflammatory cytokines. Neutrophils also release toxins that damage the alveoli, and there is formation of a hyaline membrane. Both type I and type II alveolar epithelial cells are impacted. The proliferative phase follows and is characterized by repair of the endothelial-capillary membranes and restoration of fluid balance, leading to improvements in gas exchange. The fibrotic phase follows in some patients and is more likely to occur in those on prolonged mechanical ventilation. In the fibrotic phase, there is interstitial and intraalveolar fibrosis and damage to microcapillaries.[471] Figure 15.21 demonstrates both a normal alveolus and one with ALI/ARDS.

### Clinical Manifestations

The clinical presentation is relatively uniform regardless of cause and occurs within 12 to 48 hours of the initiating event. The earliest sign of ARDS is usually an increased respiratory rate characterized by shallow, rapid breathing. Pulmonary edema, atelectasis, crackles on auscultation, and decreased lung compliance cause dyspnea, hyperventilation, and the changes observed on chest radiographs (Fig. 15.22). Unless the underlying disease is reversed rapidly, especially in the presence of sepsis (toxins in the blood), the condition quickly progresses to full-blown MODS, involving kidneys, liver, gut, CNS, and the cardiovascular system.

## MEDICAL MANAGEMENT

**DIAGNOSIS.** Diagnosis of ALI/ARDS is often delayed or missed during the critical early hours when appropriate treatment can reduce morbidity and mortality. The diagnosis is made based on a clinical history, identification of underlying medical conditions, imaging, $PaO_2/FiO_2$, and pulmonary capillary wedge pressure. Blood gas analysis is used to assess the severity of hypoxemia, and microbiologic cultures may be used to identify or exclude infection. Physicians may begin with a chest radiograph that can show diffuse opacities or a chest CT which may be more helpful in differentiating ARDS from heart failure. Clinicians are beginning to use pulmonary ultrasound at the bedside for diagnostic purposes as well.[129]

**TREATMENT.** Specific treatment is administered for any underlying conditions (e.g., sepsis or pneumonia). Lung protective strategies are employed that may include lower tidal volumes and higher respiratory rates as well as optimization of fluid balance.[252,417,418,483,484] For those with moderate to severe ARDS, prone positioning may improve mortality rates.[471]

Pharmacologic interventions have not been shown to reduce mortality.[252,471] Neuromuscular blockade and sedation may be used to improve synchrony with the ventilator, however the long-term side effects, especially from a mobility standpoint, are significant. Studies are underway to determine which sedation strategy (if any) produces better patient outcomes.

**PROGNOSIS.** The final outcome is difficult to predict at the onset of disease, but associated multiorgan dysfunction and uncontrolled infection contribute to the mortality rate for ARDS of 31% to 46%.[42] Higher mortality rates are associated with elevations in inflammatory biomarkers such as interleukin-6.[471] The major cause of death in ARDS is nonpulmonary MODS, often with sepsis. If ARDS is accompanied by sepsis, the mortality rate may reach 90%. Median survival in such cases is 2 weeks. The mortality rate increases with age, and clients older than 60 years of age have a mortality rate as high as 90%. In children, degree of hypoxia and multiple organ failure predict mortality. Mortality rates for children range between 8% and 27.5%.[417]

Survivors of ARDS may experience a myriad of issues, including muscle weakness, mobility dysfunction, memory loss, anxiety, and reduced quality of life. A new term to describe these long term effects is post intensive care syndrome or PICS (PICS-P in pediatric populations).[402] PICS is defined as a "new or worsening impairment in physical (ICU-acquired neuromuscular weakness), cognitive (thinking and judgment), or mental health status arising after critical illness and persisting beyond discharge from the acute care setting.[402] Long-term lung morbidity includes both a restrictive and obstructive pattern 1 year after discharge and a lower DLCO.[114] These patterns may be due to fibrotic changes in the lungs, as well as persistent respiratory weakness. Patients without comorbid lung disease can return to near-normal lung function with mild reductions in diffusion capacity.[214]

**SPECIAL IMPLICATIONS FOR THE THERAPIST 15.14**

### *Acute (Adult) Respiratory Distress Syndrome*

Post intensive care syndrome (PICS) refers to the musculoskeletal, cardiopulmonary, cognitive, and psychosocial impairments that persist after an ICU stay. Twenty-five percent of those discharged from

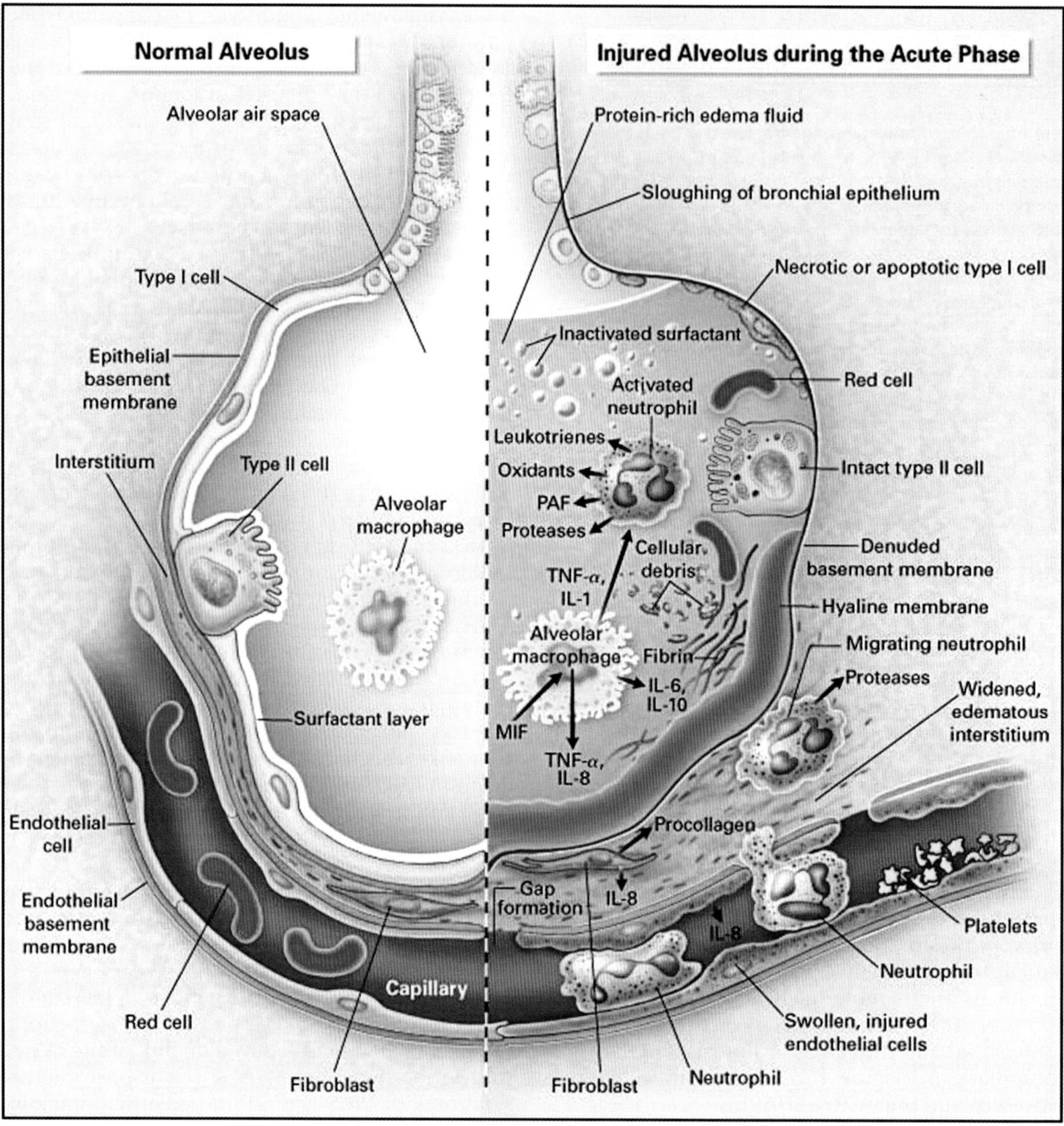


**Figure 15.21**

**Figure demonstrates both a normal alveolus and one with ALI/ARDS.**

the ICU have cognitive impairment, with another 25% also experiencing ICU acquired weakness. Up to 62% of those discharged from the ICU also develop mood disturbances, such as depression, anxiety, and posttraumatic stress disorder.[402] Muscle weakness as measured by the Medical Research Council sum score is associated with 5-year survival. Patients who are stronger at hospital discharge had improved survival.[146]

Prevention and early intervention for PICS is critical to optimize patient outcomes. Some hospitals have implemented the ABCDE bundle to prevent PICS, which includes[402]

Awakening: use of natural light in rooms, minimizing sedative medications

Breathing: use of spontaneous breathing trials when appropriate

Coordination: interprofessional communication, collaboration, and team based care

Delirium: monitoring, assessing, and early management

Early mobilization: early activity and ambulation

In the post-ICU rehabilitation setting, the 4-meter gait speed test is an excellent measure of function. Gait speed can be predictive of future hospitalizations, quality of life, and mortality. Published minimally important difference of 0.03 to 0.06 meters per second (0.067-.134 mph) can assist clinicians in determining the effectiveness of rehabilitation interventions.[110]

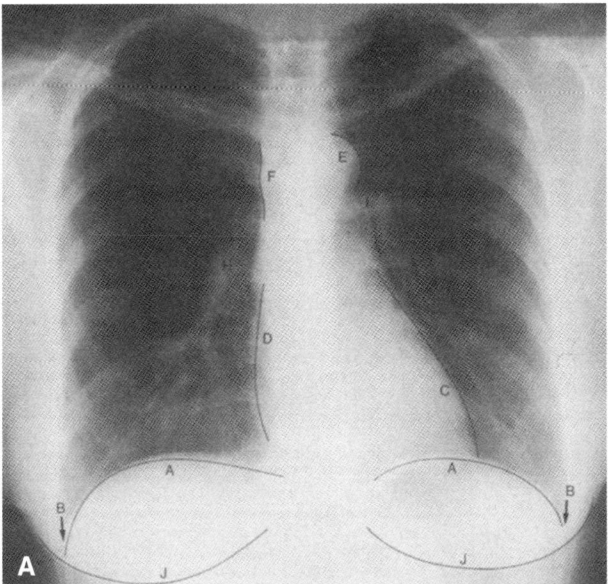


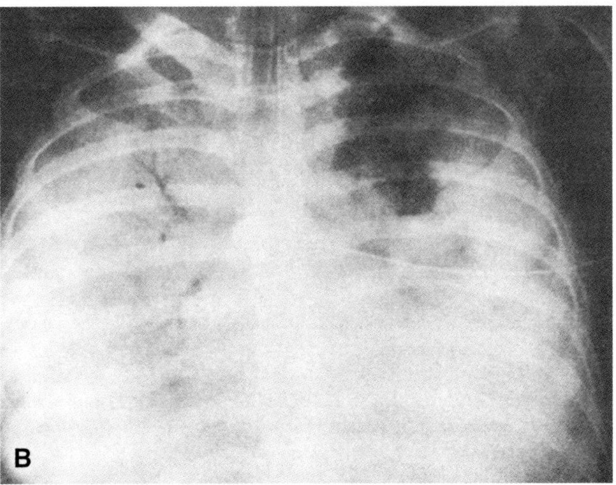


**Figure 15.22**

(A) Normal chest film taken from a posteroanterior view. The backward *L* in the upper right corner is placed on the film to indicate the left side of the chest. Some anatomic structures can be seen on the x-ray study and are outlined: *A,* diaphragm; *B,* costophrenic angle; *C,* left ventricle, *D,* right atrium; *E,* aortic arch; *F,* superior vena cava; *G,* trachea; *H,* right bronchus; *I,* left bronchus; *J,* breast shadows. (B) This chest film shows massive consolidation from pulmonary edema associated with acute (adult) respiratory distress syndrome after multisystem trauma. (A, from Black JM, Hokanson Hawks, J, editors: *Medical-surgical nursing,* ed 7, St Louis, 2005, WB Saunders; B, from Fraser RG, Paré JA, Paré PD, et al: *Diagnosis of diseases of the chest,* ed 3, Philadelphia, 1990, WB Saunders.)

### Early Mobilization

Early mobilization is becoming the standard of care in acute care inclusive of ICUs, with low reports of adverse events. In a study of over 7500 patients with 22,000 rehabilitation sessions, the incidence of adverse events was 2.6%, with less than 1% classified as having medical consequences.[357]

In addition to early mobilization, there may be a role for neuromuscular electrical stimulation or NMES. Preliminary evidence demonstrates that NMES and exercise may decrease the number of days on a mechanical ventilator compared to a control group and improve functional independence at time of ICU discharge.[148,296] There are a variety of early mobilization protocols, each of which has different indications and contraindications for initiation and termination of mobility. Many of the protocols incorporate aspects of a cognitive assessment (use of the RASS scale), stability of heart rhythm, sufficient cardiovascular reserve (HR rest is < 50% of predicted HR max), and sufficient respiratory reserve as measured by $FiO_2$ needs and oxygen saturation.[407] Other considerations include hemoglobin levels, blood glucose, and the use of invasive monitoring.

When mobilizing the patient in the ICU, therapists need to make quick clinical decisions to continue, reduce, or terminate the session based on the patient response. There are no definitive guidelines on this clinical decision-making process, however therapists should consider lowering the intensity of the intervention if:

- Pulse increases 20 to 30 beats/min above resting HR
- RR increases to greater than 30 breaths per minute and does not significantly reduce with short periods of rest
- New onset use of accessory muscles
- Mild agitation
- Reduction in oxygen saturation to 90%
- Complaints of dizziness, lightheadedness

The session should be terminated if any of the following develop:

- New onset heart rhythm that is associated with the potential for hemodynamic instability
- Drop in systolic blood pressure with activity
- Angina or new onset pain/discomfort/heaviness above the waist
- New onset or worsening of nausea
- RASS > 3
- $SpO_2 < 90\%$
- RR ≥ 40 breaths per minute
- Patient/ventilator asynchrony

## Sarcoidosis

### Definition

Sarcoidosis is a systemic disease of unknown cause involving any organ and is characterized by noncaseating granulomas present diffusely throughout the body. Its primary effects are seen in the lung and lymphatic tissues, which is why it appears in this chapter and is also referenced in infectious/inflammatory disorders.[384] The granulomas consist of a collection of macrophages surrounded by lymphocytes taking a nodular form. In fact, granulomatous inflammation of the lung is present in 90% of clients with sarcoidosis. Secondary sites include the skin, eyes, liver, spleen, heart, and small bones in the hands and feet.

### Incidence

Sarcoidosis occurs predominantly in the second through fourth decades of life, with another peak after age 50, and has a slightly higher incidence in women than men. Prevalence in the United States is estimated at 60/100,000 and is three times more likely to occur in African Americans.[377] There also seems to be an increase in diagnosis during the spring. Socioeconomic, environmental, and genetic factors appear to influence the occurrence.[126]

### Etiologic Factors and Pathogenesis

The etiologic factors and pathogenesis of sarcoidosis are unknown, but there appears to be an exaggerated cellular immune response on the part of the helper T lymphocytes to a foreign antigen whose identity remains unclear. Increasing evidence points to a triggering agent that may be genetic, infectious (bacterial or viral), immunologic, or toxic. CD4+ T cells are activated, cytokines are upregulated, and macrophages are stimulated to organize into granulomas.[377] Interferon-gamma is expressed in the lungs and other affected organs.

Granuloma formation may regress with therapy or as a result of the disease's natural course but may also progress to fibrosis and restrictive lung disease.

### Clinical Manifestations

Sarcoidosis can affect any organ, including bones, joints, muscles, and vessels. Lymph nodes are involved in 90% of patients, liver and eyes in 15% to 20%, 15% have cutaneous involvement, 2% to 7% have cardiac involvement, and 5% to 10% have CNS involvement. Initial symptoms are fever, night sweats, weight loss, fatigue, and decreased function. Lungs and thoracic lymph nodes are most often involved, with acute or insidious respiratory problems sometimes accompanied by symptoms affecting the skin, eyes, or other organs. The diverse manifestations of this disorder lend support to the hypothesis that sarcoidosis has more than one cause. The clinical impact of sarcoidosis is directly related to the extent of granulomatous inflammation and its effect on the function of vital organs.

Pulmonary sarcoidosis has a variable natural course from an asymptomatic state to a progressive life-threatening condition. Signs and symptoms may develop over a period of a few weeks to a few months and include dyspnea, nonproductive cough, fever, malaise, weight loss, skin lesions (Fig. 15.23), erythema nodosum (multiple, tender, nonulcerating nodules) and fatigue.[138]

This condition may be entirely asymptomatic, presenting with abnormal findings on routine chest radiographs. Respiratory symptoms of dry cough and dyspnea without constitutional symptoms (symptoms of systemic illness, including fatigue, weakness, malaise, weight loss, sweating, and fever) occur in more than half of all people with sarcoidosis, and up to 15% develop progressive fibrosis. Chest pain, hemoptysis, or pneumothorax may be present.

Sarcoidosis may present with extrapulmonary symptoms referable to bone marrow, skin, eyes, cranial nerves or peripheral nerves (neurosarcoidosis), liver, or heart (Box 15.10). Sarcoid arthritis with arthralgia, myopathy, chronic tissue swelling, tenosynovitis, and other periarthritic inflammatory changes occur less often but bring the affected individuals to the therapist's attention.[432]

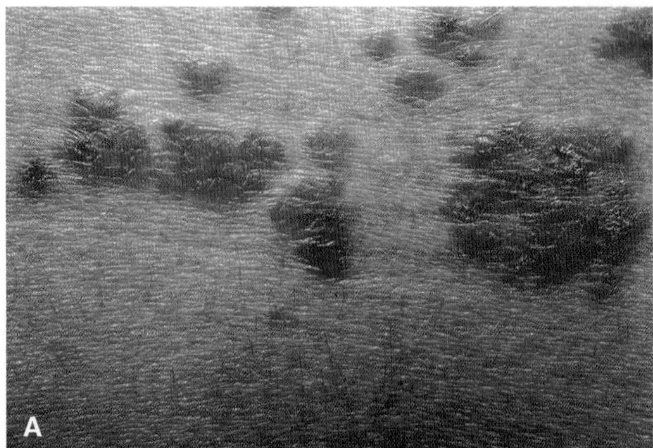


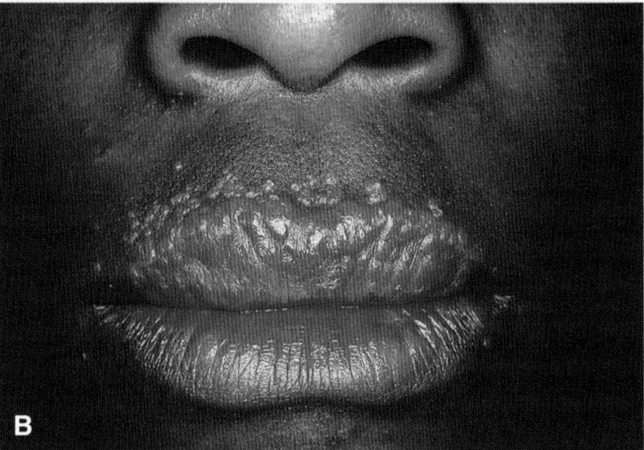


**Figure 15.23**

**Sarcoidosis.** (A) Cutaneous sarcoidosis usually consists of papules and plaques with a typical reddish-brown color. (B) Lesions often favor the lips and perioral region. (From Bolognia JL, Jorizzo JL, Rapini RP: *Dermatology*, St Louis, 2003, Mosby. Courtesy Jean Bolognia, MD. Used with permission.)

Neurosarcoidosis is uncommon but severe and sometimes life-threatening. Sarcoidosis appears to be associated with a significantly increased risk for cancer in affected organs (e.g., skin, liver, lymphoma, or lung). Chronic inflammation is the mediator of this risk.[27]

## MEDICAL MANAGEMENT

**DIAGNOSIS.** There is no specific test other than history for sarcoidosis so diagnosis is based on clinical examination, chest CT, pulmonary function, laboratory test findings, and biopsy of granulomas (e.g., skin lesions, salivary gland, or palpable lymph nodes). MRI may be used when CNS involvement is suspected and high-resolution CT may be used to identify organ disease. Other granulomatous diseases (e.g., TB, berylliosis, lymphoma, carcinoma, and fungal disease) must be ruled out.

**TREATMENT.** Treatment may not be required, especially in those clients who are asymptomatic and have an FVC greater than 70% predicted.[257] A combination of chest CT findings indicating active inflammation and decrements in FVC help determine if a watch-and-wait strategy will be used or if medication will be employed. Short-term (less than 6 months) use of inhaled steroids may improve

Box 15.10

**CLINICAL MANIFESTATIONS OF SARCOIDOSIS**

***Pulmonary***

- Asymptomatic with abnormal chest film
- Sinusitis
- Gradually progressive cough and shortness of breath
- Interstitial pneumonitis
- Pulmonary fibrosis with pulmonary insufficiency
- Laryngeal and endobronchial obstruction
- Necrotizing sarcoid granulomatosis

***Extrapulmonary***

- Löfgren syndrome: fever, arthralgia, bilateral hilar adenopathy, erythema nodosum
- Heerfordt syndrome (uveoparotid fever): fever, swelling of parotid gland and uveal tracts, seventh cranial nerve palsy
- Erythema nodosum
- Peripheral lymphadenopathy/splenomegaly
- Lymphoma
- Eyes: excessive tearing, swelling, uveitis, iritis, glaucoma, cataracts
- Integument: nodules or skin plaques (see Fig. 15.21); skin cancer
- Nervous system: peripheral and/or cranial nerve palsies (cranial neuropathy), subacute meningitis, diabetes insipidus, spinal myelopathy
- Joints: polyarticular and monarticular arthritis
- Skeletal: osteolytic lesions in phalangeal and metacarpal bones
- Cardiac: paroxysmal arrhythmias, conduction disturbances, pericarditis, myocarditis, congestive heart failure, sudden death
- Renal: hypercalcemia with nephrocalcinosis or nephrolithiasis, interstitial cystitis
- Liver: granulomatous hepatitis, liver cancer

symptoms especially in people who mainly have cough. The long-term use of corticosteroids is the treatment of choice for those clients who have impaired lung function with pulmonary granulomas. Corticosteroids are quite effective in reducing the acute granulomatous inflammation as seen on radiograph, but their efficacy in improving lung function and altering the long-term prognosis is unproven. It has been suggested that those who receive corticosteroids have a higher rate of relapse, possibly due to a decrease in ability of the body to clear the offending antigen.[257] Other treatment interventions include methotrexate or TNF-α inhibitors to suppress the immune response.[377]

Smokers are counseled to quit because, although sarcoidosis is less prevalent in smokers, those who do smoke have a quicker progression of the disease.[377]

In cases of end-stage sarcoidosis, lung transplantation has been proven successful.[293] Selection of clients with pulmonary sarcoidosis for transplantation requires that medical therapy, including the use of corticosteroids and alternative medications, has been exhausted and that other contraindicated variables are not present (see "Lung Transplantation" in Chapter 21). Sarcoidosis frequently recurs in the allograft but rarely causes symptoms or pulmonary dysfunction.[256]

**PROGNOSIS.** The prognosis is usually favorable, with complete resolution of symptoms and chest radiographic changes within 6 months to 2 years, although one-third of people have chronic issues.[377,385] Most clients do not manifest clinically significant sequelae. However, because sarcoidosis is a multisystem disease that can cause complex problems, it can have a variable prognosis ranging from spontaneous remissions to progressive lung disease with pulmonary fibrosis in active sarcoidosis. In such cases, respiratory insufficiency and cor pulmonale may eventually occur. In 65% to 70% of cases, there are no residual manifestations, 20% are left with permanent lung or ocular changes, and 10% of all cases die. Overall, sarcoidosis has a mortality rate of 1% to 6%.[138]

SPECIAL IMPLICATIONS FOR THE THERAPIST 15.15

## *Sarcoidosis*

When erythema nodosum, bihilar lymphadenopathy, and polyarthralgia occur together, it is termed Löfgren syndrome.[280] Patients may also have dyspnea, fever, and cough. Commonly, patients present with bilateral ankle arthritis of less than 2 months. While the ankles are the most common site for arthritis, issues can also arise in the hand, knee, elbow, and fingers.[280] There is also a chronic form of arthritis that is less common in sarcoidosis. Rheumatoid arthritis is typically evaluated with laboratory testing to rule it out as a causative factor. Sarcoid related arthropathy is treated with nonsteroidal antiinflammatory drugs. Low-dose steroids may also be used in patients with significant pain for functional limitations. Recently, disease-modifying antisarcoidosis drugs have begun being used, however their efficacy has not been determined.[280]

Therapists should be alert to any presenting signs or symptoms of increased disease activity associated with sarcoidosis because medical vigilance with attention to new symptoms is important in the management of sarcoidosis. Serious visceral complications (e.g., cardiac disease) may present suddenly and silently with arrhythmia. Taking vital signs routinely is especially important with this disease. Palpitations, chest pain, or progressing dyspnea require medical evaluation.

This disease presents in many and diverse patterns, but observe especially for exertional dyspnea that progresses to dyspnea at rest, chest pain, joint swelling, or increased fatigue and malaise, reducing the client's functional level or ability to participate in therapy. Muscle involvement and bone involvement are frequently underdiagnosed. Symptoms of muscle weakness, aches, tenderness, and fatigue, often accompanied by neurogenic atrophy, may indicate sarcoid myositis.[33]

Cranial nerve palsies (especially facial palsy), multiple mononeuropathy, and less commonly, symmetric polyneuropathy may all occur. Symmetric polyneuropathy can affect either motor or sensory fibers solely or both disproportionately. An unusual combination of neurologic deficits affecting the CNS or

**Table 15.11** Characteristics of Lung Cancer

| Tumor Type | Growth Rate | Metastasis | Treatment |
|---|---|---|---|
| **Small Cell Lung Cancer** | | | |
| Small cell (oat cell) | Very rapid | Very early; to mediastinum or distal area of lung | Combination chemotherapy; surgical resectability is poor |
| **Non–Small Cell Lung Cancer** | | | |
| Squamous cell (epidermal) | Slow | Localized metastasis not common or occurs late, usually to hilar lymph nodes, adrenals, liver | Surgically, resectability is good if stage I or II<br>Chemoradiation therapy is considered |
| Adenocarcinoma | Slow to moderate | Early; metastasis throughout lung and brain or to other organs | Surgical resectability is good if localized stage I or II<br>Chemotherapy or chemoradiation and surgery may be combined for stage III |
| Large cell (anaplastic) | Rapid | Early and widespread metastasis to kidney, liver, adrenals | Surgical resection is poor if involvement is widespread; better prognosis if stage I or II<br>Chemotherapy of limited use, radiation therapy is palliative |

peripheral nerves (or both) suggests sarcoidosis and should be evaluated medically. Improvement of neurologic function may occur with the use of corticosteroids.

For clients receiving steroid therapy, increased side effects of the medication should be reported to the physician. For example, long-term use of steroids lowers resistance to infection, may induce diabetes and myopathy, and is associated with weight gain, loss of potassium in the urine, osteopenia, and gastric irritation.

## Lung Cancer

### Overview

Lung cancer, a malignancy of the epithelium of the respiratory tract, is the most frequent cause of cancer death in the United States and the most common type of cancer worldwide (excluding nonmelanoma skin cancer). The term *lung cancer,* also known as bronchogenic carcinoma, excludes other pulmonary tumors, such as sarcomas, lymphomas, blastomas, hematomas, and mesotheliomas.

### Types of Lung Cancer

At least a dozen different types of tumors are included under the broad heading of lung cancer. Clinically, lung cancers are classified as small cell lung cancer (SCLC; 10%-15% of all lung cancers), and non–SCLC (NSCLC; 80%-85% of all lung cancers). Within these two broad categories, there are four major types of primary malignant lung tumors: SCLC includes small cell carcinoma (oat cell carcinoma); NSCLC includes squamous cell carcinoma, adenocarcinoma, and large cell carcinoma. Table 15.11 summarizes the characteristics of these four lung cancers.

*Adenocarcinoma,* the most common form of lung cancer in the United States, tends to arise in the periphery, usually in the upper lobes at different levels of the bronchial tree. An individual tumor may reflect the cell structure of any part of the respiratory mucosa from the large bronchi to the smallest bronchioles. Because of this, adenocarcinoma refers to a heterogeneous group of neoplasms that have in common the formation of gland-like structures. Adenocarcinoma is further subdivided into four categories: acinar, papillary, bronchioloalveolar, and solid carcinoma.

Squamous cell lung cancer occurs in 25% to 30% of people and occurs in squamous cells that line the airways. Large cell carcinomas account for 10% to 15% of lung cancers and tend to be aggressive and metastasize quickly.

### Incidence

Lung cancer remains the leading cause of cancer death in the United States, with an estimated 153,718 deaths in 2010.[93,277,478] It is one of the world's leading causes of preventable death.[249] More people die of lung cancer than of colon, breast, and prostate cancer combined.

The incidence of lung cancer has declined in men more sharply than in women.[19] Since 2010, incidence has declined in both genders, with overall mortality rates higher among men.[19]

Black males have the highest death rate and Asian/Pacific Islanders, American Indian/Alaska natives, and Hispanic males have the lowest death rate. Among women, whites have the highest mortality, whereas Asian/Pacific Islanders and Hispanic females have the lowest death rate from lung cancer.[248,478]

### Risk Factors

Risk factors for lung cancer include environment (smoking, secondhand smoke, occupational exposure, and air pollution), nutrition, and genetic factors.[273] Age, family history, and medical history (especially lung disease) also influence occurrence, morbidity, and mortality.

**Cigarette Smoking.** Cigarette smoking (more than 20 cigarettes per day) remains the greatest risk factor for lung cancer, accounting for 90% of all lung cancer deaths in men who smoke, and 80% of all lung cancer deaths in women. Of all lung cancers, 85% to 90% occur in smokers, although, remarkably, fewer than 20% of cigarette smokers develop this disease. Duration of smoking is strongly associated with lung cancer risk.[312] However, occasional smoking or lower numbers of cigarettes smoked each day also elevates risk for lung cancer.[10] Approximately 15.5% of the adult population smoke cigarettes, with a slightly higher prevalence in men (17.5%) than women (13.5%).[106] The highest smoking rates are seen in the American Indian/Alaska Native population, followed by non-Hispanic multiple race individuals, non-Hispanic blacks, and whites.[106] In 2015, e-cigarettes were the most common form of tobacco used by middle and high school students.[439]

The number of pack-years is calculated by multiplying the packs of cigarettes consumed per day by the number of years of smoking. Lung cancer risk is increased as the amount of packs smoked per year increases.

Smoking increases the risk for heart disease, stroke, lung cancer, and chronic obstructive lung disease.[101] Smoking also increases the risk for other types of cancer, such as acute myeloid leukemia and cancers of the bladder, cervix, esophagus, larynx, mouth, pharynx, stomach, and kidney. Moreover, smoking and exposure to smoke is associated with infertility, preterm delivery, low birth weight, and sudden infant death syndrome.[94]

Current smoking (any amount) is associated with an increased risk of mortality, including deaths from smoking-related cardiovascular disease, COPD, and lung cancer.[461] Former heavy smokers have a 39.1% lower risk of lung cancer within five years of smoking cessation, however, it is still three times higher than the risk to never smokers after 25 years of smoking cessation.[217] Ten years after smoking cessation, risk of dying from lung cancer is half of that compared to an active smoker.[16] The elimination of cigarette smoking would virtually eradicate SCLC. Smoking cessation also reduces the risk for coronary heart disease, stroke, and cancers of the mouth, throat, and bladder.[16]

Cigarettes contain nicotine, water, and numerous other chemicals. The substances left after removal of nicotine and water is termed "tar." Tar contains over 3500 compounds including the following major known carcinogens: polycyclic aromatic hydrocarbons, aza-arenes, *N*-nitrosamine, aromatic amines, heterocyclic aromatic amines, aldehydes, arsenic, nickel, chromium, and cadmium.[312] Tobacco smoking also results in increased exposure to ethylene oxide, aromatic amines, and other agents that cause damage to DNA.[378] For this reason, the risk of lung cancer is increased in a smoker who is also exposed to other carcinogenic agents, such as radioactive isotopes, polycyclic aromatic hydrocarbons and arsenicals, vinyl chloride, metallurgic ores, and mustard gas.

**Marijuana.** Marijuana is similar to tobacco smoke in that it contains many of the same organic and inorganic compounds that are carcinogens, cocarcinogens, or tumor promoters. Marijuana does not contain nicotine. Smokers hold the inspiration for longer periods than traditional smoke and therefore three times more tar and five times more carbon monoxide is inhaled compared to regular cigarettes.[516] Moreover, since marijuana is typically smoked without a filter, there is a higher concentration of particulates in the airways compared to cigarettes.[516] Marijuana produces inflammation, edema, and cell injury in the tracheobronchial mucosa of smokers and contributes to oxidative stress, which is a precursor for DNA mutations.[459] However, cannabinoids modulate and minimize free radical production and inhibit tumor angiogenesis. In addition, cannabinoid receptors are not found in the lung epithelial cells.[330] Cannabinoids have been shown to inhibit certain breast, lung, and brain cancers,[276] although other studies have shown an increase in head, neck, and lung cancers.[202] Respiratory symptoms such as cough, shortness of breath, sputum production, and asthma exacerbations are more frequently reported in marijuana users compared with tobacco smokers.[112]

The risk of marijuana smoking is difficult to ascertain because people often smoke both tobacco and marijuana. It is known that cannabis causes large airway inflammation, increased mucus production, increased airway resistance, and lung hyperinflation.[294] For those with low or occasional use of marijuana, early studies show little effect on $FEV_1$. However, decrements are seen in flow rates with long-term and high-volume usage.[382] Studies are largely inconclusive at this time due to methodological issues, confounding variables, and the lack of studies looking at older marijuana users compared to younger users. The relationship between smoking marijuana and lung cancer is still controversial at the time of this writing.[112,232,294]

**Environmental Tobacco Smoke.** In 1992, the EPA declared secondhand smoke or ETS to be a group A human carcinogen. ETS caused more than 7300 deaths from lung cancer each year between 2005 and 2009.[83] ETS has decreased in recent years due to legislation banning smoking in some public arenas, however exposures still exist in some public places and in homes (especially multiunit housing).

**Occupational Exposure.** Occupational exposures are associated with an increased risk for lung cancer, especially in those exposed to asbestos, silica, radon, heavy metals, and polycyclic aromatic hydrocarbons.[312] In 2013, the International Agency for Research on Cancer listed outdoor air pollution as a class I human carcinogen.[286] Exposure to vehicle exhaust is associated with an elevated risk of lung cancer, with higher exposures commonly found in urban settings.

Indoor exposure to radon, which is a colorless, odorless gas that is a product of uranium and radium produced from the decomposition of rocks and soil, is a known carcinogen and the second leading cause of lung cancer.[312] Concentrations vary geographically (more in the northern United States), and radon gas levels are highest in basements, nearest the soil.[174] Other sources of radon exposure include radioactive waste and underground mines; exposure to tobacco smoke multiplies the risk of concurrent exposure to radon.

Other occupational or environmental risk factors associated with lung cancer include diesel exhaust, coal tar fumes, untreated mineral oils, mustard gas, vinyl chloride, benzopyrenes, silica, formaldehyde, copper, chromium, cadmium, arsenic, alkylating compounds, sulfur dioxide, and ionizing radiation.

**Links Between COPD, Emphysema, and Lung Cancer.** Those with COPD have a 2- to 4-fold increase in the risk of cancer in both genders with increased risk seen in those with newly diagnosed and/or mild COPD.[428] Emphysema is also linked to an increased risk for lung cancer in both genders and regardless of smoking status.[428] Lung cancer is typically detected in areas that are affected by emphysema and not in the preserved healthy lung tissue. Genetic mutations, DNA damage with altered repair, and chronic inflammation are actively being researched as the connecting link between these conditions.

**Nutrition.** Other risk factors may include low consumption of fruits and vegetables,[196] high intake of fried or well-done red meat, reduced physical activity, and increased dietary fat (especially diets high in saturated or animal fat and cholesterol).[312] There is limited evidence that low vitamin D levels are associated with an increased risk of lung cancer

**Genetic Susceptibility.** Genomic studies have identified key chromosomal loci that may be associated with an elevated risk for lung cancer.[312] Although some of the familial risk could be from ETS exposure, a shared genetic risk is strongly suggested. Regardless, the independent effect on lung cancer risk is strongly amplified by cigarette smoking.[69,123]

## Pathogenesis

As mentioned, there is a clear relationship between cigarette smoking and the development of SCLC. The effects of smoking include structural, functional, malignant, and toxic changes. DNA-mutating agents in cigarettes produce alterations in both oncogenes and tumor-suppressor genes, as well as genes that assist with DNA repair.

The genetic basis for lung cancer is rapidly evolving, with the identification of specific genes and mutations leading to targeted treatment interventions. Several genetic and epigenetic changes are common to all lung cancer histologic types, whereas others appear to be tumor-type specific. The sequence of changes remains unknown.[273] There appears to be an interaction between estrogen receptors and epidermal growth factor in the lung that plays a role in women's susceptibility to lung cancer.[150]

There are numerous mutations in NSCLCA that are targets for new treatments. There are two main genetic lesions in NSCLC that are being explored: mutations in the epidermal growth factor receptor (EGFR) and the KRAS genes.[496] Overexpression of EGFR can be found in 62% of people with NSCLC and contributes to angiogenesis, metastasis, and inhibition of apoptosis.[496] Mutations in the RAS genes can be found in 10% to 50% of NSCLC (typically active or former smokers) and leads to rapid cellular proliferation.[165,496] Other mutations are also actively being screened and include BRAF, HER2, and MET.[223]

All lung cancers are thought to arise from a common bronchial precursor cell, with differentiation then proceeding along various histologic pathways from poorly differentiated small cell cancer to the more intermediate undifferentiated large cell tumors, to the more differentiated adenocarcinomas and squamous cell tumors. Perhaps the histologic changes (thickening of bronchial epithelium, damage to and loss of protective cilia, mucous gland hypertrophy and hypersecretion of mucus, and alveolar cell rupture) that occur more frequently in long-term smokers than nonsmokers predispose the lungs to changes. This results in a multistep process involving the development of hyperplasia, metaplasia, dysplasia, carcinoma in situ, invasive carcinoma, and metastatic carcinoma.

**Small Cell Lung Cancer.** SCLC is an aggressive cancer with a poor prognosis and is strongly associated with smoking. Less than 2% of those with SCLC are never-smokers. Genetic mutations are seen in tumor-suppressing genes (TP53, RB1) and enzymes related to chromatic remodeling.[416] When the cells become so dense that there is almost no cytoplasm present and the cells are compressed into an ovoid mass, the tumor is called small cell carcinoma or oat cell carcinoma. SCLC develops most often in the bronchial submucosa, the layer of tissue beneath the epithelium, and tends to be located centrally, most often near the hilum of the lung. These tumors can produce hormones that stimulate their own growth and the rapid growth of neighboring cells, causing bronchial obstruction and pneumonia with early intralymphatic invasion. Lymphatic and distant metastases are usually present at the time of diagnosis.

**Non–Small Cell Lung Cancer.** There are three types of non–small cell lung cancer: adenocarcinoma, squamous cell carcinoma, and large cell. Squamous cell carcinomas arise in the central portion of the lung near the hilum, projecting into the major or segmental bronchi. Although these tumors tend to grow rapidly, they often remain located within the thoracic cavity, making curative treatment more likely compared with other NSCLC types.

## Clinical Manifestations

Symptoms of early stage localized lung cancer do not differ much from pulmonary symptoms associated with chronic smoking (e.g., cough, dyspnea, and sputum production), so the person does not seek medical attention. Often times, lung cancer may be an incidental finding on a routine chest radiograph. Symptoms may include persistent cough, hemoptysis, hoarseness, weight loss, shortness of breath, fatigue, generalized weakness, and persistent pulmonary infections.[15] With metastatic lung cancer, patients may present with bone pain, headaches, balance or gait dysfunction, new onset weakness, or jaundice.[15]

**Small Cell Lung Cancer.** As with NSCLC, symptoms may not arise until the disease is widespread. Signs and symptoms of SCLC depend on the size and location of the tumor and the presence and extent of metastases. Because SCLCs most commonly arise in the central endobronchial location in people who are almost exclusively long-term smokers, typical symptoms are a result of obstructed airflow and consist of persistent, new, or changing cough, dyspnea, stridor, wheezing, hemoptysis, and chest pain.[62]

Intercostal retractions on inspiration and bulging intercostal spaces on expiration indicate obstruction. As obstruction increases, bronchopulmonary infection (obstructive pneumonitis) often occurs distal to the obstruction. Centrally located tumors cause chest pain with perivascular nerve or peribronchial involvement that can refer pain to the shoulder, scapula, upper back, or arm.

SCLC is (more often than NSCLC) associated with several paraneoplastic syndromes, including ectopic hormone production, such as with Cushing syndrome (adrenocorticotropic hormone), production of hormones by tumors of nonendocrine origin, or production of an inappropriate hormone (antidiuretic hormone or SIADH) by an endocrine gland. Neuroendocrine cells containing neurosecretory granules exist throughout the tracheobronchial tree. This phenomenon is important because resulting signs and symptoms may be the first manifestation of underlying cancer.

**Non–Small Cell Lung Cancer.** The less common peripheral pulmonary tumors (large cell) often do not produce signs or symptoms until disease progression produces localized, sharp, and severe pleural pain increased on inspiration, limiting lung expansion; cough and dyspnea are present. Pleural effusion may develop and limit lung expansion even more.

Tumors in the apex of the lung, called *Pancoast tumors,* occur both in squamous cell and adenocarcinomatous cancers. Symptoms do not occur until the tumors invade the brachial plexus. Destruction of the first and second ribs can occur. Paralysis, elevation of the hemidiaphragm, and dyspnea secondary to phrenic nerve involvement can also occur. Horner syndrome can also develop, causing drooping of an eyelid and loss of sweating on one side of the face.

Other manifestations may include digital clubbing, skin changes, joint swelling associated with hypertrophic pulmonary osteoarthropathy (see discussion of this condition in "Cystic Fibrosis" above), decreased or absent breath sounds on auscultation, or pleural rub (inflammatory response to invading tumor).

### Metastasis

The rich supply of blood vessels and lymphatics in the lungs enables the disease to metastasize rapidly. Lung cancers spread by direct extension, lymphatic invasion, and through the vasculature. Tumors spread by direct invasion in the bronchus of origin; others may invade the bronchial wall and circle and obstruct the airway. Intrapulmonary spread may lead to compression of lung structures other than airways, such as blood or lymph vessels, alveoli, and nerves.

Direct extension through the pleura can result in spread over the surface of the lung, chest wall, or diaphragm. Carcinomas of the lung of all types metastasize most frequently to the regional lymph nodes, particularly the hilar and mediastinal nodes. Supraclavicular, cervical, and abdominal channels may also be invaded. Tumors originating in the lower lobes tend to spread through the lymph channels.

Lung cancer generally has a widespread pattern of hematogenous metastases. This is caused by the invasion of the pulmonary vascular system. After tumor cells enter the pulmonary venous system, they can be carried through the heart and disseminated systemically. Tumor emboli can become lodged in areas of organ systems where vessels become too narrow for their passage or where blood flow is reduced.

The most frequent site of extranodal metastases is the adrenal gland. Lung cancer can also metastasize to the brain, bone, and liver before presenting symptomatically. Brain metastases constitute nearly one-third of all observed recurrences in people with resected NSCLC of the adenocarcinoma type. Metastases to the brain can result in CNS symptoms of confusion, gait disturbances, headaches, or personality changes.

Tumor spread intrathoracically to the mediastinum and beyond can produce superior vena cava (SVC) syndrome, with swelling of the face, neck, and arms, and neck and thoracic vein distention more common in the early morning or after being recumbent for several hours. SVC syndrome is usually a sign of advanced disease. If left untreated, SVC syndrome results in cerebral edema and possible death. Increased intracranial pressure, headaches, dizziness, visual disturbances, and alteration in mental status are signs of progressive compression. Cardiac metastasis can occur and result in arrhythmias, congestive heart failure, and pericardial tamponade.

As a form of secondary malignancy, the lungs are the most frequent site of metastases from other types of cancer. Any tumor cell dislodged from a primary neoplasm can find its way into the circulation or lymphatics, which are filtered by the lungs. Carcinomas of the kidney, breast, pancreas, colon, and uterus are especially likely to metastasize to the lungs.

## MEDICAL MANAGEMENT

PREVENTION. Prevention is the key to reducing the need for treatment of lung cancer. Targeted state and federal antitobacco programs have contributed to significant drops in cigarette consumption.

*Healthy People 2020* set a goal of reducing the lung cancer mortality rate from 50.6 per 100,000 population (1998 figure) to 45.4 per 100,000 population, representing a 10% improvement. *Healthy People 2020* outlined a systematic approach to health improvement that includes methods for lung cancer prevention through prevention of tobacco use and tobacco addiction in all age, ethnic, and socioeconomic groups. *Healthy People 2020* is available online at http://www.health.gov/healthypeople/.

Another strategy for lung cancer prevention is chemoprevention.[350] Chemoprevention involves the administration of drugs, nutraceuticals, or nutritional supplements in those with early stages of cancer aimed at absorbing free oxygen radicals and blocking or reversing carcinogenesis. Reducing exposures to workplace toxins, such as asbestos, arsenic, chromium, nickel, radon, and tar, is also another risk-reduction strategy.[297,344] Noninvasive biomarkers are being investigated, however none have sufficient validity at the time of this writing.[350]

Screening for lung cancer in current or former smokers can be employed to monitor for early signs of lung cancer. The American Cancer Society recommends annual lung cancer screening with a low-dose CT scan (LDCT) for certain people at higher risk for lung cancer who meet the following conditions: 55 to 74 years of age, current smoker or have quit smoking for the last 15 years, and have a 30 pack-year history.[18] For most people, screening to detect early lung cancer is not recommended.[20]

Other strategies for lung cancer prevention include eliminating arsenic in drinking water (the need to do so applies to smokers only), adopting a diet high in fruits and vegetables, eating foods high in carotenoids, and reducing ETS.

**DIAGNOSIS.** Many lung cancers are detected on routine chest radiographs in patients presenting for unrelated medical conditions without pulmonary symptoms, although 90% of the people with lung cancer are symptomatic at diagnosis. Many people mistake the signs of lung cancer for other common issues, such as a cold, flu, or aging. Unfortunately, chest radiographs are not sensitive enough to show tumors when they are small and operable and routine screening is not supported by evidence. A chest scan called low-dose spiral or helical CT detects tumors too small to be seen on radiographs. There are some concerns with low-dose spiral CT, such as cost, false-positive findings, unnecessary biopsies of small benign tumors, and a small risk of death from procedures that result from a (+) finding.

Despite the above limitations, a chest radiograph is usually the first diagnostic tool employed. If the patient is high risk or there is an abnormality on the radiograph, a CT may be ordered. If there is suspicion of metastasis to the spinal cord, an MRI may be indicated. Physicians may also utilize a positron emission tomography (PET) scan to detect metastatic spread. In a PET scan, a radioactive sugar substance (fluorodeoxyglucose) is injected. Cancer cells are quite metabolically active and therefore readily take up fluorodeoxyglucose, which can then be visualized in a PET scanner.

Once a tumor is found, a biopsy via bronchoscopy or fine-needle aspiration may be used to capture cells for histology. For NSCLC, specimens are tested for common mutations such as EGFR, BRAF V600e for specific targeted treatments. Other routine procedures include evaluation of serum chemistry values to look for electrolyte abnormalities (see Chapter 5), especially those associated with paraneoplastic syndrome (see Chapter 9), evaluation of renal and hepatic function, hematologic profiles, and ECG analysis.

**STAGING.** The eighth edition of the American Joint Committee on Cancer's *Cancer Staging Manual* was released in 2018. Staging of lung cancer uses the TNM or tumor, nodes, metastasis system (see explanation in Chapter 9). Clinical staging involves any information about the cancer that occurs prior to surgical resection and is indicated with a "c" and pathologic stage, includes results from the biopsy. An uppercase "C" refers to certainty and includes imaging, biopsies, and surgical resection. There are five subcomponents of "T" referring to tumor size. "M" includes metastasis outside of the thoracic cage and the presence of a malignant pleural effusion. "N" refers to nodal involvement, and a zero after the "N" or "M" indicates no nodal involvement or metasastasis.[142]

SCLC is usually not considered a surgical disease requiring staging but rather is designated as limited or extensive disease. Limited disease is defined by involvement of one lung, the mediastinum, and either or both ipsilateral and contralateral supraclavicular lymph nodes (i.e., disease that can be encompassed in a single radiation therapy port). Spread beyond the lung, mediastinum, and supraclavicular lymph nodes is considered extensive disease.

**TREATMENT.** Awareness of the influence of growth factors, oncogenes, and tumor suppressor genes, as well as signal transduction and angiogenesis pathways on the natural history of cancer cells, has led to attempts to develop new molecular-based strategies directed at interrupting tumor cell growth. Treatments using monoclonal antibodies, inhibitors, antiangiogenic substances, and gene transfer and alteration are still under investigation.[65]

In the meantime, current treatment with new agents used in combination, as well as when combined with radiation and hormones, has led to an improved response rate in the treatment of some lung cancers.[64] Photodynamic therapy is used successfully with tumors in the airways. Photochemical sensitization of the tumor precedes laser therapy that causes necrosis of the cancer.[336] Chemotherapy approaches are numerous and address different targets. Newer agents that inhibit EGFRs are showing promise alone and in combination with other drugs.[470]

***Small Cell Lung Cancer.*** For those with early stage SCLC who receive combination chemotherapy, surgery may be considered and results in high response rates (65%-85%); however, most patients present with extensive disease and are not eligible for surgery.[265]

SCLC is quite sensitive to radiation therapy, which, in conjunction with chemotherapy, is now routinely administered to those with limited disease.[47] Individuals with extensive disease usually receive combination chemotherapy initially. Other treatment options depend on the clinical manifestations and client needs (e.g., radiation therapy may be administered to the brain, bone, spine, or other sites of metastasis). Immunotherapy is on the rise as targeted intervention for many types of cancer, including lung. T cell immune checkpoint inhibitors can prolong life in early stage SCLC. Other novel interventions, such as the use of cytokines, and vaccines, are under investigation.[68]

***Non–Small Cell Lung Cancer.*** The standard treatment for stages I and II lung cancer includes surgical resection (lobectomy, segmentectomy, pneumonectomy). Anyone with positive surgical margins and mediastinal lymph node disease may also get radiation therapy and chemotherapy. Those who are poor surgical candidates receive radiotherapy or stereotactic body radiotherapy or radiofrequency ablation.[398]

For stage III NSCLC, surgery may be offered. Many tumors at this stage are unresectable or have metastasized, necessitating a combined chemoradiation approach.[398] The present regimens include platinum based chemotherapies that have a significant side-effect profile, including neuropathy. Identification of specific mutations is now a part of the clinical practice guidelines for lung cancer, enabling more precise chemotherapy regimens to be implemented.[160] Multimodal treatments can cure up to 20% of individuals with locally advanced lung cancer.[398] Approach to stage IV disease is palliative and depends on location and extent of disease and clinical manifestations. For example, clients who develop spinal cord compromise secondary to metastatic disease can be palliated effectively with short-course external-beam radiotherapy. Chemotherapy has also been useful in improving palliation and increasing survival in stage IV disease.[442]

**PROGNOSIS.** The curability of lung cancer remains poor because many people present with advanced disease. Prognosis is considerably better in cases of NSCLC than in cases of SCLC. The overall prognosis is influenced by the stage of the disease at presentation, the cell type, the treatment that can be given, and the status of the client at the time of diagnosis (e.g., people who are ambulatory respond to treatment better than those who are confined to bed more than 50% of the time). The 5-year survival rate for stage 1A1 NSCLC is 92%, which drops to 68% in stage IB, 60% in stage IIB, 36% in stage IIB, and less than 1% in stage IVB.[17] For those with SCLC and limited disease, median survival is 16 to 24 months, with a 5-year survival rate of 14%.[343] In those with extensive stage disease in SCLC, the survival is typically less than 10 months with a 1% to 5% five-year survival rate.[416]

Other factors associated with poor prognosis include weight loss of more than 10% of body weight in 6 months, generalized weakness, male gender, age older than 70 years, prior chemotherapy, elevated serum lactic dehydrogenase levels, low serum sodium, and elevated alkaline phosphatase levels. African American men and women are more likely to be diagnosed with lung cancer and to die from lung cancer.[22]

SPECIAL IMPLICATIONS FOR THE THERAPIST 15.16

### *Lung Cancer*

People with lung cancer often have concomitant lung disease and other comorbidities, which contribute to a poor performance status. In lung cancer, decreased functional performance is associated with poorer outcomes for surgery and chemotherapy. Pulmonary rehabilitation has been studied in people with lung cancer and has shown improvements in 6-minute walk test distance, quality of life, anxiety/sadness, and increased $FEV_1$.[492] Home based programs after treatment have been shown to be effective in increasing fitness and quality of life, with good adherence rates.[149] There is also evidence that prehabilitation can reduce postoperative pulmonary complications, decrease hospital length of stay, improve exercise capacity, and improve FVC, however the studies reporting these favorable findings have limitations such as risk of bias and small sample sizes.[73,352]

#### Metastasis

Metastatic spread of pulmonary tumors to the long bones and to the vertebral column, especially the thoracic vertebrae, is common, occurring in as many as 50% of all cases. Local metastases by direct extension may involve the chest wall and may even erode the first and second ribs and associated vertebrae, causing bone pain and paravertebral pain associated with involvement of sympathetic nerve ganglia. Subsequently, chest, shoulder, arm, or back pain can be the presenting symptom but usually with accompanying pulmonary symptoms.

The client may not associate the musculoskeletal symptoms with the pulmonary symptoms, so the therapist must always remember to screen for medical disease. Cases of individuals with lung cancer and shoulder pain for which no local cause could be found have been reported, and in each case, radiotherapy to the ipsilateral mediastinum eliminated symptoms. Pain referred from intrathoracic involvement of the phrenic nerve was the suspected underlying pain generator.[269] Any time a mechanical cause is not found or the client fails to progress or improve in therapy, return to the physician is recommended for further diagnostic evaluation.

Spinal cord compression from extradural metastases of lung cancer usually occurs from direct extension of vertebral metastases or through venous spread. Tumors often invade the vertebral body first, followed by the pedicles, often in the thoracic vertebra.[309] Back pain is often the first sign and may occur as progressive back pain 6 months before the diagnosis is made. The pain may be constant and aggravated by Valsalva maneuver, sneezing or coughing, movement, and lying down, and diminished by sitting up. Weakness, sensory loss, and a positive Babinski reflex may be observed.

Radiation is usually the treatment of choice for epidural metastases from lung cancer. Neurosurgical intervention may be indicated if the area of compression has been previously irradiated to maximal tolerance. Surgical decompression may also be indicated if neurologic deterioration occurs during the initiation of radiation therapy. The treatment field extends two vertebral bodies above and below the level of blockage. Corticosteroids are prescribed to reduce swelling and inflammation around the cord.[183]

Apical (Pancoast) tumors do not usually cause symptoms while confined to the pulmonary parenchyma, but once they extend into the surrounding structures, the brachial plexus (C8 to T2) may become involved, presenting as a form of thoracic outlet syndrome. This nerve involvement produces sharp pleuritic pain in the axilla, shoulder (radiating in an ulnar nerve distribution down the arm), and subscapular area of the affected side, with atrophy and weakness of the upper extremity muscles and hand intrinsics. Trigger points of the serratus anterior muscle also mimic the distribution of pain caused by C8 nerve root compression and must be ruled out by palpation, lack of neurologic deficits, and possible elimination with appropriate trigger point therapy. Pancoast tumors may also masquerade as subacromial bursitis.

## DISORDERS OF THE PULMONARY VASCULATURE

### Pulmonary Embolism and Infarction

#### Definition and Incidence

Pulmonary embolism (PE) is the lodging of a blood clot in a pulmonary artery, with subsequent obstruction of blood supply to the lung parenchyma. Although a blood clot is the most common cause of occlusion, air, fat, bone marrow (e.g., fracture), foreign intravenous material, vegetations on heart valves that develop with endocarditis, amniotic fluid, and tumor cells (tumor emboli) can also embolize and occlude the pulmonary vessels.

Venous thromboembolism is the third leading vascular disease after heart attack and stroke. Approximately 10 million cases occur annually.[400] The yearly economic burden of VTE and stroke in the United States is estimated to be 7 to 10 billion dollars.[199] In individuals over the age of 80 there is an incidence of 1 per 100 people and the annual incidence rate exponentially increases each year after 80.[211,250,400] From age 45 on, the lifetime risk of developing VTE is 8%.[41] It is the most common cause of sudden death in the hospitalized population. Recently, an observed rate of recurrence of VTE in the year after discontinuation of anticoagulation suggests a high rate of reoccurrence of VTE for up to 10 years. Khan et al.[268] found that after diagnosis of a first unprovoked VTE, 36% of patients will experience a recurrent VTE within 10 years after discontinuation of anticoagulant treatment. Thus, once VTE occurs, clinicians should always consider this as a chronic disease with a substantial long-term burden.

### Etiologic and Risk Factors

The most common cause of PE is deep vein thrombosis (DVT) originating in the proximal deep venous system primarily of the lower extremity, but 20% come from the upper extremity (see further discussion in the DVT section of Chapter 12). Risk does not differ by sex, although it seems to be two times higher in men than in women when VTE related to pregnancy and estrogen therapy are not considered.[406] PE encompasses embolism from many sources, including air, bone marrow, arthroplasty cement, amniotic fluid, tumor, and sepsis. Before the introduction of routine prophylaxis with heparin (now low-molecular-weight heparin [LMWH]) or warfarin sodium (Coumadin), the incidence of DVT after hip fracture, total hip replacement, or other surgeries involving the abdomen, pelvis, prostate, hip, or knee was extremely high.

Three major physiologic risk factors linked with PE are (1) blood stasis (e.g., immobilization caused by prolonged trips, including air travel or spinal cord injury; bed rest, such as with burn cases, pneumonia, or obstetric and gynecologic clients; orthopedic injuries requiring fracture care with casting or pinning; and older or obese populations); (2) endothelial injury (local trauma) secondary to surgical procedures (as late as 1 month postoperatively), trauma, or fractures of the legs or pelvis; and (3) hypercoagulable states (e.g., oral contraceptive use, cancer, and hereditary thrombotic disorders).

Strong risk factors for PE (DVT) include immobility, surgery, and cancer.[144] About 20% of VTE are related to cancer, whereas surgery and immobilization each account for 15% of cases.[250,472] Risk is especially high for patients undergoing major lower extremity orthopedic surgery with postoperative rates at 1% despite pharmacologic thromboprophylaxis.[245] Heredity plays a factor in the formation of VTE with the most frequent heritable risk factors besides non-O blood group are the factor V Leiden and prothrombin gene mutations, with a prevalence in the European population of 3% to 7% and 1% to 2%, respectively.[308]

### Pathogenesis

In DVT, clots form primarily in the lower extremities at the popliteal or iliofemoral arteries (50%) and deep calf veins (5%), and less frequently in the upper extremities via the subclavian vein (up to 20%). Part or all of the clot may embolize, traveling through the venous system, the right side of the heart, and into the lungs. Each embolus is a mass of fresh or organizing thrombus comprised of alternating bands of red cells, fibrin strands, and leukocytes, with a rim of fibroblasts at the periphery. Any level of the pulmonary artery, from the main trunk to the distal branches, is a site for emboli to lodge. This causes an area of blockage and ischemic necrosis to the area perfused by that vessel.

PE ranges from peripheral and clinically insignificant to massive embolism and sudden death. PE may lead to $\dot{V}/\dot{Q}$ mismatch, which leads to hypoxia. PE and DVT should be considered part of the same pathologic process, and in fact, studies showed that a large percentage of people with DVT but no symptoms of PE also had evidence of PE on lung scanning. Conversely, people with PE often have abnormalities on ultrasonographic studies of leg veins.[193]

In addition to the loss of capillary beds, pulmonary emboli cause vasoconstriction as a result of vasoactive mediators released by activated platelets, and increase pulmonary vascular resistance, pulmonary hypertension, and right ventricular failure (in severe cases).

### Clinical Manifestations

Clients may be asymptomatic in the presence of small thromboemboli or sustain cardiac arrest, depending on the size and location of the embolus and the individual's preexisting cardiopulmonary status. Common symptoms in people with PE include dyspnea (84%) or deterioration of existing dyspnea, pleuritic chest pain (74%), apprehension (59%), and cough (53%). Common signs include tachypnea greater than 16 breaths/min (92%), rales (58%), accentuated S2 gallop (53%), tachycardia (44%), and fever (43%).

Other signs and symptoms may include hemoptysis, diaphoresis, S3 or S4 gallop, lower-extremity edema, cardiac murmur, and cyanosis.[144] Many of the symptoms and signs detected in people with acute PE are also common among individuals without PE, emphasizing the need for additional evaluation.

## MEDICAL MANAGEMENT

**DIAGNOSIS.** PE is difficult to diagnose because the signs and symptoms are nonspecific. Diagnosing PE clinically is problematic because its symptoms overlap with those of other conditions and because there are numerous causes of postoperative hypoxia (e.g., hypoventilation, narcotic effects, fluid overload, and postoperative atelectasis).[31]

Clinical screening and need for further testing are conducted using Wells PE and DVT criteria and nonimaging laboratory tests (especially D-dimer, which is a by-product of fibrin crosslinks). Di Nisio et al. recommend the revised Wells PE and DVT criteria and the Revised Geneva score.[144] In patients with "likely" VTE scores by the clinical decision rule, the negative predictive value of D-dimer testing is reduced, and these patients should therefore be referred for imaging immediately.[500,501] Negative clinical assessment and D-dimer tests may limit the need for further testing. Arterial blood gases are not helpful in the physician's differential diagnosis.

Using combinations of additional tests to rule out or rule in PE to make the diagnosis is optimal. V/Q scans can rule out PE if it is normal in the presence of normal radiographs and with no other cardiopulmonary disease.[289] Those patients with revised Wells DVT scores of likely and those classified as DVT scores of unlikely but with a D-dimer higher than the conventional fixed threshold should be referred for imaging. Compression ultrasonography has replaced contrast venography as the preferred method for the diagnosis of deep vein thrombosis and is performed following two main approaches: whole-leg compression ultrasonography evaluating the entire deep vein system from the groin to the calf or only the popliteal and femoral vein segments with limited (two-point) compression ultrasonography.[144] In those patients with an initial normal test for limited-compression ultrasonography, the compression ultrasonography should be repeated after 1 week to ensure the DVT has not extended beyond the popliteal space into the proximal veins.[38]

**PREVENTION AND TREATMENT.** The management of DVT and PE has changed dramatically in the last few years. Given the mortality of PE and the difficulties involved in its clinical diagnosis, prevention of DVT and PE is crucial. Primary prevention of DVT through the prophylactic use of anticoagulants is important for persons undergoing total hip replacement, major knee surgery, abdominal or pelvic surgery, prostate surgery, and neurosurgery. All patients who are hospitalized and immobile should be evaluated for risk of PE and placed on prophylaxis as appropriate.

Treatment for VTE is by anticoagulants and is divided into three phases: the acute phase of the first 5 to 10 days after VTE diagnosis, a maintenance phase of 3 to 6 months, and an extended phase beyond this period. During the acute phase, anticoagulant treatment options include subcutaneous low-molecular-weight heparin or fondaparinux, intravenous unfractionated heparin, or the direct oral factor Xa inhibitors rivaroxaban and apixaban.[144] LMWH is a common agent for prophylaxis because it prolongs the clotting time and allows the body time to resolve the existing clot, thereby preventing further development of the thrombus; it does not reduce the immediate embolic risk or enhance clot lysis. LMWHs have fewer major bleeding complications and do not require laboratory monitoring of coagulation tests to adjust medications. Anticoagulant therapy should be continued for at least 3 months to prevent early recurrences.[263] Anticoagulant therapy reduces the risk of recurrent VTE by 80% to 90%.[264,363] Because recurrent events and anticoagulant-related major bleeding are both associated with substantial morbidity and mortality, the current approach of anticoagulant therapy should be extended beyond 3 months when the risk of recurrence exceeds the risk of major bleeding.

## A THERAPIST'S THOUGHTS*

### *Assessment of Deep Vein Thrombosis*

As a profession, physical therapists need to do a better job of assessing for a DVT to prevent the progression to a PE. From 1989 to 2006, hospital DVTs increased 3.1 times from 35 to 107/100,000 population.[448] This increase in the number of patients with DVTs is alarming. Because physical therapists are often the first health care professional to get a patient out of bed after surgery, our profession needs to take the lead in knowing what is appropriate and use an evidence-based approach in mobilizing patients that are at risk of having a DVT.

Homans sign was first mentioned in the literature in 1943 by Dr. John Homans' colleagues.[228,229] Dr. Homans called it the dorsiflexion sign in a subsequent article in 1944 and described it as passive dorsiflexion that elicits calf pain.[227] The results in this study suggest that 42% of the patients being treated for existing DVT demonstrated a positive Homans sign. This trend of insufficient data to support the use of Homans sign continued in 1962 by McLachlin et al. when Homans sign was positive in only 8% of the patients with thrombi.[326] This was also noted in a systematic review by Urbano in 2001 that reported a range of 8% to 56% positive Homans sign in patients with confirmed DVTs.[480] Urbano stated in this article, "This has led nearly all authors to declare that Homans' sign is unreliable, insensitive, and nonspecific in the diagnosis of DVT."[480] Riddle and Wells added to this in 2004 when they stated, "Studies have demonstrated that the Homans sign has essentially no diagnostic value with sensitivities on the order of 50%."[404] The author knows of no other case in which such a statement has been made about a test.

Homans sign has been declared to have no value since 2004 and yet this clinical test continues to be used by physical therapists and clinicians. This suggests that clinicians are choosing to either ignore the evidence or are unaware of the evidence. Riddle and Wells suggest the use of a clinical risk assessment as described by Wells be used for patients suspected to have a DVT in the outpatient setting.[404] Although the Wells DVT assessment tool was originally designed for the outpatient setting, slightly modified versions exist for other populations such as primary care[366,481] and inpatient, [121]and it continues to be explored in the geriatric population[437] and those patients with cancer.[260] The Wells criteria has repeatedly demonstrated good screening properties in multiple studies ranging from 96% to 100% sensitivity and 35% to 70% specificity.[441,2,423,72] Besides being highly sensitive, use of the Wells risk assessment is practical because it can be completed in less than 2 minutes in practiced individuals. Thus, it is a rapid evidence-based screening tool that helps identify appropriate referral to a physician for DVT.

Deep venous thrombosis may lead to pulmonary embolism, which may be lethal to our patients. I would advocate and invite all physical therapists to take a pledge to never again use or teach screening tools that have been demonstrated to have no diagnostic value, such as Homans sign, and to consider the evidence in support of using a clinical risk assessment such as the Wells criteria or a similar tool that is specific to the population that the therapist is serving.

*John Heick, PT, DPT, PhD, OCS, NCS, SCS

***Implantation of Filter in Inferior Vena Cava.*** Surgical implantation of a filter in the inferior vena cava (IVC) may be used to prevent PE. The indication to use an IVC filter should be carefully evaluated in each individual case, based on a clear understanding of the objectives of filter insertion and consideration of alternatives.

The generally accepted indication for IVC filter insertion is the presence of a recently diagnosed proximal DVT plus an absolute contraindication to therapeutic anticoagulation; recurrent PE even during anticoagulation therapy, and presence of anticoagulation-related complications.[391] Contraindications to therapeutic anticoagulation include:

- Current or recent active major bleeding that cannot be treated acutely.
- Frank intracranial bleeding in the past 5 days.
- Need for a major surgical procedure in the next 2 weeks.
- Severe, prolonged thrombocytopenia.[180]

As a general rule, the use of an IVC filter does not change the need for or duration of anticoagulation. Because most (or all) individuals who have IVC filters inserted have a proximal DVT, therapeutic anticoagulation should be instituted as soon as it is considered safe to do so (usually within a few days after insertion). Although IVC filters may reduce the risk of PE in individuals with DVT, they do not prevent extension of DVT, including extension through the filter. The duration of anticoagulation is the same as for individuals with DVT but without a filter.[180]

To better achieve the desired performance goals of IVC filters, it is crucially important to adhere to established criteria in selecting candidates for filter insertion. Selection criteria are clearer for the use of permanent filters as opposed to retrievable ones. A variety of both permanent and retrievable filters are available in the interventionists' armamentarium.[365] It would be important for the physician to be familiar with the particular characteristics of each device and have knowledge of comparative advantages and disadvantages.

The filter itself is a potential focus of thrombosis. IVC filters are viewed as a temporizing measure for preventing life-threatening PE.

As indicated in the case of proximal DVT, concomitant anticoagulation after filter placement is desirable when there are no contraindications, so as to prevent early IVC filter thrombosis. In the case of filter thrombosis, PE can occur either through collateral pathways or by means of propagation of caval clots through the filter. *Caval clot* is the term used to refer to an inferior vena cava filter occluded by a thrombosis.

The diagnosis of IVC filter thrombosis is based on radiologic investigations. IVC thrombosis appears to be one of the more frequent and major complications of filter placement.[465]

Inferior vena cava syndrome (IVCS) is a result of obstruction of the IVC. It can be caused by invasion or compression by a pathologic process (enlarged aorta [abdominal aortic aneurysm], the gravid uterus [aortocaval compression syndrome], and abdominal malignancies such as colorectal cancer) or by thrombosis in the vein itself. Thrombosis at the insertion site is a common complication for filter placement.[476]

IVCS presents with a wide variety of signs and symptoms, making a clinical diagnosis difficult. Primary symptoms may include edema of the lower extremities and tachycardia. Other symptoms of IVC obstruction include progressive ascites and scrotal edema.[444]

Occlusion of the IVC is considered life-threatening. Because the IVC is not centrally located, there are some asymmetries in drainage patterns. The gonadal veins and suprarenal veins drain into the IVC on the right side, but into the renal vein on the left side, which, in turn, drains into the IVC.

In one study, placement of IVC filters in individuals with advanced cancer denoted a direct correlation between the onset of kidney failure or hydronephrosis with placement of the IVC filter. The elevated pressure from obstruction may ultimately damage the kidney and can result in loss of its function.[379] It is noted that blood return with an "absent" IVC is inadequate, despite adequate collaterals, resulting in chronic venous hypertension in the lower extremities and causing venous stasis that precipitates thrombosis. "Absent" refers to a blocked or obstructed IVC (in this case caused by thrombosis under the filter, i.e., caval clot).

Essentially, the IVCS (blockage under the IVC filter) causes fluid to leak into surrounding tissue. This hypovolemia in the central circulatory system will lead to hypotension (low blood pressure), which presents significant problems for individuals with cardiac problems especially anyone with congestive heart failure.

Inferior Vena Caval Thrombosis and Treatment. Both surgical and medical options are available to treat IVC thrombosis depending on the underlying pathophysiology. Surgical therapy of IVC thrombosis encompasses caval interruption and thrombectomy. Currently, both of these modalities are being used less frequently.[163]

The goals of drug therapy center on managing the primary impact of the DVT and the impact of embolization. Medical management can include anticoagulation and thrombolytic agents.[163] However, there is the risk in use of thrombolytic agents to cause iatrogenic tear of the IVC and internal bleeding.

Prognosis with Inferior Vena Cava Filter. Knowledge of the prognosis with the IVC filter is limited. This device was designed to eliminate DVT. However, with the pending complications of IVC thrombosis and the likelihood of collateral vascularization, there is still a risk of developing DVT. In addition, even with placement of the IVC filter there is still the possibility of a proximal DVT that will not be addressed with the filter. Anticoagulation remains a therapy with placement of an IVC filter. Complications of IVCS include bilateral lower-extremity edema, which may lead to compartment syndrome.[435] Hypotension as a result of hypovolemia (secondary to fluid leak into surrounding tissue) remains a cardiac complication.

Studies have found a low rate of complications associated with use of the IVC filter. Complications such as filter migration, caval thrombosis, new venous thromboembolism, filter fragmentation, and erosion of the caval wall were thought to have minimal significance if they occurred.[425]

**PROGNOSIS.** PE is the primary cause of death for as many as 100,000 people each year (perhaps double that amount) and a contributory factor in another 100,000 deaths annually. Approximately 10% of victims die within the first hour, but prognosis for survivors (depending on underlying disease and on proper diagnosis and treatment) is generally favorable. Clients with PE who have cancer, congestive heart failure, atrial arrhythmias, or chronic lung disease have a higher risk of dying within 1 year than do clients with isolated PE.

Small emboli resolve without serious morbidity, but large or multiple emboli (especially in the presence of severe underlying cardiac or pulmonary disease) have a poorer prognosis. PE may recur despite LMWH therapy, most commonly in people with massive PE or in whom anticoagulant therapy has been inadequate. PE is the leading cause of pregnancy-related mortality in the United States.

## Pulmonary Arterial Hypertension

### Definition and Incidence

PAH is high blood pressure in the pulmonary arteries defined as a mean pulmonary artery pressure of 25 mm Hg or greater, pulmonary capillary wedge pressure of less than 15 mm Hg, and pulmonary vascular resistance above 3 Wood units.[141,327,469]

There are five categories of PAH. Group 1 refers to PAH related to genetic predisposition, drugs, connective tissue disorders, HIV infection, portal hypertension, congenital heart disease, and schistosomiasis. Group 2 refers to PAH from left heart disease inclusive of congenital inflow/outflow tract obstruction and congenital cardiomyopathy. Group 3 is PAH resulting from lung disease or hypoxia and includes COPD, interstitial lung disease, sleep-disordered breathing, hypoventilation, high altitude, and developmental lung disease. Group 4 refers to chronic thromboembolic disease. Group 5 is "miscellaneous" and includes hematologic disorders, systemic disorders such as sarcoidosis, and metabolic disorders.[181]

PAH is relatively rare, with 2 to 7.6 cases per million adults/year.[469] PAH occurs most commonly in young and middle-aged women with a mean age at onset of 45 to 65 years for idiopathic PAH and 37 years for other types of PAH.[327,469] It has no known cause (idiopathic), but is associated with systemic diseases such as scleroderma and congenital conditions.

### Pathogenesis

PAH is characterized by diffuse narrowing of the pulmonary arterioles caused by hypertrophy of smooth muscle in the vessel walls, thrombosis, inflammation, and formation of fibrous lesions in and around the vessels.[387] Every layer of the pulmonary vasculature is affected. The underlying cause of these changes is unknown, however it is now recognized that defects in endothelial function, pulmonary vascular smooth muscle cells, and platelets may all be involved in the pathogenesis and progression of PAH. Endothelial factors are altered, favoring vasoconstriction. It is likely that a combination of genetic and environmental factors contribute to this condition.[32,327,469]

In those with PAH, elevations are seen in platelet activation factors, autoantibodies, and cytokines that contribute to vasoconstriction, inflammation, and thrombosis. Endothelial cell injury may result in an imbalance in endothelium-derived mediators that reduce the production of nitrous oxide ($N_2O$), a vasodilator, from the airways resulting in vasoconstriction.

Defects in ion channel activity in smooth muscle cells in the pulmonary artery also may contribute to vasoconstriction and vascular proliferation.[236] These changes create increased resistance to the blood flow from the right side of the heart to the lungs, leading to cor pulmonale.

Secondary pulmonary hypertension is caused by any respiratory or cardiovascular disorder that increases the volume or pressure of blood entering the pulmonary arteries; narrows, obstructs, or destroys the pulmonary arteries; or increases the pressure of blood leaving the heart (pulmonary veins).

Increased volume or pressure overloads the pulmonary circulation whereas narrowing or obstruction elevates the blood pressure by increasing resistance to flow within the lungs. For example, COPD destroys alveoli and associated capillary beds, thus increasing pressure through the remaining vasculature. Left-sided heart failure causes blood to "back up" and thus resistance is increased.

With persistent PAH, there is an increase in the afterload on the right ventricle, resulting in hypertrophy. Some have adaptive RV hypertrophy and maintain adequate cardiac output, while others have maladaptive hypertrophy resulting in right heart failure (cor pulmonale).[387] Because the pediatric heart is better able to withstand this afterload, there is a better prognosis for the pediatric population.[327] In the 10% of patients with a hereditable pattern of PAH, there are mutations in transforming growth factor beta, Caveloin-1 (a membrane protein involved in cell signaling), and KCNK3 (potassium channels in pulmonary artery smooth muscle).[387]

### Risk Factors and Clinical Manifestations

Risk factors for PAH are increasing age, genetic predisposition, exposure to asbestos, parasitic infection, Down syndrome, history of DVE or PE, cocaine or amphetamine use, smoking, exposure to some chemotherapy agents, maternal use of selective serotonin reuptake inhibitors, use of weight loss drugs, clotting disorders, chronic kidney disease, hepatitis B/C infection, thyroid disease, and female gender.[346] Signs and symptoms of secondary pulmonary hypertension are difficult to recognize in the early stages when the symptoms of the underlying disease are more prominent. People may attribute their symptoms to a known underlying cardiopulmonary disorder, therefore delaying physician evaluation.

The most common symptoms of primary or secondary pulmonary hypertension are typical cardiorespiratory symptoms, such as fatigue, weakness, chest discomfort or pain, syncope, peripheral edema, abdominal distention, and unexplained SOB, beginning with exercise and later occurring with minimal activity or at rest.[36] In children, the most typical presentation includes dyspnea on exertion and syncope.[35]

#### MEDICAL MANAGEMENT

**DIAGNOSIS.** PAH can be difficult to diagnose, and there is usually a delay of 1 to 2 years between onset of symptoms and diagnosis. Patients undergo an ECG and chest radiograph. A $\dot{V}/\dot{Q}$ scan may be employed to rule out PE. Pulmonary function tests and overnight oximetry help the physician exclude diagnoses such as COPD, pulmonary fibrosis, and sleep apnea. Serologic testing for systemic diseases such as HIV, SLE, and scleroderma are also performed. The 6- minute walk test is used to assist with prognosis.[162] Patients may undergo a Doppler ultrasound and ultimately require a right heart catheterization for diagnosis.[141,469]

**TREATMENT.** Treatment includes medications targeting various pathways involved in PAH as well as supportive measures.[469] Initially patients are started on calcium channel blockers. If they don't respond sufficiently, those considered low risk are treated with combination therapy, whereas those with high risk are treated with medications that target the prostacyclin pathway.[469] If the disease worsens, patients can be considered for lung transplantation.

Prostacyclin pathway medications enhance pulmonary vasodilation and also have antiinflammatory and antiplatelet effects.[469] They can be given by IV, inhalation, or subcutaneously. Calcium channel blockers may also be used, although they are effective in only a small proportion of those with PAH. Medications impacting nitric oxide may also be used. Nitric oxide causes the smooth muscles in pulmonary arteries to relax, inducing vasodilation. The endothelin pathway can also be targeted, as endothelin is a strong vasoconstrictor.[469]

Supportive measures are also implemented to maximize heart functioning. Pharmacologic interventions include the use of diuretics, digoxin, and anticoagulants.[469] Sodium and fluid restrictions may be implemented to manage cor pulmonale. Low intensity symptom limited aerobic exercise is recommended, while keeping oxygen saturation above 90%.[469] Isometric exercises are associated with syncope and should be avoided.

**PROGNOSIS.** Median survival for PAH has improved to six years. The progression of PAH varies for each affected individual, but prognosis is poor without heart–lung transplantation. Some individuals may live 5 to 6 years from the time of diagnosis, but most people have a downhill course over a shorter period of time (2-3 years) with a fatal outcome.

The cause of death is usually right ventricular failure or sudden death; sudden death occurs late in the disease process.

Secondary PAH can be reversed if the underlying disorder is successfully treated. If the hypertension has persisted long enough for the medial smooth muscle layer to hypertrophy, secondary PAH is no longer reversible.

**SPECIAL IMPLICATIONS FOR THE THERAPIST 15.17**

*Pulmonary Hypertension*

Impairment of exercise performance is associated with PAH because pulmonary vascular resistance and pulmonary artery pressure increase dramatically with exercise. With exercise, cardiac output should rise to meet the increasing demands of the peripheral musculature. However, due to elevations in the pulmonary arteriole system and increased pulmonary vascular resistance, the right ventricle begins to fail, leading to lower volumes circulated to the lungs and to the left side of the heart. This may be especially true at the onset of exercise when a large volume of venous blood is returned to the right side of the heart. Exercise is also limited by hypoxemia and shortness of breath that results from a V/Q mismatch and early onset anaerobic muscle metabolism. With persistent low cardiac output, peripheral muscles fatigue earlier in the exercise bout.[162] For these reasons, clients with PAH must be closely monitored when participating in activities or therapy that requires increased physical stress.

Maintenance of adequate systemic blood pressure is essential, and the therapist must be familiar with the medications used and potential side effects, especially if blood pressure is altered pharmacologically. A drop in blood pressure can indicate heart failure. Inhaled $N_2O$ or prostacyclin, which are endogenous vasodilators, increase oxygen consumption at the same workload during exercise, thereby improving exercise capacity. $N_2O$ use is diminishing as a result of its toxicity and cost.[305]

Secondary PAH may occur in clients with connective tissue diseases, such as scleroderma, because the disease affects the vasculature of several organs, including the lungs (pulmonary fibrosis) and kidneys. The arterioles usually demonstrate intimal proliferation with progressive luminal occlusion. The development of hypertension often indicates the onset of an accelerated scleroderma renal crisis. Medical treatment is toward control of the blood pressure.

## Cor Pulmonale

### Definition and Incidence

*Cor pulmonale,* also called *pulmonary heart disease,* is the failure of the right ventricle (RV) due to a pulmonary cause and results in impaired ejection.[208] Right ventricular failure can occur due to increases in pressure in the pulmonary circulation, from right coronary artery occlusion and infarction, from tricuspid pathology, and from left ventricular failure. This section will focus on the pulmonary issues that result in overload and failure of the RV, which is called cor pulmonale.

Chronic cor pulmonale occurs most frequently in adult male smokers, although the incidence in women is increasing as heavy smoking in females becomes more prevalent. The actual prevalence of cor pulmonale is difficult to determine because cor pulmonale does not occur in all cases of chronic lung disease and because routine physical examination and laboratory tests are relatively insensitive to the presence of pulmonary hypertension. It has been estimated that cor pulmonale accounts for 5% to 10% of organic heart disease.

### Etiologic and Risk Factors

Pulmonary vascular diseases and respiratory diseases (e.g., emphysema or chronic bronchitis) are the primary causes of cor pulmonale. Emphysema and chronic bronchitis cause more than 50% of cases of cor pulmonale in the United States. When a PE has been sufficiently massive to obstruct 60% to 75% of the pulmonary circulation, acute cor pulmonale can occur. Cor pulmonale is frequently the cause of death in COPD.[499] Cor pulmonale can also result from pulmonary artery hypertension.

Cor pulmonale can also develop under conditions of sustained elevations in intrathoracic pressure associated with mechanical ventilation (and PEEP). The intrathoracic vessels narrow, leading to reduced cardiac output and possible cor pulmonale. Chronic widespread vasculitis, such as occurs in association with the collagen vascular disorders (e.g., rheumatoid arthritis, SLE, dermatomyositis, polymyositis, Sjögren syndrome, CREST [*c*alcinosis cutis, *R*aynaud phenomenon, *e*sophageal dysfunction, *s*clerodactyly, and *t*elangiectasis] syndrome accompanying scleroderma), can also cause chronic cor pulmonale. Occasionally, widespread radiation pneumonitis can be the underlying cause.

Other (uncommon) causes include pneumoconiosis, pulmonary fibrosis, kyphoscoliosis, pickwickian syndrome, lymphangitic infiltration from metastatic carcinoma, and obliterative pulmonary capillary changes that cause vasoconstriction and later, hypertension. The feature common to all these conditions that predisposes to cor pulmonale is hypoxia, which leads to vasoconstriction.[499]

### Pathogenesis

Sustained elevation in pulmonary arterial hypertension can be mediated through persistent vasoconstriction, abnormal vascular structural remodeling, or vessel obliteration (see "Pulmonary Arterial Hypertension" above). Cor pulmonale develops as these factors increase pulmonary vessel pressure and overload in the right ventricle. Normally, the RV is a thin-walled (heart) muscle able to meet an increase in volume and pressure, but long-term pressure overload from hypertension causes the tissue to hypertrophy. In late cor pulmonale, there is ventricular dilation, diastolic dysfunction which results in systemic edema.[208] In the case of acute cor pulmonale caused by PE, the thrombus breaks loose and lodges at or near the bifurcation of the main pulmonary artery. Whether caused by vascular abnormalities or embolic obstruction, there is a marked fall in pressure necessary to drive blood through the compromised vascular bed because the RV is compromised. Decreased output from the RV reduces the volume in the left ventricle, resulting in a reduced cardiac output, hypotension, and potentially shock.[208] Increased pressures in the RV also contribute to tricuspid regurgitation, further contributing to elevated venous pressures and systemic congestion. This systemic congestion interferes with the functioning of the kidneys, intestines, and liver.[208]

### Clinical Manifestations

Evidence of cor pulmonale may be obscured by primary respiratory disease and appear only during exercise testing. The heart appears normal at rest, but with exercise, cardiac output falls and the ECG shows right ventricular hypertrophy. Other symptoms include signs of systemic congestion, such as weight gain and jugular venous distension, a third heart sound, and signs of low cardiac output such as hypotension, tachycardia, cool extremities, and oliguria[208] (see Fig. 15.4).

With a large pulmonary embolus, sudden severe, central chest pain can occur, caused by acute dilation of the root of the pulmonary artery and secondary to ischemia. The person may lose consciousness, and death may occur within minutes if the thrombus is large and does not dislodge. If the thrombus is small or moves more peripherally, acute cor pulmonale develops rather than sudden death.

### MEDICAL MANAGEMENT

**DIAGNOSIS.** Diagnosis is made on the basis of physical examination, radiologic studies, ECG, and echocardiogram. Echocardiograms are used to characterize RV chamber size and dimensions. Right heart catheterization may be used to determine RA and RV pressures, cardiac output, and pulmonary vascular resistance.[208] PFTs may be used to characterize pulmonary disease as the cause or contributor to cor pulmonale.

**TREATMENT.** The underlying respiratory condition contributing to cor pulmonale must be addressed while simultaneously optimizing the function of the RV. Diuretics are used to optimize volume in the right ventricle, avoiding fluid overload, which worsens RV contractility. Inotropes may also be used to improve RV output. In emergent situations, norepinephrine can maintain arterial pressures as well as ECMO and ventricular assist devices.[208]

**PROGNOSIS.** Because cor pulmonale generally occurs late during the course of chronic lung diseases, the prognosis is poor. Once congestive signs appear, the average life expectancy is 2 to 5 years, but survival is significantly longer when uncomplicated emphysema is the cause. Although cor pulmonale can be caused by obstructive and restrictive lung diseases, restrictive lung diseases have a lower life expectancy once they reach the stage of cor pulmonale.

## Collagen Vascular Disease

Collagen vascular diseases, now more commonly referred to as diffuse connective tissue diseases, are diseases that have an autoimmune component and affect numerous organs, including the lungs.[247] Collagen vascular diseases include scleroderma, rheumatoid arthritis, systemic lupus erythematosus (SLE), polymyositis, dermatomyositis, and Sjögren syndrome.[247] Any part of the airway can be impacted, with pulmonary hypertension and interstitial lung disease (ILD) the most common. Prognosis for interstitial lung disease associated with collagen vascular diseases is better than for typical ILD.[247] Pulmonary issues may precede the diagnosis of collagen vascular diseases. Pulmonary hypertension is common in those with collagen vascular disease and significantly contributes to morbidity and mortality.[247] Finally, those with collagen vascular disease are at a higher risk for developing cancers such as lung cancer and liquid tumors (lymphoma, leukemia).[247]

ILD occurs in 30% to 60% of those with rheumatoid arthritis (RA).[247] People with RA may also experience airway disease, including bronchiectasis and bronchiolitis.[247] Eighty percent of those with scleroderma will have lung involvement, typically interstitial lung disease.[247] In SLE, the most common lung manifestation are pleuritis, pleural effusions, and community-acquired pneumonia.[247]

Treatment for pulmonary manifestations associated with collagen vascular diseases depends on whether this is an early manifestation or exacerbation. Some medications such as immunosuppressants and antirheumatic medications increase the risk of getting interstitial lung disease.[322] Medications may be stopped temporarily to determine if they have contributed to the onset of ILD. Treatments may also include supplemental oxygen, bronchodilators, antibiotics for infection, steroids, reflux medications, immune suppressants, biologics, or antirheumatic medications.[322] Typically, lung transplantation is ruled out due to the manifestations of the underlying collagen vascular disease.[322]

## DISORDERS OF THE PLEURAL SPACE

### Pneumothorax

#### Definition

Pneumothorax (PTX) is an accumulation of air or gas in the pleural cavity caused by a defect in the visceral pleura or chest wall. The result is collapse of the lung on the affected side. Pneumothorax is classified as primary spontaneous (no underlying lung disease), secondary spontaneous (lung disease present), or traumatic (e.g., rib fracture, puncture) (Fig. 15.24).[39] With high-resolution imaging, lung disease has been revealed in some with primary PTX, leading some to approach PTX by size and cardiovascular sequela.

#### Incidence and Risk Factors

Risk factors include tall and thin body habitus, male gender, and smoking. Two modes emerge for incidence of PTX: between the ages of 10 and 30 years and 60 to 64 years.[462] The incidence of primary spontaneous pneumothorax is 7.4 to 18 per 100,000 in males and 1.2 to 6 per 100,000 in females.[306]

The most common causes of iatrogenic pneumothorax are transthoracic needle lung biopsy, subclavian vein catheterization, thoracentesis, transbronchial lung biopsy, and positive pressure ventilation. Surgical procedures that involve the chest wall and abdomen also can precipitate pneumothorax.

#### Pathogenesis

When air enters the pleural cavity, the lung collapses and a separation between the visceral and parietal pleurae occurs (see Fig. 15.3), altering the negative pressure of the pleural space. This disruption in the normal equilibrium between the forces of elastic recoil and the chest wall causes the lung to recoil by collapsing toward the hilum. Depending on the individual's overall lung function, a loss of 40% may be present before symptoms appear.[415] The result is SOB and mediastinal shift toward the unaffected side, compressing the opposite lung. The causative pleural defect may be in the lung and visceral pleura (lung lining) or the parietal pleura (chest wall lining). After chest trauma, both air and blood are likely to escape into the pleural space. This is called *hemopneumothorax*.

*Spontaneous pneumothorax* occurs when there is an opening on the surface of the lung, allowing leakage of air from the airways or lung parenchyma into the pleural cavity. Most often this happens when an emphysematous bleb (blister-like formation) or bulla (larger vesicle) or other weakened area on the lung ruptures. Other causes include inflammation leading to degradation of the visceral pleural, bronchial tree anomaly, malnutrition and disorders of connective tissue, TB, sarcoidosis, ARDS, CF, and PCP.[306] Spontaneous pneumothorax can occur during sleep, at rest, or during exercise and can progress to become a tension pneumothorax.

*Traumatic pneumothorax* occurs when air enters the chest wall as a result of laceration, penetrating or nonpenetrating chest trauma, such as a rib fracture, stab, or bullet wound that tears the pleura.

*Open pneumothorax* is a type of traumatic pneumothorax that occurs when air pressure in the pleural space equals barometric pressure because air that is drawn into the pleural space during inspiration (through the damaged chest wall and parietal pleura or through the parietal pleura and damaged visceral pleura) is forced back out during expiration. This can rapidly lead to hypoventilation and hypoxia.

*Iatrogenic pneumothorax* develops as a result of direct puncture or laceration of the visceral pleura during attempts at central line placement, percutaneous lung aspiration, thoracentesis, or closed pleural biopsy. Direct alveolar distention can occur with anesthesia, cardiopulmonary resuscitation, or mechanical ventilation with PEEP.

*Tension pneumothorax* can result from any type of pneumothorax and is life-threatening. In tension pneumothorax, the site of pleural rupture acts as a one-way valve, permitting air to enter on inspiration but preventing its escape by closing up during expiration. Under these conditions, continuously increasing air pressure in the pleural cavity may cause progressive collapse of the lung tissue. Air pressure in the pleural space pushes against the already recoiled lung, causing compression atelectasis, and against the mediastinum, compressing and displacing the heart and great vessels. Venous return and cardiac output decrease.[510]

#### Clinical Manifestations

Dyspnea is the first and primary symptom of pneumothorax, but other symptoms may include a sudden sharp pleural chest pain, mild chest ache, fall in blood pressure, weak and rapid pulse, and cessation of normal respiratory movements on the affected side of the chest.[306] There will be diminished or absent breath sounds, and tachycardia on physical examination.

If the pneumothorax is large or if there is a tension pneumothorax, the mediastinum may shift toward the unaffected lung, causing the chest to appear asymmetric and the trachea to move to the contralateral side. The pain may be referred to the ipsilateral shoulder (corresponding shoulder on the same side as the

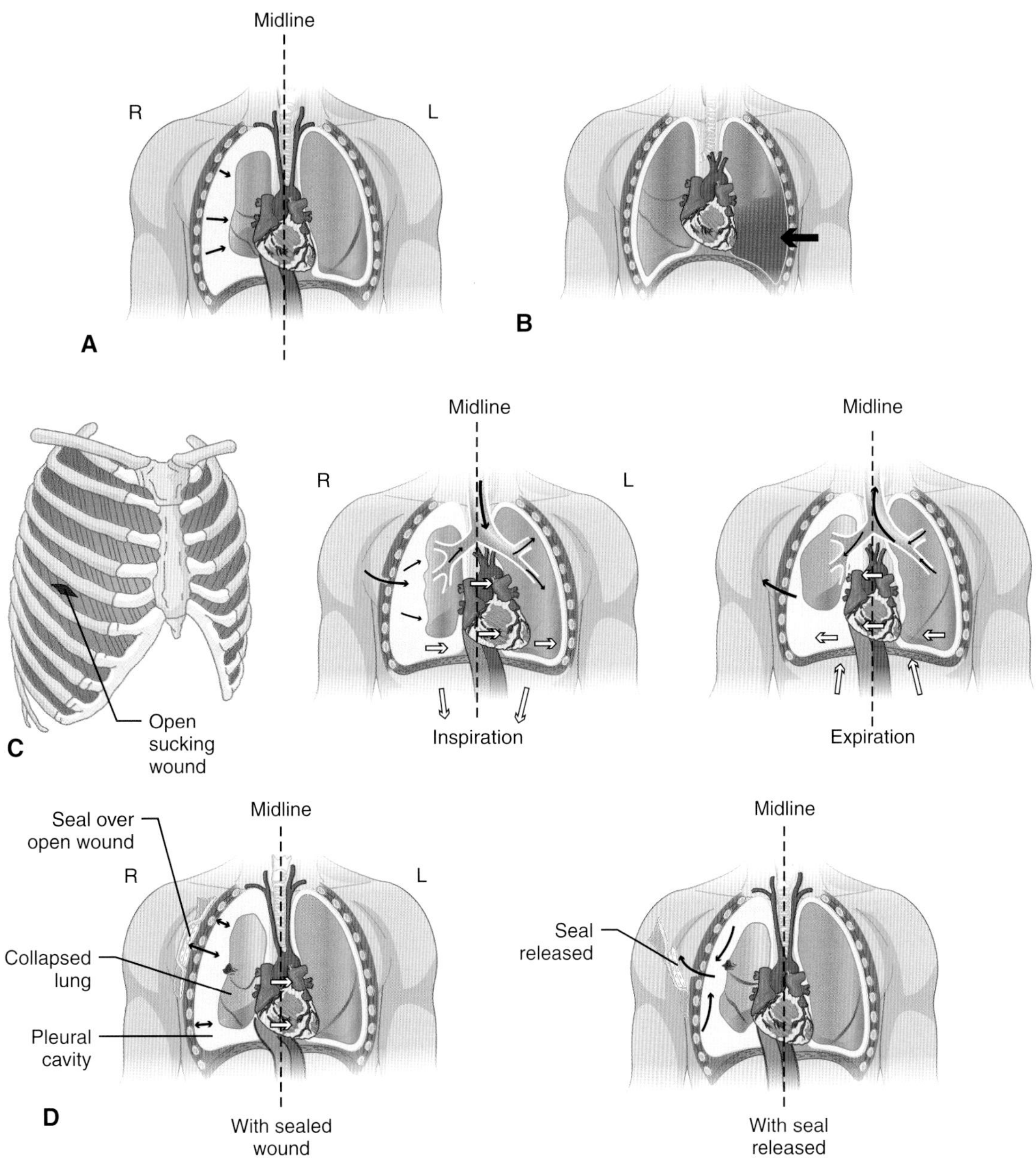


**Figure 15.24**

(A) Pneumothorax. Lung collapses as air gathers in the pleural space between the parietal and visceral pleurae. (B) Massive hemothorax, blood in the pleural space *(arrow)* below the left lung, causing collapse of lung tissue. (C) Open pneumothorax (sucking chest wound). Air movement *(solid arrows)* and structural movement *(open arrows)*. A chest wall wound connects the pleural space with atmospheric air. During inspiration, atmospheric air is sucked into the pleural space through the chest wall wound. Positive pressure in the pleural space collapses the lung on the affected side and pushes the mediastinal contents toward the unaffected side. This reduces the volume of air in the unaffected side considerably. During expiration, air escapes through the chest wall wound, lessening positive pressure in the affected side and allowing the mediastinal contents to swing back toward the affected side. Movement of mediastinal structure from side to side is called mediastinal flutter. (D) Tension pneumothorax. If an open pneumothorax is covered (e.g., with a dressing), it forms a seal, and tension pneumothorax with a mediastinal shift develops. A tear in lung structure continues to allow air into the pleural space. As positive pressure builds in the pleural space, the affected lung collapses, and the mediastinal contents shift to the unaffected side. Tension pneumothorax is corrected by removing the seal (i.e., dressing), allowing air trapped in the pleural space to escape.

pneumothorax), across the chest, or over the abdomen. With severe or large tension pneumothorax, there may be compression of the mediastinum, causing a drop in cardiac output.

Clinical manifestations of tension pneumothorax include hypoxemia, dyspnea, and hypotension (low blood pressure) in addition to the other signs and symptoms of pneumothorax already mentioned. Increased intrathoracic pressure from a tension pneumothorax may result in neck vein distention. Untreated tension pneumothorax may quickly produce life-threatening shock and bradycardia.

## MEDICAL MANAGEMENT

**DIAGNOSIS AND TREATMENT.** Diagnosis is made by chest film at inspiration. CT is replacing the standard radiograph for diagnosis because it is more sensitive and can help determine number and size of blebs.[306] Blood gas measurements indicate the degree of respiratory impairment. The presence of dyspnea, tachycardia, decrease or loss of breath sounds, percussive hyperresonance, decreased fremitus, asymmetric chest wall movement, and subcutaneous emphysema (swelling and crepitus with palpation) will assist in the diagnosis.

Depending on the size of the pneumothorax, no specific treatment is required for primary spontaneous pneumothorax of less than 20% beyond rest and the administration of oxygen to relieve dyspnea.[482] However, recurrences are frequent and associated with increased mortality in secondary spontaneous pneumothorax.

For large pneumothorax or recurrent pneumothorax, patients may have a needle aspiration of the air, placement of a chest tube, or video-assisted thoracic surgery (VATS) procedures to remove blebs with or without pleurodesis. Placement of a chest tube is standard procedure for traumatic pneumothoraces.[39] A recent systematic review demonstrated quicker resolution of the PTX with chest tubes, but a shorter length of stay with aspiration.[270]

Pneumothorax is an unwanted sequela to respiratory distress syndrome in premature infants. The use of prophylactic surfactant significantly reduces the incidence of pneumothorax in this population.[447]

It is not a good idea to travel by airplane (because of air pressure changes) or to have pulmonary function tests performed (e.g., CF) for at least 2 weeks after a pneumothorax has resolved. Encouraging smoking cessation is essential. In CF, airway clearance techniques that include positive expiratory pressure (oscillatory positive expiratory pressure) are usually held during pneumothorax and recovery as well.

**PROGNOSIS.** There is a low mortality rate with idiopathic pneumothorax, but a corresponding 15% mortality rate for pneumothorax associated with underlying lung disease. From 30% to 50% of affected persons experience a recurrence, and after one recurrence, subsequent episodes are much more likely. The physiologic events associated with tension pneumothorax are life-threatening, requiring immediate treatment.

**SPECIAL IMPLICATIONS FOR THE THERAPIST 15.18**

*Pneumothorax*

For patients with known rib fractures, therapists should observe carefully, because rib segments can shift during mobility and cause a pneumothorax, although it is not common. Lung auscultation along with vital signs and pulse oximetry can assist the therapist in determining changes to lung function as a result of movement. For patients who have invasive monitoring devices inserted or removed, therapists should await the results of a radiograph to rule out PTX prior to mobilization.

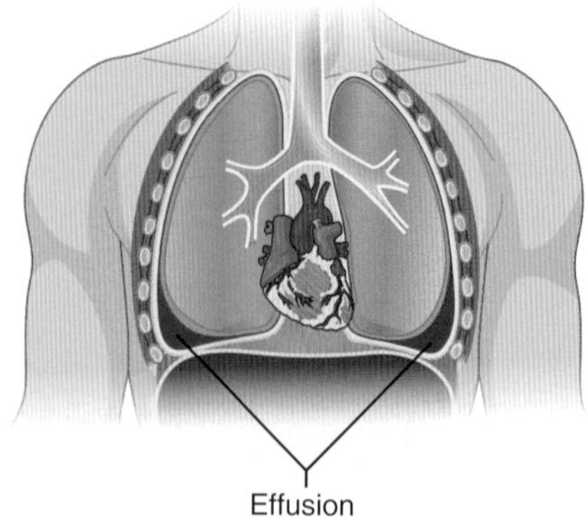


**Figure 15.25**

Pleural effusion, a collection of fluid in the pleural space between the membrane encasing the lung and the membrane lining the thoracic cavity, as seen on upright x-ray examination. Pleurisy (pleuritis) is an inflammation of the visceral and parietal pleurae. When there is an abnormal increase in the lubricating fluid between these two layers, it is called pleurisy with effusion.

## Pleurisy

### Definition and Etiologic Factors

Pleurisy (pleuritis) is an inflammation of the pleura caused by viral or bacterial infection, injury (e.g., rib fracture), or tumor (particularly malignant pleural mesothelioma). It may be a complication of lung disease, particularly of pneumonia, but also of TB, lung abscesses, influenza, SLE, rheumatoid arthritis, or pulmonary infarction.

### Clinical Manifestations

The symptoms develop suddenly, usually with a sharp chest pain that is worse on inspiration, coughing, sneezing, or movement associated with deep inspiration. Other symptoms may include cough, fever, chills, and rapid shallow breathing (tachypnea). The visceral pleurae are insensitive; pain results from inflammation of the parietal pleurae. Because the latter are innervated by the intercostal nerves, chest pain is usually felt over the site of the pleuritis, but pain may be referred to the lower chest wall, abdomen, neck, upper trapezius muscle, and shoulder. If the pleura near the diaphragm is inflamed, pain may be referred to the ipsilateral shoulder.[262] On auscultation, a pleural rub can be heard (sound caused by the rubbing together of the visceral and costal pleurae).

### Pathogenesis

There are two types of pleurisy: wet and dry. The membranous pleura that encases each lung is composed of two close-fitting layers; between these layers is a lubricating fluid. If the fluid content remains unchanged by the disease, the pleurisy is said to be dry. If the fluid increases abnormally, it is a wet pleurisy, or pleurisy with effusion (Fig. 15.25). Inflammation of the part of the pleura that covers the diaphragm is called diaphragmatic pleurisy and occurs secondary to pneumonia.

When the central portion of the diaphragmatic pleura is irritated, sharp pain may be referred to the neck, upper trapezius muscle, or shoulder. Stimulation of the peripheral portions of the diaphragmatic pleura results in sharp

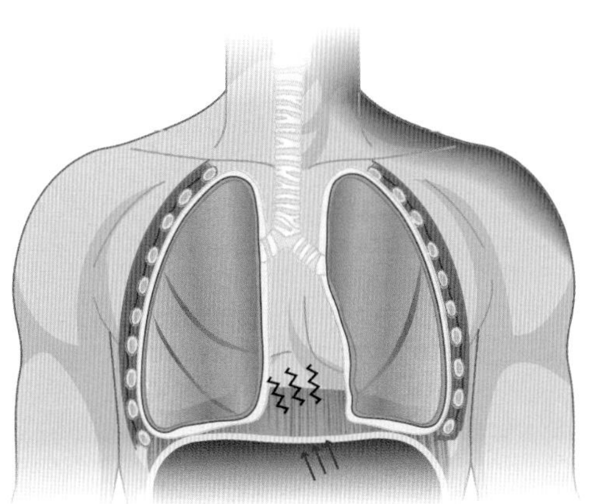

**Figure 15.26**

**Diaphragmatic pleurisy.** Irritation of the peritoneal (outside) or pleural (inside) surface of the central area of the diaphragm refers sharp pain to the neck, supraclavicular fossa, and upper trapezius muscle. The pain pattern is ipsilateral to the area of irritation. Irritation to the peripheral portion of the diaphragm refers sharp pain to the costal margins and lumbar region (not shown).

pain felt along the costal margins, which can be referred to the lumbar region by the lower thoracic somatic nerves (Fig. 15.26).

Wet pleurisy is less likely to cause pain because there usually is no chafing. The fluid may interfere with breathing by compressing the lung. If the excess fluid of wet pleurisy becomes infected with formation of pus, the condition is known as *purulent pleurisy* or *empyema*. Pleurisy causes pleurae to become reddened and covered with an exudate of lymph, fibrin, and cellular elements and may lead to pleural effusion. In dry pleurisy, the two layers of membrane may become congested and swollen and rub against each other, which is painful. Although only the outer layer causes pain (the inner layer has no pain nerves), the pain may be severe enough to require the use of a strong analgesic.

### MEDICAL MANAGEMENT

Physical examination may reveal a pleural rub or diminished breath sounds. Other pathologies should be ruled out when considering pleurisy. PE, PTX, and MI should be ruled out.[262] Diagnostic work-up may include chest radiograph or CT, ECG, and evaluation of the pleural fluid through thoracentesis.[262] Treatment is usually with nonsteroidal antiinflammatory drugs for pain management and treatment of the underlying condition. Sclerosing therapy for chronic or recurrent pleurisy may be recommended.

## Pleural Effusion

### Definition

Pleural effusion is the collection of fluid in the pleural space which exists between the parietal and visceral pleura. Typically there is slight negative pressure in this space, with a small amount of fluid that may allow the lungs to change shapes with respiration or assist with preventing atelectasis[239] (see Fig. 15.25). Pleural fluid is produced by the parietal pleura and reabsorbed by the parietal pleura and lymphatics.

### Incidence and Etiologic Factors

The causes of pleural effusions are best considered in terms of the underlying pathophysiology: transudates caused by abnormalities of hydrostatic or osmotic pressure or noninflammatory causes (e.g., congestive heart failure, cirrhosis with ascites, nephrotic syndrome, or peritoneal dialysis) and exudates resulting from increased permeability or trauma (e.g., infection, primary or secondary malignancy, PE, trauma including surgical trauma [e.g., cardiotomy]). In children, the most common causes of pleural effusion are congenital heart abnormalities and pneumonia.[515]

An exudative fluid has elevations in pleural proteins and lactate dehydrogenase levels. N-terminal pro-B-type natriuretic peptide or NT-proBNP is used to diagnose transudative fluids.[239]

Any condition that interferes with either the secretion or drainage of this fluid may lead to pleural effusion. Pleural effusion is common with heart failure and lymphatic obstruction caused by neoplasm. Less common causes include drug-induced effusion, pancreatitis, collagen vascular diseases (SLE or rheumatoid arthritis), intraabdominal abscess, or esophageal perforation. A person of any age can be affected, but it is more common in the older adult because of the increased incidence of heart failure and cancer.

### Pathogenesis

The most common mechanism of pleural effusion is migration of fluids and other blood components through the walls of intact capillaries bordering the pleura. When stimulated by biochemical mediators of inflammation, junctions in the capillary endothelium separate slightly, enabling leukocytes and plasma proteins to migrate out into affected tissues. Rupture of a blood vessel or leakage of blood from an injured vessel causes a form of pleural effusion called hemothorax (see Fig. 15.25).

Malignant pleural effusions occur in 50% of individuals with widespread cancer, largely from breast or lung cancers and lymphoma. Malignant pleural effusions produce exudative fluid from seeding of the cancer in the pleural space. The effusion can be a local effect of the tumor, such as lymphatic obstruction or bronchial obstruction with pneumonia or atelectasis. Lymphatic blockage from any cause can result in drainage of the contents of lymphatic vessels into the pleural space. It can also be a result of systemic effects of tumor elsewhere, but in either case, malignant cells in the pleural effusion of a person with lung cancer indicate an inoperable situation.

### Clinical Manifestations

Clinical manifestations of pleural effusion will depend on the amount of fluid present and the degree of lung compression. A small amount of effusion may be discovered only by chest radiograph. Large effusions cause clinical manifestations related to their volume and the rate at which they accumulate in the pleural space causing restriction of lung expansion. The diaphragm may be displaced caudally, impairing the length-tension relationship and power generation. Clients usually present with dyspnea on exertion that becomes progressive. They may develop nonspecific chest discomfort; sometimes the chest pain is pleuritic, which is a sharp, stabbing pain exacerbated by coughing or breathing and changes in position. Other symptoms characteristic of the underlying cause of pleural effusion may be the primary clinical picture (e.g., weight loss and fever with TB or cancer or signs of heart failure). Tachycardia, distant heart sounds, fixed jugular venous distention, edema of the extremities, and a paradoxical pulse may be part of the developing clinical picture.

### MEDICAL MANAGEMENT

**DIAGNOSIS.** Diagnosis begins with a chest radiograph and ultrasound, followed by CT and aspiration of pleural fluid. The pleural fluid is evaluated for pH; specific gravity; protein; stains and cultures for bacteria, TB, and fungi; eosinophilia count; and glucose concentration to aid in the differential diagnosis.[427]

**TREATMENT.** Pleural effusions, if symptomatic, are a medical emergency requiring immediate attention.[202] Treatment is different for transudative fluid as compared to exudative.[515] Transudative pleural effusions may resolve with antibiotics and treatment of the underlying medical condition. Exudative effusions, large transudative effusions, infected effusions (empyema), malignant effusions, and hemothorax require drainage. Drainage options include thoracentesis with drainage by a small- or large-bore catheter or chest tube. Those with recurrent effusions or malignant effusions may be treated with pleurodesis (sclerosing substance introduced into the pleural space to create an inflammatory response that scleroses tissues together) or a tunneled catheter to drain pleural fluid.

**PROGNOSIS.** Without treatment of the symptomatic client, cardiac function declines as venous return to the heart becomes limited by the effusion; it is essentially a restrictive heart disease. Ultimately, these individuals can go into complete circulatory shutdown. Prognosis for pleural effusion depends on the underlying cause. Those with malignant pleural effusions have a median life span of 4 to 7 months.[239] Those with empyema or recurrent pleural effusion may have long-term changes that mimic restrictive lung disease.

## Pleural Empyema

Pleural empyema (infected pleural effusion) is an accumulation of pus that occurs occasionally as a complication of pleurisy or some other respiratory disease, usually pneumonia. It is a normal response to infection but may also occur after external contamination (penetrating trauma, chest tube placement, or other surgical procedure) or esophageal perforation. Symptoms include dyspnea, coughing, ipsilateral pleural chest or shoulder pain, malaise, tachycardia, cough, and fever. In addition to radiographs, transthoracic aspiration biopsy may be done to confirm the diagnosis and determine the specific causative organism.

The condition is treated with intercostal chest tube drainage or pig-tail catheter drainage. Long-term antibiotics are generally needed, and attention must be paid to the person's nutritional status.[111] Intrapleural fibrinolytic agents may have some use in reducing need for surgery in people with empyema.[473]

## Pleural Fibrosis

Pleural fibrosis may follow inflammation (especially from asbestos), hemorrhagic effusion, and infection of the pleurae. It can present as localized plaques or diffuse. There appears to be a complex interaction of inflammatory cells, coagulation, profibrotic mediators, and growth factors in this process.[341] Early use of corticosteroids may decrease the incidence but is not effective in reducing established fibrosis. Surgical decortication can be effective in resolving symptoms.[234]

### REFERENCES

To enhance this text and add value for the reader, all references are included in the enhanced eBook on Student Consult that accompanies this textbook. The reader can view the reference source and access it online whenever possible.

CHAPTER 16

# The Gastrointestinal System

CELESTE KNIGHT PETERSON • ELIZABETH SHELLY (WOMEN'S HEALTH/PELVIC PT)

The gastrointestinal (GI) tract consists of upper and lower segments with separate functions. The upper GI tract includes the mouth, esophagus, stomach, and duodenum and aids in the ingestion and digestion of food. The lower GI tract includes the small and large intestines (Fig. 16.1). The small intestine accomplishes digestion and absorption of nutrients, whereas the large intestine absorbs water and electrolytes, storing waste products of digestion until elimination.

The enteric nervous system has become the focus of new research and discoveries in a new area of study referred to as *psychoneuroimmunology* with a subspecialty of clinical gastroenterology called *neurogastroenterology*. There are as many nerve cells in the human small intestine as there are in the human spinal cord, and the enteric nervous system can function completely independently of the central nervous system. The enteric nervous system is sometimes referred to as the "brain in the bowel."

Insight into the connections among emotions, brain function, and GI function has revolutionized our thinking about the so-called mind–body connection. New information is being discovered about the sensory functions of the intestine and how neural, hormonal, and immune signals interact. More than 30 chemicals of different classes (neuropeptides, neurotransmitters) transmit instructions to the brain, and all these chemicals are represented in the enteric nervous system.

Representatives of all the major categories of immune cells are found in the gut or can be recruited rapidly from the circulation in response to an inflammatory stimulus. The constant presence of these neurotransmitters and neuromodulators in the bowel suggests that emotional expression or active coping generates a balance in the neuropeptide-receptor network and physiologic healing beginning in the GI system. In fact, it has been suggested that because the enteric nervous system can function on its own, it is possible that the brain in the bowel can have its own psychoneuroses, such as the functional bowel syndromes discussed in this chapter (see Irritable Bowel Syndrome later).

Scientists continue to study influences of the nervous system on immune and inflammatory responses in the mucosal surfaces of the intestines along with the innervation of the immune system and the molecular communication pathways as these relate to emotions and thoughts and the GI system.[168] The gut immune system has 70% to 80% of the body's immune cells, and the protective blocking action of the secretory response in the gut is crucial to the integrity of the GI tract immune function and host defense. Studies suggest that the development and expression of the regional immune system of the GI tract is independent of systemic immunity. Nutrients have fundamental and regulatory influences on the immune response of the GI tract and therefore on host defense.

Reduction of normal bacteria in the gut after antibiotic treatment or in the presence of infection may interfere with the nutrients available for immune function in the GI tract. New understanding of intestinal disorders and new approaches to the management of these disorders are expected in the next decade.

## SIGNS AND SYMPTOMS OF GASTROINTESTINAL DISEASE

Clinical manifestations of GI disease can be caused by a variety of underlying conditions or disorders. The primary condition may be of GI origin, but some GI symptoms are part of a collection of systemic symptoms called *constitutional symptoms* and may be associated with any systemic condition (Table 16.1).

Nausea occurs when nerve endings in the stomach and other parts of the body are irritated and usually precedes vomiting. Intense pain in any part of the body can produce nausea as a result of the nausea-vomiting mechanism of the involuntary autonomic nervous system. Nausea can be caused by strong emotions and may accompany psychologic disorders; a variety of systemic disorders (e.g., acute myocardial infarction, diabetic acidosis, migraine, hepatobiliary and pancreatic disorders, Ménière syndrome, and GI disorders); and drugs such as morphine, codeine, excess alcohol, anesthetics, and anticancer drugs.

Vomiting may be caused by anything that precipitates nausea. Complications of vomiting include fluid and electrolyte imbalances, pulmonary aspiration of vomitus, gastroesophageal mucosal tear (Mallory-Weiss syndrome), malnutrition, and rupture of the esophagus.

Diarrhea (abnormal frequency, volume, or quality of stools) results in poor absorption of water and nutritive elements and electrolytes; fluid volume deficit; and

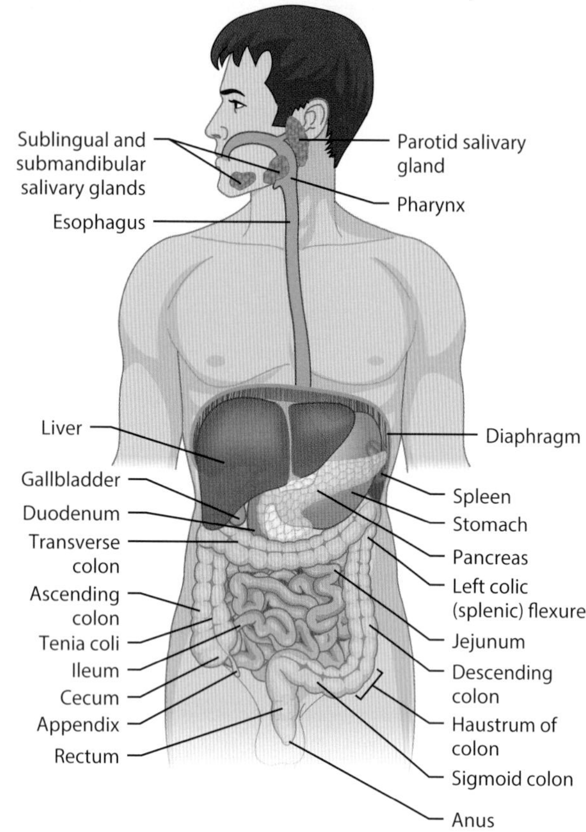


**Figure 16.1**

**The digestive system.**

**Table 16.1** Clinical Manifestations of Gastrointestinal Disease

| GI Signs and Symptoms | Constitutional Symptoms | GI Signs and Symptoms Associated With Strenuous Exercise |
|---|---|---|
| Nausea and vomiting | Nausea | Fecal urgency; diarrhea |
| Diarrhea | Vomiting | Abdominal cramps |
| Anorexia | Diarrhea | Belching |
| Constipation | Malaise | Nausea and vomiting |
| Dysphagia | Fatigue | Heartburn |
| Achalasia | Fever | |
| Heartburn | Night sweats | |
| Abdominal pain | Pallor | |
| GI bleeding: | Diaphoresis | |
| Hematemesis | Dizziness | |
| Melena | | |
| Hematochezia | | |
| Fecal incontinence | | |

*GI*, Gastrointestinal.

acidosis as a result of bicarbonate depletion, electrolyte imbalances, fluid and electrolyte imbalances, and acid–base balances. Other systemic effects of prolonged diarrhea are dehydration, electrolyte imbalance, and weight loss. The causes of diarrhea are many and varied (Table 16.2). Drug-induced diarrhea, most commonly associated with antibiotics, may not develop until 2 to 3 weeks after first ingestion of an antibiotic, but if the onset of diarrhea coincides with the use of drugs, it may resolve when the drug is discontinued.

Anorexia, diminished appetite or aversion to food, is a nonspecific symptom often associated with nausea, vomiting, and sometimes diarrhea. It may be associated with disorders of other organ systems including cancer, heart disease, and renal disease. It is the major component of eating disorders such as anorexia nervosa.

Anorexia-cachexia, a systemic response to cancer, occurs as a result of increased metabolic rate caused by the tumor cells and metabolites produced and released by tumor cells into the bloodstream. These effects of tumor cells stimulate the satiety center in the hypothalamus and produce appetite loss, gross alterations of metabolic patterns, and the profound systemic condition anorexia-cachexia. A downward spiral of symptoms occurs with appetite loss, leading to malnutrition, weight loss, muscular weakness, and a negative nitrogen balance that contributes to the development of cachectic wasting.

Constipation is a common condition affecting up to one-quarter of the American population; it is especially prevalent in women and people older than age 65 years.[132] Prevalence of constipation in nursing home residents is even higher, estimated at 67%.[192] Constipation occurs when fecal matter is too hard to pass easily or when bowel movements are so infrequent that discomfort and other symptoms interfere with daily activities. Because the definition of constipation varies among people and the condition is so common, standard criteria have been developed to better define it. The Rome IV diagnostic criteria[187] for functional constipation includes two or more of the following, present for the last 3 months and with symptom onset at least 6 months before diagnosis:

- Straining during at least 25% of defecations
- Lumpy or hard stools in at least 25% of defecations
- Sensation of incomplete evacuation for at least 25% of defecations
- Sensation of anorectal obstruction/blockage for at least 25% of defecations
- Manual maneuvers to facilitate at least 25% of defecations (e.g., digital evacuation, support of the pelvic floor)
- Fewer than three spontaneous defecations per week

Along with the above-listed criteria, constipation is diagnosed when loose stools are rarely present without laxatives and when there are insufficient symptoms to diagnose irritable bowel syndrome (IBS).

Constipation may occur as a result of many factors such as diet, dehydration (including lack of fluid intake), side effects of medication, acute or chronic diseases of the digestive system, inactivity or prolonged bed rest, emotional stress, personality, and lack of exercise (see Table 16.2).

Constipation is multifactorial, caused more often by lifestyle factors than by physiologic decline. Lifelong bowel habits, current diet, lack of fluid intake, and immobility are likely causes of constipation in adults older than 65 years.[82] Constipation may be the result of underlying

**Table 16.2** Causes of Diarrhea and Constipation

| | Diarrhea | Constipation |
|---|---|---|
| Neurogenic | Diabetic enteropathy<br>Hyperthyroidism | Irritable bowel syndrome<br>Central nervous system lesions (e.g., multiple sclerosis, Parkinson disease)<br>Dementia<br>Spinal cord tumors or lesions<br>Atomy |
| Muscular | Electrolyte imbalance<br>Endocrine disorder | Overactive or dyssynergic pelvic floor muscles<br>Obstructed defecation<br>Slow transit<br>Muscular dystrophy (Duchenne)<br>Electrolyte imbalance<br>Endocrine disorder (hypothyroidism)<br>Severe malnutrition (e.g., eating disorders, cancer)<br>Inactivity; immobility; back injury/pain |
| Mechanical | Incomplete obstruction (e.g., neoplasm, adhesions, stenosis)<br>Postoperative effect (e.g., gastrectomy, ileal bypass, intestinal resection, cholecystectomy)<br>Diverticulitis | Bowel obstruction<br>Extraalimentary tumors<br>Pregnancy |
| Other | Diet (including food allergy, lactose intolerance, food additives)<br>Supplements (creatine)<br>Malabsorption<br>Infectious/inflammatory disorders (including pelvic inflammatory disease)<br>Strenuous exercise<br>Irritable bowel syndrome<br>Caffeine<br>Medications:<br>• Antibiotics<br>• Nonprescription drugs<br>• Laxative abuse<br>• Magnesium (often found in antacids)<br>• Antihypertensive medication<br>• Nonsteroidal antiinflammatory drugs<br>• Proton pump inhibitors<br>• Antiarrhythmics | Diet (especially lack of dietary bulk or fiber, iron compounds)<br>Dehydration<br>Rectal lesions (e.g., anal fissure, hemorrhoids, abscess, rectocele, stenosis, ulcerative proctitis)<br>Psychologic variables (e.g., mental illness, busy lifestyle or ignoring the urge, emotional distress)<br>Medications:<br>• α-Adrenergic blocking agents<br>• Angiotensin-converting enzyme inhibitors<br>• Antacids with calcium carbonate or aluminum hydroxide<br>• Antiarrhythmics<br>• Anticholinergics<br>• Antiseizure drugs<br>• Antihistamines<br>• Antilipidemics<br>• Antiparkinson agents<br>• Antipsychotics<br>• Benzodiazepines<br>• Calcium channel blockers<br>• Nonsteroidal antiinflammatory drugs<br>• Opioids<br>• Antidepressants<br>• Diuretics |

Modified from DiPiro JT, Talbert RL, Yee GC, et al, editors: *Pharmacotherapy: a pathophysiologic approach*, ed 8, New York, 2011, McGraw-Hill.

organic disease or may be caused by lesions or structural abnormalities within the colon that narrow the intestines and/or rectum, slow transit alimentary canal, and defecatory disorders.

People with mechanical low back pain may develop constipation as a result of muscle guarding and splinting that causes reduced bowel motility. Pressure on sacral nerves from stored fecal content may cause an aching discomfort in the sacrum, buttocks, or thighs.[120] Individuals with a herniated disc and taking narcotic medications can be constipated, resulting in bearing down (Valsalva), which has the potential to make the herniation worse.

Constipation is typically divided into two groups: slow transit constipation and obstructed defecation. Slow transit constipation is a decrease in peristalsis, so physical therapy intervention will have little effect on this condition.

Constipation associated with obstructed defecation is the result of pelvic floor or anal sphincter dysfunction including pelvic floor dyssynergia, anismus, and disorders of increased pelvic floor muscle tone. In contrast to slow transit constipation, obstructed defecation responds well to muscle retraining.[66] In cases of obstructed defecation, the external anal sphincter contracts and tightens rather than relaxing and opening during defecation. Individuals with this type of constipation often strain to defecate and experience incomplete bowel emptying.[196]

*Dysphagia* (difficulty swallowing) produces the sensation that food is stuck somewhere in the throat or chest (esophagus). Dysphagia may be a symptom of many other disorders including neurologic conditions (e.g., stroke, Alzheimer disease, Parkinson disease), local trauma and muscle damage (including physical assault), and mechanical obstruction. Obstruction may be *intrinsic,* originating in the wall of the esophageal lumen (e.g., tumors, strictures, outpouchings called *diverticula*), or extrinsic, outside the esophageal lumen, such as a tumor or swelling that prevents the passage of food. Dysphagia caused by swelling can occur as a side effect of certain types of drugs such as antidepressants, antihypertensives, and asthma medications.

*Achalasia* is a failure to relax the smooth muscle fibers of the GI tract. This especially occurs as a result of failure of the lower esophageal sphincter (LES) to relax normally with swallowing. The affected person reports a feeling of fullness in the sternal region and progressive dysphagia.

Although the cause of achalasia is not known, the loss or absence of ganglion cells in the myenteric plexus of the esophagus appears to be a part of the cause. The myenteric plexus is the nerve plexus lying in the muscular layers of the esophagus, stomach, and intestines. Anxiety and emotional tension aggravate the condition and precipitate the attacks. Progression of the condition results in dilation of the esophagus and loss of peristalsis in the lower two-thirds of the esophagus.

*Heartburn (pyrosis)* and/or *indigestion (dyspepsia)*, characterized by a burning sensation in the esophagus usually felt in the midline below the sternum in the region of the heart, is often a symptom of gastroesophageal reflux and occur when acidic contents of the stomach regurgitate into the esophagus. Heartburn may be caused by the presence of a hiatal hernia; drugs such as alcohol and aspirin; and movements such as lifting, stooping, or bending over after a large meal. Indigestion also may be a potential manifestation of angina associated with coronary artery disease.

Certain foods act as muscle relaxants and can also bring on heartburn. For example, chocolate contains four substances that can relax the LES: caffeine, theobromine, theophylline, and fat. Fat-rich foods lower sphincter muscle pressure by release of cholecystokinin from the upper intestinal mucosa. Fat also delays emptying of the stomach, giving more opportunity for this effect to occur. Other implicated foods include spicy and highly seasoned foods, onions, alcohol, peppermint, and spearmint.

Emotional stress can stimulate the vagus nerve, which controls the secretory and motility functions of the stomach. Stimulation of this cranial nerve causes the stomach to churn, increases the flow of various gastric juices, and causes contraction and spasm of the pylorus (opening of the stomach into the duodenum). Heartburn can occur if some of the stomach contents are displaced into the esophagus during this nervous activity.

*Abdominal pain* accompanies a large number of GI diseases and may be mechanical, inflammatory, ischemic, or referred. Mechanical pain occurs because of stretching of the wall of a hollow organ or the capsule of a solid organ. *Inflammatory pain* occurs via the release of mediators such as prostaglandins, histamine, and serotonin or bradykinin that stimulate sensory nerve endings.

*Ischemic pain* occurs as tissue metabolites are released in an area of diminished blood flow. Ischemic pain may originate from decreased blood flow to organs or the abdominal muscles. Abdominal muscle trigger points can mimic pain from organ disease and can intensify visceral dysfunctions.[307] Abdominal muscle trigger points respond to physical therapy treatments.[232,269,311]

*Referred pain* usually is well localized and may be associated with hyperalgesia and muscle guarding. Pain from the spine also can be referred to the abdomen, usually as a result of nerve root irritation or compression. This type of neuromusculoskeletal pain referred to the abdomen is characteristically associated with hyperesthesia over the involved spinal dermatomes and is intensified by motions such as coughing, sneezing, or straining.

*GI bleeding* may be characterized by coffee-ground emesis (vomiting of blood that has been in contact with gastric acid), hematemesis (vomiting of bright-red blood), melena (black, tarry stools), or hematochezia (bleeding from the rectum, or maroon-colored stools), depending on the location of the lesion. Bleeding may not be clinically obvious to the client and may be diagnosed only by further testing.

The major causes of upper GI bleeding in the therapy population are erosive gastritis common in (1) severely ill people with major trauma or systemic illness, burns, or head injury; (2) peptic ulcers; (3) use of nonsteroidal antiinflammatory drugs (NSAIDs) such as aspirin or ibuprofen; and (4) chronic alcohol use. Drugs such as warfarin, heparin, and aspirin, used as anticoagulants in the treatment of pulmonary emboli, venous thrombus, or valvular abnormalities, can contribute to or exacerbate gastric erosion and subsequent bleeding.

Accumulation of blood in the GI tract is irritating and increases peristalsis, causing nausea, vomiting, or diarrhea with possible referred pain to the shoulder or back. The digestion of proteins originating from massive upper GI bleeding is reflected by an increase in blood urea nitrogen. Other complications include fatigue, postural hypotension, tachycardia, weakness, and shortness of breath on exertion. Slow, chronic blood loss may result in iron-deficiency anemia.

Fecal incontinence (inability to control bowel movements) has both psychologic and physiologic contributing factors. Psychologic factors include anxiety, confusion, disorientation, and depression. The most commonly observed physiologic causes seen in a therapy practice are neurologic sensory and motor impairment (e.g., stroke and spinal cord injury); anal sphincter damage secondary to traumatic childbirth, sexual assault, hemorrhoids, and hemorrhoidal surgery; altered levels of consciousness; and severe diarrhea. External anal sphincter damage is a disorder of decreased pelvic floor and can be improved with focused exercises.

SPECIAL IMPLICATIONS FOR THE THERAPIST 16.1

## *Signs and Symptoms of Gastrointestinal Disease*

### Fluid and Electrolyte Imbalance

Body fluid loss associated with weight loss, excessive perspiration, or chronic diarrhea and vomiting may cause an imbalance in the body chemistry (electrolyte imbalance) and may cause orthostatic changes in blood pressure (i.e., postural drops in blood pressure).

Electrolyte changes often include decreased potassium, which alters the sodium-potassium pump necessary for normal muscle function (contraction and relaxation). Muscle cramping occurs, which increases a person's risk for musculoskeletal injury during exercise.

A client with chronic diarrhea who is taking antidiarrheal agents containing bismuth subsalicylate, such as Pepto-Bismol, Bismatrol, Pink Bismuth, or Kaopectate, may report darkened or black stools. The client's tongue may also appear black.

Significant postural hypotension often reflects extracellular fluid volume depletion as occurs with excessive body fluid loss. The maintenance of arterial pressure during upright posture depends on adequate blood volume, unimpaired venous return, and an intact sympathetic nervous system. Monitoring vital signs and observing for accompanying symptoms promote safe and effective exercise for anyone with the potential for electrolyte imbalance.

In a screening interview, the therapist should always ask clients if there are any other symptoms of any kind to report. Remember to ask about the use of nutritional or other supplements (especially among athletes), as these can have adverse GI effects on some people. For example, creatine used to improve athletic performance can cause loss of appetite, diarrhea, dizziness, and cramps, presumably from dehydration.

### Pelvic Floor Muscle Rehabilitation

The specialized physical therapist can assist individuals with constipation associated with defecatory disorders involving the skeletal muscle of the pelvic floor. Pelvic floor muscle strength, tone, endurance, coordination, and breathing patterns can be assessed. Fecal incontinence related to underactive or weak pelvic floor muscles responds to pelvic floor muscle strength training. A Cochrane review concluded that pelvic floor muscle training represents an appropriate treatment for women with persistent postpartum fecal incontinence.[36] Retraining pelvic floor muscle function during evacuation is a key part of the rehabilitation process.

Clients with overactive or dyssynergic pelvic floor muscles can be trained to relax their external anal sphincter and learn to coordinate abdominal contractions to assist stool propulsion into the rectum. Toileting techniques to avoid straining during a bowel movement may help decrease the risk of developing pudendal nerve dysfunction. The therapist can be helpful in identifying ways to incorporate scheduled toileting with transfer, strength, and balance training.[80] Bathroom and safety modifications can also be made, and fiber should be added to the diet gradually.

### Exercise and Gastrointestinal Function

Inactivity appears to be related to constipation. In a recent proof-of-concept study,10 healthy young men were confined to bed rest for 35 days. During that time, 60% developed new-onset constipation.[151] However, the widely held connection between exercise and decreased constipation is based on old and conflicting research. Several older studies have suggested increasing activity in elderly patients will decrease constipation, but more recent studies have produced conflicting results. On one hand, increasing exercise and activity is beneficial for many reasons and may possibly decrease constipation. On the other hand, individuals with diarrhea can exercise but may have to take intermittent rest breaks to conserve energy and curtail activity during acute diarrhea to decrease gut motility.

During an upper quadrant screening, the therapist usually inquires whether the client has difficulty swallowing. Forward head posture or anterior disc protrusion may be a possible cause of difficulty swallowing, but a pathologic condition of the esophagus may also be the cause.

The therapist can instruct anyone with dysphagia who does not have cervical disc disease in an isometric/isotonic head lift exercise that may restore normal swallowing, thereby helping some individuals to eat normally and keep food or liquids from being aspirated into the lungs (Fig. 16.2).[206] This effect is attributed to strengthening of the suprahyoid muscles, as evidenced by comparison of electromyographic changes in muscle fatigue before and after 6 weeks of exercise.[223]

This exercise strengthens these muscles that open the upper esophageal sphincter, the "gate" that allows food or drink to slide down the esophagus to the stomach. This exercise works best for people with a weak or ineffective upper esophageal sphincter but may prove useful for other types of swallowing problems. Performance of the exercise is associated with mild muscle discomfort that resolves spontaneously after a couple of weeks.[93]

Studies document the physiologic changes in the GI system and the onset of GI symptoms during and after strenuous exercise. Intensity and duration of exercise are important factors, and lower GI symptoms predominate.[361] GI bleeding can be reduced with regular exercise, and people with limited physical activity (e.g., physical disability) are at greater risk for ulceration and GI bleeding.

### Referred Pain Patterns

An acute ulcer can manifest as thoracolumbar junction pain. Back and/or shoulder pain caused by GI bleeding and perforation associated with a long-standing ulcer may cause painful biomechanical changes in muscular contractions and spinal movement.[120,284] The clinical presentation may include objective musculoskeletal findings to support a diagnosis of back or shoulder dysfunction when in fact the symptoms may be associated with GI bleeding.

Pain in the left shoulder caused by free air or blood in the abdominal cavity is called the *Kehr sign* and may occur with perforation of viscus (e.g., stomach ulcer, diverticular disease), after laparoscopy (lasting 24 to 48 hours), or after rupture of the spleen.

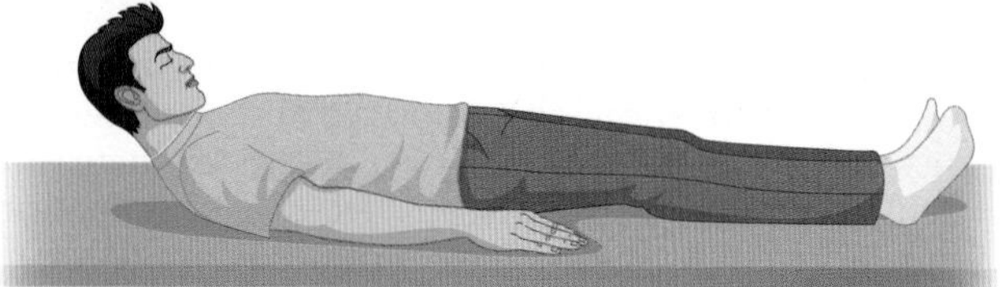

**Figure 16.2**

**The Shaker head-lifting exercise to strengthen the upper esophageal sphincter muscle.** The affected person lies in the supine position, keeping the feet, back, and shoulders and arms down. The person raises the head until the toes can be seen, pauses but does not hold the head lift, then lowers the head back down. This movement is repeated 30 times (isokinetic exercise) using a relatively constant speed of movement. The person rests for 1 minute, then raises the head and looks at the feet for 1 minute, pauses 1 minute, and repeats the long look and long rest twice more (isometric exercise). The entire sequence should be completed three times daily. These exercises can be used by anyone with dysphagia or other swallowing problems in addition to hiatal hernia and gastroesophageal reflux disease. (Exercise developed by R. Shaker, MD, Medical College of Wisconsin, Milwaukee, WI, 1998.)

## AGING AND THE GASTROINTESTINAL SYSTEM

Age-related changes in GI function begin before the age of 50 years. Oral changes may include tooth enamel and dentin wear and increasing tooth decay, causing periodontal disease and subsequent tooth loss. Sensory changes may include decreased taste buds and diminished sense of smell, resulting in altered sense of taste. These oral and sensory changes can eventually depress the appetite and make eating less pleasurable.[79] Salivary secretion often decreases, contributing to dry mouth, and when it is complicated by tooth decay or loss, chewing food and swallowing become more difficult.

The oropharynx and esophagus exhibit minor changes with age, although these changes do not contribute to significant symptoms unless disease is present. The most common problem in the stomach associated with aging is a reduction in the production of acid (hypochlorhydria). This can lead to iron malabsorption, small bowel bacterial overgrowth, and vitamin $B_{12}$ deficiency (if also associated with the loss of parietal cells, which secrete intrinsic factor). Atrophic gastritis may be the result of many possible variables including normal aging, nutritional deficiency (e.g., iron, folate, ascorbate), autoimmune mechanisms, endocrine insufficiency (e.g., thyroid, adrenal, pancreatic), or infection (usually with *Helicobacter pylori*).[156] Gastric motility and emptying remain normal, while pancreatic secretions are reduced with dysfunction of beta cells. This may contribute to the development of type 2 diabetes.[12,85,122]

The small intestine is not greatly affected by aging, allowing normal absorption of nutrients, whereas the large intestine exhibits prolonged transit time secondary to a reduction in neurotransmitters and receptors.[40] This allows increased time for water absorption and the development of constipation.

With aging, there is a change in the composition and diversity of intestinal microbiota. Intestinal microbiota are interrelated to the central nervous system, enteric nervous system, and GI tract (the gut-brain axis) by modulating and influencing neurotransmitters. This axis is bidirectional and translates chemicals from the gut into emotional and cognitive sensations and vice versa. When normal intestinal microbiota changes, there are alterations in intestinal homeostasis that can lead to a proinflammatory state and contribute to age-related GI disease.[51,234]

In addition to the effects of aging on the GI system, changes in other organ systems (e.g., endocrine, cardiovascular, and nervous systems) can affect GI structure and function, producing many variations in presentation of illness. Extraintestinal disorders, such as diabetes and the neurologic and vascular changes that occur with age, have a greater effect on the GI tract than the natural process of aging.

## THE ESOPHAGUS

### Hiatal Hernia

#### Definition and Incidence

A hiatal (or hiatus) hernia occurs when the esophageal hiatus of the diaphragm becomes enlarged, allowing the stomach to pass through the diaphragm into the thoracic cavity (Fig. 16.3). Hernias are either *congenital*, resulting from a failure of formation or fusion of the multiple developmental components of the diaphragm, or *acquired*. Acquired hernias can also be categorized as either *sliding* or *paraesophageal*. Greater than 95% of hiatal hernias are sliding, whereas only 5% are paraesophageal.

There are multiple theories as to how hiatal hernias develop. Sliding hernias form when there is widening of the hiatal tunnel surrounding the esophagus. The phrenoesophageal membrane normally surrounds and anchors the esophagus to the diaphragm. During swallowing, the longitudinal muscles of the esophagus contract, shortening the esophagus and stretching the phrenoesophageal membrane. Following swallowing, the phrenoesophageal membrane recoils, bringing the esophagus back into place. It is postulated that over time, there is wearing of the phrenoesophageal membrane due to multiple factors such as increased abdominal pressure, straining, acid reflux, vomiting, and widening of the diaphragmatic musculature. This leads to laxity and allowing the gastroesophageal junction to pass above the diaphragm. The fundus of the stomach, however, remains below the gastroesophageal junction.

Paraesophageal hernias develop secondary to surgery or trauma and are associated with laxity of the gastrophrenic and gastrocolic ligaments that normally hold the stomach in place. This allows the stomach to enter through the phrenoesophageal membrane, above the gastroesophageal junction. A paraesophageal hernia is a true hernia with formation of a hernia sac. Sometimes the defect can be large enough to allow other organs such as the colon, spleen, or small intestine to pass.

Hiatal hernia (symptomatic or asymptomatic) is common; the incidence is estimated as 5 per 1000 people. The

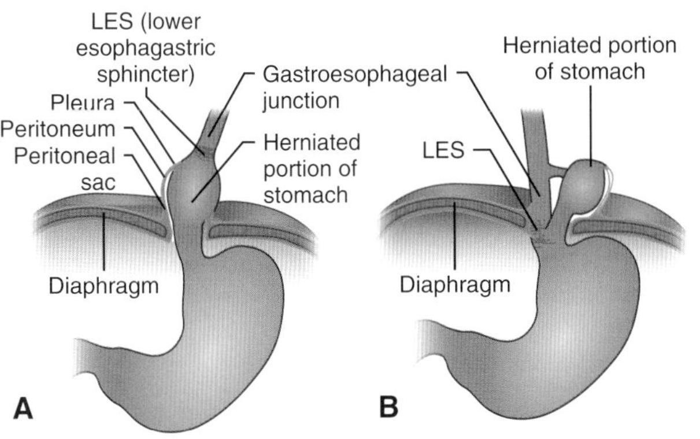


**Figure 16.3**

**Hiatal hernia.** (A) Sliding hiatal hernia. Approximately 90% of esophageal hiatal hernias are sliding hernias. The stomach and gastroesophageal junction are displaced upward into the thorax (i.e., the stomach and gastroesophageal junction slide up into the thoracic cavity, following the usual path of the esophagus through an enlarged hiatal opening in the diaphragm). (B) Rolling hiatal hernia. The remaining hiatal hernias are rolling or paraesophageal hernias. The gastroesophageal junction stays below the diaphragm, but all or part of the stomach pushes through into the thorax.

incidence increases with age and may be as high as 60% in people older than 60 years of age. Women are affected more often than men; children may have the sliding type but do not usually exhibit symptoms until they reach middle age.

### Etiologic and Risk Factors

As an acquired condition, multiple causes and risk factors exist for the development of hiatal hernia. Anything that weakens the diaphragm muscle or alters the hiatus (the opening in the diaphragm for the passage of the esophagus) and increases intraabdominal pressure can predispose a person to hiatal hernia. Muscle weakness can be congenital or caused by aging, trauma, surgery, or anything that increases intraabdominal pressure (Box 16.1).

### Pathogenesis and Clinical Manifestations

One of the most common symptoms of a hiatal hernia is heartburn or reflux. Hiatal hernias are believed to contribute to incompetence of the LES, allowing acid into the esophagus. Normally, during inspiration, diaphragmatic musculature contributes to LES tone by contracting around the LES. With widening of the musculature, there is less effect during inspiration. Also the hernia may lead to decreased LES pressures and disrupt the LES. The hernia may also "re-reflux," or not allow acid to return to the stomach when the diaphragmatic musculature "pinches" below the hernia. These factors are additive contributors to gastroesophageal reflux disease (GERD).

Symptoms vary depending on the type of hernia present and increase in the presence of tight, constrictive clothing or if the person is in a recumbent position. A sliding hernia may produce heartburn 30 to 60 minutes after a meal, especially if the person is lying down or sleeping in the supine position. Dysphagia and shortness of breath are other symptoms. Large sliding hernias with reflux may be associated with substernal pain.

**Box 16.1**

**CAUSES OF INCREASED INTRAABDOMINAL PRESSURE**

- Lifting
- Straining
- Bending over
- Prolonged sitting or standing
- Chronic or forceful cough
- Pregnancy
- Ascites
- Obesity
- Congestive heart failure
- Low-fiber diet
- Constipation (see Table 16.2)
- Delayed bowel movement
- Vigorous exercise

## MEDICAL MANAGEMENT

**DIAGNOSIS, TREATMENT, AND PROGNOSIS.** Hiatal hernias may be diagnosed by endoscopy, barium swallow, or esophageal manometry. Barium swallow may be more sensitive than endoscopy for paraesophageal hernias. Small sliding hernias (less than 2 cm) cannot be reliably diagnosed by either endoscopy or barium swallow.

The primary treatment remains symptomatic control through the use of proton pump inhibitors (PPIs) and other measures used to treat GERD (see Gastroesophageal Reflux Disease next). The prognosis is good overall with recurrences expected. Surgery or laparoscopic surgery is performed if medical management of GERD is not achieved.

**SPECIAL IMPLICATIONS FOR THE THERAPIST 16.2**

### *Hiatal Hernia*

For any client with a known hiatal hernia, the flat supine position and any exercises requiring the Valsalva maneuver (which increases intraabdominal pressure) should be avoided during therapy intervention. Before discharge, the client must be warned against activities that cause increased intraabdominal pressure and given safe lifting instructions.

A slow return to function over the next 6 to 8 weeks is advised. Postoperatively (after surgical repair of the hernia using the thoracic approach), the client may have chest tubes in place, requiring careful observation of the tubes during turning and repositioning and chest physical therapy to prevent pulmonary complications.

## Gastroesophageal Reflux Disease

### Definition

GERD may be defined as the consequences from the reflux (backward flow) of gastric contents into the esophagus accompanied by a failure of anatomic and physiologic

**Table 16.3** Causes of Gastroesophageal Reflux Disease

| Decreased Pressure of LES or Alteration in Esophageal Acid Clearance | Gastric Contents Near Junction |
|---|---|
| Foods: chocolate, peppermint, fatty foods, citrus products (including tomatoes), spicy foods, garlic, onions | Recumbency |
| Beverages: coffee (including decaffeinated), carbonated drinks, alcohol | Increased intraabdominal pressure |
| Caffeine | |
| Nicotine or cigarette smoke | |
| Central nervous system depressants (e.g., morphine, diazepam) | |
| Other medications (e.g., calcium channel blockers, nitrates, aspirin and other nonsteroidal antiinflammatory drugs, dopamine, theophylline, tricyclic antidepressants) | |
| Estrogen therapy | |
| Nasogastric intubation | |
| Scleroderma | |
| Prolonged vomiting | |
| Surgical resection (destroys sphincter) | |
| Position (right side-lying; sitting) | |
| Pregnancy (last trimester: increased progesterone relaxes sphincter) | |

*LES*, Lower esophageal sphincter.

mechanisms to protect the esophagus. Gastroesophageal reflux is a very common and chronic problem and occurs in most people on a routine basis. The disease occurs when this physiologic process causes significant symptoms or complications. GERD can occur without visible damage to the esophagus, termed nonerosive GERD, or injury can occur, causing complications (e.g., esophagitis, strictures, Barrett esophagus, or gastric cancer), which is called erosive GERD.

## Incidence and Etiologic Factors

GERD is one of the most common disorders seen in clinics. Approximately 10% to 20% of American adults have this disorder, seen equally in men and women.[244] Prevalence is often an estimate, and data vary depending on whether symptoms (i.e., heartburn) or visual inspection (i.e., via endoscopy) is used. Although any age can be affected, this condition has an increasing incidence with increasing age; older people are more likely to develop severe disease.[160,267]

It is estimated that nearly two-thirds of adults in the United States will experience significant symptoms of GERD sometime in their lives and that 15% or more of the population has daily symptoms of GERD, and as much as one-third of the population has monthly symptoms. In the United States, GERD is the most common GI-related diagnosis and accounts for substantial direct and indirect economic costs of $15 to $20 billion/year.[258,305]

A wide range of foods and lifestyle factors can contribute to GERD (Table 16.3),[249] particularly obesity and smoking. Hiatal hernia and medications are other risk factors for developing GERD. Obesity is linked to GERD,[153] which may account for the recent increase in prevalence at a time when peptic ulcer disease (PUD) is decreasing. Controversy exists as to whether *H. pylori* leads to GERD (*H. pylori* decreases the amount of acid produced in the stomach).[266,283]

If clients have typical GERD symptoms without a history of PUD, testing for *H. pylori* is not necessary. If the test is performed anyway and is positive for active infection, treatment should still be offered, understanding that GERD symptoms may not be relieved.[64]

## Pathogenesis

Three factors are involved in aiding the esophagus to remain healthy: anatomic barriers between the stomach and the esophagus, mechanisms to clear the esophagus of stomach acid, and maintaining stomach acidity and acid volume. People without GERD have episodes of reflux but do not develop disease owing to normal functioning of these mechanisms.

The most important anatomic barrier between the stomach and the esophagus is the LES. Most reflux is secondary to transient relaxation of the LES that is not related to swallowing, allowing acid to pass into the esophagus. Persons with severe disease are often found to have consistently low pressure of the LES. Hiatal hernias, where the LES and part of the stomach are above the diaphragm, create a change in the configuration of the LES, increasing susceptibility to reflux.

The esophagus uses several mechanisms to neutralize and clear acid volume. Saliva and the alkaline secretions from esophageal epithelium serve to neutralize acid. Peristalsis and gravity help move acid out of the esophagus. Medications, cigarette smoking, esophageal dysmotility disorders, and xerostomia (dry mouth) all can lead to increased acid exposure (by increasing the amount of time the esophagus is exposed and/or increasing the volume of acid), thereby causing GERD. Any of the predisposing factors listed in Table 16.3 may alter the pressure of the LES or alter protective mechanisms, resulting in reflux.

Several complications such as esophagitis, strictures, Barrett esophagus, and adenocarcinoma can occur with significant GERD.[164] Esophagitis is necrosis of the esophageal epithelial lining that leads to erosions and ulcers. Subsequent granulation of tissue causes scarring that frequently develops into esophageal strictures that narrow the esophagus, making swallowing difficult. Barrett esophagus is a precancerous change in the type of cells that line the lower end of the esophagus (columnar cells replace squamous cells). Adenocarcinoma is a cancer of the esophagus.

## Clinical Manifestations

Heartburn is the principal symptom of reflux. It is described as a burning sensation beginning at the stomach and rising up the chest. It may radiate to the chest, throat, or back. Other common symptoms include chest pain, acid regurgitation, belching, dysphagia, nausea, vomiting, early satiety, and painful swallowing.[117] Heartburn most often occurs 30 to 60 minutes after a large meal or a meal with alcohol, spicy foods, fats, and citrus. Lying down may worsen symptoms, making the night a common time to experience reflux. As chest pain is a common symptom of GERD, cardiac chest pain should be distinguished and evaluated before chest pain is assumed to be related to GERD.

Children and infants can be affected by GERD. For children, symptoms are similar to those experienced by adults; however, the diagnosis in infants can be difficult. Crying, fussiness, irritability, refusal to feed, and regurgitation are common symptoms in this age group and not specific for GERD.[208] Persistent GERD has been linked to developmental problems. Neurologic disorders and GERD can have overlapping symptoms, such as irritability associated with arching, neck extension, and abnormal muscle tone with spastic movements.

Adults older than 70 years are more likely to have atypical symptoms such as dysphagia, vomiting, respiratory difficulties, weight loss, anemia, and anorexia with or without heartburn or acid regurgitation. Older adults may also present with more severe disease because of long-standing disease with few symptoms.[160]

**Extraesophageal Manifestations.** Up to one-third of people evaluated for heartburn also exhibit symptoms separate from the esophagus.[178] The three main extraesophageal manifestations include asthma, cough, and laryngitis.[16,292] GERD is thought to cause asthma because of microaspirations of reflux material and/or vagally mediated esophago bronchial reflex. It is estimated that 30% to 90% of people diagnosed with asthma also have reflux symptoms.[177] Asthma does not respond as well as GERD to PPI medications.[219,321]

GERD accounts for approximately 13% of chronic cough cases, defined as longer than 8 weeks' duration.[265] Cough can develop from two different mechanisms. The first is a direct reflux of gastroduodenal contents (inflammation of the larynx can be seen endoscopically). The second is from an indirect vagal stimulation (inflammation is not visible). It is estimated that 35% to 75% of people with GERD-related cough do not exhibit classic symptoms of GERD.[99,195] They may describe cough during the day, while upright, or while eating. Because of the expense and discomfort of testing, a trial of PPIs is given to diagnose and treat.[58] Individuals who do not have improvement of chronic cough may undergo esophagogastroduodenoscopy (EGD)

GERD is an important cause of laryngitis. Associated symptoms include hoarseness, difficulty swallowing, repeated throat clearing, sensation of having something caught in the throat, cough, excessive phlegm, voice fatigue, and heartburn.[296]

## MEDICAL MANAGEMENT

**DIAGNOSIS.** The diagnosis of GERD is principally based on symptoms, often defined as troublesome heartburn occurring two or more times per week and/or complications associated with reflux. Frequency and severity of heartburn do not predict the severity of esophageal damage. Diagnostic tools include history, endoscopy, and esophageal pH monitoring with or without impedance (quantifying acid and reflux events with a correlation with symptoms). Impedance pH monitoring is the gold standard test for clients who partially respond to PPIs, before antireflux surgery, and for individuals with atypical symptoms. A full diagnostic evaluation is not always required when history and current symptoms clearly point to GERD. If a patient exhibits the typical symptoms of heartburn and/or regurgitation, a diagnosis is made by a trial of medication (PPIs) that relieves symptoms. Most people with just these two symptoms have normal EGD examinations. Other tests, typically EGD, are used when warning or atypical symptoms (e.g., unintentional weight loss, dysphagia, hematemesis, melena, or anemia) or symptoms that do not respond to a PPI are present.

**TREATMENT.** The goals of treatment are to alleviate symptoms, heal esophagitis if present, maintain remission of the disease, and manage any complications. Treatment options consist of medications and surgery. Endoscopic therapy has been shown to be less effective for long-term management.

***Lifestyle Modifications.*** Lifestyle modifications are recommended[9,163] including avoiding aggravating foods such as citrus, tomatoes, spicy foods, fatty or fried foods, chocolate, mint, and caffeine. Global avoidance of all foods related to GERD is not usually necessary. Clients should be aided in smoking cessation and encouraged to reduce alcohol consumption. People with GERD should remain upright for at least 3 hours after meals[111] and should avoid meals 2 to 3 hours before bedtime. Elevating the head of the bed or lying in the left lateral decubitus position can be helpful for persons with nighttime symptoms. Obese clients should be advised and given help to lose weight. Weight loss and elevation of the bed have been shown to be the most effective lifestyle modifications.[165,237]

***Medications.*** Many people will initially use nonprescription antacids to treat symptoms. Antacids work principally by buffering gastric acid for a short period of time. Other nonprescription medications include $H_2$ blockers (e.g., cimetidine, ranitidine, famotidine). These medications block histamine, which normally induces parietal cells via gastrin to secrete acid. $H_2$ blockers are more effective than antacids but less effective than PPIs. $H_2$ blockers can also develop tachyphylaxis or become less effective over time.[221]

The most effective therapy is the use of acid suppression with PPIs (e.g., omeprazole, lansoprazole, esomeprazole, rabeprazole, pantoprazole, dexlansoprazole). PPIs are currently available over-the-counter and by prescription. These medications reduce nighttime and meal-induced acid production. PPIs are superior to $H_2$ blockers in relieving symptoms and healing esophagitis. PPIs have also been found to be the most effective and cost-effective method of empirically treating GERD without warning symptoms.[114]

Treatment is for 8 weeks for symptom relief, and dosing is 30 to 60 minutes before breakfast. If symptoms are not completely relieved, the dose may be increased to twice daily. Clients who do not respond to the increase should be evaluated by EGD. Relapse is common, but $H_2$ blockers can be tried for persons who responded to 8 weeks of PPI treatment. If long-term treatment with PPIs is needed (e.g., for clients who have had erosive esophagitis), clients should receive the lowest dose possible, including as-needed or "on-demand" dosing (for clients without a history of erosive esophagitis). PPIs are well tolerated with main side effects of diarrhea and headaches. Other possible effects include vitamin $B_8$ deficiency, calcium and magnesium malabsorption, increased risk for community-acquired pneumonia (short-term use), *Clostridioides difficile* infection, osteoporosis (small increase in hip fracture for persons already at high risk[73]), and cardiovascular events. There is still controversy concerning the concomitant use of PPIs and the antiplatelet drug clopidogrel, with some studies showing an increase in risk of cardiovascular events, whereas other studies do not demonstrate adverse outcomes.[26,42,221,245]

***Surgery.*** Surgical procedures (e.g., antireflux surgery) are available for carefully selected individuals who have partially responded to PPI therapy (people who do not respond to PPIs often do not respond to surgical treatment[145]), desire or need to discontinue the use of PPIs, have symptomatic hiatal hernia, experience continued reflux despite PPIs documented by pH testing, and whose esophagitis is not healed by PPIs.[171] Clients should undergo impedance pH monitoring (by transnasal catheter or wireless capsule) before surgery. Laparoscopic fundoplication (wrapping of the fundus) is the procedure of choice and has an 80% success rate.[110] For obese clients, gastric bypass is recommended. Common adverse effects seen with antireflux surgery include gas bloat syndrome, dysphagia, diarrhea, and recurrent reflux.[281]

**PROGNOSIS.** The prognosis is good for GERD symptom resolution and reduction of complications. GERD can be a long-term disease, particularly with clients who have severe symptoms, severe esophagitis, or chronic low LES pressure. GERD frequently returns 6 months after discontinuation of therapy. GERD can contribute to asthma and vocal cord inflammation, and people who have uncontrolled acid reflux are at increased risk of developing esophageal cancer, which has a poor prognosis.[100,123]

SPECIAL IMPLICATIONS FOR THE THERAPIST 16.3

## *Gastroesophageal Reflux Disease*

Clients with GERD are often treated in a therapy practice or rehabilitation setting for orthopedic and other conditions. Occasionally, GERD manifests with atypical head and neck symptoms (e.g., sensation of a lump in the throat) without heartburn.

### Exercise and Gastroesophageal Reflux Disease

Exercise is important for anyone with GERD who is overweight. Excess abdominal fat puts pressure on the stomach; even moderate weight loss can reduce symptoms. However, people with GERD may have trouble exercising because some types of physical activity can worsen symptoms. In fact, GERD induced by strenuous exercise is extremely common among athletes. The degree of reflux is greater in activities with more body agitation such as running or aerobics than in swimming or biking.

Strenuous exercise inhibits both gastric and small intestinal emptying, which may contribute to GERD. This, combined with the potential for relaxation of the gastroesophageal sphincter, suggests the importance of avoiding high-calorie meals or fatty foods (or other triggers) immediately before exercising to avoid or minimize exercise-related GERD.[361]

The therapist can be instrumental in providing education and encouragement essential to the lifestyle modifications necessary to manage this condition and assisting the person to implement changes related to diet and exercise.

### Positioning

Any intervention requiring a supine position should be scheduled before meals and avoided just after eating. Modification of position toward a more upright posture may be required if symptoms persist during therapy. Consider a trial of the exercises to strengthen the muscles around the esophageal sphincter (see Fig. 16.2).

For nocturnal reflux, encourage the individual to sleep on the left side with a pillow in place to maintain this position. Right side-lying position makes it easier for acid to flow into the esophagus because of the effect of gravity on the esophagus (the lower esophagus bends to the left, and this straightens out with right side lying).[176] See Special Implications for the Therapist 16.2: Hiatal Hernia. Activities that increase intraabdominal pressure; constipation, which often accompanies back pain and other conditions (see Table 16.2); and tight clothing must be avoided.

The presence of GERD requires careful positioning to promote drainage of secretions without causing reflux. This is more readily accomplished when the stomach is empty. Positioning clients with GI dysfunction for breathing control and coughing maneuvers requires special attention to minimize the risk of aspiration. Although head-up positions minimize reflux by reducing intraabdominal pressure, they can promote aspiration of pharyngeal contents. Side-lying positions (especially left side-lying position) prevent regurgitation and aspiration and promote oropharyngeal accumulations and ease of suctioning.[86]

### Other Considerations

Polypharmacy (the use of multiple medications for a single disorder or for comorbidities) can result in significant toxicity and drug interactions when medications for acid-related diseases are taken. Any new or unusual symptoms reported to the therapist should be documented with notification of the physician. Fracture risk increases with prolonged use of PPIs in adults with osteoporosis. The therapist can instruct anyone taking PPIs over a long period of time in an osteoporosis prevention program.[342,379]

With postoperative complications, airway clearance techniques (formerly, chest physical therapy, pulmonary physical therapy, and pulmonary hygiene) may be indicated. In addition, coughing and bronchospasm can result from a vagally mediated reflex secondary to refluxed acid contents in the esophagus. The therapist also may observe reflux in clients who have chronic bronchitis, asthma, and pulmonary fibrosis.

## Esophageal Cancer

### Overview and Incidence

Histologically, two types of esophageal cancer exist: squamous cell carcinoma and adenocarcinoma. Squamous cell carcinoma typically develops in the middle of the esophagus, whereas adenocarcinoma is more often located in the distal portion of the esophagus. Worldwide, more than 90% of all esophageal cancers are squamous cell carcinomas. In the West, however, there has been a decline in the frequency of squamous cell carcinoma and a dramatic rise in the frequency of adenocarcinoma of the esophagus,[88] with adenocarcinoma accounting for 80% of esophageal cancer in the United States.

Esophageal cancer is relatively uncommon, accounting for only 1% of all cancers diagnosed in the United States. The cure rate is poor, however, and esophageal cancer is the sixth leading cause of cancer deaths worldwide. In 2018, the estimated number of cases was approximately 17,000, with 15,000 deaths.[174] Men are significantly more likely to develop esophageal cancer than women.

### Etiologic and Risk Factors

Esophageal cancer is known for its marked variation by geographic region, ethnic background, and gender. In the United States, adenocarcinoma of the esophagus most frequently affects middle-aged white men and often develops from Barrett esophagus, whereas squamous cell carcinoma is more common in blacks and is associated with alcohol and tobacco use.[44,75]

Other risk factors for developing squamous cell carcinoma of the esophagus include exposure to nitrosamine, corrosive injury to the esophagus (burning from chemicals), achalasia, vitamin deficiencies (selenium and zinc), and human papillomavirus infection.[125,193,215,338]

Adenocarcinoma is highly correlated with Barrett esophagus, gastroesophageal reflux, tobacco use, past thoracic radiation, increased age, diet low in fruits and vegetables, and obesity. Approximately 5% to 15% of people with GERD will develop Barrett esophagus.[306]

Barrett esophagus is a complication of GERD that can lead to adenocarcinoma. It occurs when the normal epithelial cells of the lower esophagus are replaced with columnar cells, typically seen in the intestine. This process is termed *metaplasia,* and the mechanism for this change is unknown.[236] Persons with Barrett esophagus have a 30- to 40-fold increased risk for developing cancer.[317] People with a diagnosis of Barrett esophagus are screened and placed on a surveillance program.[365]

### Clinical Manifestations

Presenting symptoms for both squamous cell carcinoma and adenocarcinoma of the esophagus are similar. The most common symptom is dysphagia, initially with solids and progressing to involve liquids. Weight loss occurs in 90% of affected people. Other symptoms include odynophagia (pain with swallowing), cough, hoarseness, chest pain, anemia, and regurgitation. Odynophagia is frequently associated with an ulcerated tumor. Most clients with early esophageal tumors are asymptomatic. Symptoms are often associated with progressive disease, such as recurrent pneumonia from the formation of an esophagorespiratory fistula or chest pain from tumor invasion into periesophageal structures.

### MEDICAL MANAGEMENT

**PREVENTION.** Primary prevention for esophageal cancer centers on modifiable risk factors such as reducing weight, alcohol intake, and smoking. Preventing GERD and Barrett esophagus is another method of reducing rates of esophageal adenocarcinoma.[54] Despite this knowledge, the rates of esophageal adenocarcinoma are increasing. There are many possible reasons for this, but the exact reason remains unclear. It is possible that GERD is underreported and undertreated in many adults, especially people older than age 65 years. Many people with GERD may have few or no symptoms, so that progression of the condition to Barrett disease and transformation to adenocarcinoma goes unnoticed until it is too late.[369] Also, obesity, a significant problem in the United States, is independently related to and increases the risk of both Barrett esophagus and adenocarcinoma.[348]

Whereas early screening and detection can reveal dysplasia (atypical, precancerous cells), there is no evidence that such screening programs actually reduce morbidity or mortality associated with this condition.[322] Studies also show that suppression of reflux does not completely protect from developing esophageal cancer. Targeted surveillance of high-risk people may be beneficial.[116,236]

Studies suggest that 40% of individuals with esophageal adenocarcinoma have no history of GERD symptoms.[149] This means that screening only individuals with known GERD will leave out a significant portion of adults who may be affected. Also, there are reports of incurable malignancies developing despite endoscopic surveillance programs.[331]

**DIAGNOSIS AND STAGING.** Diagnosis is made by endoscopy with cytology and biopsy. Following a diagnosis, staging of the disease is performed by endoscopic ultrasonography, with chest and abdominal computed tomography (CT) and positron emission tomography to determine the presence of metastatic lesions and the most appropriate treatment.[340] Stage I disease consists of superficial lesions that do not penetrate the full thickness of the esophagus. Stage II lesions are full thickness, whereas stage III disease has spread to lymph nodes (locoregional). Stage IV disease has spread distantly.

**TREATMENT.** At presentation, only 30% to 40% of people have potentially resectable disease. Clients with stage I to III disease are often treated surgically, but owing to the high recurrence rates, preoperative chemotherapy (neoadjuvant chemotherapy) and radiation have been added to most treatment regimens.[358] Chemoradiation is also used following surgery.[148] Surgery alone is currently not the preferred treatment except for the earliest stages of cancer (e.g., stage T1).

Individuals who have unresectable disease, have metastatic disease, or are poor operative candidates may receive radiation therapy, which provides short-term relief of symptoms. Other options include esophageal brachytherapy, external-beam radiation, stent placement, targeted antibodies,[274] and chemotherapy. Most treatment at this stage is palliative.

Approximately 30% of esophageal tumors overexpress the *HER2* growth factor receptor. For clients with this type of tumor, the receptor can be targeted with the anti-*HER2* monoclonal antibody trastuzumab, which can be added to chemotherapy treatment regimens. It may improve mortality by a median of 4.2 months.[356] Other distinct molecular subtypes are being analyzed to improve treatment and outcomes.[20]

**PROGNOSIS.** The first symptoms of esophageal cancer are not usually apparent until the tumor involves the entire esophageal circumference. More importantly, by that time the tumor has often invaded the deeper layers of the esophagus and adjacent structures and is unresectable. Endoscopic surveillance can detect esophageal adenocarcinomas when they are early and curable, but approximately 50%[347] of these neoplasms are detected at an advanced stage. Carcinoma of the esophagus has a high morbidity and mortality, although rates are improving. About 20% of people with esophageal carcinoma (all stages combined) survive 5 years. Five-year survival rate as reported by the National Cancer Institute Surveillance, Epidemiology, and End Results database for stage I and some stage II (localized) cancers is approximately 43%; for regional tumors (spread to lymph nodes), it is 23%, and distant spread is 5%. This is for both squamous cell carcinoma and adenocarcinoma (although adenocarcinoma may have a slightly better prognosis[335]).

Esophageal cancer metastasizes rapidly. Given the continuous nature of lymphatic vessels in the area, removal of lymph nodes with the tumor is difficult, contributing to the poor prognosis.

SPECIAL IMPLICATIONS FOR THE THERAPIST 16.4

### *Esophageal Cancer*

Lymphatic vessels of the esophagus are continuous with mediastinal structures and drain to the lymph nodes from the neck of the celiac axis. Metastasis is via this lymphatic drainage, with tumors of the upper esophagus metastasizing to the cervical, internal jugular, and supraclavicular nodes. During an upper quarter screening examination, the therapist may identify changes in lymph nodes, requiring medical referral.

The usual precautions regarding clients with cancer apply to clients with neoplasms of the GI system. The side effects of chemotherapy-induced bone marrow suppression are the primary concern. An exercise regimen including aerobic exercise at a minimal level enhances the immune system and is incorporated whenever possible. See also Cancer and Exercise in Chapter 9.

Radical surgery for thoracic esophageal cancer is highly invasive and often leads to respiratory complications; thoracoscopic surgery is a less invasive alternative but may still result in respiratory decline. Airway clearance techniques discussed in Chapter 15 may be needed postoperatively for anyone undergoing surgery for this condition.[235]

## Esophageal Varices

### Overview and Pathogenesis

Esophageal varices are one of the most serious consequences in people with cirrhosis, and approximately 50% of all individuals with cirrhosis have esophageal varices. Esophageal varices are fragile, dilated veins in the lower third of the esophagus immediately beneath the mucosa that occur in the presence of portal hypertension. Portal hypertension is an increase in pressure in the portal veins that return blood to the heart via the liver from the intestines, stomach, spleen, and pancreas. This increase in pressure is multifactorial, and the cause may be prehepatic (caused by venous thrombosis), intrahepatic (secondary to cirrhosis), or posthepatic (seen in Budd-Chiari syndrome).

In the United States the most common cause of portal hypertension is cirrhosis (90%). This is due to scar tissue and nodule formation in liver tissue (changing the anatomy and making it difficult for blood to pass through the liver), increased blood flow from dilated splanchnic vessels (secondary to an overproduction of nitrous oxide), and an imbalance between intrahepatic vasodilators and vasoconstrictors.[128] The normal anatomic reaction to portal hypertension is to decompress the portal venous system by opening up bypass veins (collaterals), most commonly around the lower esophagus and stomach.

### Clinical Manifestations

Variceal bleeding usually manifests with painless but significant hematemesis with or without melena. Associated signs range from mild postural tachycardia to profound shock, depending on the extent of blood loss and degree of hypovolemia.

### Diagnosis and Medical Management

Because of the seriousness and increased frequency of esophageal varices in people with cirrhosis, all clients with cirrhosis should be evaluated by EGD or transnasal endoscopy for the presence of esophageal varices. Once diagnosed, the class, variceal size, and appearance of the varix determine if primary prophylaxis is needed to reduce a first bleed. Prophylaxis consists of nonselective β-blockers (e.g., propranolol) or esophageal variceal band ligation.[350] Clients treated with prophylactic β-blockers do not need follow-up EGD unless bleeding develops, whereas clients who receive ligation should have EGD surveillance indefinitely. This is performed every 2 to 4 weeks until the varices are obliterated, then at 3 months, and then every 6 to 12 months thereafter.

When blood flow can no longer be counterbalanced by the variceal wall tension, the dilated veins (varices) rupture and bleed. Predictive risk factors for bleeding include severe liver disease, appearance of red markings or a "wale" on the vessels, and large variceal size (greater than 5 mm). Another important indicator of whether a variceal will bleed is the hepatic venous pressure gradient (HVPG). Varices are more likely to rupture and bleed when HVPG is greater than 12 mm Hg, with uncontrolled bleeding observed when HVPG is greater than 20 mm Hg.

Ruptured esophageal bleeding constitutes a medical emergency requiring aggressive fluid resuscitation and red blood cell transfusions to keep hemoglobin at 7 g/dL. Bleeding varices carry a high mortality of 20% at 6 weeks.[113,350] Prophylactic antibiotics given for 1 week following a bleed as well as the use of a vasoactive agent such as vasopressin or somatostatin given for 3 to 5 days have improved morbidity and mortality. Vasoactive medications aid in vasoconstricting the splanchnic venous system to reduce the amount of blood returning to the portal system and reduce portal hypertension. Following an esophageal bleed, approximately 60% of people will bleed again, with a mortality rate of 30%.[350]

For varices that are not controlled with these methods, a stent may be placed between the hepatic vein and the intrahepatic portion of the portal vein (transjugular intrahepatic portosystemic shunt). This procedure provides a means of lowering portal pressure. Liver transplantation may be considered in cases unresponsive to treatment.

SPECIAL IMPLICATIONS FOR THE THERAPIST 16.5

### *Esophageal Varices*

The primary concerns in therapy are to avoid causing rupture of varices and proper handling of clients with known GI bleeding. Carefully instruct the client in proper lifting techniques, and avoid any activities that will increase intraabdominal pressure (see Box 16.1).

For a client with known esophageal varices, observe closely for signs of behavioral or personality changes. Report increasing stupor, lethargy, hallucinations, or neuromuscular dysfunction. Watch for asterixis (involuntary jerking movements), a sign of developing hepatic encephalopathy.

To assess fluid retention, inspect the ankles and sacrum for dependent edema. To prevent skin breakdown associated with edema and pruritus, caution the client and family members caring for the client to avoid using soap when bathing the client and to use moisturizing cleansing agents instead. Precautions must be taken to handle the client gently, turning and repositioning often to keep the skin intact. Rest and good nutrition will conserve energy and decrease metabolic demands on the liver.

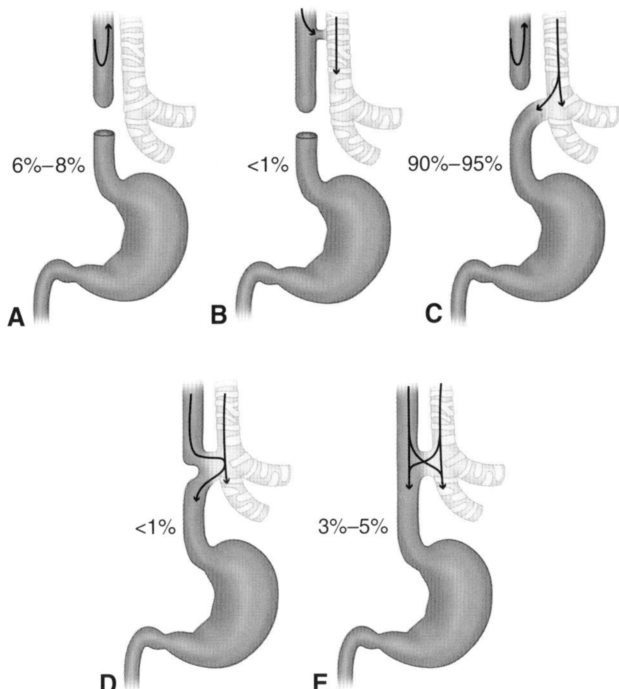


**Figure 16.4**

**Five types of esophageal atresia and tracheoesophageal fistula.** (A) Simple esophageal atresia. Proximal and distal esophageal segments end in blind pouches. Nothing enters the stomach; regurgitated food and fluid may enter the lungs. (B) Proximal and distal esophageal segments end in blind pouches, and a fistula connects the proximal esophagus to the trachea. Nothing enters the stomach; food and fluid enter the lungs. (C) Proximal esophagus ends in a blind pouch, and a fistula connects the trachea to the distal esophagus. Air enters the stomach; regurgitated gastric secretions enter the lungs through the fistula. (D) Fistula connects both proximal and distal esophageal segments to the trachea. Air, food, and fluid enter the stomach and lungs. (E) Simple tracheoesophageal fistula between otherwise normal esophagus and trachea. Air, food, and fluid enter the stomach and lungs. Between 90% and 95% of esophageal anomalies are type C; 6% to 8% are type A; 3% to 5% are type E; and less than 1% are type B or D.

## Congenital Conditions

### Esophageal Atresia and Tracheoesophageal Fistula

**Overview.** Esophageal atresia (EA) and tracheoesophageal fistula (TEF) are the most common esophageal anomalies and common congenital defects, occurring in approximately 1 in 4000 live births with equal gender distribution. EA develops when the esophagus fails to develop as a continuous passage (recanalize), and TEF forms when the lung bud fails to separate completely from the foregut, forming an abnormal communication between the lower portion of the esophagus and trachea. EA occurs as an isolated defect in only 8% of cases, while TEF occurs as an isolated defect in 4%. EA is accompanied by TEF for the remaining cases.[263]

There are typically two types of TEF, a distal-type (89%) and an H-type (3%) fistula. There are other types of TEF, but they are much more rare (Fig. 16.4). In isolated EA, the esophagus ends in a blind pouch, and the lower esophagus connects to the stomach. EA with a distal-type TEF exhibits an upper esophageal blind pouch and communication with the trachea and the lower esophagus. Other associated conditions include congenital heart disease, prematurity, and VACTERL (*v*ertebral, *a*nal, *c*ardiac, *t*racheal, *e*sophageal, *r*enal, and *l*imb) association. Specific abnormalities include imperforate anus, patent ductus arteriosus, and cardiac septal defects.

**Etiologic Factors and Pathogenesis.** Because EA and TEF are congenital malformations, the cause is unknown, but abnormalities are postulated to arise from genetic defects that prevent the trachea from separating from the esophagus during weeks 4 to 6 of embryonic development. Defective growth of endodermal cells leads to atresia (closure or absence of a normal body opening or tubular structure).

**Clinical Manifestations.** The blind end of the proximal esophagus has a capacity of only a few milliliters, so as the infant with EA swallows oral secretions, the pouch fills and overflows into the pharynx, resulting in excessive drooling and occasionally aspiration. It can often be seen prenatally as polyhydramnios because of the fetus' inability to swallow fluid.

If a fistula connects the trachea with the distal esophagus, the abdomen fills with air and becomes distended, potentially interfering with breathing. If the fistula connects the proximal esophagus to the trachea, the first feeding after birth will signal a problem. As the infant swallows, the blind end of the esophagus and the mouth fill with fluid that is aspirated into the lungs when the infant tries to take a breath. This triggers a protective cough and the choke reflex with intermittent cyanosis. Coughing, choking, and cyanosis are called the three C's of TEF and may occur especially with the H-type fistula, which may not be diagnosed for weeks to months after birth.

### MEDICAL MANAGEMENT

**DIAGNOSIS, TREATMENT, AND PROGNOSIS.** Esophageal anomalies are usually diagnosed at birth on the basis of clinical manifestations, but new technology is making in utero diagnosis more readily available. Rarely this condition escapes detection until adulthood, when recurrent pulmonary infections call attention to it. Inability to pass an orogastric catheter suggests the diagnosis of EA. Confirmation of a non–H-type fistula is made by passing a catheter into the esophagus with radiographs of the chest and abdomen taken with the tube in place to show the level of the blind pouch. Esophagography and bronchoscopy are often helpful in determining configuration of the defects.

Surgery to restore esophageal continuity and eliminate the fistula usually is performed shortly after birth. Surgical procedures may be performed in stages for infants who are premature, have multiple anomalies, or are in poor health. Antibiotics are instituted early owing to the certainty of aspiration pneumonia.

Without early diagnosis and treatment, this condition is rapidly fatal. Early detection prevents feedings until the problem is corrected; feeding can cause aspiration and its complications. The long-term survival rate is nearly 90%.

## THE STOMACH

## Peptic Ulcer Disease

### Definition and Overview

PUD may be defined as a break in the lining of the stomach or duodenum of 5 mm or more owing to a number of different causes.

Two kinds of peptic ulcer exist, although they are collectively referred to as PUD: *gastric ulcer,* which affects the lining of the stomach, and *duodenal ulcer,* which occurs in the duodenum. Approximately 95% of duodenal ulcers occur in the duodenal bulb or cap. Approximately 60% of benign gastric ulcers are located at or near the lesser curvature and most frequently on the posterior wall (Fig. 16.5). PUD may manifest as either uncomplicated gastric and/or duodenal ulcers or as a complicated ulcer. Because a small percentage of gastric ulcers are secondary to gastric carcinoma (about 5%), all gastric ulcers should be evaluated endoscopically.

*Stress ulcers,* or stress-related mucosal disease, occur in response to significant physiologic stress (e.g., severe trauma, surgery, extensive burns, brain injury). For example, gastric mucosal changes develop within 72 hours in 80% of clients with burns over more than 35% of the body. The mechanism causing stress ulcers is unknown but probably involves ischemia of the gastric mucosa, which has large oxygen requirements and low gastric pH (high acidity).

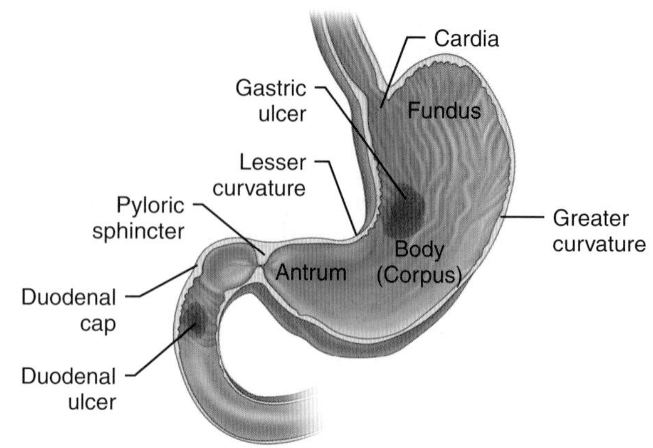


**Figure 16.5**

**Most common sites of peptic ulcers.**

Stress ulcers differ pathologically and clinically from peptic ulcers with very few symptoms and are painless until perforation and hemorrhage occur. Controversy currently exists as to which clients need prophylactic therapy,[5] what type (intravenous PPIs versus oral agents), and the role of enteral feeding in reducing the risk. Stress ulcer prophylaxis may increase the risk of nosocomial pneumonia or *C. difficile.*[19,200]

### Incidence

PUD affects approximately 6 million people per year in the United States,[102] with a prevalence rate of approximately 3.3% and a lifelong prevalence of 13.8%.[314] Incidence and prevalence have been decreasing over the past decade, presumably related to the treatment of *H. pylori.*[101,334] There are approximately 500,000 to 850,000 new cases of PUD diagnosed each year with 1 million hospitalizations, costing more than $6 billion.[55] PUD affects men and women equally.

### Etiologic and Risk Factors

NSAIDs, low-dose aspirin, and *H. pylori* bacterial infection[299] are the most common causes of peptic ulcers, accounting for approximately 90% of peptic ulcers. Other causes include Crohn disease (CD), acid hypersecretion states (such as Zollinger-Ellison syndrome), cancer, viral infections (cytomegalovirus), and drugs (cocaine). As more people are being treated with potent acid suppressants and for *H. pylori,* the incidence of uncomplicated PUD has decreased, whereas with the use of medications such as NSAIDs and low-dose aspirin, there is an increased prevalence in complicated ulcers,[233] particularly in the elderly population.[194]

Psychologic stress, diet, caffeine, tobacco use, and alcohol consumption may have some role in causing PUD, although many studies were done before the discovery of

*H. pylori*, and these factors have subsequently been found to play less of a role than once thought. Corticosteroids alone do not increase the risk for PUD,[218] although they have been found, when used with NSAIDs, to increase the risk.

### Pathogenesis

In the upper GI tract, there is a balance between mucosal insults and mucosal defenses. If there is an imbalance, an ulcer can form. Defenses include a mucous and bicarbonate layer, an epithelial barrier, prostaglandins, and adequate mucosal blood flow. Ulcers develop when this balance is changed. Some contributing insults include acid, pepsin, alcohol, bile salts, and drugs. The most common factors that cause an imbalance in the normal gastric environment and lead to ulcer formation are NSAID use and *H. pylori* infection.

Gastric acid is made by parietal cells in the stomach. There are three types of receptors on the parietal cell that stimulate production of acid: gastrin, acetylcholine, and histamine. Histamine $H_2$ receptor antagonists ($H_2$ blockers) decrease acid production by blocking histamine receptors on the parietal cells. PPIs block $H^+,K^+$-ATPase of the parietal cell and thereby block the pumping of $H^+$ and the formation of gastric acid.[309] Gastric acid production is inhibited by somatostatin and prostaglandins.

Prostaglandin deficiency can lead to the formation of ulcers. Cyclooxygenase types 1 and 2 (COX-1 and COX-2) are responsible for the production of prostaglandins. NSAIDs are known to lead to a reduction of prostaglandin production through inhibition of COX-1 and/or COX-2. This then allows for enhanced gastric motility, increased mucosal permeability, infiltration of neutrophils, and production of oxyradicals. This eventually leads to the formation of gastric lesions and ulceration.[339]

The bacterium *H. pylori* causes an inflammatory response in the gastric mucosa, with responsive production of cytokines (interleukin [IL]-8 and IL-1β). These chemicals attract neutrophils and macrophages into the area that release lysosomal enzymes, leukotrienes, and reactive oxygen species, causing a breakdown in the mucosal barrier.

*H. pylori* also has very high urease activity that produces ammonia to protect it from the acidic environment of the stomach. This local increase in alkaline ammonia triggers the epithelium to secrete somatostatin and leads to hypergastrinemia and excess acid production. The production of ammonia in large concentrations also leads to the formation of toxic chemicals such as ammonium chloride that contribute to the breakdown of the phospholipid-rich mucosal barrier that normally protects the gastric epithelium. *H. pylori* also produces phospholipases that further contribute to this breakdown. Metaplasia (changing of cell types) of duodenal epithelium must also occur, as infection with *H. pylori* is specific to gastric cells.[268]

*H. pylori* is a known carcinogen and may be involved in the development of gastric cancer and mucosa-associated lymphoid tissue (MALT) lymphoma. It is also evident that not all people who are infected with *H. pylori* go on to develop a disease (only approximately 20%).[336] Specific genes the bacteria carry may correlate not only to disease but also to drug resistance.

Other drugs may cause ulcers, including methamphetamines and cocaine. This is presumed to be due to restricted blood flow and ischemia in the stomach.

### Clinical Manifestations

There are no symptoms or physical findings specific or sensitive for PUD. Many people with NSAID-induced PUD do not have pain at diagnosis, and PUD is often discovered because of bleeding or is noted on EGD. The classic symptom of PUD, when present, is epigastric pain described as burning, gnawing, or cramping near the xiphoid or radiating to the back. Pain may be relieved with eating or occur at night. Symptoms may be nonspecific such as nausea, abdominal fullness, or early satiety.

Because gastric malignancy accounts for 5% of peptic ulcers, clients with a family history of GI cancer in the presence of symptoms that are worrisome for malignancy such as unintentional weight loss, iron deficiency, bleeding, persistent vomiting, jaundice, or left supraclavicular lymphadenopathy should undergo EGD.

### Complications

Bleeding (acute and chronic), perforation, penetration, and gastric outlet obstruction are the principal major complications seen in PUD. Bleeding, the most common complication from a peptic ulcer, is serious, requiring hospitalization, and carries a 10% mortality.[21] Bleeding may be manifested by hematochezia (bleeding per rectum), hematemesis (vomiting blood), coffee-ground emesis, or melena (dark, tarry stools secondary to blood).

Approximately 15% of people with PUD, mostly older adults, will develop bleeding. One study found that 68% of people who presented with bleeding due to PUD were older than age 60 years.[248] Elderly adults tend to have more episodes and more severe bleeding owing to higher use of aspirin, NSAIDs, antiplatelet medications, and other comorbidities.[166]

Perforation of the stomach or duodenum may occur, manifesting with sudden severe pain (thoracic spine from T6 to T10 with radiation to the right upper quadrant), associated with hemodynamic compromise. Fever may be present; bowel sounds may be absent with guarding of the abdomen. This requires immediate surgical attention and carries the highest mortality rate of the possible complications.

Penetration occurs when the ulcer erodes into adjacent organs such as the small bowel, pancreas, or liver. Pain often gradually increases in severity and frequency. Pancreatitis is a common presentation. Gastric outlet obstruction (rare) may occur because of scarring of the prepyloric region from healed ulcerations or a neoplastic process. Affected individuals may exhibit nausea, vomiting, early satiety, and weight loss.

## MEDICAL MANAGEMENT

**DIAGNOSIS.** Upper endoscopy is the test of choice for diagnosing PUD. Not only does endoscopy determine the site of ulceration, but biopsy specimens also can be obtained to evaluate for cancer and aid in diagnosing *H. pylori*. This is particularly relevant for clients older than age 55 with "alarm" symptoms such as unexplained new abdominal pain, unexplained weight loss, recurrent vomiting, or GI bleeding.

All individuals with PUD should be tested for *H. pylori*. Tests that do not require endoscopy include the fecal antigen test or urea breath test. Antibody testing (serum for IgG antibodies) is a popular method of diagnosis because of its low cost, ready availability, and quick results, although it does not determine if an infection is active (particularly in populations with a low prevalence of disease). It is also less sensitive and specific than the above-mentioned tests.

Tests performed on endoscopically obtained specimens include rapid urease test, culture, and histology. All of these tests can identify active infection.

Double-contrast barium studies of the upper GI tract can be used to diagnose an ulcer. Although these studies are less expensive than endoscopy, they are not used as frequently because of the inability to obtain biopsy specimens.

**PREVENTION AND TREATMENT.** Treatment of PUD is oriented toward the cause. If a client is taking an NSAID, it should be discontinued and an alternative analgesic implemented, or the NSAID should be taken at the lowest effective dose. PPI therapy for 8 to 12 weeks aids in healing of the ulcer. For clients needing to take aspirin to reduce stroke or acute coronary events, evidence shows that a PPI with aspirin reduces the risk of peptic ulcer bleeding.[139,355] Dual antiplatelet therapy (DAPT) is prescribed to reduce the risk of cardiac events and stroke in people who have undergone percutaneous coronary interventions. DAPT also increases the risk of GI bleeding, for which a PPI is often prescribed prophylactically. There has been controversy concerning the concomitant use of the antiplatelet medication clopidogrel as part of DAPT therapy and PPIs. Some studies show that a subset of people who concomitantly use clopidogrel and a PPI have a greater incidence of acute coronary events while others do not.[42] Care should be taken in prescribing these two medications, although it is important to note that bleeding is a serious risk with DAPT therapy, and individuals with a history of PUD or GI bleeding may benefit from PPI prophylactic use.[246,341] While PPIs have long-term consequences,[103,294] acid suppression with a PPI may be prescribed indefinitely for clients who have had a recurrence or complication from PUD or require long-term aspirin or NSAID use.[179]

If *H. pylori* is present, therapy should be directed toward the eradication of the organism. Testing and eradication can also be beneficial for clients taking long-term, low-dose aspirin and clients initiating long-term NSAIDs or antiplatelet regimens.[64] Most treatment regimens for active *H. pylori* infection include two or three antibiotics and a PPI for 7 to 14 days. Available combinations for first-line regimens are numerous. These include clarithromycin triple therapy, bismuth quadruple therapy, concomitant therapy, and sequential therapy, among others (Table 16.4). Regional drug resistance should also be taken into account, and clarithromycin-containing regimens should be used only when resistance is less than 15%.[64] Bismuth therapy has the advantage of being effective for people with previous exposure to clarithromycin.

**Table 16.4** Common First-Line Therapies for *Helicobacter pylori* Eradication

| Regimen | Drugs | Duration |
|---|---|---|
| Clarithromycin triple | Clarithromycin<br>PPI<br>Amoxicillin or metronidazole | 14 days |
| Bismuth quadruple | PPI<br>Bismuth subcitrate<br>Tetracycline<br>Metronidazole | 10–14 days |
| Concomitant | PPI<br>Clarithromycin<br>Amoxicillin<br>Nitroimidazole | 10–14 days |
| Sequential | PPI + amoxicillin<br>PPI + clarithromycin + nitroimidazole | 5–7 days<br>5–7 days |
| Hybrid | PPI + amoxicillin<br>PPI + amoxicillin + clarithromycin + nitroimidazole | 7 days<br>7 days |
| Levofloxacin triple | A PPI<br>Levofloxacin<br>Amoxicillin | 10–14 days |
| Levofloxacin sequential | PPI + amoxicillin<br>PPI + amoxicillin + levofloxacin + nitroimidazole | 5–7 days<br>5–7 days |
| LOAD | Levofloxacin<br>PPI (double dose) / omeprazole<br>Nitazoxanide (Alinia)<br>Doxycycline | 7–10 days |

*PPI*, Proton pump inhibitor.
Data from Chey WD, Leontiadis GI, Howden CW, Moss WF: ACG Clinical Guideline: Treatment of *Helicobacter pylori* Infection. *Am J Gastroenterol* 112:212–239, 2017.

Most treatments are 70% to 90% effective in the eradication of *H. pylori* and the treatment of PUD secondary to *H. pylori*.[8] Resistance to clarithromycin has reduced the effectiveness of clarithromycin-based treatments in many locations to less than 80%[64]; however, when clarithromycin triple therapy is used, it should be given for a total of 14 days. Clinical judgment should be used to identify the best regimen to eradicate *H. pylori*. Following the eradication of *H. pylori*, maintenance therapy with a PPI is usually not warranted, although confirmation of eradication is required with either the urea breath test or the fecal antigen test.[106]

Testing should be done 4 weeks following the completion of therapy and 1 to 2 weeks after discontinuing/withholding the PPI.[64] Follow-up endoscopy should be performed only when ulcers are large or complicated or when initial biopsy specimens were inadequate or yielded suspicious biopsy results. Reinfection with *H. pylori* following initial eradication is low[241]; even so, researchers are working on vaccine development[124] to prevent recurrence.

Lifestyle changes should also be addressed such as smoking cessation and reduction or elimination of alcohol use. Probiotics may also be helpful in inhibiting *H.*

*pylori* when used as an adjuvant to first-line regimens,[368,382] although many of the studies have come from China with a substantial variability in product.

Bleeding peptic ulcers are most often treated endoscopically. Injection with adrenaline/epinephrine, use of endoclips, and bipolar electrocoagulation or heater probe therapy are options, depending on what is seen endoscopically.[190] Other advances include Doppler probe–guided lesion assessment, large over-the-scope clips, and hemostatic powders.[59,156] Nearly all cases of perforation require surgical intervention/consultation. Outlet obstruction caused by scarring of the duodenum or caudal portion of the stomach typically requires endoscopic or surgical treatment.

**PROGNOSIS.** Because of improved medical treatment of PUD, including treatment of *H. pylori* and the availability of PPIs, the hospitalization rate for PUD has significantly decreased (by 21% between 1998 and 2005).[102] There has also been a significant reduction in mortality except in the older population.[319,320] Prognosis is usually good, and medical management can adequately control ulcers unless massive hemorrhage or perforation occurs, which carries a high mortality. In elderly adults, the mortality of a perforated ulcer is three to five times higher (up to 50%) than in younger people.[25] Mortality from a bleeding ulcer, around 5%, is also increased in elderly adults.[191,202] People with bleeding duodenal ulcers appear to have higher morbidity and mortality compared with people with bleeding gastric ulcers.[207,270]

SPECIAL IMPLICATIONS FOR THE THERAPIST 16.6

## *Peptic Ulcer Disease*

### Monitoring Symptoms and Vital Signs

Ulcer presentation without pain occurs more frequently in older adults and in persons taking NSAIDs for painful musculoskeletal conditions, especially arthritis. Anyone with this type of medical history should be monitored for signs and symptoms of bleeding. Observe color (pallor), activity or exercise tolerance, and fatigue level.

Vital signs should be monitored for systolic blood pressure less than 100 mm Hg, pulse rate greater than 100 beats/min, or a 10-mm Hg or greater decrease in diastolic blood pressure, with position changes accompanied by increased pulse rate, which may signal bleeding. Any client presenting with GI symptoms should be encouraged to report the symptoms to his or her physician.

### Referred Pain Patterns

Peptic ulcers located on the posterior wall of the stomach or duodenum can perforate and hemorrhage, causing back pain as the only presenting symptom. Occasionally, ulcer pain radiates to the midthoracic back and right upper quadrant including the right shoulder. Right shoulder pain alone may occur as a result of blood in the peritoneal cavity from perforation and hemorrhage.

When back pain appears to be the only presenting symptom, a careful history may reveal alternating or concomitant GI symptoms such as vomiting of bright red blood or coffee-ground vomitus. Back pain relieved by antacids is an indication of GI involvement and must be reported to the physician as well as any other indication of shoulder or back pain with accompanying GI involvement.

Musculoskeletal symptoms may recur after discontinuing NSAIDs, owing to the masking effects of these drugs. Once the drug is discontinued, painful symptoms may return in the presence of continued underlying ulcer disease. Medical follow-up is required in such situations.

### Exercise and Peptic Ulcer Disease

Researchers have reported that exercise at least three times a week greatly reduces the risk of GI bleeding. More strenuous forms of exercise such as swimming and bicycling do not provide greater protection from GI bleeding than do more moderate exercises such as walking.[63,251]

For the competitive athlete, during the acute episode, anxiety and nervousness may increase gastric secretions. This effect in combination with poor nutrition (often the athlete has not eaten at all) requires careful monitoring and maximizing the use of medications and food intake with the performance schedule. For the average adult uninvolved in competitive sports, regular exercise as part of stress reduction is essential during remission.

## Gastric Cancer

### Gastric Adenocarcinoma

**Definition and Incidence.** Gastric adenocarcinoma, a malignant neoplasm arising from the gastric mucosa, constitutes more than 90% of the malignant tumors of the stomach. Gastric cancer is the fifth most common cancer and third most common cause of cancer death in the world, with an estimate of almost 1 million new cases worldwide in 2018.[376] Most cases are diagnosed in developing countries, particularly in Asia. In the United States for 2018, 26,240 new cases and 10,800 deaths were estimated. Men are more affected than women, with incidences higher in nonwhites than whites. About 6 in 10 people diagnosed with gastric cancer are older than age 65.[175]

Gastric cancer can be classified by anatomic location, cardia or noncardia, or divided into two histologic subtypes, intestinal type or diffuse type. The intestinal type is related to environmental and dietary risk factors and is most often seen in areas with a high incidence of gastric cancer. The diffuse type is typically seen in younger people and women. Several genetic syndromes contribute to the development of gastric cancer, among them *MYH*-associated polyposis, Lynch syndrome, Li-Fraumeni syndrome, Peutz-Jeghers syndrome, and familial adenomatous polyposis (FAP). Individuals with the germline mutation in the gene *E-cadherin* have an 80% risk over their lifetime of developing gastric cancer (hereditary diffuse type). A prophylactic gastrectomy after the age of 20 is recommended.

**Etiologic and Risk Factors.** In the United States, *H. pylori* infection is associated with intestinal-type gastric cancer. Epstein-Barr virus, another infective agent that has been found in gastric tumors, may also cause gastric cancer.[147,230] Lifestyle choices that increase the risk of stomach cancer include dietary factors such as low intake of fruits and vegetables,[108] ingestion of salt[367] and salt-preserved foods, and consumption of smoked fish and meat containing nitrates.[71,154] Smoking has been linked to both types of gastric cancer. Obesity may also be a risk factor for gastric cancer, although the data are not clear.[67] Other nonenvironmental risk factors include chronic atrophic gastritis and intestinal metaplasia, pernicious anemia (which causes atrophy of the gastric mucosa),[252] previous gastric resection, and gastric adenomas.[147]

**Pathogenesis.** The development of gastric cancer is thought to be a multistep process, often requiring years, with genetic and epigenetic (DNA modifications) changes that lead to the dysregulation of the cell including cell cycle, DNA repair, signaling pathways, cell proliferation, and cell death. Both Epstein-Barr virus and *H. pylori* use epigenetic mechanisms to alter gene expression. *H. pylori* is able to quiet tumor suppressor genes, which in turn deregulates cell pathways, whereas Epstein-Barr virus–related tumors display a distinctive hypermethylation pattern. It appears that each cause of gastric cancer may have its own genetic and epigenetic alterations that, once identified, can guide a more individualized treatment. These DNA changes lead to acute and chronic gastritis, developing into atrophic gastritis, which leads to intestinal metaplasia, then dysplasia, and finally gastric carcinoma.[23,378]

**Clinical Manifestations.** The most common clinical manifestations are weight loss and abdominal pain. Other symptoms include early satiety (feeling full despite small food intake), nausea/vomiting, gastric outlet obstruction (tumors near the pyloric sphincter), and occult bleeding. Most people remain asymptomatic until the disease is advanced (80%), which results in a poorer prognosis. Typically only 50% of people are candidates for surgical resection and cure. About 5% of peptic ulcers harbor gastric cancers, making biopsies of ulcers vital. Paraneoplastic syndromes are rare clinical manifestations of gastric cancer (discussed in Chapter 9).

## MEDICAL MANAGEMENT

PREVENTION. At the present time, there is no recommendation for gastric cancer screening in the general population in the United States. In families or persons with a genetic risk factor for gastric cancer, screening endoscopy can be performed.[229] Subsequent surveillance endoscopy should also be performed for people with an adenomatous gastric polyp 1 year after removal and then every 3 to 5 years.

DIAGNOSIS AND STAGING. Diagnosis may be delayed because of a lack of symptoms or because symptomatic relief can be obtained from using nonprescription medications. Endoscopy is the first test performed with biopsies of suspicious lesions. Staging is accomplished with CT, which can determine if metastases are present, and endoscopic ultrasonography, which allows for biopsy of nodes and assesses depth of invasion and if the tumor is amenable to endoscopic mucosal resection (early, local tumor). Staging laparoscopy can be considered for clients who appear to have locoregional disease. Although all stages have subtypes, generally stage I gastric cancer confines the tumor to the stomach and to one or two nodes. Stage II confines the tumor to the stomach and three to six nodes. In stage III the tumor has grown through the stomach wall and spread in up to 16 nodes. Stage IV has metastasized to surrounding organs (liver, lungs, brain, or peritoneum).[175]

TREATMENT. A new classification from the American Joint Committee on Cancer (AJCC) defines cancers that have their epicenter 2 cm or greater into the proximal stomach from the esophagogastric junction as gastric tumors.[7a] Otherwise, tumors that are less than 2 cm are considered esophageal cancers. For stages I, II, and III, surgical therapy is still the treatment of choice for primary gastric adenocarcinoma. Chemotherapy and radiation, owing to the frequent relapse of disease with surgery alone, are also used. About two-thirds of people with gastric cancer present with stage III or IV disease, while only 10% have stage I.[24,143]

Individuals who are candidates for surgery also receive neoadjuvant chemotherapy (preoperatively) and combined adjuvant chemotherapy and radiation therapy. Persons who are not surgical candidates may receive palliative chemotherapy and stent placement for obstruction of the pylorus, but the disease is incurable. About 20% of people with gastric cancer overexpress the *HER2* growth factor receptor, which can be treated using the anti-*HER2* monoclonal antibody trastuzumab. All metastatic gastric carcinomas should be evaluated for the presence of *HER2* for possible treatment.[1] Endoscopic therapies are available for people with early disease.[316]

PROGNOSIS. Prognosis depends on the degree of gastric wall penetration, the presence of lymph node involvement, and the location of the primary site. Overall, relative 5-year survival rate is 31%, principally as a result of late stage detection.[74,129,175]

SPECIAL IMPLICATIONS FOR THE THERAPIST 16.7

### *Gastric Cancer*

Epigastric or back pain, possibly relieved by antacids, is a frequent complaint that the physician must differentiate from PUD. In general, the first manifestations of carcinoma are caused by distant metastasis when the condition is quite advanced. The therapist may palpate the left supraclavicular (Virchow) lymph node, or the client may point out an umbilical nodule.

After surgery, position changes every 2 hours, deep breathing, coughing, and incentive spirometry (use of a handheld device to provide visual feedback for voluntary maximal inspiration) may be used to prevent pulmonary complications. The semi-Fowler position (head of the bed raised 6 to 12 inches with knees slightly flexed) facilitates breathing and drainage after any type of gastrectomy.

## Congenital Conditions

### Pyloric Stenosis

**Definition and Overview.** Pyloric stenosis (PS) is an obstruction at the pyloric sphincter (the sphincter at the distal opening of the stomach into the duodenum) that occurs in 2 in 1000 live births. The pyloric sphincter is a ring of muscles that serve to close the opening from the stomach into the intestine (Fig. 16.6). Obstruction occurs as a congenital condition, or in adults, the most common causes are ulcer disease or cancer. Treatment of GERD has greatly reduced the number of acquired PS cases. When present as a congenital condition, it is known as *infantile hypertrophic pyloric stenosis (IHPS)*, which is caused by hypertrophy of the sphincter and is one of the most common surgical disorders of early infancy.

**Incidence and Etiologic Factors.** The cause of congenital hypertrophy of the pyloric sphincter is unknown. White males are affected more commonly than females in a 4:1 ratio. It is more likely to occur in a premature infant than in a full-term infant, especially a first-born child. Siblings, offspring of affected persons, and fathers and sons are at increased risk of developing PS (genetic predisposition). Administration of erythromycin and azithromycin to newborns has been reported to have a possible causal role in IHPS.[57,212]

IHPS may also be associated with other congenital conditions such as Turner syndrome, trisomy 18, intestinal malrotation, esophageal and duodenal atresia, and anorectal anomalies.

The incidence of adult idiopathic PS is unknown, but it is considered rare. Although many physicians think this condition is secondary to local disease, others think the condition in adults is the same entity as that observed in infants and children but in a milder form and later in appearance.

**Pathogenesis.** The histologic and anatomic abnormalities in adult PS are indistinguishable from those in the infantile form. Individual fibers of the pyloric sphincter thicken or hypertrophy, so the entire sphincter is grossly enlarged and inelastic.

Hyperplasia of the pyloric muscle occurs because of the extra peristaltic effort required to force the gastric contents through the narrow opening into the duodenum. This hypertrophy and hyperplasia form a palpable nodule, severely narrowing the pyloric canal between the stomach and the duodenum, causing partial obstruction.

Over time, inflammation and edema further reduce the size of the lumen, progressing to complete obstruction preventing food from passing from the stomach to the small intestine. Progressive obstruction results in complications of malnutrition and fluid and electrolyte abnormalities. This may be the result of a lack of localized nitric oxide synthase, associated with smooth muscle relaxation, or from decreased muscle neurofilaments.[181]

**Clinical Manifestations.** Projectile or forcible vomiting is the most common and dramatic early symptom and is typically seen in infants between 3 and 6 weeks of age. In the past, children were diagnosed at later stages, after developing fluid and electrolyte and nutritional problems. Infants are now diagnosed earlier before acquiring acid–base disturbances or electrolyte abnormalities.[254]

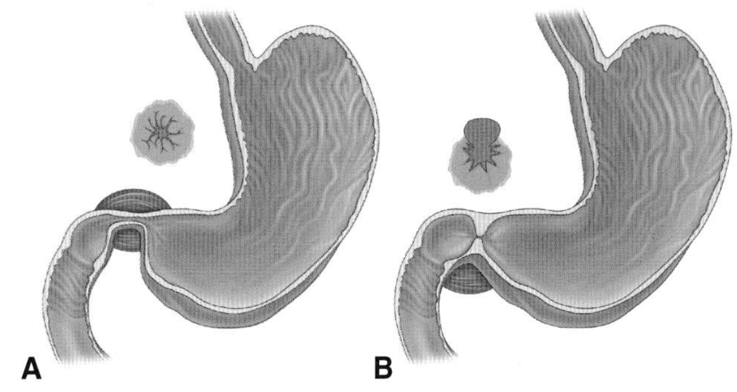


**Figure 16.6**

**Hypertrophic pyloric stenosis.** (A) Enlarged muscular area nearly obliterates the pyloric channel. (B) Longitudinal surgical division of muscle down to the submucosa or the placement of an expandable stent (not shown) establishes an adequate passageway.

The palpable nodule is firm, movable, about the size of an olive, and felt in the right upper quadrant in approximately 30% of all infants with IHPS (less than the 70% classically seen[15]). Many infants present without the typical symptoms of projectile vomiting and palpable olive but may exhibit repeated vomiting and hypochloremic metabolic acidosis.

Persistent or episodic symptoms in some adults may extend from infancy, with nausea and vomiting, epigastric pain, early satiety, weight loss, and anorexia most commonly present. In contrast to IHPS in the infant, the abdominal mass that occurs in adult PS is too small to be palpable.

### MEDICAL MANAGEMENT

DIAGNOSIS, TREATMENT, AND PROGNOSIS. In infancy, diagnosis is usually by history and recognition of the clinical presentation. Pyloric ultrasound imaging is the test of choice for the diagnosis of IHPS.

Some infants are treated with antispasmodic drugs to relax the pylorospasm and nutritional management including refeeding the infant after vomiting, waiting to see if the pylorus spontaneously opens by 6 to 8 months of age (although not usually done in the United States). Pyloromyotomy (local resection of the involved region of the pylorus), often performed laparoscopically, is typically the procedure of choice. Procedures performed laparoscopically demonstrate a 2% to 6% rate of incomplete pyloromyotomy. Endoscopic balloon dilation and pyloroplasty have been successfully used, but the recurrence rate is high. Placement of a stent at the site of obstruction is gaining popularity as an alternative intervention procedure for adults with unresectable cancer.

Postoperative vomiting is not uncommon in the pediatric population, especially during the first 24 to 48 hours. Prognosis is very good following surgery, with infants able to resume normal growth and development. Complications include persistent pyloric obstruction; partial, superficial, or total wound separation (dehiscence); or, in the case of stent implantation, stent migration.

# THE INTESTINES

## Malabsorptive Disorders

Myriad diseases have malabsorption of nutrients as a consequence. These diseases typically affect the small intestine, where the majority of nutrients are absorbed. Examples include carbohydrate malabsorption (lactose intolerance), short-bowel syndrome (secondary to a birth defect or surgery), small intestinal bacterial overgrowth (secondary to decreased acid production, changes in intestinal transit, and disruption of normal antibacterial defenses), diseases that affect pancreas function, and celiac disease.

### Celiac Disease

**Definition and Overview.** Celiac disease is an immune-mediated disorder triggered by the exposure of the digestive tract to gluten in people who are susceptible. Celiac disease was once thought to be rare, but with improved methods of detection and understanding of clinical manifestations, it has become one of the most common disorders in westernized countries. It currently affects approximately 0.5% to 1% of the population, and the incidence is increasing.[359] With westernizing of diets, more of the world will also become affected in the future.

**Risk Factors.** Celiac disease is more common in people with other autoimmune diseases, immunoglobulin A (IgA) deficiency, some genetic syndromes (e.g., Down syndrome, Turner syndrome), a family history of celiac disease, type 1 diabetes, and thyroiditis.

**Etiologic Factors.** This disorder occurs in people with a genetic predisposition. It is strongly associated with the genes *HLA-DQ2* (95%) and *HLA-DQ8*. Approximately 30% of whites carry the *DQ2* gene, although this does not mean they will develop the disease. Several other genes contribute to the development of the disease,[144] with more yet to be detected. Chronic inflammation and malabsorption of nutrients appear to be responsible for most of the complications seen in celiac disease.[49]

**Pathogenesis.** Although much progress has been made in the elucidation of the pathogenesis of celiac disease, there is still more to understand. It is thought that there is interplay between innate immunity, T cells, B cells, genes, and environment. Normal intestinal epithelium displays receptors to gliadin (a component of gluten), which bind the gliadin, bring it into the cell, and transport it to the lamina propria. It is here where the enzyme tissue transglutaminase (tTG) deamidates (removes an amide group) the glutamine residues of the gliadin and cross-links it with HLA-DQ2 and HLA-DQ8 molecules. T cells in the lamina propria have receptors specific for these HLA-gliadin complexes, which, once stimulated, lead to the production of IL-21 and interferon (IFNδ) and the activity of cytotoxic T cells. Cytotoxic T cells then cause cell death. B cells are known to form and secrete anti-tTG antibodies; however, currently the mechanism of the formation of tTG autoantibodies is uncertain. tTG-gliadin complexes may be directly presented to B cells or B cells may be stimulated by T cells are among the possibilities. The release of autoantibodies contributes to the chronic nature of celiac disease. The microbiome of the gut also plays a role and alters the normal intestinal defense barrier and triggers T-cell response to gluten.[84]

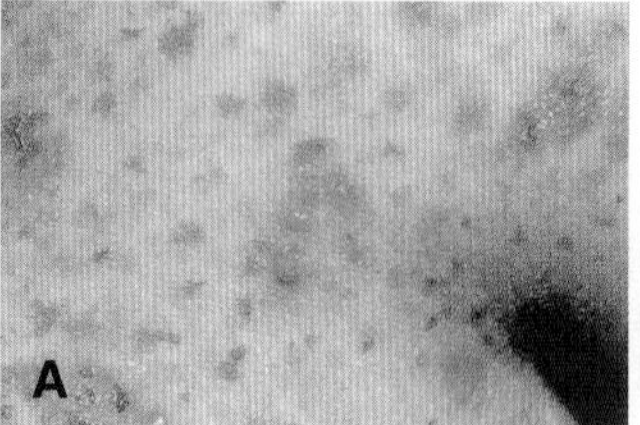


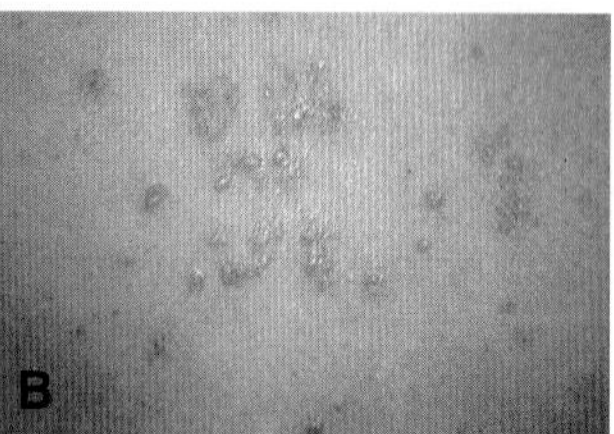


**Figure 16.7**

(A–B) Dermatitis herpetiformis. Typical grouped pruritic papulovesicles associated with skin reaction from gluten sensitivity. This skin manifestation usually appears on the buttocks, elbows, or knees. It can affect children but is more common in adults between the ages of 30 and 40 years. It is almost always a sign of celiac disease and will usually resolve in 3 to 6 months with a gluten-free diet. (A, From Feldman M, Friedman LS, Brandt LJ, editors: *Sleisenger and Fordtran's gastrointestinal and liver disease*, ed 8, Philadelphia, 2006, Saunders. Courtesy of Dr. Timothy Berger, San Francisco. B, From Noble J, editor: *Textbook of primary care medicine*, ed 3, St. Louis, 2001, Mosby. Courtesy James C. Shaw, MD.)

**Clinical Manifestations.** People with celiac disease manifest a broad array of symptoms that range from no symptoms to life-altering symptoms, making the diagnosis at times difficult. The disorder is typically characterized by diarrhea (can be severe), bloating, indigestion, flatulence, weight loss, and abdominal pain/cramping. Malabsorption and malnutrition often accompany the disease, depending on the time of diagnosis (early versus late) with associated complications. Nutrient deficiencies include folate, iron,[96] fat-soluble vitamins, and vitamin $B_{12}$.[112] Clients diagnosed with celiac disease should be evaluated for nutritional deficiencies, which should be corrected.[112]

A skin manifestation often linked to celiac disease is dermatitis herpetiformis,[50] characterized by erythema, urticarial plaques, papules, and grouped vesicles (blisters) and associated with an intense itch (Fig. 16.7).[50] Long-term complications include osteoporosis,[28] infertility, coagulation abnormalities, iron-deficiency anemia, and neurologic problems.[280] There is also a close association between type 1 diabetes mellitus and celiac disease. Whether this is a secondary autoimmune reaction is unknown, and studies are needed to define the relationship.[46] Cancer is a known complication, although it is not as prevalent as once thought.[109] Lymphoma and GI malignancies have the strongest association. The risk may be eliminated or partially reduced by following the appropriate diet.[109,121]

### MEDICAL MANAGEMENT

**DIAGNOSIS.** Serologic testing is available to diagnose celiac disease and should be performed while the client is still consuming gluten. The laboratory screening test for IgA antibodies to tTG (anti-tTG) is the recommended initial test. Testing for IgA anti-endomysial antibodies is also available but is not used as frequently as tTG. Another test identifying deamidated gliadin peptides, for the IgG class, is comparable and can be used in persons with IgA deficiency or when the diagnosis is uncertain.[201,291] A small intestine biopsy is recommended to histologically prove the diagnosis. This is typically performed by EGD. On pathology, celiac disease demonstrates an infiltration of lymphocytes, elongation of the crypts, and atrophy of the villous. A "four out of five" rule has been suggested for confirmation of the diagnosis[53]:

- Typical symptoms of celiac disease
- Positivity of serum IgA class autoantibodies at a high titer
- HLA-DQ2 and/or HLA-DQ8 genotypes (tested when clients have been on a gluten-free diet without previous confirmatory testing or other testing is uncertain or negative)
- Celiac enteropathy found on small bowel biopsy
- Response to a gluten-free diet

**TREATMENT.** Although other treatments are under investigation, the most practical consists of a diet free of gluten.[276] Rice, corn, quinoa, tapioca flour, potato starch, millet, and sorghum are other grain substitutes.[240] If the diagnosis is delayed or the diet is not adhered to, there are many complications of celiac disease caused by chronic inflammation.

**PROGNOSIS.** Most people can live asymptomatic lives if they follow the strict diet. Because celiac disease has become more common and the public has become more aware of it, more restaurants and stores are offering special food products to accommodate people with celiac disease. Many complications of the disease can be avoided with rapid diagnosis and treatment.

**Table 16.5 Symptoms Associated With Malabsorptive Disorders**

| Symptoms | Malabsorbed Nutrients |
|---|---|
| Muscle weakness, muscle wasting, paresthesia | Generalized malnutrition; fat, protein, carbohydrates |
| Osteomalacia | Fat, protein, carbohydrates, iron, water; vitamins A, D, K |
| Tetany, paresthesias, Trousseau sign, Chvostek sign | Calcium, vitamin D, magnesium, potassium |
| Numbness and tingling; neurologic damage | Vitamin $B_{12}$, vitamin B |
| Bone pain, fractures, skeletal deformities | Calcium, vitamin D, protein |
| Muscle spasms | Electrolyte imbalance, calcium, pregnancy |
| Easy bleeding or bruising | Vitamin K |
| Generalized swelling | Protein |
| Dermatitis herpetiformis (see Fig. 16.8) | Gluten induced |

SPECIAL IMPLICATIONS FOR THE THERAPIST 16.8

## *Malabsorptive Disorders*

Athletes with prolonged unexplained illnesses may have a malabsorptive disorder such as gluten intolerance or full-blown celiac disease. People with celiac disease can present with a number of different symptoms with a delay in diagnosis. A multidisciplinary approach in helping a newly diagnosed athlete with celiac disease is important to successful treatment of the disease. Athletes with celiac disease often have problems with iron absorption (leading to anemia) and/or vitamin D and calcium absorption (leading to osteoporosis and poor bone health). Even athletes with known and long-standing celiac disease need additional care and supervision in ensuring there is no disruption in their gluten-free diet, which can lead to a flare-up of symptoms or a decrease in performance.[213]

In the rehabilitation setting or for an acute care client who has not been eating solid foods, diarrhea may develop when the person begins to reestablish a normal diet. Prolonged viral conditions can wash out the enzymes normally present in the columnar epithelial cells. Reestablishing normal eating may require additional time to restore the enzymatic homeostasis in the intestines.

Paresthesia, muscle weakness, and muscle wasting accompanied by fatigue and weight loss can be signs of malnutrition (e.g., eating disorders) or malabsorbed fat, protein, or carbohydrates. Malabsorption of calcium, vitamin D, magnesium, and potassium can cause paresthesia, tetany, and positive Trousseau and Chvostek signs.

The Trousseau sign is an indication of tetany seen as carpal spasm elicited by compressing the upper arm (as occurs when taking a blood pressure measurement). The Chvostek sign is a spasm of the facial muscles elicited by tapping the facial nerve in the region of the parotid gland; it is seen in tetany.

Other effects of malabsorptive disorders possibly seen in a therapy setting include muscle spasms caused by electrolyte imbalance (especially low calcium) and pregnancy, easy bleeding or bruising as a result of vitamin K deficiency, and generalized swelling caused by protein depletion (Table 16.5).

Malabsorption of calcium, vitamin D, and protein can cause osteoporosis, bone pain with pathologic (compression) fractures, and skeletal deformities. In fact, 20% of osteoporosis is osteomalacia secondary to decreased absorption of vitamin D associated with malabsorptive conditions.[304]

Excessive absorption of vitamin D and calcium through the use of calcium carbonate for acid indigestion should be evaluated by a physician; these antacids may be used by women to obtain the daily 1500-mg calcium requirement as protection against osteoporosis. The therapist can direct education and intervention toward prevention and treatment of these related conditions.

Physicians may recommend vitamin $B_{12}$ or other vitamin B supplements for people with carpal tunnel syndrome. Malabsorption of these essential vitamins alters the structure and disrupts the function of the peripheral nerves, spinal cord, and brain and can cause numbness and tingling and permanent neurologic damage unresponsive to vitamin $B_{12}$ therapy in extreme cases.

## Vascular Diseases

Blood is supplied to the bowel by the celiac and superior and inferior mesenteric arteries. These arteries have anastomotic intercommunications at the head of the pancreas and along the transverse bowel. Obstruction of blood flow can occur as a result of atherosclerotic occlusive lesions or embolism.

### Intestinal Ischemia

Intestinal ischemia results from decreased blood supply to the bowel. Ischemia can be categorized as acute mesenteric ischemia (AMI), chronic mesenteric ischemia, or colonic ischemia.

*Acute mesenteric ischemia* is life threatening, carrying a 60% mortality, and must be treated emergently. Clients typically present with AMI in their 60s and have significant comorbidities such as atrial fibrillation, heart failure, or cardiovascular disease. It results from an occlusion (usually arterial or venous thrombosis) of the visceral branches of the abdominal aorta or secondary to previously existing atherosclerosis superimposed on a significantly decreased blood flow state. The most common vessel involved is the superior mesenteric artery, which accounts for approximately 50% of cases. Most emboli are of cardiac origin from the left ventricle or atrium, often associated with atrial fibrillation. Arterial thrombosis is more common than venous thrombosis.

Approximately 25% of individuals with AMI had symptoms of previously existing chronic mesenteric ischemia from atherosclerosis and narrowing of the vessels. Thrombosis or a low blood flow state then leads to complete obstruction or functionally occluded disease. Venous thrombosis is typically due to malignancy, use of contraceptives or estrogen-containing medications, hypercoagulable state, or abdominal or cardiac surgery. Low blood flow states, considered nonocclusive, which can result in mesenteric ischemia include heart failure; sepsis; severe hypervolemia or hypoperfusion; medications such as triptans, vasopressors, and cocaine; myocardial infarction; cardiac bypass surgery; cirrhosis; and renal failure.

The principal symptom is abdominal pain. Occult blood in the stool is common, although overt bleeding is rare. Symptoms seen later in the course include nausea, vomiting, fever, back pain, and shock. Elderly clients may have atypical symptoms including mental status changes. Key to diagnosis is a high suspicion. Pain is often initially disproportionate to the physical examination.

CT angiography is used to diagnose the involved vessel in occlusive disease. Treatment includes correction of the underlying problem and appropriate resuscitation.[222] Persons with thrombotic/embolic disease or who display peritoneal signs should undergo exploratory surgery. During surgery, necrotic tissue and perforated bowel can be removed, thrombectomy with repair of artery performed, and the abdomen lavaged. For people without peritoneal signs or venous thrombosis, thrombolytic agents can be considered. Papaverine, a nonspecific vasodilator, is frequently used in nonobstructive disease to reverse the vasoconstriction. If unsuccessful, exploratory surgery may still be warranted.

*Chronic mesenteric ischemia,* also known as intestinal angina, occurs in the setting of diffuse atherosclerotic disease of the splanchnic arteries. This leads to abdominal pain, particularly after meals (within 60 minutes), when an increased blood supply is needed during digestion but not able to adequately flow. Magnetic resonance and CT angiography are the tests of choice to make the diagnosis. Bypass surgery is the preferred treatment for lasting remission of symptoms, although percutaneous angioplasty and stenting procedures are alternative treatments.

*Colonic ischemia* is a spectrum of ischemic injury ranging from transient colitis to fulminant colitis. In contrast to AMI, mortality is low. Colonic ischemia is also more common. Factors known to contribute to colonic ischemia include aortic or cardiac bypass surgery, any event that results in hypotension, medications (oral contraceptives), drugs (cocaine), hypercoagulable states, and prolonged physical activity. The descending, sigmoid, and splenic flexure are the most commonly involved portions of the colon.

People older than age 60 years are most frequently affected. Symptoms include left lower quadrant abdominal pain, urgency to defecate, and red or maroon rectal bleeding. Diagnosis is by colonoscopy or abdominal CT, and treatment includes intravenous fluids, correction of the underlying process if possible, review and stopping of offending medications, and surgery if needed.

**SPECIAL IMPLICATIONS FOR THE THERAPIST 16.9**

*Intestinal Ischemia*

Intestinal angina as a result of atherosclerotic plaque–induced ischemia can result in intermittent back pain (usually at the thoracolumbar junction) with exertion. Clinical presentation combined with past medical history, the presence of coronary artery disease risk factors, and the presence of peripheral vascular disease may alert the therapist to the need for a medical referral if the client has not been medically diagnosed.

## Inflammatory Bowel Disease

### Overview and Definition

Inflammatory bowel disease (IBD) collectively refers to two inflammatory conditions: CD and ulcerative colitis (UC) (Table 16.6). Although the two are separate entities with their own unique pathophysiology, there are many overlapping similarities. *Crohn disease* is a chronic, lifelong inflammatory disorder that can affect any segment of the intestinal tract, although most commonly it affects the ileum and/or colon. It can affect all layers of the intestine and is characterized by diseased areas of intestine alternating with normal intestine (skip areas) with periods of exacerbation and remission. Disease may range from superficial aphthous ulcers to deep ulcers that may coalesce into a cobblestone pattern. The rectum is typically spared.

*Ulcerative colitis* is a chronic inflammatory disorder of the mucosa of the colon, typically involving the rectum, which can then advance proximally in a continuous

**Table 16.6** Comparison of Characteristics of Crohn Disease and Ulcerative Colitis

| Characteristics | Crohn Disease | Ulcerative Colitis |
|---|---|---|
| **Incidence** | | |
| Age at onset | Any age; 10–30 years most common | Any age; 10–40 years most common |
| Family history | 20%–25% | 20% |
| Gender (prevalence) | Equal in women and men | Equal in women and men |
| Cancer risk | Increased; early detection best means of prevention | Increased; preventable with bowel resection |
| **Pathogenesis** | | |
| Location of lesions | Any segment; usually small or large intestine | Rectum and left colon |
| Skip lesions | Common | Absent |
| Inflammation and ulceration | Entire intestinal wall (all layers) involved | Mucosal layers involved; submucosal involvement only in severe cases |
| Granulomas | Typical | Uncommon |
| Thickened bowel wall | Typical | Uncommon |
| Narrowed lumen and obstructed | Typical | Uncommon |
| Fissures and fistulas | Common | Absent; rare |
| **Clinical Manifestations** | | |
| Abdominal pain | Mild to severe; common | Mild to severe; less frequent |
| Diarrhea | May be absent; moderate | Typical; often severe; chronic |
| Bloody stools | Uncommon unless colon is involved | Typical |
| Abdominal mass | Common; right lower quadrant | Uncommon |
| Anorexia | Can be severe | Mild or moderate |
| Weight loss | Can be severe | Mild to moderate |
| Skin rashes | Common, mild | Common, mild |
| Joint pain | Common, mild to moderate | Common, mild to moderate |
| Growth retardation (pediatric) | Often marked | Usually mild |
| Clinical course | Remissions and exacerbations | Remissions and exacerbations |
| Complications | Cancer uncommon | Cancer fairly common |

manner to involve the entire colon. The ileum may also be involved, termed "backwash ileitis." Depending on which portion of the colon is affected, it may be more specifically referred to as *ulcerative proctitis* (involving the rectum only) or *pancolitis* (involving the entire colon).

## Incidence

Both CD and UC are bowel disorders of unknown cause involving genetic, immunologic, and environmental influences on the GI tract. These two conditions can occur in all age groups, although young people are more likely to develop CD, and men are more likely to have UC. Incidence peaks between the ages of 15 and 40 years, but CD can occur in later decades, usually after age 50. The incidence for CD has been increasing, with an incidence rate of 3.1 to 20.2 cases per 100,000 persons/year and a prevalence of 201 cases per 100,000 persons/year. UC has an incidence rate of 2.2 to 19.2 cases per 100,000 persons/year and a prevalence of 238 cases per 100,000 persons/year.[170,228,310] There are between 1 and 1.5 million people with IBD[169] in the United States. IBD is found most frequently in Northern Europe and North America, although the incidence is rising in newly industrialized countries. Asia has the fewest cases.[239]

## Etiology and Pathogenesis

Although great strides have been made in the understanding of IBD on a molecular basis, many important questions remain. IBD appears to be a polygenic disease with complex interactions between gut microbiota, host immunity, and intestinal mucosal response. Although more than 85% of people with CD do not have a family history of IBD, multiple genes have been located that are associated with IBD. Monozygotic twins and children whose parents are both affected by the disease are more likely to develop IBD. Some ethnic groups, such as Jews, have a higher risk for developing IBD. Variants in genes are specific for either CD or UC, are found in both CD and UC, or are associated with IBD and other immune-related diseases.[78] Several genes are associated with increased susceptibility to IBD, particularly in regard to developing CD.[90] Other genes are implicated in dysfunction of the epithelial barrier or in causing cellular apoptosis (cell death), whereas abnormalities in other genes may lead to defects in transcriptional regulation.

Interactions between the host immune system, the intestinal mucosa, and microorganisms in the gut appear to play a crucial role in the development of IBD. The normal intestine must be able to distinguish between toxic and infectious organisms from beneficial bacteria and food antigens. Goblet cells of the intestine not only provide a mucous protective barrier but also aid in continually transporting antigens from the lumen into the cells to begin the presentation process. These antigens are then presented to immune cells located in the lamina propria. The collection of lymphoid cells in the lamina propria and between intestinal cells is referred to as gut-associated lymphoid tissue (GALT). Myeloid cells (e.g., neutrophils, macrophages, monocytes), natural killer cells, and innate lymphoid cells have receptors (Toll-like receptors are found in macrophages and dendritic cells) that recognize certain patterns of microbes or antigens.

Macrophages and dendritic cells are antigen-presenting cells and are able to process and present an antigen along with the molecules of the major histocompatibility complex to stimulate T lymphocytes against foreign antigens. T cells recognize these molecules, and various subtypes of T cells release tumor necrosis factor, interleukins, interferon gamma, and granulocyte colony-stimulating factor, among others. A T-lymphocyte subset of cells (Th17) then responds to these factors on the mucosal surface to destroy pathologic organisms, and B cells are able to secrete specific antibodies (typically of the IgA class) to fight foreign antigens.

IBD is thought to occur when there is dysregulation of this system. This may begin with a breakdown of the normal defensive mucosal barrier. People with IBD are noted to have high numbers of bacteria in the mucus, a breakdown or alteration of the mucous barrier, or increased permeability across the intestinal barrier. An excessive number of T cells may be recruited and activated to produce increased levels of cytokines including tumor necrosis factor and interferon-gamma.[238] B cells have been found to overproduce antibodies to microbial parts and autoantibodies. Inflammation-producing neutrophils, which are normally not found in the lamina propria, are recruited or "homed" in.[39]

Changes in the intestinal microbiota can stimulate the immune system, which is demonstrated by a large number and variety of microbes in the intestines of people with IBD. Specific antibodies to microbial components, such as bacterial flagellum, are seen in individuals with CD, and microbial parts can activate signaling pathways leading to inflammatory cytokine production.[204]

More than 200 different gene loci have been implicated in the development of IBD, with about 70% of these genes shared in both UC and CD.[161] For example, several abnormalities in genes that normally code for proteins that mediate recognition of bacteria are linked to CD. Variants of genes affect immune function and cytokine pathways.[161]

Clinical complications are principally related to the overproduction of proinflammatory cytokines (such as tumor necrosis factor-$\alpha$ and IL-1$\beta$) and fibrogenic cytokines (such as transforming growth factor-$\beta$).[295] This leads to ulceration, fistula formation, and strictures.

Pathologically the inflammation associated with CD involves all layers of the bowel wall, referred to as *transmural inflammatory disease,* and the inflammatory process is discontinuous so that segments of inflamed areas are separated by normal tissue in a skip pattern. Granulomatous lesions, one of the classic differences between the two diseases, are seen in CD but not UC, although granulomas are not always seen on biopsy specimens of CD (Fig. 16.8). A combination of the granulomas, ulceration, and fibrosis results in a cobblestone appearance of the mucosal surface of the colon (Fig. 16.9). Inflammation of the mucosa associated with UC results in small erosions and subsequent ulcerations with eventual abscess formation and necrosis (Figs. 16.10 and 16.11).

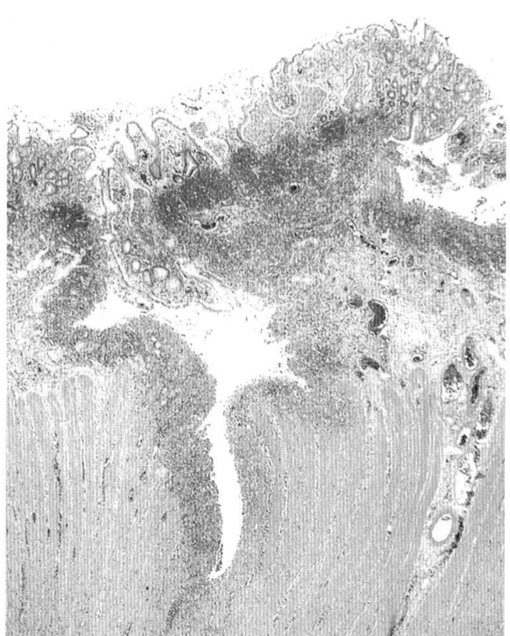

**Figure 16.8**

**Crohn disease of the colon.** A deep fissure extending into the muscle wall and a second, shallow ulcer (upper right). Abundant lymphocyte aggregates are present, evident as blue patches of cells at the interface between the mucosa and submucosa. (From Kumar V, Abbas AK, Fausto N: *Robbins and Cotran: pathologic basis of disease*, ed 7, Philadelphia, 2005, Saunders.)

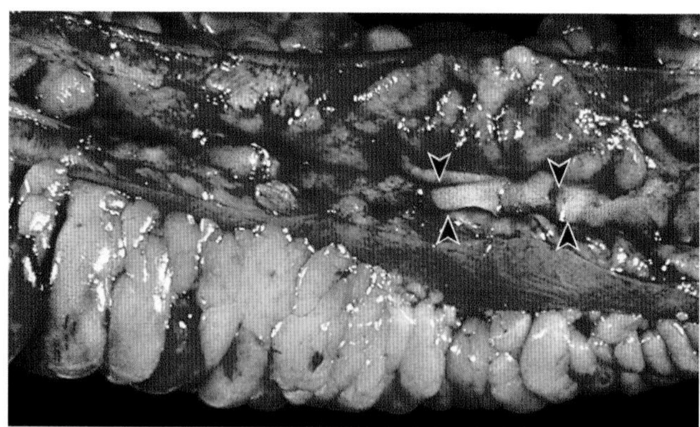

**Figure 16.9**

Crohn disease of the ileum, showing narrowing of the lumen, bowel wall thickening, serosal extension of mesenteric fat ("creeping fat"), and linear ulceration of the mucosal surface *(arrows)*. (From Kumar V, Abbas AK, Fausto N: *Robbins and Cotran: pathologic basis of disease*, ed 7, Philadelphia, 2005, Saunders.)

## Clinical Manifestations

The most common manifestations of IBD are diarrhea, abdominal pain, GI bleeding, and weight loss. The hallmark of UC is bloody diarrhea with or without mucus.[78] UC typically presents gradually, often with periods of spontaneous improvement followed by relapse of disease. Severity and location of disease often dictate symptoms. Because inflammation begins in the rectum and progressively and continuously extends toward the ileum, clients often exhibit bloody diarrhea with fecal urgency, rectal pain, fecal incontinence, and tenesmus. Constipation is not uncommon owing to rectal spasm and stasis of stool. Fever and weight loss are indicative of more severe disease.

Symptoms associated with CD depend on the location of disease but often include diarrhea, abdominal pain, and weight loss. Many symptoms of CD are shared with UC. Among people with CD, 30% have isolated small bowel disease, 40% have ileocolonic disease, and 25% have isolated large intestine inflammation. Five percent have upper GI (mouth or esophagus) or perianal disease. CD typically begins as inflammation, but with time, most people develop fistulas and strictures, which are not noted in UC. Watery diarrhea or isolated abdominal pain is more often seen in CD (small intestine or ileocolonic disease), whereas bloody diarrhea is more frequently noted in UC. For comparison of specific signs and symptoms, see Table 16.6.

**Complications.** Complications can be categorized as acute and chronic. The most serious acute problems seen in UC include severe blood loss and toxic megacolon; colon cancer is the most serious long-term complication. Risk factors for developing colon cancer associated with UC include duration of disease, degree of involvement (i.e., the greater the involvement, the more likely to develop cancer), young age at onset, severe inflammation, family history of colorectal cancer, and presence of primary sclerosing cholangitis.[78]

CD is associated with significant complications including severe bleeding; abscess formation (spontaneous and fistula associated); bowel obstruction (particularly small bowel); fistula formation with the bladder, skin, intestine, and vagina; impaired growth in children; nutritional deficiencies; and inflammation of the joints. Fistulas are seen in approximately 50% of people with CD and cause significant morbidity and quality-of-life changes (particularly perianal fistulas).[362] Fistulas also carry a high risk of abscess formation.

***Extraintestinal Manifestations.*** Approximately 10% of clients with IBD have extraintestinal manifestations, which may precede the GI symptoms. Studies demonstrate that certain antibodies have a cross-reaction with the colon and other organs of the body. This may account for extraintestinal involvement of the joints (arthritis), eyes (uveitis), skin (erythema nodosum or pyoderma gangrenosum), lungs, biliary tree (primary sclerosing cholangitis), and blood (autoimmune hemolytic anemia, thromboembolism), although studies are lacking. Involvement of the ileum can lead to vitamin $B_{12}$ deficiency and subsequent anemia.

Joint involvement ranging from arthralgia to acute arthritis is the most common extraintestinal finding in IBD. Arthritis associated with IBD is usually continuous and symmetric. Arthropathies associated with IBD (a subdivision of seronegative spondyloarthropathies) are divided into peripheral and axial involvement.[10,38] Persons with IBD may have both types.

Peripheral arthritis can be divided into type 1 and type 2 (although many rheumatologists no longer use the distinction). Type 1 is an oligoarthritis with five or fewer painful/inflamed joints, typically involving the larger joints of the

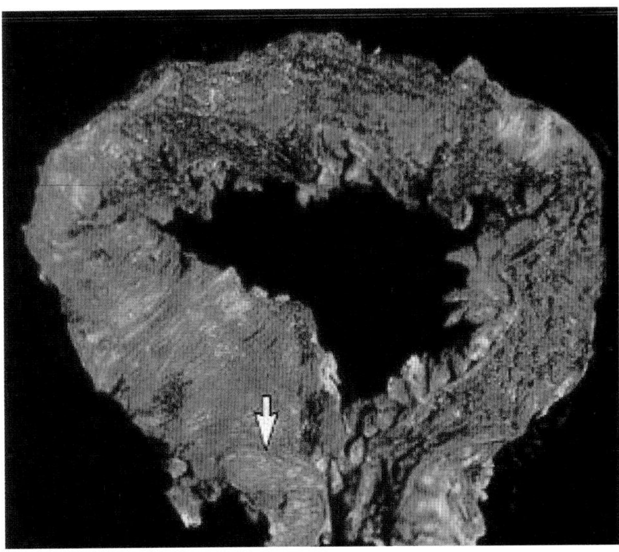

**Figure 16.11**

**Total colectomy specimen from a patient with ulcerative colitis.** The colon shows diffuse mucosal inflammation that extends proximally from the rectum without interruption to the transverse colon. The mucosal pattern in the terminal ileum and cecum *(arrow)* is normal. The distal mucosa is erythematous and friable, with many ulcers and erosions. (From Feldman M, Friedman LS, Brandt LJ, editors: *Sleisenger and Fordtran's gastrointestinal and liver disease*, ed 8, Philadelphia, 2006, Saunders. Courtesy of Feldman's GastroAtlas online, Current Medicine Group Ltd.)

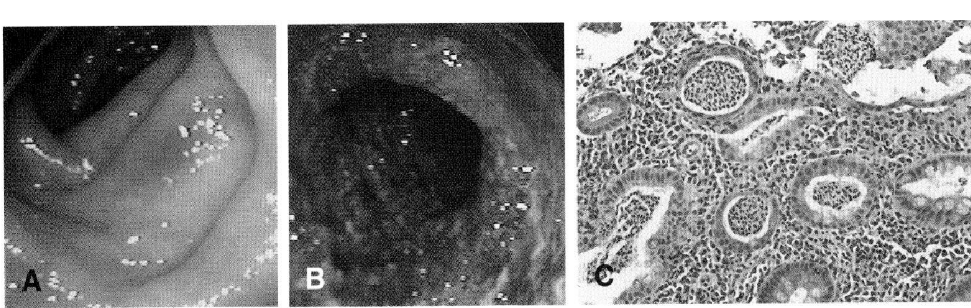


**Figure 16.10**

**Spectrum of severity of ulcerative colitis.** (A) Colonoscopic findings in mild ulcerative colitis demonstrating edema, loss of vascularity, and patchy subepithelial hemorrhage. (B) Colonoscopic findings in severe ulcerative colitis with loss of vascularity, hemorrhage, and mucopus. (C) Histologic specimen showing a severe acute and chronic inflammatory process with multiple abscesses. (From Feldman M, Friedman LS, Brandt LJ, editors: *Sleisenger and Fordtran's gastrointestinal and liver disease*, ed 8, Philadelphia, 2006, Saunders.)

lower extremity. Type 1 is usually self-limited, correlating with bowel disease activity, resolving within several months as the underlying disease is treated and without permanent sequelae or joint deformities. Type 2 is more often polyarticular, symmetric, and involving more than five joints, particularly in the small joints of the hands (metacarpophalangeal joints). Type 2 can be chronic, but similar to type 1, it is usually nondeforming. Type 2 may not parallel bowel disease. Axial arthritis often occurs independent of bowel disease activity and may include inflammatory back pain, sacroiliitis, or ankylosing spondylitis. Pathologic evaluation of the synovial fluid is nonspecific without crystals or evidence of infection. Tests for specific forms of arthritis (e.g., rheumatoid factor and antinuclear antibody) usually give negative results; test results for HLA-B27 can be positive.

## MEDICAL MANAGEMENT

**DIAGNOSIS.** The diagnosis of IBD typically requires both colonoscopy and biopsy of the colon and ileum. Because biopsy specimens include only the mucosa and not full thickness of bowel, often no distinction can be made between UC and CD. Endoscopy or colonoscopy reveals the pattern of disease and often is able to make the diagnosis between the two disorders. As parts of the small intestine are difficult to visualize by either colonoscopy or EGD, CT or magnetic resonance enterography or capsule endoscopy may add further information.

Fecal calprotectin can be used if other diagnostic tests are unrevealing. Calprotectin is a protein that is released by neutrophils secondary to inflammation and can aid in distinguishing mild inflammatory disease from noninflammatory disease. Other causes of colitis, such as *C. difficile,* should be excluded. In 10% to 15% of people, testing does not delineate between UC and CD, and this is termed "indeterminate colitis." Often a distinction is made with time and progression of the disease.

**TREATMENT.** Therapy for both UC and CD is principally medical with surgery required less frequently. Treatment is directed toward obtaining remission of disease then beginning maintenance therapy with the goal of keeping inflammation and symptoms under control.

Initial treatment for UC depends on severity and location. First-line therapy for mild to moderate UC consists of 5-aminosalicylate (5-ASA) drugs (sulfasalazine, mesalamine, olsalazine, and balsalazide) given orally or rectally (suppository or enema) or both. Topical dosing by suppository or enema is preferred because it requires decreased dosing frequency and has a quicker response compared with oral dosing. Approximately 90% of clients have an initial remission of their disease, and 75% are able to maintain the remission using a 5-ASA.

Glucocorticoids may be added orally, rectally, or, for severe disease, intravenously, although they are not effective as a maintenance agent. Budesonide is a glucocorticoid available in a controlled-release formulation that releases drug throughout the colon. This medication has the advantage of fewer glucocorticoid effects because it has a high first-pass metabolism. Maintenance drugs include immunomodulators azathioprine and 6-mercaptopurine. If an appropriate response is not obtained, a biologic agent (e.g., anti–tumor necrosis factor antibody agents such as infliximab, adalimumab, and golimumab that are approved for induction and maintenance), integrin-blocking drug (vedolizumab), or immunosuppressant (cyclosporine) can be used.[183,313]

Infrequently, colectomy may be needed for uncontrollable acute disease. In the case of UC, surgery can be curative, in contrast to CD. Time of surgery is determined based on laboratory values and symptoms.[10] There are multiple indications for surgery in the treatment of UC. Among these are failure of medical therapy, toxic megacolon, intestinal perforation, uncontrollable bleeding, intolerable side effects of medications, strictures that cannot be managed endoscopically, cancer, and growth failure in children.[68] The current surgical option of choice is a total proctocolectomy with ileal pouch–anal anastomosis, as this type of surgery preserves anal sphincter function.

The most significant complication following surgery is the development of pouchitis. This is thought to be a nonspecific inflammation of the newly formed pouch caused by antibodies toward the microflora.[377] Symptoms include increased stool frequency, urgency, incontinence, and abdominal discomfort/perianal discomfort. CD is most often treated medically; surgery is offered when needed for complications or severe, unresponsive disease. Some nonprescription medications can improve symptoms, such as fiber supplements and loperamide for diarrhea.

NSAIDs can make symptoms worse and should be avoided. Glucocorticoids are often used as initial treatment for people who need a more immediate response (significant diarrhea or abdominal pain); however, they are used for only a short time until other agents reach therapeutic dosing. Budesonide is used for clients with mild or low-risk disease. Individuals who respond to glucocorticoids should be started on an immunomodulator such as azathioprine, 6-mercaptopurine, or methotrexate while the glucocorticoids are tapered. Individuals who do not respond to glucocorticoids or have severe disease are treated with a biologic agent including anti–tumor necrosis factor inhibitors such as infliximab, adalimumab, and certolizumab.

Other options are anti-integrin antibody (leukocyte trafficking blockers vedolizumab and natalizumab) or anti–IL-12/IL-23 antibody (ustekinumab) treatments. Maintenance is often sustained with combined treatment with a biologic agent and 1 to 2 years of azathioprine. Many people with moderate to severe CD will need lifelong therapy. Ileocolonoscopy is performed 6 to 12 months after induction is achieved.[346]

Indications for surgery include severe bleeding, failure to grow (children), symptomatic fistulas, bowel obstruction, abscesses, or strictures of the intestine. Modified approaches to therapy of CD may include "deep remission" (verifying that all tissue is healed endoscopically) instead of solely clinical improvement of symptoms. This may reduce the need for hospitalization and surgery. Ensuring adequate initial therapy may also lead to less involvement of tissue and less destruction of tissue.[253]

Chemoprevention and routine screening colonoscopy are advised for the prevention of colorectal cancer associated with long-standing IBD. Several agents have been used as chemoprotective agents, although none have been shown to indisputably protect against the development of cancer. However, 5-ASAs and thiopurine analogues may be beneficial through reducing inflammation and are often already used in maintenance therapy.[61,332]

For UC involving more than the rectum and individuals with CD involving one-third of the colon, colonoscopy should be performed every 1 to 2 years after 8 to 10 years of disease with a specific biopsy protocol. The cancers associated with IBD can be flat, in contrast to sporadic colorectal carcinoma, which are typically polypoid. Flat lesions are difficult to see endoscopically and can be missed.

**PROGNOSIS.** IBD is a chronic and sometimes debilitating disease with a known increased risk of intestinal cancer. The risk for colorectal cancer is related to severity, extent of disease, and duration of disease.[287] People with UC have a 2% incidence of cancer after 10 years of disease, a 9% incidence after 20 years, and an 18% incidence after 30 years.[352,370]

CD also increases a person's risk for cancer, with a cumulative risk of 2.9% at 10 years and 8.3% at 30 years.[48] Risk factors for colorectal cancer include younger age at diagnosis of CD, duration of disease (longer duration increases risk), and greater interval between examinations.[18] Resection of disease does not prevent the development of cancer in other portions of the bowel, so screening is important.[17,70] Colorectal cancer is responsible for 20% of IBD-related mortality.

Persons with UC have a good prognosis during the first decade after diagnosis, with a low rate of colectomy as a consequence of improved medical treatment. Approximately 85% of clients with UC have mild to moderate intermittent disease managed without hospitalization. The remaining 15% demonstrate a full-blown course involving the entire colon, severe diarrhea, and systemic signs and symptoms. Approximately 30% will undergo surgery at some point to control inflammation, whether emergently, urgently, or electively.

CD is a chronic disease without cure, and most clients have an intermittent disease course. Only 13% will have an unremitting disease course, and 10% maintain a prolonged remission. Less than half of people require corticosteroids at any time, but 60% to 80% of people require at least one surgical resection in their lifetime.[52,205]

SPECIAL IMPLICATIONS FOR THE THERAPIST 16.10

## *Inflammatory Bowel Disease*

### Musculoskeletal Involvement

When terminal ileum involvement in CD produces periumbilical pain, referred pain to the corresponding low back is possible. Pain of the ileum is intermittent and perceived in the lower right quadrant with possible associated iliopsoas abscess or ureteral obstruction from an inflammatory mass, causing buttock, hip, thigh, or knee pain, often with an antalgic gait. Specific objective tests are available to rule out systemic origin of hip, thigh, or knee pain (Figs. 16.12 and 16.13).

Psoas abscesses most commonly result from direct extension of intraabdominal infections such as appendicitis, diverticulitis, and CD. Clinical manifestations of a psoas abscess include fever, lower abdominal pain, or referred pain as described. Flexion deformity of the hip may develop from reflex spasm with a positive psoas sign as shown. Symptoms are exacerbated by hip extension. A tender or painful mass may be palpated in the groin.

Approximately 25% of all clients with IBD present with migratory arthralgia, monarthritis, polyarthritis, or sacroiliitis. The joint problems and GI disorders may appear simultaneously, the joint problems may manifest first (sometimes years before bowel symptoms), or intestinal symptoms may present along with articular symptoms but are disregarded as part of the whole picture by the client.

Any time a client presents with low back, hip, or sacroiliac pain of unknown origin, the therapist must screen for medical disease by asking a few simple questions about the presence of accompanying intestinal symptoms, known personal or family history of IBD, and possible relief of symptoms after passing stool or gas.[120] Joint problems usually respond to treatment of the underlying bowel disease but in some cases require separate management. Interventions for musculoskeletal involvement follow the usual protocols for each area affected.

People with IBD are known to have low bone mineral content and a high prevalence of osteoporosis. The pathogenesis is not completely understood but is considered multifactorial at this time, including possible genetic factors,[300,304] malabsorption, corticosteroid use, and deficiency of fat-soluble vitamins including vitamin K necessary for calcium binding to bone.[298]

Low bone mineral density may be more characteristic of CD than of UC, but no consistent differentiation has been made between CD and UC in this regard.[297] The therapist can provide osteoporosis education and prevention for clients with IBD. See Osteoporosis in Chapter 24.

The therapist must always know what medications clients are taking so that the first sign of possible side effects will be recognized and the physician will be alerted. Corticosteroids are an important and effective drug for treating moderate and severe IBD but have all of the complications of prolonged high-dose steroid therapy.

### Dehydration

Hydration and nutrition are always long-term concerns with clients who have UC or CD. The client must be observed for any signs of dehydration (e.g., dry lips, dry hands, headache, brittle hair, incoordination, disorientation), in addition to any increase or pathologic change in symptoms. Any increase in painful symptoms or increased stool output or stool frequency must be reported to the physician.

### Psychologic Issues

Psychologic factors and the autonomic nervous system are implicated in the pathogenesis of IBD.[259] The chronic nature of IBD affecting persons in the prime of life often results in feelings of anger, anxiety, and possibly depression. These emotions are important factors in the client's well-being and response to treatment and in modifying the overall course of the disease.[220]

The therapist can be instrumental in acknowledging the client's feelings, validating the effects of the disease, and prescribing an exercise program to match the needs of the individual. Exercise can help moderate depression, boost immune system function, combat the effects of long-term corticosteroid use, and help improve body image.

The therapist can help individuals develop positive coping strategies and management techniques to deal with the disruptions that can occur with intermittent and unexpected bouts of diarrhea and abdominal pain. Stress management, relaxation techniques (e.g., Physiological Quieting, autogenic breathing, guided imagery) can help with visceral pain and discomfort. The therapist can help individuals find ways to improve activity and participation and not just deal with impaired body structures and functions.

**A THERAPIST'S THOUGHTS[a]**

***Stress and Pelvic Floor Activity***

According to Van der Velde and colleagues,[357] the pelvic floor muscles contract in normal subjects in response to situations perceived as threatening. The data support the idea of a general defense reaction as a mechanism of involuntary pelvic floor muscle activity. The Van der Velde study was clearly looking at skeletal muscle response. General relaxation can be helpful in treating overactivity in the pelvic floor muscle.

[a]Beth Shelly, PT, DPT, WCS, BCB-PMD

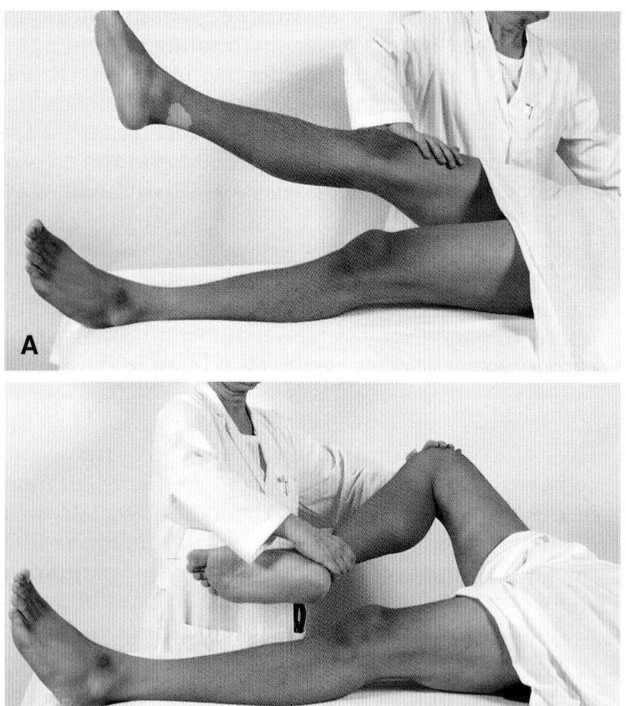

**Figure 16.12**

**Muscle tests.** (A) Iliopsoas muscle test. With the client supine, instruct the client to lift the right leg straight up; apply resistance to the distal thigh as the client tries to hold the leg up. When the test result is negative, the client feels no change; when the test result is positive (i.e., the iliopsoas muscle is inflamed or abscessed), pain is felt in the right lower quadrant. (B) Obturator muscle test. With the client supine, perform active assisted motion, flexing at the hip and knee; hold the ankle and rotate the leg internally and externally. A negative or normal response is no pain; a positive test result for inflamed obturator muscle is right lower quadrant (abdominal) pain. A physical therapist trained in internal palpation can also assess obturator dysfunction by palpating the muscle inside the vagina or rectum. (A, From Jarvis C: *Physical examination and health assessment,* ed 6, Philadelphia, 2012, Saunders. B, From Jarvis C: *Physical examination and health assessment,* ed 4, Philadelphia, 2004, Saunders, p. 586.)

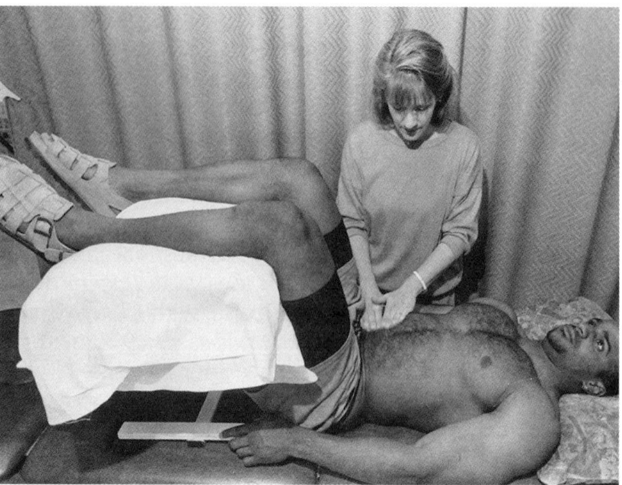

**Figure 16.13**

**Palpating the iliopsoas muscle.** In addition to assessing the McBurney point, the examiner may palpate the iliopsoas muscle by placing the client in a supine position with the hips and knees both flexed 90° and with the lower legs resting on a firm surface (a traction table stool works well for this; pillows under the lower legs may be necessary to obtain the full position). Palpate approximately one-third the distance from the anterior superior iliac spine toward the umbilicus; it may be necessary to ask the client to initiate hip flexion on that side to help isolate the muscle and avoid palpating the bowel. Palpation may produce back pain or local muscular pain from a shortened or tight muscle, indicating the need for soft tissue mobilization and stretching of the iliopsoas muscle. A positive test result for iliopsoas abscess is right lower quadrant (abdominal) pain; manual therapy (e.g., soft tissue mobilization) in this area would be contraindicated in the presence of any abdominal or pelvic inflammatory process involving the iliopsoas muscle until the infection has been treated with complete resolution.

## Antibiotic-Associated Colitis

For further discussion of this topic, see Chapter 8.

## Irritable Bowel Syndrome

### Definition and Incidence

IBS is a group of symptoms that represent one of the most common disorders of the GI system, with a worldwide prevalence of 11% (depending on region and criteria used for definition[209,323]). These symptoms include chronically reoccurring abdominal pain associated with altered bowel habits in the absence of structural, inflammatory, or biochemical abnormalities.

**SPECIAL IMPLICATIONS FOR THE THERAPIST 16.11**

***Antibiotic-Associated Colitis***

The primary concern with any client experiencing excessive watery diarrhea is fluid and electrolyte imbalance. See special implications for fluid and electrolyte imbalances discussed in Chapter 5. Because the onset of this condition may occur up to 1 month after the antibiotic has been discontinued, the client may not recognize the association between current GI symptoms and previous medications. Anytime someone taking antibiotics or recently completing a course of antibiotics develops GI symptoms, especially with joint and/or muscle involvement, encourage physician notification.

Reactive arthritis occurring after *C. difficile* infection is most common with colitis associated with antibiotic therapy. *Reactive arthritis* is defined as the occurrence of an acute, aseptic, inflammatory arthropathy arising after an infectious process but at a site remote from the primary infection.

The arthritis typically involves the large and medium joints of the lower extremities and first manifests 1 to 4 weeks after the infectious insult (see Chapter 25). Reactive arthritis may include some, but not all, of the three features associated with Reiter syndrome and is often designated incomplete Reiter syndrome.

Box 16.2

**SUBTYPING IRRITABLE BOWEL SYNDROME BY PREDOMINANT STOOL PATTERN FOLLOWING ROME IV CRITERIA AND BRISTOL STOOL FORM SCALE**

1. IBS with constipation (IBS-C): >25% of stools are hard or lumpy and <25% of stools are mushy or watery.
2. IBS with diarrhea (IBS-D): >25% of stools are mushy or watery and <25% of stools are hard or lumpy.
3. Mixed IBS (IBS-M): >25% of stools are hard or lumpy and >25% of stools are mushy or watery.
4. Unsubtyped IBS (IBS-U): Symptoms meet diagnostic criteria for IBS, but bowel habits cannot be accurately categorized.

*IBS*, Irritable bowel syndrome.
Data from Lacy BE, Mearin F, Chang L, et al: Bowel disorders. *Gastroenterology* 150:1393–1407, 2016.

Because there are no specific biomarkers or tests, it is often referred to as a functional bowel disorder. IBS is separated into four categories depending on predominant symptoms as established by the Rome IV criteria: diarrhea-predominant IBS (IBS-D), constipation-predominant IBS (IBS-C), mixed-symptom IBS, and unsubtyped IBS (Box 16.2).[107,187]

Women are affected more often than men,[107] typically between the ages of 20 and 40 years. Onset of symptoms after the age of 50 years is uncommon.[107] Many people with IBS also have other pain syndromes including migraine headaches, fibromyalgia, interstitial cystitis, chronic fatigue syndrome, and chronic pelvic pain.[97,372] IBS is costly, with direct and indirect costs estimated at $20 billion,[141] and affected people use at least 50% more health care resources than matched controls.[226]

### Etiologic Factors and Pathogenesis

IBS is considered a functional disorder because the symptoms currently cannot be attributed to any identifiable abnormality of the bowel (structural or biochemical). This terminology continues to be used, although many in the field would like to phase out the word "functional" and believe that the description "disorders of gut-brain interaction" would be more accurate.[312] Current theories regarding the cause of IBS include altered GI motor activity (clients with IBS-C have a slower transit time that increases abdominal distention and bloating),[3] increased intestinal permeability (particularly clients with IBS-D), altered intestinal microflora (IBS can develop following infectious gastroenteritis),[92] visceral hypersensitivity or hyperalgesia, and altered processing of information by the nervous system.[4,95,97,104,247,277]

Researchers continue to explore the brain (nervous system)–gut connection to better understand IBS. Studies suggest that there is an altered interaction between the nervous system and the immune system, bringing together many of the above-mentioned hypotheses.[97] An increase in intestinal permeability and abnormal intestinal flora may activate the immune system and lead to chronic, low-grade inflammation, which may alter communication with the brain. Brain imaging demonstrates altered processing of visceral stimuli, and persons with IBS exhibit a lower pain theshhold.[95] Negative emotions or stress appear to worsen symptoms, perhaps by increasing intestinal permeability.[6]

People with IBS are noted to have higher levels of serotonin,[137] a common neurotransmitter also found in the visceral nervous system. Serotonin is known to promote gut motility, visceral sensation, and secretion.[83] Studies are currently evaluating the cause for elevated serotonin levels.[185] Altered circadian rhythms (e.g., from rotating shift work) may also have a role in the pathogenesis of IBS and abdominal pain.[242]

### Clinical Manifestations

Symptoms of IBS usually begin in young adulthood and persist intermittently throughout life with variable periods of remission. For some people, IBS symptoms are annoying but manageable. Approximately 25% of Americans have symptoms consistent with IBS but do not seek medical attention. For others, IBS significantly affects quality of life and daily function.

Pain may be steady or intermittent, and there may be a dull, deep discomfort with sharp cramps in the morning or after eating. Often there is relief with evacuation of the bowels. The typical pain pattern consists of lower abdominal pain accompanied by constipation and/or diarrhea. Other symptoms may include nausea and vomiting, anorexia, sour stomach, bloating, abdominal distention, and flatus. Symptoms of IBS tend to disappear at night when the affected individual is asleep. Nocturnal GI symptoms suggest a diagnosis other than IBS.[211]

## MEDICAL MANAGEMENT

DIAGNOSIS. Diagnosis is based on history, as there are currently no definitive tests. Symptom-based criteria have been developed for the diagnosis of IBS, known as the Rome IV criteria (Box 16.3).[107,187] Diagnosis is made with a history of recurrent abdominal pain at least 1 day per week during the immediate previous 3 months, with onset at least 6 months before diagnosis. Clients should be off medications used to control symptoms to correctly make a diagnosis. In conjunction with the history, inquiries must be made concerning possible "alarm" symptoms or objective findings

Box 16.3

**ROME IV DIAGNOSTIC CRITERIA FOR IRRITABLE BOWEL SYNDROME**

Recurrent abdominal pain or discomfort (abdominal sensation not described as pain) at least 3 days a month in past 3 months (with onset >6 months prior) associated with two or more of the following:

- Related to defecation
- Associated with change in frequency of stool
- Associated with change in form (appearance) of stool

Alarm indicators that suggest other diseases:

- Age >50 years
- Short history of symptoms
- Documented weight loss
- Nocturnal symptoms
- Family history of colon cancer
- Rectal bleeding
- Recent antibiotic use

Modified from Lacy BE, Mearin F, Chang L, et al: Bowel disorders. *Gastroenterology* 150:1393–1407, 2016.

(e.g., rectal bleeding, use of antibiotics, or weight loss) that could be indications of another disease such as IBD, celiac disease, carbohydrate malabsorption (lactose and fructose intolerance), microscopic colitis, and malignancy.

Extensive studies should not be undertaken if the history is consistent with IBS and physical examination is normal. However, laboratory studies that may confirm another suspected disease may be helpful. Because anemia is an alarm sign, a complete blood count is often beneficial, as may be C-reactive protein, which may be more suggestive of IBD. For subtypes IBS-D and mixed-symptom IBS, testing for celiac disease or lactose intolerance may be appropriate. Colonoscopy should be performed only if an alarm symptom or a symptom relating to another diagnosis is present. Research is underway to identify biomarkers that are more able to reliably make the diagnosis of IBS.[47]

**TREATMENT.** As the cause of IBS is unknown, treatment is aimed at relieving symptoms. Dietary changes, medications, exercise, stress reduction, and cognitive-behavioral therapy have been advocated. Avoidance of gluten may be helpful in some people with IBS.[29] In several studies a diet restricting FODMAPs (fermentable oligosaccharides, disaccharides, monosaccharides, and polyols) was associated with improved symptoms.[77,126,324] Adding gluten restriction to a low-FODMAP diet did not show any further benefit.[30] Studies demonstrate that dietary guidance improves both health and symptoms.

Because people with IBS-C can have a slower intestinal transit time, resulting in constipation, the use of fiber supplements has been advocated, although studies are conflicting.[286,351] Soluble fiber (psyllium) showed benefit over insoluble fiber (bran), with bran exacerbating abdominal symptoms in studies.[31,94]

Although several osmotic, surfactant, and stimulant laxatives are available for the treatment of IBS-C, only polyethylene glycol has been shown to improve stool frequency and consistency (but not abdominal pain). Lubiprostone, a medication that activates type 2 chloride channels, demonstrated an overall improvement in symptoms.[89,261] Linaclotide, a guanylate cyclase C agonist, was also effective in improving abdominal and bowel symptoms.[275]

There is good evidence that antispasmodics, which act as GI smooth muscle relaxants, are effective for the treatment of all subtypes of IBS. Examples include dicyclomine, hyoscyamine, and peppermint oil. Antidepressants, particularly selective serotonin receptor inhibitors and tricyclic antidepressants, improve abdominal pain and improve other IBS symptoms.[351] Loperamide improves bowel movement frequency and consistency in clients with IBS-D, although it had no effect on other IBS symptoms. Bile acid sequestrants may also improve stool passage and consistency for clients with IBS-D.[375]

Although not completely understood, bacterial overgrowth and IBS symptoms have been linked. The use of rifaximin, an unabsorbable antibiotic, has produced significant broad improvement in clients with IBS-D. Relapse is common, and individuals can benefit from retreatment.[261,262] Probiotics, including *Bifidobacterium infantis,* can offer improvement of symptoms including pain, bloating, and flatulence.[227,373]

Therapies that augment medical treatment include a stress reduction program[381] consisting of a regular program of relaxation techniques and exercise in conjunction with cognitive-behavioral therapy[203] and biofeedback training. Behavioral therapy is focused on identifying and reducing or eliminating triggers. Hypnotherapy (hypnosis) and biofeedback therapy (relaxation training) can give some control over the muscle activity of the GI tract and the gut's sensitivity to stress and other influences.[374]

Physical activity and exercise have also been shown to be beneficial in reducing symptoms[65,158,384] and can be implemented with other treatment modalities. However, owing to bias, no guidance is available regarding which exercises are best.[11,65,384]

**PROGNOSIS.** IBS is not a life-threatening disorder, and clients should be reassured of the ability to treat symptoms through diet, medication, regular physical activity, and stress management. Future research looks to unlock the pathophysiology of IBS to treat it more effectively.

SPECIAL IMPLICATIONS FOR THE THERAPIST 16.12

## *Irritable Bowel Syndrome*

Regular physical activity helps relieve stress and assists in bowel function, particularly in people who experience constipation. It may be necessary to avoid exercises that result in jarring or jumping, as this can increase pain related to abdominal organ dysfunction. The therapist should encourage anyone with IBS to continue with the prescribed rehabilitation intervention program during symptomatic periods.

Therapists must be alert to a client with IBS who has developed breath-holding patterns or hyperventilation in response to stress. Teaching proper breathing is important for all daily activities, especially during exercise and relaxation techniques.

## Diverticular Disease

See also Meckel Diverticulum later.

### Definition and Incidence

*Diverticular disease* is the term used to describe diverticulosis and diverticulitis. Diverticulosis refers to the presence of outpouchings (diverticula) in the wall of the colon or small intestine, a condition in which the mucosa and submucosa herniate through the muscular layers of the colon to form outpouchings (Fig. 16.14). Diverticulitis is defined as inflammation/infection of the diverticula with possible complications such as perforation, abscess formation, obstruction, fistula formation, and bleeding.

This acquired deformity of the colon is rarely reversible and usually asymptomatic. The most common site in Western countries is the sigmoid colon (85% of cases), but any segment of the colon may be involved. In Asian countries, diverticular disease tends to be on the right side.

*Diverticular disease* is common and increasing in incidence in westernized countries. The disease is most common in persons older than 60 years of age, although the average age has been decreasing.[98] Diverticula are present in 10% of people older than age 45, while more than 80% of individuals older than age 85 have diverticula. About 10% to 25% develop complications including diverticulitis. Younger people with diverticular disease frequently have more aggressive disease and often require surgery after an initial episode of diverticulitis.[256]

### Etiologic and Risk Factors

It is well known that Western countries have a much higher incidence of diverticular disease than developing countries or countries where the diet is high in fiber. A lack of fiber was once thought to be the principal cause of diverticular disease; however, new studies provide conflicting data in which a diet high in fiber was not found to be protective.[257,353]

Risk factors associated with the development of diverticulosis include constipation, physical inactivity, eating red meat, obesity, smoking, and NSAID use.[134,152,329] Several connective tissue disorders also have a link with diverticular disease, including Ehlers-Danlos syndrome, Marfan syndrome, and scleroderma.[301] Genetics may also play a role, as some people are born with diverticula, probably resulting from an inherited defect in the muscular wall of the intestines. The majority of people who have diverticulosis develop it with age, indicating that both heredity and lifestyle play a role.

Clients taking chronic steroids and immunosuppressants are at a higher risk for developing diverticulitis.[364] Foods such as nuts and corn were once thought to lead to diverticulitis; however, studies have not substantiated this.[329] Fruits and vegetables, including those with small seeds, are good sources of fiber and should not be avoided.[328,344]

### Pathogenesis

Diverticular disease is a multifactorial process related to diet, structural changes in the colonic wall (alterations in musculature, collagen, elastin), and functional changes

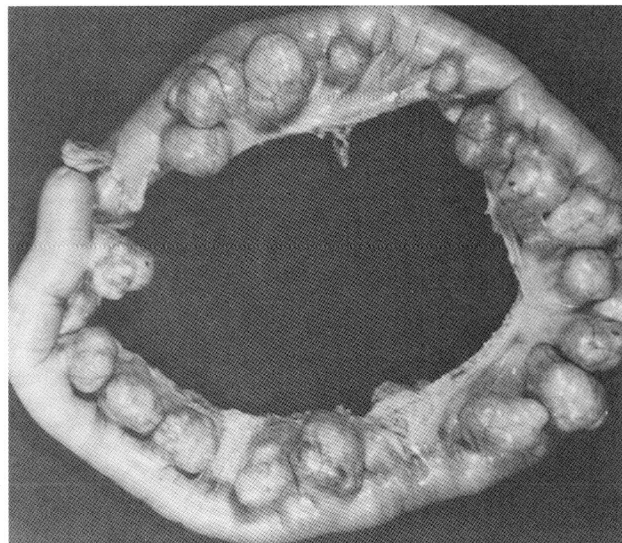

**Figure 16.14**

**Multiple diverticula in resected section of the colon.** Weak spots in the muscle layers of the intestinal wall permit the mucosa to bulge outward (herniate) into the pelvic cavity. (From Rosai J: *Ackerman's surgical pathology*, ed 7, St. Louis, 1989, Mosby.)

in the bowels (intestinal motility). As discussed earlier, a lack of dietary fiber was traditionally believed to cause diverticula. It was thought that a low-fiber diet produced small stool volumes and decreased stool transit time. This then resulted in increased intraluminal pressure that forced the mucosa and submucosa through the weakened colonic wall. However, current studies provide conflicting results, and more studies will need to be done to understand the role of fiber in the cause of diverticular disease.

Diverticula form at weak points in the colon wall, usually where arteries penetrate the muscularis. Changes in the muscular portion of the intestinal wall have been documented. The longitudinal muscle, taeniae coli, becomes thickened from aberrant deposition of elastin; the muscle cells themselves remain normal. There is also increased production of collagen.[34] The circular portion of muscle, plicae circulares, which controls peristalsis, also thickens, narrowing the lumen and increasing the intraluminal pressure.[363] These changes progress as a person ages and ultimately lead to a weakened colonic wall.

Changes in intestinal motility are also associated with diverticular disease. Based on manometric catheters, clients with diverticular disease have elevated pressures compared with persons without the disease. This is postulated to occur because the colon contracts in segments rather than a continuous tube. This increases the pressure in each fold or segment. There are documented alterations in the enteric nervous system as well, which may account for some of the abnormal motility (imbalance in excitatory versus inhibitory influences), and research is underway to determine if neurotransmitters play a role in diverticular disease.[35,157]

There is also controversy regarding the pathophysiology of diverticulitis. Diverticulitis is speculated to be secondary to fecal obstruction of the diverticulum, which then causes increased pressure within the diverticulum, resulting in local ischemia. As this process continues, ulcerations and perforations form, confounded by bacterial overgrowth. This process is similar to what occurs in appendicitis. Another more recent theory attributes diverticulitis to microperforations rather than fecal obstruction of the diverticulum.[364]

In diverticulosis, for unknown reasons, there can be weakening of blood vessels, predisposing to bleeding. Bleeding is uncommon in diverticulitis and is unrelated to infection. Recurrent diverticulitis can result in increased scarring and narrowing of the bowel lumen, potentially leading to obstruction. Perforated diverticula provide an opening through which bacteria can enter, leaving the bowel at risk for a bacterial invasion into the diverticulum with subsequent abscess formation.

### Clinical Manifestations

Diverticular disease is asymptomatic in 80% of affected people. Persons with diverticula that are not inflamed may exhibit mild, nonspecific, episodic pain. Symptoms may overlap with symptoms of IBS such as bloating, cramping, irregular bowel movements, and flatulence.

When diverticula become blocked, bacteria that are trapped inside begin to proliferate, causing infection and inflammation. Approximately 75% of diverticulitis cases are uncomplicated. Persons experience episodic or constant abdominal pain located in the left quadrant (if the sigmoid is involved) or midabdominal region, often with extension into the back. Other common symptoms include fever, change in bowel habits (usually diarrhea), nausea, vomiting, and anorexia. Bleeding is uncommon in uncomplicated diverticulitis. Approximately 10% to 15% of people will have urinary symptoms related to the close proximity of the bladder. Eating and increased intraabdominal pressure can increase pain (see Box 16.1), whereas temporary partial or complete relief may follow a bowel movement or passage of flatus.

In complicated cases, a perforation of the bowel may occur with abscess formation. A fistula may develop with the bladder (colovesical fistula). Clients may experience pneumaturia (air in the urine), fecaluria (urine in the stool), or recurrent urinary tract infections, in conjunction with fever, abdominal pain, or palpable mass.

Another entity related to diverticular disease is segmental colitis associated with diverticula. This appears to be inflammation involving tissue surrounding the diverticulum but not inside the diverticulum itself. Clinical symptoms include chronic abdominal pain (usually left-sided) associated with hematochezia (bleeding per rectum). Examination of tissue displays features similar to IBD, and some affected people have been treated with drugs used in IBD therapy.[308]

## MEDICAL MANAGEMENT

**DIAGNOSIS.** When the history and physical examination are suggestive of diverticulitis, the diagnosis can be confirmed by CT of the abdomen/pelvis. Laboratory evaluation will often demonstrate an elevated white blood cell count (in approximately 50% of cases). CT of the abdomen/pelvis can also reveal complications including fistula formation, abscess, and obstruction. Colonoscopy in the acute setting of diverticulitis is avoided because of the increased risk of perforation with air entering the abdominal cavity.

**PREVENTION AND TREATMENT.** Asymptomatic diverticular disease requires no treatment. The mainstay of treatment for uncomplicated diverticulitis is bowel rest (or clear liquids), antibiotics, and pain control. Antibiotic treatment may be given on an outpatient basis for 7 to 10 days for persons with stable vital signs, absence of fever, and no significant laboratory or CT abnormalities.

Prevention of diverticulosis is accomplished primarily through lifestyle changes, although evidence is lacking. Adherence to a high-fiber diet, decreased red meat intake, prevention of constipation with adequate fluid and fiber intake, smoking cessation, and exercise during periods of remission may decrease the risk.

Approximately one-third of people will have another acute bout of diverticulitis following an initial episode. In the past, surgery (elective sigmoidectomy) was recommended after the second episode of diverticulitis. Currently, surgery is laparoscopically performed on a case-by-case basis[288] with good outcomes.[180,272]

Hospitalization is suggested for persons who are sicker or frail and demonstrate radiographic abnormalities, fever, and leukocytosis. Symptoms should improve over 2 to 3 days, when diet may be advanced. Failure to improve should prompt reevaluation with CT and other appropriate laboratory tests. Surgical consultation should be obtained where needed. Colonoscopy should be performed 4 to 6 weeks after resolution of the initial attack to verify the presence of disease and exclude colorectal cancer or IBD.

Approximately 25% of people with diverticulitis will also develop a complication.[167] Abscesses form when a perforation is contained.[325] People with an abscess less than 3 cm can often be treated with antibiotics and bowel rest alone. Larger abscesses (greater than 3 cm) frequently require CT-guided percutaneous drainage and antibiotics. Surgery is often required once the infection is controlled.

Fistulas may form, most commonly between the colon and the bladder or vagina. This complication requires surgical management. Recurrent diverticulitis frequently leads to scarring and narrowing of the lumen with resultant obstruction. Temporary endoscopic dilation with stent placement can be performed for temporary relief until surgery is accomplished.[173] Frank perforation and peritonitis are uncommon complications but carry a high mortality (as high as 25%). Immediate surgery is required with resuscitative efforts.

**PROGNOSIS.** Prognosis is good for the person with known diverticular disease, particularly as most people remain asymptomatic. Diverticulitis can have significant complications, but the mortality remains low except in cases of frank perforation and peritonitis. Suspicion for diverticular disease should be entertained in young people because the incidence is increasing in this age group.

SPECIAL IMPLICATIONS FOR THE THERAPIST 16.13

### *Diverticular Disease*

Exercise is an important treatment component during periods of remission. Physical activity may have a protective effect on the GI system.[217] Data from a large prospective cohort suggest that vigorous physical activity lowers the risk of diverticulitis and diverticular bleeding.[330] The therapist is instrumental in helping establish an appropriate exercise program. Throughout all activity and exercise, clients with diverticular disease must be careful to avoid activities that increase intraabdominal pressure (see Box 16.1) to avoid further herniation. The therapist can provide valuable information regarding appropriate body mechanics and techniques to reduce intraabdominal pressure for all activities.

Back pain can occur as a symptom of this disease. Anyone with back pain of nontraumatic or unknown origin must be screened for medical disease including possible GI tract involvement. If infection occurs and penetrates the pelvic floor or retroperitoneal tissues (i.e., organs outside the peritoneum such as the kidneys, colon, and pancreas), abscesses may result, causing isolated referred hip or thigh pain.

A variety of objective test procedures may be employed by the therapist to assess for iliopsoas abscess formation including palpation of the McBurney point (Fig. 16.15), assessment of the pinch-an-inch test (Fig. 16.16), the iliopsoas muscle test, the obturator test, and palpation of the iliopsoas muscle (see Figs. 16.12 and 16.13).

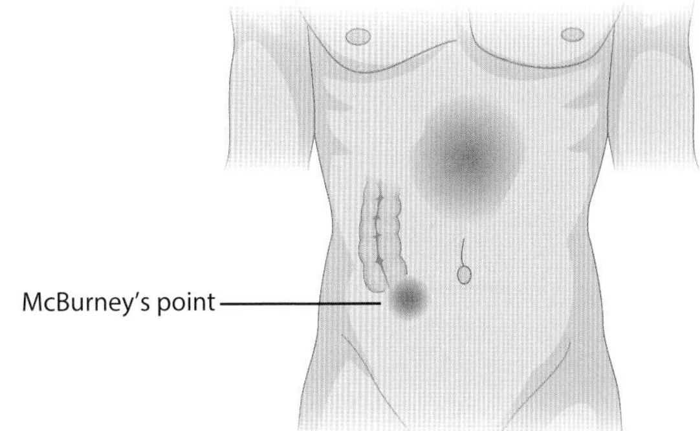


**Figure 16.15**

**Pain areas associated with appendicitis, including McBurney point.** Tenderness on palpation of this point is indicative of appendicitis. With the client supine and legs extended, isolate the anterior superior iliac spine and the umbilicus, then gently palpate approximately half the distance between those two points. A positive test produces painful symptoms in the right lower quadrant. (Modified from O'Toole M, editor: *Miller-Keane encyclopedia and dictionary of medicine, nursing, and allied health*, ed 6, Philadelphia, 1997, Saunders, p. 119.)

## Neoplasms

### Intestinal Polyps

A growth or mass protruding into the intestinal lumen from any area of mucous membrane can be termed a *polyp*. Polyps are either *neoplastic* or *nonneoplastic*. Two of the more common types of nonneoplastic polyps are hyperplastic and inflammatory. Adenomatous polyps, a neoplastic type of polyp, usually develop during middle age. More than two-thirds of the population older than 65 years old have at least one polyp. Until a polyp becomes large enough to obstruct the intestine, no symptoms are discernible. Early symptoms may be lower abdominal cramping pain, diarrhea with rectal bleeding, and passage of mucus.

Adenomatous polyps may develop into adenocarcinoma (colorectal cancer); therefore regardless of the clinical manifestations, adenomatous polyps are removed (by polypectomy, usually performed through a sigmoidoscope or colonoscope; large polyps may require removal by laparotomy). Sessile serrated polyps and traditional serrated adenomas are neoplastic and precursors to colon cancer, requiring excision. Hyperplastic polyps do not progress to become cancerous.

### Benign Tumors

The most common benign tumors of the small intestine are adenomas, leiomyomas, and lipomas. Benign tumors

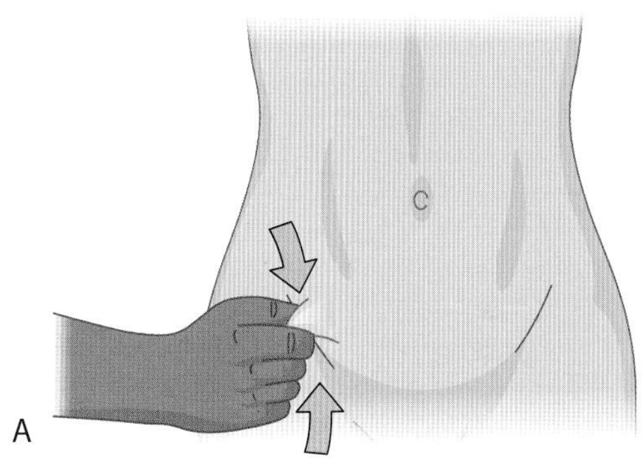


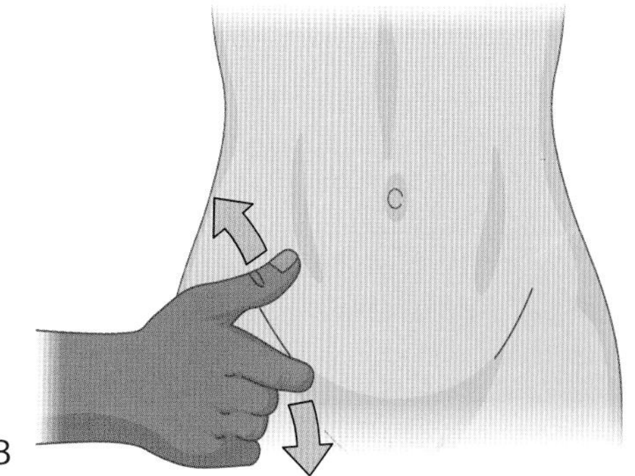


**Figure 16.16**

**Pinch-an-inch test.** To avoid the discomfort of the traditionally used (and sometimes inaccurate) rebound test, the pinch-an-inch test was developed as an alternative test for peritonitis associated with appendicitis. (A) Gently grasp and lift 2 to 3 inches of skin from over the McBurney point on the right side of the abdomen. An individual with a low threshold of pain may report pain during the initial pinch. The clinician must assess this response accordingly. (B) Quickly release the skin. A positive sign occurs if increased pain is reported when the skin returns to its position against the abdominal wall.

of the small intestine rarely become malignant and may be symptomatic or may be incidental findings at operation or autopsy.

### Malignant Tumors

The most common malignant tumors of the small intestine are metastatic through direct extension from adjacent organs (e.g., stomach, pancreas, colon). Adenocarcinoma and primary lymphoma account for the majority of bowel malignancies. Other types of tumors found in the colon including melanoma, fibrosarcoma, and other types of sarcoma are rare and are not discussed further in this book.

#### Colorectal Cancer

***Overview and Incidence.*** Colorectal cancer (cancer of the colon and/or rectum) is the fourth leading cause of cancer among American men and women, with an estimated 140,250 new cases in 2018.[243,303] It is also the second leading cause of cancer death in both men and women in the United States with an estimate of 50,630 deaths in 2018.[302] Overall incidence and mortality rates are on the decline, possibly indicating that screening is leading to earlier detection with improved survival rates. Incidence increases with age, starting at 40 years, and the disease occurs slightly more often in men and in populations of high socioeconomic status, possibly owing to dietary factors. African Americans have the highest incidence of colorectal cancer among all racial groups, with death rates approximately 30% higher than for whites. This disparity is most likely a result of differences between African Americans and whites in screening rates, early detection, and intervention.[7,267,278,371] Other reasons relate to the location and molecular abnormalities of colon cancer. African Americans are more likely to have colon cancer that develops on the right side, which carries a worse prognosis, as well as genetic abnormalities that also have worse outcomes.[62] Because of these factors, many organizations recommend screening begin for African Americans at the age of 45.

***Etiologic and Risk Factors.*** The cause of colon cancer is unknown, although a number of environmental and familial factors have been considered. Genetic syndromes are more likely to occur before age 40 years and make up less than 6% of all colorectal cancers. Approximately 75% of all colorectal cancer occurs in people with no known predisposing factors; for such individuals, the lifetime risk of developing this type of cancer is approximately 5%.

Known factors associated with increased risk of colonic cancer include increasing age, male gender, a personal history of adenomatous polyps, IBD (UC, CD), family history of colon cancer or FAP, and obesity. Cigarette smoking and excessive alcohol consumption may possibly increase risk.[186] Anyone who has first-degree relatives diagnosed with colon or rectal adenoma is twice as likely to develop colon cancer as individuals with no history of such cancer in the immediate family. The risk is even higher if the relative was younger than 50 years of age at the time of diagnosis.

Geographic distributions of highest incidence coincide with regional diets low in fiber and high in animal fat, sugar, and protein; people who emigrate tend to acquire the risk characteristics of their new environment. Eating large amounts of red or processed meat over a long period of time can increase colorectal cancer risk, but the risk from obesity and lack of exercise (inactivity) is even greater.[60]

***Pathogenesis.*** Although colon cancer is a heterogeneous disease, most cancers develop from one of three different genetic pathways.[216] The majority of cases occur secondary to a gain or loss of a chromosome or chromosomal material, leaving only one normal complementary chromosome/gene. With progressive mutations in the normal gene, including changes to tumor suppressor genes or oncogenes, malignancy can develop. This is referred to as chromosomal instability. About 70% of adenocarcinomas of the colon develop from adenomas that arise owing to this type of progression.

The second pathway is described as microsatellite instability (MSI). Microsatellites are noncoding sequences of tandomly repeated DNA with high rates of mutations. These mutations are normally corrected by enzymes produced from mismatch repair (MMR) genes. However, if there is a mutation in one or more of the MMR genes, these mutations are not repaired. When this is noted in a colon tumor, it is called MSI (if a high amount is present, it is referred to as MSI-H). Approximately 5% of colon cancer tumors express a mutation in an MMR gene, which is the key feature of tumors that are part of Lynch syndrome.

The final genetic pathway is due to alterations made to a gene itself, such as methylation of a gene's promoter region, which prevents transcription of the gene. People who have the tendency to hypermethylate genes are referred to as having CpG island methylator phenotype. This subgroup of tumor may arise through the methylation of tumor suppressor genes. These tumors often have multiple mutations and MSI. They include sessile serrated polyps and are typically poorly differentiated. About 30% of colon cancers develop from this type of genetic abnormality.

***Clinical Manifestations.*** Colon carcinoma has few early warning signs, as is the case with esophageal and stomach cancers. Common symptoms include occult blood loss (with resultant anemia and iron deficiency), melena, hematochezia, abdominal pain, weight loss, and change in bowel habits. Bright-red blood from the rectum is a cardinal sign of colon cancer, particularly rectal cancer, but must be differentiated from diverticulosis, anal fissures, and hemorrhoids, which are also common causes of bright red blood. Many cases of colon cancer are asymptomatic until metastasis has occurred, which may manifest as right upper quadrant pain (liver metastases), abdominal bloating, and early satiety. Complications include intestinal obstruction; GI bleeding; perforation; anemia; ascites; and distant metastases, to the liver most commonly but also to the lungs, bone, and brain.

## MEDICAL MANAGEMENT

**SCREENING/PREVENTION.** Because colorectal cancer is slow growing (approximately 10 to 15 years for a polyp to become a cancer), screening is very effective. Evidence exists that reductions in colorectal cancer morbidity and mortality can be achieved through screening,[13,131,198,214] early detection,[296] and removal of polyps.[380] However, approximately 22 million Americans between the ages of 50 and 75 years do not receive screening of any type, and 25,000 lives could be saved.[56,130] Many types of tests are available with advantages and disadvantages.

In 2017 the U.S. Multi-Society Task Force on Colorectal Cancer (MSTF) made recommendations for colorectal cancer screening that emphasized tiers of recommendations, providing options rather than specific tests and intervals.[279] Colonoscopy and fecal immunochemical tests (FIT) constitute the first tier of recommendations. Colonoscopy has the advantage of complete visualization of the colon (with a good bowel preparation) and the ability to obtain biopsy specimens and remove small polyps. It is, however, invasive (with associated serious outcomes such as perforation of the colon) and requires an involved colonic preparation. FIT can be done at home and tested in the health care provider's office.

Colonoscopy is greater than 90% sensitive in finding polyps larger than 1 cm and can be performed every 10 years in people who do not have polyps. Colonoscopy reduces the incidence of colorectal cancer by 67% and reduces mortality by 65%.[162] People are often more likely to be compliant with FIT[271]; however, it is not as sensitive (60% to 85%) and requires annual screening and a colonoscopy if the test is positive. People who are at increased risk for colon cancer should be offered colonoscopy, followed by FIT.

Second-tier recommendations include CT colonography every 5 years, FIT–fecal DNA every 3 years, or flexible sigmoidoscopy every 5 to 10 years. CT colonography (virtual colonoscopy) is a newer test in which the colon is inflated via a rectal tube and then CT scans are obtained of the colon in both supine and prone positions. It has a high sensitivity (95%) for lesions larger than 1 cm and is less invasive than colonoscopy. The FIT–fecal DNA test uses FIT and combines it with a test that looks for colon cancer–specific DNA in the stool. An entire bowel movement must be collected at home to be sent to the laboratory. Owing to the improved availability and decreased invasiveness, this test may be more appealing to people who have never been screened. It has an approximate sensitivity of 92% for colorectal cancer.[14] Sigmoidoscopy is sensitive for finding lesions in the descending colon but will miss proximal lesions. Similar to colonoscopy, a sigmoidoscopy is invasive, and risk for an adverse outcome is higher than other tests. Sigmoidoscopy reduces the incidence of colorectal cancer by 26% and mortality by 50%.[199,296]

Alternatively, technology has made it possible to use a tiny camera that can be swallowed for a virtual endoscopy. This test is less invasive but may not be as complete because the camera's field of view is only 140°, leaving some portions of the GI tract in blind spots. Food and other debris also can obscure lesions from view. In rare cases, the vitamin-sized capsule may get obstructed by strictures or other problems within the intestines, requiring surgical removal. Owing to a lack of evidence and difficulties in its use, capsule colonoscopy is recommended as a third-tier test every 5 years.

In April 2016 the U.S. Food and Drug Administration approved the use of a serologic test to detect circulating methylated *SEPT9* DNA, with a sensitivity of 71% to 95% (newer kits) and specificity of 81.5% to 99% for detecting colon cancer.[318] Evidence is not available to use this test for general screening, and the MSTF does not currently recommend its use in this capacity.

Colonoscopy should be performed every 10 years for persons 50 years of age and older at average risk for colorectal cancer (more frequently if abnormalities are found). For persons with special risk (e.g., UC, FAP, hereditary nonpolyposis colorectal cancer), screening should be more frequent, and each disorder has a suggested schedule. The MSTF also recommends that African Americans begin colon cancer surveillance at age 45.

The MSTF recommends discontinuing routine surveillance at age 75 if previous screening has been negative or if clients have a life expectancy of less than 10 years.[279] For people between the ages of 75 and 85 years, decisions can be tailored on a case-by-case basis,[150] particularly if they have had no prior examination and would be healthy enough to undergo treatment.

Environmental and dietary factors have been linked to colorectal cancer, either as preventable or modifiable risk factors in contributing to the development of colorectal cancer. Diets high in fruits, vegetables, and dietary fiber appear to be preventive.[146] Diets high in fat and red meat show an increased risk. An increased intake of calcium, folate, vitamin D, vitamin C, and selenium is associated with a decreased risk.[333] Obesity and a sedentary lifestyle are also associated with a higher risk for colorectal cancer.[22]

Colorectal cancer has been extensively studied in relation to physical activity, with consistent findings that adults who increase their physical activity (frequency, intensity, or duration) can reduce their risk of developing colorectal cancer by 30% to 40% relative to persons who are sedentary (regardless of age or body mass index). The greatest risk reduction occurs in persons who are most active. The protective effect appears greatest with high-intensity activity. Optimal exercise levels and duration have not yet been determined. Likewise, studies show that moderate exercise (e.g., walking 2 to 3 miles in 1 hour 6 days per week) decreases the risk of colorectal cancer recurrence by 50%.[225] Smoking and increased alcohol intake have been consistently connected with an increased risk of colorectal cancer recurrence.[290]

Individuals between the ages of 50 and 59 at high increased risk for cardiovascular disease and colorectal cancer should talk with their physicians about the preventive use of low-dose aspirin.[45,105]

**DIAGNOSIS AND STAGING.** Carcinoma of the colon should be suspected in anyone older than age 40 years who presents with occult blood in the stool, iron-deficiency anemia, overt rectal bleeding, weight loss, or alteration in bowel habits, especially if associated with abdominal discomfort or any of the risk factors mentioned earlier. Diagnostic procedures include rectal examination; colonoscopy with biopsy of lesions; and CT scans of the chest, abdomen, and pelvis. Endoscopic ultrasound is more accurate than CT for determining the staging of rectal cancer.

Laboratory tests may include evaluation for anemia, liver function tests, and screening for fecal blood. A blood test for carcinoembryonic antigen (CEA), detected in some individuals with colorectal carcinoma, is one of the most widely used tumor markers, primarily in GI cancers, especially colorectal malignancy. It is of little use in screening for colorectal cancer, but high preoperative concentrations of CEA correlate with adverse prognosis, and serial CEA measurements can detect recurrent cancer in asymptomatic clients.[91]

The AJCC TNM (tumor, node, metastasis) staging system is the standard for colorectal cancer and has replaced the Dukes classification.[315] The TNM system incorporates both clinical and pathologic staging approaches and can be applied to the preoperative evaluation of affected individuals.[72] Features associated with a risk of recurrence include obstruction or perforation at presentation, tumor adherence to adjacent organs, positive margins on the surgical specimen, pathology consistent with a poorly differentiated tumor, and the presence of lymphovascular or perineural invasion.

**TREATMENT.** Surgical removal of the tumor is the mainstay of colorectal cancer treatment. For some clients, this may be laparoscopically performed.

Using AJCC TNM staging, stage 0 disease requires local or regional excision of the tumor with wide margins. Stage 1 cancer is treated the same way, but the individual may need bowel resection and anastomosis. Stage 2 may be treated surgically or with surgery combined with adjuvant chemotherapy (depending on risk factors present predicting potential recurrence, e.g., high-grade tumor, absence of clear margins, clinical perforation/obstruction). Stage 3 disease requires surgical excision and removal and biopsy of regional lymph nodes. Regional metastasis has occurred at this stage, requiring additional regimens of adjuvant chemotherapy. Stage 4 cancer is accompanied by systemic metastasis, requiring a more comprehensive treatment regimen to address local, regional, and systemic disease.[115]

Adjuvant chemotherapy (postoperative) and/or neoadjuvant therapy (preoperative)[87] may be administered, depending on the results of the staging process for both colon and rectal cancer, to eradicate the micrometastases and improve postsurgical survival. Adjuvant chemotherapy does improve survival for resectable cancers.[27] The benefit for stage 2 is controversial, but stage 3 has survival benefit with adjuvant chemotherapy.[118,260,385] Most chemotherapy consists of 5-fluorouracil plus the reduced folate leukovorin, with some regimens including capecitabine and oxaliplatin. Even clients with limited metastatic disease can have significant improvement in their prognosis with surgical resection of metastases and adjuvant chemotherapy.

In treating rectal cancer, chemoradiation may be given before surgery (neoadjuvant therapy) to reduce the tumor size and/or after surgery to improve local control. Rectal tumors are located in a retroperitoneal position, and their location in the pelvis makes resection with wide margins difficult. Tumors in the distal rectum may require resection of the entire rectum with subsequent colostomy (a 2-cm margin is needed to perform sphincter-saving surgery).

Targeted (biologic) therapy with monoclonal antibodies (MABs) has been developed for the treatment of cancers. Even though significant controversy surrounds these agents in treating colorectal cancer, they are used for the treatment of metastatic colorectal cancer. Although designed to be given as monotherapy or accompanying chemotherapy/radiation, MABs are principally given with chemotherapy. Bevacizumab, targeted against vascular endothelial growth factor, has been shown to modestly improve outcome when used with chemotherapy in metastatic disease.[43]

The programmed death 1 receptor inhibitors, pembrolizumab and nivolumab, are effective only against colon cancers exhibiting deficient MMR, which accounts for only 1% to 2% of metastatic colorectal cancer. MABs that bind to epidermal growth factor receptors, cetuximab and panitumumab, are ineffective in 50% of cancers that express mutations in the *K-ras* and *N-ras* genes. Clients with metastatic disease should undergo tumor genotyping testing for these mutations before receiving these MABs. More research is needed to determine the optimal uses for MABs in colorectal cancer.[282,349,366]

**PROGNOSIS.** The 5-year survival for all stages combined is 64%; local (early) stages have a 90% 5-year survival; regional stages have a 69% 5-year survival; and metastatic disease (late stages) has only a 12% 5-year survival.[138] Most often, death from rectal cancer is from local recurrence rather than from distant metastasis.

Colorectal cancer survival is related closely to the clinical and pathologic stage of the disease at diagnosis. The depth of tumor penetration into the bowel wall is an important prognostic indicator. The deeper it penetrates, the worse the prognosis. Involvement of local lymph nodes is also associated with a worse prognosis. Stage-for-stage, rectal carcinoma has a poorer prognosis compared with colon cancer, owing to the location of the tumor.

CEA should be monitored every 3 to 6 months for 2 years and every 6 months for the subsequent 3 years. Follow-up colonoscopy is recommended at 1 year, with a repeat in 2 years if no lesions or polyps are present. Screening colonoscopy can then be done every 5 years. Colonoscopy is principally looking for new polyps rather than recurrence of disease (which is rare).

CT scans of the chest, abdomen, and pelvis are recommended every year for 3 years. CT is able to detect liver metastases, which, if limited and resected, can improve mortality rate by 25%. Flexible sigmoidoscopy is recommended every 3 to 6 months for 2 to 3 years for clients who are at high risk for local reoccurrence for rectal cancer. Approximately 25% of people present with evidence of hematogenous spread, and 50% will develop metastatic disease. As with most solid cancers, early detection is the key to cure.

SPECIAL IMPLICATIONS FOR THE THERAPIST 16.14

### *Colorectal Cancer*

The physical therapist's involvement may vary depending on individual comorbidities and clinical presentation. For example, a client who has a history of corticosteroid therapy or a woman who has had surgically induced menopause prematurely may be at risk for skeletal demineralization.[115]

Impaired posture can occur as a result of adaptive shortening of the abdominal musculature as a result of extensive surgical disruption and pain contributing to a stooped posture and inability to lie completely supine. Such a condition can place increased stress on the muscles of the lower back and alter body mechanics, placing the individual at increased risk for injury during lifting and risk of decreased function in other activities.[115]

The removal of lymph nodes from the abdominal/pelvic area can put a client at increased risk of lymphedema. The therapist can be instrumental in providing education regarding lymphedema risk and prevention. Many individuals are deconditioned before beginning cancer treatment. The benefits of exercise in general and especially for patients recovering from cancer treatment have been reported in the literature and are summarized in Chapter 9.

### Metastases

Tumors of the rectum can spread through the rectal wall to the prostate in men and the vagina in women. Prostate involvement can cause dull, vague, aching pain in the sacral or lumbar spine regions.

Systemic and pulmonary metastases occur through the hemorrhoidal plexus, which drains into the vena cava. Subsequent chest, shoulder, arm, or back pain can occur, usually accompanied by pulmonary symptoms; see also ***.

Liver metastasis occurs after invasion of the mesenteric veins from the left colon or the superior veins from the right colon, which empty into the portal circulation. Any time a person with low back pain reports simultaneous or alternating abdominal pain at the same level as the back pain or GI symptoms associated with back pain, a medical referral is required.

Anemia caused by intestinal bleeding associated with colon cancer requires special consideration.

### Rehabilitation

Many factors can influence whether an individual with colorectal cancer will be referred to rehabilitation services. The client's tolerance to pain, his or her ability to recover, the presence of other comorbidities, and the physician's perception of physical debilitation may play a role in the decision to refer.[76]

Complications and side effects arising from comprehensive treatment can produce impairments for which physical therapy intervention can improve quality of life, tolerance of cancer treatment, and recovery of function.[115]

The therapist may be involved in the rehabilitation of some clients with (colorectal) cancer to improve function and mobility after abdominal surgery or other medical treatments.[69]

Individuals who have had laparoscopic surgery may be able to tolerate a more aggressive approach to rehabilitation and recovery of function.[172]

Movement to stimulate the gastric system and help the flow of the abdominal contents may begin the same day as surgery, with ambulation every 4 to 6 hours on the first day.[81] The therapist may be called on to evaluate the client's needs and to instruct the staff and family in ambulation if assistance is needed.

Many people who have a colectomy without a colostomy bag have to relearn bowel control because the pelvic floor muscles are often manipulated and weakened during surgery. A program of pelvic floor rehabilitation, possibly including biofeedback and electrical stimulation, can help restore pelvic floor function (eBox 16.1).[41]

For an example of how rehabilitation might flow for someone with extensive involvement at various stages of disease based on the natural history following surgery, chemotherapy, and radiation therapy, see eBox 16.1 on the book's Student Consult site.

## Obstructive Disease

Obstruction can occur in either the small or the large intestines. Small intestinal obstruction is more common because of the narrower diameter of the lumen. Hernias, intestinal adhesions, intussusception, and volvulus account for 80% of mechanical obstructions. Tumors and infarction account for another 10% to 15%.

### Mechanical Obstruction

**Adhesion.** Adhesions are the most common cause of small and large intestine obstruction. Adhesions are caused by fibrous scars formed as a consequence of previous surgery, infections (resulting in peritonitis), and endometriosis. These fibrous bands of scar tissue create bridges through which intestine can slide and become trapped or by creating an axis around which the bowel can twist (volvulus).

**Intussusception.** Intussusception is a telescoping of the bowel into itself; that is, one part of the intestine propels into the lumen of an immediately adjacent section (Fig. 16.17). Once trapped inside the next section, continuing peristalsis forces the attached mesentery along. If left untreated, these segments compress the mesenteric vessels and can become ischemic, with resulting infarction and obstruction. There is an association between the rotavirus vaccine and intussusception in infants and young children (small increased risk).[231,345] In adults,

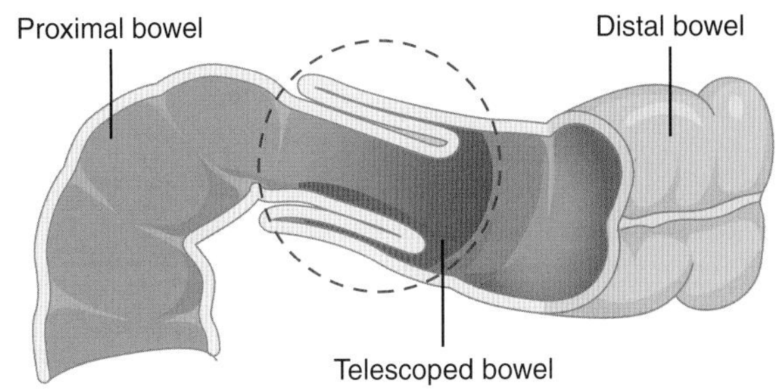


**Figure 16.17**

**Intussusception.** A portion of the bowel telescopes into adjacent (usually distal) bowel.

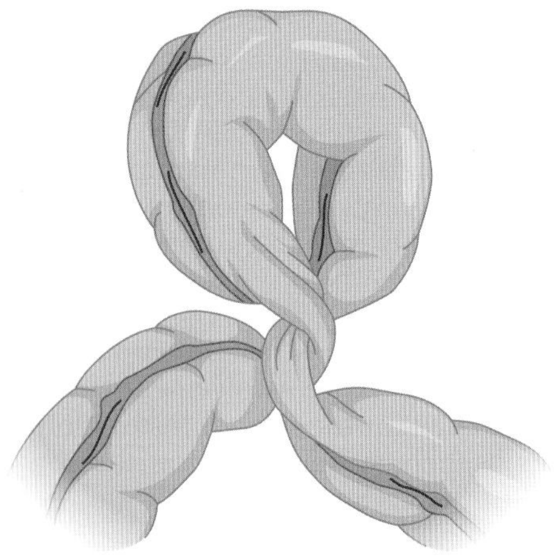

**Figure 16.18**

**Volvulus.** The intestine twists, causing obstruction and ischemia.

the leading point is due to a structural lesion and most often occurs in the small bowel. It is frequently due to neoplasm, either local or metastatic.[210]

**Volvulus.** Volvulus is a torsion of a loop of intestine, frequently redundant loops of sigmoid colon, twisted on its mesentery, kinking the bowel and interrupting the blood supply (Fig. 16.18). The cause of this phenomenon is usually a congenital abnormality, such as a malrotation of the bowel that allows excess mobility of the bowel loops and predisposes the intestine to volvulus. Nonsurgical methods are initially undertaken to detorse the intestine. It is seen in people of all ages but is rare.

Clinical manifestations include abdominal pain and distention, nausea and vomiting, constipation, and obstipation (a more significant clinical feature for obstruction). Complications include ischemia and subsequent necrosis, perforation, peritonitis, and sepsis. Usually, diagnostic testing includes rectal examination, abdominal radiography, and CT. Exploratory or therapeutic surgical intervention, either an open procedure or laparoscopic, is often required. The goal is to intervene before significant loss of tissue to ischemia. The prognosis for children and adults with this condition is good if treated early.

**Hernia**

***Definition and Incidence.*** A hernia is caused by a weakness in the peritoneal cavity through which peritoneum can slide and form a serosa-lined sac or bulge, followed by protrusion of part of an organ or tissue in the groin, abdomen, and navel (often the intestine). About 5 million Americans of all ages have some type of abdominal hernia. Hernias can occur at any age in men or women and most frequently occur in the abdominal cavity as a result of a congenital or acquired weakness of abdominal musculature.

Weakness can occur as part of the aging process, contributing to acquired hernias. As people age, muscular tissues become infiltrated by adipose and connective tissues, resulting in weakness. The most common types of hernias are inguinal (direct and indirect), femoral, umbilical, and incisional or ventral (Fig. 16.19).

***Etiologic and Risk Factors.*** When muscular weakness (congenital or acquired) is accompanied by obesity, pregnancy, heavy lifting, coughing, surgical incision, or traumatic injuries from blunt pressure, the risk of developing a hernia increases. Often, herniation is the result of a multifactorial process involving one or more of these factors. Many possible combinations of risk factors exist (Table 16.7).

Structural abnormalities account for most congenital hernias, but congenital factors do not explain the increased incidence of hernias (e.g., the direct inguinal type) with advancing age. Sudden stress, as occurs in abdominal trauma or industrial accidents, also may contribute to the development of a hernia with or without an underlying congenital defect.

Predisposing factors are equally important, such as physical stress (e.g., repetitive local trauma, strenuous physical activities), degenerative changes associated with increased abdominal pressure, the wear and tear of living, multiparity (women), and altered collagen synthesis in middle age.

***Pathogenesis.*** Structural and biochemical abnormalities and abnormalities of local collagen metabolism have been proposed as factors in the eventual appearance of a hernia. Weakness of the tissues around the *inguinal* canal leads to tears and separation of the tissues. The inguinal canal is formed by fascia to the abdominal muscles on one side and the internal oblique abdominal muscle on the other. Inside the canal is the spermatic cord in men and the round ligament in women.

Other biologic factors can affect the balance between collagen synthesis and lysis, eventually leading to the development of herniation. For example, any condition such as renal failure, diabetes mellitus, malnutrition, vitamin or mineral deficiencies, underlying systemic disease, altered immunity, or resistance to infection that can impair a person's ability to generate the proteinaceous constituents of collagen can alter collagen metabolism.

*Inguinal hernias* account for approximately 75% of all hernias and will affect approximately 25% of men in the United States sometime during their lifetime. Women also can have inguinal hernias. Indirect hernias occur in infants as the result of a congenital patency of the processus vaginalis. In adults, there is a weakening and widening of the internal ring. A peritoneal sac is then able to slip into the ring. The indirect inguinal hernia is most common in infants, young people, and males, in the last-mentioned group because it follows the tract that develops when the testes descend into the scrotum before birth. A wide space at the inguinal ligament also can contribute to the development of an inguinal hernia.

*Direct hernias,* the second most common type of hernia, occur most often as a result of a deficient number of transversus abdominis aponeurotic fibers at a site called the *Hesselbach triangle,* the area between the pubic ramus and the musculofascial components in the lower abdominal wall. The direct inguinal hernia is more common in older adults, especially in an area that is congenitally weak because of a deficient number of muscle fibers.

*Femoral hernia* is a protrusion of a loop of intestine into the femoral canal, a tubular passageway into the thigh that carries nerves and blood vessels. The pathologic anatomy present is an enlarged femoral ring with a correspondingly narrowed transversus abdominis aponeurosis. This

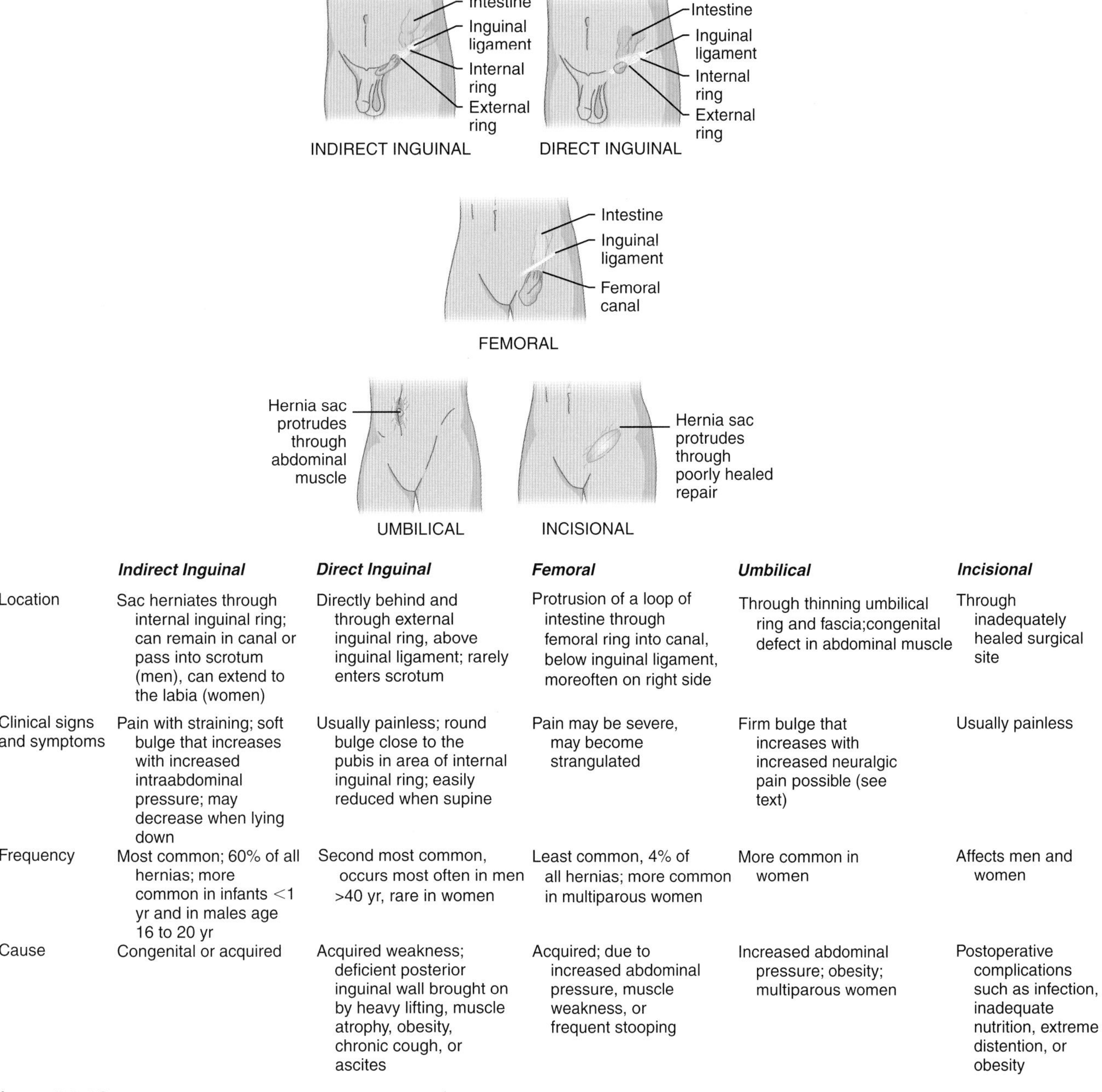


| | *Indirect Inguinal* | *Direct Inguinal* | *Femoral* | *Umbilical* | *Incisional* |
|---|---|---|---|---|---|
| Location | Sac herniates through internal inguinal ring; can remain in canal or pass into scrotum (men), can extend to the labia (women) | Directly behind and through external inguinal ring, above inguinal ligament; rarely enters scrotum | Protrusion of a loop of intestine through femoral ring into canal, below inguinal ligament, moreoften on right side | Through thinning umbilical ring and fascia;congenital defect in abdominal muscle | Through inadequately healed surgical site |
| Clinical signs and symptoms | Pain with straining; soft bulge that increases with increased intraabdominal pressure; may decrease when lying down | Usually painless; round bulge close to the pubis in area of internal inguinal ring; easily reduced when supine | Pain may be severe, may become strangulated | Firm bulge that increases with increased neuralgic pain possible (see text) | Usually painless |
| Frequency | Most common; 60% of all hernias; more common in infants <1 yr and in males age 16 to 20 yr | Second most common, occurs most often in men >40 yr, rare in women | Least common, 4% of all hernias; more common in multiparous women | More common in women | Affects men and women |
| Cause | Congenital or acquired | Acquired weakness; deficient posterior inguinal wall brought on by heavy lifting, muscle atrophy, obesity, chronic cough, or ascites | Acquired; due to increased abdominal pressure, muscle weakness, or frequent stooping | Increased abdominal pressure; obesity; multiparous women | Postoperative complications such as infection, inadequate nutrition, extreme distention, or obesity |

**Figure 16.19**

**Hernias.** (Modified from Jarvis C: *Physical examination and health assessment,* ed 3, Philadelphia, 2000, WB Saunders, p. 779.)

type occurs more often in multiparous women, acquired as a result of increased intraabdominal pressure gradually forcing more and more preperitoneal fat into the femoral canal, enlarging the femoral ring. Femoral hernias are uncommon, and the diagnosis is often difficult to make.

The pathology of *umbilical hernias* is caused by increased abdominal pressure (see discussion of risk factors) exerted against a thinning of the umbilical ring and fascia. *Incisional hernia* occurs postoperatively when the transected fibers are unable to form collagen links strong enough to hold the edges of the wound together.

*Sports hernia* is a term used to describe pain in the pubic joint of athletes and is probably multifactorial. The name is misleading, as it is not a true abdominal hernia because it does not involve bowel protrusion through the abdominal wall; a more correct term would be athletic pubalgia. The pathogenesis is not clear, but it is thought to begin initially as tendinosis (adductor longus origin or the rectus abdominis insertion). This progresses to involve muscles (rectus abdominis, internal oblique, and transversus abdominis muscles) and the pubic joint, associated with dilation of the external inguinal ring. These

**Table 16.7** Risk Factors for Hernias

| Inguinal | Femoral | Umbilical | Incisional |
|---|---|---|---|
| Advanced age<br>Prematurity<br>Positive family history<br>Abdominal wall defects<br>Undescended testis<br>Connective tissue disorders<br>Cystic fibrosis<br>Shunt for hydrocephalus<br>Ascites | Pregnancy (multiparous) | Infancy<br>Low birth weight<br>African descent<br>Congenital hypothyroidism<br>Mucopolysaccharidoses<br>Down syndrome<br>Obesity<br>Pregnancy<br>Ascites | Poor wound healing<br>Infection<br>Inadequate nutrition<br>Abdominal distention<br>Obesity<br>Prolonged use of steroids<br>Advanced age<br>Immunosuppression<br>Postoperative pulmonary complications (coughing, straining)<br>Type of incision (vertical) |

changes are called posterior inguinal wall insufficiency. Athletes who participate in sports requiring twisting and turning at high speeds (e.g., soccer, rugby, ice hockey, tennis) are at greatest risk. Insidious onset of unilateral groin pain is the most common symptom of this type of hernia.

***Clinical Manifestations.*** The most common manifestation of a hernia of any type is an intermittent or persistent bulge, accompanied by intermittent or persistent pain. Inguinal hernia usually begins as a small, marble-size soft lump under the skin. At first, it is painless and can be reduced by pushing it back into place. As pressure from the abdominal contents pushes against the weak abdominal wall, the size of the lump formed by the hernia increases, requiring surgical repair (herniorrhaphy).

The pain associated with simple hernias depends on the involved structures and whether these are compressed or irritated. The pain usually is localized and sharp, aggravated by changes in position, by physical exertion, during a bowel movement, or by any activity causing the Valsalva maneuver (bearing down with increased intraabdominal pressure such as during coughing or sneezing), and relieved by cessation of the physical activity that precipitated it.

Inguinal hernias are often more noticeable after a heavy meal or long period of standing. Pain may radiate from the groin to the testicles (males), ipsilateral thigh, flank, or hypogastrium (lowest middle abdominal region). In women, painful symptoms may be aggravated by the onset of menstruation.

The ilioinguinal nerve penetrates the abdominal wall cranially and somewhat laterally to the deep inguinal ring, passing the transverse and internal oblique muscles in a stepwise fashion. Neuralgic pain may occur when the dull inguinal hernial pain causes a local reflex increase of tone in the internal oblique and transverse muscles of the abdomen. As the nerve passes these muscles in steps, it may be exposed to pressure, giving rise to pain of the neuralgic type.

Ilioinguinal or femoral neuritis can occur, caused by nerve entrapment from sutures, adhesions, or the actual formation of a symptomatic neuroma after section of a nerve in this region. These conditions usually resolve spontaneously without specific treatment, but therapy in conjunction with local nerve blocks may be indicated if symptoms persist after the first postoperative month.

Genitofemoral neuralgia (causalgia) occurs less commonly but results in severe pain and paresthesia (or hyperesthesia) in the distribution of the genitofemoral nerve. Radiation of pain to the genitalia and upper thigh may occur, and pain is aggravated by walking, stooping, or hyperextending the hip. Recumbency and flexion of the thigh may relieve painful symptoms. This condition requires neurectomy for pain relief.

When the contents of the hernial sac can be pushed back into the abdominal cavity by manipulation, the hernia is said to be *reducible*. Hernias that cannot be reduced or replaced by manipulation are referred to as *irreducible* and *incarcerated*.

Complications occur when the protruding organ is constricted to the extent that circulation is impaired (strangulated hernia) or when the protruding organs encroach on and impair the function of other structures. When a hernia contains incarcerated or strangulated structures, the pain becomes persistent and often is associated with systemic signs or symptoms such as elevated temperature, tachycardia, vomiting, and abdominal distention.

## MEDICAL MANAGEMENT

**DIAGNOSIS.** History and physical examination remain the most important aspects of diagnosis for all types of hernia; there may be a past history of hernia. Inguinal hernias are most frequently diagnosed by noting the bulge in the inguinal canal. The diagnosis of umbilical hernia is usually obvious because of protrusion of the umbilicus confirmed by palpation of the involved structures.

Imaging (plain films and CT) is important in diagnosing sports hernias, especially to identify osteitis pubis, adductor tenoperiosteal lesions, and symphyseal instability, and to rule out hip osteoarthritis and tumors. Magnetic resonance imaging may be used to diagnose bone marrow edema about the pubic symphysis (a sign of osteitis pubis), stress fractures, avascular necrosis, labral hip tears, and articular cartilage defects that can accompany a sports hernia.[337]

**TREATMENT.** Various supports and trusses are available to contain hernias, but these offer only a temporary solution and may not prevent the hernia from getting bigger with associated complications. The use of strapping techniques is not recommended because the tape used may lead to ulceration of the thin skin covering the hernia and eventual rupture.

Watchful waiting is an acceptable treatment approach for minimally symptomatic *inguinal* hernias. Delaying surgical repair until symptoms increase is considered safe because acute hernia incarcerations rarely occur.

Surgical repair is the only curative treatment, but it is no longer recommended, as watchful waiting does not increase morbidity or mortality for asymptomatic inguinal hernias.[273] Often the size and location determine need for surgery. For example, large ventral hernias often do not require surgery because tissue does not become incarcerated/strangulated. Inguinal hernias should be repaired when examination and pain consistent with a hernia are documented. Complications of herniorrhaphy include cutaneous nerve injury, formation of seroma, bleeding, wound infection, chronic pain, and recurrence.

When surgical repair is indicated, there are several methods of correction depending on the size and location of the hernia. When repairing an inguinal hernia, choices include type of procedure (open versus laparoscopic) and use of mesh (many products available). Each type of procedure has different operative complications, recurrence rates, postoperative pain, and recovery time.[32] Ventral or incisional hernia repairs can be done through an open surgical procedure or laparoscopically, although the latter method requires further long-term studies.[293] Laparoscopic repair appears to reduce the risk of incisional wound infection and may reduce hospital stay.

**PROGNOSIS.** Prognosis varies with the type of hernia and accompanying complications. The incidence of incarceration is approximately 10% in indirect inguinal hernia and 20% in femoral hernia. Umbilical hernia in adults has a high morbidity and mortality associated with incarceration. Open and laparoscopic repairs produce excellent results; the laparoscopic procedure allows earlier return to play for athletes.

SPECIAL IMPLICATIONS FOR THE THERAPIST 16.15

## *Hernia*

### Prevention, Screening, and Referral for Hernia

Congenital muscle weakness complicated by the additional risk factors of obesity and increased intraabdominal pressure should be identified and treated. Educate clients in proper lifting techniques and precautions to avoid heavy lifting and straining, which reduce intraabdominal pressure as an additional risk factor for the development of hernias and aid in preventing worsening of an already existing hernia. The mouth-open position as a reminder to breathe properly and to prevent increased intraabdominal pressure is essential during all lifting procedures. Obesity as a cause of increased intraabdominal pressure may be addressed by weight control through exercise.

Early diagnosis is important in preventing bowel incarceration and strangulation. Ask any client experiencing chronic cough; pregnancy; or back, hip, groin, or sacroiliac pain: "Have you ever been told you have a hernia, or do you think you have a hernia now?"

Any person (especially an older client) with a known hernia complaining of pain, nausea, vomiting, or other new symptom in the anatomic vicinity of the hernia should report these symptoms to the physician to rule out a systemic condition unrelated to the herniation.

Any time a person chooses to wear a truss without prior physician evaluation, the therapist is advised to encourage that client to seek medical advice. The therapist should be aware of two complications that may occur in a client wearing a truss. In a client with a small hernia, the pressure of the overlying truss on a protruding hernial mass enhances the chances of strangulation by obstructing lymphatic and venous drainage. In a person with a large direct inguinal hernia, the constant overlying pressure of the truss pad on the margins of the hernial defect can lead to atrophy of the fascial aponeurotic structures, enlarging the hernial opening and promoting growth of the hernia, thus making subsequent surgical repair more difficult.

Although uncommon, psoas abscess still can be confused with a hernia. The therapist may perform evaluative tests to rule out a psoas abscess, but the physician must differentiate between an abscess and a hernia; see the iliopsoas and obturator muscle tests (see Fig. 16.12), iliopsoas palpation (see Fig. 16.13), and the McBurney point (see Fig. 16.15). Psoas abscess is often softer than a femoral hernia and has ill-defined borders, in contrast to the more sharply defined margins of the hernia. The major differentiating feature is the fact that a psoas abscess lies lateral to the femoral artery, not medial to it, as is the case for the femoral hernia.

### Postoperative Recovery

For most clients recovering from surgical repair of a hernia, heavy lifting and straining should be avoided for 4 to 6 weeks after surgery. This guideline may vary depending on the specific type of hernia and surgical procedure used. The therapist should read the medical record to identify these two features before beginning a postoperative rehabilitation program.

Substance abusers and cigarette smokers have an additional risk factor for delayed wound healing and dehiscence. Transient anesthesia of the skin beneath the hernial incision is a possible postoperative phenomenon. Whether in the presence of an uncorrected hernia or postoperatively, the client should avoid activities and positions that produce painful symptoms associated with the hernia.

Whereas most people do well after surgical repair, some have persistent postoperative pain or discomfort. If a person has had a previous inguinal hernial repair and now presents with painful groin or thigh pain, the physician must differentiate between ilioinguinal nerve entrapment and neuroma of a branch of the nerve severed previously.

Although most hernia surgeries are done laparoscopically, for individuals who have an open procedure, special care must be taken when there is a vertical incision. When a vertical incision transects fascial aponeurotic fibers, the incision is made perpendicular to the direction of those fibers. Simple muscle contraction, as in coughing, straining, or turning over in bed, tends to distract the wound edges. Laparoscopic repair will likely eliminate this type of surgical incision.

**Postoperative Rehabilitation**

For the most part, the guidelines for postoperative rehabilitation of herniorrhaphy presented in the literature are not evidence based.[337] Research in this area is needed. It has been suggested that postoperative rehabilitation of the athlete with an uncomplicated sports hernia can begin with isometric abdominal and adductor exercises as early as the first day after minimally invasive surgery. Progression to concentric and eccentric strengthening progresses after the end of the first week. Walking can begin during the first week after surgery. The safety of these recommendations has not been verified by randomized controlled trials.

The same authors suggest that the client can be progressed to jogging by day 10 if approved by the surgeon. Straight-line sprinting begins around day 21, with sport-specific exercises introduced gradually after that. Athletes may expect to return to full sports participation 6 to 8 weeks after open surgery (much sooner after minimally invasive surgery) unless comorbid muscle strains or unrepaired tears exist; recovery from complicated injuries can take 3 months or more. The therapist should address all aspects of pelvic flexibility, strength, and stability.

Other retrospective studies report that most athletes return to their normal sports level within 3 months after surgery.[360] A structured rehabilitation program including client education on proper posture and body mechanics and core and pelvic stabilization strengthening exercises eventually progressing to sport-specific drills is suggested as a means of maximizing the benefits of surgery, but there are no empirical data to support this recommendation.[184]

### Congenital Conditions

Intestinal atresia and stenosis, although rare, are the most frequent causes of neonatal intestinal obstruction. Either condition is diagnosed on the basis of persistent vomiting (often bilious) during the first 24 to 48 hours after birth with distention of the abdomen. Many cases are first suspected prenatally during fetal ultrasound. Surgical correction is usually successful, but coexistent anomalies often are seen and complicate treatment.

**Stenosis and Atresia.** *Stenosis* is a narrowing of intestine that leads to a partial/complete obstruction. Causes include intestinal atresia, Hirschsprung disease, malrotation of gut, volvulus, or intussusception.

Most cases of intestinal atresia are characterized by complete occlusion of the lumen, with 60% occurring in the duodenum. Of these cases, 30% involve children with a chromosomal abnormality, typically Down syndrome. Only 20% occur in the jejunum or ileum, whereas colonic atresia is uncommon accounting for only 10%. Pathogenesis depends on the location of the atresia. Duodenal atresia is believed to occur early during development when recanalization fails to occur following proliferation of endodermal cells, leaving the lumen blocked. Jejunal and ileal atresia are acquired blockages thought to be a result of vascular disruption (secondary to a volvulus, intussusception, or hernia). This leads to ischemia, necrosis, and eventually reabsorption (it is a sterile environment), leaving blind proximal and distal ends. The cause of colonic atresia is probably similar to jejunal/ileal atresia. All forms require surgery.

**Meckel Diverticulum.** Meckel diverticulum is a true diverticulum, containing all layers of the intestinal wall, located about 2 feet from the ileocecal valve. It is a remnant of the vitelline duct (connecting the midgut to the yolk sac), which normally involutes early in fetal development. Meckel diverticulum is the most common congenital malformation of the GI tract, present in about 2% of the population. Males are affected more often than females in a 2:1 ratio, with accompanying complications in the same ratio.

Meckel diverticula may be asymptomatic or produce symptoms that include abdominal pain similar to that in other conditions such as appendicitis or CD. Intestinal obstruction may occur from a herniation, volvulus, or intussusception. Diverticulitis occurs secondary to chronic inflammation and can mimic appendicitis. Painless bleeding and hemorrhage are also associated with Meckel diverticulum. Children often present with dark red stools, whereas adults demonstrate melena (due to slower transit time). Meckel diverticula frequently contain ectopic gastric mucosa that produces acid. Ulceration, bleeding, and perforation can occur downstream from the diverticulum.[326]

Diagnosis is made usually during the first 2 years, but the condition may go undetected into adulthood, when it is discovered on autopsy or during surgery for an unrelated condition. The diagnosis is made usually based on history, physical examination, and Meckel scan or mesenteric arteriography. Prognosis is good with surgical resection to remove the diverticulum.

# THE APPENDIX

## Appendicitis

### Definition and Incidence

Appendicitis is an inflammation of the vermiform appendix that often results in necrosis and perforation with subsequent localized or generalized peritonitis. On the basis of operative findings and histologic appearance, acute appendicitis is classified as simple, gangrenous, or perforated.

Appendicitis is the most common disease of the appendix, occurring at any age, with the peak incidence between the ages of 15 and 19 years, with males more often affected than females. The lifetime risk of acute appendicitis in the United States is approximately 9% for males and 7% for females.[142]

### Etiologic Factors

Approximately half of all cases of acute appendicitis have no known cause. At least one-third are caused by obstruction that prevents normal drainage. Obstruction may occur as a result of tumor, foreign body such as fecal material (fecalith) lodged in the lumen of the appendix, parasites (e.g., intestinal worms), or lymphoid hyperplasia.

Because the appendix is chiefly lymphatic tissue, an infection that produces enlarged lymph nodes elsewhere in the body also can increase the glandular tissue in the appendix and obstruct its lumen. Other causes include CD of the terminal ileum, UC when it spreads to the mucosa of the appendix, and tuberculous enteritis.

### Pathogenesis

Classically, appendicitis is thought to develop primarily from obstruction of the lumen and secondarily from bacterial infection. When the long, narrow appendiceal lumen becomes obstructed, inflammation begins in the mucosa, with swelling and hyperemia of the vermiform appendix. As mucus distends the obstructed appendix, the intraluminal pressure rises and eventually exceeds the venous pressure, causing ischemia, necrosis, and perforation. Another hypothesis considers infection to be the principal source, with bacteria or virus (such as cytomegalovirus) infiltrating mucosa resulting in ulceration.

### Clinical Manifestations

The presenting symptoms of acute appendicitis occur in a classic sequence of abdominal (epigastric, periumbilical, or right lower quadrant) pain accompanied by anorexia, nausea, vomiting, and low-grade fever in adults. High fevers in adults can be indicative of perforation. Children tend to have higher fevers. Infants and children often have a nonspecific presentation.[142] Women may experience acute pelvic pain that must be differentiated from other causes of pelvic pain (e.g., ectopic pregnancy, diverticulitis, incarcerated hernia, kidney stones).

Pain associated with appendicitis is constant and may shift within 12 hours of symptom onset to the right lower quadrant with point tenderness over the site of the appendix at McBurney point, a point between 1.5 and 2 inches superomedial to the anterior superior iliac spine on a line joining the anterior superior iliac spine and the umbilicus (see Fig. 16.15). Signs and symptoms of perforation include a white blood cell count of $20,000/mm^3$ or greater; a tense or rigid abdomen; and elevated temperature (39 °C [102 °F]).

Aggravating factors include anything that increases intraabdominal pressure (see Box 16.1) such as coughing, walking, laughing, and bending over. Older adults frequently have few or no symptoms with minimal fever and only slight tenderness until perforation occurs. Confusion or increased confusion may be the first and only presenting symptom among older adults. Although appendicitis is rare in older adults, half of all people who die as a result of a ruptured appendix are 70 years old or older.[327]

**Atypical Appendicitis.** An atypical presentation occurs in 40% to 50% of cases. Many cases of appendicitis are atypical because of the position of the tip of the appendix (Fig. 16.20); the person's age; or the presence of associated conditions, especially pregnancy, immunocompromise, AIDS. The person may not recognize the need for medical attention but may report symptoms to the therapist. Early recognition of the need for medical evaluation is imperative.

*Retrocecal appendicitis* and *retroileal appendicitis* may occur when the inflamed appendix is shielded from the anterior abdominal wall by the overlying cecum and ileum. The pain seems less intense and less localized, and less discomfort occurs with walking or coughing. The pain may not shift as expected from the epigastrium to the right lower quadrant.

*Pelvic appendicitis* may begin with pain in the epigastrium, but the pain quickly settles in the lower abdomen, commonly localized to the left side for an unknown reason. The absence of abdominal tenderness may be deceptive, but the physician will elicit this symptom on pelvic examination. *Appendicitis in the immunosuppressed individual* manifests as abdominal pain and fever without leukocytosis, but concern about other causes usually delays recognition.

Manifestation of *appendicitis in an older adult* is usually vague with minimal pain and only slight temperature elevation. Abdominal tenderness is present and localized to the right lower quadrant but is deceptively mild. *Appendicitis in pregnancy* does not present a diagnostic problem in the first trimester but later in gestation may be confused with an obstetric condition. Displacement of the appendix by the enlarged uterus may result in tenderness in the right subcostal area or adjacent to the umbilicus.

## MEDICAL MANAGEMENT

DIAGNOSIS. Acute appendicitis must be diagnosed early to prevent perforation, abscess formation, and postoperative complications, but the diagnosis is not always easy to make. Although the clinical diagnosis may be straightforward in people who present with classic signs and symptoms, atypical presentations require the physician to differentiate appendicitis from a large variety of GI, genitourinary, and gynecologic conditions.

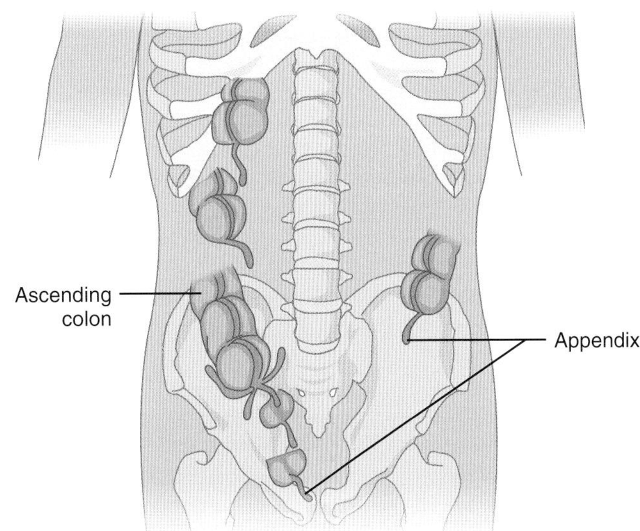


**Figure 16.20**

**Variations in the location of the vermiform appendix.** Negative test results for appendicitis using McBurney point may occur when the appendix is located somewhere other than at the end of the cecum. (From Goodman CC, Snyder TE: *Differential diagnosis for physical therapists: screening for referral*, ed 5, Philadelphia, 2013, Saunders.)

A careful history and thorough physical examination are the primary diagnostic tools. Rebound tenderness is the most accurate predictor of peritonitis associated with appendicitis[119] and is a widely used physical examination test for clients with suspected appendicitis, but the test can be very uncomfortable for the individual. Some experts prefer the pinch-an-inch test, which is a form of the rebound test in reverse and may be more comfortable to the person with peritonitis. To perform the pinch-an-inch test, a fold of abdominal skin over McBurney point is grasped and elevated away from the peritoneum. The skin is then allowed to recoil back against the peritoneum. The test is considered positive for peritonitis if there is increased pain when the skin fold strikes the peritoneum (see Fig. 16.16).[2]

An elevated white blood cell count (more than 20,000/mm$^3$; leukocytosis) suggests a ruptured appendix and peritonitis. Urinalysis reveals abnormalities in up to 40% of individuals tested.[142] Abdominal CT is more diagnostic than ultrasound and is usually done when a diagnosis cannot be made.[142] Histologic examination of the resected appendix is used to confirm the diagnosis.

**TREATMENT.** Although uncomplicated appendicitis can be treated with antibiotics alone, up to 39% of patients develop recurrent appendicitis within 2 to 5 years. Because there is no reliable method of determining who would benefit from antibiotics alone, it is recommended that all people with uncomplicated appendicitis be treated surgically.[264,289] Appendectomy, or surgical removal of the vermiform appendix, is performed as soon as possible, either by open procedure or laparoscopically; both are safe and effective in nonperforated appendicitis. Each method has pros and cons associated with it.[155] Antibiotics are administered preoperatively to decrease the incidence of postoperative wound infection and intraabdominal abscess.[142] With accurate diagnosis and early surgical removal, mortality and morbidity rates are less than 1%.

**PROGNOSIS.** Prognosis is good unless diagnosis is delayed and perforation occurs (usually more than 24 hours after initial symptoms begin). Perforation is associated with complications such as peritonitis, hypovolemia, and septic shock and carries a mortality rate of 1% to 4%, with a complication rate of 12% to 25% (such as abscess formation). Perforation is more likely in infants younger than 2 years of age and in adults older than 60 years. In up to 20% of individuals who undergo emergency appendectomy, pathologic examination of the tissue shows a normal appendix.[136]

**SPECIAL IMPLICATIONS FOR THE THERAPIST 16.16**

*Appendicitis*

When appendicitis is atypical, the client may not recognize the need for medical attention but may report the symptoms to the therapist. Early recognition of the need for medical referral is important. In an athletic training or physical therapy setting, a client with appendicitis may present with symptoms of right thigh pain, groin (testicular) pain, pelvic pain, or referred pain in the hip.

In addition to screening for the presence of constitutional symptoms, a variety of objective test procedures may be employed by the therapist. Ask the client to cough: localization of painful symptoms to the site of the appendix is typical.

Perform the iliopsoas muscle test and the obturator muscle test (see Fig. 16.12), palpate the iliopsoas muscle (see Fig. 16.13), palpate the McBurney point (see Fig. 16.15), and perform the pinch-an-inch test (see Fig. 16.16). If the result of any of these tests is positive for reproduction of symptoms in the right lower quadrant, a medical referral is necessary.

If appendicitis is suspected, medical attention must be immediate. The client should be instructed to lie down and remain as quiet as possible, taking nothing by mouth (including water); heat is contraindicated.

## PERITONEUM

### Peritonitis

#### Overview

Peritonitis, or inflammation of the serous membrane lining the walls of the abdominal cavity, is caused by a number of situations that introduce microorganisms into the peritoneal cavity. Peritonitis can occur spontaneously, meaning there is no intraabdominal known treatable source, or as a consequence of trauma, surgery, or peritoneal contamination by bowel contents (e.g., perforated duodenal ulcer or appendix), referred to as *secondary peritonitis*.

#### Etiologic Factors

Specific causes of peritonitis are many and varied. Spontaneous peritonitis is almost always associated with ascites and cirrhosis, termed *spontaneous bacterial peritonitis*. Secondary peritonitis occurs as a result of inflammation of abdominal organs; irritating substances from a perforated gallbladder, intestine, or gastric ulcer; rupture of a cyst; or irritation from blood, as in cases of internal bleeding.

Secondary peritonitis may be classified as bacterial, chemical, or metastatic. *Bacterial peritonitis* is caused by bacterial infection (*Escherichia coli, Bacteroides, Staphylococcus, Streptococcus, Pneumococcus,* gonococcus, *Mycobacterium tuberculosis*) introduced most commonly by perforation of a viscus. Such perforation can occur in the case of appendicitis, ulcer, bowel infarct, colonic diverticulum, long-term peritoneal dialysis at the site of catheter exit, and urinary infection. These bacterial organisms spread quickly throughout the abdominal cavity and may enter the bloodstream from the peritoneum, causing life-threatening septicemia.

*Chemical peritonitis* is a noninfectious inflammation caused by bile leakage, usually from a perforated gallbladder but sometimes from a needle biopsy of the liver or any breach in the GI tract wall that allows GI tract contents to spill into the abdominal cavity. Once bacteria enter the abdominal cavity, chemical peritonitis progresses quickly and develops into bacterial peritonitis.

Other causes include substances such as gastric acid, blood, or foreign material introduced by surgery (e.g., talc) and acute pancreatitis, which releases and activates lipolytic and proteolytic enzymes.

### Pathogenesis

The GI tract normally contains bacteria, but the peritoneum is sterile. Inflammation and perforation of the GI tract from appendicitis, diverticulitis, perforated gallbladder, or a peptic ulcer allow bacteria to invade the peritoneum.

Once the inflammatory process has begun, a fibrinopurulent exudate covers the peritoneal surface. The exudate becomes organized and fibrotic, forming adhesions and causing obstruction. Usually infection in the peritoneal cavity is localized as an abscess.

When a perforation drains contaminants into the peritoneal cavity, however, the ability of the peritoneum to combat the inflammatory process can be overpowered. The entire surface of the peritoneum may be involved (generalized peritonitis) or only specific sites (localized).

Peritonitis creates severe systemic effects. Circulatory alterations, fluid shifts, and respiratory problems can cause critical fluid and electrolyte imbalances. The circulatory system undergoes great stress from several sources. The inflammatory response shunts extra blood to the inflamed area of the bowel to combat the infection. Peristaltic activity of the bowel ceases, leading to a functional bowel obstruction. Fluids and air are retained within its lumen, raising pressure and increasing fluid secretion into the bowel; circulating volume diminishes.

### Clinical Manifestations

Peritonitis commonly decreases intestinal motility and causes intestinal distention with gas. At first the affected individual may feel vague, generalized abdominal pain. As peritonitis progresses, the client presents with an acute abdomen and severe abdominal pain. The abdomen becomes rigid (involuntary guarding) and sensitive to touch, with rebound tenderness. Pain is severe, increasing with movement and respirations, and can be referred to the shoulder or thoracic area. Nausea, vomiting, and high fever follow.

Without treatment, peritonitis can lead to paralytic ileus (diminished to absent peristalsis or functional obstruction), sepsis, or multiple organ dysfunction syndrome. A peritoneal abscess develops if the perforation becomes self-encased or walled off. Antibiotic therapy may mask or delay the recognition of an abscess.

In persons with underlying ascites, the signs and symptoms of peritonitis may be more subtle, with fever as the only manifestation of infection or possibly nausea, vomiting, nonspecific abdominal pain, or altered mental status.

### MEDICAL MANAGEMENT

**DIAGNOSIS, TREATMENT, AND PROGNOSIS.** Abdominal films, CT, and an abdominal tap may be used in the differential diagnosis of peritonitis. Peritonitis should be treated immediately with intravenous fluids, antibiotics to control infection, vasopressors if needed to maintain blood pressure, and correction of electrolytes. Surgery is often necessary in cases of secondary peritonitis to repair perforations or other sources of infection.

Despite treatment with antibiotics, surgical drainage and débridement, and supportive measures, generalized peritonitis is still associated with a high mortality rate and is especially dangerous in older adults.

SPECIAL IMPLICATIONS FOR THE THERAPIST 16.17

*Peritonitis*

Special considerations associated with peritonitis are related to the underlying cause (e.g., liver or kidney disease, postoperative state, cancer) and resultant complications (e.g., fluid and electrolyte imbalance, pulmonary compromise). A client with peritonitis usually is hospitalized and undergoing medical treatment. The therapist should be familiar with implications associated with the underlying cause and any complications present.

Vital signs should be regularly monitored, and a semi-Fowler position should be used to help the client breathe deeply with less pain to prevent pulmonary complications. Position changes must be accomplished with extreme caution, because the slightest movement intensifies the pain. Watch for signs of dehiscence (separation of layers of a surgical wound), such as the client reporting that something broke loose or gave way inside. Follow all safety measures such as keeping the side rails up on the bed if fever and pain disorient the client.

# THE RECTUM

## Rectal Fissure

A rectal or anal fissure is an ulceration or tear of the lining of the anal canal. An acute fissure occurs as a result of multiple factors including mechanical trauma (e.g., the passage of a large, hard bowel movement), sphincter spasm, and ischemia. The skin tear is very fragile and tends to reopen easily with the next bowel movement, prompting the person to avoid going to the bathroom for days.

Sharp pain, followed by burning, accompanies defecation. Bleeding may be noted by blood on toilet paper. Other symptoms include spasms, mucus, and itching. Anal fissures frequently heal within 1 or 2 months when treated with a combination of bran and bulk laxatives or stool softeners, sitz baths, topical anesthetics, and emollient suppositories.[188] Injection of botulinum toxin or use of 0.2% nitroglycerin or topical calcium channel blockers may help relieve spasm and ultimately aid in healing. Botulinum toxin use resulted in higher rates of recurrence than surgery.[37] Recurrence is also common if underlying factors are not addressed. Chronic fissures or acute fissures with significant pain may require surgery if other therapies have failed. Lateral internal sphincterotomy is the most studied surgical technique and the treatment of choice.[133]

## Hemorrhoids

Hemorrhoids are arteriovenous communications covered by a cushioning of connective tissue that lie just beneath the mucous membranes lining the lowest part of the rectum and anus. They can be internal, located above the dentate line, or external, located beneath the dentate line. Hemorrhoids are fairly common, affecting about 1 million people.[33]

Symptomatic hemorrhoids occur when these vessels pathologically dilate. This may result from vascular congestion or mucosal prolapse. Vascular congestion can occur from prolonged straining or increased intraabdominal pressure (ascites, obesity, or pregnancy) (see Box 16.1).

Common symptoms include burning, itching, and bleeding. In approximately 20% of cases, anal fissures are concomitantly seen with hemorrhoids. Bleeding from internal hemorrhoids is typically painless, with red blood surrounding normal stool. Other types of bleeding need immediate evaluation. Pain is not usually associated with hemorrhoids unless thrombosis has occurred, particularly in external hemorrhoids. External hemorrhoids are formed in nerve-rich tissue outside the anal canal. Internal hemorrhoids may prolapse with straining and are classified according to the degree of prolapse.

Diagnosis is made by examination. Digital, anoscopic, and sigmoidoscopic examinations may be required. Painful, thrombosed hemorrhoids should be removed. Most other hemorrhoids should be medically managed. Conservative treatment consists of local application of topical medications, sitz baths, high-fiber diet, and avoidance of constipation and other causes of increased intraabdominal pressure. A stool softener or psyllium preparation may be used when a modified diet is unsuccessful in eliminating constipation. Local topical preparations for hemorrhoids are used to reduce pain or itching. In addition, moderate aerobic exercise such as brisk walking 20 to 30 minutes daily can help stimulate bowel function.

Hemorrhoids that fail medical treatment may require rubber band ligation, sclerosing, laser surgery, or cryosurgery to destroy the affected tissue. In the case of advanced chronic hemorrhoids, recurrent bleeding and anemia may necessitate surgery (hemorrhoidectomy, stapled hemorrhoidectomy, hemorrhoidal artery ligation, or conventional hemorrhoidectomy with an advanced electrosurgical device such as the LigaSure or Harmonic scalpel.

### SPECIAL IMPLICATIONS FOR THE THERAPIST 16.18

#### *The Rectum*

Therapists may work with individuals who have an overactive external anal sphincter and pain. These individuals experience severe muscle spasm of the sphincter, resulting in groin or pelvic pain and trigger points in the pelvic floor and gluteal muscles. Any anorectal symptoms (e.g., change in bowel habits, rectal pain, bleeding) that have not been reported to the physician or are changing in pattern must be evaluated by a physician.

Clients involved in any activity requiring increased abdominal support or causing increased intraabdominal pressure should be questioned about the presence of hemorrhoids. For clients with hemorrhoids postoperatively, prone positioning or side-lying positioning supported with pillows between the knees and ankles is preferred. Supine positioning and sitting for brief periods can be accomplished with a rubber air ring under the buttocks for support. Movement, exercise, drinking plenty of fluids, and heeding the call of nature are important in the prevention of constipation-induced hemorrhoids.

In some cases the healed fissure, fistula, or surgical scar can become painful and contribute to further overactive paradoxical pelvic floor muscle contractions. Both painful scars and overactive anal sphincter tightening can be treated by specialized physical therapy.

## REFERENCES

To enhance this text and add value for the reader, all references are included in the enhanced ebook on Student Consult that accompanies this textbook. The reader can view the reference source and access it online whenever possible.

CHAPTER 17

# The Hepatic, Pancreatic, and Biliary Systems

CELESTE KNIGHT PETERSON

The *liver* has more than 500 separate digestive, endocrine, excretory, and hematologic functions. It is the sole source of albumin and other plasma proteins and also produces about 600 mL of bile each day. Conversion and excretion of bilirubin (red bile pigment, which is an end product of heme from hemoglobin in red blood cells) take place in the liver. Other important functions of the liver include production of clotting factors and storage of vitamins. The liver and gut are the key organs in nutrient absorption and metabolism.

The liver has the largest numbers of phagocytic cells and contributes to a functional immune system by reducing the amount of bacteria, viruses, and toxins that enter the body.[140] Bile acids, drugs, chemicals, and toxins undergo extensive enterohepatic circulation during the processes of metabolism. The liver also filters all of the blood from the gastrointestinal (GI) system and is therefore the primary organ for metastasis of intestinal cancer.

The *pancreas* is both an exocrine and an endocrine gland. Its primary function in digestion is exocrine secretion of digestive enzymes and pancreatic juices, transported through the pancreatic duct to the duodenum. Proteins, carbohydrates, and fats are broken down in the duodenum, aided by pancreatic and other secretions, which also help to neutralize the acidic substances passed from the stomach to the duodenum. The endocrine function involves the secretion of glucagon and insulin by islet of Langerhans cells for the regulation of carbohydrate metabolism. Pancreatic disease may result in a variety of clinical presentations, depending on whether the exocrine or endocrine function has been impaired.

The *gallbladder*, acting as a reservoir for bile, stores and concentrates the bile during fasting periods and then contracts to expel the bile into the duodenum in response to the arrival of food. Bile helps in alkalinizing the intestinal contents and plays a role in the emulsification, absorption, and digestion of fat. The signal for the gallbladder to contract comes from the release of cholecystokinin (pancreozymin), a hormone released into the bloodstream from the wall of the duodenum and upper small intestine.

## SIGNS AND SYMPTOMS OF HEPATIC DISEASE

Primary signs and symptoms of liver diseases vary and can include GI symptoms, edema/ascites, dark urine, light-colored or clay-colored feces, and right upper abdominal pain (Box 17.1). Impairment of the liver can result in *hepatic failure* (acute and chronic) when either the mass of liver cells is sufficiently diminished or their function is impaired as a result of cirrhosis, liver cancer, or infection and/or inflammation. Hepatic failure does not refer to one specific morphologic change but rather to a clinical syndrome that includes hepatic encephalopathy (HE), renal failure (hepatorenal syndrome [HRS]), endocrine changes, and jaundice.

*Dark urine* and *light stools* occur in association with jaundice (yellow pigmentation of skin, sclerae, and mucous membranes) (see Jaundice [Icterus] later) when the serum bilirubin level increases from normal (0.1 to 1.0 mg/dL) to a value of 2 or 3 mg/dL. Any damage to the liver impairs bilirubin metabolism from the blood. Normally, bile converted from bilirubin causes brown coloration of the stool. Light-colored (almost white) stools and urine the color of tea or cola indicate an inability of the liver or biliary system to excrete bilirubin properly.

*Skin changes* associated with the hepatic system include jaundice, pallor, and orange or green skin. When bilirubin reaches levels of 2 to 3 mg/dL, the sclera of the eye takes on a yellow hue. When bilirubin level reaches above 3 mg/dL, the skin becomes yellow. The changes described here in urine, stool, or skin color may be caused by hepatitis, gallbladder disease, pancreatic cancer blocking the bile duct, hepatotoxic medications, or cirrhosis. Other skin changes may include bruising, spider angiomas, and palmar erythema.

*Spider angiomas* (arterial spider, spider telangiectasis, or vascular spider) are branched dilations of superficial capillaries, which may be vascular manifestations of increased estrogen levels (hyperestrogenism). Spider angiomas and palmar erythema both occur in the presence of liver impairment as a result of increased estrogen

**Box 17.1**

**MOST COMMON SIGNS AND SYMPTOMS OF HEPATIC DISEASE**

- Gastrointestinal symptoms
- Edema/ascites (see Fig. 17.5)
- Dark urine
- Light- or clay-colored stools
- Right upper quadrant abdominal pain
- Skin changes
  - Jaundice
  - Bruising
  - Spider angioma
  - Palmar erythema
- Neurologic involvement
  - Confusion
  - Sleep disturbances
  - Muscle tremors
  - Hyperreactive reflexes
  - Asterixis (see Fig. 17.1)
- Musculoskeletal pain (see text for sites)
- Hepatic osteodystrophy

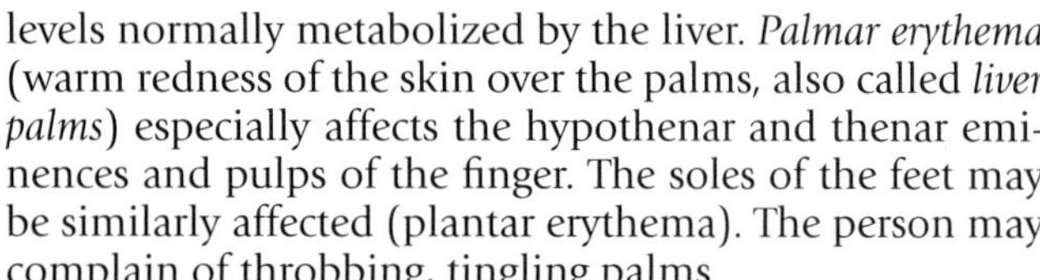

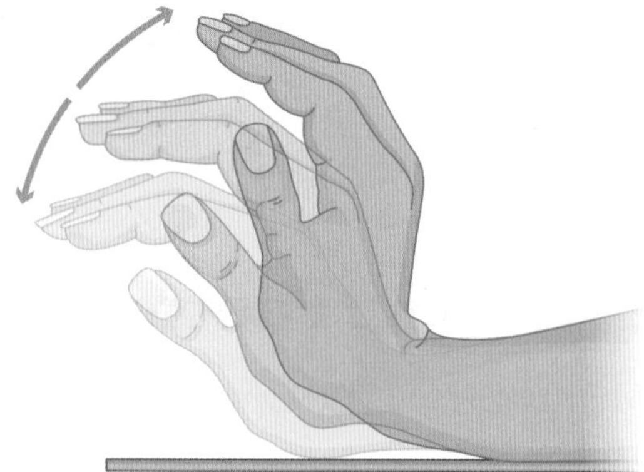

**Figure 17.1**

**Flapping tremor.** The flapping tremor elicited by attempted wrist extension while the forearm is fixed is the most common neurologic abnormality associated with liver failure. It can also be observed in uremia, respiratory failure, and severe heart failure. The tremor is absent at rest, decreased by intentional movement, and maximal on sustained posture. It is usually bilateral, although one side may be affected more than the other. (From Sherlock S, Dooley J: *Diseases of the liver and biliary system*, ed 9, Oxford, 1993, Blackwell Scientific Publications.)

levels normally metabolized by the liver. *Palmar erythema* (warm redness of the skin over the palms, also called *liver palms*) especially affects the hypothenar and thenar eminences and pulps of the finger. The soles of the feet may be similarly affected (plantar erythema). The person may complain of throbbing, tingling palms.

*Neurologic symptoms* such as confusion, sleep disturbances, muscle tremors, hyperreactive reflexes, and asterixis (see following discussion) may occur. When liver dysfunction results in increased serum ammonia and urea levels, the accumulation of neurotoxins can result in impaired peripheral nerve function. *HE* (or portosystemic encephalopathy) refers to reversible neuropsychological symptoms caused by liver failure secondary to a metabolic disturbance or buildup of metabolic toxins. Ammonia is one of the principal neurotoxins contributing to HE, although there are several factors (see Hepatic Encephalopathy later).

*Asterixis* and numbness or tingling (misinterpreted as carpal tunnel syndrome) can occur as a result of this ammonia abnormality, causing intrinsic nerve pathology. Asterixis, also called *flapping tremors* or *liver flap*, is a motor disturbance; specifically, it is the inability to maintain wrist extension with forward flexion of the upper extremities. A test for asterixis is asking the client to extend the wrist and hand with the rest of the arm supported on a firm surface or with the arms held out in front of the body. Observe for quick, irregular extensions and flexions of the wrist and fingers (Fig. 17.1). Altered neurotransmission, in the form of impaired inflow of joint and other afferent information to the brainstem reticular formation, causes the movement dysfunction.

*Musculoskeletal locations of pain* associated with the hepatic and biliary systems include thoracic pain between scapulae, right shoulder, right upper trapezius, right interscapular, or right subscapular areas. Sympathetic fibers from the biliary system are connected through the celiac and splanchnic (visceral) plexus to the hepatic fibers in the region of the dorsal spine. These connections account for the intercostal and radiating interscapular pain that accompanies gallbladder disease. Although the innervation is bilateral, most of the biliary fibers reach the cord through the right splanchnic nerves, producing pain in the right shoulder.

*Hepatic osteodystrophy,* metabolic bone disease, can occur in all forms of cholestasis (bile flow suppression) and hepatocellular disease, especially in people with primary biliary cirrhosis, primary sclerosing cholangitis (PSC), and alcoholic liver disease (ALD).[25,91] Hepatic osteodystrophy may manifest as osteomalacia or, more frequently and commonly, osteoporosis. Causes of hepatic osteoporosis are multifactorial but similar to osteoporosis seen in elderly people. Stimulation of osteoclastic differentiation and proliferation is the principal effect, while inhibition of osteoclastic activity is limited. Osteoblastic inhibition also occurs, compounding the bone disease. Contributing factors include age (greater than 65 years), alcohol, corticosteroid therapy, estrogen deficiency in postmenopausal women, vitamin D deficiency, malnutrition, and sedentary lifestyles.

Severe osteoporosis may lead to vertebral wedging, vertebral crush fractures, and kyphosis. Fractures may occur with little or no trauma. Treatment is similar for that of osteoporosis due to other etiologies. However, care must be taken when administering bisphosphonates in the presence of cirrhosis, as they may cause esophageal erosions.[284]

Osteoporosis associated with primary biliary cirrhosis and PSC parallels the severity of liver disease rather than the duration. Painful osteoarthropathy may develop in the wrists and ankles as a nonspecific complication of chronic liver disease.

*Portal hypertension, ascites,* and *HE* are three other major complications of liver disease that are discussed in greater depth in this chapter as distinct clinical conditions.

SPECIAL IMPLICATIONS FOR THE THERAPIST 17.1

### *Signs and Symptoms of Hepatic Disease*

Any client presenting with undiagnosed or untreated jaundice must be referred to the physician for follow-up. Active, intense exercise should be avoided when the liver is compromised (i.e., during jaundice or any other active liver disease) because the cornerstone of medical treatment and promotion of healing of the liver is rest. (See also Special Implications for the Therapist 17.2: Jaundice (Icterus), Special Implications for the Therapist 17.4: Portal Hypertension, Special Implications for the Therapist 17.5: Hepatic Encephalopathy, and Special Implications for the Therapist 17.6: Ascites.)

The physical therapist can be instrumental in helping the affected individual to organize self-care, pace activities, and practice relaxation techniques such as Physiological Quieting or other forms of biofeedback. At the same time, steps must be taken to prevent the potential complications of reduced activity or immobility. Identify individuals at risk for pressure ulcers and implement prevention strategies such as skin care, optimal nutrition, and hydration. Teach the client and family pressure-reducing or -relieving positions and turning strategies. Referral to a nutrition specialist may be needed.

An increased risk of coagulopathy (decreased clotting ability) also occurs with liver disease, necessitating precautions. Easy bruising and bleeding under the skin or into the joints in response to the slightest trauma can occur when coagulation is impaired. This condition necessitates extreme care in the therapy setting, especially with any intervention requiring manual therapy or the use of any equipment including modalities, resistive exercise or weight-training devices, and potentially the use of gait belts.

The most common neurologic abnormality associated with liver failure (liver flap or asterixis) (see Fig. 17.1) also can be observed in uremia, respiratory failure, and severe heart failure. The rapid flexion and extension movements at the metacarpophalangeal and wrist joints often are accompanied by lateral movements of the digits. Sometimes movement of arms, neck, and jaws; protruding tongue; retracted mouth; and tightly closed eyelids are present. The gait is ataxic. The tremor is absent at rest, decreased by intentional movement, and maximal on sustained posture. It is usually bilateral, although not bilaterally synchronous, and one side may be affected more than the other. It may be observed by gentle elevation of a limb or by the client gripping the therapist's hand. In coma, the tremor disappears.

## AGING AND THE HEPATIC SYSTEM

The liver has the incredible ability to regenerate; however, as a person ages, there are structural and functional changes that make the liver less able to withstand stress and disease. For example, with time, the volume of the liver decreases by 20% to 40%,[224,264] which is mostly a product of a decrease in the mass of each liver cell. This is accompanied by a decrease in blood flow by up to 35%.[286] These reductions lead to more time required to process substances, medications, and alcohol. Components of the liver also change such as an increase in cholesterol associated with a corresponding increase in blood levels of cholesterol and low-density lipoprotein (LDL) cholesterol. Adding to elevated blood levels of LDLs, the processing of LDL by the liver is reduced by 35%.[136]

Although more is known about liver cells and aging, less is known about the aging of Kupffer cells, hepatic sinusoidal endothelial liver cells, and other more specialized cells. Several cellular changes, however, are known to contribute to the aging of liver cells. Lipofuscin, which is composed of undegradable proteins from oxidative stress, becomes increasingly deposited, leading to the formation of reactive oxygen species and reducing the cell's viability.[115] As cells age, there is a tendency toward polyploidy with a reduction in the number and function of mitochondria and available adenosine triphosphate (ATP). Finally, there is a reduction in the amount of smooth endoplasmic reticulum with a corresponding reduction in the production of microsomal proteins.

These cellular changes contribute to the liver's difficulty in responding to stress, inflammation, and injury. The aging liver becomes less tolerant to damage and less able to repair and regenerate.[254]

### Drug Distribution and Metabolism

In the past, adjusting dosage downward based on hepatic function related to aging was not considered necessary. However, emerging data on the use of pharmacologic agents in the older population suggest that the administration of many agents may be affected by physiologic changes of the liver occurring with age.[172] As noted earlier, a reduction in blood flow and liver mass accompanies aging, decreasing the amount of drug metabolized with the first pass through the liver.[172]

Modification of drug dosage may be required with age owing to a decrease in albumin produced by the liver and to accommodate for changes in body composition. Drugs that are typically bound to albumin and rendered pharmacologically unavailable become more readily available in elderly persons with low serum albumin levels, whereas medications that are lipophilic have an increased area of distribution in older people secondary to an increase in the proportion of fat mass and decrease of lean mass. In older adults, there is variability in response to drugs depending on liver function, affecting the central nervous system (CNS) (increased sensibility to any neurologic effect of drugs), the cardiovascular system, and the renal management of water and electrolytes.

### Immune Function and Metabolism

The liver is an important immune system organ because it contains a large number of immunologically active cells (e.g., T and B lymphocytes, Kupffer cells, liver-adapted natural killer cells [pit cells], natural killer cells expressing T-cell receptor, stellate cells, sinusoidal endothelial cells, dendritic cells). The liver is the major site of production of proteins that are associated with acute inflammatory reactions. Kupffer cells have an important role in the phagocytosis that presents a barrier to invasion of pathogenic organisms from the intestine.[201] The hepatic natural killer cells and natural killer cells expressing T-cell receptor are important in resistance to tumor cell invasion.

Age-related changes in sinusoids result in substantial alterations in many immunologic functions.[201] Sinusoidal endothelial cells of the liver aid in disposal of waste molecules generated through inflammatory, immunologic, or general homeostatic processes. With time these cells become thicker, and the fenestrations (pores) become smaller.[136] Loss of these fenestrations allows a buildup of lipoprotein-like chylomicrons within the liver that negatively impacts immune system function.

The pancreas undergoes structural changes such as fibrosis, fatty acid deposits, and atrophy, but the pancreas has a large reserve capacity, and 90% of its function would have to be lost before any observable dysfunction occurs. Much remains unknown about the gallbladder in the aging process, but aging apparently has little effect on overall gallbladder function.

### Laboratory Tests

Liver function test results, such as levels of aspartate transaminase (AST), alanine transaminase (ALT), γ-glutamyl transpeptidase, alkaline phosphatase (ALP), and total serum bilirubin, remain unchanged and within normal limits established for adults. However, these tests often measure hepatic damage rather than overall function; abnormal values for these tests in older adults reflect disease rather than the effects of aging.

Box 17.2

**CLASSIFICATION OF JAUNDICE**

***Diseases Associated With Overproduction of Bilirubin***

- Hemolysis
  - Thalassemia, sickle cell anemia
  - Autoimmune hemolytic anemia
- Reabsorption of hematoma
- Blood transfusion

***Decreased Uptake or Conjugation in Bilirubin Metabolism***

- Gilbert syndrome
- Jaundice of newborns
- Medications

***Hepatocyte Dysfunction***

- Hepatitis
  - Viral
  - Alcohol-related
  - Autoimmune
  - Toxic/medication-induced
  - Ischemia
- Chronic Hepatic Disease
  - Wilson disease
  - Hemochromatosis

***Impaired Bile Flow***

- Cholelithiasis
- Primary sclerosing cholangitis
- Pancreatic cancer
- Pancreatitis

# LIVER

## Liver Disease Complications

As a result of the extraordinary number of vital functions the liver performs, severe complications result when the liver has been damaged or is no longer functioning. Jaundice is a symptom that occurs with many types of diseases and disorders (both acute and chronic). End-stage complications occur most often because of cirrhosis and include portal hypertension, HE, ascites, and HRS. Any illness, toxin, or infection that leads to end-stage liver disease can display these complications.

### Jaundice (Icterus)

Jaundice (icterus) is not a disease but is a common symptom of many different diseases and disorders (Box 17.2). It is clinically characterized by yellow discoloration of the skin, sclerae, and mucous membranes. Jaundice occurs as a result of an overproduction of bilirubin, defects in bilirubin metabolism (in uptake by the liver or conjugation), the presence of liver disease, or obstruction of bile flow.

In the normal breakdown of hemoglobin, the end product is bilirubin. In this metabolic process, the heme portion of hemoglobin is converted into biliverdin and then to bilirubin in the bone marrow and the spleen. Bilirubin is released into the bloodstream, where it binds to albumin, and is then taken up by hepatocytes to be conjugated with glucuronic acid. Once it is conjugated, it becomes water-soluble and is then released into the bile. A small percentage of conjugated bile returns to the plasma and is excreted by the kidneys. In the terminal ileum and colon, conjugated bilirubin is deconjugated and excreted as colorless urobilinogen. Diseases that result in ineffective erythropoiesis (abnormal formation of erythrocytes) produce large amounts of bilirubin as a result of chronic hemolysis or destruction of cells.

In some diseases, such as Gilbert syndrome, there are defects in the liver's ability to conjugate bilirubin. Drugs, such as rifampin, may compete with bilirubin for uptake by the liver, decreasing the quantity of bilirubin the liver can process. Diseases, toxins, infections, and ischemia can cause generalized liver disease (acute and chronic), which reduces the capability of the liver to function normally and process bilirubin. Finally, bile ducts can be obstructed by diseases, tumors, and stones, leading to an elevation in bilirubin that has been conjugated.

As mentioned, jaundice is not clinically evident (particularly in the sclera of the eyes) until the plasma level reaches 2 mg/dL. Once the level is above 3 mg/dL, the skin becomes a yellow color. Urine turns a darker color, and stool is light in color. Signs and symptoms of liver disease may also be present.

Laboratory testing can aid in the specific diagnosis of jaundice. Bilirubin can be reported as conjugated or unconjugated, which provides a more accurate measurement than direct or indirect. Direct refers to the capability of the laboratory to directly measure conjugated bilirubin, whereas indirect bilirubin refers to the unconjugated portion of bilirubin, which cannot be directly measured in the laboratory and must be subtracted from the total bilirubin present in the blood.

Conjugated and direct are not always equivalent, particularly in disorders of bilirubin metabolism. In clients with jaundice, an elevation in the conjugated bilirubin is more common than unconjugated. Elevations in liver transaminases (AST and ALT) suggest that liver disease is involved. Many other tests are available for the specific diagnosis of jaundice, depending on the suspected process, and are included in the specific disease sections in this chapter.

SPECIAL IMPLICATIONS FOR THE THERAPIST 17.2

*Jaundice (Icterus)*

With successful treatment of the underlying cause, jaundice usually begins to resolve within 4 to 6 weeks. After this time, activity and exercise can be resumed or increased per individual tolerance, depending on the overall medical condition and the presence of any complications. The return of normal stool and urine colors is an indication of resolution. (See also Special Implications for the Therapist 17.1: Signs and Symptoms of Hepatic Disease.)

## Cirrhosis

Cirrhosis is the final common pathway of chronic, progressive inflammation of the liver. It is characterized pathologically by a progressive loss of normal tissue that is replaced with fibrosis and nodular regeneration. Many diseases, medications, and toxins can damage the liver and ultimately lead to cirrhosis, but the most common in the United States include alcohol abuse, hepatitis C virus (HCV), and nonalcoholic liver disease.

Overall, in the United States, cirrhosis is the 12th leading cause of death, accounting for about 28,000 deaths a year.[113] Cirrhosis of the liver occurs when inflammation (from disease or toxin) causes liver tissue damage and/or necrosis. With continued cycles of inflammation and healing, fibrous bands of connective tissue replace normal liver cells. These fibrous bands eventually constrict and partition the liver into irregular nodules. Once 80% to 90% of the liver is replaced with scar tissue, there is also significant loss of function, associated with decompensation of homeostasis.

The signs and symptoms of cirrhosis (Figs. 17.2 and 17.3) are multiple and varied, representing interference with major functions of the liver. Some of these functions include processing dietary amino acids, carbohydrates, lipids, and vitamins; metabolizing cholesterol, hormones, vitamins, medications, and toxins; producing clotting factors and other plasma proteins; and storing glycogen.

Clients with cirrhosis exhibit fatigue, weight loss, pruritus, jaundice, coagulopathies with easy bruising or bleeding, loss of ability to metabolize drugs, and hypoalbuminemia (the remaining serious complications are discussed later). Individuals with cirrhosis can be classified as having compensated or uncompensated cirrhosis. Individuals who have vague, general symptoms or who remain asymptomatic have uncomplicated or compensated cirrhosis, whereas people with symptoms related to complications of cirrhosis (e.g., HE, spontaneous bacterial peritonitis [SBP]) are referred to as having uncompensated cirrhosis. History, physical examination, laboratory tests, and imaging tests aid in diagnosing the specific cause. Once cirrhosis has developed, it is usually not reversible, although each disease may have a specific therapy to reduce the risk of developing cirrhosis.

Typically, complications are treated on an individual basis, and transplantation provides the best therapy for long-term survival. Despite improvements in medical care for individuals with cirrhosis, mortality from infection, renal failure, HE, and hepatocellular carcinoma (HCC) remains high.[86] Life expectancy of individuals with decompensated cirrhosis who are hospitalized for an end-stage liver disease complication may be 6 months or less.[220]

SPECIAL IMPLICATIONS FOR THE THERAPIST 17.3

*Cirrhosis*

One of the most common symptoms associated with cirrhosis is ascites, an accumulation of fluid in the peritoneal cavity surrounding the intestines. The distention often occurs very slowly over a number of weeks or months and may be associated with bilateral edema of the feet and ankles. The client may be unable to put on a pair of shoes, preferring to leave the shoes unlaced or to wear slippers. In a home health or inpatient hospital setting, this change in dress may not be as noticeable as it would be in a private practice or outpatient clinic. It is always important to remain alert to these potential signs of fluid retention and to ask about any changes in health status or weight gain.

Detection of blood loss in the form of hematemesis, tarry stools, bleeding gums, frequent and heavy nosebleeds, or excessive bruising must be reported to the physician. Preventing increased intraabdominal pressure and preventing injury owing to falls require client education regarding safety precautions.

Alcohol causes whole-body and tissue-specific changes in protein metabolism. Chronic alcohol use increases nitrogen excretion and reduces skeletal muscle protein synthesis with concomitant loss of lean tissue mass. Loss of skeletal collagen contributes to alcohol-related osteoporosis. The loss of skeletal muscle protein (i.e., chronic alcoholic myopathy) occurs in up to two-thirds of all individuals with chronic alcohol use. Protein turnover changes in organs such as the heart have important implications for cardiovascular function and morbidity. Most clients with cirrhosis have significantly reduced aerobic capacity, although the exact mechanism for this has not been proved.[76,208]

Rest to reduce metabolic demands on the liver and to increase circulation often is recommended for clients with cirrhosis. Frequent rests during therapy and avoiding unnecessary fatigue are also important. Exercise limitation in cirrhosis is typically attributed to cirrhotic myopathy without impaired oxygen utilization. Chronic alcoholic myopathy affecting the proximal muscles is usually mild and results in muscle atrophy and measurable decrease in muscle strength. The therapist must remain alert to any potential medical complications in any client, regardless of the physical therapy diagnosis.

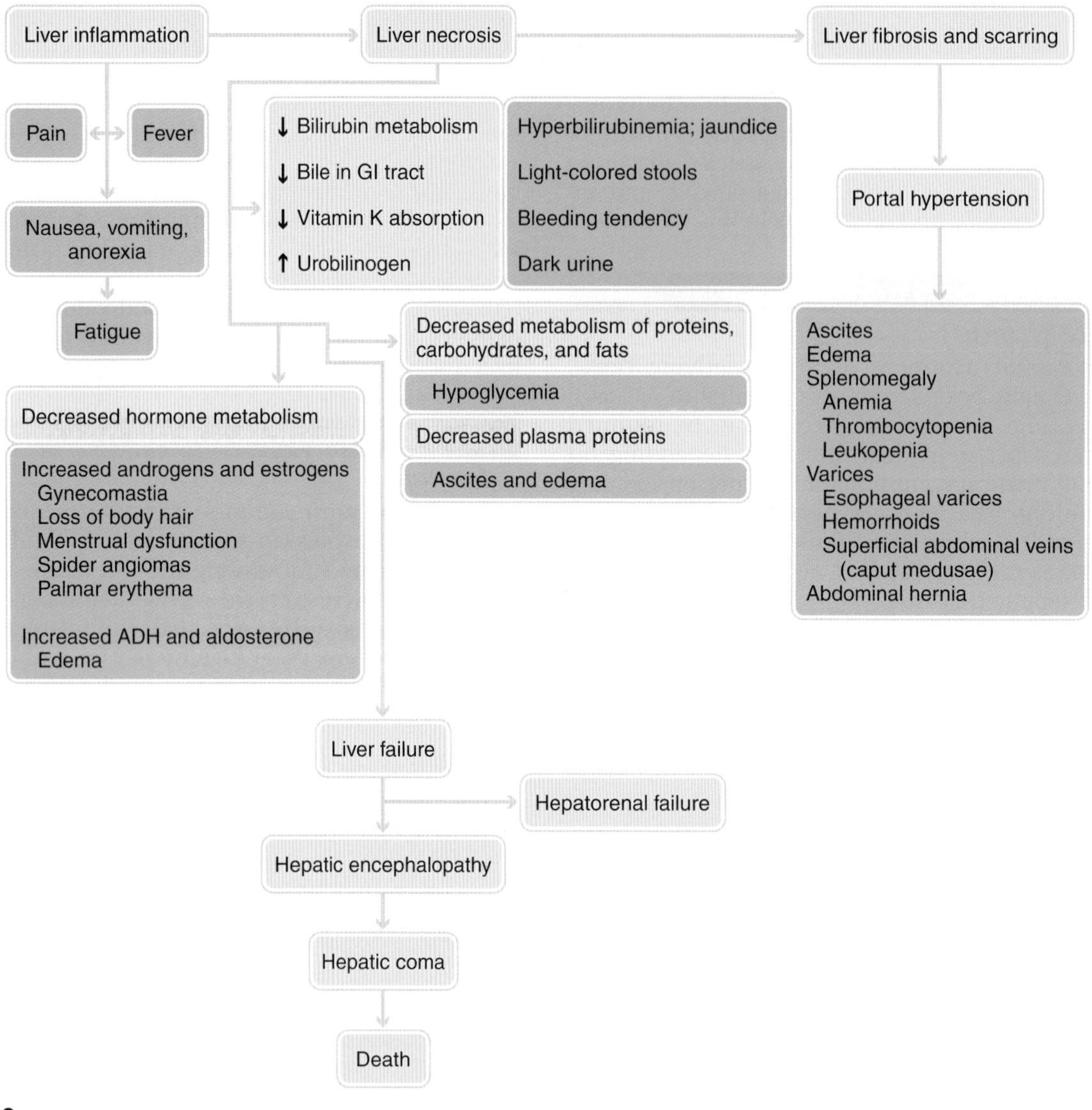


**Figure 17.2**

**Pathologic basis *(yellow boxes)* and resultant clinical manifestations *(green boxes)* associated with cirrhosis of the liver.** *ADH,* Antidiuretic hormone; *GI,* gastrointestinal.

## Portal Hypertension

Portal hypertension is defined as an increase in the portal pressure gradient greater than 6 mm Hg, although clinical complications are not normally seen until the pressure reaches 10 mm Hg or greater. Portal refers to the area where blood vessels enter into the liver. Venous blood returning from the stomach, large and small intestine, pancreas, and spleen is transported via the portal vein to the liver (the splanchnic circulation). An elevated portal pressure gradient occurs when the pressure of the blood entering the liver (portal vein) is higher than the pressure of the blood in the inferior vena cava. Most cases of portal hypertension are related to cirrhosis. Other causes include thrombus, tumor, or infection, or portal hypertension may be idiopathic. With the development of cirrhosis, two principal changes lead to portal hypertension: structural changes and hyperdynamic vascular responses. These alterations prevent the flow of blood, resulting in increased pressure and resistance in the portal circulatory system (Fig. 17.4).

Fibrosis, nodularity, and abnormal liver architecture combine to form mechanical barriers to blood flow and increase resistance. Intrahepatic blood flow is altered to favor vasoconstriction secondary to a reduction in nitric oxide release (which normally causes vasodilation) from liver endothelial cells and production of endothelins and other vasoconstrictors.

As a result of this increased portal pressure, blood that normally flows to the portal vein backs up in the stomach, esophagus, umbilicus, and rectum. This system is normally small with modest blood flow. However, in the cirrhotic state, blood volume increases in these vessels, causing dilation and expansion. These engorged vessels give rise to rectal varices, prominent vessels around the umbilicus (caput medusae), and gastroesophageal

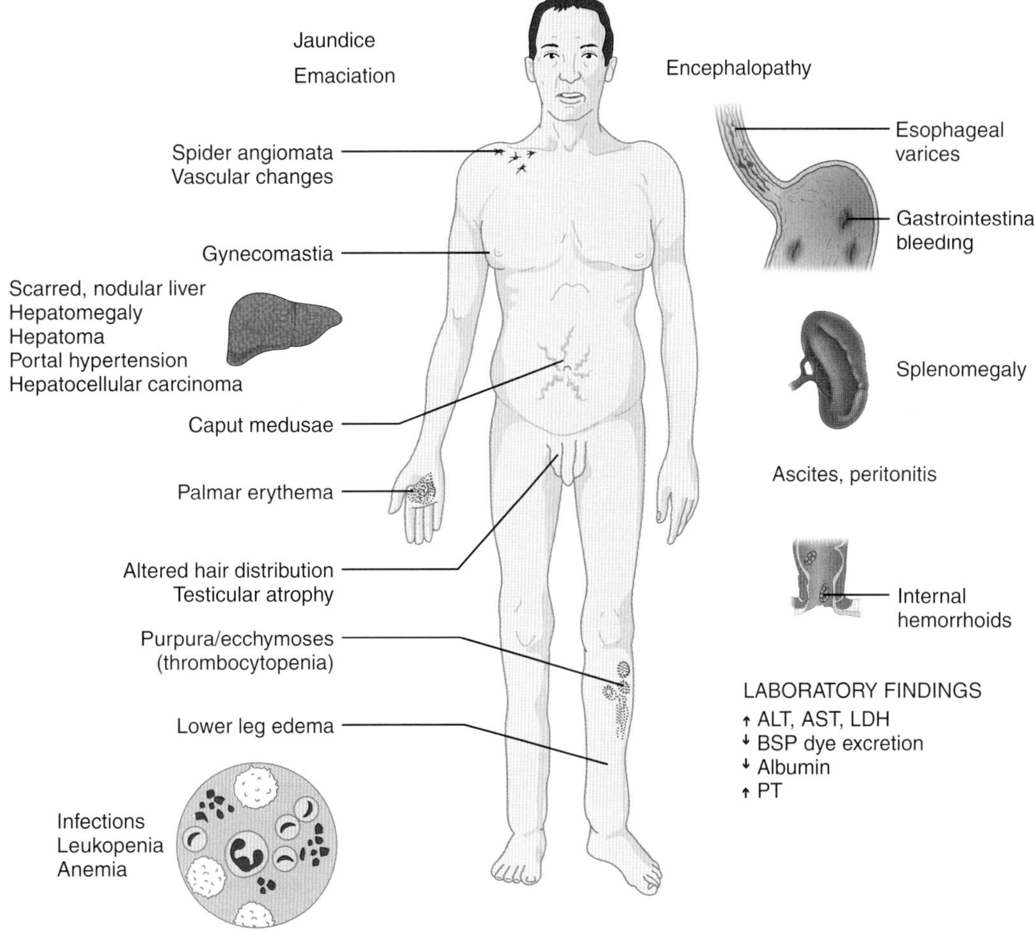


**Figure 17.3**

**Liver cirrhosis.** Clinical presentation and laboratory findings associated with liver cirrhosis. *ALT,* Alanine aminotransferase; *AST,* aspartate aminotransferase; *BSP,* sulfobromophthalein; *LDH,* lactate dehydrogenase; *PT,* prothrombin time. (From Black JM, Matassarin-Jacobs E, editors: *Medical-surgical nursing: clinical management for continuity of care,* ed 5, Philadelphia, 1997, Saunders.)

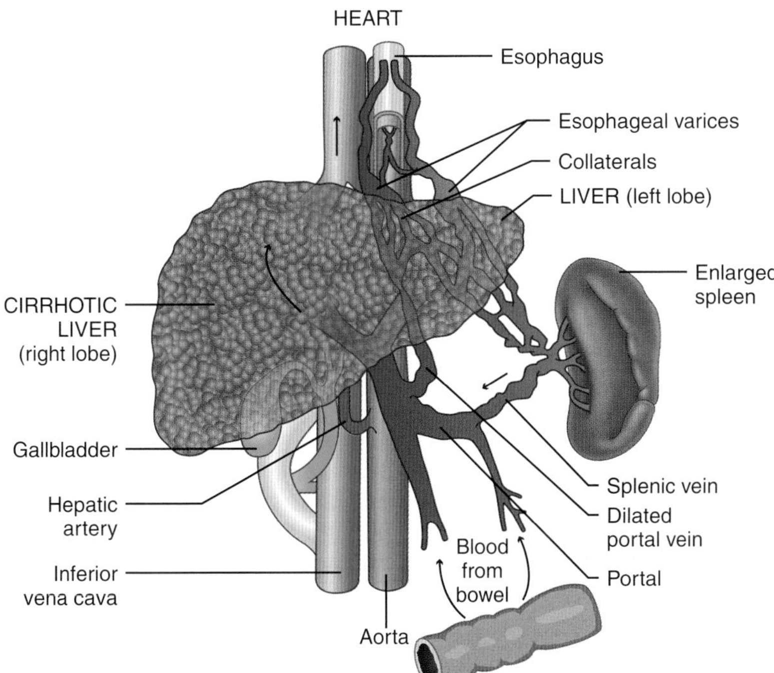


**Figure 17.4**

**Portal hypertension.** Normally, in the portal venous system (consisting of the portal veins, sinusoids, and hepatic veins), the portal veins carry blood from the gastrointestinal tract, gallbladder, pancreas, and spleen to the liver. Veins collecting from these sites form the splenic vein and superior and inferior mesenteric veins, which in turn merge to create the portal vein. Portal hypertension occurs when portal venous pressure exceeds the pressure in the nonportal abdominal veins (e.g., inferior vena cava) by at least 6 mm Hg. As portal pressure rises, increased resistance to blood flow causes blood pooling in the spleen and the development of collateral channels, which are formed in an effort to equalize pressures between these two venous systems. These collateral vessels or varices bypass the liver and cause large, tortuous veins, especially in the esophagus *(esophageal varices).*

varices. The collateral veins of the stomach and esophagus are the most likely to bleed because of a lack of communicating vessels.

*Gastroesophageal varices* (esophageal and gastric) are one of the most serious complications of portal hypertension, accounting for one-third of deaths related to cirrhosis and bleeding occurring in 25% to 40% of people with cirrhosis.[107] Clinical manifestations of gastroesophageal bleeding include hematemesis or melena (or both). The blood is usually dark red in color. More than half of bleeds stop spontaneously, and more than 90% of bleeds can be controlled with therapy. However, serious bleeding can quickly result in hypovolemia, shock, and death.

Endoscopy should be performed in all clients with cirrhosis to screen for varices. Follow-up endoscopy is scheduled depending on the presence and severity of varices. Prophylactic treatment depends on the size of the varices and whether the cirrhosis is compensated or decompensated (see Cirrhosis). If decompensation occurs, upper endoscopy should be performed for all sizes of varices. If no varices are initially noted, upper endoscopy can be repeated in 3 years. Upper endoscopy should be repeated every 2 years for small varices (smaller than 5 mm). Measures for treating small varices with red wale marks (raised, erythematous areas) include treatment with a nonselective β-blocker (such as nadolol). Large varices, measuring greater than 5 mm, can be treated with a nonselective β-blocker or endoscopic variceal ligation. Individuals who are unable to tolerate β-blockers can receive endoscopic variceal ligation. End points of β-blocker therapy are to reduce the hepatic venous pressure to less than 12 mm Hg or heart rate to less than 60 beats/min, demonstrating maximal tolerated dosage.

Therapy for acute esophageal bleeding includes initial hemodynamic resuscitation, often requiring blood transfusions, correcting coagulopathies, administering prophylactic antibiotics, and protecting the airway. Pharmacologic agents such as vasopressin and octreotide are administered to aid in stopping the bleeding. Endoscopic variceal ligation typically provides cessation of acute bleeding, although placement of a transjugular intrahepatic portosystemic shunt (TIPS) is occasionally required.[120]

Individuals who have recovered from an esophageal bleed receive endoscopic variceal ligation 1 to 2 weeks following discharge from the hospital and then every 2 to 4 weeks thereafter until the varices are eliminated. Therapy with a nonselective β-blocker is also initiated and/or continued.

Persons with recurrent bleeding despite β-blocker therapy and/or endoscopic variceal ligation can undergo placement of a TIPS.[117] This shunt provides a bypass pathway between the portal vein and the hepatic vein, reducing portal hypertension and rebleeding, although it does not improve survival.

Mortality can be as high as 20% within 6 weeks of a variceal bleed despite therapy. Prognosis is poor for clients with repeated esophageal bleeding, and liver transplantation should be pursued in individuals who are candidates.

**SPECIAL IMPLICATIONS FOR THE THERAPIST 17.4**

### *Portal Hypertension*

Portal pressure in individuals is dynamic, with highest pressures during the night; after eating; and in response to coughing, sneezing, and exercise. Such variations may combine with local factors in vessel walls to contribute to a pressure surge that can lead to a variceal bleed. The therapist can teach the individual how to modify and reduce pressure, especially anything that increases intraabdominal pressure such as coughing, straining at stool, or improper lifting. Any therapy program for a client with known varices must take this factor into account when presenting active or active-assisted exercises or unsupported gait training.[90]

## Hepatic Encephalopathy

**Definition and Overview.** HE is a complex neuropsychiatric syndrome with symptoms ranging from subtle neuropsychiatric and motor disturbances to coma and death in persons with hepatic dysfunction, portosystemic shunting of blood, or portal hypertension. It is a potentially reversible, decreased level of consciousness in people with severe liver disease. This complication can occur with both acute and chronic liver disease.[197]

**Clinical Manifestations.** HE is characterized as a spectrum of neuropsychiatric symptoms in the absence of brain disease, ranging from overt HE to minimal HE.[131] Symptoms may begin spontaneously or be precipitated by infection, medications, hypovolemia, or GI bleeding.

Mild symptoms may be noticed only by the family or with formal testing, noting changes in working memory, visuospatial abilities, and problems with attention. With progression of HE, individuals may demonstrate personality changes associated with alterations in motor function and consciousness. Clients may become disoriented, confused, disinhibited, or agitated. Asterixis may also be noted early in the course and worsens with progression of encephalopathy (although clients in a coma will no longer exhibit asterixis). Asterixis is defined as a negative myoclonus resulting in a person's inability to control posture in different body parts.[2] It can be elicited by having the person hold out their arms and extending the wrists; asterixis is present when there is flapping of the hands. This is thought to occur because of momentary motor loss in agonist muscles followed by a sudden compensatory correction in the antagonistic muscles, creating the flapping motion.[96]

Finally, the most serious expression of HE includes somnolence and coma complicated by cerebral edema. The International Society for Hepatic Encephalopathy and Nitrogen Metabolism defines overt HE as the onset of disorientation and asterixis. The classification system used most often for HE is the West Haven Criteria with scores ranging from zero (minimal HE) to 4 (being in a coma), depending on the severity of neurologic involvement (Table 17.1).[262]

**Etiology and Pathogenesis.** Although the pathologic mechanisms of HE are not well understood, they are thought to be multifactorial. Elevated levels of

**Table 17.1** Grades of Hepatic Encephalopathy

| Minimal | Grade 1 | Grade 2 | Grade 3 | Grade 4 |
|---|---|---|---|---|
| Nearly asymptomatic<br>Normal level of consciousness<br>No detectable personality or behavior changes<br>Minimal changes in memory and concentration (e.g., mildly forgetful or confused)<br>Minimal changes in executive and intellectual function | Slight personality changes, mood swings (irritability, restless)<br>Short attention span<br>Mild confusion<br>Incoordination<br>Tremor; asterixis may be observed with clinical testing (see Fig. 17.1)<br>Impaired handwriting<br>Sleep disorders (inverted sleep patterns) | Tremor progresses to asterixis<br>Resistance to passive movement<br>Myoclonus; hypoactive deep tendon reflexes<br>Lethargy or apathy<br>Unusual behavior (abusive, violent, noisy)<br>Obvious personality changes<br>Dyspraxia<br>Slow or slurred speech | Hyperventilation<br>Marked confusion, amnesia<br>Incoherent speech<br>Asterixis<br>Muscle rigidity<br>Hyperreactive deep tendon reflexes<br>Positive Babinski sign<br>Sleeps most of the time but can be aroused<br>Disorientation to time and place<br>Bizarre behavior | Comatose; unresponsive to verbal or noxious stimuli<br>No asterixis<br>Positive oculocephalic (doll's-eye) reflex<br>Decerebrate posturing<br>Dilated pupils<br>Lack of response to stimuli |

The West Haven Criteria reflected in this table is used most often to grade hepatic encephalopathy.
Modified from: Vilstrup H, Amodio P, Bajaj J, et al. Hepatic encephalopathy in chronic liver disease: 2014 practice guideline by the American Association for the Study of Liver Diseases and the European Association for the Study of the Liver. *Hepatology* 60:715–735, 2014.

ammonia are clearly involved but not likely the sole cause.[244] Ammonia is created by bacteria in the colon from the metabolism of protein and urea. Ammonia is absorbed into the portal blood system and is 5 to 10 times higher there than in the general circulatory system. The liver is typically able to metabolize ammonia into glutamine, but with liver disease and shunting of blood away from the liver (particularly to the brain), ammonia levels rise. Glutamine can also be metabolized back into ammonia and glutamate. The ammonia produced from glutamine breakdown can lead to mitochondrial dysfunction in astrocytes in the brain.[221] Glutamine can also act as an osmolyte and cause cerebral edema.

The kidneys are also a source of ammonia, which is increased in the face of diuretic use and hypokalemia. Muscles aid in ammonia removal, but cirrhosis is often accompanied by muscle wasting.

Another mechanism of HE involves the impairment of neurotransmission. Some of the alterations in neurotransmission include an increase in activation of inhibitory neurotransmitter systems (e.g., γ-aminobutyric acid and serotonin) with an accompanying impairment in excitatory pathways. There is also an increase in membrane receptors on astrocytes, perhaps secondary to exposure to ammonia, resulting in increased uptake of cholesterol and formation of neurosteroids.[197] These neurosteroids may contribute to further activation of inhibitory pathways. Changes in the quantity and function of glutamate are also considered to be associated in the development of HE. Glutamate is an excitatory neurotransmitter related to neuronal communication. It is postulated that there is a decrease in total brain glutamate (from the formation of glutamine in ammonia breakdown), while extracellular concentrations are increased. This increase in extracellular glutamate may be due to excessive neuronal release of glutamate (due to ammonia) and the inability of astrocytes to reuptake glutamate when exposed to ammonia.

The brain requires a steady supply of energy, and in HE, there are alterations in glucose metabolism. Not only is the liver unable to perform gluconeogenesis, but elevated levels of ammonia also inhibit cerebral energy metabolism. Selective changes in the transportation of amino acids (precursors to or actual neurotransmitters) through the blood-brain barrier may contribute to the development of HE.

## MEDICAL MANAGEMENT

**DIAGNOSIS, TREATMENT, AND PROGNOSIS.** The development of HE warrants a careful evaluation and correction of the cause. Serious and common causes include GI bleeding, infection (particularly SBP), hypovolemia, or electrolyte abnormalities (hypokalemia). Other common factors that may precipitate or severely aggravate HE include constipation, diuretics, and CNS depressants such as alcohol and opiates.

Lactulose (or lactitol) is a first-line pharmacologic therapy that decreases nitrogenous compounds from being absorbed from the gut and increases transit time through the intestine (the goal is two to four bowel movements a day). Ammonia-lowering therapy in suspected encephalopathy cases can be beneficial even when the ammonia level is normal, as the production is tied to other toxins. If lactulose is unable to reverse symptoms, rifaximin (a nonabsorbable antibiotic) may be added. Owing to expense, lactulose is typically the preferred initial treatment agent.[26,287]

Clients with overt HE should be treated in the intensive care unit (ICU) and monitored for cerebral edema, particularly clients with acute fulminant hepatitis.[273]

Reversal of HE is typically successful when a source is identified, corrected, and treated appropriately. Altered mental status caused by HE is a negative prognostic factor.[211] *Without* intervention, mortality is high, as the person's condition progresses into coma. Similar to most complications of end-stage liver disease, liver transplantation provides the best long-term treatment.

SPECIAL IMPLICATIONS FOR THE THERAPIST 17.5

### *Hepatic Encephalopathy*

An inpatient or homebound client with HE has difficulty ambulating and is extremely unsteady. Protective measures must be taken against falls. The home health therapist must be alert for any report of GI bleeding that will result in protein accumulation in the GI tract, exacerbating this condition (e.g., blood in stools or black or tarry stools).

The physician may prescribe lactulose in the prevention and treatment of HE,[269] but diarrhea is a side effect. A client experiencing prolonged diarrhea should be encouraged to report this information to the physician for possible follow-up. A reduced dosage may be required to prevent further electrolyte imbalance.

An immobile client who lacks reflexes is vulnerable to numerous complications requiring attention to the prevention of pneumonia and skin breakdown. Skin breakdown in a client who is malnourished from liver disease and is immobile, jaundiced, and edematous can occur in less than 24 hours. Careful attention to skin care, passive exercise, and frequent changes in position are required.

Rest between activities is advocated, and strenuous exercise is to be avoided. The therapist should watch for (and immediately report) signs of anemia (e.g., reduced hemoglobin, weakness, dyspnea on exertion, easy fatigability, skin pallor, or tachycardia), infection, and GI bleeding (e.g., melena, hematemesis, easy bruising).

Minimal HE (grade 0) in cirrhosis is associated with impaired driving skills and increased risk of motor vehicle accidents.[21] In earlier stages of HE, health care providers may identify subtle changes in mental status with impaired ability to drive. Assessments of psychometric and neurophysiologic techniques are often used to test for minimal HE to prevent driving accidents.[130] In one study, clients with cirrhosis but no evidence of HE underwent psychomotor testing; 60% were found to be unfit to drive, and 25% displayed questionable driving skills.[226] Other studies have shown similar results.[22]

A more recent review of driving fitness among people with chronic health conditions[168] concluded there is not enough evidence that clinical and neuropsychologic screening tests would lead to a reduction in motor vehicle crashes involving drivers with a chronic disability. The authors of the review stated: "It seems necessary to develop tests with proven validity for identifying high-risk drivers so that physicians can provide guidance to their patients in chronic conditions, and also to medical advisory boards working with licensing offices."[168] Until standardized driver simulation tests are available to screen effectively for individuals with cirrhosis, driving must be assessed on a case-by-case basis[168]; the therapist should keep in mind that appropriate referral for currently available testing may be needed sooner rather than later.

## Ascites

Ascites is the abnormal accumulation of fluid within the peritoneal cavity.[98] Ascites is most often caused by decompensated liver cirrhosis (85% of cases),[217] but other diseases associated with ascites include heart failure, abdominal malignancies, nephrotic syndrome, infection, and malnutrition.

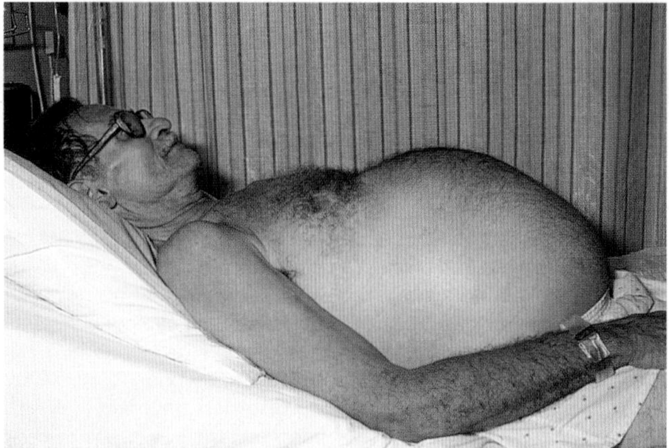

**Figure 17.5**

**Ascites in an individual with cirrhosis.** Distended abdomen, dilated upper abdominal veins, and inverted umbilicus are classic manifestations. Peripheral edema associated with developing ascites may be observed first by the therapist. (From Swartz MH: *Textbook of physical diagnosis*, ed 5, Philadelphia, 2006, Saunders.)

The mechanism for the accumulation of fluid in the case of cirrhosis is principally a result of portal hypertension. High pressure in the vessels attempting to pass blood through the cirrhotic liver leads to vasodilation of the splanchnic vessels (vessels to the gut or viscera) and reduced vascular resistance. This in turn stimulates sodium-retaining mechanisms including the renin-angiotensin-aldosterone system and secretion of antidiuretic hormone (ADH), resulting in sodium and water retention. This is accompanied by renal vascular vasoconstriction. The kidneys are unable to excrete the sodium and water load (secondary to ADH release), causing hyponatremia. Ultimately capillary permeability is altered, and a pressure gradient forms from both decreased protein and fluid overload in the splanchnic vasculature, favoring the movement of fluid from the vascular space to the peritoneal cavity.

Ascites becomes clinically detectable when more than 500 mL has accumulated, causing weight gain, abdominal distention, increased abdominal girth, and eventually peripheral edema (Fig. 17.5). Dyspnea with increased respiratory rate occurs when the fluid displaces the diaphragm.

Diagnosis of ascites is usually based on clinical manifestations in the presence of liver disease. Paracentesis is used as the initial test in people with new-onset ascites to determine the cause. Fluid is sent to the laboratory for chemical and microscopic evaluation. Abdominal ultrasonography can aid in locating pockets of ascitic fluid that may be loculated (formed or divided into small cavities or compartments).

In people with established cirrhosis, paracentesis can be diagnostic and therapeutic. Large-volume paracentesis with administration of albumin is the treatment of choice for tense ascites (i.e., when a person is no longer able to breathe or eat comfortably), followed by the use of diuretics to reduce reaccumulation of fluid.

Treatment of clients with mild ascites and urinary sodium excretion greater than 78 mEq/day includes sodium restriction. Most people, however, will also require diuretic use with spironolactone and furosemide. Fluid restriction is appropriate when the serum sodium decreases to less than 120 mEq/L. The development of refractory ascites affects 10% of individuals with advanced cirrhosis[27] and is associated with a poor prognosis. Serial large-volume paracentesis or TIPS alleviates pressure in the portal area but may induce HE caused by bypassing the liver (see Hepatic Encephalopathy earlier). Liver transplantation provides the best treatment option but is not always readily available.[218]

Over a 10-year period, 50% of individuals with previously compensated cirrhosis develop ascites. Ascites is a sign of hepatic decompensation and therefore associated with a poor prognosis. Survival is variable, depending on the presence of other coexisting cirrhotic complications such as previous bleeding esophageal varices and SBP.[98]

**Spontaneous Bacterial Peritonitis.** SBP is characterized by infection of ascitic fluid in the setting of portal hypertension. The microbial source of infection of the ascitic fluid is typically the gut, where organisms (e.g., *Escherichia coli*, streptococci [mostly pneumococci], and *Klebsiella*) are translocated to lymph nodes and into the ascitic fluid. Bacteria may also spread from a urinary tract infection, pneumonia, or skin infections. SBP is symptomatic in the majority of cases (fever, chills, abdominal pain, mental status changes, and tenderness), but symptoms can often be subtle. The diagnosis is made by paracentesis, with ascitic fluid demonstrating a neutrophil count of 250/μL or higher. Antibiotics should be administered immediately following the paracentesis, with narrowing of antibiotics once culture information is available. Mortality is high if antibiotics are not given. Individuals with SBP and renal dysfunction also benefit from albumin administration, and β-blocker medications should be discontinued. Clients at high risk for developing SBP (renal dysfunction, very low levels of ascitic protein) should be placed on prophylactic antibiotics.

SPECIAL IMPLICATIONS FOR THE THERAPIST 17.6

### *Ascites*

Most people with ascites are more comfortable in a high Fowler position (head of the bed raised 18 to 20 inches with the knees elevated). Breathing techniques are important to maintain adequate respiratory function and to prevent the development of atelectasis or pneumonia. A homebound person who has ascites should be monitored for the possible development of bacterial peritonitis. Onset of fever, chills, abdominal pain, and tenderness should be reported to the physician.

Decreases in serum albumin associated with the development of ascites are accompanied by a parallel decrease in oncotic pressure in blood vessels causing peripheral edema. Persons with serum albumin levels between 2.5 g/dL and 3.5 g/dL are at moderate risk of malnutrition, and persons whose levels are 2.5 g/dL or less are at great risk. Because albumin binds to calcium, serum albumin levels drop when serum calcium levels are low.

The edema associated with ascites may mask muscle wasting that occurs when the body does not have an adequate intake of protein to maintain structure and facilitate wound healing. The client must be encouraged to change position to maintain integrity of the skin and promote circulation. Small pillows or folded towels can be used to support the rib cage and the bulging flank while the client is lying on his or her side.

The abdominal distention associated with ascites may develop very slowly over a number of weeks or months and may be accompanied by bilateral edema of the feet and ankles. The client may be unable to put on a pair of shoes, preferring to leave the shoes unlaced or to wear slippers. In a home health, inpatient hospital, or nursing home setting, this change in dress may not be as noticeable as it would be in a private practice or outpatient clinic. It is always important to remain alert to these potential signs of fluid retention and to ask about any changes in health status or weight gain.

Aldosterone-antagonist diuretics or potassium-sparing diuretics may be prescribed to decrease fluid retention, thus slowing the development of ascites and reducing the workload of the heart. Sometimes these diuretics lose their effectiveness. Loop diuretics may be prescribed instead. The therapist must be alert to the development of this phenomenon. Symptoms of fluid overload such as weight gain, hypertension, peripheral edema, dyspnea, tachypnea, orthopnea, neck vein distention, or pulmonary crackles must be reported to the physician. Conversely, when diuretic therapy works too well, volume depletion (hypovolemia) may manifest with signs and symptoms of dehydration (e.g., hypotension, tachycardia, flat neck veins, poor skin turgor, thirst). Recognizing medical complications of this type and obtaining the necessary medical care can reduce morbidity and mortality for these individuals.[171]

Fluid intake and output are usually carefully measured and restricted, so in any setting, the therapist is encouraged to know the individual's limits and to participate in reporting measurements. This is especially important because clients frequently ask the therapist for fluids in response to perceived exertion or increased exertion after exercise or ambulation. The person who is noncompliant or in denial requests fluids because of the false belief that fluids provided but not recorded do not count. For the homebound client who is receiving diuretics, the bedroom should be close to the bathroom.

### Hepatorenal Syndrome

HRS is a severe complication of advanced cirrhosis associated with poor survival.[9,276] About 18% of people with cirrhosis and ascites develop HRS at 1 year; about 39% develop HRS at 5 years.[95] HRS develops as a consequence of abnormal hemodynamics, encompassing splanchnic system vasodilation with renin-angiotensin–activated renal vasoconstriction.[212,276] The reduction in renal perfusion also reduces glomerular filtration rate and sodium excretion.

Criteria defining the diagnosis of HRS were established by the International Ascites Club and include the presence of advanced liver disease with portal hypertension;

acute kidney injury indicated by an increase in serum creatinine of greater than 50% in 7 days; urine protein of less than 500 mg/dL and absence of microhematuria; and, most importantly, the absence of other causes for kidney involvement.[8]

Common illnesses found in people with cirrhosis that can cause renal insufficiency include infection (particularly SBP), shock, medications, and GI bleeding. Renal obstruction should be ruled out by ultrasonography. The presence of these features, along with the failure to improve after the removal of diuretics and administration of saline and albumin, suggests the diagnosis of HRS.

HRS is classified into two types. Type 1 is rapid (1 to 2 weeks) in both onset and progression to renal failure and carries a poor short-term prognosis. Type 2 is more insidious in onset, with slower progression over months; ascites resistant to diuretic therapy is often the key feature of this type.

Therapy consists of restriction of sodium and water (if hyponatremic) and discontinuing diuretics. A precipitating cause should be sought and addressed. Because of the intense vasoconstriction, treatment centers around the use of vasodilators (octreotide and midodrine) and albumin, which aid in increasing blood flow to the kidneys; this type of treatment is only 50% effective.[1,111] TIPS may also be of benefit for clients waiting for transplant.[276]

Curative treatment consists of liver transplantation, where renal function recovery is possible. Although many people with HRS will improve with medical treatment, liver transplantation should be pursued because of poor long-term prognosis.[167,275] Hemodialysis may be required as bridge treatment until a transplant is available.

## Hepatitis

Hepatitis is an acute or chronic inflammation of the liver caused by a virus, a chemical, a drug reaction, or alcohol abuse. Classifications of hepatitis discussed in this text are listed in Box 17.2. Six different identifiable hepatitis viruses (A, B, C, D, E) are responsible for more than 95% of all viral-induced cases worldwide. The letter "F" was not skipped; it represents the sixth form of hepatitis, the fulminant form, a term for any rapidly progressing form of liver inflammation resulting in HE within a few weeks of developing infection. Fulminant hepatitis is not strictly viral induced but can develop as a result of any form of hepatitis (see further discussion in Acute Liver Failure later).

Other viral causes of hepatitis include Epstein-Barr virus (mononucleosis), herpes simplex virus types 1 and 2, varicella-zoster virus, measles, and cytomegalovirus. Hepatitis from any cause produces very similar symptoms and usually requires a careful client history to establish the diagnosis.

People with mild to moderate acute hepatitis rarely require hospitalization. The emphasis is on preventing the spread of infectious agents and avoiding further liver damage when the underlying cause is drug-induced or toxic hepatitis. Persons with fulminant hepatitis (which has a severe, sudden intensity and is sometimes fatal) require special management because of the rapid progression of the disease and the potential need for urgent liver transplantation.

### Chronic Hepatitis

Chronic hepatitis comprises several diseases that are grouped together because they have common clinical manifestations and all are marked by chronic necroinflammatory injury that can lead insidiously to cirrhosis and end-stage liver disease. The disease is defined as chronic with evidence of ongoing injury for 6 months or more.

Chronic hepatitis has multiple causes including viruses, medications, metabolic abnormalities, and autoimmune disorders. Despite extensive testing, some cases cannot be attributed to any known cause. Hepatitis B (HBV) with or without hepatitis D virus (HDV), HCV, and GB virus (GBV) can progress to chronic hepatitis.

Most people with chronic hepatitis are asymptomatic, and when symptoms occur, these are nonspecific and mild, with fatigue, malaise, loss of appetite, polyarthralgias, and intermittent right upper quadrant discomfort. Some people report sleep disturbances or difficulty in concentrating. Symptoms of advanced disease or an acute exacerbation include nausea, poor appetite, weight loss, muscle weakness, itching, dark urine, and jaundice. Once cirrhosis is present, weakness, weight loss, abdominal swelling, edema, easy bruising, muscle wasting and weakness, GI bleeding, and HE with mental confusion may arise.

The diagnosis of chronic viral hepatitis is based on serologic testing; for example, the presence of positive hepatitis B antigen (HBeAg) for longer than 6 months indicates chronic hepatitis B. The diagnosis can usually be made from clinical features and blood test results alone; however, assessment of cirrhosis is typically made through noninvasive tests such as ultrasound-based elastography. While noninvasive testing is often used instead of a liver biopsy to detect cirrhosis, a liver biopsy may be helpful in assessing the activity of underlying liver disease (grade and stage) and to determine the need for antiviral treatment. Chronic hepatitis is described in diagnostic terms that include the etiology (e.g., hepatitis C), degree of active inflammation (grade 1 through 4), and extent of fibrosis (stage 1 through 4). The strict definition of chronic hepatitis (from any cause) is based on histologic features of chronic inflammatory cell infiltration in the liver. Grading/staging of liver damage chronicles the progression from inflammatory cell infiltration to hepatocellular necrosis and fibrosis.

The treatment for chronic viral hepatitis has improved substantially in the last decade. Treatment of chronic hepatitis B depends on the presence or absence of cirrhosis, the viral DNA level, and liver enzyme levels (particularly ALT). The treatment of hepatitis C now provides for the elimination of the virus and cure.[237]

The prognosis in chronic hepatitis is variable depending on the development of cirrhosis and other complications such as HCC. Male gender, moderate to severe alcohol consumption, and other coexistent liver disorders are factors that increase the rate of progression to cirrhosis. The 5-year survival rate for compensated cirrhosis is greater than 90%, but the prognosis and survival rate for decompensation (characterized by development of variceal bleeding, ascites, and HE) are extremely poor.[127]

### Acute Liver Failure

*Acute liver failure (ALF), also known as fulminant hepatic failure or fulminant hepatitis,* is the generic term for any rapidly progressing form of liver injury/inflammation without prior liver disease or cirrhosis.[150] ALF develops over days to weeks (some cases take up to 6 months to develop) and results in acute liver injury, HE (see Hepatic Encephalopathy earlier for further discussion), and associated coagulopathy.[148]

This type of hepatitis is rare, occurring in less than 1% of persons with acute viral hepatitis (approximately 2000 cases annually in the United States),[34] but can be fatal. The most common causes are acetaminophen hepatotoxicity (50% of all cases of ALF)[147]; idiosyncratic drug reaction; infections such as hepatitis A virus (HAV) and HBV, Epstein-Barr virus, cytomegalovirus, varicella-zoster virus, or herpes simplex virus; and hepatic ischemia.[253]

Encephalopathy may progress to intracranial hypertension and cerebral edema, which is the most serious complication and most common cause of death. Ammonia is one neurotoxin that can be monitored. Clients with concentrations less than 75 μM rarely progress to the development of cerebral edema, whereas individuals with levels greater than 200 μM are more likely to have intracranial hypertension.

In addition to liver failure, numerous complications can occur including infection, hypoglycemia, coagulation defects (international normalized ratio 1.5 or greater), lactic acidosis, ascites, GI hemorrhage, electrolyte disturbances, and renal insufficiency.

Diagnosis is made in the presence of a combination of HE and acute liver injury (demonstrated by elevated serum bilirubin and transaminase levels). Laboratory testing should include viral serologies for hepatitis A through E, autoimmune serologies, and ceruloplasmin levels looking for Wilson disease as well as medications (e.g., acetaminophen). Imaging studies are used to detect causes of liver injury (e.g., Budd-Chiari syndrome). Treatment should be provided in an ICU and a facility able to provide liver transplantation. Acetaminophen overdose usually responds to *N*-acetylcysteine. Therapy for ALF due to hepatitis B includes a nucleoside analogue. Hypertonic saline and osmotic agents are used to reduce cerebral edema, and hypotension is treated with careful fluid resuscitation and vasoconstrictors (e.g., norepinephrine and vasopressin).[148] However, these measures can be continued only as a bridge for individuals requiring liver transplantation. Determination of who will ultimately require a liver transplant (versus recover) is difficult. The Kings' College Hospital criteria continue to be the most reliable and clinically useful.[148,174]

The most important factors in determining recovery are the degree and severity of HE, the person's age, and cause of the injury (toxic agents versus infectious etiologies). Individuals with grade IV HE have less than a 20% chance of spontaneously recovering.[191] Clients who do not demonstrate advancement toward recovery should be immediately considered for transplantation. Short-term prognosis without treatment is very poor, and the mortality rate can be extremely high (often exceeding 90%[150]). Survival, following liver transplant however, is better than 80%.[155]

### Viral Hepatitis

**Overview.** Each of the recognized hepatitis viruses belongs to a different virus family, and each has a unique epidemiology. Table 17.2 presents the characteristics of these strains of viruses. The identification of the specific virus is made difficult by the fact that a long incubation period often occurs between acquisition of the infection and development of the first symptoms. The incubation period is 15 to 50 days for HAV, 2 to 5 months for HBV, and 2 weeks to 6 months for HCV. Not all causative agents have been identified, and because hepatitis can be easily spread before symptoms appear, morbidity is high in terms of loss of time from school or work. More than half and possibly as many as 90% of all cases go unreported because symptoms are mild or even subclinical.

HAV is transmitted by the fecal-oral route. This is typically due to poor or improper handwashing and personal hygiene, particularly after using the bathroom and then handling food for public consumption. This route of transmission also may occur through the shared used of oral utensils such as straws, silverware, and toothbrushes.

Major outbreaks of HAV occur when people consume contaminated water or food. HAV is rarely transmitted through transfused blood, and little placental transmission occurs, although the antibody is often detected in infants of infected mothers.

HAV is highly contagious, with the peak time of viral excretion and contamination occurring during the prodromal period *before* the onset of jaundice and up to 1 week after the onset of jaundice. Thus the greatest danger of transmission is during the incubation period, when a person is unaware that the virus is present. The illness can last from 4 to 8 weeks, although it may persist longer and is more severe in persons 50 years old and older or persons with underlying chronic liver disease.

HBV is transmitted percutaneously (i.e., puncture of the skin) or through mucosal contact. HBV is highly infectious. Because HBV can be transmitted through heterosexual or homosexual intercourse, it is considered a sexually transmitted disease and reportable to the U.S. Centers for Disease Control and Prevention (CDC). The incubation period is 60 to 150 days, with symptoms occurring around 90 days.[118] Although most people experience symptoms for only several weeks, others may have persistent symptoms for up to 6 months. Up to 90% of infants who become infected go on to develop chronic hepatitis B compared with only 2% to 6% of adults.

HCV is most commonly associated with injection drug use. As with HAV, the period of infectivity begins before the onset of symptoms, and the person may become a lifetime carrier of this virus. Clinically, HCV is very similar to HBV and often is asymptomatic; acute HCV infection is usually mild. Chronic HCV varies greatly in its course and outcome from asymptomatic with normal liver function to mild degree of liver injury and overall good prognosis to severe symptomatic HCV with complications of cirrhosis and end-stage liver disease.

HDV, or delta virus, is a defective single-stranded RNA that manifests as a coinfection or superinfection of HBV. This virus requires hepatitis B for its replication, so only individuals with HBV are at risk for HDV. Risk factors and transmission mode are the same as for HBV; parenteral

**Table 17.2** Types of Viral Hepatitis

| | Hepatitis A | Hepatitis B | Hepatitis C | Hepatitis D | Hepatitis E |
|---|---|---|---|---|---|
| Incidence | Overall infection rate decreased by 95% since introduction of vaccine in 1995. A number of outbreaks recently increased the incidence. 2000 cases reported in 2016, with the actual number probably around 4000 cases | Overall infection rate reduced since introduction of HBV vaccine. Over 3200 acute cases reported in 2016; actual number probably around 21,000. Injection drug use has increased the incidence since 2014. Possibly 2.2 million living with chronic HBV | About 3000 cases reported in 2016, with actual number probably over 41,000. 2.4 million live with the infection | Uncommon in United States; occurs only in people infected with HBV | Epidemic in developing countries; rare in United States; risk greatest to persons traveling to endemic regions |
| Morbidity | Results in acute infection only; does not progress to chronic hepatitis or cirrhosis; small risk of acute liver failure; lifetime immunity | 25% of people with chronic HBV die prematurely of cirrhosis or end-stage liver disease; associated with liver cancer | 75%–85% of acute infections become chronic. 10%–20% progress to cirrhosis; associated with liver cancer | Coinfection of HBV and HDV leads to more severe acute disease. Genotypes may determine outcomes | Causes acute self-limiting infection; does not progress to chronic hepatitis; high mortality in pregnant women |
| Transmission | Fecal-oral route; spread by feces, saliva, and contaminated food and water | Parenteral<br>Sexual contact<br>Vertical<br>Contact with blood or open sores | Parenteral<br>Hemodialysis<br>Vertical<br>Blood concentrates before 1987, blood transfusions or solid organ transplants before 1992 | Parenteral<br>Sexual contact (same as HBV)<br>Perinatal rare | Same as HAV; fecal-oral (contamination of water) |
| Treatment | Supportive care. Prevention with HAV vaccine. Postexposure treatment with immune globulin and vaccine (see text); most people recover within 3 months | Acute: supportive<br>Chronic: pegylated interferon and antiviral agents for chronic HBV (see text); HBIG for exposed, unvaccinated persons | Acute: supportive<br>Chronic: cure possible with combination therapy (see text) | Treatment for people with elevated HDV RNA levels and active liver disease: interferon alfa2a or b | None; preventive measures |
| Diagnosis | Blood test to identify IgM antibody; NAAT for HAV RNA | Blood tests to identify antigen and antibodies—HBsAg, HBeAg, anti-HBc HBV DNA (see text under diagnosis) | Blood test to identify antibody (anti-HCV); does not distinguish between current and past infection; hepatitis C viral RNA (qualitative and quantitative) | Blood test to detect antibody—anti-HDV; HBsAg, IgM anti-HBc | Blood test to detect anti-HEV IgM antibodies or HEV RNA |
| Vaccine | Hepatitis A vaccine available; combined HAV and HBV vaccine also available | Vaccines available: HBV as single agent or combined with HAV or DTaP or IPV (see text) | None available | Immunization against HBV can prevent HDV infection | No vaccine approved in U.S.; approved vaccine available in China (2012) |

*DTaP*, Diphtheria, tetanus, and acellular pertussis; *HAV*, hepatitis A virus; *HBcAg*, hepatitis B core antigen; *HBeAg*, hepatitis B e antigen; *HBIG*, hepatitis B immune globulin; *HBsAg*, hepatitis B surface antigen; *HBV*, hepatitis B virus; *HEV*, hepatitis E virus; *IgM*, immunoglobulin M; *IPV*, inactivated polio vaccine.

From Centers for Disease Control and Prevention (CDC): National Center for Infectious Diseases. Last updated August 2019. Available at:https://www.cdc.gov/hepatitis/. Accessed March 16, 2020.

**Table 17.3** Risk Factors for Hepatitis

| HAV | HBV | HCV | HDV | HEV |
|---|---|---|---|---|
| Household contacts or sexual contacts of infected persons | Injection drug use | Sharing needles or other equipment to inject drugs; people who use intranasal drugs | Same as HBV | Same as HAV |
| Men who have sex with men | Sex with an infected partner | | | |
| Injection/noninjection illegal drug users (regional outbreaks reported) | Incarceration in correctional facilities—adults and youths (drug use, unsafe sexual practices) | Received blood transfusion or organ transplant before July 1992 or blood clotting products made before 1987 | | |
| Living in areas with increased rates of HAV (children at greatest risk) | Contact with blood or open sores of an infected person | People with HIV infection | | |
| Travel in areas where HAV is epidemic | Travel to high-risk areas | | | |
| Persons with a blood clotting disorder | Occupational risk: morticians, dental workers, emergency medical technicians, firefighters, health care workers in contact with body fluid or blood | Occupational risk in health care workers after needlesticks | | |
| | Liver transplant recipient | Evidence of liver disease | | |
| | Infants born to mothers with HBV | Infants born to HCV-infected mothers | | |
| | Multiple blood product or blood transfusions before July 1992 | Long-term kidney dialysis (clients/staff) | | |
| | Sharing items such as razors or toothbrushes with an infected person | | | |

*HAV*, Hepatitis A virus; *HBV*, hepatitis B virus; *HCV*, hepatitis C virus; *HDV*, hepatitis D virus; *HEV*, hepatitis E virus.
From Centers for Disease Control and Prevention (CDC): National Centers for Infectious Diseases. Last reviewed 2019. Available at https://www.cdc.gov/hepatitis/. Accessed March 16, 2020.

drug users have a high incidence of HDV. The symptoms of HDV are similar to those of HBV except that clients are more likely to have ALF and to develop chronic hepatitis and cirrhosis.

*Hepatitis E virus* (HEV) is transmitted by contaminated water via the fecal-oral route and clinically resembles HAV. Hepatitis E has been considered to be a travel-associated, acute, self-limiting liver disease that causes ALF in specific high-risk groups only. It is thought to be nonfatal, although it has been clearly associated with liver damage. A 20% to 25% mortality rate exists in pregnant women from ALF. This virus tends to occur in poor socioeconomic conditions, primarily occurs in developing countries (contaminated waste water and sewage), and is rare in the United States. Although China released a recombinant vaccine, no specific treatment is available for acute HEV, and ensuring clean drinking water remains the best preventive strategy.

Two viruses have been isolated and termed *hepatitis G virus* (HGV) and GBV-C. Both are essentially identical. GBV-C is similar to HBV and is transmitted through sexual contact or transfusion of contaminated blood. Coinfection with HCV is common, and GBV-C may exert an inhibitory influence on HIV replication. GBV is found in people worldwide. GBV has been identified as the causative agent of approximately 20% of posttransfusion hepatitis cases and approximately 15% of community-acquired hepatitis cases that are not caused by HAV. However, studies fail to show conclusive evidence of clinical hepatitis after infection with GBV; this potential form of hepatitis remains under investigation.

**Incidence and Risk Factors.** Each year, approximately 500,000 Americans are infected with some form of hepatitis virus; about 15,000 persons die from complications of hepatitis virus annually. HAV is the predominant type of hepatitis, causing 40% to 60% of acute viral hepatitis cases. An estimated 4 million people are living with chronic hepatitis B or C in the United States, and many more are at risk for infection.[256]

HAV most commonly affects household contacts with people already infected, people in institutions or day care centers, men who have sex with men,[64] people experiencing homelessness, and people who live or travel in underdeveloped countries (Table 17.3). Food may become contaminated with HAV during any process in production (growing, processing, handling). Water in the United States is chlorinated to kill the virus. Because of the HAV vaccine for children, the infection rate has dramatically decreased 95% since 1995. However, since 2016, there have been widespread outbreaks in the United States in the adult population, as this population has not been widely vaccinated. More than 21,230 cases have been identified, with 12,476 hospitalizations and 203 deaths in 25 states.

In 2016, 3218 acute cases of hepatitis B were reported in the United States. Owing to underreporting and other factors, it is estimated that about 20,900 people were newly infected with HBV in 2016.[42] Similar to hepatitis A, the overall rate of hepatitis B infection declined in the period 1990–2014, particularly as a result of vaccination of children. Yet recently there has been an increase in the rate of new infections; this is thought to be secondary to an increase in injection drug use.[109] In 2015, 1715 deaths were reported to be due to hepatitis B; this is believed to be an underestimation, and the number of deaths is more likely to approach 14,000.[41,178]

Common risk factors for HBV include sexual contact with an infected partner, injection drug use, sharing needles, needlesticks, men who have sex with men, hemodialysis clients, and perinatal (vertical) transmission from mother to child. Injection drug use and intimate contact with another person with HBV are the two most frequent sources of HBV in the United States. Transfusion-related HBV is rare owing to the initiation of donor screening for HBV and the HBV vaccine. These measures have improved the incidence in people requiring blood products and hemodialysis clients and workers.

In the United States, more than 2.4 million people are infected with HCV. In 2016, 2967 acute cases were reported to the CDC, but similar to HBV, most cases go undetected and unreported.[44] It is estimated that the actual number of acute infections is 14 times the number reported, or about 41,200 cases in 2016.[114] In 2016, 18,153 deaths were reported due to HCV infection, although this is most likely underestimated.[164]

In the past, HCV infection was commonly acquired through blood transfusion (before 1992). Currently, because of donor screening, the incidence of HCV from transfusion is uncommon. People at risk for contracting HCV include those with exposures to contaminated blood, blood products, or infected body fluids such as injection drug users with needle sharing, individuals who received blood transfusions from infected donors (before 1992), persons with hemophilia who received infected clotting factor concentrates (before 1987), persons receiving hemodialysis, individuals with HIV, and children born to HCV-positive mothers. See Table 17.3 for other risk factors.

HDV is common worldwide, with more than 15 to 20 million people affected, and the incidence is increasing in the United States.[189,267] Although this incomplete RNA virus requires HBV for infection, it has been found to continue to infect hepatocytes even with the clearance of HBV.[94] It often leads to cirrhosis and increases the risk for HCC.

HEV is most common in developing countries. Risk factors for becoming infected include travel to an area where the virus is endemic and consumption of food or water that is contaminated. On the basis of serologic tests, an estimated one-third of the world's population has been infected with HEV. In India, the lifetime prevalence is more than 60%.[231]

**Pathogenesis.** The viruses associated with hepatitis are not typically cytopathic (destroy cells), yet the body's reaction to the virus often creates significant inflammation; the intensity of the disease depends on the degree of immune response.[33,215] Initially, cytokines, chemokines, and natural killer cells are employed to remove virus from the body. Later, antigen-specific T cells (maturated in the lymph tissue) enter the liver to aid in the removal of virus; antibodies prevent spread of virus and, in the case of hepatitis B, provide immunity against further infection. If these cells are unable to clear the virus and chronic disease results, the continued presence of virus-specific T cells and recruited mononuclear cells can lead to the progression of liver inflammation and eventually cirrhosis.[215] In adults with intact immunity, this initial immune response can clear the virus. However, in infants, young children, and immunosuppressed people, the immune system is unable to mount an adequate defense, and the virus continues to replicate and reside in the liver, leading to a chronic state. In these people, there is a weak response with few antigen-specific T cells.

In HCV, the virus is able to bypass the immune system in most cases. Current theories include T-cell exhaustion, T-cell dysfunction, viral escape mutations, or rapid T-cell deletion in the liver.[185] HCV has also been shown to activate natural killer lymphocytes, resulting in the loss of their receptors for immunoglobulin G (IgG). This alters the normal ability of natural killer cells to mediate the destruction of infected cells.[193] Because HCV is able to mutate, antibodies to HCV do not provide immunity against another exposure, and a vaccine is still not available.

**Clinical Manifestations.** Most cases of acute viral hepatitis are asymptomatic and never reported. Up to 70% of children younger than age 6 years remain asymptomatic with HAV infection. Infants, children younger than age 5 years, and immunosuppressed adults typically have no symptoms associated with acute HBV infection, whereas most cases of HCV infection are subclinical and not reported (about 20% to 30% of people with acute HCV become symptomatic).

Classic symptoms of acute hepatitis are often the same, regardless of the responsible virus. Most individuals present with malaise, fatigue, mild fever, nausea, vomiting, anorexia, right upper quadrant discomfort, and occasionally diarrhea. These prodromal symptoms are followed by the development of jaundice, particularly with acute HAV, HDV, HEV, and frequently HBV (30% of cases[82]). Dark urine and clay-colored stools may also be observed.

In more than 95% of adults with normal immunity, infection with HBV is self-limited; but in 5% of adults, 30% of children (younger than the age of 5), and 90% of infants as well as individuals with immunodeficiencies, the infection becomes chronic. Approximately 15% to 25% of individuals who become infected with HCV are able to clear the virus, while 75% to 85% develop chronic hepatitis C.[252] Some people may develop extrahepatic manifestations (more frequent in HCV than in HBV) such as essential mixed cryoglobulinemia, porphyria cutanea tarda, lichen planus, rheumatoid arthritis, Hodgkin lymphoma, and diabetes mellitus. Rheumatologic (arthralgias, myalgias, sicca syndrome, sensory neuropathy, paresthesias) and skin manifestations (pruritus) are the most common. Individuals with acute HBV may also demonstrate extrahepatic symptoms including rash, arthralgias, and arthritis.

HDV is a highly pathogenic virus that causes acute hepatitis, often ALF, and a rapidly progressive form of chronic viral hepatitis, leading to cirrhosis in about 70% of the cases.[81,189]

## MEDICAL MANAGEMENT

**PREVENTION.** Prevention takes place at three levels: primary, secondary, and tertiary. Primary prevention involves primary immunization (HAV, HBV, and HEV), education regarding food preparation and proper handwashing, avoiding needle punctures by contaminated needles (or other similar infective material), and practicing protective sex or avoiding sexual contact during the period of hepatitis B surface antigen (HBsAg) positivity.

Secondary prevention involves passive immunization following exposure to HAV or HBV, travel precautions when visiting areas where hepatitis is endemic (e.g., avoid drinking unbottled water or beverages served with ice, avoid eating foods rinsed in contaminated water such as fruits and vegetables, and avoid eating shellfish).

Tertiary prevention involves education of people who are infected about preventing possible infectivity to others and self-care during active infection (e.g., avoid strenuous activity and ingestion of hepatotoxins such as alcohol and acetaminophen).

***Hepatitis A.*** The HAV vaccine is routinely given to children between 12 and 23 months of age with a booster administered at least 6 months later. It may also be administered to adults wishing to obtain immunity or anyone who is at risk for infection (e.g., persons traveling to areas with intermediate to high rates of endemic HAV, persons living in communities with high endemic rates or periodic outbreaks of HAV infection, men who have sex with men, and clients with chronic liver disease.[45] HAV vaccine confers 97% to 100% protection in children and 94% to 100% in adults.

Postexposure prophylaxis refers to treatment received on exposure to the virus. If the individual has not been vaccinated, the HAV vaccine should be given within 2 weeks of exposure. In addition, for people older than age 40 years with comorbidities, immunoglobulin may also be used. When given within 2 weeks of exposure, immunoglobulin is 80% to 90% effective in preventing HAV infection. The sooner immunoglobulin is given after exposure, the more efficacious it is. People who have received the HAV vaccine at least 1 month before exposure do not require immunoglobulin.[45]

***Hepatitis B.*** HBV is a preventable disease achieved by administering an HBV vaccine. Currently, two types of vaccines are available: singe-antigen and combination vaccines. Single-antigen vaccines (Recombivax HB, Heplisav-B, and Engerix-B) protect only against hepatitis B. Combination vaccines are produced that provide protection against multiple diseases. Twinrix vaccinates for HAV and HBV in adults. Pediarix is used to vaccinate children for HBV, diphtheria and tetanus toxoids, acellular pertussis, and inactivated poliovirus. The vaccine is given in three doses over a period of 6 months. Heplisav-B can be given in two doses 1 month apart. Medical providers should attempt to use the same manufacturer's vaccine when available.[45] At least 30 years of protective immunity develops in more than 90% of healthy adults.

For health care workers or others who have been vaccinated and are exposed to an infectious source of hepatitis B (e.g., needlestick, nonintact skin exposure to blood, sexual contact), if they have adequate anti-HBs antibodies (10 mIU/mL or greater), they are protected. If their antibody titers are found not to be adequate, the person should receive one dose of hepatitis B immunoglobulin (HBIG) as soon as possible after the exposure. HBIG administers hepatitis B antibodies and offers passive immunity. The person should also be revaccinated with the HBV series at 0, 1, and 6 months. Individuals who have not been vaccinated and are exposed (the source is HBsAg positive) should receive one dose of HBIG and a dose of hepatitis B vaccine as soon as possible and complete the vaccine series. People who have not responded to the vaccine should receive two doses of HBIG (at exposure and 1 month later). For other scenarios, please visit cdc.gov/hepatitis.[223]

Once individuals begin to engage in behaviors associated with high-risk groups, they may become infected before vaccine can be given. A major obstacle in eliminating HBV is identifying persons and vaccinating them before they become infected. For this reason, in the United States, it is now recommended that all infants, health care workers, and persons in the high-risk category for HBV receive the HBV vaccine.

According to the Occupational Safety and Health Administration Bloodborne Pathogen Standard, HBV vaccination must be offered to all employees within 10 days of employment. Records related to this vaccination must be maintained. Employees who decline vaccination must sign a standardized declination form.[194]

Children younger than 5 years of age, if infected, have a high risk of developing chronic HBV infection. Testing to identify pregnant women who are HBsAg positive and providing their infants with immunoprophylaxis within 12 hours of birth (HBIG and vaccine) effectively prevents HBV transmission during the perinatal period. The World Health Organization has recommended that all countries integrate HBV vaccination into their national immunization programs, and much progress has been made toward the goal to control, eliminate, and eradicate HBV in the coming generations.[278]

***Hepatitis C.*** Currently, no vaccine is available to prevent HCV because of the rapidity of HCV mutations in adaptation to the environment, and no immunoglobulin is effective in treating exposure.[181] The only means of preventing new cases of HCV are to screen the blood supply, encourage health care professionals to take precautions when handling blood and body fluids, and educate people about high-risk behaviors (particularly injection drug users and people involved with multiple sex partners). Anyone at risk for HCV should be tested. The CDC has recommended that all adults born in the United States between 1945 and 1965 should be tested for exposure to hepatitis C because of the risk of liver disease, including liver cancer. Early diagnosis is the key to preventing serious life-threatening liver diseases.

***Hepatitis D.*** Universal HBV vaccination programs have led to a significant decline in incidence of hepatitis D in Western countries; however, HDV is not a vanishing disease. Persons with chronic hepatitis B should also be screened for hepatitis D, particularly in high-risk groups (injection drug users, men who have sex with men, and clients receiving hemodialysis).[189]

***Hepatitis E.*** A recombinant protein vaccine has been developed and shown to be effective in preventing HEV in high-risk populations.[231] The vaccine is a good option to prevent this infection that affects a large number of people in deprived geographic areas; however, it is licensed and produced in China only.

**DIAGNOSIS.** In addition to the history and clinical examination, serologic and molecular testing aid in providing an accurate diagnosis. Serology is the standard for diagnosis of viral hepatitis (see Table 17.2). A positive IgM HAV signifies acute disease, whereas IgG HAV indicates previous infection or vaccination.

Serology relating to HBV changes as the disease progresses or is contained.[43] Early in HBV infection, the serologic marker HBsAg is positive. A positive HBsAg also indicates acute infection and signifies the person is infectious. However, antibodies are negative until the body has mounted an immune response. One of the earliest antibodies to develop is the IgM antibody to hepatitis B core antigen (IgM anti-HBc) and signifies acute infection (less than 6 months). The antibody termed total hepatitis B core antibody (anti-HBc) is associated with symptoms and remains in the blood throughout life and so can represent either ongoing infection or previous infection. HBeAg is a secreted product of the hepatitis B nucleocapsid gene and represents the ongoing replication of virus associated with large quantities of virus in the blood. HBeAg is seen during the acute infection and chronic hepatitis. Conversion from e antigen to e antibody demonstrates either spontaneous conversion or conversion with medical treatment. The presence of anti-HBe predicts long-term clearance of HBV and lower levels of HBV. With recovery, there is elimination of HBsAg and the appearance of hepatitis B surface antibody (anti-HBs). This antibody is also seen in people who have been vaccinated. HBV DNA can be detected in persons with chronic infection by polymerase chain reaction techniques[161]; this information is useful in treatment and prognosis. On average, HBsAg can be found in an acutely infected person's blood about 4 weeks after infection; by 15 weeks, those who do not go on to have chronic infection will become HBsAg negative.

Chronic hepatitis B infection is marked by four phases: immune tolerant, immune active, immune control (inactive chronic HBV infection), and reactivation. The immune tolerant phase occurs in individuals who have been infected vertically (mother to child) and usually do not need treatment for 2 to 3 decades. Immune active disease is marked by elevated liver enzymes and HBV DNA greater than 20,000 IU/mL in HBe-positive disease. Immune control refers to seroconversion with loss of HBeAg and development of the antibody anti-HBe. Reactivation of HBV may result in people who are HBsAg and anti-HBc positive from a loss of immunity, such as people receiving chemotherapy or other immunosuppressive therapy. This is evident in an elevation of both HBV DNA and liver enzymes.

None of the serodiagnostic tests are able to determine the current extent of liver damage. Noninvasive ultrasound techniques and liver biopsy provide information about the severity of disease. Liver biopsy can establish grading and degree of fibrosis but is used only in cases of chronic hepatitis.

Testing for HCV should be performed in individuals who are at risk such as injection drug users or intranasal illicit drug users, clients who receive hemodialysis, and people who are infected with HIV or HBV. One-time testing for HCV is now recommended for all adults born in the United States between 1945 and 1965[242]; about 3% of this population is HCV positive and comprise 75% of all HCV-positive people. Identifying active HCV infection can be accomplished by testing for HCV RNA (initially present) and HCV antibody (which becomes positive in 1 to 3 months). For persons who seroconvert and do not become chronically infected, the HCV RNA will clear within 6 months. People who develop chronic disease will have HCV RNA and a positive HCV antibody. Because HCV mutates, a genotype should be identified, which aids in treatment. Testing for HBV and HIV should be performed, as coinfection with these viruses can speed progression toward cirrhosis. Transient elastography, magnetic resonance imaging (MRI) elastography, or liver biopsy should be done in all clients with chronic HCV to assess the liver for fibrosis.[102]

**TREATMENT.** Treatment options have expanded, and prevention methods are available for two of the six viruses. Any hepatic irritants such as alcohol, hepatotoxic medications (acetaminophen), or chemicals (e.g., occupational exposure to carbon tetrachloride) must be avoided in all types of hepatitis.

***Hepatitis A.*** Treatment for HAV is primarily symptomatic and supportive. Good sanitation and hygiene practices should be followed. Hospitalization may be required owing to excessive vomiting for administration of fluid. Rare cases of ALF occur.

***Hepatitis B.*** All people with ALF due to HBV receive treatment as well as clients with specific types of chronic disease. Individuals with immune-active hepatitis (elevated HBV DNA and liver enzymes), reactivation hepatitis, and/or cirrhosis receive the nucleoside analogues entecavir or tenofovir. Pegylated interferon may be used in select people (elevated liver enzymes, low HBV DNA levels, and without cirrhosis) for 48 weeks. Interferon has many side effects, but therapy duration is limited, and maintenance therapy is not required. Nucleoside analogues can be given orally, cost less than interferon, and have few side effects, but continued treatment is required to maintain response. Treatment goals for people with immune-active phase disease are the loss of the serologic marker HBeAg and seroconversion to anti-HBe. Individuals with reactivation disease or cirrhosis are treated indefinitely. With treatment, regression of fibrosis can occur. Because people with cirrhosis and HBV are at high risk for the development of HCC, ultrasonography of the liver or cross-sectional imaging every 6 months is advisable.

***Hepatitis C.*** All people infected with chronic HCV should receive treatment unless they are unable to tolerate the medications. HCV is treated similarly to HIV in that a combination of antiviral medications is used, each with a different mode of action. Genotype, history of previous treatment, and presence of fibrosis are factors taken into consideration for drug combinations. Cure is now possible for more than 90% of people.[6] This is defined as a negative HCV RNA test 12 weeks after completion of therapy. The HCV antibody will remain positive.

Surveillance by ultrasonography every 6 months is recommended to detect HCC in clients with higher staging fibrosis or cirrhosis, even with a negative HCV RNA test. Administration of HAV and HBV vaccine is recommended for anyone with chronic HCV because of the potential for increased severity of acute hepatitis superimposed on existing liver disease.[233] People positive for HCV and HBsAg are at increased risk for HBV reactivation while receiving direct-acting antiviral medications for HCV treatment. These individuals should be monitored during therapy. Liver transplantation should be considered for clients with decompensated cirrhosis before antiviral treatment. Although HCV recurs with transplantation, medical treatment is very successful for individuals who have not received previous therapy.

**PROGNOSIS.** Prognosis varies with each type. Chronic HBV or HCV infection is associated with increased risk of death, particularly from liver- and drug-related causes.[265] A substantial proportion of morbidity and mortality related to HBV that occurs in the health care setting can be prevented by vaccinating health care workers against HBV. In addition, health care workers must practice infection control measures.

***Hepatitis A.*** HAV is almost always a self-limited disease and rarely leads to ALF requiring transplantation (approximately 0.3% to 0.6% of cases). It does not lead to chronic hepatitis or cirrhosis. Within 3 to 6 months, greater than 90% of people fully recover and become immune to HAV.

***Hepatitis B.*** Most adults with normal immune status (94% to 98%) recover completely from newly acquired HBV infections, eliminating virus from the blood and producing neutralizing antibody that creates immunity from future infection. In immunosuppressed persons (including hemodialysis clients), infants, and young children, most newly acquired HBV infections result in chronic infection. Although the consequences of acute HBV can be severe (1% die from acute hepatitis),[42] most of the serious sequelae associated with the disease occur in persons in whom chronic infection develops. Approximately 15% of people who acquire the disease as adults and 25% of people who acquired HBV as a child die prematurely from cirrhosis or liver cancer.[173]

Despite reinfection rates, liver transplantation for cirrhosis caused by HBV provides the best treatment. The survival rate at 1 year after transplantation reaches 90%. Continued treatment of the virus with the administration of HBIG and/or antiviral therapy results in successful liver transplantation outcomes.

***Hepatitis C.*** Infection with HCV is usually not self-limiting and ends up becoming a chronic infection in up to 80% of people infected. HCV infection increases the risk of HCC and other HCV-related liver disease.[127] HCV-associated disease is a leading risk factor for HCC and a common reason for liver transplantation in the United States.[48,127] The majority of disease sequelae (e.g., leading to cirrhosis) develop within 20 to 30 years of disease onset in individuals with chronic disease. Approximately 10% to 20% of all cases of HCV progress to cirrhosis, but newer therapies now available can clear the body of HCV infection and are expected to reduce HCV-related morbidity and mortality.[257]

The progression of HCV to cirrhosis and HCC is accelerated if a person is also coinfected with HIV or HBV, misuses alcohol, has nonalcoholic liver disease, or receives immunosuppressive therapy.[270]

HDV has a high morbidity and mortality rate, rapidly leading to hepatic failure and cirrhosis when it accompanies HBV.[189]

***Hepatitis E.*** HEV is typically a self-limited acute hepatitis, usually lasting 1 to 4 weeks. Severity of symptoms increases with age. It does not progress to chronic disease. When it occurs in epidemics, it can cause substantial rates of death and complications, especially in pregnant women. The overall fatality rate is estimated to be 3%; pregnant women who develop the infection have the highest risk of acute hepatic failure.[231]

## SPECIAL IMPLICATIONS FOR THE THERAPIST 17.7

### *Viral Hepatitis*

Any direct contact with blood or body fluids of clients with HBV or HCV requires administration of immunoglobulin, a preparation of antibodies, in the early incubation period. Therapists at risk for contact with HBV because of their close contact with the blood or body fluids of carriers should receive active immunization against HBV. All therapists should follow Standard Precautions at all times to protect themselves and must wear personal protective equipment whenever appropriate. Such gear should never be worn in the car or laundered at home to avoid contamination of those sites.

Enteric precautions are required when caring for individuals with type A or E hepatitis. Any therapist working in dialysis units or providing wound care should review available infectious control guidelines.

Studies dealing with the natural history of acute hepatitis have provided perspective on the frequency of skin and joint manifestations. More than one-third of the adults studied had joint pains during the course of the illness. The frequency of arthralgia as a symptom associated with hepatitis increases with age. Joint pains affected only 18% of children compared with 45% of adults older than 30 years.

No known studies have been published regarding the benefit of physical therapy in providing symptomatic joint relief until these symptoms resolve as the person recovers from the underlying pathology. In the case of a client with undiagnosed hepatitis presenting with joint symptoms, the systemically derived arthralgia will not respond to therapy. Any time intervention fails to provide symptomatic relief or resolution of symptoms, the results must be reported to the physician for further follow-up evaluation.

Overall, in the recovery process, adequate rest to conserve energy is important. The affected individual is encouraged to gradually return to levels of activity before illness. Fatigue associated with the anicteric phase of hepatitis may interfere with activities of daily living and may persist even after the jaundice resolves. A careful balance of activity is important to avoid weakness secondary to prolonged bed rest; a reasonable activity level is more conducive to recovery than enforced bed rest. Whenever possible, rehabilitation intervention or increased activity should not be scheduled right after meals.

Affected individuals are advised by all health care professionals to avoid alcohol and to talk with a physician or pharmacist before taking any medications or nutraceuticals (e.g., herbal products, supplements).

Watch for signs of fluid shift such as weight gain and orthostasis, dehydration, pneumonia, vascular problems, and pressure ulcers and any signs of recurrence. After the diagnosis of viral hepatitis has been established, the affected individual should have regular medical checkups for at least 1 year and should avoid using any alcohol or nonprescription drugs during this period.

Interferon-α (antiviral used in the treatment of some hepatitis viruses) has bone marrow–suppressive effects requiring careful monitoring of platelet or neutrophil count. Other side effects of combination therapy may include increased fatigue, increased muscle pain and potential inflammatory myopathy, headaches, local skin irritation (site of injection), irritability and depression, hair loss, itching, sinusitis, and cough. These symptoms usually subside in the first few weeks of treatment; prolonged or intolerable side effects must be reported to the physician.

### Hepatitis B

Nosocomial transmission of HBV is a serious risk for health care workers. The risk of acquiring HBV infection from occupational exposure depends on the degree of exposure to blood and the presence of HBeAg from the source. An approximate 22% to 31% chance exists of acquiring HBV after percutaneous (needlestick) contact with an HBsAg- and HBeAg-seropositive source.[116]

HBV can be transmitted to health care workers via percutaneous injuries or by direct or indirect contact with blood from an infected client. Blood contains the highest amount of infected particles and is the most efficient means of transmission. HBV in blood is able to survive up to 1 week on environmental surfaces. The incubation period is 45 to 180 days (average 60 to 90 days).

Preexposure HBV vaccination of health care workers who are at risk (e.g., individuals who work in an area likely to have contact with blood and body fluids) is strongly recommended and can prevent acquisition of HBV. Once a health care worker has been exposed, the HBsAg status of the person and vaccination and vaccine-response status of the exposed health care worker must be determined. Postexposure prophylaxis should then be given if the health care worker is unvaccinated or nonresponsive to previous vaccine and the source is HBsAg positive.

The Occupational Safety and Health Administration bloodborne pathogen standard mandates that HBV vaccine and HBIG be made available, at the employer's expense, to all health care workers with potential occupational exposure. In addition, strict adherence to handwashing and Standard Precautions is critical in prevention of the transmission of hepatitis-contaminated body fluids. Transmission is also prevented by use of barriers during sexual activity and by not sharing personal or other items that may have blood on them.

For a health care worker who is positive for HIV, HBV, or HCV, the CDC guidelines are based on the assumption that the risk of transmission to others is greatest during invasive procedures that include (for the therapist) sharp débridement or digital palpation of a needle tip (or other sharp instrument) in a poorly visualized or highly confined anatomic site.

Any therapist performing such procedures should determine his or her own HIV and HBV DNA serum levels (rather than HBeAg status previously recommended) and HCV antigen status to monitor infectivity. HBV DNA less than 1000 IU/mL is considered "safe" for practice. Individuals who are infected should not perform the procedures unless they have obtained guidance from an expert panel about when and how they may safely do so. The CDC does not mandate restricted practice, and according to the updated guidelines, prenotification of patients/clients of a health care professional's HBV status is not required.[116] For a complete summary of the current recommendations, see Holmberg and colleagues[116] (available online at http://www.cdc.gov/mmwr/preview/mmwrhtml/rr6103a1.htm?s_cid=rr6103a1_e).

### Hepatitis and the Athlete

Great concern is often expressed over the possibility of contagion among athletes in competitive sports, particularly sports with person-to-person contact. Infectious agents including HIV and other viruses, bacteria, and fungi have been examined. No cases of HIV or HCV transmission resulting from sports participation have been reported, but two cases of HBV transmission through exposure to blood during sports participation have been documented.

For most of the infections considered, the athlete is more at risk during activities off the playing field than while competing. The main pathways of transmission of bloodborne infections in athletes are similar to those experienced in the general population. The greatest risk to an athlete for contracting any bloodborne pathogen infection is through sexual activity and parenteral drug use and not in the sporting arena.[225] One report specific to the risk of transmission among climbing athletes suggests that the transmission risk in climbing is even smaller compared with contact sports.[225]

Inclusion of immunizations against measles and HBV as a prerequisite to participation would eliminate these two diseases from the list of dangers to athletes (and all individuals). Education, rather than regulations, is the best approach in considering the risks to athletes from contagious diseases.[71,222]

Although the risk of bloodborne pathogen infection during sports is exceedingly small, good hygiene practices concerning blood are still important. The American Academy of Pediatrics has made recommendations to minimize the risk of bloodborne pathogen transmission in the context of athletic events and has issued safety precautions. The therapist in this type of setting is encouraged to review these guidelines.[5]

No evidence has been reported that intense, highly competitive training is harmful for an asymptomatic HBV-infected person, whether the disease is acute or chronic. Therefore the presence of HBV infection does not contraindicate participation in sports or athletic activities; decisions regarding play are made according to clinical signs and symptoms such as fatigue, fever, or organomegaly. Chronic HBV infection with evidence of organ impairment requires reduction in intensity and duration of activity.

### Hepatitis C

HCV is the most common etiologic agent in cases of non-A, non-B hepatitis in the United States. Seroprevalence studies among health care workers have shown a significant association between acquisition of disease and health care employment, specifically client care or laboratory work. Accidental percutaneous injuries (needlesticks or cuts with sharp instruments) are the highest-risk vehicle for transmission to health care workers from people with acute or chronic HCV.

The incubation period for HCV is 6 to 7 weeks, and nearly all individuals with acute infection will have chronic (more than 3 to 6 months' duration) HCV infection with persistent viremia and the potential for transmission to others over an extended period.

Serologic assays to detect HCV antibodies (not protective antibodies) are available and are used to determine source and health care worker status after exposure. More than 75% of all people with HCV develop chronic hepatitis, and cirrhosis may develop in up to 25% of people with chronic HCV. A risk of developing HCC (approximately 3% to 5% per year) exists, and a small percentage of people with HCV may progress to fulminant liver failure.[196]

Currently no vaccine against HCV is available. No postexposure prophylaxis can be recommended, as postexposure prophylaxis with immunoglobulin or antiviral agents does not appear to be effective in preventing HCV infection. Follow-up HCV testing should be performed to verify if seroconversion occurs.

Strict adherence to handwashing and Standard Precautions is critical in prevention of transmission of hepatitis-contaminated body fluids. Transmission is also prevented by use of barriers during sexual activity and by not sharing personal or other items that may have blood on them.

## Drug-Induced Liver Injury

### Overview and Incidence

Injury to the liver can be caused by many drugs or toxins. More than 1000 medicinal agents, chemicals, and herbal remedies are recognized as producing hepatic injury.[38,183] Although nonprescription and prescription medications are often thought to be the only agents to cause drug-induced liver injury (DILI), complementary or alternative medications such as chaparral, germander, pennyroyal oil, kava kava, mistletoe, Jin Bu Huan, and Sho-saiko-to are also known to be hepatotoxic.[38,183]

Chemicals such as carbon tetrachloride, trichloroethylene, derivatives of benzene and toluene, vinyl chloride, and organic pesticides can also lead to liver injury. Carbon tetrachloride was the most common industrial chemical considered an occupational inhalation poison until it was banned in most countries. Ingestion of poisonous mushrooms including *Amanita phalloides* and related species (rare in the United States but more common in Europe) can lead to ALF.

Although uncommon, drugs are currently the most common cause of ALF, with acetaminophen the most common cause in the United States.[149] While the hepatotoxicity related to acetaminophen is predictable, most drugs exhibit an idiosyncratic drug reaction (Box 17.3). Predictable liver damage caused by drugs is dose related (i.e., a specific toxic dose most likely will cause damage), and injury results soon after ingestion. Idiosyncratic drug reactions are unpredictable, occur without warning, are unrelated to dose, and may occur days to months after ingestion.

Medications with the most serious potential for hepatotoxicity include antibiotics (amoxicillin-clavulanate), CNS acting drugs (phenytoin and valproate), cardiovascular drugs (amiodarone and statin medications), rheumatologic agents, and antineoplastic medications (particularly azathioprine and infliximab).[31] The incidence of hepatotoxicity as a result of these agents is difficult to determine because many cases may be subclinical (i.e., mild symptoms) or misdiagnosed, leading to underreporting. One French study demonstrated a rate of 14 cases/100,000 people in the general population; 12% required hospitalization, and 6% died as a result of ALF.[228] Hepatotoxicity has also been the principal reason for removing drugs from the market.[18]

Box 17.3

**CAUSES OF CHEMICAL- AND DRUG-INDUCED HEPATITIS**

***Dose-Related (Predictable)***

- Acetaminophen[a] (Tylenol) (analgesic; suicide attempt)
- Alcohol
- *Amanita phalloides* (poisonous mushroom)
- Anabolic steroids
- Aspirin
- Benzene, toluene
- Carbon tetrachloride
- Chloroform (anesthetic)
- Methotrexate (antineoplastic agent)
- Oral contraceptives
- Organic pesticides
- Penicillin
- Tetracyclines (antibiotic)
- Trichloroethylene
- Vinyl chloride

***Idiosyncratic (Unpredictable)***

- Methyldopa (antihypertensive)
- Halothane (anesthetic)
- Isoniazid (antitubercular)
- Minocycline (antibiotic)
- Monoamine oxidase inhibitors (antidepressant)
- Nitrofurantoin
- Phenytoin (Dilantin) (anticonvulsant)
- Rifampin (antitubercular)
- Quinidine (antiarrhythmic)
- Sulfonamides (antibiotic)
- Sulindac (NSAID)[b]
- Valproate (anticonvulsant)

[a]Acetaminophen is not an NSAID. It has no antiinflammatory properties, only analgesic and antipyretic uses. It has no relationship to ibuprofen.
[b]NSAIDs as a class have the potential to cause liver injury.
*NSAID*, Nonsteroidal antiinflammatory drug.
Data from pharmacotherapy update: Tisdale JE, Miller DA, editors, *Drug-induced diseases*, ed 2, Bethesda, MD, 2010, American Society of Health-System Pharmacists; Goldman L, Schafer A, editors, *Goldman's Cecil medicine*, ed 24, Philadelphia, 2012, Saunders.

### Etiologic Risk Factors

A host of factors may enhance susceptibility to DILI including age (adults more so than children), gender (women have a higher risk than men), obesity, malnutrition, pregnancy, concurrent medication use, and history of drug reactions. An important factor is individual genetic variability of drug-processing enzymes such as cytochrome P-450 isoenzymes (one of the largest drug-metabolizing drug systems) and human leukocyte antigen (HLA) alleles.[35,263] Preexisting liver diseases appear to increase the severity and mortality associated with DILI.[50,169,251] Drugs that may increase hepatotoxicity when taken with alcohol include acetaminophen, isoniazid, methotrexate, and cocaine.

### Pathogenesis

Drugs and toxins can result in liver injury that can be described in terms of the pattern of injury (hepatocyte, bile ducts, or vascular endothelial cell damage) or the underlying process (intrinsically hepatotoxic or idiosyncratic reactions—see Overview). Intrinsic hepatocellular injury is dose dependent and predictably causes hepatocyte necrosis at certain doses. The drug or a metabolite binds to a component of the hepatocyte (DNA, proteins, etc.), hindering function or regulation of the cell, which leads to inflammation or cell death (hepatonecrosis). Acetaminophen is an example of a drug that causes hepatocellular injury.

Idiosyncratic reactions (reactions that cannot be predicted) can be classified as nonimmune (metabolic) or immune (allergic) related. Similar to intrinsic hepatotoxicity, nonimmune idiosyncratic reactions involve a metabolite of the offending drug that covalently binds to a component of the cell (e.g., DNA, proteins, enzymes, microtubules), interfering in cell structure or regulation of cell functions. This metabolite is thought to form secondary to an aberrant metabolic process that is genetically determined. Examples of drugs related to nonimmune idiosyncratic reactions include amiodarone and isoniazid.

Often the person's own immune system contributes to inflammation and necrosis of cells.[53] Although this process is not well understood, it is thought that metabolites of drugs covalently bind to cells and create a drug/protein antigen complex. This drug/protein antigen (termed *protein adduct*) is then presented by MHC surface proteins, activating helper T lymphocytes. T lymphocytes enlist the aid of B cells, natural killer cells, and cytotoxic T cells, which results in apoptosis, the creation of reactive oxygen species that damage DNA, and mitochondrial dysfunction. This immune response most likely arises in genetically susceptible people who have another process occurring such as viral hepatitis that "primes" the immune system. Once damaged cells have released necrotic components of the cell, these are recognized by Toll-like receptors on macrophages. Macrophages trigger the release of chemokines and cytokines that signal neutrophils and other inflammatory cells to move into the area, further aggravating injury.[277] Many medications have been implicated in causing immune-related hepatotoxicity, including amoxicillin-clavulanate, nitrofurantoin, and phenytoin.

### Clinical Manifestations

The manifestations of drug-related liver disease can range from mild symptoms to ALF. Vague symptoms including fatigue, nausea, and right upper quadrant pain or discomfort may be the first indications of hepatotoxicity. Other symptoms associated with liver injury are jaundice, pruritus, and dark urine. Fever, rash, joint pain, elevated white blood count, and lymphadenopathy are often present with a hypersensitivity- or immune-type reaction; this presentation is similar to infectious mononucleosis. As discussed, drugs often cause a specific pattern of injury. The most readily identifiable patterns are hepatocellular and cholestatic.

Hepatocellular liver disease frequently manifests with abdominal discomfort/pain, fatigue, and jaundice; the clinical course is acute and can be severe. Cholestatic liver disease is manifested clinically by jaundice and pruritus. In contrast to the hepatocellular pattern, cholestatic disease is often less acutely serious, but healing may be prolonged and chronic, taking weeks to months.

## MEDICAL MANAGEMENT

**DIAGNOSIS.** Because drug-induced hepatotoxicity is uncommon, people who present with symptoms consistent with liver disease should have a complete evaluation to avoid missing more common causes. This includes laboratory testing for viral hepatitis, autoimmune liver diseases, Wilson disease, hemochromatosis, and $\alpha_1$-antitrypsin deficiency. Ultrasonography, computed tomography (CT) scanning, MRI, and endoscopic retrograde cholangiopancreatography (ERCP) are useful to identify biliary obstruction. A history of heavy alcohol consumption may be consistent with alcohol-related hepatitis.

A review of medications taken, including exposures to chemicals, herbals, and nonprescription medications, may point toward DILI. Although many drugs have more immediate effects, symptoms related to unpredictable injury may not manifest for months.

Available tests detect injury only, and the diagnosis of DILI is one of exclusion. The National Institutes of Health provides an updated list of drugs with known liver toxicities that can be accessed at http://livertox.nih.gov/rucam.html.

Laboratory tests used to detect liver injury include aminotransferases (ALT, AST), bilirubin, and alkaline phosphatase (ALP). Liver injury may be principally hepatocellular, cholestatic, or mixed. DILI that causes hepatocellular injury is typically evident by elevated aminotransferases compared with ALP. Cholestatic disease usually exhibits an elevated ALP compared with aminotransferase values. Mixed injury displays an elevation in aminotransferases and ALP. Bilirubin may be abnormal in both types of injury. If abnormal liver values have been present for less than 3 months, DILI is considered to be acute. Chronic DILI is defined as abnormal enzymes for longer than 3 months. It may be difficult to determine if an elevation in liver enzymes is related to drugs or another underlying process.[250]

Significant elevations in these laboratory values are not predictive of prognosis because the liver has prodigious ability to heal.[184] The liver also has the ability to adapt to some medications. This ability is demonstrated when the introduction of a drug leads to transient elevations in liver enzyme tests, but there is no progression of injury. In these cases, the drug does not have to be stopped. For example, isoniazid often causes a transient minor increase in liver enzymes but is permanently stopped in only 1 in 1000 affected clients.[188]

**TREATMENT AND PROGNOSIS.** Treatment for drug-related hepatotoxicity most often consists of removal of the causative agent and providing supportive care.[202] Two exceptions include the usage of *N*-acetylcysteine soon after toxic ingestion of acetaminophen and intravenous carnitine for valproate-induced hepatotoxicity.[154] Reexposure or rechallenge of the offending agent should be avoided, particularly if the drug has an unpredictable liver toxicity and the hepatotoxicity was immune-related. Reexposure could lead to an even more severe and serious reaction.

Liver injury accompanied by increases in liver enzyme levels may worsen for days to weeks before improvement. In some severe cases, improvement of liver enzyme levels suggests liver failure rather than healing of injury caused by severe necrosis and loss of hepatocytes. In this setting, laboratory values indicative of liver function (e.g., prothrombin time/international normalized ratio and albumin) and symptoms (e.g., encephalopathy) are better indicators of hepatic function.

Chronic liver disease can also develop, occurring in up to 6% of drug-induced hepatotoxicity cases (principally with a cholestatic pattern of injury). Methyldopa, minocycline, and nitrofurantoin are drugs that have been associated with this problem. A poor prognosis is seen in clients who develop jaundice, impaired liver function, and encephalopathy within 26 weeks of the onset of symptoms.[202] Prognosis is the most serious and poor for people with hepatocellular damage (AST more than three times the upper limit of normal) accompanied by jaundice (bilirubin more than two times the upper limit of normal), with a mortality as high as 14% (known as the *Hy law*).[30,49] This type of injury is more likely than other types of liver injury to require liver transplantation, and mortality can be 80% in people who develop ALF and do not receive a transplant.[28]

**SPECIAL IMPLICATIONS FOR THE THERAPIST 17.8**

### *Drug-Related Hepatotoxicity*

Therapists should be alert to the possibility of drug toxicity or drug reactions in clients taking multiple medications or reactions in people who are combining prescription medications or nonprescription medications with complementary or alternative medications. Many people do not consider nonprescription drugs as medications and may take the same drug with different names or combine nonprescription drugs with prescription medications. People with memory loss or short-term memory deficits may take multiple doses in a short amount of time because they cannot remember when or whether they took their medication. Other guiding principles for the recovery process are as mentioned for viral hepatitis.

## Autoimmune Hepatitis

### Overview and Incidence

Autoimmune hepatitis (AIH) is a chronic progressive, inflammatory disorder of the liver of unknown cause. It occurs in adults and children and is characterized by the presence of abnormal liver histology, autoantibodies, elevated levels of serum immunoglobulins, and frequent association with other autoimmune diseases. AIH is one of the three major autoimmune liver diseases, along with primary biliary cholangitis (PBC) and PSC. Variant forms of AIH have been termed *overlap syndromes* because they share features of several liver diseases.

The International Autoimmune Hepatitis Group has classified two types of AIH: type 1 and type 2.[4] Both forms are more common among women than men and have similar clinical and serum biochemical features. Type 2 is rare and most often seen in childhood and in young adulthood; it is associated with more severe and advanced disease at presentation, with a poorer response to therapy. AIH is seen worldwide and in various ethnic groups, although type 2 is uncommon in the United States.

### Etiologic Factors and Pathogenesis

The cause and pathogenesis of AIH are not known. The disease appears to occur among genetically predisposed individuals on exposure to as-yet-unidentified environmental agents, triggering a cascade of T cell–mediated events directed at liver antigens.[139]

Purported triggering agents include viruses such as measles, hepatitis, cytomegalovirus, and Epstein-Barr viruses and drugs such as methyldopa, nitrofurantoin, diclofenac, minocycline, and atorvastatin.[29] It is uncertain if drugs actually trigger AIH or merely cause a drug-mediated hepatitis with features similar to AIH. Little evidence is available that supports the hypothesis that inflammation continues once a drug is discontinued, making drugs a less likely trigger for AIH. Most people with AIH, however, have no identifiable trigger. Factors that predispose an individual to AIH are not certain, but specific HLA genes (located in the MHC) have been linked to the development of AIH and probably play a major role.

Type 1 is associated with HLA-DR3 and HLA-DR4. Studies show that HLA-DR3–associated disease correlates to earlier onset, particularly in girls and young women, and more severe disease, whereas HLA-DR4 is associated with milder disease (although extrahepatic findings are more common) and better response to treatment.[139]

Autoreactive T cells and their proinflammatory response appear to cause the liver destruction seen in AIH. Research continues to identify the antigens that are targeted by T cells, but one possibility is the asialoglycoprotein receptor, which is a liver membrane protein found in hepatocytes.

Continued T-cell response with chronic liver damage may ensue because of a failure of $CD4^+CD25^+$ regulatory T (Treg) cells to regulate the response of $CD8^+$ and $CD4^+CD25^-$ cells (autoreactive T cells). Normally, Treg cells control the adaptive immune response of $CD8^+$ and $CD4^+CD25^-$ T cells by suppressing the proliferation and function of these T cells, which allows for self-tolerance maintenance. In AIH, the low number and defective function of Treg cells leads to a change in cytokine production, proliferation, and apoptosis of autoreactive T cells.[160]

Antibodies are also produced and vary depending on the type of AIH. Antinuclear antibodies, smooth muscle antibodies, atypical perinuclear antineutrophilic cytoplasmic antibodies, and antiactin antibodies are seen with type 1 AIH. Type 2 is associated with liver-kidney microsome 1 and liver cytosol 1 antibodies. Although present in the serum, there is little evidence to support the theory that these autoantibodies cause the disease.[139] Yet measurement of these antibodies can be helpful in the diagnosis of AIH.

### Clinical Manifestations

AIH is represented by a wide spectrum of clinical manifestations. Although most clients present with nonspecific, mild, or chronic liver symptoms, up to 40% present with acute symptoms of hepatitis including ALF or cirrhosis. AIH is usually progressive and chronic, although a few cases are characterized by a fluctuating course.

The most common presenting symptoms are fatigue (85%), jaundice (46%), anorexia (30%), myalgias (30%), and diarrhea (28%). Other symptoms include abdominal pain, arthralgias (particularly small joints), and malaise. Weight loss is uncommon and should prompt an evaluation for another disorder.

The presence of another autoimmune disorder such as thyroiditis, ulcerative colitis, type 1 diabetes, rheumatoid arthritis, and celiac disease is seen in one-third of affected individuals. Physical examination may be normal, but 78% of clients present with hepatomegaly. Individuals with ALF often have profound jaundice.

Complications of AIH are similar to other chronic liver diseases, particularly the development of cirrhosis. Although occurring less frequently than hepatitis associated with a virus, another serious complication is the development of HCC.

### MEDICAL MANAGEMENT

**DIAGNOSIS.** The International Autoimmune Hepatitis Group created a scoring system to aid in the diagnosis of AIH, which can be difficult because no single test is diagnostic for the disease.[158] The criteria used for scoring are based on a synthesis of clinical, biochemical, and histologic information as well as an exclusion of other liver diseases such as viral hepatitis. Laboratory findings consistent with AIH include elevated aminotransferase values, hypergammaglobulinemia, elevated bilirubin and ALP values, and the presence of autoantibodies. At presentation, aminotransferase values are typically 10 to 20 times normal, while more chronic disease exhibits less of an elevation. More than 80% of affected people have hyperbilirubinemia, although this is typically mild with values less than 3 mg/dL. Serum ALP values are usually elevated, but values twice the upper limit of normal are likely indicative of another disease. Serum globulins are elevated up to three times normal, particularly gamma globulin and IgG.

As discussed, autoantibodies are produced and can be helpful in making the diagnosis of AIH, but 10% of cases do not exhibit autoantibody production. The most common autoantibodies seen in type 1 are antinuclear and smooth muscle autoantibodies. Titers of at least 1:80 are suggestive of the diagnosis in adults.[139] Anti–liver-kidney microsome 1 and anti–liver cytosol 1 antibodies are more specific to type 2.

The magnitude of the elevations of aminotransferase and gammaglobulin does not necessarily correlate with the extent of liver damage, making liver biopsy important for diagnosis and to guide therapy, but biopsy is not always required. Although histologic appearance of AIH is not specific (can also be seen in other liver diseases), characteristic findings of AIH include a mononuclear cell infiltrate of the interface around the portal triad, particularly with plasma cells, "piecemeal necrosis" or interface hepatitis, and fibrosis.

**TREATMENT.** The mainstay of therapy is immunosuppression. More than 80% of clients achieve remission with prednisone or prednisone plus azathioprine. Serum aminotransferases and gammaglobulin levels can be used to monitor response to treatment.[110] Therapy can be withdrawn once disease is in remission (typically after 2 to 3 years),[77] but relapse is high, occurring in 50% to 90% of affected people, particularly during the first 6 months.[258] A liver biopsy, though not necessary, may be helpful in predicting which clients will have successful drug withdrawal.[69]

Therapy for relapsed disease is the same as the initial treatment and can successfully induce remission of the disease. Individuals that have several relapses following drug withdrawal should remain on maintenance therapy with azathioprine or prednisone. The risk for HCC is increased in people with AIH, so individuals with AIH should be monitored.[166]

Liver transplantation may be required for clients who develop ALF, decompensated cirrhosis, or HCC.[166] AIH recurs in approximately 17% to 40% of clients who undergo liver transplantation.[75] Treatment is similar to initial therapy with prednisone and azathioprine, although doses are typically increased.[248]

**PROGNOSIS.** Prognosis depends on the stage of disease at the time of diagnosis and initiation of therapy, but 10-year survival rates surpass 90%, even for people with cirrhosis. The 5-year survival rate after liver transplantation exceeds 75%. People who respond to treatment often have life spans similar to healthy persons[63]; individuals who choose not to receive therapy (where therapy is indicated) have a 5-year survival of 50%.

**SPECIAL IMPLICATIONS FOR THE THERAPIST 17.9**

*Autoimmune Hepatitis*

Management of a client who has an autoimmune disease with liver involvement is a challenge. Energy conservation and maintaining quiet body functions during active liver disease must be balanced by activities to prevent musculoskeletal deconditioning with accompanying loss of strength, flexibility, and/or mobility.

## Alcoholic Liver Disease

### Overview, Incidence, and Risk Factors

ALD, ranging from alcoholic steatosis (fatty liver, occurring in 90% of heavy drinkers) and alcoholic steatohepatitis to alcoholic hepatitis and cirrhosis, remains one of the most preventable diseases and a major cause of liver-related mortality in the United States and worldwide. Alcohol-related problems result in significant morbidity and mortality; more than 48% of deaths from cirrhosis are alcohol related, and 30% of HCC cases are a result of ALD.[282]

There is a clear relationship between the amount of alcohol a person consumes and the likelihood of developing ALD. However, in persons who are heavy drinkers for long periods of time, only 10% to 20% progress to develop alcoholic hepatitis or cirrhosis.[89] Research suggests that genetics may play an important role in preventing liver damage despite chronic alcohol exposure.

Women are vulnerable to developing ALD at lower daily intake levels of alcohol than men owing to a decreased production of the gastric enzyme alcohol dehydrogenase, which breaks down ethanol, and a higher body fat percentage.[88]

Some cofactors that may predispose to cirrhosis include coexisting HCV, smoking, and obesity. Although much progress has been made in understanding potential causes, many questions remain such as determining which factors lead to severe liver damage and the mechanisms that protect other heavy drinkers.

### Pathogenesis

The initial physiologic change observed in the liver with alcohol exposure is the accumulation of fat, which is reversible with abstinence. In some people, with continued exposure to alcohol, there is a progression of damage to the liver consisting of inflammation, necrosis of individual cells, and early fibrosis. With continued heavy drinking, micronodular fibrosis (small bands of fibers) can develop and eventually progress to large bands of fibrosis, creating large nodules of fibrotic liver tissue (macronodular cirrhosis).

Epidemiologic research has demonstrated that heavy quantities of alcohol can have significant detrimental effects. Many mechanisms have been described that may be responsible for liver injury caused by alcohol consumption. Damage most likely requires several of these processes to be present, and genetic factors probably play a role in prevention or progression of liver injury.

Fatty liver disease (steatosis) occurs with the accumulation of triglycerides, cholesterol, and phospholipids in hepatocytes.[73] Alcohol, through various pathways, leads to the reduction in oxidation of hepatic fatty acids associated with increased lipogenesis.

Initial injury to the liver occurs with the production of acetaldehyde from the breakdown of alcohol by alcohol dehydrogenase. Acetaldehyde can form adducts (bonding) with proteins and DNA, interfering in their function. The metabolism of alcohol also involves the microsomal enzyme oxidative system where reactive oxygen species are formed, resulting in oxidative stress to the hepatocytes. This oxidative stress can lead to cell death and the release of damage-associated molecular patterns, which are not normally seen by the immune system. Once immune cells recognize these patterns, there is a release of cytokines and recruitment of cells into the area, leaning toward a proinflammatory cycle. Chronic alcohol use results in bacterial overgrowth and disturbance of the junctions between the intestinal cells. Increased gut permeability to bacteria contributes to the persistence of inflammation by increasing the volume of presentation of bacteria-derived lipopolysaccharides to immune cells, which further stimulates the immune system and inflammation.[73]

The liver responds to inflammation and injury by forming a scar. The cells that compose this scar tissue are the same for all diseases that lead to fibrosis and scarring, with the principle cell being the hepatic stellate cell. When the liver is damaged, stellate cells become activated by cytokines from surrounding cells and begin to proliferate. They then become fibrogenic. Other products and intermediates from alcohol metabolism may also contribute to the fibrogenic activity of the stellate cells.

### Clinical Manifestations

The initial histologic change noted in heavy drinkers is fatty liver infiltrate. This is often asymptomatic and detected only on laboratory evaluation. Even clients with alcoholic hepatitis and/or cirrhosis may be asymptomatic. Others may present with nausea, vomiting, abdominal pain, jaundice, anorexia, fever, and weight loss.

The most common signs in people with alcoholic hepatitis are tender hepatomegaly, fever, and jaundice. Splenomegaly is more common as the disease worsens, and HE (related to cirrhosis) can manifest in varying degrees, ranging from mild cognitive impairment to coma. Clients with alcoholic hepatitis or cirrhosis often display muscle wasting, spider angiomata, palmar erythema, jaundice, gynecomastia, or testicular atrophy.[175]

## MEDICAL MANAGEMENT

**DIAGNOSIS.** The diagnosis of ALD is made by obtaining the appropriate history of heavy drinking (many people are not forthcoming about their actual use), laboratory values consistent with alcohol liver disease, and lack of evidence for other liver diseases (such as viral hepatitis). Because ALD can manifest similarly to other diseases, the diagnosis of ALD should not be made without a thorough evaluation. The Alcoholic Liver Disease/Nonalcoholic Fatty Liver Disease Index is available to aid in distinguishing between these two diagnoses.[47,170] Alcohol can also accelerate fibrosis in diseases such as caused by HCV.[206]

A history of heavy drinking may not be present because of client denial. Only 50% of clients who abuse alcohol are identified by their physician. People with alcoholic fatty liver disease typically present with elevated AST and ALT enzymes, which are the most common abnormal laboratory findings in ALD. Bilirubin is typically less than 3 mg/dL. Ultrasound of the liver may show steatosis (fatty liver). Individuals with alcoholic steatohepatitis demonstrate inflammation on liver biopsy (alcoholic steatohepatitis is only a histologic diagnosis). Alcoholic hepatitis, however, manifests with rapid, worsening liver disease including elevated AST and ALT (AST/ALT ratio greater than 1.5) as well as increased bilirubin greater than 3 mg/dL. About 50% of people with apparent early disease (mildly elevated liver enzymes) will actually have advanced fibrosis or cirrhosis on liver biopsy.[141] ALD is usually accompanied by malnutrition and is evident in low albumin levels and other vitamin deficiencies. Anemia and thrombocytopenia may be present, while the white blood cell count frequently is elevated. Because the diagnosis of ALD can be made using history, physical, and laboratory information, liver biopsy is needed only in cases of diagnostic uncertainty.[60] Severity and prognosis of disease can be calculated using the Maddrey discriminant function score and the Model for End-Stage Liver Disease score (MELD and MELD sodium score).[180]

**TREATMENT AND PROGNOSIS.** Treatment of alcoholic hepatitis centers on cessation of alcohol drinking, nutritional support and education, and prevention and treatment of the complications of end-stage disease. Corticosteroids, principally prednisolone, can be used for severe cases of alcoholic hepatitis. Clients may display symptoms of systemic inflammatory response syndrome, even though they may not have an infection, requiring ICU support. Alcohol withdrawal is frequently seen, and treatment is based on hospital protocols, guided by scoring systems such as the Clinical Institute Withdrawal Assessment for Alcohol, revised (CIWA-Ar) scale. Vitamin supplementation including B complex, zinc, and thiamine should be administered. End-stage complications of cirrhosis are treated similarly to other causes of cirrhosis.[239]

Clients who develop cirrhosis (but are asymptomatic) and are able to abstain from alcohol have a prognosis of 80% at 5 years. Liver transplantation is offered to clients who have end-stage liver disease and are able to stop drinking, typically for at least a period of 6 months. This often allows for sufficient improvement to the point of not requiring a liver transplant. Outcomes of transplantation for ALD are similar to other groups requiring transplantation, with a 10-year survival of 58% to 73%.[240]

Prognosis depends on the severity of disease, other coexisting illnesses (e.g., HCV), nutritional status, the client's ability to abstain from alcohol, and the presence of cirrhosis. The prognosis and severity of disease can be determined using the Maddrey Discriminant Function score; the MELD predicts survival and is often used in allocating livers for transplantation.[74] People with a Maddrey Discriminant Function score greater than 32 have a 20% to 50% mortality within 30 days.[93] Once a person has developed alcoholic cirrhosis, the risk for developing end-stage liver complications, such as ascites, portal hypertension, and HE, is 25% at 1 year and 50% at 5 years. With abstinence from alcohol, survival improves to 60% at 5 years but is only 30% for individuals that continue to drink alcohol.[124,200]

**SPECIAL IMPLICATIONS FOR THE THERAPIST 17.10**

### *Alcoholic Liver Disease*

Follow the same guidelines regarding liver protection as are discussed in Special Implications for the Therapist 17.7: Viral Hepatitis. Increased susceptibility to infections requires careful handwashing before treating the client. (See also Special Implications for the Therapist 17.3: Cirrhosis.) The presence of coagulopathy requires additional precautions. (See Special Implications for the Therapist 17.1: Signs and Symptoms of Hepatic Disease.)

## Nonalcoholic Fatty Liver Disease

Nonalcoholic fatty liver disease (NAFLD) is the most prevalent chronic liver disease in the United States and a significant cause of cirrhosis.[10,54] There is a reported prevalence of about 30% (range, 10% to 46%), typically diagnosed between the ages of 40 and 60 years.[145,274] NAFLD can be categorized into nonalcoholic fatty liver or hepatic steatosis and nonalcoholic steatohepatitis (NASH). Nonalcoholic fatty liver is defined as fatty liver disease without significant inflammation or fibrosis, whereas NASH encompasses inflammation that may lead to fibrosis and cirrhosis.

The development of NAFLD is not completely understood and most likely involves genetic, environmental, and inflammatory factors. The metabolic syndrome, consisting of insulin resistance or diabetes, hypertension, obesity, and dyslipidemia, is closely related to the development of NAFLD and particularly NASH.[62] There may be genetic factors as well, as not all people with NASH have these risk factors, and not all people with these risk factors develop NASH.[70,285] Dysregulation of the gut microbiome may also have an effect, triggering inflammation that leads to liver injury.[15,39]

Most people with NAFLD are asymptomatic, but when present, symptoms of NAFLD (usually NASH) include right upper abdominal pain, fatigue, and malaise. Hepatomegaly may be present on physical examination. NAFLD may be asymptomatic and detected only incidentally by blood liver function tests or imaging performed for other reasons. The ratio of liver enzymes AST to ALT is less than 1, whereas for ALD, the ratio is greater than 2.

The diagnosis of NAFLD is made by demonstrating hepatic steatosis on imaging and verifying a lack of significant alcohol consumption. Similar to ALD, other liver diseases must be excluded as possible causes, such as viral hepatitis or AIH. Biopsy is reserved for cases in which the diagnosis is uncertain or to determine the level of liver injury. The NAFLD fibrosis score uses clinical information to recognize individuals who are at risk for severe disease.[254a] The degree of fibrosis can be ascertained using transient elastography.

Because NAFLD is related to diabetes and insulin resistance, lifestyle changes (dietary and exercise) are the key approaches to prevention and treatment.[46] Exercise is considered a rescue treatment—restoring adipose tissue insulin sensitivity and thereby rescuing the liver from lipotoxicity.[62] Moderate- to high-intensity exercise and resistance training linked with behavioral therapy is recommended three to five times each week.[46,122] Individuals at risk and with this condition should be advised to increase all forms of physical activity (e.g., taking the stairs, walking whenever possible) as well as engage in strength training of all major muscle groups at least twice a week.[83]

Currently there are few medications that may be helpful in the treatment of NAFLD. Aspirin may be beneficial in stopping the progression of nonalcoholic fatty liver to NASH, although more studies are needed to confirm this promising result.[238] As NASH increases the risk for cardiovascular disease and heart disease is the leading cause of death in people with NASH, treatment with a statin may be indicated.[108,243] Pioglitazone and liraglutide may improve inflammation and fibrosis in persons with NASH and diabetes mellitus.[14,32] NASH is also a risk factor for HCC, and clients should undergo surveillance. Alcohol consumption should be limited for anyone with NAFLD and eliminated for anyone with NASH. Individuals with cirrhosis due to NASH are treated in the same manner as individuals with cirrhosis from other causes—managing portal hypertension, esophageal varices, and ascites. Once a person develops cirrhosis with end-stage complications, a referral should be made for liver transplantation.

## Primary Biliary Cholangitis

### Overview and Incidence

PBC, previously termed primary biliary cirrhosis, is a chronic, progressive, autoimmune liver disorder. Similar to AIH, PBC has an autoimmune basis, but in contrast to AIH, the areas of destruction involve the small bile ducts. PBC is a rare disease, although the prevalence has been increasing. This is most likely a result of earlier diagnosis and prolonged survival. PBC occurs most frequently in women (80% to 90% of cases) between the ages of 40 and 60 years.

PBC is a slowly progressive (irreversible), chronic liver disease that causes inflammatory destruction of the small intrahepatic bile ducts, decreased bile secretion, cirrhosis, and, ultimately, liver failure. An autoimmune attack against the bile duct is probably an important pathogenetic element, but the precipitating event and contribution of genetic and environmental factors are uncertain. The disease is associated with other autoimmune disorders, especially Sjögren syndrome and autoimmune thyroiditis.

### Etiologic Factors and Pathogenesis

The underlying cause of PBC has a basis in aberrant autoimmunity. People affected with PBC express antimitochondrial antibodies (90% to 95% of cases). These are specifically targeted toward large enzyme complexes associated with oxidative phosphorylation (pyruvate dehydrogenase complex-E2).[92]

Although these enzymes occur throughout the body, only the epithelial cells of the small bile ducts in the liver are affected. This may be related to how a bile duct epithelial cell processes glutathione once the bile duct cell undergoes apoptosis.[129] Autoreactive T cells then respond to these antibodies, causing inflammation. As the ducts are destroyed, toxic substances build up in the liver, intensifying the damage. Chronic inflammation leads to fibrosis, cirrhosis, and eventually, without treatment, liver failure.

Research has also been investigating factors that lead to the production of antimitochondrial antibodies. Several hypotheses are centered on molecular mimicry.[129] Evidence suggests that antibodies made against bacteria have similarities to the pyruvate dehydrogenase complex-E2 in mitochondrial cells, thus producing antibodies that target bile duct cells. Some of the bacteria proposed to play a role in this process are *E. coli*, *Novosphingobium aromaticivorans*, lactobacilli, and *Chlamydia*.[129] Other possible environmental factors include chemicals such as halogenated hydrocarbons found in pesticides and detergents, but more research is needed to verify this association.[37,152]

### Clinical Manifestations

Most people with PBC are asymptomatic (50% to 60%) at diagnosis; the remainder may present with a range from minor symptoms to advanced disease. The most common presenting symptom is fatigue, which is noted in more than 50% of affected clients at diagnosis. With progression of the disease, fatigue becomes more significant, occurring in approximately 80% of people,[84] and may be disabling.[205]

Pruritus is frequently present (20% to 70%), particularly in the perineal area and the palmar and plantar surfaces of the hands and feet, although it can be diffuse. Pruritus often worsens at night or when the environment is warm and humid. Less commonly noted is the presence of right upper quadrant pain (approximately 10%).

Other symptoms of the disease include hyperlipidemia, osteopenia, memory impairment, and the presence of other autoimmune diseases (e.g., Sjögren and autoimmune thyroid disease).[153,271] In the later stages of the disease, clients may exhibit portal hypertension, malabsorption, fat-soluble vitamin deficiencies, and steatorrhea (the result of impairment of excretion of bile into the intestine). Complications from advanced liver disease include ascites, bleeding from esophageal varices, and HE.

The physical examination is typically normal in asymptomatic people, but skin manifestations often occur as the disease progresses. Pruritus frequently leads to excoriations of the skin, and spider nevi, thickening of the skin, and increased skin pigmentation are often detected with advancement. Xanthelasmas are seen in 10% of persons with the disease (Fig. 17.6). Hepatomegaly is noted in 70% of clients, yet splenomegaly is uncommon at presentation, often developing only near the end stages of PBC. Jaundice is observed later in the illness, often months to years after diagnosis. Muscle wasting, edema, and ascites often herald liver failure.

## MEDICAL MANAGEMENT

**DIAGNOSIS.** The diagnosis of PBC is based on a triad of criteria: presence and elevation of antimitochondrial antibodies, elevated serum levels of ALP (for more than 6 months), and imaging consistent with PBC (destruction of interlobular bile ducts). A liver biopsy is needed only when the diagnosis is in question (antibody levels may not be elevated) or to aid in staging and prognosis. The degree of fibrosis can be determined using transient elastography.

The clinical course of the disease is variable, and early diagnosis is important to initiate therapeutic measures before the development of advanced disease. People, particularly women, who have first-degree relatives with PBC should be screened by checking an ALP level.

**TREATMENT.** Most people with PBC are treated with ursodeoxycholic acid (UDCA), a bile acid taken in capsules. About 40% of people taking UDCA will have normal liver enzyme tests after 1 year of therapy. Only 35% of clients do not adequately respond to UDCA and require adjuvant therapy.[58] Clients with compensated liver disease who do not tolerate UDCA can be switched to obeticholic acid, whereas the combination of UDCA and obeticholic acid is reserved for people with compensated liver disease who do not adequately respond to UDCA alone.[156,186]

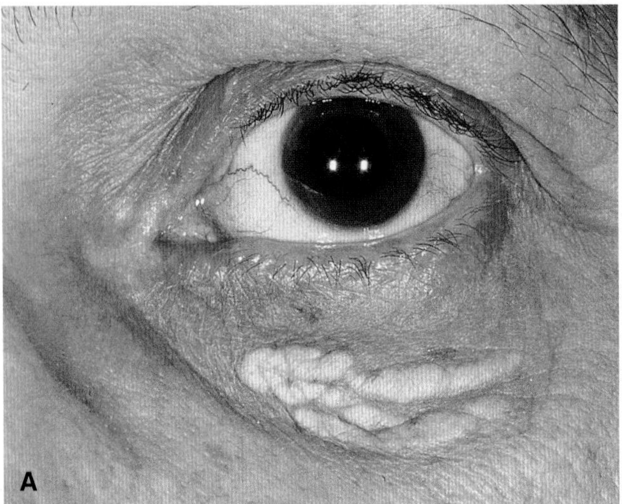


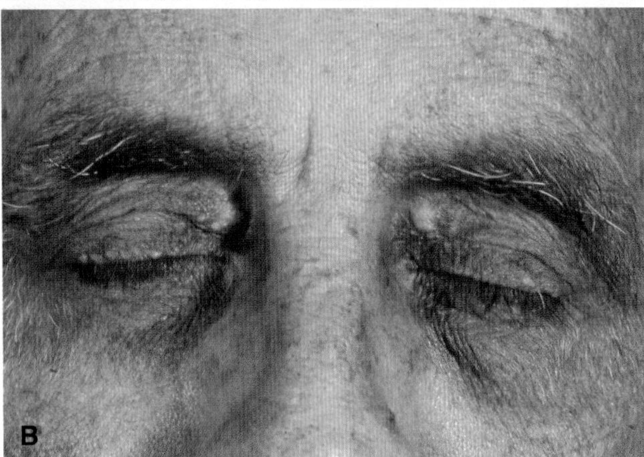


**Figure 17.6**

**Xanthelasma.** (A–B) Multiple, soft yellow plaques involving the eyelid (lower and upper). Lipid-laden foam cells seen in the dermis tend to cluster around blood vessels. Lipid deposits can also be seen along the extensor surfaces of the body (not shown) such as the heels, elbows, and dorsum of the hands. (A, From Yanoff M: *Ophthalmology*, ed 2, St. Louis, 2004, Mosby. B, From Rakel RE: *Textbook of family medicine*, ed 7, Philadelphia, 2007, Saunders.)

UDCA has also been shown to delay the progression to fibrotic disease, reducing the risk of death or need of liver transplantation.[204] It appears to be safe and has few adverse effects. UDCA has little effect in clients with advanced disease, and better options are still needed for this subgroup. Clients who have a complete response to UDCA require indefinite therapy. Progression, however, occurs in many people, requiring additional medical treatment or liver transplantation. Liver transplantation is considered for clients with bilirubin greater than 6 mg/dL, decompensated cirrhosis (i.e., HRS, diuretic-resistant edema, bleeding esophageal varices, and HE) or unacceptable quality of life caused by intractable symptoms, or anticipated death in less than 1 year.[163]

Complications of PBC such as fatigue, pruritus, osteoporosis, fat-soluble vitamin deficiencies, and hyperlipidemia also receive treatment. Fatigue is difficult to treat and can be debilitating. There is no recommended therapy, but several drugs have been studied, including modafinil.[135,236]

Cholestyramine, rifampin, and naltrexone are the principal drugs used to relieve pruritus, although side effects may not be tolerable. PBC-associated osteoporosis occurs in one-third to one-half of clients with PBC, but severe bone disease (i.e., with multiple fractures) is uncommon except in more advanced disease. Treatment with bisphosphonates is the preferred therapy. Because of a lack of bile acid secretion, the fat-soluble vitamins D, A, and K are not absorbed in the intestine. Fat-soluble vitamin deficiencies should be supplemented with parenteral or water-soluble vitamins. Many clients with PBC have significantly elevated serum lipids and may benefit from statin therapy. Planar xanthomas on the palms and soles of the feet can be painful and may be treated with plasmapheresis to decrease the serum cholesterol concentration.

**PROGNOSIS.** With the availability of treatment with UDCA, most people have a normal life expectancy. Only a minority go on to develop cirrhosis. Clients with a diagnosis of stage 1 or 2 disease typically have a better response to treatment. In one study, people with stage 1 or 2 disease who were treated with UDCA for a mean average of 8 years demonstrated a survival rate similar to healthy control subjects. However, in this same study, people with stage 3 or 4 disease were at significantly higher risk of requiring a liver transplant. The GLOBE score (https://www.globalpbc.com/globe), using clinical and laboratory information, estimates survival (without a transplantation).

Liver transplantation offers persons with liver failure improved survival. The survival rate at 1 year is 92%, and the 5-year rate is 85%. Recurrence can occur in up to 20% of clients receiving transplantation. Death is usually a result of hepatic failure or complications of portal hypertension associated with cirrhosis.

**SPECIAL IMPLICATIONS FOR THE THERAPIST 17.11**

### *Primary Biliary Cholangitis*

The most significant clinical problem for clients with PBC is bone disease characterized by impaired osteoblastic activity and accelerated osteoclastic activity. Calcium and vitamin D should be carefully monitored, and appropriate replacement should be instituted. Physical activity after an osteoporosis protocol should be encouraged but with proper pacing and energy conservation.

Occasionally, sensory neuropathy (xanthomatous neuropathy) of the hands and/or feet may occur as a result of increased serum cholesterol levels and an abnormal lipoprotein X. Cholesterol-laden macrophages accumulate in the subcutaneous tissues and create local lesions, termed *xanthomas,* around the eyelids and over skin, tendons, nerves, joints, and other locations. Treatment and precautions are as listed for this condition associated with diabetes mellitus or other etiologies.

## Pregnancy-Related Liver Diseases

Liver disorders associated with pregnancy include diseases specific to pregnancy, preexisting liver disease that is worsened by pregnancy, and disease that pregnancy may predispose to developing. Liver diseases associated with pregnancy have unique presentations, but it can be difficult differentiating these from liver diseases that happen to occur during pregnancy.[199]

Hepatobiliary diseases that are specific to pregnancy include intrahepatic cholestasis of pregnancy and acute fatty liver of pregnancy. Preeclampsia is manifested in multiple systems including the liver. Intrahepatic cholestasis (sluggish or interrupted bile flow out of the liver) of pregnancy leads to raised bile acids. The condition is characterized by pruritus and jaundice; it usually occurs in the last trimester of each pregnancy and promptly resolves after delivery. Most women present with pruritus; clinical jaundice is evident in only a minority of women. Abnormal liver tests with elevated serum bile acids are common. Intrahepatic cholestasis of pregnancy also increases the risk for a stillbirth. Although the absolute levels of bile acid where this occurs are not known, only women with total bile acids greater than 100 μmol/L had higher risks of a stillborn delivery.[195] UDCA is the treatment of choice.[19]

Acute fatty liver of pregnancy is a rare, potentially fatal complication that occurs in the third trimester (between weeks 30 and 38) or may not be noticed until the early postpartum period. Initial symptoms include nausea, emesis, epigastric pain, and malaise. Symptoms can rapidly progress to ALF if delivery is not performed. A careful history and physical examination, in conjunction with compatible laboratory and imaging results, are often sufficient to make the diagnosis, and liver biopsy is rarely indicated. The maternal outcome has improved considerably during the last decade. Prognosis of acute fatty liver of pregnancy has been radically transformed by early diagnosis, early delivery (delivery is planned at diagnosis), and treating complications.[20,268] Affected women should be evaluated for fatty acid oxidation deficits.

HELLP syndrome (hemolysis, elevated liver enzymes, and low platelets) is a rare but life-threatening complication of pregnancy. It may represent a severe manifestation of preeclampsia (hypertension and proteinuria), although 15% to 20% of women with HELLP syndrome do not have preeclampsia before developing symptoms. Most women exhibit proteinuria and hypertension. The most common symptom is colicky abdominal pain. Other nonspecific symptoms include nausea, vomiting, and malaise. Complications comprise disseminated intravascular coagulation, abruptio placentae, acute kidney injury, and rupture of hepatic hematomas. Rupture is associated with high mortality for both mother and child.[100]

## Vascular Disease of the Liver

The liver contains an extensive system of blood vessels. These vessels place the liver at risk for injury secondary to a multitude of vascular diseases or insults. Injury may occur secondary to passive congestion such as with right-sided heart failure or because of diminished perfusion, whether from thrombosis, ischemia, or obstruction.

Heart failure is the major cause of liver congestion, especially in the Western world, where ischemic heart disease is so prevalent. Right-sided heart failure leads to a passive congestion of the liver due to the inability of the heart to pump blood out of the right ventricle. The majority of clients with passive congestion remain asymptomatic. Left-sided heart failure can lead to decreased perfusion of the liver secondary to decline in cardiac output, resulting in elevation of liver enzymes.

Diminished perfusion can be a result of Budd-Chiari syndrome, hepatic infarction, sinusoidal obstruction syndrome, or ischemic hepatitis. The Budd-Chiari syndrome is an uncommon disease manifested by obstruction of hepatic veins where the veins open into the inferior vena cava (outflow obstruction). Causes may be primary, such as thrombosis of the veins, or secondary, caused by compression of the vein by cancer. Symptoms include fever, abdominal pain, ascites, lower extremity edema, and impaired liver function. Injury may be acute (with ALF), subacute, or chronic.

Hepatic infarction is a focal area of ischemia and considered separate from hepatic ischemia, which is a diffuse process. Hepatic arteries supplying the right side of the liver are the most commonly affected vessels. This may occur as an iatrogenic complication from laparoscopic cholecystectomy; thrombosis from hypercoagulable state (malignancy), atherosclerotic disease, or liver transplantation; or embolization from infective endocarditis or as part of intentional embolization for disease. Uncommon causes include polyarteritis nodosa, antiphospholipid antibody syndrome, and HELLP syndrome.

Hepatic sinusoidal obstruction syndrome is associated most commonly with early post-hematopoietic cell transplantation. The occlusion seen in sinusoidal obstruction syndrome is of the terminal hepatic venules and hepatic sinusoids, rather than the larger vessels. Weight gain, thrombocytopenia, and elevation of liver enzymes herald painful hepatomegaly and ascites. Acute kidney injury may result with 25% of clients requiring hemodialysis. Prophylactic treatment is available with UDCA or low-dose heparin. Therapy is principally supportive, though defibrotide is administered for people with severe disease.

Ischemic hepatitis or hypoxic hepatitis results when tissue of the liver does not receive adequate oxygen. This may occur in any disease process that reduces blood flow (cardiac failure, sickle cell crisis), reduces oxygen supply (respiratory failure, severe sleep apnea), or increases oxygen requirements (sepsis).

## Liver Neoplasms

Hepatic neoplasms can be divided into three groups: benign neoplasms, primary malignant neoplasms, and metastatic malignant neoplasms. Cancer arising from the liver itself is called *primary;* liver cancer that has spread from somewhere else is labeled *secondary* or *metastatic*.

Primary liver tumors may arise from hepatocytes, connective tissue, blood vessels, or bile ducts and are either benign or malignant (Table 17.4). Primary malignant cancer is almost always found in a cirrhotic liver and is considered a late complication of cirrhosis. Benign and malignant neoplasms can also occur in women taking oral contraceptives. A few rare tumors arise from the bile ducts within the liver and are associated with certain hormonal drugs and cancers. *Cholangiocarcinomas* are discussed later in this chapter.

### Benign Liver Neoplasms

**Cavernous Hemangioma.** Approximately 7% of autopsied livers contain hemangiomas, making this lesion the most common benign liver tumor. It is of unknown etiology and occurs in all age groups, more commonly among

**Table 17.4** Classification of Primary Liver Neoplasms

| Origin | Benign | Malignant |
|---|---|---|
| Hepatocytes | Adenoma | Hepatocellular carcinoma |
| Connective tissue | Fibroma | Sarcoma |
| Blood vessels | Hemangioma | Hemangioendothelioma |
| Bile ducts | Cholangioma | Cholangiocarcinoma |

women. The pathology is similar to that of hemangiomas anywhere in the body; it is a blood-filled mass of variable size (most are less than 5 cm) and can be located anywhere in the liver. Multiple lesions are observed in approximately 20% of cases.

Most hepatic hemangiomas are asymptomatic until they become large enough to cause a sense of fullness or upper abdominal pain. Hepatomegaly or an abdominal mass is the most common physical finding. Cutaneous hemangiomas may be associated with hepatic hemangiomas in children.[40] Hepatic hemangiomas are often discovered incidentally on CT scan or MRI or during laparotomy; otherwise the diagnosis is made by contrast-enhanced serial CT or MRI (particularly if small). Needle aspiration or biopsy is avoided because of the risk of hemorrhage. Larger hemangiomas (greater than 5 cm) should be followed yearly to assess the rate of growth.

Treatment is not usually recommended because most hepatic hemangiomas have a benign course with no risk of malignancy and minimal chance of spontaneous hemorrhage. Surgical resection may be performed if the hemangioma is consistently symptomatic, producing pain, or if the tumor is large enough for traumatic rupture to be considered a risk (e.g., a palpable lesion in an athlete). Other methods such as radiofrequency ablation, arterial embolization, and interferon alfa-2a have had limited success.

SPECIAL IMPLICATIONS FOR THE THERAPIST 17.12

### *Cavernous Hemangioma*

Most liver hemangiomas are small and found incidentally and require no special precautions. In the case of a known large liver hemangioma, the client must be cautioned to avoid activities and positions that will increase intraabdominal pressure to avoid risk of rupture. For the same reason, throughout therapy and especially during exercise, the client must be instructed in proper breathing techniques.

**Liver Adenomas.** Liver cell adenomas occur most commonly in the third and fourth decades, almost exclusively in women. The incidence of adenomas before the marketing of oral contraceptives was very low. Although the incidence remains low in men, oral contraceptives have significantly increased the incidence in women. Most remain asymptomatic, although with growth, right upper quadrant abdominal pain may be present. Although classified as benign tumors, they are highly vascular and carry a risk for rupture and subsequent hemorrhage. The clinical presentation is often one of acute abdominal disease because of necrosis of the tumor with hemorrhage. Pain, fever, and circulatory collapse may occur in the presence of hemorrhage. Most adenomas are evaluated with ultrasound, MRI, or CT; biopsy of lesions is not performed owing to the tendency to bleed. Liver function test results are usually within normal limits. Because of the risk of rupture and rarely malignant transformation to HCC, resection of adenomas that are greater than 5 cm or symptomatic is usually recommended. Affected women should refrain from taking oral contraceptives.

SPECIAL IMPLICATIONS FOR THE THERAPIST 17.13

### *Liver Adenomas*

The therapist is most likely to see a client with liver adenoma postoperatively after the danger of rupture and hemorrhage has passed. Standard postoperative protocols are usually sufficient.

## Malignant Liver Neoplasms

### Hepatocellular Carcinoma

***Overview and Incidence.*** HCC is the fourth leading cause of death from cancer worldwide and the fifth leading cause of cancer deaths among men in the United States[234]; it is also the most common primary liver cancer, constituting approximately 90% to 95% of primary liver cancers in adults. In Western countries, HCC is linked to cirrhosis, particularly HBV, HCV, and alcoholic-related cirrhosis. HCC is seen two times more often in men than women. Between the years 2000 and 2016, the rate of death from HCC increased by 43%, and HCC is the second most deadly cancer after pancreatic cancer.[123,126] This has been largely attributable to the increasing incidence of HCV infection,[190] although a reduction is anticipated with universal administration of the hepatitis B vaccine and hepatitis C cure.[126] Hispanics and Asians have the highest incidence and death rates (two times higher than among non-Hispanic/non-Asian whites).[235]

***Etiologic and Risk Factors.*** Although 15% of individuals with HCC have liver disease but do not have cirrhosis, there is a strong correlation between HCC and cirrhosis of any cause. Epidemiologic and laboratory studies have firmly established a strong and specific association between HCC and chronic infection with HBV and HCV. In the United States, HCV is a leading cause of HCC, particularly when associated with alcohol. Cirrhosis is typically prerequisite for HCC development in association with HCV, but not for HBV, which is directly oncogenic.

Another risk factor is dietary exposure to aflatoxin $B_1$, derived from the fungi *Aspergillus flavus* and *Aspergillus parasiticus*, a contaminate of cereals (grains) and legumes stored in hot, wet conditions. Aflatoxin $B_1$ exposure amplifies the risk of developing HCC in people already infected with HBV, making it a major concern in Africa and Asia.

Alcohol is a major risk factor for liver cancer. Tumor promotion has been linked to inflammation in the liver through alcohol-associated fibrosis and hepatitis. Even moderate amounts of alcohol increase the levels of circulating HCV in carriers of this infection. NAFLD, associated with obesity and the metabolic syndrome, is quickly becoming a significant cause of cirrhosis and HCC in the United States.[283] Other diseases, such as Wilson disease and $\alpha_1$-antitrypsin deficiency, also display an increased risk with the development of cirrhosis and subsequent HCC. Up to 10% of individuals with hemochromatosis (an iron overload disease) can develop HCC.[134]

***Pathogenesis and Clinical Manifestations.*** The exact events leading to malignant transformation of the hepatic cell remain unknown. However, the events that lead to cirrhosis, including inflammation and fibrosis, are known to predispose hepatocytes to genetic mutations. One of the most common mutations noted is in the *TERT* promoter.[227] The *TERT* promoter is also a prevailing insertion site for the HBV genome. Whether this integration is a necessary step for the transformation to HCC is still uncertain; however, it does appear that HBV is both directly and indirectly carcinogenic. HCV probably exerts both cytotoxic and immune effects.

HCC can be subdivided into proliferation and nonproliferation subclasses. The proliferation class, connected to HBV, demonstrates aggressive disease with associated activation of oncogenic pathways and immune proliferation.[261] The nonproliferation class does not express significant inflammation, and genetics are similar to normal hepatocytes. About 30% of HCCs demonstrate immune cell activation, while 25% do not.[232]

Most people who develop HCC are unaware of it until advanced stages. Right upper abdominal pain (60% to 95%) and weight loss (35% to 70%) are the most common initial symptoms. Other symptoms include weakness, fatigue, poor appetite, early satiety, abdominal fullness, diarrhea, and constipation. Jaundice is observed in only 5% to 25% of cases. Metastases occur to the bone and lungs, resulting in back pain and cough. Physical examination may demonstrate an enlarged liver, ascites, or splenomegaly. Many of these signs and symptoms may already be present because of cirrhosis and may not be distinguished as HCC.

Rarely, paraneoplastic syndromes (a result of a bioactive substance produced by the tumor) can be associated with this tumor. Hypoglycemia, caused by the defective processing of a precursor to insulin-like growth factor II, can occur early in the disease process and may be the presenting symptom. Polycythemia (an increase in erythrocytosis) occurs in less than 10% of cases of HCC but may warn of the presence of the tumor.

Uncommon complications include rupture of tumor with associated hemoperitoneum, thrombosis of portal or hepatic vein, and tumor embolism.

## MEDICAL MANAGEMENT

**DIAGNOSIS.** The widest range of therapeutic options are available to clients whose lesions are identified when 2 cm or smaller. Ultrasonography is typically used to screen high-risk people for HCC. Lesions less than 1 cm are monitored, whereas lesions larger than 1 cm require further imaging. Contrast-enhanced CT scan and MRI are the most commonly used imaging tests and have largely replaced percutaneous liver biopsy to avoid risks associated with needle biopsy (i.e., bleeding, tract seeding). CT most often is able to reveal tumor size and extent (tumor often involves the portal blood vessels). If the diagnosis is in question with imaging not meeting criteria for HCC, biopsy may be required. Definitive diagnosis is based on histologic findings in resected hepatic tumors or biopsy specimens.

Changes in liver transaminases are not helpful in distinguishing HCC from cirrhosis or other masses. One tumor marker that can be useful is serum alpha-fetoprotein. In high-risk populations, an elevation in alpha-fetoprotein is 60% sensitive and 80% specific.[159] Surveillance of high-risk clients often includes both alpha-fetoprotein and imaging.

**PREVENTION AND TREATMENT.** The use of vaccination to prevent infection with HBV has reduced the incidence of HCC associated with HBV.[51] This is the only malignancy for which an effective prophylactic immunization is available. In the meantime, early screening of high-risk populations using alpha-fetoprotein and ultrasonography remains the key to successful treatment of this malignancy.

Treatment of HCC depends on the size, location, and extent of tumor as well as the underlying liver disease and liver function. Guidelines are available to determine therapy. Surgical resection is recommended for individuals with cirrhosis but without portal hypertension or jaundice and only one lesion 5 cm or smaller. However, only 15% of cases are feasibly resectable at presentation. Liver transplantation is the most effective method to treat both the cancer and the underlying liver disease; transplantation is considered for people with cirrhosis who meet the Milan criteria and have associated portal hypertension and jaundice. Milan criteria include up to three liver lesions 3 cm or smaller or only one lesion that is smaller than 5 cm, no macrovascular invasion, and no extrahepatic spread. For clients who are not candidates for either therapy, nonsurgical locoregional treatments are offered. Radiofrequency ablation, microwave ablation, transarterial radioembolization, transarterial chemoembolization, and percutaneous injection therapy (with ethanol or acetic acid) are examples of available locoregional therapies.

Advanced disease that has not responded to other measures can be treated systemically. Sorafenib is a first-line therapy to treat people with advanced HCC.[157] Lenvatinib, a multikinase inhibitor, was approved for the treatment of HCC in 2018. Regorafenib, an oral multikinase inhibitor, and nivolumab, a humanized monoclonal antibody given intravenously, are second-line treatments.

**PROGNOSIS.** Clients who present with a solitary lesion, well-preserved liver function, and good performance status have a 60% survival at 5 years postresection. However, up to 70% of people in this group will have tumor recurrence. Liver transplantation offers a 5-year survival rate of 60% to 80% for individuals who meet Milan criteria (see Prevention and Treatment) with a recurrence rate of 15%. Symptomatic HCC has a very poor prognosis, especially in clients with multiple tumor nodules. Median survival of persons with HCC is 6 to 20 months, and the 5-year survival rate has improved from 10% to 26%, which is attributed to improved surveillance in high-risk individuals (those with hepatitis B and C and cirrhosis). Factors affecting the prognosis favorably include early detection (potentially curative at this stage[128]), tumor size (less than 5 cm), tumor location, presence of a tumor capsule, well-differentiated tumor, lack of vascular invasion, and absence of cirrhosis. However, the best hope for reduction in deaths due to HCC is through HBV vaccination, HCV cure, and surveillance programs in people with established cirrhosis.

SPECIAL IMPLICATIONS FOR THE THERAPIST 17.14

### *Primary Hepatocellular Carcinoma*

Liver tumors that cause elevation of the diaphragm can cause right shoulder pain or symptoms of respiratory involvement. Peripheral edema associated with developing ascites may be observed first by the therapist (see Ascites earlier). As the tumor grows, pain may radiate to the back (midthoracic region). Paraneoplastic syndromes (see Chapter 9) resulting from ectopic hormone may occur, including polycythemia, hypoglycemia, and hypercalcemia.

### Metastatic Malignant Tumors

The liver is one of the most common sites of metastasis from other primary cancers (e.g., colorectal, stomach, pancreas, esophagus, lung, breast, melanoma). Metastatic tumors occur 20 times more often than primary liver tumors and constitute the bulk of hepatic malignancy.

As with other types of cancers, secondary liver cancer can occur as a result of hematogenous spread, lymphatic spread, and local invasion from neighboring organs. The liver filters blood from the body, but because all blood from the digestive organs passes through the liver before joining the general circulation, the liver is the first organ to filter cancer cells released from the stomach, intestine, or pancreas.

The first symptoms of metastatic liver cancer are typically vague such as weight loss and right upper quadrant discomfort. Some primary tumors are known and have been treated before the development of metastatic disease. Others, for example, melanoma, may not be known, and workup of the liver lesion leads to the primary cancer location.

Diagnosis and treatment are dictated by the primary (original) neoplasm. Imaging, usually CT or MRI with contrast enhancement, helps verify the location and extent of disease. Biopsy may be required to confirm the diagnosis. Carcinoembryonic antigen (CEA) is elevated in some cancers such as colorectal cancer and may help identify progression of disease or response to treatment.

## Pyogenic Liver Abscess

The liver is the most common site for a visceral organ abscess. Liver abscess most often occurs among individuals with other underlying disorders such as hepatobiliary disease, pancreatic disease, abdominal infections, or liver transplantation. Other predisposing factors are diabetes mellitus and regular use of proton pump inhibitors. The most common underlying causes worldwide include *bacterial cholangitis* secondary to obstruction of the bile ducts by stone or stricture; *portal vein bacteremia* secondary to bacterial seeding via the portal vein from infected viscera following bowel inflammation or organ perforation; *liver flukes,* a parasitic infestation; or *amebiasis,* an infestation with amebae from tropical or subtropical areas.[280] In Asia, *Klebsiella pneumoniae* is an emerging pathogenic cause of liver abscess associated with colorectal cancer. It is an invasive syndrome characterized by liver abscesses and metastatic complications including bacteremia, meningitis, and necrotizing fasciitis.[241]

Clinical manifestations are commonly right-sided abdominal and shoulder pain, nausea, vomiting, weight loss, and fever. The liver's close proximity to the base of the right lung may contribute to the development of right pleural effusion. Complications of hepatic abscess relate to rupture and direct spread of infection. Pleuropulmonary involvement from the rupture of an abscess through the diaphragm and peritonitis from leakage into the abdominal cavity can occur.

The presence of an abscess is determined by contrast-enhanced CT scan or ultrasound. Most are polymicrobial and require radiologically guided needle aspiration. Treatment may consist of broad-spectrum antimicrobial therapy alone (for small abscesses less than 3 cm), or for abscesses less than 5 cm, percutaneous needle aspiration or catheter drainage can be employed. Broad-spectrum antibiotics are administered until culture and sensitivity information is available. Larger abscesses (greater than 5 cm) require catheter drainage of the abscess (usually 7 days) with antimicrobial therapy.[125] ERCP is also used to drain liver abscesses that may not be amenable to percutaneous aspiration. Surgery, open or laparoscopic, may be required to relieve biliary tract obstruction and to drain abscesses that do not respond to percutaneous drainage and antibiotics. Antibiotics are typically given for 4 to 6 weeks.

Mortality from hepatic abscess in developed countries is between 2% and 12%.[213] Amebic abscesses are an exception; when treated, the mortality rate is less than 3%. Early diagnosis and aggressive treatment can significantly reduce the mortality in some cases. Specific antibiotics are required whenever abscess is caused by amebic infestation.

SPECIAL IMPLICATIONS FOR THE THERAPIST 17.15

### *Liver Abscess*

Clients with liver abscess are very ill and usually are seen only by the therapist assigned to an ICU team. In such situations, vital signs are assessed regularly to detect high fever and rapid pulse, which are early signs of sepsis (a common complication). Movement, coughing, and deep breathing are important to prevent or limit pulmonary complications related to hepatic abscess, and skin care in the presence of high fever is essential. Careful disposal of feces and careful handwashing to avoid transmission are required when abscess is caused by amebic infestation.

# PANCREAS

## Diabetes Mellitus

The pancreas has dual functions, acting both as an endocrine gland in secreting the hormones insulin and glucagon and as an exocrine gland in producing digestive enzymes. The cells of the pancreas that

**Box 17.4**

**CONDITIONS ASSOCIATED WITH ACUTE PANCREATITIS**

- Alcohol abuse[a]
- Autoimmune diseases
- Cystic fibrosis
- Gallstones[a]
- Hereditary (familial) pancreatitis
- Hypercalcemia
- Hyperlipidemia (hypertriglyceridemia)
- Infection (bacterial, viral)
- Ischemia
- Medications (oral estrogens, antibiotics, AZT [zidovudine], thiazide diuretics, corticosteroids)
- Neoplasm (pancreatic tumors)
- Peptic ulcers
- Post endoscopic retrograde cholangiopancreatography
- Postoperative inflammation
- Pregnancy (third trimester)
- Toxins
- Blunt or penetrating trauma (including ischemia/perfusion that occurs during some surgical procedures)
- Vasculitis
- Unknown

[a]Most common causes.

function in the endocrine capacity are the islets of Langerhans, constituting 1% to 2% of the pancreatic mass. Defective endocrine function of the pancreas resulting in ineffective insulin (whether deficient or defective in action within the body) characterizes diabetes mellitus.

## Pancreatitis

Pancreatitis is a potentially serious inflammation of the pancreas and surrounding organs that may result in autodigestion of the pancreas by its own enzymes. Pancreatitis may be acute or chronic; the acute form is brief and reversible, whereas the chronic form is recurrent or persisting. Because the hormones and enzymes provided by the pancreas perform many vital functions, acute pancreatitis causes systemic problems and complications that affect the entire body. Approximately 15% of all cases of acute pancreatitis develop into chronic pancreatitis.

### Acute Pancreatitis

**Incidence and Etiologic Factors.** Acute pancreatitis is an inflammatory process of the pancreas that can involve surrounding organs as well as cause a systemic reaction. Pancreatitis can arise from a variety of factors and conditions (Box 17.4) or as a result of an unknown cause (15% to 25% of cases). About two-thirds of cases involve gallstones and chronic alcohol consumption. Yet only 3% to 7% of people with gallstones and 10% of alcoholics develop acute pancreatitis.[72] Other causes include biliary disease, hypertriglyceridemia (levels greater than 1000 mg/dL), trauma, infectious agents, ERCP, and, rarely, medications. The incidence has increased over the past few decades owing to increased obesity and gallstone disease, but the mortality rate has remained fairly constant at 5%.

Pancreatitis is classified according to the revised Atlanta classification of acute pancreatitis.[23] It can involve inflammation of the interstitium of the pancreas and peripancreatic tissue, termed *interstitial edematous pancreatitis,* or have necrosis of pancreatic tissue, called *necrotizing pancreatitis.* Interstitial pancreatitis accounts for 80% of cases and has a milder course and few complications, whereas necrotizing pancreatitis occurs in 20% of cases and can result in significant complications and higher mortality.

**Pathogenesis.** The mechanisms that lead to acute pancreatitis are not all understood and may be different depending on the inciting events or factors. Alcohol is a common factor in the development of acute pancreatitis; yet it occurs in people who have misused alcohol for years, not in people who binge drink. It is known that the risk of acute pancreatitis increases as overall consumption of alcohol increases, suggesting that alcohol and its metabolites, acetaldehyde and fatty acid ethyl esters, have a direct toxic effect on the pancreas.[12] However it is also evident that alcohol does not cause pancreatitis, but rather sensitizes the pancreatitis to multiple insults. Some of the effects include alterations in pathways such as cellular apoptosis, favoring necrosis instead of orderly cell death. Alcohol also affects zymogen release. Normally zymogens, inactive enzymes, are packaged into vacuoles and secreted out of the pancreas before being activated, but alcohol changes calcium signaling, leading to premature activation of trypsinogen to trypsin.[99] Alcohol also changes the location of secretion of the vacuoles by sensitizing the acinar cells to the effects of cholecystokinin so that the vacuoles are released in the basolateral position of the cell instead of the usual apical surface into the ducts.[56] Mitochondria are also affected. Typically mitochondria take up calcium and are induced to synthesize ATP and secrete zymogens. Alcohol interferes with calcium signaling, allowing for sustained concentrations of calcium. This in turn increases the mitochondrial membrane permeability with loss of membrane potential and eventual cell death or necrosis. ATP production is decreased, and the availability of oxidized nicotinamide adenine dincleotide is depleted. Endoplasmic reticulum normally stores calcium and is the site where proteins are folded and sent to their proper location. If the endoplasmic reticulum is stressed owing to pancreatic injury from oxidative stress, calcium imbalance, and/or buildup of misfolded proteins, this results in the unfolded protein response. Part of the unfolded protein response is the activation of pathways that promote the transcription of genes and result in necrosis and inflammation. Alcohol may also induce the production of some cytokines and chemokines that mediate inflammation.

Gallstone pancreatitis may be initiated by the reflux of bile into the pancreatic duct following the occlusion of the common bile duct with stones or sludge or blockage of the pancreatic duct at the ampulla.

Pancreatitis becomes severe when cytokines (interleukin-1, -6, and -8; tumor necrosis factor; and platelet-activating factor) and free radicals mediate a systemic response, leading to multiorgan failure and occasionally death. Severe ischemia and inflammation can disrupt the ducts, resulting in leakage of pancreatic fluid and formation of fluid collections and pseudocysts. A pseudocyst is a liquefied collection of necrotic debris and pancreatic enzymes surrounded by a rim of pancreatic tissue or adjacent tissues; it contains no true epithelial lining. Complications of pseudocysts include infection, bleeding, and rupture into the peritoneum. Infection can occur secondary to the breakdown of normal barriers in the gut because of hypoperfusion of the colon.

**Clinical Manifestations.** Symptoms in clients presenting with acute pancreatitis can vary from mild, nonspecific abdominal pain to profound pain accompanied by systemic symptoms and organ failure. Mild acute pancreatitis is defined by the absence of organ failure or local or systemic complications. Moderately severe acute pancreatitis demonstrates transient organ failure (less than 48 hours) and may have local or systemic complications. Severe acute pancreatitis exhibits persistent organ failure.[23] Most people with mild to moderate disease present with severe right upper quadrant abdominal pain, nausea, anorexia, and vomiting.

Pancreatitis related to gallstone disease is characterized by persistent, well-localized right upper quadrant pain. The pain is typically steady and at maximal intensity within 10 to 20 minutes. Pain can be triggered or made worse by eating fatty meals or drinking alcohol. Position changes may only partially alleviate the discomfort. Nausea and vomiting occur in 90% of people with pancreatitis and can be severe. Pain associated with pancreatitis caused by metabolic disorders or chronic alcohol use is not well localized, and intensity may be dull at first but can increase in quality and intensity to sharp and severe. In half of all pancreatitis cases, the pain radiates to the back.

A few cases develop into severe pancreatitis with serious complications. Symptoms that warn of worsening condition include fever, tachycardia, hypoxia, tachypnea, and changes in mental status. Complications of pancreatitis include acute peripancreatic fluid collections, pseudocysts, acute necrotic collections, and walled-off necrosis. These fluid collections can enlarge, leading to worsening pain. Bacteria can infect these collections and necrotic areas, resulting in pain, leukocytosis, fever, hypotension, and hypovolemia. Often the first sign of a complication is the failure to improve followed by unexpected deterioration. Ascites and pleural effusions are uncommon complications.

## MEDICAL MANAGEMENT

**DIAGNOSIS.** Diagnosis is based on clinical presentation, laboratory tests, and imaging studies. Early in the disease process, pancreatic enzymes released from injured acinar cells result in elevated serum amylase and lipase levels greater than three times the upper limit of normal. Amylase rises early (within 6 to 12 hours of symptom onset) but decreases quickly (within 3 to 5 days) so levels may not be very helpful unless the person seeks medical attention very early on. Amylase may also be elevated in other diseases such as celiac disease, parotitis, ulcerative colitis, and lymphoma.

Lipase levels are more specific to acute pancreatitis, rising in 4 to 8 hours, peaking around 24 hours, and staying elevated for 8 to 14 days. Lipase levels at least three times the normal range are indicative of acute pancreatitis. Elevated lipase levels are more sensitive to pancreatitis caused by alcohol than amylase.

Other tests may demonstrate hypertriglyceridemia or hypercalcemia. Imaging studies include abdominal contrast-enhanced CT scan or MRI to evaluate the pancreas (possibly serial examinations if symptoms fail to resolve with treatment) and transabdominal ultrasound to evaluate the gallbladder and cystic duct for possible gallstones. MRI is better able to diagnose early acute pancreatitis and early complications compared with CT.

In clients who have contraindications for ERCP, CT, or MRI with contrast, magnetic resonance cholangiopancreatography (MRCP), a noninvasive procedure that allows visualization of the biliary tree and pancreatic ducts without the use of contrast media, can be performed.

**TREATMENT.** For most persons (approximately 80% of cases), acute pancreatitis is a mild disease that subsides spontaneously within several days. Treatment for mild pancreatitis is largely symptomatic and designed to preserve normal pancreatic function while preventing complications and includes intravenous fluids for hydration, analgesics for pain control, and eating nothing by mouth to allow the pancreas to rest. If there is no improvement after 2 to 3 days, a CT scan should be obtained to determine whether complications are present.[255,279]

Clients are allowed to return home when the pain is under control and they are able to eat, drink, and take oral analgesics. Food intake traditionally progresses from clear liquids for 24 hours to small, soft, low-fat meals with a slow increase in quantity over several days as tolerated. If pancreatitis is secondary to gallstones, laparoscopic cholecystectomy can be performed before discharge from the hospital (if pancreatic fluid collections or other complications are not present). If fluid collections are present, surgery should be delayed until they have resolved. ERCP with endoscopic sphincterotomy may be performed preoperatively if there is a high suspicion of a bile duct stone or postoperatively if intraoperative cholangiogram demonstrates the presence of a bile duct stone.

It is important to identify clients with severe pancreatitis at admission to provide aggressive care and close observation for complications. The Acute Physiology and Chronic Health Evaluation score (APACHE II) is an accurate predictor of severity of disease, complications, and death. People admitted to the hospital with severe pancreatitis require admittance to an ICU, aggressive intravenous hydration, and pain control. Enteral nutrition (within 2 to 3 days) is preferred to parenteral feeding in most cases of severe pancreatitis because it decreases infectious complications.[87,249] Evidence fails to show a clear benefit of medications designed to improve the course of severe pancreatitis, and more research is required; some of these medications include pentoxifylline and protease inhibitors.[259,260]

Severe pancreatitis can be accompanied by significant complications including the formation of acute peripancreatic fluid collections, pseudocysts, acute necrotic collections and walled-off necrosis, bacterial cholangitis, and infected fluid collections and necrotic areas. Acute peripancreatic fluid collections typically form in less than 4 weeks from the initiation of symptoms, while pancreatic pseudocysts and walled-off necrosis occur after 4 weeks. Fluid collections should be followed by serial CT scans to verify improvement.

ERCP with sphincterotomy should be performed early in the course of severe pancreatitis caused by bile duct stones. This procedure decreases the risk for complications.[17] If the person's medical condition allows, surgery should be avoided in cases of severe pancreatitis because there is a high rate of death if done within the first few days of onset.

Fluid collections that are infected can be treated with antibiotics and drained; necrotic areas that are not infected can be watched. If necrotic areas become infected, empiric antibiotics are administered. A necrosectomy can be performed or the area can be drained percutaneously if the individual is not responding to antibiotics or is not stable.[87] Prophylactic antibiotics are not recommended for acute pancreatitis.[249]

**PROGNOSIS.** Prognosis of acute pancreatitis depends on the severity of the condition. Individuals with mild pancreatitis (80% of cases) have a better outcome than individuals with necrotizing or severe disease. The clinical course of mild disease follows a self-limiting pattern, resolving within 2 weeks of onset. Overall mortality is about 5%; individuals with interstitial pancreatitis have a mortality rate of 3%, while those with necrotizing pancreatitis have a mortality rate of 17%. In the first 2 weeks, death is often due to systemic inflammatory response syndrome; after the first 2 weeks, death is usually related to sepsis. Yet most people who experience severe pancreatitis are able to recover (recovery may take up to 2 months). Recurrences are common in alcoholic pancreatitis, particularly with continued drinking of alcohol.

SPECIAL IMPLICATIONS FOR THE THERAPIST 17.16

### *Acute Pancreatitis*

The therapist is most likely to see acute pancreatitis either when the early presentation is back pain (undiagnosed) or when acute respiratory distress syndrome develops as a complication, necessitating assisted respiration and pulmonary care. Pancreatic inflammation and scarring occurring as part of the acute pancreatic process can result in decreased spinal extension, especially of the thoracolumbar junction. This problem is difficult to treat and requires the therapist to make reasonable goals (e.g., maintain function and current range of motion), especially when the pancreatitis is in an active, ongoing phase.

Even with client compliance with treatment intervention and the subsiding of inflammation, the residual scarring is difficult to reach or affect with mobilization techniques and continues to reduce mechanical motion. Back pain associated with acute pancreatitis may be accompanied by GI symptoms such as diarrhea, pain after a meal, anorexia, and unexplained weight loss. The client may not see any connection between GI symptoms and back pain and may not report the additional symptoms.

The pain may be relieved by heat initially (decreases muscular tension); preferred positions include leaning forward, sitting up, or lying motionless on the left side in a fetal-flexed position. Promoting comfort and rest as part of the medical rehabilitation process may necessitate teaching the client positioning (side-lying, knee-chest position with a pillow pressed against the abdomen or sitting with the trunk flexed may be helpful) and relaxation techniques.

For a client who is restricted from eating or drinking to rest the GI tract and decrease pancreatic stimulation, even ice chips can stimulate enzymes and increase pain. In such cases, the therapist must be careful not to give in to the client's repeated requests for food, water, or ice chips unless approved by nursing or medical staff. Clients with acute pancreatitis are allowed to resume oral intake when all abdominal pain and tenderness have resolved.

#### Monitoring Laboratory Values

Monitor the individual with acute pancreatitis for signs and symptoms of bleeding; alert the health care team about bruising or prolonged bleeding. With acute pancreatitis, expect to see increased white blood cell count (inflammation), elevated hematocrit (associated with dehydration secondary to pancreatic necrosis), decreased hemoglobin when there is internal bleeding, tachycardia, and fever due to the inflammatory process. Mild confusion and hypoxemia are also common, so monitor pulse oximetry and ask about the need for supplemental oxygen if indicated. Monitor pain intensity levels using the same rating scale to determine changing patterns of pain and evaluate the individual's response to treatment.

## Chronic Pancreatitis

**Overview, Incidence, and Etiology.** Chronic pancreatitis is characterized by the development of irreversible changes in the pancreas secondary to chronic inflammation. Incidence and prevalence of chronic pancreatitis are low but have been increasing.[281] The principal risk factors are chronic alcohol consumption, smoking, and genetic predisposition.[165] In Western industrialized nations, the most common cause of chronic pancreatitis is alcohol misuse, accounting for about 45% of cases. Individuals who consume more than 5 drinks/day are more susceptible to chronic pancreatitis; however, only 3% of heavy alcohol users go on to develop chronic pancreatitis. Most likely, an underlying genetic variant places these people at a higher risk. Smoking significantly increases the risk of progressing from acute pancreatitis to chronic pancreatitis and increases mortality as much as five- to sixfold.[187]

Several mutations have been discovered that are associated with the disease, although the specific pathogenesis is under investigation. The *PRSS-1* gene is associated with hereditary chronic pancreatitis,[61] *SPINKI* encodes for a trypsin inhibitor, and *CFTR* is a cystic fibrosis transmembrane conductance regulator gene.

Autoimmune chronic pancreatitis occurs most frequently in the Far East and is associated with an elevated IgG level, diffuse involvement of the pancreas, a mass in the pancreas, an irregular main pancreatic duct, and the presence of autoantibodies.[192] It is occasionally related to other autoimmune diseases such as Sjögren syndrome, ulcerative colitis, and systemic lupus erythematosus.

**Pathogenesis.** The development of chronic pancreatitis is thought to result from inflammation that begins as acute pancreatitis (see Pathogenesis under Acute Pancreatitis earlier), but, instead of improving, becomes intermittent or persistent. Inflammation of chronic pancreatitis involves the activation of stellate cells, which leads to fibrosis and structural changes in pancreatic architecture as well as pancreatic function. Genetics most likely plays a major role.

**Clinical Manifestations.** Most clients with chronic pancreatitis present with abdominal pain, which is also the most significant problem. Chronic pain often leads to an abuse of opioids, decreased appetite, weight loss, and poor quality of life; it is also the most common reason for surgery in people with this disease. Pain is typically epigastric in location, often with radiation to the back. It is made worse with meals but can be relieved by bringing the knees to the chest or bending forward. Nausea and vomiting are often associated with the pain. Pain during the course of the disease varies; many people experience acute attacks followed by periods of feeling well. As attacks increase, pain becomes more chronic in nature. Other people have continual pain, which gradually increases in intensity. About 20% of clients do not experience pain, although they continue to have destruction of the pancreas and loss of pancreatic function.

The pancreas is able to compensate until greater than 90% of pancreatic function is lost. As the ability to break down fats (lipolysis) occurs before loss of the ability to break down protein (proteolysis), steatorrhea is one of the first symptoms of pancreatic insufficiency. Steatorrhea is the formation of greasy, foul-smelling stools that are difficult to flush. Endocrine function is also lost, resulting first in glucose intolerance and then, as a late complication, diabetes mellitus. In contrast to type 1 diabetes, there is destruction of both beta cells (which produce insulin) and alpha cells (which produce glucagon). This can lead to severe and prolonged hypoglycemia with the use of insulin.

History is often significant for alcohol abuse; other clients may have a history of pancreatitis or family history of chronic pancreatitis. Physical examination is usually significant for abdominal tenderness, with few other findings.

## MEDICAL MANAGEMENT

**DIAGNOSIS.** The diagnosis of chronic pancreatitis may be difficult to make, particularly in the early stages of the disease when the pancreas lacks significant functional or structural changes. Routine laboratory tests such as lipase and amylase are often not elevated except during an acute episode of pancreatitis. Steatorrhea can be diagnosed by determining fecal fat content in a 72-hour collection of stool. Owing to the difficulty of collecting 72 hours of stool, another option is to measure fecal elastase (one stool sample), which is both sensitive and specific in the early phase of the disease.

Imaging can demonstrate structural abnormalities in the pancreas. Some of the changes seen in chronic pancreatitis include pancreatic stones and calcifications, dilated pancreatic ducts (both large and small), strictures, lobularity, and atrophy. Pancreatic calcifications, which are indicative of chronic pancreatitis, are seen in only 25% of cases. Some of these changes, including atrophy and duct dilation, are seen in other diseases and with aging. Abdominal CT and MRI are most frequently used as initial diagnostic tests. If these are not diagnostic, other tests are used as needed, such as endoscopic ultrasound (EUS) or MRCP/MRI.

Genetic testing for mutations of the *PRSS-1* gene (related to hereditary pancreatitis) may be diagnostic in identifying people with hereditary chronic pancreatitis.

**TREATMENT.** The treatment of chronic pancreatitis is directed toward prevention of further pancreatic injury, pain relief, and replacement of lost endocrine/exocrine function. Intermittent attacks of severe pain are treated as acute pancreatitis. Cessation of alcohol intake is essential in the management of chronic pancreatitis in clients with alcohol-related pancreatitis. Smoking has also been linked with increased risk of mortality in people with chronic pancreatitis and should be avoided.[162] Clients should eat small, frequent meals that are low in fat.

Chronic daily pain can be treated with medications such as tramadol, low-dose tricyclic antidepressants, and gabapentin. Narcotics should be limited in their use owing to the risk of addiction. Pancreatic enzyme therapy can reduce steatorrhea, but evidence does not show a clear improvement in pain. Oral enzyme replacements are taken to correct enzyme deficiencies and to prevent malabsorption. Lipase may be used to reduce steatorrhea. Although diabetes is typically not seen until late in the disease process, insulin may be required in the case of islet cell dysfunction but should be used with care secondary to the loss of glucagon-producing cells. Nerve blocks and neurolysis have not been shown to improve long-term pain relief.

Various surgical procedures may be helpful in producing long-term pain reduction or relief. Surgical intervention to eliminate obstruction of pancreatic ducts or pseudocyst compression include lateral pancreaticojejunostomy, duodenal-preserving pancreatic head resection, and pancreaticoduodenectomy. A pancreatectomy may be performed as a last means of relieving refractory pain. People who undergo pancreatectomy can consider islet cell autotransplantation,[55] which has been successful in a small number of patients.

Care must be taken to identify other reasons for pain or change in symptoms in clients with chronic pancreatitis. The differential diagnosis may include peptic ulcer disease, pancreatic carcinoma, biliary or pancreatic duct obstruction, pancreatic stones, or expanding pseudocysts. Pancreatic cancer develops in approximately 3% to 4% of people with chronic pancreatitis and is often difficult to distinguish from chronic changes of pancreatitis.

Complications include the development of large pseudocysts, bleeding from pseudoaneurysms, splenic vein thrombosis, and fistula formation. A pseudocyst is seen in about 10% of people with chronic pancreatitis. Pseudocysts are fluid collections with well-defined walls and contain digestive enzymes. Adjacent organs such as the stomach or transverse colon may form a part of the wall. They can cause obstruction or compression on other organs or may become infected. Pseudoaneurysms are adjacent vessels that become affected by the inflammation of the pancreas. They may bleed into pseudocysts and cause rupture. Splenic vein thrombosis may develop secondary to inflammation and can lead to portal hypertension and associated gastric varices.

Uncommonly, rupture of the pancreatic duct may occur, resulting in pancreatic ascites, pleural effusions, and fistula formation.

**PROGNOSIS.** Chronic pancreatitis is a serious disease, often leading to chronic disability. Alcohol-related chronic pancreatitis has a poor prognosis without alcohol cessation, and continued alcohol use increases the risk of mortality by 60%. Overall, the 10-year survival of chronic pancreatitis is 70%, and the 20-year survival rate is 45%.[162]

**SPECIAL IMPLICATIONS FOR THE THERAPIST 17.17**

*Chronic Pancreatitis*

Back pain in the upper thoracic area or pain at the thoracolumbar junction may be the presenting symptom for some individuals with chronic pancreatitis, but past medical history including the presence of pancreatitis should raise a red flag and suggest that careful screening is required in these cases. People with alcohol-related chronic pancreatitis often have peripheral neuropathy.

The clinical presentation with aggravating and relieving factors (e.g., alcohol consumption, food intake, or positional changes noted) or failure to improve with therapy intervention adds additional red flag symptoms.[97] A person with known pancreatitis and/or pancreatectomy may need monitoring of vital signs and/or blood glucose levels depending on complications present. Education about the effects of malabsorption and associated osteoporosis should be included.

## Pancreatic Cancer

### Overview and Incidence

Pancreatic cancer represents the third leading cause of cancer mortality in the United States, with more than 45,000 deaths each year.[7,182] It also has the lowest 5-year survival rate after diagnosis (9%) of any type of cancer, being responsible for 7% of all cancer-related deaths.[7,182]

Most pancreatic neoplasms arise from exocrine cells, and about 95% are *adenocarcinoma* (75% in the proximal or head of the pancreas, 15% to 20% in the pancreas body, and 5% to 10% in the tail). The remaining primary pancreatic neoplasms include islet cell tumors and neuroendocrine tumors. Adenocarcinoma, the most aggressive type of pancreatic malignancy, is the focus of this discussion.

### Etiologic and Risk Factors

Although the specific cause of pancreatic cancer is unknown, as many as 10% of cases are possibly genetically linked to its development.[101] Some of the genes and genetic syndromes related to pancreatic cancer include the *BRACA1* and *BRACA2* genes, which also lead to breast and ovarian cancer. The *PALB2* gene is associated with both pancreatic and breast cancer. Hereditary pancreatitis develops secondary to mutations in *PRSS1* and increases the risk for pancreatic carcinoma. Lynch syndrome, familial atypical multiple mole melanoma (FAMMM) syndrome, and Peutz-Jeghers syndrome all exhibit mutations that result in increased risk of developing pancreatic cancer.

However, most people who develop pancreatic adenocarcinoma do not have a genetic or familial cause. Clear evidence has been shown of increased risk of pancreatic cancer related to advancing age with most people in their 70s and 80s at diagnosis. Pancreatic adenocarcinoma is rare in people younger than age 45 years; however, the risk increases after the age of 50 years.

Tobacco use (smoking and smokeless tobacco) accounts for 20% to 30% of cases and doubles the risk compared with nontobacco users. Chronic pancreatitis from all causes, particularly alcohol consumption and smoking, is associated with a much higher incidence and an earlier age of onset of pancreatic carcinoma.[272]

The presence of type 2 diabetes mellitus and impaired glucose tolerance are also risk factors for developing pancreatic cancer.[67] Obesity is associated with a 20% increased risk. Also, African Americans have a slightly higher risk for developing pancreatic adenocarcinoma.

### Pathogenesis

The molecular genetics of pancreatic cancer are becoming better understood, with multiple mutations noted in each adenocarcinoma. Mutations can be generally classified into three categories: alterations in genes that are oncogenic such as *KRAS;* inactivation of genes that normally suppress tumors (tumor suppressor genes) such as *CDKN2A, SMAD4,* and *TP53;* and inactivation in genes that aid in DNA repair such as *MLH1*.[121]

More than 90% of pancreatic adenocarcinomas exhibit a mutation in *KRAS,* and these mutations typically occur early. This abnormal gene produces a protein product that may be able to be targeted for early therapy. Loss of function of the *CDKN2A* gene results in the cell's inability to regulate the cell cycle. *TP53* mutations are frequently seen in pancreatic (75% to 85%) and other carcinomas. Cellular proliferation and cellular death (apoptosis) are both affected by the suppression of this gene. The *SMAD4* gene product normally transmits signals from the membrane (transforming growth factor-β receptors) to the nucleus. Inactivation of this gene results in dysfunction of this signaling pathway and is noted in about 50% of pancreatic adenocarcinomas. *BRCA2* mutations are seen principally in breast and ovarian carcinomas; however, these mutations also play a role in about 17% of pancreatic adenocarcinomas and can increase the risk 3.5- to 10-fold.[119] This gene normally functions in repairing DNA cross-linking damage.

Microscopically, adenocarcinomas contain infiltrative glands of various sizes and shapes surrounded by dense, reactive fibrous tissue. Many adenocarcinomas infiltrate into vascular spaces, lymphatic spaces, and perineural spaces. Pancreatic cancer appears to progress from flat ductal lesions to papillary ductal lesions without irregularities and then with irregularities (atypia) and finally to infiltrating adenocarcinoma.

### Clinical Manifestations

The clinical features of pancreatic cancer are initially nonspecific and vague or subtle in onset (e.g., anorexia, malaise, nausea, fatigue, pruritus), which contribute to the delay in diagnosis. Most clients are seen for abdominal pain (80% to 85%), weight loss (60%), and jaundice (47%). These symptoms suggest advanced disease. Typically, people with significant pain have a tumor in the body or tail of the pancreas, whereas jaundice and weight loss are more suggestive of a tumor in the head of the pancreas.

Pain is a common symptom of pancreatic carcinoma because of invasion of tumor into nerves. In later stages of the disease, pain may be intractable. Pain (especially night pain) is often epigastric in location, radiating to the back (thoracic or lumbar regions). Jaundice, accompanied by pruritus, dark urine, and acholic stools, occurs secondary to compression of the biliary tree by tumor. Obstruction of the portal vein results in the presence of ascites, enlarged liver, and palpable abdominal mass.

Pancreatitis may also develop from obstruction of the pancreatic duct. In some people, pancreatitis may be the first sign of the disease. The development of diabetes or glucose intolerance is common, particularly in the 36 months surrounding the diagnosis.[67] Deep venous thrombosis and pulmonary embolus can occur as a result of tumor presence.

**Metastasis.** Pancreatic adenocarcinomas metastasize first to regional lymph nodes and then via the hematologic and lymphatic systems to the liver, peritoneum, lungs and pleura, bone, and adrenal glands. These metastasized tumors may grow by direct extension, causing further involvement of the duodenum, stomach, spleen, and colon. Tumors of the body and tail of the pancreas are twice as likely to metastasize to the peritoneum compared with tumors in the head of the pancreas. Palpable metastatic cervical nodes may be present behind the medial end of the left clavicle (called the *Virchow node*) and other areas of the cervical spine.

## MEDICAL MANAGEMENT

**PREVENTION.** At the present time, the best advice to reduce the risk of pancreatic cancer is to avoid tobacco use, maintain a healthful weight, remain physically active, and limit alcohol use. Although the risk of pancreatic cancer decreases with increased activity, there is no clear dose-response relationship. Individuals who are at high risk for pancreatic adenocarcinoma may choose to undergo surveillance by either EUS or MRI to find a tumor earlier.

**DIAGNOSIS.** Pancreatic cancer is difficult to diagnose in its early stages. CT scan with intravenous contrast of the abdomen is the most common test in the initial identification of a pancreatic mass. Once a mass is located, pancreas protocol CT scans provide staging information that aids in determining resectability. EUS is helpful in viewing pancreatic tumors that may not be seen on CT and is accurate in detecting local lymph nodes. EUS is also the preferred method of obtaining a biopsy specimen for diagnostic purposes because it provides a higher diagnostic yield, is safe, and has a lower risk of seeding the peritoneum with cancer cells.

Laboratory tests can be abnormal, including elevated bilirubin level if biliary tree obstruction is present and evidence of malnutrition (low serum albumin or cholesterol level). The serum tumor marker CA 19-9 may be increased, but this is nonspecific for pancreatic cancer and should not be solely relied on as diagnostic. This marker can be useful, however, in monitoring treatment and should be obtained every 1 to 3 months during therapy. Clients should be tested for *BRCA* mutations, as a positive result will dictate and direct therapy.

**TREATMENT.** Treatment of pancreatic adenocarcinoma is based on the stage of the tumor and is often divided into three broad categories: resectable (15% to 20%), locally advanced (often encasing major blood vessels) (40% to 45%), and metastatic (40% to 45%). Surgical resection provides the only curative therapy, yet this is appropriate for only a minority of clients because even in what appears to be early-stage disease, micrometastases may have already occurred. Generally, pancreatic adenocarcinoma is thought to be resectable if the tumor does not involve blood vessels, metastatic disease is not present, and the individual is able to tolerate major surgery.[78]

There is currently no standard treatment for locally advanced disease. Therapy may include radiation therapy alone, chemoradiation, and chemotherapy alone. Some people have borderline resectable disease. These individuals may receive neoadjuvant therapy consisting of chemotherapy, with or without radiation, before surgery with the goal of reducing tumor size to increase the likelihood of complete resection at surgery.[3,112]

Metastatic disease can be treated with systemic chemotherapy, which may improve survival as well as duration of symptom-free disease. Much of the therapy offered to clients with pancreatic carcinoma is palliative to improve quality of life; therefore a palliative care consultation should be obtained. Pain control is a significant part of therapy. Long-lasting opioids and celiac plexus neurolysis can substantially improve quality of life.[13] Pancreatic enzyme replacement aids clients with malabsorption and steatorrhea problems. For clients who experience jaundice and will receive neoadjuvant therapy or may not be candidates for surgery, ERCP-guided stent placement in the biliary ducts can help relieve obstruction, or biliary bypass surgery can be performed.

**PROGNOSIS.** Survival rates for pancreatic adenocarcinoma are very low. About 23% of clients remain alive 1 year after diagnosis. The overall 5-year survival rate is only 9%. Surgical resection is currently the only treatment that provides long-term survival; yet only 37% of people with tumor deemed to be resectable are alive at 5 years[182]; this is most likely related to microfoci of tumor still present outside the main mass. For clients with locally advanced or metastatic disease, 5-year survival is only 12% or 3% respectively.[182] Long-term survival is rare, and the mortality rate is nearly 100%.

Factors associated with a more favorable outcome include tumor size less than 3 cm, lymph nodes without tumor, tumor-free surgical margins, and pathology consistent with a well-differentiated tumor.

**SPECIAL IMPLICATIONS FOR THE THERAPIST 17.18**

### *Pancreatic Cancer*

Similar to all health care professionals, the physical therapist has a role in primary prevention of pancreatic cancer through patient/client education, as smoking is the most significant reversible risk factor for this condition.

Vague back pain may be the first symptomatic presentation, and cervical lymphadenopathy (called the Virchow node) may be the first sign of distant metastases. The therapist is most likely to palpate an enlarged supraclavicular lymph node (usually left-sided), a finding that should always alert the therapist to the need to screen for medical disease.

Paraneoplastic syndrome associated with pancreatic carcinoma may manifest as neuromyopathy, dermatomyositis, or thrombophlebitis associated with abnormalities in blood coagulation (coagulopathy). The presence of coagulopathy represents a precaution in the administration of certain therapeutic interventions. (See Special Implications for the Therapist 17.1: Signs and Symptoms of Hepatic Disease.)

The therapist is most likely to be involved with a client with a diagnosis of pancreatic cancer who experiences intractable back pain. Referral to chronic pain clinics or hospice centers likely includes physical therapy services. Repeated nerve blocks may be performed after a reasonable effort to manage pain through the use of transcutaneous electrical nerve stimulation, biofeedback, analgesics, or other pain control techniques. Indwelling infusion pumps implanted to deliver analgesics directly to the site of visceral afferent nerves in the epidural or intrathecal spaces may be used for short periods (i.e., 1 to 3 months).

# BILIARY SYSTEM

See Table 17.5 for terminology related to the biliary tract.

## Cholelithiasis (Gallstone Disease)

### Overview, Definition, and Incidence

Cholelithiasis, or gallstone disease, is one of the most common GI diseases in the United States, occurring in an estimated 25 million people, or 10% to 15% of the adult population.[247] Most gallstones are asymptomatic and are detected on radiologic examinations performed for other reasons. In approximately 20% of cases, significant symptoms and complications develop because of the presence of gallstones, requiring surgery or other treatment. Age appears to play a role in the development of cholelithiasis, as gallstones are present in 20% to 35% of people by age 55 years.

Cholelithiasis occurs when stones form in the bile. These gallstones form in the gallbladder as a result of changes in the normal components of bile. Two types are classified according to composition: 75% consist primarily of cholesterol (cholesterol stones), whereas 25% are composed of bilirubin salts (e.g., calcium bilirubinate and other calcium salts), called *pigment stones* (black and brown). Symptoms occur when these stones block bile flow in any of the ducts, the most common being the cystic duct.

### Etiologic and Risk Factors

Many risk factors are associated with the development of gallstones (Box 17.5). Advancing age is a significant risk factor, markedly increasing after the age of 40. The composition of gallstones also changes with age—initially cholesterol in composition, while later in life more commonly pigmented.[247] Genetics plays a role in gallstone formation; in Native American populations in the United States, gallstone disease affects 67% of women and 30% of men.[79]

Obesity is a well-known risk factor, particularly in women. One study demonstrated a linear increase in the incidence of cholelithiasis as the body mass increased.[245] Women are also more than twice as likely to develop gallstones as men, principally owing to female sex hormones. This trend is seen until the fifth decade, when the risk for women approaches that of men, suggesting estrogen may be the principal factor. These hormones interfere with hepatic bile secretion and gallbladder function. Estrogen is noted to increase cholesterol secretion and decrease bile salt secretion, while progesterone leads to inefficient gallbladder emptying.

Because of the prevalence of gastric bypass surgery and other methods of extreme weight loss, rapid weight loss has emerged as a risk for cholelithiasis. One study demonstrated the development of gallstones in up to 50% of people within the first 6 months of gastric bypass surgery; 40% became symptomatic.[230]

People who receive total parenteral nutrition (TPN) often develop cholelithiasis; after 4 weeks of TPN, approximately 50% of people form gallbladder sludge.[105] Pregnancy is another common factor in cholelithiasis. As pregnancy progresses, the bile is more lithogenic (i.e., more prone to stone formation), and up to 5% of pregnant women develop gallstones. Many drugs contribute to the formation of gallstones. Estrogen is the most studied (i.e., oral contraceptives [excluding newer, low-dose products], estrogen replacement therapy), but reports show that the diabetic GLP-1 medications,[80] ceftriaxone, clofibrate, and octreotide are also lithogenic.[247]

Brown-pigmented stones are typically composed of unconjugated bilirubin and are seen in individuals with biliary stasis or a bacterial biliary infection. Black stones are commonly noted in people with disorders with a high hemoglobin turnover, such as chronic hemolytic anemias (e.g., sickle cell disease) and ineffective erythropoiesis. Cirrhosis and ileal inflammation (e.g., Crohn disease) also contribute to black stone formation.

**Table 17.5** Biliary Tract Terminology

| Term | Definition |
|---|---|
| Chole- | Pertaining to bile |
| Cholang- | Pertaining to bile ducts |
| Cholangiography | Radiographic study of bile ducts |
| Cholangitis | Inflammation of bile duct |
| Cholecyst- | Pertaining to gallbladder |
| Cholecystectomy | Removal of gallbladder |
| Cholecystitis | Inflammation of gallbladder |
| Cholecystography | Radiographic study of gallbladder |
| Cholecystostomy | Incision and drainage of gallbladder |
| Choledocho- | Pertaining to common bile duct |
| Choledocholithiasis | Stones in common bile duct |
| Choledochostomy | Exploration of common bile duct |
| Cholelith- | Gallstones |
| Cholelithiasis | Presence of gallstones |
| Cholescintigraphy | Radionuclide imaging of biliary system |
| Cholestasis | Stoppage or suppression of bile flow |

**Box 17.5**

**RISK FACTORS ASSOCIATED WITH GALLSTONES**

- Age (increasing incidence with increasing age)
- Genetic factors
  - Deficiency in ABCG5/G8
  - Pima women
  - Sickle cell anemia
- Decreased physical activity
- Pregnancy
- Obesity
- Diabetes mellitus
- Hypertriglyceridemia/low high-density lipoprotein cholesterol
- Rheumatoid arthritis
- Diseases of the terminal ileum
- Total parenteral nutrition
- Rapid weight loss
- Liver disease
- Biliary strictures
- Drugs
  - Clofibrate
  - Estrogen
  - Octreotide

## Pathogenesis

Gallstones are caused by changes in the composition of bile, especially bile salts, bilirubin, and cholesterol. When these solids become supersaturated in the gallbladder, gallstones may form. There are three types of gallstones: (1) soft, yellow-green stones (most common type) formed from cholesterol supersaturation in bile just mentioned; (2) small, brittle, black stones formed from high concentrations of calcium bilirubinate, usually caused by hemolytic disorders (e.g., sickle cell disease, hereditary spherocytosis), end-stage liver disease, or pancreatitis; and (3) soft, mushy, brown stones formed from calcium bilirubinate and bacterial cell bodies secondary to a bacterial infection that causes bile stasis.

Although multiple risk factors are known for the formation of gallstones, the mechanisms are not well understood. Abnormal regulation of hepatic cholesterol and bile acid synthesis with the deposition of cholesterol monohydrate crystals most likely play principal roles as well as gallbladder and sphincter of Oddi dysfunction.[216,266] Environmental and genetic factors likely affect the amount of biliary cholesterol. There are several genes that code for transporters of biliary lipids and receptors for lipoproteins. A deficiency in one of these, such as the ABCG5/G8 transporter protein, may be responsible for excess cholesterol secretion into bile.[103,104,214] Localized hypoxia, seen in severe liver disease, upregulates the gene *HIF1A*. This leads to the suppression of the secretion of water by hepatocytes and the concentration of biliary lipids, resulting in cholesterol gallstones.[16]

Gallbladder hypomotility is presumed to result from cholesterol interference in gallbladder smooth muscle (GBSM). Cholesterol inhibits spontaneous action potentials and calcium channel function in GBSM and decreases the ability of cholecystokinin to bind to receptors on GBSM. Hydrophobic bile salts also reduce gallbladder motility through activating receptors that inhibit contractility.[143] This is seen during pregnancy, after a period of rapid weight loss, in rheumatoid arthritis, and with TPN.[103,198]

Excess dietary cholesterol consumption may lead to an increase in the amount absorbed into the liver from the blood, but studies are conflicting.[177] Because of elevated levels of estrogen, pregnancy can also increase the amount of cholesterol secreted into bile and reduce bile acid production.

## Clinical Manifestations

The majority of gallstones remain asymptomatic once formed in the gallbladder. Only a minority (approximately 20%) cause painful symptoms. This occurs when the stone attempts to pass down the ducts leading to the duodenum, becoming wedged. The most common location of obstruction is the cystic duct (Fig. 17.7). This causes abdominal pain (often referred to as *biliary colic*). Pain is caused when a stone or sludge obstructs the cystic duct and the gallbladder contracts in response to a hormone or neural stimulation, increasing the pressure and distention in the gallbladder. The pain of biliary colic is typically steady, lasting from 30 minutes to 6 hours; it is usually severe and is located in the right upper quadrant just below or slightly to the right of the sternum with abdominal tenderness and muscle guarding. In more severe cases, rebound pain may be present. Painful symptoms are frequently related to meals, although not exclusively postprandial; for some clients the pain may be nocturnal. The pain often radiates to the right shoulder and upper back (60% of cases) and is associated with nausea and vomiting. Radiating pain to the midback and scapula occurs as a result of splanchnic (visceral) fibers synapsing with adjacent phrenic nerve fibers (major branch of the cervical plexus innervating the diaphragm).

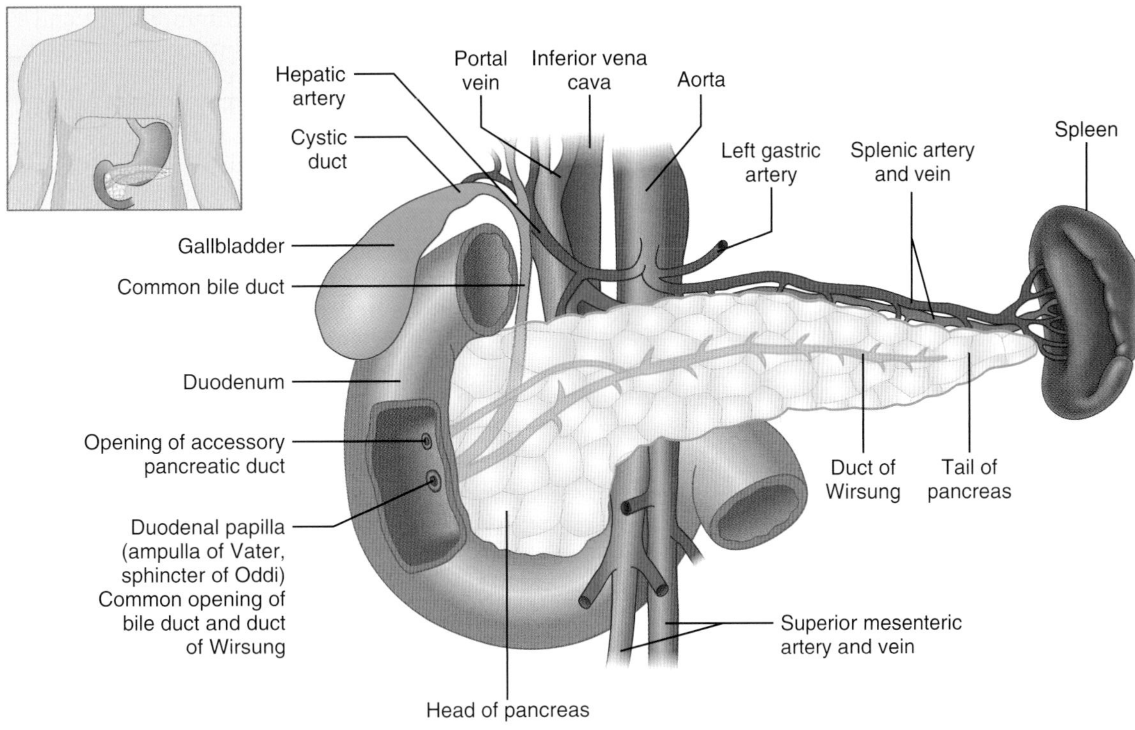


**Figure 17.7**

**The pancreas.** The pancreas (located behind the stomach) and gallbladder are anterior to the L1-L3 vertebral bodies. Attaching to the duodenum to the right, the pancreas extends horizontally across to the spleen in the left abdomen, coming in contact with the duodenum, kidneys, liver, and spleen. Obstruction of either the hepatic or the common bile duct by stone or spasm blocks the exit of bile from the liver, where it is formed, and prevents bile from ejecting into the duodenum. (From Black JM, Matassarin-Jacobs E, editors: *Luckmann and Sorensen's medical–surgical nursing*, ed 4, Philadelphia, 1993, Saunders.)

Episodes may develop daily or as infrequently as once every few years. Complicated cases often feature jaundice, fever, nausea and vomiting, and leukocytosis.

Other symptoms are vague, including heartburn, belching, flatulence, epigastric discomfort, and food intolerance (especially for fats). Gallstones in older adults may not cause pain, fever, or jaundice; instead, mental confusion may be the only manifestation of gallstones.

Serious complications occur in 20% of cases when a stone becomes lodged in the lower end of the common bile duct, causing inflammation (cholangitis), leading to bacterial infection and jaundice (indicating the stone is in the common bile duct). Sometimes acute pancreatitis develops when the duct from the pancreas that joins the common bile duct also becomes blocked (see Fig. 17.7). Approximately 15% of clients with gallstones also have stones in the common bile duct (choledocholithiasis).

## MEDICAL MANAGEMENT

**DIAGNOSIS.** Diagnosis is based on history, physical examination, and radiographic evaluation. Physical examination often reveals tenderness to palpation in the right upper quadrant of the abdomen. The radiologic test of choice is transabdominal ultrasound. Ultrasonography reveals gallstones in more than 95% of cases (when 1.5 mm or greater in size). Ultrasound can also provide information concerning the gallbladder and ducts and can aid in predicting possible technical difficulties during surgery.[203]

EUS can be used to detect stones too small for typical transabdominal ultrasound and to collect gallbladder bile for analysis. These latter tests are not routinely employed because transabdominal ultrasound is frequently sufficient for diagnosis. Other tests are available to detect the location of stones if they are not in the cystic duct and are discussed in the next section.

**TREATMENT AND PROGNOSIS.** Asymptomatic gallstones typically do not require treatment except in populations at high risk such as people at high risk for gallbladder cancer. This may include persons who have gallstones larger than 3 cm, a porcelain gallbladder (calcification of the gallbladder), or adenomas or polyps larger than 1 cm.

Once gallstones cause pain, there is a 2% to 3% annual risk of developing complications, and 65% of people with symptomatic cholelithiasis will have a recurrent episode in the next 2 years. Consequently, cholecystectomy is recommended for most symptomatic clients. Pain caused by gallstone disease can initially be treated with a nonsteroidal antiinflammatory drug.[57] Opioids are used only if the pain is not controlled. Clients who are managed as outpatients while waiting for a cholecystectomy should be reminded to seek medical attention if they experience pain longer than 4 hours, indicating a possible complication.

Laparoscopic cholecystectomy is the preferred surgical approach owing to the decreased length of hospital stay, shortened convalescence, and reduced postoperative pain compared with an open procedure. However, the procedure does have a higher risk of common bile duct injury, and some laparoscopic cholecystectomies require transitioning to an open procedure. When the gallbladder is removed, bile drains directly from the liver into the intestine, eliminating the opportunity for stone formation.

Medical treatment is used only in select clients who are unable or unwilling to undergo a cholecystectomy. Therapy is most successful for people with a functioning gallbladder, small (less than 1 cm) noncalcified stones (cholesterol stones dissolve more easily), and patent ducts. However, these characteristics are present in only about 10% of cases. Treatment consists of oral bile acid dissolution with UDCA/ursodiol. Extracorporeal shock wave lithotripsy is rarely used. Pain typically subsides after a few weeks of therapy, but multiple larger stones may require treatment for years. Even with successful medical treatment, 30% to 50% of stones recur within 5 years.

SPECIAL IMPLICATIONS FOR THE THERAPIST 17.19

### *Cholelithiasis (Gallstone Disease)*

Physical activity may play an important role in the prevention of symptomatic gallstone disease in up to one-third of all cases. Based on a limited number of studies, increasing exercise to 30 minutes of endurance-type training 5 times per week is recommended.[151] When the gallbladder has been removed (or is blocked by a stone), a small amount of less concentrated bile is still secreted into the intestine. The loss of a gallbladder itself does not appear to have an impact on physical activity and exercise.

In the past, gallbladder removal required a significant incision with muscle disruption, scarring, and frequently postoperative back pain associated with the formation of deep scar tissue. Now the closed procedure (laparoscopic cholecystectomy) can be performed as outpatient (day) surgery without these complications.

Air introduced into the abdomen during this operative technique is removed after the procedure, thereby reducing the postoperative abdominal pain. However, many individuals still experience referred pain to the right shoulder for 24 to 48 hours. Deep breathing, physical movement and activity as tolerated, and application of a heating pad to the abdomen (if approved by the surgeon) can help ease the discomfort.

The usual postoperative activities (e.g., breathing, turning, coughing, wound splinting, wearing compressive stockings, and leg exercises) for any surgical procedure apply, especially in case of complications. Early activity helps to prevent pooling of blood in the lower extremities and subsequent development of thrombosis. Early activity also assists the return of intestinal motility, so the client is encouraged to begin progressive movement and ambulation as soon as possible.

## Complications of Cholelithiasis

### Choledocholithiasis

Defined as calculi in the common bile duct, choledocholithiasis occurs in 5% to 20% of persons with gallstones and has the same etiology and pathogenesis. Common duct stones usually originate in the gallbladder, but they also may form spontaneously in the common duct and can therefore occur after a person has had a cholecystectomy (10% to 15%). Stones that occur in the absence of a gallbladder are referred to as *primary common duct stones*. Less than 50% of duct stones are symptomatic; they are typically small enough to pass through without causing an obstruction. When symptomatic, duct stones produce right upper quadrant pain, often with radiating pain to the shoulder and/or back, epigastric pain, and nausea and vomiting. Pain is often more prolonged than typical biliary colic (see Clinical Manifestations under Cholelithiasis [Gallbladder Disease] earlier). Liver enzymes are frequently elevated; in some cases the values can be similar to those seen in hepatitis. ALP and bilirubin values are usually elevated at least twofold.

Diagnosis is based on clinical picture and radiologic or endoscopic evidence of dilated bile ducts, ductal stones, or impaired bile flow. Transabdominal ultrasonography is usually the initial test and is able to stratify clients into categories of high risk, intermediate risk, and low risk of having choledocholithiasis. ERCP is frequently part of the work-up. ERCP consists of endoscopic introduction of radiopaque medium via a catheter into the opening of the common bile duct and pancreatic ducts as they enter the duodenum. This provides radiographic evidence of the patency or presence of stones. According to stratification, people at high risk can elect to undergo ERCP with stone removal and then cholecystectomy. Another option is to proceed to cholecystectomy with intraoperative cholangiography followed by ERCP to remove the stone (either intraoperatively or postoperatively). Clients found to be at intermediate risk for a common bile duct stone may choose to have EUS or MRCP or go ahead with laparoscopic cholecystectomy and intraoperative cholangiography. Clients can undergo cholecystectomy if found to be at low risk for choledocholithiasis.[59]

Complications of choledocholithiasis can be severe, including pancreatitis and cholangitis. Choledocholithiasis is currently the most common cause of pancreatitis in developed countries. Clients with mild choledocholithiasis typically will pass the stone spontaneously but require cholecystectomy to prevent another episode of pancreatitis (see Acute Pancreatitis earlier and Acute Cholangitis next).

SPECIAL IMPLICATIONS FOR THE THERAPIST 17.20

### *Choledocholithiasis*

Special considerations for the therapist are the same as for the client with cholelithiasis. When choledocholithiasis occurs in the absence of a gallbladder (primary common duct stones), the presenting symptom can be shoulder pain. The therapist must be alert to this possibility in anyone who has had a cholecystectomy. (See also Jaundice [Icterus] earlier.)

## Acute Cholangitis

Obstruction and stasis of bile from choledocholithiasis, biliary strictures, or malignancy can lead to a suppurative infection of the biliary tree, termed *acute cholangitis*. Acute cholangitis symptoms include those of biliary obstruction plus fever and jaundice. These three symptoms—pain, fever, and jaundice—are referred to as the Charcot triad and are noted in 50% to 75% of people with cholangitis. The Reynolds pentad (seen in only 14% of cases) includes the Charcot triad plus hypotension and mental confusion. In elderly individuals, hypotension may be the only presenting sign. The most common bacteria involved in acute cholangitis are those found in the GI tract: *E. coli, Klebsiella, Enterobacter,* and *Enterococcus*. Bacteria are isolated in the bile in more than 80% of cases and in the blood in 20% to 80% of cases (reports vary widely). The total bilirubin is typically elevated greater than two times normal, although it may be in the normal range early in the infection process.

Acute cholangitis can be categorized into three stages: grade I, mild; grade II, moderate; and grade III, severe. Severe acute cholangitis manifests with at least one new organ dysfunction, while people with moderate cholangitis have an elevated white blood cell count, fever, age over 75 years, hyperbilirubinemia, and hypoalbuminemia. Mild cholangitis does not meet the criteria for either severe or moderate cholangitis.[138]

Clients with the Charcot triad and elevated liver enzymes undergo ERCP for diagnosis and immediate treatment. In individuals presenting without the Charcot triad, but in whom acute cholangitis is still suspected, transabdominal ultrasonography is performed to identify stones or bile duct dilation. Abdominal CT scan, MRCA, and EUS are other tests that can be obtained if ultrasound does not demonstrate evidence of biliary tract disease. Empiric antibiotics should be given for all clients suspected to have cholangitis.

Treatment is given according to the severity of the cholangitis.[179] Clients with mild to moderate cholangitis typically respond to antibiotics and can undergo biliary decompression within 24 to 48 hours. Many clients with mild cholangitis respond to antibiotics and do not require biliary decompression. Clients who either do not respond to antibiotics or exhibit severe cholangitis should undergo biliary decompression within the first 24 hours. Endoscopic sphincterotomy with stone extraction and/or stent placement is the procedure of choice for biliary decompression and is successful in 90% to 95% of cases. EUS-guided cholangiopancreatography with biliary drainage and placement of a stent or percutaneous transhepatic biliary drainage are occasionally required when ERCP is not feasible or is unsuccessful. Surgical drainage is reserved for cases that are not amenable to endoscopic or percutaneous treatment. For clients with stones, elective cholecystectomy is later performed to prevent future attacks.

Complications of acute cholangitis include liver abscess, sepsis, and multiple organ system dysfunction. Mortality is high for untreated acute cholangitis—ranging up to 65%.[137]

## Acute Cholecystitis

Acute cholecystitis is the most common complication of gallstone disease, with 700,000 cholecystectomies performed in the United States each year. Cholecystitis, or inflammation of the gallbladder, may be acute or chronic and occurs most often as a result of impaction of gallstones in the cystic duct (see Fig. 17.7), causing obstruction to bile flow and painful distention of the gallbladder.

Acute cholecystitis caused by gallstones accounts for the majority of cases, and acalculous cholecystitis (i.e., gallstones not present) makes up the remaining 5% to 10%. Acute cholecystitis from stones is most common during middle age (particularly in women), whereas the acute acalculous form is most common among elderly men and carries a worse prognosis.

Acalculous cholecystitis is typically seen in people who are hospitalized and critically ill, such as clients who have undergone abdominal aortic reconstruction, cardiac surgery, or bone marrow transplantation. Immunosuppression, diabetes mellitus, trauma, burns, multisystem organ failure, and TPN are also risk factors.

Gallbladder disease is usually caused by gallbladder distention secondary to an obstructing stone interfering with the flow of bile. The increased pressure and stasis of bile leads to inflammation of the mucosa. For some people, inflammation results in infection and acute cholecystitis. Whereas gallbladder disease causes pain lasting less than 6 hours, acute cholecystitis causes prolonged abdominal pain lasting greater than 6 hours. The pain is characterized as steady in the right upper quadrant with tenderness, muscle guarding, or rebound pain. The pain often radiates to the upper back (between the scapulae) and into the right scapula or right shoulder. Clients may also demonstrate fever and a positive Murphy sign (interruption of deep breathing with deep palpation under the right costal arch). Accompanying GI symptoms usually include nausea, anorexia, and vomiting, and there may be signs of visceral or peritoneal inflammation (e.g., pain worse with movement and locally tender to touch).

Diagnosis is made on the basis of clinical history, physical examination, laboratory findings, and imaging. The white blood cell count is usually elevated (12,000 to 15,000/mL). Total serum bilirubin, serum aminotransferase, and ALP levels are often elevated in acute disease but may be normal or only minimally elevated. Abdominal ultrasonography is the test of choice, demonstrating stones, thickened gallbladder wall and/or edema, and pericholecystic fluid in persons with acute cholecystitis.[179] A sonographic Murphy sign may also be elicited. MRCP[179] or hepatoiminodiacetic acid (HIDA) scan is useful in demonstrating an obstructed cystic duct when ultrasound is not diagnostic.

Treatment consists of pain control, antibiotics, and cholecystectomy. Laparoscopic cholecystectomy is the procedure of choice because it is less invasive than an open procedure, and healing and hospital time are reduced. It is often performed during the first hospitalization for acute cholecystitis, although the exact timing depends on the surgeon's judgment; the presence of complications may delay surgery.[24,36,66,106,179.]

Although laparoscopic cholecystectomy offers most clients faster recovery, this procedure is also accompanied by a higher serious complication rate than open cholecystectomy. An infrequent complication of laparoscopic cholecystectomy is injury to the bile duct (0.1% to 0.2% of all cases), causing leakage of bile into the abdomen. If noted during laparoscopy (one-third of cases), the surgeon can convert the operation to an open procedure. Symptoms of unrepaired bile duct injury postoperatively include fever, abdominal pain, ascites, nausea, elevated bilirubin levels, and rarely frank jaundice. Intraperitoneal bile fluid collections can be seen on ultrasonography and CT. Prompt repair requires less treatment than delayed diagnosis, which often requires a more complex reconstruction.

Prognosis for acute cholecystitis is good with medical intervention. Complications can be serious and include gallbladder gangrene or perforation and cholangitis. The overall mortality of acute cholecystitis is 3%, but less than 1% in young, otherwise healthy people; mortality approaches 10% for older clients with complications or chronic diseases.[132]

SPECIAL IMPLICATIONS FOR THE THERAPIST 17.21

### *Cholecystitis*

Special considerations for the therapist are the same as for the client with cholelithiasis (see also Jaundice [Icterus] earlier). It is possible for a person to develop cholelithiasis cholecystitis, or inflammation of the gallbladder without gallstones. The therapist may see a clinical picture typical of gallbladder disease, including mid-upper back or scapular pain (below or between the scapulae) or right shoulder pain associated with right upper quadrant abdominal pain. Close questioning may reveal accompanying associated GI signs and symptoms.

The person may have been evaluated for gallbladder disease, but ultrasonography does not always show small stones. Unless further and more elaborate testing has been performed to examine gallbladder function, the individual may end up in therapy for treatment of the affected musculoskeletal areas. Lack of results from therapy and/or progression of symptoms corresponding to progression of disease requires further medical follow-up.

## Primary Sclerosing Cholangitis

PSC[133] is a chronic cholestatic disease of unknown etiologic origin characterized by progressive destruction of intrahepatic and extrahepatic bile ducts. It has been linked to altered immunity, toxins, ischemia, and infectious agents in people who are genetically susceptible.[144] Approximately two-thirds of cases occur in clients 20 to 40 years of age, and the incidence is thought to be rising; it is seen more commonly in men than women (3:1 ratio). Of clients with PSC, 90% also have inflammatory bowel disease, most frequently ulcerative colitis, yet only 5% of people with ulcerative colitis develop PSC.[176]

The inflammatory process associated with this disease results in hepatitis, fibrosis, and thickening of the ductal walls. This fibrosing process narrows and eventually obstructs the intrahepatic and extrahepatic bile ducts; the basic mechanisms of disease pathogenesis in PSC remain unknown.

About 50% of people are asymptomatic at the time of diagnosis. With the progression of disease, symptoms usually include pruritus and jaundice accompanied by abdominal pain, fatigue, anorexia, and weight loss.[144] Complications associated with the disease include bacterial cholangitis, pigmented bile stones, steatorrhea, malabsorption, and metabolic bone disease. Severe complications involve the development of cirrhosis and portal hypertension as well as the risk of developing cholangiocarcinoma (10% to 30% lifetime risk), HCC, and colon cancer.[207]

Diagnosis is made on the basis of clinical, laboratory, and radiologic findings. ALP is typically three to five times normal accompanied by a mild elevation in bilirubin. The diagnosis is confirmed by ERCP or MRCP, which demonstrate the characteristic "beads on a string" appearance of the bile ducts (strictures and dilation of the ducts). Liver biopsy is typically not required. Causes of secondary sclerosing cholangitis (such as chronic bacterial cholangitis and biliary neoplasms) and IgG4-associated cholangitis/autoimmune pancreatitis should also be excluded.[52]

Medical therapy is based on managing symptoms, correcting dominant strictures, and treating bacterial cholangitis when it occurs. Pruritus can be treated with bile acid–binding resins, and dominant duct strictures can be endoscopically treated (by dilation or placement of stents). Clients should receive vitamin D and calcium supplements, although select people may require bisphosphonates.

UDCA improves biliary secretion and laboratory parameters but has not been shown to significantly improve survival. Currently, liver transplantation is the only therapeutic option for people with end-stage liver disease resulting from this disorder.[144,219] Many clinical trials of medical therapy have been conducted, but none have demonstrated significant efficacy compared with liver transplantation. The results of transplantation for PSC are excellent, with 1-year survival rates of 85% and 5-year survival rates of 72%.[144] Optimal timing for liver transplantation is still not well defined, but the goal of therapy is to treat people as early as possible to prevent progression to the advanced stages of this disease or the development of cancer. Median survival without transplant is 10 to 12 years. Recurrence of PSC after liver transplantation occurs in approximately 25% of clients.[85]

SPECIAL IMPLICATIONS FOR THE THERAPIST 17.22

### *Primary Sclerosing Cholangitis*

Special considerations for the therapist are the same as for the client with cholelithiasis (see also Jaundice [Icterus] earlier in chapter).

## Neoplasms of the Gallbladder and Biliary Tract

### Benign Neoplasms

Biliary neoplasms, whether benign or malignant, are rare. Most nonmalignant tumors of the gallbladder and biliary tree are polyps. These polyps can be adenomas, pseudotumors, or hyperplastic inflammatory lesions, and most are found incidentally by ultrasonography or during cholecystectomy (for gallstone symptoms). Adenomas may be premalignant and have been associated with carcinoma in situ and invasive adenocarcinomas. Because polyps that are 1 cm or larger have a greater potential to be malignant, treatment consists of cholecystectomy.

### Malignant Neoplasms

Cancers of the biliary tract are divided into gallbladder cancer, cholangiocarcinoma, and adenocarcinoma of the ampulla of Vater. *Gallbladder cancer* is the sixth most common GI cancer, causing about 3230 deaths per year, and is the most common cancer of the biliary tree. Adenocarcinoma of the gallbladder is the most common type of gallbladder cancer (greater than 90% of cases), with squamous cell, adenosquamous, small cell, and neuroendocrine tumors accounting for the remaining cases.

Risk factors for gallbladder cancer include age (two-thirds of all cases occur in people age 65 years and older), female gender (women are more than three times more likely to develop gallbladder cancer), and gallstones (80% to 90% of people with gallbladder cancer have gallstones). Other factors include obesity, gallbladder wall calcification (porcelain gallbladder), an anomalous pancreaticobiliary junction, choledochal cysts, chronic typhoid carriers, and gallbladder polyps.[247] Gallbladder polyps larger than 10 mm are more likely to be malignant, whereas smaller polyps can be followed. However, despite these known risk factors, many cases of gallbladder cancer occur in people without obvious risk factors.

The pathogenesis of gallbladder cancer is not well understood, partly because it is often diagnosed at a late stage. Gallbladder disease is highly associated with gallbladder cancer, but gallstones are very common, whereas gallbladder cancer is very rare. It is supposed that gallstones decrease the speed at which bile empties from the gallbladder, allowing more time for inflammation and genetic mutations to occur.[142] Genes that are associated with gallstone disease are also implicated in gallbladder cancer, including the tumor suppressor gene *TP53*, the oncogene *KRAS*, the cell membrane receptor protein product of *EGFR*, and the protein product of *PIK3CA*, which is involved with signaling.[229]

Early stages of the disease include plaquelike lesions and small ulcerations in the mucosal lining of the gallbladder that progress to carcinoma in situ and then to invasive tumors.

Clinical presentation of malignant gallbladder diseases depends on the stage of disease and the location and extent of the lesion, but it is often insidious. By the time the tumor becomes symptomatic, it is often incurable. Symptoms most often mimic gallstone disease (acute and chronic cholecystitis). Right upper quadrant pain radiating to the upper back is the most common symptom (80% of cases), followed by nausea and vomiting and progressive (obstructive) jaundice (30% of cases). Weight loss, anorexia, fatty food intolerance, steatorrhea, and right upper quadrant mass (in advanced disease) may also be seen.

Pruritus and skin excoriations are commonly associated with the presence of jaundice. Gallbladder cancer is usually detected as an incidental finding at surgery thought to be gallstone disease, as a suspected tumor (because of symptoms) with the prospect of resectability, or as advanced unresectable disease. Only 10% of gallbladder cancers are discovered in the early stages due to symptoms; 20% of those found incidentally are detected early.

Ultrasonography is the most common initial test for diagnosis, although CT and MRI/MRCP are imaging tests of choice to determine the extent of disease. Disease can be metastatic to lungs and bones and usually involves the liver. Simple cholecystectomy is appropriate only for early stages; the remainder of cases require extended or radical cholecystectomy (with removal of lymph nodes, adjacent hepatic tissue, and/or portions of the extrahepatic biliary tree).[146,246]

For clients with unresectable disease and obstructive jaundice, endoscopic or surgical draining procedures may be done (stent or catheter placement). A biliary bypass (hepaticojejunostomy) can be considered if other options are not feasible. Overall prognosis is poor, with a 5-year survival rate of 18%. Cures are obtained only when all detectable tumor is surgically removed in the early stages of the disease. Localized disease has a 5-year survival rate of 61%; regional disease, 26%; and metastatic disease, 2%. Chemotherapy and radiation can be given as adjuvant therapy (after surgery) and are often used for symptom control and palliative therapy to prolong life.

Cholangiocarcinoma, or cancer of the bile ducts, is a rare tumor. Historically the term *cholangiocarcinoma* referred only to tumors of intrahepatic bile ducts; however, it now encompasses intrahepatic, perihilar, and distal extrahepatic tumors of the bile ducts. Cholangiocarcinoma occurs more frequently in people between the ages of 50 and 70 years; other risk factors include PSC, recurrent bacterial cholangitis, bile duct adenomas and papillomas, intraductal gallstones, certain infectious diseases (such as the liver fluke *Clonorchis sinensis*), and exposure in the past to the radiologic contrast agent thorium dioxide (Thorotrast).

Most tumors are located near the porta hepatis (60% to 70%), although 20% are in the distal bile duct, and 5% to 10% are intrahepatic. Affected persons most often present with jaundice secondary to obstruction of the bile duct (90% of cases) with associated acholic stool (light colored) and pruritus. Other symptoms include right upper quadrant abdominal pain, weight loss, anorexia, and fatigue. Individuals with intrahepatic tumors are less likely to develop jaundice.

On physical examination, hepatomegaly or a palpable gallbladder (Courvoisier sign) may be present with advanced disease. Laboratory values are consistent with biliary obstruction with an elevated bilirubin and ALP. CA 19-9 and CEA are elevated but nonspecific. CT scan or MRCP can detect the disease, and ERCP with brushings or biopsy may be diagnostic and relieve obstruction (a presurgical histologic diagnosis is often difficult to obtain).

Resectability is determined by a lack of metastatic disease, local invasion of the vascular structures around the liver, or the ability to completely resect the tumor. Laparoscopic surgery may be done initially to determine whether metastatic disease is present (metastatic disease is found in 25% of cases that were thought to be resectable by imaging studies). A pancreaticoduodenectomy (Whipple procedure) is performed for tumors in the distal portion of the biliary tree. However, because most cholangiocarcinomas are near the liver and large vessels, surgery must be tailored to the location of the tumor, with 35% actually resectable. Liver transplantation is a consideration for clients with hilar cholangiocarcinoma that is smaller than 3 cm and without extrahepatic metastases.

Radiation therapy and chemotherapy may be of some survival benefit.[209] Endoscopic or percutaneous stent placement for biliary decompression often relieves symptoms for clients with nonresectable disease. Cure is obtained by complete surgical resection of tumor. Survival rates are determined by extent of disease and involvement with large vessels and structures around the liver. The 5-year survival rate for resected extrahepatic cholangiocarcinoma without affected lymph nodes was 38%, while node-positive disease 5-year survival rate was only 10%. Clients with resected perihilar cholangiocarcinoma with multiple affected lymph nodes had 5-year survival rates of only 12%, while a single positive lymph node was 28%.[11] Perihilar survival has also improved with more expansive and aggressive surgical procedures. Resections with histologically clear margins with node-negative disease can have 5-year survival rates of 19% to 47%. Distal cholangiocarcinomas that are resected and do not exhibit positive nodes can have 5-year survival rates of 20% to 50%.[68]

Adenocarcinoma of the ampulla of Vater is a rare distal bile duct tumor. The ampulla of Vater is a small area (about 1 cm in diameter) located at the common opening of the pancreatic and bile ducts into the duodenum (see Fig. 17.7). This cancer has an incidence of four to six cases per 1 million people.

Risk factors include Peutz-Jeghers syndrome and familial adenomatous polyposis syndrome. Because of its location, this tumor causes obstructive jaundice early in the disease process (80% of cases). Abdominal pain (50%), weight loss (75%), and occult GI bleeding (30%) are other common symptoms.

Diagnosis can be made by transabdominal ultrasound, EUS, abdominal CT scan, and ERCP. Surgical resection, typically a pancreaticoduodenectomy, is the treatment of choice, although up to 50% of people have a recurrence without chemoradiotherapy or adjuvant chemotherapy. Resection is feasible in greater than 85% of cases with a 5-year survival of up to 50%.[65,210]

SPECIAL IMPLICATIONS FOR THE THERAPIST 17.23

### *Gallbladder and Biliary Tract Neoplasms*

Special considerations for the therapist are the same as for clients with cholelithiasis. See also Jaundice [Icterus] earlier and Special Implications for the Therapist 9.1: Oncology/Cancer in Chapter 9.

## REFERENCES

To enhance this text and add value for the reader, all references are included in the enhanced ebook on Student Consult that accompanies this textbook. The reader can view the reference source and access it online whenever possible.

CHAPTER 18

# The Renal and Urologic Systems

ELIZABETH SHELLY • G. STEPHEN MORRIS • JARED M. GOLLIE • CHARLENE MARSHALL • MICHAEL S. CASTILLO

The structures associated with the excretion of urine are (1) the kidneys and ureters, comprising the *upper urinary tract*, and (2) the bladder and urethra of the *lower urinary tract* (Fig. 18.1). The kidneys serve as both an endocrine organ and a target of endocrine action, with the aim of controlling mineral and water balance. The kidneys' main function is to filter waste products and remove excess fluid from the blood. Every day the kidneys filter 200 quarts of fluid; about 2 quarts leave the body in the form of urine, and the remainder is retained in the body.

These filtration and storage functions associated with excretion expose the kidney and bladder to carcinogens for extended periods, increasing the risk of cancer's developing in these organs compared with the other urinary tract structures. In addition, the urethra of females lies close to the vaginal and rectal openings, allowing for relative ease of bacterial transport and increased risk of infection. The shorter urethra in females also contributes to the increased incidence of urinary tract infections (UTIs) in females.

Therapists have an important role on the medical team for primary intervention for a number of renal/urinary tract disorders such as urinary incontinence (UI) and for those on dialysis or having a renal transplant. UI afflicts a significant percentage of the geriatric population, and UTIs rank second only to upper respiratory tract infections in incidence of bacterial infections. Therapists encounter these two disorders often as common comorbidities in the clinical arena.

The presence of a UTI increases the risk of infections developing elsewhere. This could occur while the therapist is treating someone for a knee injury or after cerebral vascular accident. Recognizing clinical signs and symptoms of renal/urologic problems (Box 18.1) will facilitate medical referral. Understanding how these diseases and the prescribed medical treatment can influence rehabilitative efforts is essential to help ensure a positive functional outcome.

## AGING AND THE RENAL AND UROLOGIC SYSTEMS

Aging is accompanied by a gradual reduction of blood flow to the kidneys, coupled with a reduction in nephrons (the units that extract wastes from the blood and concentrate them in the urine). As a result the kidneys become less efficient at removing waste from the blood, and the volume of urine increases somewhat with age. A tendency toward greater renal vasoconstriction in the older adult is evident, as compared with young individuals. This occurs as a result of oxidative stress in physiologic circumstances such as physical exercise, or in disease manifestations such as the effective circulatory volume depletion that develops in heart failure.[186] Physiologic changes in renal aging are associated with altered activity and responsiveness to vasoactive stimuli, such that responses to vasoconstrictor stimuli are enhanced, whereas vasodilatory responses are impa ired.[279,67,22]

Renal system changes that occur with aging cause alterations in the functional balance of fluid and electrolytes so that sodium regulation is not as effective. Mild hyponatremia is the most common electrolyte imbalance in the older population, affecting the musculoskeletal system.[140] Changes typical of the aging kidney are also accelerated when hypertension overlaps the physiologic renal process, because both aging and hypertension affect the same structure (i.e., the glomeruli).

A reduction in bladder capacity increases the number of times an individual urinates in a day and the urinary timetable also changes (i.e., length of time between episodes of bladder emptying). Although the kidneys produce most of the urine during the day in young people, a shift to night production over time makes one or two nocturnal trips to the bathroom commonplace after age 60 years.

Although specific age-related anatomic changes are not associated with urinary tract disease, certain age groups (e.g., older adults) are at significant risk of developing a variety of disorders. Hormonal changes in women, combined with the aging properties of the connective tissues, fascia, or collagen fibers, contribute to pelvic floor muscle dysfunction. Transient ischemic attacks and strokes may result in mild to severe deficits or fluctuations in muscle tone affecting the pelvic floor muscles.

The effect of multiple medications, conditions such as benign prostatic hyperplasia and pelvic floor muscle

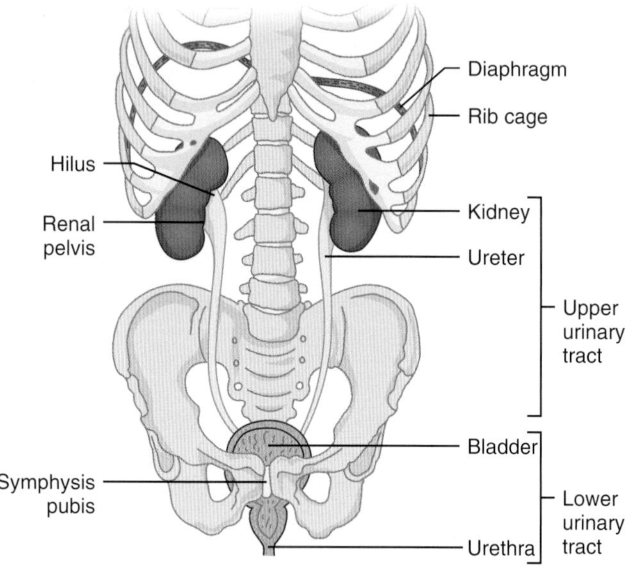


**Figure 18.1**

**Structure and function of the renal and urologic systems.** The kidneys are located in the posterior upper abdominal cavity in the retroperitoneal space (behind the peritoneum) at the vertebral level of T12 to L2. The upper portion of the kidney is in contact with the diaphragm and moves with respiration. The lower urinary tract consists of the bladder and urethra. The bladder, a membranous, muscular sac, is located directly behind the symphysis pubis and is used for storage and excretion of urine. From the renal pelvis, urine is moved by peristalsis to the ureters and into the bladder. The urethra serves as a channel through which urine is passed from the bladder to the outside of the body. (From Goodman CC, Snyder TE: *Differential diagnosis in physical therapy*, ed 3, Philadelphia, 2000, WB Saunders.)

**Box 18.1**

**MOST COMMON SIGNS AND SYMPTOMS OF URINARY TRACT PROBLEMS**

- Urinary frequency
- Urinary urgency
- Urinary incontinence
- Nocturia
- Pain (shoulder, back, flank, pelvis, lower abdomen)
- Costovertebral tenderness
- Fever and chills
- Hyperesthesia of dermatomes
- Dysuria
- Hematuria
- Pyuria
- Dyspareunia

dysfunction, and the incidence of pelvic surgeries and catheterization in the older population all increase the risk of developing urinary tract problems. A large number of adults older than age 60 years are incontinent, and many older adults require alternative living situations because of this disorder. Considering the percentage of the rehabilitation population made up by the older adult, therapists will continue to be involved in the treatment of renal/urologic disorders.

# INFECTIONS

## Urinary Tract Infections

UTIs are very common, affecting men, women, and children. Any portion of the urinary tract can become infected, although the bladder (cystitis) and urethra (urethritis) are usually involved. Bacteria may also spread to the upper portion of the urinary tract and involve the kidneys, causing a more serious infection referred to as *pyelonephritis*.

UTIs can be defined as either uncomplicated or complicated, and relapsed or recurrent. Complicated infections develop in persons with factors that can make diagnosis and treatment difficult—including diabetes, history of stroke, pregnancy, immunosuppression, structural abnormalities, or functional abnormalities of the urinary tract. The presence of such complications often requires longer treatment and further testing.[240]

Generally, UTIs in men, pregnant women, children, and clients who are hospitalized or in a long-term care setting can be considered complicated. Uncomplicated UTIs lack these factors and are more easily diagnosed and treated. UTIs may relapse or, more commonly, recur. Relapsed infections are infections that persist with the original organism without completely clearing. Recurrence of UTIs is considered a different infection that occurs after successful treatment of the initial infection, although it may be with the same organism because of repeated contamination.[240]

### Incidence and Prevalence

UTIs are among the most common bacterial infections acquired in the community and in hospitals. In individuals without anatomic or functional abnormalities, UTIs are generally self-limiting, but have a propensity to recur.[88] UTIs frequently occur in the general population, although women and older adults comprise the majority of cases. UTIs affect more than 150 million people per year worldwide,[84] By age 24, one-third of women will have had at least one physician-diagnosed UTI that is treated with prescription medication.

For those living in skilled nursing facilities, assisted living arrangements, or extended care facilities, urinary tract infection is the second most frequent type of infection and the most common cause of hospitalization.[93,127] The cost is substantial at more than $2.8 billion per year (diagnosis, treatment, and management cost). UTIs also result in restrictions in daily activities and lost days of work.

### Etiologic and Risk Factors

Most UTIs occur in adult women. The urethra in females is shorter, compared to that in males, and also close to the entrances to the vagina and rectum. The bacteria that result in most UTIs are acquired from the large bowel (fecal flora). The urethral meatus is close to the fecal reservoir and rectum.

Young, sexually active women are at higher risk of developing UTIs because it is thought that sexual intercourse can influence the movement of bacteria in the direction of the bladder. This again is because of the proximity of the urethral meatus and vagina. There are

Box 18.2

**RISK FACTORS FOR URINARY TRACT INFECTIONS**

- Age
- Immobility/inactivity
- Urinary retention
- Instrumentation; frequent urinary catheterization
- Atonic bladder (spinal cord injury; diabetic neuropathy)
- Increased sexual activity
- Spermicide associated in use with diaphragm or condoms
- Uncircumcised penis
- Obstruction
  - Renal calculi
  - Prostatic hyperplasia
  - Malformations or urinary tract abnormalities
- Constipation
- Women greater than men (see explanation in text)
  - Anatomic variations
  - Surgical or natural menopause without hormone replacement therapy
  - Pregnancy
- Kidney transplantation
- Diabetes mellitus
- Partners of Viagra (sildenafil citrate) users*
- Sexually transmitted disease (urethritis)

*This is most likely the result of increased frequency of intercourse in women older than age 35 years, who are more likely to also experience vaginal dryness.

numerous risk factors for UTIs (Box 18.2) that depend upon the characteristics of the person affected. For example, risk factors for an acute, uncomplicated UTI in a premenopausal woman may be different than those for a postmenopausal woman in a long-term care setting.

For young women, the most common risk factors include a history of a previous UTI, frequent or recent sexual activity, or the use of a spermicidal agent.[79] UTIs are also more common during pregnancy. The increased risk is from dilation of the upper urinary system, reduction of the peristaltic activity of the ureters, and displacement of the urinary bladder, which moves to a more abdominal position, thus further affecting the ureteral position.

In older women who are in a long-term care setting, the most frequently noted risk factors are advancing age and debilitation associated with conditions that impair voiding or cause poor perineal hygiene, such as dementia or stroke.[160] Healthy, community-dwelling postmenopausal women share risk factors seen in both young and older women. Sexual activity and a previous history of UTI are common risk factors for both young and postmenopausal women, while incontinence is an additional risk factor in these older women.[122] The effects of estrogen decline (dry mucosa and vaginitis) may contribute to increased risk of infection because of the change in vaginal flora, but study findings remain unclear.

People with diabetes receiving treatment are also more prone to UTIs as a consequence of immunologic impairments; the presence of glycosuria, which provides a fertile medium for bacterial growth, and voiding difficulties resulting from diabetic neuropathy (detrusor paresis).[27,183]

Another significant and common risk factor for UTI is indwelling catheterization. Placement of a urinary catheter is a leading cause of infection in the hospital setting, accounting for 40% of health care–associated infections. The reasons are clearly related to the introduction of a foreign body that provides a direct pathway for bacteria to travel from the perineum to the bladder.

Less commonly, a client may display a structural or functional abnormality that leads to a UTI. Contributing structural problems may be kidney stones, cystocele, or prostatic hyperplasia. Examples of functional problems include reflux of urine from the bladder to the kidney and neurogenic bladder from diabetes, spinal cord injury, or multiple sclerosis. Neurologic conditions that can result in low bladder tone and urine retention contributing to UTI include Parkinson disease, multiple systems atrophy, multiple sclerosis, sacral lesions, lower motor nerve conus lesions, disc disease, trauma following pelvic surgery, and diabetes mellitus.

Overactivity in the pelvic floor muscle (PFM), disorders of increased PFM tone, and interstitial cystitis can mimic symptoms of UTI.[129,225] Therapists should encourage patients to have urine tested and avoid automatic prescription of antibiotics, especially with recurrent UTI and in the presence of other pelvic pain syndromes.[129,225]

## Pathogenesis

The bacteria most often responsible for UTI are fecal-associated gram-negative organisms, with *Escherichia coli* accounting for approximately 80% of urinary tract pathogens. *Staphylococcus saprophyticus* causes 5% to 15% of UTIs, while *Enterococcus*, *Klebsiella*, and *Proteus* make up the remaining common organisms.

Hospitalized clients are more likely to become infected with *Enterobacter*, *Klebsiella*, *Proteus*, *Pseudomonas*, enterococci, and staphylococci bacteria than outpatients with UTI. *Candida* species can be seen in persons who have undergone invasive instrumental investigations or catheterizations and in children with urogenital abnormalities.

These common urinary tract pathogens are able to adhere to the urinary tract mucosa, colonize, and cause infection. Several subtypes of bacteria contain genes that allow for greater virulence and ability to colonize urothelium than other organisms, making them uropathogenic. Uropathogens have specialized characteristics, such as the production of adhesins, siderophores, and toxins that enable them to colonize and invade the urinary tract. The most common route of entry of bacteria into the urinary tract is ascending up the urethra into the bladder.[88] Although infrequent in occurrence, infections may be bloodborne (bacteria in the bloodstream) or acquired via the lymphatic system.

## Clinical Manifestations

Classic features of UTIs are evident in older children and adults and include frequency, urgency, dysuria, nocturia, and, in children, enuresis. Fever, chills, and malaise may also be present. The individual may notice cloudy, bloody, or foul-smelling urine and a burning or painful sensation during urination or intercourse.

Pain may be noted in the suprapubic, lower abdominal, groin, or flank areas, depending on the location of the infection.

In the case of kidney involvement, the diaphragm may become irritated, resulting in ipsilateral shoulder or lumbar back pain. The clinical manifestations in frail, older adults can be varied, often with malaise, anorexia, and mental status changes (especially confusion or increased confusion) as the most prominent features. Flank pain, fever, and chills often indicate an upper UTI or pyelonephritis.

Asymptomatic bacterial urine infections occur in approximately 10% of women in early pregnancy[151] (and 25%-50% in residents of long-term care facilities).[204] In elderly adults, new-onset confusion or delirium may be a sign of UTI.[75,76] Physical therapists are in a unique position to recognize this and should encourage consultation with the physician in these circumstances.

## MEDICAL MANAGEMENT

**PREVENTION.** UTIs can be prevented in some cases by drinking at least eight 8-oz glasses of water each day; urinating soon after sexual intercourse; for females, wiping from the front to back after urination[202] so that bacteria from the anal area are not pushed into the urethra;[202] changing sanitary pads often during menstruation; and washing the genital area with warm water before sexual activity to minimize the chance that bacteria can be introduced. The use of spermicidal agents with a diaphragm is associated with an increased risk for UTIs. The use of another form of birth control may be warranted if repeated UTIs become problematic.

Certain foods may also be preventative. Berry juices and products containing fermented milk may be helpful in reducing the occurrence of UTIs, although further studies are needed to verify this relationship.[147] The use of cranberry juice[166] in the prevention and treatment of UTIs has been controversial, with different studies showing positive and negative effects of cranberry juice as a preventive or therapeutic agent.[14,128] A recent database study shows that there is substantial supported evidence that the beneficial effects of cranberry against UTIs is more prophylactic by preventing infection recurrence, while at the same time the use of cranberry also shows lower effectiveness in those populations that are at an increased risk for contracting UTIs. [166,242] More studies are needed to determine efficacy, dose, and appropriate candidates for this dietary treatment. The use of probiotics to increase normal vaginal flora may be of benefit.[241] Preliminary studies are encouraging, although only certain types of *Lactobacillus* have had promising results.[78,241]

There has also been debate as to whether hormone therapy can prevent UTIs in postmenopausal women. Recent studies indicate that oral as well as vaginal hormone therapy is not preventative[28,126,210] for UTIs, but its believed detrimental effects to cardiovascular health have been closely scrutinized. Further analysis of the Women's Health Initiative shows that when started earlier in the menopausal period, some significant benefits, including protection from heart disease, reduced risk of colon cancer, and reduced risk of osteoporotic fractures, can be achieved with hormone therapy.[23,116,244]

Instrumentation and, particularly, placement of urinary catheters frequently lead to UTI. However, if a catheter is needed, intermittent catheterization is recommended. Condom catheters may reduce the risk of causing UTI compared to indwelling catheters and should be considered.[50] Preliminary studies also suggest that use of catheters coated with an antimicrobial agent may reduce the risk, but further investigations are needed.[132]

**DIAGNOSIS AND TREATMENT.** The diagnosis of a UTI is typically made based on history and urinalysis results. A bacterial count of greater than 100,000 organisms/mL of urine is a commonly accepted criterion for diagnosis. In addition to the bacterial count, the urine leukocyte count (more than 10 leukocytes/mm$^3$ of urine collected midstream) and presence of leukocyte esterase, nitrates, and protein are also helpful.

Many people demonstrate pyuria (leukocytes in the urine) without infection, and corroborating clinical and laboratory information must be evident to diagnose an infection. In clients who are healthy and without complicating features, empiric treatment with antibiotics is effective and urine cultures are not required.

Acute UTIs in healthy, nonpregnant clients are typically treated with antibiotics, as recommended by the Infectious Diseases Society of America guidelines. Because of rising resistance to antibiotics with regional differences, initial treatment must take into account local resistance patterns, as well as the health of the client. For individuals with complicating features, treatment failure could lead to severe morbidity and mortality.

Women who experience recurrent infections have several options for treatment, depending upon the clinical situation and compliance of the client. They may take antibiotics prophylactically (typically as a daily dose), they may self-treat as they recognize typical symptoms,[104,242] or in the case of sexual intercourse as a precipitating factor, women may be advised to take antibiotics just after sex. Increased fluid intake may also help relieve symptoms and signs and is often used as an adjunct to pharmacologic treatment. *Lactobacillus acidophilus*, a probiotic supplement of live, active organisms, may be recommended for anyone taking antibiotics to replace the naturally occurring bacteria in the intestines and to prevent candidiasis (yeast growth). A vaccine to prevent recurrent urinary infections of the bladder has proved successful in mice and is currently being tested in clinical trials.

For clients who develop UTIs as a result of structural or functional problems, further testing is needed to correct the abnormality. Ultrasound, radiographs, computed tomographic (CT) scans, and renal scans may be used to identify contributing factors such as obstruction. Postvoid residual and more complex tests, such as voiding cystourethrography (upper urinary system) and urodynamic testing with and without fluoroscopy determination, may be recommended for anyone at risk for urinary retention. Whenever possible, ultrasound assessment, rather than urinary catheterization, is recommended for measuring the postvoid residual.

SPECIAL IMPLICATIONS FOR THE THERAPIST 18.1

### *Urinary Tract Infections*

Depending on the severity of the infection, the person with a UTI may not be able to participate fully in a rehabilitation program until the disease is brought under control. If the client begins to complain of nausea or vomiting, or has a fever greater than 39° C (102° F), or the therapist notes a change in mental status (most often confusion), immediate contact with the client's physician is warranted. These may be indications for hospital admission.

Awareness of the symptoms and signs associated with this disease may allow the therapist to recognize the onset of infection in its early stages. The initial symptoms may be subtle enough that patients typically do not seek medical help. Early detection and treatment of this disorder are important to prevent possible permanent structural damage. In the case of insidious onset of back or shoulder pain, onset of confusion, or increased confusion, especially with a recent history of any infection, a medical screening examination may be warranted.

UTIs also increase the risk of development of infection elsewhere in the body, including osteomyelitis, pleurisy, and pericarditis. Therapists should also always be aware of their role in infection prevention and minimize their involvement as a risk factor (see Chapter 8).

Appropriate catheter care involves minimizing risks of infection. These may include: maintaining unobstructed urine flow, keeping the catheter and collecting tube free from kinking, and having the collecting bag below the level of the bladder at all times. Do not rest the bag on the floor. Changing indwelling catheters or drainage bags at routine, fixed intervals is not recommended. Rather, it is suggested to change catheters and drainage bags based on clinical indications such as infection, obstruction, or when the closed system is compromised.[10]

## Pyelonephritis

### Overview and Incidence

Pyelonephritis can be either an infectious process involving the kidneys (acute pyelonephritis) or a chronic inflammatory disease involving the kidney parenchyma and renal pelvis (chronic pyelonephritis). Acute pyelonephritis occurs in over 250,000 people per year, causing over 100,000 hospitalizations. The direct and indirect costs are estimated at $2.14 billion.[30] It typically results from bacteria ascending from the bladder to infect the kidneys.[119] Similar to UTIs, acute pyelonephritis occurs more frequently in women than men, although men have a higher complication rate.[87]

Chronic pyelonephritis is a tubulointerstitial disorder characterized by specific changes in the kidney (cortical scarring and deformation of the calices). These alterations can be a result of several diseases that can lead to renal insufficiency. Chronic pyelonephritis may be responsible for up to 25% of the population with end-stage renal disease (ESRD).

### Etiologic and Risk Factors

The majority of acute pyelonephritis cases are associated with ascending UTIs (see Box 18.2) and are caused most commonly by *E. coli* (up to 85%).[227] A smaller proportion are caused by other gram-negative organisms, such as *Proteus*, *Klebsiella*, *Enterobacter*, and *Pseudomonas* species.

Risk factors associated with increased risk for pyelonephritis in healthy, nonpregnant women include frequent sexual activity, recent UTI, recent spermicide use, diabetes, and recent incontinence.[227] There may be a genetic component for increased susceptibility to these infections; a history of upper respiratory infection in female relatives is strongly and consistently associated with UTI recurrence and pyelonephritis.[226]

In other cases, pyelonephritis can stem from bloodborne pathogens associated with infection elsewhere. People with bacterial endocarditis and miliary tuberculosis are susceptible to kidney involvement. In addition, immunocompromised people are at risk for bacterial and fungal seeding of the kidney with subsequent abscess formation.

*Chronic pyelonephritis* is the term that describes specific, abnormal renal findings. Several diseases or processes can lead to chronic pyelonephritis, such as vesicoureteral reflux (urine is forced from the urinary bladder into the ureters and kidneys), urinary obstruction, analgesic nephropathy, or bacterial infection superimposed on a structural/functional abnormality. The most common cause of chronic pyelonephritis is vesicoureteral reflux, although the renal insufficiency associated with this is most often referred to as *reflux nephropathy*.

### Pathogenesis

Although urine is typically sterile, the distal end of the urethra is commonly colonized by bacterial flora. As described under "Etiologic and Risk Factors" above, bacteria can be transported to the urinary bladder in many ways. After urination, the subsequent passage of sterile urine from the kidneys to the bladder dilutes any bacteria that may have entered the bladder. If the residual urine volume is increased, as with an atonic bladder, an accumulation of insufficiently diluted bacteria can occur. Bacteria in the bladder urine typically do not gain access to the ureters for a variety of anatomic reasons. However, people with an abnormally short passage of the ureter within the bladder muscle wall and an angle of ureter insertion into the bladder wall that is more perpendicular are at risk for reflux of urine into the ureter itself. This reflux can be of sufficient force to carry the urine and the accompanying bacteria into the renal pelvis and calices.

Chronic pyelonephritis is defined by scarring with deformity of the calices. Processes that continually cause inflammation in the kidney can lead to chronic changes. Only a few processes can cause these changes, and they can be divided into three main groups: reflux, obstruction, and idiopathic.

### Clinical Manifestations

The onset of symptoms and signs associated with acute pyelonephritis is usually abrupt. The complaints may include fever, chills, malaise, headache, and flank pain. The person may also complain of tenderness over the costovertebral angle (Murphy sign). Symptoms of bladder irritation may be present (including dysuria, urinary frequency, and urgency) but are not required for the diagnosis.

Symptoms associated with chronic pyelonephritis vary depending upon the causative process; however, symptoms may not be present. The diagnosis is made more often by laboratory detection of kidney function changes.

## MEDICAL MANAGEMENT

**DIAGNOSIS, TREATMENT, AND PROGNOSIS.** The presence of suggestive symptoms for acute pyelonephritis warrants laboratory testing and treatment. Urinalysis typically reveals pyuria, bacteriuria, and varying degrees of hematuria. A urine culture should always be obtained and often will result in the growth of the offending bacteria or fungus. In addition, the blood count usually demonstrates leukocytosis.

If the infection is severe enough or if complicating factors are present, hospital admission may be required for intravenous antibiotics and hydration. Typically, however, the condition is treated with an appropriate antibiotic medication. Symptoms typically begin disappearing within several days. If the person does not show improvement within 48 to 72 hours, contact with the physician is warranted.

If the process associated with chronic pyelonephritis continues to progress, creating worsening scarring, the result may be ESRD requiring dialysis or transplantation.

# RENAL DISORDERS

## Renal Neoplasms

### Overview and Incidence

The American Cancer Society estimates that 73,820 new cases of neoplasms of the kidney and the renal pelvis were diagnosed in this country in 2019, accounting for approximately 4% of all new cancer cases. One-sixth (n = 44,120) of the new kidney and the renal pelvis cases occurred in males and one-eighth (n = 29,700) occurred in females. The mean age at diagnosis of kidney cancers is 64 years of age and 75% of all new cases are diagnosed in those over 55, with the probability of developing a renal cancer progressively increasing after the age of 50. The average five-year survival rate is 75% but even higher (93%) when the disease is diagnosed at an earlier stage. In terms of mortality, an estimated 14,770 deaths occurred in 2019 from kidney and renal pelvis cancers (2.4% of all cancer deaths) with 9,820 of those deaths occurring in males and 4,950 occurring in females.[5]

### Overview of Renal Cell Carcinoma Subpopulations

There are several different types of kidney cancers, including renal cell carcinoma, urothelial carcinoma, renal sarcoma, Wilms tumor, and renal lymphoma. Renal cell carcinoma (RCC) is the most common adult renal neoplasm, accounting for 90% to 95% of all renal tumors (Fig. 18.2). This heterogeneous group of tumors is the result

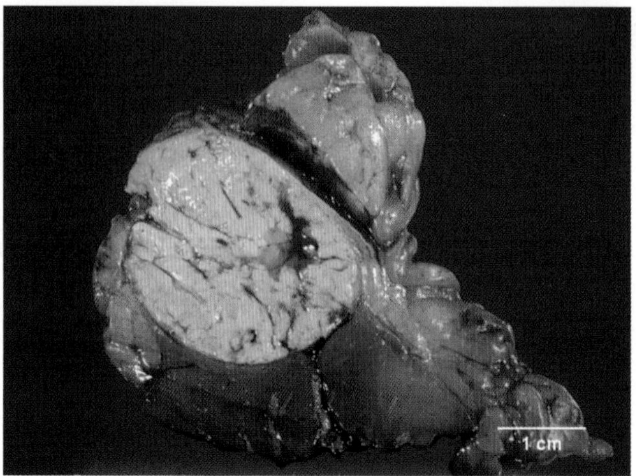


**Figure 18.2**

**Renal cell carcinoma is usually a tumor of adults with a male:female ratio of 2:1.** This partial nephrectomy specimen shows the classic appearance of renal cell carcinoma. The tumor is well circumscribed and has the characteristic golden-yellow appearance of these tumors. (Image copyright WebPathology; Dharam Ramnani, MD; used with permission.)

of accelerated growth of the cells found in the epithelial layers in the kidneys, typically the proximal renal tubular epithelium. These tumors grow over time but remain typically asymptomatic as they grow, provide few if any early warning signs, have diverse clinical manifestations and are often resistant to radiation and traditional chemotherapy, making surgery the predominant treatment intervention. Five major subtypes of RCCs are recognized with each subtype displaying differences in genetics, biology and behavior. Distinct tumors of different cell types can occasionally be seen in the same kidney. The conventional or clear cell (ccRCC) type, so named because of the clear cytoplasm found in its cells, accounts for 75% of all cases of RCCs. Papillary RCCs account for 15% to 20% of all RCC cases and arise in the renal tubular epithelium. Chromophobe RCCs account for about 5% of all RCC cases, are characterized by large tumor size, and diagnosis often occurs at an earlier stage of disease progression. Collecting duct RCCs are aggressive tumors that arise in epithelial cells found in the collecting ducts and account for less than 1% of all cases of RCC. The fifth subtype is RCC unclassified, accounting for about 2% of all RCC. This tumor type is not an RCC subtype per se but rather is a diagnostic category for tumors that do not fit into the other subgroup categories. Because of their rarity these latter three subtypes of RCC will not be discussed further.[80,198]

### Causes of RCCs

Most adult kidney cancers occur spontaneously but are associated with a number of well-recognized environmental and lifestyle risk factors including:[121]

**Age:** The risk for developing renal cancer increases with age.

**Gender:** Men are twice as likely to develop kidney cancer as women.

**Race:** African Americans have higher rates of renal cancer.

**Blood pressure:** Elevated

**Smoking tobacco:** Smoking doubles the risk of developing kidney cancer.

**Obesity:** Being overweight or obese increases the risk of developing renal cancer twofold relative to normal-weight people.[221]

**Overuse of certain medications:** Long-term use of diuretics and analgesic pain medications, such as aspirin, acetaminophen, and ibuprofen, have been linked to an increased risk for developing renal cancer.

**Occupational exposure:** Exposure to asbestos and/or cadmium (used in the production of batteries, plastics, and other industrial processes) have been linked to an increased risk for developing renal cancer.

### Chronic Kidney Disease and Long-Term Kidney Dialysis[4]

About 5% of RCCs are the result of hereditary diseases, including von Hippel-Lindau (VHL) disease (a rare autosomal dominant familial syndrome) that can lead to cysts and cancers including ccRCC, hereditary papillary renal carcinoma (an autosomal dominant disorder that can result in papillary RCC), and Birt-Hogg-Dubé syndrome (a rare autosomal dominant disorder linked to chromophobe RCCs or mixed chromophobe RCCs–oncocytomas). Risk for developing RCC is greater in people who have first-degree relatives with a history of RCC. That risk increases as the total number of those relatives increases who were under the age of 50 when diagnosed.[35,198]

As with other cancers, specific genetic abnormalities are present in the tumor cells of RCCs that drive mutagenesis. For example, mutations in the VHL (von Hippel-Lindau) gene spontaneously arise causing VHL syndrome and increased risk for ccRCC. The VHL gene is a tumor suppressor gene, which regulates cell growth. Mutations in this gene results in nonfunctional VHL protein which cannot appropriately regulate cell growth allowing tumors to grow both in cell numbers and cell size (a characteristic of all cancers). Another gene linked to RCC is the MET proto-oncogene which encodes for tyrosine kinase receptors. When these receptors bind specific ligands they influence important downstream, growth regulating processes in the cell. Mutation of this gene disrupts these growth control mechanisms, resulting in uncontrolled cell growth. This mutation is found in approximately 75% of sporadic papillary RCC cases. Mutations in the FC gene, which can be both inherited and arise spontaneously, are found in renal cells of patients with RCC. When the FC gene is defective, the cell's ability to use oxygen for energy synthesis becomes compromised and the cell becomes hypoxic, an environment that supports tumor growth and development.[35,198] Mechanisms by which risk factors cause mutagenesis are still poorly understood. The increase in risk for RCC associated with obesity appears to result from the accompanying increase in inflammatory biomarkers such as angiogenic factors, inflammatory cytokines and leptin, which both create a microenvironment that results in oncogenesis and tumor progression and suppression of tumor suppressing genes and/or growth regulating genes.[92]

### Diagnosis of RCC

Historically patients with RCC were diagnosed after presenting with a classic triad of symptoms related to RCC (i.e., flank pain, hematuria, and a palpable abdominal mass). Now, however, the majority of RCC diagnoses result from incidental findings secondary to imaging studies performed for other reasons; only 10% of patients present with the classic triad of symptoms. Diagnosis is then typically confirmed with CT imaging. It is important to again note that RCCs can remain asymptomatic for long periods of time due to the retroperitoneal position of the kidney. As a result, kidney cancers are frequently "silent" in the early stages and advanced or metastatic (spread of cancer to other parts of the body) when finally diagnosed. Metastatic disease is present in 25% to 30% of patients at the time of diagnosis, and symptoms associated with metastases are often responsible for the symptoms leading to a physician visit. Sites of RCC metastasis include the lungs (75%), regional lymph nodes (65%), bones (40%), and liver (40%).[9] RCC may also cause hematuria; episodes may be irregular and microscopic, suggesting that even a single episode of hematuria should be followed up, particularly in those with risk factors for RCC.

The primary feature of RCC is the presence of a renal parenchymal mass, which can be detected by a variety of imaging modalities. The widespread use of abdominal ultrasound, magnetic resonance imaging (MRI), and CT scanning has increased the diagnosis of incidental renal tumors. CT scans offer greater fidelity in terms of anatomic detail, and such scans provide details of neighboring organs, such as the liver, colon, spleen, and lymphatics, providing information about tumor dispersion. Ultrasonography can be used to further evaluate the renal parenchyma and detect small tumors (less than 1 cm).

Laboratory studies used for the diagnosis of RCC include the following: urinalysis (UA), complete blood cell (CBC) count with differential, electrolytes, renal profile (albumin, creatinine, glucose, blood urea nitrogen and carbon dioxide), liver function tests (LFTs; aspartate aminotransferase [AST] and alanine aminotransferase [ALT]), and serum calcium.

Potentially confusing the clinical presentation of RCC is the fact that these tumors are associated with ectopic hormone production and paraneoplastic symptoms. Tumors, including RCCs, are known to produce an array of hormones including parathyroid hormone, gonadotropins, renin, erythropoietin, glucagon, and insulin. These paraneoplastic manifestations (a set of signs and symptoms that is the consequence of the presence of a tumor in the body) of RCC include hypercalcemia, production of adrenocorticotrophic hormone (ACTH), polycythemia, hepatic dysfunction, amyloidosis, fever, and weight loss, which are present in up to 20% of patients. As discussed previously, several hereditary syndromes that predispose an individual to the development of RCC have unique signs and symptoms other than those for RCCs. For example, von Hippel-Lindau disease is associated with retinal angiomas, hemangioblastomas of the central nervous system, pheochromocytomas, and clear cell RCCs. The presence of the distinguishing features that lead to the diagnosis of these syndromes alerts clinicians to the need for regular monitoring and surveillance for the presence of RCC.[198]

**Table 18.1** TNM Staging System Category Descriptions

| Stage | Implications |
|---|---|
| Stage 0 | Abnormal cells are present but have not spread to nearby tissue. Also called carcinoma in situ, or CIS. CIS is not cancer, but it may become cancer. |
| Stage I, Stage II, Stage III | Cancer is present. The higher the number, the larger the cancer tumor and the more it has spread into nearby tissues including lymph nodes. |
| Stage V | The cancer has spread to distant parts of the body. |

Once a kidney mass has been found, determining its invasiveness (i.e., its metastatic or malignant status) becomes important. In the case of RCCs, making this determination can be difficult, often requiring surgical removal of the tumor. If hematuria is present, intravenous pyelography (IVP) may be the initial procedure to identify renal abnormalities. IVP is a radiographic test that allows for evaluation of the kidneys, ureters, and bladder. A dye injected into the bloodstream is filtered and secreted by the renal tubules. The IVP provides information, including renal size, function, position, and the presence of calculi, masses, and congenital variants.

### Staging and Grading

Part of the diagnostic workup of a patient with an RCC involves defining the stage and grade of the tumor. Tumor staging provides information about the size of the primary tumor, extent of lymph node involvement, and the presence or absence of metastatic disease (Table 18.1). The TNM staging scheme is used to stage RCCs (Table 18.2). The letter "T" in this scheme denotes the size of the primary tumor and extent of tumor infiltration into nearby tissues, with larger numbers indicating greater size and greater infiltration; "N" denotes the extent to which the cancer has invaded lymph nodes, with a larger number denoting a greater number and more distant lymph nodes containing cancer cells; and "M" refers to the presence or absence of metastatic disease. The staging of the disease is predicated on the findings from a number of diagnostic tests, including imaging studies, biopsies, and laboratory tests. Criteria for each of the TNM individual categories and the tumor stage are presented in Table 18.2.[181]

Tumors are also characterized by their histologic characteristics or appearance under the microscope (i.e., their grade). The larger the grade number (typically ranging between 1 and 4) the more disorganized the tissue and cell structure and the greater the likelihood that the tumor is fast growing and has metastasized. The smaller the grade number, the more closely the tissue and cells resemble healthy tissue and the slower the tumor growth. Tissue acquired from biopsies of the tumor provide the tissue needed for grading.[66]

## MEDICAL MANAGEMENT

The therapeutic approach to renal cell carcinoma (RCC) is guided by the probability of cure, which is related directly to the tumor stage and grade. More than 50% of patients with early-stage RCC are cured, but the prognosis for stage IV disease is poor. The principal treatment options for RCC include surgery, thermal ablation, active surveillance, radiation therapy, molecular-targeted therapy, and immunotherapy,

**Table 18.2** TNM Staging Criteria

| **Size of Primary Tumor (T) in cm** | |
|---|---|
| TX | No information available on primary tumor |
| TO | No evidence of primary tumor |
| Tis | Carcinoma in situ at primary site |
| T1 | Tumor less than 2 cm |
| T2 | Tumor 2-4 cm in diameter |
| T3 | Tumor greater than 4 cm |
| T4 | Tumor has invaded adjacent structures |
| **Lymph Node Involvement (N)** | |
| NX | Nodes not assessed |
| NO | No clinically positive nodes (not palpable) |
| N1 | Single clinically positive ipsilateral (on same side) node less than 3 cm |
| N2 | Single clinically positive ipsilateral node 3 to 6 cm; **or** Multiple ipsilateral nodes with all less than 6 cm; **or** bilateral or contralateral nodes with none greater than 6 cm |
| N3 | Node or nodes greater than 6 cm |
| **Distant Metastasis (M)** | |
| MX | Distant metastasis not assessed |
| MO | No distant metastasis |
| M1 | Distant metastasis is present |
| Stage | TNM Classification |
| 0 | Tis NO MO |
| I | T1 NO MO |
| II | T2 NO MO |
| III | T3 NO MO |
| | T1 N1 MO |
| | T2 N1 MO |
| | T3 N1 MO |
| IV | T4 NO MO |
| | T4 N1 MO |
| | Any T N2 MO |
| | Any T N3 MO |
| | Any T Any N M1 |

SURGICAL TREATMENT. Radical nephrectomy remains the only known curative treatment for localized RCC and remains the most commonly performed surgical procedure for the treatment of localized RCC. This procedure involves complete removal of the Gerota fascia and its contents, including a resection of the kidney, perirenal fat, and ipsilateral adrenal gland, with or without ipsilateral lymph node dissection. Radical nephrectomies provide a better surgical margin than simple removal of the kidney, because perinephric fat may be cancerous in some patients, making this procedure the preferred treatment if the tumor extends into the inferior vena cava. RCCs that have infiltrated adjacent structures, such as bowel, spleen, or psoas muscle, may be treated with a radical nephrectomy and en bloc excision of these structures. Radical nephrectomies may be done using open, laparoscopic, and robotic surgical techniques. Laparoscopic nephrectomy has gained acceptance as a method for reducing hospital stay and postoperative pain, and providing a faster recovery.[36,133]

Ipsilateral adrenal gland resection is no longer recommended as part of a radical nephrectomy if imaging shows it to be normal or if the tumor is not high risk based on size and location. Regional lymph node dissection is recommended for patients with palpable or enlarged lymph nodes detected on preoperative imaging tests.[106,133]

Partial nephrectomy, sometimes referred to as nephron-sparing surgery or kidney-sparing surgery, involves removal of the portion of the kidney infiltrated by a tumor. This procedure preserves some kidney function but is a more technically difficult surgery that requires an experienced surgeon and surgical team. Smaller tumors of lesser grade are more amenable to a partial nephrectomy; incidentally detected solid renal masses may be candidates for this tissue sparing surgery. Partial nephrectomy is the treatment of choice when the patient has a T1a tumor or preservation of renal function is the primary issue. Either a radical or partial nephrectomy is standard of care for managing T1b tumors. The curative therapy for TII and TIII tumors remains radical nephrectomy. The goals of nephron sparing surgery are complete removal of the malignancy and maximal preservation of renal function. Achieving these goals requires carefully balancing opposing patient needs, which makes decisions regarding kidney preserving surgery both challenging and controversial.[36]

Surgery is not always a first-line treatment strategy. Active surveillance (i.e., initial monitoring of tumors while delaying intervention) may be of benefit, particularly for elderly patients with multiple comorbidities, including poor renal function and multiple tumors, patients who are otherwise poor surgical candidates, and those with small renal masses (<2 cm). Cryo- or radiofrequency tissue ablation techniques may be combined with surveillance. These minimally invasive techniques use radiofrequency energy or cryoablation instrumentation under imaging guidance to generate a level of heat or cold in the tumor that is lethal to the tumor. Patients with tumors that are stage 1A or B are amenable to percutaneous cryoablation and can generally anticipate good outcomes. When progression is noted, more aggressive treatment may need to be considered.[106,133]

**Treatment**

***Chemotherapy.*** The word *chemotherapy* designates a drug used to treat any disease, but today this word typically refers to those drugs used to treat cancers. These drugs have been in clinical use for a long time and act by preventing cells, both cancer cells and healthy cells, from dividing and increasing in number. While used to treat a wide array of cancers, chemotherapeutic drugs including vinblastine, floxuridine, 5-fluorouracil (5-FU), capecitabine, and gemcitabine have not proven effective against RCC and so are not a standard of care for RCC. They are frequently used when other drug therapies have proven ineffective.[13]

***Targeted Therapies.*** Cell growth and cell death are carefully regulated by a complex array of cellular processes. When defects occur in these processes the result is uncontrolled and inappropriate cell growth (i.e., cancer). Certain molecules are now recognized as being responsible for regulating cell growth and death in normal cells, and defects in the genes coding for these molecules are associated with specific cancers. In the case of RCC, defects arise in the enzyme tyrosine kinase and in molecules that regulate angiogenesis. Drugs have been developed that specifically target these defective molecules in an attempt to normalize cell growth. In the case of RCC, these so-called target therapies include drugs that target tyrosine kinase, mTOR, and molecules that drive angiogenesis. Examples include Sunitinib (suntent) and pazopanib (Votrient)—both tyrosine kinase inhibitors—and bevacizumab (Avastatin) an antiangiogenic molecule. Other target therapies for treating RCC are listed in Table 18.3. These drugs shrink and slow tumor growth. They rarely effect a cure for RCC but have been approved for use because they lengthen progression-free survival time. Although they are designed to target specific molecules in cancerous cells, they are not without adverse effects (see Table 18.3) that must be recognized by rehabilitation professionals providing services to patients receiving these drugs. Sunitinib and pazopanib are considered preferred therapies for first-line treatment for RCCs.[13] In some cases sunitinib is given after surgery in an effort to reduce the risk of recurrence, a treatment strategy known as adjuvant therapy.

***Immunomodulatory Therapies.*** RCCs are among the most immunogenic tumors, that is they are particularly capable of provoking an immune response. As such, immunotherapies in the form of immune stimulating molecules called cytokines, specifically interleukin-2 (IL-2) and interferon-alpha, have been used to treat RCC for over a decade, particularly in patients who have not responded to targeted therapies. More recently, drugs called checkpoint inhibitors have become available. Many tumors secrete molecules that bind to specific receptors (checkpoints) that prevent T cells from recognizing the tumor as being foreign, allowing the tumor to escape detection by the immune system. Checkpoint inhibitors block these receptors, preventing these tumor molecules from inactivating the immune system and allowing an immune response to be initiated. Immunotherapy with checkpoint inhibitors (Table 18.4) has become a major modality for the treatment of clear cell RCC, both as an initial therapy and after antiangiogenic therapy for those initially treated with targeted agents (NCCN guidelines). Unfortunately, the untoward effects of blocking the immune system's natural inhibitory mechanisms have resulted in serious adverse effects.

***Radiation Therapy.*** Although frequently used with other solid tumors, radiation therapy is only infrequently used to treat patients with RCC. Adjuvant radiation therapy after nephrectomy does not provide benefit, even in patients with nodal involvement or incomplete tumor resection. For those patients with RCC who develop brain metastasis, whole brain radiation is recommended. Radiation therapy is considered for palliation, particularly for those with painful bone metastases, which occur in 30% to 40% of patients with advanced RCC.[133,287]

SPECIAL IMPLICATIONS FOR THE THERAPIST 18.2

## *Renal Cell Carcinoma*

### Overview

Therapists working primarily with the geriatric population need to be aware of the symptoms and signs of this disease. Questions in the history related to hematuria, unexplained weight loss, fatigue, fever, flank pain, and malaise are important, regardless of the reason or need for physical therapy care. Awareness of new onset of unexplained abdominal, flank, or back pain; cough; or other signs of pulmonary involvement should raise concern on the therapist's part and warrants communication with a physician. In addition, RCC is the most common metastatic tumor to the sternum. An onset of sternal pain or a mass in someone with a history of RCC should be quickly brought to the physician's attention.

The extensive abdominal and thoracic surgical sites may produce scarring that affects the client's posture and ability to move, increasing mechanical stress on the musculoskeletal system. Myofascial and soft tissue mobilization of the abdominal and thoracic regions may be of benefit to these people. If a history of abnormal renal function in addition to the cancer is evident, additional precautions may need to be taken by the therapist. (See the section on chronic renal failure later in this chapter.)

Persons undergoing targeted therapies for renal cancer may experience the familiar side effects of cancer treatment, such as headache, fatigue, hypertension, sore mouth and taste changes, diarrhea, nausea, and even nose bleeds. It is important that health professionals familiarize themselves with the potential side effects of the drug treatments and methods for managing these side effects.[139]

### Presenting Conditions

#### *Deconditioning*

Large numbers of survivors of kidney cancers, like Americans in general, fail to meet current exercise guidelines and are physically deconditioned at the time of diagnosis.[260,262,290] This level of deconditioning may have contributed to their diagnosis, contributes to the downstream health burdens they face, and increases their risk for disease recurrence.[139] Assessment of fitness and strength levels (6-minute walk test, graded exercise test with or without gas analysis, 1-repetition maximum) of these patients should occur as early in their care as possible, preferably at the time of diagnosis. A time lapse between diagnosis and surgery provides an opportunity for rehabilitation professionals to develop and implement a pre-habilitation program. Such programs improve surgical outcomes and positively impact hospital stays.[223] Resuming physical activity as quickly after surgery as is safe will limit further loss of conditioning and physical functional capacity during this period of recovery. Similarly, participation in an exercise training program during a multiweek course of either immune or targeted therapy can also limit further deconditioning and loss of physical functional capacity.[214] Continued participation in an exercise/physical fitness training program after completion of all treatments is also important because greater participation in moderate to vigorous physical activity is associated with a decreased risk of overall mortality in patients with renal cell cancer.[224] Guidelines to assist rehabilitation professionals in generating and implementing exercise training programs are available.[57,108,262]

#### *Increased Fall Risk*

Kidney cancer survivors, like all cancer survivors, are at increased risk for balance deficits and falls, both because of their age and because of their diagnosis.[123] Current exercise guidelines for older Americans call for both balance and fall risk assessment in these patients and implementation of a treatment plan to improve their balance. Because balance may change over the course of treatment and afterwards, balance assessments should be repeated over time.[262]

#### *Presence of Bony Metastasis*

About one-third of patients with advanced renal cell carcinoma (RCC) have bone metastases that are often osteolytic and cause substantial morbidity, such as pain, pathologic fracture, spinal cord compression, and hypercalcemia.[49] Rehabilitation professionals need to be aware of the presence of bone metastasis; the relationship between bone pain and bone "mets"; their risk for causing pathologic fractures and how to minimize that risk; and symptoms of spinal cord compression, which include spinal pain at the level of the bone lesion, muscle weakness, sensory loss, and autonomic dysfunction.[178] Participation in exercise training programs can be managed safely with careful attention to change in symptoms, particularly pain, and avoidance of exercising involved limbs.[56]

### Watchful Surveillance

National Comprehensive Cancer Network Practice Guidelines for Kidney Cancer[133] call for active surveillance as part of primary treatment for patients with stage 1A and B disease and for surveillance during adjuvant treatment. Active surveillance entails abdominal imaging (CT or MRI) and periodic metastatic surveys, including complete blood work and chest imaging for lung metastasis. For those with stage IV or relapsed disease, active surveillance occurs more frequently and involves brain scans. Given the poor conditioning status of patients with a history of kidney cancer and its impact on disease recurrence and physical functional capacity and balance, the rehabilitation professional may consider developing a functional surveillance program that periodically assesses these patients for their conditioning, strength, physical function, pain, and mobility status. Existing prospective surveillance models for identifying functional deficits[247] provide a useful blueprint that could be modified to meet the ongoing assessment and treatment needs of patients with a history of renal tumors.

**Table 18.3** Targeted Therapy Drugs, Their Clinical Use, and Adverse Effects

| TARGETED THERAPIES | | | |
|---|---|---|---|
| **Drug** | **Action** | **Approved for** | **Adverse Effects** |
| Sorafenib (Nexavar) | Tyrosine kinase inhibitor | Advanced renal cancer | Fatigue, rash, diarrhea, increased blood pressure, hand-foot syndrome |
| Sunitinib (Sutent) | Tyrosine kinase inhibitor | Advanced renal cancer | Nausea, diarrhea, changes in skin or hair color, mouth sores, weakness, myelosuppression, congestive heart failure, hand-foot syndrome |
| Temsirolimus (Torisel) | Inhibitor of mTOR which promotes cell growth and division | Advanced renal cancer | Skin rash, weakness, mouth sores, nausea, loss of appetite, peripheral edema, hyperglycemia, hypercholesterolemia |
| Everolimus (Afinitor) | Inhibitor of mTOR which promotes cell growth and division | Advanced RCC after failure of treatment with Sunitinib or Sorafenib | Mouth sores, increased risk of infections, nausea, loss of appetite, diarrhea, skin rash, peripheral edema, hyperglycemia, hypercholesterolemia |
| Bevacizumab (Avastin) | Antiangiogenic | Metastatic RCC | Hypertension, fatigue, bleeding, clotting, intestinal perferations, slow wound healing |
| Axitinib (Inlyta) | Tyrosine kinase inhibitor | Advanced RCC after failure of one prior systemic therapy | Hypertension, fatigue, bleeding, clotting, slow wound healing, hand-foot syndrome, poor appetite, voice changes |
| Axitinib (Inlyta) | Tyrosine kinase inhibitor | Advanced RCC after failure of one prior systemic therapy | Hypertension, fatigue, bleeding, clotting, slow wound healing, hand-foot syndrome, poor appetite, voice changes |
| Cabozantinib (Cabometyx) | Tyrosine kinase inhibitor | Advanced RCC | Diarrhea, fatigue, nausea and vomiting, poor appetite and weight loss, high blood pressure, hand-foot syndrome, constipation, serious bleeding, blood clots, hypertension |
| Lenvatinib (Lenvima) | Tyrosine kinase inhibitor | Advanced renal cell carcinoma following one prior antiangiogenic therapy | Diarrhea, fatigue, joint or muscle pain, loss of appetite, nausea and vomiting, mouth sores, weight loss, hypertension, peripheral edema, serious bleeding, blood clots, kidney, liver, or heart failure |

**Table 18.4** Immune Modulating Drugs, Their Clinical Use, and Adverse Effects

| IMMUNOMODULATORY DRUGS | | | |
|---|---|---|---|
| **Drug** | **Action** | **Approved For** | **Adverse Effects** |
| Interleukin-2 (Proleukin) | Recombinant form of interleukin-2 | Advanced RCC | Breathing problems, serious infections, seizures, allergic reactions, heart, problems, renal failure |
| Interferon-Alpha (Multiferon) | Stimulates B-cells and activates NK cells | Advanced RCC | Flu-like symptoms, fatigue, nausea |
| pembrolizumab (Keytruda) | Blocks PD-1 pathway | Advanced RCC | Pneumonitis, hepatitis, colitis, nephritis |
| Ipilimumab (Yervoy) | Blocks CTLA | Advanced RCC | Fatigue, diarrhea, skin rash, |
| Nivolumab (Opdivo) | Blocks PD-1 pathway | Advanced RCC | Fatigue, cough, nausea, itching, skin rash, loss of appetite, joint pain |
| Bevacizumab (Avastin) | Blocks vascular endothelial growth factor (VEGF) | Metastatic RCC | Epistaxis, hypertension, lacrimation disorder, exfoliative dermatitis |

## Pediatric Renal Cancers

### Wilms Tumor

**Overview, Incidence, and Risk Factors.** Wilms tumor, or nephroblastoma, is the most common malignant kidney neoplasm in children (Fig. 18.3). Approximately 650 new cases are reported annually in the United States. Age is the primary risk factor. The disease most commonly occurs during the first 6 years of life, with approximately 75% of cases occurring in children younger than age 5 years and the mean age at diagnosis is 44 months. Wilms tumors occur bilaterally in 5% of cases.[219]

Although these tumors develop most frequently in children without any predisposition to developing cancer, 10% of children with Wilms tumor have been reported to have congenital anomalies or syndromes. The three most common include WAGR syndrome (Wilms, aniridia, genitourinary malformation, mental retardation), Beckwith-Wiedemann syndrome, and Denys-Drash syndrome.

**Etiologic Factors and Pathogenesis.** Although the majority of cases are sporadic, approximately 1% to 3% have a family history of Wilms tumor, and up to 10% are seen in hereditary syndromes. Molecular genetics plays

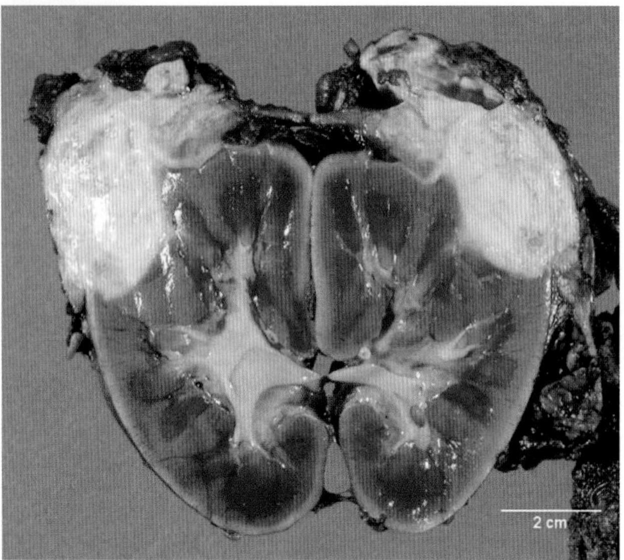


**Figure 18.3**

**The image shows a yellow-tan, soft, lobulated Wilms tumor near the upper pole of the kidney.** The tumor extends beyond the kidney and appears to be present at the inked surgical margin (Stage III; National Wilms Tumor Study). (Image courtesy of Dr. Jean-Christophe Fournet, Paris, France; humpath.com; Used with permission.)

an important role in the cause of Wilms tumor. The biologic signaling pathways determining the origin of Wilms tumor are complex, and several genes at several loci may be involved.

The most well-known and studied gene of Wilms tumor is the *WT1* suppressor gene, a complex protein that is an essential regulator of kidney development; mutations in this gene result in the formation of tumors in approximately 10% of Wilms tumor cases. These genes also are implicated in the formation of many other cancers.

Other genetic alterations, such as *WT2* and familial genetic alterations termed *FWT1* and *FWT2*, have also been located. Significant investigations are ongoing to determine how these genes and their products interact in order to understand the mechanisms in the development of Wilms tumor and provide improved therapy.

**Clinical Manifestations.** Wilms tumors can be difficult to discover early because the tumor can grow to a large size before causing symptoms. Fortunately, despite large tumor size, most Wilms tumors do not metastasize. An abdominal mass, most often detected by the parents, is the most common presenting sign. Up to 30% of children may complain of abdominal pain, malaise, loss of appetite, or nausea/vomiting. Hematuria may occur in up to 30% of cases and hypertension in up to 25% of affected children. Hypertension is present in about 25% of children at presentation which is attributed to an activation of the renin-angiotensinogen system. Congenital abnormalities may be present, particularly those associated with hereditary syndromes with a predilection for Wilms tumor (13%-28%).

## MEDICAL MANAGEMENT

**STAGING AND DIAGNOSIS.** Staging is performed according to the National Wilms Tumor Study Group (NWTSG) staging system. Tumors are staged into five groups (stages I to V), depending on tumor size and growth into surrounding structures. Histologic features are also important. Histologically, tumors can be classified as having favorable histology or unfavorable histology (anaplastic features). Approximately 40% of tumors are discovered while in stage I, whereas only 5% of cases are at stage V. Most adults with Wilms tumors are diagnosed unexpectedly following nephrectomy for presumed RCC.

Abdominal ultrasonography helps define the cystic or solid nature of the mass and helps determine whether the renal vein or vena cava is involved. CT scan of the abdomen is helpful in determining the extent of the tumor but can be difficult to perform with small children. A chest radiograph and CT of the chest are used to determine the presence of metastases to the lung. MRI may also be beneficial in determining the extent of the disease.

**TREATMENT.** Surgical resection of the tumor is the primary treatment regardless of the stage of the disease. A radical nephrectomy is the most common procedure, although a nephron-sparing procedure may be performed in clients who have lesions in both kidneys. Regional lymphadenectomy may be carried out, because lymph node involvement strongly affects the prognosis. Chemotherapy is also used for all stages of the disease, sometimes preoperatively, with radiation therapy being added to the treatment regimen for stages III and IV disease and for tumors with unfavorable histologic findings. Chemotherapeutic agents used include dactinomycin, vincristine, and doxorubicin, with cyclophosphamide for patients with stage IV tumors. Eighteen weeks of therapy is adequate for patients with stage I and II FH, and stage III and IV patients can be treated with upwards of 24 months of therapy.[199]

There are no standard treatments available for adults. A standardized approach for the management of adult Wilms tumors is proposed with the aim to limit treatment delay after surgery and encourage a uniform approach for this rare disease and thereby improve survival.[134]

**PROGNOSIS.** Prognosis depends on the histologic appearance of the lesion, stage of the disease, and age of the child. But the overall 5-year survival is very good at 90%. (32) Multimodality therapy with surgery, whole-abdomen radiotherapy, and three-drug chemotherapy delivered according to the NWTS-4 and -5 protocols resulted in excellent abdominal and systemic tumor control rates.[199]

With the development of successful treatment, emphasis is now being placed on limiting significant long-term side effects while maintaining the high cure rate in tumors with favorable histology. All children should be monitored in long-term surveillance programs for the early detection and management of therapy-related toxicities, which include subsequent malignant neoplasms, primarily digestive cancers and breast cancer neoplasms, and congestive heart failure.[199] Further, treatment options are needed for advanced tumors with unfavorable histology. Wilms tumor may recur years after the initial diagnosis.

Wilms tumors occur rarely in adults; outcome for adults is inferior compared with children, although better results are reported when treated within pediatric trials.(33) Multiple factors, including the unfamiliarity of adult oncologists and pathologists with Wilms tumors, lack of standardized treatment, and consequent delays in initiating the appropriate risk-adapted therapy, may contribute to the poor outcome.

SPECIAL IMPLICATIONS FOR THE THERAPIST 18.3

### *Wilms Tumors*

Many children with Wilms tumors are treated with vincristine, a drug known to cause peripheral neuropathy that adversely affects their gait patterns.[94] Therapists should assess children treated with this drug for sensory loss, and the Peds-mTNS scale has been developed specifically for this purpose.[95] This loss of sensation in the feet results in mobility deficits and limits conditioning secondary to loss of tibialis anterior strength. Use of an ankle-foot orthosis is effective in reducing the resulting foot drop and improving mobility.[251] It is important to note that symptoms of peripheral neuropathy can remain for upwards of 6 months.[94]

In contrast to adult survivors of kidney cancers, children are more frequently treated with chemotherapeutic agents known to cause late adverse effects and, because of their age, there is more time for these adverse effects to manifest themselves. Therapists treating adult survivors of a Wilms tumor diagnosis must be aware of the increased risk for these late effects and be prepared to screen these patients appropriately.[167]

## Renal Cystic Disease

### Overview

A renal cyst is a cavity filled with fluid or renal tubular elements making up a semisolid material. The presence of these cysts can lead to degeneration of renal tissue and obstruction of tubular flow. Renal cysts vary considerably in size, ranging from microscopic to several centimeters in diameter, and can be single or multiple, unilateral or bilateral.

Cysts in the kidney are rather common and can be classified into six categories of cystic diseases: (1) polycystic kidney disease (PKD), (2) cystic diseases of the renal medulla, (3) acquired cystic disease, (4) single cysts, (5) cystic renal dysplasia, and (6) miscellaneous renal cystic disorders.

The formation of simple cysts is the most common cystic disorder of the kidney. Simple cysts are usually less than 1 cm in diameter and do not often produce symptoms or compromise renal function. Acquired cysts may develop secondary to dialysis, diabetes mellitus, or glomerulonephritis. PKD is a leading cause of ESRD, frequently requiring dialysis and renal transplantation. Because of the seriousness and fairly common occurrence of PKD, this section principally discusses PKD. The remaining disorders constitute less-common causes of renal cysts.

### Incidence

PKD is manifested as either an autosomal dominant (ADPKD) or autosomal recessive (ARPKD) disorder. Although PKD can occur spontaneously, most cases are hereditary. ADPKD is one of the most common hereditary disorders in the United States, affecting more than 600,000 Americans (about 1 in every 500 to 1 in every 1000 persons). ARPKD is rare.

Persons with ADPKD may not manifest symptoms until the third or fourth decade of life, whereas ARPKD is evident at birth and can cause death early in life. ADPKD affects people from all races and ethnic groups. Most people with ADPKD will exhibit evidence of the disease by the age of 80 years, but only half progress to ESRD. ADPKD is the fourth leading cause of ESRD and accounts for 10% of all cases of ESRD.

### Risk Factors

Even though there is currently no way of determining which people with ADPKD will develop ESRD, there are a few risk factors that have been linked to a more rapid progression. These factors include hypertension, multiple pregnancies, male gender, and the expression of the genetic mutation PKD1.

### Etiology and Pathogenesis

Most renal cysts form from the epithelium of a preexisting renal tubule. These epithelial cells typically exhibit a reabsorptive function, but have secretory capabilities. In the case of cyst formation, epithelial cells with genetic mutations begin to secrete fluid into the tubule once stimulated by endocrine, paracrine, and autocrine regulating proteins. Such proteins may also play a role in the size and rate of growth of the cyst.

As a cyst grows, it detaches from the nephron (approximately 75% detach completely). The epithelial cells then continue to proliferate, and fibrosis develops. With time, the pressure created by the expanding, multiple cysts interrupts the function of neighboring nephrons, leading to apoptosis of noncystic nephrons. Although normal nephrons enlarge in an attempt to compensate for the loss of nephrons, this is unsuccessful in half of people with PKD.

In ADPKD, there have been several genes linked to the development of cysts. These abnormalities are located on chromosomes 16 and 4 and are called *PKD1* and *PKD2*. Other genes are likely involved as well. These genes code for proteins that function in transferring signals from the extracellular matrix into the cell to promote cellular proliferation and differentiation. Both genes need to be affected before there is the resultant development of disease.

Approximately 85% of persons with ADPKD express a mutation in *PKD1*; only 15% demonstrate a mutation in *PKD2*. A small percentage has a mutation in another gene. Although clinical manifestations are similar for people with PKD1 and PKD2, clients who exhibit the *PKD2* mutation progress to end-stage renal failure about 10 years later than those with the *PKD1* mutation.

Mutations to the gene coding for a large protein called fibrocystin on chromosome 6 lead to ARPKD. Further studies are needed in order to clearly define the role of these genes and their products in the formation of PKD.

### Clinical Manifestations

Although PKD is a hereditary disorder, only 60% of people are able to give a familial history of PKD, suggesting that spontaneous mutations occur frequently. For those families with a history of PKD, individuals can be monitored. In people who lack a familial history, cysts often are asymptomatic and found incidentally on routine urographic examination.

Symptoms associated with autosomal dominant disease may include pain, hematuria, fever, and hypertension. Abdominal or flank pain is the most common symptom in ADPKD. It can be associated with bleeding, growth of cysts, stones, infection, or, rarely, tumor. Most of these clients will have significantly enlarged kidneys that are palpable abdominally.

Associated hematuria may be gross or microscopic. Rupture of a cyst usually accounts for incidents of gross hematuria. Fever can be related to an infected cyst secondary to pyelonephritis. Hypertension is hypothesized to occur as a result of sodium and water retention because of damage to the tubules.[155,208] Hypertension also hastens the development of fibrosis and is linked with accelerated progression to ESRD.

Liver cysts are also common in clients with ADPKD; about half have liver cysts at diagnosis. Unlike the kidney cysts, liver cysts rarely lead to problems such as liver failure or portal hypertension. People with ADPKD may also be affected with other genetic abnormalities, such as thoracic and abdominal aortic aneurysms, cerebral aneurysms, mitral and aortic valve prolapse, colonic diverticular disease, and pancreatic cysts.

## MEDICAL MANAGEMENT

**DIAGNOSIS.** Ultrasonography is used to screen for PKD. People younger than 30 years of age should demonstrate at least two cysts in *one* kidney in order for PKD to be diagnosed. Persons between the ages of 30 and 59 years should have at least two cysts in *each* kidney, and people older than 60 years should demonstrate four cysts per kidney. Genetic tests can be performed to corroborate radiographic information. Simple cysts are uncommon in clients with PKD; the simultaneous presence of both large and small cysts is the norm.

CT is a useful radiographic test, distinguishing between solid and fluid-filled masses and displaying the presence of cysts of varied sizes. CT can also reveal the presence of hepatic cysts, making the diagnosis of PKD more likely. Prognostic information can also be obtained from the contrast-enhancing portion of a CT. Only the normal renal tubules will have contrast in them, revealing the degree of functioning nephrons.

MRI is often a better choice, especially for children or persons with renal dysfunction or who are in the early stages of the disease. Urinalysis may detect hematuria and proteinuria, or the clinical examination may reveal enlarged, palpable kidneys. As appropriate, other causes of renal cysts should be addressed. Occasionally, tissue biopsy or surgical exploration is necessary to make the definitive diagnosis.

**TREATMENT.** Because hypertension is a known risk factor for progression to ESRD, blood pressure should be monitored and controlled, particularly if a family history is present and the disease is diagnosed in young adults. Stimulation of the renin-angiotensin system was thought to be the cause of hypertension in ADPKD, but this has been questioned and other causes postulated. For this reason, angiotensin-converting enzyme (ACE) inhibitors and angiotensin receptor blockers (ARBs) have not been more successful than other blood pressure medications in preventing the progression of ADPKD.[170] Studies suggest that by keeping blood pressure at a normotensive level there is a slowing of progression to ESRD.[42,43,228]

Pain can be controlled through analgesics or treatment of the underlying cause (i.e., treating infections with antibiotics). Percutaneous aspiration of cystic fluid followed by injection of a sclerosing agent has helped some clients with pain from expanding cysts. Surgery and laparoscopic surgery can be performed to remove or unroof large cysts for pain relief. Infections can be difficult to treat, since the infection may be isolated in the cyst or an abscess may form. Possible associated findings, such as cerebral aneurysms, should be screened for and monitored.

**SPECIAL IMPLICATIONS FOR THE THERAPIST 18.4**

### *Renal Cystic Disease*

When treating a client with a history of renal cystic disease, therapists should be aware of symptoms and signs suggesting that the condition is worsening. The presence of any of these clinical findings warrants referral to a physician. An awareness that this population is at risk for hypertension and UTI and at increased risk of developing cerebral and aortic aneurysms and mitral valve problems is also necessary. The presentation of any symptoms or signs suggestive of the presence of these conditions again warrants referral to a physician. Lastly, the fact the kidneys may be enlarged can account for atypical findings on palpation.

## Renal Calculi

### Overview

Urinary stone disease, or nephrolithiasis, is the third most common urinary tract disorder, exceeded only by infections and prostate disease. Although a majority of the stones develop in the kidneys, once they move into the ureter they are referred to as ureteral stones (bladder stones are considered a separate disorder).

The stones, also called calculi, are crystalline and range from popcorn kernel shapes to jagged starbursts, and can cause urinary obstruction and severe pain. Urinary obstruction typically occurs at one of the following three sites: (1) the ureteropelvic junction, (2) where the ureter crosses over the iliac vessels, and (3) at the ureterovesical junction (Fig. 18.4). The four basic types of stones are calcium (oxalate and phosphate), struvite, uric acid, and cystine.

Calcium stones are by the far the most common (70% to 85%). Struvite stones are related to recurrent bacterial UTIs with organisms that produce urease. Uric acid stones (5% to 10% of nephrolithiasis cases) occur as the result of an increased level of urate in the blood and uric acid crystals in the urine, which is common in persons with gout. Cystine stones are uncommon (accounting for approximately 1% of all cases of nephrolithiasis) and caused by a hereditary disorder, cystinuria. Affected persons are unable to absorb cystine, and large amounts are excreted in the urine.

### Incidence

Nephrolithiasis occurs in approximately 5% of adults, with men being affected more frequently than women

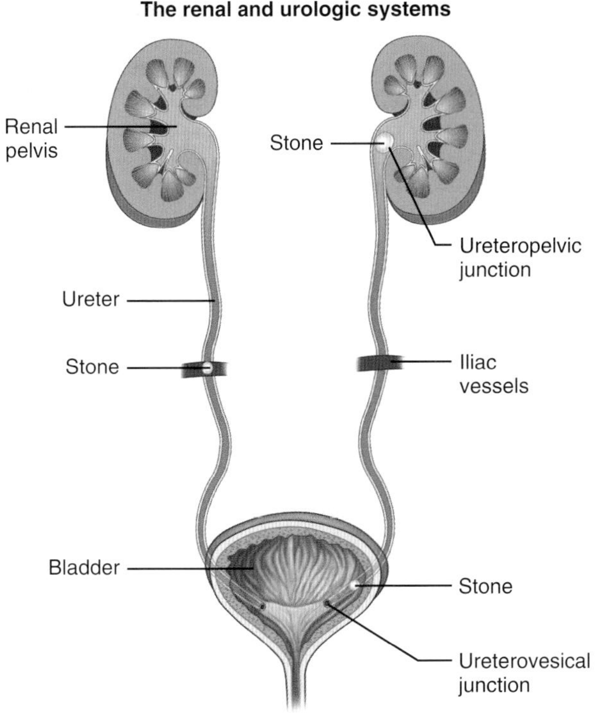


**Figure 18.4**

The three most common sites of urinary obstruction secondary to renal calculi.

(6% vs. 4%, respectively).[239] Because of the severe and debilitating pain associated with kidney stones, cost is significant, including doctor visits, hospitalizations, and lost work. In 2000, more than 2 million doctor visits annually and 177,496 hospital stays have been reported resulting from kidney stones, costing $2.07 billion.[162,248] The primary age span for the initial presentation of the disease is 30 to 60 years of age for men, and 20 to 30 years for women. A higher incidence of renal calculi occurs in industrialized countries and areas noted for high temperatures and humidity. The incidence of this disease is highest in the hot summer months.

## Etiologic and Risk Factors

With an understanding of the factors and mechanisms that lead to stone formation, risk factors are more evident and modifiable. Disorders that lead to an overexcretion and hypersaturation of calcium or oxalate can lead to stone formation. These include illnesses such as idiopathic hypercalciuria, renal tubular acidosis, primary hyperparathyroidism, and hyperoxaluria.

It is also known that low quantities of citrate (which typically binds calcium, thereby acting as an inhibitor to stone formation) can lead to nephrolithiasis. Uric acid crystals are sensitive to urine pH, coming out of solution in an acidic pH; thus an acidic urine pH can lead to uric acid stones.[232] Gout is a disorder in which excess urate is excreted into the urine, leading to a supersaturation of uric acid crystals. Chronic dehydration can lead to stone formation because of a decreased fluid content compared to crystals.

Other risk factors have been identified by epidemiologic studies but the mechanism remains unclear. For example, among persons with recurrent stone formation, it is often on one side only (unilateral). Some investigators have hypothesized that sleep posture (i.e., consistently sleeping on one side) may promote stone formation on the one side.[231] Obesity is associated with an increased incidence of urinary stone episodes in women but not in men.[206]

Excess intake of supplemental calcium, sodium, sucrose, and animal protein have been dietary risk factors implicated in stone formation. A lack of sufficient calcium and potassium in the diet can also increase risk for kidney stones.[62] Following a DASH (Dietary Approaches to Stop Hypertension)-style diet is associated with a reduced risk of kidney stones.[254]

## Pathogenesis

Several factors lead to the formation of stones—saturation, nucleation, crystal growth and aggregation, and cell/crystal interactions. Saturation refers to the amount of dissolved crystal (such as calcium oxalate or calcium phosphate) in the urine compared to volume.

Crystals are able to stay dissolved in the urine until it becomes oversaturated. Factors such as the amount of calcium, oxalate, and water excretion determine saturation. With oversaturation, crystals come out of solution (or out of the urine) into a solid and begin to grow around a particle, or nucleus. It is uncommon for urine to become so oversaturated that a new nucleus of calcium oxalate or calcium phosphate is formed. Most often, a small particle, bacteria (small nanobacteria), or other crystal already present in the urine acts as a nucleus for the crystals to grow around (i.e., stones may have a nucleus of one crystal type, but surrounded by another crystal type).

Crystals then grow at a rate depending on the saturation of the urine. The more supersaturated, the more quickly larger stones form. These stones also require enough time to enlarge, since normal flow is often sufficient to move small stones through the urinary tract. It is proposed that the growing crystal aggregate becomes attached to the urinary tract epithelium and transported into the cell membrane. Here, the cell membrane may also act as a nucleus. Investigations are ongoing to determine the significance of cell/crystal interactions.

## Clinical Manifestations

Clinical symptoms are the same for the various types of stones. The classic presentation of a kidney stone is acute "colicky" flank pain radiating to the groin or perineal areas (including the scrotum in males and labia in females) with hematuria. The pain is severe; most people are unable to find a comfortable position.

The location of the pain may vary depending on where the stone is lodged in the ureter. Abdominal pain with radiation to the groin may be more pronounced if the stone is higher in the abdomen, while a stone at the ureterovesical junction may give rise to lower quadrant abdominal pain radiating to the tip of the urethra.

Symptoms consistent with a UTI, such as urinary urgency and frequency and dysuria, are often present.

Hematuria is present in more than 90% of cases, although the absence of hematuria does not mean nephrolithiasis is not the diagnosis.[26] Nausea and vomiting may also be manifested.

## MEDICAL MANAGEMENT

**PREVENTION.** Stone disease is a highly prevalent condition associated with substantial cost and morbidity. The cost-effectiveness of a primary prevention strategy has been calculated.[162] Although preventive strategies cost more than no prevention, these strategies are at least 50% effective in preventing stones.[162]

Recurrence of calculi is common in up to 50% of people within 5 years, if preventive steps are not taken. A metabolic evaluation should be performed in clients who are willing to comply with tests and prophylactic methods (only 36%-70% of people with recurrent stones comply long-term with recommended measures).[196,266] Tests and appropriate preventive measures vary depending on the type of stone passed. Common tests include 24-hour urine collection for calcium, oxalate, uric acid, phosphate, citrate, pH, potassium, and creatinine; serum calcium; serum blood urea and creatinine; and parathyroid hormone (PTH). If a specific disorder, such as hyperparathyroidism, is identified, treatment reduces the risk for further stones.

Adequate fluid intake is essential to the prevention of stones and recurrences by reducing the saturation of stone-forming crystals. Clients should be encouraged to drink enough fluid to maintain clear-colored urine. Other dietary modifications are made according to stone type. Urinary uric acid can be reduced by decreasing the amount of protein ingested. Urine citrate can be increased by consuming more fruits and vegetables and decreasing the amount of acid-producing food (such as animal protein).[253,255] A restriction of calcium is not recommended and may be harmful.[25,61]

Medications can be helpful in certain situations if dietary means alone are insufficient to prevent stone formation. Thiazide diuretics (which increase calcium excretion), alkali, such as potassium citrate (beneficial in increasing urine citrate excretion), and allopurinol (prevents the precipitation of uric acid crystals) may be useful. Further research is needed to determine the efficacy of specific dietary changes and the best means to prevent kidney stones.

**DIAGNOSIS.** A variety of tests are used to diagnose this disease. Noncontrast helical CT scanning is the first-line imaging test for renal colic. Once a stone has been visualized on CT, a plain radiograph can help determine the type of stone. Approximately 90% of calculi are radiopaque, making them visible on an abdominal radiograph. These types of stones are composed of calcium or other minerals, whereas uric acid stones are not visible on a plain radiograph. Other traditional imaging tests (e.g., ultrasonography and IVP) can also help in the management of stone disease. Hematuria, infection, the presence of stone-forming crystals, and urine pH can be determined on urinalysis.

**TREATMENT.** The mainstay of treatment for acute nephrolithiasis includes intravenous fluids and medications to relieve nausea/vomiting and pain (narcotics or nonsteroidal antiinflammatory drugs [NSAIDs]). The α-blockers and calcium channel blockers are commonly used to treat hypertension, but both drugs also appear to flush out kidney stones by relaxing the ureter and increasing liquid pressure. Some physicians prefer α-blockers because they have fewer side effects. Most clients can be watched; however, some require immediate intervention to remove the stone.

Characteristics requiring urgent care include the presence of high-grade obstruction, anuria (no passage of urine), obstruction plus infection proximal to the stone, impending renal function deterioration, unresponsive pain or vomiting, or a solitary or transplanted kidney.[256] In these situations, percutaneous nephrostomy or ureteral stenting can be performed. Intravenous antibiotics are given for infection; *E. coli* is the most common organism.

A majority of stones less than 5 mm in diameter (a little smaller than the width of a pencil eraser) will pass spontaneously; the stones that do pass on their own do so within 4 weeks. The urine should be strained to retrieve any stones so they can be analyzed for crystal content.

Persons waiting for stones to pass should continue drinking fluid (enough to produce about 2 L/day of urine or keep the urine clear-colored instead of yellow). Fluids with sodium should be avoided; lemonade may be helpful because it increases urinary citrate and decreases calcium oxalate supersaturation.[230] A follow-up CT 3 to 4 weeks after the initial episode will verify the passage of the stone or the need for intervention if the stone is unmoved.

Clients who have kidney stones of less than 1 cm in the proximal ureter can receive shockwave lithotripsy.[272] Shockwave lithotripsy uses the transmission of shock waves (a type of sound wave) to break the calculi into fragments. Because the soft tissues of the body have similar densities, the shock waves pass through these structures with low attenuation. When the shock wave encounters a boundary between substances of differing acoustic density (i.e., a calculus in the ureter), high compressive forces are generated, causing a breakdown of the stone. The goal is to reduce the diameter to the point where spontaneous passage of the stone occurs.

Stones larger than 1 cm (and in the proximal ureter) benefit from ureteroscopy. Ureteroscopy involves passing a scope through the urethra and bladder into the ureter until the stone is reached. Then a laser is passed through the scope, the tip of the laser is placed on the stone, and the laser is discharged, producing photothermal lithotripsy.[269]

Stones located in the distal portion of the ureter can be treated with either method or with medical expulsive therapy, such as tamsulosin, the most commonly used agent, at a much lower cost.[18]

Uric acid stones are unique in their treatment. Because these stones dissolve in acid, the urine of affected clients can be acidified with potassium citrate or sodium citrate to increase the urine pH to at least 6.5. Stones are frequently not composed purely of uric acid, and further intervention may be required.

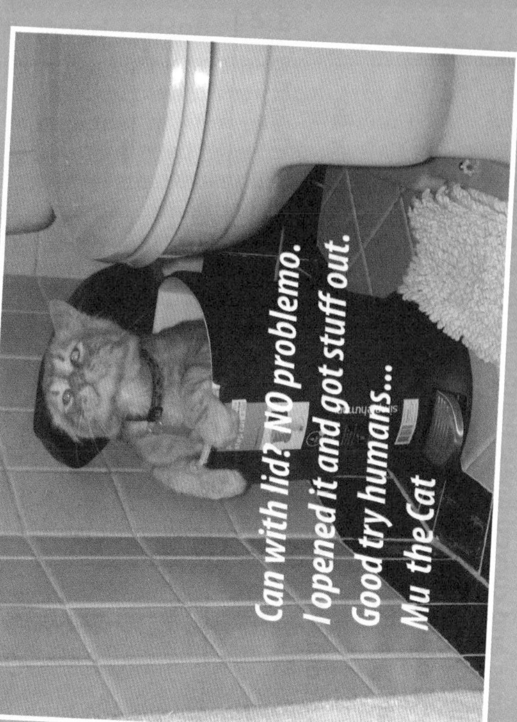


Stage 1 represents [illegible] min per 1.73 m$^2$) while stage 5 represents end-stage renal disease (ESRD) (<15 mL/min per 1.73 m$^2$) which requires kidney replacement therapy (dialysis or kidney transplantation) or conservative care (palliation or nondialytic care). The leading causes of CKD are diabetes, accounting for 30% to 50% of all CKD, and hypertension, accounting for more than a quarter of all cases.[276] The economic burden of CKD and ESRD is significant, with Medicare spending for patients with CKD ages 65 years and older exceeding $50 billion in 2013. Furthermore, spending is shown to be twice as high for patients with CKD, diabetes, and congestive heart failure all present compared to CKD alone.[39]

### Incidence

The prevalence of CKD is about 14% in the United States and is the fourteenth leading cause of death globally. Of the 661,000 Americans with kidney failure, 468,000 are on dialysis and roughly 193,000 are living with a functioning kidney transplant.[39] ESRD is 3.7 times higher among African Americans compared to Caucasians. Moreover, women (15.9%) are more likely than men (13.5%) to be diagnosed with stages 1 to 4 CKD.[39]

ESRD carries a high mortality rate, particularly in the older population. In 2013, the mortality rates for people with CKD were 117.9 per 1000, while mortality rates for those without CKD were 47.5 per 1000. More than half of all deaths in patients with ESRD were attributed to cardiovascular disease. However, since 1996 mortality rates have shown a decline for dialysis and transplant patients by 28% and 40%, respectively.[39]

**Table 18.5** Classification of CKD Stages 1-5 (Webster 2017)

| Stage | Descriptors | eGFR mL/min/1.73m$^2$ (Range) |
|---|---|---|
| G1 | Normal | ≥90 |
| G2 | Mildly decreased | 60-89 |
| G3a | Mildly to moderately decreased | 45-59 |
| G3b | Moderately to severely decreased | 30-44 |
| G4 | Severely decreased | 15-29 |
| G5 | Kidney failure | <15 |

*eGFR*, Estimated glomerular filtration rate.
From Webster AC, Nagler EV, Morton RL, Masson P: Chronic kidney disease, *Lancet* 389(10075):1238-1252, 2017.

### Etiologic and Risk Factors

The presence of a number of diseases can account for destruction of nephrons, but diabetes mellitus (principally type 2 causes diabetic nephropathy), high blood pressure, and glomerulonephritis are the leading causes of CKD. Other disorders contributing to the development of kidney failure include PKD, urinary tract obstruction, repeated infection, hereditary defects of the kidneys, toxicities, and systemic lupus erythematosus.

An increased risk of renal damage and ESRD is also associated with excessive nonprescription analgesic drug use, called *analgesic nephropathy*. This association was first noted with phenacetin-containing analgesics,[102] but is also noted with the drugs acetaminophen, aspirin, and combination analgesics (i.e., combining analgesics with codeine or caffeine).[85,113]

Heavy average intake or high cumulative intake of analgesics may increase the likelihood of developing ESRD, particularly in older people with a disorder already affecting the kidneys.[182] NSAIDs, both selective and nonselective, have significant short-term effects on the kidney, yet data have been inconsistent with regard to the risk for ESRD from NSAID use.[60,124] More research is needed to answer this question, but it may be that moderate use of NSAIDs in healthy individuals does not put them at significant increased risk for ESRD.[211]

### Pathogenesis

The basic functioning unit of the kidney is the nephron. It is composed of the glomerulus, the renal tubules, and the collecting duct (Fig. 18.5). The glomerulus is a small bundle of capillaries, surrounded by a capsule that allows fluid and electrolytes to pass through the membrane and into the tubules. The renal tubules transport electrolytes or create a gradient for fluid and electrolytes to become balanced, while the collecting tubule is responsible for the final regulation of electrolytes and water under the influence of the hormone aldosterone.

As discussed earlier, many disease processes can result in CKD. Diabetes, for example, induces kidney damage through hyperglycemia. Angiotensin II is also released, which causes vasoconstriction of the arterioles and

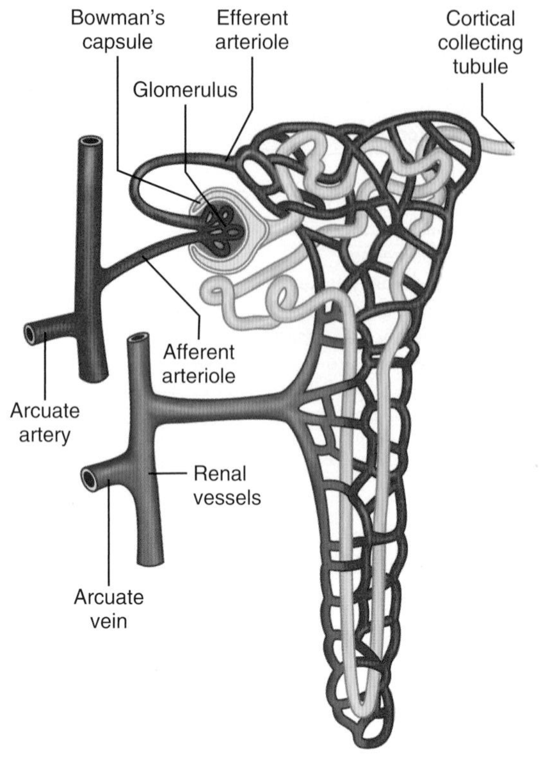


**Figure 18.5**

**Components of the nephron.** The afferent arteriole carries blood to the glomerulus for filtration through the Bowman capsule and the renal tubular system.

arteries (both in the glomerulus and systemically) in an attempt to keep the pressure adequate for filtration.

Angiotensin II release also leads to the attraction of inflammatory cells, which release cytokines and growth factors (which change the structure of the glomerulus). These changes result in mesangial expansion (a layer of cells around the glomerular capillaries), enlargement of the glomerulus, and ultimately interstitial fibrosis and glomerular sclerosis.

These processes slowly reduce the amount of surface area available for filtration to occur, thereby reducing the glomerular filtration rate (GFR). With the gradual loss of nephron function, the kidneys are unable to adequately regulate fluid, electrolytes, and pH balance or remove metabolic waste products from the blood.

The rate of nephron destruction can vary considerably, depending on the disease process. Typically, five stages mark the progression of chronic renal failure; each stage is defined by the level of the GFR (measured in milliliters per minute): (1) kidney damage with normal or increased GFR (90 mL/min or more), (2) kidney damage with mildly decreased GFR (60-89 mL/min), (3) moderately decreased GFR (30-59 mL/min), (4) severely decreased GFR (15-29 mL/min), and (5) kidney failure (ESRD; GFR of less than 15 mL/min). Systemic complications typically develop once stage 4 CKD is reached, when the GFR is less than 30 mL/min.

## Clinical Manifestations

In stage 1 of CKD, the GFR is normal or increased (hyperfiltration). No overt symptoms of impaired renal function are typically evident. Depending on the health of the person, the kidneys have tremendous adaptive and compensatory capabilities, accounting for the delay in symptoms. The unaffected nephrons undergo structural and physiologic hypertrophy in an attempt to make up for those nephrons that are no longer functioning. Results of blood tests that are indicative of kidney function, such as blood urea nitrogen (BUN) and creatinine, are typically normal.

The onset of symptoms is usually very gradual and subtle, with the continued loss of nephrons and reduction in GFR, often resulting in a delay in diagnosis. Early clinical manifestations include hypertension and anemia. Abnormalities in laboratory values include an increase in BUN and creatinine, or protein detected in the urine. Stage 1 is reversible for some people (e.g., those with diabetes who benefit from early detection and proper glycemic control). Some individuals remain in stage 1 indefinitely, whereas others progress.

During stage 2, the damaged capillaries allow small amounts of albumin to be excreted in the urine. Individuals may remain in this stage for several years with proper control of hypertension and blood glucose levels. Stage 3 is more noticeable as albumin levels increase in the urine and decrease in the blood, resulting in noticeable edema. During this stage, levels of creatinine and BUN increase, resulting in an accumulation of waste products in the blood called *azotemia*.[76]

In the final stages of CKD (stages 4 and 5, with stage 5 being ESRD), the kidney is unable to function and a multitude of complications appear with accompanying symptoms and signs. Proteinuria is the hallmark of stage 4; the kidneys are no longer able to excrete toxins, so there is a progressive increase in BUN and creatinine levels. Most people in stage 4 are hypertensive because of an increased production of renin. Hypertension accelerates the progression to stage 5 (ESRD) when the kidneys have failed to function.

Stage 5 or ESRD is heralded by a cluster of symptoms referred to as *uremia*.[197] The kidneys cannot excrete toxins; maintain fluid, pH, and electrolyte balances; or secrete important hormones (e.g., renin, vitamin D, erythropoietin). Uremia develops when poorly identified toxins are not removed from the blood. Uremia is characterized by nausea, vomiting, anorexia, lethargy, pruritus (itching), sensory and motor neuropathy, pericarditis, impaired heart function, asterixis, and seizures. Asterixis is an intermittent inability to sustain a posture, often noted when holding up the hand with the wrist flexed, creating a small "flapping-like" motion. Table 18.6 summarizes the systemic effects associated with CKD and ESRD.

**Hematologic.** Anemia is a significant hematologic problem associated with CKD. The hormone erythropoietin, primarily produced by the interstitial cells of the kidneys, has the principal function of controlling the production of red blood cells in the bone marrow. CKD leads to decreased erythropoietin production, reduced red blood cell life span, and reduced iron absorption, resulting in a subsequent decrease in red blood cells and anemia.

Anemia associated with CKD occurs most frequently in clients with a GFR of less than 60 mL/min and in persons 75 years of age or older.[9] However, a lack of

**Table 18.6** Systemic Manifestations of Kidney Failure

| Systemic Symptoms | Probable Causes |
|---|---|
| **Urinary System** | |
| Decreased urinary output<br>Abnormal urinary constituents (blood cells, protein, casts)<br>Abnormal blood serum level, such as elevated BUN and creatinine | Damaged renal tissue |
| **Cardiopulmonary** | |
| Coronary artery disease<br>Hypertension | Calcification of the arteries, other risk factors |
| Congestive heart failure<br>Pulmonary edema | Fluid overload |
| Dyspnea<br>Pericarditis | Uremic toxins irritate pericardial sac |
| **Gastrointestinal Tract** | |
| Bleeding<br>Nausea and vomiting | Platelet changes |
| Uremic breath<br>Anorexia | Uremic toxins change saliva |
| **Nervous System** | |
| ***Central*** | |
| Headache<br>Irritability<br>Impaired judgment<br>Inability to concentrate<br>Seizures<br>Lethargy/coma<br>Sleep disturbances | Effect of electrolyte and fluid changes on brain cells (usually resolves with dialysis treatment) |
| ***Peripheral*** | |
| Loss of vibratory sense and deep tendon reflexes<br>Impairment of motor nerve conduction velocity<br>Burning, tingling, paresthesias<br>Tremors | Effect of uremic toxins on peripheral nerves |
| Muscle cramps, muscle twitching<br>Foot drop<br>Weakness | Electrolyte imbalances (calcium, sodium, potassium) |
| **Integumentary (Skin)** | |
| Pruritus (itching)/excoriation (scratching) | Skin calcifications related to calcium/phosphorus imbalances |
| Hyperpigmentation | Retained uremic pigments |
| Pallor | Anemia |
| Bruising | Platelet dysfunction |
| **Eyes** | |
| Band keratopathy<br>Visual blurring | Corneal calcifications related to calcium/phosphorus imbalance |
| Dry eyes<br>Red eyes | Conjunctival calcifications related to calcium/phosphorus imbalance |
| **Endocrine** | |
| Fertility and sexual dysfunction | Effect of uremic toxins on menstrual cycles, ovulation, and sperm production |
| Hyperparathyroidism | Result of calcium/phosphorus imbalance |
| **Hematopoietic** | |
| Anemia | Decreased production of erythropoietin by kidney; destruction of red blood cells by dialysis |
| Platelet dysfunction | Uremic toxins interfere with platelet aggregation |
| **Skeletal** | |
| Renal osteodystrophy (demineralization of bones) | Related to decreased calcium absorption and resultant calcium/phosphorus imbalance |
| Joint pain<br>Myopathy | Joint calcifications |

From Goodman CC, Heick J, Lazaro R: *Differential diagnosis in physical therapy*, ed 4, Philadelphia, 2017, WB Saunders.

erythropoietin is not the only factor causing anemia in clients with CKD. Other causes, such as gastrointestinal bleeding, iron or folate deficiency, or hemolysis, may play a role and should be evaluated.

Anemia in CKD can cause significant fatigue and reduced quality of life. Another important result of anemia is the stress it places on the heart. Anemia is an independent risk factor for cardiovascular disease and should be treated aggressively (see Chapter 14 for additional information regarding anemia).[261] ESRD also leads to white blood cell dysfunction and bleeding problems caused by impaired platelet function.

**Cardiovascular.** Cardiovascular diseases often occur in people with CKD and are the leading cause of death in persons with ESRD. As the GFR decreases, the risk for cardiovascular disease increases in a graded fashion.[96,150,259] Many of the risk factors that cause CKD, such as diabetes and hypertension, also contribute to cardiovascular disease. Diseases common in clients with CKD include coronary artery disease, left ventricular hypertrophy, and congestive heart failure. Persons with CKD often have hyperlipidemia, another risk factor for coronary artery disease.

Symptoms may include chest pain (although many often have atypical or no pain), nausea, shortness of breath, and sweating. Excess fluid volume, sodium retention, and anemia associated with ESRD lead to left ventricular hypertrophy, a thickening of the left ventricle of the heart, which predisposes to congestive heart failure.

Associated clinical features include lower extremity edema and shortness of breath. Hypertension often appears early in the course of this disease because of increased angiotensin II production. Clients in stage 3 of CKD often need two or more medications to control blood pressure. Clients with CKD also have a higher incidence of stroke, peripheral vascular disease, arrhythmias, pericarditis, and heart valve abnormalities.

**Gastrointestinal.** Gastrointestinal system complaints occur often once the later stages of ESRD are reached. Azotemia (high levels of urea and other toxins in the blood) causes nausea, vomiting, and anorexia. The resultant depressed appetite contributes to malnutrition, fatigue, weakness, and malaise. Malnutrition has a high prevalence in those with advanced kidney disease, partly as a result of the therapeutic restriction on calories and proteins but also because of the metabolic reactions typical with this disease. Other clinical manifestations include gastritis, duodenitis, pancreatitis, hiccups (often difficult to control), and ascites.

**Musculoskeletal.** The skeletal changes associated with CKD are common and can occur early in the disease secondary to abnormalities in calcium, phosphate, and vitamin D metabolism. With the impairment of GFR, the body is unable to excrete phosphate or synthesize 1,25-dihydroxyvitamin D (a vitamin D derivative called *calcitriol*). Higher blood levels of phosphate lead to low ionized calcium levels. Calcitriol normally regulates calcium absorption from the gut and inhibits the parathyroid gland. But with low levels of calcitriol, hypocalcemia and increased PTH secretion result. A drop in serum calcium signals a cascade of events starting with the release of PTH, which signals the body to increase calcium resorption from bone to make up for the perceived loss (Fig. 18.6).

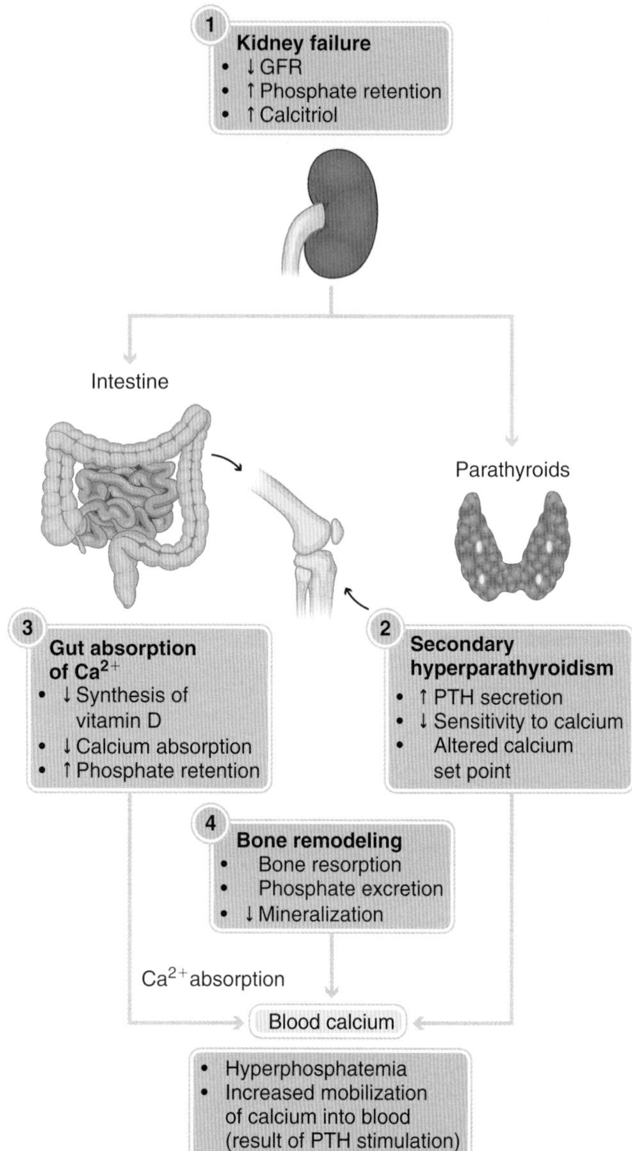


**Figure 18.6**

**Mechanisms of altered bone turnover.** (1) Renal osteodystrophy can be viewed as the result of a vicious cycle that begins with moderate to severe renal failure. As the glomerular filtration rate (GFR) decreases, phosphate excretion decreases, and calcium elimination increases. (2) The body attempts to compensate for the loss of calcitriol and reduced calcium absorption by increasing parathyroid hormone (PTH) secretion. PTH mobilizes calcium from the bones (bone reabsorption) and facilitates phosphate excretion. This release of calcium and phosphate into the blood results in hyperphosphatemia and hypercalcemia. (3) As kidney failure progresses, the damaged kidneys can no longer convert vitamin D to its active form and without active vitamin D, calcium absorption in the intestines is decreased and paradoxically facilitates phosphate retention. (4) Thus the normal process of bone mineralization with calcium and phosphate is impaired. Demineralization of the bone frees more calcium and phosphorus into the blood. As the disease progresses even more, the parathyroid gland may become unresponsive to the normal feedback system and continue to produce PTH, causing acceleration of renal osteodystrophy.

Several skeletal abnormalities result from varying types of bone turnover, collectively referred to as renal osteodystrophy. Renal osteodystrophy is a type of rickets formerly called renal rickets, and sometimes referred to as azotemic osteodystrophy. Although uncommon at one time, the incidence has risen with increased survival of people with renal disease on dialysis.

Renal osteodystrophy is characterized by varying degrees of osteomalacia, osteitis fibrosa, and adynamic bone disease. Osteomalacia occurs secondary to low bone turnover caused by aluminum deposition in the bones, with resultant increased nonmineralized bone matrix formation. Osteitis fibrosa results in inflammation and fibrosis of bone because of high bone turnover, whereas adynamic bone disease is a low bone turnover state, which may be related to excessive PTH suppression from therapy.[74]

Clients with renal osteodystrophy may present with bone pain, especially in the spine, hips, knees, or lower extremities, and fractures.[74] The pain is worse with exercise and other weight-bearing activities; the fractures occur most often in the vertebrae and long bones.[76] Increased secretion of PTH and a decreased secretion of calcitriol appear to be the cause. Metabolic acidosis may also play a role, either by increasing osteoclastic activity or by increasing the effects of PTH.[278]

Osteopenia and pseudofractures are seen most frequently in people with osteomalacia. Osteitis fibrosa is evident on radiographic films, particularly in the phalanges, skull, and distal clavicles, where there is subperiosteal bone resorption.

In addition to bone demineralization, calcification of vessels and soft tissues occurs. This calcification may be related to bone turnover and occurs during both high and low bone turnover. It is postulated that deposition of minerals may occur in extraskeletal sites because the bone is unable to incorporate them. If bone turnover is high, minerals are removed from bone and are deposited in extraskeletal sites. If bone turnover is low, minerals are also deposited in extraskeletal sites because the bone is forming abnormally or at a slow rate.

The most common sites for extraskeletal calcification include the coronary arteries, lungs, skin, peripheral arteries, joints, and cornea. Calcifications of the coronary arteries are common and may be the reason for the high death rate in CKD clients. Intraarterial calcifications can occlude vessels, leading to ischemia and gangrene.

Deposition of minerals in the skin can lead to intense pruritus (itching), and occlusion of an arteriole can cause necrosis of skin, termed *calciphylaxis*. This occurs most commonly in the lower extremities, trunk, or buttocks. Articular cartilage and joints can become calcified, causing pseudogout and arthritis symptoms.

Calcification of a tendon may lead to spontaneous rupture with minimal stress. The quadriceps tendon may rupture simply by walking, tripping, or going down stairs. Tendon ruptures can lead to pain, deformity, and disability. Other areas of commonly observed ruptures in this population include the triceps and extensor tendons of the fingers.[76] Hyperparathyroidism and metabolic acidosis are responsible for the abnormal collagen that results in weak tendons.[51,278]

Calcifications are frequently found on the cornea and conjunctiva but are typically asymptomatic. Clients who have kidney disease characterized by a slow decline in function may have more severe cases of both renal osteodystrophy and calcification of vessels and soft tissue. (Although cardiovascular manifestations were discussed earlier in this section, in view of the information here on calcification, it should be noted that vascular calcification of the arteries resulting in vascular insufficiency has been observed in nearly all individuals with ESRD by age 50 years. In fact, most people with CKD actually die from cardiovascular disease, rather than progress to the final stages of ESRD.[136,207])

Myopathy can occur with proximal muscle weakness affecting the muscles of the shoulder and pelvic girdles, leading to functional disabilities. The gluteus medius, hamstring, and psoas muscles are affected first and most severely, resulting in gait impairments and difficulty rising from low seats or accomplishing functional activities such as getting in and out of a bathtub. As the condition progresses, activities of daily living, such as combing the hair, brushing the teeth, or household tasks, become more difficult to manage independently.

**Neurologic.** Alteration of central nervous system and peripheral nervous system function often occurs in association with ESRD. Early central nervous system changes include sleeping disturbances (both getting to sleep and staying asleep) followed by daytime sleepiness and personality changes.

Uremic encephalopathy occurs when the GFR is less than 10 mL/min and is manifested by recent memory loss, inability to concentrate, perceptual errors, confusion, asterixis, and decreased alertness. These symptoms abate once dialysis is instituted. Without treatment, seizures, lethargy, obtundation, and coma develop.

The peripheral neuropathy associated with uremic toxins is characterized by a dying back of the axons of both sensory and motor nerves. These neurologic changes are typically symmetrical (stocking-glove distribution) and similar to those of any other polyneuropathy with a stocking-glove distribution. Clients can also exhibit restless leg syndrome.[105] Like central nervous system manifestations of uremia, peripheral nervous system symptoms improve with dialysis.

## MEDICAL MANAGEMENT

PREVENTION. Everyone should be screened for hypertension and diabetes, with early intervention when present. The ultimate goal and mission of the National Kidney Foundation is the eradication of diseases of the kidney. Toward that end, *Healthy People 2020* identified several goals related to kidney failure, including (1) reduce kidney failure resulting from diabetes; (2) increase the proportion of people with chronic kidney failure who receive a transplant within 3 years of registration on the waiting list; (3) increase the proportion of people with chronic kidney failure who receive counseling on nutrition, treatment choices, and cardiovascular care 12 months before the start of renal replacement therapy; (4) reduce deaths from cardiovascular disease in persons with chronic kidney failure; and (5) reduce the rate of new cases of ESRD.

Because diabetic nephropathy is the leading cause of kidney failure in the United States, prevention strategies and risk factor modification related to improving glycemic control, preventing hypertension, preventing coronary artery disease, increasing physical activity, and reducing or eliminating tobacco-related behaviors (e.g., smoking) are a large part of the prevention of renal disease. In the future, pancreas transplantation may become a part of diabetes prevention and therefore ESRD prevention.

**DIAGNOSIS.** As discussed earlier, the early stages of CKD are often without symptoms. Because of the significant morbidity and mortality associated with CKD, early detection is emphasized, with the goal of slowing progression or reversing the disease if possible. People with diabetes, hypertension, or a family history of kidney disease are at high risk for kidney disease and should be monitored for early indications of kidney disease.

Because there are many causes for CKD, multiple tests may be required to determine the cause and severity. Several laboratory tests are helpful in detecting and following progression of CKD and ESRD. Persons with diabetes should routinely be tested for microprotein in the urine (an indication of early kidney disease). GFR, BUN, and creatinine are blood tests that can indicate kidney dysfunction (GFR is actually calculated using laboratory results).

In the presence of CKD, GFR will be the first laboratory indicator of renal damage, followed by increases in BUN and creatinine with continued kidney damage. GFR not only characterizes the stage of kidney disease but also demonstrates disease progression. Urine tests may show protein or casts (abnormal protein "castings" of the tubules). For those persons with known CKD or ESRD, intact PTH (or N-terminal PTH molecule) levels should be monitored in an attempt to avoid renal osteodystrophy.

Imaging modalities may demonstrate obstruction, masses, or bilateral small kidneys (which is consistent with ESRD from a chronic disease). A kidney biopsy may be needed to confirm specific kidney pathology (such as a glomerulonephritis).

**TREATMENT.** Following the diagnosis of CKD, a referral to a nephrologist should be made. Although best outcomes occur when a referral is made early in the course of CKD, up to 40% are not referred until 3 months prior to initiating dialysis.[263] Delayed referrals lead to an increase in morbidity and mortality.

The goals of treating CKD include treating the underlying disease, modifying risk factors for cardiovascular disease, and preventing further loss of kidney function. For some diseases, treating the principal disease may involve immunosuppressive agents, such as with the treatment of membranous nephropathy. Renal artery stenosis may require angioplasty with stenting. Diabetes requires tight glycemic control.

Cardiovascular complications are common and require risk factor modification and treatment. Clients with CKD should lose weight, exercise, eliminate smoking, and modify their diet. Dyslipidemia treatment involves lifestyle modifications, and medication may be needed. Blood pressure should be strictly controlled in order to reduce cardiovascular risk and prevent further loss of renal function (although the exact range is disputed, a systolic blood pressure between 120 mm Hg and 130 mm Hg should be the goal).[156]

Measures that help prevent further loss of kidney function include avoidance of nephrotoxic drugs and radiocontrast agents, treatment of anemia, strict blood pressure control, and the use of ACE inhibitors or ARBs.[156]

For the predialysis stage, data are lacking to establish the optimal hemoglobin level to begin erythropoietin therapy. But a recommendation has been published to suggest initiation of subcutaneous erythropoietin when the hemoglobin drops below 10 g/dL, after verification of adequate iron stores and exclusion of other causes of anemia.[71] Studies demonstrate that the use of an ACE inhibitor or ARB is renoprotective beyond the ability of just lowering blood pressure.

The treatment of clients who develop ESRD continues with many of the same measures used to treat the other stages of CKD, such as blood pressure control and anemia treatment. Dietary modifications are necessary, including low-potassium, low-sodium, and low-protein diets. Excess protein can increase urea levels, and clients should not consume more than 1 g/kg per day of protein. Dietitian referrals are important, because malnutrition may occur with strict dietary regulation. Fluid intake is restricted and diuretics are needed to maintain fluid balance.

Prevention of renal osteodystrophy necessitates monitoring of calcium–phosphate balance and PTH levels. The goal is to maintain calcium at less than 9.5 mg/dL and phosphate at less than 5.5 mg/dL. This has typically been accomplished using calcium-binding agents and vitamin D sterols.

New questions have been raised, however, concerning calcification of vessels (principally the coronary arteries) and calcium/phosphate metabolism. The traditional methods of lowering calcium and phosphate may still leave levels too high to reduce calcification of the coronary arteries. A calcimimetic agent called cinacalcet, approved by the FDA in 2004, appears to treat secondary hyperparathyroidism and maintain normal calcium and phosphate levels. Further use of this drug in a larger population will determine efficacy in preventing renal osteodystrophy and cardiovascular complications.

*Renal replacement therapy* (dialysis or transplantation) is the treatment of choice for ESRD. The decision is based on the client's age, general health, donor availability, and personal preference. Dialysis can take the form of hemodialysis (HD) or peritoneal dialysis (PD) (also referred to as *continuous ambulatory peritoneal dialysis [CAPD]* and *continuous cycling peritoneal dialysis [CCPD]*). The main difference between these methods of dialysis is in their exchange schedules (daytime vs. nighttime, length of time required).

HD typically requires three sessions per week for 3 to 4 hours per session. The blood flows from an artery through the dialysis machine chambers and then back to the body's venous system, with the waste products and excess fluid and electrolytes diffusing into the dialyzing solution. HD can be done at home, although this requires specialized training, or the client can travel to a renal center. Although it is common practice that the person remains relatively immobile throughout the session, studies show that appropriately prescribed low- to moderate-intensity exercise programs done during the first 2 hours of dialysis can improve physical health, quality of life, and dialysis efficacy.[44,46,179,187,197,245] Only 1% of dialysis clients receive home HD, while 85% receive in-center treatment.

Approximately 10% of dialysis clients use PD. PD relies on the same principles as HD, but it can be done independently at home, whereas individuals on home HD must have a care partner to assist them. A catheter is implanted in the peritoneal cavity, and sterile dialyzing solution is instilled and then drained over a specific period. This process is completed four times daily or at night while the individual sleeps. With CAPD/CCPD, fewer dietary restrictions and fewer of the dramatic symptom swings associated with HD occur. Potential complications of PD include infection, catheter malfunction, dehydration, hyperglycemia, and hernia. Peritonitis occurs about once every 3 years in those undergoing PD and is the most serious potential complication. The majority of affected people are successfully treated with intraperitoneal antibiotics.

The steady improvement in the outcome of renal allografts has made kidney transplantation the treatment of choice for many people with ESRD. Transplantation is less expensive than long-term dialysis, but donor availability limits the number of transplants performed. The current contraindications for transplant include active substance abuse or noncompliance, metastatic cancer, severe arterial disease involving the iliac arteries, active infection, active ischemic cardiac and cerebrovascular disease, advanced dementia, and debility.

In adults, the renal graft is placed extraperitoneally in the iliac fossa through an oblique lower abdominal incision. In small children, the graft is located retroperitoneally with a midline abdominal incision. Complications of the procedures include renal artery thrombosis, urinary leak, and lymphocele.

**PROGNOSIS.** Despite significant advances in technologic and pharmacologic interventions, in 2016 there were 124,675 newly reported cases of ESRD; the unadjusted (crude) incidence rate was 373.4 per million/year.[264] Cardiovascular diseases remain the number one cause of death in those with all categories of renal disease, including persons with CKD, those with ESRD on dialysis, and renal transplant recipients. This is most likely a result of the presence of multiple cardiovascular risk factors (e.g., hypertension, abnormal lipids, smoking, dietary factors).[164]

## Nephrogenic Systemic Fibrosis

Nephrogenic systemic fibrosis (NSF), previously known as nephrogenic fibrosing dermopathy, was first described in literature by Cowper et al.[58] when its incidence spiked among renal dialysis patients that developed conspicuous skin conditions presenting with firm, erythematous, indurated plaques and thickening or tightening of the skin.[73]

Once believed to affect only the skin, it can also affect deeper structures, including the organs. Postmortem autopsy of affected individuals showed fibrosis and calcification of the psoas muscle, renal tubules, testes, and diaphragm. A peculiar concentration of osteoid and elastic fibers termed "lollipop bodies" are common and found to be highly specific to NSF.[258] A common presentation is skin thickening on the arms, legs, and torso while sparing the face. The skin lesions are typically symmetrical and distributed bilaterally and seem to fuse together to form hyperpigmented plaques that resemble the skin of an orange (also known as peau d'orange). These areas can have changes in pigmentation and are described as pruritic with concomitant burning pain sensation, especially when occurring on the hips or ribs.[17,258]

Medical practitioners were quick to note its similarity to scleromyxedema and called it "scleromyxedema-like cutaneous disease during dialysis." It was later differentiated from scleromyxedema by the absence of paraproteinemia and the absence of pools of dermal mucin and plasma cell infiltrates.[285] The term *nephrogenic* is a misnomer because the cause of the symptoms is not the kidney disease but the contrast agent used in the diagnostic imaging studies.[157]

The etiology of NSF remained unknown until 2006 when several patients developed NSF within weeks of receiving gadolinium for magnetic resonance angiography or contrast-enhanced MRI. MR enhanced contrast is very effective for diagnosing renal vascular disease.[2] Scientists found a strong correlation between exposure to a gadolinium-based contrast agent and NSF in individuals with kidney disease, particularly in the presence of a proinflammatory process such as major surgery, infection, or a vascular thromboembolic event.[157,180,258]

It was hypothesized that the high doses of free gadolinium ions may have caused a toxic reaction. In 2007, the United States Food and Drug Administration (FDA) issued a black box warning on all gadolinium-based contrast agents (GBCA). This drastically reduced the incidence of NSF in patients with kidney disease because it was almost malpractice for radiologists to prescribe its use as a contrast agent.[86] To clarify the offending agent and protect the public, the American College of Radiologists (ACR) put out their own classification of GBCA in regards to NSF. (See https://www.acr.org/Clinical-Resources/Contrast-Manual). The guidelines have important implications to patient care. Several types of contrast material–enhanced MR imaging in patients with impaired renal function may be safe and should remain a viable imaging option in this patient population.[6,86] Nevertheless, gadolinium-based contrast is still under close scrutiny due to its detected accumulation in the bone and brain tissue, even in patients with normal renal function.[137,157,209] More study is needed to ascertain its long-term effects, but the ACR recommends avoidance of repeated exposure to GBCAs.[2,6] Curiously, hemodialysis has had no effect on reducing risk or the incidence of NSF in CKD patients. Some patients develop NSF after several doses of GBCA, while a few acquire the symptoms after only one bout of MR enhanced GBCA.[86] There are factors that are still not clear and will need further investigation.

There is no known cure for NSF. Some cases resolve after renal transplantation and others anecdotally after extracorporeal photopheresis and intravenous sodium thiosulfate.[158] Treatment options being considered include oral and topical corticosteroids, photopheresis, ultraviolet therapy, and high dose immunoglobulin therapy.[142] The majority of affected individuals develop complications such as decreased joint mobility, flexion contractures, and resulting muscle weakness. Physical therapy is highly recommended for this population.[142] NSF is a debilitating disease and is proving to be an unwelcome burden to an already physically fragile group. Further research is needed to its cause, management, and prevention.

## A THERAPIST'S THOUGHTS*

**Nephrogenic Systemic Fibrosis**

People with kidney disease or injury are an especially challenging population when it comes to exercise prescription. They have varying sensitivities to medications, nutrition, and physical activity. Depending on the severity of their condition, these persons can have diminished activity tolerance and strength, resulting in impaired mobility status relative to comparable age-groups.[15,281] Their weakened condition can easily tip toward a vulnerable state.

Nephrogenic systemic fibrosis is a crippling condition that is afflicting this population. NSF manifestations include thickening of the skin and connective tissue, which can lead to muscle tightness and contractures. The trunk and the extremities can be equally involved. Afflicted individuals have also complained of sharp joint pains, as well as deep bone pain on the hips and ribs. These symptoms can result in progressive weakness and loss of function. It is imperative that prompt intervention is provided in order to avoid further deconditioning. Physical therapy should be instituted and be part of a comprehensive treatment program.

These individuals may benefit from joint manipulation, with connective tissue mobilization and massage. Distal joints such as those of the hands can benefit from paraffin wax treatments to increase flexibility and range of motion. Manual stretching of affected joints and skin can relieve the feeling of restricted movement. Therapeutic pool exercises and swimming have been found to be beneficial for this group. Individuals may need an assessment and instruction on the use of an assistive device or an ambulatory aid to continue their level of mobility. Both the individual and the individual's caregivers should be educated about the condition and instructed on a program to extend the management to the home setting. The physical therapist should consider all possibilities to prevent inactivity and to maintain the individual's quality-of-life.

As a result of the accompanying complaints of pain, a formal pain management program conducted by a physician-led team should be established. A special consideration brought about by the thickened skin is the difficulty in finding venous access in the extremities. Any current and potential access should be identified and kept patent for intravenous use.

Perhaps more important than the support and treatment to affected individuals is prevention of the condition. Each health professional in every setting should be vigilant about possibly exposing at-risk individuals to certain gadolinium-based agents, and should advise on its potential for causing NSF. There may be other causes for the development of NSF and it is our priority to avert any occurrence. This can only be done consistently by consciously staying informed on current applicable research.

Michael S. Castillo, PT, MHS, MPA, GCS, NCS

## SPECIAL IMPLICATIONS FOR THE THERAPIST 18.6

### *Chronic Kidney Disease*

Therapists must be aware that several specific renal syndromes may be induced by the interaction of NSAIDs and other analgesics on renal function. Although the nephrotoxicity is relatively low, the increased availability of these medications as nonprescription products and the concentration of people taking NSAIDs/analgesics in a rehabilitation setting are factors contributing to the fact that a larger percentage of these people come into contact with a therapist. Anyone with renal failure who is a regular user of acetaminophen and aspirin is at up to 2.2 times higher risk of developing CKD.[85] Analgesic nephropathy is still a real risk, but has dramatically declined as a result of the removal of phenacetin from the analgesic market, although mixed analgesics containing paracetamol, the main metabolite of phenacetin, remain popularly used.[172,173]

Older adults are especially susceptible and more likely to use these agents. Additionally, NSAID-related renal involvement is probably underrecognized, and with the FDA approval of nonprescription sale of NSAIDs (e.g., naproxen sodium, ketoprofen, ibuprofen), incidence may increase in the coming years.[168] Any time a client reports a history of prolonged and regular NSAID/analgesic use and renal symptoms, medical evaluation is required. In general, clinicians are advised to consider the risk and benefits on a case-by-case basis, with determination and consideration of the affected individual's CKD status and use of NSAIDs. The potential risk of CKD progression may be outweighed by the individual's improved quality of life.[205]

Physical therapy care of people with CKD has increased significantly in the past 20 years. Treating people with a diagnosis of CKD can be extremely challenging because of malnutrition, side effects of medications, complications from dialysis, and the number of body systems involved. The decreased alertness, inability to concentrate, and short-term memory deficits interfere with following instructions, including transfers, exercises, body mechanics, and so on.

Musculoskeletal changes occur because of abnormalities in calcium, phosphate, and vitamin D metabolism, resulting in osteomalacia, osteoporosis, and soft tissue calcification. Spontaneous tendon ruptures have been reported in the ESRD population, especially those individuals with hyperparathyroidism. Their risk is increased when treated with quinolone antibiotics and/or steroids.[16] Neuromuscular effects of CKD include both central and peripheral nervous system disorders. Kasinskas and Piazza offer consideration for a clinical pathway for clients with CKD, using the *Guide to Physical Therapist Practice* that is worth reviewing for any therapist working with this population group.[8,138]

Adverse effects of some of the medications used for renovascular hypertension may include angioedema (i.e., swelling around the face, mouth, or throat), requiring immediate medical attention. Clients should be taught to rise slowly, dangling the legs and feet before standing, and to report any unusual swelling.

Reliance on the assistance of family and other health care providers is often necessary. The fatigue and general weakness may dictate that the therapist provide rest periods during a rehabilitation session. The potential osteodystrophy requires modification of evaluation and intervention techniques, including osteoporosis education and prevention.

A number of potential renal transplantation complications that the therapist should be aware of are hypertension, lipid disorders, hepatitis, cancer, tendinopathies, and osteopenia. Lastly, corticosteroids appear to be the primary factor in the impaired bone formation found in graft recipients.

### Dialysis

Complications of dialysis are multiple and varied. Fluid shifts during dialysis can contribute to adverse neuromuscular and hemodynamic consequences that must be reported so that adjustments can be made in the dialysis fluid (dialysate). Symptoms of increased thirst and weight gain are common, and the weight gain and abdominal distention, especially with CAPD/CCPD, may cause extreme distress in the individual.

Depression among people on dialysis may be more common than is currently recognized, often masquerading as functional impairment, anorexia, or noncompliance. It has been suggested that approximately 20% to 30% of the ESRD population suffer from depression. Impaired libido, impotence, infertility, dysfunctional uterine bleeding, amenorrhea, and anovulation are very common. Altered platelet function results in bleeding tendencies in anyone with uremia.

People on dialysis have increased susceptibility to infection by various pathogens because they are immunosuppressed, and the dialysis process requires vascular access for prolonged periods of time. Infection of the vascular access site is a major concern, because signs and symptoms of local infection are often absent early on. Careful monitoring for infection or inflammation is warranted, with early medical referral. Standard precautions are essential for the individual in a dialysis unit, for those individuals dialyzing and handling the equipment at home, and for the treating therapist.

Contact transmission can be prevented by hand hygiene (i.e., handwashing or use of a waterless hand rub), glove use, and disinfection of environmental surfaces. Of these, hand hygiene is the most important. In addition, nonsterile disposable gloves provide a protective barrier for workers' hands, preventing them from becoming soiled or contaminated, and reduce the likelihood that microorganisms present on the hands of personnel will be transmitted to clients. It is important to remember to use the hand rub prior to reaching for the gloves so as to prevent contaminating the gloves in the process of putting them on. However, even with glove use, handwashing is needed, because pathogens deposited on the outer surface of gloves can be detected on hands after glove removal, possibly because of holes or defects in the gloves, leakage at the wrist, or contamination of hands during glove removal.[38]

During progressive renal failure, catabolism and anorexia lead to loss of lean body mass, but concurrent fluid retention and weight gain can mask the loss of body mass. Malnutrition, anemia, and this loss of body mass can result in significant losses in muscle strength, requiring careful assessment and rehabilitation. The mixed sensory and motor peripheral neuropathy common in people with uremia often improves symptomatically with adequate dialysis. Muscle mass will also improve with consistently good dialysis and nutrition.

Fluid retention also results in hypertension at the beginning of dialysis; alternatively, dialysis can result in dialysis hypotension when fluid is removed, too quickly or too much is removed, causing a nervous system response to the drop in blood volume. Dialysis hypotension affects up to 50% of individuals who receive this treatment. It is defined as a decrease in systolic blood pressure by more than 20 mm Hg or a decrease in mean arterial pressure by 10 mm Hg associated with any of the following signs and symptoms: abdominal discomfort, yawning, sighing, nausea, vomiting, muscle cramps, restlessness, dizziness or fainting, and/or anxiety.[194]

The therapist should ask the client about the dialysis schedule and encourage the individual not to miss any treatment. Younger clients and those who have recently started dialysis are more likely to miss treatments. This may be reflected in rising blood pressure and elevated pulse rate. Monitoring vital signs and laboratory values is essential throughout the rehabilitative process.

Chest and back pain can occur during the early days of dialysis, referred to as *first-use syndrome*. Delayed hypersensitivity reactions with mild itching and urticaria may be reported to (or observed by) the therapist. Maintaining the dialysis access site is critical, but is often difficult secondary to recurrent thromboses. Extreme caution must be given to the access site during any rehabilitation or exercise intervention. Ischemia of the arm (or leg, depending on the location of the fistula) may be the first indication of thrombosis and subsequent stenosis. Any of these signs and symptoms should be reported to the renal staff.

### Exercise Considerations for Individuals with Chronic Kidney Disease

Recent evidence suggests exercise is a safe and effective treatment to address impairments and activity limitations associated with CKD and ESRD.[3,15,40,45,111,112,120,130,236] Improvements in cardiorespiratory fitness, cardiovascular function, neuromuscular strength, and physical function have been documented in both CKD and ESRD in response to exercise. Aerobic exercise alone and combination exercise (i.e., aerobic exercise + resistance exercise) have been shown to have the greatest potential effect on improving aerobic capacity, whereas increases in neuromuscular strength seem to be best achieved with resistance exercise alone.[15,112] In addition, there is some evidence that exercise is capable of slowing the rate at which kidney function declines in individuals with CKD predialysis.[37,101,185,267] However, due to the limited available data on exercise and kidney function these findings should be interpreted with caution until larger studies are conducted confirming such findings.

Exercise capacity is severely compromised in CKD and ESRD and is inversely associated with CKD incidence.[130,143] Numerous studies have demonstrated improvements in exercise capacity in response to aerobic exercise in CKD and ESRD. For example, Van Craenenbroeck et al.[265] reported significant increases in peak oxygen consumption ($VO_{2peak}$) following 3 months of home-based aerobic cycling. Similarly, Headley et al. [110] found that 16 weeks of aerobic exercise using a variety of exercise modalities increased $VO_{2peak}$ by 8.2%. However, in both of these studies aerobic exercise did not enhance endothelial function or arterial stiffness.

In a systematic review and meta-analysis examining the effects of aerobic training on kidney and cardiovascular function in patients with CKD stages 3 to 4, aerobic exercise had favorable effects on exercise tolerance and eGFR, with no difference in changes in blood pressure.[267] In ESRD, 3 months of cycling significantly increased $VO_{2peak}$ and functional capacity.[148] Importantly, moderate-intensity exercise has not been shown to impair renal function.[222] Therefore, accumulating evidence supports aerobic exercise as a potential treatment for improving exercise capacity in CKD and ESRD.

Neuromuscular dysfunction and skeletal muscle atrophy are consequences associated with CKD and ESRD.[97,115,273] In patients with CKD stages 3b and 4, 8 weeks of progressive leg-extension resistance exercise performed at 70% one repetition maximum (1-RM) increased quadriceps CSA, volume, strength, and exercise capacity.[275] Additionally, resistance exercise has been shown to reduce inflammatory responses experienced during unaccustomed exercise.[275] Several systematic reviews and meta-analyses examining the effects of progressive resistance exercise in CKD and ESRD have demonstrated improvements in neuromuscular strength and lower extremity muscle CSA in both patients with CKD and those with ESRD.[40,45] These data underscore the potential for resistance exercise to improve neuromuscular health in CKD and ESRD.

In addition to performing aerobic and resistance exercise independently, these exercise approaches can be combined in an attempt to maximize cardiovascular and neuromuscular outcomes in parallel. Based on evidence from a systematic review conducted by Heiwe and Jacobson, combination exercise was shown to be superior to aerobic or resistance exercise alone for improving aerobic capacity.[112] However, at the time of the review there was a lack of evidence supporting combination exercise for the enhancement of neuromuscular force generation (i.e., strength). Watson et al., for example, have since demonstrated that 12weeks of combination exercise improved knee extensor strength, quadriceps volume, and rectus femoris CSA.[274] Interestingly, there is a paucity of evidence supporting the use of combination exercise for eliciting simultaneous improvements in aerobic capacity and neuromuscular strength. Despite the need for additional research in this area, combination exercise should still be considered as a viable option for health promotion in CKD and ESRD when appropriate.

For individuals with ESRD, exercise can be performed before, during, or after dialysis. Exercise during dialysis (i.e., intradialytic exercise) has been shown to be safe and effective for improving aerobic capacity, lower extremity strength, quality of life, inflammation, and hospital usage.[31,47,188,195] Compared to dialysis at rest, intradialytic dialysis significantly increases dialyzed clearance of urea.[31] Martin et al. reported that intradialytic exercise did not exacerbate inflammation in patients receiving dialysis.[169] Moreover, the proinflammatory response experienced during intradialytic exercise is shown to subside shortly after the termination of exercise. This inflammatory response to intradialytic exercise may promote anti-inflammatory adaptations, as shown in nondialysis CKD.[275]

Intradialytic exercise can be an effective approach to maximize an individual's time and health. The time spent during hemodialysis treatment, whether in an inpatient or outpatient setting, is typically viewed as a time of inactivity and exercise treatments are deferred. However, studies to verify the effectiveness of low- to moderate-intensity exercise programs done during the first 2 hours of hemodialysis have provided evidence-based protocols.[48,175,179,187,197]

Aerobic exercise during dialysis treatment is recommended to be progressed to 30 to 45 minutes per session at a moderate-intensity (11-13 on a 6-20 rating of perceived exertion scale or 55-70% of their maximal heart rate) or up to 180 minutes per week.[236] Resistance exercise should be performed on nonconsecutive days using up to 12 different muscle groups. The intensity should be at a level that allows for at least 1 set of 12 to 15 repetitions or 60% to 70% repetition maximum. When determining the appropriate exercise prescription, therapists must consider what is practical for their respective circumstances.

Intradialytic exercise also provides an easy means for medical supervision and can facilitate increased compliance and good habit forming for this cohort.[41,146] Ideal candidates will be compliant with their current dialysis, medication, and diet regimens and will have received clearance from their doctor to participate. Significant cardiovascular, neurologic, or orthopedic complications may also limit full participation. It is important to note that development of such a program in any setting requires a multidisciplinary effort. Collaboration among nephrologists, physical therapists, nurses, and dialysis technicians should occur prior to program implementation.

Finding the best schedule to maximize health and functional benefits may take a period of trial and error. For some people, functional tolerance may be lowest the day before the first and second dialysis sessions of the week. Others find it more difficult to exercise on dialysis days or even during dialysis due to decrease in blood pressure and muscle cramping.[282] Exercise during dialysis may be an option for some and usually improves the efficiency of dialysis because of better mobilization of dependent fluids and improved solute removal.[65] Clients who exercise both during dialysis and on nondialysis days have greater improvements in exercise tolerance and peak $VO_2$max compared to individuals who exercise only during dialysis or only on nondialysis days.[71] Establishing a plan of care that takes into account day-to-day differences in energy, function, and motivation may increase the chances for better outcomes.[257]

Compliance can be a big issue if the therapist is unable to convey to the client the importance of exercise and how an exercise program can really benefit that individual. Focusing on greater function and independence in day-to-day activities and gaining an increased sense of well-being or quality of life may be more important to the client than riding a bicycle 10 minutes twice each day.

Patients with CKD and ESRD often experience decrements in physical function.[189,190,249,271] Factors associated with reductions in physiologic capacities are likely to contribute to the observed functional declines.[190] The magnitude in loss of physical function increases with advances in disease severity, especially after the initiation of dialysis.[149] A prescriptive program of regular activity and exercise can improve physical functioning, exercise tolerance, and health-related quality of life.[192,193] Given the dramatic change in functional status following the initiation of dialysis, programs to maximize physiologic reserve and functional capacity prior to the start of such treatments may aid in optimizing the responses to renal replacement therapies.[234]

### Exercise Prescription

Published exercise recommendations for CKD and ESRD have been informed by exercise guidelines for older adults.[130,215,237] For aerobic exercise, it is generally recommended that individuals engage in 30 minutes or more per day of moderate-intensity activity most days of the week (5-6 on a 0-10 physical exertion scale) or 20 minutes per day of vigorous activity 3 or more days per week (7-8 on a 0-10 physical exertion scale). Examples of aerobic exercise activities include walking, cycling, rowing, or swimming.

Resistance exercise is recommended on 2 or more days per week performed on nonconsecutive days. Resistance exercise should include 8 to 10 exercises involving major muscle groups prescribed at an intensity that allows for 10 to 15 repetitions to be completed per set. When prescribing combination exercise, aerobic and resistance exercise should be alternated between exercise days. Resistance exercise can be executed using a variety of different equipment such as weight-bearing activities, elastic tubing, weight cuffs, free weights, and weight machines. Light-intensity activity for both aerobic and resistance exercise performed at lower volumes may be necessary in severely deconditioned individuals, with the goal of progressing towards the recommended dosage.

Each exercise session should include a warm-up followed by an aerobic or resistance phase, and ending with a cool-down period.[7] The warm-up should include light physical activity emphasizing the muscle group(s) to be stressed during the exercise session. Similarly, the cool-down period should also consist of light physical activity allowing for the body to gradually recover to a resting state. Low-intensity static stretching can also be performed following the cool-down period to address any range-of-motion deficits ).[7]

Prior to engaging in an exercise program, each individual should undergo a comprehensive medical review from their primary care doctor. In addition, exercise testing and evaluation should be conducted whenever possible to identify individuals at an increased risk for adverse events in response to exercise and aid in the design of individualized exercise treatments. Exercise testing and evaluation may include assessments of cardiorespiratory fitness, neuromuscular function, physical function, and body composition. Many of the risks of exercise are related more to exacerbation of comorbid conditions (e.g., arthritis, diabetes, hypertension) than to the kidney disease itself. Exercise might cause a potassium efflux from exercising muscles and may elevate blood levels, although the possibility of exercise-induced hyperkalemia and resultant cardiac arrhythmias is small.

Exercise may help control blood pressure, especially in those individuals who are hypertensive. Blood pressure should be monitored in the arm opposite the arteriovenous shunt before exercise. If blood pressure is greater than 200/100 mm Hg, the individual should not exercise. Exercise can also improve lipid levels and glucose metabolism, and increase hematocrit and hemoglobin levels. Psychosocial effects, such as improved mood and quality of life, are also possible.[131,191,192]

Anyone with diabetes should be monitored for hypoglycemia or sudden drops in blood glucose levels. In addition, the kidney is essential in the production of vitamin D, which is necessary for calcium absorption. Exercise training ameliorates the enhanced muscle protein degradation associated with chronic renal failure.

Anyone undergoing dialysis will be monitored for bone disease; strengthening exercises can help bone density, and bone density studies can provide outcome-based evidence of the value of exercise in these clients. In the case of polycystic kidney disease, moderate exercise in animal models was considered safe but did not alter bone mineral density. Additional research in this area is needed, because other benefits may be derived from exercise in this and other kidney-diseased populations.[64]

**A THERAPIST'S THOUGHTS***

**Exercise for a Patient with CKD and ESRD**

Physical therapists play a critical role in helping patients with CKD and ESRD maintain quality of life through the promotion of health and independence. While no current standardized exercise programs exist for those living with CKD and ESRD, the available evidence supports that exercise is safe when applied appropriately and under the supervision of knowledgeable professionals. Additionally, the benefits of such programs can have profound effects on health and function. The recommendations presented in this section should be used to guide clinical decision making when designing exercise treatment plans for patients with CKD and ESRD. Regardless of when the exercise is performed for this population, physical therapists must continue with their roles as educators, motivators, and facilitators for maximizing function and independence.

**Laboratory Values**

Renal failure causes metabolic waste products to accumulate in the blood, which can be measured to assess renal function. The two most commonly measured waste products are serum creatinine and BUN. Changes in creatinine and BUN levels do not usually contraindicate physical or occupational therapy intervention, but other test measures are important. Depressed serum albumin levels reflect poor nutritional status and these laboratory values should be monitored whenever available.

People with ESRD often have low levels of hemoglobin associated with anemia and poor exercise tolerance due to excessive fatigue. Dyspnea at rest or on exertion, increased fatigue, and chest pain with exertion may be signs of low hematocrit levels. Exercise guidelines based on laboratory values provided in Chapter 40 can be used with clients who have ESRD. Keep in mind that hemoglobin and hematocrit levels are usually lower for people with ESRD; potassium, creatinine, and BUN levels will be higher than normal.

*Jared Gollie, PhD, CSCS

# GLOMERULAR DISEASES

## Overview

Glomerular diseases are a group of conditions that damage the kidney's filtering units (glomeruli). Glomerulonephritis is also a group of diseases that affect the glomeruli but specifically manifest with hematuria. Glomerulonephritis is a glomerular disease, but not all glomerular diseases are termed *glomerulonephritis*. Glomerular diseases are the most common cause of ESRD worldwide, and glomerulonephritis is the third leading cause of end-stage kidney disease in the United States.

The glomeruli are tufts of capillaries connecting the afferent and efferent arterioles of the nephron (see Fig. 18.5). The capillaries are supported by a stalk made up of mesangial cells and a basement membrane and are arranged in lobules. The circulating blood is filtered in the glomeruli, with the urine filtrate being an end product. Glomerular damage produces two types of syndromes: the nephrotic syndrome and the nephritic syndrome.

*Nephrotic syndrome* is not a specific kidney disease but rather occurs as a result of any disease that causes damage to the kidney filtering units. Nephrotic syndrome is principally associated with proteinuria, which occurs with such diseases as diabetes, amyloidosis, and membranous glomerulopathy. *Nephritic syndrome* is correlated with hematuria. Glomerular diseases that result in a nephritic syndrome include lupus nephritis, immunoglobulin A (IgA) nephropathy, and acute diffuse proliferative glomerulonephritis. Overlap of the two syndromes is common, and a precise diagnosis often requires a kidney biopsy.

## Etiologic Factors

Most cases of nephritic syndrome and some cases of nephrotic syndrome have an immune origin and are part of a systemic process, such as lupus nephritis or membranoproliferative glomerulonephritis. Two different mechanisms have been proposed to account for the pathologic changes seen in glomerular diseases. The first is a result of the deposition of a circulating antigen–antibody complex into some portion of the glomerulus (the glomerular basement membrane [GBM], mesangium), followed by an inflammatory response and damage. Injury is caused via the second mechanism when an antigen is deposited into the glomerulus with subsequent antibody interaction with the antigen, followed by an inflammatory response. Antigens may be exogenous, as seen in poststreptococcal glomerulonephritis, or endogenous, as noted with lupus nephritis.

## Risk Factors

The presence of a variety of disorders can increase the risk of glomerular damage. Diabetes, principally type 2 diabetes, is a significant risk factor for CKD and the development of nephrotic syndrome. Age is another factor in the development of some diseases associated with nephrotic syndrome. For example, minimal change glomerulopathy is seen in children younger than age 10 years and accounts for more than 80% of cases of nephrotic syndrome in children. Race is also a factor in the development of glomerular disease. Focal segmental glomerulosclerosis is the most common cause of nephrotic syndrome in African Americans, whereas membranous nephropathy is seen more commonly in whites. Focal segmental glomerulosclerosis is also seen more often in persons who are obese.

## Pathogenesis

Damage to the glomerular epithelial cells or the GBM allows larger molecules, such as protein, to escape out of the circulation and into the urine, causing nephrotic syndrome. Rupture of a capillary wall or proliferation of mesangial cells leads to hematuria and nephritic syndrome. The processes that cause this damage vary depending on the underlying glomerular disease.

Nephritic syndromes are caused by antibody–antigen complexes. Damage and clinical manifestations depend on where these complexes are deposited in the glomerulus. IgA nephropathy results when circulating antibodies

(IgA antibodies) complex with an antigen (currently not defined) but are not able to be filtered through the glomerulus. These complexes stimulate an inflammatory response, accompanied by the release of cytokines and growth factors. Mesangial cell proliferation and glomerular scarring result.

Poststreptococcal glomerulonephritis occurs when antigen (streptococcal) is deposited between the glomerular epithelial cells and the GBM, resulting in an antibody response and damage to the GBM. This disruption of the GBM results in proteinuria, as well as nephritis. Lupus nephritis can result from either antigen deposition followed by antibody reaction or the deposition of antibody/antigen complexes. These depositions can also occur in several locations. Those found in the mesangium result in proliferation of mesangial cells. Complexes placed in the GBM cause proteinuria, while deposition in the subepithelial space leads to nephrosis-range proteinuria. If the antigen is chronically produced, the recurrent inflammatory reactions lead to chronic glomerulonephritis. These changes adversely affect the glomerular filtration mechanism and alter capillary permeability.

Although the nephritic syndrome results most often from depositions of immune complexes, causes of nephrotic syndrome vary, with many not well understood. For example, minimal change disease shows very few abnormalities on microscopic or electron microscopic inspection. This disease may result from damage created by a lymphocyte product. Causes of other diseases, such as membranous nephropathy, are better understood. Antigen is initially deposited in the GBM, with subsequent antibody interaction and inflammatory response. These immune complexes also trigger the complement system, causing further damage to the GBM and allowing large amounts of protein to escape from the plasma.

## Clinical Manifestations

Glomerular disease causing a nephrotic syndrome produces proteinuria (greater than 3 g in 24 hours), hypoalbuminemia, hyperlipidemia, lipiduria, and edema. The significant loss of protein from the kidney accounts for the hypoalbuminemia, which, in turn, reduces the plasma oncotic pressure in the vessels. Fluid flows to areas of greater protein concentration, which in this instance is outside the blood vessel, causing edema. The kidney perceives a loss in volume and retains both fluid and sodium, thus increasing the edema. Edema is the principal symptom that brings affected people to the physician's office. The edema can be severe enough to be disabling.

The loss of protein also stimulates the liver to produce cholesterol, leading to hypercholesterolemia (cholesterol can be as high as 300-400 mg/dL). High cholesterol not only increases atherosclerosis of the coronary arteries but also worsens existing kidney disease. Other clinical manifestations include coagulation abnormalities from the loss of coagulation proteins, resulting in a venous thrombotic event (i.e., pulmonary embolism, deep venous thrombosis, or renal vein thrombosis). Hypothyroidism may occur secondary to the loss of thyroxine, and anemia may develop because of the loss of transferrin and erythropoietin.

The nephritic syndrome is characterized by hematuria, but oliguria, hypertension, and renal insufficiency often accompany this syndrome. The urine typically contains abnormally shaped erythrocytes (sometimes called "Mickey Mouse cells"), which distinguishes the hematuria of nephritic syndromes from that of urinary or bladder sources (normally shaped erythrocytes).

Proteinuria may be present, depending on which part of the glomerulus is affected. Hematuria may be asymptomatic, as with IgA nephropathy, or clinically apparent, as with anti-GBM antibody disease. Proliferation of mesangial cells may occur. If less than 50% of the glomeruli are affected, the disease may be asymptomatic. If greater than 50% of glomeruli are involved, hematuria and proteinuria are more profound. Renal insufficiency may be mild or may lead to a rapid loss in function. This depends on the percentage of kidney involved and the severity of the disease. Epithelial crescents form when the disease involves the Bowman space. Crescent formation or extracapillary proliferation is caused by the accumulations of macrophages, fibroblasts, proliferating epithelial cells, and fibrin within the Bowman space. *Crescentic glomerulonephritis* defines a disease process that results when more than 50% of the glomeruli have crescents. Progressive disease can result in ESRD.

### MEDICAL MANAGEMENT

**DIAGNOSIS.** The diagnosis of glomerular disease requires analysis of urine, looking for protein, casts (protein, erythrocyte, or lymphocyte "castings" of the tubules), and erythrocytes. The erythrocytes are often misshaped, demonstrating the damage acquired while going through the glomerulus. A 24-hour urine collection may be required to assess the amount of proteinuria. Blood pressure is often elevated, and anemia may develop. A kidney biopsy is frequently needed to make the precise diagnosis.

**TREATMENT.** Treatment depends on the specific cause of the glomerular disease, but there are several features that may be shared and the treatment may be similar. Diseases causing nephrotic syndrome are treated with an ACE inhibitor or ARB to control blood pressure and to reduce proteinuria.

Hypercholesterolemia is usually treated with a hydroxymethylglutaryl–coenzyme A reductase inhibitor (statin). Erythropoietin can be employed if anemia is symptomatic, and vitamin D sterols may be needed to prevent a deficiency in vitamin D. Fluid is restricted, and diuretics are often used to reduce edema. Diseases with immune-associated injury often require treatment with prednisone, cyclosporine, or cytotoxic agents. Others, such as membranoproliferative glomerulonephritis, improve with treatment of the underlying disorder (i.e., treating hepatitis C–induced disease with interferon-alfa-2 with ribavirin). Some diseases progress and require dialysis or transplantation.

SPECIAL IMPLICATIONS FOR THE THERAPIST 18.7

### *Glomerular Diseases*

Therapists working with clients with a diagnosis of diabetes, systemic lupus erythematosus, vasculitis, and hypertension need to be aware of the association of glomerulonephritis with these disorders. Being vigilant for the clinical manifestations of glomerulonephritis (e.g., edema, hypertension, hematuria, oliguria) is important, and their presence warrants referral of the client to a physician.

An awareness of the side effects associated with diuretics is also important. Potential side effects include muscle weakness, fatigue, muscle cramps, headaches, increased frequency of urination with possibility of incontinence, and depression, all of which can interfere with the rehabilitation program. The onset of any of these complaints also warrants communication with a physician. Finally, many clients with glomerulonephritis progress to chronic renal failure.

# DISORDERS OF THE BLADDER AND URETHRA

## Bladder Cancer

### Overview and Incidence

The bladder is lined with transitional cells and in some places, such as at the trigone, epithelial cells. Transitional cell carcinoma is the most common type of bladder cancer, accounting for 90% of all cases. Transitional cell bladder cancer is a heterogeneous group of cancers with a wide spectrum of aggressiveness and clinical manifestations. Squamous cell carcinoma of the bladder is unusual, accounting for 8% of all cases, typically resulting from chronic inflammation. A rarer form, adenocarcinoma, accounts for the remaining 2% of cases and is thought to arise from remnants of the embryologic urachus (ligaments).

There are approximately 73,500 cases of bladder cancer each year in the United States.[235] As the fourth leading cause of cancer in men and eighth leading cause of cancer death in the United States, bladder cancer is more common than is generally appreciated.[235] Overall, the incidence of bladder cancer is increasing in industrialized countries, although the survival rate is improving. Though it is more prevalent in men, women lose more years of life and a greater fraction of their life expectancy to bladder cancer.[229,235]

### Etiology and Risk Factors

The specific cause of bladder cancer is unknown, but multiple risk factors are linked with the development of bladder cancer (Box 18.3). The strongest and most significant risk factor is *smoking*. Sixty-five percent to 75% of all individuals with bladder cancer have a strong smoking history. Cigarette smokers are twice as likely as nonsmokers to develop bladder cancer.

*Occupational exposures* are also related to bladder cancer, particularly exposure to β-naphthylamine,4-aminobiphenyl (ABP), and benzidine, used in the dye and rubber tire industries. Although these chemicals have been banned, others are currently being investigated for possible association, and those in many occupations appear to be at risk for the development of bladder cancer, such as painters, metalworkers, and truck drivers.[21,243] It is estimated that up to 20% of bladder cancer is caused by an occupational exposure.[141]

More than 90% of cases occur in people older than 55 years, making *age* another risk factor. *Whites* are twice as likely as African Americans to develop the disease, and *men* develop bladder cancer four times more often than women. A previous history of bladder cancer, previous treatment with high doses of the chemotherapy drugs cyclophosphamide or iphosphamide, and radiation to the pelvis also place people at higher risk.

Decreased fluid intake may be a risk factor because the more concentrated the urine, the more toxic irritants come in contact with the bladder mucosa. Conversely, increased fluid intake may decrease the risk of bladder cancer, leading to speculation that a more frequent urine flow decreases the time of contact between carcinogens and the bladder epithelium.[213,288]

There is evidence that food, nutrition, and physical activity are not significant factors in the development of bladder cancer. However, as to prevention, copious fruit consumption may reduce the risk for smokers by as much as 50%.[1,33] The relationship between coffee and bladder cancer remains controversial despite decades of resea rch.[68,218,252,286] Recent studies are adding to the continued

Box 18.3

**RISK FACTORS FOR BLADDER CANCER**

- Cigarette smoking
- Occupational exposures to chemicals and other toxins
  - Truck drivers (diesel exhaust)
  - Painters
  - Leather workers
  - Metal workers
- Male gender
- Age 55 years and older
- Previous treatment with cyclophosphamide or iphosphamide (chemotherapy)
- Previous pelvic radiation (e.g., ovarian cancer treatment)
- European descent
- Chronic inflammation:
  - History of chronic bladder infections (such as with spinal cord injury, stroke)
  - Kidney or bladder stones
  - Long-term catheterization (e.g., dementia, Alzheimer disease, neurologic impairment)
  - Infection with parasite causing schistosomiasis
- Neurogenic bladder
- History of previous bladder cancer
- Family history or retinoblastoma gene inheritance
- Under investigation:
  - Gene–environment interaction
  - Coffee
  - Fluid intake
  - Bacon consumption
  - Gonorrhea infection

controversy by suggesting that this relationship may be a consequence of the differential confounding effect of coffee consumption with tobacco smoking—smoking being the major risk factor for bladder cancer.[200,201,270] Individuals with some chromosomal mutations who smoke cigarettes may be at further increased risk of bladder cancers.[159]

Chronic inflammation may also contribute to an increased risk of bladder cancer. The mechanism may be that chronic irritation and inflammation cause transitional cells to undergo metaplasia and transform into malignant cells. This may also occur in areas already epithelialized with squamous cells, such as at the trigone. Chronic inflammatory irritation, such as from recurrent UTIs, kidney or bladder stones, or the parasite causing schistosomiasis, increase the risk for the development of squamous cell carcinoma of the bladder.

Long-term catheterization (e.g., in spinal cord injury) was previously thought to be a risk factor for squamous cell bladder cancer because of chronic inflammation. However, new research shows that indwelling catheters may not be the only source of increased incidence of squamous cell cancer in spinal cord patients, but the very presence of a neurogenic bladder may be a contributing factor.[135] This may be because of the interaction of the bladder mucosa with a high volume of urine commonly seen in neurogenic bladders. Whatever is the main cause, it is recommended to perform an annual cystoscopy for screening of neoplasms in this high-risk group.

Rare risk factors include uncommon birth defects such as exstrophy (where there is a defect in the abdominal wall), inheritance of the retinoblastoma gene, or a family history of bladder cancer.[63,83]

### Pathogenesis

Tumors of the urinary collecting system can arise from epithelial, mesenchymal, or hematopoietic tissues, but the majority of bladder cancers arise from the epithelium. Approximately 90% of these cancers are transitional cell carcinomas, with squamous cell carcinomas and adenocarcinomas making up the remainder. Bladder cancer is believed to develop through reversible premalignant stages followed by irreversible steps, ending in invasive cancer that can give rise to distant metastases. Variations in the clinical course suggest that different forms of bladder cancer develop along different molecular pathways, leading to tumor presentations of various malignant potential.[280]

The systemic absorption of environmental carcinogens, including cigarette smoke, followed by storage in the bladder exposes the urinary epithelium to concentrated levels of the agents for prolonged periods. This interaction of urine-soluble carcinogens with the epithelium is known as contact chemical carcinogenesis. The precise molecular events leading to the formation of bladder cancer are not known, but several genes appear to be involved. One includes the 9p21 locus (chromosome 9), which contains the CDKN2A/ARF tumor-suppressor gene.[19] Another factor may be the inability to repair deoxyribonucleic acid (DNA) following damage from carcinogens.[217] Further research is needed to determine which genes are involved and how risk factors interact in the development of bladder cancer.

### Clinical Manifestations

Painless hematuria is the most common sign of bladder cancer. Gross hematuria is present in up to 85% of people with this condition, and microscopic hematuria is present in a majority of the remainder. The onset of hematuria is often sudden, and the hematuria is frequently intermittent; the degree of hematuria is not related to the volume of tumor or its stage.[70] Clots may form and cause urethral blockage, with resultant bladder enlargement and painful spasms. The intermittent pattern of bleeding can result in a delay in diagnosis.

Other signs of voiding dysfunction may also be present, including frequency, urgency, and dysuria. Overactive bladder with or without hematuria (blood in the urine) may be a presenting symptom. This symptom is more common in women than men despite the fact that bladder cancer is more common in men than women.[91]

Lymphedema of the lower extremities may occur secondary to locally advanced masses or pelvic lymph node involvement. Obstruction of the ureter can lead to hydroureter or hydronephrosis. In the presence of advanced disease, back pain secondary to metastases to the vertebral bones may occur. Metastatic disease may also lead to liver or pulmonary symptoms.

## MEDICAL MANAGEMENT

**PREVENTION.** Although there is no specific way to prevent bladder cancer, modification of risk factors may help. Smoking cessation is the number one prevention strategy for bladder cancer. Reducing exposure to industrial or occupational carcinogens would also lower the incidence of this type of malignancy. Large total fluid intake may reduce the risk of bladder cancer by reducing the time of contact between carcinogens and the bladder epithelium.[32,289]

Vitamins and increasing consumption of fruits and vegetables initially showed benefit in reducing the risk for bladder cancer, but larger studies have not supported this relationship.[117,171]

Currently, screening of the general population for bladder cancer is not recommended, principally due to a lack of evidence for its effectiveness (large studies have not been continued for more than 10 years). But there is evidence to suggest that screening people at high risk (i.e., smokers, people with an occupational exposure) may be beneficial.[163] Early detection of bladder cancer when still superficial can reduce mortality.

The best specific tests to use to screen for bladder cancer have not been determined, but in high-risk individuals, a urine dipstick test, evaluating for the presence of hematuria, and urine cytology are economical and noninvasive. Even with the presence of intermittent symptoms, these screening tests may miss many tumors. Some experts suggest cystoscopy, which visualizes the bladder and has an increased ability to detect tumors that are intermittently symptomatic. Cystoscopy, however, is more invasive and expensive. It is probably best done for the high-risk groups, such as chronic heavy smokers or individuals with spinal cord injuries. Further research is needed to determine the most appropriate candidates and tests to screen for bladder cancer.

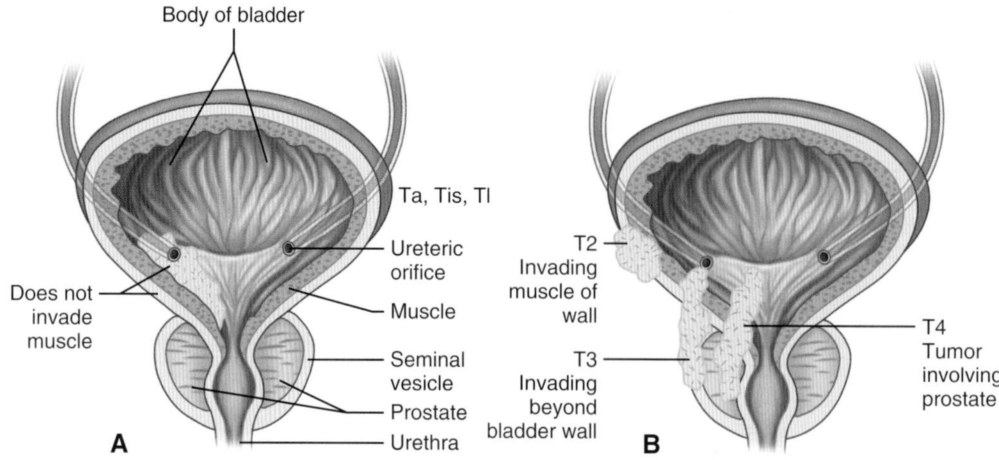


**Figure 18.7**

**Bladder cancer staging using the TNM method.** (A) In Ta, Tis, and T1 tumors, cells do not invade muscle. (B) If the muscle is involved, the tumor is staged as T2. T3 tumors invade beyond the bladder wall but do not involve other organs. T4 tumors are locally invasive to outside structures such as the prostate as shown or systemically with distant metastases (not shown).

The majority of bladder cancers are low-grade, superficial carcinomas that do not tend to metastasize. However, 50% to 90% of bladder cancers will recur, depending on the grade and stage. With recurrence, 10% to 50% will progress in stage or grade. Regular follow-up for early detection of cancer recurrence is important for anyone with a previous history of bladder cancer.

DIAGNOSIS. Bladder cancer is seldom recognized in its preclinical stage but rather is detected once symptoms present, usually hematuria. Younger people with hematuria most often have a benign cause, such as a UTI or kidney or bladder stones.

Evaluation usually consists of a history, physical examination, urinalysis, and urine culture. If the cause is not determined with these measures, further evaluation should be done. For people older than age 50 years with hematuria (gross or microscopic), a history, physical examination, urinalysis, urine cytology, and cystoscopy should be performed. It is important to note risk factors the client may have for bladder cancer.

Cystoscopy allows the urologist to view the bladder for tumor and take a biopsy and cytology washings for evaluation. The cytology samples improve the ability to detect smaller tumors (especially if they are flat), as they are difficult to distinguish from normal bladder tissue.

If tumor is noted in the biopsy specimen, depth of involvement can be determined, which aids in determining staging and treatment. Staging of the tumor may involve ultrasound, CT scan, bone scan, or other tests. A number of urine-based markers, including telomerase and nuclear matrix protein 22 (NMP22), are under investigation for their potential usefulness in diagnosing transitional cell cancer and in monitoring for recurrence.[103,144,220]

STAGING. The TNM staging system is based on the progressive depth of invasion of tumor into the bladder wall and has been used to assign treatment, assess outcomes, and predict prognosis. Cancer cells that are present along the surface of the bladder mucosa but have not yet invaded, also called in situ carcinomas, do not yet have the potential for metastasis and are classified as Tis.

Tumors that have penetrated the basement membrane and invaded into the submucosa/lamina propria but not the muscularis propria are categorized as T1. T2 tumors invade the muscularis propria, whereas T3 tumors invade through the wall into perivesical tissue. T4 tumors invade other organs and structures, such as the prostate, uterus, vagina, pelvic wall, or abdominal wall (Fig. 18.7).

Once tumor is invasive, it has the capacity to metastasize and commonly first reaches lymph nodes near the bladder. The presence of lymph node involvement, number of lymph nodes affected, and distance of involved lymph nodes from the bladder determine the N categorization (N0 for no involvement, N1 for nodes near the bladder, and N2 for nodes further away). Distant sites of metastasis include the liver, lung, and bone. The stage is determined by combining the T, N, and M status (e.g., stage 1 is T1, N0, M0). Approximately 74% of bladder cancer is diagnosed as T1 or T2 tumors; 19% is T3; and 3% is T4.

TREATMENT. Treatment of bladder cancer is determined on the basis of the stage of the tumor and the person's general health. Surgery is the principal treatment for invasive bladder cancer. The optimal treatment for noninvasive disease is not clear; more aggressive approaches, including cystectomy, systemic chemotherapy, or radiotherapy have been shown to reduce mortality.[177] Transurethral resection, surgery completed through the urethra using a rigid cystoscope called a resectoscope, is performed for early and superficial tumors. After the removal of the lesion, the tumor bed is treated either with a high-beam laser or fulguration (electric current used to destroy tumor tissue). Most clients can return home the same day or the next day. Complications include bleeding and discomfort. Long-term effects of repeated transurethral resection include fibrosis of the bladder and loss of continence.

Cystectomy is performed for invasive bladder cancer. If the tumor is small, a partial cystectomy may be performed in order to salvage functioning bladder tissue.[77] This approach is controversial, with some urologists preferring cystectomy even for selected clients with small tumor mass. A radical cystectomy is the surgery of choice for larger, invasive tumors or multiple tumors. This procedure removes the bladder and adjacent lymph nodes. The prostate is removed in men, and the uterus, ovaries, and a portion of the vagina are removed in women.

Following cystectomy, reconstructive surgery is performed to create a urine drainage system to compensate for the loss of the bladder. A urostomy procedure allows drainage of urine into a bag outside the abdomen. This is the least-preferred long-term method of draining urine. The surgery that uses a short piece of small or large intestine to create a pouch or conduit from the ureters to the outside of the body is called an ileal conduit procedure.

Another surgical option is the creation of a continent diversion. In this procedure, the reserve pouch (intestine) has a valve. This valve allows urine to be stored until a catheter is placed to drain the urine. Newer reconstructive methods create a "neobladder" from intestine, which is then attached to the urethra. This surgery allows clients the ability to urinate normally, using a Valsalva maneuver (increasing intraabdominal pressure). The surgical complications from these types of procedures include infection, urine leakage, and obstruction. Sexual side effects are common, particularly for men. Impotence has been an issue with radical cystectomies in the past, but newer techniques have reduced the risk of nerve damage. If impotence does occur, function can improve with time. Generally, younger men (younger than age 60 years) are more likely to regain function than older men.

Chemotherapy is administered in two ways: intravesically or systemically. Intravesical chemotherapy is given through a catheter into the bladder, directly affecting the lining of the bladder. Chemotherapy agents are not absorbed into the deep layers of the bladder; therefore, intravesical chemotherapy is effective only for superficial cancers. Systemic chemotherapy is usually given in combination for invasive cancer (such as methotrexate, vinblastine, doxorubicin, and cisplatin). Radiotherapy in conjunction with concurrent chemotherapy is recommended less frequently because of the long-term consequences, although it is an option for treating clients unable to tolerate surgery because of health issues.

Another therapy option for treating low-stage bladder cancer is intravesical immunotherapy with bacillus Calmette-Guérin (BCG; a bacterium sometimes used to immunize people against tuberculosis). BCG is administered through a catheter into the bladder. The immune system responds to the BCG and becomes activated. These activated cells are then believed to recognize the cancer cells as foreign and destroy them. BCG is typically administered on a weekly basis for 6 weeks. BCG may reduce the risk of recurrence by as much as 50%. Side effects include flu-like symptoms and a burning sensation in the bladder. Rarely, the bacterium can spread into the bloodstream, causing sepsis.

Stages 0 and 1 tumors are treated with transurethral resection followed by intravesical BCG. If the tumor does not respond to the BCG, intravesical chemotherapy is administered, although either BCG or intravesical chemotherapy can be used first.[90] However, more than half of the people with stage 1 tumors will have a recurrence, and 20% to 30% will have a cancer that is invasive.

Stage 2 is treated with a radical cystectomy, with or without lymph node removal. Selected people may undergo a partial cystectomy with fulguration. Systemic chemotherapy may be given prior to or after surgery to treat any small micrometastases not seen during the staging process. A radical cystectomy is also the treatment for stage 3.

Chemotherapy may be added prior to surgery (neoadjuvant) to improve survival, but further investigations are needed to determine the appropriate timing for chemotherapy.[125] Stage 4 therapy focuses on quality of life and slowing tumor growth. A radical cystectomy may be performed with chemotherapy if there are no distant metastases. Various combinations of therapy may be employed when distant metastases are present.

**PROGNOSIS.** Despite the continued increase in the number of new cases occurring each year, the mortality attributed to bladder cancer has remained fairly stable. Stage and grade of the tumor are prognostic indicators for local failure. The 5-year survival rates with treatment are 84% for white males, 71% for African American males, 76% for white females, and 51% for African American females (most likely reflecting delay in diagnosis and inadequate care because of socioeconomic issues). Individuals with T1 tumors have a 90% 5-year survival, whereas for those with muscle-invasive tumors survival at 5 years is 50%; those with deep muscle invasion will go on to have metastatic disease within 2 years.[12]

Bladder cancer is sensitive to chemotherapy and immunotherapy but also has a high incidence of local recurrence, usually within the first 2 years. In approximately 30% of cases metastasis develops during the course of the disease, and 50% of individuals with muscle-invasive disease at the time of diagnosis already have distant metastases. Although rare, long-term survival with recurrent cancer can be achieved in some individuals. Continued improvements in the management of bladder cancer will improve the prognosis in the future.

**SPECIAL IMPLICATIONS FOR THE THERAPIST 18.8**

### *Bladder Cancer*

The risk of severe late radiation sequelae is low (less than 5%), and approximately 75% of long-term survivors maintain a normally functioning bladder. The therapist may likely treat those individuals who have residual bladder control problems. The high rate of cancer recurrence requires therapists to be vigilant in observing for the onset or return of symptoms and signs suggestive of urogenital system disease or metastatic spread. Anyone reporting visible blood in the urine must be evaluated further by a physician.

Surgical management of muscle-invasive neoplasms may involve radical cystectomy (gold standard) with adjuvant chemotherapy.[55,69] Incisional considerations, pain, and reaction to medications should be considered during mobility activities. Pelvic physical therapists may be involved in the retraining of voiding patterns and pelvic floor muscle coordination for individuals after neobladder procedures. See "Pelvic Floor Muscle Dysfunction" in Chapter 27.

## Urinary Incontinence

See also "Pelvic Floor Muscle Dysfunction" in Chapter 27.

### Normal Bladder Function

Understanding the basics of normal bladder function will be helpful in understanding urinary incontinence (UI). The process of micturition and continence involves a complex interplay of nerves, smooth muscle, and skeletal muscles. Proper functioning of these structures is needed for normal voiding to occur. Normal urination involves nerve signals from the cortex of the brain, through the pons, spinal cord, peripheral autonomic system, sensory afferent innervation of the lower urinary tract, and finally to the bladder itself.

Neural control begins in the cortex, with cognitive awareness and decision making. The pontine micturition reflex center is located in the brainstem. The efferent (exiting) neurons travel down the spinal cord in the reticulospinal tract to the skeletal pelvic floor muscle and the detrusor muscle of the bladder. Parasympathetic nerves originate in the spinal cord at the level of S2, S3, and S4, and innervate the bladder wall via the pelvic nerve.

Preganglionic sympathetic nerves have their origin in the spinal cord at the levels of T10 through L2 and travel through the sympathetic chain ganglion to the bladder neck and fundus of the bladder. The bladder neck contains the internal urethral sphincter (involuntary smooth muscle). The external urethral sphincter, part of the pelvic floor muscles (PFM) (voluntary skeletal muscle), is innervated by the pudendal nerves, which originate in the spinal cord at the level of S2 through S4.

These nerve signals result in coordination of the smooth muscle of the detrusor and internal urethral sphincter and the skeletal muscle of the external urethral sphincter of the PFM. Bladder patterns in asymptomatic individuals vary greatly. Normally, the bladder is designed to hold a pint of urine for several hours. As it fills, the detrusor muscle remains relaxed to allow the bladder to stretch and accommodate more urine; the internal urethral sphincter remains contracted to prevent urine from escaping through the urethra.

Voluntary PFM support the base of the bladder and compress the urethra, further blocking the flow of urine. Stretch receptors in the bladder indicate when the bladder is full, and the person makes their way to the toilet. When positioned appropriately, urination is initiated with voluntary relaxation of the PFM. This is followed by relaxation of the internal urethral sphincter and contraction of the detrusor muscle to squeeze the urine out of the bladder.

Coordinated detrusor smooth muscle contraction with relaxation of the smooth muscle internal urethral sphincter and skeletal muscle of the external urethral sphincter is necessary to empty effectively.

Normal voiding interval is a minimum of 2 hours (often in the elderly) and usually 3 to 5 hours between voids for others. Urinating more than eight times a day is a symptom of urinary frequency. Most people feel bothersome nocturia is voiding two or more times per night. Bladder training can be used to restore normal bladder pattern and function.

### Definition and Overview

UI may be defined as a "complaint of involuntary urine loss."[107] There are currently eight categories of UI.[107] The two most common categories used to classify UI are:

1. *Stress urinary incontinence* (SUI): complaint of involuntary loss of urine on effort or physical exertion, or on sneezing or coughing. This occurs during activities that increase intraabdominal pressure.
2. *Urgency urinary incontinence* (UUI): complaint of involuntary loss of urine associated with urgency. Urgency is the report of a sudden compelling desire to urinate that is difficult to defer. UUI is often related to detrusor instability, a condition in which the bladder contracts at small volumes, often in response to triggers such as running water or arriving home. Overactive bladder syndrome (older terms include hyperreflexive bladder, or detrusor hyperreflexia) is defined as "urinary urgency, usually accompanied by frequency and nocturia, with or without UUI, in the absence of UTI or other obvious pathology."[107]

Many people have more than one type of incontinence (most often SUI and UUI together), known as *mixed* UI.

UI is common, particularly in older adults. Yet the condition is poorly understood, under-diagnosed, and often inadequately treated. Many people are embarrassed to acknowledge that they are incontinent. Only 20% to 50% of incontinent adults seek medical care.[277] Others regard incontinence as part of the normal aging process.

Estimates of the economic price tag associated with UI vary widely from $19.5 billion to $82.6 billion in 2020 in the United States, approaching the cost of treatment for osteoporosis, Alzheimer disease, and arthritis.[10] Incontinence can be a significant contributory factor related to falls in older adults,[29] pressure sores, skin breakdown, UTIs, institutionalization, depression, and isolation. Interestingly, a bidirectional relationship has been found between anxiety or depression and UI. People with anxiety or depression are twice as likely to have UI as those without depression or anxiety and those with UI are twice as likely to have anxiety or depression. Social isolation, limited work opportunities, and decreased exercise participation are also reported in association with UI.

### Prevalence

A systematic review of population-based surveys reports prevalence estimates of 1.7% to 36.4% in the United States with variations based on age and gender. UI is more prevalent in women than men and in the aging over the young. The prevalence of UI was first reported in 1988 at the National Institutes of Health Consensus Conference on Adult Urinary Incontinence. At that time, an estimated 10 million adults in the United States experienced incontinence, including 15% to 30% of community-dwelling older adults and more than 50% of nursing home residents.[54] Other groups who report a higher prevalence include athletes (e.g., gymnasts, athletes competing on trampolines, power lifters) and men after prostate surgery. Approximately 41% of female power lifters report UI at some point in their lives. Since the first consensus conference, there has been an increased awareness of and focus on the problem of UI. Until recently, the impact

Box 18.4

**RISK FACTORS FOR URINARY INCONTINENCE**

- Obesity and elevated body mass index
- Age
- Pregnancy/multiple pregnancies; childbirth/delivery (vaginal or cesarean section); episiotomy; large gestational weight
- Cystocele or uterine prolapse
- Any pelvic surgery including hysterectomy for women, prostatectomy for men
- Diabetes mellitus
- Depression
- Constipation, fecal impaction
- Tobacco use
- Medications
  - α-Adrenergic blockers (antihistamines, decongestants)
  - Antihypertensives
  - Antiparkinson agents
  - Antipsychotics
  - Diuretics
  - Narcotic analgesics
  - Tranquilizers, sedatives
  - Tricyclic antidepressants
- History of recurrent urinary tract infections
- Bladder irritation (low fluid intake, caffeine, and possibly alcohol)*
- Loss of activities of daily living skills for toileting, decreased or impaired mobility
- Impaired cognitive function
- Race (white)
- Neurologic disorder (e.g., myelomeningocele, multiple sclerosis, brain injury, Parkinson disease, cerebral palsy, spinal cord injury, stroke)
- Psychogenic (e.g., childhood and/or adult sexual trauma for both males and females, negative sexual experiences, emotional stress)
- Frequent high impact exercise[184,233]

*Bladder irritants are not likely to cause urinary incontinence without other contributing actors.

Source used for pharmacotherapy update: DiPiro JT, Talbert RL, Yee GC, Matzke GR, Wells BG, Posey LM, eds: *Pharmacotherapy. A pathophysiologic approach*, ed 8, New York, 2011, McGraw Hill.

of UI on working women employed full time, a population generally characterized as healthy, has not been the focus of research. One survey at a large university center reported that 21% of the women surveyed (age 18 years and older) reported UI at least monthly.[82]

### Risk Factors

A wide range of factors can contribute to the increased risk of developing UI (Box 18.4).[246] Some risk factors are more likely to lead to one type or another or several types of incontinence. The literature varies widely as to which risk factors are significant for different population groups.

Research constantly shows elevated body mass index is a major risk factor for both SUI and UUI. The proposed mechanisms for the association with SUI include the increased intraabdominal pressures that adversely stress the urethra, bladder, and pelvic floor, and the effect of obesity on the neuromuscular function of the genitourinary tract.[59] Studies are conflicting as to whether weight loss is associated with decreased UI symptoms.[283] Among adolescent and middle-aged women, BMI and high-impact exercises where found to be significant risk factors for UI.

Advancing age plays a significant role in the development of all forms of UI.[246] As older adults lose their mobility and manual dexterity secondary to a multitude of ailments, getting to the bathroom or commode in a timely fashion and manipulating clothing become increasingly difficult. The presence of two or more diseases significantly increases the likelihood of developing UI. Common illnesses associated with UI include diabetes, stroke, hypertension, cognitive impairment, parkinsonism, arthritis, and hearing and visual impairments.

Women are more likely than men to develop UI. This is related to structural differences, several factors associated with childbirth, and gynecologic surgery. Women who have had multiple pregnancies and deliveries (whether cesarean section or vaginal birth) have a higher incidence of UI. Hysterectomy, the presence of a cystocele, and uterine prolapse may also increase a woman's risk.

Medications commonly prescribed for other illnesses can also increase the risk of incontinence. In older adults the occurrence of medications' contribution to UI is estimated at 60%. These pharmacologic agents can interfere with conscious inhibition of voiding, induce a quick diuresis (diuretics),[174] or reduce urethral resistance to the point of stress incontinence. Tranquilizers and sedatives may impair awareness of the usual cues related to urinary urgency and may also depress the cerebral corticoregulatory tract, affecting detrusor muscle activity.[153] Laxatives, estrogen, antidepressants, and antibiotics are also associated with an increased risk for UI.[118,219]

Findings regarding the role of hormonal changes contributing to UI are inconsistent.[246] Estrogen deficiency results in changes in the urethra, which seems to predispose women to UI. Hormone replacement, including estrogen plus progestin, in healthy postmenopausal women has been linked with incontinence.[216] Topical estrogen can be used if incontinence is caused by atrophic vaginitis or severe vaginal atrophy.

High caffeine intake (more than 204 mg/day) can also contribute to the development of urge incontinence, while studies involving alcohol consumption have reported mixed results.[212] Constipation and other bowel problems increase the risk of UI, which may be related to pelvic organ prolapse.

Recurrent UTI is also an independent risk factor for developing UI. Race and socioeconomic class may also play roles in the development of UI. Smoking, COPD, and vaginal deliver are also risk factors for UI.

### Pathogenesis and Clinical Manifestations

Incontinence, as discussed earlier, is categorized depending on the cause and pathophysiology. Each type of UI has associated clinical manifestations. *UUI* is often caused by involuntary bladder (detrusor) spasms (also called detrusor overactivity) and is associated with both increased frequency and urgency. The pathophysiology of detrusor overactivity is not fully understood and may be related to irritated sensory signals from overactive PFM, bacteria of UTI, fear of leaking, and other psychologic factors.

Urge incontinence is characterized by leakage (sometimes large-volume accidents) after a sudden precipitant desire to urinate or by events such as trying to insert a key in the door, running hands under water (or hearing running water), thinking about going to the bathroom, or passing by a bathroom.

Some clinicians use the term *functional incontinence* to describe the consequence of chronic impairments of physical or cognitive function that make toileting in a timely fashion difficult (e.g., difficulty getting to the toilet on time, inability to manage pant zippers, forgetting how to get on and off the toilet).

*SUI* results from weakness or loss of tone in the PFM, internal urethral sphincter failure, hypermobility of the ureterovesical junction, or damage to the pudendal nerve (e.g., infection, tumor, childbirth). It is accompanied by leakage that is coincident with increases in intraabdominal pressure (e.g., coughing, sneezing, laughing, bending, high-impact physical activity or exercise). Someone with mixed UI will exhibit signs of both UUI and SUI.

Other clinical manifestations of UI depend on the type of incontinence and underlying pathology, but may include constant dribbling, frequency, urgency, nocturia, hesitancy, weak stream, or straining to void.

## MEDICAL MANAGEMENT

**SCREENING AND PREVENTION.** Preventive education may decrease the occurrence of incontinence. Many health care professionals advocate early education on proper PFM contraction for adolescent girls and young women before they become pregnant. Prepartum and postpartum PFM training has been shown to have immediate and long-term effects in preventing incontinence, improving quality of life, and improving sexual dysfunction.[20,176]

Modifying risk factors is also suggested to prevent UI. This might include losing weight, smoking cessation, avoiding provocative medications if possible, avoiding irritating fluids like caffeine and alcohol, and avoiding constipation through proper nutrition, adequate hydration, and responding to the need to toilet.

The therapist can establish screening programs to assess for risk factors for UI or for the presence of incontinence. All therapists can teach proper lifting techniques to minimize unnecessary increase in intraabdominal pressure, which could contribute to the occurrence of SUI and pelvic organ prolapse. Patients should be taught to contract the PFM before increased abdominal pressure (e.g., lifting, laughing, coughing, sneezing, vomiting). Anyone experiencing leaking during exercise needs a prescriptive PFM exercise program (see Chapter 27 for more information on PFM exercises) and modification of the exercise that precipitates the leaking.

**Diagnosis.** Because UI is related to a wide variety of disorders and factors, a detailed investigation may be necessary to determine the cause(s). An important part of this investigation is a bladder diary to determine the frequency, timing, and amount of voiding and to assess the numerous other risk factors potentially associated with UI. Bladder dairies are reliable and reproducible and provide a great deal of valuable information for development of treatment strategies.

A careful history will investigate medication usage, prescribed and nonprescription; past and current illnesses; and surgical and birth histories. There are many validated quality of life and symptom indexes used to quantify symptoms associated with UI and bladder dysfunction. Physical examination should include a pelvic, genitourinary, and rectal examination to evaluate for the presence of prolapse, fecal impaction, atrophic vaginitis, cystocele, PFM dysfunction, masses, prostate hypertrophy, and prostate nodule (in men).

Urinalysis may reveal hematuria or infection. In order to differentiate between UUI and urinary retention, a postvoid residual should be obtained. With a normal postvoid residual, the bladder should contain less than 50 to 100 mL of urine after voiding. Many cases of incontinence can be diagnosed without significant invasive techniques and treated by modifying reversible risk factors. The mnemonic DIAPPERS summarizes the reversible causes of incontinence: *D* for delirium, *I* for infection, *A* for atrophic urethritis/vaginitis, *P* for pharmaceutical, *P* also for psychologic disorders, *E* for excessive urine output (associated with congestive heart failure or hyperglycemia), *R* for restricted mobility, and *S* for stool impaction.[268]

Clients who have abnormal physical or laboratory findings may require further workup, particularly if surgery is planned or the diagnosis is in doubt. Cystoscopy is beneficial in the presence of hematuria to assess for bladder cancer. Urodynamic evaluation is used in select clients who may have nonspecific symptoms or for whom a more precise diagnosis of obstruction is needed.

Urodynamic studies include uroflowmetry, cystometry, urethral pressure studies, pressure-flow micturition studies, electrophysiologic studies, and video urodynamic studies. All or a portion of these tests can be performed as appropriate. One component of the urodynamic study, cystometry is used to assess bladder capacity, sensation, voluntary control, and contractility. Cystometry consists of filling the bladder with water and recording changes in intravesicular pressure, abdominal pressure, and PFM activity.

When stress incontinence is suspected, provocative stress testing is carried out. The client is asked to cough vigorously during cystometry while the examiner observes for urine loss. The test is initially done in the lithotomy position but if the result is negative, the test is repeated in a standing position. Imaging ultrasound is being used to study specific structural aspects of PFM dysfunction such as avulsion, which may be associated with stress incontinence.

**TREATMENT.** Management of UI depends on the type of incontinence and the person's age and general health, but usually falls into one of three categories: conservative, pharmacologic, and surgical. Conservative intervention is considered the first line of treatment for UI and includes a combination of:

- Education: lifestyle, dietary changes, fluid modifications, treatment of constipation, weight loss, instruction in proper lifting and exercising techniques to avoid excessive increased intraabdominal pressure, toilet position especially for children and elderly.
- Bladder training, behavioral modification, and urge deferment

- Prescriptive exercises including PFM exercises with or without facilitation (see discussion in Chapter 27), general pelvic stability exercises, specific transversus abdominal exercise, and vaginal weight training
- Environmental modifications to increase accessibility and functional mobility training to increase timely access to bathroom facilities.
- Modalities such as pelvic floor electrical stimulation, biofeedback therapy
- Support devices such as pessaries

Pessaries are devices inserted into the vagina that are designed to support the bladder and bladder neck, reducing pelvic organ prolapse and compressing the urethra to decrease UI. These devices come in a variety of shapes and sizes and are made of flexible or rigid silicone, latex, or acrylic. Some pessaries can stay in the vagina for up to 3 months before being removed, cleaned, and replaced; others are used just during exercise or sexual intercourse. A properly fitted pessary should not interfere with bowel or bladder function and should not be uncomfortable.

Physical and occupational therapists can often help improve mobility skills. For example, if physical impairments make mobility difficult, thus affecting the client's ability to reach a bathroom, appropriate devices (i.e., bedside commode) and therapy can be provided. Clothing should be easy to remove.

***Stress Urinary Incontinence.*** SUI can be treated by the conservative methods (listed above) and surgical methods. Cochrane reviews report PFM training to be effective for the treatment of SUI or mixed incontinence.[72,109,114] Electrical stimulation shows only slight improvement over placebo, while the use of vaginal weights shows no significant benefit over PFM exercises alone.[109,114] See further specific discussion of PFM training in Chapter 27.

There are many surgeries that may be used to correct pelvic floor laxity including an open retropubic colposuspension, bladder neck needle suspension, and suburethral sling procedure. The suburethral sling is the most often used technique and results in 80% to 90% success.[238] Surgical correction of pelvic organ prolapse may improve symptoms of UI. Periurethral injections with a bulking agent (such as collagen) may be administered to increase sphincter resistance in women and in men who have internal sphincter deficiency.

***Urgency Urinary Incontinence.*** Various interventions are used to treat UUI, with the primary focus being behavioral modification[250] and pharmacotherapy. Biofeedback and PFM training, along with bladder training, can significantly improve UUI. Bladder training consists of scheduled voiding (trying to increase time between each void) and urge-suppression techniques. For clients with cognitive impairment, prompted voiding can be beneficial and decrease incontinent episodes (remind every 2 hours to toilet). Clients should also be encouraged to manage constipation and avoid bladder irritants such as caffeine, alcohol, nicotine, and carbonated soft drinks.

Pharmacologic therapy is frequently used in conjunction with behavioral modifications. First-line drug therapy for UUI is the use of anticholinergics or muscarinic antagonists, which inhibit involuntary detrusor contractions.[154] The most common side effect is dry mouth. Other adverse effects include drowsiness, cognitive impairment, delirium, and hallucinations. These side effects are more likely to occur in older adults than younger clients. Therapists should be aware of medication reactions because some patients are inadvertently placed on several anticholinergics, which can result in drowsiness, dizziness, and confusion.

Other medications have shown some benefit but are not as effective as the anticholinergics/muscarinic antagonists or have off-label usage. In the past estrogen has been used to treat UI, although there is little data to support its use, and oral hormone therapy has been associated with increased incidence of incontinence. In men with symptoms of UUI and prostatic hypertrophy, α-adrenergic antagonists can be used initially. If these agents do not alleviate symptoms, obstruction should be ruled out before starting an anticholinergic agent.

**SPECIAL IMPLICATIONS FOR THE THERAPIST 18.9**

## *Urinary Incontinence*

See "Pelvic Muscle Dysfunction" in Chapter 27.

Therapists have an important direct role in the assessment and treatment of UI. Physical therapy guides the rehabilitation of muscle imbalance and pelvic alignment and promotes pelvic muscle awareness and function through biofeedback, therapeutic exercise, neuromuscular reeducation, and a behavioral management approach.[24,34,98,99] The pelvic rehabilitation program is designed to prevent recurrence of the impairment and to restore bowel, bladder, sexual, and supportive muscle functioning.

### To All Physical Therapists

Many adults think that UI is an inevitable part of aging or disease and do not report the problem. *Everyone* should be asked if they have urinary incontinence, but especially the perimenopausal or postmenopausal woman, any woman who has been pregnant, anyone (male or female) older than age 60 years (earlier if prostate or bladder infection or cancer is evident), and any person with multiple risk factors.

Anyone with onset of UI with concomitant cervical spine pain (even without a history of trauma or known cause) may be experiencing cervical disc protrusion, requiring additional screening and evaluation. Additionally, the possibility of genitourinary disorders as a result of sexual abuse or assault exists and requires careful assessment.

The generally positive rapport that develops between client and therapist may facilitate the acknowledgment that UI exists and uncover the potential underlying risk factors. Specific questions should be included in the intake history for *all* individuals to help bring this information to light, such as the following:

- Do you leak urine when you lift, cough, sneeze, or stand up?
- Do you get up at night to urinate? How often?
- Do you go to the bathroom more often than every 2 to 3 hours?
- How much water do you drink in a day?
- Are you constipated?

The therapist may be in a position to direct the patient to the appropriate physician for evaluation. Successful intervention in UI may enhance rehabilitation efforts geared to improve the client's physical and social activity level. It is helpful for physical therapists to have handouts or other resources for patients/clients to refer to. The National Association for Continence (http://www.nafc.org) offers a wide variety of information and is a very supportive organization for affected individuals, caregivers, and professionals. The Pelvic Health Academy of the American Physical Therapy Association (APTA) offers a broad range of information for patients and therapists on this topic as well.

Some physical therapists seek advanced postgraduate education and training in comprehensive treatment of PFM and pelvic dysfunction. See the section on PFM dysfunction (Chapter 27) for more on evaluating and training this skeletal muscle.

Understanding the use of medications and potential side effects for these conditions is essential; many of the same medications used to treat incontinence can also cause incontinence if used inappropriately. Medications to treat other conditions can have side effects that cause incontinence.

#### Fracture Risk and Prevention

There has been a great deal of research on the association of falls and UI. The estimated odds ration of falls with UI is 1.5 to 2.3. The exact mechanism is still under investigation but it appears that improving UI decreases fall risk.[29] An episode of UUI at least once a week increases the risk of fractures by 34% related to falls at night.[29] The therapist can perform a home assessment for the older adult with urge incontinence. Placing strategically located night lights near the bed, hallway to the bathroom, and bathroom and removing objects along the path (e.g., throw rugs) are essential preventive steps to take.

For the individual with incontinence and postural orthostatic hypotension, low blood pressure (or even use of hypertensives with the potential for hypotension as a side effect) and rising from bed quickly at night can also result in falls. Assessing for this complication and teaching prevention measures are recommended (see "Orthostatic [Postural] Hypotension" in Chapter 12).

#### Physical Therapist Intervention for Urinary Incontinence

PFM exercises can be performed to retrain and strengthen the pelvic floor musculature. Please refer to Chapter 27 for a complete review of PFM training. Continence requires the ability to suppress uninhibited detrusor contractions, especially in individuals with overactive bladder. Pelvic floor rehabilitation specifically using PFM exercises may help suppress the desire to void by reducing detrusor pressure and increasing urethral pressure, resulting in suppression of the micturition reflex.

Bladder training involves teaching the bladder to respond to a specific voiding schedule. Clients void at scheduled intervals to increase bladder capacity and decrease urinary frequency. The initial retraining interval is determined by the bladder dairy and is usually 1 to 2 hours. The voiding intervals are increased by 15 to 30 minutes using urge-suppression techniques.

Normal bladder pattern varies greatly; however, success is usually marked by voiding at 3- to 4-hour intervals, continence (perhaps measured by number of pads used), minimal sensory symptoms, and functional capacity (minimum of 300 mL of urine). In some cases increased stress and anxiety result in increased urgency. General relaxation and diaphragmatic breathing can be used to calm the autonomic nervous system and decrease urgency and detrusor pressure.

## Neurogenic Bladder Disorders

### Overview

Voiding dysfunction associated with neurologic pathology is termed a *neurogenic lower urinary tract dysfunction* (NLUTD). There are many types of voiding dysfunction that can interfere with normal urine storage and coordinated, voluntary release. Voiding dysfunctions associated with neurologic pathology are very complex and a complete discussion is beyond the scope of this text. There is no one accepted scale or category for neurogenic urinary tract dysfunction. The International Continence Society (ICS) separates storage and voiding abnormalities and expands many of the urodynamic classification categories. Abnormal bladder dysfunction includes neurogenic acontractile detrusor, neurogenic detrusor overactivity, and other variations. Conversely, abnormal sphincter dysfunction includes nonrelaxing urethral sphincter, detrusor-sphincter dyssynergia (DSD), and its variations (Box 18.5). Patients can have one or more bladder and sphincter abnormalities. It is the challenge of the medical professionals to identify all abnormalities for effective treatment. Many clients may demonstrate a mixture of sensory and motor abnormalities, and symptoms may overlap between categories.

### Prevalence

Voiding dysfunction is a common problem associated with many types of neurologic diseases. It is costly and leads to significantly decreased quality of life, particularly in the older adult when long-term care is often considered. The following gives some idea of the general prevalence of NLUTD by condition[284]:

Cerebral palsy, 36%
Dementia, 30% to 100%
Parkinson disease, 37% to 70%
Multiple systems atrophy, 73%
Multiple sclerosis, 37% to 72%
Spinal stenosis, 61% to 62%
Spinal surgery, 38% to 60%
Disc disease, 28% to 87%
Diabetes mellitus, 25% to 87%
Radical hysterectomy, 8% to 57%
Guillain-Barré, 25%

Box 18.5

**TYPES OF NEUROGENIC LOWER URINARY TRACT DYSFUNCTION**[89]

- *Neurogenic overactive bladder* is characterized by urgency, with or without urgency urinary incontinence, usually with increased daytime frequency and nocturia in the setting of a clinically relevant neurologic disorder with at least partially preserved sensation
- *Neurogenic acontractile detrusor* is one that cannot be demonstrated to contract during urodynamic studies in the setting of a clinically relevant neurologic lesion
- *Nonrelaxing urethral sphincter* is characterized by a nonrelaxing, obstructing urethral sphincter resulting in reduced urine flow.
- *Detrusor-sphincter dyssynergia (DSD)* describes a detrusor contraction concurrent with an involuntary contraction of the urethral and/or periurethral striated muscle. Occasionally flow may be prevented altogether.

## Etiologic Factors

The common disorders that can result in NLUTD include cerebrovascular accident, dementia, Parkinson disease, multiple sclerosis, and brain tumors. NLUTD can also occur secondary to spinal cord lesions, such as spinal cord injury, herniated intervertebral disc, vascular lesions, spinal cord tumors, and myelitis.

## Pathogenesis

Damage to nerves involved in micturition can result in different types of voiding dysfunction. *Supraportine lesions* (above the pontine micturition reflex center) lead to loss of voluntary inhibition of voiding and a neurogenic overactive bladder, but coordinated sphincter function is retained. This results in UUI related to urgency with good emptying. This can be seen in brain tumors, cerebral palsy, cerebrovascular accidents, dementia, Parkinson disease, pernicious anemia, and Shy-Drager syndrome.

*Lesions in the spinal cord* from the pontine micturition center to the sacral cord may take on qualities of hyperreflexic bladder seen in cerebral injuries or areflexic bladder seen in lower spinal injuries. The most dangerous dysfunction in patients with spinal cord injury is detrusor sphincter dyssynergia (DSD). In this dysfunction the sphincter remains closed while the bladder contracts resulting in urinary retention and incomplete voiding. High bladder pressure and ureteral reflux can lead to kidney damage. Diseases that can result in this type of voiding problem include anterior spinal cord lesions, ischemia, multiple sclerosis, myelodysplasia, and trauma. This type of injury also involves the sympathetic nerves and loss of sympathetic inhibition, leading to systemic sympathetic symptoms such as hypertension, facial flushing, perspiration, and headache. Because the vagal nerve is intact, bradycardia accompanies this syndrome.

*Sacral spinal cord lesions* usually lead to neurogenic acontractile detrusor and underactivity in PFM dysfunction. In this situation, both the bladder and PFM are weak. In some conditions (sacral lesions and some disc disease), the smooth muscle internal urethral sphincter is overactive; in other cases (conus lesions), the internal sphincter is underactive. The most common dysfunction in neurogenic acontractile detrusor is urinary retention, which usually manifests as overflow leakage because the bladder is so full a small increase in intraabdominal pressure will cause urine leakage. Acute transverse myelitis, diabetes, Guillain-Barré syndrome, herniated intervertebral disc, myelodysplasia, pelvic surgery, tabes dorsalis (syphilis), and trauma can cause this type of NLUTD.

*Diabetic cystopathy* occurs in over 50% of people with diabetes. The actual neurologic damage and symptoms vary among clients with diabetes and includes impaired bladder sensation, increased postvoid residuals, increased bladder capacity, and decreased bladder contractility. Diabetic bladder neuropathy occurs when other diabetic complications are apparent (e.g., diabetic retinopathy, microalbuminuria).

## Clinical Manifestations

NLUTD is manifested by a great variety of symptoms, including partial or complete urinary retention, incontinence, urgency, suprapubic pain, or frequent urination. In urinary retention the bladder fills and becomes overdistended, the pressure inside the bladder finally exceeds the maximal urethral pressure, and urine "overflows." Incontinence related to urinary retention often manifests with symptoms of stress and urge incontinence and is characterized by frequent or constant dribbling, inability to completely empty the bladder, hesitancy, weak stream, need to strain to void, bladder distention, and urinary urgency and frequent urination. Anticholinergics, narcotics, and α-adrenergic agonists can worsen these symptoms. Common complications of NLUTD include UTIs, kidney stones, and deterioration in renal function.

## MEDICAL MANAGEMENT

**Diagnosis.** The first step in assessment of NLUTD is a complete history, physical, and description of symptoms. Physical examination should include assessment of mobility, transfers, and self-care and dressing ability. Cognitive status and neurologic testing of sensation and reflexes in the area is needed. There are several outcomes measures specific to NLUTD. A measured bladder dairy and symptom record is also helpful in completely understanding the bladder dysfunction. Numerous tests can be used to assess the anatomic and physiologic status of the bladder, associated structures, and nervous system. A postvoid residual is essential to ensure complete emptying. Urodynamic testing is frequently performed to categorize abnormalities and determine cause and most appropriate treatment in individuals with neurologic deficits. Other tests can be performed as needed to diagnose other disease processes, including test of kidney function. If spinal cord or brain abnormalities are suspected, an MRI is beneficial.

TREATMENT. Accurate diagnosis is essential for effective treatment. Incorrect treatment can result in not only ineffective results but also harm to the renal system. The most important goals of treatment include preventing bladder overdistention, UTIs, and renal damage. Management of UI is also important to avoid skin damage and maximize quality of life. Treatment modalities include catheterization, pharmacologic agents, including Botox injections of the bladder, bladder training, and surgery.

*Catheterization.* Clean intermittent catheterization is a commonly employed intervention to avoid bladder overdistention in cases of urinary retention. It is usually performed at 4-hour intervals and aids in reducing the risk for vesicourethral reflux and kidney damage. Permanent indwelling catheters are used only in specific medical situations, and alternatives should be used as possible.

Although a medical necessity in certain situations, permanent indwelling catheters carry a risk. Acute and chronic UTI, stone formation, urinary leakage/incontinence, erosion of meatus and urethra, fistula formation, and reduction in bladder capacity are all associated with the use of permanent indwelling catheters in people with spinal cord injury. Although associated with fewer adverse effects, intermittent catheterization can also lead to UTI, urethral irritation, and reduced quality of life.

Catheterization is frequently used in conjunction with medications. Anticholinergic agents are used to treat voiding dysfunctions that include detrusor hyperactivity. These agents relax the bladder, reduce high pressures, and increase bladder capacity. However they must be carefully administered in patients with NLUTD and acontractile detrusor or nonrelaxing sphincter to avoid urinary retention. Side effects of anticholinergic agents include dry mouth, gastrointestinal disturbances, drowsiness, cognitive impairment, hallucinations, and delirium. Other medications can be beneficial in the treatment of other aspects of NLUTD.

*Botox Injections.* Although a relatively new treatment, botulinum toxin A injections into the detrusor muscle appear to reduce involuntary bladder contractions in people with neurogenic overactive bladder.[11,165] Long-term studies are needed to determine appropriate frequency, duration, and efficacy of treatment; however, Botox injections seem to be quite cost effective in the treatment of refractory NLUTD.

*Bladder Training.* Bladder training methods are designed to enhance bladder function and prevent complications. Patients are often encouraged to attempt urination every 2 hours. Establishing a bladder pattern can result in less UI. Sitting position on the toilet is also important for full emptying. Full relaxation of the legs (particularly the adductors and gluteals) can improve PFM relaxation and decrease residual urine. Patients may also be encouraged to double void (stand and sit immediately after voiding to allow a chance for more urine to be released). Adequate fluid intake is important for the prevention of infection and concentrated urine. With a neurogenic overactive bladder or DSD the abnormally concentrated urine can stimulate afferent nerve endings, exacerbating the bladder disorder. This could increase vesicular pressures, vesicoureteral reflux, and overflow urine leakage. Conversely, excessive fluid intake can exacerbate bladder over distention.

*Biofeedback.* Biofeedback techniques using electromyography can help the individual learn better voluntary control of PFM sphincters in conditions with incomplete nerve damage. Complete relaxation of the PFM is necessary for full bladder emptying. Research on the use of biofeedback in NLUTD is limited and mostly in patients with MS.

*Surgery.* A variety of surgical interventions for neurogenic bladder exist, although because of the invasive nature of the surgery, surgical intervention is often utilized after conservative methods have failed. Procedures include bladder augmentation cystoplasty (colon, ileus, stomach, or ureter can be used); cystectomy with or without continent diversion; ureteral and bladder neck suspension; artificial urinary sphincter implantation[152]; ileovesicostomy, ileal conduit, or placement of suprapubic catheters; denervation procedures and electrostimulation (for complete lesions); and sacral nerve neuromodulation (for incomplete lesions).

SPECIAL IMPLICATIONS FOR THE THERAPIST 18.10

### *Neurogenic Bladder Disorders*

Therapists treating patients with neurologic conditions should be aware of bladder and bowel function and include toileting functional mobility in their goals. Therapists should work on maximizing functional mobility, relaxed sitting position on the toilet, and the ability to relax the adductors. Providing handrails on the toilet can improve the feeling of security in patients with poor sitting balance and lead to better overall relaxation and better emptying. Therapists in the rehabilitation facility will need to work within established bladder schedules in scheduling therapy sessions. Coordination with nursing helps to establish a routine that allows for healthy bladder and bowel scheduling

Therapists should be familiar with complications associated with NLUTD, including the potential for UTIs, renal calculi, and renal damage. The development of any of these comorbidities can interfere with the rehabilitation process. Detection of any of these symptoms warrants communication with a physician.

Incontinence associated with any of the bladder conditions discussed here can be improved and even eliminated in many people through a program of exercise and behavioral intervention. Specialized pelvic physical therapists should be consulted if available.

## Interstitial Cystitis/Painful Bladder Syndrome

### Overview and Incidence

Painful bladder syndrome (PBS) is a term introduced in 2002 by the International Continence Society (ICS) and is now defined as "Persistent or recurrent chronic pelvic pain, pressure or discomfort perceived to be related to the urinary bladder accompanied by at least one other urinary symptom such as an urgent need to void or urinary frequency."

Interstitial cystitis (IC) is a subgroup of PBS. The terms PBS and IC are often used interchangeably; however, IC is a specific diagnosis and requires confirmation by typical cystoscopic and histologic features. Chronic prostatitis/chronic pelvic pain syndrome in men (discussed more fully in Chapter 19; see section on "Chronic Prostatitis") are terms used to describe a symptoms complex characterized by pelvic pain and voiding dysfunction without infection or obvious pathology very similar to PBS/IC. Some practitioners think they may share similar etiology.

Exact figures on the incidence of PBS/IC are unavailable because of a lack of uniform definitions and inconsistent terminology. Many individuals go undiagnosed for years. Current estimates show 2.7% to 6.5% of women in the United States report symptoms consistent with PBS/IC.[145] Most are women[53] but some practitioners believe the occurrence in men is even more severely underreported.

### Etiologic and Risk Factors

The etiology of PBS/IC has not been identified. Some genetic components have been reported. Risk factors for PBS/IC have not been identified; however, there are a number of conditions that have been found to be coexistent with PBS/IC, including gastritis, child abuse, fibromyalgia, anxiety disorder, headache, esophageal reflux, unspecified back disorder, depression, allergic reactions, vulvodynia, and irritable bowel syndrome.[52]

### Pathogenesis

The pathophysiology of PBS/IC is unclear and appears to be related to several factors, including altered permeability of the bladder wall, overactivity of the PFM and visceromuscular reflex, and hypersensitivity and neurologic irritation. Studies show overactivity of the PFM in 70% to 90% of individuals with PBS/IC.[203] Hunner lesions are superficial hemorrhages of the bladder wall seen on hydrodistention with cystoscopy. The lesions are infrequent and in those with severe presentation.

### Clinical Manifestation

PBS/IC is a syndrome with many variations. The most common symptoms are urinary urgency and frequency (in some cases up to four times per hour). Several groups of researchers are documenting subgroups of PBS/IC with very different patterns, suggesting the possibility of different etiologies.[161] Other symptoms including nocturia, pain in the bladder, urethra, or vagina, suprapubic pain, and dull low back pain are common. There may also be difficulty emptying the bladder, pressure, burning, "electric shocks," spasm, and a stabbing sensation. Symptoms may increase with physical/emotional stress, acid foods, travel, or intercourse.

## MEDICAL MANAGEMENT

**DIAGNOSIS, TREATMENT, AND PROGNOSIS.** Initial assessment is focused on ruling out other causes of the symptoms with history, physical, cystoscopy, and urinalysis with cytology. Voiding diaries and symptom indexes also help to identify impairments. Optional investigations include cystoscopy with hydrodistention to look for Hunner lesions, potassium sensitivity test to check for bladder wall permeability, urodynamics, pelvic ultrasound, and intravenous pyelogram.

Medical treatment is focused on symptom relief. Complete resolution is rare. The American Urological Guideline of IC/PBS suggests first-line treatment for all patients is education on healthy bladder habits and stress management. Second-line treatments include manual physical therapy to stretch and relax overactivity in the PFM and medications. More advanced treatment may include hydrodistention with or without intravesical therapy, neuromodulation, or in rare cases removal of the bladder with stoma placement.

**SPECIAL IMPLICATIONS FOR THE THERAPIST 18.11**

*Interstitial Cystitis*

Physical therapists are playing a larger role in conservative management of PBS/IC.

The current American Urological Association guidelines for treatment of interstitial cystitis and bladder pain syndrome list patient education, stress management, and self-help as first-line treatments. Manual therapy, including soft tissue mobilization inside the vagina or rectum, is a second-line treatment.[81] In a randomized controlled trial 57% of patients reported improved symptoms with focused myofascial release of tissues inside and outside the pelvis.[81] Relaxation training of the pelvic floor muscle (with or without biofeedback) and treatment of orthopedic dysfunctions of the pelvis are also offered to treat overactive PFM.

Myofascial restrictions are commonly found in people with interstitial cystitis involving the muscles that attach to the pelvis (e.g., adductors, gluteals, obturator internus and externus, piriformis, abdominals, and iliopsoas). Specific passive and active stretching exercises and muscle reeducation activities are progressed according to the individual's response to the soft tissue interventions. Modalities such as biofeedback, ultrasound, and electrical stimulation externally and internally along with behavioral techniques (e.g., for reducing frequency and urgency) may be employed.

A bio-psychosocial approach to pain treatment with therapeutic pain education, support, and general relaxation is also encouraged. If specialized pelvic physical therapy is not available 21% of patients have reported decreased symptoms with generalized relaxation massage.[81] Avoidance of acidic and spicy foods can also decrease irritation of the bladder lining and decrease pain and urgency.

## REFERENCES

To enhance this text and add value for the reader, all references are included in the enhanced ebook on Student Consult that accompanies this textbook. The reader can view the reference source and access it online whenever possible.

CHAPTER 19

# The Male Genital/Reproductive System

ELIZABETH SHELLY • MJ STRAUHAL • HEATHER MOKY

The male genital or reproductive system is made up of the testes, epididymis, vas deferens, seminal vesicles, prostate gland, penis, and pelvic floor muscles (PFM) (Fig. 19.1). These structures are susceptible to inflammatory disorders, neoplasms, and structural defects. Because of the incidence and nature of these disorders, an understanding of their clinical presentation is essential. Prostate cancer is the most common cancer in males in the United States, and testicular cancer, although relatively rare, is the most common cancer in males aged 15 to 35 years. Benign prostatic hyperplasia (BPH) is one of the most common disorders of the aging male population. PFM dysfunction, including weakness and spasm, is more common in women but can affect men, especially after surgical procedures or infections. Because of the high incidence of these diseases, therapists will see clients with such a history, and the disorder or prescribed medical treatment could have a profound effect on the client's clinical presentation and response to treatment.

The initial presenting symptom for some of these disorders could be urinary dysfunction or back or groin pain. An awareness of other symptoms besides pain and signs associated with urogenital system diseases may alert the therapist to other origins of the back pain. The presence of such symptoms warrants communication with a physician regarding the client's status.

Therapists have long been taught to ask clients with back pain questions regarding sexual function, the concern being the possible presence of cauda equina syndrome. An awareness of the more probable causes of sexual dysfunction helps the therapist determine the relevance and potentially urgent nature of a client's complaints. The disorders discussed in this chapter are those of the highest incidence or of greatest implications for therapists.

## AGING AND THE MALE REPRODUCTIVE STSTEM

The reproductive system undergoes degenerative changes associated with aging that can affect sexual function. The testes become smaller, with thickening of the seminiferous tubules impeding sperm production; the prostate gland enlarges, potentially affecting urine outflow; and sclerotic changes occur in the local blood vessels, possibly resulting in sexual dysfunction (erectile dysfunction [ED]/impotence).

Testosterone regulates the sex drive, adipose distribution, bone and muscle mass, and the production of red blood cells and sperm. This hormone begins to decrease gradually in the 30s. Low testosterone is diagnosed when total testosterone level is below 300 ng/dL on two separate occasions of blood test. Symptoms of low testosterone include: impaired memory; irritability; decreased motivation; decreasing sexual desire; and physical changes, including fatigue, decreased endurance, performance, strength, body mass, and bone density.[75]

The age-related decrease in male sex hormone levels (androgen deficiency) also has significant local and systemic effects. A decline in bioavailable testosterone has been correlated with age-related metabolic syndrome, central adiposity, neurodegeneration, and increased risk of cardiovascular diseases.[14] Low testosterone also appears to have an association with high levels of inflammatory markers and may be the key to pathophysiology of some conditions in men.[14] Arteriosclerosis of the blood vessels resulting in peripheral vascular disease can also affect the vessels supplying the penis. While decreases in testosterone levels, penile rigidity, and ejaculation volume are all common age-relate changes in male sexual function, sexual (erectile) dysfunction can be an indicator of ischemic heart disease and should not be ignored as a symptom requiring medical evaluation.

## DISORDERS OF THE PROSTATE

### Prostatitis

#### Overview

Prostatitis is a common condition in men and has a negative impact on quality of life.[167] Prostatitis in general is the most common urologic condition in men under 50 years

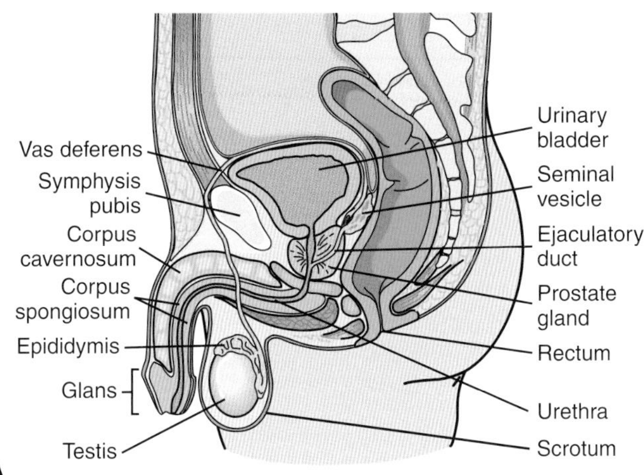


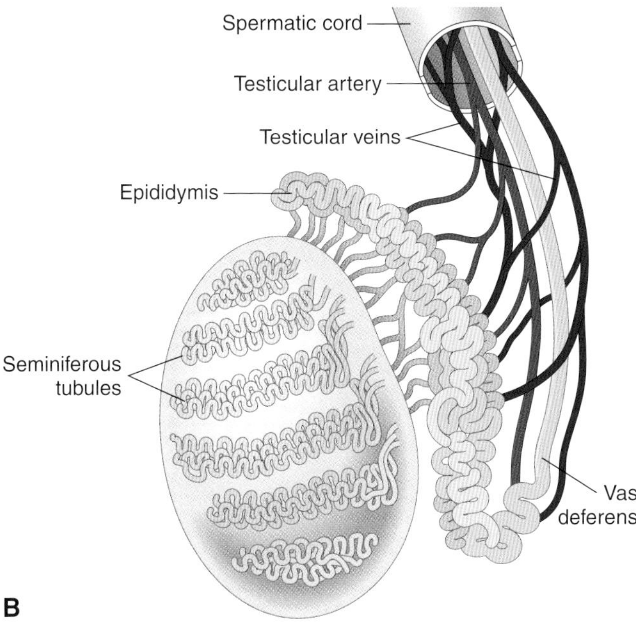


**Figure 19.1**

(A) The male reproductive system. (B) Internal structure of the testis and relationship of the testis to the epididymis. (A, From Sorrentino SA, Remmert LM: *Mosby's textbook for nursing assistants*, ed 10, St. Louis, 2021, Elsevier; B, from Chabner D: *The language of medicine*, ed 12, St. Louis, 2021, Elsevier.)

old.[113]The prevalence worldwide is 8.2% to 9.7%, with five million cases diagnosed annually.[26,76,86] In 1995, The National Institutes of Health (NIH)/National Institute of Diabetes and Digestive and Kidney Diseases devised a classification of prostatitis which is still used today (Table 19.1).[87] The term *prostatitis* refers to inflammation of the prostate, but some categories of prostatitis do not include inflammation. Inflammation of the prostate gland can be acute or chronic, bacterial or nonbacterial, symptomatic or asymptomatic. Due to the great diversity of etiology, clinical manifestations, diagnosis, and treatment, the three least common categories of prostatitis (categories I, II, and IV) will be reviewed briefly here and the most common category a physical therapist may encounter (category III, chronic pelvic pain syndrome) will be discussed in more detail later.

### Acute Bacterial Prostatitis[25,139]

Acute bacterial prostatitis (category I) is the least common of the four types but also the easiest to diagnose and treat effectively. The incidence of acute prostatitis is unknown but it is thought to account for approximately 10% of all prostatitis cases. Occurrence peaks between 20 and 40 years old and over 70 years old. Risk factors for acute bacterial infection include other genitourinary infections, sexually transmitted infections (STIs) and risky sexual behavior, immunocompromise, urethral stricture, benign prostate hyperplasia (BPH), and prostate manipulation by scope, catheter, biopsy, or surgery. Bladder outlet obstruction with urinary retention can increase bacteria grown in the bladder and subsequently allow bacteria to travel into the prostatic tissue. The pathogens associated with acute prostatitis include *E. coli* (>50% of cases), pseudomonads, enterococcus, STIs, tuberculosis, fungus, staphylococci, salmonella, and streptococci.

Clinical manifestations include irritative voiding (e.g., dysuria, urinary frequency, urinary urgency) and obstructive voiding (e.g., hesitancy, incomplete voiding, straining to urinate, weak stream). Pain can occur in a wide area, including suprapubic, rectal, sacral, low back, and perineum. In addition, painful ejaculation and painful defecation can occur. Systemic symptoms (e.g., fever, chills, nausea, emesis, arthralgia, myalgia, malaise) should alert the therapist to the possibility of sepsis.

Initial diagnosis of acute bacterial prostatitis includes a thorough history and physical examination. Midstream urinalysis and urine cultures will identify most cases of acute bacterial prostatitis, but up to 35% of urine cultures in patients with acute prostatitis will fail to grow an organism.[44] Blood cultures can be useful in these situations. Prostatic massage to express prostatic secretions, and digital rectal exam (DRE) are contraindicated in acute bacterial prostatitis due to the risk of spreading the infection and increasing sepsis. Testing for STIs would also be advised in certain circumstances, as well as postvoid residual urine volume to diagnose urinary retention. The treatment is generally a 6-week course[52] of outpatient antibiotics, with one in six men requiring hospitalization. Poor prognosis is seen in men over 65 years old with BPH, urinary retention, and a high fever. Therapists are least likely to encounter problems associated with acute prostatitis because the symptoms are usually severe enough that physician contact is initiated by the client, and rehabilitation is typically placed on hold until the antibiotic therapy is successful.

### Chronic Bacterial Prostatitis[76,114,139]

Chronic bacterial prostatitis (category II), also relatively uncommon, is chronic or recurrent infection of the prostate. Acute bacterial prostatitis can progress to a chronic infection. This may be more likely with a genetic predisposition to retrograde prostatic fluid flow or other anatomic stricture of the urethra. Autoimmunity may play a role in chronic prostatitis, because up to one-third of men with prostatitis have elevated levels of specific molecules that regulate the inflammatory response. Other risk factors are similar to those of acute prostate infections. The most

**Table 19.1** Prostatitis Classification[a]

| Category | NIDDK Classification | Description | Clinical Manifestation | Lab Findings | Treatment |
|---|---|---|---|---|---|
| I | Acute bacterial prostatitis | Bacterial infection of the prostate gland as a result of a bacteria, virus, or STD | Irritative voiding<br>Obstructive voiding<br>Pain: suprapubic, rectal, sacral, low back, and perineum<br>Systemic symptoms | WBCs and bacteria in urine | Antimicrobial medications |
| II | Chronic bacterial prostatitis | Recurrent infection of the prostate | Symptoms as for category I<br>Erectile dysfunction | WBCs and bacteria in urine | Antimicrobial medications<br>Transurethral resection of the prostate (TURP) when persistent disease is not cured with medications |
| IIIA | Inflammatory chronic prostatitis/ chronic pelvic pain syndrome (CP/CPPS) | Pain and urinary dysfunction with inflammation but without infection | Genitourinary pain:<br>Perineum, rectal<br>Testicular<br>Penis (tip)<br>Lower abdominal/pelvic<br>Low back<br>Sexual dysfunction<br>Erectile dysfunction<br>Painful ejaculation<br>Disturbed quality of life<br>Irritative voiding<br>Obstructive voiding | WBCs and other infection-fighting cells may be present in urine, semen, and prostatic fluid but without the presence of bacteria | Treatment is individual and varies; optimal treatment unknown<br>Pelvic floor reeducation; biofeedback<br>Medications |
| IIIB | Noninflammatory CP/CPPS | Pain and urinary dysfunction without inflammation or infection<br>Previously known as chronic nonbacterial prostatitis | Same as IIIA | None | Same as for CP/CPPS in IIIA |
| IV | Asymptomatic inflammatory prostatitis | | No symptoms | WBCs in semen and prostate fluid | None |

*STD*, Sexually transmitted disease; *UTI*, urinary tract infection; *WBCs*, white blood cells.
[a]Note: These are possible symptoms; not all men will have all symptoms.

commonly found pathogens associated with chronic bacterial infections are the gram-negative enterobacteria, such as *Escherichia coli, Proteus mirabilis, Klebsiella pneumoniae,* and *Pseudomonas aeruginosa*. Although controversial, other infectious agents, such as gonococci, *Ureaplasma* species, chlamydiae, and mycoplasmata, are possible etiologic factors.

Men who experience chronic bacterial prostatitis are plagued by persistent low-grade symptoms, with flare-ups of pelvic pain, voiding problems, and sexual dysfunction (e.g., erectile dysfunction, ejaculatory pain, and a decline in emotional well-being). Symptoms usually occur slowly (versus rapid onset in acute bacterial prostatitis) and last for more than 3 months. Patients rarely have a fever and may be able to function at work and home without limitations. When diagnosing chronic bacterial prostatitis a thorough history, physical examination urinalysis, analysis of an expressed prostatic specimen, and a DRE are used. Palpation of the prostate may find a normal, boggy, or tender prostate. Obtaining a urinalysis with midstream urine culture is essential to the clinical diagnosis before administering antibiotics. Blood cultures are an option if a patient has a fever because false-negative cultures can occur. Prostatic massage to extract prostatic secretions to be analyzed under a microscope for leukocytes and bacteria (Meares-Stamey 2-glass or 4-glass test) is considered a gold standard to diagnose chronic bacterial prostatitis. It is sometimes not used in practice due to time constraints and the difficulty of obtaining a sample. STI testing for *N. gonorrhoeae* and *C. trachomatis* should be considered for sexually active younger men or men who engage in high-risk sexual behavior.

Treatment of category II (chronic bacterial) prostatitis involves 4 to 12 weeks of antibiotics to eliminate the organism producing the infection. Men with frequent recurrences may be placed on antibiotic prophylaxis for 3 to 6 months and have their clinical course reassessed. Alpha blockers can also be helpful to increase urine flow and decrease urinary retention. Treatment of chronic bacterial prostatitis can be difficult because the antibiotic agents have difficulty penetrating the chronically inflamed prostate. Transurethral resection of the prostate

(TURP) may be indicated if the disease is not cured with medications.

### Asymptomatic Inflammatory Prostatitis[114]

Asymptomatic inflammatory prostatitis (category IV) is diagnosed when white blood cells and inflammatory markers are found in semen or prostate tissue in an asymptomatic man. Doctors usually diagnose this form of prostatitis when looking for causes of infertility or when testing for prostate cancer. Little is understood about the etiology or significance of category IV prostatitis. Studies are finding that it is more prevalent than originally thought. One Chinese study demonstrated an increased risk associated with category IV prostatitis and age, smoking, drinking, and lower education levels.[174] Some studies have suggested a relationship between category IV prostatitis and serum prostate specific antigen (PSA) levels.[58] There is no treatment recommendation for asymptomatic inflammatory prostatitis at this time.

### Chronic Prostatitis/Chronic Pelvic Pain Syndrome (CP/CPPS)

The remainder of this section will focus on prostatitis categories IIIA and IIIB, also known as CP/CPPS.

> **Note to Reader::** Several groups have debated the terminology used for these conditions. The International Continence Society Standard terms for chronic pelvic pain syndromes [34] recommends not using the term "chronic prostatitis" when no proven infection or other obvious pathology is present (i.e. category IIIB). The suggested term is simply "chronic pelvic pain syndrome." The term chronic pelvic pain syndrome (CPPS) may be used to describe conditions of males or females. CP/CPPS is a term specific to males.

**Overview and Incidence.** CP/CPPS is the most common (more than 90% of cases[146]) but least understood form of prostatitis. It is described as the occurrence of pelvic pain with urinary symptoms and/or sexual dysfunction without infection or other diagnosable conditions lasting 3 months over the past 6 months. Incidence is reported at 2% to 15% of men.[106,146] There is a 17% overlap between CP/CPPS and interstitial cystitis/painful bladder syndrome.[154] Irritable bowel syndrome is coexistent in 22% to 31% of men with CP/CPPS.[76] CP/CPPS is found in men of any age.

**Risk Factors.** Little is known about risk factors for CP/CPPS. One large case-controlled study of Chinese men found potential risk factors included age, nightshift work, stress, smoking status, alcohol consumption, less water intake, imbalanced diet, frequent sexual activity, delaying ejaculation and holding urine.[23] Severe pain in CP/CPPS was associated with sedentary lifestyle, caffeinated drinks, and less water intake. A large population-based study found higher physical activity associated with lower occurrence of CP/CPPS. Both moderate (brisk walking) and vigorous activity had the same benefit.[126] Anxiety disorder has also been associated with CP/CPPS in all age groups. Men in the age group of 40 to 59 years old with CP/CPPS had anxiety disorder more than twice as often as controls.[24] The European Association of Urology (EAU) guidelines on Chronic Pelvic Pain note several possible psychological risk factors, including sexual abuse.

**Etiology and Pathogenesis.** In the inflammatory form of CP/CPPS (category IIIA), urine, semen, and other fluids from the prostate show no evidence of a known infecting organism but do contain white blood cells. In the noninflammatory form (category IIIB), no evidence of infection or inflammation, including white blood cells, is present. The etiology of CP/CPPS is multifactorial and poorly understood. EAU lists several potential initiating factors, including infectious, genetic, anatomic, neuromuscular, endocrine, immune (including autoimmune), or psychological mechanisms. It has been suggested that CP/CPPS is not an organ-specific syndrome but instead may be a urogenital manifestation of regional or systemic abnormalities. Some hypothesize that the process may begin with an initial infection or trauma that affects the prostate, pelvic floor, bladder, or perineum. If not effectively treated in the early stages, it may lead to central sensitization.[167] It is also postulated that CP/CPPS may have a similar mechanism to vulvodynia in women, fibromyalgia, and other central sensitization syndromes.[45] Another hypothesis is that pelvic floor muscle (PFM) spasm, overactivity or trigger points may mimic prostate pain and prostatitis. In a 1999 study, 88% of the men with CP/CPPS had PFM trigger points and 52% had dyssynergia. A more recent study in 2008[141] found 51% of men with CP/CPPS have tenderness in either prostate, PFM or suprapubic region compared to 7% of controls. Physical therapists have also identified other pelvic joint and muscle dysfunctions in men with CP/CPPS.[68,167] It is not known whether these findings are the cause or effect of other components of the condition, but they appear to resolve with direct treatment, suggesting some causative role.

**Clinical Manifestations.** Table 19.1 contains a summary of symptoms associated with the four categories of prostatitis. The NIH classification identifies genitourinary pain as the primary component of CP/CPPS. Perineal (behind the scrotum) pain is present in 63% of patients.[76] Other areas of pain include the suprapubic region, testicles, penis (especially penile tip pain), lower back, abdomen, inguinal region/groin, and rectum. Most patients have lower urinary tract symptoms (LUTS)[87] with some combination of irritative or obstructive voiding, including painful urination (dysuria) and possibly blood in the urine. Generalized sexual dysfunction is often present with this syndrome (46% to 92%), with specific erectile dysfunction reported by 15% to 55%.[76] Some patients have intermittent symptoms which appear to be unpredictable. Pain is usually made worse by sitting, squatting, and bending and may be relieved or irritated by ejaculation. Some men find that stress, emotional factors, alcohol, spicy foods, or caffeine triggers episodes.

## MEDICAL MANAGEMENT

**DIAGNOSIS.** There is no gold standard diagnostic test for CP/CPPS. It is a diagnosis of exclusion and laboratory or imaging studies are indicated to rule out other potential causes of symptoms. Differential diagnosis includes pelvic cancer, all forms of infection, including abscess, pudendal neuralgia, bladder stone or other foreign objects, and neurologic disease affecting the bladder. Digital rectal examination is required to assess all pelvic structures, including tenderness of the PFM. Laboratory testing could include urinalysis, assessment of expressed prostatic fluid, PSA, and testing for STIs. Elevated PSA should not be attributed to CP/CPPS and warrants further investigation. Other tests for bladder function and outlet capacity could be used to rule out other treatable conditions. A diagnosis of CP/CPPS is given when testing is essentially negative or not able to explain the constellation of symptoms (grade A from EAU guidelines).[43]

A six-point clinical phenotyping system to evaluate patients with chronic urologic pelvic pain was developed and uses the acronym UPOINT.[97,123,141] The clinical domains are urinary symptoms, psychosocial dysfunction, organ-specific findings, infection, neurologic/systemic, and tenderness of muscles. Current NIH guidelines advise using the NIH Chronic Prostatitis Symptom Index (NIH-CPSI) to assess symptoms and plan treatment. The NIH-CPSI assesses the severity of symptoms and quality of life in men with CP/CPPS.[92,146]

Physical therapists have documented a number of musculoskeletal dysfunctions in patients with CP/CPPS, including dysfunction in the sacroiliac and pubic symphysis joints, poor posture (rounded shoulders), hip dysfunction (positive Faber and Thomas), and weakness and pain of the PFM rectally. Tenderness and tightness of the psoas, adductors, and abdominals is also common.[68,167]

Although not clinically feasible for making a diagnosis, functional MRI has shown alterations in the density of gray matter in pain relevant regions such as the anterior insula, which correlates to pain intensity and chroncity.[45] Psychological evaluation should be considered if symptoms are present because these conditions can have a significant impact on treatment success.[128]

**TREATMENT.** Multimodal individualized treatment is suggested by EUA guidelines. Quality research on the effect of CP/CPPS treatments is lacking, and the placebo effect is high in many studies.[47,74] In addition, efficiency of all treatments increases over time[74] and many experts suggest persistence in treatment over 32 weeks if a small effect is initially noted. A 2012 systematic review found clinical and statistical decreases in outcomes measures for multimodal treatment. This included alpha blockers, ibuprofen, thiocolchicoside (a muscle relaxant not available in the United States), mepartricin (also not available in the United States), and percutaneous tibial nerve stimulation (PTNS). Adding aerobic exercise or acupuncture significantly decreased pain scores.[74]

Despite unknown etiology, alpha blockers and antibiotics are often first line treatments for CP/CPPS. Newly diagnosed cases or those that have not been treated before may be more likely to respond to these medications compared to chronic refractory cases.[43] The systematic review found alpha blockers and antibiotics in general did not provide a significant benefit.[74] Anticonvulsants and medications to treat neuropathic pain, muscle relaxants (in some cases used rectally), ibuprophen, phytotherapies (e.g., herbal treatment with quercetin or bee pollen), tricyclic antidepressants, and antiinflammatory medications have all been considered, with varying success under specific conditions.[139] Anesthetic injection of PFM trigger points through the perineum was shown to improve pain in approximately 50% of men when used in conjunction with pelvic physical therapy.[155] Cannabis has been shown to help with symptom relief and may play a role in the complex management of CP/CPPS symptoms. However, fertility issues should be considered because regular cannabis use has been shown in multiple studies to have an effect on sperm, resulting in lower sperm concentration, lower total sperm count, and decreased sperm function.[5,38] Treatment for psychological components of CP/CPPS is also recommended, especially for anxiety disorder and in the presence of central sensitization.[162]

A review of change in treatment over 16 years reported increased treatments for psychosocial and PFM pain.[35] Many guidelines[43,76,114,146] recommend conservative management and physical therapy to include varying combinations of: biofeedback; pelvic floor reeducation and relaxation; myofascial stretching of the PFM, hips, and trunk; heat; general stretching exercises and general relaxation; and electrical stimulation for pain modulation. Research on these interventions is lacking, and most recommendations are based on consensus or case reports.[167] A recent Cochrane review found nonpharmacologic interventions, such as acupuncture and extracorporeal shockwave therapy, are likely to result in a decrease in prostatitis symptoms.[47] The report also found physical activity may have a small positive effect, but more high quality studies are needed. In an RCT not included in the Cochrane review, an 18-week aerobic exercise program resulted in more symptom improvement than stretching in men with CP/CPPS.[53] More high quality research is needed.

The Cochrane review[47] included one study on lifestyle modifications which was of poor quality and insufficient to make a strong recommendation. Most pelvic PT specialists include treatment directed at modifiable lifestyle risk factors,[23] including good sleep patterns, decreased stress, and avoidance of smoking. Patient should be educated in normal fluid intake without caffeine or alcohol and a balanced diet. A normal bladder pattern should also be adopted, without excessive urine holding. Men may also be counseled to avoid delayed ejaculation and frequent sexual activity although there is no formal recommendation of the frequency.[23]

**SPECIAL IMPLICATIONS FOR THE THERAPIST 19.1**

### *Prostatitis*

Therapists should be alert to the symptoms of prostatitis listed in Table 19.1, in particular category II and III. Prostatitis can be the cause of back and pelvic pain in young males.

Bicycle seats can aggravate prostatitis symptoms; thus, a recumbent bicycle is recommended because it puts less pressure on the perineum.

If CP/CPPS is suspected, referral to a specialized pelvic PT is recommended. All physical therapists can educate patients on a healthy lifestyle, including a general aerobic exercise program. When appropriate, correction of musculoskeletal imbalances of the pelvis with manual therapy, myofascial stretching, and exercises with special attention to the psoas, abdominal, piriformis, and adductor muscle groups should be included. Therapists should also teach diaphragmatic breathing and general relaxation and consider referral to a massage therapist for relaxation massage. Pain education can also have a great impact on chronic pain perception and is recommend by the EAU guidelines. Heat and TENS can aid in pain modulation.

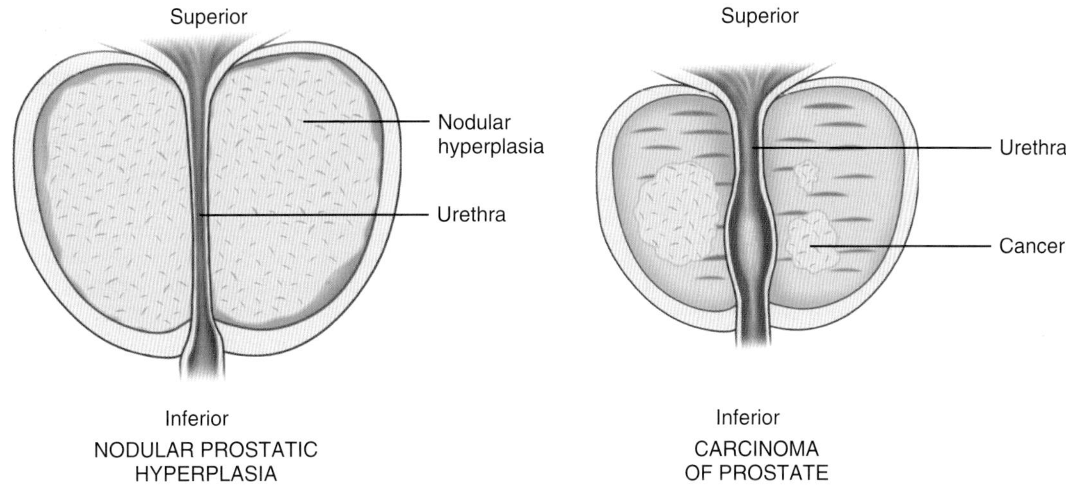


**Figure 19.2**

In benign prostatic hyperplasia (BPH), the nodules initially develop in the periurethral region, compressing the urethra. Cancer of the prostate typically develops initially in the periphery of the gland.

## Benign Prostatic Hyperplasia

### Overview

Benign prostatic hyperplasia (BPH), also called prostate gland enlargement, is an age-related, nonmalignant enlargement of the prostate gland. It is defined as a prostate volume (PV) greater than 30 mL[112] along with lower urinary tract symptoms (LUTS) and bladder outlet obstruction (BOO).

### Incidence and Risk Factors

Of men age 50 years and older, 70% experience symptoms of prostate enlargement.[90] The disease is rarely noted in men under age 40 and tends to become symptomatic after age 50 years. Data from U.S. health care plans and Medicare report that BPH is the fourth most common diagnosis in men over 50.[150] Besides age, geography and ethnicity are important factors in the incidence of this disease. BPH is found most often in the United States and western Europe and least often in the Far East. The incidence of BPH is also higher in African Americans than in whites. Markers to assess progression include the following: (1) age greater than 50 years, (2) PSA greater than 1.4 ng/mL, (3) prostate volume (PV) greater than 30 mL, and (4) International Prostate Symptom Score greater than 8.[9] These parameters are used to determine which individuals would benefit from medical therapy and possibly avoid surgery. Risk factors include age over 40, family history of BPH, diabetes, heart disease with use of beta blockers, and obesity. Exercise decreases the risk of BPH.

### Pathogenesis

The prostate gland is normally about the size and shape of a walnut, normally weighing about 20 g. This gland encircles the urethra just below the bladder (see Fig. 19.1). It consists of five lobes and produces seminal fluid to nourish and transport semen. Throughout life, the body constantly replaces old, dying prostate cells with new ones. For reasons still not completely clear, as men age the ratio of new prostate cells to old prostate cells shifts in favor of lower cell death. This increased growth of new prostate cells occurs primarily inward, encroaching on the urethra (benign prostate obstruction). By age 70 years, the hypertrophic prostate can weigh up to 200 g, resulting in significant urethral obstruction and difficulty emptying the bladder.

Although the cause is unknown, changes in hormone balance associated with aging may be responsible for the development of BPH. Other research points to the role of infection.[129] The pathologic changes are marked by *hyperplasia,* not hypertrophy. Multiple prostatic nodules develop, resulting from the proliferation of epithelial cells, smooth muscle cells, and stromal fibroblasts of the gland. These nodules initially develop in the periurethral region of the prostate as opposed to the periphery of the gland as in prostate cancer (Fig. 19.2). The enlargement of the prostate increases smooth muscle tone at the bladder neck and prostatic capsule leading to increased resistance. These effects narrow the prostatic urethra and thus diminish urinary flow. The bladder must work harder to empty urine through a narrow urethra. Over time this can result in trigone hypertrophy and thickening of the bladder wall. As urethral obstruction progresses, urinary retention and reflux into the ureters (vesicoureteral reflux) can occur. This increases the risk of developing UTIs, marked bladder distention with destructive bladder wall changes, hydroureter (dilated weakened ureter), hydronephrosis (urine-filled dilation of the renal pelvis), and destruction of renal tissue (Fig. 19.3). Ultimately, renal failure and death may occur if treatment is not initiated.

### Clinical Manifestations

Lower urinary tract symptoms occur when men experience disturbances to the urinary flow and can be related to BPH. Other causes of LUTS include UTI, prostatitis, bladder cancer, bladder stones, and overactive bladder (OAB). Differential diagnosis is essential for proper treatment. Increasing LUTS is associated with worsening quality of life although

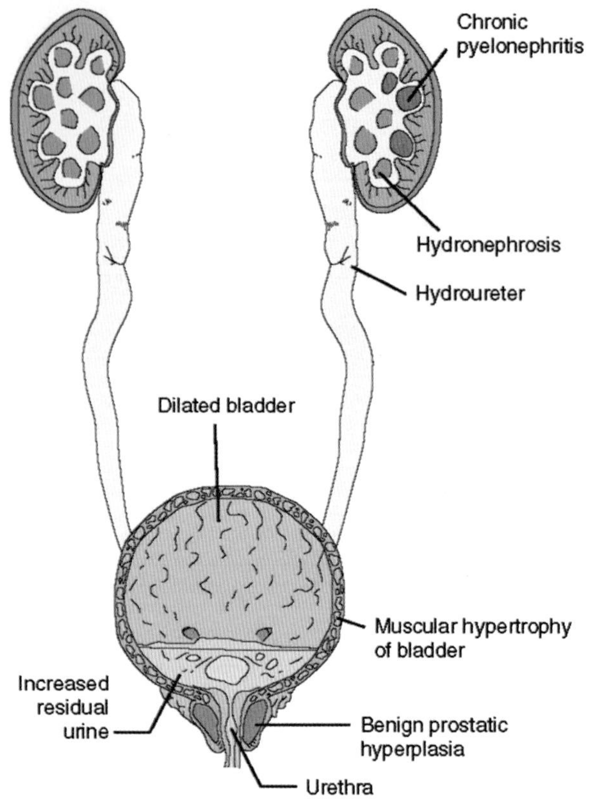


**Figure 19.3**

A cascade of destructive events potentially associated with advanced benign prostatic hyperplasia (BPH). As the prostate enlarges, the urethra becomes obstructed, interfering with the normal flow of urine, resulting in urine backing up the ureters and pooling in the kidney.

symptoms are not always reported to the physician.[150] LUTS can occur in two forms: storage (inability to store) and voiding (inability to empty) (Box 19.1). Other urinary symptoms associated with the later stages of the disease include urge incontinence, hematuria, urinary retention, and dysuria.

Box 19.1

**SYMPTOMS OF BENIGN PROSTATE HYPERPLASIA**

***Storage Dysfunction***

- Increased daytime urinary frequency: complaint that micturition occurs more frequently during waking hours than previously deemed normal
- Nocturia: complaint of interruption of sleep one or more times because of the need to void. Each void is preceded and followed by sleep.
- Urgency: complaint of a sudden, compelling desire to pass urine which is difficult to defer

***Voiding Dysfunction***

- Hesitancy: complaint of a delay in initiating micturition
- Slow stream: complaint of a urinary stream perceived as slower compared to previous performance or in comparison with others
- Intermittency: complaint of urine flow that stops and starts on one or more occasions during voiding
- Straining to void: complaint of the need to make an intensive effort (by abdominal straining, Valsalva, or suprapubic pressure) to either initiate, maintain, or improve the urinary stream
- Spraying (splitting) of urinary stream: complaint that the urine passage is a spray or split rather than a single discrete stream
- Feeling of incomplete (bladder) emptying: complaint that the bladder does not feel empty after micturition
- Need to immediately re-void: complaint that further micturition is necessary soon after passing urine
- Postmicturition leakage: complaint of a further involuntary passage of urine following the completion of micturition

Definitions are taken from The International Continence Society (ICS) report on the terminology for adult male lower urinary tract and pelvic floor symptoms and dysfunction.

D'Ancona C, Haylen B, Oelke M, et al: Standardisation Steering Committee ICS and the ICS Working Group on Terminology for Male Lower Urinary Tract & Pelvic Floor Symptoms and Dysfunction. *Neurourol Urodyn* 38(2):433-477, 2019. https://www.ncbi.nlm.nih.gov/pubmed/30681183.

## MEDICAL MANAGEMENT

**PREVENTION.** There has been some controversy over the use of saw palmetto, lycopene, and tomato products as possible antioxidant prevention of BPH.[41] The general consensus is that these natural products will not do any harm but they may not help either. Researchers are also working on a vaccination, using the theories of infection as the origin of BPH.[129]

**DIAGNOSIS.** The 2018 Canadian Urological Association guidelines on BPH reviewed previous guidelines from the American Urological Association and European Urological Association.[111] They suggest four levels of diagnostic guidelines: mandatory, recommended, optional, and not recommended (Box 19.2). Correlation of the history, palpation findings (digital rectal exam), and urinalysis typically gives rise to the diagnosis of BPH and indicates the choice of treatment. Regarding palpation, the bladder may be palpable as urinary retention progresses. In addition, a smooth, rubbery enlargement of the prostate may be noted during DRE, although the perceived size of the prostate does not always correlate with the degree of urethral compression. Special attention should be given to the presence of nodules on the prostate surface because these can sometimes indicate prostate cancer. The American Urological Association has also developed a self-administered screening tool (International Prostate Symptom Score) used to determine the frequency and severity of urinary symptoms.[9]

Prostate-specific antigen (PSA), a measure of protein in the bloodstream secreted by cells in the prostate gland, is an additional blood test that helps predict the natural course of BPH. Higher levels of PSA are linked with a greater risk of future prostate growth and subsequent complications. Urinalysis is usually done to check for hematuria and UTI. The most commonly employed urodynamic test for the assessment of BPH is uroflowmetry. The urine flow rate and the force of the urine stream are measured. It is generally agreed that a peak urine flow rate of less than 10 mL/sec is suggestive of obstruction. Uroflowmetry by itself is a screening modality, not diagnostic, because the urinary obstruction could be occurring at sites other than at the prostate gland.

**TREATMENT.** If symptoms related to BPH are mild, the condition is often only monitored because the clinical status of the disorder may stabilize or even improve. Studies

Box 19.2

**2018 CANADIAN UROLOGICAL ASSOCIATION GUIDELINES FOR ASSESSMENT OF BPH**

***Mandatory***

- History to screen for other causes of symptoms
- Physical including digital rectal exam (DRE)
- Urinalysis to rule out infection

***Recommended***

- Symptom and bother inventory: International Prostate Symptom Score (IPSS) or AUA Symptom Index (AUA-SI)
- Prostate specific antigen (PSA) blood test

***Optional***

- Urine cytology: further assess for infection
- Uroflowmetery and postvoid residual: to asses voiding dysfunction and obstruction
- Voiding diary: this can be used to inform lifestyle changes
- Serum creatinine: screen for kidney damage
- Sexual function questionnaire: to screen for further assessment and treatment needs

***Not Recommended Unless Other Symptoms are Present to Warrant Differential Diagnosis***

- Cystoscope
- Urodynamics
- X-rays of kidneys or ultrasound of prostate
- Prostate biopsy

Nickel JC, Aaron L, Barkin J, et al: Canadian Urological Association guideline on male lower urinary tract symptoms/benign prostatic hyperplasia (MLUTS/BPH): 2018 update, *Can Urol Assoc J* 12(10):303-312, 2018.

have shown that just over 50% of patients require active treatment 5 years after initiation of watchful waiting for BPH.[56] Aggressive treatment is indicated when the condition progresses to a more advanced stage. Symptoms suggesting advanced disease include urine retention, incontinence, hematuria, and chronic UTIs. The goals of treatment include providing client comfort and avoiding serious renal damage. First-line treatment for mild BPH is lifestyle changes. For those with moderate to severe symptoms, the two medical treatment approaches for BPH are pharmacologic and surgical.

***Medication.*** In most cases, symptoms associated with BPH can be controlled with medications. The Canadian Urological Association guidelines on BPH provide guidance on the use of medications.[111] In many cases combining medications produces better results than administering only one drug.

Three main pharmacologic agents are used to treat BPH: (1) medications to shrink glandular tissue (5-α-reductase inhibitors); (2) drugs to relax smooth muscle tissue of the prostate, bladder neck, and urethra (α-adrenergic blockers); and (3) antimuscarinics to address overactive bladder symptoms. The 5-α-reductase inhibitors address the hormonal causes of BPH by preventing the enzyme 5-α-reductase from converting testosterone into DHT (DHT prompts glandular tissue to develop). As a result, the prostate shrinks by as much as 20%. This is a gradual process that can take up to a year to obtain maximum benefit.

The α-adrenergic receptors are located in the muscle fibers of the adenoma and prostate capsule. The resultant smooth muscle relaxation decreases pressure on the urethra, enhancing urinary flow. Antimuscarinics block cholinergic receptors in the bladder wall to prevent bladder spasms. Antimuscarinics have been demonstrated to improve bladder capacity, increased volume at first detrusor contraction, and maximum cytometric capacity. Phytopharmaceuticals (e.g., substrates from saw palmetto and other plants) have been suggested for the management of BPH. Earlier studies in the United States showed significant effects of saw palmetto on epithelial contraction, urinary flow rates, and improved symptoms compared with placebos, but more recent studies have shown mixed results and a lack of convincing evidence. Presently, the American Urologic Association does not recommend any dietary supplement for the management of BPH. Phosphodiesterase type 5 inhibitors not only treat erectile dysfunction but also provide relief for symptoms of BPH.

***Surgery.*** Not everyone with BPH responds adequately to medications. In such cases, BPH can progress to the point where surgery is required. The goal of surgical intervention is to alleviate the obstruction to urine flow, decrease obstructive voiding symptoms and, most importantly, protect the kidneys from damage due to urinary reflux. Presently the AUA recommends surgery for men who have moderate to severe LUTS with an IPPS score of 8 or higher, acute urinary retention, or other BPH-related complications. *Transurethral resection of the prostate* (TURP) is the gold standard in surgical treatments for BPH with a prostate volume of 30 to 80 cc.[111] A rectoscope is inserted into the urethra for visual inspection of the urethra and bladder. The surgeon then trims away excess prostate tissue and enlarges the urinary channel.

TURP is very successful in relieving symptoms and improving quality of life, but some drawbacks are evident (e.g., requires a general anesthetic and hospital stay and may be accompanied by side effects such as bleeding, urinary retention, UTI, incontinence, ED, or retrograde ejaculation [in which an ejaculation goes back into the bladder]). Many less invasive procedures are reviewed in the Canadian Urological Associations guidelines.[111]

Laser Therapy. Lasers are used for rapid incision and vaporization of the prostate. Holmium laser enucleation of the prostate (HoLEP) provides significant benefits with fewer complications and shorter hospital stay than TURP.[28] Fellowship training is suggested with need for 20 to 50 practice cases. Photoselective vaporization of the prostate (Greenlight) can also provide fewer complications, shorter hospital stays, and similar outcomes to TURP.[28] This laser is suggested for treatment in men with risk factors, such as heart disease or anticoagulation therapy, or for men who do not tolerate medications well. These modalities restore spontaneous urine flow by destroying diseased prostate tissue. Diode laser and thulium laser are also used to treat BPH in men who are at high risk for surgery.

Minimally Invasive Techniques.[111] Transurethral microwave therapy (TUMT) (an outpatient procedure) is suggested for elderly men with many comorbidities. Results of long-term studies (five-year data available) are not available at this time, but short-term results demonstrate decreased LUTS symptoms. Transurethral incision of the prostate (TUIP) uses a small incision at the bladder neck to open the urethra and decrease LUTS symptoms. It is appropriate for men with a small prostate size (<30 cc) and LUTS.

Simple Prostatectomy.[111] Most procedures for BPH are performed through the urethra, thus decreasing complications and morbidity. When the prostate is larger (over 80 to 100 cc) it may be necessary to approach the prostate from the abdominal and pelvic cavities. A simple prostatectomy is removal of the inner prostatic tissue while leaving the outer capsule. This is in contrast to a radical prostatectomy which removes the entire prostate, including the capsule. Simple prostatectomy may be performed open, laparoscopically, or with robotic assistance. These procedures are more invasive, require longer hospital stays and postoperative catheter placement. Long-term complications (UI, urethral stricture) are also more common than transurethral procedures.

New and Emerging Therapies.[111] Prostatic urethral lift is an insert placed into the urethra to compress encroaching tissue and hold urethra open. Convective water vapor energy ablation uses controlled steam to ablate the excess prostate tissue. Image-guided robotic waterjet ablation is hydrodissection of excess prostate tissue, sparing blood vessels. The temporary implantable nitinol device is a temporary stent-like device designed to remodel the bladder neck and the prostatic urethra through pressure necrosis.

**PROGNOSIS.** BPH can contribute to chronic problems with lower urinary tract symptoms, ED, and decreased quality of life. Clinical progression of PBH (increase in IPPS scale of 4 or more points) occurs in 20% of men. A placebo group showed approximately 24% increase in prostate volume during a 5-year trial.[102] Over 5 years, 2.5% had urinary retention and 6% required more invasive treatment. Treatment is reserved for symptomatic presentation, but there is risk of progression and patients should be encouraged to share their symptoms with a physician and review those symptoms regularly. BPH is not a known risk factor or precursor to prostate cancer but it is possible the two coexist.[22] Prostatic tissue removed during surgical procures will be assessed for the presence of cancer cells, thus increasing the rate of incidental prostate cancer diagnosis in men undergoing surgical treatment for BPH.

**SPECIAL IMPLICATIONS FOR THE THERAPIST 19.2**

***Benign Prostatic Hyperplasia***

BPH often results in obstructed voiding with symptoms of urgency, frequency, hesitancy, intermittency, nocturia, and weak stream. Therapists conducting a medical history with men over the age of 50 years can easily include a series of four questions to help identify the presence of obstructed voiding:

- Do you urinate more than every 2 hours, or more than once during the night?
- Do you have trouble starting or continuing your urine?
- Do you have weak flow of urine or interrupted urine stream?
- Does it feel like your bladder is not emptying completely?

A *yes* answer to any of these questions warrants further medical evaluation. Painful urination; blood in the urine; or unexplained lower back, pelvis, hip, or upper thigh pain in the presence of any of these symptoms requires medical referral. Unexplained reports of sexual dysfunction warrant also communication with a physician. Men over the age of 40 years should be encouraged to get regular check-ups and report symptoms to their physician in order to prevent complications from delayed diagnosis of BPH.

Pharmacologic agents used to treat BPH are associated with numerous side effects, which the therapist should be aware of and watch out for. These include general muscle weakness, ED (inability to achieve an erection), loss of libido, gynecomastia, drowsiness, dizziness, tachycardia, and postural orthostatic hypotension. The therapist can advise clients about the possibility of falls from dizziness and loss of balance associated with these medications and take steps to institute a falls prevention program when appropriate. Any change or new onset of symptoms should be reported to the physician.

Lifestyle suggestions for BPH can be easily incorporated into the overall PT plan.[41]

- Normalize fluid intake to 50 to 70 oz per day
- Decrease caffeine and alcohol intake
- Urinate every 2 hours during the day (but try not to go more often just in case)
- Avoid constipation
- Double voiding (relax and try to urinate again)
- Add to diet flaxseed and vegetables, decrease fat and red meat [41]

Pelvic physical therapy may be appropriate for men with BPH who are experiencing urinary incontinence (UI), urgency, and/or frequency. The physical therapist can offer PFM relaxation training to increase bladder emptying during watchful waiting and PFM strength training for UI related to BPH procedures. Bladder training for overactive bladder is also helpful for symptoms of urgency and frequency.

People who answer yes to any of these questions may still be appropriate for physical therapy intervention but further evaluation is warranted and a decision made for medical referral, treat, or treat and refer.

## Prostate Cancer

### Overview

Adenocarcinoma of the prostate arises from the glandular cells and accounts for 98% of primary prostatic tumors. Ductal and transitional cell carcinomas make up the remainder of the tumors. Prostate cancer usually starts in the outer portion of the prostate and spreads inwardly and then beyond the gland, with metastases in more advanced stages.

Box 19.3

**RISK FACTORS FOR PROSTATE CANCER**

- Age >50 years
- African American
- Geography (United States and Scandinavian countries)
- Family history; inherited gene mutation
- Environmental exposure to certain chemicals
- Red meat, high-fat diet
- Obesity
- Alcohol consumption
- Microbiome and related inflammation

## Incidence

Other than skin cancer, prostate cancer is the most common cancer in American men and is the second most common cause of male death from cancer. One in six American men will develop prostate cancer. According to statistics from the American Cancer Society (ACS), approximately 174,650 new cases of prostate cancer were diagnosed in 2019 and 31,620 men died from the disease.[142] The number of new cases of prostate cancer has declined more recently due to a reduction in PSA (prostate specific antigen) screening. With PSA testing, more than 90% of prostate cancers are found early when they are highly curable. However, there is significant controversy regarding early detection because most prostate cancers are slow growing and most men will not die from it.[142] Men diagnosed with prostate cancer are typically aged 65 or older. Men less than 50 years of age make up less than 1% of those with prostate cancer. Prostate cancer incidence and mortality vary strikingly among ethnic and national groups, with a particular propensity for African Americans.[142]

In the United States, the incidence of prostate cancer is approximately 60% higher in African American men than in European American men; the mortality rate from the disease is more than twice as high among African Americans.[140] Screening rates for African American men with a positive family history of prostate cancer are significantly lower than in Caucasians, especially in older men ages 60 to 70 years.[140]

## Risk Factors and Etiology

Box 19.3 lists risk factors related to prostate cancer. Prostate cancer is a disease of the aging male, but evidence exists that genetic, environmental, and social factors contribute to observed differences in various populations. Geographically, the highest frequencies of prostate cancer are found in the United States, northwestern Europe, Australia, and the Caribbean islands, whereas the lowest are found in Asia, Central America, and South America. As mentioned, African Americans have twice the risk of non-Hispanic whites, which is attributed to socioeconomic, clinical, and pathologic factors.[140,156]

Familial history of prostate cancer is a strong risk factor.[27,40] A significant increase in risk has been estimated for men who have both a first- and second-degree relative with the disease, with higher risk if more relatives are affected. In addition, this heritable type of cancer is thought to be more aggressive, with a higher risk of mortality. Other factors with weaker associations and less evidence include diets high in fat and low in vegetable consumption, exposure to chemicals, obesity, and inflammation. Emerging evidence indicates that the human microbiome influences cancer susceptibility through the immune system, inflammatory responses, and damage to DNA.[124] Cigarette smoking is associated with higher risk of prostate cancer mortality.[166] Studies have shown a higher risk of aggressive prostate cancer in men with hypogonadism, especially men with type 2 diabetes mellitus.[95]

The precise cause of prostate cancer is unknown. The testicles manufacture most of the body's testosterone and influence the normal growth and development of the prostate. Males castrated before puberty do not develop prostate cancer or BPH. Studies looking at the racial disparity of prostate cancer have linked different levels of serum testosterone among African American and white males. The magnitude of the age-related decline in testosterone rather than levels measured at a single point is suggested to be related to the genesis of prostate cancer, and levels fall more abruptly in African American men as they age.[69]

Exercise is an environmental factor shown to influence cancer risk.[21] Systemic reviews and meta-analysis suggest that total physical activity may decrease the risk of developing prostate cancer.[21]

## Pathogenesis

Most prostatic adenocarcinomas are characterized by small- to moderate-size disorganized glands that infiltrate the stroma of the prostate. The tumors are more likely to develop initially in the periphery of the prostate, unlike BPH, in which the pathologic changes typically originate close to the urethra (see Fig. 19.2). Testosterone is important for normal cell differentiation and function in the prostate, as well as PSA production. The relationship between testosterone/androgens and prostate cancer is complex and not fully understood. In the majority of men with prostate cancer, testosterone replacement therapy (TRT) does not appear to worsen prostate cancer or increase PSA[157] and may result in lower risk of aggressive prostate cancer.[95] However, advanced androgen-responsive prostate cancer is treated with androgen deprivation therapy (ADT) to decrease the testosterone in the body and slow cancer progression.[46] Unfortunately, many of these patients progress to castration resistant prostate cancer, which may be treated with high dose testosterone replacement therapy (TRT).

The cancer invades adjacent local structures, such as the seminal vesicles and urinary bladder, and spreads to the musculoskeletal system, particularly the axial skeleton, and lungs. Lymphatic metastasis may involve the obturator, iliac, and periaortic lymph nodes, extending up through the thoracic duct.

The mechanism underlying the *organ-specific* metastasis of prostate cancer cells to the bone is still poorly understood.[134] The concept that bone provides an attractive environment that allows circulating cancer cells to survive and proliferate in bone is referred to as *seed and soil.* Different theories have been proposed that address the mechanism for metastatic progression and novel therapeutic targets are in development.

### Clinical Manifestations

The clinical presentation of prostate cancer is extremely variable and may be completely asymptomatic until the disease is advanced. In many men, the disease is noted incidentally on digital rectal exam (DRE) or discovered in fragments of prostatic tissue removed through TURP for BPH. Depending on the size and location of the lesion, the initial presenting symptom could be related to urinary obstruction, onset of pain, or constitutional symptoms such as fatigue and weight loss.

The urinary obstruction symptoms associated with cancer are similar to those associated with BPH but typically present in later stages of the disease compared with BPH. Cancer originating in the subcapsular region of the prostate as opposed to the periurethral area would account for this difference. The obstructive symptoms include urinary urgency, frequency, hesitancy, dysuria, hematuria, difficulty initiating or continuing the urine stream, and decreased urine stream. Blood in the ejaculate may also be noted.

Bony metastasis occurs via lymphatics to adjacent structures and pelvic nodes in the majority of people with metastatic disease; the spinal column is the most common site.[134] Metastases to the axial skeleton occur more often than to the appendicular skeleton, especially the ribs, sternum, femur, and pelvis. Prostate cancer is unique in that bone is often the only clinically detectable site of metastasis, and the resulting tumors tend to be osteoblastic (bone forming) rather than being osteolytic (bone lysing). Prostate cancer can also metastasize to the lungs and liver.

Pain complaints associated with prostate cancer can vary tremendously. A dull, vague ache may be noted in the rectal, sacral, or lumbar spine region, and the individual may have difficulty walking. Sacral and lumbar pain is typically associated with bony metastasis. Pain may be noted in the thoracic and shoulder girdle areas secondary to lymphatic spread of the disease or secondary to local bony metastasis. Symptoms such as fatigue, weight loss, anemia, and dyspnea have all been attributed to metastatic spread of the disease.

## MEDICAL MANAGEMENT

**PREVENTION.** Prostate cancer has a long latency period between appearance of premalignant lesions and clinically evident cancer. Prevention strategies should focus on risk reduction.

Prostate cancer growth is known to depend on androgens. Studies of predictive factors and biomarkers for chemoprevention or other agents that can interrupt the development of prostate cancer are under investigation.

A review of the literature suggests a strong link between physical activity and exercise and decreased prostate cancer risk.[21] Exercise may modulate hormone levels and can prevent obesity, while enhancing immune function and reducing oxidative stress as possible mechanisms for risk reduction.[10]

**SCREENING.** The goal of cancer screening is to identify cancer before it is symptomatic, treat it successfully, and prevent morbidity and mortality associated with more advanced cancer. Screening for prostate cancer may involve history taking and physical examination, laboratory tests, imaging, and genetic testing. Differential diagnosis includes benign prostate lesions such as adenosis (BPH), atrophy, or prostatitis.

The physical exam may include a DRE. There is no agreement on whether the DRE should be included as a screening tool for prostate cancer. Traditionally, it is performed yearly after the age of 50. Prostate cancer may be palpated as a hard area or lump on the prostate, but the DRE has been shown to detect only 25% to 50% of tumors.[107]

Laboratory tests include the blood test measuring prostate specific antigen. PSA is secreted exclusively by prostatic epithelial cells and is found in semen and blood. Levels rise slowly as a normal part of aging and are strongly correlated to prostate volume.[82] PSA is affected by age, race, BPH, prostate manipulation (DRE, biopsy), ejaculation, infection (prostatitis), medical procedures, medications, and obesity. Normal levels were established on white males and there is no clear consensus on ranges for racial or ethnic groups. Normal ranges are considered less than 4 nanograms per milliliter (ng/mL). Men with levels above 4 ng/mL may have prostate cancer; levels between 4 and 10 ng/mL poorly discriminate between BPH and cancer.[77] Studies have shown that 23% to 42% of men diagnosed with prostate cancer detected by PSA have tumors that would not result in symptoms during their lifetime.[94] Variations in PSA testing have been developed to improve accuracy in detecting clinically significant prostate cancer and include PSA velocity, percentage of free PSA, PSA density, and prostate cancer antigen 3 (PCA3). Biomarkers are a rapidly developing area of research that may help to select men who are at higher risk for clinically significant prostate cancer.[84]

Because of the significant adverse effects of cancer treatment, there is controversy regarding diagnosis with PSA. Most professional organizations endorse shared decision making between the patient and his medical provider. In 2012, the U.S. Preventive Services Task Force (USPSTF) recommended against routine screening using PSA saying that the potential harms outweighed the benefits. Urologists disagreed and predicted that prostate cancers would be diagnosed at a more advanced stage and morbidity and mortality from prostate cancers would increase. In 2018, the USPSTF reviewed the evidence and updated its recommendations to more align with the American Urological Association (AUA)[166] (Box 19.4).

**DIAGNOSIS.** Transperineal or transrectal ultrasound-guided core biopsy is still the gold standard to confirm prostate cancer in men who have abnormal DRE and PSA.[70] For transrectal ultrasound (TRUS) a small ultrasound probe is inserted into the rectum. The sound waves emitted by the probe produce a video or photographic image of the prostate. These images are used to determine the size and density of the gland and help guide needles through the rectum to the gland for a biopsy and staging. Cells taken at biopsy are given a Gleason Grade based on how they appear under a microscope, where Grade 1 and 2 are cancer cells that look almost normal and Grade 5 cells are considered haphazard and abnormal. The two areas of most abnormality are added to give a Gleason

Box 19.4

**USPSTF 2018 RECOMMENDATIONS FOR PSA SCREENING**

- 55 to 69 years old: Individual decision based on the potential benefits and harms
  - Benefit: Screening offers a small potential benefit of reducing the chance of death from prostate cancer in some men
  - Harms: False-positive results leading to additional testing, expense, and stress. Overdiagnosis and overtreatment can occur. Harms during overtreatment include incontinence and erectile dysfunction
  - Individual decision: Basis of family history, race/ethnicity, comorbid medical conditions. Balancing the benefits and harms, patient values, and other health needs
  - Clinicians should not screen men who do not express a preference for screening (C recommendation—moderate certainty that the net benefit is small)
- 70 years and older: The USPSTF recommends against PSA-based screening for prostate cancer (D recommendation—moderate to high certainty that there is no benefit or harm outweighs the benefit)

Score or Sum (Fig. 19.4) and predict the likelihood of metastases (Box 19.5).

The use of imaging to increase the accuracy of prostate biopsies and improve diagnostic sensitivity and staging is being studied.[70] This includes MRI-guided TRUS biopsy, multiparametric MRI, positron emission tomography (PET), and PET/MRI. MRI allows for evaluation of the prostate gland and regional lymph nodes. Lymph node involvement must typically be advanced (nodes larger than 1 cm) to be demonstrable. Radiographs may detect metastatic lesions, but the radionuclide bone scan, though not diagnostic, is a more sensitive modality for detection of a metabolically active lesion.

**STAGING.** There are several staging systems used at the time of diagnosis and throughout monitoring to inform the course of treatment. More recently, Gleason Groups have been developed[136] as a refinement of the Gleason Score to optimize treatment selection and outcome. The Whitmore-Jewett staging system is another commonly used method of staging for prostate cancer. With this system, the spread of prostate cancer has been divided into four stages, A through D (Fig. 19.5). The American Joint Committee on Cancer uses the TNM system of staging (Box 19.6). The National Comprehensive Cancer Network (NCCN) subdivides newly diagnosed local prostate cancer into six risk groups.[77] Groups range from very low risk (indolent, well-differentiated tumors) to very high risk (aggressive, high grade tumors that can lead to metastasis) based on TNM scores, Gleason scores, and PSA values.

**TREATMENT.** Prostate cancer management has dramatically evolved in the last decade due to advances in knowledge of disease biology and natural progression and development of new screening and treatment modalities. There has been a paradigm shift from treatment of all prostate cancers to selective identification of prostate cancers that may cause harm. The choice of treatment modalities takes into consideration the patient's age, comorbidities, life expectancy, and personal preferences. The National Comprehensive Cancer Network (NCCN) guidelines provided recommended initial therapy for six risk groups.[77] Nomograms have also been developed from studies of large groups of men to predict likelihood of prostate cancer spread and may be used in treatment decisions.[67]

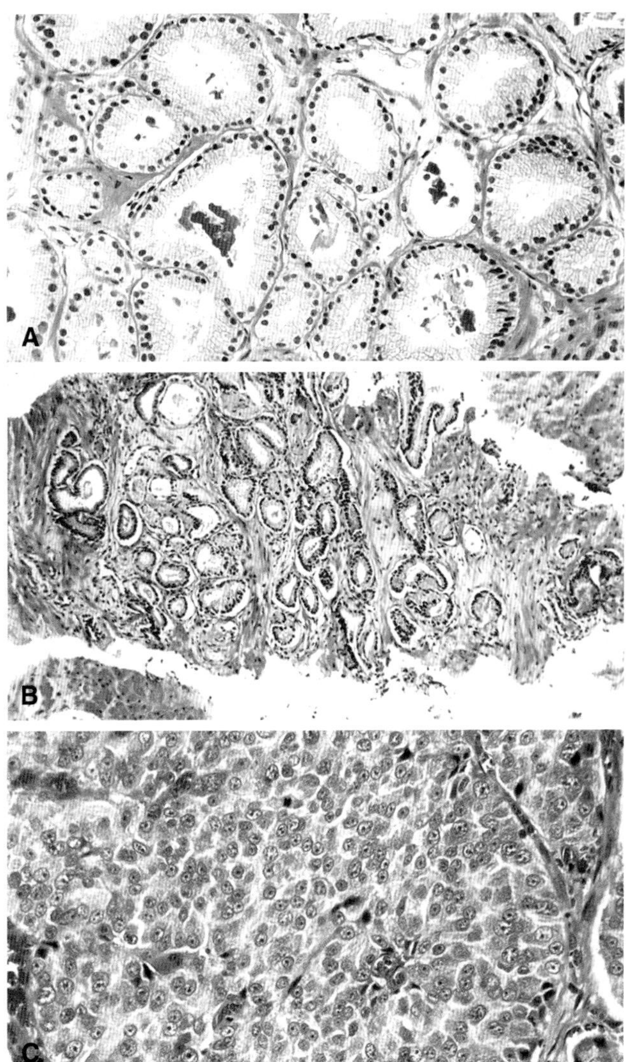


**Figure 19.4**

(A) Low-grade (Gleason score 2) prostate cancer consisting of back-to-back, uniformly sized, well-differentiated (resembling normal cells) malignant glands. (B) Variably sized, more widely dispersed glands of moderately differentiated adenocarcinoma (Gleason score 6). The higher the Gleason score, the more abnormal and poorly differentiated the cells, the more aggressive the tumor is likely to be. (C) Poorly differentiated adenocarcinoma composed of sheets of malignant cells (Gleason score 10). (From Kumar V: *Robbins and Cotran: pathologic basis of disease*, ed 8, Philadelphia, 2010, WB Saunders.)

Men with very low-risk prostate cancer may be monitored (watchful waiting) for symptoms but have minimal intervention.[171] This approach is best for older men who are likely to die from something other than prostate cancer. Repeat screening is not recommended for men who have less than a 10-year life expectancy. Active

Box 19.5

**GLEASON SCORE**

The Gleason scale score, or Gleason grading system, is used to evaluate the prognosis of men with prostate cancer. Scores are assigned based on cytologic examination and range from 2 to 10, based on how the cancerous cells look compared to normal prostate cells. The higher the Gleason score, the more likely the cancer cells will grow and spread rapidly. Pathologists often identify the two most common patterns of cells in the tissue (majority of the tumor and minority of the tumor), assign a Gleason grade from 1 to 5 to each, and add the two grades. The result is a number between 2 and 10. A Gleason score of less than 6 indicates a less aggressive cancer. A grade 7 or higher is considered more aggressive.

| Score | Interpretation |
|---|---|
| 2-4 | Unlikely to spread, good prognosis |
| 5-6 | Mildly aggressive |
| 7 | Moderately aggressive |
| 8-10 | Highly aggressive, poor prognosis |

Data from Gleason DF: The Veteran's Administration Cooperative Urologic Research Group: histologic grading and clinical staging of prostatic carcinoma. In Tannenbaum M, ed: *Urologic pathology: the prostate*, Philadelphia, 1977, Lea and Febiger, pp 171-198.

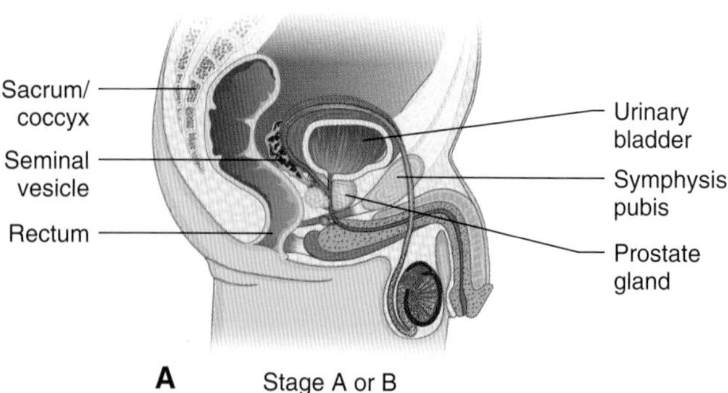


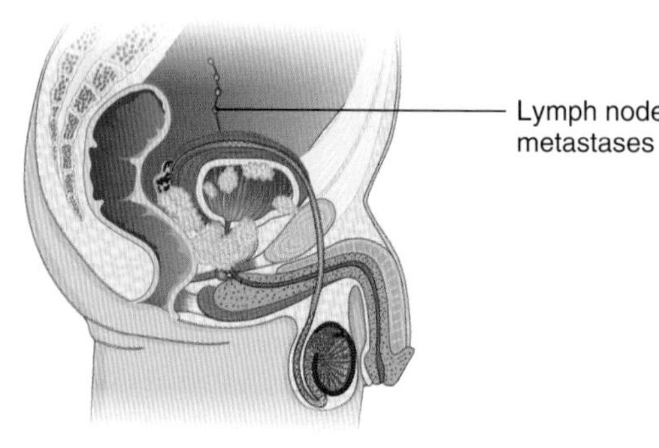


**Figure 19.5**

Prostate cancer: clinical staging using the Whitmore-Jewett staging system. (A) The tumor has not spread beyond the gland's capsule in stages A and B. (B) In stage C the tumor has spread into adjacent tissues; in stage D the disease has spread into the lymphatic system and beyond.

Box 19.6

**AMERICAN JOINT COMMITTEE ON CANCER (AJCC) DEVELOPED STAGING SYSTEM USING T, N, AND M CATEGORIES (TNM SYSTEM)**

***T Categories***

- T1 Unable to palpate or visualize the tumor with imaging such as transrectal ultrasound
  - T1a: Found incidentally during transurethral resection of the prostate (TURP)/cancer in <5% of biopsied tissue
  - T1b: Found incidentally during TURP/cancer in >5% of biopsied tissue
  - T1c: Found by needle biopsy associated with an increased PSA
- T2: Detected with DRE or imaging, confined to prostate
  - T2a: Cancer present in 1/2 or less of only one side (left or right) of the prostate
  - T2b: Cancer present in more than 1/2 of only one side of the prostate
  - T2c: Cancer present in both sides of the prostate
- T3: Cancer has spread beyond prostate
  - T3a: Cancer present beyond the prostate but not to the seminal vesicles
  - T3b: Cancer has spread to the seminal vesicles
- T4: Cancer has spread further than T3, into the urethral sphincter, the bladder/rectum, and/or pelvic wall

***N Categories***

- Presence of cancer in the lymph nodes
  - N0: No lymph node involvement
  - N1: Spread to one or more regional lymph nodes

***M Categories***

- Spread of cancer beyond the regional lymph nodes
  - M0: No spread beyond regional lymph nodes
  - M1: Spread beyond regional lymph nodes
  - M1a: Lymph nodes outside of the pelvis
  - M1b: Metastasized to the bones
  - M1c: Metastasized to other organs

surveillance involves regular DRE, PSA, and biopsy every 1 to 2 years. This approach requires careful selection and patient preference.[171]

***Surgery.*** Surgery is an option for men at any stage of prostate cancer (Fig. 19.6). The primary surgical option is a radical prostatectomy (RP). This surgery can be done as an open procedure, laparoscopically, or robotically. Open procedure can be performed using the retropubic or perineal approach. All RPs will remove the prostate and seminal vesicles, however, pelvic lymph node dissection is not done with the open perineal approach, making the open retropubic approach the gold standard.[160] Although the laparoscopic approach is minimally invasive and reduces blood loss, it only has 2-D visualization. The robotic-assisted laparoscopic radical prostatectomy (RALRP) da Vinci has 3-D visualization, which some researchers report may assist in avoidance of intraoperative injury to the cavernosal nerves and neurovascular bundle and avoidance of injury to the autonomic innervation of the bladder neck and intrapelvic branches of the pudendal nerves that innervate the rhabdosphincter of the urethra. This may lead to improved erectile and lower urinary tract function.[61] Eighty-five percent of all

Before

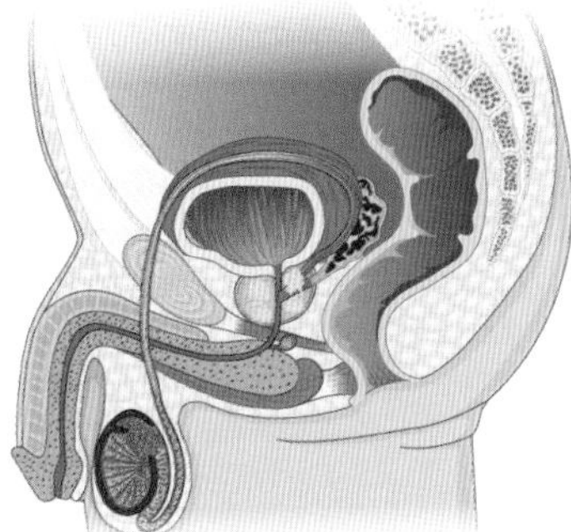

After

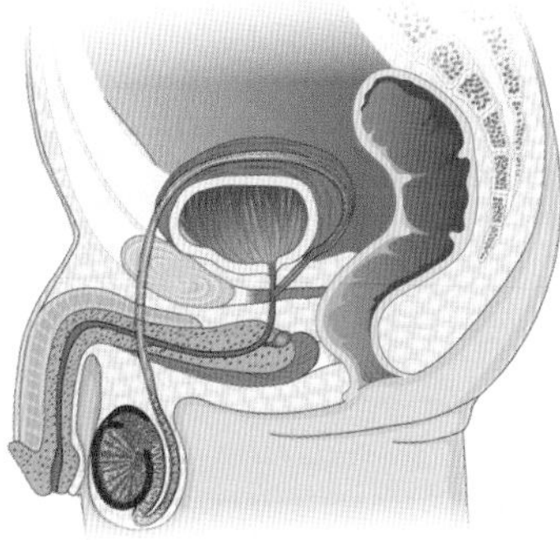

**Figure 19.6**

Before and after prostatectomy: view of male anatomy with removal of the prostate, reattachment of the urethra, and the importance of the external sphincter for continence.

RP in the United States are RALRP. A random controlled study comparing open retropubic to RALRP showed no difference in postoperative UI, ED, or bowel dysfunction.[171] Retrospective studies show that RALRP may reduce operative blood loss and improve UI and ED at 12 months compared with the open approach. There is no significant difference in oncologic outcomes such as cancer-specific mortality.[171]

In addition to surgery to remove the tumor, a pelvic lymph node dissection will be done to see if the cancer cells have left the prostate and possibly traveled elsewhere in the body. The lymph node dissection may result in lower limb lymphedema.

There is experimental and emerging data on gland preserving techniques for low to intermediate risk prostate cancer.[71,173] These focal therapies are designed to minimize treatment-related side effects and include image-guided partial gland ablation, such as partial prostatectomy/prostate gland lumpectomy, focal laser ablation, irreversible electroporation, vascular targeted photodynamic therapy, focal radiofrequency ablation, cryotherapy, and high-intensity focused ultrasound (HIFU). Long-term outcome data on these therapies is lacking.

The postoperative complications with prostatectomy include infection, UI, ED/impotence, excessive bleeding, and rectal injury with fecal incontinence. Potency may return gradually over the course of one to two years; however, after these procedures, as many as one-third of men have incontinence or urinary frequency beyond 1 year and an even greater number continue to experience ED. Collecting and interpreting data on UI and ED after RP is impeded by discrepancies in the definition of incontinence, preoperative symptoms, differences between patient and physicians reporting, and use of various outcome measures.[163] A review of research shows persistent UI occurs in 8% to 25% of men after RP.[163]

In selected individuals with prostate cancer metastases to the spine, surgical fusion, decompression, and vertebroplasty may be performed.[147] Surgical method for spinal metastasis does not appear to significantly affect survival rates but may improve quality of life.

***Radiation.*** Radiation therapy (RT) may be used to treat localized prostatic lesions as an adjunctive treatment after radical prostatectomy or for palliative effects in the presence of widespread disease.[171] Relief of pain and improvement in symptoms associated with urethral obstruction are possible benefits of this treatment modality. Potential side effects of RT include urinary frequency, burning with urination, rectal pain or burning, and diarrhea. Some men never experience these problems, but if they do, they are usually transient and clear up within days to weeks after therapy. Approximately 4.4% of men have UI more than one year after brachytherapy.[89]

Sexual dysfunction (erectile dysfunction or impotence) is a possible long-term complication and occurs in up to 50% of men treated with radiation. Age and comorbidities, such as diabetes or heart disease, can also increase this risk. Pharmacologic treatment for ED in this population is usually successful.

RT can be administered daily by external-beam radiation over a number of weeks. External beam radiation (EBRT) involves careful mapping of the tumor with imaging. Various forms include 3-D conformal RT, which conforms to the shape of the tumor; intensity-modulated RT, which directs thousands of pencil-thin radiation beams of varying intensities at the tumor from many different angles; conformal proton beam RT; and stereotactic body RT. Each type is designed to minimize the risk of postradiation bladder and bowel problems.

Brachytherapy, a specific type of RT, is the delivery of small radioactive pellets by injection directly into the prostate. This treatment provides a highly concentrated yet confined dose of radiation to the tissue in and immediately around the tumor and is used for early stage, slow growing tumors. Brachytherapy is also indicated for men with medical problems that put them at increased risk for any type of surgery or for men who do not feel comfortable with the idea of losing their prostate if there is another option. Pellets may be permanent low dose rate (LDR) administered as an outpatient procedure (the pellets remain in place after they lose their radioactivity), or temporary high dose rate (HDR) requiring a brief hospital stay. The prostate absorbs almost all of the radiation so that nerves and other tissues of the surrounding structures of the rectum, bladder, and urethra are spared, with fewer complications of ED or incontinence.

Palliative radiation therapy may be used for sites of pain secondary to bone lesions from bone metastases in men who have failed hormonal therapy. Metastases to the spine with or without spinal cord compression can be treated with external-beam radiation.

***Hormone Therapy.*** Hormone therapy is not used as a monotherapy and is most often associated with treatment of aggressive cancer phenotypes. The goal of treatment is to decrease testosterone.[171] This is also known as androgen deprivation therapy (ADT). Testosterone stimulates prostate cancer growth, so theoretically, by blocking its production, ADT shrinks or slows the progression of prostate tumors. As mentioned earlier, the relationship of testosterone and prostate cancer is very complex and not linear. Because the testes produce 95% of the circulating testosterone, orchiectomy, the removal of the testicles, is the primary method of manipulating hormone levels. Luteinizing hormone–releasing hormone agonists and antagonists suppress production of testosterone and may shrink the size of the testicles over time. Antiandrogens prevent or inhibit the effects of androgens. Estrogen therapy is used less often because of adverse effects, including gynecomastia (breast development in men), loss of libido and ED/impotence, bloating, and pedal edema. 5α-reductase inhibitors (5-ARIs) that prevent conversion of testosterone into DHT, like finasteride and dutasteride used for BPH, may be used in higher doses for prostate cancer.

The extensive use of androgen-deprivation therapy (ADT) has raised concerns about potential adverse effects such as hot flashes, osteoporosis, sexual dysfunction (e.g., loss of libido or ED/impotence), reduced body mass, insulin resistance, hyperlipidemia, and psychologic effects (e.g., depression, mood swings, or memory loss) (Box 19.7). A generalized reduction in muscle mass is not uncommon with hormone therapy. Loss of muscle mass in the pelvic floor muscle can lead to weakness, which can cause or exacerbate urinary incontinence. ADT is not usually advocated for newly diagnosed, locally contained prostate cancer because of its adverse effects. Additionally, serious cardiovascular disease, including stroke, heart attack, and deep venous thrombosis can be associated with ADT in anyone at high risk.

***Chemotherapy.*** Chemotherapy may be advised for men with advanced, metastatic prostate cancer that have relapsed after initial treatment with other modalities.[171] Chemotherapy may improve survival, delay symptoms, reduce tumor growth, or reduce PSA. Some men are treated indefinitely until unacceptable toxicity or disease progression occurs. Others are treated using an intermittent approach, with chemotherapy interrupted after the initial response. Radiopharmaceuticals are drugs containing radioactive substances that are injected into the body to treat bone metastasis and pain.

***Immunotherapy.***80. The increased availability of genomic testing has made "precision medicine" more common in the treatment of prostate and many other cancers. Many options are being investigated and many are currently available. The cancer vaccine Sipuleucel-T is an immunotherapy that is approved to treat men with advanced prostate cancer that does not respond to ADT. The National Comprehensive Cancer Network (NCCN) guidelines provide recommendations for immunotherapy.[77]

***Cryotherapy.*** Cryotherapy (CRYO) involves the insertion of needles through the perineum that can produce freezing temperatures causing tissue necrosis and destruction of the cancer cells. With this type of focal treatment, the goal is to destroy the cancer cells, with less impact on the urinary function and sexual potency of the individual. Cryotherapy typically is considered a treatment option for local recurrent prostate cancer after RT.[6] Studies have shown 75% recurrence-free survival rate 2 years after cryotherapy[172] and 57.9% after 5 years.[51] A comparative study reports brachytherapy more successful than cryotherapy.[51]

**PROGNOSIS.** Multiple sources of data show that prostate cancer incidence rates rose after the introduction of PSA testing. Unfortunately, this brought on the controversy regarding overdiagnosis and overtreatment, causing many men who might have had indolent tumors to needlessly suffer from treatment-related comorbidities such as UI and ED. When the USPSTF recommended against PSA screening, urologists lobbied that men might be diagnosed at more advanced stages of prostate cancer with increased mortality. Cancer detected earlier has a better chance of successful treatment. A comprehensive analysis of cancer found an increase of 26% in years of life lost from 2005 to 2015.[54] We are still finding a balance, but according to the American Cancer Society, relative survival rates (RSR) including all stages of prostate cancer are as follows: 5-year RSR is 99%, 10-year RSR is 98%, 15-year RSR is 96%.[3] A patient's age, overall health, comorbid conditions such as diabetes or heart disease, and stage of cancer influence survival statistics.

Currently, the rate of lymph node involvement in newly diagnosed prostate cancer is approximately 12%, but this rate is likely to increase with greater utilization of new preoperative imaging capabilities.[8] Lymph node involvement typically leads to a less favorable prognosis and these patients are considered to have stage IV disease using the National Comprehensive Cancer Network (NCCN) guidelines.[39] However, node-positive disease is different from distant metastatic prostate cancer in that some of these patients will receive aggressive treatment with improved survival.

Men who have failed ADT progress to metastatic castration-resistant prostate cancer (mCRPC) within two to three years.[159] There are many underlying mechanisms that characterize mCRPC, and new therapeutic agents are under investigation that promise to improve the prognosis. These men often have disease extending to the skeleton, which is associated with severe pain and disability, and treatment is often aimed at palliative measures.

The two major adverse effects of RP are UI and ED.[171] Predictors of recovery from these effects are younger age, normal BMI, and preoperative urinary continence.[163] Nerve sparing procedures may also improve continence and have a large role in preserving sexual function, but outcomes vary greatly.[65,83]

SPECIAL IMPLICATIONS FOR THE THERAPIST 19.3

## *Prostate Cancer*

### Screening for Referral

Considering the number of aging adult men seen in a rehabilitative setting and the incidence of prostate disease, therapists are seeing a number of clients at risk for prostate conditions. Localized prostate cancer is usually not painful and primary screening will be done by the physician using PSA and DRE. Therapists should be watchful for symptoms of metastatic disease in the axial skeleton or the periaortic lymph nodes. Nonmechanical pain in the thoracic, lumbar, or sacral area in a man over 50 years old with unknown cause of pain and with previous prostate cancer is a red flag for further medical investigation.

### Prehabilitation

An emerging field of research describes the role of preoperative PT strategies to improve treatment tolerance and overall physical and psychological recovery in men undergoing prostate surgery.[121] A Cochrane review reports moderate evidence of an overall benefit from PFMT versus control management in terms of reduction of UI in both pre- and postoperative studies, but evidence is conflicting and methodological limitations exist.[4]

It has been recommended that pelvic floor muscle training (PFMT) be considered a key element in the care pathway for patients diagnosed with prostate cancer before and after surgery.[168] A meta-analyses found that PFMT significantly increased odds of continence at 3 months, but did not significantly reduce daily pad use at 6 months post RP.[161] An RCT demonstrated that prehabilitation for men undergoing RP is feasible, safe, and has promising benefits to physical and psychological well-being with a quicker return to continence.[133] A systematic review demonstrated that PFMT significantly improved post-RP urinary continence, postmicturition dribble, and erectile function.[55] Providing interventions earlier in the care pathway may lead to better quality of life outcomes for patients during survivorship.[161]

### Physical Therapy Examination and Evaluation

All physical therapists should inquire about continence status and other urinary dysfunctions in every male patient. Patient reported outcome (PRO) measures are available for both UI and ED. Preexisting UI and ED affect prognosis. Systems review should pay specific attention to comorbid conditions, such as CVD, DM, osteoporosis, lymphedema, and general deconditioning. Performance of selected tests to identify movement disorders of the trunk and pelvic girdle that may impact coordinated and synergistic activity with the PFM should also be performed. Physical therapists with specialized training will also examine the function of the PFM externally, internally per rectum using palpation, or with imaging ultrasound and/or EMG.

### Pelvic Floor Muscle Training

Pelvic floor muscle training (PFMT) and lifestyle changes are first-line treatments for UI associated with prostate cancer treatment.[63,85,145] A 2015 Cochrane analysis evaluating conservative management of post-prostatectomy UI reports moderate evidence of overall benefit of PMFT but was unable to show which treatment (or combinations of treatment) would be most effective for this problem. Most trials were not high quality and some approaches (e.g., lifestyle changes) were not included.[4] There is substantial heterogeneity in content of exercise regimes and how they are reported.[63] This variation in content of a PFMT program likely contributes to differences in reported efficacy of PFMT post RP in men.

Beginning exercises immediately after catheter removal seems to be more effective than waiting 6 to 8 weeks after surgery. Current literature suggests that the time period toward continence after radical prostatectomy can be shortened if PFMT is initiated directly after catheter removal. More studies are needed to confirm these results. Although pelvic floor exercises help men regain continence faster, the rates of continence at the end of 1 year have been reported to be equal between the exercise groups and control groups. There is still a potential cost savings and improved quality of life with earlier return to continence.

A more recent meta-analysis[175] included more current RCTs and had several conclusions: (1) PFMT is considered economical and safe; (2) compliance and adherence is crucial for efficacy of PFMT; (3) PFMT should be under the guidance and supervision of a trained physical therapist; (4) verification of PFM performance with palpation, biofeedback, or imaging is necessary for correct and effective PFM contraction; and 5) guided PFMT could hasten the early and long-term recovery of continence post RP.[175]

Pelvic floor rehabilitation is aimed at both the striated urethral sphincter that maintains urethral resistance by drawing the urethra dorsally and the puborectalis muscles that draws the urethra ventral and elevates the bladder to prevent leakage during increased intraabdominal pressure (e.g., laughing, coughing, and lifting). According to one study, the best verbal instruction for correct PFM contraction in the male is "shorten the penis" and "hold back gas."[151] Verbal instruction of PFM contraction is not always enough[135] and many patients require imaging ultrasound to understand the proper contraction of the urethral sphincter.[178] Surface EMG can also increase awareness of PFM contraction but is not able to differentiate between the different PFM.

Continence relies on the complex coordination of both smooth and striated muscles (active component) and the integrity of fibroelastic tissue (passive component) at the bladder neck.[151] Disruption of any of these mechanisms may affect continence status. Pelvic physical therapy after prostate surgery should emphasize assessment for correct activation of PFM, precise training instructions, incorporation of patient education, and progression to functional exercise. PFMT involves repetitive contraction and relaxation of the PFM to enhance urethral closure pressure by increased muscle mass and/or improved activation amplitude and timing. PFMT may be combined with electrical stimulation and/or biofeedback, although evidence for the addition of these modalities to PFMT is lacking.[4] Promoting PFM contraction before events that cause UI may be useful, but these events vary between patients and almost 30% of men report UI for no obvious reason, even when sedentary.[105] Men often report that UI is more prominent later in the day, possibly due to decreased endurance of the PFM.

### Complications of Medical Treatment

Although reduced in recent years, delayed complications of radiation therapy can occur with increasing problems from 6 to 24 months postradiation.[37] Diarrhea, gastrointestinal or urinary bleeding, irritative voiding symptoms, ED, and tenesmus (painful spasm of the anal sphincter with straining) are all possible complications. A recent onset or worsening of any of these complications should be brought to the physician's attention.

Metastases to the pelvic lymph nodes can cause lumbar plexopathy and swelling caused by compression of veins and/or lymphatics. The development of lymphedema may be related to smoking, stage of cancer, and radiation therapy. The therapist has an important role in screening men for risk of lymphedema and early recognition/intervention for this condition.

Multiple potential side effects are associated with endocrine or hormonal manipulation (see Box 19.7). Decrease in bone mass and increase in bone turnover with a concomitant increased risk of fracture has been documented in men receiving ADT (antiandrogen deprivation therapy). Significant loss of bone mineral density occurs within 12 months of starting therapy and continues indefinitely while treatment continues; there is no recovery after treatment is stopped.

Exercise and fracture prevention are important features of treatment for anyone on androgen deprivation therapy. Up to 20% of men surviving at least 5 years after diagnosis of prostate cancer have a fracture if treated with ADT, compared with 12.6% of men not receiving ADT. Vitamin D deficiency exacerbates the development of osteoporosis. Treatment with bisphosphonates in men on ADT has been shown to prevent bone loss and increase bone mineral density, but it does not prevent fractures in this population group.

Many men on ADT for prostate cancer are not being screened or treated for osteoporosis. The therapist can assess for additional risk factors and institute an osteoporosis education and prevention plan for anyone receiving this treatment.

### Exercise and Prostate Cancer

The role of physical activity and exercise in reducing the risk of prostate cancer were discussed earlier in this chapter (see "Risk Factors" under "Prostate Cancer" above). Exercise and physical activity may be able to counter some of these side effects of ADT (e.g., fatigue, functional decline, increased body fat, loss of lean body tissue, insulin resistance, and decreased quality of life associated with these physical changes) by reducing fatigue, elevating mood, building muscle mass, and reducing body fat. Exercise may be an important component of supportive care for these men.[21,120]

The question of whether it is more efficacious to commence exercise therapy at the same time as initiating androgen deprivation is being studied. The intent is to immediately attenuate or perhaps even prevent treatment-induced adverse effects. This is in contrast to the implementation of a rehabilitative exercise program 90 days or more after the start of ADT, by which time many of the physical and psychologic problems have developed.

Moderate intensity exercise has also proven effective in reducing radiation-induced fatigue and other treatment-induced complications in men with prostate cancer. Both resistance and aerobic exercise have been shown to mitigate fatigue, increase strength, and improve quality of life in men with prostate cancer receiving radiotherapy in the short term (6 months).

Even more important is the role of exercise in decreasing cancer risk.[21] A population-based, prospective, 26-year study of approximately 50,000 men aged 40 to 75 years old found a 30% lower risk of developing advanced prostate cancer and a 25% lower risk of developing lethal prostate cancer among men in the vigorous exercise category (more than 6 MET value: jogging, running, lap swimming, squash/racquet ball, calisthenics, rowing, stair climbing).[122]

# DISORDERS OF THE TESTES

## Orchitis and Epididymitis

### Overview and Incidence

Epididymitis is an inflammation of the epididymis (Fig. 19.7A) and is more common than orchitis (inflammation of the testis). Epididymo-orchitis is the occurrence of both and accounts for about 50% of cases.[164] These infections can be acute or chronic, sexually transmitted or nonsexually transmitted. European guidelines for the management of epididymo-orchitis report an incidence of 2.45 per 1000 men in the UK.[153] Boys and men of all

**Box 19.7**

**SIDE EFFECTS OF HORMONAL MANIPULATION**

- Muscle atrophy
- Decreased bone density, osteoporosis
- Loss of libido
- Erectile dysfunction/impotence
- Hot flashes
- Gynecomastia
- Bloating and pedal edema
- Nausea and vomiting
- Diarrhea
- Weight gain/redistribution
- Myocardial infarction, cerebrovascular accident, deep venous thrombosis

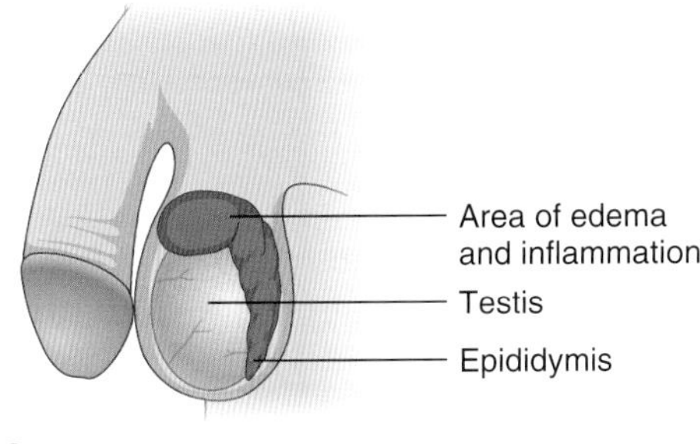


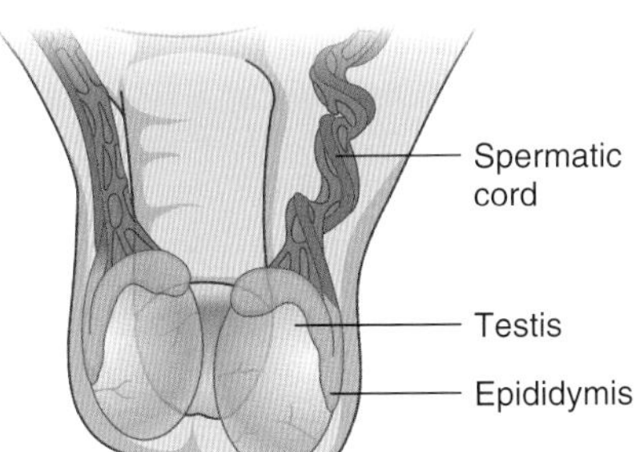


**Figure 19.7**

(A) Epididymitis: Inflammation or infection of the epididymis, the tube that holds the testicle in place. The epididymis is found along the posterolateral aspect of each testis. The tail of the epididymis becomes the vas deferens as it ascends superiorly out of the scrotum. The spermatic cord suspends the testis in the scrotum and consists of arteries, veins, nerves, lymphatics, and the vas deferens. Sperm made in the testis is stored in the epididymis, then transferred to the seminal vesicle through the vas deferens for ejaculation. (B) Testicular torsion: Testis twists on its spermatic cord, cutting off blood supply to the testis. The spermatic cord suspends the testis in the scrotum and consists of arteries, veins, nerves, lymphatics, and the vas deferens.

ages can be affected. Incidence peaks between 15 and 35 years old for sexually transmitted epididymitis and between 50 and 70 for bacterial epididymitis.[101]

### Risk Factors and Pathogenesis

The most common infectious agents are sexually transmitted infections (STI) chlamydia and gonorrhea, gram-negative bacteria (from the bladder or bowel), or viral infections (mumps). Autoimmune orchitis can occur in patients with systemic lupus.[144] The bloodstream and lymphatics can be the route of spread of infections from other body areas to the testes.[132] Reflux of infected urine into the ejaculatory ducts is most common in boys under 15 (congenital anomalies) and men over 35 (BPH, trauma).[101,132,177] Although epididymitis is relatively easy to diagnose, the route of infection is often unclear. [177]

Risk factors include primary infections of the genitourinary tract; sexually active males with multiple partners; males with indwelling catheters, and after transurethral procedures, BPH, and other causes of urethral stenosis; prolonged sitting, motorcycle or bicycle riding; trauma; mumps, or systemic lupus.[164]

### Clinical Manifestations

Epididymitis and orchitis are marked by gradual onset testicular pain and swelling. Pain usually presents as unilateral scrotal pain that may radiate to the groin or back. Fever, chills, and malaise can be present. Patient with orchitis rarely have voiding dysfunction; however, patients with epididymitis may have urethral discharge, hematuria, dysuria, and urinary frequency. Inquiry about recent change in sexual partners or urethral discharge can further clarify this diagnosis. Elevating the scrotum usually relieves the pain in patients with epididymitis (Prehn sign).[101] Patients are often uncomfortable while seated, especially on bike seats or hard surfaces.

### MEDICAL MANAGEMENT

**DIAGNOSIS.** Physical examination reveals a tender and swollen testicle and an enlarged or erythematous scrotum. Laboratory tests revealing an elevated white blood cell (WBC) count and urinalysis, urethral smear, and urine culture to determine the pathogen are an important component of the diagnostic process. Differential diagnosis would include testicular torsion and prostatitis.

**TREATMENT.** Treatment with medication is directed at the specific infection.[153] Antibiotic-resistant strains have made treatment more difficult.[132] During the acute phase, treatment includes bed rest, limiting physical activities and strain (including sexual intercourse), scrotal elevation and support, ice packs or heat packs to the affected area, sitz baths, or nonsteroidal antiinflammatory drugs (NSAIDs).[101,164] Hospitalization may be necessary if signs of sepsis or abscess formation are present or if the pain is severe. Spermatic cord block may be used to help relieve pain in severe cases. Prompt treatment is required to avoid serious complications, including abscess formation, testicular infarction, and infertility. Once treatment has been initiated, a significant decrease in pain should be noted within a week, but the scrotal edema may be present for 2 to 3 months.

## Testicular Torsion

### Overview and Incidence

Testicular torsion is an abnormal twisting of the spermatic cord as the testis rotates within the tunica vaginalis (see Fig. 19.7B). The torsion can occur intravaginally or extravaginally, but intravaginal torsion is the more common. Intravaginal torsion occurs in males 8 to 18 years of age. The condition is rarely seen after age 30 years. The extravaginal torsions occur primarily in neonates. This condition is a surgical emergency affecting 3.8 per 100,000 males younger than 18 years annually.[66,138] Incidence spikes in the neonatal period and between 12 and 18 years old. Early diagnosis and treatment (within 4 to 8 hours) is imperative to save the testis.

### Risk Factors and Pathogenesis

Risk factors include age and previous and family history of testicular torsion. Torsion of the spermatic cord is often associated with congenital abnormalities resulting in the ability of the testicle to rotate freely within the scrotum. These abnormalities include absence of the scrotal ligaments, incomplete descent of the testis, and a high attachment of the tunica vaginalis and can result in horizontal lie of the testis or bell clapper deformity. The former is more commonly associated with testicular torsion.[117] Testicular torsion can also occur after heavy physical activity, a minor injury to the testis, or while sleeping. It is more common on the left side and is most often unilateral.[117]

Normally the testes are held in a fixed position in the scrotum by the tunica vaginalis, a serous membrane that partially surrounds the testes and prevents the spermatic cord from twisting. The spermatic cord contains the vas deferens and the nerve and blood supply for the scrotal contents. Abnormal twisting of the spermatic cord during testicular torsion can result in increased venous congestion and decreased arterial blood flow, with subsequent ischemic damage.[138] Extravaginal torsion occurs most often during the fetal descent of the testes, before the tunica adheres to the scrotal wall. This allows the testis and fascial tunica to rotate around the spermatic cord above the level of the tunica vaginalis.

### Clinical Manifestations

An abrupt onset of severe unilateral testicular and scrotal pain followed by swelling suggests testicular torsion.[138] In most cases, only one testis is affected; bilateral torsion is possible but rare. The pain may extend up into the inguinal area. Cremasteric reflex (retraction of the scrotum and testicle as the skin on the same side of the inner thigh is lightly stroked) is almost always absent because nerve compression occurs when the testicle twists on its spermatic cord.[101] Urinary symptoms and fever are rare. Nausea, vomiting, tachycardia, and lightheadedness may be present, possibly because of the severity of the pain. With prolonged or complete loss of blood supply, tissue ischemia and necrosis can develop, making this condition a medical emergency. Intermittent torsion may occur, resulting in short-duration acute pain, with time between episodes varying from several hours to several months.[117]

### MEDICAL MANAGEMENT

**DIAGNOSIS.** Testicular torsion should be considered in the presence of acute testicular pain and swelling. Unfortunately the condition can be misdiagnosis as epididymitis and cause delay in treatment, resulting in testicular loss. Urgent referral to a urologist is necessary to save the testicle. Physical examination reveals a firm, tender testicle that is often positioned high and transverse in the scrotum.[101] Erythema and scrotal edema may be present. The absence of the cremasteric reflex is diagnostic. Manual elevation of the testicle usually increases pain in the presence of testicular torsion.[164] Color and power Doppler sonography make it possible to identify the absence or decrease of perfusion in the affected testis. In children, color Doppler ultrasonography has 82% specificity and 100% sensitivity for testicular torsion.[164] However, imaging should not delay emergency surgery if other diagnostic factors are present. Negative exploratory surgery is preferred to loss of the testicle due to delayed imaging. A urinalysis is performed to help rule out infection.

**TREATMENT.** Testicular torsion is considered a urologic emergency. Once the diagnosis of testicular torsion is made, emergency surgery is performed. The procedure includes detorsion and fixation of the testicle to prevent future torsion. Often both sides will undergo fixation for long-term success. An orchiectomy will be necessary if the testis is deemed nonviable. The duration of the torsion is critical regarding salvage of the testis. If the surgery is performed within 6 hours of onset, a greater than 90% salvage rate occurs. The salvage rate drops to 50% if more than 12 hours pass before the surgery.[138] Manual detorsion can be useful in the short term while arrangements are being made for surgery.

**SPECIAL IMPLICATIONS FOR THE THERAPIST 19.4**

*Testicular Torsion*

Pain extending into the groin and scrotum can occasionally be referred from muscle or joint structures, but if a client notes acute onset of scrotal pain, immediate communication with a physician is warranted. Ask the client if he has noted scrotal swelling or tenderness; feels feverish or nauseated; has any difficulties with urination, including urgency, frequency, or dysuria; or has noted any urethral discharge (indicating possible infection as opposed to torsion). If the scrotal or groin pain is associated with musculoskeletal dysfunction, it can be expected that the therapist could alter the symptoms by mechanically stressing the involved component of the musculoskeletal system. Structures to test include the genitofemoral nerve as it courses through the abdominal wall, pudendal nerve in its relationship to the obturator internus and Alcock's canal, pelvic floor muscles, adductor, and iliopsoas muscles, pubic symphysis, and the connective tissue of the scrotum and perineum in relation to scaring and adhesions.

## Testicular Cancer

### Overview

Testicular cancer occurs when cells in one or both testicles become malignant. The testicles are made up of various types of cells. The cells that make sperm are known as primordial germ cells, and more than 95% of testicular cancers start in these cells. Germ cell tumors are further divided into two histogenetic categories: seminomas and nonseminomas. The remaining neoplasms are mostly tumors of stromal or sex cord origin (sex cords develop from the gonadal ridge in embryology and later become the testis cords in males). Metastatic tumors to the testis from primary neoplasm elsewhere in the body are uncommon. Lymphoma is a common secondary testicular cancer and presents more in men over the age of 50 than primary testicular cancer.

### Incidence

Testicular cancer incidence is strongly related to age, rising steeply from around 15 to 19 years of age, peaking at about 30 to 35 years of age, and then rapidly declining. There are considerable geographic and ethnic variations in the incidence of testicular cancer. Incidence has risen in the United States and Europe in the last few decades.[115] Testicular cancer is more common among whites, Hispanics, and Native Americans, and less common among African Americans.[7] Both genetic and environmental factors in developed countries have been implicated in the increased incidence. According to statistics for 2019 from the American Cancer Society, there were 9560 new cases and 410 deaths from testicular cancer.[142]

### Risk Factors and Etiology

Personal or family history of testicular cancer significantly increases the risk for testicular cancer.[2] The most significant factor in testicular cancer is the association of cryptorchidism (undescended testes).[91] About 5% of boys born at term have an undescended testicle, but the timing of orchiopexy (surgical movement and fixation of the testicle into the scrotum) influences the risk for testicular cancer.[2] Those who undergo surgery before the age of 13 have a significantly reduced risk, suggesting a hormonal influence in the development of testicular cancer.

Prenatal or postnatal environmental estrogen exposures (e.g., endocrine-mimicking environmental pollutants, pesticides, industrial chemicals, or chemical contaminants in drinking water) may contribute to testicular cancer, but evidence is limited.[16] While some studies do not show any clear association between adulthood occupational or environmental exposure and testicular cancer[13] there is growing evidence for the "genvironmental" model that highlights the interplay between environmental and genetic factors.[93]

A history of infertility and poor semen quality have been associated with an increased risk of developing testicular cancer. Men with Klinefelter syndrome (a sex chromosome disorder characterized by low levels of male hormones, sterility, breast enlargement, and small testes) have previously been thought to be at greater risk of developing testicular cancer.[1] These men have a higher incidence of cryptorchidism and gonadal congenital alterations, but the evidence linking this condition with a higher risk of testicular cancer is controversial.

There is some association with testicular cancer and a history of infections and inflammation, such as orchitis or epididymitis.[79] There is emerging evidence of the influence of the genitourinary microbiome in the development of genitourinary malignancies.[99]

The etiology of testicular cancer is not well understood. As mentioned, there appears to be a hormonal influence. Testicular germ cell tumors (TGCTs) are considered highly heritable and multiple gene variants have been identified that strongly contribute to genetic susceptibility and predisposition.[125]

### Pathogenesis

TGCTs make up the majority of testicular cancers and the following discussion focuses solely on these tumors. It is thought that TGCTs develop from failure of the gonocytes (the earliest undifferentiated sex cell) to mature and differentiate in utero and postnatally.[12,125] These arrested gonocytes undergo oncogenic genetic adaptations that accumulate through childhood and puberty and confer susceptibility to TGCTs. A precursor lesion, termed intratubular germ cell neoplasia, develops in utero and precedes neoplastic transformation into either a seminoma or a nonseminoma. These tumor groups have a different pathogenesis, histology, clinical course, and response to treatment.[2] Seminomas grow and spread more slowly than nonseminomas and usually occur between the ages of 25 and 45. Nonseminomas usually occur earlier, between the late teens and early 30s, and have four main types: embryonal carcinoma, choriocarcinoma, yolk-sac carcinoma, and teratoma. Many nonseminomas are a mixture of these types.

### Clinical Manifestations

The most common presentation of testicular cancer is a painless nodule or swelling of the testis.[2] The condition may go undetected if no pain is experienced and the male is not periodically performing testicular self-examination. The enlargement of the testis may be accompanied by an ache in the abdomen or scrotum or a sensation of heaviness in the scrotum. A minority of patients present with back or groin pain related to metastatic disease in the retroperitoneum, or with symptoms such as a cough, chest pain, headache, or supraclavicular lymph nodes indicative of distant metastasis. Bone metastasis is a late event, often combined with metastasis to the retroperitoneal lymph nodes, lung, and liver.

Occurring during the prime of life for most men and potentially affecting sexual and reproductive capabilities, testicular cancer has a major emotional impact and can affect overall quality of life.

## MEDICAL MANAGEMENT

**SCREENING AND PREVENTION.** The U.S. Preventative Services Task Force recommends against routine screening for testicular cancer in asymptomatic men.[7] There are no known preventive strategies, but teaching and promoting testicular self-examination as a technique for early detection of this disease is recommended.[59,158] Because survival is dependent on early detection, men should be encouraged to practice testicular self-examination at least every 6 months. For optimal effect, health education programs need to take into account complexities such as cultural diversity if men are to heed vital and, in some cases, life-sustaining advice.

**DIAGNOSIS.** A thorough urologic history and physical examination are the basis for making a diagnosis of testicular cancer. A painless testicular mass is highly suggestive of testicular cancer. Blood work includes levels of creatinine, electrolytes, and liver enzymes. Serum tumor markers, including LDH (lactate dehydrogenase), AFP (alpha-fetoprotein), and beta-hCG (human chorionic gonadotropin) are assessed and used for diagnosis, staging, and prognosis.[109] These markers are elevated in a majority of cases.[100]

Diagnostic US confirms the presence of a testicular mass, and its sensitivity in detecting a testicular tumor is close to 100%.[1] US can distinguish intratesticular from extratesticular lesions and is used to explore the contralateral testis.[109] The modalities used to assess metastasis include CT scans of the abdomen and pelvis, CT scan or x-ray of the chest, MRI in select patients, and MR lymphography (used to noninvasively stage retroperitoneal lymph nodes).

**STAGING.** The NCCN guideline recommends the American Joint Committee on Cancer (AJCC) TMN staging system for testicular cancer. This uses postorchiectomy serum levels of b-hCG, LDH, and AFP and imaging studies. Various subclassifications are used to assist in clinical decision making and prognosis.

**TREATMENT.** Significant advances have been made in the treatment of local and metastatic testicular cancer.[2] A cure is achievable in 95% of patients (80% in those with metastatic disease). Radical orchiectomy is considered the primary treatment for most patients with testicular cancer. Organ sparing is done with caution and is based on tumor size.[81] If US is ambiguous, a biopsy may be performed, but that is rare.[108] Pathologic staging is performed after orchiectomy and management is based on histology, whether the tumor is a seminoma or nonseminoma, serum tumor markers (assessed before and after orchiectomy), and the presence of metastasis. Men are offered the option of sperm banking before undergoing treatment that may compromise fertility. A testicular prosthesis may be implanted at the time of orchiectomy if desired by the patient. Most men with lower stages of cancer will elect active surveillance instead of adjuvant treatment after orchiectomy.[2]

Nerve-sparing retroperitoneal lymph node dissection is an integral part of management strategies for both early and advanced-stage disease. Nerve-sparing techniques may help preserve sexual function.

Chemotherapeutic agents are used in varying combinations and dosing according to tumor type and risk stratification. Since the introduction of effective chemotherapy, radiation therapy is used less frequently, if at all.[2] Symptomatic, solitary bone lesions are responsive to chemotherapy and local radiation therapy.

**PROGNOSIS.** With early detection and appropriate intervention, more than 95% of men with newly diagnosed germ cell tumors are cured. Delay in diagnosis correlates with a higher stage at presentation for treatment.

Long-term sequelae of certain chemotherapeutic agents may include infertility, leukemia, and cardiovascular events. Chemotherapy-related cardiovascular toxicity may be the result of both direct endothelial damage and indirect hormonal and metabolic changes. There is an increased incidence of metabolic syndrome in long-term survivors that is most likely caused by the lower testosterone levels. Other chemotherapy-induced complications include chronic neurotoxicity, permanent ototoxicity (damage to the inner ear resulting in impairment of hearing and balance), renal function impairment, pulmonary fibrosis, and late relapse. There is cumulative chemotoxicity with each additional cycle of chemotherapy, and dosing is designed to achieve maximum benefit with the least toxicity.[2,108]

Most cases of metastatic TGCTs will be cured, however about 10% of patients will have refractory disease.[2] There are several options for palliative chemotherapy that might increase long-term survival.[108] Studies of molecular targeted therapies have not yet yielded positive results in testicular cancer treatment. There are ongoing investigations into immunotherapies.

SPECIAL IMPLICATIONS FOR THE THERAPIST 19.5

### *Testicular Cancer*

Therapists should be aware of the symptoms of metastatic disease in the retroperitoneum, including thoracic/lumbar pain or groin pain and symptoms such as a cough, chest pain, headache, or enlarged supraclavicular lymph nodes indicative of distant metastasis. Correlation of findings from the history and physical examination and the client's response to treatment may raise suspicion, warranting communication with a physician.

An awareness of the location of superficial lymph nodes is also important for the therapist. Observation of a mass or even a filling-in of the concavity normally found in the left supraclavicular region should alert the therapist to palpate this area. Palpation of a nodule or a positive iliopsoas sign requires medical referral.

Surgical treatment of testicular cancer also holds implications for the therapist. Postoperatively, lymph node dissection can result in compromised lymphatic flow and resultant lymphedema. The surgical scars related to orchiectomy and retroperitoneal lymph node dissection may affect the person's posture or movement mechanics of the trunk, pelvis, and hip regions. Serious adverse effects of combination chemotherapy include neuromuscular toxic effects, death from myelosuppression, pulmonary fibrosis, and Raynaud syndrome.

Damage of gonadal function and subnormal levels of testosterone are common after testicular cancer interventions and may lead to osteopenia/osteoporosis.[118] The therapist may need to include general strengthening and fall risk reduction strategies when treating testicular cancer survivors.

## DISORDERS OF THE PENIS

### Peyronie Disease

Peyronie disease is a condition of penile curvature during erection which can result in sexual dysfunction. In the acute inflammatory phase abnormal healing results in fibrotic scar tissue or plaque and a palpable hardness. This restricted tissue does not allow expansion during erection and a curvature will result. Very small and gradual curving of the penis may be a normal variant of penile shape, however, Peyronie disease results in a sharp curve often affecting function. This condition affects approximately 9% of men, most often between the ages of 55 and 60 years old and can be hereditary. It is associated with obesity, hypertension, diabetes, hyperlipidemia, smoking, Dupuytren disease, and pelvic surgery including radical prostatectomy.[96,170] Approximately 10% of men (often younger men) can recall penile injury during sexual or physical activity preceding the onset of scar tissue. About 50% of men report painful erections and many have difficulty achieving full penetrations because of the abnormal shape of the penis. In two-thirds of cases the scar tissue is located on the dorsal side of the penis resulting in an upward curve. Scar tissue on the lateral and ventral sides is more likely to affect penetration.[96] Usually within 12 months the curve stabilizes and the pain decreases as the patient enters the chronic phase. Diagnosis is largely based on physical examination of the erect penis. Doppler ultrasound is used in some cases to more fully document the condition.

The Fourth International Consultation on Sexual Medicine guidelines on Peyronie disease treatment[170] and several review articles[17,30,165] have found that conservative treatments such as penile vacuum pump, manual stretching, and scar tissue injection appear to have some effect although some studies report limited success (25% to 37% improvement in curve).[96] Surgery to decrease the curvature is the gold standard for those requesting treatment however return to previous penile length is not possible in all cases.[48,170]

## Penile Cancer

### Overview and Incidence

Penile cancer is a relatively rare malignancy, with approximately 2080 new cases and 410 deaths each year in the United States.[142] It is more common in Asia, Africa, and South America than in the United States.

### Risk Factors and Etiology

Some forms of human papillomavirus (HPV) are highly associated with risk for penile cancer.[19,152] Other risk factors include age older than 60 years (average age of diagnosis is about 68), being uncircumcised, phimosis (a congenital narrowing of the opening of the foreskin so that it cannot be retracted), poor personal hygiene, multiple sex partners, HIV, and use of tobacco products. Additionally, heavy alcohol use, lichen sclerosis, and phototherapy for psoriasis may increase the risk.

### Pathogenesis

Research has shown that two proteins made by high-risk types of HPV (E6 and E7) may block tumor suppressor gene products, allowing cells to proliferate and become cancer. Nicotine has been shown to damage the DNA of cells affecting cell growth with susceptibility to tumor growth. Phimosis is thought to produce chronic inflammation.[152]

Histopathology reveals that 95% of penile cancers are squamous cell carcinomas (SCC) that usually start on the foreskin in uncircumcised men or on the glans. These are slow growing and, with early intervention, highly curable. There are several subtypes of SCC, including basaloid, verrucous, papillary, condylomatous, and sarcomatoid. Their morphology, pathogenesis, and prognosis differ.[62] Carcinoma in situ is the earliest form of SCC when the tumor cells are found in the top layers of skin. Other types of penile cancers, but more rare, include melanomas, basal cell carcinomas, and adenocarcinomas (Paget disease of the penis).

### Clinical Manifestations

Signs and symptoms of penile cancer can include a change in the skin of the glans, foreskin, or shaft of the penis (thicker skin, change in color, rash, visible lesion or lump), foul odor and discharge or bleeding under the foreskin, and pain. There may also be a report of swelling or a mass in the inguinal node region. Because of the significantly poorer prognosis once the cancer has reached the lymph nodes, it is important to have any of these signs/symptoms addressed by a physician promptly.

## MEDICAL MANAGEMENT

**SCREENING AND PREVENTION.** There is no widely accepted screening test for penile cancer. Almost all penile cancers start in the skin, but even if a man sees a change in the skin, he may not recognize it as needing medical attention and furthermore may put off seeing a physician due to embarrassment. Early diagnosis leads to improved prognosis.

Avoiding known risk factors is the best way to prevent penile cancer. Circumcision has been recommended, but men who aren't circumcised can lower their risk by good hygiene practices. This includes retraction of the foreskin to clean the entire penis. If phimosis is present, a dorsal slit can be made in the foreskin to facilitate retraction. HPV and HIV prevention strategies and reduction of tobacco use lower the risk.

**DIAGNOSIS.** After a thorough history and physical examination are performed by a physician, a biopsy is performed to make a definitive diagnosis. Biopsies of penile tissue may be done with punch biopsy, elliptical incision, or fine needle aspiration. A sentinel lymph node biopsy in the groin may be performed to assess lymph node spread. An inguinal (groin) lymph node dissection may be performed to more accurately assess the lymph nodes, however this procedure is more invasive and is associated with wound issues and lymphedema. Imaging, including x-ray, CT scan with or without contrast, and MRI with or without contrast may be performed.

**TREATMENT.** Surgery is the most common treatment for penile cancer and is based on staging of the tumor. Surgeries attempt to limit tissue removal as much as possible to preserve urinary and sexual function. There has been a shift toward more organ-sparing and nonsurgical approaches in recent years.[127]

Circumcision may be performed for cancer confined to the foreskin, and before radiation therapy to avoid fibrosis of the tissue. Simple or wide excision of small local tumors and surrounding tissue may be appropriate. Superficial cancer may also be treated with application of topical chemo or biological therapies, laser, or cryotherapy. Mohs surgery is the most effective technique for removing SCC by stepwise excision of cancer cells from the skin, followed by detailed mapping and complete microscopic examination of the cancerous tissue and the margins surrounding it.

For invasive cancers, a glansectomy (part or all of the glans is removed) or penectomy (partial or total) may be recommended. With a total penectomy, a perineal urethrostomy is created to allow urination. Advanced penile cancer may require wide dissection and removal of surrounding tissue including the inguinal lymph nodes and the scrotum/testicles.

Radiation therapy in the form of external beam or brachytherapy can be considered as an organ-sparing option and is combined with local excision of cancer cells. RT leads to radiation fibrosis, which can impact both urinary and erectile function. The goal for all of the male genital cancers is sometimes referred to the "trifecta." The trifecta consists of cancer control (negative surgical margins) and no postoperative complications (urinary continence and normal erectile function).[15,73]

Chemotherapy is important with both local and metastatic penile cancer and during all phases of disease progression. Unfortunately, because penile cancer is rare, clinical data on the effectiveness of chemotherapy regimens for this disease are limited.[62] Recent advances have demonstrated the effectiveness of multiple drug strategies limiting the high toxicity profile of some drugs while improving the long-term survival of the patient.[137] Chemotherapy can cause peripheral neuropathy, pulmonary fibrosis, and other adverse reactions. The potential benefit of these regimens must be weighed against the remaining quality of life.

**PROGNOSIS.** Accurate survival rate data in penile cancer is limited due to its rarity. The National Cancer Institute SEER database (https://seer.cancer.gov/) tracks survival statistics in the United States. According to their database, the 5-year relative survival rate for penile cancer confined to the penis (stages 1 and 2) is approximately 85%. With spread to nearby tissue and lymph nodes (stages 3 and some 4s), the 5-year survival rate declines to 59%. With distant metastasis, the rate is 11%.

**SPECIAL IMPLICATIONS FOR THE THERAPIST 19.6**

*Penile Cancer*

Men with penile cancer may report pain and swelling in pelvis, genitals, and legs. As with screening for all types of cancer, it is important for a therapist to be able to discern if the pain arises from a musculoskeletal, neuromuscular, or visceral origin. All individuals with early stage testicular and penile cancer should engage in an exercise program to mitigate some of the effects of their treatment, especially when those treatments reduce levels of testosterone.

Urinary continence and erectile function may be improved with PFM exercises if weakness in these muscles is present. Radiation fibrosis, with the potential to cause urethral stenosis or strictures, is a long-term sequelae of RT. The therapist should ask penile cancer patients about urinary hesitancy, strength of urine flow, and other urinary symptoms as indicated. Symptoms of urinary retention or sever restriction of urine flow should be reported to the physician. Inguinal lymph node dissection increases the patient's risk for lymphedema and referral to a lymphedema specialist should be made when appropriate.

## Erectile Dysfunction

### Overview

Erectile dysfunction (also referred to as impotence) is defined by the International Continence Society as the complaint of inability to achieve and sustain an erection firm enough for satisfactory sexual performance.[31] Normal sexual function includes libido, penile erection, ejaculation, and orgasm. Difficulty in any of these areas is classified as ED. ED has a negative impact on quality of life of both the patient and his partner.[148,149] More importantly ED is a clinical marker for identification of future cardiovascular disease.[103,119]

**Box 19.8**

**RISK FACTORS FOR ERECTILE DYSFUNCTION**

- Age
- Smoking
- Excessive cycling
- Medical history
  - Diabetes mellitus
  - Coronary heart disease
  - Peripheral vascular disease
  - Hypertension
  - Metabolic syndrome
  - Psychiatric disorders
  - Multiple sclerosis
  - Parkinson disease
  - Chronic alcoholism
  - Obesity
- Surgical history
  - Prostatectomy
  - Bowel resections
  - Transurethral procedures
  - Any pelvic surgery
- Adverse effects of medications
  - Diuretics
  - Antihypertensives
  - Antidepressants
  - Antihistamines
  - NSAIDs
  - Muscle relaxants
  - Opiates
  - Anticholinergic agents

### Incidence and Risk Factors

The prevalence of ED in community studies has varied from a low of 5.1% to as high as 70.2% and increases with age.[98] There are an estimated 30 million men in the United States and 152 million men worldwide with ED, with this number expected to increase to approximately 322 million by 2025.[103,130]

Risk factors for ED are listed in Box 19.8. The most common risk factors are CAD, DM, medications, and pelvic surgery. Treatment for prostate cancer, such as prostatectomy, external radiation therapy, and brachytherapy, can also contribute to the development of ED. Neurologic conditions such as Parkinson disease and multiple sclerosis, as well as psychological conditions such as depression, can increase the risk of ED. Other modifiable risk factors include obesity, alcohol use, and smoking.[72,110,119]

### Etiologic Factors

The underlying causes of erectile dysfunction are commonly classified as organic (neurogenic, vascular, and hormonal), or psychogenic (anxiety, fear, depression, stress, fatigue).[176] Approximately 50% to 80% of men seeking treatment for sexual dysfunction have an organic cause. A psychogenic origin of ED is most common in men under 35 years old, while an organic cause is most common in men over 50 years old.

Conditions that can impede blood flow (e.g., atherosclerosis or medications) or impair nerve transmission (e.g., diabetes or surgery) are the most common organic causes.[103] Neurogenic or neurovascular ED can result from surgical or traumatic injury or radiation, to the neurovascular mechanisms that initiate erections. Prostatectomy can result in disruption of the nerve and blood supply to the penis and persistent ED.[64] Radiation may also produce ED by accelerating microvascular angiopathy, causing cavernosal fibrosis or stenosis of the pelvic arteries, leading to vascular impotence.[116] ED in individuals with poorly controlled diabetes mellitus also results from damage the nerves and blood vessels in this area.

### Pathogenesis

Coordinated interactions from the brain, the nerves, and vasculature of the penis are required for normal sexual function. Tactile stimulation and arousal begin the process of penile erection. Normal sensation in the penis and normal brain arousal function is necessary. Depression and anxiety can limit arousal capacity. Impulses from the brain and local nerves cause the smooth muscles around the spongy tissue of the penis to relax, allowing blood to flow in and fill the open spaces. As blood moves into the spongy tissue of the corpus spongiosum and corpus cavernosum the penile veins constrict to keep the penis engorged and rigid. The tunica albuginea (connective tissue) and superficial voluntary pelvic floor muscles also help trap the blood in the spongy tissue, sustaining the erection.

Disruption of the blood flow into the penis (i.e., surgery) may limit erection capacity. Conditions that stiffen the spongy tissue (radiation, arteriosclerosis) limit the ability of the penis to engorge. It is important to encourage men to address the erectile function in a timely manner when symptoms first appear. Lack of erections over time can lead to fibrosis of the spongy tissue and cause further erectile difficulties. In addition, conditions that decrease pelvic floor muscle strength result in decrease in ability to sustain an erection as the blood flows out of the penis before sexual activity is complete. Adequate circulating testosterone is also necessary for normal erectile function and conditions that decrease testosterone, including age, can result in ED.

ED can warn of ischemic heart disease and can be predictive of atherosclerosis and subsequent peripheral vascular disease.[42,72,103,119] Endothelial dysfunction is a link between ED and ischemic heart disease (IHD) and both diseases share many of same pathogenesis, as well as etiology and risk factors.[72] These links have not been fully defined or discovered, however men with ED should be tested for heart disease. Conditions resulting in arterial insufficiency can also result in local penile changes.

### Clinical Manifestations

Manifestations of erectile dysfunction include the following: need for more physical stimulation to induce an erection, less firm erections, longer time to reach orgasm, decreased force of ejaculation, fewer spontaneous erections, and erections that are lost during sexual intercourse. Most men (and their partners) experience feelings of emotional distress and/or depression associated with sexual dysfunction, especially when ED results in subsequent infertility for the couple. Quality-of-life issues are an important aspect of this disorder.[110,119] Patients can report symptoms of anxiety and depression related to sexual dysfunction, which can lead to avoidance and social isolation.[29]

## MEDICAL MANAGEMENT

**PREVENTION.** The best way to prevent ED is to prevent contributing health conditions such as coronary artery disease, hypertension, and diabetes. If these conditions occur they should be well medically managed to minimize the impact on erectile function. Few clinical trails have investigated the direct role of healthy lifestyle choices on the prevention of ED, but most authors agree this is the best preventative approach.[98] A review of lifestyle interventions for ED reports on several studies that appear to show that increased physical activity can prevent onset of ED. Healthy lifestyle includes maintaining a normal weight, good diet, and high level of physical activity. Men should also be encouraged to avoid smoking and excessive alcohol intake.[98] All health care professionals can stress to their patients the benefits of implementing a healthy lifestyle and the beneficial impact on sexual function.

## DIAGNOSIS

A commonly used instrument to evaluate the degree of ED is the International Index of Erectile Dysfunction. It is a 15-item questionnaire that has been validated in many populations and is considered a reliable standard to evaluate patients for ED.[131] Due to the sheer number of possible etiologic factors, a definitive diagnosis related to the true cause of ED can be difficult. Differentiating between an organic versus psychogenic cause is the initial challenge. The nocturnal penile tumescence test, which monitors the incidence of nocturnal erections, helps with this distinction. Men with psychogenic ED will have nocturnal erections, whereas those with an organic lesion will not.

Physical examination includes an abdominal and genital inspection and palpation, assessment of peripheral pulses and blood pressure, and DRE to evaluate prostate size. Laboratory values, including serum chemistries, complete blood cell count, fasting lipid levels, thyroid function tests, and hormone levels may help rule out systemic diseases. As a potential marker of cardiovascular risk, ED must be considered more than a benign result of aging. Its documented association with many chronic diseases and high-risk situations extends the significance of ED beyond the purely sexual domain, providing insight into general and cardiovascular health.[49,72,103,110,119]

**TREATMENT.** The goals of treatment for ED are to improve self-esteem, confidence, and overall sexual and relationship satisfaction. Medical treatment for ED varies, depending on the cause. Underlying conditions that may cause or increase ED symptoms should be addressed first. This includes good management of DM, CAD, HTN, low testosterone, and medications that contribute to ED.

*Pharmacologic treatment* with phosphodiesterase type 5 (PDE-5) inhibitors, such as sildenafil (Viagra), vardenafil (Levitra, Staxyn), avanafil (Stendra), and tadalafil (Cialis, Adcirca), will increase the blood flow to the penis by inhibiting a particular enzyme. These medications are first-line treatment for patients without heart disease. PDE-5 inhibitors can be used cautiously with α-blockers but are contraindicated in men who take any form of nitrate or nitrite medications because these drug combinations can cause serious hypotension. Interestingly, these medications are being used to treat heart disease, diabetes, and cancer.[32]

Alprostadil is indicated for those who cannot tolerate or are not satisfied with PDE-5 inhibitors. It comes in many forms; a topical gel to the head of the penis, self-injection to penis, or a suppository inserted into the urethra. Alprostadil is contraindicated in men who have a history of venous thrombosis, sickle cell anemia or sickle cell trait, thrombocytopenia, polycythemia, or multiple myeloma. Alprostadil and PDE-5 inhibitors relax the arterioles and smooth muscle of the corpus cavernosum and increase cavernous arterial blood flow, causing an erection. Testosterone injections are an option for men with documented androgen deficiency through addressing decreased libido, but may need to be used in conjunction with other treatments for sustained erection.[60]

*Penile prosthetic devices* can be implanted surgically, and men with arterial and venous deficiencies may be candidates for vascular reconstruction procedures.

*Constricting bands* placed around the base of the penis are helpful for men whose ED is associated with venous leakage. Bands may be used in conjunction with other treatments to sustain erection for improved sexual functioning. Erections can be achieved mechanically with a vacuum pump device. Pumps may also be used to maintain the elasticity of the spongy tissue in conditions of temporary ED such as post prostatectomy recovery.

*Pelvic floor muscle training* has been shown to increase the ability to obtain and maintain an erection (see following special implications box).[20,50] Referral to a pelvic PT specialist is recommended.

Patients with ED should be counseled to exercise regularly, maintain proper cholesterol levels, avoid recreational drugs and excessive alcohol, maintain an ideal body weight, and quit smoking.[88] In a meta-analysis moderate intensity aerobic exercise was shown to improve patient reported erectile dysfunction.[143] The European Association of Urologists gives lifestyle modifications a grade A recommendation.[98]

*Psychological counseling and/or behavioral therapy* is indicated for those with a psychogenic basis for the sexual dysfunction. Open communication with the sexual partner is of paramount importance in having a satisfying sexual experience.

*Gene and stem cell therapy* are currently being investigated as future treatment options for ED and sexual medicine.[57,72,176]

**PROGNOSIS.** Identifying the cause can assist in a more accurate prognosis. Successfully addressing underlying conditions and risk factors will help decrease or resolve ED. Conversely, ED may not resolve if conditions or risk factors cannot be improved. Progressive conditions will result in progressively increased ED. This is the case with radiation-induced ED because years may lapse before clinically significant ED develops.

The prognosis of ED after prostatectomy varies with age, overall health, previous erectile function, and surgical procedure. Preservation of sexual function can be difficult even among men who have been treated with nerve-sparing surgery. Younger, healthier men also may have better outcomes after surgery. Men with better erectile function before prostate surgery are more likely to return to full sexual function after surgery.[64]

SPECIAL IMPLICATIONS FOR THE THERAPIST 19.7

### *Erectile Dysfunction*

Men can be reluctant or uncomfortable discussing sexual function or dysfunction. Questions about sexual health must be culturally, ethnically, and spiritually sensitive; and nothing should be assumed. To decrease the individual's discomfort, the therapist should educate about the anatomy, importance of the topic, and correlation to cardiovascular risk and explain that these questions are routinely asked of all clients. Medical practitioners should not be embarrassed to ask patients about sexual function and dysfunction.[60] If the patient notes a sudden change in sexual function, communication with a physician is warranted.

#### Pelvic Floor Muscle Exercises

The superficial perineal muscles, specifically, the ischiocavernosus and bulbospongiosus, play a major role in gaining and maintaining penile erection. Weakness in the pelvic floor muscles may contribute to inability to maintain an erection. Focused pelvic floor muscle exercises should be offered to all men with intact nerve innervation and vascular supply as the first line of treatment for ED.[18,36,78] There is a limited amount of studies in this area, but results consistently show that pelvic floor training reeducation and rehabilitation with and without biofeedback and electrical stimulation are better than no pelvic floor exercise. Referral to a pelvic PT specialist can help ensure that the patient is properly isolating, contracting and relaxing the pelvic floor muscles so that strengthening can occur without compensation.[18,36,50,78]

## SEXUAL VICTIMIZATION IN MEN

The CDC defines sexual violence as "a sexual act committed against someone without that person's freely given consent."[11] In this definition sexual violence includes the full range of penetrative, nonpenetrative, drug-induced, and noncontact unwanted sexual experiences. Sexual victimization is another term for the same constellation of experiences. The 2010 National Intimate Partner and Sexual[104] violence survey reports 11.7% of men have experienced unwanted sexual contact, with 28.4% experiencing intimate partner violence. Also reported are the statistics of rape (1.4%, with 17.8% first rape under 10 years old), being made to penetrate someone (4.8%), and experiencing sexual coercion (6%). A more recent multination systematic review[33] reports overall occurrence of sexual victimization in men is 34%, with 6.7% occurrence of penetrative rape in the United States. Men who have experienced sexual violence have more frequent headaches, chronic pain, difficulty with sleeping, activity limitations, poor physical and mental health, asthma, irritable bowel syndrome, and diabetes than men who did not experience sexual violence.[104] It is important for physical therapists to understand the occurrence of sexual violence in men and its possible impact on health and disease.

Much of the data on men is very similar (if not redundant) to what has been written about women, including incorrect information and myth belief.[169] There does not seem to be a great deal of variation in how the abuse presents or the long-term effects of abuse between men and women. For these reasons, rather than write an extensive section on sexual abuse in men here, we refer the reader to "Domestic Violence" in Chapter 2.

## REFERENCES

To enhance this text and add value for the reader, all references are included in the enhanced ebook on Student Consult that accompanies this textbook. The reader can view the reference source and access it online whenever possible.

CHAPTER 20

# The Female Genital/Reproductive System

ELIZABETH SHELLY • MJ STRAUHAL • KAREN L. LITOS •
KAREN SNOWDEN • MARGARET E. RINEHART-AYRES

The female genital/reproductive system comprises the breasts, ovaries, fallopian tubes, uterus, vagina, and external genitalia (Fig. 20.1). The primary functions of this system are related to conception and gestation. Malfunction of this system can result in a multitude of local disorders, some benign and some life threatening, as well as widespread systemic changes secondary to hormonal influences. These conditions can greatly influence function at many stages of life.

Physical therapists are now involved in the field of urogynecology with specific evaluation and assessment tools, treatment modalities, and therapeutic interventions. Some conditions, for example, pelvic organ prolapse (POP) or postsurgical rehabilitation after mastectomy, may be the primary reason the woman is seeing the therapist. Other conditions, such as endometriosis, may be manifested solely by back or pelvic pain of unknown cause. Focus is shifting from the traditional allopathic emphasis on women's breasts and reproductive system to a more holistic view of women as unique individuals during their reproductive years and beyond, both in health and in disease.

## THE FEMALE REPRODUCTIVE SYSTEM THROUGH THE LIFE CYCLE

### Disorders of the Menstrual Cycle

The menstrual cycle is a complex process of hormonal interactions necessary for the production of oocytes and uterine preparation for pregnancy. These hormonal interactions result in a variety of symptoms each month, including changes in mood and food cravings, headaches, fatigue, abdominal bloating or pain, decline in physical performance, and enhanced risk of injury. A recent systematic review and meta-analysis reviewed 21 studies on the menstrual cycle, oral contraceptive use, and anterior cruciate ligament injury.[219] The authors concluded that there is a significant increase in ligamentous laxity in the ovulation phase of the menstrual cycle, which appears to be related to increased anterior cruciate ligament injury. Furthermore, oral contraceptives appear to provide a 20% decrease in risk of injury.[219]

Many complex physiologic processes present opportunities for dysfunction. All physical therapists should have a basic knowledge of the difference between normal and abnormal menstruation (Box 20.1). *Amenorrhea* is the absence of menstruation in women of childbearing age. *Primary amenorrhea* is the absence of menarche by age 14 to 16.[276] *Secondary amenorrhea* is the cessation of regularly established menses for 3 to 6 months. Both conditions should be fully evaluated, especially in young athletes, to avoid bone loss and skeletal injury.

Premenstrual disorders occur in approximately 12% of women, beginning at mid-cycle during the luteal phase and resolving shortly after menstruation. *Premenstrual syndrome* (PMS) includes abdominal pain, breast tenderness, and various emotional changes. *Premenstrual dysphoric disorder* has a larger psychiatric component.[224] Symptoms include abdominal bloating, breast tenderness/swelling, weight gain, fatigue, depression, irritability, headache, constipation, acne, rhinitis, edema, sleep problems, mood swings, poor concentration, noise sensitivity, and decreased motor skills. These symptoms can be disabling and are not easily resolved with over-the-counter medications or rest.

*Dysmenorrhea* is a condition of painful menstruation that can also be debilitating but is often dismissed by physicians as normal. It can be primary or secondary and occurs in greater than 45% of menstruating women. *Primary dysmenorrhea* has symptoms of pain hypersensitivity and is a risk factor for fibromyalgia.[236] Women who are young (<30 years old), thin (body mass index [BMI] <20), smoke, experienced early menarche (<12 years old), and have long or irregular cycles are more likely to experience dysmenorrhea. PMS, pelvic inflammatory disease (PID), sterilization, and history of sexual assault increase the risk of dysmenorrhea. Women who eat more fish, exercise, have more babies, and are in stable relationships are less likely to have dysmenorrhea.[291] Secondary dysmenorrhea can be associated with diseases such as infection, complications of intrauterine contraceptive device (IUD) use, endometriosis, or scarring. Symptoms include spasmodic cramping or dull aching pain over the lower abdomen, nausea, vomiting, diarrhea, urinary frequency, chills, low back pain (LBP), dizziness, syncope, heavy menstrual flow, and PMS symptoms.

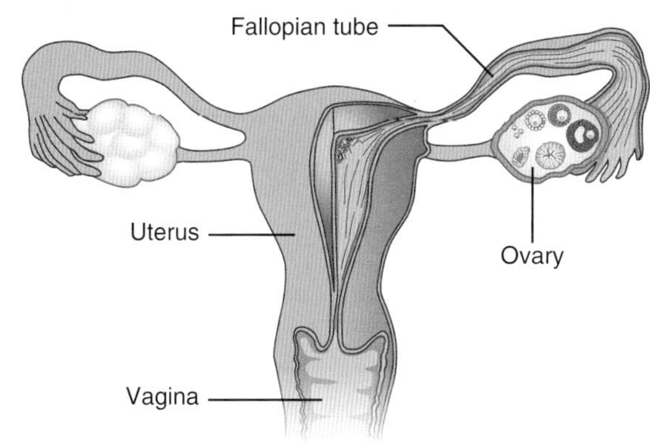


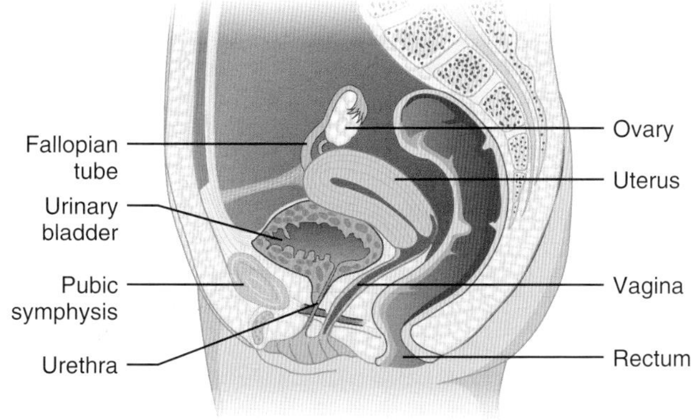


**Figure 20.1**

**Female reproductive organs.** See Figs. 27.1 and 27.2 for visual representation of the pelvic floor muscles.

## Pregnancy

### Physiologic Changes of Pregnancy

Gestation refers to the length of pregnancy, which is typically 280 days (39 to 41 weeks or 10 lunar months). The *expected date of confinement* (EDC) is the due date. Women are considered full term if they deliver 1 week before or after their EDC. *Parity (or parous)* refers to the number of pregnancies reaching a viable gestational age (includes live births and stillbirths). *Nulliparous* refers to women who have never carried a pregnancy beyond 20 weeks. Gravidity refers to pregnancies regardless of outcome. *Primigravida* describes a woman who is pregnant for the first time or has been pregnant once, whereas *multigravida* describes a woman who has been pregnant more than once.

A host of physiologic changes occur during pregnancy that affect function and performance.[64] Therapists treating women during pregnancy must understand these changes and incorporate modifications into treatment and advice. Estrogen, progesterone, and relaxin are responsible for most of these changes. Estrogen increases significantly during pregnancy and is secreted by the ovaries, adipose tissue, adrenal glands, liver, and placenta. The increase in estrogen secretion results in decreased adhesion of collagen and relaxation of ligaments, tendons, and connective tissue. Estrogen also increases water retention, prepares the breast ducts, increases the uterus size, and increases the vaginal mucosa. Relaxin also relaxes connective tissue, limits production of collagen, and increases collagen degradation. Estrogen and relaxin contribute to ligamentous laxity, which can result in musculoskeletal dysfunction during pregnancy.[111] Progesterone decreases smooth muscle excitability, increases body temperature, and prepares the breast tissue for lactation. Hormonal changes continue in the postpartum period (now referred to as the fourth trimester). Physiologic changes in the respiratory, circulatory, gastrointestinal (GI), neurologic, and urinary systems provide for fetal growth and can affect exercise, sports participation, and function (Table 20.1).[64] The American College of Obstetricians and Gynecologists (ACOG) has physical activity and exercise guidelines for women during pregnancy.[17]

Box 20.1

**COMPARISON OF NORMAL WITH ABNORMAL MENSTRUAL CYCLE[a]**

Many reproductive diseases are related to abnormal menstruation. It is helpful for physical therapists to know what is considered normal versus abnormal.

***Normal Menstrual Cycle***

- Menarche—first menstrual cycle: 11 to 15 years old.
- Length of cycle—20 to 45 days; average 28 days (day 1 is the first day of bleeding).
- It is common to have several years of irregular bleeding when menstruation starts.
- Ovulation occurs about day 14 and may be associated with a small amount of transient lower abdominal pain.
- Normal menstrual bleeding lasts about 5 days.
- Menstrual pain—abdominal cramping begins shortly before bleeding begins, peaks within 24 hours of beginning of bleeding, decreases gradually, and is gone usually within 2 days (often before bleeding ends). Normal menstrual pain does not significantly limit most functional activities.

***Abnormal Menstrual Cycle***

- Infrequent menstrual cycle—longer than 31 to 35 days apart.
- Frequent menstrual cycle—less than 2 weeks from day 1 of menstruation to day 1 of next menstruation. Both infrequent and frequent cycles can indicate the onset of menopause but should be evaluated if the woman is not of the expected menopause age (48 to 52 years old) or if there are other symptoms present, such as severe pain or heavy bleeding.
- Heavy bleeding—fills a tampon or sanitary pad after 1 or 2 hours.
- Extended bleeding—bleeding lasting longer than 7 days.
- Severe abdominal cramping—pain that limits functional activity or cannot be decreased with nonprescription medications.
- Abnormal abdominal cramping—abdominal pain occurring several days before bleeding onset, lasting longer than 3 or 4 days, increasing as bleeding decreases, or occurring mid-cycle.
- Vaginal bleeding after 12 months of menopause—may be associated with reproductive organ cancers.

[a]Information compiled from many sources.

**Table 20.1** Physiologic Changes in Pregnancy, Common Symptoms, and Exercise Implications

| Physiologic Changes | Common Symptoms During Pregnancy | Exercise Implications |
|---|---|---|
| Respiratory System<br>• Respiratory rate—minimal change<br>• Oxygen consumption—↑ 20%<br>• Tidal volume—↑ 40%<br>• Efficiency to absorb oxygen—↑<br>• Rib flare<br>  • Anteroposterior diameter—↑ 2 cm<br>  • Transverse diameter—↑ 2 cm<br>• Diaphragm—raised 4 cm with ↓ excursion<br>• Subcostal angle—100 degrees (normal = 90 degrees) | • Changes in lung capacity result in decreased expiratory reserve<br>• Shortness of breath or dyspnea on exertion<br>• Rib position changes may contribute to joint pain<br>• Nasal congestion | • Talk test used to judge acceptable level of exercise<br>• Changes in lung capacity result in decreased expiratory reserve<br>• Rib position changes may contribute to joint pain |
| Circulatory System<br>• Blood volume—↑ 40%–60%<br>  • Plasma volume—↑ 50%<br>  • RBC count—↑ 20%–30%<br>  • Anemia<br>• Cardiac output—↑ 40%<br>  • Stroke volume—↑ 30%<br>  • Resting HR—↑ 20 beats/min<br>• ECG changes<br>• Hormonal softening of blood vessels<br>• Peripheral resistance—↓<br>• Blood pressure—minimal change, ↓ diastolic<br>• Venous return—↓, pooling<br>• Femoral artery compression<br>• BMR—↑ 25% | • Supine hypotension<br>• Orthostatic hypotension<br>• Bleeding gums and nose<br>• Hemorrhoids<br>• Varicose veins—left more than right<br>• Faintness or dizziness<br>• Excessive fatigue<br>• Heat reactions/excessive warmth<br>• Palpitations<br>• Lower extremity swelling 40%, left swells in volume more than right | • Decrease intensity of exercise for obese and sedentary women<br>• HR limitations are no longer recommended. Instead women are encouraged to limit exercise to moderate on the scale of perceived exertion<br>• Avoid prolonged supine positioning to avoid supine hypotension<br>• Avoid Valsalva maneuver<br>• Rise slowly from supine to avoid orthostatic hypotension<br>• Avoid or limit exercise in outside temperatures >75° and >60% humidity to limit dangerous core temperature rise<br>• Fluid intake—before, during, and after exercise |
| Gastrointestinal System<br>• Peristalsis—↓<br>• Esophageal sphincter response—↓<br>• Upward displacement of stomach<br>• Blood sugar—↓ at rest | • Hypoglycemia<br>• Weight gain 25–30 lb<br>• Constipation<br>• Hemorrhoids<br>• Heart burn<br>• Nausea and vomiting<br>• Hyperemesis gravida (excessive vomiting during pregnancy)<br>• Excessive salivation | • Wedge for supine exercises<br>• Exercises for constipation are good<br>• Hypoglycemia—eat 2 hours before exercises<br>• Weight control is not a goal of exercise for normal-weight or underweight women<br>• Need an additional 300 cal/day<br>• Weight management through healthy diet and regular exercise to minimize additional weight gain in pregnancy may be recommended for obese women |
| Neurologic System<br>• Blind spot—↑<br>• Senses—↑ or ↓ | • Emotional and cognitive changes<br>• Visual changes<br>• Insomnia<br>• Anxiety | • Avoid uneven surfaces<br>• Be sensitive to emotional sensitivities |
| Urinary System<br>• Weakened pelvic floor muscles<br>• Bladder capacity—↓<br>• Increased urine production | • Stress incontinence<br>• Urinary frequency<br>• Pelvic organ prolapse | • Perineal or other support garments<br>• Breathing and posture exercises to engage deep core muscles<br>• Stress incontinence—pelvic floor strengthening exercise<br>• Biomechanics training to avoid Valsalva maneuver during lifting, exercise, position changes, and toileting |

*BMR*, Basal metabolic rate; *ECG*, electrocardiogram; *HR*, heart rate; *RBC*, red blood cell.

### Musculoskeletal Disorders During Pregnancy

Prevalence of *LBP* and *pelvic girdle pain* (PGP) conditions is between 70% and 85%,[199] with 10% being classified as continuing long term with severe consequences up to 11 years.[150] Many women will stop exercising because of pain or fear of harm to the pregnancy. Relatively few women report their pain to their physician,[401] and only a small percentage receive adequate education on their options for treatment and management of symptoms. Past research has reported untreated moderate to severe back and pelvic pain in pregnancy to be associated with a threefold increased risk of postpartum depression.[200] Women with recurrent or continuous back or pelvic pain during and after pregnancy have more disability and take more sick leave,[53] contributing to financial strain and stress. Understanding the physiologic changes during pregnancy[64] as well as pathologic conditions during pregnancy is necessary to provide effective treatment.

Other musculoskeletal disorders related to postural changes include rounded shoulders and forward head. These changes, potentially exacerbated by heavier breasts and general fatigue, may contribute to the occurrence of cervical pain and headaches. Changes in posture and fluid dynamics can also contribute to carpal tunnel syndrome and thoracic outlet syndrome. Thoracic pain may be related to the upward movement of the ribs by the growing fetus. Hormone-related ligamentous laxity has been considered to be a cause of joint strain and pain in women during pregnancy. Diastasis rectus abdominis is a thinning and stretching of the linea alba, with more than 2 cm distance between the rectus abdominis muscle bellies. This separation may cause a doming of the abdomen and can persist after delivery, affecting trunk stability and function long term.[294] Therapists are referred to several texts that provide more comprehensive information on the examination and treatment of women during and after pregnancy.[64,241,354]

### Disorders of Pregnancy

*Preterm labor* is the onset of labor before 37 weeks of gestation. Bed rest is considered essential to decrease uterine contractions, eliminate gravitational effects on the cervix, and prolong pregnancy, commonly seen with multiple gestation. Although bed rest is often ordered, there is no evidence that higher activity level increases the likelihood of preterm labor. Tocolytic medications may be prescribed to delay labor. Tocolysis does not appear to delay delivery beyond 1 week. Broad-spectrum antibiotics, antenatal corticosteroids, and magnesium sulfate may also be prescribed to reduce risk of neonatal mortality and morbidities.

*Cervical insufficiency* is a dysfunctional, weakened cervix that passively softens and thins (effacement) usually during the second trimester of pregnancy. The membranes may rupture, or labor may begin prematurely. A shortened cervix determined by transvaginal ultrasound is a risk factor for preterm birth. Bed rest may be ordered to decrease the physical forces causing cervical changes. Some patients require a cerclage—a stitch placed through the cervix to hold it closed to prolong pregnancy.

*Placenta previa* is a low-lying placenta that partially or completely covers the cervix and can result in sudden, massive blood loss during vaginal delivery owing to placental abruption. A partial previa present earlier in pregnancy may move from the internal os (orifice of the uterus) as the abdomen grows; however, cesarean delivery is recommended for women with partial previa still present at 36 weeks to prevent placental abruption.

*Premature rupture of membranes* is rupture in the amniotic sac leading to a slow leak or complete loss of amniotic fluid before 37 weeks of gestation. Patients remain hospitalized until labor develops, and medications are usually administered to decrease risk of infection and neonatal morbidity and mortality.

*Preeclampsia* is a pregnancy-related hypertensive disorder. It is a specific disease process occurring only in pregnancy that is diagnosed by an elevated blood pressure of 140/90 mm Hg after 20 weeks' gestation with a history of normotensive blood pressure before 20 weeks' gestation. Other diagnostic criteria include new onset of neurologic or visual symptoms, such as headache, light sensitivity, seeing spots before the eyes, pulmonary edema, thrombocytopenia, elevated liver enzymes to twice normative values, and new development of renal insufficiency. Proteinuria may or may not be present. This condition has many risks, including fetal growth restriction, premature birth, placental abruption, maternal congestive heart failure, seizures, or maternal stroke. This is a medical emergency with hospitalization for monitoring because the condition can quickly progress, requiring emergency delivery of the fetus. All therapists should monitor pregnant patients for symptoms of preeclampsia and monitor blood pressure of at risk pregnant patients during each session. The medical provider should be notified of new-onset blood pressure of 140/90 mm Hg.

Blood pressure is dependent on maternal position: lowest in side lying, highest in standing. In *supine hypotensive syndrome,* after the fourth or fifth month of pregnancy the weight of the uterus on the inferior vena cava in the supine position decreases blood flow to the fetus and maternal heart. Symptoms include shortness of breath, light-headedness, dizziness, and feeling generally uncomfortable. Patients are encouraged to move out of the supine position to alleviate symptoms. This condition occurs in approximately 11% of women.

*Gestational diabetes mellitus* (GDM) is new onset of diabetes and represents the most common medical complication in pregnancy, affecting more than 10% to 17% of pregnancies depending on source. Risk factors for developing GDM include a personal history of GDM in a previous pregnancy, history of a macrosomic (large) infant, family history of type 2 diabetes mellitus in a first-degree relative, polycystic ovarian syndrome (PCOS), severe obesity, prepregnancy diet of low fiber and high glycemic load, elevated fasting or casual blood glucose, and African American or Native American ethnicity. Risks to the mother include preterm labor, increased blood pressure, increased risk of birth complications and cesarean delivery, and development of type 2 diabetes mellitus later in life. Risks to the fetus include fetal demise, premature birth, cardiac and limb defects, respiratory distress syndrome, macrosomia, and development of long-term metabolic disorders. Women are routinely screened early for GDM and may receive dietary advice, medications, and physical therapy to improve glucose metabolism and manage weight gain through monitored exercise.

SPECIAL IMPLICATIONS FOR THE THERAPIST 20.1

### *Disorders of Pregnancy*

The Academy of Pelvic Health Physical Therapy American Physical Therapy Association (APTA) has published "Guidelines for Women's Health Content in Professional Physical Therapy Education (updated 2014)" encouraging all universities to offer comprehensive education in the assessment and treatment of the obstetric client in their physical therapy curriculum. However, the quality of obstetric education is not known and may leave the therapist ill prepared to treat this unique patient population. In addition, a survey of Canadian physical therapists found a lack of awareness of practice guidelines for pregnancy-related PGP.[143] A clinical survey found only 24% of U.S. women received treatment for pregnancy-related PGP or LBP.[199] Additional continuing education to equip the therapist in treating obstetric patients or referral to a therapist trained in obstetric physical therapy may be warranted to effectively treat more complex patients.

A more recent meta-analysis reported women with pregnancy-related LBP or PGP had a statistically significant decrease in pain and improvement in function with a supervised, core-based and/or yoga exercise program.[48] Vleeming and colleagues[528] outlined criteria for diagnosis and suggestions for treatment of PGP, including sacroiliac joint and pubic symphysis pain. More recently, the APTA Academy of Pelvic Health Physical Therapy and the Academy of Orthopedic Physical Therapy jointly released updated clinical practice guidelines for treatment of PGP in the antenatal population.[104] Obstetrics physical therapy is an emerging area of practice for therapists, who combine their base expertise in the musculoskeletal system and function with advanced training to optimize function and relieve pain for women through pregnancy, labor and delivery, and postpartum recovery. Therapists work with the health care team to provide collaborative and safe care through personalized exercise prescription, education, biomechanics training, recommendations for support garments, manual therapy for pain relief, and positioning strategies during labor and delivery to potentially reduce risk of pelvic floor injury during delivery. Continuing education courses in obstetrics and pelvic floor therapy are strongly recommended for therapists interested in treating pregnant and postpartum women effectively.

## Menopause

Menopause is a natural transition in a woman's life marked by the cessation of ovarian follicular function and reproduction. Menopause is defined retrospectively 1 year after the last menstrual period, usually occurring around age 52. Estrogen decline and other hormonal changes associated with the menopause transition (MT) induce anatomic and physiologic changes that can increase risk for certain pathologic conditions.[452]

The average reported age for menopause is 51.5 years; however, age at menopause varies, with some women experiencing early signs and symptoms of the MT starting in their late 30s. Most women experience near-complete loss of production of estrogen by their mid-50s.[452] Menopause impacts every woman who survives to middle adulthood, affecting approximately 6000 U.S. women per day and 2 million per year. There are an estimated 40 million women who are postmenopausal in the United States.[452] With the number of women in the 55-and-older age group continuing to increase in the coming years (estimates of 1.1 million women worldwide by 2025),[452] it is important for physical therapists to understand the impact of menopause.

### Physiologic Changes of Menopause

The female reproductive system including the endocrine system that supports it is fully developed in vitro, and the female fetus is born with 2 million intact ovarian follicles. About two-thirds of those follicles will degenerate by the start of menarche, occurring around ages 12 to 13, leaving a lifetime supply of approximately 200,000 follicles per ovary.[231] Monthly menstruation and ovulation are controlled by key hormones (estrogen, progesterone, follicle stimulating hormone [FSH], and luteinizing hormone [LH]) cyclically released through stimulation of the hypothalamus, anterior pituitary gland, and ovaries acting as a single neuroendocrine unit called the hypothalamic-pituitary-gonadal (HPG) axis.[231] As a woman enters her 30s, ovarian production of estrogen and progesterone begins to decline, with oocyte aging and decreased sensitivity to FSH. Initially the HPG axis responds with increased production of FSH to stimulate oocyte release that results in increasingly erratic menstrual periods, with episodes of anovulation or multiple oocyte release. Ultimately the HPG axis stops production of hormones, resulting in reduced estrogen release from the ovaries that triggers a cascade of events altering the physiology of multiple systems, leading to reproductive senescence.[231] Estrogen has effects on various target organs in the body, not just the organs of reproduction. In fact, estrogen receptor (ER) sites are found throughout the body and in all organs, including skin, blood vessels, bone, brain, heart, intestinal tract, and urinary bladder. Physiologic and physical changes associated with declining estrogen and/or hormonal imbalances include vasomotor symptoms; endometrial, vaginal, and vulvar atrophy; impaired thyroid function; altered renal function; cardiac dysfunction; insulin insensitivity; muscle atrophy; cortical bone loss; sexual dysfunctions; temporary cognitive deficits; and mood disorders.[231,452]

### Terminology

*Menopause* is the permanent cessation of menses occurring after a woman has experienced 1 full year without menstruation diagnosed retrospectively. The *menopause transition* (MT) refers to the time from when a woman experiences the initial reduction in ovarian function until she reaches menopause. *Postmenopause* refers to the years in a woman's life following menopause.[30,452]

*Natural menopause* normally occurs around age 52. *Premature natural menopause* can occur before the age of 40, resulting from *primary ovarian insufficiency*, a transient or permanent loss of ovarian function leading to amenorrhea. *Transient ovarian insufficiency* occurs when the ovaries function intermittently or are temporarily inactive, such as during chemotherapy and radiation therapy, with certain medications, or with extreme stress or excessive exercise. Spontaneous primary ovarian insufficiency results from genetic (10% to 15%), environmental, and metabolic factors and autoimmune disturbances (i.e., rheumatoid arthritis and systemic lupus erythematosus). Both prenatal exposure to smoke and current smoking is associated with ovarian aging and earlier onset of natural menopause.[493] Early diagnosis is necessary to combat the negative effects of estrogen depletion, including bone density, cognitive function, and sexual dysfunction.

*Secondary menopause* refers to premature menopause induced as a result of medical intervention, such as chemical or surgical induction, illness, or pelvic radiation. *Surgical menopause* occurs when the ovaries are removed, a procedure known as oophorectomy, and is an example of induced premature menopause.[16,314,452] If the ovaries and fallopian tubes are not removed during hysterectomy, they may continue to release reproductive hormones. In some cases the remaining ovaries stop functioning very soon after hysterectomy; in other cases they may continue to function for several more years. Estrogen levels decline quickly, and symptoms are often more severe with surgical menopause than with natural menopause. Surgical menopause increases the risk for (and severity of) several autonomic symptoms associated with menopause, including vasomotor changes (hot flashes), vaginal atrophy, and temporary cognitive deficits.[314,452]

### Menopause Transition (Perimenopause)

MT is often referred to among women as "the change before the change." For some women, MT can begin as early as 10 years before the complete cessation of the menstrual cycle. For others, it can occur just a few months before menopause. Most women report a 3- or 4-year period of time when symptoms gradually escalate. MT is the physiologic reverse of puberty. Levels of reproductive hormones start to decline gradually with sudden fluctuations on a day-to-day basis as opposed to the gradual increase that occurs during puberty.[30,452]

The intermittent variations in hormone levels account for the variations in the patterns of common symptoms women often experience during this time period. MT is further described as having two stages, early and late. Early MT is characterized by menstrual periods that continue to occur at regular intervals but with increasing distance between periods. During early MT, ovulation continues but may alternate with anovulatory periods, menstrual cycles during which the ovaries do not release an oocyte (egg), with or without menstruation as the ovaries continue to produce estrogen. Increasing irregularity of the menstrual cycle occurs in late MT, with skipped periods more common.[452]

### Postmenopause

As life expectancy continues to increase, most women can now expect to live at least one-third of their lives after menopause.[452] The physical, psychologic, and social changes associated with menopause are increasingly important for all health care practitioners to understand. The hormonal fluctuations of MT are expected to stabilize after menopause, although hormonal and symptom variations may continue during this portion of the life cycle.

### Clinical Manifestations

Thermoregulatory and vasomotor changes during menopause, especially hot flashes, also known as hot flushes, and night sweats, are considered hallmark symptoms of MT experienced by up to 85% of women. Hot flashes are a sudden sensation of extreme heat in the upper body, most often felt on the neck, face, and chest lasting 1 to 5 minutes that can occur several times a day or as frequently as several times an hour. They are associated with profuse perspiration, flushing, clamminess, chills, anxiety, and heart palpitations. Night sweats are hot flash symptoms that occur at night. Although common, intensity and frequency of hot flashes and night sweats vary, with the highest occurrence reported during perimenopause through the first 2 years postmenopause, and then symptoms usually abate. Approximately 10% to 15% of women will report severe symptoms, and symptoms may be more severe in women who smoke. Hot flashes and night sweats occur because of hormonal changes influencing the body's thermoregulatory zone, resulting in decreased tolerance to temperature changes. Serum estrogen levels are not predictive of hot flash frequency or severity, which is highly individual. Nonhormonal factors that negatively impact hot flash frequency and severity include warm environments, spicy foods, anxiety or stress, higher BMI, smoking, alcohol, certain drugs and disease conditions, and a history of total hysterectomy. Treatment is based on severity of symptoms and may include hormone replacement therapy (HRT) and dietary and lifestyle changes to avoid triggers.[329,452]

Fatigue, anxiety, sleep disturbances, difficulty with memory and concentration, reduced libido, vaginal dryness, mood swings, and irritability all are commonly reported by menopausal women (Box 20.2). Pain complaints also increase during MT, including headache, breast discomfort, and peripheral and spinal joint pain.[452] Additional signs and symptoms may occur in conjunction with the physiologic changes of menopause in the

Box 20.2

**COMMON SYMPTOMS FROM PERIMENOPAUSE THROUGH POSTMENOPAUSE**

- Hot flashes, flushing, sweats
- Vulvar or vaginal atrophy (dryness, burning, itching, dyspareunia)
- Anxiety, panic attacks, depression, mood swings, irritability
- Fatigue
- Urinary incontinence
- Insomnia, sleep disturbances
- Headache
- Decreased libido
- Prolonged bleeding, heavy bleeding, irregular menses, cessation of menses
- Heart palpitations, heart racing or pounding
- Short-term memory loss, difficulty concentrating (brain fog)
- Changes in body composition: muscle loss, weight gain, central adiposity

musculoskeletal, urologic, neurologic, cardiovascular, endocrine, GI, integumentary, and psychosocial systems. Physical changes and pathologic correlates of menopause are presented by organ system in the following sections.

**Reproductive System.** A variety of changes occur in the reproductive organs as estrogen levels decrease. The myometrium, endometrium, cervix, vagina, and labia all become atrophic to some degree. Women with endometriosis may experience relief as the endometrium volume diminishes in the postmenopausal period.[452] Pelvic ligamentous laxity contributes to the development of cystocele, rectocele, and uterine prolapse.

***Abnormal Uterine Bleeding.*** Although vaginal bleeding should stop with menopause, approximately 10% of women experience postmenopausal bleeding (vaginal bleeding that occurs 1 year or more after the last period). For most women, postmenopausal bleeding is a benign and self-limiting condition (e.g., polyps); however, there is a 10% to 15% risk for endometrial cancer, so postmenopausal bleeding always requires prompt medical evaluation.[72] Women receiving continuous combined estrogen/progestin or progesterone HRT may experience irregular spotting until the endometrium (vaginal lining) atrophies, which takes about 6 months.

***Vaginal Atrophy.*** Vaginal atrophy as well as flattening of the rugae (vaginal rugae are transverse epithelial ridges most commonly seen on the outer third of the female vagina) occurs during menopause. As a result of the surface epithelium thinning, the vaginal surface becomes friable, and bleeding is common with minimal trauma. The blood vessels in the vaginal walls narrow, and over time the vagina itself contracts and loses flexibility owing to lack of estrogen.[329,452]

***External Genitalia.*** External genitalia changes in size and integrity during menopause. The vulvar epithelium atrophies, and secretions from sebaceous glands diminish. Subcutaneous fat in the labia majora is lost and leads to shrinkage and retraction of clitoral prepuce and the urethra, fusion of the labia minora, and introital narrowing and then stenosis. As a result of these changes, the clinical symptoms associated with vulvovaginal atrophy include vaginal dryness, itching, irritation, dyspareunia during vaginal penetration, and recurrent urinary tract infections (UTIs). Vulvovaginal atrophy and dyspareunia are more common in the late stages of MT. The frequency of vaginal and bladder infections also increases with vaginal pH changes resulting from estrogen decline as well as dehydration of the vaginal and urethral tissues.[264,397,452,503]

***Pelvic Organ Prolapse.*** Menopause and aging are risk factors for POP, a condition of weakened ligamentous support for pelvic floor muscles (PFMs) causing bulging of the bowel, bladder, or uterus into the vaginal canal. Diminished estrogen causes changes in collagen, weakening the support mechanisms holding the pelvic organs in place. Symptoms of POP include aching in the vagina, lower abdomen, groin, or lower back; heaviness or pressure in the vagina or a sensation something is "falling out" of the vagina; stress urinary incontinence (SUI); frequent UTIs; and incomplete bowel or bladder emptying.[452] See further discussion of POP later in this chapter.

***Pelvic Pain.*** Some pelvic pain conditions are more common during the menopausal years. Hysterectomy is the second most common surgery among women in the United States and is common in the medical history of menopausal women. Noncyclic pelvic pain is reported in 10% to 50% of women following hysterectomy.[74] Women experiencing pelvic pain before menopause may experience a worsening of the symptoms during menopause, depending on the etiology of their pelvic pain. In particular, pelvic pain of musculoskeletal etiology may worsen during menopause as the support systems of the pelvis are weakened with changes in muscle mass and bone and connective tissue strength associated with menopause.[389,452,486] In addition, vulvar pain may increase during menopause for some women.[452,455] Pelvic pain associated with fibroids (which have ERs) may worsen in response to the naturally occurring hormone fluctuations of MT and decrease postmenopause with natural estrogen decline. Theoretically, fibroid-associated pelvic pain may also increase with HRT as a result of the estrogen stimulation, although there are no studies to support this theory.[550]

***Sexual Dysfunction.*** Sexual function is impacted by both biologic and psychosocial variables that occur during the stages of menopause. A sizable study on sexuality and menopause found that the age a woman transitions through menopause is not associated with changes in sexual intercourse, desire, arousal, or physical or emotional satisfaction.[171] Psychosocial factors reported in women in midlife associated with sexual dysfunctions include fatigue; stress; self-esteem and relationship issues; comorbidities and illness; religious, cultural, and personal beliefs about sexuality, and low libido.[170,455,456];

*Dyspareunia,* pain experienced during penetrative intercourse, is more common among women in MT and postmenopausal age groups than in women of other age groups.[452,455] The biologic effects of menopause on vaginal tone and lubrication are considered a primary etiologic factor contributing to dyspareunia among menopausal women. Blood flow to the genitalia is reduced during menopause, and painful vasocongestion is common with sexual activity. Reduced levels of testosterone and androgen and declines in estrogen contribute to genital atrophy and pain with penetration, as well as low libido, decreased sensation, and decreased sexual response.[108,452,455]

*Hypoactive sexual disorder (loss of libido)*, is a decrease/loss of sexual desire associated with aging that affects women two to three times more than men and can profoundly impact personal relationships, quality of life, and self-esteem. Women with hypoactive sexual disorder are at an increased risk for depression. The causes are both biologic and psychosocial. Relationship issues, vulvar/vaginal changes and related sexual dysfunctions, medical comorbidities, and general health and wellness concerns all are contributing factors to loss of libido.[452]

*Decreased sexual arousal* is the inability to become aroused when desire is present. *Decreased sexual response* is the inability to achieve orgasm when aroused. Both problems are more common in women older than age 45 and frequently associated with vaginal changes, hormonal changes, and decreased sensitivity in the clitoris. Over time, lack of response will often lead to lack of desire (loss of libido).[452,455] A large survey of 10,486 women close to age 60 conducted in 2012 revealed that more than half

(59%) had vulvovaginal symptoms affecting their enjoyment of sex: 55% reported vaginal dryness, 44% reported dyspareunia, and 37% reported tissue irritation.[171]

A large longitudinal study of 3167 midlife non-Hispanic white, African American, Hispanic, Chinese, and Japanese women from the Study of Women's Health Across the Nation (SWAN) compared sexual function in women who were not using HRT. The women who underwent a hysterectomy reported larger declines across the board in sexual functioning, persisting for 5 years after surgery.[29] After controlling for variables, racial and ethnic differences were also evident for decline in sexual arousal, pain, desire, and frequency of sexual intercourse. African American women reported smaller declines in sexual functioning, while Japanese women reported greater declines compared with white women in this study. Declines in function started 20 months before menopause and leveled out after a few years.[29]

Premature menopause affects reproductive status and may affect sexual identity, sexual function, and sexual relationships. Factors modulating the individual's sexual outcome after premature menopause include associated medical, psychologic, and social and sexual comorbidities. Survivors of childhood and adolescent cancers also have increased risk for negative sexual outcomes following premature menopause. The biologic basis of desire, arousal, orgasm, and vaginal receptivity are impacted by premature menopause and combine with psychosocial factors to determine a woman's response to the changes in her reproductive status and the physical changes that impact sexual function.[160]

***Fertility.*** Although fertility ends when a woman reaches menopause, many women perceive themselves as infertile when MT begins. Despite irregular menstrual bleeding and periods of anovulation, ovulation and conception can occur during MT. Contraception choices are complicated during MT, as some commonly prescribed contraceptives can increase undesirable consequences of MT, such as reduced bone mineral density (BMD). As women age, they are more likely to acquire other medical conditions, and comorbidities must be considered when contraceptives are prescribed by the appropriate health care practitioner.[329,452]

***Infertility.*** Infertility is also a concern for women during MT, as more women choose to delay marriage and childbearing until older ages. Sometimes desired pregnancy requires reproductive technologic assistance, and other times it may occur spontaneously. The risks of miscarriage and chromosomal abnormalities increase with aging oocytes. Older maternal age is associated with higher risk for cesarean delivery, GDM, pregnancy-induced hypertension, and stillbirth.[329,452] Assistive reproductive technology has allowed women age 50 and older to conceive, carry, and deliver babies safely, some even postmenopause. With oocyte donation, the uterine environment is similar to younger counterparts.[207]

***Sexually Transmitted Infections.*** Sexually transmitted infection (STI) rates are rapidly rising in midlife adults. Midlife women are at high risk for STIs because of increased exposure with new partners. Although STIs are associated with transmission through intimate contact, some STIs are bloodborne pathogens that can be transmitted by any exposure to infected blood. STIs are more easily passed from male to female than reverse. If exposed, women are twice as likely to contract human immunodeficiency virus (HIV), hepatitis B, and gonorrhea. Women are less likely to exhibit early symptoms and often receive later diagnosis after serious problems develop. Risk of bloodborne pathogen infection is highest in women with severe vaginal atrophy through vaginal skin breakdown. Women who are bisexual and women who have sex with women are also at risk; however, there are limited data available. Safe sex rules still apply in midlife, and women are advised to follow clinical guidelines of the U.S. Centers for Disease Control and Prevention (CDC).[452]

**Urologic System.** There are several changes in the urologic system during menopause, including urinary incontinence (see Chapter 18).

***Genitourinary Syndrome of Menopause.*** Genitourinary syndrome of menopause refers to a collection of symptoms that are due to changes in the urethra, pelvic floor musculature, and bladder. The female urethra, bladder, and pelvic floor musculature share the same embryologic origins as the distal vagina and possess the same ERs. Atrophic changes from estrogen decline lead to symptoms of dysuria, urethral discomfort, POP, and SUI. Common symptoms of genitourinary syndrome of menopause include genital dryness, decreased lubrication during vaginal intercourse, discomfort or pain with sexual activity, postcoital bleeding, decreased arousal or desire, irritation, burning or itching of the vulva or vagina, dysuria, and urinary urgency and frequency (overactive bladder).[264,397,452,503]

***Overactive Bladder Syndrome.*** Overactive bladder syndrome affects 19% of women ages 50 to 60, with hallmark symptoms that include urinary urge (strong sudden urge to urinate), frequency greater than seven times a day, and nocturia (voiding in the middle of the night). Other symptoms include incomplete bladder emptying, bladder spasms or painful urination, frequent UTIs, and other bacterial infections. It is associated with detrusor overactivity in 64% of affected individuals.[397,503]

***Urinary Incontinence.*** Loss of collagen from around the urethra and within the trigone of the bladder may contribute to the development of *urinary incontinence* in postmenopausal women. Women with preexisting urinary problems may experience increasing difficulty controlling urination as the decline in estrogen results in atrophic changes of the lower urinary tract, widening the urethra and decreasing resistance to the flow of urine.

Women with detrusor muscle instability or neurogenic bladder who could manage their bladder control before menopause may find themselves with an unexpected loss of control (or worsening of incontinence).[545] Urinary incontinence (when combined with even minor skin changes associated with menopause) can create major problems for women confined to a wheelchair. Attention to dry skin and hydration, strategies to manage incontinence, and pressure ulcer prevention are very important.[444a]

Physical therapists should assess for (and teach the client how to self-assess for) signs and symptoms of UTI, kidney and bladder stones, incontinence, and other changes associated with changes in kidney or bladder function.[545] See further discussion in Chapter 18.

SUI occurs in up to 47% of women ages 50 to 60 and up to 55% of women older than 60.[503] Stress incontinence is loss of urine occurring during activities with increased intraabdominal pressure, such as coughing, sneezing, laughing, jumping, lifting, or running. SUI is not considered normal aging and is underreported.[503]

Approximately one in four women with incontinence report leakage during sexual intercourse (coital urinary incontinence [CUI]). Although aging and menopause are not risk factors for CUI, SUI, obesity, hysterectomy, and POP all are significant risk factors[238] and commonly reported in midlife women. Postmenopausal women on HRT showed a numerical, but not statistically significant, decline in CUI in a review of current research.[238] Therapists should specifically ask about CUI in sexually active midlife women reporting any kind of urinary incontinence.

**Gastrointestinal System.** Bowel discomfort, abdominal pain, bloating, nausea, changes in bowel patterns (including constipation and diarrhea), and the appearance or exacerbation of inflammatory bowel disease are associated with MT and menopause. Similar patterns are reported during premenses and menses. Associations between menses, premenses, and GI symptoms provide clinical support for argument that a cause-and-effect association exists between GI symptoms and ovarian hormones. Women with comorbidities such as Crohn disease or irritable bowel syndrome (IBS) may experience worsening symptoms with hormonal changes.[452] Dietary changes, hydration, exercise, medications or supplements, and stress management may reduce the severity of menopause-associated GI symptoms.

**Integumentary System.** Age-related skin changes enhanced by the hormonal changes of menopause include thinning, reduced elasticity, hyperpigmentation (age spots), wrinkles, and itching. Collagen volume, fiber strength, and peripheral blood supply diminish during menopause. The changes in collagen integrity combine with a hormone-related reduction in subcutaneous skin volume, giving skin a looser appearance. Subcutaneous fat volume also decreases, usually more obvious in the face than in other parts of the body because the facial muscles attach to the skin's undersurface, creating facial lines. Other non–menopause-related factors contribute to the rate and degree of the signs of skin aging, including genetics and health habits. Individuals with thin, dry, fair skin usually manifest signs of skin aging earlier. Other factors associated with earlier skin aging include overexposure to sunlight, tobacco use, and alcohol use.[501]

**Endocrine System.** Even though estrogen levels decline as women age, the ovaries continue to produce significant amounts of testosterone and androstenedione after menopause. As a result, levels of testosterone may not decline sharply at menopause for women whose ovaries are intact. Testosterone preserves bone and muscle mass and alleviates menopausal symptoms, particularly the loss of libido. Androgen insufficiency can occur during menopause, reducing levels of serum testosterone. Associated symptoms include fatigue, low libido, mood changes, sarcopenia, and reduced bone mass.[452]

***Diabetes.*** Older studies associating type 1 diabetes mellitus with earlier MT have not been validated in current research.[452] Menopause is also not a risk factor for type 2 diabetes mellitus. However, lifestyle risk factors for diabetes associated with aging, including sedentary lifestyle, insulin resistance with visceral weight gain, and metabolic syndrome (MetS), are more common in postmenopausal women.[470]

***Thyroid Function.*** Thyroid function is not directly involved in pathogenesis of menopause complications but may modify clinical manifestations of certain autoimmune diseases. Hyperthyroid or hypothyroid function can worsen co morbidities of coronary atherosclerosis or osteoporosis present in postmenopausal women. Symptoms of thyroid dysfunction mimic common vasomotor symptoms of menopause, so the presence of thyroid disease should be ruled out as a possible cause first. Women taking estrogen HRT may need additional thyroxine if they also have hypothyroidism; however, the concurrence of thyroid disease is not a contraindication for HRT.[470]

***Weight Gain and Central Adiposity.*** Women typically gain 5 to 15 lb between the ages of 45 and 55 as a result of slowed metabolism and lifestyle changes. Lower circulating estrogen and progesterone reduce resting metabolism and caloric intake needs, yet appetite increases up to 67%. Body composition and fat distribution are altered during the stages of menopause, including loss of lean mass, increases in fat mass, and redistribution of fat from the periphery to the center.[452] Central adiposity (truncal obesity) is a common pattern of weight gain among menopausal women because visceral fat is a major source of estrone, a weaker form of estrogen that replaces depleted estradiol stores in the ovaries.

Central adiposity, not menopause itself, increases the risk for cardiovascular disease (CVD) and is strongly correlated with other cardiac risk factors, such as lipid and lipoprotein changes, blood pressure, and insulin level. MetS is an enzymatic or hormonal disorder of obesity triggered by food intolerance independent of caloric intake. Concomitant MetS during menopause increases the risk of CVD. Postmenopausal status increases the risk of MetS 32% to 42%, and surgical menopause is strongly linked with MetS. Women with PCOS have an increased risk of MetS during their reproductive years but a decreased risk of MetS after menopause.[365,452]

The Nutrition Science Initiative and other research support increased physical activity for weight management during MT. [365,452] As therapists develop plans of care and/or educational programs for women who are approaching or beyond MT, they should consider potential for weight gain and central adiposity as an identified health risk.

**Cardiovascular System.** Premenopausal women have a cardioprotective effect of estrogen through enhancement of high-density lipoprotein levels, the beneficial cholesterol. Cardiac risk increases exponentially when women enter postmenopause, owing to estrogen depletion. The risk for mortality associated with menopause and subsequent coronary heart disease (CHD) is significant in this age group. Menopausal symptoms are an independent risk factor for CHD in women not receiving HRT.[233] Women who experience premature or early-onset menopause are at greater risk of CHD, CVD, and mortality.[364] CHD is the cause of death for 25% of all women across age groups and is the number one killer of women (and men) in the United States.[51,407,557] More women than men die of CVD every year, and in women who survive the burden and consequences are worse than in men.[340] Heart disease is the leading cause of death for African American and white women in the United States. Among Hispanic women, heart disease and cancer cause roughly the same number of deaths each year. For American Indian, Alaska Native, Asian American, and Pacific Islander women, heart disease is second only to cancer.[217] Nearly two-thirds (64%) of women who die of heart disease have no previous symptoms.[420] Although some women have no symptoms, the National Heart, Lung, and Blood Institute reports others experience angina (dull, heavy to sharp chest pain or discomfort; pain in the neck, jaw, or throat; or pain in the upper abdomen or back. These symptoms may occur during rest, begin during physical activity, or be triggered by mental stress. High blood pressure, high low-density lipoprotein cholesterol, and smoking are key risk factors for heart disease. About half of Americans (49%) have at least one of these three risk factors.[90] Additional risk factors include diabetes, obesity, poor diet, physical inactivity, excessive alcohol use, vitamin D deficiency,[259] autoimmune disorders (systemic lupus erythematosus and rheumatoid arthritis), and history of pregnancy-related disorders (such as GDM, pregnancy-induced hypertension, and preeclampsia).[25]

**Musculoskeletal System.** Bone, muscle, and connective tissue all are affected by the physiologic changes of menopause, increasing the risk for several musculoskeletal conditions and impairments for women. A natural decline in estrogen levels during menopause causes a progressive decline in muscle mass (sarcopenia) and strength and decrease in bone density.[5,197] Sarcopenia and osteoporosis often coexist, leading to accelerated reduction in quality of life. Musculoskeletal conditions that are more common in women include Colles fracture, carpal tunnel syndrome, adhesive capsulitis, and rotator cuff tendonitis. These conditions may accelerate with menopause-related sarcopenia and kyphotic posture.[5] Researchers in Brazil found no significant association between musculoskeletal pain perception and reproductive life stage. In other words, postmenopausal women do not have more or less pain perception than younger women.[169] The occurrence of inflammatory arthritis is higher in all stages of life for women compared with men, and the risk increases with age. Estrogen has a suppressive effect on the inflammatory responses; therefore MT influences the occurrence of inflammatory arthritis.[539]

***Osteoporosis.*** Osteoporosis occurs from decreased bone mass and statistically is defined as having a BMD of 2.5 standard deviations below the average of a healthy, young woman. *Osteopenia* is BMD lower than the normal peak BMD but above the diagnostic level for osteoporosis. Estrogen limits bone resorption. During MT, declining estrogen results in faster bone resorption. Postmenopausal osteoporosis is a skeletal disease resulting in loss of trabecular bone more than cortical bone, leading to an increased risk in fractures at specific sites such as the vertebral bodies, distal radius, and hip.[492]

Vitamin D deficiency is common in the aging population, particularly among postmenopausal women, although the etiology of the deficiency is not well understood. Vitamin D deficiency is defined as a serum level of 25-hydroxyvitamin D below 10 ng/mL, whereas vitamin D insufficiency is characterized as a serum level of 25-hydroxyvitamin D of 10 to 30 ng/mL. The metabolite 25-hydroxyvitamin D is considered to be the best clinical measure of vitamin D stores.[70] Vitamin D is required for the development and maintenance of bones by assisting in calcium absorption from food in the intestine and supporting bone resorption. Vitamin D deficiency is associated with reduced calcium absorption, hyperparathyroidism, muscle weakness, and increased bone loss. Loss of bone quantity (amount of bone mass) and bone quality (microarchitecture or spatial distribution of bone mass) are both independent predictive factors for fragility fractures.[492] The daily recommended intake of vitamin D for women 50 years and older is 800 to 1000 IU daily. Calcium intake additionally protects bone loss[157] along with lifestyle choices, which can influence peak bone mass 20% to 40%.[542]

*Osteoporotic fractures* are more common than stroke, myocardial infarction, and breast cancer combined in postmenopausal women.[540] As a fracture is often the first sign of osteoporosis in women, it is important to perform a risk assessment to identify risk factors. Adequate vitamin D is an important factor in reducing the risk of osteoporosis. See Chapter 24 for more information on incidence, risk factors, prevention, diagnosis, and treatment of osteoporosis and bone health and Chapter 27 for information specific to fractures.

***Spinal Postural Deformity—Kyphosis/Hyperkyphosis.*** Kyphotic posture of the thoracic spine gradually increases in many women as vertebral height decreases in response to bone volume decrease and/or vertebral fractures during the menopausal years. Kyphotic posture can alter normal biomechanical and anatomic relationships in the shoulder girdle, cervical spine, and lumbopelvic girdle, resulting in impairments to balance reaction and gait patterns that may reduce quality of life[353] and increase fall risk.[334]

***Osteoarthritis.*** Women older than age 50 years are affected by osteoarthritis (OA) more than men, particularly OA of the hand.[538] Before age 50 years, OA is more prevalent among men than women. The role of decreased estrogen in the increase in OA that occurs among women of menopausal age is unclear, and findings are inconsistent and inconclusive, with varying explanations for the association. Menopausal women are at particularly high risk for OA of the basilar joint of the thumb.

**Nervous System.** Estrogen and progesterone both play key roles in neurologic health, with pathologic consequences possible as these hormones decline with menopause. Estradiol is a known neuroprotective factor; its effects promote attenuation of cell death and proliferation of new neurons in the face of injury and disease. Progesterone modulates well-being and cognitive and memory processes in the central nervous system both in normal physiology and in pathology.[418]

The declines in estrogen and progesterone that begin during MT are occurring simultaneously with other age-related changes in the nervous system, contributing to a cascade of neurophysiologic changes that manifest later in life as a variety of impairments and functional changes. In fact, estrogen deficiency is suggested as the initial step in the chain of causality that increases risk for impairments to affective state, cognitive function, dementia, and movement disorders, as well as hot flashes and sleep disturbances.

Early-onset menopause and surgical menopause are associated with increased risk for cognitive impairments, dementia, and Parkinson disease, implying that timing of withdrawal of sex steroids is significant in the manifestation of neurologic pathology associated with menopause. Changes to memory, reasoning, affect, and motor performance all are demonstrated to improve with HRT, reversing the sex steroid deficiency of menopause.[418]

***Psychosocial Factors.*** Women perceive menopause as a time of gains and losses.[225] During MT, women are more vulnerable to depression.[52,127,321,500] A combination of psychosocial factors in midlife combined with common symptoms of menopause (i.e., vasomotor symptoms, sleep disturbance) may complicate, co-occur, and overlap with depression. Most women in midlife who experience a major depressive episode have a prior history of depression.[321] Grief over loss of childbearing status may be more likely among women with surgical menopause who are still of natural childbearing age. Grief can affect women emotionally and psychologically following hysterectomy.[206,549]

Menopause often occurs at a time when family structures and dynamics change. Women in perimenopausal and menopausal years are often involved in managing multiple responsibilities at work, with family, and in the community. In addition to changing roles as caregiver of aging parents, social isolation when children leave home and/or midlife divorce or spousal death occurs can be challenging.[321] Midlife women who feel socially unsupported by family and their social network are at greater risk of developing depression.

Hormonal changes during natural menopause are gradual, whereas these changes are more sudden, severe, and prolonged with surgical menopause.[444] Estrogen and progesterone both have a significant influence on neural mechanisms that impact mood and behavior. Progesterone in the central nervous system modulates well-being as well as cognition and memory. Declines in estrogen trigger reductions in serotonin; serotonin and other monoamine neurotransmitters (norepinephrine and dopamine) regulate mood disorders, sleep, and vasomotor functions. As serotonin levels drop, hot flashes, anxiety, and sleep disturbance become likely; episodes of anxiety may include feelings of irritability and tension. The most common sleep-related disturbance is nocturnal awakenings, often impacting a woman's quality of life, health, and productivity.[35,36] Nocturnal hot flashes and stress are closely linked to insomnia. Insomnia increases 40% during MT[35,36] and affects 40% to 60% of women during MT.[448] Other factors disturbing sleep include disordered breathing, mood disturbance, medical conditions including periodic limb movement disorder and restless legs syndrome, and socioeconomic factors.[35,36] The shared neurotransmitter effects on vasomotor function and mood manifest as a twofold increased risk for depression among women who experience hot flashes during MT.[435] Risk factors increase for women with a history of depression (particularly PMS and postpartum depression), presence of vasomotor symptoms, surgical menopause, adverse life events, and negative attitudes toward menopause and aging.[127,527] Depression and anxiety are independent risk factors for incidence of CHD in women.[341,381]

Behaviors associated with depression include fatigue, inactivity, anhedonia (lack of enjoyment of activities that are usually enjoyable), and social isolation. As women age, changes in energy level and activity may be perceived as normal by affected individuals and their health care practitioners, a perspective that can cause difficulty in diagnosing depression. Inactivity and reduced physical mobility further increase the risk for depression. Many aging women with incontinence choose to minimize social activities as a way of managing the risk of public accidents; social isolation is a behavior exhibited by depressed individuals, as well as a behavior that can increase risk for depression.[10]

Risk for all types of *violence and abuse* (physical, emotional, sexual) is higher for women than men throughout the life span.[164] A history of sexual assault or intimate partner violence and current symptoms of posttraumatic stress disorder are associated with more intense vasomotor symptoms during menopause.[180] Specifically, independent associations have been found between emotional intimate partner violence and night sweats and dyspareunia; sexual assault has been associated with vaginal dryness.[180] Women with greater exposure to trauma throughout their life may also be at greater risk of CVD.[499] Women during MT who experience abuse within the past year, nearly 97% of which is reported as verbal/emotional abuse, report more bothersome menopause symptoms.[499] The presence of extremely bothersome menopausal symptoms may alert health care providers to screen for potential abuse, and women experiencing recent abuse may benefit from more frequent interactions with their health care providers.[518]

## MEDICAL MANAGEMENT

**DIAGNOSIS.** Blood and salivary testing are not recommended in current medical clinical guidelines to determine hormone levels because of a lack of evidence correlating either blood serum or salivary hormone levels to menopause symptoms.[452] There is weak evidence that salivary testing and capillary blood testing correlates to blood serum hormone levels if taken several times over a 24-hour period and done as an adjunct to support symptoms for bioidentical nonprescription hormone therapy.[322] Salivary and capillary blood tests determine bioavailable amounts of hormone that are significantly less than blood serum levels. Most hormone steroids in blood serum are tightly bound to proteins and not readily available for metabolism so the bioavailable hormones levels detected are much lower. Steroid hormone bioidentical assays are accurate for naturally produced hormones but not conjugated hormones from derivatives. Dosages must be monitored

**Table 20.2** Advantages and Disadvantages of Hormone Replacement Therapy

| Risks and Disadvantages | Benefits |
|---|---|
| • Increased risk of heart attack in healthy women in the first year<br>• Small (1.2%) increased risk of stroke in healthy postmenopausal women on EPT after 3 years; 4% after 7 years on ET alone<br>• Increased risk of endometrial cancer (systemic estrogen alone without progestin) in women with an intact uterus<br>• Small increased risk for breast cancer (3%) in healthy postmenopausal women on EPT after 5.6 years[329]<br>• Increased risk of gallbladder disease 6% after 5.6 years on EPT, 7 years on ET alone<br>• Small increased risk of venous thromboembolism (0.11%) after 1 year in women on EPT; 1% after 1 year in women on ET, increased to 2.8% after 7 years<br>• Increased breast density and reduced specificity and sensitivity of mammography<br>• Slight increased risk of dementia and Alzheimer disease in women >65 years<br>• Side effects (e.g., vaginal bleeding, fluid retention, weight gain, bloating, breast swelling and tenderness, headaches, mood swings, depression, skin irritation, constipation, loss of libido[a])<br>• Increased risk of ischemic CVA | • Decreased menopausal symptoms (e.g., hot flashes, night sweats, sleep disturbances, memory loss, fatigue, atrophic changes of vagina or urinary tract)<br>• Maintains skin thickness and elasticity<br>• Prevents accelerated bone loss; maintains bone density; reduces risk of fractures by 50%; clinical fracture risk reduced from 14.1% to 9.2% after 7 years in women taking ET<br>• Decreased risk of breast cancer in healthy postmenopausal women without uterus on ET alone from 2.5% to 1.5% after 7 years[329]<br>• Reduced risk of colon cancer<br>• Reduced risk of coronary artery calcification and coronary heart disease in younger, recently postmenopausal women without a uterus<br>• Prevention or delay of Alzheimer disease (mixed evidence)<br>• Decreases uterine pain<br>• Increases production or prolongs action of serotonin |

*CVA*, Cerebrovascular accident; *EPT*, estrogen progesterone/progestin therapy; *ET*, estrogen therapy.
[a]Some side effects can be managed with a reduced dose, different schedule, or changing brands. Any woman experiencing intolerable side effects should see the prescribing physician for evaluation.

and adjusted.[322] HRT is prescribed based on symptoms and a medical criteria algorithm ruling out contraindications for hormones.[452] Blood assays are used to determine thyroid function that should be assessed before starting hormone therapy because of overlap of symptoms.

**Treatment**

*Hormone Replacement Therapy.* Decisions about HRT for menopause-related symptoms and conditions are based on a thorough medical understanding of the risks and benefits of HRT and how they apply to each woman based on her individual symptoms, conditions, and risks. Table 20.2 lists the advantages and disadvantages of HRT. HRT is primarily used now as short-term therapy to manage vasomotor symptoms and vaginal atrophy and/or for osteoporosis prevention or treatment. Reevaluation of need for HRT is recommended at 6- to 12-month intervals.[329,452] Although there are potential benefits shown in research for managing other symptoms of menopause, particularly sleep disturbances, cognitive impairments (memory, concentration, decision making), and depression, HRT is not recommended as the first treatment of choice. In revised clinical guidelines from the North American Menopause Society, the individual risks versus benefits of any hormone treatment plan should be decided between the patient and her physician (Box 20.3).[329,452]

Bone-specific agents are usually considered more appropriate for long-term osteoporosis prevention or treatment (readers are referred to the discussion of osteoporosis in Chapter 24). If estrogen treatment is elected for isolated vaginal symptoms, low-dose local estrogen therapy is advised and is safe for extended treatment, with the possible exception of patients undergoing certain cancer treatments or at high risk for estrogen-driven cancers.[452,479] In those cases, nonhormone treatments are recommended as the first line of treatment.[161] The lowest effective dose for the shortest period of time is recommended for all hormone therapies by the ACOG.[18] The North American Menopause Society provides guidelines to assist women in understanding the treatment choices related to HRT and menopause.[452]

The Women's Health Initiative (WHI) research arm evaluating the effects of hormonal therapies in midlife

**Box 20.3**

**CONTRAINDICATIONS AND PRECAUTIONS FOR USE OF HORMONE REPLACEMENT THERAPY**

- History of blood clots
- Pancreatic or liver disease
- Hormone-sensitive breast or uterine cancer
- Migraine headaches that are aggravated by estrogen
- Hypertension
- Smoking, obesity, age older than 35 with oral contraceptive use[452]
- Age older than 59 or more than 10 years postmenopause[452]
- History of cardiac disease
- History of uterine fibroids
- History of endometrial cancer
- History of stroke or transient ischemic attacks
- Benign breast disease
- Current breast or endometrial cancer

women was abruptly halted in 2002 by the federal government after a review of unpublished preliminary results suggesting HRT may increase risk of breast cancer, CVD, venous thromboembolism, and cerebrovascular accidents. Millions of women stopped taking HRT overnight. A black box warning was placed on all estrogen-containing prescription drugs, although the WHI looked at only two medications, Premarin, a conjugated estrogen from mare urine, and Prempro, a combination estrogen with progestin (synthetic nonbioidentical progesterone). Newer analyses of WHI research data concluded that the original WHI data were taken out of context without reference to the subject profiles. The targeted audience in that particular study were older (average age 70) women with more health risk factors than the usual population of women prescribed HRT. Subsequent analyses of WHI and other studies showed beneficial risk ratios in younger women or women close to menopause,[288] resulting in new clinical guidelines. HRT is recommended with strong evidence for short-term relief of menopausal-related vasomotor symptoms such as hot flashes, vaginal atrophy, and other symptoms of menopause, including prevention of osteoporosis in some women..[288,329,452]

Whatever decision a woman makes should be in conjunction with her health care provider, based on the individual risks and benefits and the patient's preferences.[452] For women who cannot or prefer not to take HRT, there are alternatives for preventing osteoporosis and heart disease and for managing vasomotor and other distressing symptoms of menopause.

Women seeking pharmacologic management of vasomotor symptoms may be candidates for a trial of nonhormonal prescription off-label options. Selective estrogen reuptake modulators (SERMs)/serotonin-norepinephrine reuptake inhibitors or gabapentin, pregabalin, and clonidine may be considered.[479] These pharmaceuticals stimulate ERs in some tissues, but not in others. Ospemifene, a SERM, may be effective for women without a history of breast cancer presenting with moderate to severe dyspareunia associated with vaginal atrophy.[479] Alternatively, antidepressants can help some women with severe hot flashes. The importance of lifestyle measures such as exercising, maintaining a low-fat calcium-rich diet, and not smoking has been clearly demonstra ted.[329,452,479]

Appropriate interventions for sexual dysfunctions are usually multifactorial and must be individualized. Interventions may include HRT (testosterone or dehydroepiandrosterone), sexual or psychologic counseling, bioidenticals or other alternative or complementary therapies (see below), dietary changes, stress management, behavior modification, exercise, and pelvic floor physical therapy (see Special Implications for the Therapist 20.2).

***Alternative and Complementary Therapies.*** More than one-third of Americans report using complementary and alternative medicines (CAMs), including for treatment of vasomotor symptoms of menopause. Research indicates most patients do not tell their physician they are using over-the-counter medications or megavitamins.[452] Types of CAMs include herbals and botanicals; megadoses of vitamins; folk remedies; energy healing techniques (magnets, crystals); homeopathy; and alternative and mind/body therapies such as acupuncture, reflexology, yoga, meditation, Tai chi, Qigong, and more. The National Institutes of Health notes a shortage of well-designed research studies evaluating the effectiveness of CAMs. There is a growing body of evidence supporting mind/body practices such as yoga, Tai Chi, and meditation-based programs in reducing frequency and intensity of hot flashes, improving sleep and mood disturbances, and reducing muscle and joint pain.[373] There is little evidence supporting the use of botanicals, herbals, and megavitamins. Some may have harmful side effects or may reduce the effectiveness of other medications.[373,452] Therapists should inquire about all homeopathic and over-the-counter medications their patients may be taking.

SPECIAL IMPLICATIONS FOR THE THERAPIST 20.2

## *Menopause*

### History and Interview

Inquiring about menopause during the physical therapy examination of women who are 40 years of age or older is consistent with the expanding role of therapists in primary care.[21] Appropriate topics to cover include onset of menopause signs and symptoms being experienced, medications, alternative therapies, or behavioral strategies being used to manage the symptoms as well as the woman's attitude about the changes of menopause.

The potential pathologic correlates of menopause are important to include in the *screening and risk assessment* components of the history and interview. Obesity, osteoporosis, heart disease, diabetes mellitus, incontinence, UTIs, GI disturbances, sleep disturbance, memory impairment, depression, anxiety, falls, fractures, dental health, inflammatory arthritis, sexual function, and intimate partner violence are specific conditions to cover during screening.[34]

The therapist may wish to develop a menopause-specific questionnaire or use validated outcome tools commonly associated with menopause.[536] Use of a screening tool such as the Beck Depression Inventory[44] or Zung Scale[145] to identify depression may reveal more cases of depression than self-report through an intake questionnaire. Validated questionnaires may also be used to assess memory and cognition if answers to screening questions raise concern. Assessing attitudes about menopause are relevant, as they may increase risk for depression, anxiety, and/or altered body image. Positive screening assessments may signal to the therapist that a referral to other health care providers is appropriate to maximize the patient's rehabilitation potential.

### Physical Examination

The physical examination should be expanded beyond the requirements of the specific purpose of the therapy visit to screen for physical changes associated with menopause and aging. Height, weight, and BMI are not routinely recorded during therapy examination; however, as loss of height and weight gain are effects of aging and menopause, it is sensible to record these measurements and use the information in developing a plan of care.

Attention to spinal posture is indicated, particularly in the presence of excessive kyphotic curve, a potential sign of reduced BMD and risk factor for compression fracture and painful musculoskeletal conditions such as shoulder girdle pain (adhesive capsulitis, rotator cuff impingement, biceps tendonitis). Joint motion and muscle strength measurements provide information related to functional mobility. Tests of balance and sensation are indicated, as well as visual inspection of skin integrity and signs of neurologic or cardiovascular compromise. Assessment of weight distribution and waist circumference may identify patients with truncal obesity, which increases risks for comorbidities such as heart disease and diabetes. Blood pressure should be assessed because CVD and hypertension are common among menopausal women and frequently undiagnosed.

### Evaluation, Diagnosis, Prognosis

Identifying signs, symptoms, and risks associated with menopause informs the evaluation process so that the plan of care addresses a woman's health needs comprehensively. The woman's needs for education, consultation, and/or referral for menopause-related changes may be discovered by expanding the examination to include attention to the known correlates of MT and menopause. Menopause-associated physical impairments, functional limitations, and conditions and/or indications or contraindications for planned interventions may be discovered during the expanded examination, which will also inform the therapist's evaluation and potentially lead to modifications in the plan of care, movement diagnoses, and/or prognosis.

### Physical Activity and Exercise

Physical activity and exercise have a variety of effects that can be used therapeutically to address the changes and conditions associated with menopause. By including a physical activity prescription in the therapy plan of care, therapists can proactively assist women to respond to and/or minimize the effects of aging and estrogen decline.

*Regular physical exercise* may be prescribed to reduce the risk of obesity and its related comorbidities. Long-term benefits of exercise are reduced rates of cancer, dementia, and cognitive decline; reduction of adverse mood and anxiety; and reduction of osteoporosis, osteopenia, falls, and fractures. Additionally, exercise promotes cardiovascular fitness, muscle strength, flexibility, and balance.[195] Exercise also helps reduce menopausal side effects such as hot flashes[313] and improves quality of life during MT.[487]

Resistance exercise is recommended for sarcopenia,[115] whereas aerobic exercise has positive effects on lowering blood pressure and reducing the risk of CVD and type 2 diabetes.[27,324] Combined strength and aerobic training may be beneficial in reducing body fat in postmenopausal women.[422] Combined resistance training with high-impact or weight-bearing exercise is effective in preserving BMD.[567]

*High-intensity exercise* is recommended to reduce many of the effects of menopause and aging, including osteoporosis, CVD, and sleep disturbance.[257,359] Combined with high speed during short time intervals, in water or on the ground, power training executes explosive concentric contractions to prevent and treat postmenopausal osteoporosis. Power training has been found to be safe and effective without increased risk of pain or injury.[359] Mechanical vibration may improve bone microarchitecture, density, and strength as well as function.[359]

Many musculoskeletal disorders that increase with aging are associated with patterns of muscle imbalance and weakness (i.e., shoulder impingement). Training specificity can guide therapists in the design of prevention and wellness exercise programs for menopausal women. Exercise design needs to include focus on posture and cardiovascular and bone health, as well as prevention of diabetes.

### Pelvic Floor Muscle Rehabilitation

*PFM rehabilitation* can be a component of the therapist's plan of care for women in any of the stages of menopause. Research shows that most women do not attribute pelvic floor dysfunctions to hormonal changes with MT,[171] presenting an opportunity for therapists to educate and provide treatment. Pelvic physical therapists provide direct treatment of PFM weakness and spasm. PFM rehabilitation may also be included by all therapists as part of core stability exercise programs for women with a variety of musculoskeletal complaints and associated conditions, such as LBP, PGP, and dysfunction of the hip and shoulder girdle. Detailed information on PFM dysfunction is presented in Chapter 27.

### Postsurgical Rehabilitation (Abdominal and Pelvic Surgeries)

Gynecologic surgery often compromises abdominal and pelvic musculature with immediate and long-term effects. Restorative and preventive rehabilitation efforts after surgery focus on restoring normal neurophysiologic and biomechanical function to the muscles of the lower abdomen and pelvis.[66,129,137] Laparoscopic procedures are increasingly being used for common abdominal and gynecologic surgeries, thereby producing less muscle trauma. However, stretching or ischemic injury during surgical retraction or compression in the abdominal wall may also lead to biomechanical dysfunction, warranting inclusion of physical therapy in the postsurgical plan of care. Postsurgical physical therapy is often indicated to address problems with core stabilizing force production, secondary muscle deconditioning, and pain. Scar mobilization of myofascial restrictions from surgeries including laparoscopic procedures is helpful to address pain, pelvic floor dysfunctions, and posture dysfunctions that can occur months to years after the procedure.

### Manual Therapy

Manual therapy techniques, including myofascial release, joint mobilization, muscle energy, and thrust manipulations, are used for multiple musculoskeletal conditions by physical therapists, osteopathic physicians, chiropractors, and others. Although there are few studies specifically looking at manual therapy treatment in menopausal women, there is weak but favorable evidence in general supporting the benefits of manual therapy treatment for common musculoskeletal conditions that may worsen with aging and menopause.[102,273,472]

In addition to its use in the management of painful musculoskeletal conditions, manual therapy may also be effective in the management of other pelvic pain and urogenital conditions associated with menopause.[102,427]

### Education

Women need to better understand the physiologic processes of MT and menopause, while being educated in evidence-based strategies for managing their symptoms and associated risks secondary to physical and emotional changes occurring during this time of life. Each midlife woman should receive an individualized risk assessment, along with prevention strategies for maximizing her health. Therapists should counsel midlife women about physical activity and exercise, weight management, posture, and bone and cardiovascular health. Women may transition through menopause more easily if educated in healthy exercise and lifestyle behaviors before the onset of menopause.

### Menopause and Disability

With advances in health care, women with physical disabilities are living longer than in previous generations, and health care providers must consider how MT and menopause impact the condition and quality of life of these women. Little evidence exists describing how menopause impacts women with physical disabilities; however, attention is warranted to assess the physical and psychologic changes these women experience, whether related to menopause or aging in general. Therapists can assist these women in maximizing their function using evidence-based strategies for improving ability to perform activities of daily living, learning compensatory strategies, and implementing the use of new advances in assistive technology.[255]

Some disabilities may cause women to experience menopause at an earlier age than their able-bodied peers; therefore therapists may need to assess for early menopause.[517] A woman with a disability may have poorer general health and be at greater risk for comorbid disease. Estrogen loss compromises collagen content and vascular profusion of the skin, putting women who are wheelchair users or immobile at greater risk of skin breakdown and pressure ulcers.[139] Menopausal symptoms are similar for women with disabilities compared with the general population. One study revealed that menopause may accelerate disability in women with multiple sclerosis (MS), possibly owing to estrogen's neuroprotective effect. Most women in the study were not receiving HRT, thereby making it difficult to determine if this would make a difference. Low vitamin D levels are known to be linked to adverse MS outcomes; therefore if indicated, vitamin D supplementation may help positively influence the course of MS during menopause.[71] Evidence is limited in understanding the interaction between HRT and medications used to manage disabilities.[45]

Particular attention to the musculoskeletal system, cardiovascular system, and integumentary system is recommended for physical therapy examination of women with disabilities in MT or menopause. Cardiovascular health and fitness may be impacted by the limited mobility associated with disabilities.

Bone loss associated with perimenopause and on through the transition to menopause may be more pronounced in women with mobility impairments.[139] Whereas an able-bodied woman usually reaches peak bone mass by age 35 years, a woman with a disability may never reach that peak. The risk of bone fracture and related impairments is higher in women with disabilities, especially women who take medications that may further impair bone health (e.g., corticosteroids, tricyclic antidepressants, or anticonvulsants). Therapists can be instrumental in helping women with disabilities develop creative exercise strategies, taking into account their reduced mobility and weight-bearing status. Additional research is needed to better understand how menopause impacts women with disabilities.

## A THERAPIST'S THOUGHTS[a]

### *Menopause*

Many women who seek care from physical therapists are concurrently navigating the stages of menopause. All women of menopausal age who enter physical therapy clinics are affected in some way by the changes associated with menopause. Even if the reason they are in physical therapy is not directly related to menopause, the woman is affected by menopause physically, socially, emotionally, and/or psychologically or is at risk of being affected in the future. Therapists have a great deal to offer perimenopausal and postmenopausal women that will benefit them both short term and long term—often beyond the initial reason the patient or client sought care or consultation from the therapist. The therapist has an obligation to consider the stages of menopause when working with midlife women and how this will influence the therapist's intervention. Therapists who not only accept this responsibility but also take advantage of the opportunity will find working with this population rewarding.

Providing physical therapy care for menopausal women from a primary care approach involves intentionally and comprehensively addressing menopause and its ramifications related to overall health in addition to focusing on the particular health concern that initiated the physical therapy encounter. Taking the comprehensive, primary care approach requires some adjustment in approach to patient/client personal and family health history, interview, and physical examination to balance completeness with efficiency. A variety of resources, forms, and tools are available to assist physical therapists in setting up efficient examination procedures. By taking such a broad approach to examination, evaluation, and treatment planning, physical therapists have the opportunity to facilitate long-standing and far-reaching effects on the overall health and quality of life of menopausal women in their care.

Most of the changes associated with menopause that create difficulty and distress in women's lives are positively affected by exercise and physical activity; manual therapy is also helpful for many menopause-related symptoms. Education about menopause benefits all women no matter their age or stage of menopause. Therapists can use evidence regarding the benefits of exercise to support recommendations or prescriptions for physical activity to address osteoporosis, depression, anxiety, cardiac disease, and many other conditions associated with menopause.

As women age, health declines, and health-related decisions for both patients/clients and practitioners increase in complexity. Patient/client education, consultation, and referrals are key strategies therapists can use to maximize the information and services available to inform and support women to move with good health through the stages of menopause.

Many of the issues that arise during menopause are of an intimate or potentially embarrassing nature, requiring the therapist to assess his or her own comfort and competence addressing functional issues and impairments, including psychologic, sexual, intestinal, and urologic functions.

Referrals to other therapists or health care practitioners are often warranted, so development of a network of colleagues for consultation and referral is often necessary. Therapists also have the opportunity to create consulting roles to other practices and women in the community for non–clinic-based education and consultation related to menopause, quality of life, physical functioning, and the benefits and services offered by physical therapy. Therapists who expand their clinical skills by incorporating their knowledge of how a woman's body changes during menopause into their therapy plan of care will significantly enhance the quality of rehabilitation these women receive.

[a]Patricia (Trish) M. King, PT, PhD, OCS, MTC

## DISORDER OF THE FEMALE UPPER GENITAL TRACT

### Pelvic Inflammatory Disease

#### Overview and Incidence

PID, which refers to infection and inflammation of the female upper genital tract, comprises a variety of conditions (i.e., it is not a single entity) including endometritis, salpingitis, tuboovarian abscess, and pelvic peritonitis. Any inflammatory condition affecting the female reproductive organs (uterus, fallopian tubes, ovaries, and cervix) may come under the diagnostic label of PID. It is a common cause of infertility, chronic pelvic pain (CPP), and ectopic pregnancy.[202] Prevalence of self-reported PID is 4.4% among women of reproductive age (2.2 million women in the United States).[275] Prevalence is complicated by the wide variety of conditions and varying diagnostic criteria.

#### Etiology and Risk Factors

PID occurs as a result of multimicrobial bacteria, such as *Neisseria gonorrhoeae, Chlamydia trachomatis,* and anaerobic and mycoplasmal bacteria. Gonorrhea and chlamydia (two common STIs) acquired through vaginal, oral, or anal intercourse are the most likely causes of PID. Infection can occur when the uterus is traumatized. Infection can be introduced from the skin, vagina, or GI tract. It can be an acute, one-time episode or chronic with multiple recurrences.

PID is often associated with STIs and sexually transmitted diseases (STDs) or develops after birth or after a surgical procedure involving the reproductive tract such as an abortion or a dilation and curettage. Dilation and curettage is a procedure to scrape and collect the tissue (endometrium) from inside the uterus. Dilation is a widening of the cervix to allow instruments into the uterus; curettage is the scraping of the contents of the uterus.

Early age at first vaginal intercourse (higher prevalence for age younger than 12 years) and number of male sex partners (more than 10 lifetime partners) are two major risk factors for PID.[275] PID occurs if an STI is not treated, and even if treated, some damage to the pelvic cavity cannot be reversed. Other risk factors include bisexual and lesbian sexual activity, a sexual partner who reports symptoms or has a known history of STI, and previous pelvic infection.

#### Clinical Manifestations

Signs and symptoms of PID vary widely, making the medical diagnosis difficult. It is often asymptomatic but can manifest with vaginal bleeding and discharge and burning during urination. Constitutional symptoms associated with infection, such as fever or chills and sometimes nausea and vomiting, may be reported.

Painful intercourse (dyspareunia), painful menstruation, and back or pelvic pain are commonly reported. Moderate (dull aching) to severe back, abdominal, and/or pelvic pain are possible. If the condition progresses to PID, scarring in the pelvic organs, including the ovaries, fallopian tubes, bowel and bladder, can cause chronic pain. The woman can become infertile because of damage and scarring of the fallopian tubes.

After one episode of PID, a woman's risk of ectopic pregnancy increases sevenfold compared with the risk for women who have no history of PID.[89,88] Ectopic pregnancy can occur when a partially blocked or slightly damaged fallopian tube causes an egg to get stuck in the fallopian tube, where it is then fertilized.

### MEDICAL MANAGEMENT

**PREVENTION.** PID can be prevented by making safer choices to avoid STIs (e.g., always using barrier methods during intercourse, limiting number of sexual partners, frequent testing for treatment of STIs, choosing a partner who does not have a current or previous history of STD, and abstaining from sexual activity until an infected partner has completed treatment). If an STI does occur, all medication prescribed must be taken to prevent reinfection and progression to PID.

**DIAGNOSIS, TREATMENT, AND PROGNOSIS.** PID is diagnosed on the basis of clinical presentation, a physical and pelvic examination, and laboratory tests. Clinical presentation is often useful in identifying women who could benefit from treatment.[91] Sexually active young women with pelvic or lower abdominal pain and tenderness of the uterus, of the adnexa, or with cervical motion should be considered for initiation of treatment and possible further investigations.

A vaginal swab or urine sample is taken and sent to the laboratory. Ultrasound may be used to visualize the fallopian tubes or screen for pelvic abscess. Laparoscopic examination (a thin, flexible tube with a light at the end is inserted through a small incision in the lower abdomen) allows the surgeon to view the internal organs and take tissue samples for diagnostic purposes. Endometrial biopsy and magnetic resonance imaging (MRI) may also be used to confirm the diagnosis.

PID is curable with antibiotics; prompt treatment does not reverse any damage already done. PID may require hospitalization and can be life threatening. Complications of PID include CPP, infertility (inability or difficulty getting pregnant), and ectopic or tubal pregnancy.

The CDC recommends that all sexually active teens and young women be screened annually for STIs. Any woman who has had a new sexual partner (male or female) and women with multiple sexual partners should be screened regularly. Signs of infection or recurrence of infection should be investigated immediately and treated appropriately.[88,89]

## DISORDERS OF THE UTERUS AND FALLOPIAN TUBES

### Endometriosis

#### Overview and Incidence

Endometriosis is an estrogen-dependent disorder defined by the presence of endometrial-like tissue outside of the uterus. Usually the disorder becomes apparent in the early teen years after menses begins, and its symptoms continue until menopause, although endometriosis has been identified in women after menopause.[49,358] This is biochemically and endocrine active and responds to changes in the hormonal system. Every month during the menses, a woman with endometriosis develops a host of symptoms that depend on where the endometrial-like tissue. During menstruation, the dislocated tissue is responding just as the uterine lining, eventually forming scar tissue and irritating the affected area.

The American Society of Reproductive Medicine has classified endometriosis as follows: stage I, minimal; stage II, mild; stage III, moderate; stage IV, severe. Staging takes into account location, depth, and size of implants and the presence and severity of adhesions. Despite this classification system, a woman can have severe disease without symptoms or severe symptoms with minimal disease. Severe pelvic pain negatively affects a woman's ability to work, her family relationships, and her self-esteem.[234]

Endometriosis incidence estimates vary based on diagnostic method and are complicated by the large number of asymptomatic women. In the general population, incidence of the disease is conservatively estimated at 11%.[77] Endometriosis is found in up to 50% of all infertile women. In young women who present with pelvic pain, the retrospective incidence of endometriosis is as high as 98%.[384] Incidental endometriosis, the visualization of endometrial lesions in women undergoing procedures for unrelated conditions, is reported to be as high as 30% to 50%.[77] Similarly, 4% to 43% of asymptomatic women undergoing tubal ligation have endometrial lesions.[77]

#### Risk Factors

Any woman of childbearing age is at risk of developing endometriosis, but it is more common in women who have postponed pregnancy. In addition, other risk factors include early menarche, regular menstruation but 27-day or shorter cycles, and menstrual periods lasting 7 days or longer. The cause of endometriosis is unknown, although the high prevalence among family members suggests a genetic predisposition. A woman with a maternal history of endometriosis has twice the chance of developing endometriosis herself. Other risk factors include low birth weight, consumption of red meat and trans-unsaturated fatty acids, and exposure to endocrine-disrupting chemicals such as diethylstilbestrol.[183] A large study found no association between caffeine, alcohol, smoking, or physical activity and endometriosis.[215]

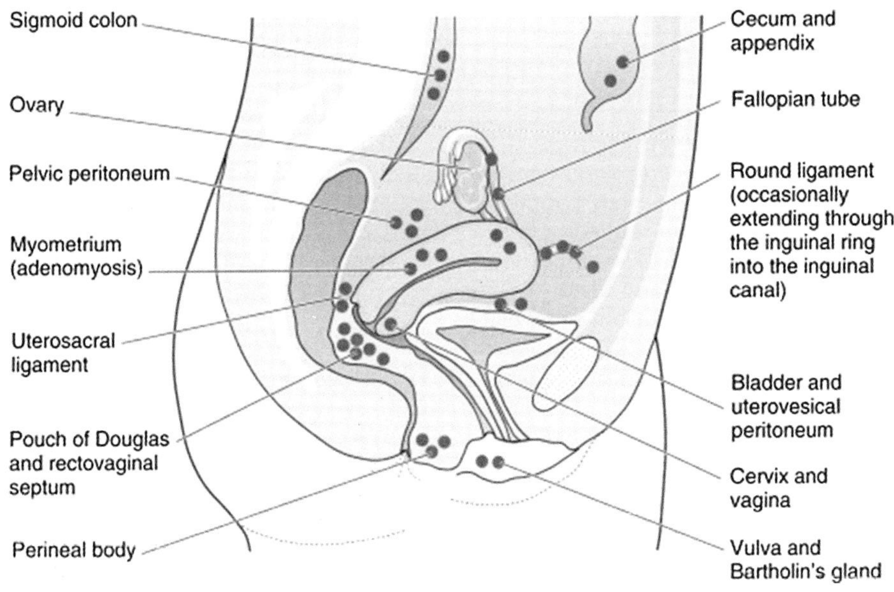


**Figure 20.2**

**Potential sites of endometrial implantation.** (From Drife J, Magowan B: *Clinical obstetrics and gynecology*, Philadelphia, 2004, Saunders.)

## Etiology and Pathogenesis

The etiology of endometriosis is still unclear despite research. Endometrial like tissue implants are found more often on posterior structures, sometimes giving rise to LBP. The most common sites of implantation include the ovaries, fallopian tubes, broad ligaments, pouch of Douglas, bladder, pelvic musculature, perineum, vulva, vagina, or intestines (Figs. 20.2 and 20.3). Although less common, endometrial tissue can also be found in the abdominal cavity and implanted on the kidneys, small bowel, appendix, diaphragm, pleura, bony elements of the spine,[158,165] and even the surface of the skin.

One strongly held hypothesis is a dysregulation or dysfunction of the immune system that allows these cells to locate and survive where they do not belong. In women with endometriosis the endometrial-like tissue located outside the uterus cells are resistant to the body's normal defense mechanisms and is not readily cleared away. Additionally, inflammation appears to play a role, but it is unclear whether inflammation predisposes women to endometriosis or is the by-product of endometriosis. Increased levels of proinflammatory cytokines have been found in several locations, including peritoneal fluid, blood, and endometrial tissue of women with endometriosis.[235]

Other theories include (1) dissemination of endometrial cells through the lymphatics or vascular system (endometrial tissue can migrate throughout the body and has been recovered from bone, lungs, and brain[184]); (2) metaplasia of the mesothelium (Meyer's theory), that is, endometrial cells change from one type of cell to another, whereby the endothelium undergoes transformation able to produce the same reproductive hormones (explains the presence of tissue in joints); (3) intraoperative implantation associated with procedures such as hysterectomy and episiotomy; (4) abnormal differentiation of precursor epithelial cells during early embryology, whereby these cells are seeded before birth (this may be related to a genetic predisposition and may explain endometriosis in girls before menstruation); and (5) central sensitization, including functional and structural changes in the central and peripheral nervous systems (these changes ultimately increase the perception of pain and may result in spread of pain to other areas; structural changes could include nerve sprouting of sensory and sympathetic nerves with branching of blood vessels.[31] A significant

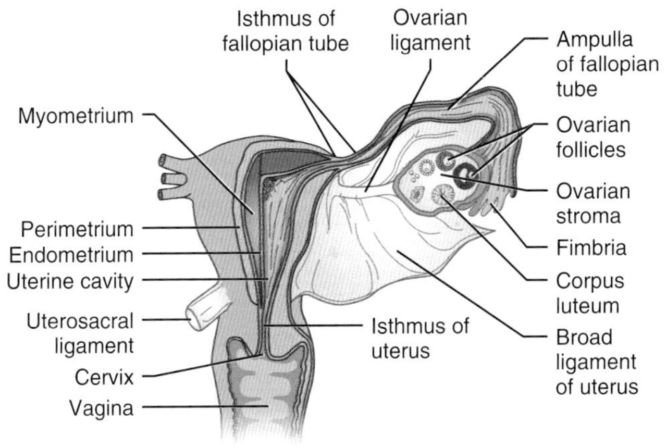


**Figure 20.3**

**Detailed anatomy of the uterus and fallopian tubes.**

positive association with endometriosis has been found with γ-hexachlorocyclohexane and β-hexachlorocyclohexane, used as insecticides and pharmaceuticals in lice and scabies treatments.[76]

Once endometrial-like tissue, can form pockets of tissue referred to as implants. These implants swell in response to the cyclic surge of estrogen and progesterone, forming cysts on the underlying organs that contain a dark, syrupy fluid composed of old blood called *chocolate cysts*. These lesions create chemical irritation, inflammation, and scarring leading to adhesions and distortion of anatomy. These changes may result in closing of the fallopian tubes or moving the ovaries away from the fallopian tubes making uptake and fertilization of the ovum difficult or impossible.

There are three primary pathologic types of endometriosis: (1) red or petechial implants are the most active, with the greatest capacity to produce prostaglandins (inflammatory mediators) and also capable of producing endometrial protein and hormones; (2) brown or intermediate implants are moderately active and precursors to powder burns; and (3) black or brown powder-burn implants are inactive with little cellular material, but are associated with adhesions that stretch organs and cause direct nerve damage through devitalization and ischemia. The powder-burn implants adhere structures together, contributing to infertility, and are sometimes referred to as a *frozen pelvis*. The severity of the disease depends on which one of these three types is present.

### Clinical Manifestations

Vercellini and colleagues[520] conducted a large study to identify correlation of endometriosis stage, location of lesions, and other factors to symptom severity. The authors found only a weak association. They listed 22 studies of the same type with similarly confusing results. At the present time there is a lack of understanding regarding how visual findings relate to symptoms.[232] The symptoms and signs associated with endometriosis depend on the location of the implants. Cyclic pelvic pain and infertility are the two major symptoms. The therapist may hear reports of intermittent, cyclic, or constant pelvic pain and/or LBP (unilateral or bilateral). Deep endometriosis is associated with very severe pain and may involve the ureter causing hydronephrosis.[271] As noted earlier, the extent of the disease does not always correlate with the intensity of the symptoms. A woman with widespread lesions may be asymptomatic, whereas a woman with few implants may have considerable pain.

Dysmenorrhea is common and results in pelvic pain, fatigue, and mood changes beginning 1 or 2 days before the onset of the menstrual flow and continuing for the duration of menses. Dyspareunia (painful intercourse) is also associated with this condition, as penile penetration can pull on adhesions. Pain during defecation can occur when there are adhesions on the large bowel.

Other symptoms include low-grade fever; diarrhea; constipation; rectal bleeding; and referred pain to the low back/sacral, groin, posterior leg, upper abdomen, or lower abdominal/suprapubic areas. Bleeding from anywhere else (e.g., nose bleeds, coughing up blood, or blood in urine or stools) is less common but still possible. Chronic abdominal pain can result in altered posture and body mechanics, particularly maintaining trunk flexion. This in turn may contribute to other musculoskeletal disorders, which add another layer to the pain syndrome.

Women with endometriosis are three times more likely to report infertility and six times more likely to take longer than 12 months to conceive.[561] It is also important to note that some endometrial lesions spontaneously regress, contributing to the confusion in whether to treat the condition aggressively.

## MEDICAL MANAGEMENT

**DIAGNOSIS.** Although the classic triad of cyclic dysmenorrhea, dyspareunia, and infertility strongly suggests the presence of endometriosis, accurate diagnosis requires direct visual examination by laparoscopy or laparotomy. One advantage of laparoscopy is that lesions can be removed immediately. However, many women do not have symptoms severe enough for invasive diagnostics, resulting in underdiagnosis. Ultrasound and MRI can be used but result in significantly lower incidence of endometriosis than visualization. Direct visualization remains the gold standard in diagnosis of endometriosis. Several biomarkers are under investigation in the hopes of early diagnosis and treatment in young women.[235]

**TREATMENT.** There is no cure for endometriosis; the goals of medical treatment are preservation of fertility and pain relief. Endometriosis can occur with other diseases of the pelvis, including IBS, vulvodynia, PID, interstitial cystitis, and fibromyalgia. In such cases, overall treatment would include treatment for associated conditions. Pregnancy appears to suppress the disease, although the condition recurs in many women.[7] In animal studies the implants disappear during pregnancy.[522] Studies assessing the success of treatment for endometriosis are difficult owing to the complexity of the disease and coexisting conditions. Placebo effect has been measured as high as 45%. Both medical and surgical treatments are effective. No studies have compared treatments. Often it is most effective to offer a combined approach in which surgery is followed by medical treatment.[496]

First-line treatment is nonsteroidal antiinflammatory drugs or other analgesics administered before or during menstruation. Many women find sufficient pain relief with these over-the-counter medications; however, a Cochrane review found insufficient data to support their widespread use.[496] Other medications are used to inhibit ovulation and lower hormone levels to prevent the cyclic stimulation of the endometrial implants. Eventually the implants will decrease in size. These medications include danazol, a combination estrogen-progesterone acetate, and leuprolide (Lupron), which is injected once per month into the muscle. Gonadotropin-releasing hormone (GnRH) is also useful in decreasing endometriosis pain. These medications act on the hypothalamus-to-pituitary interface to shut down the ovaries by blocking the ability to produce gonadotropins such as FSH and LH. Most will have side effects related to medically induced menopause including weight gain, edema, decreased breast size, acne, oily skin, headache, muscle cramps, and deepening of the voice. They can also adversely affect lipid metabolism and raise blood pressure.

Combined oral contraceptives and progesterone-only pills may be used to reduce painful symptoms and inhibit menstrual periods, which stop the growth of endometriotic implants, but these do not cause complete regression of implants already present. Once the woman stops oral contraceptive use, these implants become active again, sometimes with a rebound effect (symptoms are much worse). No medication has been shown to be superior,[496] and treatment often involves trials of medications.[485]

Surgical intervention aims to coagulate all visible endometrial liaisons, excise endometrial cysts, disrupt afferent nerves in the pelvis, cut adhesions, and restore anatomy. At the present time the optimal surgical technique has not been established. Excision of implants lowers recurrence and is effective in decreasing pain, although regrowth may occur in approximately one-third of women. Techniques include a variety of laparoscopic cauterization or laser procedures, presacral neurectomy, and uterosacral nerve ablation.[496] If the woman is older than 35 years of age, is disabled by the pain, and her childbearing is completed, a total hysterectomy, bilateral salpingo-oophorectomy (removal of ovaries and fallopian tubes), and implant removal are considered. Surgical excision of deep endometriosis provides pain relief and may improve the woman's chances of conceiving.[271]

Nontraditional therapies such as yoga, acupuncture,[541] naturopathic medicine,[426] and homeopathy may be useful adjuncts to allopathic medicine. Many women are using this type of alternative/complementary intervention combined with diet and nutrition to self-treat without medications. Numerous resources are now available in this area.[38,124,152,348]

**PROGNOSIS.** As mentioned, there is no cure for endometriosis, although pregnancy and menopause appear to arrest its continued development, with alterations in reproductive hormones.[573] Endometriosis has been linked with reproductive cancers and melanoma.[81,179] The link between endometriosis and these diseases remains unclear. A genetic predisposition and shared exposures to environmental toxins (especially dioxins) have been suggested, but the findings are inconsistent and inconclusive.[444,573]

**SPECIAL IMPLICATIONS FOR THE THERAPIST 20.3**

*Endometriosis*

Therapists may encounter endometriosis as a primary diagnosis, as a comorbidity, or as an undiagnosed condition. Many women note that their back or pelvic pain is cyclic. It is possible that the hormonal changes associated with menstruation result in ligamentous laxity, thereby stressing the joints of the pelvis and resulting in cyclic pain. This is only one possible scenario. Therapists should consider all possibilities, including pelvic disease. Troyer[507] reported on a case involving a 25-year-old woman with sudden-onset severe LBP. The patient reported pain waking her from sleep and no difference in pain from sitting to walking. In addition, the objective findings were mild and inconsistent. Further medical evaluation revealed endometriosis and an ovarian cyst, which were successfully treated with surgery, resulting in resolution of her pain. Therapists should be aware of the possibility of endometriosis in patients with pelvic pain.

Endometriosis may account for false-positive findings during the therapist's physical examination. For example, if there are endometrial implants on the psoas major muscle, local palpation and length or strength testing of the psoas may be provocative. The therapist may be led to believe the psoas is the origin of the pain complaints. Endometrial implants on PFMs and ligaments, sacroiliac ligaments, and abdominal wall muscle may lead to similar false-positive findings.

The medications commonly given to treat endometriosis can result in a variety of side effects that can account for a woman's symptoms. GI system complaints (dyspepsia, nausea) may be related to the pain or the antiinflammatory medication being taken. GnRH medications can result in hot flashes and vaginal dryness. Danazol can cause weight gain, acne, decreased breast size, and hirsutism.

Physical therapists can help women with known endometriosis pain in several ways.[350] Most effective approaches include multimodal treatment, and no one modality has been found to be superior.[97] General pain management includes (1) generalized aerobic exercise to release endorphins and maintain overall health, avoiding jarring exercises, which may increase pain in the presence of adhesions; (2) pain-relieving modalities such as transcutaneous electrical nerve stimulation[349] and continuous low-level heat[6]; (3) stress management, breathing exercises, and relaxation training[79,566]; (4) education on posture and body mechanics; and (5) therapeutic pain education.[31,311] Physical therapists can also offer evaluation and treatment for coexisting musculoskeletal disorders often related to poor posture with chronic abdominal pain. Exercise has been shown to decrease pain and improve posture in women with endometriosis,[32] thus decreasing pain from other structures such as cramped muscles and strained joints. The abdominal muscles should also be evaluated for trigger points, and treatment offered accordingly.[31] In all cases, patients/clients should have a complete home management program for further flares and progression of symptoms.

## Uterine Fibroids

### Overview

Uterine fibroids (benign tumors of the myometrial layer of the uterus) forming on the outer surface of the uterus or within the walls or lining of the uterus are common, occurring in up to 50% of all premenopausal women[319] age 35 years or older. Risk factors include age, nulliparity, obesity, smoking, PCOS, diabetes, and hypertension; incidence is higher in African American women compared with white women.[156,445] Fibroids can grow or regress,

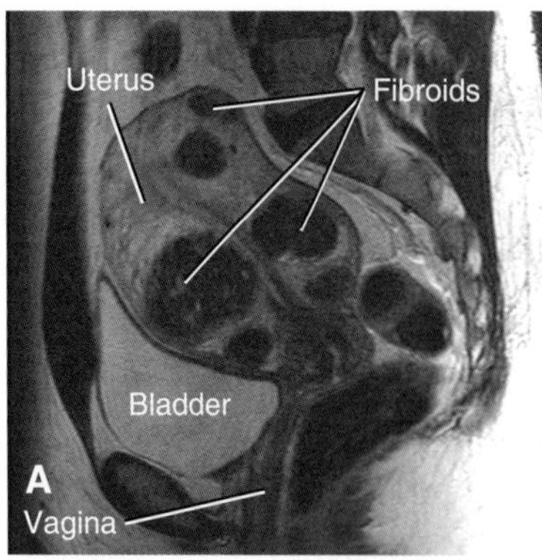


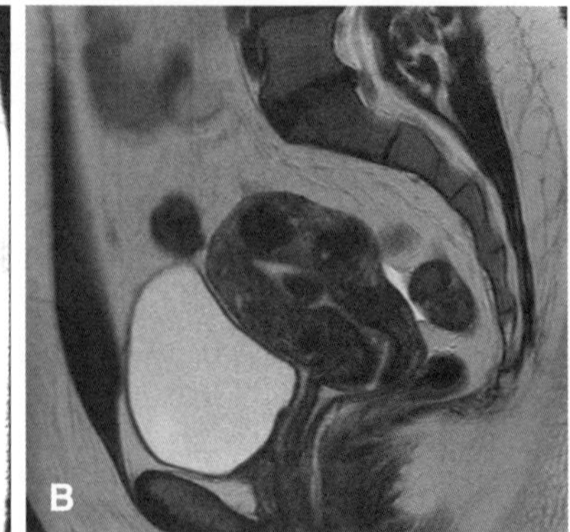


**Figure 20.4**

**Uterine fibroids.** (A) Magnetic resonance imaging of uterine fibroids. Note the position in relation to the sacrum, bladder, and pubic bone. Pressure on nerves and soft tissue in this area can cause painful pelvic, abdominal, low back, and sacral pain. (B) Magnetic resonance imaging of fibroids after uterine fibroid embolization (same individual). (Courtesy Robert L. Vogelzang, MD, Chicago, IL.)

and growth is not linear.[178] These fibroids constitute the primary reason women have hysterectomies.[471]

### Clinical Manifestations

Usually, uterine fibroids are asymptomatic, but pain, urinary or bowel discomfort, and abnormally heavy vaginal bleeding during or between menstrual periods can occur. Symptomatic women often become anemic, experiencing fatigue and weakness that contribute to an impaired lifestyle. In addition to pain and heavy bleeding, dysmenorrhea, pelvic pressure, infertility, miscarriage, and preterm labor are also associated with fibroids.[297,429]

Fibroids, also known as uterine leiomyomas, can and often do grow to the size of a grapefruit or larger. Growth is related to estrogen and progesterone; fibroids often regress after menopause and may grow again if hormone replacement is initiated. Fibroids can place pressure on the bladder, resulting in constipation, urinary frequency and urgency, and nocturia. Pressure on spinal nerves can also cause LBP (Fig. 20.4).

### Medical Management

**Diagnosis.** Diagnosis is based on history, clinical presentation, and clinical examination; uterine fibroids are frequently found incidentally during a routine pelvic examination (irregular shape of the uterus). Transvaginal ultrasonography or hysteroscopy (scope placed through the cervix into the uterus) may be used when diagnostic confirmation is needed.

**Treatment.** GnRH medications decrease estrogen in women and have been shown to shrink fibroids, decrease bleeding, and improve hemoglobin levels; they can also result in disturbing hot flushes.[297] These medications can also decrease blood loss during surgical removal of fibroids, and result in shorter surgical time and less complications. They cannot be used long term owing to bone loss. Pharmacotherapy to control fibroid-related symptoms may include nonsteroidal antiinflammatory drugs and drugs for pain control.

Surgical options include myomectomy (removing only the fibroid) or hysterectomy (removing the entire uterus). Fibroids embedded in the uterine wall usually require a laparoscopy or more invasive open abdominal surgery. Hysterectomy is considered the definitive treatment and remains the mainstay of treatment despite less invasive alternatives. There are no studies comparing the various treatment modalities for fibroids.[162,445]

A less invasive technique and alternative to hysterectomy, called *uterine fibroid embolization* or *uterine artery embolization,* may be possible for select individuals. This procedure is performed with the woman under local anesthesia and mild sedation; the radiologist inserts a catheter into the femoral artery through a small incision in the groin and then uses fluoroscopy to guide the catheter into the uterus. Tiny beadlike or small sponge particles (polyvinyl alcohol) are injected; they block the blood supply to the smaller arteries supplying the fibroids, causing them to shrink and die.

Another alternative to hysterectomy is endometrial (or balloon) ablation in which the uterine lining is destroyed (but not the uterus) through electrical energy or heat from a balloon-tipped catheter inserted in the vagina, through the cervix, into the uterus. The balloon is then filled with a sterile solution until it conforms to the shape of the uterus and is heated until the heat destroys the endometrial tissue. A conservative alternative, known as *magnetic resonance–guided focused ultrasound,* preserves the uterus and is safe and effective.[319]

Eliminating red meat and ham from the diet and eating green vegetables, fruit, and fish appear to have a protective effect. Presumably, diet influences levels of the estrogen hormone, which is known to affect fibroid growth.[98]

**SPECIAL IMPLICATIONS FOR THE THERAPIST 20.4**

### *Uterine Fibroids*

Physical therapy is not directly involved in the treatment of fibroids. Recovery after uterine fibroid procedures may require several weeks, and treatment for other conditions may need to be delayed until the woman is released to full activity. Fatigue may persist and occur rapidly without warning for the first month after the procedure. Subjectively, some women report an immediate sense of relief from pain and congestion with gradual decrease in abdominal distention. The therapist can assist in recovery in a similar way as for the treatment of endometriosis by addressing compensatory postures and gait for individuals who had pain long enough to cause such changes. The therapist can assess for abnormalities and asymmetries in muscle strength and function throughout the abdomen, trunk, pelvis, and hips. If hysterectomy is warranted, postsurgical recovery may be more extensive.

## Uterine Cancer

### Overview and Incidence

Gynecologic cancers do not get as much attention as other cancers such as breast cancer, but according to the American Cancer Society (ACS), it was estimated that more than 110,000 new cases of gynecologic cancers were diagnosed in the United States in 2018 with greater than 32,000 deaths.[11]

The uterus has a body (corpus) and cervix. Although the cervix is technically part of the uterus, uterine cancer usually means cancer of the uterine body. The body of the uterus has three distinct layers. The inner layer or lining of the uterus is called the endometrium, and cancer forming in the glandular tissue of the endometrium is called *adenocarcinoma*. Endometrial adenocarcinoma is the most common cancer of the female reproductive system and the fourth most common cancer in women. Endometrial cancer was estimated to account for approximately 63,230 new cases and 11,350 deaths in 2018.[11]

The middle layer of the uterus is a layer of smooth muscle called the myometrium. This is covered by the outer serous layer of the uterus called the perimetrium. Cancer that forms in the muscle of the uterus is called a *uterine sarcoma*, and this is much less common than endometrial carcinoma. The uterus can also develop a *carcinosarcoma* that starts in the endometrium but has features of both a carcinoma and a sarcoma.

### Risk Factors and Etiology

Endometrial carcinoma is more common in Caucasian women and in women who live in North America or Europe. The lifestyle and environmental factors associated with developed and affluent countries increase the risk of endometrial cancer.[9] Increased caloric intake and obesity, a sedentary lifestyle,[68] and a higher life expectancy influence the incidence and prevalence of endometrial cancer.[9] Postmenopausal women, generally women older than age 50, develop the disease more frequently than premenopausal women. The mean age of diagnosis is 61 years. Reproductive factors that increase exposure to estrogen increase the risk of endometrial cancer. These include younger age at menarche, late age at menopause, infertility, PCOS, nulliparity, and long-term use of unopposed (without progesterone) estrogen hormone therapy.[177] The SERMs tamoxifen and raloxifene are used to reduce the risk of breast cancer by blocking estrogen in breast cells. However, tamoxifen can enhance rather than suppress the action of estrogen in the uterus of older women, causing endometrial overgrowth and an increased risk for endometrial cancer. Family history of uterine, colon, or ovarian cancer increases the risk, as does a genetic predisposition for Lynch and Cowden syndromes. Women who inherit mutations in the *BRCA* or *PTEN* genes may be at increased risk for endometrial cancer. Hypertension, diabetes mellitus (insulin resistance), and uterine fibroids predispose women to endometrial cancer.[267] The main risk factors for uterine sarcoma include radiation therapy to the pelvic region, being African American, and a history of retinoblastoma (eye cancer).

Cigarette smoking, physical activity and exercise, and the use of hormonal contraceptives appear to decrease the risk. In fact, women who exercise are 80% less likely to develop endometrial cancer than women who do not exercise at all.[9] In postmenopausal women, taking combined estrogen and progesterone hormone therapy reduces the risk of endometrial cancer.

### Pathophysiology

Evidence points to multiple histologic subtypes of endometrial cancer based on cell type, each with distinct genetic etiology, presentation, and natural history.[280,380] These include endometrioid adenocarcinomas (called type 1), which account for approximately 85% to 90% of cases, and serous carcinomas (3% to 10%) and clear cell carcinomas (<5%) (called type 2), which are less common.[47] Uterine sarcomas, including carcinosarcomas (also considered type 2), account for approximately 9% of uterine cancers.

Type 1 is the most common type, is not very aggressive, and has the most favorable prognosis.[380] It is hormonally related (owing to unopposed estrogen stimulation) and associated with hyperplasia. Most of the risk factors listed refer to this type of endometrial carcinoma. This type of endometrial cancer arises through a series of changes at the cellular level accompanied by specific alterations in gene expression and activity.[331,513] Type 1 is further subdivided into grade 1 and 2 according to histologic tumor cell differentiation (how closely the tissue looks like normal cells under a microscope). These cells reflect more normal tissue and do not spread to other tissues very quickly. The International Federation of Gynecology and Obstetrics (FIGO) classification system[167] is used for gynecologic cancers and defines histologic differentiation of endometrial adenocarcinoma as follows: FIGO grade 1, 5% or less of tumor tissue is solid tumor growth, cells are well differentiated; FIGO grade 2, 6% to 50% of tissue is solid tumor growth, cells are moderately differentiated; FIGO grade 3, more than 50% of tissue is solid tumor growth, cells are poorly differentiated.

Type 2 endometrial cancers are more aggressive tumors that are not hormonally related. They are associated with endometrial atrophy and poorly differentiated cells. They are considered higher grade cancers (grade 3), are more likely to advance locally or metastasize, have a worse prognosis, and account for a disproportionate number of cancer deaths.[380]

PCOS and insulin sensitivity may play a role in the pathogenesis of endometrial cancer, possibly through hormone disruption. The role of the tumor suppressor gene *PTEN* in the development of endometrial cancers has been reported. Loss of *PTEN* activity is frequently observed in endometrial cancers, although the exact mechanisms for initiation and progression remain unclear.[513,560]

**Table 20.3** Symptoms of Gynecologic Cancers

| Symptoms | Uterine Cancer | Cervical Cancer | Ovarian Cancer | Vaginal Cancer | Vulvar Cancer |
|---|---|---|---|---|---|
| Abnormal bleeding not related to menstruation; any postmenopausal bleeding | X | X | X | X | |
| Abnormal vaginal discharge | X | X | X | X | |
| Feeling full too quickly or difficulty eating | | | X | | |
| Pelvic pain or pressure | X | | X | | |
| Urinary frequency and urgency | X | | X | X | |
| Dysuria (painful urination) | X | | X | | |
| Bloating | | | X | | |
| Abdominal or back pain | X | | X | | |
| Dyspareunia (painful intercourse) | X | X | X | X | |
| Mass or lump in the vagina | X | X | X | X | |
| Itching, burning, pain, tenderness at the vulva | | | | | X |

### Clinical Manifestations

Endometrial cancer has a major identifiable symptom in its early stages: abnormal bleeding (present in 90% of all cases). The most typical presentation of endometrial cancer is vaginal bleeding in a woman who is at least 12 months past menopause (cessation of menses). While not all women present with the same symptoms, Table 20.3 illustrates common symptoms associated with specific gynecologic cancers.[509] Metastases to the lymphatic system can result in abdominal or lower extremity swelling and signal more advanced disease. When metastatic spread occurs, the most common sites are lymph nodes, vagina, peritoneum, and lungs. Less typical sites include extraabdominal lymph nodes, liver, adrenals, brain, bones, and soft tissue.[280]

## MEDICAL MANAGEMENT

**PREVENTION AND SCREENING.** At the present time, the best prevention plan for any cancer is to maintain a healthy weight through diet and regular physical activity. Despite ongoing efforts, early detection of uterine cancer in women of average risk by a screen or laboratory test is not currently available. Women at increased risk, especially if a family member is found to have a gene mutation, may want to consider genetic testing. A prophylactic hysterectomy may be considered if childbearing is completed.

**DIAGNOSIS AND STAGING.** Abnormal bleeding in a woman of any age must be medically evaluated. Diagnosis of uterine cancer is based on tissue pathology, usually obtained by an endometrial biopsy, but ultrasonography of endometrial thickness and hysteroscopy have also been used. Diagnosis of a uterine sarcoma is made by pathologic examination of myomectomy or hysterectomy specimen.

Staging of cancer provides uniform terminology for better communication among health professionals. Staging refers to the extent of the cancer and reflects variation in treatment strategies.[172] For uterine cancer it is determined surgically with a hysterectomy, bilateral salpingo-oophorectomy, and bilateral pelvic lymphadenectomy using the FIGO classification.[167]

**TREATMENT.** Endometrial cancer is usually treated surgically with total laparoscopic or abdominal hysterectomy and bilateral salpingo-oophorectomy,[175] although fertility-sparing treatment is possible for some women.[176] Progestin therapy may be used in women who decline surgical intervention,[406] and hormonal therapy (including progestin and antiestrogen tamoxifen for some women) has been used with recurrent disease.

Most of these cancers are detected at an early stage when they are highly curable. Surgical pathologic findings and staging are used to determine treatment recommendations. In low-risk patients (grade 1 or 2 endometrioid tumors, lower stage), no adjuvant treatment is needed after surgery. Postoperative management of moderate- to high-risk patients (grade 1 to 3 and higher stage) is controversial. Adjuvant radiation using external-beam radiotherapy (EBRT) and vaginal brachytherapy (VBT) may be recommended.[107,198,270] Chemotherapy and hormonal therapies may be combined with radiation therapy to reduce recurrence and improve survival rates.

Women with advanced stages of endometrial cancer may not be candidates for operative intervention in the presence of tumor fixation or deeply invasive cancer. Intensive chemotherapy regimens for women with advanced or recurrent endometrial cancer are being studied.[512] Medically inoperable cases may be treated with radiotherapy alone (EBRT or VBT). Radiation may be used when the tumor spreads outside the uterus or in the case of advanced or recurrent disease after failed hormonal therapy.

An understanding of the pathogenesis of endometrial cancer at the molecular level forms the current and future focus of treatment. Efforts are underway to identify biomarkers that can be used in targeted therapies.[331,430,461] Chemopreventive agents in the form of diet (foods that contain chemicals with anticancer properties, antioxidants, and plant-based phytochemicals) also show promising but sometimes conflicting results.[414]

**PROGNOSIS.** As most cases of endometrial cancer are treated at an early stage, survival rates are high. Involvement of less than 50% of the endometrial lining is associated with 100% survival, but this drops precipitously when tumor growth involves more than half of the endometrium, especially with local or distant metastases. Recurrences occur in 15% to 20% of cases[430] and are associated with a poor prognosis.[512] Most recurrences occur within the first 3 years after surgery. Sexual dysfunction (or diminished sexual function) is prevalent following treatment for endometrial cancer; risk factors include postmenopausal status, lack of vaginal lubricant use, higher BMI, and laparotomy.[121,269]

SPECIAL IMPLICATIONS FOR THE THERAPIST 20.5

### *Uterine Cancer*

Physical activity and exercise are known to decrease the risk of uterine cancer. This is yet another area of preventive medicine in which the therapist can be instrumental in conducting a screening examination consisting of a few questions and prescribing an appropriate exercise program.

Questions may include past personal or family history of endometrial (or other) cancer, presence of menses or menopause, use of hormone therapy or nutraceutical supplements (e.g., rose hips, dong quai, or soy), presence of osteoporosis or bone density testing results, and current exercise/physical activity levels. In any woman who is at least 12 months after menopause, is not taking hormone therapy, and reports vaginal bleeding, a medical evaluation is required.

In a woman who has been treated for endometrial cancer with lymphadenectomy and/or radiation, posttreatment lymphedema and other potential side effects may require physical therapy intervention. Cardiovascular health should be monitored because these women are also at high risk for CVD, which is the leading cause of death in endometrial cancer survivors.467

## Cervical Cancer

### Overview and Incidence

The cervix is the interface between the uterus and the vagina. It is made up of two layers of epithelial cells: the endocervix, which extends into the uterus, and the ectocervix, the portion visible when the cervix is viewed from the vaginal canal. There are two main types of cervical cancer, squamous cell carcinoma (80% to 90%) and adenocarcinoma (20%).[14]

Every year in the United States, cervical cancer is diagnosed in approximately 13,240 women (half of these women have never been screened), and 4170 women die of this disease (288,000 worldwide deaths).[11] The incidence of this cancer has been reduced by 75% and mortality has declined by more than 50% in the last 50 years as a result of widespread screening with cervical cytology testing (Papanicolaou [Pap] test).[511] It is now largely a preventable disease with preventive sexual practices, regular screening, and intervention at the precancerous stage. Of new cases of cervical cancer, 25% develop in women age 65 years and older, but the prevalence appears to be increasing disproportionately in young women.

### Risk Factors and Etiology

Clinical studies confirm that the transfer of human papillomavirus (HPV), also known as papillomas or genital warts, during unprotected sexual intercourse is the primary risk factor for squamous cell cervical cancer. HPV is the most common STI in the United States, affecting more than 50% of sexually active adults. The CDC estimates that 14 million Americans become infected with HPV each year.[338] More than 200 types of HPV have been identified; 23 of these infect the cervix, and 13 types are associated with cancer. All types can interfere with host-cell mechanisms that prevent cells from growing and replicating excessively. Infection with one of these viruses does not necessarily predict cancer, but the risk of cancer is increased significantly.[511] Other risk factors are listed in Box 20.4. Use of alcohol and use of other drugs are additional risky behaviors that may play a role in young age at first sexual intercourse and having more than five sexual partners. Impaired judgment from alcohol and other drug use can lead to unsafe sexual practices and with risky partners (partners more likely to have STIs) contributing to HPV infection.[310] It is also known that the cervix is particularly vulnerable to HPV during adolescence and especially early puberty. Cervical immaturity in young girls and adolescent women is marked by inadequate cervical mucus; cervical mucus acts as a protective barrier against infectious agents. Cervical ectropion or ectopy refers to the condition in which the columnar epithelial cells of the endocervix extend into the squamous epithelium of the vagina. Cervical ectopy is a normal physiologic phenomenon in women under hormonal influence such as during puberty but may increase cervical susceptibility to infection with STIs, including HPV.[310]

### Pathophysiology

The common unifying oncogenic feature of the vast majority of cervical cancers is the presence of HPV. More than 99% of cervical cancers contain at least one high-risk

Box 20.4

**RISK FACTORS FOR CERVICAL CANCER**

- Human papillomavirus infection
- Family history of cervical cancer
- Maternal use of diethylstilbestrol (a hormonal drug given to women between 1940 and 1971 to prevent miscarriage)
- Smoking (even passive smoking)
- Long-term use of oral contraceptives
- High parity—more pregnancies regardless of outcome
- Young age (<17 years old) at first sexual encounter
- Young age (<17 years old) at first full-term pregnancy[310]
- Low socioeconomic status
- Ethnic background (African American women are disproportionately affected)[26]
- Suppressed immune system
- Multiple sexual partners[306]
- Presence of other sexually transmitted infections[11]

HPV type (16, 18, 31, 45); HPV types 16 and 18 account for approximately 66% of cervical cancers in the United States.[433] The molecular basis for oncogenesis in cervical carcinoma can be explained to a large degree by the regulation and function of the two viral oncogenes *E6* and *E7* (see discussion of oncogenes in Chapter 9). The ability of HPV to target the function of tumor suppressors is typical of DNA tumor viruses. The *E6* gene product binds to the *p53* tumor suppressor gene and induces *p53* degradation. *E7* targets another tumor suppressor that functions similar to *p53* in cell cycle control and inactivates it.[502] As a result of these molecular disruptions, dysplastic changes occur in the thin layer of cells known as the *epithelium* that covers the cervix. Cervical cancer precursors identified with a Pap test are known as cervical intraepithelial neoplasia (CIN) or dysplasia. These abnormal cells occur most commonly at the junction between the squamous epithelium of the vagina and the columnar epithelium of the endocervix, called the transformation zone.

### Clinical Manifestations

Most people never know they have had HPV because there are no symptoms and a healthy immune system clears the body of infection. When it persists, HPV can cause lesions in the cervix, vagina, or vulva. Left untreated, these lesions can progress to cancer. Early-stage cervical cancer, especially in the preinvasive stage, is usually asymptomatic. Often women have advanced disease before abnormal bleeding occurs. This can manifest as spotting between menstrual periods, longer and heavier periods, bleeding after menopause, or bleeding after sexual intercourse. Pelvic pain or LBP can also occur (see Table 20.3).

More advanced stages of cervical cancer may cause bowel and bladder problems because of pressure on the rectum or bladder or sexual difficulties because of the growth in the upper vagina causing discomfort. Ureter blockage can lead to death because of uremia (the inability of the body to excrete waste), causing uremic poisoning. The progression to this type of advanced cancer is relatively rare in developed countries.

The physical effects of cervical cancer after treatment are actually more significant. Women who have the conization procedure or loop electrosurgical excision procedure (LEEP) may experience cramping, bleeding, or a watery discharge. Hysterectomy, radiation therapy and chemotherapy, alone or combined, may all cause significant side effects. Bowel, bladder, and sexual dysfunction are not uncommon after cervical cancer treatment.

The emotional effects of cervical cancer are often significant as well. Women treated with radiation almost always lose the benefits of estrogen because the ovaries are extremely sensitive to radiation. Hormone therapy may be prescribed, but without this intervention, the emotional effects of cervical cancer can be compounded by hypoestrogenism. Some women may experience depression from no longer being able to have children.

## MEDICAL MANAGEMENT

**PREVENTION.** The most effective prevention of cervical cancer is avoidance and quick regression of HPV infections. Risk of HPV and HPV-related cases of cervical cancer can be reduced and/or prevented using barrier contraceptives, engaging in monogamous sex with a likewise monogamous partner, or practicing sexual abstinence.

Although not preventive, studies show that consistent condom use can speed the regression of the HPV-related lesions on the cervix and on the penis and shorten the time it takes to clear HPV infections.[285] The possibility of HPV infection among women who have sex with women is underestimated by both lesbians and health care providers.[537] STDs can be spread between female sex partners through the exchange of cervicovaginal fluid and direct mucosal contact. Women who have sex with women should be educated about preventive measures, including washing hands, using rubber gloves, and cleaning sex toys or using a protective barrier such as a condom, especially when partners share such devices.

Dietary factors may be protective against all types of cancer (Box 20.5). The use of IUDs do not protect against HPV, but may have a protective effect against cervical cancer among women who have not been infected with HPV.[14]

Early detection is the key to a 100% cure rate for cervical cancer. Cervical cancer screening guidelines have been established by the U.S. Preventive Services Task Force (Box 20.6).[511]

***Vaccine.*** As of 2018, there are three HPV vaccines available that have been approved by the U.S. Food and Drug Administration (FDA) (Gardasil, Gardasil 9, and Cervarix) (Box 20.7). All three vaccines prevent high-risk HPV (types 16 and 18) infections and other strains that can cause cervical cancer. Ideally the vaccine should be administered before exposure to genital HPV through sexual contact because the potential benefit is likely to diminish with an increasing number of sexual partners. Routine immunization of girls age 11 to 12 years is a controversial social issue because safe sex practices can prevent HPV and its associated complications, making universal vaccination unnecessary. Both the Advisory Committee on Immunization Practices at the CDC and the National Women's Health Network advise that the vaccine should not replace routine cervical screening or education regarding sexual practices. Vaccination is more imperative for women who do not have access to cervical cancer screening services.

Box 20.5

**DIETARY SUGGESTIONS FOR PREVENTION OF ALL TYPES OF CANCER**

***Increase***

- Plant-based foods, including a variety of vegetables, fruits, whole grains, peas, beans, and lentils
- Phytonutrients and antioxidants

***Decrease***

- High-sugar food and drinks
- Processed meats and red meats
- Alcohol
- Use of salty foods and foods processed with salt.
- Supplements for cancer prevention

Information from Foundation for Women's Cancer, The National Cancer Institute, American Institute of Cancer Research, and the American Cancer Society

**U.S. PREVENTIVE SERVICES TASK FORCE RECOMMENDATIONS FOR SCREENING FOR CERVICAL CANCER**

- Women younger than age 21 should not be screened for cervical cancer.
- Women who have had a hysterectomy with removal of the cervix without a history of high-grade precancerous lesion or cervical cancer should not be screened for cervical cancer.
- Women ages 21 to 29 should undergo screening every 3 years using a Pap test.
- Women ages 30 to 65 have 3 options for testing:
    - They can be screened using a Pap test alone every 3 years.
    - They can be tested for high-risk strains of HPV every 5 years.
    - They can undergo co-testing with both a Pap test and the HPV test every 5 years.
- Women older than age 65 do not need to be screened for cervical cancer *if* they have had adequate screening and their tests have been negative in the previous 10 years, and they do not have other risk factors.

*HPV*, Human papillomavirus.
From US Preventive Services Task Force, et al. Screening for cervical cancer: US Preventive Services Task Force Recommendation Statement. *JAMA* 320:674–686, 2018.

**DIAGNOSIS AND STAGING.** Cervical cancer is detected using a Pap test. This test is used to detect changes in the cells of the cervix that may indicate a precancerous or cancerous condition. However, Pap tests have a 15% to 25% false-negative rate for detecting cervical dysplasia and can be inconclusive, requiring further testing including HPV testing, colposcopy, punch or cone biopsy, or LEEP.

In contrast to uterine/endometrial cancer, which uses surgical staging, cervical cancer staging is based on information gathered from the physical examination, biopsies, imaging, and other tests. This is called clinical staging and is used to determine the size of the tumor, how deeply the tumor has invaded tissues within and around the cervix, and if there is metastasis to lymph nodes or distant organs. Staging is an important process and the key factor in selecting the right treatment plan. FIGO[167] staging and American Joint Committee on Cancer (AJCC) TNM staging are used for cervical cancer. Surgery may determine that the cancer has spread more than initially assessed. This new information may change the treatment plan, but it does not change the woman's FIGO stage.

*Stage 0* is the precancerous stage, and there are no gross lesions; carcinoma is limited to the mucosa and is referred to as carcinoma in situ or CIN grade 1, grade 2, or grade 3. For premalignant dysplastic changes, CIN grading is used for stage 0. Grade 1 is most likely to regress naturally and does not require treatment; grade 3 is most likely to advance to cancer. Grades 2 and 3 both require treatment.

*Stage I* is strictly confined to the cervix, and lesions are measured as less than or greater than 4 cm in size. In *stage II* the cancer extends beyond the cervix but has not extended to the pelvic wall. The vagina is minimally involved, and there may or may not be parametrial involvement.

In *stage III* the carcinoma has extended to the pelvic wall and involves the lower one-third of the vagina, and there may be kidney involvement (spread via the ureters). *Stage IV* is characterized by carcinoma that has extended beyond the true pelvis or has infiltrated adjacent organs (e.g., mucosa of the bladder or rectum). There may be metastatic spread of the growth to distant organs.

**TREATMENT.** Treatment options for cervical cancer are based on cancer stage. For precancerous (stage 0) changes (carcinoma in situ), these include cryosurgery, laser surgery, LEEP, cone biopsy, and cold knife conization. For stage I, treatment options include procedures that maintain fertility (cone biopsy and radical trachelectomy [removal of the cervix and upper vagina]) as well as procedures that do not maintain fertility (hysterectomy). Successful conception and full-term births (cesarean section delivery) occurred 6 months after radical trachelectomy in 66% of cases studied.[263] Treatment at early stages may include lymph node dissection and EBRT plus VBT.[107]

At stages II and III, a hysterectomy and lymph node dissection may be performed, but chemoradiation is the

Box 20.7

**CURRENT U.S. CENTERS FOR DISEASE CONTROL AND PREVENTION RECOMMENDATIONS FOR GARDASIL 9[a]**

- All children ages 11 to 12 should receive two doses 6 to 12 months apart.
- Adolescents who get first dose after age 15 will need three doses given over 6 months.
- Individuals ages 9 to 26 who have immunocompromising conditions need three doses.
- Young women through age 26 and young men through age 21 should receive vaccine.

[a]Gardasil 9 is the only vaccine available for use in the United States.

standard treatment. Concurrent cisplatin-based chemotherapy and radiation have shown significant improvement in survival for women with locally advanced cervical cancer. The use of hypoxic cell radiosensitizers and monoclonal antibodies that inhibit cell growth may increase numbers of malignant cells killed.[59] Biologic response modifiers are under investigation for future treatment options.

Stage IV cervical cancer has spread beyond the pelvis and is not typically considered curable. Surgery might be extensive (pelvic exenteration) depending on the area of spread. Treatment options in addition to the above-described options include targeted drugs such as angiogenesis inhibitors that deprive tumor cells from forming new blood vessels. Bevacizumab is one such drug and is considered a monoclonal antibody that targets vascular endothelial growth factor.[494]

**PROGNOSIS.** Cervical cancer is a slow-growing neoplasm with a good response rate to intervention. Almost all women with preinvasive cancer are cured. Reconstructive surgery and ovary preservation may be able to preserve childbearing status in younger women. The majority of treated women who develop recurrences do so in the first 2 years after primary therapy. Women with advanced-stage disease or with lymph node involvement have a significantly less favorable prognosis.

SPECIAL IMPLICATIONS FOR THE THERAPIST 20.6

*Cervical Cancer*

The therapist can continue to function in the role of educator and prevention specialist when conducting a personal/family history that includes questions about the consistency of Pap testing and presence of STIs (e.g., HPV or genital warts), as these relate to cervical cancer for women of all ages.

Although new, more sensitive testing is available, the majority of medical specialists agree that being screened for cervical cancer on a regular basis is more important than the availability of the latest technology. Any woman with a previous history of cervical cancer who presents with suspicious supraclavicular (or other) unusual lymph node presentation must be referred to her physician for medical evaluation.[239] Reported symptoms of vaginal bleeding and GI or genitourinary dysfunction must also be promptly investigated before initiating pelvic rehabilitation.

## Ectopic Pregnancy

### Overview

Ectopic pregnancy, also known as *tubal pregnancy,* refers to the implantation of a fertilized ovum outside the uterine cavity (Fig. 20.5). The fallopian tube is the most common site of ectopic pregnancy, with approximately 95% implanting there, but extrauterine pregnancies can occur anywhere outside the uterus (e.g., ovary, abdomen, or pelvic peritoneum). Ectopic pregnancy is a true gynecologic emergency, as a ruptured ectopic pregnancy is the cause of 4% to 10% of all maternal deaths in the United States.[328]

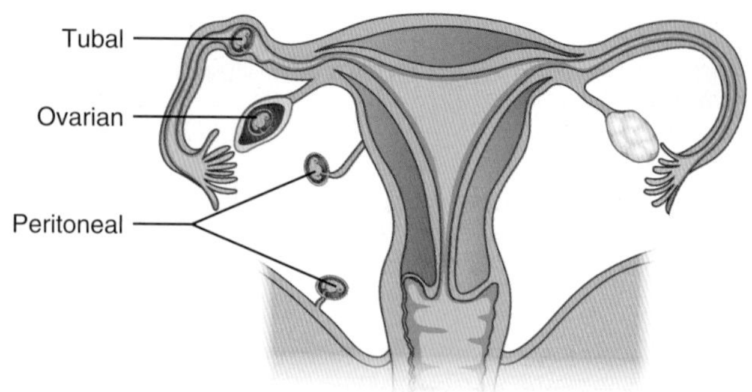


**Figure 20.5**

**Ectopic pregnancy (outside the uterus) with implantation inside the fallopian tube (tubal pregnancy), abdomen (peritoneal or abdominal), or ovary.** The majority of ectopic pregnancies (98%) are implanted inside the fallopian tube. (From Goodman CC, Snyder TE: *Differential diagnosis for the physical therapist: screening for referral*, ed 4, Philadelphia, 2007, Saunders.)

### Incidence and Risk Factors

The rate of ectopic pregnancy is stable at less than 1%[279,490] to 2.8%.[410] Risk factors include smoking, any condition that causes damage to the fallopian tubes including inflammation or infections, and prior tubal or ovarian surgery.[279] Some conditions causing damage to the fallopian tubes and increasing risk of ectopic pregnancy are STDs (especially chlamydia and gonorrhea), ruptured appendix, endometriosis, and PID. Current IUD use does not increase the risk of ectopic pregnancy, but pregnancies that occur with an IUD in place are more likely to be ectopic.[279] Other risk factors include douching[258] and previous ectopic pregnancy.[505]

### Etiologic Factors and Pathogenesis

Ectopic pregnancy is caused by delayed ovum transport secondary to decreased fallopian tube motility or distorted tubule anatomy. Advancements in diagnostic technology have revealed a number of etiologic factors, the most common being salpingitis. Salpingitis is an infection and inflammation of the fallopian tubes.

Normally the sperm fertilizes the ovum soon after the ovum enters the ampulla of the fallopian tube (about one-third of the way to the uterus). Typically 3 to 4 days are required for the fertilized ovum to travel through the fallopian tube to the uterus. The fertilized ovum is rapidly dividing and growing throughout the journey. If the journey is slowed sufficiently (decreased tubule motility), the ovum becomes too large to complete the passage through the tubule to the uterus. The trophoblasts that cover the surface of the ovum easily penetrate the mucosa and wall of the tubule, and implantation occurs in the fallopian tube.

Adhesions related to recurrent infection or endometriosis can compress the fallopian tube or distort it in such a way that passage of the ovum is impaired. In addition, a history of infertility and the use of clomiphene citrate to induce ovulation or in vitro fertilization procedures are associated with an increased risk of this condition.

The pregnancy will typically outgrow its blood supply, terminating the pregnancy. If the pregnancy does not terminate, the thin-walled tubule will no longer support the growing fetus, and rupture can occur by 12 weeks of gestation. Tubal rupture is life threatening because rapid intraabdominal hemorrhage can occur.

#### Clinical Manifestations

The classic presentation of ectopic pregnancy is marked by amenorrhea or irregular bleeding and spotting, nonspecific lower abdominal quadrant or back pain, and a pelvic mass. The woman may believe she had a menstrual period but when questioned will report the period was atypical for her. Bleeding occurs during implantation, with leakage into the pelvis and abdominal cavity.

The pain reported can be diffuse and aching or localized and will progress to a sharper, lancing acute type of pain. The pain can be sudden in onset and intermittent and may be accompanied by hemorrhage. The pain is thought to be primarily a result of the leakage of blood into the pelvic and abdominal cavity. Other symptoms include dizziness, fainting, paleness, and shock (if ectopic pregnancy bursts and causes significant bleeding).[505] Because the woman is pregnant, signs and symptoms associated with normal pregnancy may also be present, including fatigue, nausea, breast tenderness, and urinary frequency.

#### MEDICAL MANAGEMENT

**DIAGNOSIS.** Physical examination reveals a pelvic mass in approximately 50% of the cases. Pelvic ultrasound studies can reliably demonstrate a gestational sac by 5 to 6 weeks into the pregnancy. An empty uterine cavity with (slight) elevation of human chorionic gonadotropin-β subunit (HCG-β) and symptoms strongly implies an extrauterine pregnancy.[328] Blood studies may show anemia, and serum pregnancy tests (HCG-β hormonal levels) will be positive but show levels lower than expected in the presence of a normal pregnancy (lack of doubling over 2 days). Earlier diagnosis decreases mortality and preserves fertility.

**TREATMENT.** Nonsurgical management (methotrexate or watchful waiting) maybe appropriate for 15% to 40% of ectopic pregnancies. Some ectopic pregnancies resolve spontaneously. A chemotherapeutic agent, methotrexate, can be administered to dissolve the fertilized ovum and remove residual ectopic tissue after laparoscopy . This drug is also used when surgery is contraindicated or the diagnosis is made early enough that the condition is not life threatening and preserving fertility is desirable.[279]

Surgical intervention consisting of a noninvasive laparoscopic salpingostomy to remove the ectopic pregnancy is performed if the fallopian tube has not ruptured. Laparotomy is indicated if there is internal bleeding or if the ectopic site cannot be adequately visualized with the laparoscope.[279]

#### SPECIAL IMPLICATIONS FOR THE THERAPIST 20.7

*Ectopic Pregnancy*

An awareness of this potentially life-threatening condition is important for the therapist. This awareness should include knowledge of the preexisting conditions that increase the risk of ectopic pregnancy and of the symptoms associated with ectopic pregnancy. If a woman of childbearing age complains of an onset of lower abdominal, ipsilateral shoulder, or back pain, the therapist should ask questions regarding her menstrual cycle and if any of the symptoms of pregnancy are present.

In general, if the therapist suspects ectopic pregnancy, an immediate telephone call to the physician or medical referral is warranted.

If follow-up care occurs, the therapist should be aware that perinatal loss can be a profound experience for the woman (and her family). A sensitive presence and validation of the loss may be helpful. Cultural responses to perinatal loss vary; the therapist should remain alert to any intervention needed.82 Women who have an ectopic pregnancy may also have increased difficulty conceiving.57

## DISORDERS OF THE OVARIES

### Ovarian Cystic Disease

#### Overview and Incidence

Ovarian cysts, most of which are benign, are the most common form of ovarian tumor. Ovarian cysts are often categorized as functional, endometrial, or neoplastic or as PCOS.

*Functional cysts* rarely produce symptoms (unless they rupture or hemorrhage) because they develop in the course of normal ovarian activity. A *follicular cyst* develops when an egg matures but does not erupt from the follicle, but rather continues to swell as it fills with fluid. A *luteal cyst* develops from a corpus luteum when the tissue that is left after the egg has been expelled fills with blood or other fluid.

*Endometrial cysts* develop when endometrial tissue migrates to the ovaries (i.e., endometriosis), forming blood-filled cysts called *endometriomas*, or *chocolate cysts* because of the dark-brown color of the contents. Endometrial cysts can grow large enough to impair ovulation and cause pain and cramping during menstrual periods.

*Neoplastic cysts* are "new growths" considered benign in the majority of cases; only a small percentage of neoplastic cysts are cancerous or have the capacity to invade neighboring tissues and metastasize to distant sites. *Cystadenomas* (cysts forming on the surface of the ovary) are the most common type of neoplastic cyst. *Dermoid* or *teratoma cysts* are formed from embryonic tissue and contain tissue such as hair, skin, or teeth.

Ovarian cysts are one of the most common endocrine disorders in women, affecting 3% to 7% of women of childbearing age.[323] A recent study reviewed 244 cases of ovarian cysts and found 33.2% functional cysts, 10.7% endometrial cysts, 12.2% dermoid cysts, 19.3% cystadenomas, and 4.1% malignant cysts, although other studies have found more endometrial cysts.[3]

PCOS is a disorder marked by the presence of multiple cysts. This polycystic disorder is a hormonal disorder affecting premenopausal women and is one of the most common causes of infertility. The disease gets its name from the many small cysts that build up inside the ovaries, although there has been a recommendation that the name should be changed to reflect the metabolic components of the syndrome.[109,144,374] The condition is marked by hyperandrogenism, gonadotropin secretory changes, polycystic ovarian morphology, and insulin resistance. PCOS affects 6% to 20% of women in the United States.[109] Among women who seek treatment for infertility, more than 75% have some degree of PCOS. About 50% of women with PCOS are obese.[138]

### Risk Factors

Ovarian cysts can occur in females of all ages, including during fetal development and after menopause, although the most common age group affected is women of childbearing age.[3] Women who have had four or more live births are at a lower risk for ovarian cysts.[323] Other risk factors include taking infertility medications, pregnancy, endometriosis, and severe pelvic infection. Risk factors for PCOS include obesity and genetic predisposition. Several researchers have also identified possible relationships of PCOS and early onset of puberty and girls born small for gestational age.[109]

### Pathogenesis

Two types of ovarian cysts (follicular and corpus luteum) are a normal part of the reproductive cycle. At least one follicle (a sac containing an egg and fluid) matures in an ovary during each cycle. During ovulation, the follicle ruptures to release the egg. The follicular remnant, or corpus luteum, is a smaller sac containing a viscous yellow liquid. The corpus luteum releases progesterone, which promotes the development of the uterine lining in preparation for the implantation of a fertilized egg.

Ovarian cysts develop when excess circulating androgens are converted to estrone in the peripheral adipose tissue. The elevated levels of circulating estrogens stimulate the release of GnRH by the hypothalamus and inhibit the secretion of FSH by the pituitary. GnRH stimulates the pituitary, which produces LH. The increased secretion of LH stimulates the ovary to produce and secrete more androgens. This self-perpetuating cycle results in abnormal maturation of the ovarian follicles, the development of multiple follicular cysts, and a persistent anovulatory state.

The European Society of Endocrinology has published a position statement on the pathophysiology of PCOS.[109] Several genes are implicated in the pathogenesis of PCOS.[144] Researchers have discovered that many women are resistant to their own insulin. To counter this resistance, the pancreas makes extra insulin; over many years this may exhaust the ability of the pancreas to make insulin and thus lead to diabetes and subsequent cardiovascular complications. In addition, high insulin levels boost the production of androgens that may induce muscular changes, leading to reduced insulin-mediated glucose uptake creating a repeated cycle and worsening condition.[226]

### Clinical Manifestations

Most ovarian cysts are asymptomatic and resolve spontaneously.[3] The likelihood of symptoms developing often has more to do with the size and location rather than the type of ovarian cyst. As cysts grow, their weight often pulls the ovary out of its customary position, sometimes cutting off the blood supply to the ovary. Pressure from the ovary in its new position against the uterus, bladder, intestine, or vagina may result in a variety of symptoms such as abdominal heaviness or pressure; pelvic, groin, low back, or buttock pain; breast tenderness; urinary frequency or difficulty empting the bladder; dysmenorrhea; or dyspareunia. Ovarian torsion can result from larger cysts. In this case the patient may have severe pelvic pain, nausea, and vomiting. Abdominal pain is the most commonly reported symptom, reported in 58.2% of patients in one study.[3] Large cysts can impair ovarian function, reducing ovulation and causing irregular periods or infertility in premenopausal women. Sudden or sharp pain can indicate rupture or hemorrhage of a cyst or ovarian torsion.

Depending on the type of cyst, if a cyst ruptures, the contents of the sac are usually absorbed by the body. When endometriomas rupture, the contents may be distributed on the uterus, bladder, and intestines. As the immune system moves in to clean up the debris, scar tissue develops, forming adhesions, with resultant CPP. In the case of neoplastic cyst rupture, the more toxic contents can result in peritonitis.

PCOS manifests in many different ways and is characterized by physical and metabolic changes. The affected girl or woman may present with one or more of the following manifestations: weight gain and obesity, prominent facial or body hair, severe acne, thinning scalp hair, infertility, and menstrual problems. They may seek medical care with a variety of different physicians depending on the primary presenting symptom (e.g., dermatologist for skin involvement, internist for weight gain and elevated blood glucose, gynecologist for irregular periods and/or inability to get pregnant).

Of women with PCOS, 50% have amenorrhea, and another 30% have abnormal uterine bleeding. PCOS is associated with endometrial cancer because high levels of androgen interfere with ovulation, so women with PCOS do not regularly shed the endometrium. Impaired glucose tolerance is present in 40% of women with PCOS, and the subsequent risk for insulin resistance, type 2 diabetes, and heart disease has been documented.[114]

Other symptoms or conditions associated with PCOS include obstructive sleep apnea and daytime sleepiness[523] and benign breast disease (formerly fibrocystic breast disease).[118] There is a 2-fold increased risk for venous thrombosis embolism among women with PCOS who are taking combined oral contraceptives and a 1.5-fold increased risk for women with PCOS who are not taking oral contraceptives.[40] In addition, several psychological symptoms have been reported, including depression, anxiety, and general decrease in quality of life.[109]

### Medical Management

**Diagnosis and Treatment.** The history and pelvic examination lead to suspicion of cystic disease. The diagnosis is confirmed by ultrasonography or laparoscopy. Transvaginal (inserting a tampon-sized transducer into the vagina) or abdominal (moving a transducer across the lower abdomen) ultrasound may be performed and can help identify the type of cyst and whether a cyst contains solid or liquid material. Improvement and expansion of laboratory tests has occurred in the last several years.[109] Tests include a complete blood count to identify infection or anemia (heavy bleeding), testing of free testosterone, testing of sex hormone–binding globulin, carcinoembryonic antigen 125 (CA 125) test for ovarian cancer, and several others. All women with PCOS should be screened for glucose intolerance.[295]

The treatment of ovarian cysts depends on the results of the diagnostic tests and the age of the woman (preserving childbearing status). In premenopausal women, the decision whether to drain (ultrasound-guided drainage) or remove (laparotomy or laparoscopically) the cyst depends on the problems the cyst is causing (e.g., follicular or luteal cysts resolve without treatment, and endometriomas and neoplastic cysts may be removed surgically).

The treatment of PCOS is primarily hormonal, with the goal being an interruption of the persistent elevated levels of androgens. Pharmaceuticals (e.g., metformin, clomiphene citrate, antiandrogens) may be used to induce ovulation.[351,352] Oral contraceptives are also used to normalize hormonal cycles. Weight reduction is a major treatment in some forms of PCOS and can include diet and bariatric surgery.[356] If medication is not effective, laser surgery can be instituted to puncture the multiple follicles.

It is now known that the application of diabetes management techniques aimed at reducing insulin resistance and hyperinsulinemia (e.g., weight reduction, oral hypoglycemic agents, and exercise) can reverse testosterone and LH abnormalities and infertility, as well as improve glucose, insulin, and lipid profiles.

SPECIAL IMPLICATIONS FOR THE THERAPIST 20.8

*Ovarian Cystic Disease*

A history of ovarian cystic disease could account for LBP or sacral pain in a woman, but usually there is some indication in the menstrual history to suggest a gynecologic link. In women with known PCOS, elevated androgens, with the associated muscular changes that further reduce glucose uptake and elevate cholesterol, warrant the use of exercise and increased physical activity before the onset of macrovascular and microvascular symptoms.[226,272]

A meta-analysis comparing metformin with lifestyle modifications (diet and exercise in various combinations) found both decreased fasting blood sugar and risk of diabetes, but the effect on other factors such as pregnancy or hirsutism was unclear.138 Another literature review and position statement reported that adding exercise to dietary modifications improved weight loss. Reduction in adrenal androgens and improvements in hirsutism were shown with exercise in this review.[356] Optimal type and duration of exercise has not been established. Considering how common PCOS is, therapists need to be aware of the potential side effects of clomiphene citrate. These include insomnia, blurred vision, nausea, vomiting, urinary frequency, and polyuria. The onset of any of these symptoms warrants communication with the physician.

## Ovarian Cancer

### Overview and Incidence

Ovarian cancer is estimated to be the second most common female urogenital cancer and the most lethal of these cancers, largely as a result of the advanced stage at diagnosis in most women.[246] An estimated 22,240 women in the United States developed ovarian cancer in 2018 with 14,070 deaths.[11] The poor outcome is based on the difficulty of diagnosing the disease, which results in almost 70% of the women having metastatic disease at the time of diagnosis. Although there are a number of types of ovarian cancers, epithelial tumors make up approximately 90% of the cases. The incidence of epithelial tumors peaks in women during their 50s and 60s; it is rare before puberty. In the United States, white and Hawaiian women have the highest incidence of ovarian cancer, whereas Native American and black women have the lowest incidence.

### Risk Factors and Etiology

The etiology of ovarian cancer is not well understood, but hormonal, environmental, and genetic factors appear to influence the development of the disease (Box 20.8). Most important is family history of ovarian or breast cancer. Overall, more than 90% of all cases are not explained by recognized risk factors[282]; only 10% of all women with ovarian cancer have a hereditary predisposition. However, genetic variants have been shown to be a risk factor for the development of ovarian cancer.[552] The average woman has less than a 2% chance of developing ovarian cancer in her lifetime, whereas a woman with first-degree relatives with ovarian cancer or who has the *BRCA1* mutation has about a 45% lifetime chance, and for women who have the *BRCA2* mutation, the risk is approximately 25%.

The risk of ovarian cancer increases with age and is inversely proportional to the number of lifetime ovulations. Theories regarding this relationship include the incessant-ovulation theory,[521] which suggests that repeated release of an ova (egg) ruptures the ovarian epithelial surface, which then requires repair and may result in genetic alterations. This may also lead to an inflammatory reaction leading to cell damage. Other conditions associated with inflammation, such as endometriosis, PCOS, and PID, have been suggested as risk factors for ovarian cancer.[387,504] The gonadotropin theory proposes that persistent hormonal stimulation increases epithelial proliferation and mitotic activity.[417] Anything that interferes with ovulation (e.g., pregnancy, breastfeeding, hormonal contraceptives, oophorectomy) diminishes the risk of developing ovarian cancer.

Box 20.8

**RISK AND PROTECTIVE FACTORS FOR OVARIAN CANCER**

***Increased Risk for Ovarian Cancer***

- Family history of ovarian cancer or breast cancer (and other neoplasms including colorectum and endometrium)
- *BRAC1* or *BRAC2* mutation
- Lynch syndrome
- Personal history of endometrial or breast cancer
- Older age (>50 years old)
- Increased number of lifetime ovulations (findings are inconsistent and may reflect differences in definitions[412]
  - Early menarche
  - Late menopause
  - Late age (>30 years old) at first birth
  - Low parity
- Infertility
- Polycystic ovarian syndrome increases risk owing to unopposed endogenous estrogen
- Endometriosis
- Pelvic inflammatory disease
- Postmenopausal hormone replacement therapy (with unopposed estrogen)
- Higher body mass index
- Environmental factors
  - Asbestos and talcum powder exposures
  - Cigarette smoking
- Higher intake of saturated fats and meats with nitrates

***Decreased Risk for Ovarian Cancer***

- Parity (parous women have a 30% to 60% lower risk than nulliparous women)[412]
- Oral contraceptive use
  - Recent lower incidence and mortality in several high-income countries may be related to widespread oral contraceptive use in generations born after 1930
- Lactation
- Tubal ligation
- Oophorectomy (one or both ovaries removed) and salpingectomy (one or both fallopian tubes removed)
- Hysterectomy
- Diet with whole grains and higher vegetable intake
- Exercise and physical activity
- Aspirin and nonsteroidal antiinflammatory drug use
- Metformin

Data from Reid BM, Permuth JB, Sellers TA: Epidemiology of ovarian cancer: A review. *Cancer Biol Med* 14:9–32, 2017; and La Vecchia C: Ovarian cancer: Epidemiology and risk factors. *Eur J Cancer Prev* 26:55–62.

Evidence indicates that many ovarian cancers arise from precursor lesions within the epithelium of the fallopian tubes. Tubal ligation has been shown to reduce the risk of ovarian cancer, but this varies by tumor histotype.[174] Dietary fiber has also been shown to reduce ovarian cancer risk.[568]

## Pathophysiology

The ovaries have different types of cells, and the classification of ovarian tumors is based on the tissue of origin. The most common tumors (90%) are carcinomas that were originally thought to arise from the surface epithelium or covering of the ovary. Evidence indicates that most of these actually originate from the fallopian tube.[174] Epithelial ovarian cancer is further classified as *serous* (most common), *endometrioid, clear cell,* and *mucinous*. Other cell types include *stromal cells* (tumors arise from structural tissues that hold the ovary together and produce hormones) and *germ cells* (tumors arise from cells that form the ova).

Histologic subtypes have various patterns of metastasis. Epithelial ovarian cancer may initially spread within the peritoneal cavity and is found on peritoneal surfaces such as the diaphragm, bladder, and rectouterine pouch (pouch of Douglas).

## Clinical Manifestations

In the past, most ovarian cancers were considered asymptomatic or silent, presenting with symptoms so vague that the disease is advanced in many cases by the time the woman seeks care. Evidence shows that many women with early-stage disease seek medical care for symptoms including abdominal bloating, early satiety (difficulty eating/feeling full), flatulence, fatigue and malaise, gastritis, or general abdominal discomfort (see Table 20.3). Local pelvic pain is often an early symptom (1 to 6 months before diagnosis).[191] Abnormal vaginal bleeding, leg pain, pelvic mass, and LBP are less common but still reported.

Symptoms associated with metastatic spread of the disease include unexplained weight loss, weakness, pleurisy, ascites, and cachexia (general feebleness and wasting). Ascites is an accumulation of fluid within the peritoneal cavity. This can occur when there is marked increased pressure within the liver sinusoids or portal hypertension that results in serum exuding through the superficial capillaries into the peritoneal cavity.

Lymphedema associated with ovarian cancer can develop in the lower quadrants, with a prevalence of 21.8% to 38%.[205,243] The number of lymph nodes removed is a risk factor for lymphedema occurrence.[205,261] The majority of post–gynecologic surgery lymphedema occurs in the first year after surgery.[261] However, cumulative incidence of lymphedema continues to increase 10 years after surgery.[205]

*Paraneoplastic cerebellar degeneration* is a type of autoimmune syndrome that primarily affects women with gynecologic cancers. It is associated with, but not directly caused by, the cancer or its metastases. Although rare, paraneoplastic cerebellar degeneration can occur years before any discernible symptoms of malignancy, especially ovarian cancer. Paraneoplastic cerebellar degeneration can also develop following the detection and treatment of ovarian cancer. Symptoms typically include ataxic gait, truncal and appendicular ataxia, nystagmus, peripheral neuropathy, and speech impairment (dysarthria). The syndrome can be debilitating with limited treatment options.[182]

## Medical Management

**Screening and Prevention.** Screening all women for ovarian cancer is not considered practical or cost-effective and is not reliable to detect ovarian cancer in its early, most curable stages. Studies performed on asymptomatic women at average risk for ovarian cancer have not shown more benefit than harm or improved survival rates.[216,511] However, women at high risk for ovarian cancer (e.g., women with a family history of ovarian cancer) and any woman with a personal history of breast, colon, or uterine cancer should receive annual screening (see Box 20.8).

Screening high-risk women typically includes the CA 125 blood test, physical examination, and transvaginal ultrasound. The CA 125 test (a biologic marker produced by ovarian cancer cells) is elevated in about 50% of women with early-stage disease and approximately 80% of women with advanced disease. It lacks sensitivity and specificity, and results vary depending on menopausal status. It can be elevated in other conditions such as pelvic infections, fibroids, or endometriosis as well as during ovulation.[459]

There are no recommended screening tests for germ cell or stromal cell tumors. These types of tumors may release protein markers such as HCG and alpha fetoprotein, but blood tests for these markers are usually done after surgery or chemotherapy to see if treatment is working.

Researchers continue to study a symptom index that was first proposed in 2007[190] to predict ovarian cancer based on the duration and frequency of key symptoms.[450] These include pelvic/abdominal pain, increased abdominal size and bloating, difficulty eating/feeling full (early satiety), and loss of appetite/weight. The index is considered positive for ovarian cancer if any of these symptoms occur more than 12 times a month for less than 12 months.

Some women with a positive family history of ovarian cancer choose to have prophylactic oophorectomies after completing childbearing to prevent the development of this disease. This intervention is not 100% protective because the lining of the peritoneal cavity comprises the same cells as the lining of the ovaries, and development of primary peritoneal cancer after prophylactic oophorectomy can occur.[377] Hormonal contraceptives (in pill form, injectable, or patch) are recommended as cancer prevention for women with a family history of ovarian cancer, especially if the *BRCA* mutation is present. The mechanism of protection is unclear, but it is probably a result of the inhibition of ovulation; there is a potential increased risk of cervical cancer with this treatment.[417]

**Diagnosis and staging.** Despite the reputation of ovarian cancer as a silent killer, more than 90% of women with ovarian cancer (whether early or advanced) reported experiencing symptoms long before diagnosis. However, these are often nonspecific and vague and are frequently misdiagnosed as indigestion, IBS, LBP, or some other nongynecologic condition.[450] Imaging, menopausal status, and biomarkers can aid in distinguishing malignant from benign pelvic masses. A cervical smear may reveal malignant cells, and a biopsy will reveal whether the mass is benign or cancerous.[41]

*Extraovarian primary peritoneal carcinoma* (EOPPC) is a malignant epithelial tumor that arises from the peritoneal lining and may be misdiagnosed as ovarian cancer.[377] EOPPC is rare and is characterized by peritoneal carcinomatosis with minimal or no ovarian involvement and histologically similar to ovarian serous cancer. The peritoneum and ovaries share a common embryologic heritage; however, the pathologic origin of EOPPC remains unknown.

Researchers continue to investigate tumor biomarkers such as serum CA 125 to aid in earlier diagnosis.[459,571] Serum human epididymal protein 4 is being studied, but methodology is variable among studies.[247] Other studies have looked at indexes and algorithms to differentiate ovarian cancer from other pelvic masses. These include the risk of ovarian cancer algorithm or the risk of ovarian malignancy algorithm (based on age and fluctuations in CA 125 blood levels).[2,256,400,460]

Staging of ovarian cancer is usually surgical staging.[245] FIGO staging of the disease is as follows: stage I, tumor is limited to one or both ovaries; stage II, tumor involves one or both ovaries with pelvic extension/intraperitoneal extension; stage III, tumor involves one or both ovaries with extraperitoneal metastasis and lymph node involvement; stage IV, metastasis to extraabdominal organs and lymph node involvement outside the abdominal cavity. For a more comprehensive breakdown of the AJCC TNM and FIGO staging systems for ovarian cancer, see the National Comprehensive Cancer Network (NCCN) Clinical Practice Guidelines.

**Treatment.** Treatment of ovarian cancer depends on the specific tumor type.[399] For stages II through IV this usually consists of laparotomy and cytoreductive surgery that includes total abdominal hysterectomy, bilateral salpingo-oophorectomy, omentectomy (removal of supportive tissue attached to organs in the abdominal cavity), and lymphadenectomy followed by chemotherapy. Chemotherapy may be given orally, injected intravenously, and/or with an intraperitoneal catheter. Combined methods of chemotherapy may improve survival rates.[361] Radiation therapy is rarely performed in the United States for ovarian cancer.

Fertility-sparing surgery is done for any woman who desires to maintain her fertility. Women interested in more information about preserving fertility after cancer should talk to their physicians about future fertility. The ACS and NCCN offer excellent reviews of this topic.

Additional treatment options for resistant or recurrent disease include targeted drugs such as angiogenesis inhibitors that deprive tumor cells from forming new blood vessels. Other interventions under investigation include the use of molecular targeted therapy (laboratory-produced substances that find and bind to cancer cells, delivering tumor-killing agents without harming normal cells), genetic techniques (e.g., gene therapy to supply a working copy of the tumor suppressor gene *p53*), vaccines to boost a woman's immune response to ovarian tumor cells that emerge after treatment, and new combinations and sequences of currently used drug interventions.[246,361,394]

**Prognosis.** Ovarian cancer has a very poor prognosis because it is difficult to detect early and usually manifests with advanced metastases. For all ovarian cancer cell types, the 5-year survival rate is 47%. The cancer is generally responsive to treatment if found early, with a 92% 5-year survival rate. Tumor recurrence within 3 years after treatment occurs in most women. Appropriate selection of secondary debulking surgery and better chemotherapeutic response may lead to prolonged survival in patients with recurrent ovarian cancer.[468] Salvage therapy (chemotherapy to help manage symptoms and prolong survival) may be recommended if a cancer cure is not possible, but quality of life may be impaired by further aggressive therapy. Five-year survival without recurrence is a good prognostic indicator.

SPECIAL IMPLICATIONS FOR THE THERAPIST 20.9

## *Ovarian Cancer*

Therapists treating women with a history of ovarian cancer need to be cognizant of the moderate to high risk of recurrence of the disease. Ataxic gait may be the first sign of paraneoplastic cerebellar degeneration associated with gynecologic cancer. Other symptoms associated with metastases may include thoracic or shoulder girdle pain secondary to lymphadenopathy, symptoms associated with lung (dyspnea) (see Chapter 15) or liver (see Chapter 17) disease, and weight loss and fatigue. Onset of any of these symptoms warrants communication with the physician. Lymphedema associated with ovarian cancer requires ongoing surveillance for early signs and lymphedema management.[136,243]

Oophorectomy induces abrupt menopause in young women. Ovary removal (for any reason) before age 65 years increases the risk for CVD, hip fractures, and mortality.[368] Physical activity and exercise has been shown to improve cardiovascular health, quality of life, and menopausal symptoms, including hot flashes in postmenopausal women and would be appropriate to incorporate into the plan of care of any postmenopausal cancer survivor.[188] Other menopausal symptoms may include vaginal atrophy and bladder urgency/frequency (called genitourinary syndrome of menopause) negatively impacting quality of life including sexual intimacy (see Clinical Manifestations under Menopause). A referral to a qualified physical therapy specialist may be indicated.

*Chemotherapy-induced peripheral neuropathy* is a common side effect of treatment with certain drugs. Symptoms include pain, paresthesias, loss of sensation, hypoalgesia or hyperalgesia, and muscle weakness that may or may not resolve. As early detection of chemotherapy-induced peripheral neuropathy is critical to reversibility, the therapist should be vigilant about asking cancer survivors who have been treated with chemotherapy about possible symptoms (see Chapter 9). Online educational resources of interest to therapists and clients include the National Ovarian Cancer Coalition, ACS, and National Cancer Institute (NCI).

# Pelvic Congestion Syndrome

## Overview and Incidence

Pelvic congestion syndrome is an often underdiagnosed cause of CPP in which the veins of the pelvic cavity dilate, resulting in varicosities.[464] It has been diagnosed in approximately 10% of women, more than half of whom report pelvic pain.[140] Incompetent and dilated ovarian, uterine, and other pelvic veins are a common finding in asymptomatic women and a known cause of abdominal and pelvic pain in others (Fig. 20.6).[69] Ovarian varices may occur unilaterally or bilaterally, most often in women who have had children but occasionally in nonparous women.[163]

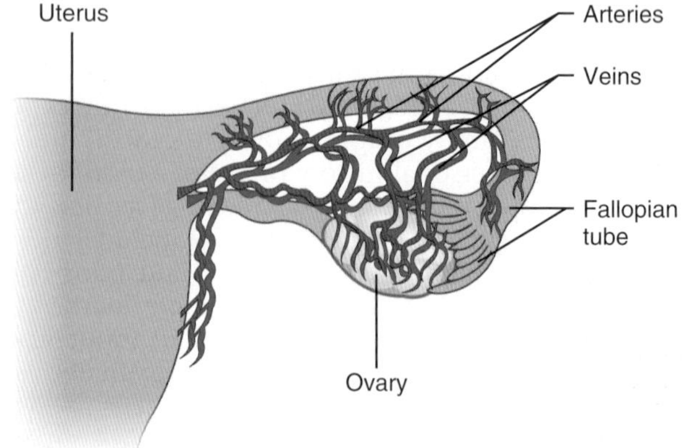


**Figure 20.6**

**Varicose veins (varicosities) of the ovary.** Ovarian varicosities associated with pelvic congestion syndrome cause chronic pelvic pain in women. This form of venous insufficiency is often accompanied by prominent varicose veins elsewhere in the lower quadrant (buttocks, thighs, calves). Men may have similar varicosities of the scrotum (not shown). (From Goodman CC, Snyder TE: *Differential diagnosis for the physical therapist: screening for referral*, ed 5, Philadelphia, 2013, Saunders.)

## Clinical Manifestations and Pathophysiology

Reported symptoms include pain that worsens toward the end of the day or after standing for a long time, pain that occurs premenstrually and after intercourse, sensations of heaviness in the pelvis, and prominent varicose veins elsewhere in the body.[473] Pain is worse during pregnancy.[69] If observed during pregnancy, these varicosities may disappear after delivery, but they become more prominent with subsequent pregnancies. Ovarian varicosities are common in patients with endometriosis.

This type of pelvic pain arises when blood pools in a distended ovarian/pelvic vein, forming a varicocele. The term *varicocele* is traditionally applied to men to describe varicose veins in the testicles, but varicoceles can also occur in the female counterparts of those organs. In fact, 10% of men experience pelvic varices of the gonadal veins manifesting as varicoceles similar to uteroovarian varices seen in women.[85]

## Medical Management

**Diagnosis and Treatment.** There are three diagnostic criteria for pelvic congestion: a tortuous pelvic vein with a diameter more than 4 mm, slow blood flow, and dilated communicating veins.[140] Ovarian vein incompetence may be suspected from the presence of vulvar varicosities. The gold standard for diagnosis is visualization with computed tomography venography. MRI and transvaginal ultrasound appear to have good sensitivity and may be more readily available.[473] Embolization of the pelvic and ovarian veins (see discussion of this technique in Uterine Fibroids) is a newer treatment but reportedly safe and effective in alleviating pain and symptoms,

**Table 20.4** Pelvic Floor Disorders

| Pelvic Floor Disorders Related to Loss of Support | Pelvic Floor Disorders Related to Pain |
|---|---|
| • Urinary incontinence (Chapter 18)<br>  • Stress urinary incontinence<br>  • Urge urinary incontinence<br>• Fecal incontinence (Chapter 16)<br>• Pelvic organ prolapse (Chapter 20)<br>  • Cystocele<br>  • Rectocele<br>  • Uterine prolapse<br>• Pelvic floor muscle dysfunction—underactive/weakness (Chapter 27) | • Organ-based conditions<br>  • Irritable bowel syndrome (Chapter 16)<br>  • Painful bladder syndrome/interstitial cystitis (Chapter 18)<br>  • Endometriosis (Chapter 20)<br>• Musculoskeletal conditions<br>  • Coccygodynia (Chapter 27)<br>  • Pelvic floor muscle dysfunction—overactive/spasm (Chapter 27)<br>• Infectious conditions<br>  • Prostatitis (Chapter 19)<br>  • Urinary tract infection (Chapter 18)<br>• Unknown origin or multiple system conditions<br>  • CP/CPPS or prostatodynia (Chapter 19)<br>  • Dyspareunia (Chapter 20) |

*CP/CPPS,* Chronic prostatitis/chronic pelvic pain syndrome.

**Table 20.5** Conditions Related to Increased Tone of the Pelvic Floor Muscles

| Diagnosis | Description | Symptoms |
|---|---|---|
| Pelvic floor muscle tension myalgia/levator ani syndrome. | Pain and spasm of pelvic floor muscles, may include obturator internus or piriformis | Perineal pain and pain with sitting |
| Vaginismus | Muscle spasm of superficial and deep muscles around the vagina | Dyspareunia |
| Anismus | Muscle spasm of superficial and deep muscles around the rectum | Obstructed defecation and coccyx pain |
| Dyspareunia | Painful penetration (which could include penis, finger, speculum, tampon, or toy) | A symptom of many other conditions |
| Vulvodynia | Refers to a large group of diseases in which perineal and vaginal pain is the major symptom; provoked vestibulodynia is a subset of vulvodynia | Dyspareunia, pain during sitting, inability to wear jeans |
| Pudendal neuralgia | Neuralgia of the pudendal nerve possibly related to compression, especially at the sacrotuberous and sacrospinous ligament crossing | Broad pelvic pain and pain with sitting |

improving sexual functioning, and reducing anxiety and depression with subsequent improved quality of life rep orted.[140,262,464]

## PELVIC FLOOR DISORDERS

Pelvic floor disorders comprise a group of conditions involving the pelvic organs and structures: bladder, bowel, uterus/prostate, muscles, ligaments, and joints. It is important for all therapists to have a basic knowledge of these conditions, symptoms, and treatments. Pelvic floor disorders can be categorized into those related to loss of support and those related to pain (Table 20.4). Pelvic floor disorders may include conditions of *PFM dysfunction*. PFM dysfunction (underactive/weakness or overactive/spasm) refers specifically to a condition of the skeletal muscle layer of the pelvic floor. Table 20.5 lists additional conditions of increased PFM tone related to overactive PFMs and spasm.

A cross-sectional survey of almost 2000 women in the United States[379] reported an overall prevalence of 23.7% for at least one pelvic floor disorder. Prevalence increased with age from 9.7% in women 20 to 39 years old to 49.7% in women older than 80. A statistically significant increase in prevalence was also seen with increasing parity, from 12.8% in women without children to 32.4% in women with three or more deliveries. Weight differences also reached statistical significance with obese women reporting pelvic floor disorders at a prevalence of 30.4% and normal-weight women reporting disorders at a prevalence of 15.1%.

A larger study of more than 4000 women[292] reported a prevalence of 37% for any one pelvic floor disorder. Individual prevalence was reported as follows: SUI 15%, overactive bladder 13%, and POP 6%. Many women reported more than one condition. This study found no association of increasing incidence with increasing age after adjusting for confounders of obesity, birth history, menopause, and hormones.

### Pelvic Pain

Pelvic pain encompasses a wide variety of conditions and pain patterns. Pelvic pain patterns are broadly categorized

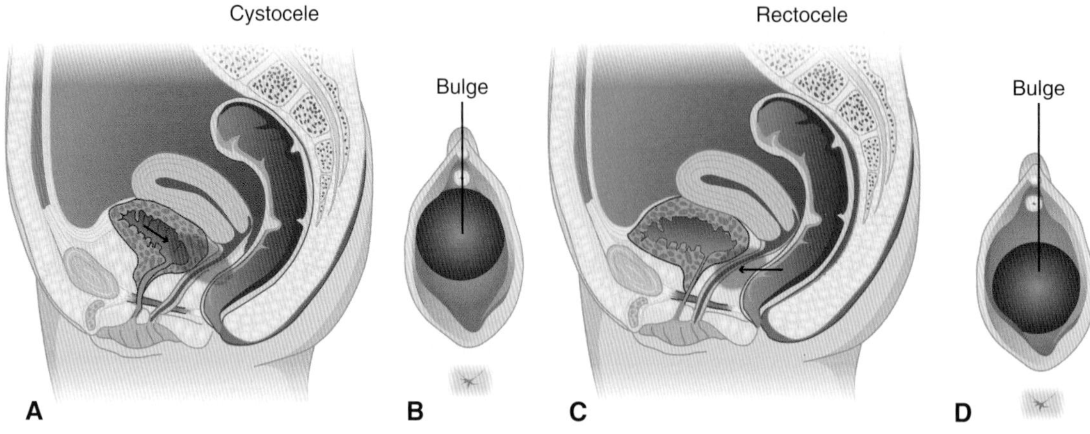


**Figure 20.7**

(A) Cystocele (sagittal view). Note the bulging of the anterior vaginal wall. The urinary bladder is displaced downward. (B) Lithotomy view. The bladder pushes the anterior vaginal wall downward into the vagina. (C) Rectocele (sagittal view). (D) Note the bulging of the posterior vaginal wall associated with rectocele (lithotomy view).

as cyclic and noncyclic.[291] CPP is pelvic pain lasting longer than 6 months. This term does not identify a cause for the pain. In some cases, there is a diagnosable cause such as IBS, interstitial cystitis, vulvodynia, or endometrioses. However, in some cases the cause or reason for the pain is not easily identified. In addition, many of these conditions are associated with central sensitization, or sensitive nervous system, making the diagnosis and treatment more difficult. Several large studies[312,330,572] have found the incidence of CPP in women 18 to 50 years of age to be between 13.6% and 24% with 6.2% listing their pain as moderate and 5% noting the pain interferes with daily life "all the time."[312] Younger women are less likely to have CPP, and women with previous pelvic trauma or surgery are more likely to have CPP.[312] Other risk factors include conditions that can be related to abdominal and pelvic adhesion such as previous miscarriage, longer menstrual flow, endometriosis, PID, and cesarean section.[291] Numerous psychologic morbidities may also contribute including abuse (childhood and sexual), anxiety, depression, and somatization.[291]

## Pelvic Organ Prolapse—Cystocele, Rectocele, and Uterine Prolapse

### Overview and Incidence

The three types of POP discussed here are cystocele, rectocele, and uterine prolapse. *Cystocele* is the loss of support of the bladder and urethra, resulting in falling of the urinary bladder and a bulging of the anterior vaginal wall into the vagina (Fig. 20.7A and B). *Rectocele* is the loss of support of the rectum, resulting in falling of the rectum and a bulging of the posterior vaginal wall into the vagina (Fig. 20.7C and D). *Uterine prolapse* is the fall of the uterus into the vagina (Fig. 20.8).

Other types of POP include cystourethrocele (bladder and urethra prolapse into the vagina), urethrocele (urethra prolapse into the vagina), enterocele (prolapse of part of the intestine into the space between the vagina and the rectum), rectal prolapse (anal and rectal canal folds over and falls out the rectum), and vaginal vault prolapse (apex of the vagina falls into the vagina, occurring sometimes after a hysterectomy).

During a gynecologic examination 30% to 76% of women are found to have some descent of the pelvic organs.[39,237] However, significantly fewer women are bothered by the condition or notice any symptoms (3% to 38%).[84,237]

### Etiology and Risk Factors

Cystocele, rectocele, and uterine prolapse are due to loss of support of the PFMs and fascial and ligamentous structures of the pelvic organs. Multiple pregnancies increase the risk of these disorders developing. There is some disagreement regarding whether there are identifiable labor or delivery parameters that contribute more to POP. Some professionals believe prolonged labor, forceps delivery, bearing down before full dilation, and forceful delivery of the placenta are possible causes of prolapse.[43] Other risk factors related to increased intraabdominal pressure include obesity, chronic pulmonary disease with prolonged coughing, prolonged heavy lifting, poor exercise technique, or excessive straining during bowel movement. Loss of ligamentous support with pelvic surgery, especially hysterectomy, can also contribute to POP.[415] Genetics may play a role, as family history of prolapse increases the individual risk of prolapse.[346] Joint hypermobility is associated with POP, and therapists treating patients with hypermobility should be aware of POP and educate patients in protection of the pelvic floor.[519] Women with loss of lumbar lordosis are 3.2 times more likely to have POP.[333]

### Pathogenesis

The uterus and other pelvic structures are maintained in their proper position by three mechanisms: suspension by intact endopelvic fascia and ligaments such as the uterosacral and cardinal ligaments; constriction by the PFMs, specifically the levator ani layer; and structural geometry of the flap valve mechanism.[544]

Overstretching, genetic weakness, and partial or full avulsion of the endopelvic fascia can result in POP.

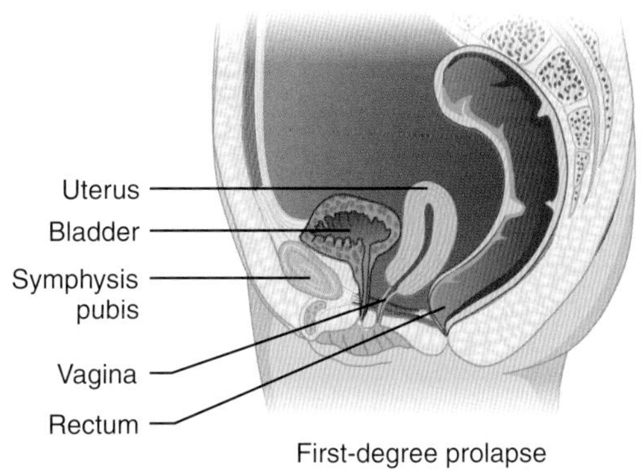


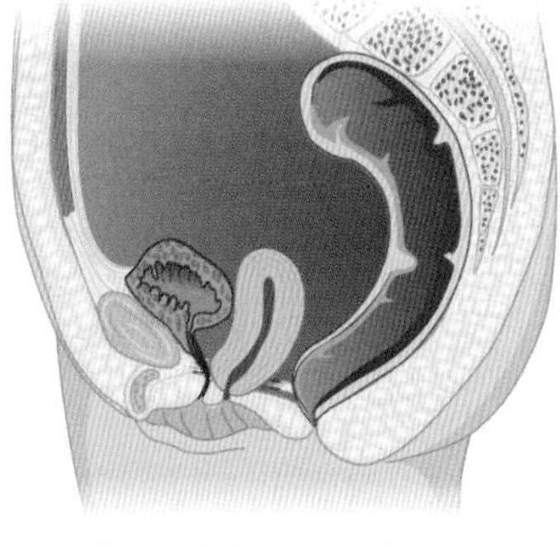


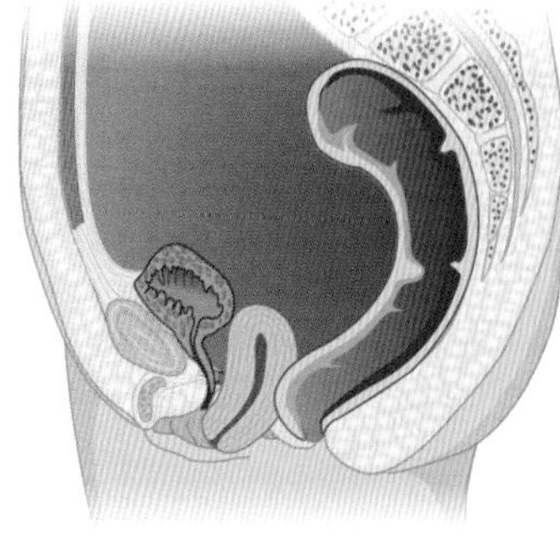


**Figure 20.8**

**Stages of uterine prolapse.** Herniation of the uterus through the pelvic floor resulting in protrusion into the vagina. *First-degree:* the cervix remains in the vagina. *Second-degree:* the cervix appears at the perineum or protrudes on straining. *Third-degree:* the entire uterus protrudes outside the body, and there is total inversion of the vagina.

Postpartum ultrasound has identified levator ani avulsion in 10% to 30% of women after vaginal delivery. Levator avulsion is significantly associated with POP.[203] The location of the weakening determines the type of prolapse: anterior endopelvic fascia weakness results in cystocele, and posterior endopelvic fascia weakness results in rectocele. The pelvic floor musculature forms a slinglike structure that supports the uterus, vagina, urinary bladder, urethra, and rectum.[130]

Multiple studies have documented the important role of the PFMs in avoiding or improving POP.[218] Similar to loss of support in the noncontractile tissue, overstretching, weakness, or partial or full avulsion of the PFMs can contribute to downward movement of the pelvic organs on POP. As the organs move downward, the canals straighten, and the flap valve mechanism is lost. The above-listed etiologic and risk factors contribute to this loss of support.

## Clinical Manifestations

The symptoms of POP vary greatly and are not related to type or severity, with some individuals having severe POP and no symptoms and others having a very small descent of the organs and significant symptoms. The most common symptom is a sense of heaviness or pressure in the perineum or lower abdomen, which is often increased after long periods of standing or upright weight-bearing postures, decreased with lying down, and may be felt by some people to be painful. Often the woman notices a lump in the vaginal area and seeks medical advice to determine the cause. Many women have more than one type of POP and thus may have many of the symptoms described next.

The symptoms associated with a cystocele include urinary frequency and urgency, difficulty in emptying the bladder, and urinary incontinence. The symptoms associated with a rectocele include a feeling of incomplete rectal emptying, constipation, and aching or pressure after a bowel movement. If the rectocele becomes large enough to trap feces, manual pressure applied to the vaginal wall may be necessary to complete a bowel movement without excessive straining (a practice called *splinting,* or *stenting,* which is usually an indication of the need for corrective surgery).

Box 20.9

**BADEN-WALKER SYSTEM FOR EVALUATION OF PELVIC ORGAN PROLAPSE**

| Grade | |
|---|---|
| 0 | Normal position |
| 1 | Descent halfway to the hymen |
| 2 | Descent to the hymen |
| 3 | Descent halfway past the hymen |
| 4 | Maximum possible descent |

Data from ACOG Practice Bulletin No. 85: Pelvic organ prolapse. *Obstet Gynecol* 110:717–729, 2007.

Primary symptoms resulting from uterine prolapse are backache and irritation and excoriation of the exposed mucous membranes of the cervix and vagina, especially from sexual intercourse and from wiping after toileting.

## Medical Management

**Diagnosis.** The diagnosis of these disorders is primarily derived from observation and the pelvic examination. The two most common grading systems are the Baden-Walker[19] (Box 20.9) and Pelvic Organ Prolapse Quantification (POP-Q) systems.[484] The POP-Q system comprises a complex set of measurements to map the shape of the vaginal walls. The Baden-Walker system is simpler and used by most gynecologists. In this system, the POP grade depends on how far the organ protrudes through the introitus (entrance to the vagina) or hymen (tissue at the introitus). A *first-degree* uterine prolapse is marked by some descent, but the cervix has not reached the introitus. A *second-degree* uterine prolapse is marked by the cervix as part of the uterus having descended to the introitus. A *third-degree* prolapse is manifested by the entire uterus protruding through the vaginal opening (see Fig. 20.8).

**Treatment.** Treatment decisions are based on intensity of symptoms (i.e., how bothersome they are to the individual) and can include surgical, mechanical, or conservative options.

Surgical procedures that can be used to correct POP include colposuspension, colporrhaphy, sacrocolpopexy, and paravaginal repair. Many women have concomitant bladder suspension or hysterectomy. There are complications with surgery, and approximately 30% of patients require another surgery for recurrence.[93] Mesh complications (CPP) and litigation have led to investigation of alternative techniques, including native tissue vaginal repairs. In addition, it has been recognized that skilled surgeons have acceptably low complication rates using mesh to support the POP.[393]

Mechanical treatments involve fitting of a pessary (a device inserted into the vagina to hold the organs in place).[326] Some women can remove their own pessary, whereas others must report to the nurse every 3 months to have the device removed, washed, and replaced. Pessaries should always be worn during recreational activities or strengthening exercises.

Conservative options are becoming more popular with new research documenting the success of conservative treatment. Rehabilitation includes PFM strengthening exercises and muscle reeducation, postural education (avoiding loss of lumbar lordosis and increased thoracic kyphosis), self-care (avoiding constipation with adequate fluid and fiber intake) and possibly biofeedback, or electrical stimulation.[480] A large multicenter randomized controlled trial reported significantly less POP symptoms among women in the PFM exercise group.[201] Many pelvic therapists think strengthening of the PFMs should be incorporated into the preoperative and postoperative rehabilitation program as well.[244] However, a more recent Cochrane review does not support the efficacy of this practice.[211]

SPECIAL IMPLICATIONS FOR THE THERAPIST 20.10

### *Cystocele, Rectocele, and Uterine Prolapse*

As with urinary incontinence, pelvic therapists can have a primary role in the treatment of POP through treatment of PFM dysfunction (see Chapter 27). Therapists will also see people with pelvic floor disorders as a comorbidity. In these cases, therapists must be vigilant to avoid increased intraabdominal pressure, such as holding the breath or bearing down, as these could exacerbate the pelvic floor condition.

Some core exercises may also exacerbate POP symptoms. Slowly adding exercises, asking patients/clients to monitor and report change in POP symptoms, and educating women against bearing down during exercise can avoid complications. Women should also be educated in proper body mechanics and avoidance of lifting in a trunk flexed position, which can exacerbate symptoms.

In addition, a woman with a second- or third-degree uterine prolapse may have difficulty tolerating extended periods of weight-bearing activities. Alternative positions for exercise may need to be incorporated into the rehabilitation program (include more sitting, reclined exercise, or pool therapy if possible).

# BREAST DISEASE

Breast disease falls into two categories: *benign breast conditions* and *breast cancer.* Most breast lumps are benign or noncancerous. These include cysts, fibroadenomas, and a number of other conditions that are characterized by lumpy and sometimes painful breasts. Because cancerous tumors of the breast cannot be distinguished from benign lesions, persistent lumps as well as breast pain should always be medically evaluated.

## Benign Breast Conditions

### Overview

*Benign breast conditions* and *benign breast changes* (also referred to as *benign breast disease*) are the preferred terms for describing a number of breast irregularities. Use of the term fibrocystic breast disease is now considered an erroneous "wastebasket" designation. Some degree of tissue nodularity (sometimes referred to as lumpiness) is normal in most younger women; tissue changes do not necessarily constitute true disease. Fibrocystic changes can be confirmed only by histologic examination. Other terms used to describe tissue nodularity include *diffuse cystic mastopathy* and *mammary dysplasia.*

### Incidence and Risk Factors

Benign breast changes, cysts, and fibroadenomas make up the majority of benign breast conditions. These changes are most often observed in women 20 to 50 years of age,[386]; breast changes associated with the menstrual cycle are estimated to occur in half of all women. It is not known if risk factors for developing breast cancer also apply to the development of benign breast disease. Cysts manifest more often in women 30 to 50 years of age,[15] and especially preceding menopause. *Cysts* are fluid-filled lumps that may fluctuate in size. Their onset may be gradual or sudden (overnight). Fibroadenomas occur most commonly in premenopausal women, with a median age of 25 years.[15] They are solid tumors that comprise glandular and fibrous connective tissue. Lumps may be easily movable under the skin, firm, painless, and rubbery with well-defined borders. They usually occur in single lumps but may be multifocal and can be bilateral. Assessment of benign breast conditions to rule out breast cancer currently accounts for more than half of all surgical procedures on the female breast.

### Etiologic Factors and Pathogenesis

Because benign breast conditions are not one disease entity, etiology is not clearly known. Variations from the normal changes associated with breast development and reproductive life (pregnancy, lactation, and involution) form the basis for most benign breast conditions. Nonproliferative tissue nodularity can be generalized, occurring in multiple areas of both breasts. Fibroadenomas are estrogen-sensitive and may be stimulated by pregnancy, lactation, and perimenopause. Cystic changes can be minimal without producing a discrete mass or can produce cysts up to 5 cm.

Hormonal factors such as the use of postmenopausal hormones or a family history of breast cancer can increase the risk of benign breast conditions.[564] The timing of certain lifestyle factors may be important in the development of benign breast conditions. Although alcohol use in adulthood does not appear to impact risk of benign

Box 20.10

**BENIGN BREAST CHANGES AND RISK FOR DEVELOPING BREAST CANCER**

***Nonproliferative Lesions***

These conditions are not linked with the overgrowth of breast tissue. They do not seem to affect breast cancer risk, or if they do, the effect is very small.

- Fibrosis
- Cysts
- Mild hyperplasia of the usual type
- Adenosis (nonsclerosing)
- Phyllodes tumor (rare; usually benign)
- Single (solitary) papilloma
- Granular cell tumor
- Fat necrosis
- Mastitis
- Duct ectasia
- Benign lumps or tumors (lipoma, hamartoma, hemangioma, hematoma, neurofibroma, adenomyoepithelioma)
- Squamous and apocrine metaplasia
- Epithelial-related calcifications

***Proliferative Lesions Without Atypia***

These conditions are linked with the growth of cells in the ducts or lobules of the breast tissue. They seem to raise a woman's risk of breast cancer slightly (1.5 to 2 times the usual risk).

- Moderate or florid ductal hyperplasia of the usual type (without atypia)
- Fibroadenoma
- Sclerosing adenosis
- Multiple papillomas or papillomatosis
- Radial scar

***Proliferative Lesions With Atypia***

These conditions are linked with the excess growth of cells in the ducts or lobules of the breast tissue, and the cells no longer look normal. They can raise breast cancer risk about 3.5 to 5 times higher than usual risk.

- Atypical ductal hyperplasia
- Atypical lobular hyperplasia

***Lobular Carcinoma In Situ***

This condition raises breast cancer risk 7 to 11 times higher than usual risk.

breast conditions, regular alcohol consumption during adolescence likely increases risk.[304]

Some types of benign breast conditions are linked to higher breast cancer risk, whereas others are not (Box 20.10).[146] Benign breast conditions can be divided into three general groups, based on whether the cells are multiplying (proliferative) and whether there are abnormal cells or patterns of cells (atypia).

- *Nonproliferative lesions* do not seem to affect cancer risk.
- *Proliferative lesions without atypia* slightly increase cancer risk.
- *Proliferative lesions with atypia* increase the risk of cancer.

## Clinical Manifestations

Clinically, benign breast conditions may manifest as:

- Nodularity (significant lumpiness; may be cyclic or not)
- Mastalgia (severe breast pain; may be cyclic or not)
- Cyclic swelling, discomfort, tenderness
- Cysts
- Nipple discharge
- Infections and inflammations (mastitis, Mondor disease, abscess)

Nodularity usually manifests bilaterally as regular, firm nodules that are mobile and may be described as bubble wrap, small gravel, or small water balloons. Masses associated with nodularity may or may not be painful. Pain, tenderness, or discomfort may occur in association with fluid retention and/or accompany hormonal changes associated with the menstrual cycle, such as during the premenstrual phase. Cysts can fluctuate in size with rapid appearance or disappearance. Fibroadenomas are typically solitary lesions about 2 to 4 cm in size when first detected. A typical fibroadenoma is nontender and easily movable under the skin, with well-defined borders.

## Medical Management

**Diagnosis and Treatment.** These benign lesions are detected on physical examination and imaging, such as mammography, ultrasound, and MRI. Because benign breast conditions are often indistinguishable from carcinomas, biopsy is often used to confirm the diagnosis. Breast ultrasound helps to differentiate cystic fluid-filled masses from solid masses. The presence of nodularity does not predispose a woman to cancer but may make diagnosis of cancerous lumps more difficult.

Treatment for benign breast conditions often takes a back seat to ruling out cancer. Palliative treatments include aspirin, mild analgesics, and local heat or cold. Dietary changes may be recommended, including salt restriction (especially during the second half of the menstrual cycle); low-fat or Mediterranean diet; and avoiding caffeine and other stimulants containing methylxanthines, which are found in coffee, chocolate, tea, and many soft drinks and energy drinks. However, current research is limited regarding the impact of dietary changes.[15]

Other recommendations with anecdotal support include evening primrose oil, use of diuretics, and vitamin and mineral supplementation (vitamins A, $B_6$, D, and E; calcium and magnesium). The use of hormones, including oral contraceptives, tamoxifen, and androgens, as well as pain medication such as danazol (Danocrine) and bromocriptine (Parlodel) may be prescribed for women with severe symptoms. Women are encouraged to wear a supportive brassiere and to use fabrics that do not irritate the breast skin. In some cases, painful cysts have been aspirated with relief of symptoms.[15,117]

# Breast Cancer

## Overview

Breast cancer is the most common malignancy in women in the United States after nonmelanoma skin cancer and accounts for one-third of all cancers diagnosed in American women. It is the second largest cause of cancer deaths in women in the United States, second only to lung cancer.[378]

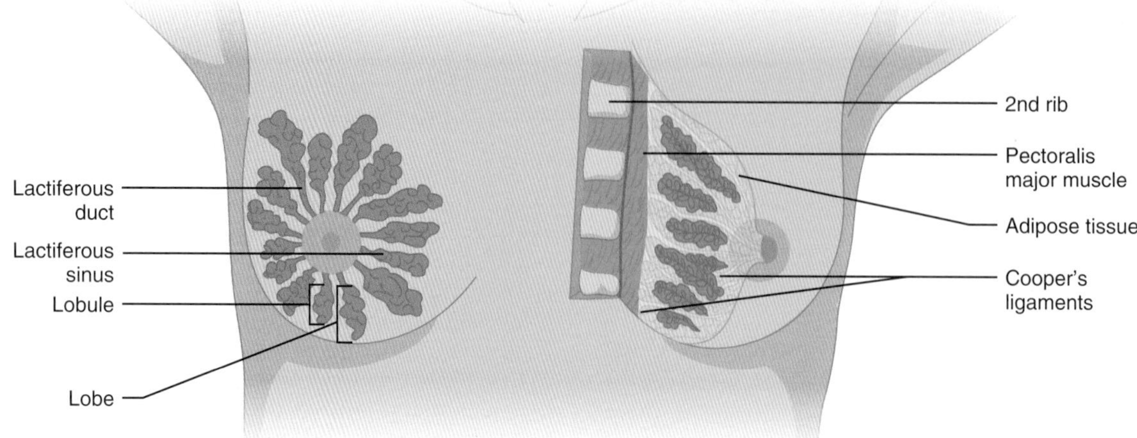


**Figure 20.9**

**Breast anatomy.** The breast is made up of glandular tissue, fibrous tissue including suspensory ligaments, and adipose tissue. Glandular tissue contains 15 to 20 lobes radiating from the nipple and made up of lobules. Within each lobe are clusters of alveoli that produce milk. Each lobe is embedded in adipose tissue and empties into a lactiferous duct. There are 15 to 20 lactiferous ducts that form a collecting duct system converging toward the nipple. These ducts form ampullae or lactiferous sinuses behind the nipple, which are reservoirs for storing milk. The lobules and ducts are surrounded by fatty and connective tissue, nerves, blood vessels, and lymphatic vessels. The suspensory ligaments (Cooper ligaments) are fibrous bands extending vertically from the surface attaching to the chest wall muscle. These support the breast tissue and become contracted in cancer of the breast, producing pits or dimples in the overlying skin. (From Jarvis C: *Physical examination and health assessment,* ed 4, Philadelphia, 2004, Saunders.)

Breasts are made up of glandular milk-producing tissue (ducts and lobules) and stromal or connective tissue. Most breast cancers are adenocarcinomas (glandular) originating in the single layer of epithelial cells that line the ductal and lobular systems of all milk ducts (Fig. 20.9).

## Categories and Classifications

Major histopathologic categories of breast cancer (based on morphologic features of the tumor) include *ductal carcinoma in situ* (DCIS), also known as *invasive carcinoma of no special type; invasive (infiltrating) ductal carcinoma* (IDC); *invasive (infiltrating) lobular carcinoma* (ILC); *inflammatory breast cancer* (IBC); and *Paget disease of the breast.*[284] Less common subtypes of IDC include *medullary, tubular, mucinous, papillary,* and *cribriform cancers* of the breast. *Lobular carcinoma in situ* is not considered a true cancer but a precancerous condition with increased risk of developing into cancer. Lobular carcinoma in situ usually occurs in more than one lobule. *Phyllodes tumors* are rare and arise in the stroma as well as the glandular tissue of the breast. They are usually benign but in rare cases can be malignant.[476] *Sarcomas* are rare cancers that start in connective tissues such as muscle tissue, fat tissue, or blood vessels.

When premalignant change or "cancer" cells multiply but remain contained within the duct, the condition is termed DCIS. IDC occurs when cancer cells break through the duct wall and enter other tissues. ILC occurs when cancer cells in the lobules break through to invade the stroma. In some cases, a single breast tumor can be a combination of these types or a mixture of invasive and in situ cancer. Rarely other kinds of cancers can occur in the breast including lymphoma, liposarcoma, angiosarcoma, and melanoma.

**Ductal carcinoma in situ** is the most common type of in situ cancer. One in 33 women will be diagnosed with breast in situ cancer (DCIS or lobular carcinoma in situ) in their lifetime; 83% of those women will have DCIS.[534] It develops at several points along a duct and appears as a cluster of microcalcifications or white flecks on a mammogram. DCIS is made up of small areas of atypical cells in an abnormal arrangement confined to the duct of the breast. For this reason, many pathologists do not consider DCIS to be true cancer. DCIS is represented by a broad continuum from slow-growing cells with little potential to be transformed into cancer to cells with more aggressive potential that may invade the duct wall and grow beyond it. It is considered to be stage 0 disease. Diagnosis and treatment of DCIS remains one of the most controversial areas in breast health medicine involving debate about potentially overly aggressive treatment.

**Invasive (infiltrating) ductal carcinoma** is the most common of the invasive breast cancers, originating in a duct, breaking through the duct wall, and invading the stromal tissue of the breast, with further possible metastasis via the lymphatic and/or circulatory systems. IDC is usually detected by mammogram or as a palpable lump during a breast examination. IDC represents 70% or more of all invasive breast cancer cases in women and 80% to 90% of all breast cancer cases in men.[534]

**Medullary, tubular, mucinous, papillary, and cribriform carcinomas** are less common subtypes of ductal carcinoma, together accounting for about 10% of breast cancers. These and other breast cancer variants present clinical challenges; because of their small numbers, treatment algorithms have relied largely on case studies and small series rather than large or randomized trials.[134] Medullary, tubular, and mucinous carcinomas are invasive but tend to have better outcomes than IDCs or ILCs.

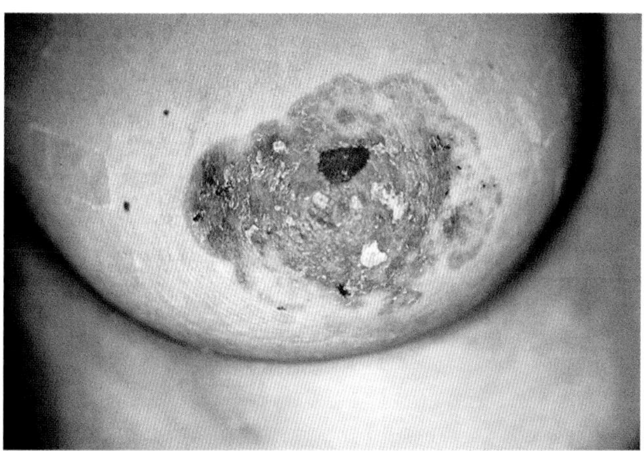

**Figure 20.10**

**Paget disease of the breast.** An erythematous plaque surrounds the nipple. (From Bolognia JL: *Dermatology*, St. Louis, 2003, Mosby.)

Papillary and cribriform carcinomas are rare and are usually associated with DCIS.

**Invasive (infiltrating) lobular carcinoma** is the second most common type of invasive breast cancer, making up 5% to 15% of invasive cancers.[141] This type of breast cancer grows through the wall of the lobule and may spread via the lymphatic or circulatory system. ILC has more of a tendency to be multifocal (discontinuous) than IDC. Because of the single-file growth pattern, ILC often is poorly imaged on mammography, with the tumor being larger than appears on mammogram or breast ultrasound.[249] Invasive lobular cancers are not typically felt as a lump; instead they may feel like an area of increased thickening, or nothing may be palpated at all.

**Inflammatory breast cancer** is a rare cancer with 1% to 5% incidence according to the NCI. It is a very aggressive, rapidly progressive form of invasive breast cancer that is not a true inflammatory process and is not usually associated with fever. In IBC, cancer cells obstruct lymphatic vessels in the breast, causing erythema and edema. IBC manifests much like mastitis or cellulitis (see Clinical Manifestations). The lymphatic blockage results in a rapid increase in breast size.[515] Because of its rarity, IBC is often misdiagnosed as mastitis or generalized dermatitis.[515]

**Paget disease of the breast** is a rare form of ductal carcinoma (1% to 3%) that is located beneath the nipple, with itching, tingling, pain, and an eczema-like rash; it can progress to crusting, ulceration, and weeping (Fig. 20.10).[142] It is usually unilateral and may involve the areola. Paget disease of the breast often occurs in conjunction with DCIS or invasive cancer. It may be dismissed at first because early symptoms are similar to those caused by some benign skin conditions.

**Male Breast Cancer.** Male breast cancer is an uncommon disease comprising less than 1% of all breast cancers. It is biologically different from female breast cancer. In men, breast cancer is most often IDC, with low incidence of lobular carcinoma. The tumors are usually hormone receptor–positive, including the androgen receptor, and there is an increased prevalence of the *BRCA2* germline mutation.[86,196] Ongoing studies show risk of genetic variations is different for men and women.[86] Involvement of the skin or chest wall is more common in male breast cancers, possibly because of the relatively small amount of breast tissue.

**Primary Molecular Subtypes.** Each classification described above will be further defined by primary molecular subtype. Currently there are four to five designations for primary molecular subtypes of different breast cancers: luminal A tumors, luminal B tumors, human epidermal growth factor receptor 2 (HER2 or HER2/neu) overexpressing tumors, basal-like tumors, and normal breast–like tumors. These classifications are based on gene profiling assays and immunohistochemical characterization of breast cancers. Assessment includes hormone receptor status, oncogene overexpression (see the discussion of oncogenes in Chapter 9), proliferative capacity, and other features.[119,409,495] See also Biomarkers under Diagnosis and Staging.)

## Incidence

Breast cancer statistics for detection, mortality, and morbidity continue to improve, with significant health focus and screening and treatment advances. Even so, breast carcinomas still account for approximately 30% of all cancers affecting women in the United States. As mentioned earlier, breast cancer is the second largest cause (after lung cancer) of female cancer deaths in the United States.

The ACS reported that for 2019 there would be an estimated 271,270 new cases of breast cancer in women and 2670 new cases in men. Projections for cancer deaths in 2019 were 41,760 deaths for women and 500 for men.[453]

## Etiology and Pathogenesis

As in every other cancer, breast cancer begins when something, an *initiator*, causes a gene to mutate. If the cell with the mutated gene survives to divide, it passes on the mutated gene to daughter cells, which in turn divide. Because they are abnormal, these cells are more vulnerable than normal cells to further mutations and may eventually become abnormal enough to be considered cancer. The immune system may recognize these cells to be abnormal and destroy them long before this happens.

The development of invasive breast cancer begins with epithelial hyperplasia, premalignant change, and in situ carcinoma, which leads to invasive carcinoma. The NCI states that in approximately 80% of breast cancers, estrogen is believed to be a key factor in promoting (rather than initiating) cancer. It may not trigger the series of genetic changes that are required to transform normal breast cells into malignant ones, but it may spur the proliferation of altered cells, increasing the likelihood that they will develop into cancer.[432] (See further discussion in Biomarkers.)

In the case of families with a strong history of breast (and often ovarian) cancer in several members with cancer at young ages, the culprit is often one of two mutated genes, altered *BRCA1* or *BRCA2*. Other genes contribute, and researchers are searching for more. *BRCA1* and *BRCA2* are tumor suppressor genes present in all humans. When working properly, they produce proteins that repair DNA and monitor cell growth. Thus mutations can render these genes inactive, making DNA vulnerable to many kinds of damage such as aging and environmental factors (i.e., environmental and medical radiation), which may increase the risk for developing breast, ovarian, and other cancers. Either of these mutated genes can pass at conception from a mother or father to a daughter or son. One abnormal gene confers significant risk of breast cancer for women with the mutation. The onset of breast cancer is at a much earlier age for these individuals as well. By age 80 approximately 72% of women with altered *BRCA1* will develop breast cancer, as will approximately 69% of women with altered *BRCA2*.[277]

Most breast cancers (90% to 95%) are not linked to identifiable hereditary factors. Mutations in oncogenes and tumor suppressor genes involved in cellular growth can be caused by external factors, such as radiation, toxins, and other factors yet to be identified.

Understanding the pathogenesis of cancer in general and breast cancer specifically is an evolving discipline (see Cancer Pathogenesis in Chapter 9). Gene mutations are the proximate cause of cancer, but mutations alone are not enough to explain the development of breast cancer. Most carcinomas develop in the glandular epithelium of the terminal duct lobular unit. In the normal breast, the milk ducts and lobules are neatly lined with epithelial cells. In the complex multistep process that leads to the development of cancer, an overproduction *(hyperplasia)* of normal-looking cells progresses to abnormal-looking cells *(atypical ductal hyperplasia or atypical lobular hyperplasia)*.

## Risk Factors for Breast Cancer in Women

Female gender, age, race/ethnicity, family history (including genetic risk factors), medical history, diet and obesity, radiation exposure, alcohol use, and environment all are factors linked to breast cancer (Box 20.11). Major risk factors for IBC include younger age at menarche and high BMI.[515]

**Gender and Hormone Exposure.** Being female is the most significant risk factor associated with this disease. Although women have many more breast cells than men, the primary reason they develop breast cancer more often is thought to be related to exposure to the growth-promoting effects of the female hormones estrogen and progesterone. The average lifetime risk for a woman in the United States to develop breast cancer is 12.4%.[453]

Endogenous estrogen exposure throughout life including in utero may have an effect on breast cancer risk. The length of a woman's total number of reproductive years including an early onset of menstruation (before age 12 years) and later cessation (menopause; after age 55 years) may affect breast cancer risk. Results from the Collaborative Group on Hormonal Factors in Breast Cancer suggest the effects of menarche and menopause may be increased by other risk factors such as obesity, with lobular cancers appearing to be more affected than ductal cancers by endogenous ovarian hormones.[106]

Of all women diagnosed with breast cancer, 80% will have ER-positive (ER+) biometrics. Tumors that are ER+ have ERs and are stimulated to grow by estrogen. Estrogen attaches to the receptor molecule and activates genes that promote cell growth. Tumors that do not have ERs are called ER-negative (ER−) and are not influenced by the hormone.

Box 20.11

### FACTORS THAT INCREASE THE RELATIVE RISK OF BREAST CANCER IN WOMEN[a]

***Relative Risk Factor; R > 4.0***

- Age (≥65 years versus <65 years, although risk increases across all ages until age 80)
- Biopsy-confirmed atypical hyperplasia
- Certain inherited genetic mutations for breast cancer (*BRCA1* and/or *BRCA2*)
- Ductal carcinoma in situ
- Lobular carcinoma in situ
- Mammographically dense breasts (compared with least dense)
- Personal history of early-onset (age <40 years) breast cancer
- Two or more first-degree relatives with breast cancer diagnosed at an early age

***Relative Risk Factor; R = 2.1–4.0***

- Personal history of breast cancer (age ≥40 years)
- High endogenous estrogen or testosterone levels (postmenopausal)
- High-dose radiation to chest
- One first-degree relative with breast cancer

***Relative Risk Factor; R = 1.1–2.0***

- Alcohol consumption
- Ashkenazi Jewish heritage
- Early menarche (age <12 years)
- Height (tall)
- High socioeconomic status
- Late age at first full-term pregnancy (age >30 years)
- Late menopause (age >55 years)
- Never breastfed a child
- No full-term pregnancies
- Obesity (postmenopausal)/adult weight gain
- One first-degree relative with breast cancer
- Personal history of endometrial or ovarian cancer
- Proliferative breast disease without atypia (usual ductal hyperplasia and fibroadenoma)
- Recent and long-term use of menopausal hormone therapy containing estrogen and progestin
- Recent oral contraceptive use

[a]See also Box 20.10: Benign Breast Changes and Risk for Developing Breast Cancer and the *Breast Cancer Risk Assessment Tool* (http://www.cancer.gov/bcrisktool/), an interactive tool developed by the National Cancer Institute and the National Surgical Adjuvant Breast and Bowel Project for health professionals to assess a woman's risk of developing invasive breast cancer. The tool has been updated to include African American, Asian American, and Pacific Islander women based on the Contraceptive and Reproductive Experiences Study (CARE) and the Asian American Breast Cancer Study (AABC).

Data from American Cancer Society. *Breast Cancer Facts and Figures, 2017-2018*. Atlanta, 2017, American Cancer Society, Inc.

Previous history of first-generation hormonal contraceptive use (higher dose formulations before 1975) and more recent prolonged use of combined HRT (estrogen-progestin) have been linked with increased risk of breast cancer, often found at a more advanced stage. According to the NCI, there is solid evidence that combination HRT is associated with an increased risk of developing breast cancer.[250] In the WHI trial, there was a 26% increase in incidence of invasive breast cancer associated with combined HRT.[423] For estrogen-only therapy, the evidence for association with breast cancer incidence is mixed.[155]

The role of estrogen in the development and progression of some breast cancers continues to be investigated to determine potential contributions from chemicals in the environment with estrogenic activity that can enter the human breast. A range of organochlorine pesticides and polychlorinated biphenyls that possess estrogen-mimicking properties have been measured in the human breast. The role of these chemicals in promoting breast cancer is not yet definitively known.[149,360]

**Age.** Age is the second most significant risk factor for the development of breast cancer; incidence increases with advancing age. The cumulative lifetime risk of developing breast cancer for women in the United States is one in eight (or 12% to 13%) based on an 80-year life span. At age 20 years the 10-year risk of developing breast cancer is quite low, 1 in 1567, with increasing risk as a woman ages. At age 50 years the 10-year risk is 1 in 43. Women age 50 years and older account for 81% of all new cases of breast cancer.[132] The median age at which a woman in the United States is diagnosed with breast cancer is 62 years.[378] There are currently an estimated 3.5 million breast cancer survivors in the United States.[347]

Women older than age 75 years are the most rapidly growing demographic of newly diagnosed breast cancers. Further research is needed to improve outcomes for women in this age group. The number of complicating comorbidities will likely be a factor in diagnosis and treatment in this age group.[23]

**Race/Ethnicity.** Racial disparities in the United States exist between groups of women developing and dying of breast cancer. White women have a higher rate of developing breast cancer than any other racial or ethnic group except for African American women younger than age 40 years. During 2005–2014, breast cancer incidence rates among African American, Hispanic, Asian American, and Pacific Islander women declined slightly, while the rates among white and American Indian/Alaska Native women remained stable.[132] According to the latest statistics, African American women and Hispanic/Latina women are more likely to be diagnosed with large tumors than white women. African American women have the highest cancer mortality rate, with a 5-year survival rate of 81%. The 5-year survival rate for white women and Asian American women is 91%; the rate for Hispanic/Latina and Pacific Islander women is 86%, and the rate for American Indian/Alaska Native women is 84%.[132,133] Among men, the risk of dying of breast cancer is almost twice as high for black men compared with white men.

Genetic mutations among specific groups have been studied extensively among Ashkenazi Jews and other groups. These studies have helped to identify both genetic and environmental contributors to the development of breast cancer.

**Personal History, Family History, and Heredity.** A personal history of breast cancer in one breast increases a woman's risk of developing a new cancer in the other breast or in another part of the same breast three- to fourfold.[12] This is not the same as a recurrence of the first cancer; it is a new cancer. Additionally, women with a personal history of uterine and ovarian cancer or a family history of breast cancer among first-degree relatives have a significantly increased risk of developing breast cancer. Benign breast disease accompanied by proliferative changes increases the risk of cancer (see Box 20.10).

Some breast cancers may be caused by inherited gene mutations. Hereditary breast cancers account for approximately 5% to 10% of all breast cancers,[12] with most of those related to altered *BRCA1* or *BRCA2*. Normally, these genes suppress cancer by making proteins that prevent cells from growing abnormally. Inheriting either mutated gene from a parent results in a significantly increased risk of breast cancer for members of some families with *BRCA* mutations. Cancer in this population tends to develop at an earlier age and has a higher rate of bilateral disease than in non-*BRCA* carriers, with *BRCA1* related to more aggressive tumors.[274] People with these mutations also have an increased risk for developing ovarian and pancreatic cancer.[187] Specific mutations of *BRCA1* and *BRCA2* are more common in women of Ashkenazi Jewish ancestry. Male carriers of *BRCA2* mutations are also at increased risk for breast cancer.[562] Other investigations related to genes include growth factor receptor genes and oncogene overexpression (e.g., *ATM, TP53, CHEK2, PTEN, CDH1,* and *STK11*).[425]

Most breast cancers (90% to 95%) are not linked to identifiable hereditary factors. Although only a small percentage of breast cancer cases are hereditary, approximately 15% of women with breast cancer have a close blood relative with this disease. Conversely, most women (more than 85%) who are diagnosed with breast cancer do not have a family history of this disease.[12] Having one first-degree relative (mother, sister, or daughter) with breast cancer doubles a woman's risk; breast cancer in two or more first-degree relatives (mother, sister, daughter) increases the risk three- to fourfold. Although the exact risk is not known, women with a family history of breast cancer in a father or brother also have an increased risk of breast cancer.[12]

**Diet, Weight Gain, and Obesity.** A recent meta-analysis suggested that there is limited evidence that plant-rich diets versus consuming animal products may lower breast cancer risk, specifically for ER– breast cancers.[553] Recommendations are for eating a healthy diet, including vegetables, fruits, fiber-rich grains, legumes, nuts, low-fat dairy products, and low amounts of refined carbohydrates.[300]

BMI, a known breast cancer risk factor, could influence breast risk through pathways related to sex hormones, insulin resistance, chronic inflammation, and altered levels of adipose-derived hormones. Current evidence shows the relationship between excess body weight and breast cancer risk to be mixed. A slightly lower risk of breast cancer has been found in overweight premenopausal women. However, postmenopausal weight gain is considered to be a significant risk factor .[497] Estrogen manufactured in adipose tissue may make the hormone available even when ovarian production of estrogen stops at menopause.[220] There is evidence to suggest that fat cells in different parts of the body metabolize differently. For example, central obesity (excess fat in the waist area) may affect risk more than the same amount of fat in the hips and thighs.[392] Elevated serum insulin levels have been linked to some cancers, including breast cancer.[254] Individuals with lifelong obesity (from childhood) seem to have less risk for developing breast cancer.[421]

**Radiation Exposure.** Exposure to ionizing radiation is a risk factor for the development of cancer. In 2004 the National Toxicology Program classified x-rays and gamma rays as known human carcinogens. X-rays, gamma rays, and materials and processes that emit x-rays and gamma rays are used in the nuclear power industry, the military, medicine, scientific research, and a variety of consumer products. Biologic damage by ionizing radiation is related to dose and dose rate.[375] Previous radiation therapy to the chest area as treatment for another cancer (such as Hodgkin disease or non-Hodgkin lymphoma) has been shown to be a significant risk factor for breast cancer in women. The risk varies with the woman's age when she had the radiation, the dose received, and the size of the radiation field. The risk of developing breast cancer from chest radiation is highest if the radiation was administered during adolescence (during the time of breast development).[8] The secondary cancer risk to women seems to increase 10 years after the initial diagnosis and treatment of Hodgkin disease; it is recommended that these women be followed for 40 years or longer.[438]

**Alcohol.** The use of alcohol is linked to an increased risk of developing breast cancer,[390] particularly in hormonally sensitive cancers (ER+) and ILC. The risk increases with the amount of alcohol consumed; there appears to be a dose-response relationship over time.[451] Breast cancer risk increases even at lower levels of consumption. After adjustment for potential confounding factors, intake of more than 30 g per day resulted in a 53% increased risk for breast cancer.[390]

Several mechanisms have been proposed. Alcohol consumption is shown to increase levels of endogenous estrogens. This hypothesis is further supported by data showing that the alcohol–breast cancer association is limited to women with IDC and ILC ER+ tumors.[33] Elevated blood concentration of acetaldehyde (a reactive metabolite of alcohol) is known to be toxic and is hypothesized to cause DNA modifications that lead to cancer.[305] The effects of alcohol may be mediated through the production of prostaglandins, lipid peroxidation, and the generation of free radicals influencing hormone levels and ERs. Alcohol also acts as a solvent, enhancing penetration of carcinogens into cells.

**Other Environmental Factors.** There is evidence that exposure to tobacco smoke increases breast cancer risk.[317] A meta-analysis suggests that there is little evidence that exposure to acrylamide in food (high levels found in potato chips, French fries, and other food products produced by high temperature cooking) is associated with breast cancer risk.[395] Evidence related to night shift work is equivocal.[506,525,543] Research is ongoing on topics of lack of sleep,[556] daughters of women who received diethylstilbestrol,[78] exposure to agricultural pesticides and herbicides,[419] radiofrequency fields,[193] and radiation exposure from accidents at nuclear power plants.[208] Scientific research thus far has been unable to establish a direct link between breast cancer and electromagnetic fields[193]; silicone breast implants[37]; abortion[131]; or chemicals in antiperspirants, deodorants, cosmetics, or hair dyes .[419]

**Protective Factors.** Factors that are considered protective against acquiring breast cancer include younger age at first live birth,[286] multiparity (more than two births),[449] and breastfeeding with an inverse relationship of length of breastfeeding and breast cancer risk.[570] The Collaborative Group on Hormonal Factors in Breast Cancer found that the relative rate of breast cancer decreases 4.3% for every 12 months of breastfeeding and 7% for each birth.[105] In addition, incorporating regular weekly physical activity appears to be protective against acquiring breast cancer. The ACS recommends at least 150 minutes of moderate physical activity each week, preferably spread throughout the week, whereas the World Cancer Research Fund/American Institute for Cancer Research (WCRF/AICR) recommends a higher level of physical activity, stating an aim of 30 minutes or more of moderate activity daily, equating to at least 210 minutes each week.[87,281] (See also Prevention later.)

### Risk Factors for Breast Cancer in Men

Age and heredity are the most common risk factors for breast cancer in men, with a mean age of 68 years at the time of detection.[230] Men who inherit altered *BRCA1* or *BRCA2* genes have an increased risk for male breast cancer at a rate of 1/100 and 6/100, respectively. .[12] As many as 40% of male breast cancers may have an altered *BRCA2* gene.[181] Because of this strong association, first-degree relatives (siblings, parents, and children) of a man diagnosed with breast cancer may choose to undergo genetic testing for *BRCA1* and *BRCA2*.

Men diagnosed with early-stage breast cancer have an 83% survival rate. Recent data suggest that compared with women, men with breast cancer were older, were more likely to be African American, and were more likely to have a more advanced stage of cancer at diagnosis.[303] Men are less likely to have lobular carcinoma but more likely to have cancers that are ER+ and progesterone receptor–positive (PR+).[194]

Other established risk factors for male breast cancer include high estrogen exposure, Klinefelter syndrome, and chest radiation.[12] Men can have high estrogen levels because of taking hormonal medications, treatment with immunosuppressant medications after organ transplantation, obesity, or estrogen exposure in the environment.[437] Nevertheless, when a man discovers a breast lump, it is usually benign unilateral gynecomastia, which can occur at any age. There is not a clear etiology, but it has been associated with medications, systemic disease, and cannabis use.[289] Fibroadenomas and cysts are rare in men.[325]

### Clinical Manifestations

Women discover 80% to 90% of breast masses that are large enough to palpate themselves. In women the mass is typically centrally located behind the areola or in the upper, outer quadrant, and in men the lump is usually centrally located behind the areola, although neoplasms can occur anywhere in the breast tissue (Fig. 20.11). Because of the single-file development of lobular cancers, areas of increased tissue density may be felt rather than a lump.

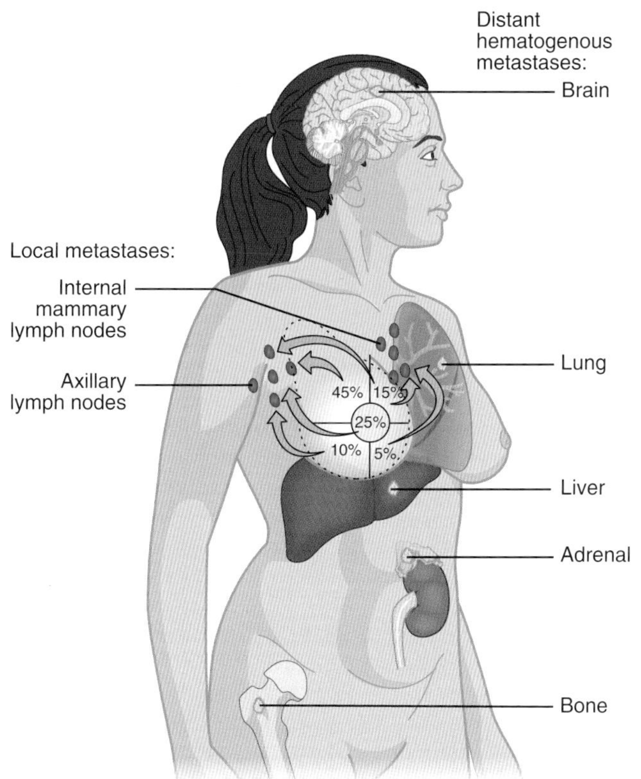


**Figure 20.11**

**The distribution of breast carcinoma and the pathway of lymphatic metastases.** Most tumors are found in the upper lateral quadrant and behind the nipple (areola) in women and behind the nipple in men. (From Damjanov I: *Pathology for the health-related professions*, ed 3, Philadelphia, 2006, Saunders.)

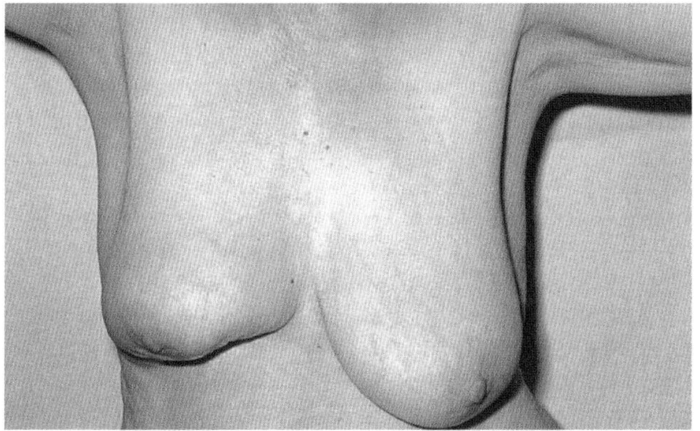

**Figure 20.12**

**Fixation.** Asymmetry, distortion, or decreased motility is observed in the woman's right breast as she lifts her arms. As cancer becomes invasive, fibrosis can fix the breast to the underlying pectoral muscle. Although at first glance, it looks as if the woman's left breast is enlarged compared with the right, in fact the woman's right breast is held against the chest wall. (From Mansel R: *Color atlas of breast diseases*, London, 1995, Mosby.)

A palpable mass tends to be firm and irregular and painless if it is a carcinoma versus smooth and rubbery if it is benign. Fixation of the breast to the underlying pectoral muscles and chest wall can cause significant asymmetry (Fig. 20.12). Other manifestations include a change in breast contour or texture, nipple discharge and retraction or inversion, local skin dimpling (Fig. 20.13), erythema, and local rash or ulceration. Lymphadenopathy (tender swollen axillary lymph nodes) may also be the initial presentation of this disease.

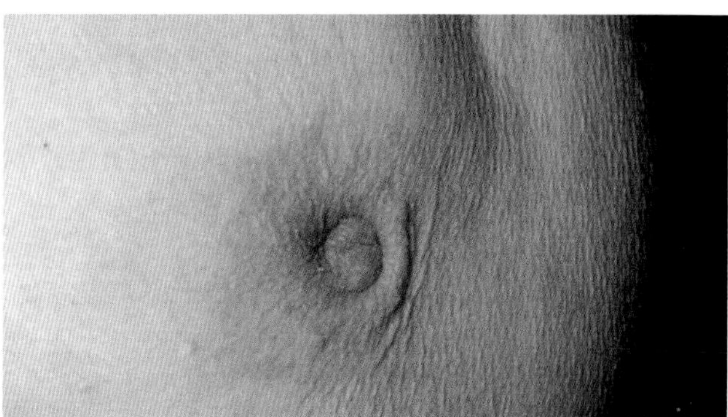

**Figure 20.13**

**Dimpling.** The shallow dimple above and slightly to the right of the nipple as viewed in this photograph shows signs of skin retraction or skin tethering. Cancer causes fibrosis, which contracts the suspensory ligaments of the breast, resulting in this clinical change in the breast tissue. The dimpling may be visible at rest, with compression, or with lifting of the arms. The fibrosis can also pull the nipple as seen by the distortion of the areola here. (From Evans AJ: Atlas of breast disease management: 50 illustrative cases, Philadelphia, 1998, Saunders.)

IBC is characterized by unilateral breast enlargement, but bilateral involvement is possible. Warmth, redness of the skin with sensation of heat, sudden swelling, itching, pain, a skin condition called *peau d'orange* (in which the skin resembles an orange peel), and nipple changes (e.g., retraction, flattening, crusting, blistering) are typical. Some women describe the presentation as a bug bite or as a bruise on the breast that does not go away. Breast color ranges from pink to red to purple, and breasts can feel heavy, thick, and congested. Symptoms can intensify over hours and days. Although a palpable tumor may not be present, lymph node involvement (metastases) to the axillary or supraclavicular lymph nodes is present in up to 81% of women at the time of diagnosis.[332]

**Cancer Recurrence.** Local recurrence means that the cancer has returned to the previously diseased breast in the case of breast conservation or along the incisional scar in the case of mastectomy. Local recurrence can manifest in the area of the lumpectomy excision or in an unrelated area of the breast. Recurrence in the scar of a mastectomy usually occurs in the skin and adipose tissue of the removed breast; it rarely includes muscle tissue. As breast cancers continue to be differentiated by molecular subtyping, recurrence rates can be reported more specifically. (See Biomarkers later.)

*Regional recurrence* means that the cancer has been now been found in the axillary, supraclavicular or internal mammary lymph nodes. Many studies investigate *locoregional recurrences.* Primary cancer involvement of the lymph nodes may predict those individuals who may be at greater risk of regional recurrence, but women without nodal metastases are still at some risk of cancer recurrence.

When comparing mastectomy alone with breast-conservation therapy (lumpectomy plus radiation therapy) for early stage disease, there is a slight benefit with mastectomy for local control. However, there appears to be a shift for improvement of overall survival rates for individuals who have breast-conservation therapy with radiation therapy.[125,367]

As breast cancers continue to be differentiated by molecular subtyping, recurrence rates can be reported with more specificity (see Biomarkers later). Current studies demonstrate that patients with luminal A tumors exhibit the lowest rates of local recurrence. Individuals with triple-negative and HER2-positive breast tumors exhibit a greater risk of local recurrence following breast-conserving therapy or mastectomy.[514,555]

**Metastases.** *Distant recurrence* is defined as cancer cells transported elsewhere in the body by the lymphatic system and/or the circulatory system. If cancer is found in lymph nodes elsewhere in the body, it suggests spread of the disease by the lymphatic system. When cancer is found in other organs, it suggests spread by the circulatory system. Metastases from a breast neoplasm typically are found first in bone and lungs. With disease progression, liver, brain and spinal cord, adrenal glands, skin, and GI system may also be involved.

The type of breast cancer must be identified not only to determine treatment but also to differentiate between cancer recurrence and a new cancer. Local metastases by direct extension of the primary disease site may involve the chest wall, ribs, pleura, pulmonary parenchyma, or bronchi. Individuals with IBC commonly present with metastases to the axillary or supraclavicular lymph nodes, and in one in three individuals there are distant metastases.[332] Metastatic spread from breast cancer rarely manifests in locations below the elbows and knees.

Symptoms associated with metastases include upper extremity edema, bone pain, jaundice, and weight loss. These are rarely the initial symptoms. Signs and symptoms of the affected system may be the first clinical indication of a problem. For example, pulmonary lesions may manifest as vague aching chest pain, hemoptysis, or unexplained dyspnea. Bone pain and fracture are the most common symptoms of bone metastases. Metastases to the liver may manifest as fatigue, jaundice, carpal tunnel syndrome, or skin changes.

**Paraneoplastic Syndrome.** *Paraneoplastic syndrome* (or *stiff person syndrome*) is a rare syndrome associated with breast cancer (and lung, ovarian, and lymphatic cancers). It is believed to be hormonally mediated and caused by tumor cell or immune response to the presence of cancer in the body, but not by the local presence of cancer cells. Sometimes the symptoms of paraneoplastic syndromes are present before the diagnosis of a malignancy. In paraneoplastic neurologic disorders, the central and/or peripheral nervous system may be affected.[366] Symptoms may include progressive symptoms of neuropathy or myelopathy with altered muscle tone.

## MEDICAL MANAGEMENT

Health care policy and scientific research on the detection, diagnosis, and treatment of breast cancer are rapidly expanding and changing with monthly and even weekly updates. The information presented here is based on current evidence. The reader is encouraged to keep abreast of new information through the following helpful websites provided for both the consumer and the therapist.

- American Cancer Society (ACS): www.cancer.org
- American Society of Clinical Oncology (ASCO): www.asco.org
- National Cancer Institute (NCI): www.cancer.gov
- National Comprehensive Cancer Network (NCCN): www.nccn.org

**Prevention.** *Healthy People* is a nationwide program devoted to health promotion and disease prevention, with comprehensive goals set by the U.S. Department of Health and Human Services.[4] *Healthy People 2020* supports continued advances in research, detection, and treatment of all cancers; it also reviews trends in cancer incidence, mortality, and survival that identify progress made toward decreasing the impact of cancer in the United States. The 2020 objectives continue to promote early detection of breast cancer by measuring the use of screening tests identified in the recommendations of the U.S. Preventive Services Task Force (USPSTF).[458] They also focus on reducing the breast cancer death rate in women and the incidence of late-stage breast cancers,[213] which are intermediate markers of cancer screening success.[371]

Breast cancer prevention includes addressing modifiable risk factors as well as protective factors. Lifestyle changes include diet and exercise, with decreased postmenopausal weight gain and avoidance of risk factors including exposure to carcinogens, limiting alcohol consumption, judicious use of HRT, and promoting long-term breastfeeding. Drug therapy for high-risk patients and precancerous conditions is being studied.

***Lifestyle Changes.*** The ACS and Institute of Medicine summary of public health recommendations based on prevention of modifiable lifestyle factors includes the following recommendations:

- Avoid unnecessary medical radiation, especially at younger ages.
- Avoid combination menopausal HRT.
- Avoid smoking (especially before first pregnancy).
- Avoid passive smoke.
- Limit alcohol consumption.
- Increase physical activity.
- Maintain healthy weight; reduce obesity.
- Limit or eliminate workplace and consumer exposure to chemicals that are plausible contributors to breast cancer risk.
- If at high risk for breast cancer, consider chemoprevention.

***Physical Activity and Exercise.*** A systematic review of epidemiologic studies found that exercise and physical activity have an established effect on breast cancer prevention, with an inverse dose-response effect in which risk decreases with increased activity level.[458] Studies support an average risk reduction for breast cancer of 25% in physically active individuals when an optimum level of moderate-intensity exercise is achieved for more than 90 minutes per day.[296] Moderate-intensity activity is recommended as opposed to low-intensity activity, and activity can be cumulative throughout the day in 10-minute increments.[398]

The NCI recommends strenuous exercise for more than 4 hours per week to reduce breast cancer risk. The ACS recommendations for Nutrition and Physical Activity for cancer prevention in adults include 150 minutes or more of moderate-intensity or 75 minutes of vigorous-intensity activity each week, or an equivalent combination, preferably spread throughout the week.[428] Examples of strenuous activity include swimming laps, aerobics/calisthenics, running, and jogging. Examples of moderate activity include brisk walking, golf, and volleyball.[135]

Research shows that physical activity in postmenopausal women reduces breast cancer risk. The relationship is not as clear in premenopausal women.[296] Possible biologic mechanisms include changes in metabolic and sex hormones, growth factors, adiposity, and immune function.[128,204] In the WHI study of postmenopausal women, 1.25 to 2.0 hours per week of brisk walking was correlated with an 18% risk reduction compared with inactive women. Ten or more hours of exercise activity per week reduced the risk even more.[339]

***Diet and Nutrition.*** There is emerging evidence that healthy dietary patterns may have a role in breast cancer risk reduction. Diets characterized by high intake of fruits and salad are shown to be associated with a slightly lower risk of breast cancer, for hormone receptor–negative breast cancer in particular.[553] Recent studies suggest that following ACS dietary recommendations, particularly limiting saturated fat, red meat, and processed foods, may decrease breast cancer risk.[122,498]

Controlling weight (especially after menopause) is associated with preventing breast cancer, the recurrence of breast cancer, and death from breast cancer.[99] It is known that MetS (which is associated with weight gain, central adiposity, elevated serum insulin and glucose levels, and insulin resistance) increases the risk of breast cancer recurrence in postmenopausal women.[391] Weight gain after treatment for breast cancer may increase the recurrence rate and mortality for breast cancer.[92]

Increased health promotion seeks to address diabetes, prediabetes, and chronic inflammation in reducing breast cancer risk. Because androgens and estrogen are elevated in obesity and are risk factors for postmenopausal breast cancer risk, weight loss may help decrease breast cancer risk in hormonally sensitive cancers by decreasing levels of serum estrogen and free testosterone.[456]

Despite conflicting or null findings of dietary interventions in numerous randomized controlled trials, results do not necessarily indicate a lack of effect of dietary factors on breast cancer risk. A combination of dietary factors (rather than single components acting in isolation) may yet show benefit. Current recommendations include approaches that are low in some kinds of fats (such as the Mediterranean diet); high in fruits, vegetables, and whole-grain carbohydrates; and low in sugar, alcohol, processed foods, and hormone-treated milk, eggs, beef, and chicken (or no animal products, strictly a plant-based diet). The impact of cholesterol is also being investigated.[335] The data seem to support reduced breast cancer risk only when weight loss accompanies a low-fat diet. Calcium, vitamin D, dietary fiber, and nut intake in adolescence is another research focus in the development of proliferative benign breast conditions and breast cancer.[481]

More research is showing a relationship between high intakes of meat, red meat, processed meat, and meat cooked at high temperatures with increased breast cancer risk. As a result, recommendations include the reduction of consumption of grilled and smoked meats cooked at high temperatures.[265]

***Alcohol.*** There is good evidence that restricting alcohol consumption reduces breast cancer risk.[390,451] Recommendations regarding acceptable levels of alcohol intake vary from no alcohol at all to less than one drink a day. (One drink equals 12 oz of beer, 5 oz of wine, or 1.5 oz of hard liquor.) There may a difference between consumption of red wine and white wine. Data suggest that red wine acts as a nutritional aromatase inhibitor.[96] More research is needed as this seems to be an area of ongoing debate.

The effect of drinking alcohol and the risk of recurrence is receiving more attention.[454] It appears that at little as 6 g of alcohol can increase the risk of breast cancer recurrence, particularly in postmenopausal women.[454] More research is needed on the relationship of reduction of alcohol-associated breast cancer risk with antioxidant and folate intake.[95,253] Consumption of alcohol in adolescence is associated with an increased risk of proliferative benign breast conditions in a dose-response relationship.[54,304]

***Childbearing and Breastfeeding.*** Reproductive factors such as late age at first birth (older than 34 years) and nulliparity are established risk factors for breast cancer. Earlier childbearing, multiple births, and breastfeeding have a protective effect on developing breast cancer. Delayed childbearing, low parity, and no or short duration of breastfeeding are increasing social trends in developed countries that are associated with higher incidence of breast cancer in these countries. Parity, early age at first full-term pregnancy, and breastfeeding have been long believed to influence the risk of breast cancer, predominantly through hormonal mechanisms that involve estrogen and progesterone. Studies confirm risk reduction for ER+ and PR+ (luminal) cancers of 25%.[286] Women younger than 20 years of age at first birth demonstrate a 27% lower risk than women in the oldest age at first birth category when adjusted for parity. Decreased risk for ER– and PR– cancers has been shown to be associated with breastfeeding, which is of particular importance, as hormone negative receptors are more common in younger women.[242] Duration of breastfeeding has shown a cumulative effect.[570]

***Hormone Replacement Therapy.*** The use of HRT should be thoroughly analyzed by individual women and their physicians. The WHI trial of combined estrogen plus progestin HRT was stopped early when health risks, which included invasive breast cancer, outweighed benefits. Not only did researchers find an increased incidence of breast cancers among women who received relatively short-term combined HRT, but these cancers were also diagnosed at a more advanced stage than in women who received placebo medication. HRT also increases the percentage of women with abnormal mammograms. These results suggest estrogen plus progestin may stimulate breast cancer growth and hinder breast cancer diagnosis.[155]

***Chemoprevention.*** In 2009 the ASCO updated its guidelines concerning the use of chemotherapeutic agents for reducing breast cancer risk.[526] The USPSTF is in the process of updating its recommendations. Recommendations include specifics on the use of SERMs such as tamoxifen and raloxifene and aromatase inhibitors (AIs). For women at high risk of developing breast cancer, treatment with tamoxifen reduces breast cancer risk for 20 years.[116] Treatment with raloxifene has a similar effect on reduction of invasive breast cancer, but appears to be less effective for prevention of noninvasive tumors.[547] Clinical tools and resources reviewing risks and benefits of breast cancer chemoprevention and summarizing recommendations are available from the ASCO.

***Other Preventive Measures.*** The influence of many types of environmental exposures on breast cancer risk requires continued scrutiny. Preventive recommendations with the strongest evidence include avoiding radiation exposure (especially the use of computed tomography in medical testing), avoiding combined postmenopausal HRT, and avoiding active smoking. Other recommendations may include limiting exposure to passive smoking and other environmental carcinogens in certain consumer products (i.e., bisphenol A, phthalates), industrial chemicals (i.e., benzene, ethylene oxide), and pesticides (i.e., sichlorodiphenyltrichloroethane/dichlorodiphenyldichloroethylene). More research is needed to establish a conclusive link of these exposures to breast cancer.[193] Increased vitamin D intake by food or supplementation as well as exposure to the sun (needed by the skin to manufacture vitamin D) may be recommended.[546] Epidemiologic studies suggest an association between vitamin D and calcium intake and breast cancer. Current research reveals a high prevalence of vitamin D deficiency and osteoporosis in individuals with breast cancer.[50]

Disturbed sleep-wake cycle with its disruption of the human circadian cycle and reduced sleep quality has been proposed as contributing to an increased risk of cancer in general and breast cancer specifically. Women in nighttime jobs or who do rotating shift work with repeated disruption of the circadian system may be at increased risk of breast cancer.[210] Achieving the recommended 7 to 8 hours of sleep per night is advocated.[327]

Prophylactic mastectomy (also referred to as risk-reduction mastectomy) for women with a *BRCA1* or *BRCA2* mutation and positive family history has proved to be extremely effective. However, testing and managing hereditary cancer risk is a complex decision-making process. A decision support tool designed for joint use by women with *BRCA* mutations and their health care providers is available online from the Stanford Medicine Cancer Institute.

**Screening and Early Detection.** Discovery of identifiable masses on mammography and ultrasound *before* a palpable lump or nodule is found is the goal of screening technologies. For decades, early detection has been considered the hallmark of effective intervention in cases of breast cancer, with the goal of finding any breast cancer when it is as small as possible. Current evidence indicates that the biology of the individual cancer is also very important. A tiny, very aggressive breast cancer may be able to spread to distant sites before it is large enough to be detected, whereas a much larger, but slow-growing cancer may present a minimal problem even if it is never detected.

In the past, women were advised to use a combination of three tools: monthly breast self-examination (BSE), clinical breast examination by a qualified health professional, and regular mammography. Routine screening mammograms for women 40 to 45 years old and the use of BSE are currently not recommended. Differing guidelines currently exist in the medical community, including guidelines from the USPTF,[355,458] ACS,[383] and other organizations.[355] A comparison of recommendations from a number of organizations is available on the CDC website. Box 20.12 presents a summary of the ACS screening recommendations.[383]

***Breast Self-Examination.*** Although mammography has been the main focus of breast cancer detection, almost half of breast cancers found in women ages 50 to 69 years are found by the women themselves or their clinicians.[424] However, because current research shows that a formal BSE plays a small role in finding breast cancer, the ACS no longer recommends that all women conduct regular BSEs (see Box 20.12). Breast cancer detection is more commonly associated with an incidental discovery of a breast lump or increased awareness of what is "normal" for an individual. Such discovery may be just as effective as a formal regimen. However, some physicians may still encourage monthly BSEs performed 1 week after menstrual bleeding begins or consistently on the same day each month in postmenopausal women. If a woman chooses to perform BSE, she should learn the correct procedure from a qualified health care professional.

Box 20.12

**RECOMMENDATIONS FOR EARLY DETECTION OF BREAST CANCER (AMERICAN CANCER SOCIETY)**

For women who have an *average* risk for breast cancer:

- For women aged 40–44 years: option to start annual breast cancer screening with mammograms if desired
- For women aged 45–54 years: should get mammograms annually
- For women aged 55 or older: option to switch mammograms every two years, or continue yearly screening, which should continue as long as the woman is in good health and expected to live 10 years or longer
- Clinical breast examination is not recommended for breast cancer screening among average-risk women at any age.

Based on data from American Cancer Society. Text Alternative for Breast Cancer Screening Guideline: American Cancer Society Recommendations for the Early Detection of Breast Cancer. https://www.cancer.org/research/infographics-gallery/breast-cancer-screening-guideline/breast-cancer-screening-guideline-text-alternative.html. Accessed May 05, 2020; Oeffinger KC, Fontham ETH, Etzioni R, et al: Breast cancer screening for women at average risk 2015 guideline update from the American Cancer Society. *JAMA* 314(15):1599-1614, 2015.

***Clinical Breast Examination.*** As with mammography there is some controversy among organizations regarding guidelines for the use of clinical breast examination as a screening tool for breast cancer. The ACS does not recommend clinical breast examination for breast cancer screening among average-risk women at any age.[383] However, the ACOG recommends offering a clinical breast examination every 1 to 3 years for women ages 25 to 39 and annually for women older than 40 years.[13] Clinicians and women need to determine the best course of action on an individual basis.

***Mammography.*** Mammography is an x-ray of the breast and is an essential tool for the detection of a lesion before the mass (cancerous or benign) is large enough to be palpable. It can detect very small lesions of 0.5 cm. The term *screening mammography* implies the mammogram is done when there is no palpable lump or any other breast findings that lead to a suspicion of cancer. The role of screening mammography in reducing breast cancer mortality has become more controversial in the past few years, particularly as there are studies that do not support a decrease in mortality rates.[151,153] Research suggests treatments have more of an impact on mortality rates than screening.[61,404] Evidence from the USPTF[376] suggests that there is a reduction in mortality with screening mammography; however, estimates of reductions are not the same in all age groups, and the most benefit is for detection of advanced cancer in women age 50 and older, hence the recommendation to begin screening at age 50.[458]

For women between the ages of 40 and 50 years, screening should be based on a shared discussion between women and their health care providers, taking into account personal circumstances and preferences. Many groups (ACOG, American College of Radiology, NCI, and NCCN) recommend that screening mammography for women at average risk of breast cancer should start at age 40 years. The ACS recommends starting annual screening at age 45.

For younger women who are at high risk for developing breast cancer the ACS recommends yearly mammograms and MRI (see Advanced Imaging Technology next). In these cases, addressing the biology of the cancer is paramount. For most of these women, screening should begin at age 30 years and continue for as long as the woman is in good health. For all high-risk women, earlier initiation of screening, screening at shorter intervals, and screening with additional modalities such as ultrasound and MRI may be advised.

*High risk* is defined as a 20% or higher chance of developing breast cancer over the course of a lifetime (as opposed to the average lifetime risk for a woman in the United States of 12% to 13%.) Persons in the high-risk group include women who have received radiation treatment to the chest between ages 10 and 30 years (e.g., for Hodgkin disease); women who are prone to breast cancer because of the presence of genetic mutations such as *BRCA1* or *BRCA2*; and women whose mothers, fathers, sisters, brothers, daughters, or sons carry those mutations. Other groups that may meet the definition of high risk include women with a personal history of breast cancer, previous atypical biopsy, dense breasts (more than 50%), and elevated risk by criteria of the Gail/Breast Cancer Risk Assessment or a number of other models available for use.[24,55,103,173,508]

The cost-effectiveness and efficacy of screening mammography in women age 75 years and older also have come under scrutiny. The ACS recommends women should continue with screening if they are in good health and their life expectancy is 10 years or more.[383]

There are limitations in the use of mammography in women with dense breast tissue. Radiologists have long known that there is decreased sensitivity of mammography in women with dense breasts and an increased risk of developing breast cancer in women with dense breasts.[531] This information has not been routinely communicated to women as part of a mammography report. There is a lack of uniform standards in the interpretation of breast densities, which may result in unnecessary surgical procedures with emotional, physical, and financial implications. As a result, legislation has been passed in more than 50% of states requiring that patients as well as providers are informed about breast density.[408]

When a lump or other breast symptom is investigated or a mammogram is read as positive, the next study is a *diagnostic mammogram* (as opposed to a screening mammogram). This is a problem-solving mammogram, which may involve additional views of the breast. Suspicious findings are usually followed by evaluation with high-frequency ultrasound and/or stereotactic biopsy.

For women with breast implants, additional mammography screening, called an *implant displacement view,* may be requested.

***Advanced Imaging Technology.*** Imaging has become increasingly important in the process of screening and diagnosis of all breast problems; even biopsies are often image-directed. The use of imaging technology for screening versus diagnosis must be distinguished. Diagnosis requires a biopsy analysis. Studies have shown that the addition of screening ultrasound or MRI to mammography in women at increased risk of breast cancer results in a higher yield of cancer detection.[214] The false-negative rate of mammography alone ranges from 25% to 59%.[309]

*Digital mammography* has a number of advantages over conventional film-screen mammography. Benefits of digital mammography include the ability to electronically store and digitally enhance images. Images can also be electronically transmitted to specialists elsewhere for consultation. Studies show that digital mammography is equal or slightly superior to film-screen mammography in detecting and describing abnormalities.[405]

Digital breast tomosynthesis (DBT), or three-dimensional mammography, uses a series of tomographic image slices through the breast that then reconstructs the breast in thin slices. DBT provides more detail about overlapping tissue, which can obscure and mimic cancer. The addition of DBT to breast screening may reduce false-positive recalls and reduce morbidity and mortality associated with breast cancer by improving early detection of tumors.[110,223]

*Ultrasound* is primarily used to differentiate a cyst from a solid lesion. It is used to help interpret a mammogram and aids in the detection of cancers that may not show on mammography (mammography-occult). Ultrasound is being used more frequently to image dense breast tissue. Breast tissue density refers to the fibroglandular composition (as opposed to fatty tissue) of the breast. High density of breast tissue is a significant and independent risk factor for breast cancer and also reduces the sensitivity of mammography, as glandular tissue masks cancer on the mammogram. It is estimated that in women with dense breasts, as many as 35% of breast cancers go undetected by mammogram. These women have an increased risk of breast cancer, with detection usually at a more advanced stage. The somo-v Automated Breast Ultrasound System (ABUS) is intended for use in combination with standard mammography in women with dense breast tissue who have a negative mammogram and no symptoms of breast cancer.[342,563]

*MRI* is an imaging technology that uses powerful magnetic field and radio waves to create images of the breast. MRI is a highly sensitive test for breast cancer and may reveal cancers missed by both mammography and ultrasound screening. However, because the cost associated with MRI is high (10 times the cost of a mammogram), MRI is not used for women at average risk for breast cancer for routine screening. Sensitivity is good, detecting 94% to 95% of invasive cancers when used in conjunction with mammogram, but specificity varies widely (30% to 90%) with frequent false-positive results. MRI is used more specifically for women at high risk for breast cancer.[483] MRI may be employed for individuals with a proven history of breast cancer and in cases where conventional imaging presents difficulties, such as individuals with ILC or when dense breast tissue precludes an accurate mammographic and physical assessment.[369]

*Elastography* is a noninvasive method in which soft tissue stiffness or strain images are used to detect or classify tumors. Elastography is currently being used with ultrasound, but some research studies are using magnetic resonance elastography and computed tomography. Use of ultrasound elastography may reduce unnecessary biopsies.[60,159]

*Thermography* is a tool that records the temperature of the breasts by measuring infrared radiation emitted. Theoretically, cancerous tissue has a higher temperature than normal tissue as a result of increased vascularity and a higher metabolic rate of the cancerous cells. Although thermography is commercially available as a screening tool for detecting breast cancer, in 2011 the FDA warned against the use of breast thermography as a substitute for mammography. Currently there is insufficient evidence to support the use of thermography in breast cancer screening or as an adjunct to mammography.[320]

***Other Imaging Methods.*** A number of other imaging methods are available for detecting breast cancer and are used mainly in research studies or to obtain more information about a tumor found by another method.[532] They have not been found to be reliable enough for routine use. *Scintigraphy* (also called *scintimammography* and *molecular breast imaging*) is used to image cellular absorption of a radioactive tracing agent. *Positron emission mammography* (PEM) measures glucose metabolism with a radioactive tracer with increased metabolism indicating the possible presence of a tumor. PEM is an advanced application of positron emission tomography that produces sharp, detailed images of breast lesions as small as 1.5 mm. PEM may be used instead of breast MRI when obesity or metal implants preclude the use of an MRI scanner. It can be helpful in individuals with breast implants and may be considered an effective tool in the evaluation of DCIS because of higher sensitivity.[343,370] *Breast-specific gamma imaging* (*sestamibi nuclear breast imaging*) involves an injected radioactive substance (technetium sestamibi) combined with another agent that makes the sestamibi collect in the breast. There has been much improvement in the ability of breast-specific gamma imaging to detect smaller cancers, and it is being used more often in conjunction with mammography.[482] Microwave imaging (MI) techniques are being studied as a diagnostic tool for early-stage breast cancer. MI techniques can be grouped as passive and active. Passive MI measures temperature differences between normal and malignant tissues, using radiometry. Active MI measures the dielectric properties contrast between healthy tissue and malignant tissue.[532,533]

***Genetic Testing.*** Genetic testing is recommended for individuals with other family members who have tested positive for *BRCA* gene mutations. Inherited mutations of *BRCA1* or *BRCA2* increase the lifetime risk of breast (and ovarian) cancer; however, having an inherited gene mutation does not mean breast cancer is inevitable, even though the first mutation has occurred by conception. Women who have a positive family history of breast cancer before the age of 40 years may want to seek genetic counseling. Testing may be advised for anyone with a family history as described previously in Incidence and Risk Factors.

Genetic testing that results in a negative test for a mutation may be difficult to interpret if the family history is unknown. Coping with the results if they are positive and weighing all the options can be challenging.[416] Although most states have genetic privacy laws to prevent discrimination by health insurers, the guidelines do not always apply to life or disability insurance. Testing is done by a simple blood test, but the test may be expensive and is not always covered by health insurance.

Breast cancer can remain dormant for years before becoming clinically apparent, so long-term follow-up is mandatory for all women, especially anyone with a previous history of breast cancer. Improvement in breast cancer screening technology such as three-dimensional mammography is a current research focus. Other investigators seek a more precise, noninvasive screening technique that does not involve the use of radiation.

**Diagnosis and Staging.** Detection of a breast abnormality occurs through physical examination or imaging studies (see Screening and Early Detection above). Diagnosis determines with certainty what the abnormality is, thus requiring biopsy and pathology examination. If the diagnosis is cancer, the physician will request additional tests for information about how extensive the cancer is *(staging)* and how it appears and behaves *(grading)* so that effective treatment can be initiated.

***Biopsy.*** Techniques used in the diagnosis of breast cancer include *core biopsy, needle biopsy, incisional biopsy,* and *excisional biopsy* (see further discussion in Diagnosis: Tissue Biopsy in Chapter 9). Sentinel lymph node mapping is used to identify metastases in invasive cancers. *Sentinel lymph node biopsy* (SLNB) consists of the removal of one to three nodes; it is now standard practice to identify and remove only the first node or nodes that cancer cells may have reached after leaving the breast. This eliminates unnecessary axillary lymph node dissection (ALND), in which more than three nodes are removed. With SLNB, radioactive blue dye is injected preoperatively to identify the first (sentinel) node of drainage from the region of the breast where the cancer is present.

SLNB (see discussion of technique in Chapter 9) has replaced ALND for the staging of clinically node-negative individuals with breast cancer, demonstrating survival equivalent to ALND for women with lymph node–negative status while resulting in reduced morbidity. ASCO guidelines now state that women with one to two metastatic sentinel lymph nodes who will undergo breast-conserving surgery and whole-breast irradiation should not undergo ALND. Women with sentinel lymph node metastases who will undergo mastectomy should be offered ALND.[185,316]

***Biomarkers.*** Breast cancers are biologically heterogeneous. Current classification of subtypes of breast cancer is based on biomarkers and gene expression profiling. Commonly measured tumor markers are hormone receptors for estrogen and progesterone. These hormone receptors are proteins that signal cell proliferation. Breast cancers are labeled ER+ if they have receptors for estrogen and PR+ if they have receptors for progesterone. Breast cancer cells (similar to normal breast cells) receive signals from estrogen and progesterone that promote growth. Hormone-positive (ER+ or PR+) cancers represent up to 80% of all breast cancers. Cancers that are ER+/PR+ have receptors for both hormones that could be supporting cancer growth and represent 60% to 65% of all breast cancers. Conversely, breast cancers without ERs or PRs are labeled hormone negative (ER−/PR−) and represent up to 25% of breast cancers.[120] Hormone receptor testing determines whether the cancer is likely to respond to hormonal therapy or other treatments. Hormonal therapy includes medications that either lower the amount of available estrogen or block estrogen from supporting the growth and function of breast cells. More research is needed to help understand cancers that are PR+.

Another biomarker that is analyzed at the time of biopsy is HER2 (also called c-erbB2 or more often ErbB2). HER2 is an oncogene that when overexpressed leads to cell proliferation. HER2-positive cancers account for approximately 15% to 20% of invasive cancers.[120]Triple-negative breast cancers (ER−/PR−/HER2-negative) represent 15% to 20% of invasive breast cancers and are considered to be more aggressive cancers with a worse prognosis.[278,388] The largest proportion of breast cancers (60% to 70%) are ER+/HER2-negative. There is a wide heterogeneity within these cancers, with some cancers having a much better prognosis than others.

**Gene expression** studies have identified five common subtypes of breast cancer: luminal A tumors, luminal B tumors, HER2 overexpressing tumors, basal-like/triple-negative tumors, and normal breast–like tumors.[120,495] Ongoing research shows variations in the occurrence of breast cancer subtypes by demographics (e.g., age, race, and ethnicity), screening detection, estimating risk of development of a second primary breast cancer in the contralateral breast, recurrence risk, and treatment and prognosis indicators (see Grading and Staging for additional information). Discoveries of additional subtypes are expected as research advances.

Several commercial tests are available for identifying different types of tumors and customizing therapies (Oncotype DX, MammaPrint, and Mammostrat). Oncotype DX samples 21 genetic markers that are used for prognosis and prediction. In women with ER+, node-negative cancers, the test has been used to predict risk of recurrence, as well as benefit from employing adjuvant chemotherapy in addition to the use of estrogen-inhibiting drugs such as tamoxifen. A low recurrence score (18 or lower) along with other favorable factors suggests that the woman can decline chemotherapy but still benefit from hormonal therapy. A high recurrence score (31 and above) suggests significant benefit from adjuvant chemotherapy. Intermediate scores of 19 to 30 require a discussion between the patient and oncologist for decision making.[524]

*Oncotype DX* has been used to predict the risk of DCIS recurrence or the development of a new invasive cancer in the same breast. Data are being used to make recommendations regarding the benefit of radiation therapy after breast-conserving surgery for DCIS. The use of Oncotype DX is being included in treatment guidelines for early-stage breast cancer by the ASCO and NCCN.

*MammaPrint* is a microarray assay. It analyzes the biology of the tumor through the activity of 70 genes and estimates the risk of recurrence for early-stage breast cancer (both hormone receptor–positive and hormone receptor–negative). The test provides a calculation of risk (low or high) for cancer recurrence that can be used to determine whether chemotherapy may reduce recurrence risk particularly for patients with ER− cancer, patients with HER2-positive cancer, and patients with positive lymph nodes.[58]

*Mammostrat* is a newer test that analyzes five immunohistochemical markers that provides a score for low risk: low, moderate, and high. It is not a true genetic test. It is used to group patients receiving tamoxifen and to inform them about prognosis and treatment choices. PAM50 (Prosigna), EndoPredict, Breast Cancer Index, and IHC4 are also used to help customize therapy.[524]

***Grading and Staging.*** Once the diagnosis of cancer is established, pathologists have a number of ways to analyze cancer cells and how they may behave. *Grading* refers to the study of cell appearance looking at differentiation as well as mitotic rate, nuclear grade, tubular formation, and other features. A *well-differentiated* cancer tends to look more like normal cells and is considered less aggressive, whereas *poorly differentiated* cancers are the opposite. A commonly used scoring system that combines these observations is the Nottingham (or Bloom Richardson) histologic score. A grade of 1 to 3 is assigned, with 3 being the most aggressive. For further discussion, see Grading and Staging in Chapter 9.

Box 20.13

**NEW CLASSIFICATION OF STAGING FOR BREAST CANCER**

The American Joint Committee on Cancer convened a multidisciplinary team of breast cancer experts to revise and update the eighth edition of the primary tumor, lymph node, and metastasis (TNM) classification. The panel felt the tumor staging should remain based on the TNM anatomic factors. However, prognosis based on biologic factors has been added to improve clinical utility.

Pathologic/anatomic stage (based on TNM staging)
- IA/IB
- IIA
- IIB
- IIIA
- IIIC

Estrogen status—positive/negative
Progesterone—positive/negative
HER2—positive/negative

From Giuliano AE, et al. Breast cancer—major changes in the American Joint Committee on Cancer Eighth Edition Cancer Staging Manual. *CA Cancer J Clin* 67:290–303, 2017.

The clinical *stage* of the tumor is ascertained to determine optimal management, including selection of candidates for adjuvant systemic therapies. A staging system is a standardized way to summarize information about how far a cancer has spread. Therapeutic decisions are formulated in part according to staging categories but primarily according to tumor size, histologic and nuclear grade of the primary tumor, proliferative capacity of the tumor, lymph node status, hormonal status (ERs and PRs), HER2 status, menopausal status, and general health of the individual.[186] Box 20.13 summarizes the staging criteria for breast cancer.

**TREATMENT.** Breast cancer is commonly treated by various combinations of surgery, radiation therapy, and systemic therapy (chemotherapy, targeted therapy, and endocrine therapy). The timing and sequencing of these interventions varies according to each individual case. Prognosis and selection of therapy may be influenced by the aforementioned clinical and pathology features. The NCCN publishes an annual update of its original 1996 NCCN Breast Cancer Treatment Guidelines.[372] The NCCN Guidelines for 2019[189] are available online for professionals with a section for patients as well. They are an important resource for keeping abreast of constant changes and recommendations regarding treatment of all stages of breast cancer.

***Cancer Removal Surgery.*** Surgery may be employed in the initial biopsy and any additional biopsies, for local control (lumpectomy or mastectomy), for accessing and analyzing the status of axillary lymph nodes, and in breast reconstruction options. Before the 1970s, *radical mastectomy*[403] was the most commonly employed procedure for surgical treatment of breast cancer. This procedure included removal of the entire breast, pectoral muscles (pectoralis major and pectoralis minor), all axillary lymph nodes, and some additional skin. Postsurgical problems included lymphedema, restricted shoulder mobility, impaired muscle function, and paresthesia. In the current era, radical mastectomy is rarely performed. The breast surgeon chooses the technique that will remove the tumor with negative or clean margins and minimal complications or negative side effects. At the time of surgery, the removed cancer and surrounding tissues are submitted to the pathologist. A pathologist report of negative, clean, or clear margins indicates that as far as can be determined, all the cancer has been successfully removed. A report of positive or dirty margins means that there are cancer cells at the edge of the removed tissue. Additional surgery is recommended when positive margins remain; however, this varies widely by surgeon and location. Surgical options to remove breast tumors include *breast-conserving therapy* (BCT) or *lumpectomy* and various forms of *mastectomy*.

Breast-Conserving Therapy. Treatment recommendations for women with stage I or II breast cancer often include BCT, also known as *breast-conserving surgery* or *lumpectomy*. More than half of women in the United States with early-stage breast cancer receive BCT and postsurgical radiation therapy (Fig. 20.14). Breast-conserving surgery followed by radiation therapy gives the same survival benefit as mastectomy for women with localized tumors. Lumpectomy may also be an option for women with larger tumors who receive neoadjuvant chemotherapy (before surgery) to shrink the tumor.

In BCT, only the tumor is removed, along with a rim of normal breast tissue, thus preserving the remaining breast. The breast cavity fills with serous fluid over time, and the breast itself is conserved. There is wide variability on lumpectomy reexcision rates. In 2014 the Society of Surgical Oncology and American Society for Radiation Oncology published guidelines on tumor-free/clean margins for breast-conserving surgery with intent to decrease the need for reexcision surgeries.[357]

Defining adequate surgical tumor clearance is an important area of research in the elimination of residual disease. A newer technology, the MarginProbe system, uses electromagnetic waves to identify possible cancerous tissue. The benefit of using this system is that the surgeon can determine intraoperatively whether more tissue needs to be removed (as opposed to waiting for pathologic analysis). MarginProbe can be used during lumpectomy for both DCIS and invasive breast cancer.[62]

The choice between breast-conserving surgery and mastectomy takes into account the balance between the need to achieve complete excision of the tumor and the woman's preferences regarding cosmetic appearance and preserving sexual sensitivity of the breast. Clinical factors that influence this choice include type, location, and spread of the tumor; multifocal disease; ratio of tumor size to breast size; and use of neoadjuvant systemic treatment. In many cases a woman chooses mastectomy for greater peace of mind, to avoid radiation therapy, and for reconstruction options. Despite recommendations for BCT, there remains concern that mastectomy (and contralateral prophylactic mastectomy) may be overused.[551]

Mastectomy. Mastectomy is usually reserved for women with more extensive disease, although mastectomy may be desirable for some women with early breast cancer as noted previously. Mastectomy is the total removal of

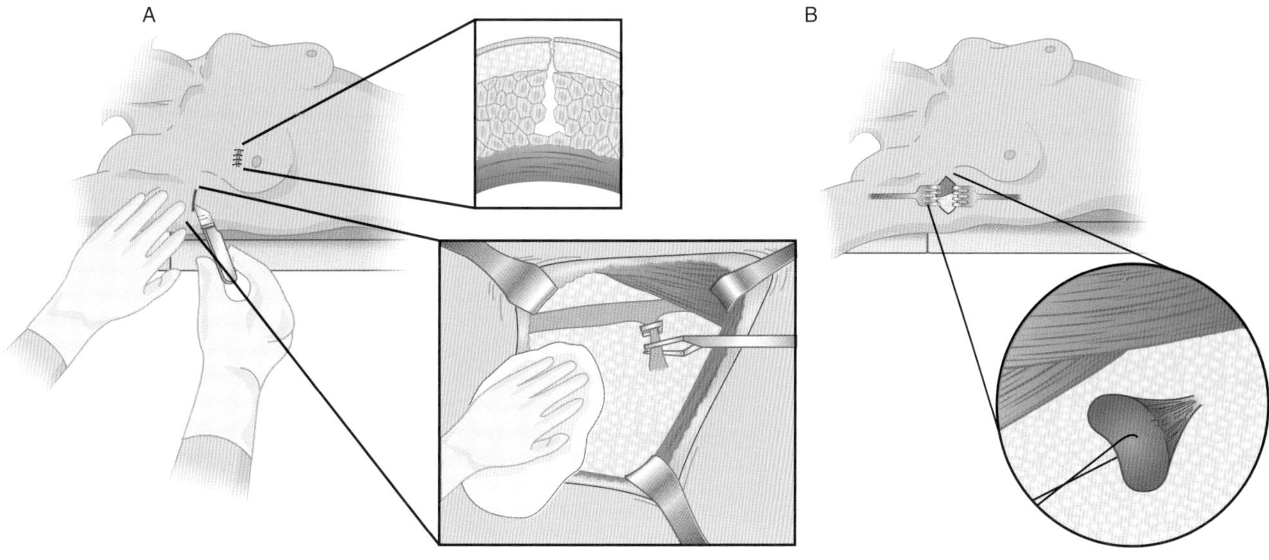


**Figure 20.14**

**Breast-conserving therapy.** (A) Incisions to remove malignant tumors are made directly over the tumor without tunneling. A transverse incision in the low axilla is used for either sentinel node biopsy or axillary dissection. The *inset* shows the excision cavity of the lumpectomy; no attempt is made to approximate the sides of the cavity, which will fill with serous fluid and gradually shrink. (B) In a sentinel node biopsy, a similar transverse incision is made and extended through the clavipectoral fascia, and the true axilla is entered. The sentinel node is located by virtue of its staining with dye or radioactivity, or both, and dissected free as a single specimen. (From Townsend CM: *Sabiston textbook of surgery*, ed 17, Philadelphia, 2004, Saunders.)

the breast. In a *simple mastectomy* (or *total mastectomy*) the entire breast is removed, including the nipple, areola, and skin. Axillary lymph nodes may or may not be removed. A *modified radical mastectomy,* or *partial mastectomy* (larger than a lumpectomy), combines a simple mastectomy with removal of the axillary lymph nodes. The pectoralis muscles are not removed .[12,11,403] In cases where immediate reconstruction is planned at the time of the mastectomy, a *skin-sparing mastectomy* retains the woman's natural breast skin, removing only the skin of the nipple, areola, and the original biopsy scar. If no immediate breast reconstruction is planned, the surgeon removes as much skin as is required to make the scar and chest surface flat. *Nipple-sparing procedures* are gaining some acceptance as well.

Lymph Node Surgery. Surgery that addresses the lymph nodes and regional metastasis has changed. For early-stage breast cancer, SLNB has replaced ALND as the standard of care for the staging of clinically node-negative individuals with breast cancer. SLNB has demonstrated survival equivalent to ALND for individuals who were lymph node–negative while resulting in reduced morbidity.

The 2017 ASCO Clinical Practice Guideline Update recommends that women without sentinel lymph node metastases should not receive ALND. Women with one or two metastatic sentinel lymph nodes who are planning to undergo breast-conserving surgery with whole-breast radiotherapy should not undergo ALND (in most cases). Women with sentinel lymph node metastases who will undergo mastectomy should be offered ALND.[316]

Breast Reconstruction Surgery. Women who have a mastectomy as part of breast cancer treatment have options. Many choose to use a breast prosthesis; others choose to go "breast-free." Breast reconstruction of one or both breasts by a plastic surgeon is increasingly chosen by women who have undergone mastectomy. Surgical reconstruction may be immediate (at the time of the mastectomy) or delayed (any time after the mastectomy, including many years later). The rate of reconstruction varies by geography, socioeconomic status (including insurance coverage), hospital type, age, and ethnicity. The number of women opting for immediate breast reconstruction continues to increase.[535] The Women's Health and Cancer Rights Act of 1998 requires all health insurance providers and health maintenance organizations that pay for mastectomy to also pay for reconstruction of the breast removed by mastectomy, surgery and reconstruction of the opposite breast to achieve symmetry, the use of a breast prosthesis, and treatment for any complications of surgery including lymphedema.

Breast reconstruction is a surgical solution to anatomic defects caused by breast cancer. Breast reconstruction can be implant-based or autologous using transplanted tissue from the woman's abdomen, back, or buttocks to create a breast mound. The 2017 statistics report from the American Society of Plastic Surgeons found that there were 106,000 reconstructive breast procedures. Almost 40% of women with breast cancer undergo breast reconstruction.[293]

Tissue Expansion. Reconstruction with an implant alone usually requires tissue expansion. This is a two-stage surgical process. First, a tissue expander is placed. The tissue expander can be placed under the chest wall muscles (pectoralis major, serratus anterior, anterior rectus fascia) or on top of the pectoralis muscle (prepectoral technique). When the expander is placed under the chest wall muscles, there is often malalignment of the pectoralis muscle/serratus anterior muscle resulting in increased postoperative pain, muscular performance deficit, and deviation of the breast mound.[529] There is a growing trend to place the tissue expander on top of the pectoralis muscle, as it does not result in malalignment of the pectoralis muscle with activity, and research demonstrates that surgical complications are similar to the dual plane technique.[94] The woman returns to the plastic surgeon's office periodically for 4 to 6 months for saline injections ("fills") through an internal valve, which gradually stretches the muscles and soft tissues. A second surgical procedure replaces the expander with the implant.

Breast Implants. Although silicone implants were once banned, their use has been reinstated. In 2011 the FDA released long-term results to date of the silicone implant monitoring program and concluded that there is no evidence that silicone implants increase the risk of breast cancer or autoimmune diseases.[510] However, recent studies suggest there is an increase in large cell lymphoma with the use of prosthetic implants.[138a]

Silicone implants have the advantage of feeling more natural than saline implants, but some surgeons prefer to use saline because of their long-term safety record. All breast implants (regardless of their intended use for augmentation or for reconstruction) have a tendency to become encapsulated in connective tissue over time. The result may be a firm breast that no longer matches the opposite breast. In these cases, additional surgery later in life may be required to address the capsular contraction.[212] Other complications that may require surgical intervention include infection, implant rupture or leaks, deflation, or pain. Outcomes assessment of breast reconstruction is complex, and revision surgery may be required.[168]

Autologous Reconstruction. Breast reconstruction with autologous transplanted tissues uses the woman's own adipose tissue, muscle, and skin that can be harvested from a number of sites to either form a breast or create a pocket for an implant.[227,443] The benefits of using abdominal and lower extremity donor sites include the absence of a foreign implant with a natural-looking result. Additionally, the breast mound ages with the woman and responds to weight loss or weight gain.[402]

The most popular of these muscle flap procedures are the *latissimus dorsi (back) flap* and the *transverse rectus abdominis myocutaneous (TRAM) flap* (Fig. 20.15).[439] A latissimus dorsi flap procedure uses a section of skin, fat, and latissimus dorsi muscle that is detached from the back region and then tunneled under the skin to the breast area (Fig. 20.16). The tissue may be shaped into a natural-looking breast and sewn into place; more commonly the latissimus muscle is used to form the base of a pocket to receive an implant to create a breast of moderate size. In these cases the latissimus flap is a combination of autologous and implant-based reconstructive surgeries.

The TRAM flap procedure can be either a pedicle flap or a free flap. In the *pedicle flap,* the tissue removed remains attached to its blood supply and is tunneled under the woman's skin into the mastectomy wound. In the case of *free flaps,* a plastic surgeon trained in microvascular technique is required. In the free TRAM procedure, muscle, fat, and skin are harvested, along with inferior epigastric vessels. This flap is separated from the abdomen and brought to the chest defect, where it is anastomosed to either the thoracodorsal or the internal mammary vessels.

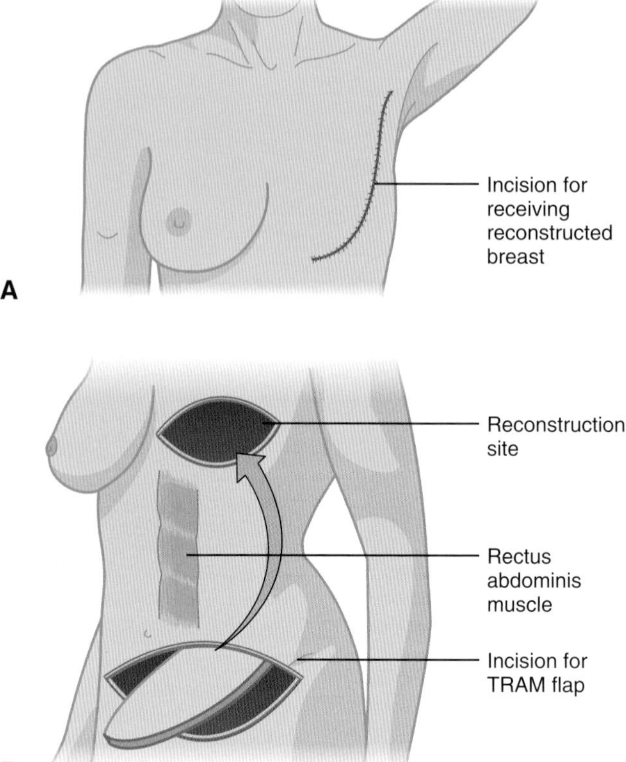


**Figure 20.15**

**Transverse rectus abdominis myocutaneous (TRAM) flap.** (A) After mastectomy of the involved breast, (B) a breast is reconstructed using the lower abdominal skin and fatty tissue. In a *pedicled* TRAM, the tissue's own blood supply remains attached, and the lower abdominal tissue is rotated into position on the chest. The tissue is tunneled under the skin to the chest area, where it is brought through the mastectomy incision. The reconstructed tissue is shaped to form a matching breast and placed in the mastectomy skin pocket. A *free* TRAM flap refers to using skin and tissue that are completely disconnected from their own blood supply, moved from the abdomen to the new site, and then reconnected to different blood vessels. A nipple and areola can be tattooed on later after healing has taken place.

Over the years, the TRAM procedure has evolved so that only a very small portion of the muscle around the required blood vessels is removed, a procedure now referred to as a *muscle-sparing TRAM*. If the blood vessels supplying the abdominal tissue are exceptionally good, no muscle tissue is required. The muscle is split rather than cut. This procedure is referred to as a *perforator flap* surgery or *DIEP* flap. Contraindications for perforator flap surgeries include a history of heavy smoking (with unfavorable vascular conditions), significant cardiopulmonary disease, history of blood clots (deep venous thrombosis or pulmonary embolus), previous surgery of the vascular territories, and allergy to anticoagulants.

Muscle-sparing free TRAM or DIEP perforator reconstructions involve a significant surgery time (4 or more hours per breast) and 3- to 5-day hospital stay because of the microvascular techniques and tissue monitoring that are required. The donor defect is repaired by *abdominoplasty* ("tummy tuck"); mesh may or may not be used. For the abdominoplasty a lower abdominal incision is made

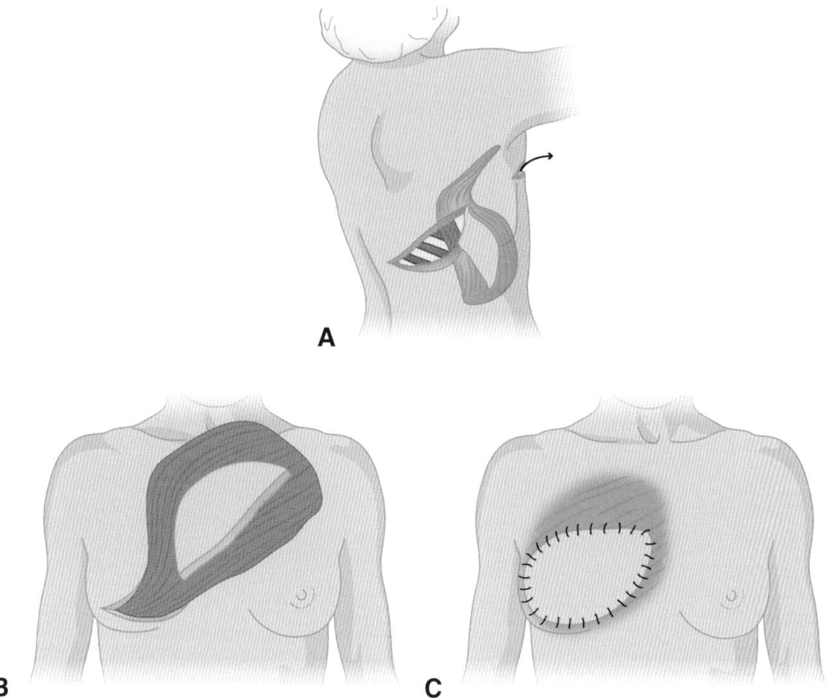


**Figure 20.16**

**Latissimus dorsi flap.** Schematic representation of latissimus dorsi flap. (A) Flap elevation. (B) Flap transposition. (C) Flap inset. (From Townsend CM: *Sabiston textbook of surgery*, ed 19, Philadelphia, 2012, Saunders.)

laterally from anterior superior iliac spine to anterior superior iliac spine (iliac crest) with removal of vascular supply, adipose tissue, and skin.[268,472] The umbilicus often requires repositioning.

The goal of the plastic surgeon is to remove as little abdominal muscle tissue as possible while still transplanting a viable flap of lower abdominal fat and overlying skin. Dissection of nerve supply is an additional area of investigation by surgeons trained in DIEP flap reconstruction. If significant rectus abdominis muscle has been removed, synthetic mesh or acellular dermal matrix may be used to repair the defect to decrease the risk of herniation. Similar to the DIEP, the *superficial inferior epigastric artery flap* transfers the same tissue from the abdomen to the chest for breast reconstruction as the TRAM flap without sacrificing the rectus abdominis muscle or fascia (Fig. 20.17).[434]

Another perforator flap used less commonly is from the buttocks: the *superior* or *inferior gluteal artery perforator* flap,[436] either of which has minimal donor-site morbidity. The *transverse upper gracilis flap* harvests muscle and tissue from the inner thigh.[113]

All of these autologous procedures are more complicated than implant surgery, requiring microvascular surgery and a longer hospital stay but with a result that is usually a softer, more natural-appearing breast. The woman often has an additional surgery (3 to 6 months later) to create a new areola and nipple on the reconstructed breast, with modification of the opposite breast if necessary to match the reconstructed breast. Tattooing or repigmentation of the nipple–areola complex is an option as well.

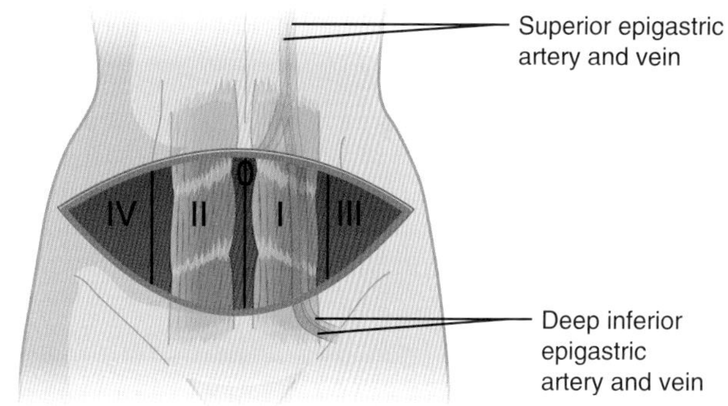


**Figure 20.17**

**Vascular territories of the abdominal wall provided by unilateral transverse rectus abdominis myocutaneous (TRAM) flap.** Studies show that the most reliable cutaneous portion is directly overlying muscle zone I, followed by zones III, II, and IV. A deep inferior epigastric perforator (DIEP) flap is an alternative procedure to the TRAM flap. A small portion of the rectus abdominis muscle is dissected to harvest the blood vessels, but the muscle is preserved because no muscle or overlying muscle fascia is used. The DIEP flap relies on blood vessels that perforate the rectus abdominis muscle (e.g., deep inferior epigastric artery and vein). (From Townsend CM: *Sabiston textbook of surgery*, ed 17, Philadelphia, 2004, Saunders.)

After surgery the treatment plan may include radiation therapy and systemic therapies, such as chemotherapy, hormone therapy, and targeted therapy or any combination of these approaches. The primary objective of these treatments is to reduce the odds of occult metastases from developing into disease.

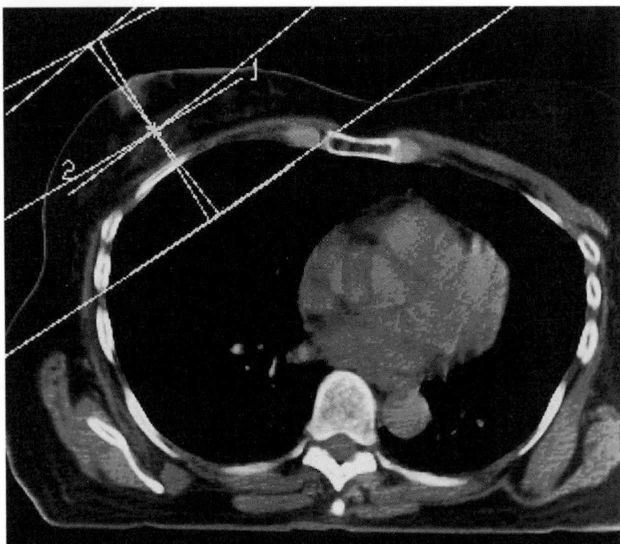

**Figure 20.18**

**Standard radiation field configuration for breast cancer.** Two tangentially directed fields encompass the breast with a minimal amount of underlying lung tissue. The contralateral breast and all of the critical structures are avoided. (From Abeloff MD: *Clinical oncology*, ed 3, Philadelphia, 2004, Churchill Livingstone.)

*Radiation Therapy.* Most women receive radiation therapy after a lumpectomy to eradicate any residual cancer cells in the affected breast or adjacent lymph nodes. Postmastectomy radiation is an increasing trend in certain groups because of the concern of local recurrence in the scar after mastectomy. These include women with large tumors, women with lymphatic vascular invasion, women with a tumor close to the rib cage or chest wall, or women with four or more positive axillary lymph nodes. Usually whole-breast radiation is delivered once a day, 5 days a week, for 5 to 6 weeks using a linear accelerator machine (Fig. 20.18). This delivery system is termed *external-beam radiation therapy* (EBRT). A later "boost" may be added by use of an external electron beam. An alternative to whole-breast radiation is *accelerated partial breast irradiation*. In 2018 the American Brachytherapy Society issued a consensus statement for accelerated partial breast irradiation regarding different techniques.[446] The techniques include the following:

- *Applicator brachytherapy* or *multicatheter interstitial brachytherapy* is delivered via balloon, often using the MammoSite (Fig. 20.19).[462]
- *Intensity-modulated radiation therapy* uses delivery of varying intensities across fields and is able to deliver a highly conformed dose to the target area, improving dose homogeneity.[80]
- *Proton therapy* uses an external proton beam to release energy in the tissue, optimizing the dose into the deep targeted tissue and reducing irradiation to the healthy tissues.[385]
- *Intraoperative radiation therapy* or *targeted intraoperative therapy* is a single dose of internal radiation therapy performed during surgery to the tumor bed after removal of the tumor .[154]

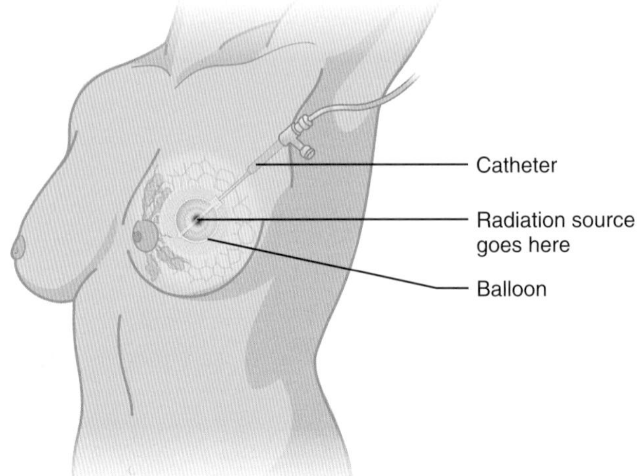


**Figure 20.19**

**Balloon brachytherapy.** The MammoSite device is approved for partial breast radiation in the treatment of early-stage breast cancer. A single-balloon catheter is inserted in the breast to deliver a site-specific, prescribed dose of radiation. The deflated balloon is placed inside the lumpectomy cavity (the space left after the tumor is removed). A tiny radioactive source (seed) is placed within the balloon by a computer-controlled machine. Because the radiation source is inside the balloon, radiation is delivered to the area of the breast where cancer is most likely to recur. Radiation exposure to the rest of the breast, skin, ribs, lungs, and heart is minimized. Once it has emitted the prescribed dose of radiation, the seed is removed. When used as primary therapy (i.e., the only form of radiation after a lumpectomy), treatments are twice a day for up to 5 days. The applicator shaft, a tube connected to the balloon, remains outside the breast. After 10 sessions in 5 days, the balloon is deflated, and the catheter is then removed.

Other approaches to radiation therapy are being explored, including three-dimensional conformal radiotherapy and CyberKnife.[192]

*Chemotherapy.* Chemotherapy is used to treat the whole body via the vascular system and is employed in patients with suspected or confirmed metastatic disease. *Adjuvant chemotherapy* is the term used for chemotherapy given at the time of breast cancer diagnosis, whereas *systemic therapy* is the term used for patients with known metastases. *Neoadjuvant chemotherapy* refers to chemotherapy given before surgical excision with the intent of shrinking the tumor size.[148]

Chemotherapy works by interfering with cell division, thus causing cell death (for further discussion, see Chapter 9). Many drugs are commonly administered as adjuvant chemotherapy for breast cancer (see Table 9.6), including cyclophosphamide (Cytoxan), methotrexate (Amethopterin, Mexate, Folex), 5-fluorouracil (Adrucil), doxorubicin (Adriamycin), epirubicin (Ellence), paclitaxel (Taxol, Abraxane), and docetaxel (Taxotere). The drugs are delivered via a vascular access device, including Hickman, Groshong, and Port-A-Cath devices. Treatment protocols developed by the oncologist and patient vary in the combination of drugs used[22] and method of delivery, usually 10 minutes to 4 hours at a time, and given in variable cycles of weeks for a total of 12 to 16 weeks.

Adjuvant chemotherapy reduces the risk of recurrence overall by one-third in individuals with breast cancer, with differential benefits based on more specific subtypes and diagnostic features.[148] For example, women with "harder-to-treat" ER– breast tumors tend to benefit more from chemotherapy than women with ER+ tumors. Increased disease-free survival time after combination chemotherapy has been noted consistently in premenopausal women with metastases to the axillary lymph nodes.

In the past, the majority of women with early-stage breast cancer received adjuvant chemotherapy. Although only a minority of women benefit from such therapy, all are affected by its toxicity. Women with ER+ early-stage breast cancers who meet certain criteria may be able to avoid chemotherapy and may be better served with hormonal therapy. Molecular profiling tests, previously discussed, assist professionals in making decisions regarding treatment. See Biomarkers for tools to evaluate risks and benefits of adjuvant therapy.

***Hormonal Therapy.*** Hormonal or endocrine therapy refers to the use of drugs in the treatment of ER+ breast cancers. These drugs work by either lowering the amount of available estrogen or blocking the action of estrogen on breast cancer cells. Hormonal therapy medications include SERMs, AIs, and ER downregulators.[240] These medications are recommended as adjuvant therapy for a period of 5 or more years to decrease risk of cancer recurrence or of cancer in the contralateral breast. They are also used as neoadjuvant therapy to reduce tumor size or for chemoprevention in individuals at high risk for breast cancer. Hormonal therapy is also used to arrest the growth of advanced hormone receptor–positive breast disease in both premenopausal and postmenopausal women.

SERMs work by blocking the effects of estrogen in the breast tissue. SERMs reduce the risk of cancer recurrence as well as the development of a new cancer in the contralateral breast by approximately 50%. They also decrease the risk of cancer mortality.[251] Tamoxifen (Nolvadex) is the best-known and most widely used SERM and has been in use for more than 30 years. When tamoxifen is taken for 5 years, studies show a lowered recurrence rate of 45% to 50% in ER+ cancers in years 0 to 4. Clinical trials continue to explore the use of tamoxifen beyond 5 years. Recent studies support recommendation of continuing hormonal medications for 10 years.[298]

The selective estrogen activation effects of tamoxifen may produce some serious, although rare, side effects including blood clots, stroke, and endometrial cancer. Other side effects that have been reported include hot flashes, fatigue, weight gain, premature menopause, leg cramps, urogynecologic symptoms (including urinary incontinence), and cataracts.[63] Raloxifene is another SERM that is less likely to promote thromboembolic events, endometrial cancer and benign uterine conditions, and cataracts.[260]

SERMs offer other health benefits unrelated to treating cancer. Even though SERMs block estrogen's action on breast cells, they activate the effect of estrogen in bone and liver cells. This results in reduced osteoporosis risk and increases heart protection by lowered cholesterol levels (higher high-density lipoprotein and lower low-density lipoprotein levels). The ongoing Co-STAR (Cognition in the Study of Tamoxifen and Raloxifene) trial is investigating effects of both medications on mood and cognitive performance.[123]

AIs work differently than SERMs. They interfere with the production of estrogen in postmenopausal women by blocking the enzyme aromatase, which converts the hormone androgen into small amounts of estrogen in the body. This results in reduced availability of estrogen to stimulate the growth of ER+ breast cancer cells. AIs are recommended as the first-choice drug in postmenopausal women. There are more benefits and fewer serious side effects than with tamoxifen. However, AIs may cause more cardiac problems, osteoporosis, and joint pain than tamoxifen. Studies show that switching to an AI after taking tamoxifen is superior to 5 years of tamoxifen alone.[148]

Selective ER degraders are another class of drugs that work by blocking estrogen in postmenopausal women with advanced ER+ breast cancer that has stopped responding to other hormonal therapy medicines.[252]

***Targeted (or Biologic) Therapy.*** Trastuzumab (Herceptin) is a highly effective drug used to treat breast tumors that are HER2-positive. HER2-positive breast cancers are more aggressive and less likely to respond to conventional therapies. Trastuzumab can be used alone or as part of a chemotherapy regimen.[248] Trastuzumab may slow or stop the growth targeting of HER2 proteins. In addition to blocking HER2 receptors, trastuzumab may facilitate the immune system in the destruction of cancer cells. It is considered an immune-targeted therapy and thus an antibody that attacks cancer at its genetic roots. Side effects from the use of trastuzumab include an increase in cardiovascular events such as left ventricular dysfunction and congestive heart disease.[363]

Bevacizumab (Avastin) is a targeted monoclonal antibody; it is an antiangiogenic agent that works by decreasing blood supply to the cancer. It is generally used along with chemotherapy in women with advanced disease. In 2011 the FDA announced that it had removed the breast cancer indication from Avastin because the drug has not been shown to be safe and effective for that use. The medicine itself was not removed from the market. Studies are ongoing to identify a subset of individuals with breast cancer who may benefit from its use.[411]

***Ovarian Ablation.*** Removing estrogens from premenopausal women by surgically removing the ovaries or using drugs to suppress ovarian function is another way of treating ER breast cancer.[166]

**PROGNOSIS.** Cancer prognosis is dependent on the age and menopausal status of the woman, the stage of the disease, type/subtype of cancer, histologic and nuclear grade of the primary tumor, biomarkers such as ER and PR status of the tumor, HER2 status, proliferative capacity of the tumor, and status of the axillary lymph nodes. A tumor's biology (hormone status, molecular subtype, and histopathology) is more important than size and how much the cancer has spread. These factors hold for both men and women, although men are typically diagnosed with later stage disease than women, with larger tumors, and with a greater likelihood of lymph node involvement and distant metastases.

When cancer characteristics (age of the individual, tumor stage, grade, nodal status, ER/PR/HER2 status) are matched, survival rates for men with breast cancer appear to be worse compared with women.[303] However, men and women with advanced breast cancer were found to have an equivalent survival rate.[554]

Other factors that influence prognosis include race/ethnicity (African American and Hispanic/Latina women are often diagnosed at later stages), activity level (sedentary individuals have poorer prognosis), and BMI (risk increased when BMI is greater than 30).

Breast tumors that lack estrogen responsiveness tend to have a poorer prognosis because of the limited response of the cancer to current antiestrogen treatments available. Individuals with tumor-negative disease (ER–/PR–/HER2-negative) represent a particular therapeutic challenge because of the lack of molecular targets. However, for these individuals, advances in conventional intravenous chemotherapy have resulted in improved survival rates.[388]

If detected early before metastases, most breast cancers are curable. According to the NCI SEER Program there has been a yearly mortality reduction of 1.8%. Five-year survival for localized cancer is 98.7%. Five-year relative survival rates (accounting for deaths from all causes) are 62% for localized cancer, 31% for regional (lymph node–positive) disease, 6% for distant metastasis, and 2% for unknown/unstaged disease. Although advancements in technology make early detection possible and new treatments are improving survival, 40,920 women died of breast cancer in 2018 As follow-up time increases, SEER data can be used to monitor and better understand the impact of how targeted therapies are contributing to reduce breast cancer mortality in the U.S. population. In another study, using SEER data, cancer prognosis was reported based on molecular subtypes and features. Patients with hormone receptor–positive subtypes have the best prognosis, whereas patients with hormone receptor–negative subtypes have the worst prognosis, especially those with triple-negative cancer.[229]

Further understanding of less common types of breast cancer and ongoing developments in molecular subtyping help to determine prognosis. For example, IBC constitutes only 2% of all breast cancers in the United States, but it represents a large percentage of locally advanced disease (this could be a consequence of late diagnosis with metastases already present rather than because of subtype). It is an extremely variable disease with a poor prognosis despite recent therapies; the survival rate for all women with IBC is 28% to 67% for 5 years and 8% to 47% for 10 years for stage III and stage IV, respectively [332].

Mortality is also important to consider when discussing prognosis. Many women experience secondary complications of the disease and its treatments including decreased quality of life, weight gain, sleep disturbances, poor body image, fatigue, increased risk for osteoporosis, CVD, premature menopause, peripheral neuropathy, cognitive changes, lymphedema, and development of other cancers.

***Recurrence.*** *Local recurrence* refers to cancer that occurs in the same breast that has been treated with BCT or in the scar of a mastectomy. A recent study found the incidence of ipsilateral breast tumor relapse in individuals who were previously treated for early-stage breast cancer by BCT and radiation therapy or by mastectomy to be close to 2.7%. Local regional recurrence is lower in patients who are younger and increased in patients with larger tumor size, hormone-negative cancers, and higher number of positive lymph nodes.[1] Differentiation between a true recurrence and a new primary tumor is necessary. Local recurrences that occur more than 5 years after initial treatment with BCT have a worse prognosis.[489]

*Regional recurrence* refers to cancer that is found in the axillary, supraclavicular, or (less commonly) internal mammary lymph nodes; this may occur after an ALND or SLNB. Risk of regional recurrence correlates with the pathologic detection of a higher number of positive lymph nodes. Although SLNB is highly accurate in predicting the status of axillary nodes in individuals with breast cancer, the procedure is associated with a low rate (up to 10%) of false-negative results. Applying mapping and operative techniques to new anatomic findings of sentinel lymphatic channels and drainage patterns may reduce this rate even more.[413] Recurrence in lymph nodes other than ipsilateral lymph nodes suggests metastasis.

*Distant recurrence* denotes disease spread to other organs; it is metastatic disease. Aalders and colleagues[1] suggest that distant metastasis is decreasing as risk of local and regional recurrence decreases. Common sites for breast cancer metastases are bone, lungs, liver, and brain. Women with advanced breast cancer (stage IV disease) may live a number of years with a good quality of life. With the continued identification of molecular subtypes of breast cancer and treatments, it is anticipated that there will be further improvements in life span.

***Contralateral Breast Cancer.*** A recent systematic review stated the annual median incidence rate of contralateral subsequent primary breast cancers is 0.5% (range, 0.2% to 0.7%).[469] There is a decrease in the global incidence rate, which may be related to more effective adjuvant therapy. Individuals with *BRCA1* and *BRCA2* mutations are at higher risk. Women without known genetic mutations who are diagnosed at a younger age (<35 years old) with ER– tumors are at higher risk for contralateral breast cancer.[307] Development of a contralateral breast cancer early (<5 years) after initial diagnosis is associated with worse survival among women younger than 70 years old at time of diagnosis compared with longer time intervals, but not among women older than 70 at time of diagnosis.[287,299]

Prophylactic approaches to reduce the risk of a second breast cancer include pharmacologic, radiotherapeutic, and surgical approaches in addition to lifestyle changes (diet, weight reduction, and exercise). The risk of developing other primary malignancies in breast cancer survivors is greater than the general population. For this reason, breast cancer survivors should undergo screening for other malignancies as well as screening for contralateral breast cancer and recurrences. The ACS and ACOG also recommend that a cancer survivorship care plan be developed that considers each patient's individual risk profile and preferences of care to address physical and psychosocial impacts.[428]

SPECIAL IMPLICATIONS FOR THE THERAPIST 20.11

## *Breast Cancer*[a]

There are many considerations for the therapist working with men and women who report upper quadrant symptoms of unknown origin or who have been diagnosed with breast cancer, both before and after treatment. Therapists who specialize in oncology rehabilitation are increasingly active in research and developing protocols for best practices. The 2012 April supplement of the journal *Cancer* is devoted to best practice rehabilitation of breast cancer.[83,337,477] The therapist should have knowledge of diagnostic categories; surgical procedures; postoperative restrictions and recommendations; and expected/adverse outcomes of surgery, chemotherapy, radiation therapy, hormonal therapy, and targeted therapies (see discussion in Chapter 9).

The therapist should be knowledgeable of time-related restrictions for performing soft tissue mobilization, risk factors for the development of lymphedema (see discussion in Chapter 13), and recommendations regarding lifestyle changes and complementary treatments. The use of complementary treatments (such as acupuncture), which take the place of medical treatments, is also an area in which the therapist can provide valuable input for the individual with breast cancer. Finally, outcome measures are an increasingly important part of clinical practice. The reader is referred to the journal *Rehabilitation Oncology* that highlights the American Physical Therapy Association–Academy of Oncologic Physical Therapy (APTA-AOPT) Task Force on Breast Cancer Outcomes recommendations on measures that can or should be used for individuals treated for breast cancer.[19a] Campbell and colleagues[83] published a prospective model of care for breast cancer rehabilitation with a rationale for the use of functional outcome measures to aid therapists in providing better rehabilitation care for breast cancer survivors.

### Screening for Disease and Cancer Recurrence

When treating a woman with a history of breast cancer, therapists should be alert to signs and symptoms that may point to local, regional, and distant metastases. Additionally, breast cancer survivors are at increased risk of developing a second primary breast cancer; it is not a recurrence, but a new cancer unrelated to the first. This may occur in either breast in a woman who has undergone BCT or mastectomy.

A local recurrence or second primary breast cancer will manifest most commonly as a new lump or mass. Masses that are painless, hard, and with irregular edges should be considered suspicious and should be evaluated. Palpation of a lump or mass in these areas or new onset of edema or swelling in the upper quadrant should raise concern for the therapist and lead to further questioning regarding the clinical findings.

Therapists examining the shoulder and shoulder girdle region need to be aware of the soft tissue structures (including breast tissue and regional lymph nodes) located in these areas. The upper, outer quadrant of the breast can extend up toward the glenohumeral joint; more cancerous masses occur in this area of the breast than in any other part of the breast. Breast tumor metastases to lymph nodes can involve the axillary, supraclavicular, infraclavicular, and internal mammary lymph nodes. Disease spread to these lymph node groups may cause compression of adjacent structures, resulting in referred pain to the shoulder, upper extremity, and/or chest wall.[336]

If the mass lies within the pectoralis major muscle, the mass should change during palpation with active muscle contraction. Metastases to the thorax are common in breast cancer, and pulmonary symptoms can be very similar to pulmonary abnormalities that occur after radiotherapy. If the therapist is in doubt regarding any reported or observed manifestations, the client should be referred for medical evaluation (see Lymphedema in Chapter 13).

Bone metastases occur in up to 70% of women with advanced breast cancer.[565] The most common sites for bone metastases are the humerus in the upper extremity and the femur in the lower extremity. Any report of new-onset or increased bone pain, especially at night and/or with weight-bearing activities, should be carefully assessed; pathologic fracture is a possibility. Positive nodal status, large tumor size, ER+ status, and age younger than 35 years are significant risk factors for bone metastases in this population. Individuals who use tobacco, have a poor diet and nutrition, report decreased physical activity, and engage in alcohol abuse are much more likely to develop metastases.

### Side Effects of Cancer Treatment

Individuals receiving neoadjuvant or adjuvant therapy (chemotherapy, radiation therapy, hormonal therapy, or targeted therapy) may experience numerous side effects that may impact rehabilitation.

## *Chemotherapy*

The vast majority of individuals receiving chemotherapy experience fatigue.[463] This is minimized to some extent with erythropoietin used to treat anemia by stimulating bone marrow production of red blood cells. Other common side effects include nausea, hair loss, mouth sores, neutropenia, and neuropathy (especially with taxanes). Less common serious side effects include sepsis, cardiac damage, and secondary leukemia.[491] Cognitive difficulties can be pronounced during treatment, but long-term cognitive deficits after chemotherapy for breast cancer are reportedly small in magnitude, most often affecting verbal ability (word finding) and visuospatial ability (getting lost more easily in unfamiliar locations.[491]

For an individual with low nadir level (lowest point of blood cell production after neutrophil and platelet count have been depressed by chemotherapy) and/or anemia, the timing of scheduled therapy visits is important to maximize productivity during the session. Exercises and functional activities may need to be paced or therapy visits adjusted to accommodate the

[a]Jane Kepics PT, DPT, Certified Lymphology Association of North America.

individual's energy level. Conditioning exercise can address the need for increased endurance for activities of daily living, family responsibilities, and occupational demands.

### *Radiotherapy*

Radiation therapy uses high-energy beams to destroy cells; both cancer and native cells are affected. Immediate radiation risks include skin redness, blistering, fatigue, and breast tenderness. Long-term effects include tissue scarring, poor wound healing, lymphedema, ischemic heart disease,[75] increased breast firmness, loss of breast volume, and permanent skin changes (e.g., telangiectasias and hyperpigmentation). Surgeons typically wait 6 months after radiotherapy to assess tissue quality for surgical options, including reconstruction.[548]

Radiotherapy to the left breast is associated with higher rates of chest pain, coronary artery disease, and myocardial infarction. Cardiotoxic drugs such as doxorubicin and trastuzumab may compound the problem. The therapist should screen individuals treated for breast cancer for cardiac symptoms and risk factors such as blood pressure and smoking. Regular cardiac surveillance is important for all breast cancer survivors regardless of whether they had radiation therapy because of the increased risk of cardiac disease with aging.[73] Tissue destruction caused by radiation therapy may include muscle damage.

### *Hormonal Therapy*

Although SERMs have a protective effect on BMD, the majority of AIs have been linked to a decrease in bone density and increased fracture risk. Baseline and follow-up bone density studies are recommended for individuals receiving AIs.[228] Drug therapy may include bisphosphonates and other medications. Education should include recommendations for adequate calcium and vitamin D supplementation and exercise.

An increased frequency of lower extremity arthralgias has been reported with the use of hormonal therapy, specifically with the use of AIs and, to a lesser degree, tamoxifen. Adverse effects include joint and muscle pain and stiffness, carpal tunnel syndrome, and trigger finger. AI-induced musculoskeletal syndrome is associated with tendon-sheath thickening and intraarticular fluid retention, with loss of grip strength.[101,301] Symptoms of arthralgias are reported in 46% of individuals receiving AIs. Intensity of symptoms is a factor in at least 20% of individuals, who choose to discontinue use of this medication.[46] The physiologic explanation of arthralgia with estrogen deprivation continues to be investigated. It is hypothesized that both systemic and local effects of estrogen deficiency may impair cartilage maintenance. The role of vitamin D is the subject of ongoing research.

A variety of therapeutic interventions for joint pain have been studied. A recent meta-analysis suggests that there is limited evidence for most interventions; however, there is some evidence that acupuncture, aerobic exercise, pharmacologic interventions, vitamin D, and omega fatty acids may provide some pain relief.[266]

## Preoperative Considerations

Preoperative evaluation of the upper quarter by a therapist is recommended for all women undergoing surgical intervention for breast cancer, whether the intervention is SLNB, ALND, lumpectomy, or mastectomy of any kind.[477] Also recommended is evaluation before breast reconstruction surgery (immediate or delayed). Educating breast surgeons, radiation oncologists, medical oncologists, and plastic surgeons regarding the benefits of preoperative assessment and postoperative therapeutic interventions is needed, as referral to a therapist may be delayed by months or years until the individual requests help with long-standing impairments.

### *Preoperative Assessment*

Preoperative assessment of an individual with breast cancer includes taking a thorough history and recording baseline measurements of both upper extremities so that any postoperative changes can be more easily detected. Radiation changes and previous surgeries are risk factors for postural compromises that contribute to movement impairments of the shoulder. The prevalence of shoulder-related dysfunction has been reported as 7% to 36% in the general population.[478]

Assessment of the individual's current physical activity level includes activities of daily living, work and leisure activities, and fitness and exercise habits and preferences. Upper quadrant motion (including biomechanics and scapulohumeral timing), posture, joint range of motion (ROM) (including accessory motions), flexibility, and soft tissue conditions should be assessed. Arthrokinematic changes of the shoulder joint and other preexisting shoulder problems present before breast cancer diagnosis and treatment may contribute to suboptimal postoperative recovery of glenohumeral and scapular motion. The therapist can address these problems before surgery or during neoadjuvant treatment, facilitating postoperative functional recovery.

### *Education*

The therapist is a key educator and care provider who may be involved before breast cancer diagnosis, throughout treatment, and during the recovery process. Preoperative education should be specific to the individual's surgery, teaching postoperative precautions and safe movement (such as log rolling), avoidance of overactivity, lymphedema prevention, and appropriate exercises in the early postoperative phase before outpatient therapy. For women who plan to undergo breast reconstruction, information about lifting and activity restriction, abdominal and chest protection, lymphedema prevention, and return to activity guidelines may be provided.

## Postoperative Considerations

Recovery after individual surgical procedures may vary. Potential complications after all types of breast cancer surgery (BCT, mastectomy, and reconstruction) include pain, sensory changes (dysesthesias and numbness), infection (cellulitis), tissue necrosis, seroma development, hematoma, and local tissue swelling. Despite the adoption of more conservative surgical approaches, pain and functional compromise after surgery remain significant clinical challenges.

Breast surgery and surgical assessment of axillary lymph nodes (either by SLNB or ALND) are commonly associated with pain, decreased shoulder ROM, weakness, movement impairment, swelling, neuropathy, fatigue, axillary web syndrome (AWS) (or cording), and lymphedema of the upper extremity and trunk. Women report upper body symptoms within the first year and at long-term follow up.[221] Functional impairments impact the ability of women to perform daily activities and work and to engage in recreational pursuits for at least a year after surgery.[67]

Therapeutic interventions employed by the oncology rehabilitation therapist address soft tissue fibrosis, deficits in muscle strength and flexibility, lymphatic insufficiency, muscle hypertonicity, and neural hypersensitivity. Proactive and preventive approaches should be employed rather than delaying treatment until problems persist. It is well known that functional impairments can persist many years after the completion of breast cancer treatment. Prospective surveillance models have been proposed for ongoing evaluation of physical functioning as opposed to a traditional model of impairment-based care.[477] This surveillance model uses therapists as experts in movement dysfunction to provide preoperative examination, education, ongoing clinical monitoring, early identification, and intervention for common conditions resulting from breast cancer treatment.

Postoperative restrictions vary with procedure and professional opinion. There is controversy regarding whether shoulder ROM, particularly shoulder abduction, should be restricted the first week after mastectomy (or drains out plus 5 days)[126] to allow lymphatic collecting vessels to regenerate and reconnect. Studies suggest early ROM does not increase seroma formation.[126,396]

The therapist must assess the biomechanics of shoulder motion after surgery and radiation therapy to provide interventions that address dysfunction of the upper quarter. Scapular and glenohumeral movement, along with cervical and thoracic spine movement, are likely to be compromised. This limited ROM is not likely to be a result of internal glenohumoral joint dysfunction but more likely external muscle and fascial tightness. Anterior chest muscle tightness and hypertonicity secondary to pain is common. Postural changes may result from efforts to protect the surgical site, which may promote further muscle and soft tissue shortening. Radiation fibrosis of the pectoral tendons and muscle sheaths may exacerbate tissue tightness. When the pectoralis major muscle is incorporated into the muscular pouch that houses breast implants (the breast implant is placed deep to the pectoralis muscle), muscle tension markedly increases, resulting in scapular protraction. Decreased shoulder ROM and pectoralis muscle spasm often result and require direct intervention. The therapist may employ soft tissue mobilization, manual therapy, and therapeutic exercises, including stretching and strengthening for endurance and proper sequencing of motor recruitment.[126] Joint manipulation or mobilization would be indicated only when decreased ROM is due to decreased accessory movements (which is not often the case in patients recovering from breast cancer treatment). Application of modalities to the shoulder should be done with caution. Heat should be avoided in patients with lymphatic compromise (node removal and/or radiation) to minimize the onset of lymphedema. Therapeutic ultrasound is contraindicated in an area where cancer might be present.

Ongoing education and support are a significant aspect of the therapist–client relationship. Most education and rehabilitation focuses on the physical performance components. While this is important, rehabilitation should also include methods to improve nonphysical issues, such as psychosocial, cognitive, occupational, and other lifestyle performance factors that will enable individuals to live with this chronic condition.[308]

### Breast-Conserving Therapy

BCT usually does not affect the pectoralis major muscle or overlying fascia; however, lobular breast cancer can progress to the chest wall, requiring deep resection. Women with BCT have not routinely been seen by therapists because the surgery is not as extensive; however, they can benefit from physical therapy interventions. Education about precautions and movement of the upper extremity is important for these women.

### Mastectomy

Mastectomy without reconstruction has different rehabilitation considerations from mastectomy with reconstruction (immediate or delayed). Women who have undergone mastectomy should be evaluated postoperatively and instructed in breathing and splinted coughing techniques to prevent pulmonary complications. Lower extremity exercises may be employed to prevent thromboemboli. Management of postoperative drains and activity modification, as well as when to begin active shoulder ROM (not too early; not too late), are important functions of the oncology rehabilitation therapist.

Up to 50% of women undergoing mastectomy or levels 1 and 2 lymph node removal experience neuropathic pain. A group from Canada[530] suggests that neuropathic pain should be called postmastectomy pain syndrome (PMPS), providing a standardized definition for research and clinical use. The proposed definition of PMPS is "pain that occurs after any breast surgery, is of at least moderate severity, possesses neuropathic qualities, is located in the ipsilateral breast/chest wall, axilla, and/or arms, lasts at least 6 months, occurs at least 50% of the time, and may be exacerbated by movements of the shoulder. Some other authors do not agree with this definition.[488] At the present time there is not an agreed-upon cause of PMPS. Tait and colleagues[488] suggest preoperative risk factors, including younger age, preoperative painful conditions and/or psychologic factors, intraoperative risk factors, including ANLD (less risk with SLNB) and/or musculoskeletal mechanics related to the pectoralis muscle, and postoperative risk factors of acute postoperative pain and/or radiation therapy. The pain occurs at the incision site, axilla, arm, or shoulder and may be experienced as burning, numbness, tingling, pins and needles, or shocklike.

Because PMPS/post–breast therapy pain syndrome seems to be increasingly reported, it is important for the clinician to inquire about postmastectomy pain. An oncology rehabilitation program to promote flexibility and prevent adhesive capsulitis and restore strength, ROM, and normal neuromuscular recruitment patterns should be employed, with a focus on functional mobility, instrumental activities of daily living, and vocational capacity. Pharmaceutical and interventional pain techniques are often used to manage the pain.

### Breast Reconstruction

#### *Autologous Reconstruction*

The surgical technique will inform decision making in physical therapy. Immediate postoperative protocols after breast reconstruction vary. Typically, room temperature is kept warm, and supplemental oxygen is provided along with tissue monitoring, including tissue oximetry to minimize risk of flap necrosis. The patient is kept in flexion (head of bed elevated, hips and knees flexed). Physicians are starting to use an enhanced recovery pathway particularly for microsurgical reconstruction to decrease length of stay, including mobilizing the patient on postoperative day 1.[65,457] Therapists are part of the team and provide guidance on proper mobilization and education regarding exercise and activities.

Altered kinesthesia and musculoskeletal mechanics following surgery require intervention. These could include altered tension of the thoracolumbar fascia and resulting back pain, substitution by the abdominal oblique muscles, and compensation of the contralateral rectus muscle. Attention should be focused on proper muscle recruitment with activities.[548]

Donor-site morbidity is more pronounced with autologous procedures that involve muscle transfer. Studies have demonstrated that incidence of fat necrosis, bulge rate, hernias, and partial flap necrosis is higher in the pedicle TRAM compared with the free TRAM and DIEP.[28,318,345] DIEP leads to less abdominal morbidity, and patients report higher satisfaction with abdominal physical well-being. Unilateral and bilateral breast reconstruction may result in an imbalance between truncal flexors and extensors. A graded postoperative abdominal muscle reeducation and strengthening program is essential to prevent further spine-related musculoskeletal complications and associated postural compromise.

Lymph vessel damage may occur during the separation of the rectus sheath from the overlying dermis, resulting in truncal lymphostasis. Truncal edema is common and can last for up to 1 year; it generally responds to lymph clearing techniques. Trauma may also produce fibrosis and tethering of the dermis to underlying tissue. Fibrosis can limit truncal extension and may result in neural entrapment, producing chronic pain. Despite the potential for functional morbidity, a significant majority of women recommended autologous reconstruction and reported enhanced health-related quality of life following the procedure.[376a]

The latissimus dorsi myocutaneous flap is another common surgery chosen particularly for bilateral reconstruction. The latissimus dorsi myocutaneous flap may be a combination of autologous and implant reconstructive surgeries. Capsular contractures are not as common, especially with use of a tissue expander.[222] A recent meta-analysis[474] suggests that during the first 3 months, shoulder flexion and abduction may be impaired, but reports there is insufficient evidence to determine long-term dysfunction 1 year after surgery Overall, women report high satisfaction with upper extremity function during daily activities after latissimus dorsi myocutaneous flap surgery.

#### *Breast Implants*

Women who receive breast implants for reconstruction after mastectomies undergo a much less extensive operation than autologous reconstructions. There is a much shorter recovery time with a breast implant than with autologous reconstruction. It does require multiple office visits during the "fill" phase before placement of the permanent implant. Patients may have postoperative restrictions related to lifting and shoulder ROM.

The most common complication of implant reconstruction is a capsular contracture where scar tissue forms around the implant, deforming or hardening the implant. Capsular contraction occurs in up to 30% of patients, although the use of AlloDerm may decrease risk.[431] Preoperative or postoperative irradiation increases the incidence of capsular contracture. Treatment for capsular contractures requires surgical intervention. Other complications include seromas and implant rupture or leakage and, less often, bruising, infection, and chronic pain.

As noted previously there may be musculoskeletal impairments because of the tissue expander if the implant is placed under the pectoralis major, serratus anterior, and anterior rectus sheaths. These include pectoral muscle spasm, splinting and guarding, chest wall tightness, scarring, and decreased shoulder ROM and function. Pectoral tightness may affect scapular retractor muscles with postural compromise.

#### *Axillary Lymph Node Dissection*

Decreased shoulder ROM, pain, and paresthesias have been reported after lymph node surgery.[466] Sensations have been described as tender, sore, pulling, aching, painful, twinge, tight, stiff, pricking, throbbing, shooting, tingling, numb, burning, hard, sharp, nagging, and deep or penetrating. These sensations many improve with time and may more quickly resolve with skilled manual therapy at the appropriate time. Numbness under the arm (axillary and medial upper arm area) is often a clue that ALND was performed. This numbness many take many months to resolve or may be permanent.

### *Axillary Web Syndrome*

AWS, also known as axillary cording or lymphatic cording, is a condition associated with surgery to the axilla. Although there is not a definitive agreement for the definition of AWS, it was first described by Moscovitz and colleagues[362] as a visible web of axillary skin overlying palpable cords of tissue that are made taut and painful by shoulder ROM. The cause of AWS remains uncertain. A recent systematic review suggested that AWS may be due to thrombosed lymphatic vessels, although the authors did report that one study suggested that the cording was secondary to disruption of both veins and lymph vessels.[559] Frequency of 6% to 80% has been reported.[559] Proximal cording into the torso and breast tissue has also been described.[290]

The cords are most visible in the axilla when the shoulder is abducted or in the antecubital space when the elbow is extended (Fig. 20.20). Common symptoms include pain radiating down the arm during shoulder abduction and limitation of shoulder abduction and/or elbow extension. Usually there are two or three palpable cords under the skin that are hard and painful, but not erythematous. AWS typically appears within 3 months of surgery and may resolve within 3 months, but it also can appear years later.[382]

The therapist may be instrumental in discovering unreported or unresolved AWS. Early recognition of symptoms (e.g., arm pain and decreased shoulder motion) and intervention may help prevent postural changes, movement dysfunction, and restriction of activities of daily living.

There is no gold standard for treatment, and there are no randomized controlled trials to describe treatment. However, clinicians report success with gentle and slow manual therapy techniques, including myofascial release, soft tissue mobilization, skin traction, cord bending, and scar massage directly to the cords and to the surrounding tissues.[315]

### *Shoulder/Upper Extremity*

Upper quarter impairments with activity and participation limitations are commonly reported in individuals receiving treatment for breast cancer. The most common complaints are pain, sensory changes, weakness in the involved extremity, decreased ROM particularly in abduction and external rotations, and impairments in functional mobility. Most arm morbidity is reported within the first year.[67,100] Two recent studies found that the severity of arm morbidity is most closely related to negative affect and perceived disability.[67,100] Chrischilles and coworkers[100] also found that health literacy as well as mastectomy with radiation therapy and upper extremity morbidity had the most impact on quality of life.

Shoulder girdle movement is affected by surgery and/or radiation. Women report more shoulder restrictions and impairments after mastectomy than

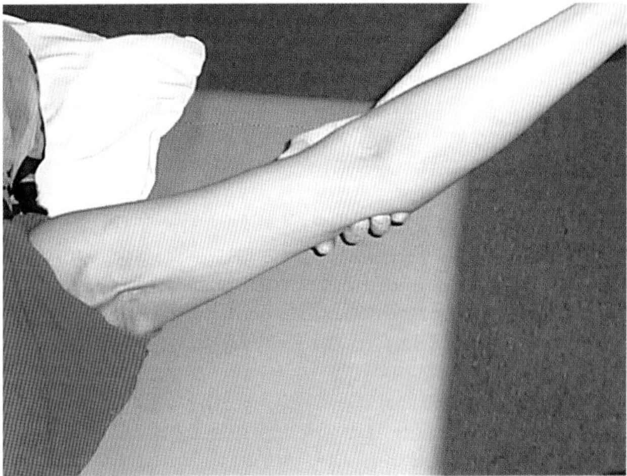

**Figure 20.20**

**Axillary cord that limits shoulder abduction.** This client had a biopsy of a swollen axillary lymph node. The biopsy was benign, but the woman had pain and limited range of motion for about 6 weeks. (Courtesy Jane Kepics, PT DPT CLT-LANA, Advance Clinician II, Lymphedema and Cancer Rehabilitation, GSPP/Penn Therapy and Fitness at Valley Forge.)

#### A THERAPIST'S THOUGHTS

While many patients undergoing axillary surgery for breast cancer or melanoma are educated about the risk of developing lymphedema, few are aware of AWS. Patients are instructed to resume activity postoperatively but become concerned and frustrated when painful cords occur, limiting their mobility. The anxiety of having cancer along with the stress of surgery, chemotherapy, and/or radiation therapy as well as a fear of cancer recurrence heightens this pain. Patients fear that they will not return to full function. Patients who concurrently receive breast implant fills as part of breast reconstruction feel even further challenged by cording. They often limit or stop exercising because of the pain.

Therapists can educate patients about this diagnosis and guide them toward good upright posture, breathing control exercises to calm them, and slow stretching to regain motion. I use soft tissue and myofascial release techniques to stretch the cords, starting in a less painful position (shoulder in slight abduction with the elbow flexed) and gradually venturing further into abduction as the patient or the cording allows. I may add manual lymph drainage if the pain is particularly acute, to help reduce inflammation. I sometimes have patients wear a light compression garment to provide a slow sustained stretch on cording. I also mobilize the chest wall at the "drain" incision. While I have not been able to corroborate this with a surgeon, I wonder if the trauma of removing the surgical drain could contribute to inflammation in this area. I often palpate cords originating at the drain site and extending into the arm. Patients say they feel better after tissue mobilization.

There is some controversy about the breaking of cords. This sometimes occurs during cord manipulation in the antecubital fossa where cords are generally thinner. The patient usually reports improved motion, less pain, and no residual issues. It is harder to do with thicker cords in the axilla—these respond better to slow stretch and nerve gliding techniques. Some studies suggest that we are breaking supporting fibrous tissue, but further research is needed in this area.

with breast-conserving surgery. Altered movement patterns of the scapula (with associated pain and dysfunction) on the side of the cancer may also impact function. Upper extremity impairments can extend beyond the acute stages of recovery and may be considered a component of chronic illness.

The role of the therapist in evaluating upper quarter dysfunction in a woman with breast cancer involves postural and arthrokinematic assessment, retraining ROM, education, and prevention. Therapists will need to follow the protocols of the individual surgeon. as there is not agreement on how soon active arm ROM should begin, especially in regard to the removal of drains. The protocol for arm mobility may be different if surgery included breast reconstruction.

Functional assessment tools should be used by therapists to monitor patient impairments and function. The AOPT (formerly known as the Oncology Section of APTA) in conjunction with the APTA has participated in the development of an Evaluation Database to Guide Effectiveness (EDGE). The purpose of this database is to improve quality measurements, with an emphasis on the psychometric properties of tests and measurements, and to promote the use of selected standard tests and measures that will improve consistency and research.

### *Lymphedema*

Education about the incidence and prevention of lymphedema, including lifetime precautions, is a primary task of the oncology rehabilitation therapist. It has been demonstrated that early diagnosis and treatment of breast cancer–related lymphedema can reduce costs and the need for intensive rehabilitation.[475] As previously mentioned, surveillance models to identify impairments at the earliest onset have been proposed as a standard of care for breast cancer treatment.[475,558] A preoperative examination to establish a baseline level of function with follow-up examinations postoperatively at 1 month and then at 3-month intervals for up to 1 year are advised rather than the traditional model of treating lymphedema with its concomitant functional limitations once it has progressed.[20,475]

Bevilacqua and colleagues[56] developed a nomogram to predict lymphedema risk for individuals who have undergone ALND. Although the nomogram has limitations, it may be a helpful tool for clinicians and patients. Factors contributing to risk of developing lymphedema include age; BMI (>30); number of chemotherapy cycles in ipsilateral arm; location of the radiation field; and development of postoperative seroma, infection, or early edema.[56] Studies show the risk of lymphedema to be least, but not nonexistent, among individuals who have undergone SLNB. More study of the association of cancer treatment and lymphedema is needed.

Secondary lymphedema of the upper quarter is a chronic and distressing condition for some women after breast cancer treatment. It is most commonly seen in the ipsilateral arm but can also affect the trunk, abdomen, and breast. Conservative therapies such as complete decongestive therapy, compression bandaging and garments, and exercise have proved effective in reducing fluid volume and improving subjective arm symptoms and quality of life.[447]

Low-level laser treatment has been approved by the FDA since 2007 for the treatment of postmastectomy lymphedema. The laser-beam pulses produce photochemical reactions at the cellular level, thereby influencing the course of metabolic processes and reducing the volume of the affected arm, extracellular fluid, and tissue hardness. Recent systematic reviews and meta-analysis suggest that low-level laser treatment is effective in reducing lymphedema; however, caution is urged secondary to low quality and generalizability of the findings.[147,465] More research is needed.

### Exercise and Breast Cancer

#### *Exercise During Cancer Treatment*

Decline in physical activity is common during treatment for breast cancer. Chemotherapy and/or radiation therapy for breast cancer may cause unfavorable changes in physical functioning, body composition, psychosocial functioning, and quality of life. Studies of aerobic or resistive exercise during adjuvant treatment for breast cancer have shown benefit in areas of self-esteem, physical fitness, fatigue,[302,516] and chemotherapy complication rate.[112] The impact of all types of aerobic exercise is significant in maintaining functional ability and reducing fatigue in women with breast cancer who are receiving chemotherapy or radiation therapy. Moderate-intensity (40% to 70% of predicted maximum heart rate) aerobic exercise is effective during adjuvant therapy for breast cancer to increase peak oxygen consumption and therefore aerobic capacity reserves.

**Note to Reader**: Throughout this text, the benefits of exercise and lifestyle changes in relation to various diseases, disorders, and conditions have been discussed, including (pertinent to the diagnosis of breast cancer) exercise and immunology (see Chapter 7), exercise and cancer from a variety of viewpoints (see Chapter 9), exercise and the cardiovascular system (see Chapter 12), and exercise and the lymphatic system (see Chapter 13). The reader is encouraged to read all of those sections to gain a perspective that takes into consideration all aspects of care throughout the lives of individuals with breast cancer.
For a full discussion of the influence of exercise and cancer and more evidence-based specifics regarding mode, intensity, frequency, and duration, see Chapter 9. This is an area of ongoing research, and the reader is advised to continue to review the literature for the most current recommendations.

#### *Exercise After Cancer Treatment*

Survivors of breast cancer are at increased risk of breast cancer recurrence, subsequent primary breast cancers, and early mortality. The ACS/ASCO Survivorship Guidelines[428] for physical activity suggest that physicians encourage patients to:

- Avoid inactivity and return to normal daily activities as soon as possible following diagnosis
- Aim for at least 150 minutes of moderate or 75 minutes of vigorous aerobic exercise per week
- Include strength training exercises at least 2 days per week; emphasize strength training for women treated with adjuvant chemotherapy or hormone therapy

Physical activity at any time after completion of primary breast cancer treatment is associated with reduced rates of mortality,[283,569] improved immune function, improved health-related quality of life, increased muscle strength, and decreased fatigue.[42,344] Most research studies have been of home-based or supervised exercise. While exercise for sedentary individuals requires behavior change, group physical activity programs can foster social support and feelings of connectedness.

### *Exercise and Breast Cancer–Related Lymphedema*

Exercise restrictions for women with or at risk for breast cancer–related lymphedema have changed as a result of updated research. Previous recommendations to avoid vigorous, repetitive, or strenuous upper body exercise (believing that such types of exercise might induce lymphedema) have been overturned. Studies of upper extremity resistance training in women after surgery for breast cancer have included teams of dragon boat racers and weight lifting. In randomized controlled trials of women at risk for lymphedema and women with stable lymphedema after breast cancer surgery, a slowly progressive weight-lifting program has shown no significant effect on developing lymphedema or exacerbating limb swelling.[209] Benefits of exercise have been shown to reduce overall symptoms and result in increased strength.[440–442] (See also Exercise and Lymphedema in Chapter 9.)

## REFERENCES

To enhance this text and add value for the reader, all references are included in the enhanced ebook on Student Consult that accompanies this textbook. The reader can view the reference source and access it online whenever possible.

CHAPTER 21

# Transplantation

CHRIS L. WELLS • SEAN T. LOWERS • BRETT KOERMER • FABRISIA AMBROSIO

Transplantation for the treatment of end-stage organ failure has been one of the major medical advances of the last 50 years. The success of this form of treatment continues to improve as surgical techniques, immunosuppressive regimen, and understanding of the rejection process become further refined.

The first successful live-donor kidney transplantation was completed in 1954 by Murray and Harrison. This transplant, performed between identical twins, provided the recipient with an additional 8 years of life, even in the absence of immunosuppressive medication.

By the end of the 1960s, further surgical and medical innovation led to the first successful heart, liver, and pancreas transplants. With the commercial introduction of the immunosuppressant cyclosporine in 1983 the world of transplantation made a remarkable stride in becoming an acceptable medical intervention for end-stage organ disease. In fact, the first successful lung transplantation was largely credited to the development of cyclosporine.[309]

In the past 3 decades we have seen great advances in the preservation of donor organs, expansion of the donor organ pool, detection of early rejection, and success of multiple-organ transplantation. More than 750,000 lives have been saved or enhanced by transplantation.[330,448]

A case study about a transplantation patient is presented in eBox 21.1 on the book's Student Consult site.

## INCIDENCE

Transplantation remains limited by a worldwide shortage of available and suitable human organs. It is estimated that every 10 minutes an individual is placed on the United Network for Organ Sharing (UNOS) waiting list for an organ transplantation, and 18 people die each day while waiting on the list. As of September 2018, there were more than 114,000 people waiting for transplants.[448] In 2016, more than 7000 people died while waiting for a suitable organ. This number has not changed significantly despite increasing public awareness of transplantation. Only 54% of U.S. adults are registered as organ donors, and only 3 in 1000 people die in a way that permits organ procurement.[185] This leads to a large disparity between the need for organ transplantation and the availability of organ donations.[448]

Each cadaveric donor can donate up to 25 organs and tissues to help as many as 50 recipients. This means up to 500,000 organs should be available for transplantation each year, but only approximately 34,000 transplantations are performed (Table 21.1).[453] Living-related donor transplants, accounting for 6200 surgeries in 2017, permit donation of a kidney or a portion of a liver, lung, or pancreas to provide an opportunity for another to survive end-stage organ disease.[330,448]

## TYPES OF TRANSPLANTATION

Many types of tissues and organs can be donated and therefore transplanted including the heart, lungs, liver, pancreas, kidneys, intestines, skin, bone and bone marrow, umbilical cord blood, veins, soft tissues, heart valves, corneas, and eyes.

Many different terms are used to describe types of transplantations (Box 21.1). *Allograft* (homograft) transplantations are between individuals of the same species (e.g., human being to human being). *Autologous* transplantations are within the same individual (e.g., skin graft from leg to hand; blood or bone marrow for own use later).

*Xenogeneic* (heterograft) transplantations are between individuals of different species (e.g., pig to human being). *Allogeneic* transplantation is one in which the source comes from a human leukocyte antigen (HLA)–matched donor (usually a sibling). *Syngeneic* transplantations are between genetically identical members of the same species (identical twins); a syngeneic transplant is also called an isograft.

*Orthotopic* homologous transplantation refers to the surgical placement (grafting) of the donor organ into the normal anatomic site. In *heterotopic homologous* transplantation, the recipient's diseased organ is left intact and the donor organ is placed in parallel with anastomoses between the two organs.

Table 21.1 National Waiting List for Organ Transplantation

| | YEAR | | | | |
|---|---|---|---|---|---|
| **Organ** | **2018** | **2014** | **2008** | **2004** | **2001** |
| Kidney | 94,954 | 100,958 | 100,597 | 61,020 | 47,574 |
| Liver | 13,233 | 15,739 | 76,089 | 16,858 | 17,889 |
| Heart | 3750 | 3996 | 2711 | 3164 | 3864 |
| Lung | 1429 | 1605 | 2016 | 3816 | 3671 |
| Heart-lung | 45 | Not reported | 91 | 169 | 207 |
| Kidney-pancreas | 1613 | 2053 | 2334 | 2362 | 3367 |
| Pancreas (including PAK) | 815 | 1188 | 1437 | 1522 | 1051 |
| Intestine | 230 | 263 | 212 | 191 | 164 |
| Total (candidates) | 113,564 | 123,101 | 100,597 | 85,170 | 76,787 |

*PAK*, Pancreas after kidney.
From U.S. Department of Health and Human Services. Health Resources and Services Administration. Organ Procurement and Transplantation Network. 2019 National Report. http://optn.transplant.hrsa.gov/data/. Accessed May 29, 2019. Figures related to active waiting list candidates are updated online daily.

Box 21.1
**TYPES OF TRANSPLANTS**

- *Allogeneic:* between individuals of the same species but of different genetic constitution (e.g., human to human)
- *Allograft* (homograft, homologous, autologous): between individuals of the same species (e.g., human to human)
- *Autologous:* within the same individual (e.g., transfer of skin from one site to another on the same body; donation of blood or bone marrow for own use later)
- *Heterologous* (heterograft, xenogeneic): between individuals of different species (e.g., pig to human)
- *Heterotopic* (autograft): transfer of organ or tissue from one part of a body of a donor to another area of the body of a recipient
- *Homologous* (homogeneous): corresponding or similar in structure, position, origin (e.g., pig heart, human heart)
- *Orthotopic:* tissue transplant grafted into its normal anatomic position
- *Syngeneic* (isograft): between genetically identical members of the same species (identical twins)
- *Xenogeneic* (heterograft): between individuals of different species (e.g., pig to human)

Box 21.2
**COMBINED ORGAN TRANSPLANTS**

- Kidney-heart
- Kidney-heart-lung
- Liver-kidney-pancreas
- Kidney-intestine
- Liver-kidney-pancreas-intestine
- Liver-pancreas-lung
- Liver-lung
- Kidney-lung
- Liver-lung-heart
- Liver-heart
- Liver-pancreas
- Liver-intestine
- Liver-pancreas-intestine
- Liver-kidney
- Pancreas-intestine
- Liver-kidney-heart

From U.S. Department of Health and Human Services. Health Resources and Services Administration. Organ Procurement and Transplantation Network. *2019 National Report.* A total of 13,340 multiple organ transplants have been performed through May 20, 2019. Comparisons by year, age, gender, ethnicity, region, and center are available online at: http://optn.transplant.hrsa.gov/latestData/step2asp?.

## Combined-Organ Transplantation

Combined-organ transplantations from a single donor are uncommon relative to single-organ transplantations (Box 21.2). Research to date generally suggests that there has been a continued increase in combined-organ transplantation, although the total numbers are low. Organ rejection is lower in cases of combined-organ transplantation compared with single-organ transplantation.[355,260] Despite the increase in surgical risk and complex posttransplant medical care, the short-term survival in combined-organ transplantation seems to be acceptable. Emerging evidence suggests that long-term survival is favorable.[28,80]

## Organ Retransplantation

Acute graft failure, chronic rejection, and recurrence of the primary disease are common reasons for organ retransplantation. In many cases, immunosuppressive medications cease to suppress the immune response, which leads to organ destruction and failure. In this circumstance, retransplantation may be a necessary life-saving procedure. Candidates for retransplantation must again meet criteria for transplantation of that specific organ.

As survival rates for all transplantations improve, the need for retransplantation will also increase; for example, since 2000 there has been a 4% increase in heart retransplantation.[449] However, there is concern about dedicating more organs for retransplantation because these recipients have lower survival rates.[22] For most organs, 3- and 5-year survivals are not as high for recipients who have undergone retransplantation.[205,206,448] For these reasons, recipients of organ retransplantation often require more aggressive monitoring for rejection.

### Pediatric Transplantation

Solid-organ transplantation has become accepted therapy for the treatment of end-stage organ dysfunction in children. As with adult organ transplantation, the supply of cadaveric pediatric organs is limited, and living-related donation is on the decline. Living-related donor transplant may offer higher immunocompatibility and improve overall outcomes.

Children can receive adult organs; in the case of the liver, only a portion of the adult donor liver is needed. Preoperative and postoperative assessment and care are very similar to adult care. Management may be complicated by infections, such as hepatitis B and cytomegalovirus (CMV). Morbidity and mortality are often attributed to the consequences of long-term immunosuppression and include graft failure, increased incidence of cancer,[141] hypertension, renal failure, and diabetes from overimmunosuppression.

There are known age-related differences in all phases of pharmacokinetics (absorption, distribution, metabolism, elimination); information specifically related to age and differences in the pharmacokinetics of immunosuppressants is very limited at the present time. Biologic and psychologic changes common during the transition from childhood to adolescence and adolescence to adulthood present some unique challenges.[200] Children receiving orthotopic liver transplantation are at risk for endocrine complications, such as growth failure, hepatic osteodystrophy, pubertal delay, adrenal insufficiency, and drug-induced diabetes.[190]

Caregiver training and education are essential components in the transplantation process. The care team pays special attention to the psychosocial and emotional needs of the child and family. Noncompliance and nonadherence are common behaviors among all age groups, but especially among adolescents. The consequences of this behavior include increased rejection, late graft loss, and death. Despite the best 1-year graft survival of any age group, the long-term transplantation outcomes in this age group are not as optimal.[130,329,364]

## ORGAN PROCUREMENT AND ALLOCATION

### Organ Distribution

With the passage of the National Organ Transplant Act in 1984 the U.S. government began the process of establishing a comprehensive framework for the development and administration of a national transplant system.[455] The Organ Procurement and Transplant Network (OPTN) (http://optn.transplant.hrsa.gov/) was created to maintain a national registry to track the process and outcomes related to organ donation and transplantation. Since 1998, more than 750,000 people have received organ transplants at 254 U.S. transplantation centers in the United States.[448]

In 2004 the Organ Donation and Recovery Improvement Act (Public Law 108-216) was signed with a legislative provision to establish a federal grant program to provide assistance to living donors for travel and other expenses. This act strengthens efforts to increase donation rates, including ways to make live donation an easier and more appealing option. Removing financial barriers from living organ donations may help expand access to transplantation for members of lower socioeconomic groups who may not be able to consider living donation.[181]

In 2006 the revision of the Uniform Anatomical Gift Act allowed individual states to develop their own donor registration process and made overriding an individual's consent to donate more difficult. This allowed organ procurement organizations (OPOs) to proceed with the donation process and prevent others from overriding donor wishes. The result of this effort was an overall 24% increase in donor registration, with multiple states exceeding a registration rate of 50%.[484] This legislation also grants money to states to promote public education, organ donor awareness, and studies of long-term effects associated with living organ donation.[490]

In 2014, vascularized composite allografts (VCAs) were added to the definition of organs covered by federal regulation and legislation. VCAs may include skin, muscle, nerve, bones, or connective tissue.

Implementation of evidence-based practice initiatives and improvements in the organ procurement process such as the use of extracorporeal support[367] have led to an increase in available organs. Surgeons are able to accept marginally suitable organs from donors who do not match general criteria, commonly referred to as an extended donor pool. Preliminary work suggests that these once discarded donor organs may have similar outcomes regarding short- and long-term recipient survival.[324,376,413] With these advancements, however, there are additional stresses placed on hospital centers to report outcomes related to length of stay and cost. Owing to increased required reporting procedures, some transplantation centers may be less likely to use organs from an extended donor pool or from donation after cardiac death or to accept high-risk transplantation candidates.[484]

#### United Network for Organ Sharing

To establish a means to procure and distribute donor organs in an appropriate and ethical manner, the United States was divided into 58 local procurement areas, ranging in population from 1 million to 12 million, and those areas were then divided into 11 regions (Fig. 21.1). Each local area has a designated OPO responsible for recovering and transporting organs to transplantation hospitals in their territories. At the present time, there are 254 transplantation centers across the United States. The local OPO also provides a wealth of medical and public education about organ transplantation and the promotion of donation.

On the national level the UNOS (www.unos.org) is a private, nonprofit organization that provides critical services in the area of organ transplantation. The UNOS administers the national organ waiting list, coordinates the matching and distribution of donor organs via the local OPO throughout the United States, tracks outcomes, establishes physician training for the medical and surgical management of transplant recipients, and provides public education. The UNOS comprises every transplantation center, tissue-matching laboratory, and OPO within the United States, all of which are required to report a massive amount of data to the UNOS. The OPTN analyzes

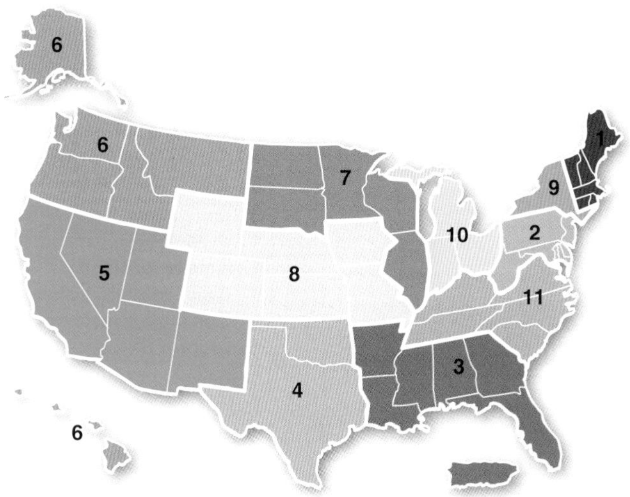


**Fig. 21.1**

**The United Network for Organ Sharing is divided into 11 geographic regions.** (Courtesy United Network for Organ Sharing, Richmond, VA.)

all data provided regarding transplantation candidates, recipients, and living and deceased donors.

The process to match candidates with a donor organ has been developed in great detail to ensure equity based on medical need. There are two large processes occurring simultaneously to match and allocate organs. One process involves the identification and management of the potential transplantation candidate (someone waiting for an organ) through the transplantation center; meanwhile the second process involves the identification and procurement of viable organs for donation.

After a thorough evaluation the transplantation center reports vital medical information about each candidate to the UNOS. When a possible deceased organ donor has been identified, the local OPO obtains and reports valuable medical information about the donor to the UNOS. The UNOS computer system will search for a suitable match between the donor and a candidate. A list of potential candidates will be provided in a priority order, and the organ is offered to the candidate who has the highest medical need, as well as the greatest likelihood of a successful outcome based on analysis of prior transplantation.

This allocation begins with the transplantation center being contacted at the local level, but if a local candidate does not match the donor organ or has a lower medical need, the organ will be offered to a candidate in the region where the donor organ was procured, then to adjacent regions, and finally nationally, with the goal to use every suitable organ.[455]

**Allocation Policy.** The UNOS has developed a status coding or allocation system to prioritize the candidates waiting for transplantation when a donor organ has been recovered. The goal of this allocation is to promote an equitable system that saves as many lives as possible. The creation of these new allocation systems has been critical to making the system more equitable for candidates who have an aggressive or highly progressive disease, such as many forms of pulmonary fibrosis. Each waiting list and the prioritization of possible candidates vary from organ to organ.

The allocation of deceased donor organs has significantly changed over the years, with the goal to ensure that people who have the most urgent medical need will be given priority despite the amount of waiting time a person has on the UNOS list.[452] In response to a perceived unfairness in organ allocation, Congress issued a final rule in 1998. The rule called for a more objective ranking of potential recipients on a waiting list and more equality in disease severity among transplant recipients across OPOs. The policy is intended to balance anticipated duration of survival on the transplantation list with length of benefit from receiving a transplant. Priority for transplanted organs will go to candidates most urgently needing a transplant and expected to receive the most survival benefit from the transplant. Waiting time is used to decide allocation if there is more than one potential candidate with equal medical urgency scores.

This distribution system is also designed to decrease the disadvantage some people have because of the progressive nature of their disease or the uneven distribution of transplantation centers within the United States. The new policy considers the waiting list urgency and transplantation benefit of each candidate, based on individual clinical diagnostic factors. The improved computerized organ-matching system has made these important changes possible. For example, it is known that an individual who is on venoarterial extracorporeal membrane oxygenation (ECMO) has a shorter life expectancy than someone who is on oral medication with compensated heart failure.[447] In this scenario, the first person would be assigned a status 1A, listed higher on the transplantation listing, and offered an organ before the second person (Box 21.3).

## Organ Donation

Organs are obtained through both deceased and living donation. Deceased organ donation continues to be the primary source for available organs and occurs when complete and irreversible loss of all brain and brainstem

Box 21.3

**UNITED NETWORK FOR ORGAN SHARING ORGAN ALLOCATION STATUS LIST**

***Heart***

- Status 1A
  - Individual admitted to listed treatment center with mechanical circulatory support (VAD, total artificial heart, intraaortic balloon pump, ECMO) for acute hemodynamic decompression; status 1A must be recertified every 14 days; an individual with total artificial heart discharge from hospital can be listed for 30 days
  - Individual with mechanical circulatory support with complications, including thromboemboli, device infection, ventricular arrhythmias
  - Individual with mechanical ventilation support
  - Individual with single high-dose inotropic medication or multiple low-dose inotropic medications with administration via a central venous line
  - Exceptions are reviewed on an individual basis
- Status 1B
  - Individuals with VAD support
  - Individuals with continuous inotrope infusion
  - Exceptions are reviewed on an individual basis
- Status 2
  - An individual waiting for transplant but does not meet the criteria for status 1A or 1B
- Status 7
  - An individual who is considered temporarily unsuitable to receive a transplant

***Lung***

Lung allocation system is a method to calculate the medical urgency of transplantation. LAS is calculated for each individual, based on certain medical items.

- Factors used to calculate LAS
  - Lung diagnosis
  - Date of birth
  - Functional status
  - Assisted ventilation
  - Height and weight
  - Diabetes
  - Supplemental oxygen
  - Percent predicted FVC
  - 6-minute walk distance
  - Serum creatinine
  - PA systolic pressure
  - Mean PAP
  - Mean pulmonary capillary wedge pressure
  - $PCO_2$
- Factors used to predict risk of death on lung transplant waitlist
  - FVC
  - Pulmonary artery systolic pressure (groups A, C, and D)
  - $O_2$ required at rest (groups A, C, and D)
  - Age
  - Body mass index
  - Diabetes
  - Functional status
  - 6-minute walk distance
  - Continuous mechanical ventilation
  - Diagnosis
  - $PaCO_2$
  - Bilirubin (current bilirubin: all groups; change in bilirubin: group B)
- Factors that predict survival after lung transplant
  - FVC (groups B and D)
  - Pulmonary capillary wedge pressure ≥20 mm Hg (group D)
  - Continuous mechanical ventilation
  - Age
  - Serum creatinine
  - Functional status
  - Diagnosis

*Group A:* Includes candidates with obstructive lung disease, including without limitation COPD, $\alpha_1$-antitrypsin deficiency, emphysema, lymphangioleiomyomatosis, bronchiectasis, and sarcoidosis with mean PAP ≤30 mm Hg

*Group B:* Includes candidates with pulmonary vascular disease, including without limitation primary pulmonary hypertension, Eisenmenger syndrome, and other uncommon pulmonary vascular diseases

*Group C:* Includes without limitation candidates with cystic fibrosis and immunodeficiency disorders such as hypogammaglobulinemia

*Group D:* Includes candidates with restrictive lung diseases including without limitation idiopathic pulmonary fibrosis, pulmonary fibrosis (other causes), sarcoidosis with mean PAP >30 mm Hg, and obliterative bronchiolitis (non-retransplant)

***Heart-Lung Transplantation***

When the candidate is eligible to receive an available heart organ, the lung shall be allocated to the heart-lung candidate from the same donor. When the candidate is eligible to receive a lung organ, the heart shall be allocated to the heart-lung candidate from the same donor if no suitable status 1A isolated heart candidates are eligible to receive the heart. ABO matching requirements for both heart and lung shall be used for heart-lung candidates.

*COPD,* Chronic obstructive pulmonary disease; *ECMO,* extracorporeal membrane oxygenation; *FVC,* forced vital capacity; *LAS,* lung allocation score; *PAP,* pulmonary arterial pressure; *VAD,* ventricular assist device.

Data from United Network for Organ Sharing (UNOS): 2018 Annual report of the U.S. Scientific Registry for Transplant Recipients and the Organ Procurement and Transplantation Network—transplant data. Richmond, VA, 2019, UNOS.

activity occurs or when the heart stops in the case of cardiac death.

The Organ Donation Breakthrough Collaborative was developed by the U.S. Department of Health and Human Services and the Health Resources and Services Administration as an attempt to unite the various agencies involved in transplantation and to define their roles and efforts to increase the identification of potential organs. This collaborative effort between 2003 and 2006 resulted in a 22.5% increase in donation, which is a fourfold increase from the precollaborative period.[392]

## Source of Organ Donations

The characteristics of what constitutes an acceptable donor, both deceased and living, have been changed over the years in an attempt to maximize the number of potential donor organs, as organ shortage is still a limiting factor. The effect of these changes on the outcome for recipients is not fully known. Early on it was typical that the deceased donor was a young individual who was declared brain dead from a traumatic brain injury. Today the majority of deceased donors are individuals aged 18 to 34 years, although an increasing number of organs are being used from older people following death by cerebral vascular injury, cardiovascular disease, or trauma.[448,484]

There is also an increased use of organs harvested from non–heart-beating deceased donors, especially in kidney transplantation. In such cases, higher incidences of graft dysfunction and organ injury have been reported, although long-term organ function and survival have been acceptable.[296] Some transplantation centers are still reluctant to transplant other organs from a non–heart-beating donor because of the risk of ischemic injury to the organs.[115] Recent studies have shown acceptable allograft function for pancreas, liver, and lung following donation after circulatory death, although heart transplantation does not appear to be a viable option after death.[296]

There has been some preliminary research that has used ECMO to support the donor and improve organ perfusion. Using ECMO for the organ recipient in the early posttransplant period is another way to support a marginal donor organ.[256] Increasing research has been devoted to the use of ex vivo perfusion techniques to improve donor organ physiology and thus increase the viability of suboptimal transplant organs. One study has suggested that transplantation of high-risk donor lungs subjected to 4 to 6 hours of ex vivo lung perfusion produces short-term outcomes similar to conventional transplantation.[108,109,264,346]

There has also been increased utilization of organs from an extended or high-risk donor pool. These are deceased donors who fall outside the general donor criteria for reasons such as advanced age, diabetes, certain forms of cancer, and positive testing for hepatitis B or C virus. Research is increasingly showing that organs from high-risk donors does not negatively affect early survival rates. Longitudinal studies are needed to examine long-term organ and recipient survivals.

Individuals previously considered unacceptable transplantation candidates may be offered a donor organ from this extended donor pool. Candidates who are seropositive for hepatitis B or C or HIV positive can now receive a transplant from a positive donor. In the past, these individuals were not considered acceptable candidates for transplantation.[70] Successful kidney transplantations have been completed from deceased donors who have a medical history of diabetes.[4]

Many so-called suboptimal organs have been discarded by centers even though people die each day while on the waiting list. Marginal organs can provide a viable solution to the organ shortage. When used with appropriate surgical techniques and immunosuppression protocols, suboptimal organs can increase the supply of donor organs by 25% to 30%.[2]

The source of organ donation is also changing in regard to the living donation. In previous years, living donation was conducted primarily between relatives, referred to as a *directed donation*. Directed donation also can be between nonrelated individuals, spouses, or friends.[330] Living donation can also occur indirectly (a nondirected donation); that is, the living donor is placed on a national living donor list and the donor's gift is anonymous to the recipient. Living donors can donate a kidney, portion of a lung, liver, intestine, and pancreas.[457] In 2017 there were just over 6000 living donors, a decrease from the high of 7000 in 2004.[25,448]

Living donors need to make a fully informed consent because of the risk to their health and life. Reports of long-term effects of living donation are currently limited. There are some studies of psychosocial and socioeconomic issues facing living kidney donors and others that indicate certain donor populations are at increased risk of developing end-stage renal disease (ESRD).[106,122] The UNOS is aware of 11 donors who donated between 1998 and 2008 (out of approximately 64,000) and were subsequently listed for kidney or liver transplantation as a consequence of complications from their donation. This report is limited to only the individuals who have registered on the UNOS. There is a poor understanding of long-term morbidity and mortality complications for living donors who never initiate transplant procedures for themselves.[122,457]

### Guidelines for Donor Candidates

General guidelines are used when determining the acceptability of a donor; criteria vary slightly, depending on organ type. These guidelines have been expanded as transplantation centers become more effective at organ procurement, surgical procedures, and medical management of transplant recipients.

Most donors are younger than 50 years of age, although this is not exclusive because of the high need for donors and advances in postoperative management. Other criteria for donors vary according to the organ being harvested. For example, a living related lung donor must not have a history of lung disease, previous thoracic surgeries, or be larger in size than the recipient (weight, height, chest size). The last requirement is necessary because only two lung lobes will support the recipient's full pulmonary function.

For all organ donations, there must be no evidence of malignancy or sepsis. Since the passage of the HOPE Act in 2013, HIV-positive to HIV-positive kidney and liver transplants have been performed.[450] Although rare, HIV transmission from a living organ donor has been documented.[47,139] To reduce the risk for transmission of HIV through living-donor organ transplantation, transplantation centers are advised to screen living donors for HIV as close to the time of organ recovery and transplantation as possible. Transplant candidates should be informed of the potential risks for disease transmission. Potential donors must be cautioned to avoid behaviors that would put them at risk for acquiring HIV before organ donation.[47]

Hepatitis B or C present in the donor is considered a precaution but not a contraindication. Transplant centers may consider organs with hepatitis B or C after risk assessment and patient consent. If the candidate already has hepatitis or is critically ill, the risk of developing hepatitis is not considered a contraindication in the decision to progress with the procedure.[208]

Body weight is an important consideration due to the risk of ischemic reperfusion injury associated with obesity.[395a] Biologically related donors with clear and altruistic motivation (as opposed to coerced by the family or guilt driven) are preferred.

Testing is performed to assess the function of each donor organ considered for procurement. For potential renal donors, urinalysis, creatinine, blood urea nitrogen, and liver function are tested. For the heart, an echocardiogram, 12-lead electrocardiogram (ECG), serial arterial blood gas measurements, and possibly a right- and left-heart catheterization are ordered. Pancreatic function is assessed with amylase and lipase studies. Serial arterial blood gases, sputum Gram stain, and bronchoscopy to inspect the airways are used to assess the function of the lungs.[329,442,455]

### Organ Recovery

Hearts and lungs can be preserved for up to 6 hours; livers and pancreata, up to 24 hours; and kidneys, up to 36 hours. This length of allowable ischemic time helps determine allowable distances between centers.

Efforts are being made to improve organ harvest and preservation techniques and the number of organs harvested. For example, eliminating physiologic abnormalities before donation through aggressive resuscitation, coagulopathy control, invasive monitoring, and dedicated intensive care unit (ICU) management while implementing a rapid brain death determination protocol has been documented as successfully increasing the number of donor organs available.[271,442,484] Technology to improve organ recovery, maintain organ perfusion, and recover normal cell metabolism is under investigation using a kidney transporter, a portable organ preservation device. The ability to maintain and monitor organ viability over an extended period of time may allow live donors to avoid traveling to the recipient's location for explant surgery. Eventually, this type of technology may be extended to include transport devices for all other organs.

Efforts to obtain consent for donation continue to improve in part owing to the Organ Donation Breakthrough Collaborative. Public education now includes National Donor Awareness Week and the choice to indicate organ donation on a driver's license. According to Health Care Financing Administration regulations, hospitals are now required to report every death and impending death to their local OPO to continue receiving Medicare benefits.[284]

Early referral of all imminent deaths to OPOs results in the OPO conferring with the medical team regarding the best medical plan of care for the recipient, including specific needs of the family as well as procedures necessary for the donor once consent is obtained. These steps help ensure that care of potential organ donors continues without premature termination.[391]

A new approach to obtaining family consent is being used. Instead of informing the family of the individual's death and at a later time discussing organ donation (referred to as *decoupling*), now most families are approached about organ donation at the time when they are making end-of-life decisions. Policies and laws have strengthened the wishes of the donor, making it easier for the OPO to begin the process of donation while discussing with the family the process and positive benefits of organ donation.[484] The discussion about organ donation has become a team approach between the OPO staff, physicians, nurses, and clergy. For families approached regarding organ donation, the current consent rate ranges from 54% to 92%.[25]

During this critical period of time assessing a potential donor, personnel from the OPO request medical evaluation from various specialists (e.g., cardiologist, pulmonologist, nephrologist, gastroenterologist, surgeon) to determine the viability of the organs that were consented for harvesting and to provide instructions for continued medical care to ensure adequate organ function until the procurement process begins.

## Criteria for Organ Candidates

Candidates for transplants are listed at one or more of the transplantation centers where they plan to have surgery. A national computerized waiting list of potential transplantation candidates in the United States is maintained by the UNOS, with active input from treatment centers. The UNOS maintains a 24-hour telephone service to aid in matching donor organs with people on the waiting list and to coordinate efforts with transplantation centers.

Each possible transplantation candidate undergoes various tests, and many of these test results, such as organ needed, blood type, body size, various organ functions, walking ability, life support need, virology, and other pertinent comorbidities, are reported to the UNOS.

There are criteria for most organs to classify candidates into levels of medical urgency or status based on the medical work-up. When a donor becomes available, the UNOS is notified, and a list of potential organ candidates for that region is identified. The UNOS notifies the OPO, which in turn notifies the transplantation center to verify that the candidate is currently medically appropriate and has consented to the transplantation process. Arrangements are then made to transport the donor organ and candidate to the transplantation center and proceed with the surgery.

Several factors are taken into consideration in identifying the best-matched candidate or candidates. In general, preference is given to candidates with the most critical status from the same geographic area as the donor because timing is a critical element in the organ procurement process. Waiting for combined-organ transplantation is much more complicated. The candidate must be listed on each organ waiting list. Once the potential candidate reaches the top of one of the organ lists and is offered an organ, the other organs from the same donor would be offered as long as there is not a higher status candidate ahead of this candidate. For example, if an individual is listed for heart-lung transplantation and has the highest lung allocation score (LAS) for the region and matches the other necessary characteristics for the organ, the individual would be offered the heart (as long as there is not another candidate who is a status 1 in that named region and who also matches the donor). This process makes multiple-organ transplantation difficult.

Box 21.4

**GENERAL CRITERIA FOR ORGAN CANDIDATES**

NOTE: This is a *general* list of criteria for potential organ recipients; considerations will vary from organ to organ among transplantation centers.

***Medical Considerations***

- Matched blood type required
- Body weight (morbid obesity [>20% of ideal body weight] contraindicated; severe malnutrition [<70% of ideal body weight] contraindicated)
- Presence of other illness or disease contraindicated
- Other end-stage organ disease
  - Irreversible renal insufficiency
  - Irreversible hepatic insufficiency
  - Severe pulmonary disease: FVC 50%, $FEV_1$ 60%
  - Fixed pulmonary hypertension
- At risk for cardiac problems (death, myocardial infarction, coronary angioplasty, bypass surgery, unstable angina)
- Uncontrolled infection or acute sepsis
- HIV
- Malignancy with metastases
- Malignancy with an expected 5-year survival of 75%
- Irreversible neuromuscular or neurologic disorder
- Severe peripheral vascular disease or cerebrovascular disease
  - Abdominal aneurysm
  - Peripheral ischemic ulceration
  - Carotid disease
- Decrease in chest wall mobility
- Nonambulatory with poor rehabilitation potential

***Nonmedical Considerations***

- History of noncompliance with medical therapy (last 5 years)
- History of ongoing alcohol or drug dependence
- Active or recent (within last 6 months) cigarette smoking (lung transplant)
- History of psychologic instability
- Financial resources available
- Family and community support available

*$FEV_1$*, Forced expiratory volume in 1 second; *FVC*, forced vital capacity.

The transplantation team bears the responsibility to conserve scarce resources for those who can benefit, requiring careful screening of potential candidates. Transplantation centers follow UNOS guidelines, but criteria may vary from center to center. Some centers require a medical evaluation for the acceptance of applicants for transplantation.

Many centers have medical and nonmedical criteria, with exclusion criteria for people with severely problematic behavior or other psychosocial risk factors (Box 21.4). There has been a recent trend toward recognizing the importance of nonmedical issues, such as psychologic stability, family support, functional status, and history of compliance or adherence to medical care when evaluating applicants because of the impact of these issues on outcomes.[121,373-375]

A history of problematic behavior, such as lack of adherence to treatment and the presence of psychiatric instability, leads to higher posttransplant mortality and morbidity.[124,251,395] Compliance issues associated with substance abuse usually include personality disorders, living arrangements, and/or global psychosocial factors. A history of substance abuse requires documentation of abstinence; ongoing drug and/or alcohol abuse can potentially impair the success of the transplantation and requires referral for treatment before placement on a transplantation waiting list.

In the case of live-donor transplantation, psychosocial risk to donors must be taken into consideration. Most published reports have indicated an improved sense of well-being and a boost in self-esteem for living donors, but there have been some reports of depression and disrupted family relationships after donation and suicide after a recipient's death.[114,217]

Medical compatibility of the donor and candidate is determined based on characteristics such as blood type, weight, and age. Illness in the recipient that cannot be treated or that will prevent transplantation success must be evaluated carefully.

Transplantation is usually not recommended if another illness is predicted to rapidly cause graft failure or impact survival in other deleterious ways after transplantation. In addition, a previous history of cancer or osteoporosis is considered carefully, as postoperative medications can greatly advance these diseases.

## Pretransplantation Evaluation

Extensive medical testing is required before a candidate is placed on the transplantation waiting list (Table 21.2). Blood and tissue typing for histocompatibility are used as some of the first eligibiity criteria for donor–candidate matching. The process of determining histocompatibility, that is, finding compatible donors and candidates, is called *tissue typing*. Before transplantation, testing in the laboratory is carried out to determine whether antibodies incompatible with the donor have been formed by the candidate (a positive crossmatch). If the crossmatch is positive, the transplant will fail; a negative test result is necessary for a successful transplant.

Predictor values for acute and chronic rejection are evaluated, such as panel reactive antibodies (a measure of the amount of antibodies circulating in the system), and offer some predictive value of hyperacute rejection. In some cases, treatment will be performed to lower the panel of reactive antibodies in a recipient to help increase the donor pool for that individual.

Other serology testing determines exposure to CMV, Epstein-Barr virus (EBV), herpes simplex viruses, and hepatitis because complications can arise related to individual exposure to viral loading (i.e., the greater the viral replication, the higher the incidence of active infection).

CMV infection may contribute to an increased incidence of chronic rejection and result in CMV syndrome (e.g., viremia [spread of virus throughout the body with fever and malaise]) or organ-specific tissue-invasive disease.[409] Herpes simplex virus is associated with an increased incidence of necrotizing pneumonitis and cervical cancer, and EBV is associated with an increase in posttransplantation lymphoproliferative diseases. Transplant recipients are placed on appropriate medications to reduce the risk of infection and undergo repeated

**Table 21.2** Referral to Transplant Center

| Blood Work | Testing[a] | Consultations[a] | Other |
|---|---|---|---|
| ABO blood type<br>Panel reactive antibodies<br>Serology<br>Liver function tests<br>Fasting lipids<br>Prostate-specific antigen<br>Prothrombin time<br>Partial prothrombin time<br>Complete blood count<br>Nicotine level<br>Drug/toxicity screen | Multigated acquisition<br>Echocardiogram<br>Transesophageal echocardiogram or transthoracic echocardiogram<br>Pulmonary function tests<br>6-Minute walk test<br>$\dot{V}/\dot{Q}$ scan<br>Arterial blood gases<br>Diffusion capacity of carbon monoxide<br>Organ catheterization (heart, kidney)<br>X-ray<br>ECG<br>Maximal or peak $VO_2$<br>Glucose testing (diabetes mellitus)<br>Peripheral vascular disease<br>DEXA scan (osteoporosis) | Surgeon<br>Pulmonologist<br>Cardiologist<br>Nephrologist<br>Transplant coordinator<br>Social services<br>Credit analysis<br>Neuropsychology<br>Physical therapy<br>Rheumatologist<br>Gynecologist<br>Dentist<br>Nutritionist | Urinalysis<br>Sputum cultures<br>Creatinine clearance<br>Purified protein derivative<br>Mammogram<br>Pap smear |

*DEXA*, Dual-energy x-ray absorptiometry; *ECG*, electrocardiogram; *$VO_2$*, oxygen consumption; $\dot{V}/\dot{Q}$ ventilation–perfusion
[a]Specific consultants and the special tests orders are determined by the type of organ transplantation planned.

serologic testing if clinical signs and symptoms suggest infection or infectious disease.

Fasting lipids, liver function studies, prostate-specific antigen levels to determine prostate function, and tests specific to the potential organ transplant are carried out. Additional tests will be completed to rule out other organ dysfunction. Functional testing and dual-energy x-ray absorptiometry scans are commonly included to determine activity tolerance and bone health, respectively.

A person with isolated end-stage organ failure with no other complications has a better chance for selection than someone with other complicating factors. In addition to all the testing procedures, the organ candidate meets with an interdisciplinary medical team (listed in Table 21.2), including, in some centers, rehabilitation staff such as physical and occupational therapists.

## ADVANCES AND RESEARCH IN TRANSPLANTATION

### Advances in Medications

Tremendous advancements have been made in the pharmacologic management of transplant recipients. Medications are used with transplant recipients to prevent or treat rejection and infection. Research is ongoing to find ways to reduce or eliminate the long-term use and adverse effects of medications, especially immunosuppressants. New discoveries in cellular immunology have led to a greater understanding of the immune system and its implications for tissue transplantation. Immunosuppressive regimens continue to improve, and newer immunomodulatory strategies are evolving. In particular, new immunosuppressive drugs may reduce or allow the recipient to overcome early or late antibody-mediated rejections.[46,142]

Induction medications are given to patients immediately after transplant and at high dosages to prevent acute rejection. Most transplant recipients are placed on a three-drug regimen to control the incidence of rejection and minimize the adverse effects that are common if any one drug is given in too high a dosage. The drug cocktail commonly consists of a second-generation calcineurin inhibitor, an antimetabolite, and a corticosteroid. New research continues to attempt to decrease the dosage and the number of immunosuppressive medications the transplant recipient is exposed to in order to promote long-term, effective graft function without the harmful side effects of these potent medications.

There has been a decline in the use of cyclosporine (Neoral) for most organs. These drugs have been replaced with the administration of tacrolimus (Prograf). Cyclosporine and tacrolimus are classified as *calcineurin inhibitors*. Calcineurin is an enzyme, protein phosphatase, that is responsible for activating the transcription of interleukin-2, which stimulates the growth and differentiation of T cells. Calcineurin is also linked to the differentiation of fiber types and hypertrophy of muscle fibers.[133]

The mechanism of action for tacrolimus and cyclosporine is similar in that they both inhibit calcineurin, although tacrolimus is more selective in its action, which may be one of the reasons its use has increased (Fig. 21.2). Both drugs bind to specific lymphoid tissues and block the production of interleukin-2, which is a critical substance in the growth and proliferation of activated T cells and other immune response cells such as natural killer (NK) cells, macrophages, and lymphocytes.[100]

The second class of drugs is the antimetabolites, including azathioprine (Imuran), mycophenolate mofetil (CellCept), and cyclophosphamide (Cytoxan). Mycophenolate mofetil is used more than the other drugs in this classification. Azathioprine works by suppressing the bone marrow (as exhibited by thrombocytopenia, leukopenia, and anemia), and mycophenolate mofetil inhibits the inflammatory response mediated by the immune system (Fig. 21.3).[256,257] Cyclophosphamide, which is typically thought of as an anticancer drug, has also been used in transplant recipients. It inhibits the replication of DNA and RNA in the lymphocytes and other key cells involved in mounting an immune response against the transplanted organ.[100]

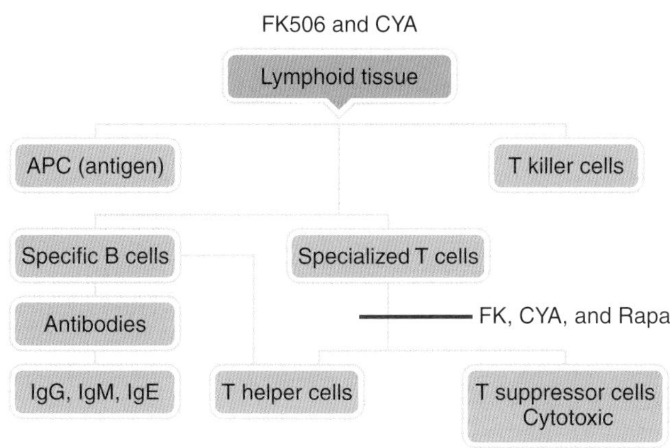


**Fig. 21.2**

**Cyclosporine (CsA, CYA, Neoral, Sandimmune) and tacrolimus (Prograf) block the sensitization of T cells.** Cyclosporine and tacrolimus inhibit calcineurin in lymphoid tissues and thus inhibit the production of immune mediators such as interleukin-2. In general, sirolimus (Rapamune) structure is similar to cyclosporine, but its action is different. It does not interfere directly with cytokine production but inhibits growth and proliferation of T and B lymphocytes by inhibiting the lymphocytes from taking action in response to stimulatory signals from certain cytokines. (Courtesy Chris L. Wells, University of Maryland Medical Center, and James H. Dauber, University of Pittsburgh Medical Center-Health Systems.)

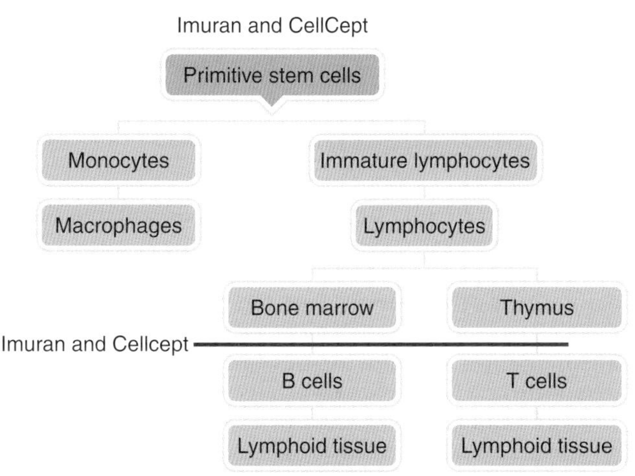


**Fig. 21.3**

**Azathioprine (Imuran) and mycophenolate mofetil (CellCept) are theorized to block lymphocytes from maturing into T cells.** This inhibits the immune-mediated inflammatory response. (Courtesy Chris L. Wells, University of Maryland School of Medicine, James H. Dauber, University of Pittsburgh Medical Center-Health Systems, and Carla Peterman, University of Maryland Medical Center.)

The third drug is prednisone, a corticosteroid with an effect at the level of the macrophages. Prednisone blocks the production of interleukin-2 in the presence of an antigen to stimulate a major histocompatibility complex (MHC), thus dampening both B-cell and T-cell responses (Fig. 21.4). Research continues to attempt to decrease the exposure to and use of corticosteroids because of the adverse effects of these medications including for diabetes, osteoporosis, muscle wasting (steroid myopathy), and fat deposition.

Sirolimus (rapamycin, Rapamune) is an immunosuppressant that inhibits cytokine-driven cell proliferation

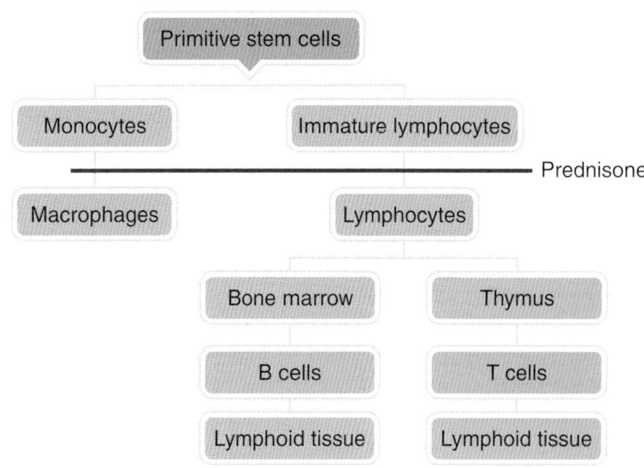


**Fig. 21.4**

**Prednisone works at the macrophage level and is theorized to block the production of interleukin-2, thus preventing the formation of major histocompatibility complexes that normally stimulate both B- and T-cell response.** (Courtesy Chris L. Wells, University of Maryland School of Medicine, and James H. Dauber, University of Pittsburgh Medical Center-Health Systems.)

and maturation. It was approved for use with renal transplants and was introduced for use with other organ transplants in the late 1990s. Sirolimus is presently being used in a low percentage of transplant recipients. It may be used in combination with a calcineurin-inhibiting drug and mycophenolate mofetil. Some centers use sirolimus and mycophenolate mofetil alone, particularly with pancreas and kidney recipients.[225,451] Some studies have reported a decrease in chronic rejection in heart transplant recipients with the use of sirolimus.[226]

In contrast to cyclosporine and tacrolimus, which prevent the body from reacting to the transplant, sirolimus "stalls the engine," disabling the body's ability to reject the transplanted organ. Because of this effect, sirolimus in combination with cyclosporine and steroids not only lowers the incidence of acute renal allograft rejection, but also permits cyclosporine sparing (reduced amounts or eventual elimination) without an increased risk of rejection.

## Medication Reduction and Withdrawal

Research is ongoing to attempt to reduce or eventually eliminate some of these potent immunosuppressive medications because of their deleterious side effects and complications, such as susceptibility to infection, diabetes, impaired muscle function, and nausea and vomiting. Withdrawal or marked reduction of corticosteroids is of particular benefit in the case of diabetes mellitus and in the presence of severe osteoporosis or aseptic necrosis of bone. Steroid withdrawal is possible in up to 70% of pancreas transplant candidates who are otherwise maintained on tacrolimus-based immunosuppression.[203,218]

Among individuals who initially received sirolimus in combination with cyclosporine and steroids, those who had steroid treatment stopped 1 month after transplantation had significantly fewer rejection episodes and were spared the numerous toxic side effects associated with long-term steroid administration.[193] Ongoing research continues to explore and support this practice as early as 4 days after transplantation.[11,14,482] Steroid withdrawal can increase the risk of acute rejection but reduces the incidence of infection. Maintaining a sufficient immunosuppressive regimen is the key to successful steroid withdrawal.

Research groups are working toward identifying the critical components on particular grafts that are seen as foreign to modify them.[57] This work will enable the graft to succeed, while simultaneously allowing the host immune response to carry out its main tasks. Strategies that teach the immune system to accept the transplanted tissue rather than attack it, a process called *chimerism*, are under investigation.[192,233,418] Chimerism involves inducing the immune system of the donor onto the candidate so that the candidate's immune system no longer rejects the organ or tissue. In bone marrow transplantation (BMT), chimerism is achieved when bone marrow and host cells exist compatibly without signs of graft-versus-host disease (GVHD).

A potential breakthrough may have been discovered in a study in which eight kidney transplant recipients were also given a mixture of stem cells from their organ donor. Five of the eight recipients were able to stop taking their immunosuppressant medications because the mixing of stem cells from the donor with the recipient helped make the recipients' immune system not recognize the donor's tissues as foreign.[252] Currently a phase II clinical trial is under way to further evaluate the role of donor hematopoietic stem cell transplantation in unrelated recipients of living donor renal allografts.[253]

Researchers studying how the developing fetus avoids destruction may be able to identify protective biologic pathways and then use this model to develop drugs to interrupt the rejection process and promote tolerance of foreign tissue.[206,444]

## Advances in Research

Advances in immunology, organ preservation, surgical technique, pharmacology, and postoperative care have permitted the rapid development of organ transplantation procedures other than traditional solid-organ transplants (e.g., heart, lung, liver, pancreas, intestine).

For example, the transplantation of pancreatic islet cells for the treatment of diabetes and ovarian preservation for later use in cases of cancer requiring ovary removal are under way. The use of hepatic segments for transplantation (either from cadavers or from living related donors) has decreased the number of people (especially children) awaiting liver transplantation.

The first transplantation of skeletal muscle cells to test whether the cells can repair damaged heart muscle took place at Temple University in the heart transplantation program in 2000. Myoblast cells taken from muscle biopsy specimens from the patient's arm were transplanted into his own heart during a surgical procedure to implant an assistive device while waiting for a heart transplant.[138]

Since then, researchers have successfully injected autologous skeletal myoblast cells into myocardial tissue in human beings undergoing concurrent coronary artery bypass grafting or ventricular assist device (VAD) implantation. This potential treatment for end-stage heart disease remains under investigation.[126,188] Patients with advanced heart failure receiving transendocardial delivery of autologous muscle–derived stem cells have demonstrated improved myocardial viability and exercise capacity.[173]

Research is under way to develop transplantable cells for the treatment of human diseases characterized by cell dysfunction or cell death and for which current treatment is inadequate or nonexistent. Scientists are also looking for a way to modulate the human immune system to prevent rejection of transplanted cells without the use of immunosuppressive drugs.[314]

Additional products under investigation include porcine neural cells for stroke, focal epilepsy, and intractable pain; porcine spinal cord cells for spinal cord injury; engineered blood vessels for use as vascular grafts; neurologic cell transfer for Parkinson disease or Huntington chorea; human liver cells for cirrhosis; and porcine retinal pigment epithelial cells for macular degeneration.[19,314]

The diverse research directions being undertaken around the world will continue to change the field of transplantation in the years to come. Gene therapy (including in utero), xenotransplantation, tissue engineering, chimerism, and new fields of study developing daily can be presented only briefly in this text but help represent the overall picture of rapid change in treatment approaches.

## Xenotransplantation

Allotransplantation remains the preferred treatment for human organ failure, but shortages of acceptable donor organs and the lack of success in developing suitable artificial organs have led researchers to investigate the use of organs from other species (xenotransplantation). Xenotransplantation is defined more fully as the interspecies transplantation of cells, tissues, and organs or ex vivo interspecies exchange between cells, tissues, and organs.[21]

Nonhuman primates are now considered an unethical and unsafe source of donor organs, so other species are being considered, in particular the pig. Baboon organs are too small to sustain human beings for long periods. The risk of transmitting deadly infectious agents from nonhuman primates is greater than from other animal species.

Physicians are already successfully using various pig components (e.g., heart valves, clotting factors, islet cells, brain cells) to treat human diseases. Researchers are now breeding genetically manipulated donor pigs whose cells, tissues, and organs could be permanently transplanted into human beings without being destroyed by the human immune system.[156] Concerns still exist about the potential for transfer of infectious agents from animals to humans and the introduction of diseases foreign to humans, leading to a possible epidemic. Scientists hope that by using modern biotechnology it may be possible to generate pigs free of threatening viruses in the future.[407]

Previously, hyperacute rejection or acute vascular rejection was the biggest disadvantage to xenotransplantation. Circulation of recipient blood through the transplanted organ caused graft failure within 24 hours. Scientific progress has eliminated this obstacle.[407] Considerable progress has been made in pig-to-primate organ xenotransplantation resulting in transplant functioning for days and weeks rather than minutes. Researchers have successfully implanted pig organs as a short-term bridge (up to 10 hours) until a human donor organ can be found and implanted.[254]

Other hurdles to xenotransplantation include anatomic, physiologic, and biochemical differences. The upright position of human beings is unique in nature. Gravity therefore exerts a different impact on the anatomic location of organs such as lung, heart, liver, and kidney. More pronounced are humoral and enzymatic differences.

Complex interactions existing in allografts are totally disturbed in xenogeneic situations. Regaining physiologic function of the graft in the foreign environment may be prevented by molecular incompatibilities between the donor and the recipient. Experts say that before xenotransplantation can become an everyday reality, safeguards must be developed to ensure the minimization of risk to the recipient and to society. The decision to proceed with clinical application of this technique depends on ethical, regulatory, and legal frameworks established by consensus.[156]

Issues yet to be resolved include the recipient's right to privacy, selection of the first recipients of xenografts, concern that the socioeconomically disadvantaged individuals will be used as test subjects for the first xenografts, and animal rights are just a few of the concerns expressed by various interest groups.[21,156,371]

## Tissue Engineering and Regenerative Medicine

**Note to Reader:** This section provides a broad overview of regenerative medicine and tissue engineering and is not intended to be comprehensive. Although these areas of research are, in many cases, still in their infancy, advances in tissue engineering and regenerative medicine are growing rapidly and offer the promise of increasingly impacting medical practice to the benefit of our patients.

Tissue engineering is a rapidly expanding industry that has the potential to address some of the aforementioned limitations in organ donation. Tissue engineering applies the principles of biology and engineering toward the development of biologic substitutes that restore, maintain, or improve tissue function. Enthusiasm and promise for the field are highlighted by the fact that biomedical engineering is offered at a number of institutions around the globe, even at the level of PhD programs. These doctoral programs are designed to train a new generation of researchers who bridge the gap across the fields of biology, medicine, and engineering, just to name a few.

The science of tissue engineering has given birth to a new clinical discipline called *regenerative medicine* aimed at replacing or regenerating living tissues so as to restore the functions of damaged, diseased, or defective tissues and organs. The reader is referred to a comprehensive review of the field, including stem cell types.[160]

Tissue engineering commonly uses cells seeded on highly porous, synthetic, biodegradable, polymer scaffolds to replace tissue function that has been lost owing to trauma or in the setting of disease. Over the past decade, the fabrication of a wide variety of tissues has been investigated, including both structural and visceral organs.

The potential applications of tissue engineering approaches are many. As an example, collagen meniscus implants are being used to regenerate or regrow new meniscus-like tissue. Stem cells are being tested for anterior cruciate ligament reconstruction,[291] with the goals of slowing down and preventing further degenerative joint disease, enhancing joint stability, providing pain relief, and returning people to activities at their desired level. Similarly, autologous chondrocyte osteochondral procedures harvest cartilage or bone tissue from a donor site, isolate and expand the cells in culture, and subsequently transplant the cells back into the area of cartilage or bone defect, respectively. Repair tissue of high quality typically requires at least 2 years to regenerate and mature.[95] A limitation of this approach, however, is donor site morbidity, which has the potential to have long-term adverse effects for the individual.

Another approach being investigated for the restoration of functional bone tissue after injury or with disease is the use of injectable hydrogels. These hydrogels may be synthetic or native and may be used as a delivery vehicle for cells or growth factors (e.g., bone morphogenetic protein). Injectable hydrogels have been shown to significantly enhance the compressive strength of bone.[397] Taken together, it is clear that tissue engineering for bone healing has great potential for many people who experience nonunion, slow-to-heal bone fractures, or traumatic bone loss associated with war injuries.[165] Indeed, bioengineered skin, bone, ligaments, tendons, and articular cartilage are already available in some clinical settings.[38]

Other examples of current progress in the area of bioengineering include implants filled with islet cells for people with diabetes to replace insulin injections, a method to generate natural breast tissue to replace saline implants, heart valves, dental tissue (gums, teeth), skeletal muscle, tissue isolated from synthetic polymers, and formation of phalanges and small joints from bovine cell sources. Tissue engineering models are also being developed to treat different conditions of the urinary bladder, such as bladder cancer, impaired contractility, and inflammatory disease.[350]

Given the vast disparity between the number of individuals on the organ transplant waiting list and the number of donor organs available, regenerative medicine scientists are also exploring the possibility of engineering organs at the laboratory bench. One method for such organ engineering involves decellularization (i.e., flushing out of all cellular components through the use of detergents) of a donor organ, often obtained from another species. This procedure allows for the maintenance of the complex, three-dimensional extracellular matrix structure of the organ, while eliminating the chance for immune rejection following transplantation. The decellularized organ may then be seeded with patient-derived stem cells, and the engineered organ is subsequently transplanted into the patient. As a proof of principle, Baptista and colleagues[35] demonstrated the potential of "humanizing" a rat liver. In their study, rat livers were harvested, decellularized, and reseeded with human cells. Incredibly, they demonstrated that these livers were metabolically functional and possessed characteristics typical of a normal liver. An important next step is to scale up these studies to human-relevant sizes. The long-term hope is to create viable donor tissue and organs for transplantation "on demand" and to develop living prosthetics (incorporating living tissue with electronics) for every organ system in the body.[249,461]

Arguably, stem cell transplantation approaches have most captured the public imagination as a potential key game changer for the future of medical practice. Embryonic stem cells, which are able to differentiate into all types of cells, have inspired many scientists in their search for novel treatments of otherwise incurable systemic diseases and tissue defects.[44,221,326] Of course, among the greatest limitations in the use of embryonic stem cells are the associated ethical concerns. In addition, the potency of embryonic stem cells raises questions about potential tumorigenicity of these cell populations. In an attempt to overcome these concerns, adult stem cells have been investigated for their regenerative potential in the context of a number of different applications. Compared with embryonic stem cells, however, adult stem cells display a more limited ability to differentiate into tissue types, thereby potentially compromising therapeutic potential. In 2006 in a seminal study, Takahashi and Yamanaki[431] demonstrated induction of embryonic stem cell–like characteristics to adult fibroblasts, called induced pluripotent stem cells, through induction of four key factors under culture conditions. Since the time of the first reports of induced pluripotent stem cells, increasing enthusiasm and clinical potential of this technology have burgeoned.

The potential applications for regenerative medicine–based therapeutics are numerous. Aging, associated with a progressive failing of tissues and organs and the leading cause of many diseases over time, is also a primary focus of regenerative medicine.[26,221] However, preclinical studies often test regenerative medicine approaches for age-associated diseases using young animals that are engineered to display a specific pathology such as cardiovascular disease. This is a limitation of the experimental paradigm, as such animal models do not take into consideration tissue-level declines associated with increasing age that may affect the overall efficacy of the intervention being tested.

Traumatic injuries represent another area in which the field of regenerative medicine is poised to make an important impact on medical practice. The military has been a major force in advancing the field as a result of the numerous traumatic and burn injuries to thousands of soldiers during the wars in Iraq and Afghanistan. In 2008 the federal government invested $85 million to create the new Armed Forces Institute of Regenerative Medicine (AFIRM). Through AFIRM, consortia including more than two dozen institutions were formed to accelerate research in the area. The goal of AFIRM was to develop cutting-edge technologies and treatments for both wounded soldiers and civilians.[116]

Given the culmination of scientific advances and the considerable investment in regenerative medicine/tissue engineering technologies, it is clear that their clinical implications are more promising than ever before. To realize the full potential of these technologies, the next crucial step is consideration of the comprehensive care program to maximize functional outcomes. This will undoubtedly require a multidisciplinary team of clinicians who work together to synergize their individual skill sets to the benefit of patients.

SPECIAL IMPLICATIONS FOR THE THERAPIST 21.1

### *Regenerative Rehabilitation*

Cell biologists, bioengineers, and developmental biologists have been among the primary drivers in the field of regenerative medicine. However, as these technologies increasingly make their way to the clinic to treat pathologies and injuries commonly encountered in rehabilitation practice, there is a need to expand communication, interaction, and collaboration across the fields of regenerative medicine and physical therapy. As a profession, physical therapists have the skills to integrate biology, biomechanics, and physiology in a way that allows for optimization of the timing and intensity of physical interventions to maximize tissue regeneration and, ultimately, functional restoration.[18] Undoubtedly, rehabilitation clinicians will be involved in designing and implementing follow-on clinical protocols aimed at maximizing function as the transplanted tissue replaces, repairs, or regenerates injured, aged, or diseased tissues.[15]

Regenerative rehabilitation has been defined as the application of rehabilitation protocols and principles together with regenerative medicine therapeutics toward the goal of optimizing functional recovery through tissue regeneration, remodeling, or repair.[359] The rationale for regenerative rehabilitation includes three main areas, as outlined below.

First, it is clear that for functional tissue regeneration to occur, resident stem cells are dependent on supporting cues from the microenvironment, or niche. These microenvironmental cues include vascularity, growth factor secretion, and neural signals, for example, all of which serve to direct stem cell fate. A strength of the rehabilitation toolset is the prescription of exercise protocols and modalities, such as ultrasound and neuromuscular electrical stimulation that optimize the healing microenvironment. With this in mind, increasing attention is being paid to the possibility of priming the donor site before transplantation (a type of "prehabilitation") to enhance the survival, proliferation, and/or differentiation of donor stem cells. Likewise, the application of rehabilitation protocols immediately after stem cell transplantation may provide a more supportive microenvironment to allow for improved donor cell survival engraftment and functional incorporation into the treated tissue.[16]

Second, in addition to being highly responsive to biochemical signals emanating from the microenvironment, stem cells themselves are also highly mechanosensitive. Stem cells "sense" static and dynamic physical aspects of their surroundings. Through a process known as mechanotransduction, or the conversion of physical stimuli into chemical responses, extrinsic signals may directly affect stem cell responses, such as gene expression and differentiation into a specific tissue lineage.[359] As an example, it has been shown that "stretching" stem cells in a cyclical manner promotes their secretion of vascular endothelial growth factor, a major growth factor involved in tissue angiogenesis.[86] These findings in a cell culture model demonstrate the ability of dynamic signals to directly affect stem cell behavior and suggest that tissue loading in the living organism (via exercise, stretching, or modalities) may similarly affect the behavior of transplanted stem cells.

Finally, differentiation of stem cells into the tissue target is often a goal of stem cell therapeutics, and physical therapy may serve as an important adjunct therapy to promote functionality of the newly formed tissue. For example, in the treatment of children with Duchenne muscular dystrophy (DMD), investigators are pursuing the transplantation of dystrophin-positive stem cells (derived from a healthy donor). DMD results from a loss of a functional dystrophin protein. The loss of dystrophin renders myofibers structurally vulnerable and highly susceptible to damage, ultimately leading to a progressive muscle weakness over time. The rationale for stem cell transplantation in DMD, then, is to promote the engraftment of donor cells into nascent dystrophin-positive myofibers that will enhance the muscle integrity and strength of the host. Future studies are needed to investigate the ability of physical therapy protocols to promote hypertrophy of the newly formed myofibers so as to maximize functional outcomes.

Clearly, physical therapists will play a major role in the success of regenerative medicine and tissue engineering approaches in the clinic, much in the same way that successful outcomes following an orthopedic procedure rely on well-defined postsurgical rehabilitation protocols. For more information about regenerative rehabilitation and to access relevant resources, the reader is referred to the American Physical Therapy Association (APTA) website (http://www.apta.org/) (type in search window: regenerative medicine for podcasts and audio conferences), and to the Alliance for Regenerative Rehabilitation Research and Training (www.ar3t.pitt.edu).

## BIOPSYCHOSOCIAL IMPLICATIONS

Many different ethical, social, moral, economic, and legal issues are associated with the procurement and allocation of living or bioengineered tissue. In addition, new information concerning the psychoneuroimmune responses in healthy tissues and organs has added new dimensions to understanding the emotional adjustment for recipients of living organ and tissue transplants.

### Legal and Ethical Considerations

Before alternative treatment methods can be fully implemented, scientific and medical communities and the general public will have to seriously consider and attempt to resolve legal and ethical issues. For example, federal law prohibits the sale of human organs in the United States, and violators are subject to fines and imprisonment. However, individuals have taken matters into their own hands and established donor-matching services on the Internet.

In some countries of continental Europe, organ donation is governed by "presumed consent" legislation. Unless legally designated otherwise, organ donation is presumed on the death of each individual. Consent legislation has had a proven and positive, sizable effect on organ donation rates.[1]

Although Western opinion is almost universally against the practice of paid organ donation and the use of organs from judicially executed prisoners, similar laws are not in place worldwide. The ethics of both issues continue to be debated.

### Bioethical Considerations

Another area of concern involves researchers growing human cells into tissues using stem cells derived from human embryos left over from attempts at artificial fertilization or following abortions. Currently in the United States, embryonic stem cell lines are being made in the private sector and in private universities that use private funding. Federal funding for stem cell research (banned under the Bush administration) has been reinstated. This change occurred after a 2010 U.S. Court of Appeals ruling upheld President Obama's executive order (2009) to allow research funding by the National Institutes of Health and Department of Health and Human Services.[262,283]

Legislation in the United States to allow federal funding for research using stem cells derived from embryos originally created for fertility treatments and willingly donated by consenting adults has been introduced and remains a debated issue. For the most part, embryonic stem cells are used only in fundamental research.

Many bioethicists and lawmakers still question the appropriateness of this research until the ethical issues and appropriate concerns can be voiced and resolved. Questions about the nature of human life and its protection, the safeguard of human dignity, and the use of genetic material have been raised. However, new discoveries in the rapidly developing field of stem cell research, such as the discovery of master stem cells replacing the use of embryonic tissue, may bypass these bioethical concerns.

Other countries, including Israel, England, and India and areas of Asia, have moved ahead in the area of stem cell research. Since January 2006, stem cell trials for the treatment of stroke, spinal cord injury, leg ischemia, and myocardial infarction have been conducted in India using bone marrow–derived stem cells.

Concerns related to animal-derived matrix proteins have also been raised. Some private bioengineering companies are proactively researching ways to develop human tissue with matrix proteins naturally secreted by the cells rather than developing tissue from animal-derived matrix proteins. In the area of animal organ transplantation (xenotransplantation), rules governing the welfare of animals bred for transplants are being formulated. Moreover, a ban on having children has been placed on all people receiving animal organ transplantation.

## Psychoemotional Considerations

### Pretransplantation

Transplant applicants face many challenges, including the obvious physical illness, complex assessment protocols, uncertainties about surgery and outcome, the possibility of relocation to obtain transplant services, and financial burden. Waiting for a transplant can be accompanied by a vast range of changing emotions, such as relief, despair, elation, depression, excitement, and apprehension.

No single attitude is common or expected; each person's reaction is a valid expression of his or her experience. Most candidates find waiting for surgery a stressful time, and, of course, the longer the wait, the greater the stress. The evaluation process itself and the wait for the results after tests and procedures require complex coping strategies, especially if the person is denied for transplantation.

When death is a possibility, candidates may worry that negative thinking will harm their health. Others are distressed that someone else must die before an organ will be available for transplantation or that receiving an available organ deprives someone else of life. Candidates are encouraged to focus on the desired outcome without completely ignoring the alternatives for themselves and outcomes for others. Counseling and support groups are often recommended.

Anxiety, depression, and feeling overwhelmed are common complications of medical illness of any kind and may interfere with the candidate's or recipient's participation in rehabilitation. Symptoms of posttraumatic stress disorder are not uncommon in the recipient or partner after organ implantation or mechanical assist device implantation followed by heart transplantation.[68,292]

Clinical symptoms of posttraumatic stress disorder, anxiety, or depression can be subtle and mimic the individual's health condition, requiring candidate or recipient self-awareness and careful screening by all members of the transplantation team to identify and treat early. The therapist can take an active role by administering simple evidence-based questionnaires to screen for the need for referral to an appropriate health provider (e.g., social work or psychology). Attention to the supporting members of the recipient's family and partners is also advised.[68] In some centers, caregivers start their own support groups while they are relocated to help with their needs during the stressful process.

A condition severe enough to require organ transplantation can sometimes impair concentration, memory, judgment, or ability to process thoughts. In particular, approximately one-third of all liver transplant candidates have severe impairment of mental abilities (i.e., hepatic encephalopathy) and may be extremely confused or even delirious at the time of transplantation. Similar mental impairment can occur with heart, lung, and kidney transplant candidates, although it is less common.

### Posttransplantation

Postoperatively, organ recipients face a long recovery period that is strongly influenced by a number of individual factors. Reintegration into family and work roles can be challenging with new lifelong stressors such as the need for drug compliance and dietary modification. Perceived success of transplantation, postoperative complications, and permanent physical changes may strongly influence an organ recipient's ability to cope and adapt.

Early identification of recipients most likely to have compliance and psychiatric problems is an important first step in providing interventions that maximize psychosocial status of recipients and improve long-term physical health outcomes.[124,426] Pretransplantation psychiatric disorders, female gender, longer hospitalization, more impaired physical function, and less social support from caregivers and family in the perioperative period are known risk factors for posttransplantation anxiety, depression, and other psychologic disorders.[123]

Stress on the family and the need for family support and counseling also affect treatment outcomes. Health care staff may observe a deterioration of family relationships after transplantation, especially between husband and wife or between partners. Support groups can be extremely helpful in these types of situations and should be recommended early by the health care team.

# POSTTRANSPLANTATION COMPLICATIONS

With advances in technology and immunology, transplantation of almost any tissue is feasible, but the clinical use of transplantation to remedy disease is still limited for many organ systems owing to potential rejection and other posttransplant complications.

Complications following organ transplantation can be classified into three broad categories: (1) complications associated with the procurement and surgical procedure, (2) complications of the transplanted organ, and (3) complications as a result of the immunosuppressive agents used to prevent rejection. Each type of organ transplantation has its own accompanying surgical risks and complications (see discussion in each section).

Following surgery, two main complications of organ transplantation are infection and organ rejection. The most serious posttransplantation complication is death, which can be caused by infection, organ toxicity, GVHD, relapse, and various other conditions (Fig. 21.5). The overall incidence of infection is 10% to 15%,[102] occurring most often (60%) in kidney transplant recipients.[235]

Infection and organ rejection are common and treatable, but prevention is the first step. For this reason, pretransplantation serologic testing is done to determine histocompatibility and to avoid transmitting infectious agents (e.g., CMV, vancomycin-resistant enterococci, hepatitis B virus, hepatitis C virus) from donor to recipient. Herpes zoster infection can be a serious complication of organ transplantation, with postherpetic neuralgia occurring in almost half of the recipients with infection. Heart and lung recipients have the highest incidence (15%), followed by renal (7.4%) and liver (5.7%) transplant recipients.[167]

With increasing survival following organ transplant, there is increased risk of other complications, such as certain forms of cancer and diabetes. Compared with the general population, recipients of a kidney, liver, heart, or lung transplant have an increased risk for diverse infection-related and unrelated cancers.[141]

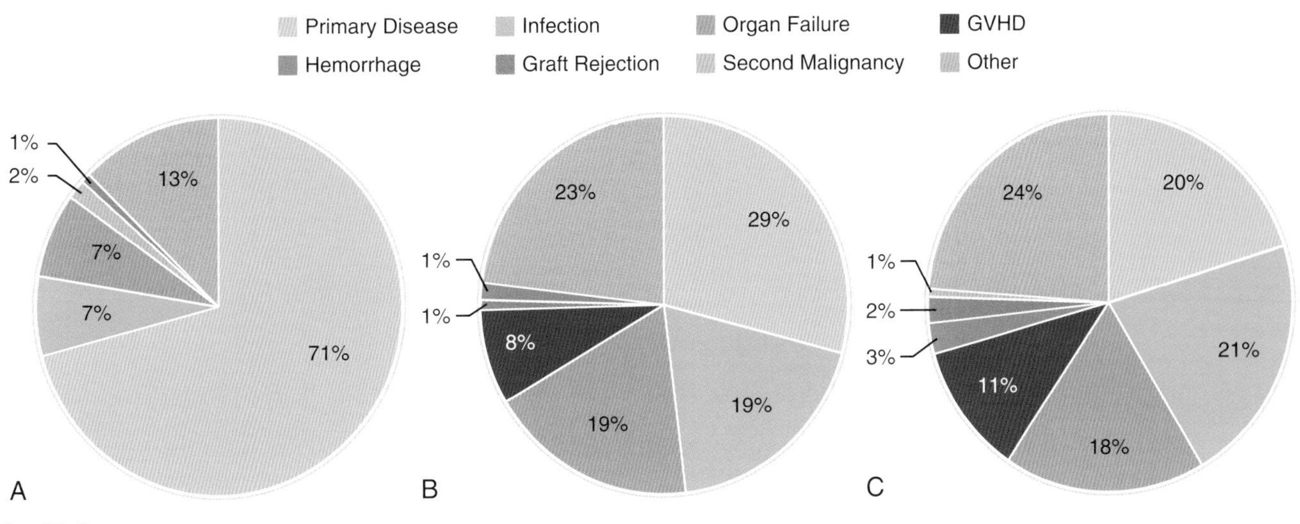


**Fig. 21.5**

**Causes of death after transplants performed in 2015–2016.** (A) The most commonly reported cause of death after an autologous hematopoietic stem cell transplantation is primary disease, accounting for 71% of deaths. (B) Among human leukocyte antigen–matched sibling transplant recipients who died within the first 100 days, 29% died of their primary disease, while 37% died of infection and organ failure. (C) Considering unrelated donor allogeneic hematopoietic stem cell transplantation recipients who died within the first 100 days, 51% of deaths were due to infection, organ failure, and graft-versus-host disease *(GVHD)*, and 48% were due to primary disease. (Courtesy Center for International Blood & Marrow Transplant Research (CIBMTR). *CIBMTR Summary Slides–HCT Trends and Survival Data.* 2018. Data from: Table D'Souza A, Fretham C. Current Uses and Outcomes of Hematopoietic Cell Transplantation (HCT): CIBMTR Summary Slides, 2018. Available athttps://www.cibmtr.org)

## Ischemic Reperfusion Injury

*Ischemic injury* occurs when normal blood and oxygen supply to the donor organ is stopped at the time of organ harvest, whereas *reperfusion injury* can occur when blood flow is returned to the organ after transplantation. The donated organ is very sensitive to the amount of time it is not being perfused or supplied with blood, which can lead to ischemia.[95] Ischemic reperfusion injury may occur with any organ transplantation; it results in the onset of the inflammatory response, which has both immediate and long-term effects on the donated organ.

After the organ has been surgically implanted, the clamps are removed to allow blood to once again perfuse the organ. It has been suggested that the abrupt return of blood to the donor organ (now transplanted into the recipient) may create further trauma to the epithelial lining of the blood vessels because the transplant recipient may be circulating blood at a higher pressure than what is tolerable for the donor organ.

This phenomenon is especially common in heart or lung transplantation in the presence of comorbid pulmonary hypertension. This results in a reperfusion injury, which leads to leukocytes and platelet aggregation, which further causes endothelial permeability and inflammatory cell activation and adherence.

Mild ischemic reperfusion injury is common, and recovery usually occurs within 3 to 5 days. If the injury is significant, reperfusion injury can contribute to graft failure and organ dysfunction. Decreased long-term survival and death of the recipient are possible. More recently it has been shown that there is a significant relationship between the presence of an ischemic reperfusion injury and development of chronic rejection via the activation of both the innate and the adaptive immune responses and organ regeneration.[59]

## Histocompatibility

In all cases of graft rejection, the cause is incompatibility of cell surface antigens. The rejection of foreign or transplanted tissue occurs because the immune system of the recipient recognizes that the surface human leukocyte antigen (HLA) proteins of the donor's tissue are different from the recipient's.

Certain antigens are more important than others for successful transplantation including ABO present on red blood cells and histocompatibility antigens, most importantly, HLAs. As expected, there is a better chance of graft acceptance with syngeneic or autologous transplants because the cell surface antigens are identical. For all categories of transplantation, minimizing HLA mismatches is associated with a significantly lower risk of graft loss.[87]

It has been shown that in a person with HLA antibodies, the antibodies are directed against the antigen of the donor kidney and will result in immediate graft failure. It also has been documented that the when specific HLA antibodies are directed against B cells, hyperacute rejection is produced, leading to graft dysfunction and possible failure.[435]

Crossmatching policies may vary by institution.

## Graft Rejection

Transplant rejection may occur for immunologic or nonimmunologic reasons. When the body recognizes the donor tissue as nonself and attempts to destroy the tissue shortly after transplantation, rejection occurs as

**Table 21.3** Clinical Manifestations of Organ Rejection

| Hyperacute Rejection | Acute (Late) Rejection | Chronic Rejections |
|---|---|---|
| Immediate reaction<br>Severe graft dysfunction or failure, then death<br>Death | Occurs days to years after transplantation<br>May be asymptomatic in early stages<br>Fever; constitutional symptoms (flu-like)<br>Loss of appetite<br>Graft tenderness<br>Blood pressure changes<br>Dyspnea<br>Fatigue<br>Peripheral edema, weight gain<br>Inflamed skin lesions<br>Reduced exercise capacity<br>Organ related-symptoms<br>• Kidney<br>  • Proteinuria<br>  • Uremia<br>  • Neurologic symptoms<br>  • Nausea and vomiting<br>• Liver<br>  • Palpable liver<br>  • Jaundice<br>  • Hematemesis (vomiting blood)<br>  • Abdominal pain<br>  • Ascites<br>  • Neurologic symptoms (see Box 21.7)<br>  • Elevated transaminase<br>  • Elevated bilirubin<br>• Heart<br>  • S3 gallop<br>  • Arrhythmias<br>  • Jugular vein distention<br>• Lung<br>  • Changes in respiratory status; breathlessness; prolonged need for ventilatory support<br>  • Fall in spirometric values (>10% change/reduction from baseline; <90% at rest)<br>  • Decreased $FEV_1$ >10%<br>  • Dry or productive cough<br>  • Change in sputum (color, amount)<br>  • Decreased oxygen saturation<br>  • Reduced vital capacity; decreased exercise capacity<br>  • Radiographic changes<br>• Pancreas<br>  • Nausea<br>  • Vomiting<br>  • Anorexia<br>  • Other gastrointestinal symptoms<br>  • Urologic symptoms | Occurs 3 months to years after transplantation<br>May be asymptomatic in early stages<br>Organ-related symptoms<br>Histologic changes<br>Graft dysfunction<br>Graft failure |

*$FEV_1$, Forced expiratory volume in 1 second.*

an immunologic phenomenon. Transplant rejection is most often caused by the degree of MHC antigen mismatch.

Nonimmunologic factors can occur as a result of the draining reperfusion process necessary in organ harvest and transplantation. Ischemic reperfusion injury is associated with an increase in acute and chronic rejection.[59]

As residual blood is drained from the transplanted organ into the host's general circulation, the body recognizes the transplanted tissue cells as foreign invaders (antigens) and immediately sets up an immune response by producing antibodies. These antibodies are capable of inhibiting metabolism of the cells within the transplanted organ and eventually actively causing their destruction.

Research to develop a reliable method to reduce the ischemic reperfusion injury is currently ongoing. Eliminating the occurrence of poor early graft function and consequently reducing the chances for rejection episodes are the primary goals of these investigations.[129,132]

### Types of Graft Rejection

There are three types of transplant rejection—*hyperacute* rejection, *acute* or late acute rejection, and *chronic* rejection—depending on the amount of time that passes between transplantation and rejection (Table 21.3).

**Hyperacute Rejection.** Hyperacute rejection (rare with antibody screening and tissue typing) is predominantly mediated by humoral responses of the immune system (natural antibodies, complement cascade) and the activation of coagulation factors. There is an immediate rejection after transplantation when the recipient has produced antibodies to donor tissue.

This reaction necessitates prompt medical action, which may include surgical removal of the transplanted tissue or the use of life support devices such as a temporary VAD or ECMO in the case of a heart or lung transplantation. These devices can be used to support blood circulation and gas exchange while the individual undergoes treatment such as plasmapheresis and immunoglobulin therapy in an attempt to remove the reactive antibodies. Medical treatment may diminish the hyperacute rejection response and allow the donor organ to recover, or it may allow time for another donor organ to be implanted.[257]

**Acute or Late Acute Rejection.** The acute or late acute rejection can appear days to years after transplantation. This type of rejection involves a combination of cellular and humoral reactions. Acute antibody-mediated rejection or vascular rejection typically occurs days to weeks posttransplantation. There is an interaction between the recipient's antibody and donor HLA or endothelial cell antigens that leads to graft vessel injury and thrombosis formation. Acute cellular rejection (ACR) is most common in the first 3 to 6 months posttransplantation and involves the proliferation and infiltration of T lymphocytes and macrophages.[189,257] Despite the early pattern of acute rejection, both humoral and cellular rejection can occur at any time.

Clinically, there may be sudden onset of organ-related signs and symptoms, such as fever, graft tenderness, fatigue, or decreased exertional tolerance; conversely, the recipient may be totally asymptomatic. Graft rejection must be differentiated from immunosuppressive toxicity.

This form of rejection can be reliably graded using a system of categories of mild, moderate, and severe rejection. Acute rejection, if detected in its early stages, can be reversed with immunosuppressive therapy. With the advancements in immunosuppressive medications and management, there has been a decline in acute rejection, which has led to an increase in 1-year graft and recipient survival.[451]

**Chronic Rejection.** Chronic rejection can occur as early as 3 months posttransplantation, but it is usually months to years before chronic rejection occurs. This type of rejection develops as a function of both cell-mediated and humoral-mediated reactions and is characterized by slow, progressive organ failure.

Growing evidence indicates that chronic rejection is the aggregate sum of irreversible immunologic and nonimmunologic injuries to the graft over time. Chronic rejection is associated with chronic vascular changes such as arteriopathy or diffuse atherosclerosis with intimal proliferative changes, depending on the type of organ. In the presence of a chronic immune/inflammatory process within the donor organ, the intimal lining of the vascular tissue undergoes fibrosis and vascular remodeling. This leads to a decrease in the lumen size and ischemia of the distal tissue and perpetuates the inflammatory reaction.[119,165]

A history of acute rejection episodes, either asymptomatic or clinically apparent, and inadequate therapeutic level of the immunosuppressive medications or poor compliance are among the most recognizable immunologic risk factors for chronic rejection.[189]

Adherence to immunosuppressive therapy is a key factor contributing to transplant failures that occur within 2 years after surgery. Financial barriers such as lack of insurance coverage are the most common reason for noncompliance or spreading out antirejection medications (i.e., taking them less often).[92] Chronic rejection results in irreversible cellular damage within the donor organ and leads to graft dysfunction and eventually failure.[184,256] Chronic rejection is rarely responsive to medical therapies.

## Immunosuppression

A primary role of the immune system is to distinguish between self and nonself (the immunologic response of the recipient to the donor's tissues), which presents a major problem for the transplant recipient. In a person with an intact immune system (immunocompetence), the recipient's immune system recognizes the transplanted tissue or organ as foreign (nonself) and produces antibodies and sensitized lymphocytes against it.

The ultimate objective of immunosuppressive therapy is to block transplantation recipient reactivity to the donor's organ while sparing other responses. Because these drugs suppress immunologic reactions, infection is a leading cause of death, particularly within the first postoperative year.[258] However, increased understanding of rejection mechanisms has made it possible to suppress specific elements of the immune response and has led to a decrease in death-related infection and rejection.[54,451]

Although lower amounts of immunosuppressive drugs are now prescribed, these drugs usually must be taken for the life of the recipient, and physical changes and other side effects remain a well-known problem.

### Side Effects of Long-Term Immunosuppression

Long-term immunosuppression can have serious consequences for the recipient, such as diabetes and accelerated hyperlipidemia, with associated atherosclerosis and subsequent cardiovascular disease.

There is a high incidence of musculoskeletal effects that will concern the therapist, such as decreased bone density and osteoporosis. Osteoporosis is diagnosed in half of all transplant recipients, and one-third of recipients have documented vertebral fractures,[263] steroid- and calcineurin inhibitor–induced myopathies, avascular necrosis, and musculoskeletal injuries.

Within the first 6 months after transplantation, the organ recipient can lose more bone density than any woman during the postmenopausal period. Osteoporosis has become a silent contributor to mortality in organ transplantation.[414] Physical therapy intervention must address this concern.

Neurotoxic reactions are manifested by a fine tremor, paresthesias, and occasionally seizures. Sensorimotor demyelinating polyradiculoneuropathy has been reported as a rare side effect in liver transplant recipients receiving tacrolimus.[266] Neuropathies and paresthesia, including footdrop (anterior tibialis weakness), can occur with this drug[476]; quadriplegia is a rare adverse event.

The individual may report difficulty with fine motor activities of daily living, such as poor handwriting and difficulty eating. These changes may be significant enough to stop some people from going out publicly or dining out in restaurants. Reports of memory loss may not be secondary to actual alterations in memory, but rather a decrease in executive function.[107,423] Most of these events are dose related and reversible.

### Cancers in Solid-Organ Transplant Recipients

Organ recipients have 3 times the incidence of various cancers, and some specific cancers are 100 times more frequent in the immunosuppressed population after transplantation than in the general population. Cancer incidence is proportional to immunosuppression drug levels, and the risk increases each year after transplantation.[115] It has been suggested that immunosuppressive agents may cause DNA damage and interfere with normal DNA repair mechanisms. Immune surveillance, which ordinarily prevents the growth and development of malignancies, may be impaired by certain immunosuppressive medications.

The most common tumors among transplant recipients (40% to 50% incidence) are squamous cell cancers of the lips and skin owing to enhanced photosensitivity. Squamous cell carcinoma is often more aggressive than in people who are not immunosuppressed, with multiple sites of presentation and frequent recurrence.[143] The incidence of basal cell carcinoma is 10% higher than in the general population, and the incidence of squamous cell carcinoma has been reported to be 250 times greater in orthotopic homologous transplantation recipients.[209]

Organ recipients are also at increased risk for some malignancies, such as Kaposi sarcoma, non-Hodgkin lymphomas and other posttransplant lymphoproliferative disorders, soft tissue sarcomas, carcinomas of the vulva and perineum, carcinomas of the kidney, and hepatobiliary tumors.[119,141,441]

Cancer risk in solid organs, such as the lung, colon, pancreas, prostate, stomach, breast, and ovary, is twofold higher in transplant recipients than in the general population, while kidney cancer risk is 15 times greater.[141,222] Malignant lymphomas occur 11.8 times more often in kidney transplant recipients compared with the general population. The majority of lymphomas occur after the first posttransplant year.[328] Exactly why kidney transplantation is more affected by these factors than other organs remains unknown.[220]

Cardiac transplant recipients have a higher incidence of cancer than other transplant recipients, perhaps because of higher levels of immunosuppression. Studies have reported an increase in lung cancer in heart transplant recipients who have a history of smoking. There is an increased incidence in posttransplant lymphoproliferative disease in heart transplant recipients who underwent $OKT_3$ induction therapy or use of antithymocyte globulin for rejection therapy.

## Gastrointestinal Problems

Gastrointestinal complications of solid-organ transplantation have been well described in the literature. Disorders of the colon and rectum are a considerable source of morbidity, especially after heart and lung transplantation. Colorectal problems occur among 7% of lung transplant recipients, 6% of heart-lung transplant recipients, and 4% of heart transplant recipients. Major complications include diverticulitis, perforation, and malignancy. More minor complications include polyps, pseudoobstruction, and benign anorectal disease.[164] Acute nausea, vomiting, weight loss, and restrictions to diet and eating can be barriers to rehabilitation; feeding tubes are often used to supplement nutrition in transplant recipients.

## Wound Healing

Advances in surgical techniques and immunosuppression have led to an appreciable reduction in postoperative complications following transplantation. However, wound complications, as one of the most common types of posttransplantation surgical complications, can still limit these improved outcomes and result in prolonged hospitalization, hospital readmission, and reoperation.[285]

Long-term immunosuppressive drug therapy impairs and prolongs wound healing, especially common among organ recipients with diabetic or neuropathic pedal ulcers. The two most important risk factors for wound complications are immunosuppression and obesity. Other risk factors include surgical and/or technical factors (e.g., type of incision, reoperation, surgeon's expertise), advancing age, diabetes mellitus, malnutrition, and uremia.[285]

Therapists should be involved in preventive management of wound complications; identifying and minimizing risk factors whenever possible is important. Therapists involved in wound therapy should inform their clients, members of the clients' families, employers of clients, and third-party payers to expect longer times in healing plantar ulcers because of long-term immunosuppressive therapy.[401]

Total-contact casting remains a highly effective and rapid method of healing neuropathic pedal ulcers in diabetic immunosuppressed clients and transplant recipients, although it may take several weeks longer than it would for individuals who are not immunocompromised. Transplant recipients who are immunocompromised appear to be no more at risk for wound failure complications when using total-contact casting as a treatment modality than individuals without these additional variables.[401]

## Posttransplantation Pain Syndromes

Reports of chronic pain among solid-organ transplant recipients were first recorded in the late 1990s.[149] Since that time, understanding of posttransplantation pain syndromes has increased. Pain associated with posttransplantation syndrome is described as burning, stabbing, or dull and may be linked with depression; a correlation between pain intensity and organ rejection has been established.[149] Primary musculoskeletal pain can occur following solid-organ transplantation often (but not always) linked with immunosuppressive medications (e.g., cyclosporine). Individuals who experience partial sympathetic reinnervation following heart transplantation may experience chest discomfort and/or shoulder and arm pain.

## ORGAN TRANSPLANTATION AND EXERCISE, ACTIVITY, AND SPORTS

Whereas some people will have a period of only a few days of physical inactivity before transplantation (e.g., toxic liver failure), the majority of organ candidates will live with their diseased organs for a prolonged period of time, often years. By the time of organ transplantation, candidates usually have experienced a period of long-term ill health, leading to end-stage organ failure accompanied by severe deconditioning and exercise intolerance.

Complications of long-term immunosuppressive therapy and the kind of organ that has failed will determine some of the problems an individual may face in relation to exercise, activities, and sports. Most transplantation candidates experience an impaired physical performance level that not only interferes with the ability to perform leisure-time exercise, but also often limits the ability to perform even simple physical tasks such as rising from a chair or climbing stairs.[230]

Weakness, dyspnea on exertion, and fatigue are often present, and there may be little motivation for exercise and sport. Finding an activity or exercise that the person can do successfully is the first step to initiating regular lifelong exercise.

Whether or not a potential candidate receives a transplant, therapy can be focused toward more function and improved quality of life. Exercise training increases work capacity as measured by increased oxygen consumption ($VO_2$), increases efficiency of oxygen utilization in the muscles, normalizes distribution of muscle fiber types, increases aerobic metabolism with delays in the onset of lactic acid buildup, and promotes modulation of the parasympathetic nervous system with more sensitive baroreceptors.[40,214] Exercise training also improves psychologic factors, such as depression in pretransplant and posttransplant individuals.[81,236,345]

An assessment of transplant candidates must take into consideration daily life and daily activities, including potential return to work requirements. For example, for a job that requires lifting, assessment of cardiovascular compliance and hemodynamic stability during lifting is needed, whereas someone at home must be able to perform activities of daily living safely.

### Pretransplantation Activity and Exercise

It has been proposed that peripheral skeletal and respiratory (in the case of thoracic involvement) muscle work capacity is reduced before transplantation and contributes to the limitations of exercise seen in the posttransplantation population.[468] Preservation of muscle strength before transplantation becomes difficult for some candidates who are acutely ill. Muscular dysfunction attributable to detraining and deconditioning is common.[245]

While a candidate waits on the transplant list, it is important that the individual participate in an exercise program with the goal to promote functional mobility. Exercise programs should be individualized to focus on the needs of each person to maintain function, self-control, and esteem. Exercises should be functional, with an emphasis on strengthening the proximal muscles of the pelvis and the lower extremities, especially the gluteal and quadriceps muscles, as well as muscles of the shoulder girdle and trunk to support upper extremity function and accessory respiratory efficiency.

Weight training to maintain or increase muscular strength may help the candidate counteract the effects of steroids on muscle and the adverse effects of immobility and chronic inflammation.[98,321,345] It has been reported by transplantation centers around the United States that transplantation candidates who take part in an exercise program before surgery are likely to recover more rapidly following transplantation. Researchers are beginning to publish data on exercise performance before and after transplantation.[84,149,183,354,408]

Educational sessions can be extremely beneficial to both the organ recipient and the caregivers with regard to the transplant process and aftercare. Preparing the potential recipient for complications such as weakness and osteoporosis before surgery and how to best treat issues when they arise can improve the individual's success in overcoming them after transplantation.

### Posttransplantation Activity and Exercise

After organ transplantation, the underlying pathophysiologic process returns to normal if the donor organ is functioning appropriately. For example, exercise performance in individuals with heart transplants increases with respect to pretransplantation performance but remains subnormal and may not improve with time after surgery.[48] The extent of recovery depends on the function of the transplanted organ, which in turn is determined by the quality and function of the organ implanted, the presence of any rejection or infection, and the development of other comorbidities.

Despite the pretransplantation physical deconditioning and exercise limitations, transplant recipients can progressively return to a normal life with return to work and even safely participate in sporting activity and exercise.[230] National and International Transplant Games, a multidisciplinary sporting event started in 1978, illustrates the degree to which organ candidates can return to exercise and sports. At the 2006 National Kidney Foundation–sponsored games in Louisville, Kentucky, transplant recipients from all 50 states, with the oldest recipient being 84 years of age, participated to celebrate the gift of life and experience competition.

Regular exercise enhances quality of life and lowers the risk of cardiovascular disease, hypertension, and diabetes. This is especially important in transplant recipients because many immunosuppressive drugs can be atherogenic and diabetogenic.[113,150,291] It is recommended that physical therapy should begin on postoperative day 1, with the goal to mobilize out of bed as soon as the recipient is medically stable. Progressive physical training should begin as soon as the recipient is up and walking.

Despite the restoration of system function that allows most recipients to experience an improved quality of life including returning to work, having and caring for children, and participating in leisure recreational activities, transplant recipients often experience a persistent limitation in peak aerobic and anaerobic capacity compared with health- and age-matched normal subjects.[286]

Heart transplant recipients have lower exercise capacity than other transplant recipients as a result of decrease in maximal and peak $VO_2$, decrease in workload, earlier onset of anaerobic threshold, and lower $VO_2$ at the anaerobic threshold.[286] There is evidence to suggest that recipients continue to have abnormalities in both central and peripheral chemoreflex mechanisms along with the adverse effects of the immunosuppressive medications that contribute to prolonged deficits of exercise capacity.[32,65]

Despite the inherent limitations caused by the posttransplantation state, exercise training after transplantation can increase exercise capacity, improve endurance, and increase muscle strength, contributing to higher quality of life after transplantation even in the presence of posttransplantation limitations.[153,193,204,210,286] Physical activity and exercise may reduce or attenuate side effects of immunosuppression. Transplant recipients tolerate progressive exercise training and can achieve near-normal and even normal levels of function.[212] There is evidence that rehabilitation can improve muscle function and exercise parameters compared with individuals who had a transplant and did not participate in rehabilitation.[279]

Various exercises have been prescribed for transplant recipients. Studies document various training programs, including aerobic programs of low-to-high intensities, muscle endurance, and resistive training. It is difficult to draw any specific conclusions about the optimal exercise program. The best recommendation that can be made is to prescribe a comprehensive exercise program that includes muscular strength and endurance training, restoring functional mobility and improving cardiopulmonary endurance.[33,170]

Gaining density in the lumbar spine is especially important because up to 35% of transplant recipients develop lumbar spine bone fractures.[63] Resistive training has been shown to restore bone density to pretransplantation levels compared with an additional 6% loss in subjects who did not participate in resistance training. Marked increase in muscle mass, strength, and exercise capacity was also observed.[421]

## Guidelines for Activity and Exercise

Whether assessing aerobic, anaerobic ability, or activities of daily living (Table 21.4), measurements of vital signs, including blood pressure, heart rate, oxygen saturation, respiratory rate, and rate pressure products (heart rate and systolic blood pressure), can provide valuable information and can be used as measurable outcomes of treatment intervention.

In general, as the intensity of activity increases, the heart rate and systolic blood pressure increase, with a concomitant return to baseline with cessation of activity. The response the transplant recipient has to exercise will depend on the type of transplant, medications taken, and present level of fitness. For example, heart transplant recipients typically have a blunted heart rate response with exercise as a result of the denervated state of the heart.

Monitoring the recovery may provide an objective measure of improvement in physical capacity. Consistent abnormal responses should be reported to the physician for further evaluation. Other considerations are determined according to the underlying pathologic condition (e.g., cardiomyopathy, congestive heart failure, renal failure, diabetes, cirrhosis) and pretransplantation treatment (e.g., VADs, medications, dialysis).

For all transplant candidates and recipients, the duration of beginning aerobic exercise should be until fatigue begins; allow for a short recovery period and repeat in an interval manner until the duration is at least 20 minutes of continuous exercise. The goal is to perform at least 30 minutes of nonstop activity daily at a moderate exertional level before reducing exercise frequency to four to five times weekly. Individuals trying to control blood pressure or lose weight should work for a longer duration, 45 to 60 minutes, at a lower intensity (e.g., 50% to 65% of predicted maximal heart rate).[147] The exercise program should consider the recipient's comorbidities and be individualized to the needs and goals of the transplant recipient.[78,230]

## Limitations on Activity and Exercise

Transplant trauma is a theoretic possibility, so organ recipients are advised not to participate in contact sports. Except for this general broad precaution, limitations on sporting and exercise must be evaluated on a case-by-case basis and may be determined by the course of the illness. For example, a person who undergoes emergency liver transplantation for acute liver failure will have relatively little secondary damage. Therefore vigorous exercise training for competition is not contraindicated for healthy transplant recipients. However, cardiorespiratory fitness and strength training should progress gradually before the client engages in more strenuous sports participation.

A client with chronic renal failure can develop renal osteodystrophy, decreased bone density, osteoporosis, reduced peak cardiac output (because of the arteriovenous fistula required for vascular access), and irreversible neuropathies and myopathies. Anyone experiencing renal failure secondary to diabetes will have multiple other secondary complications.

Many other potential limitations on sporting and exercise must be recognized and evaluated, such as the condition of the recipient at the time of transplantation and the type of organ that has failed. For example, people with severe pulmonary disease necessitating heart-lung transplantation often experience malnutrition and muscle wasting before transplantation. Liver failure can cause abnormalities of lung function, including ventilation–perfusion mismatching, pulmonary hypertension, and loss of oxygen-diffusing capacity.

### Denervation

Denervation of the transplanted heart, pancreas, liver, or kidneys results in a loss of sympathetic nerves to the organ (e.g., loss of vagal response in the heart, impaired insulin in the pancreas, and altered renin responses in the kidney) requiring some modifications in the exercise

**Table 21.4** Exercise Guidelines for Organ Candidates and Recipients[a]

Weight training has become an acceptable component of a comprehensive exercise program. It is recommended to begin strength training at low-to-moderate intensity levels along with a progressive aerobic and stretching program. It is important to assess blood pressure response during exercise and evaluate for signs and symptoms of right-sided heart failure in the presence of pulmonary hypertension. Transplant recipients should also be monitored for hemoptysis, overuse injuries, poorly regulated glucose, electrolyte and nutritional imbalances and surgical precautions. Anyone with documented pulmonary hypertension may have associated signs and symptoms (light-headedness, dizziness, angina-like pain, decreased cardiac output with exercise, or development of abnormal heart sounds with exertion) and needs to be supervised during low-level interval exercises.

Once the person is medically stable and basic level of function is restored, the therapist can more accurately prescribe a supervised exercise program by completing a symptom-limited aerobic exercise test as well as a 1 or 3 RM. As a reminder, 1 RM is defined as the heaviest weight that can be lifted safely at the weakest position in the range of motion one time. The therapist must take into account any significant impairments present and the effects of long-term steroid use, especially muscle wasting, osteoporosis, and coagulopathy. Risk for injury is higher in this group when using 1 RM.

- Select an enjoyable activity or exercise and always have a goal. Some centers target a long-term goal by organizing an annual fun run/walk or join one already organized.
- Include adequate warm-up, stretching, and cooldown periods.
- Progress activity or exercise as described in text.
- Include interval training, aerobic activity, strength training, muscular endurance training, and flexibility.
- Combine activities and/or exercise program with energy conservation techniques.
- Maintain a normal breathing pattern; breath holding may contribute to excessive elevation in blood pressure and produce associated symptoms, such as dyspnea and light-headedness.
- Exercise 4–5 days a week; allow 24–48 hours recovery time after strenuous activity and 48 hours after moderate to vigorous resistance training for involved muscles.
- Follow guidelines for neuropathy and myopathy.

**Endurance Training: High Repetitions/30–90 Seconds High-Intensity Intervals/Low to Moderate Resistance**

- Muscle endurance: 2–3 days per week
- Weights that are 50%–60% of 1 RM (to cause fatigue in 30–90 seconds)
- Perform 12–30 repetitions per set at 30- to 90-second intervals
- Perform 2–5 sets of each exercise per workout

**Strength Training: Low Repetitions/3–8 Repetitions, Moderate to High Resistance**

- Strength training 2–3 days per week
- Determine actual and predicted 1 RM
- Resistance is high with goal of 3–8 repetitions, 70%–85% of 1 RM
- Perform 3–5 sets of each exercise per workout
- Consider closed kinetic chain functional activities
- Perform each exercise through a full functional range of motion

**Aerobic Training**

- Aerobic training completed 5 days a week for minimal 30 minutes of moderate intensity or 20 minutes of vigorous intensity
- Activity should use large muscles in repetitious manner
- Intensity 40%–85% of maximal work capacity

**Weight Training: Low Repetitions/More Resistance**

- Use weights that are 40%–60% of the 1 RM[b]
- Perform 3–8 repetitions per set
- Perform 3–5 sets of each exercise per workout
- Perform each exercise through a functional range of motion

**For the Therapist**

| Maintain or Monitor | Terminate Exercise If ... |
|---|---|
| Observe client response to exercise: allow minimal to moderate dyspnea; respiratory rate should be <30 breaths/min with minimal rales heard on auscultation | Respiratory rate >40 breaths/min with increased rales |
| Allow only mild level of fatigue; use RPE (Borg scale) | 3/10 on Borg scale |
| Maintain stable vital signs (HR, blood pressure); maintain stable cardiac output (RPP, PP) | HR exceeds target zone; decrease in SBP, PP narrows (SBP − DBP), decrease in RPP (RPP = HR × SBP) |
| Maintain stable ECG | Increased incidence of arrhythmias or perceived palpitations |
| Maintain CVP | Monitor in the presence of right-sided heart failure; maintain CVP at 20 mm Hg; terminate exercise relative to other symptoms |
| Maintain PAP | Rest is indicated if PAP rises 5 mm Hg; terminate exercise if PAP rises and persists after rest and/or in the presence of other symptoms |

**Table 21.4** Exercise Guidelines for Organ Candidates and Recipients[a]—cont'd

| Maintain or Monitor | Terminate Exercise If ... |
|---|---|
| Maintain oxygen saturation 90% (this is individually determined by each center according to each person's medical status) | Oxygen saturation <90% (or saturation below prescription) |
| Monitor for signs of bleeding | See Chapter 40 |
| Maintain or expect an increase in CVP | Change in mental status (e.g., level of confusion, hostility); onset of pallor or diaphoresis; client request |

*CVP*, Central venous pressure; *DBP*, diastolic blood pressure; *ECG*, electrocardiogram; *HR*, heart rate; *PAP*, pulmonary arterial pressure; *PP*, pulse pressure; *RM*, repetition maximum; *RPE*, rate of perceived exertion; *RPP*, rate pressure product; *SBP*, systolic blood pressure.

[a]Guidelines for exercise are modified for the organ recipient, but follow *ACSM's Guidelines for Exercise Testing and Prescription*. These are only guidelines; each exercise program must be individually tailored to the organ recipient's condition and comorbidities. Progression must be according to tolerance.

[b]Intensities of 80% to 100% have been shown to produce the most rapid gain in muscle strength within the normal population. However, because of the possibility of overtraining or injury in individuals before and after transplantation, caution must be used when overloading a muscle or muscle group.[6]

program. In contrast, surgical removal of sympathetic liver nerves does not inhibit hepatic glucose production during exercise, and denervation of the lungs does not impair the ability to increase ventilation during physical exertion.[230]

The denervated lung will experience reduced tidal volumes and decreased lung compliance. There is a delay in the bronchodilation response requiring an extended warm-up period to obtain the catecholamine response necessary for organ vasodilation and thereby increased tidal volume during exercise.[71,89]

There is evidence that reinnervation does occur to some extent for some recipients. For heart transplant recipients who have some degree of autonomic nervous system function restored, there is an increase in heart rate greater than 35 beats/min, with peak exercise levels and an immediate decrease in heart rate after exercise. This restoration results in an increase in exercise capacity that is closer to healthy age-matched control subjects.[356] Without a balance in parasympathetic-sympathetic responses, heart rate variability during and after exercise is impaired. In the absence of parasympathetic activity, an increase in blood pressure may occur during exercise. For the individual who does not experience parasympathetic recovery, exercises should be performed under supervision, with close monitoring of pulse and blood pressure (and possibly ECG) during the first several exercise sessions. Arrhythmias during the acute recovery period may be an early sign of rejection.[327]

## Medications

Besides the usual exercise-related risks anyone faces, recipients have additional medication-related risks associated with the long-term immunosuppressive therapy, including exaggerated hypertensive response, myopathies, neuropathies, osteoporosis, and fractures.

The adverse effects of immunosuppressive medications on skeletal muscle, including the muscle-wasting effects of glucocorticoids are well known. It is documented that quadriceps strength of renal transplant candidates is only 70% of normal, although this side effect can be counteracted by resistance exercise training.[195,196,356] Also documented are decreased type 1 muscle fibers and decreased capillary density as a result of calcineurin-inhibitor medications.[278] Other potential side effects[363] are listed in Tables 5.3 and 5.4; see also Immunosuppression under Posttransplantation Complications.

## Chronic Rejection

Finally, transplanted organs may be exposed to chronic rejection, limiting the function of the organ. With the decline in organ function, there is a decrease in exercise tolerance. For example, in heart transplant recipients, chronic rejection is associated with a decrease in cardiac output, onset of heart failure, and accelerated atherosclerosis.[462]

With lung transplantation, the recipient experiencing chronic rejection may present with an impairment in gas exchange, leading to desaturation and increased air trapping and work of breathing. However, despite all these variables, the benefits of exercise in maintaining a healthy lifestyle and sense of well-being are much greater than the risks (e.g., rejection, respiratory impairments) imposed by organ transplantation. Exercise should be reduced in duration and intensity but not necessarily discontinued during rejection episodes.[339]

## Psychosocial Factors

Although it is assumed that transplant recipients will spontaneously increase their physical activity after transplantation, fear of harming the new organ or protective family members may discourage vigorous activity. As a member of the transplantation team, the therapist should encourage a program of regular activity immediately after transplantation and provide exercise guidelines (specifically aerobic, resistive, and core exercise) as a part of the long-term transplantation care plan.

## Education

Education regarding the need for lifelong exercise to improve endurance, strength, and function specifically to counteract the deleterious effects of the immunosuppression regimen is essential to motivate the transplant recipient to succeed. It is recommended that the recipient be referred for supervised outpatient services because many studies have documented an increase in recovery with supervised exercise as opposed to a home exercise program.[421]

## HEMATOPOIETIC CELL TRANSPLANTATION

**Note to Reader:** Hematopoietic cell transplantation (HCT) is the preferred term, but you may still see this referred to as hematopoietic stem cell transplantation. Several excellent sources for more information are suggested: Harvard Stem Cell Institute (HSCI) (www.hsci.harvard.edu); Center for International Blood and Marrow Transplant Research (CIBMTR) (www.cibmtr.org); and Be the Match, from the National Marrow Donor Program (http://bethematch.org/).

### Definition and Overview

The purpose of this section is to introduce the therapist to the process of HCT and the adverse outcomes that can accompany this procedure. Hematopoiesis is the process by which all mature, functioning blood cells develop. Central to this process are hematopoietic stem cells (HSCs), which are undifferentiated cells that reside primarily in the bone marrow. HSCs are unique in that they are self-renewing and, in response to appropriate signals, able to differentiate into all types of mature, functional blood cells (Fig. 21.6). That is, the differentiation of HSCs gives rise to all approximately $10^{11}$ to $10^{12}$ new blood cells that are produced daily across all cell lineages.

Efforts to therapeutically replace or transplant the contents of the bone marrow and specifically provide new hematopoietic cells have been ongoing for more than a century. In the mid-1950s, bone marrow was unsuccessfully transfused into several nuclear workers who had received excessive radiation exposure. In 1959 it was reported that an individual with end-stage leukemia survived for 3 months after first receiving a lethal dose of radiation followed by an infusion of bone marrow collected from the patient's identical twin.[436]

These early efforts at HCT failed because little was known about tissue rejection and immune suppression. The identification of and ability to type the MHC or HLA system in humans in the early 1960s made it possible to match donor with recipient, thus reducing graft rejection.

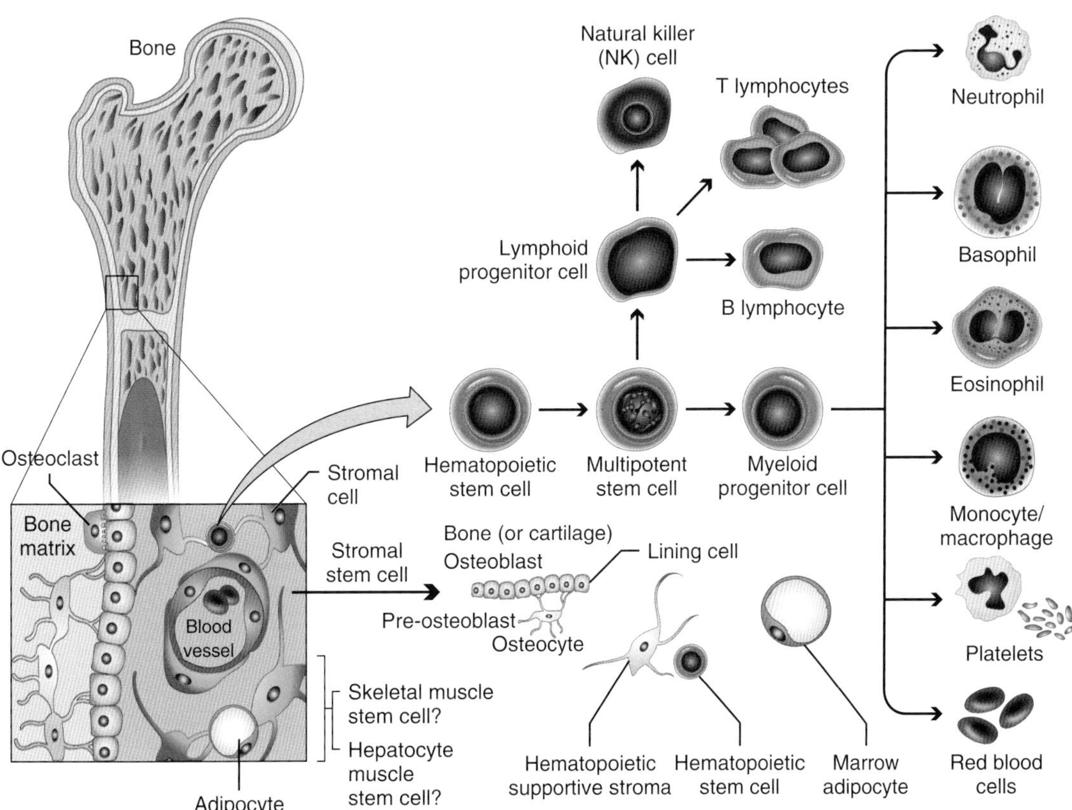


**Fig. 21.6**

**Adult stem cells.** Adult stem cells can be multipotent and have the capacity to differentiate into a limited number of different cell types, often restricted to a given tissue or organ system, as in the case of adult hematopoietic or epidermal stem cells. Two stem cell types have been isolated from adult bone marrow—the hematopoietic stem cell and the mesenchymal stem cell. Adult mesenchymal stem cells of bone marrow origin, although their range of differentiation has been shown to be broader than that of any other adult stem cell type, do not reach pluripotency (able to develop into different cells). It is thought that in some organ systems such as the gastrointestinal epithelium, a unipotent pool of progenitors exists for repopulating a rapid population turnover of only one type of cell—although it is difficult to be certain whether such progenitors can be distinguished from the overall population of fully differentiated cells in tissues with high cellular turnover. (From Goldman L, Schafer AI: *Goldman's Cecil medicine*, ed 24, Philadelphia, 2012, Saunders. Used with permission.)

This advance combined with the discovery of immunosuppression compounds such as cyclosporine reduced tissue rejection and brought about the modern era of HCT.[101]

Today, HCT is widely used to treat a number of blood diseases. Worldwide, more than 50,000 HCTs are performed annually,[483] and the number continues to increase each year, with 5-year survival rates exceeding 50% depending on the disease, age of the recipient, and source of donor material. There has been a dramatic increase of recipients older than 50 years in the last decade.[310]

## Diseases Treated by Hematopoietic Cell Transplantation

A variety of hematologic cancers are treated by HCT, including multiple myeloma, non-Hodgkin lymphoma, Hodgkin disease, acute and chronic myeloid leukemia, acute and chronic lymphocytic leukemia, and myelodysplastic syndromes. Multiple myeloma and lymphoma account for approximately 60% of all HCTs. Multiple myeloma continues to be the most common indication for autologous transplantation and acute myeloid leukemia for allogeneic transplantation.[343]

Noncancer blood diseases, including aplastic anemia, sickle cell anemia, severe combined immune deficiency, and thalassemia, may also be treated with HCT. Solid tumors, including medulloblastomas and germ cell tumors, have been treated with HCT. Age was once a limiting factor for receiving an HCT, but the introduction of less myeloablative induction regimens has allowed the transplantation of individuals older than age 70 years. Previously, HCT was used when all other treatment options had failed, but with improved outcomes HCT is increasingly used earlier in the disease process.[101]

## Sources and Types of Hematopoietic Cell Transplantations

HCTs can be of two types, depending on the source of the donated cells. If the donated cells come from the individual with the disease, the transplant is an *autologous* transplant. Candidates for this type of transplant have no demonstrable malignancy in the blood or bone marrow. Because the donated cells come from the recipient, antigenic incompatibility is reduced, resulting in lowered treatment-related morbidity and mortality rates. However, tumor relapse is more prevalent because of a lack of graft-versus-tumor effect (immunologic attack on the tumor by immunocompetent T cells and NK cells present in the donor graft) and the reinfusion of occult tumor in the graft.

Donor HSCs can also come from another individual, in which case the HCT is an *allogeneic* transplant. Preferably an allogeneic donor is an identical twin of the recipient because the twin should be genetically identical for the entire chromosome 6, the site of the HLA genes, thus reducing risk for posttransplantation morbidity. If an identical twin is not available, the search for a donor turns to individuals who are genetically related to the recipient—usually a sibling. While not perfect, such matched, related donors increase the likelihood of an optimal HLA match. Approximately 30% of HSC donors are related to the recipient.

If no related donors are available, the search turns to a matched *unrelated donor*. Such donors are found through bone marrow registries. An optimal HLA match between the donor and recipient drives donor selection so as to reduce the risk of posttransplantation morbidities including GVHD. The choice of performing a transplant using donor cells from an unrelated donor is generally determined by the urgency of the transplant.[101,159]

HSCs are collected from three different sites: bone marrow, peripheral blood, and umbilical cord blood (Fig. 21.7). In the past, HSCs collected from *bone marrow* aspirates served as the traditional source of HCTs; today, this is no longer the primary source of HSCs, now accounting for only approximately 20% of HCTs.[311]

These cells are collected from the bone marrow of the donor's superior iliac crest and require the donor to be anesthetized; a needle is inserted into the bone marrow to collect its contents. Adverse effects are generally rare and include discomfort at the harvesting site that typically lasts 1 to 2 weeks. Priming the bone marrow with granulocyte colony-stimulating factor increases the production of HSCs into the blood, reducing the required number of aspirations. Infrequently, additional collection of marrow is required for graft failure, but this is the exception not the rule.

A second (and now primary) source of HCTs comes from HSCs that circulate in the *peripheral blood*. Normally these cells are present in the blood in low numbers.

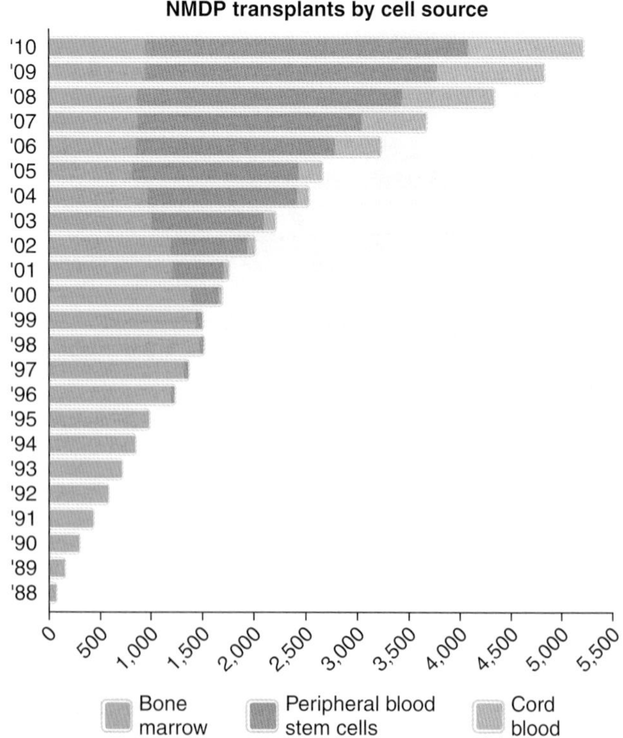


**Fig. 21.7**

**National Marrow Donor Program *(NMDP)* transplants by cell source, 2014.** (Courtesy National Marrow Donor Program. Used with permission.)

Priming the bone marrow with granulocyte colony-stimulating factor increases their number in the circulating blood. Collecting HSCs from the peripheral circulation is less complicated and more convenient than collecting bone marrow cells, which is why it has replaced bone marrow as the main source of HSCs. It is estimated mobilized peripheral blood cells account for approximately 91% of HCTs in children and 98% in adults.[343] Compared with bone marrow HSCs, those collected from the peripheral blood produce a more rapid hematopoietic reconstitution (engraftment) and a greater graft-versus-tumor effect. However, peripheral blood HSC grafts contain a greater number of T cells, increasing the risk for chronic GVHD; there is no increased risk of acute GVHD.[311]

A third source of HSCs is umbilical cord blood, the blood that remains in the *umbilical cord* and placenta after an infant is born. Use of cord blood as a source for transplantation has increased (see Fig. 21.7). This blood is rich in HSCs, which have superior proliferative capacity, but with fewer cells available compared with peripheral blood stem cells (PBSCs) and marrow. Other potential advantages include a large potential donor pool, rapid availability because the cord blood has been prescreened and tested, absence of malignant stem cells, no risk or discomfort to a donor, rare contamination by virus, and a lower risk of GVHD.

The use of cord blood requires less stringent HLA matching because mismatched cord blood cells are less likely to cause GVHD. Cord blood occurs in only small volumes, however, limiting the number of HSCs that can be collected from individual donors. In addition, hematopoietic reconstitution is slower when cord blood is used, increasing the risk for posttransplantation infection.[101,159]

## Transplantation of Hematopoietic Stem Cells

The transplantation of HSCs consists of several phases, including conditioning, harvest, infusion, preengraftment, and engraftment. *Conditioning* is a critical element in the HCT process. The primary purpose of the conditioning regimen is to render the recipient sufficiently immunosuppressed to prevent rejection of the graft and to eradicate any remaining malignant cells. Myeloablative conditioning is achieved by delivering a maximally tolerated dose of multiple chemotherapeutic agents with nonoverlapping toxicities, with or without radiation. This regimen is undertaken 7 to 10 days before transplantation; causes myelosuppression (myeloablative regimens); and has a number of potential adverse effects including mucositis, nausea, vomiting, alopecia, diarrhea, rash, peripheral neuropathies, and pulmonary and hepatic toxicity.

Nonmyeloablative preparative regimens are used in individuals with less aggressive tumors. These regimens use substantially lower doses of chemotherapy drugs and radiation than myeloablative regimens. These regimens are immunosuppressive but not myeloablative and rely on a graft-versus-tumor effect to kill tumor cells with donor T lymphocytes. They result in fewer adverse effects and are frequently used in individuals age 55 years or older and in people with notable comorbidities. All conditioning regimens result in some myelosuppression, which continues after completion of the preparative regimen. The nadir or low point in cell numbers or blood values typically occurs 5 to 7 days posttransplantation.

*Harvesting* involves the collection of HSCs and has been previously discussed. *Infusion* of the harvested cells is a relatively simple process that is performed at the bedside. HSCs are infused through a central vein over a period of several hours. The transplanted cells migrate to the bone marrow cavities by mechanisms that have not yet been fully elucidated. Once in the bone marrow, the goal is for the HSCs to begin repopulating the marrow with cells that will differentiate and mature into fully functioning blood cells.

The *preengraftment* period is the period when the transplanted cells migrate to the bone marrow and begin to populate this area. During this period recipients experience continued adverse effects of the induction strategies as white and red blood cell and platelet counts drop to their lowest value. With decline in circulating blood cell numbers, clinical manifestations can include nausea, vomiting, and hair loss, particularly if the individual has received ablative conditioning (side effects are not as likely for individuals receiving a reduced-intensity regimen).

During preengraftment, the recipient remains particularly vulnerable to infection. In fact, infection remains the primary cause of posttransplant, nonrelapse mortality. To help combat infection, some facilities keep patients in isolation rooms during this period, whereas others restrict these individuals to their units. All recipients receive antibacterial, antifungal, and antiviral prophylaxis during this period, as well as immunosuppression drugs such as tacrolimus. It is worth noting that these individuals have venous access devices in place, which further increases the risk for infection, thus requiring careful antisepsis on the part of all health care providers.

As the stem cells repopulate the bone marrow, hematopoiesis progressively improves, and circulating levels of blood cells increase. When cell numbers reach specific threshold levels, *engraftment* is said to have occurred. The time required for engraftment varies, but is generally 9 to 14 days from infusion (day 0) for PBSC, 12 to 18 days for marrow, and 25 to 56 days for cord blood transplants. Specifically, neutrophil engraftment has occurred in allogeneic transplant recipients when absolute neutrophil count exceeds 1500/mm$^3$ for 48 hours (normal values are 3000 to 7000/mm$^3$). This may take 3 to 4 weeks, but if complications occur (e.g., GVHD, infection, slow engraftment), the recipient may be hospitalized for months. A platelet count of 20,000 to 50,000 cells/mm$^3$ is a mark of platelet engraftment.

These measures suggest that the recipient now has some minimal inherent protection against infection and abnormal bleeding. Infection control prophylaxis and immunosuppression continue after engraftment has occurred. At this point, recipients may be discharged from the hospital, but at most transplantation centers, they are asked to remain within 1 to 2 hours travel time from the hospital until approximately 100 days posttransplantation. During this outpatient period, they are carefully monitored and treated for abnormal blood counts, infection, and symptom control.[159]

Box 21.5

**COMPLICATIONS ASSOCIATED WITH HEMATOPOIETIC CELL TRANSPLANTATION**

***Pretransplantation***

- Effects of immune suppression
  - Steroid myopathies, neuropathies
  - Immobility
  - Weakness
  - Renal failure
- Effects of chemotherapy and radiation therapy
  - Cognitive impairment
  - Neurologic impairment
  - Neutropenia
  - Thrombocytopenia
  - Hemorrhage
  - Anemia
  - Cardiopulmonary toxicity
    Arrhythmias
    Cardiomyopathy
    Interstitial pneumonitis
    Obstructive or restrictive disease
  - Nutritional deficits
  - Bone metastasis
  - Impaired skin integrity

***Posttransplantation***

- Infection
- Graft-versus-host disease
- Recurrence of malignancy
- Sterility
- Cystitis
- Venoocclusive liver disease
- Fatigue
- Hearing loss (ototoxic antibiotics)
- Delayed effects of radiation
  - Visual loss (cataract formation)

## Complications of Hematopoietic Cell Transplantation

Advances in transplantation techniques and supportive care strategies have resulted in significant improvement in survival for individuals who have undergone treatment. Subsequently, survivors of HCT are at risk of developing a range of long-term complications. Two-thirds of survivors of HCT develop at least one chronic health condition, and one-fifth develop severe or life-threatening conditions. HCT recipients who have survived for at least 5 years posttransplantation are at a fourfold to ninefold increased risk of late mortality for as long as 30 years after HCT, producing an estimated 30% lower life expectancy compared with the general population.[51]

Some people undergoing transplantation may already have significant multisystem damage, including cardiopulmonary, nutritional, musculoskeletal, and neurologic impairments secondary to either the underlying disease or its treatment. Bone metastasis, steroid myopathy, polyneuropathies, depleted protein stores, and impaired skin integrity are common comorbidities present before HCT (Box 21.5). Virtually all HCT recipients rapidly lose all T and B lymphocytes during and after conditioning, losing immune memory accumulated through lifetime exposure to infectious agents, environmental antigens, and vaccines.

Although not very common, neurologic complications occur in accordance with the stage of HCT. For example, during conditioning, drug-related encephalopathies and seizures or complications secondary to medical procedures are possible. During bone marrow depletion, metabolic and drug-related encephalopathies and seizures, septic cerebral infarctions, and hemorrhages may occur. The risk of neurologic complications is modest with myeloablative regimens and minimal with nonmyeloablative regimens.

Chronic immunosuppression results in infections by viruses and opportunistic organisms and late events such as central nervous system relapses of the original disease, neurologic complications of GVHD, and second primary malignancies.[238,411] Recurrence of malignancy is always a possibility. The frequency and type of neurologic complication depends on the type of HCT and the underlying disease.[382] Therapists should pay attention to altered levels of consciousness, headaches, motor or sensory deficits, visual disturbances, involuntary movements, cranial nerve palsies, or seizures, as these are clinically significant and may be a sign of neurologic complications.[232]

HCT recipients may be at an increased risk of developing hypertension, diabetes, congestive heart failure,[23] and dyslipidemia (referred to as cardiovascular risk factors), and these can potentially increase the risk of cardiovascular disease.[24] Recipients of allogeneic transplants are more likely to report diabetes and hypertension than control siblings and are more likely to report hypertension than autologous recipients.[32] Cardiac or pulmonary toxicity also may occur as a result of the irradiation and immunosuppressive drugs used to prepare candidates for the transplantation. Arrhythmias may be the first sign that a chemotherapeutic agent is becoming cardiotoxic. Interstitial pneumonitis, an inflammation of the lungs, is a common complication, especially among allogeneic transplantations, which leaves the person susceptible to obstructive small airways disease.

Infections and hemorrhagic complications during the period of bone marrow aplasia, emerging immune competence, and GVHD are the most life-threatening complications following HCT, and they may be fatal. Infections include early bacterial infections or later opportunistic infections, especially CMV interstitial lung disease. EBV-associated lymphoproliferative disorders (posttransplantation lymphoproliferative disorders) are a significant problem after stem cell transplantation from unrelated donors or mismatched family members.[186]

Other long-term complications of HCT include sterility/infertility, osteoporosis, cystitis, thyroid problems, cataract formation, cardiomyopathy, and venoocclusive liver disease. Neuromuscular changes, such as peripheral neuropathies, muscle cramping, and steroid myopathies, may also develop.[101,159] A condition known as *posttransplant distal limb syndrome* has been reported, with constant bilateral pain, bone marrow edema, and soft tissue swelling in the lower legs and ankles.[399] Decreased bone mineral density such as osteopenia has been identified in childhood survivors of BMT, which places them at higher risk for fracture or osteoporosis.[378]

The complications of PBSC transplantation are essentially the same as those of BMT, but hematologic recovery after PBSC transplantation is much more rapid (typically 11 to 14 days and as early as 9 days), thereby significantly shortening the period of postchemotherapy neutropenia (decreased neutrophils, a type of granular leukocyte used to fight infection) and thrombocytopenia (decreased platelets in peripheral blood). Faster engraftment makes PBSC transplantation a preferred procedure over BMT. However, there is no difference in overall survival between marrow and PBSCs as stem cell sources.[20]

Long-term psychologic effects of HCT on survivors are being reported, as more information becomes available from studies conducted over a period of 10 or more years. Adverse psychologic outcomes reported include anxiety, depression, somatic distress, and thoughts of suicide.[428]

## Prognosis

Enormous progress has been made in understanding the biology, therapy, and prophylaxis of transplantation and in extending the range of potential stem cell donors to include unrelated people. Dramatic advances have occurred in the prevention of serious infection, including CMV and fungal infections, formerly a significant cause of mortality.[318]

To gauge procedure-related toxicity, 100-day mortality, defined as death before 100 days after transplant, is often used. Relapse can occur in stem cell recipients as a result of the growth of residual cancer cells (e.g., leukemia) not killed by chemotherapy or radiation. Allogeneic transplants are associated with relatively high risks of GVHD, failure of engraftment, infections, and liver toxicity, resulting in high early mortality. Long-term survival rates are improved with HCT (compared with no HCT), but this type of transplantation does not confer a normal life span.[410,437]

Posttransplant toxicities with myeloablative regimens (not the case with reduced-intensity HCT) remain a major limitation to successful application of the procedure. Advancements in therapies before HCT, the conditioning regimen, and maintenance therapies have reduced the risk of posttransplant recurrence; however, primary disease recurrence continues to account for the majority of deaths in autologous transplant recipients.[318] New cancer, organ failure, and suicide are also cited as causes of death among long-term survivors after HCT. The incidence of suicide is infrequent but still higher among HCT survivors than among healthy subjects.[293,377]

Despite substantial morbidity and mortality after HCT in some cases, recipients with long-term survival are likely to experience good health. For recipients who survive more than 5 years after HCT, 93% are in good health, and 89% return to full-time work or school. Of individuals who survive 10 years after HCT, 88% report that the benefits of transplantation outweigh the side effects.[88]

Although the success rates of transplantation have been improving over time, the prognosis still depends on the underlying disease, delays in transplantation, associated risk of relapse (e.g., leukemia) and current remission state, the development of acute GVHD based on the level of match between donor and recipient, and the age of the recipient. There is no effective therapy for severe acute GVHD, and affected individuals rarely recover; however, the frequency and severity of GVHD have been declining owing to the use of high-resolution HLA typing and a decrease in total body irradiation. Research also suggests that advances in GVHD prophylaxis medications and use of bone marrow as a graft source could decrease the incidence of GVHD.[318]

With understanding of the many issues facing the individual receiving an HCT, one may wonder why anyone would agree to undergo such a challenging treatment. It may be helpful to remember that most people facing an HCT expect either certain death or a high probability of death without it. This perspective may help health care professionals working with these individuals to understand why the procedure is performed.

**SPECIAL IMPLICATIONS FOR THE THERAPIST 21.2**

### *Hematopoietic Cell Transplantation*

The therapist's subjective evaluation must include past medical and social history to assess other medical conditions; relevant past surgeries; living situation; and prior level of function, exercise, and activities.

The recipient must be asked directly about goals for therapy, and therapy should be aimed toward that goal if appropriate. Objective data may include assessment of strength; skin condition; general cognition; neuropathy and/or myopathy involvement; functional range of motion; and analysis of transfers, gait, and balance. The rate of perceived exertion (RPE) scale, oxygen saturation level, heart rate, and blood pressure in relation to activity level are also helpful tools to assess ability to function outside the hospital environment. Remember that each specific medical treatment regimen is associated with specific comorbidities.

The combination of these factors puts the person at risk for immobility and subsequent pneumonia, pressure ulcers, muscle weakness, and overall deconditioning. It is important to remember that autologous transplant recipients may receive treatment as outpatients, but allogeneic recipients may be hospitalized for 1 month or even considerably longer if complications occur.

Skin inspection and skin care are of primary importance to prevent pressure or shear injuries. Any skin opening is vulnerable to an opportunistic infection. The therapist must evaluate the need for appropriate footwear, turning schedules, specialized mattress surfaces, and chair or wheelchair cushions. The client must be instructed in self-inspection, especially when splinting is used to treat neuropathic weakness and proprioceptive loss.

In addition, long-term side effects of chemotherapy include peripheral neuropathy, and the prolonged use of steroids can induce steroid myopathy and osteoporosis. Any of these conditions places the individual at risk for falls and associated injuries.

## A THERAPIST'S THOUGHTS[A]

### *Falls Prevention*

During transplant induction and in the acute posttransplantation phase, recipients must be encouraged to remain mobile and maintain activities of daily living despite the many unpleasant symptoms present. The loss of white blood cells exposes the individual to infection, while the depletion of red blood cells reduces energy, resulting in profound fatigue and increasing the risk for falls. Oral mucositis is a painful condition that may be present as a consequence of chemotherapy and may make eating, and therefore available energy, deficient.

The increased risk of injury from falling with low platelet counts (e.g., subdural hemorrhage) makes activity and balance training and assessment during hospitalization increasingly critical. Cognitive impairment, including that due to medications such as pain medications and/or sedatives, also increases the risk of falls for these individuals.

At our facility, all HCT patients are automatically on falls precautions. We are constantly working on trying to reduce falls with our patients. There seems to be a greater risk of falls at night with toileting, whether with bed-to-commode transfers or even use of a urinal at the edge of the bed.

[a]Eva Gold, PT

### Exercise During and After Hematopoietic Cell Transplantation

**Note to Reader:** Although we report on results of studies examining the effects of physical activity and exercise on recipients during and after HCT, these studies are not all equal. Some studies specifically evaluate people receiving BMT, whereas others focus on broader HCT (which includes peripheral blood, cord blood, and bone marrow). Comparing outcomes from these various studies is a bit like comparing apples to oranges if different sources of hematopoietic cells are used in the transplantation process. So we encourage you to continue your own literature research and review based on the treatments your patients are receiving and modify your programs accordingly as new evidence becomes available.

Very early involvement of the therapist in designing an individualized and structured self-directed exercise program for recipients is of great benefit to their well-being and sense of control. There is also evidence that aerobic exercise can be safely carried out immediately after HCT and can partially prevent loss of physical performance,[127] depending on the medical and physical condition both before transplantation and after transplantation and chemotherapy.

Exercise capacity in BMT recipients is much lower when transplantation is preceded by cardiotoxic chemotherapy or irradiation. Reduced exercise endurance, reduced maximal $VO_2$, reduced rise in cardiac output during exercise, and reduced ventilatory anaerobic threshold are closely related to the potential effects of chemotherapy.[212]

Extremely abnormal responses require consultation with the physician before therapy is initiated or continued. These clients may need continuous monitoring over many therapy sessions rather than just using symptoms as a guide to exercise tolerance once a baseline is established.

Training studies of candidates before HCT to evaluate the impact of inactivity have not been performed. However, it has been demonstrated in individuals who have undergone BMT that a treadmill walking program started 18 to 42 days after transplantation results in significant improvement in maximal physical performance, walking distance, and lowered heart rate at a given workload.[131] Active exercise, muscle stretching, and treadmill walking have been shown to increase muscle strength after allogeneic BMT.[287]

Exercise in the form of 3 days/week aerobic exercise (20 to 40 minutes) plus 2 days/week of resistance training (bands or weights) performed 1 to 4 weeks before, during, and after transplantation can also help improve cancer-related fatigue, physical capacity, overall physical function, anger/hostility, pain, and global distress.[180,478] Interestingly, the EXIST (EXercise Intervention after Stem cell Transplant) study demonstrated no significant benefit of a high-intensity strength and interval training program on physical fitness or fatigue. However, major critiques of this article include concern for control group contamination as well as poor timing of patient education and intervention.[348]

Aerobic exercise improves the physical performance of peripheral stem cell recipients who have undergone high-dose chemotherapy. To reduce fatigue, this group of individuals should be counseled to increase physical activity rather than rest after treatment.[76] The therapist should be aware of potential side effects of cytokine growth factors used to mobilize peripheral stem cells, including bone pain, myalgias, and flu-like symptoms; some people may develop a low-grade fever.[306]

Pulmonary conditioning with inspiratory muscle training, muscular strengthening, and endurance exercises is important to help maintain mobility but must be balanced with pacing, prioritizing, and other energy conservation techniques as an important part of treatment.

Range of motion, supervised or assisted ambulation, and resistive or endurance exercises can be used. Active assisted and passive range of motion is sometimes required for joint disuse and stiffness. Resistive exercises in the form of functional activities, such as bridging, transfers, and walking, are individually prescribed.[103] Resistance training may also help offset the decreased bone mineral density observed in childhood survivors of BMT by increasing fat-free mass and decreasing the fat mass index (kg of fat mass/height [$m^2$]).[378]

Interval activity training combined with energy-conservation techniques is an important component of therapy because the client's blood counts drop (including hemoglobin count, resulting in anemia), thereby reducing the body's capacity for exertion or aerobic activity.

Decreased platelet counts increase the person's susceptibility to bleeding from minor injuries. The amount of resistance and the use of equipment to provide resistance depend on platelet count. The therapist must monitor blood values to avoid causing joint hemorrhage. Safety education is important, and assistive devices may be needed.

### A THERAPIST'S THOUGHTS[a]

***Physical Activity, Exercise, and Hematopoietic Cell Transplantation***

**From Eva Gold, PT**

The discussion of exercise is often a challenge with HCT recipients. To most of them, it does not make sense to exercise when they are sicker than they ever have been and are fighting for their life. So at our hospital we use the term "activity" whenever possible, and we do as much activity as possible with all HCT recipients, even though many are on experimental protocols and profoundly ill.

Our program ranges from supine exercises to treadmill and stationary biking, sometimes at very slow pace but often following Dimeo's interval idea (http://frankdimeofitnesss.blogspot.com/2013/03/how-to-do-interval-training.html), although trying to encourage hospitalized patients to exercise for 30 continuous minutes is typically challenging and probably inappropriate. We use the Borg Rating of Perceived Exertion. We encourage patients to work out in the rate of perceived exertion range of 11 (fairly light) to 13 (somewhat hard). With aerobic (treadmill, bike, or even walking in the halls) intervals, we encourage them to build up during the warm-up to 11, then push it toward 13, then back to 11, and up to 13—back and forth as tolerated. We have even had some lower-level patients walk on the treadmill, then sit in a chair on the stopped treadmill, then start up again.

Functional and energy levels vary so widely between patients and even with the same patient over time that we need to be quite creative and adjust with each treatment. Some patients who were very active before diagnosis may have a treadmill or bike in their room and use it frequently. It is important to ensure that these patients do not overdo their workouts.

**From Cyd Dashkoff, PT-CSLT**

During the recipient's stay in a hospital setting, the physical therapy and occupational therapy staff attempt to keep recipients active. We teach them how to follow daily blood counts, monitor their heart rate, and adjust activities accordingly. They are instructed not to allow their heart rate to get above a target heart rate determined by the formula: 220 − recipient's age × 60%.

[a]Eva Gold, PT, and Cyd Dashkoff, PT-CSLT

### Infection

Myelosuppression as a result of specific chemotherapeutic agents or drug combinations is the number one factor that predisposes the person to infection. Until bone marrow function returns, the HCT recipient is extremely susceptible to life-threatening infection, which requires all staff to practice interventions to minimize or prevent infection, such as good handwashing technique. Some facilities require surgical scrubbing and mask when going into a recipient's room.

Preventing infections among HCT recipients is preferable to treating infections. Any therapist working with this population is advised to obtain the guidelines for preventing opportunistic infections among HCT recipients available from the U.S. Centers for Disease Control and Prevention.[440]

Therapists and nursing staff must work closely together to prevent infection, recognize early signs of infection or rejection, and reinforce the educational program, which is complex and is often taught in a short time under less-than-ideal conditions. Very early on, therapists instruct recipients on deep breathing exercises, ventilatory strategies, and airway clearance including effective coughing technique as important ways of minimizing infections.

### Monitoring Vital Signs

Vital signs must be monitored before, during, and after exercise to assess each HCT recipient for an abnormal response. Monitoring responses over time during the recovery process can alert the therapist to any developing cardiopulmonary compromise. RPE and heart rate can also be used to monitor patients during exercise and activity, with a goal of keeping the RPE between 11 (fairly light) and 13 (somewhat hard) on the 6 to 20 scale. This scale correlates with expected heart rates, so adding a zero behind the RPE gives the likely heart rate at that level of exertion in healthy individuals.

The concept of routine monitoring applies to anyone who is seemingly healthy after transplantation and may also provide helpful information about when to advance an exercise program. Knowledge of past medical history and preexisting conditions that could affect physical conditioning is essential. Preexisting conditions in the presence of extended periods of inactivity can contribute to further physical deconditioning.

Normal changes in vital signs include an increased heart rate and increased systolic blood pressure proportional to the workload, with minimal change in diastolic blood pressure (no more than 10 mm Hg). Hypertension or the use of antihypertensive medications (or other medications) can alter the normal response of blood pressure to exercise. Recipients may be deconditioned with a less than normal (sluggish) blood pressure response.

### Monitoring Laboratory Values

In addition to monitoring vital signs, the therapist must be aware of daily laboratory values for red blood cells, white blood cells, and platelets. Each facility will have its own guidelines for activity and exercise based on blood counts. For example, in some facilities, absolute neutrophil count must be more than $500/mm^3$ on 3 consecutive days for allogeneic HCT recipients before ambulating in the hallway while wearing a high-efficiency particulate air filter mask. Individuals with platelets less than 10,000 $cells/mm^3$ may require transfusion before activity and exercise can be resumed or progressed. Resistive bands are used only if platelets are 20,000 $cells/mm^3$ or more. Exercise tolerance is not based on white blood cell count unless the count is elevated owing to infection with accompanying fever and elevated heart rate.[161]

Often symptoms are used as the primary measure of acceptable activity. Neutropenia precautions may be in effect, limiting activity outside the individual's room and requiring an N-95 (respirator and dust) mask whenever leaving the room. Platelet levels must be evaluated (thrombocytopenia) before chest percussion is performed.

aEva Gold, PT, and Cyd Dashkoff, PT-CSLT

# GRAFT-VERSUS-HOST DISEASE

## Overview

**Note to Reader:** Although GVHD is a complication of the use of HCT in bone marrow–depleted or immunodeficient patients, it is presented here as an independent section (rather than a subsection of Posttransplantation Complications) because of the impact it has on recipients. GVHD remains a major obstacle in the curative potential of allogeneic HCT. Recipients may find their underlying disease (e.g., leukemia) cured by HCT, only to die of the complications of GVHD.

The use of HCT in bone marrow–depleted or immunodeficient patients has resulted in the complication of GVHD. GVHD remains a major obstacle in the curative potential of allogeneic HCT.

GVHD does not occur with organ transplantation. In organ transplantation, it is host-versus-graft disease when the recipient recognizes the transplanted organ as foreign and rejects it because the recipient has a competent immune system. In individuals who receive HCT, there is no longer a competent immune system; HCT is the infusion of immunocompetent cells, which begin to recognize the recipient as foreign. In other words, GVHD occurs when immunocompetent T lymphocytes in the grafted material (donated stem cells) recognize foreign antigens in the recipient (person receiving cells), thus initiating an immune response against the recipient's tissues and rejection of the host/recipient.

GVHD may be acute, typically occurring within the first 100 days after transplantation, or chronic, usually developing 3 to 6 months after transplantation.[91] Chronic GVHD is associated with a reduced risk of relapse, mediated by graft-versus-tumor effect (Fig. 21.8). Acute GVHD remains the most significant complication of HCT, with survival dependent on the response to therapy. To date, it has not been possible to dissociate detrimental chronic GVHD and beneficial graft-versus-disease effect.[97,42,105,479]

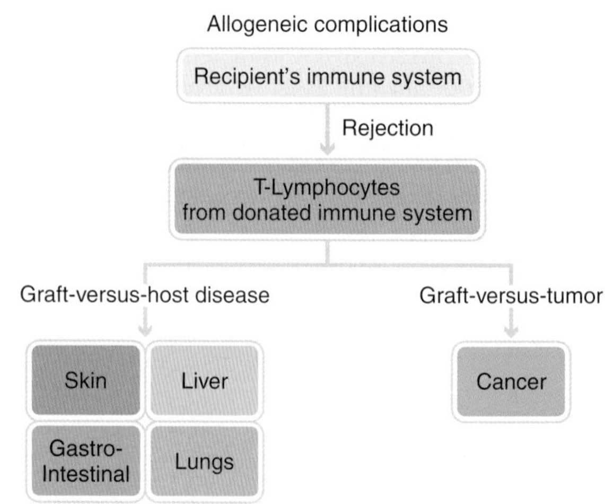


**Fig. 21.8**

**Several forces are at work inside a recipient's body when undergoing an allogeneic stem cell transplant.** First, remnants of the recipient's own immune system may attack the donated immune system, which is called *rejection*. Factors that help prevent rejection include finding the best possible match, total-body irradiation, and chemotherapy conditioning. A second complication occurs when the donated immune system T cells attack the recipient's own body, which is defined as graft-versus-host disease (GVHD). GVHD is not desirable in and of itself. However, if the donated immune system attacks the cancerous cells and destroys them, there is less chance of relapse and better long-term survival; this is a desirable situation. This effect is called graft-versus-tumor. Researchers are looking for ways to promote the graft-versus-tumor effect without causing GVHD. (Courtesy Linda M. Tripp, PT, University of Minnesota Medical Center, Fairview–University Campus, Minneapolis, MN. Used with permission.)

## Risk Factors

Key risk factors for the development of GVHD include older age of donor or recipient, source of allogeneic stem cells (higher risk for chronic GVHD with PBSCs than marrow and with marrow than cord blood), and degree of HLA disparity.[91] Donor/recipient sex mismatch increases the risk of GVHD; a female donor into a male recipient increases the risk over same-sex transplants.

Conditioning regimens containing total-body irradiation are associated with higher incidence and severity of GVHD compared with regimens involving only chemotherapy.[10] The disease state and the intensity of the conditioning regimen also influence the risk of developing GVHD. The fact that individuals prepared with low-dose conditioning regimens and transplanted with cells from HLA-identical siblings have an incidence of acute GVHD of 40% speaks to the biologic challenges of HCT.[42,105]

## Clinical Manifestations

### Acute Graft-Versus-Host Disease

Acute GVHD primarily involves the skin, with the liver and gastrointestinal tract being secondary sites. Diagnosis may be challenging and require tissue-based diagnosis because posttransplant infections, diarrhea, or other transplant-related toxicities could be the causative agent, rather than acute GVHD. Signs and symptoms of GVHD include fever, skin rash (first affecting the palms, soles of the feet, back of the neck, and shoulders but with eventual spread throughout the body possible), hepatitis, diarrhea, abdominal pain, ileus, vomiting, and weight loss. Ocular involvement may also occur.

If acute GVHD progresses, skin involvement may advance from 25% or less of the integument to spread over the entire body. The skin rash may progress to skin blistering, desquamation, and erythema. The presence of a damaged integument increases the risk of infection with normal skin flora; for individuals with severe skin involvement, medical management is similar to that used to care for severe burns.

Diagnosis of hepatic GVHD is graded primarily on serum bilirubin levels, but in the absence of specific tests for liver involvement, diagnosing hepatic GVHD may be questionable. Gastrointestinal GVHD may cause nausea, anorexia, pain, and watery secretory diarrhea. Endoscopy and mucosal biopsy are used to diagnose gut GVHD. Fluid loss may be high in these patients making frequent monitoring of electrolytes and intake/output measurements essential.[42,105,479]

Low-level GVHD (grades 1 and 2 acute GVHD) does not typically substantially impair quality of life. However, grades 3 and 4 acute GVHD have a poorer prognosis.

### Chronic Graft-Versus-Host Disease

Chronic GVHD affects upwards of 70% of recipients who survive 100 days beyond HCT. Chronic GVHD manifests similarly to an autoimmune disease. Common characteristics include scleroderma-like hardening of skin, muscle pain or weakness, and joint contractures that may severely decrease function.[344]

Gastrointestinal symptoms may include mucositis of the oral mucosa, progressing into the remainder of the gastrointestinal tract with esophageal narrowing and dysphagia, chronic diarrhea, and malabsorption. The patient may develop dyspnea and nonproductive cough (constrictive bronchiolitis, formerly known as bronchiolitis obliterans). Hepatitis and cholestasis are also common symptoms (Box 21.6).

Generalized polyneuropathy coincident with the occurrence of GVHD has been reported. The neuropathy affects proximal and distal muscles and demonstrates hyporeflexia or areflexia. Electrophysiologic studies do not meet strict criteria for demyelination. The signs of neuropathy may improve after immunosuppressive treatment has been completed or simultaneously with the resolution of GVHD.

There is some evidence that individuals with cancer who undergo HCT are at risk for cognitive deficits. Patients with cumulative clinical risk factors (e.g., length of hospital stay, history of cranial irradiation, intrathecal chemotherapy, allogeneic transplantation, unrelated donor, and post-HCT complications such as severity of mucositis and enteritis as well as GVHD) are more likely to demonstrate cognitive decline and diminished neuropsychologic recovery over time than recipients who have fewer risk factors. Individuals who have a complicated clinical course should be referred for evaluation and management of cognitive deficits.[216]

Box 21.6

**SIGNS AND SYMPTOMS OF GRAFT-VERSUS-HOST DISEASE**

***Gastrointestinal***

- Mucositis
- Esophageal inflammatory changes (esophageal narrowing, dysphagia)
- Abdominal cramping
- Nausea, vomiting
- Diarrhea, malabsorption
- Anorexia
- Ileus
- Hepatic injury (hepatitis, cholestasis)

***Pulmonary***

- Constrictive bronchiolitis (formerly bronchiolitis obliterans)
  - Wheezing
  - Rapid, shallow breathing
  - Nonproductive cough
  - Skin and soft tissue retractions during respirations
  - Fever
  - Cyanosis
  - Dehydration
  - Respiratory failure
- Progressive dyspnea

***Integument***

- Hypopigmentation or hyperpigmentation of the skin
- Progressive maculopapular rash
- Sclerodermatous changes
- Pressure ulcer formation
- Alopecia
- Photosensitivity
- Keratoconjunctival sicca

***Neuromusculoskeletal***

- Generalized polyneuropathy
- Muscle wasting and weakness
- Distal joint pain and stiffness
- Joint contractures (chronic graft-versus-host disease)
- Changes in deep tendon reflexes (hyporeflexia or areflexia)
- Guillain-Barré syndrome (rare)
- Polymyositis (rare)

***Other***

- Hemorrhage
- Infection
- Vision changes (dry eyes, blurred or double vision)
- Severe headaches

## MEDICAL MANAGEMENT

**Prevention and Treatment.** GVHD is a multisystem alloimmune disorder characterized by immune dysregulation, immunodeficiency, impaired organ function, and decreased survival. Virtually all organs and organ systems in the body are adversely impacted by chronic GVHD, and management is focused largely on immunosuppression therapies.[56] The therapy regimen is not standardized and varies by individual institution.

Mitigating the risk of GVHD can be done by finding the best match possible for allogeneic cells, depleting T lymphocytes in the donated stem cells, and using prophylactic immunosuppressives (e.g., cyclosporine or tacrolimus). Although antirejection drugs such as tacrolimus and cyclosporine are given prophylactically, approximately 40% to 90% of individuals receiving HCT still develop acute GVHD.[42,56,105,479] Untreated GVHD is often fatal as a result of hemorrhage and infection.

High-dose corticosteroids are the preferred treatment for acute GVHD. The dosages of steroids used to treat GVHD as well as pulmonary hemorrhage and engraftment syndrome in patients following HCT are significantly greater than the dosages used in treating rejection in organ transplantation. Additionally, steroids have their own adverse effects (avascular necrosis, osteoporosis, steroid myopathy, diabetes, and glaucoma) further adding to the symptom burden of these patients.

Treatment with immunosuppressive therapy, including prednisone, cyclosporine, tacrolimus, thalidomide, or a combination of these agents, has improved the long-term prognosis for people with chronic GVHD. Even so, high-dose corticosteroids increase the risk of infection and myopathy, and there is a high mortality rate. Chronic GVHD may resolve slowly (sometimes taking years) with gradual restoration of cell-mediated and humoral immunity function.

GVHD plays an important role in function and overall quality of life. Fatigue, dyspnea, gastrointestinal side effects, worries/anxieties, and skin problems can create severe impairments of quality of life in survivors of HCT with GVHD. Taking into account that the prevalence of GVHD might be higher in patients after PBSC transplantation compared with recipients after BMT, PBSC transplantation may lead to more severe impairments of quality of life than BMT.[341,353]

**Future Trends.** Many other treatment strategies are under investigation, such as donor lymphocyte infusion, tandem transplants, and use of NK cells.

*Donor lymphocyte infusion* is an important therapeutic intervention for treating individuals who have relapsed or developed refractory disease following allogeneic HCT. The procedure, involves, infusing peripheral lymphocytes collected from the original HCT donor with the goal of hastening or intensifying the graft-versus-disease (in the case of leukemia, graft-versus-leukemia) reaction.[304] Donor lymphocyte infusion has proven to be most effective against chronic myeloid leukemia but with some success against other leukemias, multiple myeloma, and lymphomas. Despite the utility of donor lymphocyte infusion, postinfusion development of GVHD remains a significant problem.[117]

*Tandem transplants* are used in clinical trials in an effort to increase survival in select individuals with multiple myeloma and other types of cancer. This process of tandem stem cell transplants involves receiving two autologous stem cell transplants weeks apart or an autologous transplant followed by reduced-intensity conditioning and an allogeneic stem cell transplant.[305,317]

*NK cells* are components of the innate immune system, capable of recognizing targets without prior sensitization in order to recognize and attack malignant cells. They provide a first line of defense against malignant cells and virally infected cells. In an effort to make use of the anticancer properties, NK cells can be collected and infused to try to kill tumor cells. NK cell therapy can be used as a stand-alone treatment in individuals with lymphoma, breast cancer, or ovarian cancer.

NK cells may be infused before HCT to achieve remission in relapsed acute myelogenous leukemia with a poor prognosis or with umbilical cord transplant for relapsed leukemia. They may be infused after HCT in an effort to kill remaining tumor cells, prevent relapse, promote engraftment, and mediate control of infections without inducing GVHD.

Treatment precautions for individuals receiving NK cells are based on the protocol, the specific concerns of the physician for that patient, and other factors. Precautions may vary from clinical site to site, but these individuals usually are permitted to ambulate in the halls, even though their absolute neutrophil count is below 500 cells/mm$^3$, as long as they wear an N-95 mask. In other facilities, such patients may not be permitted to leave their rooms to walk in the hallways even with a mask.[148]

SPECIAL IMPLICATIONS FOR THE THERAPIST 21.3

### *Graft-Versus-Host Disease*

Early symptoms of GVHD (see previous discussion in this chapter) usually appear within 10 to 30 days after transplantation and may include rash, dryness of eyes, blurred or double vision, severe headaches, distal joint pain and stiffness, hepatomegaly, persistent nausea and vomiting, stomach cramps, and diarrhea. For a video of an assessment protocol for chronic GVHD[82] see http://www.fhcrc.org/en/labs/clinical/projects/gvhd.html.

Although some cardiopulmonary abnormalities can be detected only by echocardiography, early warning symptoms of cardiopulmonary complications, such as progressive dyspnea, sensation of heart palpitations, irregular heartbeats, chest pain or discomfort, or increasing fatigue, may be reported by the recipient or observed by the therapist. The physician must be notified of such changes, and modifications must be made to the exercise program for mildly to moderately abnormal responses.

In most centers, there is no waiting period for exercising in individuals undergoing HCT. Stationary bikes in isolation rooms can be provided. Strengthening exercises for large proximal muscle groups are prescribed. Manual therapy, exercise, and education are aimed at improving functional mobility and quality of life. Modification of activities, home safety, and ambulation devices when warranted are included. The therapist should watch for steroid myopathy. An extended period of time may be required before normal strength and function return owing to the combination of fatigue and steroid myopathy.

**From the National Marrow Donor Program**

The National Marrow Donor Program has resources that can be very useful for clinicians as well as recipients. To view their Allogeneic and Autologous Transplant Guidelines, visit https://bethematchclinical.org/Resources-and-Education/Materials-Catalog/HCT-Guidelines-for-Referral-Timing-and-Post-Transplant-Care/. These are available in a mobile application, online, and in print. The posttransplant guidelines toolkit contains posttransplant care recommendations for late effects and screening for GVHD.

## ORGAN TRANSPLANTATION

### Kidney Transplantation

#### Overview

The first kidney transplantation, performed in 1954 by Joseph Murray, resulted in a successful graft and provided the recipient with an additional 8 years of life. It was the first organ transplantation of any kind ever performed, with the success largely credited to the live donor (adult twin brother). Kidney transplantation remains the most common type of solid-organ transplant (see Table 21.1).

As people older than age 65 years become the fastest growing segment of the population, the number of cases of ESRD requiring kidney transplantation will continue to increase. Diabetes is now the most common cause of ESRD.[348] Almost half of adults undergoing transplantation already have diabetes.[451]

Kidney transplant remains the most successful form of treatment for ESRD and, in the case of diabetes, offers an opportunity to eliminate dependence on dialysis and exogenous insulin. Simultaneous kidney-pancreas transplantation has become a safe and effective method to treat advanced diabetic nephropathy and results in stable metabolic function, reduced cholesterol, and improved blood pressure control.[427]

Until recently, almost all candidates for renal transplantation had been treated for months or years with hemodialysis; now it is possible to plan a kidney transplant before the complete shutdown of the kidney or kidneys, avoiding dialysis completely. Studies show that when dialysis is used, peritoneal dialysis is associated with a lower incidence of delayed graft function and may be preferred over hemodialysis.[52,464]

Continuous ambulatory peritoneal dialysis is a maintenance system of dialysis in which an indwelling catheter permits fluid to drain into and out of the peritoneal cavity by gravity. The individual is able to complete this type of dialysis three or four times per day while at home rather than coming to a hemodialysis clinic three or four times per week for 3 or 4 hours at a time while the blood is filtered through a dialysis machine.

Receiving a kidney transplant without prior experience of the burden of hemodialysis or peritoneal dialysis may lead to fixation on the side effects of antirejection drugs and potential complications of surgery. Conversely, a person receiving a kidney transplant with a prior history of dialysis may view liberation from dialysis as a welcome relief.

## Indications and Incidence

As mentioned, the primary indication for renal transplantation is type 1 diabetes with ESRD, which occurs in more than one-third of all cases of type 1 diabetes.[169] Cardiac autonomic neuropathy develops as a result of uremia and diabetes, with severe cardiac dysfunction when these conditions are present at the same time. Both kidney transplantation and kidney-pancreas transplantation result in improved cardiac autonomic function and modulation of heart rate.[64]

A less common indication for kidney transplantation is polycystic kidney disease, especially when combined with polycystic liver disease. As of 2018, more than 95,000 people were waitlisted for kidney-alone transplant, while just over 19,000 transplants were performed in the prior year.[448]

## Transplantation Candidacy

For updated guidelines describing general recommendations for kidney transplant candidacy please visit the Kidney Disease: Improving Global Outcomes (KDIGO) organization website at https://kdigo.org/mission/. It should be noted that these guidelines serve as general recommendations rather than a protocol or standard of care. These guidelines recommend the consideration of all individuals with chronic kidney disease grades 4 and 5 (glomerular filtration rate <30 mL/min/1.73 m$^2$) who are expected to progress to end-stage renal disease for kidney transplantation. for kidney transplantation. However, known psychiatric disorder impairing decision making, medical nonadherence, multiple myeloma, light chain deposition disease, active malignancy, end-stage lung disease, systemic amyloid, nonhealing extremity wounds with active infection, and progressive neurodegenerative disease may preclude referral for transplant evaluation.[227]

While recipient age is an important consideration for many transplant surgeries, recent studies suggest a survival advantage in elderly adults treated with kidney transplant versus maintenance dialysis therapy, even with the use of ECD organs.[294] Individuals with type 1 diabetes younger than 45 years of age with little or no atherosclerotic vascular disease are ideal candidates for a combined kidney-pancreas transplantation. The addition of a pancreas transplant is associated with greater morbidity and may require higher levels of immunosuppression but can result in stabilization of neuropathy and improved quality of life.[32]

Some renal transplant candidates are at high risk for sometimes fatal cardiac events. Analysis of the clinical risk factors (including age at least 50 years, type 1 diabetes mellitus, and abnormal ECG) may assist in identifying candidates who may be at risk for cardiac death.[255]

## Transplantation Procedure

Kidney grafts may be positioned intraperitoneally, anastomosed to the iliac vessels, and then drained into the bladder (Fig. 21.9); extraperitoneally in the iliac fossa through an oblique lower abdominal incision; or, in small children, retroperitoneally with a midline abdominal incision. The diseased or damaged kidney may or may not be removed from the patient. The new kidney will usually start to work right away, but it may not start producing urine for 10 to 14 days.

More recently, a procedure called *laparoscopic nephrectomy* was introduced to remove the live-donor kidney. Four small incisions called ports are made in the abdomen. The ports allow the surgeon to insert the laparoscope and other instruments used in the procedure to clamp off arteries and the ureter and cut the kidney loose.

## Complications

As with other solid-organ transplantation, renal recipients experience graft dysfunction, organ-related infection, and graft rejection as the three most common complications. Surgical complications include renal artery thrombosis, urinary leak, and lymphocele, although chronic rejection accounts for most renal allograft losses after the first year following transplantation. Donor organ quality, delayed graft function, and other donor and recipient variables leading to reduced nephron mass are nonimmunologic factors that contribute to the progressive deterioration of renal graft function.[295]

Cardiovascular and cerebrovascular diseases are major causes of morbidity and mortality after kidney transplantation. Extensive carotid vascular wall abnormalities increase significantly despite kidney and pancreas

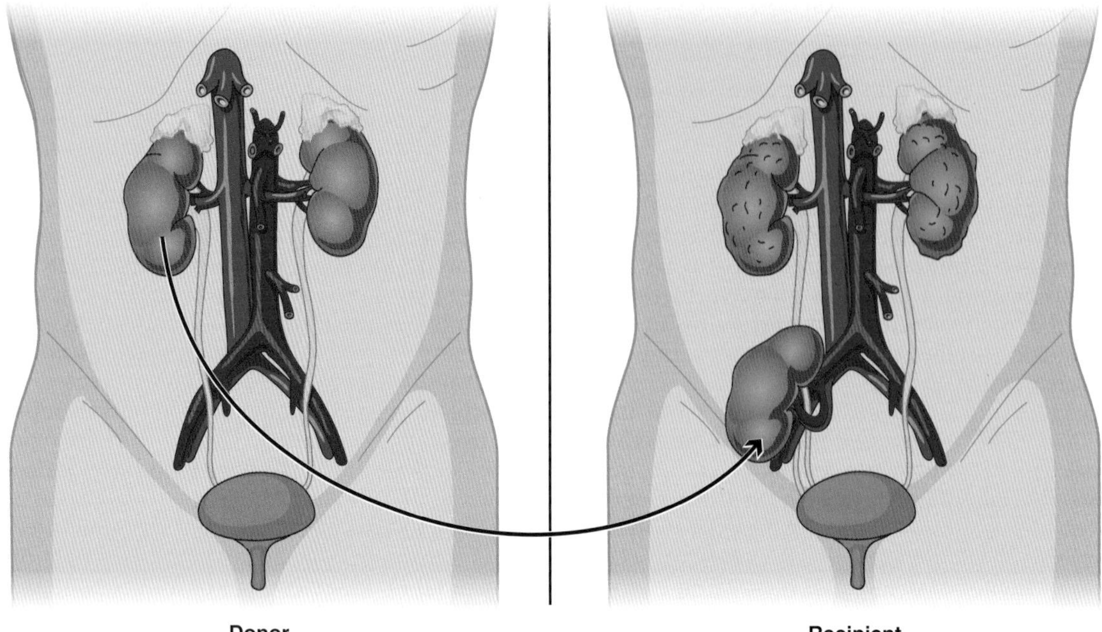


**Fig. 21.9**

**In a minimally invasive live-donor kidney transplantation, surgeons remove the donor's kidney through a 3- to 4-inch incision below the donor's umbilicus.** For the recipient, blood vessels of the donor kidney are attached to the major abdominal blood vessels. The ureter of the donor kidney is attached to the recipient's bladder. The donor kidney begins working immediately. The recipient's own malfunctioning kidney is not always removed.

transplantation in individuals with type 1 diabetes mellitus and progressive uremia. Although initiation of plaque development is related to systemic factors, progression of established plaque is largely influenced by local factors within the arterial wall and therefore unaffected by organ transplantation.[302] In fact, research shows an association between CMV infection and atherosclerotic plaque formation in coronary heart disease, a finding that has also been reported in posttransplant cardiac complications in kidney recipients with CMV.[202]

Other complications may include renal dysfunction with prolonged use of cyclosporine, hypertension, lipid disorders, hepatitis, cancer, and osteopenia. Hypertension occurs in up to 80% of renal graft recipients. In developed countries, approximately 8% of kidney transplant recipients are infected with hepatitis C virus.[384,390] There is a high degree of impaired bone formation associated with renal grafts, resulting in severe osteoporosis compared with other organ transplantations.

Basal cell and squamous cell carcinomas, Kaposi sarcoma, lymphomas, and posttransplant lymphoproliferative disease are 20 times more frequent in this population. Kidney cancer is 15 times more common after kidney transplantation compared with the general population. Melanoma, leukemia, hepatobiliary tumors, and cervical and vulvovaginal tumors are five times more likely compared with the general population. Testicular and bladder cancers are three times more common.[220]

Pelvic congestion syndrome can occur in a kidney donor or recipient when removal of the kidney ligates the ovarian vein. Retrograde flow in the ovarian vein causing ovarian varicosities (varicose veins of the ovaries) with venous stasis produces congestion and chronic pelvic pain in some women.[41] Imaging studies have verified the fact that there are very few venous valves in the blood vessels of the pelvic area.[140,188,432] Any compromise of the valves or blood vessels in the area can result in pelvic congestion syndrome.

## Prognosis

According to 2008–2015 data from the OPTN, patient survival rates for cadaveric and living kidney donation at 1 year and 5 years are 93.2% versus 97.5% and 74.4% versus 85.6%, respectively. Per the U.S. Renal Data System Report in 2016, the 10-year survival rate remains high but is similarly influenced by whether the transplant was received from a living or deceased donor. The probability of returning to dialysis or undergoing retransplantation is much less now for all donated sources.[459]

While living donor kidney transplant recipients generally demonstrate superior survival, expanded criteria for donor kidneys are not associated with increased mortality or transplant failure in recipients older than 70 years. For all types of donors, the persistent association between living donor kidneys and lower all-cause mortality across all ages suggests that, if possible, elderly recipients gain longevity from living donor kidney transplant.[294]

The National Kidney Foundation reports average survival rates of kidney-pancreas transplants to be 95% at 1 year and 92.5% at 3 years after transplantation.[308] The success rates are good for combined kidney-pancreas transplants from deceased donors, but the best results are usually achieved with a closely matched kidney from a living donor (usually from a sibling). The next best results are achieved with a kidney from a less closely matched living donor (such as a spouse or friend).[307]

## Future Trends

The renal research community has made great strides in improving client outcomes on dialysis and following organ transplantation. However, only a small fraction of individuals with ESRD undergo transplantation because of a lack of donor organs. As a result, novel innovations that aim to increase organ availability or treat primary disease are needed. , requiring continued research to find other methods of successful treatment. For example, preserving donor organs more effectively may ensure better graft survival rates. Alternatively, preserving donor organs more effectively may ensure better graft survival rates. Because both glomerular and tubular functions are inhibited at temperatures below 18°C (64.4°F), efforts to improve organ preservation techniques are under way.[339,424] Research is also ongoing to use stem cell therapy in the treatment of acute kidney injury associated with diabetes, vascular disease, or chronic kidney disease.[439]

New directions in dialysis research include cheaper treatments, home-based therapies, and simpler methods of blood purification toward the goal of ambulatory dialysis. Innovations in the field of artificial kidney include the use of miniaturization, microfluidics, and nanotechnology, research that may lead to a new era of transportable, wearable dialysis. Some wearable ultrafiltration systems and wearable artificial kidneys use extracorporeal blood cleansing as a method of blood purification, whereas others use peritoneal dialysis as a treatment modality.[369] A wearable artificial kidney worn as a belt has demonstrated safety and feasibility over short duration in clinical trials.[172,338] This unit can provide continuous dialysis, weighs about 10 lb, and runs on two 9-volt batteries. The wearable artificial kidney would allow individuals to continue with normal daily activities while providing gentle dialysis that mimics normal kidney function more closely than standard dialysis.[113,369]

A complete system for hemofiltration in neonates and infants (referred to as CA.R.PE.DI.E.M. [CArdio-Renal PEdiatric DIalysis Emergency Machine]) has been developed. The miniaturization of a dialysis circuit for acute

**SPECIAL IMPLICATIONS FOR THE THERAPIST 21.4**

### *Kidney Transplantation*

As an increasing number of studies document the effectiveness of exercise in disease prevention and prevention of transplant complications, timely and effective rehabilitation programs will be implemented. Physical and occupational therapy can offer a great deal to aid renal rehabilitation, especially to increase endurance and physical strength and to improve function and independence.

Given the high rate of malignancies in this population, the therapist should continue to work with the recipients in cancer education and prevention. Cancer screening is an important ongoing feature of any physical therapy examination and evaluation with this population. Skin protection and tobacco use cessation should be emphasized as part of patient education by all health care professionals, including physical therapists.

#### Acute Care Phase

Most kidney recipients are discharged about 5 days after surgery and are not seen by the therapist until later in the recovery process (or perhaps not at all) as an outpatient, approximately 1 month postoperatively. At that time, the recipient will most likely still be monitoring both blood pressure and blood glucose levels. The therapist should pay close attention to both measurements as the rehabilitation component is added.

#### Exercise

Kidney transplants have been performed longer than any other organ transplant, providing a greater number of retrospective studies to assess the influence of exercise on kidney transplantation. It has been shown that pretransplantation and posttransplantation exercise training improves lipid profile, increases hematocrit level, normalizes insulin sensitivity, and lowers the requirement for antihypertensive medication.[162,163] Posttransplantation exercise in kidney recipients has been associated with improved $VO_2$ peak and quality of life; however, it appears to have no direct influence on allograft function.[323]

Although a kidney transplant recipient may be normotensive at rest, there is an elevated blood pressure response to exercise, possibly caused by altered function of blood pressure control and by the effects of cyclosporine. This requires careful monitoring and documentation of vital signs in exercise program planning and assessment.

Training effectively modifies factors known to be associated with atherogenesis and cardiac disease in hemodialysis clients. However, exercise training alone after renal transplantation is not enough to modify the cardiovascular risk profile. Research to determine the effects of multiple risk interventions is needed.[340]

Before transplantation, clients with kidney disease, especially those receiving hemodialysis, are susceptible to bone loss as a result of altered vitamin $D_3$ function and its role in calcium absorption. Resistive exercises can help increase bone density (in the general population and in all organ transplantations) and should be initiated before transplantation or as early after transplantation as possible.[62,247,297]

Overuse tendon injuries occur at a high rate in kidney transplant recipients[7,299]; whether the mechanism for this is immunologic, metabolic, or medication induced remains unclear. The use of fluoroquinolones (potent oral antibiotics such as levofloxacin, ciprofloxacin, and norfloxacin) has been linked as a responsible factor.[271,286,488] The Achilles is the most commonly reported tendon injury, but injury can occur in the upper extremities as well. For anyone taking fluoroquinolones, care should be taken to avoid overloading tendons, as dramatic ruptures following even small trauma have been reported.[406]

The deep inferior epigastric artery, which feeds the lower rectus abdominis muscle, is usually transected in kidney transplantation. The therapist will have to take this into account when prescribing exercises and addressing core strength. Studies investigating whether preservation of the deep inferior epigastric artery can prevent lower rectus abdominis muscle atrophy show that this is possible.[210] The therapist should read the operative report to determine the status of the lower rectus abdominis muscle before beginning rehabilitative efforts.

**Table 21.5** Liver Transplantation

| Indications | Possible Contraindications |
|---|---|
| Primary biliary cirrhosis | Sepsis |
| Neoplasm (selected cases) | Hepatic lymphoma |
| Acute fulminant liver failure | AIDS |
| Inborn errors of metabolism | Poor client understanding |
| Alcoholic cirrhosis after documented treatment and recovery | Alcoholic cirrhosis (documented continued abuse) |
| Drug-induced liver disease | Cirrhosis secondary to drug abuse |
| Chronic active hepatitis (see text) | Chronic active (type B) hepatitis |
| Neonatal cholestasis (bile suppression) | Advanced cardiopulmonary disease |
| Biliary atresia | Inability to follow up with treatment |
| Sclerosing cholangitis | |
| Budd-Chiari syndrome | |
| Congenital hepatic fibrosis | |
| Cystic fibrosis | |

kidney injury in pediatric patients may help reduce the high mortality rate (more than 50%) for these patients.[368]

## Liver Transplantation

### Overview

The first human liver transplantation was performed in 1963. In 1989, surgeons at the University of Chicago developed the live-donor transplant that requires only a lobe or small piece of the liver. While this technique permits for expanded live-donor organ donation,[69] it is less frequently used, owing to health concerns for the living donor.[3,300,443] More than 160,000 liver transplantations have been performed.[452]

### Indications

Orthotopic liver transplantation has become an established therapy for end-stage liver disease (e.g., cirrhosis caused by alcoholism, hepatitis C), acute liver failure, and primary biliary cirrhosis or primary sclerosing cholangitis, as well as for nonalcoholic cirrhosis and hepatic or biliary malignancy.

Biliary atresia (bile ducts not formed normally) is the most common indication for pediatric liver transplantation. There are 500 pediatric liver transplants performed annually; more than half are for biliary atresia. Other indications include neonatal cholestasis (children born with liver failure for unknown reasons), metabolic error leading to liver failure, and acute liver failure for any reason (e.g., viral infection, drug overdose, tumor, cirrhosis).

Theoretically, anyone with advanced, irreversible liver disease with certain mortality may be considered for a liver transplant, provided that the disease can be corrected by liver transplantation (Table 21.5).

Hepatitis B is not eliminated by transplantation, but its recurrence and the damage it can cause may be substantially reduced by giving the patient hepatitis B globulin. Hepatitis recurs in the majority of liver transplants, but the damage to the new liver is slow, so many years of symptom-free living can occur. Novel treatments seek to eliminate rather than suppress the virus by specifically targeting covalently closed circular DNA.[93]

With the exception of metastatic malignancy and hepatic lymphoma, there are few absolute contraindications to liver transplantation. Liver transplantation for large primary liver cancers is very limited; transplantation remains the best treatment for small tumors (less than 5 cm) in a liver that is already cirrhotic.[481]

People with metastatic disease that has spread to the liver are no longer treated with liver transplantation because of the poor outcome. The exception is a small group of people whose liver cancer is characterized by neuroendocrine tumors that are very slow growing. The results of transplantation in this group are not as good as for individuals with benign disease but acceptable enough to qualify for transplantation.

Some metabolic disorders (e.g., familial hypercholesterolemia) that arise in the liver but produce damage elsewhere in the body can be cured if the liver is replaced with a liver from a healthy individual. Many inborn errors of liver metabolism are benign and are not associated with end-stage liver disease. Acute fulminant liver failure secondary to severe hepatitis owing to a virus, toxin, or poison can be life threatening and requires liver transplantation to prevent death.

### Transplantation Candidates

Historically, liver transplant candidacy was determined subjectively by the medical team based on perceived "best use" of the donor organ.[66,357,385,438] This led to worse outcomes secondary to increased frequency of multiorgan failure at time of transplant, owing to poor consideration of donor and recipient characteristics.[301,312,313,369,385,415,454] Many centers worldwide have adopted more objective evaluation methods, by which organ allocation is based on disease severity.[134,385]

One of the first tools developed to objectively assess mortality in liver transplantation was the Model for End-Stage Liver Disease (MELD) score. It was initially used to predict survival in patients undergoing transjugular intrahepatic portosystemic shunt but is now routinely used in liver transplant work-up.[272,351,388] The logarithmic score, ranging from 6 (less severe) to 40 (more severe), is calculated through the use of an equation that considers serum creatinine, bilirubin, and international normalized ratio. Generally, patients with a MELD score ≥15 with worsening organ function should be considered for transplant.[272] A phenomenon of underestimation of mortality in patients with a lower MELD score has been identified,[34,53,207] which is partially attributed to the absence of a physical or functional outcome measure in composite scoring.[178,315] A separate Pediatric End-Stage Liver Disease (PELD) score has also been developed for children younger than 12 years old.[446]

Adult and pediatric clinical practice guidelines were produced by the American Association for the Study of Liver Diseases (AASLD) in 2013[272] and 2014,[416] respectively, to further assist clinicians in the determination of liver transplant candidacy.

For adults, no formal age cutoff for liver transplant exists; however, persons older than 70 years of age with significant comorbidities demonstrate inferior outcomes compared with younger recipients.[259,416] For persons with a body mass index ≥40, liver transplant is relatively contraindicated. Alcoholic cirrhosis is not a contraindication, pending 6 months alcohol abstinence before

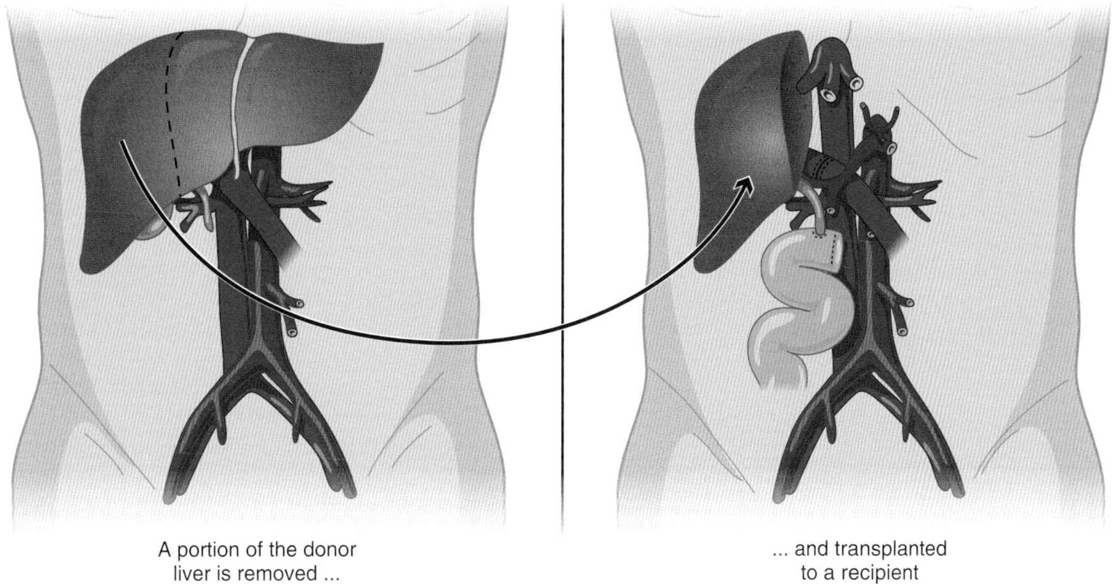


**Fig. 21.10**

**In a minimally invasive live-donor liver transplant, an incision is made just under the donor's rib cage.** A portion of the liver is removed; the donor's liver will grow back to a normal size within a few weeks. For the recipient, the diseased liver is removed through an incision in the upper abdomen. The donor liver is placed into the abdomen, and blood vessels are reattached to the new liver. The bile duct of the donor liver is attached to the recipient's bile duct or to a segment of intestine so the bile can drain into the small intestine.

transplant.[259] In pediatric patients, surgeons may defer surgery in small-birth-weight infants until significant growth has occurred, owing to technical difficulty of the procedure.[416] In all cases, severe cardiac or pulmonary disease, ongoing drug abuse, uncontrolled sepsis, extrahepatic malignancy, and lack of adequate social support may contraindicate liver transplantation.[272,416]

## Transplantation Procedure

The liver from the cadaveric donor is removed through a midline incision from the jugular notch to the pubis including a median sternotomy, with particular care to avoid hepatic injury or portal vein transection. The iliac artery and vein are also harvested in the event that vascular reconstruction is required.

Living-related transplantation requires a much less extensive operative opening, and the reduced-size graft is usually taken from the donor's left lobe (Fig. 21.10). In some situations (e.g., presence of metabolic abnormalities) the autologous graft is placed in an anatomically altered site, thereby preserving the orthotopic position for future use in the case of graft failure; this technique is not possible with disorders leading to portal hypertension.

Successful engraftment of the donor organ requires a recipient hepatectomy to remove the diseased liver, a procedure that can be difficult when there is severe portal hypertension and excessive collateral formation. In many centers the recipient is placed on heart-lung bypass to avoid congestion of the portal circulation and improve venous return to the heart during implantation, thus improving hemodynamic stability.

The implantation procedure begins with anastomoses, that is, surgical formation of a connection between the donor and the recipient's suprahepatic and then infrahepatic vena cava. Alternatively the donor vena cava can be anastomosed side-to-side with the recipient vena cava if it is left in situ during the recipient hepatectomy (piggyback technique). The operation then proceeds to the portal anastomosis. After all venous connections are made, the liver is reperfused.

## Complications

Transplantation of the liver differs from renal, lung, or heart transplantation because there is no intervening assistance from an artificial liver; the technical aspects of liver transplantation require precise connection of the hepatic artery, the hepatic and portal veins, and the bile duct. In the case of a living donor, there is a risk of hemorrhage and death if an artery is accidentally severed.

Rejection is the most common cause of liver dysfunction after transplantation, most likely after the first week and during the first 3 postoperative months.[118,474] As with all organ transplantation procedures, the chance of organ rejection requires the use of immunosuppressants with their associated complications, especially suppression of the body's natural defenses, making infections a common complication and cause of graft dysfunction.

Each person is also placed on prophylactic medications and preemptive therapy for a period of time to decrease the risk of opportunistic infection.[298] CMV, a common infectious process, can occur early after liver transplantation. CMV remains a major cause of morbidity but is no longer a major cause of mortality after liver transplantation.

Extrahepatic complications may include renal failure, neurologic disorders, and pulmonary involvement (e.g.,

Box 21.7

**CENTRAL NERVOUS SYSTEM COMPLICATIONS OF LIVER TRANSPLANTATION**

- Focal seizures
- Encephalopathy
- Central pontine myelinolysis
- Hemorrhages, infarcts, or both (intracranial, intracerebral, subarachnoid)
- Confusion
- Coma
- Psychosis
- Cortical blindness
- Quadriplegia
- Tremors
- Alzheimer type II astrocytosis
- Central nervous system aspergillosis (fungal infection)
- Cytomegalovirus (viral infection)

pneumonia, atelectasis, respiratory distress syndrome, pleural effusion). Hepatocellular carcinoma, hepatitis B, and Budd-Chiari syndrome may recur in the transplanted liver, but other chronic liver diseases do not recur.

In Budd-Chiari syndrome, occlusion of the hepatic veins impairs blood flow out of the liver, producing massive ascites and hepatomegaly. It is associated with any condition that obstructs the hepatic vein (e.g., abdominal trauma, use of oral contraceptives, polycythemia vera, paroxysmal nocturnal hemoglobinuria, other hypercoagulable states, congenital webs of the vena cava).

Mechanical postoperative complications include biliary strictures; nonfunction of the graft (i.e., the transplanted liver does not function); hemorrhage; and vascular thrombosis of the hepatic artery, portal vein, or hepatic veins. Mononeuropathy of the ulnar and peroneal nerves occurs in approximately 5% to 10% of orthotopic liver transplantations, primarily attributed to intraoperative compression (tilting of the surgical table) or postoperative trauma. Poor nutritional status, use of intermittent pneumatic compression devices, and body shape (tall and slender) are other potential contributing factors to peroneal neuropathy following liver transplantation.[404,486] Other upper extremity mononeuropathies may occur as a result of vascular cannulations (flexible tube inserted to deliver medication or drain fluid).[79]

Other clinically significant neurologic events occur in a substantial percentage of adult liver transplant recipients. Central nervous system complications after liver transplantation may be a consequence of liver disease itself, may be caused by the adrenergic effects of immunosuppressants (e.g., tacrolimus, cyclosporine), or may result from a wide array of metabolic abnormalities or vascular insults occurring in the early postoperative period.

Box 21.7 lists the most common central nervous system complications. The therapist is likely to be familiar with most of these terms, with the possible exception of central pontine myelinosis, which is demyelination of the central pons that causes a locked-in syndrome characterized by paralysis of the limbs and lower cranial nerves with intact consciousness.

Children receiving orthotopic liver transplantation are at risk for endocrine complications, such as growth failure, hepatic osteodystrophy, pubertal delay, adrenal insufficiency, and drug-induced diabetes. Other potential complications include bone fractures caused by malnutrition, malabsorption, and osteodystrophy. Low spine bone mineral density is associated with lumbar spine fractures and chronic pain. An excellent article reviewing endocrine and skeletal complications with preventive screening recommendations is available for physical therapists working with pediatric patients.[191]

### Prognosis

Factors determining survival include the underlying cause of liver failure (e.g., poorer prognosis for advanced cirrhosis); the person's ability to stop the intake of alcohol in the case of alcoholic cirrhosis; and the presence of complications or symptoms of hematemesis, jaundice, and ascites. Continued advances in the use of immunosuppressant-steroid combinations have increased survival rates through effective immunosuppression with minimal toxicity.

In the case of liver transplantation, survival rates correlate with the number of liver transplantation procedures performed in transplantation centers. Overall 1-year survival rates have improved from 70% 10 years ago to more than 85% in many high-volume centers.[135]

More than 50% of recipients of liver transplants survive 20 years and report improved quality of life compared with people who have liver disease.[405] Unadjusted deceased-donor transplant survival at 1, 3, and 5 years is 91.2%, 82.8%, and 75%, respectively, while live-donor survival at the same intervals is 92.3%, 88.4%, and 83.9%, although far fewer live-donor transplants are performed.[448,329] Survival after emergency liver transplantation for acute liver failure is less because such clients are seriously ill at the time of the operation.

The expected 1-year survival rate after a second or subsequent liver transplantation has improved drastically in the past decade to approximately 78.6%.[448] Individuals with serious postoperative complications because of mechanical failure or rejection and those who have a slow, progressive course of chronic hepatic dysfunction, usually caused by rejection or recurrence of primary disease, may qualify for liver retransplantation.

Risk factors have been identified to help predict graft failure in retransplantation. These include recipient age older than 55 years, donor age older than 45 years, MELD score greater than 27, history of more than one previous liver transplant, and need for mechanical ventilation before retransplantation.[194]

### Future Trends

Current animal research is centered on identifying and harvesting specific stem cells from the bone marrow that, under special conditions, will convert into functioning liver tissue.[349] In human research, a new procedure called *hepatocyte transplantation* is being pioneered. In this procedure, billions of donor liver cells are injected by intravenous infusion into the blood with the hope that the cells will correct life-threatening liver problems that would otherwise require a liver transplant.[171,201,366]

Other research efforts include working toward the development of bioartificial liver devices to provide detoxification and synthetic function during liver failure. Efforts are under way to develop artificial liver support that can stimulate the regeneration of injured liver cells and increase the likelihood of spontaneous recovery.[319]

Bioartificial liver devices are not purely mechanical devices, but rather cell-based biologic devices; they create a flow of blood through an extracorporeal circuit lined with healthy hepatocytes.[248] An effective temporary extracorporeal liver support system could improve the chance of survival with or without transplantation as the final treatment.[157] A randomized controlled trial using an extracorporeal liver assist device demonstrated improved 91-day survival rates in patients with alcohol-induced liver decompensation with MELD scores ≤28 treated with the extracorporeal liver assist device, but long-term benefit has yet to be identified.[438] No device has been developed that can perform all the necessary functions of a healthy liver; researchers are trying to develop liver cells that will perform as many of these tasks as possible.[83,90,319]

**SPECIAL IMPLICATIONS FOR THE THERAPIST 21.5**

## *Liver Transplantation*

The majority of transplanted livers begin to function well within minutes to hours after the vascular clamps are released. The client must be closely monitored for signs of respiratory compromise, bleeding, infection, rejection, and fluid or electrolyte imbalance. Vital signs must be monitored as activities are slowly resumed with physician approval and according to the client's tolerance levels.

### Acute Care Phase

Postoperatively the client will have multiple intravenous lines, drains, and a Foley catheter, as well as a painful abdomen with a large abdominal incision and a 4- to 5-inch left axillary incision (bypass procedure) restricted by staples and dressings. Standing postoperative orders are usually followed in the ICU.

The typical ICU stay is 24 to 48 hours, with ventilatory support for the first 24 hours. The patient must relax and let the machine breathe for him or her. The patient cannot talk and may be very anxious. The staff should make every effort to keep the patient informed about what is going on and help the patient communicate.

The large incisions are contraindications for resistive exercises; gradual low-resistance training can be introduced according to the physician's protocol, and abdominal precautions may be implemented. Physical therapy orders for nonspecific out-of-bed activity and mobility begin by postoperative day 1. The therapist can inspect joint motion, observe for thrombosis or infection, begin thrombosis prevention, and assess potential discharge needs. Falls prevention is an important aspect of rehabilitation postoperatively. A multidisciplinary approach to mobility coordinated by the therapist may help with falls prevention as well as reduce length of stay and increase the rate of return home.[448,465]

Any signs or symptoms of infection should be reported immediately. This may include headache, fever, skin rash or red streaks, change in pulse rate, confusion, burning with urination, or other constitutional symptoms. Mild signs and symptoms of rejection are present during the first few days to weeks but are controlled in most cases. The patient may report pain caused by the liver, fever, fatigue, and change in color of stool (gray) or urine (tea color). In terms of morbidity or mortality after liver transplantation, infection is usually a much greater concern than rejection.

Upper extremity range-of-motion exercises and client education for prevention of adhesive capsulitis (i.e., frozen shoulder) are important concerns. Coughing and deep breathing with a pillow splint are taught early. Liver recipients may be reluctant to cough, and respiratory infection is a hazard to avoid.

Often postoperative ascites is a significant problem, making functional training (e.g., bed mobility training, transfers) more difficult in the presence of an altered center of gravity. Hand, pedal, and, in men, scrotal edema from dependent positioning frequently develops, requiring active-range-of-motion exercises and bed mobility training as soon as possible.

Assisted ambulation should occur as soon as the client is stable in the upright position; placement of the gait belt can be problematic because the T-tube to drain bile is placed in the right lower abdomen and this area should be avoided. The gait belt can be tried around the upper trunk instead.

Once the telemetry is removed, rehabilitation can progress rapidly. Ascites and associated edema usually resolve within 3 to 4 weeks, but if edema persists, comprehensive lymphedema therapy may be required.

### Outpatient Phase

Outpatient therapy continues for approximately 8 weeks postoperatively. A liver transplant recipient with healthy heart and lungs can usually function well at home and resume independent activities of daily living. Rest and energy conservation balanced with nutrition, exercise, and correct, consistent lifelong drug self-administration all are considered important features of the rehabilitation process.

Pretransplant hepatic encephalopathy usually resolves slowly in the posttransplant period if the donor organ is functioning well; the client and therapist will see a reduction or cessation of associated signs and symptoms.

Common problems during the outpatient phase are centered around balance and coordination. Fatigue and reduced endurance add to the client's instability. Contributing to fatigue, sleep disturbance may occur as a side effect of medications.

The therapist must be alert to any self-medicating or use of nonprescription drugs by the client; the client should be encouraged to check with the physician before continuing unmonitored drug use. Steroid usage in older women can cause posttransplant mental confusion; the woman may become uncooperative and disoriented to time and place and experience hallucinations.[402] Observe for steroid myopathy in all recipients.

The therapist should be aware of incisional precautions because of the abdominal incision. Often surgeons place weight-lifting restrictions for a period of time (usually 6 to 8 weeks if the incision is healing well).

The abdominal scar may result in a kyphotic posture and altered breathing. Some people continue to use an assistive device. The therapist may be able to assist in improving posture, strength, balance, coordination, and fatigue levels. Exercise is an extremely valuable part of the postoperative recovery phase.

### Exercise

Extreme weakness and fatigue reducing activity levels are common in many liver transplant candidates with chronic liver disease. Low maximal $VO_2$ is common in pretransplant candidates with primary biliary or alcoholic cirrhosis, along with alcohol-induced myopathy contributing to exercise limitations.

Improvement in exercise capacity with training before transplantation has been demonstrated, and new studies confirm the same outcome after liver transplantation on physical fitness, muscle strength, and functional performance in candidates treated for chronic liver disease.[49,50] There is emerging evidence to suggest maximal oxygen uptake as demonstrated by cardiopulmonary exercise testing may be prognostic for liver transplant mortality, highlighting the potential role of the therapist in both preoperative and postoperative conditioning.

Compliance with a home program of exercise and activity may be a problem. Fatigue and quality of life are cited most often for poor adherence. Education is the key, as both of these symptoms can be improved with exercise.[237,273,370,405,463]

The liver plays an important role in providing glucose for oxidation and the maintenance of glucose homeostasis during physical exercise. Denervation of the liver does not alter the release of glucose during physical activity. Consequently, liver transplant candidates can perform quite heavy exercise and maintain acceptable glucose levels.

## Heart Transplantation

### Overview

In 1905, Carrel and Guthrie began to perform experimental procedures to prove heart transplantation was possible. In 1946, Demikhov performed the first heterotrophic heart transplantation in a dog. In 1960, Lower and Shumway developed the technique for heart transplantation that remains the basis of standard clinical surgical transplantation technique worldwide. The first human heart procedure was performed in South Africa by Christiaan Barnard (1967), followed shortly by the first U.S. transplant by Norman Shumway at Stanford in 1968.[154] Between January 1988 and December 20, 2018, more than 72,000 heart transplantations were performed, with the majority occurring for people between 50 and 65 years of age.[333]

### Incidence and Prevalence

There has been an increase in available donor hearts, which have exceeded 3000 since 2016. At the present time more than 72,000 individuals have received a heart transplant, with the largest donor age group being 18 to 34 years of age. The primary recipient group comprises individuals between 50 and 65 years of age. In 2017, 3244 heart transplants were done, with approximately 13% of transplants being completed in pediatric recipients (age 17 years or younger).[333]

Currently there are more than 3800 individuals waiting for a heart transplantation, with the range for median wait time being 72 to 415 days in 2011–2014. The wait period depends on the medical condition of the potential candidate, body size and blood match between the candidate and donor, and geography (i.e., the distance the candidate and transplant center is from the donor). During this wait period the candidate is constantly monitored and medically managed to ensure proper candidacy and accurate UNOS listing and to minimize the adverse effects of any further progression of the heart failure or the onset of new medical issues.

Over the past 4 years there have been some other subtle changes in the characteristics of candidates for a heart transplantation. There has been a 3% increase of candidates among minorities but no increase in the number of women receiving transplantation, with men receiving approximately 71.5% of transplants. The primary diagnosis of coronary disease and congenital disorders continues to be the leading diagnosis for heart transplantation in adults and children, respectively.[333]

### Indications

Potential candidates for cardiac transplantation must have end-stage heart disease with severe or advanced heart failure (New York Heart Association class III or IV end-stage heart disease) with a life expectancy of less than 1 year. The most common underlying cause of heart failure leading to cardiac transplantation is cardiomyopathy because of either end-stage ischemic coronary heart disease or nonischemic dilated cardiomyopathy. Other, less common cardiac diseases that may be treated with heart transplantation include sarcoidosis, restrictive cardiomyopathy, hypertrophic cardiomyopathy, and congenital heart disease. In the pediatric population, cardiomyopathy is the leading reason for the need for transplantation. All pediatric cardiomyopathies are considered nonischemic, but classification of the disease is a very complex process because up to 68% of patients present with a mixture of disease features.[489]

### Transplantation Candidates

The selection of candidates for heart transplantation involves the use of multiple prognostic variables (Box 21.8) in conjunction with medical urgency criteria established through UNOS status listings (see Box 21.3). People accepted as candidates for heart transplantation are expected to have a limited survival if they do not undergo transplantation and to have exhausted other medical or surgical options that could extend the individual's life or improve their physical capacity.

Box 21.8

**INDICATIONS AND REQUIREMENTS FOR HEART TRANSPLANTATION**

- Cardiogenic shock or low cardiac output state requiring mechanical support
- Low cardiac output or refractory heart failure requiring inotropic support
- ESHD with NYHA class III or IV not responding to medical intervention
- Intractable severe angina not amenable to intervention
- Life expectancy <50% of expected survival at 1 year that includes:
  - LVEF <20%
  - Maximal $VO_2$ <12 mL/min/kg
  - Peak $VO_2$ <10 mL/min/kg
  - Ventricular arrhythmias not responsive to medical therapy
  - Cardiac index <2.0 L/min/$m^2$
  - Pulmonary capillary wedge pressure >16 mm Hg
- Age typically <65 years old
- No irreversible organ dysfunction
- No irreversible pulmonary hypertension
- Free of cancer (time of remission depends on type of cancer)
- Free from substance abuse (minimally >6 months)
- Diabetes mellitus with peripheral end-stage organ complications
- No active infections
- Good compliance
- HIV negative
- Psychologic stability
- Financial support
- Family support

*ESHD*, End-stage heart disease; *LVEF*, left ventricular ejection fraction; *NYHA*, New York Heart Association; *$VO_2$*, oxygen consumption.

The candidate needs stable social support and financial resources to cover medications and follow-up care. Ideally, the candidate should be younger than 70 years of age and have no other disease, such as cancer, that would shorten the life of the individual or limit the life expectancy of the transplantation.[460] Age cutoff is also controversial and has increased over the past decade; although the upper age limit for transplantation candidates is currently 70 years, age over 70 years is considered a relative contraindication.[67]

Pediatric listings differ from adults. Status 1A characterizes a child less than 18 years of age who requires a mechanical ventilator, a mechanical assist device, or a balloon pump or a child younger than 6 months of age with a congenital or acquired heart disease exhibiting reactive pulmonary arterial pressure greater than 50% of systolic pressure, who requires infusion or a single high-dose intravenous inotrope or multiple intravenous inotropes, or who has a life expectancy without a heart transplant of less than 14 days. Status 1B candidates require infusion of one or more inotropic agents that does not qualify for status 1A, are less than 6 months of age and diagnosed with hypertrophic or restrictive cardiomyopathy and do not meet the criteria for status 1A, or show growth failure less than 5th percentile or 1.5 or more standard deviations below expected height growth or weight growth. Status 2 includes all actively listed children who do not meet the criteria of status 1. Risk factors in the adult heart transplant candidate must be assessed to provide guidelines about the timing of placing a person on the UNOS waiting list and when to perform the transplantation. The measure of exercise $VO_2$ has become an indicator of prognosis in advanced heart failure and is currently being used as a major criterion in many centers for the selection of candidates for heart transplantation.[331]

As part of the cardiac assessment the individual will undergo an extensive work-up, including an exercise test to assess maximal $VO_2$. Individuals with a maximal $VO_2$ of less than 12 mL/min/kg have a lower survival rate unless treated successfully with transplantation. However, $VO_2$ can be affected by age, gender, muscle mass, and conditioning status. The multiple factors that affect exercise capacity may explain why some people with congestive heart failure and a peak $VO_2$ of less than 14 mL/min/kg have a favorable prognosis even when transplantation is deferred.[45,73,267,358]

Ejection fraction, cardiac index, and diabetes status are also used to assess transplantation needs. Anyone with an ejection fraction of less than 20% and a cardiac index of less than 2 L/min/$m^2$ is also considered a potential candidate for transplantation. Ejection fraction is the amount of blood the ventricle ejects; the normal ejection fraction is approximately 60% to 75%. A decreased ejection fraction is a hallmark finding of ventricular failure. Normal cardiac index ranges from 2.5 to 4 L/min/$m^2$.

### Transplantation Procedure

An allograft transplant procedure is used for heart transplantation. Almost all heart transplantations done at this time are orthotopic; that is, the diseased heart is removed, and the donor heart is grafted into the normal anatomic site. There are three surgical procedures that can be used to implant the heart: biatrial, bicaval, and total procedure. The bicaval approach is the most common because it decreases the incidence of atrial arrhythmias and improves atrial function. The bicaval procedure involves the anastomoses of the superior and inferior venae cavae.[67,166,372]

In rare cases a heterotopic cardiac transplantation can be performed in which the recipient's diseased heart is left intact and the donor heart is placed in parallel with anastomoses between the two right atria, pulmonary arteries, left atria, and aorta. In heterotopic transplantation, the donor heart assists the diseased heart. This type of procedure may be performed in an individual with fixed pulmonary hypertension or someone who is physically very large, requiring a higher cardiac output than a donor heart from an average-size donor. With the use of left ventricular assist devices (LVADs) to manage pulmonary hypertension, more candidates are qualified for orthotopic transplantation.[242]

One of the effects of an orthotopic transplantation is the denervation of the heart, which means the loss of the autonomic nervous system influence on cardiac function. This means the transplant recipient has lost the fight-or-flight response, and the heart relies on its own intrinsic properties for sufficient contractility and cardiac output at rest.

In general, the recipient will have an elevated heart rate at rest because of the loss of the parasympathetic input and the downregulation of the sympathetic nervous system, a decrease in compliance (the heart's ability to relax to completely fill), and a blunted heart rate response with exertion because of the loss of the sympathetic nervous system. The heart relies on the release of catecholamines to increase rate and contractility, and there is a delay in recovery of this function following transplantation. The therapist should also expect a delay in recovery until the body processes the released hormones. In general, the recipient has an exercise capacity of 65% to 70% of predicted $VO_2$.[189,417] There is promising evidence that partial normalization of heart rate can be achieved by 12 months after transplant, but this is very variable.[320]

### Complications

One of the most common posttransplantation complications is rejection. Rejection can be classified as hyperacute, acute, and chronic rejection. With blood and antigen typing techniques, hyperacute rejection is rare. This type of rejection occurs within minutes to hours postimplantation and involves a catastrophic immune response from the interaction between the recipient's circulating antibodies and donor antigens that contributes to graft failure.[154,256] Primary graft failure occurs in 3.8% of transplantations and carries a 96% mortality rate unless retransplantation is an option.[281]

**Acute Rejection.** Acute rejection can occur at any time after transplantation. Within the first year posttransplantation, 25% of recipients will experience acute rejection, accounting for a 12% mortality rate.[466] Depending on the type and severity of acute rejection, recipients can present with signs and symptoms such as fever, malaise, heart rate alteration or arrhythmias, jugular vein distention, decreased exercise tolerance, or heart failure. Rejection can also be asymptomatic.[189,261,292,412]

ACR is characterized by inflammatory lymphocytic infiltrates along with the presence of macrophages and eosinophils and myocardial necrosis. It is important for routine biopsies to be performed because ACR is commonly asymptomatic.[281,466]

Acute mediated rejection is associated with antibodies developed against the capillary endothelium layer leading to a complex immune response and the activation of cytotoxic T cells, B cells, and NK cells, resulting in the destruction of interstitial and vascular graft tissue.[281,466]

**Cardiac Allograft Vasculopathy or Transplant Coronary Artery Disease.** Chronic rejection or cardiac allograft vasculopathy (CAV) is a medical condition that a recipient may experience months to years after transplantation. Although still under investigation, CAV is suspected to have an immune-mediated and a nonimmune response and to be correlated with persistent inflammation directed at the vasculature of the donor heart. This leads to a diffuse proliferation of smooth muscle cells, concentric intimal narrowing, and accelerated diffuse obliterative atherosclerosis of both intramyocardial and epicardial arteries and veins (Figs. 21.11 and 21.12).[134,168,357] It accounts for 14% mortality at 5 to 10 years posttransplantation.[412] CAV is associated with severe ACR and death, with survival reduced by 10% to 12%.[412]

Recipients with CAV may initially be asymptomatic, but as the disease progresses the recipient will present with signs and symptoms of heart failure. These signs and symptoms include dyspnea, syncope, jugular vein distention, peripheral edema, malaise, low-grade fever, general fatigue, and variable arrhythmias (most likely atrial tachycardia arrhythmias).

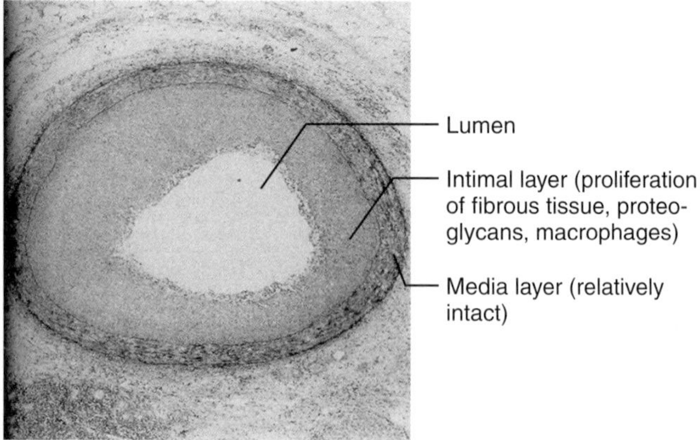


**Fig. 21.11**

**Transplant coronary artery disease.** Proliferation of the intimal layer of the epicardial coronary artery from a 14-year-old cardiac transplant recipient 1 year after transplant. This condition produces a significant reduction in diameter of the arterial lumen that will compromise blood flow to the myocardium. (Reprinted from Gajarski RJ: Update on pediatric heart transplant: long-term complications. *Tex Heart Inst J* 24:260–268, 1997.)

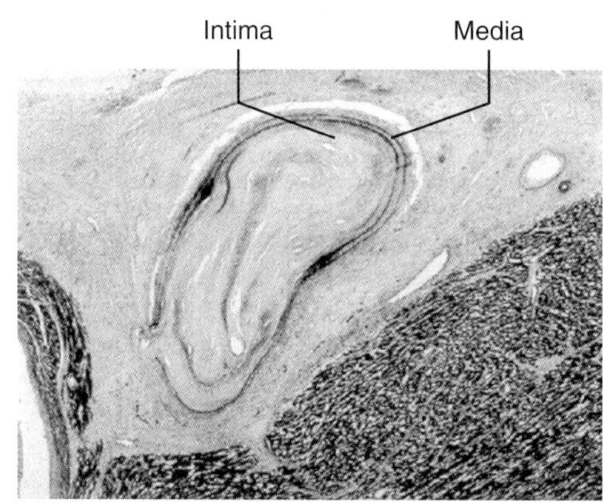


**Fig. 21.12**

**Transplant coronary artery disease resulting in complete occlusion of epicardial coronary artery in an 11-year-old heart transplant recipient 4 years after transplantation.** The lumen is obstructed with dense fibrous tissue with thinning and fibrosis of the media layer. (Reprinted from Gajarski RJ: Update on pediatric heart transplant: long-term complications. *Tex Heart Inst J* 24:260–268, 1997.)

With the denervation of the donor heart, many recipients will not experience angina despite the atherosclerosis and decrease in myocardial perfusion associated with CAV. Symptoms of angina cannot be ignored because it is now recognized that a portion of recipients will obtain some degree of sympathetic nervous reinnervation.[43,128,189] The classic diagnosis by angiography is not as useful for diagnostic purposes for CAV because CAV is more diffuse, with small arterial disease initially. Cardiovascular magnetic resonance imaging has predictive value in monitoring cardiac function in the presence of CAV. Dobutamine stress echocardiography is limited in predictive value for early diagnosis of CAV. Computed tomography scan has a high sensitivity and specificity and predictive value for CAV, but its use is limited by concern regarding dye exposure and risk to renal function.[211] Intravascular ultrasound is particularly effective in diagnosing early CAV by assessing the entire cardiac arterial tree and assessing the hyperplasia of the intimal layer of the arteries.[386]

**Infection.** The severe consequence of infection has a high impact on mortality and morbidity because of the need for immunosuppressant medications. Non-CMV infections account for 13.4% and 31% of deaths in the first postoperative month and first year, respectively. There has been a continuous decrease in infection-related mortality after the first year, but infection still accounts for 10% to 13% of mortality per year (see Figs. 21.11 and 21.12).[281]

The incidence of infection has improved because of the improvement in immunosuppressive medications, less induction therapy, further development of antimicrobial medications, and improved prophylactic management.[176]

The most common site for infection is the respiratory system, and respiratory system infection is associated with a high incidence of death, particularly in the first 3 months. The most common pathogens are *Aspergillus fumigatus*, CMV, and *Pneumocystis jirovecii* with an associated 30% mortality rate.[281] Infections can be divided into three time periods: infections occurring within the first month are typically related to either the donor or the recipient and are complicated by the higher immunosuppressive medication dosages; infections occurring 1 to 6 months posttransplantation are typically caused by opportunistic organisms such as *Pneumocystis*, *Toxoplasma gondii*, and mycobacteria; infections occurring after 6 months are commonly urinary tract infections and community-acquired pneumonia.[412]

Viral infections, including CMV, herpes simplex virus, and EBV, have also decreased as a result of prophylactic management but continue to require close monitoring and intervention. This is especially true for a recipient who was negative for viral exposure and mismatched with a seropositive donor.[176] Fungal infections such as *Aspergillus* and *Candida* are also a concern, but there has been a significant decrease in invasive *Aspergillus* infections in the past decade.

**Primary Graft Dysfunction.** In the early postoperative phase, the donor heart may not sufficiently support the circulatory demand of the body, and this is associated with early morbidity and mortality. The dysfunction of the graft may be related to an ischemic injury sustained in the procurement process. There may be a reperfusion injury sustained at the time when the circulation is reestablished through the donor heart. Finally, primary graft dysfunction (PGD) may be the result of acute right ventricular failure because the right ventricle is not accustomed to contracting against the elevated pulmonary arterial pressures within the recipient's pulmonary vascular resistance. Within the first 30 days posttransplantation, primary graft failure has a 3% incidence, and mortality is up to 80%.[211,466]

**Neuromuscular Dysfunction.** There has been a rise in neuromuscular dysfunction over the past decade. The increased incidence has been attributed to the larger percentage of individuals with pretransplant polyneuropathies (30%) associated with diabetes and renal dysfunction, which increases to 70% posttransplant. The rate of cerebrovascular accident ranges from 10% to 30% with 20% mortality for heart transplant recipients. Postoperative delirium occurs in 9% of recipients. Up to 37% experience chronic pain and depression that limit function and quality of life.[281]

**Musculoskeletal Conditions.** There has been an increased incidence of frailty (approximately 33%), which is related to the increased number of transplantations in candidates >65 years of age and candidates with higher burden of comorbidities. Moderate to severe frailty is an independent predictor of all-cause mortality. Heart transplantation is also associated with a decrease in muscle mass and strength from effects of immobility, chronic effects of elevated inflammatory response associated with heart failure, and effects of immunosuppressive medications.[280] Tacrolimus and cyclosporine inhibit and transform myosin heavy chain and oxidative enzymes from fast to slow muscle twitch. There is also a decrease in skeletal muscle perfusion because of the increased sensitivity of peripheral chemoreceptors.[98,412]

Osteopenia and osteoporosis are significant complications for transplant recipients of all ages. Osteopenia has been reported to affect 20% to 49% of candidates waiting for transplantation and accounts for 14% of vertebral compression fractures.[235] The risk of bone disease increases after transplantation with the use of immunosuppressive medications and renal dysfunction, with the greatest degree of bone loss in the first year posttransplantation. Osteoporosis rates are 15% and 25% for the spine and hip, respectively, and up to 36% of vertebral compression fractures are reported within the first year posttransplantation.[239]

The adverse effect on bone density is multifactorial. Corticosteroids inhibit bone formation proliferation and function by decreasing the levels of type I collagen. Corticosteroids also reduce intestinal calcium, stimulating an increase in osteoclastic activity, and have adverse effects on skeletal muscles that further contribute to decreased bone density. Calcineurin inhibitors, cyclosporine, and tacrolimus directly decrease bone density by increasing osteoclastic activity and indirectly decrease bone density by altering T-cell function and impairing renal function. Tacrolimus and cyclosporine also have adverse effects on skeletal muscles.[61,239,240,263]

**Cancer.** The incidence of cancer is proportional to the drug levels of the immunosuppressive medications and survival time posttransplantation; in general, average onset of malignancy is between 2.5 and 4 years posttransplantation, with 28% incidence within 10 years posttransplantation. By 15 years after transplantation, some form of malignancy is diagnosed in almost 50% of recipients. Skin cancer is the most common form of cancer present, at a rate of 18% (basal cell more often than squamous cell carcinoma).[281,420] In 2% of cases, cancer is diagnosed with a malignant lymphoma that leads to death. Other types of cancer associated with heart transplantation include prostate cancer, lung cancer, Kaposi sarcoma, breast cancer, cervical cancer, colon cancer, and renal cancer.[281]

**Other Complications.** Other complications occur as a result of long-term use of immunosuppressive medications and their adverse effects. It has been reported that 50% to 95% of recipients are treated for hypertension caused by medications and renal insufficiency and that 60% to 80% of recipients develop hyperlipidemia. Approximately 35% to 40% develop diabetes.[420]

Half of recipients have renal dysfunction, with approximately 6% progressing to ESRD and requiring hemodialysis or renal transplantation.[281] Cyclosporine- or tacrolimus-induced hyperuricemia, along with renal insufficiency and use of loop diuretics, can lead to an increase in gout. Gout is characterized by early symptoms, including arthralgias and monarthritis affecting the first metatarsophalangeal joint, knees, ankles, heels, and insteps. Over time, upper extremity joints become involved, progressing to polyarticular chronic arthritis. Treatment is the same as for primary gout.[412]

## Prognosis

In general, people tolerate the transplantation procedure well, and the graft resumes normal function promptly. Recipients are often extubated and out of bed into a chair 1 to 2 days after surgery. Median survival rate is 11 years.[67]

The UNOS National Data for 2018[333] reported continued improvement in survival rates after cardiac transplantation. Survival rates are excellent, with 1-year, 3-year, and 5-year survival rates of 90.5%, 85.3%, and 77.7%, respectively. Survival rates for African American recipients have significantly improved in the last decade, closely matching Caucasian recipients, 73.4% and 78.3%, respectively, at 5 years. Age difference in regard to survival no longer is significantly different at 5 years posttransplantation with a range of 72.3% to 78.3% for adult recipients at 75% to 84.2% in pediatric recipients.

## Current Trends

**VENTRICULAR ASSIST DEVICES.** VADs have become an accepted surgical intervention for the management of heart failure, with 2018 devices implanted in the United States in 2017.[234] Since the early 1990s, VADs have been used as a bridge to transplant when an individual was not expected to survive the wait time for a heart transplant. More recently with significant engineering advances in VADs, implantation has become an option for patients who are not transplant candidates (i.e., destination therapy). Kormos and colleagues[234] reported that 49% of individuals implanted with a VAD were registered for destination therapy in 2017.

In many cases, VAD implantation is used as a rescue device to save a medically unstable patient, which often leads to complications, prolonged hospitalization, and higher mortality. However, ideally the VAD should be implanted before irreversible dysfunction of other organs (renal, liver, and cardiac cachexia).[60,244]

VADs have significantly changed in the last decade. Many of the devices are smaller and easier to operate now. The most common devices provide continuous blood flow, thus reducing or eliminating the moving parts in the pump. This has led to an increase in durability and thus made the option of destination therapy possible. VADs are most commonly implanted for left-heart failure and account for 90% of the VADs that were implanted in 2017.[234] Currently the most commonly implanted devices for left-heart failure are the HeartMate 3 (Abbott, Abbott Park, IL) (Fig. 21.13) and the HeartWare HVAD (Medtronic, Minneapolis, MN) (Fig. 21.14).

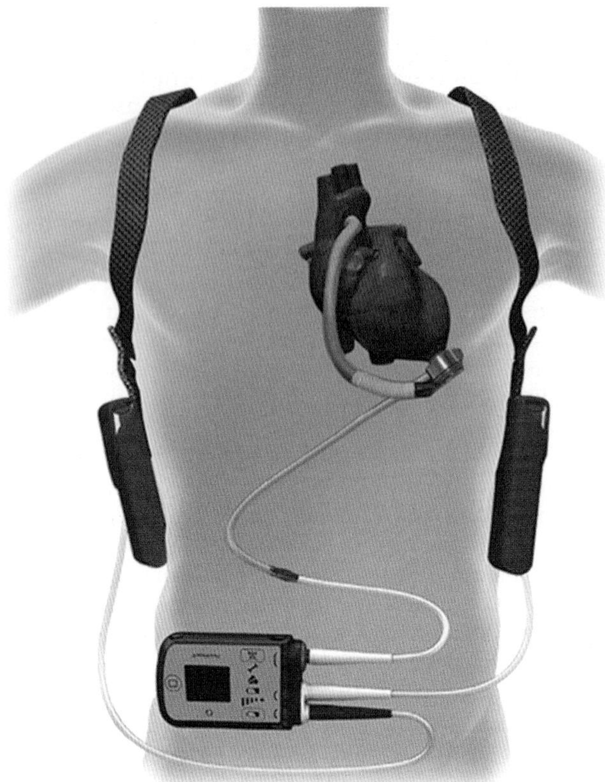

**Fig. 21.13**

HeartMate 3 is a nonpulsatile left ventricular assist device that works in parallel with the native heart to support systemic circulation. (Courtesy Abbott.)

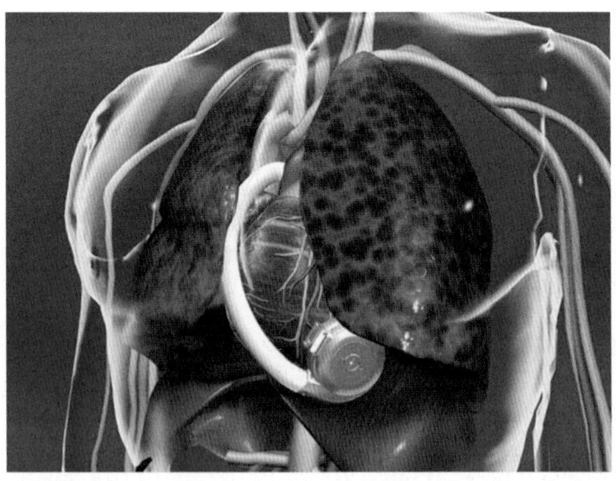

**Fig. 21.14**

**HeartWare HVAD is a centrifugal nonpulsatile left ventricular assist device that provides continuous systemic circulation.** The components of the device include a pump that is implanted intrathoracically, a very short inflow conduit or cannula, and an outflow conduit or cannula. Additional components not shown in the image are the percutaneous lead (driveline), controller, and power source. Blood circulates from the left ventricle through the inflow cannula into the pump that continuously delivers blood forward to the ascending aorta via the outflow cannula. (Reproduced with permission of Medtronic. All rights reserved.)

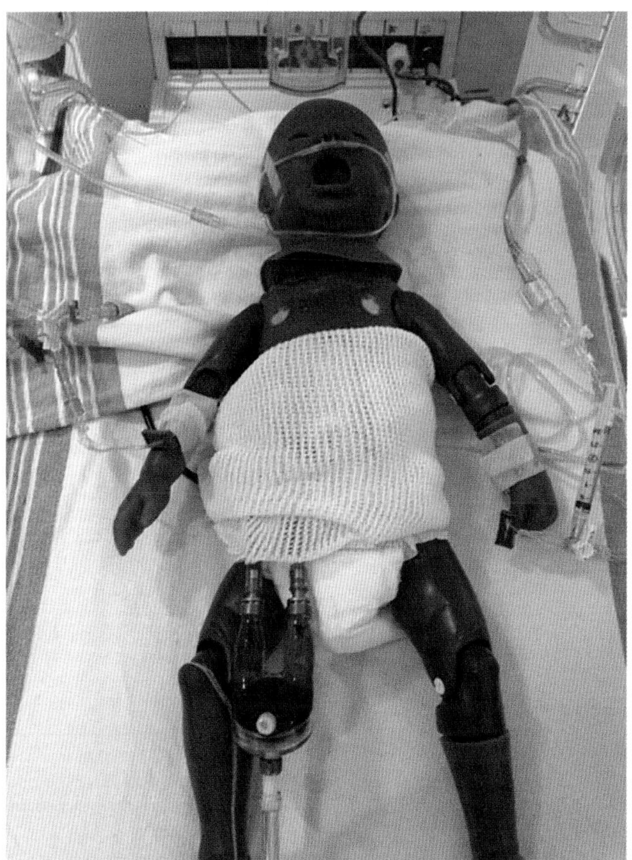

**Fig. 21.15**

**The Berlin Heart is a pneumatically driven ventricular assist device shown here with various cannulation options.** ((From Villa CR et al: Pediatric ventricular assist device simulation: constructing a situ simulation training program to facilitate education and competency, *Progress in Pediatric Cardiology*, 47:34-36, 2017.)

At the present time there is no VAD similar to the LVAD designed for right-heart failure, although the Thoratec pVAD (Abbott) can provide long-term right ventricle support and has been implanted in approximately 900 individuals.[234] Surgeons have implanted the HeartWare LVAD off-label for isolated right ventricular failure and for biventricular failure.[120,396] For biventricular failure, the most common long-term devices are the Thoratec pVAD (Fig. 21.15) and the SynCardia temporary Total Artificial Heart (TAH) (SynCardia Systems, Tucson, AZ). The SynCardia temporary TAH is a true replacement of the person's native ventricles. The diseased ventricles are excised, and two mechanical ventricles are sewn to the native atria. Since 2006, the TAH has been implanted in 339 patients.[234]

VADs are designed to support heart function and can be described as pulsatile or nonpulsatile or continuous flow depending on how the device circulates blood. VADs can be classified as providing short-term or long-term support. Pulsatile pumps such as Thoratec pVAD or Syncardia temporary Total Artificial Heart (TAH) (Syncardiac Systems, Tucson, AZ) mimic heart function in that the atrium fills the VAD, which then pumps the blood out into systemic circulation. Currently nonpulsatile LVADs are the most commonly used VAD, owing to their small size and improved longevity, thus promoting discharge from the hospital. Because these devices circulate blood continuously, the patient may or may not have a palpable pulse or auscultatory blood pressure, depending on how fast the VAD is circulating blood and how much underlying heart function exists. The faster the VAD circulates blood, the less likely traditional methods for monitoring a patient's vital signs will be possible.

**Indications for Ventricular Assist Device.** As mentioned, the use of VADs in the management of heart failure has significantly changed in the last decade. In 2017, 41% of VADs were classified as a bridge to transplant for individuals who had optimized medical therapy and required additional support while a suitable organ was found. Over the past 5 years, roughly 26% of patients were classified as a bridge to decision at the time of implantation.[234] The implantation of a VAD allows the transplant center and potential candidate to address medical or psychosocial issues to transform the VAD recipient into a more suitable heart transplant candidate. Less than 1% of individuals are able to be weaned from a device once the native heart recovers from the cause of the acute dysfunction.[234]

The largest growing sector for VAD utilization comprises patients who are implanted for lifelong support of heart failure, with no intention to receive a transplantation. In these cases, the VAD is a substitute for cardiac transplantation and is referred to as destination therapy. The use of a VAD as destination therapy accounted for 49% of VAD implantations in 2017; this figure was less than 2% in 2006.[234]

In the United States the two most commonly used LVADs are the HeartWare HVAD and the HeartMate 3. These two pumps are referred to as third-generation VADs; they continuously circulate blood using a centrifugal flow pattern, which means the flow enters the pump at a perpendicular direction and then the blood leaves the pump. Both of these pumps are implanted intrathoracically, so there is no longer a need for the surgeon to make a pump pocket in the abdominal cavity, which had been a site for infectious complications.

There has been an increase in the number of published reports regarding exercise tolerance and quality of life for patients on LVAD support over the past 5 years. Individuals benefit from participation in formal cardiac rehabilitation with improvements in exercise capacity, 6-minute walk test, and quality-of-life measures. Although there are positive improvements, Schmidt and colleagues[387] reported decreased exercise capacity and walking tolerance in patients compared with age-match control subjects. More research is needed to determine optimal timing for implantation, particularly for the destination therapy group, as well as the best format and exercise prescription to optimize recovery and outcomes after implantation.

**Precautions and Considerations.** There are several common components of all VADs that the physical therapist should understand (e.g., what they are, what their function is, and how to manage each component if an alarm is activated). There is a surgically implanted pump with cannulas (tubes) that circulate blood forward. The pump can be implanted internally or external to the body and is connected to a controller that is external to the body via a driveline. The driveline typically exits the body at the abdominal wall, where it connects to the controller and power sources.

It is critical that the therapist makes sure the driveline is covered with a dressing and is secured to the body with an adhesive anchor or abdominal binder. If the tissue around

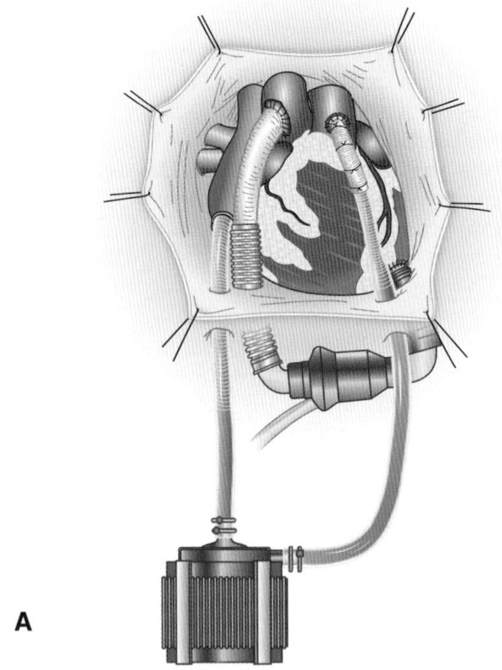


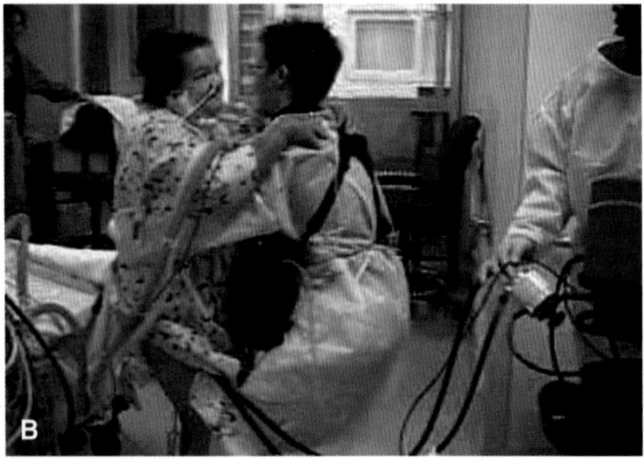


**Fig. 21.16**

(A) Thoratec CentriMag is a ventricular assist device (VAD) that is designed to provide emergent and temporary (up to 14 days) right, left, or biventricular support with the goal to achieve hemodynamic stability. (B) A patient is initiating gait training while being supported by a right VAD (CentriMag), another more long-term left VAD (VentrAssist), and mechanical ventilation. (B, Courtesy Chris L. Wells, University of Maryland Medical Center, Baltimore, MD.)

the driveline is disrupted, there is a significant likelihood that an infection could occur; it is very difficult to eradicate the infection once it contaminates the driveline. In general, the controller is the computer that is programmed by the engineer to operate the pump and monitors the function of the pump. Finally, there is some type of power source. Most VADs can operate on AC power or portable batteries, and some can run on DC power. For some VADs, there is a computer monitor or console that allows the therapist to monitor the function of the VAD, and some VADs display critical information including the type of alarm and action to correct the alarm on the face of the controller. The VAD team can use the computer to make programming changes as indicated. See Fig. 21.13 (HeartMate II) for an example of the common VAD components.

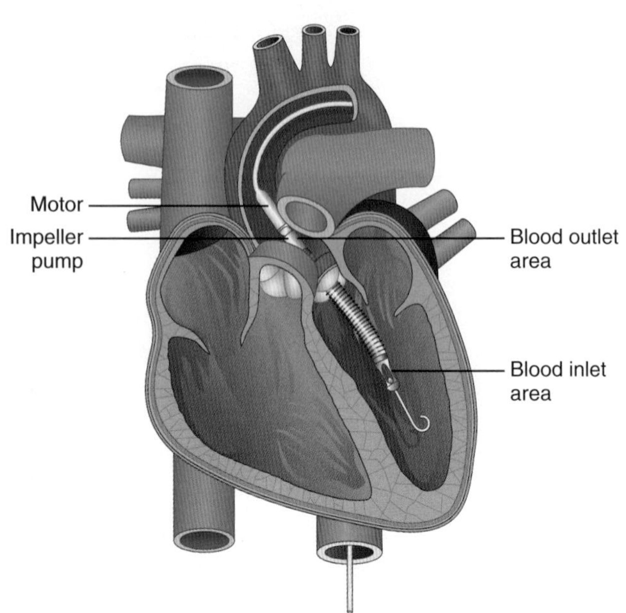


**Fig. 21.17**

**Abiomed's Impella 5.0.** Impella is the world's smallest heart pump. This pump is positioned across the aortic valve, which allows continuous flow of blood from the left ventricle to the aorta. This pump can provide peak flows of up to 5 L/min. (Courtesy Abiomed, Danvers, MA.)

Besides the development of nonpulsatile pumps, short-term VADs have been developed. These pumps have become important because they can provide right ventricular, left ventricular, or biventricular support for days or weeks. These short-term devices have also become extremely useful to temporarily support cardiac function for a transplanted heart that initially is not functioning properly. These VADs provide circulatory support while also supporting the donor heart with the goal for recovery. The most common devices for short-term support are the CentriMag (Abbott) (Fig. 21.16A), Abiomed Impella LP 5.0 (Fig. 21.17), and TandemHeart (LivaNova, London, UK).

**Extracorporeal Membranous Oxygenation.** Another option for short-term management of patients with end-stage heart failure who are in cardiogenic shock is the use of venoarterial ECMO. ECMO is similar to cardiopulmonary bypass machines used in operating rooms. ECMO allows for emergent cardiopulmonary circulatory support for a patient who becomes hemodynamically unstable, with the goal to support circulation and decompress the heart while the medical team decides the best plan of care.

Venoarterial ECMO supports circulation through continuous flow similar to nonpulsatile VADs, but ECMO also provides management of gas exchange to preserve tissue cellular function. Blood flows out of the body via a venous cannula to a pump that creates blood flow. The blood then goes to the membranous oxygenator, where gas exchange occurs. Then the oxygenated blood is returned to the body via an arterial cannula. This configuration allows for full cardiopulmonary support. Cannulation of the patient can be done in various ways to support circulation. Common cannulation configurations include femoral venous to femoral arterial, femoral vein to axillary or subclavian artery, or central cannulation, where the cannulas are placed in the right atrium to return blood to the aorta.

More recently ECMO is being considered for short-term bridge to heart transplantation. Placing someone on ECMO is less expensive than implanting a VAD, and it can be done at the bedside if necessary. With the trend to decrease the use of sedation to permit more patient engagement, rehabilitation including functional strengthening, muscular endurance training, and function restoration including ambulating is safe and feasible.[471]

## SPECIAL IMPLICATIONS FOR THE THERAPIST 21.6

### *Heart Transplantation*

The therapist has an important role in the heart transplant team. In the pretransplant period, the role of the therapist may be focusing on conducting outcome measures to determine frailty as part of the transplant work-up. The acute care therapist may be restoring function and increasing strength and endurance for the hospitalized individual to prepare for discharge and a successful transfer to outpatient services. A community-based therapist may treat these clients in the outpatient setting to further promote muscle strength and aerobic and anaerobic exercise capacity. Goals are to improve function, strength, and exercise capacity either to make the client a stronger candidate for transplantation or to assist the transplantation team in determining timing for transplantation listing or timing for other medical or surgical interventions. Potential transplant recipients should be educated on the role of physical therapy during the pretransplantation and posttransplantation periods. For the posttransplant period, the therapist will focus on restoring function, instructing the patient in any restrictions related to the mediastinal surgical procedures, and preparing for discharge. Physical therapy in the post–acute care setting should address advancing exercise capacity and assisting the patient in return to their pre-illness work and leisure activities if appropriate.

Outcome measures should be a standard part of the assessment throughout the continuum of care. Gait speed, sit to stand, short physical performance battery, hand grip, and the 6-minute walk test provide a clinical assessment tool that is useful in developing an effective rehabilitation program and offers the therapist some guidelines for recommending someone as a potential transplantation candidate.[77]

General criteria required before initiating an aerobic exercise program include (1) resting heart rate below 120 beats/min, (2) ability to speak comfortably while exercising, (3) respiratory rate below 30 breaths/min, and (4) reports of no more than moderate fatigue. For inpatients with a pulmonary artery catheter or invasive monitoring, the cardiac index should be greater than or equal to 2 L/min/m$^2$, or central venous pressure must be less than 12 mm Hg.[69] It is vital that the therapist consider these as guidelines to complete a comprehensive assessment of activity tolerance and discuss physiologic differences with the medical team to individualize the rehabilitation plan of care. In the acute care setting more articles are being published that demonstrate the safety and feasibility of mobilization of patients with various ICU lines and devices. Patients can be safely mobilized, including walking in the presence of a pulmonary artery catheter, femoral arterial lines, various vasoactive drugs, temporary VADs, and ECMO.[145,282,347] For suggested guidelines regarding mobilization of individuals who have a pulmonary artery catheter in place, see eBox 21.2 on the book's Student Consult site.

In the acute postoperative period the therapist's goal is to prepare for discharge, which often means addressing airway clearance and general strengthening and restoration of basic functional mobility as important aspects of the plan of care. See Table 21.6 for an overall plan of care. Part of restoring function is modifying functional mobility to accommodate any sternal precautions. Recent published work supports the ability of allowing patients to use their upper extremities to promote basic functional recovery without increasing the risk of sternal complications.[6,12]

During each therapy session the therapist should be monitoring the patient. The patient may experience chest pain or discomfort that may be related to musculoskeletal impairments, muscle soreness, or medical conditions such as pericarditis or pleural effusion. In the first 6 months the patient's chest pain is unlikely to be caused by myocardial ischemia, owing to the fact that the heart is denervated. Any other symptoms that

**Table 21.6** Physical Therapy Management

| Acute | Outpatient |
|---|---|
| Progress functional mobility<br>Sternal precaution training<br>Airway clearance techniques<br>Monitor hemodynamics<br>Monitor anticoagulation/ antiplatelet levels<br>Monitor for dysfunction<br>OHTx: infections and rejection<br>VAD: pump dysfunction<br>Assess for neuromuscular changes, especially for patient with VAD support<br>Education:<br>• Side effects of medications<br>• Vital response to exercise<br>Self-monitoring:<br>• Signs of infection/ rejection/VAD alarms<br>• Home exercise program | Exercise capacity testing and/or functional field testing<br>Monitor vital signs<br>Functional strengthening program and general stretching<br>Reentry into community (work, recreational, leisure activities)<br>Monitor anticoagulation/ antiplatelet levels<br>Monitor for dysfunction<br>OHTx: infections and rejection<br>VAD: pump dysfunction<br>Assess for neuromuscular changes, especially for patient with VAD support<br>Education:<br>• Side effects of medications<br>• Vital response to exercise<br>Self-monitoring:<br>• Signs of infection/ rejection/VAD alarms<br>• Home exercise program: osteoporosis care (weight-bearing activities, spine care, scar management) |

*OHTx*, Orthotopic heart transplantation; *VAD*, ventricular assist device.

may be associated with ischemia (e.g., dyspnea, lightheadedness, faintness, or increase in perceived exertion) should be attended to and reported. These signs or symptoms could be related to infection, rejection, or organ dysfunction.

Heart transplant recipients should be highly encouraged to participate in a routine exercise program using the rate of perceived exertion scale to monitor intensity. The recommended goal is for the recipient to progress to 30 minutes of aerobic exercise at moderate intensity 5 days a week.[365,17] The patient needs to be thoroughly instructed in the use of the rate of perceived exertion scale or Borg scale, as heart rate is no longer a viable means to indicate intensity. It is recommended to begin at a low intensity level (2 to 3 out of 10 on the modified rate of perceived exertion scale or 12 to 13 out of 20) and then progress to 16 out of 20 (equivalent to 75% to 85% of predicted heart rate).

Strength training should be a key portion of posttransplantation rehabilitation to address the chronic decrease of muscular strength. For the upper extremities, resistive training will need to be consistent with sternal precautions and should be progressed once the surgeon has lifted the activity restrictions. Lower extremity resistive training can be prescribed when the recipient is hemodynamically stable and should focus on functional activities, such as closed-chain exercises, sit to stand, and step-ups. Resistive training should be prescribed at 50% of 1 maximal repetition for 8 to 15 repetitions, 1 to 3 sets, and include 4 to 10 exercises that are repeated twice a week.[199,417]

### Discharge Planning

Many topics of clinical education need to be disseminated to the recipient before discharge and continued in outpatient services. The therapist should educate the recipient on the adverse effects of the immunosuppressant medications on the neuromuscular and musculoskeletal system and how to minimize some of these effects with exercise and activity modifications.

The recipient also needs to know how to monitor heart rate, blood pressure, and the Borg Rate of Perceived Exertion Scale at rest and during exercise. The therapist should work with the medical team to reinforce healthy living behaviors and continue to reduce cardiac risk factors, including proper nutrition, healthy weight management, smoking cessation, medication adherence, and maintaining a routine exercise program. The recipient can even continue to exercise during bouts of rejection as long as there are no signs of unstable heart failure and vital signs are stable.[417]

By the time of discharge, the recipient and caregiver should be able to independently monitor vital signs and perform proper handwashing. They should demonstrate knowledge of signs and symptoms of infection and transplant rejection and be able to articulate what action to take when they suspect changes in health. This is an important topic for the therapist to assist the transplant team with, especially as these clinical health changes may be noticed first during exercise with a decrease in exercise tolerance, fatigue or an increase in fatigue, and abnormal changes in vital signs. Finally, the recipient and caregiver should be independent in basic functional mobility and be able to comply with sternal precautions during mobility and activities.

### Outpatient Rehabilitation

Rehabilitation should continue on discharge, with the focus on restoring functional independence, increasing muscle mass and strength, and increasing exercise capacity. If the patient has muscle atrophy and decrease in muscle strength and endurance and is taking corticosteroids, it is advised for the patient to be referred to outpatient physical therapy for comprehensive muscular strength and muscular endurance training, advanced balance, coordination, and community entry activities.[183]

Outpatient services should also continue to address osteoporosis rehabilitation and introduce scar management. After completion of outpatient physical therapy, the individual should be referred to outpatient cardiac rehabilitation to increase aerobic capacity. Typically, cardiac rehabilitation programs focus on aerobic training, and therefore it is important that the recipient see a therapist for a comprehensive exercise program to reach muscle mass, muscular endurance, and strength potential as described.

Although assessing work capacity is important, performing an assessment of transplant recipients must take into consideration daily life and daily activities first. Assessing potential for return to work and work requirements may occur as early as 3 to 4 months posttransplantation, depending on the recipient's occupation.

For more physical jobs (e.g., manual labor, any job that requires lifting, carrying, or repetitive load), work assessment typically does not occur until 6 to 12 months after transplantation. For example, a job that involves lifting requires assessment of cardiovascular compliance and hemodynamic stability during lifting. The team will assess hemodynamic status; the therapist will make objective assessments of the recipient's hemodynamic responses to activity and exercise.

### Exercise

Individuals undergoing heart transplantation, similar to individuals undergoing coronary artery bypass surgery, are affected by preoperative inactivity, the adverse systemic effects of heart failure, postoperative deconditioning, and medication effects. These individuals can benefit greatly from exercise rehabilitation. Heart transplant recipients can experience significant improvements with exercise. Exercise can improve hemodynamics and assist in managing blood glucose level, hypertension, and weight management.[90]

There are many reasons why a heart transplant recipient demonstrates a decrease in exercise tolerance, but the appropriately prescribed exercise program and adherence can potentially minimize these adverse effects. Reasons for limitation include cardiac denervation, diastolic dysfunction, lack of pericardium, use of corticosteroids and immunosuppressant medications, deconditioning and muscle atrophy, decrease in arteriovenous oxygen difference, and chronic stress effects of

Box 21.9

**EFFECTS OF CARDIAC DENERVATION**

- Heart rate
  - Elevated at rest
  - Blunted rise with exertion
- Stroke volume: blunted rise with exertion
- Cardiac output: 70%–75% of predicted
- $VO_2$: 70%–80% of predicted
- PAP
  - Elevated at rest
  - Marked rise with exertion
- Anticipatory effect: lost
- Abnormal diffusion capacity
- Ventilation: increased response to exertion
- Loss of anginal pain as a warning sign of myocardial ischemia during early years of denervation

***Clinical Meaning***

- Need for extensive warm-up
- Decrease in exercise capacity
- Marked blood pressure response
- Rely on other data to detect ischemia

*PAP*, Pulmonary arterial pressure; *$VO_2$*, oxygen consumption.
Modified from Braith RW: Exercise training in patients with congestive heart failure and heart transplant recipients. *Med Sci Sports Exerc* 30:S367–S378, 1998.

skeletal muscles related to heart failure.[183,199,417] With a comprehensive rehabilitation program, the heart transplant recipient can increase muscle mass and strength, increase $VO_2$, improve arteriovenous oxygen difference, improve quality of life, and experience a decrease in anxiety and depression.[96,100,417]

### Effects of Denervation

Heart transplantation results in a denervated myocardium and an impaired ability by the autonomic nervous system to regulate cardiac function (Box 21.9). The resting heart rate after transplantation is higher than normal (usually in the range of 90 to 115 beats/min); an external pacemaker may be used if there is not an efficient heart rate to sustain cardiac output. Besides the effect of organ denervation on heart rate, most recipients are on antihypertensive medications that will further delay or blunt an increase in heart rate in response to exercise.

Persisting denervation and sympathetic vasoconstriction inducing functional vascular abnormalities prevent adequate increase in blood flow to exercising limbs and may contribute to decreased exercise performance.[48] Residual abnormalities of ventilatory and gas exchange responses to exercise following heart transplantation are also attributed to the chronotropic incompetence associated with denervation.[336] "Chronotropic incompetence" is a term used to describe the reduced heart rate response to exercise in heart transplant recipients.[40]

Decreased peripheral blood flow is only one variable to consider. Reduced oxygen extraction and utilization, differences in muscle fiber type, and decrease in oxidative enzymes may also contribute to reduced exercise tolerance.[85,417]

In addition to reduced cardiac and skeletal muscle performance, it is likely that the mood state of the individual; level of depression and anxiety; and decreases in cognitive function, such as attention, concentration, and mental flexibility, may affect the individual's ability to participate in activity by affecting frequency, intensity, and duration of exercise.[85,107]

Over time some recipients may regain partial reinnervation, in which case the individual should be able to exercise at higher workloads, have fewer exertional symptoms related to cardiac limitation, and have an increase in heart rate that may surpass 35 beats/min.[149] Partial reinnervation can be recognized when there is an increase in heart rate for each minute during a graded exercise test and when the heart rate decreases every minute during the recovery phase.[417] This phenomenon of reinnervation may begin months to years posttransplantation; the magnitude of reinnervation is variable.[417]

Studies show a functional significance during exercise in people with marked reinnervation, including a higher maximal heart rate, increased peak oxygen uptake, increased oxygen pulse, and earlier heart rate recovery after cessation of exercise (and falling more rapidly) than in cases without reinnervation.[223,224,433,453,477]

### Importance of Warm-Up and Cooldown

In the denervated myocardium, peak heart rate will (on average) increase only 15 to 25 beats/min from the resting level during moderate to high submaximal exercise. The therapist needs to remember that the recipient is catecholamine dependent, which means a minimal of 5 minutes is needed to warm up and allow the body to release catecholamines. Catecholamines will allow a minimal increase in heart rate and contractility, thus increasing cardiac output. Exercise should include large muscle groups to promote venous return, thereby maximizing filling of the ventricles.[58,289]

If the recipient does not warm up sufficiently, the feeling of fatigue and stress (similar to an athlete "hitting the wall") is experienced because of the inability to increase cardiac output to meet demands. The recipient is functioning in anaerobic metabolism.

The physiologic changes unique to heart transplant recipients require a thorough warm-up before exercise to stimulate catecholamine release (epinephrine, norepinephrine) and to give the heart necessary time to prepare for peak activity. The warm-up period should be mild and long to prevent a large oxygen deficiency. Each step in the exercise protocol should be prolonged for up to 5 minutes to allow for a steady state of heart rate.[77]

Likewise, a cooldown period is essential after cessation of exercise to allow for the decrease in blood pressure and return to baseline. The recipient's heart rate can remain elevated for several minutes to an hour as a result of the loss of parasympathetic input and high levels of circulating catecholamines combined with an adrenergic hypersensitivity.

Individuals must be monitored for intensity and tolerance according to symptoms and by rate of perceived exertion scale while working within an acceptable range for heart rate response. Remember that a rise in heart rate of more than 35 beats/min with a moderate to high level of exertion should not be observed during the early posttransplantation period. If this occurs, the person should be monitored closely for rejection.

Although denervation eliminates the sympathetic and parasympathetic nervous system input to the heart, the Bainbridge reflex, catecholamine response, and the Starling law allow for increased stroke volume. The Bainbridge reflex causes the heart rate to increase as venous return to the heart stimulates volume receptors in the atria to trigger an increased heart rate. Release of catecholamines such as epinephrine and norepinephrine results in sympathetic stimulation to increase rate and force of muscular contraction of the heart. The net effect is to increase heart rate and stroke volume, thus increasing cardiac output. At the same time, peripheral blood vessels constrict, resulting in elevated blood pressure.

The Starling law states that the greater the myocardial fiber length (or stretch), the greater will be its force of contraction. The more the left ventricle fills with blood, the greater will be the quantity of blood ejected into the aorta. This is like a rubber band: the more it is stretched, the stronger it recoils or snaps back. Thus a direct relationship exists between the volume of blood in the heart at the end of diastole (the length of the muscle fibers) and the force of contraction during the next systole.

With the start of an activity there will be an increase in venous return associated with large muscle contraction that is responsible for early increases in heart rate; within 5 to 6 minutes after warm-up, catecholamines are activated and heart rate continues to increase. The heart rate may remain elevated after exercise secondary to remaining circulating catecholamines. Some recipients, particularly those with insufficient reinnervation, will achieve peak heart rate response after exercise rather than during exercise.[417]

A similar catecholamine response is not observed during isometric or isotonic contractions; thus it is very important to incorporate a sufficient warm-up or design an exercise program that includes evenly spaced short bouts of aerobic training (8 to 10 minutes) interspersed among the strength training component of the exercise program to allow the recipient's cardiovascular system to adjust to the new demands. The recipient may increase tolerance to strength, power, and muscle endurance training, which may improve compliance.[85,417]

With the loss of autonomic nervous system input over time, diastolic dysfunction occurs. The ventricles hypertrophy because of a loss of compliance and from working against elevated pulmonary and systemic pressures. These changes, combined with the reduced cardiac output, altered kidney function, and use of antihypertensive medications, lead to a reduction in cardiac reserve, or the ability to increase output from rest to exertion. This reduced reserve will be most evident during exercise, requiring close monitoring for exertional hypertension.

### Importance of Monitoring Vital Signs

With the loss of vagal innervation, hypotension can be a problem, especially if there has not been an adequate warm-up or cooldown period. It is not uncommon to see a change in diastolic blood pressure (increase or decrease by 10 to 15 mm Hg) during exertion. Each transplantation center typically has guidelines for blood pressure parameters. In general, an increase or decrease in diastolic pressure greater than 20 mm Hg from baseline, a drop in systolic pressure greater than 10 mm Hg or rise greater than 40 mm Hg above baseline, or a peak pressure of 180 to 200 mm Hg warrants notification of the physician and adjustments to workload intensity or duration.

Following heart transplantation, there may be allograft vasculopathy, a manifestation of chronic rejection, which will cause increasing ischemia of the transplanted heart during increasing activity and exercise. CAV can contribute to reduced oxygen uptake and a ventilation–perfusion mismatch, limiting exercise capacity.[389] With insufficient reinnervation, this ischemic condition may not be detected except through the monitoring of vital signs and diagnostic testing.[182,386]

If the recipient has concomitant pulmonary involvement, abnormal diffusion capacities with altered ventilation responses may occur. These pulmonary components can cause a decrease in cardiac function, with possible myocardial ischemia and possible mild desaturation.

Although there have been some documented cases of angina, most of these clients will not experience ischemia-induced angina as an early warning sign of cardiac impairment. This is another reason the therapist must follow appropriate exercise guidelines, which includes providing sufficient warm-up aerobic stimulation to stimulate a catecholamine response and monitor vital signs to assess cardiac function. The signs of decreasing activity tolerance should be reported to the transplant center because it may be associated with CAV.

### Isometric Exercise

Isometric exercise, exercises where the intensity is high enough to cause a breath hold, puts a volume stress rather than a pressure stress on the heart. This section is not considering such common exercises as quadriceps or gluteal muscle isometric contractions. In the acute care phase, the recipient's heart is very volume or preload dependent; consequently, aggressive isometric exercise that can lead to decrease in preload should be avoided. The acute care therapist should modify functional activities to avoid the Valsalva maneuver.

When introducing isometric exercises in the post–acute care phase of recovery, the therapist should be involved to closely monitor the patient. A dynamic warm-up should be completed to produce a gradual rise in heart rate, and blood pressure response should be monitored closely to avoid excessive hypertensive responses. Before introducing these stressful activities, the patient should be instructed in breath control exercises and ventilatory strategies. Ventilatory strategies involve matching the phase of breathing with the biomechanical movement of the spine: doing activities like reaching overhead should be coupled with inhalation and when lowering something to the ground the patient should exhale. If the patient cannot complete the activity without breath holding, the therapist should help modify the task and teach the patient how to independently modify activities.

### Rehabilitation of Individuals With Ventricular Assist Device Support

Patients with acute decompensation as a consequence of myocardial ischemia and heart failure may be placed on an intraaortic balloon pump. This device improves myocardial perfusion and decreases left ventricular afterload. The catheter or balloon is typically inserted into the aorta via the femoral artery. If the patient is stable, low-level strengthening, range of motion, modified bed mobility, and airway clearance activities can be prescribed. The principal restriction is typically no hip flexion beyond 30 degrees. The therapist should monitor peripheral perfusion of the involved extremity and perform skin inspection for signs of limb ischemia or wound development. If the catheter is placed in the upper extremity, more functional mobility and reconditioning can be prescribed during time of support. More recently the intraaortic balloon pump catheter is being placed in the upper extremity to allow for ambulation.

The key to the rehabilitation of patients being supported on a VAD is for the therapist to be competent in the operation and management of any alarms. With nonpulsatile VADs, the therapist will need to modify how the patient is monitored because it is common for these individuals not to have a palpable pulse; the typical blood pressure method and use of pulse oximetry are commonly inaccurate or cannot be obtained. It is important that the patient fully understands how to use a subjective scale so that the therapist can monitor the recipient's tolerance during the therapy sessions.

One of the benefits of VAD support is that the patient is no longer restricted by activity tolerance because of low cardiac output. This means that a comprehensive and aggressive rehabilitation program can be instituted, including functional strengthening, functional mobility, and aerobic and anaerobic reconditioning. The therapist should monitor the patient and VAD function closely during exercise and report findings to the VAD team in case they need to make adjustments in the VAD setting to optimize VAD performance. Many of these patients can be discharged home within 2 weeks after implantation. Besides monitoring VAD function, the rehabilitation goals and procedures are very common to what has been discussed earlier in this chapter for heart transplant recipients.

The therapist should monitor the patient for any VAD alarms and complications. The most common complications include bleeding in the early postoperative period, infections, thrombus formation, and stroke. It is advised that the therapist know and teach the patient to auscultate the VAD so that the patient knows what the sound should be normally. The sound of the VAD may change if there is pump dysfunction or thrombus. With nonpulsatile pumps the sound will change from a hum to a knocking if the patient is hypovolemic and a grinding sound if there is thrombus formation within the pump.

The therapist should always follow the strict guidelines on driveline care to minimize the risk of driveline infection. If the pathogen gets seeded on the device, the VAD may need to be explanted to address the infection, and this typically leads to a high mortality rate. Finally, because stroke is still a major concern for patients being supported by a VAD, the therapist should conduct thorough neurologic screening, including cranial nerve, coordination, and functional testing. This is important to obtain a functional baseline for the individual in case a problem arises.

The prognosis for patients with VAD support is still under investigation and depends on the reason for VAD implantation and medical status of the patient. For patients receiving nonpulsatile VADs as destination therapy, in general the 1-year survival rate is 83% and 5-year survival is 50%.[234]

SPECIAL IMPLICATIONS FOR THE THERAPIST 21.7

### *Mechanical Circulatory Support*

An increasing number of centers nationwide are routinely implanting mechanical circulatory support devices, and there has been an increase in clinical trials to use VADs as a destination therapy, allowing patients to be discharged home with these devices. Therefore, it is likely that therapists in a variety of settings will encounter clients with these devices and become involved in evaluation and treatment progression. For a therapist's thoughts regarding mobilizing individuals who have a pulmonary artery catheter in place while listed for heart and/or lung transplantation and mobilization of individuals on ECMO, see eBoxes 21.2 and 21.3, respectively, on the book's Student Consult site.

Throughout the rehabilitation process, the therapist must monitor international normalized ratio values for bleeding risk monitor drivelines during transfer training to avoid torsion or pulling, monitor VAD pump rate and pump output at rest and during exercise, observe for volume overload or dehydration, assess for neurologic and musculoskeletal complications, and observe for any signs of infection. In addition, there is a high incidence of orthostatic hypotension in this population, requiring monitoring of vital signs.

## Lung Transplantation

### Overview

Lung transplantation has become a viable option for the treatment of various end-stage lung diseases, with the most prevalent disease categories being chronic obstructive lung disease, interstitial pulmonary fibrosis, and pulmonary arterial hypertension.[175] Lung transplantation is performed in pediatric patients for treatment of congenital defects and pulmonary arterial hypertension.[334]

The first lung transplant was performed in 1963 in a 58-year-old man with bronchogenic carcinoma; he survived for 18 days. Limited success of early lung transplantation was the result of lung rejection, anastomotic complications, or infection in transplant recipients. A monumental breakthrough in transplantation came in 1965 with the discovery of chemical immunosuppression, but it would be another 15 years before the world saw the first successful heart-lung transplantation in 1981 for the treatment of pulmonary vascular disease, followed by the first double-lung transplantation in 1983.[372,472]

Despite all the advances in procurement procedures, surgical techniques, and pharmaceutical discoveries and utilization, it remains difficult to preserve the lung's function during harvest and reimplantation. The donor lung is extremely vulnerable to multiple conditions. Many donor organs come from patients who have been declared brain dead, which implies organ preservation, but as part of the physiologic cascade of brain death the body releases large amounts of catecholamines, which leads to the disruption of the pulmonary capillary beds. The consequence is pulmonary edema and difficulty with ventilation and oxygenation.[146,250] This response can lead to ventilatory acquired trauma, along with risk of pulmonary contusion and aspiration of the donor lung, which can significantly decrease the number of suitable donor lungs available for transplantation. There is also an increased risk of lung injury because of pulmonary contusion if the death of the donor was traumatic, as well as the risk of aspiration and ventilatory-related trauma and pneumonia.[175,250,372]

Thus only approximately 20% to 30% of donors have lungs classified as suitable for transplantation, although it is estimated that as many as 40% are suitable if advanced care is provided to the donor and recipient.[175] In 2018 the OPTN reported that only 2542 lungs were recovered, and 2530 individuals underwent a lung transplant procedure, while there were approximately 1500 candidates waiting for a suitable donor lung.[334]

Suitable donor lungs are from a donor ideally less than 55 years of age with a ratio of partial pressure of oxygen in arterial blood ($PaO_2$)/fraction of inspired oxygen ($FiO_2$) ≥300 mm Hg, which is an indication of good gas exchange function of the lungs, and minimal to no smoking. If the donor has been declared brain dead, great care is needed to maintain hemodynamic stability and endocrine function and provide protective mechanical ventilation to avoid barotrauma.[250] More experienced centers are accepting organs that extend beyond the ideal parameters to increase the number of transplants that can be done and decrease the death rate while waiting. There has been improvement in infection and circulatory support of recipients who may have received a less ideal organ, which has allowed for an increase in transplantation.[250,445]

The type of lung transplantation depends on many factors, including candidate factors such as age, disease process and progression rate, expected time of waiting list, other organ function, surgical preference, and organ availability. Currently single-lung transplantation accounts for 25% of all adult lung transplant procedures and 3% of pediatric procedures.[445] The majority of surgeons prefer to perform a bilateral lung transplant procedure because the recipient has a greater chance of achieving higher lung function as well as decreased future infection and other lung dysfunction secondary to leaving a native diseased lung and thus an increased median survival rate.[334] In the United States the performance of living related lobar transplantation is very rare, with only two cases reported in 2 years,[334] and this decrease has contributed to the implementation of the lung allocation system and LAS. However, in Japan this type of transplant procedure is commonly done for interstitial pulmonary fibrosis, constrictive bronchiolitis, and GVHD with a 5-year survival rate of 45%, which is similar to single lung transplantation.[112]

### Indications

At the present time there are approximately 70 active lung transplantation centers in the United States.[332] Over the past 25 years there has been an expansion in the number of diseases that can be successfully treated by lung transplantation. In the past decade with the new lung allocation system and LAS, there has been a change in the distribution of recipients based on their primary disease.

In 2001, 53.3% of lung transplant recipients had chronic obstructive pulmonary disease (usually smoking-related emphysema, but also including emphysema caused by $\alpha_1$-antitrypsin deficiency). In 2018 this percentage had been reduced to 19% with an increase in transplants occurring as a result of pulmonary fibrosis from 16.2% to 35.6%. Other common indications include cystic fibrosis, idiopathic pulmonary hypertension, and secondary hypertension as a result of congenital diseases.[335]

Less frequent indications include lymphangioleiomyomatosis, eosinophilic granuloma, drug-induced and radiation-induced pulmonary fibrosis, and occupation-induced pulmonary diseases such as silica farmer's lung that lead to pneumonitis and pulmonary fibrosis. Pulmonary disease arising from an underlying collagen vascular disorder, such as scleroderma and lupus, can also lead to end-stage lung disease.

Although lung cancer has traditionally represented an absolute contraindication to transplantation, successful transplantation for bronchoalveolar carcinoma has been documented.[8,29,467]

### Transplantation Candidates

Many factors are analyzed in the determination of a lung transplantation candidate because of the potential complications associated with these factors (see Box 21.4). Some of these variables include the presence of severe osteoporosis, the degree of systemic and pulmonary hypertension, diabetes mellitus, and coronary artery disease that may worsen after transplantation; severe gastroesophageal reflux disease (GERD), obesity, and mechanical ventilation at the time of transplantation (higher mortality rate); underlying collagen vascular disease; presence of antibiotic-resistant infections, especially *Burkholderia cepacia* (a multiresistant bacterial respiratory infection associated with severe and often lethal postoperative infections); and previous thoracic surgery.[219,429]

It is both science and art to determine the best time to list a person for transplantation based on the disease process and its progression, blood type, and other medical conditions, as well as the activity level of the transplantation center. The important thing is to list a potential candidate for transplantation when the data suggest that the person can survive the expected waiting time for transplantation without developing other contraindications to transplantation.

Contraindications may include irreversible damage to other organs (unless a multiorgan transplant would be appropriate), certain types of infection, dependency on mechanical ventilation, cancer within at least 2 years from listing, chronic extrapulmonary infections from such viruses as HIV or hepatitis, untreatable psychiatric disorder, severe chest wall/spinal deformity, and documented poor adherence to medical care.[104,196,219] The candidate must be free of clinically significant cardiac, renal, or hepatic impairment. Some relative contraindications include severe functional limitations, mechanical ventilator support, ECMO, obesity, and severe osteoporosis.[155,290]

**Lung Allocation System.** In 2005 the Lung Allocation System was adopted to improve the survival for individuals on the transplantation waitlist. The LAS is calculated based on the following measures: (1) expected number of days lived without a transplant during an additional year on the waitlist; (2) expected number of days lived during the first year posttransplantation; (3) the transplantation benefit measure, which is calculated by posttransplantation survival minus the waitlist urgency measure (urgency – survival).[175] The LAS is based on the previous 6 months of medical information. Box 21.10 presents the International Guidelines for criteria for timing to list for transplant candidates. The goal is to perform transplantation in the most appropriate candidate at the most appropriate time to maximize outcomes and decrease the rate of deaths while waiting for a suitable organ to be found.[175] See Box 21.3 for the LAS formula and the variables that are factored in to calculate the waitlist urgency and the posttransplantation benefit.

General categories to cluster diseases have been created to allow factors such as degree of pulmonary systolic pressure and amount of supplemental oxygen to be more sensitive as predictors in the LAS formula based on the disease. Each candidate is assigned an LAS; the procurement centers then allocate donor organs based on LAS. The LAS is assigned as 0 to 100, and the higher the LAS, the higher the probability of receiving an offer. The LAS can be updated as the candidate's state of heath changes (see Box 21.3).

Allocation is based on several factors. For lung allocation, determination depends on survival benefit, medical urgency, waiting time, distance from donor hospital, and pediatric status.[456] Medical urgency may include a patient with respiratory failure as defined as a need for mechanical ventilation, ECMO support, or using an $FiO_2$ greater than 50% pro sufficient saturation or having a $PaO_2$ less than 50 mm Hg or a partial pressure of carbon dioxide ($PCO_2$) greater than 56 mm Hg. Medical urgency may also be related to severe pulmonary hypertension with cardiac index less than 2 L/min/m$^2$.[174] For pediatric patients younger than 12 years of age, an LAS is not assigned to determine prioritization; the above-mentioned medical urgency criteria are used to assign a pediatric patient a priority 1 status, and all other conditions would assign the pediatric patient a priority 2 status. When a child turns 12, an LAS is calculated and is used for lung allocation in place of the pediatric priority system.[458]

Since implementation of the LAS, it appears that there has been a decrease in waiting time on the lung transplant list and decrease in mortality rates on the waitlist; however, sicker patients are undergoing transplantation, which may complicate posttransplantation management, and 90-day and 1-year survival rates are lower. After 1 year there appears to be no difference in long-term survival. The lung allocation system has not seemed to benefit patients with pulmonary fibrosis as well as patients with other types of pulmonary disease.[175,458]

Currently there are between 1400 and 1500 people waiting for a lung transplantation. The median wait time ranges from 234 to 307 days for pediatric patients and 73 to 226 days for adults, with the individuals older than 65 years of age waiting the least amount of time.[336] In 2018, 47 people died while waiting for a lung transplantation; the leading primary diagnosis was idiopathic pulmonary fibrosis. National data reports provided by the

Box 21.10

**INTERNATIONAL SELECTION CRITERIA FOR LUNG TRANSPLANTATION**

***General Criteria***

- Candidate should meet criteria listed in Box 21.4

***Chronic Obstructive Pulmonary Disease:***

- BODE Index ≥7
- $FEV_1$ <20%
- ≥3 severe exacerbations during previous year
- 1 severe $PaCO_2$ respiratory failure
- Moderate to severe pulmonary arterial hypertension

***Cystic Fibrosis***

- Chronic respiratory failure with
  - Hypoxia with $PaO_2$ <60 mm Hg
  - Hypercapnia with $PaCO_2$ >50 mm Hg
  - Long-term use of noninvasive mechanical ventilation
  - Pulmonary arterial hypertension
  - Frequent hospitalization
  - Rapid decline in functional mobility
  - World Health Organization Functional Class IV

***Pulmonary Vascular Disease***

- NYHA class III or IV despite trial or 3 months of combination therapy including prostanoids
- Cardiac index <2 L/min/m$^2$
- Mean central venous pressure >15 mm Hg
- 6-Minute walk test <350 m
- Presence of hemoptysis, pericardial effusion, right heart failure with renal insufficiency, elevated bilirubin, brain natriuretic peptides, or recurrent ascites

***Interstitial Pulmonary Fibrosis***

- FVC <80% with 10% decline in last 6 months
- DLCO <40% with >15% in last 6 months
- Desaturation <88% or <250 m during 6-minute walk test or decrease >50 m in last 6 months
- Pulmonary arterial hypertension
- Hospitalization with respiratory failure, pneumothorax, or acute exacerbation

*BODE*, Body mass index, airflow Obstruction, Dyspnea, Exercise; *DLCO*, diffusing capacity of lung for carbon monoxide; *FEV*$_1$, forced expiratory volume in 1 second; *FVC*, forced vital capacity; *NYHA*, New York Heart Association.

Data from Hachem RR: Lung transplantation: General guidelines for recipient selection. Trulock EP, Hollingswood H, eds. *UpToDate*. Waltham MA: UpToDate Inc. https://www.uptodate.com/contents/lung-transplantation-general-guidelines-for-recipient-selection

OPTN indicate a steady increase in the number of lung transplantations occurring in the United States. In 2018, 2530 lung transplantations occurred, with the largest number in patients between the ages of 50 and 64; the 65 and older age group has become the second largest age group since the implementation of the lung allocation system.[24,337]

### Transplantation Procedure

The four major surgical approaches to lung transplantation are single-lung transplantation, bilateral sequential transplantation, heart-lung transplantation, and transplantation of lobes from living donors. Since 2002, bilateral lung transplantations have exceeded the number of single-lung transplants. Bilateral lung transplantations account for 75% and 97% of adult and pediatric transplantations, respectively, completed at the current time,[445] with very few living related transplantations done owing to the implementation of the LAS.[112]

Single-lung transplantation typically requires a posterolateral thoracotomy, but some surgeons use an anterior approach, whereas bilateral lung transplantations are typically done through bilateral anterior thoracotomies and a horizontal disruption of the sternum, referred to as a clamshell. The clamshell approach allows good visibility of the mediastinum. The heart-lung procedure is still generally performed through a mediastinotomy.

In general, donor lungs should be the same size or just slightly larger than the recipient's lungs so that the donor lobes fill each hemithorax, avoiding persistent pleural space problems in the recipient. However, donor lungs must have a lung volume similar to (or less than) that of the intended recipient; larger lungs in single-lung transplantation can be placed on the left side, where the diaphragm has the potential to descend because of the absence of the liver under the left hemidiaphragm. In living related donations, a lobe (generally the right or left lower lobe) is removed from each of the two donor lungs and is used to replace the lungs of the recipient.

**Denervation.** The lung loses autonomic nervous system innervation below the bronchial anastomosis. This results in a loss of the cough reflex of the donor lung. There is a delay in bronchial dilation during exertion and impairment of ciliary function. These neurologic deficits increase the recipient's risk for sputum retention and pneumonia.

### Complications

Postoperative complications of primary lung transplantation vary based on the time from transplantation, with graft failure, bleeding, and dysfunction of the bronchial and/or vascular anastomoses occurring in the early postoperative period, whereas infections and varying types of rejection can occur throughout the lifetime of the transplant recipient. Moreover, patients with long-term survival may face complications, such as cancer, hypertension, renal failure, and diabetes.

**Primary Graft Dysfunction or Failure.** PGD is defined as graft dysfunction or failure that occurs within the first 72 hours posttransplantation and is associated with diffuse allograft edema and infiltrates. The severity of PGD is measured by the $PaO_2/FiO_2$ ratio, with mild PGD having a ratio greater than 300 and severe PGD have a less than 200. Approximately one-third of all recipients experience some level of PGD, and PGD accounts for 25% of recipients within the first 30 days posttransplantation.[175,290] PGD is associated with oxidative radicals, proinflammatory cytokines, and cellular ischemia and necrosis.[429] Risk factors associated with PGD include non–cardiac-related pulmonary edema, pulmonary hypertension, issues with proper organ procurement, donor or recipient infection, need for ECMO during the operative procedures, and presence of ischemic reperfusion injury.[219,487]

There are donor- and recipient-related risk factors associated with PGD. Donor-related factors include age, African American ethnicity, female gender, history of smoking, prolonged mechanical ventilation, aspiration pneumonitis/pneumonia, trauma, and hemodynamic instability. Recipient-related risk factors include idiopathic pulmonary hypertension, use of cardiopulmonary bypass, and large blood transfusion.[55]

**Rejection.** The lung transplant recipient needs to be continuously monitored for rejection, as 37% of all recipients experience at least one episode of rejection within the first year.[97] Hyperacute rejection is predominantly an antibody-mediated response that occurs immediately after revascularization and leads to a massive immune response, thrombus formation, and destruction to the donor lung. Treatments may include plasmapheresis, intravenous immunoglobulin therapy, and augmented B lymphocyte–targeted therapy such as mycophenolate mofetil or azathioprine. Patients may be so critically ill with a $PaO_2/FiO_2$ ratio of less than 300 that they require ECMO (see The Medically Complex Patient: Critical Illness in Chapter 5). There is a high mortality rate for individuals who experience hyperacute rejection.[229,250,316,472,480]

Acute rejection is generally a T cell–mediated response. Class 1 HLAs located in all nucleated cells are recognized by CD8 recipient cells that mediate the immune response, whereas class 2 HLAs are found in endothelial cells that activate CD4 T lymphocytes. Both T cell–mediated responses lead to the activation and proliferation of the recipient's immune response, including perivascular and peribronchial lymphocytic infiltrates and donor-specific antibodies.[229,316,480]

Some people experiencing acute rejection will be asymptomatic; when a person experiencing rejection is symptomatic, he or she may present with dyspnea, fatigue, fever and chills, oxygen desaturation, decreased exercise tolerance, and changes in x-ray findings. The recipient may experience significant respiratory distress or even respiratory failure, requiring mechanical ventilator support.[155] Recipients should use a home spirometer daily to check for expiratory indices (e.g., forced expiratory volume in 1 second), and monitor exercise tolerance, which will show a decline because of acute rejection. Infection control should be heightened when any recipient is being treated for rejection because the primary treatment is to increase the immunosuppressant medications, which increases the risk of infection. Careful handwashing and use of a surgical mask may be recommended.

Chronic rejection, which used to be referred to as bronchiolitis obliterans syndrome, is now called chronic lung allograft dysfunction (CLAD). CLAD accounts for 30% of deaths in the first year posttransplantation and is the leading cause of death after 3 years.[175,290] CLAD is the fibrotic occlusion of small airways as a result of the adverse effects of rejection on the donor lung and is diagnosed with biopsy. It is defined as a 20% decrease in the best postoperative forced expiratory volume in 1 second with an identifiable cause such as ACR or an infection. The recipient can present with the more classic obstructive pattern, which has associated risk factors such as PGD, ACR, and lymphocytic bronchitis, or a more restrictive pulmonary function pattern, referred to as resistive allograft syndrome, which is associated with younger recipients, female recipients, late onset of diffuse alveolar dysfunction, CMV mismatch, underlying pulmonary fibrosis, and increased incidence of bronchoalveolar neutrophil infiltrates. Resistive allograft syndrome is associated with a worse prognosis.[290,487] CLAD is the primary limiting factor to long-term survival and limits 5-year survival to 56%.[487]

**Infection.** The absence of the cough reflex and diminished mucociliary function in the denervated lung leads to insufficient mucus clearance and contributes to the elevated frequency of pulmonary infection (at least three times more common than in heart transplant recipients). Pulmonary infection is also related to the increased level of immunosuppressive medications required posttransplantation, poor nutritional status, and the fact that the lung is exposed to environmental factors. Signs and symptoms of infection may be very difficult to distinguish from acute rejection (fever, tachycardia, tachypnea, fatigue, malaise, decrease in exercise tolerance, oxygen desaturation, and respiratory failure) except that there is an increase in sputum production with a productive cough in most cases.

Infections are associated with a significant negative impact on transplantation outcomes. Infections account for 35% of deaths in the first year and 20% in subsequent years. Lung transplant recipients may develop a viral infection; these infections peak within the first 3 months after transplantation and typically involve CMV or EBV. CMV infections account for 2.5% mortality within the first year.[2,97,175]

The donor and recipient are tested for viral infections so that proper medications can be administered to decrease the risk of infection. Finally, the recipient may develop a fungal infection, commonly *Candida* or *Aspergillus,* although mortality and morbidity rates associated with fungal infections have decreased with the availability of new antifungal medications. It is critical for the recipient to practice good hand hygiene, be cautious of infectious exposures associated with social gatherings and travel, and be aware of the infectious risk depending on the where they live or may be visiting.

**Bone Density Loss.** Glucocorticoid-induced changes in bone density are a significant medical complication after lung transplantation. In fact, in contrast to other transplant recipients who develop osteoporosis after surgery from antirejection drugs, lung transplant recipients are more at risk for osteopenia or osteoporosis as a result of decreased muscle mass before transplantation; exposure to acute, high-dosage, or long-term use of corticosteroids; and lack of weight-bearing activities.

Besides pretransplantation exposure to corticosteroids, lung transplant candidates commonly have poor absorption of nutrients associated with the underlying disease process (e.g., cystic fibrosis, collagen vascular diseases). Malabsorption deficits and deficits of enzymes needed to use vitamin D further increase the risk for bone loss in individuals with these pathologies.

Immunosuppressive medications such as cyclosporine, mycophenolate mofetil, and azathioprine may be used in the pretransplantation period for management of interstitial lung disease and autoimmune diseases such as scleroderma and lupus, which can result in further bone loss. The incidence of osteoporosis of the vertebral spine is 29% in lung candidates before transplantation; bone loss continues after transplantation at a rate of 2% to 5% in the first year, with up to 20% of recipients having a significant progression of osteoporosis. The incidence of fractures has been reported as high as 37% within the first year posttransplantation, primarily related to the adverse effects of immunosuppressive drugs on bone remodeling and bone quality.[61,94,240,407]

Lung transplant recipients are more likely to be exposed to higher immunosuppressive levels and longer exposure to corticosteroids than other organ transplant recipients as a result of the highly vascular and immunogenic nature of the lung, which further compromises the health of bone.[470,472]

**Gastrointestinal Disorders.** Gastrointestinal problems are a considerable source of morbidity for lung transplant recipients, often because of the poor absorption patterns of nutrients previously mentioned in association with the underlying pathologies such as cystic fibrosis. The most common major complication is diverticulitis, requiring colectomy. Malignancy occurs slightly less often; minor problems such as polyps and benign anorectal disease have also been reported.[164]

**Nutrition/Swallowing.** Many recipients fail initial swallow studies after transplantation as a result of vocal cord injury or weakness, which accounts for 25% of the cases. Many recipients are also kept NPO (nothing by mouth) because of severe GERD, which is reported in the past medical history of 30% to 70% of transplant recipients.[403] This requires a nasogastrojejunostomy tube for nutrition during NPO status. The therapist should be alert to the diet requirements of the individual, specifically whether the patient is cleared to take oral medications, liquids, and solid foods, or whether the liquids need to be thickened to prevent aspiration. This is especially important if the individual has diabetes and requires quick increases of blood glucose but is unable to take juice or glucose tablets by mouth.

**Diabetes Management.** Of lung transplant recipients, 34% develop steroid-induced diabetes in the early postoperative phase. Lung transplant recipients should be trained to check and manage their blood glucose; the therapist needs to be aware of the individual's glucose status before and during exercise. Patients should be encouraged to bring their glucometers to rehabilitation in case it is necessary to check glucose status. The therapist should be aware of the facility guidelines and policies regarding blood glucose and exercise and be able to assist patients as needed to maintain blood glucose in an acceptable range for exercise.

**Pulmonary Problems.** The transplanted lung may have deficiencies in lymphatic drainage, especially in the early period after transplantation. Ventilation and ventilation–perfusion may be impaired if effusion is clinically significant. If effusion is persistent, affected by dietary intake, and cloudy in appearance, the patient should be evaluated for a chylothorax. Disruption of the lymphatic system appears to be restored 3 to 6 weeks after transplantation, and mucociliary function may be depressed for up to 16 weeks.[403]

Other pulmonary complications include surgical trauma to the phrenic nerve, anastomosis dysfunction, pneumothorax, pulmonary embolus, and native lung hyperinflation. Although phrenic neuropathy is an infrequent complication of lung transplantation, the therapist may see evidence of it with subsequent diaphragmatic dysfunction. Clinical evidence of phrenic nerve damage may include atelectasis, pneumonia, elevated hemidiaphragm, and prolonged ventilatory support and is reported in up to 30% of lung transplant recipients.

Narrowing of the bronchus can occur from the formation of granulation tissue or fibrosis or owing to malacia. A laser procedure can be done to remove the obstruction and a custom-fitted stent can be placed within the airway to stabilize the lumen and allow for sufficient air flow.[9,155,445]

In individuals with an underlying obstructive disease (most commonly emphysema) who undergo a single-lung transplant, either acutely or chronically, the native lung can develop further hyperinflation because of increased lung compliance and the presence of bullous disease. The lung can displace the mediastinum away from the native lung; can lead to a decrease in pulmonary function, dyspnea, tachycardia, and flattening of the diaphragm; and, if severe, can alter the flow of blood through the cardiac system.[9]

Gastric reflux and dysphasia are receiving increased attention. One report indicates that up to 70% of lung transplant recipients have an abnormal swallow on diagnosis testing. Dysphasia can lead to aspiration, pneumonitis, and an increased risk of pneumonia.[155] It is theorized that dysphasia is the result of intubation and the transesophageal echocardiogram probe placed during the surgery and dysfunction of thoracoabdominal pressure regulation.[277]

**Other Complications.** Lung transplant recipients are at risk for other complications, as previously discussed in other transplantation sections of this chapter. These complications significantly reduce quality of life and increase mortality and morbidity rates. For example, cancer accounts for one-third of deaths in the first 5 years posttransplantation and up to 18% of recipient deaths after 5 years.[325] Renal dysfunction is present in 62% of recipients. There is a high prevalence of cardiac risk factors as well, with 57% of recipients with a diagnosis of hyperlipidemia, 39% with diabetes, and almost 83% with systemic hypertension.[97,325] Slightly more than 9% of deaths after 10 years are related to cardiovascular disease.[97,155]

### Prognosis

The leading causes of death for lung transplant recipients vary based on the time posttransplantation. Causes of death within the first 30 days include non-CMV infections, which account for 20% of the deaths, and other complications such as coagulopathy, disruption of one of the anastomoses, and ventilatory-induced injury.[97] In the case of acute PGD, ventilation needs may exceed the parameters of standard mechanical ventilation and ECMO may be required, in which case gas exchange takes place entirely or in part outside the body (Fig. 21.19). See further discussion in Future Trends.

The leading cause of death within the first year posttransplantation is non-CMV infections (35.3%) followed by graft failure and other complications such as bronchial anastomosis dysfunction. After 3 years, the primary cause of death is related to CLAD, and deaths associated with renal failure, cancer, and complications of diabetes are increased.[97,111,425,470]

Survival rates for lung transplantation continue to improve as surgical techniques and postoperative care improve despite the fact that the recipients are older and there has been an expansion of the medical criteria for donor lungs. The median survival rate for single-lung and bilateral lung transplantation is 4.6 years and 6.9 years, respectively. The 1-, 3-, and 5-year survival rates range from 83% to 89% for adults and 74% to 89% for pediatric patients at 1 year to 45% to 59% for adults and 49% to 75% for pediatric patients at 5 years.[336] There are differences in survival rates based on primary pulmonary diagnosis and age.

Only a few heart-lung transplantations are performed annually. Despite the complexity of candidate medical status, the technical surgical issues, and the management of both heart and pulmonary function, the current 5-year survival rates are similar to lung transplantation.[336]

### Future Trends

With the increasing history of lung transplantation there is much research to be done to fully understand and assess the effects of transplantation. Research should continue in the assessment of survival rates based on new advances in procurement and candidate selection and pretransplant management. Beyond these topics, research needs to expand in the area of postoperative management, including further studies in dysphasia and dysfunction of other neuromotor structures such as the phrenic nerve and vagus nerve that may impact mortality and morbidity. Research is needed in the areas of quality of life, rehabilitation, and community reentrance for these recipients.

**Extracorporeal Membrane Oxygenation.** One of the most exciting areas of pretransplantation management is the use of ECMO as a bridge to transplantation (see Fig. 21.18). Once thought of as an extreme medical intervention to salvage an individual for possible transplantation, which was very controversial, ECMO is becoming more common in the management of

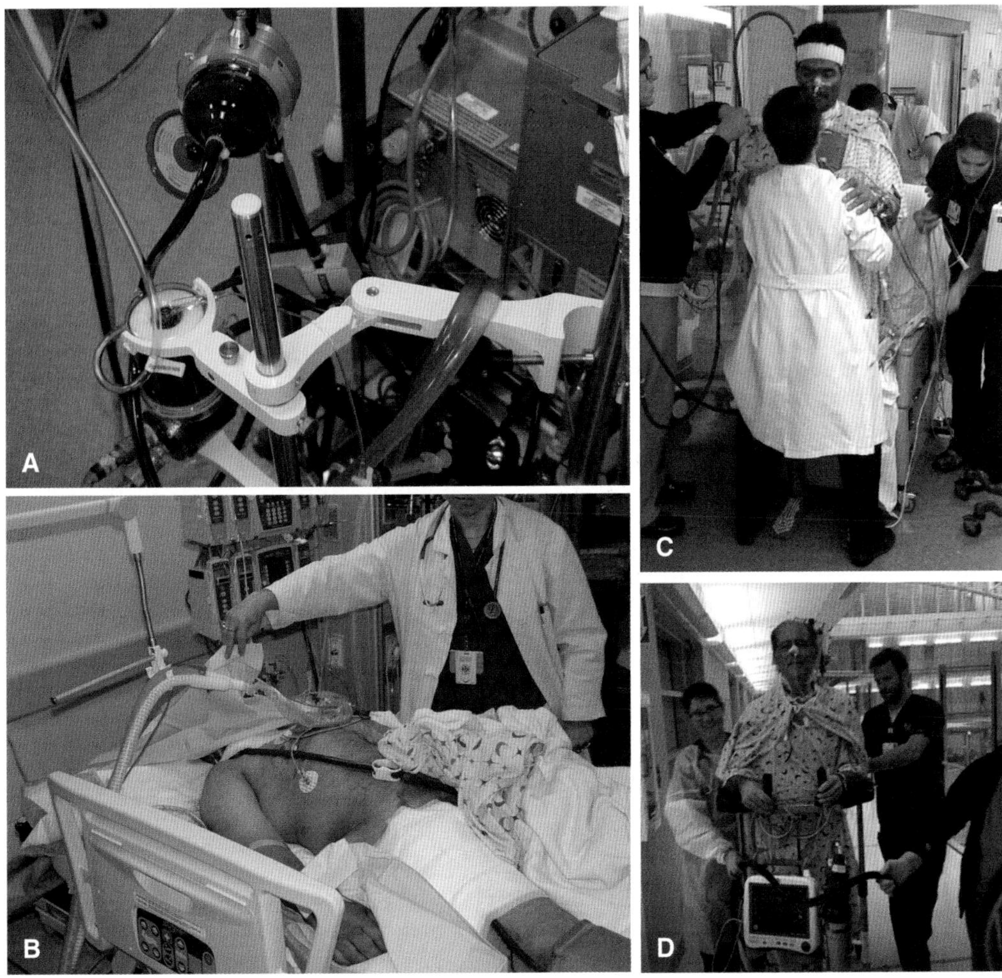

**Fig. 21.18**

**Extracorporeal membrane oxygenation (ECMO).** (A) ECMO is used to support the cardiopulmonary system by controlling gas exchange and assisting the heart in blood circulation. With ECMO, venous blood is circulated through a $CO_2$ scrubber and membrane oxygenator (white canister) and returned to the body via a centrifuge pump (red and silver machine) as oxygenated blood with a desired $PaCO_2$ and $PaO_2$. (B) Depending on how the machine is cannulated to the patient, ECMO can assist or control cardiopulmonary function. The cannulation sites in this individual are the femoral vein and artery. In more critically ill patients the cannulas can be inserted in the inferior vena cava or the right atrium and the aorta, primarily bypassing cardiopulmonary function. This photo illustrates traditional nonambulatory ECMO. (C–D) With advances in ECMO technology in the oxygenator, cannulations, and pump, patients can be mobilized early including advancing to ambulation, even with femoral cannulations. (A–D, Courtesy Chris L. Wells, University of Maryland Medical Center, Baltimore, MD.)

individuals with refractory hypoxemia as a bridge to transplantation.

ECMO is a device that allows gas exchange to occur outside the body to aid or replace the function of the lungs that no longer can properly regulate the body's pH by performing adequate gas exchange. ECMO could interface with the body via venovenous or venoarterial circulation. In venovenous circulation, the common cannula sites are the femoral and jugular veins, and these sites are commonly used as a bridge to lung transplantation. Venoarterial ECMO cannulas are typically femoral vein to femoral artery or right atria to pulmonary trunk or left atria for cardiac support.

New advances in the oxygenator, the ECMO device, and the flexibility of the cannulas have resulted in this new use of ECMO as a bridge to transplantation. These advances along with the focus of early rehabilitation of critically ill patients to prevent the iatrogenic effects of immobility has placed rehabilitation services as a key part of the critical care and transplant team to prepare these individuals for transplantation. It is now possible to progress these individuals to ambulatory status (see Fig. 21.19).[471]

These advances have allowed individuals to be placed on ECMO earlier to decrease the additional organ complications of hypoxemia and prolonged mechanical ventilation. In many cases patients can be weaned from mechanical ventilation, which has decreased the risk of pneumonia and decreased the burden to the medical team when mobilizing the patient. Progressing functional training while on ECMO support has been shown to result in no difference in transplant outcomes for patients on ECMO compared with patients not on ECMO[290] and better outcomes compared with patients on mechanical ventilation.[174] One study reported significant outcomes in patients supported by venovenous ECMO compared with patients supported by mechanical ventilation.[152] These patients had a 30% reduction in mortality, 23% reduction in days on mechanical ventilation posttransplantation, and a decrease in ICU stay and length of hospital stay by 21 days and 29 days, respectively.[241]

The ECMO device is also being used more in the postoperative period for the management of PGD. Marasco[270] reported increased success of using ECMO within the first 48 hours posttransplantation for PGD. His group reported success in supporting the patient and the new donor lungs through the initial period of PGD to allow for healing and medical intervention.[179,246,270] This allowed for a significant reduction in the patient requiring emergent retransplantation. Marasco[270] also reported that patients' outcomes were poor when ECMO was introduced after postoperative day 7 for reasons of graft failure that may have been infectious or rejection.

**Artificial Lung.** Work continues in the area of developing an artificial lung device that would further allow function and improve quality of life for the treatment of end-stage lung disease. Investigators are currently attempting to create a wearable artificial lung, similar to a VAD, which would allow patients to be more mobile in the community while they waited for a viable lung to be found for them. The Paracorporeal Ambulatory Assist Lung (PAAL) (Breethe, Baltimore, MD) is one such experimental device.

The potential benefits in using either an artificial lung device or ambulatory ECMO device are significant and include a more effective way of oxygenating the individual while preventing the adverse effects of immobility.

## SPECIAL IMPLICATIONS FOR THE THERAPIST 21.8

### *Lung Transplantation*

#### Preoperative Phase

Transplantation candidates may have a life expectancy of less than 2 years. In the preoperative therapy program, functional goals are the primary focus, with attention directed toward increasing functional mobility, maintaining or improving strength and muscle endurance, improving breathing patterns whenever possible, and educating the recipient and the caregiver regarding the transplant process.

Many people with end-stage lung diseases can improve their aerobic capacity, especially with aggressive rehabilitation before lung transplantation. Supplemental oxygen should be increased as needed to achieve an oxygen saturation as measured by pulse oximetry of at least 88% with exercise. The therapist should stay in close communication with the transplant team if a potential recipient is requiring more oxygen to complete the same level of exercise or if the person's performance declines significantly for several days in a row. Prompt assessment by the transplant pulmonologist is recommended if the individual is exhibiting signs and symptoms of exacerbation of lung disease.

The psychosocial elements of care, especially management of depression and anxiety, are an important aspect of intervention. Helping the recipient manage anxiety during rehabilitation in the preoperative phase is extremely important and often requires referral to a psychologist, social worker, or psychiatrist. Often there is significant anxiety posttransplantation; the more the recipient can deal with it preoperatively, the better the recipient can manage it after surgery. This is especially true given that maximizing psychosocial status improves long-term physical health outcomes in patients undergoing transplantation.[121,373]

More recent studies are supporting the benefits of rehabilitation with patients with pulmonary fibrosis and pulmonary arterial hypertension.[381,430] The pulmonary rehabilitation studies have reported promising results with improvements in 6-minute walk test, decreased dyspnea and anxiety, and improvement in various quality-of-life measures.[177] Caution must be taken in these patient groups to provide sufficient oxygen delivery and a slow progressive, interval exercise program and to monitor closely for severe desaturation, arrhythmias, and signs of heart failure.

#### Acute Care Phase

Following the initial surgery, the ICU plan will focus on supporting respiratory function and initiating airway clearance techniques to minimize the risk of infections and resolve atelectasis, stabilize hemodynamics, and begin functional restoration. During this acute phase the patient should be monitored closely for ischemic reperfusion injury and rejection.

It is important that the therapist monitor vital signs, including oxygen saturation and breathing patterns. A few centers place these patients on reverse isolation, but in most centers the medical staff will follow standard precautions. Therapy may be initiated on postoperative day 1 and may range from positioning for skin care and pulmonary management to beginning functional mobility.

Posttransplantation pulmonary blood flow and ventilation are variable and may be affected by the function of the graft, function of the native lung, presence of pulmonary hypertension, a change in cardiac output, or diaphragmatic function. For the patient who is having difficulty with ventilation and perfusion, the therapist will need to assess oxygenation and breathing patterns to determine the optimal position to maximize respiratory function.

#### Positioning

In the early postoperative period the therapist can be instrumental in positioning the patient to maximize breathing pattern and ventilation and perfusion. In a single-lung transplant recipient who is experiencing oxygenation issues, a trial of side lying may improve saturation. The therapist may need to trial both side lying positions to determine which is more effective. This can be dependent on degree of ventilation–perfusion matching, pleural effusions, type of underlying disease, and secretions.

The client may be weaned from a ventilator within 24 to 48 hours if the organ is functioning well and the patient is able to clear the airway effectively, but some people may remain on a ventilator longer. Supplemental oxygen is usually no longer necessary by the time of hospital discharge. Client education, including various airway clearance techniques, handwashing skills, strength training, and breathing exercises, is initiated early in the recipient's recovery.

### Airway Clearance and Breathing Techniques

The therapist will need to assess respiratory function along with a complete evaluation to determine the best airway clearance techniques (ACTs) and breathing techniques that promote deep breathing and coughing to maximize ventilation and oxygenation in the early postoperative period. Traditional chest physical therapy and early mobilization can be completed early in the postoperative period if the person is hemodynamically stable.

The therapist must consider the risks and benefits of completing percussion and vibration in Trendelenburg positions and should consider modifying the position or the techniques, especially with the high incidence of GERD and dysphasia in the lung transplant recipients and the association of silent aspiration and worsening pulmonary function.[27,74,75,403]

If the therapist does position the person in a Trendelenburg position, the therapist should not complete the treatment right after feeding. The postpyloric position of the feeding tube should be documented, and feeding should be stopped a minimum of 30 minutes before treatment, or treatment should be delayed at least 30 minutes until after the person has consumed food or beverages. Many transplant patients experience delayed gastric emptying and stomach contents remain for longer than normal. The therapist should also coordinate ACT with pain medications and ventilation weaning protocols.

Before and after every manual ACT, the therapist should inspect the chest tube sites to rule out air leak and subcutaneous emphysema. Care should be taken not to apply any ACT directly over the insertion site. The recipient will have a decrease in coughing and efficient breathing because the lung is denervated (Box 21.11). Pain, anxiety, and any decrease in mental alertness need to be considered when selecting an ACT for the recipient.

*Conditioned breathlessness* is a term that applies to the lung transplant recipient. These clients often need to relearn how to normalize the breathing pattern and to understand that the feeling of breathlessness does not necessarily indicate a lack of oxygen, infection, or rejection, but is instead a function of anxiety and muscle fatigue. Exertional dyspnea and tachypnea may be seen for several weeks to months postoperatively. Teaching recipients the use of the Modified Borg Scale of Dyspnea is important, as well as teaching them to understand their dyspnea and how far they can push themselves without having an anxiety or panic attack. It is also important to teach breath control strategies, such as pursed-lip, inspiratory hold, or stack breathing strategies, so that they can obtain and maintain controlled breathing. It is important to teach these techniques at rest so they can be readily implemented at times of stress.

The therapist should determine in what positions the recipients have the most energy-efficient breathing pattern so that they can fully rest. It is ideal to position them in a position that maximizes diaphragmatic breathing to decrease the work of breathing and improve ventilation to the lower lobes. If the therapist notices the patient cannot recruit the diaphragm, the patient has an elevated diaphragm on x-ray, or the patient is having difficulty with weaning from the ventilator, diagnostic ultrasound should be obtained to determine if the phrenic nerve was damaged at the time of surgery, which has been reported in up to 30% of heart-lung and lung transplantation cases.

Soft tissue and joint mobilization to the thoracic spine, rib cage, and abdominal wall can be effective manual techniques to improve chest wall mobility and therefore decrease the work of breathing. Once the surgical incision is healed, scar management should begin, to avoid soft tissue restriction, decreased rib mobility, and chronic pain.

Finally, upper extremity muscle endurance exercises should focus on improving accessory respiratory function. Strengthening of scapula and thoracic spine musculature should be addressed to further improve scapular stabilization, which will improve the breathing pattern and decrease dyspnea.[39,274]

Anxiety can be a barrier to rehabilitation and ventilation management if the person does not have a sufficient coping mechanism.[125] Patients need to learn to trust that the therapist will not push them with such intensity that will cause a panic attack. The therapist needs to remember that shortness of breath to many recipients means something is seriously wrong. Telling the client to "slow your breathing down" is not an effective instructional or biofeedback technique. Instructing the individual to use breath control strategies such as pursed-lip breathing with a pause at the top of inspiration and then an inspiratory hold before exhaling is an effective means of decreasing the respiratory rate and aids in gas diffusion. There are several

**Box 21.11**

**EFFECTS OF LUNG DENERVATION**

- Decreased tidal volume
- Decreased lung compliance
- Decreased chest wall compliance
- Delay in bronchodilation
- Impairment of mucociliary blanket
- No cough reflex
- Decreased breath holding
- Loss of Hering-Breuer reflex[a]
- Increased work of breathing
- Increased dyspnea
- Exercise
  - Decreased tidal volume
  - Decreased minute ventilation
  - Increased respiratory rate

[a]Increased volume on inspiration will reflexively decrease respiratory rate, with a period of apnea (cessation of breathing).

excellent resources to guide the therapist in establishing specific therapeutic exercises to improve respiration and phonation.[151,187,275,276]

It is important for the therapist to monitor vital signs and signs and symptoms of rejection and infections, as well as critical complications such as pulmonary embolus and pneumothorax. A decrease in exercise tolerance and desaturation may be the first identified symptoms during exercise. Subtle desaturation may also be related to insufficient warm-up periods before exertion. Saturation levels should normally be above 93%; supplemental oxygen may be needed when saturation levels are at or below 90% (see Table 21.4). Any changes in exercise tolerance and vital signs should be reported to the transplantation center for further investigation.

Rehabilitation in the early postoperative period should focus on airway clearance, functional strength, and functional mobility training. Once basic functional mobility is restored, therapy should focus on progressing muscular strength, muscular endurance tolerance, and finally aerobic exercises. Once rehabilitation goals are met, the recipient should begin to increase cardiovascular and pulmonary endurance and continue toward completing their muscular training. If pulmonary function is insufficient for extubation, functional mobility training and strengthening should progress as appropriate with proper mechanical ventilation support, including supplemental oxygen to help the person progress and contribute to the weaning process.

### Outpatient Phase

Client education regarding the importance of consistently following an at-home or community-based program to increase and maintain metabolic equivalent level (multiples of resting oxygen consumption) with exercise is essential. There is some evidence that recipients with poorer caregiver relationships and greater psychologic distress may need additional support to perform the self-care behaviors expected after lung transplantation. Recognition of problems in this area may require consultation with the case worker or discussion with the transplant team to plan intervention before discharge.[121]

It is recommended that the recipient be referred to outpatient physical therapy immediately after hospital discharge for further strength and muscular endurance and functional training, with the goal of improving muscular strength and endurance along with aerobic capacity, so that the person can maximize the benefits from traditional pulmonary rehabilitation and participate easily in community-based activities without fatigue. Recipient should be able to self-monitor and progress through the exercise program independently by the time they are discharged from the supervised rehabilitation program.

A traditional pulmonary rehabilitation program is an effective therapy for recipients whose primary limitations are decreased aerobic capacity and muscle weakness and who would benefit from extensive client education and support. The majority of people should participate in a walking program to help minimize weight gain, muscle atrophy, osteoporosis, and edema. In addition, resistance exercise, especially for the lower extremities, is essential to improving strength and function. The therapist should verify on a weekly basis that the recipient is compliant with self-monitoring of blood pressure, blood glucose, and spirometry volumes and report any changes to the physician's office.

The peak effect of transplantation on lung function is typically within 3 to 6 months, at which point the limiting effects of surgically related factors (e.g., postoperative pain, altered chest wall mechanics, respiratory muscle dysfunction, acute lung injury) have dissipated. After double-lung replacement, normal pulmonary function is usually achieved. Communication with the transplant team, especially the transplant coordinator, is important during the outpatient phase of rehabilitation, particularly when complications arise. It is essential to keep the transplant team informed of the patient's progress with rehabilitation and any deficits that are noted.

#### Exercise

Before lung transplantation, candidates are characterized by very low exercise capacity (maximal $VO_2$ 14 mL/min/kg) because of the restricted oxygen uptake caused by reduced ventilatory capacity, ventilation–perfusion mismatching, or decreased diffusion capacity and/or blood shunting.[269]

After transplantation, overall pulmonary function improves and exercise capacity increases because the lungs can now perform improved oxygen uptake and maintain oxygen saturation levels greater than 90% during submaximal $VO_2$. An aerobic endurance training program improves submaximal and peak exercise performance significantly in lung transplant recipients.[422,425] Muscular endurance and strength training has shown improvements in strength or muscle function and improvements in bone density.[473]

By the end of the first year after transplantation, approximately 80% of recipients report no limitations in activity; exercise is not limited by ventilation despite a decrease in tidal volume and increased respiratory rate with exercise.[362] However, the recipients reach only 40% to 60% of predicted $VO_2$ capacity.[9,168,197,473] The therapist should continue to follow the guidelines outlined in Table 21.4.

Despite these improvements, cardiopulmonary exercise testing consistently shows that maximal $VO_2$ in recipients of single- and double-lung transplants is still lower than sedentary, healthy, matched control subjects.[158,475] Maximal $VO_2$ is depressed despite the absence of clinically significant cardiac or ventilatory limitations on exercise. There is evidence that the continued decrease in exercise capacity is related to deficits in oxygen extraction, abnormal microcirculation oxygen delivery, anemia, and alterations in muscle fiber type and oxidative enzymes.[9,168,245,362] Evidence shows, however, that posttransplantation rehabilitation can improve aerobic capacity closer to predicted levels.[279]

A number of studies show that lower limb skeletal muscle dysfunction may be a major factor in exercise limitation. Clients report lower extremity fatigue rather than dyspnea as the main reason for exercise intolerance. There may be an intrinsic abnormality of the skeletal muscle in recipients of transplants. An in-depth summary of exercise limitations in this population is available.[473] It is essential to emphasize to all lung transplant recipients the importance of lifelong exercise to improve and maintain function and well-being. In addition, the therapist should convey to the patient that it may take much longer to achieve optimal strengthening and endurance capabilities compared with people without transplants as a consequence of the many factors discussed in this section.

## Pancreas Transplantation

### Overview

Pancreas transplantation has become an accepted therapeutic approach to treat type 1 diabetes, which is caused by the autoimmune destruction of pancreatic islet β cells, thereby successfully restoring normoglycemia. Pancreas transplantation is mainly performed for individuals with type 1 diabetes mellitus.

Although whole-pancreas transplantation represents a physiologic approach to reverse diabetes mellitus, a new technique of pancreas islet β-cell transplantation is now available for carefully selected individuals with severe, unstable type 1 diabetes. Islet transplantation remains an experimental procedure in the United States and awaits formal results of ongoing phase III trials to justify biologic licensure and transition to standard of care. Transplanting insulin-secreting cells is a low-invasive procedure, with the possibility of modulating graft immune response before transplantation, allowing reduced or minimized immunosuppressive medications.[469]

In June 2000 the *New England Journal of Medicine* prereleased the findings of a report (the Edmonton protocol) from researchers injecting pancreas cells near the liver in eight people with type 1 diabetes. The cells took up residence in the liver and began producing insulin.[394]

Since that time continued advancement has occurred through extensive collaboration between key centers.[243] For example, the Collaborative Islet Transplant Registry (CITR) reports continued improvement in efficacy and safety outcomes of islet transplantation with fewer islet infusions and adverse events per recipient.[36]

A clinical trial was completed in 2017 by the Clinical Islet Transplantation Consortium, in which islet cells are transplanted into two groups: islet-alone treatment in individuals with type 1 diabetes with severe hypoglycemia unawareness and islet after kidney transplant in patients with prior successful kidney transplant.[213] Formal results of this study have not yet been published.

To date more than 1500 patients have been treated with islet transplantations worldwide according to the CITR 10th Annual Report. There are still limitations with this approach, but newer pharmacotherapies and interventions designed to promote islet survival, prevent apoptosis, promote islet growth, and prevent immunologic injury are approaching clinical trial status.[288]

### Indications

In contrast to heart, lung, or liver transplantations, pancreas transplantations are not an immediately life-saving procedure. Recipients have to be carefully selected to reduce morbidity and mortality; investigation of myocardial and cerebral vascularity is essential.

Even with these guidelines, pancreas transplantation has become a routine treatment for patients with type 1 diabetes with uremia and for patients who previously received a kidney transplant. Pancreas transplantation at the same time as a renal transplant is now considered more frequently especially if the diabetes has been difficult to control.[380]

Although the recipient must remain on lifelong immunosuppressive medications, 80% to 90% 1-year survival rates are considered very acceptable given the alternatives of insulin therapy, dietary restrictions, hypoglycemic and hyperglycemic episodes, dialysis, and potential long-term complications associated with diabetes mellitus.[99] Recent research shows that pancreas transplants can provide excellent glucose control in recipients with type 2 diabetes as well.[303,383]

Diabetic nephropathy is the leading cause of kidney failure in people with type 1 diabetes. Successful pancreas transplantation leads to normal glycemic control in people with type 1 diabetes, but historically this type of transplantation has been limited to people with both kidney failure and diabetes. Pancreas transplantation does not reverse the advanced complications (e.g., diabetic retinopathy, vascular sclerosis) present with long-term diabetes. However, pancreas transplantation has the potential to reverse neuropathy (i.e., improved nerve action and potential amplitudes).[13]

Despite the difficulty of this surgical procedure and the many potential complications, pancreas transplantation before the development and progression of diabetic nephropathy is being suggested.[198,419] However, this is a controversial subject because others believe that in the absence of end-stage renal failure, there is no justification for pancreas transplants alone except in cases where diabetes itself poses a greater risk to life than the transplantation procedure.

Individuals with diabetes and renal involvement and individuals with unstable diabetes may be helped with an islet or pancreas transplant, but this approach is still considered experimental. Such transplantation may speed up the need for a kidney replacement. For individuals with well-controlled diabetes and intact function, pancreas or islet transplantation may not be advised given the risks of immunosuppression following transplantation.[380]

Simultaneous pancreas-kidney transplantation is an accepted treatment for carefully selected candidates with type 1 diabetes and ESRD and in a individuals with uncontrolled severe metabolic problems.[393]

### Transplant Candidates

Many centers consider pancreas transplantation contraindicated in people with cardiovascular disease, especially atherosclerotic vascular disease and congestive heart failure, because of the poor outcome after pancreas transplantation when either of these risk factors is present.

Some centers may consider transplantation in cases of atherosclerotic vascular disease if coronary lesions are corrected before transplantation. Other risk factors include age older than 45 years, obesity, and hepatitis C.[268]

### Transplantation Procedure

The donor pancreas is most often placed extraperitoneally on the right side using the recipient's (native) vessels. It is necessary to drain the pancreatic exocrine secretions by channeling them to the urinary bladder or into the stomach. This may be accomplished with a variety of surgical techniques.

In the case of pancreas islet cell transplantation, cells removed from a cadaver are injected into the blood vessel leading to the liver (portal vein). Because development of these procedures is in its infancy, they presently require the cells from two pancreases, matched for blood type, to produce an apparent cure. Better methods for extracting cells from the donated pancreas or a way to grow the cells in the laboratory are being investigated.

### Complications

Surgical complications remain the primary source of morbidity after pancreas transplantation (especially when combined with a simultaneous kidney transplantation), affecting approximately 35% of studied cases.[361] This may change with continued advances in surgical techniques, but data are limited at this time. Specific complications include graft vascular thrombosis, pancreatic hemorrhage, intraabdominal bleeding or infection, allograft failure, and urologic problems associated with the bladder drainage surgical technique.

Other nonsurgical complications may include post-transplant pancreatitis possibly secondary to ischemic reperfusion microvascular injury and the more typical transplantation complications associated with other solid organs such as infection and side effects of prolonged immunosuppression.

Complications of pancreatic islet cell transplantation are minimal, but long-term safety and effectiveness of this technique remain to be proven. The recipients must take a combination of three immunosuppressive medications to prevent the body from rejecting the transplanted cells. The increased risk of cancer, infection, and other long-term side effects associated with these medications has been discussed.

### Prognosis

Over the past 20 years there has been a progressive improvement in outcomes after pancreas transplantation alone, simultaneous pancreas-kidney transplantation, and pancreas after kidney transplantation.[169] Vascular disease remains the major cause of both morbidity and mortality after transplantation in recipients who have diabetes and is correlated with the degree of vascular disease before transplantation. Graft and recipient survival rates in diabetic recipients are higher when the recipient receives simultaneous pancreas-kidney transplantation. These survival rates are even higher when the kidney donor is a living related donor.[360]

Compared with other abdominal transplantations, pancreas transplants have had the highest incidence of surgical complications. This trend may be reversing owing to identification of donor and candidate risk factors, better prophylaxis regimens, refinements in surgical technique, and improved immunosuppressive regimens.[228] Steroid withdrawal is possible in up to 70% of pancreas transplant recipients as long as the person is maintained on some form of immunosuppression (usually tacrolimus).[204,218]

Even with surgical complications, survival rates of pancreas transplant recipients are 96% to 98% at 1 year and 92% at 3 years.[30,169] Data on survival rates following islet transplantation are limited given the recent development of this technique and the scarcity of donor islet cells. Of people who have received autotransplants worldwide following total or subtotal pancreatectomy, insulin independence has been achieved in 40%. Islet allotransplantations have demonstrated improved metabolic control in more than 50% of cases and insulin independence in approximately 20%.[322]

### Future Trends

More widespread application of pancreas transplantation is expected in the future, with earlier transplantation indicated in the course of diabetic disease.[133] Successful transplantation of human fetal pancreatic tissue into recipients who have type 1 diabetes is under investigation.[45] Strategies to reduce the metabolic consequences of hyperglycemia on nerves and to enhance axonal regeneration are being studied.[342,352,485]

As previously mentioned, pancreatic islet β-cell transplantation may replace whole-organ transplantation or may be used in combination with kidney transplantation or after pancreas transplantation failure. Xenogeneic sources of cells, engineered islet cells with genes that induce immunoprotection, some form of β-cell replacement therapy, and sustaining populations of transplanted β cells all are part of current research.[136,137,379]

Artificial pancreas systems, with the ability to automate insulin delivery based on continuous glucose monitoring data while taking into consideration exercise and meals, have been developed. In fact, the U.S. Food and Drug Administration recently approved the first artificial pancreas system for use in individuals older than 14 years of age with type 1 diabetes.

## Skin Transplantation

Human cadaver allograft skin is widely used for covering excised burn wounds when skin donor sites are limited or the overall client condition does not permit immediate grafting with autologous skin. However, recurring problems are associated with human cadaver allograft skin, including limited supply, variable quality, ultimate immune rejection, and the potential for bacterial and viral disease transmission.

Several biotechnology companies are working on tissue-engineered skin substitutes that could revolutionize the treatment of severe burns as well as pressure ulcers and other serious wounds. Engineers can now mass produce postcard-size sheets of durable, uniform tissue that the body readily accepts. Cells can be grown on biodegradable lattices to produce the functional equivalent of dermis and epidermis.

The Food and Drug Administration has approved products for use in burn cases requiring immediate closure of wounds but where there is not enough undamaged skin to be used as autografts. These products are also approved in Europe for plastic and reconstructive surgery and for the treatment of excisional wounds.

One type of patch is made up of two layers; the chemicals within the bottom layer help the new cells form a pattern similar to the normal dermis instead of the normally developing pattern of scar tissue. As dermis cells regenerate, blood vessels grow into this microscopic scaffolding over a 7- to 10-day period.

Within 3 weeks, the scaffolding dissolves as the new dermis grows in under the top layer of silicone. Acting as a pseudoepidermis, these patches close the burn injury to invading bacteria much like a normal skin graft would do.[72] Later, the top silicone layer can be pulled away easily for skin grafting.

Another type of newly developing artificial skin product is dermal fibroblast cells (connective tissue in the skin that produces collagen and elastic fibers) constructed from the foreskin of newborns and cultured onto a mesh that serves as the scaffolding. During the formation of tissue, the fibroblasts proliferate within the mesh, where they secrete human dermal collagen, matrix proteins, and growth factors.

One foreskin the size of a postage stamp can produce as many as 200,000 grafts. The separation process discards the immune stimulating cells and saves the fibroblasts (stimulate growth and regeneration of the dermis) and keratinocytes (provide protective epidermis). It takes approximately 6 days for the layer of dermis to grow, at which time the keratinocytes are added, forming the tough outer layer known as the *stratum corneum,* which is capable of resisting injury and infection. The complete process takes approximately 20 days.

In both types of artificial skin products, the patches act as a template or scaffolding on which new dermis cells can form, allowing early wound excision and immediate wound closure with control of fluid loss. Reduced cases of rejection and reduced risk of infection and disease transmission potentially allow for early ambulation, earlier rehabilitation, and faster recovery.

Recognizing wound infection after graft application can be challenging because the graft appears white or yellow after hydration with wound fluid. Any change from baseline at the wound site; in the amount or type of edema, erythema, drainage, odor, and warmth; unexplained fever; or pain should be reported to the physician.

Normal skin grafting is still necessary for burns, but the new developing dermis allows surgeons to place over the wound a thinner, smaller skin graft from donor sites that heal within 1 week. Temporary skin replacement for excised burn wounds before autografting has been attached as long as 74 days without rejection and without hypertrophic scarring.

The drawbacks to this procedure are the cost and patch fragility, making the grafts difficult to work with and more easily dislodged than skin grafts. Researchers are continuing to explore the concept of an off-the-shelf full-thickness skin product that would be a permanent replacement for skin.

Stem cell–based therapy in the area of burns and wound healing has been explored over the last few years. One study demonstrated improved closure by applying a topical treatment of mesenchymal stem cells to patients with chronic skin wounds.[31] In another study, patients treated with bone marrow–derived mesenchymal stem cells demonstrated improved healing of their chronic lower extremity ulcers and reduced pain.[110] Mesenchymal stem cells have also been studied in an application of fibrin/thrombin spray, which accelerates wound closure.[144,160]

In addition to wound healing, burn wounds represent a major clinical challenge because of loss of large areas of skin, but stem cell therapy has not played a large clinical role to date. However, trials are ongoing using bioreactors, which serve to grow cells in a three-dimensional environment to isolate and grow skin stem cells from the patient and then apply them to burned areas of skin using a spray gun for maximal coverage and healing.[116]

## Intestine Transplantation

Intestinal transplants are performed relatively infrequently, with the OPTN reporting just over 3000 performed to date since 1990.[448] This is in part due to the high lymphatic load within the intestine, which makes it an immunologically reactive graft. Indications for transplant may include mesenteric infarction, Crohn's disease, acute volvulus, motility disorders, malignancy, and congenital defects. Waitlist mortality is high in adult intestinal transplant candidates, with 19.6 deaths per waitlist year.

## Face Transplantation

Advances in reconstructive procedures now permit partial to near-total face transplant. The first partial face transplantation was performed in 2005 and the first near-total face transplant performed at Cleveland Clinic in 2008. To date, approximately 40 face transplants have been performed worldwide.

Candidates for face transplant have typically experienced a burn or trauma injury and present with severe facial deformities and functional limitations. They may or may not have had previous reconstructive surgeries. Choosing candidates for face transplantation is particularly difficult owing to the ethics of performing a non–life-saving surgery and subjecting the patient to lifelong immunosuppression and its related complications. Face transplants are a type of VCA, which may include transplantation of skin, muscle, nerve, bone, vasculature, and connective tissue as well as facial features such as the lips, nose, ears, and eyelids.

Sensory recovery is first reported about 3 months posttransplantation and is generally complete between 8 and 12 months. Motor recovery begins later in the healing process, usually at 6 months, and can continue for up to 2 years. Maximizing motor function in the new face requires participation in physical therapy. Patient compliance with rehabilitation also contributes to an acceptable aesthetic outcome. Other factors affecting aesthetics posttransplantation include time since injury, age, gender, and matching of facial features between donor and recipient. As with other transplant patients, face transplant recipients have to start an immunosuppression regimen and can experience the same complications postoperatively including rejection, diabetes, delayed wound healing, infection, and psychologic disturbances.[400]

## Hand Transplantation

The first single hand transplant was performed in 1964; however, the patient experienced acute rejection and required amputation 3 weeks posttransplantation.[400] Advances in immunosuppression post-VCA led to the first hand transplant in recent years in 1998. Since this time, more than 110 hand transplantations have been performed.

Indications for transplant include bilateral or dominant hand loss or amputation distal to mid-forearm. In younger patients, amputation is usually a result of a congenital anomaly, trauma, or infection, whereas amputation in older patients is more frequently associated with medication toxicity or vascular disease.[265]

Besides meeting criteria similar to candidates for solid-organ transplantation, a candidate for hand transplantation must be prepared to accept the morbidity associated with immunosuppression medications given that the transplant is elective, as well as the intensive rehabilitation required to restore sensation, motor control, and proprioception for functional use of the hand. Therapy sessions are usually 3 to 6 hours, 5 days per week, for 3 to 6 months.[265]

Outcomes are generally good, with most patients developing protective sensation and experiencing return of intrinsic and extrinsic function with ability to perform activities of daily living and improved quality of life.[215,398]

## REFERENCES

To enhance this text and add value for the reader, all references are included in the enhanced ebook on Student Consult that accompanies this textbook. The reader can view the reference source and access it online whenever possible.

# SECTION 3 PATHOLOGY OF THE MUSCULOSKELETAL SYSTEM

## CHAPTER 22

# Introduction to Pathology of the Musculoskeletal System

KEVIN HELGESON

A musculoskeletal condition or injury can significantly affect an individual's ability to participate in daily activities, work, and recreation. Physical therapists must understand how a musculoskeletal condition impacts the individual across a spectrum of participation and tasks down to the cellular and genetic levels. The study of genomics is providing an increasing understanding of the molecular basis for disease and injury. The understanding of genomics has led to the identification of phenotypes, which describes how an individual's characteristics are a result of their genotype interacting with the environment. Phenotypes can provide a more effective method for grouping patients so that they receive treatments that are specific to their genetic makeup. Phenotypes has been identified for individuals with osteoarthritis, fibromyalgia, and central pain processing.[21] This new knowledge is changing the approach for health care intervention in many areas including the musculoskeletal system.[12]

The ability to document the influence and effects of exercise at the molecular and cellular levels has resulted in early functional rehabilitation, preventive exercise programs, and the use of exercise as a first-line intervention for many conditions. Maintaining good musculoskeletal health and recovering quickly from musculoskeletal injury or disease contribute to an individual's overall health, welfare, and quality of life. The skeletal system with its associated soft tissues provides a protective covering for important structures such as the brain and heart and essentially makes up the limbs, putting this system at risk for traumatic and repetitive insults and injuries (Box 22.1).

Better technology has made it possible to measure what happens to muscle with age without invasive muscle biopsies. Imaging methods can measure fatty infiltration of skeletal muscle, a contributor to metabolic problems and muscle dysfunction with aging. Magnetic resonance spectroscopy and computed tomography are being used to characterize this fatty infiltration. Scientists are looking for ways to reduce the risk of falls, fractures, and disability from changes in the supportive and protective skeletal muscle.[20]

Preclinical disability is defined as progressive and detectable but unrecognized decline in physical function in older adults.[8] Early signs of decline in physical function are observed in the ability to perform mobility tasks and activities of daily living needed to maintain an independent living status. Preclinical disability may be seen as an increased time to complete a task, modification of a task, or decrease in the frequency with which a task is performed.[9] Individuals with preclinical disability are at increased risk for progression to more severe disability; early identification of decline in physical function is important if intervention to stop the decline is possible.

Similar to all other body systems, the musculoskeletal system does not function in isolation. Therefore primary disease of the musculoskeletal system can significantly affect other body systems and vice versa. In addition, certain diseases are systemic, meaning that all body systems including the musculoskeletal system can be involved to some degree. The challenge to develop an effective rehabilitation program is heightened when one is faced with complex, multisystem disorders (see Chapter 5).

The purpose of this section is to provide an overview of the musculoskeletal system, keeping in mind the biologic response to trauma discussed in Chapter 6 and examples of how primary diseases in other organs affect the musculoskeletal system and vice versa, and to begin to examine the local (musculoskeletal) and systemic (e.g., immune system, endocrine system, gastrointestinal system) effects of exercise. An approach that assesses all the systems and considers underlying pathology is essential when identifying the source of impairments.

## ADVANCES IN MUSCULOSKELETAL BIOTECHNOLOGY AND REGENERATIVE MEDICINE

Advances in molecular biology techniques have extended the potential for understanding musculoskeletal disorders from the microscopic (histologic) level down to the molecular level of gene expression within individual cells. These advances are initiating new avenues of research and, ultimately, novel clinical interventions. Orthopedic surgery has been revolutionized by tissue engineering, use of synthetic material as skeletal substitutes, transplantation and fabrication of avascular tissue (e.g., meniscus, articular cartilage), and joint restoration instead of joint replacement.[44]

Box 22.1

**COMMON MUSCULOSKELETAL DISORDERS**

- Fracture
- Dislocation
- Subluxation
- Contusion
- Hematoma
- Repetitive overuse, microtrauma
- Strain, sprain
- Degenerative disease

Other technologic advances under scientific investigation include bone implants to stimulate bone development and prevent limb loss associated with cancer[43]; injectable degradable scaffolds used as bone substitute for bone defects, to strengthen osteoporotic vertebral bodies, or to heal compression and nonunion fractures[25]; and new materials and plastics, making it possible to replace spinal discs or extend joint replacements by an additional 10 years or more.

In addition, the first nerve tubes for the repair and regeneration of peripheral nerves are now available for clinical use.[6] Biodegradable polymer scaffolds to support axonal regeneration in the transected spinal cord are being investigated in animal studies. Multichannel scaffolds are seeded with neural stem cells and Schwann cells needed to facilitate regeneration across the cord. The hope is to have such treatment available immediately for anyone with a spinal cord injury.

## AGING AND THE MUSCULOSKELETAL SYSTEM

Much has been written about the effects of aging on the musculoskeletal system, especially in light of exercise as an effective intervention for so many diseases and conditions. Participation in a regular exercise program is an effective intervention to reduce or prevent a number of functional declines associated with aging.

Endurance training can help maintain and improve various aspects of cardiovascular function (as measured by maximal $VO_2$, cardiac output, and arteriovenous oxygen difference) and enhance submaximal performance. Importantly, reductions in risk factors associated with disease states (e.g., heart disease, diabetes) improve health status and contribute to an increase in life expectancy.[10]

Strength training helps offset the loss in muscle mass and strength typically associated with normal aging. Additional benefits from regular exercise include improved bone health and therefore reduction in risk for osteoporosis; improved postural stability, thereby reducing the risk of falling and associated injuries and fractures; and increased flexibility and range of motion.

Although not as abundant, evidence also suggests that involvement in regular exercise can provide a number of psychologic benefits related to preserved cognitive function, alleviation of depressive symptoms and behavior, and an improved concept of personal control and self-determination.[17]

### Muscle

#### Sarcopenia

**Overview and Definition.** Age-related loss in muscle mass, strength, and endurance accompanied by changes in the metabolic quality of skeletal muscle is termed *sarcopenia*. Sarcopenia involves the reduction of muscle mass and/or function as well as the impairment of the muscle's capacity to regenerate.[27]

Muscle mass is lost at a rate of 4% to 6% per decade starting at age 40 in women and age 60 in men.[19] The greatest decline in both men and women occurs with inactivity, acute illness, and after age 70, at which time the mean loss of muscle mass has been measured as 1% per year. At all ages, females appear to be more vulnerable to loss of lean tissue than males; however, in men and women, muscle strength can be maintained through exercise well into the eighth decade.

**Etiology.** The etiology is multifactorial, involving changes in muscle metabolism, endocrine changes (e.g., low testosterone levels), nutritional factors, and mitochondrial and genetic factors.[27] It remains uncertain how much age-related loss of muscle function is an inevitable consequence of aging; nutritional status; or dysregulation of neurologic, hormonal, and/or immunologic homeostasis.

Likewise, it remains unknown how much sarcopenia reflects a decline in physical activity and exercise capacity and, as part of a broad cycle, whether this decline is a function of age, lack of motivation, decline in neuromuscular function from disuse or loss of motoneurons, age-associated decreases in metabolism, or other factors such as anemia or high levels of inflammatory markers.[11]

**Pathogenesis.** Animal studies suggest that myofiber regeneration in sarcopenic muscle is halted at the point where reinnervation is critical for the final differentiation into mature myofibers. Studies of humans and animals point to a decreased capacity among motoneurons to innervate regenerating fibers. Changes are also observed in the expression of several cytokines known to play important roles in establishing and maintaining neuromuscular connectivity during development and adulthood.[14] The decline in muscle mass previously thought to be the result of proteins breaking down faster than they were being created and restored may be linked instead to other potential reasons such as diet and nutrition, the body's ability to use protein from food, and hormonal changes.

Loss of muscle function appears to be due to a combination of decreased total fibers, decreased muscle fiber size, impaired excitation-contraction coupling mechanism, and decreased high-threshold motor units. Selective loss of motor unit number or atrophy (particularly after 70 years of age) of fast twitch (type IIa) muscle fibers may occur. Some researchers suggest that no preferential loss of type I or type II muscle fibers occurs with age but rather both types are equally affected and type II fiber cross-sectional area is reduced, which accounts for the significant decrease in muscle strength.[2] Other studies have shown that type II fibers are preferentially affected by aging and that fiber II atrophy is associated with a decline in satellite cells (essential for skeletal muscle growth and repair).[40]

Other researchers hypothesize an extrinsic apoptotic pathway to explain how type II fiber–containing skeletal muscles may be more susceptible to muscle mass losses.[31] However it occurs, the clinical significance of this loss is that it leads to diminished strength and exercise capacity.

**Effects of Sarcopenia.** From a clinical perspective, loss in muscle mass accounts for the age-associated decreases in basal metabolic rate contributing to metabolic disorders such as type 2 diabetes mellitus and decreases in muscle strength and activity levels, which in turn are the cause of the decreased energy requirements of the aging adult. Loss of muscle mass (i.e., atrophy) and loss of muscle function resulting in subsequent muscle weakness are implicated in difficulty accomplishing activities of daily living (e.g., rising from a chair, climbing stairs, carrying groceries), slow gait speed, impaired balance reactions, and increased risk of vertebral compression (and other) fractures.[27]

**Exercise and Sarcopenia.** See also The Musculoskeletal System, Aging, and Exercise later. Appropriate exercise can alter, slow, or even partially reverse some of the age-related physiologic changes that occur in skeletal muscle, including sarcopenia. Skeletal muscle adaptations in response to strength training in older adults occur with progressive resistance training or high-intensity training (e.g., two to six sets of eight repetitions at approximately 80% of the person's one-repetition maximum).[42]

Understanding muscle fiber types and the impact of physical therapy interventions on muscle fiber type conversions is important in geriatric clinical practice. An excellent review of these concepts is available.[7] We know, for example, that age-related changes can be counteracted and physical function improved by increased physical activity of a resistive nature. Mechanical load on muscle can increase the cross-sectional area of the remaining fibers but does not restore fiber numbers characteristic of young muscle.

Strength training has been shown to improve insulin-stimulated glucose uptake both in healthy older adults and in individuals with diabetes. Strength training also improves muscle strength in healthy adults and adults with chronic diseases. Increased strength leads to improved function and a decreased risk for falls, injuries, and fractures.[39] These results also promote increased independence and improved quality of life.

High-resistance-training exercise has been of significant benefit to sarcopenia. In fact, after 6 months of exercise training, resistance exercise has been shown to reverse mitochondrial dysfunction for genes that are affected by both age and exercise.[28] Combinations of resistance exercise, aerobic exercise, and stretching have shown beneficial effects on sarcopenia, but the optimal regimen for older adults remains unclear.[7]

Many older adults would like to be more physically active but do not have the experience or knowledge to develop and build up an exercise regimen without appropriate supervision such as a physical therapist can offer. Others have participated in athletics throughout adulthood and continue to train and remain in good health.[36] The therapist can help educate older adults about the importance of maintaining strength training and endurance with the emphasis on strength, which decreases more rapidly than endurance.

## Joint and Connective Tissue

At the same time as changes in bone and muscle are taking place, a progressive loss of flexibility and changes in connective tissue starts contributing to an increased incidence of joint problems beginning in middle age and progressing through old age. Loss of flexibility also contributes to increased risk of falls and other injuries. Connective or periarticular tissues including fascia, articular cartilage, ligaments, and tendons become less extensible, with resultant decreased active and passive range of motion.

### Increased Stiffness and Decreased Flexibility

Decreased flexibility within muscle occurs with a combination of biologic aging, inactivity, structural and biochemical changes, and degenerative diseases. The extracellular matrix of skeletal muscle will undergo changes that increase the concentration of collagen, changes in the composition of elastic fibers, and changes that increase the infiltration of fat within the matrix. These changes will have a significant effect on increasing muscle stiffness and limiting muscle force generation.[22]

Others have shown that aging collagen has increased cross-links between molecules, increasing the mechanical stability of collagen but also contributing to increased tissue stiffness.[24] Increased collagen content in the endomysium of animal intramuscular connective tissue has been shown to correlate with increased stiffness of the whole muscle.

Another possible source of extracellular matrix changes is related to fibrinogen, produced in the liver and converted to fibrin, which constantly circulates throughout the body to serve as a clotting mechanism (with superglue-like effects) should an injury occur. Fibrinogen normally leaks out of the vasculature in small amounts into the intracellular space and then adheres to cellular structures, causing microfibrinous adhesions among the cells. Activity and movement normally break down these adhesions along with macrophage activity to dissolve unused fibrinogen and fibrin. In the aging process, less fibrinogen and fewer (less efficient) macrophages are available. These factors, along with less physical activity and movement, allow these microadhesions to accumulate in muscle and fascia, resulting in an increased sense of overall stiffness.[23]

Regardless of the exact physiologic mechanism for the gradual increase in stiffness associated with aging, physical activity is important in alleviating stiffness. Further research is needed to understand how and what kind of physical activity influences or possibly prevents stiffness.[5]

### Changes in Articular Cartilage

Articular cartilage, which cushions the subchondral bone and provides a low-friction surface necessary for free movement, contains few cells, is aneural and avascular, and often starts to break down with increasing age.[26] The main proteoglycan in articular cartilage (aggrecan) binds with hyaluronan to form massive aggregates that expand the collagen matrix of the tissue to provide it with its compressive and tensile strength. With age, proteoglycan aggregation is reduced, and smaller proteoglycans are synthesized with an increase in keratin sulfate and reduced chondroitin sulfate content. The hydrophilic proteoglycans have been shown to become shorter in aged tissue and therefore lose their ability to hold water in the matrix. Dehydrated articular cartilage may have a reduced ability to dissipate forces across the joint.

Degeneration and thinning or damage of articular cartilage with loss of water content contribute to a significant increase in incidence of osteoarthritis with aging. By age 60, as much as 80% of the population shows evidence of osteoarthritis, although only about 15% present with symptoms.[13] Knowledge of these changes has resulted in a variety of interventions for osteoarthritis (see Chapter 27).[35] With or without a symptomatic presentation, educating adults about the importance of joint protection is an important role of the physical therapist.

#### Tendons

Tendons exhibit a lower metabolic activity associated with aging that has implications for injury and healing in the aging population.[38] A reduction in the stiffness of tendons with aging will affect the contractile properties of a musculotendinous structure, reducing maximal force production and the slower transmission of forces. Also an age-related decrease occurs in the tensile strength of some tendons and ligament–bone interfaces, and loss of integrity of some joint capsules occurs.[29] For example, rotator cuff impairment with loss of joint function is common in older people. A gradual loss of connective tissue resistance to calcium crystal formation occurs in older adults, leading to an increase in the incidence of crystal-related arthropathies (e.g., gout, pseudogout) (see Chapter 27).

#### Proprioception

Joint proprioception, described as sensations generated to increase awareness of joint orientation at rest and in motion, declines with age, especially in the knee and ankle.[34] Joint proprioception provides both a sense of joint position and a sense of joint movement. Mechanoreceptors located in the joint capsules, ligaments, muscles, tendons, and skin provide the sensory information needed for a sense of joint position. The presence of osteoarthritis seems to make joint proprioception even worse, though it is unclear whether impaired joint sense promotes arthritic change or whether arthritic change causes the sensory loss.

### Bone

The skeletal system serves numerous functions in the human body throughout the life span. Bone is the primary storage depot for calcium, phosphate, sodium, and magnesium. Bones are the hosts for the hematopoietic bone marrow (growth and development of elements of blood). Bones also serve important mechanical functions such as protection of components of the nervous system and visceral organs, provision of rigid internal support for the trunk and extremities, and provision of attachment sites for numerous soft tissue structures.

Bone is remodeling constantly throughout life. While osteoclasts resorb the existing bone, new bone is being formed by osteoblasts. Three primary influences affect this remodeling process: (1) mechanical stresses; (2) calcium and phosphate levels in the extracellular fluid; and (3) hormonal levels of parathyroid hormone, calcitonin, vitamin D, cortisol, growth hormone, thyroid hormone, and sex hormones.[41] Aging adversely affects the quality of bone, both the stiffness and the strength. These effects are caused by factors such as architectural changes, compositional changes, physiochemical changes, changes at the micromechanical level, and the degree of prior in vivo microdamage.

The bone density of the skeleton reaches its peak during an adult's late 20s and remains stable for about 2 decades. Around the time of menopause for women, resorption, the process by which bone is broken down and calcium is released from the bone for use by the body, increases, whereas formation, the bone-rebuilding process, fails to keep pace. This imbalance, which is triggered by declining estrogen levels, leads to rapid bone loss during the first decade after menopause, with moderate bone loss thereafter. In women with low peak bone mass, it can result in osteoporosis with the increased potential for vertebral, hip, or other fracture.[32]

The same progressive decrease of calcium can occur in men, only at a reduced and slowed rate. In women, loss occurs at a rate of approximately 1% per year after age 35 with acceleration especially during the first 5 years after menopause, amounting to about 20% by age 65 and 30% by age 80. In both genders, by age 65, bone loss generally has progressed to a point where the older adult is predisposed to fractures.[41]

## THE MUSCULOSKELETAL SYSTEM, AGING, AND EXERCISE

By 2030, 70 million people in the United States will be 65 years old or older; people 85 years old and older will be the fastest-growing segment of the population. As more individuals live longer, the importance of exercise and physical activity to improve health, functional capacity, quality of life, and independence will increase in this country.[10,17]

Strength training is considered a promising intervention for reversing the loss of muscle function and the deterioration of muscle structure that is associated with advanced age. The capacity of older men and women to adapt to increased levels of physical activity is preserved, even in the most aged adult.[15]

Regularly performed exercise can affect nutritional needs and functional capacity in the older adult, contributing a preventive effect. Combining knowledge of exercise principles with nutrition is important for all people but especially older adults; disabled individuals; athletes; adolescents; and anyone with a medical condition, disease, or illness.

### Muscle

The distribution of muscle fiber types is thought to be an inherited characteristic. Although distribution varies among individuals, the average ratio of fast-to slow-twitch fibers is 50:50. Individuals trained in endurance activities usually have a higher proportion of slow-twitch fibers, and those trained for high-intensity, high-speed activities have more fast-twitch fibers. The oxidative capacity of both fibers can be increased greatly by endurance training, but the glycolic capacity and contractile properties are not modified.[33]

Muscle function can be described in terms of strength and endurance, which is also how we focus training of muscle. Strength can be defined in several ways depending on the specific method of measurement but is usually related to the diameter of the muscle fiber, which has been consistently shown to increase with strength training.

Endurance can be measured as the ability to work over time; local muscle endurance is distinguished from general body endurance as the ability of an isolated muscle group to continue a prescribed task rather than the ability to continue an activity such as running, swimming, or jogging for an extended period of time. As a result of specificity of training and the need for maintaining muscular strength and endurance and flexibility of the major muscle groups, a well-rounded training program including aerobic and resistance (strength and endurance) training and flexibility exercises is recommended.

### Strength Training

Strength training refers to exercise directed at improving the maximum force-generating capacity of muscle. There is evidence that strength training has a positive effect on aging skeletal muscle.[42]

Collectively, studies indicate that strength training in the older adult (1) produces substantial increases in the strength, mass, power, and quality of skeletal muscle; (2) can increase endurance performance; (3) normalizes blood pressure in those with high-normal values; (4) reduces insulin resistance; (5) decreases both total and intraabdominal fat; (6) increases resting metabolic rate in older men; (7) prevents the loss of bone mineral density with age; (8) reduces risk factors for falls; and (9) may reduce pain and improve function in those with osteoarthritis in the knee.[17]

Significant strength gains are possible in all populations including older adults when exposed to an adequate strength training program. Strength gains occur from enhanced neuromuscular activation over the initial 8 weeks and from increased fiber density and hypertrophy during subsequent weeks. Considerable evidence exists that sarcopenia can be prevented, reduced, and reversed with prescriptive strength training programs that emphasize gradual, progressive, high-intensity resistance exercises (e.g., high load/low repetition) for the upper and lower extremities.[42]

Resistance training significantly increases muscle size and increases energy requirements and insulin action in adults older than age 65 years. A program of once- or twice-weekly resistance exercise (carried out at a level described as "reasonably difficult" or "difficult") achieves muscle strength gains similar to 3 days/week training in older adults and is associated with improved neuromuscular performance. The goal is to design a program for each individual to provide the proper amount of physical activity and exercise to attain maximal benefit at the lowest risk.[3]

Strength training does not increase maximal oxygen uptake beyond normal (i.e., individuals attain the same maximal $VO_2$ before and after training). In postmenopausal women, muscle performance, muscle mass, and muscle composition are improved by hormone replacement therapy. The beneficial effects of hormone replacement therapy combined with high-impact physical training appear to exceed the effects of hormone replacement therapy alone.[39]

### Endurance Training

Endurance training refers to exercise directed at improving stamina (the duration that a person can maintain strenuous activity) and aerobic capacity ($VO_{2max}$). Endurance training places a high metabolic demand on the muscle and will increase the oxidative capacity of all muscle fiber types.[33] Endurance exercise can reverse the decline in physical conditioning associated with aging. An endurance training program using relatively modest intensity of training can reverse 100% of the loss of cardiovascular capacity, returning some healthy older adults to levels of aerobic power present in young adulthood. Even an older person who has failed to maintain fitness over time can benefit from an exercise program.

In middle-aged adults, the mechanism responsible for decline in cardiovascular capacity appears to be a reduced plasticity of heart muscle; improved aerobic power after training appears to be directly related to peripheral oxygen extraction (i.e., the muscles' ability to take up and use oxygen).[10]

## Joint

As discussed earlier, tendons, ligaments, and muscles around the joints have less water content, resulting in increased stiffness, with increasing age. Articular cartilage has less tensile strength, and the biochemical composition changes, often leading to osteoarthritis. Joint changes with deterioration of subchondral bone and atrophy of the synovium also can occur. Well-regulated exercise does not produce or exacerbate joint symptoms and actually may improve symptoms.[16] This concept is discussed in greater detail in Osteoarthritis in Chapter 27.

## Bone

The relationship between bone mass and activity is well established. Complete immobilization and weightlessness result in rapid onset of accelerated bone resorption; bone mass recovers when activity resumes, but whether bone loss is completely reversible is unknown. Immobilization also leads to changes in collagen, ligaments, and the musculotendinous junction at the joint, causing reduced range of motion.[41] Osteopenia, osteomalacia, and osteoporosis affect the mineralization of bone matrix and can impact the bone health of the aging adult. Older adults are at greater risk for osteoporosis-related fractures, both age related for all adults and postmenopause related for women. Fractures are discussed in more detail in Chapter 27.

## Specific Exercise Guidelines

Resistance training is an integral component in the comprehensive health program promoted by major health organizations such as the American Heart Association, American College of Sports Medicine, and Surgeon

General's office.[10,4,1] Population-specific guidelines have been published, and the current research indicates that for healthy people of all ages and many people with chronic diseases, single-set programs of up to 15 repetitions performed a minimum of two times per week are recommended.

Each workout session should consist of 8 to 10 different exercises that train the major muscle groups. Single-set programs are less time-consuming and generally result in greater compliance. The goal of this type of program is to develop and maintain a significant amount of muscle mass, endurance, and strength to contribute to overall fitness and health.

Although age in itself is not a limiting factor to exercise training, a more gradual approach in applying prescriptive exercise at older ages may be necessary, because exercise programs also can cause injury, especially in the presence of comorbidities such as arthritis, obesity, neurologic disease, postural instability, cardiovascular impairment, previous joint injuries, joint deformity, or other musculoskeletal complications such as tendinitis or shoulder impingement syndrome. High-intensity resistance training (>60% of the one-repetition maximum) has been demonstrated to cause large increases in strength in older adults (older than 65 years).[30]

People with chronic diseases may have to limit range of motion for some exercises and use lighter weights with more repetitions. Otherwise, older adults do not have to "take it easy" when performing exercise. The presence of heart disease, diabetes, cancer, or other comorbidities may require some initial progression in the prescribed program.[42]

Overall, therapists should pay careful attention to finding exercise intensities that are optimally suited to induce the desired training effects. Skeletal muscle of older people is more easily damaged with the loading that occurs during training compared with skeletal muscle of younger adults. Care should be taken to monitor soreness and prevent muscle injuries after exercise.[42]

Recommendations for the quantity and quality of exercise for developing and maintaining cardiorespiratory and muscular fitness and flexibility in healthy adults also have been published. A certain combination of *frequency* (3 to 5 days/week), *intensity* (55% to 90% of maximum heart rate or 40% to 85% of $VO_{2max}$) and *duration* (20 to 60 minutes continuously or 10-minute bouts intermittently throughout the day) of exercise performed consistently over time has been found effective for producing a training effect.[10]

Fatigue, the inability to continue to maintain a given activity, may develop as a result of depletion of muscle and liver glycogen, decreases in blood glucose, dehydration, and increases in body temperature. In a strength training program for adults older than age 65 years, repeated maximum voluntary contractions resulting in fatigue may differ from those for younger populations. This may be relevant for designing optimal strength training programs for older adults specifically requiring closer supervision to ensure that each repetition is completed without substitution or incomplete range of motion and to adjust rest times between contractions. Alternatively, electrical stimulation may provide more consistent muscle activation during strength training in this age group.[37]

Exercise guidelines for the very old (age >85 years) population have recommended a *frequency* of at least 2 days/week, preferably 3 days; *intensity* of 40% to 60% of heart rate reserve; and *duration* of at least 20 minutes. Walking, leg/arm ergometry, seated stepping machines, and water exercises are recommended.[18]

Additional recommendations for resistance training include two to three sets of 8 to 12 repetitions performed with good form and through the entire range of motion for each exercise performed on each training day (one set may be sufficient); some standing postures with free weights and balance training should be included. When 12 repetitions can be completed without difficulty (observe for increased respiration, extremity tremors, facial grimacing), the weight can be increased by 5% with a lower number of repetitions to begin a new training cycle.

## REFERENCES

To enhance this text and add value for the reader, all references are included in the enhanced ebook on Student Consult that accompanies this textbook. The reader can view the reference source and access it online whenever possible.

# CHAPTER 23

# Genetic and Developmental Disorders

ALLAN M. GLANZMAN • ANN HARRINGTON • JAMILA ABERDEEN • IAN M. LEAHY

Pediatric diseases and disorders comprise a large number of conditions. Entire volumes have been devoted just to pediatric pathologies. Given the format of this book and space limitations, this chapter includes as many of the more commonly encountered genetic and developmental disorders as possible. Cerebral palsy will be discussed separately as a neurologic condition in Chapter 35.

A brief discussion of several other rare but important diagnoses also is included. Because physical and occupational therapy intervention is not the focus here, the reader is referred to other, more appropriate resources for specific and thorough intervention guidelines for these conditions.[48,175,281,335,349]

## DOWN SYNDROME

### Definition and Incidence

Down syndrome was the first genetic disorder attributed to a chromosomal aberration and is referred to as trisomy 21. Down syndrome is characterized by muscle hypotonia, intellectual disability, dysmorphic facial features, and other distinctive physical abnormalities affecting multiple systems of the body.

Down syndrome is the most common inherited chromosomal disorder, occurring approximately once in every 700 live births. The incidence of Down syndrome rises with maternal age. Before maternal age 30 years the incidence is 1 in 2000 births; it is 1 in 50 for mothers age 35 to 39 years, and 1 in 20 for mothers older than 40 years. There is a 2% risk of recurrence for a couple who have had a child with Down syndrome. The prevalence has been increasing because of a number of factors and at birth is 11.8 to 12.8 per 10,000 inf ants.[206,271,329]

### Etiologic Factors and Pathogenesis

The actual cause of the phenotype in Down syndrome is not yet known; however, some hints have begun to emerge as researchers continue to explore gene mapping and develop genetic models for Down syndrome.[16] Evidence from cytogenetic and epidemiologic studies supports multiple causality.[63]

#### Chromosomal Abnormality

Trisomy 21 produces three copies of chromosome 21 instead of the normal two because of faulty meiosis (cell division by which reproductive cells are formed) of the ovum or, sometimes, the sperm. This results in a karyotype (chromosomal constitution of the cell nucleus) of 47 chromosomes instead of the normal 46.[180] The faulty cell division can also occur after fertilization, leading to only a portion of cells being affected, with a milder clinical picture. This situation is referred to as mosaicism. Because of the positive correlation between increasing age and Down syndrome, it is hypothesized that deterioration of the oocyte (immature ovum) or environmental factors such as radiation and viruses may cause a predisposition to mistakes in meiosis and the resulting chromosomal abnormality. In a small number of cases, Down syndrome occurs as a result of a translocation of chromosome 15, 21, or 22 (i.e., the long arm of the chromosome breaks off and attaches to another chromosome). Chromosomal translocation can be hereditary or associated with advanced parental age. Although Down syndrome usually is attributed to the aging woman, evidence suggests that in 5% to 10% of cases Down syndrome correlates with paternal age.[319,353,399]

The third copy of chromosome 21 is the cause of the phenotypic characteristics that are observed in people with Down syndrome. Some of the genes are dosage sensitive and contribute to the Down syndrome phenotype; however, this is complicated by the fact that there might be downstream effects in some cases that impact the expression of genes on other chromosomes. The 21st chromosome is the smallest, and there are approximately 305 coding genes that are present in triplicate in individuals with Down syndrome. Another possible cause for some features of the phenotype might be not only elevated expression of specific genes, but the elevated expression of groups of genes and a resulting lack of genetic stability.[274] Only a few specific genes have been identified as causative of specific pathology in Down syndrome and the specific causative factors that contribute to the Down syndrome phenotype are still being considered.

**Table 23.1** Down Syndrome: Clinical Characteristics

| Most Frequently Observed Manifestations | Associated Manifestations |
|---|---|
| Flattened nasal bridge (90%)<br>Almond eye shape<br>Flat occiput<br>Muscle hypotonia and joint hyperextensibility<br>Congenital heart disease<br>Language and cognitive delay<br>Short limbs, short broad hands and feet<br>Epicanthal folds<br>High arched palate; protruding, fissured tongue<br>Delayed acquisition of gross motor skills<br>Simian line (transverse palmar crease) | Other congenital anomalies<br>• Absence of kidney<br>• Duodenal atresia<br>• Tracheoesophageal fistula<br>• Feeding difficulties<br>Atlantoaxial instability<br>Sensory impairment<br>• Hearing loss (conductive)<br>• Visual impairment<br>  • Strabismus<br>  • Myopia<br>  • Nystagmus<br>  • Cataracts<br>  • Conjunctivitis<br>Delayed growth and sexual development<br>Obesity<br>Diabetes mellitus |

It is likely that there will emerge a more comprehensive model of phenotypic causation in the future.

## Clinical Manifestations

Children with Down syndrome are readily identified by their flattened nasal bridges, up-slanting palpebral fissures, epicanthic folds, short broad hands, transverse palm crease, and mild to moderate hypotonia. Table 23.1 lists the most frequently observed clinical characteristics. The phenotypic presentation in individuals with Down syndrome includes delayed motor development and hypotonia, intellectual disability, and early onset Alzheimer disease. There is an increased incidence of ophthalmologic disorders (35%), thyroid dysfunction (25-60%), and gastrointestinal anomalies, with associated constipation (13%). The risk of leukemia (10 to 20 times typical) and congenital heart disease in this population is also elevated, while coronary artery disease and arterial hypertension risk is diminished when compared to the general population. Other associated clinical manifestations may also be present. For example, people with Down syndrome have altered immune function. They tend to exhibit increased susceptibility to infections[219,288] such as respiratory infection and otitis media (ear infection); they are more likely to contract hepatitis B if exposed; and there is a decreased antibody response to immunization.

### Congenital Heart Disease

Congenital heart disease (CHD) has an incidence of 50% in those with Down syndrome, though it is somewhat lower when there is a mosaic presentation, and is also impacted by the increased use of prenatal ultrasound diagnosis and surgical decision making. The most common defect is atrioventricular septal with atrial septal and ventriculoseptal defects as well as tetralogy of Fallot also significantly more common than in the general population, with the specific incidence varying to a great degree by race. Overexpression of genes (*DSCAM* and *DSCR1*) on chromosome 21 in addition to the presence of specific chromosome 21 alleles and various other genetic characteristics on chromosomes other than 21 play a role, though still unclear, in the increased susceptibility to CHD.[20,270] The presence of CHD in these patients is further complicated by the systemic hypotonia and resultant risk of pulmonary obstructive disease with associated pulmonary arterial hypertension of the newborn, which is between 10 and 50 times more common than in the non–Down syndrome newborns, with early surgical repair recommended for prevention of pulmonary hypertension in the newborn. On the whole, infants with Down syndrome fare better than the general population when it comes to repair of CHD, and they tend to have lower mortality rates and lower rates of second surgeries.[270]

Coronary artery disease in this population is less common. There are a number of genes on chromosome 21 that may contribute to this finding. Heart-type fatty acid binding protein function is diminished (it typically acts to regulate mitochondrial function in the heart and aid in importation of long chain fatty acids from the cell membrane into the cell[373]) and adiponectin may have a protective effect stemming from its antiinflammatory and vascular protective effects when levels of adiponectin are increased.[66]

### Endocrine Dysfunction

Bone mineral density seems to more rapidly diminish with age and vitamin D levels may be more decreased when compared with the general population.[49] However, there is considerable controversy owing to diminished stature and the resulting bone density measurement impacts this creates. When monitoring for height and weight it is important to use Down syndrome–specific growth charts and to consider this when using dual energy x-ray absorptiometry for bone density measurement. Puberty can be expected to progress as in the general population. Although rates of hypogonadism are significant and progresses into adulthood, some individuals are fertile[286] and able to bear children. The underlying dysfunction in males with trisomy 21 may rely in defective spermatogenesis and testosterone production. Sertoli cells of the testis typically function during spermatogenesis and are abnormal from infancy. In the case of the interstitial cells of Leydig, which act in testosterone production, the functional deficit is more mild and the production of testosterone more typical.[121]

Thyroid disease is more common in those with Down syndrome[184] and can be autoimmune or congenital, with hypothyroidism present subclinically in a quarter or more of patients.[170] In addition to autoimmune thyroid disease, type 1 diabetes is more common in individuals with Down syndrome, though its cause is still uncertain. Pancreatic anatomy appears intact in these patients though there is an elevated incidence of auto-antibodies, which may be related to the presence of the *AIRE* gene on chromosome 21 which regulates T cell function.[286]

## Alzheimer Disease

Alzheimer disease is also more common in people with Down syndrome, occurring at an earlier age than that of the Alzheimer population in general. By the age of 40 years, symptoms of Alzheimer disease can be seen in almost everyone with Down syndrome. The increased rate of Alzheimer disease in individuals with Down syndrome is a result of abnormally high production of β-amyloid that makes up the extracellular plaques seen in individuals with Down syndrome. This results from the increased expression of the amyloid precursor protein (*AAP*) gene, which not only increases β-amyloid but also impairs mitochondrial function in Down syndrome. This effect of *AAP* gene expression is also found in familial Alzheimer disease.[311]

Amyloid precursor protein is processed through a variety of enzymatically driven steps, with the ultimate aggregate being pathogenic. The extra copy of *AAP* in those with Down syndrome impairs cellular endocytic protein recycling and autophagic protein degradation within the cell by altering the lysosomal pH through the β-cleaved carboxy terminal fragment of *APP*, impairing the activity of the lysosome.[269,398] In addition, extracellular plaques, intracellular tangles, and striated neutrophil threads are found within the cell, which result from a hyperphosphorylation of protein tau, a protein that contributes to the cytoskeleton of the cell and acts to stabilize the microtubule infrastructure of the cell. The *AAP* gene expression also has an impact on energy metabolism in the mitochondria. This phenomenon, and the fact that the gene for superoxide dismutase (an important free radical defense) is also found on the long arm of chromosome 21, suggests a role in the neuropathology of Down syndrome through the action of free radical–induced damage, which may be additive in diminishing lysosomal function. Although superoxide dismutase shows normal expression in the fetuses of individuals with Down syndrome, it is overexpressed in the brains of adults with Down syndrome and declines as symptoms of dementia appear. There is also an imbalance between superoxide dismutase and glutathione peroxidase activity, and this imbalance relates to the presence of free radicals in the brain. This suggests that the imbalance may play a role in the developmental brain abnormalities and is likely secondary to chronic oxidative injury as opposed to an underlying primary cause.[251,266,274]

The resulting gross pathology observed in the brains of people with Down syndrome is an overall reduction in brain weight with a reduced size of the cerebral and cerebellar hemispheres, the hippocampus, the pons, and the mammillary bodies. Additional abnormal findings may include smaller convolutions within the brain, structural abnormalities in the dendritic spines of the pyramidal neurons of the motor cortex, and abnormalities of the pyramidal system as a whole, including decreased pyramidal neurons in the hippocampus. This last finding and the decreased size of the amygdala in people with Down syndrome who develop Alzheimer disease have particular significance because these factors are associated with the increased incidence of Alzheimer disease symptoms in older adults with Down syndrome.[12]

Both acute lymphoblastic (ALL) and acute myeloid leukemia (AML)[210,318] and a few other cancers (germ cell, testicular, gastric, and liver) occur at elevated rates in people with Down syndrome. ALL and AML are between 7 and 18 times more common than in the typically developing population. One theory underlying the increased cancer risk is the immune surveillance theory that proposes the immune system acts as an early detection system in the face of nascent cancer cells, protecting the body by removing them. This is an attractive theory, but many other cancers occur at reduced rates in people with Down syndrome, arguing against this as the foundation for ALL and AML heightened risk.

Children with Down syndrome frequently present with a variety of musculoskeletal or orthopedic problems[236] thought to be acquired secondary to soft tissue laxity and muscle hypotonia. Some of the more common findings include recurrent patellar dislocation, excessive pes planus, scoliosis, slipped capital femoral epiphyses, and late hip dislocation (after 2 years of age).

Atlantoaxial or occipitocervical instability of the cervical spine is found in 10% to 15% of children[236,280] with Down syndrome. This instability is thought to be secondary to ligamentous laxity, odontoid maldevelopment, or defect in the formation of the posterior arch. Atlantoaxial displacement is identified on plane radiographs with anterior–posterior, lateral, mouth open, and flexion–extension views. Occipitocervical instability is harder to identify on plain radiographs because of overlap of the bony structures at the base of the skull; an MRI with supervised flexion and extension might be needed. Anyone with instability should be educated on symptomatology to watch for and instructed in activity modification. For example, they should avoid contact sports, gymnastics, and diving, and should be followed closely by a medical team.[236] The majority of cases are asymptomatic; however, clinical changes indicative of symptomatic spinal compression include hyperreflexia, clonus, positive Babinski sign, torticollis, progressive weakness, changes in sensation, loss of established bladder and bowel control, and a decrease in motor skills.

Children with Down syndrome often present with feeding difficulties and delayed acquisition of motor skills. These skills, however, improve with age. Because of the hypotonia, midline upper extremity movement is difficult and emerges later in development than would be expected. Gait[61,65] usually is characterized by a smaller step length, decreased knee flexion at heel contact, and knee hyperextension in stance. There is also a decreased single-limb support time, and a decreased push off at terminal stance. Individuals with Down syndrome present with slower reaction times and postural reactions and altered biomechanics at the initiation of gait. Movement patterns are typically characterized by increased variability, which is often magnified[334] with advancing age. Secondary disorders often develop after age 30 or 35 years, including obesity, diabetes mellitus, and cardiovascular disease. Other significant problems can include osteoarthritic degeneration of the spine and osteoporosis,[125] in addition to vertebral or long bone fractures.

## MEDICAL MANAGEMENT[370]

**DIAGNOSIS.** Measurement of α-fetoprotein (AFP), human chorionic gonadotropin, and unconjugated estrogen in maternal serum (triple screen) allows detection of an estimated 60% to 70% of fetuses with Down syndrome. Using this screening test, prenatal diagnosis may be made during the second trimester (between 15.5 and 20 weeks' gestation).

Nuchal translucency ultrasound at 10 to 14 weeks' gestation provides a good way to identify the fetus with Down syndrome. Ultrasound carries a 6% false-positive rate and will identify only 77% of affected fetuses.[209]

Postnatal diagnosis usually begins with suspected physical findings at birth. Genetic studies showing the chromosomal abnormality can confirm the diagnosis. Specific diagnostic testing for the secondary problems discussed earlier varies depending on the involved organ systems suspected of dysfunction.

**TREATMENT.** Treatment focuses on specific medical problems (e.g., antibiotics for infection, cardiac surgery, monitoring/treatment of thyroid function, and monitoring for development of Alzheimer disease). The overall goal of treatment intervention is to help affected children develop to their full potential. This involves a team of experts, including therapists.

**PROGNOSIS.** The improved life expectancy of people with Down syndrome is a result of the greater availability of surgery, particularly for congenital cardiac defects, but life expectancy remains lower than that for the general population.[160,192,283]

The presence of congenital malformations, especially of the heart and gastrointestinal tract, can result in high mortality rates in the affected population[109]; lack of mobility and poor eating skills are also predictors of early death.[92] Respiratory tract infections are very common and contribute significantly to morbidity and to some extent to mortality.[136]

Significant health problems contributing to mortality have been reported in the adult population with Down syndrome, including untreated congenital heart anomalies, acquired cardiac disease, pulmonary hypertension, recurrent respiratory infections, aspiration leading to chronic interstitial lung disease, and complications from Alzheimer disease.

Over the last 40 years, the life span of those with Down syndrome has increased significantly. In 1968, the average age of death was 2 years of age; by 1997, it had increased to 50 years of age. Unfortunately, this degree of improvement has not occurred for everyone with Down syndrome. There is a significant disparity that exists based on race, with Caucasians with Down syndrome enjoying a significantly longer life span than some other races.[51,176]

### SPECIAL IMPLICATIONS FOR THE THERAPIST 23.1

### *Down Syndrome*

#### Precautions

Because atlantoaxial instability is a potential problem, activities that could result in a direct downward, traction, or translational force on the cervical area require caution and may be contraindicated if screening for atlantoaxial instability is positive. Some examples that may be limited include manual therapy; gymnastics/trampoline; swimming butterfly stroke or diving; horseback riding; pentathlon/high jump; and contact sports such as football, soccer, martial arts, and rugby. Positioning precautions for surgery, especially head and neck surgery, are also important to be aware of. Transportation in a car or bus or bicycle may be considered a potentially risky activity requiring specific support. Likewise, riding carnival-type rides such as fast-moving carousels, roller coasters, and so on should be discussed with the family.

Some disagreement exists on the degree of screening and restriction that is required. The Committee on Sports Medicine and Fitness of the American Academy of Pediatrics as well as the Sport and Exercise Medicine, English Institute of Sport, and British Gymnastics have published position papers on atlantoaxial instability in children with Down syndrome.[42,356] Plain radiographs are somewhat technically problematic and do not predict which children are at increased risk and cannot assure that children will not develop problems in the future; other sources favor radiologic examinations of the cervical spine of children with Down syndrome.[285] The therapist is an important source of information for increasing family and community awareness regarding the potential precautions and contraindications associated with atlantoaxial instability. Symptomatic children should have radiographs taken in the neutral position, with further evaluation based on the initial result and referral as needed.

Decreased muscle tone compromises respiratory expansion. In addition, the underdeveloped nasal bone causes a chronic problem of inadequate drainage of mucus. The constant stuffy nose forces the child to breathe by mouth, and dries the oropharyngeal membranes. These anatomic differences, as well as immunologic factors, increase the individual's susceptibility to upper respiratory tract infections and ear infections.

Low oral motor tone and a protruding tongue can interfere with feeding, especially solid foods. Children with Down syndrome have between a 50% and 80% incidence of feeding problems, the etiology of which is varied and complex. In addition to the presence of low tone, the oral motor anatomy may be unique and the development over time of periodontal disease creates limitations in mastication. In addition, refusal and retention can be issues along with abnormalities in all phases of swallowing. Beyond the incoordination of oral motor function, esophageal peristalsis and lower sphincter can also be limited. The reflux this creates is often uncomfortable and, along with the poor oral motor control, avoidance behavior around feeding often develops. A multimodal approach, including therapists, psychologist, and physicians can optimally address these issues.[10]

### Gross and Fine Motor Development

The therapist concerned with motor development as well as other clinical, educational, psychosocial, or vocational issues relevant to people with Down syndrome is referred to other more intervention-oriented resources and community supports.[37,137,389]

### Physical Activity and Exercise

Developing an active lifestyle early in childhood is important given the risk factors for the development of obesity, dyslipidemia,[204] diabetes mellitus, and cardiovascular disease in this group. The presence of cardiac defects may affect the client's overall level of activity, fitness, and endurance training, especially in the school setting.

Some evidence suggests that individuals with Down syndrome physiologically work harder when engaged in physical activity or exercise (e.g., higher heart rate, greater oxygen consumption, and minute ventilation) compared to peers who are without impairment or who are developmentally delayed but do not have Down syndrome.[94]

Anyone with Down syndrome interested in participating in competitive sports activities must work closely with the therapist, support staff, and physician to establish guidelines for safety. When prescribing an aerobic conditioning plan, the frequency, intensity, and duration must be modified from the general recommendations of the American College of Sports Medicine (ACSM) based on the characteristics and exercise response of the patient. When designing a program it should be remembered that a similar degree of walking speed (treadmill or over ground) results in higher $VO_2$ as compared to typically developing individuals. Vital signs should be monitored throughout the exercise program as a means of determining workload levels and progressing the activity or exercise.

# SCOLIOSIS

## Definition

Scoliosis is an abnormal lateral curvature of the spine. The curvature may be toward the right (more common in thoracic curves) or the left (more common in lumbar curves). Rotation of the vertebral column around its axis occurs and causes an associated rib cage deformity. Scoliosis is often associated with kyphosis and lordosis.

## Overview and Incidence

Scoliosis is classified as idiopathic (unknown cause; 60% of all cases[299]), osteopathic (as a result of spinal disease or bony abnormality), myopathic (as a result of muscle weakness), or neuropathic (as a result of a central nervous system [CNS] disorder), with the latter two often being combined and denoted as a neuromuscular scoliosis.

Age of onset can vary from birth onward and is referred to as infantile (0-3 years), juvenile (ages 3-10 years), adolescent (age 10 until bone maturity at between 18 and 20 years of age), or adult (after skeletal maturation). Between 0.4% and 5.5% of children may present with some type of scoliosis,[339] with one in four of those requiring some type of treatment intervention. The incidence is increased with associated neuromuscular impairments, such as cerebral palsy, spina bifida, neurofibromatosis, and muscular dystrophy, with one-third of all cases of scoliosis occurring in the context of a primary neuromuscular disorder.[299]

The overwhelming majority of cases of progressive idiopathic scoliosis are found in the adolescent age group when the growth velocity of the spine increases after the relatively slow growth period between the ages of 5 and 11 years for girls and up to age 13 years for boys.[54]

Infantile idiopathic scoliosis (rare in the United States) accounts for 1% of cases.[299] It is characterized by curvatures that are most often thoracic and toward the left, and most commonly affects males. Juvenile idiopathic scoliosis is characterized most often by a right thoracic curvature and can be rapidly progressive. This type of scoliosis has a much more variable natural history and can lead to significant deformity if left untreated.[182] Adolescent idiopathic scoliosis of greater than 30 degrees is seen most often in females without any neurologic impairments in a 10:1 female-to-male ratio.[382] In its milder forms (10-degree curve or less), scoliosis affects boys and girls equally, but girls are more likely to develop more severe curvatures requiring intervention.

Adult scoliosis (curves greater than 30 degrees) affects approximately 500,000 people in the United States, and the prevalence of scoliosis in adults older than age 50 years is reportedly between 6% and 10% (based on routine radiographs).[32]

## Etiologic Factors

Scoliosis may be functional or structural. Functional or postural scoliosis may be caused by factors other than vertebral involvement, such as pain, poor posture, leg length discrepancy, or muscle spasm induced by a herniated disk or spondylolisthesis. These curves disappear when the cause is remedied. Functional scoliosis can become structural if untreated.

Structural scoliosis is a fixed curvature of the spine associated with vertebral rotation and asymmetry of the ligamentous supporting structures. It can be caused by deformity of the vertebral bodies and may be congenital (e.g., wedge vertebrae, fused ribs or vertebrae, hemivertebrae), musculoskeletal (e.g., osteoporosis, spinal tuberculosis, rheumatoid arthritis), neuromuscular (e.g., cerebral palsy, polio, myelomeningocele, muscular dystrophy), or, most commonly, idiopathic.

At the present time, despite extensive study, the cause of idiopathic scoliosis remains unknown. Researchers hypothesize that this type of scoliosis relates to the maturation disturbances of the CNS, including neurohormonal transmitters or neuromodulators secondary to genetic defect.[203] These, in addition to the aforementioned causes of scoliosis, lead to a triggering effect, such as lateral wedging of the vertebrae, which in turn results in the "vicious cycle" theory, creating spinal curvature, asymmetrical loading, and therefore asymmetrical growth.[342]

Multiple areas of research, including abnormalities of connective tissue, neuromotor mechanisms, neurohormonal imbalances (e.g., melatonin, calmodulin), and biomechanics (e.g., the importance of the erect posture) have been explored for a potential relationship to the cause of idiopathic scoliosis. However, no clear evidence supports any one area as an etiologic factor of this disorder; rather, it appears to be multifactorial.[199] Genetic studies have identified a genetic predisposition to some types of scoliosis[391]; and polymorphisms that contribute to susceptibility are actively being investigated.[157,338]

## Pathogenesis

The pathogenesis of scoliosis remains unclear but may be better understood in relation to the underlying cause. Abnormal embryonic formation and segmentation of the spinal column are possible pathologic pathways in congenital scoliosis. Neuromuscular scoliosis is often the result of an imbalance or asymmetry of muscle activity through the trunk and spine.

The earliest pathologic changes associated with idiopathic scoliosis occur in the soft tissues as the muscles, ligaments, and other tissues become shortened on the concave side of the curve. Some hypothesize[339] that scoliosis sets up abnormal forces across the spine as a consequence of the differences in length–tension relationships, with the muscles on the convexity being in a lengthened position and those on the concavity positioned in a relatively shortened state, and as a result a muscle imbalance is present.

Evidence establishes the existence of hypertrophy of the muscles on the side of the convexity[191]; however, the muscles on the concavity still are at a mechanical advantage and facilitate the progression of a curve once it is established. In time, bone deformities occur, as compression forces on one side of the vertebral bodies apply asymmetric forces to the epiphyseal ossification center, resulting in increased bone density on that side. The compressive force is greatest on the vertebrae in the apex of the concavity, so the apical vertebrae become most deformed (Fig. 23.1). Vertebral torsional deformities also begin to form in two distinct ways: mechanical torsion and geometric torsion. Mechanical torsion refers to the twisting of the spine about its own axis without changing the shape of the spinal column. Geometric torsion is the twisting with a translation, thus changing the shape of the spinal column.[343]

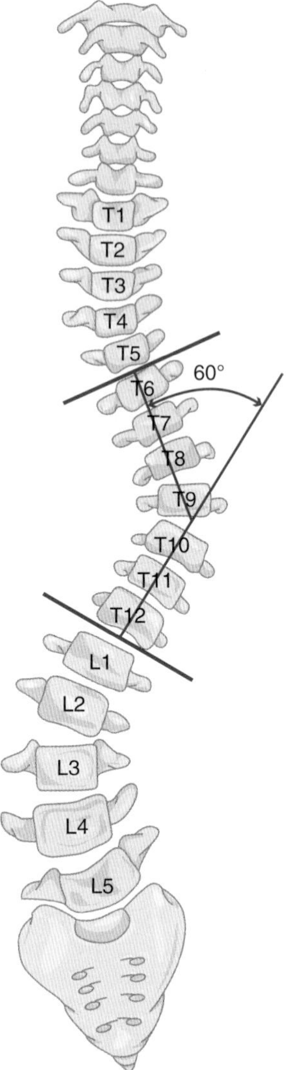


**Figure 23.1**

**The Cobb method of measuring scoliosis.** The top vertebra used in the measurement is identified as the uppermost vertebra whose upper surface tilts toward the curvature's concave side (the superior surface of the vertebra that is most tilted). The bottom vertebra is the lowest vertebra whose inferior surface tilts most toward the curvature's concave side. A line is drawn parallel to each of these vertebrae. The angle formed by the two perpendicular lines drawn to each of these lines creates the angle of the curvature.

## Clinical Manifestations

Curvatures of less than 20 degrees (mild scoliosis) rarely cause significant problems. Severe untreated scoliosis (curvatures greater than 60 degrees) may produce pulmonary insufficiency and reduced lung capacity, back pain, degenerative spinal arthritis, disk disease, vertebral subluxation, or sciatica.

Back pain is not typical in children or adolescents with mild scoliosis[69] and should be evaluated by a physician who can rule out spondylolisthesis, tumor, infection, or occult trauma. Back pain may be associated with curve progression after institution of brace treatment for idiopathic scoliosis.[290] The adult with scoliosis often presents with back pain that is considered multifactorial, arising from muscle fatigue, trunk imbalance, facet arthropathy, spinal stenosis, degenerative disk disease, and radiculopathy. Back pain in adults with scoliosis occurs more frequently[69] than in the general population; the pain is typically greater and more persistent,[32] affecting function and disability level measures.[69]

Common characteristics of scoliosis are asymmetric shoulder and pelvic position, often identified when clothes do not hang evenly. Curves are designated as right or left, depending on the convexity (e.g., right thoracic scoliosis describes a curve in the thoracic spine with convexity to the right). Usually one primary curvature exists with a secondary

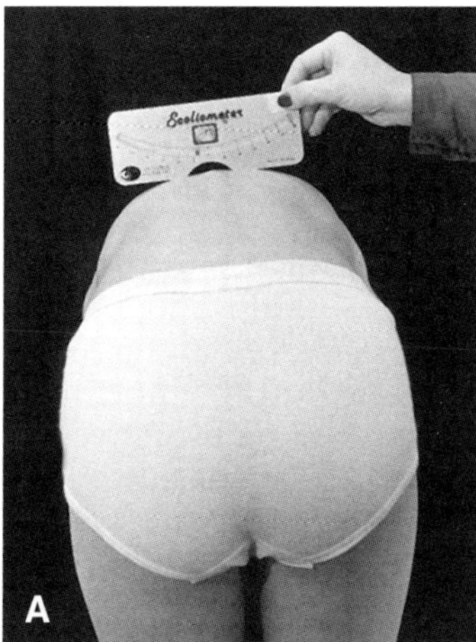


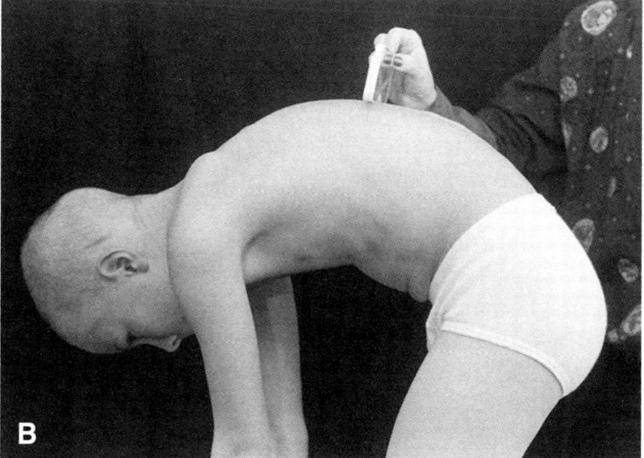

**Figure 23.2**

**The scoliometer.** This device can be used by any health care worker trained to screen for scoliosis. Some medical personnel also use this device to monitor curvatures over time, thereby avoiding unnecessary radiographs. Ask the client to bend forward slowly (the Adam position), stopping when the shoulders are level with the hips. View the client from both the front and back, keeping your eyes at the same level as the back. Before measuring with the scoliometer, adjust the height of the person's bending position to the level where the deformity of the spine is most pronounced. This position varies from one person to another depending upon the location of the curvature (e.g., a low lumbar curvature requires further bending than an upper thoracic curvature). Lay the scoliometer across the deformity with the 0 mark over the top of the spinous process. A measurement of 5 degrees or more in the screening test is considered positive and requires medical followup. Visually observe for asymmetry of the ribs or paravertebral muscles. In this child, hamstring tightness (greater on the left) accounts for the positional shift to the left. The scoliometer reading was zero. (Courtesy Todd Goodrich, University of Montana, Missoula.)

or compensatory curvature that develops to balance the body. Two primary curvatures may exist (usually right thoracic and left lumbar). If the curvatures of the spine are balanced (compensated), the head is centered over the center of the pelvis; if the spinal alignment is uncompensated, the head is shifted to one side. Rotational deformity on the convex side is observed as a rib hump sometimes seen in the upright position, but always apparent in the forward bend position, commonly known as the Adam test.

## MEDICAL MANAGEMENT

**DIAGNOSIS.** Diagnosis by clinical examination requires the client to bend forward 90 degrees with the hands joined in the midline as if taking a dive into a swimming pool. A scoliometer also can be used to measure the angle of trunk rotation (Fig. 23.2).

An abnormal finding includes asymmetry of the height of the ribs or paravertebral muscles on one side. The examiner also checks for leg length discrepancy and other asymmetries and for the presence of hair patches, nevi, pits, or areas of abnormal skin pigmentation in the midline indicating possible underlying spinal abnormality.

Differential diagnosis is important in determining whether the scoliosis is structural or functional. Structural curvatures are defined by positive findings of a rotational prominence during forward bending, a spinous process line that is not linear, disruption of normal flexion of the spine as seen from a lateral view, and radiographic findings of spinal curvature greater than 10 degrees. Functional curvatures straighten when placed in a forward bend position. The physician also performs a neurologic examination to rule out an underlying neurologic disorder, especially in the presence of left thoracic curvature.

Full-length radiographs of the spine, using posteroanterior views instead of anteroposterior views can reduce breast radiation dosage[81] by 20 times. The radiographs are evaluated using the Cobb method (see Fig. 23.1) to measure the degree of curvatures. The use of EOS imaging has also been shown to provide a reliable 3D quantitative analysis of scoliotic deformities,[154] while administering one-tenth the amount of radiation as an x-ray and one-thousandth the amount of radiation of a CT scan.

The Risser sign is also determined from the film as an indication of maturation and is used as a prognostic predictor of progression.[275] Typically, the iliac crest ossifies from anterior to posterior. Risser divided the crest into four quarters according to ossification, grading the ossification from 1 to 4, with a grade 5 indicating that the whole apophysis has ossified and is fused to the iliac crest. More recently the use of hand and finger growth plates have also been used as a predictor of progression.[313]

Neuroimaging beyond plain films may be necessary. For example, bone scan may be used to rule out neoplasms, infections, spondylolysis, or compression fractures as the underlying cause. Magnetic resonance imaging (MRI) is used to differentiate cord lesions, disk herniations, neoplasms, infections, spondylolysis, spinal stenosis, and compression fractures.

**TREATMENT.** Prevention of postural or idiopathic structural scoliosis is the key to management of the majority of scoliosis cases. Early detection allows for early treatment without surgical intervention and with good long-term results. Overall goals of management are to prevent severe and progressive deformities that might lead to decreased cardiorespiratory function.

Conservative care in the past has included exercise and electrical stimulation; however, this has not been shown to be efficacious.[254] Based on the Scoliosis Research Society, observation and monitoring every 4 to 6 months for curvatures less than 25 degrees, spinal orthoses for curvatures 25 to 45 degrees (Table 23.2), and surgery for curvatures greater than 45 degrees is recommended.[241,295] The goal of using spinal orthoses is to serve as a passive restraint system to maintain curvatures within 5 degrees of the curve measurement at the time of initial application. This

**Table 23.2** Scoliosis: Bracing Options

| Brace | Use |
|---|---|
| Milwaukee (cervicothoracolumbosacral orthosis) | Best with curvature at T8 or above |
| Boston (thoracolumbosacral orthosis) | Best with curvature apex lower than T9 or T10 |
| Lyon | For idiopathic scoliosis with thoracic hypokyphosis |
| Charleston | For idiopathic curves fabricated in maximum side-bend correction |

is accomplished successfully in 85% to 88% of cases.[387] Curves with an apex between T8 and L2 and compensated thoracolumbar curves respond the most favorably to bracing,[275] whereas curves with an apex at T6 or above have the poorest outcome. More recently, the Society of Scoliosis Orthopedic Rehabilitation and Treatment (SOSORT) has included the use of physiotherapy scoliosis specific exercises (PSSE) as part of their treatment algorithm for curves in both observation and bracing ranges.

Research into the use of PSSE has continued to be a growing topic of interest in the management of adolescent idiopathic scoliosis. In 2012, a Cochrane review[178] was published which showed low quality of evidence in physical therapy directly related to objective measures such as Cobb angle, trunk rotation, and pain. However, numerous randomized controlled trials[178,238,243,388] have been published showing strong evidence of effective management of AIS using PSSE. Orthotic regimens have varied for late-onset idiopathic scoliosis, but typically bracing is indicated for curves greater than 20 degrees in the skeletally immature individual, or earlier if progression has been noted.[32] Bracing is now recognized as the mainstay of nonsurgical intervention, as evidenced by the Bracing in Adolescent Idiopathic Scoliosis Trial (BRAIST), a prospective, randomized, controlled trial.[383] It demonstrated a 72% treatment success after bracing in the treatment group compared to 48% after observation for curves less than 50 degrees. In addition, the relative risk of progression was decreased by over 50%. Newer braces such as the Rigo Cheneau brace are showing even better results of slowing progression of the curve due to their three-dimensional correction of the curvature.[238]

Interventions in the adult with scoliosis should follow a conservative nonsurgical course of physical therapy to improve aerobic capacity, strengthen muscles, and improve flexibility and joint motion. In addition, nonnarcotic analgesics, nutritional counseling, smoking (or tobacco-use) cessation, nerve root blocks, facet injections, and epidural steroid injections should be considered to address the problem of pain before surgery (if pain is the primary concern). Bracing has never been shown to have an effect on the natural history of adult scoliosis, but may be used symptomatically for certain people who are not surgery candidates.[32]

Surgical intervention (e.g., fusion with posterior segmental spinal instrumentation) may be necessary for curvatures greater than 45 degrees, in the presence of chronic pain, or when the curvature appears to be causing neurologic changes. Surgical goals are to halt progression of the curvature, improve alignment, decrease deformity, prevent pulmonary problems, and eliminate pain. The surgical options include a variety of segmental instrumentation systems. These are combined with a posterior fusion and, in more severe cases, anterior fusion. In children and adolescents who are not skeletally mature, instrumented fusion is not possible and either growing rods or a vertical expandable prosthetic titanium rib is considered. These methods of instrumentation allow the spine and thoracic cavity to continue to grow while providing internal stabilization for the scoliosis until a final spine fusion can be completed.[289,396]

Minimally invasive surgery can be used in the population who need an anterior release along with a spinal fusion to decrease the morbidity associated with open thoracotomy. This procedure is designed to maximize the stability of the spine. This technique is still evolving and long-term data are needed but it may result in faster recovery, fewer complications, and less pain along with adequate alignment.[278,317]

**PROGNOSIS.** Postural curvatures resolve as the primary problem is treated. Structural curvatures are not eliminated but rather increase during periods of rapid skeletal growth. If the curvature is less than 40 degrees at skeletal maturity, the risk of progression is small. In curvatures greater than 50 degrees, the spine is biomechanically unstable, and the curvature will likely continue to progress at a rate of 1 degree/yr throughout life.[32]

Poor seating can contribute to this progression.[174] In severe kyphoscoliosis, pain and the inability to achieve comfortable positioning can complicate care, and ultimately pulmonary compromise can lead to death.

**SPECIAL IMPLICATIONS FOR THE THERAPIST 23.2**

## *Scoliosis*

### Intervention

Now that there is more evidence regarding the effectiveness of PSSE in the management of scoliosis, it is imperative for a clinician to understand the goals of the rehabilitation process for an individual with scoliosis to decrease the asymmetrical loading of the spine caused by the scoliotic posture. There is a flexible, postural component of scoliosis that can be influenced by exercise. Postural changes made in rehab thus create a change in spinal proprioception. Rehabilitation must aim to change the corporal schema of the patient, creating a new "normal" posture. Once this new posture can be achieved independently, strengthening in this new position will then allow the patient to hold the corrected posture effectively through their daily lives. These exercises and the ability to "feel" a change in posture are also important when removing the brace to avoid return to the baseline scoliotic posture.

The aim of nonsurgical treatment of scoliosis is to stop progression, improve 3D trunk shape and global posture, improve general health, cope with body deformity and treatment, and diminish functional limitations.[384]

### Postoperative

During the hospital stay after surgery the therapy and nursing staff must check sensation, color, and blood supply in all extremities to document neurovascular status. A serious complication following spinal surgery that is monitored for intraoperatively is neurovascular compromise.

Initially, the person should be log-rolled and deep-breathing exercises encouraged to prevent the development of pulmonary complications. For those who are ambulatory, mobilization can begin within 24 to 48 hours, depending on the surgeon's protocol. Adults are treated with antiembolic stockings and sequential compression devices until they are ambulatory, and most patients (depending on the instrumentation used) are fitted soon after surgery with a custom-molded, lightweight plastic thoracolumbosacral orthosis. The brace is to be worn full-time when out of bed; in some cases, a progressive tolerance schedule may be required initially to achieve this. A vigilant preventive skin care program is also important.

Activities of daily living (brushing the hair or teeth) and active range of motion exercises of the extremities help maintain circulation and muscle strength. Clients should be instructed in quadriceps setting, ankle pumps, and other range-of-motion exercises. These should be performed frequently on their own throughout the day.

Cast syndrome (superior mesenteric artery syndrome) is a rare but serious complication that can follow spinal surgery and application of a body cast that is infrequently used for immobilization. It is characterized by nausea, abdominal pressure, vomiting, and vague abdominal pain; cast syndrome probably results from hyperextension of the spine. This hyperextension accentuates lumbar lordosis, with compression of a portion of the duodenum between the superior mesenteric artery and the aorta and vertebral column posteriorly. The therapist encountering anyone in a body jacket, localizer cast, or high hip spica cast must be aware of this condition, because it can develop as late as several weeks to months after application of the cast. Medical treatment is necessary for this condition.

The incidence of other postsurgical complications is low but may include infection at the surgical site, dislodgment or fracture of instrumentation, failure of fusion, and urinary tract infection, among other common postoperative complications. Osteophytes and foraminal narrowing in the concavity of the lumbar curvature may develop in older clients, causing nerve root impingement and radicular pain. Recovery in the adult may take 6 to 12 months, with improvement continuing for up to 2 years.[32]

### Precautions

Precautions after spinal fusion depend on the type of fusion, segmental stabilization versus Harrington rod, and physician preference. Segmental stabilization provides some advantages over the traditional Harrington rod, including the ability to get out of bed on the first or second day after surgery and go home from the hospital a few days after surgery. The more rigid segmental stabilization may make osteoporosis more likely to occur; however, the rate of pseudarthrosis is lower.[161]

Segmental instrumentation provides a better correction of the scoliosis, and postoperative casting or bracing often is not required. Precautions generally include avoiding excessive bending, trunk rotation, or hyperextension. Lifting limitations are often imposed, depending on type of fusion. These precautions are to help prevent breaking or dislodging of the hardware while promoting bony union in the corrected position.

Functional mobility is severely limited for the first 4 weeks after surgery. After 3 months any type of noncontact sport is acceptable, including aerobic exercise such as walking or stationary bicycling; swimming especially is encouraged and can be started once the incision is healed after some types of fusions; however, diving is contraindicated. Vigorous activities and contact sports usually are avoided unless the client is directed otherwise by the physician. Restrictions can vary from one physician to another and with various types of fixation devices.

Skin care and prevention of breakdown are essential for anyone wearing a cast or spinal orthosis or brace. The client should be taught good skin care and how to recognize signs of irritation that can lead to lesions. For individuals with neuromuscular scoliosis who are not ambulatory, it is important to be aware of the degree of residual pelvic obliquity and accommodate this in wheelchair seating systems while monitoring skin tolerance.

## KYPHOSCOLIOSIS

### Overview and Etiologic Factors

Scheuermann disease (juvenile kyphosis, vertebral epiphysitis) is a structural deformity classically characterized by anterior wedging of 5 degrees or more of three adjacent thoracic bodies, affecting adolescents between the ages of 12 and 16 years. Scheuermann disease is the most common cause of structural kyphosis in adolescence with an incidence of between 4% and 8%.[362] The mode of inheritance is likely autosomal dominant, but the etiologic factors and pathogenesis of this excessive kyphosis remain unknown.

Scheuermann originally proposed that a vascular disturbance of the vertebral epiphyses during periods of rapid growth was the underlying cause; however, this has not been subsequently supported. Scheuermann disease also has been associated with increased levels of growth hormone, and individuals with this disease are frequently taller than average.

In the aging population, kyphoscoliosis (adult round back) is more likely to develop as a result of poor posture, degeneration of the intervertebral disks, vertebral compression fractures or osteoporotic collapse of the vertebrae. In addition, endocrine disorders (e.g., hyperparathyroidism, Cushing disease), arthritis, Paget disease, metastatic tumor, or tuberculosis can also result in kyphosis.

## Clinical Manifestations

Adolescent kyphosis is usually asymptomatic despite the prominent vertebral spinous processes. Some adolescents experience mild pain at the apex of the curvature in addition to fatigue, and tenderness or stiffness in the involved area or along the entire spine. The pectoral, hamstring, and hip flexor muscles are often tight, producing a crouched posture with anterior pelvic tilt and lumbar lordosis. Signs and symptoms associated with adult kyphosis are similar to those of the adolescent form, but rarely produce local tenderness, unless caused by vertebral compression fractures.

In both adolescent kyphoscoliosis (Scheuermann disease) and adult kyphosis, the vertebrae are wedged anteriorly and disk lesions called Schmorl nodes develop. Schmorl nodes are localized extrusions of the nucleus propulsus material through the cartilaginous plates and into the spongy bone of the vertebral bodies. The cancellous bone reacts by encapsulating the herniated tissue within a wall of fibrous tissue and bone, producing the Schmorl node.

### MEDICAL MANAGEMENT

DIAGNOSIS. Adolescents may be referred for medical evaluation as a result of school screening, or they may present because of concerns over posture and appearance. Adults more commonly present because of increased pain. Diagnosis is based on clinical examination and confirmed by radiographic findings, including Schmorl nodes, endplate narrowing, and irregular endplates.

TREATMENT. Indications for treatment remain controversial, because the true natural history of this disease has not been clearly defined. Presently, the choice of treatment in Scheuermann kyphosis is based on the severity and progression of the curve, the age of the individual, and the symptomatology present.

Bracing appears to be very effective if the diagnosis is made early in adolescents who have not reached skeletal maturity and have curves of less than 50 to 65 degrees, where a correction of more than 15 degrees can be achieved in the brace.[198,362] Surgical management is warranted in those with more severe curves and in adults who continue to show progression of the curve or who have progressive neurologic symptoms or unmanageable pain.

SPECIAL IMPLICATIONS FOR THE THERAPIST 23.3

*Kyphoscoliosis*

Scheuermann kyphosis usually responds to physical therapy intervention combined with antiinflammatory medications and behavioral modifications.[359] Exercises (e.g., postural exercises, hamstring stretching, and core stability exercises) are helpful to maintain flexibility and improve strength in the thoracic musculature.

Precautions and implications for postoperative care are discussed in the previous section (see "Special Implications for the Therapist 23.2: Scoliosis"). Physical load capacity after extensive surgical correction and spinal fusion for Scheuermann kyphosis is unknown; an individualized decision must be made in each case.

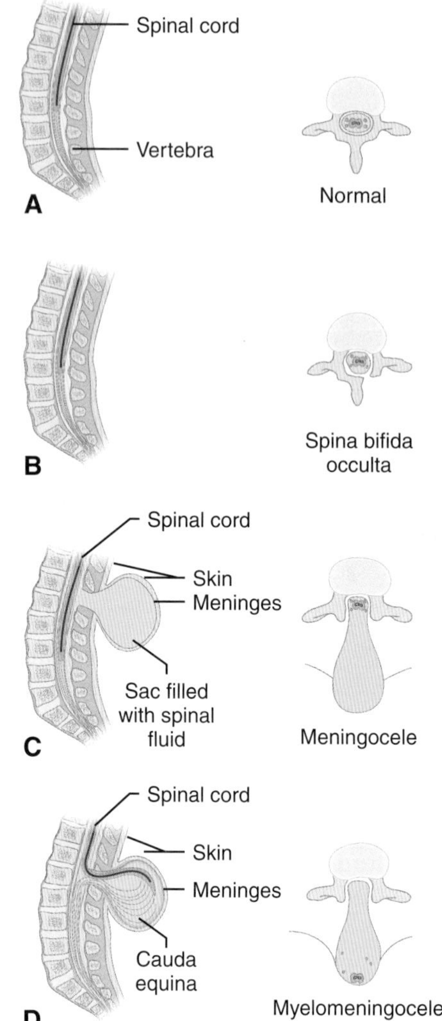


**Figure 23.3**

**Various degrees of spina bifida.** (A) Normal anatomic structure. (B) Spina bifida occulta results in only a bony defect, with the spinal cord, meninges, and spinal fluid intact. (C) Meningocele involves the bifid vertebra, with only a cerebrospinal fluid (CSF)–filled sac protruding; the spinal cord or cauda equina (depending on the level of the lesion) remains intact. (D) Myelomeningocele is the most severe form because the spine is open and the protruding sac contains CSF, the meninges, and the spinal cord or cauda equina.

# SPINA BIFIDA OCCULTA, MENINGOCELE, MYELOMENINGOCELE

## Definition

Congenital neural tube defects (NTDs) encompass a variety of abnormalities. The term *spina bifida* is the one most often used to describe the more common congenital defects of neural tube closure. Normally, the spinal cord and cauda equina are encased in a protective sheath of bone and meninges (Fig. 23.3). Failure of neural tube closure during development produces defects that may involve the entire length of the neural tube or may be restricted to a small area.

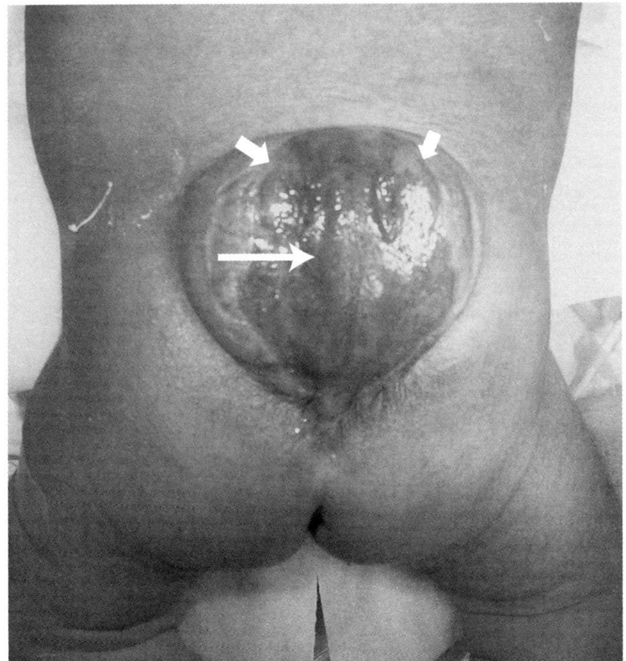

**Figure 23.4**

**Myelomeningocele in a newborn.** The neural placode is visible at the surface (*long arrow*) in this lumbosacral myelomeningocele. A placode is an area of thickening in the embryonic epithelial layer where the spinal cord develops later. Abnormal epithelium lines the edges of the cerebrospinal fluid–filled cyst (*short arrows*). (From Burg FD, Ingelfinger JR, Polin RA, et al: *Current pediatric therapy*, ed 18, Philadelphia, 2006, WB Saunders.)

The three most common NTDs—spina bifida occulta (incomplete fusion of the posterior vertebral arch), meningocele (external protrusion of the meninges), and myelomeningocele (protrusion of the meninges and spinal cord)—are presented here. Generally, these defects occur in the lumbosacral area but also may be found in the sacral, thoracic, and cervical areas (Fig. 23.4).

## Incidence and Etiologic Factors

The incidence of NTDs varies by ethnic background, geographic area, and socioeconomic status, with variable prevalence data depending upon the inclusion of anencephaly and encephalocele in the category of NTDs.[153] NTDs are estimated to occur in 1 in 1000 pregnancies[9,240] and are estimated at 3.4 per 10,000 livebirths.[30,262] Regional variations are significant, but the approximate ratio of males to females is 1:1.[9]

The overall incidence of spina bifida appears to be declining.[183,397] Termination of pregnancies as a result of the wider availability of maternal serum screening in addition to better nutrition and prenatal vitamins containing folic acid have contributed to this decline. Folic acid, also known as vitamin $B_9$, is found chiefly in green leafy vegetables, legumes, egg yolks, baker's yeast, and bread products, which are now fortified with folic acid. Multivitamins containing folic acid taken when planning a pregnancy and during at least the first 6 weeks of pregnancy prevent 50% to 70% of NTDs.[50,242] Women must be cautioned that half of all pregnancies are not planned and that folic acid must be taken before conception to be effective. While a proportion of NTDs occur despite folic acid supplementation,[246,142] taking supplements containing folic acid is the safest and most effective way of preventing NTDs.[237]

Evidence supports the hypothesis that the etiology of NTDs is multifactorial and related to the interaction of a genetic predisposition, teratogenic exposure (i.e., substances or agents that can interfere with normal embryonic development), and an essential folic acid deficiency or folic acid metabolic disorder. Genetic factors are considered important in the pathogenesis of spina bifida. Couples who have had one child with spina bifida have a recurrence rate of 3% to 8%.[195] Several individual genes have been identified in the folate–homocysteine metabolism pathway and have been linked to elevated risk.[239] There is interest in developing genetic risk profiles based on alterations in different metabolic pathways that have been proposed as underlying factors in the alteration of risk in different groups with similar ethnic backgrounds. In the Hispanic population, it has been proposed that alterations in the groups of genes that govern various steps in purine biosynthesis may be at the root of an elevation of basal risk level, while in the non-Hispanic white population genes that govern homocysteine metabolism may underlie alterations in risk.[217] Increased rates of spina bifida are found in individuals with trisomies 13 and 18 and in the case of triploid (having three times the number of normal chromosomes in the cell nucleus),[76] and in chromosome 13q deletion syndrome.[197,323]

Teratogenic exposure and epigenetic influences also are associated with an increased incidence of NTDs. Exposure to vitamin A, valproic acid, solvents, lead, herbicides, glycol ether, clomiphene, carbamazepine, aminopterin, and alcohol is linked to increased rates of NTDs. A number of occupations have also been linked to NTDs, presumably because of teratogenic exposure. Finally, insulin-dependent diabetes is associated with increased risk of NTDs in addition to maternal obesity, weight gain, and elevation of glycemic index in nondiabetic women.[130,300]

## Pathogenesis

Normally, about 20 days after conception, the embryo develops a neural groove in the dorsal ectoderm. The neural groove deepens as the two edges fuse to form the neural tube. By about day 23 this tube is completely closed except for an opening at each end. The upper end closes on day 25 and continues to fold and develop, forming the brain, whereas the bottom end closes on day 27 and forms the spinal cord.

The neural groove is formed by both cell proliferation and the production of a hyaluronic acid extracellular matrix. The first opportunity for failure of vertebral architecture to develop and close normally is through abnormalities in the hyaluronic acid matrix or the actin microfilaments that support elevation of the neural crest. A second opportunity for failed closure is slightly later in development, when an abnormal overgrowth at the caudal end may develop, causing closure to fail. Just before closure of the neural tube surface glycoproteins are produced by the ectoderm and act as the glue that holds the

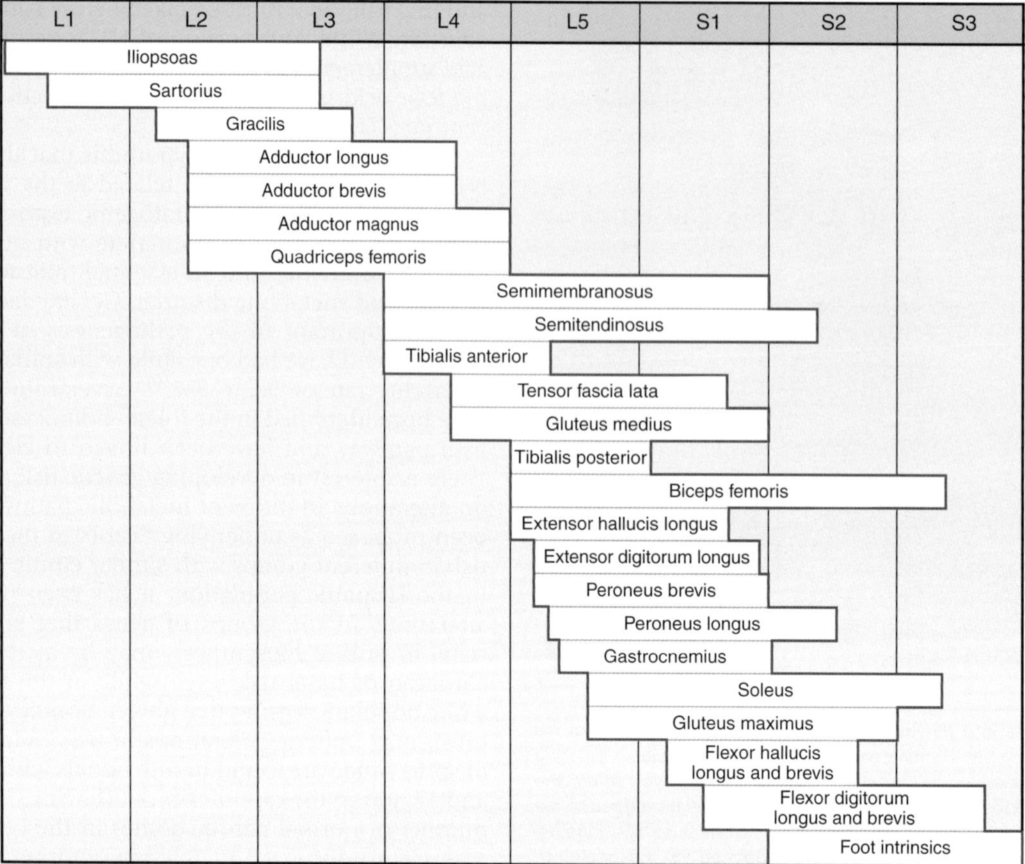


**Figure 23.5**

**Normal lumbar and sacral segmental innervation.** For the child with myelomeningocele, once the level of the lesion has been identified, the therapist can begin to assess muscle involvement above and below that level. (From Sharrard WJ: The segmental innervation of the lower limb muscles in man, *Ann R Coll Surg Engl* 35:106-122, 1964.)

cells together. A third opportunity for failed closure is abnormal production of these glycoproteins, leading to failure of the neural tube to close. A final possible genesis of myelomeningocele is the rupture of the neural tube after its closure as a result of cerebral spinal fluid (CSF) pressure. In this case development of Chiari II malformation occurs, in which the cerebellar tonsils develop below the foramen magnum or are forced through the foramen magnum because of pressure leading to increased CSF pressure and forcing the neural tube open. The defect in myelomeningocele can be identified by the eighth week of gestation and is complete by the 12th week.[14]

Some animal models support the presence of a defect in homocysteine metabolism in the pathogenesis of NTD, which correlates with an increased risk of NTD in some populations.[214] Plasma homocysteine levels and folic acid levels show an inverse relationship, and current research is focusing on the metabolism of folic acid and its genetic determinants,[242] in addition to the importance of these genetic defects in spina bifida. It appears that the genetics of NTDs are multifactorial.

## Clinical Manifestations

NTDs are typically divided into two groups: occulta (hidden) and aperta (visible). Approximately 75% of vertebral defects are located in the lumbosacral region, most commonly at the L5 to S1 level. Motor dysfunction depends on the level of involvement and sparing of sensory and motor innervation (Fig. 23.5 and Table 23.3).

The loss of motor function is not evenly distributed over the limbs and spine, resulting in muscle imbalance contributing to the development of scoliosis and various musculoskeletal deformities and contractures that are related to the specific denervated muscles and the resulting imbalance across the joint. Table 23.4 lists the clinical features and other associated characteristics of NTD.

### Spina Bifida Occulta

Spina bifida occulta does not protrude visibly but is often accompanied by a depression or dimple in the skin, a tuft of dark hair, soft fatty deposits (subcutaneous lipomas or dermoid cyst), port-wine nevi, or a combination of these abnormalities on the skin at the level of the underlying lesion. Spina bifida occulta usually does not cause neurologic dysfunction, but occasionally bowel and bladder disturbances or foot weakness occurs.

### Spina Bifida Aperta

In spina bifida aperta (meningocele and myelomeningocele), a sac-like cyst protrudes outside the spine. Like spina bifida occulta, a meningocele rarely causes

**Table 23.3** Myelomeningocele: Functional Mobility

| Motor Level Spinal Cord Segment | Critical Motor Function Present | Bracing/External Support For Ambulation | Typical Functional Activity |
|---|---|---|---|
| ≤T10<br>T12 | No LE movement<br>Strong trunk<br>No LE movement | Standing brace or equipment<br>HKAFOs<br>Sometimes with thoracic corset | Supported sitting[a]<br>Sliding board transfers<br>Good sitting balance[a]<br>Therapeutic ambulation<br>Independent wheelchair mobility |
| L1-L2 | Unopposed hip flexion, some adduction | Standing brace or equipment<br>HKAPOs, KAFOs, or RGOs<br>Crutches once ambulating with walker | Household ambulation[a]<br>May community ambulate if motivated |
| L3-L4 | Quadriceps[b]<br>Medial hamstrings<br>Anterior tibialis | KAFOs<br>Crutches<br>Floor reaction<br>AFOs/twister cables | Household and short community ambulation[a]<br>Wheelchair for long distances |
| L5 | Weak toe activity | KAFOs<br>Crutches (yes and no)<br>Floor reaction<br>AFOs (yes and no) | Household and short community ambulation[a]<br>Community ambulation[c] |
| S1 | Lateral hamstring<br>Peroneals | Usually no AFOs or upper limb support | Community ambulation |
| S2-S3 | Mild intrinsic foot weakness | Possible crutch or cane with increased age | Community ambulation |

*AFO*, Ankle-foot orthosis; *HKAFO*, hip-knee-ankle-foot orthosis; *KAFO*, knee-ankle-foot orthosis; *LE*, lower extremity; *RGO*, reciprocating gait orthosis.
[a]Do not usually walk as adults.
[b]Approximately 50% probability of long-distance ambulation with muscle grades 4/5.
[c]Able to use ambulation as the primary means of locomotion outside the home.

**Table 23.4** Myelomeningocele: Clinical Features and Associated Characteristics

| Clinical Features | Associated Characteristics |
|---|---|
| Hydrocephalus | 90% have intelligence within the normal range (IQ >80)<br>Increased incidence of learning disabilities<br>10%-30% risk of seizures<br>Increased cerebrospinal fluid pressure |
| Arnold-Chiari malformation | Weakness, pain, sensory changes, vertigo, ataxia, diplopia |
| Bowel and bladder incontinence | Small spastic bladder: reflux<br>Large flaccid bladder: residual urine, infection |
| Sensory impairment below the lesion | Lack of response to pain and touch<br>Trophic ulcers of the sacrum and/or lower limbs |
| Flaccid paralysis below the lesion | 0-2 years: truncal hypotonia<br>Delayed automatic reactions<br>Vasomotor insufficiency<br>Obesity |
| Absence of deep tendon reflexes | |
| Clubfoot (talipes equinovarus) | Altered biomechanics |
| Hip subluxation/dislocation | 30% demonstrate decreased ambulation status by age 12 years |
| Scoliosis | Late childhood and early adolescence: kyphoscoliosis |

neurologic deficits, whereas myelomeningocele is associated with permanent neurologic impairment the severity of which is correlated with the level of involvement.

**Myelomeningocele.** Myelomeningocele is typically accompanied by flaccid or, less often, spastic paralysis, as well as various combinations of bowel and bladder incontinence, musculoskeletal deformities (e.g., scoliosis, hip dysplasia, hip dislocation, clubfoot [talipes equinovarus], hip and knee contractures), hydrocephalus, and sometimes intellectual developmental disorder. During the first 2 years of life, children with myelomeningocele often present with various degrees of truncal hypotonia and delayed automatic postural reactions. With prenatal (fetal) repair (intrauterine corrective surgery) there is some amelioration of the motor phenotype and improvement in ambulatory ability, which can be detected by the age of 2.5 years. There are also risks associated with prenatal repair, including inducement of premature labor and uterine rupture.

Between 83% and 90% of children born with this condition have an associated hydrocephalus if closure is completed after birth (Box 23.1). Between 40% and 54% of those who have an in utero closure of the myelomeningocele have hydrocephalus.[2,35] Hydrocephalus accompanying myelomeningocele usually occurs in the presence of a type I or type II Arnold-Chiari malformation; that is, the cerebellar tonsils are displaced through the foramen magnum (Fig. 23.6), resulting in obstruction of CSF flow and increased CSF pressure and hydrocephalus.

Generally speaking, most children with myelomeningocele have some degree of type II Arnold-Chiari

Box 23.1

**SIGNS AND SYMPTOMS OF HYDROCEPHALUS**

- Full, bulging, tense soft spot (fontanel) on top of the child's head
- Large, prominent veins in the scalp
- Setting sun sign (child appears to only look downward; the whites of the eyes are obvious above the colored portion of the eyes)
- Behavioral changes (e.g., irritability, lethargy)
- High-pitched cry
- Seizures
- Vomiting or change in appetite

malformation, regardless of the presence of hydrocephalus. This picture has been altered by the advent of fetal repair. The Arnold-Chiari malformation may be reversed after repair, and lower rates of hydrocephalus are noted after fetal closure.[3,36,239,365] Even though an Arnold-Chiari malformation may be present radiographically, it may not be symptomatic.

Tethered cord syndrome is also a common comorbidity following surgical closure of the primary lesion and can occur at any time during growth. As the child grows, the spinal cord can become tethered or bound down, which may result in progressive neurologic compromise. The presenting features are consistent with neurologic compromise and include incontinence, progressive weakness, and back pain. Tethered cord syndrome occurs in 3% to 5% of children with spina bifida.[159]

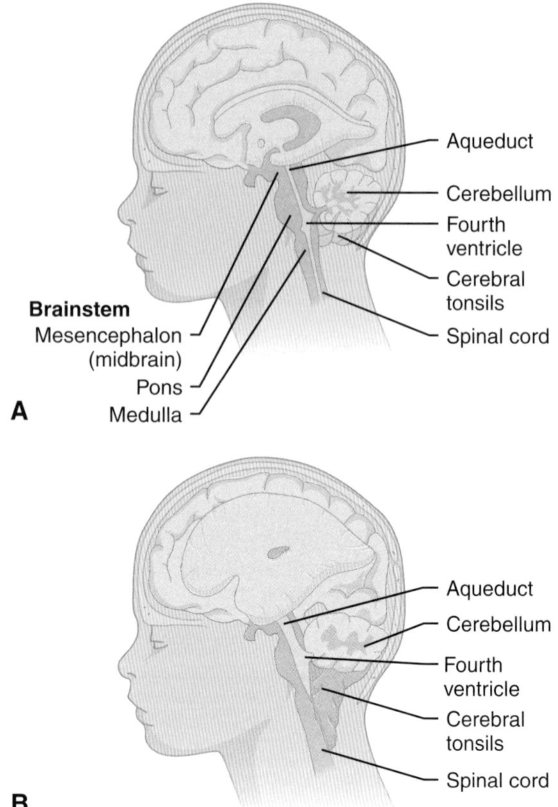


**Figure 23.6**

**Arnold-Chiari malformation.** (A) Normal brain with patent cerebrospinal fluid (CSF) circulation. (B) Arnold-Chiari type II malformation with enlarged ventricles, which predisposes a child with myelomeningocele to hydrocephalus. The brainstem, fourth ventricle, part of the cerebellum, and the cerebral tonsils are displaced downward through the foramen magnum, leading to blockage of CSF flow. Additionally, pressure on the brainstem housing the cranial nerves may result in nerve palsies.

## Syringomyelia

Syringomyelia, a cavity or syrinx, present within the spinal cord or medulla also can be present. This can progress, with increased pressure impinging on the surrounding tissue. Severe Arnold-Chiari malformations and syrinxes are rare, but can lead to potentially fatal consequences. Because of the location of the respiratory centers of the brainstem, central apnea can be serious, can necessitate the use of mechanical ventilation, and can potentially result in death. Sleep problems, including hypersomnolence, sleep fragmentation, choking, snoring, and morning headaches, are all potential clinical findings.[29] Cranial nerve involvement with resulting feeding difficulties, choking, pooling of secretions, aspiration, and stridor is also a common finding. Vertigo, ataxia, or spasticity, as well as pain, progressive weakness, or diplopia, can also be presenting findings in the older child.

## Integumentary

Sensory disturbances usually parallel motor dysfunction. Pressure ulcers at the sacrum, ischial tuberosities, knees, and the dorsum of the feet can be a significant comorbidity, resulting in increased medical costs associated with hospitalization.[79] Box 23.2 lists the factors that contribute to pressure ulcers in this population. Many of these same risk factors are present in other conditions prone to pressure ulcers. As may be expected, individuals with greater motor impairment and sensory loss are at greater risk for skin breakdown, with up to 30.7% of patients with thoracic-level lesions having pressure ulcers.[346]

Box 23.2

**FACTORS CONTRIBUTING TO PRESSURE ULCERS IN MYELOMENINGOCELE**

- Ammonia from urine burns
- Friction burns (feet and knees of young active children)
- Pressure from casts or splints
- Bony prominences
- Vascular problems
- Poor transfer skills
- Obesity
- Asymmetric weight bearing or posture (scoliosis, orthopedic deformities)

## Urologic

Bladder (and bowel) problems are present in virtually all children with myelomeningocele because these functions are controlled at the S2 to S4 levels. Even children with sacral lesions and normal leg movement often have bowel and bladder problems.

Problems with urinary incontinence and infection can occur if the bladder is small and spastic (bladder holds little urine) or large and hypotonic (incomplete emptying of the bladder and ureteral reflux). Bladder dyssynergy occurs with either a flaccid or spastic sphincter. Normally, when the bladder contracts, the sphincter relaxes, allowing urine to flow. In a dyssynergistic state, the bladder and sphincter contract together, predisposing the child to urethral reflux. Bowel and bladder incontinence is an ongoing concern for adults with spina bifida, as is the risk of kidney dysfunction from urinary retention.[352]

## MEDICAL MANAGEMENT

**DIAGNOSIS.** Frequently, NTDs are detected prenatally with ultrasonic scanning and serum AFP testing. Elevated AFP usually occurs by 14 weeks' gestation in the presence of NTDs. This type of screening will not detect skin-covered (closed) neural defects such as spina bifida occulta. The potential for false-positive results with this test may result in unnecessary intervention.

Additionally, as the incidence of this condition continues to decrease, the test becomes less reliable because the positive predictive value of the AFP test is dependent on the prevalence of the disease in a population. The less prevalent the disease, the less accurate laboratory results may be.

Amniocentesis can detect only open NTDs and is recommended for pregnant women who have previously had children with NTDs or in the case of a large lesion noted with ultrasonic scanning. The need for more accurate, noninvasive imaging of the CNS is recognized, and fetal MRI is an effective, noninvasive means of assessing fetal CNS anatomy with superior ability to resolve posterior fossa anatomy over ultrasonography. However, to date fetal MRI has not surpassed ultrasonography in evaluating hydrocephalus and the level and nature of the spinal lesion.[41,212]

Postnatally, meningocele and myelomeningocele are obvious on examination. Transillumination of the protruding sac usually can distinguish between these two conditions. In meningocele, the sac with its CSF contents is transilluminated (light shines through the sac); in myelomeningocele, the light does not shine through the neural bundle that is present. Spinal films can be used to detect bony defects, and the computerized tomographic scan or MRI demonstrates the presence of hydrocephalus. Other laboratory tests may include urinalysis, urine cultures, and tests for renal function.

**Treatment.** Timing of the closure is important. Prenatal diagnosis has made planned cesarean sections, fetal repair,[17] and therapeutic abortion possible. A cesarean section is the preferred method of birth to avoid trauma to the neural sac that occurs during vaginal delivery. Prenatal closure is now available by fetal surgery and has been found to decrease the incidence of shunt-dependent hydrocephalus and Arnold-Chiari malformation from above 90% in each case to 59% and 38%, respectively.[36,365] By interrupting the flow of CSF during gestation, intrauterine repair enables the cerebellum and brainstem to resume a normal (or nearly normal) configuration.

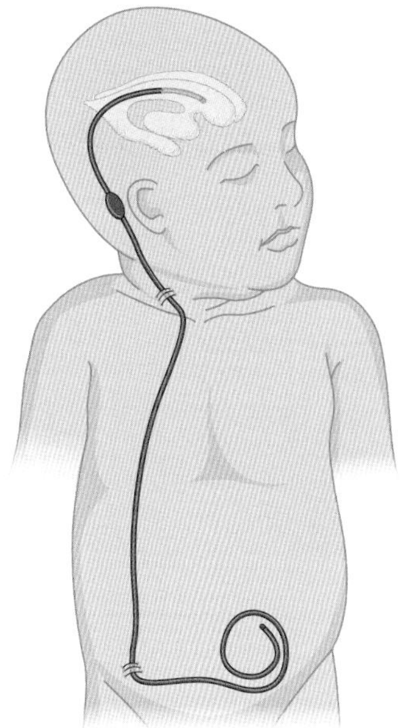

**Figure 23.7**

**Ventriculoperitoneal shunt.** This shunt provides primary drainage of cerebrospinal fluid from the ventricles to an extracranial compartment (usually either the heart [ventriculoatrial] or the abdominal or peritoneal [ventriculoperitoneal] cavity, as shown here). Extra tubing is left in the extracranial site to uncoil as the child grows. A unidirectional valve designed to open at a predetermined intraventricular pressure and close when the pressure falls below that level prevents backflow of fluid.

Prospective parents should be cautioned not to expect improvement in leg function as a result of this surgery. The potential benefits of surgery must be weighed carefully against the potential risks of preterm labor and delivery, potential infection, and blood loss.[364] If postnatal closure is chosen, infection and drying of the nerve roots can lead to further loss of function and necessitates surgical closure within 48 hours of birth. Ventriculoperitoneal shunting (Figs. 23.7 and 23.8) is recommended in the presence of hydrocephalus; shunt revision is often required as the child grows or if the shunt becomes obstructed, infected, or separated. Hydrocephalus in children with myelomeningocele is most commonly addressed by ventriculoperitoneal shunting (77% of[352] individuals with myelomeningocele in the national patient registry) with a smaller proportion being candidates for endoscopic third ventriculostomy.[70]

A variety of orthopedic surgical interventions may be required throughout the child's growing years. Surgical correction for hip dislocation rarely is indicated, except in the case of ambulatory clients with unilateral dislocation.[107,109] Investigation shows that a level pelvis and good range of motion of the hips are more important for ambulation than is reduction of bilateral hip dislocation.[139]

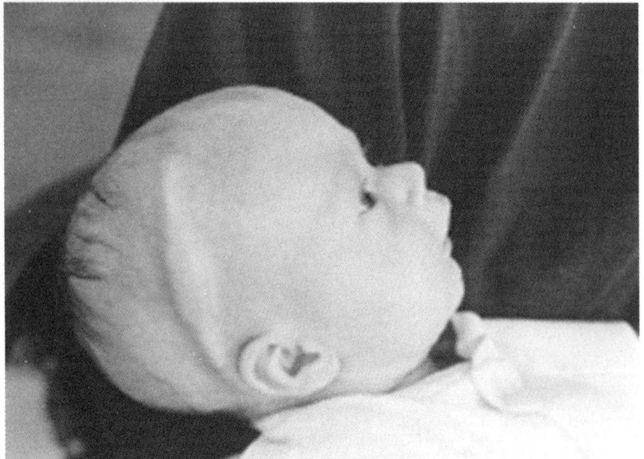

**Figure 23.8**

**Placement of the shunt.** The shunt is placed very superficially, necessitating caution when handling the infant. The therapist must be careful to avoid placing pressure over the shunt, stretching the neck, or placing the child in the head-down position. Parents may be distressed initially by the cosmetic appearance of the shunt, but as the child grows, and with hair growth, the shunt is no longer visible. See Fig. 23.10 of this same child with no obvious signs of a shunt. (Courtesy Todd Goodrich, University of Montana, Missoula.)

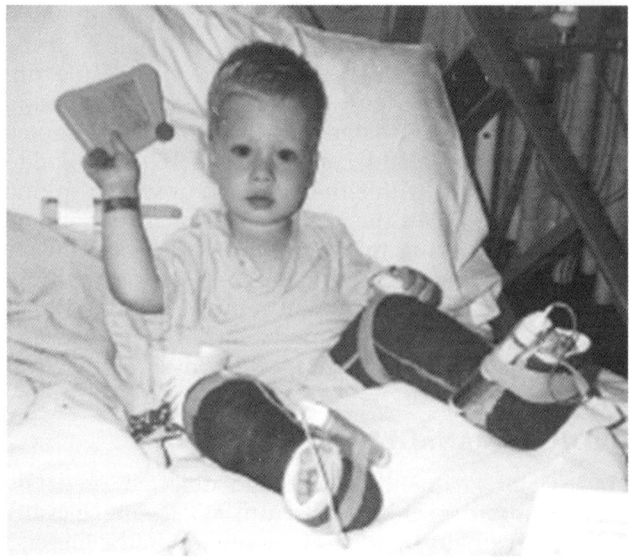

**Figure 23.10**

**Postoperative inpatient after orthopedic reconstructive surgery for congenital vertical talus deformity.** Drainage tubes directly from the incision sites were used for 12 hours. (Courtesy Zane and Dianna Kuhnhenn, Missoula, MT.)

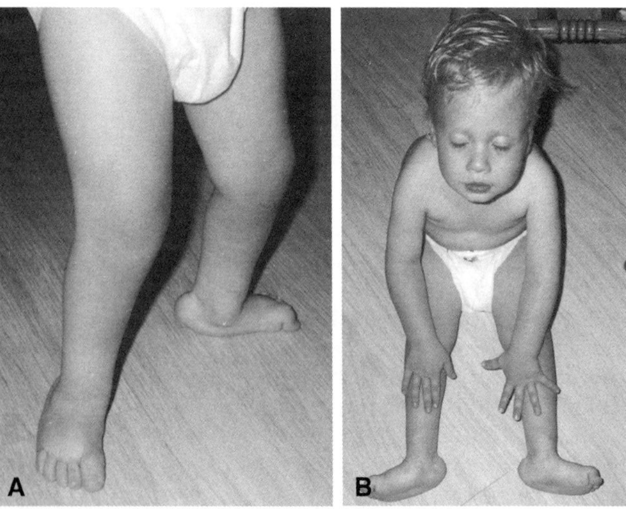


**Figure 23.9**

**Orthopedic involvement.** (A) Three-year-old boy with bilateral congenital vertical talus resulting in rocker-bottom foot deformities caused by an L4 to L5 myelomeningocele. Note the compensatory knee flexion and genu valgus along with developing toe flexion contractures (the latter from loss of motor control). (B) Rocker-bottom foot deformity seen more clearly in the non–weight-bearing position. (Courtesy Zane and Dianna Kuhnhenn, Missoula, MT.)

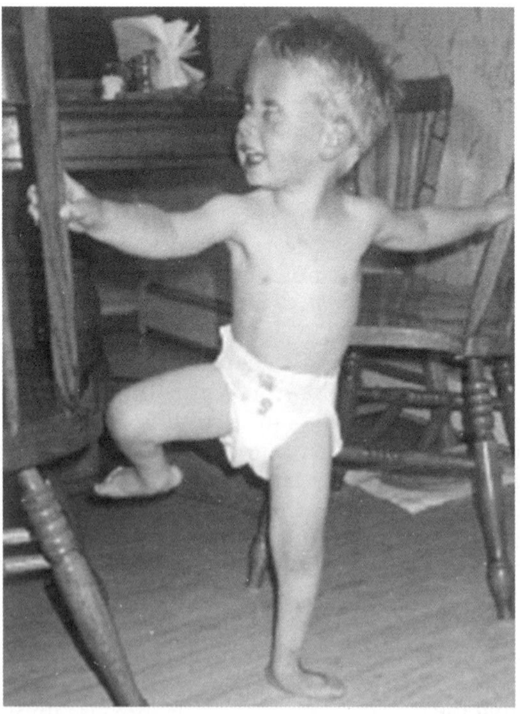

**Figure 23.11**

**Postoperative result.** Risk for skin breakdown is reduced around the great toe (no longer contracted into flexion), and base of support is improved for ambulation and allows the child to stand on one leg with support (note the more neutral alignment of lower extremity, especially the knee). The child wears ankle-foot orthoses to maintain proper alignment; there may be some regression of alignment in time because of the continued lack of motor control. (Courtesy Zane and Dianna Kuhnhenn, Missoula, MT.)

Spinal fusion for kyphotic deformity of the spine has had mixed results and frequent complications. Hip flexion and knee flexion contractures often are addressed with muscle releases, and foot deformity correction often is achieved with soft tissue procedures and in more-severe cases with bony procedures (Figs. 23.9 through 23.11).

Medical management of the bowel and bladder dysfunction is of critical importance from both a medical and social standpoint. The muscles of the bladder can show either spasticity or flaccidity, leading to either a condition where the bladder is small and under high pressure from urine or large and stretched out and under low pressure. However, during early childhood neurologic status is not always stable and can be volatile in the context of a tethered cord and subsequent release. As a result, urologic function should be monitored serially with urodynamic and upper tract evaluations.[249]

In children with spastic bladders under high pressure, vesicoureteral reflux and decreased bladder volume and compliance are critical factors. These factors together contribute to damage to the upper urinary tract and kidneys if not managed effectively.

Children with hypotonic bladders often have more residual urine and are more prone to infection. Infection is treated prophylactically in most children with spina bifida, with antibiotics and high fluid intake as a critical part of an overall management program. Kidney damage is unusual in children with hypotonic bladders because bladder urine is under low pressure and reflux is less of a problem.

Complete bladder emptying using clean intermittent catheterization provides a means to manage urine flow and avoid elevated pressures; in addition, the use of anticholinergic medication can also help avoid elevated pressures by increasing bladder capacity. Manual pressure on the bladder (the Credé method) is used less often because of its tendency to cause reflux. Implantation of an artificial urinary sphincter has been used in the older child or adolescent,[277] and bladder augmentation or urinary diversion are options for the child with high pressures and insufficient volume.

Artificial urinary sphincters can also be implanted to accomplish the opening and closing of the bladder outlet by use of a cuff placed around the outlet. The cuff can be constricted to close the outlet or relaxed to open the outlet and allow urine to flow; however, these devices come with a relatively high complication rate.[249] Intravesical electrical stimulation remains controversial; however, it has been employed at some centers, with the benefits of increased bladder compliance and increased bladder volume being the most common positive outcomes.[164] Renal function can lead to significant morbidity or mortality in this population and should be monitored regularly.[296]

Stool incontinence is managed most commonly by a program to regulate bowel movements using diet, timed enemas, or suppositories. In some centers, the Malone antegrade continence enema procedure is being used to aid in bowel control. This procedure places a cecostomy, bringing the cecum to the abdominal wall in a procedure similar to the placement of a percutaneous endoscopic gastrostomy tube. Antegrade enemas are then used to control bowel function.[75]

**PROGNOSIS.** Early, aggressive care of NTDs has now improved the overall prognosis associated with this condition. Prognosis varies with the degree of accompanying neurologic deficit. At present, prognosis is poorest for those children who have total paralysis below the lesion, kyphoscoliosis, hydrocephalus, and progressive loss of renal function secondary to chronic infection and reflux.

At present, survival to adulthood is approximately 85%; most deaths occur before age 4 years. Overall adjustment of the parents and siblings to having a family member with myelomeningocele can be stressful and should not be overlooked in terms of its impact of the affected individual or family as a whole. Often either depression or anxiety, in addition to impairments in social functioning, can be challenges that children with myelomeningocele face and should be addressed with psychologic support.[148]

Approximately two-thirds of children with myelomeningocele and shunted hydrocephalus have intelligence that falls in the normal range. The remaining one-third fall into the range for intellectual developmental disorder, usually mild. Irrespective of IQ, children with spina bifida often have difficulties in perceptual and organizational abilities, attention, speed of motor response, memory, and hand function, in addition to mental flexibility, efficiency of processing, conceptualization, and problem solving. Overall cognitive delays occur less often as a result of improved medical treatment for these children.

Adult outcome data are incomplete and evolving[296] as individuals cared for in different time periods age. Most adults older than 50 years of age survived the preshunt era of the 1950s and are without hydrocephalus, whereas adults now in their 30s include people with more severe disabilities who benefited from the advances in medical and surgical management.

Adults with myelomeningocele continue to need therapy and medical management secondary to joint and spinal deformities, joint pain, pressure ulcers, neurologic deterioration, depression, and poor social interaction and adjustment.

***Prognosis for Motor Function.*** The child's motor abilities vary according to the level of the lesion, but delay in achieving ambulation can be expected in all children with spina bifida, including those with low neurosegment-level lesions. Approximately 45% of individuals with myelomeningocele are community ambulators.[31]

A child's ability to walk outdoors and use a wheelchair by age 7 years usually suggests a good ambulation prognosis.[84] If functional ambulation is not present by 7 to 9 years of age, it is unlikely to occur subsequently.[11,97] A third of all people with myelomeningocele demonstrate a decline in ambulatory status with increasing age, usually around age 12 years. These losses in ambulatory status often correlate with a variety of adolescent changes, including increasing body size and composition, loss of upper- and lower extremity strength potentially related to preference for sedentary activities, or immobilization for varied periods of time secondary to musculoskeletal surgery or fracture healing. Adult ambulatory status in spina bifida is highly influenced by two variables, including motor level and sitting balance. Overall ambulation status declines over time.

SPECIAL IMPLICATIONS FOR THE THERAPIST 23.4

## *Spina Bifida Occulta, Meningocele, Myelomeningocele*

Throughout the life span of an individual with any of these conditions, the therapist participates actively in providing direct intervention, preventive care that can reduce complications and morbidity (and the associated costs of these), adaptive equipment, and client and family education. The therapist participates in both preoperative and postoperative care throughout the life of the individual. Functional rehabilitation provided by the therapist facilitates functional outcomes.

A helpful resource to the therapist and family with practical advice regarding the physical, emotional, and cognitive growth of the individual with spina bifida is available.[201] Areas for consideration beyond the scope of this text are also covered in this resource (e.g., legal issues, financial planning, vocational assessment).

### Neonatal Intensive Care Unit

Before surgery to repair the meningocele, pressure of any kind against the sac must be avoided. Whenever holding the (unrepaired) infant, the spine must be maintained in good alignment without tension in the area of the defect. The infant must be kept in the prone position to minimize tension on the sac and to reduce the risk of trauma.

The prone position allows for optimal positioning of the legs, especially in cases of associated hip dysplasia. The infant is placed flat with the hips slightly flexed to reduce tension on the defect. The legs are maintained in abduction with a pad (a folded diaper or towel) between the knees, and a small diaper roll is placed under the ankles to maintain a neutral foot position.

The prone position is maintained after operative closure, although many neurosurgeons allow a side-lying or partial side-lying position unless it aggravates a coexisting hip dysplasia (see "Developmental Dysplasia of the Hip" below) or permits undesirable hip flexion. The side-lying positioning offers an opportunity for position changes, which reduces the risk of pressure sores and facilitates feeding.

In all handling procedures, care must be taken to avoid pressure on the sac preoperatively or on the operative site postoperatively. If permitted, the infant can be held upright against the body. For the infant with hydrocephalus, until the shunt is in place and draining well, activities that position the head above the body tend to decrease intracranial pressure. Activities that position the head below the body increase intracranial pressure; as a result, care should be taken with handling. In the older child, positional headaches may be indicative of shunt malfunction.

In children who have undergone fetal repair of the NTD, physical therapists evaluate motor function and joint position in the neonate. Education on positioning, range-of-motion exercises, and developmental activities and referral to early intervention is important as part of this role.

### Skin Care

Areas of sensory and motor impairment are subject to skin breakdown and require close attention. The loss of skin sensation accompanied by lack of pain can lead to injury and pressure ulcers. Inadequate circulation increases the problem, because wounds do not heal properly.

Placing the infant on a soft foam or fleece pad reduces pressure on the knees and ankles. Periodic cleansing, application of lotion, and gentle massage can aid circulation, which often is compromised. Bath water must be tested prior to submerging the child to protect against burns because the child cannot feel the water temperature. The family should be advised to use sunscreen to prevent sunburn and to assure that shoes and braces fit appropriately, as these can also be a source of pressure resulting in skin breakdown. The skin should be checked daily for red areas that do not disappear readily when the pressure is removed.

### Early and Ongoing Intervention Precautions

Passive range-of-motion exercises must be performed slowly and cautiously given the tendency toward fracture in this population. When the hip joints are unstable, stretching into hip flexion or adduction may aggravate a tendency toward subluxation. For this reason, the prone hip extension test for measuring hip extension is the method of choice over the traditional Thomas test.[144] An early role of the therapist in assessment is to assist in establishing baseline information regarding the level of initially available muscle function and sensation. Information regarding strength assessment specific to this population is available.[144]

Ongoing assessment includes an awareness of signs and symptoms associated with changes resulting from increased CSF pressure in the presence of hydrocephalus with or without a shunt (Box 23.3). A shunting mechanism is used for hydrocephalus associated with a variety of conditions other than myelomeningocele. Depending on the underlying condition, shunts can become obstructed or stop functioning for many reasons (e.g., occlusion resulting from blood clots or brain fragments, tumor cell aggregates, bacterial colonization, or other debris; the tube itself can become kinked or blocked at the tip; or growth of the infant or child or physical activities can result in disconnection of the shunt components or withdrawal of a distal catheter from its intended drainage site). Shunt systems also may fail because of mechanical malfunction, including fracture of the catheters, leading to underdrainage or overdrainage.

Infants do not show typical signs of increased intracranial pressure, because skull suture lines are not fully closed. In this age group, a bulging fontanelle is the most obvious sign of pathology. Once the skull bones have fused and the anterior fontanelle is no longer palpable (9-16 months of age), pressure can build inside the closed space, resulting in a variety of symptoms, including headache, vomiting, and irritability.

Tethering of the spinal cord may develop with myelodysplasia. The cord becomes caught or tethered from scar tissue and is stretched as the vertebral canal continues to elongate (Box 23.4). Other causes of a tethered cord include meningomyelocele repair, obstructed CSF shunt, syringomyelia, benign tumor, and spinal cord hypoplasia (i.e., the cord is progressively shorter than the canal and pulled as a result).

Box 23.3

**SIGNS AND SYMPTOMS OF SHUNT MALFUNCTION**

- Congestion of scalp veins
- Firm or tense soft spot on cranium (fontanel)
- Listlessness, drowsiness, irritability
- Vomiting, change in appetite
- Marked depression of the anterior fontanel (overdrainage)
- Disturbance in urinary and bowel patterns
- Increasing head circumference
- Swelling along the shunt
- Seizures
- Nuchal (nape of the neck) rigidity
- Additional symptoms for older children and adults:
  - Gradual personality change
  - Headaches
  - Blurring vision
  - Memory loss
  - Progressive coordination problems
  - Declining school or work performance
  - Decrease in sensory or motor functions

Box 23.4

**SIGNS AND SYMPTOMS OF TETHERED CORD SYNDROME**

- Changes in bowel and bladder function
- Scoliosis
- Increased spasticity
- Increased asymmetric postures or movement
- Altered gait pattern
- Decreased upper extremity coordination
- Changes in muscle strength (at or below the lesion)
- Back pain

Likewise, children with spina bifida have been identified as having the greatest risk of becoming allergic to latex.[128] Typical symptoms include watery eyes, wheezing, hives, rash, swelling, and, in severe cases, anaphylaxis, a life-threatening reaction. These responses occur when items containing latex touch the skin, mucous membranes (mouth, genitals, bladder, or rectum), or open areas.

The therapist must avoid using toys, feeding utensils, or other items made of latex that the infant or child might put in the mouth. Parents must be advised to read all labels and avoid products, especially toys and utensils, containing latex. If latex content is not indicated, the manufacturer should be contacted for verification before purchase or use of the item.

### Controversies

The timing of the operative repair of the lesion remains under heavy debate. Some centers are repairing the defect before birth and are having good results. In most centers, children undergoing postnatal repair have early closure (within the first 24-48 hours after birth), and care is taken to prevent local infection, avoid trauma to the exposed tissues, and avoid stretching of other nerve roots, with the goal of preventing further motor impairment.[220]

A variety of surgical procedures can be used for skin closure. The goal is to place the sac and its contents back in the body with good skin coverage of the lesion and careful closure. Excision of the membranous covering or removal of any portion of the sac may damage functioning neural tissue and is avoided. Although this corrective procedure may prevent an infection of the spinal cord or brain, the goal of surgery is not an improvement in neurologic function.

Philosophic differences exist regarding the necessary characteristics of management programs for children with myelomeningocele. Children whose programs emphasize upright activities and ambulation show better outcomes in terms of bone density, lower extremity fracture risk, pressure ulcer risk, transfer skills (even after they have stopped ambulating) compared with children whose programs focus primarily on wheelchair mobility.[222,228] High-level lesions do not preclude ambulation; however, this may be a relatively energy-intensive activity as compared with wheeled mobility and may have a negative impact on some aspects of school performance. This needs to be balanced with the long-term benefits noted above related to an emphasis on ambulation in the early years.[105]

Controversy also exists regarding the best choice of lower extremity bracing and ambulation method. One area of contention involves the hip-knee-ankle-foot orthosis (HKAFO) for swing-through gait only versus the reciprocating gait orthosis (RGO), which allows the individual options of a swing-to, swing-through, or reciprocating gait. Precautions when considering HKAFO or RGO include severe spinal deformity, spasticity, decreased upper extremity strength, moderate obesity, knee flexion or plantar flexion contractures greater than 15 to 20 degrees, and hip flexion contracture greater than 35 degrees. The weight of the brace components may also impact clinical decision making.

Another area of bracing controversy is whether to brace high and provide a more normal- appearing pattern and protect against progressive orthopedic deformity or to brace low and allow more freedom of movement. Given the many improvements and number of bracing options available, the key to maintaining ambulatory status is good lower extremity range of motion and a level pelvis. The choice of bracing depends on a careful evaluation of the individual's range of motion, strength, and gait pattern.

## DEVELOPMENTAL DYSPLASIA OF THE HIP

### Overview

Developmental dysplasia of the hip (DDH), previously known as congenital hip dysplasia or dislocation, is a common hip disorder affecting infants and children. The change in name reflects the fact that DDH is a developmental process occurring dynamically in utero and during the first year of life; this condition is not necessarily present at birth as the word *congenital* implies.

DDH can be unilateral or bilateral and occurs in three forms of varying severity: (1) unstable hip dysplasia, in which the hip is positioned normally but can be dislocated by manipulation; (2) subluxation or incomplete dislocation, in which the femoral head remains in contact with the acetabulum but the head of the femur is partially displaced or uncovered; and (3) complete dislocation, in which the femoral head is totally outside the acetabulum.

## Incidence and Risk Factors

The incidence of DDH is between 8.6 and 11.5 per 1000 live births and 15% of infants have instability or immature structural hip development with many milder cases resolving without treatment.[190,327] Approximately 85% of affected infants are females. The risk of hip dysplasia increases dramatically in the presence of certain obstetric conditions (e.g., breech delivery, large neonate, twin or multiple births) and other conditions such as idiopathic scoliosis, myelomeningocele (spina bifida), arthrogryposis, and cerebral palsy. The presence of other musculoskeletal deformities such as torticollis,[376] metatarsus adductus, and calcaneal valgus deformity should alert the medical practitioner to the need for further evaluation. Other risk factors include family history, first pregnancies, multiple fetuses, and oligohydramnios (deficient volume of amniotic fluid limiting fetal movement). Certain ethnic groups (Eastern Europeans, Lapps, and Native Americans) also have an increased risk of DDH and certain genetic markers are also associated with increased risk.[401] One-fourth of all cases involve both hips; when only one hip is involved, the left hip is affected three times more often than the right.

## Etiologic Factors

The cause varies depending on the associated condition but is usually the result of mechanical, physiologic, or environmental factors. Hormonally derived (maternal hormone relaxin may affect the child in utero and during the neonatal period) or hereditary laxity of the ligaments about the joint and positioning are possible etiologic factors.

Infant positioning, both prenatally and postnatally, may affect the formation of the acetabular cup and hip stability because the acetabulum is formed as a result of contact with the femoral head, and this is thought to be one possible cause of DDH.[83]

Cultural customs of how babies are carried affect rates of DDH; those cultures that swaddle infants with the hips in extension and adduction are at greater risk of DDH. Conversely, carrying the infant or young child with hips and lower extremities abducted, flexed, and externally rotated may increase stability of the femoral head in relation to the acetabulum.

## Pathogenesis

DDH can affect the acetabulum, the femoral head, and the relationship of the femoral head to the acetabulum.

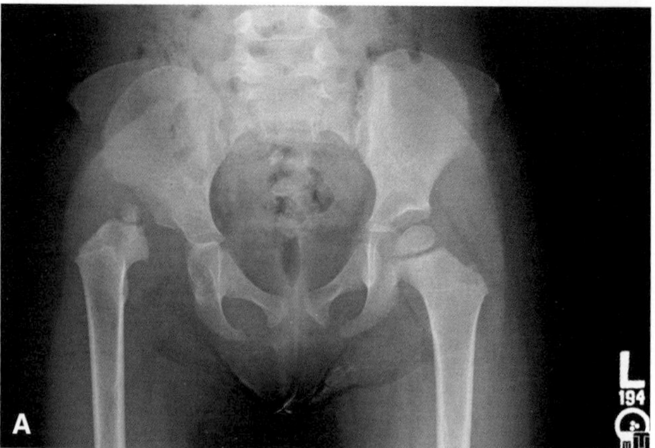


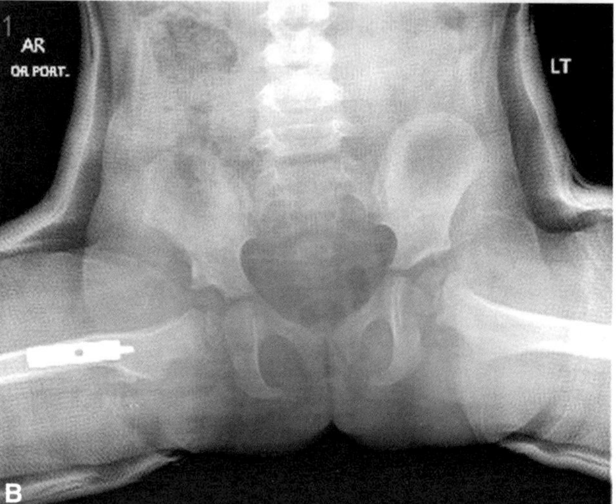


**Figure 23.12**

**Developmental dysplasia of the hip.** Three-year-old child with unilateral developmentally dysplastic hip. (A) Note the head of the femur sitting lateral to the acetabulum. The roof of the acetabulum appears dysplastic and the proximal femur somewhat valgus. (B) Postoperative: the femur has been relocated in the acetabulum and a varus derotation osteotomy performed. A wedge is cut from the femoral shaft, then internally rotated and positioned in varus to correct the femoral anteversion and valgus. It is also common when there is acetabular insufficiency for a portion of the iliac crest to be removed and used as a wedge above the acetabulum to deepen the acetabulum. (Courtesy Allan Glanzman, The Children's Hospital of Philadelphia, PA.)

The femur, acetabulum, and hip joint capsule usually are well developed by approximately 10 weeks' gestation but continue to enlarge throughout gestation and develop through contact between the femoral head and acetabulum. Most dislocations result in a progressive deformation of the femoral head and acetabulum during gestation.[83]

The subluxated hip maintains contact with the acetabulum but is not well seated within the hip joint. Often this occurs because the acetabulum is shallow, with the roof of the acetabulum sloping at an increased angle (acetabular index) in hips with DDH, rather than showing a normal cup shape. The dislocated hip has no contact between the femoral head and the acetabulum, the femoral head sits on the iliac wing and the ligamentum teres is elongated and taut (Fig. 23.12).

If the dislocation is not diagnosed and treated early, secondary changes in both soft tissues and bony

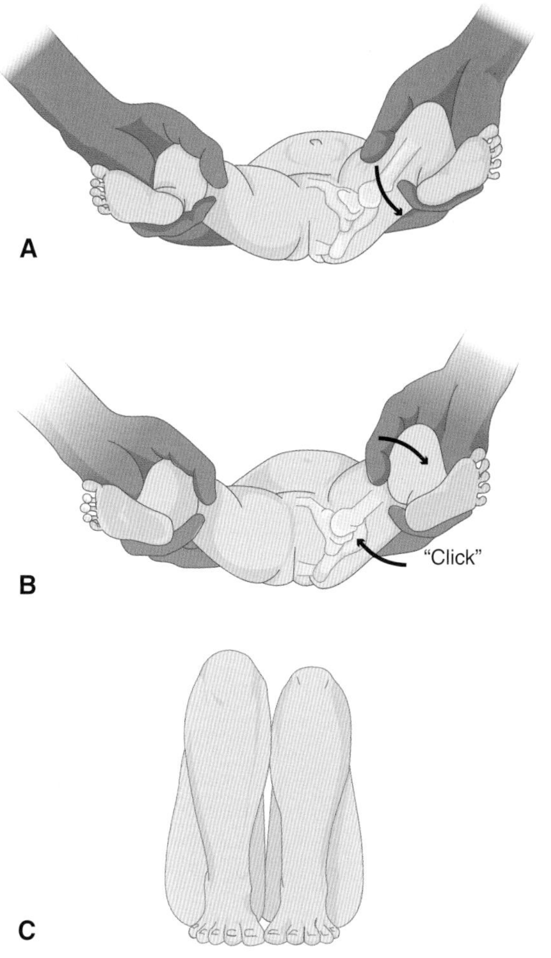


**Figure 23.13**

**Signs of hip dislocation.** (A) Ortolani maneuver No. 1 (also the second part of the Barlow test): hip flexion and adduction with downward pressure dislocates the hip. (B) Ortolani maneuver No. 2: gentle hip flexion, abduction, and slight traction reduce the hip with a discernible click or clunk, and increased hip abduction is possible in a positive test. This test is valid only for the first few weeks after birth. (C) Galeazzi test (the Allis sign): in the supine position, with hips and knees flexed and feet flat on the floor, the knee is lower on the dislocated side, indicating that the head of the femur is positioned posterior or superior to the rim of the acetabulum. This test is used to assess unilateral hip dislocation and can be used in older children (from 3 months on).

structures occur. The longer the dislocation has been present, the greater the secondary changes that occur. These changes include stretching of the hip capsule, contracture and shortening of the structures of the hip joint, changes in the blood supply to the hip, flattening of the femoral head, and acetabular dysplasia, sometimes with development of a false acetabulum while reduction allows for remodeling of the acetabulum and improved hip stability.[5]

## Clinical Manifestations

Clinical manifestations of DDH vary with age. In the newborn and nonambulatory period up to 12 months of age, one or more positive signs may be present; Ortolani or Barlow signs, or in asymmetric cases a positive Galeazzie

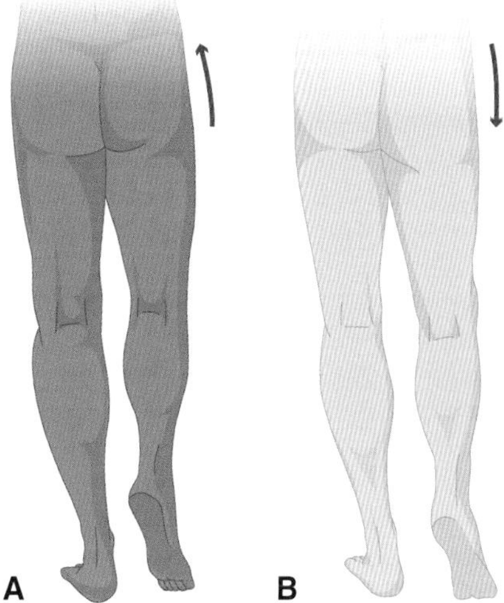


**Figure 23.14**

Trendelenburg sign.(A) Negative: with the weight on one leg, the pelvis on the opposite side is slightly elevated (observed from behind the client). (B) Positive: with weight on one leg, the pelvis drops on the opposite side because of muscle weakness or pain in the hip joint on the stance side. The Trendelenburg sign measures weakness of the hip abductor muscles, especially the gluteus medius.

sign (Fig. 23.13). Any observed physical asymmetries in range of motion (even as little as 10 degrees is considered significant, especially as a limitation of hip abduction), asymmetry in the buttock or gluteal fold (higher on the affected side), extra thigh skin folds, or leg length discrepancy requires medical evaluation.

In the ambulating child, uncorrected bilateral dysplasia may cause a characteristic gait pattern known as a compensated Trendelenburg gait. As the child leans the torso to the side on weight bearing to compensate for an ineffective gluteus medius, the child assumes a waddling gait pattern.

Unilateral dysplasia usually is characterized by a limp with a positive Trendelenburg sign during the stance phase of gait on the involved side (Fig. 23.14). A flexion contracture on the involved side(s) develops as a result of posterior displacement of the hips, which then contributes to marked lumbar lordosis.

## MEDICAL MANAGEMENT

**DIAGNOSIS.** In the newborn period, clinical examination is the most important diagnostic tool and continues to be the standard screening tool. A positive Ortolani or Barlow click confirms DDH in the first month of life, with a specificity of greater than 99% but a sensitivity of only 60% (see Fig. 23.13).[325] These tests are considered significantly less diagnostic past 2 to 4 weeks.[122] As ligamentous structures become stronger or if the joints become stretched and worn, it is more difficult to elicit the characteristic popping in and out described. A positive Barlow on adduction is indicative of a hip that has pathologic instability and easily subluxes, while in the case of a positive Ortolani the hip is resting out of the socket and relocates on abduction.[394]

In some cases, dislocation is not diagnosed by these standard tests, and the disorder may not be apparent at birth. Because a normal neonatal examination cannot guarantee that a hip will not become dysplastic, serial examination throughout infancy is essential. Well-baby checkups should include hip examination until the child begins to walk with a normal gait pattern.

The Galeazzi sign becomes positive in the older infant in symmetric cases once shortening of the thigh becomes apparent. Radiographic examination is unreliable in the infant and is used more commonly in older infants and children. Plain radiographs are not able to image the hip adequately until the head is ossified and may not confirm the diagnosis if the unstable hip is in the reduced position at the time the film is taken.

For this reason, ultrasonography is suggested in cases of suspected but unconfirmed DDH. Ultrasonography by the Graf method allows visualization of the bony acetabular roof and rim and the cartilaginous roof of the acetabulum, with a score of 1 to 4 assigned. A dynamic assessment to assess stability of the hip involves a Barlow maneuver under ultrasound guidance and is graded as normal, subluxed, or dislocated.[325] It is especially accurate during the first 4.5 to 6 months of life; however, its use as a screening tool remains controversial.[122,330,394]

**TREATMENT.** The goal of treatment for DDH is to ensure stability of the femoral head in the acetabulum, thereby encouraging the development of a normally shaped socket and femoral head. This is accomplished by replacing the head of the femur into the acetabulum with no intervening soft tissue. The proper position then must be maintained for a period of time sufficient for the bony and cartilaginous structures to develop sufficient stability so that the hip does not subluxate or dislocate with normal movement. Lack of contact of the femoral head in the acetabulum will allow the persistence of acetabular dysplasia. Treatment depends on the age of the child and the severity and duration of the dysplasia.

The most common treatment in the infant is placement of the hip in a position of 100 to 110 degrees flexion and 40 to 60 degrees abduction until the joint capsule tightens and the acetabulum is molded to assume a cup shape. This can be accomplished through the use of a hip harness such as the Pavlik harness (Fig. 23.15). The former standard of treatment with triple diapering is no longer recommended, because it is ineffective and proper positioning cannot be ensured. Although the current standard improves this risk there are still reports of avascular necrosis that range between 0 and 60% in the literature, with a higher risk found when there is delay in the onset of treatment and with increased severity of the underlying hip dysplasia.[325,327] The infant must wear the apparatus continuously for 3 to 9 months to stabilize the hip in the correct alignment. The infant is gradually weaned from the harness so it's used at nighttime only before the infant's final discharge. Criteria for discontinuation of the harness are not standard. Some physicians advocate complete removal of the harness 6 weeks after the hip can no longer be moved in and out of the acetabulum. Others recommend discontinuation when ultrasound or radiographic findings confirm hip stabilization.

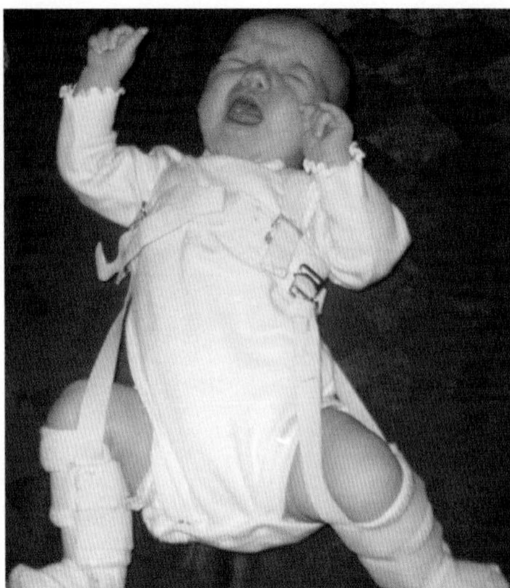

**Figure 23.15**

**Pavlik harness.** A 7-month-old with developmental hip dysplasia wearing a Pavlik harness that holds her legs in flexion and abduction. The harness is worn 23 hours a day, removed only for bathing and diaper changes. The goal of treatment is to keep the femoral head in good contact with the acetabulum. A stable hip encourages the development of a normally shaped socket and rounded head of the femur. The proper hip position must be maintained for enough time to stabilize the joint. The hip should be flexed to 95 degrees and abducted (apart) at least 90 degrees. This position keeps the femoral head in the best position and allows the ligaments and joint capsule to tighten up. (Courtesy Allan Glanzman, The Children's Hospital of Philadelphia, PA.)

In the child treated between ages 6 months and 2 years, a closed reduction is used, often with an adductor release and psoas tenotomy. An arthrogram can be used to confirm the reduction followed by 3 to 5 months in a hip spica cast. Treatment after the age of 18 months requires surgical reduction, often with both femoral varus derotational osteotomy and pelvic osteotomies to augment the acetabulum in addition to tenotomy of contracted muscles (see Fig. 23.12B) depending on the clinical presentation. Traction can be used before closed reduction by some in an attempt to aid in reducing the dislocation by applying a distractive force to the joint to loosen the surrounding tissue before the closed reduction. Overall there is considerable variability in recommendations at decision making inflection points across the development of the child and evolution of the hip joint.[7]

**PROGNOSIS.** Outcome is directly related to the child's age at initiation of treatment and severity of the anatomic deformity. If the dislocation is corrected in the first few weeks of life, the dysplasia is completely reversible and a normal hip can develop, with rates of success as high as 95%.[211] If surgical reduction is required, 86% have a satisfactory outcome with rates of long-term osteoarthritis of 25% in those individuals who required a closed reduction and 49% in those needing an open reduction.[325] When the condition is untreated, long-term problems can include degenerative joint disease, hip pain, antalgic gait, scoliosis, back pain, or the need for total hip replacement.

SPECIAL IMPLICATIONS FOR THE THERAPIST 23.5

### *Developmental Dysplasia of the Hip*

Often therapists are involved early and regularly in managing a child's program for some condition other than hip dysplasia and may be the first health care workers to observe signs of hip pathology. An awareness of quick screening strategies for hip dysplasia is critical (Box 23.5).

Physical therapy preoperatively and postoperatively is often a vital part of the rehabilitation process. Preoperative intervention may include lower extremity and trunk strengthening and parent/caregiver education. Positioning and handling techniques are an important aspect of the child's care both before and after surgery. Postoperatively, the therapist can participate in reviewing cast or orthotic care; transfers; or traction/ care with the child's family/caregivers.

#### Precautions

Positioning and splinting strategies focus on hip abduction and external rotation. Care must be taken not to set the harness in too much flexion (more than 120 degrees) or abduction (more than 70 degrees) secondary to the potential for impingement on the vascular supply to the femoral head. Force should not be used in flexing and abducting the hip because the excessive pressure can cause avascular necrosis. The ideal "safe zone" for the hip in the harness should be 100 to 110 degrees of flexion and 40 to 60 degrees of abduction.[385]

Positions to avoid include lower extremity adduction and flexion as occurs in the side-lying position, especially with one lower extremity drifting across the midline.[48] Tests for hip subluxation or dislocation (see Fig. 23.13) should not be repeated too often, because they can result in persistent laxity, articular damage to the head of the femur, and dislocation.

When transferring a child immediately after casting, make sure the casts are dry; plaster casts typically need 1 to 2 hours to completely air dry, whereas fiberglass will cure faster. Use the palms to avoid making dents in the cast as indentations in the cast can predispose the child to pressure ulcers. Check capillary refill, color, sensation, and motion of the child's legs and feet periodically while the cast is in place and notify the physician immediately if delayed capillary refill or dusky, cool, or numb toes is noted.

#### Motor Development

The widely abducted position of the lower extremities limits opportunities to initiate or continue development of low back and hip extension, especially in the absence of the prone position. Likewise, the widely abducted base of support in sitting decreases opportunities for the use of trunk rotation necessary for transitioning in and out of positions such as sitting and lying prone. The therapist must closely monitor overall progression of motor development during this time and provide as many opportunities as possible for the development of these important skills.

Box 23.5

**HIP DYSPLASIA: QUICK SCREEN**

History
- Breech delivery
- Family history
- Female

Lower extremity examination
- Foot alignment
- Hip range of motion (asymmetry, limited abduction)
- Asymmetric skin folds (thigh, gluteal)
- Buttocks appear flattened
- Leg-length discrepancy

Hip stability (only one positive test required)
- Ortolani sign
- Barlow sign
- Galeazzi sign

Gait (if ambulating)
- Abnormal (waddling gait, limp)
- Positive Trendelenburg sign
- Pain

Typical posture
- Lower extremity hip flexion, adduction, internal rotation
- Asymmetric head and neck alignment when associated with torticollis

## NEUROMUSCULAR DISORDERS

Neuromuscular disorders, including the muscular dystrophies, congenital myopathies, and spinal muscular atrophy, are presented in this chapter. Other neuromuscular disorders, such as Charcot-Marie-Tooth disease, amyotrophic lateral sclerosis, Guillain-Barré polyneuritis, and chronic inflammatory demyelinating polyneuropathy, are discussed in other chapters in this text.

### The Muscular Dystrophies

#### Definition and Overview

The muscular dystrophies (MDs) comprise the largest and most common group of inherited progressive neuromuscular disorders of childhood. They affect all population types, even animals. Signs of MD can occur at any point in the life span. These disorders, in general, have a genetic origin and are characterized by ongoing, typically symmetric, muscle wasting with increasing deformity and disability. Paradoxically, in some forms (e.g., Duchenne, Becker) wasted muscles tend to hypertrophy because of connective tissue, muscle inflammation, and fat deposits, giving the visual appearance of muscle strength. Six major types of MD are included in this text discussion: (1) Duchenne muscular dystrophy (DMD), (2) Becker muscular dystrophy (BMD), (3) facioscapulohumeral (Landouzy-Dejerine) dystrophy (FSHD), (4) limb-girdle dystrophy (LGMD), (5) myotonic dystrophy, and (6) congenital muscular dystrophy (CMD), also known as muscular dystrophy congenita. These forms of MD involve a primary degeneration of muscle with a gradual loss of strength, but each type differs as to which muscle groups are affected, age of onset, and rapidity of progression (Fig. 23.16).

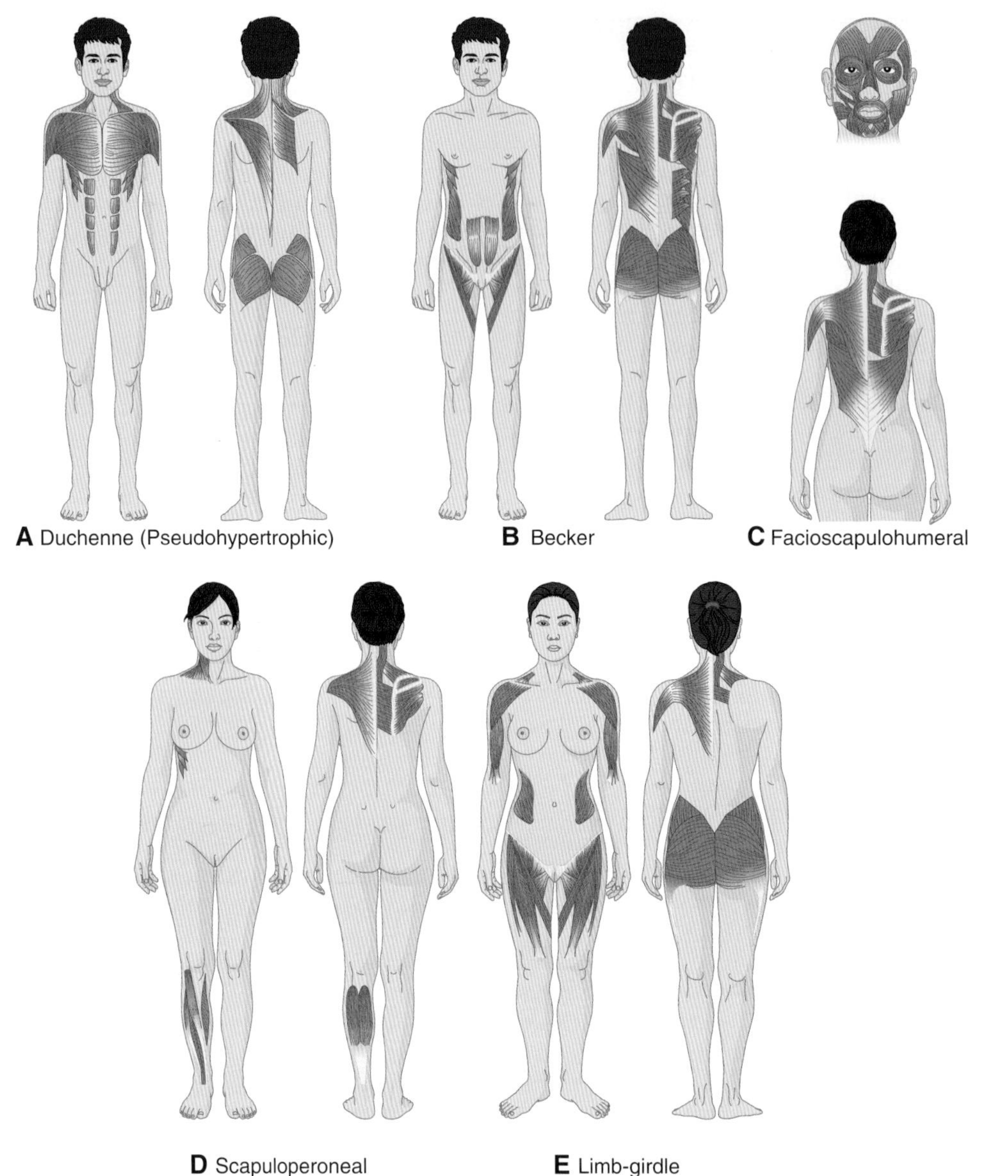


**Figure 23.16**

**Muscle groups involved in muscular dystrophies.** These are presented in relative terms; that is, unlike spinal cord injury with definitive muscle involvement, in muscular dystrophy, proximal or distal muscle groups are affected in varying ways, with individual differences noted. For example, in the facioscapulohumeral form, the lower erector spinae is featured here but may be spared, and in limb-girdle dystrophy, the lower abdominal muscles may be involved but are not shown in this illustration. (A) Duchenne: shoulder girdle (trapezius, levator scapulae, rhomboids, serratus anterior), pectoral muscles, deltoid, rectus abdominis, gluteals, hamstrings, calf muscles. (B) Becker: neck, trunk, pelvic and shoulder girdle. (C) Facioscapulohumeral: muscles of the face and shoulder girdle. (D) Scapuloperoneal: muscles of the legs below the knees (first), shoulder girdle (later). (E) Limb-girdle: upper arm (biceps and deltoid) and pelvic girdle.

## Incidence and Etiologic Factors

The incidence of DMD is approximately 1 in 3500 live births. Rates of occurrence for each type are listed in Table 23.5. DMD and BMD are X-linked recessive disorders caused by mutations in the dystrophin gene *Xp21* that codes for the muscle protein dystrophin. The affected gene on the short arm of the X chromosome *(Xp21)* is one of the largest genes in the human genome. In these two forms of MD, males are affected clinically and females are typically carriers. Male offspring have a 50% chance of being affected and females have a 50% chance of being carriers.

FSHD is primarily an autosomal dominant disorder with onset most typically in adolescence but with variable presentation. The son or daughter of a person affected with FSHD is at 50% risk of inheriting the defective gene. FSHD occurs with an incidence that is variable across populations of between 1 in 8000 to 22,000.[379]

LGMD may be inherited in several ways depending on the type. LGMD type 2 (A through Z are often labeled by the instigating protein defect) disorders are autosomal recessive disorders of late childhood or adolescence and type 1 LGMDs are autosomal dominant disorders also labeled with type 1 and the accompanying letter or with

**Table 23.5** Disorders of Muscle

| Type | Incidence | Onset | Inheritance | Course |
|---|---|---|---|---|
| Duchenne (DMD) (pseudohypertrophic) | 20-30 in 100,000 live male births; female carrier | Becomes apparent at age 2-4 years | X-linked; recessive; mutation in the dystrophin gene; 30% arise from mutation | Rapidly progressive; loss of walking by 9-10 years; death in 20s |
| Becker (BMD) | 5 in 100,000 livebirths; female carrier | Variable, initial diagnosis 5-10 years | X-linked; recessive; mutation in the dystrophin gene | Slowly progressive; walking maintained past early teens; life span until adulthood |
| Facioscapulohumeral (FSHD) | 5 in 100,000 live births (males more often affected than females); female carrier | Any age: usually early adolescence | Autosomal dominant; 10%-30% arise from mutation | Slowly progressive; loss of walking in later life; variable life expectancy |
| Limb-girdle (LGMD) | 1 in more than 100,000 live births | Late adolescence: early childhood | Autosomal recessive or dominant | Slowly progressive; mild impairment |
| Myotonic dystrophy | 1 in 5000 to 1 in 50,000 live births Variable by population founder effect | Variable onset classically adolescence | Autosomal dominant | Rate of progression dependent on age of onset; mild involvement, greater functional independence, greater longevity |
| Congenital muscular dystrophy | 4.65 in 100,000 live births | Birth or shortly after | Autosomal recessive or de novo autosomal dominant | Progressive; death for some in first years, others more slowly progressive and achieve ambulation |
| Congenital myopathies | 2 in 100,000 live births (Nemaline) | Onset at birth | Autosomal recessive or dominant | Initial improvement, static to slowly progressive |

the protein. The dominant LGMDs only account for 10% to 14% of all cases. Dominant disorders have a 50% risk of inheritance if one parent is affected; recessive disorders carry a 25% risk of disease when both parents are carriers and a 50% chance of carrier status. Overall, the prevalence of LGMD is 1 in 100,000 individuals and the prevalence of various types is often dependent on ethnic background.[297] The incidence of the sarcoglycanopathies can be quite variable by population.[173]

Myotonic dystrophy has an incidence that varies between 1 in 5000 and 1 in 50,000 births, with rates in some populations that approach 1 in 550 because of local founder effects.[400] A founder effect occurs when there is a loss of genetic variation in a population. For example, when the population is isolated or reduced in size because of environmental or social factors the genes of the "founders" of the smaller population are disproportionately frequent. Myotonic dystrophy demonstrates an autosomal dominant inheritance pattern, with each generation being somewhat more severely affected than the last. This increase in the phenotypic severity of the disease state with succeeding generations is referred to as anticipation and can be correlated with an expansion in the size of the triple-repeat genetic enlargement that is the causative factor in this disease.[186]

CMD represents a group of recessively inherited disorders that can be divided into two groups based on the presence of brain involvement. Only the most common forms are included here. The overall incidence has been placed at 4.65 per 100,000 in the Italian population.[247] In Japan, however, Fukuyama MD, one form of CMD, is as common as DMD.

A number of classification schemes have been proposed for the CMDs. For our purposes we will use a biochemical classification that divides the disorders based on the location of the abnormality in the muscle. In this way, CMDs can be divided into (1) those that are the result of protein deficits found in the extracellular matrix including merosin negative (Laminin alpha 2-LAMA2) and Ullrich (collagen VI) CMD; (2) defects in the endoplasmic reticulum including Selenoprotein 1 (SEPN1); and (3) defects of glycosylation of dystroglycan including Walker-Warburg syndrome (WWS), muscle-eye-brain disease (MEB), Fukutin and Fukutin-related protein defects (FKRP), and like-glycosyltransferase (LARGE) defects making up the final group.[253]

## Pathogenesis

Knowledge of the MDs and an understanding of their complexities has escalated dramatically since the late 1980s, when the protein dystrophin was identified as the causative factor in DMD and BMD.[146] Subsequently, other members of the dystrophin glycoprotein transmembrane complex have been identified as causative factors in many other forms of MD.

In addition to transmembrane proteins of the dystrophin glycoprotein complex, there have been proteins in the extracellular matrix, sarcomere, and nuclear membrane identified as causative factors in various forms of MD (Fig. 23.17). Recently, it has become apparent that in addition to structural proteins, enzymatic defects in glycosylation (the posttranscriptional modification of proteins by the addition of sugars) can also create other forms of

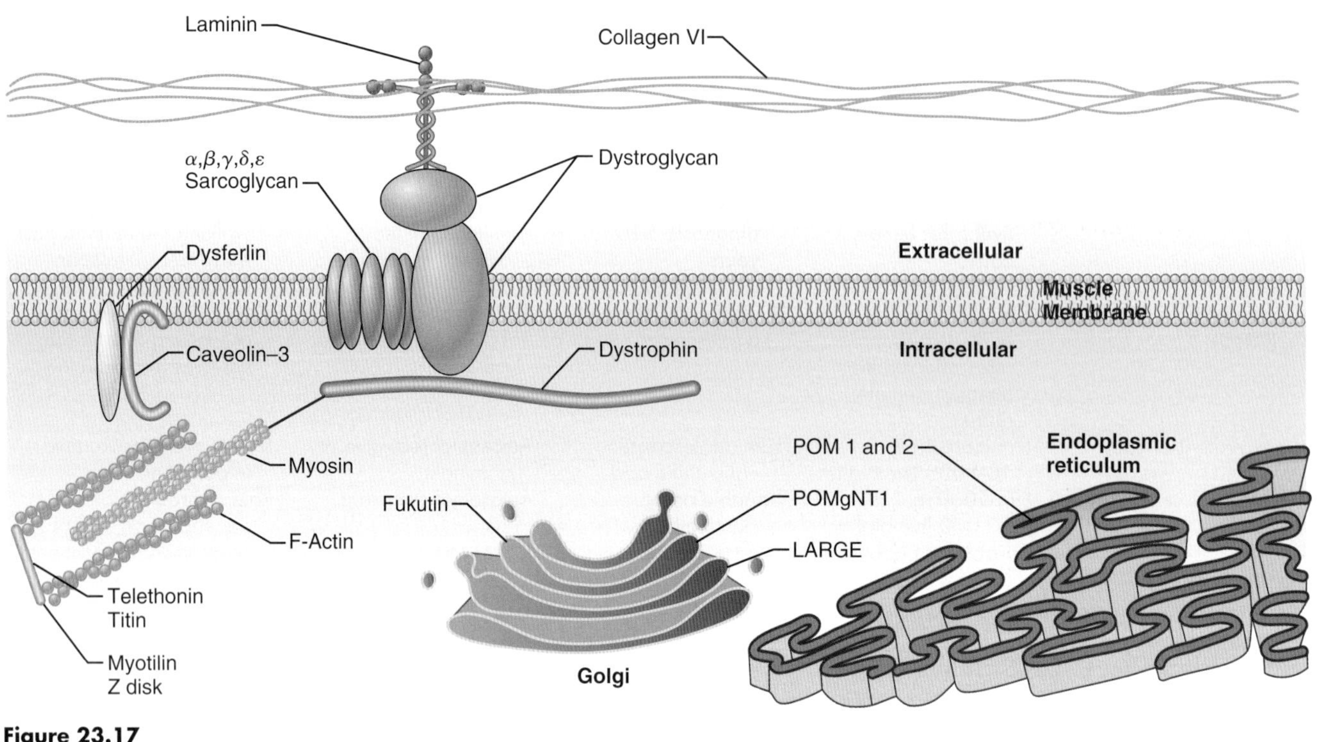


**Figure 23.17**

**Diagram showing the most common muscle protein defects that lead to muscle disease.** The dystroglycan complex spans the muscle membrane and connects dystrophin and the myosin/F-actin contractile mechanism to the extracellular matrix. The Golgi complex and endoplasmic reticulum are also displayed with the causative factors related to glycosylation defects. (Courtesy Allan Glanzman, The Children's Hospital of Philadelphia, PA.)

MD. These discoveries, along with advances in genetic testing, have brought new information on the molecular pathogenesis of these disorders, including the genetic and molecular characterization of many forms of MD.

**Duchenne and Becker Muscular Dystrophies.** The affected gene in DMD/BMD encodes for the protein dystrophin, which, along with its binding partners, is needed for incorporation of the dystroglycan complex in the muscle membrane and the resulting membrane stability that it conveys. Muscle membrane lesions play a fundamental role in the pathogenesis of DMD/BMD, involving skeletal, cardiac, and smooth muscle membranes.

Dystrophin is the protein that links the muscle membrane (sarcolemma) with the contractile muscle protein (actin). Lack of normal dystrophin makes the sarcolemma susceptible to damage during contraction–relaxation cycles. Disruption of the muscle membrane and muscle fiber necrosis are initiated by muscle contraction, especially eccentric contraction.[276] In addition the dystroglycan complex, which is dependent on the proximal attachment with dystrophin to integrate properly in the membrane, is important not only for structural stability of the membrane but also for its role in cell signaling. Cell signaling is accomplished through the detection of mechanical strain and its regulation of satellite cell recruitment, modulation of protein turnover, and control of blood flow to the muscle.[185] The underlying biochemical defect in all types of MD does not necessarily disrupt the integration of dystrophin in the membrane. While the absence of some sarcoglycan molecules in LGMD (see "Limb-Girdle Muscular Dystrophy" below) can lead to susceptibility to mechanical trauma, the absence of other muscle-based proteins does not.[123]

The absence of dystrophin creates an impairment in the connection between the extracellular matrix and the actin and myosin contractile apparatus. Dystrophin is an exceedingly large protein, with domains on either end that allow for interaction with its binding partners and a central domain of 24 spectrin repeats that fold and unfold to act as a shock absorber during muscle contraction.[188] In the absence of dystrophin the transmembrane dystroglycan complex fails to integrate properly and results in a destabilized membrane, allowing the uncontrolled influx of $Ca^{2+}$. This action triggers the destruction of the cell from the inside through the activation of calpain, a calcium-activated proteinase.[264] This process is accompanied by inflammation and oxidative stress that occurs over successive 2-week degeneration regeneration cycles, establishing a chronic inflammatory environment and ultimately impacts the pathogenesis of muscle damage.[185] The inflammatory state following the initial mechanical damage exposes the body's immune system to the cell's cytoplasmic contents, chronically activating an immune response and initiating a secondary process of necrosis and apoptosis. These actions may also impact the satellite cells and their differentiation into myoblasts,[185,298] impairing the muscles' ability to regenerate and altering the differentiation of satellite cells through the production of TGF-β-activating enzymes from fibro-adipogenic progenitors to favor fibroblasts or adipocytes with Ly6C-$^{pos}$ macrophages facilitating the production of type 1 collagen.[162] Muscle cells are replaced by fatty and connective tissues, and contractures develop. Fat cells then continue to accumulate between damaged muscle fibers as a response to the ongoing muscle atrophy. Disorganization of tendinous insertions represents areas of greater muscle pathology and associated fat accumulation.[60,149]

Males with undetectable levels of dystrophin typically have DMD, whereas those with dystrophin of an abnormal size or structure or with lower levels of dystrophin typically have BMD. The division between BMD and DMD, however, is determined by the age that ambulation is lost. Those who lose ambulation prior to 13 years of age fall into the DMD group, and those who walk past age 16 years fall into the BMD group, with the middle group defined as intermediate.

**Limb-Girdle Muscular Dystrophy.** LGMD represents a collection of genetically heterogeneous disorders currently with over 34 different protein origins that can be broadly divided based on genetic inheritance into an X-linked group, dominantly inherited group LGMD type 1, and a recessively inherited group LGMD type 2. Here we will discuss many of the more common forms of LGMD. Some of the forms of LGMD are the result of proteins that are part of the sarcoglycan transmembrane complex, others are related to extracellular collagen, and still others are related to the nuclear membrane. Often, in these cases, not only will the primary protein be absent but many of the protein's binding partners will not integrate properly and will be diminished as well. Although there is little data on the impact of exercise in children with LGMD, an understanding of the protein structure allows one to be more conservative with those forms of LGMD that might limit the full integration of the transmembrane glycoprotein complex where contraction-induced muscle cell damage has been demonstrated in animal models.

LGMD type 1A (5q31.2) is the result of the absence of myotilin and is very rare, resulting a myofibrillar myopathy. Myotilin (MYOT) is a thin filament protein associated with the Z disk and involved in assembly of the contractile mechanism of the cell.[303,309]

LGMD1B (Lamin A/C or LMNA) (1q21) results from the absence of lamin A and lamin C. Lamins A and C are both produced from the same gene, which is spliced in different ways to produce these two similar proteins that function in the nuclear membrane. They are found in the inner nuclear membrane and function in nuclear stability, cell differentiation, gene expression modulation, and cell signaling.[124,194]

LGMD1C results from the absence of Caveolin 3 (CAV3) (3p25). Caveolin 3 is found as part of the muscle membrane and acts in cell signaling related to glucose management and glycogen formation in the muscle.[74]

LGMD1D is caused by mutations in the *DNAJB6* gene (7q36), which codes for one of a class of proteins called "J" proteins that act as modulatory proteins or cochaperones. The mutations found in *DNAJB6* result in an impairment of inhibition of toxic protein folding, assembly, aggregation, and protein turnover within the cell.[360]

LGMD1E is related to an abnormality in the gene for DESMIN (DES) (2q35) and is located on chromosome 2q35.[120] Desmin, a filament protein, is needed for organization of the cytoskeleton within the cell acting as both a transport system within the cell and providing physical stability to the cell to keep it from collapsing. This is especially important in muscle cells where physical demands are significant. Desmin has been proposed as an integral player in the mechanochemical signaling apparatus of the cytoskeleton.[395] In addition, the connections are important for signaling between the nucleus, the sarcolemma, and the actin and myosin of the cell. Additionally connections with the extracellular matrix aid the overall structural composition and alignment of the Z disks within the muscle cell. Finally, there is an interaction with mitochondria to facilitate its localization adjacent to the contractile mechanism of the muscle so that sufficient energy is available. This interruption in the desmin filamentous network of the cell is also seen in other disorders of cardiac or skeletal muscle and comprises a group of disorders sometimes referred to as desmin-related myopathies or myofibrillar myopathies.[228]

LGMD1F (chromosome 7q32.1)(TNPO3), G (chromosome 4q21)(HNRNPDL), and H (chromosome 3p25.1-p23) have been identified in single families and are not discussed in detail here. The reader is referred to the primary descriptions.[24,267]

The second group of LGMDs (2A through 2O and 2Q) are more common than the dominant forms and are inherited recessively. LGMD2A is one of the most common, with an estimated carrier frequency of 1 in 103.[279] The underlying defect in LGMD2A is that of a cellular regulatory enzyme P94, calpain 3 (*CAPN3*) gene (15q15.1), one of the calpain family of molecules (calcium-activated protein enzymes). The function of calpain 3 is not well understood, but it appears to play a role in the organization of the muscle cell as it forms during the regenerative process, its function is Ca2+ dependent, and it is likely involved in sarcomere remodeling following exercise.[111,138,264] *CAPN3* is attached to the structural protein titin, as well as possibly to parts of the sarcomere, and becomes activated with exercise over a certain threshold when it interacts with myosin light chain 1. In addition, *CAPN3* is involved in the muscle membrane repair[138] and some have suggested that *CAPN3* is necessary to protect against exercise-induced muscle damage. This theory is based on animal models of LGMD2A that show exercise-induced muscle damage and abnormal adaptation of the muscle architecture following the stress of exercise.[260]

LGMD2B is caused by an absence of dysferlin (2p13.2). This is also the protein defect found in Miyoshi myopathy. Miyoshi myopathy presents with a distal dystrophic phenotype in contrast to the proximal LGMD2B proximal phenotype.[381] Dysferlin acts as a membrane repair molecule in the initial stages of "emergency" membrane repair; it also interacts with other molecules[47] (Mitsugumin 53, annexin, and calpain) at the muscle membrane to execute membrane repair by a calcium-mediated process of intracellular vesicle aggregation that involves the attachment of lysosomes at the site of membrane damage and subsequent vesicle fusion with the sarcolemma[15] acting as the initial stage of membrane repair. For a review of membrane repair see Barthélémy.[15] In addition, the pathology of LGMD2B is accompanied by a significant inflammatory response in the muscle secondary to the impaired muscle repair.[133]

The absent genes in LGMD2C through F include γ-sarcoglycan (13q12) (2C), α-sarcoglycan (17q21.33) (2D), β-sarcoglycan (14q11)(2E), and δ-sarcoglycan (5q33.3)(2F), all code for a specific proteins in the sarcoglycan–glycoprotein complex and as a group can be referred to as sarcoglycanopathies. There are six sarcoglycan proteins, the absence of four of which; γ2C, α(2D), β(2E), and δ(2F) represent the four sarcoglycanopathies (ε and ζ abnormalities have not been found to cause muscle pathology). The γ-, β-, and δ-sarcoglycans are type II proteins with C-terminal extracellular domains, while α-sarcoglycan is a type I protein with an extracellular N-terminal domain; all four have phosphorylation sites intracellularly. These proteins are found in close association with dystrophin in the muscle membrane and act to stabilize the membrane and through the dystroglycan complex along with costameres attach the subsarcolemmal cytoskeleton with the sarcomere and extracellular matrix. Sarcoglycan-deficient muscle is sensitive to eccentric, contraction-induced disruption of the plasma membrane. δ-Sarcoglycan is strongly associated with β-sarcoglycan and β-dystroglycan,[173] and forms the core of this group of proteins additionally stabilized by sarcospan. In the absence of these core proteins, none of the members of this group of proteins integrate properly. Reduced levels of other sarcoglycans (e.g., γ, α, β) also appear to be involved with the stability at the muscle membrane but do not as significantly account for contraction-induced muscle injury as those in the core of the complex.[361] Additional binding partners of the sarcoglycans include nNOS, α-dystrobrevin and syntrophin; the association with nNOS as well as posttranscriptional modification of some subunits in response to mechanical stress indicate a potential signaling role for the complex.[82]

LGMD2G is the result of a genetic defect on the seventeenth chromosome (17q12), which codes for the protein telethonin (or titin-cap). Telethonin is a protein that acts together with titin (discussed later) in the formation of the muscle cell sarcomere acting to join two titan domains together with other proteins of the Z disk. In the adult muscle (and cardiac muscle), it is found at the Z disk in the sarcomere.[245] Telethonin also plays a role in interactions between the contractile apparatus of the muscle cell and the membrane in sensing the degree of stretch that the sarcomere is experiencing.[40]

LGMD2H results from the absence of the tripartite-motif–containing (*TRIM 32*) gene (9q33), which belongs to a large family of over 70 similar proteins that regulate other cellular cascades. *TRIM 32* acts in conjunction with ubiquitin and other enzymes in the muscle to facilitate proteasome-mediated breakdown of various proteins such as actin and α-actin, as well as desmin, tropomyosin, dysbindin, various enzymes, and cell cycle regulators. *TRIM 32* is found to be upregulated in situations where muscle remodeling is occurring, as is the case when changes in weight bearing or nutrition occur.[187] In addition, it is found in increased levels when muscle cells are differentiating and is expressed in animal models of myogenic stem cells. It impacts differentiation through the modulation of c-Myc, a regulator gene that modulates transcription.[257] *TRIM 32* is also found associated with the thick myosin filaments and the z disk of the sarcomere.[177]

LGMD2I is a common form of LGMD caused by a mutation in the FKRP gene (19q13.3). FKRP encodes for an enzyme that is involved in glycosylation of α-dystroglycan and can be referred to along with the other LGMDs and CMDs that involve proteins that impair O-glycosylation as dystroglycanopathies.[357] Glycosylation is a process by which a protein is modified after it is transcribed by the addition of a carbohydrate to a portion of the protein. In this case both α- and β-dystroglycan are produced by the same gene and function differently because of alternative patterns of glycosylation. α-Dystroglycan (and β) is a component of the dystrophin glycoprotein complex and the o-glycan portion of α-ystroglycan binds to laminin α2. The glycosylation process provides the structure of the extracellular binding site with laminin α2, which provides a structural connection to the extracellular matrix, and through the cell membrane by the dystroglycan complex for signaling purposes.[207,244]

LGMD2J results from a mutation at 2q31.2 in the Titin gene. Titin is a large intracellular protein that reaches from the Z-disk to the M-line,[302] where it binds obscurin and small ankyrin.[302] It is responsible for elasticity through its Ig-like domains and stability, preventing linear tensile damage of the sarcomere as well as playing a signaling role related to sensing mechanical stress through its kinase domain, which results in serial addition of sarcomeres,[302,315] as seen in serial casting.[171] In addition, it plays a role in the assembly of the sarcomere in the developing muscle cell. Clinically titinopathies can present as LGMD2J when there is homozygous mutation (mutations on both alleles) and in this case there is also a secondary absence of calpain-3. When there is a heterozygous mutation (only one allele affected) the phenotype is milder and presents as tibial MD.[366]

LGMD2K (POMT1) (9q34) codes for O-mannosyltransferase 1, an enzyme participating in the first step in posttranscriptional α-dystroglycan glycosylation and represents the LGMD form of one of the disorders of glycosylation. LGMD2K can also present in a more severe form as a CMD (see discussion below).

LGMD 2L anoctamin 5 (*ANO5* or TMEM16E) (11p14) was thought to code for a segment of a calcium-activated chloride channel as the other ANO genes do; however, ANO5 is a paralog whose protein is found intracellularly and has been proposed to facilitate $ca^{2+}$ activated phospholipid scrambling (PLS), moving phospholipids along the membrane, that are associated with nonselective ion flows. PLS plays a role in the cell fusion of muscle progenitor cells during muscle repair, however the relationship of ANO5 to muscle repair via muscle progenitor fusion still needs further investigation.[78,386] Recessive loss of function mutations result in this LGMD phenotype, whereas dominant gain of function mutations result in gnathodiaphyseal dysplasia, a sclerotic disorder of bone.[143]

LGMD 2M is the designation for another one of the dystroglycanopathies that results from abnormalities in Fukutin (9q31). This LGMD form is a milder presentation for what was originally identified as a Fukuyama CMD (see below) and later found to present also in this milder form. In the Japanese population this is one of the more common neuromuscular disorders.[145]

LGMD 2N POMT2 (14q24) is an uncommon, mild presentation of this dystroglycanopathy (see below for discussion).

LGMD 2O POMGnT1 (1p32) is an uncommon LGMD presentation of one of the dystroglycanopathies that typically presents as a CMD (see below).

LGMD 2Q plectin 1f (8q24) results in an abnormality in the connection between the sarcomere and muscle cell membrane, with additional abnormalities noted in overall sarcomeric structure.[129]

LGMD2S transport protein particle complex 11 (TRAPPC11) (4q35.1) functions intracellularly in antitrade membrane transport between the endoplasmic reticulum and Golgi.[26]

LGMD2T GMPPB dystroglycanopathy resulting from abnormal glycosylation of α-dystroglycan.

**Congenital Muscular Dystrophy.** The first group of CMDs are disorders of glycosylation that present to varying degrees with muscle, brain, and eye involvement. Glycosylation is the addition of sugars or chains of sugars (glycans) to proteins. In this case we will focus on the diseases resulting from abnormal glycosylation of the proteins coded for by the DAF1 gene (dystrophin-associated glycoprotein 1) which produces the precursor that is split to form both α-dystroglycan and β-dystroglycan. The types of glycosylation can be grouped into N-glycans and O-glycans based on their binding characteristics. This process takes place in the endoplasmic reticulum and Golgi complex and is regulated by a series of enzymes (glycosyltransferases) that control the addition of glycans. Glycan chains are thought to be important in signaling between cells and intracellular signaling, as well as the establishment of the proper folded structure of the proteins.[89,328]

O-mannose glycans develop sequentially in the endoplasmic reticulum, with each step facilitated by an enzymatic transferase into very complicated structures which are carried by α-dystroglycan and closely associated with β-dystroglycan. These represent an integral part of the dystrophin-associated protein complex, with important associations in muscle with the actin contractile apparatus and laminin 2 in the extracellular matrix and in brain development.[328]

Five of the CMDs are linked to mutations in the process of glycosylation, and in all there are at least 19 different genes that have been implicated in either α-dystroglycan or glycosyltransferases that facilitate posttranscriptional protein modification. Different mutations in these genes can produce a wide range of phenotypic severity, which in some cases results from the varied amounts of residual enzyme activity.[287]

WWS (POMT1) (9q34) is the most severe CMD, though there is also an LGMD phenotype of the POMT1 gene. This is the result of defects in the first step in the glycosylation process of α-dystroglycan where O-mannose is added to α-dystroglycan. This is caused by the absence of O-mannosyltransferase 1 that facilitates this reaction. The gene that is responsible is the POMT1 gene. WWS is a phenotypic diagnosis and POMT1 is only responsible for approximately 20% of the cases. An additional 10% of cases may also be contributed by abnormalities in ISPD (7p21.2) whose absence affects O-mannosylation. Mutations in POMT2 and the enzyme O-mannosyltransferase 2 is also a cause of WWS, and the combination of these two genes in the endoplasmic reticulum modulates glycosylation.[380]

MEB can be caused by mutations in the *POMGnT1* gene (1p34.1) that encodes for the transferase in the next step in the O-mannosyl glycosylation pathway. Clinically MEB represents a spectrum of phenotypic expression from mild (those who will live into adulthood) to severe; in general, MEB presents a phenotype that is less severe than WWS. Because of this variability, other factors are presumed to affect the severity of the presenting phenotype.

Fukuyama CMD is caused by a mutation in the fukutin gene (9q31.2); the products are expressed in muscle in the same location as dystroglycan. Fukutin is found in the *cis*-Golgi, but beyond that its function has not been established, although it is thought to participate in glycosylation of α-dystroglycan. The pathology of the CNS that is seen is that of a cobblestone lissencephaly where the layering of the cerebrum is disrupted as the result of abnormal neuronal migration. Fukutin is likely involved in both neuronal migration and synapse function in addition to formation of the basement membrane, the glia limitans, which separates the cerebral cortex and the pia mater of the meninges.[393]

CMD resulting from a mutation in LARGE can present phenotypically as MEB, WWS, or more mildly with intellectual disability and only mild weakness. LARGE is found in the Golgi complex and is the rate-limiting step in the glycosylation of α-dystroglycan. When it is overexpressed, α-dystroglycan is hyperglycosylated in animal models. Despite this knowledge, its exact function still remains unclear. The potent effect of LARGE makes it an ideal target for drug development as its overexpression can rescue both in vitro and in vivo models of a variety of glycosylation-based MDs.[108]

Merosin-negative CMD results from a mutation in the laminin alpha-2 *(LAMA2)* gene (6q22-23) and in deficiency or absence of merosin (also known as laminin), the protein affected in merosin-negative CMD.[172] The underlying pathophysiology is not well understood, but the function of laminin 2 is primarily one of cell adhesion. It is found as a three-chained structure composed of three subunits: $\alpha_2$, $\beta_1$, and $\gamma_1$. It binds to dystroglycan (as well as integrin) and provides structural support for the basement membrane protecting the cell from contraction-induced damage.[112]

Ullrich CMD (and Bethlem myopathy; see below) is one of the more common CMDs and is the result of a defect in the extracellular matrix protein collagen type VI. Collagen type VI is made up of three strands, COL6 A1, A2, and A3, These three strands are coded for on 21q22.3 or 2q37.3 and form a triple helix, which then associates into a dimeric structure consisting of two associated subunits that are aligned in an antiparallel "head-to-toe fashion." Finally, two of these dimeric proteins become aligned in a parallel fashion, creating a tetrameric four-protein complex, which is then the final product and is transported out of the cell and becomes a component of the extracellular matrix. It is found both near the basement membrane and within tendons surrounding fibroblasts, which is the cell of origin of COL6. The underlying structural defect that leads to poor force transmission might relate to interaction with the muscle cell membrane and biglycan, which might provide an intermediate connection to the membrane because it binds with both COL6 and the dystrophin-associated transmembrane protein complex, but the exact function still remains unclear.[28]

**Facioscapulohumeral Dystrophy.** The genetic defect has been found at 4q35 in 90% to 95% of individuals with FSHD.[45,369] FSHD occurs as the result of a decrease in the typical number of tandem repeats on chromosome 4q35 to less than 10, which allows chromatin changes and a decrease in methylation; however, the pathogenesis of this is impacted by the presence of a pLAM1 polyadenylation site distal to the gene on the fourth chromosome. This combination of factors allows transcription of the double home box protein 4 (DUX4) gene,[380] which is normally not produced in healthy subjects. The presence of DUX4 alters the expression of many other genes, particularly in the germline or early embryonic stages of development. There are many different functional pathways that are impacted and the exact causative mechanism for the resulting muscle pathology remains to be detailed.[156] The muscle in FSHD shows a characteristic inflammatory pattern, with the resulting phenotype likely the result of an immune-mediated process. The presence of DUX4 ultimately causes the symptomatology associated with FSHD. This is in contrast to most other genetic disorders where the absence of a protein is the disease-causing factor. Here the presence of a previously silent gene that has been turned on produces a protein that causes phenotypic expression. The remaining 5% of patients have FSHD2 that results from a series of genes that impact methylation of D4Z4, resulting in a similar phenotype but as the result of digenic inheritance.[379]

**Myotonic Dystrophy.** There are three forms of myotonic dystrophy. The major form of myotonic dystrophy is known as Steinert type or MD11 myotonic dystrophy with protein kinase *(DMPK)* gene (9q13.3) being the identified abnormality, and it represents 98% of the cases. A second type of myotonic dystrophy has been identified, which is myotonic dystrophy type 2 (MD2) zinc finger protein (ZNF9) (3q21.3).[231] In MD1, the underlying defect of the gene is a trinucleotide repeat in which cytosine, thymine, and guanine are repeated an abnormally large number of times. With succeeding generations this defect expands, a condition known as anticipation, also seen in other triple-repeat disorders. In diseases that demonstrate anticipation, each succeeding generation is more affected than the last.[186]

The precise pathophysiology remains poorly understood, but the triple repeat results in abnormal splicing of RNA. There are two similar RNA binding proteins, CUG-BP and MBNL-1 that mediate a subset of splicing events that are impaired in MD1. This results in abnormalities involving the creation of abnormal RNA transcript processing and alterations in other genes, some of which code for the chloride channel,[23] the insulin receptor, and microtubule-associated protein tau, each related to a portion of the underlying phenotype (myotonia, risk of diabetes mellitus, and cognitive delay).[22] In myotonic dystrophy muscle fibers demonstrate altered resting muscle membrane potentials, possibly resulting from a dysregulation of ion channel function.[19]

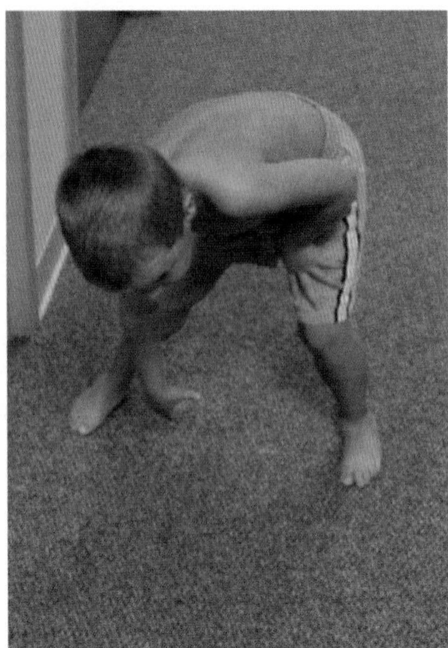

**Figure 23.18**

**The Gowers sign.** This boy adopts the typical movement seen with proximal weakness, such as myopathies, when arising from the floor, a chair, or even when climbing stairs. During the Gowers maneuver, the client places the hands on the thighs and walks up the legs with the hands until the weight of the trunk can be placed posterior to the hip joint. This sign is characteristic of weakness of the lumbar and gluteal muscles. (Courtesy Allan Glanzman, The Children's Hospital of Philadelphia, PA.)

## Clinical Manifestations

**Duchenne Muscular Dystrophy.** DMD is usually identified when the child has difficulty getting up off the floor (the Gowers sign; Fig. 23.18), falls frequently, has difficulty climbing stairs, and starts to walk with a waddling gait (proximal muscle weakness) and an increased lumbar lordosis (compensation for abdominal and hip extensor weakness). At the same time, the child begins to walk on the toes because of contracture of the posterior calf musculature and weakness of the anterior tibial, peroneal, and proximal muscles.

Hip abductor weakness produces a positive Trendelenburg sign (see Fig. 23.14), which eventually changes to a compensated Trendelenburg emblematic of the gluteus medius weakness. Classically ambulation continues to deteriorate up to the age of 7 to 12 years, at which time the majority of people with DMD lose the ability to walk.[33,227,336] However, treatment with prednisone or deflazacort may delay the cessation of ambulation for 2 to 5 years, allowing children to continue to walk until an older age.[250]

The shoulder girdle becomes involved, with excessive scapular winging, which is made more prominent by the presence of an excessive lumbar lordosis (Fig. 23.19). Shoulder girdle weakness and the need to maintain the weight line posterior to the hips and anterior to the knees to enhance stability at those joints often prevents the use of crutches or a walker to support the body weight.

Weakness of the shoulder girdle also causes difficulty in performing overhead activities related to hygiene and

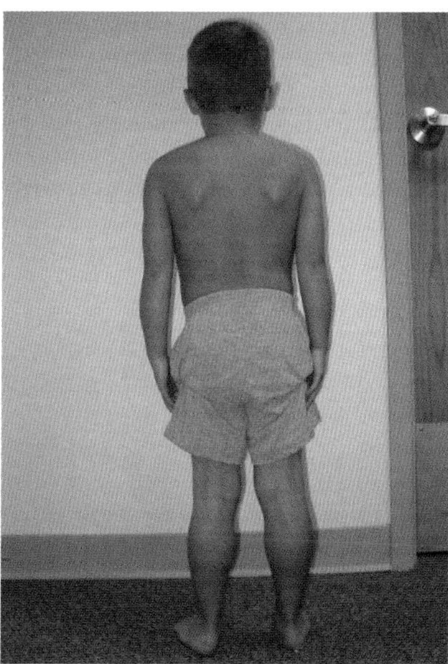

**Figure 23.19**

**Duchenne muscular dystrophy with pseudohypertrophy of calves and lordotic posture that places the weight of the trunk behind the hip joint.** Even though weakness occurs symmetrically, habitual standing postures may create asymmetries in flexibility in some cases. (Courtesy Allan Glanzman, The Children's Hospital of Philadelphia, PA.)

work. Biceps tendinitis, subacromial bursitis or other impingement disorders at the shoulder occur as the children get older as the result of weakness and the repeated manual lifts that become necessary for transfers. Muscle imbalances create biomechanical dysfunction, and weakness impairs the ability to stabilize the shoulder girdle, contributing to shoulder problems.

With the progression of weakness, scoliosis occurs at a rate of 80% to 90% in individuals who are untreated with corticosteroids and less than 27% in those treated.[223] Scoliosis usually progresses more rapidly after the person is wheelchair bound. Spinal fusion is usually considered when the spinal curve approaches 40 degrees. Early fusion, when a good correction and level pelvis can be obtained, and when the individual's respiratory status is relatively more intact, produces the best result.

Common comorbidities associated with DMD include variable cognitive, respiratory, cardiac, and gastrointestinal dysfunction. The average IQ of individuals with DMD is 1 standard deviation below the mean, with specific reading disorders noted irrespective of IQ. Even so, many children with DMD have normal or above-normal intelligence.

Children with DMD develop a progressive restrictive respiratory impairment secondary to weakness and contracture of the respiratory muscles. Respiratory problems become more of a problem after the children become wheelchair bound. Nocturnal hypoventilation is one of the earlier manifestations of respiratory involvement and is usually accompanied by morning headaches, sleep disturbance, or nightmares. Chest muscle deterioration combined with joint contractures and spinal scoliosis results in diminished ventilation and ability to produce pressure to cough up secretions, leading to upper respiratory infections or pneumonia.[221]

Dilated cardiac myopathy and, less frequently, conduction abnormalities can be life-threatening, and with the improvements in pulmonary care this has often become the life-limiting impairment.

Gastrointestinal problems are common in patients with DMA; gastrointestinal transport and motility, however, are not tightly correlated with the observation of constipation, pseudoobstruction, and gastric dilation in patients that can result from the smooth muscle deterioration.[196]

**Becker Muscular Dystrophy.** Signs and symptoms of BMD resemble those of DMD but with a slower progression and longer life expectancy. Ambulation is preserved into midadolescence or later, but often is marked by toe walking, with bilateral calf muscle hypertrophy and contracture.

Proximal muscles tend to be affected to a greater degree and before the involvement of the distal musculature, with primary effects observed in the neck (relatively preserved in BMD versus DMD), trunk, pelvis, and shoulder girdle. Muscle cramps are a common complaint in late childhood and early adolescence. Scoliosis and contractures (elbow flexors, forearm pronators, and wrist flexors in the upper extremity and plantar flexors, knee flexors, and hip abductors in the lower extremity) and other comorbidities also found in DMD are common; however, these occur less frequently and with less severity in the BMD type.

**Limb-Girdle Muscular Dystrophy.** LGMD affects proximal more than distal muscles and follows a steady progressive course, although the course can vary widely even in a given family in some forms. Early symptoms develop as a result of muscle weakness in the pelvic and shoulder girdle muscles; usually the first symptoms are noticed in adolescence or early adulthood. Winging of the scapulae, lumbar lordosis, abdominal protrusion, waddling gait, poor balance, and inability to raise the arms may also develop.

LGMD1A (myotilin), also known as a myofibrillar myopathy, has a typical age of onset in adulthood as late as the seventh decade of life. Some individuals have cardiac involvement, and there is an associated neuropathy that is axonal in character associated with LGMD1A. As a result, some people with this type will have prominent distal weakness superimposed on the proximal LGMD phenotype.[321]

LGMD1B (lamin A/C or LMNA) has a wide variability in phenotype depending on mutation type. This ranges from severe Emery-Dreifuss muscular dystrophy to a somewhat less-aggressive LGMD-type phenotype. Cardiac conduction defects are common and need to be aggressively managed. In addition, the development of dilated cardiomyopathy is also seen in this population.[55] The contracture pattern in this population includes the development of severe elbow flexion and ankle plantar flexion contractures, along with trunk and cervical extension contractures, with relative sparing of the quadriceps muscle strength in most cases.[252]

LGMD1C (caveolin 3) is one of a number of ways that abnormalities in caveolin 3 can present. In this form, first symptoms are typically seen in the first decade, with proximal weakness and the Gowers sign. In addition, calf hypertrophy similar to DMD and postexercise soreness is common. Caveolin 3 can also present with isolated elevated creatine kinase without weakness, rippling muscle disease (percussion-induced muscle contraction), or as an isolated hypertrophic cardiomyopathy.[39]

LGMD1D (DNAJB6) onset is typically between the third and sixth decade of life and ambulation is typically preserved, with functional deficits characterized by problems climbing steps and running. Contracture is not a prominent feature in LGMD1D. The distribution of weakness of the legs is characterized by proximal weakness in addition to posterior compartment (hamstring more than quadriceps) weakness with inconsistent involvement of the arms, with a smaller group presenting with distal weakness. Creatine kinase is typically mildly elevated, ranging between normal and 10 times normal.[312,316,360]

LGMD1E (desmin) also falls in the group of myopathies known as myofibrillar myopathies typically present between the second and sixth decade of life, with the distribution of weakness in a typical LGMD distribution or more distally in a scapuloperoneal pattern. Affected individuals can develop respiratory, as well as oral, motor dysfunction. Cardiac findings are common in this population and may be the presenting symptom, with the rod domain of the gene typically a mixed skeletal and cardiac muscle presentation and the tail domain most often showing a predominant cardiac phenotype.[134,322,395]

Clinical manifestations of LGMD2A calpain-3 (p94 protein) (CAPN3) include phenotypic variability from first decade of life onset and rapid progression to later onset and slower progression. Approximately 70% of affected individuals present between ages 6 and 18 years.[255] The typical pattern of involvement is that of a classic limb-girdle pattern, with the gluteal muscles most affected. The average age of ambulation loss varies considerably (5-39 years) and is related to age of onset. The underlying genetics seems to be related to the phenotypic severity. Individuals with two null mutations are much more homogeneous, with an average age of presentation of 15 years.[294]

The phenotypic presentation of LGMD2B (Dysferlin) can be that of classic LGMD (61% of patients) or, alternatively, either a Miyoshi myopathy phenotype (31% of patients), which presents with gastrocsoleus involvement as the defining factor, or as a more rapidly progressive wasting of the anterior tibialis. [132] However these are not distinct syndromes because there is significant phenotypic overlap as the disease progresses. One out of four patients presents with symptoms prior to the teen years but there is significant variability in age of onset, with initial symptoms being recognized as late as the 70s in one patient and reports on congenital onset in others.[181]

The typical presentation of LGMD2C-F sarcoglycan (gamma 13q12, alpha 17q21.33, beta 4q11, delta 5q33.3) is in the later first decade of life with proximal weakness similar to that of DMD. However, there is significantly more variability and some individuals present later in the second decade of life or even in adulthood. Cardiomyopathy is most common in individuals with β and δ sarcoglycanopathies. Respiratory failure is also a concern in a pattern similar to that found in DMD, although with somewhat more variability in onset. The contracture pattern[173] associated with this form includes plantarflexion contractures.

LGMD2G (telethonin) presents primarily as an LGMD pattern of skeletal muscle weakness; however, there are some reports of congenital presentation or hypertrophic cardiomyopathic presentation.[95] The muscle atrophy pattern is one of proximal predominance, primarily in the anterior compartment of the legs with foot drop, with first symptoms in childhood and ambulation loss by 40% of patients by the fourth decade. Contractures and pseudohypertrophy of the gastric soleus can be noted. Dominant mutations with a cardiac phenotype have also been reported.[40]

LGMD2H (TRIM32) presents with significant variability between groups of individuals and with typically proximal weakness that ranges from nonprogressive to slowly progressive.[354] In its mildest form patients can have only a chronic increase in CK with no detectable muscle weakness, while the phenotype can extend to weakness that limits ambulation with onset in the teens or twenties and a slow progression of disease, with some losing ambulation in their 50s and beyond.[306]

LGMD2I (FKRP) or the fukutin-related protein gene is one of the dystroglycanopathies. Its clinical presentation is widely distributed, ranging from mild, late-onset disease with onset in the teens or twenties as is found in the LGMD2I phenotype to a severe form of CMD with brain and eye abnormalities in addition to severe weakness at birth, with more than a third of patients presenting in the first decade, many with pain on exertion in addition to weakness.[27,207] Both cardiac and respiratory symptoms are also common with FKRP. The severity of the phenotype is dependent on the efficacy of the underlying protein that is produced in the glycosylation of dystroglycan. Many of the genes implicated have both more-severe and less-severe forms, depending on the specific mutation characteristics and how severely the final protein is affected in terms of its function in the glycosylation process.[344]

LGMD2J (titin) can present in two phenotypic varieties, some with concomitant dilated cardiomyopathy. When there is a mutation on one allele (with dominant inheritance), the phenotype is one of a tibial muscular dystrophy, with anterior tibialis and long toe extensor weakness as the first symptoms beginning in the fourth to sixth decade, which may progress to proximal weakness in old age. When there is a mutation to the gene on both alleles (either homozygous or compound heterozygous recessive inheritance), the phenotypic picture is often one of LGMD2J and dilated cardiac myopathy, sometimes without skeletal muscle involvement owing to different splicing in skeletal and cardiac muscle.[366] The recessive compound heterozygous phenotype can present a number of different ways, depending on the second novel mutation. These phenotypes include proximal lower extremity weakness, early onset distal myopathy, primary heart disease with congenital myopathy, and two contracture phenotypes with myopathy, one presenting congenitally (arthrogryposis) and the other with a progressive Emery-Dreyfuss–like picture that includes contracture (elbow/achilles), proximal weakness (neck flexor), rigidity (limited flexion), scoliosis, and respiratory impairment.[129]

LGMD2K has been designated to identify the milder phenotypic variants of POMT1 gene mutations at 9q34.13. This is the same mutation that is found in some of the more severe CMD cases with WWS. This form of

LGMD is one of the only forms that includes intellectual developmental disorder as a component. There are some intermediate forms that fall between LGMD and WWS. Like the other glycosylation defects found in FKRP, there is a spectrum of severity found in people with POMT1 mutations. This is likely the result of modifying factors that remain incompletely discribed.[67]

Proximal weakness is the most common presentation of LGMD2L, which represents mutations in anoctamin 5 (ANO5) and occurs between the ages of 20 and 50 years. A less-common form is phenotypically similar to Miyoshi myopathy where the calf is first involved. In both cases, males are more severely affected.[143]

LGMD2M is the phenotype seen in people with the LGMD form of Fukuyama congenital muscular dystrophy, which has a very broad spectrum of phenotype ranging from the severe CMD presentation to that of isolated hypercalcemia, all resulting from the same FKTN gene.[377]

LGMD2N is a rare LGMD presentation of Walker-Warberg CMD.

LGMD2O is the LGMD milder presentation of MEB.

LGMD2Q presents with early onset of weakness and delayed motor skills in the first years of life followed by a plateau with a continuation of ambulation until the third decade (ages 20-30 years).[127]

In LGMD2S transport protein particle complex 11 (TRAPPC11) (4q35.1) the clinical phenotype can range from a classical LGMD phenotype to forms that include intellectual disability and movement disorder. Typical onset is in childhood, with a slowly progressive phenotype.[26]

LGMD2T GMPPB gene that encodes guanosine-diphosphate-mannose has a wide disease spectrum ranging from isolated elevated CK, mild adult onset LGMD to Walker-Warberg syndrome in addition to a congenital myasthenic phenotype. Patients can also have associated arthrogryposis, cognitive delay, autism-spectrum disorder, ataxia, or seizures.[126]

## A THERAPIST'S THOUGHTS*

### *Clinical Phenotypes*

The details of clinical phenotyping as described in these sections may be easy to skip over but this information is important for the physical therapist when establishing a plan of care in the absence of a known natural history. Therapists need to provide anticipatory guidance and treatment in the context of progression that is expected.

To expand on this point further, remember that clinical features are often dependent on the specific underlying LGMD type and even then the severity of presentation can be quite variable between individuals, making this type of MD more difficult to diagnose. Identification of the specific type of LGMD should be pursued to provide the best guidance for the client and to allow the therapist and physician to treat the person proactively, with full knowledge of the natural history of the specific disorder rather than approaching the case reactively. For example, an understanding of the natural history of the specific form of LGMD will aid in anticipating the pattern of potential contracture and weakness in addition to the anticipated functional course and typical timing of functional decline.

*Allan Glanzman, PT, DPT, PCS

**Congenital Muscular Dystrophy.** CMD represents a spectrum of disease states that most commonly present at the more severe end of the spectrum in infancy, with rapidly progressive muscle strength loss and progressive respiratory symptoms. The first group includes those with disorders of glycosylation. Affected individuals demonstrate a mixed central and peripheral picture, with involvement of both the brain and muscle in addition to involvement of the visual system.

WWS is the most severe of the CMDs and presents at birth with a rapidly progressive course, with death most commonly occurring prior to 1 year of age. Ocular impairments include retinal abnormalities, microphthalmia glaucoma, cataracts, and anterior chamber abnormalities. The CNS complications include a cobblestone lissencephaly[77] with polymicrogyria. Cerebellar abnormalities are also present and include hypoplasia in addition to fourth ventricular dilation. MEB has similar clinical findings to WWS but a wider range of phenotypic presentations.

Fukuyama MD can also present as a CMD but is more often found in its milder LGMD form. Common phenotypic presentation includes onset at or shortly after birth, with weakness and delayed gross motor skills with progressive contractures and weakness, with very few individuals achieving ambulation and a typical loss of ambulation by the age of 10 years. Cognitive impairment is common and often severe, with MRI findings somewhat similar to those found in WWS.

Ullrich CMD can present along a spectrum of severity, with its milder form, Bethlem myopathy, representing the mildest presentation. In its more severe forms, children have significant weakness that either prevents ambulation or allows them to walk only for a short time prior to adolescence.[234] The most prominent feature of the phenotype is the distal laxity mixed with proximal contractures, particularly of the knee and the elbow, with prominent shoulder protraction resulting from contracture of the pectoral muscles. The distal laxity in the Achilles tendon can contribute to a crouched gait pattern or the gastrocsoleus and posterior tibialis can present with contracture and a plano varus foot position in standing.

Merosin-negative CMD typically presents with weakness at birth. However, most infants attain the ability to sit, and a spectrum of severity exists, including an LGMD phenotype that has been reported, with the milder phenotypes, including the ability to ambulate in childhood in those patients with partial merosin deficiency.[172] Contracture pattern includes limitation in neck flexion and early development of hip flexion contractures. Muscle strength of the quadriceps is typically relatively spared. Respiratory insufficiency develops, typically in the first decade.

**Facioscapulohumeral Dystrophy.** FSHD begins with weakness and atrophy of the facial muscles and shoulder girdle, usually presenting in the second decade of life; however, there is significant variability even within families. Phenotypic expression is more common in males than in females (95% vs. 69%), with more females being carriers. Inability to close the eyes may be the earliest sign; facial expressions are limited even when laughing or crying, forward shoulders and scapular winging is a prominent feature, as is difficulty raising the arms overhead

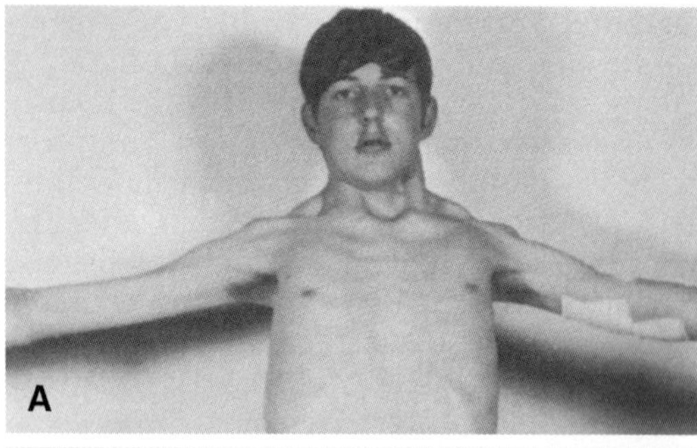


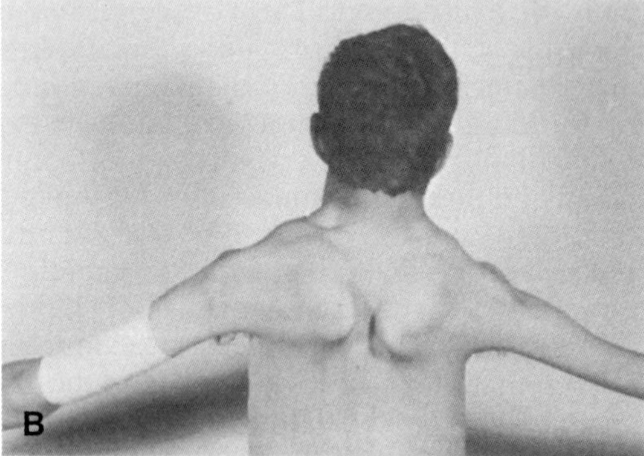


**Figure 23.20**

**Facioscapulohumeral dystrophy.** Weakness of subscapular musculature makes it difficult to perform overhead activities; wasting also causes the clavicles to jut forward and the shoulders to have a drooping appearance. During humeral movement, the scapulae wing and ride up over the thorax. (From Morgan-Hughes JA: Diseases of striated muscle. In Asbury AK, McKhann GM, McDonald WI, editors: *Diseases of the nervous system: clinical neurobiology*, ed 2, Philadelphia, 1992, WB Saunders, p. 170.)

(Fig. 23.20). Age of diagnosis and fewer D4Z4 repeats are associated with more severe disease.

Other changes in the face include diffuse facial flattening, a pouting lower lip, and inability to pucker the mouth to whistle. Progression is descending, with subsequent involvement of either the distal anterior leg (quadriceps and anterior tibialis) or hip girdle muscles.[348] Weakness of the lower extremities may be delayed for many years. Contractures, skeletal deformities, and hypertrophy of the muscles are uncommon.

There is wide variability in age at onset, disease severity, and side-to-side symmetry, even within affected members of the same family. Associated non–skeletal muscle manifestations include high-frequency hearing loss and retinal telangiectasias, both of which are usually asymptomatic.[348,369]

**Myotonic Dystrophy.** The clinical presentation of myotonic dystrophy represents a spectrum of disease severity that is based on the size of the genetic triple repeat. Three phenotypes have been identified. The most severe is congenital myotonic dystrophy, with weakness and myotonia at birth. The classic form is characterized by weakness and some degree of disability, with mild myotonia and cataracts.

The clinical symptomatology of myotonic dystrophy includes muscle weakness and wasting, with a delayed relaxation of the muscle and increased excitability. Ocular cataracts are also a defining feature; cardiac conduction defects represent a serious comorbidity. A wide variety of other symptoms, including sensorineural hearing loss, hypersomnia, testicular atrophy (and sterility), and endocrine dysfunction, are also found in myotonic dystrophy.[19] People with myotonic dystrophy have muscular weakness, wasting, and hypotonia.

## MEDICAL MANAGEMENT

DIAGNOSIS. Researchers continue to develop noninvasive imaging procedures for evaluating the localization, extent, subtype, and mechanisms of skeletal muscle damage in MD. Diagnosis is currently based on clinical presentation, family history, and diagnostic testing, such as muscle ultrasound or MRI, genetic testing, electromyography (EMG), muscle biopsy, and serum enzymes. The use of these five diagnostic tests with each of the major types of MD is presented briefly in this section.

***Duchenne and Becker Muscular Dystrophy.*** Most cases of Duchenne are identified with the onset of weakness and decline in motor function in the preschool years. Chorionic villi sampling and amniocentesis and preimplantation screening are prenatal diagnostic techniques in which deoxyribonucleic acid (DNA) is removed during gestation to determine the presence or absence of the defective gene. Currently, standard laboratory genetic testing can detect large deletions and duplications of the dystrophin gene in approximately 65% of cases. Most of the remaining 35% of cases represent point mutations and are more difficult to identify but can be found by sequencing the gene or are easily identifiable if the specific mutation that is present in the family is known. New mutations cause 30% of cases of DMD. Mothers who are carriers of a dystrophin gene mutation will pass on the mutated gene to 50% of their daughters (making them carriers) and 50% of sons, who will be affected by DMD.[44]

EMG studies in DMD/BMD demonstrate the presence of fibrillation potentials, positive sharp waves (more in DMD), and long-duration polyphasic motor unit action potentials (MUAPs) (more in BMD) with full recruitment at low force. Nerve conduction velocities are normal in both DMD and BMD.[85] A muscle biopsy specimen shows variation in the size of muscle fibers; central nuclei, inflammatory cells, and fat and connective tissue deposits are prominent characteristics of the biopsy specimen. In DMD the muscle stains negative for dystrophin antibodies, whereas in BMD levels of dystrophin vary.

Serum enzyme levels are used to identify the presence of active muscle breakdown. Levels are extremely high in the first years of life before the onset of clinical weakness and persist as symptoms develop. Eventually, after replacement of muscle substance has become chronic and extensive, the creatinine kinase (CK) level may be only mildly elevated (less than five times normal). Approximately 50% to 60% of female carriers of DMD/BMD have elevated CK. Males affected by DMD/BMD present with CK levels that are approximately 2 to 10 times normal, reflecting active muscle damage.

***Limb-Girdle Muscular Dystrophy.*** LGMD presents with markedly increased levels of CK, however, often not to the same magnitude seen in DMD. EMG and muscle biopsy results demonstrate myopathic changes. EMG findings reveal positive sharp waves, and fibrillation potentials are absent in some individuals and increased in others. Short-duration, small-amplitude MUAPs and an increased number of MUAPs are characteristic of LGMD.[85]

Muscle biopsy specimens present with variable fiber size and atrophy alternating with hypertrophy; in the later stages connective tissue is increased. Muscle in LGMD can be stained for a variety of components of the sarcoglycan complex as well as many other known protein defects. In the context of a suspected sarcoglycanopathy, this often does not provide a specific diagnosis, because defects in one sarcoglycan can affect incorporation of the others; however, the clues provided can lead to appropriate genetic testing to confirm the diagnosis.[361]

*Congenital Muscular Dystrophy.* A good clinical examination will provide insight into the basis of an infant's hypotonia and determine if it is thought to be central in origin (based on soft neurologic signs) or peripheral. However, most of the disorders of glycosylation show a mixed central and peripheral picture, which can complicate the interpretation of the examination. Initial CK will be increased in CMD, and a muscle biopsy specimen will present as an active dystrophic process with a variation in fiber size, fiber splitting, some increase in central nuclei, degenerating fibers, and basophilic staining of regenerating fibers. Combined MUAPs will be diminished, and in merosin-deficient CMD, a mixed picture may be noted, including demyelination.

*Facioscapulohumeral Dystrophy.* In FSHD, serum CK is elevated in 75% of affected individuals. Electrodiagnostic testing demonstrates a myopathic pattern, with positive sharp waves and fibrillation potentials often noted; however, these are less prominent than in DMD. The most striking characteristic in FSHD is short-duration, small-amplitude, polyphasic MUAPs.[85]

Muscle biopsy findings are somewhat dependent on which muscle is biopsied, with variable fiber size and necrotic and regenerating fibers being common; central nuclei and inflammatory infiltrates can also be noted. Analysis for the underlying genetic defect 4q35 can be used to confirm the diagnosis.

*Myotonic Dystrophy.* In myotonic dystrophy microscopic evaluation of muscle and nerve demonstrates alterations. In the muscle, selective atrophy of the type I fibers is noted, with central nuclei and hypertrophic fibers and increased connective tissue present. Nerve biopsy results show a variable degree of demyelination, particularly in large fibers, in addition to regenerating fibers characteristic of axonal neuropathy.[378] EMG is used to document myotonia, with the unmistakable "dive bomber" sound produced by a myotonic discharge.

**TREATMENT.** The improvement in our understanding of the pathogenesis of these diseases has presented the real possibility that some will have effective treatments in the near future.[205,324,375] Current intervention is for the most part directed toward maintaining function in unaffected muscle groups for as long as possible, utilizing supportive measures such as physical and occupational therapy, orthopedic appliances, orthopedic surgery, and pharmaceuticals (corticosteroids for DMD). Children who remain active as long as possible avoid complications (e.g., contractures, pressure ulcers, infections) and deconditioning that are common once they are wheelchair bound.

It is important to remember that there is an active muscle degeneration underlying some of the MDs. Strengthening, especially eccentric exercise, is not helpful and may cause increased weakness, particularly in DMD and other disorders that impact the muscle membrane. Contracture management is the focus of treatment for the therapist and is important in maintaining function in those with MD. Splinting, stretching, serial casting, and assistive technology are mainstays of treatment in this group and should be considered when approaching these clients.

Glucocorticoid therapy (e.g., prednisone and deflazacort) has been used to slow the progression of DMD and BMD. The use of glucocorticoids has become the mainstay of treatment for many individuals with these forms of dystrophy. The use of glucocorticoids has been demonstrated to increase myogenic differentiation, myoblast fusion, and laminin expression in animal models[8] and has been shown to improve muscle force and function in children with DMD.[62] The functional advantage of this medical treatment is the child's ability to maintain independent ambulation, respiratory function, and spinal alignment for longer periods of time.

Stem cell and gene therapy for MD are currently under investigation. Investigators are exploring a variety of ways to exogenously deliver healthy copies of the dystrophin gene to dystrophic muscles[189,229] or to pharmacologically treat the effects of this disease.[53] Experiments in the MDX mouse have investigated gene therapy techniques through the use of viruses to implant a miniversion of the dystrophin gene into dystrophin-deficient muscles to delay or stop muscle degeneration. The main obstacle has been immunologic; however, human trials are on the horizon.

In other research models, attempts have been made to inject skeletal muscles with donor cells, a gene transfer method referred to as myoblast transfer therapy. These myoblasts fuse with diseased muscle fibers and provide the missing gene to replace dystrophin. However, this has not produced a viable treatment approach for clinical application to date.[248,337,374]

There are also treatments on the horizon for specific genetic defects. DMD is the end result of a variety of different genetic mutations in the dystrophin gene. Most people with DMD have large mutations; others have point mutations, duplications, or early stop codon mutations. There is the potential that some of these may be amenable to drug treatments, either to reestablish the reading frame or to facilitate read-through in the case of a premature stop codon.

In a small portion of people (up to 15%) with DMD and other genetic disorders, the underlying genetic defect is a premature stop codon or nonsense mutation (a stop codon normally stops ribosome reading at the appropriate time). The inability to read the genetic material and produce dystrophin in these individuals potentially can be suppressed by compounds that induce read-through.[226]

People with point mutations might be amenable to a treatment with antisense oligonucleotides designed to induce exon skipping. Genes are read in sets of three base pairs. When someone has a point mutation, if it is an out-of-frame mutation, everything after the mutation is shifted and the groups of three base pairs do not produce the appropriate amino acids. These drugs cause

RNA to skip over the exon where the point mutation is present during the transcription process when the introns are removed and the messenger RNA is formed. In this way, the affected exon is removed and the gene is allowed to continue reading in sets of three base pairs with the remaining exons being assembled appropriately.[1,104]

**PROGNOSIS.** Prognosis varies with the type of muscle disease present. As a general rule, the earlier the clinical signs appear the more rapid, progressive, and disabling, though congenital myopathies are a notable exception in some cases. Puberty and the onset of middle age often create the tipping points for functional decline in muscle disease in general because of the rapid change in body size with puberty and the loss of muscle mass that comes with middle age. DMD presents with obvious functional concerns during early childhood with a relatively rapid progression of symptoms and results in death, often in the third or fourth decade of life. Pulmonary complications, resulting from respiratory muscle dysfunction, and cardiac dysfunction in the form of conduction defects or dilated cardiomyopathy are the common sources of morbidity and mortality, although the use of noninvasive ventilation has made cardiac dysfunction the primary cause of mortality in DMD. People with BMD usually live into the fifth decade (their forties) or beyond; mortality is most often related to cardiac dysfunction.

SPECIAL IMPLICATIONS FOR THE THERAPIST 23.6

## *Muscular Dystrophy*

### Precautions

When people with MD become ill or injured and are on bed rest (at home or in the hospital) even for a few days, they may lose many of their functional abilities. For example, a child who falls and breaks a leg and is on bed rest or otherwise immobilized will lose muscle strength and may never regain the ability to ambulate. These children should be encouraged to be as mobile as possible, and, if possible, ambulate for even a few minutes every day during the course of any illness.

Although activity helps individuals maintain functional abilities, strenuous exercise may facilitate the breakdown of muscle fibers, especially in those disorders that involve the integrity of the muscle membrane, so that exercise must be approached cautiously. Low-repetition maximum weightlifting, especially eccentric strengthening, is not recommended. Exercise is best done in the pool or on a bike, where exercise is concentric. Any exercise program should be submaximal, with no postexercise soreness, because the amount of damage to the muscle membrane with exercise is related directly to the magnitude of the stress placed on it during contraction and is related to the degree of postexercise soreness noted.

Respiratory involvement requires careful monitoring of breathing techniques, respiratory movements, and oxygen saturation levels. Monitoring oxygen saturation and/or heart rate during the initiation of an exercise program is recommended. Airway clearance techniques, including the use of percussion and postural drainage and mechanical coughalator or insufflator–exsufflator for assisted cough, are especially useful during illness and to maintain the flexibility of the thoracic cavity.[52]

In the later stages of respiratory compromise nighttime mechanical ventilation (e.g., continuous positive airway pressure or bilevel positive airway pressure delivered by face mask) is an intervention used to rest the respiratory muscles and assure there is not $CO_2$ retention during sleep when the respiratory drive is diminished. Early signs of nighttime hypoventilation include morning headache, nighttime arousals/nightmares, and daytime somnolence; symptomatic children should be referred for evaluation. A major priority for these children is safety during sleep in addition to avoiding or delaying the need for intubation and full-time mechanical ventilation; these noninvasive methods can aid in this goal.[72]

### Therapy Interventions

For individuals with the more disabling forms of MD such as DMD, the therapist can provide anticipatory guidance about the course of the disease and valuable information regarding the use of various types of adaptive equipment. Initially, grab bars provide for safety, but eventually a rolling commode or combination commode and bath chair is needed. As DMD progresses, a power wheelchair provides functional mobility once ambulation is no longer possible.

Eventually, adapted controls (mini-joystick, touch pad, or fiberoptic switches) may be required for the power chair to accommodate the severe weakness and contracture that develop in the later stages of DMD. Power Tilt-In-Space wheelchair systems allow for pressure relief where air or gel cushions are no longer sufficient.

In the individual who no longer has access to a computer for school or work secondary to severe weakness, environmental control systems allow computer access by inferred link and mouse emulation to allow control of the mouse from the wheelchair control or completely hands-free control through the use of voice recognition software.

Overhead slings and mobile arm supports are helpful with feeding and other upper extremity activities, especially after spinal surgery, when axial flexibility is removed and greater active range of motion is required for these functional tasks.

Splinting and night positioning in addition to active and passive range-of-motion exercises will aid in delaying the onset of contractures and reducing the associated morbidity. Once the formation of contractures has occurred serial casting can be considered if ambulation has not progressed to end stage and the person is still strong enough to rise from the floor independently, though it is important to retain the ground reaction force of the gastrocnemius following casting and to only cast to a function range (5 to 10 degrees of dorsiflexion).[115] Home environmental assessment and careful family and client interviews are important in planning out the appropriate adaptive equipment and home modifications.

Both children and adults can benefit from ambulation, bike, and pool therapy programs aimed at improving endurance. For a more in-depth discussion of the direct intervention protocols for this condition, the reader is referred to other resources.[48,73,282]

Inspiratory muscle training improves both force and endurance of the respiratory muscles in this population. These training-related improvements in inspiratory muscle performance are more likely to occur in those who are less severely affected by the disease. In those clients who have disease to the extent that they are already retaining carbon dioxide, little change may occur in respiratory muscle force or endurance with training.[225]

## Congenital Myopathy

### Definition and Overview

Congenital myopathy describes a group of disorders with somewhat similar phenotypic course, including central core disease, nemaline myopathy, multicore-minicore disease, and myotubular myopathy/centronuclear myopathy. The nomenclature of congenital myopathies has traditionally been one driven by the histopathology of the muscle and here we will largely adhere to this while attempting to put it in the context of what is significant genetic overlap between histopathology. A full appreciation of the natural history of each disease in the context of both genetics and histopathologic diagnosis is necessary for treatment planning. As a group they are characterized by weakness at birth or shortly thereafter, with a course that is relatively stable or slowly progressive. Often there are developmental gains made early in the course of the disease while the natural developmental progression of the child is in full force. Later the child might lose skills, as muscle strength does not keep up with the gain in body size; or contractures interfere with function; or where the natural aging process through middle age is accompanied by a decline in muscle strength.

### Incidence

Nemaline myopathy is the most common of these diseases and occurs at a rate of 2 per 100,000 live births.[38] The remaining types each account for a smaller incidence but greater total number of cases (prevalence).

### Pathogenesis

Nemaline myopathy is a heterogeneous disease defined by the appearance of nemaline bodies or rods on muscle biopsy. There are a number of genetic loci identified. The genes, loci, and protein products responsible for the resulting pathology include nebulin (2q21-22, NEB), α-tropomyosin slow (1q22-23, TPM3), β-tropomyosin (p13.2, TPM2), troponin 1 (19q13.4, TNNT1), and α-actin (1q42.1, ACTA1). These genes can have either autosomal dominant loss of function, dominant negative or recessive mutations. The pathophysiology of nemaline myopathy is connected to the abnormality of the actin thin filament or its interaction with myosin and the inevitable abnormality in force production of the contractile potential of the muscle. The genes associated with nemaline myopathy code for proteins either integral to the actin filament; its interaction with myosin; or which act in the regulation, localization, or turnover of actin.[116]

Central core myopathy appears on biopsy with areas of clearing within the cytoplasm, representing areas devoid of mitochondria and replaced by myofibrillar disorganization. This most commonly is the result of a mutation in the ryanodine receptor protein (RYR1) gene (19q13.1) with a defect in the ryanodine receptor and can be inherited both as a recessive (more severe) or dominant gene (less severe). RYR1 functions as part of a calcium release channel. It sits between the T-tubule and the sarcoplasmic reticulum and is integral to the process of excitation-contraction coupling through its regulation of cytosolic calcium homeostasis.[116]

Multicore-minicore myopathy can be the result of a mutation in Selenoprotein N1 *(SEPN1)* gene (1p36), which is inherited recessively, or it can have the same mutation as central core disease (RYR1). Both central core and multicore-minicore myopathy are named because of the characteristics of the muscle biopsy findings. In multicore-minicore myopathy there are several intracellular collections within the muscle cell. In central core, there is one larger collection. These cores occur in type I fibers and lack oxidative enzyme activity. Early in the course of a ryanodine receptor defect, the muscle biopsy specimen can present with multiple intracellular cores. As the disease progresses it may be that these cores coalesce and form one central core, which accounts for the overlap in the genetics of these two diseases. RYR1 codes for a calcium channel on the terminal sarcoplasmic reticulum and results in aberrant release of calcium during excitation-contraction coupling.[116]

Myotubular (centronuclear) myopathy is X-linked and caused by a mutation in the myotubularin gene *(MTM1)* located on Xq28.[38] There are also causative mutations (both dominant and recessive) in a number of other genes ($DNM_2$, $BIN_1$, $RYR_1$, TTN, $MTMR_{14}$, SPEG, and $CCDC_{78}$) that can result in the centronuclear histopathologic presentation defined by the presence of central nuclei, by convention greater than 25%, found in the muscle biopsy. Myotubularin is involved in membrane trafficking and remodeling related to the formation of the excitation contraction coupling apparatus and neuromuscular junction, including the T-tubules and sarcoplasmic reticulum.[116]

### Clinical Manifestations

**Nemaline Myopathy.** Nemaline myopathy presents in a phenotypically heterogeneous way with five types identified. Type 1 is the severe congenital form, type 2 the intermediate form, type 3 the most typical, and types 4 and 5 present in childhood or adulthood, respectively.

The typical form presents in infancy and is characterized by hypotonia throughout the body, including the face. Feeding difficulties, including aspiration and respiratory insufficiency, initially present at night and are common comorbidities. Contractures and spinal rigidity are also common; there is both weakness of the extremities and a lack of flexibility of the trunk, especially in flexion. Rigid spine presentation is typical in individuals who have selenoprotein defects.

**Central Core Myopathy.** Central core myopathy as the result of recessive mutations typically presents in infancy but can also present later when it is the result of a dominant mutation. CK levels are usually normal or only mildly elevated. Common comorbidities include congenital hip dislocation, scoliosis, and talipes equinovarus. Because there is often variable penetrance, members of the same family can have varied phenotypic presentations. Anyone with central core disease is at risk for malignant hyperthermia, a severe and life-threatening reaction to certain anesthetics.

**Multicore-Minicore Myopathy.** Four groups of multicore-minicore myopathy have been identified. The classic form is characterized by proximal weakness and scoliosis, as well as pulmonary insufficiency. Distal joint laxity is a common finding. Myopia is a common visual finding. Individuals with group II have ophthalmoplegia and severe facial weakness in addition to more global weakness. Individuals classified as having group III disease also have arthrogryposis and early onset.

**Myotubular (Centronuclear) Myopathy.** Myotubular myopathy is very phenotypically variable, with a range of presentations possible. The severe neonatal form is the most common type and can lead to death in the first year of life. Despite the fact that many have life-threatening pulmonary involvement, those who receive intensive ventilatory support can survive past the first year, gain strength, and show improvement in their respiratory status as they progress past the first year. Even so, upper respiratory infections remain significant challenges for many affected individuals. A less-common form presents with a milder course and survival into adulthood.[38,347]

## MEDICAL MANAGEMENT

DIAGNOSIS. Diagnosis of congenital myopathy is made first by clinical examination. The differentiation of central versus peripheral causes of the hypotonia will help guide the physician's workup. These factors include deep tendon reflexes, upper motor neuron signs, and cognitive status.

If a peripheral process is suspected, one must include spinal muscular atrophy (discussed below) on the differential for weak infants since it is treatable and can be ruled out by genetic testing or EMG can differentiate a neurogenic versus myogenic process with a subsequent muscle biopsy performed to evaluate the histopathologic characteristics of the muscle. Special stains or electron microscopy can be ordered to further narrow the possible diagnoses with genetic testing to confirm the genetics of the diagnosis.

TREATMENT. Treatment is primarily symptomatic. Management of contractures is important in maintaining function, and supportive pulmonary care is important, especially in those clients who develop nocturnal hypoventilation. Cardiac monitoring is important for those with a propensity toward cardiac symptoms.

## Spinal Muscular Atrophy

### Overview and Incidence

Spinal muscular atrophy (SMA) is a neuromuscular disease characterized by progressive weakness and wasting of skeletal muscles resulting from anterior horn cell degeneration. SMA is the second most common fatal autosomal recessive disorder after cystic fibrosis. The overall incidence is 1 in 6000 to 1 in 10,000 live births, and 1 in 40 to 1 in 60 individuals carry the genetic defect with sub-Saharin African and some other isolated populations having higher or lower carrier frequencies[372] (Table 23.6).

SMA in the untreated natural history represents a phenotype that is accompanied by slowly progressive loss of function. The earlier the first symptoms are noted the more severe the weakness and more rapid the progression. The recent approval of Nusinersen,[98,232] and the promise of other medications still in clinical trials,[230,292] has provided an altered natural history of SMA. Many patients, with treatment, now show functional improvement over time that is propelled by an increase in underlying muscle strength.

Childhood SMA is classically divided into SMA type I, SMA type II, and SMA type III, with some also including a type 0 and type IV for fetal and adult onset presentations. There are also a group of disorders genetically distinct from the most common form; these represent a motor only nerve disease that some authors include under the SMA umbrella, while many others classify these with Charcot-Marie-Tooth disease.[165] Here we will discuss only the most common form that results from homozygous deletion of the survival of motor neuron gene (*SMN1*) on the fifth chromosome. SMA type I, the more severe or acute form, is referred to as Werdnig-Hoffmann disease and causes respiratory failure and early death, typically in the first few years of life, if left untreated; type 0 is an even more severe presentation, with weakness evident at birth. Kugelberg-Welander disease, or type III SMA, is the mild form (with type IV even milder and later onset). These individuals learn to walk without assistance; a relatively slow progression of weakness is noted in type III. SMA type II represents an intermediate form; affected individuals demonstrate the ability to sit independently at some point, but significant functional impairment and reliance on power mobility is typical when left untreated (see Table 23.6). Despite the classification system that divides SMA into three types based on the maximal independent motor skill achieved, SMA really represents a continuous spectrum of severity, and with the approval of disease modifying therapies[98] the division of SMA into subgroups based on function seems somewhat artificial as many children will be diagnosed and classified in one group and will progress and require reclassification as they gain skills, which is rarely the case in the untreated natural history.

### Etiologic Factors and Pathogenesis

The basis of this recessively inherited motor neuron disease is a genetic mutation in the *SMN1* gene found on the long arm of chromosome 5 (5q13.1).[113] The *SMN1* gene is defective in 99% of all cases of SMA and is the cause of SMA. The *NAIP* gene is defective in 45% of the more severely involved type I individuals, and it has been proposed that an NAIP deletion is associated with SMA severity.[4,158] The *SMN1* gene has a homologous gene, which is an inverted duplicated centromeric copy, termed

**Table 23.6** Spinal Muscular Atrophy

| Type | Incidence | Onset | Inheritance | Features | Course |
|---|---|---|---|---|---|
| SMA type I (Werdnig-Hoffmann; acute or severe form) | Overall incidence for all types of SMA is 1 in 6000-10,000 live births[272,273] | 0-3 mo | Autosomal recessive | LEs flexed, abducted, and externally rotated (frog position)<br>UEs abducted, externally rotated, unable to move to midline against gravity<br>Poor head control<br>Significantly decreased muscle tone/weakness<br>Decreased newborn movements, decreased diaphragmatic movements<br>High risk of scoliosis<br>Proximal muscle weakness greater than distal weakness<br>Weak cry and cough<br>Normal sensation and intellect | Rapidly progressive<br>Severe hypotonia<br>65% survive 4th year[265] but only 28% of those with less than 16 hours of ventilation.<br>50% survive 10 years but only 16% of those with less than 16 hours of ventilation[265] |
| SMA type II (intermediate form) | 27% of SMA Dx is type II | Before 18 months | Autosomal recessive | LEs flexed, abducted, and externally rotated<br>Limited trunk control<br>Weakness<br>Increased risk of scoliosis<br>Normal sensation and intellect | Progressive but stabilizes<br>Moderate to severe hypotonia<br>Shortened life span,[242] although a 100% survival has been reported to 10 years of age[213]<br>Attain the ability to sit at some point<br>Reliance on power mobility |
| SMA type III (Kugelberg-Welander; mild form) | 13% of SMA Dx is type III | Present after 18 months | Autosomal recessive | Proximal weakness (greatest with trunk, hip, knee extension)<br>Trendelenburg gait, especially with running<br>Slow continued development progression; sits independently<br>Walks independently (lumbar lordosis, waddling gait, genu recurvatum, protuberant abdomen)<br>Wheelchair bound early adulthood (dependent on age of onset)<br>Good UE strength | Slowly progressive<br>Attain the ability to ambulate at some point<br>Wheelchair dependence determined by age of onset: with onset prior to 2 years of age, 50% lose ambulation ability by 12 years of age; with onset after 2 years of age, 50% lose ambulation by 44 years of age[304] |

*LE*, Lower extremity; *UE*, upper extremity.

*SMN2*, that can compensate for the absence of *SMN1* by producing survival motor neuron (SMN) protein, although in reduced quantities. *SMN2* can be present in multiple copies; the more copies of *SMN2* present, the more SMN protein is produced, and the milder the phenotype becomes.[332]

Although SMA is now recognized to be a multisystem disease, developmental arrest, dysfunction, and progressive degeneration of anterior horn cells of the spinal cord is the most functionally impactful pathologic result. In the remaining motor neurons, axonal sprouting occurs, resulting in enlarged motor units. The underlying pathogenesis of anterior horn cell loss appears to be the persistence of programmed cell death in the anterior horn cells[331]; however, motor neuron and neuromuscular junction dysfunction are also important components of the impairment of neuromuscular function. Diminished motor neuron drive from the proprioceptive portion of the reflex arc influences motor neuron function. Abnormalities in microtubule structure that underlies mitochondrial axonal transport impacts overall neuronal health and acyl choline management at the neuromuscular junction that results in abnormalities in acetylcholine distribution and abnormal endocytic function limiting acetylcholine handling appear to underlie the dysfunction of existing motor neurons. This is characterized in part by increased input resistance created as the result of sustained depolarization and the resulting sodium channel inactivation.[56,80,101]

The SMN protein has a number of isoforms. The main SMN isoform is full-length protein and is ubiquitously expressed at the highest levels early in development and is localized primarily to the nucleus and cytoplasm in addition to axons, dendrites, and synapses. There are a number of other isoforms of SMN that represent shortened SMN proteins with developmentally or tissue-specific expression, while the function characteristics of other isoforms has yet to be elucidated.[56]

The *SMN1* gene mutation decreases intracellular levels of SMN protein present in the cytoplasm and nucleus of all cells. SMN protein functions as part of the splicing mechanism during protein production, ultimately preventing motor neuron cell death.[169] The variability of phenotype in SMA is related to the presence of multiple copies of the *SMN2* gene. *SMN2* is an almost identical copy of *SMN1* except for a difference in exon 7, where there is a single base pair C>T change which diminishes the likelihood of inclusion of exon 7 through the impairment of an exonic splicing enhancer at the pre–messenger RNA stage.[46,345] The partial splicing alteration results from the formation of a portion of *SMN2* mRNA that is impaired in producing the gene product SMN. Only 10% of the protein that *SMN1* produces occurs as a result of the altered splicing.[93] This results in various intracellular levels of SMN that are dependent on how many copies of the *SMN2* gene are present.

From the many animal models of SMA that have been produced, it is known that SMN is found in the nucleus and cytoplasm of all cells and is needed functionally for all cells. SMN functions in the nucleus as part of the spliceosome in U12 splicing dependent genes. U12 dependent splicing represents a minority of protein production in the body, with the U2 mechanism accounting for most of the body's protein formation. In order for SMN to act in the splicing mechanism, it first needs to be assembled into its functional protein complex, and is trafficked out of the nucleus where it binds with Unrip and seven Gemin proteins.[326] This complex facilitates the formation of small nuclear ribonucleoproteins that are important in the structure of the spliceosome once the complex is transported back into the nucleus, where it colocalizes with Gems and coiled (cajal) bodies which are associated with RNA processing, splicing, and ribosomal formation.[179] The spliceosome functions in the removal of the introns and the assembly of the exons in preparation for formation of amino acids by the ribosome.[93]

The spinal alpha motor neurons are specifically sensitive to low levels of SMN, and the result is a reduced pool of anterior horn cells. In addition, in the remaining anterior horn cell pool there is an alteration of the structure and function of the existing motor neurons.[93] Ultimately children with SMA have a diminished number of poorly functioning anterior horn cells that create a diminished neuronal output.

### Clinical Manifestations

The natural history of SMA is characterized by progressive atrophy of skeletal muscles resulting from the partial denervation, there is a variable degree of weakness, and fatigue is reported as the primary phenotypic characteristics of SMA. Often restrictive lung disease is present and this is the major source of mortality in the most severe forms. Initial weakness and loss of motor strength in the natural history is noted around the time of presentation but muscle strength can remain stable over long periods of time and medical intervention with SMN modulating therapies can improve strength and function over time.[98,232] That said, the natural history is characterized by a slowly progressive loss of motor function that is detectable only over years as well as contracture formation that limits functional progression.[308] Explanations for this loss of function remain undetermined, but decrease in motor function could be caused by factors such as increased body size.[152]

Children with SMA type I present with features of this disorder within the first days or few months of life. Hypotonia and severe generalized weakness is characteristic and infants with SMA type I are unable to sit unsupported. Children with type II present before age 18 months with chronic weakness and attain independent sitting but never walk without assistance. Individuals with type III SMA are able to ambulate independently at some point in their lives, although they often require the use of a wheelchair by puberty or middle age, with the rate of progression dependent on the age of the onset of symptoms. Clinical problems associated with the muscle weakness seen in SMA include feeding and nutrition, respiratory, and orthopedic, including scoliosis.

## MEDICAL MANAGEMENT

**DIAGNOSIS.** The diagnosis may be made at birth on the basis of newborn screening or is suspected on the basis of clinical manifestations, muscle biopsy, or EMG in which a neuropathic pattern is found. Nerve conduction velocities should be normal; combined motor action potentials are decreased in magnitude.

Clinically, the first symptom noted is the presence of weakness that should be evaluated in the context of the rapidity of onset and the child's age. Deep tendon reflexes are typically absent, suggesting a disorder of the peripheral nerve, and sensation will be intact, including vibratory sense. Fasciculations may also be noted in the tongue and more reliably will be seen on muscle ultrasound.

On needle EMG, fibrillations and sharp waves (hyperexcitability caused by denervation) are usually present and action potentials are high amplitude (showing large motor units) with polyphasic morphology (indicating denervation/reinnervation).[344] Muscle biopsy specimens show groups of small atrophic fibers, representing those without anterior horn cells and those with anterior horn cells, alternating with large hypertrophic fibers. Genetic testing for a homozygous deletion of the *SMN1* gene confirms the diagnosis.

**TREATMENT.** Treatment is symptomatic and preventive, primarily building strength, preventing pulmonary infection, and treating or preventing secondary orthopedic problems, including contracture and scoliosis. Feeding problems are common, especially in cases with bulbar muscle weakness; gastrostomy tube feedings are often necessary to optimally manage nutrition.[233]

Respiratory problems (involvement of the intercostals) are common in the type 1 population. Oronasal suctioning, percussion and postural drainage, and treatments with an in-exsufflator (also known as coughalator) will help in the removal of bronchial secretions

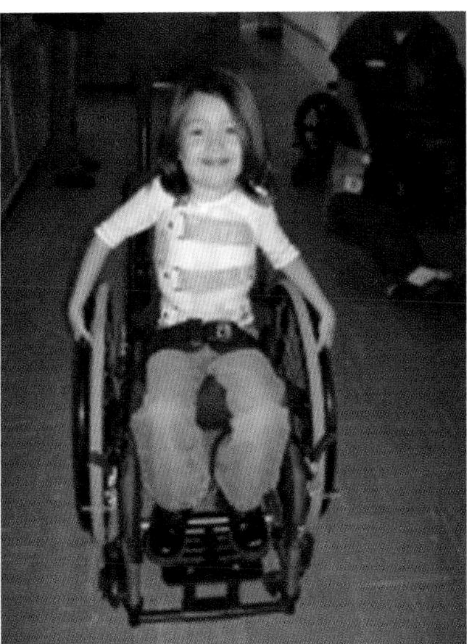

**Figure 23.21**

**Spinal muscular atrophy (SMA).** This 4-year-old child with SMA type II is fitted with a one-piece body jacket or thoracolumbosacral orthosis (TLSO). The TLSO offers support and control of the trunk and lower spine for improved sitting posture, balance, and greater stability. Full body jackets of this type may increase the work of breathing; an abdominal cutout (not present in this body jacket) to allow diaphragmatic excursion is typically provided for individuals with SMA who rely on diaphragmatic respiration due to the pattern of muscular weakness. The chair is a titanium ultralight wheelchair, which this child can propel for independent mobility. (Courtesy Tamara Kittelson-Aldred, Access Therapy Services, Missoula, MT. Used with permission.)

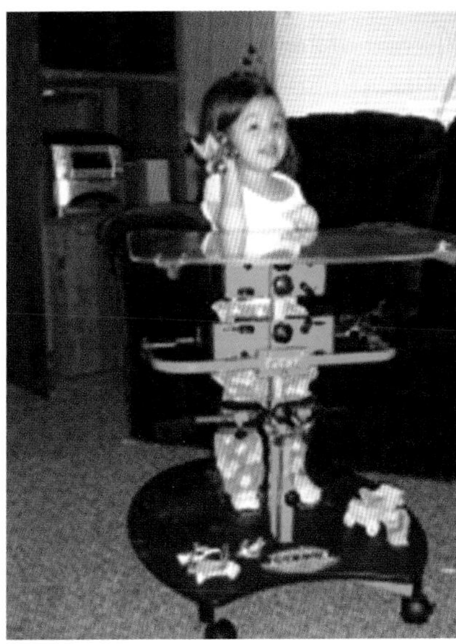

**Figure 23.22**

**Static vertical standing frame provides support and stability in the upright position for the child with spinal muscular atrophy.** Ankle-foot orthoses provide support for weight bearing through the lower extremities. (Courtesy Tamara Kittelson-Aldred, Access Therapy Services, Missoula, MT. Used with permission.)

from the respiratory tract and can aid in airway clearance, especially during intercurrent illness, and will maintain flexibility of the chest wall with chronic use. Positive-pressure ventilatory support, typically by noninvasive bilevel positive airway pressure (initially at night), can extend the life span in the most severely involved individuals.[99]

The majority of people with SMA type I or II develop some degree of scoliosis; individuals with SMA type III who become nonambulatory are also at risk for the development of scoliosis. Bracing has not been found to delay the progression of scoliosis but might help with sitting balance and posture (Fig. 23.21). Care should be taken to allow good diaphragmatic movement and not create increased respiratory effort if a soft spinal orthosis is chosen to manage sitting posture. There are a variety of flexible garments, some with semirigid stays to provide additional stability and others with a more rigid plastic shell that can aid in sitting posture.

Spinal fusion is the primary means of management for scoliosis. Although fusion is often necessary, there is some consequence to function. Many will not return completely to their prior functional level.[110] In addition, the thorax no longer grows once a fusion is complete and as a result ultimate vital capacity is diminished. Two types of spinal instrumentation (growing rods and vertical expandable prosthetic titanium ribs) allow the thorax to continue to grow when scoliosis is noted at a young age so a spinal fusion can be delayed till the majority of growth is complete at 12 years of age. Individuals with type II SMA can also develop hip subluxation or dislocation, but this is not typically painful, and the literature on surgical correction is mixed.

Individuals with type II SMA should participate in a standing program (Fig. 23.22). Knee-ankle-foot orthoses (KAFOs) with ischial weight bearing or parapodiums are ideal for this in the younger age group and standers for older children may be best. However, as contractures develop, standing will become more difficult despite the most aggressive splinting, range-of-motion, and serial casting program. SMA type III clients initially ambulate, although the natural history is that about half of this group loses ambulatory skills in childhood or adolescence.

**PROGNOSIS.** Prognosis varies according to age of onset or type of SMA (see Table 23.6). The earlier the disease occurs, the faster the progression of muscle weakness and the poorer the prognosis without medical intervention. The presence of respiratory distress also contributes to a poorer prognosis. Earlier treatment with disease modifying therapies typically provides for a better prognosis, with progressive improvement over time.[100]

SMA type I is the most severe with death likely in the first years of life as a result of respiratory insufficiency or infection without medical attention. Most children with this form of SMA do not survive past 3 years without the aid of mechanical ventilation. Clients with type III (with onset after 2 years of age) typically remain independently ambulatory into adult life; if onset is before 2 years, loss of ambulatory ability at an average age of 12 years is typical and patients with type 2 have an intermediate course.[304]

SPECIAL IMPLICATIONS FOR THE THERAPIST 23.7

## *Spinal Muscular Atrophy*

### Precautions

The infant or child with SMA who lacks independent mobility requires frequent changes of position to prevent skin problems and other complications, especially pneumonia. Suctioning to remove secretions in the more severe cases may be required, and feeding must be carried out slowly and carefully with good positioning to prevent aspiration in those individuals with oral motor involvement. The involvement of a therapist with specialization in feeding (usually an occupational therapist or speech-language pathologist) is essential for these children.

Respiratory weakness or diminished head control may prevent the child from tolerating prone positioning. This is especially problematic when the child cannot lift the head to clear the airway. The use of prone positioning must be evaluated and monitored carefully by the therapist because children with SMA breathe primarily with the diaphragm and prone position restricts abdominal expansion. In addition, changes of position in the more severe patients prompt the movement of secretions within the pulmonary system and need to be managed with coughalator and suctioning. Vertical positions (sitting and standing) tend to be the most functional, primarily for biomechanical reasons because the head is balanced above the trunk and the strength required is less than in prone or quadruped; however, they might be more challenging than horizontal from a respiratory standpoint.

Monitoring oxygen saturation levels may be necessary in evaluating programming effectiveness, especially in the person with type I SMA. Observe how much work is required to breathe, and whenever possible use a pulse oximeter to measure oxygen saturation noninvasively.

### Therapy Intervention

Specific treatment protocols for this condition are beyond the scope of this book. The therapist is referred to a more appropriate resource.[48,231,349] An overall management program should include positioning to encourage head and trunk control and to promote functional strengthening, in addition to splinting and stretching to maintain range of motion. Assistive technology can provide the maximum possible independence for children with SMA.

Power mobility for the child with SMA who has no independent mobility is essential and should be considered in the child as young as 18 months to 2 years of age (Fig. 23.23); however, in the context of improving strength as children age and receive medical treatment, an assessment of the potential for manual wheelchair mobility must be considered as well.[350] Low-technology solutions, such as "slings and springs," mobile arm supports, or body weight support systems for exercise also may be very liberating for the child who has limited antigravity movement by providing a wide variety of exploratory opportunities and to provide the potential to exercise beyond the range available with the full impact of gravity.

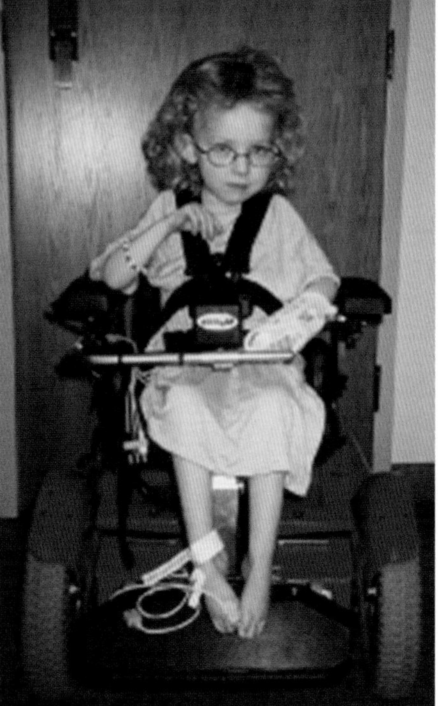

**Figure 23.23**

**Spinal muscular atrophy (SMA).** Three-year-old with SMA in her power wheelchair, which allows her to adjust the seat height so that she can be on the floor to aid with transfers or at eye level with her peers. The adjustable seat allows the child to participate in activities at elevated surfaces (e.g., counter or table heights), retrieve objects from a shelf, or help decorate the tree at Christmas. (Courtesy Allan Glanzman, The Children's Hospital of Philadelphia, PA.)

Facilitation and active assistive work toward standing and ambulation can be effective in increasing strength through closed chain exercise, and standing can help reduce the incidence of contracture and build strength. More severely involved clients may benefit from positioning in a standing frame or KAFOs.

Inspiratory muscle training also has been found to be effective in neuromuscular disorders in improving maximal voluntary ventilation, maximal inspiratory mouth pressure, as well as respiratory load perception,[118,390] and should be considered in this population.

Aquatic therapy can be a valuable adjunct to traditional intervention strategies for people at all levels of the SMA continuum. By using the physical properties of water, such as buoyancy, hydrostatic pressure, viscosity, and turbulence, the therapist provides additional tools for intervention, especially in the case of extreme weakness characteristic of this disorder.[96, 98]

# TORTICOLLIS

## Definition and Overview

*Torticollis* (congenital muscular torticollis [CMT]; wry neck) means twisted neck and is a contracted state of the sternocleidomastoid muscle (SCM), producing head tilt toward the shortened SCM, with rotation of the chin to the

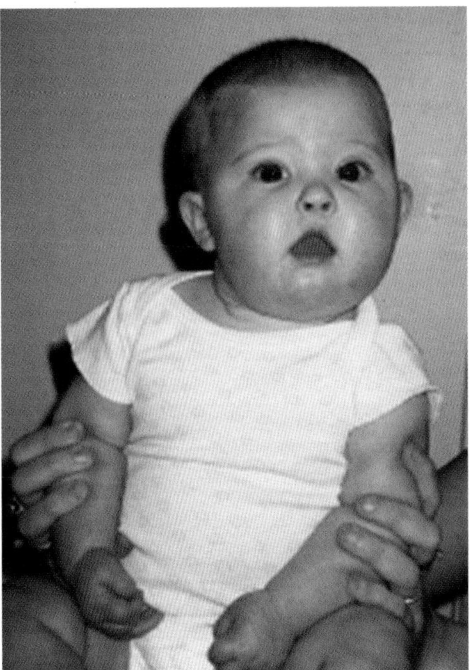

**Figure 23.24**

**Torticollis.** Five-month-old with torticollis (head tilt toward the involved side and rotation away from the involved side). (Courtesy Allan Glanzman, The Children's Hospital of Philadelphia, PA.)

**Table 23.7** Classification of Torticollis

| Nonparoxysmal (Nondynamic) Torticollis | Paroxysmal (Dynamic) Torticollis |
|---|---|
| 1. Congenital muscular torticollis<br>Intrauterine constraint<br>Birth trauma<br>2. Osseous torticollis<br>Congenial<br>Traumatic<br>Inflammatory<br>3. Central nervous system/ peripheral nervous system torticollis<br>Brain<br>Posterior fossa<br>Basal ganglia<br>Spinal cord<br>Spinal nerve root/ peripheral nerve<br>4. Ocular torticollis<br>Superior oblique muscle palsy<br>Other ocular deviations<br>Spasmus nutans<br>5. Nonmuscular, soft tissue torticollis Infectious | 1. Benign paroxysmal torticollis<br>2. Spasmodic (cervical dystonia)<br>Primary<br>Secondary<br>3. Sandifer syndrome<br>4. Drug-induced torticollis<br>5. Torticollis from increased intracranial pressure<br>6. Torticollis as a conversion disorder |

From Tomczak K, Rosman P: Torticollis, *J Child Neurol* 28(3):365-378, 2012.

opposite side (Fig. 23.24). It can develop prenatally (congenital) or postnatally (acquired) and can be accompanied by cranial and facial asymmetries. These asymmetries are rarely seen when torticollis is postnatally acquired.[155] Four types of muscle abnormalities have been identified on ultrasonography: 15% have a fibrotic mass in the SCM (type 1), 77% have diffuse fibrosis mixed with normal muscle (type II), 5% have fibrotic tissue without normal muscle (type III), and the last group (type IV) present with a fibrotic cord and represent only 3% of the population.

Traditionally medical classification of torticollis has been divided into congenital and acquired types but there are instances when a particular cause can be prenatal, perinatal, or postnatal. Instead, recent[261] classification divides torticollis into two main categories: nonparoxysmal (static) and paroxysmal (dynamic or episodic) (Table 23.7).[355] In a recent clinical practice guideline published by the Pediatric Academy of the American Physical Therapists Association, CMT is subcategorized as postural, muscular, and SCM mass.[163] This most common form of torticollis, CMT (musculoskeletal phenomenon), is the focus of this section. In addition to the aforementioned classifications, it should be noted that there are multiple taxonomies that exist for CMT in the literature, including based on severity of ROM limitations.[59] Cervical dystonia, though often confused with CMT, is a dynamic form of torticollis (movement disorder) and is presented separately in this text (see "Dystonia" in Chapter 31).

## Incidence and Etiologic Factors

The incidence of CMT ranges from 3.92%[257] to 16%[340] of newborns, with a 3:2 male predominance.[4,140] The two most frequently cited causes of CMT are intrauterine malposition and birth trauma.[355] Other theories on etiology include overcrowding (first born or one of multiple births) during intrauterine life that causes a contracture and development of a compartment syndrome in the SCM from prolonged time in the birth canal.[140] Exact etiology remains unknown.

Incidence is increased in breech (19%) and forceps (6%) delivery, vacuum extraction (30.5%), and cesarean section (17.9%).[58] Predisposing factors can include poor muscle tone or cervical-vertebral abnormalities. Heredity may also account for CMT.[57,91]

## Pathogenesis

The possible pathogenesis of the muscular fibrosis seen in CMT has been explored experimentally in animal models and has been produced through venous occlusion, and this, in addition to arterial occlusion, has been proposed as the possible pathogenesis.[147]

One theory postulates that the malposition of the head potentially leads to a compartment syndrome. In this scenario, the SCM is not stretched or torn, but rather kinked or compressed. With the head and neck in a position of forward flexion, lateral bend, and rotation, the ipsilateral SCM kinks, causing an ischemic injury and subsequent edema.[71]

## Clinical Manifestations

The first sign of CMT identified in only a portion of affected children is a firm, nontender, palpable enlargement of the

SCM often referred to as a sternocleidomastoid tumor of infancy. A portion of cases demonstrate bulbous fibrotic tissue in the inferior third[140] of the involved SCM. This local lesion usually reaches its maximal size by 1 month and then slowly regresses within 4 to 8 months and does not always result in torticollis.[363] The typical position observed of lateral head tilt and rotation to the opposite side predominates regardless of whether a fibrotic mass is present (estimated in 15%-66% of cases[147,151]) or no mass is palpated and the muscle is uniformly fibrotic and shortened.

If the torticollis is left untreated the deformity can become severe, and the infant's face, ear, and head flatten from resting on the affected side, a condition referred to as plagiocephaly ("oblique head"); this cranial asymmetry gradually worsens. The infant's chin turns away from the side of the shortened muscle, the head tilts to the shortened side, and the shoulder is elevated on the affected side, further limiting cervical movement. Plagiocephaly (best observed by looking down on the head from above) is usually marked by the side of the flattened forehead, which is accompanied by the contralateral occipital flattening. When torticollis and plagiocephaly occur together, this condition is referred to as plagiocephaly–torticollis deformation sequence (Fig. 23.25).

The incidence of other deformities, such as developmental dysplasia of the hip, hip dislocation, and clubfoot is elevated in cases of CMT.[58,140] Subluxation or bony anomalies of the cervical spine can also be associated with CMT and should be ruled out by cervical spine radiographs.[147,333]

## MEDICAL MANAGEMENT

**DIAGNOSIS.** Clinical examination combined with the history forms the basis of the initial diagnostic process. Medical evaluation including radiographic studies of the spine is always indicated to rule out congenital deformities of the cervical spine, ocular disorders, and, less frequently, tumors or other CNS pathology in children with presumed torticollis. Ultrasonography has been shown to be useful for evaluating neck masses in children; it has high sensitivity and facilitates easier follow up and reevaluation after treatment.[57]

PT examination should include documentation of asymmetries of the skull and face. One of the most clinically feasible tools is the classification scales by Argenta.[371] If available, other more reliable tools such as plagiocephalometry and the modified Severity Scale for Assessment of Plagiocephaly should be used.[263,371]

**TREATMENT.** The primary treatment of CMT is physical therapy to correct the contracture in the SCM. First choice of interventions should include neck passive range of motion, neck and trunk active range of motion, development of symmetrical movement, environmental adaptations, and parent/caregiver education.[163] Passive range of motion should be performed twice daily to stretch the shortened muscle; stabilization of the proximal attachment of the SCM and trapezius is important to ensure appropriate elongation of the muscle. Positioning/environmental adaptations are important to encourage erect and midline head posture. Strengthening activities should also be included, both active and active assistive exercises, in addition to the incorporation of postural reactions in treatment when these reactions begin to develop.[166]

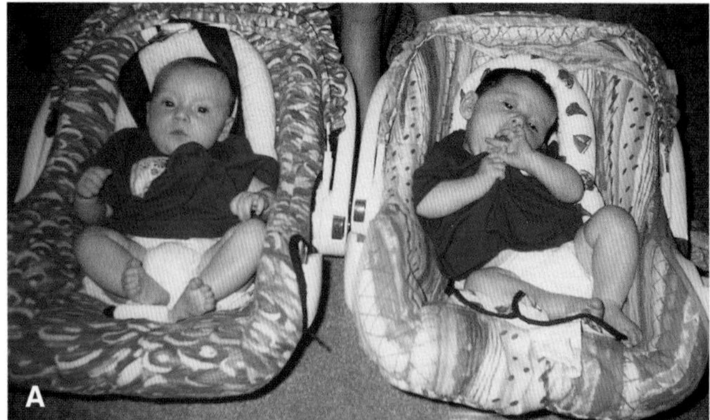

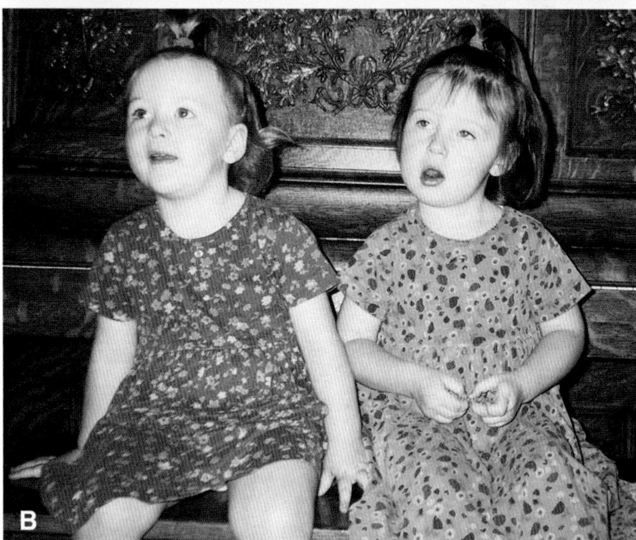

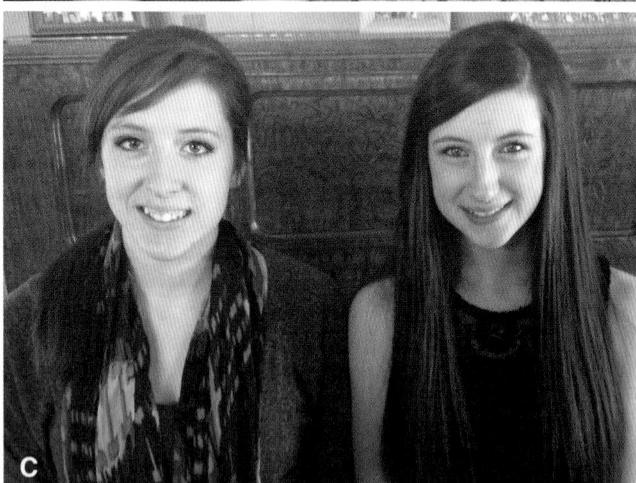

**Figure 23.25**

**Plagiocephaly–torticollis deformation.** (A) Four-month-old fraternal twins: the child on the right has marked untreated congenital muscular torticollis (CMT) with plagiocephaly. Note the positional pelvic asymmetry from placement in a car seat. (B) The same twins (2 years old) after physical therapy (PT) intervention at age 6 months for the child on the right. PT intervention over a 3-month period of time included passive range of motion, facilitated active range of motion, positioning, and a cervical collar. A home exercise program was prescribed with periodic rechecks. Eventually the use of a helmet was instituted to remodel craniofacial asymmetry (see Fig. 23.27). Some craniofacial asymmetry persists, although full active and passive range of motion are present. (C) The same twins as teenagers in high school. (Courtesy Laurie Matteson, Great Falls, MT. Used with permission.)

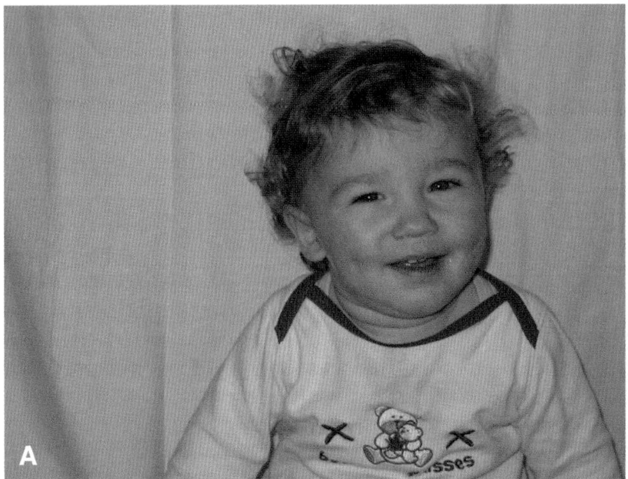

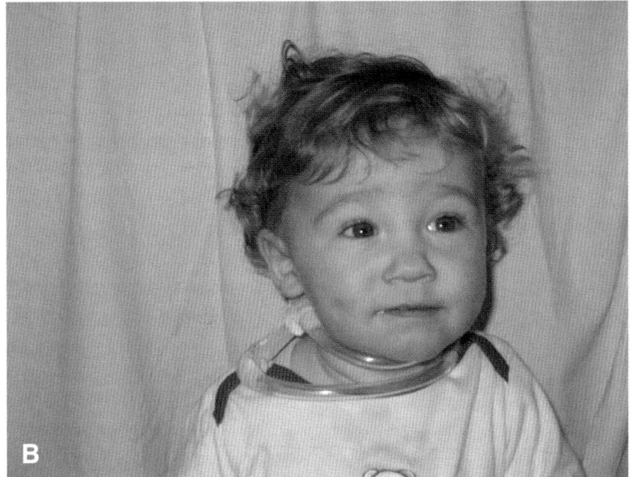

**Figure 23.26**

**Congenital torticollis.** (A) Note the head tilt in this toddler with right-sided congenital torticollis. Despite his full range of motion, he has an occasional residual head tilt to the right and turn to the left. (B) The same child wearing a TOT Collar (tubular orthosis for torticollis) to encourage a more vertical head position. (Courtesy Allan Glanzman, The Children's Hospital of Philadelphia, PA.)

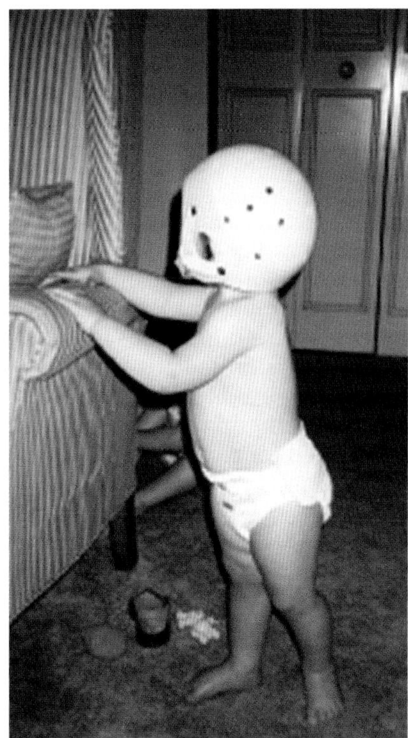

**Figure 23.27**

**Fourteen-month-old girl wearing a polypropylene helmet lined with durometer foam.** This helmet placed remodeling pressure on the cranium to reshape unresolved craniofacial asymmetry that persisted as a result of delayed medical intervention and inconsistent use of a cervical collar. The helmet was accepted readily by the child and worn at all times (except for bathing) for approximately 4 months. Pressure was applied to the right posterior occiput to bring the head and neck into midline alignment, while space was created where the skull was flattened in the left posterior occipital area to allow for bony growth in that area. See Fig. 23.25B, for intervention outcome. (Courtesy Laurie Matteson, Great Falls, MT. Used with permission.)

Splinting has been advocated by some for older children (older than 4 months) who continue to demonstrate head tilt.[155] A cervical collar or tubular orthosis for torticollis can be helpful in providing tactile cueing for movement in the direction opposite the lateral tilt. Usually these collars are the most effective at a time that is compatible with active head control in supported sitting and more than 5 or 6 degrees of head tilt. (Fig. 23.26).[167]

In cases of delayed treatment or where craniofacial asymmetry persists, nonsurgical remodeling of the skull using externally applied pressure can be used (Fig. 23.27). With advances in computer software and technology (e.g., pressure scanners), researchers are determining the pressure per square inch (psi) that applies the appropriate force needed to achieve the remodeling process for each individual head diameter, volume, and topography.[367,368] It is recommend that if little improvement is seen after 6 to 8 weeks of repositioning and physical therapy, then cranial orthotic therapy should be considered while there is still enough head growth to allow for correction.[119]

In patients younger than 1 year of age who do not respond to a manual therapy course, botulinum toxin A injection has been shown to have some benefit.[140,193] Surgical intervention is rare (e.g., SCM tenotomy, plastic surgery for craniofacial asymmetry) and is considered only if the individual continues to demonstrate significant motion restrictions of 30 degrees after 6 months of age or the deformity persists past 12 months of age. A unipolar release of the sternal or clavicular heads of the SCM is the most common surgical intervention for children younger than 3 years of age.[140] Increased thickening of the SCM or increased deformity are also indications to consider surgical intervention.[166]

**PROGNOSIS.** CMT usually resolves with conservative treatment. Complete recovery, including full passive range of motion, can be expected to take approximately 3 to 12 months; the earlier intervention is started typically results in shorter duration of treatment.[163] However, recurrence with growth is sometimes seen and a period of follow up after resolution is warranted. Fewer than 16% of children presenting in the first year ultimately require surgery.[87] Left untreated or poorly managed, chronic, unresolved torticollis can result in persistent deformity and asymmetry of the head shape and position.

SPECIAL IMPLICATIONS FOR THE THERAPIST 23.8

*Torticollis*

Physical therapists should discontinue direct PT services when 5 criteria are met: PROM within 5 degrees of the nonaffected side, symmetrical active movement patterns, age appropriate motor development, no visible head tilt, and the parents/caregivers understand what to monitor as the child grows.[163] When parents are provided with more precise information about the length of treatment, parents may be more willing to adhere to the exercise program.[88] Torticollis that does not respond to physical therapy may have a nonmuscular cause, such as bony anomaly or ocular disorders, and may require further medical evaluation and should be referred for reevaluation if a child does not respond to therapy.

**Postoperative**

After surgery for this condition, postoperative bracing to position the lengthened muscle on stretch has been advocated to allow the muscle to heal in the lengthened position.[155] Standard postoperative monitoring of vital signs and skin condition is recommended. Relapse is common if postoperative rehabilitation is inadequate.[140]

# BRACHIAL PLEXUS BIRTH PALSY

## Definition and Overview

Brachial plexus injury at birth can be divided into a number of categories. Erb palsy is a paralysis of the upper limb typically resulting from a traction injury to the brachial plexus at birth. Erb palsy actually is made up of three distinct types of brachial plexus palsies: (1) Erb-Duchenne palsy affecting the C5 to C6 nerve roots (95%-99% of all cases), (2) whole-arm palsy affecting C5 to T1, and (3) Klumpke palsy affecting the C8 and T1 (lower plexus) nerve roots.

## Incidence

The incidence of brachial plexus injuries has decreased secondary to improved obstetric management of difficult labors. Traction injuries are most common in newborns, occurring in 0.1% of spontaneous, 1.2% of breech, and 1.3% of forceps deliveries. Overall, the incidence of birth-related traction injuries is between 0.4 and 4 per 1000 live births.[258]

## Etiologic and Risk Factors

The major contributing factor to these injuries has been attributed to stretching of the brachial plexus when the head is laterally flexed to deliver the shoulder during the birth process.

The lower plexus injury resulting in Klumpke palsy usually is caused by manipulation during delivery resulting from hyperabduction of the arm at the shoulder; that is, the trunk remains relatively immobile in the mother's pelvis while the upper extremity is stretched. However, some question remains about the role of the obstetrician as compared with the position of the infant and the forces encountered in the canal before birth. Evidence suggests that the propulsive nature of the birth process, when stretching of the involved nerves occurs, is something over which the birth attendant does not have full control.[314]

Obstetric history associated with Erb palsy is characterized by high birth weight or vertex delivery with shoulder dystocia (i.e., during delivery the baby's shoulder impinges on the mother's symphysis pubis). Klumpke palsy more commonly is associated with heavy sedation, difficult breech delivery, and brow or face presentation. Rarely, neoplasm present at birth results in brachial plexus palsy. The absence of signs of a traumatic injury accompanied by the onset of weakness and progressive course in the first few days of life should be investigated by MRI.[6]

## Pathogenesis

Plexus injury during birth is usually the result of a stretch or avulsion of the plexus. A mild lesion is characterized by stretching of the nerve fibers, whereas a moderate injury involves some nerve fibers being stretched and others actually torn. A more severe injury is characterized by a complete rupture of the plexus trunks, with avulsion of the roots from the spinal cord. The degree of disability depends on the site and severity of injury. Diaphragmatic and serratus anterior paralysis suggests an avulsion injury as indicated by the location of the nerves with respect to the plexus. Persisting disability in neonatal brachial plexus palsy is partly a result of impaired motor unit activation. This impairment may be a form of developmental apraxia caused by defective motor programming in early infancy.[34] Persistent limitations are found in between 19% and 36% of patients treated conservatively, and early referral to a specialized multidisciplinary team will allow appropriate monitoring and surgical referral if needed.[258]

## Clinical Manifestations

Children with brachial plexus injuries are unlikely to demonstrate postural or placing responses with the involved upper extremity when tested. In Erb palsy the arm is maintained in adduction and internal rotation at the shoulder, with the lower arm pronated and fingers flexed, assuming the waiter's tip position (Fig. 23.28). Children with this type have difficulty with activities such as hand-to-mouth, hand-to-head, and hand–to–back of neck movements but usually have control of the wrist and fingers.

In Klumpke palsy, paralysis of the small muscles of the hand and wrist flexors causes a claw hand appearance. Proximal shoulder control is good, but voluntary wrist and hand control is difficult. In severe forms of brachial palsy (whole-arm palsy), the whole plexus can be affected but to a varying degree (Fig. 23.29). In this case careful examination is necessary to identify affected muscles. In all three cases (Erb, Klumpke, and whole-arm palsy) normal sensation is diminished; however, gross pain sensation may not be decreased to the same degree as movement.

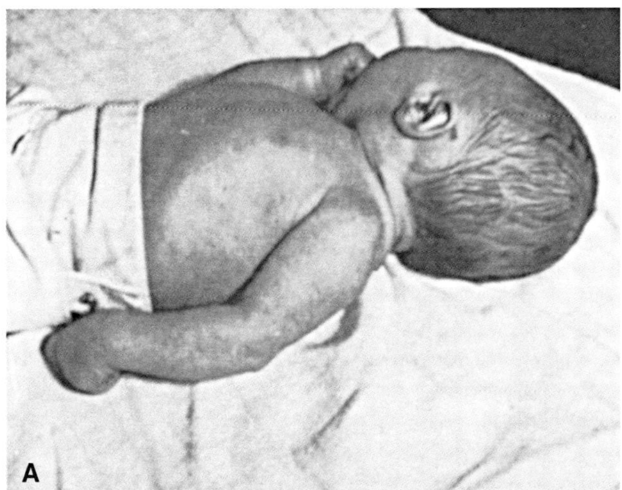


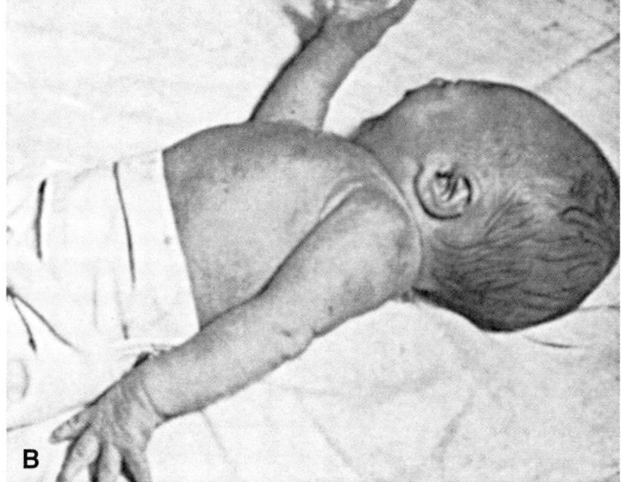


**Figure 23.28**

**Erb palsy.** (A) In this infant with Erb palsy, the arm is maintained in a position of adduction and internal rotation at the shoulder with the lower arm pronated and fingers flexed. (B) Same infant demonstrating an asymmetric Moro reflex with opening of the left hand but still in the "waiter's tip" position. (From Behrman RE, Kliegman RM, Jenson HB: *Nelson textbook of pediatrics,* ed 17, Philadelphia, 2004, WB Saunders.)

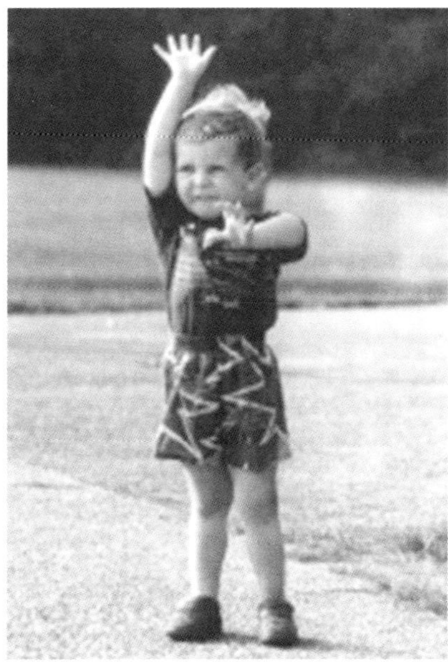

**Figure 23.29**

**Brachial plexus palsy.** Child with limited shoulder external rotation and abduction of the left arm associated with whole-arm palsy. Full motion of the upper extremity is demonstrated on the right side. (From Green DP, Hotchkiss RN, Pederson WC: *Green's operative hand surgery,* ed 5, London, 2005, Churchill Livingstone.)

Table 23.8 summarizes the clinical characteristics of brachial plexus injury.

## MEDICAL MANAGEMENT

DIAGNOSIS. Some injuries are recognizable readily at or soon after birth. Radiographs may be taken to rule out associated fractures of the clavicle. Imaging of the brachial plexus using MRI is not invasive and can demonstrate proximal and distal lesions.

MRI can be used to detect nerve root avulsions, nerve ruptures, brachial plexus scarring, posttraumatic neuroma, brachial plexus edema, spinal cord damage, abnormalities of the shoulder joint, trauma, neoplasms, and infection. This type of imaging allows diagnosis and careful preoperative evaluation of children with brachial plexus injuries.[21]

EMG can be used to delineate the extent of injury and aid in the prognosis and assist the surgeon in identifying appropriate surgical procedures. EMG usually is delayed until 4 to 6 weeks after birth and may be followed serially over time to track recovery. Conduction studies can aid in separating actual axonal loss from conduction block. Needle EMG can help determine the portion of the plexus damaged as well as the severity of the damage.[85]

TREATMENT. Treatment is often delivered as part of a multidisciplinary team that includes a neurologist, surgeon, and therapist. The therapy approach is typically one that follows the strategies outlined in Table 23.8. Microneurosurgical intervention including distal nerve transfer, single nerve transfers, and sural nerve graft reconstruction[259] at an early stage can improve the outcome in some cases, especially in more severe cases where acceptable recovery is not anticipated (C5-T1 global injury without some recovery by 8-10 weeks of age). For example, some children have no chance of recovery unless they undergo early aggressive surgical reconstruction of the injured brachial plexus. In children with global or total paralysis, surgery is performed by 3 to 4 months to maximize ultimate extremity function and minimize disability, however timing recommendations vary from site to site.[123,351,64]

Options for surgical care include tendon transfers considered after a plateau in recovery has occurred or microneurosurgery. The latter procedure is best considered between the ages of 6 months and 12 months for optimal functional results.[305] The role of surgery in those individuals affected at the C5 to C6 and C5 to C7 levels is less clear. There are a number of predictive models that can be used at 3 months to anticipate the degree of recovery that can be expected and aid in treatment planning. In many cases, referral for microsurgical intervention is initiated too late for primary nerve surgery, which has the best outcomes when surgery is performed at the proper stage in development. Secondary reconstructive procedures at a later date can still improve the outcome in many cases.[168]

**Table 23.8** Brachial Plexus Injury: Clinical Characteristics

| Type | Typical Posture | Strength Losses | Sensory Losses | Skeletal Changes | Treatment Strategies |
|---|---|---|---|---|---|
| Erb palsy (C5-C6) | Shoulder IR, adduction, finger flexion (difficulty with hand to mouth, hand to head, and hand to back of neck) | Deltoid, supraspinatus, infraspinatus, teres minor, biceps, brachialis, brachioradialis, supinator | C5-C6 deficits | Flattening of glenoid fossa/humeral head<br>Elongating deformity of coracoid process hooking down and lateral<br>Scapular winging potential<br>Posterior shoulder dislocation | Active/active assistive exercise: shoulder abduction; elbow flexion; forearm supination and shoulder ER |
| Klumpke (C8-T1) | Pronation, elbow flexion contractures; no grasp reflex | Wrist flexors, long finger flexors; hand intrinsics | Diminished sensation | Hypertrophy of olecranon and coronoid process: elbow flexion contracture; posterior dislocation of radial head (25%) | Active/active assistive exercise: forearm supination, elbow extension, finger flexion<br>Positional splint to assist with elbow extension; combined with UE weight bearing |
| Total plexus injury (whole arm) | Combinations of above | Combination of Erb and Klumpke types | Moderate losses | Posterior glenohumeral dislocation | Combination of above |

*ER*, External rotation; *IR*, internal rotation; *UE*, upper extremity.

**Table 23.9** Key Indicators of Recovery of Motor Control*

| Predictors of Good Recovery | Predictors of Poor Recovery |
|---|---|
| Return of biceps function by 3 months of age<br>C5-6 involvement only | Minimal bicep and deltoid function at age 6 months<br>C7 involvement with lack of improvement between ages 3 and 6 months<br>Global palsy or lower plexus involvement |

Data from Ruchelsman DE, Pettrone S, Price AE, Grossman JA: Brachial plexus birth palsy: an overview of early treatment considerations, *Bull NYU Hosp Jt Dis* 67(1):83-89, 2009.

**PROGNOSIS.** In most instances full recovery can be expected, with 53% recovering normal or near-normal function and an additional 39% achieving good functional recovery, though between 19% and 36% will have residual impairment without surgical intervention.[258] Erb palsy has the best rate of recovery, with up to 90% of cases demonstrating spontaneous recovery with the rate and onset of recovery related to outcome. If C7 is involved in an Erb palsy, poor outcome is more likely, with the lower plexus palsies having the poorest prognosis.[301] Some children do have long-term disability as an outcome and require careful followup to prevent the development of contractures and to facilitate active motor control.

The first muscles to return are the elbow, wrist, and finger extensors, followed by the deltoid and biceps and later the external rotators. The timely recovery of these muscles (beginning at 6 weeks and continuing through 3 months) is prognostic of good functional recovery, with the lack of antigravity elbow flexion at 3 months predicting poor recovery.[85]

The long-term prognosis for recovery of motor control is poor beyond 18 months (Table 23.9), and probably 15% of infants experience significant disability, with reports showing a wide range of long-term impairments.[305]

SPECIAL IMPLICATIONS FOR THE THERAPIST 23.9

### *Brachial Plexus Birth Palsy*

An integrated team approach to congenital brachial plexus injuries is imperative. Each child must be carefully evaluated, therapy interventions maximized, and the surgical approach (when required) individualized to obtain the best outcome.

An aggressive and integrated physical and occupational therapy program is essential in the treatment of these injuries. The therapist uses a problem-solving approach and adjusts the interventions based on each child's unique needs. The maintenance of full passive range of motion through the use of splinting and range of motion during the period of neurologic recovery is essential for normal joint development and optimal long-term recovery.

Early surgical correction of shoulder contractures and subluxations reduces permanent disability. Postoperative rehabilitative therapy can preserve and build on gains made possible by medical or surgical interventions.[284,291]

Treatment should focus on activities that encourage active and active assistive movement and that maintain the normal joint kinematics. The shoulder requires particular attention to maintain the normal scapulohumeral and scapulothoracic relationships in addition to maintaining the normal "roll and glide" of the glenohumeral joint and preventing subluxation.

Some strategies used to maintain functional upper extremity range of motion, prevent subluxation, and improve active movement include neuromuscular electrical stimulation, biofeedback, joint mobilization, and positioning using splints. Scapulothoracic stabilization for winging of the scapula using taping may be helpful if there is scapulothoracic weakness.

Passive range-of-motion exercises should be performed to help prevent the development of contractures, and a well-thought-out home program is an integral part of the therapy program with the intensity of the program determined by the clinical course. When splints are used, careful follow-up and family education by the therapist is necessary, especially if sensory impairment is present.

# OSTEOGENESIS IMPERFECTA

## Overview and Incidence

Osteogenesis imperfecta (OI) or brittle bone disease is a generalized connective tissue disorder that has major manifestations in bone, leading to skeletal fragility and growth deficiency. OI was previously described as an autosomal dominant disorder caused by the most abundant protein of bone, skin, and tendon extracellular matrices and included four phenotypes (I-IV) involving COL1A1 and COL1A2 mutations. The disorder is now more fully understood as a predominantly collagen-related disorder. The 1979 Sillence classification divided OI into four types on the basis of clinical and radiographic features. The classification has since evolved with new genetic discoveries. However, the latter has the disadvantage of an evolving list and causes confusion and inability to correlate a specific genetic defect with the clinical presentation. As a result, the initial clinical classification continues to be used but types are now characterized by Arabic rather than Latin numerals. Type 5 was added because it has radiographic features distinct from all the other types.[358]

A functional metabolic classification is thought to have the broadest usefulness and still allow retention of genetic type numeration.[102]

OI occurs worldwide without gender preference.[218] The clinical spectrum of the disease is broad, ranging from the severe form which can present as stillbirth to a mild phenotype diagnosed later in life[358] (Table 23.10). Clinical features vary widely between types, within types, and even within the same family. Studies from Europe and United States have found a birth incidence of 0.3 to 0.7 per 10,000 births and it is estimated that between 25,000 and 50,000 people have OI in the United States. These birth cohort analyses reflect more severe types of OI and do not include more subtle types that become more apparent after birth.[215] In populations with a high level of consanguinity or a high number of carriers, the incidence of OI is higher than in outbred populations.

## Etiologic Factors and Pathogenesis

Most children with OI inherit the disorder from a parent (autosomal dominant inheritance). However, genetic counseling requires recognition that the mutations can be the result of a de novo change in the child, a parent can be a carrier of the dominant gene by parental mosaicism (i.e., the parent carries the mutation in a portion of the parent's germ cells), and in as many as 15% of cases the phenotype may result from recessive inheritance.[106]

The majority of mutations that underlie the cause of OI rest on the original 2 genes identified in the early 1980s that code for the 2 chains of the type I collagen heterotrimer which is extensively modified during its posttranscriptional formation.[268] Many different mutations have been identified in association with OI.[208,256,268] Around 90% of cases are caused by two primary groups of mutations that result in autosomal dominant OI. These genetic defects reduce the amount of type 1 collagen (quantitative defects) and tend to have milder phenotypic presentation or affect its structure (qualitative defects) and present with a more severe phenotype. The rest of the cases are caused by genetic defects in genes involved in the posttranslational modification and intracellular trafficking of type 1 collagen or genes associated with osteoblast differentiation and function. Those generally result in a moderate to severe phenotype.[358]

The quantitative defect group is composed of either nonsense mutation (premature stop codon) or frame-shift mutation (an alteration of the three base pair sequence) both resulting in haploinsufficiency, where one allele does not produce functional protein and the other allele produces insufficient quantity for the biologic demands. The qualitative defect group of mutations produces proteins with structural abnormalities. The most typical are mutations that replace glycine in the triple helical structure of collagen with a different amino acid and alter its function with respect to both its stability and communication with the extracellular matrix. These mutations tend to have more severe phenotypes, with almost all of those with type I OI and 80% of those with moderate to severe OI having the most common dominantly inherited gene impacted.[18,268] Type I collagen is found in the extracellular matrix of bone, skin, and tendon and is the major structural protein (scaffolding) of these tissues. Autosomal dominant mutations of IFITM5 are responsible for a distinctive form of OI, type 5, with hypertrophic callus formation and calcification of the interosseous membranes.

In endochondral and intramembranous bone formation the final structure of bone is similar, despite different mechanics of formation. However, bone modeling in OI appears to be defective and the resulting fragility is complex and not easily understood. Patients tend to have low areal bone mineral density (BMD), associated with lower bone size and volumetric BMD. Histomorphometry studies have indicated low cortical width and trabecular bone volume. In each OI type, baseline histology was characterized by decreased cancellous bone volume due to a 41% to 57% decrease in trabecular number and decreased cortical width. Trabecular thickness was decreased by 15% to 27%.[218] Increased cortical porosity has also been indicated.

The smaller cross-sectional area observed and thinner cortex noted in the long bones lead to diminished strength.

**Table 23.10** Sillence Classification of Osteogenesis Imperfecta (OI)*

| Type | Severity | Description |
|---|---|---|
| I (most common form) | Mildest form of OI | Dominantly inherited with blue sclerae |
| | | Mild to moderate fragility without deformity Most fractures occur before puberty |
| | | Associated with blue sclerae, triangular face, hearing loss (beginning in 20s or 30s); easy bruising |
| II | Most severe form (perinatal lethal) | Stillbirth or death during infancy or early childhood |
| | | Extreme fragility of connective tissue |
| | | Multiple in utero fractures |
| | | Usually intrauterine growth retardation |
| | | Severe bone deformity |
| | | Soft, large cranium |
| | | Micromelia: long bones crumpled and bowed; ribs beaded |
| III | Moderately severe | Progressive deformities |
| | | Scoliosis |
| | | Triangular-shaped face, large skull |
| | | Severe osteoporosis |
| | | Severe fragility of bones; usually in utero fractures |
| | | Fractures heal with deformity and bowing |
| | | Normal sclerae |
| | | Extreme short stature |
| | | Usually wheelchair bound by teenage years |
| IV | Variable but usually milder course; normal or near-normal life span | Mild to moderate skeletal fragility and osteoporosis (more severe than type I); dominant inheritance |
| | | Associated with bowing of long bones |
| | | Barrel-shape rib cage |
| | | Bone fracture easily before puberty; some children improve at puberty |
| | | Light or normal sclerae; may or may not have moderate short stature and joint hyperextensibility |

*Note:* As mentioned in the text, classifications of OI are currently under expansion and/or revision. For this edition, the original Sillence classification, as presented here, was not replaced with one of the emerging classifications that have been proposed as no consensus has been reached regarding updated changes. The reader is advised to seek additional information regarding any future proposed (or actual) changes made.
Adapted from Sillence DO, Senn A, Danks DM: Genetic heterogeneity in osteogenesis imperfecta, *J Med Genet* 16(2):101-116, 1979.

The overall mass of cancellous bone is also decreased in OI, and cancellous bone volume does not increase with age as it does in children who do not have OI.

The rate at which matrix is laid down in these three types of OI is slowed when compared with the normal rate. Because this slowing is uniform across types I, III, and IV of OI, severity probably is not related to the decreased rate of matrix production.[293]

The underlying causes of the bony abnormalities seen in people with OI are not entirely understood but probably result from one or a combination of factors. These factors have a potential role in the ultimate phenotypic expression in OI and include the unique structural characteristics of the abnormal collagen created by the mutation; the absence of other connective tissue proteins that impact the assembly of the extracellular matrix; and the degree to which the collagen is incorporated into that matrix.[86,216]

## Clinical Manifestations

This disease has a wide range of clinical presentations ranging from a normal appearance with occasional fractures to severe involvement with growth retardation and long bone and spinal deformities (Fig 23.30; see Table 23.10). In its severe forms, OI is evident at birth because of the fractures and deformity that have occurred in utero.

The less-severe forms may not become evident until the child begins to walk and fractures develop. The tendency to fracture declines after puberty when cortical bone density increases despite trabecular density remaining low. The fracture rate in women increases after menopause. Some children with OI can be mistaken for abused children until the diagnosis is made.

Shortened stature is common in children with OI. This is partly caused by the abnormal development of epiphyseal growth plates, deformity after fractures, osteoporosis, and vertebral collapse, which contribute to loss of height with increasing age. Lower extremities tend to be more involved than upper extremities. These children often bruise easily, and ligaments tend to show increased laxity.

Additional clinical features may include thin skin, joint hypermobility, deformity of bony auditory structures with subsequent hearing impairment, scoliosis, pectus deformity, deformed teeth, a tendency toward recurrent epistaxis, excess diaphoresis, cardiovascular complications (e.g., aortic and mitral valve insufficiency, aortic

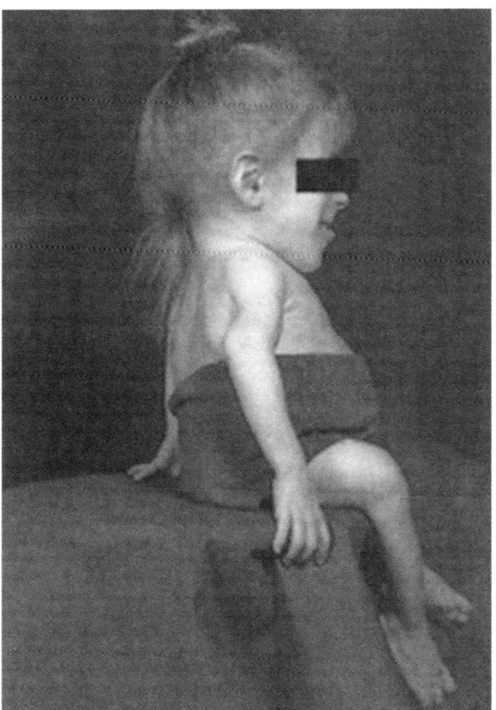

**Figure 23.30**

**Child with osteogenesis imperfecta type III.** This shows defect of all four limbs and increased anteroposterior diameter of the chest. Note the spinal deformity. (From Bullough PG: *Bullough and Vigorita's orthopaedic pathology*, ed 3, St Louis, 1997, Mosby, p. 133.)

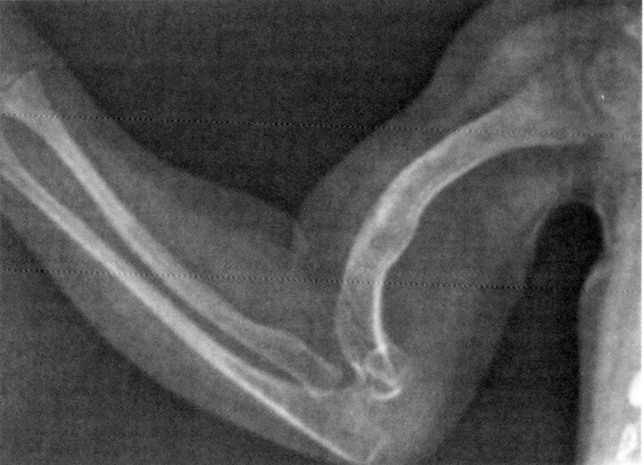

**Figure 23.31**

**Radiograph of upper extremity in a person with osteogenesis imperfecta.** This radiograph shows severe osteoporosis, slender bones, and multiple healed fractures. (From Bullough PG: *Bullough and Vigorita's orthopaedic pathology*, ed 3, St Louis, 1997, Mosby, p. 134.)

dissection), and metabolic defects (e.g., elevated serum pyrophosphate, decreased platelet aggregation). Children with type III or IV OI are born with a dysmorphic facies, a feature that makes them easily identifiable.

Blue or tinted (purple, gray) sclerae are present. The sclerae are blue or tinted because they are abnormally translucent like thin skin, and consequently they filter the red color of the underlying choroid plexus of blood vessels, just as a bruise or a subcutaneous hematoma appears blue through thin translucent skin.[310]

Developmental motor skills often are delayed because of mild weakness, hypermobility and contracture of joints, and multiple fractures requiring immobilization. The majority of children with type I OI ambulate either as functional or household ambulators, and approximately 50% walk without any type of assistive device as community ambulators.

Almost half of children with type III OI are dependent on power mobility, with only 27% becoming household ambulators. Of those children with type IV disease, 26% are community ambulators and 57% household ambulators. The best predictors of ambulatory status are disease type and the ability to sit by 9 or 10 months of age.[68,90]

## MEDICAL MANAGEMENT

DIAGNOSIS. Diagnosis of OI is based on clinical manifestations and skin biopsy that looks at collagen. The collagen defect is used to determine what type of OI the person has according to the Sillence classification. Bone scans and x-ray films show evidence of multiple old fractures and skeletal deformities. Skull radiographs show wide sutures with small, irregularly shaped islands of bone called wormian bones.

TREATMENT. Orthopedic management is central to the overall care of symptomatic OI. Fracture prevention and control are the primary focus; careful positioning and handling are required to prevent fractures in the neonate. Lightweight hip-knee-ankle-foot orthoses and splints also may be used to help support the limbs, prevent fractures, and aid in ambulation. Hip-knee-ankle-foot orthoses are used more often than KAFOs because KAFOs have a longer lever arm for rotational force, resulting in greater risk for proximal femur fractures.[114]

Fracture immobilization is as minimal as possible to prevent disuse atrophy. A repeated cycle of fractures-immobilization of the same bone can inhibit progress in mobility and the development of strength (Fig. 23.31). The use of intramedullary rods is one way of managing recurring fractures (Fig. 23.32). Telescoping intramedullary rods are used to stabilize the bones, elongating as the bone grows, although this procedure is not without risk.[341]

The reoperation rate is significant, with complications related to osteopenia that occurs around the rods (greater around thicker rods), rod migration, and bony growth even beyond the available expansion. Osteotomies also are performed to help control rotational deformities, with appropriate bracing to prolong the time period between potential surgeries.

Medical management has included the use of bisphosphonates, a class of medications (including pamidronate) that inhibit osteoclast function, improve bone mineral density, and decrease the incidence of fractures. Some data exist on the use of growth hormone in OI, but reports of an increased rate of fractures have prevented the use of growth hormone as a first-line drug in the treatment of OI.[392]

Initial reports of allogeneic bone marrow transplantation of mesenchymal cells (progenitors of osteoblasts) have been promising, with increased bone mineral content and histologic evidence of new bone formation 3

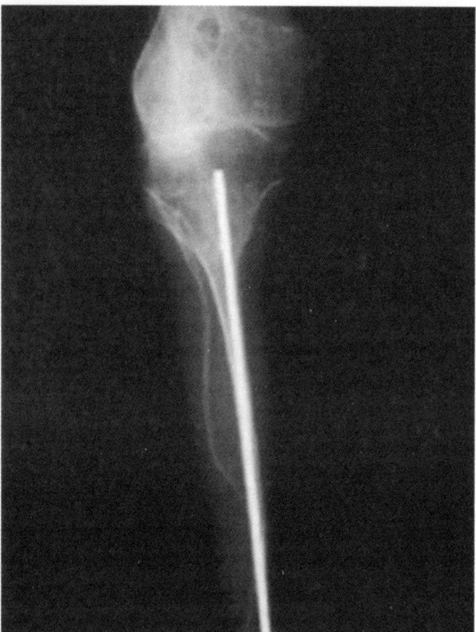

**Figure 23.32**

**Radiograph of the leg of an individual with severe clinical osteogenesis imperfecta that has been treated by rodding of the tibia.** The extreme ribbon-like quality of the bones is apparent in the fibula. (From Bullough PG: *Bullough and Vigorita's orthopaedic pathology,* ed 3, St Louis, 1997, Mosby, p. 135.)

months after engraftment.[150,307] Studies in cell cultures and in mice have raised the possibility that several additional strategies may be developed to treat OI through the use of gene therapy; a review of current gene therapy strategies under investigation is available.[103] At present, no effective treatment exists for type II (perinatal lethal) OI.

PROGNOSIS. People with OI types I and IV have a milder course and live a relatively normal life span. In type III OI, mortality can be related to cardiorespiratory failure stemming from kyphoscoliotic deformity. A significant risk also exists of basilar invagination of the skull and intracranial bleeding.[224]

Incomplete and relatively painless fractures after birth that receive no treatment can produce deformities from bones healing in poor alignment. Short stature and deformities give some individuals with OI the appearance of having achondroplasia. Milder forms of this condition have fewer clinical problems, and these children survive into adulthood.

SPECIAL IMPLICATIONS FOR THE THERAPIST 23.10

## *Osteogenesis Imperfecta*

### Precautions

Infants and children with this disorder require careful handling to prevent fractures. They must be supported when they are being turned, positioned, moved, burped, and cuddled or held. Diaper changing must be carried out gently, never lifting the legs by the ankles but rather by gently lifting the buttocks.

With the older child, passive range-of-motion exercises (especially to obtain hip extension) can be used with caution and are considered safe if used in moderation. Rotational forces are contraindicated, but gentle stretching in straight planes and myofascial stretching are acceptable if done carefully and with the client's participation.

The child must be encouraged to use full active range of motion without force. Strengthening activities should avoid placing weight near joint lines, and if manual resistance is applied, long lever arms should be avoided.

### Family Education

Educational material and information can be obtained from the Osteogenesis Imperfecta Foundation (www.oif.org). The family must be instructed in handling and positioning techniques. Precautions should be given to avoid lifting the child under the arms or by the hands. The young child should not be tossed into the air or be involved in roughhouse play.

At the same time, families should be encouraged to hold and play with their child appropriately and to help the child develop interests that do not require strenuous physical activity. Fine motor skills are encouraged, and activities of daily living modifications for personal hygiene may be necessary.

Swimming frequently is recommended, but the child must be monitored carefully to avoid falls in the shower and pool area. Nonskid aquatic shoes can be worn (by the child or by the caregiver carrying a nonambulatory child in the aquatic area) to assist with this precaution.

Family members must also be instructed to assess for fractures daily. The child may bruise easily, but it is common for a child to have no bruises around the fracture site. Symptoms to look for include limited use of an extremity, malposition of an extremity, focal swelling or tenderness, or crying when a body part is moved or when the child attempts to move.

In the case of diagnosed OI involving child abuse allegations, the parents are encouraged to carry a letter from the primary care physician documenting the diagnosis. Even so, any suspicion of actual abuse in the case of a child with OI requires careful documentation and appropriate referral.

### Therapy Intervention

Therapy helps to prevent disuse weakness or loss of bone stock and strengthens muscles and builds bone density. Light resistance to exercise or movement can be used; aquatic programs are especially helpful in allowing exercise with light resistance.

Strengthening programs emphasize hip extension, hip abduction, trunk extension, and abdominal muscles. A hip extension, hip abduction, and spinal muscular strengthening program complemented by a swimming program two times per week correlates with an increased ability to assume and maintain an upright position and subsequent ambulation.[25]

Positioning is a significant part of the overall management program for these children. Positioning emphasizes a neutral position of the head, trunk, and lower extremities; neutral hip rotation; and hip extension. In fragile cases, the prone position should be avoided except when fully supported or while being supported in the swimming pool.

The ability to stand is important and should be implemented at approximately 10 to 14 months chronologic age.

Standing can be initiated in a standing frame for 30 minutes twice daily. Special care must be taken to avoid fractures when placing and securing the child in the stander. Aquatic therapy also can be used as a medium for initiating standing activities in more-severe cases. Throughout any standing activity the therapist must continue to monitor for lower extremity bowing secondary to bone instability.

### Mobility

The therapist may have to use a significant amount of creativity to adapt ambulating devices and to accommodate for various musculoskeletal deficiencies while fostering the skills necessary for independent mobility. If ambulation is unlikely, the therapist should not hesitate to move quickly toward a wheelchair as the child's primary means of mobility.

When upper extremities are not involved (or minimally affected), manual propulsion chairs offer a functional means of strengthening. Wheelchair fit is extremely important, because bones can bow around supporting surfaces such as armrests. Although children as young as 2 years old cognitively can use and benefit from powered mobility,[350] whenever possible, powered mobility is delayed in this population until the child is older (e.g., 5 or 6 years).

**Box 23.6**

**ARTHROGRYPOSIS: CLINICAL PICTURE**

- Speech, cognition usually within average limits
- Facial asymmetry
- Oral-motor: hypotonia, congenitally absent muscles, jaw stiffness contribute to oral-motor difficulties
- Trunk: thoracolumbar scoliosis (20%), rigid movement, slow responses, minimal rotation, all affecting equilibrium and balance
- Lower extremity jackknife posture (55%)
  - Flexed dislocated hips with extended knees
  - Clubfeet (talipes equinovarus)
- Lower extremity frog posture (45%)
  - Abducted, externally rotated hips
  - Knee flexion
  - Clubfeet (talipes equinovarus)
- Upper extremity posture
  - Shoulder adduction and internal rotation
  - Extended elbow, wrist ulnar deviation
  - Flexed wrists with stiff straight fingers; poor thumb control
- Functional reach impaired, requiring multiple muscle substitution, co-contraction of flexors and extensors, use of opposite arm or hand to assist
- Delayed motor development
  - Sitting independently: approximately 15 months
  - Ambulation: approximately 2 to 3 years if musculoskeletal limitations allow

## ARTHROGRYPOSIS MULTIPLEX CONGENITA

### Definition and Overview

Arthrogryposis multiplex congenita (AMC) is the presence at birth of multiple congenital contractures (2 or more body areas)[131,202] resulting from decreased fetal movement in an intact skeleton. Contracture can result from any number of underlying pathologies. Contractures may occur either in flexion or extension and be primarily distal or proximal in character.

AMC can be subdivided into three broad groupings: (1) contracture syndromes, which typically have a central nervous system etiology, (2) amyoplasia (lack of muscle formation or development), and (3) distal arthrogryposis, primarily affecting the hands and feet.[235] Occasionally, the child presents with associated abnormalities, such as cleft palate, cardiac lesions, urinary tract malformations, and cryptorchidism (failure of testes to descend into the scrotum); however, their presence or absence depends on the underlying cause of the arthrogryposis.

### Incidence and Etiologic Factors

AMC affects 1 in 4300 individuals[200] and can result from any condition that limits fetal movement. Various investigations have attributed the basic defect to an abnormality of muscle, CNS, lower motor neuron, or fetal environment. Hereditary factors have been identified in a number of isolated cases of AMC, with autosomal dominant, recessive, X-linked recessive, and mitochondrial inheritance patterns being identified.[117,131] AMC also is associated with a variety of CNS disorders, including migrational brain disorders and neurodegenerative disorders. CMD also is associated with a smaller percentage of cases of AMC. Other possible causes are prenatal viral infection, drugs, maternal hyperthermia, vascular compromise between mother and fetus, and decreased amniotic fluid in utero (oligohydramnios) limiting fetal movement. The joint deformities present in AMC appear to be secondary to the lack of active motion during intrauterine development, the presence of joint contractures, and forces across the joint.

### Pathogenesis

The underlying cause of AMC is unknown and the contracture phenotype is the result of potentially many different causes; however, the underlying condition in all cases results in decreased fetal movement.[43]

### Clinical Manifestations

The dominant features of AMC include joint contracture, articular rigidity, muscle weakness, and in some cases replacement of the muscle with fibrous and fatty tissue. Arthrogryposis can affect all joints of the body but tends to have a preference for the feet, hips, wrists, knees, elbows, and shoulders (in order of decreasing frequency). Box 23.6 outlines a typical clinical picture of a child with arthrogryposis.

Because many of these children demonstrate normal intelligence, they are able to accommodate for loss of motion with a variety of alternative mobility patterns, such as scooting in sitting or rolling. Typical postures include hip flexion with knee extension or a "jackknife" posture, which affects the child's ability to attain certain developmental postures, including prone, quadruped, short sit, and ring sit, because of the contractures. Those children with fixed knee flexion and hip external rotation are typically slower to roll but quicker to sit and scoot. Many of the children are unable to

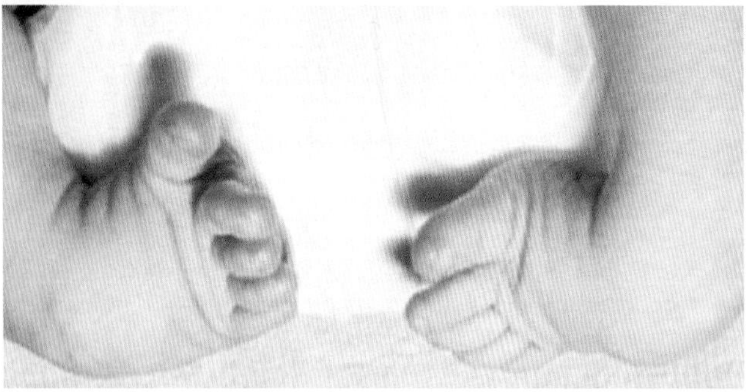

**Figure 23.33**

**Clubfoot deformity, talipes equinovarus (bilateral deviation).** This 4-month-old child was diagnosed with spina bifida, hemivertebrae, and clubfoot. Early intervention can include serial casting to provide stretch to the contracted structures and to provide a more normal plantigrade foot position. Clubfoot is a common morbidity found in children with spina bifida. The casts are typically changed every 1 to 2 weeks and followed by the use of a molded ankle-foot orthosis to maintain the corrected position. Often, as the child grows, surgical releases and osteotomies also are required to provide an optimal correction. (From Zitelli BJ, Davis HW: *Atlas of pediatric physical diagnosis*, ed 4, St Louis, 2002, Mosby.)

make the transition from sitting to standing and can't maintain a standing position once placed upright, often because of hip extension weakness and hip flexion contractures.

As adults, arthritis is a common comorbidity in a variety of different joints as a result of overuse and the abnormal stresses that are placed across the joints. Many affected individuals will benefit from some type of wheeled or powered mobility for long distances, either because of the wear and tear on malaligned joints or the amount of energy required to move in a malaligned position to improve their functional mobility.

## MEDICAL MANAGEMENT

DIAGNOSIS. Prenatal diagnosis may be made by ultrasonic examination based on diminished fetal movement and detection of joint contractures. These findings usually do not become evident until 16 to 18 weeks' gestation.[320] A definitive diagnosis is made by neonatal examination and, if needed, radiographs. However, congenital joint contractures may be secondary to many conditions, requiring differential diagnosis.

TREATMENT AND PROGNOSIS. Physical therapy and occupational therapy are the mainstays of early treatment, with passive mobilization and splinting of the joints, positioning, strengthening, and enhancement of functional adaptation skills (e.g., prevention of falls, mobility training, movement up and down stairs or on uneven terrain).

Orthopedic surgery often is used to address the many musculoskeletal limitations associated with AMC and often is combined with serial casting. The most common proximal contracture pattern that is apparent is a flexed abducted and externally rotated hip, with some patients alternately fixed in hip extension; knee posture can be in flexion or in extension; and the club foot deformity can occur with or without congenital vertical talus.[135] Management varies significantly across surgeons, with the general goal of achieving joint congruency, maintaining strength, and improving flexibility.

Clubfoot deformity (Fig. 23.33) (80-90% of children) often is treated first of all the contractures with various adaptations of the Ponseti method of serial casting followed by a heel cord lengthening, limited posterior release, and a talar procedure if needed to achieve a good correction.[135]

Hip contractures and dislocations (56-90% of children) are often treated with open reduction, proximal femoral (pelvic) osteotomy, and fascial releases to maintain muscle strength, avoiding tenotomies if possible.[135]

Knee flexion contracture may be addressed with serial casting, posterior release, guided growth, or external fixation. Knee extension contracture surgical rectus lengthening or rectus and quadricepsplasty may be performed, although some surgeons prefer to wait to address this at older ages, with fascial surgery related to concern for the preservation of quadriceps strength.[135]

Upper extremity impairment is found in 56% of patients, with the most common position one of internal rotation, elbow extension, wrist flexion, and ulnar deviation with the thumb in palm. Proximal upper extremity procedures are less common and it is difficult to achieve active shoulder external rotation and elevation. Improved upper extremity position can come with an external rotation osteotomy. Elbow flexion range of motion can be achieved with stretching and splinting and active flexion by muscle transfer (latissimus dorsi, long head triceps, or pectoralis). The flexion contracture of the wrist may require osteotomy but transfer of the extensor carpi ulnaris to extensor carpi radialis brevis with fascial release may allow improved passive and active extension along with thenar release with or without transfer, though this is not uniformly possible.

SPECIAL IMPLICATIONS FOR THE THERAPIST 23.11

### *Arthrogryposis Multiplex Congenita*

**Therapeutic Intervention**

Management of range of motion from birth is vital in achieving optimal functional outcomes. During growth spurts more intensive therapy or additional orthopedic intervention or casting may be necessary, always with functional goals related to optimal functional mobility and activities of daily living. Strengthening programs focus on weak muscles or movement in opposition to typical resting postures and should include a home program with optimal frequency and intensity to maintain and improve strength.

Bracing and splinting are recommended for positioning to maintain muscle length. These should be worn a minimum of 6 to 8 hours per day and preferably up to 22 hours per day if they don't interrupt sleep. In children who are nonambulatory, power mobility should be considered as early as 2 years of age if the underlying weakness or contractures make functional ambulation or manual wheelchair mobility impractical. A variety of adaptive equipment (including powered and nonpowered feeding devices)[13,141] is available to aid in the completion of activities of daily living.

## REFERENCES

To enhance this text and add value for the reader, all references are included in the enhanced ebook on Student Consult that accompanies this textbook. The reader can view the reference source and access it online whenever possible.

# CHAPTER 24

# Metabolic Disorders

KEVIN HELGESON

Metabolic disorders occur from abnormal physiologic processes of the endocrine and nervous systems. Metabolic disorders primarily affecting the skeletal system are the focus of this chapter. Primary metabolic diseases and their implications for the therapist are discussed in Chapter 11.

The skeleton is a metabolically active organ that undergoes continuous remodeling throughout life with an annual turnover of cortical and trabecular bone of about 10% of the adult skeleton. Remodeling of bony tissues through resorption and laying down of new osteocytes is necessary both to maintain the structural integrity of the skeleton and to serve the metabolic function as a storehouse of calcium and phosphorus. These dual functions can come into conflict under conditions of changing mechanical forces or metabolic and nutritional stress.[37]

Clinical disorders in which bone resorption is increased are common and include osteoporosis and the secondary effects of cancers such as occur in myeloma and metastases from breast or prostate cancer. Paget's disease results in abnormal bone turnover, resulting in focal areas of increased and decreased bone formations.[3] Clinical disorders of reduced bone resorption resulting in osteopetrosis are less common and have a genetic basis.

Metabolic bone diseases are primarily characterized by diffuse loss of bone density and bone strength. Significant disability from postural deformities and fractures can occur secondary to the loss of bone density. The commonly observed accentuated thoracic spine kyphosis in clients with vertebral collapse secondary to osteoporosis can compromise cardiopulmonary function, affecting the person's ability to participate in a rehabilitation program.[53]

The most serious, potentially life-threatening and costly complication of metabolic bone disease is fracture (see "Fractures" in Chapter 27). Osteoporosis is a risk factor for fractures, with two million fractures annually attributed to this factor, and is why 1 in 2 caucasian women older than 50 years of age experience an osteoporosis-related fracture in their lifetime. Fractures of the proximal femur, distal forearm, and vertebrae are the most common sites of these fractures. The monetary cost of these fractures is estimated to reach 25 billion dollars by 2025.[19]

Therapists have an important role in the prevention of disabilities secondary to the complications of metabolic bone diseases. Client education regarding habitual postures, body mechanics, and proper exercise is an important component of these prevention programs. Physical therapy interventions are also a vital part of the rehabilitation of clients disabled by the resulting postural deformities that can accompany these diseases. Therapists also treat many clients who have experienced traumatic injury precipitated by the presence of metabolic bone disease or, conversely, people who are experiencing the metabolic consequences of trauma.

Finally, therapists treat many people with a primary diagnosis of low-back, knee, or shoulder conditions with osteoporosis as a comorbidity. The presence of such a disease may influence the therapist's choice of examination tests and choice of interventions and exercise parameters. A thorough understanding of this disease process will enable the therapist to treat clients safely and effectively.[53]

## OSTEOPOROSIS

### Definition and Overview

Osteoporosis is a chronic, progressive disease characterized by low bone mass, impaired bone quality, decreased bone strength, and enhanced risk of fractures.[19] Signs of decreased bone density found on radiographic images should be described as osteopenia. Osteoporosis can be classified as primary or secondary, depending on the underlying etiology. *Primary osteoporosis,* the most common, is associated with aging-related physiologic changes. Significant loss of bone density secondary to diseases, medications, or other conditions is referred to as *secondary osteoporosis* (Box 24.1).

### Incidence

Osteoporosis is by far the most common metabolic bone disease, affecting approximately 10 million people living in the United States. An additional 43 million Americans already have low bone mass (osteopenia) that places them at increased risk of osteoporosis. With the aging of America, osteoporosis is expected to increase in prevalence.[19]

The disease is much more common in women, especially postmenopausal women who are estrogen deficient. However, osteoporosis in men over 70 years of age represents a major public health problem, which until

Box 24.1

**RISK FACTORS AND CONDITIONS ASSOCIATED WITH OSTEOPOROSIS**

***Risk Factors***

*Nonmodifiable*

- Age 50 years and older
- Caucasian/Asian
- Northern European ancestry
- Menopausal (occurs early in those <45 years and can be surgically induced through bilateral oophorectomy)
- Family history of osteoporosis; personal history of fragility fracture; fragility fracture in first-degree relative
- Long periods of inactivity, immobilization, long-term care
- Depression
- Lactose intolerance
- Femoral neck BMD

*Risk Factors for Which Intervention Might Reduce Incidence of Osteoporosis and Fractures*

- Inactivity or sedentary lifestyle
- Excess intake of:
  - Alcohol (>2 drinks/d)
  - Tobacco (active or passive)
  - Caffeine[a] (equivalent to >3 cups caffeinated coffee/d)
- Amenorrhea (abnormal absence of menses)
- Estrogen deficiency (women)/testosterone deficiency (men)
- Medications (>6 months)
  - Corticosteroids/steroids
  - Immunosuppressants
  - Anticoagulants (Heparin; Coumadin)
  - Nonthiazide diuretics (furosemide)[b]
  - Methotrexate (MTX)
  - Cisplatin (chemotherapy)
  - Aromatase inhibiters (breast cancer treatment)
  - Antacids (containing aluminum)
  - Laxatives
  - Anticonvulsants
  - Benzodiazepines (Valium, Librium, Xanax)
  - Some antibiotics (e.g., tetracycline derivatives)
  - Buffered aspirin
  - Excessive thyroid hormones
  - Lithium
  - Androgen deprivation (prostate cancer)
  - Depo-Provera (contraceptive)
  - Gonadotropin-releasing hormone agonists
- Low body weight and body mass index, thin, small body frame
- Diet and nutrition
  - Calcium and magnesium deficiency
  - Vitamin D deficiency
  - Vitamin C deficiency (helps with calcium absorption)
  - High ratio of animal to vegetable protein intake
  - High-fat diet (reduces calcium absorption in the gut)
  - Excessive sugar (depletes phosphorus)
  - High intake of low-calcium beverages such as coffee and carbonated soft drinks
  - Eating disorders (bulimia, anorexia nervosa, binge eating)
  - Repeated crash dieting or "yo-yo" dieting

*Associated Diseases and Disorders*

- Endocrine disorders
  - Hyperthyroidism
  - Hyperparathyroidism
  - Type 2 diabetes mellitus
  - Cushing disease
  - Male hypogonadism (testosterone deficiency)
- Malabsorption
  - Celiac disease
  - GI disease; gastric surgery
  - Hepatic disease
- Medication related
  - Organ transplantation
  - Chronic pulmonary disease
  - Rheumatic diseases, including juvenile idiopathic arthritis
- Chronic renal failure
- Osteogenesis imperfecta
- Sickle cell disease
- Cancer and cancer treatment (children and adults), skeletal metastasis
- Eating disorders
- Spinal cord injury
- Cerebrovascular accident or stroke
- Acid–balance imbalance (metabolic acidosis)
- Depression
- Erectile dysfunction
- Hypogonadal states
- HIV/AIDS

[a]Caffeine from any source in excess of 300 mg/d should be avoided.
[b]Some diuretics such as the nonthiazide diuretics have calcium-retaining properties with reduced incidence of hip fracture with long-term use.
*GI*, Gastrointestinal; *HIV/AIDS*, human immunodeficiency virus/acquired immunodeficiency syndrome.

recently has received little recognition. Approximately 2 million men are affected by osteoporosis, and another 12 million are at risk as a result of low bone mass.[19]

Half of women older than 50 years of age with osteoporosis will experience fractures due to loss of bone density.[36] One in 4 men with osteoporosis will also experience these types of fractures. Because men are older at the time they sustain these fractures, men have a higher morbidity and mortality than that of women.[34,29]

## Etiologic Factors

The origin of *primary osteoporosis* is unknown but is attributed to the factors of aging, prolonged negative calcium balance, declining gonadal and adrenal function, progressive estrogen deficiency, and sedentary lifestyle. *Secondary osteoporosis* is caused by conditions and/or medications that interfere with the attainment of bone mass or result in accelerated rates of bone loss.[34] (see Box 24.1).

## Risk Factors

Bone mass reaches peak levels between the ages of 25 and 35 years; after this time the rate of bone resorption begins to exceed the rate of bone formation. This physiologic mismatch can progress to a point at which osteopenia (Box 24.2) may be noted radiographically and bone mineral density can be measured with a DEXA scan (Fig. 24.1).

Box 24.2

**TERMINOLOGY OF METABOLIC BONE DISEASE**

**Osteomalacia:** Softening of the bones
**Osteopenia:** Low bone mass
**Osteopetrosis:** Increased bone density
**Osteoporosis:** Systemic disease that decreases bone density

Osteoporosis is contrasted from osteopenia (low bone mass) by its characterization as "low bone mass, microarchitectural deterioration of bone tissue and decreased bone strength with bone fragility and consequent increase in fracture risk" [as defined by the National Osteoporosis Foundation].

Assessment of bone mineral density is recommended for women at age 65 and for men at age 70. Individuals assessed to have a greater risk for osteoporosis may need this assessment at an earlier age.

Box 24.1 lists the risk factors and medical conditions or diseases associated with primary and secondary osteoporosis. Osteoporosis is related to other risk factors for fractures. Estrogen status, heredity, and ethnicity are important risk factors for osteoporosis in women; alcoholism, cigarette smoking, steroid therapy, and hypogonadism or androgen withdrawal therapy for prostate cancer are the most common factors for men.[105] Age is a risk factor for both men and women; the 10-year fracture risk at age 50 years quadruples by age 80 years; although women are affected earlier in the decades compared to men, the associated mortality and morbidity is much greater for men.[1]

## Hormonal Status

Postmenopausal women are at higher risk to develop the disease due to the decreased production of estrogen, leading to estrogen deficiencies. Estrogen has the physiologic effect of inhibiting bone resorption, thus estrogen deficiencies will result in an increased rate of bone resorption.[55] Estrogen deficiency is linked mostly to the loss of cancellous bone, which is linked to the increased risk for fractures. Decreased intestinal calcium absorption, increased bone resorption to compensate for low calcium levels, and impaired osteoblastic activity have all been associated with estrogen deficiency.[55]

Women normally lose bone at the rate of 1% per year after peak bone density is achieved, usually around the age of 30. Bone loss will accelerate to a varying degree for about 5 to 8 years after menopause, increasing the risk for the development of osteopenia and osteoporosis. Researchers report a wide range from 2% to 11% loss for the 10 years after menopause, slowing after that to about 0.5% to 1% of bone mass per year.[56] Women with a family history of osteoporosis are at high risk of developing osteoporotic fractures.[84]

Men experience a gradual slowing of testosterone production with age, and below-normal testosterone levels have been associated with loss of bone mineral mass. The outward signs of this phenomenon (e.g., loss of muscle strength, fatigue, and a decreased interest in sex) are often attributed to aging without considering the accompanying osteoporosis that ensues. Other risk factors include androgen-deprivation treatment for prostate cancer and hypogonadism associated with erectile dysfunction.[11] Low serum testosterone levels have also been documented in men treated with corticosteroids for chronic inflammatory conditions such as sarcoidosis.[1]

## Genetics

Numerous genes have been linked to peak bone density and the risk of osteoporosis. Gene variations can affect bone mineral density through osteoblast development, osteoblastic synthesis of new bone, and osteoclastic activity.[100,18] Further identification of genetic pathways involved with bone formation will lead to more specific treatments for patients with different forms of osteoporosis.

Bone density also has a strong connection to the receptors for parathyroid hormone (PTHR1). This hormone plays a crucial role in determining the level of calcium in the blood. Genetic differences in the levels of receptors for PTH in the blood may determine bone density.[28]

Peak bone density is partly genetically determined as evidenced by the varying bone densities among different racial and ethnic groups and individual differences among people of the same ethnic background. A lower prevalence of osteoporosis has been found in African American populations compared to white and Hispanic populations.[15] The implications for different racial and ethnic variables have not been well standardized to allow for identification of specific factors that link these variables to bone development and risks for osteoporosis.[63,57]

Body frame size is related to bone density. Older women who weigh less than 127 pounds tend to have less cortical bone and are therefore at greater risk of fractures. Obesity, by increasing the mechanical strain on bone, may result in increased peak bone mass, reducing the risk for osteoporosis. In addition, obesity increases the amount of biologically available estrogen stored in adipose cells, protecting against fracture.[84]

## Physical Inactivity

Inactivity and immobilization of a limb have been associated with decreased bone formation. Prolonged inactivity results in reduced gravitational and muscular forces acting on the skeletal system. The decreased mechanical stress on bony structures alters bone physiology, resulting in decreased bone mass.

Disuse osteopenia, which is caused by immobilization (e.g., cast, bed rest, long-term care, or neurologic impairment), results from a change in osteocyte cellular function or an increase in the recruitment of osteoclasts.[5] The difference in the quality of bone produced is in the decreased number of trabeculae and in increased osteoclastic performance. Residents in nursing home or long-term care facilities have a 5- to 10-fold greater fracture risk than community dwellers.[30]

## Tobacco

Cigarette smoking is associated with a reduction of bone mass and is a well-known risk factor for spinal and hip fractures. Evidence suggests that cigarette smoke may affect bone progenitor cells, thereby directly contributing to the development of osteoporosis.[26] Smokeless tobacco

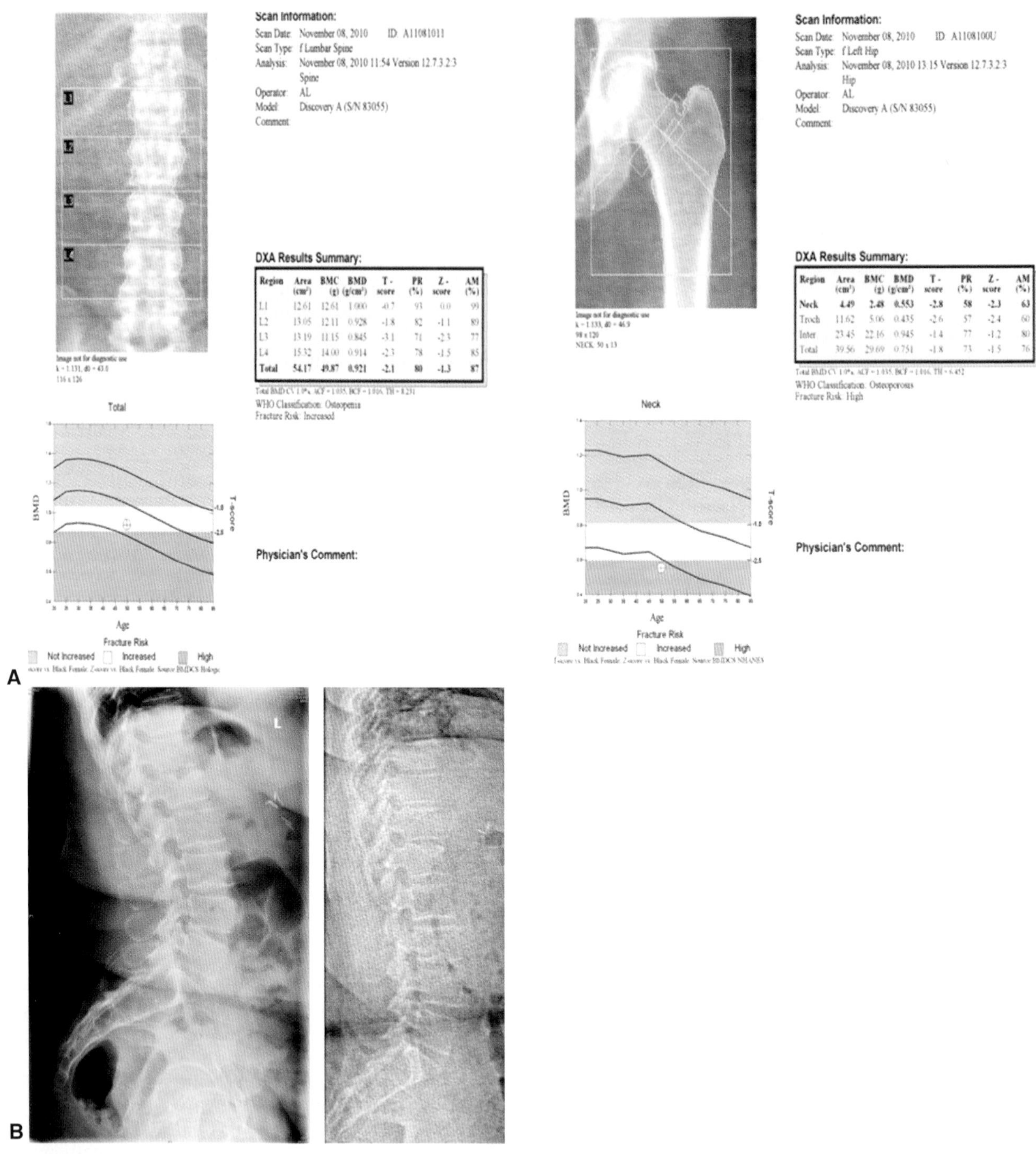


**Figure 24.1**

**Example of DEXA scan results.** (From Chun KJ: Bone densitometry. *Semin Nucl Med* 41(3): 220–228, 2011.)

has been found to accelerate loss of bone mineral density in females over the age of 60 years.[78]

## Alcohol

More than two "units" of alcohol per day is a risk factor for osteoporosis.[50] A unit is defined as one 12-oz beer, one 5-oz glass of wine, or 1.5 oz of hard liquor. Excessive alcohol intake during adolescents and young adulthood alters osteoblast gene expression and matrix synthesis, thereby reducing peak bone mineral density. Chronic alcohol use can reduce intestinal absorption and increase renal excretion of calcium and disrupt the production of vitamin D. Alcoholism is associated with poorer overall nutrition and increased likelihood of a fall.[61] In men, consuming large amounts of alcohol is a major independent risk factor for hip fractures.[41]

## Medications

Long-term use of medications, especially corticosteroids, has been associated with the development of secondary osteoporosis. Patients with a wide variety of conditions use corticosteroid medications to control inflammation and symptoms. Most bone loss occurs during the first 6 months of corticosteroid therapy. Loss of 10% to 15% of spinal trabecular bone mass is possible; after that, bone loss averages 1% to 2% annually.[101] Corticosteroids impair osteoblastic activity and the maturation of preosteoblastic cells to osteoblasts, increase osteoclastic activity, and impair vitamin D–dependent intestinal calcium absorption, which can result in secondary hyperparathyroidism.[13] The hyperparathyroidism increases bone resorption and decreases renal resorption of calcium, thereby increasing the amount of calcium excretion.

Other medications have also been implicated for the development of secondary osteoporosis (see Box 24.1). Selective serotonin reuptake inhibitors (SSRIs) have been linked to the increased risk of fracture for those older than age 50 years, but the link to the development of osteoporosis has not been definitely made.[12,103]

### Depression

Depression has been proposed as an independent source for immune and endocrine changes that can produce loss of bone and is recognized as a risk factor for osteoporosis.[17]Depressive disorders are associated with physiologic, behavioral, and medical treatments that are potential contributory factors to bone loss. Individuals with a history of a major depressive disorder are more likely to have lower levels of vitamin D and higher levels of parathyroid hormone and cortisol than people without depression, regardless of physical activity levels.[67]

### Diet and Nutrition

Nutrition is a key component for the optimal development of bone density during early life and helps determine the peak bone mass for each individual. Nutritional intake of calcium, vitamin D, and protein have the greatest effect for the development and maintenance of bone health.

Calcium is the primary mineral component of bone and is essential for bone rigidity. A healthy diet that includes high levels of calcium intake has been shown to limit bone loss in adulthood and is a protective mechanism for bone mineral content after menopause. Childhood intake of calcium-rich foods has been associated with elevated levels of bone mineral content. Calcium ingested as part of a healthy diet has been shown to be more effective than calcium supplements alone.[83,104]

Vitamin D serves as a regulator for levels of calcium in the body. Vitamin D is found in dietary foods and synthesized from sunlight exposure. The role of vitamin D supplementation for older adults is not as well supported as calcium supplements. Current recommendations include measuring serum levels of vitamin D before recommending supplements to prevent the onset of osteoporosis. Recent studies have noted improvements in bone mineral content with vitamin D supplements for young women.[104]

Protein is a key building block for bone formation. Diets low in protein content have been found to be detrimental to good bone formation, but diets with high levels of protein have only made small improvements in bone mineral densities in the lumbar vertebrae and femoral neck.[104,86] A clear connection between supplementing protein intake and fracture prevention has not been established.[104,86]

Bone density is decreased in anorexic and bulimic women and is possibly the result of estrogen deficiency, low intake of nutrients, low body weight, early onset and long duration of amenorrhea, low calcium intake, reduced physical activity, and hypercortisolism. This type of reduced bone density is associated with a significantly increased risk of fracture even at a young age.[66] The female athlete triad describes the combination of disordered eating, amenorrhea, and osteoporosis, which is a situation that often goes unrecognized and untreated.[69,96]

A significant number of people with osteoporosis also have celiac disease, a gastrointestinal (GI) disorder that impairs the absorption of calcium, various nutrients, and vitamin D needed for maintaining healthy bones. Identification of and effective dietary therapy for celiac disease can lead to improved absorption of vital nutrients and potentially reverse the decline in bone mineral density.[100] Celiac disease increases the risk of fractures and complications related to these fractures due to the limitation on the ability to absorb calcium and nutrients for fracture healing.[107] Serum screening for celiac disease in anyone with osteopenia or osteoporosis is advised because dietary changes can restore normal absorption of dietary nutrients in this group, including calcium and vitamin D, contributing to a reversal in the decline of BMD associated with osteoporosis.[95]

## Pathogenesis

Bone is composed of osteocytes with a meshwork of collagen fibers inlaid with calcium and phosphate. These minerals are mixed with water to form a hard, cement-like substance called *hydroxyapatite*. Sodium, magnesium, and potassium are also present in smaller amounts. The human skeleton is composed of the denser outer surface of cortical bone and the less-dense inner layers of cancellous bone. Bone strength is based on two factors: bone density and bone quality. Bone density refers to how many bone cells are present in a square millimeter. Bone quality reflects the health of the bone cells present. The quality of the cells, tissues, and minerals that make up bone, the density of all these bony tissues, and the architecture of the cortical and cancellous bone all make up this entity we call bone quality.

Bone mineral density (BMD) indicates the amount of calcium, phosphate, and other mineral deposited amongst the meshwork of bony tissues. BMD is a measurement of the mass of minerals per volume of bone, usually reported as grams per centimeters.[3] BMD increases during growth and development to enhance the bone density and bone quality. Peak bone mass is achieved during the third decade of life. This amount of bony tissues serves as the bone bank for the rest of a person's life. An individual with a high peak bone mass who starts to lose bone later in life and loses it slowly is unlikely to sustain osteoporotic fractures, whereas someone with suboptimal peak bone mass who starts to lose bone earlier in life or loses bone rapidly is more likely to develop osteoporosis with fractures.

The onset for normal bone loss and the subsequent rate of bone loss is influenced by genetic factors. Bone loss increases at the time of menopause because of the marked reduction in the circulating concentrations of

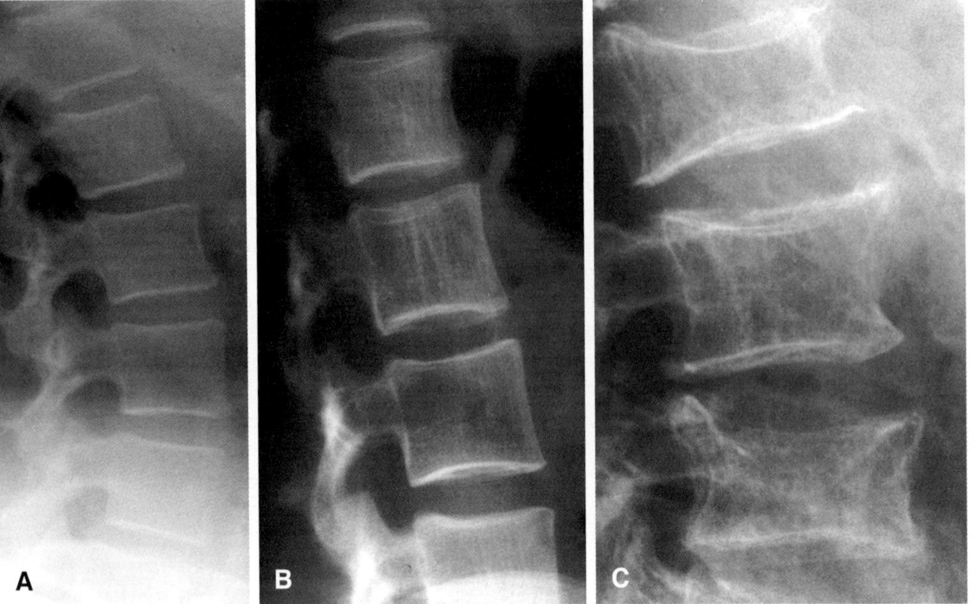


**Figure 24.2**

**Osteoporosis. A** , Lateral lumbar spine radiograph showing normal vertebrae and intact end plates. **B**, An early feature of spinal osteoporosis is the presence of prominent vertical striations due to loss of secondary horizontal trabeculae. **C**, Multiple vertebral fractures are shown in this image. (From Pope TL, Bloem HL, Beltran J, et al: *Musculoskeletal imaging*, ed 2, Philadelphia, 2015, Saunders.)

estradiol and progesterone (Fig. 24.2).[19] Small deficits in bone formation remaining at the complfetion of a normal remodeling cycle accumulate and contribute to age-related losses in bone mass. Thus the bone that experiences the greatest number of remodeling cycles is at the highest risk for age-related losses in mass. Maintenance of adult skeletal mass is controlled not only by changes in the production of osteoclasts and osteoblas ts but also by altering the duration of their respective life spans through regulated apoptosis (programmed cell death). During bone remodeling, disruption of the rate of supply of new osteoblasts and osteoclasts and the timing of this supply by apoptosis may be an important mechanism behind the deranged bone turnover found in most metabolic disorders of the adult skeleton.[46]

### Mechanical Stimuli

Mechanical stimuli may be the only type of stimuli capable of inducing modeling in mature bone; emphasizing the importance of physical activity and exercise in the adolescent and young adult.[31] Physical activity transmits mechanical loads to the skeleton through gravitational forces and muscular pull at sites of attachment. In the absence of mechanical forces (space flight or prolonged bed rest), urinary calcium excretion increases and bone density decreases. BMD changes induced by loading are not maintained long term, which is why regular site-specific and weight-bearing exercises must be done routinely to prevent osteoporosis and reduce bone fracture risk.[102] Subsequently, hormonal levels, physical activity, and nutrition are the key factors that facilitate bone growth because they regulate the osteoblastic and osteoclastic remodeling cycles, initiate a natural cycle of microscopic bone damage and subsequent repair, and foster solid bone architecture.[76]

## Clinical Manifestations

Loss of height, postural changes, back pain, and fracture are the most common presenting features of osteoporosis. Marked thoracic spine kyphosis and loss of overall body height are common findings, especially after a vertebral compression fracture.[53,51,6]

Muscular pain and trigger points can occur in the lower back paravertebral muscles and rhomboid muscles, as can burning pain in the midthoracic region lateral to the spine because of excess stretch placed on the rhomboid muscles from the compensatory forward rotation of the scapulae. Similar muscle imbalance and muscular symptoms are observed or reported in the lower quadrant with involvement of the lumbosacral and sacroiliac joints and surrounding musculature.[47]

### Fractures

The vertebral bodies, hip, ribs, radius, and femur are the most common fracture sites (in that order), although any bone in the body can be affected. A first fracture is a risk factor for a second fracture, which, in turn, increases the risk of death.[10] Fractures are often "silent" compression fractures of vertebral bodies, sacral insufficiency fractures, or complete fractures of the spine or femoral neck. Metatarsal insufficiency stress fractures in both men and women may be an unrecognized early sign of osteoporosis.[97]

Vertebral compression fractures are the most common osteoporosis-related spinal fractures, presenting with clinical symptoms of back pain, posture change, loss of height, functional impairment, disability, and diminished quality of life (Fig. 24.3). These can occur without injury and are believed to occur with excessive compression onto the vertebral body from hyperkyphotic postures, lifting

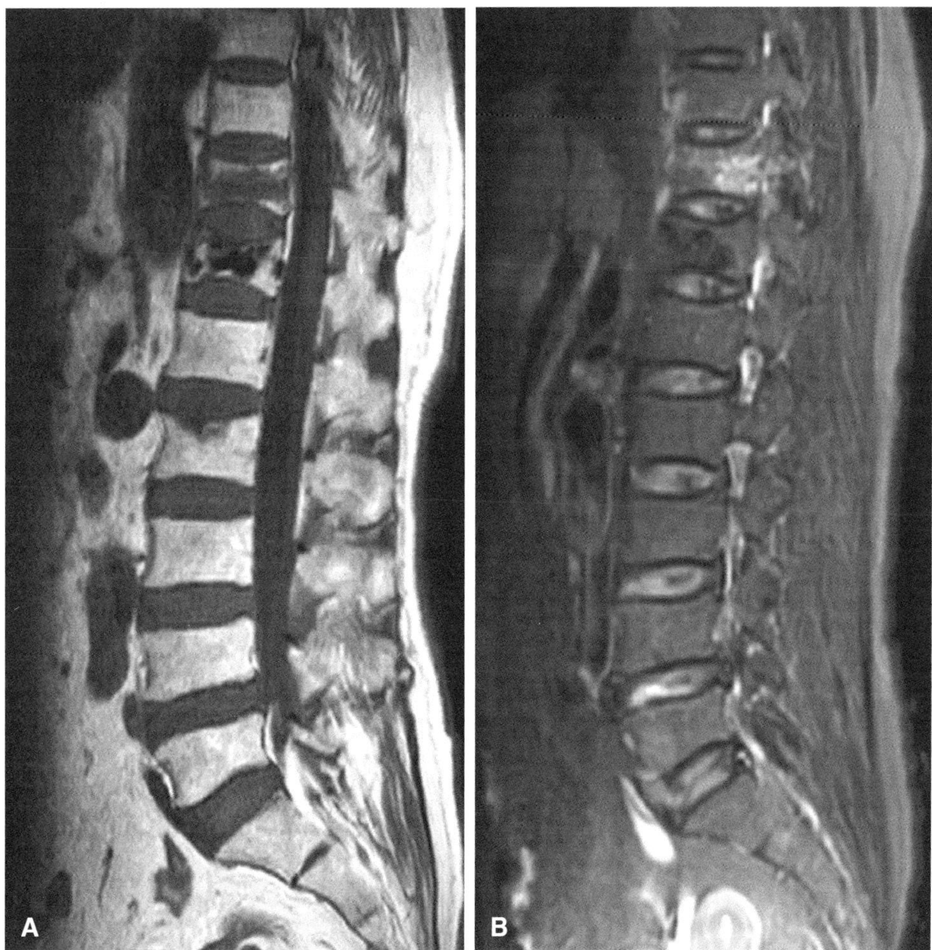


**Figure 24.3**

**Vertebral compression fracture. A,** T1-weighted magnetic resonance imaging showing dark signal change of T11 indicating recent compression fracture. **B,** Bright signal change of T11 vertebral body is shown. (From Bae JS, Park JH, Kim KJ, Kim HS, Jang I: Analysis of risk factors for secondary new vertebral compression fracture following percutaneous vertebroplasty in patients with osteoporosis. *World Neurosurg* 99: 387–394, 2016.)

of heavy objects or increased intrathoracic pressure from coughing and sneezing[62] (see "Fractures" in Chapter 27).

The prevalence of vertebral fractures increases steadily with age, ranging between 20% for 50-year-old postmenopausal women and 64% for older women. The majority of vertebral fractures are not connected with severe trauma, and only one in three is diagnosed clinically. Patients with a vertebral compression fracture are at a significant risk for suffering another compression fracture and for fractures at other sites.[62] Almost 20% of women will experience another fracture within 1 year after a vertebral fracture.

Pain associated with vertebral compression fractures is usually severe and localized to the site of fracture, typically midthoracic, lower thoracic, and lumbar spine. Tenderness to palpation over the fracture is common in both symptomatic and otherwise asymptomatic cases. Pain may radiate to the abdomen or flanks and is aggravated by prolonged sitting or standing, bending, or performing a Valsalva maneuver. Side lying with hips and knees flexed may alleviate the pain. Generalized bone pain is more suggestive of metastatic carcinoma or osteomalacia. Neurologic symptoms may not occur immediately but rather develop insidiously over days to months.[62,70]

## MEDICAL MANAGEMENT

PREVENTION. The National Osteoporosis Foundation has developed universal recommendations for the prevention of osteoporosis.[19]Individuals with a family history of osteoporosis and other risk factors need to receive counseling and recommendations to prevent the development of osteoporosis. Since no cure is available for osteoporosis, prevention and, more effectively, early intervention, even in utero, is essential for everyone (men, women, young, and old) but especially for those at risk (Box 24.3).[106] By minimizing modifiable risk factors, people at high risk for developing osteoporosis may be able to achieve higher peak bone mass in the hope of delaying or preventing the onset of osteoporosis.[19] Because peak adult bone density depends on factors during growth and development, preventing osteoporosis in the aging adult begins by providing necessary dietary calcium intake during bone development and calcification in childhood and adolescence (Table 24.1).

***Calcium.*** Peak bone mass is attained around age 30 years, at which time the pattern of bone building and bone loss is reversed, with more calcium loss than deposit. Regular exercise and physical activity, combined with adequate calcium, is considered both a prophylactic

Box 24.3
**MANAGEMENT OF OSTEOPOROSIS**

| ***Prevention*** | ***Management*** |
|---|---|
| Client education<br>Optimize calcium and magnesium intake (see Table 24.1)<br>Exposure to sunlight; vitamin D therapy<br>Regular physical activity (weight bearing) and prescriptive exercise<br>Other lifestyle changes (e.g., reduce or eliminate alcohol and tobacco)<br>Maintenance of menstrual cycles from youth through adulthood<br>Minimize intake of carbonated soft drinks and caffeine<br>Minimize use of medication(s) known to cause bone loss<br>Recognize and treat any medical conditions that can affect bone health<br>Adequate nutrition and calories; avoid chronic dieting or "yo-yo" dieting<br>Reduce animal sources of protein; increase vegetable sources of protein<br>Phytoestrogens (under investigation)<br>Psychosocial support | Same as for Prevention<br>Pharmacotherapy (single or combination)<br>• Bisphosphonates<br>  • Intravenous: pamidronate (Aredia); zoledronate (Zometa)<br>  • Oral: risedronate (Actonel); ibandronate (Boniva); etidronate (Didronel); alendronate (Fosamax sodium); tiludronate (Skelid)<br>  • Oral/IV: clodronic acid<br>• Hormonal therapy (ERT/HRT for women, testosterone for men)<br>• Estrogen agonists/antagonists (Raloxifene/Evista)<br>• Calcitonin (nasal or injection):<br>  • Miacalcin<br>  • Calcimar<br>• Parathyroid hormone (PTH; rhPTH: teriparatide/Forteo)<br>• Osteoprotegerin (OPG)<br>Osteoporosis education, balance assessment, and falls prevention<br>Psychosocial support<br>Falls and fracture prevention (see Chapter 27) |

*IV*, Intravenous; *ERT*, estrogen replacement therapy; *HRT*, hormone replacement therapy; ESTROGEN AGONIST/ANTAGONIST s, selective estrogen receptor modulators; *PTH*, parathyroid hormone; *rhPTH*, recombinant human PTH; *OPG*, osteoprotegerin.

and treatment measure for osteoporosis from childhood through the adult years. The American Academy of Pediatrics has endorsed recommendations for dietary intake of calcium and vitamin D to promote healthy bone development.[35] Low-fat dairy and other calcium- and magnesium-rich foods (e.g., broccoli or kale, sardines or salmon with the bones, fresh or dried apricots, figs, turnip greens, oranges or calcium-enriched orange juice, or tofu) and calcium supplements are the primary means of achieving an adequate calcium intake.[14]

***Vitamin D.*** Vitamin D helps the body absorb, synthesize, and transport calcium within the body, therefore necessitating adequate sunshine each day. Vitamin D requirements vary by geographic location and age. In northern areas (above the 42-degree latitude parallel; in the United States, imagine a line stretching from the California–Oregon border to Boston), the sunlight in winter limits the exposure to ultraviolet light needed for the production of adequate vitamin D levels. Daily intake of 800 to 1000 IU of vitamin D (food and supplementation) is recommended for individuals age 50 and older; many calcium supplements also contain vitamin D.[19]

Individuals with high risk for developing osteoporosis should consider a combination of dietary modifications and supplements. For women, baseline BMD tests performed at the time of menopause (cessation of menstrual flow) or even earlier (during the perimenopausal phase) can provide a baseline assessment for future reference. Falls prevention (as a means of fracture prevention) is a separate component of osteoporosis management but not necessarily osteoporosis prevention (see "Falls Preventions" in Chapter 27).

**SCREENING.** Whereas osteoporosis was once called a "silent disease" because it was not recognized until a fracture signaled its presence, the widespread availability of technology to measure bone density has made it possible to identify people at risk for osteoporosis before fractures are imminent. The NOF recommends that all men and postmenopausal women age 50 and older should be assessed for their risk of osteoporosis and related fractures. A BMD test is recommended or women at age 65 and older and men age 70 and older. For men and women ages 50 to 69, a BMD test is recommended for those with high risk factors or who have had a recent fracture.[19]

Until evidence supports the cost-effectiveness of routine screening or the efficacy of early initiation of preventive drugs, an individualized approach has been recommended. There is accumulating evidence that more and more younger adults are developing osteoporosis at an earlier age (ages 50–70), suggesting that baseline screening should begin even earlier. Therapists treating anyone with fragility fractures, vertebral compression fractures, or fractures anywhere in a postmenopausal woman should advise these individuals to ask their physician about medical screening for osteoporosis, including dual energy x-ray absorptiometry (previously DEXA, now DXA) scans and blood tests for metabolic bone markers (e.g., vitamin D, calcium, parathyroid hormone).[27]

**DIAGNOSIS.** Careful evaluation of the osteoporotic person is essential in developing a comprehensive plan that reduces fracture risk and improves quality of life. Examination of the individual with osteoporosis includes history and physical examination, laboratory testing, and imaging studies. Diagnosis and intervention are based on bone density and risk assessment; in the case of secondary osteoporosis, the specific underlying cause must be determined through the diagnostic process before intervention can be initiated.[20]

***History.*** The medical history should contain the personal and family history of fractures, lifestyle, intake of substances such as vitamin D, calcium, corticosteroids, and other medications. Clinicians should be aware of problems with vitamin D measurement, including seasonal variation, variability among laboratories, and the desirable

**Table 24.1** Daily Calcium Requirements

| Age Group | Minimum Daily Requirements (mg of elemental calcium) | Comments on Calcium Administration |
|---|---|---|
| Birth to 6 mo | 200 mg | Calcium supplements come in several preparations (e.g., acetate, carbonate, citrate, gluconate, glucarate, glubionate, lactate, phosphate). Recommended daily requirements refer to elemental or actual calcium. Check the label in the % Daily Value and note how many tablets or capsules are required to obtain this amount. |
| 6 mo to 1 y | 260 mg | The body can absorb 500 mg of calcium at a time. Spread calcium intake (food or supplements) over the course of a day. Separate calcium supplements from foods high in calcium or vitamins with calcium added. |
| 1–3 y | 700 mg | Beware of foods containing wheat bran or oxalic acid (e.g., chocolate, cauliflower, rhubarb, beet greens, brussels sprouts) that interfere with calcium absorption. Take calcium supplements apart from these foods. |
| 4–8 y | 1000 mg | Calcium can interfere with the effectiveness of a variety of tetracycline antibiotics and fluoroquinolones such as Cipro, Floxin, Levaquin, Avelox, Factive, Vibramycin, and Minocin. Avoid consuming calcium (food or supplements) within 2–4 hours of taking these drugs. |
| 9–18 y | 1300 mg | Calcium, especially in antacids, may interfere with certain calcium channel- and beta-blockers and thyroid medication (Thyroxine). Check with prescribing physician about how to take calcium. |
| 19–50 y | 1000 mg | Calcium can interfere with bisphosphonate absorption. If taking bisphosphonates, delay consuming calcium (food or supplements) at least 30 minutes.<br>Spend at least 10 minutes daily in the sun (longer if using sunscreen) to obtain vitamin D necessary for calcium absorption and bone formation. |
| 51–70 y | 1000 mg for males<br>1200 mg for females | For every ounce over 4 oz of animal protein, an additional 100 mg of calcium is required to stay even. |
| >70 y | 1200 mg | Take calcium supplements with a meal rather than on an empty stomach, unless the foods contain significant amounts of calcium. |
| Pregnant or lactating females | 1000–1300 mg | Extra-strength antacid made with calcium-carbonate in tablet form (e.g., Tums) is used by some people to obtain calcium. Beware of this antacid; decreased stomach acid alters calcium and absorption. For the individual with reduced stomach acid and especially the older adult, this may not be a good choice. |

For anyone with osteoporosis (or trying to prevent osteoporosis), the RDA of calcium is as stated for his or her age group in the table above.
Data from National Women's Health Information Center, Department of Health and Human Services, 2000; Swan KG et al. Osteoporosis in men: a serious but under-recognized problem, *J Musculoskelet Med* 18(6):310–316, 2001; Institute of Medicine of the National Academies. Dietary reference intakes (DRIs): recommended dietary allowances and adequate intakes, elements. In: Ross CA, Taylor CL, Yaktine AL, Del Valle HB, editors. DRI: *Dietary Reference Intakes.* Calcium, Vitamin D. Washington (DC): The National Academies Press: 2011;1108; DiPiro JT, Talbert RL, Yee GC, Matzke GR, Wells BG, Posey LM, editors. *Pharmacotherapy. A Pathophysiologic Approach.* 8th ed. New York (NY): McGraw Hill; 2011.

therapeutic range. The physical examination can reveal relevant information such as height loss and risk of falls.[19]

***Bone Mineral Density Testing.*** A BMD test is the best way to assess for osteoporosis. Without this test, most people are unaware they have osteoporosis until a fracture occurs, although some fractures can be painless, or the pain may be mistaken for arthritis, delaying diagnosis. BMD is a measurement of the mineral content of bone in grams per square centimeter (g/cm$^2$) for the area of the body that has been scanned. A person's BMD measurement is compared to norm values of those of the same age and sex (called a Z score) or can be compared to estimated peak bone mass of the same sex (T score) (see Table 24.2). The T score is usually reported to the patient and is most commonly used as a reference for tracking bone mineral densities. A "normal" level is a BMD within one standard deviation of young adult (T score at 1.0 or above), the "osteopenia" level is a BMD between 1.0 and 2.5 standard deviations below a young adult, and "osteoporosis" being a BMD is 2.5 standard deviations or more below a young adult.[19] For premenopausal women and men under age 50, a Z score adjusted for ethnicity of 2.0 standard deviations below the mean along with an assessment of their risk factors are used to make the diagnosis of osteoporosis.

**Table 24.2** WHO Classification for Bone Mineral Density

| T Score | Significance |
|---|---|
| −1.0 or higher | Normal; low risk for fracture |
| −1.0 to −2.5[a] | Osteopenia (low bone mass) |
| −2.5 or lower[b] | Osteoporosis |

[a]Half of fragility fractures occur in this group.
[b]The National Osteoporosis Foundation (NOF) suggests that anyone with a T score of −2.0 or less or −1.5 or less with at least 1 risk factor should be treated to reduce fracture risk.
From World Health Organization Study Group: Assessment of fracture risk and its application to screening for postmenopausal osteoporosis, Tech Rep Series, No 843, Geneva 1994, The Organization. Update to Cosman F, de Beur SJ, LeBoff MS, et al. Clinician's Guide to Prevention and Treatment of Osteoporosis. *Osteoporos Int* 25:2359–81, 2014.

DXA is used to measure bone densities of the spine, hip, or total body density. The DXA uses two beams of low-level ionizing radiation to assess the attenuation of the beams due to the bony structures. Peripheral DXA (pDXA) measures bony structures for smaller regions such as the wrist and ankle. Alternative methods include quantitative ultrasound (QUS) using sound waves to measure calcaneal, tibial, or patellar density or peripheral computed tomography (pCT). These methods are not interchangeable and do not provide equivalent information. DXA is the preferred procedure because it measures bone density at the femoral neck and lumbar vertebral bodies, where bone loss occurs more rapidly with aging[45] (Table 24.2). The Trabecular Bone Score (TBS) is an assessment of the bone texture correlated with bone microarchitecture. This score independently and in combination with BMD has been shown to be an accurate assessment of fracture risk. Assessment of bone texture can be an important for assessing fracture risk for patients with early onset of osteoporosis or for secondary osteoporosis.[39]

***Predicting Fracture Risk.*** The World Health Organization has developed a computerized tool called the *Fracture Risk Assessment* or FRAX to calculate the 10-year risk of sustaining a fracture.[19,49] Fracture risk is calculated based on an individual patient's age, weight, gender, smoking history, alcohol use, medications, medical history, fracture history, and BMD T score. The FRAX score is then used to assess the individual's need for active management of osteoporosis and fracture prevention.

***Laboratory Testing.*** Laboratory testing can detect other risk factors and can provide clues to etiology for patients suspected of developing osteoporosis.[2] Selection of laboratory tests should be individualized because there is no consensus regarding which tests are optimal. Biochemical markers of bone turnover (e.g., alkaline phosphatase, osteocalcin, urinary hydroxyproline, urinary deoxypyridinoline, urinary *N*-telopeptide, and others) reflect the rate of bone remodeling and may be helpful in assessing for fracture risk and for effectiveness of the treatment regimen but are not widely used at present. Levels of serum total testosterone may be obtained for men.

TREATMENT. Osteoporosis is not curable, but there is evidence that interventions can slow the progression of bone loss and prevent further morbidity. The guidelines published by the National Osteoporosis Foundation recommend a comprehensive plan of care for managing primary and secondary osteoporosis. Management of primary and secondary osteoporosis in the adult should include lifestyle measures to reduce bone loss such as a high calcium intake, smoking cessation, reducing alcohol intake, and physical activity and exercise. Management of secondary osteoporosis will focus on addressing the primary condition resulting in bone loss. Fall prevention is an important intervention for anyone with low bone mass and high risk factors.

***Medications.*** Pharmacotherapy to reduce fracture risk is initiated when the T score is at or below 2.5 at the femoral neck or lumbar spine, or when there is a history of hip or vertebral fractures, or in postmenopausal women and men over 50 with T scores between 1.0 and 2.5. in the absence of risk factors or below 1.5 if other risk factors are present.[19] Screening individuals for osteopenia (low bone mass but without the microarchitectural bone changes seen in osteoporosis) is important because there are increasing numbers of people who are osteopenic and who do experience bone fracture.[90] Medications for osteoporosis include bisphosphonates, calcitonin, estrogen therapies, parathyroid hormone, and Denosumab, a drug that inhibits osteoclast formation.

Bisphosphonates are a family of drugs that are called antiresorptives, as they inhibit osteoclasts to slow bone resorption and actually reverse bone loss. These drugs are used in various bone conditions involving increased levels of bone resorption such as osteoporosis from a variety of clinical causes, glucocorticoid-induced bone loss, hypercalcemia of cancer, and Paget disease of bone. The use of bisphosphonates in reducing bone pain associated with cancer is described in Chapter 26. Calcitonin is a hormone produced by the thyroid gland and is involved in the regulation of calcium and phosphate levels in the bloodstream. Although calcitonin is not approved for prevention, it is approved for treatment because it acts directly on osteoclasts, suppressing activity.[59]

Postmenopausal women need estrogen replacement with estrogen agonist/antagonist which maximizes the beneficial effect of estrogen on bone and minimizes or antagonizes the deleterious effects on the breast and endometrium. Estrogen and estrogen plus progestogen supplementation has been found to reduce the risk of fractures, but once discontinued, within 1 year, fracture risk resumes at a level similar to that in women who have not received such therapy.[59] Estrogen agonist/antagonists and bisphosphonates have been shown to increase BMD and decrease fracture risk.[59] Raloxifene (Evista) is a commonly prescribed estrogen agonist/antagonist used for the treatment and prevention of osteoporosis. It is the first compound with selective estrogen agonist activity in bone but with estrogen antagonist activity or no activity in reproductive tissues and breast.

The use of agents that stimulate new bone formation, such as Teriparatide, a recombinant human parathyroid hormone, can be used alone and in combination with antiresorptive agents. Teriparatide acts as an anabolic bone-building agent and is best used in individuals with bone loss associated with long term use of systemic glucocorticoid therapy. Use of these injections is limited to 18–24 months and need to be replaced by other medications to maintain bone mass.[19,59]

***Exercise.*** Exercise that includes strengthening components and weight-bearing activities should be a component for the prevention and treatment of osteoporosis.[19] Exactly how much benefit can be gained from given levels or types of exercise remains unclear, but the consensus is that regular exercise has a positive effect on bone mass levels. Weight-bearing exercises (against gravity), such as walking and jogging, stress the skeletal system and are associated with greater changes in bone remodeling and result in larger bone mass, although the effects on bone mass differ in premenopausal versus postmenopausal women. For those with osteoporosis, exercises that include progressive strengthening and balance activities are recommended for the prevention of falling.[54,88] Exercises combined with bracing or other rehabilitative measures aimed at reducing the anterior translation of the cervicothoracic spine and thoracic hyperkyphosis may be beneficial in reducing the risk or occurrence of osteoporotic fractures.[44]

*Surgery.* Because of the challenges of reconstruction of osteoporotic bone, open surgical management is reserved only for those rare cases that involve neurologic deficits or an unstable spine.[87] New minimally invasive procedures for management of acute vertebral fractures, vertebroplasty, and kyphoplasty, which involve the injection of bone cement into the fractured vertebra, are discussed in Chapter 27.

**Prognosis.** Osteoporosis, once thought to be a natural part of aging among women, is no longer considered age- or gender-dependent. Although osteoporosis is one of the greatest deterrents to women's health and accounts for significant morbidity and mortality, it is largely preventable because of the remarkable progress in the scientific understanding of its causes, diagnosis, and treatment. As mentioned, a first fracture has a 2- to 4-fold increased risk of a second fracture with associated morbidity and mortality. The exact mechanism for increased fracture-associated mortality is unclear. It could be secondary to the underlying (poor) health of the affected individual (e.g., poor nutrition, dementia, weakness, deconditioning, low bone density).[9]

Medical treatment for osteoporosis has been shown to decrease the incidence of vertebral fractures by 40% to 60% after just 1 year of treatment. The occurrence of a single vertebral fracture substantially increases the likelihood of future fractures and progressive kyphotic deformity.[59] Even so, only half of women with vertebral compression fractures diagnosed incidentally with chest radiographs are started on any pharmacologic treatment, and limited a number of patients admitted with an osteoporotic hip fracture are referred for osteoporosis treatment.[65] Vertebral fractures are accompanied by increased mortality, with the relative risk of death after such a fracture being almost 9 times higher than the person without osteoporosis-associated vertebral fracture.[9] Low bone density at the hip is a strong and independent predictor of all-cause and cardiovascular mortality in older men age 65 years and older.[98]

Adherence to osteoporosis medications is relatively poor, with up to 30% of individuals suspending their treatment within 6 to 12 months of initiating therapy. Poor adherence is usually attributed to drug-induced adverse effects and results in increased risk of fracture and hospitalization.[73] There are number of drugs and combinations of treatment available to patients who may not tolerate oral bisphosphonate medication.

SPECIAL IMPLICATIONS FOR THE THERAPIST 24.1

### *Osteoporosis*

Physical therapists may initially see someone with osteoporosis for problems that are secondary to this condition. Medical diagnoses and impairments can include cervical and thoracic pain from hyperkyphotic postures, vertebral fractures and degenerative disc disease, and falls from balance disorders. There may be additional activity limitations as well. All older adults need to be asked about their history of bone health and for known results of prior tests for bone mineral densities such as with a DXA scan. These individuals may have been given their DXA scan T scores but may not have been assessed for risk of fracture using the newer FRAX assessments. Therapists should keep in mind that the diagnosis of osteoporosis has implications for the quality of movement, independence with daily activities, and risk for other disease conditions.

Treatment programs for osteoporosis and osteoporosis-related conditions should be designed to address the common impairments found with these individuals and to prevent problems associated with falls and vertebral fractures. The goals for a treatment program need to be set at 3 to 6 months in length in order to see key changes in impairments and activities limitations. The treatment program should be designed to be continued by the patient/client independently for up to a year before a reevaluation will be needed. A long-term commitment to any program is required. No immediate benefit may be perceived, especially when the individual is asymptomatic and has an overall lack of appreciation of the seriousness of the problem. Older adults experiencing cognitive decline and forgetfulness are also at risk for nonadherence. Management goals are centered on stabilizing or increasing bone mass, preventing fractures and falls and managing symptoms, especially in the presence of pain from fractures and deformity.[53,85,8]

#### Screening Assessment

The clinical implications of osteoporosis are varied, numerous, and significant. Considering the prevalence of primary and secondary osteoporosis, therapists will encounter this disease frequently. A patient with a first osteoporotic-induced or low-trauma fracture should be screened for lower extremity weakness and level of physical activity. The Osteoporosis Assessment Questionnaire and the health-related quality of life (HR-QOL) can be used to assess the functional levels of individuals with osteoporosis.[89,72]

#### Postural Assessment

Older adults should be routinely assessed for postural changes secondary to osteoporosis. The assessment of posture in supine and prone position may reveal problems not seen in standing, including tightness in pectoral and hip flexor muscles and weaknesses in the extensor muscles of the trunk and hips. A hyperkyphotic posture may be associated with movement dysfunctions at the shoulder, as well as limiting pulmonary function. Older individuals with hyperkyphosis may choose to limit their walking patterns and activities to prevent falling episodes and may not report this as a problem or concern. The assessment of balance, functional activities, and walking speed may show deficits compared to age-matched norms.[53,52]

The therapist should also be aware of the potential side effects common to osteoporosis medications. For example, calcium can cause constipation, calcitonin may be accompanied by nausea and flushing, bisphosphonates may cause leg cramps and are associated with GI intolerance and/or esophagitis. Side effects of estrogen replacement therapy are listed in Box 24.4.

Numerous medications (e.g., antihypertensives, sedatives, psychotropics, diuretics, narcotics, antidepressants, and antipsychotics) can contribute to a loss of balance and falls. A balance and fall assessment and falls prevention program is essential for anyone at risk for osteoporosis, anyone with diagnosed osteoporosis, or anyone with a history of fragility fractures associated with osteoporosis.

### Exercise and Osteoporosis

Therapists have an important role in the promotion of exercise as a preventive measure for osteoporosis. As mentioned, exercise is considered to have an important role in maintaining and possibly increasing peak bone mass. Exercise should be started early in life to increase peak bone mass and should be maintained across the life span to minimize the risks of osteoporosis. Exercise not only improves musculoskeletal health but also reduces the chronic pain syndrome and decreases depression associated with osteoporosis.[92]

The American College of Sports Medicine and the National Osteoporosis Foundation have published position stands on physical activity and bone health, including suggestions for exercise prescription for children and adolescents and for adults (Table 24.3).[104,4] Some evidence that exercise-induced gains in bone mass in children are maintained into adulthood suggests that physical activity habits during childhood may have long-lasting benefits on bone health. Quantitative dose-response studies are still lacking in this area, so the guidelines offered are suggestions based on best evidence.

**Box 24.4**

**SIDE EFFECTS OF ESTROGENS**

- Sudden onset of or change in headache, coordination, vision, breathing, speech, or extremity strength or sensation[a]
- Chest pain
- Groin or calf pain
- Change in vaginal bleeding
- Urinary incontinence
- Increased blood pressure
- Breast discharge or lumps
- Skin rash
- Extremity edema
- Jaundice
- Abdominal pain ss
- Tremors

[a]The above side effects warrant communication with a physician. Those marked with an "a" call for *immediate* communication.

### Exercise for Adults

The results of numerous studies of exercise and bone health as they are presented here represent four different exercise-related issues: (1) building bone mass, (2) slowing the decline of BMD, (3) preventing fracture, and (4) maintaining muscle mass and strength. Summaries of studies for specific types of exercise in differing populations are available.[54,71]

Although the effect of exercise on slowing the decline of BMD later in life is modest, studies have shown that the factors associated with falls such as balance, strength, and mobility are improved with moderate-level exercise program.[43,48] The level of exercise must be maintained because the benefits are lost if exercise is discontinued. A physical therapist understands the musculoskeletal system and the underlying pathologies and comorbidities and can implement an effective intervention plan that takes these variables into consideration.

Weighted exercise combined with calcium citrate supplementation has been shown in the Bone Estrogen Strength Training (BEST) study to increase bone density even in women who did not take HRT. Exercises such as leg presses, seated rows, wall squats, and back extensions and latissimus pull downs improved bone in the wrist, hip, and spine by 1% to 2% even in women who did not take a hormone replacement.[22]

**Table 24.3** ACSM Position Stand: Physical Activity and Bone Health

| Parameter | Children and Adolescents | Adults |
|---|---|---|
| Mode | Impact activities<br>• Gymnastics<br>• Plyometrics<br>• Jumping<br>Resistance training (moderate intensity)<br>Participation in aerobic sports (involving running and jumping) | Weight-bearing endurance activities<br>• Tennis<br>• Stair-climbing<br>• Walking/Jogging<br>Jumping<br>• Basketball<br>• Jump rope<br>• Volleyball<br>Resistance exercise (weight training) |
| Intensity | High intensity required for bone loading<br>Resistance training: less than 60% of 1 repetition maximum (1-RM) advised for this population (safety considerations) | Moderate to high intensity required for bone loading |
| Frequency | At least 3 times/wk<br>5–7 times/wk preferred | Weight-bearing endurance activities: at least 3–5 times/wk; 5–7 preferred<br>Resistance exercise: at least 2 times/wk |
| Duration | At least 10 minutes/session<br>Two sessions per day preferred when time is limited to 10–20 minutes/session | 30–60 minutes of combined weight-bearing endurance activities, jumping, and resistance training that targets all major muscle groups |

Data from Kohrt WM: Physical activity and bone health. American College of Sports Medicine Position Stand. *Med Sci Sports Exerc* 36(11):1985–1996, 2004.

### Type of Exercise

Exercises to build bone density must be directed at the muscles supporting or attached to the affected bone. Both aerobic and resistance training exercise can provide weight-bearing stimulus to bone, but research indicates that resistance training has a more profound site-specific effect (directed at the areas that demonstrate bone loss) than aerobic exercise. Numerous studies have shown a direct, positive relationship between the effects of resistance training and bone density.[71,108,109,60]

For the more active adult with osteoporosis, activity assessment is important to avoid flexed postures and forceful movements that compress the spinal column. For those with vertebral osteoporosis or previous history of vertebral fractures, activities such as golfing, bowling, biking, rowing, sit-ups, or other exercise with a major component of spinal flexion, side bending, or spinal rotation should be excluded. Swimming is an excellent physical activity, especially for those individuals with arthritis or other joint involvement, but without a weight-bearing component, it is not beneficial to offset the complications of osteoporosis, nor does it build bone density. Intervention modalities may include therapeutic exercise, resistance bands, foam rolls or balance balls, electrotherapy modalities, spinal orthoses or corsets, and soft tissue mobilization.[8]

### Exercise Prescription

Similar to muscle strengthening, the intensity of the load on the bone must be gradually increased and exceed the level of load to which the bone has already adapted. The program then must be progressed over a number of months to allow for the bone remodeling process to develop increased bone density. The amount of loading on the bone needs to be above what occurs with daily activities in order to stimulate osteoclastic activity. The therapist can choose high-loading activities performed infrequently or low-loading activities performed more frequently based on the patient's tolerance to these activities. The remodeling process seems to respond best to changes in the distribution of strain, suggesting that exercise should be diverse, involve different loading situations, and involve strains imposed at fast rates, with few repetitions needed to obtain the maximal osteogenic effect.[71]

The therapist will need to determine the overall needs of the patient to determine how to prescribe exercises that address the primary problems of osteoporosis as well as the secondary problems of muscle weakness, postural correction, balance, and flexibility. Site-specific extensor isometric stabilization exercises are key to the prescriptive exercise program but must be augmented by a total program of reducing risks; implementing postural correction and scapular stabilization; and improving weight-bearing patterns, strength, balance, and flexibility (Box 24.5).[53,54] To minimize the risk of development of musculoskeletal repetitive overuse syndromes, education regarding the proper use of exercise equipment, proper body mechanics, variety in the exercise program, and awareness of warning signs of overuse injuries is essential.

**Box 24.5**

**EXERCISE PRESCRIPTION GUIDELINES**

The following guidelines are used in providing prescriptive exercise:

- **Specificity:** Activities selected for osteogenic effects should stress those skeletal sites at risk for osteoporotic fractures.
- **Overload:** Progressive increase in the intensity of the exercise for continued improvement must be evident, but applied skeletal loads must be within the structural capacity of the bone to sustain the given stress.
- **Initial Values:** Those with the lowest bone mass and weakest muscles will have the greatest improvement; those with average or above-average bone mass and muscle strength will have the least.
- **Diminishing Returns:** A biologic ceiling for exercise-induced improvement in the functioning of any physiologic system is evident. As this ceiling is approached, more effort is required to attain smaller gains.
- **Maintenance:** Exercise to maintain healthy bone and muscle is a lifelong endeavor; once peak bone mass has been reached, regular physical activity, aerobic exercise, and site-specific exercise are required to maintain strength.
- **Reversibility:** The positive effect of exercise on bone and muscle will be lost if the exercise program is discontinued. It takes longer to build bone than to lose it.

Data from National Osteoporosis Foundation (NOF): *Clinicians Guide to Prevention and Treatment of Osteoporosis* (2009).

### Aquatic Therapy

Although swimmers have been shown to have higher mineral densities than those of control groups, the protective effect of swimming as an effective exercise against osteoporosis and subsequent fractures has not been demonstrated. Activities with substantial muscular involvement but without gravitational forces are associated with lower BMD than those with a weight-bearing component.[23]

Although swimming and aquatic therapy limit weight bearing on bone and therefore are not preventive, they still help maintain range of motion, build strength, and increase cardiovascular fitness with minimal stress on bones and joints. Patients with comorbidities of rheumatic diseases may benefit from forms of aquatic therapy to allow for safe movements. Walking in the water against the resistive force of the water is a better alternative for those individuals participating in an aquatic exercise program. There was significant improvement in the physical functioning, vitality, social functioning, and mental health for the intervention group. Water-based programs for older adults may also improve the psychosocial domains from the benefits of increased activity, effects of the water, or the group interaction and socialization.[24]

### Fracture Prevention

Therapists also have a role in the prevention of the most serious complication associated with osteoporosis: fracture. A prescriptive exercise program designed to improve flexibility, balance, and strength may help prevent osteoporosis, fractures, and falls. Based on our understanding now that there is a link between depression and osteoporosis, the therapist's intervention for people who are experiencing major depression should include fracture prevention.[67] (See "Depression" in Chapter 3.)

A physical therapist can design an exercise program that can help increase bone density with proper strengthening and weight-bearing exercises; lessen stress on bones through improved balance, posture, and body mechanics; and identify potential hazards in the home or workplace environment that could lead to fractures in those with osteoporosis. Choosing the appropriate gait-assistive device and teaching the person how to use the walker, cane, and other aids properly could also prevent injury. Educating the individual and family regarding home ambulatory hazards, such as throw rugs and faulty footwear, is important for fall prevention. (See extensive discussion of this topic in "Fracture" in Chapter 27.)

#### Quality of Life

Because of the costs involved in treating osteoporosis and the potential benefits offered by exercise, a need exists to expand the evaluation of exercise programs to include other relevant endpoints, such as quality of life and general fitness and well-being. Among older women who have exceeded average life expectancy, quality of life is profoundly threatened by falls and hip fractures. Any loss of ability to live independently in the community has a considerable detrimental effect on their quality of life. A study of women age 70 to 80 years found that two-thirds had moderate to high concerns about falling and have self-limited participation in social activities due to concerns of falling.[74]

#### Precautions and Considerations

In people with known osteoporosis or those at high risk of having the disease, caution should be taken with examination and treatment techniques. Manual therapy techniques that place pressure across the thorax may need to be modified to limit stress on the rib cage and lessen the risk of a fracture of the ribs. Thoracic spine mobilizations in a seated position have been used as part of a successful rehabilitation program to attenuate thoracic kyphosis in elderly women with osteoporosis. Although it is important that provocation and mobility information be collected and joint dysfunction be treated to improve functional abilities, precautions must be taken, including using other techniques or altering the person's position (e.g., side lying or sitting) so that the anterior thorax is not stabilized.[7]

As with other metabolic bone diseases, delayed healing and poor retention of internal fixation devices after fracture can occur in clients with osteoporosis. Postoperatively, the response to rehabilitation may be slowed, and adjustments may have to be made in the program to protect the injured area as recovery takes place. Close communication with the physician is called for to ensure safety.

BMD of the spine is correlated with the strength of spine extensors, so maintaining muscular strength of the spine muscles is important.[42,93] Reduction of back extension strength is correlated with increasing age and body mass index in both men and women, although men have a greater loss than women with increasing age. In both genders, more loss of back extension strength than appendicular muscle strength occurs.[91] Trunk flexion stresses need to be minimized for patients with osteoporosis. Anterior compressive forces associated with forward flexion of the spine can contribute to vertebral compression fractures. Posterior pelvic tilt and partial sit-ups (minimal abdominal crunches, lifting the head and upper torso only to the level of T6) do not appear to cause any anterior compressive force.[53]

## OSTEOMALACIA

### Definition

In contrast to osteoporosis, which results in a loss of bone mass and brittle bones, osteomalacia is a progressive disease in which lack of mineralization of the bone matrix results in a softening of bone without the loss of the bone matrix. Osteomalacia is a generalized bone condition in which insufficient mineralization of the bone matrix results from deficiency of calcium, vitamin D, and/or phosphate. The disease is sometimes referred to as the adult form of *rickets*, with the absence of epiphyseal plates in adults precluding the epiphyseal plate changes seen in rickets.

### Etiologic Factors

The two primary causes of osteomalacia are insufficient intestinal calcium absorption and increased renal phosphorus losses. The insufficient calcium absorption occurs because of either a lack of calcium or a resistance to the action of vitamin D. Excessive levels of the fibroblast growth factor-23 will inhibit reabsorption of phosphate in the renal tubules.[33] Increased renal phosphorus losses can also occur associated with renal osteodystrophy (see "Chronic Renal Failure" in Chapter 18) and renal tubular insufficiency. In addition, the long-term use of antacids, which contain aluminum hydroxide that bind with dietary forms of phosphate to prevent GI absorption, and the presence of long-standing hyperparathyroidism can lead to phosphate deficiencies, contributing to the development of osteomalacia.[68]

The dietary deficiency type of osteomalacia has been eradicated in the United States for the most part by the widespread supplementation of dairy products with vitamin D. However, osteomalacia does occur in the malnourished aging adult who may not receive adequate nutrition or enough exposure to sunlight.

### Incidence and Risk Factors

Osteomalacia is essentially a histologic diagnosis, so little information on its overall prevalence in the adult population is available. Diseases of the small intestine, cholestatic disorders of the liver, biliary obstruction, and chronic pancreatic insufficiency increase the risk

Box 24.6

**RISK FACTORS ASSOCIATED WITH OSTEOMALACIA**

- Old age
- Residence in cold geographic area
- Vitamin D deficiency
- Gastrectomy
- Intestinal malabsorption associated with:
  - Diseases of the small intestine
  - Cholangiolitic disorders of the liver
  - Biliary obstruction
  - Chronic pancreatic insufficiency
- Long-term use of:
  - Anticonvulsants
  - Barbiturates
  - Antacids, especially those containing aluminum
  - Lithium
  - Etidronate
  - Sodium fluoride
  - Acetazolamide
- History of:
  - Hyperparathyroidism
  - Chronic renal failure
  - Renal tubular defects (decreased reabsorption of phosphate)

of developing osteomalacia. Osteomalacia is common in the aged adult because of calcium- and vitamin D–deficient diets and decreased sunlight exposure. This situation is worsened by the intestinal malabsorption problems associated with aging or the presence of SLE that usually requires avoidance of sunlight to prevent ultraviolet-induced flare-ups.[68] The incidence of osteomalacia is believed to be greater in the world's colder regions, which is related to decreased exposure to sunlight, affecting vitamin D levels.

Long-term use of commonly prescribed medications also increases the risk of developing osteomalacia. Anticonvulsant medications, such as phenobarbital and phenytoin, accelerate breakdown of the active forms of vitamin D by inducing hepatic hydroxylases.[38] As mentioned, antacids can cause phosphate deficiency. Box 24.6 summarizes the risk factors associated with osteomalacia.

## Pathogenesis

Osteomalacia develops from the lack of calcium salts depositing in the bony matrix resulting in an increase in the extent of the uncalcified or osteoid matrix (Fig. 24.4). The structure of the bone is unchanged but is greatly weakened from the lack of mineralized content. The radiographic appearance of osteomalacia is characterized by changes of the cortical bone that creates Looser zones. These zones or seams appear as radiolucent bands that run transverse to the cortical margins of long bones. These seams occur because of the excessive time lag between collagen deposition and the appearance of the calcium salt. These zones can be referred to as pseudofractures or insufficiency fractures. Looser zones or pseudofractures occur most commonly on the concave side of long bones

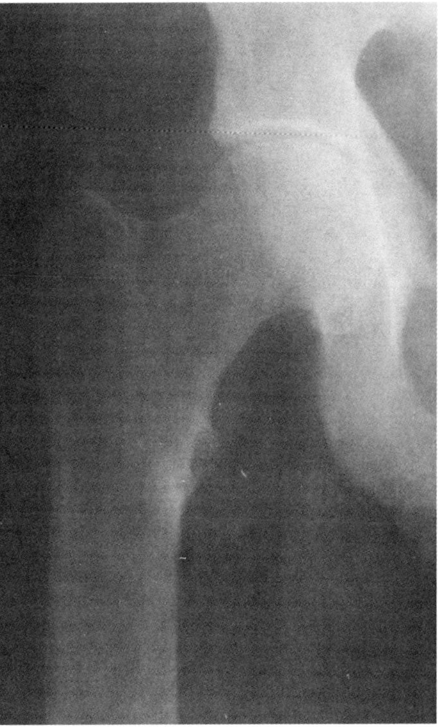

**Figure 24.4**

**Osteomalacia of the femur.** Note the loss of the sharp interface between cortical bone and cancellous bone caused by demineralization of the cortex. (From Richardson JK, Iglarsh ZA: *Clinical orthopaedic physical therapy,* Philadelphia, 1994, WB Saunders.)

such as the femur and ulna, pelvic bones, and the ribs (Fig. 24.5).[16]

## Clinical Manifestations

The diagnosis of osteomalacia is difficult and often delayed because many people present initially with diffuse, generalized aching and fatigue in the presence of anorexia and weight loss.[32] Proximal myopathy and sensory polyneuropathy may also be present, resulting in a confusing clinical presentation. Bone pain and periarticular tenderness can occur in the spine, ribs, pelvis, and proximal extremities.[81]

The combination of muscle weakness and softening of bone contributes to postural deformities, including increased thoracic kyphosis, a heart-shaped pelvis, and marked bowing of the femurs and tibias. The muscular weakness (proximal myopathy) may lead to a waddling gait and difficulties with transitional movements such as rising from sitting to standing, climbing stairs, or moving into and out of bed.[99] Occasionally, the hypocalcemia associated with osteomalacia leads to latent tetany, with paresthesias of the hands and around the mouth, muscle cramps, and positive Chvostek and Trousseau signs.

### MEDICAL MANAGEMENT

DIAGNOSIS. Osteomalacia may present with a variety of clinical and radiographic signs mimicking other musculoskeletal disorders (e.g., fibromyalgia or polymyalgia

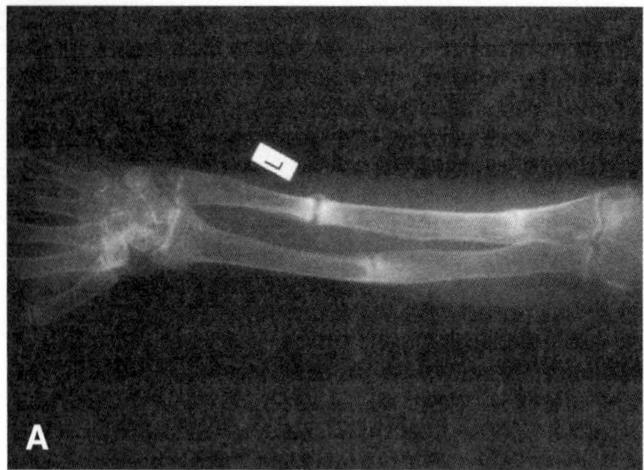


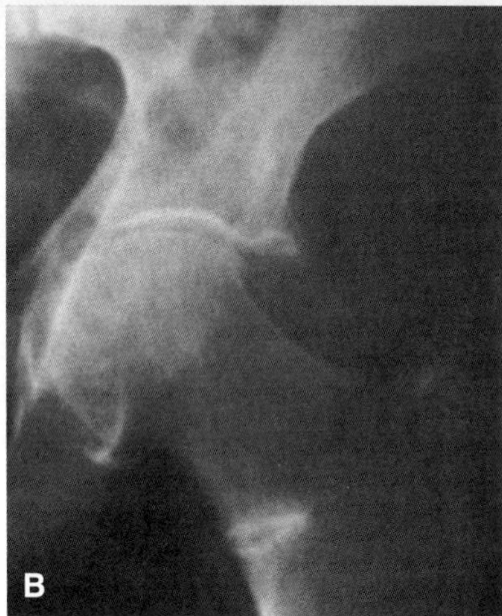


**Figure 24.5**

Osteomalacia. **A,** Forearm and **B,** femoral neck. Looser zones are seen as translucent zones with sclerotic margins. Usual sites include the medial femoral neck, pubic rami, lateral borders of the scapulae, and ribs. Complete fractures can extend through Looser zones; these will heal with appropriate treatment. (From Bullough P: *Orthopaedic pathology,* ed 3, London, 1997, Mosby-Wolfe.)

rheumatica). For this reason, numerous methods are used to diagnose osteomalacia, including radiographs, bone scan, bone biopsy, and a laboratory workup. Blood serum levels of calcium, albumin, phosphate, alkaline phosphatase, and PTH are obtained and urine is collected to assess calcium and phosphate excretion rates.[99,82] Radiographically, osteomalacia, like osteoporosis, may appear as osteopenia. Besides osteopenia, radiolucent bands in the bone cortex (Looser zones) may be revealed radiographically (see Fig. 24.5). A bone biopsy at the site of osteopenia will evaluate the calcification levels of the bone matrix.

**TREATMENT.** The treatment of osteomalacia depends primarily on the cause. If inadequate nutrition is the problem, strengthening the dietary regimen with calcium and vitamin D is necessary. This step may be sufficient to improve the calcification of the organic matrix and thereby result in healing of the pseudofractures and strengthening the bones in general. If osteomalacia is a result of intestinal malabsorption, treatment is directed to correct the primary disease. Phosphate supplementation can be prescribed in the presence of renal phosphate wasting. If used, vitamin D must be given to enhance calcium absorption impaired by the phosphate.[77]

**SPECIAL IMPLICATIONS FOR THE THERAPIST 24.2**

### *Osteomalacia*

See "Special Implications for the Therapist 24.1: Osteoporosis" above.

Considerable overlap occurs between osteomalacia and osteoporosis regarding implications for the therapist. The reader is directed to the section associated with osteoporosis for the discussion of client injury during examination and intervention, recognition of possible fracture, postoperative care, and side effects of calcium agents. See Chapter 27 for a discussion of prevention of fracture.

# PAGET DISEASE

## Definition

Paget disease (also known as *osteitis deformans*) is the second most common metabolic bone disease after osteoporosis. The disease is a progressive disorder of the adult skeletal system, characterized by increased bone resorption by osteoclasts and excessive, unorganized new bone formation by osteoblasts. Eventually, the normal bone marrow is replaced by vascular and fibrous tissue. Although Paget disease is a state of high bone turnover, the excess bone that is formed lacks the structural stability of normal bone (enlarged bone but weakened), leading to complications such as deformity, fracture, arthritis, and pain. The disease may involve one or more sites.

## Incidence and Prevalence

Paget disease is a common disease of the aging adult population, rarely presenting before age 35 years, with increasing prevalence among adults over age 50 years. Approximately 3% of the population over age 50 years and 10% of those over age 70 years may be affected, with the prevalence decreasing over the past 50 years.[64] Men and women are both affected, although a slight increased prevalence is evident among men. The disease is often familial and has an unusual geographic distribution.[21] Populations of the British Isles and countries where migration from Britain occurred (the United States, Australia, New Zealand, and Canada) have a greater incidence.

## Etiologic Factors

The cause of Paget disease is unknown. Paget disease is often inherited in an autosomal dominant pattern, but the genetic basis of the condition is not well understood.[79,75] Family studies have localized gene susceptibility to Paget disease at three different chromosomal regions, although these defects do not appear to account for the majority of cases. Because of the late age of onset of this disease, finding large families with a number of generations with the disease has been difficult and has hindered progress in research.

Environmental factors, specifically slow viruses that take years to progress to a point where symptoms become evident, may play a role in the development of Paget disease; the hereditary factor may be the reason family members are susceptible to the suspected virus.[21] Exactly how the viruses affect osteoclasts remains unknown. Paget disease has become less prevalent and people are presenting even later and with less severe disease than before; thus, environmental factors may be an important etiologic factor in this disease.

## Pathogenesis

Paget disease has been considered a disorder of the osteoclasts. However, osteoblasts are major regulators of osteoclast development and function, and a tightly coupled pathway of communication and collaboration is evident between these two groups of cells. The exact mechanism by which these two cell types contribute to the formation of Paget disease is unclear.

An initial resorptive phase where abnormal osteoclasts proliferate unrestrained is evident. The bone resorption is so rapid that osteoblastic activity cannot keep up and fibrous tissue replaces bone. Radiographically, the resultant lytic areas are sharply defined and appear as flame- or wedge-shaped. The initial resorption stage is followed by abnormal regeneration called the *osteoblastic sclerotic phase.*

The mixed phase occurs with the rapid increase in osteoblastic activity, but the normal cancellous architecture is replaced by coarse, thickened struts of trabecular bone, and the cortical bone is irregularly thickened, rough, and pitted. The abnormal arrangement of the lamellar bone, separated by so-called cement lines, gives the bone the look of a mosaic. Although heavily calcified, the bone is now enlarged but weakened, with a chaotic woven pattern, rather than the well-organized lamellar structure seen in normal bone.

Involvement of the vertebral bodies presents with a picture-frame appearance radiographically as the cortical shell and endplates become greatly exaggerated in comparison to the coarse, cancellous bone portion of the vertebral body. The final stage of the disease is characterized by little cellular activity.[75]

## Clinical Manifestations

Paget disease begins insidiously and progresses slowly. In mild cases, a person may have a few symptoms or may be symptom free over a very long period, eventually presenting with bone pain and skeletal deformities. When Paget disease is active in several bones, overactive osteoclasts can release enough calcium into the blood to cause hypercalcemia, resulting in fatigue, weakness, loss of appetite, abdominal pain, and constipation.[75]

### Musculoskeletal

The progressive deossification that weakens the bony structure primarily affects the axial skeleton. The lesions occur at multiple sites, particularly the skull, spine, pelvis,

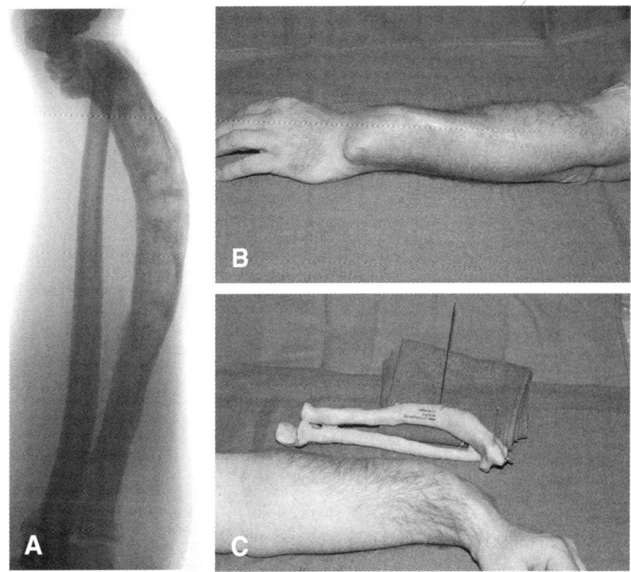


**Figure 24.6**

**Paget disease.** A complex malunion of the radius in a 62-year-old man after several fractures. **A,** The presenting lateral radiograph of the severe deformity. **B,** The clinical appearance. **C,** A bone model made from computed tomographic scans and used for preoperative planning for correction of the deformity. (From Browner BD: *Skeletal trauma: basic science, management, and reconstruction,* ed 3, Philadelphia, 2003, WB Saunders.)

femurs, and tibias. Pathologic fractures can occur in any bone (Fig. 24.6), especially in the radius, proximal femurs, pelvis, and lumbar spine.

Affected bones change in size, shape, and alignment, resulting in bone pain, deformities, fractures, and arthritis (Box 24.7). The most common manifestation is pain, which may be of a headache, radicular, osteoarthritic, muscular, or other skeletal origin. Pain from periosteal irritation of involved bones is deep and boring, worse at night, and reduced but not eliminated with activity. In some people, this pain may be referred to nearby muscles and joints.

Clients may also experience fatigue, lightheadedness, and general stiffness. New onset of pain may be related to pathologic fracture of the vertebral bodies, pelvis, or long bones. Damage to the cartilage of joints adjacent to the affected bone and distortion of the normal joint alignment from bony changes may lead to osteoarthritis. The osteoarthritis is often more disabling than the Paget disease itself and will not respond to treatment of the underlying bone disease.[95]

Clinical findings also include postural deformities such as increased thoracic kyphosis and bowing of the femurs and tibias (Fig. 24.7). Bony softening of the femoral neck can cause coxa vara (reduced angle of the femoral neck) and may result in a waddling gait. These changes may produce increased local mechanical stresses resulting in pain.[75]

### Neurologic

Paget disease of the skull and spinal column can produce neurologic complications as a result of either direct impingement (myelopathy) or ischemia related to a

Box 24.7

**CLINICAL MANIFESTATIONS OF PAGET DISEASE**

***Pain***

- Headache
- Muscular
- Osteoarthritis
- Radicular
- Skeletal

***Skeletal***

- Pain (bone pain that may be referred to nearby joints and muscles)
- Deformities
  - Kyphoscoliosis
  - Bone thickening or enlargement (including skull)
  - Bowing (outward bowed femur, forward bowed tibia)
  - Coxa varus (waddling gait); acetabular protrusion
  - Vertebral compression or collapse
- Fractures
- Osteoarthritis

***Muscular***

- Pain (myalgia)
- Stiffness

***Neurologic***

- Nerve compression syndromes (including cranial, spinal, and peripheral nerves)
- Mental confusion, deterioration in cognitive function
- Sensorineural hearing loss

***Cardiovascular***

- Increased cardiac output
- Increased vascularity (increased skin temperature over involved bone)
- Heart failure

***Miscellaneous***

- Fatigue
- Tinnitus
- Lightheadedness, dizziness, vertigo

*pagetic steal syndrome* (hypervascular pagetic bone "steals" blood from the neural tissue). Affected individuals also report tinnitus, vertigo, and hearing loss. Typical neurologic deficits include eighth cranial nerve involvement with hearing loss related to involvement of the ossicles or bony foraminal encroachment. Headaches may occur if the skull is involved, and the forehead may enlarge as the amount of bone in the skull expands and the foramen for the cranial nerves becomes smaller (Fig. 24.8).

Other nerve or spinal cord compression syndromes may occur as enlarged pagetic bones put pressure on various nerve structures. Findings may include myelopathy, spinal stenosis, radiculoneuropathy, cauda equina syndrome, peripheral nerve entrapment, carpal and tarsal tunnel syndromes, and any of the effects of cranial nerve compression.[75]

## Cardiovascular

Other findings may include mental deterioration (Paget disease causes reduced blood flow to the brain) and cardiovascular disease (rare). The cardiovascular disease is

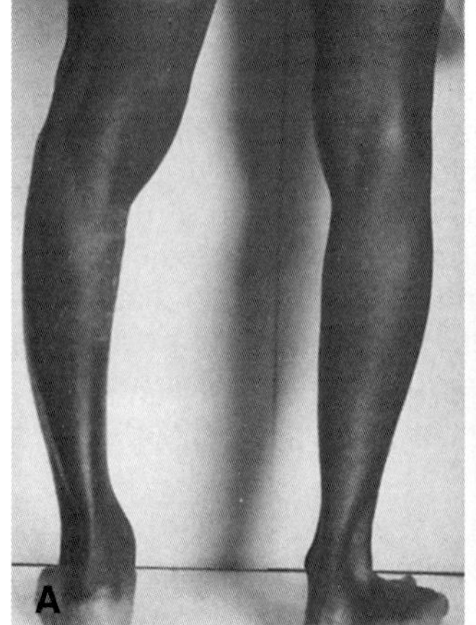


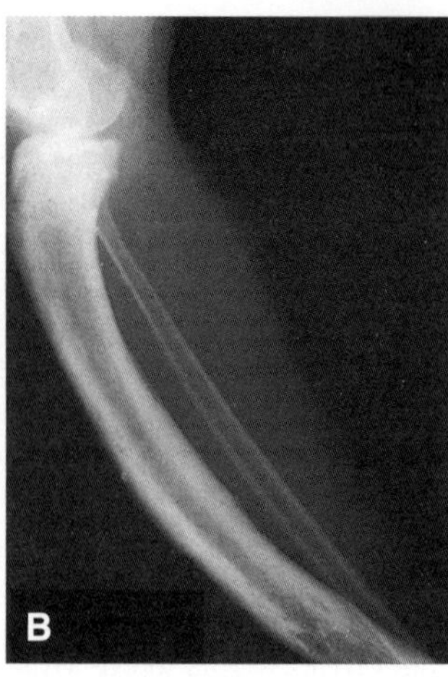


**Figure 24.7**

**A,** Bowing of the leg is often seen in Paget disease. **B,** Radiograph of a person with Paget disease affecting the tibia (but not the fibula). Overgrowth has resulted in an increase in length of the tibia, associated with bowing. Irregularity of both the periosteal and endosteal surfaces is shown. (From Bullough P: *Orthopaedic pathology,* ed 3, London, 1997, Mosby-Wolfe.)

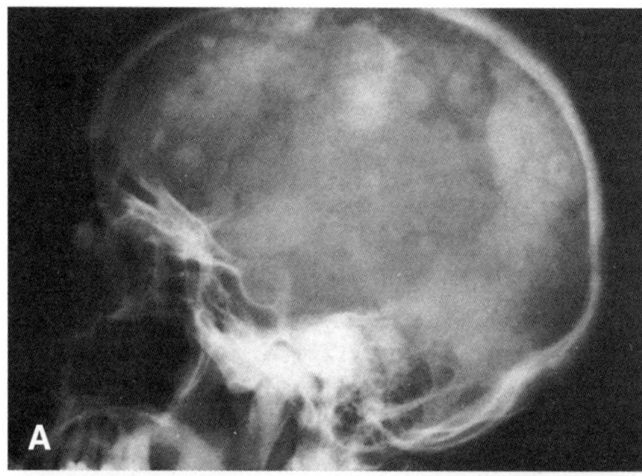


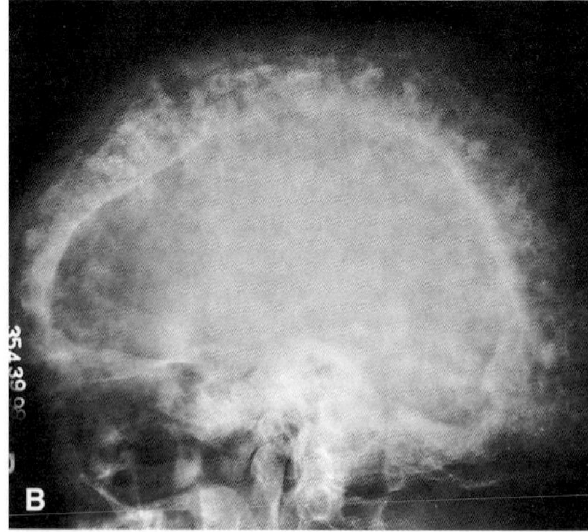


**Figure 24.8**

**Clinical radiographs of the skull in later stages of Paget disease. A,** Marked patchy sclerosis appears in the bone, the organized architecture is lost, and the bone becomes extremely thick, on occasion several times thicker than normal. **B,** Advanced involvement of the skull with marked thickening of the entire vault, areas of osteolysis, and patchy new bone formation, resulting in a "cotton-wool" appearance called *osteoporosis circumscripta cranii.* This person experienced progressive hearing loss. (**A** from Bullough P: *Orthopaedic pathology,* ed 3, London, 1997, Mosby-Wolfe; **B** from Goldman L: *Cecil textbook of medicine,* ed 22, Philadelphia, 2004, WB Saunders.)

due to vasodilation of blood vessels in the bones and skin and subcutaneous tissues overlying the affected bones. When one-third to one-half of the skeleton is involved, an increase in cardiac output may be severe enough to cause heart failure. This is the most common cause of death in people with advanced Paget disease.[75]

## MEDICAL MANAGEMENT

**DIAGNOSIS.** Because Paget disease progresses slowly and the severity of the disease varies considerably among individuals, it may be many years before a diagnosis is made or the person may be misdiagnosed with arthritis or other disorders. In fact, the diagnosis is often made incidentally on the basis of radiographs after a fracture or laboratory tests done for other conditions.

A screening test that measures alkaline phosphate blood levels can be used to detect those at risk of Paget disease. Alkaline phosphatase is an enzyme that is produced by bone cells and overproduced by pagetic bone. Siblings and children of those with Paget disease may have a standard alkaline phosphatase blood test every 2 or 3 years. Alkaline phosphatase levels can also be used to diagnose Paget disease and to monitor response to therapy. If the alkaline phosphatase level is above normal, other tests, such as the bone-specific alkaline phosphatase test, bone scan, or radiographic examination, can be performed.

The diagnosis is usually based on the characteristic bone deformities and radiologic bony changes. Radiographic signs of osteopenia will be found during the early resorptive phase, with pockets of sclerotic and osteopenic changes within cancellous bone found during the later phases of the disease process. Bone scans are positive only if the disease is active and marked by rapid bone turnover but provide information that helps determine the extent and activity of the condition. Bone scans must be confirmed by radiographic examination, as other conditions are also accompanied by a metabolically active lesion. A bone biopsy may be performed for a medical differential diagnosis to rule out hyperparathyroidism, bone metastasis, multiple myeloma, and fibrous dysplasia.[75]

**TREATMENT.** The goal of treatment is to normalize bone health for a prolonged period. Inhibitors of bone resorption, nitrogen-containing bisphosphonates such as oral alendronate or risedronate, are the first line of treatment.[80] These pharmacologic agents (see Box 24.3) decrease bone turnover through the inhibition of osteoclastic activity to improve bone density, and reduce fracture incidence. These pharmacologic agents have a long-lasting effect on biochemical processes and provide long-lasting remissions in the majority of people.

Treatment response is assessed by the extent of reduction of the biochemical markers of bone turnover, especially plasma total alkaline phosphatase. The goal of treatment is to induce full remission through normal levels of alkaline phosphatase and prevention of complications of the disease.[21] Some experts in the field are recommending treatment of asymptomatic people who have active disease at sites where complications are likely to develop, although no data are available at this time to prove that complications can be prevented by pharmacologic intervention.[80]

Management of Paget disease depends on the degree of pain and extent of the pathologic changes. Nonsteroidal and other antiinflammatory agents are used to control the pain. Surgical intervention may include fracture repairs, occipital craniectomy to relieve basilar and nerve compression, tibial osteotomy if the deformity is severe, and joint replacement(s) if severe degenerative joint disease is present.

**PROGNOSIS.** The course of Paget disease varies widely from stable and asymptomatic, to rapid progressions of signs and symptoms. The outlook is generally good, particularly if treatment is given before major changes have occurred. Biochemical remission with bisphosphonates is achievable in a majority of individuals.[94] Paget disease is accompanied by osteogenic sarcoma in less than 1% of all cases but represents an increase in risk that is several thousand-fold higher than the general population.[40]

Prognosis for individuals with Paget sarcoma is poor and is unrelated to the site or stage of presentation. Little progress has occurred in the treatment of Paget sarcoma over the years despite improvement in the treatment of standard osteosarcoma.[25] See Chapter 26 for an overview of osteogenic sarcoma.

### SPECIAL IMPLICATIONS FOR THE THERAPIST 24.3

#### *Paget Disease*

Although Paget disease and osteoporosis can occur in the same person, these are completely different disorders, with different causes. However, despite their marked differences, considerable overlap is evident between Paget disease and osteoporosis regarding interventions and implications for the therapist (see "Osteoporosis" above). The overlap includes the discussion of client injury during examination and treatment, recognition of possible fracture, and postoperative care. For a discussion of fractures and fracture prevention see Chapter 27.

#### *Screening Assessment*

Therapists need to be aware of the symptoms and signs of Paget disease. Because pain is often the initial symptom and is usually a vague diffuse ache, difficulty in distinguishing this disease from degenerative joint disease of the lumbar spine, hips, or knees can be evident. Clients with diffuse headaches may present to the therapist with undiagnosed Paget disease. These clients may report hearing loss, tinnitus, incontinence, diplopia, or swallowing difficulties. Slurring of speech or the onset of signs or symptoms associated with heart disease is evident. The presentation of any of the above clinical manifestations warrants communication with a physician.[75] Clients with fractures should have their radiographs assessed for the appearance and contrast of the cancellous bone. Again, if any of these signs or symptoms are reported to the therapist, communication with a physician is warranted.

#### *Exercise and Paget Disease*

Exercise is very important in maintaining skeletal health and is recommended for people with Paget disease. Joints adjacent to involved bone may function at a mechanical disadvantage, causing muscular pain that can be reduced with exercise. Strengthening muscles can also help minimize skeletal complications of Paget disease with its mechanical stresses and resultant structural abnormalities of bone.

The pain associated with Paget disease often leads to less physical activity in daily life. Loss of muscle strength, joint motion, and cardiovascular endurance occur, leading to functional limitations such as slower walking and shorter distances.[58] Exercise helps with weight control, improving cardiovascular function and cardiac output, and maintains muscular strength and joint motion. Severity of Paget disease will determine the exercise program. Stretching, strengthening, endurance, aerobics, balance, and coordination exercises are all important. Some types of exercise should be avoided such as jogging, running, jumping, and if the spine is affected, forward bending and twisting exercises.

Complications of orthopedic surgery on pagetic bone include hemorrhage, infection, pathologic fracture, delayed union or nonunion, and aseptic loosening of the hardware. The therapist may be involved in management of extremity deformities requiring management with orthotics.

## REFERENCES

To enhance this text and add value for the reader, all references are included in the enhanced ebook on Student Consult that accompanies this textbook. The reader can view the reference source and access it online whenever possible.

# CHAPTER 25

# Infectious Diseases of the Musculoskeletal System

KEVIN HELGESON

Understanding the epidemiology, pathogenesis, and treatment of musculoskeletal infections will allow the clinician to play an active role in all phases of diagnosis and intervention. From early detection of signs and symptoms that identify clients who are at risk and need further medical evaluation to the rehabilitation of clients who undergo surgical intervention for musculoskeletal infections, the role of therapists and their impact on the outcome of treatment cannot be underestimated.

The use of temporary and permanent implants and prosthetic materials including bioprosthetic implants is now commonplace. Therapists often treat clients with biomaterial implants. Joint replacements, heart valves, vascular prostheses, artificial disk replacements, shunts, dental implants, baclofen/insulin/pain pumps, sutures, catheters, and allografts are a few of the devices that can harbor infections. Musculoskeletal infections can require drastic measures to treat and prevent morbidity. For example, infection after total joint replacement often requires removal of the hardware, and joint sepsis may require extensive surgical débridement.

Only the most common infectious diseases seen in a therapy practice are included in this chapter (e.g., osteomyelitis, diskitis, infectious arthritis, and tuberculosis [TB]). Necrotizing fasciitis, streptococcal myositis, and soft tissue infection leading to gangrene are discussed in Chapter 8; cellulitis is discussed in Chapters 8 and 10.

## OSTEOMYELITIS

### Overview

Osteomyelitis is an inflammation of bone caused by an infectious organism such as bacteria, but fungi, parasites, and viruses can also cause skeletal infections (see Chapter 8). Areas affected most often include the spine, pelvis, and arms or legs.[15] The pathophysiology of osteomyelitis is complex and poorly understood. Key factors include the virulence of the infecting organism; the individual's immune status; any comorbidities; and the type, location, and vascularity of the involved bone.

*Acute osteomyelitis* is the clinical term for a new infection in bone. It is a rapidly destructive pyogenic infection often seen in children, older adults, and intravenous (IV) drug abusers. The infectious agent enters the body through an open wound or the gastrointestinal (GI) tract. The infection has the capability to spread quickly through the bloodstream, resulting in septicemia or a septic infectious joint. In adults, osteomyelitis is usually a subacute or chronic infection that develops secondary to an open injury to bone and surrounding soft tissue. *Chronic osteomyelitis* is often the result of a persistent bone infection or acute disease remaining undiagnosed.[24]

### Incidence

Acute osteomyelitis is a relatively uncommon but potentially serious disease occurring more often in children than adults and affecting boys more often than girls. Acute hematogenous osteomyelitis is the most common type and is usually seen in children. Chronic osteomyelitis is more common in adults and immunocompromised people. The incidence of osteomyelitis was expected to decline with more widespread availability of antibiotics. However, with the presence of drug-resistant organisms, the number of IV drug abusers, and the increased use of implantable prosthetic devices, osteomyelitis is actually becoming more common.[40,1]

### Etiologic Factors

*Staphylococcus aureus* is the usual causative agent of acute osteomyelitis. It has the ability to bind to cartilage, produce a protective glycocalyx, and stimulate the release of endotoxins. Glycocalyx is the glycoprotein and polysaccharide covering that surrounds many cells; in bacterial cells, the glycocalyx forms masses of fibers that extend from the bacterial cell and are the means by which the bacteria adhere to surfaces.[24]

Other organisms such as group B streptococcus, pneumococcus, *Pseudomonas aeruginosa, Haemophilus influenzae,* and *Escherichia coli* also produce bone infections.[32] In people with sickle cell anemia, *Salmonella* infection is associated with osteomyelitis. Osteomyelitis can be acquired from exogenous or hematogenous sources.

*Exogenous osteomyelitis* is acquired by invasion of the bone by direct extension from the outside as a result of inoculation into the bone by a penetrating or puncture wound, extension from an overlying abscess or burn, or other trauma such as an open fracture.[6] Surgical procedures, open

Box 25.1

**STATES ASSOCIATED WITH MUSCULOSKELETAL INFECTION**

***Congenital***

- Chronic granulomatous disease
- Hemophilia
- Hypogammaglobulinemia
- Sickle cell hemoglobinopathy

***Acquired***

- Diabetes mellitus
- Hematologic malignancy
- HIV infection
- Pharmacologic immunosuppression
  - Organ transplantation
  - Collagen-vascular diseases
- Uremia
- Myelopathy (spinal cord injury)
- Alcoholism
- Malnutrition; poor nutritional status

Data from Brennan PJ, DeGirolamo MP: Musculoskeletal infections in immunocompromised hosts. *Orthop Clin North Am* 22:390, 1991; Berbari BF, Steckelberg JM, Osmon DR.: Osteomyelitis. In Mandell GL, Bennett JE, Dolin R, editors: *Principles and practice of infectious diseases*, ed 7, Philadelphia, 2009, Elsevier; Matteson EL, Osmon DR: Infections of bursae, joints, and bones. In Goldman L, Schafer AI, editors: *Cecil medicine*, ed 24, Philadelphia, 2011, Saunders.

fractures, and implanted orthopedic devices are common sources of acute osteomyelitis infection. These examples of osteomyelitis secondary to a contiguous area of infection are common in immunocompromised people and in people with diabetes or severe vascular insufficiency.[75]

*Hematogenous osteomyelitis* is acquired from spread of organisms from preexisting infections such as occur in impetigo; furunculosis (persistent boils); infected lesions of varicella (chickenpox); and sinus, ear, dental, soft tissue, respiratory (through alveoli when an upper respiratory infection is present), and genitourinary infections. Vaginal, uterine, ovarian, bladder, and intestinal infections can lead to iliac or sacral osteomyelitis.[34]

Osteomyelitis of the arm and hand bones may occur in drug abusers, and vertebral osteomyelitis is seen in adults from hematogenous spread from pelvic or urinary tract infections. The lumbar spine is the most commonly involved area. In children the infection is spread hematogenously and usually develops in the metaphyseal regions of the long bones, adjacent to the growth plates (e.g., distal femur, proximal tibia, humerus, and radius).[40]

## Risk Factors

In general, anyone who is chronically ill (e.g., diabetes or alcoholism) or who receives large doses of steroids or immunosuppressive drugs is particularly susceptible to osteomyelitis (Box 25.1). Infection with methicillin-resistant *S. aureus* increases the risk of developing osteomyelitis.[64]

Risk factors for osteomyelitis of the foot in individuals with diabetes include ulceration, sausage toe, or visible or palpable bone. Infected or nonhealing ulcers following several weeks of appropriate care and off-loading pressure increase the risk of osteomyelitis. Ulcer areas deeper than 3 mm, over bony prominences, and larger than 2 $cm^2$ are additional risk factors.[64]

Older adults with additional preexisting medical conditions, such as malignancy, malnutrition, and renal or hepatic failure, are also at a greater risk. Individuals with spinal cord injury with complete motor and sensory paralysis at the paraplegic level appear to be at risk for vertebral osteomyelitis.[55]

Nutritional status is an often overlooked variable in acute and chronic illness. Anyone who is at risk for malnutrition or is compromised by poor nutritional status is at risk for infection, slowed tissue healing, and an increased incidence of postsurgical complications.

Infection is the second most common cause of prosthetic joint failure, after mechanical loosening. Some cases of prosthetic joint infection may be misclassified as aseptic loosening. The incidence of prosthetic joint infection is higher after a revision.[65]

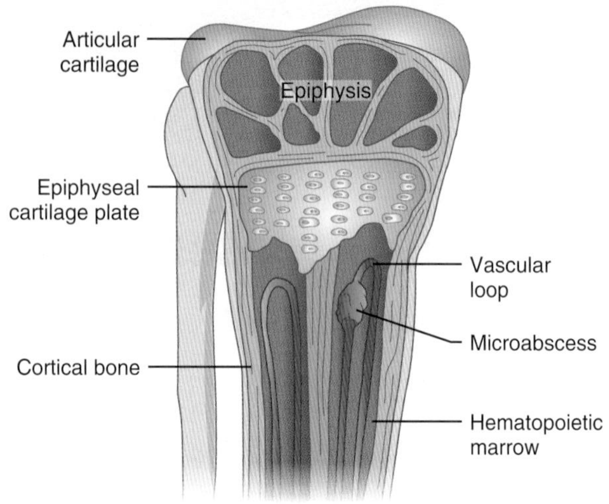


**Figure. 25.1**

The vascular loop in growing bone is a common initial site of bacterial seeding.

## Pathogenesis

The pathophysiology of osteomyelitis is complex and poorly understood. Key factors include the virulence of the infecting organism; the person's immune status; any underlying disease; and the type, location, and vascularity of the involved bone. Regardless of the source of the pathogen, the pathogenesis of bone infection initially involves an inflammatory response. Acute osteomyelitis may develop in the metaphysis of long bones because of the decreased amount of phagocytosis and/or slower rate of blood flow in the terminal arterioles. The vascular loop in growing bone is a common site of bacterial seeding because the arterioles form a loop and then drain into the medullary cavity without establishing a capillary bed (Fig. 25.1). Trauma, including microtrauma, may also increase susceptibility to infection by slowing the blood flow.[24]

The metaphysis of long bones is very porous, allowing exudate from the infection to spread easily. As the organisms

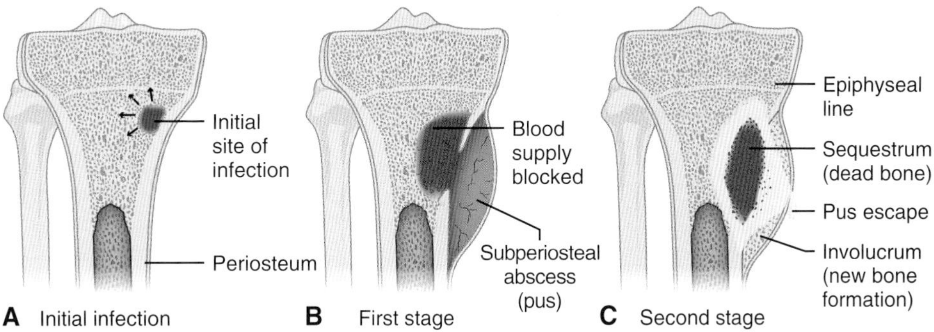


**Figure. 25.2**

**Osteomyelitis.** (A) Initial infection. The bacteria reach the metaphysis through the nutrient artery. (B) First stage: bacterial growth results in bone destruction and formation of an abscess. (C) Second stage: from the abscess cavity, the pus spreads between the trabeculae into the medulla, through the cartilage into the joint, or through the haversian canals of the compact bones to the outside. These sinuses traversing the bone persist for a long time and heal slowly. The pus destroys the bone and sequesters part of it in the abscess cavity. Reactive new bone is formed around the focus of inflammation. (From Damjanov I: *Pathology for the health-related professions*, ed 3, Philadelphia, 2006, Saunders.)

grow and form pus within the bone, tension builds within the rigid medullary cavity, forcing pus through the haversian canals. Haversian canals contain blood, lymph vessels, and nerves. Once bacteria gain access to these channels, they are able to proliferate unimpeded, forming a subperiosteal abscess that deprives the bone of its blood supply and eventually may cause necrosis. Necrotic cells then become a fertile bed for the organisms to multiply. Because sensory nerve endings are absent in cancellous bone, this process can progress without pain. Necrosis then stimulates the periosteum to create new bone.

A sheath of new bone, called an *involucrum,* forms around the *sequestrum* of necrotic tissue that has become separated from the surrounding bone (Fig. 25.2). By the time the sequestrum forms, the osteomyelitis is considered to be chronic. In adults, this complication is rare because the periosteum is firmly attached to the cortex and resists displacement. Instead, infection disrupts and weakens the cortex, which predisposes the bone to pathologic fracture.[64]

In vertebral osteomyelitis, the infection is first found in the metaphysis or cartilaginous endplates and quickly spreads to the intervertebral disk. Abscess formation is common through direct extension of the infection to adjacent tissues. The abscesses can advance posteriorly to involve the epidural area or anteriorly to produce a paravertebral abscess that can extend to the psoas muscle, producing hip pain.[71]

## Clinical Manifestations

The primary manifestations of osteomyelitis vary between adults and children. Back pain is typically the chief complaint in adults, but once the infection becomes systemic (as opposed to an abscess), a low-grade fever may be present. Children are more likely to present with acute, severe complaints such as high fever and intense pain, but in some cases, local manifestations will predominate such as edema, erythema, and tenderness. These signs are easier to detect in the extremities, in contrast to vertebral osteomyelitis, where the infected structures lie much deeper.[2]

In the initial phases of the infection, pain may not be a factor because of the lack of pain fibers in cancellous bone. This makes diagnosis and intervention difficult because of the potential rapid spread of the infectious agent, which is facilitated by the delay in administration of appropriate antibiotics. When the infection extends into the periosteum, increased joint pain; diminished function; and systemic signs such as fever, swelling, and malaise may rapidly develop.

The pain will likely be described as deep and constant, increasing with weight bearing when the infection is anywhere in the lower extremity. Clients presenting with chronic osteomyelitis complain of local pain and swelling and may limp but otherwise are often asymptomatic. The clinical sign of sausage toe has been used to detect underlying pedal osteomyelitis. This clinical sign has been demonstrated to have good sensitivity and specificity in clients with diabetes.[34]

Once present, spinal osteomyelitis can produce intermittent or constant back pain. The pain can be aggravated by motion but is also present regardless of activity level in some individuals and throbbing at rest. It may radiate in a radicular distribution and is commonly accompanied by spinal tenderness and rigidity; accessory motions of the spine are often difficult to perform. As mentioned, pyogenic vertebral osteomyelitis may result in a psoas abscess, causing painful hip extension and/or an antalgic limp. Cervical abscess formation may lead to torticollis or dysphagia.[71]

Radiculopathy, myelopathy, or even complete paralysis can occur with neural compression as a result of abscess, instability, or spinal deformity associated with vertebral osteomyelitis. Direct spread of the infection into the epidural space can cause meningitis.[65]

Sacroiliac osteomyelitis is usually characterized by severe, local pain with tenderness and an antalgic gait. The pain may radiate to the buttocks or abdomen. The history will be a recent onset of localized pain. Besides pain, other symptoms may include fever, local tenderness, and swelling. Any unexplained cellulitis should be considered a sign of osteomyelitis in children, even if no other contributing signs or symptoms are evident.

### MEDICAL MANAGEMENT

**PREVENTION.** Because chronic osteomyelitis is also recognized as a complication of treatment of open fractures, prevention of infection is important. The risks can be minimized if the wound is thoroughly débrided, irrigated, and left open for delayed primary closure. Delayed primary closure allows the wound bed to be inspected, and further débridement can be carried out if necessary.

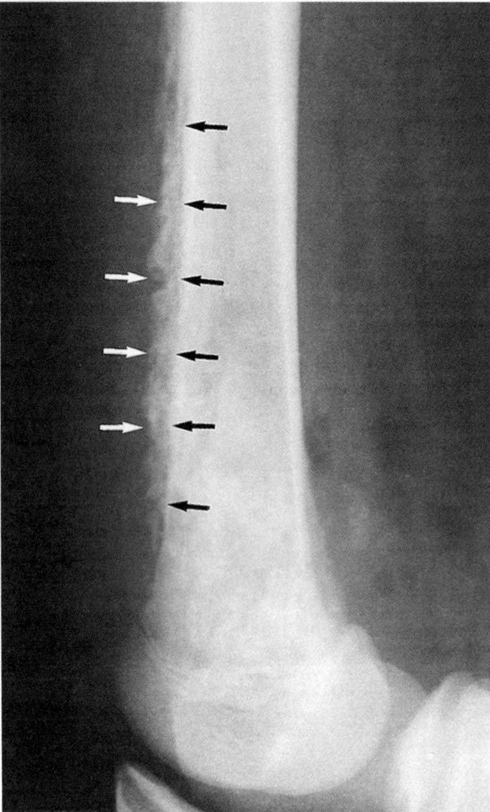

**Figure. 25.3**

**Chronic osteomyelitis.** A lateral view of the knee shows the periosteal reaction *(arrows)* suggestive of chronic osteomyelitis. The bone of the distal femur has a mottled appearance as a result of the infection. (From Mettler FA: *Essentials of radiology*, ed 2, Philadelphia, 2005, Saunders.)

Clients with any of the conditions listed in Box 25.1 or with any additional risk factors should be taught proper preventive measures and be aware of early warning signs. As mentioned, nutritional status plays a critical role in the prevention of infection and the body's ability to combat infection once it occurs. Anyone with biomaterial implants will have an increased risk of infection, especially in the immediate postoperative period. Although rare, late infections occurring 1 year postoperatively have been reported.[68]

**SCREENING.** Although diagnosing infectious diseases is outside the scope of the therapist's practice, screening is still appropriate, using a thorough history and a review of systems to help identify pathologies that require further medical evaluation. For screening purposes, the presence of a fever, unexplained weight loss, history of cancer, and failure to respond to adequate treatment are good indicators of more serious pathology.[34]

Disturbances in the sleep pattern, such as awakening with pain, requiring sleep medications, or inability to fall asleep, along with symptoms that increase with walking, have been found to be associated with serious back problems. In other areas of the body, localized pain in the presence of other risk factors may raise suspicion.

**DIAGNOSIS.** Medical diagnosis is often delayed because of the lack of specific signs and symptoms, especially in chronic osteomyelitis. Signs and symptoms that are generally associated with infection may be masked by (or mistaken for) normal postoperative changes. Laboratory values and radiographs are often negative in the early stages. Positive cultures are obtained in only half of the cases; however, this is improving because of advancements in molecular techniques.[12] Any unexplained cellulitis in children is suggested to be considered as a possible indicator of underlying osteomyelitis.[4]

Radiographs are recommended for initial imaging of suspected infections, but they may not detect bony abnormality with an acute infection.[8] Lytic lesions may be demonstrable on radiographs within 2 weeks of onset of the disease A periosteal reaction develops later (Fig. 25.3). Magnetic resonance imaging (MRI) with contrast is the procedure of choice in delineating the anatomic extent of disease. Imaging tests are often used to localize or confirm the presence of infection. MRI is sensitive and provides valuable details of septic arthritis, spinal osteomyelitis, and diabetic foot infections.[59] Computed tomography (CT) scans may be used if MRI is contraindicated. Radionuclide bone scan can detect early-stage disease and is helpful in detecting and identifying multiple sites of involvement.

Nuclear medicine imaging techniques such as tomography scans provide accurate localization of infection and/or source of fever of undetermined origin, thereby guiding additional testing. Tomography helps diagnose spinal osteomyelitis and can be useful in measuring the extent of disease and monitoring response to treatment.[59,48,78]

Identification of the infectious pathogen is of utmost importance because the type of medication used often depends on the infecting microorganism. Specimens are obtained for culture or stains by aspiration, needle biopsy, or swab. Accurate identification is often difficult because of the technical problems of obtaining an acceptable sample. Image-enhanced needle biopsy can improve the specimen quality.[64]

Early acute postoperative prosthetic joint infection in most cases occurs in the first 3 months after surgery. Chronic, postoperative prosthetic joint infection is characterized by more subtle signs of inflammation, chronic persistent postoperative pain, and/or early loosening of the implant. Differentiating late postoperative prosthetic joint infection from aseptic implant failure can be challenging.

**TREATMENT.** Immediate treatment is indicated, especially in acute osteomyelitis. Sequential IV and high-dose antibiotic therapy is now an accepted modality and has lessened the role of surgery in these infections. The choice of antibiotics is based primarily on the culture results as well as the client's age and health status, site of infection, and previous antimicrobial therapy.[34]

Antibiotics are delivered intravenously to hasten their effect when faced with serious infection that can progress rapidly. Evaluation of response to treatment by monitoring C-reactive protein levels has decreased the average duration of therapy to 3 to 4 weeks with few relapses.[7,44]

Surgery is indicated if the infection has spread to the joints, as this is considered an orthopedic emergency. Articular cartilage can be damaged in a matter of hours. The goal of surgery is to drain exudate or pus from the bone or joint. Often extensive débridement of both bone and surrounding soft tissue is required. Various reconstructive procedures may be considered once the infection is eliminated. These include soft tissue procedures to provide well-vascularized soft tissue coverage of defects and revascularized bone for stabilization of the affected area. In adults, both surgery and antibiotics are often required.[64]

The goals for treatment of chronic osteomyelitis are to eliminate the infection by use of antibiotics if possible or by surgically removing infected tissue. If surgery is indicated, the current trend is toward more radical surgery rather than serial débridements. In general, chronic osteomyelitis is more difficult to treat than the acute type because it is difficult to eradicate completely. Exacerbations may respond well to treatment with rest and antibiotics, only to flare up again months later.

In the spine, surgery may be necessary to treat the infection and to address spinal deformity. Deformity of the spine from the infection or subsequent surgery may lead to pain or neurologic compromise. If surgery is not indicated, the person may be treated with short-term bed rest or the use of a brace for immobilization.

The use of appropriate antibiotics prophylactically is standard for some procedures such as total joint replacements and in open wounds that are contaminated. Antibiotic bead chains can be implanted in the infected area to achieve concentrated levels of antibiotics in the local tissue without raising serum levels to toxic ranges. These bead chains can be an effective method of prophylaxis and treatment of established infections.[14]

**PROGNOSIS.** There is a small risk of death for the majority of individuals with acute osteomyelitis, but treatment remains a challenge. With early medical interventions, an infection arrest rate of 70% to 90% can be expected; a permanent loss of bone structure and changes to the surrounding soft tissues almost always occur.[75] When osteomyelitis is diagnosed in the early clinical stages and treated with antibiotics, the prognosis for regaining function of the involved tissues is excellent. For skeletally immature children and adolescents, there is a greater possibility of an infection, resulting in a growth abnormality in the affected bony structures.

When osteomyelitis persists for a long period of time, infected necrotic bone serves as an isolated reservoir for infection that will not respond well to systemic antibiotics. Reduced blood flow will facilitate the likelihood that an infection will be established and the pharmacologic agent will be prevented from reaching the locus of infection. The comorbidities of diabetes and peripheral vascular disease increase the risk of a recurring infection.[7] The emergence of antibiotic resistance, particularly resistance to methicillin and vancomycin by *S. aureus* organisms, contributes to long-term sequelae and morbidity.[75]

Chronic osteomyelitis has a poor prognosis, even when treated surgically. People with chronic osteomyelitis are often in great pain, require prolonged medical care, and may rarely require amputation of an extremity. In the older adult population, the recurrence of chronic osteomyelitis ranges from 3% to 40%, and the mortality rate is reported to be less than 5%.[75] The bottom line is that the best way to minimize the mortality and morbidity observed in osteomyelitis is to practice preventive measures and reduce the time between the onset of the infection and the initiation of an appropriate intervention.

**SPECIAL IMPLICATIONS FOR THE THERAPIST 25.1**

## *Osteomyelitis*

### Surgery

If surgery is indicated, current resection and débridement techniques may result in soft tissue and bony defects that require secondary microsurgical reconstruction with split-thickness skin grafting, muscle flaps, or bone grafting. If the infection has affected the articular cartilage, controlling weight-bearing and compressive forces with exercise should be a priority.[18] For example, weight bearing on the affected leg may be restricted, and crutches may not be advised when arms and legs are affected simultaneously until sufficient healing occurs to avoid pathologic fractures.

Often, surgery and initial management are performed without adequate consideration for adjacent joints. Prolonged immobilization or limited mobility and weight bearing with external fixators may lead to significant impairment of previously uninvolved joints and muscles. Attention must not be focused on the infection site to the exclusion of the rest of the limb. Important elements of successful rehabilitation include minimizing the original effects of the trauma or disease process and preventing as many complications as possible.

### Preventing Complications

Therapists should first recognize the possible side effects of medical intervention that may lead to complications such as contractures, atrophy, impaired joint mechanics, and loss of function. In addition to the musculoskeletal problems, the therapist should consider other involved organ systems such as the cardiovascular system and what impact the comorbidities may have on healing, rehabilitation, and return to a high level of function. Strict aseptic technique must be used when changing dressings and performing wound care. Reconstructive surgery to cover bone or soft tissue defects requires careful monitoring, dressing changes, and protection. If the client is in skeletal traction for fractures, the insertion points of pin tracks should be covered with small, dry dressings.

Pins used in external fixators also warrant close inspection. Therapist and client must avoid touching the skin around the pins and wires. Assess vital signs, wound appearance, and any new pain daily for signs of secondary infection. During the acute phase of this illness, any movement of the affected limb will cause discomfort or pain. The affected limb should be firmly supported and kept level with the body.

Active, active assisted, and passive range-of-motion (ROM) exercises of adjacent joints are essential. Good skin care is essential, with proper positioning including frequent (but careful and gentle) position changes (at least every 2 hours) and skin assessment for any signs of developing pressure ulcers. Techniques that can possibly spread the infection through mechanical means should be avoided.

# INFECTIONS OF PROSTHESES AND IMPLANTS

## Overview

Over the past decades, joint replacement surgery has become commonplace, which is largely attributed to the success of these procedures in restoring function to people with disabling arthritis. Implant infection remains the primary cause of prosthetic failure, occurring either acutely within the first month postoperatively or months to years after the joint replacement.[69] Nearly 80% of these infections are caused by staphylococcus organisms, which enter by perioperative, hematogenous, or contiguous means. Perioperative infections occur around the time of surgery and are probably caused by contaminated instruments at the surgical site. Hematogenous infections occur as a result of a primary infection somewhere else in the body. Contiguous infections occur secondary to a nearby infection.[30]

Other types of prostheses or implants susceptible to infection include internal fixation of the spine, breast implants, penile implants, dental implants, cardiac implants, other orthopedic devices and hardware, shunts, and even contact lenses (external to epithelial surfaces that can give rise to serious life-threatening infections).

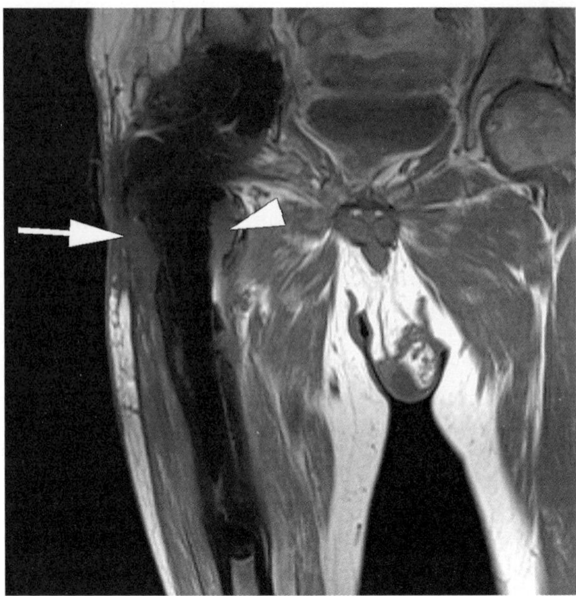

**Figure. 25.4**

**Infected prosthesis.** Magnetic resonance imaging showing infected femoral prosthesis with osteomyelitis along the medial aspect *(arrowhead)* and infection along the iliotibial tract *(arrow)*. (From Cahir JG, Toms AP: CT and MRI of hip replacements. *Orthop Trauma* 23:101–108, 2009.)

## Incidence

The successful development of synthetic materials and the introduction of artificial devices into nearly all body systems have been accompanied by the adaptation of microorganisms to the opportunities these devices provide for eluding defenses and invading the host. With improvements in surgical procedures and prophylactic antibiotics, the incidence of infection has been reduced to less than 1.5%.[69] The incidence of infection increases with longer procedures and revisions. However, as the number of people undergoing replacements has grown, reoperations have become increasingly common.[42] Multiple reoperations carry a higher risk of infection. Likewise, as the population ages, revision is required for an increasing number of total hip, knee, shoulder, elbow, wrist, and finger arthroplasties.

Infection of a prosthetic joint causes loosening of the prosthesis and sepsis, with significant mortality and morbidity. Two-thirds of prosthetic joint infections occur within 1 year of surgery and are the result of intraoperative inoculations of bacteria into the new joint or postoperative bacteremias. Early infections have been substantially reduced by preoperative use of antibiotics, the use of laminar flow in operating rooms, and improved surgical technique.[42]

## Risk Factors

Certain groups have been identified to be predisposed to infection of their prosthetic joints, including people with prior surgery at the site of the prosthesis, rheumatoid arthritis, corticosteroid therapy, diabetes mellitus, poor nutritional status, low albumin, obesity, and extremely advanced age.[45]

Any factor that delays or impairs wound healing increases the risk of infection. Psoriasis, steroids, diabetes mellitus, and immunodeficiency increase the risk of prosthetic infection. Immunodeficiency can be either local (e.g., wear debris from the implant) or systemic. Risk factors for infection of spinal instrumentation may include IV drug use, paraplegia with neurogenic bladder, and pyelonephritis secondary to renal calculi.

## Etiologic Factors and Pathogenesis

Locally introduced forms of infection account for most prosthetic joint infections and occur as a result of wound infection next to the prosthesis or operative contamination.[73] Operative contamination may be a result of direct implantation at the time of the operation by the operating team, from environmental sources, or from contaminated implant materials. Holes in the implants (e.g., press-fit acetabular cups) are potential pathways through which debris can gain access to the implant–bone interface, resulting in infection, creating periprosthetic bone loss, and potentially initiating loosening. In general, these infections are caused by a single pathogen, but polymicrobial sepsis can occur (Fig. 25.4).[58,54] Staphylococci (coagulase-negative staphylococci and *S. aureus*) are the principal causative agents of joint prosthesis infection (approximately 40% and 20%, respectively); aerobic streptococci and gram-negative bacilli are each responsible for 10% and 5% of cases, mixed flora constitutes 10%, and anaerobes are involved in about 5% of infections. No organism is found in about 10% of cases.[73] Rarely, latent foci of chronic, nonactive osteomyelitis are reactivated by the disruption of tissue associated with prosthetic surgery. Previous *S. aureus* and *Mycobacterium tuberculosis* infections can recur postoperatively.

Bacteria adhere tightly to the implant surface by adhesins, which recognize specific host proteins absorbed on the material surface. They also use biofilms, a type of slime that protects bacterial colonies from destruction by phagocytes. Multiple layers of biofilm allow staphylococci to cling to the surface of the implant and avoid both immune system defenses and antibiotic diffusion. The biofilms can even alter the host's immune capability and increase antibiotic resistance. Bacteria can lie dormant on the prosthetic device for years until the person becomes immunocompromised from aging or other health issues.[60]

In the presence of prosthetic or implantable devices, many bacteria form a fibrous material called *glycocalyx*. Organisms can reproduce within this matrix and form a thick biofilm that is protected in part from host defense mechanisms. Biofilms are an important issue for surgery involving prosthetic or implantable devices. For example, only 32% of infections caused by slime-producing staphylococci resolved with antibiotics compared with 100% recovery in non–slime-producing strains.[73]

The implant and its adherent biofilm must be removed for the infection to resolve, because recurrent, acute infections or disseminated, persistent infection may develop if these reservoirs are allowed to continue. Meticulous protocols for sterilization of implants should be followed, because biofilms may be an important mechanism of antibiotic resistance.

## Clinical Manifestations

Persistent joint pain may be the only symptom, with no clinical signs of infection at all. Staphylococcus infections are usually characterized by symptoms similar to wound infection such as edema, hematoma, fever, and local pain. Late-onset or delayed infection usually manifests as increasing joint pain followed by rapid onset of systemic symptoms.[73]

Prosthetic joint infections can be divided into the following three categories: early (infection that develops less than 3 months after surgery), delayed (3 to 24 months after surgery), and late (more than 24 months). Clients with early infections typically present with acute symptoms such as fever, joint pain, warmth, and redness. These individuals may form a sinus tract from the prosthesis to the skin with purulent drainage. Virulent organisms such as *S. aureus* or gram-negative bacilli are usually responsible for early infections.[73]

People who present with delayed infections often lack systemic symptoms, making diagnosis difficult. These individuals display joint pain and/or joint loosening. Organisms responsible for these infections are less virulent, such as coagulase-negative staphylococci (particularly *Staphylococcus epidermidis*) and *Propionibacterium acnes*. Early and delayed infections are typically acquired at the time of surgery, whereas late infections develop from hematogenous seeding.

When a bloodborne infection arises in a prosthetic joint several months or years after implantation surgery, the fully healed connective tissue often is capable of restricting the septic process to a relatively small focus at the bone–cement interface. Joint pain is the principal symptom of deep tissue infection, regardless of mode of presentation, and suggests either acute inflammation of the periarticular tissue or loosening of the prosthesis caused by subacute erosion of bone at the bone–cement interface.

### MEDICAL MANAGEMENT

**PREVENTION.** Sterilization and attention to infection control guidelines reduces the risk of infection. Surgical helmets and body suits have been developed to reduce the risk of infection transmission from surgical team members.[82] Researchers are working to design self-sterilizing materials and more effective infection-resistant materials.

**DIAGNOSIS.** Clinical manifestations of joint pain, swelling, erythema, and warmth all reflect an underlying inflammatory process in the surrounding tissues but are not specific for infection. When a painful prosthesis is accompanied by fever or purulent drainage from overlying cutaneous sinuses, infection is likely. The physician must differentiate infection from aseptic and mechanical problems (e.g., hemarthrosis, mechanical loosening, or dislocation). Constant joint pain is suggestive of infection, whereas mechanical loosening commonly causes pain only with motion or weight bearing.[73]

The diagnosis of joint prosthesis infection is dependent on isolation of the pathogen by aspiration of joint fluid or by obtaining tissue at arthrotomy. Gram stain and culture will typically identify the responsible organism in most cases.[54] Special media may be required if fungus or atypical organisms are suspected. Culture of sinus tract drainage or overlying skin should be avoided. Elevated serum leukocyte count, erythrocyte sedimentation rate, and C-reactive protein level are suggestive, but not diagnostic, of joint infection. Ultrasound-guided and fluoroscopy-guided aspiration techniques are used in cases of suspected sepsis of arthroplasty to determine the type of pathogen.[61]

Radiographs of the involved joint will identify noninfectious causes for symptoms that may mimic an infection or indicate the need for other types of imaging. Radiologic abnormalities may be helpful when changes are noted over serial radiographs. When both the distal and the proximal components of a prosthetic joint demonstrate pathology on radiography, infection is more likely than simple mechanical loosening.

A three-phase bone scan is most commonly used for the identification of a prosthetic joint infection. A bone scan will demonstrate increased uptake in areas of bone with enhanced blood supply or increased metabolic activity. Positive scans at 6 months after implantation are abnormal but do not differentiate among inflammation, possible loosening, and infection. A CT scan can identify the signs of infection in the periprosthetic tissues but is not as accurate as a bone scan for identifying all of the signs for an infection. Positron emission tomography scan and scintigraphy with radioisotope-labeled leukocyte and bone marrow have also been used to identify prosthetic joint infections.[73,77]

**TREATMENT.** Successful treatment requires a combination of surgical intervention (usually removal and replacement of the entire implant) and long-term antimicrobial therapy.[72] Prosthesis removal, extensive and meticulous surgical débridement of surrounding tissue, and effective antimicrobial therapy are usually necessary to treat deep infections, especially infections involving the interface between prosthesis and bone. Surgical débridement with retention of the prosthesis followed by a course of antibiotics may be appropriate for a limited and select group of people.[35]

For more predictably effective treatment of prosthetic joint replacement sepsis, complete removal of all foreign materials (metallic prosthesis, cement, and any accompanying biofilm) is essential. This can be done in a one- or two-stage exchange. The most successful protocol incorporates standardized antimicrobial therapy with a two-stage surgical procedure: (1) removal of prosthesis and cement and placement of an antibiotic-impregnated cement spacer, followed by a 6-week course of bactericidal antibiotic therapy and (2) reimplantation of a new prosthesis using cement impregnated with an antibiotic at the conclusion of the 6-week antibiotic course.[66] Cementless two-stage hip procedures may result in infection rates similar to total hip arthroplasties done with cemented components.[73,51]

Sometimes surgical intervention is not possible because of a medical or surgical condition or refusal on the part of the affected individual. in such cases, lifelong oral antibiotic treatment may be required to suppress the infection and retain function of the joint. Serial radiographs are needed to monitor progressive bone resorption at the bone–cement interface. In such cases, the localized septic process may still extend into adjacent tissue compartments or become a systemic infection, or the person may develop side effects of long-term antibiotic administration.

**PROGNOSIS.** Infection associated with prostheses and implants can produce significant morbidity and occasionally death. Early recognition and prompt therapy for infection in any location is critical to reducing the risk of seeding the joint implant hematogenously. Situations likely to cause bacteremia should be avoided.[76]

The American Academy of Orthopedic Surgeons currently recommends routine use of microbial prophylaxis for anyone undergoing joint replacements, and the American Dental Association advises that a single dose of prophylactic antibiotic be given to selected individuals undergoing dental procedures associated with significant bleeding and potential hematologic bacterial contamination.[66] The selected populations include people with inflammatory arthropathies, immunosuppression, diabetes mellitus, malnutrition, hemophilia, or previous prosthetic joint infection and anyone undergoing these dental procedures within 2 years after joint replacement.

Perioperative antibiotic prophylaxis has been shown to reduce deep wound infection effectively in total joint replacement surgery. Cephalosporins continue to be the antibiotic of choice for orthopedic surgeons because of the broad spectrum of activity against the most common pathogens. The antibiotic is given before the incision is made, and if the procedure is long, another dose is administered during surgery. The medication is then continued for 24 hours after surgery.[59] Although the percentage of prostheses that become infected within 10 years after implantation is very low, there is considerable risk of morbidity (e.g., hospitalization, amputation, or disability) and even death.[58]

**SPECIAL IMPLICATIONS FOR THE THERAPIST 25.2**

## *Infections of Prostheses and Implants*

Many cases of infection after instrumentation or prosthetic implantation occur months to years after the surgery. The therapist must be aware of existing hardware and must include questions in the interview to elicit this information. A recent history of infection from dental caries, pulmonary or upper respiratory tract, GI tract, or genitourinary tract in such a person should be considered for a patient reporting discomfort over a joint with a prosthesis. Any spontaneous drainage from previous scars or sites of surgery may be a sign of infection, and the person must immediately be referred.

Anyone with implants of any kind with onset of increasing musculoskeletal symptoms (especially in the area of the surgery) must be screened for the possibility of infection. A recent normal radiograph of the joint does not rule out the presence of a joint prosthesis infection. Knowing the risk factors for developing an antibiotic-resistant infection (e.g., multiple surgical procedures, previous *S. aureus* infection, or multiple antibiotics) and recognizing red flag symptoms of infection can help the therapist in recognizing the need for persistence in obtaining follow-up medical care.

### Breast Implantation

See also Breast Reconstruction in Chapter 20. Silicone breast implants are medical devices implanted subcutaneously or subpectorally for cosmetic breast augmentation or reconstruction after mastectomy. Postoperative infection can occur in up to 35% of postmastectomy reconstructions and in up to 2.5% of breast augmentation procedures.[46,79] Factors that increase the risk for infection have not been well studied, but surgical technique and underlying disease appear to be the principal reasons.

Women who undergo reconstruction with placement of an implant after mastectomy for cancer are up to 10 times more likely to develop an infection than women receiving cosmetic augmentation. This is often the result of the side effects of chemotherapy and radiation therapy required with surgery.[46] Two-thirds of infections occur during the acute postsurgical period, whereas one-third appear months to years later. Infections that develop months to years later most likely result from organisms seeded from a distant location.

Other complications of breast implants include hematomas, seromas, visible wrinkles or folds, scarring, asymmetry or displacement of the implant, capsular contracture, implant leak or rupture, silicone gel bleed, or prolonged pain of the breast. Implants may interfere with mammography, causing some women to discover breast cancer at later stages. Some studies have shown that silicone devices can prolong wound healing and delay formation of granulation tissue.[46]

## SPONDYLODISKITIS

### Overview and Incidence

Spondylodiskitis is an infection that affects the vertebral spine components. The intervertebral disk is the most common site for a spinal infection, with the infection affecting the annulus, the nucleus, or the vertebral endplates.[23]

### Etiologic and Risk Factors

Spondylodiskitis is the most common complication after a diskectomy. The infection may involve the adjacent vertebrae and spread to the disk through the cartilaginous endplates. Other procedures capable of directly inoculating the disk, such as diskography, also carry the risk of infection. Direct inoculation is the only method by which an infection can arise from within the disk.

### Pathogenesis

A bacterial organism is usually the cause of the infection. *S. aureus* is commonly found, but in some cases, no organism can be isolated. *M. tuberculosis* is also detected in disk infections. The origin of the infection in children may be traumatic, but the source of infection is more likely to be the hematogenous spread of a bacterial infection preceding the diskitis, such as in the upper respiratory tract or urinary tract.[3] Fungal or yeast infections can also lead to spondylodiskitis.[13] An infection extending to the disk from the cartilaginous plate can spread to cause an epidural abscess posteriorly or a paravertebral abscess anteriorly. The pathogenesis of infection formation is described later in this chapter (see Pathogenesis under Infectious Arthritis).

### Clinical Manifestations

Diskitis manifests in different ways at different ages, but fever and spinal pain are classic symptoms in children. In very young children, back pain or a refusal to walk and pain with hip extension may be the first symptoms and must be taken seriously. Abdominal pain and weight loss may occur, and the child may not be able to flex the lower back. In children presenting with diskitis the concern is whether the diagnosis is actually vertebral osteomyelitis.[43] However, children with vertebral osteomyelitis often appear more ill and febrile.[13]

In adults, disk infection after spinal procedures usually is noted within a few days, whereas those developing from an infection at a distant site may not be evident for months. Spinal pain is common and sometimes severe, with radiation of the pain into the lower extremities. The lower extremity pain is not usually radicular; instead, it may involve multiple nerve levels. Adults may present with unusual postures and movement patterns. In both children and adults, back pain may range from mild to severe. The client will often report that the pain is made worse with activity and that rest does not relieve the pain.[3]

#### MEDICAL MANAGEMENT

**DIAGNOSIS.** Inflammatory markers may be elevated, but often laboratory tests are inconclusive, and cultures of blood and disk tissue are negative. Plain radiographs should be taken for anyone suspected to have spinal infection. Disk space narrowing, endplate irregularity, and a loss of lumbar lordosis may be visualized. Bone scans are also used for initial evaluation.[13] However, MRI is essential in providing the differential diagnosis when vertebral osteomyelitis is a possibility; MRI reduces diagnostic delay and may help avoid the need for a biopsy.[13]

In adults, MRI in conjunction with bone scans using gadolinium enhancement has been found to be useful in differentiating nonpyogenic inflammation changes from changes caused by infection. MRI is most useful in determining the extent of the infection and the required duration of oral antibiotic therapy after initial IV antibiotics but less valuable in demonstrating the type of infection (e.g., pyogenic versus tuberculous). Sclerosis present later in the disease course may be confused with a benign degenerative process or even with metastatic disease. MRI and biopsy may be used to differentiate chronic cases.[23,67]

**TREATMENT.** Treatment may consist of bed rest and a removable body jacket that can be used along with specific or empiric antibiotic therapy. The use of prophylactic antibiotics is common after spinal surgery in adults to prevent this condition from developing. Antifungal agents may first be tried for *Candida* diskitis. Surgery will be necessary in 10% to 20% of all cases.[13]

**PROGNOSIS.** In both adults and children the prognosis is good, although pain may persist for several months up to several years. In children, long-term follow-up care has shown a resolution of the pain despite persistent radiographic changes.[3]

Late radiographic changes in adults include vertebral collapse, kyphosis, and eventually bony ankylosis, which can take up to 2 years to run its course. Adults can expect similar spontaneous healing to occur, especially in individuals with a strong immune response.

Complications can arise when the infection spreads or when an abscess forms. An epidural abscess can result in paralysis and is noted in older people, in people who have involvement of the cervical region, and in people with associated medical problems such as diabetes.

## INFECTIOUS ARTHRITIS

### Overview and Incidence

This section discusses bacterial arthritis (also called *septic* or *infectious arthritis*) (Box 25.2), which differs from reactive arthritis. *Bacterial arthritis* is a local response with joint destruction and sepsis, whereas *reactive arthritis* occurs in a joint that has been affected by the inflammatory markers produced by a distant infection site. Some of the other infectious causes of arthritis are discussed in other chapters (see Chapter 8 for Lyme disease and Epstein-Barr virus, Chapter 12 for rheumatic fever, and Chapter 7 for HIV).

### Etiologic and Risk Factors

Bacteria, viruses, and fungi all are capable of infecting a joint by invading and inflaming the synovial membrane.[57] *S. aureus, Streptococcus pneumoniae, Kingella*

Box 25.2

**CAUSATIVE AGENTS OF INFECTIOUS (SEPTIC) ARTHRITIS**

***Bacterial***

- Gonococcal
- Infectious endocarditis
- Lyme disease
- Syphilis
- Tuberculosis

***Fungal***

- Candida

***Viral***

- Epstein-Barr virus
- Hepatitis
- HIV
- Mumps
- Rubella

***Reactive***

- Acute rheumatic fever
- Chlamydial infection
- Enteric infection
- Reiter syndrome

Box 25.3

**PREDISPOSING FACTORS IN ADULT SEPTIC ARTHRITIS[a]**

- Immunosuppression/immunodeficiency
  - Systemic corticosteroid use
  - Chemotherapy
  - Radiation therapy
  - HIV
- Preexisting arthritis
- Arthrocentesis
- Diabetes mellitus (poorly controlled)
- Sickle cell disease
- Alcohol or drug abuse
- Trauma
- Other infectious diseases
- Chronic renal failure
- Unknown or none

[a]More than one factor may exist.
From Esterhai J, Gelb I: Adult septic arthritis. *Orthop Clin North Am* 22:504, 1991.

*kingae*, and *Neisseria gonorrhoeae* are the most common organisms responsible for infectious arthritis.[33] Direct penetrating trauma, joint arthroplasty, and chronic joint damage as seen in diseases such as rheumatoid arthritis are also considered to put a joint at risk.[25] Predisposing factors for development of septic arthritis are listed in Box 25.3. Microorganisms can be introduced into the joint by direct inoculation, by direct extension, or by hematogenous (through the bloodstream) spread, which is the most common route (Box 25.4).

The primary risk factor for septic arthritis is an abnormal synovium from rheumatoid or degenerative conditions. Conditions that result in immunosuppression

Box 25.4

**INTRODUCTION OF BACTERIAL ARTHRITIS**

- Hematogenous spread (via bloodstream)
- Direct inoculation and penetrating injury
  - Penetrating or puncture wound; fracture; human bite
  - Surgery
  - Arthrocentesis
  - Arthroscopy
  - Total joint arthroplasty
- Direct extension
  - Periarticular osteomyelitis
  - Contiguous soft tissue infection, abscess, cellulitis

From Esterhai J, Gelb I: Adult septic arthritis. *Orthop Clin North Am* 22:504, 1991.

increase the likelihood of having an infectious joint that becomes septic. Although nongonococcal infectious arthritis can affect individuals across the life span, infants, children, and older adults are at greatest risk. Risk factors for poor outcomes after septic arthritis include delayed diagnosis, onset earlier than 3 months, osteomyelitis, and methicillin-resistive *S. aureus* as the underlying organism.[9]

## Pathogenesis

Bacteria that enter a joint capsule rapidly multiply in the liquid culture medium of the synovial fluid and are phagocytosed by synovial lining cells. Bacteria are either killed by the synovial cells or form an abscess within the synovial membrane. Organisms that reach the synovium through the bloodstream multiply in this abscess until they break into the articular cavity.

Bacterial products such as endotoxins and cell wall fragments stimulate synovial cells to release tumor necrosis factor and interleukin-1. These cytokines upregulate expression of adhesion ligands in synovial membrane vessel endothelial cells, resulting in leukocyte attachment and migration into synovial fluid and articular tissues. Bacterial fragments form antigen–antibody complexes that activate the classic pathway of complement, and bacterial toxins activate the alternative complement pathway to produce proinflammatory products (see Chapter 6).

The phagocytosis of bacteria also results in autolysis of neutrophils with release of lysosomal enzymes into the joint, which causes synovial, ligament, and cartilage damage. Cellular immune mechanisms also appear to play a role in acute joint infection. After 48 hours of synovial infection, T lymphocytes infiltrate the synovium, interleukin-6 levels are increased, and B-cell activation results in immunoglobulin G antibody production.

Bacterial toxins also activate the coagulation system, causing intravascular thrombosis in the subsynovial vessels and fibrin deposition on the surface of the synovium and articular cartilage. This layer of fibrin provides a gelatinous nidus for bacterial replication. Microvascular obstruction leads to ischemia and necrosis, further permitting abscess formation, destroying the cartilage matrix.

Finally, after the acute necrotic inflammatory synovitis, the synovial membrane proliferates, forming an inflammatory exudate called *pannus* that erodes articular cartilage of the joint capsule and subchondral bone. Joint destruction can take place within a few weeks, underscoring the need for urgency in detection and intervention in septic arthritis.[37] A chronic inflammatory synovitis may persist even after antibiotics have eradicated the infection.

## Clinical Manifestations

People with infectious arthritis can be any age and can present with an acute onset of joint pain, swelling, tenderness, and loss of motion. Fever, chills, and other systemic symptoms depend on the stage of the illness. Physical examination may reveal the classic signs of infection such as increased temperature of the joint, swelling, redness, and loss of function. Pus may drain outside through a sinus formed from the joint to the outside. Only the severity and the nature of these signs will differentiate the septic joint from more mundane causes such as tendonitis and other noninfectious inflammatory diseases.[37]

A child with a septic joint will often refuse to bear weight on the affected leg or use the affected arm; there may be extreme tenderness to palpation at the joint and along the metaphysis. Destruction of the joints can proceed rapidly and have long-lasting effects, with pathologic fracture, growth arrest in children, deformity, and joint dislocation.[10] In addition to the infection, white blood cells that enter the joint to combat the infection release enzymes that have a deleterious effect on articular cartilage. In more severe cases, septic shock, multiorgan disease, pericarditis, or pyelonephritis can develop, especially if diagnosis and treatment have been delayed. Long-term complications of septic arthritis in children include joint instabilities and lower extremity deformities.[41]

In adults, *S. aureus* produces a monarticular sepsis, usually at the hip or knee. In children the ankle and elbow are also common sites.[33] Although not as common, shoulder septic arthritis and polyarticular involvement have been reported.[9] *Gonococcus* affects mostly women and may produce skin lesions, tenosynovitis, and polyarthralgias, in addition to systemic symptoms. Prosthetic joints are also sites of infection, which is probably introduced at the time of surgery. *S. epidermidis* is often the cause.

In general, the coexistence of fever and the signs and symptoms of an acute exacerbation of arthritis must arouse suspicions of a septic joint and be managed as a medical emergency until proved otherwise.[41]

### MEDICAL MANAGEMENT

**DIAGNOSIS.** After a detailed history and physical examination, the diagnosis is confirmed by analysis of the joint fluid obtained by aspiration. The decision to aspirate the joint, however, is made on the basis of the history and physical examination. The method to obtain a sample of the aspirate depends on the joint that is involved. Needle aspiration, when possible, is often considered the method of choice. Aspiration of the sacroiliac and hip joints is difficult and may be aided by the use of fluoroscopy (real-time x-ray). Imaging studies such as x-rays, contrast MRI (arthrograms), and ultrasonography may be done before joint aspiration. Decisions regarding treatment and appropriate antibiotics are aided by the results of cultures, stains, and laboratory studies such as the white blood cell count, C-reactive protein, and erythrocyte sedimentation rate.[54]

**TREATMENT.** As already mentioned, any joint infection is considered a medical emergency. Admission to the hospital for treatment with specific IV antibiotics is required. Continued treatment with oral medication for an additional 2 to 3 weeks is standard. The combined use of antibiotics along with corticosteroid medications such as dexamethasone has been shown to produce a chondroprotective response, speed recovery, and reduce hospitalization time.[33,41] Aspiration of the joint is critical. Besides needle aspiration, more aggressive techniques of tidal irrigation, arthroscopy, or arthrotomy may be used depending on the situation.[41] Surgical drainage may be indicated for hip or shoulder joint infections. In prosthetic joints the infection may require removal of the hardware and cement, along with a more prolonged course of antibiotics.

Early in the course of intervention, the joint should be rested. This may be accomplished by splinting, traction, or casting. Care in application of the splint will preserve function, and the splint should be removed periodically for ROM exercise. The importance of these simple ROM exercises cannot be overlooked, because the risk for joint contracture as a complication of immobilization is a concern, especially in an older adult. More vigorous types of exercise and aggressive mobilization activities are performed when signs of infection have resolved.[38]

The aggressiveness of intervention is dictated by the specific organism, the joint involved, the duration of symptoms, and the health of the individual. Surgical drainage is often required to preserve function and prevent complications. In some cases, joint instability (e.g., chronic or repeated hip subluxation) may require more extensive surgical intervention.

**PROGNOSIS.** As for other infectious diseases, prompt treatment is key to a successful outcome. If treatment is initiated within 5 to 7 days of onset, a good or excellent long-term result can be expected. Currently the mortality rate has dropped considerably for infections caused by nongonococcal agents; however, sequelae in the form of destructive changes in the bone or joint can result in significant functional limitations.[9]

Mortality is higher in older adults (increases after age 65 years) even with quick and correct interventions. Overall mortality from septic arthritis ranges from 10% to 25%, and permanent joint disability occurs in 25% to 50% of survivors. Septic arthritis of the knee is associated with better outcomes than that of the hip or shoulder.[9] More common complications include osteomyelitis, abscess formation, and permanent loss of joint motion and joint instability. If the infection is not controlled, toxemia and septicemia can cause death. The risk of morbidity and mortality is increased when there are multiple sites of infection and when the individual has multiple comorbidities.[25]

SPECIAL IMPLICATIONS FOR THE THERAPIST 25.3

### *Infectious Arthritis*

Immediate referral of a client with a suspected septic joint to a specialist may save the joint from unnecessary destruction. Being aware of client history and potential risk factors and assessing for signs and symptoms of infection are essential. Including joint infection in the differential diagnosis of some clients with joint pain may expedite early intervention. This is important because the prognosis is related to the time between onset of symptoms and definitive treatment (Fig 25.5).

Treatment of hip infections within 4 days of symptomatic presentation can result in preservation of the joint and complete resolution of the infection. However, delayed intervention can result in serious complications, leading to total hip replacement.[4] Even with prompt and appropriate intervention, the chance of some degree of joint dysfunction is likely.[10,41]

The age of the client and the previous condition of the joint are also important factors. An older adult, who often has additional joint pathology such as degenerative joint disease, rheumatoid arthritis, or complications from diabetes, may not recover full function of the joint. The presence of associated joint pathology also tends to confound the diagnosis of sepsis, which further diminishes the chances of a favorable outcome and may result in a significant amount of residual impairment (e.g., contractures or fibrous ankylosis), especially among older adults.

# INFECTIOUS (INFLAMMATORY) MUSCLE DISEASE

## Myositis

### Overview

Myositis is a general term used to describe inflammation of the muscles, which can be an autoimmune condition or directly caused by viral, bacterial, and parasitic agents. Infection-induced myositis is most often caused by *S. aureus* and parasites such as trichinella and the tapeworm larva *Taenia solium*.

When affecting skeletal muscle, these infectious agents result in inflammatory changes with sequela, ranging from significant functional losses to a minor self-limiting condition. Autoimmune conditions can be activated or aggravated by infections, which may explain the link between myositis, infections, and autoimmune processes.

The most common forms are inclusion body myositis (IBM), dermatomyositis (DM), and polymyositis (PM) (Box 25.5). DM appears to occur more often in children and older adults.

Box 25.5

**TYPES OF MYOSITIS**

- Dermatomyositis (see Chapter 10)
- Polymyositis
- Inclusion body myositis
- Myositis ossificans (see Chapter 27)
- Idiopathic inflammatory myopathies (see Chapter 27)
- Rhabdomyolysis (see Chapter 27)
- Pyomyositis

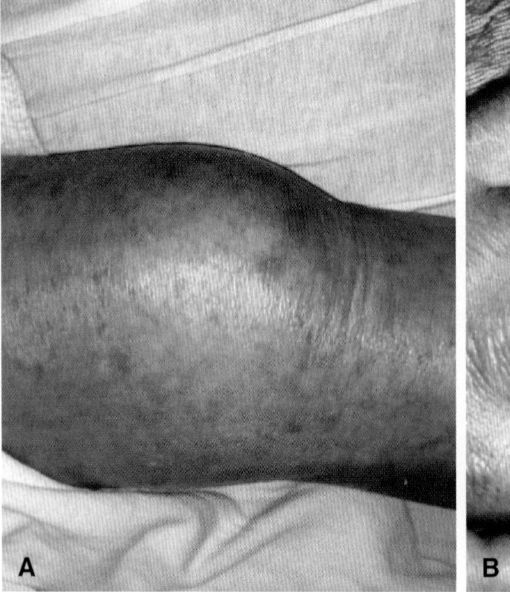


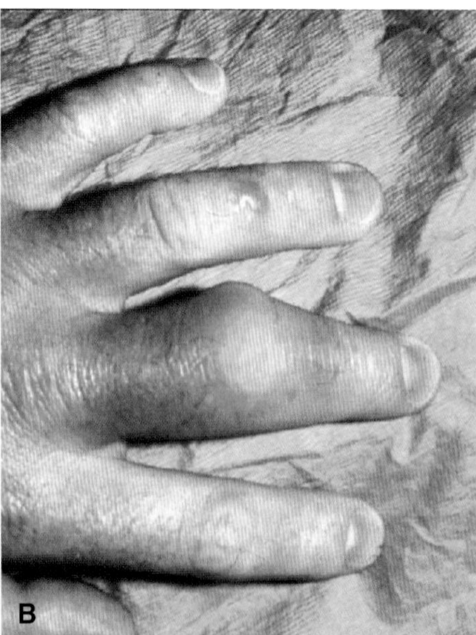


**Figure. 25.5**

**Infectious arthritis.** (A) Bacterial infection of the knee with signs of joint effusion. (B) Septic arthritis of the third proximal interphalangeal joint with signs of swelling and redness. (From Bennett JE, Dolin R, Martin JB: *Mandell, Douglas, and Bennett's principles and practice of infectious diseases*, ed 9, Philadelphia, 2020, Elsevier.)

### Incidence

IBM is the most common acquired muscle disease in adults older than age 50 years and is often misdiagnosed. Myositis is diagnosed in 1 in 100,000 people a year, although some experts suspect that many cases may go unidentified because it is so often mistaken for the symptoms of aging or, in women, depression.[63]

### Etiology and Pathogenesis

The primary pathology is from intra–muscle fiber degeneration that leads to muscle fiber destruction and severe weakness. This form is often progressive and debilitating and often does not respond to available treatments.[2,22] Inflammation is a major cause of the muscle damage. Numerous drugs may induce myopathies, including cholesterol-lowering statins. Lipid-lowering drugs associated with myotoxicity can cause symptoms ranging in severity from myalgias to rhabdomyolysis, resulting in renal failure and death (discussed in Chapter 27).[5,50] Myositis caused by parasites is considered a relatively uncommon condition; however, the parasitic infection trichinosis is reported to affect up to 4% of the population.[21]

Myositis can be the first sign of a malignancy. Some experts theorize that the autoimmune rheumatic diseases that occur in people older than age 40 years may reflect an anticancer immune response in a large number of people. Studies have quantified the risk, finding that people with DM face a threefold risk of cancer, whereas individuals with PM face a 40% increase in risk.[28]

The antigens that produce the immune response are present in normal muscle tissue but at low levels. They are much more prevalent in myositis cells of individuals with autoimmune myositis and in muscle cells that are regenerating such as those that occur after an injury. It is hypothesized that a feed-forward loop occurs when damaged muscle cells start to repair themselves. These cells express higher amounts of the antigens, causing the immune system to respond; the immune response causes further damage to the muscle, which in turn repairs itself, its regenerating cells expressing even more antigens and continuing the feed-forward cycle.[11]

IBM appears to be autoimmune-mediated by cytotoxic T cells and deposits of amyloid-related proteins. There is a strong association of IBM with human leukocyte antigens class I and II. IBM tends to develop in individuals with other autoimmune disorders or immunodeficiency.[17,49] A small number of IBM cases may be hereditary, but most are sporadic, meaning there is not a direct genetic link.[27]

### Clinical Manifestations

The commonly observed signs and symptoms for this family of conditions are characterized by muscle swelling and tenderness, with fever and lethargy. The inflammatory response found in PM and DM is focused in connective tissues and muscle fibers. There is a risk of tissue necrosis and extensive muscle tissue damage with atrophy and weakness, especially if left untreated. Other clinical features of myositis are dysphagia, decreased esophageal motility, vasculitis, Raynaud phenomenon, cardiomyopathy, and interstitial pulmonary fibrosis. A purple skin rash and eyelid edema are often associated with DM. The distribution of the rash includes the eyelids, face, chest, and extensor surfaces of the extremities. In adults, subcutaneous calcium deposits are a sign of severe long-term DM.[63,27]

In most cases, IBM progresses slowly over months or years and is characterized by muscle weakness, resulting in falling episodes, difficulty climbing stairs, or difficulty standing from a seated position. Drop foot and subsequent tripping may be reported. Weak grip, difficulty swallowing, and muscle atrophy and weakness are often accompanied by functional decline and pain or discomfort secondary to weakness.

## MEDICAL MANAGEMENT

**DIAGNOSIS.** A careful and thorough history will indicate an inflammatory condition, and a muscle biopsy is the primary diagnostic tool. A differential diagnosis requires muscle biopsy, electromyography, and blood laboratory values. The muscle biopsy will make the differentiation between PM, DM, and IBM and exclude other myotonic disease. Electromyography will demonstrate muscle irritability and myopathic changes. Because of the associated release of creatine kinase into the blood with skeletal muscle damage, this enzyme can be a useful measure of the extent of the infection. Creatine kinase levels are 5 to 10 times higher than normal in PM but only mildly increased in IBM.[27] The International Myositis Assessment and Clinical Studies Group has developed a set of measures for the level of disease activity, extent of tissue damage, and patient-reported outcomes.[56]

**TREATMENT AND PROGNOSIS.** Aggressive early treatment of any of these conditions is needed to control the inflammatory processes. Treatment of PM and DM often includes immunosuppressive therapy and corticosteroids. There is no established treatment that consistently improves or slows the progression of IBM, and IBM has been resistant to treatments with antiinflammatory, immunosuppressant, or immunomodulating agents.[19] Treatments that block myostatin pathways and improve protein homeostasis are being studied.[63] Because of the resulting muscle weakness and possible extensive skeletal muscle damage associated with myositis, the client must be prepared for an aggressive and prolonged rehabilitative process. The role of the physical and occupational therapist should not be underestimated in the attainment of a successful outcome. Submaximal exercise has been shown to be effective, although eccentric or intense exercise is not recommended.[56,19,39]

**SPECIAL IMPLICATIONS FOR THE THERAPIST 25.4**

*Myositis*

Muscle pain and weakness in anyone at risk for myositis and especially for individuals taking lipid-lowering statins should be a red flag for the therapist. Underlying neuromuscular diseases may become clinically apparent during statin therapy and may predispose the individual to myotoxicity. Exercise may be an additional risk factor for the symptomatic presentation of myotoxicity. The alert therapist will recognize this potential condition and make an appropriate medical referral sooner rather than later.[74]

## Infections of Bursae and Tendons

### Overview and Incidence

Acute infections affecting the bursae and tendons are uncommon and must be treated appropriately to avoid complications. The hand is very susceptible to scratches and bites that lead to infections. Hand infection can range from cellulitis to tenosynovitis. Because of the superficial nature of these tissues and the potential for dysfunction, hand infections are given special attention in this section.

### Etiologic and Risk Factors

The bursae and tendons that lie close to the skin surface are most susceptible to infection from direct contact with microorganisms. Trauma to the elbow and knee is common, especially in sports such as wrestling. The bacteria enter the body by direct inoculation through a local skin abrasion, with anaerobic bacteria most commonly found in these wounds. *S. aureus* is the most common organism isolated and may cause up to 80% of infections.

### Pathogenesis

Infection in the hand can spread along synovial sheaths, along fascial planes, and via lymphatic channels. Bursae are lined with a membrane similar to synovium and are therefore subject to the same pathologic processes, namely, inflammatory conditions caused by acute or chronic infections. (See Pathogenesis under Infectious Arthritis earlier.)

### Clinical Manifestations

The olecranon and prepatellar bursae can be sites of localized infection. An olecranon bursal infection will cause localized swelling with pain, erythema, warmth, and loss of function. Infections of other bursae, such as the prepatellar and subdeltoid bursae, have similar presentations.[62] Tendon sheaths of the extremities can also become infected. As mentioned earlier, the hand is a common site because of its susceptibility to minor trauma. The anatomy of the hand determines the nature and presentation of the infection. For example, the tendon sheaths of the thumb and small finger extend proximally to the wrist, whereas the sheaths of the index, long, and ring fingers stop at the proximal pulley. Common signs associated with an infectious tenosynovitis include a finger maintained in slight flexion; fusiform (spindle-shaped) swelling; pain on extension (passive or active); and tenderness along the tendon sheath into the palm.[29]

### MEDICAL MANAGEMENT

**DIAGNOSIS, TREATMENT, AND PROGNOSIS.** In most joints, examination will identify a localized swelling, not a joint effusion. Aspiration of fluid for laboratory analysis is performed before treatment. The use of antibiotics is often adequate, but surgical incision and drainage are sometimes required; occasionally, bursectomy is required. Prompt treatment with drainage, irrigation, and antibiotics is crucial.[62]

Appropriate treatment of hand infections is based on an accurate identification by culture of the organism causing the infection. In addition to the appropriate antibiotic, the hand is immobilized and elevated, and surgical drainage is often necessary. Necrotic tissue is cautiously débrided, and the wound is left open to drain.[53]

Early and aggressive rehabilitation is essential, especially for a structure as complicated and integrated as the hand. Both physical and occupational therapists may play a role in this process. Given the potential complications of surgery and immobilization and the potential for tissue loss, a comprehensive rehabilitation program is necessary to maximize function.

**SPECIAL IMPLICATIONS FOR THE THERAPIST 25.5**

### *Infections of Bursae and Tendons*

Treatment of hand injuries has developed into a subspecialty, and rightfully so, not only for the orthopedic surgeon but also for the therapist. Clients recovering from infection and surgery must be monitored carefully, and their treatment should be adjusted often. Splinting of the hand is an important feature throughout the course of treatment.

Early immobilization must be done with eventual recovery and function in mind. The wrist should be placed in 30° to 50° of extension, the metacarpophalangeal joints in 75° to 90° of flexion, and the interphalangeal joints in full extension. Active ROM exercise is initiated early, as soon as the infection begins to subside and treatment appears to be successful, which is often within 48 hours.

Prognosis depends on the extent of the infection and how soon treatment was initiated. Delayed intervention usually requires more extensive surgical débridement with an increased chance of scar tissue formation, the need for possible skin grafts, and prolonged rehabilitation to maximize function.

### *Extrapulmonary Tuberculosis*

TB is an acute or chronic infection caused by *M. tuberculosis* that can affect multiple organ systems via lymphatic and hematogenous spread during the initial pulmonary infection (see Chapter 15). Disseminated or miliary TB involves not only the lungs but also most other organ systems. The pulmonary, genitourinary, musculoskeletal, and lymphatic systems may be involved. Of these, the lymphatic system is most commonly involved in immunocompromised hosts such as people with HIV.[26]

Extrapulmonary TB is more difficult to diagnose and treat than pulmonary TB. This is due in part to clinicians' lack of familiarity with the condition. In addition, extrapulmonary TB is often in inaccessible areas, which makes aspiration or biopsy, and therefore diagnosis, more difficult. Also, smaller numbers of bacilli can cause extensive damage to joints but are harder to detect. TB involving the bone is usually transferred hematogenously from some other organ, usually the lung. Only one-fourth of people with skeletal TB have a known history of TB.[70]

## Skeletal Tuberculosis

### Overview and Incidence

Because skeletal TB is relatively uncommon, delays in diagnosis are frequent. After a 40-year decline, the incidence of TB has increased over the past several decades. The World Health Organization estimates that more than 10 million new cases of TB occur annually, and approximately 1.6 million individuals die of TB and associated complications every year.[81] More than 15 million people in the United States are estimated to be infected with TB. TB is a leading cause of death for patients with AIDS. The causes for this change in number of active cases of TB are discussed at length in Chapter 15. Skeletal TB is uncommon, but infection rates have held constant over the years. Of TB cases, 10% to 15% are extrapulmonary, and only 10% of extrapulmonary TB cases are skeletal.[80]

### Pathogenesis and Clinical Manifestations

Extrapulmonary TB is spread hematogenously from other organs. In adults the onset of skeletal TB is insidious, developing 2 to 3 years after the primary infection. Early signs and symptoms include pain and stiffness; the pain may be localized or referred. The lower thoracic and lumbar spine is commonly involved (Pott disease), but other sites (e.g., weight-bearing joints or elbows) have been reported.[16] Systemic signs such as fever, chills, weight loss, and fatigue are not common in the early phase. Joint effusion often occurs with TB arthritis and has been shown to affect muscles and nerves around the joint.[47]

In the case of spine involvement (5% in the cervical spine, 25% in the thoracic spine, and 20% in the lumbar and lumbosacral spine), infection begins in the cancellous bone of the vertebral body and eventually spreads to the intervertebral disk and adjacent vertebrae. As the disease progresses, nerve root irritation, pressure from abscess, and collapse of the vertebral body will cause a progressive increase in pain and protective spasm, with cord compression and possible paraplegia.[65] The abscess may extend from the lumbar region to the psoas muscle, producing hip pain.

### MEDICAL MANAGEMENT

**DIAGNOSIS.** Early diagnosis is very helpful in preserving articular cartilage and the joint space but is often delayed for several months to years after the initial presentation because there are no symptoms pathognomonic of extrapulmonary TB. Conventional radiographs and bone scans are important in the initial detection, and CT and MRI can assist in further evaluation.[31] Confirmation of skeletal TB requires microbiologic assessment with smear and culture. In the spine, this confirmation can be accomplished with fine-needle aspiration. Tissue biopsy is more often required for extrapulmonary disease.[52]

**TREATMENT AND PROGNOSIS.** Treatment does not differ for pulmonary and extrapulmonary TB. Although surgical débridement is sometimes necessary, usually pharmacologic treatment is sufficient. (See Chapter 15 for discussion of medical management of TB.) Chemotherapy is the mainstay in the management of TB spondylitis, but decompressive surgery may be required in the presence of Pott paraplegia.[36]

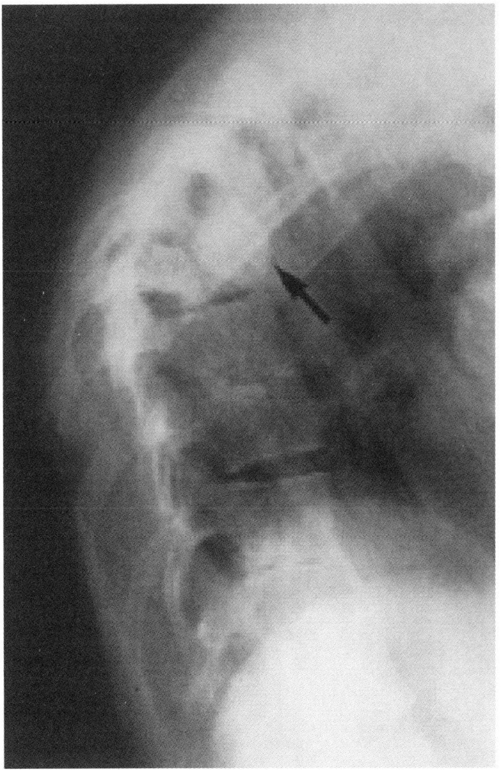

**Figure. 25.6**

**Tuberculous spondylitis.** Involvement at multiple levels. Gibbus deformity is seen in the upper thoracic region *(arrow)*. (From Yao D, Sartoris D: Musculoskeletal tuberculosis. *Radiol Clin North Am* 33:681, 1995.)

Rehabilitation after surgery for TB of the spine or extremities follows standard orthopedic principles. Medical intervention and subsequent rehabilitation are individualized based on the extent of the infection. Surgical treatment of joint infection may include arthrotomy, synovectomy, and treatment of articular erosions.

Extraarticular infections can sometimes be treated with curettage and bone grafting. For more advanced infections, resection of bones and joints, arthrodesis, and limb salvage or amputation may be indicated. Factors to be considered include the affected bone; extent of surgical excision; and involvement of soft tissue, articular cartilage, or bone. Weight bearing is often limited, but active movement is often encouraged.

In the spine, surgery is more often needed to address nerve compression or deformity secondary to collapse of the vertebral body rather than the infection. The resultant deformity often includes a marked kyphotic curve with a gibbus formation (Fig. 25.6). Paralysis can be a serious complication of vertebral TB and can be a result of the disease process or a secondary spinal deformity. Paralysis persisting longer than 6 months is unlikely to improve, and late paralysis with inactive disease and significant kyphosis is much less responsive to treatment.[20]

In the joint, if TB is diagnosed early when the infection is confined to the synovium, rest, medication, and joint protection may be adequate. In advanced disease with

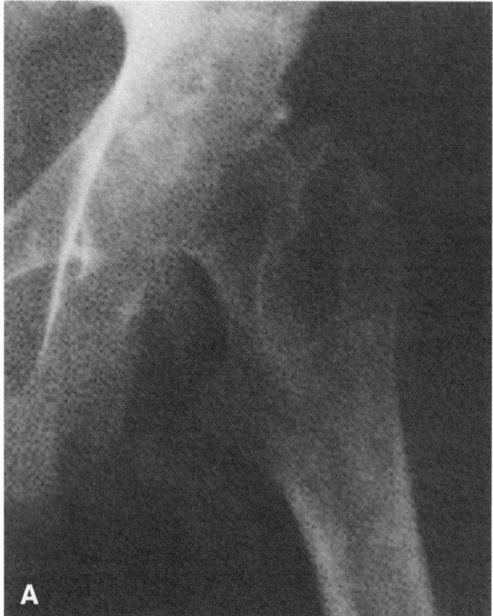


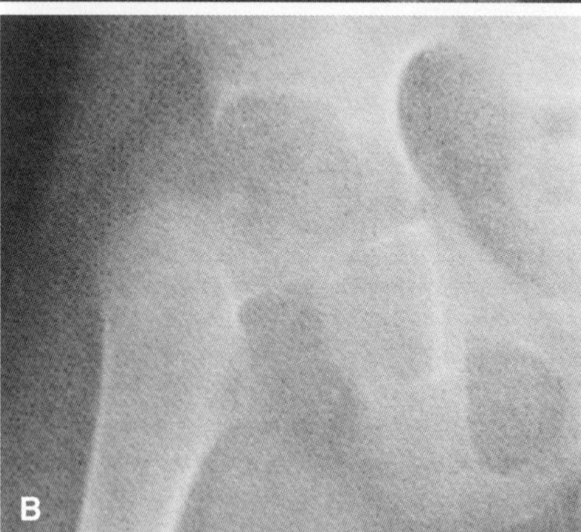


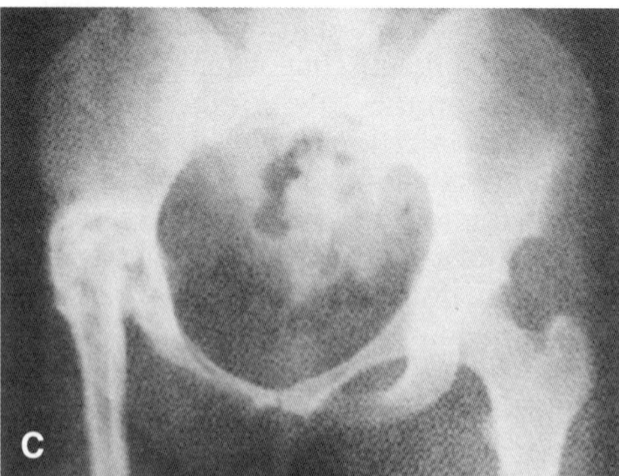


**Figure. 25.7**

**Tuberculous arthritis.** (A) Bony erosion of acetabulum and femoral head with joint space loss. There also is evidence of periarticular osteopenia. (B) Similar findings to (A) but with further destruction of the femoral head and acetabulum. (C) Advanced tuberculosis of the hip with superior displacement and ankylosis of the right hip joint. (From Yao D, Sartoris D: Musculoskeletal tuberculosis. *Radiol Clin North Am* 33:687, 1995.)

caseation, fibrosis, and scarring, the vascularity is reduced (Fig. 25.7), which makes medications less effective. Surgical excision or curettage of the affected areas may be necessary. In joints the granulomatous tissue acts to separate the articular cartilage from the underlying bone.[47]

SPECIAL IMPLICATIONS FOR THE THERAPIST 25.6

### *Extrapulmonary and Skeletal Tuberculosis*

Extrapulmonary (skeletal) TB is not often seen in a physical therapy practice but can manifest as arthritis or other musculoskeletal manifestations of unknown cause. Anyone with this type of clinical presentation with a compromised immune system, especially HIV/AIDS; past or recent release from incarceration; a history of immigration to the United States from an area where TB is endemic; or any other risk factor for TB listed in Chapter 15 should be screened for medical disease.

Therapists may provide treatment to clients with pulmonary TB including postural drainage and percussion to remove secretions from the lung. Care must be taken with clients' sputum. All health care professionals working with people who have TB must be aware of the risk to themselves of contracting or spreading the infection to others. This is equally important for extrapulmonary TB. Although it is thought that once the client is started on appropriate medical therapy the risk of transmission decreases in as little as 2 weeks, there are types of drug-resistant TB that may be infectious for longer periods.

In addition to the obvious orthopedic concerns that will evolve during the treatment of skeletal TB, therapists should be aware of psychosocial issues that may develop. Clients undergoing long-term treatment for infectious diseases will undoubtedly have some difficulties in managing their disease. Chronic pain, repeated hospitalizations, frequent setbacks, fear of long-term disability, and loss of independence all may contribute to a number of abnormal, but expected, illness behaviors. A multidisciplinary team that includes physical and occupational therapists, psychologists, community health nurses, and others will be useful in achieving functional goals.

## SUMMARY OF SPECIAL IMPLICATIONS FOR THE THERAPIST

Rehabilitation after medical interventions for infectious diseases must proceed in a comprehensive and coordinated fashion. The pathology of each type of infectious disease process and the medical decisions made for treatment will have some bearing on the rehabilitation plan. The patient's goals and expectations, general health, and potential for repair of the affected bone and structures must be considered in the rehabilitation plan.

Early in the course of intervention, rest and protection of healing tissues will be the primary objective. All health care providers must be made aware of the potentially adverse effects of apparently simple movements. For example, using a bedpan and performing isometric exercises produce acetabular contact pressure close to that of walking. Therefore clinicians should not assume that a client who is on bed rest is not producing elevated joint compressive forces. Clients must be instructed in proper methods of moving, transferring, and positioning themselves.

Active ROM exercise is often the first type of supervised exercise permitted. These movements must be done while noting limits set by pain, spasm, or apprehension. Active hip flexion has been found to increase acetabular contact pressure similar to that of full weight bearing. However, passive ROM exercise has been found to have a beneficial effect on healing joints. Restoring full ROM may not be as realistic or as necessary as obtaining the ROM required to restore function. Continuous passive ROM is a means of early mobilization in a postoperative rehabilitation regimen that may improve early motion and decrease postoperative pain.

Once the client is ambulatory, his or her weight-bearing status must be determined and monitored. This will depend on the type of infection, surgical procedure, stage of recovery, and extent of joint destruction. Articular cartilage heals very slowly, and the cartilage on weight-bearing surfaces should be protected from undue compressive or shear forces.

Exercise after prolonged immobilization should take these factors into consideration. Often a non–weight-bearing status is used with the intention of minimally loading the joint. In fact, the compressive forces may actually increase compared with those of a touch-down, weight-bearing gait pattern. Other factors such as the weight of the limb and muscular contraction must be considered. Long-term use of an ambulatory aid may be indicated for a 2- to 3-year period.

## REFERENCES

To enhance this text and add value for the reader, all references are included in the enhanced ebook on Student Consult that accompanies this textbook. The reader can view the reference source and access it online whenever possible.

# CHAPTER 26

# Musculoskeletal Neoplasms

KEVIN HELGESON

The term *neoplasm* is defined as a new or abnormal growth of cells and is often used interchangeably with *tumor,* which means any swelling or mass. Neoplasms are divided into two broad categories: benign and malignant. Benign neoplasms show no tendency to metastasize, are noninvasive, and are usually slow growing. A malignant neoplasm is one that can be invasive or can metastasize. Although neoplasms represent a small portion of the spectrum of pathology seen in clinics, their severity and potential for serious consequences necessitate an understanding of their detection and treatment.

The purpose of this chapter is to review the characteristics of primary and secondary musculoskeletal neoplasms. The neoplasms that may be detected during an encounter with a therapist are highlighted.

## PRIMARY TUMORS

### Overview

#### Description

Primary musculoskeletal tumors are tumors that have developed from or within tissue in a localized area. Primary musculoskeletal neoplasms can be benign or malignant, soft tissue or bone. A soft tissue tumor may originate from muscle, cartilage, nerve, collagen, adipose, lymph or blood vessels, and skin. Common sites in the body and location within the bone vary depending on the type of tumor (Table 26.1 and Fig. 26.1).

Modern classification of soft tissue tumors recognizes more than 200 benign and approximately 70 malignant (sarcomatous) lesions with a ratio of benign tumors to malignant sarcomas of 100:1. The focus of this chapter will be on the most common bone and soft tissue tumors encountered in the physical therapist's practice. Other soft or connective tissue tumors (e.g., skin, heart, myeloma, lymphatic, hematologic, neurologic) are discussed elsewhere in this text.

#### Benign Neoplasm

Benign tumors are made of well-differentiated cells, resemble normal tissue, rarely invade locally, and have low potential for autonomous growth. However, benign does not necessarily mean innocuous, as their growth can encroach on surrounding tissues. For example, osteoblastomas in the spine may produce serious neurologic problems requiring resection, with additional complications possible from the surgical procedure.

Some benign bone tumors pose difficult evaluation and management decisions and can result in a significant level of impairment. For example, large fibrous defects in weight-bearing bones can cause pathologic fractures. A *pathologic fracture* refers to bone that has been weakened by local destruction (osteoclastic resorption) from any cause; bone with this type of impairment is more readily fractured than normal bone.

Although rare, some benign lesions can develop into a malignancy. Benign lesions are usually not associated with the constant, severe pain that is commonly present with progressive malignant disease, but benign tumors can impair blood supply or compress nerve tissue.

#### Malignant Neoplasm

Malignant primary tumors by definition have the capacity to spread to other sites and often do so aggressively by invading locally and destroying adjacent tissues and by metastasizing to distant sites. Skeletal neoplasms often metastasize to the lungs through the bloodstream.

Malignant tumors are not as common as benign lesions; however, there are many rare types that have made it difficult to standardize treatment interventions and management.

#### Incidence

Primary tumors of the musculoskeletal system are uncommon, although the incidence is difficult to determine, as many benign tumors do not become symptomatic (Table 26.2). Primary bone neoplasms account for less than 0.2% of all tumors diagnosed per year. Bone tumors are diagnosed in men 1.5 times more frequently than in women.

#### Risk Factors

Although genetic links to the development of different types of bone tumors have been found, the risk factors involved in the etiopathogenesis of malignant bone tumors are not well understood. Though bone tumors

**Table 26.1** Classification of Soft Tissue Tumors

| Tissue of Origin | Benign Tumor | Malignant Tumor |
|---|---|---|
| **Connective Tissue** | | |
| Fibrous | Fibroma | Fibrosarcoma<br>Malignant fibrous histiocytoma |
| Cartilage | Chondroma<br>Enchondroma<br>Chondroblastoma<br>Osteochondroma | Chondrosarcoma |
| Bone (osteogenic) | Osteoma; osteoblastoma (giant osteoid osteoma) | Osteosarcoma (osteogenic sarcoma) |
| Bone marrow (myelogenic) | | Leukemia<br>Multiple myeloma<br>Ewing sarcoma<br>Hodgkin lymphoma of bone |
| Adipose (fat) | Lipoma | Liposarcoma |
| Synovium | Ganglion, giant cell of tendon sheath | Synovial sarcoma |
| **Muscle** | | |
| Smooth muscle | Leiomyoma | Leiomyosarcoma (uterus, gastrointestinal system) |
| Striated muscle | Rhabdomyoma | Rhabdomyosarcoma (can occur anywhere) |
| **Endothelium (Vascular/Lymphatic)** | | |
| Lymph vessels | Lymphangioma | Lymphangiosarcoma<br>Kaposi sarcoma<br>Lymphosarcoma (lymphoma) |
| Blood vessels (angiogenic) | Angioma<br>Hemangioma | Angiosarcoma<br>Hemangiosarcoma |
| **Neural Tissue** | | |
| Nerve fibers and sheaths | Neurofibroma<br>Neuroma<br>Neurinoma (neurilemmoma) | Neurofibrosarcoma<br>Neurogenic sarcoma (also known as neurosarcoma or schwannoma) |
| Glial tissue | Gliosis | Glioma |
| **Epithelium** | | |
| Skin and mucous membrane | Papilloma<br>Polyp | Squamous cell carcinoma<br>Basal cell carcinoma |
| Glandular epithelium | Adenoma | Adenocarcinoma |

may have a predilection for certain sites, age groups, and gender, most causes of osteosarcoma are unknown. The main factors implicated are Paget disease, Li-Fraumeni syndrome, antineoplastic drugs, ionizing radiation, and hereditary retinoblastoma.[40]

Exposure to alkylating chemotherapeutic agents such as cyclophosphamide, used in the treatment of acute lymphocytic leukemia, has been associated with subsequent development of osteosarcoma in a small percentage of cases. Several genetic conditions are related to the development of soft tissue sarcoma (e.g., neurofibromatosis, tuberous sclerosis, basal cell nevus syndrome), but this is only a small number of cases. Soft tissue tumors also may be associated with high doses of radiation or exposure to toxic chemicals in the workplace (e.g., herbicides, dioxin, preservatives, and so on).

### Etiologic Factors and Pathogenesis

**Bone Tumors.** To grasp the concepts of bone tumor formation, one must understand that bone metabolism is a balancing act of bone formation and resorption. The coupling of these two processes usually results in a balance of bone resorption and formation. When metabolic bone disease and neoplastic formations occur, this balance is upset. Under normal circumstances, bone remodeling involves a fine balance between osteoblast activity, which promotes new bone synthesis, and osteoclasts, which stimulate bone resorption. This balance is disrupted by the presence of malignant cells, resulting in uncoupling of the process of remodeling. A variety of paracrine factors including tumor necrosis factor-α, tumor necrosis factor-β, interleukin-1, and prostaglandins are released during the remodeling process and may ultimately contribute to growth of the metastatic cells.[72]

Cortical bone is most abundant in the outer walls of the shafts of long bones and is quite dense. The haversian canal system, which refers to the concentric rings of lamellae, is found in cortical bone. Cortical bone surrounds the trabecular or cancellous bone, which is the honeycomb-like bone found in the ends of long bones. Trabeculae are aligned with applied stresses in the bone. The metabolic activity is higher in cancellous bone than cortical bone, which

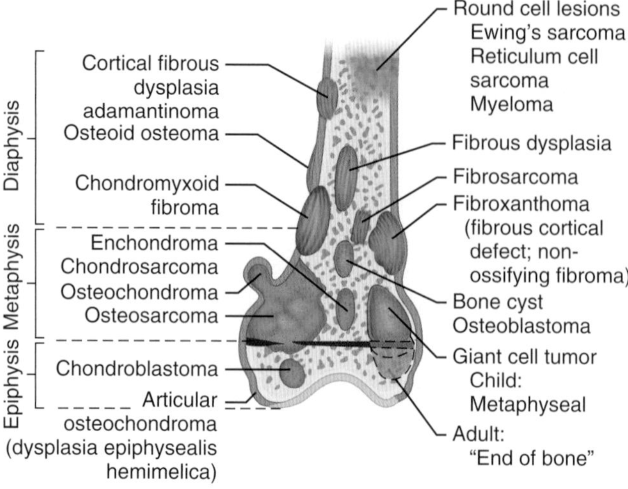


**Figure 26.1**

**Composite diagram illustrating frequent sites of bone tumors.** The diagram depicts the end of a long bone that has been divided into the epiphysis, metaphysis, and diaphysis. The epiphysis refers to the articular end of the long bones, which is primarily cartilaginous in the growing child. The metaphysis is the wider part of the shaft of the long bone. The diaphysis refers to the shaft itself. The typical sites of common primary bone tumors are labeled. (From Madewell JE, Ragsdale BD, Sweet DE: Radiologic and pathologic analysis of solitary bone lesions: I. Internal margins. *Radiol Clin North Am* 19:715, 1981.)

accounts for why many disorders that create disturbances in metabolic activity are first noted in cancellous bone.

Bone tumors are considered to be either osteoblastic or osteolytic, although most have characteristics of both processes. The osteoblastic process can be preceded by tumor cells or by normal cells in the host bone reacting to the tumor. Because the host bone continues with the normal process of resorption and bone formation, there will likely be a variety of cell types within the lesion. This makes histologic interpretation difficult.

Neoplastic cells do not themselves destroy bone, but their presence incites local osteoclastic resorption of bone. The cells of certain neoplasms also incite local osteoblastic deposition of normal bone, referred to as reactive bone. The neoplastic cells of the osteogenic group of neoplasms are capable of producing osteoid (young bone that has not undergone calcification) and bone, which are then referred to as tumor bone or neoplastic bone. The radiographic appearance of lesions affecting bone reflects varying proportions of bone resorption (osteolysis) and bone deposition (osteosclerosis)—some of the latter being reactive bone and some being neoplastic bone.[72]

**Soft Tissue Tumors.** Four types of genetic disorders underlying soft tissue sarcomas have been identified: translocations, gene amplifications, mutations, and complex genetic imbalances. Detection of these molecular changes can guide treatment and may predict response to treatment. Techniques used to detect translocations are very sensitive and in some cases may be used to detect microscopic metastasis.[41]

Soft tissue sarcomas have a predictable growth pattern, beginning as small masses and often growing in a centripetal pattern. The leading edge of the tumor (reactive zone) contains edema, fibrous tissue, inflammatory cells, and tumor cells. Uncontrolled growth often causes loss of blood supply at the center of the tumor.

**Table 26.2** Relative Frequency of Primary Bone Tumors[a]

| | |
|---|---|
| **Benign** | |
| Osteochondroma | 35% of benign tumors; 10% of all bone tumors |
| Osteoid osteoma | 10%–12% of benign bone tumors |
| Enchondroma | 10% of benign bone tumors; some report as high as 24% |
| Osteoblastoma | 1%–2% of benign bone tumors |
| Chondroblastoma | <1% of all bone tumors |
| Hemangioma | <1% of all bone tumors |
| **Malignant** | |
| Metastatic neoplasm | Most common form of bone malignancy; *secondary* neoplasm of bone |
| Multiple myeloma | Most common *primary* neoplasm of bone; plasma cell malignancy (bone marrow) |
| Osteosarcoma | Most common form of primary bone tumor; 35% of all malignant bone tumors; 15%–20% of primary sarcomas (excluding multiple myeloma) |
| Chondrosarcoma | 25% of malignant bone tumors (excluding multiple myeloma) |
| Ewing sarcoma | 16% of malignant bone tumors; second most common in children; fourth overall *primary* bone tumor for adults and children (after myeloma) |
| Malignant fibrous histiocytoma | 2%–5% of malignant bone tumors (excluding multiple myeloma) |
| Chordoma | 1%–4% of all malignant tumors; slow-growing but locally aggressive |
| Angiosarcoma | 14% of malignant bone tumors (excluding multiple myeloma) |

[a]Listed by decreasing order of frequency; with the exception of metastatic neoplasm listed, these statistics refer to primary bone tumors. Primary neoplasms of the skeleton are rare, amounting to only 0.2% of the overall primary bone tumors.

Data from Dorfman HD, Czerniak B: Bone cancers. *Cancer* 75:203–10, 1995; Zhang PJ: *Essentials in bone and soft tissue pathology*, New York, 2010, Springer; Sundaresan N: Primary malignant tumors of the spine. *Orthop Clin North Am* 40:21–36, 2009; Fletcher C: *Pathology and genetics of tumours of soft tissue and bone*, ed 4, Geneva, 2013, World Health Organization; International Association [IARC]/World Health Organization [WHO]: WHO Classification of Bone Tumours (2006). Available online at http://www.iarc.fr/en/publications/pdfs-online/pat-gen/bb5/bb5-classifbone.pdf [Accessed October 8, 2012].

Benign soft tissue tumors also have a centripetal growth pattern, but the expansion is more controlled and much slower. Benign lesions tend to be more superficially located compared with malignant lesions, which often grow within tissues under the deep fascia.[33] Soft tissue tumors found in the trunk tend to be larger in size and result in poorer outcomes than tumors in the extremities.[13]

## Clinical Manifestations

The clinical features must be well understood to ensure that the diagnostic evaluation proceeds expeditiously.

Many tumors are not diagnosed on their initial presentation. This is due to the ambiguous presentation of most tumors in their early stages; rarely does one actually find the case that is described as typical for a given lesion. This may be true regarding benign or malignant tumors, the initial presentation, and the appearance of the lesion.

**Pain.** Pain is a hallmark of tumor development, especially with malignant lesions. With bone tumors, intense pain is more likely to occur with rapidly growing lesions caused by pressure or tension on the sensitive periosteum and endosteum. Constant pain that is not dependent on position or activity and is increased with weight-bearing activities is a red flag symptom. The presence of night pain is considered an additional important finding. When the client reports night pain, further questioning is required.

The therapist should ensure that the client is reporting true night pain, which awakens the person from sleep, rather than a pain that makes it difficult to fall asleep. Ask the individual if rolling onto the involved side or painful area awakens him or her. Ascertain whether the pain subsides with movement and change in position, possibly indicating mechanical ischemia or positioning as the cause of the night pain.

Because pain is the overriding symptom in many people who seek treatment, a great deal of information should be obtained concerning the pain. Onset, progression, nature, quality, intensity, and aggravating factors are some of the factors that may be important in identifying a tumor in the early stages.[76]

Keep in mind that with cancer, pain is not always a measure of disease progression. Some tumors can progress to advanced stages without causing significant pain. Soft tissue tumors can occur in any anatomic region, although most develop in the extremities, usually the legs. These tumors may progress with relatively little pain because the soft tissue allows the growth to occur without putting undue pressure on nerve endings. Any swelling present is often attributed to a minor injury, delaying medical examination.

In fact, clients often report a recent history of trauma, although no scientific evidence directly connects such injury to the inception of soft tissue or bone sarcomas. Instead, such traumatic episodes are thought to call attention to a specific body part or location, thereby increasing the likelihood of detecting an otherwise painless and often innocuous soft tissue mass or bone lesion.

**Fractures.** Pathologic fractures are rare in primary neoplasms, but if the lytic process affects a significant portion of the cortex (more than 50%) or occupies 60% of the bone diameter, the risk of fracture increases. A relatively small lytic lesion in the femoral neck that destroys the inferior cortex of the femoral neck also places the client at increased risk. In benign lesions, no other symptoms may warn of the impending fracture.

A history of sudden onset of severe pain may be an indication of a pathologic fracture. Solitary bone cysts, fibrous dysplasia, nonossifying fibroma, and enchondromas may be detected only after presentation with a pathologic fracture. In addition to the tumor itself, other factors such as disuse, treatment (biopsy, radiation), and other health problems (osteoporosis) may increase the risk of pathologic fracture.[97]

**Miscellaneous.** Other signs and symptoms often encountered include swelling, fever, and the presence of a mass. Other factors that are useful in screening for serious pathology include unexplained weight loss, failure of rest to provide pain relief, age, and history of cancer. The history will often give more meaningful information regarding the possibility of skeletal neoplasms than the physical examination.[33]

**Swelling.** Swelling surrounding a tumor may not be detectable in a bone tumor, but with soft tissue tumors close to the skin surface, swelling may be one of the first presenting signs. The nature of swelling, including the location, amount, temperature, and tenderness, is somewhat dependent on the vascularity of the lesion.

**Mass.** A careful physical examination may reveal a mass or other signs of an inflammatory process. The presence of a mass should raise questions concerning the location, mobility, tenderness, dimensions, and recent changes in any of these factors. As with pain, the size of the mass is not indicative of the severity of the lesion but is one factor to consider. Any change in size, appearance, or other characteristics of a lump, local swelling, or lesion of any kind within the previous 6 weeks to 6 months should be referred to a physician.

**Metastases.** Sarcomas spread by hematogenous routes rather than through the lymphatics. The most common site of metastases for individuals with extremity sarcomas is the lung, followed by liver and other bone sites. Anyone diagnosed with soft tissue sarcoma has an approximately 50% chance of local recurrence, because these tumors spread along tissue planes and involve adjacent tissue. Lymph node involvement is uncommon and is often associated with poor prognosis.[72]

## MEDICAL MANAGEMENT

DIAGNOSIS. Physical examination, imaging studies (e.g., x-rays, computed tomography [CT], magnetic resonance imaging [MRI]), and biopsy are the primary diagnostic tools.

*Physical Examination.* Many tumors cannot be observed or palpated during the physical examination, but if a mass is present, its characteristics must be noted. The presence of café au lait spots (associated with neurofibromatosis), skin ulceration, or neurologic findings (e.g., footdrop, calf pain) may be significant.

Because synovial sarcoma, rhabdomyosarcoma, and epithelioid sarcoma can metastasize via the lymphatics, examination of the lymph nodes is essential. A tumor overlying bone and muscle can be evaluated by contracting the muscle and checking for movement or change in consistency of the tumor.

*Radiographic Examination.* Radiographs also help differentiate between bone and soft tissue involvement. Plain radiographs are a mainstay in the detection and evaluation of many skeletal tumors. In many cases, skeletal tumors are found incidentally on routine radiographs for associated injuries. The radiograph provides unique information concerning skeletal tumors.[10] MRI has emerged as the most useful imaging tool for evaluating soft tissue tumors, although biopsy is essential for a definitive histologic diagnosis.[95]

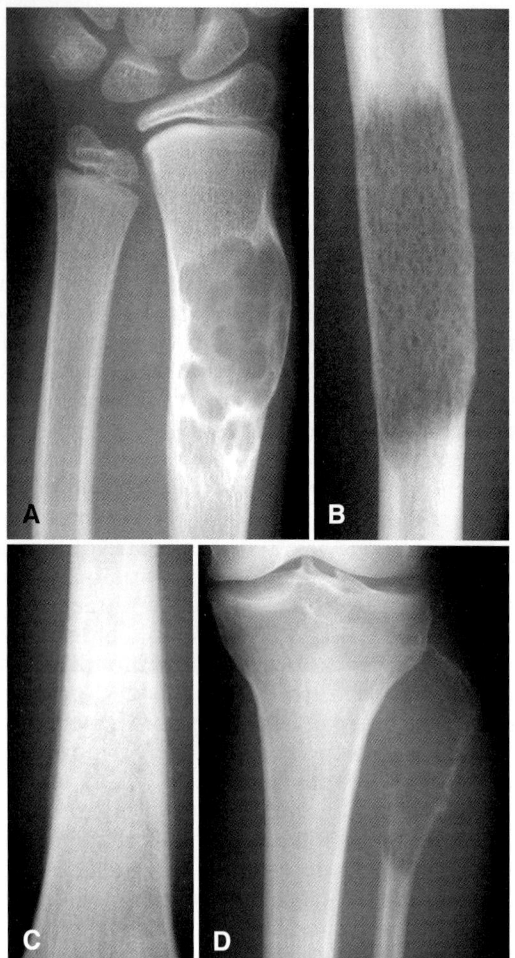


**Figure 26.2**

**Patterns of bone destruction.** (A) Anteroposterior (AP) radiograph of the distal radius in a patient with nonossifying fibroma, demonstrating the sharp, "geographic" margin indicating slow growth. Endosteal scalloping and bone expansion with an intact overlying cortex are additional features of slow growth. (B) AP radiograph of the humerus showing a moth-eaten appearance caused by the coalescence of multiple small lytic areas in a patient with renal carcinoma metastasis. (C) AP radiograph of the distal femur showing a permeative pattern of bone destruction in a patient with primary bone lymphoma. (D) AP radiograph of the fibula showing a lytic lesion with expansion and destruction of the cortex indicating an aggressive growth pattern. (From Adam A: *Grainger & Allison's diagnostic radiology*, Philadelphia, 2008, Churchill Livingstone.)

The location of the tumor will give many clues to the type of lesion (see Fig. 26.1). Some tumors develop exclusively in the epiphysis, whereas others develop in the diaphysis of long bones. Bone tumors tend to predominate in the ends of long bones that undergo the greatest growth and remodeling and hence have the greatest number of cells and amount of cell activity (shoulder and knee regions).

When small tumors, presumably detected early, are analyzed, preferential sites of tumor origin become apparent within each bone, as shown in Fig. 26.1. This suggests a relationship between the type of tumor and the anatomic site affected. In general, a tumor of a given cell type arises in the field in which the homologous normal cells are most active. These regional variations suggest that the composition of the tumor is affected or may be determined by the metabolic field in which it arises.

The effect that the tumor has on bone is described as destructive or lytic if the normal bone pattern is disrupted (Fig. 26.2). Approximately 50% of the bone must be destroyed before the lesion can be detected. This may be evident by an irregular, erosive border surrounding the lesion; loss of trabeculae; or disruption of the cortex.[57]

The response of surrounding bone to the tumor is another important feature to note on plain radiographs. Sclerotic borders give an indication of the growth characteristics of the tumor. A well-defined border with definite sclerotic margins is seen with a slow-growing lesion.

A tumor with a permeated or moth-eaten appearance (i.e., an area with multiple holes with irregular edges randomly distributed) with an expansive cortical shell indicates an aggressive malignant lesion. Codman triangle, a triangular-shaped area of reactive bone, is formed when the neoplasm has eroded the cortex, elevating the periosteum and producing reactive bone in the angle where it is still attached (Fig. 26.3).

The tumor's location, its effect on bone, and the local bone response to the lesion are just some of the radiographic features to be noted and will help in planning the rest of the evaluation.

***Imaging.*** Radionuclide bone scan (scintigraphy), CT, MRI, angiography, and ultrasonography all have a place in the evaluation of bone lesions. *Bone scans* help locate skip metastases and the presence of bone metastases as well as metastatic bone lesions, and they assess tumor activity by the amount of radioisotope uptake in and around the tumor. Greater uptake indicates a more aggressive and malignant tumor. *CT scans* allow for good visualization of the tumor's location, matrix, and responses of the surrounding tissues to the tumor. CT is also good for detecting pulmonary metastases. *MRI* is more valuable for determining the extent of the marrow involvement and soft tissue masses outside the bone.[40,55] The surgical team uses the information provided by MRI to help visualize the involvement of the tumor and to plan limb salvage techniques.[8,1]

*Angiography* plays an important role when limb-sparing surgery is being considered by providing information regarding the neovascularity of the tumor and mapping the vascular anatomy. *Ultrasonography* is a noninvasive imaging method that can be used to determine the size and consistency of a soft tissue mass and the need for other imaging studies. It may be used to establish intraarterial access for subsequent chemotherapy.

***Biopsy.*** A biopsy is the definitive diagnostic procedure in both bone and soft tissue tumors and is usually performed after physical examination and imaging. This procedure can take many forms. The decision to do an open or incisional biopsy, core needle or fine-needle biopsy, or excisional biopsy is based on the location and type of tumor.

***Laboratory Tests.*** Various laboratory studies are used to detect, diagnose, and differentiate musculoskeletal neoplasms. Laboratory tests that may be of value include complete blood count, urinalysis, erythrocyte sedimentation rate (elevated in Ewing sarcoma), serum calcium (elevated in metastatic bone disease), phosphorus (decreased with brown tumors associated with hyperthyroidism),

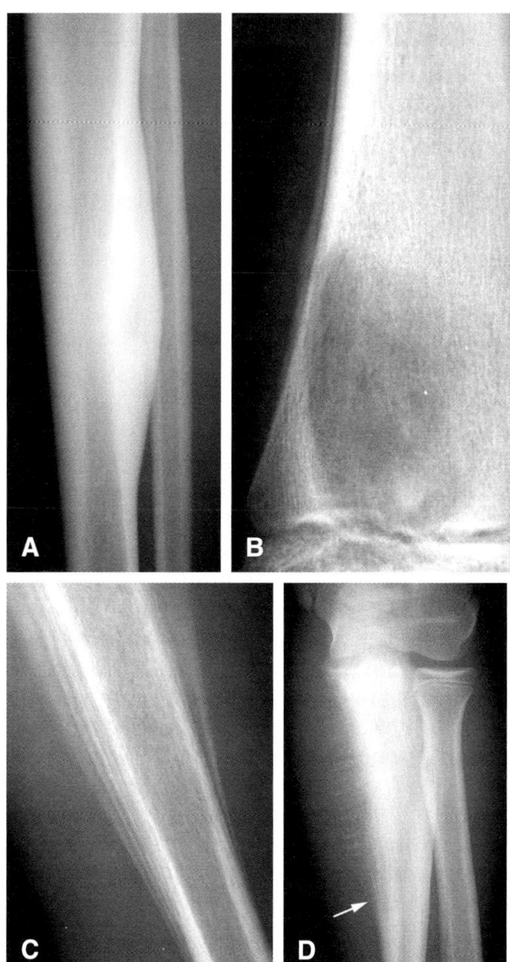


**Figure 26.3**

**Patterns of periosteal reaction.** (A) Lateral radiograph of the tibia showing a solid periosteal reaction due to osteoid osteoma. (B) Anteroposterior (AP) radiograph of the distal tibia showing a single, laminated periosteal reaction associated with a Brodie abscess. (C) AP radiograph of the humerus showing a multilaminated periosteal reaction associated with Ewing sarcoma. (D) AP radiograph of the proximal ulna showing a "hair-on-end" type of vertical periosteal reaction associated with Ewing sarcoma. Note also the Codman triangle *(arrow)*. (From Adam A: *Grainger & Allison's diagnostic radiology*, Philadelphia, 2008, Churchill Livingstone.)

alkaline phosphatase (elevated in osteosarcoma and Paget disease), and serum protein electrophoresis (abnormal in metastatic bone disease). Elevated alkaline phosphatase and lactic dehydrogenase also occur with osteosarcoma. Serum levels of alkaline phosphatase and calcium are often elevated with metastatic diseases.

**Staging and grading.** The purpose of much of the extensive workup once a tumor is identified is to determine the grade and stage of the tumor. Grading determines the histologic characteristics such as the extent of anaplasia or differentiation of the cells from grade I, indicating cells that are very differentiated, to grade IV, indicating cells that are undifferentiated.

Staging of a tumor is concerned with the extent of its growth, both local and distant. The tumor, node, metastasis staging system reflects the degree of local extension at the primary tumor site, involvement of local nodes, and presence of metastasis. This classification group is strongly correlated with survival.

The relative rarity of soft tissue sarcomas, the anatomic heterogeneity of these lesions, and the presence of more than 30 recognized histologic subtypes of variable grade have made it difficult to establish a functional system that can accurately stage all forms of this disease.[84] The staging system of the American Joint Committee on Cancer (AJCC) is the most widely employed staging classification for soft tissue sarcomas.[88] Staging helps in planning and standardizing the intervention strategy for these neoplasms.

TREATMENT. Once a tumor has been identified and staged, decisions about management and intervention can be considered. Treatment ranges from *observation* in the case of some benign bone tumors to *surgical interventions* for potentially malignant tumors. The age and health of the patient will also determine the most appropriate treatment pathway for management of the tumor.[70] Multimodal measures are needed for a long-term successful outcome, as chemotherapy or surgery alone cures few patients.[62]

Complete tumor resection is the best surgical strategy and is attempted whenever possible. A marginal excision removes the tumor at its border, resulting in some of the tumor remaining. A wide excision (sometimes referred to as an en bloc incision) removes some of the normal surrounding tissue, leaving none of the tumor. Soft tissue sarcomas often require wide excision to reduce the recurrence rate. Radical resection may be required in which the entire involved bone and all the tissue compartments adjacent to the tumor are removed.

The spine, sacrum, pelvis, ankle, hand, mediastinum, and chest wall are just a few examples of bone cancer locations that make surgery difficult. When local excision has positive margins (not all the cancer was removed), local control may be increased with radiation and chemotherapy regimens.

Limb salvage or limb-sparing procedures have largely replaced amputation as the principal method to eradicate primary sarcomas.[68] The three phases to any limb-sparing procedure are (1) resection of the tumor, (2) reconstruction of the skeletal area involved, and (3) soft tissue and muscle transfer to complete the reconstruction. Obtaining a wide surgical margin while preserving limb viability and function remains the challenge to the medical team, requiring close coordination of surgical, medical, and oncologic staff. Often, soft tissue reconstruction is necessary to provide wound coverage after tumor removal.[17]

*Radiation therapy* is used to kill tumor cells and to assist in slowing or stopping the growth of the tumor. Reducing the size of a bone tumor may provide pain relief and provide for a clearer margin between tumor and normal tissues in preparation for surgical excisions. Radiation therapy is recommended for some primary bone tumors such as Ewing sarcoma and myeloma, but many malignant tumors, such as chondrosarcomas, are not affected by radiation. For some soft tissue tumors, adjunctive radiation is used in an attempt to limit the degree of surgical excision needed.

In general, radiation is not recommended for benign conditions.

Because hematogenous spread occurs early in musculoskeletal tumors, *chemotherapy* is used to prevent the spread of malignant tumors elsewhere in the body. Combination of chemotherapy drugs has resulted in increased survival rates in clients with Ewing sarcoma and rhabdomyosarcomas. Chemotherapy is combined with other modalities such as surgery and radiation to best treat bone and soft tissue tumors.[70]

As discussed in Chapter 9, modern clinical oncology is moving toward tailored therapy according to genetic profiling. Treatment can be stratified with different intensities prescribed based on the genetic and epigenetic characteristics of the individual.[59] Individuals with a poor prognosis may do better with a combination of treatments to best arrest the primary tumor and control the potential for secondary tumors. Immunotherapies have found few successes for the treatment of bone and soft tissue neoplasms, but this may improve as understanding of the immune response to sarcomas and their microenvironments advances.[62]

**PROGNOSIS.** The prognosis is based in part on the type of tumor and whether it is benign or malignant. Survival is influenced by the grade of malignancy, tumor stage, and achieved surgical margins. A high grade and evidence of metastasis are associated with a poor prognosis for all neoplasms of bone or soft tissue regardless of the staging system that is used. Tumor extensions into both the spinal column and the skull are correlated with a poor outcome. Incomplete resections are more likely to result in tumor recurrence with subsequent surgeries and increased risk for complications and poor outcome.

Slow-growing tumors should be followed for prolonged periods to determine the natural history and to identify the ultimate prognosis. Prognosis can vary from 3- to 5-year survival rates for clients with sarcomas and myeloma to tumors that are asymptomatic. Successfully treated individuals may develop severe late effects including second cancers (e.g., radiation-induced sarcomas or treatment-related leukemia), particularly after high-dose therapy with an alkylating agent, and chemotherapy-induced cardiomyopathy.[37]

**RECURRENCE.** People with recurrent disease generally have a poor prognosis but need to undergo a complete reevaluation of the extent of the disease to determine this more specifically. The prognosis depends on the type of therapy given previously, duration of remission, and extent of metastases. The lung is the most common initial site of distant metastases for the majority of soft tissue and bone sarcomas. Other sites may include distant osseous sites, bone marrow, and lymph nodes.

## PRIMARY BENIGN BONE TUMORS

### Bone Island

#### Overview and Incidence

Bone islands, also known as enostoses (singular: enostosis), are oval, usually small, sclerotic lesions of bone.

**SPECIAL IMPLICATIONS FOR THE THERAPIST 26.1**

### *Primary Tumors*

#### Screening Assessment

A therapist's involvement with clients with musculoskeletal neoplasms should begin with increased efforts directed toward early detection and education. Although many musculoskeletal tumors produce symptoms that are also present with more mundane conditions, careful examination and monitoring of a client's response to intervention may lead to earlier detection and treatment.

Assessing for past history of cancer, family history, and risk factors may alert the therapist to the need to screen further for medical disease. This is especially true in the case of musculoskeletal symptoms of unknown cause or when the individual does not respond to physical therapy intervention as expected for a musculoskeletal problem.

The presence of suspicious lymph nodes or aberrant soft tissue masses can be identified by the therapist but must be further evaluated by a physician. By including the possibility of a primary musculoskeletal tumor in the differential diagnosis of clients who have continued pain despite appropriate rest and treatment, further medical evaluation may be recommended, which may help reveal other pathology.

#### Rehabilitation

An achievable goal for the majority of people with soft tissue and bone sarcomas is freedom from disease with long-term resumption of nearly normal function. Therapists are key to the successful attainment of this goal for individuals who are undergoing treatment for primary musculoskeletal neoplasms.[32] A comprehensive approach should be used to ensure that both psychosocial-spiritual aspects and physical problems are addressed. Occupational status, family structure, and age all are important factors.[86]

Communication among team members including social workers, rehabilitation counselors, physicians, nurses, and therapists cannot be overemphasized. Communication is essential to coordination and follow-through in the treatment and rehabilitation program. A detailed approach to evaluation and treatment of clients with cancer should be formulated.

Therapists must understand the pathology of the tumor to understand the entire management plan. Specific interventions and goals can be developed with a thorough understanding of the pathology and the medical treatment being undertaken.[85]

Early postoperative mobilization is essential to prevent complications such as pressure ulcers, deep venous thrombosis, lymphedema, pneumonia, muscle wasting, and generalized weakness associated with prolonged bed rest. Surgical procedures will have an effect on multiple organ systems, as will chemotherapy and radiation therapy. A detailed assessment and description of pain is always indicated, as described in Chapter 9, because pain control is a critical component in successful acute rehabilitation.

Many other factors to consider before implementing a treatment plan following orthopedic procedures include controlling compressive forces and weight bearing. Wolf's law demonstrates bone strength to increase in response to imposed mechanical stress, such as the pulling force of muscles and the pressures of weight bearing. When bone resorption exceeds bone formation, osteopenia develops.

After excision of cancerous bone (sometimes accompanied by muscle resection), mechanical weakening and resultant bone instability may limit or contraindicate weight bearing and use of the involved extremity. Remaining muscles should be strengthened, and substitution patterns of muscle control should be implemented and encouraged where necessary.[78]

Other considerations in the rehabilitative process may include rehabilitation for the amputee, evaluation of adaptive equipment needs, ambulation devices, use of orthoses to support involved extremities, wound care management, environmental adaptations (e.g., access ramps, accessible doorways, bathroom grab bars), work site modifications, and quality-of-life issues. Client education is essential regarding proper body mechanics; energy conservation; side effects of treatment; and prevention and recognition of complications such as infection, deep vein thrombosis, skin breakdown, lymphedema, scar formation, and loss of flexibility, strength, balance, or endurance.

### Prescriptive Exercise

As discussed, treatment of tumors can result in amputation (sometimes as extensive as a hemipelvectomy),[59] prolonged immobilization, bone or muscle resection, or extensive surgical reconstruction, all of which require consideration of postoperative complications (e.g., ischemia, infection) and the involvement of many different types of rehabilitation.

Limb-sparing techniques (instead of amputation and/or disarticulation) such as endoprosthetic replacement (distal femoral replacement with rotating hinge device, expandable for pediatric patients) continue to undergo modification and refinement. Surgeons are attempting to minimize muscle resection, maintain mechanical function, and successfully reattach the muscles to the endoprostheses or to surrounding soft tissue structures, thereby reducing functional impairment.[42,27] An individualized program of exercise that takes into account the diagnosis, underlying pathology, physical condition of the individual, effects of various interventions, strength deficits, and structural instability is essential. Toward this end, the therapist should be aware that studies are underway concerning the long-term effects of prosthetic knee replacement after wide resection, risk factors for prosthetic failure, and the most effective rehabilitative strategies after limb salvage procedures for bone tumors.

Rehabilitation techniques for these clients remain conjectural. Despite loss of range of motion (ROM) and muscle power, most clients report good limb function (depending on their definition of "good"). Early gait training and weight bearing with active assisted range are indicated, and isometric exercises about the joint are recommended.[81]

General principles regarding energy conservation and exercise for a person with cancer, especially following chemotherapy or radiotherapy, are discussed in Chapter 9. Additionally, the therapist must keep in mind safety guidelines for the use of laboratory values as discussed in Chapter 40 and in Special Implications for the Therapist 26.9: Metastatic Tumors.

They are one of the most common benign bone lesions. Bone islands have been observed in all bones and may be solitary or multiple lesions. The lesion is well defined and made up of cortical bone with a well-developed haversian canal system. The borders blend in with the surrounding bone. The presence of spicules of cortical bone extending from the margins to the surrounding trabeculae is characteristic.[64]

The true frequency of these lesions remains unknown, but the estimated prevalence of bone islands of the pelvic bone is about 1%. In the spine, enostoses may be apparent in 1% to 14% of people. Bone islands are seen in both men and women and in all age groups, with perhaps a lower frequency in children. Any osseous site can be affected, but the lesions have a predilection for the pelvis, proximal femur, and ribs.

### Clinical Manifestations

Bone islands do not usually cause any symptoms, although there have been isolated reports of mild arthralgias and/or skin lesions. They are seen on radiographs as incidental findings.

## MEDICAL MANAGEMENT

When the bone islands are small (less than 1 cm), diagnosis with plain radiographs is adequate. They are usually oblong and align themselves with the axis of the bone. The emphasis is not on intervention but on the judicious use of diagnostic tools. Biopsies should be avoided, as they are usually unnecessary. Although some bone islands can enlarge, they do not transform into malignant lesions.

**SPECIAL IMPLICATIONS FOR THE THERAPIST 26.2**

*Bone Islands*

Bone islands are seen in radiographs of clients with a variety of musculoskeletal traumas. If clients are aware of these lesions, they should be reassured that they pose no significant health concern. Many physicians do not inform clients that bone islands are present. Care must be taken not to alarm the client. The word *tumor* is foreboding and should be used sparingly.

## Osteoid Osteoma

### Overview, Incidence, and Etiologic Factors

Osteoid osteoma is a rare benign vascular osteoblastic lesion. The lesion usually manifests as an osteoid nidus within loose vascular tissues found in the cortex of long bones such as the femur and tibia. Spine and

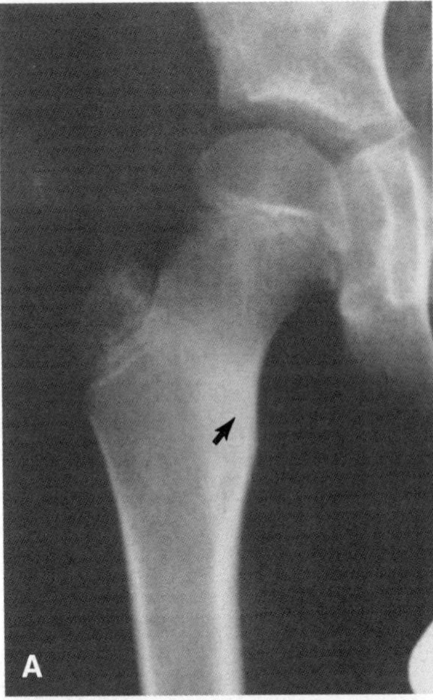


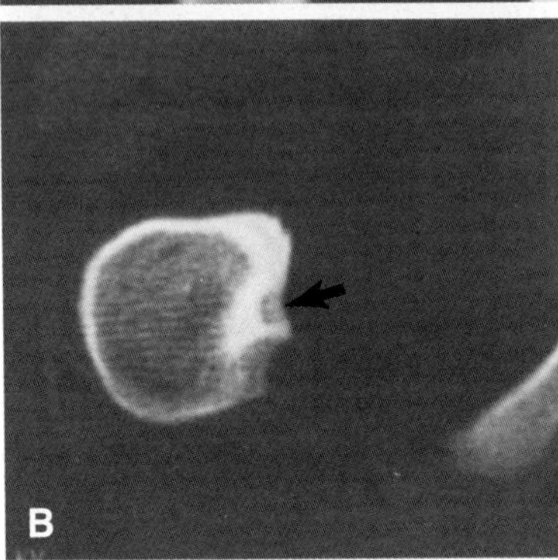


**Figure 26.4**

**Osteoid osteoma.** (A) Bony sclerosis with cortical thickening is seen in this person with pain in the proximal femur. A faint lucency *(arrow)* can be seen in the area of sclerosis, which is the nidus of an osteoid osteoma. (B) A computed tomography (CT) scan through the nidus shows it to lie just dorsal to the lesser trochanter *(arrow)*. This is a characteristic appearance of an osteoid osteoma on CT. (From Helms C: *Fundamentals of skeletal radiology: benign cystic lesions*, Philadelphia, 1989, WB Saunders.)

pelvis may also be affected, but osteoid osteomas can occur in almost any bone except the skull. The tumors occur near the end of the diaphysis (Fig. 26.4).[11] Osteoid osteomas have been reported to be found in the acromion and hip acetabulum but are rare. Osteoid osteoma accounts for about 10% to 12% of benign bone tumors. Most of these lesions are found in men younger than age 25 years. The cause of osteoid osteoma remains unknown.[83]

### Pathogenesis

Pathologic study shows areas of immature bone surrounded by prominent osteoblasts and osteoclasts. The lesion is vascular, but no cartilage is present. Osteoid osteoma is probably a reactive bone-forming lesion rather than a true neoplasm, consisting of a small, round nidus (nest) of osteoid tissue surrounded by reactive bone sclerosis. Soft tissue and bone changes are caused by local secretion of prostaglandins by the tumor.

The zone of sclerosis is not an integral part of the tumor and represents a secondary reversible change that gradually disappears after the removal of the nidus. Osteoid osteomas are not progressive and rarely grow larger than 1 cm in diameter. They are uncalcified and therefore radiolucent.

### Clinical Manifestations

Gradually increasing and persistent local pain in the area of the tumor, described as a dull ache progressing to intense pain, is the primary complaint. The pain is often worse during rest and at night and is characteristically relieved by aspirin and other nonsteroidal antiinflammatory drugs (NSAIDs). Pain relief may be due to the inhibitory effect on prostaglandins produced by osteoid osteomas. Systemic symptoms are uncommon with normal blood and chemistry tests. Left untreated, an osteoid osteoma can be symptomatic over a 2- to 3-year period, followed by a recovery period lasting 3 to 7 years needed for ossification of the osteoid nidus.[11]

When the lesion is located near a joint, synovial effusion may develop and interfere with joint function, with local muscle atrophy developing.[44] A significant leg length discrepancy can occur, caused by the increased growth rate of affected bone in young individuals with open growth plates.

Though osteoid osteomas occur rarely in the spine, if present, they are found in the lower thoracic or lumbar spine located in the posterior vertebral arch. The tumor can lead to joint pain and dysfunction, often delaying the diagnosis by masquerading as a more common problem such as an overuse syndrome.[66]

Spine involvement may result in an unexplained backache or painful type of scoliosis with unilateral spasticity of spinal muscles. Some people with vertebral lesions may have clinical symptoms suggestive of a neurologic disorder, lumbar disc disease, or both. In the case of spine involvement, neurologic deficits can be caused by extradural compression.[66]

## MEDICAL MANAGEMENT

**DIAGNOSIS.** Radiographs can be diagnostic for osteoid osteoma, although these are often normal early in the course. Later, a small (less than 1 cm) translucency or nidus forms, surrounded by sclerotic bone. Lesions in the cortex of the bone may appear with a reactive sclerosis that will make visualization of the lucent nidus difficult. When the tumor is not easily identified on radiographs (e.g., vertebral nidus), further testing is required, such as a bone scan (scintigraphy), which will show a focal uptake of the radiotracer. Plain films may not be adequate when the tumor is intraarticular; in such cases, CT or MRI can be used to accurately locate the nidus. The use of percutaneous needle biopsy will confirm only half of the cases.

**TREATMENT AND PROGNOSIS.** Initial treatment of this condition is to control symptoms with use of aspirin or NSAIDs, with most people having some relief of symptoms. Follow-up radiographs at 3- to 6-month intervals will determine if the nidus is growing or starting to show signs of recovery. Osteoid osteomas have no potential for malignant transformation.[66]

Because this condition is primarily found in young men wanting active lifestyles, most will choose a surgical excision of the nidus. Surgical excisions can be performed with an en bloc resection if the lesion is found in a long bone; otherwise, a curettage method will be used to preserve the bone tissue surrounding the nidus. A surgical excision is usually a curative treatment for an osteoid osteoma, with the incidence of a recurrence being rare. Lesions that are found in the spine or near joint surfaces can be treated with use of percutaneous needle excisions. Radiofrequency or laser ablation can also be used for difficult-to-localize lesions. These treatments have a one-third rate of incomplete resection and greater potential for persistent symptoms and recurrence of the osteoma.[66]

**SPECIAL IMPLICATIONS FOR THE THERAPIST 26.3**

*Osteoid Osteoma*

The size and extent of the resection may mandate some activity restrictions or weight-bearing limitations if the risk of fracture exists. Monitoring bone healing with serial radiographs may help guide the weight-bearing progression. Intraarticular lesions require more extensive rehabilitation for restoration of normal function.

## Osteoblastoma

### Overview

Osteoblastoma is a benign bone lesion similar to osteoid osteoma, only larger, with a tendency to expand. Some aggressive forms of osteoblastoma have been recognized. In contrast to osteoid osteoma, osteoblastomas are often found in the spine, sacrum, and flat bones. Osteoblastomas involve the spine in approximately 35% of affected individuals, with the cervical spine affected in up to 39% of these individuals (Fig. 26.5).[34]

Lesions found in the long bones are usually in the diaphysis, although as with most tumors, they can be seen elsewhere (Fig. 26.6). The histologic makeup of osteoblastoma is very similar to that of an osteoid osteoma. In fact, sometimes it is size alone that differentiates the two, with osteoblastoma being the larger. The lesions are osteolytic and have a sclerotic border.

### Incidence

Osteoblastoma occurs most often in men younger than 30 years of age, but cases have been reported in children as young as 2 years old and adults in their 70s. Osteoblastoma is a rare osteoblastic tumor that makes up only 1% to 2% of all benign bone tumors.[34]

### Clinical Manifestations

A dull, aching pain that is poorly localized is a common presentation for an osteoblastoma.[74] In general, the pain of osteoblastoma is not as severe as with osteoid osteoma and will not be relieved with NSAIDs. Larger tumors will become tender to palpation, and symptoms will be more localized to the diaphysis of the bone or pedicles of the spine. Spinal tumors may result in a functional scoliosis and produce neurologic deficits secondary to nerve compressions. Metastases and death have been reported with the aggressive variant, which can behave in a fashion similar to that of osteosarcoma.

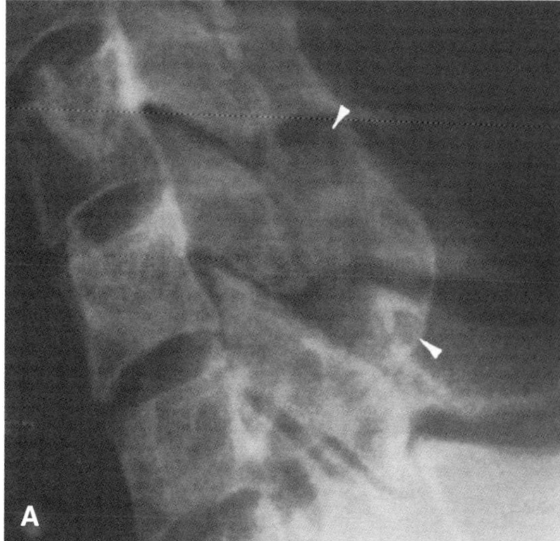


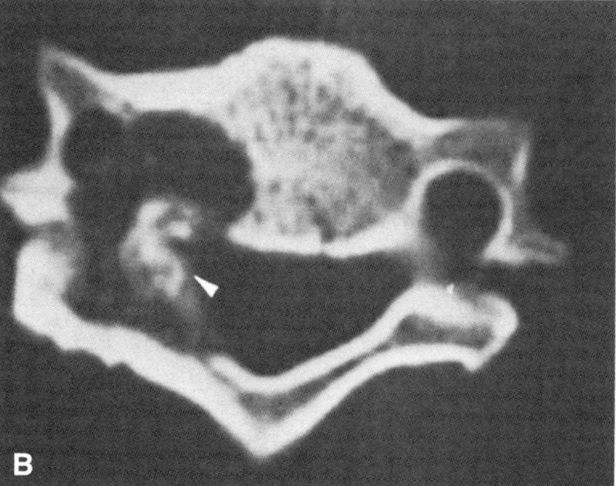


**Figure 26.5**

**Osteoblastoma of the spine.** (A) An expansile lesion *(arrowheads)* in the lamina of the fifth cervical vertebra is evident. (B) Note an osteolytic lesion containing calcification or ossification *(arrowhead)* affecting the body, transverse and costal elements, and lamina of a cervical vertebra as depicted on a transaxial computed tomography scan. (From Resnick D: *Bone and joint imaging*, ed 3, Philadelphia, 2005, Saunders.)

### MEDICAL MANAGEMENT

DIAGNOSIS. Osteoblastoma is seen on plain radiographs, but when it is located in the spine, other imaging techniques are also useful. The lesion can have variations in its appearance. Often it looks like a large osteoid osteoma with a well-defined radiolucency in the central portion and a thin, sclerotic border. It also can be similar to an aneurysmal bone cyst that is expansile and lytic with a soap bubble appearance (see Fig. 26.3). CT and MRI are valuable in localizing the tumor and determining the extent of tissue involved. An aggressive lesion can expand beyond the cortex and involve soft tissue.

TREATMENT. In the long bones, curettage (scraping to remove the contents of the bone cavity) is often adequate.

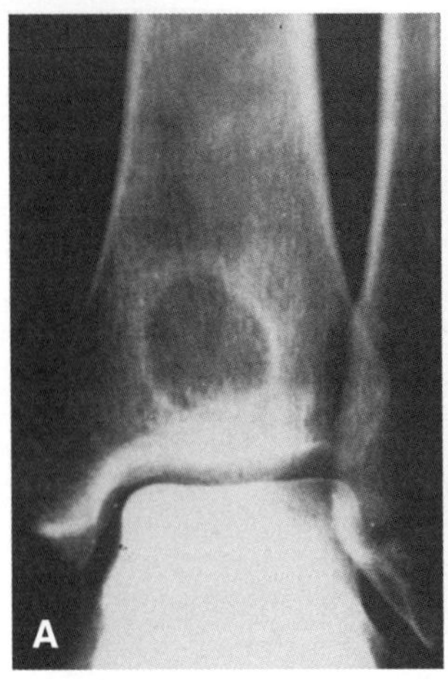


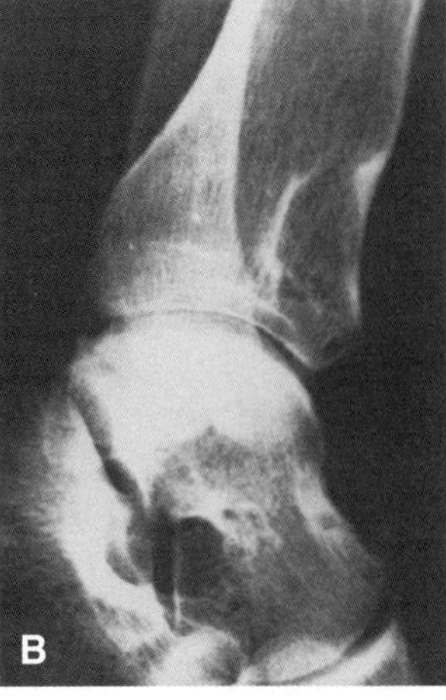


**Figure 26.6**

**Genuine (conventional) osteoblastoma of the tibia in a 24-year-old woman.** Anteroposterior (A) and lateral (B) radiographs show a round radiolucent lesion with slightly sclerotic borders at the lower and anterior aspect of the tibia. (From Gitelis S, Schajowicz F: Osteoid osteoma and osteoblastoma. *Orthop Clin* 20:320, 1989.)

A wider excision is sometimes recommended because of the unpredictable nature of osteoblastoma and high recurrence rate (up to 15%). Recurrence is often attributed to incomplete resection.[29]

Extramarginal excisions can result in the need to perform reconstructive procedures using autografts or allografts and internal fixation when the tumor is located in the diaphysis of long bones. If the joint is affected, implants may be needed. In the spine, removal of the tumor may lead to instability, which may require fusion and internal fixation.

In the cervical spine, their presence so close to neurovascular structures (e.g., vital blood vessels and the spinal cord) makes treatment of this problem very complex. Embolization (either partial or complete) may be done first before surgery. Embolization is a nonsurgical, minimally invasive procedure using metal sponges or other devices to purposefully block blood flow. Surgery to remove the tumor is then done within 24 hours of the embolization. When necessary, bone defect filling and instrumented fusion may be done.[29]

**PROGNOSIS.** Most osteoblastomas are cured by the initial treatment, but even with careful removal of the tumors, they recur in about 10% to 20% of affected individuals.[7] There is a risk of malignant transformation into an osteosarcoma, which can be avoided with early interventions. Appropriate intervention with adjunctive chemotherapy or radiation is the current standard of care. Embolization before marginal resection may reduce the rate of recurrence.

SPECIAL IMPLICATIONS FOR THE THERAPIST 26.4

### *Osteoblastoma*

Surgical excision may be extensive. In the long bones, the risk of pathologic fracture is often present. The use of external fixation, allografts, immobilization, and limited weight bearing is common.

# PRIMARY MALIGNANT BONE TUMORS

Primary malignant bone tumors are relatively rare, representing about 6% to 7% of all pediatric neoplasms. They can be broadly categorized into low-grade (chordoma, chondrosarcoma) and high-grade (osteosarcoma, Ewing sarcoma) tumors.[87] Osteosarcomas are the most frequent type, followed by chondrosarcoma and then Ewing sarcoma. Osteosarcomas make up more than half of all malignant bone tumors; Ewing sarcomas account for one-third of all primary malignant bone tumors (Table 26.3).

## Osteosarcoma

### Overview

Osteosarcoma, also known as *osteogenic sarcoma,* is an extremely malignant tumor with destructive lesions and abundant sclerosis, both from the tumor itself and from reactive bone formation. Most deaths associated with osteosarcomas are from metastatic pulmonary diseases. A characteristic of osteosarcoma is the production of osteoid by malignant, neoplastic cells. This is seen on photomicrographs and is one of the features used to help differentiate this tumor. Resected specimens usually show that the cortex has been broken by the destructive tumor.[72] Although various types of osteosarcoma exist, including parosteal, periosteal, telangiectatic, and small cell, only the most common, conventional or classic intramedullary osteosarcoma is discussed here.

### Incidence

Osteosarcoma is the second most frequent malignant condition of bone, accounting for 15% to 20% of all primary bone tumors; only myeloma is seen more often. It is fairly rare, occurring most often in male children, adolescents, and adults younger than age 30, with a peak frequency during the adolescent growth spurt when there is rapid bone turnover and another smaller peak in people older than 50 years.

Osteosarcoma can develop in many bones but is more common in long bones, the site of the most active epiphyseal growth. The distal femur (knee) is the most common site, followed by the proximal tibia and proximal fibula (50% are located in the knee region), proximal humerus, and pelvis and occasionally the mandible, vertebrae, or scapula.[39]

### Etiologic and Risk Factors

Osteosarcomas can be primary or secondary. Certain genetic or acquired conditions increase the risk of osteosarcoma (e.g., retinoblastoma, Paget disease of bone, enchondromatosis, ionizing radiation). Alterations of multiple chromosomes and their extra copies have been demonstrated but only in distinct clinical subsets of osteosarcoma. Secondary osteosarcomas develop from other lesions such as Paget disease, chronic osteomyelitis, osteoblastoma, or giant cell tumor.

### Pathogenesis

The mechanisms involved in the development of osteosarcomas are still obscure. Osteosarcoma originates

**Table 26.3** Bone Tumors Presentation and Treatment

| Tumor | Type | Clinical Manifestations | Medical Treatment |
|---|---|---|---|
| Bone islands | Benign | Incidental finding | No treatment recommended |
| Osteoid osteoma | Benign | Local, persistent pain at diaphysis | Excision of nidus and monitoring |
| Osteoblastoma | Benign | Localized pain near metaphysis | Excision of tumor |
| Giant cell tumor | Low-grade malignant | Pain along long bones, fractures | Radiation or chemotherapy/ excision and bone grafting |
| Enchondroma | Benign | Local swelling at metaphysis | Curettage/bone grafting |
| Osteochondroma | Benign | Lump or swelling near the physis (similar to a chondrosarcoma) | Monitoring/removal if symptomatic |
| Osteosarcoma | Malignant | Pain and swelling near metaphysis | Chemotherapy/excision and limb salvage procedure |
| Chondrosarcoma | Malignant | Swelling and hard growth off of the metaphysis | Wide resection with limb salvage |
| Ewing sarcoma | Malignant | Pain and swelling along shaft of long bones | Multimodal treatment plan |
| Chordoma | Malignant | Pain and swelling along midline of sacrum or cervical spine | Chemotherapy and resection |

from primitive (poorly differentiated) cells from the osteoblasts of the mesenchyme. This suggests that early osteoprogenitor cells with the ability for chondroblastic differentiation are affected in the development of osteosarcoma.[72]

Osteosarcoma grows rapidly and is locally destructive. It may be osteosclerotic (producing considerable neoplastic or tumor bone), or it may arise from more primitive cells and remain predominantly osteolytic, eroding the cortex of the metaphyseal region and resulting in pathologic fracture. As it continues to grow beyond the confines of the bone, the tumor lifts the periosteum, resulting in the formation of reactive bone in the angle between elevated periosteum and bone called the *Codman triangle* (see Fig. 26.3).

### Clinical Manifestations

Osteosarcoma seems to appear in bones undergoing an active growth phase and is often located in the metaphysis but does not cross the physis. The long bones such as the distal femur, proximal humerus, and proximal tibia have a relatively more active growth period than other bones, which makes them more vulnerable (Fig. 26.7).

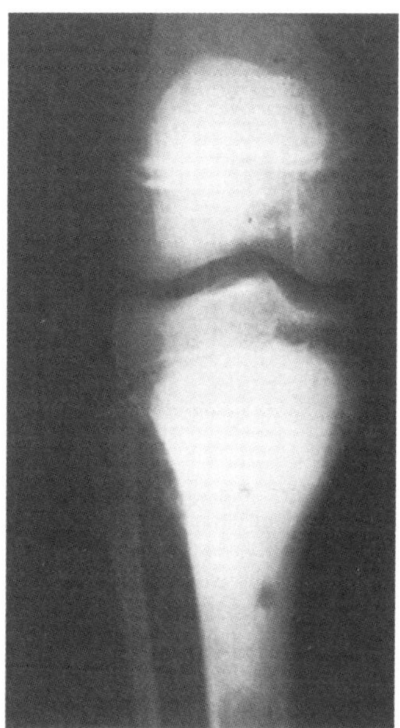

**Figure 26.7**

**Osteosarcoma.** An extremely sclerotic lesion in the proximal tibia of a child is noted, which is characteristic of an osteogenic sarcoma. (From Helms C: *Fundamentals of skeletal radiology: benign cystic lesions*, Philadelphia, 1989, Saunders.)

Pain near a joint line that has continued for several weeks to months is the presenting symptom. Joint pain and tenderness can be present as the lesion penetrates the cortex and invades the joint capsule, also spreading to other nearby structures (e.g., tendons, fat, muscles).

The pain increases, and swelling may develop in just a few weeks, accompanied by some limitation of motion. Systemic symptoms are rare, although occasional fever may occur. This aggressive neoplasm is very vascular, and the overlying skin is usually warm. Metastases are found in 20% to 25% of cases at the time of presentation, with most of these found in the lung.[39]

## MEDICAL MANAGEMENT

**DIAGNOSIS.** Dull, aching pain and night pain that persist over many months' duration and become more severe are common presentations that lead to the suspicion of a tumor. There may be a delay in care given to adolescents, as lower extremity pain at night may be interpreted to be normal growing pains. Localized swelling, tenderness, and limited joint motion may also be present. Plain radiographs will demonstrate dramatic changes and obvious tumor formation with poorly defined margins and a permeated or moth-eaten appearance in the lytic area.

CT scans and especially MRI are used to evaluate the extent of disease. In Fig. 26.8, plain films of a pelvis demonstrate minimal changes that could easily be dismissed as insignificant. CT scan, however, reveals a

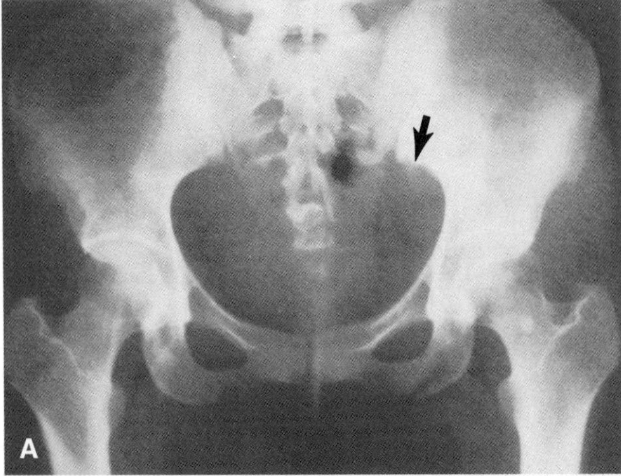


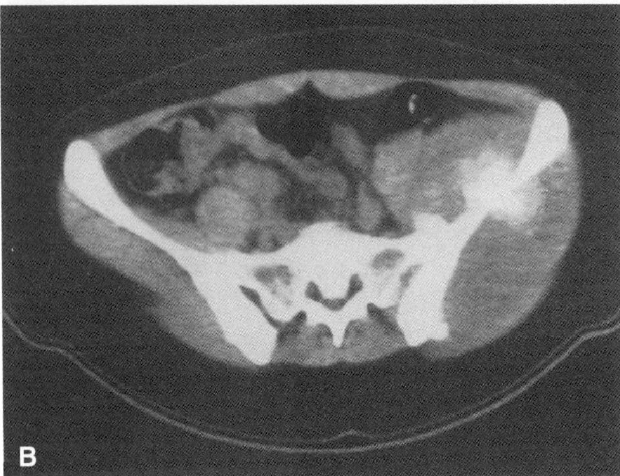


**Figure 26.8**

**Osteosarcoma.** (A) A subtle sclerotic lesion is seen in the left ilium adjacent to the sacroiliac joint that was initially diagnosed as osteitis condensans ilii, a benign entity. Because of persistent pain, the person returned for a follow-up visit, and a small amount of cortical destruction on the pelvic brim was noted *(arrow)*. (B) A computed tomography scan was performed, which showed a large tissue mass and new bone tumor around the ilium, which is characteristic of an osteogenic sarcoma. (From Helms C: *Fundamentals of skeletal radiology: benign cystic lesions*, Philadelphia, 1989, Saunders.)

large osteosarcoma involving the ilium. The development of positron emission tomography/CT imaging has allowed for better visualization and assessment of metabolic activity in a region and is used for monitoring treatment responses and surveillance to detect recurrence.[72]

A biopsy is performed to determine the histologic makeup of the lesion. The level of vascular endothelial growth factor at the time of diagnosis may be prognostic for the risk of metastasis and the 5-year survival rate for individuals with osteosarcomas.[69] Serum alkaline phosphatase level is often elevated, but this is not diagnostic.

TREATMENT. Many factors such as age, remaining growth, expected functional outcome, and prognosis are considered in making the best treatment choices for osteosarcoma. Treatment protocols will involve neoadjuvant chemotherapy treatments, followed by surgical resection of the involved bone and follow-up chemotherapy treatments. Chemotherapy that effectively creates necrosis of the tumor will slow the growth of the tumor and lessen the chance of metastases to other regions of the body leading to a greater chance of survival.[39] Limb amputation and joint fusion techniques may be needed for patients with advanced destruction of limb bone and connective tissues.

***Surgical Excision and Salvage.*** Surgical removal of the tumor with wide margins is the definitive treatment for an osteosarcoma. Some osteosarcomas result in limb amputation, but most are treated using limb salvage techniques to insure complete tumor removal followed by reconstruction of a functional extremity.[35] Limb salvage options include reconstruction using allograft bone and/or endoprosthesis and the use of tissue regeneration methods.

***Endoprosthesis.*** The use of a noninvasive expandable prosthesis is the preferred method for treating skeletally immature children and adolescents following limb salvage surgeries (Fig. 26.9). Prostheses allow better local tumor control and improved cosmesis, with the potential for equal limb length at skeletal maturity; however, more revisions may be required over time with this approach. An expandable metal rod prosthesis for pediatric osteosarcoma can be used to replace the bone and does not require repeated procedures to lengthen as the child's other leg grows. Painless electromagnetic rays are used to expand the rod slowly without compromise to the surrounding skin and muscle.

PROGNOSIS. The use of adjunctive (preoperative) chemotherapy with surgery has resulted in 5-year cure rates of 60% to 78% for local disease if there are no known metastases at the time of diagnosis. The expected 10-year survival rate is only 20% to 30% when there are clinically detectable metastases.[3]

Osteosarcoma survivors have received significant chemotherapy and have undergone substantial surgeries, which can have an impact on very long-term outcomes. Childhood osteosarcoma survivors reportedly do relatively well, considering their extensive treatment, but are at risk of experiencing chronic medical conditions, activity limitations, and adverse health status. Survivors warrant lifelong follow-up.[61] In older people, osteosarcoma may develop as a complication of Paget disease, in which case the prognosis is extremely grave.

SPECIAL IMPLICATIONS FOR THE THERAPIST 26.5

## *Osteosarcoma*

See previous discussion and Special Implications for the Therapist 26.1: Primary Tumors. Many survivors of cancer experience lasting, adverse effects caused by either their disease or its treatment. Physical therapy interventions can reverse or ameliorate the impairments (body function and structure) found in these individuals, improving their ability to carry out daily tasks and actions (activity) and to participate in life situations (participation). Measuring the efficacy of physical therapy interventions in each of these dimensions is challenging but essential for developing and delivering optimal care. An *International Classification*

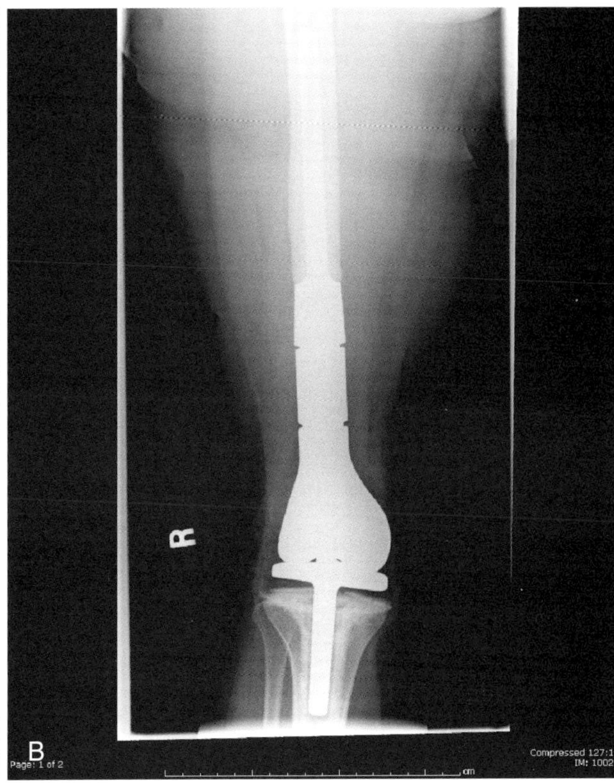


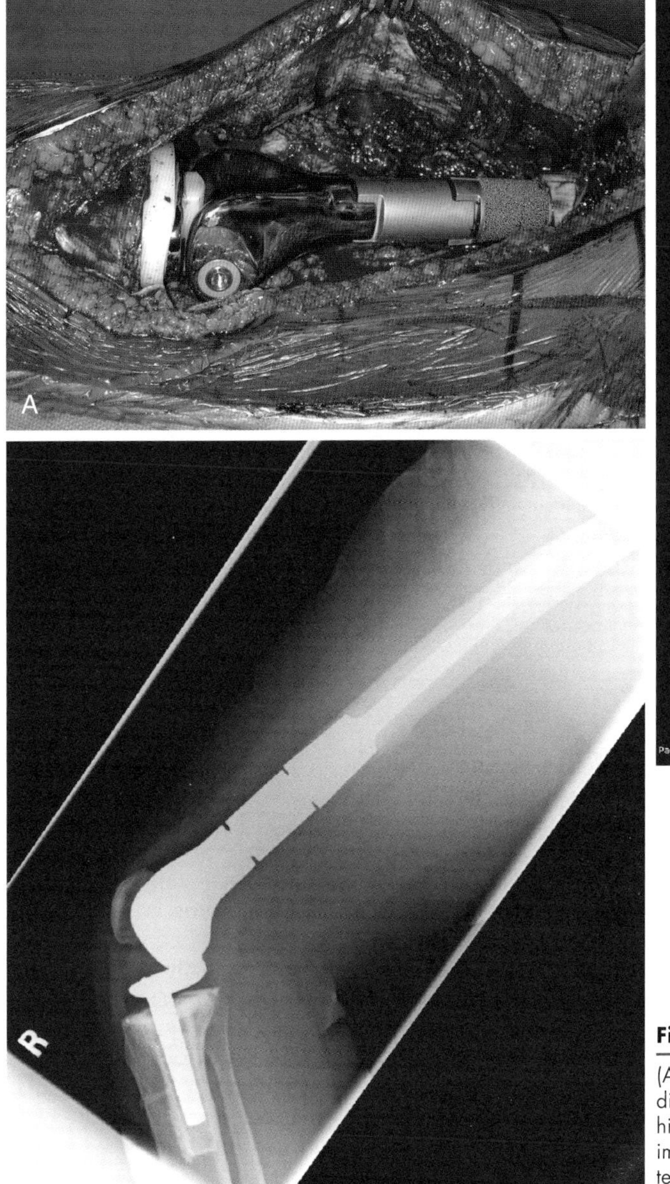


**Figure 26.9**

(A) Intraoperative photograph of a modular endoprosthesis for the distal femur. This prosthesis is cemented in place and has a rotating hinge knee design. The prosthetic stem is roughened near the femur implantation site to allow for tissue ingrowth. (B and C) Anteroposterior and lateral postoperative radiographs of the prosthesis shown above. (From Abeloff MD: *Abeloff's clinical oncology*, ed 4, Philadelphia, 2008, Churchill Livingstone.)

*of Functioning, Disability and Health* framework for the physical therapist's assessment in oncology rehabilitation is available.[32]

Malignant neoplasms usually necessitate aggressive intervention, and therefore rehabilitation is more intensive, prolonged, and individualized. Extensive surgery such as limb-sparing techniques has provided therapists with an opportunity to assist these clients in maximizing their function (Fig. 26.10). When musculoskeletal structures are involved, it is important to be aware of reduced tensile strength of malignant tissue compared with uninvolved bone tissue. Studies also show that ROM correlates with functional mobility and quality of life in individuals with lower extremity sarcoma after limb-sparing surgery. ROM exercises are an important component of a physical therapy program for children and adolescents with this condition.[53]

### Preoperative Assessment

People who have been diagnosed with cancer and are faced with the impending amputation of a leg find themselves in a state of shock and grief. Parents of children who are born with a lower limb difference experience similar emotions. Under these circumstances, it is difficult to talk openly with a surgeon about amputation and to meet with a prosthetist to discuss future prosthetic needs. The fact that the majority of these clients are children, teenagers, and young adults only increases the level of anxiety. Yet beneath the surface of these painful conversations are seeds of hope: amputation can save a person's life, preoperative consultations can help people make better decisions, and children who are fitted early with a prosthesis can lead very active lives. Knowing what the options are before surgery

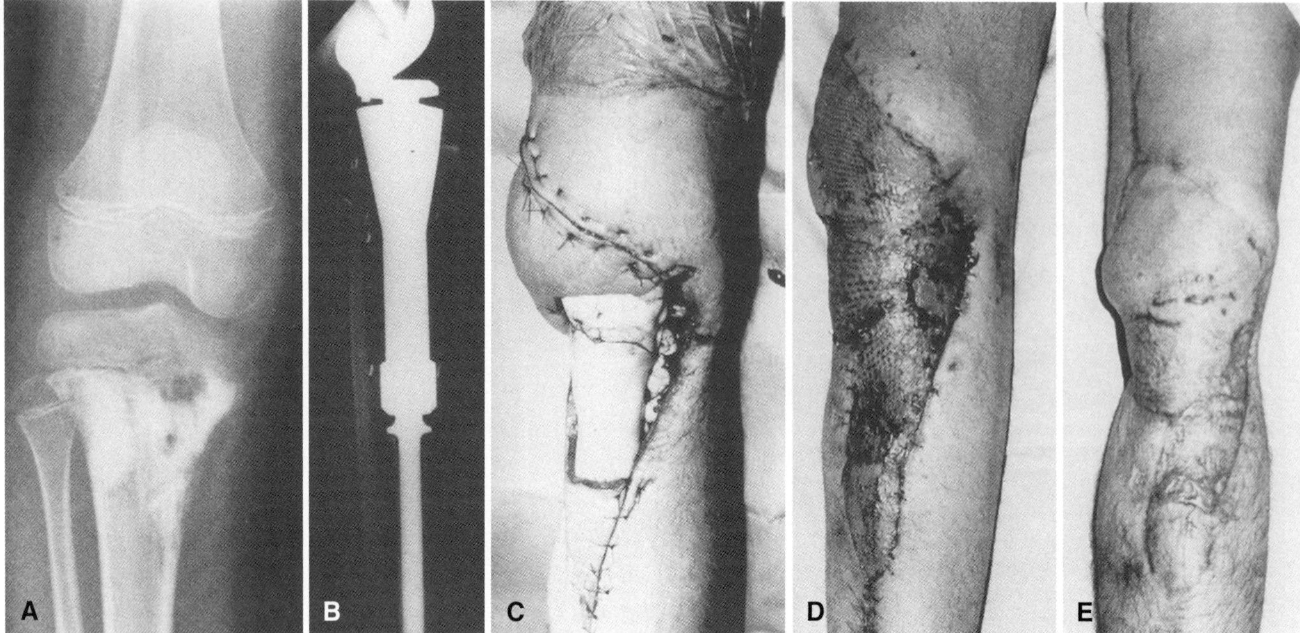


**Figure 26.10**

**Use of a free muscle transfer to salvage an infected massive prosthesis.** (A) Preoperative radiograph of a 9-year-old boy with an osteosarcoma. (B) After radical resection, an expandable prosthesis was inserted. (C) When infection occurred, with subsequent breakdown of the wound, the prosthesis was removed, and the area was widely débrided. A spacer of antibiotic-impregnated methacrylate was inserted. (D) Infection was controlled, and the knee was reconstructed with another prosthesis and a free latissimus transfer. (E) A satisfactory result was obtained, sparing the leg. (From Hausman M: Microvascular applications in limb-sparing tumor surgery. *Orthop Clin* 20:434, 1989.)

can enable individuals and their families to make the best choice for each specific situation.

### Postoperative Rehabilitation

Because these tumors are treated at regional medical centers, the initial phases of rehabilitation may be implemented by therapists with a great deal of experience working with clients with malignant neoplasms and those who have undergone various reconstructive surgical procedures. When the client returns home, a local therapist may be called on to continue the rehabilitation program. Communication with the therapist at the regional medical center to confirm the initial management plan, progression, and prognosis is recommended.

The Functional Mobility Assessment tool with reference values has been examined in clients with lower extremity sarcoma. Functional Mobility Assessment requires the individual to physically perform functional mobility tasks and provides a reliable and valid measure of objective functional outcome and may help therapists guide children and adolescents in returning to daily activities.[51,52]

## Chondrosarcoma

### Overview and Incidence

Chondrosarcoma is usually a relatively slow-growing malignant neoplasm that arises either spontaneously in previously normal bone or as the result of malignant change in a preexisting nonmalignant lesion, such as an osteochondroma or an enchondroma. The pelvic and shoulder girdles are common sites of tumor and related pain, as are the proximal and distal femur, proximal humerus, and ribs.

Chondrosarcoma is the second most common solid malignant tumor of bone in adults (after osteosarcoma, third after myeloma). Primary chondrosarcomas are more common, but their origin is idiopathic. Secondary tumors are those that arise from previously benign cartilaginous tumors or from a preexisting condition such as Paget disease. Men in their 40s to 60s are most likely to be affected by primary chondrosarcoma.[72]

### Pathogenesis

In general, chondrosarcomas develop from cells committed to cartilaginous differentiation. The neoplastic cartilaginous cells produce cartilage rather than the osteoid seen with osteosarcoma. Alterations of programmed cell death (apoptosis) may play a significant role in the pathogenesis of low- to intermediate-grade chondrosarcomas, whereas high-grade lesions most likely develop by means of a multistep mechanism involving multiple transforming genes and tumor suppressor genes.

The lesion can range from a slow-growing lesion to an aggressive malignancy capable of metastasizing to other organs. The metastatic potential of chondrosarcoma is less than for osteosarcoma. The majority of chondrosarcomas are grade I or II, which rarely metastasize. When metastasis occurs, it is via the hematogenous route to the lungs, other bones, or organs.[19]

Chondrosarcoma is classified by location of the lesion: central, peripheral, or juxtacortical. With *central chondrosarcoma,* the neoplastic tissue is compressed inside the bone, and areas of necrosis, cystic change, and

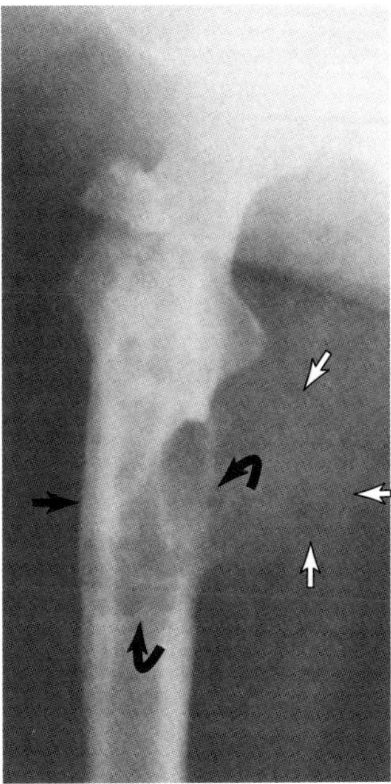

**Figure 26.11**

Characteristic radiographic features of chondrosarcoma include thickening of the cortex *(black arrow)*, destruction of the medullary and cortical bone *(curved arrows)*, and soft tissue mass *(white arrows)*. Note the characteristic punctate calcifications in the proximal part of the tumor. (From Greenspan A: Tumors of cartilage origin. *Orthop Clin* 20:359, 1989.)

hemorrhage are common. *Peripheral chondrosarcoma* arises outside the bone and then invades the bone. A *juxtacortical chondrosarcoma* is thought to be periosteal (affecting the periosteum) or parosteal (affecting the outer surface of the periosteum) in origin. Chondrosarcomas can be graded based on their microscopic appearance. The presence of a chondroid matrix, extent of necrosis, and type of cells are some of the grading standards used.

### Clinical Manifestations

Pain is the most common presenting symptom, although as this is a slow-growing tumor, in some cases the tumor can exist for years without symptoms. Tumors may affect joint structures and surrounding soft tissues, creating symptoms secondary to a space-occupying lesion.

### MEDICAL MANAGEMENT

DIAGNOSIS. On radiograph, the tumor often shows an expansile lesion in the diaphysis of long bones with cortical thickening and destruction of the medullary bone (Fig. 26.11). The appearance is variable depending on the rate of growth and the host bone response. Biopsy is important not only for accurate diagnosis but also for guiding treatment. Chondrosarcoma can develop on the surface of bone or be multicentric, involving several bones.

TREATMENT. Treatment of chondrosarcoma is surgical, with complete tumor removal. Wide resections or limb-sparing procedures are often required, and internal fixation after tumor removal to prevent fracture may be recommended. Because of the slow-growing nature of this malignancy, radiation therapy and chemotherapy have limited effectiveness.[72]

PROGNOSIS. The prognosis is dependent on the aggressiveness and stage of the lesion. For example, a grade I lesion is unlikely to metastasize, and if it is completely resected, a good prognosis follows, with 80% to 90% chance of survival. A grade III lesion is much more likely to metastasize. Undifferentiated lesions found in the pelvis or any bone where complete resection is difficult have a poorer prognosis.[4] Secondary chondrosarcomas are usually of a low-grade malignancy and have a good prognosis with adequate intervention; metastasis is rare.[19]

## Ewing Sarcoma

### Overview and Incidence

Ewing sarcoma is a malignant nonosteogenic primary tumor that can arise in bone or soft tissue. It is the third most common primary malignant bone tumor of children, adolescents, and young adults and the fourth most common overall, although it accounts for only approximately 3% of all pediatric malignancies.[48] Most tumors of this type (80%) occur in people younger than 20 years of age. The pelvis and lower extremity are the most common sites. In contrast to many tumors, no predilection for a certain part of the bone is evident.

SPECIAL IMPLICATIONS FOR THE THERAPIST 26.6

### *Chondrosarcoma*

Recovery and restrictions may vary depending on the size and location of the tumor and postoperative condition (once the tumor and surrounding bone have been removed). The postoperative protocol may vary from institution to institution and surgeon to surgeon. Common precautions include no driving for 6 weeks, no lifting for 3 months, and no work (depending on type of occupation) for 3 months. Shoulder motion is restricted at first to below 90° when the upper extremity is affected. Use of the hand below the elbow may be allowed for writing and other functional activities in the first few days to week. Food and meal preparation is not allowed until the arm can be moved above 90°.

More complex chondrosarcomas with wide surgical excision may require longer recovery time because of reconstruction, allografts, hardware, or prosthetic implants. Rehabilitation may be further compromised by adjunct therapy such as chemotherapy and/or radiotherapy. The therapist is advised to read the surgical report and consult with the surgeon when formulating a specific plan of care for each individual.

### Risk Factors, Etiologic Factors, and Pathogenesis

Based on different levels of scientific evidence, the main risk factors related to Ewing sarcoma include Caucasian race, parental occupation (exposure to pesticides, herbicides, fertilizers), and parental smoking.[25] Cytogenetic studies show that 95% of these tumors are derived from a specific genetic translocation between chromosomes 11 and 22, although the molecular oncogenesis remains unknown.[63]

Ewing sarcoma is composed of sheets of small, uniformly round cells of neuroectodermal origin. The tumor is characterized by cells with low differentiation. These morphologic

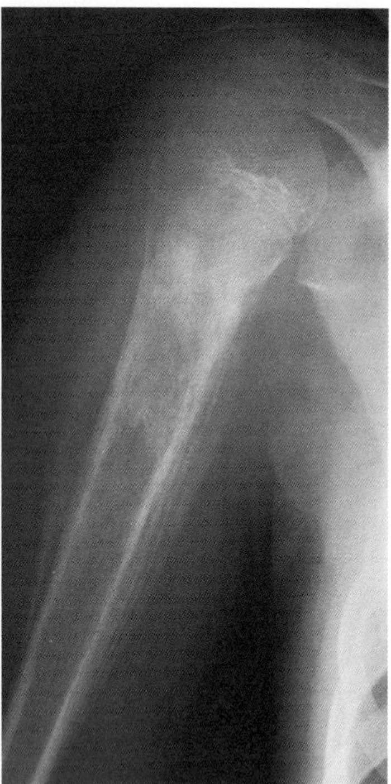

**Figure 26.12**

**Ewing sarcoma of the humerus.** Bone destruction is seen in the proximal metadiaphysis. The cortex is infiltrated, and a multilaminar periosteal reaction with an onion-skin appearance is present medially; Codman triangles are present on the lateral aspect. (From Grainger RG, Allison D: *Grainger and Allison's diagnostic radiology: a textbook of medical imaging,* ed 4, Philadelphia, 2001, Churchill Livingstone.)

features are characteristic enough to serve as useful diagnostic markers. The most common sites for a primary tumor are the lower extremities and the pelvis, with extraosseous tumors primarily starting in the trunk and extremities.[63,9]

The tumor is soft, sometimes viscous, with hemorrhagic necrosis caused by the rapid tumor growth outpacing its blood supply. The cortical bone is affected through the haversian canals. The medullary cavity is affected, and infiltration of the bone marrow can progress extensively without radiographic evidence of bone destruction. When the tumor perforates the cortex of the bone shaft and elevates the periosteum, the consequent reactive bone formation causes layered calcification referred to as an onion-skin appearance seen radiographically (Fig. 26.12). T2-weighted magnetic resonance images will demonstrate high signal intensity for the extent of the tumor within bone and surrounding soft tissues.[63,9]

## Clinical Manifestations

As with other malignant bone tumors, local bone pain is the most common presenting symptom after an injury (e.g., sports-related injury), a factor that sometimes delays diagnosis. Ewing sarcoma presents most often in the long (tubular) bones (e.g., femur, tibia, fibula, humerus) and the pelvis. Less often, the ribs, scapula, vertebrae, feet, and craniofacial bones are involved.

Swelling occurs in approximately 70% of all cases, and both pain and swelling are usually progressive. The pain may be intermittent, which also delays diagnosis. There may be a palpable or observable mass. Pathologic fractures occur at the site of the tumor in long bones in 5% to 10% of cases. In young children, flu-like symptoms including a low-grade fever may be present, which may lead to the mistaken diagnosis of osteomyelitis.[9]

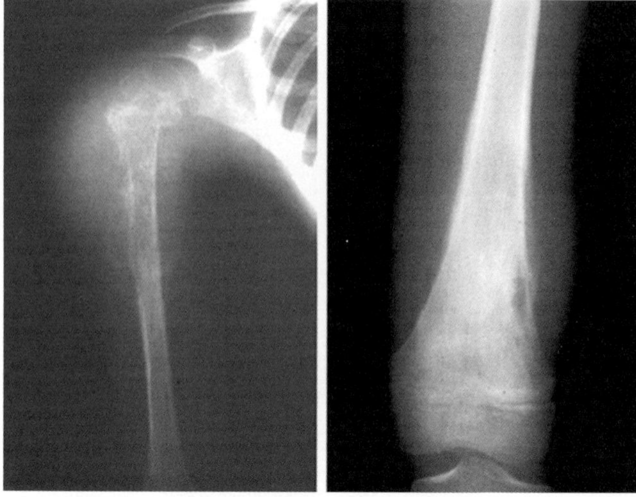

**Figure 26.13**

**Ewing sarcoma.** Radiographs of the left humerus *(left)* and right distal femur *(right)* show destructive permeative lesions with soft tissue extension. (From Weidner N: *Modern surgical pathology*, ed 2, Philadelphia, 2009, Saunders.)

Ewing sarcoma frequently metastasizes to other bones, especially late in the course of the disease.

## MEDICAL MANAGEMENT

**DIAGNOSIS.** Anyone suspected to have Ewing sarcoma is staged for both local and metastatic disease. Radiographs show an obvious lytic process with a moth-eaten appearance involving a diffuse area of bone and soft tissue extension (Fig. 26.13). As mentioned, an onion-skin formation may be seen, which is due to layers of reactive bone (see Fig. 26.12). On radiographs, the appearance may not differentiate this lesion from osteomyelitis or osteosarcoma.[63,55]

CT, MRI, and bone scans can help diagnose and define the extent of the tumor. MRI is more sensitive than CT scan in assessing soft tissue involvement and bone marrow spread. MRI or CT scan is repeated after several cycles of chemotherapy to better assess the response to chemotherapy and help plan further treatment of the local site with radiation or surgery. An elevated erythrocyte sedimentation rate may be noted but is not diagnostic.

Metastatic disease is evaluated at the time of presentation with chest x-ray or chest CT scan looking for pulmonary metastases. Bone scan to detect bone metastases, bone marrow aspirate at a site far from the local tumor site, and tumor biopsy are used to assess the spread of the disease and help with staging and treatment planning.

**TREATMENT.** The treatment plan is individualized based on the stage and resectability of the primary tumor. Multimodal treatment can include multiagent chemotherapy, radiotherapy, immunotherapy or biotherapy, embolization, and surgery.[9,30]

Presurgical chemotherapy and radiation therapy can result in a minimally sized tumor, which will result in a less invasive surgical procedure and a better chance of survival. Local tumors are very responsive to high-dose radiation. Effective repeated cycles of combination chemotherapy over a period of 6 months to 1 year have been developed to eradicate distant metastases.

Surgery in the treatment of primary Ewing sarcoma can result in amputation, but the development of limb-sparing techniques has reduced amputations considerably. The choice of method is individualized based on many factors including age; the location and extent of the tumor; preferences of the client or, in the case of a child, the family; the availability of surgical facilities and expertise; and the cost of the procedure.

New targets for treatment have focused on the oncogene associated with Ewing sarcoma in children and factors that control the microenvironment of the tumor's blood supply and ability to resist detection by the immune system.[30]

**PROGNOSIS.** Although Ewing sarcoma is extremely malignant, with a high frequency of both metastatic spread and local recurrence, the prognosis for clients with this tumor is improving steadily with improved treatment. The 5-year survival rate is as high as 80% if metastasis has not occurred at the time of diagnosis and treatment. Delay between symptom onset and diagnosis is common and a negative prognostic factor with a survival rate of less than 30% for individuals with metastatic disease.[48]

Long-term survival is determined by the presence or absence of metastasis and the site and extent of the local tumor. Smaller tumors at an early stage of development are easier to treat and have a low risk for developing metastasis. Individuals with isolated pulmonary metastasis have a greater chance of survival, whereas more than four metastatic nodules is a poor prognostic indicator. Recurrence of a sarcoma or other cancer-related diseases is associated with a poor prognosis.[30] People with Ewing sarcoma of distal sites such as the bones of the hands and feet have a much better prognosis than people with lesions in central sites such as the pelvis and sacrum. The presence of uncommon sites of metastasis confers a worse prognosis. With the increase in long-term survival rates from improved treatment protocols, the therapist should be aware of the secondary effects of radiation and chemotherapy and of the signs of recurrence of a sarcoma and occult metastasis.[50]

## Chordoma

### Overview and Incidence

Chordomas develop from the remnants of the primitive notochord along the vertebral column and primarily begin in the sacrococcygeal or sphenooccipital regions. Chordomas are usually slow-growing but locally aggressive malignant neoplasms and account for 1% to 4% of all malignant bone tumors, primarily affecting older adults.[96]

Chordomas do not have a capsule and tend to infiltrate into neighboring soft tissues. Metastases can occur to the liver, lungs, lymph nodes, peritoneum, skin, heart, brain, and distant regions of the spine but often remain asymptomatic and are discovered only on postmortem examination. Metastases occur most often when there is local recurrence of the primary tumor.[56]

**SPECIAL IMPLICATIONS FOR THE THERAPIST 26.7**

*Ewing Sarcoma*

As with osteosarcoma, initial intervention is aggressive, involving chemotherapy and/or radiation therapy, surgical resection, limb salvage procedures, and sometimes amputation. After that, rehabilitation becomes the focus, including recovery of function, social reintegration, and return to work.[90]

Analysis of rehabilitation suggests that clients with cemented modular oncologic endoprostheses recover normal function faster than individuals treated using other procedures. The level of functional performance may differ depending on the treatment plan chosen. For example, sparing the extremity may lead to greater functional impairment in people compared with some people undergoing amputation who are provided with a modern prosthesis.

Some of the newer amputation surgeries and reconstructive techniques provide greater function but possibly less cosmetically acceptable results for some people. Some clients complete the entire course of rehabilitation but eventually decide that an amputation will provide greater functionality.

### Clinical Manifestations

Most chordomas arise in the midline of the body, involving the clivus (central skull base) in half of cases. One-third of all chordomas occur in the sacrum and account for half of all sacral tumors, with the remaining found in the cervical and lumbar spine. The high cervical region, especially C2, is affected most often. Clival chordomas are frequently midline lesions whose posterior growth may breach the dura and invaginate the brainstem.[74]

Clinical manifestations based on the biologic behavior of chordoma appear to differ from person to person. The most common presenting symptom is pain; generally, symptoms depend on the location of the tumor. Clival chordomas may cause headaches, visual disturbances, dysphagia, muscle weakness, and even hemiparesis. People with sacral tumors often present with nonspecific symptoms such as low back pain, sacrococcygeal pain, or referred buttock or leg (sciatica) pain.[32]

Night pain or pain at rest that is not relieved by analgesics is a red flag finding. Other symptoms include bowel and/or bladder dysfunction, gait disturbances, and motor impairment.

### MEDICAL MANAGEMENT

**TREATMENT.** The mainstay of treatment for chordoma is aggressive surgical resection preceded by chemotherapy to stabilize the tumor. Complete resection of the tumor is not always possible, especially when it is located in the high cervical region. Adjuvant therapy (radiation and/or chemotherapy) may be administered before and/or after surgery. Recurrence is seen, often requiring subsequent treatment. Metastases require resection and chemotherapy unless the metastases are too extensive for systemic treatment.[56,92]

**PROGNOSIS.** Although chordoma is a relatively slow-growing tumor, it has a high incidence of local recurrence and a poor long-term prognosis. Cancer recurrence often necessitates repeat surgical procedures with risk for complications. The 5-year survival rate for a chordoma has been estimated to be 50%. Metastases are becoming more common as people with chordomas live longer as a result of more aggressive surgical and adjuvant treatments.[92]

## Giant Cell Tumor

### Overview and incidence

Giant cell tumor of bone (also known as giant cell myeloma) is a distinct, locally aggressive neoplasm that accounts for approximately 5% of all primary bone tumors. Although classically considered benign, these tumors are now considered a low-grade (malignant) sarcoma because of their high rate of recurrence and potential for malignant transformation with metastases to the lungs.[82]

The tumor most frequently involves the epiphyseal ends of long tubular bones in skeletally mature adults between 20 and 55 years of age, with a peak age incidence in the third decade of life. Of tumors, 60% occur around the knee; 10% to 12% involve the distal radius. The bones of the hand and wrist are rarely affected.[42] Giant cell tumors are the second most frequent primary tumor involving bone in the sacrum; this type of tumor is extremely rare in the vertebrae.

### Etiology and Pathogenesis

The etiology of giant cell tumors is unknown. The tumor is classified based on its local aggressiveness and risk for local recurrence. Pathologic examination of the neoplasm reveals a tumor that is soft, friable (easily breaks apart), fleshy, and red-brown with yellow areas. The tumor usually extends to, but not into, the articular cartilage. Destruction of the bone cortex with expansion into soft tissue can occur (Fig. 26.14). Hemorrhage, cyst formation, and necrosis can be seen on gross pathology. Hemorrhage and necrosis (often accompanied by pathologic fracture) occur often in the weight-bearing bones. The tumors can be locally invasive (into bone and soft tissue) with extensive bone destruction and cortical expansion.[82] Pulmonary metastases referred to as benign pulmonary implants occur in 1% of cases.

### Clinical Manifestations

Symptoms depend on the location, but pain on weight bearing with pathologic fracture may be the presenting clinical feature when tumors occur in the weight-bearing bones. People with sacral tumors may present with localized pain in the low back radiating to one or both of the legs. Abdominal discomfort and bowel and bladder symptoms may be present.

### MEDICAL MANAGEMENT

Diagnosis is by radiographs and confirmed by histologic assessment, with findings typical of this particular type of tumor observed. Treatment is with surgical excision; bone grafting to fill the cavity and further reconstruction may be needed.[80] Radiation or chemotherapy may be used in cases of surgically inaccessible or incompletely resectable lesions. The use of adjuvant treatment such as chemotherapy and radiotherapy is debated.

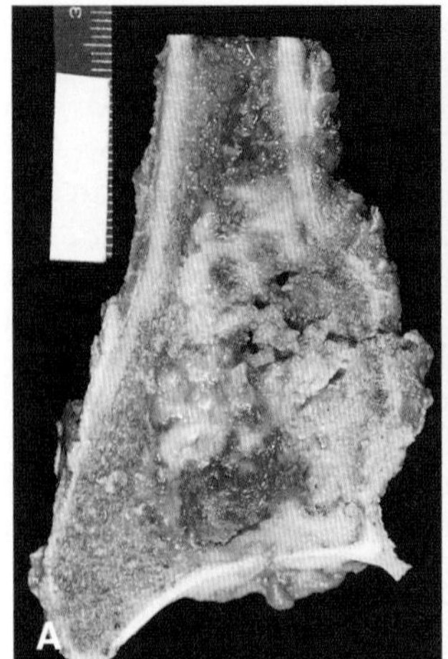


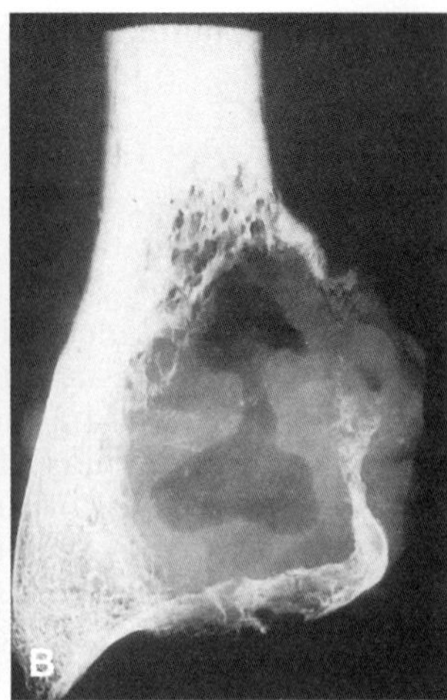


**Figure 26.14**

**Giant cell tumor.** Gross morphologic features of giant cell tumor. (A) Bisected distal end of radius with well-demarcated tumor mass expanding bone contour. Tumor tissue is red-brown with yellow septations. (B) Radiographic presentation of tumor showing focal destruction of cortex. (From Dorfman HD, Czerniak B: *Bone tumors*, St. Louis, 1998, Mosby.)

# MULTIPLE MYELOMA

Multiple myeloma is a hematopoietic neoplasm involving bone marrow. It is a primary bone cancer with plasma cell proliferation and is one of a group of disorders called *plasma cell dyscrasias*.

Skeletal involvement is most common in the spine, pelvis, and skull because bone marrow is found in high concentrations in these structures. Deep bone pain is often present clinically, and radiographs may demonstrate osteopenia and punched-out areas of bone with sclerotic borders (in flat bones) (Fig. 26.15).[65]

# PRIMARY SOFT TISSUE TUMORS

## Benign Soft Tissue Tumors

Common benign soft tissue tumors include lipoma, ganglia, popliteal cyst (Baker cyst), nerve sheath tumor (neurofibroma and schwannoma), and desmoid tumors.

*Lipoma* is the most common soft tissue tumor, generally occurring in middle-aged and older adults and composed of mature fat cells. These tumors are usually superficially located in the subcutaneous tissue and remain asymptomatic. Occasionally a lipoma of the breast will grow large enough to cause tenderness and block lymphatic drainage, requiring removal. Even without surgical excision, lipomas are unlikely to ever undergo malignant transformation, but recurrence is possible if the lesion, including microscopic cells, is not completely removed.

*Ganglion cysts* arise from a joint capsule or tendon sheath, usually on the dorsal aspect of the wrist but sometimes on the volar aspect of the wrist or on the lower extremity. Pain or tenderness may or may not be present; pressure on a nerve can cause focal neurologic symptoms.

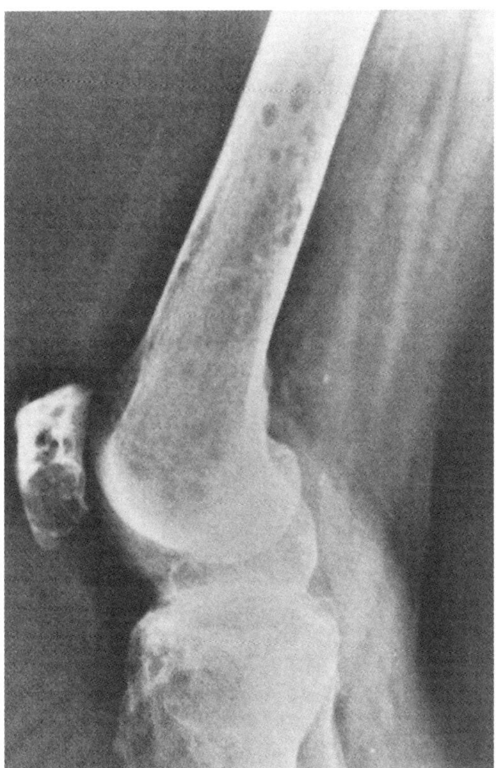

**Figure 26.15**

**Multiple myeloma.** Small lucencies in the distal femur, proximal tibia, and patella. (From Ghelman B: Radiology of bone tumors. *Orthop Clin* 20:307, 1989.)

*Popliteal cyst,* more commonly referred to as a *Baker cyst,* is a subtype of ganglion that often communicates with a joint space. A Baker cyst is most often palpated behind the knee in older adults with osteoarthritis. Rupture of the cyst or hemorrhage from the joint into the cyst causes episodes of severe pain.[36] Swelling distal to the lesion (calf and foot) may also occur.

*Nerve sheath tumor* is a tumor of the nerve sheath arising in a peripheral nerve and growing concentrically from the center of the nerve. Neurofibromas infiltrate the nerve and splay apart the individual nerve fibers. They are usually superficially located, painless, and benign but can sometimes degenerate into cancer.

*Neurofibromas* can occur as a single lesion or in greater numbers as part of a collection of symptoms in association with von Recklinghausen disease (neurofibromatosis) and schwannomas. Neurofibromas contain cells and features of Schwann cells but also contain fibroblasts and perineural cells. Both neurofibromas and schwannomas are benign, grow slowly, and can be cured surgically.[38]

*Schwannomas* and neurofibromas arise from the coverings of peripheral and cranial nerves. Schwannomas arise from Schwann cells as the name suggests. Schwannoma is a rare tumor of the sheath or lining around the peripheral nerves. It starts in the Schwann cells, which is how it gets its name. Schwann cells help form the cover around the nerves called the myelin sheath. Schwannomas can be benign or malignant. The malignant type is called *neurosarcoma* or *neurogenic sarcoma.*

In the benign form, growth is slow and painless. The tumor stays on the outside of the nerve. The benign form does not spread to other areas and is not likely to cause death. However, if it grows large enough to put pressure on the nerve, pain, numbness, and paralysis can occur.

Schwannomas can arise from Schwann cells covering the vestibular portion of cranial nerve VIII, causing benign acoustic neurinomas. Although the tumors grow slowly and are considered benign, they can compress cranial nerve VIII, resulting in hearing loss and tinnitus. Vestibular function is lost but slowly enough that the body compensates; for this reason, vertigo is uncommon with acoustic neuromas. Large tumors can compress the cerebellum and brainstem, resulting in ataxia and hydrocephalus. The affected individual may also experience facial paralysis if the trigeminal nerve is compressed.[18]

Schwannomas can also occur as intradural extramedullary tumors, most often in individuals with neurofibromatosis. Multiple schwannomas in this population group are common. The tumors often extend through the intervertebral foramen into the abdomen or thoracic cavity. Compression causes local or radicular pain and may progress to include symptoms of spinal cord compression (e.g., motor weakness, sensory disturbances, autonomic changes). As with all benign schwannomas, surgical resection is curative.

## Malignant Soft Tissue Tumors

### Overview and Incidence

Soft tissue sarcomas are a heterogeneous group of rare tumors that arise predominantly from the embryonic mesoderm and manifest most often as an asymptomatic mass. They can occur anywhere in the body, but most originate in the extremities (59%), trunk (19%), retroperitoneum (15%), or head and neck (9%).[86] Sarcomas account for 1% of all newly diagnosed adult cancers. The incidence is much higher in children, constituting 15% of annual pediatric malignancies.[77]

**Types of Soft Tissue Sarcomas.** More than 50 histologic types of soft tissue sarcoma have been identified. The most common are malignant fibrous histiocytoma, leiomyosarcoma, liposarcoma, synovial sarcoma, and malignant peripheral nerve sheath tumors. Rhabdomyosarcoma is the most common soft tissue sarcoma of childhood (Table 26.4).[20]

*Malignant schwannoma,* also known as *neurosarcoma* or *neurogenic sarcoma,* is a rare nerve sheath tumor of the peripheral nerves arising from Schwann cells or within existing neurofibromas. They can occur anywhere in the body but are often located on the flexor surface of the extremities. They are usually slow growing and painless and are often present for years. When pressure is placed on the involved nerve, pain, paresthesia, and paralysis may occur.

*Rhabdomyosarcomas* constitute more than half of all soft tissue sarcomas in children younger than 15 years of age. Occurrence in adults is possible but relatively rare. Eighty percent of affected individuals are white. Boys are affected slightly more than girls; approximately 250 children in the United States are diagnosed each year with rhabdomyosarcoma.[24]

Table 26.4 Soft Tissue Sarcoma[a]

| Tumor | Age | Sex Ratio | Common Sites |
|---|---|---|---|
| Malignant fibrous histiocytoma | 50–70 years | 3:1 (M/F) | Leg, thigh, retroperitoneum; extremities (lower > upper) |
| Liposarcoma | 40–60 years | 1:1 | Any site of adipose tissue; extremity, trunk, retroperitoneum, breast |
| Rhabdomyosarcoma | Children <15 years 2 peaks: 2–6 years and 15–19 years | 1.4:1 (M/F) | Any site; four main areas: head and neck, genitourinary (bladder, prostate, testes), extremities, trunk |
| Leiomyosarcoma | 50–70 years | Women > men | Skin, deep soft tissues of the extremities, retroperitoneum, uterus |
| Malignant schwannoma | 20–50 years; can occur at any age | Men > women | Peripheral nerves, any site; flexor surface extremities |
| Synovial sarcoma | Young adult, 15–40 years | Men > women | Extremity, knee (popliteal area), feet, hands, forearm |
| Epithelioid sarcoma (rare) | Young adult | Men > women | Extensor surface of extremities, tendon sheath, joint capsule (shoulder), hands, feet |
| Clear cell sarcoma (rare) | Young adult | Women > men | Deep to dermis; tendon, aponeuroses; spinal nerve root (rare) |
| Fibrosarcoma (rare) | 35–55 years | Men > women | Fibrous connective tissue (thigh, posterior knee); scars, subcutaneous fibrous tissue, deep connective tissue, around tendons or nerve sheaths, ligaments, muscle fascia; can occur as bone tumors (periosteum) |

[a]Listed in approximate descending order of prevalence. Most soft tissue sarcomas are rare; some (as labeled) are extremely rare.
*F*, Female; *M*, male.
Data from Pisters PWT: Soft tissue sarcomas, *Cancer management*, ed 14, CancerNetwork, 2011. Available online at: http://www.cancernetwork.com/cancer-management/soft tissue-sarcomas/article/10165/1802713; Zhang PJ: *Essentials in bone and soft tissue pathology*, New York, 2010, Springer; Fletcher C: *Pathology and genetics of tumours of soft tissue and bone*, ed 4, Geneva, 2013, World Health Organization.

Rhabdomyosarcoma is a malignancy of striated muscle but can occur sporadically at any site in the body (e.g., bladder, prostate, head and neck, limbs, testes, muscle), and the cause is unknown. Symptoms are site dependent, but the tumor manifests as a painless mass in the soft tissues. About one-third of all people with rhabdomyosarcoma have readily resectable tumors, one-half do not, and in about half of all cases, regional lymphatic spread at diagnosis is evident, with a much less favorable prognosis. Diagnosis is often delayed, as lesions are frequently attributed to sports-related trauma.[24]

Other sites of metastases include the lungs, bone, and bone marrow. Tumors are aggressive and must be excised whenever possible. If tumors are too large to remove surgically, preoperative chemotherapy is used first to shrink the tumor. This allows for the possibility of complete resection and possibly a lower dose of radiation to achieve local control.

Other common soft tissue sarcomas include malignant fibrous histiocytoma, liposarcoma, synovial sarcoma, epithelioid sarcoma, and clear cell sarcoma. *Malignant fibrous histiocytoma* is now recognized as the most common (although still occurring rarely) soft tissue sarcoma in adults, primarily affecting men 50 to 70 years old. Malignant fibrous histiocytoma occurs as a deep-seated mass that typically enlarges to 5 cm or more by the time of diagnosis and is usually located on the leg, especially the thigh.

*Liposarcoma* is a soft tissue malignancy with a peak incidence between 40 and 60 years of age. These are slow-growing lesions that can achieve a large size (10 to 15 cm), usually located in the thigh but occasionally retroperitoneally, causing pain and weight loss. *Synovial sarcoma* occurs most often in a young adult as a slow-growing mass of the extremities, often located near the knee. These lesions are painful and tender to palpation and often present similarly to a Baker cyst or ganglion. Reclassification of this sarcoma will eventually reflect the fact that the synovium is not involved in this type of sarcoma.[22]

*Epithelioid sarcoma,* a small, firm, slow-growing mass, typically occurs in young adults on the extensor surface of an extremity but can also occur on the shoulder. These can develop deep enough to be undetectable on physical examination. Epithelioid sarcoma can look like a rheumatoid nodule, ganglion, or draining abscess and is often confused with a benign lesion.[6]

*Clear cell sarcoma* arises deep to the dermis, has a uniform growth pattern, and is often located on tendons or aponeuroses. In rare cases, this type of tumor can also originate in the spinal nerve roots with dissemination to the vertebral bodies, resulting in cauda equina. In approximately 20% of individuals, the tumor has a dark appearance resulting from production of melanin, and it is often confused with benign soft tissue tumors.[21]

## Etiology and Risk Factors

Most soft tissue sarcomas will develop without an identifiable cause. Specific inherited genetic alterations are primarily associated with an increased risk of soft tissue sarcomas. Distinct chromosomal translocations that code for oncoproteins are associated with certain histiologic subtypes of soft tissue sarcomas.[20] Risk factors for soft tissue sarcomas include radiation therapy for cancer of the breast, cervix, testes, or lymphatic system with a mean latency period of approximately 10 years. Other risk factors include occupational exposure to chemicals including herbicides and wood preservatives. Chronic lymphedema following axillary dissection is an additional risk factor for the development of lymphangiosarcoma.[20]

### Pathogenesis

All sarcomas share a mesodermal cellular origin, but research has not been able to completely identify the pathogenesis involved. Sarcomas probably do not originate from normal tissue but arise from aberrant differentiated and proliferative malignant mesenchymal cell formations. Some genetic origins have been specifically identified for individual sarcoma types. Many sarcoma-linked oncogenes appear to be triggered by viruses; sequencing of these viruses may eventually allow for the development of specific antibodies against oncogenic activation.[20]

### Clinical Manifestations

Soft tissue sarcomas manifest most often as painless, asymptomatic masses. They can grow quite large before being observed but do not usually produce pain when compressing surrounding structures. Metastasis occurs primarily hematogenously, with lymph node dissemination in rare cases.[79]

## MEDICAL MANAGEMENT

DIAGNOSIS. Diagnostic imaging, fine-needle aspiration, biopsy, and clinical studies are the mainstay of diagnosis. X-rays are used to look for lung metastases; CT scans and contrast-enhanced techniques provide details of high-grade lesions and large tumors and assess the extent of tumor burden and proximity to vital structures. MRI is the preferred imaging modality for sarcomas of the extremities.[79,58]

Staging of soft tissue sarcomas follows the AJCC method of staging based on anatomic location (depth), grade, size of the tumor, and presence of distant or nodal metastases (nodal status). Metastases occur to the lungs first, but also to the bone, brain, and liver. Intracompartmental or extracompartmental extension of extremity sarcomas is important for surgical decision making and planning.

TREATMENT. Treatments are based on the type of tumor, stage, and location. Surgery is the primary treatment for tumors that are small and well contained. Surgical excision with clear margins is combined with radiation or chemotherapy to attain good local control of most tumors. The ongoing challenge is to prevent metastasis to surrounding and systemic tissues. Low survival rates remain a significant problem, especially for individuals who have sarcomas at sites other than the extremities. High-grade sarcomas may result in amputation if surgical excision methods cannot conserve enough tissue to allow for limb-sparing techniques.[26]

Chemotherapies are effective only for certain histologic subtypes of sarcomas. The adverse toxic side effects in individuals who do not respond to chemotherapy negate the routine use of this form of treatment. Many studies have now shown that chemotherapy does not improve the chance for a disease-free status and overall survival in people with soft tissue sarcomas.[20,79]

PROGNOSIS. The overall 5-year survival rate for soft tissue sarcomas of all stages remains about 60% to 80%. Death from recurrence and metastatic complications occurs within 2 to 3 years of the initial diagnosis in 80% of cases. Despite improvements in local control rates, individuals with high-risk soft tissue sarcomas have poor long-term results. There is some evidence that individuals who had limb-sparing surgery display superior functional outcomes over those who have amputations.[79] Pain and perceiving that the cancer negatively influenced opportunities have been associated with poor outcomes.[89]

Advanced, metastatic sarcomas are always incurable; management is palliative. Individuals with leiomyosarcomas, clear cell sarcomas, and malignant fibrous histiocytomas may have a poorer survival rate compared with individuals who have fibrosarcomas, liposarcomas, and neurofibrosarcomas.[20]

Current 5-year survival in rhabdomyosarcoma is 60% to 80% in cases without metastasis but remains less than 30% in cases with metastasis. Over the last 30 years, the prognosis for children with rhabdomyosarcoma has improved dramatically with the use of multiagent chemotherapy, aggressive surgery for local disease, and more precise delivery of radiation therapy. Prognosis depends on the type of gross residual tumor (histology), location of the tumor, and presence and number of metastases at the time of diagnosis. Age and completeness of resection are additional prognostic factors.[24,71]

## Cartilaginous Tumors

Many tumors of cartilaginous origin can occur. Three of the more common cartilaginous tumors are enchondroma, osteochondroma, and chondrosarcoma. Cartilaginous tumors involving some parts of the skeleton (e.g., small bones of the hands and feet) are almost always benign, whereas cartilaginous lesions of the ribs, sternum, and flat bones such as the pelvis and scapula are more likely to be aggressive.[15]

### Benign Cartilaginous Tumors

#### ENCHONDROMA

***Overview and Incidence.*** Enchondroma is a common, benign tumor arising from residual islands of cartilage in the metaphysis of bones (Fig. 26.16). The tubular bones of the hands and feet (phalanges, metacarpals, metatarsals) are common sites, although the long tubular bones (femur, humerus) can be affected. They are rarely seen in sites most commonly affected by chondrosarcoma (trunk bones). Enchondromas account for approximately 10% of benign skeletal tumors. They are seen in people between the ages of 20 and 40 but can occur at any age in both men and women.[60]

***Pathogenesis and Clinical Manifestations.*** Cartilaginous tumors are lesions in which cartilage is produced, rather than osteoid as in osteosarcomas. These lesions are classified as chondromas. Enchondral ossification is the process by which most bones in the skeleton are formed—that is,

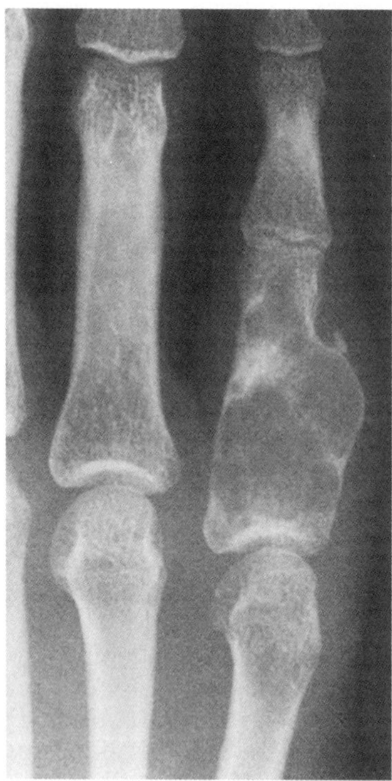

**Figure 26.16**

**Enchondroma of the proximal phalanx of the small finger in a 27-year-old woman.** Note radiolucent, expansile lesion that resulted in attenuation and thinning of the cortex. (From Greenspan A: Tumors of cartilage origin. *Orthop Clin* 20:351, 1989.)

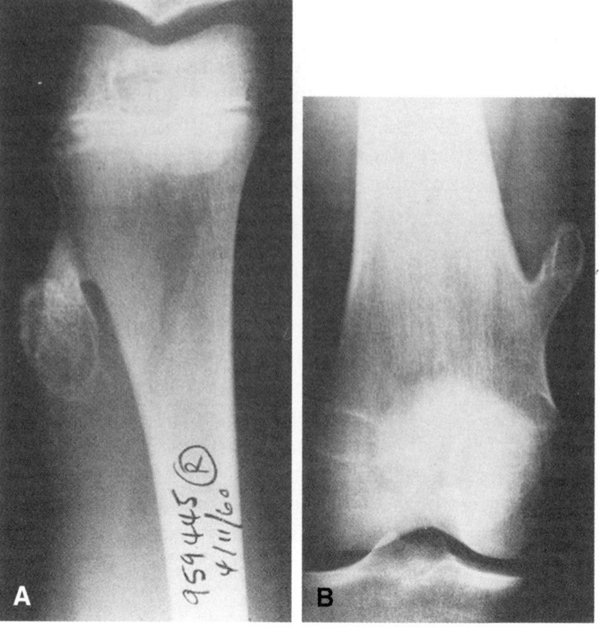


**Figure 26.17**

**Osteochondroma.** (A–B) Two radiographs showing mature osteochondroma: stalked lesion pointing toward the diaphysis and away from the growth plate. (From Bogumill G, Schwamm H: *Orthopaedic pathology*, Philadelphia, 1984, Saunders.)

bone is slowly absorbed from the inner cortex while periosteal reactive bone is deposited on the outer surface. A cartilaginous model exists as a precursor to mature bone. A tumor may then develop from cartilage islands displaced from the growth plate during development. This is thought to occur perhaps secondary to trauma or to an abnormality in the growth plate.

Histologically, enchondroma consists of hyaline cartilage appearing as lobules rimmed with a narrow band of reactive bone. These may be difficult to differentiate from a slow-growing chondrosarcoma, and in a small percentage of cases, a single enchondroma (usually in a large long bone) undergoes malignant change to become a chondrosarcoma.

Enchondromas may be asymptomatic. In some cases, some swelling may occur. When present in the hands, pain may be a symptom of pathologic stress fracture.[46]

## MEDICAL MANAGEMENT

DIAGNOSIS. In cases in which no symptoms are present, the tumor is an incidental finding on plain radiographs or bone scans performed for other reasons. Once detected, differentiating the lesion from a chondrosarcoma is crucial. The radiograph and clinical history, not the histologic makeup, are the most informative. Radiographs of enchondromas do not show cortical destruction. Pain without evidence of a fracture is also suspicious of malignancy rather than enchondroma.[60]

TREATMENT AND PROGNOSIS. Curettage is a common form of treatment, with or without spongy bone grafting, depending on the size and location of the lesion. Clients with enchondromas in the hand may develop stress fractures, which often respond to splinting. Recurrence of enchondromas after curettage is less than 5%, and malignant transformation occurs in 2% of all cases (usually adults).[27]

### OSTEOCHONDROMA

***Overview and Incidence.*** Osteochondroma is the most common primary benign neoplasm of bone, accounting for 90% of all benign bone tumors. A continuous osseous outgrowth of bone with a cartilaginous cap is characteristic (Fig. 26.17). The outgrowth arises from the metaphysis of long bones and extends away from the nearest epiphysis. The metaphyses of long bones, especially the distal femur, proximal humerus, and proximal tibia, are common sites. The flat bones of the ilium and scapula can also be involved.[54]

The incidence of osteochondroma is unknown. Some reports indicate that men are affected more often, but this may be due to the fact that it is often an incidental finding, and men may be more likely to have a radiograph taken during the second decade of life, when the lesion is usually seen.

***Pathogenesis.*** Osteochondromas appear to result from aberrant epiphyseal development. They are an extension of normal bone capped by cartilage that forms a prominent "tumor" (lump, swelling), sometimes referred to as *osteocartilaginous exostosis.* The younger the individual, the larger is the cartilage cap, because during the growing years, an osteochondroma has its own epiphyseal plate from which it grows.[54]

The lesion will usually cease growing when the individual reaches skeletal maturity. The central portion of

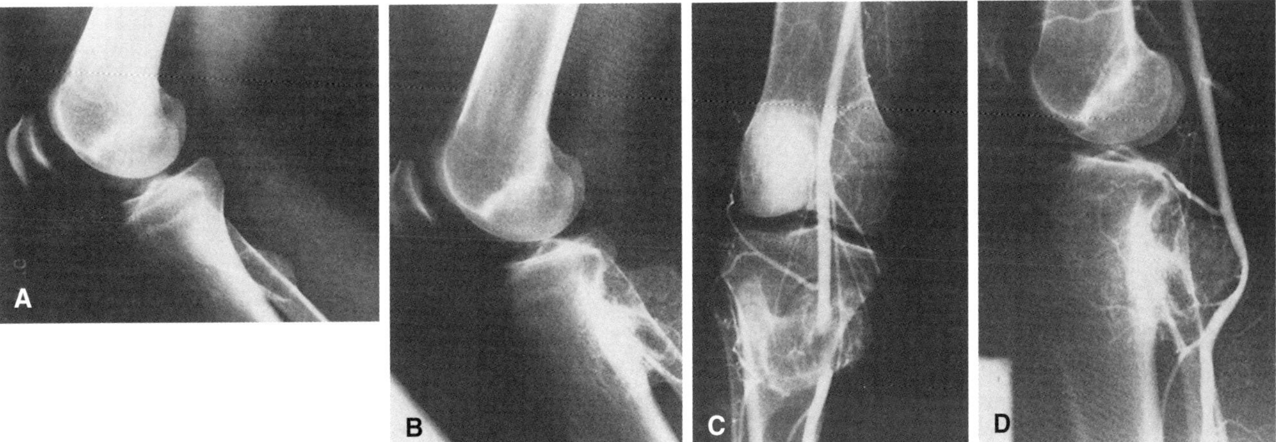


**Figure 26.18**

**Osteochondroma of the proximal fibula in a young man.** (A) Lateral radiograph of the right knee obtained when the patient was 17 years old demonstrates an exophytic lesion arising from the proximal fibula. (B) Lateral radiograph obtained 8 years later shows considerable interim growth of the osteochondroma, although a smooth outline is maintained. (C) Anteroposterior and (D) lateral angiograms demonstrate displacement and marked narrowing of the distal popliteal artery by the tumor. (From Guidici M, Moser R, Kransdorf M: Cartilaginous bone tumors. *Radiol Clin North Am* 31:247, 1993.)

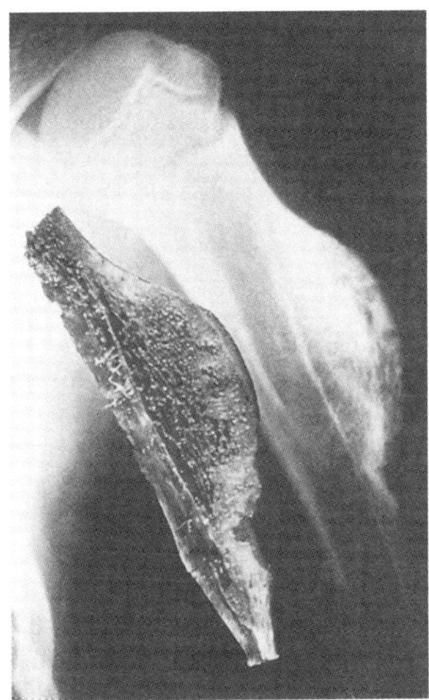

**Figure 26.19**

**Osteochondroma.** Radiograph and gross specimen of sessile osteochondroma. Note the cartilaginous component causing the radiographic defect in the distal portion. Note also incorporation of hematopoietic tissue into the base of the osteochondroma. (From Bogumill G, Schwamm H: *Orthopaedic pathology*, Philadelphia, 1984, Saunders.)

the lesion is normal medullary bone. The lesion may begin as a displaced fragment of epiphyseal cartilage that penetrates a cortical defect and continues to grow.

***Clinical Manifestations.*** In some people, a hard mass will be detected, sometimes present for many years. When the tumor is palpable, it may, owing to the cartilaginous cap, feel much larger than is apparent on radiographs.

Osteochondromas are not painful lesions in themselves, but they may interfere with the function of surrounding soft tissues such as tendons, nerves, or bursae. Blood vessels can also be compromised by the tumors (Fig. 26.18), and if tumors are sufficiently large, they may even limit joint motion.[54] Synovial osteochondromatosis can occur secondary to benign proliferation of the synovium and manifests as multiple loose bodies within a joint.

## MEDICAL MANAGEMENT

DIAGNOSIS. Plain radiographs may show a slender stalk of bone directed away from the nearest growth plate. This is referred to as a *pedunculated osteochondroma.* A sessile osteochondroma has a broad base of attachment (Fig. 26.19). In both types, the most important feature to note is the continuity of the cortex between the host bone and the tumor.[54]

CT and MRI are not commonly used in the diagnostic workup of benign lesions, but if atypical clinical manifestations or recent changes in the appearance of the lesion on plain radiographs are evident, MRI may be indicated. For example, MRI can demonstrate the continuity of the marrow between the tumor and the host bone, thereby ruling out a periosteal osteosarcoma.

TREATMENT AND PROGNOSIS. Because osteochondromas usually cease their growth at skeletal maturity, no intervention is needed unless they are symptomatic or interfere with normal limb function. Removal of the lesion is sometimes required when symptoms such as vascular compromise, chronic bursitis, or pain develop secondarily.[54] Rarely an osteochondroma can transform into a chondrosarcoma. Symptomatic lesions that are removed have a very low recurrence rate.

### Malignant Cartilaginous Tumors

**Chondrosarcoma.** *Chondrosarcoma* is defined as a malignant tumor of cartilage in which the matrix formed is uniformly or entirely chondroid in nature.[60] These tumors are classified as malignant bone tumors and therefore are discussed in Primary Malignant Bone Tumors.

## Fibrous Lesions

### Overview

Fibrous (fibroosseous) lesions (also referred to as fibrous dysplasia) within bone are a common osseous anomaly of mesenchymal tissue. They are usually solitary lesions found in the femur, skull, humerus, and tibia. Adolescents and young adults are affected. These lesions vary from small, fibrous cortical defects to larger fibrous dysplasias. Although most are benign, fibrosarcoma has many of the features of osteosarcoma. Many children have defects in the metaphysis, but most resolve spontaneously. Those that persist are seen in young men. The distal femur and tibia are common sites.

SPECIAL IMPLICATIONS FOR THE THERAPIST 26.8

*Cartilaginous Tumors*

With *enchondromas,* as with benign neoplasms of bone, limitations on early function may be needed depending on the size and location of the tumor. Because *osteochondroma* is a benign tumor and will likely require only symptomatic, if any, intervention, the role of the therapist is to educate clients and alleviate any anxiety that may be present. The special implications of *chondrosarcoma* for the therapist are similar to those of other malignant neoplasms such as osteosarcoma.

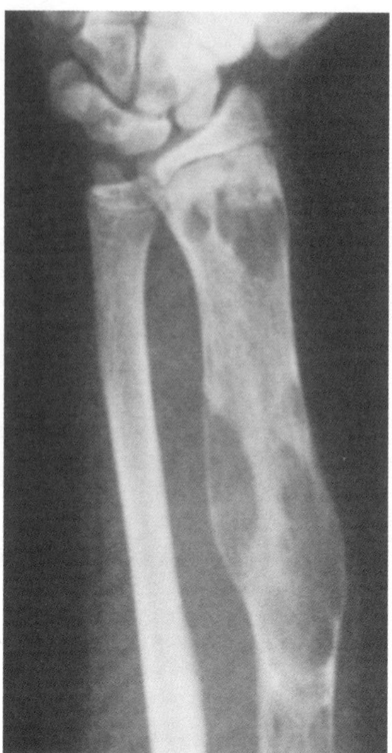

**Figure 26.20**

**Fibrous dysplasia.** A predominantly lytic lesion with some sclerosis and expansion is seen in the distal half of the radius in a child. Expansion and bone deformity are commonly seen in fibrous dysplasia. The sclerotic areas are described as having a ground-glass appearance. (From Helms C: *Fundamentals of skeletal radiology: benign cystic lesions,* Philadelphia, 1989, Saunders.)

### Pathogenesis and Clinical Manifestations

The hallmark of this disease is the inability of bone-forming tissue to produce mature bone. The process is arrested at the level of woven bone; even if a large amount of osteoid tissue is produced, it cannot or does not mature to lamellar bone. The pathogenesis is unknown, but it appears the underlying molecular mechanism involves the fundamental cell differentiation process.[5]

Although the defect occurs in the metaphysis, during normal bone growth, the defect may be displaced into the diaphysis. Microscopic examination reveals disorganized, haphazard deposits characteristic of woven bone, sometimes accompanied by local hemorrhage and serous fluid accumulation. Growth of lesions is often stabilized during puberty.

Most fibrous defects are asymptomatic. Some individuals experience mild to moderate pain with swelling or deformity of the affected site. The more extensive the disease, the earlier the onset of symptoms. Pathologic fractures may be the initial symptom and occur where large lesions exist. Depending on the specific form of dysplasia, affected bones include ribs; craniofacial bones; long, tubular bones; and pelvis.[5]

There may be associated extraskeletal symptoms such as hyperpigmentation of the skin (café au lait spots corresponding to the site of musculoskeletal involvement) or endocrine dysfunction (e.g., early menarche in girls, acromegaly, hyperthyroidism, hyperparathyroidism, Cushing syndrome).

#### MEDICAL MANAGEMENT

Plain radiographs are usually diagnostic, with lesions usually an incidental finding on radiographs obtained for other reasons. The appearance of the lesion depends on the amount of mineralized and fibrous tissues, with most lesions having an irregular shape with a thin sclerotic border (Fig. 26.20). Most fibrous lesions are treated with observation, but patients may benefit from bisphosphonates to inhibit osteoclastic resorption of bony tissues. For fibrous lesions that do not resolve spontaneously, treatment sometimes requires surgery. When the dysplasia thins the cortex of a weight-bearing bone or occupies more than half of the diameter of the bone, the risk of pathologic fracture increases. Benign fibrous defects generally have a good prognosis.[28] Implications for the therapist are similar to those with other benign bone tumors.

# METASTATIC TUMORS

## Overview

Cancer commonly metastasizes to bone; skeletal involvement represents the third most common site of metastatic spread (after lung and liver). *Secondary* or *metastatic neoplasms* refer to lesions that originate in other organs of the body. All malignant tumors have the capability to spread to bone. Malignant tumors that have metastasized to the bone are the most common neoplasm of the bone.

Although all the factors that affect the timing and location of metastasis are not known, bone tissue contains a number of growth factors that can stimulate the proliferation of tumor cells that may metastasize to these sites. Cancer metastases (both carcinomas and sarcomas) to bone are a common clinical problem because the cancers that cause them are prevalent and often metastasize.

Primary cancers responsible for 75% of all bone metastases include prostate, breast, lung, kidney, gastrointestinal, and melanoma.[31]

Common sites for *breast* cancer to metastasize include the pelvis, ribs, vertebrae, and proximal femur. *Lung* cancer can metastasize to the bone early in the disease, remaining asymptomatic until widespread dissemination has taken place; therefore treatment is often unsuccessful. Neoplasms in the *kidney* metastasize to the vertebrae, pelvis, and proximal femur in about 40% of cases. The *prostate* is the most common source of skeletal metastases in men.[97]

Early detection is important for successful intervention. Therapists should be aware of this possible cause of lumbar spine and hip pain, especially in men older than age 50. Cancer of the thyroid is uncommon but does metastasize to bone. Women are affected by bone metastases from the thyroid three times more often than men. Therapists should remember that the development of metastasis may be delayed and may even occur after removal of a cancerous thyroid. For discussions of specific primary cancers, see the relevant chapters.

## Incidence and Etiology

Metastatic bone neoplasms are much more common than primary bone lesions; about half of all individuals with cancer (except skin cancer) will develop bone metastases at some point. Incidence increases to 80% of individuals with advanced cancer. The incidence of bone metastasis is expected to increase with the prolonged survival associated with improved antineoplastic therapies now available. The spine is the site most commonly affected, with more than 50% of metastases involving the spine, usually the thoracic or lumbar spine.[31]

In the spine, the size of the vertebral body may influence the distribution of metastases. The larger lumbar vertebral bodies are more commonly affected than the smaller thoracic or cervical vertebrae. Neurologic compromise is more likely to occur when metastatic lesions affect the thoracic spine because of the smaller ratio between the diameter of the spinal canal and the spinal cord within the thoracic spine.[93]

## Risk Factors

Risk factors are those related to the primary cancer. For some cancers, the risk factors are well documented, and efforts to educate individuals on health risks should be stressed. Adequate exercise, proper diet and nutrition, and avoidance of tobacco use are the primary preventive measures. It is likely that the increase in incidence of spinal (and other) metastases can be attributed to the improving survival of clients with cancer.[93]

## Pathogenesis

The pathophysiology of metastasis is not completely understood (see Invasion and Metastases in Chapter 9). The development of metastatic disease, regardless of the eventual target organ, usually follows a common pathway. Cancer can spread through the bloodstream, through the lymphatic system, or by direct extension into adjacent tissue. Hematogenous spread of the cancer is most common, and therefore skeletal metastases are found in areas of bones with a good blood supply. These include the vertebrae, ribs, skull, and proximal femur and humerus.

The skeletal vasculature represents a significant proportion of the body's total vasculature. At the same time, the vertebral plexus of veins has no valves, so that the retrograde venous pressure is often increased in the abdominal and chest regions. This enables the retrograde blood flow to bypass the caval system, reaching the bones of the vertebral column instead via the extradural Batson venous plexus. Batson plexus may be the route by which breast cancer cells metastasize directly to the thoracic spine.[31,93]

The unique vasculature of the spine contributes to the high rate of spinal involvement in metastatic disease. The vertebral venous system is a valveless channel that extends from the sacrum to the skull. Venous connections to this system exist from the breasts, lungs, thyroid gland, kidneys, and prostate gland. Cells from the primary tumor mass enter the circulation by traversing either the walls of small blood vessels in normal tissue or the walls of vessels induced by the tumor itself. Once having gained access to the vertebral vein system, tumor cells can travel to distant organ sites. There are also direct connections to the vertebrae, ribs, pelvis, skull, and the shoulder and pelvic girdles.

From a biologic point of view, it is very unlikely that the abundance of the vascular network within the bone is the only factor that predisposes to metastasis, because metastases rarely develop in other tissues that have an equally rich vascular supply. It is proposed that the biologic conditions of bone tissue must be important factors in promoting the growth of tumor cells that reach the marrow through the venous and arterial blood network.[31]

The development of skeletal metastasis involves a series of events that begins when a tumor cell separates from the primary site, enters the blood system, and then extravasates from the blood vessel to the secondary site.[40] Adhesion molecules control separation and clustering of cancerous cells. The presence or absence of certain molecules controls the ability of cells to metastasize. Various types of adhesion molecules have been implicated. Cadherins, integrins, and selectins each have distinct properties that can regulate the propensity for a primary lesion to metastasize to a specific organ.

Metastasis to bone often results in osteolysis because cancer cells secrete a number of paracrine factors that stimulate osteoclast function. The cancer tries to destroy the bone (lytic process), and in response, the bone attempts to grow new bone (blastic process) to surround the cancer. If the cancer overwhelms the bone, it becomes weak and fractures easily. Bone metastases may be lytic (most common), blastic, or mixed. Lesions originating from the breast, lung, kidney, and thyroid are usually lytic. Blastic metastases are commonly associated with advanced carcinomas of the prostate and sometimes the breast.[97]

## Clinical Manifestations

Although as many as 50% of people with breast or prostate metastasis have no bone pain, pain remains the most common presenting symptom, often characterized as sharp, severe, worse at night, and transient or intermittent in the early course but eventually constant in more advanced stages.

Bone pain of a mechanical nature associated with skeletal metastases occurs as a result of significant bone destruction, joint instability, mechanical insufficiency, and fracture. It is often incapacitating and persistent despite local and systemic therapies. Long bone or vertebral fractures with or without spinal cord compression may be the first indication of advanced disease. Spinal cord compression, the most serious complication of bone metastasis, occurs secondary to increased pressure on the spinal cord or as a result of vertebral collapse. Classic signs and symptoms of cord compression include pain, numbness, and/or paralysis.[2]

Pain may also arise from a biologic origin for a number of reasons. It may occur as a result of rapid growth of the tumor, stretching the periosteum. Increased blood flow or angiogenesis (sometimes giving a throbbing or pulsatile sensation) and the release of cytokines at the site of the metastases gives rise to bone pain. Also, neuropeptides elaborated by or acting on bone-associated nerves in the endosteum can result in bone pain. Because the skeleton provides both form and support, growing tumors that deform the cortical bone contribute to activity-associated pain. This type of pain is often intermittent and related to weight bearing and movement.[91]

Bone often functions as a metastatic conduit for peripheral nerves, as bone metastases travel hematogenously from distal body parts to the central nervous system. Therefore bone tumor growth and invasion into surrounding tissues can result in neuritic pain syndromes, plexopathies, and spinal cord compression.

These pain syndromes contribute to increasing loss of mobility and bed rest, the effects of which are increasing generalized weakness, risk of thromboembolism, hypercalcemia, atelectasis, and pneumonia. The latter occur particularly in anyone with painful rib metastases. Mechanical failure or pathologic bone fracture may occur as a result of prolonged immobilization (osteoporosis). As with primary tumors, pathologic fractures can occur directly from the tumor itself or from the secondary effects of intervention.[91]

Metabolic changes can also occur as a result of the disease or the treatment, increasing the risk of fracture. In people with multiple metastases, the resultant hypercalcemia may cause anorexia, nausea, vomiting, general weakness, and depression. Unexplained weight loss is typically a late sign of metastatic disease.

Left untreated, hypercalcemia may lead to diffuse osteoporosis, renal insufficiency, and dehydration. These symptoms may be relieved (and possibly prevented) by the use of bisphosphonates (e.g., intravenous pamidronate [Aredia] and clodronate; oral ibandronate and clodronate), small molecules that inhibit osteoclast-induced bone resorption. The reactive bone formation stimulated by these lesions accounts for the elevation of serum alkaline phosphatase.[31]

## MEDICAL MANAGEMENT

**DIAGNOSIS.** A history of malignancy raises the suspicion of recurrent disease or a metastatic lesion. The evaluation of an individual with a previous history of cancer or a current malignancy and bone pain begins with a physical examination and basic radiographic studies.[57] Because much of the bone matrix must be destroyed before the lytic process is noted on radiographs, plain films are not useful in early detection, but they are important in staging and treatment planning. Spinal metastasis may be evident by the loss of the vertebral pedicle or with a pathologic fracture of a long bone.

Whole-body bone scans are much more sensitive for early detection of skeletal metastasis but are not useful in predicting fractures. Approximately one-third of people with skeletal metastatic disease have positive bone scan findings yet negative radiographic results. Scans are also used to determine the extent of dissemination.

CT and MRI also have roles in delineating various types of metastasis and assessing the size and extent of the lesion. More advanced technology using single-photon emission tomography allows for better determination of anatomic location of the areas of radioisotope uptake.[93] Biopsy is sometimes necessary to confirm a diagnosis when the primary source is not known. CT-guided biopsy is used to assess spinal lesions; diagnostic accuracy is greater for lytic lesions (93%) compared with sclerotic lesions (76%).[45]

Other diagnostic tests may include serum chemistries, urinalysis, serum protein electrophoresis, and prostate-specific antigen determination (for men). Biochemical markers of bone turnover such as N-telopeptide and pyridinium cross-links (pyridinoline and deoxypyridinoline) may provide information on bone dynamics that reflect disease activity in bone.

Several studies have shown bone turnover markers to be correlated with the extent of metastatic disease and the number of skeletal sites involved. Increases in such markers may be the first indication of bone involvement and possibly a useful early diagnostic sign of progression. Markers of bone turnover may be helpful in identifying individuals likely to respond to bisphosphonate treatment and as a means of monitoring the effectiveness of bisphosphonate therapy in the management of bone metastases.[43]

**TREATMENT.** Therapeutic interventions may depend, in part, on the extent of involvement. A person with localized disease may be offered potentially curative therapy, whereas an individual with extensive skeletal and visceral involvement may benefit only from palliative treatment.[97,85]

Treatment of bone metastasis is problematic, costly, and primarily palliative. Prolonging survival is not always possible, so improving function with pain relief, local control of disease, and bone stability is often the primary goal. This is becoming more important as treatment for primary cancers improves. Individuals may die as a result of the primary tumor or the metastasis (e.g., breast cancer). When survival rates and longevity increase, the likelihood of skeletal metastasis increases.

Intervention for skeletal neoplasms requires a multidisciplinary approach to optimize therapy options and coordinate their sequencing. Intervention modalities may include endocrine therapy (for breast and prostate cancer), chemotherapy, biotherapy (immunotherapy), use of bone-seeking radioisotopes (a therapy that has analgesic

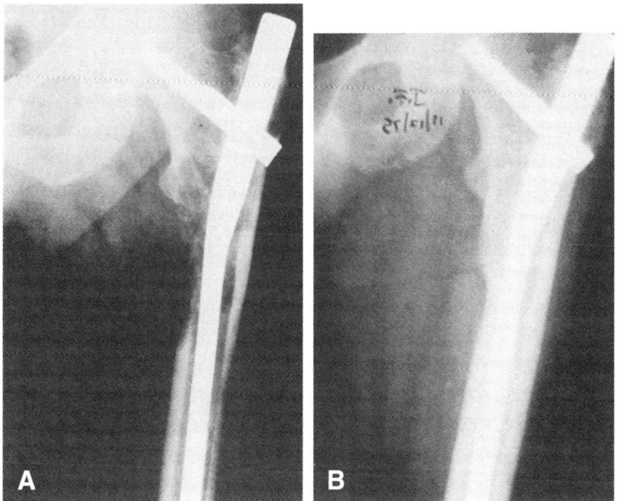

**Figure 26.21**

(A) Prophylactic fixation in a 63-year-old woman with an impending fracture secondary to breast metastasis treated by Zickel nailing. (B) Complete healing of this subtrochanteric lesion 5 months after radiation and chemotherapy. (From Habermann E, Lopez R: Metastatic disease of bone and treatment of pathologic fracture, *Orthop Clin* 20:475, 1989.)

and antitumor effects), and bisphosphonates to suppress bone resorption. These are often combined with other localized interventions such as surgery and site-directed radiation therapy.[31]

Surgery is rarely curative but can be an effective therapy to decompress neural tissue for resolution of symptoms and/or restoration of function (especially ambulation), reduce anxiety, improve mobility and function, facilitate nursing care, preempt fracture (i.e., repair bony lesions before they fracture), and control local tumor when nonsurgical therapies fail.[31]

Pathologic fractures that occur in the femur and humerus often require surgical stabilization. Intramedullary fixation with interlocking devices to limit motion at the fracture site is indicated in many instances. The desire to restore normal anatomy must be weighed against the reality that the individual may have a terminal disease. An estimated life expectancy of at least 6 months is desirable before extensive joint reconstructive procedures are carried out.

Where the risk of fracture is great, as when more than 50% of the cortex is destroyed, prophylactic nailing of the femur may be indicated (Fig. 26.21).

Spinal metastases can cause severe pain, instability, and spinal cord compression with neurologic compromise. Management of metastatic spinal cord compression is challenging, as affected individuals have widely different symptoms, comorbidities, adjuvant therapies, and tumor prognosis. For example, people with metastatic breast cancer often survive longer than people with metastatic spinal disease from lung cancer; aggressive surgical options may be pursued depending on the type of primary cancer.[16]

Pathologic fractures of the spine can be immobilized in an appropriate spinal brace, but a progressive neurologic deficit is an indication for surgical intervention. Surgery can take the form of decompression, posterior stabilization, excision, and reconstruction or prosthetic replacement.[67] Vertebroplasty or kyphoplasty may be considered for a person with a vertebral compression fracture and minimal bone deformity. The decision to pursue surgery to prolong ambulation is an individual one and must take into consideration the person's health status, individual prognosis, attitudes, and expectations.[16]

**Prognosis.** Although management of a skeletal metastasis may be successful in terms of restoring stability to a pathologic fracture, the prognosis for the primary cancer is still guarded. Only rarely is the skeletal metastasis actually the cause of death. Skeletal morbidity includes bone pain, hypercalcemia, pathologic fracture, spinal cord or nerve root compression, and immobility, all of which can impact mortality rates.[31]

The median survival for people with tumors that have metastasized to the bone is determined by the type of tumor. The overall median survival after detection of bone metastases is approximately 19 months; this significant amount of time allows for interventions that can dramatically improve a person's quality of life and functional independence.[47] Metastases to the vertebrae with epidural spinal cord compression can increase morbidity and hasten mortality. Loss of function, poor quality of life, and poor survival rates accompany spinal metastases.[16]

Favorable prognostic factors include indolent nature of the primary lesion (e.g., prostate cancer); well-differentiated tumor on histologic examination; a long recurrence-free survival (greater than 3 years); sclerotic lesion on radiograph as opposed to a lytic lesion, especially after treatment; a single bone lesion; a single system involved with metastatic disease; low tumor markers; no vital organ involvement; and general good condition of the individual.

Unfavorable prognostic factors include an aggressive primary tumor, lytic bone lesions, multiple bone lesions, and poor health of the patient.[31,47]

The risk of pathologic fracture is greater in osteolytic lesions of the long bones. A direct relationship exists between the degree of cortical destruction and the risk of pathologic fracture. When cortical destruction is less than 25% to 35%, the risk for fracture is low. Destruction greater than 50% correlates with a much higher risk for pathologic fracture. The presence of pain with weight-bearing activities indicates compromised structural integrity and therefore also places the individual at greater risk of fracture.

SPECIAL IMPLICATIONS FOR THE THERAPIST 26.9

## *Metastatic Tumors*

### Early Detection

Metastases to the skeleton are important to the therapist because the presence of musculoskeletal pain may be the initial symptom of an undetected primary carcinoma or an occult metastasis. Early detection is essential for effective interventions. A thorough history and a high index of suspicion can lead to timely referral or consultation with a physician. In people with a history of cancer, the clinician should be vigilant regarding the likelihood and common sites of metastasis. Bone metastases are commonly found in the vertebrae, pelvis, femur, and bones of the upper extremity. Metastases distal to the elbow or knee are rare; when they do occur, the kidney is most likely the site of the primary tumor.[31]

### Preoperative Intervention

Exercise is recommended for individuals with bone metastases before and after surgery, focusing on increasing muscle strength and endurance while maintaining bone protection. Exercise programs directed at strengthening and stretching are often needed; high-impact and high-torsion activities should be avoided.[14]

An understanding of common postoperative impairments helps in treatment planning, preventing or minimizing length of hospitalization, and fostering an early return to independence. Chemotherapy for some cancers includes the use of steroids that can lead to muscle atrophy, especially of the type II fibers. Isometric exercises may prevent marked atrophy. Radiation therapy can lead to contracture of soft tissues, and clients should be taught to stretch and self-mobilize the soft tissues of susceptible areas before treatment.

Instruction in fall prevention strategies, including optimal body mechanics and exercises to maintain strength and balance, is essential before and after surgery. This is especially true for anyone taking pain medication that causes drowsiness and decreased coordination.

### Rehabilitation

People who have had a pathologic fracture stabilized are often referred for rehabilitation. Hypercalcemia is common in the acute or subacute phase and occurs when bone resorption is greater than new bone formation. Osteolysis that occurs with bone metastasis is one cause of hypercalcemia.[12]

Treatment of the primary cancer with chemotherapy and/or radiation therapy often provides additional challenges, such as fatigue and increased risk of infection. For a client with lung cancer, baseline pulmonary status should be established, and proper breathing techniques should be taught. Management of clients with metastatic disease is challenging, because in addition to these complications, clients often need extensive rehabilitation after medical treatment.[23]

Management of skeletal metastasis including fracture is aimed at improving or restoring function, especially maintaining ambulatory function to preserve quality of life and prevent the negative sequelae of immobility.[32] If the bone has been compromised or fractures have occurred, surgical intervention will attempt to stabilize the defect.

After surgery, early mobilization including gait training, bed mobility, and transfers is essential. Maximizing functional independence is the driving force behind all rehabilitation efforts. Safety and bone protection are important during mobility and strengthening activities. Evaluation of upper extremity function and coexisting upper extremity metastases before allowing weight bearing through the arms is important.

There is a reluctance to allow walking activities with clients who are at risk of pathologic fracture because a measure of risk has not been developed, but in fact, an active rehabilitation program may not place a client at increased risk of fracture. The risk of producing pathologic fractures in clients with cancer by increasing mobility and function is low. Many individuals with skeletal metastases and pathologic fracture have been shown to be good candidates for intensive rehabilitation programs if they do not have hypercalcemia caused by lytic metastases or pain severe enough to require parenteral narcotics.[78,12]

Because many people with metastatic disease are at risk for pathologic fractures, the risk of falling must be considered when planning for ambulation training, especially among older adults. Assessments of mental status, balance, strength, ROM, endurance, vision, ambulation history, and symptoms of dizziness are all important and will help plan ambulation training. Even with the most critical analysis of the risks and benefits, therapists who work with individuals who have serious medical conditions such as metastatic lesions and pathologic fractures must be prepared for setbacks and unexpected events to occur when attempting to preserve or maximize function.[78,49]

Rehabilitative decision making in this area requires collaboration between the therapist and the medical staff (e.g., oncologist, surgeon) and takes into primary consideration the degree of cortical involvement. It is very helpful if the therapist has access to imaging studies with accurate information about the extent of involvement, specific levels affected, and knowledge of stability (or instability) of spinal segments to assist in treatment planning.[75,73,94]

Generally for clients with invasion of less than 25% of the cortex, submaximal isometrics and gentle aerobics (e.g., bicycling at low resistance, aquatics if approved by the physician for clients with wounds or fractures that are healing) are generally permitted, and the involved limb most typically is cleared for weight bearing as tolerated. When cortical involvement increases to 25% to 50%, restrictions tighten and allow for gentle ROM without pressure into the end ROM and limb offloading to partial weight bearing. Finally, with greater than 50% cortical involvement, exercise may need to be deferred and the limb maintained non–weight bearing. See Chapter 9 for other exercise guidelines for the client with cancer and Special Implications for the Therapist 26.1: Primary Tumors.

## REFERENCES

To enhance this text and add value for the reader, all references are included in the enhanced ebook on Student Consult that accompanies this textbook. The reader can view the reference source and access it online whenever possible.

# CHAPTER 27

# Soft Tissue, Joint, and Bone Disorders

KEVIN HELGESON • ELIZABETH SHELLY • JAN DOMMERHOLT • NATHAN MAYBERRY

People presenting with muscle, joint, and bone disorders make up a significant percentage of the therapist's practice. These conditions are primarily manifested by pain, deformity, and loss of mobility and function. Many of the people seen by therapists have these conditions secondary to trauma or repetitive overuse; these conditions are local in terms of the involved tissues and nonprogressive in nature.

Therapists may treat impairment in other regions of the body to reduce the mechanical stresses on the involved region, but the disorder itself (i.e., degenerative joint disease, bursitis, tendinitis) does not spread to other body regions. This is in contrast to rheumatic diseases and systemic disorders, which can be manifested not only by local joint or muscle pain and impairments but also by additional symptoms associated with other body systems.

Although this book is primarily a compilation of diseases and conditions of all systems, this chapter contains both orthopedic and systemic conditions that affect the bones, joints, or muscles that may not fall into any other category. Because the focus of this text is not orthopedics, many orthopedic conditions have not been included. For the most part, conditions with a more generalized effect or accompanied by a systemic component are included here. The concepts presented in Chapter 22 are especially important to the discussion of this chapter and should be reviewed or read along with this chapter.

This chapter is divided into three distinct anatomic areas—soft tissue, joint, and bone—with conditions and diseases placed in the area most notably affected. Frequently there is overlap, and one condition affecting more than one area is found in a single section. As always, the reader is encouraged to keep a broad perspective whenever studying an isolated condition or anatomic area.

## SOFT TISSUE

### Soft Tissue Injuries

Soft tissue injuries such as strains and sprains, lacerations, tendon ruptures, muscle injuries, myofascial compartment syndromes, dislocations, and subluxations are described briefly in this introductory section. Strains refer to stretching or tearing of the musculotendinous unit; they may be partial or full tears. The musculotendinous junction is a region of highly folded basement membranes between the end of the muscle fiber and the tendon. These involutions maximize surface area for force transmission but contain a transition zone where the compliant muscle fibers become relatively noncompliant tendon, placing this junction at increased risk for injury. The sarcolemma of the muscle fiber is the usual site for the initial injury from an excessive stretching force.

Strains can be classified as mild, moderate, or severe (complete) tears or as injuries of first, second, or third degree depending on the severity of tissue damage. Stretching or minor tearing of a few fibers without loss of integrity is classified as *first degree* (mild), with only minor swelling and discomfort accompanied by no or only minimal loss of strength and restriction of movement.[182]

*Second-degree* (moderate) strain refers to partial tearing of muscle tissue with clear loss in function (ability to contract). Pain, moderate disabilities, point tenderness, swelling, localized hemorrhaging, and slightly to moderately abnormal motion are typical.

A *third-degree* (severe) strain refers to complete loss of structural or biomechanical integrity extending across the entire cross section of the muscle and usually requires surgical repair. An alternative classification scheme uses three grades of injury (I, II, III). Common sites for this type of injury include the ankle, knee, and fingers.

The tendon is most vulnerable to injury (*tendinitis, tendon rupture*) when it is tense or the attached muscle is maximally contracted, with tension applied excessively or from shearing forces across the tendon. Tendon injuries can also be created by extrinsic forces that excessively cause compression or a frictioning on the tendon. Tendinosis or tendinopathy reflects more of a chronic condition, with minimal or no inflammatory process detected histologically. Changes have been documented at the cellular level, with expansion of local cells and thinner collagen fibrils resulting in a chronic inflammatory condition.[287]

*Muscle contusion* (bruising with intact skin) is common in contact sports and incites an inflammatory response, sometimes involving hematoma formation. The clinical manifestations of this soft tissue injury are local pain, edema, increased local tissue temperature, ecchymosis, hypermobility or instability, and loss of function.

*Myofascial compartment syndromes* develop when increased interstitial pressure within a closed myofascial compartment compromises the functions of the nerves, muscles, and vessels within the compartment. Compartment syndromes may be acute or chronic and are most likely to occur within the "envelopes" of the lower leg, forearm, thigh, and foot where the fascia cannot give or expand.

Many clinical conditions predispose to the development of compartment syndromes, including fractures, severe contusions, crush injuries, excessive skeletal traction, and reperfusion injuries and trauma. Other risk factors may include burns, circumferential wraps or restrictive dressings, or a cast or other unyielding immobilizer. Ischemia and irreversible muscle loss can occur, resulting in functional disability (and even potential loss of limb) if the condition is left untreated.[176]

The earliest clinical symptom of impending acute compartment ischemia is pain disproportionate to that expected from the injury. The pain is described as deep, throbbing pressure. There may be sensory deficit or paresthesia within the region distal to the area of involvement. In severe compartment syndromes, objective signs are visible, such as a swollen extremity with smooth, shiny, or red skin. The extremity is tense on palpation, and passive stretch increases the pain.[357] Prompt surgical decompression is the standard intervention.

Injury to the *growth cartilage* can occur in skeletally immature children and adolescents. During adolescent growth spurts the cartilage cells of the physis become more active and more prone to injury. Hypertrophy and weakening of the hypertrophic zone of cartilage are thought to be the cause.[119]

The three areas of growing cartilage in a skeletally immature individual include the physis (growth plate), articular cartilage of joint surfaces, and major bone–tendon attachments (apophyses). These sites account for a large number of sports injuries in young athletes, including osteochondritis dissecans (articular surface) and Osgood-Schlatter disease (apophysis); both conditions are discussed later in this chapter.

The terms *subluxation* and *dislocation* relate to joint integrity. Subluxation is partial disruption of the anatomic relationship within a joint. The glenohumeral, acromioclavicular, sacroiliac, and atlantoaxial joints are at most risk for subluxation. Once the joint condition has stabilized, rehabilitation should address local muscle imbalances and adjacent joint hypomobility, which could increase mechanical stresses at the joint.

Dislocation implies complete loss of joint integrity, with loss of anatomic relationships. Often significant ligamentous damage occurs with this type of injury. Dislocations most often occur at the glenohumeral joint. Congenital dislocations are most frequently seen at the hip joints (see Developmental Dysplasia in Chapter 23).

Joint dislocation can also be a late manifestation of chronic disease, such as rheumatoid arthritis (RA), paralysis, and neuromuscular disease. In the presence of a joint dislocation, the integrity of nerve and vascular tissue must be assessed. If compromise is suspected, timely reduction is essential to prevent serious complications.

**SPECIAL IMPLICATIONS FOR THE THERAPIST 27.1**

## *Soft Tissue Injuries*

Immediate stabilization is required with soft tissue injuries to avoid excessive scar formation and prevent rerupture at the injury site. Both further retraction of the ruptured muscle stumps and hematoma size can be minimized by placing the injured extremity in a resting position. Immobilization of the tissues appears to provide the new granulation tissue with the needed tensile strength to withstand the forces created by muscle contractions. Strict immobilization should not extend beyond the first few days following the injury.

Early mobilization for the treatment of acute soft-tissue injuries has proven effective, especially in treating injured athletes. Early mobilization induces rapid and intensive capillary ingrowth into the injured area, with better repair of muscle fibers and more parallel orientation of the regenerating myofibers compared with immobilization. Early mobilization has the added benefit in muscle of improved biomechanical strength, which returns to the level of uninjured muscle more rapidly using active mobilization.[124]

The therapist can guide the injured individual in following a recovery protocol to enhance healing. Crutches may be advised with severe lower extremity muscle injuries, especially injuries where adequate early immobilization is difficult to achieve (e.g., groin area). Movement during the first 3 to 7 days should be done with care to avoid stretching the injured muscle.

### Preventing Effects of Immobilization

The therapist can be very helpful in treating soft tissue injuries by preventing the detrimental effects of immobilization by promoting tissue flexibility and strength, by minimizing inflammation, and by enhancing tissue healing.

Between 7 and 10 days after an injury the therapist can gradually progress the individual in using the injured muscle more actively, using pain and tolerance as a guide to setting limits. All rehabilitation activities should begin with a warm-up of the injured muscle, as warming up reduces muscle viscosity and relaxes muscles neurally. Stimulated, warm muscles absorb more energy than unstimulated muscles and can better withstand loading. Combining a warm-up with stretching can improve the elasticity of injured muscle.[167]

Isometric training should be started first and progressed to isotonic training; isotonic strengthening begins without a resisting load–counterload, which is then progressively added. All exercises should be done within the limits of the client's pain. When the individual can complete isometric and isotonic exercises without pain, isokinetic training with minimal load can begin.

The effects of loading on the musculotendinous unit during rehabilitative exercise are increased tendon size, tensile strength, and enhanced collagen fiber organization of newly formed collagen. Restoring kinesthetic and proprioceptive awareness at the site of injury and restoring mobility and strength are also important elements of the rehabilitation program. A protocol of eccentric contraction is advocated for chronic tendinopathies, especially for the Achilles tendon.[118]

### Fluoroquinolones

The therapist should guide athletes who are taking fluoroquinolones in reducing intensity and volume of training routines until the antibiotic has been completed. Gradual return to full level of physical activity, exercise, training, and competitive play must be delayed until the full antibiotic course is completed. All athletic activity should be stopped if any adverse reactions are experienced. Monitoring for any complication (e.g., cardiac arrhythmia, photosensitivity, rashes, tendinopathies, central nervous system disorders, and hepatic and renal dysfunction) is advised for a full month after cessation of the antibiotic.[146]

Fluoroquinolone-associated tendon disorders are more common in people older than 60 years of age, especially individuals who are also taking oral corticosteroids.[347] Therapists should monitor for tendon injuries in people with previous history of tendinopathy, magnesium deficiency, hyperparathyroidism, diuretic use, peripheral vascular disease, RA, or diabetes mellitus.

### Injury Prevention

Overuse injuries from repetitive stresses and microtrauma are common among children and adults, especially children participating in organized sports. The therapist working with young athletes from any sport can emphasize injury prevention by educating both the athletes and their parents and encouraging coaches to emphasize injury prevention.

Prevention begins with conditioning, especially at the beginning of the season for one-sport athletes who do not play year round. Training errors, variable skeletal and muscle growth rates, anatomic malalignment, and faulty equipment are just a few of the key factors that contribute to injury. For individuals involved in multiple sports, volume and intensity of athletic involvement combined with inadequate time for recovery after injuries of any kind are key issues.[50]

Learning and practicing the basic skills (e.g., sliding into bases correctly, making a tackle in football, learning how to head-butt the ball in soccer) and understanding the fundamentals for each sport activity are essential. Many more injuries occur during practice than during actual competitive play, as more time is spent in practice. Early participation in organized sports at younger ages often results in overuse injuries, likely because of strength and flexibility imbalances.

The therapist can help identify and correct such risk factors before they translate into injury. Early detection of risk factors and injuries can help minimize the severity of injury and reduce long-term consequences of soft tissue damage. Everyone should be encouraged to think about injury prevention during practices, as well as during competitions.

## Heterotopic Ossification

### Overview and Definition

Heterotopic ossification (HO) is defined as bone formation in nonosseous tissues (usually muscles and other soft tissue areas). It is considered a benign condition of abnormal bone formation in soft tissue that occurs most commonly after trauma, such as fractures, surgical procedures (especially total hip replacements), spinal cord and traumatic brain injuries, burns, and amputations. Classification of HO is based on the anatomic location and effect on functional motion. A number of classification systems are available based on the location of the ossifications and history of the patient (Box 27.1). In addition to acquired forms of HO, there are forms that result from hereditary causes such as osteodystrophy. These conditions are extremely rare but provide helpful information on the pathophysiology of the condition.[348]

*HO* and *myositis ossificans* are terms often used interchangeably. Both conditions represent the deposition of mature lamellar bone and share radiographic and histologic characteristics, but they occur in different locations. HO develops in nonosseous tissues, whereas myositis ossificans forms in bruised, damaged, or inflamed muscle.[52]

HO in people with spinal cord injuries is often referred to as *neurogenic HO*. Neurogenic HO appears to be related more to the degree of completeness of spinal cord injury than the level involved; individuals with complete

Box 27.1

**CLASSIFICATIONS OF HETEROTOPIC OSSIFICATION**

***Hastings Classification of Heterotopic Ossification***[a]

| | |
|---|---|
| Class I | Presence of heterotopic ossification but without functional range-of-motion limitations |
| Class II | Heterotopic ossification with limitations in all planes of motion |
| Class III | Heterotopic ossification with ankylosis preventing motion |

***Brooker Classification of Heterotopic Ossification***[b]

| | |
|---|---|
| Class I | Islands of bone within soft tissues of any size |
| Class II | Bone spurs from pelvis or femur, leaving at least 1 cm between opposing bone surfaces |
| Class III | Same as class II but space between opposing bone surfaces reduced to less than 1 cm |
| Class IV | Ankylosis of involved joint |

[a]Data from Hastings H: Classification and treatment of heterotopic ossification about the elbow and forearm. *Hand Clin* 10:417–437, 1994.

[b]Data from Della Valle AG et al. Heterotopic ossification after total hip arthroplasty: a critical analysis of the Brooker classification and proposal of a simplified rating system. *J Arthroplasty* 17:870–875, 2002.

transverse spinal cord injuries are more likely to develop HO compared with individuals with incomplete spinal cord injuries.[24]

### Risk Factors

Risk factors for HO include a serious traumatic injury, previous history of HO, hypertrophic osteoarthritis (OA), ankylosing spondylitis (AS), and diffuse idiopathic skeletal hyperostosis (DISH). Men seem to be at higher risk for HO than women. Other risk factors include Paget disease, RA, posttraumatic arthritis, neural axis and thermal injuries, and osteonecrosis.[52]

Surgery-related factors may contribute to the formation of HO. Surgeries of the hip region may pose additional risk for the development of HO.[350] HO is the most common complication of total hip arthroplasty.[54] Individuals who have undergone multiple surgical interventions over a short period of time are at increased risk of HO. This may be attributed to the extensive damage to soft tissues, presence of disseminated bone dust, or formation of hematoma.

HO occurs in 1% to 3% of individuals with burn injuries. It appears to be related more to the degree of thermal injury than to the location of the burn. Individuals with third-degree burns affecting more than 20% of the total body surface are at greatest risk for the development of HO. Systemic physiologic factors in conjunction with local factors are the likely underlying etiology.[58]

### Etiology and Pathogenesis

The initiating factor for HO is debatable. Direct trauma is the most common cause of heterotopic bone formation in the elbow. There appears to be a link between the severity of injury and the amount of ectopic bone formation that develops. A person who sustains a massive traumatic injury is very likely to develop HO; HO is five times more likely in cases of both fracture and dislocation of the elbow.[52] There is an increased incidence of HO among military personnel with blast injuries. The extreme force destroys bone, muscles, and tendons, resulting in amputation. Bones grow into long spikes or develop more like cobwebs.

It is most likely that pluripotent mesenchymal (stem) cells that could differentiate into cartilage, bone, or tendon/ligament become osteoblasts instead. Differentiation begins early after surgery and peaks at 32 hours, possibly induced by a bone-inducing substance such as bone morphogenetic protein. The stimulus and mechanism that cause this to happen in soft tissues after trauma have not been determined. There may be local factors such as mechanical stress (e.g., articular disruption, muscle damage) and/or systemic factors.[184]

Individuals with traumatic brain injury are predisposed to HO, most likely because of osteoinductive factors released at the site of the brain injury, although little is known about this process.[256] In the case of bone fracture or reaming of the bone during joint replacements, bone marrow, which is capable of forming bone, may spread into well-vascularized muscle tissue. Bone marrow combined with growth factors from traumatized tissues may set off a series of steps leading to bone development and HO.[27]

Histologically, in the acute phase the inflammatory process results in edema and degeneration of muscle tissue. After a few weeks, the inflamed tissue is replaced with cartilage and bone, and the bone undergoes intensive turnover. This process cannot be distinguished histologically from the formation of bone callus in fractures.

There are histologic differences between normal bone and the ectopic (displaced) bone formed in HO. In normal bone the periosteal layer covering the external surface of the bone has an inner vascular cambium layer surrounded by an outer fibrosis layer. In HO the ectopic bone is not enveloped by periosteum. Instead there are three zones. The center is made up of dense cells and is surrounded by a layer of osteoid. The outermost layer consists of highly organized bone, although ectopic bone has twice the number of osteoclasts compared with normal bone and a higher number of osteoblasts.[29]

### Clinical Manifestations

The hallmark sign of HO is a progressive loss of range of motion at a time when posttraumatic inflammation should be resolving. Muscle pain and loss of motion are the most common presenting symptoms, often within 2 weeks of the precipitating trauma, surgery, burn, or neurologic insult. Swelling, warmth, erythema, and tenderness mimic a low-grade infection or, in the case of surgery, the normal postoperative inflammation that is often present.

As the ectopic ossification advances, the acute symptoms described may subside, but motion continues to decrease, even with intervention such as dynamic and/or static progressive splinting. Over the next 3 to 6 months, the HO matures and the individual develops a rigid or abrupt end feel with pain at the end range of motion. Delayed nerve palsy is common when the elbow is affected.[52]

Areas of calcification and bone spurs may progress to ankylosis. Sites affected most often include the hip, elbow, knee, shoulder, and temporomandibular joints. Pressure from the bone formation can result in pressure ulcers and interfere with skin grafts. Loss of motion can have serious consequences for daily function, especially for individuals who are already neurologically compromised.

Different classification schemes are used depending on the site affected. Most schemes grade the condition based on a scale from 0 to 3 or 0 to 4. Grade 0 denotes no islands of bone visible on x-ray. The final grade is bony ankylosis, with progressive involvement between the lowest and highest grade (e.g., bone spurs, periarticular bone formation).[349]

## MEDICAL MANAGEMENT

**PREVENTION.** Measures can be taken to prevent HO, including radiation treatment and pharmaceuticals (e.g., nonsteroidal antiinflammatory drugs [NSAIDs], diphosphonates).[192] Diphosphonates inhibit osteoid cells from calcifying, thereby preventing HO. The effect lasts only as long as the drug is taken. Gastrointestinal disturbance and osteomalacia are adverse side effects of this treatment, making it less than optimal.

NSAIDs such as indomethacin and rofecoxib are effective in reducing the frequency and magnitude of ectopic bone formation in some areas (e.g., hip). Used during the first 3 weeks postoperatively, NSAIDs inhibit precursor (undifferentiated) cells from developing into osteoblasts.[192]

Low-dose external-beam radiation is another effective preventive measure. Fractionated radiation of the pluripotent mesenchymal cells has been shown to be effective in preventing HO from developing when delivered within 72 hours after surgery.[297] Prevention is recommended for individuals at high risk of ectopic ossification, including individuals with neurologic injury, burns, past history of HO, or a previous history of other conditions previously mentioned. The best prevention for HO is to minimize soft tissue trauma, especially in high-risk individuals undergoing surgery of any kind. Complete wound lavage and the removal of all bone debris and reamings may help prevent HO.

**DIAGNOSIS.** Radiographs of the involved region may be the initial imaging choice to rule out other possible sources of the symptoms and loss of motion. Radiographic evidence of mineralization will be observed 4 to 6 weeks after the trauma (sometimes as early as 2 weeks after the incident event). Radiographs show the location, extent, and maturity of pathologic bone. HO must be differentiated from metastatic calcification, most often associated with hypercalcemia, and from dystrophic calcifications in tumors and may require a muscle biopsy.[358] Computed tomography (CT) scan will complement radiographic images in determining the extent of the ossification. Ultrasound may prove useful in diagnosing HO around the hip or elbow and distinguishing HO from a deep vein thrombosis in a patient with a spinal cord injury.[90] Laboratory tests to measure the serum alkaline phosphatase level are sometimes used, but they are not consistently accurate.

**TREATMENT AND PROGNOSIS.** Initial treatment should focus on controlling the development of a hematoma with use of rest, compression, elevation, and cryotherapy. NSAIDs and bisphosphonates may be useful for controlling inflammation and limiting ossification. Radiation applied to the damaged limb site within a few days after the injury may be useful, but there is always a risk of impaired healing for individuals with bone fractures. Surgical resection is delayed until the bone matures and develops a distinct fibrous capsule to minimize trauma to the tissues and reduce the risk of recurrence and may be done only in cases where activities of daily living (ADLs) are compromised by loss of motion.[358]

Indication for surgery may not be just the presence of HO, but rather the severity of functional restriction when loss of motion prevents the individual from using the affected extremity. A comprehensive rehabilitation program is needed to maximize motion, restore function, and reduce the risk of developing ankylosis. After surgical removal, radiation and NSAIDs are continued to prevent recurrence.

**SPECIAL IMPLICATIONS FOR THE THERAPIST 27.2**

### *Heterotopic Ossification*

The therapist's management of HO has evolved based on knowledge of the condition. Traditional thinking that any passive range of motion is contraindicated with HO has been abandoned. There was concern that passive range of motion could lead to further bone growth, but this has not proven accurate. Forcible muscle stretching can lead to muscle tears and ossification within the muscle and is contraindicated but should not be confused with passive range-of-motion exercises, which can be effective in preventing loss of motion and ankylosis.[52]

A specific program of physical therapy intervention can be planned based on the timing of the referral. During the acute and edematous phase (first 1 to 2 weeks postoperatively), proper measures are taken to reduce swelling, minimize scar formation, and provide pain management to allow for maximum participation in the program. Range-of-motion exercises (passive and active) can begin but must take into account the type and extent of injury present (e.g., fracture, joint instability).

Phase 2 occurs during the inflammatory stage approximately 2 to 6 weeks after the injury or incident event. Unorganized scar tissue forms during this phase but remains soft and deformable so that range-of-motion gains can be made. The soft tissues still respond to various modalities, and self-passive stretching with weighted stretches and/or dynamic or static progressive splinting is most likely to recapture lost motion. Specific recommendations for HO affecting the elbow are available.[52]

The therapist should continue to encourage functional use of affected areas, including strengthening when appropriate and emphasize motion throughout all motions, even if x-rays show HO developing around weeks 4 to 6 in this phase. By week 6, bone fractures are typically healed, allowing for more aggressive splinting. Scar tissue is fully formed but still malleable during this third (fibrotic) phase from 6 to 12 weeks. Splinting and resistive exercises can continue to maximize gains in motion.

Finally, during the last phase, 3 to 6 months after injury or surgery, scar tissue is organized and fibrotic. The individual may continue to make small gains, but often motion has reached a plateau, and splints are discontinued gradually. Clients should be encouraged to continue a home strengthening program for at least another 6 months.[52]

## Connective Tissue Disease

### Overview and Incidence

Connective tissue disease may manifest as a single entity or may have features of multiple autoimmune diseases. Mixed connective tissue disease (MCTD) or overlap connective tissue disease (OCTD) refers to at least two connective tissue diseases in a patient that occur at the same time or in different time frames. OCTD frequently includes overlapping features of systemic lupus erythematosus (SLE), scleroderma, or polymyositis. The incidence of this disease is unknown, but adults, particularly women, are predominantly affected.[266,174]

There is also a condition termed *undifferentiated connective tissue syndrome,* in which the clinical and serologic characteristics of multiple autoimmune diseases such RA, SLE, polymyositis, dermatomyositis, and Sjögren syndrome are present, which makes the differential diagnosis for single connective tissue disease difficult.[246]

#### Etiology and Risk Factors

The cause of OCTD is unknown, but hypotheses implicating self-antigens and infectious agents in the pathogenesis of OCTD have been proposed. Persons with this condition will frequently be found to have a specific autoantibody implicating OCTD as a single clinical entity and not necessarily a combination or mixture of other more defined rheumatic conditions.[174] Patients with this condition will have higher levels of the antibody to ribonucleoprotein, but this has not been implicated as a primary factor for developing this condition. OCTD is most commonly found in women younger than 50 years of age.

#### Clinical Manifestations

OCTD combines features of SLE (rash, Raynaud phenomenon, arthritis, arthralgia); scleroderma (swollen hands, esophageal hypomotility, pulmonary interstitial disease); polymyositis (inflammatory myositis); and, in most people, polyarthralgias. RA is present in 75% of cases. Proximal muscle weakness with or without tenderness is common.

Pulmonary, cardiac, and renal involvement as well as Sjögren syndrome, Hashimoto thyroiditis, fever, lymphadenopathy, splenomegaly, hepatomegaly, intestinal involvement, and persistent hoarseness may occur. Neurologic abnormalities including organic mental syndrome, aseptic meningitis, seizures, multiple peripheral neuropathies, and cerebral infarction or hemorrhage occur in approximately 10% of people with OCTD. A trigeminal sensory neuropathy appears to occur much more frequently in MCTD/OCTD than in other rheumatic diseases.[266]

### MEDICAL MANAGEMENT

**DIAGNOSIS, TREATMENT, AND PROGNOSIS.** The diagnosis is considered when additional overlapping features are present in persons appearing to have SLE, scleroderma, polymyositis, RA, juvenile idiopathic arthritis (JIA), Sjögren syndrome, vasculitis, idiopathic thrombocytopenic purpura, or lymphoma. High titers of serum antibodies to U1 small nuclear ribonucleoprotein 70 kDa are a characteristic serologic finding seen much more often with OCTD than with any other rheumatic disease.

General medical management and drug therapy are similar to the approach used in SLE. Most persons are responsive to immunosuppression with corticosteroids, especially if administered early in the course of the disease. Mild disease often is controlled by salicylates, other NSAIDs, antimalarials, or very low doses of corticosteroids. High doses of steroids may be used in combination with cytotoxic drugs when the disease is progressive and widespread. People with this condition should be encouraged to develop regular exercise habits and participate in an active lifestyle.[266,174]

The overall mortality has been reported as 13%, with the mean disease duration varying from 6 to 12 years. Individuals who respond well to steroid therapy have a good prognosis. Pulmonary and cardiac complications (e.g., pulmonary hypertension) are the most common cause of death in MCTD.

## Polymyalgia Rheumatica

#### Overview

Polymyalgia rheumatica (PMR) is a disorder marked by diffuse pain and stiffness in multiple muscle groups that primarily affects the shoulder and pelvic girdle musculature. This condition is significant in that diagnosis is difficult and often delayed; severe disability can occur unless proper intervention is initiated. PMR may be the first manifestation of a condition called giant cell arteritis, an endocrine disorder, malignancy, or an infection.[134]

The initial symptoms associated with PMR are often subtle and of gradual onset, resulting in the person delaying in seeking care. The symptoms also may be localized to one shoulder, leading to an initial diagnosis of a localized orthopedic condition such as bursitis. As the disease progresses, carrying out ADLs becomes increasingly difficult. Bed mobility and sit-to-stand transfers are among the functional activities affected.

Finally, a significant number (15% to 20%) of people with PMR also develop giant cell arteritis, a condition characterized by inflammation in the arteries of the head and neck. The risk related to giant cell arteritis is blindness, secondary to obstruction of the ciliary and ophthalmic arteries from inflammation-associated swelling.[197]

#### Incidence and Risk Factors

Female gender, age, and race are the three primary risk factors associated with PMR. Women are affected twice as often as men, and the disease is rare before age 50 years; most cases occur after age 70 years. White women are more commonly affected than women of other ethnicities. PMR is a relatively common condition, with incidence estimated at 1 in 200 for the general population.[361]

#### Etiologic Factors and Pathogenesis

The cause of PMR is unknown, but genetic factors, infection, or an autoimmune malfunction may play a role. There is a genetic predisposition for individuals with the immune system genetic marker HLA-DR4. Tumor necrosis factor (TNF) appears to influence susceptibility to both PMR and giant cell arteritis.[134]

Despite complaints of pain and stiffness in the muscles, PMR is not associated with any histologic abnormalities. Serum creatinine kinase levels, electromyograms, and muscle biopsy results are negative in this population. Rather, the aching and stiffness typical of this condition are caused by joint inflammation.[361]

A number of imaging studies can be used to image the effects of this condition, with ultrasound and scintigraphy the most promising techniques. Magnetic resonance imaging (MRI) studies show that subacromial and subdeltoid bursitis of the shoulders, iliopectineal bursitis, and hip synovitis are the predominant and most frequently observed lesions in active PMR.[47] The inflammation of the bursa associated with glenohumeral synovitis, bicipital tenosynovitis, and hip synovitis may explain the diffuse discomfort and morning stiffness.

### Clinical Manifestations

PMR may begin gradually, taking days or weeks for symptoms to become fully evident, but more often it develops suddenly, and the person wakes up one morning feeling stiff and sore for no apparent reason. Getting out of bed in the morning can be the biggest challenge for individuals with PMR before initiating drug therapy.

Even though the initial muscle pain and stiffness may occur unilaterally, the symptoms are often bilateral and symmetric, affecting the neck, sternoclavicular joints, shoulders, hips, low back, and buttocks. Painful stiffness lasts more than 1 hour in the morning on arising and is a hallmark feature of this disorder. Flu-like symptoms such as fever, malaise, and weight loss are not uncommon.[134]

Peripheral manifestations (e.g., wrists or metacarpophalangeal joints) are present in approximately 50% of all cases of PMR and include joint synovitis, diffuse swelling of the distal extremities with or without pitting edema, tenosynovitis, and carpal tunnel syndrome. Many people are misdiagnosed with fibromyalgia, myositis, tendinitis, thyroid problems, or depression and spend months searching for answers and help before the correct diagnosis is made.

Despite difficulties with bed mobility, sit-to-stand maneuvers, and accomplishing ADLs such as combing the hair or brushing the teeth, muscle weakness is not the problem. Pain and stiffness are the primary issues. Local tenderness of the involved muscles is noted with palpation. In addition, fever, malaise, unexplained weight loss, and depression may occur.[134]

The person may be anemic and present with an elevated erythrocyte sedimentation rate (ESR) (measure of viscosity); lowered hemoglobin and elevated platelet count (indicators of inflammation); and elevated C-reactive protein (indicator of current disease activity).[248]

For individuals with concomitant giant cell arteritis, additional symptoms of headache, jaw pain, scalp tenderness, fever, fatigue, weight loss, anemia, or blurred or double vision can occur.

## MEDICAL MANAGEMENT

**DIAGNOSIS.** Because there are no definitive tests to identify PMR, the diagnosis is often based on the presence of a constellation of findings and the person's rapid response to a trial of prednisone.

The current diagnostic criteria include as a requirement an ESR higher than 30 or 40 mm/h.[248] However, several reports indicate that a large number of people with PMR (7% to 22%) have a normal or slightly increased ESR at the time of diagnosis, supporting the notion that an increased ESR should not be an absolute requirement for the diagnosis of PMR. This subset is characterized by younger age, less marked predominance of females, lower frequency of constitutional symptoms (e.g., weight loss, fever), and a longer diagnostic delay.[230]

The lack of rheumatoid factor, the presence of antinuclear antibodies, and the lack of histologic changes in the muscles contribute to the diagnosis by excluding other conditions. MRI or ultrasonography of the joint or joints may facilitate diagnosis in individuals with typical proximal symptoms of PMR who also have normal ESR values.[248]

**TREATMENT AND PROGNOSIS.** Untreated, PMR can result in significant disability. It is imperative that the individual be checked for giant cell arteritis, a frequently concurrent condition that can cause irreversible blindness. Treatment is with corticosteroids (e.g., prednisone); the response is dramatic. In fact, if dramatic improvement is not noted within 1 week of starting the prednisone, the diagnosis of PMR is questioned, and the person must be reevaluated.

The slow tapering of prednisone dosage, the rate of which is based on clinical symptoms and some laboratory parameters, begins 2 to 4 weeks after symptoms are controlled. Most people require a maintenance dosage of prednisone for 6 months to 3 years that is gradually tapered to the lowest effective dose required to control symptoms. Treatment may take up to 5 years or longer before complete clinical remission occurs.[345] Methotrexate (MTX) is not as effective as steroids but may be used for or in combination with corticosteroids for individuals who develop a dependency on corticosteroids to decrease the corticosteroid load.

PMR is not life threatening, but it can limit daily activities, decrease restful sleep with nighttime awakenings and difficulty turning in bed, and decrease a sense of well-being and quality of life. With proper treatment, the prognosis is good, as the disease is self-limiting in many people with resolution within a period of 1.5 to 2 years; however, recurrence can be as high as 30% in people who received treatment for 1 to 2 years. Individuals with temporal arteritis are at increased risk for stroke or blindness.[134]

**SPECIAL IMPLICATIONS FOR THE THERAPIST 27.3**

### *Polymyalgia Rheumatica*

When treating someone with a history of PMR, the therapist must be aware of the potential risk of giant cell or temporal arteritis. An adult older than age 65 years with sudden onset of temporal headaches, exquisite tenderness over the temporal artery, scalp sensitivity, or visual complaints should be seen by a physician immediately, as this vasculitis is associated with stroke and blindness.[345]

Increased complaints of muscle pain and stiffness should direct the therapist to ask if the client is still taking the prednisone as directed. Because of the dramatic relief obtained with prednisone, clients may quit taking it prematurely. Careful monitoring of the dosage level is necessary for proper tapering of the medication. Communication with the primary physician is warranted in this situation.

Potential side effects of prednisone include weight gain, mood swings, cataracts, glaucoma, diabetes, easy bruising, rounding of the face, difficulty sleeping, and hypertension. Side effects are less likely to occur at low doses; any of these side effects must be evaluated by the physician. Accelerated bone loss and compression fractures are important concerns. The therapist can be very instrumental in client education about preserving bone strength through the use of calcium, vitamin D, and exercise (see Osteopenia and Osteoporosis in Chapter 24).

Because PMR is an inflammatory response involving bursitis and tenosynovitis, therapy intervention can begin with this pathogenesis in mind. For example, the use of ultrasound as a deep heating agent in the presence of inflammation should be reconsidered when approaching this type of problem.[247]

Box 27.2
**CAUSES OF RHABDOMYOLYSIS**

*Physical*

- Prolonged high fever; hyperthermia
- Electrical current (electrical and lightning injuries)
- Excessive physical exertion (push-ups, cycling, marathon running)

*Mechanical*

- Crush injury
- Burns (including electrical injuries)
- Compression (e.g., tourniquet left on too long)
- Compartment syndrome

*Chemical*

- Medications (e.g., antibiotics, statins, first-generation $H_1$-receptor antagonists)
- Herbal supplements containing ephedra (rare)
- Excessive alcohol use
- Electrolyte abnormalities
- Infections
- Endocrine disorders
- Heritable muscle enzyme deficiencies
- Mushroom poisoning (rare)

## Rhabdomyolysis

### Overview and Definition

Rhabdomyolysis is the rapid breakdown of skeletal muscle tissue as a consequence of a mechanical, physical, or chemical traumatic injury (Box 27.2). The injury results in a large release of the creatine phosphokinase enzymes, myoglobin, and other cell by-products into the blood system. Accumulation of these muscle breakdown products can lead to acute renal failure.[284]

### Etiology and Risk Factors

Strenuous exercise including marathon running, biking, and exercises such as push-ups, sit-ups, and pull-ups can result in damage to skeletal muscle cells, a process known as exertional rhabdomyolysis. Rhabdomyolysis also has been reported in performance athletes taking herbal supplements containing ephedra and weight-loss herbal supplements.[229] Underlying neuromuscular diseases may become clinically apparent during statin therapy and may predispose to myotoxicity.

Rhabdomyolysis can also result as a side effect from high-dose statins (cholesterol-lowering medications).[338] The exact mechanism for statin-induced rhabdomyolysis is unknown. There may be a drug influence on DNA, an enzyme deficiency, or autoimmune reaction triggered by the drug. Less than 5% of adults who take statins develop this problem. However, with more than 15 million Americans taking these drugs, the prevalence is on the rise.[339]

### Clinical Manifestations

People with exertional rhabdomyolysis will report excessive fatigue and inability to recover from a strenuous event. The individual may report muscle pain (myalgia) and weakness ranging from mild to severe. Individuals who report a change in color of the urine, most often tea colored or the color of cola soft drinks, should be immediately referred to an emergency department.[284]

The therapist is most likely to encounter this condition in military recruits or marathon runners who have been exercising in hot and humid weather or individuals who have taken analgesics, had a viral or bacterial infection, and/or have a preexisting condition.[72] Acute excessive consumption of alcohol exacerbated by a hot environment and dehydration can also predispose individuals competing in athletic events to exercise-induced rhabdomyolysis.

Massive skeletal muscle necrosis can also occur, further complicating the situation with reduced plasma volumes leading to shock and reduced blood flow to the kidneys resulting in acute renal failure. As the injured muscle leaks potassium, hyperkalemia may cause fatal disruptions in heart rhythm.

## MEDICAL MANAGEMENT

**DIAGNOSIS, TREATMENT, AND PROGNOSIS.** The diagnosis is typically made by history and clinical presentation and confirmed by laboratory studies when abnormal renal function and elevated creatine phosphokinase are observed. To distinguish the causes, a careful medication history is useful. Often the diagnosis is suspected when a urine dipstick test is positive for blood, but no cells are seen on microscopic analysis. This suggests myoglobinuria and usually prompts a blood sample for serum creatine phosphokinase, which confirms the diagnosis.[269]

Treatment is directed toward rehydration and correction of electrolyte imbalances by administering intravenous fluids; in the case of renal failure, dialysis may be necessary. In most cases of rhabdomyolysis, especially in cases of exertional rhabdomyolysis, damage to skeletal muscle cells resolves without consequence. Clinically significant rhabdomyolysis is uncommon but can be life threatening when present.[269]

SPECIAL IMPLICATIONS FOR THE THERAPIST 27.4

### *Rhabdomyolysis*

Patients with a history of exertional rhabdomyolysis should be cautioned regarding participation in extreme exertional activities and events. Hydration and electrolyte replacement during training and events need to be carefully planned to ensure full recovery periods. A risk assessment based on the patient's family and medical history should be done as part of a return-to-sport plan.[21]

Recovery from statin-induced rhabdomyolysis occurs with cessation of the medication, but there may be some evidence that muscle training can speed up the recovery process. The presence of peripheral rhabdomyolysis should prompt the therapist to assess the individual for impaired muscle performance, especially proximal muscle weakness including the inspiratory muscles. Changes in cardiorespiratory function in individuals taking statins and presenting with muscle weakness anywhere in the body should be investigated more closely.[339]

Box 27.3

**CLASSIFICATION OF MYOPATHIES**

***Hereditary***

- Muscular dystrophy
- Congenital myopathy
- Myotonia
- Metabolic myopathy
- Mitochondrial myopathy (e.g., zidovudine [AZT] myopathy [rare])
- Neurologic (e.g., Charcot-Marie-Tooth disease)

***Acquired***

- Inflammatory myopathy
  - Idiopathic
  - Dermatomyositis, polymyositis
  - Rheumatoid arthritis
  - Autoimmune diseases
  - HIV-associated myopathy
- Endocrine myopathy
  - Diabetes mellitus
  - Thyroid disease
- Myopathy associated with systemic illness
  - Renal impairment
  - Cancer
  - Acute lung injury
  - Acute respiratory distress syndrome
  - Septic inflammatory response syndrome
- Drug-induced or toxic myopathy
  - Corticosteroids
  - Alcohol
  - Statins (cholesterol-lowering drugs)

Data from Goldman L, Schafer AI. *Goldman's Cecil medicine, expert consult premium edition*, ed 24, Philadelphia, 2011, Saunders; and McDonald CM: Myopathic disorders. In Braddom R, editor: *Physical medicine and rehabilitation*, ed 4, St. Louis, 2012, Elsevier.

# Myopathy

## Definition and Overview

*Myopathy* is a term used to describe nonspecific muscle weakness secondary to an identifiable disease or condition. The term *myositis* is also used to describe idiopathic inflammatory myopathies. Many metabolic and hormonal diseases and autoimmune diseases can cause muscle weakness.[226] Myopathies are usually classified as either hereditary or acquired (Box 27.3).

The disorder *critical illness myopathy (CIM)* is associated with prolonged stays in intensive care units (ICUs). CIM is a nonnecrotizing myopathy accompanied by fiber atrophy, fatty degeneration of muscle fibers, and fibrosis. As improvements in medical technology and medical management of patients with severe illness continue to occur, the incidence of CIM is expected to rise.[108]

Myopathy (myositis) associated with infectious causes is mentioned briefly in Chapter 25. Information about other sources of muscle pain not discussed in this chapter and their neurophysiologic basis is also available.

## Etiologic Factors and Pathogenesis

Idiopathic inflammatory myopathies are thought to be immune-mediated processes that are triggered by environmental factors in genetically susceptible individuals. The pathogenesis of acquired myopathies and their course are highly variable and depend on the underlying cause. For example, in thyrotoxicosis, the high metabolic rate reduces the muscle stores of nutrients, whereas in hypothyroidism, the entire metabolism, including the energy-generating metabolism of muscles, is slowed down. Expression of proinflammatory cytokines such as interleukin (IL)-1 on endothelial cells and expression of major histocompatibility complex class I antigens on muscle fibers are associated with muscle weakness in individuals with active and chronic disease.[226]

Diabetes is associated with myopathy of three origins: vascular, neurogenic, and metabolic. Diabetes affects the small blood vessels and is associated with chronic hypoperfusion of muscles with blood. Diabetes also affects the peripheral nerves and causes neurogenic muscle atrophy and weakness. The disturbances of carbohydrate and lipid metabolism caused by insulin deficiency or insulin resistance adversely affect muscle function.[243] Acquired myopathy can also occur as part of a paraneoplastic syndrome (see discussion in Chapter 9). Tumors may produce muscle weakness with or without inflammation.

Medications such as the cholesterol-lowering statins are associated with tendinitis and muscle abnormalities. Use of systemic corticosteroids combined with prolonged exposure to neuromuscular blocking (paralytic) agents during the treatment of various critical illnesses in the ICU mentioned above may be the key risk factor for this type of acute myopathy. Septic inflammatory response syndrome may be another risk factor.[108]

## Clinical Manifestations

Myopathy is characterized by progressive proximal muscle weakness with varying degrees of pain and tenderness. Distal involvement is possible but is more common with myositis. During the early stages of disease, the muscles may be acutely inflamed and painful to move and touch. Muscle weakness and easy fatigability eventually compromise aerobic capacity and affect the person's endurance and ability to work, socialize, and complete ADLs. Other symptoms of systemic illness may be present, including fever, fatigue, morning stiffness, and anorexia.[226] Statin-induced myopathy can produce respiratory myopathy with impaired inspiratory muscle performance characterized by fatigue, muscle pain, and weakness.[55]

## MEDICAL MANAGEMENT

DIAGNOSIS. The management of myopathy is determined by the underlying cause. Muscle biopsy, electromyography, and laboratory findings (measurement of muscle enzymes) are essential to ensure diagnostic accuracy, especially in the case of idiopathic myopathy. Electromyography can allow differentiation between myopathy and neuropathy and can localize the site of the neuropathic condition. The typical laboratory profile reveals mild to marked elevations in muscle enzymes, including creatine kinase and aldolase.[226,209]

Some imaging techniques of muscles such as MRI and magnetic resonance spectroscopy can assess changes in local inflammatory activity.[114] Changes in protein and gene expression patterns in repeated biopsy specimens provide molecular information that may lead to a more precise disease classification scheme and improved treatment, but these are research tools at this time.

**TREATMENT AND PROGNOSIS.** Inflammatory myopathies may respond to pharmacologic treatment, especially corticosteroids but also immunosuppressives and antimalarial agents. Oral creatine supplements combined with exercise have proven effective for improving muscle function without adverse effects in adults with inflammatory myopathies.[68]

Prognosis is variable, with some people responding well to medical therapy and rehabilitation and others continuing to decline. Long-standing disability is not uncommon despite aggressive immunosuppressive treatment; the reasons for the persisting disability are unknown. Additionally, corticosteroid-related complications can have a significant impact.

Factors associated with poor survival include onset after age 45 years, delayed diagnosis and intervention, severe weakness and pharyngeal dysphagia, malignancy, myocardial involvement, and interstitial lung disease.[228] CIM is reversible, but there is often considerable morbidity (e.g., persistent pain and weakness, HO with frozen joints). ICU-acquired myopathy prolongs hospitalization because of the need for extensive rehabilitation. Even with rehabilitation, many affected individuals remain heavily dependent on others for personal care and ADLs.[108]

SPECIAL IMPLICATIONS FOR THE THERAPIST 27.5

## *Myopathy*

Reduced muscle strength, endurance, and coordination accompanied by fatigue are commonly reported with myopathies. Myalgia occurs at rest and with exercise in one-half or more of all affected individuals in all stages of the disease. Left untreated, most cases of muscle weakness associated with inflammatory myopathies progress slowly over months and result in further decline of muscle strength and endurance.[14] Limited evidence is available to guide decision making for patients with critical illness myopathy.[240]

### Acute Care

Therapists in the acute care setting frequently see the effects of bed rest, even without associated injury and after only as little as 1 week, as disuse atrophy causes decrease in muscle mass. Often this occurs in the older adult population who have already experienced significant decline in muscle mass.[241] The effects of ICU-acquired myopathy are even more pronounced in persons who are both on bed rest and critically ill. CIM is also often accompanied by critical illness polyneuropathy, a disorder of the peripheral nerves triggered by the same events as CIM.

Patients with the combination of these two conditions have difficulty weaning from the ventilator. Once the individual is alert and less sedated, weakness and atrophy of the limbs becomes more readily apparent. Severe flaccid tetraparesis may even be observed. Muscles innervated by the cranial nerves appear to be spared. Whereas critical illness polyneuropathy can affect all limbs and muscle groups, distal weakness and sensory changes are more common. CIM typically affects larger, more proximal muscle groups; sensation is not impaired.[38]

Recovery can be delayed by weeks to months. Further details regarding intervention and prognosis are available in Chapter 5. The therapist is a key member of the rehabilitation team, recognizing the need for psychologic and emotional support of the patient and the family. Understanding that the patient is not just deconditioned and has a complex pathologic condition can help facilitate appropriate referrals to other disciplines (e.g., occupational therapy, psychology, social work, physiatry, speech pathology).

### Exercise and Myopathy

Early rehabilitation is important in the course of myopathy, with careful application of rest and exercise (rest during the active inflammatory phase; rebuilding of muscle strength during remission). During periods of severe inflammation, bed rest and passive range of motion are recommended; active range-of-motion exercises are contraindicated.[85]

It is important to design a rehabilitation program according to the type, stage, and severity of myopathy. Muscle assessment and functional evaluation are prerequisites to determining an appropriate intervention program. In extremely acute cases, a tilt table may be necessary to reacclimatize the cardiovascular system and assist with balance training in individuals who have been on bed rest.

The exercise program begins in the acute phase with stretching and passive range of motion and progresses throughout the recovery process according to the person's tolerance to include isometric, isotonic, and low-intensity aerobic activities. Moist heat applied before stretching inflamed or sore muscles may be helpful. Performing exercises in a gravity-eliminated environment (aquatic program) or gravity-eliminated position may be necessary in the beginning.[160] Attention to the muscles of respiration and breathing assessment are also important, and a patient with cardiac involvement must be evaluated before initiating an aerobic program.

Concern about stressing the already inflamed muscles with a resultant increase in creatine phosphokinase level has traditionally prevented the use of strengthening exercises in individuals with inflammatory myopathies. However, exercise itself can cause elevated serum creatine kinase levels in healthy individuals, and studies have shown that people with stable active disease can perform isometric exercise without causing a sustained rise in creatine phosphokinase level.[13]

The effects of exercise training on inflammatory myopathies have determined the potential role of exercise as a method for lowering systemic inflammation markers.[251] Studies show improvement in adults with stable myopathies after a 12-week program of 20 minutes of home exercise combined with 15 minutes of walking 5 days per week. Improvement was measured as reduced impairment and reduced activity limitation/participation restriction.[12]

Similar results have been reported for individuals with active myopathies performing an intensive resistive exercise program.[11] People in a variety of exercise programs including stair climbing, stationary cycling, strength training, group exercise in a pool or at a gym, and outdoor walking using a wide range of frequency, intensity, and duration have shown improvement in fatigue and aerobic fitness while serum creatine kinase levels remain unchanged.[14] Experts advise a general recommendation of daily physical activity for 30 minutes 5 to 7 days each week. Supervised continuous aquatic exercise adapted to the individual's disease level and disability is also recommended.[14]

A home program, including heat modalities, prescriptive exercise, and assistive devices, assists the individual to manage with functional disability. Upper extremity splinting and lower extremity bracing may be necessary to prevent contractures, prolong mobility, and enhance functional skills. A weak quadriceps mechanism combined with footdrop or a shuffling gait can contribute to increased falls, necessitating an assessment of muscle strength and balance, and risk for falls with necessary intervention.

Client education about this condition is important and should include energy conservation and joint protection. Serious side effects can accompany high-dose corticosteroid therapy, compounding the functional difficulties already present with the myopathy.

## Myofascial Pain Syndrome

### Overview

Myofascial pain syndrome (MPS) and trigger points (TrPs) have been described for centuries, but they are not always recognized or even acknowledged as a valid pathology or clinical entity other than by pain management specialists. Travell and Simons are credited with conceptualizing TrPs in an organized and coherent manner starting in the 1950s.[179] The recent surge in interest in dry needling as a treatment technique of TrPs has increased awareness among clinicians. TrPs have been described concomitant with other pain diagnoses, such as fibromyalgia, arthritis, migraines and tension-type headaches, epicondylalgia and carpal tunnel syndrome, shoulder problems including subacromial pain syndrome, pelvic pain conditions, and whiplash injuries, among others. The most broadly accepted definition describes TrPs as "hyperirritable spots in a taut band of a skeletal muscle that is painful on compression, stretch, overload or contraction of the tissue, which usually responds with a referred pain that is perceived distant from the spot."[179] When Travell, who was a cardiologist and pharmacologist at Cornell University, started exploring muscle referred pain, she realized that skeletal muscles often harbor TrPs with typical referred pain patterns. In just a few years, she shifted her attention from cardiology to muscle pain and dysfunction. In 1952, she published common referred pain patterns for 32 muscles and their TrPs.[340] Clinically, referred pain phenomena can be confusing for clinicians and patients, as the location of the pain symptom usually does not match the source of the pain; for example, pain in the medial aspect of the patella and knee may be due to TrPs in the adductor longus or psoas major muscles, and retroorbital headaches may originate in TrPs in the sternocleidomastoid or trapezius muscle.

TrPs are classified as active when they cause spontaneous local and referred pain and as latent when they cause pain only on stimulation. Active TrPs are more sensitized, feature more endplate noise, involve a greater area of a muscle, and have a significantly altered chemical milieu and significantly lower pain thresholds with electrical stimulation in the muscle and the overlying cutaneous and subcutaneous tissues than latent TrPs and non-TrP muscle tissue.[97] Nevertheless, research has confirmed that latent TrPs also provide nociceptive input into the dorsal horn even though they are not spontaneously painful. Whether a TrP is considered active or latent depends at least partially on the degree of sensitization. It is often assumed that TrPs represent strictly local muscle phenomena, but it is now known that TrPs are peripheral sources of persistent nociceptive input, leading to peripheral and central sensitization and primary and secondary hyperalgesia, also known as referred pain.[113,100] Both active and latent TrPs can cause allodynia and primary and secondary hyperalgesia, which implies that afferent fibers from TrP nociceptors can make new effective connections with dorsal horn neurons that normally process information only from remote body regions. Recently, 60 experts in MPS from 12 different countries agreed that the preferred term is *referred sensation*.[112] Several recent studies have confirmed that the interrater reliability of identifying TrPs ranges from moderate to excellent, depending on the muscle.[236,83]

### Etiologic and Risk Factors

TrPs have been reported in all age groups except infants. There is evolving evidence that they develop following various forms of muscle overload, including unaccustomed eccentric and concentric loading, as well as with low-load repetitive tasks and sustained postures.[128] In addition to mechanical overload, TrPs may develop in association with visceral pain and dysfunction, such as endometriosis, interstitial cystitis, irritable bowel syndrome, and prostadynia; with psychologic or emotional conditions; or even with respiratory stress such as overbreathing, or hyperventilation.[97] In other words, any sustained or repetitive activity may contribute to TrPs. According to Travell, mechanical and structural factors, including anatomic variations such as forward head posture, significant leg-length deficiencies, or scoliosis that impact or overload muscles must be identified, resolved, or alleviated.[179] In the current thinking, such mechanical factors are not always considered as relevant. The attention has shifted more toward biopsychosocial factors.

### Pathogenesis

The formation of TrPs follows the development of contractured muscle fibers, commonly referred to as a "taut band," which is not always painful. The exact mechanisms of the formation of taut bands and TrP remain enigmatic but are thought to be the result of an excessive nonquantal release of acetylcholine (ACh) at the motor endplate combined with an inhibition of acetylcholine esterase (AChE) and an upregulation of nicotinic acetylcholine receptors.[128] This local endplate dysfunction does not require an electrical activation of the α-motor neuron, as demonstrated in multiple human and animal studies. The excessive release of ACh can be attributed to a wide variety of possible causes, including an insufficiency of AChE, an acidic pH, hypoxia, a lack of adenosine phosphate, certain genetic mutations, and particular chemicals such as calcitonin gene-related peptide (CGRP).[128,239,98] Injections with botulinum toxin, which blocks the release of ACh and CGRP from presynaptic cholinergic nerve endings, are often effective in deactivating TrPs. The abnormal spontaneous release of ACh correlates with the occurrence of endplate noise, which is now considered a gold standard in TrP research.[110] Of particular interest is that dry needling of TrPs can also decrease ACh levels, reduce the sensitivity of acetylcholine receptors, and increase the concentrations of AChE in rats.[216]

The development of TrPs is best expressed in the *integrated TrP hypothesis* originally developed by Simons, Travell, and Simons and frequently updated based on emerging research and new evidence.[179,128,239,181] According to the integrated TrP hypothesis, abnormal depolarization of the postjunctional membrane of motor endplates causes a localized hypoxic energy crisis associated with sensory and autonomic reflex arcs that are sustained by complex sensitization mechanisms.[179,239] Low oxygen levels immediately reduce the pH of the tissue. In the immediate vicinity of active TrPs the pH can be as low as 4.5, which is far below the level required to excite and activate pH-sensitive transient receptor potential vanilloid receptors and acid-sensing ion channels, among many others. These receptors play an important role in initiating and maintaining central sensitization and hyperalgesia. An acidic pH inhibits AChE but stimulates the release of adenosine triphosphate (ATP) and bradykinin, which is one of the many chemicals found in the immediate vicinity of active TrPs, along with TNF-α, ILs, serotonin, norepinephrine, bradykinin, substance P, and CGRP. There are many positive feedback links between these chemicals. The combination of ATP and a low pH increase the pH sensitivity of the ASIC3 receptor. The chemicals found near active TrPs not only sensitize and activate muscle nociceptors but also can activate microglia cells.[100,110]

Nociceptors are dynamic structures that can be modified depending on the local tissue environment. They play an active role in the maintenance of normal tissue homeostasis by sensing the peripheral biochemical milieu and by mediating the vascular supply to peripheral tissue. Nociceptive input from muscles is particularly effective in inducing neuroplastic changes in the dorsal horn and is partially responsible for the referred pain phenomena associated with TrPs. The mechanisms of TrP referred pain have been described in detail and involve an expansion of the receptive fields of spinal neurons and sensitization.[100,98,110]

TrPs can also develop with low-level submaximal contractions, for example, in the upper trapezius muscles of computer operators or in the forearm muscles of musicians, which is best explained with the Cinderella hypothesis.[132] With low-level muscle contractions, smaller motor units are recruited before and de-recruited after larger motor units, which means that smaller type 1 fibers are continuously activated. This can lead to muscle fiber degeneration, an increase in $Ca^{2+}$ release, energy depletion, and the release of various cytokines, which were found near active TrPs.[98]

Jafri[181] expanded on the integrated TrP hypothesis incorporating the role of reactive oxygen species (ROS). His hypothesis centers on the excessive release of $Ca^{2+}$ in muscles through the process of X-ROS signaling. During mechanical stress of the microtubule network, as in muscle overload, there is an activation of nicotinamide adenine dinucleotide phosphate oxidase 2 (NOX2), which produces ROS. As a result, ROS oxidizes ryanodine receptors, leading to an increased release of $Ca^{2+}$ from the sarcoplasmic reticulum.[100,98,181] In skeletal muscle, this process sensitizes $Ca^{2+}$-permeable sarcolemmal transient receptor potential, which may be a source of nociceptive input and inflammatory pain. Expanding on this hypothesis, Gerwin and Shannon[286] postulated that dysfunctional ATP-sensitive sodium channels ($K_{ATP}$ receptor channels) may influence the influx of $Ca^{2+}$ and formation of ROS. Excessive ACh concentrations may not be the only mechanism leading to intense sarcomere contractures.

### Clinical Manifestations

Clinically a detailed history and physical examination are required. The clinician needs to explore the occurrence of possible precipitating events, habits, or activities that may have caused muscle overload. Knowledge of typical referred pain patterns is necessary to link the history to clinically relevant TrPs, as the location of the pain symptom rarely matches the location of the responsible TrPs. The term *referred pain* should be interpreted broadly, as this term encompasses not only pain but also other paresthesias, such as tingling, burning, and numbness.[112] The history taking should also consider the presence of muscle pain and TrPs secondary to visceral pathology. The physical examination needs to include a biomechanical assessment with appreciation of which muscles could potentially be subjected to repetitive or sustained overload and an assessment of any compensatory movement strategies. Unusual asymmetries and abnormal breathing patterns should be noted. Range of motion of clinically relevant joints must be assessed before and after TrP inactivation. It is common to see an immediate improvement in range of motion, muscle strength, movement coordination, and pain levels. Palpation of relevant muscles is the last step in the process and starts with the identification of the taut bands, after which this taut band is further assessed for the presence of TrPs. They are usually painful to touch, and palpation often results in verbal reactions, body movements, and recognition by the patient of the familiar pain symptom. TrPs can restrict range of motion, alter movement activation patterns, cause local and referred pain, and cause weakness, which perhaps is better classified as inhibitory patterns without signs of atrophy.[100]

## MEDICAL MANAGEMENT

In general, myofascial pain is recognized as a legitimate clinical entity with a degree of consensus among expert clinicians and researchers despite a lack of uniformly accepted diagnostic criteria.[112,45,127,169,249] The most relevant criteria for the identification of TrPs include the presence of a taut band in a relevant muscle, the presence of a TrP in that band, and referred pain.[112] The medical diagnosis is made based on history and physical examination. The problem may be confined to just a few muscles or may be more widespread, regional, or generalized. Although taut bands and TrPs can be visualized with MRI and sonoelastography, these tests have no clinical utility at the present time. TrPs can be located and treated with shockwave technology, but owing to the high costs, few clinicians use shockwave therapy in the diagnosis and management of myofascial pain.

Clinicians should evaluate patients for any possible underlying causes or contributing factors, such as structural or mechanical perpetuating factors; localized or widespread joint hypermobility (i.e., classical or hypermobile-type Ehlers-Danlos syndrome, Marfan syndrome, and hypermobility spectrum disorders); and nutritional, metabolic, or systemic perpetuating factors. Some of the factors impair the ability of muscles to respond appropriately to common stressors, leading to overload issues.[285] Although randomized controlled double-blind studies and even epidemiologic correlational studies verifying the clinical observations that certain metabolic and nutritional factors are relevant in the treatment of patients with myofascial pain are lacking, clinical observations are part of the accepted hierarchy of evidence-based medicine and should be considered. The most common metabolic and hormonal factors in myofascial pain are hypothyroidism; gonadal hormone conditions; other hormonal imbalances; protozoal infestations (i.e., amebiasis, fascioliasis, and giardiasis, among others); and iron, magnesium, vitamin $B_{12}$, vitamin D, estrogen, and testosterone insufficiencies or deficiencies.[285] Possible side effects of medications, such as statin drugs, may include widespread myalgias.[99] Physical therapists, occupational therapists, and other clinicians need to be familiar with the most common perpetuating factors and communicate with patients' physicians when they suspect any underlying problems.

**TREATMENT.** The medical management must include addressing any contributing and perpetuating factors and possible comorbidities based on common differential diagnostic considerations. Pain, depression, anxiety, and poor sleep hygiene must be addressed using contemporary approaches, including pharmacologic interventions. As many patients with persistent pain have poor sleep hygiene, sleep studies may be needed. Referral to other health care providers may be indicated, including physical therapists, cognitive-behavioral psychologists, or clinical social workers.

**PROGNOSIS.** The prognosis of myofascial pain is directly related to clinicians' awareness of the current scientific literature and their training and experience. Well-trained health care providers are able to provide effective treatments, inactivate TrPs, and return patients to full functional status. Unfortunately, few medical and physical therapy schools include extensive course work in myofascial pain and TrPs in their curricula.

**SPECIAL IMPLICATIONS FOR THE THERAPIST 27.6**

### *Myofascial Pain Syndrome*

When properly identified, TrPs can be treated very effectively with manual techniques, dry needling, and injections as part of a comprehensive management strategy.[97] Perpetuating factors must be addressed.[349] Of particular interest during these techniques is the phenomenon of a local twitch response (LTR). The LTR is a localized spinal cord reflex of muscle fibers in a taut band. Eliciting LTRs is an important component of inactivating TrPs, as it has been positively correlated with decreasing endplate noise and the concentration of inflammatory mediators. From a clinical perspective, eliciting LTRs produces superior patient outcomes.[100]

There is some evidence that laser, high-power ultrasound, and some electrotherapy modalities may be useful, but not all studies support this. Conventional ultrasound had only a temporary antinociceptive effect. Many patients with MPS present with inadequate posture, including forward head posture, which must be addressed through education and proprioceptive training.[117] Physical therapists can also contribute to improved sleep patterns. Once pain levels are reduced and TrPs have been inactivated, physical therapy should include common treatment interventions, such as strengthening, flexibility, and cardiovascular conditioning, among others.

**A THERAPIST'S THOUGHTS**

Although the textbooks by Simons, Travell, and Simons are among the best sold medical texts in the world with translations in many languages, it is striking that awareness of the existence and implications of TrPs is not widely integrated in the thought process of health care providers. Very few schools of physical therapy cover the assessment and treatment of TrPs in their curriculum, despite overwhelming scientific evidence from many different sources. The growing interest in dry needling is pushing TrPs to the foreground, but it seems that the intrigue is more focused on the "new modality" than on the evidence-informed use of it to help patients reduce or eliminate their pain and regain function. There is still strong opposition by some physical therapy groups, even though in exchanges on websites and blogs it is obvious that most opponents of TrP concepts are not familiar with the surge in scientific studies and do not really have a basis for their concerns. Some argue that "pain is produced by the brain" and that therefore a focus on muscle pain would be counterproductive. Yet, TrPs should be considered as persistent sources of peripheral nociceptive input within the context of contemporary pain sciences. It is our hope that in the near future, schools of physical therapy will seriously explore the current scientific knowledge base and incorporate TrP concepts throughout their curricula. In the end, patients and society at large will benefit from this change in direction and focus.

## Pelvic Floor Muscle Dysfunction

### Overview

The pelvic floor muscles (PFMs) are a collection of voluntary skeletal internal muscles stretching like a sling from the pubic bone to the coccyx and surrounding

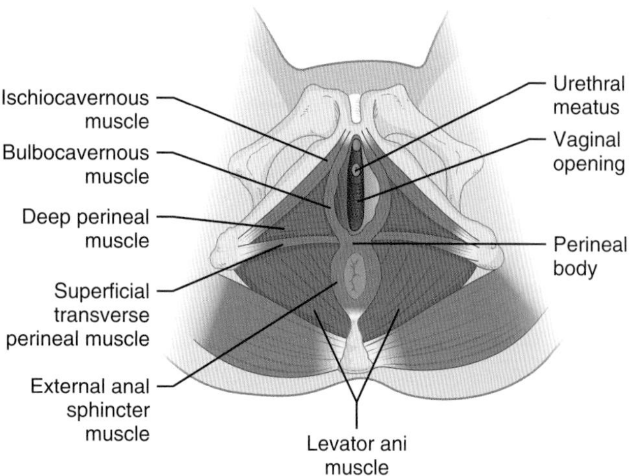


**Figure 27.1**

**Pelvic floor muscles (PFMs).** There are three layers of the PFMs from superficial to deep; the most superficial layer of the PFMs include the external anal sphincter for control of gas and feces, the sexual muscle (bulbocavernous and ischiocavernous), and the superficial transverse perineal muscles. The second layer, sometimes referred to as the *urogenital diaphragm,* includes the sphincter urethra and urethrovaginal sphincter and participates in urinary continence. (From Myers RS: *Saunders manual of physical therapy,* Philadelphia, 1995, Saunders.)

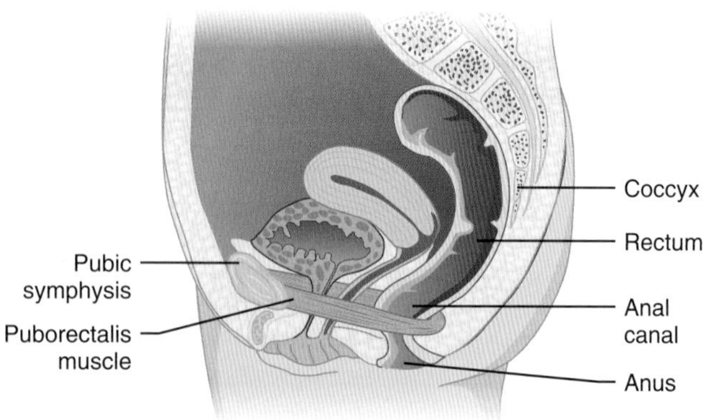


**Figure 27.2**

**Pelvic floor muscles.** The deepest layer is collectively known as the levator ani muscles. The levator ani muscle is made up of four muscles—the puborectalis, pubococcygeus, coccygeus, and ischiococcygeus muscles (not shown)—and supports the pelvic viscera in both males and females. (From Myers RS: *Saunders manual of physical therapy,* Philadelphia, 1995, Saunders.)

the vagina, urethra, and rectum (Fig. 27.1). They work together to support the internal pelvic organs and close off the urethra and rectum to maintain continence (Fig. 27.2). These muscles also participate in sexual arousal and orgasm. The nomenclature of the skeletal muscles in this area is not consistent throughout the literature.[183] In this section, PFMs refers to all the skeletal muscles of the pelvic floor.

PFM dysfunction is the specific dysfunction of the skeletal muscle layer in the pelvic floor (Table 27.1). Therapists who have expertise in skeletal muscle dysfunction have a great deal to offer individuals with these dysfunctions.

## Prevalence

The overall prevalence of PFM dysfunction is unknown, but it is considered a common problem among women of reproductive age, many of whom have never been diagnosed. Levator avulsion is associated with under activity of the PFM. Although the definition of levator avulsion is debated, one CT study reports a prevalence of 6.4%.[89] Prevalence is available for the pathologies of PFM dysfunction, such as urinary and fecal incontinence (see discussion in Chapter 18) and pelvic organ prolapse. The lack of a consensus on the definition of chronic pelvic pain and lack of a classification scheme hinder epidemiologic studies. A recent systematic review reported chronic pelvic pain prevalence in females to between 5.7% and 26.6% worldwide.[8] Although the majority of these conditions affect women, men can also be affected.

## Etiology and Pathogenesis

PFM dysfunction can be due to a number of causes; the most common etiologies are covered in this section.

*Under activity of the PFM* is reflected in decreased strength and endurance and poor PFM coordination during increased intraabdominal pressure, such as coughing and sneezing. Under activity of the PFM is associated with urinary incontinence and pelvic organ prolapse. Birth-related trauma is the most common factor in under activity of the PFM. PFM avulsion, overstretching of the muscle and connective tissue, and damage to the pudendal nerve all are implicated as possible causes of PFM weakness and loss of support. Forceps, episiotomy, and long pushing stage appear to contribute to the trauma.[89,53] See Box 27.4 for other factors that contribute to PFM dysfunction.

*Over activity of the PFM* is characterized by an increase in PFM tension, active spasm, or incoordination causing musculoskeletal pain or dysfunction of the urogenital and/or colorectal system. The pathogenesis of over activity of the PFM and chronic pelvic pain remains poorly understood, and laparoscopic investigation often reveals no obvious cause for pain. Injury to the pudendal nerve or coccyx, pelvic asymmetry, childbirth, sexual assault, or bowel/bladder dysfunction may account for some cases of chronic pelvic pain. Origin of dysfunction can be categorized as tissue-based/nociceptive or neuropathic/central sensitization. Current evidence points to the occurrence of central sensitization as the primary origin of pain in some conditions of chronic pelvic pain.[161] In these cases, there will be little tissue impairment, and treatments should be directed at the hypersensitive nervous system.

## Clinical Manifestations

Clinical manifestations of PFM dysfunction are determined by the underlying etiologic factors and pathologic findings. For example, the primary presentation of someone with under activity of the PFM can vary from urinary incontinence to perineal pressure of pelvic organ prolapse.

Clinically, individuals with over activity of the PFM present with pain, pressure, or ache, usually poorly localized in the perivaginal, perirectal, and lower abdominal quadrants and pelvis (suprapubic or coccyx regions) and sometimes radiating down the posterior aspect of the thigh. Symptoms of over activity of the PFM are often reproduced by manual palpation and examination of the

**Table 27.1** Pelvic Floor Muscle Disorders

| Name of Condition | Description | Symptoms/Diagnosis | Signs/Impairments |
|---|---|---|---|
| Normal PFM | PFM is able to contract and relax on command and in response to increased intraabdominal pressure as appropriate | Normal urinary, bowel, and sexual functioning | Normal voluntary and involuntary contraction and relaxation of PFM |
| Under activity of the PFM | PFM is unable to contract when needed | Urinary or fecal incontinence, pelvic organ prolapse | Absent or weak voluntary PFM contraction; noncontracting PFM |
| Over activity of the PFM | PFM is unable to relax and may contract during functions such as defecation or micturition | Obstructive voiding or defecation, dyspareunia, pelvic pain | Absent or incomplete voluntary PFM relaxation; nonrelaxing PFM |

*PFM*, Pelvic floor muscle.
Based on data from Haylen BT: An International Urogynecological Association (IUGA)/International Continence Society (ICS) joint report on the terminology for female pelvic floor dysfunction. *Int Urogynecol J* 21:5–26, 2010.

**Box 27.4**

**CAUSES OF PELVIC FLOOR MUSCLE DYSFUNCTION**

***Under Activity of the PFM***

- Pregnancy alone and/or birth-related trauma
- Abdominal or pelvic surgery
- Chronic increased intraabdominal pressure: obesity, chronic constipation, chronic coughing, poor exercise and lifting techniques
- Psychogenic origin
- Spinal cord injury or other neurologic condition (e.g., stroke, Parkinson disease, multiple sclerosis)

***Over Activity of the PFM***

Research has been unable to clearly identify causation. This list represents conditions that appear with or precede over activity of the PFM:

- Musculoskeletal injury or trauma (back, sacrum, sacroiliac area, hip, pelvis)
- Habitual postural dysfunction
- Fibromyalgia, chronic fatigue syndrome
- Nerve entrapment or injury, nerve root irritation
- Myofascial pain syndrome, trigger points
- Abdominal or pelvic surgery
- Childbirth trauma and episiotomy
- Pain related to rectal hemorrhoids, rectal fissures
- Psychogenic origin
- Sexual assault, sexual abuse, or negative sexual experiences
- Bowel and bladder disorders, including endometriosis, interstitial cystitis, diverticulitis, constipation, irritable bowel syndrome, regional enteritis (Crohn disease)
- Unknown cause

*PFM*, Pelvic floor muscle.

PFMs. Other symptoms of over activity of the PFM dysfunction may include low back pain that is intermittent and unpredictable, changes location often, and is difficult to reproduce; sharp, fleeting rectal pain; painful intercourse or inability to penetrate; extreme rectal pressure; and pubic bone pain or tenderness (Table 27.2).

## MEDICAL MANAGEMENT

DIAGNOSIS. Diagnosis and diagnostic testing depend on history and clinical presentation. Evaluation of PFM dysfunction involves a detailed history and documentation of symptoms; physical examination of the PFM vaginally and/or rectally; and examination of external structures of the pelvic bones, joints, and muscles.

PFM examination can include electromyography, manometery, ultrasound imaging, dynamometry, and digital palpation. Although there is some disagreement as to the reliability and reproducibility of muscle grading (absent, weak, moderate, strong), most experienced clinicians agree that digital palpation of the PFM contraction inside the vaginal canal is of great value in assessing the ability to perform a correct PFM contraction.[40] Some physicians have developed skill in diagnosis and examination of PFM dysfunction, but most physicians recognize PFM weakness or pain when screening for other pathology and disease and refer the patient to a pelvic physical therapist for more definitive examination.

PFM tenderness on vaginal/rectal palpation and a positive Patrick or FABER (flexion, abduction, external rotation) test with overpressure results in 100% specificity in identifying women with chronic pelvic pain related to musculoskeletal dysfunction, including over activity of the PFM.[254] These screening tests are suggested in an effort to correctly identify individuals with chronic pelvic pain who would benefit from a physical therapy referral. A comprehensive musculoskeletal evaluation would be performed by the physical therapist to identify specific tissue dysfunction and to develop an effective treatment plan. Comprehensive diagnosis of patients with PFM dysfunction includes testing to rule out pelvic floor organ dysfunction such as CT, MRI, laparoscopy, ultrasound, and urinalysis for infection.

TREATMENT. Specific medical intervention can be employed in cases of known and treatable causes, but more often, medical management has been limited to treatment of symptoms using pharmacologic and hormonal agents and surgical intervention, with variable results.

Physical therapy intervention is quickly becoming the first-line therapy of choice for many causes of PFM dysfunction. Working with a counselor or other skilled professional is recommended when treating someone with a past (or current) history of abuse.

Proper instruction in PFM exercise is an important part of prevention and treatment. Although the lay public refers to them as Kegel exercises, the preferred term is *PFM exercises*. Brief verbal or written instruction in performing a PFM contraction is not adequate for 14% to

**Table 27.2** Over Activity of the Pelvic Floor Muscle Diagnoses

| Name of Disorder | Brief Description and Major Symptoms |
|---|---|
| Levator ani syndrome/ tension myalgia | Pain and spasm of PFM, may also involve other local muscles such as obturator internus or piriformis. Symptoms include perianal pain and pain with sitting |
| Vaginismus | Muscle spasm of superficial and deep muscles around the vagina. Technically a psychologic diagnosis, but the physical components are becoming more recognized. Symptom is dyspareunia. This condition is difficult to distinguish from vulvodynia |
| Anismus | Muscle spasm of the superficial and deep muscles around the rectum. Symptoms include obstructed defecation and coccyx pain |
| Coccygodynia | Technically means pain in the coccyx and does not specify the origin of the pain, which is often over activity of the PFM or trigger points of the PFM. May also include sacrococcygeal joint dysfunction. Symptom is painful sitting |
| Dyspareunia | Refers to painful penetration (which could include penis, finger, speculum, tampon, or toy). Is a symptom of many other disorders |
| Vulvodynia | Refers to a large group of disorders in which perineal and vaginal pain is the major symptom. Provoked vestibulodynia is a subset of vulvodynia. Major symptoms are dyspareunia and pain during sitting |
| Pudendal neuralgia | As the name implies, disorder is related to neuralgia of the pudendal nerve possibly related to compression, especially at the sacrotuberous and sacrospinous ligament crossing. Symptoms include broad pelvic pain and pain with sitting |
| Chronic prostatitis/ chronic pelvic pain syndrome | Pain in the area of the prostate usually related to over activity of the PFM and confused with prostatitis owing to symptoms of urgency and frequency |
| Chronic pelvic pain | Continuous or intermittent pelvic pain lasting for 6 months or more. Symptoms vary and may include difficulty with sitting, walking, or other functions |
| Interstitial cystitis/ painful bladder syndrome | Pain in the area of the bladder associated with over activity of the PFM with symptoms of urgency, frequency, and pain |

*PFM*, Pelvic floor muscle.

50% of cases investigated.[155] A properly performed PFM exercise should result in a significant increase in the force of the urethral closure without an appreciable Valsalva effort. Improperly done, the PFM exercise technique can potentially promote incontinence.

The best time to explain a PFM contraction is during a pelvic examination. The medical practitioner can describe the exercise and verify that it is done correctly during digital palpation of the muscle inside the vagina or rectum. A trained practitioner such as a physical therapist can also provide follow-up assessment and training with necessary biofeedback to ensure the success of a properly performed exercise program. This may be particularly helpful in older adults, who often have a difficult time localizing pelvic muscles. Other treatments for under activity of the PFM include biofeedback, electrical stimulation, vaginal weights, facilitated exercises, and functional exercises.

Tissue-based treatments for over activity of the PFM would include joint mobilization, myofascial release, exercise and education, modalities, PFM relaxation/biofeedback, and vaginal/rectal dilators. Treatments to decrease sensitivity to the nervous system also benefit over activity of the PFM conditions and include aerobic exercise, breathing, pain education, transcutaneous electrical nerve stimulation, and relaxation training.

SPECIAL IMPLICATIONS FOR THE THERAPIST 27.7

## *Pelvic Floor Muscle Dysfunction*

### Prevention and Education

The International Consultation on Incontinence concludes that PFM exercises prevent urinary incontinence in pregnant and postpartum women, and education for community-dwelling elderly individuals can prevent urinary incontinence.[96] It is imperative that women (including adolescent girls) receive education about the functions and dysfunctions of the pelvic floor complex to promote preventive exercises rather than waiting for the need for restorative pelvic floor exercise. Exercises for the pelvic floor should be part of every woman's fitness regimen, either as prevention or specific to the type of PFM dysfunction and its causes.

Therapists should routinely ask women questions about pelvic floor function (e.g., presence of urinary incontinence, pain with sexual intercourse or other sexual dysfunction, presence of known reproductive organ or pelvic floor dysfunction, and past history) and provide education and exercise programs for these muscles, making a medical referral when appropriate.

### Physical Therapist Intervention

Intervention must be determined based on examination, including external assessment and, in the case of therapists with additional training, internal PFM examination. Patients may be instructed to visualize the perineal area in a mirror or palpate lightly to sense an inward movement of the area during PFM contraction. Internal vaginal assessment by a skilled physical therapist would be recommended if there is outward movement or no movement or if the person is unsure of the proper technique, as many individuals cannot perform PFM exercises correctly with only verbal instructions.[155]

Any unspoken behaviors or indication of discomfort on the part of the client should prompt the physical therapist to stop and communicate with the client before continuing or discontinuing. Issues of childhood incest or sexual assault or adult sexual issues may be a significant contributing factor, requiring combined pelvic muscle rehabilitation and psychotherapy or sexual abuse counseling.

Special considerations include cultural differences in modesty, the possibility of current substance use or abuse, and past (or present) sexual abuse or sexual dysfunction.

### Pelvic Floor Muscle Training

To date, many systematic reviews, Cochrane reviews, and meta-analyses have documented the benefits of PFM exercises for female stress urinary incontinence. Comparing PFM training with no treatment,[235] women with stress urinary incontinence who were treated were 17 times more likely to report cure or improvement and were 5 to 16 times more likely to be continent on pad test.[102] Dumoulin and colleagues[102] concluded that it is "no longer a question of whether PFM training programs work but what components and combinations thereof are most effective."

Men, children, older adults, and individuals with neurologic dysfunction can also benefit from specialized PFM training and conservative management provided by a pelvic physical therapist.[49] PFM training should be tailored to the needs of the individual and may include increasing PFM force and endurance, decreasing PFM resting tone, and coordinating the PFM to contract and relax when needed.[39]

Therapists are encouraged to provide instructions and monitor results. The patient should be referred to a specialized physical therapist if expected improvements are not reported.[102] A skilled evaluation is needed to fully identify each person's needs and is beyond the scope of this text; however, a brief review of PFM strengthening is included here.

### Exercise Prescription

PFM exercises can be prescribed in several modes: active assistive, active, and resistive.

### Active Assistive Pelvic Floor Muscle Exercises

Active assistive PFM exercises include exercises with overflow facilitation. The adductors, gluteals, and external rotators are thought to assist in strengthening the PFMs.[102,342] Contraction of overflow muscles such as squeezing a ball between the knees or pushing the knees apart against elastic band resistance can decrease urinary incontinence symptoms, especially in the elderly and pediatric populations. A recent study shows bird-dog, plank, and leg lifts elevate the PFM and close the urogenital hiatus and may also be useful as facilitation exercises.[315]

### Active Pelvic Floor Muscle Exercises

Active PFM exercises form the bulk of training and have been studied and reported most often. These exercises can be combined with several forms of biofeedback (manometry or electromyography). Despite expert opinion, multiple randomized controlled trials have failed to show a statistically significant difference between outcomes with and without electromyography training as long as the exposure to individual PFM training is the same.[158]

Individualized PFM training includes attention to several factors. Components of the PFM training program would include determining the *number of seconds* the PFM contraction is held and the amount of rest between contractions. *Number of repetitions* performed and *number of times the set is repeated* during the day would also be determined.

Exercise prescription would also include choosing the *position* (supine, sitting, or standing) used for static exercises. Likewise, consideration is given to selecting positions used during PFM training for dynamic activities (such as lifting and bending) and PFM training in combination with abdominal muscle contraction.[187] "The Knack" is a technique in which the individual practices squeezing the PFM before sneezing and coughing and can result in 98% decrease in urinary incontinence. Attention is also given to breathing phase to restore normal intraabdominal pressure and avoid bearing down.[187,165]

### Resistive Pelvic Floor Muscle Exercises

Resistive PFM exercises include insertion of a vaginal weight or changing to upright position for exercises. Some practitioners believe that exercises done in an upright position (sitting or standing) provide gravity resistance and are more difficult. However, at least one randomized study comparing supine-only PFM exercises with supine and upright PFM exercises showed no significant difference in decreasing urinary incontinence.[42] Still most physical therapists start exercises in the supine position and add upright exercises as needed. Vaginal weights can result in decreased urinary incontinence, but comparison studies do not show a significant advantage over PFM exercises alone.[41,157]

There is some research to show optimal *frequency* of supervised PFM training. Dumoulin and colleagues[102] reported training carried out under supervision more than two times per month to be the most effective. *Individual versus group training* is another decision that must be made when planning prescriptive training exercise for PFMs. In a study comparing individual PFM training with group PFM training, participants undergoing individual training were dryer on pad test, but otherwise both groups had improvement in strength, quality of life, and personal satisfaction (86% in both groups). Group PFM exercises are significantly better than no treatment.[102]

Studies on long-term effects of PFM training found that adherence was a significant predictor of success both during the period of therapy and thereafter.[103] A meta-analysis of PFM training showed that the program must last for at least 6 weeks (*duration*).[63] There is no standard agreement on maintenance; this aspect of the plan of care should be individualized for each person.

### Under Activity of the Pelvic Floor Muscles

In addition to the PFM exercise training discussed above, intervention for under activity of the PFM may focus on postural education to place the pelvic floor in the most optimal position for strengthening and function and motor learning techniques (e.g., use of a Swiss ball) and behavioral training. Principles of motor learning guide the therapist in incorporating pelvic muscle function with breathing (work of the diaphragm muscle), the abdominal muscles, and the low back muscles. This is an important step in creating sensory awareness of the pelvic floor, which takes time and repetition. Restoring normal pelvic floor strength and bladder control is essential before resuming vigorous physical activity or exercise.

The therapist is instrumental in teaching contraction of the appropriate muscles without contraction of the gluteal muscles and with complete relaxation of the pelvic muscles between contractions. With verbal and manual cues or biofeedback (auditory, visual, or electronic), clients can be taught to contract the PFMs while maintaining decreased activity in other hip and trunk muscles. Patients are also taught to maintain PFM tone while avoiding a Valsalva maneuver.

**Over Activity of the Pelvic Floor Muscles**

Interventions for over activity of the PFMs may focus on postural education to place the pelvis and the PFMs in the most optimal position for relaxation and function and aerobic exercise to mobilize the pelvis. Manual therapy techniques could include joint alignment; soft tissue, scar, and/or visceral mobilization; myofascial release therapy; and stretching for the adductors, iliopsoas, piriformis, obturator internus, abdominals, and other muscles as determined by the assessment. Biofeedback and relaxation training can enhance normalization of overactive tone, and dilators may be used to stretch the vaginal tissues and train the PFMs to relax during intercourse. Education on the physiology of pain and cognitive-behavioral therapy may also contribute to success in individuals with chronic pelvic pain syndromes.

## Coccygodynia

### Overview and Etiology

Coccygodynia (also coccydynia) describes pain related to the coccyx and the muscles attached to the coccyx. Causes are often unclear, but fall into several categories: musculoskeletal, direct trauma related to childbirth or direct fall, inflammation related to trauma or sacrococcygeal calcium deposits, infections, referred pain from visceral sources in the pelvis, neoplasm (sacral chordoma), or centralized pain syndrome.[290,273] Musculoskeletal causes include poor sitting posture, pelvic asymmetry/malalignment, PFM spasm, sacrococcygeal luxation or hypermobility, coccygeal spicule (hook on end of coccyx), and lumbosacral disk degeneration.[62]

Sacral chordoma is a rare, slow-growing tumor that should be considered in the medical differential diagnosis, especially when there are neurologic symptoms present. Overactivity of the ganglion impar (ganglion impar is the location where two pelvic sympathetic trunks converge, ending in a ganglion at the front of the coccyx) can also cause chronic coccyx pain.[278]

### Clinical Manifestations

Symptoms are primarily related to pain with sitting, transfer from sit to stand, and defecation. Pain with transfer from sit to stand is often related to the musculoskeletal causes of coccyx pain and is often amenable to manual therapy of the inferior gluteal muscles. In addition, palpation of the PFMs rectally may identify TrPs, over activity of the PFMs, and decreased ability to relax the PFMs.

### Medical Management

Medical examination includes radiography in standing and lateral sitting positions,[224] which could reveal posterior luxation, hypermobility in flexion, coccygeal spicule, and/or crystal deposits in the sacrococcygeal or intercoccygeal joints.[290,278]

Medical treatments include medications (e.g., oral analgesics and NSAIDs) as a first-line treatment. A short course of oral corticosteroids for calcific deposits may be recommended.[290] Corticosteroid injection (with or without anesthesia) can result in 60% to 65% improvement in some musculoskeletal cases.[273] Local anesthetic injections to block ganglion impar often produces 42.9% to 61.9% relief of coccyx pain.[307]

Partial or total coccygectomy is not recommended based on a review in the pain literature, while the same procedure is recommended by a systematic review published in the orthopedic literature.[273,193] Studies supporting the use of this type of surgical intervention are levels 3 and 4 and report 54% to 96% success with overall complication rate of 11% related to infections. Removal of the distal segment of a nonunion coccyx fracture appears to provide some surgical success. Chordoma and other sacral tumors are curable with surgery, and early diagnosis may lead to preservation of bladder, bowel, motor, and sexual function.

**SPECIAL IMPLICATIONS FOR THE THERAPIST 27.8**

*Coccygodynia*

Physical therapy treatments include manipulations of the coccyx, massage to levator ani muscles, and manual treatment of pelvic joint malalignment. The therapist assesses and treats muscle imbalances and prescribes exercises to address biomechanical dysfunction of the PFMs. The therapist also provides patient/client education on sitting posture, use of appropriate cushions, and avoidance of aggravating factors such as lifting and constipation.[168,306]

# JOINT

## Chondrolysis

### Overview

Chondrolysis is a process of rapid cartilage degeneration resulting in narrowing of the joint space and loss of motion. This process is associated with infection, trauma, and prolonged immobilization. Trauma can also include orthopedic procedures such as arthroscopic meniscectomy, shoulder arthroscopy, anterior cruciate ligament reconstruction, and thermal capsulorrhaphy.[150]

The hip is the most likely location for chondrolysis to occur, especially associated with slipped capital epiphysis, but cases have been reported affecting the knee, shoulder, and ankle. Spontaneous chondrolysis without known risk factors occurs occasionally, most commonly in adolescent girls. Chondrolysis occurs five times more often in females than in males, and adolescence is the most common period of onset.[281]

#### Etiology and Pathogenesis

The etiology is unknown; many theories have been proposed including nutritional abnormalities, mechanical injury, use of intraarticular pain pumps during surgery, ischemia, abnormal chondrocyte metabolism, ischemia, and abnormal intracapsular pressure. There may be some evidence to support an autoimmune mechanism responsible for the cartilage destruction.[150,281]

Various studies have implicated IL-1, which has chondrolytic action by stimulating the release of inflammatory mediators, enhancing the breakdown of cartilage proteoglycans. Clearly, some disruption of the cartilage extracellular matrix occurs leading to chondrolysis, but the key to the process has not been discovered.

#### Clinical Manifestations

Regardless of the underlying cause of this condition, the affected individual presents with progressive joint stiffness, with progressive loss of motion and pain. Chondrolysis of the hip causes anterior hip and/or groin pain accompanied by an antalgic gait. Soft tissue contracture can result in an apparent leg-length discrepancy and pelvic obliquity with muscle atrophy. Painful ankylosis may develop in some individuals, whereas others experience an improvement in pain and range of motion.[115]

### MEDICAL MANAGEMENT

DIAGNOSIS, TREATMENT, AND PROGNOSIS. Imaging studies are used to make the diagnosis. Plain radiographs may exhibit signs of joint narrowing, erosions of subchondral bone, or even signs of osteopenia. For advanced cases the definitive diagnosis may be made on the basis of scintigraphy and/or MRI.

Treatment is with NSAIDs to control synovial inflammation. Protected weight bearing and maintenance of joint motion are important components of the treatment plan. Surgery may be indicated (e.g., capsulectomy, tendon release of the adductor and iliopsoas), but the best course of operative treatment is unknown.[151]

## Osteoarthritis

#### Overview

Osteoarthritis (OA), or degenerative joint disease, is a slowly evolving articular disease that appears to originate in the cartilage and affects the underlying bone, soft tissues, and synovial fluid. OA is divided into two classifications: primary and secondary. The cause of primary OA is unknown, and the cascade of joint degeneration events associated with it is thought to be related to a defect in the articular cartilage. Secondary OA has a known cause, which may be trauma, infection, hemarthrosis, osteonecrosis, or some other condition.

OA is present worldwide as a heterogeneous group of conditions that lead to slow, progressive degeneration of joint structures with defective integrity of articular cartilage in addition to related changes in the underlying bone at the joint margins. OA can lead to loss of mobility, chronic pain, deformity, and loss of function.

#### Incidence

OA is the most common joint disease, with an estimated prevalence of 60% in men and 70% in women after age 65 years, affecting an estimated 30 million people in the United States.[353] Before age 50 years, the prevalence of OA in most joints is higher in men than in women, but this pattern changes after age 65 years. In fact, OA is the most common musculoskeletal disorder worldwide affecting the hands and large weight-bearing joints such as the hip and knee and causing disability. The development of OA is a risk factor for also developing cardiovascular disease. The risk appears to more prevalent in women with an early onset of knee OA.[203] The overall prevalence of OA is expected to increase dramatically over the next 20 years as the population ages.

#### Etiologic and Risk Factors

The etiology of OA is multifactorial, including many components of biomechanics and biochemistry. There is a strong association of genetics as a risk factor for OA, with a number of loci within the human genome found to increase this association. Numerous phenotypes have been identified for the development of OA, which will determine the progression of the disease for each individual. These phenotypes describe how an individual's genotypes interact with attributes such as nutrition and weight control, estrogen deficiency (menopause), bone density, immune system response, and local biomechanical factors.[353] Injuries to joint ligaments and meniscus, joint malalignments, and subsequent decreases in muscle strength are strong predictors for the onset and progression of OA. Labral tears and femoroacetabular impingement are risk factors for the development of hip OA.[353]

Participation in occupations and sports that require prolonged stresses on joints has been associated with a greater risk of OA. Football players, soccer players, hockey players, and baseball pitchers are especially at increased risk.[2] Regular, moderate running and similar activities have not been associated with progression of OA and may provide some reduction in risk based on preventive factors associated with lower body weight and better cardiovascular health. Participation in sports that require high levels of physical activity such as snowboarding, mountain biking, and aggressive in-line skating, with the increased incidence of repeated impact or joint injuries, may be risk factors for OA developing earlier in life, requiring a hip or knee replacement.[185]

Generalized ligamentous laxity and hypermobility joint syndrome are from a dominant inherited connective tissue disorder. Hypermobility syndrome is characterized by excessive laxity of multiple joints, a condition that is separate from the generalized hypermobility associated with disorders such as Ehlers-Danlos syndrome, RA, SLE, or Marfan syndrome.[365] Hypermobility syndrome appears to be a systemic collagen abnormality with a decreased ratio of type I to type III collagen. Women with this syndrome may develop OA earlier than the norm. Muscle weakness in anyone can also cause joint changes leading to OA, such as occurs with prolonged immobilization, polymyositis, multiple sclerosis, or any of the myopathies listed in Box 27.3.[365]

#### Pathogenesis

The progression of OA is characterized by a process of joint tissue destruction and aberrant repair because of alterations in cellular function. Inflammatory and procatabolic mediators affect the function of chondrocytes within the articular cartilage, creating hypertrophic differentiation and early cell death. Age-related changes within the collagen and proteoglycans of the cartilage along with lifestyle choices can further enhance this inflammatory response, creating more changes to the articular cartilage.[242] The synovial lining of the joint undergoes hyperplasia, secreting excess synovial fluid. The extra fluid creates a joint effusion that activates joint mechanoreceptors that through a spinal reflex inhibit muscles crossing the joint and affect joint nociceptors.[109] People with OA may have a general tendency toward increased bone metabolic activity, resulting in remodeling of subchondral bone.[5]

As OA develops, there is a loss of hyaline cartilage, hypertrophic changes in neighboring bone and joint capsule, synovial inflammation, and focal calcifications of the cartilage. Articular cartilage has an important role in joint physiology by providing a smooth, relatively friction-free surface between the bony ends making up the joint. In addition, the cartilage attenuates the mechanical load transmitted through the joint. OA changes lead to a mechanopathology where abnormal loading on regions of articular cartilage allows for further damage and dysfunctional movements.[109] With progressive loss of cartilage, inflammation develops, with resultant bony overgrowth, ligament laxity, and progressive muscle weakness and atrophy accompanied by joint pain.

The joint space narrows as the cartilage thins, and sclerosis of the subchondral bone occurs as new bone is formed in response to the now excessive mechanical load. New bone also forms at the joint margins (osteophytes) (Fig. 27.3) with the end result being mechanical joint failure and varying degrees of loss of joint function. Once the cartilage begins to break down, excessive mechanical stress begins to fall on other joint structures. Eventually, fissuring and eburnation appear in the cartilage, which is a thinning of the articular cartilage resulting in exposure of the subchondral bone.[242]

### Clinical Manifestations

The most common symptoms of OA include bony enlargement, limited range of motion, crepitus on motion, tenderness on pressure, joint effusion, malalignment, and joint deformity. Inflammation is a prominent sign that plays a role in symptom generation. Soft tissue inflammation and edema are observed during acute exacerbations. The most commonly involved joints associated with this disorder are the weight-bearing joints, especially the hip and knee but also the shoulder, lumbar and cervical spine, and first carpometacarpal and metatarsophalangeal joints.[147]

The onset of symptoms related to OA can occur insidiously or suddenly. For most people, the pain symptoms progress slowly and gradually related to their activities. In the early stages of OA the predominant cause of joint pain is attributed to a breakdown in the mechanics of movement rather than inflammation. The pain is often described as a deep ache that is worse with activity and

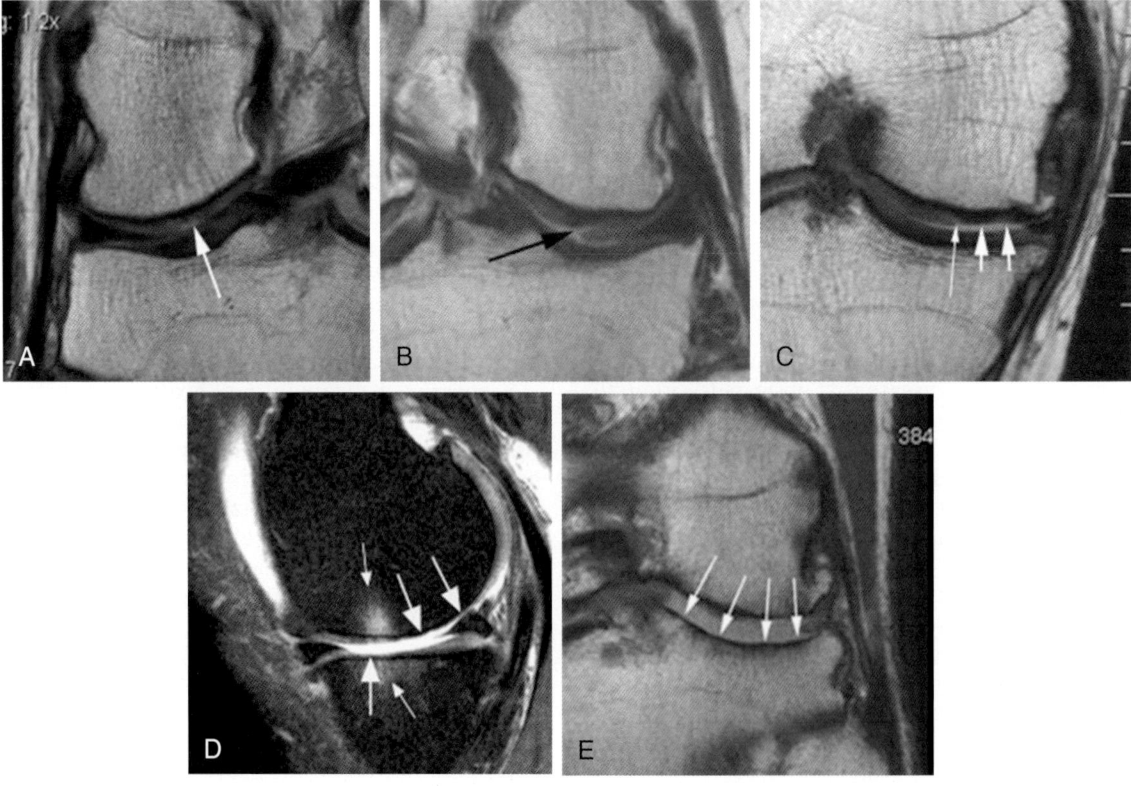


**Figure 27.3**

**Magnetic resonance imaging of knee osteoarthritis.** (A–E) Defects in the articular cartilage are demonstrated with *arrows* in the images. (From Roemer FW, et al: An illustrative overview of semi-quantitative MRI scoring of knee osteoarthritis: lessons learned from longitudinal observational studies. *Osteoarthritis Cartilage* 24:274–289, 2015.)

better after rest. Later the pain can become unpredictable, without an obvious preceding activity to trigger the response. The pain will become more persistent, even with rest and at night.[109]

Stiffness over the involved joint for a short duration (less than 30 minutes) can occur after periods of inactivity, including sitting and sleeping. Morning stiffness usually lasts only 5 to 10 minutes after awakening. Movement and activity dissipate this stiffness until the individual sits or rests for a long period of time. This differs from RA, in which the morning stiffness or gelling can last until noon or even midafternoon. Swelling, if present, is mild and localized to the joint. Loss of flexibility is usually associated with significant disease and can occur secondary to soft tissue contractures, intraarticular loose bodies, large osteophytes, and loss of joint surface congruity.[109]

Crepitus (audible crackling or grating sensation produced when roughened articular or extraarticular surfaces rub together during movement) may be noted on physical examination, and enlarged joint surfaces including osteophytes may be palpable. Although many people have physical and radiographic findings of OA, they may not have symptoms, whereas others with minimal changes observed develop significant symptoms. The reasons for this are unknown.

For many women, OA typically develops within a few years of menopause and is often associated with mild inflammation for the first year or two that a particular joint is involved. The joints may intermittently be warm and tender. The disease is strikingly symmetric, although the degree of involvement may vary.[147]

OA of the hands affects the distal interphalangeal and proximal interphalangeal joints and occurs most often in women. The gradual loss of joint motion can assume major significance, with the person finding it difficult to grasp small objects. After 1 or 2 years of inflammation, the joints enlarge with osteophyte (spur) formation, referred to as Heberden nodes (affecting the distal interphalangeal joints) and Bouchard nodes (affecting the proximal interphalangeal joints) (Fig. 27.4) and become unsightly. Pain may also be noted with loss of joint articular cartilage. Lateral deformities of the joints are common, with stretching of the collateral ligaments and bone resorption. This leads to overlapping of the fingers and considerable loss of functional ability.[214]

Some individuals experience OA of the carpometacarpal joint. With advanced disease, individuals with carpometacarpal involvement may develop joint subluxation as the metacarpal flexes and adducts, leaving the metacarpal base prominent. Axial loading (e.g., pinching) and rotation characteristically reproduce symptoms and cause crepitus.[326]

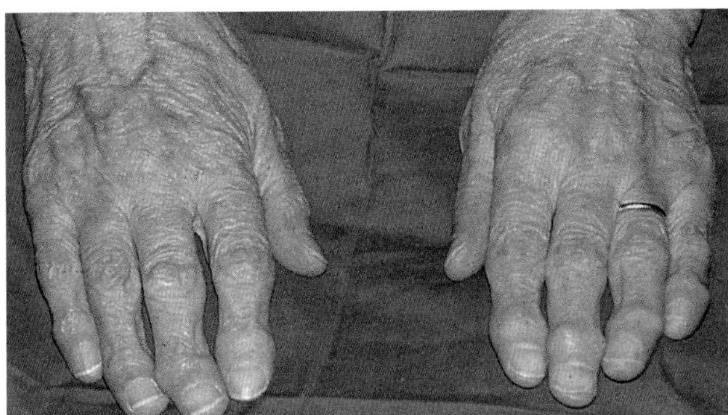

**Figure 27.4**

**Typical hand deformities in osteoarthritis.** Heberden nodes are seen on the distal interphalangeal joints, and Bouchard nodes are on the proximal interphalangeal joints. (From Forbes CD, Jackson WF: *Color atlas and text of clinical medicine*, ed 3, London, 2003, Mosby.)

## MEDICAL MANAGEMENT

**PREVENTION.** Research is providing a growing body of knowledge about OA, but there are gaps in the understanding that limit the use of effective methods to prevent and treat OA. Slowing the progression of the disease with a combination of drug and behavioral interventions is the current best method for managing this condition. Education is a cornerstone of prevention and management for this condition. A healthy lifestyle helps prevent OA, and exercise can lessen disability if OA has developed. Exercise programs should be personalized for each individual with OA to best adjust their phenotypes for the progression of OA.[125]

Prevention of joint injuries is a key factor for eliminating the onset of OA. Early diagnosis and intervention with complete rehabilitation of joint injuries can decrease the risk of subsequent OA. In the future, biomarkers found in joint fluid, blood, or urine that indicate changes in bone or cartilage may help identify people at risk for OA, allowing for prevention of disease progression and early intervention.[242]

**DIAGNOSIS.** OA is diagnosed through the combination of history, radiologic findings (Figs. 27.5 and 27.6), physical examination, and laboratory tests, which rule out rheumatic disease. Box 27.5 lists radiographic changes associated with OA. The history of location of symptoms,

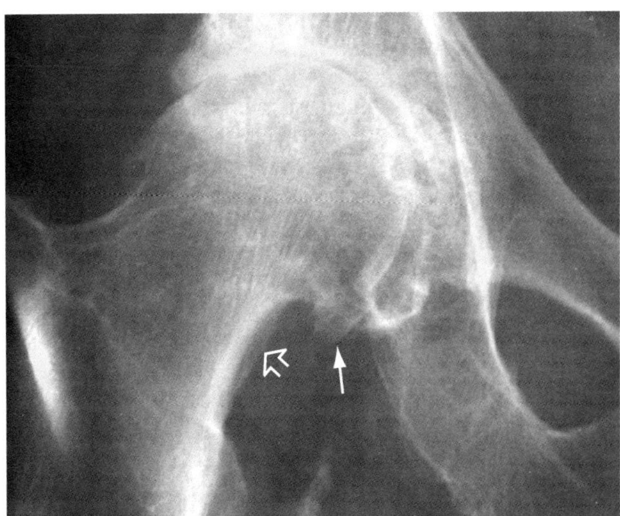

**Figure 27.5**

**Osteoarthritis of the hip.** Anteroposterior view of the hip shows complete cartilage space loss superiorly. There is osteophytic lipping from the femoral head, especially medially *(arrow)*, and buttressing bone *(open arrow)* is present along the femoral neck. (From Harris ED: *Kelley's textbook of rheumatology*, ed 7, Philadelphia, 2005, Saunders.)

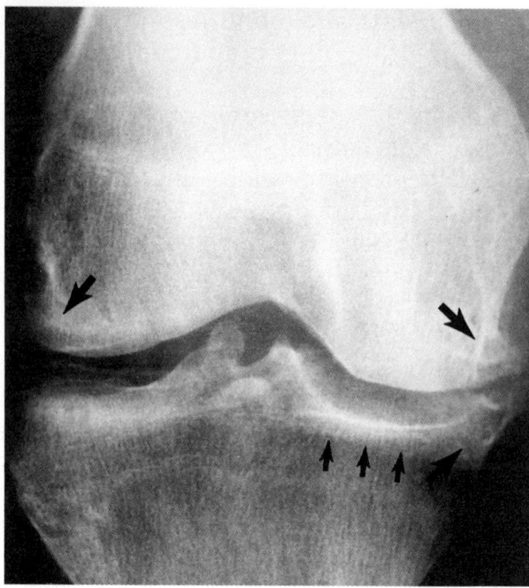

**Figure 27.6**

**Osteoarthritis of the knee.** Proliferative marginal osteophytes *(larger arrows)*, narrowing of the medial weight-bearing joint space, and eburnation (exposure of the subchondral bone; surface becomes smooth and polished as it wears down) *(smaller arrows)*. (From Noble J: *Textbook of primary care medicine*, ed 3, St. Louis, 2001, Mosby.)

**Box 27.5**

**OSTEOARTHRITIS: RADIOGRAPHIC FINDINGS[a]**

- Joint space widening (early evidence)
- Subchondral bone sclerosis
- Subchondral bone cysts
- Osteophytes
- Joint space narrowing

[a]Listed in order of progression.

symptom duration, functional limitations, trauma, medical comorbidities, and family history helps guide the physician in making the diagnosis.

The American College of Rheumatology (ACR) guidelines for the clinical diagnosis of knee OA were originally published in 1986 and were revised in 2012 with recommendation for therapies. The guidelines continue to include knee pain with at least three of the following: age older than 50 years, morning stiffness lasting less than 30 minutes or crepitus on motion, bony tenderness, bony enlargement, and no palpable warmth over the knee joint. These clinical findings along with radiographic signs of degeneration are most commonly used to make the diagnosis of knee OA. Guidelines for the diagnosis of hip OA are similar, while the signs of OA of the hand are typically seen first in the more distal interphalangeal joints.[163,164]

The physician also relies on findings from the physical examination, such as joint line or bony tenderness, joint effusion, joint giving way sensations, muscle atrophy, unsteadiness on uneven surfaces or stairs, varus or valgus deformity (knee), and any abnormalities such as Heberden nodes. Laboratory evaluation may include ESR and rheumatoid factor, but generally these tests are not needed.

OA is classified based on clinical information and radiologic evidence. The classification system proposed by Kellgren and Lawrence uses radiographic images and

**Box 27.6**

**KELLGREN AND LAWRENCE GRADING SYSTEM FOR THE KNEE**

| Grade | Radiographic Findings |
|---|---|
| 1 | Possible osteophytes; no joint space narrowing |
| 2 | Definite osteophytes; possible narrowing of joint space |
| 3 | Moderate multiple osteophytes; definite joint space narrowing; some sclerosis and possible deformity of bone ends |
| 4 | Large osteophytes; marked joint space narrowing; severe sclerosis and definite deformity of bone ends |

Data from Kellgren J, Lawrence J: Radiologic assessment of osteoarthritis. *Ann Rheum Dis* 16:494–501, 1957.

is used to classify stages of OA and to determine progression of the disease. The classification is based on grades of 0 to 4, using the criteria of joint space narrowing and changes to bony structures (Box 27.6).Grade 4 changes include large osteophytes, severe joint space narrowing, bony sclerosis, and bone exposure.[105]

MRI is helpful in determining OA pathology because of its ability to show the condition of cartilage and the surrounding soft tissues. MRI is used to identify the presence of bone marrow lesions, synovitis, and periarticular inflammation that can be the source of chronic pain for patients with OA.[152]

TREATMENT. OA is managed on an individual basis, and treatment consists of a combination of nonsurgical and surgical options. Treatment is modified based on response and should begin with conservative care, including education, weight loss, exercise, orthotics and/or braces, medications, and complementary, alternative, and integrative therapy approaches. There are also treatments that may be beneficial for controlling symptoms in some individuals, but their appropriateness is uncertain.[237]

The combination of modest weight loss and moderate exercise provides better overall improvements in function, pain, and mobility in older adults who are overweight or obese with knee OA. Greater improvements in function and preservation of articular cartilage have been observed in older obese adults with the most weight loss.[126,354] Surgery is avoided and is considered only when debilitating pain and major limitation of function interfere with walking and daily activities or impair ability to sleep or work.

***Pharmacotherapy.*** Acetaminophen is recommended as a first-line treatment. Topical capsaicin and glucosamine/chondroitin should also be considered for symptom relief. NSAIDs and cyclooxygenase-2 inhibitors should be tried if acetaminophen is ineffective. Current recommendations for treatment with NSAIDs include using the lowest effective dose for the shortest possible period to reduce pain and preserve mobility. Newly discovered information about the pathophysiology of OA is paving the way for researchers to design medical therapy that targets specific sites of pathophysiologic pathways involved in the pathogenesis of OA. Medical attention has shifted from easing the pain of OA to slowing the progression of the disorder or preventing it.

Research on cytokines, growth factors, and signaling pathways that was started in the 1990s is now producing new concepts for disease-modifying OA drugs, similar to the disease-modifying drugs developed and now available for RA.[170]

Antiresorptive drugs aimed at altering the increased metabolic states of the subchondral bone may have an effect in altering damage done to the overlying cartilage. This approach is based on the hypothesis that the underlying subchondral bone, either indirectly through biomechanical effects or directly via release of cytokines, is responsible for driving the release of degradative enzymes and, ultimately, the destruction of overlying cartilage.[367]

Injection of *viscosupplementation* has been proposed for individuals in whom standard conservative treatments for knee OA have been inadequate or ineffective. This intervention involves direct injections into the knee of substances derived from sodium hyaluronate, a principal component of natural synovial fluid. The injections can also include a corticosteroid medication. These injections were proposed to help restore some of the viscosity and elasticity of the diseased joint fluid and offer pain relief for 6 to 12 months.[275]

The injection of platelet-rich plasma into joints with OA has been proposed as a method to use growth factors with the plasma to stimulate healing processes. These processes are thought to result in less pain and in improvements in joint function. Studies of these injections have found few complications and consistent improvements in pain levels and measures of daily function.[78]

***Education.*** Multimodal treatment should include client education and self-management. The Arthritis Foundation website contains information on consumer education and self-management of OA. Behavioral interventions directed toward enhancing self-management are important, including prevention diet and weight control and low-impact exercise. More attention to psychosocial problems (e.g., isolation, depression) that may influence the person's perception of pain and to exercise is recommended.

***Complementary, Alternative, and Integrative Therapy.*** Complementary and integrative medicine may be recommended or may have been found to be successful for certain individuals with OA. The evidence suggests that treatments such as acupuncture, several herbal preparations (e.g., devil's claw root, white willow bark, frankincense), and capsaicin cream are not sufficient to recommend to most patients, but there is no evidence to conclude they are not effective for all patients with OA, a chronic disease that results in pain, joint dysfunction, and disability.[237,86]

Nutraceuticals are foods or food products that have potential treatment or preventive benefits for a disease process. Glucosamine and chondroitin sulfate are components of articular cartilage. Glucosamine is derived from the shells of lobster, shrimp, and crabs; chondroitin sulfate is derived from cow cartilage. These can be taken orally with potential effects of decreasing joint inflammation, inhibiting proteolytic enzymes that break down cartilage and stimulating the synthesis of proteoglycans and hyaluronic acid.

Long-term use of these agents may provide symptom-modifying effects but has not been found to significantly affect joint function or overall disability.[316] Most individuals taking glucosamine and chondroitin take 1500 mg of glucosamine and 1200 mg of chondroitin daily; individuals weighing more than 200 lb should increase the dosage to 2000 mg of glucosamine and 1600 mg of chondroitin sulfate.[159]

***Surgery.*** Surgical intervention is considered when pain and loss of function are severe. Arthroscopic management, including subchondral penetration procedures such as drilling and microfracture, and matrix-induced chondrogenesis, may benefit some individuals, potentially delaying reconstructive procedures Each of these procedures is under investigation for efficacy and long-term results.[260,121]

PROGNOSIS. OA is a major contributor to functional limitations and reduced independence in adults older than 65 years of age. It is a chronic condition with unpredictable symptoms that often cause fluctuations in pain and function.

Mobility disability, defined as needing help walking or climbing stairs, is common for people with hip and/or knee OA. The social burden in terms of personal suffering and use of health resources is expected to increase with the increasing prevalence of obesity and the aging of the U.S. population.[163]

Although there is no known cure for OA, by following the guidelines for lifestyle changes, pain management, and self-management incorporating exercise and weight loss, affected individuals can substantially decrease the pain and dysfunction associated with OA.[237]

SPECIAL IMPLICATIONS FOR THE THERAPIST 27.9

## *Osteoarthritis*

Therapists need to be aware of the potential poor correlation between the extent of radiographic degenerative changes and the presence of symptoms. It should not be assumed that a person with significant, extensive joint degeneration will not improve until a thorough rehabilitation program has been attempted.

Conversely, it should not be assumed that an individual with minor radiographic degenerative changes is not experiencing severe, intense pain. Comorbidities and other factors may create central sensitization changes for pain perception. Therapists should rely primarily on the clinical examination findings for direction regarding the prognosis (including development of the plan of care) and intervention.

### Medications and Nutraceuticals

The medications commonly prescribed for OA have significant potential side effects. NSAIDs have ulcerogenic potential, especially when taken with nonprescription drugs. Gastric irritation can result from inhibition of prostaglandin production, which can reduce mucus and bicarbonate production and decrease local blood flow. Peptic ulcer disease can be manifested by a multitude of symptoms, including indigestion, nausea, vomiting, thoracic pain, and melena (black tarry stools). The onset of any of these symptoms calls for communication with a physician.[237]

Nutraceuticals such as chondroitin can also cause problems in some individuals. Chondroitin may increase the risk of bleeding in patients with a clotting disorder or who are taking heparin. Individuals taking these supplements who present with unexplained back or shoulder pain or excessive bruising or bleeding from any part of the body (nose, gums, vagina, urine, and rectum) must be evaluated by a physician.

### Joint Protection

People with symptoms associated with OA must understand their role in minimizing the mechanical stresses on the involved joint or joints. The diseased joints need to be protected from excessive mechanical forces. Educating the client on how to reduce the daily wear and tear on the joint is essential. This may include the use of postural supports, knee braces, and orthoses during an exercise program to vary the stresses to which the involved joints are exposed.

Proper posture and avoidance of prolonged stressful postures, use of supports, varying of physical activities to vary the stresses (i.e., alternating biking with swimming or walking), and following through with a flexibility and strengthening exercise program all are components under the affected individual's control.

Wearing shoes that fit properly and are appropriate for the activity may help avoid injury. Good alignment of the joints is important, especially in the knee. Evaluating the need for an assistive ambulatory device, a shock-absorbent shoe insert or heel wedge, brace, or other orthotic device is important to unload the pressure on affected joints. A simple lateral wedge insole of 5 or 10 degrees directly reduces the knee varus torque in individuals with medial knee OA and can interrupt the OA cycle, slowing the progression of the disease and disability.[341]

### Exercise and Osteoarthritis

Since the realization that structured exercise programs can improve function without exacerbating symptoms, exercise and joint protection techniques have become mainstays of treatment. In fact, attempts to alleviate pain through pharmacologic or physical modalities may not improve symptoms unless accompanied by some form of physical conditioning.[360] The plan of care for a person with OA is dictated by the extent of the disease and the joints involved, but everyone with OA should be encouraged to continue exercising, including strength training and low-intensity aerobic components.

### General Concepts

Physical therapy has been shown to be effective in OA of the knee to reduce pain; improve physical function; increase isometric muscle strength, gait speed, and stride length; and improve quality of life. A combination of manual physical therapy and supervised exercise provides beneficial effects that are still present 1 year later and delays or prevents the need for surgical intervention, with fewer joint replacements reported.[92,1] Such supervised exercise/manual therapy programs have been shown to increase improvement and provide greater symptomatic relief compared with a similar unsupervised home exercise program (Fig. 27.7).[91]

In the presence of mild joint swelling, the client should be taught to use ice before exercise and to incorporate a program of submaximal exercise to warm up before beginning the prescribed exercise program. If there is joint effusion, the surrounding muscles cannot contract maximally because of reflex inhibition caused by joint distention. Submaximal exercise for 3 or 4 minutes on a swollen joint decreases this inhibition mechanism, allowing for continued strength training. Moderate to severe joint effusion may require additional physical therapy intervention, such as electrical stimulation.

Resistance and low-intensity aerobic exercise may reduce the incidence of disability related to ADLs and prolong autonomy in adults older than 60 years of age, specifically those with knee OA. The lowest risks for disability related to ADLs were found for participants with the highest compliance to the exercise program. Lower extremity balance exercise programs significantly improve postural sway in older adults, thereby improving lower extremity stability.[218]

Clients should be encouraged to exercise to the extent that they are capable. Many older adults are more likely to adhere to a program that comprises short, frequent episodes of exercise rather than long, once-a-day programs. Educating, motivating, and providing prescriptive exercise are important roles the therapist plays to help maximize function and prevent significant recurrence of symptoms. The therapist should take into account psychosocial factors, especially self-efficacy, which is an important variable in the rehabilitation process predictive of physical function.[149] See further discussion of self-efficacy in Chapter 2.

Sometimes increasing physical activity does cause increased pain, but studies show this is short-lived. The therapist can help clients get over the "pain hump" by assuring them that this response is normal and temporary.[116] Older adults may become more motivated to exercise if they understand the benefits. Teach them the overall health benefits of exercise in preventing chronic conditions such as diabetes, heart disease, osteoporosis, and cancer. The therapist can help educate older adults about how exercise can help reduce their risk factors for OA as well as decrease risk for falls with a program of balance and gait training.

### Specific Exercise Training

Muscles have been shown repeatedly to be the major shock-absorbing mechanism of joints, especially the knee. Eccentric muscle performance serves this shock-absorbing function, supporting the idea that rehabilitation programs should include activities to enhance eccentric function, especially of the quadriceps muscle. The quadriceps muscle group must absorb the force and decelerate the increasing load as the weight-bearing limb stabilizes under the walking load. Overloading the bones' capacity to accept force may be what leads to osteoarthritic changes and/or pain in the knee.[355]

For patients with knee OA, the strength of the quadriceps can be enhanced with a variety of clinical and home exercise methods. Open chain quadriceps-strengthening exercises pose a risk for exercise-induced arthralgias in this population and generally should be avoided. It is likely that the loss of joint proprioception associated with OA may contribute to gait alterations, muscle imbalances, repetitive microtrauma, loss of coordination, and, ultimately, excessive joint loading.[48] Closed chain kinetic strengthening exercises (e.g., leg press, wall slide) can be effective for quadriceps strengthening and are usually well tolerated when performed correctly.[261] Exercises to facilitate proprioception and closed kinetic chain exercises for knee OA have both been shown to improve functional score, walking speed, and muscle strength.[322] Research on strengthening exercises for people with hip OA is not as abundant as for people with knee OA, but the evidence supports a similar approach.[299]

#### Aquatic Physical Therapy

Aquatic physical therapy is used often in the management of individuals with hip and knee OA. Patients who experience increased symptoms with weight-bearing activities can use aquatic therapy to begin activities to promote joint motion without overloading the joint structures. Studies to confirm the efficacy of this treatment and the long-term outcomes yield inconsistent results, with reduced disability levels, but no significant effects on long-term pain relief.[360]

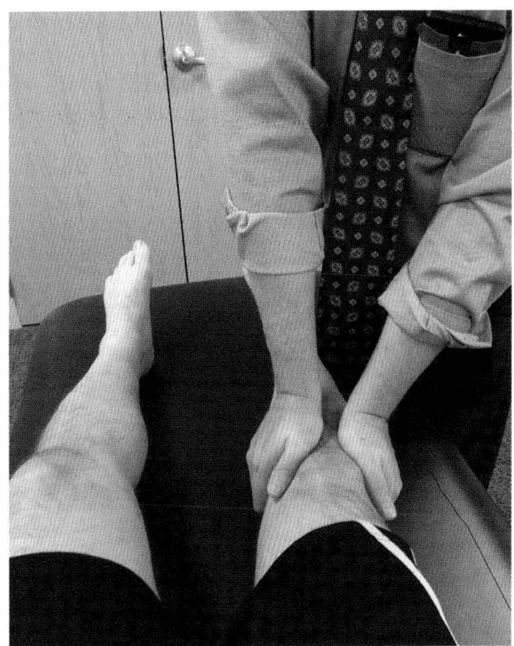

**Figure 27.7**

**Manual therapy for knee osteoarthritis.** Maintaining joint mobility is important for the management of joint range of motion and minimizing joint pain.

## Degenerative Intervertebral Disk Disease

### Overview and Definition

Degenerative intervertebral disk disease is a common condition that frequently results in neck and low back pain. The condition is related to age-related changes in the intervertebral disk materials that can produce radiculopathy, limited spinal stability, and disability. The process of disk degeneration has been described as an aberrant, cell-mediated response to progressive structural failure.[4]

### Incidence

This disease and resulting condition can occur before age 20 years, usually in a familiar pattern or in elite athletes who have been exposed to repetitive physical loading of the spine from frequent trunk rotations, frequent kicking or jumping, or repeated spinal flexion and extension. Lumbar disk degeneration begins early in life, with macroscopic changes being visible from the age of 30 years onward. Half of all Americans older than age 40 years are affected by degenerative disk disease (DDD). Men present with sciatica owing to disk herniation approximately 1.5 to 3 times more often than women, but it is not clear if this is a true difference in prevalence of DDD or can be attributed to anatomic and mechanical factors that contribute to nerve root compression.[10]

### Risk Factors

The greatest risk factor for disk degeneration is familial aggregation including genetic inheritance, which accounts for approximately 50% to 70% of the variability in disk degeneration between identical twins.[32] Individual genes associated with disk degeneration have been identified (e.g., aggrecan, collagen type IX, matrix metalloproteinase-3, vitamin D receptor). Age and body weight appear to be two other significant risk factors for DDD.[189]

There has been a prevailing view that DDD occurs as a result of excessive forces, particularly from the cumulative effects of repeated loading from occupational physical demands such as manual material handling. Results of research to confirm or refute this hypothesis have been mixed; some studies find a correlation between disk degeneration and physical demands, while other do not.[31] Results of the Finnish Twin Cohort suggest that routine (daily) physical loading of the spine may actually have a training (rather than detrimental) effect. Occupational lifting or repeated loading of the spine from physical activity may benefit the disks, as cyclic mechanical stresses may increase the growth rate and collagen fibers of the nucleus pulposus.[189]

Body height has been suggested, but not consistently found in all studies, to be a risk factor; the link between DDD and obesity and smoking also is controversial. The role of psychosocial factors has also been investigated, and psychosocial factors have been found to have a positive link as risk factors for disk herniation, which can lead to further DDD. Atherosclerosis is another potential risk factor. Obstruction in the abdominal aorta and lumbar and middle arteries can lead to ischemia in the lumbar spine, resulting in hypoxia and tissue dysfunction with eventual disk degeneration.[195]

### Etiology and Pathogenesis

A number of events can contribute to age-related disk degeneration (Box 27.7). The most important event appears to be decreased cellular function and concentration. The progressive decline in arterial supply to the periphery of the disk and the impairment of nutrient delivery across the cartilaginous endplate contribute to the reduced nutritional supply to the cells, affecting cellular function. In addition, the impaired cartilaginous endplate diffusion results in reduced cellular waste product removal and an increased lactic acid concentration.

Box 27.7

**DISK DEGENERATION**

***Three Stages of Disk Degeneration***

- Dysfunction
  - Circumferential and radial tears in the disk annulus
  - Localized synovitis and hypermobility of the facet joints
- Instability
  - Internal disruption of the disk
  - Progressive disk resorption
  - Degeneration of the facet joints, with capsular laxity
  - Subluxation
  - Erosion
- Stabilization
  - Osteophytosis (bone spur formation)
  - Spinal stenosis

***Events Leading to Disk Degeneration***

- Impaired cellular nutrition
- Reduced cellular viability
- Cellular senescence
- Accumulation of degraded matrix macromolecules
- Fatigue failure of the matrix

***Risk Factors for Disk Degeneration***

- Age
- Body mass index
- Heredity
- Physical loading[a]
- Occupational (repetitive) lifting

[a]New evidence suggests that these factors may not be as strongly linked with degenerative disk disease as previously thought. Regular physical activity may benefit the disks. Age, body weight, and hereditary factors may be the greatest risk factors for degenerative disk disease.[4,493]

Data from Schoenfeld AJ, et al: Incidence and risk factors for lumbar degenerative disc disease in the United States military 1999–2008. *Mil Med* 176:1320–1324, 2011; and Beattie PF: Current understanding of lumbar intervertebral disc degeneration: a review with emphasis upon etiology, pathophysiology, and lumbar magnetic resonance imaging findings. *J Orthop Sports Phys Ther* 38:329–340, 2008.

The resultant decreased pH level compromises cellular metabolism and biosynthesis and can lead to cell death. The reduced biosynthesis can adversely affect the biomechanical properties of the matrix over an extended period of time.[120,359]

Besides the internal events affecting the general health of the intervertebral disk, repetitive external mechanical loading on the structure can lead to fatigue failure of the matrix. When enough structural breakdown occurs, what once were normal mechanical loads acting on a normal disk are now excessive loads on a compromised disk. At this point the degenerative process is accelerated.[141]

Collapse of the inner annulus into the nucleus is a common feature in the disks of older adults, with the anterior annulus being affected more than the posterior annulus (Fig. 27.8). This could be caused by nucleus decompression following endplate fracture. In many older disks, the cartilage endplate becomes detached from the underlying bone, presumably because the high internal pressure that presses it against the bone in young disks has been lost.[4]

Associated with intervertebral disk degeneration are spinal stenosis and degenerative spondylolisthesis, two common conditions in adults older than age 65 years.[304,308] As the intervertebral disk loses height, the annulus may bulge circumferentially, and the ligamentum flavum can buckle. Both encroach on the spinal canal, subarticular (facet) recesses, and lateral intervertebral foramina. With a loss of disk height, compressive force increases on the neural arch, causing OA of the facet (apophyseal) joints and osteophytes around the margins of the vertebral bodies (Fig. 27.9). In addition, concurrent osteophyte formation on the vertebral bodies or articular processes may occur, compounding the stenosis.

Degenerative spondylolisthesis as a result of disk degeneration and degenerative changes of the posterior facet joint is marked by anterior slippage of one vertebra over another, with an intact posterior neural arch. The L4-L5 spinal segment is the most common site where this occurs (Fig. 27.10). Lytic or isthmic spondylolisthesis (a separate etiology from degenerative spondylolisthesis and more common in younger groups) is marked by anterior slippage of one vertebra over another with a defective

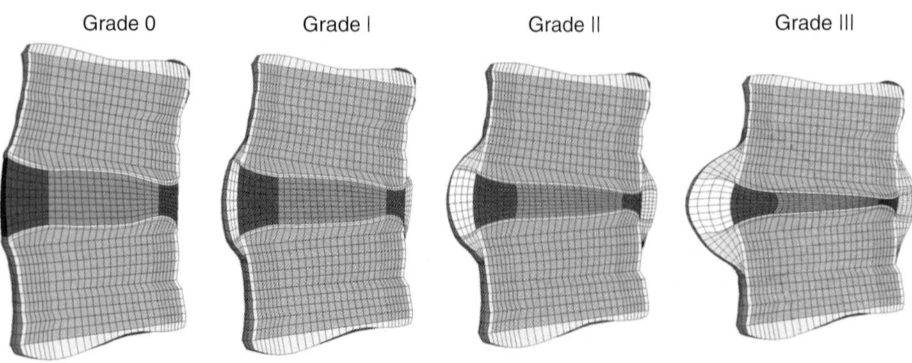


**Figure 27.8**

**Stages of disk degeneration.** (From Schmidt H, et al: The risk of disc prolapses with complex loading in different degrees of disc degeneration—a finite element analysis. *Clin Biomech (Bristol, Avon)* 22:988–998, 2007.)

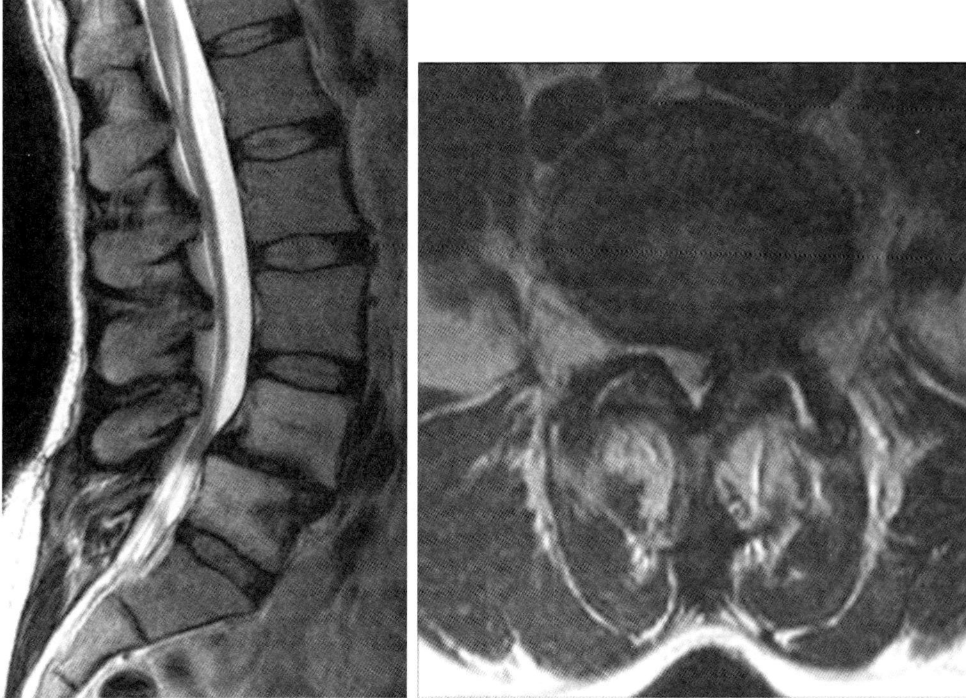

**Figure 27.9**

**Degenerative spondylolisthesis with disc space narrowing and spinal stenosis at the L4-5 level.** (From Lee JYB, Patel A: Lumbar spinal stenosis and degenerative spondylolisthesis. *Semin Spine Surg* 25:256–262, 2013.)

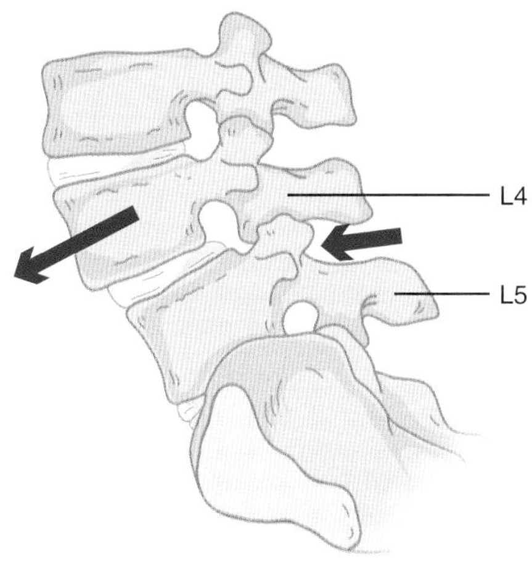


**Figure 27.10**

**Degenerative spondylolisthesis at L4-L5.** Loss of disc structures and fluids results in spinal instability. (From DeRosa C, Porterfield JA: Lumbar spine and pelvis. In Richardson JK, Iglarsh ZA, editors: *Clinical orthopaedic physical therapy*, Philadelphia, 1994, Saunders, p 144.)

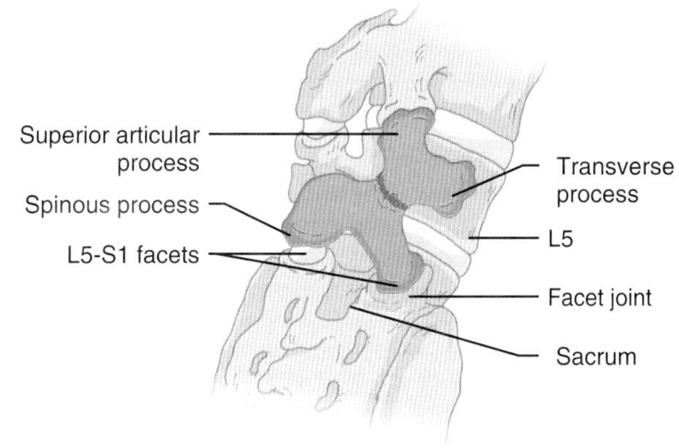


**Figure 27.11**

**Spondylolysis or posterior arch defect, which can lead to a lytic spondylolisthesis.** The Scottie dog with a collar, which is visible on the radiograph (posterior oblique view), is outlined. (From Magee D: *Orthopedic physical assessment*, ed 5, Philadelphia, 2008, Saunders.)

posterior neural arch (Fig. 27.11). The L5-S1 spinal segment is the most common site for lytic spondylolisthesis to occur. The loss of disk height associated with degeneration allows for a buckling of the annulus and ligamentum flavum, slackening them somewhat. This allows the vertebrae to migrate anteriorly in response to the shear forces inherent to the lumbar lordosis.[308]

In contrast to the L5-S1 segment, the facet joint orientation at the L4-L5 segment tends to be more in the sagittal plane, so there is no structural bar to anterior slippage. The facet joint orientation at L5-S1 tends to be more in the frontal plane, making anterior migration of L5 difficult unless there is a structural defect in the posterior neural arch. Stenosis can be caused by the displacement of one vertebra over another, as well as by the concurrent buckling of the annulus and ligamentum flavum.

## Clinical Manifestations

Low back pain is often the first symptom, but DDD is asymptomatic in up to one-third of all affected individuals. Most people with DDD have a gradual onset of increasingly severe midline lower back pain. At first, symptoms last only a few days. This type of back pain is often intermittent but recurring over the years. Each time it occurs, the pain may seem worse than the time before. Eventually the pain may spread into the buttocks or thighs, and it may take longer to subside. Although there is not a 100% correlation between the presence of DDD and pain, the structural alterations will decrease motion and alter the mechanical properties of the spine.[65]

In the lumbar spine, radiculopathy causing sciatic pain and restricted straight leg raise may occur as the sheath of the nerve root is compressed or as a result of inflammatory irritation from chemicals released by the damaged disk. Centralization of radiating pain is characteristic of sciatica from disk protrusion or herniation. Specifically, leg pain routinely reduces or "retreats" to the lumbar midline before the disappearance of back pain.

Other signs of disk herniation include ankle dorsiflexion weakness; great toe extensor weakness; impaired ankle reflexes; loss of light touch sensation in the medial, dorsal, and lateral aspects of the foot; and positive ipsilateral or crossed straight leg raise test. These six neurologic tests allow detection of most instances of clinically significant nerve root compromise resulting from L4-L5 or L5-S1 disk herniations.[364]

Gait abnormality, muscle weakness, sensory changes such as numbness and tingling, and bowel or bladder dysfunction can occur as a result of myelopathy associated with either disk herniation or degeneration. In the case of cervical disk involvement, difficulty swallowing, hand numbness, the Lhermitte sign, and hoarseness or voice difficulties may occur. MRI findings of disk degeneration and herniation are poorly correlated with clinical signs and symptoms. On one hand, a large, extruded disk may be clinically tolerable if the spinal canal is large and the spinal nerve roots are not compressed. On the other hand, a focal, contained subligamentous herniation may produce severe symptoms if it occurs in the foramen adjacent to the dorsal root ganglion of the affected nerve.[317]

Degeneration of the intervertebral disks in the lumbar spine may create enough instability or a spondylolisthesis. There is not a clear consensus that low back pain is associated with spondylolisthesis. In the case of disk degeneration associated with stenosis and spondylolisthesis, the person can be asymptomatic, even when moderate to severe changes are observed on imaging studies. Conversely, early or mild changes can be accompanied by severe pain and neurologic symptoms.[190]

## MEDICAL MANAGEMENT

**DIAGNOSIS.** The diagnosis of DDD is made based on the history of the person's condition, physical examination, and imaging studies. Standard radiographs of the lumbar spine can demonstrate disk space narrowing and the presence of spondylophytes along the margins of the vertebral bodies, which are common signs of degenerating vertebral disk. MRI is the best choice for the visualization and grading of the degenerating disk material. MRI will also allow for the assessment of the surrounding soft tissues, adjacent facet joints, and possible effects on the spinal nerves. CT scans may be a better tool for the assessment of spondylolysis and spondylolisthesis.[190,225]

**TREATMENT.** Conservative care including NSAIDs, mild analgesics for short-term pain control, physical therapy, cognitive-behavioral therapy, lifestyle changes (e.g., smoking cessation, weight loss, fitness program), and aerobic conditioning are the first line of treatment for painful DDD.[194] The goal is to reduce painful symptoms and enable the person to return to normal activities as soon as possible. Bed rest is no longer the standard of care.

***Surgery.*** Surgery to remove the disk or disk fragments (diskectomy), laminectomy, and/or spinal fusion may be considered if conservative care has been unsuccessful and/or neurologic symptoms persist. The use of surgical procedures for the treatment of lumbar spine conditions is controversial, as long-term outcomes have not proven to be significantly better than conservative management approaches.[194] Surgical procedures can be appropriately used to avoid permanent nerve damage and footdrop.

A number of procedures have been proposed to address the effects of a degenerating vertebral disk. Injection of steroid, denervating, and anesthetic agents into the disk or adjacent facet joints has been used to diminish local inflammation and decrease nociceptor activity. Electrothermal and radiofrequency energy have been used to induce shrinkage of disk material or to destroy pain receptors surrounding the disk. Many of these methods have provided short-term relief of pain associated with DDD, but have not demonstrated consistent long-term benefits.[65]

For some individuals, artificial disk replacement (ADR) is an alternative to spinal fusion. After removing what is left of the damaged or worn-out disk, the ADR device is inserted in the space between two lumbar vertebrae. The goal is to replace the diseased disk while maintaining normal spinal motion. ADR devices are not designed at this time for the treatment of herniated disks but for one or two levels of DDD. Cervical arthroplasty is also available, with primary indications for the treatment of radiculopathy and myelopathy at one or two levels.[194]

The advantages of this treatment over spinal fusion are maintenance of spinal movement, disk height, and neural foramina, thus simulating a more normal spinal alignment, angulation, and mechanics. Immobilization is avoided with ADR, and early return of function is possible. An additional advantage is prevention of adjacent-segment deterioration that can occur after spinal fusion.

**PROGNOSIS.** Disk structural failure is irreversible, always progresses by physical and biologic mechanisms, and is closely associated with mechanical dysfunction and pain. The potential for recovery varies based on the size of the protrusion, the size of the canal, the person's age and activity level, the extent of disk disruption, and similar parameters related to spondylolisthesis and stenosis.[204] Levels of disability during episodes of back pain, maladaptive coping behaviors, and genetic factors have also been identified as important for recovery of DDD and return to function.[194]

SPECIAL IMPLICATIONS FOR THE THERAPIST 27.10

### *Degenerative Intervertebral Disk Disease*

Degenerative changes of the spine affecting the intervertebral disks often occur concomitantly with other spinal degenerative and osteoarthritic changes, such as spinal stenosis and with the effects of vascular occlusion from atherosclerosis. Two additional conditions are associated with spinal stenosis: cauda equina syndrome and vascular/neurogenic claudication.

Cauda equina syndrome is characterized by pain in the upper sacrum, with paresthesias of the buttocks and genitalia, possibly resulting in bowel or bladder incontinence or sexual dysfunction (difficulty achieving orgasm or inability to achieve or maintain an erection). Numerous conditions may lead to these manifestations, including spinal canal stenosis. Therapists working with clients with back or neck pain should ask about these symptoms, and if any are present, immediate communication with a physician is recommended.[327]

Even with the local degenerative changes in the spine, stenosis may be marked primarily by lower extremity symptoms (neurogenic claudication) as opposed to back pain. The symptoms may include pain, altered sensation, or muscle weakness.

The symptoms are typically brought on by walking and are relieved by prolonged rest (sitting or lying down) or by flexion of the spine. When a person is upright and walking, the lumbar spine is in a relatively backward-bent position, which further reduces the size of the foramina and subarticular recesses. When the spine is flexed, the foramina are opened, relieving pressure on the nerves. Similar symptoms are noted with vascular claudication (tissue ischemia secondary to vascular insufficiency) except that vascular symptoms are not dependent on the position of the spine but rather on the level of activity.

Functionally, people with neurogenic claudication lack the backward-bending range of motion to tolerate walking. If the therapist can improve overall backward-bending range of motion by mobilizing the thoracic and upper lumbar regions and by stretching the hip flexors, the affected individual may be able to assume an upright posture without reaching the end range of motion at the involved segments where the nerve compression is occurring. If this can be accomplished, walking tolerance should improve.[16]

#### Exercise and Degenerative Disk Disease

There is some evidence supporting the efficacy of exercise therapy.[153,35] Most guidelines recommend early stability and motor control exercises for effective treatments for DDD.[145,88] Compared with mobilization treatment, stabilization exercises improved pain and function significantly more than mobilization. More studies are needed to identify the exact type of exercise along with frequency, duration, and intensity. Predictive factors for outcome need to be identified along with identification of candidates most likely to improve with exercise therapy (or type of exercise needed for each person).

Aerobic conditioning is an important feature of the exercise program, especially to address the vascular component of this condition. Walking, swimming and/or water aerobics, and stationary cycling are some possible choices. Each individual's lifestyle and overall physical condition will dictate the most likely course of action to prescribe or suggest.

## Rheumatic Diseases

Rheumatic disorders are systemic diseases encompassing more than 100 different diseases divided into 10 classification categories. The pathogenesis and progression of these disorders can affect all body systems. The onset of joint pain and loss of function may be accompanied by fever, rash, diarrhea, scleritis, or neuritis symptoms that are not typically associated with joint or muscle conditions normally brought on by repetitive overuse or trauma.

Rheumatic disorders are also often marked by periods of exacerbation and remission. During a period of exacerbation the therapist will often need to modify the treatment approach considerably. In addition, aggressive medical intervention (i.e., dose) may need to be initiated to prevent or minimize the tissue destruction that can occur with these disorders. Many rheumatic conditions are chronic and progressive, requiring long-term rehabilitation and ongoing adjustment of functional goals.

Therapists must be able to differentiate the presentation between degenerative joint disease (OA) and rheumatic joint conditions (Table 27.3). If there is any suspicion of the presence of a rheumatic disorder, immediate referral to a physician is warranted. When someone with RA presents with systemic symptoms or if existing symptoms worsen, communication with a physician is advised. An understanding of the diseases discussed in this chapter will assist the therapist regarding this clinical decision-making process.

### Rheumatoid Arthritis

**Overview.** RA is a chronic systemic inflammatory disease that manifests with a wide range of articular and extraarticular findings. Chronic polyarthritis, which perpetuates a gradual destruction of joint tissues, can result in severe deformity and disability. Systems that may be involved include the cardiovascular, pulmonary, and gastrointestinal systems. Eye lesions, infection, and osteoporosis are other potential extraarticular manifestations. RA is a major subclassification within the category of diffuse connective tissue diseases that also includes juvenile arthritis, SLE, progressive systemic sclerosis (scleroderma), polymyositis, and dermatomyositis.[196]

**Incidence and Risk Factors.** RA has a worldwide distribution and affects all races. Approximately 1% to 2% of U.S. adults have RA, which is the second most prevalent form of arthritis after OA. Age and female gender are the two primary risk factors associated with RA. Although the onset of the disorder can occur at any age, the peak onset is usually between 30 and 60 years; with the aging of the U.S. population, the prevalence of RA is

**Table 27.3** Osteoarthritis and Rheumatoid Arthritis

| | **Osteoarthritis** | **Rheumatoid Arthritis** |
|---|---|---|
| Onset | Usually begins at age 40 years<br>Gradual onset over many years; affects majority of adults older than age 65 years | Initially develops between ages 25 and 50 years<br>Onset may be sudden over several weeks to months; intermittent exacerbation and remission |
| Incidence | 12% of U.S. adults age 60 years and older | 1% of U.S. adults; 600,000 men and 1.5 million women; estimated prevalence rate of juvenile RA in children younger than 16 years is 30,000–50,000 |
| Gender | Most common in men before age 45 years; more common among women after age 45 years | Affects women 3 times as often as men, but more disabling and severe when present in men |
| Etiology | Etiology is unknown; immunologic reaction with massive inflammatory response; possible genetic and environmental triggers | Multifactorial; local biomechanical factors, biochemistry, previous injury, inherited predisposition |
| Manifestations | Usually begins in joints on one side of the body | Symmetric simultaneous joint distribution |
| | Primarily affects hips, knees, spine, hands, and feet | Can affect any joint (large or small); predilection for upper extremities |
| | Inflammation with redness, warmth, and swelling in 10% of cases | Inflammation almost always present |
| | Brief morning stiffness that is decreased by physical movement | Prolonged morning stiffness lasting 1 hour or more |
| Associated signs and symptoms | No systemic symptoms; possible associated trigger points | Systemic presentation with constitutional symptoms (e.g., fatigue, malaise, weight loss, fever) |
| Laboratory values | Effusions infrequent; synovial fluid has low WBC and high viscosity | Synovial fluid has high WBC and low viscosity |
| | ESR may be mildly to moderately increased | ESR markedly increased in the presence of an inflammatory process but not specifically diagnostic for RA |
| | Rheumatoid factor absent | Rheumatoid factor usually present but is not specific or diagnostic for RA (can be elevated C-reactive protein) |
| | Numerous biomarkers for inflammation and matrix destruction with uCTX-II and sCOMP being most consistently found | C-reactive protein, a true indicator of systemic inflammation and strong predictor of disease outcome. Numerous possible biomarkers for bone, synovium, and cartilage destruction have been identified |

*ESR*, Erythrocyte sedimentation rate; *RA*, rheumatoid arthritis; *WBC*, white blood cell count.

expected to rise. Women are affected nearly three times more frequently than men; although it is less common, children can also develop the disorder (see Juvenile Idiopathic Arthritis later).

An association between autoimmune thyroid diseases and rheumatic diseases has been established, although the precise mechanism is unclear. For example, RA often occurs in association with Graves disease and Hashimoto thyroiditis. In these individuals, there is a significant presence of antithyroid autoantibodies.[292]

**Etiologic Factors.** The exact pathogenesis of RA is unknown except that joint inflammation is a consequence of massive infiltration of immune cells, especially T lymphocytes, into the synovial fluid. Genetic predisposition and environmental triggers such as bacteria (e.g., *Mycoplasma fermentans*) are both considered possible etiologic factors in the stimulation of T cells.[66,87]

**Pathogenesis.** The cause of RA is unknown, but it is most likely a combination of genetic and environmental factors. Some genetic markers have been identified for the disease, but not all persons with RA have these genes. Approximately 80% of people with RA are rheumatoid factor–positive.[87,131]

Rheumatoid factors are autoantibodies that react with immunoglobulin antibodies found in the blood. Rheumatoid factor has also been found in the synovial fluid and synovial membranes of individuals with the disease. It is hypothesized that the interaction between rheumatoid factor and the immunoglobulin triggers events that initiate an inflammatory reaction. RA begins attacking the joint in the synovium. The normal synovial membrane consists of loose connective tissue that contains blood vessels and is covered by a layer of synovial lining consisting of macrophages and synoviocytes and is only minimally infiltrated by lymphocytes. In RA the cells of the synovial lining multiply, there is an influx of leukocytes from the peripheral circulation, and the synovium becomes edematous. The synovial lining thickens, resulting in the clinical synovitis that is seen so often.[238]

These changes can result in the development of thickened synovium, a destructive vascular granulation tissue called *pannus*. The inflammatory cells found within the pannus are destructive, preventing the synovium from performing its two primary functions: lubricating the joint and providing nutrients to the avascular articular

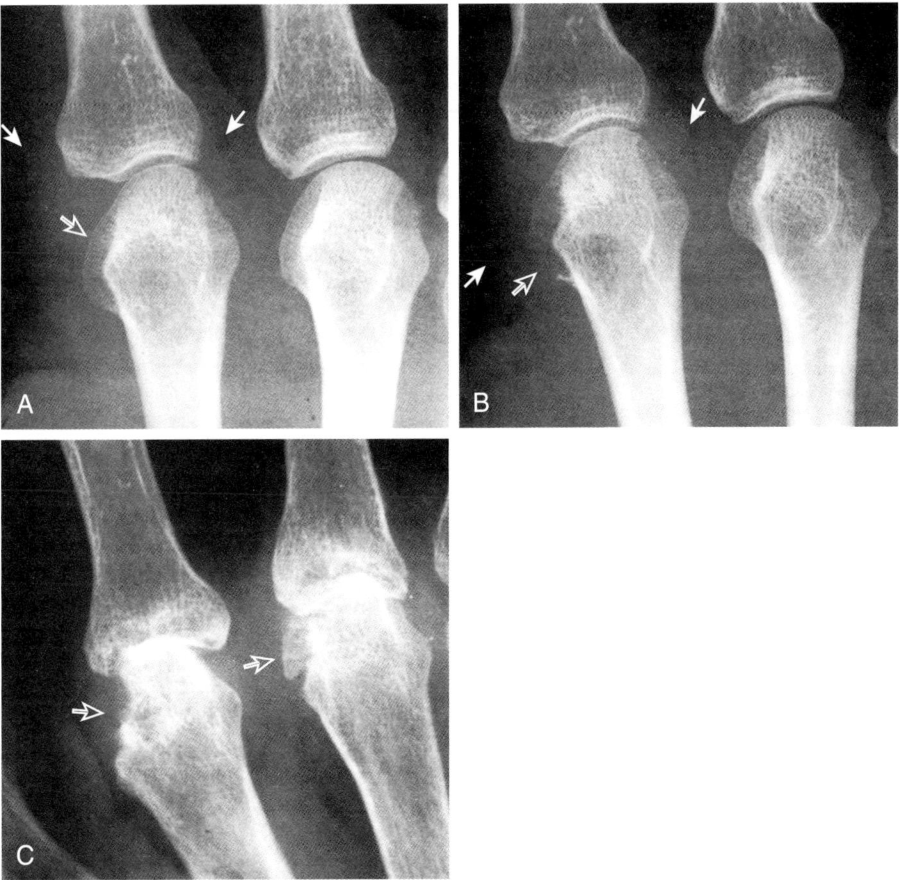


**Figure 27.12**

**Changes seen in rheumatoid arthritis.** (A) In the early stages, swelling of the soft tissue *(solid arrows)*, beginning joint space narrowing, and changes in the metacarpal head *(open arrow)* can be seen. (B) Increase in soft tissue swelling *(arrows)* can be seen including osteoporosis secondary to erosion to the margins of the metacarpal heads *(open arrow)*. (C) In the later stages, the articular space is completely obliterated, and osseous erosions *(open arrows)* are evident. (From Resnick D: *Diagnosis of bone and joint disorders*, ed 4, Philadelphia, 2002, Saunders.)

cartilage. As this tissue proliferates, encroaching on the joint space at the margins where the hyaline cartilage and synovial lining do not adequately cover the bone, it dissolves collagen, cartilage, subchondral bone, and other periarticular tissues in its path (Fig. 27.12).

Although the cause of RA remains unknown, recent advances in molecular techniques have allowed for identification of distinct cell subtypes, surface markers, and products that may initiate and propagate the inflammatory and destructive components of the disease. Cytokines, TNF-α, IL-1, and IL-6, found in abundance in the rheumatoid synovium, appear to play a major role in the pathophysiologic process of RA.[66]

The interaction of cytokines and immune and nonimmune cells (e.g., synovial fibroblasts and osteoclasts) prompts a massive inflammatory response. As the attracted leukocytes, monocytes, and lymphocytes phagocytize the immune complexes, these cytokines stimulate the secretion of matrix metalloproteinases (protein-degrading enzymes that lyse the cartilage and destroy the joint), leading to articular cartilage destruction and synovial hyperplasia with local tenderness, swelling, and intense joint pain. Elevated cytokines also inhibit bone formation and induce bone resorption by directly or indirectly activating osteoclasts. Elevated levels of IL-6 contribute to anemia and fatigue associated with RA by disrupting iron homeostasis and stimulating the hypothalamic-pituitary-adrenal axis, respectively.

The synovial changes that occur in RA can result in irreversible joint instability, joint deformity, or ankylosis (adhesions and fibrous or bony fusion of the joint). Joint destruction eventually leads to laxity of the tendons and ligaments, which contributes to the altered biomechanics and deformities frequently observed. The wide range of extraarticular problems is also probably a result of local inflammatory injury induced by the immune complexes traveling through the circulatory system.

**Clinical Manifestations.** RA is a systemic disease typically manifested by articular and extraarticular symptoms (Box 27.8). The symptoms usually begin insidiously and progress slowly as the disease process moves from cartilage degradation to ligamentous laxity and, finally, synovial expansion with erosion. Patients often initially present with symptoms of fatigue, weight loss, weakness, and general, diffuse musculoskeletal pain. Deconditioning and depression are common complications of this disease.[188]

The course of RA can vary considerably from mild to severely disabling and is difficult to predict, but it appears

Box 27.8

**ARTICULAR AND EXTRAARTICULAR MANIFESTATIONS OF RHEUMATOID ARTHRITIS**

***Cardiac***

- Conduction defects (usually asymptomatic)
- Pericarditis
- Interstitial myocarditis
- Coronary arteritis
- Vasculitis
- Aortitis

***Hematologic***

- Anemia of chronic disease
- Felty syndrome (splenomegaly, neutropenia)
- Lymphoma, leukemia

***Musculoskeletal***

- Osteopenia, osteoporosis (associated fractures)
- Joint pain (reflects severity of synovitis; may not be present at rest)
- Joint stiffness (present in most cases, especially after inactivity; duration reflects degree of synovial inflammation; improves with physical activity)
- Joint contracture (extension of involved joints most commonly affected)
- Swelling (synovial tissue)
- Muscle atrophy (hands, feet; occurs rapidly in severe disease)
- Muscle weakness; often out of proportion to degree of muscular atrophy
- Tenosynovitis, tendinitis, tendon triggering, tendon rupture
- Joint deformity

***Neurologic***

- Compression neuropathies; nerve entrapment syndromes (e.g., carpal tunnel syndrome, tarsal tunnel syndrome)
- Polyneuropathy
- Peripheral neuropathy (mononeuritis multiplex, stocking-glove peripheral neuropathy)
- Myelopathy; subluxation or instability of C1-C2
- Lhermitte sign (upper extremity paresthesias that increase with neck flexion)

***Integumentary***

- Nodulosis (subcutaneous nodules, especially over olecranon and proximal ulna, extensor surfaces of fingers, Achilles tendon ["pump bumps"]) (see Fig. 27.15)
- Nodules can occur in tendon, bone; sclerae; over pinna or ear; and in visceral organs, especially lung
- Palmar erythema (identical to changes found in liver disease and pregnancy; persists even in remission)
- Sweet syndrome
- Vasculitis

***Ocular***

- Episcleritis (inflammation of superficial sclera and conjunctiva)
- Scleritis (inflammation of sclera)
- Sicca syndrome (dry eyes)

***Psychologic***

- Depression (common); other mood disorders

***Pulmonary***

- Effusions
- Interstitial pneumonia
- Interstitial fibrosis
- Nodules (rheumatoid nodulosis)
- Pleurisy, pleuritis
- Empyema
- Pulmonary hypertension

***Renal***

- Interstitial nephritis, nephritic syndrome
- Vasculitis

***Vascular***

- Skin changes (rash, ulcers, purpura, bullae)
- Infarctions (brain, viscera, nail folds)
- Digital gangrene
- Medium vessel arteritis
- Small vessel vasculitis

***Other***

- Unexplained weight loss, anorexia
- Malaise, fatigue
- Lymphadenopathy (lymph node enlargement; more common in men)
- Colon cancer

Data from McInnes IB, O'Dell JR. State-of-the-art: rheumatoid arthritis. *Ann Rheum Dis* 69:1898–1906, 2010; and Clinical manifestations of rheumatoid arthritis. Available at: https://www.uptodate.com/contents/clinical-manifestations-of-rheumatoid-arthritis. Accessed September 6, 2019.

that adults with RA today have less severe symptoms and less functional disability than even a decade ago. This positive trend and more favorable course of disease may be attributed to earlier diagnosis with a shorter duration of symptoms at the time of diagnosis and more aggressive use of drug therapy.[323]

*Joint.* The musculoskeletal symptoms gradually localize to specific or target joints. Multiple joints are usually involved, with symmetric, bilateral presentation. The most frequently involved joints are the wrist; knee; and joints of the fingers, hands, and feet; however, RA can affect any joint, including the temporomandibular joints. The metacarpophalangeal and proximal interphalangeal joints of the hand are involved early. The involved joints can be edematous, warm, painful, and stiff. After periods of rest (e.g., prolonged sitting, sleeping), intense joint pain and stiffness may last 30 minutes to several hours as activity is initiated.[323]

As the disease progresses, joint deformity can occur, including subluxation. Deformities in the fingers are common, including ulnar deviation, swan neck deformity, and boutonnière deformity. The ulnar deviation occurs as the extensor tendons slip to the ulnar aspect of the metacarpal head. The swan neck deformity comprises hyperextension of the proximal interphalangeal joint and partial flexion of the distal interphalangeal joint (Fig. 27.13). The boutonnière deformity is marked by flexion of the proximal interphalangeal joint and hyperextension of the distal interphalangeal joint (Fig. 27.14).

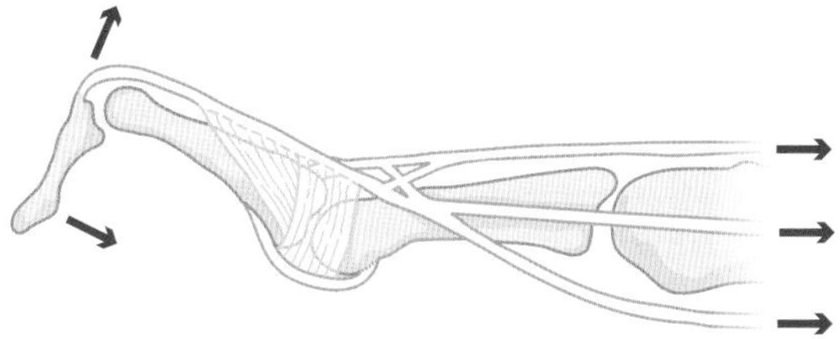

**Figure 27.13**

**Swan neck deformity.** Note the characteristic flexion deformity at the distal interphalangeal joint with hyperextension at the proximal interphalangeal joint. (From Jacobs JL: Hand and wrist. In Richardson JK, Iglarsh ZA, editors: *Clinical orthopaedic physical therapy*, Philadelphia, 1994, Saunders, p 309.)

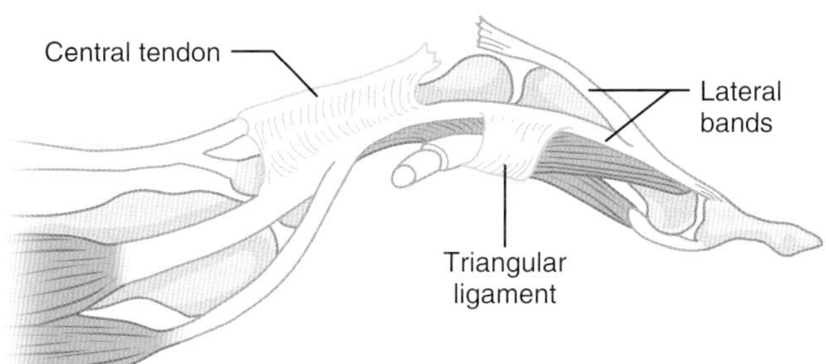


**Figure 27.14**

**Boutonnière deformity.** Note the characteristic flexion deformity of the proximal interphalangeal joint. (From Jacobs JL: Hand and wrist. In Richardson JK, Iglarsh ZA, editors: *Clinical orthopaedic physical therapy*, Philadelphia, 1994, Saunders, p 664.)

*Soft Tissue.* Soft tissue manifestations of RA include synovitis, bursitis, tendinitis, fasciitis, neuritis, and vasculitis. These problems are often overlooked but can be very debilitating. Soft tissue imbalance combined with joint involvement can result in significant deformity, especially in the hands and feet.

*Spine.* Early involvement of the spinal column is common and typically limited to the cervical spine, with deep, aching cervical pain radiating into the occipital, retroorbital, or temporal areas reported in 40% to 88% of persons.[202] Neck movements aggravate cervical pain; facial and ear pain and occipital headaches occur frequently, with active disease from irritation of the C2 nerve root supply to the spinal trigeminal tract, greater auricular nerve, or greater occipital nerve.

There is a potential for atlantoaxial subluxation (usually anterior) and brainstem or spinal cord compression. The upper cervical spine is affected most commonly because the occiput-C1 and the C1-C2 articulations are purely synovial and are thus primary targets for rheumatoid involvement. In addition, because the C1 and C2 facets are oriented in the axial plane, there is no bony interlocking to prevent subluxation in the face of ligamentous destruction. Asymmetric destruction of the lateral atlantoaxial joints may result in a clinical presentation of head tilt down and to one side. When the neck is flexed, the spinous process of the axis may be prominent.[202,227]

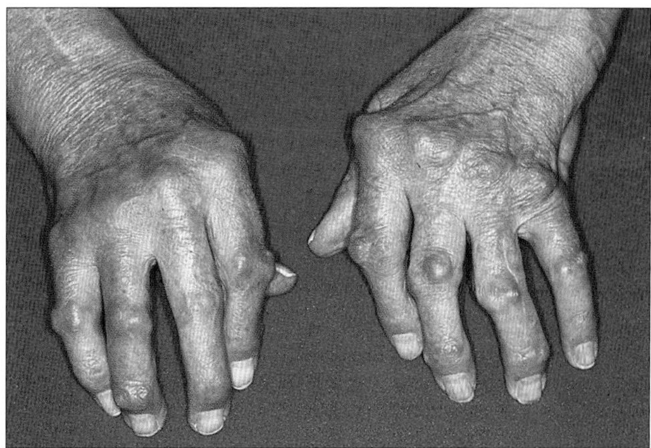

**Figure 27.15**

**Rheumatoid nodules of the digits.** (From Hochberg MC, et al: *Rheumatology*, ed 7, Philadelphia, 2019, Mosby.)

The natural history of cervical instability in people with RA is variable, and only some develop cervical myelopathy.[259] Symptoms of C1-C2 subluxation include a sensation of the head falling forward with neck flexion, loss of consciousness or syncope, dysphagia, vertigo, seizures, hemiplegia, dysarthria, nystagmus, peripheral paresthesias, and loss of dexterity of the hands. Urinary retention and later incontinence are symptoms of more severe involvement of myelopathy. Sleep apnea may be caused by brainstem compression associated with atlantoaxial impaction.[310]

There may be a positive Lhermitte sign with shocklike sensations of the torso or extremities with neck flexion. Atlantoaxial instability may result in vertebrobasilar insufficiency with visual disturbances, loss of equilibrium, vertigo, tinnitus, and dysphagia. These symptoms can also be caused by mechanical compression of the cervicomedullary junction or brainstem.[202]

*Cutaneous.* The visible rheumatoid nodule is a characteristic skin finding in RA, occurring in approximately 25% of all cases. These granulomatous lesions usually occur in areas of repeated mechanical pressure such as over the extensor surface of the elbow, Achilles tendon, and extensor surface of the fingers (Fig. 27.15). Nodules are usually asymptomatic, but they can become tender or cause skin breakdown and become infected. Nodules that cannot be seen visibly can also occur in the heart, lungs, and gastrointestinal tract, causing serious problems such as heart arrhythmias and respiratory failure.

*Neurologic.* One-third of adults with RA have cervical spine involvement leading to compressive cervical myelopathy manifested as neck pain and stiffness, the Lhermitte sign, weakness of the upper or lower extremities, hyperactive distal tendon reflexes, and presence of the Babinski sign. In severe cases, urinary and fecal incontinence and paralysis can occur.[202]

Chronic inflammation of the atlantoaxial joint can lead to laxity of the transverse ligament, which normally keeps the dens closely abutted against the anterior arch of the atlas. With loss of integrity of the ligament, the dens moves backward and presses against the spinal cord

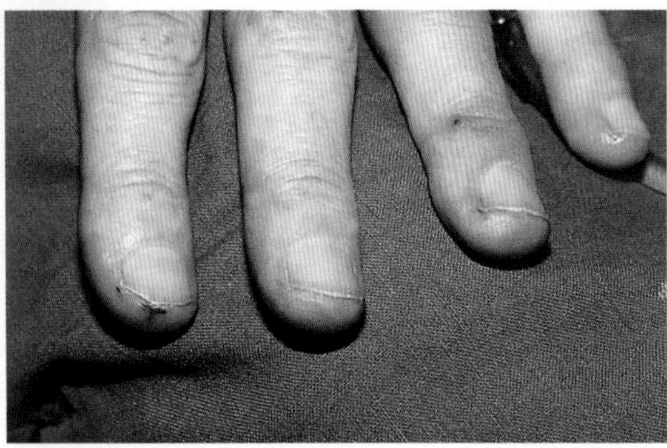

**Figure 27.16**

**Small vessel vasculitis secondary to rheumatoid arthritis.** Small brown infarcts are found in the palm and fingers of patients with chronic rheumatoid arthritis. (From Glynn M, Drake WM: *Hutchison's clinical methods*, ed 24, St. Louis, 2018, Elsevier.)

during forward neck flexion. The individual experiences a shocklike sensation and numbness down the arms with forward flexion of the neck (the Lhermitte sign, previously mentioned). Arthritic changes with erosive involvement of the lower cervical spine facet (zygapophyseal) joints can also lead to compressive myelopathy or radiculopathy.

Peripheral neuropathies are common as the nerves become compressed by inflamed synovia in tight compartments. Pain, dysesthesias, motor loss, and muscle atrophy can occur, leading to dysfunction and disability. Rheumatoid vasculitis involving medium-sized arteries to the muscles can lead to mononeuritis multiplex, while small vessel vasculitis causes stocking-glove peripheral neuropathy.[202]

***Extraarticular.*** The extraarticular manifestations are numerous and affect men and women equally (Fig. 27.16; see Box 27.8). Many of these manifestations impair cardiopulmonary function, restrict activity, decrease endurance, and are disabling; some are life threatening. They could easily hamper rehabilitation efforts, delaying or preventing progress. See Chapters 12 and 15 for descriptions of the cardiovascular and pulmonary manifestations, respectively.

Sjögren syndrome (discussed later) is marked by lymphocytic and plasma cell infiltration of the lacrimal and parotid glands. This can result in diminished salivary and lacrimal secretions. Felty syndrome is marked by splenomegaly and leukopenia. Mood disorders, especially depression, are common.[221]

Individuals with RA are also at increased risk for severe infection, including tuberculosis requiring hospitalization.[30,101] There is also a greater risk of cardiovascular and cerebrovascular morbidity and mortality among adults with RA compared with adults with OA.

The increased risk of myocardial infarction, congestive heart failure, and cerebrovascular accident is not explained by traditional cardiovascular risk factors, but the mechanism for this association is unknown at the present time. Altered immunologic function may possibly explain the increased association, but other factors such as the new biotherapies for RA (e.g., TNF-α blockers) may be at work as well.[101,257]

## MEDICAL MANAGEMENT

**DIAGNOSIS.** In the early stages of RA the diagnosis can be difficult because of the gradual, subtle onset of symptoms. The symptoms may wax and wane, delaying a visit to a physician's office. Early diagnosis can help prevent or reduce erosive and irreversible joint damage as well as reduce morbidity and mortality associated with this chronic disease. The diagnosis is ultimately based on a combination of history, physical examination, imaging studies, and laboratory tests, with careful exclusion of other disorders. Most individuals will be symptomatic for a long period before seeing a physician. At least half of all adults with RA are not referred for rheumatologic consultation until they have had the disease for at least 6 months (sometimes more than 1 year).

The American Academy of Rheumatology has transitioned from endorsing diagnostic criteria for rheumatoid diseases to classification criteria.[7] Classification criteria allow for better specificity in identifying patients with similar attributes and provide for more homogeneous groups of patients for comparison of treatment results. The use of classification criteria has better utility for research purposes but does not have treatment implications for individual patients.

Table 27.4 lists the 2010 Rheumatoid Arthritis Classification adopted by the ACR.[3] The classification is based on the presence of synovitis in at least one joint that cannot be accounted for by an alternative diagnosis, with a score of 6 or higher in four individual score domains of the ACR criteria. The presence of serum rheumatoid factor supports the diagnosis but can also be found in healthy persons. Synovial fluid analysis will reveal an elevated white blood cell count, protein content, and protein antibodies. Also, a decrease in synovial fluid volume and poor viscosity and an increased turbidity may be noted (see Table 27.3). C-reactive protein, an acute-phase reactant, may be helpful when obtained in a series over time to predict individuals who are at increased risk for joint deterioration and as a measure of response to treatment. Persistent elevation in C-reactive protein is a predictive factor for cervical spine subluxation.[369]

Conventional radiography, ultrasonography, and MRI allow for an accurate assessment of the joints with rheumatic changes.[336] The earliest joint changes (periarticular swelling and cortical thinning with erosion at the margins of the articular cartilage and joint space narrowing) are seen on plain radiographs (Fig. 27.17). Screening cervical spine radiographs should be considered for all individuals with RA, but especially for persons with advanced peripheral joint disease.

MRI is more sensitive than conventional radiography for detecting early signs of RA and can show lesions of the synovium and cartilage as well as joint effusions. MRI has the ability to visualize synovitis and detect bone edema, which is emerging as a predictor of future erosive bone changes. Ultrasonography enables the visualization of small superficial structures and can reveal synovial inflammation and tenosynovitis, as well as effusions and bone erosions.[336]

**Table 27.4** 2010 American College of Rheumatology/European League Against Rheumatism Classification Criteria for Rheumatoid Arthritis

Target population (who should be tested):
1. Individuals who have at least 1 joint with definite clinical synovitis (swelling)
2. Individuals with synovitis not better explained by another disease

Classification criteria for RA (score-based algorithm: add score of categories A–D; a score of ≥6/10 is needed for classification of a person as having definite RA)

| | Score |
|---|---|
| A. Joint involvement | |
| 1 large joint | 0 |
| 2–10 large joints | 1 |
| 1–3 small joints (with or without involvement of large joints) | 2 |
| 4–10 small joints (with or without involvement of large joints) | 3 |
| >10 joints (at least 1 small joint) | 5 |
| B. Serology (at least 1 test result is needed for classification) | |
| Negative RF and negative ACPA | 0 |
| Low-positive RF or low-positive ACPA | 2 |
| High-positive RF or high-positive ACPA | 3 |
| C. Acute-phase reactants (at least 1 test result is needed for classification) | |
| Normal CRP and normal ESR | 0 |
| Abnormal CRP or abnormal ESR | 1 |
| D. Duration of symptoms | |
| <6 weeks | 0 |
| ≥6 weeks | 1 |

*ACPA*, Anticytoplasmic antibody; *CRP*, C-reactive protein; *ESR*, erythrocyte sedimentation rate; *RF*, rheumatoid factor.

From Aletaha D, Neogi T, Silman AJ, et al: 2010 Rheumatoid arthritis classification criteria: an American College of Rheumatology/European League Against Rheumatism collaborative initiative. *Arthritis Rheum* 62:2569–2581, 2010.

**TREATMENT.** The primary goal for treatment of RA is to reduce the signs and symptoms to a state of remission. A process described as "treating to target" is used to customize the use of pharmacologic agents and other therapeutic measures to reach this goal for each patient with RA.[324] Early treatment of RA is critical to improving long-term outcomes, as clinical evidence clearly shows that joint destruction in RA begins early in the disease. The treatment goals for patients with RA are to reduce pain; maintain mobility; and minimize stiffness, edema, and joint destruction. Aggressive combination drug therapy (Box 27.9) in conjunction with other management techniques including physical therapy is the mainstay of treatment.[74]

The management approach is individualized, especially in the presence of extraarticular manifestation. The physician has a challenging task trying to optimize the pharmacologic management when there is no way to identify which people will need aggressive therapy. The physician must balance the need for conservative care without being too conservative to avoid unchecked inflammation and joint damage, while avoiding being too aggressive, leading to exposure to potentially toxic medications when less expensive, safer drugs would be just as effective.[324]

The chronic nature of the disease makes client education and continual adherence to the treatment program vital. Because the inflammatory process results in progressive joint destruction, controlling inflammation is a primary goal. Medications, rest, ambulatory assistive devices, orthoses, and ice can be used during the acute phase.

***Pharmacotherapy.*** Many medications are available now to help in the management of RA (see Box 27.9). MTX has become the standard medication for patients with newly diagnosed RA with low disease activity and is the most widely used immunosuppressant for RA management because of its long-term efficacy. Although its exact mechanism is unknown, MTX allows for rapid

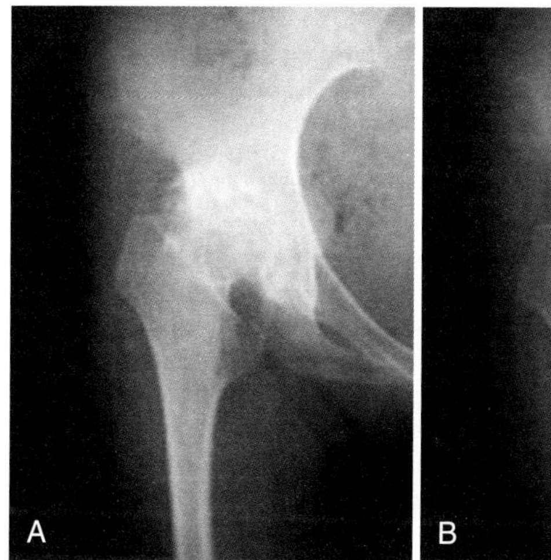

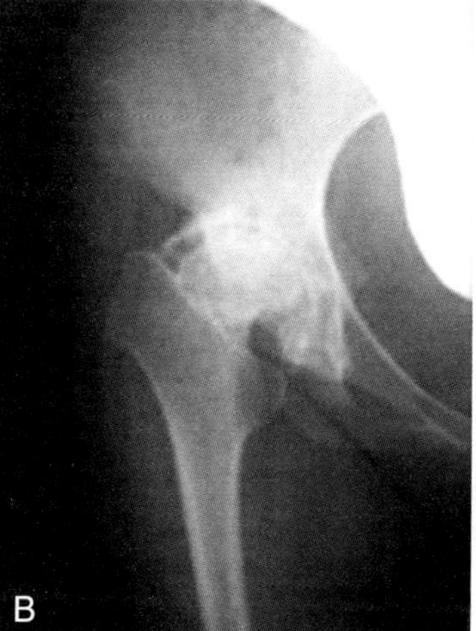

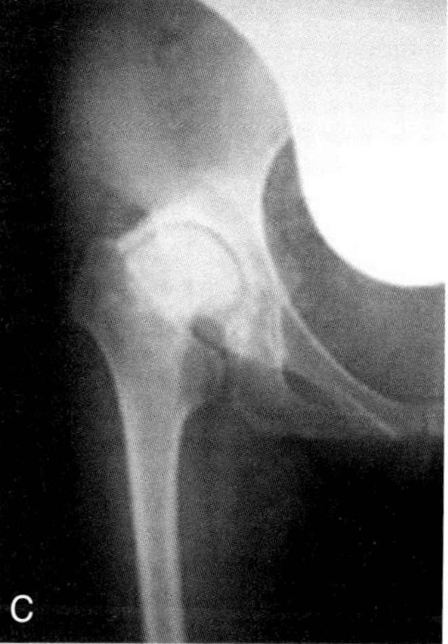


**Figure 27.17**

(A–C) Radiographs showing progression of degeneration of the hip joint secondary to rheumatoid arthritis over a 10-year period. (From Sakuma Y, Ikari K, Iwamoto T, Tokita A, Momohara S. Reparative radiological changes of the hip joint in rheumatoid arthritis: Do these findings indicate the true repair of the joint? *Joint Bone Spine* 77:278–279, 2010.)

Box 27.9

**PHARMACOTHERAPY FOR RHEUMATOID ARTHRITIS**

***Analgesics***

- Various nonprescription and prescription drugs, including acetaminophen (Tylenol), tramadol (Ultram), and codeine

***Nonsteroidal Antiinflammatory Drugs (NSAIDs)***

- Nonprescription and prescription formulas, including aspirin, ibuprofen (Advil, Motrin), naproxen (Aleve, Anaprox, Naprelan, Naprosyn), ketoprofen (Orudis, Oruvail), diclofenac (Voltaren), diflunisal (Dolobid), and indomethacin (Indocin)

***Corticosteroids***

- Oral or injection formulas including prednisone (Cortan, Deltasone, Meticorten), methylprednisolone (Medrol)

***Disease-Modifying Antirheumatic Drugs (DMARDs)***

- Antimalarials (hydroxychloroquine [Plaquenil])
- Nonantibiotic sulfonamides (sulfasalazine [Azulfidine], minocycline [Minocin, Dynacin])
- Injectable and oral gold (Ridaura)
- D-penicillamine (Depen, Cuprimine)
- Methotrexate (Amethopterin, Rheumatrex)
- Immunosuppressants (azathioprine [Imuran], cyclophosphamide [Cytoxan], cyclosporine [Neoral, Sandimmune], leflunomide [Arava])

***Cytokine Inhibitors***[a]

- TNF inhibitors[b] (etanercept [Enbrel], infliximab [Remicade], adalimumab [Humira])
- Interleukin-1 inhibitor (anakinra [Kineret])
- Golimumab (Simponi; human monoclonal antibody to TNF-α)
- Certolizumab (Cimzia; human monoclonal antibody to TNF-α)

***Lymphocyte Inhibitors***

- Rituximab (Rituxan; antibody originally developed for the treatment of B-cell lymphoma)
- Abatacept (Orencia; interrupts the activation of T cells, leading to T-cell anergy and apoptosis)
- Belimumab (Benlysta; inhibits B-cell growth and survival)

[a]Pegylation is a new way to deliver anti–TNF-α agents that are site specific. Polyethylene glycol is added to enhance the pharmacokinetic properties of a molecule, decreasing its volume of distribution and clearance and increasing its half-life.

[b]May also be referred to as TNF-α antagonists.

*TNF,* Tumor necrosis factor.

Data from Yazici Y, Abramson SB: Bright future for RA therapies. *J Musculoskelet Med Suppl* S32–S35, 2006; and McInnes IB, O'Dell JR: State-of-the-art: rheumatoid arthritis. *Ann Rheum Dis* 69:1898–1906, 2010.

remission of joint pain and stiffness found in the early stages of the disease process. Effects tend to plateau after 3 to 6 months, and side effects can be numerous; regular serum monitoring of liver and renal function is required.[325]

Disease-modifying antirheumatic drugs (DMARDs), also known as biologic DMARDs, are used in combination with analgesics, antiinflammatories, and steroids to alter the course and clinical presentation of RA. Some DMARDs block the activity of a protein (TNF) that triggers and prolongs the inflammatory process, leading to joint destruction. Others block IL-1, a protein present in excess in people with RA, thus inhibiting inflammation and cartilage damage.

DMARDs, often used in combination (double or triple therapy), are started for patients with moderate or high levels of disease activity to reduce or prevent joint damage. These drugs take weeks to months to begin working and must be monitored carefully for adverse side effects. DMARDs are often given along with a steroid, which quiets inflammation and improves symptoms while the individual is waiting for the DMARD to take effect. The steroid is then withdrawn slowly.[325]

NSAIDs are effective for pain and swelling associated with inflamed joints caused by RA, but these pharmacologic agents do not affect disease progression. Corticosteroids may be prescribed in addition to DMARDs and NSAIDs to relieve pain and in clients with unremitting disease with extraarticular manifestations. Intraarticular injections can provide relief of acute inflammation. Administration of these drugs for 3 to 6 months is often necessary for benefit to be noted.[123]

Cytokine inhibitors have had an important role in treating individuals with RA. Targeting TNF-α, an important proinflammatory cytokine present in the rheumatoid synovium, has been a great help in treating this disease. IL-1 has several actions that overlap those of TNF-α; TNF-α appears to be more important in early inflammation, while IL-1 may be more important in erosive arthritis. Cytokine targets such as IL-6, IL-12, and IL-18 remain under investigation.[201]

Anti-TNF biologic drugs were developed to target the interaction sites in the pathologic pathway blocking the action of TNF-α, which initiates the inflammatory response, thereby suppressing inflammation more effectively. Etanercept (Enbrel) is a genetically engineered (recombinant) version of a receptor for TNF that helps bind and inactivate excess TNF, thereby reducing the inflammatory response (cytokine inhibitor). When used in combination with MTX, results are superior to those of MTX alone.[191] Non-TNF biologic drugs are for patients with moderate and high levels of disease activity to inhibit the immune response of B and T cells. These drugs can be used in combination with DMARDs and anti-TNF biologics.[332]

Osteoprotegerin is a protein that plays a key role in the physiologic regulation of osteoclastic bone resorption, counteracting the destruction and bone degradation caused by the cytokine-induced inflammatory process. Osteoprotegerin might represent an effective therapeutic option for diseases such as RA that are associated with excessive osteoclastic activity. Other drugs under investigation block protein signals that cause inflammation.[332] Reducing the number of these proteins or blocking the receptors that receive their signals might help control RA.

***Surgery.*** Surgery may be indicated if conservative care is insufficient in achieving acceptable pain control and level of function. Synovectomy to reduce pain and joint damage is the primary operation for the wrist. Total joint replacement procedures are performed at the shoulder, hip, knee, wrist, and fingers. The most common soft tissue procedure is tenosynovectomy of the hand. Studies support prophylactic stabilization of the rheumatoid cervical spine to prevent paralysis in high-risk individuals.[252]

***Complementary, Alternative, and Integrative Therapy.*** Complementary and alternative therapy approaches such as acupuncture and autogenic training have been advocated by some in the treatment of RA but have not shown adequate efficacy for the management of RA.[220] Nutraceuticals such as fish and plant oils and vitamin, mineral, and other supplements (e.g., S-adenosylmethionine) have also been advocated for individuals with RA. Safety and effectiveness have not yet been proven in long-term studies. Physical therapists may be more involved in studying the effects of movement therapies such as Tai chi, Qigong, and yoga.

PROGNOSIS. There is no known cure for RA at the present time, and joint changes are usually irreversible. Restrictions in the ability to perform specific actions and difficulty in performing ADLs can result in functional limitations and disability. It is now established that the longer a person has RA, the greater the likelihood of having cervical spine disease. More specific predictors of neurologic recovery from brainstem or spinal cord compression include location of the disease (basilar invagination has a poorer prognosis than isolated atlantoaxial or subaxial instability), degree of preoperative neurologic deficit, and spinal canal diameter.[202]

Knowledge of the natural history of RA affecting the cervical spine is limited. Studies are small in size and limited in scope. Transition from reducible subluxation to irreducible subluxation often accompanies atlantoaxial impaction an average of 6 years after atlantoaxial subluxation. Up to 80% of individuals with rheumatoid subluxations demonstrate radiologic progression but may not experience corresponding clinical symptoms.[200]

Quality-of-life issues are central to this disease when people in early adulthood who are expected to be active and productive are severely incapacitated. The natural history of RA varies considerably, but people who present to a physician at an early stage and receive early intervention continue to do well years later, with reduced joint pain and inflammation and preservation of function.[140]

Mortality in adults with extraarticular manifestations of RA is significantly greater than in adults whose disease is limited to the joints; in many people the extraarticular manifestations are more debilitating than the arthritis itself. Death from complications associated with RA and its treatment can occur. These complications include subluxation of the upper cervical spine; infections; gastrointestinal hemorrhage and perforation; and renal, heart, and lung disease. The same factors that contribute to joint inflammation also accelerate atherosclerosis and heart disease; early death resulting from coronary artery disease will be the focus of future treatment efforts.[140]

As the complex pathogenesis is better understood, new disease-modifying and biologic drugs that can interrupt tissue and joint destruction without interfering with host defense mechanisms or causing other adverse effects may be developed to stop the progression of this disease.

### Juvenile Idiopathic Arthritis

**Overview and Incidence.** Although the term *juvenile idiopathic arthritis* brings to mind a single disease similar to adult RA, JIA actually comprises a heterogeneous group of arthritides (Box 27.11) of unknown cause beginning in children up to 18 years of age and occurring for at least 6 weeks. Each classification of JIA has a different presentation, genetic background, and

SPECIAL IMPLICATIONS FOR THE THERAPIST 27.11

#### *Rheumatoid Arthritis*

#### Medical Screening of Joint Pain

Therapists must be aware of the symptoms and signs associated with RA. The patient's history will help identify the cause of joint pain. Joint pain and stiffness that is persistent and more bothersome in the morning may indicate symptoms consistent with RA. The distribution of joint involvement is an important clue. RA usually affects the small joints of the feet and hands symmetrically; generalized pain ("I hurt all over") is not characteristic of RA.[3]

Quick, aggressive medical treatment is necessary to minimize joint destruction. Unexplained joint pain for 1 month or more, especially accompanied by systemic symptoms, skin rash, or extensor nodules, no matter how mild, should raise concern on the therapist's part. Cervical pain with reports of urinary retention or incontinence warrants immediate medical evaluation. Also, insidious onset of polyarthritis or joint pain within 6 weeks of an infectious disease or taking a new medication should raise suspicion regarding the nature of the pain symptoms. Any of these red flags suggests the need for a medical referral if a physician has not recently evaluated the affected individual.

When distinguishing articular pain from periarticular involvement, remember that true arthritis produces pain and limitation during both active and passive range of motion, while limitation from tendinitis is much worse during active motion than during passive motion. Inflammatory joint involvement typically produces warmth, erythema, and tenderness. Frequently, there is bogginess related to underlying synovitis or effusion. These indicators are not present with joint pain of a mechanical cause.

#### Patient/Client Education

Helping individuals affected by RA understand the disease, disease process, treatment, possible outcomes, and role of exercise and self-care is a major part of the therapist's task. Self-management includes learning pacing, joint protection, and energy conservation; monitoring symptoms; and maintaining or progressing an exercise program.[337]

Each person must be taught ways to minimize trauma to inflamed joints by unloading joints and reducing mechanical joint stresses. This can be done through modification of activities (e.g., using assistive devices to open doors and jars) and avoiding excessive weight bearing on inflamed joints by reducing movements such as bending and stooping. Energy conservation should become a way of life for anyone with acute or subacute disease. The systemic nature of this disease produces global fatigue; the demand for energy to move joints may increase if biomechanics are altered.[235]

The need for frequent rest breaks, change in level of activity, and change in positions throughout the day should be taught and their use encouraged, but they should be balanced by the need to avoid muscle wasting and weakness from immobilization. Range of motion, stretching, and isometric exercises must be taught, monitored, and reinforced for as long as the therapist follows the individual, always teaching the client how to modify the program during periods of active inflammation.

### Cervical Spine Involvement

Cervical collars may be used for comfort but do not protect against progressive subluxation or neurologic compromise. Rigid cervical collars can partially limit anterior atlantoaxial subluxation, but they also prevent reduction of the deformity in extension. Rigid orthoses are also poorly tolerated in these individuals because of skin sensitivity and temporomandibular joint involvement. Anyone with cervical spine involvement should be taught to avoid cervical flexion. The therapist can focus on isometric strengthening of neck muscles and overall postural training.

In the case of conservative intervention with nonsurgical management, the therapist must observe for (and teach the client to observe for) gradual deterioration in function that may indicate the development of subtle myelopathy (see Clinical Manifestations above).

### Rehabilitation

RA is a chronic, progressive disease requiring an interdisciplinary team approach that is individual to the client and comprehensive, with long-range planning that extends beyond the initial acute phase. The role of the therapist in the management of RA is well established, especially with the renewed focus on outcome-based intervention.[215,173] The ACR developed criteria for classification of functional status for individuals with RA that may help guide the therapist in designing and monitoring the results of an appropriate plan of care (Box 27.10).[18]

The Ottawa Panel identified nine goals in the rehabilitation of individuals with RA, including decreasing pain, effusion (swelling), and stiffness; correcting or preventing joint deformity; increasing motion and muscle force (decreasing weakness); improving mobility and walking; increasing physical fitness; reducing fatigue; and increasing functional status.[268]

Before initiating any rehabilitation program for this group of individuals, a thorough limb and joint examination must be done to provide an objective way to assess and document disease activity and progression or, conversely, remission and improved function. Physical therapy examination should also include assessments of activities and tasks that are noted to be limited by the patient and an overall assessment of ADLs.

Complete bed rest is rarely indicated and is reserved for individuals with severe, uncontrolled inflammation. For many people, a rest period of up to 2 hours during the day is important for dealing with general body fatigue and protection of involved joints. Splints can be applied to rest involved joints, prevent excessive movement, and reduce mechanical stresses. Crutches, canes, or walkers can be used to reduce weight-bearing stresses and enhance balance.

Adaptations may be necessary (e.g., platform crutches) because of upper extremity involvement. A home program of self-management will include instruction in proper body mechanics, positioning, joint protection, and energy conservation. Adaptive equipment designed to make tasks easier may include large key handle attachments allowing the person to use the whole palm to turn a key, spring-open scissors with big loops for anyone with hand involvement, jar openers and electric can openers, clip-on bottle openers, and ergonomic kitchen utensils with large handles and ergonomically angled handles.[34]

Instability at any joint, particularly at the atlantoaxial segment, requires caution on the therapist's part. Such a joint may demonstrate a marked reduction in range of motion, such as the shoulder or neck feeling stuck or caught with a certain movement. A history of periods of significant loss of range of motion alternating

**Box 27.10**

**CLASSIFICATION OF GLOBAL FUNCTIONAL STATUS IN RHEUMATOID ARTHRITIS**

| | |
|---|---|
| Class I | Completely able to perform usual activities of daily living (self-care, vocational, avocational)[a] |
| Class II | Able to perform usual self-care and vocational activities, but limited in avocational activities |
| Class III | Able to perform usual self-care activities, but limited in vocational and avocational activities |
| Class IV | Limited in ability to perform usual self-care, vocational, and avocational activities |

[a]Usual self-care activities include dressing, feeding, bathing, grooming, and toileting. Vocational (work, school, homemaking) and avocational (recreational and/or leisure) activities are patient-desired and age- and sex-specific.

From American College of Rheumatology. Available at: https://www.rheumatology.org/Practice-Quality/Clinical-Support/Criteria/ACR-Endorsed-Criteria. Accessed September 9, 2019.

with full range of motion suggests joint hypermobility. Restoration of mobility is an important goal, but choosing techniques that are gentle or applying traction while stretching is necessary.

Extraarticular problems may affect the rehabilitation program. For example, if fatigue is present, the therapist may have to allow periods of rest during the treatment session. During periods of symptom exacerbation there is a fine line between overextending the client and maximizing activity. There are times when active exercise may have to be curtailed, but passive stretching remains important to prevent contractures.

### Remission

The primary goal for RA treatments is to attain and maintain a long period of remission. Physical therapists should regularly assess a patient's functional abilities and joint mobility as assessment for the remission of the inflammatory process. The complete absence of tender or swollen joints is the most important sign of remission.[9] An absence of joint symptoms for 2 consecutive months is needed to determine a remission, but a definitive timeline has not been established.

### Postoperative Care

Surgical treatment of RA is often complicated by the client's generalized debilitated condition. Joint replacements may be performed to diminish persistent target joint symptoms, improve function, and improve the appearance of a joint deformity.[231] People with RA tend to have poor skin condition, poorly healing wounds, and osteopenic bone. Generalized bone loss occurs early in the course of RA and correlates with disease activity. This condition is further affected by the use of corticosteroids.

Poor nutritional status has been associated with higher complication rates, including infection following surgery. Following Standard Precautions with adequate handwashing is important. Likewise, promoting respiration with good breathing techniques is an important component of the therapist's postoperative intervention.

Clients with RA should be taught early on that if surgery is ever indicated, a program of isometric and range-of-motion exercises before surgery is advised. Review dislocation precautions and restrictions before the surgical procedure. After arthroplasty, correction of deformity and relief of pain are typical, but recurrence of deformity is possible even with appropriate rehabilitation. Many clients are still very satisfied with the improved cosmesis, reduced pain, and improved function. Maximum benefit from arthroplasty may not occur for up to 1 year after surgery.[258]

The postoperative rehabilitation regimen must be tailored to the specific needs of each individual. The surgeon's intraoperative assessment of the quality of tissues, component stability, and any associated repairs is critical to the rehabilitation protocol selected. Specific motion limitations vary depending on intraoperative repairs made, complications, and adverse events (e.g., infection, wound dehiscence, dislocation, implant fracture or failure, nerve damage).

### Exercise and Rheumatoid Arthritis

Therapeutic exercises, including specific functional strengthening and whole-body functional activities, are a beneficial intervention for individuals with RA. The benefits may vary depending on the stage of disease (acute, subacute, inactive) but include reduced pain, improved overall function, and decreased number of sick leaves.[268,171,178]

Whereas rest has often been the treatment of choice, a balance must be attained between rest required during acute flare-ups and activity necessary to prevent the deconditioning effects of prolonged rest, immobilization, and inactivity. Education regarding the efficacy of exercise and its proper use in self-management of RA has been shown to be effective in reducing stiffness and improving function in as little as 4 hours of a community-based physical therapy intervention delivered over a period of 6 weeks.[37]

To date, there is no evidence that active exercise beneficially affects the inflammatory processes associated with adult RA, but it has been shown that a short-term intensive exercise program in active RA is more effective in improving muscle strength than a conservative exercise program and does not have deleterious effects on disease activity.[171,26]

Studies of long-term intensive exercise have not shown an increase in joint swelling or pain with such a regimen. In fact, people with RA who exercise rigorously at least twice a week for 1 hour show more improvement in physical abilities such as stair climbing and reduced psychologic distress compared with individuals who received standard care.[84]

### General Concepts

Exercises to prevent contractures, improve strength and flexibility, and enhance cardiorespiratory or aerobic conditioning are important components of the rehabilitation program.[294] Joint pain leads to a reflex inhibition of muscle surrounding the joints, causing disuse atrophy of these muscles. Use of corticosteroids may lead to an additional decrease in strength and function.

The feet are often overlooked in people with RA, but foot involvement occurs frequently, can impair gait, and can prevent safe participation in an exercise program. Foot involvement resembles that of the hand, with one important difference being that alterations in biomechanics may cause excessive stress to proximal lower extremity joints and to the spine areas forced to compensate for the altered gait.

Careful assessment of the feet may reveal uneven or pathologic weight-bearing patterns. Gait analysis and assessment of shoe wear can provide additional significant information regarding altered biomechanics. Providing assistive devices or orthotics before initiating an exercise program may be essential.[25,156]

Range-of-motion exercises should begin with low repetitions several times throughout the day. Isometric exercises with short holds (4 to 6 seconds) have been suggested, again using low repetitions (start with one or two and build up gradually to four to six).

Range-of-motion exercises can be increased up to 8 to 10 repetitions in subacute cases, with the addition of dynamic strengthening exercises. Stable, quiescent, or inactive disease makes it possible to add an aerobic component such as walking, aquatics, or biking for at least 15 minutes each day, three times a week. Range of motion and strengthening can be continued and monitored.

During active exercise programs the therapist should monitor fatigue levels and should avoid overtraining. For individuals with active (acute) disease, adequate sleep is essential for controlling mood, fatigue, and pain levels. Encourage 8 to 10 hours of rest each night.[177]

### Exercise Prescription

A helpful guide in establishing the level of acceptable exercise intensity is as follows: Acute pain during exercise indicates a need to modify the program; if joint pain persists for more than 1 hour after exercise is completed, the exercise was probably excessive. Engaging in moderate-level exercise for 30 minutes per day 4 or 5 days per week appears to substantially increase physical fitness, even for older adults. Exercise spaced out over the course of the day can help loosen up stiff, achy joints while still providing cardiovascular benefits.[331]

The Arthritis Foundation website describes the benefits and types of exercises, how to start, and how to keep going. This website educates people about the possible effects of not exercising (e.g., increased joint stiffness, muscle weakness, muscle atrophy, increased risk of fracture and deformity). The foundation also provides valuable exercise tips for before, during, and after exercise.[106]

Currently the National Arthritis Foundation offers the largest standardized exercise program to individuals with arthritis through two community-based programs: an on-land exercise program called the Arthritis Foundation Exercise Program and an aquatic exercise program called the Arthritis Foundation Aquatic Program. The Arthritis Foundation Exercise Program is led by a certified instructor using a variety exercises to improve motion, strength, endurance, balance, coordination, posture, and body mechanics.[20]

### Strength Training

Dynamic strengthening (gradually increasing resistance) through the full available range of motion helps stabilize joints, reducing erosive wear and tear on the structures. Regular, dynamic strength training combined with endurance-type physical activities improves muscle strength and physical function, but not bone mineral density, in adults with early and long-standing RA, without causing detrimental effects on disease activity.[26,143]

Low-load resistive muscle training has been shown to increase functional capacity and is a clinically safe form of exercise in mild to moderate RA. Moderate- or high-intensity strength training programs have better training effects on muscle strength in RA. It is essential to maintain the training routine to obtain long-term benefits.[144] Strengthening in some cases of RA can be difficult because exercise may lead to increased joint swelling and subsequent joint destruction. Persons with RA may be hesitant to participate in a regular exercise program.[352]

### Aerobic Exercise

Aerobic exercise in this population is necessary to help reduce weight and improve cardiovascular fitness without increasing pain.[302] Aerobic exercises are safe to perform during the subacute and inactive stages of RA. Aerobic capacity can be estimated using a single-stage submaximal treadmill test. Training programs begin at 50% (and work toward 80%) of maximal oxygen uptake based on the baseline test results. Without baseline testing, the therapist can rely on (and teach the client to use) the Borg scale for rate of perceived exertion. Heart rate monitors are also helpful in enabling clients to track their cardiovascular responses.

Screening for unknown coronary artery disease is recommended before initiating resistance or aerobic exercise. RA can also affect the bony structures of the rib cage and cause a decrease in chest expansion. The usual precautions for cardiopulmonary screening still apply based on the individual's age, risk factors, and health history (especially heart health history).

People with RA may have normal pulmonary function tests but reduced respiratory muscle strength and endurance with reduced aerobic capacity compared with adults without RA.[70] Assessment of respiration and intervention to improve breathing patterns are important components of the rehabilitation program.

### Aquatic Therapy

Aquatic therapy may be beneficial for conditioning, strengthening, and flexibility while reducing mechanical stress on the joints. Water exercise provides the means by which people with RA can reach needed training levels in a comfortable environment. The Arthritis Foundation Aquatic Program consists of 72 exercises similar to the PACE (personalized aerobics for cardiovascular enhancement) program that can be done in water with decreased joint loading, a reduced effect of gravity, increased buoyancy, and increased circulation.[20]

### Modalities and Rheumatoid Arthritis

Various modalities provide temporary pain relief and may be used for effectively and safely controlling symptoms of the acute inflammatory phase of RA. Information on the rationale for use and effectiveness of the various physical modalities is available.[19] Although cold may be more suitable in acute inflammation, people with RA usually prefer heat. Superficial heat (e.g., paraffin baths, moist hot packs, hydrotherapy, or aquatic therapy) is recommended for palliative treatments of acute flare-ups. Caution must be used with prolonged or deep heat because it may increase intraarticular temperature, leading to increased collagenase activity, possibly contributing to joint destruction.[293]

Electrotherapeutic modalities and thermotherapy physical agents are often used as part of a rehabilitation program mainly to obtain pain relief, to control inflammation, and to reduce joint stiffness. Therapeutic ultrasound, thermotherapies, electrical stimulation, and transcutaneous electrical nerve stimulation have been used as adjuncts to the management of RA.[172] These modalities are considered to be preparatory for the initiation of active exercises and manual therapies.

### Medications

Because of the long-term nature of RA, interventions are an ongoing process. Numerous other side effects can occur with any of the pharmacologic agents used in the management of RA. The therapist should be aware of the potential side effects with any medications the client is taking. NSAIDs and other medications are potentially ulcerogenic, and prolonged use of corticosteroids can lead to osteoporosis. Periodic screening of each of the body systems is imperative when working with this population; a patient taking DMARDs but still having joint pain and swelling should be reevaluated by the rheumatologist.

prognosis. The ACR currently uses three major classifications for JIA: pauciarticular, polyarticular. and systemic. The International League of Associations for Rheumatology recently revised their classifications system.[311,232]

Many other forms of arthritis (e.g., SLE, dermatomyositis, scleroderma) that affect adults occur less frequently in children. Approximately 30,000 to 50,000 children in the United States are affected by one of the classifications discussed here (Fig. 27.18). The general classification of JIA is based on the number of involved joints and the presence of systemic signs and symptoms.[311]

*Pauciarticular or oligoarticular* (meaning "few joints") JIA generally affects four or fewer joints during the first 6 months of disease, usually in an asymmetric pattern, and most commonly involves the knees, elbows, wrists, and ankles. Girls are affected more often than boys, usually between the ages of 1 and 5 years. This type of JIA is relatively mild with few extraarticular features. Parents may notice a swollen joint and limp or abnormal gait, usually early after the child wakes up in the morning. Leg-length discrepancy is common. Pain is not a central feature at first, and the disease rarely manifests any constitutional symptoms.

Pauciarticular JIA is the most common type of JIA, accounting for half of all JIA cases; it has three subtypes. The first is characterized by the presence of antinuclear antibodies and a high risk of uveitis, a potentially dangerous inflammation of the eye resulting in irreversible damage and blindness. The second subtype affects the spine as well as other joints, although spinal involvement may not occur until the child reaches late adolescence. Children with this subtype may test positive for the HLA-B27 genetic marker, which is common in adults with AS (this subtype is sometimes referred to as juvenile AS). In the third subtype, joint involvement is the extent of the disease. Usually pauciarticular JIA has a benign course; up to 20% of children experience recurrences, most often during the first year but possibly delayed by as much as 5 years after the initial diagnosis. Some children develop persistent joint disease, referred to as extended oligoarthritis.[76]

*Polyarticular* JIA affects five or more joints, most commonly including large and small joints (wrists, cervical spine, temporomandibular joint, small joints of the hands and feet as well as knees, ankles, and hips). Joint involvement is usually symmetric and is most like that of adult RA, with the potential for severe, destructive arthropathy.

Polyarticular JIA comprises 40% of all cases of JIA and affects girls more often than boys. There are two subtypes depending on whether children are rheumatoid factor–positive or rheumatoid factor–negative. The rheumatoid factor–positive subtype is characterized by the presence of rheumatoid factor (a type of autoantibody found in the blood of adults with RA) and the *DR4* genetic type, also common in adults with RA. Subcutaneous nodules, cervical spine fusion, chronic uveitis, and destructive hip disease can occur in this type of polyarticular JIA.[76]

The second subtype is characterized only by joint involvement, usually less severe. Children with this subtype do not test positive for rheumatoid factor. Morning

**Box 27.11**

**SUBCATEGORIES OF JUVENILE IDIOPATHIC ARTHRITIS**

- Pauciarticular JIA (oligoarthritis)
- Polyarthritis JIA (RF+)
- Polyarthritis JIA (RF–)
- Systemic-onset JIA
- Psoriatic JIA
- Enthesitis-related arthritis
- Other (undefined)

*JIA*, Juvenile idiopathic arthritis; *RF+*, rheumatoid factor–positive; *RF–*, rheumatoid factor–negative.

Data from Petty RE: ILAR classification of JIA: second revision, Edmonton 2001. *J Rheumatol* 31:390, 2004.

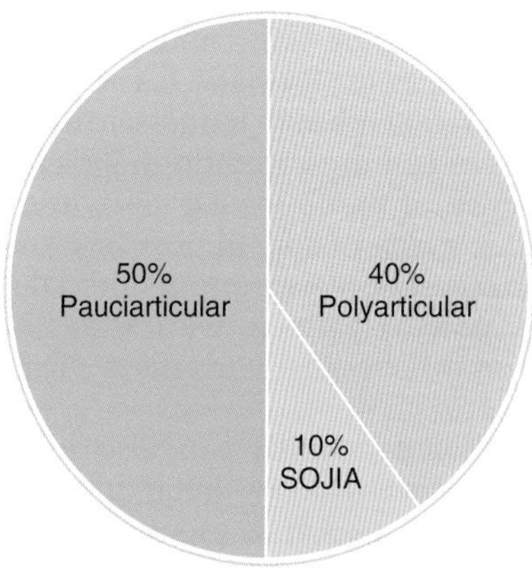


**Figure 27.18**

**Breakdown in types of juvenile idiopathic arthritis.** *SOJIA*, Systemic-onset juvenile idiopathic arthritis.

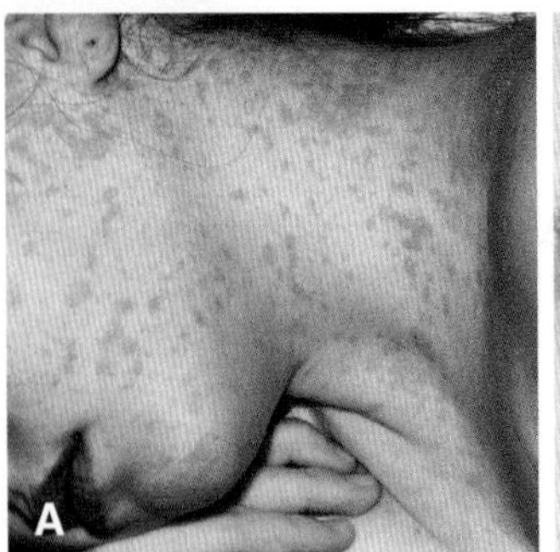

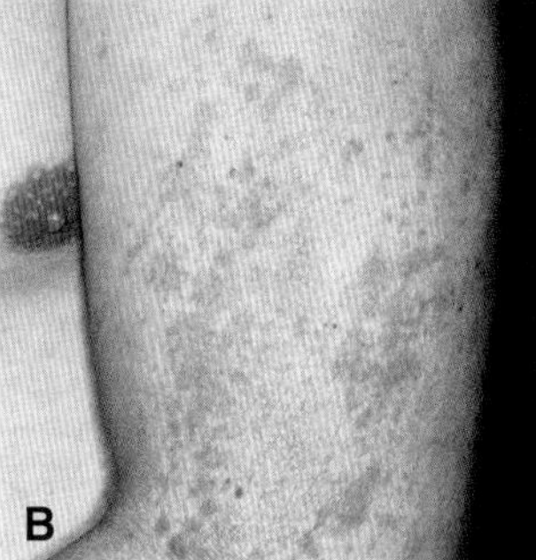


**Figure 27.19**

(A–B) Skin rash associated with juvenile idiopathic arthritis. (A, From Paller AS, Mancini AJ: *Hurwitz clinical pediatric dermatology: a textbook of skin disorders of childhood adolescence*, ed 3, Philadelphia, 2006, Saunders. B, From James WD, et al: *Andrews' diseases of the skin: clinical dermatology*, ed 10, Philadelphia, 2006, Saunders.)

stiffness and fatigue with possible low-grade fever are common clinical manifestations of this type of JIA.

*Systemic-onset* JIA (also called Still disease; sometimes also affecting adults, although rare) affects boys and girls equally, with involvement of any number of joints. This subtype has the most severe extraarticular manifestations, affecting many body systems, and comprises 10% of all cases of JIA. It often begins with a high-spiking fever and chills that appear intermittently for weeks and may be accompanied by a rash on the thighs and chest that often goes away within a few hours (Fig. 27.19). The fever pattern is marked by spikes exceeding 39 °C (102 °F) and periods between the spikes during which the child feels much better.[69]

Inflammatory arthritis typically develops at some point, and 95% of the children have joint symptoms within 1 year of the initial presenting symptoms. Approximately one-half of the children who have systemic-onset JIA recover almost entirely; one-third of affected children remain ill, with persistent inflammation manifesting as fever, rash, and chronic destructive arthritis.

In addition to inflamed joints, the child may experience macrophage activation syndrome and lymphadenopathy; inflammation of the liver, spleen, heart, and surrounding tissues; and anemia. Box 27.12 lists clinical manifestations associated with Still disease.[298]

Psoriasis is a chronic skin condition associated with autoimmune processes. Psoriatic JIA is the inclusion of joint swelling along with skin redness, irritation, and scaling. Psoriatic JIA is more common in girls and manifests with at least two of the following: dactylitis, nail abnormalities, and a family history of psoriasis. Diagnosis may be delayed because joint symptoms precede skin manifestations by years. Treatment with aggressive immunosuppressives may be required; uveitis is a feature in some cases.[70]

Enthesitis-related arthritis can also occur in childhood and is characterized by inflammation of the tendon attachments to the bone, especially along the spine and Achilles tendon. This type of arthritis is classified by presentation of these symptoms along with any two of the following: sacroiliac joint tenderness, inflammatory spinal pain, the presence of HLA-B27, positive family history, acute uveitis, and pauciarticular or polyarticular arthritis in boys older than 8 years.[6]

**Box 27.12**

**CLINICAL MANIFESTATIONS ASSOCIATED WITH STILL DISEASE**

***Systemic***

- Fever
- Rash
- Lymphadenopathy
- Polyarthritis
- Pericarditis
- Pleuritis
- Peptic ulcer disease
- Hepatitis
- Anemia
- Anorexia
- Weight loss

***Musculoskeletal***

- Polyarthritis, polyarthralgias
- Myalgia, myositis
- Tenosynovitis
- Skeletal growth disturbances (short stature, failure to thrive)

Data from Bagnari V, Colina M, Ciancio G, Govoni M, Trotta F. Adult-onset Still's disease. *Rheumatol Int* 30:855–862, 2010.

## Pathogenesis and Risk Factors

The cause is still poorly understood, but JIA may be triggered by infection (viral or bacterial) and environmental factors in children with a genetic predisposition. Genomic studies hope to identify genetic traits that will predict disease risk and other characteristics, such as disease course, age of onset, and disease severity. Researchers may eventually be able to identify pathogenetic pathways to help diagnose and target treatment for this group of arthritides.[291]

JIA can occur in boys or girls of any age (girls more often than boys) and most commonly begins during the toddler or early adolescent period. The pathogenesis is similar to that of adult RA, with immune cells mistakenly attacking the joints and organs, causing inflammation, destruction, fatigue, and other local and systemic effects. TNF, IL-1, and IL-6 seem to be the primary cytokines responsible for many systemic features. These cytokines increase collagenase activity, osteoclast activation, body temperature, and muscle and fat breakdown as well as acute-phase reactants.

## MEDICAL MANAGEMENT

**DIAGNOSIS.** Early disease recognition is needed to help improve the clinical outcome, but symptoms of rheumatic disease are often mistaken for a persistent infectious diseases or growing pains, delaying diagnosis by many months. Diagnosis involves a medical history; physical examination; and laboratory tests including serum evaluation to measure inflammation and to detect antinuclear antibodies, rheumatoid factor, or sometimes HLA-B27.[291]

For a diagnosis of JIA, signs of arthritis must be seen in one or more joints for at least 6 weeks in children younger than 16 years; it may take up to 6 months to determine which subtype is present. Pain is often dull and aching and less severe, but presents in the morning and early during the day rather than the more common presentation of growing pains at night. The systemic features in systemic-onset JIA are more readily diagnosed.

**TREATMENT AND PROGNOSIS.** There are a number of treatment options for individuals with JIA, which include medications to decrease cytokines and inflammatory mediators within the affected joints. The goal of treatment is to control pain, preserve joint motion and function, minimize systemic complications, and assist in normal growth and development.[328]

Early use of DMARDs such as MTX are replacing the previous gradual add-on approach to treatment (i.e., start with one drug and slowly add another and another to gain the desired effects without too many side effects). TNF inhibitors have been shown to be very beneficial for individuals with JIA. IL-1 blockade is used for patients with macrophage activation syndrome as a complication of systemic JIA. Medications are administered to control the systemic and articular symptoms and, in some cases, halt the progression of the disease.

Adverse effects from taking anti-TNF agents (e.g., neurologic disorders, weight gain, severe infection, hemorrhagic diarrhea) have been reported and should be monitored for carefully. In systemic JIA, approximately 50% respond to anti-TNF agents, but in many children, the response is not sustained. Corticosteroids and other antiinflammatory drugs are indicated if severe anemia, unrelenting fever, or vasculitis is present. Bone marrow transplantation may be used in cases of JIA that are resistant to standard medical management.[328]

The prognosis for children with JIA has greatly improved as a result of substantial progress in early detection and in disease management matching medications with the classification type of JIA. Early-onset, progressive forms of JIA have a guarded prognosis. Many children attain long periods of remission but still have symptoms that extend into adulthood. Mortality risk is increased for individuals with severe forms of systemic JIA secondary to complications and need for stem cell transplants.[82] Autologous and allogeneic stem cell transplantation is used for some individuals whose disease is refractory to MTX and other DMARDs. Complete remission is possible for up to half of patients receiving autologous stem cell transplantation, with improvement reported in individuals who are not resistant. Infections are a common morbidity associated with this treatment.[180]

**SPECIAL IMPLICATIONS FOR THE THERAPIST 27.12**

### *Juvenile Idiopathic Arthritis*

Children with JIA may have no disability, especially if they have the oligoarticular form of the disease. Severe disability is seen most often in cases of rheumatoid factor–positive polyarticular and systemic disease, followed by rheumatoid factor–negative polyarthritis, enthesitis-related arthritis, and psoriatic arthritis. Physical therapy is an important adjunctive therapy for JIA.[136]

Physical therapy and occupational therapy are used for pain control, facilitation of mobility, and function. Equally important is the role of exercise in improving strength, endurance, and aerobic capacity.[138] Resistive exercise produces a change in the immune response, with significantly lower levels of cytokines and higher levels of antiinflammatory compounds compared with subjects who did not exercise. Loss of joint motion is the strongest indicator of functional disability in children with systemic JIA, and loss of joint motion has a greater effect on lower limb function than on upper limb function.[36] By the time children become adults, only 20% of them have moderate to severe limitations.

The therapist should keep in mind the significant impact JIA has on children and their families. Psychosocial-spiritual and quality-of-life issues should also be addressed by the rehabilitation team.[136] Appearance and body image are affected directly by JIA (e.g., generalized growth failure, local growth anomalies such as micrognathia), side effects of drug therapy, surgical scars, and severity of pain and fatigue. The therapist may be the first to recognize overall problems with adjustment, as reflected by anxiety, depression, and/or social withdrawal. For children with JIA who reach adulthood, significant problems can result from arthritis and uveitis, medication morbidity, and the lifelong costs associated with disability.[130]

#### Exercise and Juvenile Idiopathic Arthritis

Exercise programs prescribed for patients with JIA are generally well tolerated, but the lack of high-quality studies limits the ability to provide specific recommendations for each classification of JIA. A recent systematic review found 10 quality studies of exercise programs prescribed or led by a physical therapist.[206] Aquatic physical therapy is an excellent way to complete exercises while providing joint protection and engaging the child in a fun activity. A study of children 5 to 13 years of age with JIA in a supervised aquatic training program found the program to be well tolerated with no worsening health status and symptoms, suggesting that swimming is a safe exercise program.[333]

Strengthening programs for children with rheumatic disease can be part of the exercise program, even for children younger than 6 years of age. Short sessions distributed throughout the day are advised. A strengthening program using play-related activities of jump roping and lower extremity weight-bearing activities has been shown to be well tolerated and resulted in improved muscle strength in a study of children and adolescents with JIA.[300]

Active exercise is not advised during flare-ups when joints are inflamed, but most children usually self-limit their physical activity according to symptoms. Passive stretching and modified aquatic physical therapy are better choices during exacerbations. Parents and children should be educated on the importance of avoiding forced or deep flexion of inflamed joints. Some activities may need to be modified or avoided.

Children with quiescent JIA can participate in some sports activities. With improved medical therapies, children with JIA are able to lead a more active lifestyle than similar children were able to do even 10 years ago.[212] The therapist can be helpful in assessing each child for abnormal biomechanics that can place the child at increased risk for injury or future articular damage. Neuromuscular training to improve neuromuscular function and biomechanics has been described for a young athlete with JIA. Proper technical performance during athletics may allow children with JIA to use joint-loading techniques (e.g., during jumping and landing) in a safe and controlled manner.[250]

Low bone mineral density is a common secondary condition associated with JIA. Weight-bearing exercise programs to reduce the risk of low bone mineral density are safe and effective for children with JIA who are healthy and should be included in the plan of care. More research is needed to determine the amount, duration, and frequency of weight-bearing activity needed to reduce the risk for low bone mineral density in this population.[301]

The role of physical activity and an active lifestyle in cardiorespiratory fitness has been documented, but long-term follow-up is still needed to show if such a program protects from loss of aerobic fitness in this population group.[334] The 6-minute walk test has been shown to be a good test for measuring functional exercise capacity in a small study of children 7 to 17 years of age (boys and girls) with JIA. Exercise programs for patients with JIA can include aerobic activities, but need to be assessed for patient tolerance, progressed based on the patient's fitness, and age appropriate.

## Spondyloarthropathies

Spondyloarthropathies (SpAs), a group of disorders formerly considered variants of RA, are in fact distinct entities with similar features affecting the spine (Box 27.13). SpAs are characterized by inflammation of the joints of the spine and include several distinct entities: AS, Sjögren syndrome, psoriatic arthritis, reactive arthritis including arthritides that accompany inflammatory bowel disease (known as enteric arthritides), and Reiter syndrome. Inflammatory eye disease (e.g., uveitis, conjunctivitis, iritis) occurs in approximately 25% of clients.[3]

Box 27.13

**COMMON FEATURES OF THE SPONDYLOARTHROPATHIES**

- Chronic inflammation of the axial skeleton and sacroiliac joints
- Asymmetric involvement of a small number of peripheral joints
- Young males (late teens, early adulthood) most commonly affected
- Familial predisposition
- Inflammation at sites of ligament, tendon, and fascial insertion into bone
- Seronegativity for rheumatoid factor, but an association with histocompatibility antigens including HLA-B27
- Extraarticular involvement of eyes, skin, genitourinary tract, cardiac system

Enteropathic arthritis (arthritis associated with inflammatory bowel disease) occurs in approximately 20% of clients who have inflammatory bowel disease (e.g., Crohn disease, ulcerative colitis) and is discussed further in Chapter 16. Arthritic symptoms flare with inflammatory bowel disease and usually affect the lower extremities in an asymmetric pattern. Vasculitis, clubbing of the fingers, and skin changes may be present.

Biomarkers for SpAs include matrix metalloproteinases, collagen neoepitopes, and the presence of IL-6. Specific changes in the cells of the synovial tissue correspond to treatment with TNF blockers. Biopsy specimens of synovial tissue taken after treatment, showing changes in synovial macrophages, polymorphonuclear leukocyte levels, and expression of matrix metalloproteinase-3, which are thought to play a role in the degradation of collagen, may lead scientists to use these same biomarkers for early identification and treatment of RA.[57]

### Ankylosing Spondylitis

***Overview and Incidence.*** AS, sometimes referred to as Marie-Strümpell disease, is an inflammatory arthropathy of the axial skeleton including the sacroiliac joints, apophyseal joints, costovertebral joints, and intervertebral disk articulations. This results in both erosive osteopenia and bony overgrowth within these involved joints. Approximately one-third of individuals with AS have asymmetric involvement of the large peripheral joints, including the hip, knee, and shoulder. Fig. 27.20 shows the most commonly involved joints. The disorder can ultimately lead to fibrosis, calcification, and ossification with fusion of the involved joints. The pain, resultant postural deformities, and complications associated with this disease can be disabling.[320]

Prevalence of AS is up to 0.5% in the U.S. general population. Nearly 2 million people in the United States have this condition, making it almost as common as RA. It is higher in white men and some Native Americans than in African Americans, Asians, or other nonwhite groups. AS typically affects young people, beginning between the ages of 15 and 30 years (rarely after age 40 years). This differs from back pain of mechanical origin, which is much more likely to develop between 30 and 65 years of age. Men are affected two to three times more often than women, although this disorder may be just as prevalent in women but diagnosed less often because of a milder disease course with fewer spinal problems and more involvement of joints such as the knees and ankles.

***Etiologic and Risk Factors.*** AS is a rheumatologic condition that potentially develops from genetic factors, environmental triggers, and biomechanical stresses. Approximately 90% of individuals with AS are positive for the antigen HLA-B27, but of all people with this antigen, less than 5% develop AS. However, in individuals with inflammatory back pain and HLA-B27, the risk of AS significantly increases.[289] Studies of genome-wide associations have found other genes, *IL23R* and *ERAP1*, that are associated with the development of AS. Immune pathways that affect the development of ILs and controlling CD8 and CD4 T cells have been implicated for inflammatory processes responsible for AS. Environmental factors

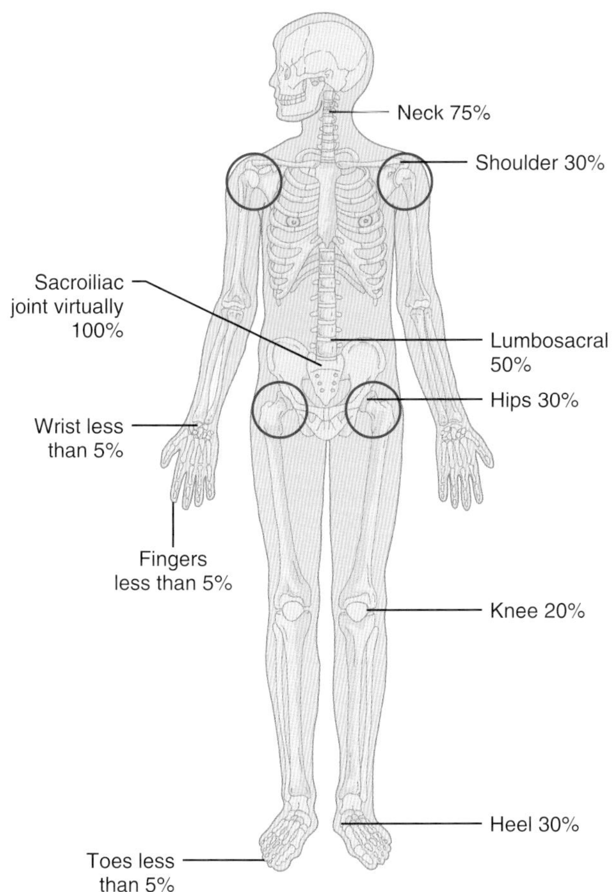


**Figure 27.20**

**Joints most commonly involved in ankylosing spondylitis and incidence of involvement.**

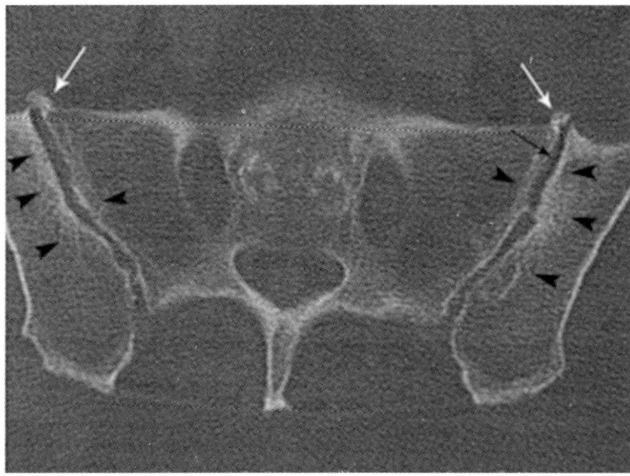

**Figure 27.21**

Computed tomography scan of the sacroiliac joints demonstrating joint space narrowing, subchondral sclerosis *(black arrowheads)*, interarticular gas *(black arrow)*, and osteophytes *(white arrows)*. (From Kotsenas AL: Imaging of posterior element axial pain generators. *Radiol Clin North Am* 50:705–730, 2012.)

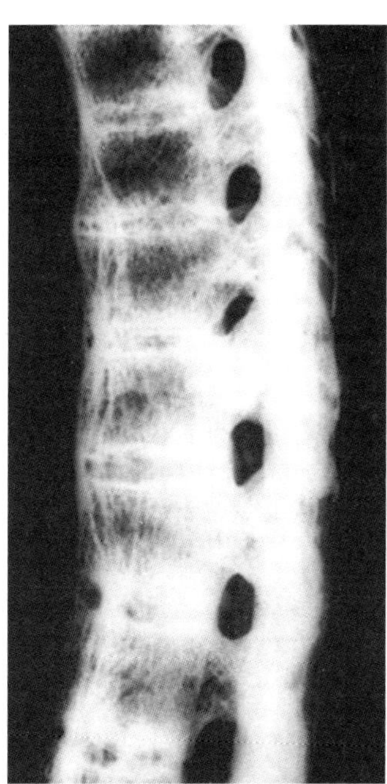

**Figure 27.22**

**Radiograph of a sagittal vertebral column in a person with ankylosing spondylitis.** There is complete fusion of the spine, accentuated kyphosis, and loss of lumbar and cervical lordosis. There is also complete fusion of the intervertebral disk spaces. (From Bullough PG: *Orthopaedic pathology*, ed 3, London, 1997, Mosby-Wolfe, p 301.)

such as infectious microbes have been found to play a role in the development of AS.[320]

*Pathogenesis.* The pathogenesis of AS is poorly understood, but the fundamental lesion appears to be chronic inflammation at sites of attachment of cartilage, tendons, ligaments, and synovium to the bone. AS is marked by a chronic nongranulomatous inflammation at the area where the ligaments attach to the vertebrae (an area called the enthesis), initially in the lumbar spine and then in the sacroiliac joint. Disruption of this ligamentous–osseous junction results, and reactive bone formation occurs as part of the repair process. Cartilage of the sacroiliac joints may also be involved (Fig. 27.21). The replacement of inflamed cartilaginous structures by bone contributes to progressive ossification with bony growth between the vertebrae, leading to a fused, rigid, or bamboo spine, characteristic of end-stage disease (Fig. 27.22).[320]

*Clinical Manifestations.* Low back, buttock, or hip pain and stiffness with insidious onset and lasting for at least 3 months are often the initial presenting symptoms. Symptoms occurring during childhood often go unrecognized as indicating the onset of AS. Onset of symptoms leading to a diagnosis occurs most often during early adulthood. At first the pain is described as a dull ache that is poorly localized; over time, pain becomes more severe and constant. Many patients report symptoms will increase with prolonged rest and are relieved with active movements. Coughing, sneezing, and twisting may worsen the pain. Pain may radiate to the thighs but does not usually extend below the knee. Significant morning stiffness, lasting more than 1 hour, is often present. There may be tenderness over the spinous processes and sacroiliac areas, with associated paraspinal spasms.[329]

Enthesitis (inflammation of the tendons, ligaments, and capsular attachments to bone) may produce tenderness, pain and/or stiffness, and restricted mobility in the costosternal, costovertebral, and manubriosternal joints; iliac crest; ischial tuberosities; greater trochanters; spinous processes; or ligamentous attachments at the calcaneus. Other clinical features include early loss of normal lumbar lordosis with accompanying increased kyphosis of the thoracic spine, painful limitation of cervical joint motion, and loss of spine mobility (flexibility) in all planes of motion.[329]

In some cases the initial symptoms may occur in the extremities. Shoulder symptoms and loss of shoulder mobility are common but are rarely disabling. Involvement of the shoulder joints is associated with involvement of other peripheral joints. Hip flexion contractures are often present bilaterally and can lead to loss of hip mobility and reduced functional abilities.

Loss of chest wall excursion is an indicator of decreased axial skeleton mobility because of involvement of the thoracic spine and the costovertebral and costosternal joints. If the ligaments that attach the ribs to the spine (costovertebral junction) become ossified, the chest may be unable to expand, compromising breathing.

***Complications.*** Long-standing AS is associated with skeletal complications, including osteoporosis, fracture, atlantoaxial subluxation, and spinal stenosis. In the most severe cases the spine becomes so completely fused that the person may become locked in a rigid upright or stooped position, unable to move the neck or back in any direction. Flexion contractures, rigid gait, and flexing at the knees to maintain an upright position are common findings.

The stiff and osteoporotic spinal column is prone to fracture from even a minor insult; a significant proportion of individuals with AS experience thoracic or lumbar vertebral fracture during the course of the disease.[343] Fractures can also occur in the cervical spine from the effect of osteoporosis, spinal stiffness, and cervical kyphotic deformity. These fractures result in significant loss of functional mobility and may be unstable enough to result in neurologic changes in the spinal cord and cervical nerve roots. These fractures may result in surgical fixations and correction of the kyphotic deformity.

The atlantoaxial segment is one of the last areas of the axial skeleton to fuse. Because of the inherent mobility of C1 and C2 and the immobility of the remainder of the cervical spine secondary to the disease, attempts to move the head could result in subluxation. Spinal stenosis can result from the proliferation of bony tissue from the spinal ligaments and facet joints, creating neurogenic claudication and cauda equina syndrome.

AS may be accompanied by inflammatory bowel syndrome with fever, fatigue, loss of appetite, weight loss, and other extraarticular complications. These clinical features distinguish AS from mechanical pain. The most common extraarticular manifestation is uveitis, occurring in 20% to 30% of affected individuals.[135] Cardiomegaly, pericarditis, aortic regurgitation or insufficiency, amyloidosis (rare), and pulmonary complications may also occur. Pulmonary problems include upper lobe fibrosis and decreased total lung capacity and vital capacity (late stages of AS).

## MEDICAL MANAGEMENT

**DIAGNOSIS.** Diagnosis is usually based on identification of the clinical manifestations and radiographic findings. Intraarticular inflammation, early cartilage changes, and underlying bone marrow edema and otitis can be seen with MRI short tau inversion recovery sequences. In the physical examination, mobility tests of the thoracic and lumbar spine such as the Schober test can help assess for loss of motion and to document a baseline measurement. Measurements of chest expansion can also document motion of the rib cage with the thoracic spine.[280]

Radiographic findings of symmetric, bilateral sacroiliitis include blurring of joint margins, juxtaarticular sclerosis, erosions, and joint space narrowing. The replacement of ligamentous tissue by bone at the site where the annulus fibrosus of the intervertebral disk inserts into the vertebral body results in a characteristic square-shaped vertebral body. In addition, as bony tissue bridges the vertebral bodies and posterior arches, the thoracic and lumbar spine takes on the appearance of a bamboo spine on radiographs (see Fig. 27.22).[329]

No laboratory test is diagnostic of AS; laboratory tests assist primarily by ruling out other diseases. The presence of HLA-B27 is a useful adjunct to the diagnosis but is not diagnostic itself, as individuals with other causes of back pain also are HLA-B27–positive. ESR and C-reactive protein are elevated in 75% of affected individuals and may correlate with disease activity in some people, but these levels can be normal even in individuals with active disease.[280]

Several classification schemes are used in the diagnosis of AS. The Assessment of SpondyloArthritis International Society classification criteria apply to individuals who are younger than 45 years of age with back pain for more than 3 months. A diagnosis of AS can be made in a patient with signs of sacroiliitis on imaging plus one or more features of a spondyloarthritis or in a patient with HLA-B27 antigen plus two or more features.[296] Features can include enthesis, uveitis, dactylitis, psoriasis, Crohn disease, family history of AS, and elevated levels of C-reactive protein. These diagnostic criteria have allowed for earlier identification and treatment of AS.[280]

The modified New York criteria for classification of AS include the signs of sacroiliitis, limited lumbar spine motion in three planes, and decreased chest expansion. The European Spondyloarthropathy Study group criteria for the classification of SpA list inflammatory back pain or synovitis in the lower extremities accompanied by at least one of key features.[329,280]

**TREATMENT.** The primary focus of intervention is to maximize health-related quality of life through control of inflammation and stiffness in the joints, maintaining mobility and proper postural alignment of the spine to prevent structural damage while providing pain relief.[329] Effective education is essential because much of the management requires lifestyle adjustments and cooperation, especially compliance with the exercise program.[309]

Joint involvement can be managed with NSAIDs, but in some cases DMARDs such as MTX or sulfasalazine may be used for peripheral disease. After a 3-month period, persistent symptoms of spinal involvement, peripheral arthritis, or enthesitis unresponsive to NSAIDs or DMARDs can be managed with biologic agents such as TNF-α antagonists (e.g., etanercept, infliximab, adalimumab). These agents are effective in preventing the progression of disease by reducing disease activity, decreasing inflammation, and improving spinal mobility.

A new monoclonal antibody that inhibits IL-17, secukinumab, can be used as a second-line biologic therapy.[280] Other targeted therapies may be needed to treat specific organ involvement, such as eye inflammation. To avoid long-term complications associated with severe postural deformities, a lifetime commitment to exercise is important.[329]

Surgery has a limited role in the management of AS and is most appropriate for individuals with a severe deformity that impedes vision, walking, eating, abdominal expansion, or respiratory function. Spondylodiskitis or spinal fracture may require surgical intervention. Spinal fusion may be needed but is not routinely recommended. The most valuable surgical intervention is total joint arthroplasty, especially a total hip replacement. It is expected that with the new biologic therapies, the need for surgical intervention will become rare.

**PROGNOSIS.** The extent of disability in people with AS varies considerably, but few experience complete remission, and more than 80% experience daily pain. Periods of exacerbation and remission are common during the course of the disease. It is thought that the use of biologic therapies has provided some patients with a slower progression of joint degeneration and to experience less disability.[329,344]

The severity of symptoms during the first decade indicates the long-term severity and disabling nature of the disorder. Severe disease is usually marked by peripheral joint and extraarticular manifestations. The onset of hip disease in a person with AS at any stage of the disease is a major prognostic marker for long-term severe disease and is more common in people with onset at a young age.[46]

Individuals with AS have an increased mortality rate. The impact of this disease can be seen in various aspects of workforce participation such as needing more assistance, withdrawal from the workforce, and reduced quality of life. Early diagnosis and management will likely help prevent functional disability and improve outcomes.

## SPECIAL IMPLICATIONS FOR THE THERAPIST 27.13

### *Ankylosing Spondylitis*

AS should be considered to be a "do not miss" condition for any young adult with low back pain. The diagnosis of AS should be considered in a person with significant spinal pain with rest that eases with movement and limitations in thoracolumbar mobility. An early referral to a rheumatologist will allow for a complete evaluation of the condition and allow for early treatment to control for inflammation.

Treating a client with a diagnosis of AS requires that the therapist keep in mind different considerations. If the client reports sharp pain associated with a fall, sneeze, or lifting a moderately heavy object, one must consider the possibility of a fracture.[267] With osteoporosis being a potential complication, technique modification is warranted.

Management should follow guidelines similar to those outlined for fibromyalgia (see Chapter 7). With the fragility of the spine in AS and the risk of fractures from even a minor injury or fall, prevention of falls is also important. This is an area for careful attention because a number of people with AS experience neurologic deficit after injury, especially spinal fracture.[162]

Trunk range-of-motion and strengthening exercises to minimize thoracic kyphosis are essential. The more severe the kyphosis, the more hindered pulmonary function will be and the more pronounced the compensatory forward head posture. Postural deformities contribute to cervical pain and headaches and may also affect balance. Avoiding obesity is recommended to reduce stress on weight-bearing joints and the cardiopulmonary system.[309]

Finally, smoking should be discouraged because of its adverse effects on the cardiopulmonary system. The therapist can also monitor clients taking NSAIDs for early signs of gastrointestinal bleeding or other adverse side effects (see Chapter 6).

Slowing the progress of AS is possible in the majority of individuals taking TNF-α blockers. These drugs are used to treat arthritis of the joints, as well as the spinal arthritis associated with AS. One drawback with TNF-α blockers that the therapist should be aware of is an increased risk of infections. Any sign of infection (even a sore throat) should be reported to the physician, as the drug therapy may have to be suspended because of the involved immunosuppression.[280]

#### Exercise and Ankylosing Spondylitis

Therapists play a potentially important role in the rehabilitation of these patients. Although more studies are available now than ever before in this area, there still is insufficient evidence to base recommendations for or against specific physical therapy interventions.[274,77] A summary of the available scientific evidence on the effectiveness of physical therapy interventions in the management of AS is presented here.

#### General Concepts

Although exercise is a commonly recommended intervention for AS, little is known about the effectiveness of unsupervised recreational and back exercises. Most studies suggest that exercise improves pain, stiffness, and function when performed at least 30 minutes per day, with back exercises performed at least 5 days per week, although these effects vary with the duration of AS. There may be an optimal duration for exercise performed independently over a weekly period, but consistency rather than quantity appears to be a much more significant variable. Patients who experience loss of function early in the disease process may be more motivated to maintain a regular exercise program than individuals with well-regulated symptoms.[107]

#### Exercise Prescription

A multimodal physical therapy program, including aerobic, stretching, and pulmonary exercises along with routine medical management, has been shown to yield greater improvements in spinal mobility, work capacity, and chest expansion compared with medical care alone.[176] After 3 months, individuals who participated in a 50-minute, three-times-a-week multimodal exercise program were significantly improved in chest expansion, chin-to-chest distance, occiput-to-wall distance, and modified Schober flexion test.

Functional and breathing capacity as well as balance should be assessed and developed. Stretching of the shortened muscles and chest expansion exercises should be encouraged. Improving and/or maintaining cardiovascular fitness is important. Strengthening of the trunk extensors is equally important, so that if and when spinal fusion occurs, the spine is aligned in the most functional position possible. This requires a coordinated effort among all team members, including the affected individual and family.[111]

High-impact and flexion exercises should be avoided, whereas low-impact aerobic exercise with extension and rotational components can be emphasized. Each individual will need to identify personal limitations and safe levels of participation.

In general, contact sports and high-risk activities such as downhill skiing, horseback riding, boxing, football, soccer, and water skiing should be avoided; aquatic therapy is an excellent option for most people, provided that extension principles are emphasized. In the presence of spinal fusion and osteoporosis, other activities requiring high levels of balance, agility, and coordination (e.g., bicycling, ice skating, rollerblading) can result in falls and fractures.

Overexercising can be potentially harmful and can exacerbate the inflammatory process; principles of relaxation, proper body mechanics, and energy conservation should be a part of the education program offered, including assessment of ADLs and providing necessary aids or devices such as long-handled reaching tools, adaptations for the car, special garden tools, or elastic shoelaces. Learning and using proper breathing techniques throughout all activities will help maintain chest expansion, improve oxygenation, and minimize muscle fatigue.

At the present time, aggressive but careful stretching to address the areas of hypomobility and the muscle imbalances is purported to help maintain as optimal a posture as possible.[362] An exercise program focusing on specific strengthening and flexibility exercises of the shortened muscle chains offers promising short-term and long-term results in the management of this condition.

#### Positioning

The affected individual may need help modifying home or work situations. Appropriate footwear advice should be provided; some people benefit from functional foot orthoses. Resting in the prone position is advised to help avoid hip and spine flexion contractures. The Spondylitis Association of America recommends a firm, supportive sleeping surface to maintain good spinal alignment. Soft mattresses or waterbeds can contribute to excessive flexion and stooped postures.

The therapist can provide additional recommendations for the use of pillows or towel rolls for proper alignment in the various positions. The person may not stay positioned all night, but with time and training, changing positions and realigning props can be incorporated into the sleep cycle at least part of the time.

Proper lifting techniques can be demonstrated, with return demonstration provided by the client. The therapist should assess the work area or instruct the individual in appropriate ergonomics, given the diagnosis of AS.

#### Outcome Measurements

Mobility tests to establish a baseline and measure the effectiveness of short-term intensive physical therapy and exercise on spinal, hip, and shoulder motion have been evaluated.

Finger-to-floor distance, thoracolumbar rotation, and thoracolumbar lateral flexion are the most sensitive tests to detect improvements (or progression) in short-term clinical trials, whereas the Schober test, thoracolumbar flexion, and occiput-to-wall distance are insensitive measures of improvement. Hip internal rotation, shoulder flexion, and abduction measurements are also sensitive, although more suitable for individuals with articular symptoms. Thoracolumbar rotation and hip rotation are the only measurements that correlate with disease duration, but not with age.[154]

The Bath Ankylosing Spondylitis Functional Index (BASFI), Dougados Functional Index score, Bath Ankylosing Spondylitis Metrology Index, Bath Ankylosing Spondylitis Disease Activity Index (BASDAI), and miniBASDAI are self-assessment tools that can be used both by the therapist and by the client to establish a baseline and document improvement or decline.[370]

The therapist must be vigilant for an exacerbation of the inflammatory process. Assess (and periodically reassess) the spine and peripheral joints for mobility, range of motion, and strength. Modalities such as ultrasound, heat and cold, and electrotherapy may be effective during the acute phase if used judiciously.

### Diffuse Idiopathic Skeletal Hyperostosis

**Overview and Definition.** DISH is considered to be an idiopathic variant of OA and is also called Forestier disease. The condition results in ossification of ligaments, especially the longitudinal ligaments of the spine, causing stiffness and back pain. The ossification of the anterior longitudinal ligament leads to the development of a lengthy and complex, paravertebral mass along the anterior aspect of the vertebral column (Fig. 27.23). The condition more commonly affects men than women (2:1), with individuals presenting between the ages of 50 and 70 years.[166]

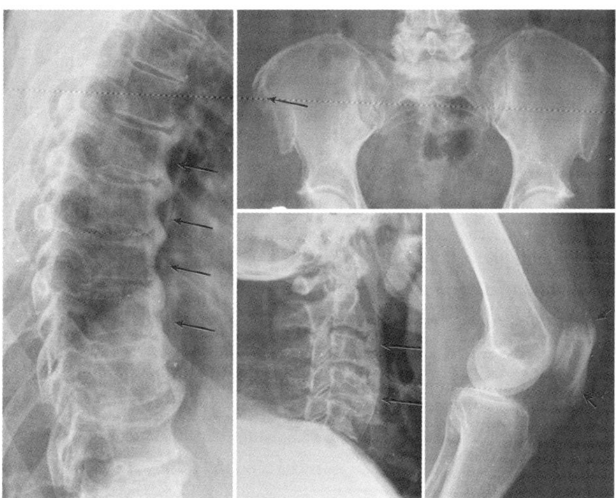

**Figure 27.23**

**Diffuse idiopathic skeletal hyperostosis (DISH).** DISH is seen in older individuals, predominantly involving the thoracic spine with flowing anterior ossification (at least four levels), associated with enthesophytes elsewhere (especially the pelvis). Patients are at increased risk for heterotopic bone formation after joint replacement. DISH is differentiated from ankylosing spondylitis by age (older), location (cervical, thoracic spine > lumbar spine, no sacroiliac involvement), and morphology (loosely flowing ossification on lateral view). (From Morrison WM, Sanders TG: *Problem solving in musculoskeletal imaging*, St. Louis, 2008, Mosby.)

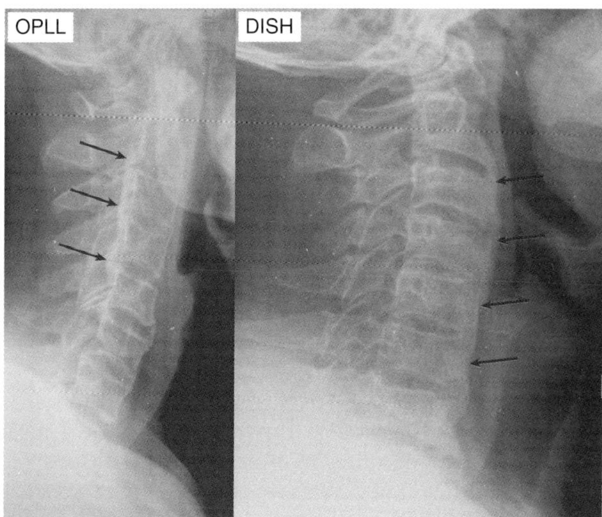


**Figure 27.24**

**Contrast findings of ankylosing spondylitis with ossification of the posterior longitudinal ligament *(OPLL)* and diffuse idiopathic skeletal hyperostosis *(DISH)*.** In OPLL, note linear ossification along the posterior vertebral bodies, and in DISH, note undulating anterior ossification. Occasionally, there is overlap of these disorders. (From Morrison WM, Sanders TG: *Problem solving in musculoskeletal imaging*, St. Louis, 2008, Mosby.)

The thoracic spine is most commonly affected by the ossification of the anterior longitudinal ligament. Ossification of ligaments in the lumbar and lower cervical spine are usually found with ossification extending into the thoracic spine. In contrast to OA, the condition does not directly result in degeneration of vertebral facet joints, joint space narrowing, or spondylophytes (lipping of vertebral bodies); instead, it manifests with syndesmophytes (bony outgrowths attached to ligaments), resulting in decreased mobility of the spine, especially the lumbar spine. The condition can aggravate the effects of OA and other degenerative conditions of the spine.

Extraspinal forms of this condition have been identified for the large synovial joints of the upper and lower extremities.[223]

**Risk Factors.** Diseases that produce endothelial cell damage, causing aggregation of platelet-derived growth factor, will stimulate osteoblast production that may be the genesis of the hyperostosis. The disease processes associated with hypertension, coronary artery disease, diabetes mellitus, AS, and metabolic diseases such as Paget disease and hyperparathyroidism have been hypothesized to be precursors to the development of DISH.

DISH has been found in individuals with high levels of uric acid, type 2 diabetes, severe atherosclerotic cardiovascular diseases, and high body mass index levels.[222] People who have undergone surgical procedures using periosteal stripping or who have experienced blunt trauma to the spine and peripheral joints have subsequently developed DISH. Genetic influences have been investigated, as with other seronegative SpAs, but no specific genetic factors have been identified.

**Etiology and Pathogenesis.** DISH is characterized by ossifications starting at the insertion of ligaments, tendons, and joint capsule insertion points (entheses) to bone. The ossification usually starts along the body of a vertebra, extending along the longitudinal ligaments. The ossification process is separate from the subjacent vertebral body and any sclerotic changes occurring along the vertebral disk. Fusion of cortical bone of the vertebrae with the ossification of ligament has been observed only with advanced cases of the disease.[166]

The etiology of DISH has not yet been identified. A number of disease processes as well as genetic, environmental, and anatomic causes have been investigated without a clear cause found for why the ossification process develops in some individuals. The presence of elevated endogenous insulin, the serum matrix Gls protein, and other growth factors have been identified as possible stimuli to ossification. AS is a similar condition resulting in proliferation of bony growths in the spine that has been linked to the presence of the HLA-B27 antigen (Fig. 27.24). No definitive relationship has been established between individuals with DISH and the presence of this antigen.[262]

**Clinical Manifestations.** This condition begins and develops asymptomatically and is usually identified inadvertently from radiographs taken for other conditions. Individuals with this condition will have spinal and joint mobility that is normal for their age and may not find any limitations in their daily functions or recreational activities during the early stages of the disease.

Symptoms are usually dull pain and stiffness in the spine following prolonged periods of rest/sleep (e.g., on waking in the morning) or with activities that require spinal bending or twisting motions. The symptoms will usually subside with rest and the use of NSAIDs. Patients with extensive hyperostosis formations along the anterior surface of the cervical spine may present with symptoms of hoarseness, stridor/snoring, or difficulties swallowing (dysphagia).[351] As the condition progresses to more extensive calcifications along the spine or peripheral joints, an individual will experience more persistent symptoms, limitations in joint mobility, and abnormal spinal posture.

Individuals with advanced cases of DISH are more susceptible to sustaining vertebral fractures of the cervical and thoracic spine that can lead to neurologic complications.[93] In some cases, extra bone growth around the spinal cord can also cause loss of sensation and even paralysis.

## MEDICAL MANAGEMENT

DIAGNOSIS. DISH is most commonly identified from radiographic findings of a "flowing" ossification along the anterolateral margins of the vertebral column (see Figs. 27.23 and 27.24). The ossification along at least four contiguous vertebral bodies, preservation of disk height, and absence of facet joint ankyloses are the criteria for the diagnosis of DISH of the spine. For extraspinal cases, calcification is found along the attachment sites for ligaments and tendons of the joint.[223] Uniform classification criteria for diffuse idiopathic skeletal exostosis do not exist. A number of criteria have been used to study the condition, which has resulted in a lack of consensus for the best treatments for this condition.[207]

Further evaluation for the extent and effects of the ossifications can be made using CT and MRI. Radiographic findings of DISH are indications for further work-up of other rheumatologic conditions, especially AS, is performed. All persons with signs of cardiovascular and metabolic syndrome associated with DISH should be evaluated and treated for these conditions.[222]

The use of imaging will determine the extent of the ligamentous ossifications and risks for spinal fractures. The presence of hyperostosis along peripheral joints can be well visualized with radiographic views. CT scan can provide accurate visualization of spinal ossifications with sagittal and coronal views with good resolution to assess the facet apophyseal joints.

The lower segments of the *cervical spine* are more commonly involved, with ossifications extending to the atlantoaxial joint and occiput. Progression of hyperostosis along the cervical spine can restrict function of the larynx and pharynx, which may require swallowing studies. For the *thoracic spine,* there is usually more ossification along the right lateral aspect of the spine, with advanced cases having hyperostosis extending to the posterior aspect of the ribs. Involvement of the *lumbar spine* will usually affect the upper segments, with advanced conditions extending to the posterior ligaments of the spine.

Individuals who have sustained a vertebral fracture secondary to DISH will need extensive imaging studies to determine the extent of the fracture and to plan surgical procedures to treat the fracture and possibly remove the ossifications along the spinal column.[335]

TREATMENT. For individuals identified in the early stages of DISH, a conservative approach that treats symptoms of pain and stiffness using pharmaceuticals such as NSAIDs and exercise is warranted. Ongoing evaluation of hyperostosis is also advised. Many of these people are at risk for coronary artery disease, type 2 diabetes, and other metabolic diseases and will need further medical evaluation and preventive measures for these conditions.[224]

Individuals with cervical hyperostosis that affects swallowing or breathing function will need imaging and fiberoptic laryngoscopy to assess the extent of the ossifications. A rehabilitation approach may be possible using modifications to diet and compensations to improve swallowing function to allow for satisfactory management of this problem. For advanced cases, surgical procedures to remove the ossifications from the cervical spine allow for a return to normal breathing and swallowing functions.

SPECIAL IMPLICATIONS FOR THE THERAPIST 27.14

### *Diffuse Idiopathic Skeletal Hyperostosis*

Therapeutic exercise programs for this condition have been employed with the goals of diminishing back pain, improving spinal range of motion, and decreasing disability. Al-Herz and colleagues[15] reported on the use of a daily program of trunk and hip stabilization exercises, active trunk range of motion, and stretching for the hamstrings and lumbar spine. After 6 months, participants demonstrated improvements in trunk mobility but had inconsistent improvements in symptoms and disability levels.

Therapists should develop an individualized plan to address mobility and symptoms for individuals with DISH. A multimodal approach of modalities, spinal mobility and stretching, postural exercises, and aerobic exercises should be considered to best address symptoms and activity limitations.

### Sjögren Syndrome

**Overview.** Sjögren syndrome is a chronic autoimmune disease that causes arthritis-related effects in several organs, most commonly the moisture-producing glands (e.g., mouth, eyes) but also joints, lungs, kidneys, or liver. The syndrome may be a primary condition occurring alone or secondary to other autoimmune diseases, such as RA or lupus.[282]

**Incidence and Risk Factors.** Sjögren syndrome is the second most common autoimmune rheumatic disease, affecting an estimated 2 million to 4 million Americans, developing most often in postmenopausal women, with women affected nine times more often than men. Secondary Sjögren syndrome has been associated with SLE, other autoimmune disease, or having a family member with Sjögren syndrome.

**Etiologic Factors and Pathogenesis.** The primary symptoms of Sjögren syndrome are the result of exocrine gland (mainly salivary and lacrimal gland) destruction by focal T-lymphocytic infiltrates. The infiltrating T and B cells interfere with glandular function at several points. Additional potential contributing factors are B-cell hyperreactivity (these locally produce immunoglobulins having autoantibody reactivity) and long-term immune system stimulation. Evidence supports a genetic component in its etiology, but there is no strong evidence for a specific candidate gene.[44]

Neurogenic regulation of the salivary gland is impaired, with structural abnormalities of the secretory acinar apparatus. The acinar basement membrane is abnormal, as it lacks the laminin $\alpha_1$ chain; this loss may impair its ability to induce stem cells to differentiate into acinar cells.

Significantly lower basal adrenocorticotropic hormone and cortisol levels have been found in individuals with Sjögren syndrome, implicating blunted pituitary and adrenal responses with interactions between the neuroendocrine and immune systems.[186]

**Clinical Manifestations.** The hallmark symptoms of Sjögren syndrome are dry eyes and dry mouth. This syndrome may also cause dryness in other areas, such as the kidneys, gastrointestinal tract, blood vessels, sinuses, respiratory tract, liver, pancreas, and central nervous system.

Other clinical manifestations vary according to the systemic problems present from integumentary, respiratory, renal, hepatic, neurologic, and vascular involvement. Associated symptoms may include extremely dry throat, esophagitis, gastritis, and dental cavities from a lack of saliva; vaginal dryness with painful sexual intercourse; fatigue; joint and muscle pain; joint and muscle stiffness; swelling; rashes (vasculitis); numbness (peripheral neuropathy as a consequence of small vessel vasculitis); Raynaud phenomenon; B-cell lymphoma; and inflammation of the lungs, kidneys, or liver.[282]

Some of the problems (e.g., recurrent bronchitis or sinusitis) arise from exocrine dysfunction in other organs, while other problems (e.g., interstitial lung disease, interstitial nephritis) occur as a result of extraglandular spread of lymphocytic infiltration discussed in the pathogenesis of this disease. Primary Sjögren syndrome causes salivary gland swelling and tenderness. The dry eyes (keratoconjunctivitis sicca) are described as the feeling of sand or a burning sensation in the eyes, with decreased secretion of tears. Dry mouth (xerostomia) and dry cough make it difficult for affected individuals to chew and swallow food or speak continuously.

Depression, anxiety, thyroiditis, and fibromyalgia are frequent comorbid illnesses requiring a comprehensive management approach to this condition. Quality of life is decreased by complications such as sleep loss, loss of teeth and poorly fitting dentures, loss of vision, profound fatigue, musculoskeletal pain, and morning stiffness.[255]

## MEDICAL MANAGEMENT

DIAGNOSIS. Many conditions manifest similarly to Sjögren syndrome with dry eyes and dry mouth, such as lupus, vasculitis, thyroid disease, and scleroderma. Side effects of some medications (e.g., tricyclic antidepressants, antihistamines, radiation treatments of the head and neck) can mimic Sjögren syndrome. Sjögren syndrome is a systemic disease with the potential to affect almost every organ system in the body, so the proper diagnosis is important.

Diagnosis is based on the medical history and tests such as a slit-lamp test to detect damage to the surface of the eye by using a dye that exposes eroded areas of the conjunctiva (the membrane that covers the eye and lines the inside of the eyelids), Schirmer test to assess degree of dryness in the eyes, lip biopsy to show inflammation of the salivary glands, and blood tests to detect antibodies (e.g., rheumatoid factor, antinuclear antibody, anti–Sjögren syndrome A antibody, and anti–Sjögren syndrome B antibody) that are associated with primary Sjögren syndrome.[312]

Many serum and salivary biomarkers for Sjögren syndrome have been proposed, but none has been specific enough for diagnostic purposes or correlated with disease activity measures. Modern genomic investigation is looking for candidate biomarkers and possible etiopathologic mechanisms underlying this disorder.

TREATMENT. There is no cure for Sjögren syndrome, but it can be managed effectively. Ocular involvement is managed with local and systemic stimulators of tear secretion. Treatment of oral manifestations includes intense oral hygiene and prevention and treatment of oral infections. The use of saliva stimulants and mouth lubricants can help with the dryness. Avoiding situations and activities that contribute to dryness and moisturizing other areas of dryness such as the skin and vagina (women) are advised.[283]

Intervention typically involves medications (e.g., corticosteroids such as prednisone, NSAIDs, or hydroxychloroquine [Plaquenil]) to help reduce joint pain and stiffness and ease fatigue and muscle pain, as well as other palliative measures for symptomatic relief. Exercise and proper nutrition may help with fatigue and joint symptoms.[59]

Mild cases of peripheral neuropathy can remit spontaneously, but usually symptomatic treatment (e.g., gabapentin) is needed. More severe involvement affecting ambulation may require the use of steroids, azathioprine, or intravenous gammaglobulin or cyclophosphamide. Direct and indirect B cell–targeted therapy is the best biologic agent for primary Sjögren syndrome, especially for glandular and extraglandular manifestations such as glomerulonephritis or vasculitis. 44

PROGNOSIS. Sjögren syndrome progresses slowly, with the interval between first symptoms and diagnosis ranging from 2 to 8 years. Left untreated, dryness of the eyes can lead to eye infections and may result in damage to the cornea and visual loss.

Sjögren syndrome is a benign disease that affects quality of life. When extraoral and extraocular exocrine gland dysfunction or lymphocyte-mediated tissue destruction involves other organs, significant morbidity and mortality can occur. There is a high risk of malignant transformation that requires close follow-up.

SPECIAL IMPLICATIONS FOR THE THERAPIST 27.15

### *Sjögren Syndrome*

Special implications and preferred practice patterns are determined by the presenting clinical features but follow the general guidelines for RA. See Special Implications for the Therapist 27.11: Rheumatoid Arthritis.

Physical capacity is reduced in Sjögren syndrome, and fatigue is a dominating and disabling symptom.[255] Evidence-based studies on the effect of exercise in Sjögren syndrome are limited, with small sample sizes. The available studies indicate that clients with Sjögren syndrome can benefit from moderate- to high-intensity levels of exercise, with positive effects on aerobic capacity, fatigue, physical function, and depression (mood).[330,81]

## Psoriatic Arthritis

**Overview and Incidence.** Psoriatic arthritis is a seronegative inflammatory joint disease affecting a small percentage of people who have psoriasis. This joint disorder is associated with radiographic evidence of periarticular bone erosions and occasional significant joint destruction. Psoriatic arthritis tends to progress slowly, and for most affected individuals, it is more a nuisance than a disabling condition.[133]

Approximately 1% of the population of the United States has psoriasis. Psoriatic arthritis occurs in approximately 20% of people with psoriasis and more often in people with severe psoriasis. Uncomplicated psoriasis typically manifests during the second and third decades of life, with the onset of arthritis occurring up to 20 years later. The disease can occur in children, with onset typically between the ages of 9 and 12 years. Psoriatic arthritis does not appear to have a strong predilection for one gender.

**Etiologic and Risk Factors.** A strong familial association has been noted with this disease. Although specific marker genes have not been discovered, there is general agreement that a genetic predisposition exists for psoriatic arthritis. There is approximately an 80% to 90% chance of contracting psoriatic arthritis if one has a first-degree relative with the disorder.[73]

**Pathogenesis.** An inflammatory synovitis results in the joint changes associated with psoriatic arthritis. Lymphocyte infiltration into the synovium occurs. Initially the synovium is pale, with edematous granulation tissue extending along the contiguous bone. The synovium later becomes thickened with villous hypertrophy. Eroded articular margins begin to appear at this time. In severe cases, the joint space tends to be filled in with dense fibrous tissue.[73]

**Clinical Manifestations.** The arthritis can be oligoarticular or polyarticular. There is a predilection for the distal interphalangeal joints of the hands. Other joints of the digits may be involved. The joint changes may lead to significant hand deformities, including claw deformity. The digital joint changes and associated flexor tenosynovitis can result in an edematous, thickened digit.

Joints of the axial skeleton can also be affected but typically become involved several years after the onset of the peripheral joint disease. The sacroiliitis is usually unilateral, in contrast to that in AS. Sacroiliitis can occur in 20% to 40% of clients.

Although not as common as in RA or Reiter syndrome, extraarticular manifestations can occur with psoriatic arthritis. Inflammatory eye disease including conjunctivitis and iritis, renal disease, mitral valve prolapse, and aortic regurgitation are associated with this disorder. Pitting of the nails and onycholysis (Fig. 27.25) are also commonly associated with psoriatic arthritis.

There are some differences in the manifestations of this disease between children and adults. A slight predilection for girls is noted in children. In addition, the arthritis may appear before the skin manifestations in a number of children. Compared with adults, the onset of arthritis tends to be more acute in children, with the involvement of multiple asymmetric joints. The hip joint is much more commonly involved in children.

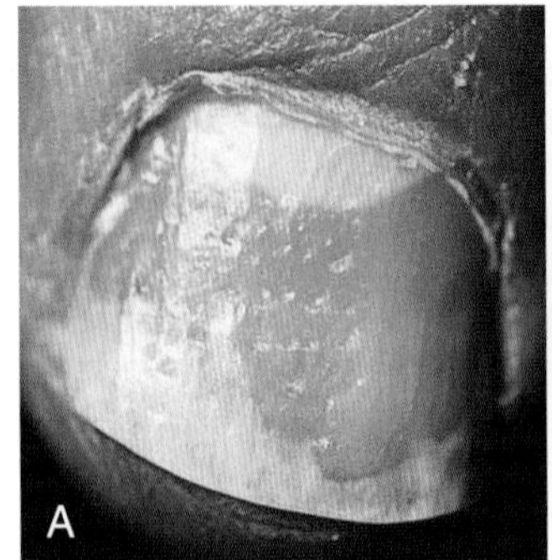


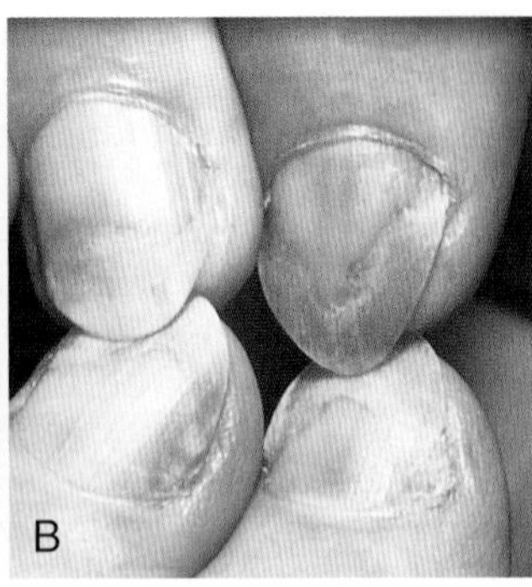


**Figure 27.25**

**Nail changes associated with various forms of arthritis.** (A) Pitting of the nail beds associated with psoriasis. (B) Onycholysis associated with reactive arthritis, a separation of the nail plate from the nail bed beginning at the free margin and progressing inward. (A, From James WD, et al: *Andrews' diseases of the skin: clinical dermatology*, ed 10, Philadelphia, 2006, Saunders. B, From Arndt KA: *Primary care dermatology*, Philadelphia, 1997, Saunders.)

**Box 27.14**

**RADIOGRAPHIC FEATURES OF PSORIATIC ARTHRITIS**

- Asymmetric oligoarticular distribution of disease
- Relative absence of osteopenia
- Involvement of distal interphalangeal joints
- Involvement of sacroiliac joint (unilateral)

Data from Amrami KK: Imaging of the seronegative spondyloarthropathies. *Radiol Clin North Am* 50:841–854, 2012.

## MEDICAL MANAGEMENT

DIAGNOSIS. The diagnosis of psoriatic arthritis is usually easily made because of the onset of inflammatory arthritis in the presence of obvious psoriasis. Differential diagnosis can be difficult, however, if the psoriasis is absent or equivocal. Laboratory tests do not help except to rule out RA. Box 27.14 lists common radiographic findings in psoriatic arthritis.[17]

TREATMENT AND PROGNOSIS. There is currently no cure for psoriasis or psoriatic arthritis. People with mild arthritis are treated symptomatically with NSAIDs. If there is an acute flare of only one or two joints, local corticosteroid injections may help. Anyone with more aggressive disease may benefit from DMARD therapy with MTX, sulfasalazine, and TNF-$\alpha$ antagonists.[73]

Because of the association between severe skin involvement and severe arthritis, treatment of the psoriasis is emphasized with the hope of reducing the arthritis. Multiple medications have been used in an attempt to control progressive psoriatic arthritis but with equivocal results. As noted earlier, for most persons with psoriatic arthritis, the disease is mild, not destructive.

SPECIAL IMPLICATIONS FOR THE THERAPIST 27.16

### *Psoriatic Arthritis*

See Special Implications for the Therapist 27.11: Rheumatoid Arthritis.

The goals for therapy are to prevent the development of joint degeneration while increasing functional abilities and improving quality of life. With the goal of early remission of the disease, a team approach of working with a rheumatologist, dermatologist, occupational therapist, and psychologist will provide the best outcome for these people. Because a person with this disease can present with a variety of inflammatory conditions in the axial skeleton and the extremities, the therapist will need to develop a treatment plan that is specific to each individual.[219] If a flare-up of the skin condition is noted, encourage the client to see his or her physician. If the joint inflammation worsens, prompt communication with the physician should occur so the client can be placed on an appropriate medication regimen.

## Reactive Arthritis

**Overview.** Reactive arthritis is defined as the occurrence of an acute, *aseptic,* inflammatory arthropathy arising after an infectious process but at a site remote from the primary infection, which differs from bacterial arthritis, a local response with joint destruction and sepsis.[122] The borderline between reactive arthritis and true septic arthritis may be obscure, as several organisms can cause both, with overlapping symptoms and laboratory features. Other infectious causes of arthritis are discussed in other chapters (e.g., HIV in Chapter 7, Lyme disease and Epstein-Barr virus in Chapter 8, and rheumatic fever in Chapter 12).

**Etiologic and Risk Factors and Pathogenesis.** Reactive arthritis is a recognized sequela of infection with a number of enteric pathogens such as *Campylobacter jejuni* (gastrointestinal tract), *Salmonella typhimurium, Shigella* (dysentery), *Chlamydia trachomatis* (genitourinary tract), *Chlamydia pneumoniae* (respiratory tract), *Yersinia, M. fermentans,* and *Clostridium difficile* (colitis associated with antibiotic therapy), with chlamydiae the most common cause of reactive arthritis.[51]

The overall prevalence of reactive arthritis has declined, although an increase has been seen in intravenous drug users with AIDS. Reactive arthritis is most common in young, sexually active adults, especially men who have been infected with *C. trachomatis.* However, children and older adults of both genders are affected by the postenteric form. Reactive arthritis following urogenital infection is underdiagnosed in women. The tendency for chlamydial infection to be subclinical or asymptomatic and the relative infrequency of pelvic examinations are contributing factors.

The major histocompatibility complex class I antigen HLA-B27 is well recognized as a genetic marker of susceptibility to reactive arthritis. Bacteria in the joint may stimulate the immune system to produce antibodies and protein factors (cytokines), several of which produce local inflammation and tissue damage, leading to an arthritic joint.

**Clinical Manifestations.** The arthritis first manifests 1 to 4 weeks after the infectious insult and is usually asymmetric affecting more than one joint, typically the large and medium joints of the lower extremities. Sacroiliac joint involvement occurs in approximately 10% of acute cases and 30% of chronic cases. The clinical picture varies from mild arthralgia and arthritis to incapacitating illness that may result in bed rest for several weeks. Joint pain may be minimal with no signs of inflammation, but stiffness, pain, tenderness, and loss of motion are often present.[51]

Associated findings may include uveitis, enthesitis (inflammation involving the sites of bony insertion of tendons and ligaments), sacroiliitis, urethritis, and conjunctivitis. Reactive arthritis encompasses a subgroup that demonstrates the classic clinical triad of arthritis, urethritis, and conjunctivitis, which is called Reiter syndrome (see further discussion in the next section). Reactive arthritis is a broader category that includes some, but not all, of the more restrictive features associated with Reiter syndrome. The distinction between these two conditions is somewhat arbitrary.

Extraarticular manifestations of reactive arthritis may include onycholysis of the fingernails or toenails, dactylitis (sausage-like swelling of the toes and fingers because of joint and tenosynovium inflammation), painless mucosal ulcers in the mouth, discharge from the vagina or penis, urologic symptoms (urgency, frequency, difficulty starting or continuing a flow of urine), or various types of skin lesions. Rarely, neurologic or cardiac involvement occurs secondary to inflammatory and fibrotic lesions.

### MEDICAL MANAGEMENT

DIAGNOSIS. There is considerable clinical overlap among the various types of inflammatory arthritides. Usually a careful clinical and family history and physical examination will lead to the diagnosis. Laboratory evaluation, synovial fluid aspiration, cultures for bacteria, antibody testing, measurement of serum immunoglobulin, and imaging studies contribute to the differential diagnosis.[51]

TREATMENT AND PROGNOSIS. NSAIDs and disease-modifying drugs are the basis of medical management. A short course of corticosteroids may be necessary in some cases, and antirheumatic agents may be beneficial in chronic reactive arthritis. Antibiotics are recommended if the infection is identified.

The overall prognosis for reactive arthritis is good even in severe cases, but full recovery does not always occur. Many people experience some form of persisting symptoms, with degeneration of lower extremity joints that can lead to chronic disability.[122]

Recurrence is possible, and a chronic form of this condition can develop, characterized by recurring arthritis that is accompanied by tendinitis or tenosynovitis. Sacroiliitis and spondylitis may not resolve but may persist with ongoing pain and stiffness of the neck and back.

**SPECIAL IMPLICATIONS FOR THE THERAPIST 27.17**

### *Reactive Arthritis*

See Special Implications for the Therapist 27.11: Rheumatoid Arthritis.

The relationship of infections of the gastrointestinal or genitourinary system to the joint is well documented (see Arthritis and Inflammatory Intestinal Diseases in Chapter 16), and anyone with new onset of joint involvement must be medically evaluated for an underlying bacterial or infectious cause.

Past medical history may reveal a recent infectious process, use of antibiotics, presence of a sexually transmitted disease, or bowel disease to alert the physician. The presence of joint involvement accompanied by (or alternating with) gastrointestinal signs and symptoms such as diarrhea, abdominal pain or bloating, constitutional symptoms (e.g., fever, night sweats), or positive iliopsoas or obturator sign must be reported to the physician.

Anyone taking NSAIDs for reactive arthritis must take them as prescribed and not just for analgesia or occasionally. The therapist can help educate affected individuals that a stoic attitude of enduring the pain and restricted mobility with a refusal to "take pills" will result in less optimal and delayed recovery.

Physical therapy intervention is very valuable during convalescence to regain full motion, strength, and function. Temporary splinting may be advised in the most painful cases, but muscle atrophy can be rapid, and therefore immobilization should be minimized. If new symptoms develop or the person does not respond to therapy, medical evaluation is advised; modification of medications may be needed.

## Reiter Syndrome

**Overview.** Reiter syndrome is one of the most common examples of reactive arthritis. Reiter syndrome usually follows venereal disease or an episode of bacillary dysentery (enteric infection) and is associated with typical extraarticular manifestations. The prevalence and incidence of Reiter syndrome are difficult to establish because of (1) the lack of consensus regarding diagnostic criteria, (2) the nomadic nature of the young target population, (3) the underreporting of venereal disease, and (4) the asymptomatic or milder course in affected women.[366]

**Etiologic and Risk Factors.** The most common microbial pathogens are *Shigella, Salmonella, Yersinia, Campylobacter,* and *Chlamydia* species. Age, gender, and medical history are important risk factors associated with Reiter syndrome. The peak onset of this disorder occurs during the third decade of life, although children and older adults can also develop this disease. Individuals with the HLA-B27 antigen have been found to have more severe symptoms.

Men are more commonly affected than women but not to the extent once thought. The incidence in women is potentially underestimated because clinical manifestations in women are less severe than clinical manifestations in men, and women are more prone to occult genitourinary disease, leading to misdiagnosis.

A history of infection, especially venereal or dysenteric, is associated with increased risk of developing this condition. Men and women are equally affected by enteric infections. Reiter syndrome is the most common form of reactive arthritis observed in HIV-infected adults and appears to be more strongly associated with male homosexuality than with injection drug use or other risky behaviors.

**Pathogenesis.** Reiter syndrome is believed to be due to a combination of immune and infectious causes and is primarily marked by inflammatory synovitis and inflammatory erosion at the insertion sites of ligaments and tendons (enthesitis). Heterotopic bone formation can occur at these sites. Synovial findings include edema, cellular invasion (lymphocytes, neutrophils, plasma cells), and vascular changes. Extensive pannus formation is rare, in contrast to in RA.[366]

**Clinical Manifestations.** The triad of symptoms classically associated with Reiter syndrome includes urethritis, conjunctivitis, and arthritis. The urethritis and conjunctivitis often occur early in the disease. Other ocular manifestations include uveitis and keratitis (fungal infection of the cornea).[366]

Three musculoskeletal manifestations are acute inflammatory arthritis, inflammatory back pain, and enthesitis. Only about one-third of individuals with Reiter syndrome have all three. Low back pain is found in 50% of people with the syndrome, with signs of decreased lumbar flexion. As discussed in the previous section, the arthritis is usually asymmetric; is often acute; and typically involves joints of the lower extremity, including the knees, ankles, and first metatarsophalangeal joints. Isolated hand joints can be involved. Although most of the symptoms and signs disappear within days or weeks, the arthritis may last for months or years.

Extraarticular manifestations are as previously mentioned for reactive arthritis. The skin lesions may be indistinguishable from lesions of psoriasis. Low back pain is also a common symptom. The arthritis can progress and spread to the spine and even to the upper extremities.

### MEDICAL MANAGEMENT

DIAGNOSIS. The diagnosis of Reiter syndrome may require months to establish because the various manifestations can occur at different times. The combination of peripheral arthritis with urethritis lasting longer than 1 month is necessary before the diagnosis can be confirmed.

Laboratory tests typically reveal an aggressive inflammatory process. Elevated ESR and C-reactive protein are detected, and thrombocytosis and leukocytosis are common findings. Urine samples, genital swabs, and stool cultures are useful laboratory tests for identifying the triggering infection.

Up to 70% of people with established Reiter syndrome may have radiographic abnormalities including (1) asymmetric involvement of the lower extremity diarthroses, amphiarthroses, symphyses, and entheses; (2) ill-defined bony erosions with adjacent bony proliferation; and (3) paravertebral ossification.[366]

**TREATMENT AND PROGNOSIS.** Although Reiter syndrome is precipitated by an infection, there is no evidence that antibiotic therapy changes the course of the disorder. Treatment in general is largely symptomatic, with NSAIDs being the primary intervention.

If the arthritis persists, joint protection and maintenance of function become important. Immobilization and inactivity are usually discouraged, whereas range-of-motion and stretching exercises are emphasized. TNF-α antagonists may improve the outcome, but no controlled trials have been performed. Typically the arthritis resolves in 3 to 12 months, but it can recur. Chronic articular or spinal disease affects 30% of the population affected; severe disability occurs in less than 15% of affected individuals.

SPECIAL IMPLICATIONS FOR THE THERAPIST 27.18

### *Reiter Syndrome*

See Special Implications for the Therapist 27.11: Rheumatoid Arthritis.

Questions related to the presence and treatment of current and past infection should be asked during the history taking. Also inquire into the person's general health, both current and before the onset of the presenting pain symptoms. Typically the onset of joint pain associated with concurrent systemic symptoms would raise suspicion.

New-onset inflammatory joint disease with a history of recent enteric or venereal infection or new sexual contact strongly suggests a systemic origin of symptoms. Reiter syndrome is one condition in which past medical history and general health status may provide the most important information.

If the client has not received a diagnosis or has not yet been seen by a physician, medical evaluation is required. See also Reactive Arthritis and Special Implications for the Therapist 27.17: Reactive Arthritis.

## Gout

**Overview.** Gout comprises a heterogeneous group of metabolic disorders marked by an elevated level of serum uric acid and the deposition of urate crystals in the joints, soft tissues, and kidneys. Gout is the most common crystallopathy (crystal-induced arthritis) in the United States.

Hyperuricemia and gout are generally classified into one of three groups. *Primary hyperuricemia* is an inherited disorder of uric acid metabolism. *Secondary hyperuricemia* occurs as a result of some other metabolic problem such as glucose-6-phosphatase dehydrogenase deficiency, reduced renal function (from any number of causes), certain medications that block uric acid excretion, or neoplasms. The third category, *idiopathic hyperuricemia,* encompasses conditions that do not fit into either of the other categories.[79]

Although gout is a metabolic disorder and could be presented in Chapter 24 as such, it is predominantly viewed as a form of arthritis because of its clinical presentation (gout can be manifested as a joint disorder characterized by acute or chronic arthritis) and so is included here instead. Crystals other than uric acid crystals can also form inside joints, such as occurs in a condition called *pseudogout* when calcium pyrophosphate dihydrate (CPPD) crystals are present.

The presence of CPPD crystals in the synovial fluid can cause symptoms identical to symptoms of acute gout. In contrast to gout, however, CPPD most often affects the knees of older women and may have polyarticular involvement. Pseudogout, also known as chondrocalcinosis, is associated with a number of metabolic disorders such as hypothyroidism, hemochromatosis, hyperparathyroidism, and diabetes mellitus.

**Incidence.** Primary gout is predominantly associated with middle-aged men, with a peak incidence during the fifth decade of life. It is the most common inflammatory disease in men older than 30 years, generally becoming symptomatic after a period of hyperuricemia lasting 10 to 20 years. New cases of gout have doubled in the last few decades.[208]

Gout is rare in children, and less than 10% of the cases occur in women. Most women with gout have been postmenopausal for 15 years or more (longer for women taking hormone replacement therapy); estrogen deficiency for a few years is necessary before gout becomes evident in this population).[142]

**Etiologic and Risk Factors.** A family history of gout increases the risk of developing the disorder. The prevalence of gout increases with increasing serum urate concentration and age. With the aging of the American population, decreased renal function is becoming more prevalent, accompanied by a rise in the number of cases of gout.

Secondary hyperuricemia (gout) can be a result of urate overproduction or decreased urinary excretion of uric acid. People with a history of leukemia, lymphoma, psoriasis, or hemolytic disorders and people receiving chemotherapy for cancer are at risk for urate overproduction.

Heavy alcohol consumption (especially beer), obesity, fasting, medications (e.g., thiazide diuretics, levodopa, and salicylates), renal insufficiency, hypertension, hypothyroidism, and hyperparathyroidism all can lead to decreased excretion of uric acid. Among the associated factors, age, duration of hyperuricemia, genetic predisposition, heavy alcohol consumption, obesity, thiazide drugs, and lead toxicity contribute the most to the conversion from asymptomatic hyperuricemia to acute gouty arthritis.[64]

A diet rich in purines (nitrogen-containing compounds found in foods such as shellfish, trout, sardines, anchovies, meat [especially organ meats], asparagus, beans, peas, spinach) can increase the risk of gout or make gout attacks more severe. Ingestion of fructose-sweetened foods and beverages has also been implicated with an increased risk of hyperuricemia and gout. Fructose is the only sugar known to elevate serum uric acid levels. Conversely, there is a lower prevalence of gout in vegetarians and with supplemental vitamin C intake.[64]

In many cases of primary gout, the specific biochemical defect responsible for hyperuricemia is unknown. Most cases probably result from an unexplained impairment in uric acid excretion by the kidneys. This impairment could result from decreased renal filtration, increased reabsorption, or decreased urate excretion by the renal tubules.

**Pathogenesis.** Uric acid is a substance that normally forms when the body breaks down cellular waste products called *purines*. In healthy people, uric acid dissolves in the blood, passes through the kidneys, and is then excreted through the urine. If the body produces more uric acid than the kidneys can process or if the kidneys are unable to handle normal levels of uric acid, the acid level in the blood rises.

When the uric acid in the blood reaches high levels, it may precipitate out and accumulate in body tissues, forming supersaturated body fluids, including in the joints and kidneys. These crystals frequently collect on articular cartilage, epiphyseal bone, and periarticular structures. The crystal aggregates trigger an inflammatory response, resulting in local tissue necrosis and a proliferation of fibrous tissue secondary to an inflammatory foreign-body reaction. The genetics of gout are under investigation; there is some evidence that genetic variants of urate transporters that aid in the excretion of urate may contribute to altered serum uric acid levels.

**Clinical Manifestations.** The disease occurs in four stages: asymptomatic hyperuricemia (defined as serum urate of more than 7 mg/dL), acute gouty arthritis, intercritical gout, and chronic tophaceous gout. Many people with elevated uric acid levels for a prolonged period of time never develop signs or symptoms.[366]

The most common clinical presentation is acute, monarticular, inflammatory arthritis manifested by exquisite joint pain occurring suddenly at night. Although the first metatarsophalangeal joint (i.e., the big toe) is a common site of pain, the ankle, instep, knee, wrist, elbow (olecranon bursa), and finger all can be the site of the initial attack (Fig. 27.26). Besides local, intense pain of quick onset, erythema, warmth, and extreme tenderness and hypersensitivity are typically present. Chills, fever, and tachycardia may accompany the joint symptoms.

After recovering from the initial episode the person enters an asymptomatic phase called the *intercritical period*. This period can last months or years despite persistent hyperuricemia and synovial fluid that contains monosodium urate crystals.

Gouty attacks return suddenly with increasing frequency and severity and often in different joints. These attacks may be precipitated by trauma, surgery, alcohol consumption, or overindulgence in foods with high purine content. The arthritis can enter the chronic phase up to a decade after the initial attack, characterized by joint damage, functional loss, and disability. Deposits of monosodium urate crystals in soft tissue (tophi) and bone abnormalities are the hallmarks of chronic disease (Fig. 27.27). Tophi can be located in tendons, ligaments, cartilage, subchondral bone, bursa, synovium, and subcutaneous tissue around the joints. Common sites of these hard, sometimes ulcerated masses that extrude chalky material include the helix of the ear, forearm, knee, and foot.[263]

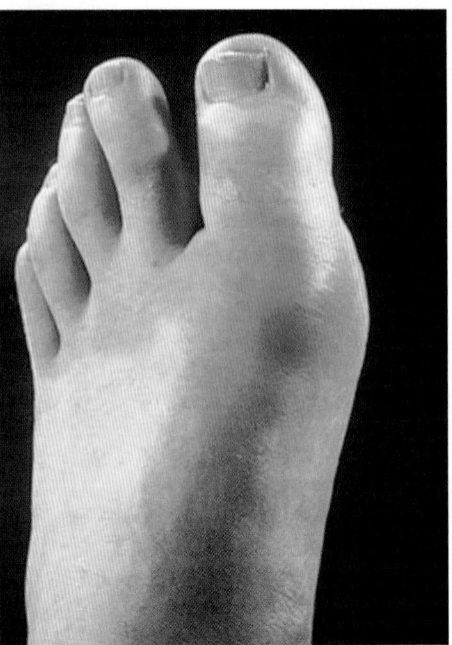

**Figure 27.26**

**Gout of the first metatarsophalangeal joint.** (From Ralson SH, et al, editors: *Davidson's Principles and Practice of Medicine*, ed 23, Edinburgh, 2018, Elsevier.)

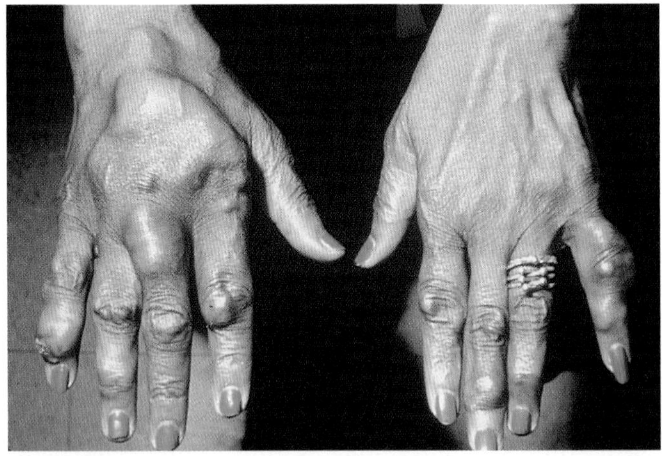

**Figure 27.27**

**Gout tophus on digits.** (From Swartz MH et al: *Textbook of physical diagnosis: History and examination*, ed 8, St. Louis, 2021, Elsevier.)

## MEDICAL MANAGEMENT

DIAGNOSIS. Often called the "great imitator," gout may masquerade as septic arthritis, RA, or neoplasm. The diagnosis can be delayed for weeks or months. A definitive diagnosis of gout is made when monosodium urate crystals (tophi) are found in synovial fluid, connective tissue, or articular cartilage.

Serum uric acid levels are elevated in approximately 10% of the affected population (more than 6 mg/dL); the presence of hyperuricemia alone does not equal a diagnosis of gout, nor does a normal serum level exclude its presence. The diagnosis is made most often on the basis of the triad of acute monarticular arthritis, hyperuricemia, and prompt response to drug therapy.[79]

Bone abnormalities seen on imaging studies (e.g., calcification, overhanging edges of bone erosions with sclerotic margins but with normal bone density) may be present in a small number of affected individuals. These are usually late findings in the disease process, occurring most often in the chronic phase.[263]

Musculoskeletal ultrasonography is another imaging method used to evaluate gouty joints. This noninvasive technique shows where the crystals have been deposited in the joint. Ultrasound pictures show the hyaline cartilage—the cartilage that coats the ends of the bones to protect them.

Ultrasonography can also show the *double contour sign*. This sign looks like a top covering or extra coating of the joint surface when crystals are deposited in the hyaline cartilage. Ultrasound studies do not replace fluid removal and examination under a microscope because ultrasound does not confirm infection.

**TREATMENT AND PROGNOSIS.** The goals of intervention are twofold: (1) to end acute attacks and prevent recurrent attacks and (2) to correct hyperuricemia. The ACR have established treatment guidelines for pharmacologic and nonpharmacologic treatments. The guidelines are based on the acute and chronic presentation of this disease.[198]

The first line of pharmacologic treatments is the use of a xanthine oxidase inhibitor (e.g., allopurinol) to lower the level of urate in the bloodstream. These agents should lessen the level of symptoms and can prevent or lessen future gout attacks by slowing the rate at which the body makes uric acid in cases of excess uric acid production.

NSAIDs are effective in treating the pain and inflammation of an acute attack. Occasionally intraarticular injection of corticosteroids is used to manage acute attacks. These pharmacologic agents must be taken on a continuous basis to maintain a lower concentration of uric acid in the blood. Colchicine with its antiinflammatory effects is another medication given during the acute phase but is less commonly used now because of its narrow therapeutic range and numerous side effects. Involved joints should also be rested, elevated, and protected (e.g., crutches, foot cradle, assistive devices, orthoses, proper shoe wear).

Once the acute attack has been relieved, the hyperuricemia may be treated, especially in the case of recurrent attacks of acute gouty arthritis or chronic gout. This requires lifelong management, and compliance is absolutely necessary. Dietary changes, weight loss, and moderation of alcohol intake all are important. Controlling hyperuricemia is the key to preventing this disease from becoming chronic and disabling.

New understanding of the exact mechanisms behind gout has led to the development of new agents for individuals with *refractory* gout. Refractory means the symptoms are not resolved with standard treatment and the condition has become chronic and unmanageable.[271]

**SPECIAL IMPLICATIONS FOR THE THERAPIST 27.19**

### *Gout*

Education on the causes and risk factors for gout will be the keystone treatment for gout. Individuals who are obese will need a well-monitored exercise program to improve physical health and to promote weight loss. The onset of severe joint pain with a swollen, hot joint should always concern the therapist. Gout, infection, and hemarthrosis all are conditions that could account for this clinical scenario. Gout may be associated with fever and malaise, making it difficult to distinguish clinically from a septic joint.

People with long-term gout often develop numerous complications, including orthopedic conditions of the foot and lower extremities, diabetes, and cardiovascular diseases. These individuals report poor quality of life, including physical and mental health issues. The therapist's plan of care should include interventions to address these comorbidities and to address quality-of-life issues.[305]

A septic joint is an orthopedic emergency, so when a red, hot painful joint is observed without prior medical diagnosis, immediate medical evaluation is necessary. Quick diagnosis and initiation of intervention are necessary to control or prevent damage to the joint structures.

Sometimes individuals with gout experience a flare-up after taking urate-lowering agents. This reaction can come as a surprise, as the expectation is that the pain and swelling will get better. Flares of this kind occur when old deposits of crystals stored in the tissues are being released. The increase in symptoms is not a sign that new crystals are forming. The affected individual should not stop taking prescribed medications without first checking with the physician. Getting rid of the old crystals can help protect the joint from further damage.

## Neuroarthropathy

Neuroarthropathy, or neuropathic arthropathy, is an articular abnormality related to neurologic deficits, regardless of the nature of the primary disease. Other terms applied to this disorder are Charcot joint, neurotropic or neuropathic joint disease, and neuropathic osteoarthropathy. Many underlying diseases or conditions can cause neuropathy, such as syphilis, syringomyelia, meningomyelocele, injury or trauma, multiple sclerosis, congenital vascular anomalies, diabetes mellitus, alcoholism, amyloidosis, infection (e.g., tuberculosis, leprosy), pernicious anemia, and intraarticular or systemic administration of corticosteroids. See the individual discussions of each condition.[205]

Early joint changes as seen on imaging studies may look very similar to those of OA. When present, advanced neuroarthropathy is more clearly defined, with enlarging and persistent effusion and minimal subluxation, fracture, or fragmentation. Microfractures can progress quickly into gross fragmentation, and the joint may appear to deteriorate quickly over a period of days to weeks.

Malalignment with angular deformity, subluxation, or dislocation leads to increased stress on the articular bone, contributing to sclerosis and fractures. Fracture lines can originate in the subchondral region and extend in an extraarticular direction. Management with arthrodesis or arthroplasty is often unsuccessful. More specific intervention approaches are discussed with each individual underlying condition.

# BONE

## Fracture

### Overview

A fracture is any defect in the continuity of a bone, ranging from a small crack to a complex fracture with multiple segments. Fractures can be classified into four general categories: (1) fracture by sudden impact (traumatic), (2) stress or fatigue fracture, (3) insufficiency fracture, and (4) pathologic fracture.

A *stress* or *fatigue* fracture, sometimes referred to as a stress reaction or bone stress injury, is defined as a partial break (reaction) or complete break (fracture) in the bone caused by the bone's inability to withstand stress applied in a rhythmic, repeated, microtraumatic fashion. More simply stated, a fatigue fracture occurs if normal bone is exposed to repeated abnormal stress, and an insufficiency fracture occurs if normal stress is applied to abnormal bone.

These types of overuse stress or fatigue fractures are most common in track and field athletes, distance runners, and soldiers in training. Most occur in the lower extremity and affect the tibial shaft and metatarsal bones, but they can also occur at the pubic ramus, femoral neck, or fibula; an increasing number of stress fractures have been reported in the knee (tibial plateau, proximal tibial shaft, femoral condyles).[303]

The two kinds of stress fractures are compressive and distractive. Compressive stress fractures occur as a result of forceful heel strike during prolonged marching or running. Distractive stress reactions occur as a result of muscle pull and can become more serious if displacement occurs.

*Insufficiency* fractures (sometimes referred to as insufficiency stress fractures) result from a normal stress or force acting on bone that has deficient elastic resistance or has been weakened by decreased mineralization. Reduced bone integrity can result from many factors but occurs most commonly from the effects of radiation, postmenopausal or corticosteroid-induced osteoporosis, or other underlying metabolic bone disease (e.g., hyperparathyroidism, osteomalacia, rickets, and osteodystrophy). Insufficiency fractures arise insidiously or as a result of minor trauma. It has been proposed that weight bearing alone can be enough to transmit a traumatic force to the compromised spine.[233]

*Pathologic fracture* is a term used to describe a fracture that occurs in bone rendered abnormally fragile by neoplastic or other disease conditions. Insufficiency fractures can be thought of as a subset of pathologic fractures, occurring in bones with structural alterations owing to osteopenia, osteoporosis, or disorders of calcium metabolism. A complete fracture extends through the entire bone; a greenstick fracture does not. A greenstick fracture often has to be completed before effective healing occurs. Other incomplete fractures may be called torus (or buckle), crack, or hairline fractures.

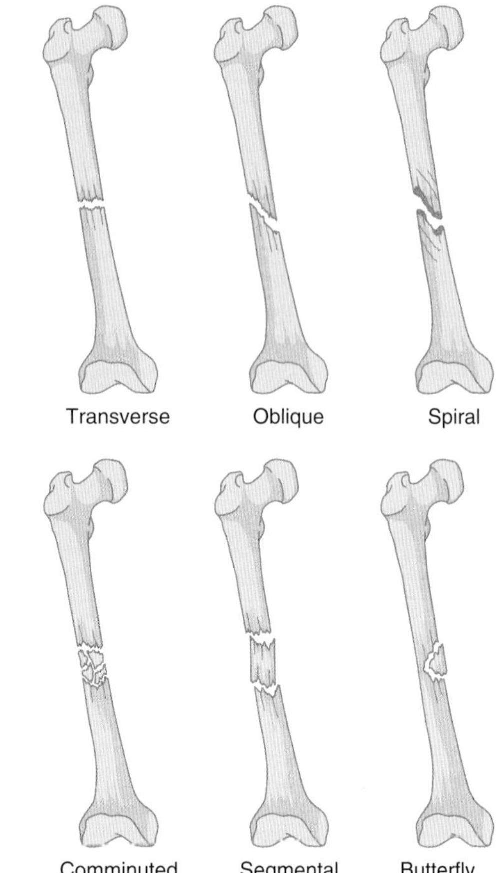


**Figure 27.28**

**Classification of fractures.** In a transverse fracture the fracture line is at a right angle to the long axis of the bone; this fracture is usually produced by shearing force. An oblique or spiral fracture occurs following a twisting or torsional force; fragments displace easily in the oblique fracture, whereas nonunion rarely occurs in a spiral fracture because of the wide area of surface contact. A fracture is comminuted if the bone is broken into more than two fragments and segmental if a fragment of the free bone is present between the main fragments. The separation of a wedge-shaped piece of bone is called a butterfly fracture. See Box 27.15 for other types of fractures and their definitions.

Fractures can be described for the orientation of the fracture line through the bone. Transverse, oblique, and spiral fracture lines are commonly found from traumatic causes of bone fractures. Comminution describes a fracture with multiple fragments at the fracture site and can be associated with different fracture lines. Fractures can also be described by the orientation of the fracture fragment ends and the long axis of the bones to describe if they are in a position and alignment that will allow for normal healing of the fracture. Fig. 27.28 and Box 27.15 show the classification, types, and definitions of fractures. Displaced, open fractures are more likely to be unstable. Compressive or shear forces can cause stable fractures to

Box 27.15

**TYPES AND DEFINITIONS OF SOME FRACTURES**

- **Colles fracture:** fracture of the distal radius and ulnar styloid in which the lower fragment is displaced posteriorly, usually from a fall on an outstretched hand
- **Galeazzi fracture:** fracture of the middle third and distal third of the radius accompanied by dislocation of the distal radioulnar joint at the wrist
- **Jones fracture:** fracture of the base of the fifth metatarsal
- **Maisonneuve fracture:** tear of the anterior and interosseous tibiofibular ligaments and a fracture (usually oblique) of the fibula 3 or 4 inches above the ankle mortise
- **Monteggia fracture:** fracture of the proximal third of the ulna with dislocation of the radial head
- **Nightstick fracture:** fracture of the ulna alone, usually midshaft
- **Piedmont fracture:** fracture of the radial shaft (rare)
- **Pott fracture:** oblique fracture of the lateral malleolus and transverse fracture of the medial malleolus; the talus may be displaced posteriorly (avulsion)
- **Torus fracture:** sometimes referred to as a "buckle" fracture; a fracture in which there is localized cortical expansion but little or no displacement; most common in young children when a compression fracture may merely "buckle" the thin cortex surrounding the cancellous bone

shift, becoming unstable. Unstable fractures are more likely to require surgery to stabilize them.

An *epiphyseal* fracture occurs in the growth centers of children and adolescents, located in the long bones. Growth can be arrested or altered in this type of fracture, and immediate intervention is required. An *articular* fracture occurs on or near a joint and is described by the course of the fracture line (e.g., T- or Y-shaped, transcondylar, supracondylar, intercondylar).

*Pelvic* and *sacral* fractures were traditionally classified according to stability, but with improvements in orthopedic procedures, these types of fractures are more often classified based on causative force vectors; this system is more appropriate, as the force vectors direct surgical fixation. The mechanisms of force vectors from the injury include anteroposterior compression, lateral compression, vertical shear, and combined/mixed mechanisms.[318]

Pelvic and sacral fractures may include a single pubic or ischial ramus, ipsilateral pubic and ischial rami, pelvic wing of the ilium (Duverney fracture), or fracture of the sacrum or coccyx. If the injury results only in a slight widening of the symphysis pubis or the anterior sacroiliac joint and the pelvic ligaments are intact, the fracture is considered stable. Unstable pelvic fractures can cause rotational instability, vertical instability, or both.

Vertically unstable pelvic fractures occur when a vertical force is exerted on the pelvis such as occurs when an individual falls from a height onto extended legs or is struck from above by a falling object. Disruption of the ligaments (posterior sacroiliac, sacrospinous, and sacrotuberous) is usually complete, and the hemipelvis is displaced anteriorly and posteriorly through the symphysis pubis.

Sacral fractures occur from stress transmitted through the pelvic ring to the sacrum. Lateral compression fractures are seen most often in motor vehicle accidents. Direct stress to the sacrum from a high fall onto the buttocks occurs less often and produces a transverse, rather than vertical, fracture.

*Vertebral compression fracture* (VCF) is one of the most common osteoporosis-related fragility fractures. VCFs often occur with only minor trauma. Only 20% to 25% of people who sustain a VCF develop symptoms severe enough to seek medical attention. VCFs are classified as wedge, crush, or biconcave according to their morphologic appearance. The greater prevalence of wedge fractures may be related to DDD, a condition that causes normal intradiscal pressure to shift and concentrate load to the peripheral aspects of the vertebral body.[270]

## Etiology

Bone mass is known to reach its maximum size and density (peak bone mass) by the time an adult reaches age 30 years. Women have a tendency to lose bone mass sooner than men, often beginning in their late 30s during the perimenopausal years. Bone loss is accelerated for women during and after menopause; men are more likely to experience bone loss in their mid- to late 60s.

## Risk Factors and Incidence

By far the most common traumatic fractures are those associated with sudden impact such as occurs with assault, abuse, traumatic falls, or motor vehicle accidents. Motor vehicle accidents involve fractures of the skull, nasal bone, and mandible most often; high-velocity injuries, including automobile or motorcycle accidents, often result in open fractures of the lower extremity. In the general population, radius and/or ulna fractures comprise the largest proportion of upper extremity fractures. The most affected age group is children ages 5 to 14 years as a result of accidental falls at home.

Age is an important risk factor for fractures. The rate of hip fracture increases at age 50 years, doubling every 5 to 6 years. Increasing age and low bone mineral density (BMD) are the two most important independent risk factors for an initial vertebral or nonvertebral fracture.[279]

Decreased BMD associated with osteoporosis accounts for the largest number of fractures among older adults (see Osteoporosis in Chapter 24). In fact, a fracture may be the first sign of an underlying diagnosis of osteoporosis, and a serious fracture is a risk factor itself for future fractures in high-risk groups. There are an estimated 1.5 million osteoporosis-related fragility fractures in the United States each year.[28] One in every two women older than 50 years of age will experience fragility fractures secondary to osteoporosis.

VCFs are the most common osteoporosis-related fractures, accounting for approximately 700,000 injuries. The incidence increases with age and with decreasing bone density. Factors that increase the risk of a first vertebral fracture include previous nonspine fracture, low BMD at all sites, low body mass index, current smoking, low milk consumption during pregnancy, low levels of daily physical activity, previous fall, and regular use of aluminum-containing antacids.[270]

Fractures at the hip were most common, accounting for 38% of the fractures identified. The proximal humerus, distal radius/ulna, and ankle also were common fracture sites. Fractures distal to the elbow or knee had only small increases in incidence with age older than 65 years. Women have higher fracture rates than men of the same race, and whites generally have higher rates than blacks of the same gender. Men are less likely to develop osteoporosis and subsequent fracture, but they are not immune to this condition and are frequently undertreated for osteoporosis even after a fracture. Fracture risk has been consistently associated with a history of falls, including falls to the side and attributes of bone geometry such as tallness, hip axis, and femur length.[343] Box 27.16 lists other risk factors for fracture; see also Box 27.17 for risk factors for falls. Some risk factors for fracture, such as age, low body mass index, and low levels of physical activity, probably affect fracture incidence through their effects on bone density and propensity to fall and inability to absorb impact.

**Stress Fractures.** In the case of stress reactions and fractures, an abrupt increase in the intensity or duration of training (i.e., military trainees, athletes preparing for marathons) is often an additional risk factor. Female recruits are at increased risk for pelvic and sacral stress fractures. The generally increased risk of bone stress injuries among women has been explained by anatomic (wide pelvis, coxa vara, genu valgum), hormonal, and nutritional factors.[234]

## Pathogenesis

The repair or regeneration of bone involves a complex sequence of cellular activities, beginning with acute hematoma formation and early inflammatory response and followed by granulation tissue infiltration, recruitment, proliferation, and differentiation of osteogenic and often chondrogenic cells; matrix formation and mineralization; and eventual remodeling.

The process is orchestrated and guided by a series of biologic and mechanical signals. Molecular signaling cascades and nutrition are key factors in the success of bone repair or regeneration. Bone response to injury and the phases of the reparative process are discussed in greater detail in Chapter 6.

When a bone is fractured, its normal blood supply is disrupted. Osteocytes (bone cells) will die from the trauma and the resulting ischemia. Bone macrophages will remove the dead bone cells and the damaged bone. A precursor fibrocartilaginous growth of tissue occurs before the laying down of primary bone, eventually followed by the laying down and remodeling of normal adult bone.

This complex process of fracture healing can be broken down into five stages: (1) hematoma formation, (2) cellular proliferation, (3) callous formation, (4) ossification, and (5) consolidation and remodeling. Some resources describe the phases of bone healing more succinctly as inflammatory, reparative, and remodeling.[104]

During the initial 48 to 72 hours after fracture, hematoma formation occurs as clotting factors from the blood initiate the formation of a fibrin meshwork. This meshwork is the framework for the ingrowth of fibroblasts and capillary buds around and between the bony ends.

During the cellular proliferation phase, osteogenic cells proliferate and eventually form a fibrocartilage collar around the fracture site. Eventually the collars and the ends of the bones unite. The cartilage is eventually replaced by bone as osteoblasts continue to move into the site (callous formation and ossification). Finally, the excessive bony callus is resorbed, and the bone remodels in response to the mechanical stresses placed on it.

**Box 27.16**

**RISK FACTORS FOR FRACTURES**

- Trauma
  - Motor vehicle accidents
  - Industrial or work-related accidents
  - Assault
  - History of falls; risk factors for falls
  - Overuse (marathon runners, military); sudden changes in training (duration, intensity)
  - Participation in sports including dance (recreational or competitive)
- Advanced age
- Women: postmenopausal osteoporosis; military: stress fractures
- Men: hypogonadism (erectile dysfunction, prostate cancer)
- Any insufficiency[a] or fragility fractures, especially vertebral fractures
- Residence in a long-term care facility
- Poor self-rated health
- Low physical function
  - Slow gait speed; gait disorders or movement dysfunction; low levels of physical activity
  - Difficulty in turning while walking; inability to pivot
  - Use of a walking aid (cane, walker)
  - Decreased quadriceps strength (e.g., inability to rise from chair without using arms)
  - Increased postural (body) sway[b]
  - Impaired cognition, dementia
- Physical attributes
  - Low physical fitness
  - Decreased bone mineral density
  - Bone geometry (see text description)
  - Leg-length discrepancy
  - Height
  - Low body mass index; low muscle mass
  - Poor nutrition; eating disorder; vitamin D deficiency
- Alcohol and/or substance use
- Other diseases or conditions
  - Osteoporosis; failure to treat or undertreatment of osteoporosis
  - Osteogenesis imperfecta
  - Osteonecrosis
  - Neoplasm; skeletal metastases; surgical resection for tumor
- Radiation treatment
- High-dose, long-term use of proton pump inhibitors

[a]Fracture in bones with nontumorous disease (e.g., rheumatoid arthritis, osteoporosis, following radiation) at normal load.[256]

[b]Postural sway is a corrective mechanism associated with staying upright and can be used as a measure of balance. Postural sway increases with age (reflecting decreased balance) and with the use of benzodiazepines.[698]

## Clinical Manifestations

The primary manifestations of fracture include pain and tenderness, increased pain on weight bearing, edema, ecchymosis, loss of mobility, and loss of function of the

Box 27.17

**RISK FACTORS FOR FALLS**

***Age Changes***

- Muscle weakness; loss of joint motion (especially lower extremities)
- Abnormal gait
- Impaired or abnormal balance
- Impaired proprioception or sensation
- Delayed muscle response/increased reaction time
- Decreased systolic blood pressure (<140 mm Hg in adults older than age 65 years)
- Stooped or forward bent posture
- Hearing loss

***Environmental/Living Conditions***

- Living alone
- Poor lighting
- Throw rugs, loose carpet, complex carpet designs, pets underfoot
- Cluster of electrical wires or cords
- Stairs without handrails
- Bathroom without grab bars
- Slippery floors (water, urine, floor surface, ice); icy sidewalks, stairs, or streets
- Restraints
- Use of alcohol or other drugs
- Footwear, especially slippers

***Pathologic Conditions***

- Vestibular disorders; episodes of dizziness or vertigo from any cause
- Orthostatic hypotension (especially before breakfast)
- Chronic pain condition
- Neuropathies
- Cervical myelopathy
- Osteoarthritis; rheumatoid arthritis
- Visual or hearing impairment; multifocal eyeglasses; change in perception of color; loss of depth perception; decreased contrast sensitivity
- Cardiovascular disease
- Urinary incontinence
- Central nervous system disorders (e.g., stroke, Parkinson disease, multiple sclerosis)
- Motor disturbance
- Osteopenia, osteoporosis
- Pathologic fractures
- Any mobility impairments (e.g., amputation, neuropathy, deformity)
- Cognitive impairment; dementia; depression

***Medications***

- Antianxiety; benzodiazepines
- Anticonvulsants
- Antidepressants
- Antihypertensives
- Antipsychotics
- Diuretics
- Narcotics
- Sedative-hypnotics
- Phenothiazines
- Use of more than four medications (polypharmacy/hyperpharmacotherapy)

***Other***

- History of falls
- Female sex; postmenopausal status
- Elder abuse/assault
- Nonambulatory status (requiring transfers)
- Gait changes (decreased stride length or speed)
- Postural instability; reduced postural control
- Fear of falling; history of falls
- Dehydration from any cause
- Recent surgery (general anesthesia, epidural)
- Sleep disorder/disturbance; sleep deprivation; daytime drowsiness; brief disorientation after waking up from a nap

From Goodman CC, Snyder TE: *Differential diagnosis for physical therapists: screening for referral*, ed 5, Philadelphia, 2012, Saunders. Used with permission.

involved body part. Point tenderness over the site of the fracture is usually present, but not all fractures are equally painful. Insufficiency fractures of the spine, pelvis, or sacrum often manifest with nonspecific low back, groin, or pelvic pain, mimicking other clinical conditions such as local tumor or metastatic disease or disk disease.

With many fractures, attempts to move the injured limb will provoke severe pain, but in the presence of a fatigue fracture (stress reaction) active movement is typically painless. Resistive motions or repetitive weight bearing will cause pain, and the area will be exquisitely tender to local palpation. Edema may be observed in the area of the fracture. Clinical manifestations are most severe when the fracture is unstable.

VCFs are often painless but are associated with height loss and respiratory dysfunction. When painful, the initial pain may be sharp and severe, but after a few days it may become dull and achy. The pain may be reproducible on examination with pressure over the spinous process of the involved level. Pain associated with VCFs tends to be postural (i.e., worse with spinal extension or even standing up straight); it can be debilitating enough to confine some older adults to a wheelchair or bed.

## Complications

The deformity associated with an extremity fracture is often obvious, but the deformity of a spinal fracture is not always so. For example, a compression fracture of a thoracic vertebral body may result in an anterior wedging of the body but only a mildly accentuated thoracic kyphosis. When thoracic kyphosis does occur, decreased trunk strength and decreased pulmonary function are possible.[199]

Occasionally in an adolescent or young adult who has not achieved mature bone growth, a persistent but painless prominence may occur 1 to 3 months after a minimally displaced fracture. It is located on the compression side of the fracture within the newly formed subperiosteal bone (intracortical) as a result of encapsulation or calcification of a hematoma. This transient postfracture cyst is benign, but must be medically diagnosed as such, as it cannot be distinguished clinically from infection or tumors.[295]

The healing of a fracture can be abnormal in one of several ways. The fracture may heal in the expected amount of time but in an unsatisfactory position, with residual bony deformity called *malunion*. The fracture may heal, but this may take considerably longer than the expected time *(delayed union)*, or the fracture may fail to heal *(nonunion)* with resultant formation of either a fibrous union or a false joint *(pseudarthrosis)*.

Loss of blood supply to the fracture fragments may impede healing by preventing adequate revascularization. Motion at the fracture site or an excessively wide gap can also contribute to nonunion. Individuals with nonunion often have pain, heat, and tenderness at the fracture site.

Other complications may include associated soft tissue injury, complications secondary to treatment, infection, skin ulceration, growth disturbances, posttraumatic degenerative arthritis, soft tissue or connective tissue adhesions, arthrodesis, myositis ossificans, osteomyelitis, refracture, nerve injury and neurologic complications, and vascular compromise.

## MEDICAL MANAGEMENT

**PREVENTION.** Therapists have a key role in the prevention of falls. Education and risk evaluation are two important variables in preventing fractures from occurring. Combining BMD with fracture assessment (e.g., use of dual x-ray absorptiometry to assess vertebral fractures) has a positive impact on lowering repeat fractures.[75] Fall prevention is important in adults older than 60 years of age (Box 27.18). High-risk groups can be identified (e.g., long-term care residents) and treated with low-cost interventions (e.g., calcium plus vitamin D or external padded hip protectors). Use of hip protectors (padded, convex plastic shields worn inside specially designed undergarments) to prevent hip fracture for people at risk has met with mixed results. The use of hip protectors has been advocated for institutionalized individuals. Instead of relying on hip protectors, older adults should be encouraged to increase bone mass through nutrition and physical activity and take extra care with medications that cause dizziness.

Fracture prevention in athletes begins with assessment of the athlete's past history, training variables, biomechanical factors, and shoe wear. In the military population, most bone stress injuries occur during the 8-week basic training period; injury-prevention programs to target this group are advised.[234]

**DIAGNOSIS.** Fractures are often diagnosed by visual inspection and confirmed by plain radiographs. Fractures can often involve surrounding soft tissue, vascular, and neurologic structures, requiring careful assessment at the time of injury. In the case of stress reactions (stress fractures), conventional x-rays are usually inadequate; often the lag time between manifestation of symptoms and detection of positive radiographic findings ranges from 1 week to several months. Up to 35% of sacral fractures are undetected on plain radiographs; cross-sectional imaging such as CT or MRI may be needed to identify and confirm sacral fractures. MRI is the gold standard for identifying bone stress injuries of the lower extremities, especially during the early stages of developing injury. CT is the imaging technique of choice to identify pathologic fractures.[276]

**Box 27.18**

**PREVENTION OF FALLS**

- Wear low-heeled, closed footwear with rubber soles or good gripping ability; avoid smooth-bottomed shoes or boots. This applies to slippers; wear slippers or shoes when getting out of bed at night.
- Provide adequate lighting for hallways, stairways, bathrooms; use a flashlight outdoors. Wear glasses at night when getting out of bed for any reason.
- Conduct a home safety evaluation. Remove loose cords, slippery throw rugs; repair uneven stairs, steps, sidewalks.
- Avoid oversedation; carefully monitor medications (especially sleep medications, antidepressants) and drink alcohol in moderation (never drink alcohol without your physician's approval if taking medications).
- Provide sturdy handrails on both sides of stairways.
- Provide grab bars on bathroom walls and nonskid strips on mats in tub or shower and beside tub or shower.
- Avoid going outdoors when it is wet, icy, or slippery; wear footwear with good traction or clip-on ice grippers; avoid walking on wet leaves or garden or yard clippings or debris.
- Carry items close to the body and leave one hand free to grasp railings or for balance.
- Know the location of pets before walking through a room or area of the house or apartment; maintain floors free of clutter and small objects.
- Use an appropriate assistive device as recommended by the therapist (e.g., cane, walking stick, walker); walkers equipped with a seat work well for people with limited endurance.
- Participate in a program of physical activity and exercise that is attainable.
- Avoid changing position quickly such as when getting out of a chair or bed. Stand for a moment to see if you are dizzy so that you can sit down again if necessary. See discussion of postural hypotension for prevention strategies (see Chapter 12).
- Keep items on shelves in the kitchen and elsewhere within reach. Do not stand on a chair or stepladder to reach items. Consider the consequences of a fall and broken hip if you are tempted and if you are thinking, "Nothing will happen, I will be fine."

**TREATMENT.** The medical approach to management of fractures is based on the location of the fracture, assessment of fracture type, need for reduction, presence of instability after reduction, and functional requirements of the affected individual. For example, stress fractures are usually uncomplicated and can be managed by rest and restriction from activity, whereas an unstable fracture of any bone may require immediate surgical intervention.

Individual factors such as the person's age, activity level, and general health and overall condition and the presence of any other injuries must also be taken into consideration. The goal of treatment is to promote hemostasis, hemodynamic stability, comfort, and early mobilization to prevent potential complications from immobility (e.g., constipation, deep vein thrombosis, pulmonary embolism, pneumonia). In the case of stress fractures, the initial period of rest is followed by a gradual return to activity. The progression of return to sports is based on symptomatic response to increasing activity.

The presence of osteoporosis complicates the need for immobilization or spinal fusion. Nonoperative treatment for VCFs includes activity modification, bracing, assistive devices, pharmacology (e.g., narcotic analgesics, calcitonin), and physical therapy. Hospital admission and bed rest is required for up to 20% of the population for whom conservative care is not possible or adequate.[319]

The debilitating effects of immobilization and keeping older adults bed bound are well recognized, with increased risks for developing pulmonary complications, pressure ulcers, deep vein thrombosis, and urinary tract infections. BMD is further reduced by immobility and bed rest, thereby increasing the risk of additional VCFs and other fragility fractures.

***Surgery.*** Surgical intervention may be required for VCFs, including bone grafts or bone graft substitutes, internal fixation (e.g., metal plating, wiring, screws), traction, or reduction and casting or immobilization. Minimally invasive procedures for the management of acute vertebral fracture have been developed. Direct injection of polymethyl methacrylate bone cement into the fractured vertebra is known as *vertebroplasty*. Insertion of a balloon to expand a collapsed vertebra followed by bone cement to stabilize the vertebral body is known as *kyphoplasty*.[22]

A similar technique is used for the treatment of complex fractures of the distal radius with calcium phosphate bone cement injected into the trabecular defect of the fracture site. Using a gene transfer vector, this remodelable bone cement allows for earlier removal (at 2 weeks instead of 6 weeks or more) of the cast or splint and early mobilization.[253] Results have been very encouraging, with better clinical and radiologic results than with conventional treatment. The use of this cement on other bones such as the calcaneus and in cranial reconstruction has been explored.

***Rehabilitation and Fractures.*** With or without surgical intervention, following bone fracture there is usually a period of immobilization (casting or splinting, fracture brace) to remove longitudinal stress. This period allows for the phagocytic removal of necrotic bone tissue and the initial deposition of the fibrocartilaginous callus.

For any type of fracture, management during the perifracture period is directed toward blood clot prevention (mechanical and/or pharmacologic), the avoidance of substances that inhibit fracture repair (e.g., nicotine, corticosteroids), and the possible need for supplemental caloric intake. Treatment should be initiated for anyone with osteoporosis, including calcium and vitamin D supplements, oral bisphosphonates, selective estrogen receptor modulators, calcitonin, and teriparatide (see discussion of treatment of osteoporosis in Chapter 24).

Gradually progressive stress will be applied to stimulate fracture callus formation and healing. In the case of pelvic or lower extremity fractures, the timing and extent of mobilization depend on the type of fixation used. For example, if an external fixation is applied for fracture stabilization, mobilization can occur within tolerance of the person's symptoms almost immediately.

***Modalities and Fractures.*** Many studies on the effect of ultrasound waves on fracture healing show that bone heals faster when it responds to applied pressure. Low-intensity (0.1 W/cm$^2$) pulsed ultrasound (2-ms bursts of sine waves of 1.0 MHz [frequency]; duration of 20 minutes daily) is an established therapy for fracture repair.[211] The mechanism by which ultrasound achieves these outcomes is not clear. One possible mechanism is direct stimulation of bone formation. Ultrasound has a direct effect on blood flow distribution around a fracture site, resulting in greater callus formation. This increased circulation serves as a principal factor facilitating the acceleration of fracture healing by ultrasound.

***Bone Grafting.*** Bone grafting to enhance bone repair can be applied during the repair stage of bone formation. Autogenous bone grafting takes bone from another part of the body and implants it in the bony defect that requires healing. The graft is most often taken from the iliac crest or fibula and contains all the components needed for bone healing. Donor site pain is a common complaint and the primary reason why some people prefer to use allogeneic bone graft material from a donor (bone bank).

Tissue engineering of bone has emerged as a new treatment alternative in bone repair and regeneration.[94,60] Porous scaffolds and biodegradable plastics have been developed to provide scaffolding for the regrowth of tissue, with the potential for healing fractures and repairing bone lost to tumors, osteoporosis, trauma, and other disorders. The use of osteoconductive scaffolds, growth factors, and osteoprogenitor cells has been proposed as methods for inducing bone formation when blood supply and osteoporotic conditions are present.

Commercially available demineralized bone matrix can be used to enhance bone healing, especially in people with nonunions or after the removal of bone cysts or fibrous lesions. Demineralized bone matrix still retains some of the original trabecular structure, which can function as a scaffold for osteoconduction.[137]

PROGNOSIS. In general, fractures in children heal in 4 to 6 weeks, in adolescents in 6 to 8 weeks, and in adults in 10 to 18 weeks. The process from fracture to full restoration of the bone will take weeks to months, depending on the type of fracture, location, vascular supply, health, and age of the individual. Nonunion or delayed union is more likely to occur in adults and occurs in up to 10% of all fractures. Older adults who have sustained a hip fracture have the highest rate of nonunion complications (15% to 30%). These individuals are almost four times more likely to die in the first year after fracture compared with individuals without fracture. Delay of surgery after hip fracture increases mortality and risk for complications of pneumonia and pressure ulcers significantly. Older women (older than 65 years) who survive the first year after a hip fracture may be at increased risk of death up to 15 years after the injury.[356]

Many people are at high risk for premature death or loss of independence following fracture; mortality after fracture is higher among men than among women. Less than 50% of older adults with a hip fracture will regain their prior level of function, with approximately half experiencing at least one fall in the year after their fracture.[217]

The inability to stand up, sit down, or walk 2 weeks after surgery is the strongest predictor for mortality among older adults with surgically repaired hip fractures.[264]

A person's condition before fracture (especially older adults with hip fractures) has important prognostic implications. Older adults who fall within 6 months following a hip fracture are more likely to demonstrate poorer balance, slower gait speed, and greater decline in ADLs from the prefracture level than older adults who do not fall.[313]

Healthy functional status contributes to faster recovery time with fewer complications and reduced medical expenses. Negative predictors for healing include medications such as calcium channel blockers and NSAIDs, renal or vascular insufficiency, smoking, alcoholism, and diabetes mellitus. Treatment can also affect healing via inadequate reduction, poor stabilization and fixation, distraction damage to blood supply, and postoperative infection.

## SPECIAL IMPLICATIONS FOR THE THERAPIST 27.20

### *Fracture*

The therapist managing patients with fractures should consider the patient's orthopedic intervention, expected time frames for healing along with rehabilitation considerations and precautions, and patient goals. For the older adult, there are many potential consequences of fractures. These include biomechanical, functional, and psychologic effects that can limit function and result in considerable disability. Biomechanical consequences can include anorexia and weight loss, compression of abdominal contents and decreased lung function from kyphotic posture, and the risk of more fractures.

Chronic, debilitating pain and increased dependence on family and friends occur as part of the functional consequences. Often there is a significant decrease in the individual's ability to perform ADLs because of impaired physical function. These factors, combined with depression and anxiety (and sleep disorders in some people), result in psychologic consequences. The therapist must remain alert to all of these potential consequences when evaluating each client and planning the best approach to clinical management.

#### Acute Care and Complications

Complications of fractures require vigilance on the therapist's part and possibly quick action. Significant swelling can occur around the fracture site, and if the swelling is contained within a closed soft tissue compartment, compartmental syndrome may occur (see Soft Tissue Injuries). Because of the progressively increased intracompartmental pressure, nerve and circulatory compromise can occur. This condition may be acute or chronic. The compartment becomes exquisitely painful.[276]

A thorough sensory and motor examination may be warranted. If the therapist notes skin changes, decreased motor function, burning, paresthesia, or diminished reflexes, physician contact is necessary. Permanent damage and loss of function may result if this condition is not treated. The therapist's examination may be helpful in establishing the extent of the injury and baseline function.

Another complication associated with fractures is fat embolism, a potentially fatal event. The risk of developing this condition is related to fracture of long bones and the bony pelvis, which contain the most marrow. The fat globules from the bone marrow (or from the subcutaneous tissue at the fracture site) migrate to the lung parenchyma and can block pulmonary vessels, decreasing alveolar diffusion of oxygen.[244]

The initial symptoms typically appear 1 to 3 days after injury, but this complication can occur up to a week later. Subtle changes in behavior and orientation occur if there are emboli in the cerebral circulation. There may also be symptoms of dyspnea and chest pain, diaphoresis, pallor, or cyanosis. A rash on the anterior chest wall, neck, axillae, and shoulders may develop. The onset of any of these symptoms warrants immediate physician contact.

The therapist must be alert to other complications that can occur following fracture, such as breakage of wires, displacement of screws, loss of fixation, refracture, delayed union and malunion, and infection. Individuals on bed rest are at risk for complications from immobility, including constipation, deep vein thrombosis, pulmonary embolism, and pneumonia.

#### Fracture Rehabilitation

Similar to medical treatment, fracture rehabilitation is shaped by fracture type, need for reduction, presence of instability after reduction, and functional requirements of the affected individual. Postoperative rehabilitation can begin immediately to within 1 week after surgery, depending on the physician's protocol.

There are some widely accepted guidelines and rehabilitation protocols for various types of fractures. The American Academy of Orthopaedic Surgeons offers guidelines for the rehabilitation of many different types of fractures.[139] Early mobilization accompanied by transfer training and maintaining strength and range of motion after fracture surgery are essential to reduce the risk of deep vein thromboembolism, pulmonary or infectious complications, skin breakdown, and decline in mental status.

Following a fracture in the lower extremity (including the hip), some orthopedic surgeons advocate unrestricted weight bearing, advising the client to decide himself or herself how much weight to put on the leg. Stable fractures can usually tolerate weight bearing. Rotationally stable but potentially long unstable femur fractures may be allowed toe-touch weight bearing. Clients with vertically and rotationally unstable femoral fractures may be restricted to non–weight-bearing status, using a wheelchair or electric scooter (if not in a spica hip cast). Although immediate weight bearing may cause initial bone loss, the long-term success of achieving bone growth remains unchanged, and the short-term benefits of functional recovery and quicker return to independent living that accompany unrestricted weight bearing are important.[272,321]

Again, depending on the type of fracture, some movements may be restricted to allow for proper fracture consolidation. Most importantly, a non–weight-bearing status can actually place greater forces on the hip as a result of the biomechanics involved in maintaining correct positioning of the lower extremity. In the case of femoral neck or intertrochanteric fractures, there is little biomechanical justification for restricted weight bearing; indeed, there is far greater pressure generated from performing a hip bridge while using a bedpan (almost equivalent to the effect of unsupported ambulation).

Partial weight bearing is usually considered 30% to 50% of body weight. Touch or touchdown weight bearing is 10% of body weight, but this is a subjective decision that is not easily determined. Allowing for unrestricted weight bearing according to the client's tolerance is less restrictive, but the therapist must assess for intact cognition and decision-making abilities, intact sensation, upper body strength, vestibular function and balance, and proprioception before allowing unsupervised weight bearing as tolerated.

Early fracture repair and physical therapy reduce hospital stays, increase chances of returning home (rather than being discharged to a nursing facility or rehabilitation facility), reduce complications, and improve functional mobility and independence at discharge and are associated with higher rates of 6-month survival.[23] There are usually impairments that will require continued strength and functional interventions for 7 to 9 months after fractures.

## Osteochondroses

A number of clinical disorders of ossification centers (epiphyses) in growing children share the common denominator of avascular necrosis and its sequelae. These disorders are grouped together and referred to as *osteochondroses,* with multiple synonyms (epiphysitis, osteochondritis, aseptic necrosis, ischemic epiphyseal necrosis). There are additional eponyms based on the name of the person or persons who described the disorder as well, such as Köhler disease (tarsal navicular bone disease), Osgood-Schlatter disease, and Legg-Calvé-Perthes disease.[80]

The underlying etiologic factors and pathogenesis are similar in all these entities, and the clinical manifestations are determined by the stresses and strains present. The most susceptible areas are the epiphyses, which are entirely covered by articular cartilage and therefore poorly vascularized.

## Osteochondritis Dissecans

Osteochondritis dissecans is a disorder of one or more ossification sites, with localized subchondral necrosis followed by recalcification. This condition affects the subchondral bone and the adjacent layer of articular cartilage; a piece of articular cartilage and fragment of bone separate and pull away from the underlying bone. These fragments can become loose bodies in the joint; the most common sites of involvement are the concave surfaces of synovial joint, such as the medial femoral condyle, talar head, and capitellum of the humerus.

Osteochondritis dissecans is caused by repetitive microtrauma resulting in ischemia and disruption of the subchondral growth. The articular cartilage softens, and fragment separation leads to cartilage injury that can progress to form a crater. Activity-related pain, swelling, and giving way are common symptoms. Pain is increased with passive knee extension and tibial internal rotation and relieved with tibial external rotation (Wilson sign).[346]

Signs of osteochondritis dissecans can be seen on a plain radiographs with MRI used to determine if the lesion is stable or unstable. Management varies with the person's age and the severity of the lesion and includes nonoperative management for stable lesions (activity modification, protected weight bearing, immobilization for 4 to 6 weeks). Arthroscopic procedures can be used to fixate the lesion, débride tissues from the defect, and implant tissues to stimulate healing.[33]

## Osteonecrosis

### Overview and Incidence

The term *osteonecrosis* refers to the death of bone and bone marrow cellular components as a result of loss of blood supply in the absence of infection. *Avascular necrosis* and *aseptic necrosis* are synonyms for this condition.

The femoral head is the most common site of this disorder (sometimes called Chandler disease), but other sites can include the scaphoid, talus, proximal humerus, tibial plateau, and small bones of the wrist and foot. Avascular necrosis is the underlying cause for approximately 10% of total hip replacement surgeries and overall affects approximately 20,000 people annually, often between the second and fifth decades of life.[67]

### Etiologic and Risk Factors

Osteocytic necrosis results from tissue ischemia brought on by the impairment of blood-conducting vessels. A minimum of 2 hours of complete ischemia and anoxia is necessary for permanent loss of bone tissue. The bony ischemia may be secondary to trauma disrupting the arterial supply or to thrombosis disrupting the microcirculation.

Bones or portions of bones that have limited collateral circulation and few vascular foramina are susceptible to avascular necrosis. Box 27.19 lists conditions associated with osteonecrosis. A number of these conditions are linked to osteonecrosis by the development of fat emboli (caused by altered fat metabolism) in the vascular tree of the involved bone.

Conditions associated with the development of fat emboli include alcoholism, obesity, pregnancy, pancreatitis, medications (e.g., oral contraceptives, corticosteroids), and unrelated fractures. Many cases of femoral head osteonecrosis are idiopathic (i.e., no known cause or risk factor can be identified).

Osteonecrosis has also been recognized as a complication in HIV-positive individuals; in fact, individuals who are HIV-positive have a 100-fold greater risk of developing osteonecrosis than the general population.[245] The exact mechanism for this remains unknown. It may be caused by hyperlipidemia secondary to the use of protease inhibitors; however, avascular necrosis was reported before the era of highly active antiretroviral therapy.

Box 27.19

**CONDITIONS ASSOCIATED WITH OSTEONECROSIS**

- Idiopathic
- Trauma (e.g., fall)
- Systemic lupus erythematosus
- Pancreatitis
- Diabetes mellitus
- Hyperlipidemia
- Cushing disease
- Gout
- Sickle cell disease
- Alcoholism
- Obesity
- Pregnancy
- Medications
  - Oral contraceptives
  - Corticosteroids
  - Bisphosphonates (under investigation)
- Organ transplantation (medication related)
- HIV infection
- Radiation therapy (less common)
- Dysbaric disease (deep sea diving; rare)

***Investigational Drugs (in Clinical Trials)***

- HuMax-CD20 (antibody that targets B cells)
- Atacicept (inhibits B-cell growth and survival)
- Tocilizumab (Actemra) (anti–interleukin-6 receptor monoclonal antibody)

More recently, the use of bisphosphonates that are prescribed for conditions related to osteoporosis has been linked with osteonecrosis of the jaw, especially after trauma to the teeth or bones of the jaw such as occurs with dental surgery (e.g., tooth extraction). The jaw has a high rate of bone renewal in response to stress via generation of an inflammatory response by the gums and teeth; bisphosphonates keep osteoclasts from reabsorbing damaged bone cells in the jaw that eventually may result in osteonecrosis.[265]

## Pathogenesis

Certain bones are more vulnerable to osteonecrosis than others. These bones are covered extensively by cartilage, have few vascular foramina, and have limited collateral circulation. The femoral head is a prime example of a bone at risk. The superolateral two-thirds of the femoral head receives its blood supply almost entirely from the lateral epiphyseal branches of the medial femoral circumflex artery (Fig. 27.29).

The only other source of blood for the femoral head is the medial epiphyseal artery (contained within the ligamentum teres), which has limited anastomoses with the lateral epiphyseal vessels. Hip dislocation or fracture of the neck of the femur can compromise the precarious vascular supply to the head of the femur. The talus, scaphoid, and proximal humerus are also susceptible to osteonecrosis.

As the ischemia progresses, repair processes occur but are not capable of preventing necrosis and deformation of the bone, such as flattening and collapse of the femoral head (Fig 27.30). The articular cartilage and acetabulum are usually spared until late in the disease process, but the articular cartilage may be lifted off the underlying bone, resulting in irreparable damage to the joint. The entire process extends over many years, and in contrast to osteochondrosis of immature bone (e.g., Legg-Calvé-Perthes disease), spontaneous healing never occurs.

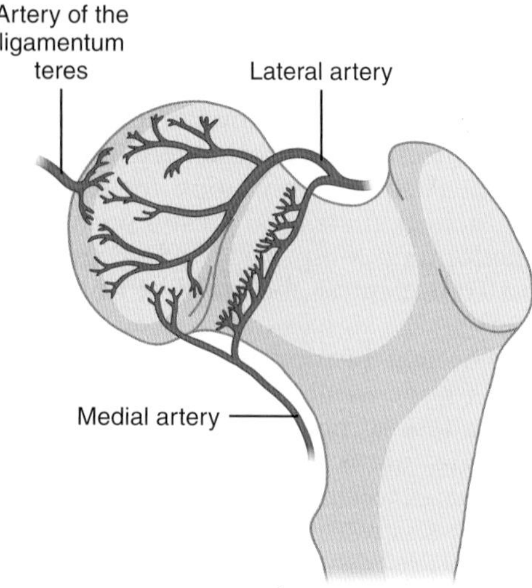


**Figure 27.29**

**Blood supply to the femoral head in a child.** (From Bullough PG: *Orthopaedic pathology*, ed 3, London, 1997, Mosby-Wolfe, p 263.)

## Clinical Manifestations

Often no symptoms are observed during the initial development of osteonecrosis even though an ischemic condition of the bone exists. Hip pain is the usual initial presenting complaint, with a gradual onset, sometimes of many weeks' duration, before diagnosis. The pain may be mild and intermittent initially but will progress to become severe, especially during weight-bearing activities.

If the femur is involved, the pain may be noted in the groin, thigh, or medial knee area. An antalgic gait is noted, and pain provocation occurs with weight-bearing activities and hip range-of-motion exercises, especially internal rotation and flexion and adduction. The affected individual will report a slowly progressive stiffening of the joint. When fracture occurs, it is usually at the junction between necrotic bone and reparative bone, possibly extending down through the reparative interface to the healthy inferior cortex of the femoral neck. Eventually degenerative joint changes and osteoarthrosis occur at the involved hip joint; the pathologic process is often relentless, with collapse of the femoral head imminent despite medical intervention.[67]

Osteonecrosis of the jaw is characterized by exposed bone in the mouth, numbness or heaviness in the jaw, pain, swelling, infection, and loose teeth. Delayed or poor wound healing after dental surgery may be the first indication of a problem. Crepitus as the jaw opens and closes may be present and is often described as similar to the sound of someone walking on ice.[288]

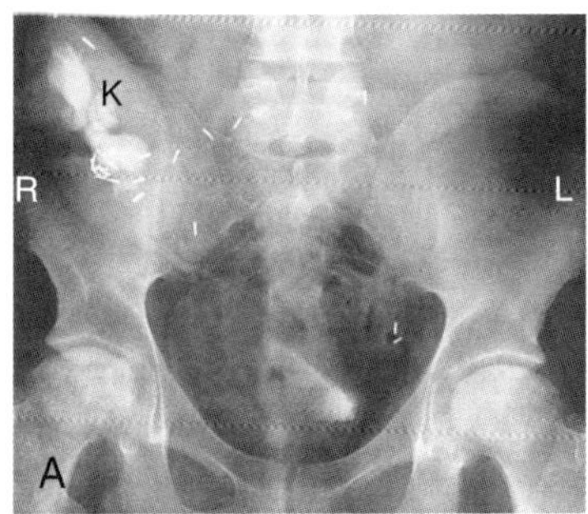

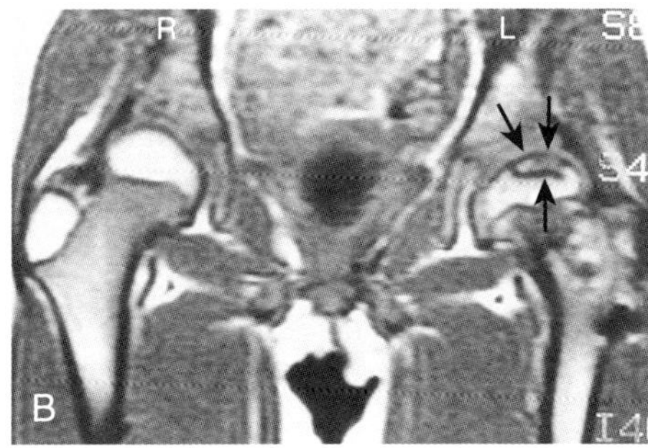


**Figure 27.30**

**Aseptic necrosis of the hip joints.** (A) Anteroposterior radiograph shows a patient with a history of steroid use with bilateral aseptic necrosis. (B) Magnetic resonance image shows a patient with signs of an aseptic necrosis in the left femoral head. (From Mettler FA, editor: *Primary care radiology*, Philadelphia, 2000, Saunders.)

## MEDICAL MANAGEMENT

DIAGNOSIS. Plain films may be normal initially. Bone scan, MRI, and CT are much more sensitive procedures and detect subtle bony changes.

TREATMENT. The choice between conservative and surgical intervention depends on the size of the lesion, how early the diagnosis is made, and whether bony collapse has occurred. If surgery is not indicated, protected weight bearing is essential to prevent collapse of the lesion.[67]

Surgical intervention may consist of core decompression for small lesions without evidence of structural collapse (most common procedure in early diagnosis) to relieve pain and delay or prevent structural collapse, hemiarthroplasty, or total joint replacement. An osteotomy may be performed to shift the site to where maximal weight bearing occurs on a particular joint surface. Core decompression removes a core of bone from the femoral head and neck in an attempt to relieve intermedullary pressure, thereby promoting revascularization and allow for bone grafting. Joint replacement may be required if femoral head collapse occurs or to prevent this complication. However, this procedure is limited by young age and high activity level as well as the limited life expectancy of the prosthesis.[368]

PROGNOSIS. The prognosis depends on the extent of damage that has occurred before diagnosis in the case of nontraumatic disease. Many cases are diagnosed in an advanced stage of disease, when minimally invasive surgical procedures are no longer helpful. Early intervention (both surgical and nonsurgical) has definitely improved the outcome, but many people with femoral head osteonecrosis experience irreversible damage to the joint and will need total arthroplasty.

SPECIAL IMPLICATIONS FOR THE THERAPIST 27.21

### *Osteonecrosis*

Therapists are always advised to obtain a thorough and complete history from clients, especially in the presence of musculoskeletal manifestations of apparently unknown cause. Because osteonecrosis is difficult to identify early, knowledge of causative factors (see Box 27.19) is important. Differential diagnosis of lumbar, hip, thigh, groin, or knee pain is essential because osteonecrosis may manifest with referred pain and symptoms as if coming from any one of these.

When treating people at risk for osteonecrosis, therapists must consider the possibility of fracture if there is a sudden worsening of pain symptoms followed by a sudden, dramatic loss in range of motion. Once the diagnosis is made, close communication with the physician is important for safe progression of weight bearing and exercise.

Following surgical intervention, the usual postoperative precautions and indications apply for minimization of complications (e.g., deep vein thrombosis), early mobilization, assessment for gait-assistive devices, gait training, demonstration of motion restrictions, and pain management.

In the case of microvascular bone transplantation, some physicians caution clients to avoid high-impact activities such as jumping, skiing, competitive tennis, and carrying more than 100 lb, although long-term studies of these stresses on repaired or reconstructed bones have not been carried out.

## Legg-Calvé-Perthes Disease

### Definition and Overview

Legg-Calvé-Perthes disease, also known as *coxa plana* (flat hip) and *osteochondritis deformans juvenilis,* is epiphyseal aseptic necrosis (or avascular necrosis) of the proximal end of the femur. It is a self-limiting disorder characterized by avascular necrosis of the capital femoral epiphysis (the center of ossification of the femoral head). Complete revascularization of the avascular epiphysis occurs over a period of time without any treatment.

This condition occurs in approximately 1 in 1200 children, primarily boys (5:1 ratio of boys to girls) usually between 5 and 8 years of age, making it the most common of the osteochondroses. Legg-Calvé-Perthes disease occurs 10 times more often in whites than in blacks.[95]

Deformation of the epiphysis with changes in the shape of the femoral head and the acetabulum occur during the process of revascularization in a significant portion of affected individuals. This may lead to degenerative

**Table 27.5** Stages of Legg-Calvé-Perthes Disease

| Stage | Time Period | Pathogenesis |
|---|---|---|
| Avascular (stage 1) | 1–2 weeks | Quiet phase: spontaneous vascular interruption to the epiphysis causes necrosis of the femoral head with degenerative changes; hip synovium and joint capsule are swollen, edematous, and hyperemic; joint space widens; cells of the epiphysis die, but bone remains unchanged |
| Revascularization (stage 2; fragmentation stage) | 6–12 months | Vascular reaction: new blood supply causes bone resorption and deposition of new bone cells; deformity from pressure on weakened area occurs; the entire or anterior one-half of the epiphysis of the femoral head is necrotic; increased blood supply and decalcification of bone cause softening at the junction of the femoral neck and the capital epiphyseal plate; granulation tissue and blood vessels invade the dead bone now detectable on radiographic examination |
| Reparative (stage 3; residual stage) | 2–3 years | New bone replaces necrotic bone; femoral head is replaced or is surrounded by new bone, with flattening of the femoral head causing the femoral neck to become short and wide with subluxation, progressive deformity, and even fracture possible |
| Regenerative (intravascular) | Final months | Completion of healing or regeneration gradually reforms the head of the femur into live spongy bone; restoration of the femoral head to a normal shape is more likely in younger children and only if the anterior epiphysis was involved; residual deformity may exist in some cases that can lead to gradual development of joint disease (osteoarthritis) |

Adapted from Perthes Kid Foundation: Symptoms & Stages. Available at: http://www.pertheskids.org/stages. Accessed September 6, 2019.

arthritis in young adulthood. Stulberg's classification used five classes to describe the shape and size of the femoral head, configuration of the acetabulum, and congruency of the joint surfaces. Individuals with classes I and II have retained a spherical femoral head. Class III is an ovoid femoral head. Classes IV and V have a flattened or irregular femoral head.[213]

### Etiologic Factors

The direct cause is a reduction in blood flow to the femoral leading to ischemia. This will occur after at least two episodes of ischemia, with the loss of blood flow potentially caused by a number of factors that include microtrauma, exposure to smoking, prenatal factors, delayed formation of the circumflex femoral artery, and hypercoagulability of the blood. Delay in bone age relative to the child's chronologic age suggests a possible general disorder of skeletal growth, with focal expression in the hip. Mechanisms proposed to explain the delay in bone maturation include genetic, endocrine, nutritional, and socioeconomic factors.[213]

### Pathogenesis

The disease process consists of four stages lasting from 2 to 5 years (Table 27.5). Because the growth plate of the femoral head lies above the insertion of the capsule of the hip joint in children and because the epiphyseal plate acts as a firm barrier to blood flow between the metaphysis and epiphysis, the femoral head depends on vessels that track along the surface of the neck of the femur to enter the epiphysis above the growth plate. The most important vessels supplying the epiphysis are the lateral epiphyseal vessels. These vessels are vulnerable to interruption of blood flow by trauma or by increased intraarticular pressure. It is possible that in Legg-Calvé-Perthes disease the ischemic events are episodic in nature and result from increased intraarticular pressure.[175]

Delays in bone maturation observed with this disease are correlated with the stage of the disease. The decrease in bone age delay in the later stages of the disease indicates that as the disease progresses, bone maturation accelerates and tries to catch up with the chronologic age. This phenomenon is referred to as *bone maturation acceleration*. This process occurs earlier in the epiphyses of the lower ends of the radius and ulna and short bones of the hands compared with the carpal bones.[210]

### Clinical Manifestations

Legg-Calvé-Perthes disease is characterized by insidious onset, initially manifesting as the intermittent appearance of a limp on the involved side, with hip pain described as soreness or aching with accompanying stiffness. The pain may be present in the groin and along the entire length of the thigh following the path of the obturator nerve or referred pain just in the area of the knee. There is usually pinpoint tenderness over the hip capsule.

Painful symptoms are aggravated by activity and fatigue and relieved somewhat by rest. Mild Legg-Calvé-Perthes disease is characterized by partial femoral head collapse, retention of a full range of hip abduction and rotation, and lack of subluxation on radiographic examination.[56]

Delay in bone maturation is a common feature of this condition. Skeletal development is unevenly timed in the growing bones, with the maximum delay occurring in the distal limb segments. As the condition progresses, there are decreases in active and passive range of motion, as well as limited physiologic (accessory) motion affecting walking and running.

Severe Legg-Calvé-Perthes disease begins later and involves collapse of the whole femoral head, stiffness, and subluxation. Atrophy of the thigh musculature and restriction of hip abduction and rotation may develop. Short stature may develop as a result of epiphyseal dysplasia, and in individuals who are left untreated, a flat femoral head will develop that is prone to degenerative joint disease.

Late complications in adults with a childhood history of Legg-Calvé-Perthes disease include early OA of the hip and acetabular labral tears. Hip, groin, or back pain may be the first symptom in affected adults. Postural asymmetry, leg-length discrepancy, decreased range of motion, and decreased strength may be accompanied by an abnormal gait pattern.[213]

## MEDICAL MANAGEMENT

**DIAGNOSIS.** Physical examination, clinical history, and radiographic examination (Fig. 27.31) confirm the diagnosis. MRI is widely accepted as the imaging method of choice, allowing early diagnosis and providing staging information necessary for adequate management.

Several different classifications are used to determine severity of disease and prognosis. The Catterall classification specifies four different groups defined by radiographic appearance during the period of greatest bone loss.[213]

The Salter-Thomson classification simplifies the Catterall classification by reducing it down to two groups: group A (Catterall I, II), in which less than 50% of the ball is involved, and group B (Catterall III, IV), in which more than 50% of the ball is involved. Both classifications share the view that if less than 50% of the ball is involved, the prognosis is good, while more than 50% involvement indicates a potentially poor prognosis.

The Herring classification studies the integrity of the lateral pillar of the ball. In lateral pillar group A there is no loss of height in the lateral third of the head and little density change. In lateral pillar group B there is a lucency and loss of height of less than 50% of the lateral height. Sometimes the ball is beginning to extrude the socket. In lateral pillar group C there is more than 50% loss of lateral height.

**TREATMENT.** The goal of treatment is to limit deformity and preserve the integrity of the femoral head. Mild disease may not require intervention, but careful follow-up with radiographic examination every 3 months is needed to observe for deterioration and progression of the disease.

Current methods of treatment attempt to prevent deformation of the femoral head and restore the spherical and congruent femoral head contour of the acetabulum. This is done by ensuring that the vulnerable anterolateral part of the avascular capital femoral epiphysis is contained within the acetabulum, a process called *containment*. The femoral head can be molded to a normal shape as it heals. The idea is to accomplish this while the bone is biologically plastic and before it is irreparably deformed.[213]

The closer to normal the femoral head is when growth stops, the better the hip will function in later life. The way that surgeons achieve this goal is through containment. In the past, weight bearing was minimized, but more recent therapy allows the child to continue weight bearing with the femur in an abducted and internally rotated position. Keeping the head of the femur well seated in the acetabulum decreases focal areas of increased load and minimizes distortion, thereby maintaining range of motion and preventing deformity.[314]

The femoral head must be held in the joint socket (acetabulum) as much as possible. It is better if the hip is allowed to move and is not held completely still in the joint socket. Joint motion is necessary for nutrition of the cartilage and for healthy growth of the joint. All treatment options for Legg-Calvé-Perthes disease try to position and hold the hip in the acetabulum as much as possible. This healing process can take several years.

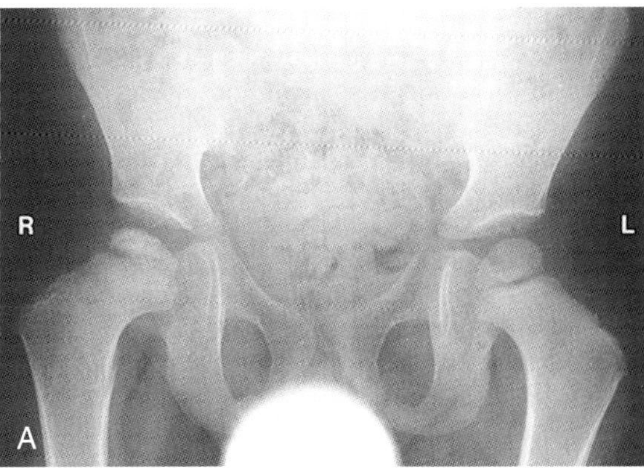


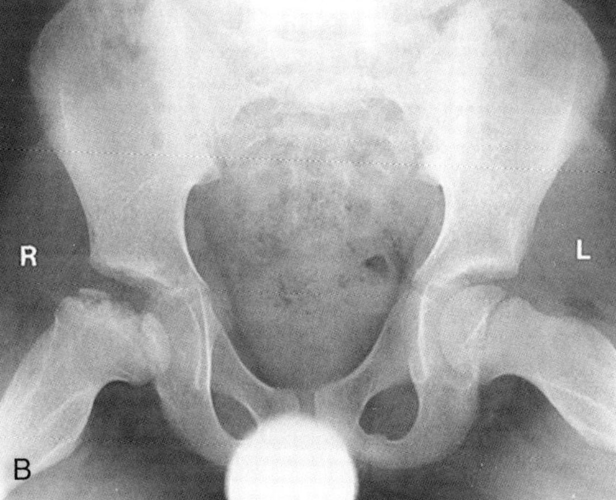


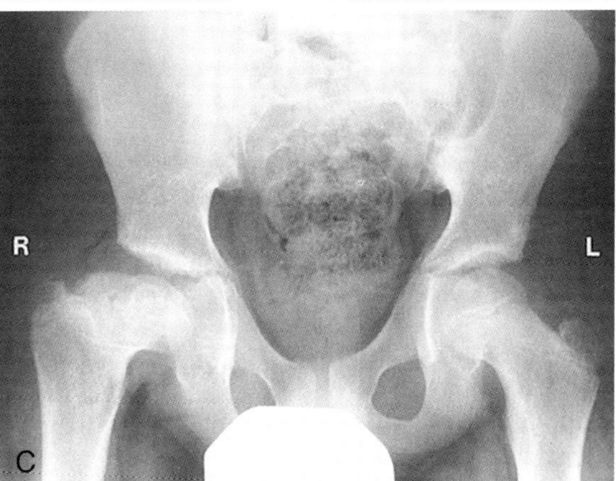


**Figure 27.31**

**Legg-Calvé-Perthes disease.** (A) Anterior view of the pelvis demonstrates fragmentation and sclerosis of the right femoral epiphysis *(arrow)* in a 6-year-old boy. (B) Follow-up film obtained 8 years later shows continuing deformity resulting from osteonecrosis. (C) The child developed significant degenerative arthritis by age 12 years. (From Mettler FA: *Primary care radiology*, Philadelphia, 2000, Saunders.)

Conservative care is usually continued for 2 to 4 years. A variety of splints, braces, and positional devices may be used to maintain the proper position.[148] When lack of motion has become a problem, the child may be admitted to the hospital and placed in traction. Traction is used to quiet the inflammation. Antiinflammatory medications may be prescribed. Physical therapy is used to restore the hip motion as the inflammation comes under control. Home traction may also be an option.

In some cases, surgery will be required to obtain adequate containment. Sometimes, adequate motion cannot be regained with traction and physical therapy alone. If the condition is long-standing, the muscles may have contracted or shrunk and cannot be stretched back out.

To help restore motion, the surgeon may recommend a *tenotomy* of the contracted muscles. When a tenotomy is performed, the tendon of the muscle that is overly tight is cut and lengthened. This is a simple procedure that requires only a small incision. The tendon eventually scars down in the lengthened position, and no functional loss is noticeable.

Surgical treatment for containment may be best in older children who are not compliant with brace treatment or where the psychologic effects of wearing braces may outweigh the benefits. Surgical containment does not require long-term use of braces or casts. Once the procedure has been performed and the bones have healed, the child can pursue normal activities as tolerated.

Surgical treatment for containment usually consists of procedures that realign the femur (thighbone), the acetabulum (hip socket), or both. Realignment of the femur is called a *femoral osteotomy*. This procedure changes the angle of the femoral neck so that the femoral head points more toward the socket.[213]

To perform this procedure, an incision is made in the side of the thigh. The bone of the femur is cut and realigned in a new position. A large metal plate and screws are then inserted to hold the bones in the new position until the bone has healed. The plate and screws may need to be removed once the bone has healed.

Realignment of the acetabulum is called a *pelvic osteotomy*. This procedure changes the angle of the acetabulum (socket) so that it covers or contains more of the femoral head. To perform this procedure, an incision is made in the side of the buttock. The bone of the pelvis is cut and realigned in a new position. Large metal pins or screws are then inserted to hold the bones in the new position until the bone has healed. The pins usually must be removed once the bone has healed.[213]

If there is a serious structural change in the anatomy of the hip, there may need to be further surgery to restore the alignment closer to normal. This is usually not considered until growth stops. As a child grows, there will be some remodeling that occurs in the hip joint. This may improve the situation such that further surgery is unnecessary.

In severe cases, both femoral osteotomy and pelvic osteotomy may be combined to obtain even more containment.

**PROGNOSIS.** Legg-Calvé-Perthes disease may vary in severity from a mild self-healing problem with no sequelae to a condition that will destroy the hip unless serious action is taken. Early on, it may be difficult to determine which course the disease will follow. Radiographic signs for the involvement of the femoral capital epiphysis, metaphyseal changes, and subluxations of the femoral head with acetabulum will determine the probable outcome of treatment.[363,61]

Even though the disease is self-limiting, the prognosis varies according to the age of onset (better prognosis in children whose onset is before age 5 years). Children older than age 8 years at the time of onset have a better outcome with surgical treatment than with nonoperative care. There is some evidence to suggest that early delay in bone age (stage I of the disease) is linked with more severe disease.[210]

Older age, complete involvement of the femoral head, and noncompliance with treatment contribute to a poorer prognosis. Although girls are less likely to develop Legg-Calvé-Perthes disease compared with boys, they often have a poorer prognosis. The reason for this difference is unknown.

A delay in bone age maturation of more than 2 years in stage I of the disease has been linked with greater severity of the disease. However, children with Legg-Calvé-Perthes disease have a normal onset of puberty, and by the time they are 12 to 15 years old, their stature and bone age are the same as those of their peers.[213]

**SPECIAL IMPLICATIONS FOR THE THERAPIST 27.22**

*Legg-Calvé-Perthes Disease*

Therapists may be involved in gait training, aquatic therapy, and range-of-motion exercises during this period. It should be emphasized to the child and family that Legg-Calvé-Perthes disease is a long-term problem, with treatment aimed at minimizing damage while the disease runs its course. Performing exercises daily is essential during the healing process to ensure that the femur and hip socket have a perfectly smooth interface.[43] This will minimize the long-term effects of the disease. As individuals age, problems in the knee and back can arise as a result of the abnormal posture and stride adopted to protect the affected joint.

Surgery may be performed to contain the femoral head in the acetabulum, especially in children older than 6 years with serious involvement of the femoral head. Hip replacements are relatively common during the sixth decade, as the already damaged hip suffers routine wear; this varies from individual to individual.

## Osgood-Schlatter Disease

### Overview

Osgood-Schlatter disease (osteochondrosis) results from fibers of the patellar tendon pulling small bits of immature bone from the tibial tuberosity. In the past, Osgood-Schlatter disease was considered a form of osteochondritis (inflammation of bone and cartilage), but more recent thinking suggests that the process is one part of the spectrum of mechanical problems related to the extensor mechanism. Rather than being an actual degenerative disease, Osgood-Schlatter is considered a form of tendinitis of the patellar tendon.[129]

It is most commonly seen in active adolescent boys 10 to 15 years of age, but can also affect girls ages 8 to

13 years. The ratio of boys to girls affected by Osgood-Schlatter disease is 3:1. It is estimated that 20% of adolescents actively involved in sports have some symptoms of Osgood-Schlatter disease, with an equal number of military recruits experiencing symptoms that affect kneeling and squatting during military training.[277]

### Etiologic Factors and Pathogenesis

Osgood-Schlatter disease is probably the result of indirect trauma (force produced by the sudden, powerful contraction of the quadriceps muscle during an activity) or repetitive stress (repeated knee flexion against a tight quadriceps muscle) before complete fusion of the epiphysis to the main bone has occurred. It is further aggravated by the longitudinal traction associated with bone growth in adolescents and the presence of external tibial torsion. Long-standing tension on the patella and patellar tendons during rapid growth spurts sets up an imbalance between the femur and the anterior structures of the knee.

Another possible cause of Osgood-Schlatter lesions is abnormal alignment in the lower extremities. Children with genu valgum and children who are flatfooted seem to be most prone to the condition. These postures place more tension on the bone growth plate of the tibial tuberosity, increasing the chances for an Osgood-Schlatter lesion to develop. A high-riding patella, called *patella alta,* is also thought to contribute to development of Osgood-Schlatter lesions.[129]

In young athletes, the tendon is attached to prebone, which is weaker than normal adult bone. With excessive stresses on the tendon from running and jumping, the structure becomes irritated, and a tendinitis begins. Often fragments representing cartilage or bone formations are found on the surface of the patellar tendon and are a potential cause of pain. These patellar tendon fibers can actually pull fragments away from the tibial epiphysis. This process is described as avulsion of the secondary ossification center of the tibial tuberosity (Fig. 27.32).[129]

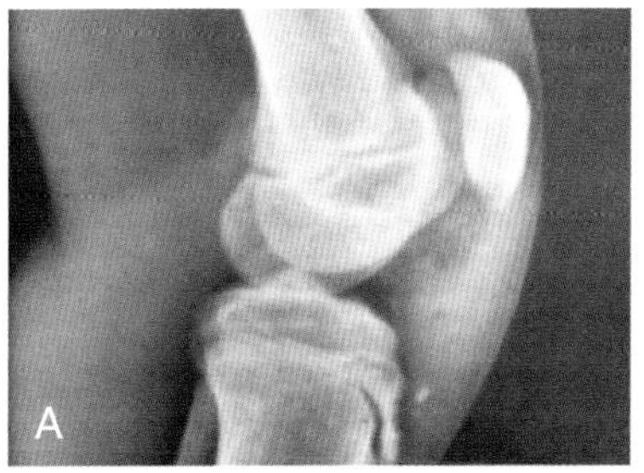


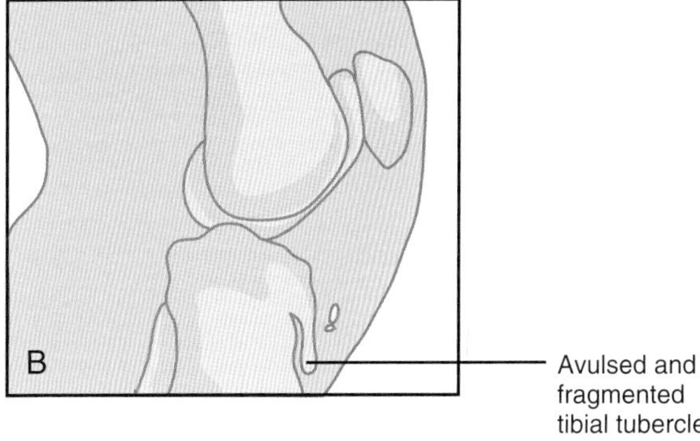


**Figure 27.32**

**Clinical radiograph of the knee in a 12-year-old child shows fragmentation and avulsion of the tibial tubercle.** Swelling below the knee and an enlarged tibial tuberosity may be observed clinically. This condition, known as Osgood-Schlatter disease, is probably posttraumatic. (From Bullough PG: *Orthopaedic pathology*, ed 3, London, 1997, Mosby-Wolfe, p 98.)

### Clinical Manifestations

Clinically, clients report constant aching and pain at the site of the tibial tubercle (just below the kneecap), which is often enlarged on visual examination. Symptoms are aggravated by any activity that causes forceful contraction of the patellar tendon against the tubercle, such as active knee extension or resisted knee flexion (e.g., going up or down stairs, running, jumping, biking, hiking, kneeling, squatting).

Besides the obvious soft tissue swelling, there may be localized heat and tenderness, the latter elicited with direct pressure over the anterior aspect of the proximal tibial tubercle. Many children with this condition also have significant tightness in the hamstrings, iliotibial band, triceps surae (bellies of the gastrocnemius and soleus), and quadriceps muscles. Tightness in these areas can potentially increase the flexion moment and subsequent stresses at the tibial tubercle.

## MEDICAL MANAGEMENT

DIAGNOSIS. On physical examination, the examiner is able to palpate tenderness at the tibial tubercle; later there will be a bony bump at that site that distinguishes this problem from other conditions affecting the knee.

Clinical diagnosis may be confirmed by radiography (or ultrasonography to avoid exposure to x-ray), as many conditions are very similar (e.g., patellar tendinitis, chondromalacia patella, synovial plica). Although the films may be normal, epiphyseal separation, soft tissue swelling, and bone fragmentation can be visualized in many cases.

TREATMENT AND PROGNOSIS. Rest from aggravating activities and/or activity modification/restriction is recommended until symptoms have subsided. This time frame ranges from 2 to 3 weeks in some individuals to 2 to 3 months or longer in others. Enough time must be allowed for revascularization, healing, and ossification of the tibial tubercle before resumption of unrestricted athletic participation. NSAIDs and ice are used regularly.[129]

Treatment should include exercises to address the mechanical inefficiencies of the extensor mechanism, stretching for any areas of inflexibility, and strengthening areas of weakness (e.g., ankle dorsiflexion, pain-free quadriceps strengthening).

Balance and coordination should be assessed and rehabilitation provided as appropriate. Support may be provided through the use of a knee sleeve, brace, or narrow strap around the leg, placing pressure over the tibial tubercle. This latter device is used to reduce the pulling stresses of the patellar tendon on the tubercle and subsequently reduce pain.

Approximately 90% of children with this condition respond well to nonoperative treatment. Complete recovery is expected with closure of the tibial growth plate, but 60% of affected individuals report discomfort with kneeling long after skeletal maturity. Conservative measures are usually sufficient to provide pain relief and resolution of local swelling.

When conservative care fails to resolve painful symptoms, full-extension immobilization of the leg through reinforced elastic knee support, cast, or splint may be prescribed for 6 to 8 weeks. In chronic, unresolved cases (rare), surgery may be necessary to remove the prominent tibial tubercle and any epiphyseal ossicles that have formed in the tendon. Sometimes ossicle removal without tibial tubercle excision is performed. In extreme cases the epiphysis may be removed or holes drilled into the tibial tubercle to facilitate revascularization of the area. Response to surgical treatment for symptomatic unresolved disease in skeletally mature adults is reportedly good to excellent, with resolution of pain and return to daily activities including unrestricted sports participation. Pain on kneeling remains a persistent problem.[277]

## REFERENCES

To enhance this text and add value for the reader, all references are included in the enhanced ebook on Student Consult that accompanies this textbook. The reader can view the reference source and access it online whenever possible.

# CHAPTER 28

# Introduction to Central Nervous System Disorders

KAREN L. MCCULLOCH • KENDA S. FULLER

## OVERVIEW

The central nervous system (CNS) controls and regulates all mental and physical functions. The nervous system is unparalleled among organ systems in terms of diversity of cellular constituents. It is composed of a network of neural tissue that includes both receptors and transmitters. There is a complex interaction among the areas that control both thought and movement; dysfunction in one area will cause changes in the other. Disease or trauma of the CNS may affect the nervous system through damage to several types of tissues in a local area, such as in stroke, or it may cause dysfunction in one type of tissue throughout many areas of the CNS, such as in multiple sclerosis (MS). Dysfunction of the neurons in particular areas of the brain can disrupt the complex organization of neuronal firing, resulting in abnormal perception of the environment, uncoordinated movement, loss of force production, or dysfunction in cognition.

Behavior is shaped by the interplay between genes and the environment. There are genes that control entry into the cell cycle where cells synthesize DNA and undergo mitosis. Proliferation can be triggered by internal signals or in response to external growth factor stimulation. There is a complex spectrum of alterations produced by aging, disease, exposure to environmental factors, and neoplastic transformation. Mutations of genes cause changes in cell growth, differentiation, and death. A set of genes appears to inhibit cellular proliferation; these genes are the "brakes" of the cell cycle, and loss of these genes may lead to neoplastic, or tumor, growth.[28]

Inherited patterns of DNA expression may cause a predisposition for neurologic disease and affect the ability to repair damage from an insult in the nervous system. Genetic information is stored in the chromosomes within each individual cell in the body; about 80,000 genes are represented and arranged in a precise order. More than one-third of the genes are expressed as messenger RNA in the brain, more than in any other part of the body. An anomaly or alternative gene version is referred to as an *allele*. Single-gene mutations or alleles have been identified and can be associated with degenerative neurologic disease, such as Huntington disease. However, for most chronic disorders, there appear to be multiple abnormalities, and it is clear that environmental conditions and exposures have an effect on how the abnormalities are manifested.[2] Pathologic derangements of normal cellular processes are a way of looking at possible causes of disease.

The following chapters describe typical neurologic disorders and the differential diagnosis to identify each. The incidence, risk, and etiologic factors are described in each chapter. With ongoing research, it is increasingly clear that there is overlap in the pathologic processes for neurologic conditions. Symptoms can be both similar and distinguishing. Treatment for one disorder may have some of the same components as another, with pharmacologic interventions often targeting neurotransmitters or pathophysiologic effects. In general, science is discovering the value of nutrition, exercise, and mindfulness as contributing to what is termed *neuroprotection*.

## PATHOGENESIS

### Cellular Dysfunction

Neuronal cell death is a hallmark of many disorders of the nervous system through the processes of necrosis and apoptosis, or programmed cell death. The intensity of cellular injury determines whether the cell dies or is able to survive. Very severe injury leads to the passive process of necrosis, less severe but irreparable injury leads to the active process of apoptosis, and survivable injury leads to reactive changes such as gliosis or scarring.

Apoptosis is a type of cellular suicide, but apoptosis does not cause inflammatory responses. It is a more organized process with fragmentation of the cells and degradation of the DNA. It is common during the development of cells to eliminate the overproduction of one cell type. The biochemical pathway is present in all cells of the body and is used normally in the maturation and regulation of the nervous system, with systematic removal of neurons from the brain. In apoptosis the cell is removed by macrophages and leaves no residual damage to other components of the CNS. If the cell sustains genetic damage through neurodegenerative disease or injury and cannot be repaired by the system, the cell dies. Damage to the CNS can cause excessive apoptosis through the process of trophic factor withdrawal, oxidative insults, metabolic compromise, overactivation of glutamate receptors, and exposure to bacterial toxins.[63] Both necrosis and apoptosis underlie diseases as diverse as stroke, trauma, demyelinating disorders, infections, and neurodegenerative disorders.

When cell death is caused by necrosis, there is cellular swelling, fragmentation, and cell disintegration. Necrosis causes the internal structure of the cell to swell as water enters the cell through osmosis, causing cell membranes to rupture. Lymphocytes and polynuclear cells can cause inflammatory cells to surround the necrotic debris, resulting in release of cytotoxic compounds that cause destruction of neighboring cells. Excitotoxicity results from the inappropriate activation of excitatory amino acid receptors, leading to the entry of calcium ions into the cell. The calcium activates intracellular function. Damaged cells release excitotoxins that cause further destruction within surrounding cells.[28]

Free radical formation is a by-product of excitotoxicity. Free radicals are capable of destroying cellular components and triggering apoptosis. Free radicals are molecules with an odd number of electrons. The odd, or unpaired, electron is highly reactive as it seeks to pair with another free electron. Free radicals are generated during oxidative metabolism and energy production in the body. Free radicals are related to normal metabolism but can also be a cause of oxidative stress in brain injury and disease. Oxidative stress refers to cells and tissues that have been altered by exposure to oxidants. Oxidation of lipids, proteins, and DNA leads to tissue injury. Nitrogen monoxide (nitric oxide) is a free radical generated by nitric oxide synthase. This enzyme modulates physiologic responses, such as vasodilation or signaling in the brain. Oxidative stress, rather than being the primary cause, appears to be a secondary complication in many progressive disorders, such as Alzheimer disease, Parkinson disease, and amyotrophic lateral sclerosis (ALS), as well as disorders of mental status. Enhanced antioxidant status is associated with reduced risk of several diseases.[78]

The extracellular environment is critical to the function of the neurons. The blood-brain barrier is made from endothelial cells and has tight junctions that block diffusion so that substances can pass only through the cell and not in between cells. This process is regulatory in nature and not completely protective. Entry into the CNS is determined by lipid solubility. Glucose and amino acids cross the endothelial cell barrier via protein transporters.[88]

The ependymal cells line the ventricles and spinal canal and regulate metabolism between the channels of the extracellular space and the ventricles. The ependyma forms the basis of the blood-brain barrier. There is movement of molecules through the extracellular space, with the possibility of long-range and relatively diffuse actions of neurotransmitters released into the extracellular space. This type of signaling is known as *volume transmission* and may have a major role in setting large-scale neuronal excitability or inhibition.[28]

Dysfunction within the nervous system can affect either or both of the two main classes of cells: the glial cells and the neurons. Stem cells create new glia and new neurons. The region immediately beneath the ependymal cell layer produces new cells at a very low rate in the adult compared with the amount created during neurogenesis in early development. The cells migrate widely through the brain and conform phenotypically to the regions where they end up.

## Glial Cells

Aside from neurons, macroglia and microglia are the two primary cell types located throughout the CNS. The macroglia are derived from a nerve cell lineage and are classified into three distinct subtypes: astrocytes, oligodendrocytes, and Schwann cells. These macroglia are the most populous cells of the CNS and support and maintain neuronal plasticity throughout the CNS. Glial cells are often implicated in disease processes that affect brain tissue.[49]

Microglia are the resident immune cells of the brain. Microglia are interspersed throughout the brain and represent approximately 10% of the CNS population of cells. Microglia differ from the macroglia because they are derived from a monocyte cell lineage. Microglia respond to CNS insult by diffuse proliferation and infiltration of CNS tissue. Microglia are pivotal in innate immune activation and function to modulate neuroinflammatory signals throughout the brain. In the absence of a stimulus indicating inflammation, microglia are dormant. Inflammatory cytokines produced within the CNS target neuronal substrates, triggering responses of fever, increased sleep, reduced appetite, and lethargy. Collectively, these behavioral symptoms of sickness are evolutionarily conserved and function to increase the metabolic demand for clearance of pathogens via the microglia.[36] Active microglia show macrophage-like activities, including scavenging, phagocytosis, antigen presentation, and inflammatory cytokine production. Activated microglia and monocytes coming in from the bloodstream can assume the form of macrophages. Microglia recruit and activate astrocytes to propagate inflammatory signals further. Normally, neuroinflammatory changes are transient and beneficial, with microglia returning to the dormant state after the resolution of the immune challenge. However, nearby neurons may be damaged by toxins released from activated macrophages and microglia. Aging provides a brain environment in which microglia activation is not resolved, leading to a heightened sensitivity of immune activation; this lack of resolution may also contribute to the pathogenesis of neurologic disease.[95]

Astrocytes, another type of glial cell, are so named because they look like star cells. They are the most numerous cells in the brain and outnumber neurons 10 to 1. Fig. 28.1 shows the relationship of the glial cell to the neuron. The glial cells provide support and structure for the CNS and fulfill the role that connective tissue plays in other parts of the body. The neurons communicate information to one another to process sensory information, program motor and emotional responses, and store information through memory. In addition to their support function, the cells serve a nutritive function, as they connect to the capillary wall and to the nerve cell. Astrocytes are permeable to potassium and therefore are involved in maintaining the correct potassium balance in the extracellular space. Astroglia have the ability to monitor and remove extracellular glutamate and other residual neuronal debris after brain injury and can seal off damaged brain tissue.[49,90]

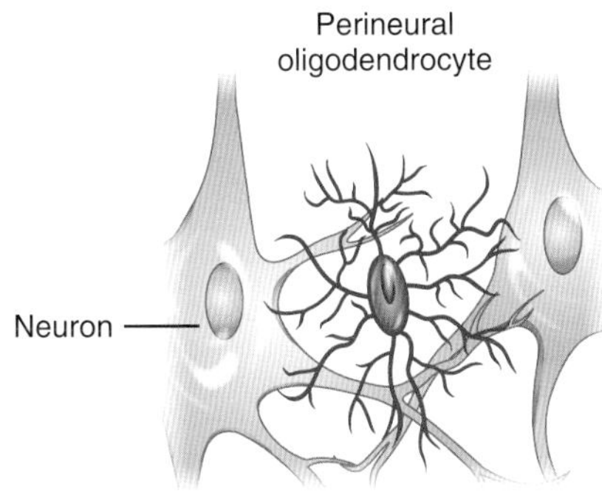


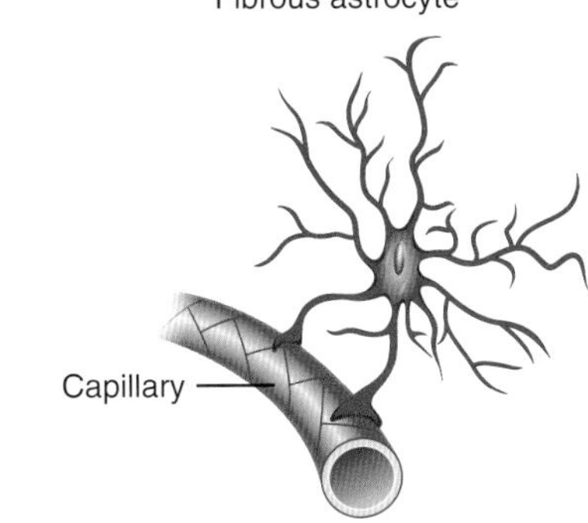


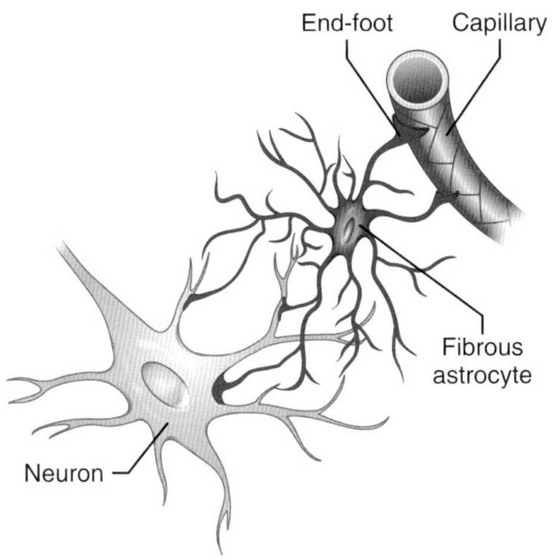


**Figure 28.1**

**The relationship of the glial cells (astrocytes, oligodendrocytes) to the neurons and capillaries.** (From Kandel ER, Schwartz JH: *Principles of neural science*, ed 2, New York, 1985, Elsevier.)

When the astroglial cells become dysfunctional as part of an injury or degenerative process, neuronal damage may proliferate. Astroglial changes are widely recognized to be one of the earliest and most remarkable cellular responses to CNS injury via both hypertrophy and regeneration.[73] Astrocyte swelling is a common pathologic finding and is often seen at the interface with the vascular system. Astrocytes are involved in creating glial scarring, or fibrillary gliosis.[72] Astrocytes may alter their gene expression in response to brain injury. Astroglial cell tissue can also be the site of neoplastic disorders that disrupt nerve cell function by compressing the neurons and blood supply in the surrounding area (see Chapter 30).

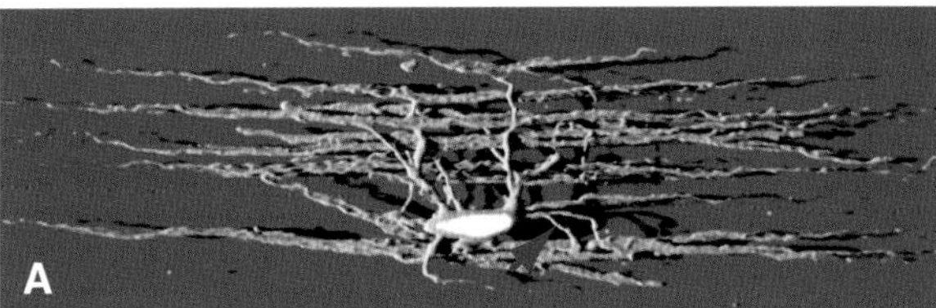


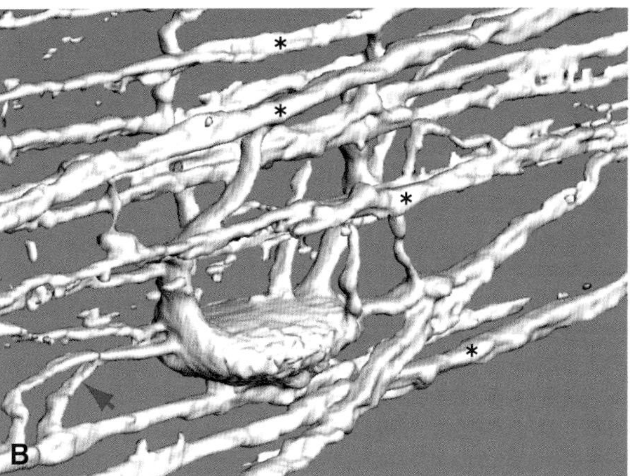


**Figure 28.2**

(A) Single oligodendrocyte from a rat. (B) More magnified view showing the process as the oligodendrocytes emerge from the cell body. (From Nolte J: *The human brain: an introduction to its functional anatomy*, ed 5, St. Louis, 2002, Mosby. Courtesy Dr. Peter S. Eggli, Institute of Anatomy, University of Bern, Bern, Switzerland.)

Pain was classically viewed as being mediated solely by neurons, as are other sensory phenomena. It is clear now that spinal cord glia amplify pain and are activated by certain sensory signals arriving from the periphery. These glia express characteristics in common with immune cells in that they respond to viruses and bacteria, releasing proinflammatory cytokines, which create pathologic pain. (See Chapter 7 for more information about interactions between the immune system and the CNS.) An apparently discrete CNS lesion may lead to glia activation throughout the pain neuraxis, and systemic rather than localized treatment may be required to effectively treat neuropathic pain. Modulation of glia activity is the goal, as a total block leads to anesthesia and adverse neurologic side effects.[39]

The two other glial cell types, the oligodendrocyte, a part of the CNS, and the Schwann cell, found in the peripheral nervous system, are responsible for the production of the myelin sheath, which surrounds the axon. (See Chapter 39 for information on the peripheral disorders that are associated.) Demyelinating disorders that target the CNS such as MS are often the result of disrupted function of the oligodendrocyte.[1] This process is further described in Multiple Sclerosis in Chapter 31. Figs. 28.2 and 28.3 show the oligodendrocyte and describe the process of myelination.[73]

## Nerve Cells

Communication between nerve cells is related to the structure and function of each cell type. The location in the nervous system, the input cells, and the target cells will determine how a cell communicates. The cell body

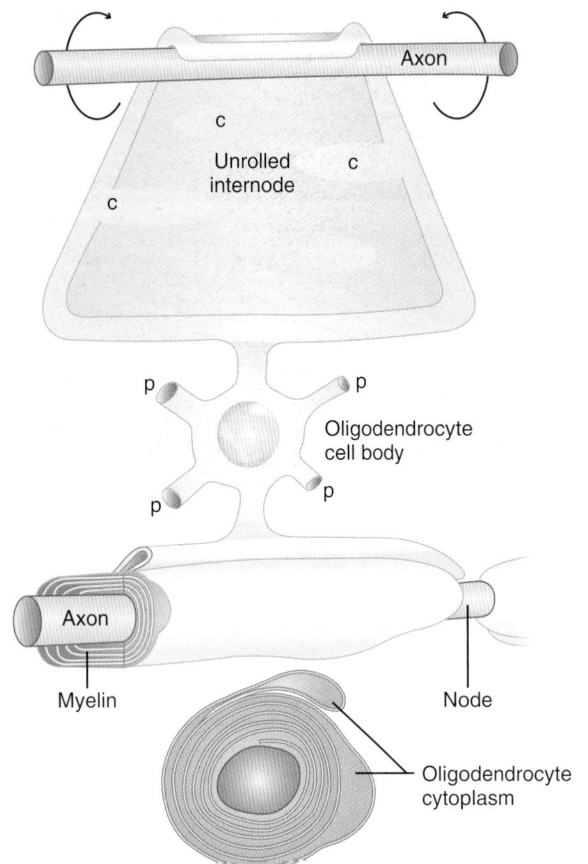


**Figure 28.3**

**Schematic diagram of the formation of myelin in the central nervous system.** (From Nolte J: *The human brain: an introduction to its functional anatomy*, ed 5, St. Louis, 2002, Mosby. Redrawn from Krstié RV: *Illustrated encyclopedia of human histology*, Berlin, 1984, Springer-Verlag.)

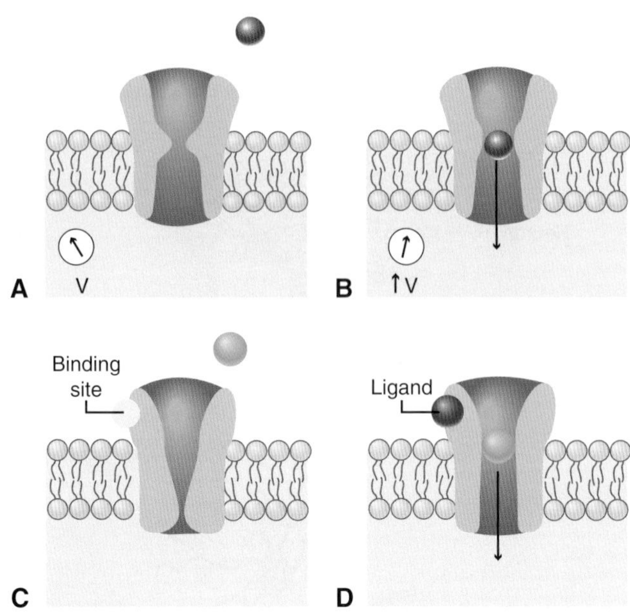


**Figure 28.4**

**Ion channels respond to the changes in voltage.** (A) represents the closed state, and (B) represents the open state that allows neurotransmitters to gain entry into the cell. (C and D) represent the opening based on the ligand attaching to the protein that causes the channel to open. (From Nolte J: *The human brain: an introduction to its functional anatomy*, ed 5, St Louis, 2002, Mosby.)

size as well as the shape and configuration of dendrites and axons will also affect the method of communication. However, almost all neurons will typically fire through a manner that can be described schematically. Essentially, the chemical information encoded by a gene within one nerve cell is delivered to the appropriate postsynaptic genome through a series of molecular reactions.[96] Information is transferred via electrical signals that travel along the neuron and is carried to the next neuron through a series of biochemical events that will influence the behavior of the second-order neuron.

The cell body of the neuron is the metabolic center of the neuron and includes the nucleus where the genetic material is located. The gene expressed in a cell directs the manufacture of proteins that determine the structure, function, and regulation of the neural circuits. Mutation, or changes in the structure of the DNA, can lead to the production of abnormal proteins that can be associated with vulnerability to neurologic disease. Abnormalities within the gene structure leading to predisposition for mutations can be inherited. Toxicity or abuse of drugs can also affect the ability of the DNA to replicate in a normal manner and can cause long-term dysfunction of the nervous system. Cell body inclusions are growths that occur within the cell body as a part of aging, such as Lewy bodies, but can also be a part of a disease process and can cause loss of function of the cell as a result of damage to the nucleus of the cell.[78]

The cell body generates electrical activity through action potentials. A transient increase in sodium permeability is the molecular foundation of the action potential. The increase in sodium permeability causes this ion to be dominant and establishes the membrane potential as +40 mV, expressed as an action potential. This quickly changes as potassium channels open and resting potential is restored.

Ion channels are proteins that span the cell membrane and are able to conduct ions through the membrane. The ion channels recognize and select specific ions for transfer. They are able to open and close in response to specific electrical, mechanical, or chemical signals. Fig. 28.4 describes these gating properties.[72] Sodium channel blockers bind the outer axonal surface of the channel and prevent the flux of sodium. The nerve cells sequentially generate four different signals at different sites within the cell: an input signal, a trigger signal, a conducting signal, and an output signal. The input signal depolarizes the cell membrane. Dendrites are typically the site for receiving incoming signals from other neurons. In the trigger zone on the initial segment of the axon the receptor signals are summed, and with sufficient input the neuron then fires an action potential through the length of the axon. The intensity of the conducting signals is determined by the frequency of individual action potentials. As the action potential reaches the neuron's terminal, it stimulates the release of a chemical neurotransmitter cell through the presynaptic terminals.[49] Fig. 28.5 shows the processes

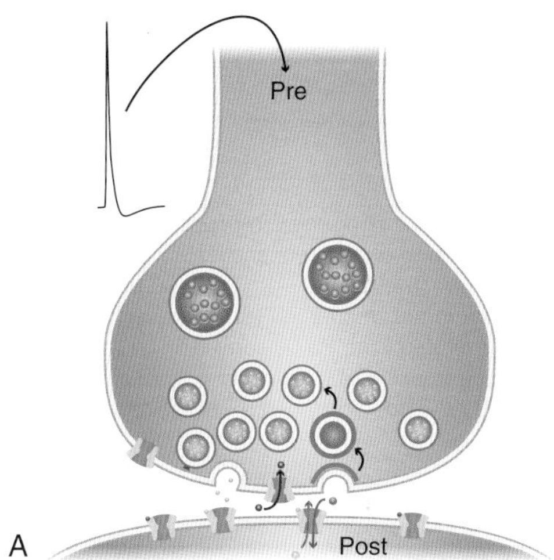


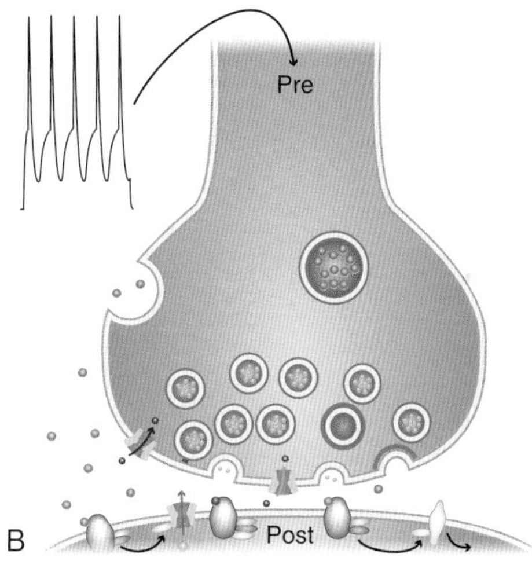


**Figure 28.5**

(A) Depolarization of the terminal causes sodium influx and opening of the channels in the postsynaptic neuron. (B) Release of transmitters from large and small vesicles; the status of the postsynaptic proteins will affect the binding capability. (From Nolte J: *The human brain: an introduction to its functional anatomy*, ed 5, St. Louis, 2002, Mosby.)

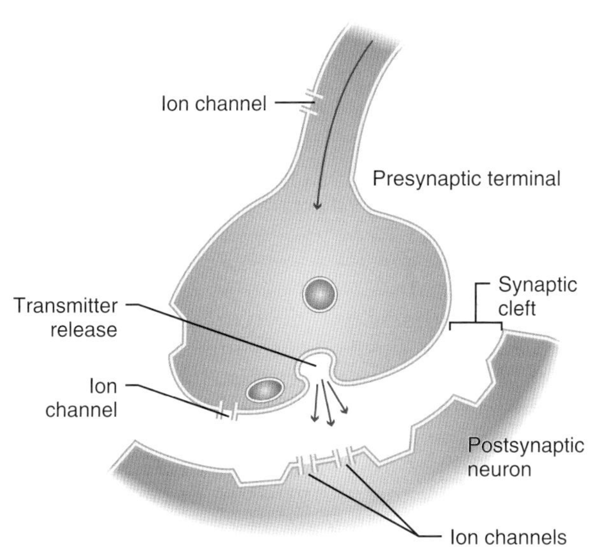


**Figure 28.6**

**Schematic representation of the postsynaptic neuron and the presynaptic terminal.** Transmitter substances are synthesized in presynaptic terminals, released into the synaptic cleft, and occupied in the postsynaptic terminal.

related to transmitter release.[72] Excitatory synapses are distributed distally in the dendritic receptive field, and inhibitory synapses exist in the proximal dendritic field or on the cell body. The combination of excitation and inhibition modulates input.

The axon serves as the entry route of a number of pathogens and toxins and presents a large target as a result of its large volume. The axon of the nerve can be selectively damaged, without destruction of the cell body, causing a decrease or loss of presynaptic activity. For instance, stretch damage to axons is responsible for the abnormal or delayed firing associated with brain injury. Axonal spheroid formation is a reaction to injury resulting in formation of axon retraction balls and can be seen in radiation necrosis and traumatic brain injury. It is clear now that axon degeneration plays a part in secondary and primary progressive MS.[28]

## Neurotransmission

By means of its axonal terminals, one neuron contacts and transmits information to the receptive surface of another neuron. The release of neurotransmitter from the presynaptic terminal and the uptake of that substance in the postsynaptic receptor are known as a synapse. A simplified diagram is shown in Fig. 28.6. Virtually all communication between neurons occurs via chemicals. The chemical communication involved in this process is universally known as either neurotransmission or neuromodulation.[50] Changes in neurotransmitter substances in the space surrounding the neurons have been implicated in many nervous system disease processes.

Neurotransmitters are synthesized within each neuron, stored in presynaptic vesicles, and released from depolarized nerve terminals. They bind specifically to presynaptic or postsynaptic receptors, which recognize the chemical conformation of the neurotransmitter. A single neuron can release several different neurotransmitter substances, and a single neuron can be selectively receptive to different types of neurotransmitters because of the differences in ion channels.[97] Activation of a receptor in response to neurotransmitters can cause changes in a variety of molecules. Modification, or modulation, of the system can take place presynaptically, postsynaptically, or within the cell body.

Changes in a target cell can cause abnormal responses even with normal levels of transmitters. The amount of neurotransmitter released in the synaptic cleft is determined by the neuronal firing rate, the quantity of transmitter in the nerve terminal, and the cumulative regulatory actions of excitatory and inhibitory neurotransmitters. These biochemical actions alter the electrical activity of the postsynaptic neurons. One aspect of chemical transmission that is extremely important in signaling

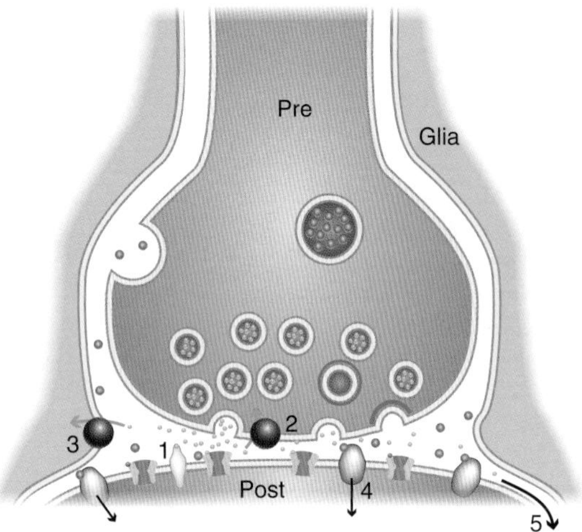


**Figure 28.7**

The transmitter substances can be removed by (1) enzymatic inactivation of neurotransmitter, (2) reuptake of the neurotransmitter by the presynaptic terminal, (3) removal by the nearby glial cells, or (4) uptake by the postsynaptic terminal, or (5) it may just move out of the synaptic space into adjoining spaces. (From Nolte J: *The human brain: an introduction to its functional anatomy*, ed 5, St. Louis, 2002, Mosby.)

is the time course of the transmitter in the synaptic cleft. The breakdown of a transmitter is an important variable and can change the concentration of the substance in the synaptic cleft.[40] Control of the neurotransmitter in the synaptic cleft is the basis for pharmacologic treatment in degenerative neurologic disease. Fig. 28.7 diagrams the various ways that the substances in the synaptic cleft can be removed.[72] An important concept for all neurotransmitters is that the final result of either hyperpolarization or depolarization depends on both the transmitter and its receptor. Whether facilitation or inhibition occurs at a synapse relates not so much to the neurotransmitter as to the interaction between neurotransmitter and receptors at a particular synapse.

A wide range of substances make up the neurotransmitter substances used by the nervous system. In some cases, they can coexist in the same neuron. Box 28.1 presents some typical substances that act as neurotransmitters. These substances can be used by neurons in different ways, according to the function of the specific neuron. To be used as a neurotransmitter, these substances are packaged in vesicles within the neuron and respond to particular enzymes that are specific to that neuron.[97]

**Amino Acids.** Amino acid neurotransmitters include γ-aminobutyric acid (GABA), glycine, glutamate and aspartate. One of the small-molecule neurotransmitters, glutamate is an excitatory amino acid transmitter active throughout the brain and spinal cord. It is an intermediate transmitter in cellular metabolism, so the presence of glutamate in a cell does not necessarily suggest neurologic activity. Glutamate functions with its receptors in an excitatory or depolarizing system at primary afferent nerve endings, granule cells of the cerebellum, dentate gyrus, and corticostriatal and subthalamopallidal pathways important to basal ganglia function. When levels of glutamate rise above normal,

**Box 28.1**

**SELECT NEUROTRANSMITTERS AND ASSOCIATED RESPONSES**

***Amines***

- Acetylcholine: decreases in production associated with diseases such as Alzheimer disease and myasthenia gravis
- Catecholamines
  - Dopamine: decreased levels responsible for symptoms associated with Parkinsonism
  - Norepinephrine: related to cocaine or amphetamine
- Serotonin: involved in control of mood and anxiety

***Amino Acids***

- GABA: increasing GABA activity decreases incidence of seizure activity
- Glutamate: degenerative diseases such as Parkinson disease, ALS, or Alzheimer disease may be related to increases in glutamate; increased levels contribute to secondary damage associated with stroke and spinal cord injury
- Glycine: more active in the spinal cord than cortex

***Neuroactive Peptides[a]***

- Enkephalins and β-endorphins: pain control achieved by use of drugs (opiates) that bind to endorphin and enkephalin receptors
- Substance P: involved in pain pathways

*ALS*, Amyotrophic lateral sclerosis; *CNS*, central nervous system; *GABA*, γ-aminobutyric acid.

[a] More than 50 neuroactive peptides have been identified; these are most typical.

glutamate excitotoxicity can occur and may cause cell death. Glutamate opens ion channels to bring calcium into the cell. In the case of excess glutamate, too much calcium is allowed into the cell, and the calcium eventually destroys the cell. Excess glutamate can be an effect of neuronal injury, as in stroke, and brain or spinal cord injury. It appears that the genes in the nerve cell body may trigger this excitotoxic mechanism, resulting in release of excess glutamate that may lead to the degenerative processes associated with diseases such as ALS, Alzheimer disease, Huntington disease, and Parkinson disease.[75] Part of the activation of seizure is due to glutamate receptors. Toxins or drug abuse can also trigger an excitotoxic level of glutamate.[96]

GABA is a tiny amino acid that serves both as a neurotransmitter and as an intermediate metabolite in the normal function of cells and is active in the spinal cord, cerebellum, basal ganglia, and cortex. GABA is synthesized from glutamate by way of the vitamin $B_6$–dependent enzyme glutamate decarboxylase. GABA is the major transmitter for brief inhibitory synapses. Loss of GABAergic neurons that inhibit glutamate results in increased excitation. Glycine is another amino acid neurotransmitter that is the transmitter at some inhibitory CNS synapses. The distributions of GABA and glycine synapses overlap, but glycine is more prominent in the spinal cord.[72]

*N*-methyl-D-aspartate (NMDA) receptor has a complex process using glutamate and glycine activation at the same time but also requiring membrane polarization to remove magnesium from inside the cell, so that the cell can allow sodium to be active within the cell. NMDA receptors are widely distributed throughout the neocortex, hippocampus, and anterior horn motor neurons. The NMDA response thus works when the membrane bearing the receptor has already been depolarized by another stimulus, so it prolongs or augments the initial depolarization. This activity supports learning and memorization. During cellular energy failure induced by ischemia, there is collapse of membrane potentials (depolarization) and uncontrolled synaptic and transmembrane release of excitatory amino acids into the extracellular space. NMDA receptors open and allow calcium into the intracellular space, causing damage to the mitochondria, limiting the production of adenosine triphosphate (ATP). Drugs that are NMDA receptor antagonists include ketamine and eliprodil. Antiepileptic drugs such as felbamate and lamotrigine block glutamate and glycine activity at the NMDA receptors.[28]

**Amines.** Amines include acetylcholine, the catecholamines dopamine and norepinephrine, epinephrine, serotonin, and histamine. Acetylcholine was the first neurotransmitter discovered and has primary activity at the level of the peripheral nervous system. It is the transmitter released by the motor neurons at neuromuscular junctions and within the autonomic nervous system at preganglionic neurons of sympathetic ganglia and postganglionic parasympathetic neurons. Disorders related to acetylcholine are discussed in Chapter 39. Cholinergic neurons play two different roles in the nervous system: in peripheral nervous system activity and within the CNS in the regulation of the general level of activity. Cholinergic systems can be mapped to the medial cortex and to the areas responsible for information flow to the hypothalamus and amygdala through the reticular formation. The cholinergic and biogenic amine systems appear to establish the activity set-point of the cortex and basal ganglia rather than point-to-point neural firing.[28] Biogenic amines are synthesized from amino acid precursors, dopamine, serotonin, and norepinephrine.

Dopamine is synthesized in multiple major CNS pathways. The most important and most widely understood is the nigrostriatal pathway of the basal ganglia. Dopaminergic function is decreased in individuals with Parkinson disease and attention disorders affecting the frontal lobe.

Norepinephrine is a neurotransmitter found in the hypothalamus and the locus coeruleus in the brainstem. It is synthesized from dopamine and therefore shares the same enzymes, including the rate-limiting tyrosine hydroxylase. Similar to dopamine, norepinephrine is removed from the synapse by active reuptake into the presynaptic cell and then is metabolized by two enzymes, monoamine oxidase (MAO) and catechol-*O*-methyltransferase (COMT).[37] Norepinephrine is associated with control of activity, mood, and wakefulness.

The catecholamines appear to have an important role in working memory. The cholinergic system appears to be critical for the acquisition of long-term declarative memory. Cholinergic function decreases somewhat with age and greatly in individuals with Alzheimer disease, and these changes may contribute importantly to corresponding reductions in memory ability. Centrally acting cholinesterase inhibitors are marketed for improvement of memory.

Serotonin has its main cell bodies in the dorsal raphe nucleus of the brainstem as well as the spinal cord, hippocampus, and cerebellum. Serotonergic pathways are inhibitory in nature, projecting from the brainstem to the brain and spinal cord, and are associated with mood, pain, and sleep. Similar to the catecholamines, serotonin is metabolized by active reuptake into the presynaptic cell and then metabolism by MAO. Serotonin is removed from the synaptic cleft by reuptake pumps rather than by degradation. Antidepressant medications work by inhibiting this reuptake.[28] Fig. 28.8 illustrates the pathways for multiple neurotransmitter systems associated with cognitive and motor function.

**Neuropeptides.** Neurons can secrete hormones, or neuropeptides, and most or all of them can function as neurotransmitters. Neuropeptides are metabolically difficult for cells to make and transport and can be effective at very low concentrations. Synthesis of neuropeptides begins in the nucleus of the cell, where the gene is transcribed into RNA. See Chapter 2 for epigenetic factors that influence emotion as well as the variety of mechanisms and factors (such as stress) that modify these effects.[9]

**Gaseous Neurotransmitters and Others.** Nitrous oxide (NO) is a gas that can diffuse easily through neuronal membranes and can influence subsequent transmitter release. Astrocytes may be the target, mediating cell-to-cell communication between vessel endothelium and smooth muscle, and are critical in vasomotor control, inflammation, and neuronal communication. NO released from endothelial cells acts on vascular smooth muscle, causing vasodilation. NO released from inflammatory cells occurs in high concentrations and kills cells. NO may play a role in neurodegeneration, and acute elevations may contribute to damage in ischemia and trauma. NO synthesis is augmented by NMDA receptor activation by glutamate; therefore NO may synergize excitotoxity.[50]

Neurotrophic factors are essential to maintenance and survival of neurons and their terminals but are produced by the body in a limited supply. Four major neurotrophins have been identified in humans: nerve growth factor, brain-derived neurotrophic factor, neurotrophin 3, and neurotrophin 4/5. Neurotrophins interact with receptor cells to prolong the life of the neuron. Although this class of substances is also not fully understood, it is clear that neurotrophins play a role in the development of the nervous system and also support the health of the nervous system and plastic changes that occur following injury or disease. They appear to work by suppressing the pathway that leads to apoptosis.[49] Aerobic exercise increases the presence of neurotrophic factors such as brain-derived neurotrophic factor and may provide a way to maintain or improve brain health (see Chapter 3).

It is well known that vigorous physical activity is related to lower stress levels, and exercise releases brain-derived neurotrophic factor, a substance that improves brain health. Exercise increases the number of serotonin neurotransmitter receptors in the hippocampus via stimulation of neurogenesis. The release of endorphins during aerobic exercise and the reduction cortisol levels in

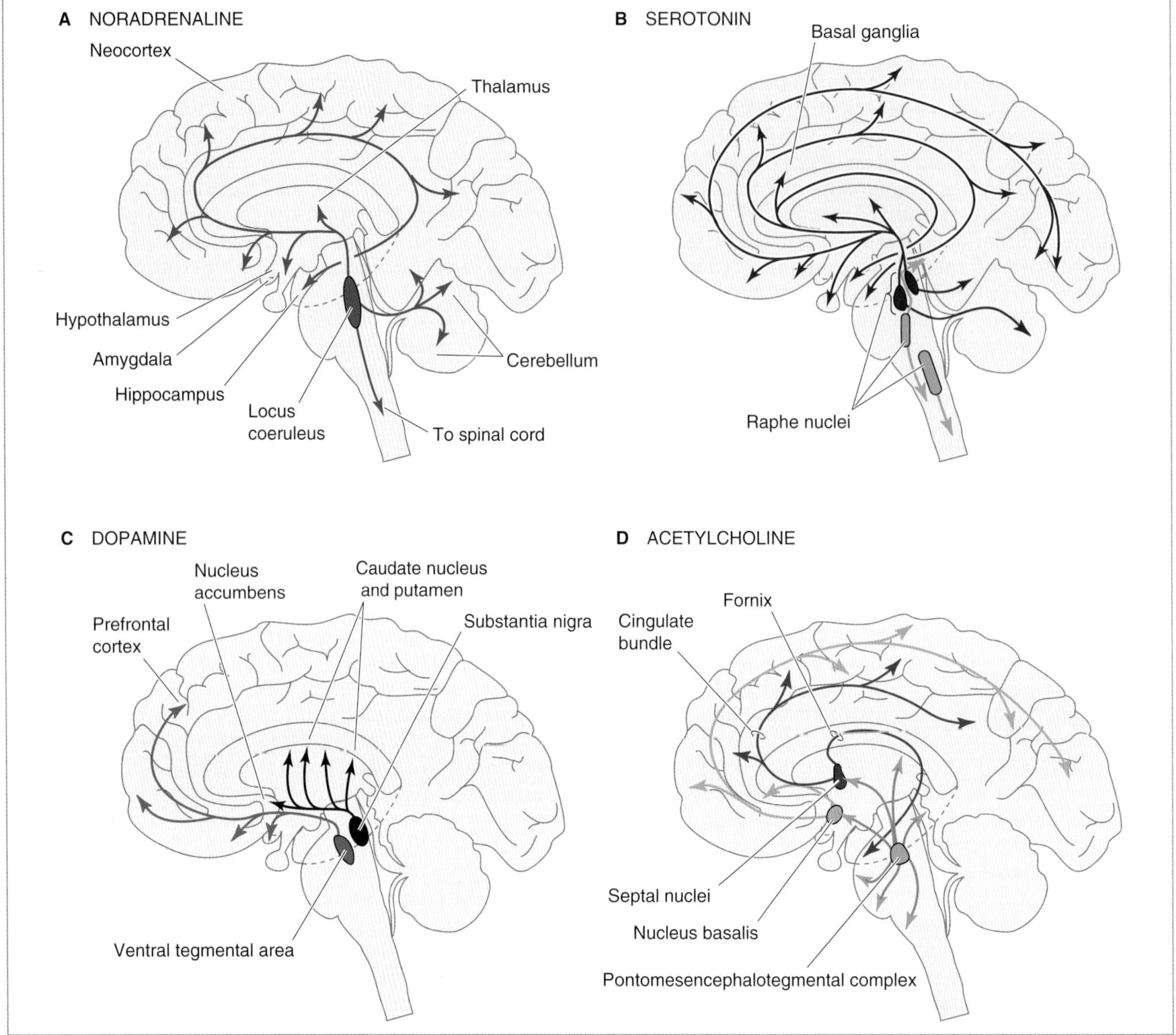


**Figure 28.8**

**Sagittal sections of the brain, indicating simplified versions of major pathways of central neurons using important neurotransmitters** (A) Noradrenaline. (B) Serotonin (5-HT). (C) Dopamine. (D) Acetylcholine. (From Boron WF, Boulpaep EL. *Medical physiology: a cellular and molecular approach. Updated ed*, Philadelphia, 2005, Saunders.)

the bloodstream elevate mood, reduce pain, and mediate stress reactions. Many of the special implications for physical therapists in this chapter include the psychologic benefits of exercise.[81]

## CLINICAL MANIFESTATIONS

### Sensory Disturbances

The skin, muscles, and joints contain a variety of receptors that create electrical activity as described previously[12,94] (and described in more detail in Chapter 39). Electrical input is carried to the CNS through *afferent axons* to cell bodies in the dorsal root ganglia that lie adjacent to the spinal cord. These afferent fibers are arranged somatotopically in the spinal column and ascend to the brainstem and the sensory cortex. Fig. 28.9 shows the simplified synapse.[72] A characteristic of the fibers that run in the dorsal column of the spinal cord is that they synapse at the level of the brainstem nuclei, where they cross over to the contralateral (opposite) hemisphere of the brain. This phenomenon is illustrated in Fig. 28.10.[72] When there is a disorder of the brain that affects the afferent system above the level of the brainstem, symptoms occur on the side contralateral to the lesion.[49,72]

The brainstem receives information from specialized senses. For example, vestibular information is received via cranial nerve VIII and integrated through the brainstem nuclei, contributing to postural control and locomotion. Disorders of the afferent nerve, dorsal columns of the spinal cord, and brainstem result in loss or change in sensory input. This can manifest as lack of cutaneous

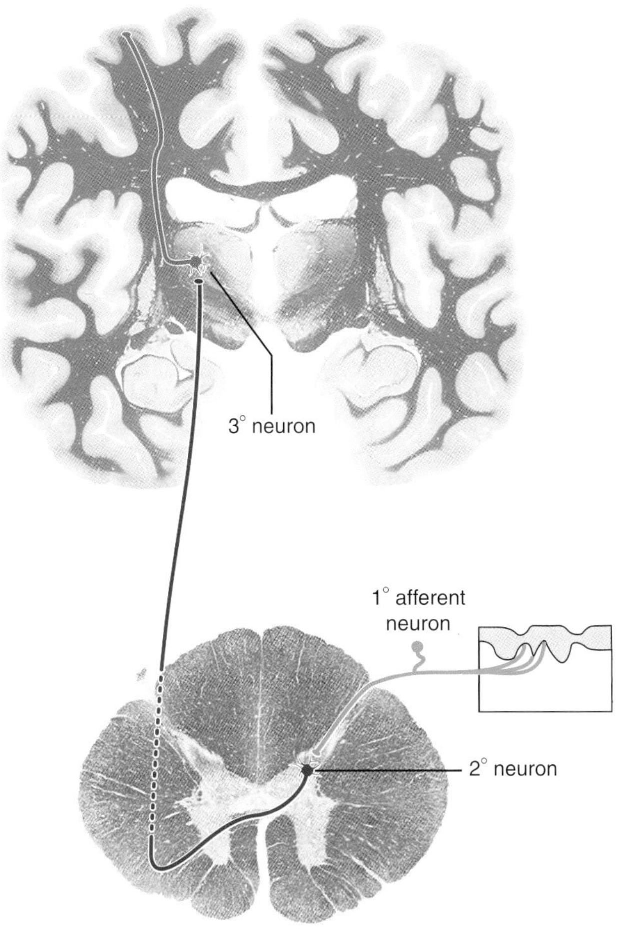


**Figure 28.9**

**The minimum sensory pathway from the periphery to the cerebral cortex.** (From Nolte J: *The human brain: an introduction to its functional anatomy*, ed 5, St. Louis, 2002, Mosby.)

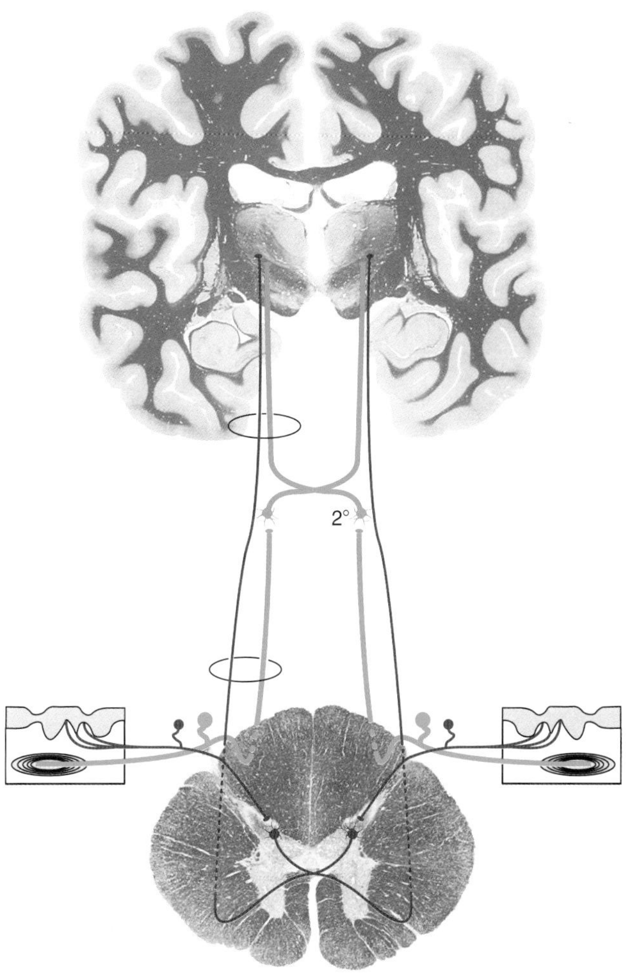


**Figure 28.10**

(A) In the spinal cord, a lesion would result in decreased touch on the same side of the lesion and decreased pain sensation on the contralateral side. (B) A lesion above the medulla would cause decreased touch and pain on the contralateral side. (From Nolte J: *The human brain: an introduction to its functional anatomy*, ed 5, St. Louis, 2002, Mosby.)

sensation, numbness, tingling, paresthesias, or dysesthesias in the distribution of the nerves affected. Sensory input from the joints and muscles is known as *proprioception*. When this sensory function is lost or disturbed, the person will have difficulty maintaining the body in the appropriate position for the voluntary and involuntary movements necessary for functional activities, especially those required for postural control. Movements become uncoordinated because of the loss of feedback on position from the joints.[3]

The nervous system has several pain-control pathways available, some of which suppress and some of which facilitate the experience of pain. Modulation of noxious stimuli is directed by the reticular formation. Noxious stimuli can be experienced as more or less painful, depending on the individual's circumstances. When a lesion affects the midbrain areas that modulate and interpret sensory input, such as the thalamus, the result can cause exaggeration of sensory stimuli.

Disruption of the sensory input provided by the optic nerve is evident in some disorders of the brain and will result in loss of vision in some or all of a field of view. Visual-field cuts are common with stroke (see Chapter 32). Visual hallucinations can also be part of a CNS disorder when the optic radiations or occipital lobe is damaged, which may also be caused by a degenerative disease such as Lewy body dementia.

Our survival instincts are driven by sensory inputs of smell, taste, vision, hearing, and vestibular balance. They are the first signals for the motor responses of behaviors important for survival, triggering other autonomic responses to allow the body to "fight, flight, or freeze."

## Movement Disorders

Control of movement is accomplished by the cooperative effort of many brain structures.[12,94] Abnormal movement patterns in neurologic disorders can result from lesions of the CNS at many levels. A simplified representation of the typical synaptic flow of neurons and interneurons is shown in Fig. 28.11. It is important to recognize that there are many synapses not represented here in the levels of the brainstem and central modulation centers of the basal ganglia and limbic system. Activity initiated in the cerebral cortex triggers interneurons that regulate

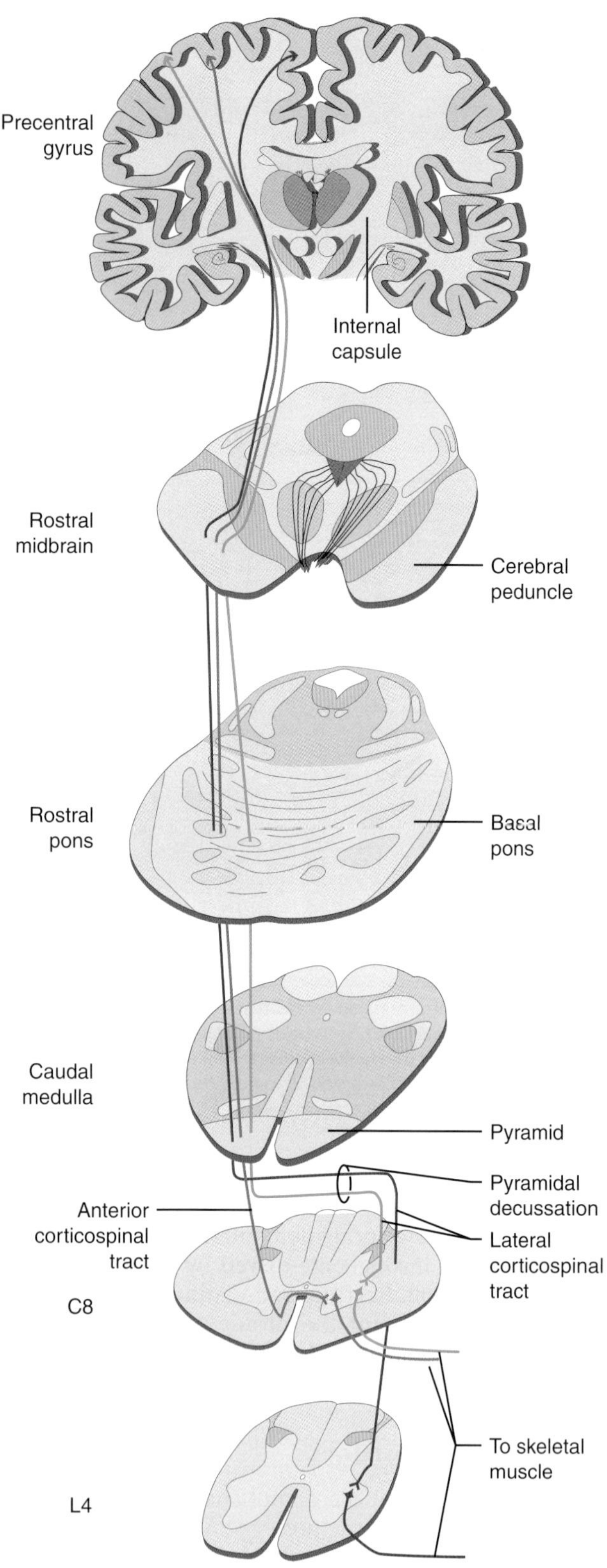


**Figure 28.11**

**Pathway of the motor system from the cortex to the skeletal muscle as it courses through the brainstem structures and spinal cord.** (From Nolte J: *The human brain: an introduction to its functional anatomy*, ed 5, St. Louis, 2002, Mosby.)

interaction of the lower motor neurons. The parietal and premotor areas of the cerebral cortex are involved in identifying targets in space, determining a course of action, and creating motor programs. The cortex determines strategies for movement. The brainstem and spinal cord are responsible for the execution of the task. The same signal may be processed simultaneously by many different brain structures for different purposes, showing parallel distributed processing.

Various areas of the brain such as the cerebellum and basal ganglia interact to establish a motor program that modifies the hierarchic information going from the cortex to the spinal cord. For example, parietal and premotor regions together with basal ganglia–sustained activation underlie the special skill of handwriting with the dominant hand.[45] The reticulospinal and corticospinal pathways work in parallel to generate a large repertoire of diverse, coordinated movement in the hand. The reticulospinal pathway may become a therapeutic target when the corticospinal tract is damaged or injured.[44] During motor adaptation, goal locations and movement vectors are differentially remapped, and separate motor plans based on these features are effectively averaged during motor execution.[109]

## Disorders of Coordinated Movement

Lack of coordinated movement known as ataxia can occur with damage to a variety of structures of the nervous system including sensory neuropathies, but is most commonly associated with cerebellar dysfunction. Input regarding the position of the head, trunk, and extremities comes from the spinal cord to compare the resulting activity with the intended motor output. This input comes in rapidly because the relay involves only a few synapses. The input comes through the climbing fibers that connect the inferior olive to the Purkinje cell or from mossy fibers that relay the remaining information.[5] The deep cerebellar nuclei are the structures that communicate information from the Purkinje cell to the various nuclei of the brainstem and thalamus.[49] The cerebellum has no direct synapse with the spinal cord but exerts its influence through the action on interneurons within the nuclei of the brainstem.

The medial region known as the *vestibulocerebellum* connects with the cortex and brainstem through both its ascending and its descending projections. The cerebellum has influence on movement through the vestibulospinal and reticulospinal tracts. Lesions result in the inability to coordinate eye and head movement, increased postural sway, and delayed equilibrium responses.[5] Postural tremor is present in some individuals with vestibulocerebellar lesions.

The spinocerebellum connects to the somatosensory tracts of the spinal cord. It receives input from the cortex regarding ongoing motor commands. Control of proximal musculature is achieved via the connections to the motor cortex. Lesions of the spinocerebellum can cause hypotonia and disruption of rhythmic patterns associated with walking. Precision of voluntary movements is lost when this area is dysfunctional.[66]

The anterior lobe of the cerebellum is implicated in disorders of gait, with loss of balance noted in stance. Proprioception may be impaired because the cerebellar relays become disrupted. Long loop reflexes lose adaptability and are unable to trigger appropriate responses in the lower leg to maintain balance when the body sways or the surface is moving. The ability to modify reflexes is lost during repeated trials.[101]

In the cerebrocerebellum, or posterior lobes, connections are made to the cortex through the pons. The posterior lobes are involved in complex motor, perceptual, and cognitive tasks. Lesions of the cerebrocerebellum lead to a decomposition of movement and timing.

*Hypotonicity,* or decreased muscle tone, can occur on the side of the lesion or bilaterally if the lesion is central and is seen primarily in the proximal muscle groups. A person with hypotonicity is unable to fixate the limb posturally, leading to incoordination with movement. *Asthenia,* or generalized weakness, is sometimes seen in persons with cerebellar lesions. Hypotonicity and asthenia, however, do not always occur together. It is believed that both disorders represent loss of input from the cerebellum to the cerebral cortex, but they may represent loss of input to different areas of the cortex.

*Dysmetria,* the underestimation or overestimation of a necessary movement toward a target, is commonly seen with cerebellar disorders. There is an error in the production of force necessary to perform an intended movement. The initiation of movement is prolonged compared with normal, and the ability to change directions rapidly is impaired. The resulting overshoot and undershoot during movement are known as an *intention tremor*. *Dysdiadochokinesia,* the inability to perform rapidly alternating movements, is related to the inability to stop ongoing movement. The movement becomes slow, without smooth rhythm or consistency. It is common to observe muscular cocontraction as a means to stabilize an extremity and reduce distal dysmetria.

Decomposition of movement, termed *dyssynergia,* is seen in persons with cerebellar dysfunction. Instead of performing a movement in one smooth motion, the person will move in distinct sequences to accomplish the motion. Multijoint movements are more affected than single-joint movements. Disruption in force and extent of movement will result in difficulty with grip control and maintaining static hold against resistance. When the resistance is removed, for example, the extremity will oscillate because of lack of feedback regarding position and force needed to maintain static hold.

*Scanning speech* is a component of cerebellar dysfunction representing complexity of the motor activity. Word selection is not affected, but the words are pronounced slowly and without melody, tone, or rhythm. This reflects the incoordination or hypotonicity of the muscles of the larynx in controlling the voice.

Eye movements are disrupted in persons with cerebellar dysfunction, both in a static head and eye position and with movement of the head. *Gaze-evoked nystagmus,* or nonvoluntary rhythmic oscillation of the eye, occurs when the cerebellum is unable to hold the gaze on an object, especially in a lateral position. When looking at a lateral target, the eyes drift back toward midline and then immediately back to the target. Eyes flickering on and off the target, eyes fluttering around the target, or spastic bursts of eye oscillations may be present with brainstem or midline cerebellar lesions.

*Ocular dysmetria* is similar to the dysmetria seen in the extremities. This dysmetria is seen in cerebellar lesions when the eyes are moving from one target to another (known as *saccadic movement*) or when attempting to follow a target (known as *smooth pursuit*).

Vestibuloocular function is disrupted in medial cerebellar lesions, and the ability to maintain eye stability during head movement is affected. See Vestibular Dysfunction in Chapter 38 for more information on vestibuloocular dysfunction.

Gait disturbance is another disorder related to dysfunction of the cerebellum. Gait becomes wide based and staggering, with uneven step length and width, with the feet often lifted higher than necessary, and without typical arm swing. Stance and swing become irregular, challenging adaptation to changes in terrain. It becomes difficult to perform heel-to-toe walking or walking a straight line. In some people, there is a surprising ability to avoid falling, although standing balance is abnormal.[35] Impedance control, the ability to adjust the mechanical behavior of limbs to account for instability, allows adaptation to environmental disturbances such as responding to unexpected starts or stops while using public transportation. The ability to selectively modulate the end point stiffness of the arms adjusting for varying directions of environmental disturbances is affected in cerebellar injury.[34]

The cerebellum plays a major role in motor learning. The cerebellum is vital in anticipatory, or feed-forward, activity and modifications of response.[55] The cerebellum learns or memorizes small movements that are integrated into complex activity. During the acquisition phase of motor learning, the cerebellum is active.[42] Increased activity has also been noted during mental imagery or mental rehearsal of a motor program.[85] The cerebellum is active during cognitive and emotional processes, and lesions can cause difficulty in shifting attention from one sensory or thought domain to another.

## Deficits of Higher Brain Function

The cortex has a great deal to do with the abilities and activities that are a part of the highest development in humans, including language and abstract thinking. Perception, movement, and adaptive response to the outside world depend on an intact cerebral cortex. Crystallized intelligence refers to the knowledge and skills that are accumulated over a lifetime. This intelligence (wisdom) tends to increase with age. Fluid intelligence involves the ability to reason, think flexibly, and make sense of abstract information. Fluid intelligence is important for problem solving and learning and is thought to degrade with aging. Both types of intelligence can be compromised as a result of damage to the processes of the cortex and deeper components of the brain. The cortex is subdivided for ease of understanding the separate functions, although structure and function have considerable overlap. Fig. 28.12 shows some of the functional specialization of the brain. Fig. 28.13 shows the lobar relationship to the cerebellum and brainstem.

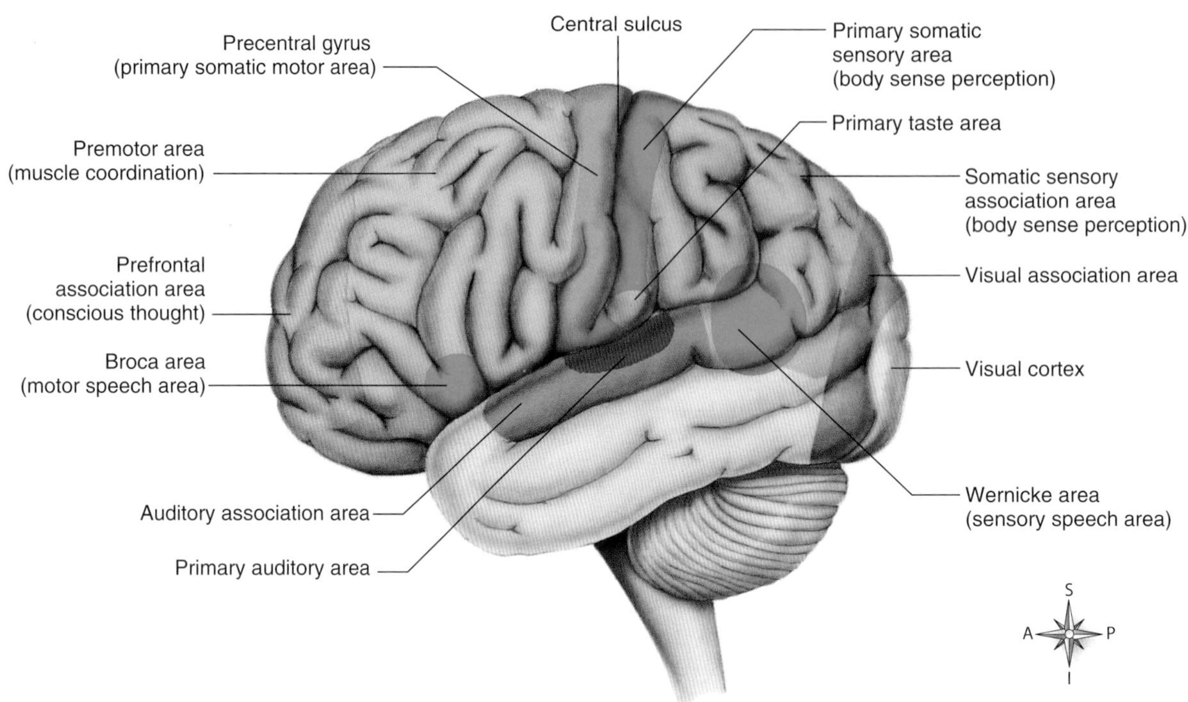


**Figure 28.12**

**Schematic representation of functional specialization in the cortex.** (From Patton KT, Thibodeau GA: *The human body in health and disease*, ed 7, St. Louis, 2018, Elsevier.)

The *frontal lobe* is the largest single area of the brain, constituting nearly one-third of the brain's cortical surface. It is phylogenetically the youngest area of the brain and has major connections with all other areas of the brain. The frontal lobe is responsible for the highest levels of cognitive processing, control of emotion, and behavior. An individual's personality is established as a frontal lobe function, and one of the most disturbing deficits seen with lesions affecting the frontal lobe is change from the person's premorbid personality. A person's character and temperament are changed by damage to the frontal lobe. Slow processing of information, lack of judgment based on known consequences, withdrawal, and irritability can be the result of an insult to the frontal lobe. Lack of inhibition and apathy are common clinical problems related to frontal lobe damage. A person with a frontal lobe disorder may lack insight into these deficits, and therefore behavior can be difficult to control.

*Right hemisphere syndrome* is associated with an inability to appropriately orient the body in external space and generate typical motor responses for postural and limb control. Hemineglect is one of the most common deficits seen with right hemisphere lesions. The individual does not respond to sensory stimuli on the left side of the body and does not respond to the environment surrounding the left side. Hemineglect is evident in the involved extremities and trunk during mobility and self-care activities. The ability to draw in two and three dimensions is often impaired, along with other drawing skills such as perspective and accurate copying. Spatial disorientation can result, with the person losing familiarity with the environment and becoming lost in areas that should be familiar. Inability to read and follow a map can be an indication of right hemisphere deficit.[25]

Disorders of emotional adjustment often follow a lesion in the right hemisphere. These disorders are primarily in the affective domain of interpersonal relationships and socialization. Cortical control of the limbic system is believed to be responsible, but the exact mechanism of control of more complex emotional behavior is not completely understood. There appears to be hemispheric lateralization of emotions, with suggestions that the right hemisphere is the dominant hemisphere in controlling emotions.

Language is one of the higher functions of the brain that is affected in many disorders of the CNS. Speech is a more elementary capacity than language and refers to the mechanical act of uttering words using the neuromuscular structures responsible for articulation. *Dysarthria,* a disturbance in articulation, and *anarthria,* the lack of ability to produce speech, are disorders of speech not language. Individuals with dysarthria may also have *dysphagia,* or difficulty coordinating the muscles used in swallowing. *Aphasia* is a term used to describe language impairments and may affect the ability to understand and/or generate language. One common language disorder is *expressive aphasia,* a deficit in language output, accompanied by a deficit in communication, in which speech comes out as garbled or inappropriate words. It is important to differentiate a problem with motor speech

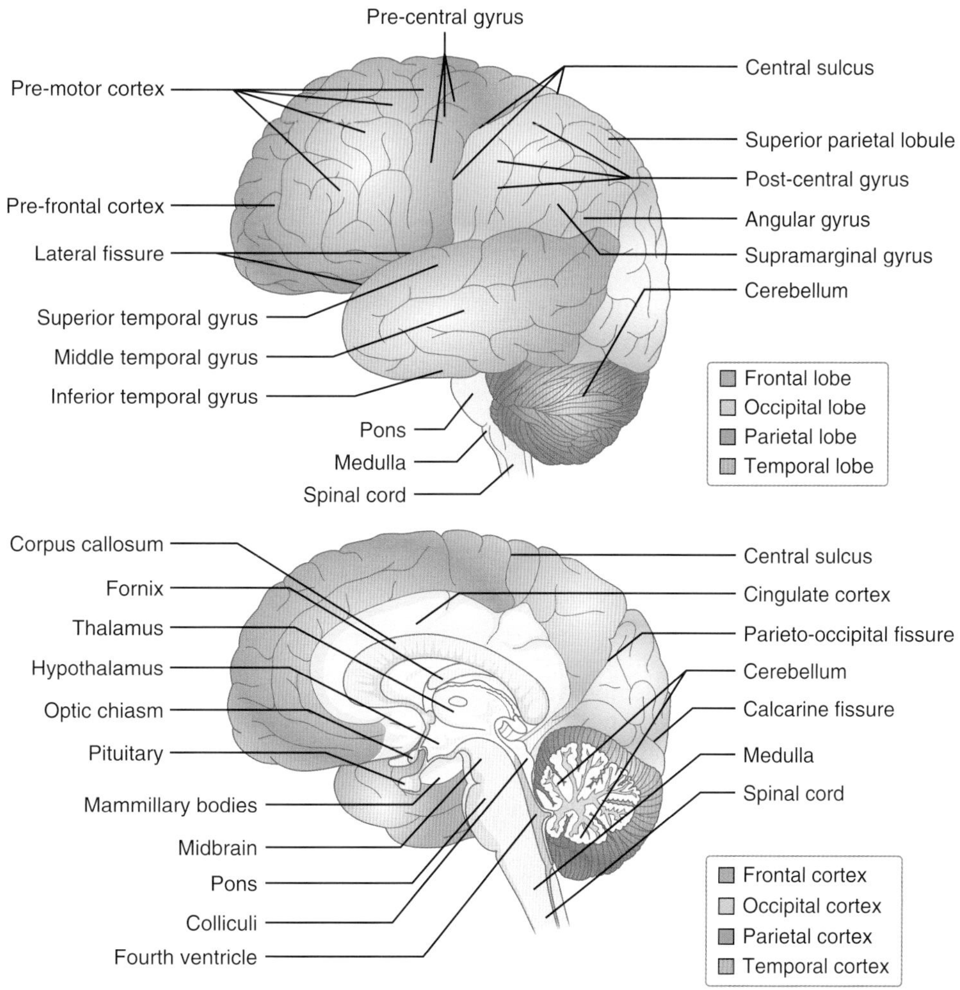


**Figure 28.13**

**The lobes of the cortex and their relationship to the cerebellum, midbrain, and brainstem.** (From Farber SD: *Neurorehabilitation: a multisensory approach*, Philadelphia, 1982, Saunders.)

or articulation from a language deficit. Individuals with articulation problems may understand speech and form perfectly normal thoughts they wish to express, but they are difficult to understand and so may use a communication board to spell out what they wish to "say." In contrast, a patient with an expressive or receptive language difficulty may need gestures and demonstration to interact because they have difficulty with generating or understanding language.

Localization of speech production in the left frontal lobe and impaired language comprehension in the temporal lobe demonstrate how higher functions can be related to brain regions. However, language control may be in different areas for different persons, and therefore damage to the same area of the brain may produce aphasia in some individuals, while others may be spared. Left hand–dominant people may have right hemisphere dominance for language.[57]

*Alexia* is another symptom of higher brain dysfunction. It is the acquired inability to read. Alexia is typically caused by lesions in the left occipital lobe and the corpus callosum that prevent incoming visual information from reaching the angular gyrus for linguistic interpretation. *Agraphia* can be caused by lesions located anywhere in the cerebrum. Because writing is a motor skill, lesions of the corticospinal tract, basal ganglia, and cerebellum; myopathies; and peripheral nerve injuries all can cause abnormal or clumsy writing. These disorders may be seen in addition to neurobehavioral syndromes. Typically the features of agraphia tend to parallel the characteristics of aphasia, so that writing does not serve as a feasible way to compensate for a language deficit.

*Apraxia* is an disorder of skilled purposeful movement that is not a result of paresis, akinesia, ataxia, sensory loss, or comprehension. Apraxia can be acquired following a brain injury or stroke or can be a congenital problem, typically described as developmental coordination disorder. *Ideomotor apraxia* is the most common type and represents the inability to carry out a motor act on verbal command. Ideomotor apraxia appears to be caused by a lesion in the arcuate fasciculus. The anterior connection from the left parietal lobe may be disrupted, preventing the motor system from receiving the command to act. A lesion in the left premotor area can cause apraxia by directly interrupting the motor act. Damage to the anterior corpus callosum can lead to apraxia that is evident in the left hand only. *Ideational apraxia* is failure to perform a sequential act even though each part of the act can be performed individually. The lesion causing ideational apraxia appears to be in the left parietal lobe, as in hemiparesis, or in the frontal lobe, as in Alzheimer disease. The syndrome is also seen with diffuse cortical damage associated with degenerative dementia.

*Agnosia*, most commonly occurring with vision, is the inability to recognize an object; thus the shape, color, and other visual features of an object can no longer be interpreted to name that object. A similar difficulty can occur with tactile sensation, described as stereognosis, or lack of ability to identify an object by feeling it in one's hand. Agnosias are associated with lesions of the sensory cortices involved with seeing, hearing, and feeling, so not the primary senses that are used to gather information, but rather how that information is interpreted cortically. These deficits are difficult to identify because the person is often easily able to compensate by using senses and processing that remain intact. For example, the ability to recognize a peach by vision may be impaired, but the ability to identify a peach by feeling, smell, or taste is retained.

Anosognosia is a lack of awareness of a disability one has and occurs as result of parietal or frontotemporoparietal lesions. Individuals with anosognosia do not recognize deficits that they have in motor function and may be at significant safety risk, as they perceive their abilities to be unimpaired, and therefore they may attempt tasks that they are not safe to do without assistance.

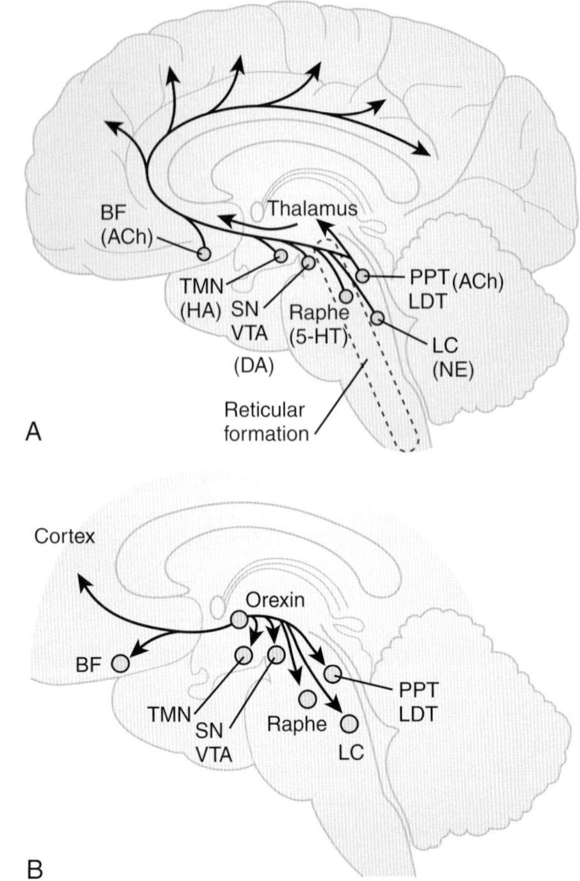


**Figure 28.14**

**Reticular activation system networks that influence sleep and wakefulness.** (A) Sagittal view of a brain providing an overview of the reticular activating system (wake-control networks). The upper brainstem, posterior and lateral hypothalamus, and basal forebrain *(BF)* contain groups of neurons with identified phenotypes with arousal-inducing properties. These clusters include neurons expressing serotonin *(5-HT)*, norepinephrine *(NE)*, acetylcholine *(ACh)* in both pontomesencephalic and basal forebrain clusters, dopamine *(DA)*, and histamine *(HA)*. (B) Sagittal view of brainstem and diencephalon showing localization of orexin-containing neurons and their projections to both forebrain and brainstem. All of these groups facilitate electroencephalography arousal (waking and rapid eye movement sleep) and/or motor-behavioral arousal (waking). The arousal systems facilitate forebrain electroencephalography activation both through the thalamus and the basal forebrain and through direct projections to neocortex. Arousal systems also facilitate motor-behavioral arousal through descending pathways. *LC,* Locus coeruleus; *LDT,* lateral dorsal tegmental; *PPT,* pedunculopontine; *SN,* substantia nigra; *TMN,* tuberomammillary nucleus; *VTA,* ventral tegmental area. (From Kryger M, Roth T, Dement WC: *Principles and practice of sleep medicine*, ed 6, Philadelphia, 2017, Elsevier.)

## Disorders of Consciousness

Alteration of consciousness is not considered an independent disease entity but rather a reflection of some underlying disease or abnormal state of brain function. The human brain possesses a mechanism that allows a waking and sleeping state (arousal), as well as a separate ability to focus awareness on relevant environmental stimuli (attention).[25,65] To achieve a state of consciousness the cerebral cortex must be activated by the ascending reticular formation fibers in the brainstem. The fibers extend to the thalamus, limbic system, and cortex. The upper part of this system acts as an on/off switch for consciousness and controls the normal sleep-wake cycle. The lower part controls respiration. Fig. 28.14 illustrates pathways related to sleep-wake cycles from the reticular formation.

Disturbances of arousal and attention can range from coma after brainstem injury, to minimally conscious state following recovery from traumatic brain injury, to confusional states caused by drug intoxication. Metabolic or systemic disorders generally cause depressed consciousness without focal neurologic findings.[100] CNS disorders may or may not have concomitant focal signs. Table 28.1 compares metabolic and drug-induced coma with coma caused by space-occupying lesions, such as those caused by hemorrhagic stroke or increased swelling within the brain after trauma.

Clinical disorders of arousal may result in hyperarousal states and can appear as restlessness, agitation, or confusion. This is presumably a result of the loss of hemispheric inhibition of brainstem function. Hypoarousal can be described on a spectrum ranging from drowsiness to stupor to coma. Stupor is a state of unresponsiveness that requires vigorous stimulation to bring about arousal. Coma is a state of unarousable unresponsiveness, so that eyes remain closed. Small, restricted lesions of the brainstem can result in stupor. Larger brainstem-level lesions or massive bilateral hemispheric lesions are necessary to cause coma. Table 28.2 identifies the brainstem reflexes in coma.

Damage to the cerebral cortex can be caused by loss of blood flow, subarachnoid hemorrhage, anesthetic toxicity, hypoglycemia, hypothermia, or status epilepticus (see

**Table 28.1** Characteristics of Comas

| Manifestations | Metabolic and Drug-Induced | From Space-Occupying Lesions |
|---|---|---|
| Onset | Behavioral changes, decreased attention and arousal | Usually severe headache, focal seizures |
| Pain response | Present and equal | May be different on each side |
| Reflexes | Intact deep tendon reflexes equal responses | Deep tendon reflexes may be unequal; positive Babinski sign (UMN lesion) |
| Pupillary reaction | Bilateral normal response | May be unequal |
| Size of pupil | May be at midpoint with anticholinergics; pinpoint from opiates; dilated from anoxia | Midbrain lesion—midpoint<br>Pons lesion—pinpoint<br>Herniation to brainstem—large |
| Corneal reflex | Bilateral, intact | Unequal, may be absent |
| Eye movement | Spontaneous movement without intention; no reaction to VOR | May have paresis of lateral gaze with CN III compression |
| Decorticate or decerebrate posturing | Absent; movement is normal | Posturing may be present depending on level of lesion |
| Extremity movement | Equal movement on both sides | Paresis may be unilateral |

*CN III*, Third cranial (oculomotor) nerve; *UMN*, upper motor neuron; *VOR*, vestibuloocular reflex.

**Table 28.2** Brainstem Reflexes in the Comatose Patient

| | Examination Technique | Normal Response | Afferent Pathway | Brainstem | Efferent Pathway |
|---|---|---|---|---|---|
| Pupils | Response to light | Direct and consensual pupillary constriction | Retina, optic nerve, chiasm, optic tract | Edinger-Westphal nucleus (midbrain) | Oculomotor nerve, sympathetic fibers |
| Oculocephalic | Turn head from side to side | Eyes move conjugately in direction opposite to head | Semicircular canals, vestibular nerve | Vestibular nucleus; medial longitudinal fasciculus; parapontine reticular formation (pons) | Oculomotor and abducens nerves |
| Vestibulooculocephalic | Irrigate external auditory canal with cold water | Nystagmus with fast component beating away from stimulus | Semicircular canals, vestibular nerve | Vestibular nucleus; medial longitudinal fasciculus; parapontine reticular formation (pons) | Oculomotor and abducens nerves |
| Corneal reflex | Stimulation of cornea | Eyelid closure | Trigeminal nerve | Trigeminal and facial nuclei (pons) | Facial nerve |
| Cough reflex | Stimulation of carina | Cough | Glossopharyngeal and vagus nerves | Medullary cough center | Glossopharyngeal and vagus nerves |
| Gag reflex | Stimulation of soft palate | Symmetric elevation of soft palate | Glossopharyngeal and vagus nerves | Medulla | Glossopharyngeal and vagus nerves |

Chapter 36). Following serious brain injury that results in coma, if cortical links to the brainstem are damaged, the person may progress to a wakeful unresponsive (or vegetative) state, where eyes are open in sleep/wake cycles, but no voluntary responses are observed. Progression beyond wakeful unresponsiveness may include a minimally conscious state, where some level of ability to interact (e.g., verbalization, eye tracking, response to sounds) occurs. As further improvement of consciousness occurs, a posttraumatic confusional period may occur where cognitive ability is impaired. See Chapter 33 for more detail about disorders of consciousness. Akinetic mutism occurs with damage to the mediofrontal lobe and results in lack of motivation to perform any motor or mental activity (abulia). In *locked-in syndrome,* there is damage to the pons, resulting most often from thrombosis of the basilar artery. This is a rare but remarkable impairment involving normal consciousness but complete body paralysis with the exception of the ability to blink and move the eyes vertically. The recognition of consciousness with such marked lack of movement abilities requires very careful observation to confirm eye responses that are conveying meaning.

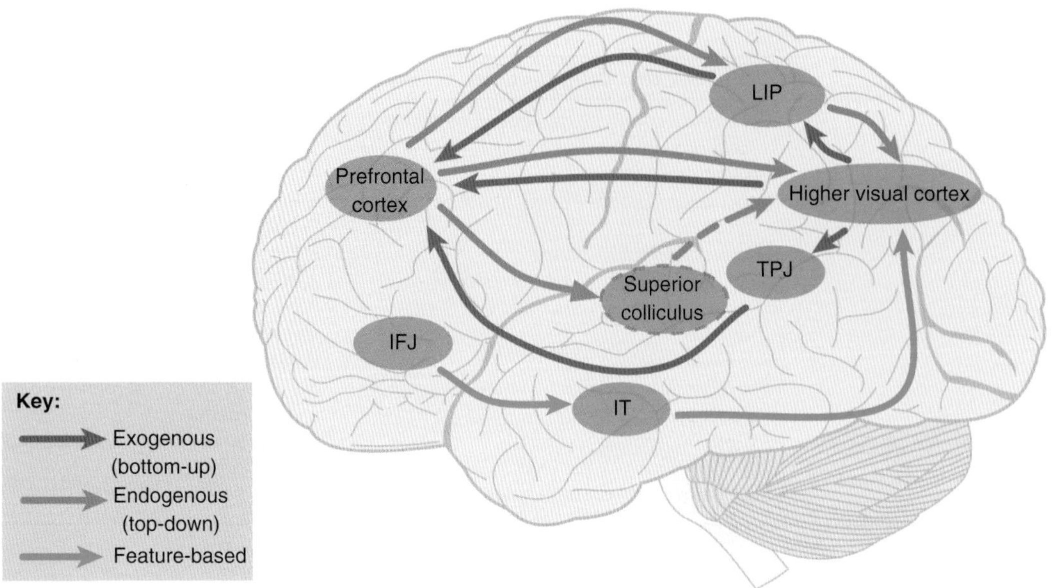


**Figure 28.15**

**Structures involved in visual attention.** Selective attention networks in the primate brain. This schematic combines results from human and nonhuman primates. *Blue arrows* indicate the flow of endogenous spatial information. Signals from the superior colliculus reach higher visual cortex by way of the thalamus *(broken line)*. *Red arrows* denote exogenous signals. *Green arrows* denote feature-based signals. *IFJ,* Inferior frontal junction; *IT,* inferotemporal cortex; *LIP,* lateral intraparietal cortex (in humans this is more generally referred to as middle intraparietal sulcus); *TPJ,* temporoparietal junction. (From Mueller A, et al: Linking ADHD to the neural circuitry of attention. *Trends Cogn Sci* 21:474–488, 2017.)

Supratentorial lesions that cause increased pressure such as hemorrhage, cerebral edema, or neoplasm can cause coma by producing tentorial herniation and subsequent compression of the brainstem. There is usually a hemiparesis with a dilated pupil on the side of the lesion because of central compression involving cranial nerve III by the herniation.

In infratentorial lesions, brainstem damage can be related to drugs, hemorrhage, infarction, or compression from the posterior fossa. Disruption of ocular movements is an early sign of brainstem involvement.[106] There is loss of the pupillary reaction to light, while the corneal reflex remains intact.

Brain death relates to destruction of both the upper and the lower parts of the reticular formation in the brainstem, which will eventually lead to death without the use of ventilator support to continue respiration. Cortical electrical activity and spinal reflexes may be preserved, but these are of no consequence because they are unable to be used for thought or movement.

The acute confusional state is one of the most common neurologic disorders encountered, where a deficit in attention is a typical symptom. Attention is more difficult to relate to a specific brain structure than arousal, as the network of brain structures active during attention tasks is distributed throughout the brain, and the structures vary based on the type of attention required (e.g., visual, auditory, tactile, cognitive processing). As an example, the network identified for visual attention tasks by Posner includes structures that span multiple brain structures throughout the brain (Fig. 28.15). Frontal and prefrontal areas of the brain are responsible for mental control, concentration, vigilance, and performance of meaningful activity.

Cognition and emotional control are established by extensive white matter connections between the frontal lobes and the remainder of the cerebrum.[93] Diseases that affect the white matter such as MS can affect the level of attention without decreasing arousal. Psychiatric disease often affects both arousal and attention.[65] The acute confusional state may be the result of a number of causes. Intoxicants, metabolic disorders, infections, epilepsy, blood flow disorders, traumatic injuries, and neoplasms all can be responsible for change in orientation or attention. Older adults have a particular susceptibility to develop *delirium,* which is a transient confusional state that may occur as result of physiologic stressors (e.g., developing infection, abnormal blood sugar levels) or from medication side effects; if delirium is identified and treated, the confusion resolves. If an older adult also has problems with depression or dementia, it may be difficult to determine which condition is driving cognitive impairments.[21]

## Emotional Instability

The orbital prefrontal region is especially expanded in the right cortex and is important for selective attention to facial expressions. It has extensive connections with limbic and subcortical regions, important in regulation of emotional information and mediation of pleasure and pain. Muscles of the head and neck represent a unique relationship to the primary senses. Humans have more facial muscles than any other species, and the connections to the limbic lobe reflect emotion. Maternal–infant connection and bonding and social-emotional connection

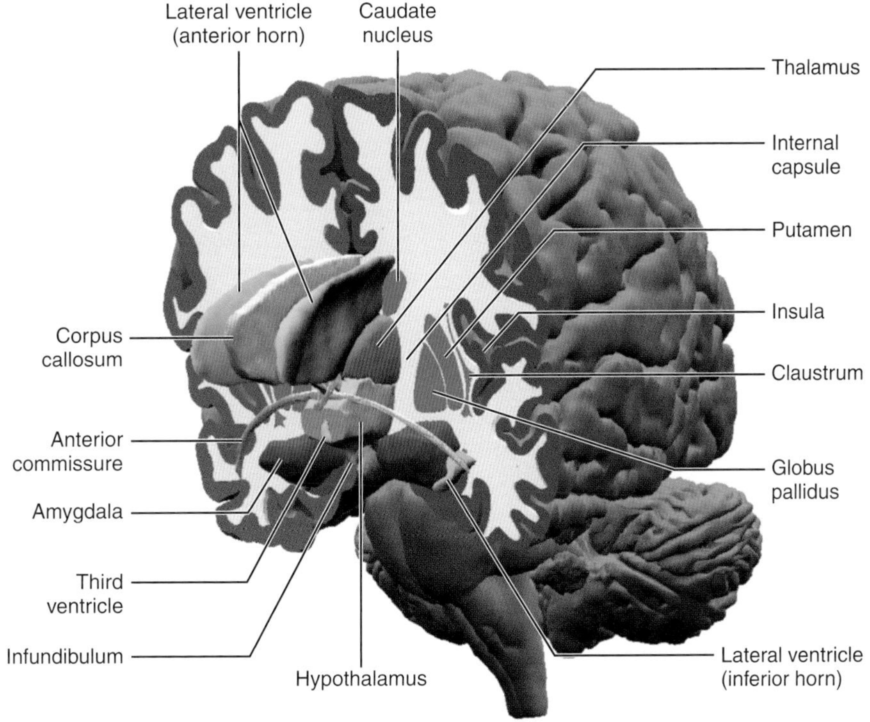


**Figure 28.16**

**Three-dimensional representation of the structures of, and those surrounding, the limbic lobe.** (From Nolte J: *The human brain: an introduction to its functional anatomy*, ed 5, St. Louis, 2002, Mosby.)

between individuals depend on facial expression. Primitive emotions that serve fundamental motivational and social communication functions and nonverbal affects are spontaneously expressed on the face. Psychic systems process unconscious information. Empathetic cognition and the perception of the emotional states of other human beings are developed within the first 3 years of life. Control of vital functions enable the individual to cope actively with stress and environmental challenge. Self-regulation functions are learned through this region.[91]

The thalamus is a two-lobed medial structure that sits just above the brainstem and is bounded on its dorsal surface by the lateral ventricles. The thalamus consists of multiple nuclei that receive input from sensory receptors and brainstem arousal systems and relay information to the frontal cortex, cingulate gyrus, amygdala, and hippocampus. With the exception of olfaction, all sensory input goes through thalamic nuclei before being sent onto the cortex. The thalamus affects the quantity and quality of sensory processing. The fact that basic sensory information and arousal signals converge in the thalamus explains why even basic sensory signals can be distorted under conditions of high arousal. Although moderate arousal may facilitate transmission, conditions of high stress likely will distort or hinder transmissions to target structures throughout the brain.

Although the limbic system defies exact definition, it is recognized as the area of control of human behavior and is widely studied in behavioral neurology. The limbic system, sometimes referred to as the limbic lobe, is generally considered to encompass part of the cortical, diencephalon, and brainstem structures. This system includes the orbitofrontal cortex, hippocampus, parahippocampal gyrus, cingulate gyrus, dentate gyrus, amygdala, septal area, hypothalamus, and portions of the thalamus. The limbic lobe structures are seen in Fig. 28.16.[72] Working together, these structures provide the essential, need-directed motor activity necessary for survival. This is the area that integrates motivation and intentional drive to trigger a motor act. Both the automatic and the somatic systems are influenced by the limbic system.[105] Limbic syndromes involve the primary emotions, which are those associated with pain, pleasure, anger, and fear. The limbic system is critical in assuring emotionally charged experiences will be more easily remembered than experiences with less emotional.[25] In lower animals the limbic system is concerned primarily with the sense of smell, and it is a common observation that smells can trigger a strong emotional response in humans.

The amygdala are nuclei located in the medial temporal lobe anterior to the hippocampus as illustrated in Fig. 28.17. The amygdala is involved in sensory processing and determining the value of the information received. Patterns of emotional memories are formed here, and this is the area that links anxiety and panic or pleasure that is unconsciously related to an experience that may or may not be remembered.[3] The amygdala is richly connected with the prefrontal cortex, the thalamus, hypothalamus, and brainstem as seen in Fig. 28.18.[72] Not represented here is the influence that the prefrontal cortex has on the amygdala, which is thought to be inhibitory. The amygdala is the central structure associated with the learning of fear, fearful responding, and associated autonomic and behavioral responses.

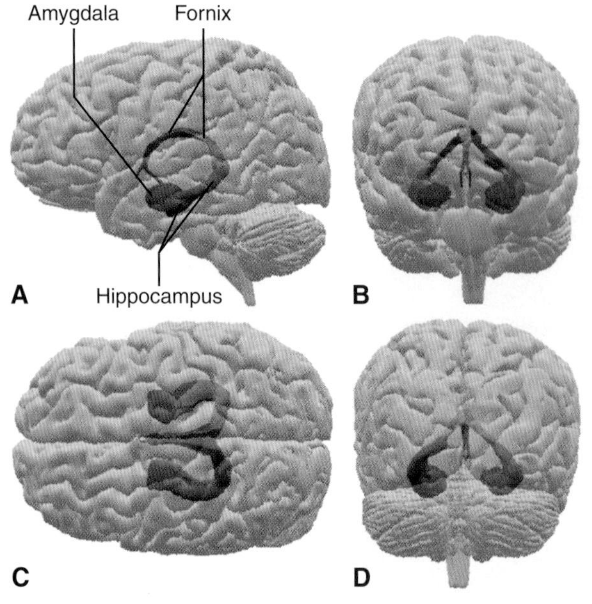


**Figure 28.17**

Placement of the main structures of the limbic lobe as seen from left (A), back (B), above (C), and behind (D). (From Nolte J: *The human brain: an introduction to its functional anatomy*, ed 5, St. Louis, 2002, Mosby.)

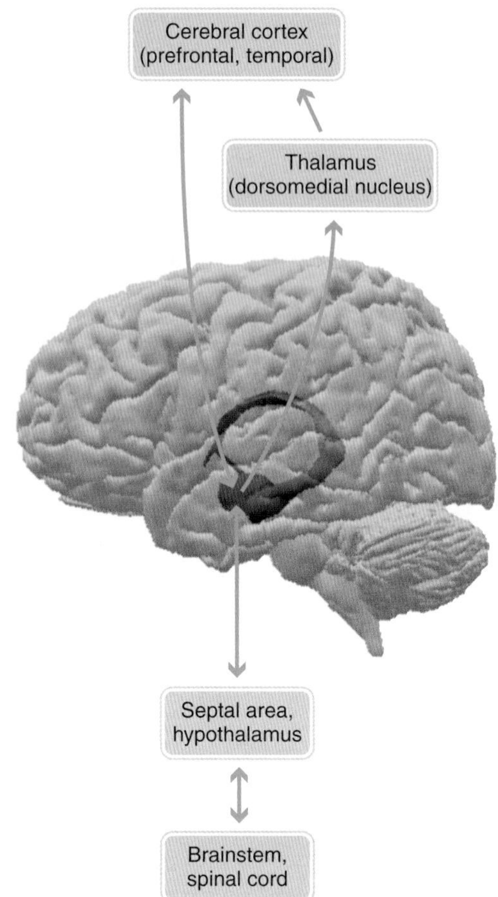


**Figure 28.18**

**The limbic lobe gives input directed toward the cerebral cortex and the hypothalamus, brainstem, and spinal cord.** (From Nolte J: *The human brain: an introduction to its functional anatomy*, ed 5, St. Louis, 2002, Mosby.)

*Kindling* is a term originally used to describe how subthreshold seizure activity becomes increasingly active and severe with successive seizures. Partial kindling also can occur in the amygdala, and it appears to be related to increased defensive responses and anxiety-like behavior in animals. In humans the amygdala is involved in integrating emotional and contextual information that is part of the human stress response. Amygdaloidal lesions result in hampered fear conditioning, whereas amygdaloidal stimulation results in classic fear responses, such as defensive and aggressive behavior and autonomic reactivity. It has been demonstrated that the amygdala plays a role in conditioned fear responding in general and the startle response in particular.

Perhaps the best example of an anxiety disorder that seems to follow the classic fear-conditioning model is posttraumatic stress disorder (PTSD). Greater amygdala activations were identified in persons with PTSD than in healthy control subjects. Activations in the amygdala correlated with weakened activation of the medial prefrontal cortex and hippocampus.[68] The prefrontal cortex is thought to be hypoactivated in PTSD, particularly during trauma memory activation. See Chapter 3 for more details about the role of the hypothalamic-pituitary-adrenal axis and its role in PTSD. The amygdala and the hippocampus play a crucial role in the pathophysiology of social phobia.

Dissociative symptoms are common among survivors of trauma, and maladaptive levels of dissociation can develop alongside other pathologic responses to trauma. Dissociation is defined as a disruption in the usually integrated functions of consciousness, memory, identity, or perception of the environment, and the term *dissociative symptoms* in the literature has been used to capture a range of symptoms that can include changes in time perception, altered sensory perception, flashbacks, psychogenic amnesia, reduction in awareness, affective blunting, feelings of detachment, depersonalization, multiple identities, and derealization.[27,52]

Although severe disturbances in sensory processing may occur under conditions of extreme stress, more subtle changes may occur even at baseline. The thalamus has rich bidirectional connections with the cingulate gyrus and the frontal cortex, two of the structures responsible for the prioritization and shifting of attention. During the extreme stress of an actual trauma, it is likely that the thalamus impairs rather than facilitates the processing of environmental stimuli. In this sense the thalamus has a role to play in amnesia for traumatic events. For example, disruption in the relay of contextual and traumatic information could contribute to the fragmentation and inaccuracies associated with traumatic memory. In contrast to the role the hippocampus might play in fragmenting sensory elements of the memory, however, thalamic interference would result in an initial interference with basic stimulus encoding.[52]

Levels of emotion that are generated and advanced by the limbic system, or more specifically the amygdala, can be described on a continuum. An emotion can be

**Table 28.3** Terms Commonly Used to Describe Psychogenic Disorders and Their Implications[a]

| Psychogenic Disorder | Implication |
|---|---|
| Psychogenic | Suggests psychologic causation |
| Conversion disorder | Operationalized within *DSM-IV*: requires an identified psychologic triggering factor for diagnosis |
| Somatization disorder | Operationalized within *DSM-IV*: requires presence of multiple physical symptoms, including one conversion neurologic symptom |
| Medically unexplained symptoms | Suggests that a medical explanation might one day be apparent<br>Could refer to many medical symptoms that are not thought to be psychogenic but still do not have a known cause |
| Functional | Broad term suggesting a functional rather than a structural deficit, which could apply to several neurologic disorders not regarded as psychogenic but where structural pathology is absent (e.g., migraine) |
| Hysteria | Historical term that carries substantial stigma in society and implies a link between symptoms and the uterus |
| Nonorganic | Defines the condition by what it is not; the term organic is itself not well defined |

[a]Some terms such as psychogenic, conversion, or somatization directly suggest that the cause of physical symptoms is psychologically mediated. Conversion and somatization are operationalized diagnoses that specifically need the presence of a psychological triggering factor and exclusion of feigning. However, for most movement disorder specialists, the presence of a psychologic triggering factor is not a requirement for diagnosing a patient with a functional movement disorder, and the difficulties of routinely excluding feigning in clinical practice are complex.

*DSM-IV, Diagnostic and Statistical Manual of Mental Disorders* (Fourth Edition).

From Edwards MJ: Functional (psychogenic) movement disorders: merging mind and brain. *Lancet Neurol* 11:250–260, 2012.

triggered as fear or frustration, which when heightened can manifest as anger. If the neurochemical activity continues to build and leads to internal chaos or conflict, it becomes rage. The motor response will become violent if there is a sufficient trigger. Genetics and environmental history will lead to differences in how a person moves from fear to violence. When there is damage to the area of the limbic lobe that results from injury or disease, there can be an increase in rage and easy progression to violence. The diffuse axonal damage with brain injury can cause a tendency to become easily frustrated or to have unsubstantiated fears.[104] Fear conditioning is a fast process, with a long-lasting effect, but repeated exposure to the conditioned stimulus in the absence of the unconditioned stimulus can lead to extinction. Extinction reduces the likelihood that the conditioned stimulus will elicit the fear response. The medial prefrontal and anterior cingulate cortices have been implicated in extinction learning. Understanding how learned fears are diminished and how extinction learning is changed in individuals who have anxiety disorders might be an important step in translating neurobiologic research to diagnosis and treatment of these individuals.

Functional (psychogenic) movement disorders are part of the spectrum of functional neurologic disorders, which are some of the most prevalent disorders seen in neurologic practice. In common with other functional disorders, appropriate provision of health services for individuals with functional movement disorders, as well as research interest, is lacking despite the prevalence of these disorders. Functional movement disorders occupy a gray area between neurology and psychiatry. The key clinical feature that separates patients with functional movement disorders from patients with organic movement disorders is that the movements have features that one would usually associate with voluntary movement (distractibility, resolution with placebo, and presence of premovement potentials), but patients report them as being involuntary and not under their control. There seem to be just two logical explanations for this feature: either movements are deliberately feigned or there must be a brain mechanism that allows voluntary movement to occur but to be experienced subjectively as involuntary. Understanding this mechanism would seem to be key to understanding the development of symptoms and their treatment. Table 28.3 presents terms used to describe the various psychogenic disorders.[23]

The symptom dimensions of obsessive-compulsive disorder and other anxiety disorders are likely to share common neural substrates dedicated to general threat detection and emotional arousal because these reactions are adaptive and useful to deal with different kinds of threats. Research suggests that syndrome-specific neural substrates may have evolved to deal with specific threats. In evolutionary terms, general anxiety, which is common to individuals who have obsessive-compulsive disorder and other anxiety disorders, may have evolved to deal with nonspecific threats; for example, cleanliness is important for protection against infections. Likewise, harming obsessions and checking rituals relate to safety, and hoarding may help people survive periods of scarcity; however, when manifested outside of such threats, these responses may create functional problems. Neuroimaging findings showing increased activation of limbic and ventral frontostriatal regions in obsessive-compulsive disorder could reflect exaggerations of normal emotional responses to biologically relevant stimuli rather than fundamentally abnormal neuronal responses.[62]

Borderline personality disorders, including affective dysregulation, identity disturbance, and self-mutilating behaviors, were originally thought to involve a disorder of character. In more recent studies, it appears that individuals with borderline personality disorder are compromised significantly in executive skill and/or other frontal lobe functions, visuomotor speed, attention, and verbal memory. These fairly consistent neuropsychologic findings in

**Table 28.4** Correlation of Anatomic Site to Disorders of Memory and Other Neurologic Findings

| Anatomic Site of Damage | Memory Finding | Other Neurologic and Medical Findings |
|---|---|---|
| Frontal lobe | Lateralized deficit in working memory. Right spatial defects, left verbal defects, impaired recall with spared recognition | Personality change<br>Perseveration<br>Chorea, dystonia<br>Bradykinesia, tremor, rigidity |
| Basal forebrain | Declarative memory deficit | |
| Ventromedial cortex | Frontal lobe–type declarative memory deficit | Upper visual field defects |
| Hippocampus and parahippocampal cortex | Bilateral lesions yield global amnesia, unilateral lesions show lateralization of deficit<br>Left: verbal deficit; right: spatial deficit | Myoclonus<br>Depressed level of consciousness<br>Cortical blindness<br>Autonomations |
| Fornix | Global amnesia | |
| Mammillary bodies | Declarative memory deficit | Confabulation, ataxia, nystagmus, signs of alcohol withdrawal |
| Dorsal and medial dorsal nucleus thalamus | Declarative memory deficit | Confabulation |
| Anterior thalamus | Declarative memory deficit | |
| Lateral temporal cortex | Deficit in autobiographic memory | |

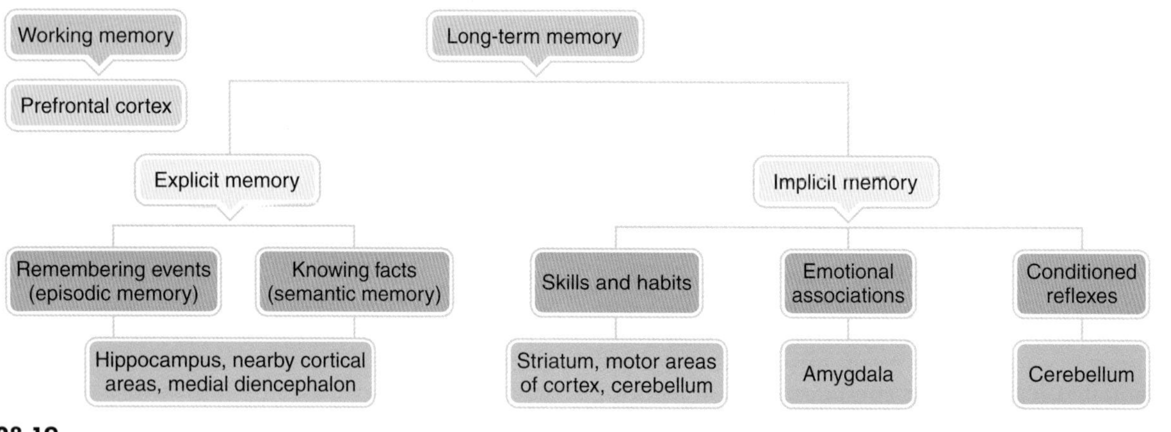


**Figure 28.19**

**Anatomic correlates for explicit and implicit learning.** (From Nolte J: *The human brain: an introduction to its functional anatomy*, ed 5, St. Louis, 2002, Mosby.)

adults are supported by developmental studies of children with borderline features. These children appear to have greater difficulty with executive skills, including planning, organizing, and sequencing; perceptual motor functioning; and memory proficiency.[68]

## Memory Problems

Memory is associated with various areas of the brain, and a particular area may be responsible for different aspects of memory. The hippocampus, thalamus, and basal forebrain are critical for the formation of declarative memory (Table 28.4). Fig. 28.19 shows the relationship of types of memory, learning, and associated brain regions. For immediate auditory memory, left and right temporoparietal cortices mediate auditory verbal and nonverbal material. Neurogenesis has been observed in the dentate gyrus of the hippocampus throughout the lives of many species including humans. Not all newly generated hippocampal neurons survive, but hippocampal-dependent memory tasks can enhance the survival of these neurons.[37] Inflammatory cytokines reduce hippocampal neurogenesis and impair the ability to maintain long-term potentiation in the hippocampus, which is a critical physiologic process involved in memory consolidation.[36]

*Working memory*, the ability to hold information in short-term storage while permitting other cognitive operations to take place, appears to depend on the prefrontal cortex. This capacity to manipulate bits of information (typical capacity of 7 plus or minus 2 items) is important for cognitive processing such as that used in remembering an email address, performing arithmetic, or following a conversation. Keeping a spatial location in mind may involve a right frontal area that directs the maintenance of that information in a right parietal area, whereas keeping a word in mind may involve a left frontal area that directs the maintenance of that information in a left temporal or parietal area. Specific basal ganglia and cerebellar areas appear to support the working memory capacity of particular frontal regions. It appears that the brain performs problem solving based on working memory that is found and lost in the course of a task. This fluid memory, related to reasoning, is maintained with active use and can be improved with practice in many cases. Essentially the goal is to expand the work space of the brain. This is the area that is being explored in relation to "brain training"; however, current evidence demonstrating that cognitive training using computer games and applications causes functional improvements or delays cognitive decline in older adults is limited.[31–33]

Disorders of memory, known as *amnesia*, are a significant neurobehavioral phenomenon and common in persons after traumatic brain injury. *Declarative memory* is retention of facts and events of a prior experience or the memory of what has occurred and is related to explicit learning. *Procedural memory* describes the learning of skills and habits, or how something is done. Implicit learning is based on procedural memory. The relationship to memory and relearning motor skills is discussed in Special Implications for the Physical Therapist 28.1: Motor Learning Strategies.

*Anterograde amnesia* is the failure of new learning or formation of new memory and is synonymous with posttraumatic amnesia when it occurs after brain injury. *Retrograde amnesia* is the loss of ability to recall events before the traumatic event. When individuals have dementia, the ability to recall more recent events is typically lost before more remote events. This loss of recent memory continues to increase so that memory of one's children may be lost, but the ability to reminisce about early years is intact. The inability to remember is often accompanied by *confabulation*, the fabrication of information in response to questioning that may be an adaptive way to save face in the presence of diminishing memory abilities. *Traumatic amnesia* refers to an individual's inability to recall significant aspects of their traumatic experience. Traumatic memories are reported to be fragmented, compartmentalized, and disintegrated, suggesting that the hippocampus still may have a role to play in the phenomenon of traumatic amnesia. Dysregulation in the hippocampal system has the potential to generate narratives of traumatic events that are spotty and unreliable.

Neuromodulators such as norepinephrine have the potential to affect hippocampal functioning in a more dynamic fashion. For example, the locus coeruleus, located in the brainstem, projects directly to the hippocampus and modulates its functioning through norepinephrine release. The effects of such a network are unclear, although the implications are that stress-related memory alterations might occur on a split-second basis, and deficient or extreme locus coeruleus input may severely disrupt normal hippocampal processing. Given that the hippocampus plays a role in integrating input from diverse sources when encoding memory, disruptions in its functioning may lead to memories that seem fragmented and nonlinear. Over time, fragments of the memory may become consolidated, vivid, and easily recalled, while other fragments rarely are accessed.[52]

Several chronic neurologic disease states such as Alzheimer disease and Parkinson disease are associated with elevated secretion of stress hormones, which results from overactivity of the hypothalamic-pituitary-adrenal axis. Stress or perceived threat activates the hypothalamus, triggering release of hormones that cause increased adrenal output of cortisol and glucocorticoids.[87] Stress hormones also can decrease natural recovery in acute neurotrauma. Elevated glucocorticoids negatively influence neuroplasticity associated with both acquired brain trauma and degenerative neurologic disorders. Abnormal regulation of glucocorticoid release is associated with many affective disorders, such as depression and PTSD (see Chapter 3) that are overrepresented in populations with neurologic disease; Parkinson disease is a prime example. Acute and sustained glucocorticoid release also can precipitate changes in peripheral and central immune signaling, resulting in cytokine profiles that may be deleterious for functional recovery in the face of neurologic challenge.[41]

Accumulation of risk is another concept that plays a pivotal role in the life-course model of chronic diseases. Allostasis is defined as the ability to achieve stability through change. The price of this accommodation to stress has been defined as the allostatic load. It follows that acute stress (the "fight, flight, or freeze" response) and chronic stress resulting from the cumulative load of minor day-to-day stresses can add to the allostatic load and have long-term consequences. Subacute stress is defined as an accumulation of stressful life events over a duration of months and includes emotional factors such as hostility and anger, as well as affective disorders such as major depression and anxiety disorders. Chronic stressors include factors such as low social support, work stress, marital stress, and caregiver strain and manifest as feelings of fatigue, lack of energy, irritability, and demoralization.

The link between chronic psychologic distress and adverse behaviors such as overeating may be centrally mediated. Normally, glucocorticoids help end acute stress responses by exerting negative feedback on the hypothalamic-pituitary-adrenal axis. The combination of chronic stress and high glucocorticoid levels seems to stimulate a preferential desire to ingest sweet and fatty foods, presumably by affecting dopaminergic transmission in areas of the brain associated with motivation and reward.[30]

Brain areas associated with reward are linked with areas that sense physical pain. Chronic pain can cause depression, and depression can increase pain. Most individuals who have depression also present with physical symptoms. Studies using functional magnetic resonance imaging (fMRI) have shown that social rejection activates brain areas that are also key regions in the response to physical pain. The area of the anterior cingulate cortex that is activated by visceral pain is also activated in response to social rejection.

Disturbances of neurologic function can result in behavioral disturbances that mimic disturbances of mental function in psychiatric disorders. *Delusions*, or fixed false beliefs, have been reported in a great variety of neurologic conditions and appear to be associated with the limbic system. Paranoid delusions are common in disorders of the medial temporal lobe or a combination of the frontal and right parietal lobes. *Hallucinations* are sensory experiences without external stimulation. Visual hallucinations generally suggest neurologic involvement such as Lewy body dementia; auditory hallucinations imply psychiatric disease. Midbrain lesions in the cerebral peduncles can cause hallucinations involving animals. Temporal lesions can cause recurrent auditory experiences.[25]

Box 28.2

**RAPID EYE MOVEMENT SLEEP BEHAVIOR DISORDER AND RELATED BRAINSTEM STRUCTURES**

- Substantia nigra (midbrain-dopaminergic)
- Locus coeruleus (brainstem-noradrenergic)
- Pedunculopontine nucleus (pons-cerebellum)
- Dorsal vagus nucleus
- Dorsal raphe nucleus (involved in serotonin pathways)
- Gigantocellular reticular nucleus (control of arousal)

Modified from Gagnon JF: Rapid-eye-movement sleep behaviour disorder and neurodegenerative diseases. *Neurology* 5:424–432, 2006.

Rapid eye movement sleep behavior disorder is characterized by loss of muscular atonia and prominent motor behaviors during rapid eye movement sleep. Sleep behavior disorder can cause sleep disruption. The disorder is strongly associated with neurodegenerative diseases, such as multiple-system atrophy, Parkinson disease, Lewy body dementia, and progressive supranuclear palsy. The symptoms of sleep behavior disorder precede other symptoms of these neurodegenerative disorders by several years. Furthermore, several recent studies have shown that sleep behavior disorder is associated with abnormalities of electroencephalography (EEG) activity; cerebral blood flow; and cognitive, perceptual, and autonomic functions. Sleep behavior disorder might be a stage in the development of neurodegenerative disorder. Box 28.2 lists the areas of the brain that play a role in sleep behavior.[29]

Lesions of the hemispheres or lobes may cause loss of the functions that each hemisphere controls. Because diseases and damage caused by trauma will often affect one area of the brain, the associated syndromes for the main areas of the brain are described.[59]

## Brainstem Dysfunction

The brainstem contains the lower motor neurons for the muscles of the head and does the initial processing of general afferent information concerning the head. The cranial nerves enter the system at the brainstem through the respective nuclei and provide sensation and motor control of the head and neck.[72] The sensory and motor functions of the cranial nerves are outlined in Table 28.5. A working knowledge of the attributes of the cranial nerves assists in the understanding of the level and impact of lesions within the CNS.

Distinctive brainstem functions include a conduit for spinal cord activity in both ascending sensory tracts and descending motor tracts. The nuclei in the brainstem provide relay functions to divert the information to the appropriate higher level structures for further modification.

The brainstem has been divided into three major subdivisions related to a characteristic set of features: the medulla, pons, and midbrain. The medulla, attached directly to the spinal cord, houses the inferior olivary nucleus that has direct output connections to the cerebellum and gets direct input from the spinal cord and cerebellum. The pons extends from the medulla and is attached to the cerebellum through both the middle and the superior cerebellar peduncles, receiving major outflow from the cerebellum. Vestibular nuclei sit within the pons, making it the center for integration of vestibular input. The midbrain contains the red nucleus with fibers that connect the cerebellum to the thalamus. The substantia nigra found here connects to the basal ganglia structures and shares the dopamine pathway related to the initiation and control of movement. It is also connected to the cortex through the cerebral peduncle, containing descending fibers.

The reticular formation is a diffuse network of neurons, extending through the brainstem to higher levels, and is important in influencing movement. The reticular regions are closely related to the cerebellum, basal ganglia, vestibular nuclei, and substantia nigra and involved with complex movement patterns. It is through the reticular formation that there is inhibition of flexor reflexes, so that only noxious stimulus can evoke the flexor response, such as the reflexive pulling a hand away from a hot stove.

This is a brief reflection of the complexity of the brainstem and is not intended to be comprehensive. However, it is clear that advanced knowledge of the interface and connections of the brainstem helps the therapist understand the functions that are described throughout this text.

## Autonomic Nervous System Dysfunction

The term *autonomic nervous system* was introduced to describe the system of nerves that controls the unstriated tissue, the cardiac muscle, and the glandular tissue of mammals involved in the control of autonomic function. The autonomic nervous system neurons are located at many levels from the cerebral cortex to the spinal cord. Efferent autonomic pathways are organized in two major outflows: the sympathetic and parasympathetic. Finally, the enteric nervous system, which is considered a separate and independent division of the autonomic nervous system, is located in the walls of the gut. A schematic diagram of the autonomic nervous system is shown in Fig. 28.20.

Neurons in the cerebral cortex, basal forebrain, hypothalamus, midbrain, pons, and medulla participate in autonomic control. The central autonomic network integrates visceral, humoral, and environmental information to produce coordinated autonomic, neuroendocrine, and behavioral responses to external or internal stimuli. A coordinated response is generated through interconnections among the amygdala and the neocortex, forebrain, hypothalamus, and autonomic and somatic motor nuclei of the brainstem. The insular and medial prefrontal cortices (paralimbic areas) and nuclei of the amygdala are the higher centers involved in the processing of visceral information and the initiation of integrated autonomic responses. The central nucleus of the amygdala projects to the hypothalamus, periaqueductal gray (PAG), and autonomic nuclei of the brainstem to integrate autonomic, endocrine, and motor responses to emotionally relevant stimuli. See Chapter 3 for information on self-regulation and the role of the ANS.

The hypothalamus integrates the autonomic and endocrine responses that are critical for homeostasis. The PAG of the midbrain is the site of integrated autonomic,

**Table 28.5** Cranial Nerves and Their Functions

| Cranial Nerve | Component | Function |
|---|---|---|
| I—Olfactory | S | Olfaction |
| II—Optic | S | Vision |
| III—Oculomotor | M | Innervation of inferior oblique muscle and medial, inferior, and superior rectus muscles of eye |
| | A | Innervation of ciliary ganglion, which regulates papillary constriction (papillary constrictor muscle) and accommodation to near vision (ciliary muscle) |
| IV—Trochlear | M | Innervation of superior oblique muscle of eye |
| V—Trigeminal | S | Sensation (epicritic, protopathic) from face, nose, mouth, nasal, and oral mucosa, anterior two-thirds of tongue, and meningeal sensation, through all three divisions (ophthalmic, maxillary, mandibular) |
| | M | Innervation of muscles of mastication and tensor tympani muscle (through mandibular division only) |
| VI—Abducens | M | Innervation of lateral rectus muscle of eye |
| VII—Facial | S | Taste from anterior two-thirds of tongue |
| | M | Innervation of muscles of facial expression and stapedius muscle |
| | A | Innervation of pterygopalatine ganglion, which innervates lacrimal and nasal mucosal glands, and submandibular ganglion, which innervates submandibular and sublingual salivary glands |
| VIII—Vestibulocochlear | S | Hearing (cochlear division); linear and angular acceleration, or head position in space (vestibular division) |
| IX—Glossopharyngeal | S | Taste and general sensation from posterior one-third tongue; sensation (epicritic, protopathic) from pharynx, soft palate, tonsils; chemoreception from carotid body and baroreception from carotid sinus (unconscious reflex sensory information) |
| | M | Innervation of pharyngeal muscles |
| | A | Innervation of otic ganglion, which supplies parotid gland |
| X—Vagus | S | Visceral sensation (excluding pain) from heart, bronchi, trachea, larynx, pharynx, GI tract to level of descending colon; general sensation of external ear; taste from epiglottis |
| | M | Innervation of pharyngeal and laryngeal muscles and muscles at base of tongue |
| | A | Innervation of local visceral ganglia, which supply smooth muscles in respiratory, cardiovascular, and GI tract to level of descending colon |
| XI—Spinal accessory | M | Innervation of trapezius and sternocleidomastoid muscles |
| XII—Hypoglossal | M | Innervation of muscles of tongue |

*A*, Autonomic nervous system; *GI*, gastrointestinal; *M*, motor nervous system; *S*, sensory nervous system.
From Felten DL, Felten SY: A regional and systemic overview of functional neuroanatomy. In Farber SD: *Neurorehabilitation: a multisensory approach*, Philadelphia, 1982, Saunders, pp 53–54.

behavioral, and antinociceptive stress responses. It is organized into separate columns that control specific patterns of response to stress. The lateral PAG mediates sympathoexcitation, opioid-independent analgesia, and motor responses consistent with the fight-or-flight reaction. The ventrolateral PAG is associated with sympathoinhibition, opioid-dependent analgesia, and motor inhibition.

Neurons in the medulla are critical for the control of cardiovascular, respiratory, and gastrointestinal functions. The medullary nucleus of the solitary tract is the first relay station for the arterial baroreceptors and chemoreceptors, as well as cardiopulmonary and gastrointestinal afferents.

Preganglionic sympathetic neurons are organized into different functional units that control blood flow to the skin and muscles, secretion of sweat glands, skin hair follicles, and systemic blood flow, as well as the function of viscera. Selectivity is refined by the release of different neurotransmitters.

Visceral afferents transmit conscious sensations (e.g., gut distention and cardiac ischemia) and unconscious visceral sensations (e.g., blood pressure and chemical composition of the blood). Their most important function is to initiate autonomic reflexes at the local, ganglion, spinal, and supraspinal levels. Visceral sensation is carried primarily by the spinothalamic and spinoreticular pathways, which transmit visceral pain and sexual sensations. Brainstem visceral afferents are carried by the vagus and glossopharyngeal nerves. Brainstem visceral afferents are important in complex automatic motor acts, such as swallowing, vomiting, and coughing.[37] Sensory messages from the visceral organs travel back to the medulla and the limbic lobe. This may be the explanation for the term "gut feeling." The walls of the intestinal organs contain independent nerve cell clusters that operate independently from the vagus nerve and use the same neurotransmitters as the brain.[86]

Traumatic spinal cord injury, particularly injury above the T5 level, is associated with severe and disabling cardiovascular, gastrointestinal, bladder, and sexual dysfunction. These individuals have both supine and orthostatic hypotension and are at risk of developing bradycardia and cardiac arrest during tracheal suction or other maneuvers that activate the vagovagal reflexes. A life-threatening condition, autonomic dysreflexia, occurs in this same group of patients. See Chapter 34 for details about this condition.

In the physical therapy context, problems with autonomic regulation are commonly observed in response to body position changes and physical exercise. Signs of autonomic dysfunction, such as diaphoresis and flushing of the skin, may be evident in addition to subjective symptoms of lightheadedness, intolerance for exercise, and gastrointestinal problems. During physical therapy, impairment of regulation of heart rate and blood pressure is a significant concern, and thus careful monitoring of blood pressure during position changes is advised. The use of supplemental indicators of the appropriateness of exercise, including ratings of perceived exertion and pulse oximetry, may prove more valuable than traditional heart rate measurement.

Pure autonomic failure with no other neurologic deficits is rare. More often, autonomic failure occurs in combination with other neurologic disorders, such as Guillain-Barré syndrome and multiple system atrophy. Autonomic failure also occurs in individuals with some peripheral neuropathies, such as those associated with diabetes. Because autonomic failure may be caused by lesions at different levels of the nervous system, a history of secondary trauma, cerebrovascular disease, tumors, infections, or demyelinating diseases should be established. Additionally, because the most frequent type of autonomic dysfunction encountered in medical practice is pharmacologic, there should be a thorough review of medication use, especially antihypertensive and psychotropic drugs.

Some conditions may be confused with autonomic failure, including neurally mediated syncope, which is referred to as vasovagal, vasodepressor, or reflex syncope. This condition is caused by a paroxysmal reversal of the normal pattern of autonomic activation that maintains blood pressure in the standing position; these individuals do not have autonomic failure. A detailed history is important to differentiate this disorder. In contrast to

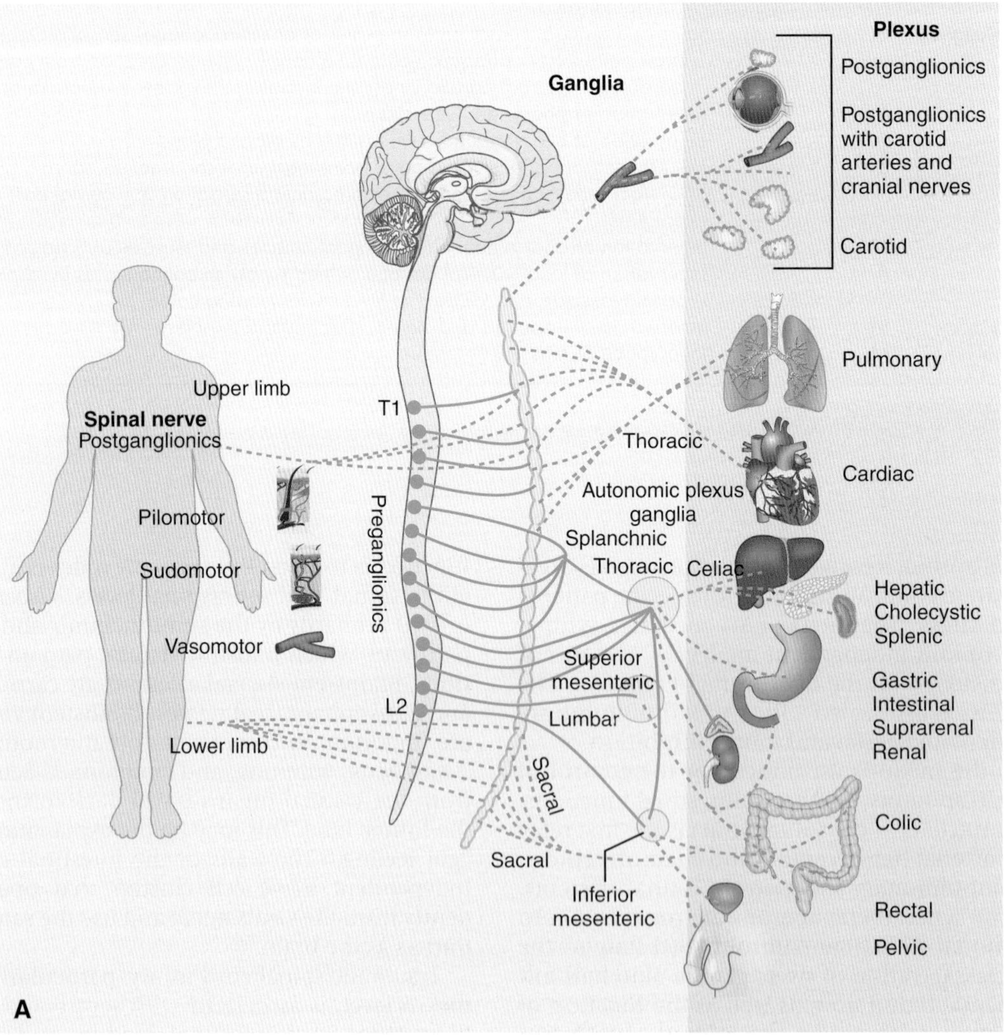


**Figure 28.20**

Sympathetic (A) and parasympathetic. (B) divisions of the autonomic nervous system: efferent systems. (From Levy MN, Koeppen BM: *Berne and Levy principles of physiology*, ed 4, St. Louis, 2006, Mosby.)

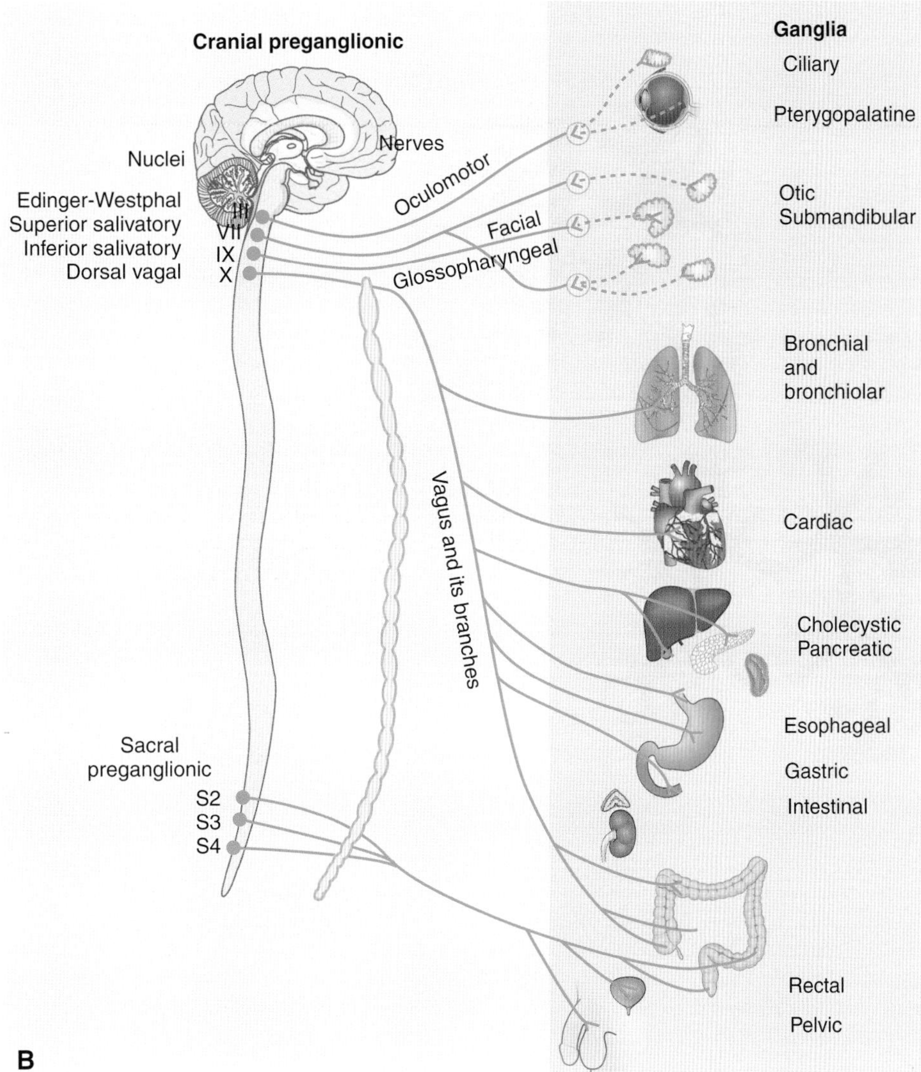


**Figure 28.20, cont'd**

individuals with chronic autonomic failure in whom syncope appears as a gradual fading of vision and loss of awareness, individuals with neurally mediated syncope often have signs and symptoms of autonomic overactivity, such as diaphoresis and nausea before the event. This distinction and the episodic nature of neurally mediated syncope should be part of a thorough clinical history.

The complexity of the nervous system cannot be overstated. The information provided in this overview of the components of the CNS is meant to illuminate the many facets of the system that can be affected by pathologic processes. Fig. 28.21 shows the relationship of the areas that have been described here.[44] Familiarity with this relationship is the basis of attempting to understand the neural pathologies that will be considered in subsequent chapters. To understand pathology, one must have a good working knowledge of brain structure and function. The Whole Brain Atlas website provides dynamic images of the brain, integrating imaging techniques that link anatomy and pathology.[107]

## Aging and the Central Nervous System

Senescence, or aging, results from changes in DNA, RNA, and proteins. Errors in the duplication of DNA increase with age because of random damage over time. There may be a specific genetic program for senescence. Fibroblasts from an older individual double fewer times than fibroblasts of an embryo.

Age-related reduction in adult brain weight represents loss of brain tissue. There is highly selective atrophy of brain tissue in the aging CNS. It is not clear how much of the change represents actual loss of nerve cells, as the changes in vascular tissue and glial cells may represent some of the loss. Simple loss of cells is common. Nerve cell shrinking, causing possible changes in functional efficiency, may be a more important effect of old age than

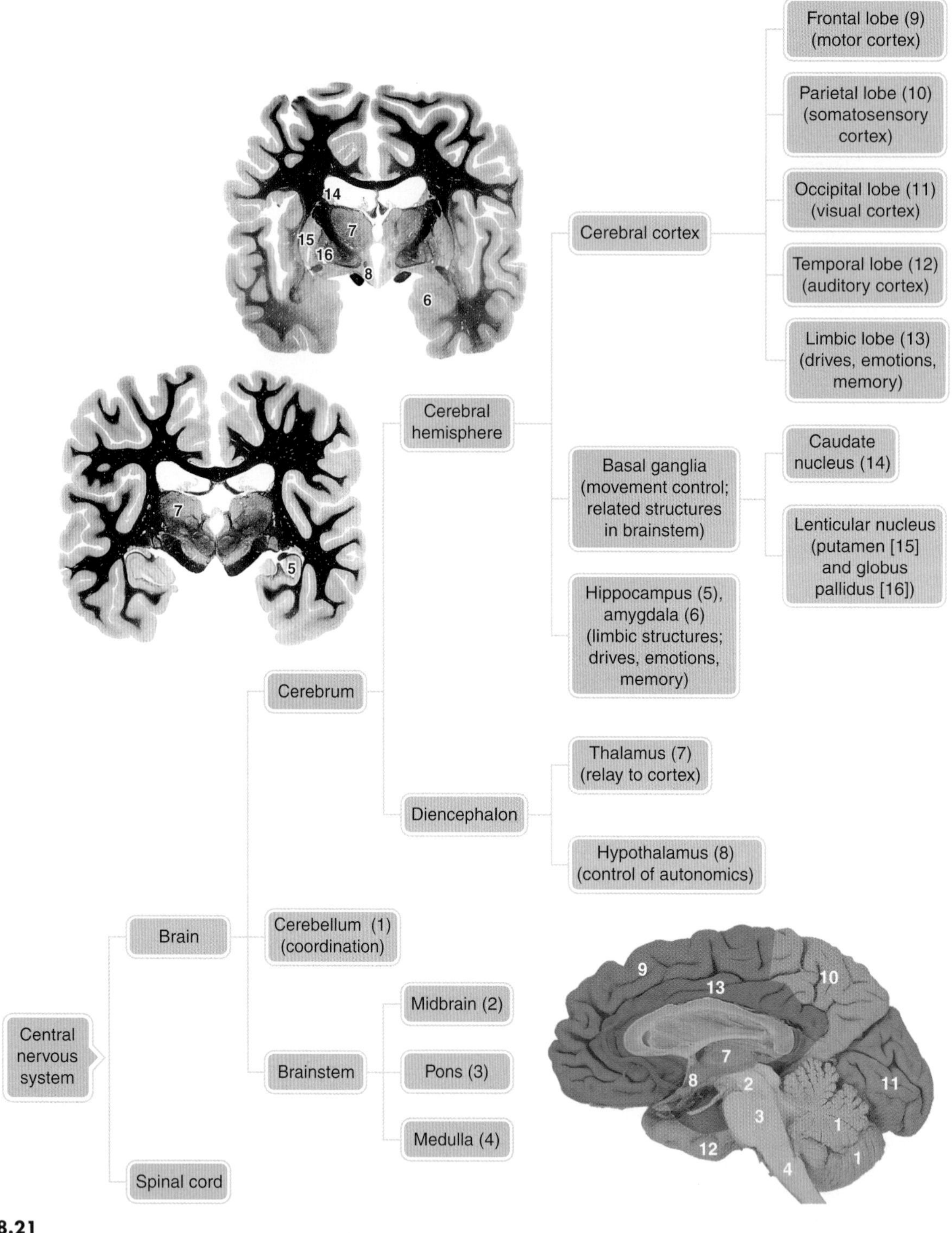


**Figure 28.21**

**Overview of the subdivisions of the central nervous system.** (From Nolte J: *The human brain: an introduction to its functional anatomy*, ed 5, St. Louis, 2002, Mosby.)

cell loss. Nerve conduction velocity decreases with age in both the motor and the sensory systems. By the eighth decade, there is an average loss of 15% of the velocity in the myelinated fibers.[58]

The inner structure of the nerve cell changes with aging. The presence of lipofuscin, or wear and tear pigment, a pigmented lipid found in the cytoplasm, may interfere with normal cell function via pressure on the cell nucleus. Damage to an axon close to the neuronal cell body results in changes in the area of the cell body and is referred to as an axonal reaction. The mechanism and relationship to dysfunction are still not clearly understood. The deposition of amyloid-β protein creating plaques in the cerebral cortex is found in many, but not all, older people. Neuritic, or senile, plaques are found outside the neuron filled with degenerating axons, dendrites, astrocytes, and amyloid. They represent damage to brain tissue. The neuritic plaques are thought to occur most often in the cortex and hippocampus and have been associated with dementia and Alzheimer disease.[26]

Neurofibrillary tangles, or abnormal neurologic fibers that displace and distort the cell body, are found in higher concentrations in the older brain. Neurofibrillary tangles and amyloid are also found in higher concentrations in people with Alzheimer disease (see Chapter 31), although these substances can also be present without signs of dementia.

Overall blood supply also diminishes during aging, with a net reduction of 10% to 15%. The relationship of cerebral blood flow, the resultant decrease in the glucose supply to the brain, and decreased metabolism are not well established as to cause and effect. All three are noted in the aging brain.[78]

Morphologic changes in the aging brain are accompanied by neurochemical changes. Aging has a more deleterious effect on myelinated primary afferents than their unmyelinated counterparts. Neuronal atrophy, axonal lesions, loss of peripheral nerve endings, receptor organs, and centrally projecting nerve terminals represent large myelinated primary afferent neurons. An inability to maintain appropriate neuronal function in senescence may result from a disturbance in the trophic signaling between neurons and their target cell. There is a decreased capacity of peripheral target tissues, such as skeletal muscle and skin, to synthesize neurotrophic factors of the nerve growth factor family of neurotrophins. Neurotrophins have been shown to regulate the expression of neurofilaments, which affect neural plasticity. Neurotrophins also influence the capacity of neurons to withstand the damaging effects of free radicals. Decreased neurotrophin signaling may be related to abnormal neuropeptide and other neurotransmitter substances that influence important functional aspects of primary sensory neurons, as it affects sensory neurons.[22] Changes in these neurotransmitters may be reflected in decreased control over visceral functions, emotions, and attention. Serotonin, involved in central regulatory activities of respiration, thermoregulation, sleep, and memory, appears to be reduced in the older brain. Depression in older adults may be related to increased production of MAO, which breaks down catecholamines and results in a loss of the feeling of well-being.[50]

Other changes in the brain related to neurotransmission are described in the chapters that follow. Mood and depressive symptoms also are common in elderly individuals who are ill and are associated with increased morbidity and mortality. A growing body of data suggests that hyperactivation of the immune system has been implicated in the pathophysiology of major depressive disorder. Several proinflammatory cytokines, such as tumor necrosis factor-α and interleukin-1, have been found to be significantly increased in patients with major depressive disorder.[51] Age-associated alterations in immunity are apparent in the innate immune cells of the brain. There is an elevated inflammatory profile in the aging brain consisting of an increased population of reactive glia. A potential consequence of a reactive glial cell population in the brain is an exaggerated inflammatory response to innate immune activation. Even in the absence of detectable disease, the glia population undergoes an age-related transformation that creates a more sensitive brain environment.

An amplified and prolonged inflammatory response in the aging brain promotes protracted behavioral and cognitive impairments, and the behavioral consequences of illness and infection in elderly individuals, if prolonged, can have deleterious effects on mental health. There is an increased prevalence of delirium in elderly individuals who present to the emergency department as a result of infections unrelated to the CNS. Viral or bacterial pneumonia in older adults frequently manifests clinically as delirium, even in the absence of classic pneumonia symptoms.[36]

Both neurophysiologic and neuropsychologic investigations support the general concept that the speed of central processing is reduced with advancing age.[74] The central mechanisms that are involved in the control of balance do not appear to change excessively with age but are more likely to be affected by degenerative neurologic diseases such as Parkinson disease or Alzheimer disease. Age-related changes in the peripheral vestibular system include hair cell receptors that begin to decrease at the age of 30 years, and by age 55 to 60 years there is a loss of the vestibular receptor ganglion cells. The myelinated nerve cells of the vestibular system show up to a 40% loss. Partial loss of vestibular function in the older population can lead to symptoms of dizziness, with less ability of the nervous system to accommodate the loss compared with younger people.

In addition to vestibular losses, there is concomitant loss of other sensory inputs relating to balance and mobility, including vision and somatosensation. Maintaining equilibrium, or balance, requires a multimodal system integrating vestibular, visual, and somatosensory signals. The integration of these signals in the CNS coordinates multiple output responses, including eye movement, postural correction, motor skill, and conscious awareness of spatial orientation. There are longer response latencies and delayed reaction times. Vision changes include loss of acuity, decreased peripheral fields, and loss of depth perception. The loss of input from this combination is slow, with compensation developing through the years.[16] Eventually a loss of functional reserve, or redundant function, that is normally present in virtually all physiologic systems is seen with aging. There is an apparent decrease in the ability to integrate conflicting sensory information to determine appropriate postural responses. Changes occur as well in motor output that may contribute to the loss of balance and mobility.[14] Although the response patterns are the same in young and old people, with responses being activated in the stretched ankle muscle and radiating up to the thigh, this response is disrupted in some older people, with the proximal muscles being activated before the distal muscles. In the older person there appears to be more cocontraction of muscles around the ankle as a result of perturbation.[92]

There are data showing alterations in peripheral and central autonomic nerve activity and decreases in neurotransmitter receptor action that lead to diminished autonomic reactivity with decreased control of blood pressure and cerebral blood flow regulation and poorly coordinated autonomic discharge required for bladder function. Strategies for autonomic function improvement and increasing cortical blood flow include walking and somatic afferent stimulation through activities including stroking skin or acupuncture to increase sympathetic, parasympathetic, and central cholinergic activity.[46]

Neurologic disease is more prevalent in older persons, as is the risk of neurologic sequelae as a result of intracranial hemorrhage, subdural hematoma, and neoplasms. Awareness of the signs and symptoms of these disorders is essential. The therapist may be able to identify a disease or the potential for a disorder that may manifest during a treatment session.

## DIAGNOSIS

### Clinical Localization

Clinical localization is the first step to differential diagnosis for an individual with neurologic disease. Coupling the time course of the illness with the clinical localization is the essence of neurology. The history of the onset and nature of the symptoms is critical to establish the diagnosis related to the neurologic disorder. In many cases the clinician is able to generate a hypothesis based on the history and symptoms regarding the site in the nervous system that has been affected and the nature of the lesion. A complete history of the nature of the symptoms is also critical to determining which diagnostic tools will provide the most accurate differential diagnosis and best determine the cause.

The examination of a client with neurologic dysfunction often begins with mental status changes. Alterations of consciousness and disturbances of higher brain function give the clinician clues about the nature of the disease process and the location of damage within the brain (Table 28.6).[100]

Motor and sensory changes will also reflect the type, level, and extent of damage to the system in the case of both disease and trauma. Understanding the typical motor and sensory changes associated with a particular disease or disorder directs the evaluation. For example, knowing that ALS involves both upper and lower motor signs may help the clinician when an individual with this otherwise perplexing condition presents in the clinic. Understanding the functional deficits related to each condition can also lead the clinician to a diagnosis. Gait disorders are often representative of the level or location of damage within the nervous system.

The diagnosis of neurologic disorders remains a clinical specialty, although the use of sophisticated imaging and measurement of neural function provides insight into the pathologic state of the nervous system. With the development of imaging such as fMRI and noninvasive brain stimulation techniques, there is hope for new strategies focused on enhancing neurologic recovery and functional ability, even in chronic conditions.[10] The following are examples of diagnostic tests currently performed.

### Computed Tomography

Computed tomography (CT) scans provide a rapid and relatively inexpensive snapshot of the CNS, and damage within tissue can be identified. Disorders affecting blood flow, MS, neoplasm, and infection can be identified with these scans. CT is an excellent study to evaluate for acute intracranial hemorrhage, particularly in the subarachnoid space. Active bleeding may be detected in either epidural or subdural hemorrhages as a relative lucency, which is commonly referred to as the "swirl" sign. Edema from excitotoxic damage associated with infarct or diffuse anoxia can be seen representing intracellular fluid, and vasogenic edema is the abnormal accumulation of extracellular fluid in the white matter that looks like fingers following the white matter tracts. Evaluation of ventricular size and symmetry can be done by CT. Enlargement of the temporal horns out of proportion to the lateral ventricular bodies is helpful in recognizing early hydrocephalus. CT can be helpful to follow ventricular size after shunting.

CT is very useful for detecting intracranial calcifications, such as those seen in congenital infections, vascular lesions, and metabolic disease. The location and distribution of calcifications is helpful in differentiating these various causes. The identification of calcification in a neoplasm aids in differential diagnosis.[37]

### Magnetic Resonance Imaging

Magnetic resonance imaging (MRI) signal patterns are recognizable with common diseases, such as cerebral edema, neoplasm, abscess, infarcts, or demyelinating processes. MRI is the study of choice to evaluate all lesions in the brain and spine. However, CT is more sensitive than MRI for the evaluation of calcifications and subtle fractures and remains pivotal in the diagnosis of acute subarachnoid hemorrhage. MRI is the modality of choice for detecting congenital malformations. Infection of the spine is also better evaluated by MRI.

MRI cannot be performed in individuals who have intraorbital foreign bodies, pacemakers, or non–MRI-compatible implants, such as artificial heart valves, vascular clips, cochlear implants, or ventilators. To obtain valid images, a patient must lie still in the scanner, which may require sedation for some individuals with cognitive impairment or intolerance for small spaces.

### Functional Magnetic Resonance Imaging

fMRI is based on blood oxygenation level–dependent imaging of the brain and provides evidence of cerebral activation during any given task (e.g., motor, visual, or cognitive), typically in contrast to a resting or control state. fMRI shows both neuroanatomy and functions of the brain and is a brain-mapping tool for clinicians, researchers, and basic scientists. A noninvasive procedure with no known risks, fMRI is used for presurgical mapping of motor, language, and memory functions and allows neurosurgeons to be aware of, and to navigate, the precise location of cortices and structural anomalies from space-occupying lesions.[43]

### Positron Emission Tomography

Positron emission tomography (PET) and single photon emission CT can show cellular activity via regional blood

**Table 28.6** Useful Studies in the Evaluation of Disorder of Level of Consciousness

| Syndrome | Neuroimaging | Electrophysiology | Fluid and Tissue Analysis | Neuropsychologic Tests |
|---|---|---|---|---|
| Bilateral cortical dysfunction; confusion and delirium | Usually normal; may show atrophy; rarely bilateral chronic subdural hematoma or evidence of herpes simplex encephalitis; dural enhancement in meningitis, especially neoplastic meningitides | Diffuse slowing; often, FIRDA; in herpes simplex encephalitis, PLEDS | Blood or urine analyses may reveal etiology; CSF may show evidence of infection or neoplastic cells | In mild cases, difficulty with attention (e.g., trail making tests); in more severe cases, formal testing is not possible |
| Diencephalic dysfunction | Lesion(s) in or displacement of diencephalon; also displays mass displacing the diencephalon | Usually, diffuse slowing; rarely, FIRDA; in displacement syndromes, effect of the mass producing displacement (e.g., focal delta activity, loss of faster rhythms) | Usually not helpful | Usually not obtained |
| Midbrain dysfunction | Lesion(s) in the midbrain or displacing it | Usually, diffuse slowing; alpha coma; evoked response testing may demonstrate failure of conduction above the lesion | Rarely, platelet or coagulation abnormalities | Usually not performed |
| Pontine dysfunction | Lesion(s) producing syndrome; thrombosis of basilar artery | EEG: usually normal; evoked responses usually normal | Rarely, platelet or coagulation abnormalities | Usually not performed |
| Medullary dysfunction | Lesion(s) producing dysfunction | EEG: normal; brainstem auditory and somatosensory evoked responses may show conduction abnormalities | Rarely, platelet or coagulation abnormalities | Usually not performed |
| Herniation syndromes | Lesion(s) producing herniation; appearance of perimesencephalic cistern | Findings related to etiology | Findings related to etiology | Usually not performed |
| Locked-in syndrome | Infarction of basis pontis | EEG and evoked potential studies: normal | Findings related to etiology | Usually not performed |
| Death by brain criteria | Absence of intracranial blood flow above foramen magnum | EEG: electrocerebral silence; evoked potential studies may show peripheral components (e.g., wave I of brainstem auditory evoked response) but no central conduction | Absence of hypnosedative drugs | Not done |
| Psychogenic unresponsiveness | Normal | Normal | Normal | Helpful after patient "awakens" |

*CSF*, Cerebrospinal fluid; *EEG*, electroencephalography; *FIRDA*, frontally predominant intermittent rhythmic delta activity; *PLEDS*, periodic lateralized epileptiform activity.

From Koenigsberg RA, et al: Neuroimaging. In Goetz CG: *Textbook of Clinical Neurology*, ed 2, Philadelphia, 2003, Saunders.

flow in the brain and are used to monitor changes in the brain with functional activity. Both techniques can be used to depict the regional density of a number of neurotransmitters, allowing researchers to better understand the role of different parts of the brain during activity. PET and combined PET/CT provide powerful metabolic and anatomic information together in a single examination.[67] Table 28.7 describes the use of various neuroimaging techniques correlated to anatomic site.

## DaTSCAN

Routine clinical studies with single photon emission CT markers of the presynaptic dopamine transporter

**Table 28.7** Neuroimaging Applications in Diagnosis and Therapy

| Technique | Diffuse or Multifocal Cerebral | Focal Cerebral | Subcortical | Brainstem | Spinal Cord |
|---|---|---|---|---|---|
| Plain film | Neoplasm<br>Metabolic<br>Congenital | Neoplasm | Not useful | Not useful | Trauma<br>Neoplasm<br>Degenerative |
| CT | Hemorrhage<br>Calcification<br>Infarct<br>Neoplasm<br>Inflammation<br>Vascular | Hemorrhage<br>Calcification<br>Infarct<br>Neoplasm<br>Inflammation<br>Vascular | Hemorrhage<br>Calcification<br>Infarct<br>Neoplasm<br>Inflammation<br>Vascular | Hemorrhage<br>Calcification<br>Infarct<br>Neoplasm<br>Inflammation<br>Vascular | Hemorrhage<br>Calcification<br>Neoplasm<br>Inflammation |
| MRI | Neoplasm<br>Inflammation<br>Hemorrhage<br>Vascular<br>White matter disease<br>Congenital<br>Infarct | Neoplasm<br>Inflammation<br>Hemorrhage<br>Vascular<br>White matter disease<br>Congenital<br>Infarct | Neoplasm<br>Inflammation<br>Hemorrhage<br>Vascular<br>White matter disease<br>Infarct | Neoplasm<br>Inflammatory<br>Hemorrhage<br>Vascular<br>White matter disease<br>Infarct | Neoplasm<br>Inflammatory<br>Hemorrhage<br>Vascular<br>White matter disease<br>Infarct |
| Myelography | Not useful | Not useful | Not useful | Not useful | Degenerative<br>Neoplasm<br>Hematoma<br>Inflammatory<br>Vascular<br>Congenital |
| Angiography | Mass effect<br>Vasculopathy<br>Atherosclerosis | AVM tumor<br>Aneurysm<br>Atherosclerosis | AVM tumor<br>Aneurysm<br>Atherosclerosis | AVM tumor<br>Aneurysm<br>Atherosclerosis | AVM |
| Ultrasonography | Hemorrhage (neonatal)<br>Congenital<br>Neoplasm<br>Infection<br>Vascular | Hemorrhage (neonatal)<br>Congenital<br>Neoplasm<br>Infection<br>Vascular | Hemorrhage (neonatal)<br>Congenital<br>Neoplasm | Congenital<br>Neoplasm | Congenital<br>Neoplasm |
| PET-SPECT | Vascular<br>Neoplasm<br>Infection<br>Degenerative<br>Trauma | Vascular<br>Neoplasm<br>Infection<br>Degenerative<br>Trauma | Vascular<br>Neoplasm<br>Infection<br>Degenerative<br>Trauma | Not useful | Not useful |

*AVM*, Arteriovenous malformation; *CT*, computed tomography; *MRI*, magnetic resonance imaging *PET-SPECT*, positron emission tomography–single photon emission computed tomography.

system (DaT) allow differential diagnosis of neurologic conditions affecting the basal ganglia. Two radiopharmaceuticals, both cocaine analogs labeled with iodine-123, are commercially available under the name of DaTSCAN and demonstrate excellent ability to distinguish patients with Parkinson disease from normal control subjects and other patients with nonparkinsonian tremor, particularly benign essential tremor. The DaT radiotracers show specific uptake in the striatum within the caudate nucleus and putamen, with almost homogeneous distribution in normal control subjects. Patients with benign essential tremor demonstrate similar findings, whereas in individuals with idiopathic Parkinson disease there is marked reduction of tracer uptake in the putamen contralateral to the more affected body side (Fig. 28.22). In patients with dopa-responsive dystonia, the striatal uptake of DaT ligands is clearly normal and distinct from patients with early-onset Parkinson disease.

## Diffusion Tensor Imaging

Diffusion tensor imaging is capable of quantifying anisotropy of diffusion of water in white matter, allowing analysis of structural integrity of white matter tracts. Diffusion is *isotropic* when it occurs with the same intensity in all directions. It is *anisotropic* when it occurs preferentially in one direction, as along the longitudinal axis of axons, and will do so at higher levels if all the axons are intact. In normal white matter, diffusion anisotropy is high because diffusion is greatest parallel to the course of the nerve fiber tracts. These images can also be color coded based on the direction a fiber is traveling (e.g., anterior to posterior, medial to lateral), allowing for spectacular visualization of nerve fiber tracts (Fig. 28.23). Any disruption of a given nerve fiber tract (e.g., MS, trauma, gliosis) will reduce anisotropy, and the disruption of the white matter tract can be visualized.

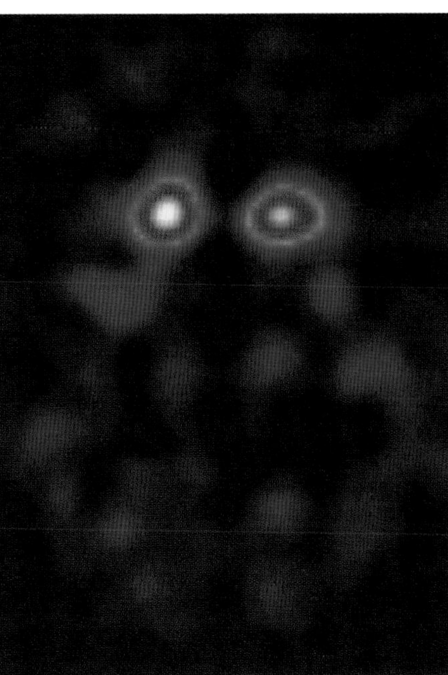

**Figure 28.22**

**Transverse slice from a single photon emission computed tomography study with β-FP-CIT in a 61-year-old patient with idiopathic Parkinson disease.** There is marked reduction of the tracer uptake in the putamen, worse in the left hemisphere contralateral to the more affected body side. (From Ell PJ, Gambhir S: *Nuclear medicine in clinical diagnosis and treatment*, ed 3, London, 2004, Churchill Livingstone.)

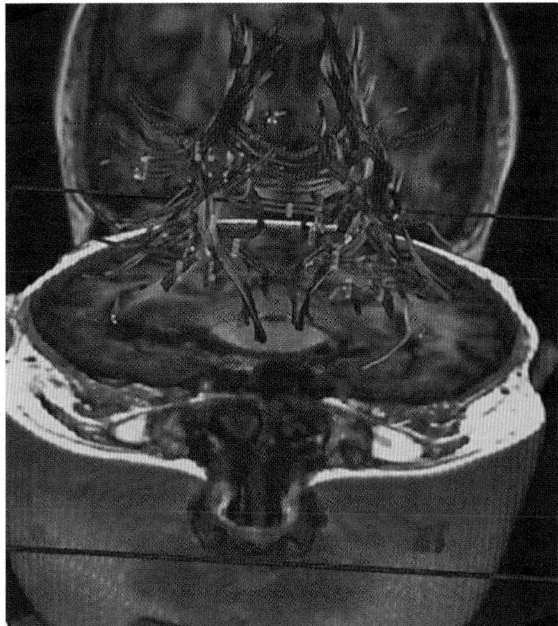

**Figure 28.23**

**Diffusion tensor image obtained with a 3-Tesla scanner.** (From Daroff RB: *Bradley's neurology in clinical practice*, ed 6, Philadelphia, 2012, Saunders.)

## Electroencephalography

Cerebral ischemia produces neuronal dysfunction, leading to slowing of frequencies or reduced amplitude in the EEG tracing. These changes may be generalized (global ischemia) or regional (focal ischemia). The depth of ischemia is associated with the severity of EEG changes. EEG cannot assess the whole cerebral cortex, however, and is less reliable at assessing subcortical structures. Chapter 36 further describes the uses of EEG in recording brain activity.

## Evoked Potentials

Electrophysiologic evoked potentials measure brain responses to various forms of stimulation (somatosensory, auditory, visual) and are used as a diagnostic adjunct to more conventional imaging for various neurologic conditions.[84] Motor evoked potentials are also used during surgical interventions to monitor motor pathways that are at risk of damage during a procedure. In addition, stimulation centrally at the cortex or spinal cord may be used to evaluate motor responses. Table 28.8 provides a summary of the features and uses of various evoked potential tests. These tests are used to test the integrity of peripheral nervous system and CNS pathways, as typical amplitudes and latencies for various forms of stimulation are well known. However, many other diagnostic tests are easier to conduct, so these tests are typically used in circumstances that present challenges, such as when MRI cannot be used (metal implants) or when a patient is nonresponsive (e.g., coma), or may be used to clarify impairments in demyelinating or degenerative diseases (e.g., MS, ALS) or in spinal cord lesions that affect sensory and motor pathways (e.g., spinal stenosis, transverse myelitis, syringomyelia). The use of vestibular evoked myogenic potentials is a growing area to diagnose of vestibular nerve impairment, and testing is often conducted by audiologists. Vestibular evoked myogenic potential testing targets the otolith organs of the inner ear specifically and so may be a part of the diagnostic work-up for patients who are referred for vestibular rehabilitation.[110]

## Transcranial Doppler Ultrasonography

Transcranial Doppler ultrasonography uniquely measures local blood flow velocity in the proximal portions of large intracranial arteries. Hemodynamic compromise is inferred when there is reduction in mean flow velocities or when there is slow flow acceleration. In addition, transcranial Doppler ultrasonography can detect cerebral microembolic signals, reflecting the presence of gaseous or particulate matter in the cerebral artery. Solid, fat, gas, or air materials in flowing blood are larger and of different composition and have different acoustic impedance than surrounding red blood cells. Thus the Doppler ultrasound beam is both reflected and scattered at the interface between the embolus and blood, resulting in an increased intensity of the received Doppler signal. A completely accurate and reliable characterization of embolus size and composition, however, is not yet possible with current technology.

## Near-Infrared Spectroscopy

In brain tissue the venous oxygen saturation predominates (70% to 80%), and cerebral oximetry relies on this fact.

**Table 28.8** Evoked Potentials

| Type of Evoked Potential | Purpose and Anatomic Targets | Examples of Diagnostic or Other Purposes |
|---|---|---|
| Somatosensory evoked potentials (SEPs or SSEPs)[a] | Assess integrity of peripheral or central proprioceptive pathways (dorsal column/medical lemniscus) by providing a sensory input (electrical stimulation) and measuring response at cortex | Spinal cord integrity testing (spinal stenosis, spinal tumor); chronic inflammatory sensory polyradiculopathy; to determine prognosis in postanoxic coma |
| Visual evoked potentials (VEPs)[b] | Stimulation of visual fields with the use of a shifting checkerboard stimulus, recording P100 responses in the occipital cortex, targets central visual pathways | Optic chiasm lesions; optic neuritis in MS; may identify functional impairments in conductivity vs. identifying MRI lesion; less expensive than MRI |
| Brainstem evoked potentials (BAEPs)[c] | Assess peripheral and central auditory pathways by delivering click in one ear that activates CN VIII, cochlear nucleus, superior olivary nucleus, lateral lemniscus, inferior colliculus | Multiple waveforms are produced in auditory cortex for hearing loss testing in infants, CNS lesions in auditory CN VIII, pathways in brainstem; can be used in nonresponsive patients (infants, coma); acoustic neuroma |
| Motor evoked potentials (MEPs)[d] | Commonly used to monitor central motor pathways that are at risk during surgery, may provide stimulation centrally (cortex or spinal cord) and measure motor responses to examine brain circuitry | May be used for diagnosis of demyelinating or degenerative diseases (MS, Parkinson disease, ALS, transverse myelitis) |
| Vestibular evoked myogenic potentials (VEMPs)[e] | Presentation of acoustic stimulus results in motor responses of 2 types: cervical VEMPs (cVEMPs) stimulate saccule with muscle response at ipsilateral sternocleidomastoid; ocular VEMPs (oVEMPs) stimulates utricle response at contralateral inferior orbit; tests vestibular labyrinth, otolith organs, and vestibular nerve | Differentiates superior vs. inferior vestibular nerve function or damage |

[a]SSEP/SEP Watson JC, Carter JL Somatosensory evoked potentials. In Rubin DI, Daube JR: *Clinical neurophysiology*, ed 4, Oxford, 2016, Oxford University Press.
[b]VEP. Carter JL Visual evoked potentials. In Rubin DI, Daube JR: *Clinical neurophysiology*, ed 4, Oxford, 2016, Oxford University Press.
[c]BAEP in Central Disorders Carter JL Central disorders. In Rubin DI, Daube JR: *Clinical neurophysiology*, ed 4, Oxford, 2016, Oxford University Press.
[d]MEP Strommen JA, Boon AJ Motor evoked potentials. In Rubin DI, Daube JR: *Clinical neurophysiology*, ed 4, Oxford, 2016, Oxford University Press.
[e]Vertigo and Imbalance Zapala DA Vertigo and imbalance. In Rubin DI, Daube JR: *Clinical neurophysiology*, ed 4, Oxford, 2016, Oxford University Press.
*ALS*, Amyotrophic lateral sclerosis; *CN VIII*, eighth cranial (vestibulocochlear) nerve; *CNS*, central nervous system; *MRI*, magnetic resonance imaging; *MS*, multiple sclerosis.

Near-infrared spectroscopy uses light optical spectroscopy in the near-infrared range to evaluate brain oxygen saturation by measuring regional cerebral venous oxygen saturation.

### Transcranial Magnetic Stimulation

Transcranial magnetic stimulation is a brain stimulation technique that allows study of the physiology of the CNS, identifying the functional role of specific brain structures and, more recently, exploring large-scale network dynamics. Transcranial magnetic stimulation has diagnostic value as well as therapeutic potential for several neuropsychiatric disorders. The stimulation involves restricted cortical and subcortical regions and, when used in combination with a visually guided technique, results in improved accuracy to target specific areas, including functional maps of the motor and visual cortex. New combinations of these techniques in conjunction with neuroimaging will further advance the utility of their application.[18,83]

While technological advances continue to offer greater resolution and sensitivity with imaging and electrophysiologic techniques (e.g., transcranial magnetic stimulation) as methods to stimulate brain responses, many techniques are used in a research context, as the time and expense to conduct such tests preclude their routine use in clinical practice. If additional testing is used, it is often to complement structural imaging (MRI) that is increasingly able to identify abnormalities in the CNS.

## INTERVENTION

Intervention is based on an understanding of the level and type of neuronal dysfunction, the current phase of the condition, prognosis for improvement, and the needs and wishes of the patient and family. Condition-specific interventions will be described in subsequent chapters; however, treatments that address methods to control CNS damage will be reviewed.

### Methods to Control Central Nervous System Damage

Damage or disease of the nervous system often results in changes in the production and uptake of neurotransmitters. Many important drugs that alter nervous system function act by selective interaction with neurotransmitter receptors. Drugs that act at synapses either enhance or block the action of these neurotransmitters. Most neurotransmitters with a prominent role in brain function produce very brief receptor-mediated actions at specific groups of synapses. A few neurotransmitters are more prolonged and act more widely throughout the extracellular space. The combined action of both a briefly acting neurotransmitter and a more enduring neurotransmitter produces a modulation of postsynaptic neuronal activity. Pharmacologic strategies are aimed at modulation of neurotransmitter synthesis, release, reuptake, and degradation.[48] Some drugs mediate inhibition of neurotransmitter release by acting at presynaptic receptors. Opiates are one group of drugs that act by the inhibition of neurotransmitter release. Drugs used to control excessive tone in specific muscle groups often work by inhibiting neurotransmitter release. Anesthetic drugs modify the actions of neurotransmitter receptors by changing the membranes of cells on or within which the receptors are located.[19]

Drug therapy can stimulate neurotransmitter release. Drugs aimed at maintaining neurotransmitter activity in the synaptic cleft can be useful in neuromuscular junction diseases. Another way to regulate the level of neurotransmitters is to influence the rate of chemical degradation. Drugs can inhibit the breakdown of certain elements that may be broken down by natural processes such as oxidation. One action of these drugs is to prolong the efficacy of released neurotransmitters by inhibiting their degradation.[102] An example of this process is the regulation of dopamine. Dopamine activity can be increased by four mechanisms: increased synthesis, increased release, prolonged neurotransmitter activity and direct receptor simulation.

Synthesis of the neurotransmitter can be increased by giving levo dopa because it is the product beyond the rate-limiting enzyme, and there is ordinarily an abundant amount of aromatic amino acid decarboxylase in the CNS. When levo dopa is combined with a peripherally active decarboxylase inhibitor, it is delivered across the blood-brain barrier and can be used to synthesize central dopamine. Drugs such as amphetamine and methylphenidate can increase release.

The normal metabolism of dopamine involves reuptake of dopamine into the presynaptic cell, with subsequent metabolism by two enzymes, MAO and COMT. Prolongation of dopamine activity can be affected by blocking reuptake or altering enzyme activity. Amantadine and possibly some tricyclic antidepressant medications operate on the dopaminergic system through blockade of reuptake. MAO inhibitors and COMT inhibitors for human use also increase dopaminergic activity. Finally, direct activation of the dopamine receptors on the striatal cell can be induced by agonists such as bromocriptine, pergolide, and other drugs. Importantly, orally administered dopamine itself has no place in altering the CNS dopamine levels because, being a positively charged molecule, it cannot cross the blood-brain barrier.[37]

Other drugs protect the cell membrane in the presence of toxins that act on the membrane, such as the toxic effects of the free radicals produced in brain tissue after hypoxia, ischemia, and seizures. Damage to the neuron occurs when the free radical is allowed to penetrate the membrane.[79]

The best defense is to prevent free radical penetrance. Antioxidant therapies are being tested for a variety of neurodegenerative disorders and the sequelae of stroke and spinal cord injury. Oxidative stress has been consistently linked to aging-related neurodegenerative diseases. As oxidative stress invariably contributes to various forms of cell death, a better understanding of how antioxidant defenses are maintained in particular brain cells will probably help to develop protective strategies in degenerative insults specifically affecting these cells.[38] Optimal functioning of the CNS and peripheral nervous system depends on a constant supply of appropriate nutrients.[54] Ongoing studies are looking at the above-mentioned natural substances, as well as manufactured substances that will provide antioxidant effects or increase free radical scavenging. There is great hope that substances that will slow down the destruction related to oxidative stress will prove to be curative for progressive diseases of the CNS, as well as other degenerative processes associated with connective tissue, neoplasm, and aging.[8] There are similar cellular mechanisms underlying neuronal loss, neurodegeneration, and disease that share common mechanisms, such as protein aggregation, oxidative injury, inflammation, apoptosis, and mitochondrial injury.

Although cerebrovascular disease has different causes than the neurodegenerative disorders, many of the same pathophysiology mechanisms come into play following a stroke. Novel therapies that target each of these mechanisms may be effective in decreasing the risk of disease, abating symptoms, or slowing down their progression. Although most of these therapies are experimental and require further investigation, a few seem to offer promise.[98] Brain training, specialized exercises designed to keep the brain functioning at the highest levels possible, is gaining momentum in controlling the effects of aging and has potential to impact the training to maximize brain activity after injury or in relationship to progressive disease.

*Stem cells* are unspecialized living cells that have the capacity to renew themselves for long periods of time through cell division. Under certain physiologic or experimental conditions, they can be induced to become cells with special functions, such as the beating cells of the heart muscle or the insulin-producing cells of the pancreas. *Embryonic stem cells* are derived from embryos that develop from eggs that have been fertilized in vitro and then donated for research purposes with the informed consent of the donors. The embryos from which human embryonic stem cells are derived are typically 4 or 5 days old and consist of a hollow microscopic collection of cells called the *blastocyst.* An *adult stem cell* is an undifferentiated cell found among differentiated cells in a tissue or organ. The primary roles of adult stem cells in a living organism are to maintain and repair the tissue in which they are found. Some researchers now use the term *somatic stem cell* instead of adult stem cell. In contrast to embryonic stem cells, which are defined by their origin, the origin of adult stem cells in mature tissues is unknown. A single adult stem cell could have the ability to generate a line of genetically identical cells, or *clones*.[2]

There is evidence for the impact of immune system dysfunction in these diseases despite the blood-brain barrier protection of the CNS from the direct effects of autoimmune responses. Identification of immune system elements is leading researchers toward an understanding of the role of the immune system in diseases such as MS, ALS, Parkinson disease, and Alzheimer disease.

Use of catheters to deliver drugs directly into the cerebrospinal fluid or brain tissue has enhanced the ability to deliver drugs that act directly on the neuron. This approach has been well refined, for instance, in the use of intrathecal baclofen delivered through a pump implanted in the patient's abdomen that is used for intractable problems with spasticity after spinal cord injury, cerebral palsy, and brain injury. Although more sophisticated catheters have been developed that can deliver the drugs in measured doses, the maintenance of such systems requires careful and consistent medical follow-up.

### Treatment of Nonneural Dysfunction

Many drugs used to treat neurologic disorders influence nonneural tissue, including cerebral blood vessels and glia. Cerebral edema can increase the permeability of the blood-brain barrier, causing an increase in fluid within the brain. The resulting compression of brain tissue can be life threatening. Drugs such as mannitol that control cerebral edema or drugs that provide diuresis can help preserve neuronal function. In demyelinating disease, antiinflammatory and immunosuppressive drugs are used to preserve the function of the glial cells that produce the myelin sheath.

For some viruses that invade the CNS, there is replication of cells in nonneural tissue. Use of drugs that inhibit RNA or DNA synthesis can prevent viral replication without disrupting neuronal integrity. Acyclovir, used in the treatment of herpes encephalitis, is an example of this type of drug.

In infants and children, drug metabolism is altered, which must be considered whenever administering drugs that act on the nervous system. Concomitant illness and fever will further alter drug metabolism. An immature blood-brain barrier can also affect the absorption of drugs into brain tissue. When anticonvulsants are administered, close monitoring of blood levels is necessary.

## PROGNOSIS

Prognosis is the keystone to management of neurologic disorders because it links diagnosis to outcomes and identifies need for treatment. Prognostic studies can also identify if available treatment is ineffective. In addition, these studies can indicate which diseases have an important impact on function or disability.[60]

Disability resulting from neurologic disease and trauma can be extensive, and care of these clients often requires use of limited resources (i.e., time and money). With the tremendous advances made in the emergent medical care of trauma victims and people with significant neurologic disease, the number of people living with a neurologic disorder is increasing at a steady rate.[6]

Permanent or progressive impairments can be demoralizing to clients and their families. Clients must reorganize their perspectives to learn alternative ways of regaining as much control as possible over life activities. Success builds a sense of efficacy, and failure undermines self-worth. Tackling challenges in successive attainable steps will lead to further competencies in associated tasks. When individuals see others with similar disabilities perform successfully, they may have increased confidence in their own abilities. The persuasion of health care providers and caregivers can boost effort but must be realistic. Perceived self-efficacy can influence the course of health outcomes and functional status. The prognosis for an individual should consider both the social and the cognitive status of the individual in relationship to the diagnosis.[4]

The economic evaluation of health care reflects the complexity of the disease treatment process and the value of health effects. Policy makers are demanding information about the economic outcomes of diseases and their treatments. Research methodologies oriented toward cost-of-illness and cost-benefit analysis have emerged. Clinicians should be involved in this analysis to maintain perspective, especially in catastrophic and degenerative processes.[55]

Several chronic neurologic disease states, such as Alzheimer disease, are associated with elevated secretion of stress hormones such as cortisol. Stress also can trigger or exacerbate symptom onset and perhaps progression of chronic illness, such as Parkinson disease. Thus neurologic disease states can occur within a context of elevated glucocorticoids, which may have profound influences on recovery and neuroplasticity. In addition, abnormal regulation of glucocorticoid release is associated with many affective disorders, such as depression and PTSD, that are overrepresented in populations with neurologic disease. Release of glucocorticoids, however, also can occur in anticipation of adverse events. Anticipatory release of glucocorticoids occurs in the absence of a frank physical stimulus, keyed by memories or instinctual predispositions.[86]

The use of common outcome measures for patient management is an important element of neurologic practice. The Academy of Neurologic Physical Therapy (ANPT) has advocated a common set of measures for use with neurologic patients as a starting point to address the gait and balance impairments that are often the focus of intervention. Disease-specific measures have also been reviewed by ANPT task force groups in multiple areas, with specific recommendations for measures made based on clinical setting, phase or chronicity of condition, and functional status. Measures of health-related quality of life address the impact of health on physical, social, and psychologic aspects of life. The particular scale may address issues related to a specific population or may be sensitive to a clinical intervention. The therapist should be familiar with the measurement tools typically used during intervention for a condition or disease. These tools are described in the subsequent chapters in this section.[6]

## Physiologic Basis for the Recovery of Function

After injury to the nervous system, there are changes in the structure and function of the neurons. In some instances, the changes can lead to further damage, whereas other changes facilitate recovery.

*Diaschisis*, or neural shock, occurs when there is injury to a nerve and disruption of the neural pathway that extends a distance from the site of injury. When the neurons distal to the injury regain function, which may be soon after the injury, partial function may return.

Injury may be secondary to either swelling of the axon or edema in the surrounding tissue that blocks *synaptic activity* in the injured neurons, as well as that in the surrounding area. With reduction of the edema, function may return. This is the reason that medications that reduce edema are often given in the context of diffuse brain swelling.

When there is a loss of presynaptic function in one area, the postsynaptic target cells for that area may become more sensitive to neurotransmitters that are now produced in lower concentrations. The compensatory mechanism is known as *denervation supersensitivity*. *Regenerative synaptogenesis* occurs when injured axons begin sprouting. *Collateral sprouting* is the process of neighboring axons sprouting to connect with sites that were previously innervated by the injured axon.

Suppression of a response to a stimulus is considered habituation, whereas sensitization is an increased response to a stimulus, usually related to noxious stimuli or pain. Adaptation is the ability to modify a motor response based on changes in the sensory environment or input received.

Long-term potentiation occurs when a weak input and a strong input arrive at a dendrite at the same time. The weak stimulus is enhanced by the strong stimulus. With repeated activation of combined stimuli, there is an increase in the presynaptic transmitter associated with the stimulus. After the long-term potentiation has been established, the weak input will elicit a stronger response than it had initially.[57] Long-term potentiation is a key element for change in learning and also thought to drive structural change.

The characteristics of a lesion will have a profound effect on recovery from a brain injury. Small lesions in a location where there is little nervous system redundancy, such as the brainstem, may in fact be as devastating as large lesions of the cerebral cortex, where adjacent structures or contralesional structures may be able to take over functions. Cerebellar damage can affect both learning and memory of movements. Lesions that occur gradually, such as a slow-growing tumor, allow the nervous system to gradually compensate for change and thereby cause less disruption of function than lesions that occur all at once, such as a massive ischemic stroke. Advanced age will adversely affect the return of function. Studies show that a person's prior level of activity and environment will affect the rate and extent of recovery. An enriched environment will positively affect recovery when it is available, either before the insult or during the recovery period.

Redistribution of cortical mapping is seen after a lesion in the brain.[13] These changes may involve unmasking of previously nonfunctional synaptic connections from adjacent areas or result in neighboring structures taking on function. It is clear that both sensory and motor maps in the cortex are constantly changing according to input from the environment. In addition, the brain appears to increase use of ipsilateral pathways after a lesion that affects one side.[80]

Neural modifiability or adaptation may be seen as a change in the organization of connections among neurons and is often referred to as plasticity.[92] The above-described elements are active in this process, including genetic coding, neuronal networks, individual synapses, and neurotransmitters. Physiologic studies suggest that motor relearning and recovery of function may be accomplished through the same neural mechanisms and reflect the plasticity of the brain. Learning alters our capability to perform an appropriate motor act by changing the effectiveness of the neural pathways used and may also modify the anatomic connections to accomplish the activity.

Learning involves storage of memory and can occur in all parts of the brain, with both parallel and hierarchic processing. The area of representation within the brain becomes specialized for both inputs and outputs. Areas of the brain used during the early phase of learning movement are different from those used once a skill is learned. Initially, more areas of the brain are active, as skill develops both the number of neurons firing and location of activity change. The use of sensory input is increased in the early stages of learning. The prefrontal areas are also more active in the learning phase and become less active during automatic movements.[13] The stimuli repeatedly excite cortical neuron populations, and the neurons progressively grow in numbers. Repetition will lead to greater specificity, and the responses become stronger. With skill acquisition, sensory feedback appears to be less critical.

Control of learning comes from many areas of the CNS working together. The area involved may depend on a number of variables associated with the type of learning taking place and is influenced by the environment. The cortex is involved in learning through sensorimotor integration. It is theorized that distributed groups of neurons act as a cortical engram, or memory trace, and are composed of multiple functional groupings. Thus when an activity is repeated and stored in memory, the engrams trigger groups of cells that fire synchronously during movement. These engrams appear to influence the precision, speed, and accuracy of movement and may be described as a motor program.[57]

The limbic system is critical to the learning phase because it generates need-directed motor activity and communicates the intent to the rest of the brain. The limbic system is a critical part of the neural representation necessary for memory that includes the cortex and thalamus.

The cerebellum is active during procedural learning. A possible mechanism is through the influence of the climbing fibers on the mossy fibers with eventual change in the output fibers, the Purkinje fibers.[99] The lateral cerebellum affects cognition through its relationship to the frontal areas active during cognitive processes.[69,85]

The basal ganglia appear to be highly involved in the cognitive aspects of motor behavior, although the level of contribution remains unclear. Habit formation appears to be associated with functions of the basal ganglia, and the control of internally generated movement here appears to be a part of the motor learning continuum.[57]

SPECIAL IMPLICATIONS FOR THE THERAPIST 28.1

## *Motor Learning Strategies: Neuroplasticity*

Comorbid impairments should always be considered, as well as the individual's prior health status, age, motivation, and established life practices. In every case, it is important to remember that the focus of intervention should not be so much on the condition that the person has, but rather on the person who has the condition. For maximal effectiveness, CNS injury should be treated as soon as possible beyond the initial injury phase, when the chance of exacerbating cellular damage has passed. The location of the injury should drive the intervention. The interaction between the client with neurologic dysfunction and the therapist is critical for optimal motor learning to take place. To elicit the highest level of function within the motor system and allow insight regarding the program, goal-directed activities must be included.[103,108]

During the examination and evaluation of disability the therapist should recognize the impairments that contribute to abnormal motor control.[17,71,89,92] Force production, speed of motion, coordination of movement, sensation, and cognition are often affected in neurologic disorders. Identification and modification of environments that can alter responses should be made early in the management process. Difficulty with bowel and bladder control can affect progress with recovery and should be managed with either physical or medical means. Management of nonneural tissue changes secondary to weakness or changes in tone may improve overall outcome. Compensation through the use of substitution devices, assistive devices, and environmental changes should be considered when it is clear that the client will not recover from specific impairments. Reintegration into social and personal roles is of prime importance to clients with neurologic dysfunction. Functional status is the critical outcome marker, and therapists are able to positively influence outcomes in this area. Analysis of the relationships between impairment, functional limitation, and lack of activity/participation is paramount in the rehabilitation process. Intervention focused on task specificity to address underlying impairments that affect function typically improve activity and participation abilities.[56]

The recovery of function after CNS injury involves the reacquisition of complex tasks. Inherent in the recovery of function that has been lost secondary to a neurologic insult is the process of motor relearning, which can be defined as the process of acquisition or modification of movement.[16,92] Motor learning is a modification of behavior by experience and includes perceiving, remembering, thinking, and acting. Behaviorally important inputs are trained through specialization. Interaction and integration of critical systems can facilitate improvement in movement despite anatomic or physiologic deficits in the CNS. Learning-based activities drive reorganization, stimulate neurons from adjacent areas, create new synapses, and may activate neurons in uninjured areas of the brain. Changes in the cortical synaptic structure and function, with increases in dendritic activity as the result of learning, are seen both in the course of child development and after behavioral training in adults. Memory is the retention of these modifications; therefore memory plays a critical role in motor learning.[57] Memory for motor behaviors is developed through explicit and implicit learning and involves different brain regions. Memory associated with fear or other emotional stimuli is thought to involve the amygdala. Memory established through operant conditioning requires the striatum and cerebellum. Memory acquired through classical conditioning and habituation involves changes in the sensory and motor systems included in the learning. Input to the brain is processed into short-term working memory before it is transformed into a more permanent long-term storage.[37]

Motor learning, or the precision of movement, takes place as the client determines the optimal strategy of movement to perform a motor task. There are several models that incorporate defined stages of motor learning involved in skill acquisition. The Fitts and Posner model includes the *cognitive stage* as the first stage, which requires a great deal of thought, experimentation, and intervention. Performance is variable, as is seen in the first attempts to walk after brain injury. In the cognitive stage, the treatment environment is highly structured to allow clients to think and focus on a task. Feedback is given more frequently and may involve more sensory systems. Problem solving is focused on the movement strategies necessary to complete the task. The task may be broken down at this time to work on component parts of the total movement and practiced with repetition.[87,89]

The second stage of skill acquisition is the *associative stage,* represented by refining of the skill. Fewer errors of performance are experienced, and the motor programs elicited are more consistent and efficient. Feedback can be given in a summary format, often after a few trials. The individual will use trial and error to fine-tune the movement. The final stage is the *autonomous stage,* in which the movement is efficient and the need for attention to the activity is decreased. The motor program has been integrated by the basal ganglia, and each component is initiated with little thought. This activity can now be performed in conjunction with another activity.

The need for feedback during each stage of learning is different. The therapist can enhance treatment by providing the correct amount of feedback for the client attempting to perform a task. For a skill to be acquired, learning principles that promote associative and automatic phases need to be incorporated in the intervention. This appears to be related to the practice conditions. It is clear that repetition is required in every stage. Initially blocked or serial practice is used until the learner understands the dynamics of the task. When cognition or memory is limited, it may be better to keep to a blocked practice schedule longer. For a skill to become learned or transferred to other activities, random practice is more effective. Part-task training can be beneficial if the task can naturally be broken down into component parts that create the whole movement when put back together. Differences in input sources, including afferent activity from different components of sensory systems, may create different representational activities within the thalamic nuclei and associated cortical areas. Representation changes can occur as a result of environmental interaction and purposeful behavioral practice.[47,82] Motor learning is reflected in changes to the brain's functional organization as a result of experience, and motor learning also changes sensory systems.[70] Integrated motor imagery practice has been shown to improve function in many areas and shows functional carryover.[20] Use of imagery can be effective throughout the rehabilitation process, especially when tolerance for physical activity is limited.

## Neuroprotection

Aging and neurodegenerative conditions such as Alzheimer disease and Parkinson disease are characterized by tissue and mitochondrial changes that compromise brain function. Alterations can include increased reactive oxygen species production and impaired antioxidant capacity, with a consequent increase in oxidative damage, mitochondrial dysfunction that compromises brain ATP production, and ultimately increases in apoptotic signaling and neuronal death. Among several nonpharmacologic strategies to prevent brain degeneration, physical exercise is an effective strategy to counter mitochondrial dysfunction that is damaging to brain tissue.[61] Forced exercise appears to increase cerebral glycolysis even more than voluntary exercise via increased cerebral metabolism.[53,77]

Animal studies have shown efficacy in neuroprotection related to hippocampal cell survival and further maturation and neurogenesis.[7,11,24] Exercise interventions in individuals with Parkinson disease incorporate goal-based motor skill training to engage cognitive circuitry important in motor learning. With this exercise approach, physical therapy helps with learning through instruction and feedback (reinforcement) and encouragement to perform beyond self-perceived capability.[15,64,76]

The general idea is that exercise that incorporates goal-based motor skill learning improves motor skill performance and can be enhanced through cognitive engagement. Studies suggest that with combined goal-based and aerobic training, improving automatic cognitive motor control may be possible, reducing the attention demands of walking. Aerobic exercise may contribute to more general improvement in brain health and repair through the recruitment of the immune system and/or increasing blood flow and trophic factor signaling. These aerobic exercise benefits are likely to impact connectivity through *priming* the brain environment conducive for promoting synaptic neuroplasticity, leading to altered circuitry. Exercise can restore important circuits in motor behavior by modulating glutamate neurotransmission as well as influencing general brain health. Fig. 28.24 shows the process that is considered to explain the concept of neuroprotection with exercise.

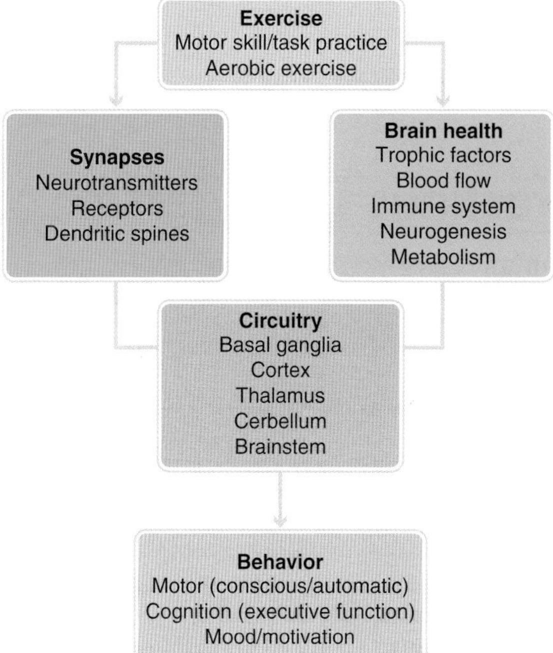


**Figure 28.24**

**Exercise and neuroplasticity in Parkinson disease.** Clinical and basic research studies support the effects of exercise on neuroplasticity in Parkinson disease. Neuroplasticity is a process by which the brain encodes experiences and learns new behaviors and is defined as the modification of existing neural networks by adding or modifying synapses. Evidence is accumulating that both goal-directed and aerobic exercise may strengthen and improve motor circuitry through mechanisms that include, but are not limited to, alterations in dopamine and glutamate neurotransmission, as well as structural modifications of synapses. In addition, exercise may promote neuroprotection of substantia nigra neurons and their existing connections. Finally, exercise-induced alterations in blood flow and general brain health may promote conditions for neuroplasticity important for facilitating motor skill learning, including cognitive and automatic motor control and overall behavioral performance. Although more studies are needed, taken together these findings are supportive of a disease-modifying effect of exercise in Parkinson disease. (Adapted from Petzinger GM, et al: Exercise-enhanced neuroplasticity targeting motor and cognitive circuitry in Parkinson's disease. *Lancet Neurol* 12:716–726, 2013.)

## REFERENCES

To enhance this text and add value for the reader, all references are included in the enhanced ebook on Student Consult that accompanies this textbook. The reader can view the reference source and access it online whenever possible.

# CHAPTER 29

# Infectious Disorders of the Central Nervous System

APRIL M. XAYAVONG • KENDA S. FULLER

## OVERVIEW

Infection of the central nervous system (CNS) remains relatively rare in that many protective responses limit the access of harmful organisms to the nervous tissue. However, neurologic infections are a major cause of mortality and morbidity worldwide. Bacterial infections can be serious and life-threatening. Biologic adaptations of infectious agents and altered modes of transmission present new challenges. Drug-resistant strains create new threats, and travel has increased the exposure to both viruses and bacteria that can cause infection of the nervous system.[20,43]

Despite protective mechanisms, once there is access to the brain, viruses produce a large range of neuropathologic conditions, including oncogenic states producing astrocytomas.[65] CNS infections can affect the brain parenchyma, directly causing abscess. Remote infectious processes such as bacterial endocarditis resulting in infected emboli can cause infectious intracranial aneurysms.[50] Sepsis can cause diffuse, multifactorial involvement of the CNS, including invasion of the meninges with resulting meningitis.[64] The cerebrospinal fluid (CSF) can be contaminated when an object penetrates the meninges. This is often a result of trauma or a neurosurgical procedure.[11] Trauma to the front of the face that causes damage or fracture of nasal structures or the cribriform plate can lead to infection in the CSF. Infection of the inner ear can spread to the brain via the CSF.[53] Disease spread by mosquitoes has been linked to neurologic conditions such as microcephaly and Guillain-Barré syndrome (GBS).[75] Prion diseases can be spread to humans by infected meat products, resulting in abnormal folding of proteins in the brain.[34]

## MENINGITIS

### Definition

In meningitis the meninges of the brain and spinal cord become inflamed. The three layers of the meningeal membranes (dura mater, arachnoid, and pia mater) can be involved. The relationship of the meninges to the brain tissue is shown in Fig. 29.1. The pia mater and arachnoid become congested and opaque. The inflammation extends into the first and second layers of the cortex and spinal cord and can produce thrombosis of the cortical veins. There is an increased chance of infarction, and the scar tissue can restrict the flow of CSF, especially around the base of the brain. This block of CSF can result in hydrocephalus or a subarachnoid cyst. Stretch or pressure on the meninges will cause the cardinal sign of headache.[2]

### Incidence

The estimated incidence of meningitis is 2 to 6 per 100,000 adults per year in developed countries and is up to 10 times higher in less-developed countries. The incidence of bacterial meningitis is highest among children younger than 1 year of age. Extremely high rates are found in Native Americans, Alaskan Natives, and Australian aboriginals, suggesting that genetic factors play a role in susceptibility. Other risk factors include acquired or congenital immunodeficiencies; hemoglobinopathies such as sickle cell disease; functional or anatomic asplenia; and crowding such as occurs in some households, day care centers, or college and military dormitories. A CSF leak resulting from a congenital anomaly or following a basilar skull fracture increases the risk of meningitis, especially infection caused by *Streptococcus pneumoniae*.

Enteroviruses cause meningitis, with peaks during summer and fall. Enteroviruses are a group of RNA viruses that typically start in the gastrointestinal tract and at times spread to the CNS. These infections are more prevalent among people of low socioeconomic status, young children, and immunocompromised persons. The prevalence of arboviral meningitis is determined by geographic distribution and seasonal activity of the arthropod (mosquito) vectors. An arbovirus refers to any group of viruses that is spread by mosquitoes, ticks, or other arthropods. In the United States, most arboviral infections occur during the late spring to fall.[42]

### Etiologic and Risk Factors

Vaccines developed in the past 30 years to protect against the development of meningitis, primarily against *Haemophilus influenzae* type B (Hib) infection, have

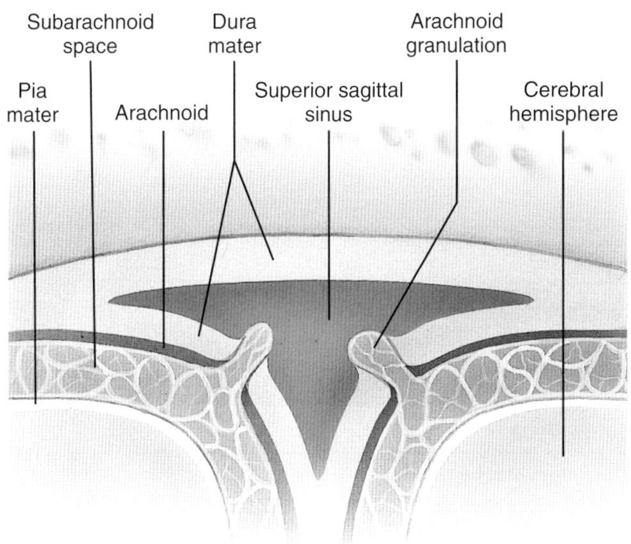


**Figure 29.1**

**The meninges, showing the relationship of the dura, arachnoid, subarachnoid space, pia, and brain tissue.** (From Lundy-Ekman L: *Neuroscience: fundamentals for rehabilitation*, ed 3, Philadelphia, 2007, Saunders.)

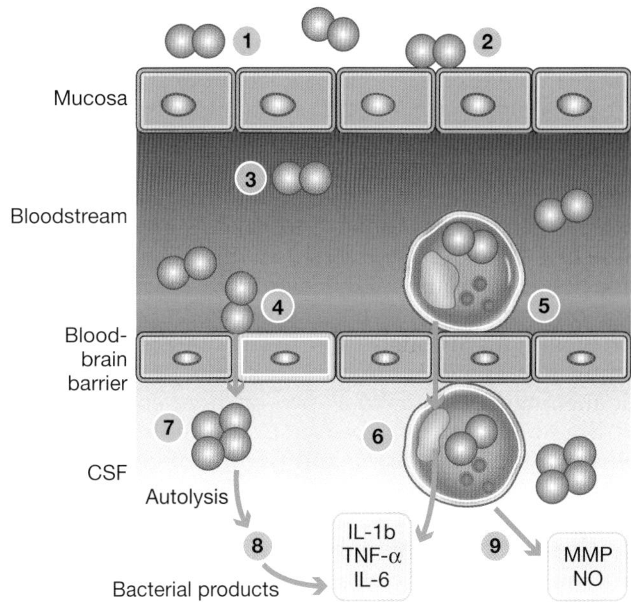


**Figure 29.2**

**Pathogenesis of bacterial meningitis.** *(1)* Adherence and colonization of mucosa; *(2)* invasion of bloodstream; *(3)* multiplication in bloodstream; *(4)* increased permeability of the blood-brain barrier, and bacteria cross the blood-brain barrier; *(5)* infiltration of cerebrospinal fluid *(CSF)* by white cells; *(6)* release of proinflammatory cytokines; *(7)* uncontrolled replication of bacteria in sanctuary site, CSF; *(8)* bacterial products stimulate inflammatory cascade; *(9)* activated leukocytes lead to production of matrix metalloproteinase *(MMP)* and oxidants. *IL,* Interleukin; *NO,* nitric oxide; *TNF-α,* tumor necrosis factor alpha. (From Magill AJ, Ryan ET, Hill D, et al: *Hunter's tropical medicine and emerging infectious disease*, ed 9, Philadelphia, 2012, Saunders.)

dramatically decreased the incidence in countries where there is access to the vaccine. There appears to be a second period of increased susceptibility during late adolescence. In adulthood, bacterial meningitis is mostly associated with conditions that affect the defense mechanisms of the host.[20] Individuals with compromised immune function related to other conditions such as HIV remain at high risk to develop meningitis.[43] When the spleen is damaged or removed, a person becomes more susceptible to pneumococcal disease. Otitis, mastoiditis, and sinusitis are common predisposing conditions that may need specialized treatment. Neoplastic meningitis is a complication that occurs infrequently but is characterized by neurologic signs and symptoms and has a poor outcome.[21] It is caused by the infiltration of subarachnoid space by cancerous cells and occurs in 1% to 8% of patients with cancer.[47] Meningitis associated with cutaneous anthrax became an urgent health concern with the 2001 bioterrorism threat. There is meningeal involvement in only 5% of persons exposed, and there has not been a global threat to humans in recent years.

## Pathogenesis

The most common bacteria causing acute bacterial meningitis *(S. pneumoniae, Neisseria meningitidis,* and *H. influenzae)* have neurotropic potential, which allows them to invade the host mucosal epithelium, multiply in the bloodstream, and cross the blood-brain barrier into the CSF.[64] Fig. 29.2 shows the process that allows access into the CNS. Young children mount inadequate immune responses to bacterial capsular polysaccharides, rendering them particularly vulnerable to these infections.[41]

Once there is penetration of the blood-brain barrier and infectious agents move into the CSF and parenchyma of the brain, there is less immune protection than in the rest of the body. The CSF has about {1/200} the amount of antibody as blood, and the number of white blood cells is very low compared with the blood. The brain lacks a lymphatic system to fight infection, despite the fact that the level of leukocytes in the brain increases.[19] Cytokines, chemokines, macrophages, and microglia respond to viral and bacterial infections. The polymorphonuclear cells recruited to the infection cause damage to the surrounding brain tissue by the release of cytotoxic free radicals and excitatory amino acids such as glutamate. Neuronal cell death occurs mainly in the hippocampus through apoptosis and in the cortex through necrosis. White matter injury also occurs secondary to small vessel vasculitis, focal ischemia, or venous thrombosis. Oxidative stress may be responsible for apoptosis in the hippocampus. Vasculitis can lead to infarction and decreases in cerebral blood flow, causing a drop in the glucose level of the CSF. Responses to inflammation in the brain can block CSF, resulting in hydrocephalus, edema, and increased intracranial pressure.[9,59]

### Aseptic (Viral) Meningitis

Viral infection is the most common cause of inflammation of the CNS. Viral meningitis is an acute febrile illness with signs and symptoms of meningeal irritation, usually with a lymphocytic pleocytosis of the CSF and negative CSF bacterial stains and cultures. Aseptic meningitis most often is caused by enteroviruses, which are the major cause of meningitis in 40% of adults 30 to 60 years old.[24] Other causes of meningitis include the mumps virus, herpes simplex virus 2, measles virus, influenza virus, and arboviruses such as West Nile virus. Epstein-Barr virus can also be responsible and is more often seen in late adolescence and early adulthood. Systemic lupus erythematosus, a disorder of connective tissue, can cause aseptic meningitis. Sarcoid tumors and other intracranial tumors or cysts can lead to aseptic meningitis through rupture.[4] Often the meningitis occurs days or weeks after the exposure. Recurrent aseptic meningitis is defined as two or more episodes with a disease-free interval between. This must be distinguished from the waxing and waning of chronic meningitis.[21] Certain medications or chemicals can cause aseptic meningitis. The medications most commonly involved are nonsteroidal antiinflammatory drugs. Chemicals can cause direct meningeal irritation and are often related to surgical procedures that expose the chemical.

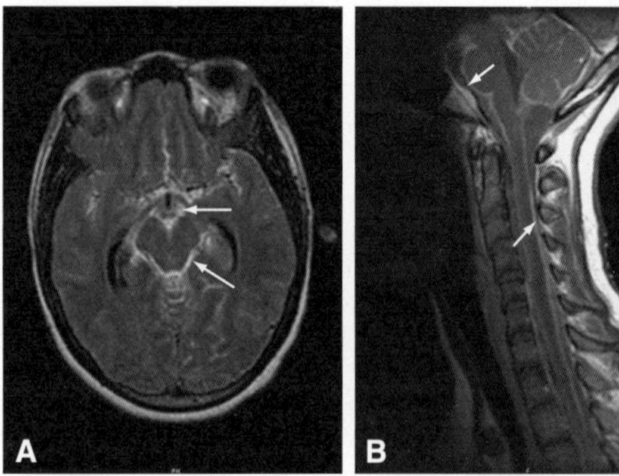


**Figure 29.3**

**Tuberculous meningitis.** (A) T1-weighted transverse magnetic resonance imaging (MRI) of the brain. (B) Sagittal MRI of base of brain and spinal cord in a patient with tuberculous meningitis. Note enhanced meninges *(arrows)* in basilar regions of brain, brainstem, and spinal cord. (From Vincent J, Abraham E, Kochanek P, et al: *Textbook of critical care*, ed 6, Philadelphia, 2011, Saunders.)

## Tuberculous Meningitis

Tuberculous meningitis is a severe form of extrapulmonary tuberculosis. It is rare (0.9% to 5.8%) but is associated with high mortality and disability among survivors.[33] Tuberculous meningitis is an infection by *Mycobacterium tuberculosis,* which enters the body by inhalation.[20,71] CNS involvement includes abscess or spinal cord disease. The hallmark pathologic processes are meningeal inflammation, basal exudates, vasculitis, and hydrocephalus. Diagnosis is based on the characteristic clinical picture, neuroimaging abnormalities, and CSF changes (increased protein, low glucose, and mononuclear cell pleocytosis). CSF smear examination, mycobacterial culture, or polymerase chain reaction (PCR) is mandatory for bacteriologic confirmation. Prompt diagnosis and early treatment are crucial. The decision to start antituberculous treatment is often empiric. The World Health Organization (WHO) guidelines recommend a 6-month course of antituberculous treatment; however, other guidelines recommend prolonged treatment extended to 9 or 12 months. Corticosteroids reduce the number of deaths. Resistance to antituberculous drugs is associated with a high mortality. Patients with hydrocephalus may need ventriculoperitoneal shunting. Bacillus Calmette-Guérin vaccination protects to some degree against tuberculous meningitis in children.[27,26]

Tuberculous brain abscesses may produce mass effect and edema. CSF may demonstrate formation of multiple cysts, with lymphocytes and elevated protein. Infected bacilli enter the subarachnoid space to cause diffuse meningitis.[46] Magnetic resonance imaging (MRI) of a tuberculoma is shown in Fig. 29.3.[45]

## Bacterial Meningitis

The organisms generally responsible for bacterial meningitis are those found in mucosal surfaces in the upper respiratory tract. Bacteria in the birth canal can be transferred from the mother to the infant during birth. Group B streptococcus, *Escherichia coli,* and *Listeria monocytogenes* are bacteria that can cause infection in the neonate, although antibodies are passed through the placenta. As these antibodies decline, the susceptibility to Hib, pneumococcus, and meningococcus increases, especially in the second half of the first year of life. On the other end of the spectrum, *S. pneumoniae* and *N. meningitidis* are the most common bacteria causing infection in the adult and elderly populations.[49,59]

In bacterial meningitis, inflammation initially is confined to the subarachnoid space, then spreads to the adjacent brain parenchyma. Vasculitis starts in the small subarachnoid vessels. Thrombotic obstruction of vessels and decreased cerebral perfusion pressure can lead to focal ischemic lesions. Veins are more frequently affected than arteries, probably because of their thinner vessel walls and the slower blood flow. Damage to the cell bodies causes the production of amyloid beta precursor protein that is carried through the axon and accumulates within terminal axonal swellings, or spheroids. This axonal pathology contributes to neurologic sequelae seen after bacterial meningitis.

## Fungal Meningitis

*Cryptococcus neoformans* infections are very rare among healthy people but are more commonly the cause of fungal meningitis in people with weakened immune systems, with an estimated 220,000 cases worldwide each year. Fungal meningitis is caused by the spread of fungus through the blood to the brain or spinal cord. The most common cause of fungal meningitis for people living with HIV/AIDS is cryptococcal meningitis (70% of cases).[14] Diagnosis is based on prompt lumbar puncture, with measurement of CSF opening pressure and rapid cryptococcal antigen assay. Fungal meningitis is treated with long courses of high-dose intravenous antifungal medications.[13]

### Spirochetal Meningitis (Neurosyphilis and Lyme Disease)

Syphilis was first documented as a disease in the 1500s, but it was not until 1912 that it was confirmed that the spirochete *Treponema pallidum* was the cause of syphilis. Syphilis is spread sexually and can be passed from a pregnant woman to her infant. In 2017 there were 101,567 reported new diagnoses of syphilis. An infected pregnant woman is at high risk for delivering a stillborn infant. If an infant is born alive with syphilis infection, the infant may have no signs or symptoms of the disease initially. The infant is at risk for seizures, developmental delays, or death. Without treatment, syphilis can spread to the brain (neurosyphilis), typically 10 to 30 years after the syphilis infection began, but spread to the brain may occur at any stage of syphilis. Symptoms of neurosyphilis include severe headache, incoordination, paralysis, numbness, and dementia. Two types of blood tests are necessary to confirm a diagnosis of syphilis: (1) nontreponemal tests and (2) treponemal tests. Syphilis is treated with an intramuscular dose of antibiotics, typically benzathine penicillin G.[13,78]

Lyme disease, a tick-borne zoonosis caused by spirochetes in the *Borrelia burgdorferi* sensu lato complex, can affect multiple human organ systems. The blacklegged tick, *Ixodes scapularis,* is the vector of Lyme disease in the eastern and upper Midwestern United States; the western blacklegged tick, *Ixodes pacificus,* is the vector of Lyme disease on the Pacific Coast. It has been a notifiable condition since the early 1990s. If left untreated, Lyme disease can spread to the brain and cause meningitis. The neurologic manifestation of Lyme disease, known as neuroborreliosis, is caused by a systemic infection of spirochetes of the genus *Borrelia*. Between 2001 and 2016, 2% of confirmed cases of Lyme disease resulted in meningitis/encephalitis.[13] Lyme disease peaks among children aged 5 to 9 years and adults aged 50 to 55 years, with illness onset most prevalent in spring and summer. The majority of Lyme disease cases occur in the Northeast, mid-Atlantic, and upper Midwest regions. Neurologic manifestation occurs in approximately 12.5% of cases, with only 1.3% of cases resulting in meningitis. In most cases, diagnosis can be made based on clinical presentation and serology, without a CSF sample. CSF can be tested if there is clinical doubt and serology results are pending. Symptoms typically start several weeks after inoculation, so antibodies should be present in an immunoassay. However, if neuroborreliosis remains a clinical concern with a negative immunoassay, retesting at 1 month is indicated. If symptoms have been present for more than 4 weeks, immunoglobulin G (IgG) Western blot alone is recommended, as it is highly sensitive for Lyme disease of more than 4 weeks' duration. Serologic testing is highly sensitive for patients with neurologic manifestations at the time of presentation (≥80%).[58] If there is strong clinical concern for neuroborreliosis, clinicians should consider treatment with appropriate antibiotics immediately while awaiting serology results.[57,58]

## Clinical Manifestations

Headache, vomiting, meningeal signs, focal deficits, vision loss, cranial nerve palsies, and raised intracranial pressure are dominant clinical features in tuberculous meningitis. Symptoms of spirochetal meningitis include severe headache, incoordination, paralysis, numbness, and dementia. Adults with acute bacterial meningitis usually present with features of fever, neck stiffness, and altered mental status. More advanced disease may include opisthotonos, focal neurologic deficit, seizures, and reduced level of consciousness. One clinical sign of suspected meningitis is a headache accentuated by the patient rotating his or her head two or three times in a second, referred to as the jolt accentuation of headache (JAH).[1] Pain in the lumbar area and the posterior aspects of the thigh or pain with combined hip flexion and knee extension is identified as the Kernig sign. As the inflammation progresses, flexion of the neck will produce flexion of the hips and knees; this is known as a positive Brudzinski sign.[60] The positions for Kernig and Brudzinski tests are shown in Fig. 29.4. JAH is better at ruling out meningitis, with the highest sensitivity of the three tests. The sensitivity for JAH, Kernig, and Brudzinski tests is 84.4%, 55.5%, and 53.3%. The Kernig and Brudzinski tests are better at ruling in meningitis. The specificity of JAH, Kernig, and Brudzinski tests is 65.3%, 89.3%, and 90.6%.[1] It is important that the clinician look at multiple clinical signs, as well as patient symptoms on presentation. If the infection remains undetected or untreated, the brainstem centers may be affected. The individual may then experience seizures and coma, vomiting, and papilledema. Focal neurologic signs including cranial nerve palsies and deafness can also be seen when the brainstem is affected.

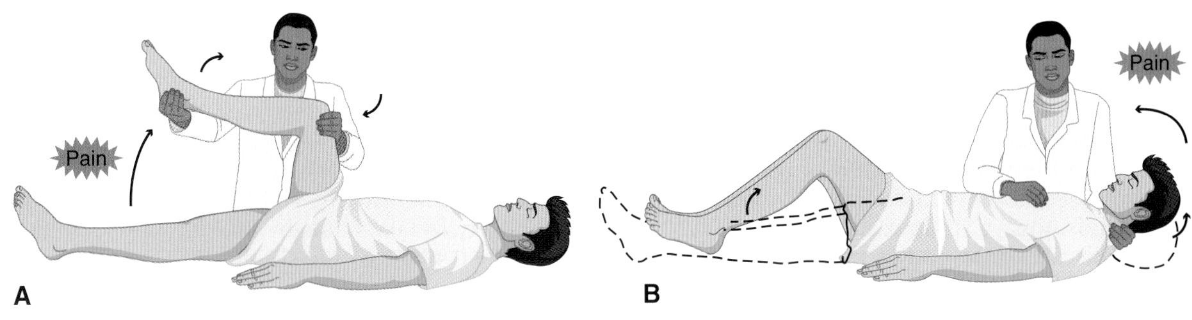


**Figure 29.4**

**Assessing a client with meningeal irritation.** (A) Kernig sign. (B) Brudzinski sign. (From Black JM: Medical-surgical nursing: clinical management for positive outcomes, ed 7, Philadelphia, 2004, Saunders.)

## MEDICAL MANAGEMENT

**DIAGNOSIS.** Early symptoms of meningitis and septicemia often resemble viral illnesses such as influenza, making the condition difficult to diagnose. Classic symptoms such as a nonblanching rash and a stiff neck are often late symptoms of the disease, and neck stiffness is rarer in infants and young children. The presence of ear or upper respiratory tract infections does not necessarily exclude a diagnosis of meningitis. The emphasis should therefore be on regular, close monitoring of an ill child and assessment of the vital signs. Awareness of the recognized red flag symptoms of septicemia—cold hands and feet, limb pain, and pale or mottled skin—could also aid earlier diagnosis and hence potentially improve prognosis.[35]

Lumbar puncture is the only absolute means of confirming a diagnosis of meningitis. The viruses causing viral meningitis can be isolated in CSF and include enteroviruses, lymphocytic choriomeningitis, and herpes simplex virus. Lumbar puncture reveals mononuclear cells in the hundreds, a normal glucose level, a mild increase in protein, and absence of bacterial organisms (see Laboratory Values in Chapter 40). Radiographs may be taken to rule out fracture, sinusitis, and mastoiditis. Computed tomography (CT) scan or MRI will reveal evidence of brain abscess or infarction that may be responsible for the symptoms. Fig. 29.3 shows evidence of abnormal MRI with tuberculous meningitis.

Viral infection is the most common cause of inflammation of the CNS in children. Differentiation from bacterial infection of the CNS is made on the basis of signs and symptoms and CSF changes. Clinical symptoms consistent with meningeal involvement are milder but overlap with symptoms of bacterial infection.[49]

Prompt diagnosis is critical in bacterial meningitis because death can occur without antibiotic treatment. Because determining the bacterial etiology can take up to 48 hours with CSF cultures, an alternative diagnostic test should be considered. Gram stain examination of CSF is recommended when meningitis is suspected. It is fast, inexpensive, and accurate up to 90% of the time. PCR is useful for excluding a diagnosis of bacterial meningitis and may eventually, with further refinement, be used for determining etiology.[19]

When CSF findings suggest bacterial meningitis, but Gram stain and culture results are negative, a combination of laboratory tests is necessary to distinguish bacterial from viral meningitis. In bacterial meningitis, the opening pressure generally is between 200 and 500 mm $H_2O$ (lower in children), white blood cell count and protein concentration are elevated, glucose concentration may be low, and there may be a neutrophil or lymphocyte predominance.[65]

When there is a neoplasm or brain tumor, the infection may be the result of pleomorphic manifestations of neoplastic meningitis and co-occurrence of disease at other sites. Useful tests to establish diagnosis and guide treatment include MRI of the brain and spine, CSF cytology, and radioisotope CSF flow studies. Assessment of the extent of disease of the CNS is valuable because large volume subarachnoid disease or CSF flow obstruction is prognostically significant.[30]

Spirochetal meningitis results in CSF with leukocytosis (10 to 1000/mm$^3$), but CSF may be normal, especially early in the course. CSF protein concentrations are usually higher than seen in other acute infections, without the reduction in glucose concentration seen in tuberculous meningitis. There are often unmatched CSF oligoclonal IgG bands.[57,58] The time course after onset of the disease indicates the type of organism involved. Viral meningitis is hyperacute, with symptoms developing within hours. Acute pyogenic bacterial meningitis can also develop in 4 to 24 hours. Individuals with fungal meningitis or tuberculous meningitis develop symptoms over days to weeks. In spirochetal meningitis, symptoms may develop weeks or even decades after inoculation. It is difficult to identify the tuberculosis bacterium, so clinical signs are important to follow.[17]

**TREATMENT.** Guidelines for the diagnosis and treatment of bacterial meningitis from the Infectious Diseases Society of America (IDSA) are updated on a regular basis. Prompt treatment of bacterial meningitis with an appropriate antibiotic is essential. Optimal antimicrobial treatment of bacterial meningitis requires bactericidal agents able to penetrate the blood-brain barrier, with efficacy in CSF. Several new antibiotics have been introduced for the treatment of meningitis caused by resistant bacteria, but their use in human studies has been limited. More complete understanding of the microbial and host interactions that are involved in the pathogenesis of bacterial meningitis and associated neurologic sequelae is likely to help in developing new strategies for the prevention and treatment of bacterial meningitis.[63,70]

When acute bacterial meningitis is suspected, treatment with an antimicrobial and a steroid should begin as soon as possible. Bacterial meningitis is a neurologic emergency; progression to more severe disease reduces the likelihood of a full recovery. Targeted antimicrobial therapy can begin in adults following a positive CSF Gram stain result. Antibiotic therapy should not be delayed pending the results of Gram stain or other diagnostic tests. Antimicrobial therapy should be modified as soon as the pathogen has been isolated. Duration of therapy depends on individual responses.[65,72]

Suspected bacterial meningitis in a child or infant is considered a medical emergency. The general picture involves fever, decreased feeding, vomiting, bulging fontanel (in infants), seizures, and a high-pitched cry. In neonates with meningitis caused by gram-negative bacilli, the duration of therapy should be determined in part by repeated lumbar punctures documenting CSF sterilization. If there is no response after 48 hours of appropriate therapy, repeat CSF analysis may be necessary. Because any complications of bacterial meningitis usually occur within the first 2 or 3 days of treatment, outpatient management requires close follow-up. Criteria for outpatient therapy are inpatient antimicrobial therapy for 6 or more days; no fever for at least 24 to 48 hours; no significant neurologic dysfunction, focal findings, or seizure activity; stable or improving condition; and ability to take fluids by mouth. There should be an established plan for physician and nurse visits, laboratory monitoring, and emergencies. Seizures can be controlled with antiseizure medications. As the infection is controlled, the seizures are resolved, so a short course is all that is usually necessary.[65]

The addition of dexamethasone can reduce the subarachnoid space inflammatory response that is related to morbidity and mortality and may therefore alleviate many of the pathologic consequences of bacterial and tuberculous meningitis related to cerebral edema or cerebral vasculitis. Change in cerebral blood flow, increase in intracranial pressure, and neuronal injury can be controlled by judicious steroid use.[78]

Radiologic treatment is effective with neoplastic meningitis. Because neoplastic meningitis affects the entire neuraxis, chemotherapy can include intra-CSF fluid. Neoplastic meningitis is often a part of a progressive systemic disease, and consequently treatment is palliative.[30]

Usual treatment for viral meningitis is symptomatic. Medication is given for headache and nausea. The prognosis in viral meningitis is excellent, and most individuals recover within 1 to 2 weeks. Treatment of acute episodes of herpes meningitis with acyclovir has been shown to decrease the duration and severity of symptoms. It may work as well for prophylactic control of episodes. Tuberculous meningitis is managed with drugs given to treat the tuberculosis. In addition, adjunctive therapy with corticosteroids may reduce mortality and decrease neurologic sequelae in severe meningitis. Drugs that scavenge for free radicals and the use of *N*-methyl-D-aspartate receptor blockers can help reduce tissue injury.[65]

**PROGNOSIS.** Mortality ranges from 5% to 25% depending on the infecting bacteria and the health and age of the person infected. At least one neurologic complication, such as impairment of consciousness, seizures, or focal neurologic abnormalities, typically develops in 75% of individuals with bacterial meningitis. Systemic complications, cardiorespiratory failure, and sepsis are also common and found about 40% of the time. Hyponatremia occurs about 30% of the time, with an average duration of 3 days, and is well managed by fluid restriction.

Cranial nerve palsies occur about 30% of the time, with hearing impairment during hospitalization a common symptom, but more than half of patients have full return of hearing. The severity of hearing loss has been graded as mild one-third of the time, moderate one-third of the time, and profound one-third of the time. When there is hearing loss, it is more likely to be bilateral than unilateral.[76]

In children, long-term neurologic consequences of bacterial meningitis include developmental impairment, hearing loss, blindness, hydrocephalus, hypothalamic dysfunction, hemiparesis, and tetraparesis. There is a 30% mortality rate, with increasing death in individuals older than 60 years. Most deaths occur within 2 weeks as a result of both systemic and neurologic complications. Aseptic or viral meningitis is usually self-limiting, and there is not the same degree of neurologic sequelae involvement. Neoplastic meningitis is considered terminal, with a median survival of 4 to 6 weeks, which may be improved to 3 to 6 months with treatment, including intrathecal chemotherapeutics and radiation therapy.[47] Mortality rates for tuberculous meningitis range from 20% to 50%, and survivors may have neurologic sequelae similar to those seen in acute bacterial meningitis.[37,38] With better understanding of the role of cytokines, therapies targeting these processes are being studied and show promise. These therapies may help to further control damage to the nervous system during the infectious or inflammatory process.[9,68] Poor outcome is significantly associated with severe disturbance of consciousness and the presence of intracranial brain swelling, seizure, cerebral hemorrhage, or pneumonia.[62]

# ENCEPHALITIS

## Definition

Encephalitis is an acute inflammatory disease of the parenchyma, or tissue of the brain, caused by direct viral invasion or hypersensitivity initiated by a virus. Encephalitis is characterized by inflammation primarily in the gray matter of the CNS. Neuronal death can result in cerebral edema. There can also be damage to the vascular system and inflammation of the arachnoid and pia mater.[3] Viruses carried by mosquitoes or ticks are responsible for most of the worldwide known cases of primary CNS infection. In many cases, such as those involving West Nile virus, Lyme disease, and herpes simplex virus, the individual can develop either encephalitis or meningitis. This is reflected in the different levels of impairment that may be experienced after exposure.

## Incidence

Before 1994, outbreaks of West Nile virus were sporadic and occurred primarily in the Mediterranean region, Africa, and eastern Europe. Since 1994, outbreaks have occurred with a higher incidence of severe human disease, particularly affecting the nervous system. Incidence peaked around 2002, but then decreased. By 2017, incidence dropped to less than 4 per 100,000 population in the Midwest. There have been almost 23,000 human neuroinvasive disease cases and more than 2000 deaths reported in the contiguous United States since 1999. Incidence is highest in the Midwest from mid-July to early September. West Nile fever develops in approximately 20% of those infected, clinical severity varies greatly, and symptoms may be prolonged. The virus has caused meningitis, encephalitis, and poliomyelitis.[28] Of infected people, 1 in 150 experience permanent neurologic damage or die.[8,13,51]

## Etiologic and Risk Factors

West Nile virus is a flavivirus that was originally isolated in 1937 from the blood of a febrile woman in the West Nile province of Uganda. The virus is widely distributed in Africa, Europe, Australia, and Asia, and since 1999, it has spread throughout the Western Hemisphere including the United States, Canada, Mexico, and the Caribbean and into parts of Central and South America.

Acute viral encephalitides such as eastern and western equine encephalitis, St. Louis encephalitis virus, California encephalitis virus, and West Nile virus depend on mosquitoes for transmission and tend to occur in mid- to late summer. The eastern variety is the least common but most deadly. It occurs in outbreaks along the entire east coast of the United States. It is rapidly progressive, with lesions in the basal ganglia. It carries high mortality and morbidity rates. The western version has a much lower mortality but appears to be particularly severe in infants and children.[16] Fig. 29.5 illustrates the West Nile virus transmission cycle and factors that influence its effects.

## Pathogenesis

Encephalitis produces an inflammatory response and pathologic changes in the brain. Ballooning of infected cells and degeneration of the cellular nuclei can lead to cell death. Plasma membranes are destroyed, and cells form multinucleated giant cells. There is perivascular cuffing, causing damage to the lining of a vessel and hemorrhagic necrosis. The oligodendrocytes are affected, creating gliosis or scarring. Widespread destruction of white matter can occur through inflammation and thrombosis of perforating vessels. Focal damage can affect discrete areas such as the optic nerve.[29]

West Nile virus is thought to initially replicate in dendritic cells after the host has been bitten by an infected mosquito. The infection then spreads to regional lymph nodes and into the bloodstream. The way in which the virus invades the nervous system is still unknown; retrograde transport along peripheral nerve axons has been proposed. Histologic CNS findings of West Nile virus infection are usually characterized by perivascular lymphoplasmacytic infiltration, microglia, astrocytes, necrosis, and neuronal loss, with predilection to structures such as the thalamus, brainstem, and cerebellar Purkinje cells. This variable anatomic involvement explains different clinical presentations.[36]

Herpes simplex virus is found in neonates and appears to arise from maternal genital infection with the virus. It is acquired as the infant passes through the birth canal. Of infants who contract herpes simplex virus, 50% will develop CNS disease, whereas others may develop only skin, eye, and mouth disease. Herpes simplex encephalitis is found after the age of 3 months and is often a latent infection found in the gray matter of the temporal lobe and surrounding structures of the limbic system and the frontal lobe. It is the most common cause of sporadic nonepidemic encephalitis in the United States. Possible genetic factors are being studied, and in animal studies, there appears to be a connection to the $\gamma_1 34.5$ gene.[2]

Encephalomyelitis can result from viral infections such as measles, mumps, rubella, rabies, Ebola, or varicella. Mumps is usually benign and self-limited, but it can trigger encephalitis and other CNS complications such as acute hydrocephalus, ataxia, transverse myelitis, and deafness.[67] Vaccines that contain neuronal antigens have been known to precede these infections, particularly for rabies or smallpox. When there is an illness at the time of vaccination, the risk of developing infection increases. Neurologic problems typically occur within 3 weeks of the illness or vaccination.[4]

Epstein-Barr virus and hepatitis A have been associated with CNS disorders of an infectious nature. Acute toxic encephalitis occurs during the course of a systemic infection with a common virus. Parasites, bacteria, and toxic

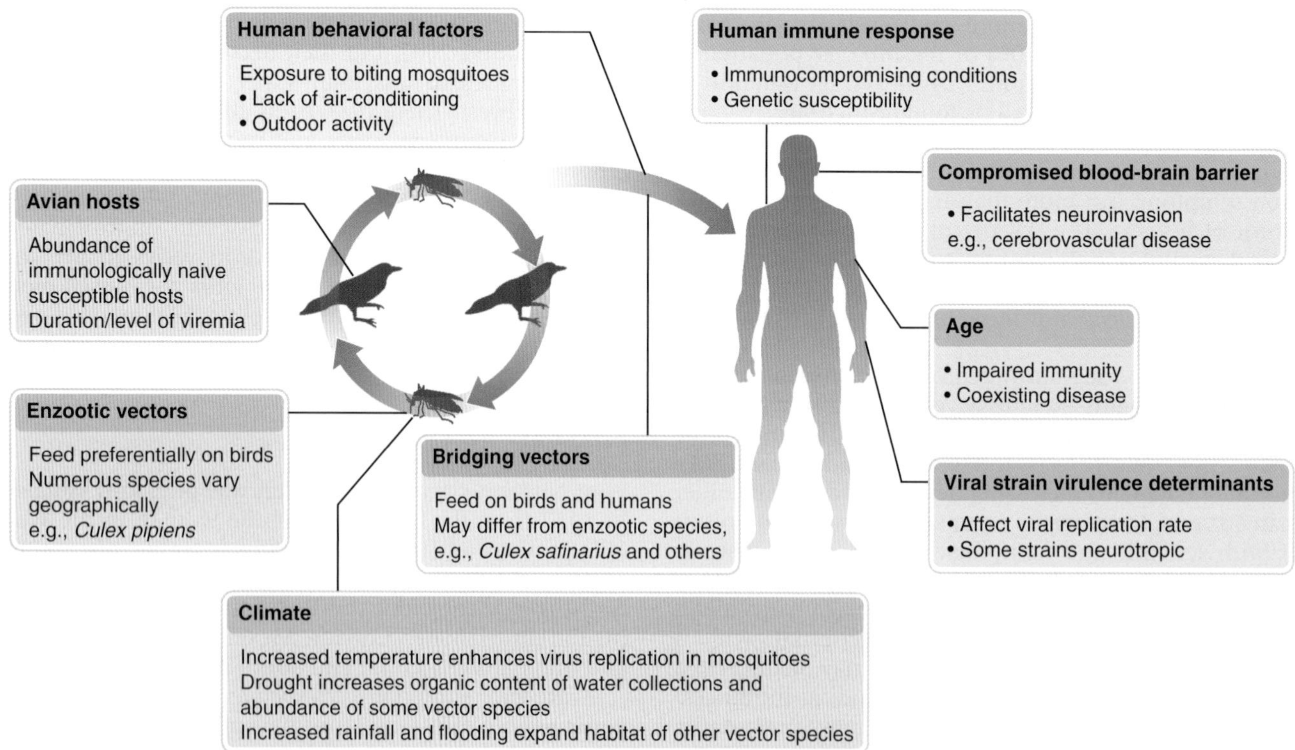


**Figure 29.5**

**West Nile virus transmission cycle and examples of modifying climatologic, vertebrate, mosquito, and human factors on infection and illness.** (From Tsai TF, Vaughn DW, Solomon T: Flaviviruses. In Mandell GL, Bennett JE, Dolin R, eds: *Principles and practice of infectious diseases*, ed 6, New York, 2005, Churchill Livingstone.)

drug reactions can lead to infection of the brain and cause encephalitis or encephalopathy.

## Clinical Manifestations

Signs and symptoms of encephalitis depend on the etiologic agent, but in general, headache, nausea, and vomiting are followed by altered consciousness. If the person becomes comatose, the coma may persist for days or weeks. Agitation can be associated with the degree of infection and may be associated with abnormal sensory processing. Depending on the area of the brain involved, there may be focal neurologic signs with hemiparesis, aphasia, ataxia, or disorders of limb movement. There can be symptoms of meningeal irritation with stiffness of the back and neck. With herpes simplex encephalitis, repeated seizure activity, hallucinations, and disturbance of memory may occur, reflecting involvement of the temporal lobe.[53]

Many individuals infected with West Nile virus are asymptomatic; however, symptoms develop in approximately 20% of infected people. The incubation period is 2 to 14 days before symptom onset. Most individuals present with flu-like symptoms. West Nile virus is characterized by fever, headache, malaise, myalgia, fatigue, skin rash, lymphadenopathy, vomiting, and diarrhea. Kernig and Brudzinski signs may be found on physical examination. Less than 1% of infected individuals develop severe neuroinvasive diseases. West Nile meningitis usually manifests with fever and signs of meningeal irritation, such as headache, stiff neck, nuchal rigidity, and photophobia. Box 29.1 lists the findings that are most critical to watch for to determine the potential for high level of disability or death. In addition, West Nile virus can manifest as acute flaccid paralysis. The lesion of spinal anterior horns results in a paralysis similar to polio and reaches a plateau within hours. Deep tendon reflex can be diminished in severely paralyzed limbs. Reports of substantial muscle ache in the lower back and bowel and bladder functions are common. There is minimal or no sensory disturbance.[36,73]

Encephalitic lesions appear to alter sleep patterns as sequelae of brain–immune interactions. Responses of the immune system to invading pathogens are detected by the CNS, which responds by orchestrating complex changes in behavior and physiology. Sleep is one of the behaviors altered in response to immune challenge. Cytokines may play an active role in infectious challenge by regulating sleep.[48]

### MEDICAL MANAGEMENT

**DIAGNOSIS.** The etiologic agent of encephalitis often cannot be determined. The IDSA reports that an etiologic agent was determined definite or probably in only 16% of immunocompetent patients. Diagnosis usually rests on detection of IgM antibody in serum or CSF. Differential diagnosis of the types of infections of the brain has improved with the use of MRI and PCR to diagnose herpes simplex encephalitis. The electroencephalogram (EEG) will show seizure activity in the temporal lobe in herpes simplex virus. In general, lumbar puncture is abnormal, with increased proteins. The glucose level, however, may be normal or moderately increased. CT scans do not show much until the damage is extensive. MRI shows cerebral edema and vascular damage earlier in the process and leads to earlier detection.[2] In West Nile virus, lesions can sometimes be seen in the white matter, pons, substantia

Box 29.1

**CLINICAL CHARACTERISTICS OF NONFATAL AND FATAL HOSPITALIZED WEST NILE VIRUS–INFECTED PATIENTS**

***Signs and Symptoms Most Likely Related to Death***

- Fever >38°C (>100.4°F)
- Headache
- Mental status changes
- Nausea
- Vomiting
- Chills
- Muscle weakness
- Confusion
- Fatigue
- Lethargy
- Abdominal pain

***Underlying Conditions That Have Potential to Increase Risk of Complications***

- Diabetes
- Hypertension
- Chronic obstructive pulmonary disease
- Dementia
- Coronary artery disease
- Alcoholism
- Asthma
- Cancer
- Immunosuppression

***Other Common Signs and Symptoms***

- Decreased appetite
- Diarrhea
- Myalgia
- Malaise
- Neck stiffness
- Skin rash
- Shortness of breath
- Cough
- Dizziness
- Increased sleepiness
- Balance problems
- Photophobia
- Back pain
- Joint pain (arthralgia)
- Tremor
- Weight loss
- Slurred speech
- Neck pain
- Sore throat
- Seizures
- Blurred vision
- Coma
- Numbness
- Flaccid paralysis
- Lymphadenopathy
- Paresthesias

From Mazurek JM: The epidemiology and early clinical features of West Nile virus infection. *Am J Emerg Med* 23:536–543, 2005.

nigra, and thalamus. An important MRI finding is the focal abnormal signal intensity within the anterior horns; the level of abnormal spinal MRI findings corresponds to the paralysis. Change can be seen in the spinal roots, possibly a result of axonal degeneration secondary to spinal motor neuron loss or wallerian degeneration in the spinal roots.

West Nile virus infection begins with nonspecific symptoms, making early clinical diagnosis challenging. IgM antibodies against the virus (usually by enzyme-linked immunosorbent assay) are generally indicative of a recent West Nile virus infection. Blood samples that are collected between 8 and 21 days after onset are likely to give the best yield. IgM antibodies are only detectable 8 days after symptom onset. There may be a negative result from a blood sample obtained before the 8th day after symptom onset. After the 21st day, the titer of IgM could decline. The lymphocyte count, particularly the degree of relative lymphopenia, is a readily available test; the degree of relative lymphopenia (≥10%) appears to have prognostic importance in West Nile encephalitis. Clinicians should maintain a high index of suspicion for West Nile virus infection during the epidemic season, particularly when evaluating elderly adults with neurologic or gastrointestinal symptoms.[17,44]

West Nile meningitis and encephalitis have similar degrees of pleocytosis, or multiple cystic lesions. However, West Nile encephalitis tends to create higher concentrations of total protein in the CSF and leads to a more severe outcome. Electrophysiologic studies are helpful for the diagnosis of paralysis induced by West Nile virus. Motor nerve conduction studies may reveal severely reduced amplitudes of compound muscle action potentials in symptomatic limbs. However, if the nerve conduction study is done in the early phase of the illness, compound muscle action potentials can be normal because wallerian degeneration can take 7 to 10 days to complete. Nerve conduction velocities are usually preserved, and sensory nerve conduction is typically normal. Needle electromyography shows severe denervation in muscles of weak limbs and corresponding paraspinal muscles. Taken together, these abnormalities in the paralyzed limbs localize the lesions to the anterior horn motor neurons or their ventral nerve roots. The localization is typically consistent with the MRI findings. Individuals presenting with an otherwise unexplained facial palsy during the summer should be tested not only for neuroborreliosis but also for West Nile virus. West Nile encephalitis may manifest with cranial nerve abnormalities involving cranial nerves VI or VII.[18,36]

**TREATMENT.** Treatment varies with the infectious agent. No antiviral treatment is available for encephalitis except for that caused by herpes simplex virus. Acyclovir appears to improve the outcome in herpes simplex encephalitis. Close monitoring of symptoms is critical, especially with the complication of cerebral edema, which may require surgical decompression, hyperventilation, or administration of mannitol. The use of corticosteroids is controversial because of the potential suppression of antibody protection within the CNS. Human vaccines for flavivirus infections are currently available only for yellow fever, Japanese encephalitis, and tick-borne encephalitis.[16] For West Nile virus, treatment is supportive; no licensed human vaccine exists. Prevention uses an integrated pest management approach, which focuses on surveillance, elimination of mosquito breeding sites, and larval and adult mosquito management using pesticides to keep mosquito populations low. During outbreaks or impending outbreaks, emphasis shifts to aggressive adult mosquito control to reduce the abundance of infected, biting mosquitoes. Pesticide exposure and adverse human health events following adult mosquito control operations for West Nile virus appear negligible.

**PROGNOSIS.** The prognosis depends on the infectious agent. The rate of recovery can range from 10% to 50% even in individuals who may have been very ill at the onset. Individuals with mumps meningoencephalitis and Venezuelan equine encephalitis have an excellent prognosis. Other encephalitides such as western equine, St. Louis, and California encephalitis viruses and West Nile virus have a moderate-to-good rate of survival. Although with the use of medication herpes simplex encephalitis has a moderately good outcome (20% mortality), neurologic sequelae are common in 50% of people.[3,16] Recovery for paralysis is remarkably variable. The variation may be caused by different degrees of motor neuron or motor unit loss.[36]

Some recovery is complete within weeks, but outcome is highly variable. The severity of the original illness does not always predict the final outcome. Prediction of post–West Nile virus poliomyelitis syndrome similar to post-polio syndrome is not yet possible. Permanent cerebral problems are more likely to occur in infants. Young children will take longer to recover than adults with similar infections. Anti–West Nile virus IgM can persist for 1 year or longer.

Development of West Nile virus vaccines has been explored, including immunization of animals with recombinant viral proteins, inactivated West Nile virus, DNA that expresses viral antigens, or attenuated West Nile virus isolates.[36]

# BRAIN ABSCESS

## Definition

Brain abscess is an uncommon disorder accounting for only 2% of intracranial mass lesions. CNS abscesses are circumscribed, enlarging, focal infections that produce symptoms and findings similar to those of other space-occupying lesions such as brain tumors. Brain abscesses, however, often progress more rapidly than tumors and more frequently affect meningeal structures. Brain abscesses occur when microorganisms reach the brain and cause a local infection. There may be only one area of abscess, or many areas may be infected because of spread by bloodborne pathogens. Although the site and size of the abscess influence the initial symptoms, evidence of increased intracranial pressure is common.[64]

## Risk Factors and Pathogenesis

Persons with a compromised immune system receiving steroids, immunosuppressants, or cytotoxic chemotherapy or persons with a systemic illness such as HIV infection have an increased risk of developing a brain abscess. Whereas viruses tend to cause diffuse brain infections as described previously, most bacteria, fungi, and other parasites cause localized brain disease. Brain abscesses may develop from other infections in the cranium such as sinusitis or mastoiditis.

Infections leading to brain abscess can come from extracerebral locations; bloodborne metastases; infection from lung or heart; or infections within the cranium such as otitis, cranial osteomyelitis, and sinusitis. Recent or remote head trauma or neurosurgical procedures may be the cause. Bloodborne infections seed the brain and spread and produce abscesses in brain regions in proportion to the blood flow; accordingly, parietal lobe abscesses predominate. Extension of infection from otitis and mastoiditis involves contiguous brain regions of the temporal lobe and cerebellum, whereas abscesses resulting from sinusitis affect the frontal and temporal lobes. Neurologic complications develop in nearly one-third of patients with infective endocarditis, and neurologic manifestations can be the initial symptom. Infective endocarditis should always be considered in a patient with a fever and stroke.[23]

Subdural empyema is an infection in the space between the dura and the arachnoid. It usually results from infected paranasal sinuses and rarely from infected mastoid sinuses by extension of thrombophlebitis from the sinuses into the subdural space. The infection is most commonly unilateral because bilateral spread is prevented by the falx. The empyema may evolve to cause cortical vein thrombosis, cerebral abscesses, or purulent meningitis.

Most brain abscesses evolve over a number of stages, with involvement of the cerebrum occurring during the first 1 to 3 days. Inflammatory infiltrates of polymorphonuclear cells, lymphocytes, and plasma cells follow within 24 hours. By 3 days, the surrounding area shows an increase in perivascular inflammation. The late cerebritis phase develops approximately 4 to 9 days after infection, during which time the center becomes necrotic, containing a mixture of debris and inflammatory cells. Early reactive astrocytes surround the zone of infection and proceed to early capsule formation between approximately 10 and 13 days. At this time, the necrotic center shrinks slightly, and a well-developed peripheral fibroblast layer evolves. The late capsule stage continues to evolve between 14 days and 5 weeks, with continual shrinking of the necrotic center and a relative decrease in the inflammatory cells. The capsule thickens with astrocyte scarring.[64]

If the infection is carried in the blood from another site in the body, the abscess will usually develop at the junction of the gray and white matter. Anaerobic bacteria are found in more than one-half of brain abscesses. The infection usually begins as local encephalitis with necrosis and inflammation of the neurons and glial cells. As the process continues, a capsule wall is formed by the proliferation of fibroblasts. There is usually an area of cerebral edema around the abscess. Bacterial and fungal abscesses will continue to grow until they become lethal. Abscesses caused by other parasites are usually self-limiting.[53]

## Clinical Manifestations

Normal body temperature is common, and white cell counts are not always high. Neck stiffness is rare in the absence of increased intracranial pressure. Otherwise the presenting features resemble those of any expanding intracranial mass such as a slow-growing neoplasm, or it may be rapid and progress to possible herniation and brainstem compression, causing death. A headache of recent onset is the most common symptom, representing distortion or irritation of pain-sensitive structures within the cranial vault, especially those of the great venous sinuses and the dura mater about the base of the brain. If the process continues untreated, isolated headache increases in severity and is accompanied by focal signs, such as hemiparesis or aphasia, followed by obtundation and coma. The period of evolution may range from hours to many days to weeks with more indolent organisms. Seizures may occur with abscesses that involve the cortical gray matter.[64] Lethargy and confusion progress with the increased intracranial pressure present with the growing mass. Focal signs reflect the area of the brain that is affected, with paresis resulting from frontal and parietal lesions and visual disturbances noted with occipital lobe dysfunction.[53] Table 29.1 lists typical manifestations of brain abscess.

The most common symptoms of subdural empyema are headache, fever, neurologic deficit, and stiff neck. However, subdural empyema may progress and cause signs of raised intracranial pressure, such as vomiting, altered level of consciousness, seizures, and papilledema. A high degree of suspicion is needed to establish the diagnosis early in the course of the illness. In patients with sinusitis, the symptoms of subdural empyema may be incorrectly attributed to the sinusitis.

### MEDICAL MANAGEMENT

**DIAGNOSIS.** A history of infection or immunosuppression will lead to suspicion of abscess rather than neoplasm. Imaging plays an important role in the diagnosis and treatment of brain abscess, pyogenic infection, and encephalitis. MRI can detect early changes such as brain edema and is preferable to CT. The area of cerebritis that is seen initially as an ill-defined area with low signal intensity later progresses to a central cavity with slightly higher signal intensity than CSF, surrounded by edema that is slightly hypointense compared with

**Table 29.1** Manifestations of Brain Abscess

| | |
|---|---|
| Headache | 55% |
| Disturbed consciousness | 48% |
| Fever | 58% |
| Nuchal rigidity | 29% |
| Nausea, vomiting | 32% |
| Seizures | 19% |
| Visual disturbance | 15% |
| Dysarthria | 20% |
| Hemiparesis | 48% |
| Sepsis | 17% |

Data from Lu CH, Chang WN, Lin YC, et al: Bacterial brain abscess: microbiological features, epidemiological trends and therapeutic outcomes. *Q J Med* 95:501–509, 2002.

brain parenchyma. Later stages of infection show central necrosis and formation of a rim of slightly high signal intensity on T1-weighted imaging.[56] Gadolinium administration shows a ring-enhancing lesion. Diffusion-weighted imaging helps differentiate abscesses from brain tumors; an abscess cavity demonstrates high signal with decreased apparent diffusion coefficient values, whereas necrotic tumor cavities demonstrate the opposite.[31] When combined with CSF, serologic studies, and patient history, imaging findings can suggest the cause of encephalitis.[5] Fig. 29.6 shows the effect seen on MRI. Although the early signs are similar to those of meningitis, the focal signs of compression in one area of the brain distinguish the abscess over time. EEG is often abnormal.[29]

**TREATMENT.** An appropriate and timely antibiotic protocol and surgical drainage are required to reduce the mass effect. Careful clinical observation is necessary with multiple abscesses, and CT scans should be repeated often to determine if the abscess continues to expand. Initially, corticosteroids may be used to control the cerebral edema caused by the abscess, but these are used for a short time only because of their interference with capsule formation and immunosuppressive action in the brain. Treatment of patients with infective endocarditis and cerebral emboli requires prevention of embolization, with appropriate antibiotic therapy and sometimes cardiac surgery. Anticoagulation is contraindicated in patients with cerebral infarcts and septic emboli because of the high risk for complications from intracerebral bleeding.

Medical treatment alone is not generally advocated, although it may be considered if a patient is too sick to undergo surgical therapy. Medical therapy alone is more likely to be successful if treatment is begun in the cerebritis stage before a capsule forms (generally within 10 days of symptom onset), if the lesions are small (<3 mm), and if patients show definite clinical improvement in the first week. Surgery should be avoided if the location is surgically inaccessible or if the surgical approach would traverse eloquent tissue or the ventricular system, if there is concomitant meningitis or ependymitis, or if the patient has hydrocephalus requiring a shunt that could become infected during the operative procedure. Surgical excision of an abscess can be done only if the abscess is encapsulated (usually after 10 days of symptom onset) but can dramatically reduce the length of antibiotic therapy to as short as 2 weeks. If an abscess is larger than 3 cm or if a patient is deteriorating clinically, surgical therapy should be initiated. Two surgical options currently in use are aspiration and excision. Stereotactic aspiration can be done under local anesthesia if necessary. Because of the limited space in the posterior fossa and the mild clinical deficits associated with removal of cerebellar tissue, cerebellar abscesses should be managed surgically unless the patient cannot tolerate surgery, owing to excessive bleeding risk. Fig. 29.7 shows the process of determining care that might be followed to decide the best clinical action to take.

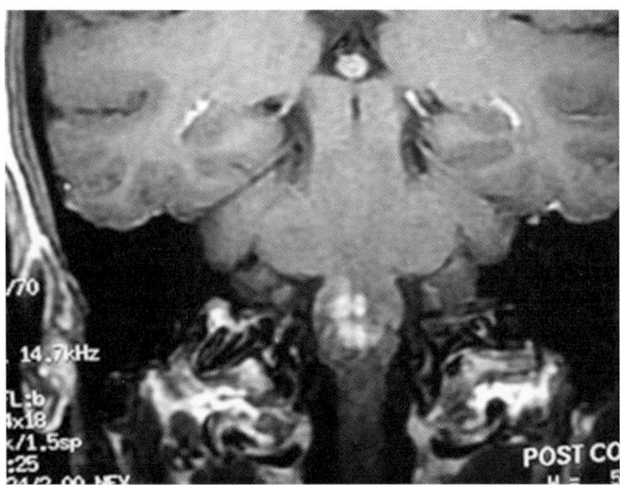


**Figure 29.6**

**Brainstem abscess.** Magnetic resonance imaging with gadolinium shows an enhancing lesion in the brainstem caused by *Listeria* infection. (From Goldman L, Schafer AI: *Goldman's Cecil medicine*, ed 24, St. Louis, 2011, Saunders.)

For supportive therapy, patients need to be hospitalized to initiate intravenous antibiotics, and a neurosurgeon should be involved in the patient's care. The hemodynamic and respiratory status of the patient may need to be supported. Steroids can be considered in patients who have clinical deterioration secondary to vasogenic edema surrounding the abscess. The use of steroids is not advocated in all patients because it may reduce the penetration of antibiotics into the abscess, and steroids may increase the risk of rupture into the ventricle. The use of steroids can slow the reduction of capsule formation and may reduce the amount of contrast enhancement on CT, so when these patients undergo follow-up CT, it is important to not consider the lessening degree of contrast enhancement as a sign of improvement. Serial CT scans (once every 1 to 2 weeks) should show decrease in the size of the abscess. If the patient develops seizures, an antiepileptic medication should be started. The role of prophylactic anticonvulsant therapy is controversial, but such therapy is likely not to be of benefit in cerebellar or deep cerebral abscesses.[79]

**PROGNOSIS.** Mortality from brain abscess can be reduced from 65% to 30% with control of the infection with antibiotics and surgery. Nearly one-half of clients are left with some neurologic sequelae, which may include focal signs and seizure activity.[64]

Mortality rates in patients with infective endocarditis and cerebral emboli range from 30% to 80%. Mortality is high if there is hemorrhagic transformation of the infarct. Mortality in patients with ruptured mycotic aneurysms is 80%, and patients with unruptured aneurysms have a mortality rate of 30%.

## ZIKA

### Definition

Zika virus is a positive-sense single-stranded RNA virus in the family *Flaviviridae*. It is spread primarily through the bite of an infected *Aedes aegypti* or *Aedes albopictus* mosquito. Zika was first discovered in 1947 in Uganda in a

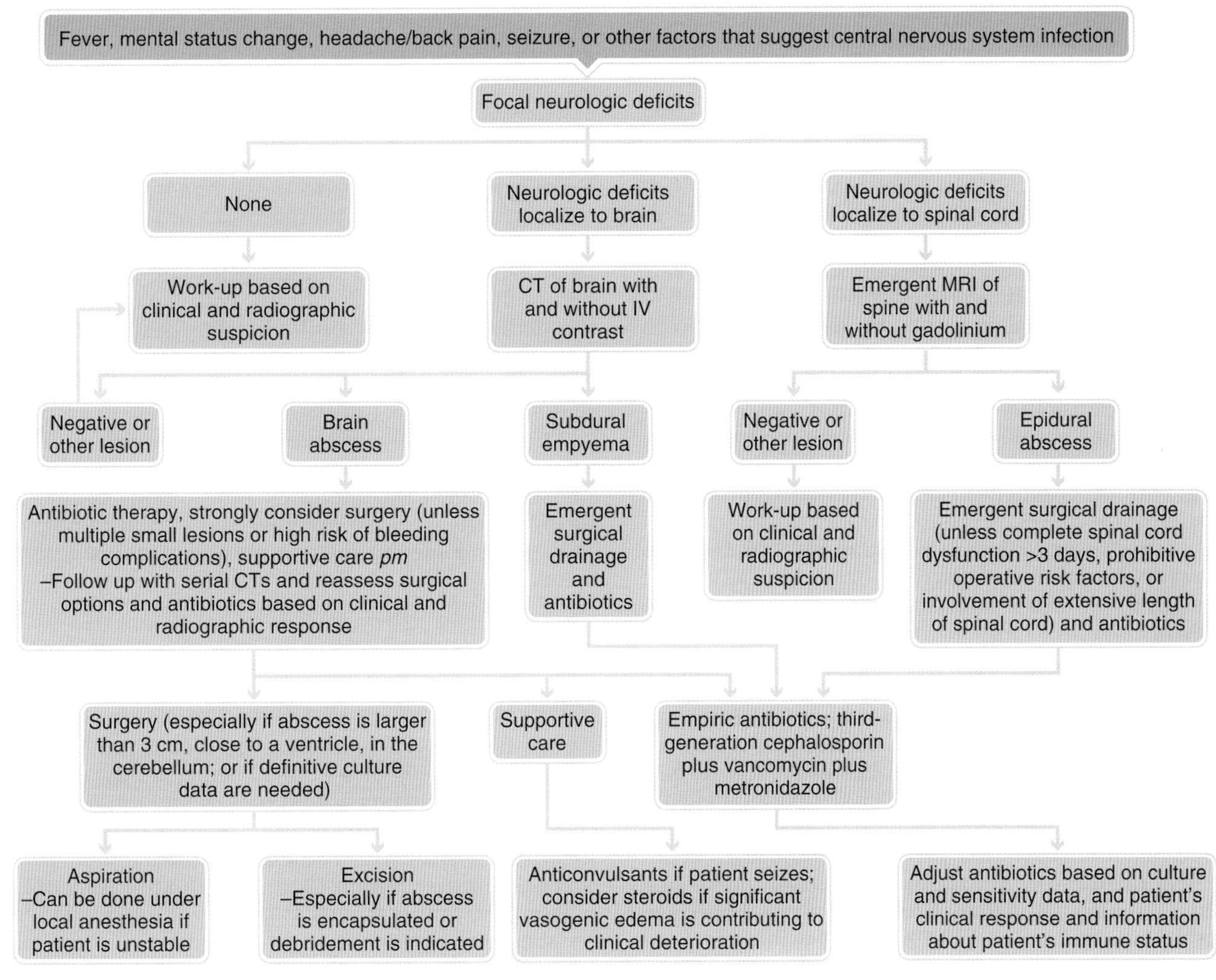


**Figure 29.7**

**Approach to a patient with possible brain abscess or parameningeal infection.** *CT,* Computed tomography; *IV,* intravenous; *MRI,* magnetic resonance imaging. (From Wright W: Brain abscess and parameningeal infection. In Johnson RT, et al, editors: *Current therapy in neurologic disease,* ed 7, St. Louis, 2008, Mosby.)

monkey and in 1952 in humans. Rare yet documented cases occurred in Africa, Southeast Asia, and the Pacific Islands. Between 2015 and 2016, Zika became a public health concern when clusters of microcephaly and other neurologic manifestations of Zika occurred in many countries and territories.

## Risk Factors and Pathogenesis

Although Zika virus is primarily spread through mosquito bites, it can also be spread from a pregnant woman to her fetus, sexually, via laboratory exposure, through blood transfusions, and possibly through animal bites. Zika is an arbovirus, arthropod-borne virus, and a member of the family *Flaviviridae* and the genus *Flavivirus,* with an enveloped, icosahedral virion 40 to 50 nm in diameter, containing the nonsegmented, single-stranded, positive-sense RNA genome. *Aedes* mosquitoes usually bite during the day, peaking during early morning and late afternoon/evening. They breed in small collections of water around homes, schools, and work sites. This is the same mosquito that transmits dengue, chikungunya, and yellow fever. After mosquito inoculation of a human host, the virus enters skin cells through cellular receptors, enabling migration to the lymph nodes and bloodstream. Zika can be transmitted sexually from a man or woman. There is particular concern regarding sexually transmitted Zika because of the severity of the risk to a fetus if Zika is transmitted from an infected woman to the fetus. The virus can remain in a man's sperm for months. Therefore for prevention of sexually transmitted Zika virus, the WHO recommends practicing safer sex or abstinence for 6 months for men and 2 months for women who are returning from areas of active Zika transmission.[52] If Zika virus is transmitted from a pregnant woman to her fetus, there is increased risk of microcephaly and other congenital brain malformations. Studies with mice have found that the Zika virus replicates efficiently in embryonic mouse brain and causes cell-cycle arrest, apoptosis, and inhibition of neural precursor cell differentiation, leading to cortical thinning and microcephaly.[66,75]

### Clinical Manifestation

The incubation period from mosquito bite to symptom onset is typically around 3 to 12 days. Approximately 80% of people infected with Zika will remain asymptomatic. Symptoms that develop are typically mild and may include fever, headache, rash, joint pain, muscle pain, or conjunctivitis. Zika infection has been associated with neurologic implications, including a link to increased incidence of GBS in adults and children and congenital microcephaly in newborns. In extremely rare cases, Zika has been linked to encephalitis and meningitis. Reports indicate that 1.23% of people infected with Zika develop GBS, which is typically preceded by symptoms of infectious illness. It has been suggested that the immune response that occurs in people with symptomatic Zika virus[34] results in damage to the myelin sheath, resulting in prevention of nerve signal transmission to the brain, with involvement of peripheral nerves and nerve roots.[34,52]

Evidence suggests that there is a causal link between Zika virus infection and microcephaly, especially if the fetus is infected in the first trimester.[75] An estimated 2% to 3% of newborns have microcephaly when the mother is infected with Zika virus.[10] Microcephaly is a neurologic condition in which the brain of an infant is smaller than normal, which is defined as a head circumference less than the third percentile for the age and sex of the infant, or 2 standard deviations below average size. It can cause cognitive and motor dysfunction. Infants with mild microcephaly may present with no symptoms other than a smaller than normal head size. Severe microcephaly may manifest as developmental delays, intellectual delays, seizures, impaired motor control, dysphagia, hearing loss, and visual deficits. Fig. 29.8 illustrates the presentation of infant signs and imaging findings associated with Zika.

#### MEDICAL MANAGEMENT

**DIAGNOSIS.** Zika virus may be detected in whole blood, urine, amniotic fluid, urine, saliva, and CSF. Testing algorithms suggest clinical evaluation, blood, and urine testing for Zika diagnosis. Clinical evaluation alone is not sufficient, as the history and symptoms are similar between Zika virus and other arboviruses such as yellow fever and dengue. If a patient is symptomatic and is living in or has traveled to a location with Zika, testing serum or plasma to detect virus, viral nucleic acid, or virus-specific IgM and neutralizing antibodies is recommended. Several countries that have seen Zika outbreaks have also reported an increased incidence of GBS, which is a rapid-onset muscle weakness caused by the immune system damaging the peripheral nervous system. Lumbar puncture, electromyography, and nerve conduction studies assist in diagnosis of GBS.[13,52,78]

Testing should be offered to all pregnant women who have traveled to areas with ongoing Zika virus transmission. If a pregnant woman has confirmed Zika infection during laboratory testing, serial ultrasound scans should be considered every 3 to 4 weeks during pregnancy to monitor fetal growth and anatomy. Serologic tests and reverse transcriptase PCR assays are recommended in infants whose mothers have had a risk of Zika virus exposure during pregnancy. If microcephaly is not diagnosed during pregnancy, it can be diagnosed after an infant is born by measuring head size.

**TREATMENT AND PROGNOSIS.** There is no treatment for Zika virus other than symptom management and supportive care. The main way to avoid infection is to prevent Zika exposure with aggressive mosquito control and limiting potential exposure. In the rare instance when an adult or a child has an immune response to Zika virus and develops GBS, there is no cure for GBS. Plasma exchange (plasmapheresis) and immunoglobulin therapy may reduce the severity of the illness. Plasmapheresis may rid the plasma of certain antibodies that contribute to the immune system's attack on the peripheral nerves. High doses of immunoglobulin block the damaging antibodies that may contribute to GBS.

Microcephaly is a lifelong condition without a cure or standard treatment protocol. Treatment is based on management of the clinical manifestations of the condition, such as developmental services, rehabilitation therapy, and medications to control seizures or other symptoms.

## PRION DISEASE

### Definition

Rare forms of encephalopathies include the prion diseases of sporadic genetic or acquired Creutzfeldt-Jakob disease (CJD). The incubation period is slow and can be up to 5 to 8 years.[15] Classic CJD is a rare, fatal, and degenerative neurologic disease with a long asymptomatic latent period that was first described in 1920. The causative agent of CJD is thought by most experts to be a prion protein (PrPsc), an abnormal conformation of a normal cellular protein (PrPc) that can recruit additional PrPc to PrPsc, resulting in deposition of insoluble precipitates in neural tissue. CJD is one of a variety of prion diseases of humans that occur spontaneously at a rate of approximately 1.5 cases per 1 million throughout the world and can be transmitted vertically in familial conditions, such as Gerstmann-Sträussler-Scheinker syndrome or fatal familial insomnia.[54]

Similar to classic CJD, variant CJD (vCJD) is a fatal, degenerative neurologic disease, although it occurs in younger persons and has distinctive clinical, histopathologic, and biochemical features, including the presence of readily detectable prion protein in non-CNS lymphoreticular tissues such as appendix, spleen, tonsil, and lymph nodes. In contrast to classic CJD, vCJD disease is new, first reported in the United Kingdom in 1996. The causative agent of vCJD, a prion, is the same agent that causes *bovine spongiform encephalopathy* (BSE), or "mad cow disease." A massive epidemic of BSE occurred in Great Britain in the 1980s and early 1990s as a result of the recycling and processing of material from dead sheep and cattle into food meal for cattle. Although this practice was stopped in the mid-1990s after massive fear of the vCJD epidemic, an estimated 250,000 cattle had already been infected with BSE. Transmission of the BSE prions to humans occurred by oral consumption of beef and other cattle products containing reticular endothelial or neural tissue, resulting in a delayed outbreak of vCJD in the United Kingdom.[25]

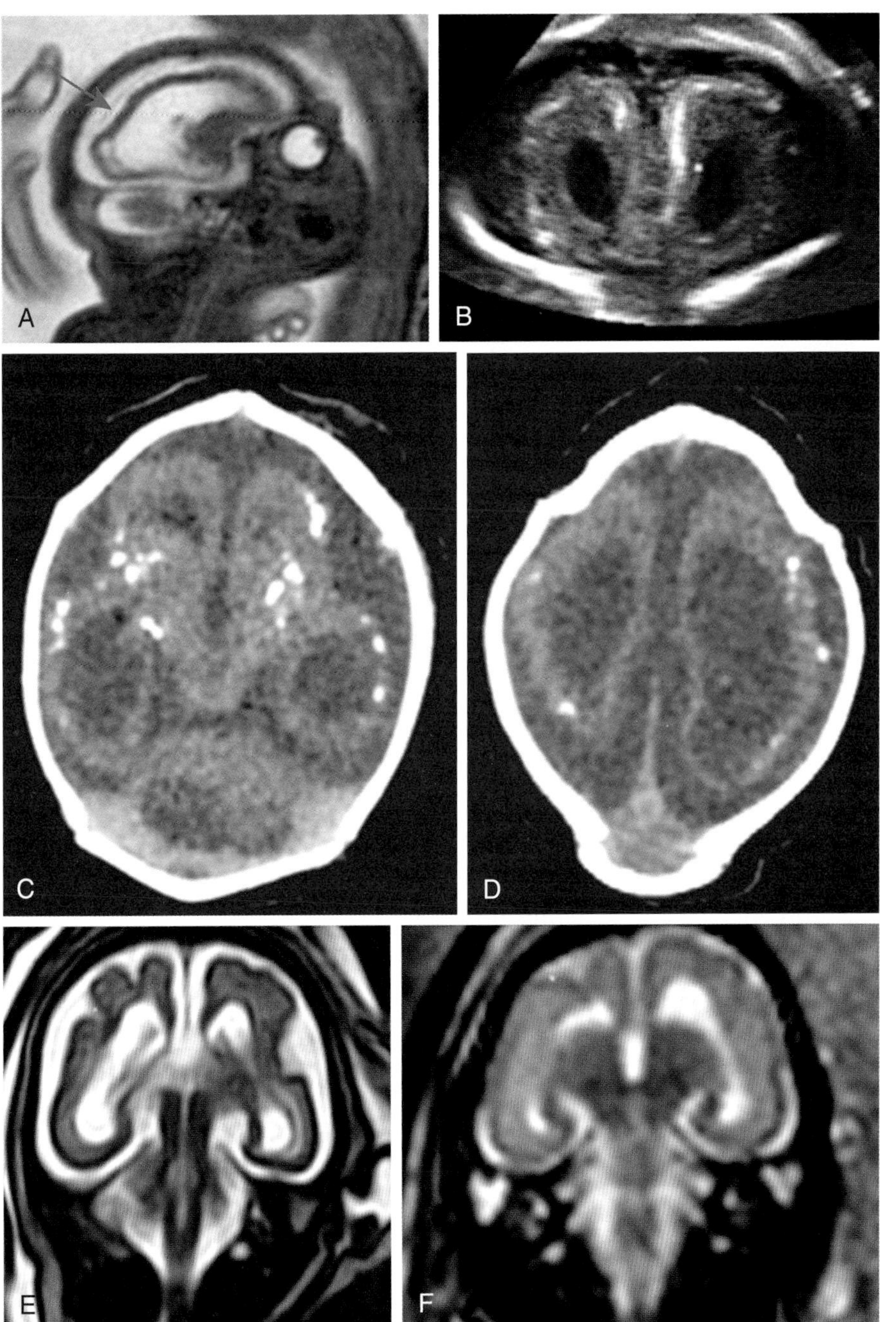


**Figure 29.8**

**Brain findings and clinical features in congenital Zika virus syndrome.** A and B, MRI T2 weighted images show parenchymal bone loss and abnormal brain sulcation (*arrows*). C and D, Abnormalities seen on a computed tomography (CT) scan include reduced volume of cortical brain parenchyma, cortical and subcortical calcifications, simplified gyral pattern and ventriculomegaly. E and F, Neonates show microcephaly, clubbed feet with malpositioned lower extremities. (A,B, E, and F from Sanz Cortes M, Rivera AM, Yepez M, et al: Clinical assessment and brain findings in a cohort of mothers, fetuses and infants infected with ZIKA virus, *American Journal of Obstetrics and Gynecology* 218(4):440.e1–440.e36, 2018; C and D from Barreto de Araujo et al: Association between Zika virus infection and microcephaly in Brazil, January to May, 2016: preliminary report of a case-control study, *The Lancet Infections Diseases* 16(12):1356–1363,2016.

## Incidence and Etiologic and Risk Factors

The annual incidence of all human prion diseases is generally reported to be about 1.5 cases per 1 million individuals worldwide. The incidence increases with age to 3.4 cases per 1 million in persons older than 50 years of age.[13]

The classic forms, sCJD MM1 and sCJD MV1, are by far the most common, accounting for 85% of sporadic prion diseases.[13] In Italy the incidence of genetic transmissible spongiform encephalopathy diseases is the second highest among European countries.[24] Infection with BSE-derived or vCJD-derived prions depends on the host's genetic makeup, which means that there could be a substantial number of symptom-free human carriers of these infectious agents. There is now evidence that vCJD prions can be transmitted through blood transfusion and other iatrogenic routes.[6,7]

Iatrogenic transmission has occurred via corneal and dural transplants and depth cerebral electrodes. Hormone therapy using human pituitary products can be a cause. Transmission of prion disease is also possible through ingesting nervous system products that contain infected material. Eating nervous system products of beef that had been fed rendered protein led to the increased incidence in the United Kingdom in the 1990s.[61] Skeletal muscle tissue from CWD-infected deer has shown prion infectivity; however, the implications of these findings for human beings are unclear. Studies are looking at the role of the PrP encoding gene *(PRNP)* in conferring susceptibility to human prion diseases.[32] It is very difficult, if not impossible, to predict how prions from one species will behave when they transit species barriers; however, studies are ongoing.[55,69]

## Pathogenesis

In the prion formation mechanism, a pathogenic protein is generated from its normal isoform through a change in conformation. The prion is a substance that contains no nucleic acid but can replicate within the nervous system. Prions and other alternatively folded proteins might also be involved in normal cell function, including the formation of biochemical memory at the synapse. Therefore the term *prion* currently applies not only to a disease-specific pathogen but also to a mechanism that could have a wide and crucial role in pathologic and physiologic processes.[54] Similar to oncogenes, mutations of the normal cellular prion protein gene cause disease.

Abnormal prion protein differs from oncogene products in that the prion protein programs its own creation from normal cellular proteins and then instructs the normal protein to change so that it is functionally similar to the abnormal protein. The microscopic alterations consist of spongy change in neuropil, neuronal loss, and gliosis. The spongiform change is similar to that seen after anoxia and in some cases of Alzheimer disease. There appears to be accelerated death of Purkinje cells, resulting in the ataxia that is commonly seen.[22]

## Clinical Manifestations

Prion disease occurs most commonly in people between 50 and 80 years of age and shows rapidly progressive multidomain cognitive impairment and confusion, occasionally accompanied by cortical visual disturbances, ataxia, focal weakness or sensory symptoms, and spontaneous or induced myoclonus. It is common to see a gaze that expresses apprehension or fear and shows heightened reactivity to external stimuli. This syndrome is frequently preceded by mild psychiatric symptoms such as malaise, apathy, anxiety, mood changes, anorexia, and diminished ability to concentrate. Extrapyramidal and cerebellar signs occasionally occur at onset, but the neurologic examination can also be unremarkable. Less common presentations include a prominent ataxia eclipsing the cognitive impairment; concomitant epilepsy; and visual deficits such as field defects, distortion, and cortical blindness. Neurologic signs can be unilateral. Fig. 29.9 illustrates imaging findings of patients with CJD.

Movement progressively becomes abnormal, with dementia that also worsens over time. Sleep-wake symptoms develop with severe sleep EEG abnormalities with loss of sleep spindles, very low sleep efficiency, and virtual absence of rapid eye movement (REM) sleep.[39] Akinetic mutism will eventually develop, with overriding startle myoclonic jerks when an auditory or sensory stimulus is introduced, particularly during later stages of the disease.[40]

### MEDICAL MANAGEMENT

**DIAGNOSIS.** Human prion diseases present a formidable diagnostic challenge to clinicians, mainly because of their rarity and varied manifestations. The heterogeneity of human prion diseases is attributable to the presence of three forms with distinct causes—sporadic, inherited, and acquired by infection. Detection of spongy change alone is not sufficient for the neuropathologic diagnosis of prion disease but must be corroborated with Western blot testing. If familial prion proteinopathy is suspected, molecular genetic analysis of DNA from lymphocytes can be performed.[22] For the practical purpose of enabling a prompt diagnosis, sporadic prion diseases can be separated into three groups: the cognitive subtypes including sCJD MM1 and sCJD MV1, sCJD MM2, and sCJD VV1; the ataxic subtypes including sCJD VV2 and sCJD MV2; and sporadic prion diseases with non-CJD phenotypes.[54]

**TREATMENT AND PROGNOSIS.** Once diagnosed, prion diseases are rapidly progressive and eventually fatal, typically within 6 to 12 months. The key barrier to effective therapy is that these disorders manifest clinically when neuronal loss is advanced and irreversible. Current treatments are almost all directed at modifying symptoms; few address underlying pathogenic mechanisms and are inevitably delivered too late to rescue dying neurons. A new therapeutic target for prion disease, effective animal studies, lends further insight into mechanisms of prion neurotoxicity, with the possibility for a window of reversibility in neuronal damage characterized as neuronal rescue. Using lentivirally mediated RNA interference (RNAi) against native prion protein (PrP) interventions results in prevention of symptoms and increased survival in mice with established prion disease. The treatment prevents the formation of the neurotoxic prion agent at a point when diseased neurons can still be saved from death; however, the target and the timing of the intervention appear to be critical.[28,74,77]

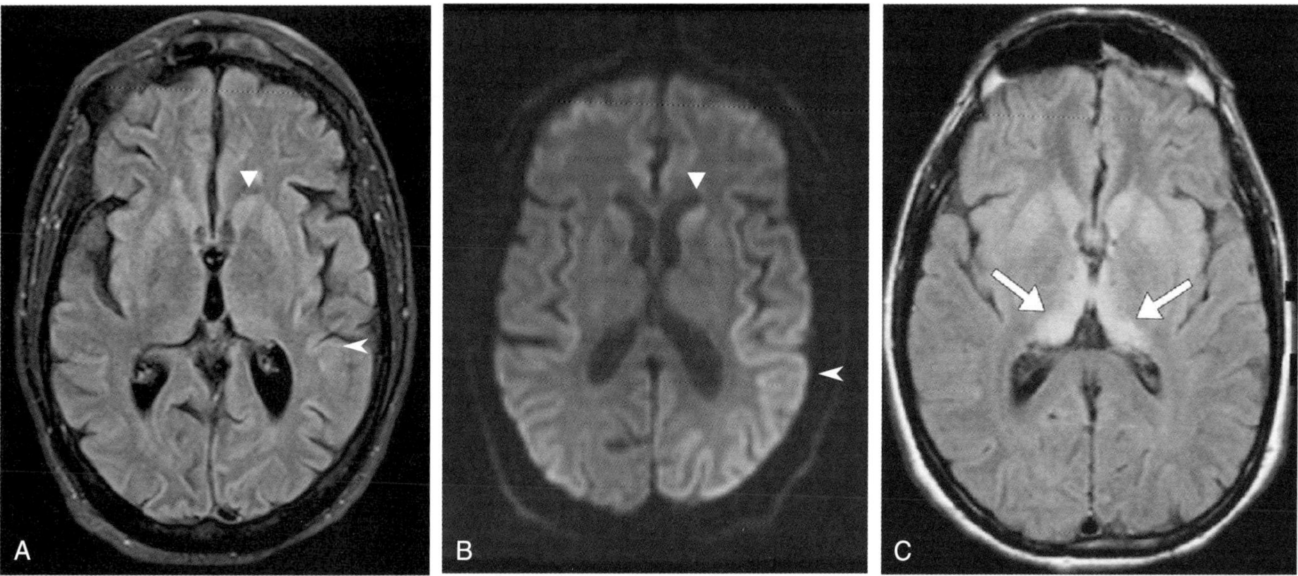


**Figure 29.9**

**Magnetic resonance imaging appearance of prion disease.** (A–B) Fluid-attenuated inversion recovery (FLAIR) (A) and diffusion-weighted imaging (DWI) (B) from a 63-year-old man with sporadic Creutzfeldt-Jakob disease (CJD). There is subtle hyperintensity in the cortical ribbon *(arrowhead)* and head of the caudate *(triangle)*, seen more clearly on DWI than on FLAIR. (C) FLAIR from a patient with variant CJD displays hyperintensity in the posterior thalamus *(arrows)*, the so-called pulvinar sign that is characteristic of this form of CJD. (A–B, From Bennett JE, Dolin R, Blaser MJ: *Mandell, Douglas, and Bennett's principles and practice of infectious diseases*, ed 9, Philadelphia, 2020, Elsevier. C, From Tschampa HJ, Zerr I, Urbach H. Radiological assessment of Creutzfeldt-Jakob disease. *Eur Radiol.* 17:1200–1211, 2007.)

SPECIAL IMPLICATIONS FOR THE THERAPIST 29.1

## *Infectious Disorders of the Central Nervous System*

The therapist must understand and observe all isolation procedures. Often the treatment of these clients begins in the intensive care unit. Monitoring vital signs throughout the treatment session may be necessary when the client is in the acute stage. The client may demonstrate symptoms that are similar to many noninfectious brain disorders. The clinical picture may represent the diffuse disorders typical of brain trauma, or there may be only focal neurologic symptoms that may appear similar to stroke or neoplasm.[60]

Initially, when the inflammatory response is greatest, there may be a profound alteration of consciousness. The therapist should be familiar with the scales used to monitor levels of consciousness such as the Glasgow Coma Scale. The client may be agitated, with difficulty in processing sensory input resulting in increased sensitivity to sound and light. Cognitive and perceptual disorders with memory deficits probably represent the involvement of the brain in the area of the ventricles.[53] It is essential that the therapist understand the behavioral changes that accompany diffuse brain disorders. See Chapter 33 for further details.

Sensory dysfunction should be thoroughly evaluated. If the client has a history of instability of heart rate, blood pressure, or respiration, these should be monitored during the evaluation of sensation because sensory input may aggravate responses in some individuals. Cutaneous sensation may be affected in different distributions, depending on whether the damage is diffuse or deep in one area of the brain. Distorted or absent sensory input can affect mobility and functional status in a dramatic way. See Chapter 32 for a further description of sensory and motor deficits related to specific areas of damage.

Movement disorders also reflect the nature and depth of the insult to the brain. Abnormal posturing of the client in the acute phase may be noted, and abnormal postural reflexes may be present. Decorticate posturing and decerebrate posturing are often seen in the early stages of these brain disorders.[12] Positioning and range-of-motion exercises are critical in the early phases because the stiffness of the back and neck can exacerbate the pain. Often, maintaining a darkened and quiet environment during treatment will decrease headache symptoms. Understanding motor learning strategies is important because movement often must be relearned in the context of residual damage or agitated behaviors (see Special Implications for the Therapist 28.1: Motor Learning Strategies in Chapter 28).

When interacting with the client and family, it is important to be familiar with the acute, subacute, and chronic prognosis related to the type of infection causing the brain injury. Knowing there may be a good outcome will be encouraging during the acute and devastating onset of the infections. Neurologic recovery will continue for many years if the brain remains stimulated as a course of appropriate physical rehabilitation.[53] If the prognosis is less favorable, focusing on preventive measures (range-of-motion teaching, optimizing positioning, pressure relief), compensatory strategies (alternative means for mobilization and locomotion), and family training (bed mobility, lift training, transfer training) is indicated as opposed to restorative rehabilitation. The degree of patient participation in therapy will depend on the level of consciousness and the presence and degree of persistent neurologic deficits. During the late summer season, the therapist should be aware of the manifestations of mosquito- or tick-borne illnesses. Changes in clients that are consistent with infections should be monitored, and a referral should be made to the appropriate health care provider when necessary.

## A THERAPIST'S THOUGHTS[a]

"Until the therapist determines that the vital functions, such as rate of respiration, heart rate, and blood pressure vary appropriately with the demands of the intervention, these factors should be monitored."

[a]Judith A. Dewane, PT, Dsc, NCS

## REFERENCES

To enhance this text and add value for the reader, all references are included in the enhanced ebook on Student Consult that accompanies this textbook. The reader can view the reference source and access it online whenever possible.

# CHAPTER 30

# Central Nervous System Neoplasms

KORRE L. SCOTT

## INTRODUCTION

Several categories of neoplasia affect the central nervous system (CNS). *Primary* tumors, which may be either benign or malignant, may develop in the brain, spinal cord, or surrounding structures. Secondary, or *metastatic,* tumors may spread to the CNS from another site, such as the lung or breast. *Paraneoplastic syndromes* may occur because of remote or indirect effects on the CNS from cancer elsewhere in the body. Additionally, and less commonly, *leptomeningeal carcinomatosis* may occur, in which carcinoma metastasizes to the pia mater and arachnoid, with multiple lesions to the meninges and cerebrospinal fluid (CSF) pathways of the brain and/or spinal cord.

The presence of any CNS tumor is cause for concern because of the vital functions of the brain and spinal cord. The critical areas and confined spaces in the CNS make it vulnerable to a space-occupying lesion. Most primary malignant CNS tumors are locally invasive and cause significant morbidity and mortality.[97]

The early effects of a CNS tumor are related to mechanical displacement of brain or spinal cord tissue or a mild block in CSF circulation, causing increased intracranial pressure (ICP). As a tumor grows, compression or destruction of local brain or nerve tissue may occur, resulting in specific neurologic deficits. Symptoms of brain tumors may range from minimal such as mild lethargy to marked such as seizures, blindness, and paralysis as the tumor progresses. Likewise, symptoms of spinal cord tumors may range from mild to severe and include pain, sensory impairments, weakness, and paralysis. Although primary CNS tumors typically do not metastasize outside the CNS because of the lack of a CNS lymphatic system to transport cancer cells, some tumors such as medulloblastoma may infrequently travel through the CSF to the spinal cord as "drop metastasis" and cause spinal cord complications. Hematogenous dissemination of a primary brain tumor to a site outside the skull does not usually occur.

The diagnosis of a CNS tumor, with its threat of significant loss of neurologic and cognitive function, is devastating to the client and family. A CNS tumor robs a person of independence and dignity and is viewed as a humbling and inextricably fatal process.[87] Difficult decisions about treatment options and quality-of-life issues add stress for the client and family. In children with brain tumors, the diagnosis creates parental fear and emotional upheaval and requires adjusting and decision making for the different needs at varying stages of the illness.[50] Caregiving and financial struggles frequently are encountered with both brain and spinal cord tumors.

Despite the inescapable realities of these difficult issues, the situation is improving, with dramatic new advances in radiologic imaging, neurosurgery, and adjuvant therapy. At the present time, approximately 50% of patients with CNS tumors, including patients with both benign and malignant tumors, can be successfully treated and have an excellent long-term prognosis.[162] Knowledge and awareness of current treatment advances provide the health professional with the information and skills to care for the client and family in a sensitive, compassionate, and hopeful but realistic manner.

### Classification

The major purpose of tumor classification is to facilitate communication about tumor behavior and treatment and to design studies to learn more about the tumors.[174] Primary brain tumors are classified by light microscopy according to their predominant cell type.[92] The World Health Organization (WHO) classification system, which incorporates the Ringerz system for astrocytomas, is becoming the most commonly accepted system, making it easier for clinicians to accurately compare the effects of treatment.[21,38,92,111] It is a three-tiered system based on neuroembryonal origin, that is, naming a tumor by the most likely cell of origin, and adding qualifying phrases to describe its behavior.[174] An update to the WHO classification system in 2016 included molecular parameters, which changed the classification of several tumor families and brings more precision for clinical, experimental, and epidemiologic purposes.[93]

Table 30.1 presents the 2016 WHO classification of primary tumors. The grading, from I to IV, indicates the aggressiveness of the tumor, with grade IV being the most aggressive. The St. Anne–Mayo (Daumas-Duport)[128] system is another classification system in use. It is four-tiered, based on the presence or absence of four major criteria (nuclear atypia, mitoses [cells in a state of division], endothelial proliferation, and necrosis), with grade I having none of these features, grade II having one feature, grade III having two features, and grade IV having three or

**Table 30.1** World Health Organization Classification of Primary Brain Tumors According to Histology and Molecular Parameters

| Tumor Group | Common Tumor Types | WHO Grade |
|---|---|---|
| Diffuse astrocytic and oligodendroglial tumors | Diffuse astrocytoma | II |
| | Anaplastic astrocytoma | III |
| | Glioblastoma | IV |
| | Oligodendroglioma | II |
| | Anaplastic oligodendroglioma | III |
| Other astrocytic tumors | Pilocytic astrocytoma | I |
| | Subependymal giant cell astrocytoma | I |
| | Pleomorphic xanthoastrocytoma | II |
| | Anaplastic pleomorphic xanthoastrocytoma | III |
| Ependymal tumors | Subependymoma | I |
| | Myxopapillary ependymoma | I |
| | Ependymoma | II |
| | Anaplastic ependymoma | III |
| Other gliomas | Angiocentric glioma | I |
| | Chordoid glioma of third ventricle | II |
| Choroid plexus tumors | Choroid plexus papilloma | I |
| | Atypical choroid plexus papilloma | II |
| | Choroid plexus carcinoma | III |
| Neuronal and mixed neuronal-glial tumors | Dysembryoplastic neuroepithelial tumor | I |
| | Gangliocytoma | I |
| | Ganglioglioma | I |
| | Anaplastic ganglioglioma | III |
| | Dysplastic gangliocytoma of cerebellum (Lhermitte-Duclos disease) | I |
| | Desmoplastic infantile astrocytoma and ganglioglioma | I |
| | Papillary glioneuronal tumor | I |
| | Rosette-forming glioneuronal tumor | I |
| | Central neurocytoma | II |
| | Extraventricular neurocytoma | II |
| | Cerebellar liponeurocytoma | II |
| Tumors of the pineal region | Pineocytoma | I |
| | Pineal parenchymal tumor of intermediate differentiation | II or III |
| | Pineoblastoma | IV |
| | Papillary tumor of the pineal region | II or III |
| Embryonal tumors | Medulloblastoma (all subtypes) | IV |
| | Embryonal tumor with multilayered rosettes | IV |
| | Medulloepithelioma | IV |
| | CNS embryonal tumor | IV |
| | Atypical teratoid/rhabdoid tumor | IV |
| | CNS embryonal tumor with rhabdoid features | IV |
| Tumors of the cranial and paraspinal nerves | Schwannoma | I |
| | Neurofibroma | I |
| | Perineurioma | I |
| | Malignant peripheral nerve sheath tumor | I, II, or III |
| Meningiomas | Meningioma | I |
| | Atypical meningioma | II |
| | Anaplastic (malignant) meningioma | III |
| Mesenchymal, nonmeningothelial tumors | Solitary fibrous tumor/hemangiopericytoma | I, II, or III |
| | Hemangioblastoma | I |
| Tumors of the sellar region | Craniopharyngioma | I |
| | Granular cell tumor | I |
| | Pituicytoma | I |
| | Spinal cell oncocytoma | I |

*CNS*, Central nervous system; *WHO*, World Health Organization.
Adapted from Louis DN, et al: The 2016 World Health Organization Classification of Tumors of the Central Nervous System: a summary. *Acta Neuropathol* 131:803–820, 2016.

four features. Various other systems exist, based on a number of distinguishing criteria, as follows: neuroembryonal origin, primary versus secondary, benign versus malignant, histologic grade, anatomic location, and childhood versus adult tumors. The multiplicity of grading systems has been confusing, making it difficult for clinicians to accurately compare the effects of treatment,[128] so the acceptance of one system would be beneficial.

Primary brain tumors originate from the various cells and structures normally found within the brain.

Secondary or metastatic brain tumors originate from structures outside the brain, most often from primary tumors of the lungs, breast, gastrointestinal tract, or genitourinary tract[63] or from melanoma.[170]

Primary CNS tumors, also may be subdivided into *malignant* tumors, such as astrocytomas, and so-called *benign tumors*, such as meningiomas, neurinomas, and hemangioblastomas. A histologically benign tumor has a slow growth rate and is relatively noninvasive. However, because of space-occupying properties in vital tissue with a resultant high threat of functional limitation, the use of the term *benign* is somewhat misleading. Some authors insist that because of location even a very slow-growing CNS tumor should be considered basically malignant.[49,92] The histologically benign tumor may be surgically inaccessible or located in a vital area, such as the pons or medulla, and will continue to grow, thereby causing an increase in ICP, neurologic deficits, herniation syndromes, and, finally, death.

Malignant CNS tumors typically have a high growth rate and are invasive and infiltrative. They are capable of modulating the surrounding extracellular matrix by secretion of substances that allow for invasion of surrounding tissue by the tumor cells.[128] Tumors also have the ability to create new blood vessels to sustain the tumor, a process called *angiogenesis*.

Anatomic brain tumor location refers to the location of the lesion in reference to the tentorium or cerebral tissue. Knowing the anatomic location helps to predict probable deficits based on the function of that particular area in the brain. Box 30.1 lists the anatomic location of the most common CNS tumors.

There are other typically recognized subdivisions. The two main groups of primary tumors in the brain are *gliomas*, which are the most common type and include astrocytomas and glioblastomas, and tumors arising from supporting structures, such as meningiomas, neurinomas, and pituitary adenomas. A third group arising from embryonal undifferentiated nerve cells has been termed *primitive neuroectodermal tumors (PNETs)*[58]; these arise more frequently in children. Examples of primary tumors in the spinal cord include the more common neurinomas (schwannomas or neurilemomas) and the less frequent gliomas and meningiomas.

Further subgroups of gliomas have been established based on cellular atypism, the presence of mitotic figures, the incidence of endothelial hyperplasia, and the presence of necrotic areas. It is hoped that newer techniques of molecular biology, such as the ability to identify growth factors and inhibitors necessary for cell growth and differentiation, may lead to a more sophisticated subclassification. Molecular and genetic signatures may predict brain tumor behavior and may soon guide not only tumor classification and diagnosis but also tumor-specific treatment strategies.[45]

Because the clinical presentation, treatment, and prognosis are heavily dependent on the location of involvement and whether the tumor is primary or metastatic, this discussion is divided into four parts: (1) primary brain tumors, (2) primary intraspinal tumors, (3) metastatic tumors, and (4) childhood brain tumors.

Box 30.1

**ANATOMIC SITES OF THE MOST COMMON CENTRAL NERVOUS SYSTEM TUMORS**

***Supratentorial Tumors***

- Cerebral hemispheres
  - Metastases
  - Meningiomas
  - Gliomas (malignant gliomas: anaplastic astrocytoma and glioblastoma multiforme, astrocytoma, oligodendroglioma)

***Midline Tumors***

- Pituitary adenomas
- Pineal tumors
- Craniopharyngiomas

***Infratentorial Tumors***

- Adults
  - Acoustic schwannomas (neurinomas, neurilemomas)
  - Metastases
  - Meningiomas
  - Hemangioblastomas
- Children
  - Cerebellar astrocytomas
  - Medulloblastomas
  - Ependymomas
  - Brainstem gliomas

***Spinal Cord Tumors***

- Extradural
- Metastases
- Intradural
- Extramedullary
  Meningiomas
  Schwannomas, neurofibromas
- Intramedullary
  Ependymomas
  Astrocytomas

Adapted from Weiss HD: Neoplasms. In Samuels MA, ed: *Manual of neurologic therapeutics*, ed 5, Boston, 1995, Little, Brown, p 225.

# PRIMARY BRAIN TUMORS

## Incidence and Prevalence

Tumors of the CNS are not uncommon. The National Cancer Institute (NCI) projected that 23,888 new *malignant primary* tumors of the brain and nervous system would be diagnosed in 2018 in the United States.[7] According to data from the NCI Surveillance, Epidemiology, and End Results (SEER), in 2015 there were approximately 166,039 people alive with a history of CNS cancer. The mean age at diagnosis of brain and nervous system cancer is 58 years. The overall 5-year relative survival rate for 2008–2014 was reported to be 33.2%. It was estimated that 23,880 new cases of brain and nervous system cancer would occur and that 16,830 men and women would die from these cancers in 2018.[3,7,107]

*Benign primary* brain tumors add to the total incidence. The American Brain Tumor Association reported a combined estimate of 80,000 new primary malignant and benign brain tumors in 2018, the most recent estimate available.[4,5] The number of people living with either a benign or malignant brain tumor (prevalence) in the

United States in 2018 was estimated to be greater than 700,000.4 An estimated 32% of all brain and CNS tumors are malignant.[2]

Although malignant brain tumors accounted for a small percentage of the approximately 1.7 million new cases of *all* types of cancer, brain tumors kill more Americans each year than multiple sclerosis and Hodgkin disease combined.[150] For all intracranial diseases, death from intracranial neoplasms is second only to death from stroke.[58] Approximately 16,000 deaths each year in the United States are caused by primary brain and nervous system tumors.[5] The incidence of primary brain and nervous system tumors peaks in the pediatric population, then increases by approximately 1.2% per year until it plateaus in the population older than 70 years of age.[128] Primary brain tumors are the second most common form of cancer in children,[13,106] and primary CNS tumors are the leading cause of death from cancer in children, resulting in more deaths than leukemia in a 2016 study. Gliomas account for approximately 50% of CNS tumors. The average age of onset for all primary brain tumors is 60 years.[127] Table 30.2 summarizes the frequency of primary CNS tumors.[2]

More than 60% of tumors in adults are supratentorial, or located in the cerebral hemispheres above the tentorium. The tentorium is a flap of meninges separating the cerebral hemispheres from the posterior fossa structures. The majority of pediatric tumors are infratentorial, involving primarily the cerebellum and brainstem.[34] Certain tumor types have a predilection for specific areas of the brain, although they may arise elsewhere in the brain. Fig. 30.1 illustrates the topologic distribution and preferred sites of primary CNS tumors.

## Pathogenesis

Brain tumors affect the brain through compression of cerebral tissue, including brain substance and cranial nerves, invasion or infiltration of cerebral tissue, and sometimes erosion of bone.[63] These mechanisms precipitate pathophysiologic changes, such as cerebral edema and increased ICP.

In most brain tumors, vasogenic edema develops in the surrounding tissue of the tumor because of compression and obstruction of CSF pathways, moving CSF across ventricular walls.[58] Substances released from tumor cells altering the blood-brain barrier also may cause rapid cerebral edema. Increased permeability of the capillary endothelial cells of the white matter impairs cellular activity and causes electrochemical instability, resulting in seizures. As the edema continues to develop, signs and symptoms of increased ICP become more apparent.

Initially the brain may have a surprising tolerance to the compressive and infiltrative effects of brain tumors, particularly with slow-growing tumors, and early symptoms may be few. Compensatory mechanisms to accommodate the edema and maintain normal ICP are limited. When the brain can no longer compensate, the resultant increase in ICP leads to more evident signs and symptoms. Intracranial herniation and herniation through the foramen magnum are potential results of serious ICP elevation. Fig. 30.2 illustrates intracranial herniation syndromes evoked by supratentorial masses.

## Clinical Manifestations

The particular clinical presentation of a brain tumor depends on the compression or infiltration of specific cerebral tissue, the related cerebral edema, and the development of increased ICP.[63] Cerebral edema surrounding the tumor results from the inflammatory response of tissues to the tumor and contributes to the increase in ICP. Box 30.2 lists common signs and symptoms of brain tumors.

The initial clinical signs of an intracranial tumor are related to the generalized effect of an increase in ICP. Headache is commonly present (in one-third to one-half of cases), is typically generalized or retroorbital, and is typically worse in the morning and better later in the day.

**Table 30.2** Frequency of Primary Central Nervous System Tumors

| CHILDREN (AGE 0–14 YEARS) | | ADULTS (AGE ≥15 YEARS) | |
|---|---|---|---|
| **Type** | **Percentage** | **Type** | **Percentage** |
| Glioblastoma | 20 | Glioblastoma | 50 |
| Astrocytoma | 21 | Astrocytoma | 10 |
| Ependymoma | 7 | Ependymoma | 2 |
| Oligodendroglioma | 1 | Oligodendroglioma | 3 |
| Medulloblastoma | 24 | Medulloblastoma | 2 |
| Neuroblastoma | 3 | Pituitary adenoma | 4 |
| Neurinoma | 1 | Neurinoma | 2 |
| Craniopharyngioma | 5 | Craniopharyngioma | 1 |
| Meningioma | 5 | Meningioma | 17 |
| Teratoma | 2 | Teratoma | — |
| Pinealoma | 2 | Pinealoma | 1 |
| Hemangioma | 3 | Hemangioma | 2 |
| Sarcoma | 1 | Sarcoma | 1 |
| Others | 5 | Others | 5 |
| Total | 100 | Total | 100 |

Adapted from Janus TJ, Yung WKA: Primary neurological tumors. In Goetz CG, ed: *Textbook of clinical neurology*, ed 2, Philadelphia, 2003, Saunders.

The headache is intensified or precipitated by any activity that tends to raise the ICP, such as stooping, straining, coughing, or exercising. Irritation, compression, or traction of pain-sensitive structures, such as the dura mater and blood vessels, causes the headache.[131] Although tension-type headache is more common, migraine-type and other types may be exhibited.[172] The sixth cranial nerve (abducens) is highly susceptible to elevated ICP because of its local anatomic relationships as the basis pontis slips caudally during transtentorial herniation, not, as previously believed, because of its long intracranial path.[60] This causes weakness in the lateral rectus muscle and diplopia. Nausea and vomiting are common, often caused by increased ICP. About one-third of patients with glioblastoma multiforme (GBM) experience nausea and vomiting. Box 30.3 lists signs and symptoms of intracranial hypertension.

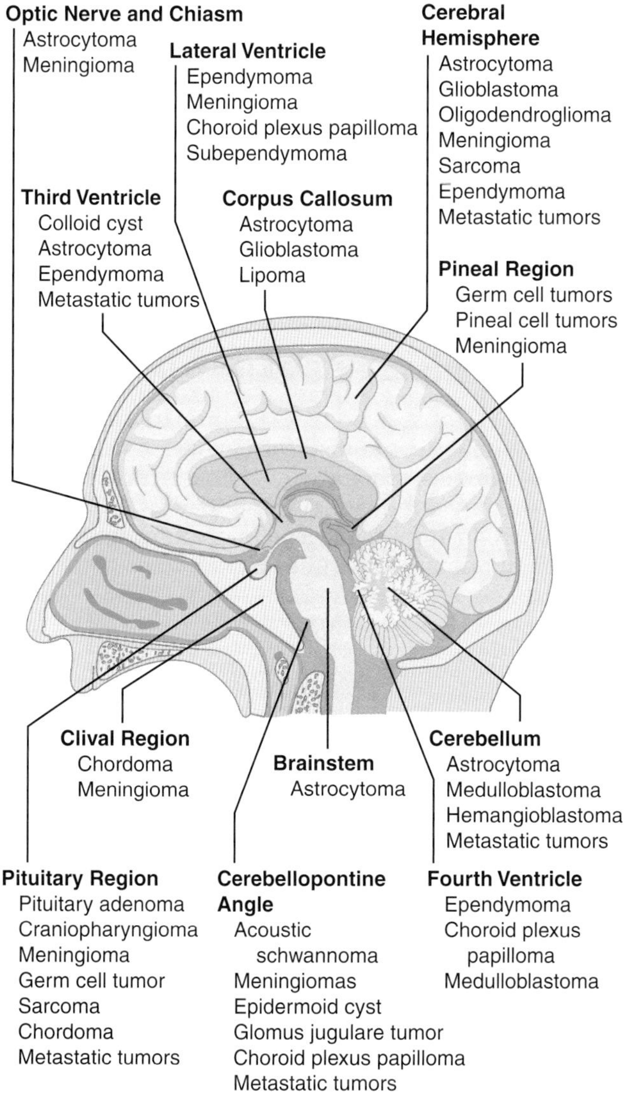


**Fig. 30.1**

**Topologic distribution and preferred sites of primary central nervous system tumors.** (Adapted from Burger PC, et al: *Surgical pathology of the nervous system and its coverings*, ed 3, New York, 1991, Churchill Livingstone.)

Other common initial signs are mental clouding, lethargy, alterations in consciousness and cognition, syncope (fainting), and easy fatigability. Behavioral changes may include irritability, flat affect, emotional lability, and lack of initiative and spontaneity. Increasing intracranial CSF pressure may precipitate an increase in perioptic pressure, which in turn impedes venous drainage from the optic head area and retina, causing papilledema, or edema of the optic disc. Papilledema, present in approximately 70% to 75% of patients with brain tumors, is associated with visual changes, such as decreased visual acuity, an enlarged blind spot, diplopia, and deficits in the visual fields. Often deterioration in vision may be the precipitating factor that leads the patient to seek an appointment with an optometrist or ophthalmologist. A dilated ophthalmologic examination showing papilledema is important to the diagnosis when it is not straightforward.

Approximately 20% to 50% of adults with brain tumors develop seizure activity.[28] The cerebral edema causes hyperactive cells, which produce abnormal, paroxysmal discharges or seizure activity.[134] Seizures may be the first presenting sign of a tumor. In patients presenting with seizures, detection of low-grade gliomas is becoming increasingly frequent with magnetic resonance imaging (MRI). Fig. 30.3 shows an MRI scan of a low-grade glioma manifesting with a seizure. In the later stages of illness, seizure activity is present in 70% of patients.[117] A common feature of a tumor-related seizure is its repetitive

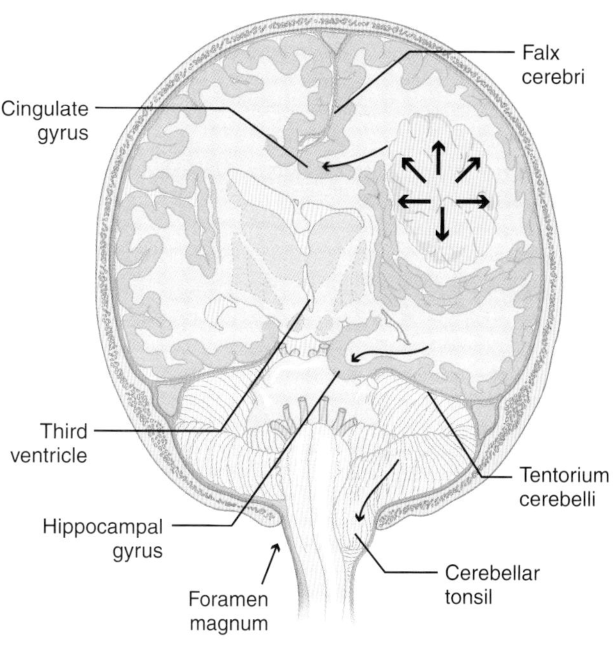


**Fig. 30.2**

**Intracranial herniation syndromes evoked by supratentorial masses.** The tumor and its edema *(arrows)* have produced the following *(curved arrows)*: cingulated gyrus herniation under the falx cerebri; diencephalic herniation across the midline, compressing the ipsilateral ventricle and producing hydrocephalus in the contralateral ventricle; hippocampal gyrus herniation through the tentorial notch compressing the posterior cerebral artery and brainstem; and herniation of the cerebellar tonsils through the foramen magnum. (From Abeloff MD, et al: *Clinical oncology*, ed 3, Philadelphia, 2004, Churchill Livingstone; and adapted from Plum F, Posner JB: *The diagnosis of stupor and coma*, ed 2, Philadelphia, 1980, FA Davis.)

Box 30.2

**SIGNS AND SYMPTOMS OF BRAIN TUMORS**

- Headache
- Visual changes (double vision, blurred vision)
- Nausea
- Vomiting
- Cognitive changes—impairment of memory, judgment, personality
- Lethargy
- Behavioral changes
- Seizures
- Syncope
- Weakness
- Hemiparesis, hemiplegia
- Apraxia
- Cortical sensory deficits (graphesthesia, stereognosis difficulties)
- Sensory impairments (tingling, spatial orientation changes)
- Cranial nerve palsies
- Aphasia
- Facial numbness
- Hearing disturbances
- Anosmia
- Swallowing difficulties
- Paralysis of outward gaze (sixth cranial nerve)
- Papilledema
- Incoordination
- Ataxia
- In children, diastases of cranial sutures and enlarging head size

Box 30.3

**SIGNS AND SYMPTOMS OF INTRACRANIAL HYPERTENSION**

***Common***

- Headache
- Tinnitus
- Vomiting (with or without nausea)
- Visual obscurations, visual loss, photopsias
- Papilledema
- Diplopia
- Lethargy and increased sleep
- Psychomotor retardation
- Pain on eye movement

***Less Common***

- Hearing distortion or loss
- Vertigo
- Facial weakness
- Shoulder or arm pain
- Neck pain or rigidity
- Ataxia
- Paresthesias of extremities
- Anosmia
- Trigeminal neuralgia

Adapted from DeAngelis LM: Tumors of the central nervous system. In Goldman LM, Ausiello D, eds: *Cecil textbook of medicine*, ed 22, Philadelphia, 2004, Saunders.

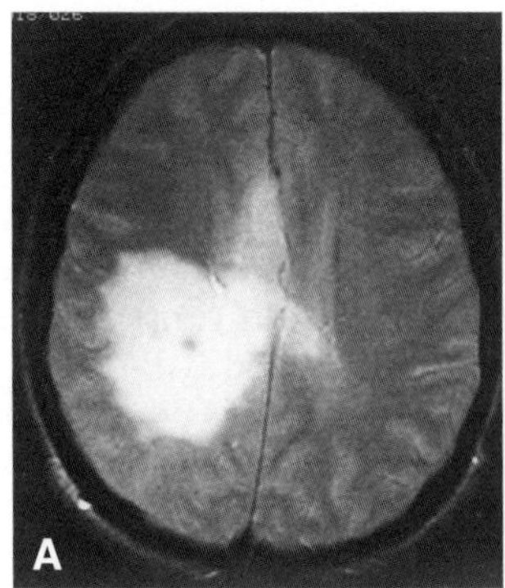


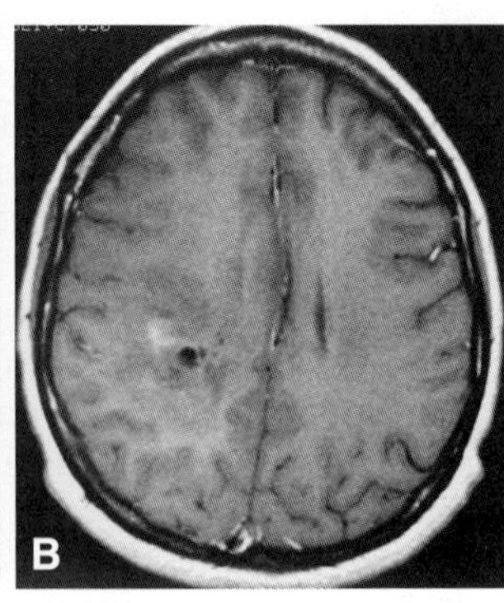


**Fig. 30.3**

**Magnetic resonance imaging (MRI) of a low-grade glioma.** (A) T2-weighted image. (B) T1-weighted image, gadolinium contrast with minimum enhancement. The images are typical of this tumor, which is being detected with increasing frequency by MRI in patients with seizure disorders. Many are invisible on computed tomography scans. (From Goldman LM, Ausiello D, eds: *Cecil textbook of medicine*, ed 22, Philadelphia, 2004, Saunders.)

nature, with seizures being very stereotypical in a given patient.[172]

As the tumor grows, causing progressive destruction or dysfunction of tissue, locally referable signs may occur (hemiparesis, specific cranial nerve dysfunction, aphasia, visual symptoms, ataxia), which may help to localize the tumor site. Table 30.3 lists signs associated with localized brain lesions.

## SPECIFIC PRIMARY BRAIN TUMORS

A wide variety of specific types of primary brain tumor exist, with similarities in medical management and implications for physical therapy. Therefore the specific tumors are first presented individually, followed by a discussion of diagnosis, medical management, and therapy implications for all primary brain tumors.

### Gliomas

#### Overview and Incidence

Gliomas are the most common primary brain tumors, accounting for 30% to 40% of all brain tumors, with men more frequently affected than women in a 3:2 ratio.[4] Gliomas are divided into *benign* or *low-grade gliomas,* such as low-grade astrocytomas, and *malignant gliomas,* such as anaplastic astrocytomas and GBMs. Other gliomas are oligodendrogliomas, ependymomas, and medulloblastomas. Terms such as *brainstem glioma* and *optic nerve glioma* refer to the location of these tumors. Only a tissue sample will give the specific diagnosis.

Low-grade astrocytomas account for 7% to 10% of primary brain tumors[1,4] and are the most common type of intracranial tumor in children. Malignant astrocytomas (anaplastic astrocytoma and GBM) are much more common in adults than low-grade astrocytomas, making up 20% to 30% of primary brain tumors. Oligodendrogliomas and ependymomas make up another 5% to 7%. Medulloblastomas, sometimes termed *embryonal tumors* or *PNETs,* make up approximately 1% of primary brain

**Table 30.3** Signs Associated With Localized Brain Lesions

| Location of Lesion | Associated Signs |
|---|---|
| Prefrontal area | Loss of judgment, failure of memory, inappropriate behavior, apathy, poor attention span, easily distracted, release phenomena |
| Frontal eye fields | Failure to sustain gaze to opposite side, saccadic eye movements, impersistence, seizures with forced deviation of the eyes to the opposite side |
| Precentral gyrus | Partial motor seizures, jacksonian seizures, generalized seizures, hemiparesis |
| Superficial parietal lobe | Partial sensory seizures, loss of cortical sensation including two-point discrimination, tactile localization, stereognosis, and graphism |
| Angular gyrus | Agraphia, acalculia, finger agnosia, allochiria (right-left confusion) (Gerstmann syndrome) |
| Broca area | Motor dysphasia |
| Superior temporal gyrus | Receptive dysphasia |
| Midbrain | Early hydrocephalus; loss of upward gaze; pupillary abnormalities; third nerve involvement—ptosis, external strabismus, diplopia; ipsilateral cerebellar signs; contralateral hemiparesis; parkinsonism; akinetic mutism |
| Cerebellar hemisphere | Ipsilateral cerebellar ataxia with hypotonia, dysmetria, intention tremor, nystagmus to side of lesion |
| Pons | Sixth nerve involvement—diplopia, internal strabismus; seventh nerve involvement—ipsilateral facial paralysis; contralateral hemiparesis; contralateral hemisensory loss; ipsilateral cerebellar ataxia; locked-in syndrome |
| Medial surface of frontal lobe | Apraxia of gait, urinary incontinence |
| Corpus callosum | Left-hand apraxia and agraphia, generalized tonic-clonic seizures |
| Thalamus | Contralateral thalamic pain, contralateral hemisensory loss |
| Temporal lobe | Partial complex seizures, contralateral homonymous upper quadrantanopsia |
| Paracentral lobule | Progressive spastic paraparesis, urgency of micturition, incontinence |
| Deep parietal lobe | Autotopagnosia, anosognosia, contralateral homonymous lower quadrantanopsia |
| Third ventricle | Paroxysmal headache, hydrocephalus |
| Fourth ventricle | Hydrocephalus, progressive cerebellar ataxia, progressive spastic hemiparesis or quadriparesis |
| Cerebellopontine angle | Hearing loss, tinnitus, cerebellar ataxia, facial pain, facial weakness, dysphagia, dysarthria |
| Olfactory groove | Ipsilateral anosmia, ipsilateral optic atrophy, contralateral papilledema (Foster Kennedy syndrome) |
| Optic chiasm | Incongruous bitemporal field defects, bitemporal hemianopsia, optic atrophy |
| Orbital surface frontal lobe | Partial complex seizures, paroxysmal atrial tachycardia |
| Optic nerve | Visual failure of one eye, optic atrophy |
| Uncus | Partial complex seizures with olfactory hallucinations (uncinate fits) |
| Basal ganglia | Contralateral choreoathetosis, contralateral dystonia |
| Internal capsule | Contralateral hemiplegia, hemisensory loss, and homonymous hemianopsia |
| Pineal gland | Loss of upward gaze (Parinaud syndrome), early hydrocephalus, lid retraction, pupillary abnormalities |
| Occipital lobe | Partial seizures with elementary visual phenomena, homonymous hemianopsia with macular sparing |
| Hypothalamus, pituitary | Precocious puberty (children), impotence, amenorrhea, galactorrhea, hypothyroidism, hypopituitarism, diabetes insipidus, cachexia, diencephalic autonomic seizures |

From Gilroy J: *Basic neurology*, ed 2, Elmsford, NY, 1990, Pergamon Press, 228–229.

tumors. Brainstem gliomas often affect children between 5 and 10 years of age but can also occur in adults between 30 and 40 years of age. Most optic gliomas occur in children younger than age 10 years. Table 30.4 lists the types of primary brain tumors, the cell of origin, and the distribution of primary CNS tumors by histologic type. The age of peak incidence is 45 to 55 years in adults and 2 to 10 years in children.[168]

Gliomas are tumors of the glial cells, the group of cells that support, insulate, and metabolically assist the neurons. Glial cells are derived from glioblasts. It is of interest to note that neurons, despite their prevalence in the CNS (100 billion in the adult brain, according to some authors), are rarely the cellular basis of neoplastic transformation.

Glial cells, which numerically exceed the number of neurons, are subdivided into astrocytes (star-shaped cells, sometimes termed *long arms*), which provide nutrition for neurons; oligodendrocytes (glial cells with few processes, sometimes termed *short arms*), which produce the myelin sheath of the axonal projections of neurons; and ependymal cells, which line the ventricles and produce CSF.[63] Gliomas are subdivided into *astrocytomas, oligodendrogliomas,* and *ependymomas,* named for the cell of origin of the tumor. A combination glial cell tumor may occur as well, such as an oligoastrocytoma. *Medulloblastomas* are tumors of the vermis of the cerebellum and are classified by some authors as gliomas and by others as PNETs or embryonal tumors. Medulloblastoma is grouped with the PNETs because of common features, but some pathologists and clinicians prefer to distinguish these two; currently the debate continues.[127]

Astrocytomas are given histologic grades of I through IV to indicate the rate of cell division (mitosis), nuclear atypia, endothelial proliferation, and necrosis. Grade I and II astrocytomas are the slowest-growing tumors, and grade III and IV astrocytomas are progressively faster growing with higher rates of mitosis.[122] Astrocytomas are capable at any time of converting to a higher grade.[114] See Table 30.1.

**Table 30.4** Cell of Origin and Distribution of Primary Central Nervous System Tumors by Histologic Type

| Tumor | Cell of Origin | Frequency (%) |
|---|---|---|
| Meningioma | Arachnoidal fibroblast | 36.4 |
| Glioblastoma | Astrocyte | 15.1 |
| Astrocytoma | Astrocyte | 11.3 |
| Ependymoma | Ependymal cell | 1.9 |
| Oligodendroglioma | Oligodendrocyte | 2.5 |
| Embryonal including PNET/medulloblastoma | Unknown[a] | 1.1 |
| Pituitary adenoma | Pituitary | 6.6 |
| Craniopharyngioma | Rathke pouch | 0.8 |
| Nerve sheath | Schwann cell | 8.1 |
| Lymphoma | Lymphocyte | 2.0 |
| All others | | 12.6 |
| Choroid plexus papilloma or carcinoma | Choroid epithelial cell | |
| Hemangioblastoma | Endothelial cell | |
| Germ cell tumor | Primitive germ cell | |
| Pineocytoma | Pineal parenchymal cell | |
| Chordoma | Notochordal remnant | |

[a]Average annual age-adjusted incidence rate.

*PNET,* Primary neuroectodermal tumor.

Data from Ostrom QT, et al: CBTRUS Statistical Report: Primary Brain and Central Nervous System Tumors Diagnosed in the United States in 2008-2012. *Neuro Oncol* 17(Suppl 4):iv1–62, 2015; and Abeloff MD, et al, eds: *Clinical oncology: a clinical perspective balanced with relevant basic science,* ed 3, Philadelphia, 2004, Churchill Livingstone.

## Etiologic and Risk Factors

Relatively little is known about the cause of gliomas. They are characterized by a significant genetic heterogeneity, which makes the basic biology of glial neoplasms difficult to understand. A relationship may exist with chromosome abnormalities. Advances in the fields of molecular biology have allowed identification of mutated genes that increase the cell's susceptibility to the development of certain cancers.[114] These mutated genes that lead to the development of cancer are known as *oncogenes* (see Chapter 9).[128] Another type of chromosome abnormality leads to deletion of the cell's defense mechanism or its normal tumor-suppressing activity. This tumor suppressor gene, when altered, is unable to inhibit or is limited in its normal ability to inhibit cellular proliferation.[128] The presence of an oncogene and/or the absence of a tumor suppressor gene may be only one step toward tumor formation. Tumorigenesis is thought to be a multistep process, with other contributing factors in addition to chromosome abnormalities.[27]

Certain specific chromosome abnormalities have been linked to specific brain tumor types.[150] The oncogene *c-sis* has been identified with GBM. The oncogene *C-erb*B has been identified in 30% of malignant gliomas and is associated with the transforming growth factor receptor. Chromosome 17 abnormalities are present in all grades of astrocytomas.[150] Oncogenes may have some bearing on other genetic disorders associated with brain tumors. Neurofibromatosis, or von Recklinghausen disease (a familial condition involving the nervous system, muscles, bones, and skin and characterized by multiple soft tumors over the entire body associated with areas of pigmentation), is associated with spinal neuromas, acoustic neuromas, meningiomas, and gliomas. Tuberous sclerosis is associated with astrocytomas.[48] von Hippel–Lindau disease, a hereditary condition characterized by angiomatosis of the retina and cerebellum, is associated with hemangioblastomas.[168] The best-described tumor suppressor genes are Rb and p53, associated with retinoblastoma and Li-Fraumeni syndrome, a familial breast cancer associated with soft tissue sarcomas and other tumors.

No risk factors have been identified for the development of brain tumors, other than exposure to ionizing radiation.[130,140,174] The effects of carcinogenic viruses or agents are unclear. Associations have been made between certain viruses and brain tumors, such as Epstein-Barr virus and primary central nervous system lymphoma (PCNSL), but they are insufficient to constitute direct cause-and-effect relationships. Sustained exposure to certain pesticides, vinyl chloride, nitrosoureas, and polycyclic hydrocarbons has been implicated in astrocytic tumors, but epidemiologic surveys of workers in the farming, petrochemical, and rubber industries have produced conflicting results.[162] Certain industries, such as synthetic rubber processing, vinyl chloride production, and petrochemical and oil refining, do show increased risk.[127,153] Infection, trauma, and immunosuppression are other suspected triggers. Radiation treatment for scalp ringworm in children is associated with an increased rate of developing brain tumors late in life.[55] A history of frequent exposure to full-mouth dental x-rays, particularly at an early age, also is associated with certain brain tumors.[27] Most of the extensive research in the area of nonionizing radiation exposure such as that from cellular phones, household appliances, and high-voltage electrical lines does not support an association with cancer.[6] Although some studies may show an association with exposure to electromagnetic fields, either many other confounding variables such as exposure to other carcinogens may account for the association[27] or a direct causal relationship cannot be proven (see Chapter 4).[127] An increased risk of childhood tumors is also associated with maternal diet, including consumption of cured meats containing nitrites during pregnancy.[27,127]

## Low-Grade Astrocytoma—Grades I and II

**Incidence.** Low-grade astrocytomas account for 10% to 12% of primary brain tumors in adults.

**Pathogenesis.** Low-grade astrocytomas include WHO grades I and II. Grade I includes pilocytic astrocytoma (composed of fiber-shaped cells), sometimes termed *juvenile astrocytoma,* and is considered benign by some authors and malignant by others.[90,135] Grade I astrocytoma grows slowly and often becomes cystic. It is composed of astrocytes with densely staining nuclei and scanty cytoplasm and is usually relatively acellular. The cells are uniform and closely resemble mature resting or reactive nonanaplastic astrocytes (well differentiated). Mitoses are absent or very rare.[73,90] Although these are slow-growing tumors, they may become large.[5] Fig. 30.4 shows a well-differentiated astrocytoma. Grade II astrocytomas may be diffuse, infiltrative, and/or fibrillary and have more anaplastic features. *Fibrillary* refers to the neuroglial fibrils. Other types are protoplasmic (cells that consist largely of protoplasm) and gemistocytic (large, densely packed cells with a globoid appearance).[135] There is moderate cell density. Fig. 30.5 shows computed tomography (CT) and MRI scans of astrocytomas with and without the use of contrast material. The contrast agent, such as gadolinium, distinguishes the edema from the actual tumor. The larger the extent of the edema after administration of an intravenous contrast agent, the more malignant the lesion is likely to be.[106] Cerebral astrocytoma appears as a solid, gray mass with indistinct boundaries. Differentiation falls somewhere within a spectrum from well-differentiated (grade I) tumors to more anaplastic (grade II) tumors.[55] Astrocytomas in the cerebellum are often cystic and well circumscribed.

**Clinical Manifestations.** In adults, astrocytomas typically occur in the third and fourth decades of life and are usually located in the cerebrum, most commonly in the frontal lobes, but also may be found in the temporal lobes, parietal lobes, basal ganglia, and occipital lobes. Astrocytomas usually appear in the cerebellum in children.

In adults, typical initial symptoms are unilateral or focal headaches that become generalized as ICP increases. Frontal lobe tumors may produce personality disorders, with changes in behavior and emotional state. Parietal and temporal lobe tumors may cause seizures on one side of the body. Occipital lobe tumors produce visual changes. Involvement of the optic apparatus or optic pathways also may produce visual changes. See Table 30.3 for more signs associated with tumor location. Over time, astrocytomas, similar to other gliomas, tend to become more malignant. In children, cerebellar astrocytomas lead to symptoms of unilateral cerebellar ataxia involving the limbs and trunk, followed by signs of increased ICP.

**Prognosis.** Individuals with low-grade astrocytomas treated optimally have 5- to 10-year survival rates of 100% for completely excised lesions and 60% 5-year survival and 35% 10-year survival for partially excised lesions with radiation therapy. For many individuals there will be an average 5- to 7-year period of relative clinical stability.[124,135] Untreated low-grade astrocytomas have a 5-year survival rate of 32% and a 10-year survival rate of 11%.[162] Despite the benign categorization, astrocytomas are nearly always infiltrative lesions and are generally progressive. Conversion of a low-grade astrocytoma to a higher-grade lesion over the years is a common phenomenon.[105]

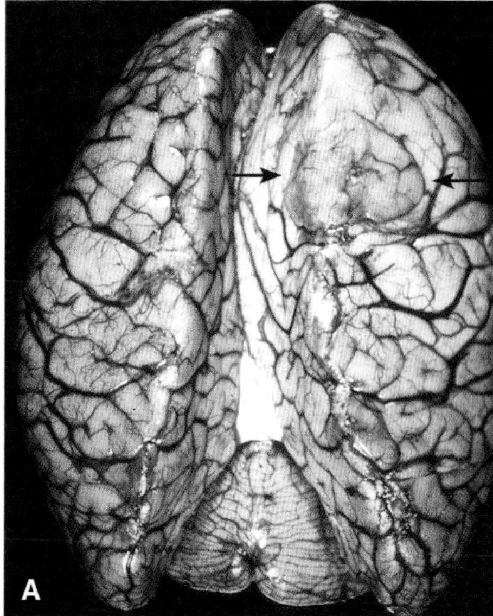


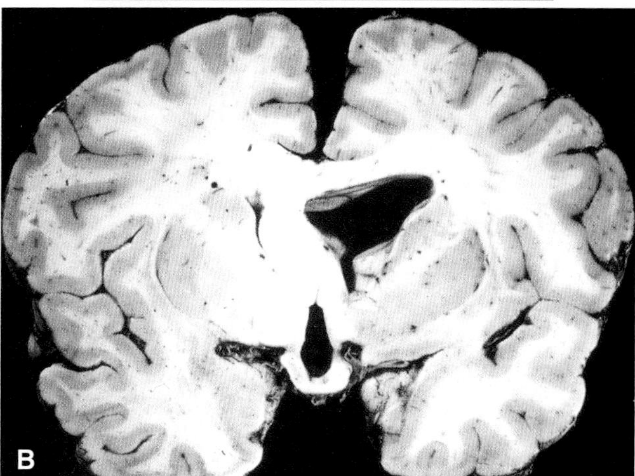


**Fig. 30.4**

**Well-differentiated astrocytoma.** (A) The right frontal tumor has expanded gyri, which led to flattening *(arrows).* (B) Expanded white matter of the left cerebral hemisphere and thickened corpus callosum and fornices. (From Kumar V, et al, eds: *Robbins and Cotran pathologic basis of disease,* ed 7, Philadelphia, 2005, Saunders.)

## High-Grade Astrocytoma—Grades III and IV

**Incidence.** High-grade malignant astrocytomas, WHO grades III and IV, are much more common in adults than low-grade astrocytomas. Grade III astrocytoma is often termed anaplastic astrocytoma, and grade IV is termed GBM, although both are highly anaplastic. Grade III and IV astrocytomas make up 20% to 35% of primary brain tumors.

**Pathogenesis.** Anaplastic astrocytomas, grades III and IV, are diffusely infiltrative tumors that invade the cerebral

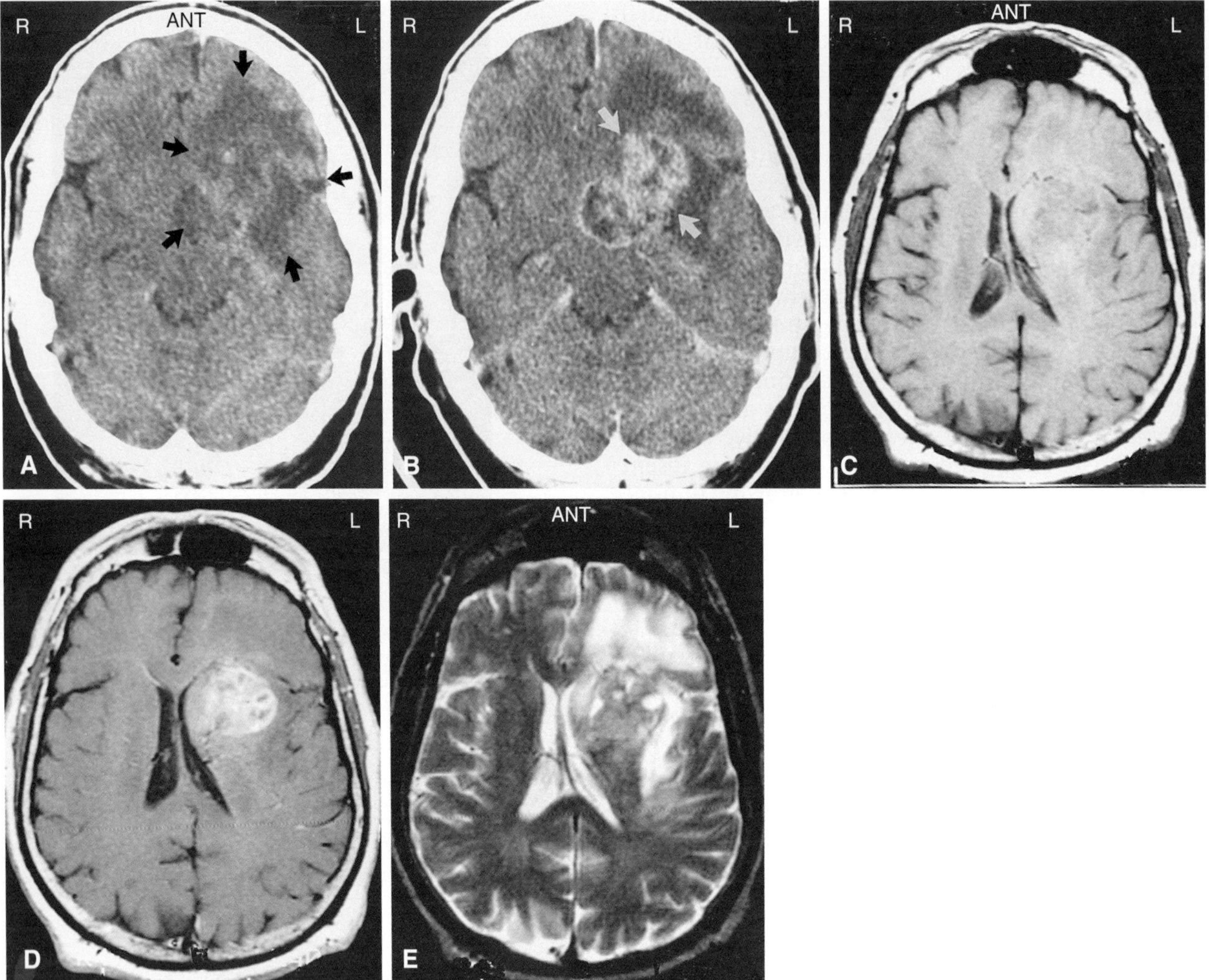


**Fig. 30.5**

**Astrocytoma.** Contrast and noncontrast computed tomography (CT) and magnetic resonance imaging (MRI) scans were obtained in the same patient and demonstrate a left astrocytoma with a large amount of surrounding edema. (A) Noncontrast CT shows only a large area of low density that represents the tumor and edema *(arrows)*. (B) Contrast CT shows enhancement of the tumor *(arrows)* surrounded by the dark or low-density area of edema. (C) Noncontrast T1-weighted MRI clearly shows a mass effect caused by impression of the tumor on the left lateral ventricle and some midline shift. (D) Gadolinium-enhanced T1-weighted MRI clearly outlines the tumor, but the edema is difficult to see. (E) T2-weighted MRI shows the tumor poorly, but the surrounding edema is easily seen as an area of increased signal *(white)*. (From Mettler FA Jr: *Essentials of radiology*, ed 2, Philadelphia, 2005, Saunders.)

parenchyma. They typically involve the white matter of the cerebral hemispheres.[18] They often contain a mix of cells and cell grades but are graded by the highest-grade cell seen in the tumor. GBM is a particularly rapidly growing, aggressive, infiltrative tumor that tends to invade both cerebral hemispheres via the corpus callosum. Fig. 30.6 shows MRI and intraoperative pictures of a GBM. GBM is a pinkish-gray or multicolored, well-demarcated mass with scattered areas of grossly visible hemorrhage. The blood vessels show endothelial proliferation: it is a highly vascular tumor, with vascular endothelial growth factor implicated, suggesting that the malignant progression from low-grade astrocytoma to GBM includes an "angiogenic switch."[18] The histologic distinction of an anaplastic astrocytoma from a glioblastoma is based largely on the absence or presence of tumor necrosis[168] and microvascular proliferation.[18] Microscopically the tumor is pleomorphic (having various distinct forms) and hypercellular, with the cells showing hyperchromatic nuclei. There are many mitoses, giant cells, and young glial forms.

Of interest is the advance in molecular genetics in astrocytoma. Two moderately common genetic alterations are found to occur: inactivation of the *TP53* tumor suppressor gene and loss of chromosome 22q.[88] Further inactivation of tumor suppressor genes on chromosomes 9p, 13q, and 19q leads to anaplastic astrocytomas.[88] The EphA receptor is overexpressed in GBM and is a functional, targetable receptor that can be altered for treatment.[39] Many further mutations occur, and an understanding of the complexity of these mutations is beginning to suggest methods to intervene therapeutically. Also, understanding tumor stem cells that are responsible for populating and repopulating the tumors may have therapeutic implications, as

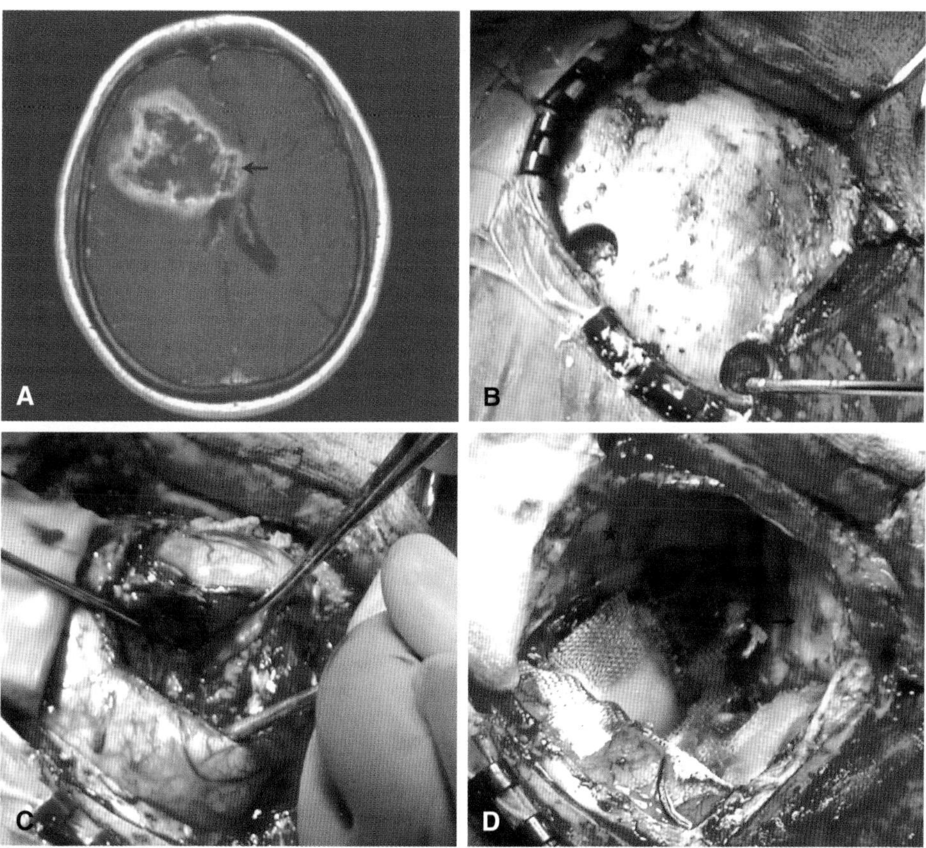


**Fig. 30.6**

**Magnetic resonance imaging (MRI) and intraoperative pictures of a patient with a right frontal glioblastoma multiforme.** (A) Axial T1-weighted MRI. The enhancing lesion demonstrates central necrosis and is causing mass effect. Infiltration along the corpus callosum is also shown *(arrow)*. (B) A frontal craniotomy is being performed. Burr holes have been placed and will be connected for bony removal. (C) The brain has been incised, and the tumor is being removed using a combination of suction and blunt dissection. (D) The tumor and frontal lobe have been resected. The cut edge of the brain is seen at the lower left. The resection cavity has been lined with carmustine polymer (Gliadel) wafers and covered with a layer of Surgicel for hemostasis. (From Townsend CM Jr: *Sabiston textbook of surgery*, ed 17, Philadelphia, 2004, Saunders.)

therapies that do not ablate the tumor stem cells will be ineffective in eradicating the tumor.[18,51,91,94]

**Clinical Manifestations.** Anaplastic astrocytoma and GBM most frequently arise in the frontal and temporal lobes, with the cerebellum, brainstem, and spinal cord being rare sites for adults. They most frequently occur in the fifth and sixth decades of life. Signs and symptoms progress rapidly, with grade IV GBM being particularly aggressive. Patients may present with unilateral headache that is followed by generalized headache, indicating an increase in ICP. The development of seizures is not unusual. Lethargy, memory loss, motor weakness, and personality changes may occur.

**Prognosis.** All malignant astrocytomas will eventually recur. With optimal treatment (excision, radiation therapy), clients with anaplastic astrocytoma (grade III) have a 64% 1-year survival rate, a 46% 2-year survival rate, and a 30% 5-year survival rate. GBM (grade IV) has a poorer prognosis with a 40% 1-year survival rate, a 18% 2-year survival rate, and rare long-term survival, with a 5-year survival rate at less than 7%.[132,162] The relationship between genetic alterations and prognosis is complex and may be age dependent.[18,67] For patients younger than 50 years, the most significant prognostic factor is histology, with median survival for anaplastic astrocytoma of 49.4 months and for GBM of 13.7 months. For patients older than 50 years, the most significant prognostic factor is the performance status. Patients with an anaplastic astrocytoma or a GBM with a high performance status live a median of 10.3 months compared with 5.3 months for patients with a lower performance status.[113,127]

## Oligodendroglioma

**Incidence.** Oligodendrogliomas make up 10% to 15% of gliomas.[4] It is not uncommon to have a combination of cell types such as astrocytes, creating a mixed oligodendroglioma/astrocytoma, or oligoastrocytoma. Oligodendrogliomas occur most frequently in young and middle-aged adults but can also be found in children.[2]

**Pathogenesis.** Oligodendroglioma is a slow-growing, solid, calcified tumor arising from oligodendrocytes, the myelin-producing cells of the CNS. It stains for myelin basic protein. It can be either a low-grade (grade II) tumor or a high-grade (grade III) tumor. It is a gray-pink to red cystic area in the brain and has a honeycomb appearance at low microscopic power because of the presence of a fibrovascular stroma. On higher power the cells have a uniform appearance, with a central nucleus surrounded by a clear cytoplasm, or a fried egg appearance. Mitotic figures are infrequent. Approximately 70% of these tumors show some evidence of calcification. There is a high chemosensitivity to nitrosourea-based compounds when the loss or deletion of chromosomes 1p and 19q occurs.[71]

**Clinical Manifestations.** Oligodendrogliomas are located predominantly in the cerebral hemispheres, often in the frontal lobes. They expand toward the cortex and may spread through it and eventually attach to the dura.[55] A history of partial or generalized seizures, usually of long duration and sometimes with chronic headache, is the typical presentation pattern of oligodendrogliomas. They tend to bleed spontaneously and may manifest with a strokelike syndrome.[150] The hallmark of this tumor radiologically is calcification, which can be identified on CT in the vast majority of people. It is usually nonenhancing with gadolinium, meaning that the surrounding edema is limited.[135] If an oligodendroglioma contains astrocytoma cells, it is graded at the highest level of anaplasia present.

**Prognosis.** With optimal treatment, 5- and 10-year survival rates are 80% to 100% and 45% to 55%, respectively. The median overall survival is 17 years.[116] Radiotherapy alone is no longer considered the primary treatment choice.[104] Although a long interval of quiescence may occur after treatment, oligodendrogliomas eventually recur, often as a more aggressive tumor with progressing symptoms.[162]

## Ependymoma

**Incidence.** Ependymomas have a low incidence, accounting for only approximately 2% to 3% of gliomas.[4] Ependymoma is much more prevalent in children than adults and is the third most frequent posterior fossa neoplasm of children.[7]

**Pathogenesis.** An ependymoma is a neoplasm derived from the ependymal cell lining of the ventricular system and the central canal of the spinal cord. It is graded I to IV, depending on the degree of anaplasia. It is usually reddish, lobulated, and well circumscribed, resembling a cauliflower in shape. Pseudorosette formation, in which the cells are arranged about a clear space or a blood vessel, may occur, and blepharoplasts (small round or rod-shaped intracytoplasmic bodies) may be seen.

**Clinical Manifestations.** Ependymoma is more common in the fourth ventricle and is likely to be detected early because of the signs and symptoms of increased ICP in the posterior fossa (e.g., headache, nausea, vomiting, and papilledema). Many of the symptoms and eventually survival depend on the grade and location of the tumor. In a recent series, 69% were supratentorial, and 31% were infratentorial.[32] Mortality for ependymoma is greatest in patients receiving subtotal resection, regardless of whether or not radiation therapy is employed after surgery. Radiation therapy can be avoided even in anaplastic tumors if total resection is achieved.[167] However, supratentorial ependymomas often grow large before detection. Fig. 30.7 shows an ependymoma of the fourth ventricle.

**Prognosis.** The prognosis for ependymomas is improving: 5-year survival rates exceed 80%, and 10-year survival rates are 40% to 60%.[162]

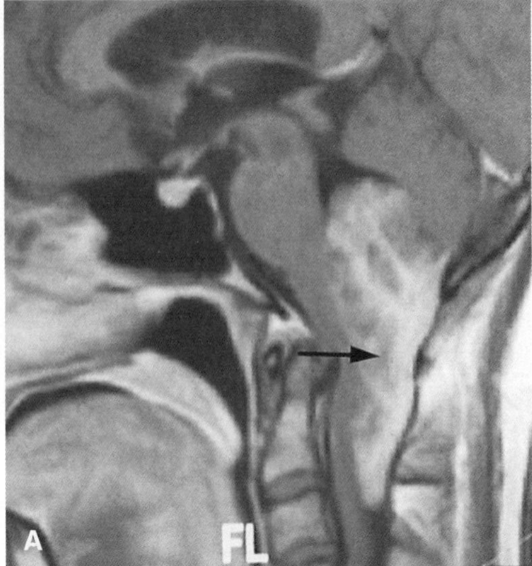


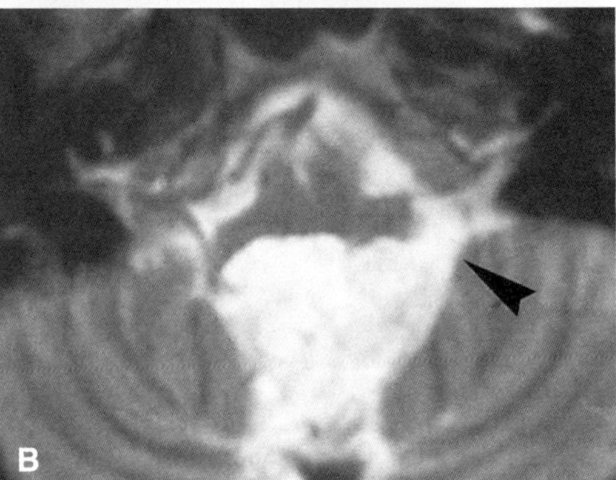


**Fig. 30.7**

**Ependymoma of the fourth ventricle.** Sagittal gadolinium-enhanced T1-weighted (A) and axial T2-weighted (B) magnetic resonance imaging. A heterogeneously enhanced mass *(arrow)* fills the lower half of the fourth ventricle and extends through the foramina of Luschka *(arrowhead)* and Magendie to lie posterior to the medulla oblongata and upper cervical spinal cord, which are compressed from behind. There is obstructive hydrocephalus. (From Grainger RG, et al, eds: *Grainger and Allison's diagnostic radiology: a textbook of medical imaging*, ed 4, Philadelphia, 2001, Churchill Livingstone.)

## Medulloblastoma

**Incidence.** Medulloblastomas account for less than 2% of primary brain tumors.[4] The age of peak incidence is 20 to 45 years in adults. In children, the tumor occurs mainly between the ages of 1 and 10 years. Medulloblastoma is the most common malignant primary CNS tumor in children and the second most common posterior fossa tumor in children.[2]

**Pathogenesis.** Medulloblastoma is typically a rapidly growing malignant tumor. The cell of origin is unknown, but it is presumed to arise from the embryonal external granular layer of the cerebellum. It is considered to belong to a group of tumors known as PNETs. It has a tendency to metastasize to the surface of the remaining CNS via the subarachnoid spaces. Grossly it is red and soft and is composed of many closely packed cells, with oval nuclei and many mitoses. Pseudorosette formations are common. It is highly vascular, containing numerous small blood vessels.[162] Four separate types of medulloblastoma can be classified: classic, large cell (anaplastic), desmoplastic, and nodular.[175]

**Clinical Manifestations.** Medulloblastoma often develops in the cerebellar vermis and is very aggressive in younger children. Because of its proximity to the fourth ventricle, early development of hydrocephalus is common, along with other signs of cerebellar dysfunction, such as ataxia. Medulloblastomas tend to metastasize through CSF pathways, more predominantly into the spine but also into the supratentorial compartment. Drop metastases to the spinal subarachnoid space, causing cord compression and possible paraplegia, are a common enough complication that close monitoring is warranted.

**Prognosis.** Early in the 20th century medulloblastomas were uniformly fatal tumors. Improvements in therapeutic strategies during the past 30 years have dramatically improved the prognosis.[157] Favorable prognostic factors include age older than 2 years, undisseminated local disease, and greater than 75% tumor resection. In these individuals, the 5-year disease-free survival rate exceeds 60% to 70% in most studies.[62,162] In cases with poorer prognostic factors the 5-year disease-free survival rate is approximately 45%.[162] After recurrence, the survival rate at 1 year is 22%, but 0% at 3 years.[99]

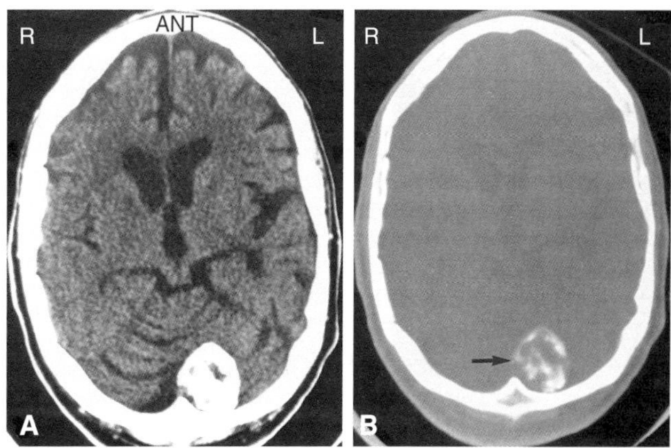


**Fig. 30.8**

**Meningioma.** (A) Noncontrast computed tomography scan shows a very dense, peripherally based lesion in the left cerebellar area. (B) Bone window image obtained at the same level shows that the density is caused by calcification within this lesion. (From Mettler FA Jr: *Essentials of radiology*, ed 2, Philadelphia, 2005, Saunders.)

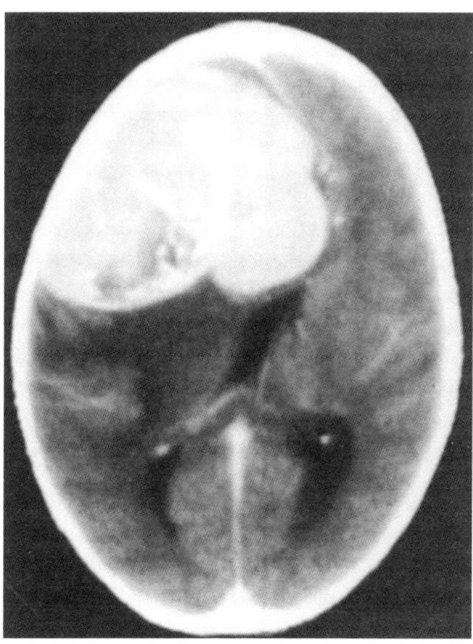

**Fig. 30.9**

Computed tomography (CT) scan with contrast of a meningioma in a patient who presented with mild cognitive deficits, illustrative of the size a slow-growing tumor can attain in the brain. The tumor was completely resected. (From Goldman LM, Ausiello D, eds: *Cecil textbook of medicine*, ed 22, Philadelphia, 2004, Saunders.)

## Tumors Arising From Supporting Structures in the Brain

### Meningioma

**Overview.** Meningiomas are slow-growing, usually benign lesions that occur most commonly along the dural folds and cerebral convexities, although they may occur in the spinal cord as well. The WHO classification recognizes three groups: grade I or benign, grade II or atypical, and grade III or malignant (anaplastic).[47,162] Although 90% of meningiomas are grade I, making their prognosis favorable in many cases, complete resection is possible in less than 50% of patients.[47]

**Incidence.** Meningiomas represent approximately 36% of all intracranial neoplasms and are the second most common primary intracranial tumor in adults and the most common of benign brain neoplasms.[5] Of meningiomas, 90% are considered benign, and approximately 2% to 3% are grade III. Most are single lesions, but multiple meningiomas also occur. They are most common between the ages of 40 and 70 years and are two to three times more prevalent in women than in men.[162] They are increased in neurofibromatosis, in women who use postmenopausal hormone replacement therapy, and in patients who have had breast cancer.[2]

**Pathogenesis.** Meningiomas originate in the arachnoid layer of the meninges and are believed to be derived from the cells and vascular elements of the meninges. Cytogenetic analysis demonstrates multiple deletions on chromosome 22 in most people with meningiomas. Gene downregulation is observed in recurrent and advanced cases, and this gene repression may be caused by gene promotion hypermethylation, suggesting that this type of epigenetic event may play an important role in meningioma progression or recurrence.[121] Tumors are most often located between or over the cerebral hemispheres, at the skull base, or in the posterior fossa. Meningiomas are typically well-circumscribed globular masses. They may infiltrate the dura, dural sinuses, or bone, but generally do not invade the underlying brain parenchyma. Figs. 30.8 and 30.9 show CT scans of meningiomas. Most meningiomas grow as well-encapsulated tumors, but others develop in relatively thin sheets along the dura.

Because of their proximity to or invasion of the bone, meningiomas are known to provoke a local osteoblastic response termed *hyperostosis*. This may cause a profuse local thickening of the skull. Fig. 30.10 shows diffuse reactive hyperostosis, as well as facial distortion from the growing meningioma.

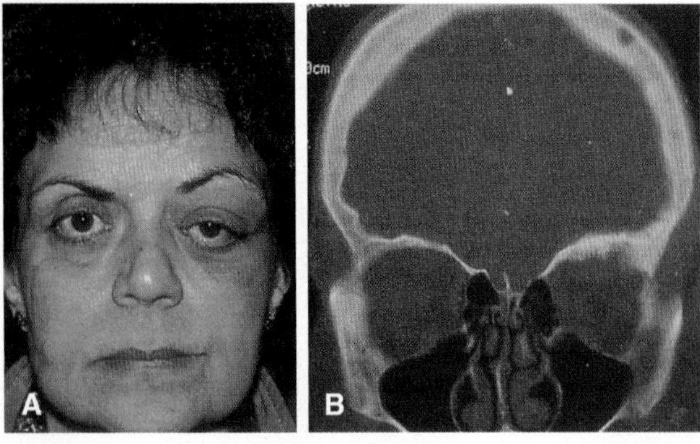


**Fig. 30.10**

(A) Upper eyelid edema, mild proptosis, and downward displacement of the eye as a result of en plaque sphenoid wing meningioma. (B) CT scan of the same patient demonstrating lytic bone lesions and diffuse reactive hyperostosis as a result of bone infiltration by meningioma. (From Abeloff MD, et al: *Clinical oncology*, ed 3, Philadelphia, 2004, Churchill Livingstone.)

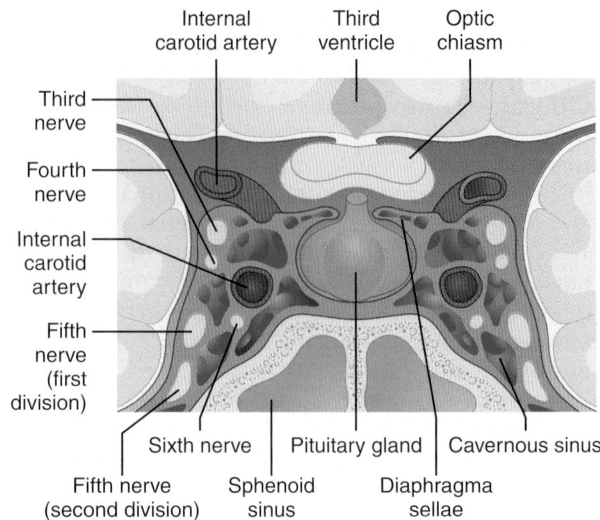


**Fig. 30.11**

**Anatomic relationships of pituitary gland and surrounding parasellar structures.** (Adapted from Warwick R: *The orbital vessels.* In Warwick L, ed: *Eugene Wolff's anatomy of the eye and orbit*, ed 7, Philadelphia, 1976, Saunders.)

**Clinical Manifestations.** Meningiomas are more common in the later years of life and are more frequent in women. Because they are slow growing, abnormal signs and symptoms may evolve over a period of many years. When located in silent brain areas, some meningiomas can become very large before causing clinical symptoms. Also, they can be discovered incidentally as masses that show little or no growth over time. Neurologic abnormalities depend on the location of the tumor; seizures are a common finding with skull base lesions.

**Prognosis.** Meningiomas, when completely resected (surgical accessibility determines excision capabilities), have excellent prospects of long-term cure. Patients with completely excised lesions experience a 10-year survival rate of 80% to 90%. Partially resected meningiomas have a 50% to 70% 10-year progression-free survival. Malignant meningiomas, approximately 1% to 10% of meningiomas, have a shorter disease-free interval[162] and a tendency to recur.

### Pituitary Adenoma

**Overview.** Pituitary adenomas are benign tumors derived from cells of the anterior portion of the pituitary gland. The pituitary gland, located at the base of the brain, sits in the sella turcica, the saddle-shaped transverse depression on the superior surface of the body of the sphenoid bone. Fig. 30.11 depicts the anatomic relationships of the pituitary gland, optic chiasm, and surrounding parasellar structures. Although pituitary adenomas are the most common pituitary tumors, infrequently other types of pituitary tumors may occur in the location of the pituitary gland and may be primary or metastatic. (See also Pituitary Gland in Chapter 11.)

**Incidence.** Pituitary adenomas are common lesions, accounting for approximately 12% of all intracranial tumors, making them the third most common primary brain tumor in adults after meningiomas and the gliomas.[111] They are usually found in middle-aged or older people. Women are affected more often than men, particularly during childbearing years. Almost 70% are functional, or secreting, tumors, and these tend to occur in younger adults. Nonfunctioning tumors (nonsecreting), also called nonfunctioning adenomas, tend to occur in older adults.[2]

**Pathogenesis.** With recent advances in molecular techniques, genetic abnormalities associated with pituitary tumors are becoming clearer. The great majority of pituitary adenomas are monoclonal in origin, suggesting that most arise from a single somatic cell. Additional molecular abnormalities occur in aggressive pituitary adenomas and include mutations of the Ras oncogene and overexpression of the c-Myc oncogene, which suggests that these genetic events are linked to disease progression. Small lesions of the pituitary gland, called *microadenomas,* are less than 10 mm in diameter and may be asymptomatic. Most grow in the front two-thirds of the pituitary gland. Larger tumors, or macroadenomas, may compress the adjacent normal pituitary gland. Fig. 30.12 shows a pituitary tumor extension down into the sphenoid sinus. Extension of the tumor above the sella turcica compresses the optic chiasm.

**Clinical Manifestations.** In the majority of pituitary tumors, the release of excess pituitary hormones or pituitary insufficiency results in dramatic and unique clinical syndromes. Galactorrhea and amenorrhea, gigantism and acromegaly, and the symptoms of Cushing disease (hypertension, facial and truncal obesity, osteoporosis, muscle weakness, menstrual abnormalities, and female hirsutism) are among the hormonal symptoms. Pituitary insufficiency, or hypopituitarism, can lead to symptoms such as fatigue, weakness, and hypogonadism. A second pattern of presentation consists of regression of secondary sexual characteristics and hypothyroidism. The third pattern of presentation is one of neurologic findings, including headache, bitemporal visual loss, and ocular palsy. Fig. 30.13 depicts localization of masses, such as a pituitary tumor

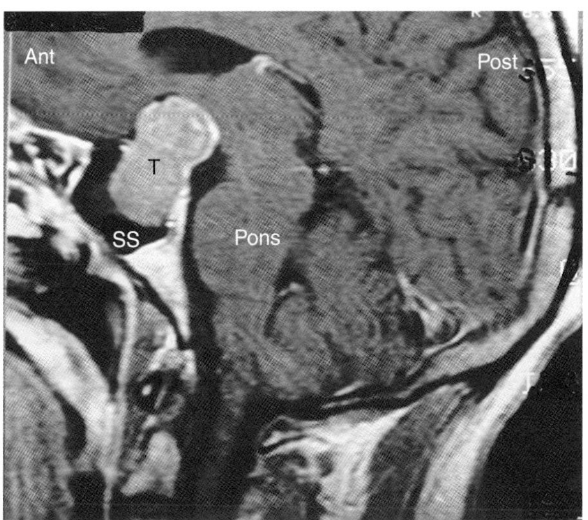


**Fig. 30.12**

**Pituitary adenoma.** Sagittal view of the base of the brain on T1-weighted magnetic resonance imaging shows the pituitary tumor *(T)* and its extension down into the sphenoid sinus *(SS)*. (From Mettler FA Jr: *Essentials of radiology*, ed 2, Philadelphia, 2005, Saunders.)

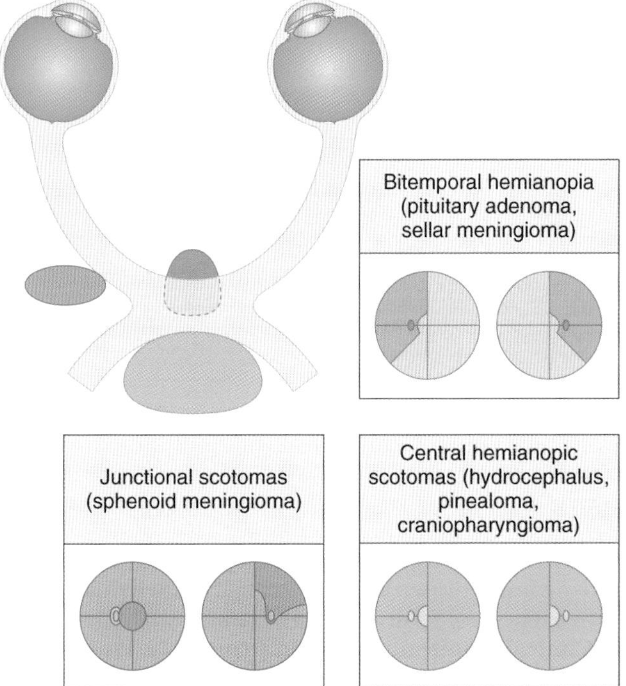


**Fig. 30.13**

**Localization and probable identification of masses by pattern of field loss.** Junctional scotomas occur with compression of the anterior angle of the chiasm (sphenoid meningioma). Bitemporal hemianopia results from compression of the body of the chiasm from below (e.g., because of pituitary adenoma, sellar meningioma). Compression of the posterior chiasm and its decussating nasal fibers may cause central bitemporal hemianopic scotomas (e.g., because of hydrocephalus, pinealoma, craniopharyngioma). (From Yanoff M, et al., eds: *Ophthalmology*, ed 2, St. Louis, 2004, Mosby.)

by the pattern of visual field loss. Fig. 30.14 illustrates the local effects of an expanding pituitary tumor causing visual field defects.

## MEDICAL MANAGEMENT

Nonfunctioning tumors usually require no treatment. Functional tumors may respond to hormonal therapy. Malignant tumor treatment is by surgery (the transsphenoidal approach is employed when possible) and conventional and stereotactic radiotherapy.[78] A multicenter study demonstrated good results with Gamma Knife (Elekta, Stockholm, Sweden) radiosurgery for the management of nonfunctioning pituitary adenomas.[147]

**PROGNOSIS.** Tumors of the pituitary are very treatable, with the majority of people achieving long-term survival or cure. Because visual compromise is a complicating feature of many pituitary tumors, serial recording of visual field deficits can document disease progression in addition to responses to treatment.

### Neurinoma/Neuroma

**Overview and Incidence.** Neurinomas are slow-growing, benign tumors originating from Schwann cells. In the brain they most commonly develop on the vestibular component of the eighth cranial nerve and are also called *acoustic neurinomas, acoustic neuromas,* or *schwannomas.* Acoustic neurinomas account for approximately 8% of all brain tumors.[111] They occur mainly in adults in the fourth to sixth decades of life, with a 2:1 female-to-male ratio. Approximately 5% occur in the context of neurofibromatosis. Bilateral lesions are most likely to occur in neurofibromatosis.[2]

**Pathogenesis.** Acoustic neurinomas typically originate in the internal auditory canal in the transition zone of the oligodendroglial cells and peripheral nervous system Schwann cells. Neurinomas also may be found attached to other cranial nerves, such as the trigeminal nerve. The tumor grows into the cerebellopontine angle, eventually compressing the facial nerve, and encroaches on the brainstem. Some lesions may remain relatively quiescent for long periods of time, but the majority are slow-growing, progressive lesions. The tumor is thickly encapsulated, is often highly vascular, and microscopically consists of spindle-shaped cells, with rod-shaped nuclei often lying in parallel rows.

**Clinical Manifestations.** Individuals with acoustic neurinomas typically present with progressive unilateral sensorineural hearing loss. Other symptoms include tinnitus, vertigo, and unsteadiness. Facial numbness, difficulty swallowing, impaired eye movement, and taste disturbances may occur. Weakness of the facial muscles is generally a late feature. Deformity and obstruction of the fourth ventricle leads to hydrocephalus, with headache, vomiting, and other symptoms of increased ICP. Fig. 30.15 provides a surgical view of a large acoustic neuroma.

**Prognosis.** In the majority of cases, cure is achieved with surgical resection. Stereotactic radiotherapy may be possible, reducing surgical side effects.[8] On one hand, as acoustic neurinomas are slow growing, and surgery often accelerates hearing loss, surgery may be delayed until absolutely necessary. On the other hand, because

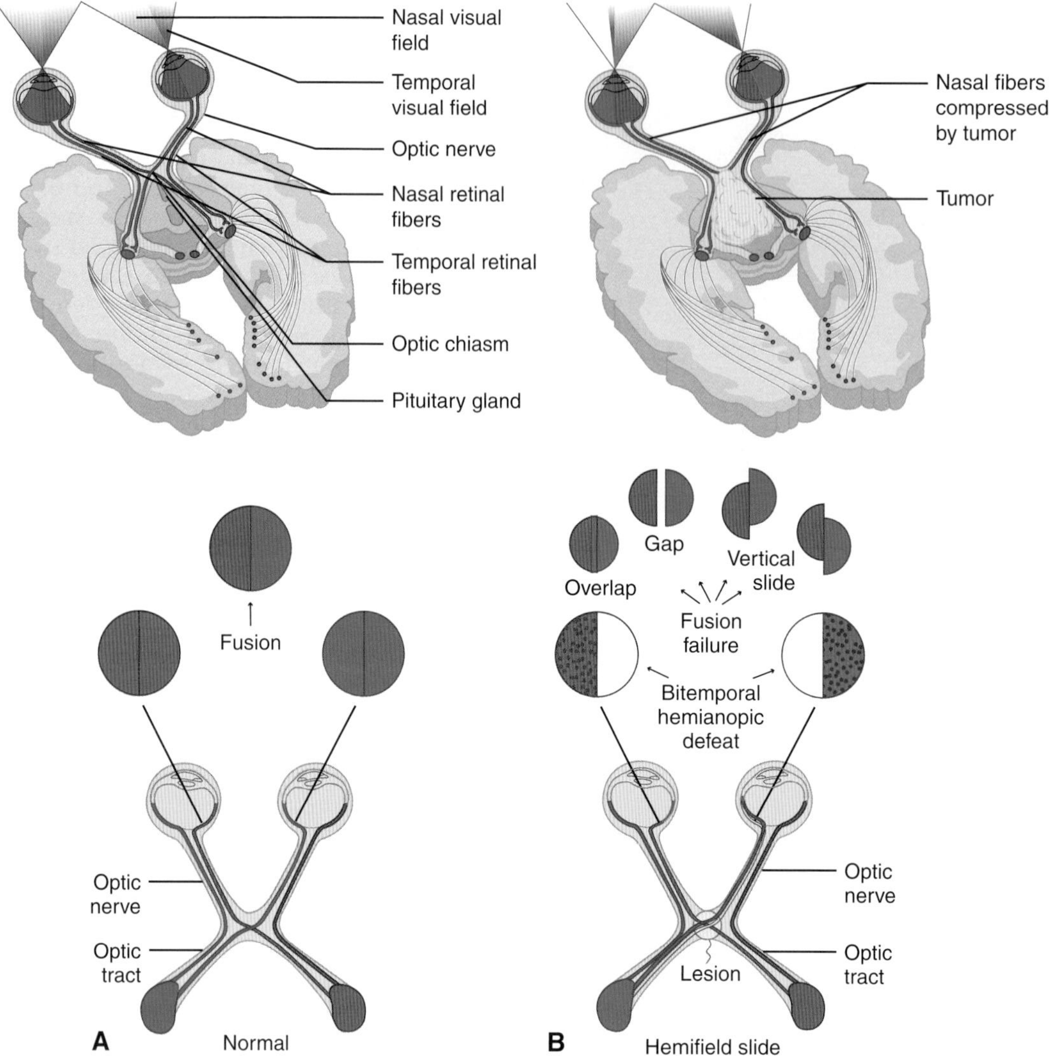


**Fig. 30.14**

**Local effects of an expanding pituitary tumor causing visual field defects.** (A) Normal vision. (B) Bitemporal hemianopsia. The nasal and temporal fields lose their linkage, resulting in overlap of the preserved visual field. (From Larsen PR, et al, eds: *Williams textbook of endocrinology*, ed 10, Philadelphia, 2003, Saunders.)

the likelihood of hearing retention is greatest when the tumor is small, surgery may be done as soon as possible.

### Choroid Plexus Papilloma

Choroid plexus papilloma is a low-grade neoplasm of the choroid plexus, the vascular coat along the ventricles carrying blood vessels within the pia mater to each ventricle. It is relatively rare and usually is found in children. It often is associated with overproduction of CSF and hydrocephalus. Complete removal of the tumor usually results in an excellent prognosis and resolution of the hydrocephalus. The prognosis for choroid plexus carcinoma, another variation of a choroid plexus tumor, is dismal.

### Pinealoma

**Overview and Incidence.** Pineal region (posterior to the third ventricle) tumors are rare (1% of all intracranial tumors), more common in children, and more common in males than females. They tend to occur in adults between 20 and 40 years of age. These are a heterogeneous group of tumors. Germ cell pinealomas have an embryonal basis, and although some are very radiosensitive, others are aggressive, highly malignant, and generally incurable. Germinomatous tumors have a survival rate of 98%; nongerminomatous tumors do not fare as well and are less radiosensitive.[108] Pineal parenchymal tumors have a tendency to disseminate craniospinally.

**Clinical Manifestations and Prognosis.** Pineal region tumors typically result in obstructive hydrocephalus because of the proximity of the pineal gland to the ventricular system. Symptoms include headache, nausea, vomiting, and ocular abnormalities. Management is by shunting the hydrocephalus, if present; radiation therapy; and surgical excision. Individuals with responsive tumors have a 5-year survival rate of 70%.[162] Those with nonresponsive tumors have a 1-year survival rate of only 33%.

### Craniopharyngiomas

**Overview.** Craniopharyngiomas are histologically benign congenital tumors and occur most commonly in

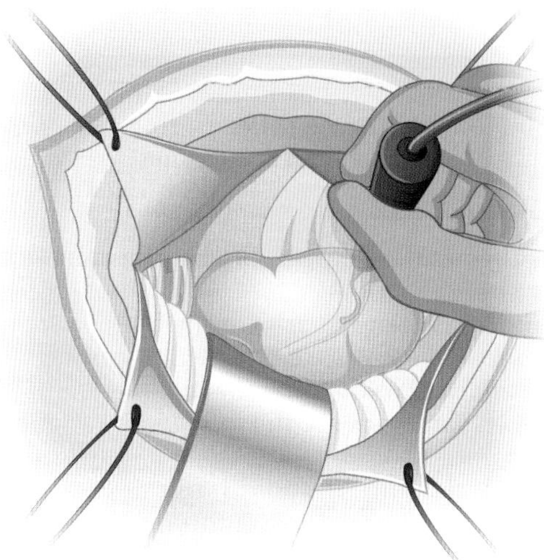

**Fig. 30.15**

**Surgical view of large acoustic neuroma (retrosigmoid approach) showing use of a flexible-tipped probe to locate the facial nerve on the medial surface of the tumor out of direct view.** Early identification of the facial nerve "around the corner" on the ventral surface of the tumor helps speed the procedure by allowing rapid removal of the remaining capsule. The tumor is drawn as if transparent to show details of anatomy on the hidden surface. (From Yingling CD, Gardi JN: Intraoperative monitoring of facial and cochlear nerves during acoustic neuroma surgery. *Otolaryngol Clin North Am* 25:413–448, 1992.)

the suprasellar region in the pituitary stalk adjacent to the optic chiasm.

**Incidence.** Craniopharyngiomas are rare and account for 1% to 3% of all intracranial tumors.[30] They are the third most common intracranial tumor in children, accounting for 10% of all intracranial tumors in this age group.

**Pathogenesis.** Craniopharyngiomas presumably arise from embryonic remnants of Rathke pouch and grow slowly from birth. They vary in size from small, solid, well-circumscribed masses to huge multilocular cysts that invade the sella turcica, reaching a large size before they are diagnosed. They often involve the pituitary gland, optic nerve, and third ventricle. Two basic histologic subtypes have been described: adamantinomatous and papillary.[66] Of tumors, 60% to 80% of tumors are calcified.

**Clinical Manifestations.** Based on the location, craniopharyngiomas can compromise a number of important intracranial structures and produce multiple signs and symptoms. The most common presentations are pituitary hypofunction, visual difficulties, and severe headaches. Other signs are increased ICP, neuroendocrine disorders, hypothalamus involvement, cranial nerve palsies, hydrocephalus, and progressive dementia. Sexual dysfunction is the most common endocrine problem in adults, with 90% of men experiencing erectile dysfunction and most women having amenorrhea. Depression may occur, presumably because of extension of the tumor into the frontal lobes, striocapsulothalamic areas, or limbic system.[136]

**Prognosis.** Optimal treatment is controversial, but radiation and surgical resection are used. Intracavitary radiation is used in select tumors. With complete resections or resections followed by radiation therapy, 10-year survival rates of 78% have been reported. Recurrence rates are higher in patients receiving less than 54 Gy of radiation. The tumors have a tendency to recur, and even though histologically they are benign, they may be better thought of as low-grade malignancies.

## Epidermoid and Dermoid Tumors (Cysts)

**Incidence.** Epidermoid and dermoid tumors are rare benign tumors that arise from imperfect embryogenesis of the CNS and account for 2% of intracranial tumors. The most common cysts in the brain are epidermoid, arachnoid, colloid, and dermoid.

**Pathogenesis.** Cysts are fluid-filled spheres composed of desquamated epidermal cellular debris, keratin, and cholesterol. During embryologic development, groups of cells are diverted from the areas of the face or skin to the neural tube. They grow in basal regions of the brain and tend to enlarge along CSF pathways. Most cysts are benign and grow slowly and may not cause symptoms for many years.

The epidermoid cyst often contains remnants of skin cells or tiny pieces of cartilage and occurs near the cerebellopontine angle or the pituitary gland. The arachnoid cyst is found in the subarachnoid space, often in the Sylvian fissure, the cerebellopontine angle, the cisterna magna, or the suprasellar region of the brain, and may cause increased ICP. The colloid cyst is most frequently found in the third ventricle and may block CSF, causing headache, seizures, and increased ICP. The dermoid tumor has epidermal cellular debris, but it is mixed with additional dermal elements such as hair, hair follicles, sweat glands, and sebaceous glands. Dermoid cysts are usually located in the posterior fossa or the adjacent meninges or in the lower spine.

**Prognosis.** In most cases, complete surgical excision of the tumor capsule and contents is curative.[162] If the tumor is unable to be totally removed, it may recur, although growth is slow.[3]

## Hemangioblastoma

**Incidence.** Hemangiomas make up 2% of all intracranial tumors, are the most common adult intraaxial tumor of the posterior fossa, and occur more frequently in men. They most commonly occur in people about 40 years old.

**Pathogenesis.** Hemangiomas are benign, slow-growing tumors typically arising in the posterior fossa, primarily in the cerebellar vermis or pons, as solitary lesions with clearly indicated borders. The origin is thought to be cells in the blood vessel lining. Hemangioblastomas are a vascular conglomerate of endothelial cells, pericytes (found wrapped about precapillary arterioles), and stromal cells. These highly vascular tumors attached to the wall of a surrounding cyst are often associated with von Hippel–Lindau syndrome.[133]

**Clinical Manifestations and Prognosis.** Blockage of the CSF results in ICP and hydrocephalus. Common symptoms include headache, nausea and vomiting, balance and gait disturbances, and poor coordination. Complete surgical excision for tumors arising in the cerebellum is curative.

### Chordoma

Chordomas rarely arise in the brain and represent less than 1% of all intracranial neoplasms. They are much more typical in the axial skeleton, preferring the clivus (in the posterior cranial fossa) and sacrum. They are tumors of bone, presumed to arise from the embryonal notochord remnants. They are considered histologically benign but have a locally destructive nature, progressive course, and occasionally metastatic behavior.[162] Cranial chordomas typically involve the skull base, with a destructive process that invades rostrally into the optic chiasm, into the brainstem, or ventrally into the sinuses. Because of surgical inaccessibility, curative resections are difficult, if not impossible. Median survival is approximately 7.7 years; 5- and 10-year survival rates are 72% and 45%, respectively.[149]

### Primary Central Nervous System Lymphoma

**Overview and Incidence.** PCNSL is a non-Hodgkin lymphoma and occurs in the absence of systemic lymphoma. It is also called an extranodal lymphoma. This tumor was formerly quite rare, but between 1973 and 1985 it tripled in frequency in immunocompetent patients and increased in the immunosuppressed population—that is, in clients with AIDS and collagen vascular disorders, organ transplant recipients, and individuals with congenital immunodeficiency.[5,168] There was a decrease in incidence in young men and patients with AIDS between 1995 and 1998, which was explained by the introduction of highly active antiretroviral therapy for patients with HIV infection.[171] PCNSL in patients with AIDS continues to decrease in incidence owing to highly active antiretroviral therapy.[56] It currently accounts for 4% to 7% of all primary brain tumors.[1,30,32,61,96]

**Pathogenesis.** The pathophysiologic basis for development of these tumors is unclear, particularly in immunocompetent patients. PCNSL most commonly originates from B lymphocytes and is associated with cytokines. In immunosuppressed patients, it is almost always associated with latent infection of neoplastic B cells by Epstein-Barr virus.[61] The lymphoma cells typically assume a periventricular pattern, involving the deep white matter, basal ganglia, corpus callosum, and thalamus. PCNSL may also involve the CSF, the eyes, or the spinal cord. Lesions may be multiple. Lesions in immunocompetent patients more often may be a single brain lesion, in a supratentorial location, and with frontoparietal lobe involvement. The diagnostic procedure of choice is a stereotactic (x-ray–guided) biopsy, as patients derive little clinical benefit from surgical resection.[72]

**Clinical Manifestations.** Symptoms and signs generally evolve over several months and include personality and behavioral changes, confusion, generalized seizures, and symptoms associated with increased ICP (headaches, nausea and vomiting). The most frequent presenting symptom in 30% to 40% of patients is impaired cognition.[40] Focal neurologic signs, such as hemiparesis or blurred or double vision, may occur. The appearance on MRI or CT of multiple deep cerebral and periventricular lesions, along with an immunodeficient state, suggests the diagnosis.[83] Differential diagnosis includes infections, other tumors, and inflammatory disorders.

**Prognosis.** The prognosis is generally poor, with median survival of 10 to 14 months, although adding systemic chemotherapy (methotrexate and cytosine arabinoside) to radiation has improved median survival to 32 to 60 months.[72,162] Age affects prognosis significantly; younger patients have better outcomes.

### Other Miscellaneous Brain Tumor Types

Other infrequent brain tumors bearing mention are as follows:

- **Chondromas** tend to arise at the base of the skull, are slow growing, and are composed of cartilage-like cells often attached to the dura mater.
- **Chondrosarcomas** are the malignant variant of chondromas.
- **Atypical teratoid rhabdoid tumors** are high-grade tumors occurring most commonly in the cerebellum in children and are aggressive, with frequent metastasis through the CNS.
- **Dysembryoplastic neuroepithelial tumors** are slow-growing, benign, grade I tumors, often containing a mix of neurons and glial cells, and typically found in the temporal or frontal lobe.
- **Gangliocytomas** and **gangliogliomas** arise from ganglia-type cells (groups of neurons) and are most commonly located in the temporal lobe and third ventricle.
- **Germ cell tumors** include germinoma, teratoma, embryonal carcinoma and yolk sac tumors, and choriocarcinoma. These tend to arise in the pineal or suprasellar regions and occur primarily in children and young adults. Teratomas are composed of various tissue types within the tumor, often containing calcium, cysts, fat, and other soft tissues.

More details on these CNS tumors as well as further information on the numerous other infrequent CNS tumors are available in various references.[1,6,22,73,84,97]

## Diagnosis of Primary Brain Tumors

When a brain tumor is suspected on clinical evaluation, a thorough neurologic examination and brain imaging studies are done to confirm its presence and exact location.

MRI has evolved as the most informative brain imaging study because of its superior imaging capabilities and lack of artifact from the temporal bones. With the addition of gadolinium contrast enhancement, which distinguishes tumor from surrounding edema, MRI can detect tumors a few millimeters in size. MRI also defines critical anatomic relationships between the tumor and surrounding neurovascular structures. The multiplanar capability of MRI allows optimal visualization of the anatomy. MRI is particularly useful in visualizing the brainstem and other posterior fossa structures.[168] New MRI techniques are being developed to investigate the biochemical basis of tumors, such as proton magnetic resonance spectroscopy, which measures the signals from nuclei other than water.[127]

Although MRI has many advantages over CT, CT scanning is widely accessible, convenient, and effective in revealing most brain tumors if they are large enough. The increased vessel formation or neovascularization accounts for the enhancement of these tumors and allows them to be visualized. Although the brain imaging capabilities of CT are inferior to MRI, CT can identify cerebral edema, midline shift, and ventricular compression of obstructive hydrocephalus. In intraventricular masses, CT is highly sensitive in detecting calcification. CT also is better than MRI for demonstrating bone destruction. CT imaging may be needed when a patient has precautions for a magnetic study (e.g., pacemaker or other metallic implants). Intravenous contrast agents greatly increase the sensitivity of CT scan for brain tumors.

Once a tumor has been detected with MRI or CT, other particular parameters may help to characterize it further. For example, establishing the location of an intracranial neoplasm in either the extraaxial or the intraaxial compartment is valuable in differential diagnosis.[168] For example, astrocytomas are intraaxial, and meningiomas are extraaxial. MRI or CT may detect a cleft between the brain parenchyma and the tumor, which indicates a possible extraaxial mass such as a meningioma. Resting functional MRI and connectivity mapping, a relatively new technique, demonstrate the connections between motor, premotor, and somatosensory cortex and can be used in the presurgical evaluation of patients.[96]

There are numerous new techniques to image tumors. Single photon emission CT imaging uses preoperative thallium-201 emission CT, in which the maximum uptake area of the brain tumor distinguishes benign from malignant tumors and localizes the area for biopsy. Iodine-123-α-methyl-L-tyrosine single photon emission tomography uses a radioisotope to distinguish glioma recurrence from benign posttherapeutic change. Positron emission tomography (PET) is able to localize the areas of maximum glucose utilization within a tumor, guiding the neurosurgeon to perform biopsy of locations with the most aggressive biologic behavior and differentiating viable tumor from necrosis.[34,58,127] The PET scan also maps functional areas of the brain before surgery or radiation to minimize injury to eloquent areas.[168] Fluorodeoxyglucose PET measures glucose utilization and helps to differentiate recurrent tumor from radiation necrosis. It also is not influenced by corticosteroid therapy.

Echo planar MRI is a new technique of functional MRI that provides maps of tumor blood flow and may allow better resolution of tumor versus surrounding edema at the tumor borders. Magnetic resonance spectroscopy may show pathologic spectra outside the area of contrast enhancement, suggesting infiltrative lesions.[115,134] More recent imaging developments include the use of diffusion tensor imaging, functional MRI, and magnetic resonance spectroscopy.[82]

Additional tests may be indicated to further delineate the tumor and identify possible surgical hazards. Cerebral angiography delineates the vascularity within the brain and can help determine the best surgical approach. Visual field and funduscopic examination identifies visual defects that are specific to a particular area. Audiometric studies determine hearing loss. Chest films help to rule out lung cancer with metastatic lesions to the brain, and other studies are used to rule out a primary lesion outside the brain when a metastatic lesion is suspected. Endocrine studies are done when a pituitary adenoma or craniopharyngioma is suspected.[63,112] A needle biopsy using CT-guided stereotactic (x-ray–guided) technique through a burr hole in the cranium may be performed to identify the specific tumor type and grade. A needle biopsy may not be possible, however, with vascular tumors or tumors near vital centers, for fear of precipitating bleeding or respiratory distress. As tumors may have variation in grading throughout the tumor, a needle biopsy may potentially miss the higher-graded area, limiting the accuracy of the diagnosis.

## MEDICAL MANAGEMENT

Surgery, radiation therapy, chemotherapy, and immunotherapy are the treatment options for brain tumors. Management of symptoms and side effects is a major component of medical management.

### TREATMENT

***Surgery.*** Surgical excision is the most important form of initial therapy because it provides histologic confirmation of the tumor and a basis for determining the treatment and prognosis. Stereotactic neurosurgical techniques have had a profound impact on efficacy and safety of neurosurgery. Intraoperative magnification and the operating microscope have allowed stereoscopic visualization of otherwise inaccessible tissues and have reduced the morbidity and mortality of brain surgery.[127] MRI combined with computer-aided navigation tools helps the neurosurgeon map the exact tumor location and track its removal during the procedure. Surgery reduces tumor load and quickly relieves the ICP and mass effect, thereby reducing symptoms and improving neurologic function. The surgical cytoreduction also enhances the effectiveness of adjuvant therapy (e.g., radiation therapy).

A traditional operative technique is *craniotomy*, a resection of the skull overlying the tumor, removal of the tumor, and replacement of the bone flap (Fig. 30.16). *Stereotactic biopsy* of the lesion without craniotomy is used when deep mass lesions are surgically unresectable or when the risk of craniotomy outweighs the benefits. Stereotactic procedures involve creating a burr hole in the brain at an exact location using a computer, radiologic equipment, and a special head-fixation device.

The technologic and conceptual advances in neurosurgery (e.g., intraoperative magnification, ultrasonic aspirators, microinstrumentation, computer-based stereotactic resection procedures) have allowed safer and more precise approaches to previously inaccessible tumors.[151,162] Awake cortical mapping before and during surgery identifies critical areas of brain functioning to avoid and/or reduce damage to these areas.[24,46,96] Endoscopic surgery for pituitary adenomas, tumors of the orbit, vestibular (acoustic) neuromas, meningiomas, and other skull base tumors uses endoscopes attached to an endocamera and a video monitor system.[152] Transsphenoidal resections, which avoid an external craniotomy, are possible through the nose (transnasal) (Fig. 30.17). Short videos of actual endoscopic brain surgeries are available for viewing on the Internet.[77] As Fig. 30.18 shows, facial craniotomy or endoscopy uses incisions positioned between facial cosmetic subunits.

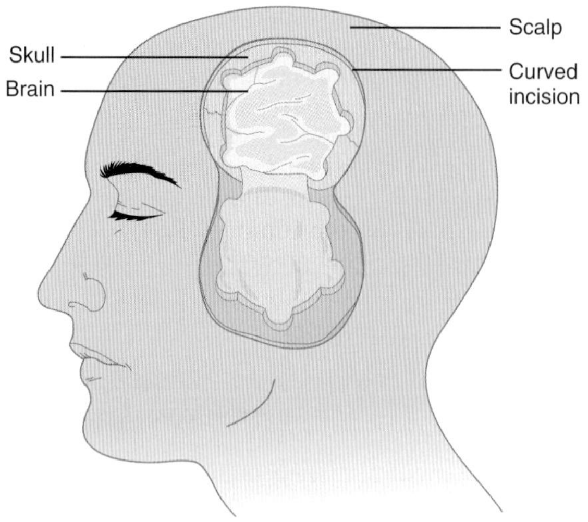


**Fig. 30.16**

**Craniotomy with osteoplastic bone flap.** (From Schnell SS: Nursing care of clients with cerebral disorders. In Black JM, Matassarin-Jacobs E, eds: *Luckmann and Sorensen's medical-surgical nursing*, ed 4, Philadelphia, 1993, Saunders, p 734.)

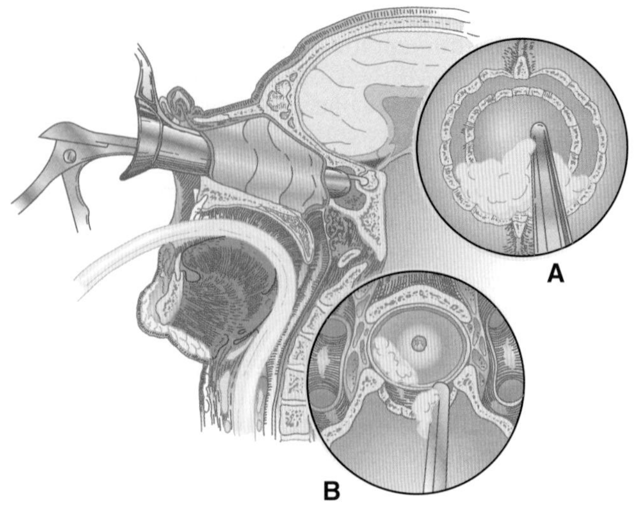


**Fig. 30.17**

**Endonasal transsphenoidal resection of the pituitary tumor.** (A) Removal of the sella floor with small rongeurs. (B) Exposed inferior aspect of a pituitary adenoma. (From Tindall GT, Barrow DL: *Disorders of the pituitary*, St. Louis, 1986, Mosby.)

The goal of surgery is total excision, while minimizing trauma to vital neural structures. The survival rates of patients undergoing total resections for brain tumors are significantly higher than those of patients undergoing partial resections.[113] In infiltrative intraaxial lesions, in which total excision is not possible, the goal is to provide a measure of temporary control by reducing mass effect and ICP. If the preoperative neurologic deficit is caused by destruction of brain tissue by tumor, surgical resection will not improve the situation. In the case of many benign extraaxial tumors (e.g., meningiomas, schwannomas, pituitary adenomas), cure can be achieved.

Operative complications include hemorrhage, infection, seizures, hydrocephalus resulting from an impairment of CSF absorption, and neuroendocrine disturbances, especially if surgery is in the region of the pituitary. Brain edema, usually present before surgery, may be severely aggravated during surgery. Corticosteroids usually are given for several days before craniotomy to reduce preoperative edema. Improved surgical techniques have reduced the complications of hemorrhage, infection, and permanent neurologic injury to less than 10% of cases.[162] Postoperative survival is prolonged, but complication risks increase in patients who undergo multiple cranial surgeries for brain tumors.[65]

***Radiation Therapy.*** Radiation therapy following surgical resection is of proven effectiveness for most malignant brain tumors.[41,80] Various brain tumors have different susceptibilities to radiation therapy, but the survival advantage is unquestionable. A greater degree of tumor anaplasia and younger age may result in a better response to radiation.[16] Unresectable or incompletely resected tumors in particular are candidates for radiation therapy. Established radiation doses that avoid exceeding thresholds of CNS tolerance are in the range of 40 to 60 Gy (4000 to 6000 rad). Radiation using a linear accelerator is typically given in fractionated doses five times a week over 34 to 36 weeks.

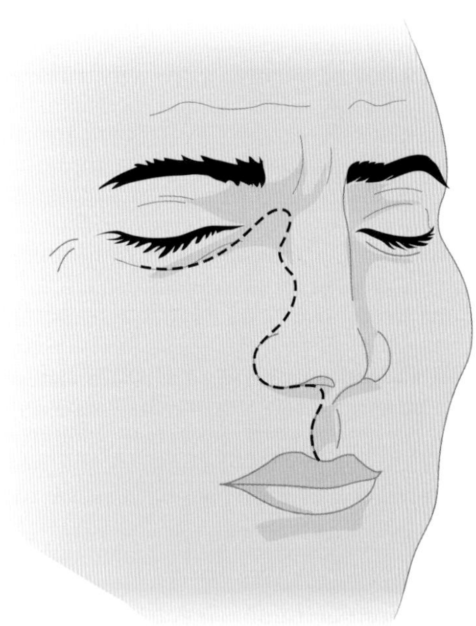

**Fig. 30.18**

**Illustration of standard location for facial incisions, with craniofacial resection completed using traditional methods.** These incisions are positioned between facial cosmetic subunits *(dashed lines)*. (From Cummings CW Jr, et al, eds: *Cummings otolaryngology—head and neck surgery*, ed 4, Philadelphia, 2005, Mosby.)

Radiation is delivered to a localized area of the brain to minimize the volume of tissue irradiated. Acute reactions to radiation are a result of acute brain swelling, occur during or immediately after radiation, and manifest as an increase in neurologic deficit or increased ICP. Steroid therapy is given to reduce this effect during radiation therapy. A similar delayed postirradiation syndrome 1 to 3 months after radiation also can be controlled by steroids. A third brain reaction known as *radiation necrosis* may occur months to years after irradiation and is severe and irreversible.[81,156] It is presumed to be the result of direct toxic effects on the brain and its microvasculature (Fig. 30.19). There is progressive deterioration, dementia, and focal neurologic signs.

As survival time increases, other long-term complications of irradiation are of concern. Hypopituitarism, radiation-induced occlusive disease of cerebral vessels, radiation-induced oncogenesis, leukoencephalopathy, and myelopathies from spinal axis irradiation are included in these complications (Fig. 30.20). White matter injuries correlate significantly with radiation dose in long-term survivors (longer than 18 months). These changes correlate with functional neurologic status,[38] including altered mental status, speech impairments, motor deficit, cranial nerve deficit, personality changes, altered memory, and other neurologic signs.[9]

Advances in radiation therapy have led to newer methods of radiation delivery. Interstitial radiation therapy, or *brachytherapy,* involves the placement of the radiation source, such as radium seeds, within the tumor for a period of several days. Brachytherapy has shown promise in treating GBM and other primary brain tumors.

*Stereotactic radiosurgery* is a technique to deliver a large single fraction of highly focal radiation to a brain tumor.[89] It originally was used to treat functional disorders (e.g., pain and movement disorders) but is now being used in the treatment of primary and metastatic brain tumors.[146] There are several methods. The linear accelerator–based systems, which are the most widely available, deliver high-energy photon beams using converging arcs that intersect at the target site. Various modifications in the linear accelerator are available. Three-dimensional conformal radiation therapy allows shaping of the radiation beams to match the tumor's contours. Intensity-modulated radiation therapy is a refinement of three-dimensional conformal radiation therapy; it ensures that maximum intensity is directed at a specific site, reducing the dose to the surrounding tissues. Gamma Knife radiosurgery uses high-energy photon beams from cobalt-201 sources, each directed at a specific isocenter. A halo device is attached to the skull, and the patient's head is positioned in a collimator that delivers focused gamma beams to the targeted tumor.

*Synchrocyclotron proton beam therapy* delivers heavy charged particle beams through a small number of portals in the skull.[162] The CyberKnife (Accuray, Sunnyvale, California) is a frameless robotic radiosurgical device with increased fractionation flexibility and the ability to treat extracranial lesions. It is capable of changing the target of the beam delivery instantaneously.[137,146]

In some specific primary and metastatic brain cancers, radiosurgery, instead of surgery, may be the first line of treatment. The advantages of radiosurgery compared with surgery are avoiding the risk of hemorrhage, infection, and tumor seeding; linking treatment directly to three-dimensional visualization, which reduces the chances of a marginal miss; and requiring minimal hospitalization.[69,146] The use of pegylated gold nanoparticles in animals increases survival, increases tumor cell radiosensitization, and preferentially targets tumor-associated vasculature that may be of future benefit.[75] Although Gamma Knife, proton beam, and CyberKnife equipment are expensive, and treatment requires collaboration between radiation oncologists and neurosurgeons, the use of these modalities is rapidly increasing, and data on their effectiveness

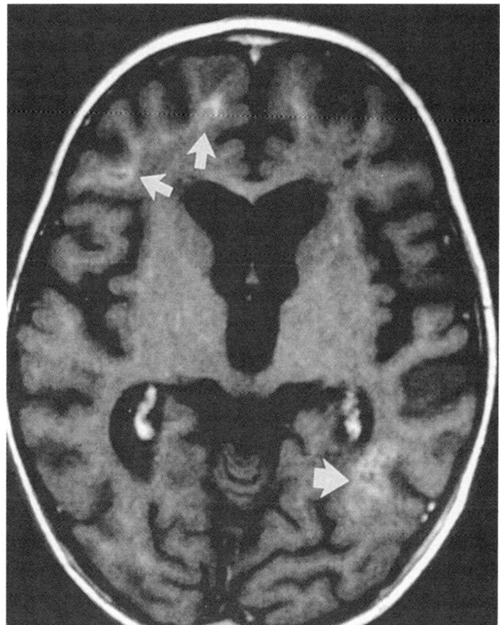

**Fig. 30.19**

**Generalized brain changes after radiotherapy.** T1-weighted magnetic resonance imaging of a child shows both central and cortical atrophy, as well as high-signal areas *(arrows)* owing to mineralizing microangiopathy. (From Behrman RE, et al, eds: *Nelson textbook of pediatrics,* ed 17, Philadelphia, 2004, Saunders.)

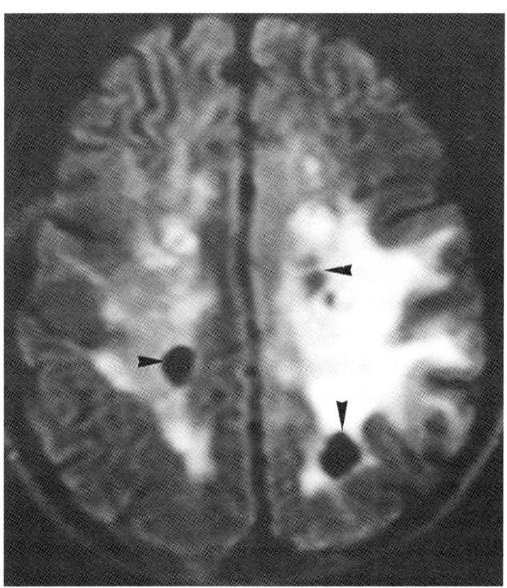

**Fig. 30.20**

**Postradiotherapy encephalopathy.** Axial fluid attenuated inversion recovery magnetic resonance imaging. Extensive high signal in the white matter of both cerebral hemispheres is caused by radiation-induced leukoencephalopathy. There are also areas of cystic necrosis in this case *(arrowheads).* (From Adam A, et al, eds: *Grainger and Allison's diagnostic radiology: a textbook of medical imaging,* ed 4, Philadelphia, 2001, Churchill Livingstone.)

and neurotoxicity are becoming available. Radiotherapy may prove increasingly to be a beneficial modality of client care[119] as it becomes more available and easier to deliver. Brain metastases are ideal lesions to be treated with stereotactic radiation because they can be optimally covered by the radiation distribution, which can be easily designed by careful treatment planning.[6,37,164] In time, technologic modifications will allow treatment at other sites, such as the spine.

***Chemotherapy.*** Chemotherapy has been extensively studied in brain tumors and may have an impact on both survival and quality of life in individuals who have primary brain tumors, particularly for certain pediatric neoplasms such as medulloblastoma.[162] The early studies in the 1960s involved the nitrosoureas (carmustine [BCNU] and lomustine [CCNU]) and hydroxyurea because of their in vitro sensitivity and lipophilic characteristics allowing them to cross the blood-brain barrier. BCNU has been the most effective cytotoxic agent against malignant glioma.[168]

Newer agents with antitumor activity include diaziquone, procarbazine, imidazole carboxamide (DTIC), vincristine, cisplatin, carboplatin, tamoxifen, irinotecan (CPT-11 or Camptosar), and temozolomide (TMZ or Temodar).[127,168] TMZ is the chemotherapy drug of choice for high-grade gliomas in the adjuvant setting; it is associated with significant improvements in median progression-free survival.[11,70,154,155,161] It is thought that TMZ may be especially useful for elderly patients with glioblastomas as an alternative to radiation therapy to maintain a reasonable performance status.[26] A three-drug regimen of procarbazine, lomustine, and vincristine also benefits patients with anaplastic glioma, but offers no survival benefit for patients with GBM.[127] Clinical trials are investigating paclitaxel (Taxol), phenylacetic acid, and other novel techniques, such as the thymidine-kinase gene, continuous infusion chemotherapy, and the use of antiangiogenesis drugs such as thalidomide. Trials of intracavitary placement of carmustine polymer wafers (Gliadel) are demonstrating prolonged survival without the systemic side effects of chemotherapy.[168] Targeting vascular endothelial cell growth factor with agents such as bevacizumab has demonstrated promising results.[133] To bypass the blood-brain barrier, intrathecal delivery (through an Ommaya reservoir surgically placed in the scalp with its tube inserted into the lateral ventricle) can be done. Another technique is an intraarterial (intracarotid) delivery allowing much higher concentration of drugs such as methotrexate, vincristine, or cisplatin than intravenous injection allows, which overcomes molecular resistance. Intrathecal chemotherapy may be given when leptomeningeal involvement occurs with tumor or to increase the CSF concentration. Addition of chemotherapy to surgery and irradiation for malignant gliomas provide some increases in 24-month survival, up to 23.4% from 15.9%.[162]

***Hormonal Therapy.*** Hormonal therapy is often used to treat functioning pituitary tumors. Dopamine agonists are used to control the production of prolactin. Somatostatin analogues are used to reduce growth hormone levels and relieve the associated symptoms. If satisfactory results are achieved, surgery and/or radiation may not be necessary.

***Immunotherapy.*** Immunotherapy or biotherapy is the most infrequently used and least-proven therapy for brain tumors. Immunotherapy, originally the use of donor serum containing preformed antibodies, now includes the use of interferons and interleukin-2 (see Interferons in Chapter 7 and Immunotherapy in Chapter 9) to boost immune function.[63] The depressed immunocompetence of clients with malignant glioma gives at least a theoretical basis for the potential roles of biologic response modifiers in the treatment of these tumors. Preliminary studies show some promise.[162] Many advances have occurred in immunotherapy and hold promise, as advances in surgery, radiation therapy, and chemotherapy have been modest.[12]

***Symptom Management.*** Brain tumors lead to edema of tissue surrounding the tumor, and brain swelling can be massive and extend the neurologic deficits caused by the tumor alone. Antiinflammatory drugs (corticosteroids, e.g., dexamethasone [Decadron], prednisone, hydrocortisone) are used to provide prompt and effective reduction in peritumoral edema. Improvement in symptoms of ICP and in focal neurologic signs begins within 24 to 48 hours after steroid initiation, and by the fourth and fifth day the maximum degree of improvement is obtained.[168]

Corticosteroids generally are used perioperatively and are tapered gradually after tumor resection because long-term high-dose corticosteroids precipitate undesirable side effects. Corticosteroids also may be used periirradiation because radiation also precipitates edema. On tumor recurrence or progression, corticosteroids may again be instituted to temporarily maximize residual neurologic function.

It is possible for a brain tumor to cause an acute increase in ICP that may be life threatening because of imminent cerebral herniation. Emergency treatment is required if ICP reaches 20 mm Hg or more. Quick-acting agents are needed to lower the pressure. Mannitol is used as a temporary agent to quickly reduce brain water and relieve the pressure. Steroids are used in conjunction with mannitol to decrease edema. Table 30.5 lists emergency treatments for elevated ICP in acutely decompensating patients.

Anticonvulsants also may be needed to prevent or control seizure activity. These drugs also are used before and after surgery to control symptoms and are continued as long as they are indicated.[34] One of the most common anticonvulsant therapies used today in patients with brain tumors is phenytoin (Dilantin).[117]

Brain tumors also cause a variety of motor, speech, hearing, visual, and other neurologic signs and symptoms. Although control of the tumor and edema through medical management is the first priority, residual neurologic problems can significantly lower the quality of life. Timely referral to rehabilitation specialists for management of these functional deficits can improve performance status and quality of life. Strengthening, motor and balance evaluation and training, splinting, bracing, fatigue and pain management, incontinence training, home adaptation, activities of daily living retraining, speech therapy, hearing adaptations, auditory retraining,

**Table 30.5** Emergency Treatment of Elevated Intracranial Pressure in Acutely Decompensating Patients

| Therapy | Treatment | Onset (Duration of Action) | Other |
|---|---|---|---|
| Hyperventilation | Lower $PaCO_2$ to 25–30 mm Hg | Seconds (minutes) | Usually requires intubation and mechanical ventilation |
| Osmotherapy | Mannitol 0.5–2 g/kg IV, repeat as necessary | Minutes (hours) | Brisk diuresis<br>Requires Foley catheter<br>Strict attention to electrolytes |
| Corticosteroids | Dexamethasone 50–100 mg IV, followed by 50–100 mg/day in divided doses | Hours (days) | Most effective on vasogenic edema (tumors, abscesses)<br>Less effective on cytotoxic edema (stroke) |

*IV*, Intravenous; *$PaCO_2$*, arterial partial pressure of carbon dioxide.
From DeAngelis LM: Tumors of the central nervous system. In Goldman LM, Ausiello D, eds: *Cecil textbook of medicine*, ed 22, Philadelphia, 2004, Saunders.

and vision programs are available to improve and alleviate these functional deficits.

Other specialists are also part of the rehabilitation team. Pharmacists provide assistance with pain management; the oncology nurse provides symptom management, psychosocial support, and education; the nutritionist provides diet and nutrition counseling; the social worker assists with community resources and placement in settings for necessary further care; and clergy provide assistance with personal and spiritual issues.

The psychosocial implications of brain tumors are enormous. Referral to psychooncology specialists for alleviation of psychologic distress and family disruption and promotion of role reorganization and adaptation are often of great value. Brain tumor support groups, psychotropic medications, oncology educational classes for the client and family, and enrollment in one-on-one support programs can be very helpful. Survivors of childhood tumors may experience neurocognitive effects that may manifest after many years; surveillance for these problems is paramount.[29]

## SPECIAL IMPLICATIONS FOR THE THERAPIST 30.1

### *More Attention is Being Paid to Primary Brain Tumors*

#### Rehabilitation Referrals

Therapists will undoubtedly encounter clients with brain tumors in any practice arena because of the significant neuromuscular and cardiopulmonary impairments. Neurologic or orthopedic practices may see patients with brain tumors presenting with gait and balance instability or cervical pain. When the signs and symptoms of a yet undiagnosed brain tumor bring the person to therapy (e.g., unsteady gait and poor balance, weakness), differential diagnosis skills are needed by the therapist to determine a cluster of signs and symptoms indicating a possible tumor, such as headache, nausea and vomiting, lethargy, and others (see Boxes 30.2 and 30.3 and Table 30.3) or a progression of symptoms despite physical therapy intervention requiring referral to the physician.

#### Knowledge Needed for Rehabilitation

Brain tumor studies are beginning to demonstrate rehabilitation effectiveness.[20,57] As the survival of patients with brain tumors increases, rehabilitation needs become more prominent.[20] A general knowledge of primary brain tumor and medical treatment is needed to provide the therapist with skills for differential diagnosis, examination and evaluation, treatment planning, and goal setting. Knowledge of malignant versus benign status, disease progression, expectations, complications, prognosis, and need for precautions, such as for seizures and deep vein thromboses (DVTs), is needed to plan intervention and establish goals. The therapist should also be aware of expected focal symptoms in relation to tumor location to anticipate functional changes that may require treatment modifications, as well as possible paraneoplastic syndromes that may complicate rehabilitation. In geriatric populations, managing a patient with brain cancer may require comprehensive geriatric assessment to identify comorbidities.[13,14]

It is important to be able to distinguish between a meningioma (a benign, potentially curable tumor) and a malignant glioma (a rapidly growing fatal tumor) to set goals, to interact with the family, and to provide appropriate intervention. The advancements in brain tumor medical management (e.g., the promising effectiveness of TMZ for malignant gliomas) and the developing preciseness of radiation therapy brings longer survival and opportunities for better quality of life.[154] The therapist must be aware, prepared, and hopeful that, as the demand for rehabilitation grows, the rehabilitation outcomes will improve.

In addition, knowledge of medical treatment complications from surgery, radiation, chemotherapy, and other interventions will give the therapist the ability to adjust the rehabilitation program as needed, to accommodate, for example, myelosuppression from chemotherapy or fatigue from radiation therapy. Overall, the fact that there are no existing randomized or controlled clinical trials for best evidence to support multidisciplinary rehabilitation after treatment of brain tumors highlights the challenge of design, rigor, and outcome measurements in this population.[79]

### Acute Postoperative Management

When a referral is received for acute postoperative rehabilitation therapy, awareness of general postoperative complications, including atelectasis, pneumonia, cardiac arrhythmias, fluid and electrolyte imbalances, infection, meningitis, intracranial hemorrhage, and renal and gastrointestinal disorders, is important. Potential symptoms after brain surgery include confusion, pain, weakness, and headache. Observing the client closely during therapy intervention for any significant signs and symptoms and making appropriate adaptations during therapy are part of the role of the therapist.[142]

### Postoperative Complications of Intracranial Surgery

Potential complications of intracranial surgery may be very serious and even fatal because of the significant functions performed by the structures involved. Some postoperative complications may improve; however, others may be permanent.

Increased ICP (resulting from cerebral edema or bleeding) is the major complication of intracranial surgery. Findings may include decreased level of consciousness, with headaches, visual and speech disturbances, muscle weakness or paralysis, pupil changes, seizures, vomiting, and respiratory changes (see Box 30.3). Approximately 50% of primary pediatric brain tumors will manifest with hydrocephalus; shunting is often necessary during surgical resection.[173]

In at-risk patients, several methods can be used to continuously measure ICP, including intraventricular catheters, subarachnoid or subdural screws or bolts, epidural sensors, and intraparenchymal catheters. Other monitored parameters include mixed venous oxygen saturation and jugular oxygen saturation, which reflects oxygen saturation of the blood returning from the brain. Normal ICP ranges from 0 to 15 mm Hg, with a midrange of 8 mm Hg and fluctuations occurring with active movement of the extremities and trunk, coughing, suctioning, noxious touch, and other physical stress maneuvers. Use of pleasant sensations such as music and therapeutic touch to reduce ICP are being investigated. Sustained ICP above 20 mm Hg requires emergency treatment. A therapist noting a rise in ICP above 15 mm Hg should contact the nurse or physician.

Because of increased ICP, further surgical intervention may be needed to release excess fluid. A catheter may be inserted to drain excess fluid from a ventricle or other fluid-filled space, called a shunt, or a Jackson-Pratt suction drain may be needed. CSF postoperative leaks are evidenced by saturation of the surgical head dressing or leaking of a clear, thin fluid from the ear or nose that dries in concentric circles.

Management of the postoperative client with increased ICP typically includes, among other things, elevation of the head to about 20 to 30 degrees. The client should be protected from any position that allows stasis of the CSF drainage and should be taught to observe the drainage and to be aware of signs of infection. The client also should be instructed against coughing, sneezing, or blowing the nose. An erratic body temperature may occur after intracranial surgery. Either hypothermia or hyperthermia may be present. The therapist should check with the nursing staff before beginning therapy if concern exists regarding abnormal temperature.

DVT occurs in one-third of patients who have surgery. Seizures,[64] CSF leakage, and wound infection are also risks. Periocular edema is common, as are temporary visual field deficits. Patients may have other temporary deficits resulting from cerebral edema such as communication, motor, and sensory deficits; diminished gag and swallowing reflexes; diplopia; loss of corneal reflex; and personality changes.[63] *Pneumocystis carinii* pneumonia (PCP) is a life-threatening opportunistic infection that occurs in immunocompromised hosts, such as with corticosteroid use. Signs of PCP are fever and dyspnea with or without a prominent dry cough, though the onset may be subtle. The risk of PCP is increased while steroids are being tapered.[117,141]

Meningitis also may occur, caused by irritation of the meninges by infection or blood in the subarachnoid space. If it develops, meningitis typically appears 2 or 3 days after surgery. Chills, fever, nuchal rigidity, headache, irritability, increased sensitivity to light, and decreased level of consciousness are signs of meningitis. Other signs to be aware of include ecchymosis, stress ulcer, swallowing difficulties and aspiration, and impaired airway. Respiratory changes should be monitored carefully. An abnormal respiratory rate and depth may indicate rising ICP. By carefully observing the client during therapy, protecting the client from harm, and alerting medical staff of seizure activity or other adverse signs and symptoms, the therapist can provide a valuable adjunct to postoperative care.

### Positioning in the Acute Postoperative Phase

If there is any question about positioning of a client during therapy, the therapist should communicate with the nursing staff. Incorrect positioning may have serious, possibly fatal, consequences. In the acute phase after surgery above the tentorium, orders may be given to avoid lowering the head, to avoid extreme flexion of the legs, and to keep the neck in a neutral position. After surgery below the tentorium, the client may be kept flat and turned every 2 hours or have orders for elevation of the head of the bed. It is recommended that the neck not be angulated anteriorly or laterally, but there are usually no restrictions placed on turning. For infratentorial tumors that may cause dizziness on arising, elevating the head of bed gradually while concurrently monitoring vital signs is recommended. The dizziness is caused by transient edema in the area of the eighth cranial nerve. For posterior fossa surgery, the client is typically positioned on the side with a pillow under the head. This protects the operative site from pressure and minimizes tension on the suture line.[63]

If a bone flap was removed for decompression, the orders may be to place the client only on the nonoperated side or the back. This facilitates brain expansion. If a large tumor has been removed from a cerebral hemisphere, there may be an order to avoid positioning on the operative site to prevent shifting of the cranial contents because of gravity.

If a client is neurologically unstable, and with ICP in a critical range (more than 20 mm Hg), therapy procedures that require a flat position (e.g., lowering the head of the bed for range-of-motion exercises) should be avoided. Placing a pillow under the head facilitates good venous outflow. When the client is in a side-lying position, protecting the hips from sharp flexion avoids an increase in intrathoracic pressure, which can in turn increase cerebral ICP.

### Intervention Preparation

Before physical therapy intervention, examination should include a review of the medical chart. If indicated, physicians should be contacted for pertinent information and guidelines. Hematologic values may be of critical importance for exercise training plans. Anemia causes fatigue, leukopenia increases infection susceptibility, and thrombocytopenia increases bleeding susceptibility and is of particular concern because it may lead to intracranial hemorrhage.[115,117]

Familiarity with cancer terminology and the behavior of the particular tumor aids communication with others on the team. For example, interdisciplinary care planning and intervention are facilitated by knowledge of tumor staging and grading; the prognosis; and the medical management including the surgical procedure, presence of an Ommaya reservoir, and the various types of central lines and monitoring devices. Knowledge of the Karnofsky Performance Scale (KPS), a functional performance scale used by many oncologists to indicate the client's activity level in the hospital, home, or community, is helpful. It can facilitate communication among the team on issues such as a client's candidacy for home discharge with home health assistance or need for more supervised care. The Eastern Cooperative Oncology Group performance status (Table 30.6) is another, simpler scale that may be used to identify functional performance and can help determine a patient's ability to tolerate various cancer therapies.

Initial outcomes expected for clients with brain surgery include full range of motion, active where possible, of all extremities and optimal functioning of respiratory, cardiovascular, and other systems within the precautions indicated. When the client's condition is stable, functional outcomes include independent bed mobility and transfers, ambulation, and self-care skills (activities of daily living).

### Rehabilitation Examination for Postoperative Care

During the acute postoperative phase, a thorough examination within the constraints of the precautions, including strength, joint range of motion, sensory and perceptual status, neurologic signs, pain patterns, presence of fatigue, and mobility, helps to identify treatable impairments that affect function.[100] During examination and intervention, the therapist should avoid any Valsalva maneuver that would increase intrathoracic pressure, thus increasing ICP.

**Table 30.6** Eastern Cooperative Oncology Group Performance Status

| Performance Status | Definition |
|---|---|
| 0 | Fully active; no performance restrictions |
| 1 | Strenuous physical activity restricted; fully ambulatory and able to carry out light work |
| 2 | Capable of all self-care but unable to carry out any work activities. Up and about >50% of waking hours |
| 3 | Capable of only limited self-care; confined to bed or chair >50% of waking hours |
| 4 | Completely disabled; cannot carry out any self-care; totally confined to bed or chair |

Adapted from Oken MM, et al: Toxicity and response criteria of the Eastern Cooperative Oncology Group. *Am J Clin Oncol* 5:649, 1982.

### Rehabilitation Intervention

After intracranial surgery, bed rest precautions may be initiated, usually for 24 hours, and should be observed by the therapist. If the client is stable, passive range-of-motion exercises may begin.

Position changes are important, and use of a draw sheet and adequate help ensure that the patient will not strain with position change and increase ICP. When movement to the bedside chair is safe but ICP precautions preclude active supine-to-sitting movements, lifting the client to a reclining chair by a draw sheet with the help of several caregivers or use of lift equipment and then gradually raising the client's back and head in the chair protects him or her from straining. Bedside sit-and-dangle exercises also may be requested. Blood pressure checks for postural hypotension; close assessment for dizziness and faintness; and monitoring of respiratory rate, heart rate, and ICP during activities are essential. General conditioning activities early in the recovery process are valuable to address the fatigue cycle typical of cancer.

### Subacute and Ambulatory Rehabilitation

As the patient becomes more stable and is moved into lower levels of acuity, including inpatient and ambulatory care, continued monitoring is imperative. The therapist must monitor vital signs and observe for any neurologic change; any adverse indications such as seizures, bleeding at the operative site, or signs of a DVT; or sudden changes in mental status.

Medical treatment modalities and side effects have a pronounced effect on the client's participation in therapy. Chemotherapeutic and radiation side effects such as myelosuppression, nausea, and fatigue may temporarily lower energy levels, requiring adjustment of the therapy program. Irradiated areas should be protected against skin injury. No heat or cold or topical agents should be used in the irradiated area during the treatment series or for several weeks after the treatment series until the skin damage has cleared. The radiation oncologist will determine the topical agents to be used. If persistent trophic change occurs to the skin with obvious circulatory impairment, heat or cold should not be applied over the site because of poor dissipation effects.

Examination and intervention are based on the impairments and disabilities identified. Safety in mobility, gait and balance training, protection from falls, strengthening, equipment decisions, functional training, and aerobic capacity training are important rehabilitation interventions.[166] Written educational materials are increasingly requested.

The efficacy of increasing the activity level has been demonstrated, and functional training, gait training, and exercise are well-accepted postoperative interventions.[129] Long-term management may include family training and education and more advanced treatment aimed at self-care and safety, return to family roles, and work and leisure activity.

More attention is being paid at the present time to cancer-related fatigue, identifying possible causes such as myelosuppression, anorexia, pain, sleep deprivation, and somnolence. Treatment modalities, including surgery, radiation therapy, and chemotherapy, are associated with fatigue. Understanding fatigue and the ameliorating factors is increasingly becoming the subject of studies. In a recent study on glioblastoma, fatigue was associated with decreases in almost all aspects of quality of life.[95] Addressing fatigue with a structured progressive exercise program has some efficacy.[43,44,109,143] Although there is no consensus on the ideal type of exercise, frequency, intensity, duration, or mode, there is good cardiopulmonary response to interval training at 50% to 70% of heart rate reserve or working at an exertion level of 11 to 14 on the 6-to-20 rate of perceived exertion scale. While treatment is being given, most studies recommend decreasing the intensity to the lower end of the heart rate range.[35] Some studies suggest careful monitoring to avoid overstressing the immune system.[120] Other problems associated with fatigue should be addressed as they occur.[138] Throughout the rehabilitation process, activities that increase ICP, such as vigorous resistive exercises or isometrics, should be avoided.

Studies support the benefits of comprehensive and interdisciplinary rehabilitation for patients with primary and metastatic brain tumors.[65,110,117] Patients who have a malignant brain tumor can make functional gains in both the inpatient and the outpatient rehabilitation settings.[145] Outcomes of physical therapy intervention may be measured by a variety of standardized tools, such as KPS, European Organisation for Research and Treatment of Cancer (EORTC) QLQ-C30, Psychosocial Adjustment to Illness Scale, Functional Living Index–Cancer (FLIC) Scale, Functional Assessment of Cancer Therapy–Brain, and Functional Assessment of Chronic Illness Therapy (FACIT) Scale. Considerations of quality of life are increasingly part of medical oncologic studies. Specific tools have been developed and validated for assessing health-related quality of life in patients with brain cancer, including EORTC QLQ-BN20, Functional Assessment of Cancer Therapy–Brain (FACT-Br),[53,98] and MD Anderson Symptom Inventory Brain Tumor Module (MDASI-BT).[160] Fatigue measures include the 1-to-10 analog scale, Brief Fatigue Inventory (BFI),[25] Piper Fatigue Scale, and numerous other newer fatigue measures. Some studies have used the Functional Independence Measure (FIM) to evaluate changes in function with inpatient rehabilitation[68,98,110,115] and have demonstrated improvements.

### Steroid Effects

Corticosteroids are prescribed during surgery and again during radiation to reduce cerebral edema. Long-term effects include many adverse problems, including proximal weakness, behavioral changes, osteoporosis, increased appetite, bloating, hypertension, and many more. Long-term steroid use is avoided, and the drugs are typically discontinued after the acute surgical or radiation management is completed. However, with steroid tapering and discontinuation, there may be a possible increase in cerebral edema and a recurrence of symptoms previously present before surgery or radiation. For example, a person receiving brain radiation taking dexamethasone during the radiation series may demonstrate improved hemiparesis as a result of the steroid. However, when radiation therapy is completed and steroid therapy is tapered and discontinued, the hemiparesis may worsen. The therapist needs to be aware of decreasing function related to steroid tapering during this time and report it to the physician. The decision may be made to continue the steroid at a low dose. If corticosteroids are tapered too rapidly after surgery or radiation therapy, causing peritumoral edema, a bolus dose of dexamethasone followed by a more gradual weaning schedule may alleviate the symptoms.[54] Edema fluctuations from the tumor effect itself may cause a puzzling improvement and regression in neurologic status. Mobility issues and goals should be planned with the client and family, keeping in mind this potential of variable symptoms from edema fluctuations. The therapist must avoid creating either false hope or pessimism when patient performance varies because of edema fluctuations.

### Psychosocial Impact

The impact of the diagnosis may be difficult for the client to comprehend. The client who does comprehend may demonstrate extreme behavioral responses or a profound sense of hopelessness. The client should be encouraged to ask questions and express his or her feelings about the situation. Depression is difficult to distinguish from apathy caused by the brain tumor,[74] but a differential diagnosis, if possible, through depression testing is important to help the therapist to advocate for improved management of depression. Managing cognitive effects of radiation therapy is difficult for the client and family.[31,138] The caregiver's support, realistic reassurance, and inclusion of the client and family in the decision-making process will have a positive impact on the quality of life.[63]

Because the diagnosis of a brain tumor is so devastating to the client and family, causing fear and uncertainty, the therapist must have sufficient maturity and psychosocial skills to be supportive and understanding. The challenge is not necessarily to provide solutions to these psychosocial problems but rather to provide support and validation and to facilitate referrals to appropriate professionals while addressing the physical problem for which the person was referred.

### Rehabilitation Team

The therapist involved in rehabilitation of a person with a brain tumor is part of a rehabilitation team of professionals. The team consists of the patient and the patient's family and may include representatives from the physician office staff, nursing, nutrition services, pharmacy occupational therapy, speech therapy, recreational therapy, respiratory therapy, social work, psychology, the chaplain's office, durable medical equipment suppliers, hospice staff, and complementary or volunteer services, such as massage and music therapy. An interdisciplinary approach allows access to needed resources and allows for a continuum of care.

The therapist must understand that the term *cancer rehabilitation* is used by many specialists and community programs that provide services for people with cancer and may mean different things in different contexts. Cancer rehabilitation has grown exponentially over the past decade, with multiple cancer programs considering rehabilitation to be a crucial component of cancer care.[148] Oncology nurses are increasingly supportive of cancer rehabilitation and an interdisciplinary approach[101] and include symptom control and psychosocial issues in their definition of rehabilitation. Many local groups, such as church and synagogue support groups, provide another aspect of rehabilitation. The NCI has identified four objectives for cancer rehabilitation: psychologic support, optimal physical functioning, vocational counseling, and optimal social functioning.[103] Financial issues, nutrition, spousal relationships, sexual counseling, vocational rehabilitation, employment opportunities, physician–patient communication, patient education, and coping skills are broader aspects of rehabilitation.

In some acute care and outpatient settings, the therapist may be part of a more formalized cancer rehabilitation program that includes these facets of rehabilitation. The advantages for the client with access to such a program include early and appropriate referrals to skilled professionals and resources, coordination of care and information, and a smooth transition across the continuum of care. Other benefits include enhancement of program development resulting from collaboration of professionals, outcome studies that will improve the quality of care, and the potential for rehabilitation research.

## PRIMARY INTRASPINAL TUMORS

Primary spinal cord tumors are about one-sixth as common as primary brain tumors. The histologic types of tumor cells in the spinal cord are the same as those found in the brain, although the prevalence of certain types may differ. The most common tumor in the spinal cord is schwannoma or neurinoma, followed by meningioma and glioma.[106]

A convenient anatomic classification system of spinal cord tumors is based on the relationship of the tumor to the spinal cord and dura. Fig. 30.21 diagrams the location and relative incidence of spinal tumors. Intradural–intramedullary tumors arise within the spinal cord substance. Intradural–extramedullary tumors arise outside the spinal cord but within the dura. Extradural spinal cord tumors arise outside the spinal cord and the dura (Fig. 30.22).[162] The specific spinal cord tumor types and their incidence are discussed first, followed by clinical presentation and medical management.

### Intradural–Intramedullary Tumors

#### Incidence

Intradural–intramedullary (within the dura, within the cord) tumors are the least common type of primary intraspinal tumors in adults, but the most common type in children. These tumors account for 5% to 10% of intraspinal tumors. The dominant tumor types are astrocytomas and ependymomas.[169]

#### Pathogenesis

Because they are located within the cord itself, intradural–intramedullary tumors generally are derived from the cellular substrate of the spinal cord such as the astrocytes and ependymal cells or from the primitive embryonal cells. Astrocytomas may occur anywhere along the spinal cord and may span several cord segments longitudinally. In children they may run the entire length of the cord.

Although all astrocytomas are infiltrative, most are low grade and slow growing in the spinal cord. Ependymomas are generally slow growing as well and less infiltrative and therefore more amenable to surgical excision. Other, less frequent types of intradural–intramedullary tumors are hemangiomas, epidermoid and dermoid cysts, teratomas, lipomas, and neurenteric cysts. Of interest to therapists is chemical meningitis, with its significant chronic pain that can occur when epidermoid or dermoid cysts leak debris into the CSF. Very infrequently, a primary intramedullary spinal lymphoma (PCNSL) may occur.[19,163]

### Intradural–Extramedullary Tumors

#### Incidence

Intradural–extramedullary (within the dura, outside the cord) tumors are the most common type of primary intraspinal tumor in adults, and they account for approximately 45% of all spinal tumors. Neurinomas (schwannomas) and meningiomas are the dominant tumors in this group. Meningiomas occur in middle age and are 10 times more common in women than in men.[169]

#### Pathogenesis

Intradural–extramedullary tumors are primarily derived from the supporting elements of the CNS, including the meninges and nerve sheath. Tumors in this compartment occasionally are carried down as drop metastases by the CSF from malignant brain tumors (medulloblastomas, less commonly ependymomas and PNETs). Fig. 30.23 shows a PNET in the brain and spinal cord surfaces.

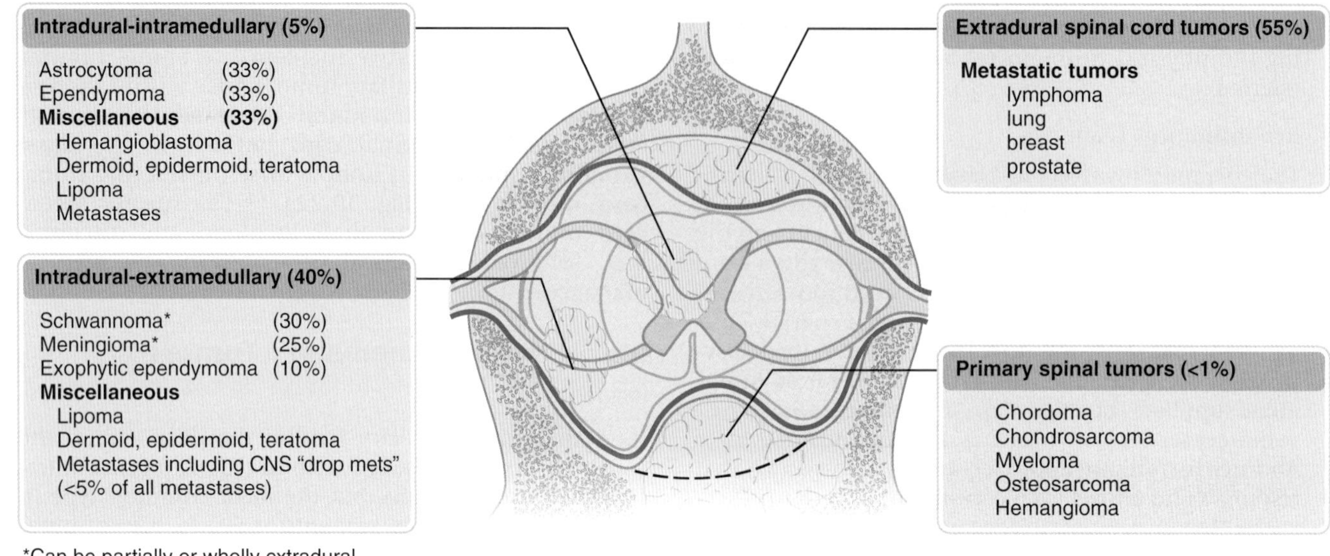


**Fig. 30.21**

**Primary and metastatic tumors of the spine and spinal cord.** (Adapted from Poirier J, et al: *Manual of basic neuropathology*, ed 2, Philadelphia, 1990, Saunders.)

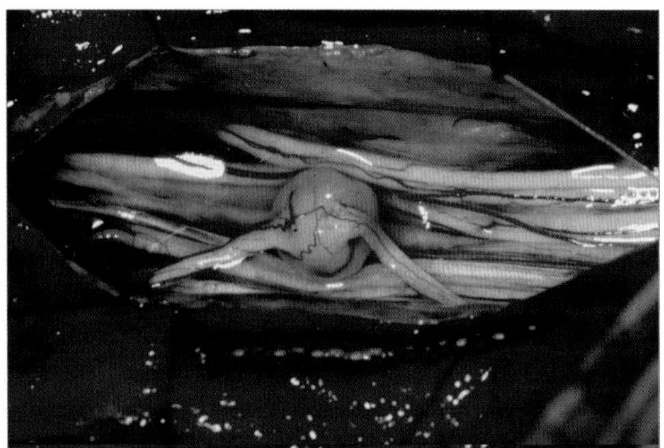

**Fig. 30.22**

**Spinal cord neoplasms are extradural or intradural tumors according to their relationship to the thecal sac.** (Copyright © 2007 Michael English/ Custom Medical Stock Photo/Science Photo Library.)

Intradural–extramedullary tumors cause compression of the spinal cord, rather than invasion of the cord. Neurinomas are soft, globular masses that arise at the sensory or dorsal nerve root. Occasionally they may straddle the intervertebral foramen and extend outside the foramen, in the so-called *dumbbell configuration.* Spinal meningiomas are benign, slow-growing globular tumors that often grow in the thoracic, cervical, and foramen magnum regions. They may be present for many years before symptoms occur.

## Extradural–Extramedullary Tumors

### Incidence

Extradural–extramedullary tumors are most often metastatic tumors and are addressed later in Metastatic Tumors. Extradural–extramedullary tumors represent approximately 45% of all spinal cord tumors. An occasional meningioma, neurinoma (schwannoma), or spinal chordoma arises extradurally. Spinal chordomas represent less than 1% of spinal cord tumors.[169]

### Pathogenesis

Spinal chordomas are primary tumors that arise from the vertebral bodies, usually in the cervical or sacral regions of the axial skeleton. They are prone to metastasize outside the spinal column. Lesions are characterized by expansive destruction of the bone, for example, the sacrum, or by varying degrees of vertebral collapse. Box 30.4 summarizes the type and location of spinal tumors.

### Clinical Manifestations of Primary Intraspinal Tumors

Spontaneous pain caused by nerve root irritation is a common clinical feature of primary spinal tumors and is usually worse at night. Intramedullary tumors give rise to a poorly localized, deep, burning type of pain in the spinal region. Extramedullary tumors produce a knifelike radicular type of pain typically radiating to the periphery of the nerve, often aggravated by coughing, sneezing, or straining. The association of asymmetry of reflexes with nerve root pain and an insidious onset is strongly suggestive of a spinal cord tumor.

Nerve root pain may be followed by motor weakness of muscles supplied by the nerve. The motor changes of intramedullary tumors include lower motor neuron changes at the level of the lesion and may also include upper motor neuron changes at lower levels. The motor changes of extramedullary lesions begin with segmental weakness at the lesion site and may progress to Brown-Séquard syndrome or later to a transverse cord syndrome.[162] The

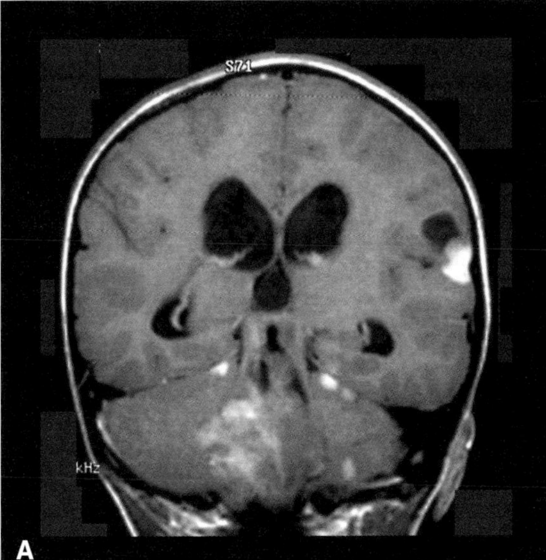


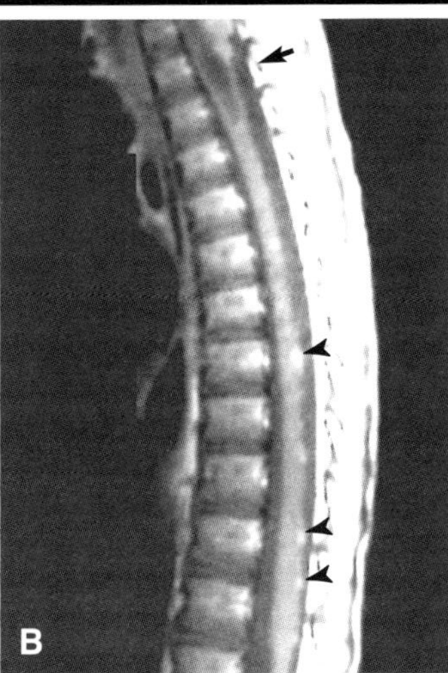


**Fig. 30.23**

**Primitive neuroectodermal tumor.** (A) T1-weighted coronal magnetic resonance imaging (MRI) after injection of contrast medium in a 5-year-old boy. There is a large multifocal tumor in the posterior fossa causing hydrocephalus. There are multiple smaller, contrast-enhancing tumors along the surface of cerebellum and in the cerebrum. (B) T1-weighted sagittal postcontrast MRI of the spinal canal shows a large mass *(arrow)* in the junction of the cervical and thoracic spine with a syrinx and multiple small enhancing nodules *(arrowheads)* over the surface of the spinal cord. (From Adam A, et al, eds: *Grainger and Allison's diagnostic radiology: a textbook of medical imaging*, ed 4, Philadelphia, 2001, Churchill Livingstone.)

weakness is characterized by upper motor neuron signs, including spasticity. Sphincter weakness, increasing urinary frequency, and urgency may develop. In men, the development of sphincter disturbances frequently is followed by impotence.

Sensory changes in extramedullary tumors are usually along the distribution of the involved nerve roots. Intramedullary tumors result in dissociated sensory disturbances in the limbs below the level of the lesion because of their growth pattern of crossing fibers of the spinothalamic tract. People often report a feeling of temperature change, particularly a feeling of cold below the level of the lesion. Pain and temperature sensation are compromised, but proprioception and light touch may be preserved.

Syringomyelia-like symptoms of loss of pain and temperature sensation below the level of the lesion on one or both sides of the body may occur from damage to the decussating lateral spinothalamic fibers. This often is accompanied by progressive spastic paraparesis caused by pressure on the descending corticospinal tracts. Anterior growth of the tumor produces anterior horn signs, such as muscle weakness, wasting, and fasciculations in the muscles supplied by the anterior horn cells.

Other symptoms of intramedullary cord tumors are papilledema, hydrocephalus, and elevations in ICP. The reason for development of papilledema is unclear, but it is more common with tumors of the thoracic and lumbosacral regions. Box 30.5 lists signs and symptoms of spinal cord tumors.

Box 30.4

**SPINAL TUMORS**

***Extradural***

- Metastasis
- Primary bone tumors arising in the spine

***Intradural and Extramedullary***

- Meningiomas
- Neurofibromas
- Neurinomas (schwannomas)
- Lipomas
- Arachnoid cysts
- Epidermoid cysts
- Metastasis

***Intramedullary***

- Ependymoma
- Glioma
- Hemangioblastoma
- Lipoma
- Metastasis

From DeAngelis LM: Tumors of the central nervous system. In Goldman LM, Ausiello D, eds: *Cecil textbook of medicine*, ed 22, Philadelphia, 2004, Saunders.

## MEDICAL MANAGEMENT

DIAGNOSIS. After a history and neurologic examination, MRI is the method of choice for the identification of spinal cord tumors. Gadolinium-enhanced MRI is helpful to differentiate between edema and tumor. Plain films occasionally may be helpful in treatment planning. Lumbar puncture and CSF examination are no longer used as diagnostic tools.

TREATMENT AND PROGNOSIS. Surgery is the principal treatment for all primary intraspinal tumors. Complete and curative resection is the objective. Radiation therapy is not required when lesions are completely excised. Intraspinal astrocytomas have a lower rate of cure, although surgery and radiation may prolong the disease-free survival. Childhood astrocytomas, however, have a more favorable prognosis, with a 5-year survival rate of 90%.

SPECIAL IMPLICATIONS FOR THE THERAPIST 30.2

### *Primary Intraspinal Tumors*

**Alertness to Signs and Symptoms**

As specialists in motor function, therapists may be involved even before a diagnosis of cancer has been made in observing and identifying the signs of spinal cord tumors. Clients referred to physical therapy because of back pain symptoms who have intractable pain that worsens with recumbency and is not relieved by physical therapy should raise the suspicion of an intraspinal tumor. Progressive neurologic signs should alert the therapist to the need for medical referral and MRI or CT scan to elicit the diagnosis. A thorough initial examination and evaluation of any person with back pain, including symptoms; pain patterns; strength assessment; and other neurologic signs, such as impaired bowel and bladder function, changes in deep tendon reflexes, and signs of spasticity, should be the standard of practice to rule out tumors and other systemic disorders.

**Rehabilitation Referrals**

Neurologic deficits from primary spinal cord tumors may result in impairments such as spinal pain, weakness in the extremities and trunk, sensory loss, bowel and bladder dysfunction, spinal instability, and impaired aerobic capacity. Functional impairments for bed mobility and transfers, impaired balance, gait instability, knowledge deficit regarding spinal safety, decreased independence with self-care, equipment issues, and difficulties in returning to work, community activities, and leisure activities all require rehabilitation therapy. Because of a favorable prognosis with completely excised primary tumors, the approach of the therapist should be toward achieving maximal function and support of the client and family toward long-term goals. Many patients will survive their tumors, but residual deficits and functional limitations are common. Medical management, including surgery (resections, kyphoplasty, fusions), chemotherapy, and radiation therapy, causes complications over a prolonged time period that require rehabilitation intervention at numerous time points during recovery.

**Knowledge Needed for Rehabilitation**

As with primary brain tumors, therapists should know the medical management plan, the prognostic expectations, the side effects of treatment, and precautions to prepare for the rehabilitative approach to a client with an intraspinal tumor. Knowledge of the most common intraspinal tumors, their patterns of growth, and neurologic changes assists the therapist in assessing the patient accurately, setting goals, and providing intervention.

**Rehabilitation Evaluation**

A thorough examination of the neurologic and musculoskeletal systems is very important to identify impairments that affect function. For example, an anterior tibialis muscle weakness or a lower extremity paraparesis may be the impairment that limits mobility and may be amenable to therapy. The therapist should review medical records, laboratory and radiologic reports, and other studies. If the treatment is provided on an outpatient basis, blood value determinations should be requested to assist the therapist in planning exercise programs. Communicating with the oncologist, surgeon, and nurse; keeping abreast of imaging reports and other diagnostic tests; and being alert to other medical management, such as the effect of steroids and chemotherapy, allow the therapist to be more effective in treatment. Postoperative precautions may include protection from spinal torsion and use of an external support. Protection of irradiated skin follows the same guidelines as given in Primary Brain Tumors.

## METASTATIC TUMORS

The extended survival in all types of cancer has allowed time for metastasis to occur from primary tumors elsewhere in the body. Metastatic complications are an escalating problem. Metastases to the brain and spinal cord are among the most serious complications of metastatic cancer.[21,162]

### Incidence

The incidence of metastatic CNS tumors is estimated to be 150,000 to 180,000 per year, although exact figures are difficult to ascertain.[4] The number of metastatic brain tumors is estimated to be 150,000 per year, and the number of metastatic spinal cord tumors is estimated to be approximately 80,000 per year.[4] These tumors are the most common intracranial tumors in adults.[169] The incidence of metastatic CNS tumors is on the rise as a result

**Box 30.5**

**SIGNS AND SYMPTOMS OF SPINAL CORD TUMORS**

- Pain
- Weakness
- Sensory changes
- Urinary frequency
- Urinary urgency
- Sphincter disturbances
- Syringomyelia-like symptoms
- Brown-Séquard syndrome–like symptoms
- Hydrocephalus
- Increased intracranial pressure
- Papilledema
- Atrophy
- Hyporeflexia
- Spasticity
- Hyperreflexia
- Gait disturbances
- Sexual dysfunction

of improved life expectancies from advances in cancer treatment. These tumors find a safe haven behind the blood-brain barrier through which many chemotherapeutic agents for the primary cancer cannot pass. The blood-brain barrier restricts passage of high-molecular-weight compounds through its tight capillary endothelial junctions.[128] The brain is a metastatic site in approximately 20% of people with primary cancer elsewhere, and the spinal cord is a metastatic site for 10% of primary cancers.[162]

## Pathogenesis

Metastatic tumors reach the brain generally through the arterial blood system.[10] A smaller number arise by direct extension from extracranial sites, such as the neck or paranasal sinuses. The cascade of events for formation of a metastasis includes tumor cells at the primary site reaching a critical volume in proximity to a blood vessel; dislodging from the primary tumor and entering blood vessels; and embolizing, traveling, extravasating from the blood vessel, and growing in parenchyma of another organs.[49,21] Most metastatic tumors arise in the distribution area of the middle cerebral artery to the cerebral hemispheres, with most lesions located in the parietal or frontal lobes. Approximately 20% are found in the posterior fossa, primarily the cerebellum. About half of cases include multiple metastatic lesions in the brain (Fig. 30.24).

Metastatic tumors reach the spine and spinal cord through direct arterial dissemination to the vertebral body, by retrograde spread via the vertebral venous plexus as it perforates into the epidural space and vertebral bodies, or by direct invasion from a paravertebral tumor to the epidural space via the intervertebral foramen. The majority of spinal metastases are extradural–extramedullary, although in less than 5% of cases the location is intramedullary. The thoracic spine is the most frequent site of metastasis (70%), followed by the lumbosacral spine (20%) and the cervical area (10%).[162]

The most common cancers resulting in brain metastases are lung cancers, especially small cell carcinoma; cancers of the breast, kidney, and gastrointestinal tract; and melanoma. Fig. 30.25 shows dural metastasis from breast cancer. The most common cancers metastasizing to the spinal column are lung, breast, prostate, and kidney cancers and lymphomas. In approximately 10% of cases, the primary tumor is never found.

## Clinical Manifestations of Brain Metastasis

Persons with metastatic brain tumors present with headache, seizures, elevated ICP, and similar signs of primary tumors. Table 30.7 provides a more complete list of presenting signs and symptoms. However, symptoms may progress much more rapidly, often in days to weeks, as a result of the significant edema that accompanies a metastasis. Cerebellar metastases may cause obstructive hydrocephalus and abrupt deterioration.

# MEDICAL MANAGEMENT

DIAGNOSIS, TREATMENT, AND PROGNOSIS. MRI is the diagnostic procedure of choice because it is the most sensitive in revealing multiple small lesions. A review of the chest film is often enough to give a presumptive diagnosis of lung cancer. With a history of cancer elsewhere in the body, a solitary brain lesion has approximately a 90% certainty of being a metastatic deposit.[162] Because meningiomas have a high prevalence in people

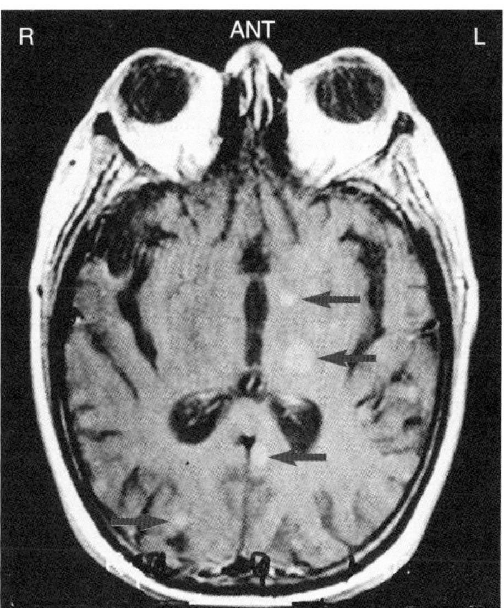


**Fig. 30.24**

**Metastatic disease in the brain.** Gadolinium-enhanced T1-weighted magnetic resonance imaging shows multiple metastases as areas of increased signal *(arrows)*. (From Mettler FA Jr: *Essentials of radiology*, ed 2, Philadelphia, 2005, Saunders.)

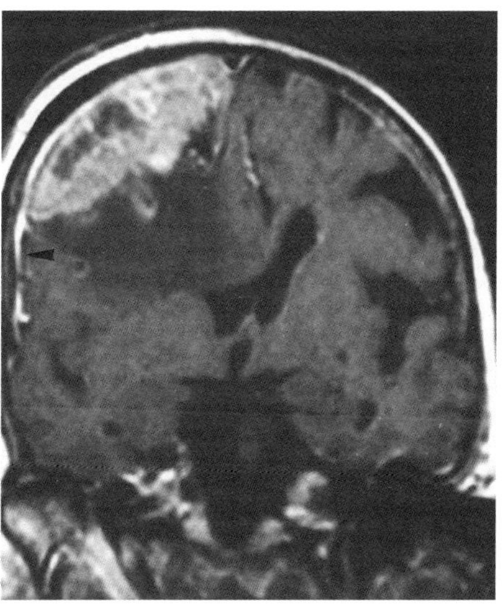

**Fig. 30.25**

**Dural metastasis from breast carcinoma.** Coronal T1-weighted postcontrast magnetic resonance imaging. There is a heterogeneously enhancing mass with an irregular surface that arises from the dura over the right cerebral convexity. It displaces the underlying brain and causes considerable low-signal edema within it. There is a dural tail extending away from the tumor *(arrowhead)*. (From Adam A, et al, eds: *Grainger and Allison's diagnostic radiology: a textbook of medical imaging*, ed 4, Philadelphia, 2001, Churchill Livingstone.)

**Table 30.7** Presenting Symptoms and Signs of Brain Metastasis

| Symptoms | Common Signs |
|---|---|
| Headache | Focal weakness or unexplained falls |
| Mental status change | Focal sensory deficits |
| Altered level of consciousness | Speech difficulty |
| Seizures occurring when older than 35 years of age | Aphasia, focal weakness |
| Papilledema or visual obscurations | Ataxia |
| Visual complaints or unexplained motor vehicle accidents | Visual field defect |

From Goetz CG, ed: *Textbook of clinical neurology*, ed 2, Philadelphia, 2003, Saunders.

with breast cancer, metastatic breast lesions in the brain must be differentiated pathologically from meningiomas for optimal treatment.

Medical management includes corticosteroids, surgical excision when solitary or small numbers of metastases are accessible, and irradiation in almost all cases. Of solitary brain metastases associated with non–small cell lung cancer, up to one-third may be cured with surgery followed by radiation therapy. Steroids have a dramatic effect in relieving symptoms caused by the significant peritumoral swelling. Radiotherapy provides adequate palliation for many people because death occurs from the primary cancer, not the brain metastasis.[76] Brain metastases from breast cancer are increasing in incidence.[158] The treatment of brain metastases with stereotactic Gamma Knife radiosurgery provides an average survival time of 8 months.[144] In general, the prognosis for people with brain metastasis is poor because the metastasis indicates that the primary cancer has already escaped control.

### Clinical Manifestations of Spinal Metastasis

Back pain is the most common and prominent symptom of metastasis to the spinal column and cord and is present in 95% of cases. Anyone with a known cancer history who presents with new-onset back pain of unknown etiology should be considered to have spinal metastasis until proven otherwise.[131] Pain is caused by stretching of the periosteum, tension or traction on the spinal nerve roots and cord, or compression of the cord and meninges. It is usually a dull ache, worse at night in the recumbent position, and may be local in the spine or may be a radicular pain. Intradural–intramedullary metastases are less common than primary tumors in this location, and overall their occurrence is rare.[169]

Without treatment, pain progresses in weeks or months (sometimes days) to weakness, sensory loss, and bowel and bladder sphincter disturbance. These tumors characteristically progress quickly after onset of weakness to cause paraplegia and permanent loss of sphincter control. Diagnosing and treating the metastasis early is important because people treated while still ambulatory are likely to remain so, but people who have reached the stage of paraplegia and sphincter loss do not typically regain function.

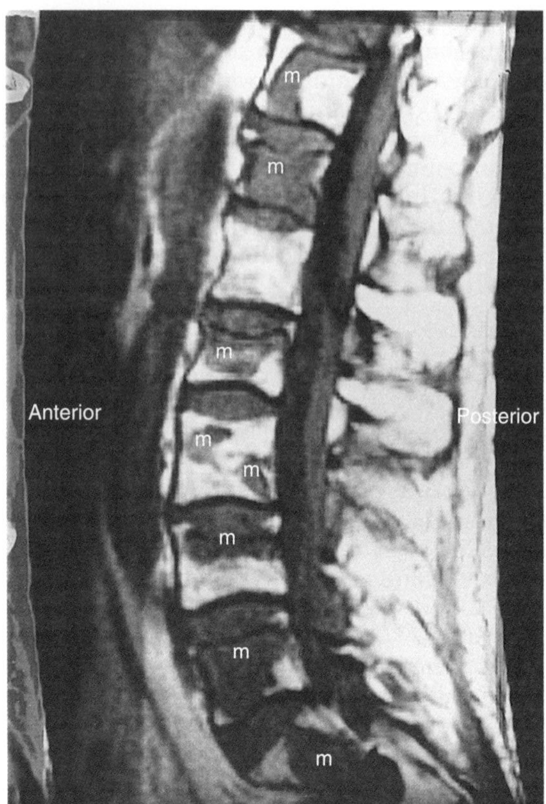


**Fig. 30.26**

**Focal spine metastases.** Sagittal, or lateral, T1-weighted magnetic resonance imaging of the lumbar spine shows the normal white or high signal in fat within the bone marrow. In many of the vertebral bodies, the high signal of normal marrow has been replaced by dark areas of metastatic deposits *(m)*. (From Mettler FA Jr: *Essentials of radiology*, ed 2, Philadelphia, 2005, Saunders.)

## MEDICAL MANAGEMENT

**DIAGNOSIS.** A careful neurologic examination, followed by plain films of the spine, is an important first approach and results in a diagnosis in the majority of cases. The most common findings are pedicular erosion, vertebral collapse, pathologic fracture-dislocation, and a soft tissue shadow suggestive of a paraspinal mass.[162] Bone scans are the next test of choice. If results of any of these tests are positive, MRI or CT is performed for more definitive imaging of the lesion. This will also determine whether the tumor is intramedullary and can be performed in the absence of vertebral disease. Fig. 30.26 shows MRI depicting focal spine metastases.

**TREATMENT.** Radiotherapy is typically the treatment of choice for spinal metastasis to reduce pain, reduce tumor compression, and restore neurologic function. Radiotherapy and/or chemotherapy is also helpful in preserving spinal stability. For tumors that are sensitive to chemotherapy, urgent management with chemotherapy is indicated to preserve spinal integrity.

Surgery is reserved for patients with a worsening neurologic deficit during radiation therapy, patients with spinal instability causing cord compression, patients with tumors known to be radioresistant, and patients who already have received the maximum radiation.

Past attempts at surgical decompression with laminectomy have proved to be disappointing, with neurologic improvement occurring in only 30% of cases.[162] Surgical access via laminectomy to the typically anterior tumors compressing the cord from a ventral direction is technically difficult. Evidence exists that very high doses of corticosteroids relieve local spinal edema. Current practice is to initiate very large doses of corticosteroids as soon as spinal cord compression from metastatic tumor is diagnosed. This dose is continued for several days and then reduced, allowing time for decisions to be made for radiation or surgery.[168]

**PROGNOSIS.** Prognosis for return of neurologic function is based on the degree of loss before radiotherapy. With radiotherapy, 80% of clients who are ambulatory at the time of treatment remain so, and 30% who are nonambulatory regain gait.[162] Pain and neurologic function improve in the majority of people. Because the metastasis indicates loss of containment of the primary tumor, cure is beyond expectation. However, early diagnosis and treatment lead to the optimal result, the prevention of paraplegia.

Radiation to the spinal cord may cause complications of myelopathy. Although radiation has no acute effects on the cord, an early delayed radiation myelopathy after irradiation of the neck is common. The Lhermitte sign (a sudden electric shock sensation radiating down the back and lower extremities brought on by neck flexion), the hallmark of this radiation myelopathy, is present for several months and then abates. It is not a predictor of late delayed radiation spinal cord injury.[42] A late effect of radiation to the cord, occurring between 6 and 36 months after radiation, is a chronic progressive myelopathy that begins as Brown-Séquard syndrome and progresses over weeks or months to spastic paresis. No effective medical treatment exists, but the therapist can provide mobility management, skin precautions, and safety education for these clients.

SPECIAL IMPLICATIONS FOR THE THERAPIST 30.3

### *Primary Intraspinal Tumors*

#### Rehabilitation Referrals

Neurologic deficits resulting from metastatic CNS tumors in the brain or spinal cord often require physical and occupational therapy. Neurologic impairments from either intracranial or intraspinal tumors may include weakness, paralysis, decreased sensation, and pain leading to loss of mobility and self-care skills. Paraplegia from spinal metastasis requires much rehabilitative intervention. The incidence of metastatic CNS tumors is increasing.

#### Prediagnosis Alertness to Signs and Symptoms

Because therapists are often in a position to observe the mobility and neurologic status of clients before a diagnosis of a CNS metastasis is made, being alert to abnormal neurologic signs in any client with a history of cancer is vital. In someone with a cancer history, any signs of intracranial metastasis such as visual symptoms or mental status changes should be reported immediately to the physician. Knowing the signs and symptoms of an intraspinal metastasis and immediately referring the client to the physician cannot be overemphasized. Spinal cord compression can progress in a matter of hours or days to paraplegia. Spinal pain symptoms particularly in the thoracic spine, progressive strength changes, sensory changes, and bowel or bladder function changes in a patient with a cancer history are red flags. A therapist who refers the patient to the physician in time may prevent irreversible paraplegia and sphincter function loss.

#### Knowledge Needed for Rehabilitation

As with primary CNS tumors, therapists need to know the medical management plan, the prognostic expectations, and the hematologic guidelines for exercise. Goal setting needs to be realistic for noncurable disease, yet not without hope for good management.[23] Families and caregivers may need to have an even greater role in goal setting and training. As with primary brain tumors, the psychosocial implications have a profound impact on the client and family, and the therapist can provide support as well as be a sounding board for decision making. It is helpful to realize that in some cases, paraplegia from a metastatic spinal cord tumor may respond to irradiation and improve enough for some return of function such as limited ambulation. The physical therapist must be alert to any neurologic improvement.

#### Rehabilitation Precautions

As with primary CNS tumors, clients and their families must have an awareness of the side effects of the various treatment modalities. Postoperative acute care precautions are discussed in Primary Brain Tumors. A general knowledge of metastatic spread and behavior is helpful.[10,102] Myelosuppression, fatigue, nausea, and precautions need to be understood. Avoiding modalities such as heat or cold or any topical agents over skin being irradiated is important for skin protection because poor circulation inhibits normal heat and cold dissipation. Once the irradiation sessions are completed and the skin has healed and depending on skin integrity and adequate circulation, modalities such as heat or cold or transcutaneous nerve stimulation may be used. Although ultrasound is not usually recommended for pain management because of concerns about tumor growth, its use for palliation of pain in end-stage disease may be allowed.

## PARANEOPLASTIC SYNDROMES

Cancer may cause effects on the nervous system that are not directly related to the primary tumor mass or a metastasis. These so-called remote effects, or paraneoplastic syndromes (see Chapter 9), include paraneoplastic cerebellar degeneration, brainstem encephalitis, myelitis of the spinal cord, and motor neuron disease.[52] Paraneoplastic syndromes are also termed paraneoplastic neurologic disorders. The cause of most paraneoplastic syndromes is unknown, although an immune mechanism is the most likely hypothesis. The response of the immune system to the antigen may be misdirected and cause neurologic dysfunction. Paraneoplastic syndromes may be the first sign of the presence of cancer.[17,126,139]

Although paraneoplastic syndromes involving the CNS are rare, they are often severe, associated with an inflammatory CSF, and leave the person with severe neurologic disability. Treatment effectiveness has been limited. Some syndromes are associated with particular tumors, such as paraneoplastic cerebellar degeneration with lung cancer. In this syndrome, the early symptoms are a slight incoordination in walking, with progressive gait ataxia; incoordination of arms, legs, and trunk; dysarthria; and often nystagmus. After a few months the illness reaches its peak and stabilizes. By this time, most clients must have assistance to walk, handwriting is impossible, many cannot sit unsupported, and speech requires great effort.

It is not within the scope of this chapter to elaborate on CNS paraneoplastic syndromes. However, it is helpful for the therapist to have an acquaintance with these syndromes because they appear in the practice of caring for people with CNS neoplasms.[21]

## LEPTOMENINGEAL CARCINOMATOSIS

Infiltration of the meninges and CSF pathways of the CNS by neoplastic cells is a less common complication of cancer and is known as *leptomeningeal carcinomatosis*. This metastatic seeding of the meninges can be widespread and multifocal. Neurologic signs will depend on location. Brain symptoms may include headache, change in mental status, seizures, double vision, abducens palsy, and hemiparesis; spinal symptoms include radicular pain, numbness, and weakness.[127] Meningeal carcinomatosis occurs in approximately 5% of patients with cancer, but it is being diagnosed with increasing frequency as patients live longer and as neuroimaging studies improve.[59,126] Cancers of the breast and lung, non-Hodgkin lymphoma, melanomas, and adult acute leukemias are the most common primary tumors responsible for leptomeningeal carcinomatosis. Diagnosis is by CSF studies, which show malignant cells in most cases. MRI is also done to assess bulky disease in the brain or spine. Current therapy includes radiotherapy to symptomatic sites, with concurrent intrathecal chemotherapy.[162] Survival is measured in months from treatment.

## PEDIATRIC TUMORS

### Incidence and Pathogenesis

An estimated 3720 brain and other CNS tumors were expected to be diagnosed in 2019.[33] The incidence of primary brain and nervous system tumors peaks in the pediatric population from age 0 to 6 years, drops at age 7 to 10 years, remains steady until age 18 years, then drops. In infants and young children age 0 to 14 years, brain and other CNS tumors (malignant and nonmalignant) are the most common form of cancer, followed by leukemia.[118] The peak incidence of these tumors occurs between birth and age 6 years. Brain tumors are the second leading cause of cancer-related deaths in children younger than age 15 years. Table 30.2 compares the frequency of childhood tumors with the frequency of adult tumors.[33]

The etiology of pediatric brain tumors is not well understood. Cranial exposure to radiation and possible evidence of a heritable syndrome are causes. Other factors being studied include maternal diet and intake of vitamins during pregnancy.

The most frequently encountered types of intracranial tumors in children are astrocytoma, medulloblastoma, ependymoma, and brainstem glioma, which collectively account for approximately one-half of all CNS tumors in the pediatric population.[48,86] Brain tumors in children are typically located infratentorially, primarily in the cerebellum and brainstem, although they may occur at any location. Fig. 30.27 shows the relative frequency and location of brain tumors.

Astrocytomas are the most common type of pediatric intracranial tumor, accounting for approximately 47% of all brain tumors in children. They are usually well-differentiated grade I tumors. About half of them occur supratentorially, most commonly in the frontal lobes, but also in the temporal and parietal lobes. The cerebellum is the most common infratentorial site of astrocytomas in children. Cerebellar astrocytoma is more common in males and usually occurs in the first 2 decades of life, with the median incidence at age 18 years. Children with grade I astrocytomas are known to have an excellent 10-year postoperative survival rate and can have a 20-year overall survival rate of up to 87%.[15] Infrequently, high-grade astrocytomas occur, with a poorer prognosis.

Medulloblastomas account for 20% to 25% of childhood brain tumors and are the most common malignant tumor in children. These aggressive tumors are more common in males than females and have a peak incidence between the ages of 5 and 9 years in children. Evolution of therapeutic strategies, including multimodal chemotherapy followed by surgery, has dramatically improved the outlook for children with medulloblastomas.[162] Medulloblastomas belong to the group of tumors known as *PNETs* and arise in the fourth ventricle. Medulloblastomas have a predilection for meningeal seeding. The 5-year survival rate is approximately 50%, with patients with diagnosis at a young age having a significantly poorer prognosis.[125]

Ependymomas usually arise in children from the floor of the fourth ventricle and make up less than 10% of childhood tumors. There is a peak incidence in early childhood, with 25% to 40% of diagnoses occurring in children less than 2 years old. Recurrences are common postoperatively, with a 10-year overall survival of approximately 50% to 70%.[165]

Brainstem gliomas may be of several tumor types; the most common is astrocytoma, but they also may be glioblastomas or ependymomas. The overall prognosis for brainstem tumors is relatively poor, but occasionally gratifying treatment results are obtained.[162]

### Clinical Manifestations

Clinical manifestations of CNS neoplasms in children are more difficult to evaluate because children are less able to

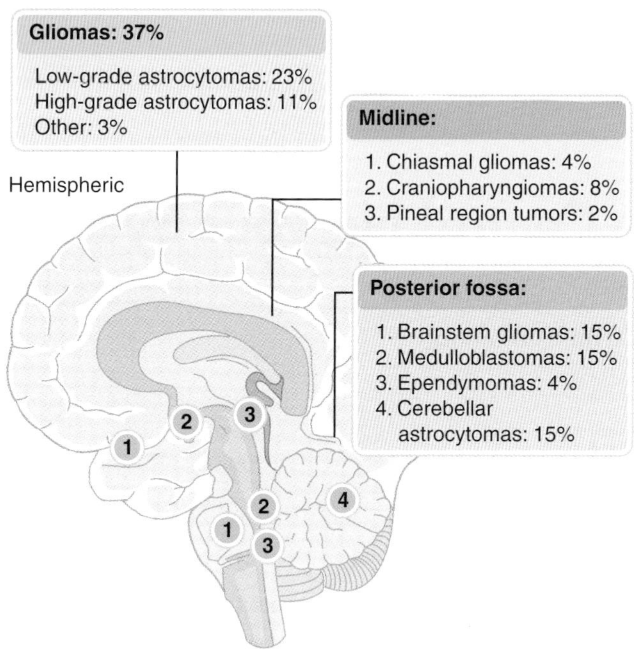


**Fig. 30.27**

**Childhood brain tumors occur at any location within the central nervous system.** The relative frequency of brain tumor histologic types and the anatomic distribution are shown. (From Kliegman RM, Behrmann RE: *Nelson textbook of pediatrics*, ed 18, Philadelphia, 2007, Saunders.)

relate and report symptoms. Parents, teachers, and caretakers may notice problems before the child is aware of a change. Most supratentorial astrocytomas initially manifest with seizures. Cerebellar astrocytomas produce typical cerebellar findings such as ataxia, and many produce symptoms of increased ICP. Tumors of the cerebral aqueduct or the fourth ventricle such as an ependymoma or medulloblastoma typically manifest at an early stage with headache, nausea, and cranial nerve palsies but also may produce long-tract signs such as hemiparesis. Hydrocephalus is a complication in patients with ependymoma and medulloblastoma and a late manifestation of brainstem gliomas.[55]

## MEDICAL MANAGEMENT

**DIAGNOSIS AND TREATMENT.** Diagnosis is by MRI or CT, although CT may not be adequate to detect the early stages of brainstem or fourth ventricle tumors. Early treatment includes high-dose dexamethasone, emergency ventricular drainage in the case of hydrocephalus, and surgical resection. Radiation is the principal form of treatment for brainstem gliomas. Postoperative radiation is indicated for medulloblastomas and may be helpful for ependymomas and gliomas. Chemotherapy, although generally not beneficial, has been helpful for medulloblastomas.

The risks of radiation therapy to the brain in children are of great concern. The effects of radiation may include learning disabilities, hypopituitarism, occlusive disease of cerebral vessels, and radiation-induced secondary tumors. Because myelinization of the CNS is not generally complete until 2 to 3 years of age, radiation therapy performed before this age can be especially devastating and is not usually done.[162] Long-term effects from childhood tumors and treatment have been reported by Packer.[79,119]

Spinal cord tumors rarely occur in children. Spinal ependymoma is the most prominent primary intraspinal tumor and has a predilection for the lumbosacral spine. It is treated with resection and radiation therapy. The risks of radiation therapy in children include myelopathy and spinal deformities.

Metastatic spinal cord tumors in children arise most commonly from sarcomas and less often from neuroblastomas, lymphomas, and leukemias. Metastatic tumors in children occur principally by direct extension from an adjacent primary cancer[162] and can be the presenting feature of the primary cancer. This is in contrast to adult spinal tumors, in which access is by a vascular route and usually occurs in the setting of an advanced malignancy.

Because pediatric metastatic spinal cord tumors usually are not associated with extensive vertebral column destruction, they generally can be removed through a simple laminectomy. An aggressive approach to metastatic spinal tumors in children results in a more favorable outcome in children than in adults.[162] Approximately 96% of children have improvement or stabilization of neurologic deficits, and 60% of nonambulatory children regain the ability to walk after treatment.

**PROGNOSIS.** According to data from the NCI SEER program, 70% of children with brain tumors will be long-term survivors.[85,90] At least half of these survivors will experience chronic problems, such as focal motor and sensory abnormalities, seizures, cognitive deficits, and neuroendocrine deficiencies, including hypothyroidism. Another study showed long-term sequelae in adult survivors of childhood brain tumor, such as hearing loss, blindness, and coordination and motor control problems.[85] Rehabilitation can be helpful with functional outcomes.[123]

## ACKNOWLEDGMENT

The author and editors would like to express their deepest gratitude to Dr. Stephen A. Gudas, PT, PhD, who helped develop this chapter in the previous edition of the text.

## REFERENCES

To enhance this text and add value for the reader, all references are included in the enhanced ebook on Student Consult that accompanies this textbook. The reader can view the reference source and access it online whenever possible.

# CHAPTER 31

# Degenerative Diseases of the Central Nervous System

KAREN L. MCCULLOCH (ALS, AD, HD) • ERICA DEMARCH (PD) • AUDREY C. CZEJKOWSKI (MS) • CATHERINE HAMILTON (MS) • PATRICIA A. WINKLER (DYSTONIA)

Degenerative diseases of the central nervous system (CNS) can affect gray matter, white matter, or both. The neurodegenerative disorders are characterized by loss of functionally related groups of neurons. The pattern of neuronal loss is selective, affecting one or more groups of neurons while leaving others intact. The cause of the neuronal loss is unknown but is clearly multifactorial. The diseases appear to arise without any clear inciting event in individuals without previous neurologic deficits. The clinical symptoms produced depend on which neuronal populations are lost. Degenerative changes in gray matter diseases interfere with the function of the neuronal cell bodies and synapses. The diseases can affect the cortex, the spinal cord, or both. The most common factor in this group of diseases is the slow deterioration of body functions controlled by the brain and spinal cord.

The neuropathologic findings observed in the degenerative diseases reflect changes in different components. In some disorders there are intracellular abnormalities, such as Lewy bodies and neurofibrillary tangles, whereas in others there is a primary loss of neurons. Some degenerative diseases have prominent involvement of the cerebral cortex, such as Alzheimer disease; others are more restricted to subcortical areas and may present with movement disorders such as tremors and dyskinesias, such as Parkinson disease. Demyelination has a major impact on other disorders, such as multiple sclerosis. Through genetic and molecular studies of these diseases it is becoming clearer that there are many shared features across the disorders.

Cellular stress is a major component of neurodegenerative disease. When the cell is stressed, the proteins that form filaments and microtubules creating the cytoskeleton can collapse and form perinuclear bundles or clumps of protein aggregates. If the stress experienced by the cell is not lethal, the cell adapts and manufactures several proteins that may restore functional activity of partially denatured proteins. If the proteins cannot be restored, then a process begins to destroy the proteins. If the proteins do not fully degrade, they become clumped together to form intracellular inclusions. The inclusions in neurodegenerative disorders are examples of such aggregates. The aggregated proteins are generally cytotoxic, but the mechanisms by which protein aggregation is linked to cell death may be different in these various diseases. The histologic characteristics of the inclusions often form the diagnostic hallmarks of these different diseases.

Disorders of movement associated with gray matter destruction are reflected in functional loss and decreased fractionation of movement. Dementia can be present and always represents a pathologic process; dementia, despite popular belief, is not part of normal aging. The majority of the degenerative diseases that affect the basal ganglia are associated with involuntary movements. Disruption of smooth coordination of muscles can be seen in diseases affecting the cerebellum and brainstem. Many of the disorders appear later in life and mimic deterioration of the nervous system that comes with aging.

The cost of care for people with degenerative neurologic disease is significant as a consequence of the protracted time of disability before death and the extent of the disability. Although medical science has made tremendous progress in the recent years, degenerative disorders continue to be a challenge to health care providers and a scourge to modern society.

## AMYOTROPHIC LATERAL SCLEROSIS

### Overview and Definition

Amyotrophic lateral sclerosis (ALS) is a disorder that is generally recognized as an adult-onset progressive motor neuron disease, but is also a complex disease process underlying a multisystem illness. The first detailed description was by Jean Martin Charcot in 1869, in which he discussed the clinical and pathologic characteristics of "la sclérose latérale amyotrophique," a disorder of muscle wasting (amyotrophy) and gliotic hardening (sclerosis) of the anterior and lateral corticospinal tracts involving both upper and lower motor neurons. It is the most physically devastating of the neurodegenerative diseases. Peripheral nerve changes result in muscle fiber atrophy or amyotrophy. The resulting weakness causes profound limitation of movement. Executive dysfunction, characterized by deficiencies in attention, language comprehension, planning, and abstract reasoning, also occur as a result of cortical involvement.

## Incidence and Etiologic and Risk Factors

The incidence of ALS is approximately 2 per 100,000 adults in Europe and in adults of European descent. Approximately 90%[60] of cases of ALS occur sporadically and are clinically manifest in the fifth decade or later. The cause is still unknown. Known risk factors include the presence of genetic mutations associated with familial ALS, family history, age, gender (male greater risk than female), white, non-Hispanic, and geographic area (Europe, North America, New Zealand). Possible risk factors include chronic exposure to heavy metals, such as lead or mercury, pesticides or solvents; history of vigorous physical exercise (athletes, military service); lifestyle factors (cigarette smoking, alcohol intake, diet), although clear mechanisms for possible risks are not established. ALS occurs predominantly in men, although bulbar onset occurs more often in women.

Familial ALS (FALS) is an inherited autosomal trait. It occurs in 5% to 10% of all ALS cases. The identification of at least one additional family member with ALS in successive generations is essential for the diagnosis of FALS. Most FALS is inherited in an autosomal dominant pattern and is characterized by an early onset. Family linkage may be missed if there was a death of a family member before the usual age of onset. A genetic mutation can be linked to ALS in 60% to 80% of patients with familial ALS, with C9orf72 (40%), SOD1 (20%), FUS/TLS (1-5%), and TARBDP (1-5%) being the most common genes identified.[103]

## Pathogenesis

The pathologic hallmarks of ALS are the degeneration and loss of motor neurons, with astrocytic gliosis and microglial proliferation in the presence of intraneuronal inclusions in degenerating neurons and glial cells. Upper motor neuron cell loss occurs in the motor cortex, with loss of Betz cells from Brodmann area 4, frontotemporal cortex, hippocampus, thalamus, and substantia nigra. Astrocytic gliosis with axonal loss occurs in corticospinal tracts. There is loss of lower motor neuron axons in the brainstem and spinal cord, spinocerebellar tracts, and dorsal columns.

Eighty percent of FALS cases have degeneration of the spinocerebellar tract. Dementia result from changes in the frontotemporal cortices or in the substantia nigra (basal ganglia). Some histologic changes seen in ALS are consistent with those in other lower motor neuron diseases. Destruction of large motor neurons of the anterior horn cells is greatest in the cervical and lumbar regions of the cord and between the internal capsule and the bulbar pyramids. Critical neurons are sparse, and the dendrites are shortened, fragmented, and disorganized. Microscopic examination demonstrates a reduction in the number of anterior horn neurons throughout the length of the spinal cord, with associated reactive gliosis and loss of anterior root myelinated fibers. There are similar findings in the cranial nerve nuclei in bulbar manifestations. Diffuse and patchy loss of myelin appears in all areas of the spinal cord except the posterior columns, allowing for preservation of sensation.

A number of genes associated with FALS are also implicated in sporadic ALS, including C9orf72, TBK1, and NEK. More than 30 genes have an association with the disease. SOD1 was the first gene associated with ALS and was used in the first mouse model of the disease. The TARDBP gene codes for the protein TDP-43 that is important in regulating gene expression, and contributes to RNA processing deficits. TDP-43 deposits within cells appear to be part of the ALS disease pathway.[62] The aggregation of protein into inclusion bodies in cells has been described in many other neurodegenerative disorders, including Parkinson disease, Huntington disease, and Alzheimer disease. It is still unclear whether protein aggregation is directly toxic to cells or is a defense mechanism to reduce intracellular aggregation of toxic proteins.

Immune processes are active in the pathogenesis, if not the initiation, of ALS. Immune complexes have been identified in gut and renal tissue from patients with ALS. Antibodies have been found in some cases of ALS that may indicate involvement of hormones in the immune process; however, there appears to be a poor response to immunologic treatment.

Glutamate, the principal excitatory neurotransmitter in the human motor system, can cause excitotoxic damage when extracellular glutamate concentration increases as a result of reduced glutamate upake and other factors driven by genetic tendencies (Fig. 31.1). Plasma glutamate levels in individuals with motor neuron disease can be twice that of normal. This may be related to a defect in the transport and breakdown of excitatory amino acids, predisposing the person to neurotoxicity. Astrocytic glutamate transporter, termed *GLT1* or *EAAT2*, is markedly reduced in the motor cortex and anterior horn cells of patients with ALS, resulting in significantly raised levels of glutamate in cerebrospinal fluid (CSF) in ALS. Environmental toxins may act as excitotoxins.

Oxidative damage appears to play a role in the damage to nerve cells in ALS. Calcium-mediated excitotoxicity can generate free radicals. In FALS, the mutated SOD1 appears to cause increased reactivity to hydrogen peroxide and leads to an increase in free radicals. Copper ions in a reduced state will cause this process to become harmful to the neuron. Oxidative damage and glutamate toxicity may interact or potentiate each other. They may also contribute to other mechanisms of motor neuron degeneration, including axon transport abnormalities and apoptosis.

The death of the peripheral motor neuron in the brainstem and spinal cord leads to denervation and atrophy of the corresponding muscle fibers. In the early phases of the illness, denervated muscle may be reinnervated by sprouting of preserved nearby distal motor axon terminals, although reinnervation in this disease is less extensive than in other chronic neurologic disorders.

There is remarkable selectivity of neuronal cell death, involving motor neurons of the brainstem and spinal

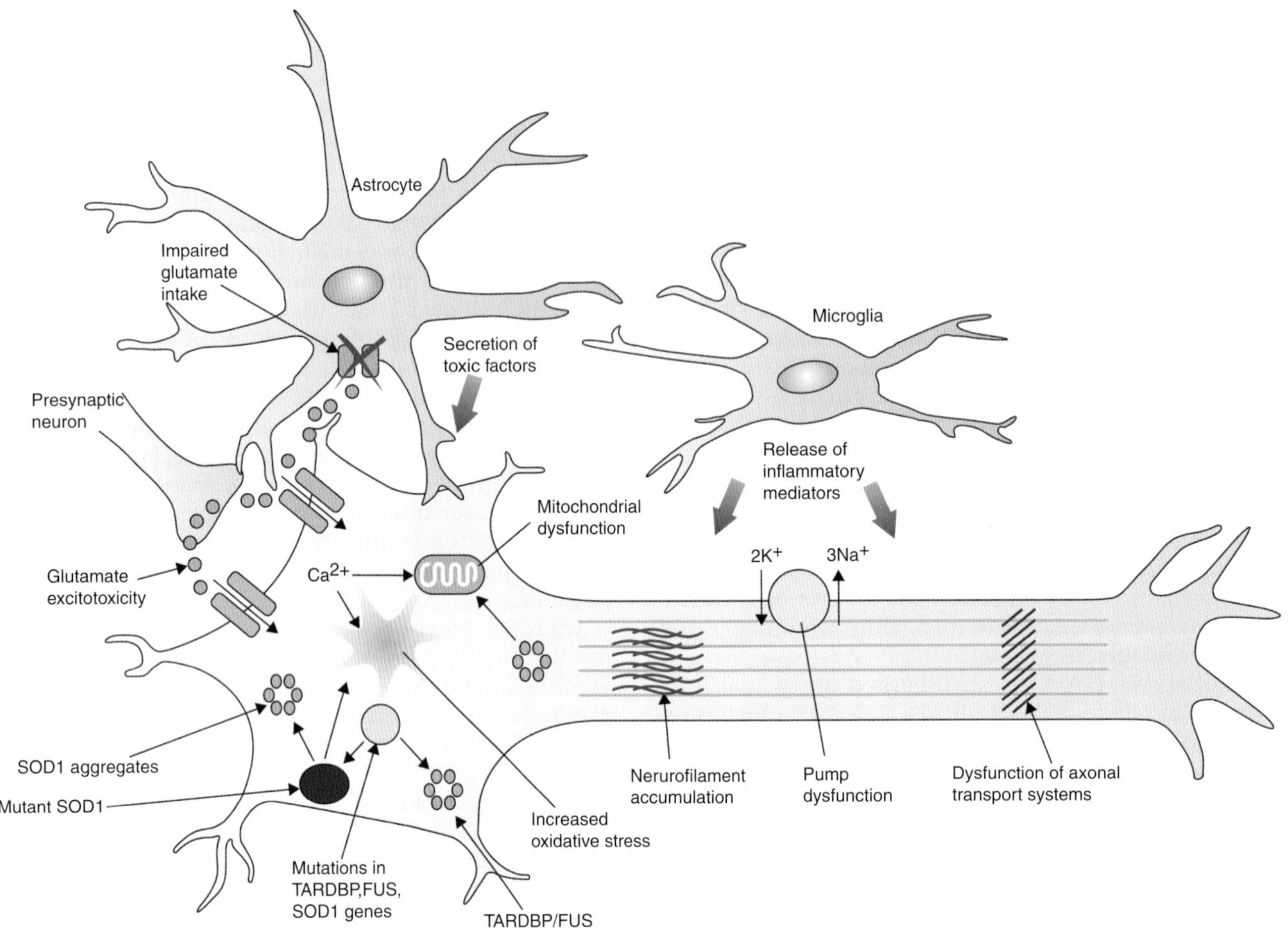


**Figure 31.1**

**Amyotrophic lateral sclerosis (ALS) appears to be mediated by a complex interaction between molecular and genetic pathways.** Reduced uptake of glutamate from the synaptic cleft, leading to glutamate excitotoxicity, is mediated by dysfunction of the astrocytic excitatory amino acid transporter 2 (EAAT2). The resulting glutamate-induced excitotoxicity induces neurodegeneration through activation of $Ca^{2+}$-dependent enzymatic pathways. Mutations in the c9orf72, TDP-43 and fused in sarcoma (FUS) genes result in dysregulated RNA metabolism leading to abnormalities of translation and formation of intracellular neuronal aggregates. Mutations in the superoxide dismutase-1 (SOD-1) gene increases oxidative stress, induces mitochondrial dysfunction, and leads to intracellular aggregates and defective axonal transportation. Separately, microglia activation results in secretion of proinflammatory cytokines and neurotoxicity. (From Kiernan MC, et al: Amyotrophic lateral sclerosis, *Lancet* 377(9769):942 –955, 2011.)

cord, with relative sparing of the oculomotor nuclei. There is eventual spread into the prefrontal, parietal, and temporal areas, as well as into the subthalamic nuclei and reticular formation. In persons kept breathing with ventilatory support, there may eventually be sensory system changes.

## Clinical Manifestations

Cognitive impairments are noted in up to 50% of individuals with ALS.[64] With careful assessment, these deficiencies can be noted early on. Executive function deficits can be found in visual attention, working memory, cognitive flexibility, problem solving, and visual-perceptual skills. Verbal fluency declines before dysarthria develops. The cognitive deficits are a result of changes in frontal lobe function and may be related to frontotemporal dementia (FTD); in fact, the suggestion that ALS and FTD may represent a spectrum of disease is supported by the development of criteria to characterize cognitive impairment in both disorders using the same items,[94] linking the two in ALS-frontotemporal spectrum disorder. Bulbar onset is more predictive of cognitive impairment than limb onset. Pseudobulbar affect, resulting in emotional lability, emotional outbursts, and pathologic laughing or crying, is not related to a psychologic or psychiatric condition and is not a part of FTD.

The motor control manifestations of ALS vary depending on whether upper or lower motor neurons are predominantly involved. With lower motor neuron cell death and early denervation, the first evidence of the disease typically is insidiously developing asymmetric weakness, usually of the distal aspect of one limb progressing to weakness of the contiguous muscles. Extensor muscles become weaker than flexor muscles, especially in the hands. Cervical extensor weakness develops and can lead to drooping of the head and pain associated with overstretched muscles. Increased lumbar lordosis occurs as part of the compensatory strategy to attempt to right the head and bring the eyes level.

The neurons innervating muscles controlling articulation, chewing, and swallowing originate in the medulla, or the "bulb," and any weaknesses in these muscles are considered bulbar signs. In the lower motor or flaccid component, facial muscles are affected. Inability to hold the eye closed against pressure is a standard test. Weakness around the mouth develops, and air leaks out. The movement of the tongue is decreased, and atrophy is present. Fasciculations in the tongue are present, with lower motor neuron dysfunction. Dysarthria associated with lower motor neuron involvement is reflected by inability to shout or sing, a hoarse or whispering quality of the voice, and nasal tone. Manipulating food inside the mouth becomes difficult. Eventually, weak swallowing may trigger reflex coughing.

Individuals with ALS complain of drooling because of the absence of automatic swallowing, which is made worse by the forward head position. Breathing becomes difficult, and accessory breathing replaces diaphragmatic breathing. Respiratory distress can occur when sleeping, especially on the back.

Deformities of the extremities are common, especially since weakness causes shortening of the extensor muscles. Clawhand develops as the weakness of lumbricals and interossei hinders metacarpal flexion and tenodesis flexes the distal joints. Figure 31.2 shows the hands of an individual with ALS.

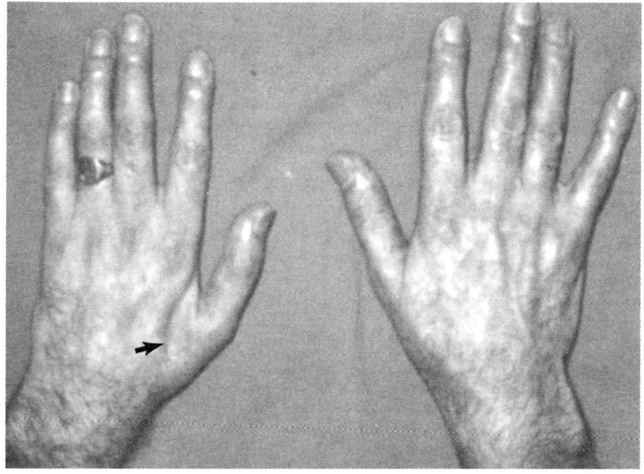

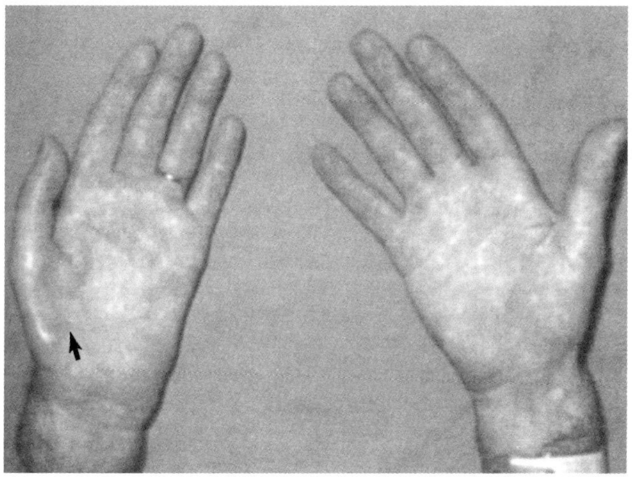

**Figure 31.2**

**Wasting of hand muscles in amyotrophic lateral sclerosis.** (From Parsons M: *Color atlas of clinical neurology*, London, 1993, Wolfe.)

Weakness caused by denervation is associated with progressive wasting and atrophy of muscles. Cramping with volitional movement in the early morning is often reported, with complaints of stiffness. Muscle cramps indicate lower motor neuron dysfunction. It may be related to hyperexcitability of distal motor axons. Early in the disease there are fasciculations, or spontaneous twitching of muscle fibers. Fasciculations are the result of spontaneous contractions of a group of muscle fibers belonging to a single motor unit. The impulse for the fasciculation appears to arise from hyperexcitable distal motor axons. This is random in time and in muscles affected. It should be noted that both muscle cramping and fasciculations are found in healthy adults and should not be taken alone as an indication of ALS.

Upper motor neuron symptoms are characterized by loss of inhibition and the resulting lack of dexterity and spasticity. Muscle strength is decreased consistent with upper motor neuron pattern. Extensor muscles of the upper extremity and flexor muscles of the lower extremity are weakened, as spasticity develops as the result of loss of brainstem control of the vestibulospinal and reticular formation control. As in other upper motor lesions, spasticity can limit the ability to accurately assess muscle strength.

Spastic bulbar palsy occurs when upper motor neurons and the corticobulbar fibers controlling speech, mastication, and swallowing are affected. This is termed *pseudobulbar palsy* and differs from the palsy associated with lower motor neuron loss in the brainstem. Pseudobulbar affect may manifest as inappropriate laughter, irritability, anger, and tearfulness.

The tendon, or muscle stretch, reflexes become hyperactive based on the loss of the Ia inhibitory reflex. This also extends to the development of clonus, in which manual quick stretch of a muscle induces repeated rhythmic muscle contractions. The Babinski response is positive, characterized by extension of the great toe, often accompanied by fanning of the other toes in response to stroking the outer edge of the ipsilateral sole upward from the heel with a blunt object. With sufficient wasting of the dorsiflexors, the Babinski response may appear to be flexor despite upper motor neuron involvement.

It is characteristic of ALS that, regardless of whether the initial disease involves upper or lower motor neurons, both categories are eventually demonstrated. In most persons with ALS, the Babinski and Hoffmann signs are present and the tendon jerks are disproportionately active. Throughout the course of the disease, eye movements and sensory, bowel, and bladder functions are typically preserved.

ALS is characterized by differing areas of CNS involvement and has been categorized in terms of four major groups of symptoms listed below. Figure 31.3 shows the levels of dysfunction associated with the terms that describe them.

1. *Pseudobulbar palsy* reflects damage in the corticobulbar tract.
2. *Progressive bulbar palsy* is a result of cranial nerve nuclei involvement. There is weakness of the muscles involved in swallowing, chewing, and facial gestures. Fasciculations of the tongue are typical. With early bulbar

involvement, there can be difficulty with respiration before weakness of the limbs. Dysarthria and exaggeration of the expression of emotion, or pseudobulbar affect, indicate involvement of the corticobulbar tract. The oculomotor system is usually not involved, and eye movement remains normal.

3. *Primary lateral sclerosis* results in neuronal loss in the cortex. Signs of corticospinal tract involvement include hyperactivity of tendon reflexes with spasticity, causing difficulty with active movement. Weakness and spasticity of specific muscles represent the level and progression of the disease along the corticospinal tracts. There is no muscle atrophy, and fasciculations are not present. This form of ALS is rare.
4. In *progressive spinal muscular atrophy* there is progressive loss of motor neurons in the anterior horns of the spinal cord, often beginning in the cervical area. There is progressive weakness, wasting, and fasciculations involving the small muscles of the hands. Other levels of the spinal cord can be the site of the initial disease process, with symptoms reflecting the level involved. These areas of weakness can be present without evidence of higher-level corticospinal involvement, such as spasticity.

ALS with probable upper motor neuron signs is a condition in which there are no overt upper motor neuron signs, but involvement of the corticospinal tracts is indicated by the incongruous presence of active tendon reflexes in limbs with weak, wasted, and twitching muscles. Upper and lower limbs are usually affected first, with progression to facial symptoms and respiratory failure.

## MEDICAL MANAGEMENT

**DIAGNOSIS.** Diagnosis is predominantly made by the combination of clinical presentation and electromyogram (EMG). The time to diagnosis differs, typically according to the first presenting symptoms. With upper limb onset the time to diagnosis is approximately 15 months, with lower extremity onset it is 21 months, and with bulbar involvement as the first sign it is approximately 17 months. Box 31.1 describes diagnostic findings that suggest abnormalities that could indicate ALS.

In 1990 the World Federation of Neurology El Escorial criteria for the diagnosis of ALS were established,

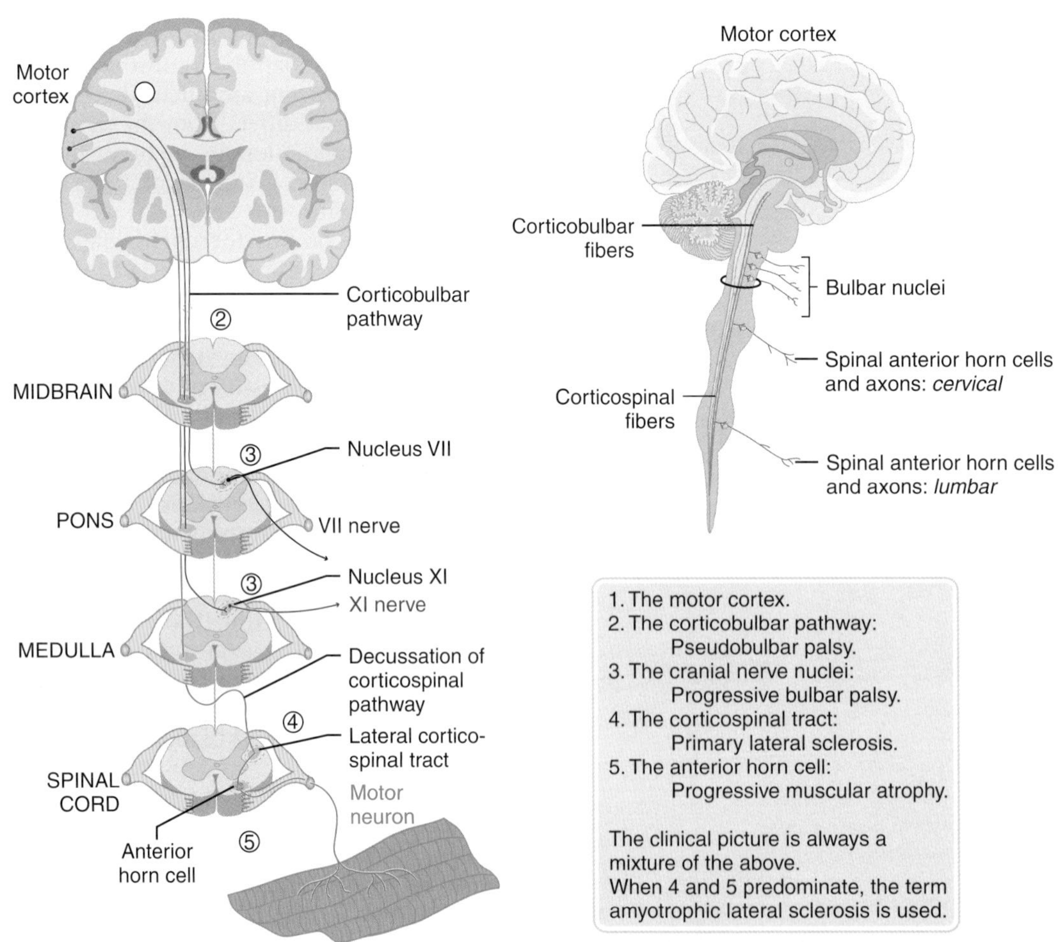


**Figure 31.3**

**Areas of damage in the central and peripheral nervous system as a result of amyotrophic lateral sclerosis.** (From Lindsay KW, Bone I, Callander R: *Neurology and neurosurgery illustrated,* New York, 1986, Churchill Livingstone. Insert from Noble J: *Textbook of primary care medicine,* ed 3, Copyright 2001, Mosby, Inc., and borrowed from Pryse-Phillips WM, Murray TJ: *Essentials of neurology: a concise textbook,* New York, 1992, Medical Examination Publisher, p 660.)

and four categories of ALS were outlined (Box 31.2). In general the diagnosis is made based on the exclusion of other possible causes of symptoms or conditions that could mimic ALS. The diagnosis requires at least one of these conditions: (1) progressive upper and lower motor neurologic deficits in at least one limb or region OR (2) lower motor neuron deficits observed by clinical examination (one region) and/or by EMG in two body regions (bulbar, cervical, thoracic, lumbosacral). The diagnostic criteria include clinically definite ALS, clinically probable ALS, and clinically possible ALS.

Suspected ALS is characterized by lower motor neuron signs alone in two or more regions, to which might be added upper motor neuron signs on the basis of the clinical examination. Possible ALS is defined as upper and/or lower motor neuron signs in only one region, possibly with a grouping of upper or lower motor neuron signs in other regions. Exclusion of structural lesions and other possible causes would be a focus. Probable ALS is considered if there are upper and lower motor neuron signs in two regions, and the upper motor neuron signs are above the lower motor neuron signs. Structural lesions must be definitely ruled out by imaging studies. Definite ALS requires lower motor neuron signs to be present in addition to upper motor neuron signs in three CNS regions concomitantly with upper or lower motor neuron signs in other regions, with structural lesions excluded. Definite EMG signs of lower motor neuron degeneration require the presence of evidence of acute denervation with fibrillations or positive sharp waves and chronic denervation represented by large-amplitude and long-duration motor unit potentials, as well as reduced recruitment in each muscle.

Symptoms are generally first reported to a primary care physician, which may result in a greater delay in reaching the diagnosis. The use of EMG is advocated to facilitate an earlier diagnosis of the disease, so involvement of a neurologist in assessing early symptoms increases the likelihood of EMG testing and the use of other diagnostic procedures. Often in the early cases and those that are progressing slowly, there may be minimal abnormality on the first EMG, and the changes that lead to diagnosis may not appear for 6 to 12 months. Rapidly progressive ALS shows different changes on the EMG compared with slowly progressive ALS. It is thought that some of these differences come from the adaptation and sprouting that occur early in the process. This adaptation cannot be sustained as the disease progresses.

EMG studies include the muscles of the extremities and trunk, and are selected based on the propensity for weakness in ALS. EMG criteria for the definitive diagnosis of ALS include the presence of LMN and UMN signs reflected by fibrillation potentials, positive sharp waves, fasciculations, and motor unit potential changes in multiple nerve root distributions in at least three regions (bulbar or cervical, thoracic, or lumbosacral spinal regions). These changes occur without change in sensory responses.

There are several disorders that resemble ALS that are treatable. ALS must be differentiated from other conditions that produce a combination of upper and lower motor neuron lesions. Lymphoma and Lyme disease can cause diffuse lower motor axonal neuropathy. Disorders of the cervical cord, such as skull base deformities, syringomyelia, cord tumors, and cervical spondylosis, must be ruled out. Box 31.3 describes disorders that can mimic ALS and are important considerations in differential diagnosis.

In such cases, however, there should not be any evidence of anterior horn cell involvement in the legs or trunk, but only in the upper limbs. Cervical myelopathy can look like ALS if cord compression is combined with root involvement. The lower motor neuron findings are only in the arms, an important diagnostic feature, and this situation

Box 31.1

**ABNORMAL DIAGNOSTIC FINDINGS IN AMYOTROPHIC LATERAL SCLEROSIS**

- Clinical features of weakness, atrophy, and fatigue
- EMG: shows fibrillations and fasciculations
- Unstable motor units (in rapidly progressing ALS)
- Increased duration/amplitudes (in slowly progressing ALS)
- Low-amplitude polyphasic motor unit potentials
- Muscle biopsy: shows denervation atrophy
- Muscle enzymes, such as creatine phosphokinase, elevated
- CSF normal
- No changes on myelogram

Box 31.2

**WORLD FEDERATION OF NEUROLOGY EL ESCORIAL CRITERIA FOR DIAGNOSIS OF AMYOTROPHIC LATERAL SCLEROSIS (ALS)**

| WEAKNESS/ATROPHY/HYPERREFLEXIA/PLASTICITY EMG/NCV/NEUROIMAGING | | | |
|---|---|---|---|
| **Suspected ALS** | **Possible ALS** | **Probable ALS** | **Definite ALS** |
| LMN signs in more than two regions | UMN + LMN signs in one region | UMN + LMN signs in two regions | UMN + LMN signs in three regions |
| UMN signs in more than one region | UMN + LMN signs in more than two regions<br>Add LMN signs to UMN regions<br>Add UMN signs to LMN regions<br>Exclude structural lesions (Exclude other causes) | UMN + LMN signs in more than two regions<br>Add LMN signs to UMN regions<br>Add LMN signs to UMN regions<br>Exclude structural lesions (Exclude other causes) | UMN + LMN signs in more than three regions(Discern from ALS plus, ALS LAUS, ALS mimics)<br>Exclude structural lesions<br>(Exclude other causes) |

*( )*, Proposal to add this category to diagnostic criteria for ALS, WFN El Escorial Revisited; *EMG*, electromyography; *LAUS*, laboratory abnormalities of uncertain significance; *LMN*, lower motor neuron; *NCV*, nerve conduction velocity; *UMN*, upper motor neuron.

Data from Brooks BR: Introduction: defining optimal management in ALS: from first symptoms to announcement, *Neurology* 53(Suppl 5):S1–S3, 1999.

Box 31.3

**DISORDERS THAT CAN MIMIC AMYOTROPHIC LATERAL SCLEROSIS**

- Myasthenia gravis
- Cervical myelopathy
- Multifocal motor neuropathy
- Hypoparathyroidism
- Inclusion body myositis
- Bulbospinal neuronopathy
- Lymphoma
- Radiation-induced effects

can be confirmed by imaging of the cervical cord and use of EMG to determine if there are fasciculations in the legs. Any signs of disease caused by a lesion above the foramen magnum, such as bulbar signs or cranial nerve V or VII involvement, would rule out a cervical cause. Lower motor neuron lesions may be predominant with spinal arachnoiditis (usually syphilitic) and radiculitis, cervical ribs, and peripheral nerve lesions, including postpolio syndrome. Weakness and wasting are typical of all forms of hereditary motor neuropathy, some of which occur first in adult life, and in hereditary motor and sensory neuropathy. The same findings, although without fasciculations, are also seen in primary muscle disease, rheumatoid arthritis, and myotonic dystrophy. If there is doubt about evidence of anterior horn cell disease in the trunk or legs, EMG should be able to demonstrate that which cannot be seen clinically.

Weight loss may suggest carcinoma, and investigations should be undertaken to rule out underlying malignancy if there is any atypical feature on examination or investigation, such as marked slowing of motor nerve conduction velocities. Most other mimics can be excluded by inquiring about history of hereditary neuropathy, prior gastrectomy, polio, or electrical injury. Dyspnea may suggest chronic obstructive pulmonary disease or heart failure. Thorough examination will reveal hyperthyroidism or acromegaly. Laboratory tests will reveal lead or other metal poisoning. ALS symptoms may mimic nonneurologic diseases, and neurologic signs may be missed. Involvement of the sensory system or conduction block with evoked potential testing may indicate other neurodegenerative disease processes.

The El Escorial criteria for ALS diagnosis were reconsidered in 2015[58] with recommendations made to replace the categories of probable and definite ALS by a validated staging system for the disease that characterizes the impairments and functional limitations, similar to those used for clinical trial enrollment. Two such staging systems have been proposed, demonstrating complementary abilities to characterize early to mid-disease progression (King's staging system) and later disease progression (Milano-Torino or MiToS functional staging).[26] King's stages include 1: involvement of 1 clinical region, 2: involvement of a second clinical region, 3: involvement of a third clinical region, 4: nutritional or respiratory failure, 5: death. The MiToS system focuses on functional ability loss with stage 0: functional involvement, 1: loss of independence in 1 domain, 2: loss of independence in 2 domains, 3: loss of independence in 3 domains, 4: loss of independence in 4 domains, 5: death.

**TREATMENT.** Riluzole was the first Food and Drug Administration (FDA)–approved drug for ALS. Riluzole has a broad range of pharmacologic effects, including inhibition of glutamate release, postsynaptic glutamate receptor activation, and voltage-sensitive sodium channel inactivation. Riluzole appears to be neuroprotective and slows the disease course by approximately 10% to 15%, but it is not curative. There is controversy over the best time to begin therapy with riluzole. Neuroprotective effects would be more extensive when there are more motor units intact to preserve, and this argument supports early treatment. Asthenia and gastrointestinal side effects are common, and the long-term neurotoxic effects are unknown.

In 2018 the FDA approved Radicava (edaravone) for use with ALS. Edaravone is an infusion medication (28 day cycle, with infusions for 14-10 days at the start of each cycle) that targets oxidative stress thought to accentuate degenerative changes in ALS.[98] Specific subsets of patients, those with definite or probable ALS and disease duration of less than 2 years and without respiratory dysfunction, received 6 cycles of the medication, resulting in 33% less decline in ALSFRS-R for the treated group versus the placebo group. Additional clinical trials are underway to understand its optimal use. An oral form of the medication is also in development.

Although neuroinflammation occurs in the brainstem and spinal cord of individuals with ALS, suggesting that antiinflammatory agents may be effective in treating this disease, use of medications directed toward inflammation has not proved to change the course of ALS.

The high metabolic load of motor neurons and the consequent dependence of these cells on oxidative phosphorylation may make them particularly vulnerable to the loss of mitochondrial function. Coenzyme Q10 is an antioxidant and an essential mitochondrial cofactor facilitating electron transfer in the respiratory chain. Studies have not proven significant changes when given after diagnosis is made. Use of vitamin E as an antioxidant early in the course has been advocated, but studies show limited effect. The impetus for studying and treating individuals with antioxidant therapy is its role in protecting against motor neuron injury.

Oxidative stress appears to put people at risk for ALS comparable to that found in those with Alzheimer disease. People at risk for ALS might be identified by use of bioassays showing increased oxidative damage comparable to that in individuals with diagnosed disease. These assays could lead to early intervention and primary prevention. A ketogenic diet similar to the one employed to control epilepsy may be of some effect, as ketones have the ability to alter mitochondrial function and have a positive effect in ALS based on animal studies. Although no medication can stop the disease, much can be done in the form of symptomatic therapy. Health care providers should emphasize the value of maintaining the highest level of function throughout the course of the disease, providing education and support to prepare for the rapid decline in function. Symptomatic measures

**Table 31.1** Symptomatic Treatment in Amyotrophic Lateral Sclerosis

| Symptoms | Pharmacotherapy | Other Therapy |
|---|---|---|
| Fatigue | Pyridostigmine bromide<br>Antidepressants<br>Methylphenidate<br>Amantadine<br>Modafinil | Energy conservation, work modification<br>Sleep study: BiPAP if abnormal |
| Spasticity | Baclofen<br>Tizanidine<br>Dantrolene sodium<br>Diazepam | Movement to inhibit tone, Botox injections |
| Jaw clenching | Benzodiazepines | Botulinum toxin injections into masseters |
| Cramps | Quinine sulfate<br>Baclofen<br>Vitamin E<br>Clonazepam | Massage<br>Physical therapy |
| Fasciculations | Carbamazepine | Assurance |
| Sialorrhea | Hyoscyamine sulphate<br>Diphenhydramine<br>Scopolamine patch<br>Glycopyrrolate<br>Atropine<br>TCAs | Suction machine<br>Botox injection into salivary glands<br>Parotid gland radiation therapy<br>Steam inhalation<br>Nebulization<br>Dark grape juice |
| Pseudobulbar laughing or crying | TCAs<br>SSRIs<br>Levodopa/carbidopa<br>Lithium<br>Mirtazapine<br>Venlafaxine<br>Quinidine/dextromethorphan | |
| Thick phlegm | Guaifenesin<br>Nebulized *N*-acetylcysteine<br>Nebulized saline<br>Propranolol | Insufflation–exsufflation<br>High-flow chest wall oscillation therapy<br>Cool mist humidifier<br>Rehydration<br>Pineapple or papaya juice<br>Reduced intake of dairy products, caffeine, alcohol |
| Aspiration | Cisapride | Modified food consistency, tracheostomy, modified laryngectomy, and tracheal diversion |
| Joint pains | Antiinflammatory drugs<br>Analgesics | Range-of-motion exercise, warmth-generating modalities |
| Depression | TCAs<br>SSRIs, venlafaxine, mirtazapine, bupropion | Counseling<br>Support group meetings, psychiatry |
| Insomnia | Zolpidem tartrate<br>Lorazepam<br>Opioids<br>TCAs | Pressure air pad/gel mattress<br>Noninvasive positive pressure ventilation where appropriate |
| Laryngospasm | Sublingual lorazepam | |
| Respiratory failure | Bronchodilators<br>Morphine sulfate | Hospital bed<br>Nocturnal noninvasive ventilator IPPB |
| Constipation | Increase oral liquid<br>Metamucil<br>Dulcolax suppositories<br>Lactulose and other laxative | Exercise<br>"Power pudding": prune juice, prunes, applesauce, bran |

*BiPAP*, Bilevel positive airway pressure; *IPPB*, intermittent positive-pressure breathing; *SSRI*, selective serotonin reuptake inhibitor; *TCA*, tricyclic antidepressant.
From Daroff RB, Fenichel GM, Jankovic J, Mazziotta JC: *Bradley's neurology in clinical practice*, ed 6, Philadelphia, 2012, WB Saunders, Table 74.4.

may include the use of anticholinergic drugs to control drooling and baclofen or diazepam to control spasticity. Dextromethorphan-quinidine, commonly used for coughs, shows benefit in the treatment of pseudobulbar emotional lability. Table 31.1 lists medications used for symptomatic control.

Maintenance of nutrition is a significant problem because of the difficulty chewing and swallowing. Weakness of jaw movement, loss of tongue mobility, and difficulty in lip closure, in addition to impairment of the swallowing reflex, are common. This may lead to respiratory complications from aspiration. By modifying the consistency and texture of food and fluids, the risk of aspiration is reduced. Percutaneous endoscopic gastrostomy is used to provide nutrition when eating is no longer possible. The inability to speak is also an eventual deficit, but through work with a speech-language pathologist it is possible to "voice bank" one's typical voice for use in an augmentative communication system. The use of eye movement to interact with a computer system is a viable alternative for most patients, but requires practice and guidance to achieve a functional system.

On the horizon are therapies that attempt to modify the disease through the use of stem cell therapies, with mesenchymal stem cells that have the ability to secrete neurotrophic factors showing promise in animal models when administered through thecal or intraspinal injection.[76] Case studies in humans suggest this intervention is tolerable and may have benefits.[27] Fetal neural tissue stem cell lines have been injected directly into anterior horn cells with positive results.[30,66] Intrathecal injection of antisense oligonucleotides that inhibit SOD1 expression or prevent protein aggregation is also being tested in clinical trials.[29,43,69]

Noninvasive ventilation should be considered to treat respiratory insufficiency in order to lengthen survival and to slow the decline of forced vital capacity. Noninvasive ventilation may be considered to improve quality of life. Early initiation of noninvasive ventilation may increase compliance and insufflation–exsufflation may be considered to help clear secretions.

Multidisciplinary ALS clinics provide coordinated care. Survival has been found to be longer for individuals with bulbar symptoms; the use of aids and appliances was greater and the mental quality of life was better for the individuals with ALS who were treated at multidisciplinary clinics than for individuals who did not receive specialty clinic care. With focused care, up to 80% of individuals with ALS can die at home.

**PROGNOSIS.** The course of ALS is relentlessly progressive. It appears that earlier onset (younger than 50 years of age) has a longer course, as exemplified by some well-known individuals with ALS (e.g., Stephen Hawking). Death from the adult-onset sporadic type usually occurs within 2 to 5 years, resulting mainly from pneumonia caused by respiratory compromise, although individuals who choose to go on ventilator support may survive for longer. In general, those with bulbar palsy have a more rapid course than those with primary lateral sclerosis, in whom the prognosis is markedly better. Respiratory failure and inability to eat are part of the final stages of ALS. Tube feeding and use of a respirator may be options to prolong life. Individual and family wishes concerning these procedures should be discussed as early as possible in the course of the disease, because some clients may experience a rapid decline in function at any time.

## DEMENTIAS INCLUDING ALZHEIMER DISEASE

Dementia is a cognitive impairment that affects the ability to think, remember, and reason. The most common

SPECIAL IMPLICATIONS FOR THE THERAPIST 31.1

### *Amyotrophic Lateral Sclerosis*

The ALS-Specific Quality of Life Instrument (ALSSQOL) is based on the McGill Quality of Life Questionnaire (MQOL), modified by changes in format and by adding questions on religiousness and spirituality. A 59-item tool with a completion time averaging 15 minutes, it is a practical tool for the assessment of overall quality of life in individuals with ALS and appears to be valid and useful across large samples. Validation studies of a shortened version are now under way.

The ALS Functional Rating Scale (ALSFRS-R), which can be found at and downloaded from https://www.alspathways.com/hcp/monitoring-als/#the-alsfrs-r-scale, is a functional scale that can be used to follow the progression of ALS. Six months are needed to detect changes in the ALSFRS-R score because of variability, due principally to differing rates of progression among patients.

The relationship between verbal associative fluency, verbal abstract reasoning, and judgment in ALS can be evaluated using a 20-minute screening evaluation. Deficiencies in these measures were found in 20% to 35% of patients with limb-onset ALS and in 37% to 60% of patients with bulbar-onset ALS. This simple screen identifies deficits that affect discussions of treatment interventions and end-of-life issues.

Muscle strength declines in an overall linear progression throughout the course of the disease. Staging of ALS helps the therapist to prioritize interventions based on the current functional status and on the predicted progression of the disease. Table 31.2 describes interventions associated with progression of the disease. Moderate exercise programs can be safely adapted to abilities, interests, specific response to exercise, accessibility, and family support.

The rate of loss is stable within a broad range after the first year, but during the first year there is fluctuation of strength that may be a result of the potential for adaptation within the CNS. At this point, the goal of therapy is to maintain general physical activity and muscular tone. Regular exercise in moderation can help alleviate fatigue and have a beneficial effect on the client's general well-being. Complaints of diffuse pain will start in the early stages, related to joint stiffness and decreases in muscle control in the limbs or trunk. Spasticity contributes to complaints of weakness. Consistent slow stretching that decreases tone may be of benefit. Cramps, which can be a source of pain, also respond to a daily stretching routine.

Changes in gait are significant, and gait analysis is necessary to assess the need for assistive devices. Falls caused by weakness are a major problem. Ankle dorsiflexion is lost before strength in plantar flexion. Hamstring strength appears to correlate with walking, and the decrease parallels the loss of walking ability. Isometric muscle strength as a percentage of normal shows a dramatic decrease late in the course of the disease when fewer muscle fibers are available. This is when the greatest functional losses

**Table 31.2** Exercise and Rehabilitation Programs for Clients with Amyotrophic Lateral Sclerosis

| Stage | Treatment |
|---|---|
| **Phase I (Independent)** | |
| ***Stage I:*** | |
| Patient characteristics<br>• Mild weakness<br>• Clumsiness<br>• Ambulatory<br>• Independent in ADL | • Continue normal activities or increase activities if sedentary to prevent disuse atrophy<br>• Begin program of ROM exercises (stretching, yoga, tai chi)<br>• Add strengthening program of gentle resistance exercises to all musculature with caution not to cause overwork fatigue<br>• Provide psychologic support as needed |
| ***Stage II:*** | |
| Patient characteristics<br>• Moderate, selective weakness<br>• Slightly decreased independence in ADL<br>• Difficulty climbing stairs<br>• Difficulty raising arms<br>• Difficulty buttoning clothing<br>• Ambulatory | • Continue stretching to avoid contractures<br>• Continue cautious strengthening of muscles with MMT grades above F+ (3+); monitor for overwork fatigue<br>• Consider orthotic support (i.e., AFOs, wrist, thumb splints)<br>• Use adaptive equipment to facilitate ADL |
| ***Stage III:*** | |
| Patient characteristics | • Continue stage II program as tolerated; caution not to fatigue to point of decreasing patient's ADL independence<br>• Keep patient physically independent as long as possible through pleasurable activities, walking<br>• Encourage deep-breathing exercises, chest stretching, postural drainage if needed<br>• • Prescribe standard or motorized wheelchair with modifications to allow eventual reclining back with head rest, elevating legs |
| **Phase II (Practically Independent)** | |
| ***Stage IV:*** | |
| Patient characteristics | • Active assisted passive ROM exercises to the weakly supported joint—caution to support, rotate shoulder during abduction and joint accessory motions<br>• Encourage isometric contractions of all musculature to tolerance<br>• Try arm slings, overhead slings, or wheelchair arm supports<br>• Motorize chair if patient wants to be independently mobile; adapt controls as needed |
| ***Stage V:*** | |
| Patient characteristics<br>• Severe lower-extremity weakness<br>• Moderate to severe upper-extremity weakness<br>• Wheelchair-dependent<br>• Increasingly dependent in ADL<br>• Possible skin breakdown secondary to poor mobility | • Encourage family to learn proper transfer, positioning principles, turning techniques<br>• Encourage modifications at home to aid patient's mobility and independence<br>• Electric hospital bed with antipressure mattress<br>• If patient elects HMV, adapt chair to hold respiratory unit |
| **Phase III (Dependent)** | |
| ***Stage VI:*** | |
| Patient characteristics<br>• Bedridden<br>• Completely dependent in ADL | • For dysphagia: soft diet, long spoons, tube feeding, percutaneous gastrostomy<br>• To decrease flow of accumulated saliva: medication, suction, surgery<br>• For dysarthria: palatal lifts, electronic speech amplification, eye pointing<br>• For breathing difficulty: clear airway, tracheostomy, respiratory if HMV elected<br>• Medications to decrease impact of dyspnea |

*ADL*, Activities of daily living; *AFOs*, ankle-foot orthoses; *HMV*, home mechanical ventilation; *MMT*, manual muscle test; *ROM*, range of motion.
Modified from Sinaki M: Exercise and rehabilitation measures in amyotrophic lateral sclerosis. In Yase Y, Tsubaki T: *Amyotrophic lateral sclerosis: recent advances in research and treatment:* Amsterdam, 1988, Elsevier.

are noted. A surprisingly small amount of muscle activity is necessary across the joints to allow normal function of a joint. Some movement and joint stability are maintained until the degeneration causes atrophy of muscle activity to less than 20% of normal. The weakness and wasting often produce painful subluxation of the scapulohumeral joint, and the arm should be supported. Contractures should be routinely stretched, taking care to support the joints, because there is minimal control of muscle activity in the late stages. Complaints of pain may begin when the client is unable to shift weight in bed or in sitting, necessitating a pressure-relieving wheelchair cushion and mattress. Caregivers need to be educated in this aspect of care.

Braces, other assistive devices, and motorized scooters or wheelchairs help to maintain mobility and freedom, although consideration of the timeline to obtain equipment is critical so that the motor function of the patient remains consistent with the ability to use the device. Borrowing equipment from loaner closets may be a reasonable alternative if such resources are available. Many upper extremity devices are available to maintain joint alignment at rest, make daily activities easier to perform, and support mobility when it is lost. Braces for the lower extremity can extend the time of upright walking, but they must be lightweight, given the weakness that is typically present. Braces for the back and neck may assist with head and trunk control. Pain is often a complaint brought to the therapist. Thermal modalities and transcutaneous electrical nerve stimulation can help the pain associated with muscle shortening, joint stiffness, and muscle cramping.

Evaluation of the home environment, providing rails, mechanical lifts, or supports; eliminating stairs where possible; and advising on helpful devices for feeding, shaving, and dressing is essential as the individual becomes limited to household mobility. Posture for activities of daily living may be improved with a collar, a brace, or spring-loaded splints. Special beds can be leased or borrowed. The legs should be elevated and elastic stockings used if leg swelling is a problem.

Frustration and boredom are common. Family and volunteers can be mobilized from neighborhood groups, such as church or social groups, to visit to talk, listen, play cards, turn pages or read, or just to be there for a while.

Sexual frustration is common and is not often discussed. The clinician should do so freely and without embarrassment with both the patient and spouse; the problems are mainly matters of method. The partner may need counseling to understand that he or she needs to take the active role and to learn effective techniques that overcome weakness and muscle spasms.

Respiratory changes cause the most disability and eventually lead to death. Respiratory distress is a mechanical problem because of lack of muscle support. From the earliest stages of care of the client with ALS, prevention of respiratory complications should be emphasized.

Early evidence of respiratory involvement may be shortness of breath, poor cough reflex, and headache. Some clients can be taught to use their abdominal muscles to increase inspiration and expiration when the muscles of the diaphragm and intercostal muscles become weak. Swallowing becomes difficult and should be evaluated by a speech pathologist. Pseudobulbar affect causing uncontrolled laughing or crying decreases the capacity to regulate breathing and increases risk of shortness of breath. Aspiration is common, and techniques to control this can be taught. Mechanical ventilation is an option to prolong the ability to breathe. Individuals with a relatively slow disease progression, and those with spinal onset, might benefit more from treatment with noninvasive ventilation than patients with rapid disease progression or bulbar onset. Noninvasive positive pressure ventilation improves the patient's quality of life, despite progression of ALS, and without increasing the caregiver burden or stress. In addition, suction, intermittent positive pressure breathing, and postural drainage appear to be useful in maintaining bronchial hygiene. Only 5% of individuals choose long-term, invasive ventilation because of the restriction of activity, caregiver involvement, and overall cost. Communication becomes limited, again because of loss of oral muscle control and breath support. Communication strategies can be taught, and augmentative equipment is available. In all cases, the individual becomes dependent over time. In the terminal stages, the comfort of the patient is the therapeutic goal.

As patients with ALS weaken, the decisions facing the patient progress from issues of morbidity to mortality. Traditionally, the neurologist and other therapeutic support staff have deferred to the wishes of the patient and family members in determining level of support in response to progressive physical decline. Impairments in judgment have potentially significant clinical implications that should be considered by health care providers and caregivers when discussing treatment interventions and end-of-life issues with patients.

All patients with ALS and their families have to come to grips with the many end-of-life decisions that confront them. These include the need to get the many events in life in order, come to terms with relationships, and decide how forthcoming disabilities will be handled. Decisions regarding care at home versus in a nursing facility should be made as early as possible. Information about advance directives, living wills, and power of attorney should be available. Patients may raise the question of suicide or assisted suicide, and the caregivers should be comfortable not only talking about these issues but also calling on others who may have more expertise and experience in discussing these issues. It makes things more difficult for the patient and family if the caregivers avoid these sensitive areas and talk only about the disease and medical management. Psychologic and emotional support for the individual and the family is critical. A direct and informative approach is appreciated; giving false hope should be avoided.

Box 31.4

**POSSIBLE CAUSES OF ACUTE CONFUSION (DELIRIUM)**

D—Drugs, dehydration, detox, deficiencies, discomfort (pain)
E—Electrolytes, elimination abnormalities, environment
L—Lungs (hypoxia), liver, lack of sleep, long ED stay
I—Infection, iatrogenic events, infarction (cardiac, cerebral)
R—Restraints, restricted movement/mobility, renal failure
I—Injury, impaired sensory input, intoxication
U—UTI, unfamiliar environment
M—Metabolic abnormalities (glucose, thyroid), metastasis (brain), medications

form of dementia, Alzheimer disease, is a progressive condition. It is also possible to have dementia as a result of multiple brain infarcts that occur from stroke, but the pattern of onset may be more sudden or step-wise as infarcts occur. The cognitive changes associated with dementia can also occur acutely driven by factors that may be easily treatable, in which case the term *delirium* is more appropriate. Common causes of delirium are summarized in Box 31.4 with a mnemonic.

## Overview and Definition

In 1907, Alois Alzheimer described the case of a 51-year-old woman who presented with a relatively rapidly deteriorating memory along with psychiatric disturbances, resulting in death 4 years later. Alzheimer disease (AD), as it is now labeled, is described by the hallmark pathology of neurofibrillary tangle and continues with progressive neurologic deterioration.

*Dementia* is a general term for a decline in intellectual functioning severe enough to interfere with a person's relationships and ability to carry out daily activities. A significant decline in memory is a hallmark of dementia, but is not the only characteristic. Age-associated memory impairment, or benign senescent forgetfulness, is a decline in short-term memory that does not progress to other mental or intellectual impairments. Other causes of dementia must be carefully ruled out, and there are syndromes that mimic AD in relationship to the dementia but have different neurologic causes.

AD is the most common cause of dementia overall, making up 60% to 80% of cases. It is one of the principal causes of disability and decreased quality of life among older adults. Progress in clinical knowledge of AD has led to more reliable diagnostic criteria and accuracy; the earliest manifestations and even the presymptomatic phases of the disease may soon be identifiable. Table 31.3 lists definitions related to dementia.

## Incidence and Etiologic and Risk Factors

There are approximately 24 million people with AD worldwide, 5 million in the United States. The prevalence of AD rises with each decade of age. The known prevalence is 6% in people older than 65 years of age, 20% in people older than 80 years of age, and more than 95% in those older than 95 years of age.

**Table 31.3 Key Definitions Related to Dementia**

| Term | Definition |
|---|---|
| Delirium | A condition of severe confusion and rapid changes in brain function, not a disease but a cluster of symptoms that result from a disease or other clinical process. It is often the result of a treatable and therefore transient physical or mental illness. |
| Cognitively impaired, no dementia (CIND) | A clinical syndrome with deficits in memory or other cognitive abilities that have minimal impact on day-to-day functioning and does not meet criteria for dementia |
| Mild cognitive impairment (MCI) | A clinical subsyndrome of CIND. Amnestic or nonamnestic |
| Dementia | A clinical syndrome consisting of global cognitive decline, memory deficits plus 1 other area of cognition, and significant effect on day-to-day functioning. Not delirium |
| Alzheimer dementia | A dementia syndrome that has gradual onset and slow progression and is best explained as caused by Alzheimer disease |
| Alzheimer disease | A brain disease characterized by plaques, tangles, and neuronal loss |

From Nowrangi MA, Rao V, Lyketsos CG: Epidemiology, assessment, and treatment of dementia. *Psychiatr Clin North Am* 34(2):275–294, 2011, Table 1.

Data from Alzheimer's Disease International forecast that the prevalence of AD worldwide will almost double every 20 years, to 75 million by 2030 and 131.5 million by 2050, with higher increases in low and middle income countries as compared to higher income countries. Because life expectancy continues to rise, so does the potential for more individuals to be afflicted. It is thought that many individuals with the symptoms go undiagnosed and untreated. The cause of AD remains unknown, but there appears to be a relationship among genetic predisposition; the abnormal processing of a normal cellular substance, amyloid; and advanced age. Lifetime risk of developing AD is estimated to be between 12% and 17%. Known risk factors for development of AD include prior head injury in males, older age, diabetes mellitus, smoking, and lower levels of social activity. Protective factors include the use of statins, light to moderate alcohol consumption, Mediterranean diet, higher educational level, APOE ε2 gene, and engagement in stimulating physical and cognitive activities.[41]

The apolipoprotein E (*APOE*) gene, on chromosome 19, is the major genetic source of the common forms of late-onset AD. The APOE ε4 allele is associated with increased risk. Individuals inherit a copy of one type of allele from each parent, but AD is not inevitable, even in people with two copies of the APOE ε4 allele. People without APOE ε4 have an estimated risk of between 9% and 20% for developing AD by age 85 years. In people with one copy of the gene, the risk is between 25% and 60%. In people with two copies, the risk ranges from

50% to 90%. But only 2% of the population carries two copies of the APOE ε4 allele. No evidence exists that these mutations play a role in the more common, sporadic, nonfamilial form of late-onset AD. However, there is a subtype of early onset AD seen in families with histories of late-onset disease. The exact genetic abnormality and transmission are still unclear. APOE ε4 accounts for only part of the genetic risk for Alzheimer disease. A family history of dementia, regardless of APOE ε4 status, can also increase the risk of developing the disorder. Specifically, persons with a first-degree relative with dementia have a 10% to 30% increased risk of developing AD.

The underlying mechanism through which *APOE* influences AD risk has not yet been determined. Scientists have explored several possibilities, including the idea that *APOE* may play a role in cholesterol transport, neuronal integrity, and amyloid deposition.

The amyloid precursor protein (APP) gene is located on chromosome 21. Studies report the greatest deposits of β-amyloid in people with APOE4. It appears that the APOE protein removes β-amyloid but that the APOE ε4 variant does so less efficiently than other APOE types. Genetic mutations in the genes that control APP are also being targeted as causes of early onset AD. In the genetic disease Down syndrome, for example, β-APP, the source of β-amyloid, is overproduced, which almost always leads to early AD.

Mutations in genes known as presenilin 1 and presenilin 2 account for most cases of early onset inherited AD. The defective genes appear to accelerate β-amyloid plaque formation and apoptosis, a natural process by which cells self-destruct.

Mutations of these and other genes have been identified and provide strong support for the "amyloid cascade hypothesis" of AD (Fig. 31.4). Although the amyloid cascade is currently considered by many researchers as a key contributor to the pathogenesis of AD, some researchers have challenged this assertion and have proposed that β-amyloid occurs secondary to neuron stress and functions as a protective adaptation to the disease rather than causing cell death.

The same genes may have different effects depending on the ethnic population. Dietary and other cultural factors that increase the risk for hypertension and unhealthy cholesterol levels may also play a role. For example, a study of Japanese men showed that their risk increased if they emigrated to America. And the disease is much less common in West Africa than in African Americans, whose risk is the same as or higher than that of white Americans.

Some studies have reported an association between AD and systolic hypertension. Furthermore, some studies report a lower risk for AD in individuals whose blood pressure was reduced. Nevertheless, although hypertension is strongly linked to memory and mental difficulties, stronger evidence is needed to prove any causal relationship between hypertension and AD.

Cardiovascular risk factors increase the risk for AD, including stroke, hypertension, diabetes, and hyperlipidemia. Cardiovascular factors influence the integrity of the blood-brain barrier, setting up conditions that trigger physiologic changes conducive to neuronal injury, inflammation, and protein deposition (amyloid). Clearing of such depositions occurs during deep sleep, which may also be reduced with cardiovascular dysfunction.[36] A number of recent studies support the link between AD and cholesterol by suggesting that certain cholesterol-lowering drugs known as statins may be protective against AD. The APOE genotype is linked with both atherosclerosis and AD. The APOE ε4 genotype reflects abnormal cholesterol transport.

Highly educated (or highly intelligent) people typically have a higher cognitive reserve, allowing longer and more effective adaptation to declining brain function. People with less education (often less wealthy), may be at higher risk because of exposure to malnutrition and noxious substances early in life. Some studies suggest that depression is a risk factor for dementia. Additional studies revealing the true mechanism could eventually lead to more specific treatments for AD. Indeed, studies of asymptomatic APOE ε4 carriers show that these persons are more likely to display subtle abnormalities on brain scans, such as positron emission tomography (PET) or magnetic resonance imaging (MRI) scans. Combining information on APOE ε4 carrier status with other informative biologic marker data is a promising research strategy for detecting individuals who might be candidates for AD prevention strategies. Box 31.5 outlines some of the key risk factors, as well as possible protective factors related to AD.

## Pathogenesis

Like other degenerative conditions, AD has no single identified cause. The loss of neurons is thought to be a consequence of the breakdown of several processes necessary for sustaining brain cells. There are several neuropathologic hallmarks of AD. There is progressive accumulation of an insoluble fibrous protein, amyloid. Described as "plaques," extracellular amyloid is found in higher concentrations in the brains of individuals with AD than in normal aging brains. β-amyloid protein is a natural substance that is required to maintain fibroblasts and cell function. Components of this protein occur typically as a by-product of neuron function. Normally, the β-amyloid dissolves and is reabsorbed by the brain tissue. When it remains in the fluid surrounding the neurons, the β-amyloid protein may deform its shape by folding in on itself. This abnormal protein then sticks together with other β-amyloid material, forming a sheet of connected proteins; the result is a plaque. The amyloid plaque may also include fragmented axons, altered glial cells, and cellular debris. This plaque triggers an inflammatory response, resulting in increased free radicals that cause damage to the nervous system.

APP is a large nerve-protecting protein that is the source of β-amyloid. In AD, certain enzymes, particularly those called γ-secretases, snip APP into β-amyloid pieces. This process is controlled by presenilin proteins. An additional protein in the areas of the brain affected by AD is endoplasmic reticulum–associated binding protein, and it appears to combine with β-amyloid, which in turn attracts new β-amyloid from outside the cells. High amounts of endoplasmic reticulum–associated binding protein may also enhance the toxicity of β-amyloid. It appears that the amyloid plaque, when it

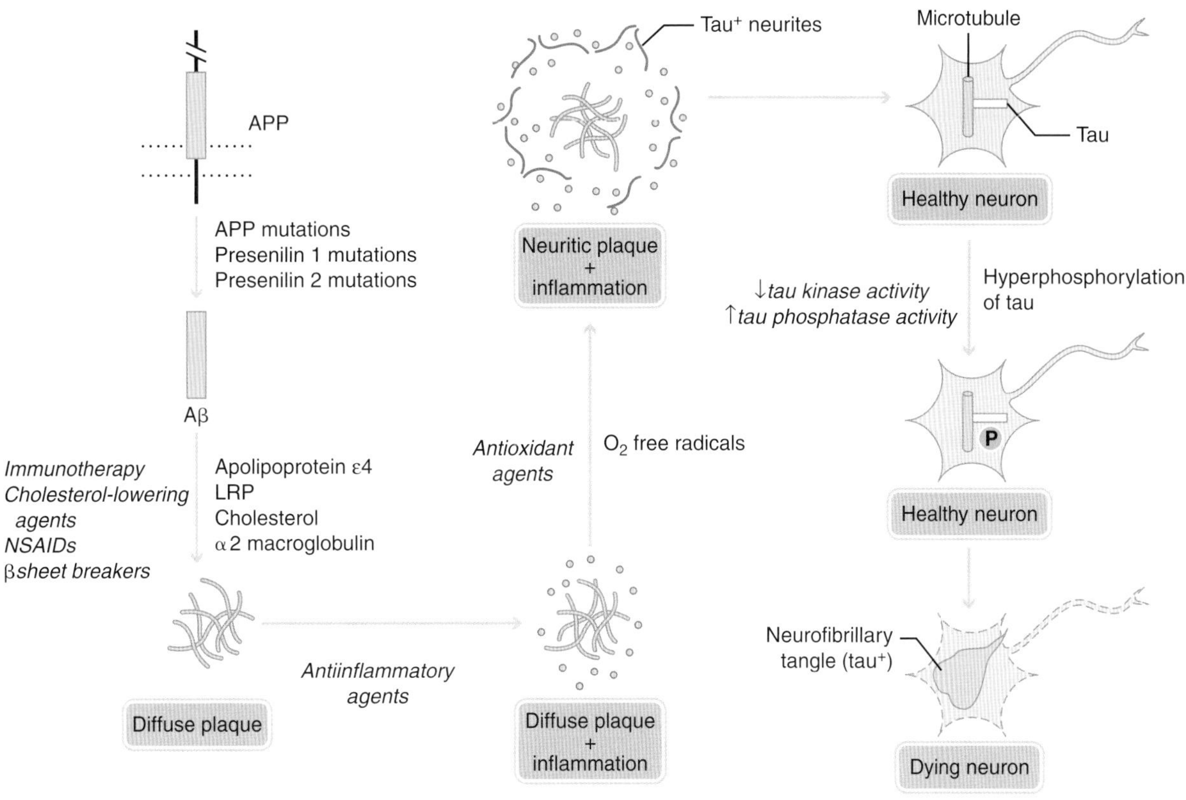


**Figure 31.4**

**The amyloid cascade hypothesis of Alzheimer disease pathogenesis and potential therapeutic targets.** (From Goetz CG: *Textbook of clinical neurology,* ed 3, Philadelphia, 2007, WB Saunders.)

**Box 31.5**

**KEY RISK FACTORS AND PROTECTIVE FACTORS FOR ALZHEIMER DISEASE**

- Primary risk factors: age; family history; genetic markers such as apolipoprotein E ε4 gene (late form AD); trisomy 21; mutations in APP, presenilins 1 and 2 (early AD); female gender after 80 years of age; cardiovascular risk factors such as stroke, hypertension, type 2 diabetes, obesity, and hypercholesterolemia
- Possible risk factors: head injury; depression; progression of Parkinson-like signs in older adults; lower thyroid-stimulating hormone level within the normal range; hyperhomocysteinemia; folate or vitamin D deficiency; hyperinsulinemia; low educational attainment; widowhood status; prolonged stress; sleep disorders; smoking
- Possible protective factors: apolipoprotein E ε2 gene; regular fish consumption; regular consumption of omega-3 fatty acids; high educational level; regular exercise; nonsteroidal antiinflammatory drug therapy; moderate alcohol intake; adequate intake of vitamins C, E, $B_6$, and $B_{12}$, D, and folate

From Desai AK: Diagnosis and treatment of Alzheimer's disease, *Neurology* 64(12 Suppl 3):S34–S39, 2005; and Silva MVF, et al: Alzheimer's disease: risk factors and potentially protective measures, *J Biomed Sci* 26(1):33, 2019.

comes in contact with a neuron, causes chemical changes that may lead to the destruction and destabilization of microtubules, the structural components of the neural cells. A protein molecule called tau, normally responsible for holding the microtubules together, detaches and causes the microtubule to disintegrate. This process may be caused by an enzyme that escapes its normal restraints and breaks down the tau. As the microtubule disintegrates, neurofibrillary "tangles" form and remain in the system. The overall effects are decreased cell division and loss of axonal transport of neurotransmitters. Figure 31.5 shows a typical neuritic plaque and neurofibrillary tangle.

AD is characterized by disruptions in multiple major neurotransmitters, of which cholinergic abnormalities are the most prominent. Acetylcholine is an important neurotransmitter in areas of the brain involved in memory formation, and loss of acetylcholine activity correlates with the severity of AD. The reduction in the number of acetylcholine receptors precedes other pathologic changes, and these receptors are reduced significantly in late AD, particularly in the basal forebrain. There is selective loss of nicotinic receptor subtypes in the hippocampus and cortex. Presynaptic nicotinic receptors control the release of neurotransmitters important for memory and mood, such as acetylcholine, glutamate, serotonin, and norepinephrine. There is still some question whether this plays a primary role in the disease or is a secondary reaction.

Glutaminergic neurons appear to be prone to formation of neurofibrillary tangles. The most vulnerable group of cortical neurons are pyramidal cells with corticocortical and hippocampal projections. Other subgroups of

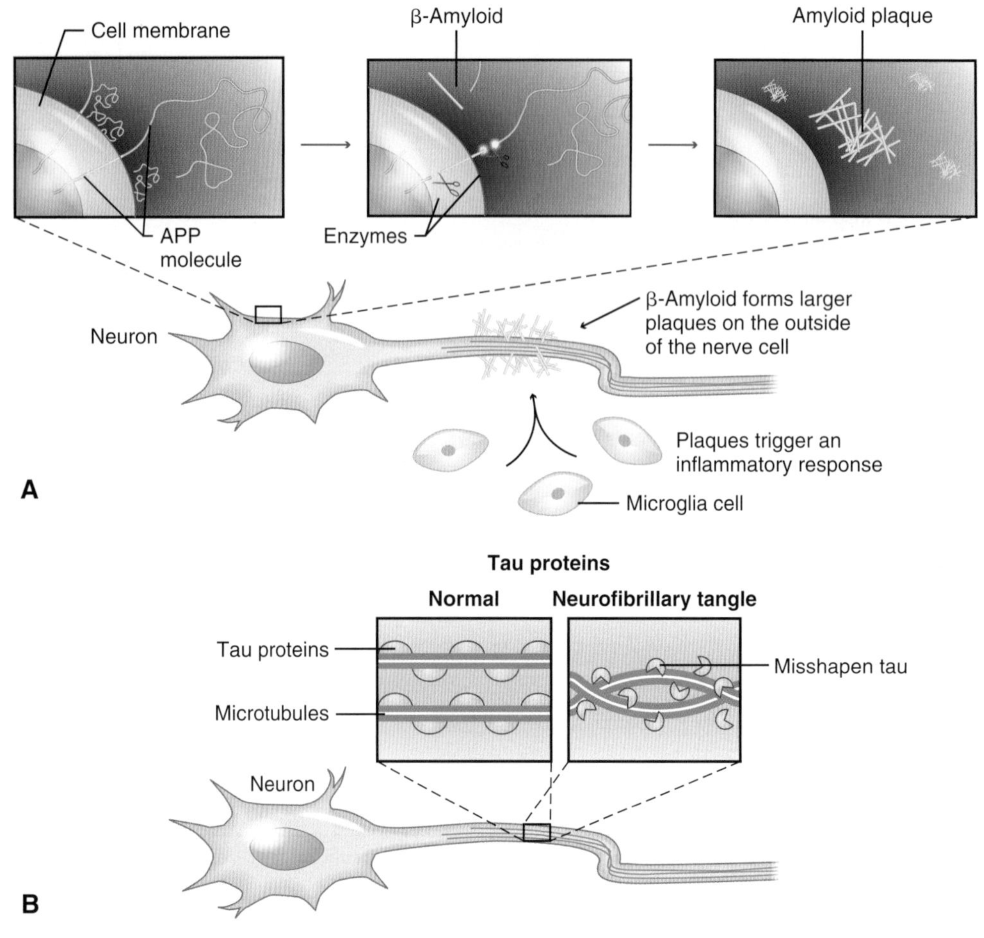


**Figure 31.5**

**Current etiologic theories for the development of Alzheimer disease.** (A) Abnormal amounts of β-amyloid are cleaved from the amyloid precursor protein (APP) and released into the circulation. The β-amyloid fragments come together in clumps to form plaques that attach to the neuron. Microglia react to the plaque, and an inflammatory response results. (B) Tau proteins provide structural support for the neuron microtubules. Chemical changes in the neuron produce structural changes in tau proteins. This results in twisting and tangling (neurofibrillary tangles). (From Lewis SM: *Medical-surgical nursing: assessment and management of clinical problems*, ed 8, St Louis, 2011, Mosby.)

neurons are resistant to the degenerative process, such as the projections from primary sensory to adjacent secondary sensory areas. Increased excitotoxicity resulting from increased glutamatergic stimulation of *N*-methyl-D-aspartate (NMDA) receptors results in abnormally high levels of intracellular calcium and may ultimately lead to cell death. Synaptic loss is the best pathologic correlate of cognitive decline, and synaptic dysfunction is evident long before synapses and neurons are lost. Once synaptic function stops there may be little chance of changing the disease process.

There appears to be a hierarchy of cortical connection systems that are affected differently during the course of AD. A progression of the neurofibrillary tangles seems to move from the entorhinal cortex and hippocampus to the limbic system to the cortex, including the frontal, temporal parietal, and occipital cortices. One study suggests that the effect of AD on hippocampal volume equals the effect of roughly 17 years of aging. This may correlate with the changes seen in memory, behavior, and motor skills as the disease progresses. The distribution of the lesions in the cerebral cortex may be different in AD compared with that in other disease processes that cause dementia.

Cerebral amyloid angiopathy may predispose an individual to develop AD. Cerebral amyloid angiopathy is an important feature of senile dementia and AD along with senile plaques, neurofibrillary tangles, neutrophil threads, and synapse loss. Amyloid gradually causes atrophy of the medial smooth muscle cells of the arteries of the brain that weakens them, causing predisposition to hemorrhage. There is a strong relationship between stroke history and risk for development of AD (see Chapter 32). Abnormalities have been reported in fibroblasts, red and white blood cells, and platelets. Alterations in blood proteins have been observed.

Protein kinase R (PKR) plays a role in recognizing and signaling viral infection, and is altered in several neurologic disorders in which it negatively modulates memory and can become toxic. PKR accumulates in the brain of patients with AD and can indirectly induce the phosphorylation of tau, inducing the death of neurons. PKR levels in the CSF and the activity of PKR in the brain are highly elevated in patients with AD.

Box 31.6

**10 WARNING SIGNS OF ALZHEIMER DISEASE**

1. **Memory loss that disrupts daily life.** One of the most common signs of AD is memory loss, especially forgetting recently learned information. Others include forgetting important dates or events; asking for the same information repeatedly; increasingly needing to rely on memory aids (e.g., reminder notes or electronic devices) or family members for things they used to handle on their own.
2. **Challenges in planning or solving problems.** Some people may experience changes in their ability to develop and follow a plan or work with numbers. They may have trouble following a familiar recipe or keeping track of monthly bills. They may have difficulty concentrating and take much longer to do things than they did before.
3. **Difficulty completing familiar tasks at home, at work or at leisure.** People with AD often find it hard to complete daily tasks. Sometimes, people may have trouble driving to a familiar location, managing a budget at work, or remembering the rules of a favorite game.
4. **Confusion with time or place.** People with AD can lose track of dates, seasons, and the passage of time. They may have trouble understanding something if it is not happening immediately. Sometimes they may forget where they are or how they got there.
5. **Trouble understanding visual images and spatial relationships.** For some people, having vision problems is a sign of AD. They may have difficulty reading, judging distance, and determining color or contrast, which may cause problems with driving.
6. **New problems with words in speaking or writing.** People with AD may have trouble following or joining a conversation. They may stop in the middle of a conversation and have no idea how to continue or they may repeat themselves. They may struggle with vocabulary, have problems finding the right word or call things by the wrong name (e.g., calling a "watch" a "hand-clock").
7. **Misplacing things and losing the ability to retrace steps.** A person with AD may put things in unusual places. They may lose things and be unable to go back over their steps to find them again. Sometimes, they may accuse others of stealing. This may occur more frequently over time.
8. **Decreased or poor judgment.** People with AD may experience changes in judgment or decision making. For example, they may use poor judgment when dealing with money, giving large amounts to telemarketers. They may pay less attention to grooming or keeping themselves clean.
9. **Withdrawal from work or social activities.** A person with AD may start to remove themselves from hobbies, social activities, work projects, or sports. They may have trouble keeping up with a favorite sports team or remembering how to complete a favorite hobby. They may also avoid being social because of the changes they have experienced.
10. **Changes in mood and personality.** The mood and personalities of people with AD can change. They can become confused, suspicious, depressed, fearful, or anxious. They may be easily upset at home, at work, with friends, or in places where they are out of their comfort zone.

From Alzheimer's Association: 10 Early Signs and Symptoms of Alzheimer's. Available at: http://www.alz.org/alzheimers_disease_10_signs_of_alzheimers.asp. Accessed July 17, 2020.

## Clinical Manifestations

The early symptoms of AD may be overlooked because they resemble signs of natural aging. However, older adults who begin to notice a persistent mild memory loss for recent events may have a condition called mild cognitive impairment. Mild cognitive impairment is now thought to be a significant sign of early-stage AD in older people. Studies suggest that older individuals who experience such mild memory abnormalities convert to AD at a rate of approximately 10% to 15% per year. The therapist should be familiar with the warning signs of AD. Because the disease mimics other signs of old age, the symptoms may go unreported. It is often the spouse who asks questions regarding the possibility of the client's developing AD. Information regarding the types of symptoms related to the disease can be helpful to the family in deciding whether more evaluation is needed. The 10 most common signs of AD development are provided in Box 31.6.

Disorders of function are found in the person with AD that correlate with the level of damage in the various components of the cortex as described earlier. Visuospatial deficits are an early clinical finding. Navigating the environment, cooking, and fixing or manipulating mechanical objects in the home are all visuospatial tasks that often are impaired in the first stages of AD. Drawing is abnormal; the ability to draw a three-dimensional object is often lost. The loss of executive functions such as the ability to solve mathematical problems and handle money is typical in the early stages of AD. Judgment is impaired, and safety in driving is diminished.

Subtle personality changes occur in AD, such as indifference, egocentricity, impulsivity, and irritability. People with AD may become withdrawn and anxious. Memory is affected, and this is seen as inability to recall current events. Studies show that particular memory subsystems are relatively more or less vulnerable to diffuse cortical pathologies. People with AD seem to retain higher capacity in implicit memory than was originally thought. Eventually AD causes loss of older memories, so that recall of events from early life fades. Language declines in a characteristic progression. Word-finding difficulty is first, followed by inability to remember names (anomia), and finally diminished comprehension. Social situations become difficult, and mood swings are common. Between 40% and 60% of individuals with late-onset AD suffer from psychotic symptoms, which may include hallucinations, delusions, and dramatic verbal, emotional, or physical outbursts. This is a severe form of AD, with a genetic basis, that has a more rapid and aggressive course. Table 31.4 describes the difference between normal aging and AD.

Major depression is uncommon, but many persons with AD have periods of depressed mood associated with feelings of inadequacy and hopelessness. AD-associated depression is often more modifiable by environmental manipulation than depressions not associated with AD.

**Table 31.4** Differences Between Normal Signs of Aging and Dementia

| Normal | Dementia |
|---|---|
| **Early Signs of Alzheimer Disease** | |
| ***Memory and Concentration*** | |
| • Periodic minor memory lapses or forgetfulness of part of an experience<br>• Occasional lapses in attention or lapses in attention or concentration | • Misplacement of important items<br>• Confusion about how to perform simple tasks<br>• Trouble with simple arithmetic problems<br>• Difficulty making routine decisions<br>• Confusion about month or season |
| ***Mood and Behavior*** | |
| • Temporary sadness or anxiety based on appropriate and specific cause<br>• Changing interests<br>• Increasingly cautious behavior | • Unpredictable mood changes<br>• Increasing loss of outside interests<br>• Depression, anger, or confusion in response to change<br>• Denial of symptoms |
| **Later Signs of Alzheimer Disease** | |
| ***Language and Speech*** | |
| • Unimpaired language skills. | • Difficulty completing sentences or finding the right words.<br>• Inability to understand the meaning of words.<br>• Reduced and/or irrelevant conversation. |
| ***Movement/Coordination*** | |
| • Increasing caution in movement.<br>• Slower reaction times. | • Visibly impaired movement or coordination, including slowing of movements, halting gait, and reduced sense of balance. |
| ***Other Symptoms*** | |
| • Normal sense of smell. No abnormal weight changes in either men or women. | • Impaired sense of smell. Severe weight loss, particularly in female patients. |

Data from Alzheimer's disease: early warning signs and diagnostic resources, The Junior League of NYC, Inc, 1988.

Abnormal motor signs are common, related to the area of the brain that is involved, and perhaps caused by the type of neurotransmitter dysfunction. A relationship between the motor impairments and levels of function can be seen. Presence of tremor appears to be associated with increased risk for cognitive decline, presence of bradykinesia with increased risk for functional decline, and presence of postural-gait impairments with increased risk for institutionalization and death. Disorders of sleep, eating, and sexual behavior are common. The electroencephalogram shows more awake time in bed, longer latencies to rapid eye movement sleep, and losses in slow-wave sleep.

## MEDICAL MANAGEMENT

**DIAGNOSIS.** The most important diagnostic step in evaluating dementias is to determine whether a chronic encephalopathy results from a potentially reversible cause. Interaction of multiple medications can also trigger dementia and should be assessed.

A decline from previous levels of functioning and impairment in multiple cognitive domains beyond memory are critical in establishing dementia. Determining the rate of change is useful, since abrupt changes are not consistent with AD. The progression is usually continuous and does not fluctuate or improve. Box 31.7 shows the Global Deterioration Scale. Information obtained from family members or caregivers can provide data when there seems to be lack of insight from the client. The Functional Activities Questionnaire is a useful informant-based measure.

Clinical screening tests, such as the Short Test of Mental Status, the Mini-Mental State Examination, the Montreal Cognitive Assessment, and Mattis Dementia Rating Scale, provide a baseline for monitoring the course of cognitive impairment over time and document multiple cognitive impairments.

Neuropsychologic tests can accurately predict the probability of conversion to incident AD after 5 or 10 years. Clues on physical examination include a variety of findings that may be common in elderly individuals but are not part of the typical picture of AD, such as ataxia, hyperreflexia, and tremulousness. Depression can be difficult to distinguish from dementia, and it can coexist with dementia.

Ruling out a partially or completely reversible dementia by performing a blood count, chest radiography, and general neurologic examination is critical in the diagnostic evaluation of a person with suspected AD. Autoimmune and paraneoplastic serologic studies may be helpful in such individuals as well.

Forming a complete differential diagnosis requires ruling out other potential causes of disease. The American Academy of Neurology recommends serum analyses that include thyroid function tests, hepatic panels, metabolic panel, complete blood count, vitamin $B_{12}$ levels, and folate levels. In addition, heavy metal screens, syphilis serology, urine or serum toxicology, electrocardiogram, and chest radiograph may be considered. Brain imaging may include either noncontrast head computed tomography, brain MRI, or PET based on clinical findings. Other biomarkers, such as CSF tau, β-amyloid levels, and genetic screening for APOE4, continue to be used in research but may soon be used in the clinical setting.

Use of neuroimaging can be beneficial in the diagnosis of AD. Both MRI and computed tomography (CT) can identify the changes in brain size that are associated with AD. Diagnostic criteria are based on the measurement of medial temporal lobe atrophy or on the volumetric measurement of the entorhinal cortex and hippocampus. The brain demonstrates atrophy with normal aging, so this is not the only diagnostic test.

Single-photon emission computed tomography (SPECT) can be used to determine brain activity, especially in areas where information is processed for

Box 31.7

**GLOBAL DETERIORATION SCALE**

***Stage 1***

NO COGNITIVE DECLINE: During the first of the dementia stages, there is no subjective complaint of memory deficit. No memory deficit evident on clinical interview.

***Stage 2***

VERY MILD COGNITIVE DECLINE (Age Associated Memory Impairment): Subjective complaints of memory deficit, most frequently in following areas: (a) forgetting where one has placed familiar objects; (b) forgetting names one formerly knew well. No objective evidence of memory deficit on clinical interview. No objective deficits in employment or social situations. Appropriate concern with respect to symptomatology.

***Stage 3***

MILD COGNITIVE DECLINE (Mild Cognitive Impairment): During this stage of the dementia stages, one might observe clear-cut deficits. Manifestations in more than one of the following areas: (a) patient may have gotten lost when traveling to an unfamiliar location; (b) coworkers become aware of patient's relatively poor performance; (c) word and name finding deficit becomes evident to intimates; (d) patient may read a passage or a book and retain relatively little material; (e) patient may demonstrate decreased facility in remembering names upon introduction to new people; (f) patient may have lost or misplaced an object of value; (g) concentration deficit may be evident on clinical testing. Objective evidence of memory deficit obtained only with an intensive interview. Decreased performance in demanding employment and social settings. Denial begins to become manifest in patient. Mild to moderate anxiety accompanies symptoms.

***Stage 4***

MODERATE COGNITIVE DECLINE (Mild Dementia): Clear-cut deficit on careful clinical interview. Deficit manifest in following areas: (a) decreased knowledge of current and recent events; (b) may exhibit some deficit in memory of one's personal history; (c) concentration deficit elicited on serial subtractions; (d) decreased ability to travel, handle finances, etc. Frequently no deficit in following areas: (a) orientation to time and place; (b) recognition of familiar persons and faces; (c) ability to travel to familiar locations. Inability to perform complex tasks. Denial is dominant defense mechanism. Flattening of affect and withdrawal from challenging situations frequently occur.

***Stage 5***

MODERATELY SEVERE COGNITIVE DECLINE (Moderate Dementia): Patient can no longer survive without some assistance. Patient is unable during interview to recall a major relevant aspect of their current lives, for example, an address or telephone number of many years, the names of close family members (such as grandchildren), the name of the high school or college from which they graduated. Frequently some disorientation to time (date, day of week, season, etc.) or to place. An educated person may have difficulty counting back from 40 by 4s or from 20 by 2s. Persons at this stage retain knowledge of many major facts regarding themselves and others. They invariably know their own names and generally know their spouses' and children's names. They require no assistance with toileting and eating, but may have some difficulty choosing the proper clothing to wear.

***Stage 6***

SEVERE COGNITIVE DECLINE (Moderately Severe Dementia): May occasionally forget the name of the spouse upon whom they are entirely dependent for survival. Will be largely unaware of all recent events and experiences. Retain some knowledge of their past, but this is very sketchy. Generally unaware of their surroundings, the year, the season, etc. May have difficulty counting from 10, both backward and, sometimes, forward. Will require some assistance with activities of daily living, for example, may become incontinent, will require travel assistance but occasionally will be able to travel to familiar locations. Diurnal rhythm frequently disturbed. Almost always recall their own name. Frequently continue to be able to distinguish familiar from unfamiliar persons in their environment. Personality and emotional changes occur. These are quite variable and include: (a) delusional behavior, for example, patients may accuse their spouse of being an impostor, may talk to imaginary figures in the environment, or to their own reflection in the mirror; (b) obsessive symptoms, for example, person may continually repeat simple cleaning activities; (c) anxiety symptoms, agitation, and even previously nonexistent violent behavior may occur; (d) cognitive abulia, that is, loss of willpower, because an individual cannot carry a thought long enough to determine a purposeful course of action.

***Stage 7***

VERY SEVERE COGNITIVE DECLINE (Severe Dementia): Here in the last stage of the dementia stages all verbal abilities are lost over the course of this stage. Frequently there is no speech at all—only unintelligible utterances and rare emergence of seemingly forgotten words and phrases. Incontinent of urine, requires assistance toileting and feeding. Basic psychomotor skills, for example, ability to walk, are lost with the progression of this stage. The brain appears to no longer be able to tell the body what to do. Generalized rigidity and developmental neurologic reflexes are frequently present.

Information compiled from http://7dementia-stages.com/dementiastages. Accessed June 10, 2013; and https://www.dementiacarecentral.com/aboutdementia/facts/stages/#reisberg. Accessed July 17, 2020.

memory functions. This may be used in the future to predict potential for development of AD. Fluorodeoxyglucose PET imaging reveals a patient's pathology, and provides a marker of clinical status and disease progression. Hippocampal atrophy, decreased CSF amyloid, and decreased brain glucose metabolism when present together in a patient appear to lead to development of AD.

Researchers are looking at different components of the human brain cell to identify molecular changes in deoxyribonucleic acid (DNA) and RNA seen in individuals with dementia and AD. Approaches are widespread, as it is clear that the disease is multifactorial. Patients with AD typically have a selective reduction in CSF β-amyloid 42, the brain effectively acting as a "sink" for the molecule. Conversely, tau and phosphorylated tau are excessively *released* from the brain and into the CSF in patients with AD, with an increase in total tau representing neuronal damage and increased phosphorylated tau reflecting neurofibrillary tangle formation.

Disease states that can mimic AD include vascular dementia, dementia with Lewy bodies, and frontotemporal dementia. Dementia that emerges later in Parkinson disease is described later in this chapter.

***Vascular Dementia.*** The second most common type of dementia after AD, vascular dementia, or multi-infarct dementia is a possible cause of cognitive impairment in those with a history of cardiovascular disease, transient ischemic attacks or stroke. The cognitive dysfunction results from multiple small vessel infarcts that affect deep brain structures, strategic infarcts that affect brain regions critical for cognition, hemorrhage or hypoperfusion. The presentation of symptoms may be more step-wise and variable, paralleling cardiovascular events in contrast with the gradual progression of AD, and may also include other focal neurologic impairments associated with stroke.

***Lewy Body Dementia.*** This disorder exhibits highly variable clinical and neuropathologic overlap with AD and Parkinson disease, and is often under- or misdiagnosed. It occurs before or concurrently with parkinsonism and is unresponsive to standard medications for other types of dementia, therefore correct diagnosis of LBD is important. Cognitive impairments are manifest attention, executive function, and visuospatial abilities. There also may be fluctuations in cognitive impairment (periods of decreased attention, frequent naps), REM sleep behavior disorder, and visual hallucinations. Cellular changes include presence of the Lewy bodies, misfolded protein a-synuclein, neurofibrillary tangles, senile plaques, and granulovacuolar degeneration similar to those in AD. Motor presentation includes resting tremor (but less pronounced than with Parkinson), stooped posture, bradykinesia, and postural instability. The presence of hallucinations may drive development of delusions and paranoia.

***Frontotemporal Dementia.*** Frontotemporal dementia was first described by Arnold Pick in 1892, so for many years was known as Pick's disease. FTD is a term now used to describe the various progressive disorders that have a predilection for the frontal lobes, the most common of which (behavioral variant) results in impairments in executive function and behavioral changes. This presentation may be confused with psychiatric issues. Two other variants affect language to a greater degree: semantic dementia and progressive nonfluent aphasia. The development of motor symptoms can occur that are parkinsonian, are consistent with corticobasal syndrome, or that overlap with progressive supranuclear palsy (covered later in this chapter).

The diagnosis of dementia type is not always clear. It is important to recognize that individuals could have multiple dementia types co-occuring, as there is overlap in the risk factors. Clarity on a diagnosis is helpful to the individual and their family, however, to understand the ways that the individual with dementia is changing, anticipate future care needs, and seek appropriate interventions.

TREATMENT. There is currently no cure for AD or other dementia types. Current treatment focuses on establishing an early accurate clinical diagnosis, early institution of cholinesterase inhibitors, and/or NMDA receptor–targeted therapy. Treating medical comorbidities and dementia-related complications, ensuring that appropriate services are provided, addressing the long-term well-being of caregivers, and treating behavioral and psychologic symptoms with appropriate nonpharmacologic and pharmacologic interventions also are important. Individuals who are genetically predisposed to AD are advised to closely control their blood pressure because hypertension was recently shown to interact with the *APOE* ε4 genotype to increase amyloid deposition in cognitively healthy middle-aged and older adults.

The importance of defining factors that may delay the onset, slow the progression, or even prevent AD and cognitive decline cannot be overestimated. With the aging of world populations, the burden of individuals with all degrees of cognitive impairment on societies will be enormous. A great deal of research has been conducted concerning these factors over the past decades. Although it is true that there are no definitive interventions that have been defined to prevent or slow the cognitive decline in aging, there are very strong trends in the literature. The available evidence suggests that physical activity, intellectual activity, and social engagement are the most helpful factors at reducing AD and cognitive decline. These same factors are helpful for enhancing quality of life. There is optimism in the field with respect to possible disease-modifying effects that can be achieved through a variety of nutritional, pharmacologic, and lifestyle modifications. Box 31.8 outlines the medications commonly in use.

Treatment oriented at preventing the breakdown of tau, or the formation of plaques, is being tested now and

Box 31.8

**COMMON MEDICATIONS USED IN ALZHEIMER DISEASE**

- **Donepezil** (Aricept) has only modest benefits, but it does help slow loss of function and reduce caregiver burden. It works equally in patients with and without *APOE* ε4. It may even have some advantage for patients with moderate to severe AD.
- **Rivastigmine** (Exelon) targets two enzymes (the major one, acetylcholinesterase, and butyrylcholinesterase). This agent may be particularly beneficial for patients with rapidly progressing disease. This drug has slowed or slightly improved disease status even in patients with advanced disease. (Rivastigmine may cause significantly more side effects than donepezil, including nausea, vomiting, and headache.)
- **Galantamine** (Reminyl) not only protects the cholinergic system but also acts on nicotine receptors, which are also depleted in AD. It improves daily living, behavior, and mental functioning, including in patients with mild to advanced-moderate AD and those with a mix of AD and vascular dementia. Some studies have suggested that the effects of galantamine may persist for a year or longer and even strengthen over time.
- **Tacrine** (Cognex) has only modest benefits and has no benefits for patients who carry the *APOE* ε4 gene. In high dosages, it can also injure the liver. In general, newer cholinergic-protective drugs that do not pose as great a risk for the liver are now used for AD.
- **Memantine** (Namenda), targeted at the NMDA receptor, is used for moderate to severe AD.
- **Selegiline** (Eldepryl) is used for treatment of Parkinson disease, and it appears to increase the time before advancement to the next stage of disability.

shows promise. The treatment of those persons identified as at high risk may someday be protective gene therapy. Combining information on *APOE4* carrier status with other informative biologic marker data is a promising research strategy for detecting individuals who might be candidates for AD prevention strategies.

A management model for AD that incorporates a diagnostic protocol to identify and assess people with possible dementia and care management addressing individual function, caregiver support, medical treatment, psychosocial needs, nutritional needs, and advance directives planning is critical. To improve end-of-life care for people with AD, any treatment model should also incorporate patient-centered care and palliative care from the initial diagnosis of AD through its terminal stages. Short-term intensive counseling can significantly reduce the long-term risk for depression among those who care for spouses or partners with AD.

Management of the client with AD is a challenge to health providers and to the family who become caregivers. Manipulation of the environment can be effective. It is difficult to manage aggressive behavior in the home, and long-term care in a facility with a special Alzheimer unit is often the most appropriate place for that client. In many individuals with AD, treating comorbid conditions such as depression, hearing or vision impairment, congestive heart failure, symptomatic urinary tract infection, or hypothyroidism may produce a greater benefit than focusing treatment only on AD. Cardiovascular disease may influence the expression and clinical manifestations of the disease.

There is compelling evidence for the important role of regular physical activity. Exercise training combined with behavioral management techniques can improve physical health and depression in individuals with AD. Leisure-time physical activity at midlife is associated with a decreased risk of dementia and AD later in life. Regular physical activity may reduce the risk or delay the onset of dementia and AD, especially among genetically susceptible individuals.

Diet in midlife shows potential for neuroprotection, and findings can be generalized to a combination of the following: consumption of a diet low in fat, high in omega-3 oils, and high in dark vegetables and fruits; use of soy (for women only); supplementation with vitamin C, coenzyme Q10, and folate; and moderate alcohol intake. The relationship of diet and exercise to cardiovascular health and reducing risk factors known to be associated with dementia is difficult to differentiate. It appears that no single item creates the protection, but the foods and supplements may work together to lower risk.

The mutations in APP, presenilin 1, and presenilin 2 allow genetic screening to be used in suspected cases of familial AD with early onset and for appropriate genetic counseling and support. Although preimplantation genetic diagnosis of the embryo, prenatal diagnosis, preimplantation embryo selection, and presymptomatic testing have been offered to families of individuals who have early onset familial AD, complex legal and ethical issues surrounding these interventions must be addressed before these interventions can be routinely recommended.

**PROGNOSIS.** AD is the fourth leading cause of death in adults. The period from onset to death typically is 7 to 11 years. Initially, deficits in higher cortical function are the most noticeable. Motor signs may reflect higher burden or different type or more biologically detrimental localization of neuropathology. The association of different aspects of motor signs with different outcomes may reflect varying underlying neurotransmitter systems being affected. For example, in Parkinson disease, tremor and bradykinesia are viewed as representing more purely dopaminergic manifestations, whereas posture, balance, and gait disorders may be mediated by other neurotransmitter systems in addition to dopamine. Changes caused by the dementia may advance relentlessly over many years, creating not only deep emotional and psychologic distress, but also practical problems related to caregiving that can overwhelm affected families. During the middle stages of the disease, the client often develops behavioral and motor problems. Finally, the client becomes mute and unable to comprehend. Death is often secondary to dehydration or infection.

## SPECIAL IMPLICATIONS FOR THE THERAPIST 31.2

### *Alzheimer Disease*

Dementia syndromes almost always affect ability to independently perform activities of daily living, such as grooming, toileting, and eating. Instrumental activities of daily living include complex activities such as meal preparation, banking, driving, and decision making.

Cognitive decline consistent with the diagnosis of primary degenerative dementia is a unique clinical syndrome with characteristic phenomena and progression. The Global Deterioration Scale (see Box 31.7) can be used for the assessment of degenerative dementia and delineation of its stages.

Use of a comprehensive cognitive stimulation program in AD patients enhances neuroplasticity, reduces cognitive loss, and helps the patient to stretch functional independence through better cognitive performance. Remarkable effects have been observed also in the areas of mood and behavior. Behavioral disturbances influence caregiver burden and institutionalization as well as being associated with patient and caregiver distress. Increase in social attention and interaction improves mood and behavior in demented elderly. Important mood benefits are reported from stimulation programs predominantly aimed at cognition. Changes in functional abilities correlate with cognitive deficits and prognosticate clinical course because they significantly affect caregiver burden and rates of institutionalization. Tools to be used are the Functional Activities Questionnaire and the Assessment of Motor and Processing Skills.

Cognitive rehabilitation programs can minimize demands on executive control systems in favor of structured tasks that are designed to exploit implicit memory. Appropriate feedback is critical because there is increased agitation and anxiety when mistakes are recognized. Nonverbal cues can be helpful when language is the source of confusion. Moving through parts of a task with guidance can facilitate understanding and promote confidence to proceed. When the experience is more pleasurable, the response is improved, as the stress of the task may be reduced.

The client with AD has generalized weakness that is increased by general inactivity and may demonstrate abnormality of movement. Movements become more stereotyped and rigid. Postural reflexes are diminished, and the incidence of falls increases. Falls occur in approximately 30% of clients with AD, which may be attributable to their lack of perception of where their bodies are in space or an inability to navigate around objects. Reducing obstacles may decrease falls. The use of increased lighting, especially in the early evening, will decrease the agitation often referred to as *sundowning*.

The therapist often sees a client with AD in a structured living environment, since many people become difficult to maintain at home. Movement and exercise can provide the client with an activity that the client can succeed in, as well as maintain mobility, good breathing patterns, and endurance. Restlessness and wandering are typical of the client with AD, and a structured exercise program appears to decrease restlessness. Daytime exercise can also help control nighttime pacing and the resulting daytime drowsiness. Some residential programs have set up areas that the client can access without wandering out of the facility. The use of these areas may decrease agitation and allow individuals to pace safely.

Group therapy with simple exercises that use images rather than commands is most effective. The use of music may also be beneficial to encourage movement. Storytelling integrated into the exercise program helps to stimulate thinking as well as movement. Clients need to be able to attend to an activity for at least 5 minutes, and the group therapy session must not provide more stimulation than clients are able to tolerate. Exercises should be short and simple and done in the same order each day. Repetition and reassurance can help keep clients engaged. The exercise program should include group interaction with physical touching, such as holding hands or working in pairs. Use of exercise bands, balls to kick and throw, and light weights works well. Community-dwelling individuals with Alzheimer disease and sleep problems can benefit from walking and increased light exposure, alone or in combination, but these interventions must be implemented with caregiver assistance.

Word fluency scores appear to improve with community-based walking. A multimodal exercise program is associated with a reduction in the neuropsychiatric symptoms of patients with AD and contributes to the attenuation of the impairment in the performance of instrumental activities of daily living in elderly women with AD. The Preventing Loss of Independence through Exercise (PLIÉ) program combines elements of Eastern and Western exercise traditions, including yoga, tai chi, Feldenkrais, physical therapy, occupational therapy, mindfulness, and dance movement therapy. PLIÉ instructors have patients sit in a circle, which promotes group movement and social interaction. Conversations tend to build and become more complex in this setting.

In working with the individual with AD, knowing something about the individual enables the therapist to use words and terms that are more familiar. Approach to the person should be slow and from the front. Always identify yourself and use the person's name before intervention begins. Identifying pain during activity is important, because pain may trigger agitation or aggression. Use of modalities to decrease the client's pain may result in improved behavior. The Alzheimer's discomfort rating scale is useful.

Intervention should be based on the individual's stage of progression. In the early stages, work on high-level balance and gait activities will help to maintain mobility and balance. Strength gains have been reported to be significant in older persons in a strengthening program, and strength is an important component of balance. Maintaining range of motion, especially in the trunk and distal extremities, will help to maintain function. Caregiver training is important for consistent follow-through with activities and provision of appropriate cues. When assistance is needed for mobility, caregiver training on transfers, contracture management, and assistance with gait is included in the intervention. Choosing the appropriate orthotic, assistive device, and wheelchair can be a challenge as dementia develops. Walkers have been designed for the AD client to use on flat surfaces with appropriate support and safety.

# DYSTONIA

## Definition and Overview

Dystonia is a movement disorder characterized by sustained or intermittent muscle contractions causing abnormal, often repetitive, movements, postures, or both. Dystonic movements are typically patterned, twisting, and may be tremulous. It is frequently initiated or worsened by voluntary action and associated with overflow muscle activation. It is most likely a group of disorders with differing neurophysiologic pathology along the sensory-motor brain networks.[44,45]

Multiple methods of classifying dystonia exist. In 2013, the consensus update by the International Consensus Committee of the European Federation of Neurologic Societies clarified terminology to improve clinician diagnosis, prognosis, and treatment and is used for this chapter. Recommendations include two divisions to classify dystonia. The first is clinical characteristics which comprise four categories: (1) age of onset, (2) area of the body involved, (3) temporal course of dystonia and, (4) whether it is isolated or combined with other features. Etiology

Box 31.9

**CAUSES OF DYSTONIA RELATED TO CAUSES THAT ARE NONGENETIC**

- Drugs, including neuroleptics, dopamine agonists, anticonvulsants, antimalarial drugs
- Intramedullary lesions of the cervical cord
- After hemiplegia: often a delayed reaction to stroke
- Focal brain lesions: vascular malformation, tumor, abscess
- Demyelinating lesions, such as with multiple sclerosis
- Traumatic brain injury with lesion to contralateral basal ganglia or thalamus
- Encephalitis
- Environmental toxins: manganese, carbon monoxide, methanol
- Hypoparathyroidism
- Degenerative disease: Parkinson disease, Huntington disease, Wilson disease, progressive supranuclear palsy, multiple system atrophy
- Cerebral palsy

is the second division and contains three categories: (1) nervous system pathology, (2) heritability and, (3) idiopathic.[46] Each of the subcategories of the two major divisions are defined as follows:

A. Clinical characteristics
  1. Age of onset
     - Infancy (birth to 2 years)
     - Childhood (3-12 years)
     - Adolescence (13-20 years)
     - Early adulthood (21-40 years)
     - Late adulthood (>40 years)

  The average age of onset of primary or genetic dystonia is 12 years old. For focal dystonias, the age of onset is between 30 and 50 years.
  2. Body distribution of symptoms
     - Focal. Limited to one body segment. Examples are cervical dystonia, writer's cramp, and blepharospasm
     - Segmental. Affects adjacent body parts. An example is cranial dystonia, which involves blepharospasm with jaw involvement.
     - Multifocal. Involves two or more noncontiguous body regions. An example is the right arm and left leg.
     - Generalized. Affects the trunk and at least two other body parts.
     - Hemidystonia. Mainly affects one side of the body.
  3. **Temporal pattern** describes the disease course which can be static, progressive, variable, persistent, action-specific, diurnal, or paroxysmal.
  4. Associated features
     - Isolated
     - Combined with other neurologic or systemic disorders

  The divisions help the clinician with narrowing causes and assist with focusing diagnostic testing.[45] For example, the age division category would help as follows: dystonia that begins in the first year of life is often an inherited metabolic disorder that suggests a poor prognosis. Dystonia manifesting between 2 and 6 years of age is consistent with dystonic cerebral palsy. Dopa-responsive dystonias tend to manifest between 6 and 14 years of age. Focal dystonia usually occurs after 50 years of age.

B. The second major classification of dystonia is based on its *etiology*. It is as follows:
  1. Nervous System Pathology
     - Degenerative
     - Structural (lesions)
     - Not degenerative or structural lesions
  2. Heritability
     - Inherited (autosomal, dominant or recessive, mitochondrial)
  3. Idiopathic
     - Sporadic
     - Familial
  4. Acquired
     - Perinatal brain injury
     - Infection
     - Drug/toxic
     - Vascular
     - Neoplastic
     - Brain injury
     - Psychogenic

Functional (psychogenic) dystonia (FD) is a common disorder.[22a] Two types of FD are identified: (1) a group with fixed abnormal posture usually affecting the extremities with onset in mid 30s and, (2) a later onset with intermittent contraction that mainly affects cranial and neck areas. Characteristics of FD include inconsistency in the history and neurologic exam, inconsistent movements or posture during distraction, unusual age of onset for the particular phenotype and robust responses to placebo.[78] The two categories cover secondary conditions in the acquired dystonias categories.

Nonmotor features of dystonia have been delineated. They vary depending on the type of dystonia, but include cognitive decline and psychiatric symptoms in some of the degenerative categories. Finally, *cervical dystonia* is a separate entity from spasmodic torticollis. Torticollis is a musculoskeletal phenomenon treated as an orthopedic condition.

## Incidence

The world-wide estimate for primary dystonia is about 16.4 per 100,000.[93] There is no significant difference in prevalence between men and women.

## Etiologic and Risk Factors

### Genetic

Genetic nomenclature (DYTs) has changed due to expanded findings from next-generation sequencing. The new nomenclature uses DYT for dystonia followed by the gene name, so DYT1 dystonia is now DYT-TOR1A. Isolated dystonia has three established genes: (1) DYT-TOR1A, early onset; (2) DYT-THAP1, adolescent onset; and (3) DYT-GNAL, adult onset segmental dystonia. These are found in less than 5% of patients. Genes for the combined dystonia with dopa-responsive (dystonia-parkinsonism symptoms) include DYT-GCH1,

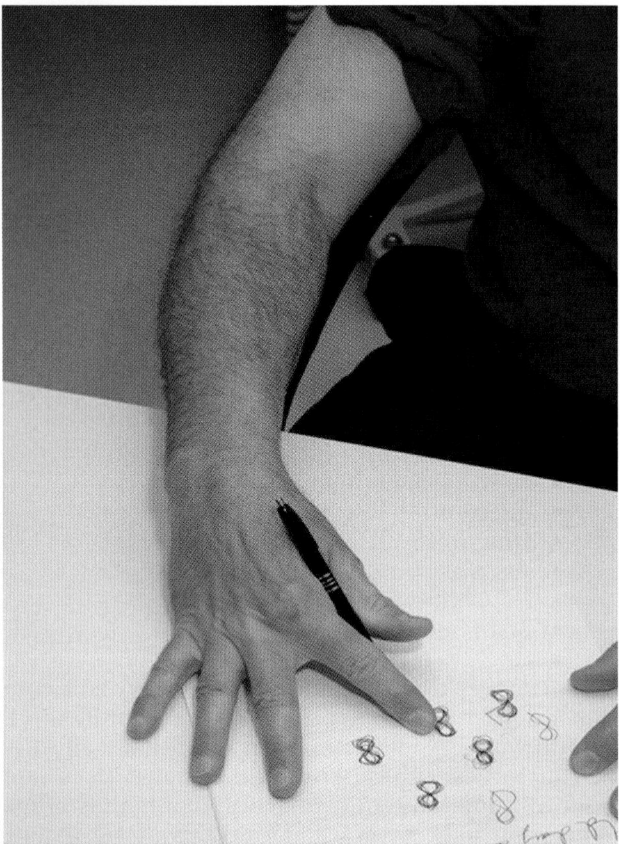

**Figure 31.6**

Focal hand dystonia. (From Lin PL, Hallet M: The pathophysiology of focal hand dystonia, *J Hand Therapy* 22(2):109 –114, 2009.)

and DTY-ATP1A3. DTY-SGCE gene is associated with myoclonus dystonia. Many additional genes may be contributory to dystonia (over 100) and often accompany developmental delays. See Lohmann and Klein[56] or Shaikh et al.[89] for a review of genes and complications identifying causal factors. People with generalized dystonia carry a different gene than those with focal dystonias.

Patterns and types of motor use may be the final key in developing dystonia. Clinical symptoms (penetrance) of dystonia are only present in 30% of those with the DYTTOR1A gene and in 60% of those with the DYTTHAP1 gene. Because several types of dystonia do not appear to have a genetic basis, an environmental "use-dependent" factor is also proposed (with or without a genetic basis) for many dystonias, particularly focal dystonias. Use-dependent environmental factors like peripheral injury or repetitive and precise movement training, may trigger dystonic movement development in people with abnormal neuroplasticity.[102] Both somatosensory cortex and somatotopic representation at the thalamus degrade in individuals with dystonia, suggesting that the somatosensory cortex may function abnormally, contributing to the altered motor output. Studies of musicians and writers with hand dystonia, also known as writer's cramp (Fig. 31.6) show somatosensory degradations in the involved hand of graphesthesia and stereognosis.[55]

Although generally listed as idiopathic, recent evidence supports a genetic basis, at least in some cases of focal dystonia.

### Drug-induced Dystonia

Drug-induced dystonia (DID) is a common side effect associated with antipsychotic drugs (neuroleptics). This results in various acute and chronic dystonias, such as blepharospasm (difficulty in opening the eyelids), torticollis, or retrocollis (involuntary extension of the neck). Second-generation antipsychotics have an incidence that varies from 1.4% (quetiapine) to 15.3% (L-sulpiride).[63]

Children also are susceptible to dystonia from antipsychotic drugs; however, based on emergency room visits for DID, gastrointestinal medications produce the highest rate of DID in children.[104] The fact that β-blocking agents are effective in reducing symptoms in DID cases points to the possibility that neuroleptic drugs increase the activity of β-adrenergic transmitters.

### Acquired Dystonia

Traumatic dystonias-both post-traumatic brain injury-usually accompanied by unconsciousness, and peripheral nerve injuries can result in dystonia.[27b]

## Pathogenesis

Three neurophysiologic deficits underlie the abnormal motor output associated with dystonia:

1. Loss of inhibition of motor programs arising from a relative overactivity of the direct pathway in the basal ganglia and defective surround inhibition leading to abnormal involuntary movements,
2. Abnormal sensorimotor integration as evidenced by defective temporal and spatial discrimination on testing and the effect of sensory tricks in altering dystonic movements, and
3. Abnormal homeostatic plasticity as evidenced by experiments using repetitive transcranial magnetic stimulation (TMS).

Dystonia varies widely in body area(s) affected, progression, age of onset, and outcome. The heterogeneous nature of dystonia suggests a pathogenesis based on a network model (disruption anywhere along the sensory-motor pathways) rather than a specific localized pathology model.[28,45]

Abnormal neuroplasticity is present in many dystonias and especially in focal dystonias. An in-depth review of research and discussion of striatal basis for dystonia is available.[80]

A defect in the body's ability to locally process inhibitory neurotransmitters, such as γ-aminobutyric acid (GABA), dopamine, acetylcholine, norepinephrine, and serotonin, may contribute to poor inhibition of motor control. Dysfunction of the lenticulothalamic neuronal circuit seems to be related to the development of dystonia following head trauma. The striatum also has strong thalamocortical somatosensory connections as well as cerebellar connections, with potential to disrupt normal sensory processing along the neuronetworks.[3]

Cervical dystonia may be a neural integrator problem in pathways of the interstitial nucleus of Cajal (INC) versus dystonia seen in Parkinson disease, which appears basal ganglia related.[88,89] A summary of the mechanisms of cervical dystonia is presented by Sedov et al.[88] The integrative networks of the brainstem, cerebellum, and basal ganglia can cause dystonia when the basal ganglia output reflects abnormal neural integration based on faulty input from the other systems. The basal ganglia abnormality is secondary, due to impaired network feedback. Additional support comes from monkey studies showing that cervical dystonia occurs when the INC is either inhibited or facilitated.[89] The INC converts head velocity to angle (acting as a neural integrator) and continuously provides input to maintain cervical posture from bilateral sensory inputs. While vision and vestibular information play a role in maintaining head position, proprioception is a critical input component.[80] Sedov[88] found a strong correlation with firing of cells between the globus pallidius and cervical muscles. These results suggest that cervical dystonia is caused by a bihemispheric asymmetry in feedback, resulting in asymmetric dysfunction in the neural integrator causing head turning.

## MEDICAL MANAGEMENT

DIAGNOSIS. Dystonia is a clinical diagnosis except for cases that have a genetic basis. Testing for genetic forms of dystonia is recommended. Testing to rule out other neurologic diseases is important (Box 31.9). Most often, there is no definitive test for dystonia, and the diagnosis of idiopathic dystonia is often delayed a year or more. The clinical presentation of dystonic movements, such as head deviation or neck pain, may be the first sign.

Five features of dystonia that guide diagnosis are:

1. Dystonic postures—a body part is flexed or twisted along its longitudinal axis and sensation of rigidity and traction is present.
2. Dystonic movements—movement is of a twisting or pulling nature in a preferred direction, repetitive and patterned attitude (consistent and predictable).
3. Geste antagoniste (sensory trick) —alleviation of dystonia occurs during the geste movement, which may or may not last through the entire movement. The geste movement is natural (never forceful) so it does not push or pull the affected body part, but is a sensory input. (A common geste is a light touch to the chin for people with cervical dystonia.)
4. Mirror dystonia—mirror movements are observed in the opposite body side.
5. Overflow dystonia—dystonic movement or postures extend beyond the commonly involved body region. Observed at peak of dystonic movement.

Determining that there is no evidence for other neurologic disorders or secondary dystonia is essential in the diagnosis of idiopathic dystonia.

TREATMENT. Treatment includes deep brain stimulation, drug therapy, including botulinum toxin type A and type B injections Figure 31.7, transmagnetic stimulation, physical and occupational therapy, and sometimes surgery.

Deep brain stimulation of the globus pallidus internus has also been successful in some patients, especially in children and people with genetic-based generalized dystonia; however, several review articles show it varies in its effectiveness[23] based on type of dystonia. It is less effective for patients with dystonia as part of other neurologic disease processes.

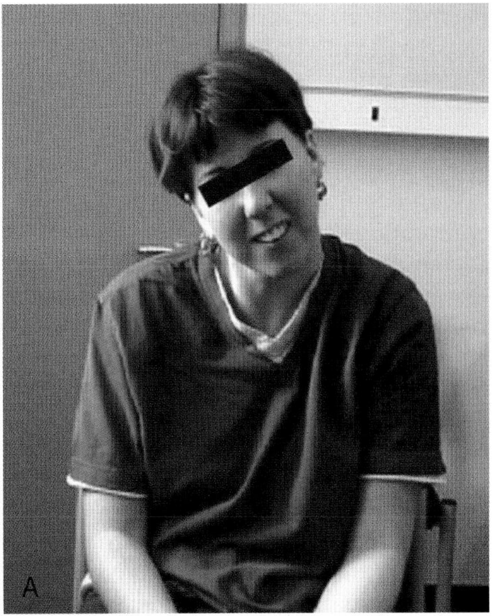


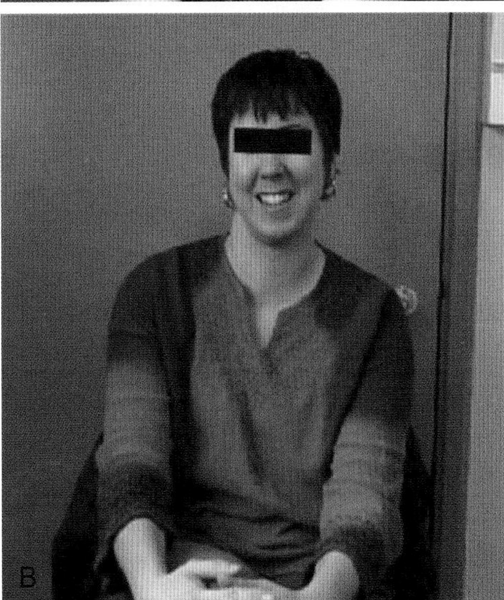


**Figure 31.7**

Cervical dystonia. (A) Dystonia before treatment. (B) Dystonia after intervention wtih BoTox. (From Hu M: Other movement disorders, *Medicine* 36(12):636 –639, 2008.)

Anticholinergics such as trihexyphenidyl (Artane) have been the most widely used medications to decrease acetylcholine and correct a cholinergic imbalance in the basal ganglia. Side effects of these drugs vary but the medication is effective. Baclofen and other muscle relaxants are used occasionally for relief.

Botulinum toxin types A and B, injected intramuscularly, have emerged as a safe and effective symptomatic treatment, particularly for focal dystonias involving a limited number of muscles. These injections are effective in improving postural deviation and pain in approximately 80% to 90% of people with cervical dystonias (see Fig. 31.7). Response occurs in 3 to 7 days and lasts 3 to 4 months. Muscle weakness can result from this treatment. Dysphagia is the most serious side effect, but can be decreased in incidence and severity by injecting lower doses, particularly into the sternocleidomastoid. The need to continue indefinitely with repeat injections approximately every 3 months is a major drawback.

Surgery may be considered only when other treatments are no longer effective, although surgical intervention may also lose its effect over time, providing only temporary symptomatic relief. Surgeries to interrupt the pathways or foci responsible for the abnormal movements can be effective. Thalamotomy is the destruction of a portion of the thalamus. Pallidotomy is a destructive operation on the globus pallidus. Rhizotomy involves the surgical resection of the anterior cervical spinal nerve roots and is not as commonly used since deep brain stimulation has been developed.

**PROGNOSIS.** Age of onset is the best predictor of prognosis. If dystonia starts at or near birth and affects other members of the family, it tends to get progressively worse over the years. If the condition starts in childhood and is secondary to cerebral palsy or other brain injury close to the time of birth, the dystonia tends to remain static for many years. In one-third of cases of adult-onset focal dystonia there is progression to segmental dystonia, although there is less than a 20% chance that the disease will progress to generalized dystonia.

Spontaneous remission occurs in some cases within the first year, but the majority of clients show steady progression of their dystonia, with maximal disability occurring after 5 years. Neck pain, occurring in 70% to 80% of clients, contributes significantly to disability. Cervical dystonia has important psychosocial consequences, since many people with this condition withdraw from their jobs and social activities.

## SPECIAL IMPLICATIONS FOR THE THERAPIST 31.3

### *Dystonia*

#### Testing

The Toronto Western Spasmodic Torticollis Rating Scale (TWSTRS) and the Tsui are two commonly used impairment and disability scales for rating the severity of cervical dystonia. The TWSTRS is more involved but has good reliability and validity. The Barry-Albright Dystonia Scale is used for dystonia associated with other neurologic diseases. Range of motion, pain, and descriptions of active motion, as well as limitations in functional activities, are also useful measurements. Outcomes can be measured with life satisfaction scales, such as the SF-36 (Short Form-36 General Health Survey).

### *Intervention*

The therapist should address all aspects of functional ability with the client who has been affected by dystonia, including stress and pain management, energy conservation, adaptive equipment, mobility, and selective splinting, which can improve or deteriorate symptoms depending on the type of dystonia. It is important not to do repetitive stereotyped movements during retraining.

Physical and occupational therapy may have a much greater role in the future based on new concepts of the neurobiology for dystonia. As different mechanisms are elucidated for different types of dystonia, interventions can be more effective. For example, Popa[80] et al., Shaikh,[89] and Sedov[88] present evidence that abnormal cerebellar processing of the neck proprioceptive information drives dysfunctions of the integrator in cervical dystonia. Therefore retraining neck proprioception through current published techniques has potential for treatment.[77]

Additionally, intervention using TMS has shown promise in several types of dystonia but the research in this area is still very basic and limited.[49]

Sensory processing abnormalities, as discussed under pathogenesis, may be involved in the abnormal movements of dystonia and can provide some direction for intervention. In owl monkeys, who developed dystonic movements of the hand fingers in response to a high number of repetitive movements of the forearm and hand, the sensory cortex and thalamus had reorganized hand representation to be much less organized and precise (dedifferentiation). For treatment, the same laboratory demonstrated recovery of the cortical representation and redifferentiation using sensory stimulation therapy rather than motor retraining.[11,12,84] A case series using sensory retraining demonstrated success with this method in humans who had writer's cramp, a focal dystonia.

A sensory discrimination retraining program should include:[11]

- Subjective grading of stimuli (texture, objects)
- Programs that employ principles of direct, repeated sensory practice
- Comparison of sensation between sides
- Verbalization of sensation
- Need to focus on interpretation of stimuli to induce plasticity

Other sensory approaches, such as EMG biofeedback, have the potential to improve dystonia also. Theoretically, visual input provides an alternate, functional route for sensory input to reach the motor output system through the surface EMG visual feedback. The primary motor cortex, which is responsible for initiating motor tasks, receives highly processed visual information from cortical areas other than the somatosensory cortex (i.e., parietal lobe, basal ganglia). These pathways may be able to override the malfunctioning input systems. Surface EMG feedback is effective in reducing symptoms in persons with focal hand dystonia. Trials using surface EMG for hand dystonia demonstrated results in as few as five sessions, although long-term retention is questionable. Several studies, using a series of cases, demonstrate EMG biofeedback is effective for treatment of patients with cervical dystonia. Other studies of EMG biofeedback do not appear to be as effective, especially studies using EMG as a relaxation training technique.

There is weak support for modalities, stretching, and strengthening alone. However, Tassorelli et al[98a] reported success using physical therapy of stretching, strengthening, postural control, and balance exercises along with surface EMG biofeedback, in a study comparing outcomes of two groups, one receiving Botox (BTX) only and the other receiving BTX and physical therapy. The group given physical therapy and BTX showed significantly better outcomes than the BTX-only group.

Task-oriented treatment, rather than more traditional strengthening and stretching exercises, has better potential for improving function. Having clients do highly skilled tasks in treatment that are challenging and stimulating improves learning. A combination of treatments often is most effective. For example, a client with right lower-extremity dystonia of 8 years' duration used a combination of surface EMG feedback on the anterior tibialis and gastrocnemius during stepping to targets and using the foot to identify and manipulate small objects in order to normalize motion. BTX type A injections into the hip flexor and gastrocnemius were done later to assist in reducing the abnormal hip flexor component of walking. The outcome was a normal gait pattern.

When the jaw, tongue, or lips are involved, gentle pressure on the lips or teeth may lessen spasm. Exerting slight pressure against the jaw on the side to which the head is rotated may decrease or inhibit muscle spasm, although this is an immediate and short-term reaction. Guidelines for chewing and swallowing may be helpful for the client with oral mandibular dystonia.

Aquatic therapy can be especially helpful in reducing discomfort and facilitating movement.

In some cases of dystonia, splinting has been effective for improving function.

Aggressive strengthening and range-of-motion treatments may increase the symptoms of dystonia; any treatment should be carried out within the client's tolerance and without increasing the manifestations of the dystonia. Because dystonia originates in the CNS, passive techniques such as massage provide only temporary relief from symptoms and do not affect the underlying movement disorder. Likewise, focal dystonia does not respond to facilitatory or inhibitory techniques used for modulating spasticity. When relief of spasm allows the client to assume a more normal or correct posture, underlying tight soft tissues may benefit from short-term use of physical therapy modalities and soft-tissue mobilization to restore full range of motion.

# HUNTINGTON DISEASE

## Overview and Definition

Huntington disease (HD) is a progressive hereditary disorder characterized by abnormalities of movement, personality disturbances, and dementia. Known also as Huntington chorea, it is most often associated with choreic movement that is brief, purposeless, involuntary, and random. These movements begin as random fidgety movements in the distal extremities but progress to involve more proximal muscles and ballistic movements. Over time chorea may "burn out" to result in more disabling movement problems, including bradykinesia, dystonia, rigidity, and ataxia. The progression of the disease continues over an average of 20 years, includes cognitive impairment, and ultimately is fatal.[105] HD is a disorder of the CNS and is classified as a neurologic disorder, but because it is a condition with complex effects, management requires a multidisciplinary approach.

## Incidence and Etiologic and Risk Factors

The prevalence of HD in North America ranges from 4 to 8 per 100,000 persons. It is estimated that there are 25,000 cases in the United States. HD may begin at any time after infancy but usually starts in middle age. Twenty-five percent of persons with HD have disease of late onset, which is defined as onset of motor symptoms after age 50 years. There is almost always a history of an affected parent. There is a 50% risk in each child of an affected adult. Transmission of the juvenile form of HD (onset before age 20 years) appears to be primarily from the father. With adult onset there is more equal transmission from both parents.

HD is an autosomal dominant disease with the IT15 or HD genetic marker found on the tip of chromosome 4. In a subset of cases, the junctophilin-3 gene is responsible for the HD genotype. All the people who inherit the gene will develop symptoms of the disease if they do not die prematurely. Because there is no cure for HD, there is an ethical dilemma associated with testing prior to symptom onset. Studies are underway to determine the psychiatric and social problems that may result from the knowledge that one will develop HD.

## Pathogenesis

Although the cause remains unknown, pathologic findings show a consistent pattern of tissue changes in the brain. The ventricles are enlarged as a result of atrophy of the adjacent basal ganglia, specifically the caudate nucleus and putamen (collectively the striatum) (Fig. 31.8). This is a result of extensive loss of small and medium-sized neurons. The volume of the brain can decrease by as much as 20%. Caudate atrophy correlates with a measured decline in Mini-Mental State Examination scores, but not with the severity or duration of neurologic symptoms. It is the atrophy of the putamen that correlates with neurologic symptoms. The atrophy of the cortices appears to occur at the same rate as that of the striatum. White matter degeneration in the frontal cortex appears to be associated with the course of the disease. Slower disease progression appears to be correlated with more white matter changes, with more aggressive progression with less white matter loss and more striatal damage. Other subtle changes occur in the cortex and cerebellum, including both loss of neurons and production of glial cells that inhibit neural transmission.

As with other progressive diseases, there is selective vulnerability of neurons in a particular region with preservation of others. In the early and middle stages of HD, neurons projecting from the striatum to the substantia nigra are depleted. This reduces the amount of neurotransmitters, including GABA, acetylcholine, and

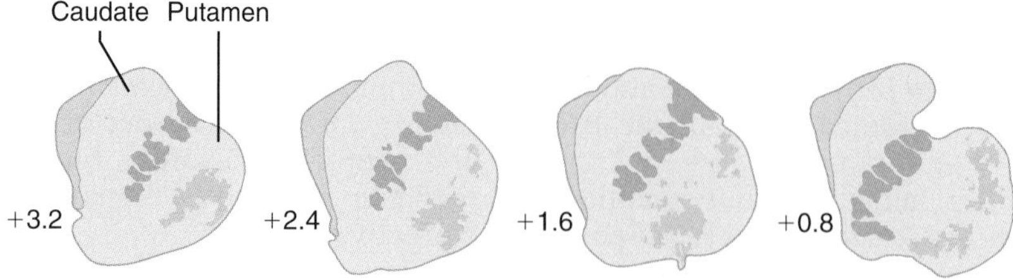


**Figure 31.8**

**Atrophy seen in the caudate and putamen in a person with Huntington disease.** As the disease progresses there is a change in the caudate at the interface with the ventricle. The outline becomes more and more concave, representing the progressive atrophy.

metenkephalin. This leaves relatively higher concentrations of other neurotransmitters, such as dopamine and norepinephrine. The normal balance of inhibition and excitation responses in the complex organization of the basal ganglia and thalamus that allows for smooth, controlled movement is disrupted. The result is an excess of dopamine and excessive excitation of the thalamocortical pathway. This may explain the excessive abnormal involuntary movements described as chorea.

In the later stages of HD, there is a loss of the direct inhibitory substance that causes more inhibition of the thalamocortical output, with resultant rigidity and bradykinesia, or slowness of movement. By the late stages of HD, virtually all the caudate nucleus projection neurons are affected. The mechanism of neuronal loss is not known. One hypothesis is that an excitotoxin causes the cell death noted in the basal ganglia.

## Clinical Manifestations

### Movement Disorders

Many individuals with suspected early HD will show almost no neurologic abnormality on routine examination other than minor choreic movements. The movements may be suppressed during the examination as they can often be integrated into a purposeful movement, such as raising the hand to the head as if to smooth the hair. Early in the course the involuntary movements may appear to be no more than an exaggeration of normal restlessness, usually involving the upper limbs and face. The chorea is increased by mental concentration, emotional stimuli, performance of complex motor tasks, and walking. Problems with voluntary movement may be detected by asking for rapid tongue movements or finger-to-thumb tapping, or testing for dysdiadochokinesia, the inability to make rapid alternating movements.

Assessment of muscle strength will usually be normal in early cases but eventually may be affected by bradykinesia or general motor disturbance. Tone will usually be normal initially, but rigidity becomes part of the clinical picture in many cases as the disease progresses. The tendon reflexes are usually normal.

Abnormalities in eye movement are common in HD. The ability to execute a saccade, a rapid movement of the eyes from one target to another in order to move the visual focus rapidly to different objects, is disturbed. There is often a decrease in the velocity of eye movement, an undershooting of the target, or latency in initiation of movement. Gaze fixation abnormalities have been noted; that is, inability to fix on a light source without the intrusion of small saccadic movements. Smooth pursuit, or tracking of the eye to follow a moving object, is interrupted by the same small, jerky saccadic movements. There is often an inability to suppress reflex saccades to a visual stimulus, which leads to visual distractibility.

The term *chorea* is derived from the Greek word for dance, and gait abnormalities are common in HD. When chorea is a predominant sign, persons walk with a wide-based, staggering gait. Those persons with bradykinesia and hypertonicity may walk with a slow, stiff, unsteady gait.

Dysarthria, reflected as a decrease in the rate and rhythm of speech, may be mild in the early course with progression to the point that speech may become unintelligible. In addition to the mechanical problems, neuron loss disrupts linguistic abilities, resulting in reduced vocabulary and syntactic errors. Some persons become mute at a stage before motor disability is severe.

Abnormalities of swallowing, or dysphagia, can cause choking and asphyxia. Dysphagia may involve multiple abnormalities of ingestion, including inappropriate food choices, abnormal rate of eating, poor bolus formation, inadequate respiratory control, weight loss, and aspiration.

Cachexia, or the wasting of muscle with weight loss, is found despite an adequate diet. This appears to be independent of the hyperkinesia and is found in persons with rigidity as well.

Sleep disorders become a progressive problem throughout the course of HD. An increased latent period before sleep and increased periods of wakefulness are common in moderately affected persons. Sleep reversal—daytime somnolence and nighttime restlessness—is seen in severely affected persons and is probably related to the dementia. Choreic movements are reduced during the deepest part of sleep.

Urinary incontinence is often a problem. This could be related to cognitive impairment, depression, decreased mobility, or hyperreflexia of the muscles that control urine output. There can be a concomitant increase in the incidence of urinary tract infections.

### Cognitive Impairment

Cognitive deficits can be detected prior to motor symptoms, with impairments in information processing speed, attention, executive function, and memory retrieval. Individuals with HD also may have limited insight into their deficits, making management more difficult for caregivers and families. There is difficulty with organization, planning, and sequencing, even when all the information is provided. Other prominent abnormalities include visuospatial deficits, impaired judgment, and ideomotor apraxia, the inability to perform previously learned tasks despite intact elementary motor function.

Loss of awareness of deficits in HD is associated with the severity of the disease in terms of CAG repeats, functional decline, motor dysfunction, and cognitive impairment, including memory deficits and executive dysfunction.

### Neuropsychologic and Psychiatric Disorders

Early mental disturbances in persons with HD include personality and behavioral changes, such as irritability, apathy, depression, decreased work performance, violence, impulsivity, and emotional lability. Patterns of psychiatric disorder may relate to the pattern of brain damage with depression, OCD, and emotional regulation related to striatal circuits to the frontal lobe and thalamic nuclei (ventral anterior, medial dorsal). Disinhibition and apathy is likely related to medial prefrontal, anterior cingulate, and anterior temporal paralimbic cortex involvement. Intellectual decline usually follows the personality changes.

More than one-third of persons with HD will develop an affective disorder. Depression is the most common psychiatric condition and does not appear to be simply a reaction to a fatal illness. Evidence for this is the fact that mood disorders are not randomly distributed but occur in subsets of families with HD.

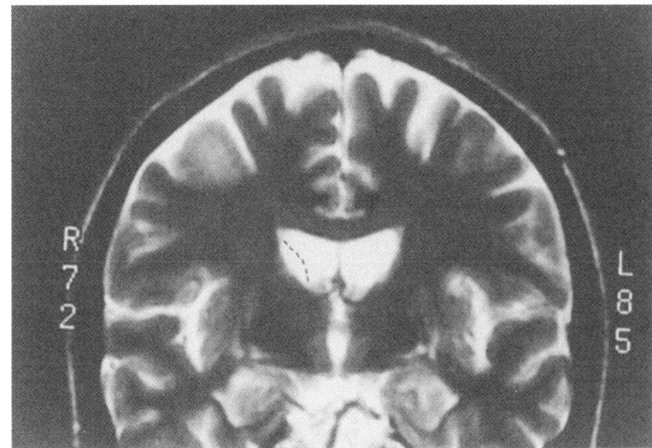


**Figure 31.9**

**Magnetic resonance scan showing the degeneration of the caudate in a person with Huntington disease (HD).** The *dotted lines* show where the tissue would be in a person without HD. (From Ramsey R: *Neuroradiology*, Philadelphia, 1994, WB Saunders.)

## MEDICAL MANAGEMENT

DIAGNOSIS. The clinical diagnosis of HD depends on recognition of patterns of symptoms given in the client's history and clinical signs, and the family history. Difficulties in diagnosis arise when the family history appears negative. Some families deny the presence of cognitive or psychiatric disease. Understanding of the clinical signs must take into account the fact that signs change during the course of the illness. Different patterns may be observed depending on the age of onset. PREDICT-HD found cognitive changes decades before the expected date of motor diagnosis.

MRI demonstrates atrophy of the striatum that is most easily appreciated as enlargement of the frontal horn of the lateral ventricles. Figure 31.9 shows this change in brain structure. This is not of great diagnostic value unless it is very pronounced, given the normal reduction in brain mass with age and the occurrence of atrophy in other disorders that might be confused with HD. PET will also show atrophy, but its value as a diagnostic tool has the same limitations as MRI.

In addition to genetic linkage analysis, which requires testing of family members, it is now possible to evaluate the DNA of an individual to identify specific components that are diagnostic for HD. This eliminates the need to compare DNA of affected family members, but there are still problems with this method, because there is a small percentage of affected individuals who do not display the characteristics on the specific gene and there are nonaffected individuals who carry the gene. Identification of easily obtainable, reliable, and robust biomarkers of HD progression will be important for the development and evaluation of disease-modifying treatments.

Recognition of HD in older persons is critical to establish the genetic link for future generations. Often the diagnosis is overlooked in favor of the label of senile chorea, because there are minimal changes in behavior and cognition. The differential diagnosis of HD in the older population includes various degenerative, systemic, and drug-related conditions. An individual treated with neuroleptics for a psychiatric presentation of HD, for example, may go on to develop movement disorders, and these may be confused with the typical side effects of the medication.

TREATMENT. Management of HD requires a team approach, including medical and social services. Education of clients and their families about the implications of the disease is important. Genetic, psychologic, and social counseling are started as soon as the diagnosis is confirmed. Organizations designed to help families with HD are often of great help. There are two medications that are FDA approved for treatment of chorea, first tetrabenazine (TBZ), and later deutetrabenazine, both that target the dopamine pathway. TBZ is a reversible inhibitor of the vesicle monoamine transporter type 2. It inhibits primarily dopamine and to a lesser degree serotonin and norepinephrine. Side effects include parkinsonism and depression. TBZ had a black box warning for an increased suicide risk, but deutetrabenazine has an improved pharmokinetic profile. Additional medications may be used off label that target excitotoxicity, protein aggregation, translation of the mHtt, and mitochondrial dysfunction, which have shown efficacy in human trials. Numerous other medications have shown efficacy in rodent models, but have not been tested in humans.[82]

A phase 1-2a clinical trial testing IONIS-HTT$_{RX,}$ an antisense oligonucleotide designed to reduce HTT messenger RNA and reduce the presence of mutant huntingtin shows promising results. This medication is delivered intrathecally, with the primary focus being to assure that the treatment was safe. No one enrolled had significant adverse events aside from headaches associated with intrathecal administration, and a dose-dependent relationship of mutant huntingtin was observed in CSF. Functional

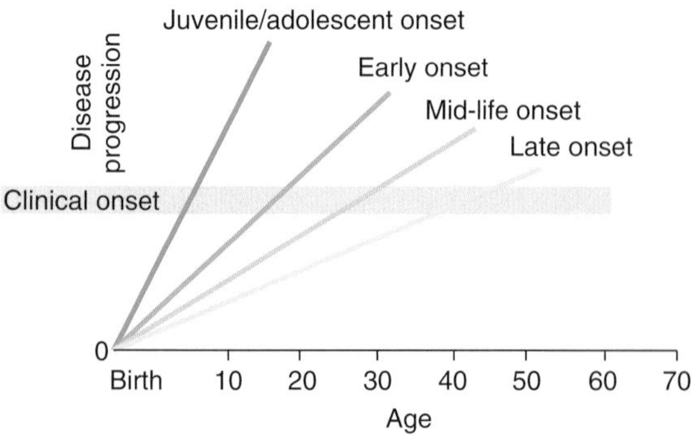


**Figure 31.10**

**Progression of HD related to age at onset.** (From Fahn: *Principles and practice of movement disorders*, ed 2, Philadelphia, 2011, WB Saunders.)

changes were not significant between the placebo and treatment groups, but further trials are underway.[95]

Other medical treatment is primarily symptomatic. Drugs that block dopamine transmission, including anticonvulsants and antipsychotics, may be used off label for the symptomatic relief of chorea. They can also help with the emotional outbursts, paranoia, psychosis, and irritability seen in HD. Drug therapy for chorea should be held in reserve if the abnormal movements are slight. There is a high incidence of side effects with the drugs, including acute dystonias, pseudoparkinsonism, and akathisia, which is characterized by uncontrollable physical restlessness. The most serious effect is chronic tardive dyskinesia resulting in involuntary movement of the face, tongue, and lips. Another adverse reaction is neuroleptic malignant hyperpyrexic syndrome, characterized by fever and rigidity.

Surgical procedures to remove the medial globus pallidus, thought to be overexcited by neuronal loss in the striatum, have been tried with mixed results. A number of case reports of deep brain stimulation to the pallidum and subthalamic nucleus have been published,[33] but not all with positive results.[91] Implantation of adrenal medullary grafts has not been encouraging; the improvement appears to be transient. The use of stem cell transplantation has been studied extensively in animal models of HD, but application to humans is reserved to a few case reports demonstrating disease progression 4 to 6 years post-transplant with the presence of mutant huntingin in the grafts, suggesting this avenue of treatment is not ready for application in people.[5,6,17]

**PROGNOSIS.** It is characteristic of the disease that younger people, with onset of symptoms at age 15 to 40 years, will experience a more severe form of the disease than older people, with onset in their 50s and 60s. The advance of the disease is slow, with death occurring on average 15 to 20 years after onset. Survival into the 80s is not uncommon, and persons living to past 90 years old have been recorded. Age at onset and age at death frequently show a familial correlation. Clinicopathologic studies demonstrate a strong inverse correlation between the age at onset and the severity of striatal degeneration. Figure 31.10 shows the relationship of time of onset to progression of disease.

Increasing disability from involuntary movements and mental changes often results in death from intercurrent infection. Suicide accounts for approximately 6% of deaths, and 25% of persons with HD attempt suicide at least once.

**SPECIAL IMPLICATIONS FOR THE THERAPIST 31.4**

### *Huntington Disease*

Education of the client and family about movement disorders, including gait and safety in mobility, is the basis for therapeutic intervention. *Apraxia*, the inability to perform skilled or purposeful movements, may become severe.This impairment may lead to significant disability in performance of activities of daily living. The client may lose the ability to dress and do self-care activities, such as grooming, regardless of cues provided by caregivers. Positioning to prevent soft-tissue deformities and safety in transfers should be taught according to the current movement disorder identified. Both the therapist and the family should understand that these techniques may need to be changed as the movement disorder progresses. The therapist should be aware that it is possible that chorea and bradykinesia are manifested in the patient at the same time, owing to the progressive neuronal loss in the basal ganglia described earlier. In clients whose bradykinesia is predominant, there is a propensity to freeze, especially in confined spaces, and this may precipitate falls.

Clients with HD do fall, but it is surprising that mobility is maintained despite the seemingly precarious arrangements of the limbs and trunk. As the disease progresses, postural stability becomes impaired and axial chorea may throw the client off balance. Lower scores on the Tinetti mobility test and younger age were significant predictors of falls. Use of a metronome to drive modulation of gait may have a training effect to increase gait speed. Intensive rehabilitation treatments may positively influence the maintenance of functional and motor performance in patients with HD and may last as long as 3 years.

The ability to intervene with neurotherapeutic techniques, including motor learning, may be limited in the face of the concomitant decline in mental function as the motor system impairments progress. Participation in typical activities declines. Role changes, sense of isolation, and concerns for children are commonly described by individuals with HD and therefore should be addressed.

# MULTIPLE SCLEROSIS

## Overview

Multiple sclerosis (MS) is a chronic neurodegenerative disorder of the central nervous system (CNS). The name is descriptive of the sclerotic plaques disseminated throughout the CNS that are the hallmark of the disease. Lesions can be found throughout the brain, spinal cord, and optic nerves. These lesions slow or block neural transmission, resulting in weakness, sensory loss, visual dysfunction, and other symptoms. The course of MS is highly variable and benefits from a multidisciplinary approach to optimize care for individuals with MS. There are many clinical courses (phenotypes) of MS: radiologically isolated syndrome (RIS), clinically isolated syndrome (CIS), relapsing-remitting (RRMS), secondary progressive (SPMS), and primary progressive (PPMS).[57] RIS lacks clinical manifestations but demonstrates abnormal imaging. CIS involves a clinical attack but may or may not be diagnosed as MS depending on dissemination. RRMS is the most common type of MS. It is characterized by relapses or attacks, which are periods of neurologic dysfunction lasting at least 24 hours and followed by full or partial recovery. New symptoms must be at least 30 days apart to qualify as a new attack. RRMS is seen in approximately 85% of newly diagnosed individuals. After presenting with a pattern of RRMS early in the disease course, many patients go on to develop fewer acute relapses and over time develop a more insidious progression of neurologic decline called SPMS. Approximately 60% of patients progress to this stage within 2 decades from onset of disease. PPMS is a steady decline in neurologic function from the onset, with episodes of minimal recovery. PPMS is seen in approximately 15% of newly diagnosed individuals and affects men and women equally. More recently, additional descriptors are recommended to characterize the disease course. The terms active and nonactive should also be used to describe all phenotypes, based upon clinical relapses and MRI activity. Additionally, progressing and nonprogressing should be utilized to specify advancing clinical findings for those with SPMS and PPMS.

## Incidence

MS is typically diagnosed between the ages of 20 and 50 years of age. It affects women more than men, with a 3:1 ratio. Pediatric MS as well as late onset MS can both occur but with much less frequency. There are "cluster" areas where MS is more commonly found, including temperate zones of the United States, Scandinavian countries, northern Europe, southern Canada, New Zealand, and southern Australia. MS can occur in any ethnicity but predominantly affects Caucasians. There are more than 2.3 million persons affected worldwide with an estimated incidence of 3.6 per 100,000 persons.[1] In the United States, it is estimated that nearly 1,000,000 people are living with MS, with about 10,000 new cases per year.[70] Figure 31.11 shows the incidence rates worldwide.

## Etiologic and Risk Factors

The cause of MS remains unknown. It is theorized that MS is triggered by a combination of multiple factors, including infection, immunologic response, genetics, and environmental factors. One theorized cause is an abnormal autoimmune response triggered by an infection or virus, with ongoing research on the Epstein-Barr virus and human herpes virus 6 and their association with MS. Repeated studies suggest that infection with Epstein-Barr virus (EBV) increases a person's risk of developing MS. An increase in immunoglobulin and oligoclonal bands

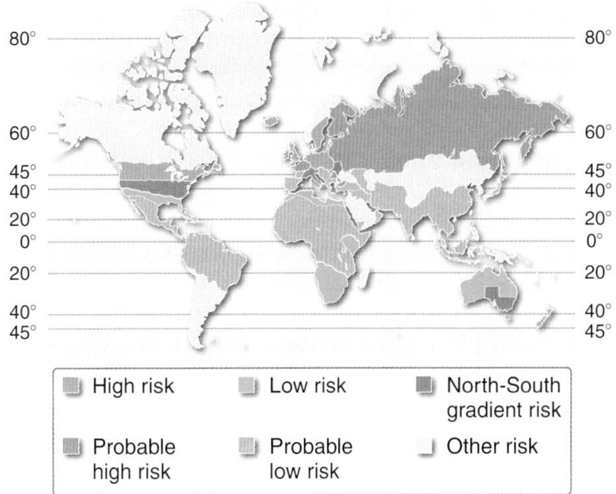


**Figure 31.11**

**World map showing the relative incidence of multiple sclerosis.** Areas of greatest risk are in the northern latitudes. (Adapted from National Institute of Neurological and Communicative Disorders and Stroke: *Multiple sclerosis: hope through research*. Publication no. 79-75, Washington, DC, 1981, National Institutes of Health. In Umphred DA: *Neurological rehabilitation*, ed 5, St Louis, 2007, Mosby.)

in the cerebrospinal fluid, used as a diagnostic indicator, supports the role of infection as a factor in disease development. In addition, viral infection often precipitates an attack of MS, infection being the only natural event that unequivocally increases the risk of a relapse of MS. Less than 10% of infections are followed by relapses, but more than one-third of the relapses are proceeded by infection.

There is a clear genetic component in the risk of developing MS. When one parent is affected, especially if that parent developed MS before 20 years of age, a child has a fivefold higher risk of developing MS. Absence of the inhibitory *KIR2DL3* gene has been associated with the development of MS, but there does not seem to be an association between the presence or absence of *KIR* genes with clinical disease parameters. There have been more than 100 MS genetic risk loci identified in research, but these only explain a part of the heritability of the disease. Many of these genes are associated with immune-response proteins that are active in the pathophysiology of the disease.[7] The human leukocyte antigen (HLA) region (HLA-DRB1) is clearly associated with MS. However, interactions with other genes that increase risk are complex and may involve multiple weak links that are difficult to identify using current research methods. In Scotland, where risk of developing MS is high, there is an increase in the incidence of the HLA-DR2 allele in the population, which has a proven association with MS. A variety of genes have been associated with the disease, including interleukin-1b receptor, interleukin-1 receptor antagonist, and immunoglobulin Fc receptor. Twin studies shed light on genetic components as well as the importance of other factors that may or may not cause MS. For example, an identical twin with the same genetic make-up of someone with MS has a 25% chance of developing the disease. Genetic studies have shown that major histocompatibility complex (MHC) proteins are linked with MS.

Coexisting autoimmune disorders are seen in a majority of individuals, such as Hashimoto thyroiditis, psoriasis, inflammatory bowel disease, and rheumatoid arthritis. Families with a history of MS have autoimmune disorders in greater than 65% of first-degree relatives. Hashimoto thyroiditis, psoriasis, and inflammatory bowel disease are the most common disorders also occurring in family members. The presence of various immune disorders in families with several members with MS suggests that the disease might arise on a background of a generalized susceptibility to autoimmune disorders. The impact of hormone levels is also being investigated. Relapse rates may decline 70% in the third trimester of pregnancy, most likely from circulating levels of estriol. This suggests a complex hormonal modulation of the immune system.

Environmental factors can increase susceptibility to developing MS and affect its disease course. There is an inverse correlation between vitamin D levels and the risk of developing MS, which may explain the impact of geographic location and the development of MS. Smoking and obesity are additional factors that increase risk of an MS diagnosis, as well as negatively impact prognosis.

## Pathogenesis

MS is the classic example of a primary demyelinating disorder, but demyelination alone does not account for the persistent functional disturbances that characterize the disease as it progresses. After myelin is damaged, nerve conduction properties, initially abnormal, can recover, in part related to redistribution of sodium channels. Myelin loss occurs initially around the small veins and venules in the brain and spinal cord. Focal abnormalities referred to as plaques are disseminated throughout the CNS, especially in the white matter surrounding the ventricles, the optic nerves, and the brainstem. However, MS is not a disease of the white matter only—MS plaques may also affect the gray matter, and MS affects CNS tissue outside of the plaques. The corpus callosum is usually involved in MS. Spinal cord pathology has been hypothesized to be an important factor in disease progression in primary progressive MS but is not always predictive.

The pathologic conditions that occur in MS include inflammation, demyelination, axon loss, and gliosis. MS has traditionally been considered a predominantly T cell–mediated inflammatory disorder, but there is increasing evidence that B cell–mediated autoimmunity is an important mechanism in CNS tissue damage in MS. Demyelination can result from either direct damage to neuronal myelin by immune-mediated mechanisms, or indirectly because of the extracellular environment. This demyelination can cause neurons to be more susceptible to apoptosis. Although demyelination may lead to clinical relapses that occur during the disease, long-term disability is primarily caused by irreversible axon loss and cell death.

The initial event in MS may be priming of autoreactive, peripheral T cells against myelin antigens by an infectious agent. It is thought that preexisting autoreactive T cells are activated outside the CNS by foreign microbes, self-proteins, or microbial superantigens. Activated T cells cross the blood-brain barrier through a multistep process. In this trafficking process, lymphocytes attached to endothelial cells proceed to pass through the endothelial cell cytoplasm (transcellular route) or through the inter-endothelial junctions (paracellular route). Chemokines, like cytokines, are secreted polypeptides that can induce increased production of integrin molecules by lymphocytes and switch these integrin molecules into a higher affinity state that allows lymphocytes to transmigrate more effectively across CNS endothelium. The activated T cells secrete cytokines that stimulate microglial cells and astrocytes, recruit additional inflammatory cells, and induce antibody production by plasma cells. Antimyelin antibodies, activated macrophages or microglial cells, and tumor necrosis factor are thought to cooperate in producing demyelination. The oligodendrocyte produces the myelin that wraps around the axon of the nerve cell. The myelin sheath increases the speed of the action potential and is critical for smooth and rapid movement. In the inflammatory milieu, excessive amounts of glutamate are released by lymphocytes, microglia, and macrophages. The glutamate activates various glutamate receptors, causing the influx of calcium through ion channels associated with toxic damage to oligodendrocytes and axons. Multiple factors other than glutamate-mediated mechanisms contribute to axonal loss in MS. Axonal loss in MS is present from the onset of disease, and with accumulation over time, it is responsible for progression in disability. An illustration of the mechanisms of the disease is provided in Figure 31.12.

Brain atrophy is a clinically relevant component in MS and begins early in the disease course. The caudate nucleus (part of the basal ganglia) can be smaller in volume and also have changes in shape. Cortical demyelination may influence dendrite and axon function and decrease neuronal viability, which may further activate disease progression. Axonotmesis as a result of inflammation in MS lesions can lead to retrograde neuronal degeneration and apoptosis. In chronic lesions, demyelinated axons undergo a slow, disseminating Wallerian degeneration along neural tracts away from the initial site of injury, contributing to long-term disability.

New plaques frequently appear at new sites or within or at the edges of previously stable lesions. New lesions can form within or overlap shadow plaques (areas of thin remyelination) and may contribute to failed remyelination or the conversion of shadow plaques into classic demyelinated plaques. Thus some lesions may appear to be quite large.

The plaques may be acute or chronic lesions. The acute plaques are small, circumscribed areas of hypercellularity, demyelination, and axonal loss. Astrogliosis, resulting in scar tissue formation, is more severe in MS lesions than in most other neuropathologic conditions. Inflammatory infiltrates consisting of macrophages, T cells, B cells, and microglia fill the plaque. Axons passing through may be spared, but there seems to be more and more evidence of axon loss within the plaques. New active plaques are pink, with faint borders that exhibit an intense inflammatory response. Old inactive plaques are gray and firm, with sharp edges with a gliotic background crossed by axons but lacking oligodendrocytes.

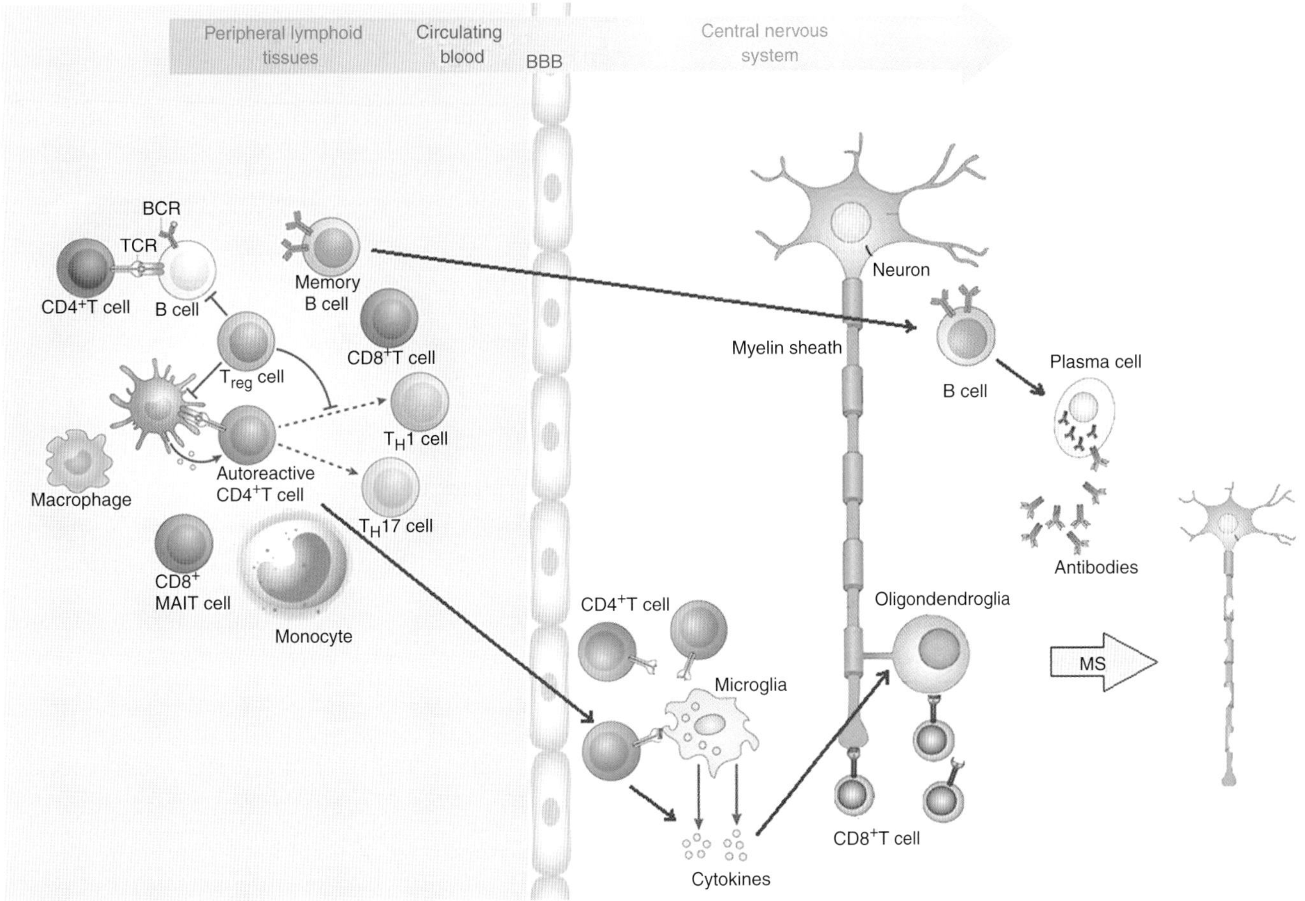


**Figure 31.12**

**Pathophysiology of multiple sclerosis.** (From Dolati S, et al: Multiple sclerosis: therapeutic applications of advancing drug delivery systems, *Biomed Pharmacother* 86:343–353, 2017)

A variety of pathogenic mechanisms may be involved in the development of MS plaques, which occur as a result of diversity in the sequence of events that causes the condition to arise. The features of the lesions, including the amount and nature of T cell–, macrophage-, and immunoglobulin-related damage, seem to vary from individual to individual, but there is much less variation among the active lesions within an individual. For example, the survival of oligodendrocytes varies among individuals. In some individuals, it appears that oligodendrocyte dystrophy and apoptosis are the primary cause of demyelination. In others, the presence of immunoglobulins suggests that demyelinating antibodies have a pathogenic role. As with demyelination, axonal destruction could result from direct immunologic attack or inflammatory mediators or from secondary effects of chronic demyelination. As in other chronic inflammatory diseases of the CNS, vascular pathology is profound in the brains of patients with MS, seen both within the lesions and in normal-appearing white matter. Inflammatory changes occur in the perivascular space. Dysfunction of the blood-brain barrier is shown by changes in endothelial tight junctions. In chronic lesions, vascular fibrosis is common. The relation between inflammation, blood-brain barrier damage, and structural vascular pathology is complex. Serum protein leakage from vessels is seen in early stages of the disease and seems to decrease with progression. Widespread hypoperfusion in normal-appearing white matter and in cortical and deep gray matter has been recorded in patients with relapsing-remitting MS and progressive MS.

## Clinical Manifestations

An individual with MS will have symptoms based on the location of the MS lesion(s). Common initial clinical presentations are optic neuritis, sensory changes, and weakness. Symptoms are often unpredictable and can be visible or invisible. An interdisciplinary approach should be used to manage the variety of symptoms.

In most individuals, MS is characterized by progressive disability over time, but the amount of accumulated disability varies widely. A benign course may affect up to 10% of individuals and is characterized by an abrupt onset, with one or a few relapses followed by complete or near complete remitting periods. These individuals experience little or no permanent disability and remain relatively symptom free. This is a designation that can only be made with certainty retrospectively as there are no perfect prognostic markers. More recent MRI scan data suggest that even in individuals with benign MS there is the likelihood for progression of lesions. Each individual's CNS appears to have a different threshold for producing symptoms and signs reflecting the affected regions of the CNS. This threshold, or the capacity of the individual's brain to adapt to the lesions, will determine the severity of the clinical manifestations.

### Visual Changes

Optic neuritis is often the first manifestation of MS. The optic nerve is an extension of the cerebral cortex, virtually a tract of the CNS, and is therefore subject to the effects of demyelination, with the syndrome of optic neuritis. Optic neuritis typically presents as a unilateral, painful decrease or loss of vision. It is commonly associated with visual field defects, decreased color vision, and reduced clarity of vision. Individuals with optic neuritis must be carefully evaluated for an ocular mobility abnormality to determine the possibility of a second anatomically distinct lesion, because the symptoms of blurring may be caused by an eye movement disorder.

There can also be gaze palsies, the loss of active control of eye movement, and nystagmus, involuntary rhythmic movement of the eye. Intranuclear ophthalmoplegia (INO) is the most common gaze palsy, resulting in lateral gaze paralysis, and is caused by demyelination of the pontine medial longitudinal fasciculus, an area of the brain's white matter involved in the control of eye movement. Other lesions in the brainstem and reticular formation can cause other palsies, resulting in difficulty with conjugate gaze and ipsilateral gaze palsy.

Other abnormalities of ocular mobility, such as instability of fixation or inability to suppress the vestibulo-ocular response, are related to lesions involving brainstem nuclei and tracts. Vertigo, the sensation of spinning, may appear suddenly and in dramatic fashion, with gait unsteadiness and vomiting. In MS, this reflects a brainstem rather than end organ vestibular disorder; a careful look at associated brainstem symptoms will help to distinguish the cause.

### Sensory Changes

Sensory changes are also common initial complaints. This is often a paresthesia or dysesthesia noted in one extremity or in the head and face. Often these symptoms are transient and may not be reported. It is usually when multiple symptoms occur or the symptoms are unchanging that a person seeks medical attention. Dorsal column symptoms include paresthesias (tingling, pricking) and hypoesthesia (diminished sensitivity). These may begin in an extremity and ascend over hours or several days to include the rest of the leg or arm, the perineum, the trunk, and perhaps other body areas. Other sensory complaints include a feeling of swelling, of wetness, sometimes itching, or that the body part is tightly wrapped. Involvement of a cord level is diagnostically helpful in distinguishing this attack from a peripheral neuropathologic incident. Other positive dorsal column signs are loss of vibration and position sense. Sensory complaints are often not substantiated by objective findings, especially if the symptoms are mild or remission has already begun before the individual is examined. For example, the feeling of numbness may not result in a loss of response to pinprick.

### Pain

Pain is common in MS, occurring in over 50% of individuals. The pain usually is a burning neuropathic type but can also be musculoskeletal in nature. The distribution of the pain may not follow any recognizable neurologic distribution. It can be paroxysmal in nature but often is fairly constant. Trigeminal neuralgia is a common example of this type of painful, paroxysmal symptom. This lancinating, electrical sensation along the distribution of a branch of the trigeminal nerve can be terribly disabling. It may be a standalone problem in some individuals, but is also a symptom associated with MS. Another clinical symptom is Lhermitte's sign, a momentary electricity-like sensation in the spine and lower extremities evoked by neck flexion or cough.

### Weakness/Motor Control

Weakness in MS usually is a result of demyelination and axonal loss. Signs of muscle weakness secondary to damage of the motor cortex and tracts reflect the loss of orderly recruitment and rate modulation of motor neurons. Muscle activation patterns and agonist–antagonist relationships are disturbed. The use of excessive resistive exercises may contribute to fatigue and give the appearance of increasing weakness. Heat, either from increased ambient temperature or from fever, often increases weakness. This may be the result of a conduction block. Uhthoff phenomenon, or a pseudoexacerbation, is a temporary worsening of neurologic symptoms that can occur when one's core temperature increases, but it does not increase disease activity. Avoidance of heat or use of cooling devices/environments often allows more efficient conduction and improved strength if there is appropriate innervation. Spasm or weakness of facial muscles can also be seen. Dysarthria, abnormal speech resulting from poor control of the muscles of speech, and dysphagia, including signs of gurgling, coughing, weight loss, pneumonia, choking, or a weak voice, can present as a result of brainstem involvement.

### Coordination

Coordination (ataxia) problems and tremor are among the most difficult symptoms to manage. Compensatory techniques via exercise can be helpful. Cerebellar syndrome deficits may be symmetric, with all four limbs involved, or asymmetric, with only one side affected. Manifestations include ataxia, hypotonia, and truncal weakness, causing postural and movement disorders. Dysarthria of cerebellar origin (scanning speech, producing abnormalities in the rhythm of speech) is common. Cerebellar signs are often associated with the progressive phases of the illness.

### Fatigue

The most common and often most disabling symptom of MS is fatigue. Many patients recall that fatigue often preceded diagnosis or the occurrence of identifiable neurologic lesions by several years. Fatigue is typically present in midafternoon and may take the form of increased motor weakness with effort, mental fatigue, and sleepiness. MS-related fatigue presents as an overwhelming feeling of tiredness in those who have not exerted themselves and are not depressed. Neuromuscular or short-circuiting fatigue is common and can be central in origin. The demyelinated nerve fires again and again until it shorts when it is called upon to do a repetitive task. Short breaks with energy conservation, can make this fatigue less prominent.

Sleep dysfunction is related to fatigue in MS. Excessive limb movements, nocturia, and pain are the main symptoms resulting in fragmented sleep and poor sleep efficiency in MS. Insomnia is a common complaint, with pain and discomfort being linked to sleep initiation insomnia, and nocturia being linked to sleep maintenance insomnia.

### Tone and Spasticity

Spasticity, velocity-dependent stiffness about a joint, is an extremely common problem with MS, caused by abnormal firing of the ascending and descending excitatory and inhibitory pathways in the brain and spinal cord. It can vary from nonexistent to severe, even in the same person, and from moment to moment, making its management challenging. GABA and other neurotransmitters are involved. Those who have significant spasticity and weakness may use their spasticity to walk, transfer, and manage their daily living. Treatment becomes a consideration if the spasticity is causing discomfort, pain, or problems with daily living. Pain, either from an injury or from a bladder infection, exacerbates spasticity. Thus, the management of spasticity begins with the removal of noxious stimuli. In some individuals, spasticity can be intractable. The high doses of medications necessitated by this circumstance sedate and cause disability on their own. Spasms may accompany the spasticity and usually are more severe and frequent at night. They often interrupt the sleep cycle, even in those who do not recognize their awakenings. This may lead to severe fatigue the next day; thus, minimizing nocturnal spasms is important.

### Speech and Swallowing

Speech impairments may include dysarthria and dysphonia and are often related to muscle weakness. Swallowing impairments (i.e., dysphagia) are often due to impaired coordination of tongue and oral muscles. Individuals with more advanced MS with dysphagia may be at risk for developing aspiration pneumonia, a serious medical condition that can lead to death.

### Cognitive Dysfunction

Cognitive impairments can occur in any stage of MS and may affect more than 50% of those with MS. Changes may include decreased attention, concentration, memory, impaired executive function, and slowed processing speed. The ability to perform dual tasks and sustain divided attention can be reduced in individuals with MS.

### Affective Changes

Depression is a primary symptom of MS, occurring because of actual changes in the brain and its chemistry. Depression can occur as a direct result of the MS plaques or as a reaction to the diagnosis or disability. Depression may lead to greater disability than that caused by the level of neurologic impairment. Medication use for other symptoms may contribute to the cognitive problems with sedation and confusion; thus, these must be reviewed regularly in those who have dulled cognition. Depression may be an additive culprit and is treatable if recognized. There is no question that reactive (exogenous) depression occurs frequently in MS and is amenable to counseling and other nonpharmacologic techniques, but the brain disease seen in MS clearly leads to chemical (endogenous) depression in many. The suicide rate for MS seems greater than that for many other neurologic diseases. Pseudobulbar affect can be found in individuals with more progressive disability.

### Bladder and Bowel Dysfunction

Bladder and bowel symptoms are common and usually occur when the spinal cord is involved. Bladder urgency, frequency, and incontinence associated with an overactive bladder are often seen early in the disease and generally precede incontinence. Bladder issues are prominent in those who have MS. Bladder impairment can be manifest with frequency, urgency, hesitancy, and incontinence with differing mechanisms. Most frequent is the small, failure-to-store bladder characterized by a low postvoid residual, often with uncontrolled contractions. This can be measured by catheterization or ultrasound.

More problematic from a management point of view is the large, failure-to-empty bladder. It overfills with residuals from 200 to 900 mL and presents with similar symptomatology despite looking different anatomically and physiologically. Frequently, there is a dyssynergia between the bladder and the urinary sphincter, causing similar symptoms from yet another mechanism. Residual urine after emptying, with subsequent overflow incontinence and heightened risk of urinary tract infections, is a problem for 50% of persons with MS, especially later in the course of the disease. This may require intermittent or chronic catheterization, or use of the Credé method (manual pressure on the bladder to express urine).

Neurogenic disorders may also impair bowel function, resulting in incontinence or constipation. Bowel function is affected less than bladder function but can be problematic. Irritable bowel is a common associated problem, and regulating the bowel often means changing treatments, depending on the circumstances. It is better to be slightly constipated than slightly loose.

### Sexual Dysfunction

Sexual expression may require special attention in MS, considering its impact on relationships. Men may experience erectile dysfunction, decreased sensation, difficulty with ejaculation, and loss of libido. Females may experience vaginal dryness, decreased or altered sensation in the vaginal area, loss of libido, and difficulty in achieving orgasms. Although pregnancy may affect relapse rates as previously mentioned, no studies have found MS to have a negative impact on fertility and sustaining a healthy pregnancy.

## MEDICAL MANAGEMENT

DIAGNOSIS. The McDonald Criteria of the International Panel on Diagnosis of MS, updated in 2017, is used to diagnose MS (Table 31.5).[99] The diagnosis of MS must show evidence of dissemination in time and space. The

**Table 31.5** The 2017 McDonald Criteria for Diagnosis of MS Clinical Presentation and Additional Data Needed for MS Diagnosis

| Number of Clinical Attacks | Number of Lesions with Objective Physical Evidence | Additional Data Needed for MS Diagnosis |
|---|---|---|
| ≥2 | ≥2 | None[a] |
| ≥2 | 1 (as well as clear-cut historical evidence of a previous attack involving a lesion in a distinct anatomic location) | None[a] |
| ≥2 | 1 | Dissemination in space demonstrated by an additional clinical attack implicating a different CNS site or by MRI[b] |
| 1 | ≥2 | Dissemination in time demonstrated by an additional clinical attack or by MRI[b] OR demonstration of CSF-specific oligoclonal bands |
| 1 | 1 | Dissemination in space demonstrated by an additional clinical attack implicating a different CNS site or by MRI[c] AND Dissemination in time demonstrated by an additional clinical attack or by MRI OR demonstration of CSF-specific oligoclonal bands |

If the 2017 McDonald criteria are fulfilled and there is no better explanation for the clinical presentation, the diagnosis is MS. If MS is suspected by virtue of a clinically isolated syndrome but the criteria are not completely met, the diagnosis is possible MS. If another diagnosis arises during the evaluation that better explains the clinical presentation, then the diagnosis is not MS.

[a]An attack (relapse; exacerbation) is defined as patient-reported or objectively observed events typical of an acute inflammatory demyelinating event in the CNS, current or historical, with duration of at least 24 hours, in the absence of fever or infection. It should be documented by contemporaneous neurologic examination, but some historical events with symptoms and evolution characteristic for MS, but for which no objective neurologic findings are documented, can provide reasonable evidence of a prior demyelinating event. However, reports of paroxysmal symptoms (historical or current) should consist of multiple episodes occurring over not less than 24 hours. Before a definite diagnosis of MS can be made, at least one attack must be corroborated by findings on neurologic examination, visual evoked potential response in patients reporting prior visual disturbance, or MRI consistent with demyelination in the area of the CNS implicated in the historical report of neurologic symptoms.

[b]No additional tests are required to demonstrate dissemination in space and time. However, unless MRI is not possible, brain MRI should be obtained in all patients in whom the diagnosis of MS is being considered. Spinal cord MRI or CSF examination should be considered in patients with insufficient clinical and MRI evidence supporting MS. If imaging and other tests are undertaken and are negative, caution needs to be taken before making a diagnosis of MS, and alternative diagnoses should be considered.

[c]Clinical diagnosis based on objective clinical findings for two attacks is most secure. Reasonable historical evidence for one past attack, in the absence of documented objective neurologic findings, can include historical events with symptoms and evolution characteristics for a prior inflammatory demyelinating event; at least one attack, however, must be supported by objective findings.

From Sheremata W, Tornes L: Multiple sclerosis and the spinal cord, *Neurol Clin* 31(1):55–77, 2013.

presence of both gadolinium-enhancing and nonenhancing lesions on the baseline MRI can substitute for a follow-up scan to confirm dissemination in time, as long as it can be reliably determined that the gadolinium-enhancing lesion is not due to non-MS pathology.[99] Box 31.10 shows some examples of diseases for which differential screening should be done. In addition to MRI, lumbar puncture assessing for oligoclonal bands in the CSF can be used for dissemination in time. Evoked potentials can detect slowing of conduction, suggesting demyelination.

Gray matter lesions are different from white matter lesions, showing little T cell inflammation or disruption of the blood-brain barrier but with leakage of plasma proteins. Cortical demyelination might be primarily related to meningeal inflammation. Within the white matter, glutamate excitotoxicity and mitochondrial dysfunction have the potential to cause axonal damage with secondary effects in the cortex.

MS is associated with lesions within the spinal cord. The spinal cord may be abnormal when the brain MRI is normal. However, an abnormal spinal cord is found more than half the time when there are nine or more brain lesions.

The whole spinal cord can be imaged with high resolution and phased-array coils, showing abnormalities in 80% to 90% of individuals with MS, usually without accompanying neurologic symptoms or signs. Incidental spinal cord lesions do not occur with aging and are rarely reported in other immune-mediated disorders. Most individuals with early MS have lesions within the spinal cord. But imaging may not be performed, so they may not be dentified. Spinal cord lesions tend to increase as the number of brain lesions rises; this is associated with higher risk for a second attack and a diagnosis of clinical MS. Ultimately, abnormal brain MRI scans are present in more than 90% of individuals with clinically definite MS. Normal brain MRI scans may represent disease that is relatively restricted to the spinal cord. Reductions in nerve fiber density are seen in the spinal cord, including in otherwise normal-appearing tissue, and are likely related to permanent disability. Axonal loss can be profound in later stages of disease.

Figure 31.13 shows the plaques seen on MRI. The lesions do not always correlate with the clinical signs, and there can be evidence of focal lesions in the absence of disease. In fact, the vast majority of enhancing lesions are considered to be asymptomatic when they first appear on the brain scan. However, there is a correlation between periods of clinical worsening of the disease and increases in the total number of lesions, the number of new lesions, and the total area of enhancement on MRI. Thus, enhanced lesions on brain MRI after a first event

Box 31.10

**DIFFERENTIAL DIAGNOSIS OF MULTIPLE SCLEROSIS**

***Other Inflammatory Demyelinating Central Nervous Symptom Conditions***

- Acute disseminated encephalomyelitis
- Neuromyelitis optica

***Systemic or Organ-Specific Inflammatory Diseases***

- Systemic lupus erythematosus
- Sjögren syndrome
- Inflammatory bowel disease
- Vasculitis
- Periarteritis nodosa
- Primary central nervous sytem angitis
- Susac syndrome
- Eales disease
- Granulomatous diseases
- Sarcoidosis

***Infectious Disorders***

- Lyme neuroborreliosis
- Syphilis
- Viral myelitis
- Progressive multifocal leukoencephalitis
- Subacute sclerosing panencephalitis

***Cerebrovascular Disorders***

- Multiple emboli
- Hypercoaguable states
- Sneddon's syndrome
- Neoplasms
- Metastasis
- Lymphoma
- Paraneoplastic syndromes

***Metabolic Disorders***

- Vitamin $B_{12}$ deficiency
- Vitamin E deficiency
- Central (or extra) pontine myelinolysis
- Leukodystrophies (especially adrenomyleoneuropathy)
- Leber hereditary optic neuropathy

***Structural Lesions***

- Spinal cord compression
- Chiari malformation
- Syringomyelia/syringobulbia
- Foramen magnum lesions
- Spinal arteriovenous malformation/dural fistula

***Degenerative Diseases***

- Hereditary spastic paraparesis
- Spinocerebellar degeneration
- Olivopontocerebellar atrophy

***Psychiatric Disorders***

- Conversion reactions
- Malingering

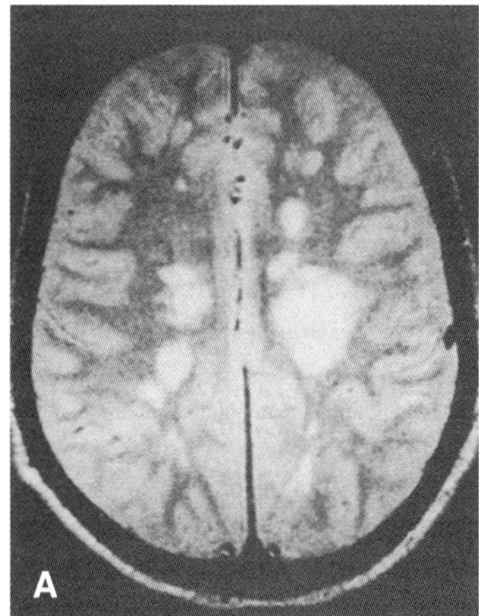

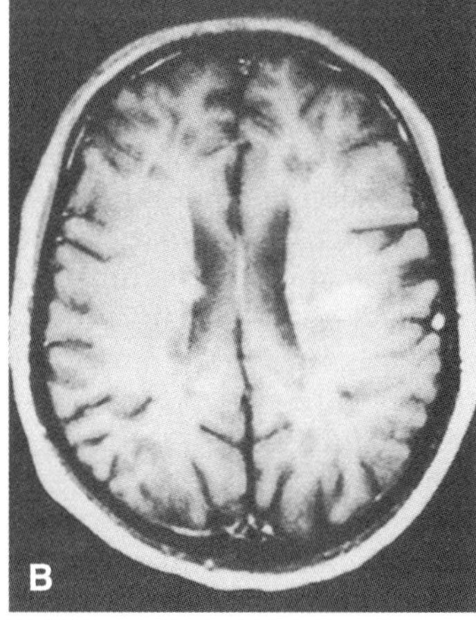

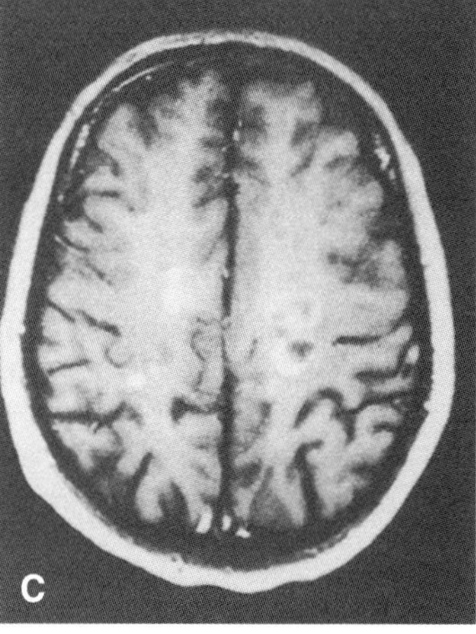


**Figure 31.13**

(A) Typical scattered, variably sized plaques in the brain associated with the diagnosis of multiple sclerosis (MS). (B) Contrast-enhanced magnetic resonance imaging reveals scattered area of solid and ring-shaped enhancement. (C) Note the atrophy, greater than would be expected for the person's age, a common finding in MS. (From Ramsey R: *Neuroradiology,* Philadelphia, 1994, WB Saunders.)

is highly prognostic of development of clinically definite MS. Figure 31.14 shows an example of aggressive MS over 2 years revealed in MRI imaging.

Contrast enhancement in CT and MRI suggests inflammation but is more accurately a measure of leakage of moderate-size molecules across the damaged tight junctions of the CNS endothelium. The enhancement pattern (size, shape, solid versus ring) may be variable within and more so between individuals, which reflects a heterogeneous pathology. Ring enhancement, for example, may suggest a more severe pathology. Figure 31.15 demonstrates the development of a T2-weighted hyperintense lesion by serial MRI. Monitoring serial MRI studies with enhancement helps to identify agents that may be active against the early inflammatory stage of MS. Figure 31.16 shows changes related to progressive forms of MS. Functional MRI maps the brain areas activated using a task paradigm. Functional disturbances have

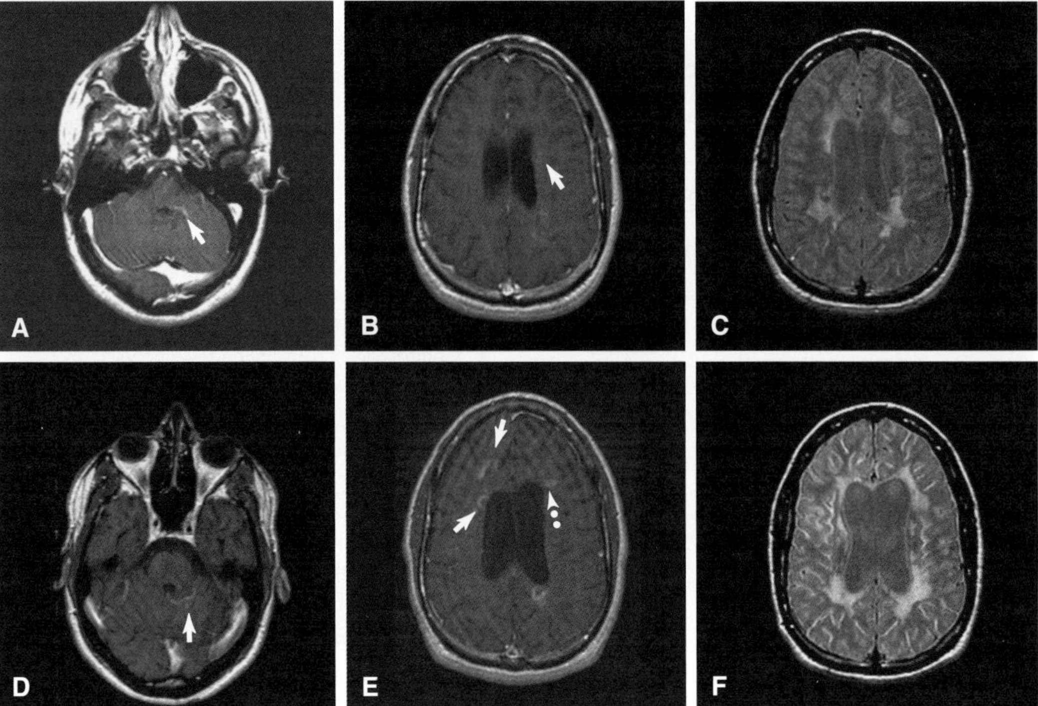


**Figure 31.14**

**Aggressive multiple sclerosis over 2 years.** Disease was initially relapsing-remitting but converted relatively quickly to secondary progressive MS. *Top row:* Contrast-enhanced left pons (A) and left frontal-parietal white matter (B), both showing a relatively rare edge enhancement pattern *(arrows)*. Typical confluent T2 hyperintensities and mild-moderate volume loss based on lateral ventricle size (C). *Bottom row:* Two years later magnetic resonance image shows different edge-enhancing lesions *(arrows)* in posterior fossa (D) and both edge enhancement *(arrows)* and ring enhancement *(dotted arrow)* in deep white matter along the lateral ventricles (E). Progressive volume loss based on moderately large lateral ventricles and more extensive confluent T2 hyperintensity is seen in (F). (From Simon JH: Update on Multiple Sclerosis, *Radiologic Clinics of North America* 44(1):79-100, 2006.)

been the basis for hypotheses suggesting that compensatory mechanisms develop in early MS, which initially may mask injury and delay the appearance of dysfunction. Functional disturbance may only become apparent after exhaustion of these adaptive mechanisms. Fatigue severity is correlated with the reduction in thalamic and cerebellar activation. Although abnormal functional MRI patterns may be observed in given individuals with MS, their interpretation may not be straightforward. Functional MRI findings reflect functional adaptation, they do not necessarily serve as direct evidence for gray matter pathology.

Functional MRI appears to identify sensorimotor and cognitive disturbances in MS. The most consistent finding by functional MRI studies in populations of individuals with MS is impairment in sensorimotor activation indicated by abnormally increased contralateral blood oxygenation level and ipsilateral supplementary motor activation. Sensorimotor functional MRI is sensitive even in the early stages of disease.

Measures of regional brain atrophy are useful to determine neuropsychologic dysfunction. Imaging data suggest that neuropsychologic impairment in MS is related, in part, to atrophy of gray matter regions and in the juxtacortical areas. Gray matter atrophy is associated with impairments in verbal memory, euphoria, and disinhibition.

Whole-brain atrophy reflects the destructive aspects of the disease. The data linking brain atrophy to clinical impairments suggest that irreversible tissue destruction is a major determinant of disease progression, whereas white matter lesion activity has less correlation. The strongest correlations between MRI measures and disability may be those provided by atrophy measures. Confounding factors must be considered when assessing whether loss of brain volume directly indicates tissue atrophy. Secondary progressive disease causes significantly more atrophy of both white matter and gray matter and a significantly higher lesion load than relapsing-remitting disease. Primary progressive disorders show decreased numbers and volume of enhancing lesions, related to the less intense inflammation.

PET scans and functional MRI show widespread cerebral hypometabolism and selective hypometabolism in the bifrontal and basal ganglial regions in MS. The regional analysis of deep and cortical gray matter atrophy suggests an association between the neurodegenerative process taking place in the striatum–thalamus–frontal cortex pathway and the development of fatigue in relapsing-remitting MS. The inclusion of the posterior parietal cortex as one of the best predictors of the modified fatigue impact scale cognitive domain suggests the major role of the posterior attentional system in determining cognitive fatigue in relapsing-remitting MS.

CSF analysis often shows increased mononuclear cell pleocytosis, an elevation in total immunoglobulins, and the presence of oligoclonal bands. These responses suggest an inflammatory response in the CNS. In 85%

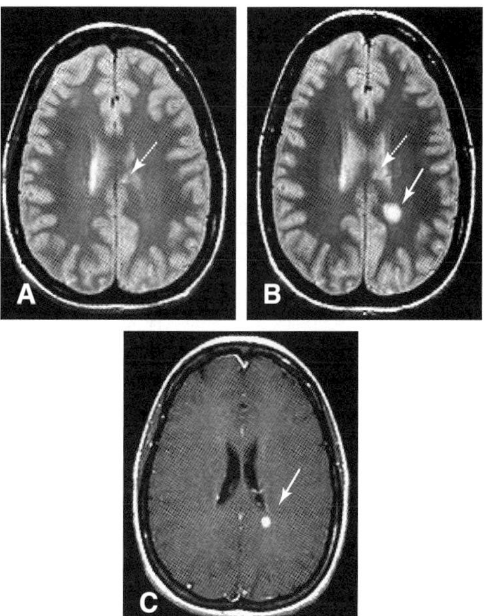


**Figure 31.15**

**Development of a T2 hyperintense lesion by serial magnetic resonance imaging.** (A) Case of relapsing multiple sclerosis with low T2 hyperintense lesion burden, including chronic lesions in the corpus callosum *(arrow)*. (B) One month later, a new T2 hyperintense lesion develops in the left parietal-occipital white matter *(solid arrow)*, whereas the corpus callosum lesions remain stable *(dotted arrow)*. (C) Corresponding enhancement in acute lesion *(arrow)* from blood-brain barrier breakdown and concurrent inflammation. (From Simon JH: Update on Multiple Sclerosis, *Radiologic Clinics of North America* 44(1):79-100, 2006.)

to 95% of individuals with clinically definite MS, these values are abnormal. In people with suspected MS, the number is much lower. Abnormal values, including oligoclonal bands, also may be seen in a smaller percentage of those with a variety of disorders, especially other inflammatory or infectious disorders that may affect the CNS. Metabolites from the breakdown of myelin may also be detected in CSF but are very nonspecific.

Evoked potential response testing may detect slowed or abnormal conduction in visual, auditory, somatosensory, or motor pathways. These tests employ computer averaging techniques to record the electrical response evoked in the nervous system following repetitive sensory or motor stimuli. Evoked potentials are abnormal in up to 90% of individuals who have clinically definite MS. Testing can provide evidence of a second lesion in an individual with a single clinically apparent lesion, or it can demonstrate an objective abnormality in an individual with subjective complaints and a normal examination.

Myelography and CT are both insensitive to the pathologic changes in MS and should not be used where the diagnosis of MS is a possibility. Both may still be used to rule out other disorders that mimic MS symptoms.

**PHARMACOLOGIC TREATMENT.** Pharmacologic management for MS may include disease modifying agents for the MS disease course and reduce relapse rates, treatment for management of relapses, and symptom management. The availability of MS-specific agents has expanded in recent years, summarized in Table 31.6.

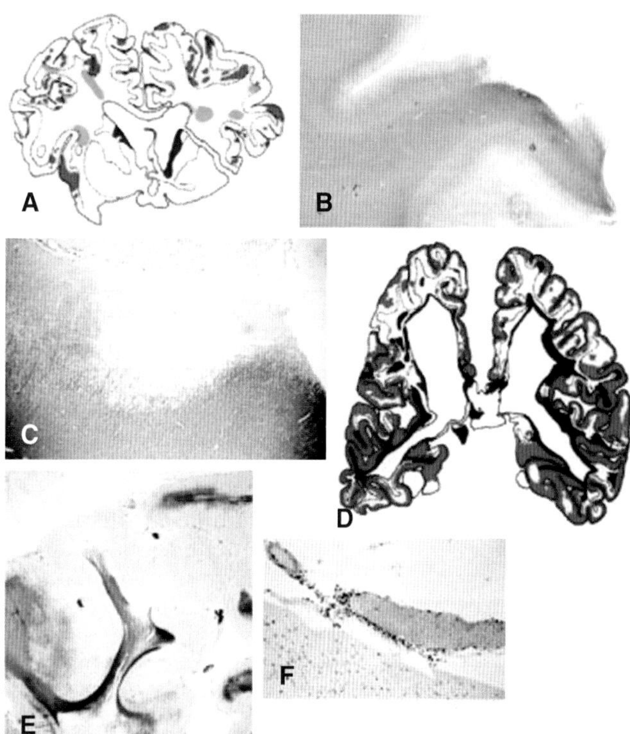


**Figure 31.16**

**Cortical plaques in progressive forms of multiple sclerosis (MS).** Cortical demyelination and diffuse white matter inflammation are hallmarks of primary progressive MS (PPMS) and secondary progressive MS (SPMS). (A and D) Schematic lesion maps based on whole hemispheric sections from two archival cases of progressive MS. Case A (PPMS): A 37-year-old man with a history of gradually progressive hemiparesis (left greater than right), sphincter dysfunction, and dysarthria, requiring use of a wheelchair within 6 years of disease onset. Patient died at age 72 of aspiration pneumonia and acute myocardial infarction. Case D (SPMS): A 33-year-old woman initially presenting with diplopia and hemiataxia that partially resolved following short course of corticosteroids. Subsequent course characterized by gradually progressive dysarthria, dysphagia, ophthalmoplegia, and limb and gait ataxia, requiring use of a wheelchair within 7 years of disease onset. She also developed a focal seizure disorder 4 years prior to death and died at age 46 of aspiration pneumonia. (B and C) Subpial cortical demyelination is demonstrated in case A at low (B) and high (C) magnification. (E) Extensive subpial demyelination involving multiple gyri is illustrated in case D at low magnification. (F) Meningeal inflammation may be prominent, often in close proximity to areas with subpial cortical demyelination. Proteolipid protein immunocytochemistry; *green* = focal demyelinated plaques in the white matter; *orange* = cortical demyelination; *blue* = demyelinated lesions in the deep gray matter. (From Pirko I: Gray matter involvement in multiple sclerosis, *Neurology* 68[9]:634–642, 2007.)

***Disease-modifying Treatments.*** Disease-modifying drugs significantly decrease new lesion development and cortical atrophy progression and can reduce relapse rates, disability progression, and transition to secondary progressive MS. Different steps of the pathologic cascade in MS may eventually be targeted therapeutically for optimal treatment of MS. Understanding the inflammatory process in MS is important because inflammation includes destructive components that should be targeted for inactivation and potentially beneficial mechanisms that should be enhanced or not disturbed by treatment. Despite earnest research efforts, there is no cure for or immunization against MS. Currently, there are injectable therapies, oral therapies, and intravenous infusion therapies.

**Table 31.6** Common Disease-Modifying Medications Used for MS

| Injectable Treatments | Oral Medications | IV Infusion |
|---|---|---|
| Avonex (interferon beta-1a) | Aubagio (teriflunomide) | Lemtrada (alemtuzumab) |
| Betaseron (interferon beta-1b) | Gilenya (finglomod) | Novantrone (mitoxantrone) |
| Copaxone (glatiramer acetate) | Mavenclad (cladribine) | Ocrevus (ocrelizumab) |
| Extavia (interferon beta-1b) | Mayzent (siponimod) | Tysabri (natalizumab) |
| Glatiramer acetate injection (generic equivalent of Copaxone) | Tecfidera (dimethyl fumarate) | |
| Glatopa (generic equivalent of Copaxone) | | |
| Plegridy (perinterferon beta-1a) | | |
| Rebif (interferon beta-1a) | | |

Injectable Therapies. First-generation injectable disease-modifying therapies, including interferon (IFN)-β-1b, IFN-β-1a, and glatiramer acetate, have more similarities than differences. All these agents reduce the rate of exacerbations by approximately 30%. In addition, these medications reduce the risk of new MRI activity. IFN-β-1a IM/SC was also shown to reduce the risk of sustained disability progression. In general, the injectable disease-modifying therapies are safe and well tolerated. Because of the risk of hematologic abnormalities and hepatotoxicity, a blood count and liver function tests should be monitored with the IFN therapies.

Initially described as the "ABC" drugs, based on the three immunomodulator drugs available for MS starting with those letters (Avonex, Betaseron, Copaxone), now there are many other medications that have been developed for MS. A is for IFN-β-1a (Avonex, Biogen Idec), and B is for IFN-β-1b (Betaseron, Berlex Laboratories). The higher the dose of interferon, the more potent is the response. Rebif, another INF-β-1a drug, is used in higher doses. Rebif is given subcutaneously at a 46% higher dose three times weekly, for a total of 4.4 times as much drug as Avonex. Plegridy (peginterferon beta-1a, Biogen Idec) is another injectable therapy. Peginterferon beta-1a is a "pegylated" form of interferon, which means that polyethylene glycol is attached to the interferon molecules. This allows them to maintain effects in the body for a longer duration with less frequent dosing. In one larger study, Plegridy demonstrated a reduction in relapse rates by 35.6%, up to 67% reduction in new brain lesions on MRI scans, and reduction in disability progression by 38%.[13] The potent antiinflammatory effects of interferons have an effect on the MRI scans, with decreased contrast-enhancing lesions. INF-β-1a also has been shown in relapsing individuals with MS to slow progression of disability, brain atrophy, and cognitive dysfunction. Given the complex mode of action of INF-β in MS, the clinically meaningful treatment effect can be delayed by at least several months. Proposed mechanisms by which INF-β might also limit brain atrophy include increasing nerve growth factors, limiting immune-mediated destructive inflammation, and limiting toxic mechanisms such as pathologic iron deposition.

The C drug, glatiramer acetate (Copaxone, Teva Pharmaceutical Industries), is a polypeptide that appears to fool the immune system. It seems to decrease the attack by blocking immune cells headed toward myelin and thereby preventing damage. The principal effect may be a shift from a proinflammatory cell bias to an antiinflammatory cell bias. It also has a partial and delayed but significant effect of limiting the rate of brain atrophy in relapsing-remitting MS and there are fewer occurrences of the flulike symptoms that are associated with the interferons. Glatiramer acetate has shown beneficial effects on MS-related fatigue. Glatiramer acetate occasionally induces a systemic reaction. This rare, but real, symptom complex presents with a feeling of panic, chest discomfort, shortness of breath, and a feeling of doom and gloom. It usually lasts for 20 minutes and then clears rapidly, but if panic sets in and an emergency is called, the issue may be magnified and complicated. The treatment is to realize that the problem is associated with the medication and requires resting for the duration of the symptoms to allow them to abate on their own. This usually is not a recurrent problem but occasionally can repeat.

The aggressive use of immune-modulating agents to slow down the actual disease process has contributed to the development of a whole new set of symptoms that the clinician must recognize and manage. Interferon initiation often brings about a fever, which may be disabling to the person who has MS. It often is recommended that interferon be administered in the evening before going to bed. This allows for the impact of the fever overnight, when it may be less disabling to activities of living. Antipyretic medications (ibuprofen or acetaminophen) may be administered 30 minutes before the injection, at the time of injection, and then, if necessary, 4 hours after the injection.

Subcutaneous injections can lead to immune reactions within the skin, with inflammation, redness, and significant irritation. Good injection technique involves icing the area before injecting, avoiding a shallow injection, and may require use of cortisone or local anesthetic. Improved injection devices have decreased many of these side effects. Rotation of the injection sites is an absolute necessity to preserve as much skin area as possible and allow healing between injections. With some treatments, pain can linger after the injection. Cooling can offer symptomatic relief.

Oral Therapies. Fingolimod (Gilenya) is an oral immunomodulating agent/relative immunosuppressant. Its final effect is also to reduce the normal circulation and trafficking of leukocytes. It was shown to reduce the relapse rate by about 50%, to reduce the number of new or enlarging T2W lesions on brain MRI by about 70%, and also reduced the risk of disability progression.[47]

Teriflunomide (Aubagio) is another oral immunomodulating agent. The exact mechanism of action in individuals with MS is unknown but may include impacting the interaction between T cells and antigen-presenting cells, thereby reducing T cell activation. Its efficacy is comparable to injectable therapies. Its effects lasted 9 years, the relapse rates were reduced by 31%, and the risk of 3-month disability worsening was reduced by 30%.[74,100]

Dimethyl fumarate (Tecfidera) is the other oral therapy option for individuals with MS. It also is an immunomodulatory agent with antiinflammatory properties. The mechanism of dimethyl fumarate is unknown, but it likely inhibits immune cells and may be protective against CNS damage. It is taken twice daily and has been shown to reduce MS relapses, progression of disease/disability, and new MRI lesions. The occurrence of PML is uncommon but can occur.[100]

Infusion Therapies. Mitoxantrone (Novantrone, Immunex) is used to modify relapsing and secondary progressive MS. Mitoxantrone is the only drug approved for treatment of secondary progressive MS in the United States. Of note, Betaferon is also labeled for SPMS in Europe. Mitoxantrone is administered intravenously every 3 months. Mitoxantrone presumably works by depression of T cell counts and removal of activated T cells from the immune repertoire. Because of potential side effects, its use is being limited at present to individuals whose MS is clearly advancing in spite of other aggressive therapy or some selected patients who are in a secondary progressive phase.

Natalizumab (Tysabri) is a monoclonal antibody that prevents immune cells from moving from the blood to the CNS. It was originally approved by the FDA based on a dramatic lowering of relapse rate and a 50% reduction in the development of a sustained increase in disability. This treatment is a once-monthly intravenous infusion. One serious potential side effect from Tysabri is the development of progressive multifocal leukoencephalopathy (PML), an often fatal viral disease. This risk is mitigated by testing for the JC virus. If an individual is JC virus positive, the risk of developing PML is higher. Individuals who may begin taking medications that increase the risk of developing PML (i.e., Tysabri, fingolimod, and dimethyl fumarate) should have blood tests prior to taking the medication and approximately every 6 months to ensure they haven't developed the JC virus.

Alemtuzumab (Lemtrada) is a recombinant, humanized monoclonal antibody that targets the CD52 cell surface antigen expressed on B and T lymphocytes.[100] Alemtuzumab is administered over two courses; a five-day IV course followed one year later by a three-day IV course. Comparative studies have shown improvements related to reduction in relapse rates, new lesions on MRI, and disease progression with alemtuzumab versus those who were unsuccessful with interferon beta-1a.[18] Relapse rates were reduced by 55.6% and disease progression was reduced by 22% versus 9%.[19] Both medications were efficacious in reducing new or increasing T2 lesions and contrast-enhancing T1 lesions on MRI, as well as brain volume loss. There are many potential side effects, but most concerning is the potential increase in risk of developing secondary autoimmunity which may occur in up to 47.7% of patients treated with alemtuzumab.[101]

Ocrelizumab (Ocrevus) is another humanized, recombinant monoclonal antibody but targets CD20 positive B lymphocytes. Ocrelizumab is the first medication to show benefits and be FDA approved for either relapsing or primary progressive MS. It is administered intravenously every 6 months. It doesn't impose the risk of autoimmunity because the antibody doesn't bind to stem cells or plasma cells and therefore preserves immune function. Studies have identified improvements for both patients with RRMS and progressive MS. With RRMS, annualized relapse rate was reduced by 46%, disease progression by 40%, and T1 gadolinium-enhancing lesions per T1 weighted MRI scans by 95%.[38] Compared to placebo, studies have found potential reduction in disability progression by 24% and have also found positive effects on brain MRI lesions.[71] Further investigation of harmful side effects is warranted, such as depletion of B cell depletion over time, as well as its potential to increase neoplasms.

***Relapse Management.*** Corticosteroids remain the first-line treatment for acute exacerbations. There is no consensus regarding optimal dosing; however, a regimen of 1000 mg intravenous (IV) methylprednisolone daily for 3 to 5 days is considered standard. It is typically thought that oral corticosteroids are equal in efficacy, but the key is that one must use high-dose steroids. Corticosteroids can alter almost every aspect of the immune system. Corticosteroid-induced restoration of the blood-brain barrier, and has an antiedema benefit. Decreased activity of the macrophages and lymphocytes results in less damage to the myelin in response to steroid therapy. Individuals with severe demyelination who do not respond to corticosteroids may improve with plasma exchange.

***Symptomatic Treatment.*** Despite the time and effort given to slow the disease, the bulk of current intervention is devoted to symptomatic management. Improvement in the ability to control symptoms through therapy and medications can enhance quality of life in the individual with MS.

Dalfampridine (Ampyra) is a broad-spectrum potassium channel blocker, and is thought to enhance signal conduction in the nerves by blocking potassium leaks. Studies show increased walking speed in persons with MS after taking dalfampridine. History of seizure or kidney disease is a contraindication for this medication.

Amantadine, pemoline, modafinil, and armodafinil can reduce fatigue in MS. Modafinil is a popular and relatively safe drug, with the most common side effect being headache, and is considered first line for MS-related fatigue that is associated with daily sleepiness. Amantadine produced small but statistically significant improvements in fatigue related to energy level, concentration, problem solving, and sense of well-being. Given the strong coexistence of depression and fatigue in MS, treatment with antidepressants, such as selective serotonin reuptake inhibitors, monoamine oxidase inhibitors, tricyclic antidepressants, selective serotonin-norepinephrine reuptake inhibitors, and dopamine-norepinephrine reuptake inhibitors, is considered, although there are few systematic studies assessing their efficacy in MS-related fatigue as a separate symptom.

Centrally acting and peripherally acting muscle relaxants, such as baclofen (Lioresal), tizanidine, and dantrolene, decrease hypertonicity and leg spasms. Anticonvulsants and antidepressant medicines are used to treat pain. Intrathecal baclofen pumps reduce severe spasticity. Focal injections of Botox can be helpful in decreasing muscle spasticity. Repetitive transcranial magnetic stimulation may improve spasticity in MS. The antiepileptic agents and antidepressant treatments often are effective in modulating the painful symptoms. Gabapentin in relatively high doses often is necessary for the desired effect. Paroxysmal tonic spasms typically respond to antiepileptic medications such as carbamazepine.

Sleep disorders may contribute to fatigue and must be recognized and treated appropriately. Amitriptyline is helpful, especially at night, as it can sedate and provide pain relief. Clonazepam, given at bedtime, can aid in sleep initiation and decrease spasms with minimum side effects. Diazepam has a similar effect. Dose escalation should be avoided. Dopamine agonists and dopamine itself also may be used for restless leg syndrome. All of these treatments require adjustment from time to time to maintain some relief.

Oxybutynin and tolterodine, solifenacin, mirabegron, and fesoterodine fumarate diminish bladder hyperactivity. All medications currently available to control symptoms of MS have potential side effects and therefore must be used judiciously.

**PROGNOSIS.** The average frequency of attacks of MS is approximately one per year. The attacks vary in severity; therefore close observation is required to reliably track the attack frequency. Attacks tend to be most common in the early years of MS and become less frequent in later years, regardless of the disability. The risk for rapid development of moderate disability may be greater in persons in whom the frequency of attacks is higher than average.

Multiple factors may predict a severe course, such as motor and cerebellar symptoms, disability after the first attack, and short time interval between attacks. Numerous relapses within the first year negatively influence the clinical course. Conversely, sensory symptoms, infrequent attacks, full neurologic recovery after a relapse, and a low level of disability after 5 to 7 years may be associated with an improved prognosis.

Burden of disease on MRI scans may be the strongest predictor of clinical outcomes. Over 14 years, there was no significant disability accrued in individuals with normal MRI findings at the time of diagnosis, whereas MRI scans with greater than 10 lesions predicted that individuals would require a cane for walking within that same time frame. A change in lesion load within the first year also is a negative predictor of outcome. Late-onset MS is not necessarily associated with a worse outcome. Progression of primary progressive and relapsing MS differed little between late-onset and early adult-onset disease. The individuals with late-onset disease were older when reaching an Expanded Disability Status Scale score of 6.

Because disability is often significant in individuals with MS, lifestyle changes are frequently necessary. Movement impairment is frequently associated with MS, and difficulty in walking is a major disability. If MS is untreated, 15 years after diagnosis 50% of individuals with MS will require the use of an assistive device to walk, and at 20 years 50% will be wheelchair bound. About one-fourth of persons with MS will require human assistance with activities of daily living.

It is the coexistence of physical and cognitive impairments together with emotional and social issues in a disease with an uncertain course that makes MS rehabilitation unique and challenging. Individual rehabilitation improves functional independence but has only limited success in improving the level of neurologic impairment. Severely disabled people derive as much as or more benefit than those who are less disabled, but cognitive problems and ataxia tend to be refractory. Cost and utility are significantly correlated with functional capacity. There is now good evidence that exercise can improve fitness and function for those with mild or moderate MS-related disability and helps to maintain function for those with moderate to severe disability. Several different forms of exercise have been investigated. For most individuals, aerobic exercise that incorporates a degree of balance training and socialization is most effective. Time constraints, access, impairment level, personal preferences, motivations, and funding sources influence the prescription for exercise and other components of rehabilitation. Rehabilitation in MS should be viewed as an ongoing process to maintain and restore maximum function and quality of life.

Life expectancy is reduced by a modest amount in MS; the risk of dying of MS is strongly associated with severe disability. The death rate in persons who are unable to stand or walk is more than four times that in persons the same age without MS. In mildly disabled individuals, the death rate is approximately 1.5 times that of the age-matched population. Persons with more frequent initial episodes, with rapidly developing disability, have a poorer long-term outcome. Individuals with primary progressive disease also have decreased life expectancy. Suicide is more than seven times more common than in age-matched controls, and depression must be treated aggressively.

## SPECIAL IMPLICATIONS FOR THE THERAPIST 31.5

### *Multiple Sclerosis*

Because MS is typically progressive, it is expected that individuals will need to access the medical community with greater needs over time. Maintaining function in the household and community is a typical rehabilitation goal. Although people with MS are advised to be as active as possible in all ways of life, there is no consensus on the best method to attain that goal. Activity carried out in accordance with individual strength and abilities, avoiding exhaustion, will help to prevent or diminish the complications leading to disability. Skin breakdown following sensory loss and immobility is a common problem that can be controlled by appropriate skin care and positioning.

Fatigue and weakness are common impairments reported to therapists. The Modified Fatigue Index is a self-report scale to monitor changes in the level of fatigue. This can be helpful for therapists to measure changes associated with interventions or to describe changes in function following a relapse. Exercise has a beneficial effect on both physiologic and psychological factors leading to reduced fatigue in those with MS.[40] Interval training is well tolerated and allows for greater improvements in aerobic capacity, mobility, strength, and fatigue.[72]

The replacement of oral spasticity medications with intrathecal baclofen has become more routine, and the therapist can be involved in the dosing and management. Any spasticity the individual is using for activities of daily living may be altered. Thus, transferring techniques may require a different approach. The perception of strength that may be given by stiffness may disappear, giving the perception of weakness. Determining the appropriate muscle for use of Botox should also be done with the therapist who is most familiar with the individual's functional status.

In establishing a training program for endurance and strengthening, careful consideration of the neurologic changes is critical. Careful monitoring of exercise appears to be necessary because of impaired cardiopulmonary systems. Respiratory muscle dysfunction may impair an individual's tolerance to exercise. Interval training has been found to be a beneficial training technique for individuals with MS. Exercising just prior to fatigue and then resting may allow the individual to overall perform more work. Repetitive submaximal strength training appears to be of benefit to most people, with an increase in both peak torque generated and a decrease in the reported perception of fatigue. Changes achieved in strength and endurance are probably the result of the normal physiologic changes that are associated with this type of training. Individuals with MS demonstrating increased reflex activity with exertion will need a longer time to recover after fatigue and may notice increased extensor tone and difficulty with flexion. Use of cooling vests to lower core temperature during exercise can be beneficial to those who have heat intolerance. It is important to realize that for most people with MS, fatigue will exacerbate symptoms. Nonpharmacologic measures for managing fatigue are more consistently beneficial in patients with MS-related fatigue. The cumulative evidence supports the theory that exercise training is associated with a small improvement in quality of life among individuals with MS.

Understanding movement disorders common to lesions in specific brain regions and the spinal column is essential for the therapist. Analysis of movement is the most critical skill necessary to determine sensory and motor deficits that may be contributing to loss of postural control and mobility. The therapist must be able to identify the specific impairments to establish the appropriate stretching, strengthening, and balance exercises. A successful exercise program depends on a number of factors essential to motor learning, including practice, adequate feedback, and knowledge of results. Therapy has the potential to reduce falls risk for individuals with MS.[35] Individuals with MS may be restricted in practice by neurologic fatigue and by impairments that disrupt sensory feedback, attention, memory, and motivation. The therapist will need to carefully identify the individual's resources and abilities and capitalize on them to minimize the level of disability. Establishing individually designed fitness programs is an important role of the physical therapist. Models for such programs can lead the therapist in the appropriate direction and provide protocols taking into consideration the common concerns associated with MS.

The day-to-day variation in MS makes determination of an appropriate training program challenging. Use of both impairment and disability scales will assist in monitoring changes. The scales show the relative improvement after intervention or overall decline regardless of intervention. The scales are useful in tracking the disease process for both the individual and the health care provider. Therapists making decisions regarding the need for adaptive equipment can use the scales to establish trends in the course of the disease. A common disability scale used by rehabilitation professionals and researchers working with patients with MS is the Kurtzke Expanded Disability Status Scale (Box 31.11). It is used to monitor changes in global disability levels and has value in determining prognosis. Therapists working with this patient population should become adept at using this tool. The Academy of Neurologic Physical Therapy MS Task Force highly recommended various measures for physical therapist use in acute, inpatient, and outpatient rehabilitation, summarized in Table 31.7.

Box 31.11

**KURTZKE EXPANDED DISABILITY STATUS SCALE**

| | |
|---|---|
| 0.0 | Normal neurologic examination |
| 1.0 | No disability, minimal symptoms |
| 1.5 | No disability, minimal signs in more than one functional level |
| 2.0 | Slightly greater disability in one functional system |
| 2.5 | Slightly greater disability in two functional systems |
| 3.0 | Moderate disability in one functional system; fully ambulatory |
| 3.5 | Fully ambulatory but with moderate disability in one functional system and more than minimal disability in several others |

**Box 31.11**

**KURTZKE EXPANDED DISABILITY STATUS SCALE—cont'd**

| | |
|---|---|
| 4.0 | Fully ambulatory without aid, self-sufficient, up and about 12 hr/day despite relatively severe disability; able to walk about 500 m without aid or rest |
| 4.5 | Fully ambulatory without aid, up and about much of the day, able to work a full day; may otherwise have some limitation of full activity or require minimal assistance; characterized by relatively severe disability; able to walk about 300 m without aid or rest |
| 5.0 | Ambulatory for about 200 m without aid or rest; disability severe enough to impair full daily activities (e.g., to work a full day without special provisions) |
| 5.5 | Ambulatory for about 100 m without aid or rest; disability severe enough to preclude full daily activities |
| 6.0 | Intermittent or unilateral constant assistance (cane, crutch, brace) required to walk about 100 m with or without resting |
| 6.5 | Constant bilateral assistance (canes, crutches, braces) required to walk about 20 m without resting |
| 7.0 | Unable to walk beyond approximately 5 m with aid; essentially restricted to a wheelchair; wheels self in standard wheelchair and transfers alone; up and about in wheelchair 12 hr/day |
| 7.5 | Unable to take more than a few steps; restricted to wheelchair; may need aid in transfer; wheels self but cannot carry on in standard wheelchair a full day; may require motorized wheelchair |
| 8.0 | Essentially restricted to bed or chair or perambulated in wheelchair but may be out of bed itself much of the day; retains many self-care functions; generally has effective use of arms |
| 8.5 | Essentially restricted to bed much of the day; has some effective use of arm or arms; retains some self-care functions |
| 9.0 | Helpless bed patient; can communicate and eat |
| 9.5 | Totally helpless bed patient; unable to communicate effectively, eat, or swallow |
| 10.0 | Death from multiple sclerosis |

Modified from Kurtzke J: Rating neurological impairment in multiple sclerosis: an expanded disability status scale (EDSS), *Neurology* 33:1444, 1983.

**Table 31.7** Outcome Measures Recommended for Use with Patients with MS by the Academy of Physical Therapy MS EDGE Task Force

**Outcome Measures Highly Recommended for Use in Acute, Inpatient (IPR) and Outpatient Rehabilitation (OPR)**

Upper extremity control
- 9 hole peg test

Balance
- Berg Balance Scale
- (OPR) Dizziness Handicap Index

Gait
- 12 item MS walking scale
- Timed 25 foot walk
- TUG (with cognitive and manual)
- (OPR) 6 minute walk test

Global and quality of life measures
- MS Impact Scale (MSIS-29)
- (IPR/OPR) MS QOL-54
- (OPR only) MS Functional Composite

Note: Many additional measures are also recommended for use with patients with MS; these are those with the highest level of recommended based on the evidence available in 2010–2011 when the task force did its work. Other recommendations and any updates regarding revisions to these recommendations are accessible on www.neuropt.org.

# PARKINSONISM AND PARKINSON DISEASE

## Overview and Definition

Atrophy of the brain leading to degeneration of neurons in the basal ganglia can be caused by a variety of disorders that are not well understood. These include multiple system atrophy, progressive supranuclear palsy, corticobasal ganglionic degeneration, and diffuse Lewy body disease. Parkinsonian features can be manifested as a part of other diseases affecting the CNS, such as atherosclerosis, ALS, and HD.

Parkinson disease (PD), or idiopathic parkinsonism, is a chronic progressive disease of the CNS, characterized by rigidity, tremor, bradykinesia, and postural instability. The disease is thought to result from a complex interaction between multiple predisposing genes and environmental effects, although these interactions are still poorly understood. PD is still regarded as a sporadic neurodegenerative disorder, characterized by the loss of midbrain dopamine neurons and presence of Lewy body inclusions.

## Incidence

PD, following AD, is the second most common neurodegenerative disorder in the United States. Parkinsonism, including PD, affects more than 800,000 adults in the United States, with prevalence rates of 350 per 100,000 adults. Approximately 42% of parkinsonism is related to PD. The lifetime risk of developing parkinsonism is 7.5% according to a Mayo study. There appears to be a higher rate among white Americans and Europeans compared with black Africans. Black persons in America and Chinese in Taiwan have higher rates of the disease than their counterparts in West Africa or China. Parkinson disease is about 1.4 times more frequent in men than women. PD becomes increasingly common with advancing age, affecting more than 1 person in every 100 older than age 75 years. A possible explanation of the correlation between age and prevalence may be the age-related neuronal vulnerability. Because of the increase in life expectancy, the aging of the baby boomers, and the precision of diagnosis, the incidence of PD is expected to rise. In 2016, 6.1 million individuals had Parkinson disease globally, compared with 2.5 million in 1990.[31] It is estimated that approximately 630,000 people in the United States were diagnosed with PD in 2010, and The Parkinson's Foundation Prevalence Project estimates that number will rise to 930,000 by the year 2020 and to 1.2 million by 2030.[61] The national economic burden of PD exceeds $14.4 billion in 2010 (approximately $22,800 per patient). The majority of cases begin between the ages of 50 and 79 years. Approximately 10% will develop initial symptoms before the age of 40 years.

## Etiologic and Risk Factors

An increasing number of chromosomal features linked to familial parkinsonism have been found, notably PARK1 to PARK11. There are 27 genes reported in the literature since 1997, associated either with autosomal dominant (AD): LRRK2, SNCA, VPS35, GCH1, ATXN2, DNAJC13, TMEM230, GIGYF2, HTRA2, RIC3, EIF4G1, UCHL1, CHCHD2, and GBA; or autosomal recessive (AR) inheritance: PRKN, PINK1, DJ1, ATP13A2, PLA2G6, FBXO7, DNAJC6, SYNJ1, SPG11, VPS13C, PODXL, and PTRHD1; or an X-linked transmission: RAB39B.[59] Autosomal dominant parkinsonism (*synuclein, UCHL1, NURR1, LRRK2*) means one copy of an altered gene in each cell is sufficient to cause the disorder. In most cases, an affected person has one parent who has both the condition and three altered genes that cause autosomal recessive disease (*DJ1, PINK1, parkin*). This type of inheritance means that two copies of the gene in each cell are altered. Most often, the parents of an individual with autosomal recessive PD each carry one copy of the altered gene but do not show signs and symptoms of the disorder. These provide insights into the molecular pathogenesis of the disease, but genetic testing for these mutations is of little clinical relevance. The chance of identifying parkin mutations is less than 5% in sporadic cases with onset at younger than 45 years. The probability is much greater in those with onset at younger than 30 years of age and in those with an affected sibling. Confirmation of this recessive form of disease might be helpful in genetic counseling, because it renders transmission to the subsequent generation very unlikely. Given the late onset of typical PD, it is likely that by the time individuals become symptomatic, many first-degree relatives are deceased from other causes. Some Parkinson mutations are more prevalent in certain groups. SNCA is more prevalent in a small number of European families with a greater likelihood of disease and earlier onset. Mutations in LRRK2 account for a much greater number of PD cases in Ashkenazi Jewish, North African Arab Berbers, and Basque populations than in the general population, with a moderate likelihood of disease, which increases with age. GBA is more prevalent in people of Ashkenazi Jewish descent, very common but with lower likelihood of disease, and is a major PD risk factor often associated with dementia. PRKN, PINK1, and DJ1 cases present with typical early onset PD with slow progression, whereas other AR genes present severe atypical parkinsonism. The Parkinson Progression Marker Initiative,[34,52] started in 2010, was designed to identify PD progression biomarkers both to improve understanding of disease etiology and course and to provide crucial tools to enhance the likelihood of success of PD disease-modifying therapeutic trials.

Many potential exposures have been cited as possible risk factors for PD. Three major groups include toxic exposures, infection exposures, and a heterogenic group of miscellaneous exposures. Some toxic agents, such as carbon monoxide, manganese, cyanide, and methanol, can damage the basal ganglia and produce parkinsonian symptoms. A rapidly developing Parkinson-like disease has been linked to the use of MPTP (1-methyl-4-phenyl-1,2,3,6-tetrahydropyridine), a synthetic narcotic related to heroin. Some neuroleptics can produce a parkinsonian syndrome. In drug-induced parkinsonism, the symptoms can usually be reversed by withdrawal of the drug.

The link to infection exposure remains unresolved, despite years of study. There may still be a possibility that infection plays a role, based on observations of serum antibody titers for measles virus, rubella virus, herpes simplex virus types 1 and 2, and cytomegalovirus in persons with PD. Pesticides and herbicides may be environmental causes and are likely to produce between 2% and 25% increased risk. If some individuals are determined to be particularly susceptible to low environmental exposure, then pesticides may pose a more serious risk.) Long-term exposure to either manganese or copper has been linked to an increased incidence of parkinsonism.[8] More years of formal education appear to increase the risk of PD. Physicians are at significantly increased risk of PD when occupational data are used. By contrast, four occupational groups show a significantly decreased risk of PD according to one source: construction and extractive workers (miners, oil well drillers), production workers (machine operators, fabricators), metalworkers, and engineers.

There is a relatively well-established relationship between PD and a history of smoking. Individuals with a history of smoking seem to have a lower risk of developing PD. Coffee and tea drinking as well as caffeine consumption are also associated with a lower risk of PD.[75]

High levels of physical exercise may lower PD risk. The risk of PD appears to be lower among women who report strenuous exercise during early adulthood. Physical exercise can promote secretion of growth factors in the CNS that in turn may contribute to the survival and neuroplasticity of dopaminergic neurons. Moreover, exercise decreases the ratio between dopamine transporter and vesicular monoamine transporter; a decrease in this ratio may lower the susceptibility of dopaminergic neurons to neurotoxins and reduce dopamine oxidation. Finally, physical exercise may activate the dopaminergic system and increase dopamine availability in the striatum. Any of these or other mechanisms may be responsible for the beneficial effects of forced exercise in animal experiments. In the rat model of PD, forced exercise prior to chemically induced parkinsonism caused a significant increase of glial-derived neurotrophic factor that has neuroprotective effects for dopaminergic neurons. Studies to determine if results found in animal studies are relevant to neuroprotective effects of physical exercise in human PD pathogenesis are ongoing.

## Pathogenesis

Parkinsonian symptoms come primarily from dysfunction within the subcortical gray matter in the basal ganglia. Physiologic studies have shown the basal ganglia to be actively involved in almost all types of movement, including postural responses, alternating movements, and spontaneously occurring movements. The basal ganglia are active prior to recorded EMG activity in the muscles involved in a movement. Lesions do not produce paralysis or weakness, but rather change the character of movement, leading to loss of adaptive control, slowing of movement, and poor coordination. The motor loop that determines the initiation and scaling of motor activity derives its input from the premotor, motor, and somatosensory cortices. This is the process of preparation for forthcoming movement, and when disrupted it can cause a reduction in size and speed of the movement.

Basal ganglia–cerebral cortex interactions are disrupted by the abnormal function of the basal ganglia. This reflects a delay in motor programming related to the unconscious initiation of motor preparation, or lack of "response set" or readiness to move. The complex loop that includes the basal ganglia is involved in motivation and in planning global aspects of behavior. The basal ganglia interact with the frontal cortex and with the limbic system, including the hippocampus and amygdala, and therefore have a role in cognitive and emotional function. The basal ganglia, in association with the frontal lobe, appear to play an important role in the integration of sensory information. It is now recognized that diffuse neuronal loss in the cerebral cortex may also contribute to changes observed in PD.

The basal ganglia are large subcortical structures that are interconnected and functionally interposed between the cortex and the thalamus. They also have direct connections to the limbic lobe, frontal cortex, and brainstem. It is likely that the fundamental principles that will be described here in relationship to the cortex–basal ganglia–thalamus–cortex system can also explain the disorders related to the connections between the basal ganglia and the frontal cortex, limbic lobe, and brainstem. The failure to facilitate desired behaviors and simultaneously inhibit unwanted behaviors may be responsible for the cognitive, emotional, and memory problems that coexist with movement disorders.

The signs and symptoms of parkinsonism are neurochemical in origin. The pathologic hallmark is the degeneration of a nucleus that is part of the basal ganglia, the substantia nigra. It loses its ability to produce dopamine, a neurotransmitter necessary to normal function of basal ganglia neurons. Although the degeneration of the dopaminergic pigmented neurons in the SN is the most consistent neuropathologic feature found in many clinical parkinsonian neurodegenerative conditions, the pattern of dopamine cell loss in the SN is distinctive for PD, with the most severe loss found in the ventrolateral region of the SN, whereas dopaminergic neurons in the nearby ventral tegmental area are nearly entirely spared.[37] A depletion of 70% to 80% of the dopamine is estimated to occur before clinical signs of the disease are noted. Initially, the system adapts, and there is increased efficiency in the pathways that depend on dopamine, but over time, as the dopamine depletion continues, function declines.

Abnormal protein breakdown, which may occur spontaneously or in relationship to a gene mutation, contributes to the neurodegeneration of PD. It appears that there are many possible triggers for the programmed cell death that results in mitochondrial dysfunction and oxidative stress. Despite significant research in this area, many observations are correlative in nature, and a precise process has not been identified. The inherited, early onset forms of the disease may have a mutation that causes degradation of protein that may mimic the changes found in those individuals with sporadic, later-onset disorder. The changes in neurochemistry and protein are both consistent with aging. There is some overlap of degeneration similar to the processes seen in the dementias, including AD.

Free radical or oxidative stress appears to also have a role in the dysfunction of the basal ganglia. Compared to the rest of the brain, the substantia nigra is exposed to higher levels of oxidative stress. Evidence of inflammation is typically found in the area of the substantia nigra pars compacta in conjunction with programmed cell death. It is proposed that neuroinflammation does not initiate PD but can promote progression and add to the worsening of symptoms. Recent animal study findings appear to support the "dying back" hypothesis of PD, which proposes that the tyrosine-hydroxylase-positive terminal loss in the striatum is the first neurodegenerative event in PD, which later induces neuronal degeneration in the substantia nigra.

Although Lewy body pathology, impaired protein turnover, and mitochondrial dysfunction may all play a role in PD pathogenesis, none of these mechanisms explains the most characteristic feature of the disease: selective neuronal vulnerability. Only a small subset of neurons in the brain ever degenerates in PD or shows other signs of pathology. One theory is that the pattern of pathology is dictated by the spread of a prion-like strain of alpha-synuclein and that this spread is determined by the brain connectome. An alternative theory is that neurons at risk in PD have a preexisting phenotype that renders them vulnerable to the PD triumvirate of alpha-synuclein aggregates, mitochondrial dysfunction, and defective protein turnover.[75]

### Shedding Light on Early Parkinson Disease Pathology

The motor pattern generators, thoughts and behaviors, and processes for memory are all initiated through the cerebral cortex. The parietal-occipital-temporal lobes, prefrontal areas, thalamic nuclei, limbic lobe, amygdala, and hippocampus use glutamate projections into the striatum (caudate and putamen). The input into the striatum comes in a topographic organization that is maintained to some degree throughout the basal ganglia.

Dopamine is produced in the substantia nigra pars compacta. Dopamine has more than one configuration, and the $D_1$ configuration either increases the efficiency or decreases the effect of cortical input to the striatum, depending on the context of the desired movement. $D_2$ primarily decreases the effect of cortical input to the striatum. The striatum (caudate and putamen) has medium spiny neurons that project outside of the striatum. Dopamine input to the striatum terminates largely on the shafts of these dendritic spines and is able to modulate transmission from the cerebral cortex to the striatum. Cholinergic interneurons and GABA interneurons also synapse on these dendrites. Although there are fewer GABA interneurons, they have a powerful inhibitory effect. Through long-term potentiation and long-term depression, dopamine may be involved in the neural mechanism of habit learning. Depletion of dopamine in the striatum impairs the learning of new movement sequences.

$D_1$ dopamine goes from the striatum primarily to the internal globus pallidus and substantia nigra pars reticulata. (These two groups of neurons are functionally related and often grouped together.) The second population contains GABA and enkephalin and expresses $D_2$ dopamine receptors. These neurons project to the external globus pallidus. The external globus pallidus sends inhibitory input via GABA receptors to the internal globus pallidus.

The primary basal ganglia output comes from the internal globus pallidus, representing the body below the neck, and the substantia nigra pars reticulata, representing the head and eyes. The output is to the thalamus and, via several additional pathways, eventually to the brainstem and spinal cord. The output to the brainstem and spinal cord is through GABA neurotransmitters and is inhibitory.

There is another parallel circuit via the subthalamic nucleus. Excitatory input using glutamate via the hyperdirect pathway comes from the frontal lobe and motor areas and goes directly to the subthalamic nucleus, forming a somatotopic organization. There also appears to be a topographic separation of motor and cognitive inputs to the subthalamic nucleus. The output of the subthalamic nucleus is excitatory, using glutamate, and facilitates the external globus pallidus and the substantia nigra pars reticulata, producing a GABA inhibition to the thalamus.

The subthalamic nucleus also participates in a third or indirect pathway. This pathway involves signaling from the striatum (caudate and putamen) to the external globus pallidus to the subthalamic nucleus to the basal ganglia outputs.

The basal ganglia intrinsic circuitry is complex, with the direct pathway through the striatum (caudate and putamen) and a hyperdirect pathway through the subthalamic nucleus to the basal ganglia outputs. The hyperdirect pathway through the subthalamic nucleus is excitatory and fast, and the direct pathway through the striatum (caudate and putamen) is slower and inhibitory but more powerful.

The cumulative inhibitory output of the basal ganglia acts as a brake on the motor pattern generators in the cerebral cortex and brainstem. The interaction among these pathways allows for a planned movement to be executed while competing movements are prevented, thereby increasing the precision of the movement without losing the power necessary to perform an activity. This is thought also to allow one part of a movement sequence to be activated in order for another sequence to begin. Through these mechanisms, movement and thought can be adapted quickly when the environment requires a different response.

When dopamine stimulation is decreased or withdrawn from the cycle, the overall effect is increased inhibition of input into the thalamus. The final effect of increased inhibition of the thalamus decreases the ability of the thalamus to send excitatory input back to the frontal cortex. So the ultimate outcome is less activity in the cortex, resulting in slowed movement and less power generated through the musculoskeletal system (Fig. 31.17).

These abnormal responses also influence the pathways to the brainstem that travel through the superior colliculus to the nucleus raphe magnus, resulting in abnormal facial expression, blinking, and eye and eyelid movements. Although less clearly understood, abnormal firing or sequencing to the pedunculopontine tegmental nucleus can influence locomotion, sleep cycle regulation, attention, arousal, and startle.

Although the relationship of the substantia nigra and the striatum (caudate and putamen) are foremost in the disorder of parkinsonism, neuropathologic findings can be found in many other dopaminergic and nondopaminergic cell groups. The pathway responsible for postural stability may be affected outside of the basal ganglia. Changes in cerebellar circuits and in interactions between the cerebellum and the basal ganglia are now also recognized to be important in the case of parkinsonian tremor.[14]

## Clinical Manifestations

Movement disorder is the hallmark of parkinsonism, although other symptoms are evident and may actually precede the impairment of movement. The ability to move is not lost, but there is a problem with movement activation and loss of reflexive or automatic movement. Movement becomes reliant on cortical control. The ability to perform known tasks, such as walking, changing direction, writing, and basic activities of daily living, is diminished. The considerable variation among individuals in the clinical manifestations and the level of deterioration in movement over time can be explained by the complex mechanism of dysfunction defined in "Pathogenesis" above.

The tremor of PD, the most common initial manifestation, often appears unilaterally and may be confined to one upper limb for months or even years. It is first seen as a rhythmic, back-and-forth motion of the thumb and finger, referred to as the pill-rolling tremor. It is most obvious when the arm is at rest or during stressful periods. The tremor starts unilaterally but can eventually spread to all four limbs, as well as neck and facial muscles. Tension or exertion will cause the tremor to increase, and it will disappear during sleep. Tremor does not usually impact the functioning of the individual.

Rigidity is an increased response to muscle stretch that appears in both antagonist and agonist muscle groups. Rigidity, like tremor, usually appears unilaterally and proximally in an upper limb and then spreads to the other extremities and trunk. One of the earliest signs of rigidity is the loss of associated movements of the arms when walking. Rigidity is identified when another person is trying to passively move the extremity and there is a jerky response (tremor under rigidity), known as cogwheel rigidity, or a slow and sustained resistance, known as lead-pipe rigidity. Rigidity does not appear to have a direct effect on volitional movement. Axial rigidity usually limits rotation and extension of the trunk and spine and contributes to the characteristic "en bloc" trunk motions, which can decrease the ability to make adjustments of the extremities during functional tasks, such as transfers, reaching, and bed mobility, as well as gait. Postural instability and an increased risk for falls are more frequent in patients with PD, with axial rigidity and worse trunk mobility.[2,15] Reduced variability and less adaptation of

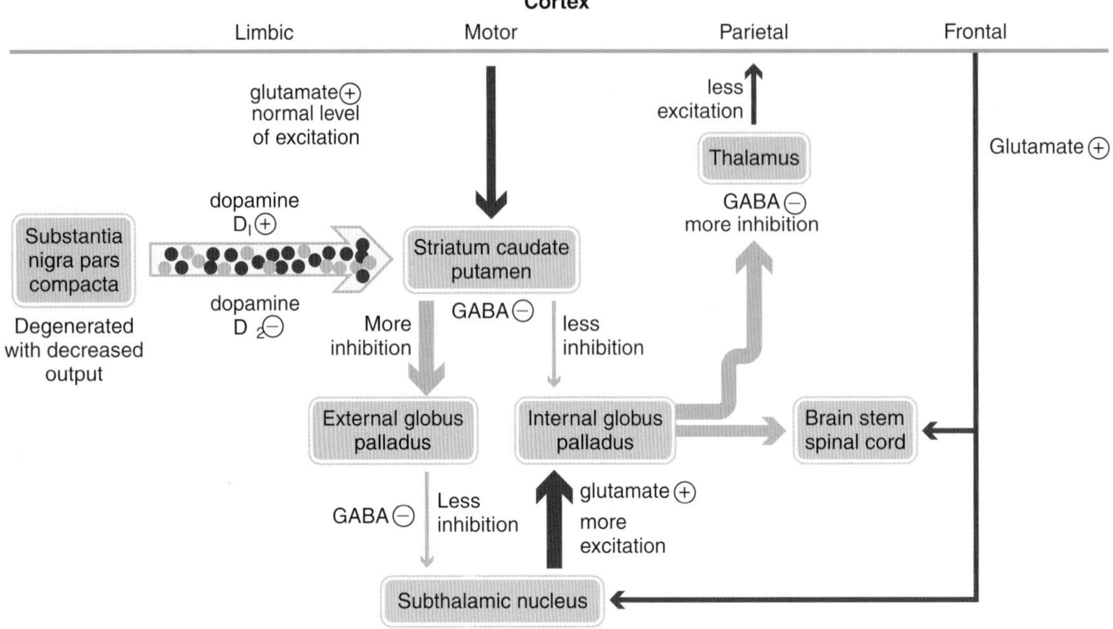


**Figure 31.17**

**How the loss of dopamine production in the substantia nigra causes the eventual decrease in excitation of the cortex in the motor loop that involves the basal ganglia.** Glutamate (positive transmission) is *red* and GABA (negative transmission) is *blue*. The decreased dopamine causes less than normal inhibition of the striatum (caudate/putamen), so there is more output to the internal globus pallidus. This output is inhibitory, so the cycle of inhibition is already started. Because the internal globus pallidus has been inhibited, there is less output, resulting in less inhibition of the subthalamic nucleus. This results in increased output of the subthalamic nucleus, this time causing more facilitation of the external globus pallidus. The increased output of the external globus pallidus, because it is inhibitory, causes greater inhibition of the thalamus, and the final end result is decreased excitation of the frontal or motor cortex. So the movement coming out of the cortex is less forceful than intended.Note the other available pathway from the frontal cortex directly to the subthalamic nucleus. The subthalamic nucleus then facilitates the external globus pallidus, and the output of the external globus pallidus is inhibitory to the internal globus pallidus. The output of the internal globus pallidus is inhibitory to the thalamus, as well as the brainstem and spinal cord. In this case, because of the double inhibition (sometimes referred to as disinhibition) the final output is excitatory. This pathway is not dependent on dopamine, but because it sends signals to the same nuclei that have already been affected by the decreases in dopamine, the system gets out of balance and the result is loss of normal modulation. Note also the pathway out of the basal ganglia to the brainstem and spinal cord.

movement between thoracic rotation and pelvic motion appears early in the onset of PD. One of the most common musculoskeletal complaints is shoulder stiffness, sometimes diagnosed as frozen shoulder; in fact, this may be the first sign of PD and should be screened further for other symptoms of PD.

Bradykinesia is the slowness of movement seen in parkinsonism. Impairment of the normal mechanisms that scale the output of agonist muscles causes the inability to produce, modulate, and terminate quick movements. Persons diagnosed with PD show relatively small EMG bursts in agonist muscles and move the legs in a series of small steps rather than in a single movement. Bradykinesia results from disruption of the neurotransmitter from the internal globus pallidus to the motor cortical regions known as the supplementary motor area and the primary motor cortex.

The slowing of lip and tongue movements during talking causes a garbled speech pattern. There is loss of fine motor skills, with the gradual development of small, cramped writing, or micrographia. Parkinsonism is accompanied often by diminished efficiency of pursuit eye movements, so that small accelerations of eye movement (saccades) are required to catch up with a moving target, which causes smooth pursuit eye movements to be jerky instead of smooth. Eye movement in the vertical plane may be reduced.

Hypokinesia refers to decreasing range and size of movement. Small gestures associated with expression are reduced. The face is mask-like, with infrequent blinking and lack of expression. Akinesia is a disorder of movement initiation and is seen in parkinsonism as a paucity of natural and automatic movements, such as crossing the legs or folding the arms. Freezing, or gait akinesia, is the sudden cessation of movement in the middle of an action sequence, as if the foot is stuck to the floor. Sometimes it is the environment that seems to trigger freezing, such as when the individual walks through a doorway or over a change in surface, like stepping from a carpet to a hard floor. Freezing most often affects walking turning, and dual-task performance is a common trigger. It can also affect speech, arm movements, and blinking. Freezing is uncommon in the early phase but increases over time. Research shows "reduced connectivity of the pedunculopontine nucleus with the cerebellum, thalamus, and multiple regions of the frontal cortex. These results support the notion that freezing of gait is strongly related to structural deficits in the right hemisphere's locomotor network, involving prefrontal cortical areas involved in executive inhibition function."[6a,27a]

The gait pattern in parkinsonism is highly stereotyped and characterized by impoverished movement, with distinctive features of stooped posture, narrow-based, short shuffling steps, foot drags or "catches," reduced arm swing, difficulty initiating walking or turning, and slowness. People with PD are unstable with 90-degree turns when asked to walk and turn faster than their preferred speed.[68] Range of motion in the joints of the lower extremity is often limited. In gait, there is a loss of heel strike, reduced toe elevation, reduced movement at the knee joints, loss of dynamic vertical force, reversal of ankle flexion–extension movement, and loss of backward-directed shear force. Trunk, pelvic, and hip movements are diminished, resulting in a decreased step length and reciprocal arm swing. Decreased maximal hip extension in terminal stance reduces force generation by the gastrocnemius in preswing, which affects gait speed. Increased left/right gait asymmetry and diminished bilateral coordination occurs with a loss of ability to produce a steady gait rhythm.

As the disease progresses, a shuffling pattern emerges, with a tendency for retropulsion and/or propulsion. Festination is common when attempting to stop or change direction; the stride becomes smaller but more rapid, and instead of stopping, the individual actually increases speed and is usually stopped by running into something or by falling. Preparatory postural responses to move from a bipedal to single-limb stance are frequently absent for induced steps, which may increase instability during first step. There is reduced ability to adapt to changes of environments or to perform new tasks. Difficulty with "ambulation" is a "clinical red flag" that marks emerging disability. Longitudinal studies reveal an overall decline in walking ability in PD, with a reduction in the average number of steps taken per day and a reduction in moderate-intensity steps (100 steps per minute). Rehabilitation aimed at improving gait, with an emphasis on intensity, is important for optimizing function and reducing disability.[16,96]

The posture in PD is characterized by flexion of the neck, trunk, hips, and knees, with elbows bent and arms adducted (Fig. 31.18). Other postural abnormalities include extreme neck flexion (antecoli), increased lateral flexion of the trunk (Pisa syndrome), or abnormal posture of the trunk in the anteroposterior plane, with marked flexion of the thoracolumbar spine. Kyphosis, or extensive flexion of the spine, is the most common postural deformity. Scoliosis, an abnormal lateral curvature of the spine, can result from the unequal distribution of rigidity in posture.

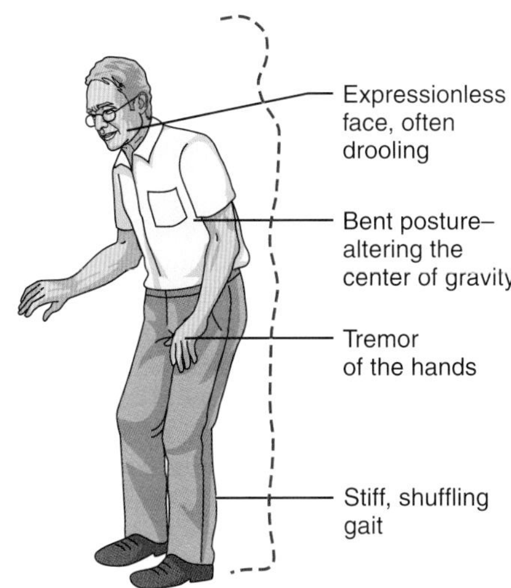


**Figure 31.18**

Typical posture that results from Parkinson disease.

Postural instability in people with PD is a result of impairments of multiple systems. Musculoskeletal constraints of persistent posturing of a forward head and trunk, decreased joint mobility, narrow foot stance, and axial rigidity tend to pull the center of gravity forward and reduce functional limits of stability, especially in the backward direction. Central motor drive is impaired, causing bradykinetic movements, poorly timed and scaled anticipatory postural adjustments. Feedforward control to stabilize posture before and during voluntary movements is compromised. Abnormal patterns of postural responses, including excessive antagonist activity, results in coactivation of distal and proximal muscles. Adapting to changing support conditions is less efficient in individuals with PD. The ability to sequence motor activity appears to have an impact on postural correction. During posterior perturbations, lack of stability appears to be the result of lack of appropriate knee flexion.

Most people with PD experience weakness and fatigue once the disease becomes generalized. The person has difficulty sustaining activity and experiences increasing weakness and lethargy as the day progresses. Repetitive motor acts may start out strong but decrease in strength as the activity progresses. This compounds bradykinesia and increases immobility. Performing dual tasks causes more slowing in individuals who have parkinsonism. Smooth performance of sequential motor tasks is broken down into distinct components. The functions of the basal ganglia incorporate motor program selection and adaptation, which involves maintenance of coordination between body parts, task-specific adjustments of movement, and quick shifts from one task to the next. Changing the "set" for an activity is more difficult for the individual with parkinsonism when the context or environment requires a sudden change in activity.

Nonmotor symptoms, such as those related to autonomic dysfunction, are common and potentially disabling manifestations of the disease. Loss of neurons in the sympathetic ganglia may cause autonomic dysfunction. This results in excessive sweating, excessive salivation, incontinence, and disabling orthostatic hypotension. There is a greasy appearance to the skin of the face and occasional drooling because of loss of the swallowing movements that normally dispose of saliva. Olfactory dysfunction is an early sign of PD in most individuals, and overlaps with multiple system atrophy and progressive supranuclear palsy. Many visual problems can affect PD patients, such as visual acuity, alterations in the blink pattern, contrast sensitivity, color discrimination, vergence eye movements/ocular motilities and visual field sensitivity, and visual processing speeds. Individuals with PD have a higher prevalence of convergence insufficiency and symptomatology (double vision, fatigue, blurred vision, tearing when reading).[42]

Rapid eye movement sleep behavior disorders result in lack of the normal muscle atonia and jerking of body

**Box 31.12**

**CAUSES OF BALANCE IMPAIRMENT IN PARKINSON DISEASE**

- Loss of postural reflexes
- Visuospatial deficits
- Central vestibular processing deficit
- Impaired anticipatory postural adjusments
- Retropulsion
- Start hesitation
- Freezing
- Festinating gait
- Orthostatic hypotension
- True vertigo

and limbs, causing disrupted sleep. Restless leg syndrome appears to be associated, mostly because of the similarities in treatment response. Abnormal sleep patterns may also contribute to the daily fatigue.

Fatigue is related to other nonmotor features, such as depression and excessive daytime sleepiness. In more than half of the individuals, mental fatigue is persistent and seems to be an independent symptom that develops parallel to the progressive neurodegenerative disorder of PD.

Dysfunction of the basal ganglia also influences sensory integration. The inability to distinguish self-movement from movement in the environment can contribute to abnormal balance reactions. There is an increased dependence on visual information for motor control. There is strong visual dependency for balance, resulting in the inability to choose a balance strategy based on vestibular information, even when the visual surround is unavailable for visual stability. Visual verticality perception is deviated already in early stages.[86] Spatial organization is often disturbed, resulting in difficulty with orientation to the environment. People with PD have difficulty rapidly changing sensory weighting for different balance situations.[87] Box 31.12 outlines some of the contributions to imbalance seen in individuals with parkinsonism

Pain syndromes and discomfort in PD usually arise from one of five causes: (1) a musculoskeletal problem related to poor posture, awkward mechanical function, or physical wear and tear; (2) nerve or root pain, often related to neck or back arthritis; (3) pain from dystonia, the sustained twisting or posturing of a muscle group or body part; (4) discomfort caused by extreme restlessness; and (5) a rare pain syndrome known as "primary" or "central" pain, arising from the brain.

Cognitive impairment in PD varies in its severity, rate of progression, and affected cognitive function. Progression to dementia does not always occur but develops in about 80% of patients with PD durations longer than 20 years. Cognitive deficits in PD typically affect executive functions, attention, visuospatial function, and processing speed. Bradyphrenia, a slowing of thought processes, with lack of concentration and attention, may also occur. REM sleep behavior disorder is closely related to PD cognitive impairment, and greater daytime sleepiness has been associated with worse cognition in PD.[32] Coexisting AD, organic brain disease, and vascular compromise may also contribute to the dementia.

**Table 31.8** Hoehn and Yahr Classification of Disability

| Stage | Character of Disability |
|---|---|
| I | Minimal or absent; unilateral if present |
| II | Minimal bilateral or midline involvement; balance not impaired |
| III | Impaired righting reflexes; unsteadiness when turning or rising from chair; some activities restricted but patient can live independently and continue some forms of employment |
| IV | All symptoms present and severe; standing and walking possible only with assistance |
| V | Confined to bed or wheelchair |

Modified from Hoehn MM, Yahr MD: Parkinsonism: onset, progression and mortality, *Neurology* 17:427, 1967.

Depression is common and is probably related to the dopamine depletion. Loss of serotonin in the brainstem and limbic lobes has been found using PET studies. Behavioral changes, such as apathy, lack of ambition, indecisiveness, and anhedonia, are common and may be related to depression. Depressive episodes or panic attacks can precede onset of motor symptoms.

Although reduced motor activity by itself would not seem to be a functional disorder, many of the small automatic muscular adjustments are important for successfully carrying out functional activities. For example, in attempting to rise from a chair a person may fail to make the small initial adjustments of legs that are crucial to standing up and fail to be able to get from sitting to standing without an assist.

The person with PD typically becomes deconditioned. Rapid heart rate and difficulty breathing are common. Vital capacity is reduced as the kyphosis increases and the intercostal muscles develop rigidity. Respiratory complications are the leading cause of death. The Hoehn and Yahr classification (Table 31.8) is a common scale used to define the level of disability associated with PD.

## MEDICAL MANAGEMENT

**DIAGNOSIS.** There is no single blood or imaging test that can definitively diagnose PD. In most cases, the diagnosis is made on the basis of the classic triad of signs (tremor, rigidity, and akinesia), a typical medical history, and characteristic findings on physical examination. The combination of asymmetry of symptoms and signs, the presence of a resting tremor, and a good response to levodopa best differentiates PD from parkinsonism as a result of other causes. Diagnostic problems may occur in mild cases. New clinical criteria for PD diagnosis does not include dementia any longer as an exclusion criterion and accepts the diagnosis of PD independent of when dementia arises.[81] Other movement disorders that do not fall under the category of parkinsonism need to be recognized by clinicians to establish a differential diagnosis. Box 31.13 lists features of parkinsonism as a result of causes other than PD. Imaging may be helpful, especially if specific MRI changes precede satisfaction of clinical criteria, but accuracy of diagnosis based on MRI findings

Box 31.13

**ATYPICAL PARKINSONIAN SYNDROMES**

| Multiple System Atrophy—Parkinsonian Type | Multiple System Atrophy—Cerebellar Type |
|---|---|
| Symmetrical onset | Cerebellar limb, gait ataxia |
| Rapid symptom progression | Early gait instability, falls |
| Jerky, myoclonic, postural/action tremor | Dysarthria (scanning, ataxic) |
| Contractures of hands and feet | Dysphagia |
| Anterocollis, axial dystonia (camptocormia ± lateral flexion, or Pisa syndrome) | Gaze impairment (hypo/hyperkinetic saccades) |
| Early gait difficulty, falls | Lower and upper motor neuron signs |
| Severe dysphonia, dysarthria | Emotionality, depression, anxiety |
| New/increased snoring, sleep apnea | Progressive dementia |
| Respiratory/laryngeal stridor | No family history of ataxia or parkinsonsism |
| Hyperreflexia, Babinski's | |
| Pseudobulbar affect (emotional lability) | |
| Cold hands/feet | |
| Dysautonomia (69% vs 5% in PD) | |
| Poor/unsustained levodopa response (≈30%) | |
| Orofacial dyskinesia/dystonia | |

From McFarland NR. Diagnostic approach to atypical parkinsonian syndromes *Continuum* 22(4):1134, 2016. doi: 10.1212/CON.0000000000000348.

and PET/single-photon emission computerized tomography (SPECT) imaging is not higher than clinical expertise. Whereas structural changes are mild in PD, changes in PSP and parkinsonian-type multiple system atrophy are largely more evident including atrophy, increased iron load, increased diffusivity, and signal changes in specific brain regions. In PSP, the most prominent changes are seen in the midbrain, the superior cerebellar peduncles, and less so in the basal ganglia. In parkinsonian-type multiple system atrophy, changes predominate in the basal ganglia, pons, and cerebellum.[75]

Depression, with its associated expressionless face, poorly modulated voice, and reduction in voluntary activity, may be difficult to distinguish from mild parkinsonism. Olfaction is frequently impaired in PD, suggesting that deficiencies in smell may be a potentially useful test to distinguish PD from related disorders.

CT or MRI is not helpful in diagnosis of PD but can identify other causes of symptoms, such as Wilson disease, or mass effects causing disruption of the basal ganglia function, such as stroke or hydrocephalus. Additional conditions that have similar symptoms and presentations are presented in Box 31.14. In 2011, the United States Food and Drug Administration approved the use of DaTSCAN for detecting images of the level of dopamine transporters in the brains of people with suspected parkinsonian syndromes. DaTSCAN binds to the presynaptic dopamine active transporter (DAT) on neurons that communicate with areas controlling movement, including the striatum. The DaTSCAN SPECT is

Box 31.14

**CONDITIONS WITH SIMILAR SYMPTOMS TO PARKINSON DISEASE**

***Dementia with Lewy Bodies***

- Dementia: cognitive impairments (attention, executive function, visuospatial skills)
- At least one the following:
  - Parkinsonian syndrome onset after or at most 12 months before onset of dementia
  - Fluctuations in alertness and attention
  - Repeated visual hallucinations

***Multisystem Atrophy***

- Dysautonomia: urinary incontinence, erectile dysfunction, orthostatic hypotension
- At least one of the following:
  - Parkinsonian syndrome: bradykinesia with rigidity, tremor, or postural instability
  - Cerebellar syndrome: gait ataxia with cerebellar dysarthria, limb ataxia, or cerebellar oculmotor dysfunction
- **Progressive Supranuclear Palsy** (includes presentation variations that are diagnosed with late-onset of vertical supranuclear gaze palsy)
  - PSP-RS (40% of cases): symmetric axial-oriented, akinetic rigidity, levodopa resistant Parkinson syndrome with early postural instability and vertical supranuclear gaze palsy
  - PSP-P (20% of cases): asymmetric, limb-predominant, levodopa-responsive parkinsonian syndrome with late-onset of vertical supranuclear gaze palsy
  - Behavioral variant of frontotemporal dementia (15% of cases): apathy and impaired executive functions, late-onset of vertical supranuclear gaze palsy
  - Corticobasal syndrome (10% of cases): at least one cortical symptom (apraxia, loss of cortical sensitivity, alien limb phenomenon) and at least one extrapyramidal symptom (akinesia, rigidity, dystonia, myoclonus)
  - Progressive nonfluent aphasia (5% of cases): nonfluent speech production with agrammatism but spared single word comprehension
  - Pure akinesia with gait freezing (< 5%): gait freezing without rigidity, without tremor, late-onset of vertical supranuclear gaze palsy

***Corticobasal Degeneration***

A neuropathological diagnosis, so may include other clinical syndromes from PSP category

- Corticobasal syndrome (25%): at least one cortical symptom (apraxia, loss of cortical sensitivity, alien limb phenomenon) and at least one extrapyramidal symptom (akinesia, rigidity, dystonia, myoclonus)
- Frontal behavioral spatial syndrome (10%): executive dysfunction, behavioral or personality changes, visuospatial deficits
- Richardson's syndrome (40%—see description above)
- Progressive nonfluent aphasia (<5%—see description above)

Information compiled from Levin J, Kurz A, Arzberger T, Glese A, et al: The differential diagnosis and treatment of atypical Parkinsonism, *Dtsch Arzlebl Int* 113:61-69, 2016; and Lang AE, Lozano AM: Parkinson's disease, *N Engl J Med* 339(15):1044-1053, 1998.

Box 31.15

**MOVEMENT DISORDERS SOCIETY CLINICAL DIAGNOSTIC CRITERIA FOR PD**

| Supportive | Red Flags | Exclusionary |
|---|---|---|
| Cardinal features: rest tremor, rigidity, bradykinesia (documented) | Rapid progression of gait impairment, requiring a wheelchair within 5 yrs of onset | Unequivocal cerebellar abnormalities (e.g., cerebellar gait, limb ataxia, oculomotor abnormalities) |
| Clear response to dopaminergic therapy (subjective or >30% change in UPDRS III with treatment) | Absence of progression of motor symptoms or signs over 5 yrs or more (absent treatment) | Downward vertical supranuclear gaze palsy or selective slowing of vertical saccades |
| Marked on/off fluctuations, end-dose wearing off<br>Presence of levodopa-induced dyskinesias | Early bulbar dysfunction (< 5 yrs from onset) | Probable behavioral variant FTD or PPA within <5 yrs onset |
| Olfactory loss | Inspiratory respiratory dysfunction (stridor, frequent sighs) | Restriction of parkinsonism to lower extremities >3 yrs |
| Cardiac sympathetic denervation on MIBG scintigraphy | Severe autonomic failure (< 5 yrs from onset) | Drug-induced parkinsonism (documented prior use and link to drug, i.e., antipsychotic, etc.) |
| | Recurrent (>1/yr) falls from imbalance within 3 yrs of onset | Absence of response to high-dose levodopa |
| | Anterocollis or limb contractures within 10 yrs of onset | Cortical sensory loss (evidence of graphesthesia, astereognosis) ideomotor apraxia, or primary aphasia |
| | Absence of common nonmotor features (sleep dysfunction, RBD, RLS/PLMS, daytime somnolence, autonomic dysfunction, hyposmia, mood disturbance) | Normal dopamine transporter imaging (presynaptic) |
| | Otherwise unexplained pyramidal tract signs | Documentation of an alternative condition |
| | Bilateral symmetric parkinsonism | |

Adapted with permission from Postuma RB, et al: MDS clinical diagnostic criteria for Parkinson's disease, *Mov Disord* 30:1591–1601, 2015and McFarland NR, Hess CW: Recognizing atypical Parkinsonisms: "red flags" and therapeutic approaches, *Semin Neurol* 37(2):215–227, 2017.

most helpful in differentiating between PD and essential tremor, drug-induced parkinsonism, and psychogenic parkinsonism. It is not able to differentiate between PD, progressive supranuclear palsy, multiple systems atrophy, and other neurodegenerative diseases affecting the dopamine neurons in the brain. For the classic motor symptoms of PD to be present, typically 50% or more of these neurons must be lost. DaTSCAN is able to detect this decreased activity early in the course of PD, when the diagnosis may still be uncertain. Neither DaTSCAN nor a doctor's examination is a perfect (gold standard) method for diagnosing PD. Both methods will occasionally miss actual cases of PD, while misdiagnosing other diseases that resemble PD. Only an autopsy can conclusively determine whether a person's brain exhibits PD pathology. Box 31.15 provides diagnostic criteria that support or exclude PD as a diagnosis.

Functional imaging through PET is highly sensitive to regional changes in brain metabolism and receptor binding associated with movement disorders. SPECT shows differences in the posterior putamen, contralateral to the predominantly affected limb. Asymmetric scan findings have been observed in individuals with mild, newly recognized symptoms. Unilateral disease produces a significant difference in striatal uptake between the ipsilateral and contralateral sides in both the caudate and putamen nuclei. One explanation is that there is a preceding unequal functional reactivity of the basal ganglia, which results in an asymmetrical clinical response.

Altropane (a close cousin of cocaine), a component of radioactive technetium-99m, is a compound that can measure the concentration of dopamine transporters imaged by SPECT. This may lead to diagnosis of PD based on identifying decreasing levels in the brains of persons when only mild symptoms appear.

Assessing progression of PD using clinical rating scales such as the United Parkinson's Disease Rating Scale is a common way to track progression. However, the progression may be masked by medication, and because of the multitude of symptoms that may change at different rates, it is hard to determine a change in the course of the disease. Research is ongoing to continue to develop better tests to diagnose and track PD. New imaging scans include selective alpha-synuclein brain scan in human trials. Noninvasive tests include projects looking at the retina, sweat, and facial expression.[79] Wearable devices such as smartwatches, sensors, and phone apps are researching different ways to track symptoms.[24]

**TREATMENT.** Overall, the treatment is to preserve a patient's independence and quality of life. The current therapeutic approach to PD is symptomatic; major studies to determine possible therapeutic neuroprotection are still being researched, but no single intervention has proven to be disease modifying. Drug therapy is adapted to the person's needs, which may vary with the stage of the disease and the predominant manifestations. When mobility becomes affected to the degree that walking and self-care activities become difficult, medications improve the control of movement. As the disease progresses over time, the effectiveness of medication changes, leaving the individual with a shorter "on" time during which symptoms are reduced and more rigidity during "off" times when symptoms are active. Long-term use of medication can also increase the dyskinesia or chorea-like movement resulting from the change in activity in the basal ganglia. Side effects can become more problematic as the dosages needed to control symptoms are increased. The management of these medications becomes the focus of intervention.

Levodopa (L-dopa), which is taken up by remaining dopaminergic neurons in the basal ganglia and converted to dopamine, improves most of the major features of parkinsonism, including tremor, rigidity, bradykinesia, and walking problems. Initially it leads to nearly complete reversal of symptoms, with effects lasting up to 2 weeks, known as long-duration levodopa response. As the disease progresses, the length of the effect becomes shorter, it takes longer for the effect to be noticed after dosing, and symptoms increase during the end of the dose period. Eventually there is dose failure or lack of any effect at all. Levodopa can cause dyskinesias that produce chorea, athetosis, dystonia, tics, and myoclonus. Predictable fluctuations include a wearing-off effect and early morning akinesia. The duration of effect of each dose becomes shorter and will often match the drug's half-life of less than 2 hours. Protein in food uses the same mechanism as levodopa for crossing the blood-brain barrier. When levodopa is given with protein, the protein blocks the ability of the levodopa to cross the blood-brain barrier. This is usually managed by having the individual eat most of the daily protein in the evening, when immobility will cause the least inconvenience. Caffeine administered before levodopa may improve its pharmacokinetics in some individuals with parkinsonian symptoms. Levodopa should be avoided in persons with malignant melanoma and in persons with active peptic ulcers, which may bleed.

Carbidopa (Sinemet) inhibits the breakdown of levodopa and is often used in combination with levodopa. Carbidopa reduces the amount of levodopa required daily for beneficial effects and is often combined with levodopa in a single preparation (Sinemet). New formulations of levodopa and novel delivery systems designed to smooth out the motor fluctuations and reduce dyskinesia have been developed. Rytary is an extended-release combination of carbidopa-levodopa designed to maintain a steady level of relief and minimize on and off periods. Carbidopa-levodopa enteral suspension (Duopa®) is a carboxymethylcellulose aqueous gel form of the carbidopa-levodopa medication delivered continuously to the proximal jejunum via a percutaneous gastrojejunostomy tube connected to a portable infusion pump. Since the gel medication bypasses the stomach, it allows the medication to be more predictably and consistently absorbed throughout the day, which reduces fluctuations and the frustrating effects that can come during off periods. A new sublingual apomorphine formulation (APL-130277) and an inhaled levodopa are under FDA review to provide a convenient and rapid method for treating off episodes.[54,83] Catechol-*O*-methyl transferase (COMT) inhibitors slow the breakdown of dopamine in the body. Of these, entacapone (Comtan) and tolcapone (Tasmar) reduce the off time, and allow for decreased dosing of levodopa. Liver function must be monitored regularly with the use of tolcapone. Tolcapone must be used with levodopa but can decrease the amount of levodopa needed. A combination pill called Stalevo combines carbidopa/levodopa and entacapone.

Dopamine agonists act directly on dopamine receptors. Bromocriptine (Parlodel) seems to be the best tolerated, and its use in parkinsonism is associated with a lower incidence of response fluctuations. It is often given in combination with levodopa and carbidopa. Pramipexole (Mirapex) or ropinirole (Requip) can be used either to delay starting levodopa or to decrease the amount needed. Transdermal application of dopamine agonists can be provided with rotigotine (Neupro Patch) and lisuride. Apomorphine (Apokyn) is injected under the skin to provide quick action, typically 20 minutes, and is used for rescue treatment when wearing off is abrupt or unpredictable. Another novel means of drug delivery under development in Europe is a nasal spray version of apomorphine. Researchers have developed a new drug that is in the early phases of research called dopamine D2/3 receptor agonist that may limit the progression of Parkinson disease while providing better symptom relief.[53] One possible adverse effect of dopamine agonists is sedation, sleep attacks, and the occurrence of drug-induced compulsive behaviors (shopping, gambling, eating, hypersexuality).

Monoamine oxidase type B (MAO-B) inhibitors (selegiline (Eldepryl) and rasagiline (Azilect) and Xadago) block the effect of the enzyme MAO-B that naturally breaks down several chemicals in our brain, including dopamine, allowing more dopamine to be available.[9] These inhibitors are usually used early in treatment when symptoms are mild and can be added when problems with wearing off occur and symptoms return between medication doses. Research has shown the neuroprotective functions of rasagiline and selegiline with an increase in glial-derived neurotrophic factor and brain-derived neurotrophic factor.

Persons with mild symptoms but no disability may be helped by amantadine (Osmolex ER (amantadine extended-release), Symmetrel (immediate-release amantadine), and Gocovri (extended-release amantadine). Gocovri (extended-release amantadine) is the only medication that is FDA approved to reduce dyskinesia. Coadministration of levodopa and amantadine controls dyskinesia without disrupting the effect of levodopa.[25]

In the striatum the low level of dopamine is accompanied by increased cholinergic transmission. Anticholinergic drugs help reduce rest tremor only and are not used to treat other motor symptoms. The side effects of the anticholinergic medications, including sedation, confusion, and psychosis, limit their usefulness, especially with advancing age. MAO-B inhibitors have replaced the use of anticholinergics in treatment of PD.

Antioxidants have been studied for neuroprotection, such as coenzyme Q10, which helps stabilize mitochondria and appears to decrease the worsening of symptoms. Trophic factors, antiinflammatories, antiapoptotics, and antioxidants have been identified by the National Institutes of Health for further study for control of neuronal death.

Deep brain stimulation uses a pacemaker-like device surgically implanted with electrodes in the nuclei of choice and a pulse generator implanted in the chest. The generator is controlled externally through a magnetic field. Stimulation through the electrodes can be applied to the internal globus pallidus and the subthalamic nucleus or thalamus. Thalamic stimulation is most effective for tremor, with less effect on dyskinesia and rigidity. Electrode implantation in the globus pallidus appears to have good initial effect; however, there is a chance of psychosis and punding activity over time. Most centers are now stimulating the subthalamic nucleus bilaterally, but the individual's profile leads the decision. Although the picture is not yet clear on the issue of target choice, the subthalamic nucleus does seem to provide more medication reduction, whereas the globus pallidus may be slightly safer for language and cognition. Preoperative response to levodopa predicts better outcome after deep brain stimulation of the subthalamic nucleus. Recent developments in the field of DBS surgery include high-field MRI for target identification, intraoperative MR localization to help electrode placement, and the performance of DBS procedures under general anesthesia. Stimulation can increase on time and decrease off time, as well as the severity of the off periods. Dyskinesia typically improves over time, either as a result in medication reduction or as an effect of stimulation. The ability to perform activities of daily living is improved, and there is typically improved sleep time. Apathy and abulia can occur over time; this may be related to withdrawal of levodopa. There can be an increase in sadness or the opposite response with excessive hilarity that may be related to stimulation of the surrounding area or change in subthalamic limbic activity. Edema around the electrode may contribute to the psychotropic effects. The implant is thought to last approximately 5 years and can be removed if another more effective type of treatment is found. Bilateral subthalamic stimulation, alone or in combination with levodopa, causes improvement in axial signs for posture and postural stability.

Although there is little evidence for drug effect on postural stability and gait disorders, researchers in motor control are making progress in identifying the nature of the abnormal responses both inside and outside of the basal ganglia. Based on the strong evidence that relates prior exercise and activity status to risk of PD, and the recent knowledge gained about neuroplasticity in the brain, it is likely that changes in postural control may come through interventions that drive neuroplastic changes.

Although orthostatic hypotension affects less than 20% of individuals with parkinsonism, it can limit activity. Use of midodrine (ProAmatine), fludrocortisone (Florinef), and pyridostigmine (Mestinon) can be helpful in maintaining normal blood pressure. Supine hypertension may result and must be monitored. Urinary dysfunction is treated via antimuscarinic agents or α-agonists. Anticholinergics or scopolamine patches may be helpful for drooling, and use of intraparotid injection of botulinum toxin-A (Xeomin) can help. Constipation is common and may precede the motor symptoms in PD; it is usually managed by fluids, fiber, stool softeners, and exercise.

Depression is found in more than 40% of individuals with PD. Medication interactions must be looked at carefully. Use of serotonin uptake inhibitors may interact with selegiline. Tricyclics can be useful, but the central effects must be monitored more carefully than in the healthy younger population.

Respiratory complications, which are the leading cause of death, can be prevented to some extent with an early aggressive aerobic exercise program, followed by regular moderate activity as the disease progresses. Control of breathing can be facilitated using verbal and tactile stimuli and should be integrated into any intervention.

Behavioral abnormalities can be associated with high doses of dopaminergic replacement therapy, including the phenomenon of punding, characterized by fascination with technical equipment and excessive sorting of objects, grooming, hoarding, or use of a computer. This may be related to the impaired frontal lobe function and a result of psychomotor stimulation. Other abnormalities in reward-seeking behavior related to dopamine are hypersexuality and excessive gambling. Reducing the level of medication is helpful, and some neuroleptics such as clozapine will lessen symptoms of psychosis.

Experimental therapeutics targeted at improving dopaminergic drugs to increase selectivity for various receptor subtypes and at controlling the uptake of dopamine are currently under study. Improved plasma stability is achieved through transdermal application, which bypasses the fluctuations in gastric release. Studies are aimed at potential substances that evoke antiparkinsonism through neurotransmitter systems outside of dopamine. Pharmacologic manipulation of glutamate and GABA neurotransmission includes the drug istradefylline, which completed phase III trials. In Japan, istradefylline is approved to use in the adjunctive treatment of PD, but is still not an FDA-approved drug in the United States. Opiate, serotonin, and histamine receptors are possible sites for intervention. A more careful look at the cholinergic system may help to manage the issues of dementia and find possibilities for reducing the apparent dysfunction at the level of the brainstem that affects sleep-wake cycles and orthostasis. Droxidopa can help patients with neurogenic orthostatic hypotension. It augments norepinephrine levels, which should lead to improved cerebral perfusion following orthostatic challenge, thereby reducing rapid drop in blood pressure and symptoms of dizziness, fainting, and falls.[39,48]

Researchers found that the compound MCC950, a potent inhibitor of the NLRP3 inflammasome, given orally once a day could stop neuroinflammation. MCC950 arrested the effects of PD in several animal models of the disease, leading to reduced brain neuron loss and higher levels of dopamine. A team at Harvard Medical School is developing a therapy using induced pluripotent stem cells (iPSCs) to replace midbrain cells that produce dopamine. The goal is to reduce or prevent the motor symptoms of PD, along with medication-induced dyskinesias. At McGill University, scientists are looking for compounds that activate parkin, which could be developed into drugs for PD. Loss of parkin activity is associated with both familial PD through inherited genetic mutations, as well as idiopathic PD.[97] Cell transplantation of grafted dopaminergic neurons in PD continues to hold promise. The striatum (caudate and putamen) are primary targets for the implants.[10]

**PROGNOSIS.** In general, all the clinical manifestations in PD worsen progressively, although not to the same extent. Tremor as a presenting symptom may be used to predict a more benign course and longer therapeutic benefit to levodopa. In individuals with newly diagnosed PD, older age at onset and rigidity/hypokinesia as an initial symptom can be used to predict more rapid rate of motor progression.

The presence of associated comorbidities, stroke, auditory deficits, and visual impairments as well as male sex may be used to predict faster rate of motor progression. Older age at onset and initial hypokinesia/rigidity may be used to predict earlier development of cognitive decline and dementia. Older age at onset, dementia, and decreased dopamine responsiveness may be used to predict earlier nursing home placement as well as decreased survival. Lack of mobility, loss of balance reactions, and weakness result in more falls than in an age-matched normal population. Osteoporosis can result from prolonged inactivity and may be present secondary to advanced age at onset. Falls more often lead to fractures, owing to the prevalence of osteoporosis. Fracture healing may be delayed. Posture and gait abnormalities are the most difficult to control in advanced cases.

PD does not significantly reduce life span in most persons who develop the generalized form between 50 and 60 years of age. However, because there is progressive neuronal loss despite the response to treatment, deterioration continues until death occurs, often from infection or other conditions associated with debilitation.

As the onset of disease is typically in the fifth or sixth decade of life and is progressive despite medication, the economic cost of the disease can be quite high because of loss of income and costs of drugs, assistive devices, and assisted living. Pain, fatigue, and depression also adversely affect the quality of life compared with that of age-matched normal subjects.

## SPECIAL IMPLICATIONS FOR THE THERAPIST 31.6

### *Parkinson Disease*

There are clearly various and separate components of the movement disorders related to parkinsonism, especially in PD. As we become better able to identify the relationship between specific impairment and the resulting function, intervention by the therapist will have more impact on ability to participate in typical activities. Each individual's needs and goals must be addressed and programs modified as the movement disorders change as the disease progresses. Skills are learned most effectively when they are practiced repeatedly in relation to meaningful goals. The benefits of exercise are well established for people with PD, but long-term compliance is limited. Research is now studying how to promote increased activity/exercise/walking in the community. The use of community-based wellness exercise classes, a virtual exercise coach, pedometers, and tandem bikes are all being explored.

Of course, we understand the benefits of exercise "use it or lose it" theory, but educating and improving our patient's confidence is important for them to adhere to a program and make life-long changes in exercise and physical activity habits. Low outcome expectation from exercise, lack of time to exercise, and fear of falling appear to be important perceived barriers to engaging in exercise in people who have PD, are ambulatory, and dwell in the community. These may be important issues for physical therapists to target in people who have PD and do not exercise regularly.

Following the World Health Organization in the International Classification of Functioning, Disability, and Health (ICF) model intervention should address all of the ICF categories: body structure and function (directly related to PD: tremor, bradykinesia, rigidity, akinesia, postural instability; indirectly related to PD: decreased flexibility decreased endurance), activity (gait, transfers, bed mobility) and participation (ability to work and interact socially, self-care, recreational sports, quality of life). Environmental factors (home and community settings) and personal factors (resources, personal attitudes, self-efficacy, emotions and feelings) all need to be considered. In addition, understanding the timing and effects of their medication and collaborating with the multidisciplinary team will optimize the benefits of your treatment plan. The elements of repetition, intensity, and challenge, together with skilled training, will lead to improved goal-directed motor skill learning. The SPARX trial was the first dose-response study in people who have PD and are not yet on medications to show high-intensity treadmill exercise may be feasible and prescribed safely and may slow symptoms of PD. Over a 6-month period, patients who were assigned to the high-intensity treadmill exercise group (4 days per week, 80 to 85% maximum heart rate) had lower mean changes in their Unified Parkinson's Disease Rating Scale motor score, signifying less progression of motor symptoms as compared to the moderate-intensity (4 days per week, 60% to 65% maximum heart rate), and no-exercise control group.[85]

#### Exercises to Address Rigidity

Spinal flexibility or axial mobility contributes to function. It can impact ability to perform many of the components of tasks, including functional reach, movement in bed, and turning while walking. Exercises should minimize co-contraction (i.e., by performing rhythmic and alternating movements), promote axial rotation, lengthen the flexor muscles, strengthen the extensor muscles, promote erect posture, and teach relaxation strategies.

#### Exercises to Address Bradykinesia

Bradykinesia is associated with slow and weak postural responses to perturbations and anticipatory adjustments. Slowed rate of muscle activation patterns occurs. "Because bradykinesia is due to impaired central neural drive, rehabilitation to reduce bradykinesia should focus on teaching patients to increase speed, amplitude, and temporal pacing of their self-initiated and reactive limb and body center of mass movements."[50]

#### Exercises to Improve Balance/Postural Stability

More research is looking at how balance control relies on the interaction of several physiologic systems (the musculoskeletal, neuromuscular, cognitive, sensory systems) with environmental factors and the performed task. Exercises need to improve sensory integration of the vestibular and somatosensory system and decrease visual dependency, improve timing and amplitude, and improve task-specific adaptation. Whole-body coordination, the ability to shift between different tasks and control center of mass and base of support to increase functional limits of stability should be a part of the exercise regimen in those with fall risk. Each component of balance needs to be progressed in difficulty and complexity. Meta-analyses show that physical therapy is effective in decreasing fall risk and improving gait and balance.[51,90,106]

Tai chi, yoga, tango dancing, and boxing and theoretically based, highly challenging, and progressive exercise programs have all shown improvements in postural stability.[92,51,22]

### Exercises to Improve Gait

The use of external cues is effective in replacing the absent internal control that disturbs automatic and repetitive movements and allows movement to be directly controlled by cortical control. The use of rhythmic auditory stimulation in persons with PD leads to an increase in gait velocity, cadence, and stride length associated with an increase in the EMG activity around the ankle. Complexity of task appears to be related to gait. Individuals with moderate disability associated with PD experience considerable difficulty when they are required to walk while attending to complex visuomotor tasks involving the upper limbs. Visual cueing for improved gait appears to have the most effect on stride length and decreases time spent in double stance during walking but has shown limited retention. Walking speed, arm swing amplitude, and step length can be increased by verbal instructional sets, using cognitive strategies. Many studies support the benefits of treadmill training to improve gait speed, stride length, walking distance, and quality of life. Treadmill training offers opportunity for a lot of practice; high number of reps may facilitate retention, and external cue to provide rhythmic and somatosensory feedback, used with external cues (auditory) paired with attentional strategy, maximizes benefits. Gait training strategies and goals will vary according the progression of the disease.

Managing the home environment is critical, as most falls occur at home. The training of a caregiver to give the appropriate verbal and visual cues can be beneficial. Use of grab bars can be valuable, especially if there is a bathtub, since stepping over the edge requires significant weight shift. A vertical grab bar or counterbalancing reminder next to doors can help individuals with retropulsion. Recognizing areas that may induce freezing (doorways, narrow spaces) may decrease the fall risk in those areas. Keeping a diary of falls can be helpful. Strategies mentioned earlier can work by means of bypassing the basal ganglia and making use of the supplementary motor area. External feedback can be effective in improving movement when it cannot be controlled from internal organization. Use of virtual reality has been shown to be effective in persons with parkinsonism. Until the time that it is readily available, techniques employed by persons with PD to trigger movement or to "unfreeze" are used by most individuals with PD. Parkinsonian syndromes studies are limited but are starting to be researched more than case studies. Findings support the use of balance and eye movement exercises to improve gaze control in progressive supranuclear palsy. Another study involved audio-biofeedback to improve balance.[73]

Nonmotor symptoms may have an effect on therapy. Anxiety, apathy, and/or depression can cause low energy, fear, poor motivation, poor compliance, and contribute to gait disorders.[4] Cognitive impairment may impact the ability of individuals with PD to learn new motor skills and/or answer questions. Pathways leading to and from the frontal cortex, limbic lobe, and hippocampus are affected in PD. Learning strategies and environments that best eliminate stress need to be identified. Decreased attention (shifting or selecting and decreased concentration (increased distractibility) may require a quiet environment, redirection, simple commands, and repetition. Decreased executive functioning may decrease problem solving and cause poor self-analysis and self-correction. Decreased organizational ability may need lists, reminders, timers, and simplification. Decreased multitasking or dual-tasking may need to begin with one task at a time before adding increased cognitive and motor loads. Sleep disturbances may cause fatigue and/or low energy. Bladder urgency and frequency may shift focus from the task at hand. Orthostatic hypotension may cause dizziness, unsteadiness, and/or falls. Pain or paresthesia may limit activity level and cause fear. Dyskinesia may increase instability, and safety and compensatory techniques may need to be taught. Medication side effects may impact the client's ability to participate in therapy, and modifications may be necessary if the medication level drops during the session. Caregivers can be trained to assist in mobility during "off" periods.

Intervention strategies have been established and can be used to establish programs. Clinical trials with randomized approaches are under way to provide evidence of interventions addressing the movement disorders discussed here. This will assist therapists the most when the components studied can be extrapolated into functional tasks. Disease-modifying aspects of exercise show strong promise. Future research may look at the complexity of the motor skills and degree of protection.

## Secondary Parkinson Syndrome

Parkinsonian syndromes, also called *atypical parkinsonism* or *Parkinson plus syndromes,* are a family of neurodegenerative disorders that result from neuronal loss in different components of the basal ganglia, the brain system of which the dopaminergic midbrain neurons affected in PD are a part. All of these disorders can be difficult to differentiate from PD early in the course of the illness. These disorders have distinctive clinical features, which may emerge only after the onset of parkinsonism. Important clinical clues that one of these disorders is present are symmetric onset of parkinsonism, absence of typical resting tremor, early autonomic dysfunction, prominent dystonia, significant early cognitive impairment, and prominent early falls.

Iatrogenic parkinsonism or drug-induced parkinsonism results from the use of pharmacologic agents that block dopamine effects or interfere with dopamine metabolism. The most common causes of drug-induced parkinsonism are dopamine antagonist antipsychotic medications. The risk of drug-induced parkinsonism is reduced significantly with newer atypical antipsychotic agents. Another group of drugs that can cause drug-induced parkinsonism is older (non–serotonin antagonist) dopamine antagonist antiemetics. Agents interfering with dopamine production or synaptic vesicular storage can cause drug-induced parkinsonism. These include methyl-para-tyrosine, methyldopa, and reserpine. Flunarizine and cinnarizine, when they are used as vestibular suppressants or cerebral vasodilators, can cause parkinsonism. Sodium valproate may cause tremor that can progress to parkinsonism. Features of iatrogenic parkinsonism are bilateral onset and predominant bradykinesia, with increased involvement in the arms compared to the legs in the younger population, but more consistent with PD in older individuals. If drug-induced parkinsonism is suspected, the suspected offending agent is withdrawn, and the individual should improve. With dopamine antagonists or reserpine, improvements can occur within days to weeks after medication withdrawal, but there is sometimes a prolonged latency of months before marked improvement occurs.

Vascular parkinsonism involves primarily the lower extremities. It is associated with lacunar infarcts (see Chapter 32) and probably represents small infarcts in the basal ganglia or corticobasilar pathways. A stroke in the region of the striatum (caudate and putamen) and hemiparesis of the arm is common. Systemic lupus erythematosus may also cause cerebral vasculitis. Vascular parkinsonism presents typically with start hesitation, a broad-based shuffling gait (rather than the narrow-based gait associated with PD), and frequent falls. Depending on the level of damage and the cause, the response to levodopa will vary.

Infectious causes of parkinsonism are suspected when the symptoms develop during the acute or recovery phase of an illness with fever. Cases of parkinsonism have been reported as a result of West Nile virus infection and have historically been associated with encephalitis. Human immunodeficiency virus (HIV) infection can cause parkinsonism via the viral damage in encephalopathy or opportunistic infections.

Toxicity, often related to manganese accumulation in the substantia nigra, can cause parkinsonism and dystonia, seen in miners, factory workers making dry cell batteries, and those exposed to some fungicides.

## Disorders with Parkinsonian Characteristics

### Benign Essential Tremor

Benign essential tremor is not associated with any underlying cause, is common after the age of 50 years, and is usually hereditary. This tremor is of a different character, and there is a lack of other neurologic signs.

### Progressive Supranuclear Palsy

Progressive supranuclear palsy (PSP) has symptoms of bradykinesia, rigidity, and postural instability similar to those of PD and is frequently misdiagnosed as PD. The main pathology in PSP is the accumulation of hyperphosphorylated tau throughout the brain, as well as in distinctive regions. The hallmark of PSP is the tufted astrocyte, but the pathology includes also neurofibrillary tangles, pretangles, and coiled bodies.[67] Postural instability is the most pronounced symptom, with early falls that are not associated with obstacles or change in surface.[20] Falls in PSP are likely to be multifactorial, central sensory integration deficits. Patients with PSP have an inability to perceive backward tilt of the surface or body, abnormal otolith-mediated reflexes, impaired proprioceptive sensory inputs, cognitive deficits, and axial rigidity, all likely contributing to PSP falls.[21] Motor recklessness may occur, such as getting abruptly out of a chair. There is usually lack of tremor, progressive onset of symmetric symptoms, gait freezing, and apraxia. Dysarthria and dysphagia are on a continuum, with dysphagia typically occurring later than 2 years after onset. Visual symptoms are also a hallmark of PSP. These include blurred vision, photosensitivity, diplopia, and difficulty reading due to both the inability to look down and due to convergence insufficiency. Downgaze impairment is the most sensitive predictor for PSP. Inhibition of eyelid opening and closure, or blepharospasm, can cause functional blindness. Inability to perform vestibulo-ocular reflex cancellation is lost. Apathy, intellectual slowing, and impairment of executive function progress, and there can be pseudobulbar features (emotional lability, dysarthria, dysphagia). The autonomic nervous system maintains near-normal function.

Levodopa and deep brain stimulation are effective for the movement disorder, and Botox can help to improve blepharospasm, dystonic posturing of the neck and limbs, and eye-opening apraxia. Brain imaging has been the most useful adjunctive diagnostic tool for PSP to date. The midbrain and superior cerebellar peduncles are typically atrophied in PSP, which can help distinguish it from other parkinsonian disorders.[67]

### Multiple System Atrophy

There is extreme clinical variability within the multiple system atrophy group of disorders that is primarily familial but can be sporadic. Neuronal atrophy is seen to a variable degree in the brainstem, cerebellum, spinal cord, and peripheral nerves. The differential pathology is associated with gliosis and cytoplasmic inclusion in the glia. Multiple system atrophy (MSA) typically has its onset in the fifth to seventh decade, and parkinsonism is the primary condition; however, there is more evidence of cerebellar involvement, and autonomic dysfunction is greater and more disabling than that found in PD. Levodopa is used in the treatment, but with less success than when it is used in PD. Cerebellar and autonomic nervous system dysfunction respond poorly to anticholinergics. Large European studies are underway to examine pathogenesis and intervention strategies. There are different types of MSA. MSA-A, sometimes called Shy-Drager syndrome, is characterized by akinetic rigid parkinsonism with early onset severe postural hypotension not related to drugs. Autonomic abnormalities are predominant and include bowel and bladder dysfunction, impotence, upper airway obstruction, cardiac

## A THERAPIST'S THOUGHTS*

### *Parkinson Disease*

Every patient with PD should be educated on neuroprotection and neuroplasticity, and the earlier they are educated, the better. In treating those diagnosed with a progressive disorder, you want to empower them on how they can change their brain and maximize the benefits of their exercise program. The intensity, difficulty, complexity, and specificity of exercises need to be explained and incorporated in their exercise routine. Although they may consider themselves "active," their intensity may not be at a sufficient level to promote the most benefits. An easy way to assess the intensity of their walking is to count their steps per minute and use a metronome or music to maintain their speed and/or increase it (100 steps/min would be considered moderate intensity). Your role as a therapist is to increase the intensity level of practice beyond their self-selected energy expenditure. Many of my patients report therapists do not work them hard enough and give in to their complaints. Make sure you always try to motivate and work your patient to their fullest ability; help them understand they are capable of moving more than they think.

Besides the intensity of exercise, the quality of movement maintained during repetitive movements is very important. One of the main movement problems due to basal ganglia disorder is the failure to automatically maintain an appropriate amplitude and timing of sequential movements. Training should include the awareness of complete muscle activation, attention to effort, and amplitude of movement. Use of auditory cues (music or metronome while walking on a treadmill), visual or tactile cues (touching a target to maintain range of motion during calf raises) will immediately enhance the size and timing of their movement and therefore maximize overall performance.

You should become aware of your patient's goals and interests (i.e., sports, hiking, dancing) and incorporate task-specific exercises to help improve outcomes and compliance. For example, if your patient plays tennis, incorporate the racket in your session during reaching and stepping exercises.

*Erica DeMarch, PT, MS

arrhythmia, disturbances of sweating and temperature regulation, and pilary changes. MSA with predominant parkinsonism (MSA-P) is defined as MSA where extrapyramidal features predominate. The term striatonigral degeneration, parkinsonian variant, is sometimes used for this category of MSA. MSA-C is defined as MSA where cerebellar ataxia predominates. It is sometimes termed sporadic olivopontocerebellar atrophy.

Olivopontocerebellar atrophy is one of the most common and variable of the non-PD parkinsonian conditions. Neuronal loss with gross atrophy is concentrated in the pons, medullary olives, and cerebellum. Ataxia, rigidity, spasticity, and oculomotor movement disturbances are present in variable degrees and combinations. The intracytoplasmic inclusions are predominantly oligodendrocytic, and there is modest tau and synuclein immunoreactivity. Tremor in MSA-P is often higher in frequency and lower in amplitude, with a jerky, stimulus-sensitive myoclonic postural/action component differentiated from the typical pill-rolling type of tremor typically seen in PD. Compared to PD, parkinsonism in MSA is more symmetrical in appearance, with dystonia (axial and appendicular), early dysarthria/dysphonia, gait and postural instability (though later compared to that in PSP), rapid progression, and autonomic dysfunction.[67]

### Wilson Disease

Wilson disease, or progressive hepatolenticular degeneration, is rare but also represents degeneration of the basal ganglia and is related to excess deposition of copper. Cysts or cavities form in the basal ganglia with necrosis. The lateral ventricles can be enlarged with associated brain atrophy. This can be imaged using MRI, PET, or SPECT studies. Cerebellar and brainstem damage is common, and there can be spheroid bodies in the cerebral cortex. The symptoms of Wilson disease go far beyond movement disorder mimicking PD and include profound affective disorders. Ophthalmologic signs of brownish or greenish rings in the periphery of the cornea are a hallmark. The disorder is treated via copper chelating.

### Restless Leg Syndrome

Restless leg syndrome is reported as the desire to move the extremities associated with paresthesia, motor restlessness with worsening of symptoms at rest (typically at night), and relief with activity or sensory stimulation. It is familial in 60% of cases, and the effect is related to reduced iron stores in the substantia nigra. There is no loss of dopaminergic neurons as is seen in PD, but the dysfunction lies within the presynaptic and postsynaptic junction of dopaminergic neurons. Levodopa is the traditional treatment, and it is effective when movement is the most problematic symptom. Opioids such as methadone can help when dopamine agents are not effective. For the individual with pain or dysesthesia, neuroleptics can be of benefit.

## REFERENCES

To enhance this text and add value for the reader, all references are included in the enhanced ebook on Student Consult that accompanies this textbook. The reader can view the reference source and access it online whenever possible.

# CHAPTER 32

# Stroke

VICKI STEMMONS MERCER • KENDA S. FULLER

## OVERVIEW

Stroke often occurs in well-appearing adults as a sudden, devastating focal vascular event that results in destruction of surrounding brain tissue. Stroke is primarily a consequence of changes in both the function of the heart and the integrity of the vessels supplying blood to the brain. See Chapter 12 for cardiac structure and function and related pathogenesis.

*Transient ischemic attack* (TIA) has been defined historically based on complete resolution of all symptoms within 24 hours of onset. However, this time-based definition has been questioned in light of findings of relevant ischemic lesions in a large percentage of individuals with presumed TIA.[20] Because clinical management and outcomes of TIA are similar to those of minor ischemic stroke, these diagnoses are commonly used interchangeably.

Stroke is a major global health problem that will continue to increase over the next 20 years as the population ages. Although stroke mortality rates have declined in recent years, stroke is the second leading global cause of death behind heart disease, accounting for 11.8% of deaths worldwide.[6] Stroke is also a leading cause of serious long-term disability. The absolute number of people affected by, or who remain disabled from, stroke is increasing, especially in low-income and middle-income countries, which bear the majority of the global stroke burden.[33] Stroke affects workplace productivity, not only of the survivors, but also of their caregivers. Work is often interrupted or abandoned based on the need to provide care for a family member.[118] Attempts to decrease the stroke burden related to intrinsic damage at onset, and control of recurrence, underlie most current studies. Effective rehabilitation strategies are also at the forefront of research.

## INCIDENCE

Of the 16.9 million people worldwide who have a first-time stroke each year, approximately 11 million survive, adding to the growing pool of stroke survivors.[41] The prevalence of stroke survivors is estimated to reach 77 million by the year 2030.[104] The average incidence rate of first strokes is 114 per 100,000 persons, which accounts for approximately 800,000 new or recurrent strokes that occur each year in the United States. First strokes account for about 75% of acute events, and recurrent strokes account for about 25%.

Incidence of stroke is increased with a family history of stroke, with both paternal and maternal influence.[51] There are several stroke types with different etiology and risk factors; therefore, management is driven by the stroke subtype. Figure 32.1 shows the prevalence of stroke types.

## RISK FACTORS

Cerebrovascular disease, the primary cause of stroke, is caused by one of several pathologic processes involving the blood vessels of the brain. The damage may be intrinsic to the vessel, or the damage may originate remotely, such as when an embolus from the heart or extracranial circulation lodges in an intracranial vessel. The stroke may result from the rupture of a vessel in the subarachnoid space or intracerebral tissue. Figure 32.2 shows the effects of different types of stroke on brain tissue.[106]

Risk factors for stroke can be divided into those that are potentially modifiable and those that are not. Among the nonmodifiable risk factors (age, race, and sex), age constitutes the greatest risk. The incidence of stroke doubles with every decade after age 55 years.[86] With regard to race, annual age-adjusted incidence for first-ever stroke is higher in black individuals than white individuals.[6] In 2015, age-adjusted stroke death rates remained higher among non-Hispanic blacks than among all other racial/ethnic groups.[6] Sex is another nonmodifiable risk factor, with women having a higher lifetime risk of stroke than men. This is largely because women live longer than men. In the Framingham Heart Study, lifetime risk of stroke among those 55 to 75 years of age was 1 in 5 for women and approximately 1 in 6 for men.[96] Although age-specific incidence rates are substantially lower in young and middle-aged women compared to men, these differences narrow with aging, so that in the oldest age groups, incidence rates in women are similar to or even higher than in men.[6]

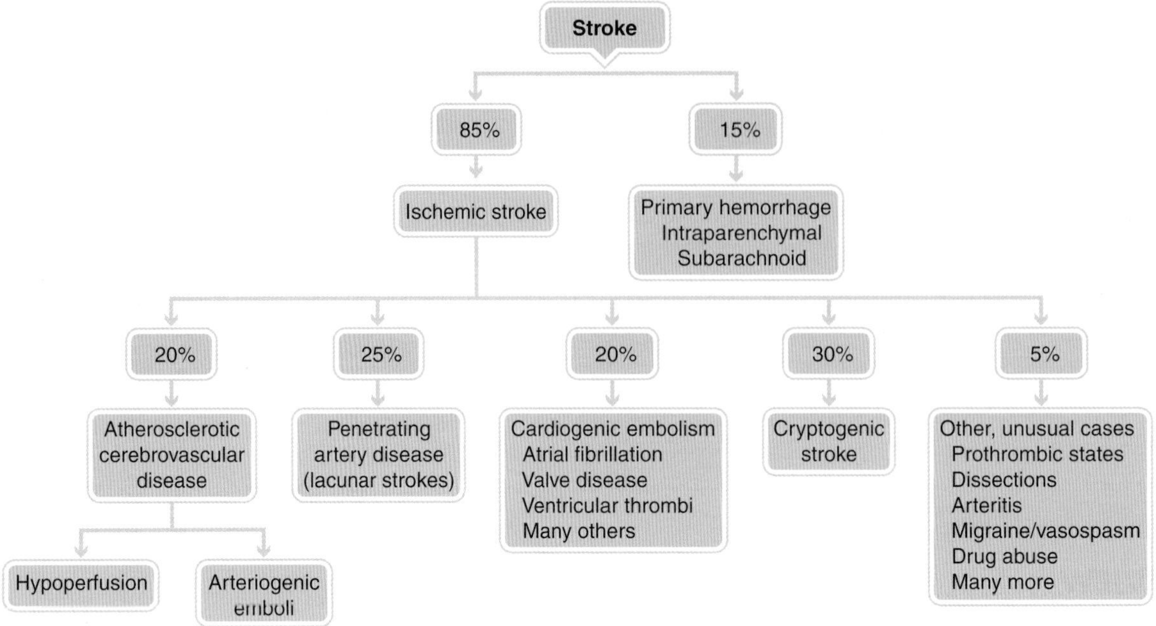


**Figure 32.1**

Percentage of strokes caused by different etiologies. (Reprinted from Townsend CM: *Sabiston textbook of surgery*, ed 17, Philadelphia, 2004, Saunders.)

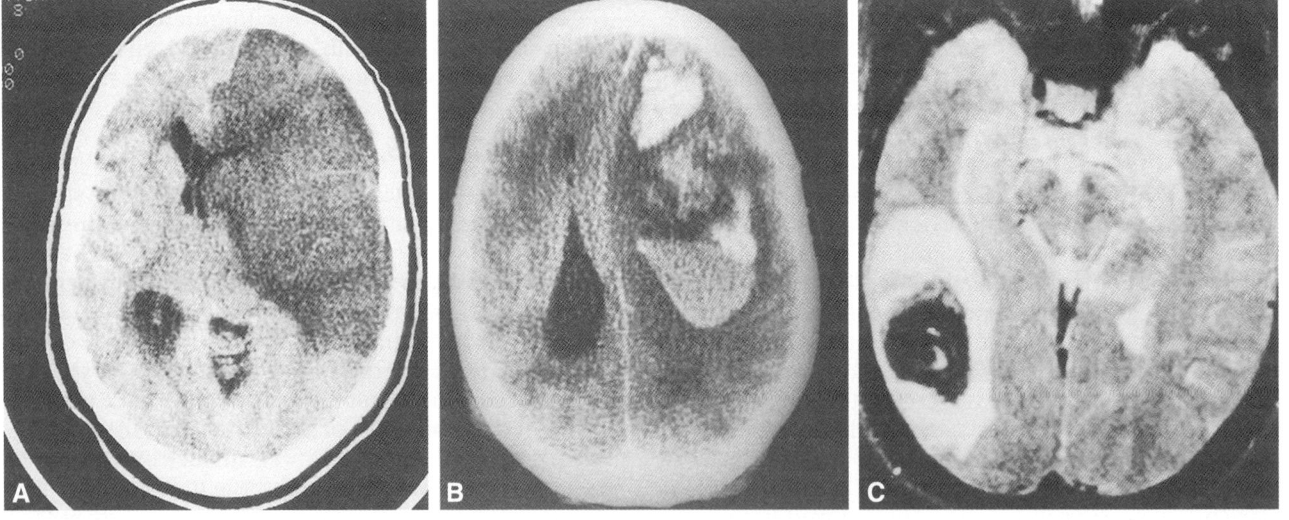


**Figure 32.2**

**Radiographic images of the brain after stroke.** (A) An acute infarct with mass effect and compression of the ventricle. (B) An acute intracerebral hemorrhage in the hemisphere. (C) Amyloid angiopathy with acute hemorrhage; the edema surrounding the area results in a slight mass effect on the midbrain. (Reprinted from Ramsey R: *Neuroradiology*, Philadelphia, 1994, WB Saunders.)

## Genetic Factors

Stroke is a heterogeneous multifactorial disorder, but epidemiologic data provide substantial evidence for a genetic component. Several genetic loci (e.g., *ALDH2*) have been associated with ischemic stroke and its subtypes.[41] This has implications for both stroke prevention and treatment. Two gene regions (*PITX2* and *ZFHX3*) are associated with cardioembolic stroke, two others (*HDAC9* and *TSPAN2*) with large-vessel stroke, and an area near the *FOXF2* gene with small-vessel disease.[78,81] Studies of sickle cell disease have drawn attention to the importance of modifier genes and of gene-gene interactions in determining stroke risk. There are probably many alleles with small effect sizes associated with multifactorial stroke. Genetic association studies on a wide range of candidate pathways are currently underway. Figure 32.3 shows the interaction of genetics, disease, and environment.[24]

## Hypertension and Cardiovascular Disease

Blood pressure has a strong, direct, and linear relationship with stroke risk; consequently, hypertension is the most important modifiable risk factor for stroke.[7] In the INTERSTROKE study, the proportion of strokes in the population attributable to hypertension was 54%.[85]

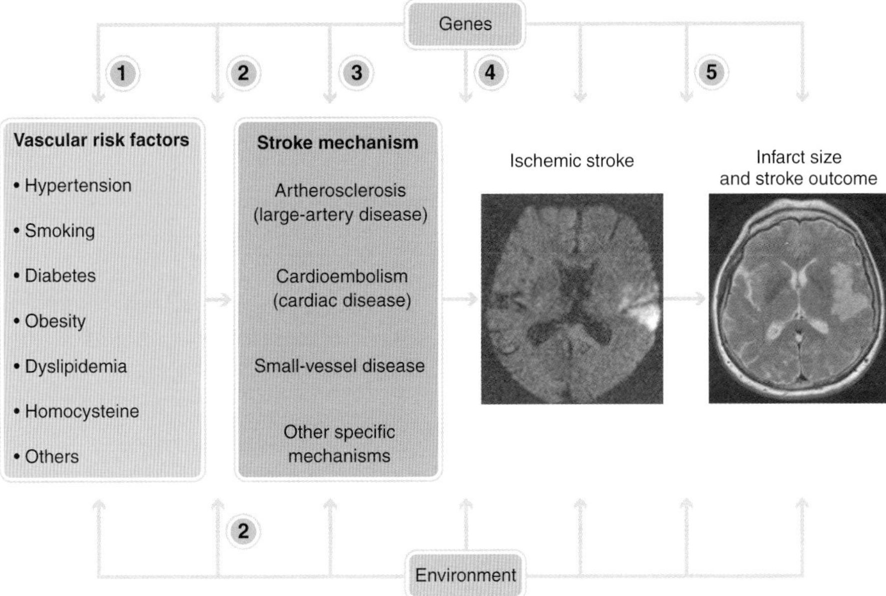


**Figure 32.3**

**Genetic factors and ischemic stroke.** Genetic factors may affect stroke risk at various levels. They could act through conventional risk factors *(1)*, interact with conventional and environmental risk factors *(2)*, or contribute directly to an established stroke mechanism such as atherosclerosis or small vessel disease *(3)*. Genetic factors could further affect the latency to stroke *(4)* or infarct size and stroke outcome *(5)*. Similarly, environmental factors and interactions between genes and the environment could occur at various levels. (Reprinted from Dichgans M: Genetics of ischaemic stroke, *Lancet Neurol* 6:149–161, 2007.)

A decrease in blood pressure of 10 mm Hg systolic or 5 mm Hg diastolic is associated with a 40% reduction in stroke risk, an effect that is present even when blood pressure levels are within the normal range, down to 110 mm Hg systolic and 60 mm Hg diastolic.[7]

Various cardiac diseases have been shown to increase risk of stroke, including coronary heart disease, left ventricular hypertrophy, and cardiac failure. The stroke risk increases with the degree of stenosis. Death is more often from fatal coronary artery disease than stroke. The risk of stroke is increased after myocardial infarction (MI), although reported stroke rates vary widely among studies. The risk appears highest early after MI.[119] If cerebral microembolism occurs after MI, the risk of an embolic event increases.[75] Development of neurologic deficits preceded by brief focal symptoms in the same vascular territory usually suggests atherothrombosis as the vascular mechanism. Cardiac valve abnormalities such as mitral stenosis and mitral annular calcification are moderate risk factors. Structural abnormalities of the heart such as patent foramen ovale and atrial septal aneurysm increase risk.

Atrial fibrillation has long been recognized as a major stroke risk factor. This risk factor is becoming more prominent with the aging of the United States population, with the incidence of stroke related to atrial fibrillation nearly tripling in the past three decades.[7] The association between atrial fibrillation and stroke has been assumed to be the result of stasis of blood in the fibrillating left atrium, causing thrombus formation and embolization to the brain. However, this assumption has been challenged in light of evidence suggesting that atrial tissue substrate, as well as cardiac rhythm, may play a role.[7]

Fibrinogen is a coagulation factor that has been associated with increased stroke risk. Fibrinogen plays a crucial role in platelet aggregation. Platelets initiate thrombosis by attracting fibrin and other clot-forming substances. Conditions associated with increased fibrin deposition or increased blood viscosity are rheumatic heart disease, endocarditis, atherosclerosis, polycythemia, and thrombocytosis.

## Diabetes

Diabetes mellitus, a common endocrine disorder, is another well-known risk factor for stroke. Individuals with diabetes have a two-fold increase in risk of stroke, and stroke accounts for approximately 20% of deaths among people with diabetes.[7] Diabetes is known to cause large artery atherosclerosis, increased cholesterol levels, and plaque formation. Duration of diabetes also is associated with stroke risk, with a marked increase in risk for individuals with diabetes for 10 years or longer.[5] The ability of the cerebral arterioles to dilate is reduced in longstanding type 2 diabetes.[48]

## Lifestyle Factors

Lifestyle choices have a significant effect on several of the risk factors for stroke, and a large body of research is focused on targeted lifestyle modification to reduce stroke risk. Healthy lifestyle behaviors such as maintaining a healthy diet, exercising regularly, and abstaining from tobacco should begin in childhood and continue throughout one's life. Cholesterol level has long been considered a part of the stroke risk profile; however, the relation between dyslipidemia and stroke is complex.[7,102] High total cholesterol levels create increased risk of ischemic stroke, including the large artery and lacunar stroke subtypes that have atherosclerotic pathogeneses, but may actually decrease the risk of hemorrhagic stroke. Younger individuals and those with low high-density lipoprotein (HDL) levels are at greater risk; higher levels of HDL cholesterol are associated with decreased risk of ischemic stroke. Low-density lipoprotein (LDL) cholesterol levels currently are thought to be biochemical predictors of coronary artery disease associated with carotid atherosclerosis.[109]

Dietary factors that increase LDL cholesterol include saturated fatty acids, *trans*-fatty acids, and dietary cholesterol. Soluble fiber as is present in foods such as beans, oats, barley, and some fruits and vegetables reduces LDL cholesterol through decreased absorption of cholesterol and bile acids. The potential for soy protein to decrease serum cholesterol levels has been studied extensively, with recent meta-analyses demonstrating that 30 to 50 g per day of soy protein can reduce LDL cholesterol by 3% to 5%.

Phytosterols are cholesterol-like compounds that are found mostly in vegetable oils, nuts, and legumes. When included in the diet, they inhibit cholesterol absorption by displacing cholesterol from mixed micelles, as opposed to statin drugs, which inhibit cholesterol synthesis. Phytosterols create additional lipid lowering when combined with a heart-healthy diet using other LDL-lowering strategies. Carotenoids in carrots, pumpkin, apricots, spinach, and broccoli are recommended in conjunction with consuming phytosterols. Phytosterols can also be used with statins for greater LDL cholesterol lowering and may be preferable to doubling the statin dose. See statins in "Treatment" below.[49]

Lipid-modifying medications can also substantially reduce the risk of stroke. Treatment with statins is associated with the reduction in the risk of a first stroke in various populations of patients at increased risk of cardiovascular events. National Cholesterol Education Program III guidelines recommend statins for the management of patients who have not had a stroke and who have elevated total cholesterol or elevated non–HDL cholesterol in the presence of hypertriglyceridemia.

High plasma homocysteine levels and low levels of folate and vitamin $B_6$ have been thought to be associated with increased risk of carotid disease and heart attack. Homocysteine is a sulfur-containing acid formed during the metabolism of methionine. The use of folic acid, pyridoxine, and vitamin $B_{12}$ has been reported to lower levels of homocysteine in the blood. However, homocysteine was only weakly correlated with risk of cardiovascular disease in meta-analysis.[62] Cardioprotective benefits have been found with consumption of even modest amounts of omega-3 fatty acids provided by an average intake of 1 to 2 ounces of fish daily.[91]

Many countries in the Mediterranean region have distinct dietary patterns with an overlap of similar characteristics. The Mediterranean diet is associated with a low incidence of cardiovascular disease, which is attributed in part to a high consumption of olive oil and low consumption of saturated fat. Box 32.1 outlines the common characteristics of the diet.

Obesity is a risk factor for stroke, although the mechanisms underlying this relationship are not clear. Results of a large meta-analysis indicated that 76% of the effect of obesity, as measured by body mass index (BMI), on stroke risk was mediated by blood pressure, cholesterol, and glucose levels.[37] Increased abdominal adiposity, as measured by the waist-to-hip ratio, is increasingly recognized as a greater contributor to stroke risk than BMI. Weight loss provides approximately 10% effect on lipid lowering and improves glycemic control, decreases blood pressure, reduces inflammation, and improves fibrinolysis. In addition, sustained weight loss may increase life expectancy.

The protective effect of physical activity may be related to its role in controlling other risk factors such as hypertension, diabetes mellitus, and obesity. Regular aerobic exercise can induce favorable changes in triglycerides and HDL cholesterol, as well as beneficial changes in the activity of lipoprotein lipase, which is increased following aerobic exercise. The beneficial effect of physical activity appears to be more apparent for men than women.

Cigarette smoking nearly doubles the risk of stroke; the risk is directly related to pack-years. Secondhand smoke also has been implicated in stroke. In the REGARDS study, risk of stroke was 30% higher for individuals who had been exposed to secondhand smoke compared to those who had not, after accounting for other stroke risk factors.[67] The relationship between alcohol consumption and stroke risk appears to depend on stroke type. For ischemic stroke, this relationship is J-shaped, with light-to-moderate alcohol consumption being protective against stroke, and heavy drinking associated with increased risk.[7] For hemorrhagic stroke, a more direct

Box 32.1

**THE MEDITERRANEAN DIET**

The International Conference on the Diet of the Mediterranean summarized the key dietary components in 1993. They are:

1. An abundance of plant foods (e.g., fruits, vegetables, potatoes, breads, grains, beans, nuts, and seeds)
2. Minimally processed and, whenever possible, seasonally fresh foods
3. Fresh fruits as the typical daily dessert
4. Olive oil as the principal source of dietary fat
5. Dairy, poultry, and fish in low to moderate amounts
6. Fewer than five eggs per week
7. Red meat in low frequency and amounts
8. Wine in low to moderate amounts (one to two glasses per day for men and one glass per day for women)

The Mediterranean diet, being largely plant based, also includes a high intake of fiber and phytosterols (≈400 mg per day).

From Katcher HI: Lifestyle approaches and dietary strategies to lower LDL-cholesterol and triglycerides and raise HDL-cholesterol. *Endocrinol Metab Clin North Am* 38:45–78, 2009.

dose-dependent effect exists. Light to moderate drinking may have beneficial effects in relation to ischemic stroke risk by increasing HDL cholesterol levels and decreasing platelet aggregation and fibrinogen levels. Heavy consumption of alcohol—more than 14 drinks per week or more than 4 drinks per occasion in men and more than 7 drinks per week or more than 3 drinks per occasion in women—causes increased risk through hypertension, hypercoagulable states, arrhythmia, and decreased cerebral blood flow.

Cocaine use is associated with hemorrhagic stroke by increased risk related to focal arterial vasoconstriction and occasionally to inflammatory vasculitis. Although the evidence remains inconclusive, other recreational drugs such as marijuana are thought to increase the risk. Some concern exists regarding the use of over-the-counter cold medications, diet pills, ephedrine, and pseudoephedrine.

Young women have a low absolute risk of stroke, and use of oral contraceptives seems to be insignificant. However, the absolute risk of stroke is much greater in postmenopausal women simply because they are older. In older women, a modest relative increase in stroke risk when using oral contraceptives may produce a much larger absolute increase in risk of stroke. Thus, differences in prescribing estrogen-containing compounds to premenopausal versus postmenopausal women appear to be justified. Women with hypertension or a history of smoking have a higher absolute risk. Individuals who have had an ischemic stroke are at risk of a second stroke. Thus, oral contraceptive use should be discouraged in women with prior stroke and should certainly be stopped in women who have had a stroke while taking oral contraceptives.

Recognition of the multiple risk factors that can interact to increase the probability of stroke is important. Use of risk profiles, such as the one established as a part of the Framingham study, can assist in the ability to predict stroke in a single individual.[120] The percentage of individuals with "no known risk factors" is declining, and the prevalence of high blood pressure, type 2 diabetes, and obesity is increasing.

## PATHOGENESIS

Energy failure following a reduction in blood flow induces a region of cell death known as the *infarct* and a surrounding area of damaged tissue called the *penumbra*. Inflammatory processes in the penumbra exacerbate the infarct. Endothelial and glial cells become activated, releasing free radicals, cytokines, and chemokines, in addition to increasing the production of enzymes causing neuronal cell death and changes in the blood-brain barrier, leading to leukocyte infiltration. Inflammatory processes are further activated by the C-reactive protein and cytokine-induced functions. Cytokines also signal the CNS, thereby initiating brain-mediated defenses such as fever. Uncontrolled or excessive inflammatory responses to injury can have devastating results in the CNS, where tissues lack the capacity to regenerate (Fig. 32.4). Damage related to the different stroke subtypes varies and is discussed further in each section.

## CLINICAL MANIFESTATIONS

The first indication of the onset of stroke may be transient with focal symptoms. Early warning signs are listed

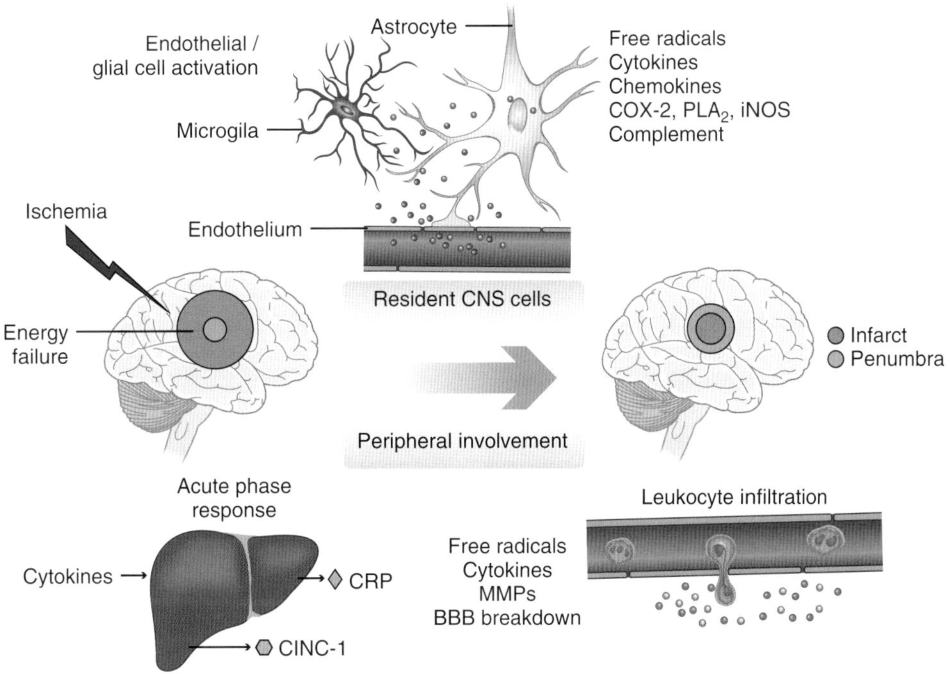


**Figure 32.4**

Immune/inflammatory responses and their contribution to ischemic injury after stroke. (From Skinner R, Georgiou R, Thornton P, Rothwell N: Psychoneuroimmunology of stroke. *Immunol Allergy Clin North Am* 29[2]:359–379, 2009.)

in Box 32.2. Although the risk factors and early warning signs have been well publicized, individuals at highest risk do not appear to be aware of warning signs and may not consult a physician when the symptoms occur. Clinical manifestations are related to the type of stroke that occurs and are addressed later in the chapter in the individual stroke subtypes.

## TREATMENT

The chain of events favoring good functional outcome from an acute ischemic stroke begins with the recognition of stroke when it occurs. Despite public educational campaigns for stroke awareness, such as the "Face, Arm, Speech, Time" (FAST) campaign, the public's knowledge of stroke warning signs remains poor. Interviews of patients and bystanders indicate poor recall and use of the FAST assessments and lack of appreciation of the need for urgent action.[13,70] This lack of knowledge often leads to delays between symptom onset and hospital arrival, with resultant decreased access to and/or benefits of thrombolysis.

Compared with care provided in general wards, organized inpatient care in a stroke unit reduces death and dependence and increases the likelihood of discharge to home.[41] Processes of care associated with decreased mortality include review by a stroke consultant within 24 hours of admission, nutrition screening and formal swallow assessment within 72 hours, and antiplatelet therapy and adequate fluid and nutrition for the first 72 hours.[12] Antihypertensive medications are considered in extreme hypertension with systolic blood pressure 220 mm Hg or greater. Hypoglycemia, with levels less than 60 mg/dL, is frequently found in patients with stroke-like symptoms; thus, prehospital glucose testing is critical.[44]

Extensive and growing evidence implicates inflammatory and immune processes in the occurrence of stroke and particularly in the subsequent injury. Trials of many neuroprotective drugs for the treatment of acute stroke, including citicoline, high-dose albumin, and magnesium sulfate, have failed to show functional benefits. However, several preclinical and clinical studies suggest that therapies that target inhibition of interleukin-1, a family of regulatory and inflammatory cytokines, may be effective for both ischemic and hemorrhagic stroke.[100]

Box 32.2

**WARNING SIGNS OF STROKE**

- Sudden weakness or numbness of the face, arm, or leg
- Sudden dimness or loss of vision, particularly in one eye
- Sudden difficulty speaking or understanding speech
- Sudden severe headache with no known cause
- Unexplained dizziness, unsteadiness, or sudden falls

## PROGNOSIS

Various clinical risk prediction scores have been developed to help physicians stratify risk of progression to a stroke with greater consequences (Box 32.3). The ABCD2 score is one of the most validated triage tools for predicting stroke risk after TIA or minor stroke. In an effort to further improve risk stratification, the ABCD3-I was introduced to include dual TIA, vascular findings, and brain imaging in addition to the ABCD2. Without treatment, risk of second stroke after TIA or minor stroke is about 10% at 1 week, 15% at 1 month, and 18% at 3 months. The risk is greater among individuals with recent symptomatic atherosclerosis and

Box 32.3

**ABCD SCORES FOR PREDICTING PROGRESSION OF STROKE[52]**

| | ABCD2 Score | ABCD3 Score | ABCD3-I Score | ABCD3-I(d, c/i) Score | ABCD3-I(c/i) Score |
|---|---|---|---|---|---|
| Age ≥ 60 years | 1 | 1 | 1 | 1 | 1 |
| Blood pressure ≥ 140/90 | 1 | 1 | 1 | 1 | 1 |
| Clinical Features | | | | | |
| Speech impairment without weakness | 1 | 1 | 1 | 1 | 1 |
| Unilateral weakness | 2 | 2 | 2 | 2 | 2 |
| Duration | | | | | |
| 10–59 minutes | 1 | 1 | 1 | 1 | 1 |
| ≥ 60 minutes | 2 | 2 | 2 | 2 | 2 |
| Diabetes mellitus present | 1 | 1 | 1 | 1 | 1 |
| Dual TIA[a] | NA | 2 | 2 | 2 | 2 |
| Imaging | | | | | |
| Ipsilateral ≥ 50% stenosis of internal carotid artery | NA | NA | 2 | NA | NA |
| Acute diffusion weighted imaging hyperintensity | NA | NA | 2 | 2 | NA |
| MAXIMUM SCORE | 0–7 | 0–9 | 0–13 | 0–13 | 0–11 |

[a]TIA prompting medical attention plus at least one other TIA in the preceding 7 days.

NA, Not applicable.

From Kiyohara T, Kamouchi M, Kumai Y, et al. ABCD3 and ABCD3-I scores are superior to ABCD2 score in the prediction of short- and long-term risks of stroke after transient ischemic attack. *Stroke* 45(2):418-425, 2014.

high ABCD3-I and recurrence risk estimator scores. Urgent assessment and appropriate intervention lowers the risk of recurrent stroke by 80%.[41]

Living with stroke can be a challenge, with the onset of impairments causing limited mobility, difficulty eating, urinary incontinence, and difficulty speaking or understanding language. Hemiparesis remains a long-term consequence in almost half of stroke survivors. Cognitive changes, anxiety, and confusion can be very disturbing for the individual and add to caregiver stress. Quality of life often is reported as poor.

Concomitant diseases of aging such as arthritis, diabetes, and osteoporosis, along with the decreased plasticity of the nervous system associated with aging, can increase the challenge of recovery from stroke. Medical complications occur in up to 85% of stroke survivors and present potential barriers to optimal recovery. Infections occur in almost 25% of stroke survivors, primarily in the urinary tract and chest. Incidence of deep vein thrombosis and pulmonary emboli is increased. Falls resulting from impaired mobility are also prevalent, with serious injury reported in 5% of the reported falls. Approximately 75% of stroke survivors will have a fall within the first 6 months after stroke. Pain and depression are reported in more than 30% of stroke survivors.[58] Presence of urinary incontinence after stroke indicates a poorer prognosis for both survival and functional recovery.

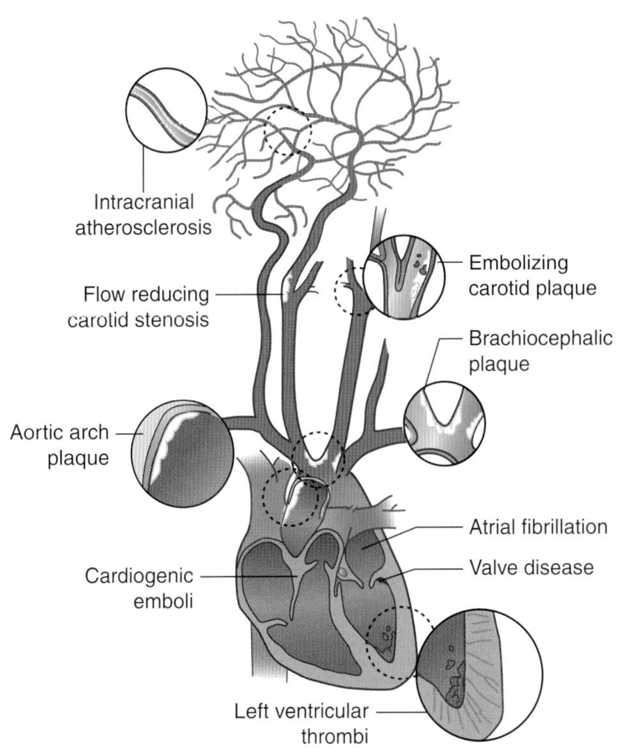


**Figure 32.5**

Cardiogenic and arterial atherosclerotic sources for stroke. (Reprinted from Townsend CM: *Sabiston textbook of surgery*, ed 17, Philadelphia, 2004, Saunders.)

## ISCHEMIC STROKE

### Pathogenesis

#### Occlusion of Major Arteries

Thrombosis and embolic occlusion of a major vessel are the most common causes of ischemic stroke. The heart is the most common source of embolic material, as a result of damage to heart tissue from atherothrombotic disease. Atrial fibrillation is thought to cause thrombus formation in the fibrillating atrium. Left ventricular MI can be a source of emboli, especially in the first few weeks following the event when thrombus formation is most prevalent.[47] Mitral valve prolapse or congenital septal defects are also sources of emboli. Formation of emboli during or after coronary artery surgery or intracardiac surgery is a well-recognized complication.

Artery-to-artery embolism, usually arising from an atherothrombotic lesion in the carotid or vertebrobasilar system, may lead to stroke. The emboli from this lesion may travel along the course of circulation and may cause occlusion in the smaller branches. The proximal internal carotid artery is the most common site of atherosclerosis and atherothrombosis leading to stroke. Other causes may be fat or cholesterol emboli in the blood, tumor emboli from a neoplastic process and, very rarely, amniotic fluid emboli in the maternal venous circulation.[69] Sources of emboli are shown in Figure 32.5.

Changes in the collateral pathways of the circle of Willis are apparent in response to internal carotid artery obstruction that may provide some protection against neurologic damage associated with occlusion. Deficient blood supply from the internal carotid artery leads to chronic blood flow compensation by secondary collaterals such as the ipsilateral ophthalmic artery, ipsilateral posterior communicating artery, anterior communicating artery and pia mater collaterals.[124] Figure 32.6 shows the distribution of the circle of Willis.

#### Secondary Vascular Responses

When a cerebral artery is occluded, the formation of thromboemboli probably begins in the distal vessels of that artery. These presumed microvascular occlusions progressively increase in number and continue to impair blood flow in the brain. Cell death surrounding the area of blocked blood flow may be due to the squeezing effects of microvessels by the swelling of the *astrocyte*, one of the cellular support structures of the nervous system. Astroglial swelling is one of the earliest cell changes induced by single-artery occlusion. The formation of fibrin in the gray matter surrounding the occluded vessel also may contribute to microvascular occlusion. Other factors may include sustained pericyte contraction, microcirculatory clogging, and disruption of the integrity of the blood-brain barrier.[22] The narrowed lumina of the microvessels are filled with entrapped erythrocytes and, to a lesser extent, leukocytes and fibrin-platelet deposits.

#### Secondary Neuronal Damage

The tissue of the brain, or the *parenchyma*, is highly vulnerable to an interruption in its blood supply. When the cerebral blood flow (CBF) falls below 20 mL/100 mg of tissue per minute, neuronal functioning is impaired. Neuronal

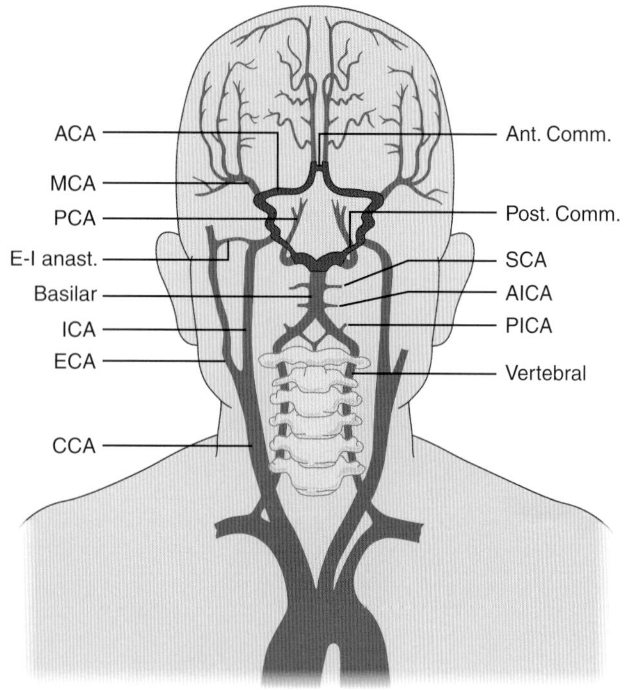


**Figure 32.6**

**Extracranial and intracranial arterial supply to the brain.** Vessels forming the circle of Willis are highlighted. *ACA*, Anterior cerebral artery; *AICA*, anterior inferior cerebellar artery; *Ant. Comm.*, anterior communicating artery; *CCA*, common carotid artery; *ECA*, external carotid artery; *E-I anast.*, extracranial-intracranial anastomosis; *ICA*, internal carotid artery; *MCA*, middle cerebral artery; *PCA*, posterior cerebral artery; *PICA*, posterior inferior cerebellar artery; *Post. Comm.*, posterior communicating artery; *SCA*, superior cerebellar artery. (Modified from Lord R: *Surgery of occlusive cerebrovascular disease*, St Louis, 1986, C.V. Mosby.)

death, or infarction, occurs when CBF is less than 8 to 10 mL/100 mg/min. Frequently, in an acute infarction, a portion of the affected brain receives no blood, and is not salvageable. This is the *ischemic core.* A surrounding area may have low CBF but high or preserved cerebral blood volume. This hypoxic, but potentially salvageable, territory has been termed the *ischemic penumbra.*[46] The major injury to the neurons in the brain is the hypoxia-ischemia related to the occlusion of the artery, causing cell death near the core. Further damage to the brain tissue and neurons occurs as a secondary response. There is decreased perfusion relative to the necessary oxygen requirements, causing decreased metabolism in the infarcted area. If blood flow to this ischemic area is restored before irreversible damage occurs, then the tissue will likely recover and resume normal function.

After an ischemic event, the cells that normally clear excess glutamate are compromised, and excess glutamate is found in the extracellular space. Depolarization of the postsynaptic cell occurs in response to this increase in glutamate. Excess glutamate allows abnormally high entry of calcium ions into the cells. Excessive numbers of calcium ions begin the process that causes cell death. Catabolic enzymes are activated by the release of calcium ions and can cause damage of the proteins that support neurons, the glial cells. During the ischemic process, other mechanisms result in excess calcium that, with excess glutamate, contributes to dysfunction of the electrochemical gradient in the damaged membrane.

Apoptosis, or programmed cell death, occurs in response to hypoxic damage.[64] The changes in the perfusion pressure associated with hypoxia can also cause the endothelial cells to trigger the release of neurotoxic substances, such as free radicals. Oxygen free radicals can initiate many destructive processes in the brain tissue. The overall result of the hypoxic event is a chain of reactions, some that occur simultaneously, extending the damage and death of brain tissue beyond the area of vascular supply. Figure 32.7 shows the cascade of destruction after ischemia. See Chapter 28 for further information on apoptosis and free radicals.

Distant from the ischemic and stroke sites are regions that also show alterations in metabolism despite being normal on anatomic imaging studies, such as CT or MRI. There appears to be an uncoupling of oxygen consumption and glucose use that may reflect a change in brain metabolism caused by deafferentation, while other areas are hypometabolic after a cortical infarct. This decline in oxygen metabolism in the unaffected hemisphere from the acute to the subacute stage suggests a delayed effect. Neurologic recovery appears to be influenced by prefrontal metabolism, possibly because this region is part of a network that has an important compensatory role in motor recovery.[79]

## Clinical Manifestations

### Vascular Syndromes

Disruption of blood flow in specific areas of the brain produces syndromes that are named according to the arteries supplying the specific areas. The syndrome can be partial or complete. When the blockage is in the more proximal component of the artery, the resulting area of hypoxia is greater than if the clot is lodged in a more distal part of the artery. Because of the collateral circulation provided by the circle of Willis, some areas of the brain are supplied by more than one artery. When one artery is blocked, circulation is provided to the tissues through the blood supply of other arteries. In these cases, the clinical syndromes are not as extensive. The actual configuration of arteries is different in each individual, so the syndromes described here are not all-encompassing. This is an overview of the types of symptoms that might be encountered when a particular artery is blocked.

**Middle Cerebral Artery Syndrome.** If the entire middle cerebral artery is occluded at its stem, blocking both the penetrating and cortical branches, the clinical findings are contralateral *hemiplegia* and *hemianesthesia*, or the loss of movement and sensation on one-half of the body. If the dominant hemisphere is affected, *global aphasia*, or the loss of fluency, ability to name objects, comprehend auditory information, and repeat language, is the result. (See "Parietal Lobe Syndromes" in Chapter 28.)

Partial syndromes resulting from embolic occlusion of a single branch include brachial syndrome, or weakness of the upper extremity, and frontal opercular syndrome, or facial weakness with motor aphasia, with or without arm weakness. A combination of sensory disturbance,

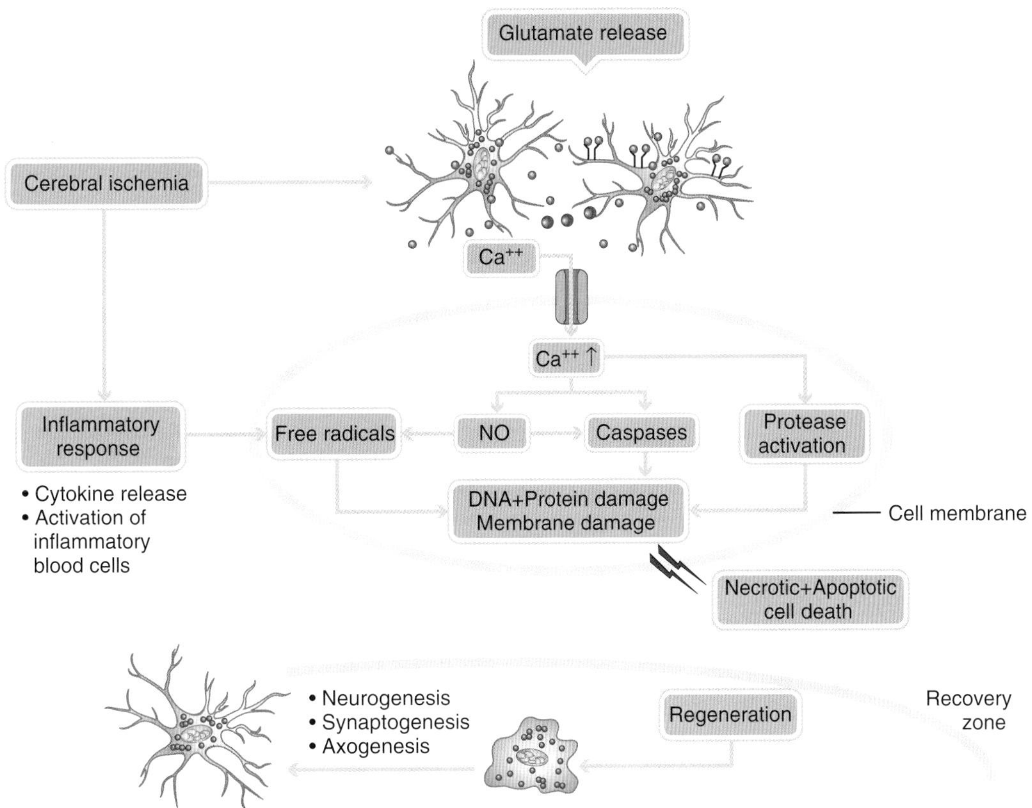


**Figure 32.7**

**Depiction of the major events that encompass the ischemic cascade of cellular injury.** *DNA*, Deoxyribonucleic acid; *NO*, nitric oxide. (Courtesy Dr. Wolf-Rudiger Schaebitz. Creager: *Vascular medicine: a companion to Braunwald's heart disease*, ed 2, Philadelphia, 2012, Saunders.)

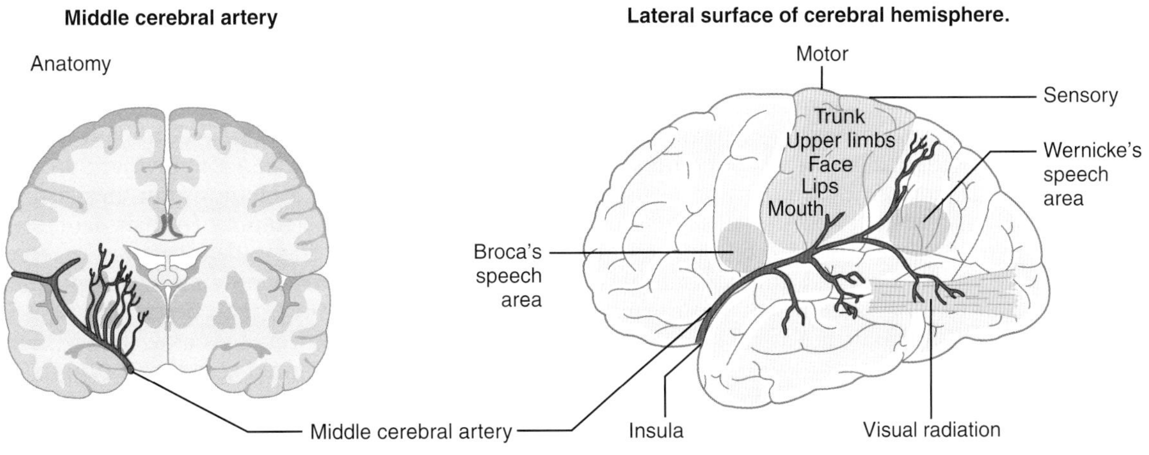


**Figure 32.8**

The middle cerebral artery is the largest branch of the internal carotid artery and the most common site of emboli. Its deep branches feed the internal capsule and basal ganglia. On the lateral surface, the branches feed areas of the parietal, frontal, and temporal lobes. (Reprinted from Lindsay KW, Bone I, Callander R: *Neurology and neurosurgery illustrated*, New York, 1986, Churchill Livingstone.)

motor weakness, and motor aphasia suggests that an embolus has occluded the proximal superior division branch and has infarcted large portions of the frontal and parietal cortices.

If fluent (Wernicke) aphasia occurs without weakness, the inferior division of the middle cerebral artery supplying the temporal cortex of the dominant hemisphere has been occluded. Jargon speech and an inability to comprehend written and oral language are prominent features. Hemiplegia or spatial agnosia without weakness indicates that the inferior division of the middle cerebral artery in the nondominant hemisphere is involved. Figure 32.8 represents the area of the middle cerebral artery.

**Anterior Cerebral Artery Syndrome.** Infarction in the territory of the anterior cerebral artery is uncommon and is more often the result of embolism than

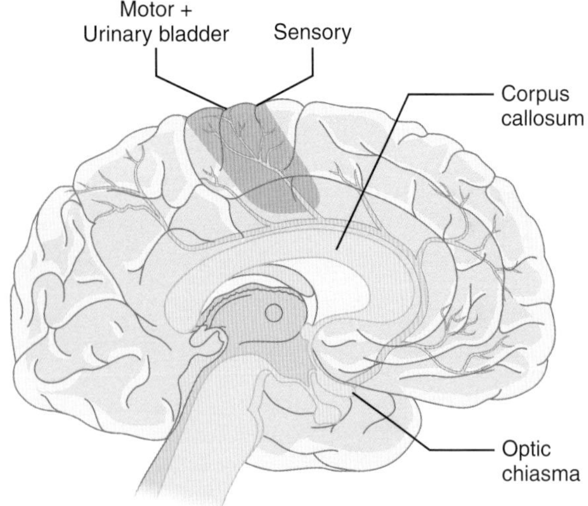


**Figure 32.9**

**The anterior cerebral artery branches from the internal carotid.** Deep branches supply the internal capsule and basal ganglia. Superficial branches supply the frontal and parietal lobes. (Reprinted from Lindsay KW, Bone I, Callander R: *Neurology and neurosurgery illustrated*, New York, 1986, Churchill Livingstone.)

atherothrombosis. Collateral flow is able to compensate for most occlusion of the artery so that dysfunction is minimal. If both segments of the artery arise from a single anterior cerebral stem, the occlusion affects both hemispheres. Contralateral hemiparesis and sensory loss are usually seen, with the lower extremity more involved. Profound *abulia*, a lack of willpower for movement or other action, is common. Akinetic mutism also can result in significant disability. Figure 32.9 represents the area of blood flow of the anterior cerebral artery.

**Internal Carotid Artery Syndrome.** The clinical picture of internal carotid occlusion varies depending on whether the cause of ischemia is thrombus, embolus, or low flow. The cortex supplied by the middle cerebral territory is affected most often. Occasionally, the origins of both the anterior and middle cerebral arteries are occluded at the top of the carotid artery. Symptoms consistent with both syndromes result. With a competent circle of Willis producing adequate collateral circulation, the occlusion can be asymptomatic.

**Posterior Cerebral Artery Syndrome.** If the proximal posterior cerebral artery is occluded, including penetrating branches, the areas of the brain that are affected are the subthalamus, medial thalamus, and ipsilateral (same side) cerebral peduncle and midbrain. Signs include thalamic syndrome, including abnormal sensation of pain, temperature, proprioception, and touch. Sensations may be exaggerated and light pressure stimuli may be interpreted as painful. This may develop into intractable, searing pain, which can be incapacitating. The anterior pattern consists mainly of perseverations and superimposition of unrelated information, apathy, and amnesia. After paramedian infarct, the most frequent features are disinhibition syndromes with personality changes, loss of self-activation, amnesia and, in the case of extensive lesions, thalamic dementia; this pattern may often be difficult to distinguish from primary psychiatric disorders, especially when neurologic dysfunction is lacking. After inferolateral lesion, executive dysfunction may develop but is often overlooked, although it may occasionally lead to severe long-term disability. After posterior lesion, cognitive dysfunction with neglect and aphasia are well known.[17]

If the posterior cerebral artery is completely occluded at its origin, hemiplegia results from infarction of the cerebral peduncle. Involvement of the red nucleus or dentatorubrothalamic tract can produce contralateral ataxia. When palsy of cranial nerve III occurs with contralateral ataxia, it is known as Claude syndrome. Third nerve palsy occurring with contralateral hemiplegia is known as Weber syndrome. Hemiballismus, or flailing of the extremity, usually results from a deep penetrating vessel causing infarct in the contralateral subthalamic nucleus. Ocular movement disorders (including paresis of upward gaze), drowsiness, dysarthria/aphasia, amnesia, and abulia can be attributed to occlusion of the artery of Percheron.[114] If the posterior cerebral stem is occluded, there can be infarction of the subthalamus; coma and decerebrate rigidity may result.

Peripheral supply of the posterior cerebral artery includes the temporal and occipital lobes. Occlusion of this component of the artery often affects the occipital lobe with homonymous hemianopsia, in which the visual field defect is on the side opposite to the lesion. Cortical blindness, the inability of the brain to record an image although the optic nerve is intact, is one of the visual disturbances seen with infarcts in this region.

Medial temporal lobe involvement (including the hippocampus) can cause an acute disturbance in memory, particularly if it occurs in the dominant hemisphere. This typically resolves because memory has dual representation. Memory is represented on both sides of the brain; if one area is affected, the intact side can compensate to a considerable extent. If the dominant hemisphere is affected and the infarct extends to involve the corpus callosum, the individual may demonstrate alexia (impairment of reading) without agraphia (impairment of writing). Agnosia, or difficulty in identification or recognition, affecting the ability to identify faces, objects, mathematical symbols, and colors, may occur. Anomia, impaired ability to identify objects by name, and visual hallucinations of brightly colored scenes and objects can occur with peripheral posterior cerebral infarction. Embolic occlusion of the top of the basilar artery can produce a clinical picture that includes any or all of the central or peripheral territory symptoms. Figure 32.10 represents the area of blood flow of the posterior cerebral artery.

**Vertebral and Posterior Inferior Cerebellar Artery Syndrome.** Blood supply to the brainstem, medulla, and cerebellum is provided by the vertebral and posterior cerebellar arteries. Collateral circulation is provided by the bilateral component of the vertebral artery so that ischemia often is not manifested in the presence of atherothrombosis.

Wallenberg syndrome is related to the lateral medulla and the posteroinferior cerebellum and is characterized by vertigo, nausea, hoarseness, and dysphagia (difficulty swallowing). Other symptoms can include ipsilateral

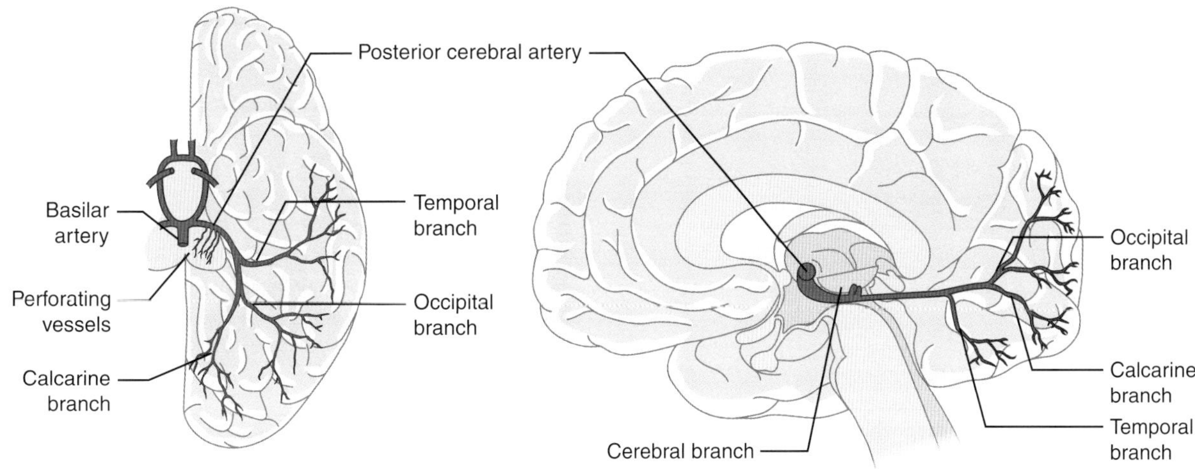


**Figure 32.10**

**The posterior cerebral arteries branch from the basilar artery.** The small perforating branches supply the midbrain structures and posterior thalamus. The temporal branch supplies the temporal lobe, and the occipital and calcarine supply the occipital lobe, including the visual cortex. (Reprinted from Lindsay KW, Bone I, Callander R: *Neurology and neurosurgery illustrated*, New York, 1986, Churchill Livingstone.)

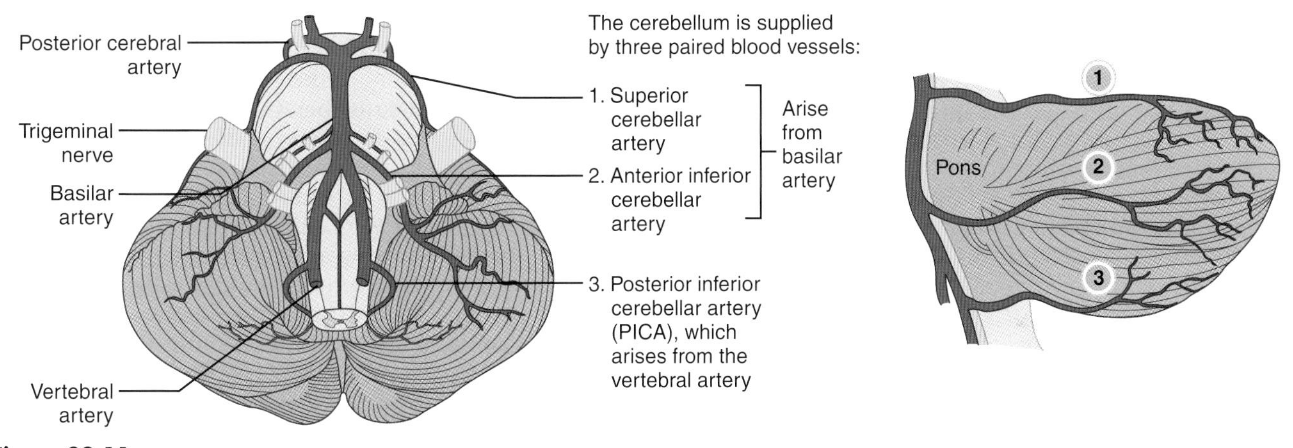


**Figure 32.11**

A lesion in the cerebellar territory will produce both cerebellar and brainstem signs and symptoms. (Reprinted from Lindsay KW, Bone I, Callander R: *Neurology and neurosurgery illustrated*, New York, 1986, Churchill Livingstone.)

ataxia (uncoordinated movement), ipsilateral body lateropulsion, ptosis (eyelid droop), and sensory deficits affecting the ipsilateral side of the face and the contralateral trunk and extremities.[77] Individuals with lateral medullary infarction may report numbness, burning, and cold in the face and limbs, reflecting involvement of the spinothalamic tract. In these cases, the onset of symptoms may be delayed for several days or longer.[77]

A medial medullary infarction of the pyramid can result in contralateral hemiparesis of the arm and leg, sparing the face. If the medial lemniscus and the hypoglossal nerve fibers are involved, loss of joint position sense and ipsilateral tongue weakness can occur.

The edema associated with cerebellar infarction can cause sudden respiratory arrest from high intracranial pressure (ICP) in the posterior fossa. Gait unsteadiness, dizziness, nausea, and vomiting may be the only early symptoms. Figure 32.11 shows the area of distribution of the superior cerebellar, anterior inferior cerebellar, and posterior inferior cerebellar arteries.

**Basilar Artery Syndrome.** Atheromatous lesions can occur anywhere along the basilar trunk, but they occur most often in the proximal basilar and distal vertebral area. Ischemia as a result of occlusion of the basilar artery can affect the brainstem, including the corticospinal tracts, corticobulbar tracts, medial and superior cerebellar peduncles, spinothalamic tracts, and cranial nerve nuclei.

If the basilar artery is occluded, the brainstem symptoms are bilateral. When a branch of the basilar artery is occluded, the symptoms are unilateral, involving the sensory and motor aspects of the cranial nerves.

**Superior Cerebellar Artery Syndrome.** Occlusion of the superior cerebellar artery results in severe ipsilateral cerebellar ataxia, nausea and vomiting, and dysarthria, or slurring of speech. Scanning speech, a drawn-out and monotone speech pattern, reflects damage to the cerebellum. Loss of pain and temperature in the contralateral extremities, torso, and face occurs. Dysmetria, characterized by the inability to place the extremity at a precise

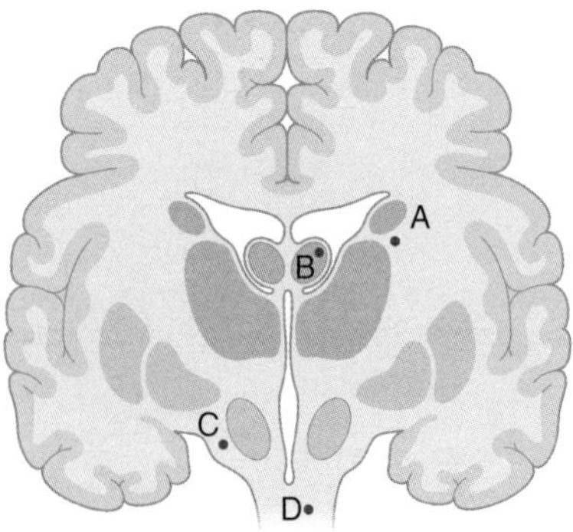


**Figure 32.12**

**Usual sites of lacunar infarcts in the deep white matter.** (A) Internal capsule/putamen. (B) Thalamus. (C) Mesencephalon. (D) Pons. (Reprinted from Pryse-Phillips W, Murray TJ: *Essential neurology: a concise textbook*, ed 4, New York, 1992, Medical Examination Publishing.)

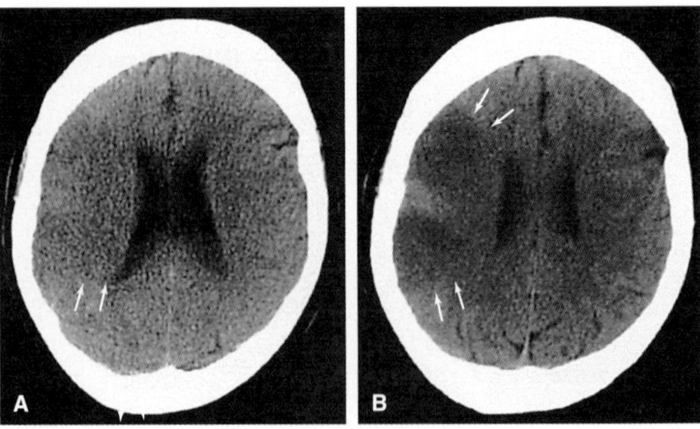


**Figure 32.13**

(A) CT scan taken 2 hours 50 minutes after large right middle cerebral artery occlusion. There are subtle, ultra-early ischemic changes, including loss of the gray-white interface *(arrows)* and subtle evidence of sulcal effacement. (B) CT scan of same patient approximately 8 hours after symptom onset shows acute hypodensity *(arrows)* and more prominent sulcal effacement. (Reprinted from Marx JA: Rosen's emergency medicine: concepts and clinical practice, ed 6, St Louis, 2006, Mosby.)

point in space, is common, affecting the ipsilateral upper extremity.

**Anterior Inferior Cerebellar Artery Syndrome.** Principal symptoms include ipsilateral deafness, facial weakness, vertigo, nausea and vomiting, *nystagmus* (rhythmic oscillations of the eye), and ataxia. *Horner syndrome*, characterized by ptosis, miosis (constriction of the pupil), and loss of sweating over the ipsilateral side of the face, may occur. A paresis of lateral gaze may be seen. Pain and temperature sensation are lost on the contralateral side of the body.

**Lacunar Syndrome.** Lacunar infarcts are small subcortical lesions caused by occlusion of a penetrating artery from a large cerebral artery, typically from the Circle of Willis. Lacunar infarcts are found most commonly in the basal ganglia, pons, and subcortical white matter structures (internal capsule and corona radiata). A small chronic cavity (lacune) surrounded by astrocytic gliosis represents the healed phase of lacunar infarction.[112] These small cystic spaces are common in individuals with hypertension or diabetes. A large majority are asymptomatic, but in about 20% of cases a stroke syndrome occurs with a slowly progressive (over 24-36 hours) dysfunction of the cells in the area of the lacunae.[72] The lacunar syndrome is representative of the area of infarct in which the lacunae are predominant in the deep structures of the brain and have their effect often on white matter. If the posterior limb of the internal capsule is affected, a pure motor deficit may result; in the anterior limb of the internal capsule, weakness of the face and dysarthria may occur. If the posterolateral thalamus is affected, there is a pure sensory stroke. When the lacunae occur predominantly in the pons, ataxia, clumsiness, and weakness may be seen. Parkinsonism can manifest due to involvement of the basal ganglia, as can subcortical dementia. Figure 32.12 shows the areas of predilection for lacunae to develop.

## MEDICAL MANAGEMENT

DIAGNOSIS. History of the neurologic event should be obtained, including timing, pattern of onset, and course. An embolic stroke occurs rapidly, with no warning. A more progressive and uneven onset is typical with thrombosis. The presenting symptoms will help to determine the location of the lesion. Information about the nature and severity of the ischemic insult may be just as important as the "time" of the ischemic event for predicting outcome and making therapeutic judgments.

*The National Institutes of Health Stroke Scale (NIHSS)* is a valuable clinical tool for assessing stroke severity, and is recommended for use in emergency departments.[56] The scale includes 15 items for initial and serial examination of impairments following acute stroke. A higher number on the NIHSS indicates a more severe stroke.

Neuroimaging of the brain has become a standard procedure in the diagnosis of stroke. In the acute stroke setting, there is a trade-off between the increased information provided by perfusion imaging and the increased time needed to acquire additional imaging sequences. The performance of these additional imaging sequences should not unduly delay treatment with intravenous recombinant tissue plasminogen activator (rt-PA) in the 4.5-hour-or-less window in appropriate patients. Non–contrast-enhanced computed tomography (NECT) remains sufficient for identification of contraindications to fibrinolysis and allows patients with ischemic stroke to receive timely intravenous fibrinolytic therapy; imaging should be performed within 25 minutes of the patient's arrival.

CT scan is the fastest, most convenient, and widely available test to use for the diagnosis and early treatment of acute stroke. However, CT scans may be normal in the acute stage of an embolic stroke. CT can rule out other pathologies and help determine the extent of the lesion. It can also determine if there is hemorrhage, which would prevent the use of clot-busting drugs. Figure 32.13 shows how an acute stroke looks on CT. Displacement of brain structures, such as the ventricles, by edema sometimes can be seen early in a large infarct. In ischemic stroke, CT scans reveal the area of decreased density and loss of gray/white matter differentiation resulting from edema. Cortical lesions appear wedge shaped, and deeper lesions appear to be round or oval.

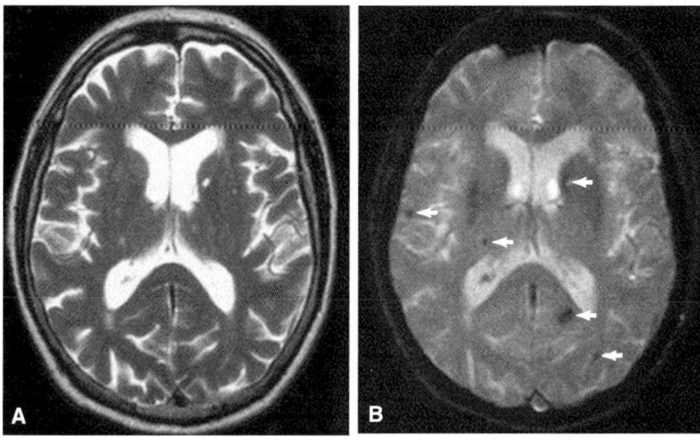


**Figure 32.14**

In these images, the left side of the brain is on the right of the panel. Axial T2-weighted fast spin-echo sequence (A) and corresponding axial T2*-weighted gradient echo sequence (B) from a 57-year-old man who presented with a left lacunar syndrome; his risk factors included hypertension and smoking. The T2-weighted fast spin-echo sequence shows several hyperintense foci in the cerebral white matter and basal ganglia but no microbleeds. The T2*-weighted gradient echo image shows several areas of focal signal loss consistent with microbleeds *(arrows)* in the right frontal lobe, right thalamus, left parietal lobe, and left caudate nucleus. (Reprinted from Werring DJ, Coward LJ, Losseff NA, et al: Cerebral microbleeds are common in ischemic stroke but rare in TIA, *Neurology* 65(12):1914–1918, 2005.)

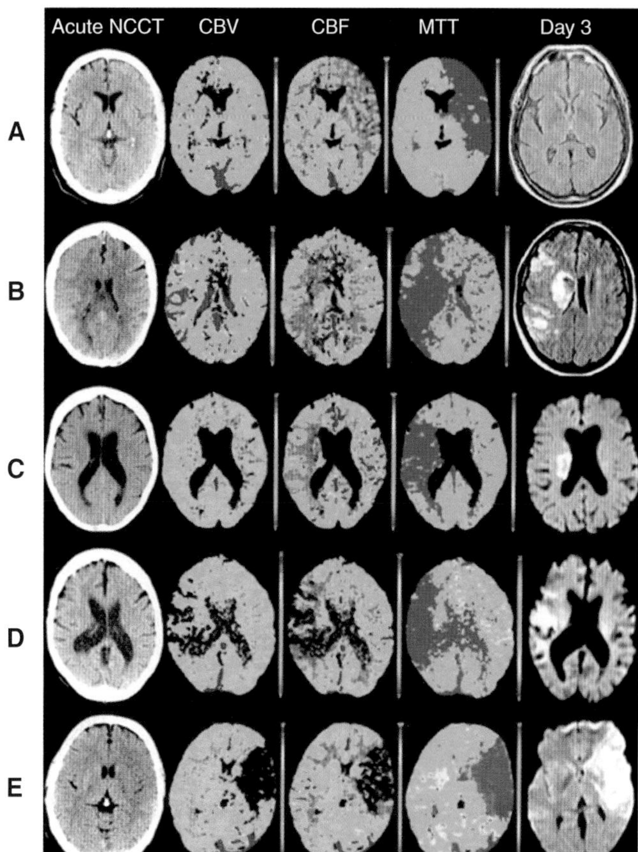


**Figure 32.15**

*Patient A:* Isolated focal swelling (IFS) on noncontrast CT (NCCT), hypoperfusion on mean transit time (MTT), and increased cerebral blood volume (CBV) on acute CT perfusion (CTP) maps, and no progression to infarction with subsequent major reperfusion. *Patient B:* IFS on NCCT, hypoperfusion on MTT, and increased CBV on acute CTP maps, but progression to infarction occurred without major reperfusion. *Patient C:* Hypoperfusion on MTT and increased CBV on acute CTP maps without any change apparent on acute NCCT. No infarction in cortical regions on follow-up with major reperfusion. *Patient D:* Hypoperfusion on MTT and decreased CBV on acute CTP maps without any apparent change on NCCT. Subsequent infarction present in reduced CBV regions on follow-up MRI. *Patient E:* Profound decrease in CBV and CBF on acute CTP maps with associated parenchymal hypoattenuation on NCCT. Extensive infarction on follow-up MRI. (Reprinted from Parsons M, Pepper EM, Bateman GA, et al: Identification of the penumbra and infarct core on hyperacute noncontrast and perfusion CT. *Neurology* 68:730–736, 2007.)

Potential for hemorrhagic transformation of the ischemic infarct can often be seen on CT.[89] Lacunar infarcts are sometimes visible on CT scans as small, punched-out, hypodense areas. Images of lacunae can be seen in Figure 32.14. Identification of the penumbra and infarct core on hyperacute noncontrast and perfusion-weighted CT may lead to potentially more aggressive treatments related to reperfusion and to arrest progression of stroke damage in the early part of the stroke.[46,88] Figure 32.15 demonstrates how the use of new imaging techniques may assist in this goal.

MRI allows for the identification of an ischemic event within 2 to 6 hours of onset. The soft tissue contrast and multiplanar imaging capability offered by MRI have led to its wide acceptance as the method of choice for high-resolution brain imaging. Diffusion-weighted MRI (DWI) provides an indication of the brain tissue's physiologic response to ischemia and can document the evolution of stroke. Because halting the evolution of the stroke is the therapeutic goal, DWI may be useful in the evaluation of therapeutic effectiveness. Two major approaches, both involving use of a contrast agent and a sequence of rapid MRI scans to detect the passage of the agent through the brain tissue, are used to measure cerebral perfusion with MRI. The first involves application of an exogenous, intravascular, nondiffusible contrast agent, usually gadolinium-based, that emphasizes either the susceptibility effects on the signal echo (dynamic susceptibility or DSC MR perfusion) or the relaxivity effects on the signal echo (dynamic contrast-enhanced or DCE MR perfusion). The second is application of an endogenous contrast agent using magnetically labeled arterial blood water as a diffusible flow tracer in arterial spin labeling or ASL MR perfusion.[31] MRI stroke sequences can be used as a measure of ischemic penumbra and can help pinpoint potentially salvageable brain tissue, helping to identify who is going to be a good candidate for the later window of intervention using thrombolysis and who is not.[46,95]

Positron emission tomographic (PET) imaging has been of great benefit in advancing the understanding of the pathophysiology of cerebrovascular disorders. PET imaging allows for the detection of stroke earlier and with higher sensitivity than anatomic imaging with either MRI or CT. Furthermore, PET imaging has been useful in evaluating the extent of the functional damage because areas not immediately affected by the infarct may show hypometabolism or decreased blood flow. Initial stroke severity has been shown to correlate with the initially affected volume as determined by PET,

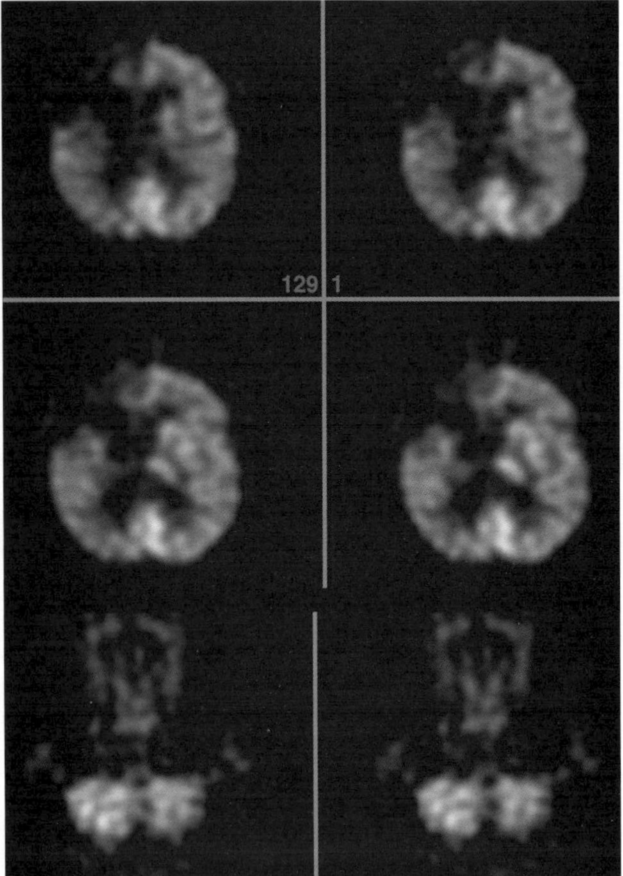


**Figure 32.16**

**Fluorodeoxyglucose PET scan of a patient after embolic stroke in the distribution of the right anterior cerebral artery.** There is severely decreased metabolism in the right frontal lobe extending to the midline. There is also crossed cerebellar diaschisis with decreased metabolism in the left cerebellum. (Reprinted from Newburg AB, Alavi A: The role of PET imaging in the management of patients with central nervous system disorders. *Radiol Clin North Am* 43:49–65, 2005.)

whereas neurologic deterioration during the first week after stroke correlates with the proportion of the initially affected volume that infarcted, and functional outcome correlates with the final infarct volume. Crossed cerebellar diaschisis (inhibition of function of an area at some distance from the acute injury, but connected by fiber tracts) is seen as hypometabolism and hypoperfusion in the cerebellar cortex contralateral to the site of the infarct and usually occurs during the first 2 months after infarction (Fig. 32.16).[79]

Studies of the carotid artery and vertebral arteries are performed using ultrasound evaluation. Doppler ultrasound looks at the flow velocity of the blood through the artery. Plaque accumulation and ulceration can be identified by Doppler. Doppler studies are used to determine the need for carotid endarterectomy.[39] Cerebral angiography can be used in the absence of CT or MRI but is an invasive procedure and is used only when other forms of imaging are not appropriate.

All acute stroke patients should undergo cardiovascular evaluation, both for determination of the cause of the stroke and to optimize immediate and long-term management. This cardiac assessment should not delay reperfusion strategies. Atrial fibrillation may be seen on an admission electrocardiogram; however, its absence does not exclude the possibility of atrial fibrillation as the cause of the event. Thus, ongoing monitoring of cardiac rhythm on telemetry or by Holter monitoring is indicated in some patients.

**TREATMENT.** The American Stroke Association recommends that blood pressure be kept less than 180/105 mm Hg after infusion of IV rt-PA and that permissive hypertension up to a systolic blood pressure of 220 mm Hg and diastolic blood pressure of 120 mm Hg be allowed for those who do not receive thrombolysis unless there is a compelling indication otherwise.[44] An excessive rise in blood pressure may cause an increase in edema. Cerebral edema occurs in all infarcts. The goal of medical interventions for cerebral edema is to prevent significant increases in intracranial pressure (ICP). Interventions may include restriction of free water, avoidance of excess glucose administration, minimization of hypoxemia and hypercarbia, treatment of hyperthermia, avoidance of anti-hypertensive medications, and elevation of the head of the bed to 20 to 30 degrees.[44] If cerebral edema leads to increased ICP, management strategies similar to those used for traumatic brain injury (e.g., administration of osmotic diuretics), may be implemented.

Delayed deterioration caused by edema of the infarcted tissue is a common poststroke complication. This is especially common after large-volume infarcts. Proximal large-vessel occlusion, such as occlusion of the internal carotid artery or proximal middle cerebral artery, causes infarction of a large portion of the hemisphere. These types of infarctions, as well as those involving the cerebellum, are associated with increased risk of herniation and brainstem compression. Clinical deterioration often occurs rapidly in these cases, and mortality can be as high as 50% to 70%. Although decompression surgery can dramatically reduce mortality, survivors may have severe disability.[66]

Thrombolytic and antithrombotic agents form the cornerstone of ischemic stroke treatment and prevention.[1,66] Intravenous alteplase (rtPA) is used for the emergent care of embolic stroke. Alteplase activates plasminogen to form plasmin, which actively digests fibrin strands, and is effective in dissolving the thrombosis or blood clot responsible for the blockage.[2,117]

By promoting early recanalization of occluded vessels and early reperfusion of ischemic fields, there is potential to salvage penumbral neuronal tissue. If it is received within 4.5 hours after the initial stroke, the person is significantly more likely to recover function.[40] Recently, IV rt-PA has been used for up to 6 hours after the onset of symptoms.[34] The risk of brain hemorrhage with IV t-PA is about 5% in stroke patients, and its inappropriate use in a stroke that is hemorrhagic will increase that risk. It must be determined on CT that the stroke is purely embolic; guidelines are established by the National Institute of Neurological Disorders and Stroke study.[36] With the use of DWI imaging and further understanding of the status of the ischemic penumbra, the window of opportunity may become larger and therapies more effective.

Thrombolysis reduces the overall risk of dependency in the long term, although the incidence of fatal intracranial hemorrhage is increased.[116]

Several prognostic factors must be considered for selecting candidates for intravenous thrombolysis. Younger age, absence of cardiac disease or diabetes, lower blood pressure on admission, lower neurologic score, absence of early ischemic parenchymal changes, large artery thrombus visible on baseline brain CT, and a developed collateral circulation are all factors associated with a more favorable outcome. Risk factors for developing brain hemorrhage include time to treatment, dose of thrombolytics, blood pressure level, severity of neurologic deficit, and severity of ischemia. Besides hemorrhage, potential complications of thrombolysis include reperfusion injury, arterial reocclusion, and secondary embolization due to thrombus fragmentation. Thus, adequate hospital facilities and personnel are required for administration of thrombolytic therapy, as well as for monitoring and managing potential complications. Following t-PA administration, blood pressure should be closely monitored and kept at less than 180/105 mm Hg and antithrombotic agents should be avoided for 24 hours.

Intracranial clot retrieval is now possible with endovascular thrombectomy. Endovascular thromboaspiration, sonothrombolysis, angioplasty, or stent placement can be performed. Most stroke centers are now offering these options, with trials done up to 8 hours after symptom onset when used with very large clots.[99] Several RCTs have shown that endovascular thrombectomy results in complete vessel recanalization in three of four treated patients, producing outcomes superior to those of intravenous alteplase in selected patients with large proximal artery occlusions.[97] In addition, a comprehensive systematic review and meta-analysis of eight randomized controlled trials that included data from a total of 2049 patients confirmed an increased likelihood of good outcome with mechanical thrombectomy as compared to standard alteplase treatment.[18]

Acute ischemic stroke is recognized as the third leading cause of death in the United States; improved treatments for management are important to reduce disability and death. The standard of care of acute stroke therapy has been reperfusion/recanalization of the occluded vessels using pharmacologic management, endovascular management, or a combination approach. Significant improvements have been made in management with the use of endovascular therapy.

### *Prophylaxis*

Anticoagulation. Anticoagulation therapy has played a prominent role in the prevention of acute infarction for several decades, and current research supports its use in high-risk individuals. The prevention of cardioembolic stroke is best accomplished with oral anticoagulation, barring any contraindications. Antiplatelets such as aspirin are used to decrease risk of second MI and may reduce the chance of stroke after MI.

Aspirin has become the antiplatelet standard for individuals with acute ischemic stroke. The American Heart Association/American Stroke Association evidence-based guidelines for patients with acute ischemic stroke recommend oral administration of aspirin within 24 to 48 hours of stroke onset for most patients, although those who have had intravenous fibrinolysis should not be given aspirin or other antiplatelet agents for 24 hours after receiving t-PA.[44]

Anticoagulation should not be used with high blood pressure or other risk factors of hemorrhagic stroke. Studies are underway to determine use in acute post-stroke management. Heparin can be used prophylactically against deep venous thrombosis and pulmonary embolism.[66]

In patients with atrial fibrillation, oral anticoagulation with vitamin K antagonists, such as warfarin, decreases the odds of recurrent stroke by two-thirds.[41] For patients with nonvalvular atrial fibrillation, direct oral anticoagulants that inhibit thrombin (dabigatran etexilate) and factor Xa (rivaroxaban, apixaban, and edoxaban) are preferred over warfarin. These anticoagulants reduce recurrent stroke and systemic embolism by about a sixth, without increasing major bleeding. Because it does not require laboratory monitoring, dabigatran therapy is less complicated than warfarin therapy, but it costs significantly more.[15] Dabigatran is not as effective or safe as warfarin in patients with mechanical heart valves.

Lipid-Lowering Agents. Cholesterol-lowering agents such as statins decrease the risk of stroke after MI. Studies show that the antistroke effects may be separate from the lipid-lowering properties through changes in the endothelium, inflammatory response, plaque stabilization, and thrombus formation. Several organizations have endorsed the use of statins for stroke prevention. The FDA has added ischemic stroke as an indication for statin therapy. The use of statins, in accordance with National Cholesterol Education Program Adult Treatment Panel III guidelines, is endorsed by the American Heart Association and American Academy of Neurology for both primary and secondary prevention of stroke.[98]

Despite the success of the statins, a second class of agents, cholesterol absorption transport inhibitors, also has been developed and approved for LDL cholesterol lowering. Ezetimibe is one of these medications that provides excellent tolerability and safety, along with moderate reductions in LDL cholesterol of approximately 18%. Reductions in LDL cholesterol of 44% or more can be achieved with combination therapy (e.g., ezetimibe plus simvastatin).[10,101]

PET studies have been used to monitor the success of various treatment regimens, including the effects of thrombolytic therapy in acute stroke. Results of these studies indicate that critically hypoperfused tissue can be preserved by early reperfusion, and that large infarcts can be prevented by early reperfusion of viable tissue. In the future, functional imaging modalities that could eventually include tracers for neuronal integrity may be used to help in the selection of individuals for thrombolytic therapy, possibly permitting the extension of the critical time period for inclusion of individuals to aggressive stroke management strategies.[79]

Neuroprotection. Medications aimed at creating neuroprotection to decrease ischemic cell death within the penumbra are the focus of much ongoing research. Researchers have targeted key factors, including excitotoxicity, oxidative and nitrosative stress, and inflammation.[18] However, results continue to be limited.

Excitotoxicity has been a widely investigated area in stroke. Excitotoxicity refers to the rapid and massive release and decreased uptake of the excitatory amino acid glutamate, which produces a surge in calcium influx and resultant elevation of intracellular free calcium. Even transient exposure to excess excitatory amino acids is toxic to cultured neurons, and altered neuronal energy balance increases the vulnerability of neurons to excitotoxic damage, even in the presence of physiologic concentrations of excitatory amino acids.[51] Evidence that this process progresses for several hours after the ischemic insult highlights a potential role for neuroprotective strategies administered during the critical window before irreversible loss, although the exact duration of this window in humans remains unknown. These anti-excitotoxic therapies may be suitable for either hemorrhagic or ischemic stroke.

Many different approaches have been used to try to decrease excitotoxic damage after stroke. Compounds that decrease glutamate levels or interfere with its binding to the *N*-methyl-D-aspartate receptor have been the focus of many studies.[107] Unfortunately, clinical trials of a long list of drugs with various mechanisms of action on glutamate receptors have not identified any with efficacious outcomes.[18] More recent investigations have studied methods of removing glutamate from the blood via plasma glutamate dialysis, as well as methods of modulating calcium influx by administration of calcium channel antagonists.[18] Promising early results of some of these investigations will require validation in future research.

Another potential therapeutic strategy is the neutralization of oxidative and nitrosative stresses. Reactive oxygen species (ROS) and reactive nitrogen species (RNS), which are generated primarily in the ischemic penumbra, trigger detrimental cellular responses in acute stroke. Uric acid, a compound that accounts for much of the total antioxidant capacity of plasma, has been shown in animal models to suppress ROS and RNS, reduce infarct volume, and improve functional outcome.[18] Randomized controlled trials in human beings of administration of uric acid, sometimes in combination with thrombolytics, have demonstrated reduced expansion of the infarct and improved functional outcomes in some patient subgroups. Responses to treatment with uric acid appear to be more favorable in women than men.

Neurotrophic Factors. Animal studies have shown that providing treatment with bone marrow stromal cells ameliorates neurologic functional deficits after stroke. Nerve growth factor is a neurotrophic factor that supports the survival and growth of neural cells. Noggin, an antagonist of bone morphogenetic protein, promotes the differentiation of stem cells into neurons. Treatment of stroke with a combination of transfection of nerve growth factor and noggin in bone marrow stromal cells induced a synergistic effect on improved neurologic functional outcome.[25]

Animal studies also have demonstrated that brain-derived neurotrophic factor (BDNF) is beneficial for neuronal survival via anti-apoptotic pathways, such as inhibition of intracellular calcium overload and upregulated expression of anti-apoptotic proteins.[126] In humans, a lower concentration of BDNF in the acute stroke phase has been associated with poorer functional status 90 days after stroke onset. However, other studies have shown a lack of correlation between serum BDNF levels and lesion size or recovery in stroke patients.[126] An important factor to consider in interpreting this research is that serum BDNF levels may not be an accurate representation of BDNF concentrations in the brain.

Surgical Intervention. Carotid revascularization, by means of carotid artery endarterectomy or carotid artery stenting, is recommended for symptomatic patients who have more than 50% stenosis or asymptomatic patients who have more than 70% stenosis.[82] In comparing the two carotid revascularization procedures, recent meta-analyses appear to support the superiority of carotid endarterectomy over carotid artery stenting in the periprocedural period, but show inconclusive results for long-term outcomes.[82] Careful selection of candidates for surgery is essential, as it takes an experienced team of surgeons and other health care providers to manage the postoperative course. Because carotid revascularization procedures have risks of complications and medical therapy has improved, controversy surrounds surgical management of asymptomatic patients. Nonsurgical medical management, including antiplatelet drugs, antihypertensive agents, and statins, can go beyond stabilizing atherosclerotic lesions to actually breaking down the plaque.

Control of Symptoms. Pharmacotherapy of spasticity in stroke is controversial. Weakness of the extremities can result, and if the spasticity is contributing to stability, that may be lost with use of medications. Baclofen and benzodiazepines work at the level of the spinal cord; dantrolene works on the muscle fibers.

Treatment with botulinum toxin to decrease the firing of specific muscles gives more discrete control of treatment effects and leads to significant improvements in muscle tone in patients with poststroke upper or lower limb spasticity.[45] However, investigations of improvements in voluntary motor function and reduction in pain with botulinum toxin injections have not produced robust results. Choosing the appropriate muscle or group of muscles is critical for successful outcomes. The effects of botulinum toxin are temporary, usually lasting for approximately 3 to 6 months.[105]

Urinary incontinence can be a disabling consequence of stroke. Urge incontinence is treated with behavioral therapy and anticholinergics. An areflexic bladder can be managed with self-catheterization or use of a Foley catheter.

Depression after stroke is common and does not appear to be related to the area of the lesion. Depression after stroke responds to treatment and should be guided by the other concomitant medical conditions and the side effects of the particular medication. Use of selective serotonin (5-hydroxytriptamine, 5-HT) reuptake inhibitors (SSRIs) has been beneficial in preventing and treating poststroke depression, although the effects of these medications have not been demonstrated unequivocally, and they may cause bleeding and intracerebral hemorrhage.[113] SSRIs are preferred over tricyclic antidepressants because they have fewer side effects. The longer the duration of treatment, the greater the improvement in depressive symptoms, especially after 3 to 4 months.[113]

**PROGNOSIS.** The prognosis for survival after cerebral infarction is better than after intracerebral infarct or subarachnoid hemorrhage (SAH). Loss of consciousness after an ischemic stroke implies a poorer prognosis than remaining conscious. Individuals with ischemic stroke are at risk for other strokes or MIs. The risk factors and type of damage related to the stroke syndrome relate to degree of disability and mortality.

Recovery from stroke is the fastest in the first few weeks after onset, with the most measurable neurologic recovery in the first 3 months.[61] However, movement patterns can continue to be influenced by intervention with goal-directed activities, and repetition of movement appears to improve the speed and control of the movement in the individual up to 5 or more years after stroke. (See "Special Implications for the Therapist 32.1: Stroke Rehabilitation" below.)

## INTRACEREBRAL HEMORRHAGE

### Overview and Definition

Intracerebral hemorrhage (ICH) is bleeding from an arterial source into brain parenchyma (often referred to as an *intraparenchymal hemorrhage*) and is regarded as the most deadly of stroke subtypes. Primary ICH describes spontaneous bleeding in the absence of a readily identifiable precipitant and is usually attributable to microvascular disease associated with hypertension or aging. Secondary ICH occurs most often in association with trauma, impaired coagulation, toxin exposure, or an anatomic lesion. Hemorrhagic transformation, or conversion of an ischemic cerebral infarction, refers to secondary bleeding thought to occur either with early reperfusion into a damaged vascular bed with impaired autoregulation or as a result of development of collateral circulation into the same vascular bed.

Chronic hypertension causes fibrinoid necrosis in the penetrating and subcortical arteries, weakening of the arterial walls, and formation of small aneurysmal outpouchings, or microaneurysms, that predispose to spontaneous ICH. Bleeding usually arises from the deep penetrating arteries of the circle of Willis, including the lenticulostriate, thalamogeniculate, and thalamoperforating arteries and perforators of the basilar artery. Acute rises in blood pressure and blood flow can also precipitate ICH even in the absence of preexisting severe hypertension. A ruptured vascular malformation is the second most common cause of ICH.

Bleeding is limited by the resistance of tissue pressure in the surrounding brain structures. If a hematoma is large, distortion of structures and increased ICP cause headache, vomiting, and decreased alertness. Because the cranial cavity is a closed system, enlargement of a hematoma or development of severe edema may shift brain tissues into another compartment, causing deterioration in the clinical condition.

Supratentorial ICH, so named because it occurs above the cerebellar tentorium, is classified as being lobar (i.e., involving the hemispheres of the cerebrum) or deep (i.e., implying involvement of subcortical structures, such as the thalamus, putamen, or caudate nucleus). Infratentorial, below the tentorium, refers to involvement of either the brainstem, most commonly the pons, or the cerebellum.[94]

### Incidence

ICH accounts for 10% to 20% of all strokes, but is associated with the highest mortality rate (40-50%) of all stroke subtypes.[3] The incidence of ICH increases with advanced age, with an increase in relative risk of 1.97 per decade.[30] ICH tends to occur more frequently in men. In the United States, African Americans are more likely to have an ICH than are Caucasians. In one population-based study, the incidence of ICH per 100,000 person-years was 48.9 for African Americans compared to 26.6 for Caucasians.[3] Worldwide rates are higher in Asian populations than in Western populations. Locations of hypertensive ICHs include the basal ganglia, thalamus, cerebellum, pontine tegmentum, and deep lobar white matter.[30] Figures 32.17 and 32.18 represent the areas most likely to be involved in ICH.

Spontaneous ICH can also occur in association with the prescription of anticoagulants, primary or metastatic brain tumors or granulomas, and use of sympathomimetic drugs.

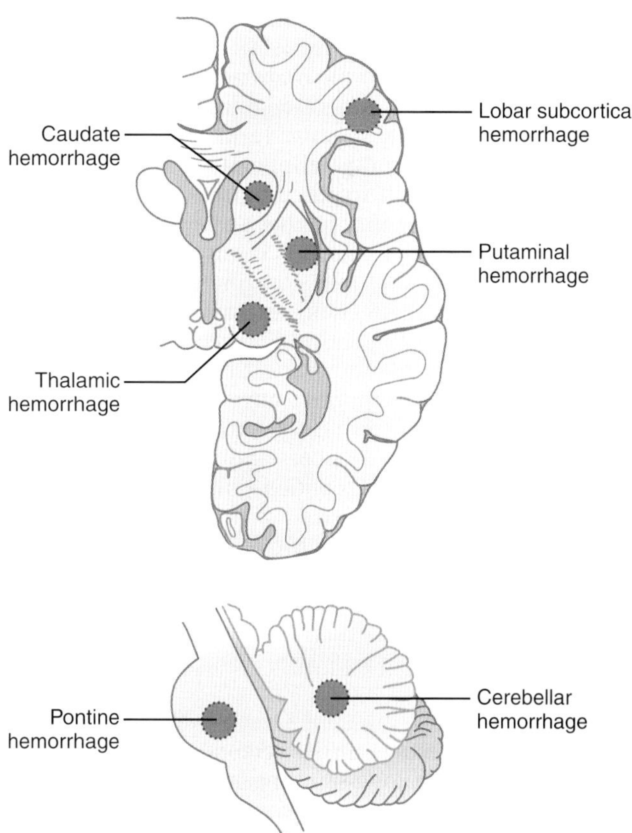


**Figure 32.17**

Horizontal cerebral section *(top)* and sagittal brainstem section *(bottom)* showing most common sites of ICH. (Modified from Caplan LR: *Caplan's stroke: a clinical approach*, ed 3, Boston, 2000, Butterworth-Heinemann.)

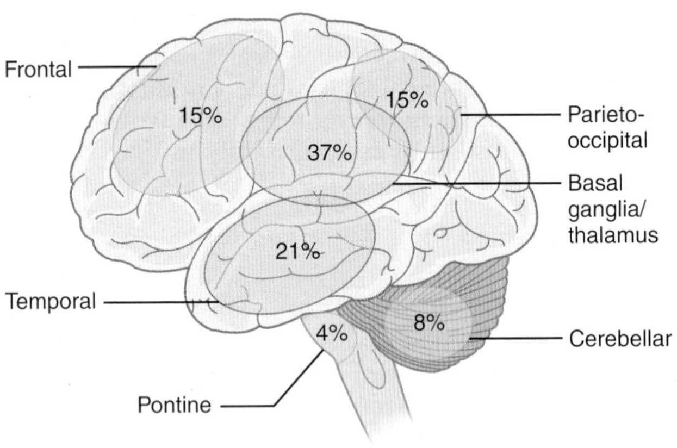


**Figure 32.18**

Sites of predilection of ICH. (Modified from Lindsay KW, Bone I, Callander R: *Neurology and neurosurgery illustrated*, New York, 1986, Churchill Livingstone.)

Aneurysms rarely bleed only into the brain, but when they do, they cause a local hematoma near the brain surface.

## Etiologic and Risk Factors

Spontaneous ICH in the parenchyma of the brain usually is from an anomaly of the vessel structure or changes brought on by hypertension. Hypertension represents the single most important modifiable risk factor for ICH. Cerebral amyloid angiopathy (CAA) causing abnormal changes in the vessels of the brain accounts for approximately 10% of ICHs. CAA is recognized as an important cause of ICH in elderly persons. Hemorrhages caused by CAA typically occur in the peripheral lobar white matter near the gray and white matter interface.[30]

Excessive use of alcohol has been associated with massive spontaneous ICH. Alcohol has a number of acute and chronic effects that may contribute to hemorrhagic stroke, such as direct effects on cerebral vessels, hypertension, and impaired coagulation. Cigarette smoking also is a major modifiable risk factor for ICH.

ICH is the most important adverse effect of thrombolytic therapy. Hemorrhage from fibrinolytic agents typically occurs within 24 hours and in already-infarcted brain tissue.[125] Long-term anticoagulant therapy also is associated with an increased risk for ICH. Individuals using warfarin have a two- to five-fold increase in the risk of ICH.[3] The incidence of anticoagulation-related ICH is increasing because of the increased use of oral anticoagulation in older adults.

## Pathogenesis

Histopathologic changes in the cerebral microvasculature of individuals with long-standing hypertension include processes that affect both the contents and the walls of the blood vessels of the brain. These changes are seen in small cerebral arteries and arterioles where they branch, and they are more severe in the small penetrating vessels in the deep white matter than in cortical vessels of similar size. Changes are more severe distally than proximally. Smooth muscle cells are progressively replaced by collagen (hyalinization). Altered permeability of the vessel wall leads to fibrinoid necrosis of the subendothelium, with microaneurysms and focal dilatations in some individuals.[3]

Individuals with hypertension have a substantial reduction in the percentage of smooth muscle in the vessel wall. This decrease in smooth muscle most likely represents structural weakening, increasing the likelihood of rupture and hemorrhage. Necrosis of the endothelium may be a result of vessel ischemia. The changes in smooth muscle and the thickening of the intimal wall increase the metabolic requirements and impede the flow of oxygen to the outermost part of the vessel wall.

Whereas lipohyalinosis, prominently related to hypertension, is most often found in nonlobar ICH, CAA is relatively more common in lobar ICH.[3] CAA is characterized by protein fibrils in the arterioles and small cerebral arteries and is formed by aberrant protein synthesis. Amyloid-β peptide replaces smooth muscle in the media separating the elastic membranes. Lymphocytic infiltrates, hyaline arteriole degeneration, and fibrinoid necrosis are characteristic changes in the vessel wall. The parenchymal changes seen in CAA reflect the consequences of the vascular pathology and direct deposition of amyloid in the brain tissue.

In drug-related ICH, some underlying vascular pathologic lesion may be present, such as an arteriovenous malformation (AVM) or chronic vasculitis. The ICH occurs as a result of a sudden increase in blood pressure triggered by the drug. The effects of excessive alcohol consumption may differ according to underlying vessel pathology. Alcohol appears to have a more prominent effect on arteriosclerotic processes involving deeply located cerebral small vessels; heavy alcohol intake has been associated with increased risk for deep, but not lobar, ICH.[19]

When hemorrhage occurs, it spreads along a path of least resistance, primarily following the fiber tracts of the white matter. Gray matter, with its dense cell structure, is more resistant to the shearing forces of the growing hematoma and is more likely than white matter to be compressed rather than infiltrated by the spreading hematoma. Edema forms in the parenchyma surrounding the hematoma. Blood is reabsorbed by macrophages at the periphery of the hemorrhage, leaving a cavity surrounded by necrotic tissue.

## Clinical Manifestations

Neurologic symptoms of ICH usually develop gradually over minutes to a few hours, representing the expansion of the hematoma.[3] In some cases (approximately 30%), onset is sudden. The earliest signs relate to blood issuing into parenchymatous structures. For example, a hematoma in the left putamen and internal capsule would first cause weakness of the right limbs; a cerebellar hematoma would cause gait ataxia. As the hematoma enlarges, the focal symptoms increase. If the hematoma becomes large enough to raise ICP, headache, vomiting, and decreased alertness develop. Some hematomas remain small and the only symptoms relate to the focal collection of blood. Once the condition is stabilized, the symptoms improve in parallel with the resorption of the hematoma.

**Table 32.1** Signs in Patients with Intracerebral Hemorrhages at Various Sites

| Location | Motor/Sensory | Eye Movements | Pupils | Other Signs |
|---|---|---|---|---|
| Putamen or internal capsule | Contralateral hemiparesis and hemisensory loss | Ipsilateral conjugate deviation | Normal | Left: aphasia<br>Right: left-sided neglect |
| Thalamus | Contralateral hemisensory loss | Down and in upgaze palsy | Small; react poorly | Somnolence, decreased alertness; left: aphasia |
| Cerebellum | Gait ataxia, ipsilateral limb hypotonia | Ipsilateral gaze or cranial nerve VI paresis | Small | Vomiting, inability to walk, tilt when sitting |
| Pons | Quadriparesis | Bilateral horizontal gaze paresis, ocular bobbing | Small; reactive | Coma |
| Caudate | None or slight contralateral hemiparesis | None | Normal | Abulia, agitation, poor memory |
| **Lobar** | | | | |
| Frontal | Contralateral limb weakness | Ipsilateral conjugate gaze | Normal | Abulia |
| Temporal | None | None | | Hemianopia<br>Left: aphasia |
| Occipital | None | None | | Hemianopia |
| Parietal | Slight contralateral hemiparesis and hemisensory loss | | | Hemianopia; left: aphasia; right: left neglect; poor drawing and copying |

Although headache is an important symptom of ICH, it is present in severe form in only 30% to 40% of cases. Headache is most common as a sign of superficial and large hemorrhages.

The location of the hemorrhage influences the likelihood of seizures. Cerebral cortex hemorrhage is most likely to result in seizure activity. Two-thirds of the seizures are generalized and one-third are focal. Focal seizures affect the body on the contralateral side (see Chapter 36). The level of consciousness at onset is unrelated to the occurrence of seizure.

## Syndromes

Syndromes associated with ICH are representative of the area of bleed and reflect brain activity of the particular site.[54] Table 32.1 gives typical signs in individuals with ICHs at various sites.

**Putamen.** The putamen is the most common location of hypertensive ICH. Contralateral sensorimotor deficit results from the proximity of the putamen to the internal capsule. If putaminal ICH affects the dominant hemisphere, a transcortical type of aphasia may occur. If the nondominant hemisphere is affected, contralateral neglect or constructional apraxia may result. Pupillary abnormalities, visual field loss, and oculomotor deficits are common. Conjugate gaze deviation toward the side of the lesion may be present if frontopontine fibers are involved.[54]

**Thalamus.** Sensory losses or dysesthesias are common with thalamic hemorrhage, and some motor deficit occurs secondary to internal capsular involvement. An ICH involving the dorsolateral thalami may produce prominent ataxia because of the loss of proprioceptive inputs to this region. Oculomotor dysfunction also is seen, the most frequent abnormalities being vertical gaze palsies, often with downward eye deviation and convergence spasm. Constriction (miosis) of the pupil is seen in 50% of cases. In dominant hemisphere thalamic lesions, aphasia, disorientation, and memory disturbances may be seen. With nondominant lesions, apraxia (impairment of a learned motor activity) may exist. Midline hematomas are associated with alterations in the level of consciousness during the acute phase followed by prefrontal signs, such as change in character, speaking to oneself, memory disturbance, and impaired learning.

**Cerebellum.** A hallmark of cerebellar hemorrhages is ataxia. Additional symptoms may include vertigo, dysmetria, hypotonia, nausea, vomiting, and nystagmus. The vertiginous symptoms typically are more severe than those associated with a peripheral vestibular problem. The individual may be dysarthric. Brainstem signs, such as facial paresis, can be present with a hemorrhage that extends to the brainstem. The signs of cerebellar hemorrhage should be carefully monitored, as the progression to compression of vital structures in the region of the fourth ventricle and medulla can be rapid and can produce life-threatening changes.

**Pons.** Brainstem hemorrhages commonly arise in the midline of the pons, leading to coma, quadriparesis, and nonreactive pupils with absent horizontal eye movement. Lateral pontine hemorrhage can result in extraocular paresis with deviation away from the side of the lesion. Quick, downward jerks of the eye occur with a slow, upward drift, a phenomenon known as "ocular bobbing." Pupils are small (pinpoint) but reactive. Contralateral sensory and motor symptoms and ipsilateral cerebellar signs also are seen. In some cases, patients with pontine ICH have paroxysmal autonomic instability with dystonia (PAID) or diffuse, uncontrolled activation ("storming") of the sympathetic nervous system.[54]

**Caudate.** Caudate hemorrhages can rupture into the ventricles and therefore have a presentation like that of an SAH. Headache, neck stiffness, and neurobehavioral changes are common presenting symptoms. Loss of consciousness may occur. Caudate hemorrhages are more likely to affect the anterior limb of the internal capsule than the posterior limb; consequently, neurobehavioral changes are more prominent than motor or sensory abnormalities.

**Lobar.** Lobar hematomas are centered in the immediate subcortical white matter. The most common cause of lobar hemorrhage in elderly persons is CAA. Symptoms of lobar hemorrhages are lobe-specific (see "Clinical Manifestations" in "Ischemic Stroke" above and "Higher Brain Disorders" in Chapter 28). Patients with CAA-associated ICH often have some degree of cognitive dysfunction, with the cognitive changes preceding the ICH in some cases.[3,54] Seizures are more common with lobar hemorrhages than with deeper bleeds.

## MEDICAL MANAGEMENT

DIAGNOSIS. The availability of CT allows for prompt diagnosis of ICH. The specific area of damage can be imaged and the amount of blood identified. CT accurately documents the size and location of the hematoma, the presence and extent of any mass effect, and the presence of hydrocephalus and intraventricular hemorrhage. CT scans should be performed immediately in individuals suspected of having an ICH. Follow-up CT scans are utilized when there is a change in clinical signs or state of alertness in order to monitor changes in the size of the lesion and ventricular system and to detect important pressure shifts. If the clinical syndrome and CT findings are typical of hypertensive hemorrhage in the basal ganglia, caudate nucleus, thalamus, pons, or cerebellum, angiography is usually not necessary. If the hemorrhage is in an atypical location, and the individual is young and not hypertensive, angiography is indicated to exclude an AVM, aneurysm, vasculitis, or tumor. Individuals who have ICH after cocaine use have a high likelihood of vascular malformations and aneurysms that need angiography. Particular attention should be directed to the presence of a coagulopathy. A drug screen should be obtained to evaluate use of sympathomimetics if substance abuse is suspected. Increased sympathetic outflow due to the hemorrhage may lead to an increase in dysrhythmias. Dysrhythmias also may signal impending brainstem compression from an expanding hemorrhage.

MRI can provide multiplanar views and can discriminate subtle tissue changes and rapidly flowing blood. However, it is of limited usefulness in the first 24 hours after ICH. MRI has the capability to detect previous hemorrhage, and can image the posterior fossa more clearly than can CT.

Prothrombin time, partial thromboplastin time, and platelet count should be performed in all individuals to rule out a bleeding disorder. Coagulation factor deficiencies can be detected by evaluation of liver enzymes. Bleeding time, platelet aggregation studies, and fibrinogen assay also can be indicators of disorders related to possible repeat hemorrhage.

The differential diagnosis for ICH is similar to that of ischemic stroke and includes migraine, seizure, tumor, abscess, hypertensive encephalopathy, and trauma. Hypertensive encephalopathy and migraine also can present with headache, nausea, and vomiting. Although focal neurologic signs are uncommon, they may occur with these entities. With hypertensive encephalopathy, individuals usually have marked elevation in blood pressure and other evidence of end-organ injury, including proteinuria, cardiomegaly, papilledema, and malignant hypertensive retinopathy. These individuals usually improve significantly with treatment of hypertension. Migraines often are associated with an aura, and the individual often has a history of similar headaches.

The difference between ICH and labyrinthitis can be especially difficult to determine in the elderly. The abrupt onset of vertigo, vomiting, and nystagmus can represent a peripheral process, such as labyrinthitis, or a central process, such as cerebellar or brainstem infarct or hemorrhage. Age older than 40 years and a history of hypertension or other risk factors for ICH increase the possibility of a cerebellar hemorrhage. Findings specifically referable to the brainstem must be sought; these include hiccups, diplopia, facial numbness, dysphagia, and ataxia. Vertiginous individuals often have a strong desire to remain immobile with their eyes closed, but this must not preclude a thorough cranial nerve and cerebellar examination, including gait. Gross ataxia is present with cerebellar stroke and absent with labyrinthine disease. A head CT scan should be strongly considered in individuals older than age 40 years to assist in differentiating labyrinthitis and cerebellar hemorrhage.

Acquired immunodeficiency syndrome should be considered as a possible cause of ICH. Biopsy of brain tissue can be diagnostic of CAA, cerebral vasculitis, and neoplasm. Evaluation of cerebrospinal fluid may indicate levels of toxicity; however, individuals with increased ICP are at risk during the procedure for possible herniation, causing compression of the brainstem.

**Treatment.** A number of clinical trials have been conducted to identify new treatments to minimize early hematoma expansion. Research has produced conflicting results as to whether elevated blood pressure contributes to hematoma expansion. Intensive blood pressure reduction after ICH, to a systolic target of less than 140 mm Hg, may not be safe for all patients, and may not be more effective in reducing mortality and disability than a target of less than 180 mm Hg.[41] For ICH not associated with thrombolytic therapy, recombinant activated factor VII was found to decrease hematoma expansion, but with no effects on functional outcome, and with an associated increase in thromboembolic events. For spontaneous ICH associated with anticoagulation therapy, reversal of the INR to less than 1.3 and reduction of systolic blood pressure to less than 160 mm Hg within 4 hours is associated with decreased hematoma expansion. Four-factor prothrombin complex concentrate is preferred over fresh frozen plasma for normalizing the INR and reducing hematoma growth.[41] A major issue in the management of ICH is control of edema (see "Treatment" under

"Ischemic Stroke" above). Anticonvulsant therapy should be considered with lobar hemorrhage.

An individual with a potential ICH requires rapid assessment and transport to a facility that has CT scanning capability and intensive care management. The prehospital management is similar to that for ischemic stroke. The circumstances surrounding the event and other concomitant medical conditions also should be ascertained. An evaluation of the initial level of consciousness, Glasgow Coma Scale, any gross focal deficits, difficulty with speech, clumsiness, gait disturbance, or facial asymmetry should be noted. The NIHSS described earlier in this chapter is a helpful tool for measuring stroke-related neurologic deficit.[56]

Supportive care involving attention to airway management and perfusion is of the highest priority. Individuals with hemorrhagic stroke are more likely to have an altered level of consciousness that may progress rapidly to unresponsiveness, requiring emergent endotracheal intubation. Intravenous access and cardiac monitoring should be initiated. Evaluation of blood glucose and appropriate dextrose and naloxone administration should be considered in any patient with altered mental status.

There is disagreement regarding optimal blood pressure management in an individual with ICH. Hypertension may cause deterioration by increasing ICP and potentiating further bleeding from small arteries or arterioles. Hypotension may decrease cerebral blood flow, worsening brain injury. In general, recommendations for treatment of hypertension in individuals with ICH are more aggressive than those for individuals with ischemic stroke. The current consensus for ICH is to recommend antihypertensive treatment with parenteral agents for systolic pressures greater than 160 to 180 mm Hg or diastolic pressures greater than 105 mm Hg. In order to avoid overshoot hypotension, elevated blood pressures should be treated with medications that have a short half-life, such as labetalol or nicardipine. Hydralazine and nitroprusside may be associated with increased intracranial pressure, and consequently should not be used.[74]

Elevation of the head to 30 degrees, adequate sedation, and avoidance of hyponatremia are mainstays of management of increased ICP. Hyperosmolar therapy with agents such as mannitol may be useful for reducing cerebral edema in the acute setting, and should be considered in patients at risk for transtentorial herniation.[74] The problem with hyperosmolar therapy is that rebound swelling can occur and worsen the individual's clinical status. These agents also can cause dehydration and lead to hypotension. The use of steroids in cerebral hemorrhage, previously a common practice, may be harmful and is not recommended.

Seizure activity can cause neuronal injury, elevations in ICP, and destabilization of an already critically ill individual. Risk of seizures is higher in individuals with lobar hemorrhage or medical complications.[74] However, because some data suggest that phenytoin may worsen outcome, prophylactic antiepileptic therapy is not recommended. Only individuals with evidence of seizures should receive antiepileptic drugs.

Selected individuals with sizable lobar hemorrhage and progressive neurologic deterioration may benefit from surgical drainage. Surgery is more efficacious in individuals with cerebellar hemorrhage. The clinical course in cerebellar hemorrhage is notoriously unpredictable. Individuals with minimal findings may deteriorate suddenly to coma and death with little warning. For this reason, most neurosurgeons consider emergent surgery for individuals with cerebellar hemorrhage within 48 hours of onset.

**PROGNOSIS.** Although the overall mortality from ICH is high, functional recovery among survivors is also high. The most important predictor of mortality is hemorrhage size. The individuals who are comatose at onset or who have a wide spectrum of neurologic deficits tend to do poorly compared with those who remain alert and have focal neurologic symptoms. Survival depends on the location, size, and rapidity of development of the hematoma. ICHs are at first soft and dissect along white matter fiber tracts. If the individual survives the initial changes in ICP, blood is absorbed and a cavity or slit forms that may disconnect brain pathways. Individuals with small hematomas located deep and near midline structures often develop secondary herniation and mass effect and have a high mortality rate. Survivors invariably have severe neurologic deficits. In individuals with medium-sized hematomas, the deficit varies with the location and size of the hematomas. Most individuals survive with some residual neurologic signs. Survival for individuals with hemorrhage in the posterior fossa is more dependent on location of hemorrhage than size. Midline pontine hemorrhage is often fatal, whereas lateral hemorrhages carry a better prognosis.

## SUBARACHNOID HEMORRHAGE

### Overview and Definition

SAH can begin with the sudden onset of a severe headache that reaches maximal intensity in seconds (a "thunderclap" headache); sometimes the headache begins with exertion. SAH results in frank blood in the subarachnoid space between the arachnoid and the pia, which are contiguous membranes that surround the brain tissue. SAH can be spontaneous, is often seen in normotensive persons, and results in searing pain that patients describe as "the worst headache of my life."[60] One percent to 4% of all individuals presenting to the emergency department with a headache have an SAH.

### Etiologic and Risk Factors

Aneurysm and vascular malformations are responsible for most SAHs. SAH can be the result of trauma, developmental defects, neoplasm, or infections that cause rupture into the subarachnoid space. Hypertension may be seen in 32% and fever in 5%. Vascular malformations are responsible for approximately 6% of hemorrhages into the subarachnoid space. Included in vascular malformations are venous malformation, AVM, and cavernous malformation. Risk factors for SAH include smoking, excessive alcohol consumption, and hypertension. Genetic associations are being studied. A total of 9 suggestive linkage regions have been identified, with 2 that have appeared in several populations: the 7q11.2, also known as the intracranial berry aneurysm-1 (*ANIB1*) and the region at chromosome 19q13.3.[72]

First-degree relatives of persons who have experienced an SAH have a threefold to sevenfold increased risk of an SAH. If transmitted genetically, the effect is most likely related to connective tissue. Aneurysms are also more common among individuals with hereditary connective tissue disorders. Individuals with hemorrhage resulting from an aneurysm tend to be younger than those with hemorrhage secondary to hypertension.

Individuals with fibromuscular dysplasia, polycystic kidney disease, or connective tissue diseases have a higher incidence of aneurysms. Embolization, often from endocarditis, can cause mycotic aneurysms. Fungi or tumor tissue can travel to the brain. About one-fifth of individuals with aneurysms have more than one vascular anomaly or other aneurysms.

## Types of Subarachnoid Hemorrhage

*Berry aneurysm* is a congenital abnormal distention of a local vessel that occurs at a bifurcation, where the medial layer of the vessel is the weakest. About 90% of SAHs are due to berry aneurysms. Aneurysms are probably caused by a combination of congenital defects in the vascular wall and degenerative changes. Aneurysms usually occur at branching sites on the large arteries of the circle of Willis at the base of the brain. When an aneurysm ruptures, blood is released under arterial pressure into the subarachnoid space and quickly spreads through the cerebrospinal fluid around the brain and spinal cord. Aneurysms are less often caused by arterial dissection through the adventitia of arterial walls, embolism of infected material of distal cerebral arteries (mycotic aneurysms), and degenerative elongation and tortuosity of arteries (dolichoectasia). Figure 32.19 shows the typical formations of berry aneurysms.

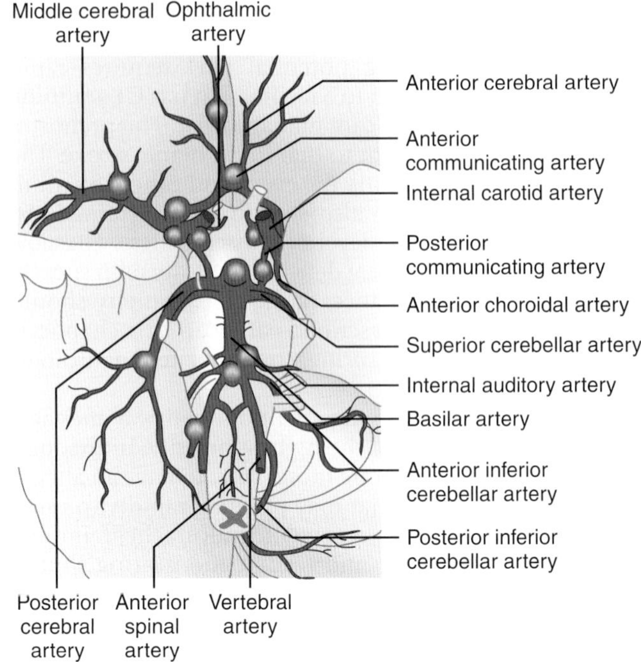


**Figure 32.19**

Berry aneurysms typically develop at the bifurcations of arteries on the undersurface of the brain. (Reprinted from Goldman L: *Cecil textbook of medicine*, ed 22, Philadelphia, 2004, WB Saunders.)

*Venous malformations* are composed entirely of veins, which are usually thickened and hyalinized, with minimal elastic tissue or smooth muscle. The veins converge on a draining vein. Normal brain parenchyma is interspersed among the vessels. Venous malformation is the most common form of vascular malformation, constituting approximately 50% of malformations. The risk of hemorrhage from venous malformation has been estimated at 20% per year. Individuals with a cerebellar malformation have the greatest risk of hemorrhage. Occasionally, seizures may be associated with venous malformations. Headaches and focal neurologic deficits are manifested according to the area of the brain that is disrupted.

*Arteriovenous malformation* is characterized by direct artery-to-vein communication without an intervening capillary bed. The blood vessel contains elastin and smooth muscle cells. Brain parenchyma is found within the AVM, and it is usually gliotic and nonfunctional. AVMs are the result of abnormal fetal development at approximately 3 weeks' gestation. More than 90% of AVMs occur in the cerebral hemispheres. Most AVMs are sporadic, but familial AVMs occur; these appear to have an autosomal-dominant inheritance with incomplete penetrance.

In recent research, the annual risk of bleeding from an unruptured brain AVM was 1.3%; the risk of recurrent hemorrhage was four times higher, at 4.8%.[23] The risk of rebleeding is particularly high within the first year from ictus. AVMs result in an SAH more than 50% of the time. Seizures, headache, or an audible bruit may precede a hemorrhage. Progressive focal neurologic deficits develop in some individuals, and cognitive decline may also precede a hemorrhage. AVM-associated hemorrhages occur predominantly in the third and fourth decades of life.

Malformations less than 3 cm in diameter are more likely to bleed than are larger AVMs because arterial pressure is higher in the smaller vessels. A single draining vein, obstructed drainage, or a periventricular or intraventricular location increases the risk of hemorrhage.

Angiography is the definitive diagnostic procedure for an AVM. CT scanning is diagnostic for a dense lesion in the brain. Suspicion of an AVM arises when an area of decreased density is seen around the hematoma and heterogeneous densities appear within the hematoma. MRI is not useful in the diagnosis; however, AVM can be suspected based on MRI with evidence of intravascular moving blood. An AVM should be suspected as a cause of hemorrhage in persons younger than 40 years, especially if they are normotensive. Figures 32.20 and 32.21 represent the vascular disorder and its appearance on imaging.[92]

Neuroradiologic embolization, stereotactic radiotherapy, and surgery are the current treatments for AVM. These techniques are used alone or in combination, depending

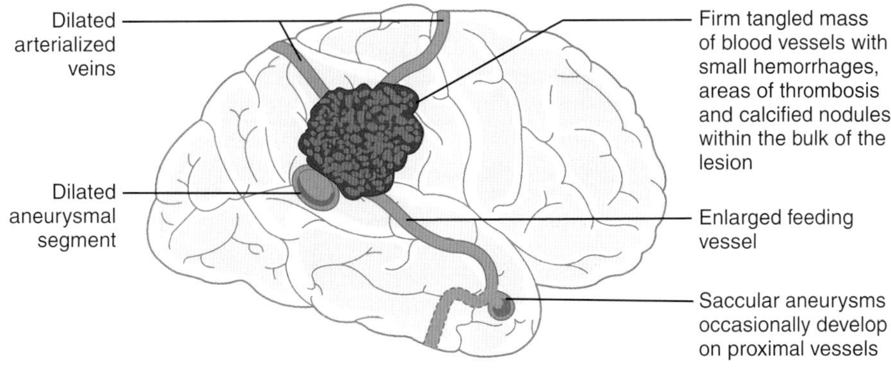


**Figure 32.20**

Typical deformation of blood vessels and brain tissue in relation to an AVM. (Reprinted from Lindsay KW, Bone I, Callander R: *Neurology and neurosurgery illustrated*, New York, 1986, Churchill Livingstone.)

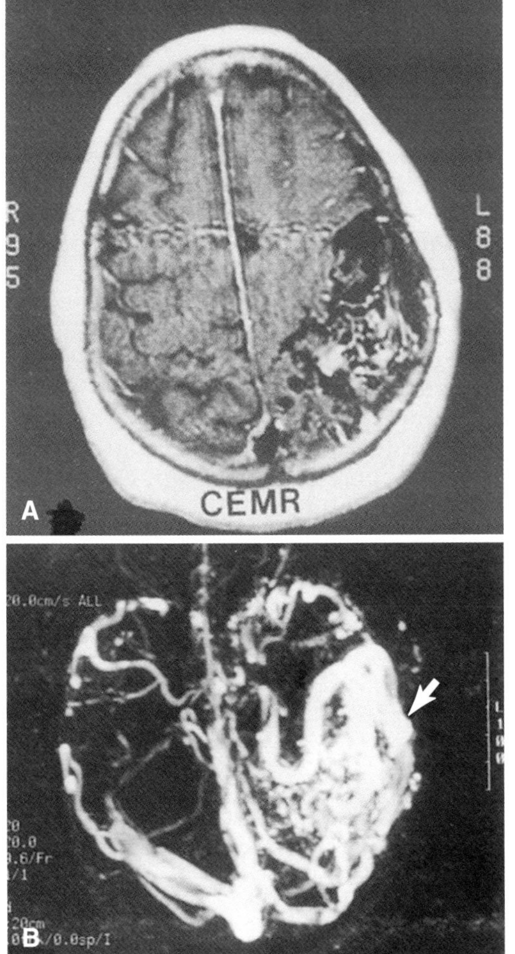


**Figure 32.21**

The AVM as seen with MRI (A) and MR angiography (B). *Arrow* points to enlarged vessel in periphery of AVM. (Reprinted from Ramsey R: *Neuroradiology*, Philadelphia, 1994, WB Saunders.)

on the size and site of the lesion. The goal of treatment is complete obliteration of the AVM; noncurative treatment exposes patients to treatment risks but does not lower or eliminate the risk of hemorrhage.[23]

*Cavernous malformations* consist of dilated, endothelium-lined, fibrous channels. No smooth muscle or elastin is present in the vascular walls. Neural tissue is present only at the periphery of the lesion. Thrombosis and calcification within the malformation occur, and gliosis (scarring) often surrounds the malformation.

Cavernous malformations represent approximately 10% of vascular malformations. Multiple malformations can occur in the same person. It is thought that cavernous malformations are inherited through autosomal dominance, with close to 100% penetration. Hispanics are at particular risk for the familial disorder. No apparent relation exists between malformation size and age and the likelihood of hemorrhage. Women tend to be more susceptible to hemorrhage than men. Subclinical bleeding frequently occurs around the malformation.

MRI is the imaging procedure of choice for visualizing cavernous malformations. The malformation appears as a well-defined region with a central area of mixed signal intensity surrounded by a rim of hypointensity.

The majority of individuals recover from a cavernous malformation hemorrhage, and the risk of repeat bleeding is low. Spontaneous rupture of a venous malformation is not common, and the resulting hemorrhage is often not of great consequence. Surgery is the treatment of choice for malformations that have hemorrhaged and are in an accessible part of the brain.

Syndromes are associated with the location of the hemorrhage, as they are in ICH. (See section above.)

## Clinical Manifestations

Forty percent of individuals who have SAH present with a sentinel headache. A sentinel headache results from a minor aneurysm leak that precedes rupture by days or weeks. Individuals who experience a sentinel headache typically report headache as the only symptom and have a normal physical examination

Common associated symptoms at the time of the rupture include nausea and vomiting (75%), syncope (36%), neck pain (24%), coma (17%), confusion (16%), lethargy (12%), and seizures (7%). Physical examination in individuals who have SAH can have variable findings. For example, nuchal rigidity may take several hours to develop and is present in only 35% to 52% of individuals. Thirty-six percent have a normal level of consciousness, whereas 28% are somnolent or confused. Focal motor weakness is detected in only 10%, and cranial nerve palsies are seen in 9%. Alteration of consciousness, drowsiness, restlessness, and agitation are especially common. Severe focal neurologic signs, such as hemiplegia and hemianopia, are absent at onset unless the aneurysm also bleeds into the brain.

### MEDICAL MANAGEMENT

**DIAGNOSIS.** Up to 38% of individuals who have an SAH are misdiagnosed initially. Misdiagnosis of SAH is associated with increased morbidity and mortality. The most common misdiagnoses for SAH are viral meningitis, migraine, and headache of uncertain etiology. Often individuals have subtle presentations and normal neurologic examinations. It is important to realize that the headache of SAH may occur in any location, may be mild, may resolve spontaneously, or may be relieved by analgesics. Prominent vomiting may lead to a misdiagnosis of viral syndrome, gastroenteritis, influenza, or viral meningitis. The presence of blood irritating the cervical or lumbar theca may lead to a misdiagnosis of cervical strain or sciatica.

A CT scan of the head without intravenous contrast is the diagnostic modality of choice in individuals suspected of having SAH. The sensitivity of CT for SAH is approximately 90% to 95%. The longer the duration is from onset of symptoms, the lower is the sensitivity of CT for SAH. Therefore, a lumbar puncture should be performed in all individuals suspected of having an SAH when the CT scan is negative or inadequate. The hematoma caused by an aneurysm tends to be of a different character than that caused by hypertension. The location of hemorrhage is also a clue to the diagnosis of aneurysm. Primary sites for hematoma resulting from aneurysms are in the area of the corpus callosum and anterior horns, the frontal lobe, and the temporal lobes. Angiography is required to establish that an intracerebral hematoma has been caused by a ruptured aneurysm.

**TREATMENT.** Once the diagnosis of SAH is made, a neurosurgical consultation and arrangement for transport to the closest emergency department is critical. The treatment of individuals with SAH involves the prevention and management of the relatively common secondary complications of SAH: rebleeding, vasospasm, hydrocephalus, hyponatremia, and seizures. About one-half of individuals with SAH have vasospasm, and this problem may resolve or progress to cerebral infarction. Fifteen percent to 20% of individuals with vasospasm die despite maximal therapy. Angiographic vasospasm has a typical temporal course: onset between 3 and 5 days after hemorrhage, maximal narrowing at 5 to 14 days, and gradual resolution over 2 to 4 weeks. Decreasing the risk of delayed cerebral ischemia involves maintenance of appropriate fluids, avoidance of antihypertensive drugs, and administration of the calcium-channel blocker nimodipine.[60,110]

The International Subarachnoid Aneurysm Trial confirmed endovascular treatment as the treatment of choice for intracranial berry aneurysms. Isolating the aneurysm or rupture site from the circulation is the primary goal of treatment via coiling or clipping. Spontaneous rupture of a venous malformation is not common, and the resulting bleed is often not of great consequence. Surgical resection of the hematoma may be necessary if it is significantly extensive. With evacuation of the hematoma, the malformation is left intact in most cases.

**PROGNOSIS.** Mortality rate from SAH is high in elderly persons. Functional outcomes are poor, and few individuals 75 years or older are able to live independently at discharge. Early aggressive surgical treatment of elderly individuals admitted in good condition may lead to better outcomes. Seizure-like episodes occur in 25% of individuals after SAH.

If the resulting hematoma is less than 3 cm, the prognosis is good. Evacuation of hematomas that are larger should include resection of the causative aneurysm. Prompt removal may result in dramatic and early improvement of neurologic function. Repeat hemorrhage is more likely to occur if the hematoma is evacuated without treatment of the ruptured aneurysm.[60]

## SUBDURAL HEMORRHAGE

A subdural hemorrhage, or hematoma, is most often the result of tearing of the bridging veins between the brain surface and dural sinus. It results in accumulation of blood in the dural space. If it is a small amount, the body can reabsorb the fluid; if the blood is of great enough volume, as can occur with trauma, it becomes a space-occupying lesion. The lesion is reflected in the area of the hemorrhage and the result can be herniation of the cortex into the adjoining spaces. Figure 32.22 illustrates the actual spaces and potential spaces in the cranial meninges. Compression of the brain tissue can result in both localized lesions and general decrease in the level of consciousness. Figure 32.23 represents the pressures on the brain that accompany a subdural hemorrhage. Chronic subdural hematoma (CSH) is defined as a subdural hemorrhage that is more than

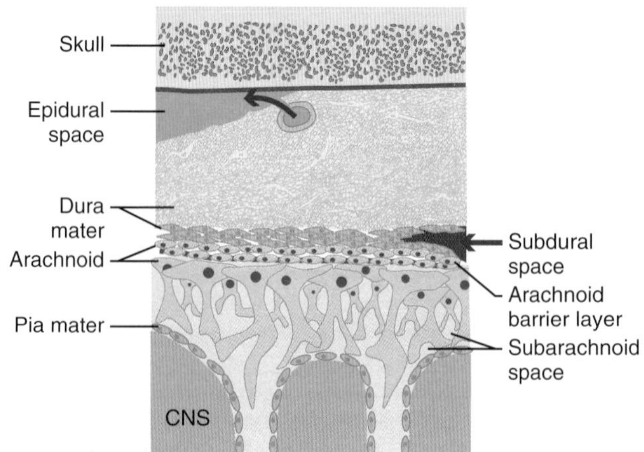


**Figure 32.22**

**Actual spaces and potential spaces in the cranial meninges.** Epidural space between dura and skull can be opened up by blood from a ruptured meningeal artery. Subdural space may be opened up by blood from a vein that tears as it crosses the arachnoid to enter a dural sinus. (Reprinted from Nolte J: *The human brain*, St Louis, 2002, Mosby.)

20 days old. The peak incidence for CSH occurs in the sixth and seventh decades, with up to 80% occurring in elderly men. In elderly persons, CSH often is caused by minor trauma, especially falls. In the majority of cases, there is no underlying brain injury. Fragility of the bridging veins and cerebral atrophy allow increased movement of the brain within the skull, thereby predisposing elderly individuals to CSH. Anticoagulant therapy is a recognized risk factor for CSH.

Elderly individuals who have CSH typically present with a complaint of headache and/or changes in mental status.[115] Mild generalized headache is present in up to 90% of individuals who have CSH. Any elderly individual who has headache, especially with a change in mental or functional status, should be evaluated for CSH. The diagnostic modality of choice for CSH is a non–contrast-enhanced CT scan of the head. When a hematoma is dense, delayed contrast-enhanced CT scan or MRI may be helpful. Once the diagnosis is confirmed, the physician should consult a neurosurgeon promptly, and the individual should be transported rapidly to the closest emergency department.

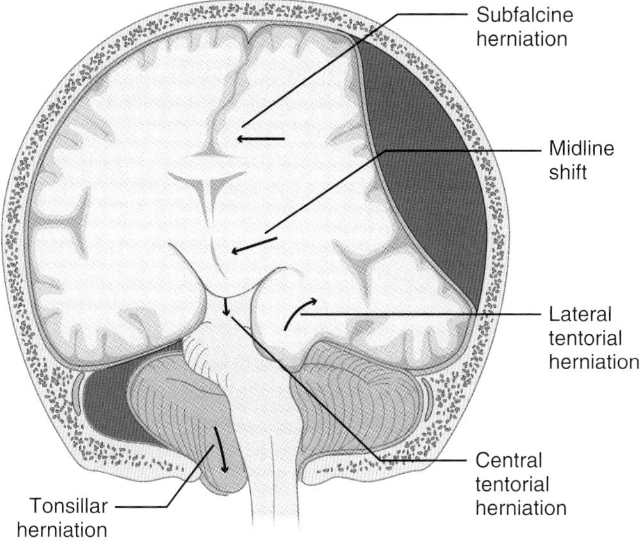


**Figure 32.23**

Compression of brain tissue with herniation into adjacent structures produced by the subdural hemorrhage. (Reprinted from Lindsay KW, Bone I, Callander R: *Neurology and neurosurgery illustrated*, New York, 1986, Churchill Livingstone.)

## EPIDURAL HEMATOMA

The meningeal arteries run in the periosteal layer of the dura. They can be torn during a traumatic skull injury, leading to bleeding between the periosteum and the skull and formation of an epidural hematoma. The damage comes from compression of the brain. Because there is potential for extensive pooling of blood, an epidural hematoma is considered a medical emergency and should be evacuated immediately to prevent compression of the posterior structures, which may cause death. Figure 32.24 presents an MRI showing an epidural hematoma.

## VASCULAR DISORDERS OF THE SPINAL CORD

Vascular disorders of the spinal cord are rare; however, vascular disorders of the brain and spinal cord have many common factors. Because of anatomic differences, some special issues must be considered in vascular disorders of the spinal cord. Infarctions in the spinal cord can be a result of any of the same causes as those in the brain; however, some of the symptoms appear to affect the lower motor neuron at the site of the anterior horn, and the result may be flaccid extremities and muscle atrophy.

An AVM in the spine can cause pain and burning below the level of the lesion, with progressive spastic paraparesis, with or without lower motor neuron lesion. Bowel

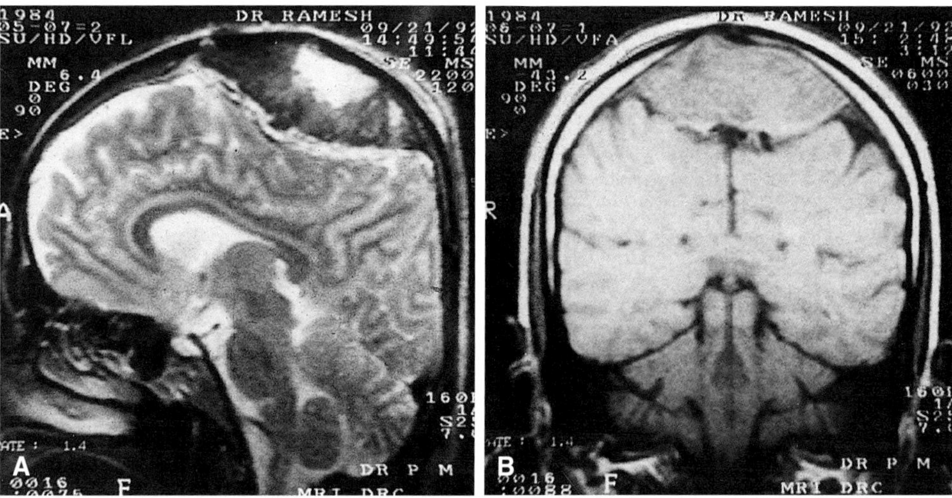


**Figure 32.24**

**Epidural hematoma seen on MRI.** (A) Sagittal view. (B) Coronal view. (Reprinted from Ramesh VG, Sivakumar S: Extradural hematoma at the vertex: a case report. *Surg Neurol* 43:138, 1995.)

and bladder dysfunction are seen when the AVM occurs in the lumbar region.

Transverse myelitis, the dysfunction of both halves of the spinal cord in a transverse section, can be related to vascular disorders. In addition to congenital vascular malformation, transverse myelitis can be caused by viral infection, multiple sclerosis, and degenerative disorders. Necrosis of the spinal cord often occurs at several levels, resulting in sensory and motor loss and pain. The lesion may involve nerve roots or just the central structures. The majority of individuals with transverse myelitis experience some degree of recovery (see also Chapter 34).

Box 32.4

**MOVEMENT PROBLEMS ASSOCIATED WITH STROKE**

- Decreased force production
- Sensory impairments
- Abnormal synergistic organization of movement
- Altered temporal sequencing of muscle contractions
- Impaired regulation of force control
- Delayed responses
- Abnormal muscle tone
- Loss of range of motion
- Altered biomechanical alignment

SPECIAL IMPLICATIONS FOR THE THERAPIST 32.1

## *Stroke Rehabilitation*

The disability resulting from stroke is a major problem for the stroke survivor, the family, and health care providers. A team of professionals is necessary to address the multitude of problems present after stroke. Therapists play a key role on this team, and there is now stronger evidence relating therapeutic intervention to decreased levels of disability. Stroke is highly heterogeneous in its effects, and each individual must be managed according to the particular impairment and disability that remains in the aftermath of stroke.[84]

The organization of movement changes after stroke. Mobility can be limited by a number of impairments. Basic reflex patterns can change as a result of disruption of the balance of supraspinal inhibitory and excitatory inputs directed to the spinal cord.[111] In addition to hyperexcitable stretch reflexes, secondary soft tissue changes in the paretic limbs can occur, further increasing resistance to passive movement. The hypertonia attributable to these soft tissue changes is often referred to as nonreflex hypertonia or intrinsic hypertonia. Limb mobilization may be critical for preventing and treating both spasticity (velocity-dependent increases in stretch reflexes) and nonreflex hypertonia.[111] On the other hand, spasticity may not always require treatment, and may in fact be useful for body support during stance and locomotion.[14]

Another factor that may contribute to spasticity is a decrease in transmitter depletion at the synapse of group Ia afferents with the motoneuron, a phenomenon known as homosynaptic depression. When group Ia afferents are activated repetitively at low frequencies, the release of excitatory transmitter at the synapse on the motoneuron is depressed. When these changes occur in reflex pathways, the resulting decreases in transmitter release contribute to the "habituation" of reflexes. A decrease in homosynaptic depression has been a consistent finding in patients with spasticity, and this abnormality is associated with the degree of spasticity and does not occur on the nonparetic side.[14] Box 32.4 gives examples of typical motor impairments after stroke.

Poststroke fatigue differs from the normal fatigue caused by exertion that resolves with rest. Rather it is described as pervasive, abnormal, persistent, and excessive weariness not consistent with the amount of energy expended. Physical activity has been linked with the IL-6 system, and through this system regular activity influences mood, performance, and cognitive function. The IL-6 processing, related to inflammatory responses, is one of the mechanisms that become abnormal after stroke. Stroke is also associated with increased mental fatigue, resulting in poor concentration, memory difficulties, irritability, and emotional lability. Poststroke fatigue results in decreased functional independence, institutionalization, and mortality even after adjustment for age.

### Examination

Identification of which impairments may be causing an inability to perform functional activities and cause disability is critical. Despite the spontaneous recovery that occurs after stroke, some degree of impairment typically persists over time. A solid understanding of the characteristics of the different stroke syndromes is critical to establishing the appropriate strategies for intervention. Figure 32.25 represents areas of brain damage and associated clinical signs.

Qualitative as well as quantitative measures should show sensitivity to change over time and identify relevant issues for the stroke survivor, including quality of life.[73] Many measures are currently used and there are efforts to benchmark levels of function that can help determine rehabilitation potential as early in the process as possible.[27,42]

Upper limb recovery after stroke appears to be related to the early ability to shrug or abduct the shoulder and perform at least synergistic hand movement.[50,42] In addition, the presence of active finger extension at 7 days after stroke predicts better hand function at 6 months as measured by the 9-hole peg test, Fugl-Meyer assessment, and Motricity Index.[42] Individuals who have some voluntary shoulder abduction and finger extension within 72 hours after stroke have a probability of 0.98 of regaining functional dexterity at 6 months.[80]

The prognosis for recovery of ambulation after stroke is fairly good, with 70% to 80% of chronic stroke survivors having the ability to walk.[42] However, only 30% to 50% return to community ambulation. Gait speed is a key determinant of ambulatory function, and an important measurement to include in physical therapy examination of individuals poststroke.[84] The use of functional walking categories (e.g., physiological

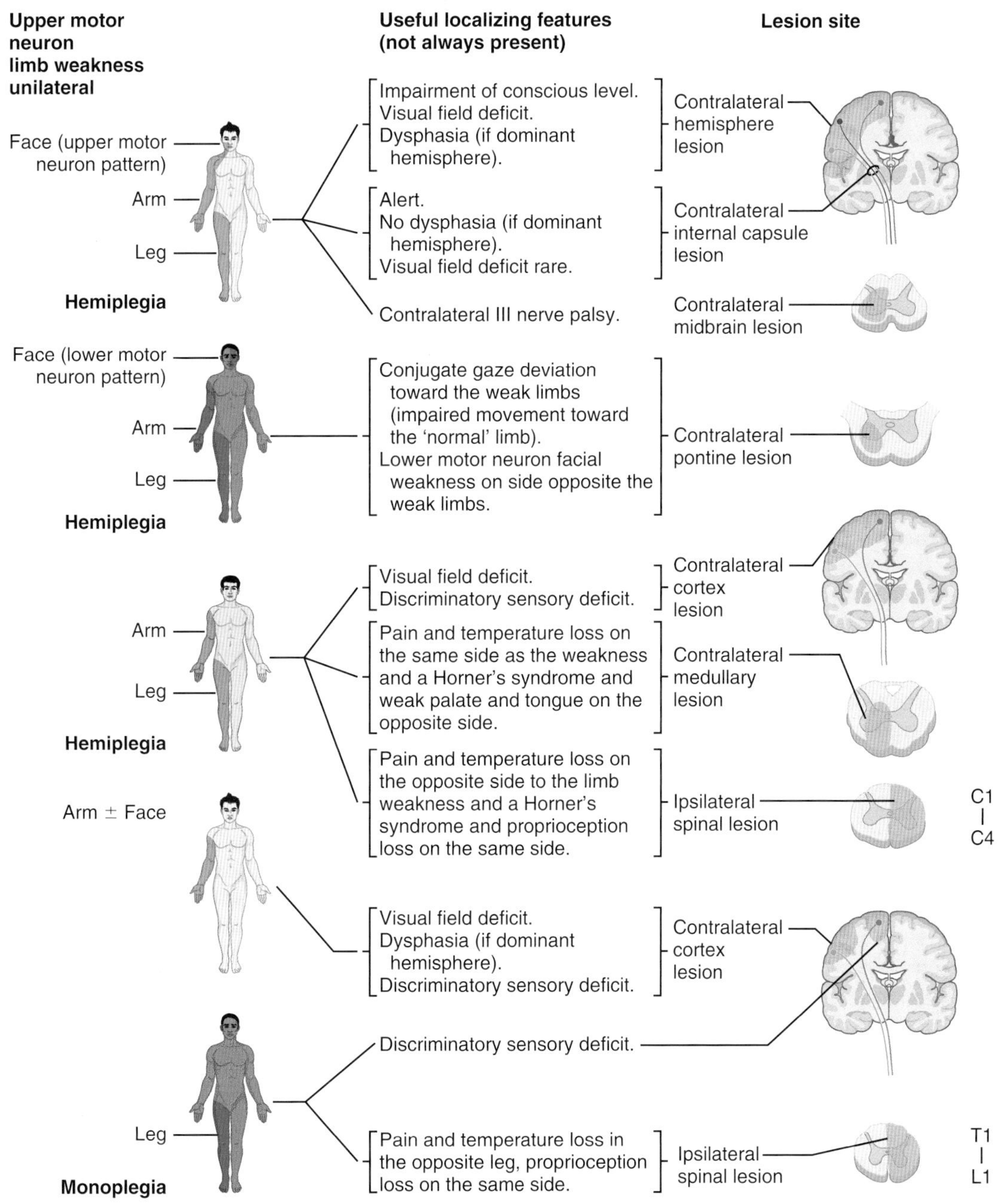


**Figure 32.25**

Localizing features of damage to specific areas of the brain and spinal cord. (Reprinted from Lindsay KW, Bone I, Callander R: *Neurology and neurosurgery illustrated*, New York, 1986, Churchill Livingstone.)

walker, unlimited household walker) can be helpful for identifying and communicating with other health care providers about the individual's customary level of walking at home and in the community.

Interest in the use of transcranial magnetic stimulation (TMS) for predicting motor outcomes has been growing in recent years.[42] TMS can be used to measure the integrity or conductivity of motor pathways in the CNS. Although some evidence suggests that the absence of TMS-induced motor-evoked potentials in the tibialis anterior muscle of the paretic leg predicts poor recovery of transfer and walking ability, additional research is needed to validate these findings.

## Intervention

Brain reorganization after neural injury is of great interest to therapists, as understanding the relation between alterations in neural structure and functional recovery are critical to the interventions chosen for each individual. It appears that the nature of the infarct may drive the plasticity related to recovery, and while recovery after a small infarct may result in reorganization around the area of the infarct, a large lesion may require more extensive changes in remote metabolism, blood flow, neurotransmitter function, and axonal sprouting that may not follow the same pattern of plasticity. Inherent in the processes of rehabilitation-dependent motor recovery are restoration and reorganization of motor maps within the cortex surrounding the lesion.[35,83,103]

Skill acquisition for recovery of function is the main goal in movement retraining. Increased knowledge of neural plasticity will lead to more precision in determining the optimal task practice for motor learning. Problem solving is critical for improving skill, but impairments of motor control, such as decreased force production, increased tone, and poor control of degrees of freedom in movement, must be adequately addressed. Implicit motor learning also depends on a neural network that can be affected in the pathogenesis of stroke.[11,53]

Many interventions are based on the manipulation of the environment to both guide and induce adaptive changes in brain function. In some cases, the therapy sets out to trick the brain into activity. For example, there is evidence for the effectiveness of mirror therapy for improving both upper extremity motor function and activities of daily living and decreasing pain, at least as an adjunct to usual rehabilitation for patients after stroke.[108] Significant gains in voluntary strength and muscle activation on the untrained, more-affected side after stroke can be invoked through training the opposite limb. Residual plasticity existing many years after stroke requires the clinical application of the cross-education effect when training the more-affected limb is not initially possible.[26] Bilateral arm training allows for greater force generated at movement initiation. Distributed constraint-induced therapy, a modified version of constraint-induced movement therapy (CIMT), leads to higher functional ability and better performance in the amount and quality of use of the affected arm.[122] Procedures involving shaping, repetitive exercises, and instructions for behavioral change appear to be the most important components of CIMT.[57] Movement of the upper extremity facilitated with electromyography-triggered stimulus and use of electrical stimulation orthoses continues to be studied with positive effects on movement and functional use of the upper extremity.[4]

Gait impairments that limit walking distance and speed are common after stroke, and reduce the quality of life of stroke survivors. Physical therapy interventions to optimize walking have received considerable research attention.[121] Task-specific locomotor training, including treadmill training with and without partial body weight support and various types of over-ground locomotor training, have been reported to produce improvements in gait speed, with effect sizes ranging from 0.25 to 3.00.[121] In the LEAPS trial, Nadeau and colleagues[76] found similar gait improvements, compared to a usual care group, for participants receiving clinic-based walking training on a treadmill and over ground and those receiving home-based strength and balance exercises.

A growing body of evidence supports the efficacy and relevance of incorporating robotic devices and brain-machine interfaces in stroke rehabilitation.[32,63] Advances in technology have led to development of devices for robot-assisted rehabilitation of both the upper and lower limb in stroke survivors. Wearable robots that assist three-dimensional movement show success because they mimic the trajectories of human movement.[55] Robot-assisted upper limb therapy is safe and significantly decreases motor impairments of the targeted segments; however, there is insufficient evidence to conclude that these impairment-level changes lead to meaningful functional improvements.[68] For lower limb rehabilitation, researchers have developed treadmill-based robotics, in which braces attached to the patient's legs produce the mechanics of gait on a treadmill. Powered robotic exoskeletons are similar in structure to treadmill-based robotics, but have control strategies that require active participation from the user for gait subtasks such as swing initiation and foot placement.[63] Active subject participation in robot-driven gait therapy is vital to many of the potential recovery pathways and is therefore an important feature of gait training. Higher levels of participation and activity may be achieved when designs allow sufficient degrees of freedom to facilitate other aspects of gait, such as balance.[123] Because powered exoskeletons are used for over-ground walking, the user has responsibility for maintaining trunk and balance control and for navigating over various surfaces. Clinical trials suggest that exoskeletal gait training is equivalent to conventional therapy during the chronic phase of stroke recovery, but may provide additional benefits in the subacute phase.[63] The expense of these systems typically restricts their use to institutional environments.

Virtual reality applications are being developed with a focus on attention, executive function, memory, and spatial ability. Functional training for activities such as crossing the street, driving, preparing meals, and navigating by wheelchair are possible with virtual reality.[21,93] Although virtual reality interventions appear efficacious as part of upper limb training programs, more research is needed to determine whether these interventions are beneficial for improving lower limb function, gait, and cognitive function.[59]

Brain stimulation techniques designed to augment traditional neurorehabilitation hold promise for reducing the burden of stroke-related disability. Repetitive transcranial magnetic stimulation (rTMS), transcranial direct current stimulation, and epidural cortical stimulation can enhance neural plasticity in the motor cortex poststroke.[29] rTMS has been shown to have a positive effect on motor recovery in patients with stroke, especially for those with subcortical stroke. Low-frequency rTMS over the unaffected hemisphere may be more beneficial than high-frequency rTMS over the affected hemisphere.[43]

Fall prevention is always a primary goal for the individual sustaining a stroke. Falls are frequent, and in more than 5% of cases result in significant injury. Because falls are common during the transition from sit to stand, researchers have studied the kinematics of this activity in relation to falls. Evidence shows that people who fall take more time to rise and to sit down and demonstrate increased mediolateral center of pressure displacement. They also exhibit significantly greater weight bearing through the nonparetic than the paretic leg during the activity.[9] Physical therapy interventions, such as balance retraining with center of pressure feedback, produce more symmetric weight distribution and faster task performance.[90] Placing the paretic foot posterior to the nonparetic foot helps to increase weight bearing through the paretic lower extremity and increases activation of the tibialis anterior and quadriceps muscles on the paretic side.[9]

Although a therapeutic goal is often to move clients out of assistive devices, studies show that for some parameters of gait the orthosis or assistive device still provides control over some of the critical components of gait. Orthoses and electrical stimulation orthotic substitute devices can both be effective in improving self-selected and fast gait speeds, 6-minute walk distance, and balance performance after stroke.[8] Although electrical stimulation orthotic substitute devices do not appear to be superior to ankle-foot orthoses for improving gait, patient satisfaction with these devices tends to be higher.[8]

Cardiovascular endurance training is indicated for stroke survivors; programs incorporating such activities should be part of rehabilitation programs. Treadmill training has been shown to reduce the energy expenditure and cardiovascular demands of gait within the stroke population.[65,87] Ergometers also can be used for aerobic training after stroke. Research is ongoing to establish the parameters of cardiovascular training within the limits created by neurologic deficits.

Failure to maintain functional gains after the course of therapy is a concern for all individuals involved in the management of poststroke rehabilitation. Functional exercise done on a regular basis has been shown to have a positive impact on recovery.[28] Early and consistent involvement of the family or primary caretakers is paramount, as is the follow-through of a home management program of activity and exercise. Exercise adherence of stroke survivors and caregivers continues to be less than ideal, despite efforts toward better education.[71] The functional consequences of fatigue for participation in physical, professional, and social activities should be considered.[38]

Several secondary conditions may arise after stroke. The clinician and family should watch for symptoms related to angina, peripheral vascular disease, and deep vein thrombosis. Bone loss, typically limited to the paretic side and more evident in the upper extremity, is a known consequence of stroke.[16] Factors that may influence bone mass in stroke survivors include the degree of muscle weakness, gait disability, and duration of immobilization. Interventions to preserve bone mass and prevent fractures should be included as a part of a standard protocol.[16]

## REFERENCES

To enhance this text and add value for the reader, all references are included in the enhanced ebook on Student Consult that accompanies this textbook. The reader can view the reference source and access it online whenever possible.

# CHAPTER 33

# Traumatic Brain Injury

KAREN L. MCCULLOCH • KENDA S. FULLER

## TRAUMATIC BRAIN INJURY

### Overview and Definition

Traumatic brain injury (TBI) is damage that impairs brain function, resulting from external physical force. The severity of brain injury varies widely, with the majority of injuries in the mild category. Concussion is a subset of mild traumatic brain injury (mTBI) that is generally self-limited and at the less-severe end of the brain injury spectrum but still involves a complex pathophysiological process. Moderate to severe injuries most often have significantly worse outcomes. Regardless of the severity of injury, there is a diminished or altered state of consciousness, at least initially. Impairment of cognition and physical function are common and may be temporary or permanent. Changes may be seen in behavior and emotional control. Functional disability or psychological maladjustment can be persistent and can have a devastating impact on lifestyle. Differences in recovery are seen in people who appear to have similar injuries.

### Incidence and Risk Factors[16]

The Centers for Disease Control National Injury Prevention Center reported 2.87 million U.S. emergency department (ED) visits, hospitalizations, and deaths in 2014 as a result of brain injury. The majority (87%) of these injuries required emergency department visits and discharge and were milder TBI or concussion that occurred as a result of falls (47.9%), being struck by or against an object (17%), and motor vehicle crashes (13.2%).[17] Of the total number of injuries, only 11% required hospitalization and 2% resulted in death. TBI contributes to a third of all injury-related deaths in the United States.[18]

The CDC numbers are likely a significant underestimation of the total number of injuries that occur. Unreported and untreated injuries, individuals who seek treatment in outpatient or office settings, and those who are treated in federal facilities (active duty military, veterans) are not included in CDC emergency-based surveillance. From 2006 to 2014 ED visits increased 53% while more severe injuries and deaths remained stable, likely resulting from increased awareness of the importance of reporting and seeking care for concussion. The CDC is undertaking efforts to develop a national concussion surveillance system that will clarify the extent of this injury and its effects.

Concussion has been publicized as an injury that requires careful attention, and can occur as a result of falls, motor vehicle crashes, being hit in the head with or against an object, violence, and as a result of recreational and sport injury. Concussions occur in all sports, with the highest incidence in organized sports that involve possible collisions. Sports that involve more participants, such as football, basketball, and soccer, have more total injuries, but the risk for injury remains higher in lacrosse, rugby, hockey, wrestling, and sports that could involve a collision with another player or object, in contrast with noncontact sports.

The reported incidence of concussion is higher in female athletes than in male athletes despite similar playing rules in most sports. This difference in incidence may be a result of weaker female neck strength, greater female acknowledgment of injury, or other factors. Certain sports, positions, and individual playing styles have a greater risk of concussion. Preinjury mood disorder, learning disability, attention-deficit disorder, and migraine headache complicate diagnosis and management of a concussion.[43] Early posttraumatic headache, history of headaches, fatigue/fogginess, amnesia, alteration in mental status, or disorientation lead to prolonged symptoms.[50] Concussion may occur in sports and situations not typically thought to put the athlete at risk and not necessarily during games. Concussion most commonly occurs *without* a loss of consciousness, rather with an alteration in mental status, such as feeling disoriented or confused. A single concussion does not necessarily lead to long-term impairment, but individuals who have had previous concussion are more likely to have future concussions with longer recovery times. In fact, a history of concussion is a highly probable risk factor for recurrent concussion, with particular susceptibility in the 10 days after an initial concussion.[45] Concussion has also been associated with other subsequent injuries after return to play.[47] For these reasons, return to play postconcussion is carefully monitored.

The leading causes of brain injury–associated hospitalization are falls (52%) and motor vehicle–related incidents (20.4%),[19] whereas causes of death are most commonly intentional self-harm (32.5%), falls (28.1%), and motor vehicle crashes (18.7%).[20] TBI peaks at three points across the lifespan. The first peak occurs in early childhood at age 1 to 2 years and is related most often to child abuse or falls that occur with early mobility. The second peak occurs in late adolescence and early adulthood between ages 15 and 24 years and may be related to risk-taking behaviors, and is associated most often with motor vehicle crashes. Adolescent sports concussion is common given the prevalence of youth sport participation. The importance of safety in nonorganized sports and recreation cannot be underestimated. Younger children sustain injuries during playground activities, and bicycling is one of the most widespread causes of injury among young people. High-speed sports that could result in a fall, such as skiing, snowboarding, and skateboarding, can result in serious injury. Wearing an appropriate helmet reduces the risk of severe brain injury by 88%.[6]

The third peak in TBI occurs in those 75 years of age and over and is related most often to falls. This group is the most likely to be hospitalized, and death is more likely, at rates of 79.3%, 42.5%, and 10.7% for severe, moderate, and mild TBI, respectively.[63] Although elderly individuals account for less than 15% of trauma admissions due to falls, they account for half of deaths due to falls. There is more susceptibility with age to tearing of the bridging vessels over the surface of the brain. In addition, there seems to be a significant, age-related decline in cerebrovascular autoregulation that may partially explain the poor outcomes seen in elderly individuals with TBI.[2]

Of those who sustain severe brain injury, many are injured in high-velocity motor vehicle crashes. Required seatbelt use, widespread availability of air bags, and graduated driving privileges have resulted in fewer injuries in recent years. Pedestrians injured by automobiles represent some of the most seriously injured individuals after trauma. The elderly are at particular risk for being struck as pedestrians because of slower ambulation, impaired reflexes, and impairments in visual, auditory, and gait abilities. Misjudgment of crossings may result, as elderly individuals are frequently struck within marked crosswalks or walk directly into the path of an oncoming vehicle. In the elderly, there are significantly increased mortality rates, with a majority of deaths occurring at the scene or at the emergency department.[2] Brain injury due to firearms is associated most often with attempted suicide.[53] The incidence of penetrating TBI from gunshot wounds is increasing, and in some urban communities is now the most common type of injury seen.[28] Alcohol use and abuse are frequently associated with brain trauma. Fifty percent of people admitted into hospitals with head trauma are intoxicated at the time. Brain injury may be two to four times higher in alcoholics than in the general population.[38]

A significant decline in TBI mortality from motor vehicle crashes from 2006 to 2013 affected by preventive measures such as speed limits, seatbelt laws, and airbag protection has been countered by an increase in mortality from self-harm and falls. The decline in mortality in high-velocity injuries has paralleled an understanding of the secondary injury process and an appreciation that all neurologic damage does not occur at the moment of insult but evolves over the ensuing hours and days from various biochemical and molecular derangements. As a result, acute medical management minimizes secondary injury more effectively. Appropriate management of the brain injury results in improved outcome from trauma.[42]

The CDC estimates that there are 3.2 to 5.3 million people living in the United States with TBI-related disability. These individuals who survive TBI often experience persistent morbidity, with reduced participation and productivity driving the need for ongoing supports for them and their families.

## Etiologic Factors

TBIs can occur with open or closed injury to the head. With an open head injury, the meninges have been breached, leaving the brain exposed. Penetrating missile injuries create localized, focal lesions that, when not fatal, cause limited damage to the brain. It is not the size of a missile but its velocity that generally determines the extent of damage. Penetrating injury also causes vascular injury, including disruption or the formation of aneurysms or pseudoaneurysms.[54] (Fig. 33.1A) shows the kind of damage that can occur from a gunshot wound, with subsequent intracranial bleeding (Fig. 33.1B).

A closed head injury occurs when there is no skull fracture or laceration of the brain itself, but the soft tissue of the brain is forced into contact with the hard, bony, outer covering of the brain, the skull. Injuries that occur with TBI can be both focal and diffuse. For instance, the anterior and inferior surfaces of the frontal and temporal lobes are particularly susceptible to contact with the inner surface of the skull, sometimes resulting in focal damage to those areas. If the head is struck by an object, under the point of impact a contusion, another manifestation of focal injury, may occur (termed the "coup" injury); then, as the brain decelerates and contacts the contralateral skull, injury occurs to tissue on the opposite side (the "contre-coup"). Such contre-coup injury is frequently worse than the injury underlying the impact. During brain injury, there are often torsional or rotational forces exerted throughout the brain, transmitting shear forces to the brain that may cause axonal disruption throughout the cortex and the brainstem. Small (petechial) hemorrhages may occur at the juncture of gray and white matter as a result of these forces, indicating the diffuse nature of the injury throughout the brain. Rotational forces are the most likely forces to cause diffuse axonal injury (DAI), including damage to brainstem structures, such as the reticular activating system.

Loss of consciousness does not always occur, although an altered state of consciousness is a hallmark of brain injury. Mild brain injury can occur after a severe neck injury, without the head actually striking any surface. The symptoms are typically worse when there is a rotational component to the injury in addition to the back-and-forth jarring.[29] Subdural and subarachnoid hemorrhage can occur in the presence of diffuse injury and rupture of veins bridging the brain to the venous sinuses.

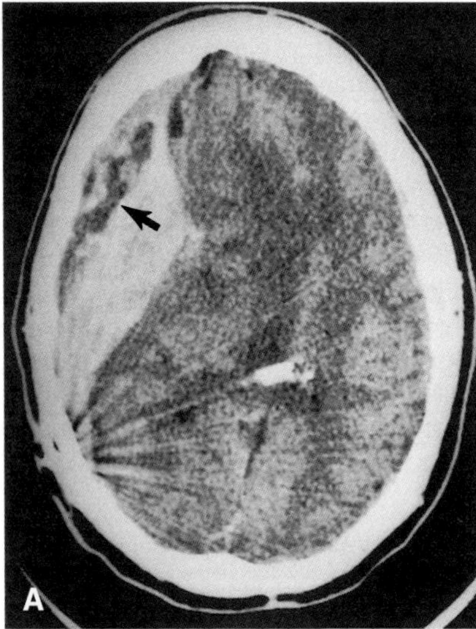


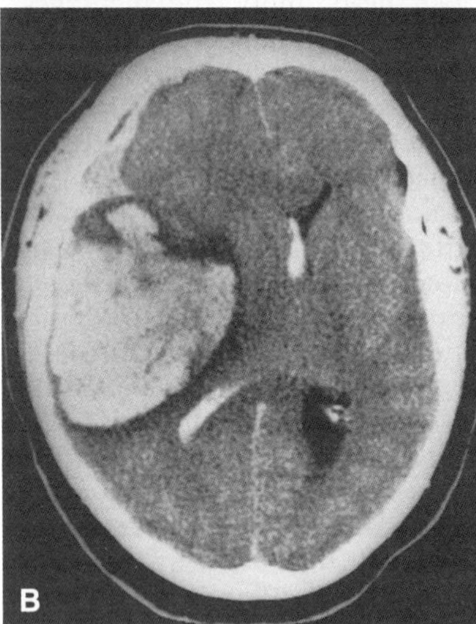


**Figure 33.1**

Gunshot wound resulting in both intracerebral and epidural hemorrhage.(A) The bullet is shown on CT scan resting in a midline position with streaking effect of fragments also seen. The *arrow* points to an area of decreased density thought to be epidural bleeding. (B) Large intracerebral hemorrhage is noted, with blood present in the ventricle. (Reprinted from Ramsey R: *Neuroradiology*, Philadelphia, 1994, WB Saunders: 407.)

Severe head injury may cause significant bruising and bleeding within the brain. Approximately 25% of people with a normal initial computed tomographic (CT) scan will develop late hemorrhages or evidence of contusion. The presence of an epidural hematoma, commonly a result of middle meningeal artery hemorrhage with skull fracture, is an emergent condition that may require surgical evacuation of the rapidly progressing arterial bleeding. Subdural hematomas are more likely to have a venous source, expanding less rapidly.

Contusions are usually more severe in persons with skull fracture than in those without fracture. Although contusion is a common occurrence in TBI, severe or even fatal damage to the brain can occur without contusion.[8]

## Pathogenesis

Primary injury is the result of forces exerted on the brain at impact. Secondary injury refers to changes compromising brain function in the hours, days, and weeks following the initial injury and results from the brain's reaction to trauma or other system failure, such as brain swelling and impaired cerebral perfusion (Fig. 33.2). Secondary injury effects are more pronounced, with more severe injury.

### Vascular Changes

Internal or extremity injuries caused by trauma can cause excessive bleeding and decreased blood pressure, which if persistent can cause hypoperfusion to the brain, accentuating secondary injury. Vascular damage can lead to ischemia and infarction within the cortical gray matter. Typically, contusions occur at the poles and on the inferior surfaces of the frontal and temporal lobes. Occipital blows are more likely to produce contusions than are frontal or lateral blows. With fracture of the cranial vault, there may be damage to the superficial epidural vessels and, particularly in the case of falls, there can be rupture of the bridging vessels between hemispheres.[69] Fig. 33.3 shows CT scan images of changes seen after TBI, with the presence of epidural and subdural hematomas.

TBI can be associated with other forms of vascular change. Gliding contusions, or hemorrhagic lesions in the cortex, may be the result of movement of the cortical gray matter in relation to the underlying white matter, causing shear strains that damage the penetrating vessels found at the gray and white matter interface.[87] Fig. 33.4 shows the effects of shear injury as seen on CT scan. Subarachnoid hemorrhage is common because of the rupture of pial vessels within the subarachnoid space. This may trigger vasospasm that can lead to reduced regional blood flow. Injury to the vessels within the white matter can also cause significant neurologic consequences, especially if it is in the area of the basal ganglia.[41]

An increase in cranial blood volume is considered to be the most important cause of increased intracranial pressure (ICP) after trauma. There can be bleeding into the epidural compartment, creating a mass effect that can displace the brain and increase ICP. The shear and tensile forces of traumatic injury can also create a subdural hematoma by disruption of the bridging veins. Acute hydrocephalus occurs when blood accumulates in the ventricular system, expanding the size of the ventricles and causing increased pressure on brain tissue being compressed between the skull and the fluid-filled ventricles.[27] Vascular volume can increase if venous outflow is blocked or increased cerebral blood flow (CBF) increases passively because of loss of autoregulation. Cerebrospinal fluid volume increases may be the result of blockage of outflow pathways or interference with reabsorption. When CSF volume of one compartment changes slowly, compensatory decreases in the volume of other compartments may prevent a rise in ICP. When the volume change is rapid or the compensatory mechanisms are exhausted or dysfunctional, the ICP goes up.[21] Methods to keep ICP under 20 mm Hg are a target of acute management.

The overall result of these vascular changes is the decreased ability of the cerebral vessels to maintain necessary

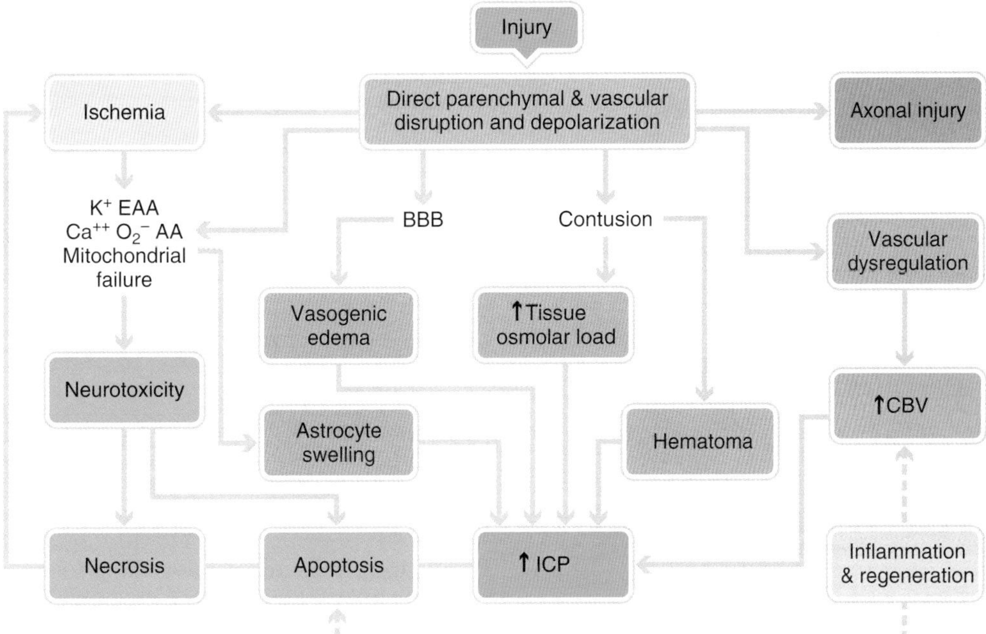


**Figure 33.2**

Categories of mechanisms proposed to be involved in the evolution of secondary damage after severe TBI from biochemical and molecular substrates of the secondary injury cascade. (From Kochanek PM, Clark RSB, Jenkins LW: Pathobiology of secondary brain injury. In Salaman M, ed: *Current techniques in neurosurgery*, ed 2, Philadelphia, 1993, Current Medicine.)

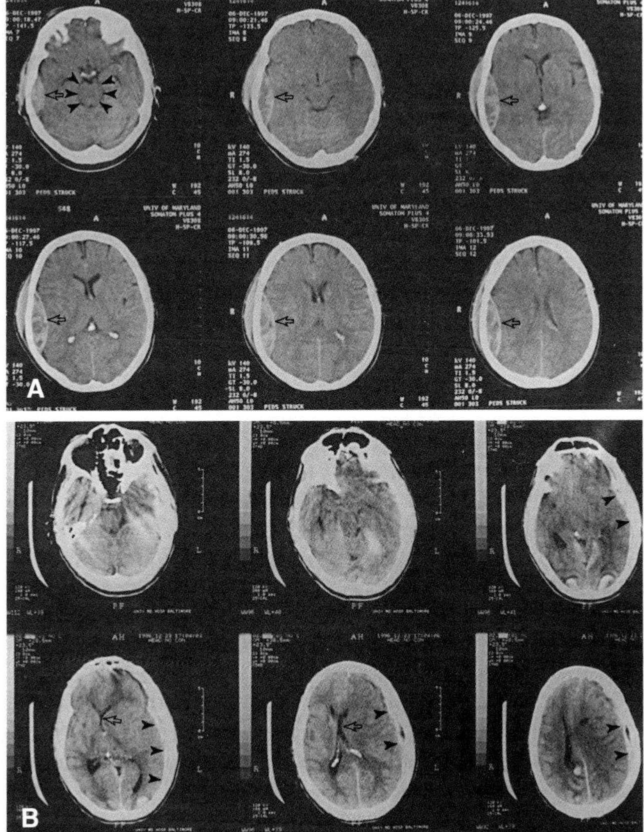

**Figure 33.3**

**CT scans of two patients with brain injury.(A) This patient has a right temporal epidural hematoma (*arrows*). The mesencephalic cisterns are patent in the top left, indicating a lack of brainstem compression despite mass (*arrowheads*). (B) This patient has suffered an acute left subdural hematoma (*arrowheads*) with midline shift (*arrows*).** (Reprinted from Townsend CM: *Sabiston textbook of surgery*, ed 17, Philadelphia, 2004, Saunders.)

homeostasis in the face of changing blood pressure or blood gas composition. Initially, within the first few hours after severe injury, there is decreased CBF both globally and at the impact site, which can induce ischemia. Within 24 hours, the blood flow can be at normal or above-normal levels.[41] The management of brain perfusion can conflict with therapeutic goals focusing on problems with infection, ventilation, renal function, or even systemic circulation. For this reason, integration of brain and systemic care is critical on all levels, from understanding the pathophysiologic principles to treatment through interdisciplinary communication.[21]

**Hypoxia.** Hypotension (systolic blood pressure less than 90 mm Hg) occurring between injury and resuscitation occurs in one-third of severe TBI victims. It can be caused by blockages resulting in decreased blood in the brain, by decreased oxygen in the blood due to concomitant pulmonary insult, or by internal bleeding or extremity injuries that cause excessive blood loss. It is associated with doubling of mortality rate and a significant increase in morbidity. Early hypotension is also a strong predictor of poor outcome.[70]

**Hypertension.** Intracranial hypertension or increased ICP is an important factor for critical care management. Following severe TBI, ICP is commonly monitored with a ventricular catheter or other device, some of which allow draining of CSF to reduce ICP. Under normal circumstances, cerebral pressure autoregulation maintains constant CBF to ensure tissue oxygenation. Following trauma, this relationship may be partially or totally disrupted. ICP is typically maintained below a target of 20 mm Hg for adults, because persistence of higher levels of ICP are associated with morbidity and death. 12,52 Specific strategies for management of severe TBI in children are also available.[52]

Impaired vascular responsiveness of blood gas changes after brain injury results in abnormal arteriolar vasoconstriction in the presence of carbon dioxide. Vascular volume

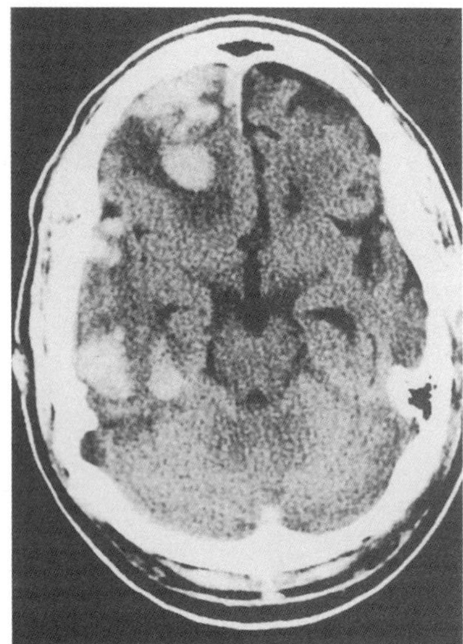

**Figure 33.4**

**Contusion with shearing injury.** CT scan shows multiple rounded areas of blood density, with surrounding edema. Many of these areas are at the junction of gray and white matter, consistent with shear injury. (Reprinted from Ramsey R: *Neuroradiology*, Philadelphia, 1994, WB Saunders, 409.)

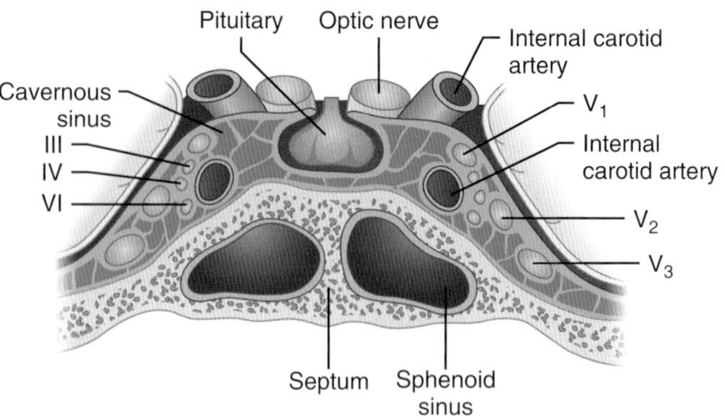


**Figure 33.5**

**Diagram showing the proximity of the intracavernous internal carotid artery and the sphenoid sinus.** (Reprinted from Cummings CW, Haughey BH, Thomas R, et al: *Cummings otolaryngology: head and neck surgery*, ed 4, St Louis, 2004, Mosby.)

in the skull can increase if venous outflow is blocked or increased CBF is recruited for metabolic reasons (e.g., seizures, pyrexia) or if loss of autoregulation occurs.

Posttraumatic aneurysms of the intracavernous internal carotid artery can be associated with delayed and sometimes lethal massive epistaxis. This can be a result of basal skull fractures in the region of the carotid canal or cavernous sinus and/or orbital fractures and compromise of the optical nerves. Knowledge of these risk factors and early diagnosis can minimize the high mortality risk. Fig. 33.5 demonstrates the proximity of these structures. It can take from days to years for artery weakening to develop, with an average time of 3 weeks. Because of the close anatomic relationship of the intracavernous portion of the internal cerebral artery to the oculomotor, optic, abducens, trochlear, and trigeminal nerves, these structures may also be damaged during the aneurysm development, resulting in effects such as blindness, facial numbness, and/or oculomotor palsy.[31]

There appears to be a change in the endothelium, or walls, of the blood vessels following brain injury. In the normal brain, neurotransmitters such as acetylcholine induce dilation of the vessels through the release of endothelium-derived releasing factor, causing relaxation of the smooth muscle in the vessel wall. In the injured brain this reaction can be missing, resulting in abnormal vasoconstriction.[26] Additional changes at the level of the endothelium result in a disturbed blood-brain barrier in the injured brain. This results in leakage of serum proteins and neurotransmitters into the parenchyma, causing edema. The effects of edema in the brain are described in Chapters 28 and 32.

## Parenchymal Changes

Axonal injury is a consistent feature of the traumatic event. Shear and tensile forces disrupt the axolemma. The distal axon segment can detach and trigger Wallerian degeneration. This triggers reactive axonal swelling, forming retraction balls that are full of axon material. In animal models these structures can be detected in the injured brain within 12 hours of injury. The myelin sheath pulls away from the axon. These axonal changes may be distributed throughout the brain regardless of site of impact. The damage is different from that of stroke or tumor, which produces a more complete but local deafferentation. Typically, with DAI, there remain intact axons interspersed with the damaged axons.

Primary injury triggers a metabolic cascade (see Fig. 33.2) that is a critical driver of secondary injury through excitotoxicity and free radical formation. Secondary cell death by necrosis of the cellular membrane results from edema. Apoptosis, or programmed cell death from within the cell through changes in the DNA, can result in cell loss that occurs days, weeks, or months after injury.[60] There is evidence of the potential for recovery of function based on the possible sprouting of undamaged axons to reoccupy the areas left vacant by degenerating axons.

Excitotoxicity is a common occurrence with diffuse brain injury and results in an increase in extracellular neurotransmitters and increased potassium, causing a massive depolarization of the injured brain. The excitatory neurotransmitter glutamate rises to abnormal amounts following brain injury. Glutamate is neurotoxic when concentrations increase. A complex interaction of the various amino acids and neurotransmitters may affect postsynaptic functions, resulting in secondary injury of the neural mechanisms of the brain. Inhibition function of the synaptic receptors can be altered and may relate to both functional and behavioral changes. See Chapter 28 for information on the damage to the nervous system associated with glutamate.

Free radicals are generated by TBI. Extensive membrane depolarization, induced by trauma, allows for a nonselective opening of the voltage-sensitive calcium channels and an abnormal accumulation of calcium within neurons and glia. Such calcium shifts are associated with activation of lipolytic and proteolytic enzymes, protein kinases, protein phosphatases, dissolution of microtubules, and altered gene expression.[28]

The possibility of parenchymal changes occurs even in milder injury with the presence of the metabolic cascade that may trigger an energy deficiency, and which may be related to extreme fatigue observed after a concussion. As the brain works to regain homeostasis, a period of rest is necessary to counter this energy deficiency.

### Compressive Damage

Intracranial hypertension and mass bleeding inside the skull can produce herniation, causing shifts from the normal brain symmetry. The most common herniation is transtentorial and downward, at the lateral tentorial membrane separating the cerebral hemispheres from the posterior fossa. This shift may cause compression of the brainstem, the pituitary, or other delicate brain structures. Because the brainstem controls the body's major visceral functions, brainstem involvement may result in paralysis or death. In less severe situations, increased pressure in the area may cause autonomic nervous system symptoms with changes in pulse and respiratory rates and regularity, temperature elevations, blood pressure changes, excessive sweating, salivation, tearing, and sebum secretion. Because the adult brain is surrounded by the rigid skull, swelling of the brain or pooling of blood pushes tissue through openings in the base of the skull, resulting in cerebellar tonsillar herniation through the foramen magnum. Figs.33.6 and 32-23 show the herniation possible with epidural bleeding. Table 33.1 lists the possible signs of intracranial hypertension and associated herniation syndromes. In the more flexible infant skull, open injuries that result in skull fracture, or surgical decompressive craniectomy may accommodate swelling to a greater degree. The use of surgical decompression after severe TBI is a second-tier approach to allow brain swelling to occur to avoid catastrophic outcomes with uncontrolled swelling and herniation.[52]

Although brain injury etiologies, risk factors, and aspects of pathogenesis are similar regardless of the severity of an injury, there are distinct differences in the clinical manifestations and management of moderate to severe TBI and milder injury or concussion. This necessitates addressing these two categories of brain injury separately. Additional considerations for managing children with TBI will also be summarized.

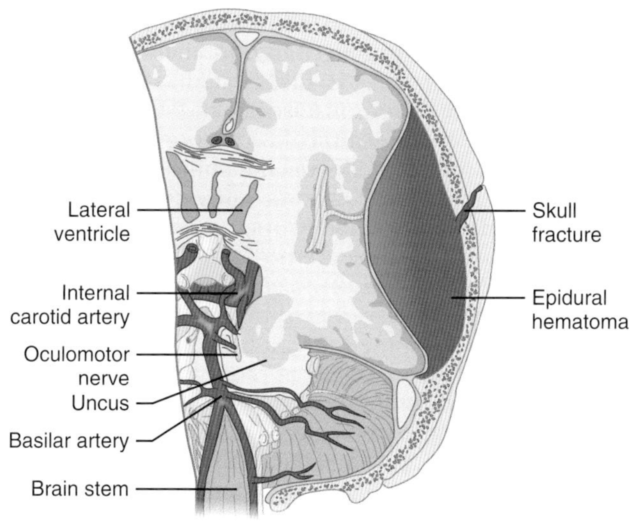


**Figure 33.6**

**Anterior view of transtentorial herniation caused by large epidural hematoma.** Skull fracture overlies hematoma. (Reprinted from Rockswold GL: Head injury. In Tintinalli JE et al, eds: *Emergency medicine*, New York, 2004, ed 6, McGraw-Hill, p 915.)

## Clinical Manifestations of Moderate to Severe TBI

Moderate TBI often involves structural injury such as hemorrhage or contusion. Epidural hematomas frequently result from skull fractures with subsequent laceration of the middle meningeal artery. Classically, epidural hematoma leads to an initial loss of consciousness, which is followed by recovery of consciousness and a lucid period. The individual then progressively deteriorates neurologically, with development of headache, a decline in mental status, and focal neurologic findings such as contralateral weakness or numbness, pupillary reflex abnormalities, or facial asymmetry. This injury results from rapid accumulation of pressure from arterial blood, often the middle meningeal artery, that if not recognized and treated can result in death. Severe TBI generally results in some form of cognitive and/or physical disability or in death, especially with very low Glasgow Coma Scale (GCS) scores.[28]

### Disorders of Consciousness

Altered level of consciousness is a state that can occur with diffuse or focal head injury, or when there is a

**Table 33.1** Signs of Intracranial Hypertension and Associated Herniation Syndromes

| Sign | Mechanism | Type of Herniation |
|---|---|---|
| Coma | Compression of midbrain tegmentum | Uncal, central |
| Pupillary dilation | Compression of ipsilateral third nerve | Uncal |
| Miosis | Compression of the midbrain | Central |
| Lateral gaze palsy | Stretching of the sixth nerves | Central |
| Hemiparesis[a] | Compression of contralateral cerebral peduncle against tentorium | Uncal |
| Decerebrate posturing | Compression of the midbrain | Central, uncal |
| Hypertension, bradycardia | Compression of the medulla | Central, uncal, cerebellar (tonsillar) |
| Abnormal breathing patterns | Compression of the pons or medulla | Central, uncal, cerebellar (tonsillar) |
| Posterior cerebral artery infarction | Vascular compression | Uncal |
| Anterior cerebral artery infarction | Vascular compression | Subfalcine (cingulate) |

[a]Hemiparesis will occur ipsilateral to the hemispheric lesion (false localizing sign).

Box 33.1
**GLASGOW COMA SCALE**

| ***Eye Opening*** | ***E*** |
|---|---|
| spontaneous | 4 |
| to speech | 3 |
| to pain | 2 |
| no response | 1 |
| ***Best Motor Response*** | ***M*** |
| To Verbal Command: | |
| obeys | 6 |
| To Painful Stimulus: | |
| localizes pain | 5 |
| flexion-withdrawal | 4 |
| flexion-abnormal | 3 |
| extension | 2 |
| no response | 1 |
| ***Best Verbal Response*** | ***V*** |
| oriented and converses | 5 |
| disoriented and converses | 4 |
| inappropriate words | 3 |
| incomprehensible sounds | 2 |
| no response | 1 |

***E+M+V = 3 to 15***

- Severe injury GCS ≤8, coma determined by whether eyes are open or not. Scores in severe injury range highly influenced by motor score, motor score "ceiling" at GCS sum of 13
- Moderate injury 9-12
- Mild injury 13-15
- Sum scores in 7-12 range are highly influenced by verbal and eye scores. Eye scores floor - 8, ceiling -14; verbal scores floor - 7, ceiling - 15.[71]

https://www.glasgowcomascale.org/downloads/GCS-Assessment-Aid-English.pdf?v=3
Adapted from Teasdale G, Jennett B: Assessment of coma and impaired consciousness: a practical scale, *Lancet* 304(7872):81-84, 1974.

combination of the two types of injury. This can be a result of diffuse bilateral cerebral hemispheric damage or a smaller lesion that affects the brainstem. In moderate or severe brain injury, unconsciousness can be prolonged or persistent. Arousal that is associated with wakefulness depends on an intact reticular formation and upper brainstem.

Coma is regarded as the lowest level of consciousness and is characterized by not obeying commands, not uttering words, not opening the eyes—a complete state of unresponsiveness. This indicates advanced brain failure, with bilateral cerebral hemispheric or direct involvement of the brainstem. Coma rarely lasts longer than 4 weeks. The GCS is the most widely used instrument for determining level of consciousness; it is used in the acute setting to determine current status and potential for improvement (Box 33.1). In rehabilitation contexts, individuals with disorders of consciousness are best examined using the Coma Recovery Scale–Revised (CSR-R), because it allows for more detailed assessment of responses to various sensory stimuli and basic functions that are observed when emerging from coma.[15]

*Wakeful unresponsiveness* (also sometimes described as vegetative state) is characterized by periods of appearing awake but with no evident cerebral cortical function. Eye opening with resumption of sleep-wake cycles and respiration, observed in this phase are controlled at a subcortical level. Eyes may open spontaneously, but do not track or fix gaze. There is no purposeful movement or communication, although startle reactions, sounds made especially with tight muscle stretch, and facial expressions unrelated to the environmental context may be observed. This behavioral state results from diffuse cerebral hypoxia or from severe, diffuse white matter impact damage, but the brainstem is usually relatively intact. *Wakeful unresponsiveness* may be characterized as persistent if present for more than a year after a traumatic injury or following months if the injury involved anoxia (near drowning, cardiac arrest, etc).

The *minimally conscious state* is a progression from wakeful unresponsiveness but has some similarities. Individuals in the minimally conscious state demonstrate eye-opening, sleep-wake cycles, and often will track objects visually. The hallmark of the minimally conscious state is an inconsistent but clearly observable ability to sometimes follow simple commands, communicate (yes or no, by talking or gesture), show appropriate emotion, or reach for or hold an object appropriately. Because the ability to do these tasks is inconsistent, differentiating between wakeful unresponsiveness and the minimally conscious state can be difficult. The use of the CRS-R for serial assessments improves the ability to track these inconsistent responses. Once an individual can consistently communicate, follow instructions, or use an object (e.g., brush or pen), they are no longer in a minimally conscious state. The use of imaging techniques to measure brain responses to verbal information is also gaining ground to identify some individuals who are minimally conscious but have limited motor abilities, but this approach is not in widespread clinical use.[1]

As a patient progresses in consciousness, they may demonstrate a confused state marked by disorientation, severe cognitive deficits (e.g., memory, attention), inconsistent arousal from drowsy to restlessness, sleep disturbances, and delusions or hallucinations. This confusion may be further characterized by exhibiting signs of appropriate or inappropriate behavior or communication. Fatigue or other triggers during the course of a day may cause someone to display aspects of appropriate and inappropriate behavior at different times or as they emerge from being more or less confused about their environment and surroundings.

A rare but alternative form of injury associated with injury to the ventral pons is "locked-in syndrome" that involves quadriplegia but preserved awareness and arousal.[28] Locked in syndrome typically spares vertical eye movements and the ability to blink, so these movements can be used to communicate.

Disordered breathing patterns associated with injury to brainstem respiratory centers are also common. Respiratory abnormalities associated with brain injury include *Cheyne-Stokes breathing*, a rhythmic pattern of alternating rapid breathing and momentary stopping of breathing, associated with hemispheric lesions that are bilateral or diencephalon; *hyperventilation*, with pontine or midbrain lesions; *apneustic breathing*, characterized by a prolonged pause at the end of inspiration, associated with lesions of the mid- and caudal portions of the pons; and *ataxic breathing*, irregular in both rate and tidal volume, seen with damage to the medulla.

### Cognitive and Behavioral Impairments

Residual cognitive and behavioral deficits often remain despite a return to full consciousness, including problems with slower information processing and deficits in attention, memory, and executive function. Disorders of learning, memory, information processing, abstract thinking, and complex problem solving reflect the prefrontal cortex pathology associated with TBI. It is important to take into account any focal lesions evident on imaging that may result in impairments resembling those observed in stroke based on the brain tissue affected by the focal insult. These focal deficits may occur in addition to more global deficits from the brain injury.

Loss of executive functions that regulate, control, and coordinate cognitive processes (planning, problem solving, inhibition, mental flexibility, task switching, initiation, and monitoring of actions) are observed when the dorsolateral prefrontal cortex is damaged.

When the damage is in the orbitofrontal area, behavior may be excessive and disinhibited. Inappropriate social and interpersonal behaviors, including inappropriate sexual behavior, occur with lesions in this area. Mood disturbances may include depression and anxiety. Septal area lesions result in irritability and rage. Pseudobulbar injuries can result in emotional lability, including euphoria, involuntary laughing, or crying that is not associated with negative emotions.

Cognitive deficits are not always directly observable, but observation of behavior provides information regarding the ability to integrate cognitive processes and adjust to the environment. Typical behaviors include erratic wandering; motor, sensory, and verbal perseveration; imitation of gestures; restlessness; refusal to cooperate; and striking out in response to a stimulus or in a random fashion. An individual may attempt to run away from the institution or home. Impulsivity, hyperactivity, and difficulty sustaining attention may occur. Behavioral changes can be present without cognitive or physical deficits.[79] Table 33.2 includes some of the behavioral disturbances and their manifestations in people with TBI.

Memory function is dispersed throughout the brain (see Chapter 28). After TBI memory is commonly impaired, which may be compounded by attention and executive function deficits. In order to remember things, one must pay attention and also use semantic organizational strategies to remember something by associating it with relevant cues. Complaints of memory problems are associated with poor performance on tests of speed, reaction time, attention tasks, and complex perceptual-motor abilities. Language deficits are often seen as word- and name-finding problems. However, recovery of language function appears to surpass that of memory in individuals with minor head injury.[25]

Impairment of memory common with head injury includes retrograde amnesia, the partial or total loss of ability to recall events that occurred during the period immediately preceding head injury. Posttraumatic amnesia is the time lapse between the injury and the point at which functional memory returns.[13] During this time, there may be improvement in automatic activities, but a lack of carryover of tasks requiring memory or learning. The duration of posttraumatic amnesia is an indicator of the severity of the injury.[64] Anterograde amnesia is the in ability to form new memory. Anterograde amnesia is common and manifests as decreased attention or inaccurate perception. The capacity for amnesia anterograde memory is frequently the last function to return following recovery from loss of consciousness.

TBI is associated with several neuropsychiatric disturbances that can range from subtle deficits to severe disturbances, including cognitive deficits; mood disorders, including depression, anxiety disorders, psychosis; and behavioral problems. More than 50% of individuals with TBI develop psychiatric sequelae.[68]

### Pain

Pain is a common complaint after brain injury, with complex interactions of physical and neuropsychological function. Subdural hematomas can result in headaches that are nonspecific and that can be mild to severe, paroxysmal or constant, and bilateral or unilateral.[28] The presence of pain or headache can affect the ability to sleep, which leads to daytime lethargy, and contributes to emotional reactions such as anxiety and depression.[72]

Neuropathic pain can result from the aberrant somatosensory processing in the peripheral or central nervous system, most commonly with damage in the area of the thalamus. Myofascial pain is common with trigger points, stiffness, and weakness. Fibromyalgia can develop, because it is related to sleep disturbances, anxiety, and depression. Another component of pain is suffering, in which the intensity is dependent on the person's mood, life experience, and level of social support. The result can often be that the cycle of pain and limitation of central processing can lead to a condition that mimics chronic pain syndrome. Chronic pain can have an impact on the neuropsychological function as part of a vicious cycle. Managing this syndrome in the individual with brain injury can be challenging and warrants good decisions regarding both the pharmacologic and neuropsychological approaches.[25]

### Cranial Nerve Damage

Focal damage in the brainstem can be reflected in the loss of cranial nerve function, as cranial nerves emerge throughout the brainstem and are also at risk of damage with trauma or herniation syndromes. Refer to Table 28.5 for specifics about the functions of each cranial nerve. Impairments particular to TBI will be reviewed.[36,73] Examination of the eyes may yield valuable information about the level of brainstem disease causing coma, given the proximity of centers governing eye movement, pupillary function, and elements of the reticular activating system. Completely normal pupillary function and eye movements suggest that the lesion causing coma is rostral to the midbrain.

The olfactory nerve (CN I) is well protected in the cribriform plate, but shearing of the fibers to the extent

Table 33.2 A Typology of Behavioral Disturbances After Traumatic Brain Injury

| Symptom | Description |
|---|---|
| **Behavioral Excesses** | |
| Inappropriate abrupt physical action | Responds to a situation too quickly without thinking about the adequacy or consequences of the behavior: doing before thinking. Does not include verbal interruptions |
| Tangential verbal output | Expresses one thought after another in disconnected or unrelated sequences: rambling speech, unable to get to the point |
| Excessive verbal output | Provides too much information; content may be overly detailed or redundant; may be unaware of conversational turn exchange signals or unable to terminate conversation. |
| Verbal interruptions | Inserts comments that disrupt the flow of conversation or the task at hand; may force other person to relinquish conversational turn before completing the thought. |
| Inappropriate topic selection | Poor discrimination of appropriate topics for the social context. Revealing statements about personal matters, relationships, feelings that are inappropriate for the social context or level of relationship: excessive self-disclosure. |
| Inappropriate word choice | Use of profanity or emotionally charged words that are inappropriate for the social context. Overly explicit descriptions and explanations. |
| Physical proximity violation | Positions body within a spatial proximity of another person that is inappropriate for the level of relationship or social context: violating personal space. |
| Sexual inappropriateness | Acts with intent to develop intimate or sexual contacts or relationships inappropriate for the level of relationship or in violation of social mores (e.g., with adolescent minors); conversation contains sexual innuendos or lewd comments. May misinterpret others' expression of friendship as sexual advances, and responds as above. |
| Poor social judgment | Unaware of or does not apply rules governing social behavior; does not consider personal safety or safety of others in social context: rude, immature, coarse, tactless. Violates rules of etiquette. |
| Irritability | Feelings of annoyance or impatience; may accompany restlessness; easily provoked but generally does not escalate into an anger outburst. Tends to be a constant state, usually neither improving nor worsening by a significant degree. |
| Lability of affect | Magnitude of affect displayed is disproportionate to the antecedent event or social context and does not necessarily reflect the true nature or extent of feelings. |
| Anxious affect and rumination | Feelings of worry, tenseness, fearfulness, uncertainty about the future. Complains or verbalizes concern over trivia. |
| Angry transition—verbal | An escalation of verbal output, where pitch, volume, or speaking rate increases, dysfluency occurs, aggressive content is delivered. Still within the realm of appropriate. A building-up phase before an outburst. |
| Angry transition—behavioral | Facial flush; posture threatening; personal space may be violated, body positions exaggerated; agitation behavior is evident such as hair pulling, wringing of hands, clutching the fist. |
| Anger outburst—verbal | Explosive speech, screaming, abusive language, forceful or harmful content, self-deprecating content, or threats toward another person. |
| Anger outburst—behavioral | Hitting objects, striking out, exaggerated motions, forceful actions. |
| **Behavioral Deficits** | |
| Absence of or decrease in self-directed action | Decrease in spontaneous behaviors, requires prompts for behavioral action. |
| Depressed mood | Downcast facial expression, tearfulness, verbalizations of sadness, hopelessness, helplessness, low self-esteem; paucity of interest in pleasant events. |
| Restricted affect | Display of affect less than proportional to the event; face expressionless; voice monotonous; movement fails to reflect stated feelings. |

Modified from Vomoto JM: Neuropsychological assessment and rehabilitation after brain injury. In Berrol S, editor: *Physical medicine and rehabilitation clinics of North America. Traumatic brain injury*, Philadelphia, 1992, WB Saunders, 307.

of damage occurs in about 7% of brain injuries, with a higher likelihood of injury in moderate to severe injury (19-25%). The olfactory nerve is the only cranial nerve that is commonly injured in concussion, and should be suspected with frontal vault fracture, frontal or occipital blows that may cause damage of olfactory bulbs across the cribriform plate, and CSF rhinorrhea. There are no established treatments for this disorder, but resolution may occur within 2 years of the injury.

The optic nerve (CN II) is not a true cranial nerve but rather a direct extension of the brain and may be damaged as a result of injury to the globe itself or circulatory impairment that results from injury. These injuries occur in approximately 5% of brain injuries and are typically permanent. The most vulnerable component of the optic nerve in people with head injury is the portion of the nerve located within the optic canal. Damage to this portion can result in monocular blindness, a dilated pupil with an absent, direct pupillary response, and a brisk, consensual response to light. Partial visual defects may take the form of scotomata, peripheral visual field sector defects, and upper or lower hemianopia. These may result from damage to optic tracts in the brain itself as opposed to the cranial nerve.

The oculomotor nerve (CN III) works in conjunction with the trochlear (CN IV) and abducens (CN VI) nerves to move the eyeball in the orbit to maintain gaze stability and scanning. Extraocular movement testing reveals difficulty with conjugate movement control. Oculomotor palsies occur in 17% of people with brain injury, resulting in a characteristic outward turning of the affected eye that results in double vision. In addition, there is ptosis associated with lack of eyelid control, lack of accommodation because of ciliary muscle involvement, and if a complete palsy, pupillary dilation.

It is important to understand the difference between peripheral damage to the oculomotor system and the abnormal movement that represents damage of a central nature that affects eye movements. Conjugate lateral deviation of the eyes is a sign either of an ipsilateral hemisphere lesion, a contralateral hemisphere seizure focus, or damage involving the contralateral pontine horizontal gaze center. Lateral gaze palsy may signal central herniation, with compression of bilateral sixth nerves. Tonic downward deviation of gaze is suggestive of injury or compression involving the thalamus or dorsal midbrain, such as may occur with acute obstructive hydrocephalus or midline thalamic hemorrhage. Tonic upward gaze has been associated with bilateral hemispheric damage. Ocular bobbing, a rapid downward jerk followed by a slow return to midposition, is indicative of pontine lesions. Rapid intermittent horizontal eye movements suggest seizure activity.[28]

Trochlear nerve injury (CN IV) occurs less than 2% of the time in brain injury. Damage is usually in the form of contusion or stretching. With severe frontal blows, there can be direct damage to the fourth nerve or hemorrhage of the tentorial incisura. There can be a vertical diplopia mimicking a third nerve palsy. This injury is detected with attempts to look downward with the eye adducted, which is not feasible with this injury. The prognosis for recovery in fourth nerve palsy is poor because the nerve is so slender and its course is long, so trauma results in avulsion.

The most common form of trigeminal nerve (CN V) injury after head trauma involves the supraorbital and supratrochlear nerves as they emerge from the orbit, occurring in 2% or fewer of individuals with TBI. Damage results in anesthesia of a portion of the nose, eyebrow, and forehead. Lack of corneal sensation and drying may occur. Facial trauma may extend the sensory deficits to the cheek, upper lip, gums, teeth, and hard palate. In deep coma, the eyelids can be opened easily, and the corneal reflex (indicating fifth nerve palsy) is often absent.

The abducens nerve (CN VI) is often injured when the head is crushed in an anteroposterior plane, with resultant lateral expansion and distortion of the skull and is estimated to occur in up to 4% of cases. It can also be damaged in fractures of the petrous bone. Vertical movement of the brainstem may severely stretch the sixth nerve as it leaves the pons. There can also be damage in relation to the CN III and IV in the orbital fissure. There is failure of the eye to abduct, so at rest the eye may be positioned inward, causing double vision. Abnormal wandering eye movements are present in midbrain lesions, and they usually disappear when the person regains consciousness.

Trauma to the facial nerve (CN VII) is common in head injury, second only to olfactory nerve damage. With fracture of the temporal bone, swelling of the nerve, or external compression caused by hematoma, symptoms of facial nerve palsy may occur. Loss of tear production, saliva secretion, and taste in the anterior two-thirds of the tongue and loss of stapedius muscle function may be noted. An ipsilateral CN VII injury results in ipsilateral weakness of all face muscles, including those that activate forehead muscles.

Hearing and vestibular dysfunction occur in brain injuries. Transverse fractures of the temporal bone commonly disrupt the auditory and vestibular end organs or result in transient eighth nerve dysfunction (vestibulocochlear nerve, CN VIII). Symptom complaints include vertigo, tinnitus, and hearing loss. A blow to the head creates a pressure wave that is transmitted through the petrous bone to the cochlea, resulting in hair cell damage and degeneration of cochlear nerves. For further information on dizziness and vertigo, see Chapter 38.

The glossopharyngeal (CN IX), vagus (CN X), spinal accessory (CN XI), and hypoglossal (CN XII) cranial nerves pass through the jugular foramen at the base of the skull. The twelfth nerve passes through the hypoglossal foramen nearby. If trauma affects one of these cranial nerves, it often affects others, given their close proximity. Injury is most often from a missile wound, but fractures of the occipital condyle can also produce lower cranial nerve palsies. Symptoms include cardiac irregularities, excessive salivation, loss of sensation and gag reflex of the palate, loss of taste on the posterior third of the tongue, hoarse voice, dysphagia, and deviation of the tongue to the side of the lesion.

### Motor Deficits

Abnormalities of movement are dependent on the area of the brain injured, with more focal lesions resulting in involvement of a single limb or hemiplegia with abnormal reflexes. The specific manifestations of hemiparesis may include loss of selective motor control, sensory loss, and abnormal balance reactions. Cerebellar damage may result in ataxia and may be on one side of the body or more global in presentation. Basal ganglia dysfunction can result in tremor or bradykinesia. See Chapter 32 for further information regarding focal damage to the brain associated with specific areas of infarct.

Often there is *flaccidity*, the absence of motor responses, at the onset of brain injury, which is gradually replaced by increased tone, spasticity, and rigidity. *Decorticate posturing*, or hyperactive flexor reflexes in the upper extremities and hyperactive extensor response in the lower extremities, is common initially and reflects the loss of cortical control with motor patterns similar to those seen in a cortical stroke. *Decerebrate posturing*, or hyperactive extensor reflexes in both the upper and lower extremities, reflects injury at the superior border of the pons, resulting in the loss of inhibitory control of the cortex and basal ganglia.[6,57] The progression from decorticate to decerebrate posturing in the acute phase of care is seen as a negative sign, as lower levels of the brain are affected.

Direct trauma to subcortical and substantia nigral neurons can result in movement disorders occurring shortly after an injury. Movement disorders occurring months following the injury have been hypothesized to be related to sprouting, remyelination, inflammatory changes, oxidative reactions, and central synaptic reorganization. Peripheral trauma that precedes the development of a movement disorder may alter sensory input, leading to central cortical and subcortical reorganization.

Postural and kinetic tremor can be due to direct traumatic lesions of the dentatothalamic circuit. Postural-kinetic tremors of the arms, legs, or head may occur within weeks of mild TBI, even without loss of consciousness. Peripheral trauma can induce tremor, which can occur along with complex regional pain syndrome, dystonia, and myoclonus. Myoclonus, dystonia, and athetosis may be present in individuals with posttraumatic tremors.

Contralateral dystonia can be due to a lesion in the striatum, particularly the putamen. The onset of dystonia may have a latency period from 1 month to 9 years. Spastic dystonia due to pyramidal and extrapyramidal injury and paroxysmal nocturnal dystonia are variants of posttraumatic dystonia. Individuals may develop posttraumatic dystonia as a delayed sequela of severe TBI, initially characterized by coma and quadriplegia. After the individual awakens and the movement improves, severe action dystonia develops.[28]

### Heterotopic Ossification

Another complication associated with head injury is the formation of *heterotopic ossification* (HO), or abnormal bone growth in the periarticular tissue. The cause and pathogenesis of HO is unknown, but is associated with trauma around a joint, immobility, and increased tone. Bone scans show evidence of increased uptake reflecting osteogenic activity with elevation of alkaline phosphatase.

The onset of HO is usually 4 to 12 weeks after the head injury, and it is first detected with a loss of range of motion. Local tenderness and a palpable mass eventually can be detected, and there can be erythema, swelling, and pain with movement. HO in the hip area can mimic deep vein thrombosis. Peripheral nerve compression will sometimes develop, especially if the HO is in the elbow. HO can also result in vascular compression and possible lymphedema.[82]

### Medical Complications

Multiple medical complications can also occur after TBI. Following severe injury, severe autonomic dysfunction may occur, sometimes described as "storming" but more accurately termed paroxysmal sympathetic hyperactivity (PSH), reported in 62% to as many as 92% of patients admitted to ICU.[4] A hypersympathetic response is observed, with increases in heart rate, blood pressure, respiratory rate, temperature, sweating, and motor posturing.[3] Triggers for episodes of PSH may include noxious stimuli (pain, suctioning, passive movement, constipation, etc.) that initiate cycles of sympathetic overactivity, but responses may also be exaggerated to stimuli that are typically not considered painful. The presence of PSH typically resolves several months after injury, but overactivity to external stimuli could persist in more subtle ways beyond the acute period.

Cardiovascular effects of TBI include neurogenic hypertension and cardiac dysrhythmias. Respiratory complications such as neurogenic pulmonary edema, aspiration pneumonia, and pulmonary emboli usually caused by deep venous thrombosis are common. Other complications include disseminated intravascular coagulation, hyponatremia, diabetes insipidus, and stress gastritis. Iatrogenic infections are common.

## MEDICAL MANAGEMENT

**Diagnosis.** When a person sustains a severe head injury, the GCS is used to assess level of consciousness and injury severity. Consideration of whether alcohol or drugs were in use by the injured person is important, because GCS scores may appear lower until the effects of substance use have resolved. Using this scale, three aspects of response are observed independently: eye opening, verbal response, and best motor response. Factors that could influence responses are checked first (under influence of alcohol or other substances, unable to speak because of intubation), followed by observation for spontaneous eye opening, speech, and movement. Stimulation in the form of noxious stimuli (e.g., nailbed pressure) or verbal commands is provided to determine the best response in each area. Eye opening is scored from 1 to 4, verbal response from 1 to 5, and motor response from 1 to 6. Scores in each area are summed to range from 3 to 15, with scores 8 or below indicating a severe brain injury. GCS scores are very commonly used in acute settings to reflect injury severity and as such relate to long-term outcomes. Once a patient survives the acute phase of care, GCS scores have limited value as an outcome measure, given the basic nature of the items tested.

Oculomotor and pupillary signs are valuable in assisting with the diagnosis, localizing brainstem damage, and determining the depth of coma. Pupillary examination should document size and reactivity to light. Greater than 1 mm difference in size or asymmetry should be considered abnormal. Once the baseline neurologic status has been determined, repeated evaluations are critical to monitor improvement, provide prognostic data, or detect deterioration (e.g., "blown pupil" sign of herniation), which should be addressed immediately. Symptoms of focal neurologic deficits, lethargy, or skull fractures should be monitored. A mental status examination is important for all individuals with brain injury. Subtle abnormalities may be indicators of significant intracranial injury.

Higher GCS scores are associated with greater than normal cardiac index responses and better tissue oxygenation. Poor outcomes are related to low GCS, hypertension, mild tachycardia, normal pulmonary function, and reduced tissue oxygenation.[66]

Diagnostic imaging can provide significant information, which can guide the intervention and allow a more accurate prognosis. CT is the primary imaging modality for the initial diagnosis and management of the person with brain injury. CT scanning of the head reveals the presence of hemorrhage, swelling, or infarction rapidly and less expensively to rule out the need for surgical intervention. In individuals with traumatic coma, patterns on CT that have been associated with worse neurologic outcome include lesions in the brainstem, encroachment of the basal cisterns, and diffuse axonal injury (DAI) (Fig. 33.7).[80]

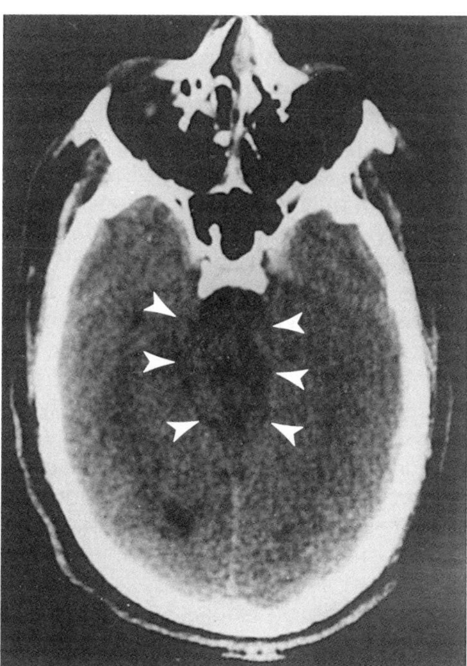

**Figure 33.7**

**CT scan of the head in a patient with a closed head injury.** Severe compression of mesencephalic cisterns is seen, indicating midbrain compression. (Reprinted from Townsend CM: *Sabiston textbook of surgery*, ed 17, Philadelphia, 2004, Saunders.)

DAI is a pathologic correlate of severe TBI associated with poor outcome.[32] DAI typically occurs throughout the brain as a result of translational, rotational, or angular acceleration forces. These forces stretch and damage blood vessels, cause axonal damage, and areas where brain structures have different densities, such as white-gray matter junctions, are susceptible to injury. The rostral brainstem is also at risk, given the extent of the brain positioned above it. With sufficient acceleration forces exerted on the brain, shear forces can cause axonal damage throughout the brainstem. Axotomy in the initial injury combined with oxidative stress can trigger secondary axotomy and additional damage. As a result, severe DAI may not be visible with imaging immediately after injury. Eventually these diffuse lesions may be observed on imaging via multiple punctate hemorrhages in the deep white matter or white-gray matter junctions, along the corpus callosum, and the brainstem. DAI may also occur as a result of mild TBI and may culminate in subtle types of cognitive deficits. DAI may be detectable on CT in more severe cases, but MRI offers a more sensitive means for detecting DAI.

In severe TBI, a CT is routine because it can be done quickly to identify possible intracranial bleeding. If arterial bleeding occurs, an epidural hematoma can progress very rapidly and cause herniation. In the presence of extracranial or intracranial vascular disruptions, angiography may be useful.[28]

Warning signs that may portend the need for urgent intervention include vomiting, restlessness, any GCS score decrease, severe headache, confusion, and injuries with a focal temporal blow.[23] Vomiting may also be associated with individuals with migraine familial characteristics, so this should also be considered.[24] It is important to realize that a CT scan that doesn't show damage does not confirm lack of injury, because the presence of abnormal tissue change evolves over time.

MRI is complementary to CT and is used in conjunction with, not as a replacement for, CT. The multiplanar capabilities of MRI are important to better demonstrate extra-axial hemorrhage located subfrontally, subtemporally, or along the tentorium. Lesions in the posterior fossa, as well as shear injury, are better demonstrated on MRI than on CT. MRI can also detect small hemorrhages in the corpus callosum, intraventricular hemorrhages, or effacement of basal cisternal structures in the absence of brain shift or mass lesions.[40] MRI is often used to identify the degree of tissue damage after a patient has stabilized. Positron emission tomography can be used to identify both structural and functional consequences and is valuable for identifying activation patterns after mild head injury, but it is primarily used in a research context. Prediction of outcome should not be based on imaging in isolation from other physical markers.[37]

Electrophysiologic tests that have been used for predicting coma outcomes include somatosensory evoked potentials, transcranial motor evoked potentials, brainstem auditory evoked potentials, and event-related potentials. Visual, auditory, and somatosensory evoked potentials test the integrity of sensory circuits relaying information to the brain and can be used to document changes in a lesion, and therefore may aid in prognosis, but they are not routinely used in isolation.

Approximately 5% to 10% of individuals with severe TBI have an associated spine and/or spinal cord injury. Initial head injury evaluation and management thus require simultaneous evaluation and management for potential spinal injuries. The majority of individuals with severe TBI have multisystem injury. Possibility of other significant and potentially life-threatening injuries should be evaluated and the proper treatment priorities accordingly established.

**Treatment.** Treatment of TBI requires coordinated care and service from the onset of injury through the person's lifetime. Prehospital management of the person with severe TBI includes rapid triage, resuscitation, and transport. Survival and medical management with the goal of stabilization and prevention of secondary complications are the primary medical focus. In the face of hypoxia, determining if the upper airway is obstructed, and clearing the airway, is the first treatment administered. Intubation and ventilation are critical procedures, with positive-pressure breathing techniques supplemented by 100% oxygen and early intervention.[40] Hypotension (systolic blood pressure less than 90 mm Hg) and hypoxia ($PaO_2$ less than 60 mm Hg or oxygen saturation of less than 90%) should be avoided if possible and corrected if present.

Emergency department treatment includes determination of head injury severity, identification of persons at risk of deterioration, and control of hypoxia and hypotension. Prevention of secondary brain damage caused by edema, increased intracranial pressure (ICP), or bleeding should be addressed. Treatment of the medical complications of the trauma is paramount but not discussed here; the focus of this chapter is on the control and treatment of neurologic sequelae. Close clinical observation remains the best tool for neurologic monitoring in the early stages of brain injury.

Surgical intervention is critical in the presence of hemorrhage to prevent neurologic compromise and can improve both short- and long-term outcomes. Uncal, transtentorial, or tonsillar herniation can occur with hematomas. In some cases, the individual may be lucid after the injury and, then, in the presence of undetected hematoma, lapse into coma and die.

Injury to the dural sinus can occur with a depressed fracture over a major sinus and requires evacuation. Decompression of the skull is warranted in the presence of significant cerebral edema or subdural hematoma. Decompressive craniectomy may be considered to counter the effects of intractable increased ICP, but it does not appear to improve outcomes.

The Brain Trauma Foundation provides clinical practice guidelines for acute management of severe TBI.[8,12,13,52] Normal ICP for adults ranges from 7 to 15 mm Hg. ICP monitoring is recommended for adults with severe TBI (GCS score 3-8) and an abnormal CT scan. Additional consideration for ICP monitoring includes individuals with two or more of the following: age greater than 40 years, presence of unilateral or bilateral limb posturing, and systolic BP less than 90 mm Hg.[52]

ICP monitoring in children is also suggested to improve overall outcomes.[52] Guidelines are to maintain ICP below 22 mm Hg for adults and below 20 mm Hg for children.[12,52] A ventricular catheter is used to measure ICP, and its presence also allows the draining of cerebrospinal fluid in order to reduce ICP. Health of brain tissue is dependent on receiving sufficient oxygen, which is contingent on sufficiently high cerebral perfusion pressure (CPP). CPP is calculated by subtracting ICP from mean arterial pressure, with target CPP values for adults of 60 to 70 mm Hg. Recommended CPP values for children are 40 to 50 mm Hg, with variation in acceptable values for infants and adolescents.

If ICP increases, the level of systemic arterial pressure may be increased with medications to maintain healthy levels of CPP. Monitoring of ICP can be accomplished in a number of ways. The ventriculostomy catheter allows monitoring and drainage of cerebrospinal fluid, but it is the most invasive method and is associated with risk of infection. The epidural catheter, hollow subarachnoid bolt, and subarachnoid fiberoptic catheter are other options. All must be surgically placed. The noninvasive Doppler waveform can also provide information regarding ICP. If an ICP monitor is in place, the drainage of cerebrospinal fluid may have significant therapeutic benefits.

Cerebral fluid volume can be reduced pharmacologically. Mannitol is used to reduce blood viscosity and thereby improve circulation to brain tissue. Hyperventilation has been used as a mechanism for controlling cerebral blood volume by increases in $PaCO_2$, resulting in vasoconstriction of the central vessels and reduced CBF. This must be considered a short-term procedure to be used judiciously because the cerebral vasoconstriction induced may produce ischemia; therefore, it is not recommended in the first 24 to 48 hours after injury and then only used on a short-term basis to reduce ICP.

Blood pressure control is important in brain-injured clients, and systolic blood pressure should be kept at a minimum of 90 mm Hg. If fluid management cannot keep the blood pressure at an adequate level, then vasopressor drugs are used. Phenylephrine is effective at maintaining stability. In clinical studies, the use of mild hypothermia does not improve outcomes, so is not recommended for use in adults. In children, hypothermia may be considered for management of increased ICP. Interventions that reduce morbidity or mortality in the acute period do not always result in improved longer-term outcomes.

Glucocorticoids have been used to treat cerebral edema in other conditions, but after severe TBI their use is not recommended because of increased mortality associated with their use. The management of severe TBI remains subject to practice standards established in facilities based on physician expertise, however, so variations from published guidelines may occur in cases in which response to recommended interventions is limited.

Management of secondary injury is as critical in TBI as it is in other brain disorders. A promising agent that may offer reduction of secondary injury is progesterone, a hormone that is present in the brain of men and women in similar concentrations. In animal studies, progesterone has reduced brain edema and damaging excitotoxicity, while enhancing antioxidant activity. Initial human trials of progesterone in the acute environment demonstrated reduced mortality and disability without adverse effects; however, two larger randomized controlled trials did not result in significant differences in the mortality or the Glasgow Outcome Scale–Extended, the primary outcome measure.[58,76,85] The reasons for these failed trials may relate to differences in dose and administration of progesterone, but the lack of ability to clearly characterize the complexity of TBI and relatively gross outcome measurements may also have played a role.[46,74,78] Study of various neurotrophic and antioxidant agents show benefits in animals, but the transfer of these benefits to humans has been limited. A clinical trial of mesenchymal stem cell (SB623) implantation post-TBI to address motor deficits specifically is underway, involving sites around the world.

An active area of TBI research is the area of molecular genetics. It has been noted that certain genes are upregulated, whereas others are downregulated, after both trauma and ischemia. Particular attention has been focused on the apolipoprotein E gene (ApoE) and its various alleles. This gene is associated with susceptibility for late-onset and familial Alzheimer disease and also has been linked to greater risk of CTE in boxers. Certain alleles have been associated with an increased susceptibility and severity of brain injury, and others have been linked to improved recoveries after TBI. Availability of genetic information may inform prognosis in the future.

In addition to attempting to maintain homeostasis in the brain, management of the other sequelae of brain injury is important. Spasticity is controlled by the administration of baclofen, dantrolene, or tizanidine. These medications must be used carefully because of their side effects, which include increased weakness, lethargy, and drowsiness. Abnormal muscle tone can also be controlled by nerve and motor point blocks or by the administration of botulinum toxin directly into the muscle belly.[40]

**Table 33.3** Rancho Los Amigos Scale for Levels of Cognitive Functioning

| Level | Behaviors Typically Demonstrated |
|---|---|
| I. | No response: Client appears to be in a deep sleep and is completely unresponsive to any stimuli. |
| II. | Generalized response: Client reacts inconsistently and nonpurposefully to stimuli in a nonspecific manner. Responses are limited and are often the same regardless of stimulus presented. Responses may be physiologic changes, gross body movements, or vocalization. |
| III. | Localized response: Client reacts specifically but inconsistently to stimuli. Responses are directly related to the type of stimulus presented. May follow simple commands in an inconsistent, delayed manner, such as closing eyes or squeezing hand. |
| IV. | Confused—agitated: Client is in heightened state of activity. Behavior is bizarre and nonpurposeful relative to immediate environment. Does not discriminate among persons or objects; is unable to cooperate directly with treatment efforts. Verbalizations frequently are incoherent or inappropriate to the environment; confabulation may be present. Gross attention to environment is very brief; selective attention is often nonexistent. Client lacks short-term and long-term recall. |
| V. | Confused—inappropriate: Client is able to respond to simple commands fairly consistently. However, with increased complexity of commands or lack of any external structure, responses are nonpurposeful, random, or fragmented. Demonstrates gross attention to the environment, but is highly distractible and lacks ability to focus attention on a specific task. With structure, may be able to converse on a social-automatic level for short periods of time. Verbalization is often inappropriate and confabulatory. Memory is severely impaired, often shows inappropriate use of objects; may perform previously learned tasks with structure but is unable to learn new information. |
| VI. | Confused—appropriate: Client shows goal-directed behavior but is dependent on external input for direction. Follows simple directions consistently and shows carryover for relearned tasks with little or no carryover for new tasks. Responses may be incorrect because of memory problems but appropriate to the situation; past memories show more depth and detail than recent memory. |
| VII. | Automatic—appropriate: Client appears appropriate and oriented within hospital and home settings; goes through daily routine automatically, but frequently robot-like with minimal-to-absent confusion; has shallow recall of activities. Shows carryover for new learning, but at a decreased rate. With structure is able to initiate social or recreational activities; judgment remains impaired. |
| VIII. | Purposeful—appropriate: Client is able to recall and integrate past and recent events and is aware of and responsive to environment. Shows carryover for new learning and needs no supervision once activities are learned. May continue to show a decreased ability relative to premorbid abilities, abstract reasoning, tolerance for stress, and judgment in emergencies or unusual circumstances. |

Modified from Hagen C, Malkmus D, Durham P: Levels of cognitive functioning. In *Rehabilitation of the head injured adult: comprehensive physical management*, Downey, CA, 1979, Professional Staff Association of Rancho Los Amigos Hospital, pp 87-88.

Intrathecal baclofen can be used to decrease tone with a baclofen pump, and the overall side effects are decreased, but this intervention is only initiated when other strategies have failed.

Control of seizures is provided by the use of medication such as valproate or carbamazepine. If the thalamus is affected, there can be abnormal sensations or intractable pain. The use of antiseizure medications is effective but carries high side effects and is often not tolerated by the individual, whose system is already compromised. Attempts to control aggressive behavior through use of carbamazepine and propranolol have had limited success. The nontricyclic antidepressants seem to be the most effective when the person is depressed.[33] Rehabilitation of the person with brain injury targets a return to optimal function once medical status is stable. Highly skilled, specially trained interdisciplinary teams provide an organized approach to the complex deficits encountered after head injury. Rehabilitation management of the individual is dependent on the cognitive and behavioral level of function of the individual. A useful tool to assess behaviors as a function of cognitive recovery is the Rancho Los Amigos Levels of Cognitive Function Scale (Table 33.3). This scale was developed in the late 1970s, so some of the terminology currently in use in clinical practice is not included. The Braintree Neurologic Stages of Recovery from Diffuse TBI (Box 33.2) scale provides more contemporary terminology and corresponding Rancho stages. Cognitive and motor abilities may progress at different rates, such that some patients may be close to preinjury level in one area and remain very impaired in another, with diverse presentations. Cognitive impairment is the primary contributor to disability with moderate to severe brain injury, where test results are used to determine areas where rehabilitation or compensatory strategies may be necessary.[44]

Restoration of mobility, self-care, employment, and recreational activities are important, goals, each depending on the level of sensorimotor impairment, as well as cognitive status. See "Special Implications for the Therapist 33.1: Traumatic Brain Injury," below.

Community-based programs for the person with brain injury that enhance the transition from rehabilitation unit to independent living have become less available, given that funding for such programs is limited. However, therapists still play a significant role addressing the need for intervention as the individual transitions to community living. To return to a lifestyle that may include work or school, the person with TBI needs to learn how to cope with the multiple demands on his or her attention that are part of that lifestyle. The person with TBI will have difficulty with executive functions, such as organizing time and information, self-monitoring, and self-correcting. Self-motivation is often lacking, and structure is necessary

Box 33.2

**RECOVERY FROM DIFFUSE TBI AND CORRESPONDING RANCHO LOS AMIGOS SCALE LEVELS**

1. *Coma*: unresponsive, eyes closed, no sign of wakefulness (Rancho Level I) (emergency medical services; acute inpatient hospital)
2. *Vegetative state (VS)/wakeful unresponsiveness:* no cognitive awareness; transition marked by beginning spontaneous eye opening and sleep-wake cycles (Rancho Level II) (acute hospital, long term care facility)
3. *Minimally conscious state (MCS):* Inconsistent, simply purposeful behavior, inconsistent response to commands begin; transition can be documented using Coma Recovery Scale–Revised (CRS-R) subscale criteria for minimally conscious state (47); often mute (Rancho Level III) (acute hospital; acute inpatient rehabilitation; subacute rehabilitation, long term care facility)
4. *Post-Confusional state*: Interactive communication and appropriate object use begin; transition can be documented using CRS-R subscale criteria for emergence from minimally conscious state (47); but may continue to be amnesic (PTA), severe basic attentional deficits, hypokinetic or agitated, labile behavior; later more appropriate goal-directed behavior, with continuing anterograde amnesia (Rancho Levels IV, V, and partly VI) (acute inpatient rehabilitation; acute hospital)
5. *Emerging independence*: marked by resolution of PTA; transition can be marked with improvement of cognition, the ability to develop more independence is possible; may continue with cognitive impairments in higher level attention, memory retrieval, and executive functioning; deficits in self-awareness, social awareness, behavioral and emotional regulation; achieving functional independence in daily self-care; improving social interaction; developing independence at home (Rancho Level VI and VII) (acute inpatient rehabilitation, subacute inpatient rehabilitation, outpatient rehabilitation, residential treatment, outpatient day hospital, community based programs)
6. *Social competence/community reentry*: with further cognitive improvement, resumption of basic household independence and ability to be left home unsupervised for the better part of a day; developing independence (may include school or work); recovering higher level cognitive abilities (divided attention, cognitive speed, executive functioning), self-awareness, and social skills; developing effective adaptation and compensation for residual problems (Rancho Levels VII and VIII) (outpatient community reentry programs, community-based services—vocational, special education, supported living services, mental health services)

Based on data from Model Systems Knowledge Transition Center, TBI Factsheets, https://msktc.org/tbi/factsheets/understanding-tbi/the-recovery-process-for-traumatic-brain-injury, 2020 and Katz DI, Zasler NC, Zafonte RD: Clinical continuum of care and natural history. In Zasler ND, Katz DI, Zafonte RD (eds): *Brain injury medicine: principles and practice*, ed 2, New York, 2013, Demos Medical.

to ensure follow-through on assigned activities. Use of checklists, devices that provide reminders, and environmental cues are helpful when attempting to reintegrate the client into the community.

Individuals with high-level physical skills and moderate- or low-level cognition skills are often the most difficult to reintegrate into the family and society. Family and coworker expectations are high because physical function appears at the preinjury level, but cognitive and behavioral deficits can severely limit safety and the ability to participate in life roles. In general, it is cognitive function that makes one more successful in society. Aggressive counseling should start as soon as the behavioral and cognitive impairments are identified. Neuropsychologists and counselors can suggest interventions that help with cognitive functions, especially techniques to deal with memory loss, decreased attention span, and inappropriate behavior.

Significant deficits in motor skills but higher levels of cognitive skills generally lead to a higher quality of life. There are numerous upper and lower extremity adaptive devices to help perform activities of daily living. Power wheelchairs controlled by the head, mouth, or hand and lifts for vans, as well as hand controls for driving, can assist with mobility. Computerized communications systems can improve interactions when speech is disrupted and cognition is intact.

The lack of motivation associated with TBI becomes a challenge for the therapist. Lack of internal initiation and decreased ability to learn may persist despite cues from the external environment. Setting goals that are meaningful to the client, even though they may seem to be unrealistic, is the first step in motivating the individual.

Alterations in attention span can be detrimental to progress in therapy. Reducing distracting stimuli can be helpful initially; distractions can be reintroduced as the ability to manage multiple inputs improves. In most cases, the family of the survivor needs help understanding their family member's social and behavioral changes.[77]

**Prognosis.** TBI accounts for a disproportionate share of morbidity and mortality across the life span. Of these, 3% (approximately 52,000) die, 16% (275,000) are hospitalized; and 81% (1.365 million) are seen in the emergency room and then released. The incidence of severe long-term disability is small.[28]

Factors that affect outcome can be categorized in three major areas: injury severity, preinjury factors, and postinjury factors.[9,67] Injury severity is the area that has been most studied. The depth of impaired responsiveness and the duration of altered consciousness is related to outcome.[50] In addition, the duration of posttraumatic amnesia has been used as a predictor of severity of the brain injury. Other aspects of neurologic functioning that indicate injury severity are also correlated with outcome.

Loss of pupillary light reflexes reflects significant damage to the brainstem and portends a poor prognosis. Oculomotor deficits often signal concomitant cerebral damage, resulting in severe cognitive deficits. The degree of hypoxemia and hypotension encountered in the early stages can also have an effect on the long-term prognosis.[75]

CT has increased the ability to predict outcome when there are lesions of the brain parenchyma, intercranial hematoma, subdural hematoma, or massive hemispheric swelling. Acute hemispheric swelling with an extracerebral hematoma is associated with the worst prognosis. Unilateral brain contusion and DAI also carry a poor prognosis. A midline shift of brain structures, absent or compressed basal cisterns (indicating rising ICP), and subarachnoid hemorrhage will increase the risk of death or remaining in a vegetative state.[80]

Box 33.3

**SYMPTOMS SELF-REPORTED POST-CONCUSSION BY CATEGORY**

| Somatic/Sensory | Affective | Cognitive |
|---|---|---|
| Feeling dizzy | Headaches | Poor concentration |
| Loss of balance | Fatigue, loss of energy | Forgetfulness, can't remember things |
| Poor coordination/ clumsy | Difficulty falling or staying asleep | Difficulty making decisions |
| Nausea | Feeling anxious or tense | Slowed thinking |
| Vision problems, blurring, trouble seeing | Feeling depressed or sad | |
| Sensitivity to light | Irritability, easily annoyed | |
| Hearing difficulty | Poor frustration tolerance | |
| Sensitivity to noise | | |
| Numbness | | |
| Changes in taste/ smell | | |
| Loss of appetite or increased appetite | | |

Factor analytic studies of postconcussion self-report measures have demonstrated 2-4 factors represented in patient responses. The factors listed here are based on the Neurobehavioral Symptom Inventory in a military population, derived from a study done by Caplan et al.[11] These self-report measures are not unidimensional and therefore a total score is not as meaningful as considering items in each factor area based on a study with the same population and the same self-report measure.

From factor analysis by Caplan LJ, Ivins B, Poole JH, et al: The structure of postconcussive symptoms in 3 US military samples, *J Head Trauma Rehabil* 25(6):447-458, 2010. https://doi.org/10.1097/HTR.0b013e3181d5bdbd.

With severe injury, the possibility of cognitive and behavioral deficits increases. Cognitive deficits that affect motivation, attention, emotion, memory, or learning will limit recovery. A lack of awareness of deficits and lack of social skills reduces the ability to reintegrate into the community.[81]

Epilepsy occurring within 7 days is often related to severe injury, depressed fracture, penetrating injury, or intracranial hemorrhage. Posttraumatic epilepsy may emerge months or years following brain trauma and is more common after severe brain injury. Late epilepsy occurs most often as grand mal seizures or temporal lobe seizures.[38] Further information on seizures is available in Chapter 36.

Many studies of outcome relate injury severity to mortality as an important indicator. Once a person survives an injury, factors that affect outcome are complex but include preinjury characteristics and postinjury factors. Neuropsychologic dysfunction appears greater in people who sustain injury over the age of 30 years and those with less education. History of substance abuse, low educational level, prior brain injury, and psychiatric disorders can also limit success. Social and family problems are common and can cause isolation and poor quality of life.[56]

Postinjury factors such as access to appropriate care and adequate supports are critical to optimize recovery. A multidisciplinary rehabilitation team is effective in facilitating TBI recovery. However, it is important that the individual is able to be active in the rehabilitation process to take full advantage of the benefits. If an individual has a disorder of consciousness, more intense rehabilitation may be more effective once consciousness resumes. Family and social supports are key factors in recovery. Families require education and support in order to understand how to best help their family member. Often it becomes difficult to sustain relationships that were stable before the injury. Working with professionals who recognize these deficits and are trained to treat them will improve the chances of increasing quality of life after brain injury. Because change in functional abilities is common with moderate and severe injury, supports that will allow for community-based treatment and living are important, but are not always available.

Measures that address global functioning/outcome are the Glasgow Outcome Scale–Extended and the Disability Rating Scale (http://tbims.org/combi/drs/index.html). These scales measure function from coma to community reintegration, so they capture gross abilities. As a result, they are not very sensitive to small changes in function or for those with milder injuries. The Mayo-Portland Adaptability Inventory may be more useful for considering common obstacles to community reintegration, including physical, cognitive, emotional, behavioral, and social factors (http://tbims.org/combi/mpai/index.html). For specific recommendations of outcome measures for use in physical therapy practice across a range of clinical practice settings, refer to the TBIEDGE recommendations developed by a task force from the APTA Neurology Section. These recommendations are available on the neuropt.org site and are also shared on the https://www.sralab.org/rehabilitation-measuressite.[83]

## Clinical Manifestations of Mild TBI or Concussion

### Signs and Symptoms

Acute clinical symptoms of concussion largely reflect a functional disturbance rather than a structural injury, with rapid onset of short-lived impairment of neurologic function that resolves spontaneously. Symptoms usually associated with concussion are headache, dizziness, nausea, and changes in attention. These symptoms are commonly queried with a postconcussion checklist, including items that are summarized in Box 33.3, although some checklist items are uncommonly reported. However, even with a mild injury, there is some level of trauma. Head and neck pain is common with whiplash. Pain can cause a persistent distraction that pulls the individual's attention away from activity and can decrease the ability to concentrate. The client may be irritable or distractible and have difficulty with reading and memory. Sleep may be significantly disrupted (insomnia or somnolence). These symptoms typically resolve in the month following injury, but may persist in more complicated injuries. A single concussion does not typically result in long-term neuropsychologic or cognitive complications.

Prediction of which individuals will experience persistent postconcussive symptoms is difficult. Factors that may increase recovery time include prior psychiatric or migraine history and symptom burden acutely and subacutely. Learning disability and ADHD may influence the baseline abilities of an individual with concussion, but not necessarily prolong recovery.[48] Nonspecific psychological symptoms such as anxiety and depression are reported by more than one-half of individuals within 3 months of mild TBI. Fatigue and disruption of sleep patterns are often reported. Ongoing clinical symptoms associated with persistent neurocognitive impairments can be demonstrated on objective testing. Animal and human studies support the concept of postconcussive vulnerability, meaning that a second blow sustained prior to brain recovery results in worsening metabolic changes. Experimental evidence suggests the concussed brain is less responsive to usual neural activation, and when excessive cognitive or physical activity occurs in the acute period after injury, the brain may be vulnerable to prolonged dysfunction.[55]

*Second impact syndrome* has been described as a rare but catastrophic reaction to a second concussion that occurs before recovery from a previous concussion. The existence of this condition is controversial—having been documented in case reports—and its actual incidence is unclear. The theory is that the second injury causes rapid and severe lack of cerebral autoregulation, loss of consciousness, and rapid progression to severe disability or death if not identified and treated emergently. Second impact syndrome has been suspected primarily in the sport-related deaths of adolescents, underscoring the importance of identifying every concussion in middle or high school sports to reduce risk of this catastrophic condition that could occur with a second exposure.[61]

Current research suggests that damage from multiple concussive blows over a lifetime may be associated with chronic traumatic encephalopathy (CTE), even though the incidence and cause(s) of CTE is unclear. An association between blows to the head and neurodegenerative changes was first described as "punch-drunk" in 1928, based on impairments observed in boxers, and was characterized by degenerative motor symptoms (parkinsonism, dysarthria, ataxia, and incoordination). In recent years the possibility of repetitive injuries in football resulting in CTE has captured the interest of the press, even though association does not equate to cause.[7,30,49] CTE has been documented in well-publicized cases of college and professional athletes who have a history of repetitive exposure to concussive and subconcussive forces during sport, mostly who were retired, but one athlete as young as 18 years. The diagnostic characteristics of CTE have been identified on autopsy as phosphorylated tau in sulci and perivascular areas, microgliosis, and astrocytosis, but this pathology is not universally agreed upon and has not been clearly linked to clinical presentations.

Individuals diagnosed with CTE post mortem have often been football players who demonstrated neuropsychiatric behaviors, including behavioral (depression, aggression, apathy, delusions, suicidality) and/or cognitive deterioration (deficits in attention, concentration, memory, executive function, and language) leading to presentations that are similar to various types of dementia.[10,35,59] Individuals who demonstrate these behaviors and their families have sought pathologic analysis, sometimes following the individual's suicide. However, these individuals represent a biased sample, as there may be others who have similar brain tissue findings who don't request autopsy evaluation because they did not have the behavioral presentation associated with CTE. In fact, there are studies that demonstrate a lack of CTE in populations that one might presume to be at high risk, yet these studies are not typically covered in the press.

Unfortunately, repeated concussion has been implicated by the media as the cause of CTE, when the full clinical history of these individuals has not been examined in detail. Factors such as a single more severe brain injury, chronic steroid use, substance abuse, psychiatric response to chronic pain, chronic health conditions, and genetic predisposition to dementia could also contribute to signs and symptoms associated with CTE. Careful study of athletes who exhibit cognitive and behavioral changes is necessary to clarify the role of repeated concussion to long-term cognitive deficits. Parents and athletes should manage recovery from concussion carefully after an injury, and follow medical advice in deciding to continue in a sport with high concussion risk after one or more injuries has occurred.[35]

Brain injury during military conflict is increasingly a result of blast exposure associated with improvised explosive devices or repeated exposure to explosive weaponry.. The injuries that result from proximity to an explosion include damage to fluid- and air-filled cavities from the pressure wave, injury from projectiles or being thrown by the force of the blast, and the potential for toxic exposure to fumes that could affect tissue oxygenation. Polytrauma may occur that affects systemic blood supply and adds to potential ischemia in the brain. If the injury is severe, the need for state-of-the-art field medicine and immediate transport for ongoing care is clear. Mild injury is more difficult to detect. A service member may underreport symptoms in the face of more seriously injured colleagues. Injury in a combat situation is very different from that on the playing field, as the risk to life is clear. Acute stress reactions and long-term posttraumatic stress co-occurs with TBI and share common symptoms. Careful assessment by an interdisciplinary professional team accustomed to working with service members may be necessary to determine what symptoms result from TBI versus other behavioral health conditions, so that appropriate treatment can be chosen.

Headache is the most common complaint following mild TBI. Migraine headaches with and without aura can develop in the hours to weeks after a concussion. Immediately after mild TBI in sports such as soccer, football, rugby, and boxing, children, adolescents, and young adults may have a first-time migraine with aura. Cluster headaches can develop after mild TBI. Refer to Chapter 37 for information about characterizing and treating headache from a PT perspective.

## MEDICAL MANAGEMENT

**DIAGNOSIS AND INTERVENTION** Concussion remains a clinical diagnosis ideally made by a health care provider familiar with the individual and knowledgeable in the recognition and evaluation of concussion. Every concussive event should be reported and maintained as part of an individual's medical record. Recognition and initial assessment of a concussion should be guided by neurologic physical examination to rule out more serious concerns, and then followed by an age-appropriate symptom checklist to determine the effects of the injury. The SCAT-5 is a common sideline assessment or the MACE-2 in a military context that may prove useful if contact is made acutely post injury to confirm concussion has occurred.[60]

Individuals who have sustained a concussion should be advised to rest for 24 to 48 hours to avoid potential additional injury and to allow the brain to recover. Education should encourage an expectation of recovery and guidance regarding reasons to contact primary care (e.g., red or yellow "flags"). Following the initial period of rest, gradual resumption of activity is advisable as tolerated. Guidance for staged return to activities in sport or military service is available.[5,62] Recovery from injury commonly occurs without specific intervention, but specific guidance may be required for return to learning, play, work, military duty, or to resume risky activities. Younger children and older adults may require particular guidance to assure that activity levels are appropriate and activity progression is progressing as expected. Referral to rehabilitation disciplines to manage persistent problems with dizziness, cervical dysfunction, vision, headache, posttraumatic stress, cognitive impairment, or other troublesome symptoms may prolong intervention and recovery.

Graded symptom checklists are commonly used with athletes and military service members to provide a self-report of a variety of symptoms related to concussion, while also tracking the severity of those symptoms over serial evaluations. Such generic self-report measures that span many impairments may prove less useful in a rehabilitation context than self-report measures focused on residual impairments (e.g., vestibular, cervical or headache symptoms) that may be more sensitive to specific complaints. Performance-based measures that provide objective evidence of system impairments (e.g., balance and vestibular measures) are also useful to counter over- or underreporting that can occur with self-reports. There should be no same-day return to play for an athlete or to demanding activity for other individuals with possible concussion because they should be monitored for changes in physical or mental status, and avoidance of another injury is important.

## A THERAPIST'S THOUGHTS*

### *Concussion in Youth and Adolescents*

Concussion is often referred to as an invisible injury with obscure subjective symptoms, such as dizziness, unsteadiness, head pressure, and mental fog. A thorough PT examination must include a comprehensive patient and family interview related to the daily activities specific to the individual child or adolescent, incorporating age-appropriate questions to describe symptoms disrupting participation. Those who experience protracted recovery may have underlying genetic, neuroinflammatory, immunologic, sensorimotor processing or developmental factors that are not clinically obvious but can influence the response to interventions.

Using child-appropriate language to determine whether head pressure (feeling like wearing a hat or headband that is too tight) or dizziness is present can be enlightening to a parent who may not know their child has symptoms of postconcussion syndrome. Frequently, the most prominent symptom a parent will report involves behavior issues such as tantrums, outbursts, excessive tears, or anxiety because the younger child or adolescent will not have vocabulary or knowledge to connect symptoms to daily struggles. Vestibular dysfunction typically involves an underlying sense of motion at rest (motion sickness) with eyes closed, where sensory conflict cannot be resolved by utilizing visual fixation. A child can be asked if they feel frozen, as if playing freeze tag, or if their body is moving while seated in a firm chair. Injuries that occur during critical periods of growth and development evolve and change, and prolonged recovery can be heavily influenced by fatigue.

*Nicole Miranda, PT, DPT

Many blood serum biomarkers are under study for use in helping diagnose concussion or to determine the need to order imaging for a suspected bleed.[34] The level of diagnostic accuracy of single biomarkers is not sufficient to warrant their routine use in clinical practice, but panels of biomarkers are showing promise as adjuncts to support a concussion diagnosis. Imaging with CT or magnetic resonance imaging (MRI) does not permit quantification of neural injury that occurs after a concussion. Advanced neuroimaging techniques such as proton magnetic resonance spectroscopy may be sensitive to neurochemical damage from a cerebral concussion by monitoring *N*-acetyl-L-aspartate levels over time. *N*-acetyl-L-aspartate diminution appears linked to a general mitochondrial dysfunction, providing a possible surrogate marker of metabolic recovery. Other imaging approaches that show promise for demonstrating damage as a result of concussion include functional MRI, positron emission tomography, diffusion tensor imaging, and functional connectivity techniques; however, these are not routinely used in practice. The use of multifaceted data collection with metabolic data, physiologic data, and clinical observations is the current standard to identify concussion and monitor recovery from the injury.[55]

Neuropsychological tests are an objective measure of brain-behavior relationships and are more sensitive for subtle cognitive impairment than clinical exam. The evaluation consists of a series of cognitive challenges given to the individual, including assessment of sensorimotor status, attention span, memory, language, sequencing, problem solving, and verbal and spatial integration tasks. An example computerized test protocol that is used in some settings as a baseline test for athletes who play contact sports with high risk of concussion is seen in Fig. 33.8. If an injury occurs, postinjury testing aids in determining resolution of injury impairments. Such postinjury tests (or comparison to healthy control norms) must be interpreted with recognition of the reliable change index, baseline variability, and false-positive and false-negative rates for components of the protocol, and never used in isolation of other indications of severity. Some athletes may intentionally perform poorly on baseline tests in order to minimize their time out of play. Interpretation of standardized cognitive test results should be done by a neuropsychologist or speech-language pathologist and in the context of the individual's current situation. Previous tests of intellectual function, including IQ tests and achievement tests, can be helpful for comparison.

Athletes may require neuropsychological evaluation if recovery does not occur in the first several weeks postinjury, although the timing of this evaluation is advocated after the initial recovery period and resumption of typical activities, including return to school for adolescent athletes and children. Postural stability testing may also be undertaken for adjunctive data in determination of concussion severity with the use of computerized balance testing systems (Sensory Organization Test) or more simple clinical tests in standing (Balance Evaluation Scoring System). Collegiate and some high school athletic programs have preseason testing programs that compare baseline cognitive and balance scores to postinjury results when a concussion occurs. Although this is commonplace in larger schools, increasingly there are questions

## Sample Clinical Report

ImPACT™ Clinical Report

Sample Student

| Exam Type | Baseline | Post-Injury 1 | Post-Injury 2 | | |
|---|---|---|---|---|---|
| Date Tested | 07/14/2009 | 08/25/2010 | 08/31/2010 | | |
| Last Concussion | | 08/23/2010 | 08/23/2010 | | |
| Exam Language | English | English | English | | |
| Test Version | 2.0 | 2.0 | 2.0 | | |

| Composite Scores | | | | | |
|---|---|---|---|---|---|
| Memory composite (verbal) | 90 80% | **72** 17% | 94 88% | | |
| Memory composite (visual) | 79 69% | **55** 8% | 71 39% | | |
| Visual motor speed composite | 29.08 33% | **19.65** <1% | 33.17 34% | | |
| Reaction time composite | 0.55 93% | **0.79** 4% | 0.59 56% | | |
| Impulse control composite | 8 | 13 | 13 | | |
| Total Symptom Score | 0 | **31** | 0 | | |

Scores in **bold RED** type exceed the Reliable Change Index (RCI) when compared to the baseline score. However, scores that do not exceed to RCI index may still be clinically significant. Percentile scores if available are listed in small type.

**Figure 33.8**

**Baseline and postinjury neurocognitive tests.** (From The ImPACT Test, ImPACT Applications, Inc., Pittsburgh, Pennsylvania [https://impacttest.com/about/])

about whether the cost of extensive baseline testing is justifiable, given the small number of concussions that may occur. A baseline testing approach is not always possible because a concussion can happen to anyone, including those who are not part of any organized sports activity.

Mild TBI or concussion is a topic of significant interest as a result of media attention on sports-related injury and the frequency of brain injury during the recent military conflicts in Iraq and Afghanistan. The American Academy of Neurology and the Consensus Conference on Concussion in Sport[60] provide guidance for management of concussion in the sports context. Although 80% to 90% of those who sustain sports concussion will recover fully in 7 to 10 days, this timeline for recovery may be longer for younger athletes.

Individuals with suspected concussion should be removed immediately from play and not be allowed to return to play on the same day. The Berlin guidelines for progression of return to activity after injury has not been well studied, but conventional practice encourages rest for 24 to 48 hours after injury, followed by activity that is tolerated without increasing symptom complaints. For school-aged athletes, return to school is recommended first, with a part-time schedule initially if necessary, with resumption of typical routines while monitoring responses to the cognitive and activity demands of a usual day. If well tolerated, a graded return to sport activity is recommended as described in the Berlin guidelines[60] (Table 33.4). Components of the concept are as follows:

- *RETURN TO CLASS:* Students may require cognitive rest and may require academic accommodations, such as reduced workload and extended time for tests while recovering from a concussion.
- *RETURN TO PLAY* (RTP): Concussion symptoms should be largely resolved at rest before returning to exercise. An RTP progression involves a gradual, stepwise increase in physical demands, sports-specific activities, and ongoing assessment to determine readiness for contact drills and eventually full participation. If symptoms increase with activity, the progression should be halted and restarted at the preceding step. Full RTP in competition should occur only with medical clearance from a licensed health care provider trained in the evaluation and management of concussions. The primary concern with early RTP is decreased reaction time, with increased risk of a repeat concussion or other injury and exacerbation or prolongation of symptoms.
- *DISQUALIFICATION FROM SPORT:* There are no evidence-based guidelines for disqualifying/retiring an athlete from a sport after a concussion. Each case should be carefully deliberated and an individualized approach to determining disqualification taken.

**Table 33.4** Common Principles in Advancing Activity Post-Concussion

| GRADUATED RETURN TO SPORT OR MILITARY ACTIVITY | | |
|---|---|---|
| **Rehabilitation Stage** | **Functional Exercise** | **Objective of Each Stage** |
| 1. Brief period of rest (24–48 hours) with symptom-limited activity | Daily activities that do not provoke symptoms, including extremely light activities/ADLs | Allow brief rest to promote recovery, but resume light basic activities if tolerated |
| 2. Light routine activity and aerobic exercise | Introduce and promote limited effort activities (walk, treadmill, stationary bike) at slow to medium pace. No resistance training | Increase HR using symptom response as a guide for progression |
| 3. Light occupation-oriented or sport-specific exercise | Running or skating drills. No head-impact activities | Full-body movement progressing in complexity related to duty or sport goals |
| 4. Moderate-level training, including noncontact training drills for sport | Harder training drills, incorporating cognitive demands. May start progressive resistance training (sub-maximal level) | Exercise, coordination, and increased thinking |
| 5. Intensive-level training, including full-contact practice for sport | Participate in normal training activities for sport- or duty-related roles | Restore confidence and assess functional skills to judge readiness to return to competitive play in sport or duty roles in the military |
| 6. Return to play | Normal game-play | |

Note: An initial period of 24-48 hours of both relative physical rest and cognitive rest is recommended before progressing with activity challenges. Typical staged progressions require 24 hours (or longer) for each step of the progression. If any symptoms worsen during progression to a new stage, regression to the previous step is recommended. Resistance training should be added only in the later stages (stage 3 or 4 at the earliest). If symptoms are persistent (more than 10-14 days in adults or more than 1 month in children), referral to a healthcare professional who is an expert in the management of concussion is recommended.

Based on date from Concussion in Sport Group Consensus Guidelines for Progressive Return to Activity After Concussion, 2016 and Defense and Veterans Progressive Return to Activity Clinical Recommendations for Mild Traumatic Brain Injury, 2014.

• *EDUCATION:* Greater efforts are needed to educate involved parties, including athletes, parents, coaches, officials, school administrators, and health care providers to improve concussion recognition, management, and prevention.[55]

The Symptom Wheel lists common symptoms that guide progression of activity in the classroom first, and then, if desired, field of play.

In the military context, past history of mild TBI and current symptoms influence the duration of rest that is recommended after exposure to blast or injury where concussion is suspected. Clinical recommendations developed through the Defense and Veterans Brain Injury Center and Defense Centers of Excellence for Psychological Health and Traumatic Brain Injury direct military physicians and therapists in strategies to manage concussion complaints and maintain health of service members with brain injury (see https://dvbic.dcoe.mil/material/progressive-return-activity-following-acute-concussionmild-tbi-clinical-suite).

Many more patients report to emergency departments each year as a result of concussion from falls, recreational injury, motor vehicle crashes, and other accidents than sports concussion. These patients may need assistance in returning to their daily activities including school, work, driving, recreation, and daily activities.

In 2020 a clinical practice guideline for the PT management of a concussive event was published to address the needs for individuals across the lifespan that sustain a concussion and have physical symptoms that may respond to PT. This guideline emphasizes the strong likelihood that someone who sustains a concussion could have other injuries that occur because of the mechanism of injury and forces involved, so that physical therapists should screen carefully for cervical, vestibular, exertional, and functional mobility impairments that could result from the injury. Consideration of the type and degree of symptom irritability, as well as careful sequencing of intervention, is often necessary in order for the patient to tolerate rehabilitation and progress to preinjury levels.

Cognitive and behavioral dysfunctions caused by brain injury are similar to posttraumatic stress syndrome, conversion or hysterical reactions, malingering, depression, and anxiety. Therefore each individual should be carefully evaluated to determine cause(s) of symptoms. Trauma occurring at the time of the injury may trigger posttraumatic stress reactions or other psychoses in susceptible individuals with history of prior trauma.

## TRAUMATIC BRAIN INJURY IN CHILDREN

TBI is one of the leading causes of death and disability in children of all ages.[65] Nonaccidental injury is a common cause of brain injury in infants and toddlers and is often the result of the battered child or shaken baby syndrome. Injury is caused by shaking or striking the child.

Although the pathology of the brain injury in the child reflects damage similar to that in the adult, there are differences. Infants typically have tears in the white matter of the temporal and orbitofrontal lobes. The infant will more often sustain a subdural or epidural hemorrhage than an older child but is less likely to have skull fracture because of the pliancy of the skull.

Drowning is the third leading cause of death in children aged 1 to 4 years. Peak incidences occur in 1- to

Box 33.4

**PEDIATRIC GLASGOW COMA SCALE**

| Rating | Criterion | 2 years or older | Less than 2 years |
|---|---|---|---|
| ***Eye opening*** | | | |
| 4 | Open before stimulus | Spontaneous | Spontaneous |
| 3 | After spoken or shouted request | To sound | To sound |
| 2 | After physical stimulation | To pressure | To pressure |
| 1 | No opening at any time, no interfering factor | None | None |
| NT | Closed by interfering factor | NT | NT |
| ***Verbal response*** | | | |
| 5 | Correctly gives name, place, date or produces words or phrases normal for chronological age | Oriented; words/phrases normal for chronological age | Babbles/coos; words/ phrases normal for chronological age |
| 4 | Not oriented but communicating coherently; produces some words or phrases but not normal for chronological age | Confused; some words/ phrases, not normal for chronological age | Some words/ phrases, not normal for chronological age |
| 3 | Intelligible single words | Words | Inconsolable crying |
| 2 | Only moans or groans | Sounds | Sounds |
| ***Eye opening*** | | | |
| 1 | No audible response, no interfering factors | None | None |
| NT | Factor interfering with verbal communication | NT | NT |
| ***Motor response*** | | | |
| 6 | Obeys 2-part request or request appropriate for chronologic age | Obeys commands | Normal spontaneous movement |
| 5 | Brings hands above clavicle for stimulus on head or neck | Localizing | Rapidly withdraws extremity to stimulation |
| 4 | Bends arm at elbow rapidly, but features not predominantly abnormal | Normal flexion | Normal flexion |
| 3 | Bends arm at elbow, features clearly abnormal | Abnormal flexion | Abnormal flexion |
| 2 | | Extension | Extension |
| 1 | | None | None |
| NT | Extends arm at elbow No movement in arms/ legs, no interfering factor | NT | NT |

Reprinted from Kirschen MP, Snyder M, Smith K, et al.: Inter-rater reliability between critical care nurses performing a pediatric modification to the Glasgow Coma Scale,* *Pediatr Crit Care Med* 20(7):660-666, 2019. https://doi.org/10.1097/PCC.0000000000001938.

4-year-olds and in adolescent boys. Boys are three times more likely to be injured. Rapid resuscitation leads to better outcomes, with poor outcome associated with near-drowning. As in adults, motor activity return and pupillary light response are prognosticators of outcome.

A modified version of the Glasgow Coma Scale has been developed for use in children (Box 33.4). This version differentiates eye, motor and verbal responses that can be observed in children younger than 2 and provides guidance for scoring responses in older children so that the familiar scale of 3 to 15 is used for any age.

Early management of the infant or child with TBI is similar to that of the adult, with some difference in the child's ability to tolerate the medications used. Late seizures are less common with children than with adults, so the need to be maintained on seizure medication is less.[51]

Rehabilitation goals for the child are similar to those of the adult, although play is more critical during therapy. Orthotic and assistive devices are more critical frequently but for a shorter time than for adults. Agitation is common and is often difficult for the parents and siblings to handle. Aggression, decreased attention span, hyperactivity, and socially inappropriate behavior are seen. These children often require a great deal of behavior modification.

Community reintegration can be as difficult for the child as it is for the adult. Schools are better prepared to handle cognitive delays than abnormal behaviors. Cognitive status may return in one area and remain defective in another. Attention and memory deficits may produce the greatest obstacles to learning. Children who recover from TBI may continue to need assistance as they progress in school, especially as academic demands increase. Professionals who understand the unique cognitive and behavioral challenges of brain injury are pivotal in facilitating strategies for academic success.

SPECIAL IMPLICATIONS FOR THE THERAPIST 33.1

## *Traumatic Brain Injury*

Rehabilitation of the brain-injured person involves the therapist at many different levels and in different settings. Typical progression through the system of care is illustrated in Fig. 33.9. Understanding the deficits common in acute injury and the natural recovery patterns of the brain dependent on the site and type of injury is paramount for the therapist treating brain injury. The therapist working with individuals with brain injury must understand the interaction between the deficits related to cognitive and social behaviors and the ability to learn to move.[84] Cognitive rehabilitation and physical rehabilitation are closely related. Functional outcomes are limited by the cognitive status, and understanding of the techniques that foster

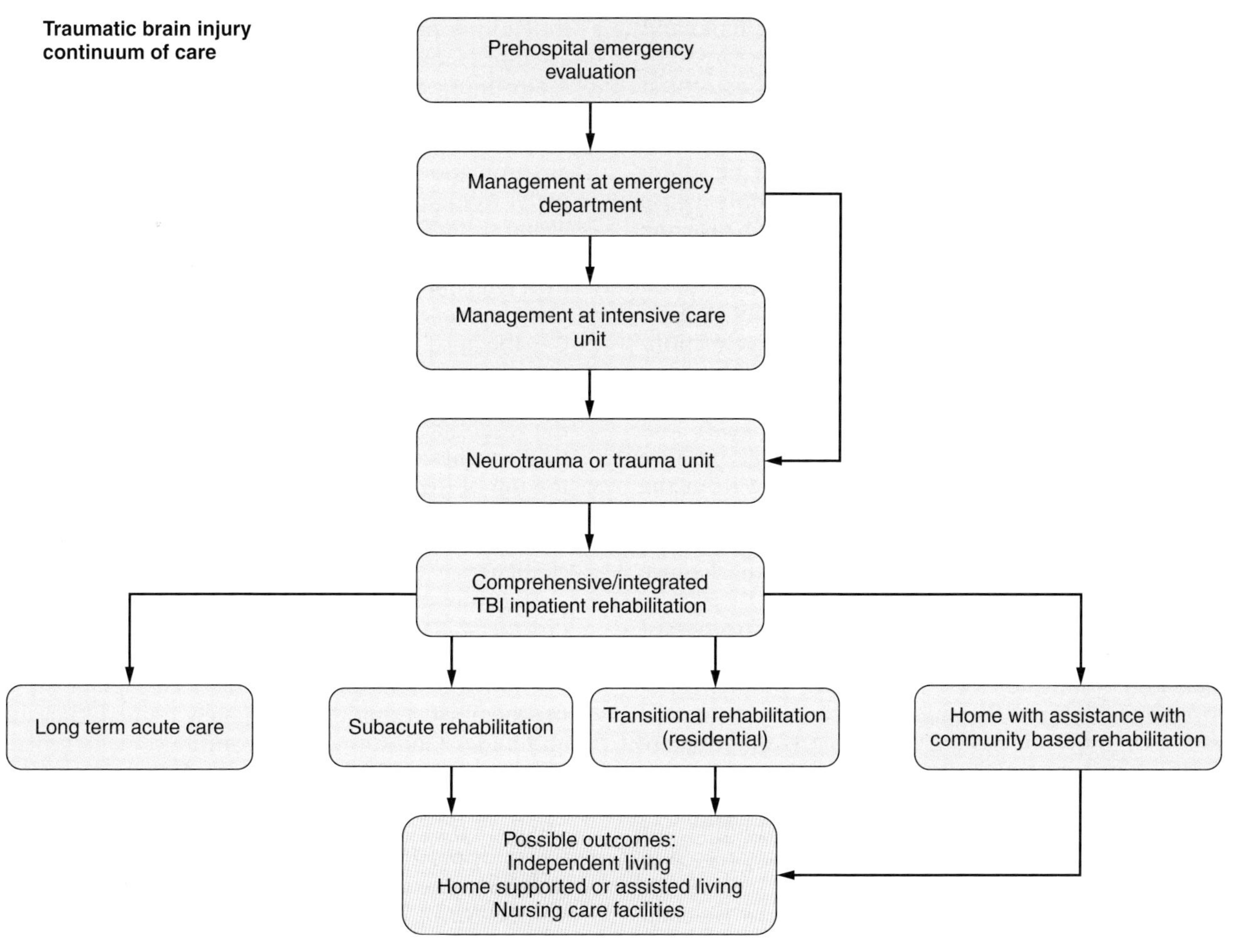


**Figure 33.9**

**Typical flow of patients through the continuum of care.** (From Reina-Guerra SG, Lazaro RT, Quiben MU: *Umphred's neurological rehabilitation*, ed 7, St. Louis, 2020, Elsevier.)

behavioral modification and learning should be used by the therapist during motor skill acquisition.[79] Occupational therapists assess individuals with brain injury in functional contexts to observe for the ability to integrate motor, sensory, and cognitive function in common activities of daily life. In some settings, occupational therapists may test components of cognitive and perceptual abilities. Language and cognitive problems are examined as well by speech pathologists and can include naming tests, aphasia examinations, as well as tests of auditory comprehension and speed of comprehension. Speech-language pathologists also assess for oral-motor control difficulties such as dysphagia (difficulty swallowing) and dysarthria (difficulty with articulation for speech).

Often the therapist will be involved in a dedicated brain injury unit or in a community based program. Even in a more general setting, the therapist is often responsible for intervention with individuals sustaining brain injury, often acutely, or when an individual has been through a rehabilitation setting and is referred for follow-up based on residual deficits. Provision of therapy in the long-term care setting involves care for individuals in the minimally conscious state, or with behavioral deficits precluding independent living.[14]

In the acute care setting, the therapist is responsible for the evaluation of neurologic function in conjunction with physicians and nurses. One role may be consistent monitoring of cranial nerve function. In addition, the therapist is involved in monitoring reflexive and voluntary motor behaviors. The treatment plan often includes pulmonary care, positioning, range-of-motion exercises, and relaxation techniques. Movement facilitation begins early in the treatment and continues throughout rehabilitation in many cases. Because treatment starts while the individual is still in the intensive care unit, a discussion of life-sustaining equipment follows.

Chest tubes are common with a pneumothorax or hemothorax. The drainage tube should be kept below the level of the chest at all times. Upper extremity movement should be monitored so as not to interfere with the tube. Nasogastric tube feeding is also common initially, and when a tube is in place, the head of the bed should be placed at 30 degrees to avoid aspiration. It is important that cerebral venous blood volume be controlled in head injury. Maintaining the head in a neutral nonrotated position and at a 20- to 40-degree tilt will usually provide adequate drainage. However, compression of venous drainage from tracheal ties and collars and extreme neck flexion or extension can occur if precautions are not followed. Lines such as central venous pressure catheters, pulmonary or arterial lines, and ICP monitors can be compromised during movement, and often the movement will trigger an alarm that can be upsetting for the client and family. Close communication with the nursing staff will give the therapist confidence in moving the person in the intensive care setting.

Pulmonary management is another critical area. Techniques such as percussion, vibration, and suctioning are used to keep the airway clear but must be done with caution and may be contraindicated in the presence of increased ICP. Monitoring blood gases and oxygen saturation is critical in some clients, because movement may alter these values. Weaning from the ventilator is an individual endeavor. Some clients are able to continue to incorporate activity during weaning, but for others it may mean a decrease in tolerance to movement.[39]

Management of decreased range of motion from spasticity or HO is another intervention provided by therapists. Joint contractures are a secondary problem produced by inability of the muscle to return to its normal resting length. Serial casting and dynamic splinting are used to maintain joint motion in the presence of spasticity, rigidity, or HO.[8] Managing excessive muscle and reflex activity through movement and positioning begins in the acute phase and often must still be addressed in the rehabilitative phase.

Similar concepts apply to decisions for wheelchair seating and positioning in the nonambulatory individual. Prevention of secondary joint disorders, pain, and disfigurement is facilitated by provision of support in the anatomically proper position. Materials and equipment that are lightweight and provide total contact provide the most comfortable support.[22]

Swallowing deficits and related problems with respiration or coughing occur in approximately one-third of persons with head injury. Head, neck, and trunk control affect the ability to swallow. Intervention based on lack of strength and mobility of the perioral structures often starts in the acute phase. Sensation, dentition, tongue control, and laryngeal control are assessed to determine the level of impairment relating to disability of speech and swallowing.[86]

Hemiplegia often persists and is seen in more than 50% of individuals with brain injury 6 months after onset. Diffuse damage to the central white matter tracts and midbrain with loss of integration of reflexes can have a devastating effect on function.

Because somatosensory, visual, and vestibular inputs can be disrupted after TBI, dizziness and imbalance is common. A thorough evaluation of sensory integration function is necessary in order to design intervention. Therapists must be knowledgeable about the effects of brain injury so as to intervene without overstimulating, and attend to cognitive and behavioral aspects of the brain injury to ensure adherence to therapy. Visual stimulation may be disorienting, so the client may prefer to maintain an environment without peripheral visual stimuli, have difficulty reading, and avoid situations with fluorescent lighting. The individual may be hypervigilant in regard to the vestibular input and is already overstimulated by the time he or she reaches the therapist. Often there is a sensation of moving when at rest that is uncovered by sitting with the eyes closed. This can be an indication of maladaptation of the vestibular system. Settling techniques, such as putting weights on the shoulders, or pressing down on the top of the head can increase somatosensory input. Sensitivity to vestibular input can be decreased with activities that gradually increase exposure to vestibular challenges.

The individual with TBI will have complex movement disorders related to force production, timing, reaction time, and fatigue, and movements may be too slow for function. Sensory disturbances are significant, and the therapist should be adequately trained to evaluate and understand the sensory contributions to function. Learning new tasks is difficult, as described previously in relation to central dysfunction, and cognitive deficits can limit progress. However, there are many opportunities to work with patients on high levels of balance and mobility function. The High-level Mobility Assessment Test (HiMAT) is an outcome measure developed specifically to monitor progress in people with brain injury who have the potential to return to running (http://tbims.org/combi/himat/index.html).

The therapist should understand that with repetition of appropriate activities, these individuals can make significant gains. Although recovery may be rapid closer to the time of injury, small incremental changes can continue over months and years post injury. The use of appropriate environmental supports may be necessary to compensate for abilities that are lost, but quality of life can be restored. There are excellent resources available to assist the therapist in treatment. Many therapists have special expertise, and institutions are focused on management of the individual with brain injury.

Thank you to Nicole Miranda for her review and contributions to the information regarding concussion.

## REFERENCES

To enhance this text and add value for the reader, all references are included in the enhanced ebook on Student Consult that accompanies this textbook. The reader can view the reference source and access it online whenever possible.

# CHAPTER 34

# Traumatic Spinal Cord Injury

KAREN L. MCCULLOCH • CANDY TEFERTILLER

## SPINAL CORD INJURY

Spinal cord injury (SCI) is a catastrophic event of low incidence and high cost that most often affects highly active persons. Within a matter of seconds, the person sustaining a severe traumatic SCI may become dependent on others or on assistive devices to perform even the most basic activities of self-care. SCI rarely occurs in isolation, and more than 75% of these individuals have some other systemic injury. In 10% to 15%, there is an associated head injury. This concern has led to the widely quoted clinical maxim that all trauma patients or any patient with a severe head injury should be presumed to have a spine injury or SCI until proven otherwise.[58]

### Incidence and Risk Factors

Males account for more than 78% of all cases of traumatic SCI. Traditionally SCI occurred mostly in young people, but the mean age of people with SCI increased in the 1990s and is now recorded at 43. There is now a higher survival rate in the geriatric population; in addition, the mean age of the general population also has increased. It is estimated that there are approximately 54 cases per 1 million persons on an annual basis, with an additional 6 to 8 deaths per 1 million occurring before hospitalization; however, the number of deaths occurring before hospitalization is decreasing. The number of individuals living with SCI is approximately 291,000, with 12,000 new cases each year.[97]

The primary cause of SCI is motor vehicle accidents, which account for nearly 39% of SCIs. Falls are the second most common cause, accounting for 32%. Approximately 13.5% of SCIs are caused by violence; these include job-related injuries to security guards and policemen, workers shot during robberies, victims of violent crimes, and others. The likelihood of SCI from a gunshot wound appears to be higher among individuals who have had previous gunshot wounds (30%) or who have had prior involvement in the criminal justice system (52%). In contrast to sports injuries, which peak nationwide during the summer months, the incidence of penetrating wounds of the spine remains the same throughout the year, and 40% occur on a Saturday or Sunday.[48]

Sports-related injuries account for 8% of total SCIs. Accidents resulting in SCI are most prevalent in the contact sports of football and wrestling, high-speed sports such as snow skiing and surfing, and sports in which injuries can involve a fall from a height, such as a trampoline or a horse. Fig. 34.1 shows a breakdown of the incidence of injury types based on 2019 data.

Approximately 39% of all persons with SCIs have paraplegia, and 61% have tetraplegia. Of all thoracic and lumbar cord injuries, 24% are complete lesions, and 18.7% of cervical injuries are complete lesions. For penetrating wounds of the spine, however, a significantly greater proportion are complete, with more thoracic spinal injuries compared with injuries of the neck or lumbar spine.[96,121]

### Definition and Etiologic Factors

*Traumatic SCI* is classified as concussion, contusion, or laceration. A *concussion* is an injury caused by a blow or violent shaking and results in temporary loss of function, similar to the cerebral concussion associated with head injury. In *contusion* injury the glial tissue and spinal cord surface remain intact. There may be a loss of central gray and white matter, which creates a cavity that is surrounded by a rim of intact white matter at the periphery of the spinal cord. *Laceration* or *maceration* of the cord occurs with more severe injuries, in which the glia is disrupted and the spinal cord tissue may be torn. Occasionally this can result in complete transection of the cord. Gunshot wounds, knife wounds, and puncture injuries fall into this category.

Hemorrhages into the dura are common, although they rarely become large enough to compromise the spinal cord. Subarachnoid hemorrhages, caused by contusion and laceration of the cord, are frequent and can cause further compression of the cord.

The mechanism of injury influences the type and degree of the spinal cord lesion. Fig. 34.2 shows the flexion damage that is referred to as hangman's fracture, related to

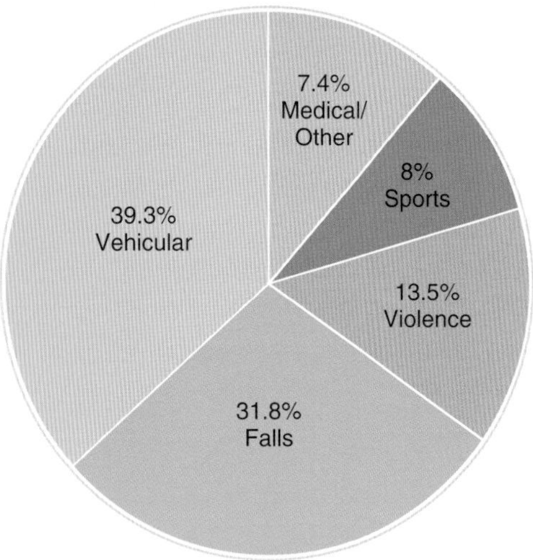


**Fig. 34.1**

**Approximate causes of traumatic spinal cord injury in 2019.** (Data from National Spinal Cord Injury Statistical Center: Facts and figures at a glance. University of Alabama at Birmingham. Available online at www.nscisc.uab.edu. Accessed January 10, 2020.)

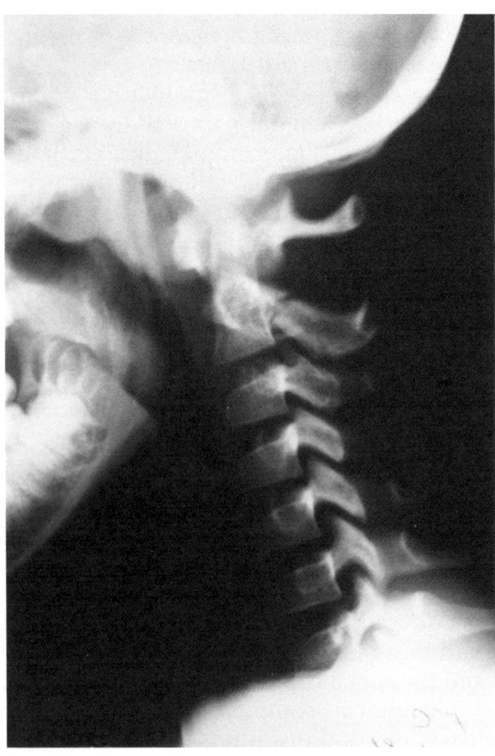

**Fig. 34.2**

**Fracture of C2 (hangman's fracture).** (From Green NB, Swiontkowski MF, eds: *Skeletal trauma in children*, ed 3, Philadelphia, 2003, Saunders.)

excessive flexion. Approximately 50% of injuries come from excessive flexion of the spinal column that results in a severe neurologic disorder.[24] Fig. 34.3 shows how extension can cause SCI in elderly patients. Fig. 34.4 illustrates how vascular change may result from displacement of spinal components. The spinal cord is often violently displaced or compressed momentarily during an injury with forceful flexion, extension, or rotation of the spine.

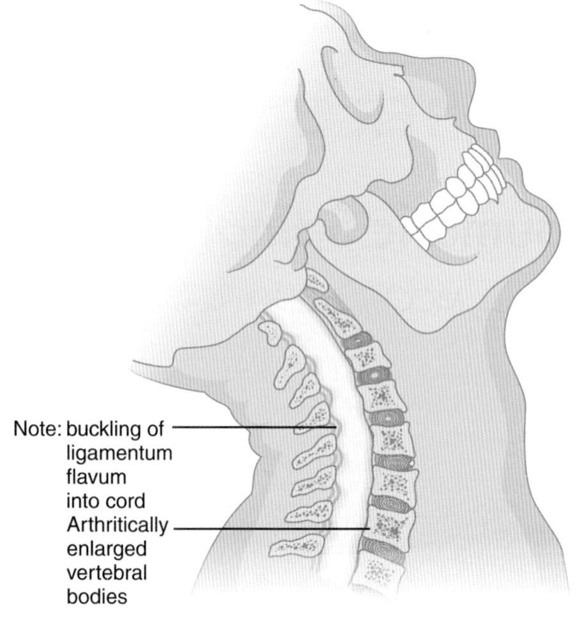


**Fig. 34.3**

Elderly patients subjected to extension forces can sustain cervical spinal cord injury as a result of compression of the spinal cord between the posterior hypertrophic ligamentum flavum and the arthritically enlarged anterior vertebral bodies. (From Marx JA, ed: *Rosen's emergency medicine: concepts and clinical practice*, ed 6, Philadelphia, 2006, Mosby.)

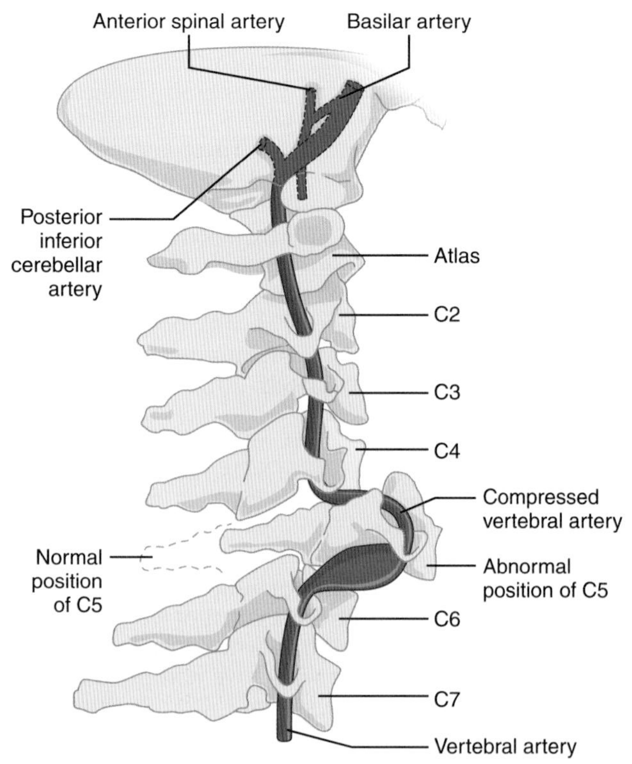


**Fig. 34.4**

**Mechanism of vascular injury of the spinal cord resulting from cervical vertebral injury.** (From Marx JA, ed: *Rosen's emergency medicine: concepts and clinical practice*, ed 6, Philadelphia, 2006, Mosby.)

The vertebral body can burst and cause pressure or scatter bone fragments into the spinal cord. Fig. 34.5 illustrates this phenomenon. Complete spinal cord lesions occur in about one-third of flexion injuries. With crush fractures of the vertebrae, there is a 75% chance of a complete spinal cord lesion.

The majority of patients with SCI have at least one other system injury. Occasionally these injuries take precedence in evaluation and treatment. If one level of bony injury has been identified, it is necessary to survey the entire spine because there is a 10% to 15% incidence of spinal injury at other levels.[58]

The difference between a complete and an incomplete spinal cord lesion depends on the survival of a small fraction of the axons in the spinal cord. Evidence of axonal conduction across the lesion site has been found in individuals with clinical neurologic diagnoses of complete SCI at that level. The surviving axons may be injured and therefore have a decreased response to stimuli. The injured axon conducts slowly and fatigues rapidly.[129]

## Pathogenesis

The development of the spinal lesion occurs over time and in a neuroanatomic distribution. In the first 18 hours, there is necrotic death of axons that were directly disrupted by the trauma. In the following weeks, there is further progression of tissue injury in both directions from the lesion. The immune system probably plays a major role during this phase. It appears that immune cells such as monocytes and macrophages emit chemical signals, including cytokines and chemokines, that trigger apoptosis, or programmed cell death. This breakdown of cell function can occur distal from the lesion site, as far away as four spinal segments.[22]

The pathophysiology of SCI may be divided into phases. *Primary injury* refers to structural damage occurring instantly after the traumatic event. Trauma to the spinal cord results in primary destruction of neurons at the level of the injury by disruption of the membrane, hemorrhage, and vascular damage. More extensive primary injury may occur, however, if an injured spine is not adequately immobilized. A critical aspect of these lesions is that even after severe injuries, a small peripheral rim of spared tissue and axons often remains. Spared descending systems play an important role in recovery. In paraplegia the amount of spared rim correlates with the level of locomotor function.[9,120]

*Secondary injury* refers to a pathophysiologic cascade initiated shortly after injury. Ischemia and hypoxia occur, with gray matter being more prone to damage because of increased capillary density and neurons with higher metabolic demand. Release of cytoplasmic content causes an increase in glutamate excitotoxicity and triggers an inflammatory response that may increase neural damage. Excitotoxicity increases protein degradation and oxidative stress on the area, which in turn triggers apoptotic cell death. Swelling and edema exacerbate ion imbalance and increase axonal susceptibility to damage.[101] See Chapter 28 for information regarding the effects of these disturbances. These processes are initiated with injury and extend for hours, days, or weeks.[3,6,]3 Fig. 34.6 shows the changes that can result from SCI. Because it is extremely rare for the primary injury to cause transection of the spinal cord, and it has been shown that less than 10% of the cross-sectional area of the spinal cord supports locomotion, it is very important to focus clinical attention on the secondary injury process. Injury results in ischemia, edema formation, membrane destruction, cell death, and eventually permanent neurologic deficits.[58] The relationship of mechanisms of damage leading to cell death is shown in Fig. 34.7.

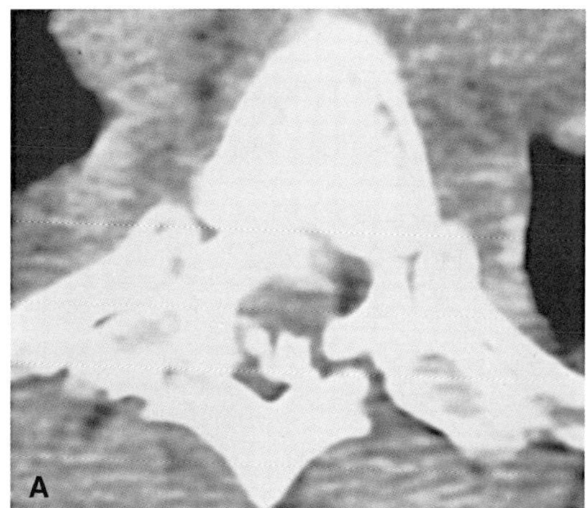


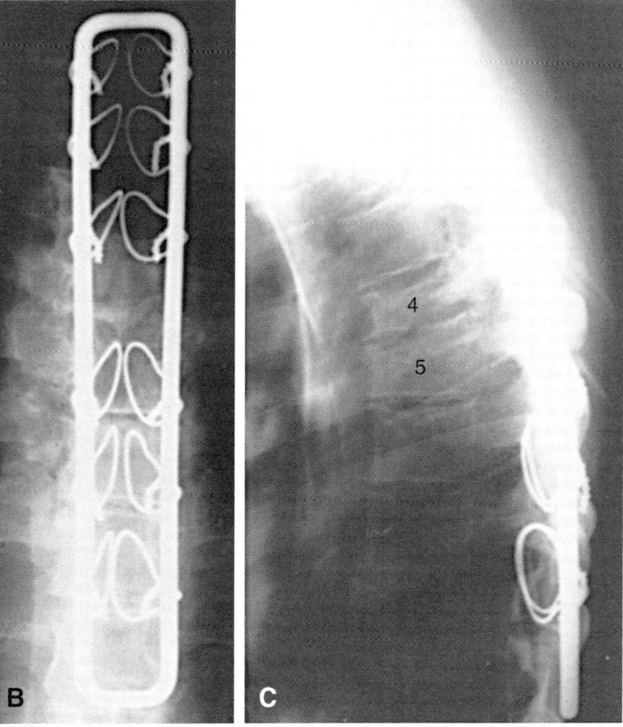


**Fig. 34.5**

**A T4-T5 fracture-dislocation resulted in a complete spinal cord injury in a 30-year-old man.** (A) Computed tomography scan through the injured level demonstrates marked displacement and comminution at T4-T5, with multiple bone fragments within the canal. (B) Postoperative anteroposterior radiograph shows stabilization with a Luque rectangle and sublaminar wires. This instrumentation provided rigid fixation and allowed early mobilization, with minimal external support. The strength of fixation could have been improved with the use of double wires around the lamina bilaterally. (C) Postoperative lateral radiograph. (From Browner BD, et al: *Skeletal trauma: basic science, management, and reconstruction*, ed 3, Philadelphia, 2003, Saunders.)

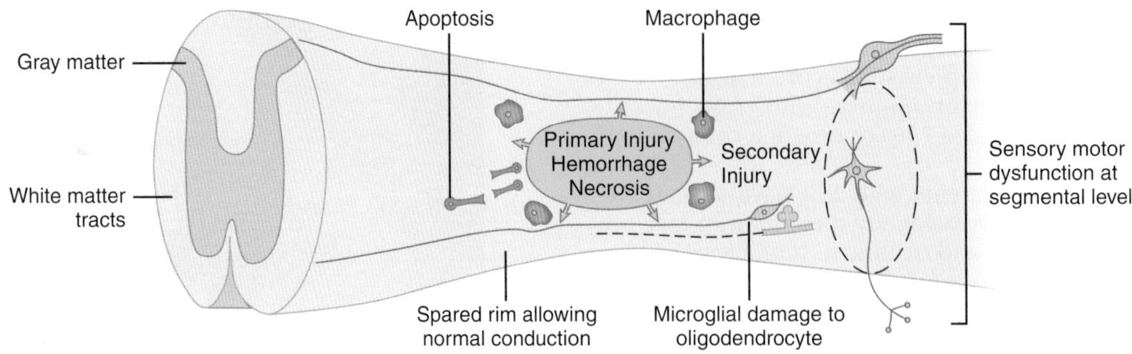


**Fig. 34.6**

Spinal cord contusion lesions are characterized by a primary area created by hemorrhage of blood vessels causing necrosis of cells. This area eventually spreads because of secondary injury associated with apoptosis (programmed cell death), macrophages acting as immune mediators, and microglia causing damage to oligodendrocytes. The secondary damage may continue for days to weeks and move along the segmental levels, causing sensory and motor dysfunction. The spared rim may allow normal processing and preservation of function.

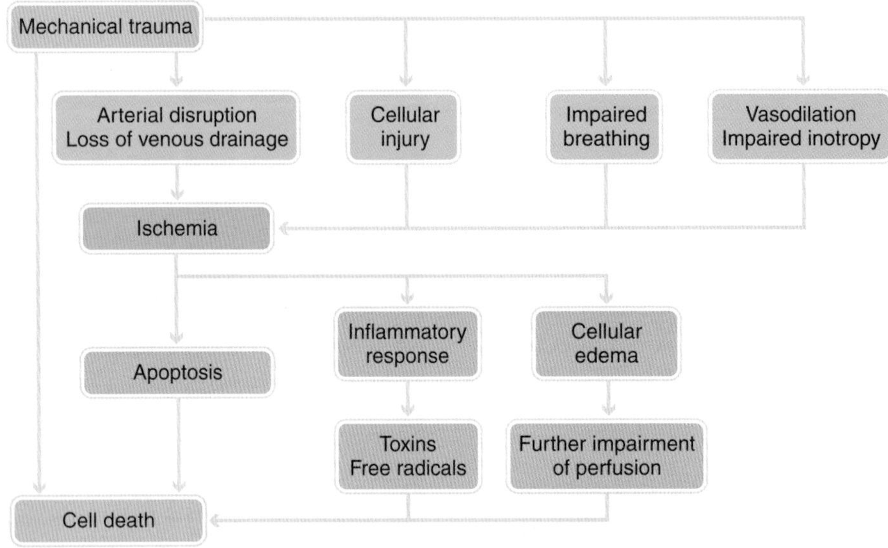


**Fig. 34.7**

**Mechanisms of spinal cord injury.** Mechanical trauma to the spinal cord is exacerbated by systemic hypoperfusion or hypoxia. (From Miller RD, ed: *Miller's anesthesia*, ed 6, New York, 2005, Churchill Livingstone. Redrawn from Dutton RP: Spinal cord injury. *Int Anesthesiol Clin* 40:109, 2002.)

## Blood Flow Changes

Ischemia related to reduced blood flow is a very prominent feature of post-SCI events. Damage to blood vessels and microhemorrhage in the central gray matter spread radially and axially. The resulting hypoxic and ischemic events deprive gray and white matter of oxygen and nutrients necessary for neural cell survival and function. Ischemia in the area of injury may be due to the presence of norepinephrine, serotonin, histamine, and prostaglandins, all of which cause vasoconstriction. This ischemia may be compounded by loss of the normal autoregulatory response of the spinal cord vasculature.

Autoregulation of circulation is dysfunctional at the injury site. Systemic pressure changes may be responsible for changes in spinal blood flow, which may cause nervous tissue damage by direct effects. The changes in blood flow may reflect rather than cause secondary injury.[62]

After several hours, gross hemorrhages may appear, preceded by endothelial breakdown and pathologic coagulation products in the blood vessels. Macrophages enter the lesion and begin to digest the necrotic debris, converting the complex myelin lipids to neutral fat. Axonal swelling and increased permeability of blood vessels result in a visibly swollen spinal cord. Glial cells become active after about 6 days, and astrocytic fibers form scarlike tissue that lines the cavities created by the necrosis.

## Inflammation

Inflammation is a process that has both positive and negative effects on recovery. In the days after injury, microglia, astrocytes, and neutrophils migrate to the injury site and cause antigen-triggered activation of B and T lymphocytes. $CD4^+$ helper T cells produce cytokines that stimulate B-cell antibodies that trigger phagocytes; these antibodies also increase inflammation that is damaging to neural tissue. Astrocytes, neutrophils, microglia, and macrophages all play roles in increasing inflammation, which can be damaging to existing tissue, but these cells can also have neuroprotective or regenerative qualities under specific conditions. Research to determine how to trigger these facilitatory processes is under way in preclinical studies.[3]

### Demyelination

Demyelination results in a reduced rate of axonal firing in the injured spinal cord. The demyelination is due to direct trauma to the oligodendroglial cells that produce myelin. Lymphocytes and macrophages invade the lesion site by way of the disrupted blood-brain barrier as part of the inflammatory response. The myelin sheath becomes thin between the nodes, and this causes a decrease in the peak currents along the axon. Loss of a single segment of myelin renders an axon dysfunctional; therefore a large subset of axons crossing the lesion eventually become nonfunctional despite the axons remaining physically intact.

Changes in white matter begin with wallerian degeneration in the ascending posterior columns above the level of the lesion and in the descending corticospinal tracts. Wallerian degeneration may be triggered by microglial activation and by the destruction of the oligodendrocytes via the release of cytokines or other neurotropic factors.[76] The immune system appears also to trigger the release of nerve growth factor, which can be neuroprotective to some cells while being toxic to other cells in the spinal cord.

A prominent feature of SCI is the maturation of a scar around the lesion. The glial scar consists of astrocytes, oligodendrocyte precursor cells, microglia, fibroblasts, and pericytes. This scar serves a protective role in preventing immune cells within the central nonneural lesion core from spreading to nearby tissue, but also may inhibit repair and regeneration across to the lesion core. Just beyond the scar is an area of spared reactive neural tissue that includes reactive astrocytes, microglia, and oligodendrocyte precursor cells. This area continues to react with functioning neurons and is a target for triggering synaptic and circuit plasticity after injury. This area of reactive neural tissue may also cause maladaptive change, such as the development of spasticity and neuropathic pain.[3]

### Gray Matter

Typically the loss of central gray matter is confined to between 1 and 1½ segmental levels of the spinal cord, causing central cavitation. The result is a fluid-filled cyst or syrinx (described in more detail later), or the cord collapses around the loss of tissue in an hourglass shape, with the minimal diameter located at the spinal segment of the original injury.

### Dural Scarring

Scarring of the dura can cause a permanent connection of the cord to the overlying dura. Because the cord is normally freely mobile within the spinal canal, restricted motion attributable to dural scarring produces unusual forces on the cord as a result of neck bending, normal breathing, or the cardiac cycle. These forces can produce microscopic injury, which may limit optimal regeneration and recovery.

### Neural Function

Neural activity below the injury level is related to passive and active limb movements and sensory stimuli from the moving limbs. Substantial reduction of neural activity limits the body's ability to maintain the cellular functions of the spinal cord circuitry. Slow progressive loss of function is normal in chronic SCI. It is thought that the injured central nervous system (CNS) undergoes accelerated aging, with abnormal cell production and impairments in mechanisms of cellular repair. The cellular mechanisms important for regeneration may be limited as a part of this process.

Animal models of SCI suggest that areas of the brain involved in sensorimotor control undergo atrophy after spinal cord transection. A significant decrease in the size and number of corticospinal neurons has been demonstrated in the rat brain. Atrophy may occur in the subacute phase (5 to 10 weeks), with cell death occurring in the chronic phase (months to years). In the somatosensory system, shrinkage of the dorsal column nuclei and thalamus has been demonstrated in primates following upper limb deafferentation. Thus both the somatosensory system and the motor system are susceptible to atrophy after nervous system damage.[75]

### Neurapraxia

The syndrome of neurapraxia is of special concern after athletic injury. Affected individuals experience dramatic, although transient, neurologic deficits, including tetraplegia. Transient tetraplegia most commonly occurs as a result of axial loading of the spine. In athletes with narrowing of the anteroposterior diameter of the spinal canal, both hyperextension and hyperflexion can lead to cord compression. This is referred to as the pincer mechanism. In an already stenotic canal, hyperextension compresses the cord between the posteroinferior margin of the superior vertebral body and the anterosuperior aspect of the spinolaminar line of the subjacent vertebra. Conversely, in hyperflexion the cord is compressed between the anterosuperior aspect of the spinolaminar line of the superior vertebra and the posterosuperior margin of the inferior vertebra. In both cases, this sudden decrease in the anteroposterior diameter of the spinal canal results in compression of the spinal cord. Many attempts have been made to quantify the level of risk to these individuals of continued athletic participation; however, considerable controversy still exists.[49]

### Syringomyelia

One type of pathologic condition that can appear over time in the spinal cord related to trauma is syringomyelia. This is a clinical syndrome that results from cystic cavitation and gliosis of the spinal cord. It is reported to occur in close to 2% of persons with paraplegia and in 0.2% of persons with quadriplegia. In the chronic spinal cord lesion, the cysts may continue to develop, become tubular in shape similar to a syrinx, and extend over several spinal levels (Fig. 34.8). Posttraumatic syringomyelia can develop up to 30 years after the initial lesion, but most

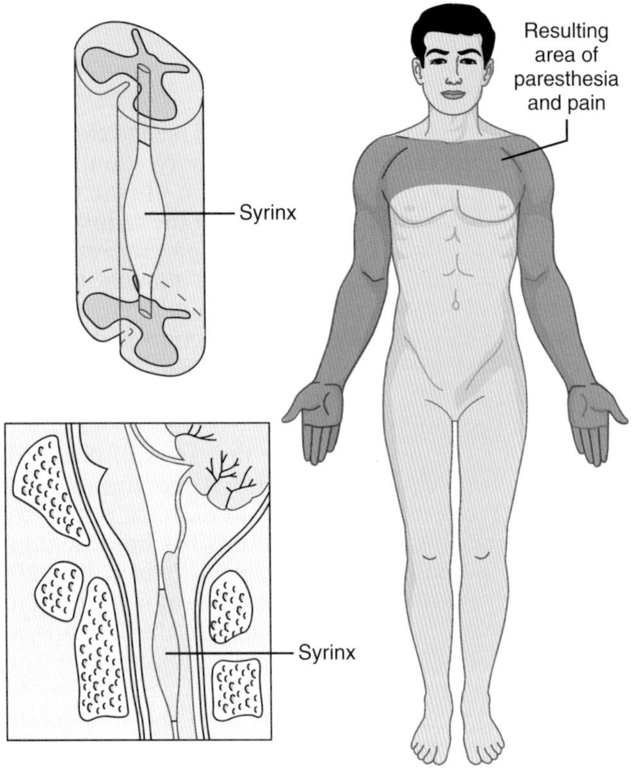


**Fig. 34.8**

A syrinx formed in the late stages of spinal cord injury as a part of syringomyelia.

commonly occurs 4 to 9 years after trauma. One mechanism of syrinx formation is an initial hematomyelia, followed by resorption and formation of a cyst cavity.[58]

In some cases there are multiple cavities. The cavity may occupy almost the entire cross-sectional area of the cord, compressing the posterior columns. As a cyst develops, usually below the level of the initial lesion, there can be significant pain as a result of the compromise of the central spinal cord structures, such as the substantia gelatinosa and the posterior root entry zone.[122] The spinothalamic tracts are involved, which can result in sharp pain that is often the first presenting symptom. There can be lower motor neuron dysfunction, causing weakness, atrophy, and loss of reflex activity. Sensory loss is common, and the sympathetic nervous system can become involved, resulting in conditions such as Horner syndrome.[85]

The thoracic area of the spine is the most common site for the syrinx to develop, with descending and ascending fibers running in the walls of the cavitated lesions. The size and extent of the syrinx are related to symptoms, but because the location is below the site of the lesion, changes are not easily recognized. Syringomyelia may be responsible for spasms, phantom sensations, reflex changes, and autonomic visceral phenomena. Scoliosis can result from the loss of input to the paraspinals.[76] Anything that blocks the free flow of cerebrospinal fluid (CSF) can keep this fluid from moving normally in and out of the head. Pressure can build up in the syrinx, causing expansion and possible rupture, damaging normal spinal cord tissue and injuring nerve cells. Many people with posttraumatic syringomyelia do not develop any symptoms until midlife or later.[60]

Syringomyelia can be a very disabling condition. Spasms, phantom sensations, and autonomic visceral (organ) changes can occur. Sexual dysfunction, muscle spasticity, and loss of bowel or bladder control can develop. The first symptom may be sharp pain. Muscle atrophy, stiffness, and weakness of the neck, back, shoulders, arms, or legs, along with loss of reflexes, are common. Symptoms may be distributed like a cape over the shoulders and back. Headaches and loss of sensation (pinprick and temperature) in the hands may be reported. The symptoms may occur on only one side of the body, depending on where the syrinx develops.

## Clinical Manifestations

### Level of Injury

SCIs are named according to the level of neurologic impairment. Differences may exist in the motor versus sensory levels identified. The International Standards for Neurological Classification of Spinal Cord Injury is widely used for assessment and classification (Fig. 34.9). The American Spinal Injury Association (ASIA) distributes and maintains the ISNCSCI, a multidimensional approach to categorize motor and sensory impairment in individuals with SCI (ASIA 2019). Currently in its eighth edition, it identifies sensory and motor levels indicative of the most rostral spinal levels demonstrating "unimpaired" function. Twenty-eight dermatomes are assessed bilaterally using pinprick and light touch sensation, and 10 key muscles are assessed bilaterally with manual muscle testing. The results are summed to produce overall sensory and motor scores and are used in combination with evaluation of anal sensory and motor function as a basis for the determination of AIS classification.

A clinical examination is conducted to rate sensation as follows: 0 = absent; 1 = impaired; 2 = normal. Muscle function is rated from 0 (total paralysis) to 5 (normal—active movement, full range of motion [ROM] against significant resistance). The presence of anal sensation and voluntary anal contraction are assessed as a yes/no. Bilateral motor and sensory levels and the AIS are based on the results of these examinations. The AIS (5-point ordinal scale)[69] classifies individuals from A (complete SCI) to E (normal sensory and motor function). Preservation of function in the sacral segments (S4-S5) is key for determining the AIS score. The AIS scores are clearly defined and understood by most clinicians working with individuals with SCI.[113]

Lesions are reported as *complete* when there is complete loss of sensory and motor function below the level of the lesion. Complete lesions are a result of spinal cord transection, severe compression or contusion, or extensive vascular dysfunction.

*Incomplete* lesions are the partial loss of sensory and motor function below the level of the injury. Incomplete lesions often occur when there is contusion produced by bony fragments, soft tissue, or edema within the spinal canal. The resulting motor or sensory function is called *sparing*.

ASIA AMERICAN SPINAL INJURY ASSOCIATION — INTERNATIONAL STANDARDS FOR NEUROLOGICAL CLASSIFICATION OF SPINAL CORD INJURY (ISNCSCI) — ISCOS INTERNATIONAL SPINAL CORD SOCIETY

Patient Name________________ Date/Time of Exam ________________

Examiner Name________________ Signature ________________

**RIGHT** — MOTOR KEY MUSCLES — SENSORY KEY SENSORY POINTS: Light Touch (LTR), Pin Prick (PPR)

**LEFT** — SENSORY KEY SENSORY POINTS: Light Touch (LTL), Pin Prick (PPL) — MOTOR KEY MUSCLES

C2, C3, C4

**UER** (Upper Extremity Right) / **UEL** (Upper Extremity Left)

- C5 Elbow flexors
- C6 Wrist extensors
- C7 Elbow extensors
- C8 Finger flexors
- T1 Finger abductors (little finger)

Comments (Non-key Muscle? Reason for NT? Pain? Non-SCI condition?):

T2, T3, T4, T5, T6, T7, T8, T9, T10, T11, T12, L1

**MOTOR** (SCORING ON REVERSE SIDE)

0 = Total paralysis
1 = Palpable or visible contraction
2 = Active movement, gravity eliminated
3 = Active movement, against gravity
4 = Active movement, against some resistance
5 = Active movement, against full resistance
NT = Not testable
0*, 1*, 2*, 3*, 4*, NT* = Non-SCI condition present

**SENSORY** (SCORING ON REVERSE SIDE)

0 = Absent; 1 = Altered; 2 = Normal; NT = Not testable; 0*, 1*, NT* = Non-SCI condition present

C2 C3 C4 C5 C6 T1 T2 T3 T4 T5 T6 T7 T8 T9 T10 T11 T12 L1 L2 L3 L4 L5 S1 S2 S3 S4-5 Dorsum Palm • Key Sensory Points

**LER** (Lower Extremity Right) / **LEL** (Lower Extremity Left)

- L2 Hip flexors
- L3 Knee extensors
- L4 Ankle dorsiflexors
- L5 Long toe extensors
- S1 Ankle plantar flexors

S2, S3, S4-5

(VAC) Voluntary Anal Contraction (Yes/No)

(DAP) Deep Anal Pressure (Yes/No)

RIGHT TOTALS (MAXIMUM) (50) (56) (56)

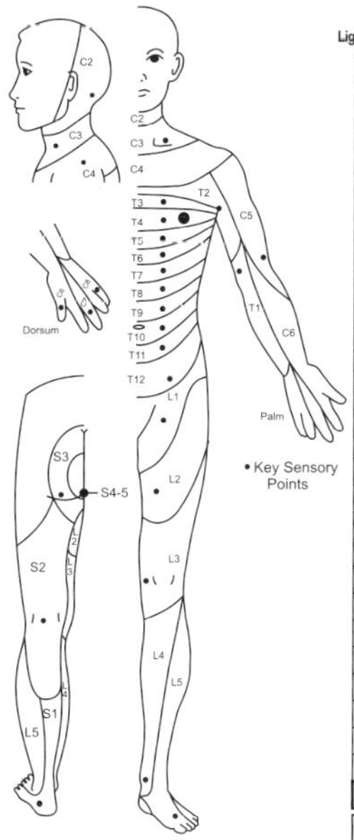

LEFT TOTALS (MAXIMUM) (56) (56) (50)

MOTOR SUBSCORES

UER ___ + UEL ___ = UEMS TOTAL ___ MAX (25) (25) (50)

LER ___ + LEL ___ = LEMS TOTAL ___ MAX (25) (25) (50)

SENSORY SUBSCORES

LTR ___ + LTL ___ = LT TOTAL ___ MAX (56) (56) (112)

PPR ___ + PPL ___ = PP TOTAL ___ MAX (56) (56) (112)

NEUROLOGICAL LEVELS (Steps 1-6 for classification as on reverse) R L — 1. SENSORY 2. MOTOR

3. NEUROLOGICAL LEVEL OF INJURY (NLI)

4. COMPLETE OR INCOMPLETE? Incomplete = Any sensory or motor function in S4-5

5. ASIA IMPAIRMENT SCALE (AIS)

6. ZONE OF PARTIAL PRESERVATION (In injuries with absent motor OR sensory function in S4-5 only) Most caudal levels with any innervation — R L SENSORY MOTOR

Page 1/2 This form may be copied freely but should not be altered without permission from the American Spinal Injury Association. REV 04/19

## Muscle Function Grading

0 = Total paralysis

1 = Palpable or visible contraction

2 = Active movement, full range of motion (ROM) with gravity eliminated

3 = Active movement, full ROM against gravity

4 = Active movement, full ROM against gravity and moderate resistance in a muscle specific position

5 = (Normal) active movement, full ROM against gravity and full resistance in a functional muscle position expected from an otherwise unimpaired person

NT = Not testable (i.e. due to immobilization, severe pain such that the patient cannot be graded, amputation of limb, or contracture of > 50% of the normal ROM)

0*, 1*, 2*, 3*, 4*, NT* = Non-SCI condition present [a]

## Sensory Grading

0 = Absent 1 = Altered, either decreased/impaired sensation or hypersensitivity

2 = Normal NT = Not testable

0*, 1*, NT* = Non-SCI condition present [a]

[a] Note: Abnormal motor and sensory scores should be tagged with a '*' to indicate an impairment due to a non-SCI condition. The non-SCI condition should be explained in the comments box together with information about how the score is rated for classification purposes (at least normal / not normal for classification).

## When to Test Non-Key Muscles:

In a patient with an apparent AIS B classification, non-key muscle functions more than 3 levels below the motor level on each side should be tested to most accurately classify the injury (differentiate between AIS B and C).

| Movement | Root level |
|---|---|
| **Shoulder:** Flexion, extension, adbuction, adduction, internal and external rotation<br>**Elbow:** Supination | C5 |
| **Elbow:** Pronation<br>**Wrist:** Flexion | C6 |
| **Finger:** Flexion at proximal joint, extension<br>**Thumb:** Flexion, extension and abduction in plane of thumb | C7 |
| **Finger:** Flexion at MCP joint<br>**Thumb:** Opposition, adduction and abduction perpendicular to palm | C8 |
| **Finger:** Abduction of the index finger | T1 |
| **Hip:** Adduction | L2 |
| **Hip:** External rotation | L3 |
| **Hip:** Extension, abduction, internal rotation<br>**Knee:** Flexion<br>**Ankle:** Inversion and eversion<br>**Toe:** MP and IP extension | L4 |
| **Hallux and Toe:** DIP and PIP flexion and abduction | L5 |
| **Hallux:** Adduction | S1 |

## ASIA Impairment Scale (AIS)

**A = Complete.** No sensory or motor function is preserved in the sacral segments S4-5.

**B = Sensory Incomplete.** Sensory but not motor function is preserved below the neurological level and includes the sacral segments S4-5 (light touch or pin prick at S4-5 or deep anal pressure) AND no motor function is preserved more than three levels below the motor level on either side of the body.

**C = Motor Incomplete.** Motor function is preserved at the most caudal sacral segments for voluntary anal contraction (VAC) OR the patient meets the criteria for sensory incomplete status (sensory function preserved at the most caudal sacral segments S4-5 by LT, PP or DAP), and has some sparing of motor function more than three levels below the ipsilateral motor level on either side of the body.
(This includes key or non-key muscle functions to determine motor incomplete status.) For AIS C – less than half of key muscle functions below the single NLI have a muscle grade ≥ 3.

**D = Motor Incomplete.** Motor incomplete status as defined above, with at least half (half or more) of key muscle functions below the single NLI having a muscle grade ≥ 3.

**E = Normal.** If sensation and motor function as tested with the ISNCSCI are graded as normal in all segments, and the patient had prior deficits, then the AIS grade is E. Someone without an initial SCI does not receive an AIS grade.

**Using ND:** To document the sensory, motor and NLI levels, the ASIA Impairment Scale grade, and/or the zone of partial preservation (ZPP) when they are unable to be determined based on the examination results.

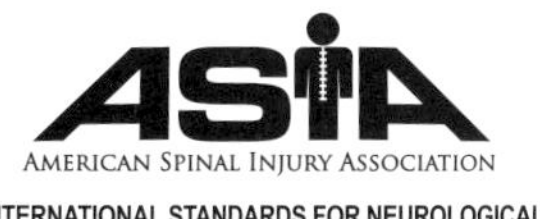


INTERNATIONAL STANDARDS FOR NEUROLOGICAL CLASSIFICATION OF SPINAL CORD INJURY

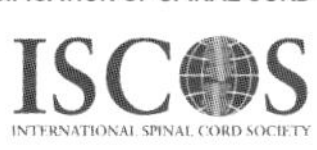


Page 2/2

## Steps in Classification

The following order is recommended for determining the classification of individuals with SCI.

**1. Determine sensory levels for right and left sides.**
*The sensory level is the most caudal, intact dermatome for both pin prick and light touch sensation.*

**2. Determine motor levels for right and left sides.**
*Defined by the lowest key muscle function that has a grade of at least 3 (on supine testing), providing the key muscle functions represented by segments above that level are judged to be intact (graded as a 5).*
*Note: in regions where there is no myotome to test, the motor level is presumed to be the same as the sensory level, if testable motor function above that level is also normal.*

**3. Determine the neurological level of injury (NLI).**
*This refers to the most caudal segment of the cord with intact sensation and antigravity (3 or more) muscle function strength, provided that there is normal (intact) sensory and motor function rostrally respectively.*
*The NLI is the most cephalad of the sensory and motor levels determined in steps 1 and 2.*

**4. Determine whether the injury is Complete or Incomplete.**
*(i.e. absence or presence of sacral sparing)*
*If voluntary anal contraction = **No** AND all S4-5 sensory scores = **0** AND deep anal pressure = **No**, then injury is **Complete**.*
*Otherwise, injury is **Incomplete**.*

**5. Determine ASIA Impairment Scale (AIS) Grade.**
**Is injury Complete? If YES, AIS=A**
**NO ↓**

**Is injury Motor Complete? If YES, AIS=B**
**NO ↓** (No=voluntary anal contraction OR motor function more than three levels below the motor level on a given side, if the patient has sensory incomplete classification)

**Are at least half (half or more) of the key muscles below the neurological level of injury graded 3 or better?**
**NO ↓ AIS=C** **YES ↓ AIS=D**

**If sensation and motor function is normal in all segments, AIS=E**
*Note: AIS E is used in follow-up testing when an individual with a documented SCI has recovered normal function. If at initial testing no deficits are found, the individual is neurologically intact and the ASIA Impairment Scale does not apply.*

**6. Determine the zone of partial preservation (ZPP).**
*The ZPP is used only in injuries with absent motor (no VAC) OR sensory function (no DAP, no LT and no PP sensation) in the lowest sacral segments S4-5, and refers to those dermatomes and myotomes caudal to the sensory and motor levels that remain partially innervated. With sacral sparing of sensory function, the sensory ZPP is not applicable and therefore "NA" is recorded in the block of the worksheet. Accordingly, if VAC is present, the motor ZPP is not applicable and is noted as "NA".*

**Fig. 34.9 American Spinal Injury Association (ASIA) Motor Assessment Form.** (© 2020 American Spinal Injury Association. Reprinted with permission.)

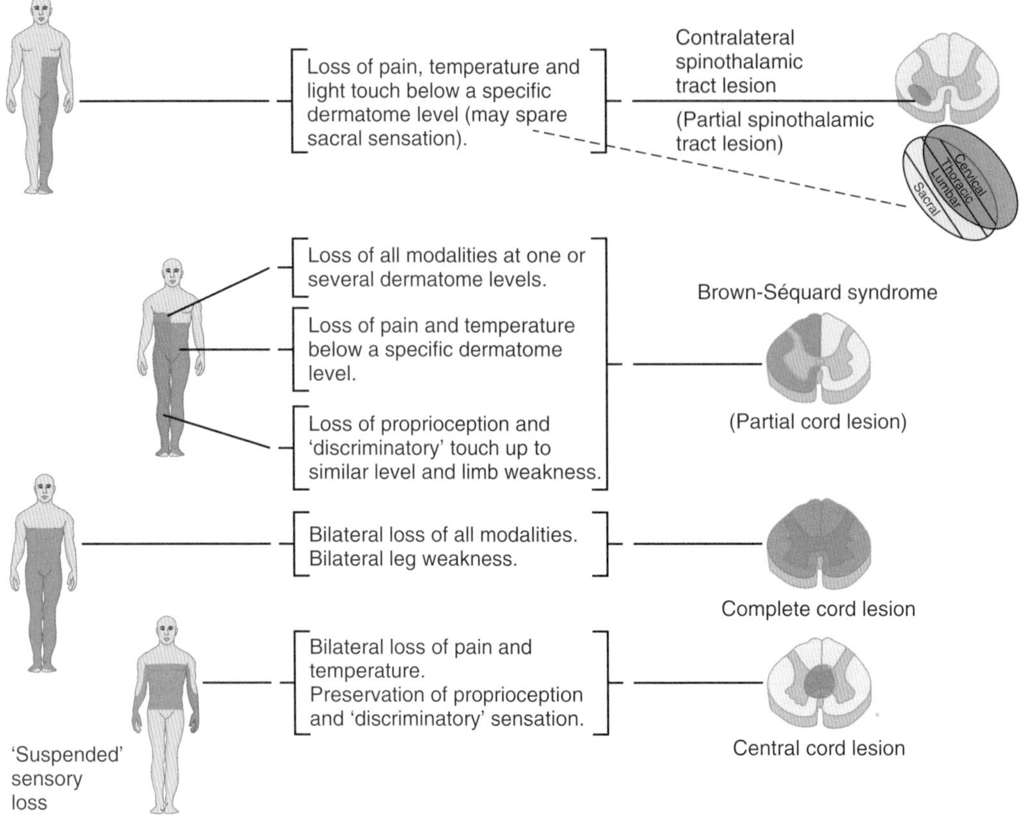


**Fig. 34.10**

**Spinal cord syndromes.** Patterns of sensory loss and weakness. (From Lindsey KW, et al: *Neurology and neurosurgery illustrated*, New York, 1986, Churchill Livingstone, p 188.)

## Spinal Cord Injury Syndromes

Incomplete spinal cord lesions include several recognizable syndromes, as illustrated in Fig. 34.10.*Brown-Séquard syndrome* is characterized by damage to one side of the spinal cord. The most common causes are stab and gunshot wounds. Loss of the entire hemisection of the spinal cord is rare; a natural lesion is irregular. There is weakness ipsilateral to the lesion. Lateral column damage results in abnormal reflexes, including a positive Babinski sign and clonus. Often there is ipsilateral spasticity in the muscles innervated below the lesion. As a result of dorsal column damage, there is loss of proprioception, kinesthesia, and vibratory sense. On the contralateral (opposite) side, there is pain and temperature loss starting a few levels below the lesion. The lateral spinothalamic tract ascends on the same side for several segments before crossing, giving rise to the discrepancy between the level and contralateral signs.

*Anterior cord syndrome* is frequently associated with flexion injuries, such as a backward fall when the head is struck and flexed forward, and is often the result of loss of supply from the anterior spinal artery. Damage to the anterior and anterolateral aspect of the cord results in bilateral loss of motor function and pain and temperature sensation because of interruption of the anterior and lateral spinothalamic tracts and corticospinal tract.

*Central cord syndrome* is a result of damage to the central aspect of the spinal cord, often caused by hyperextension injuries in the cervical region. Neurologic involvement is characteristically more severe in the upper extremities than in the lower extremities. Peripherally located fibers may not be as severely affected, and therefore function may be retained or recovered in the thoracic, lumbar, and sacral regions, including the bowel, bladder, and genitalia.

*Posterior cord syndrome* is extremely rare, with preservation of motor function, pain, and light touch sensation. There is loss of proprioception below the level of the lesion, leading to severe gait deviations.

*Conus medullaris syndrome* and *cauda equina syndrome* reflect damage at the base of the spinal cord and generally result in flaccid lower limb paralysis, flaccid bowel and bladder sphincters, resulting in difficulty with bowel accidents and bladder leakage, and lack of penile erection in men.

The site of spinal cord damage determines the extent of the physical impairments. Injury of the cord in the cervical region results in tetraplegia, or paralysis of all four limbs. In addition to the limbs, the trunk and muscles of respiration are involved. Damage in the thoracic or lumbar region results in paraplegia or paraparesis involving only the lower extremities and generally the lower trunk.

## Changes in Muscle Tone

When the spinal cord is transected, all cord functions below the transection become substantially depressed; this is referred to as *spinal shock*. Spinal shock involves the loss of deep tendon reflexes and voluntary control as well

Box 34.1

**COMMON SYMPTOMS THAT APPEAR DURING SPINAL SHOCK**

- *Arterial blood pressure may fall significantly,* indicating that the output of the *sympathetic* nervous system is completely interrupted.
- *All skeletal muscle reflexes are nonfunctional.* In humans, 2 weeks to several months may be required for reflex activity to return to normal. If the transection is incomplete and some descending pathways remain intact, some reflexes become hyperactive.
- *Sacral autonomic reflexes that regulate bladder and bowel function may be suppressed for several weeks.*

From Hall JE: Spinal cord transection and spinal shock. In: *Pocket companion to Guyton and Hall textbook of medical physiology,* ed 12, St. Louis, 2011, Saunders, p 665.

as flaccidity below the level of the lesion. The condition may persist for a few hours, days, or weeks. It is thought to represent a period during which the excitability of spinal neurons is dramatically reduced owing to the loss of all descending projections. Autonomic symptoms, including sweating and reflex incontinence of bladder and rectum, follow. As is the case in other areas of the nervous system, the affected neurons gradually regain their excitability as they reorganize and adapt to the new levels of reduced synaptic input.[61] Box 34.1 outlines the common physiologic events related to spinal shock.

Spasticity is an inevitable consequence of spinal cord lesions. There is an essential or basic spasticity, which may be of some benefit to the individual when emptying the bladder or flexing the hip and knee. Excess spasticity is triggered by afferent stimuli. Spasticity can be made worse by the presence of constipation, infection, fracture, or a pressure sore below the level of the lesion, and it can be exacerbated by a sudden change in temperature or by physical or emotional stress. Typically the flaccid condition lasts longer and spasticity comes later in a cervical injury compared with a thoracic injury.[68,77]

The Spinal Cord Injury–Spasticity Evaluation Tool (SCI-SET) assesses the impact of spasticity on daily life in people with SCI. It requires participants to recall the past 7 days when rating spasticity on a 7-point scale ranging from −3 (extremely problematic) to +3 (extremely helpful). The SCI-SET assesses the impact of spasticity on daily life in people with SCI.[1] The Penn Spasm Frequency Scale (PSFS) is a self-report measure of the frequency of reported muscle spasms that is commonly used to quantify spasticity. The PSFS is a two-component self-report scale developed to augment clinical ratings of spasticity and provide a more comprehensive understanding of an individual's spasticity status. The first component is a 5-point scale assessing the frequency with which spasms occur, ranging from 0 (no spasms) to 4 (spontaneous spasms occurring more than 10 times per hour). The second component is a 3-point scale assessing the severity of spasms, ranging from 1 (mild) to 3 (severe). The second component is not answered if the person indicates they have no spasms in part 1.[103]

The Spinal Cord Assessment Tool for Spastic Reflexes (SCATS) is a physiologically based measure for spastic reflexes for use in individuals with SCI. It was developed in response to the demand for a standardized, simple clinical measure that encompasses the primary spastic reaction in the SCI population. The SCATS is split into three subscales, each addressing a separate spasm: clonus, lower extremity flexor, and lower extremity extensor. For each subscale, a spasm is triggered with rapid stretch or pinprick stimulus and then rated with a score ranging from 0 to 3.[13]

### Autonomic Nervous System Changes

Autonomic dysreflexia (AD) can occur with a lesion above T6 and is the result of impaired function of the autonomic nervous system (ANS) caused by simultaneous sympathetic and parasympathetic activity. The ANS regulates body functions, such as heart rate, blood pressure, and gland activity. Noxious stimuli, such as overextended bladder or bowel, pain, or other visceral stimuli, will typically elicit a sympathetic response, resulting in vasoconstriction below the level of injury, which leads to an increase in blood pressure. In the healthy spinal cord, descending parasympathetic output compensates for this increase in blood pressure by causing vasodilation to bring blood pressure to a more normal level. Following SCI, sensory nerves below the level of the injury continue to transmit excitatory impulses, causing vasoconstriction and increased blood pressure. In a fully functioning ANS system, rising blood pressure is modified by slower heart rate and vasodilation via parasympathetic feedback loops. As inhibition of sympathetic output below the lesion is blocked, blood pressure keeps rising unchecked. Secretions of neurotransmitters, such as norepinephrine, epinephrine, and dopamine, lead to parasympathetic stimulation to slow the heart rate (bradycardia) through stimulation of the vagus nerve. However, heart rate slowing is insufficient to reduce blood pressure, and vasoconstriction below the lesion persists. Vasodilation occurs above the level of the lesion and results in profuse sweating and skin flushing. A severe pounding headache may follow, with sweating and chills without fever. The increase in blood pressure makes the person susceptible to subarachnoid hemorrhage, renal or retinal hemorrhage, and seizure or myocardial infarction. AD should be handled as a medical emergency.[4,50] Box 34.2 lists signs and triggers of AD.[130]

Loss of thermoregulation below the level of the spinal cord lesion is a result of the disruption of the autonomic pathways from the hypothalamus, resulting in subnormal body temperature in a normal ambient environment. Vasoconstriction and the ability to sweat are lost. Thus the body temperature is greatly influenced by the external environment, and sensory feedback from the head and neck must be used to assist in regulating body temperature. The higher the lesion, the more severe the problem becomes.

### Skeletal Changes

Joint ankylosis caused by heterotopic ossification or ectopic bone formation in the soft tissue such as the tendons and connective tissue can limit ROM, cause pain, and

Box 34.2

**SIGNS AND TRIGGERS OF AUTONOMIC DYSREFLEXIA**

***Signs***

- Sudden and significant (>20 mm Hg) increase in both systolic and diastolic blood pressure above normal (Normal blood pressure when the lesion is above T6 may be 90 to 110 mm Hg systolic and 50 to 60 mm Hg diastolic)
- Onset of a sudden throbbing or pounding headache
- Sweating and flushing of the face, neck, or shoulders
- Goose bumps above the level of the lesion
- Blurred vision
- Visual field changes
- Nasal congestion
- Increased anxiety and apprehension without cause
- Changes in heart rhythm, such as arrhythmias, fibrillation, premature ventricular contractions, bradycardia (relative slowing, may still be in normal range)

***Triggers***

- Urinary system: full bladder, blocked catheter, catheterization, urologic tests, infection, bladder or kidney stones
- GI system: bowel distention/impaction, gastritis, ulcers, hemorrhoids
- Integumentary system: Tight clothing/shoes, contact with hard/sharp objects, blisters, burns, ingrown toenail, insect bites, pressure sores
- Reproductive system: intercourse, sexually transmitted diseases
- Men—ejaculation, scrotal compression, epididymitis; Women—menstruation, pregnancy (especially labor and delivery), vaginitis
- Other systemic causes: deep vein thrombosis, pulmonary emboli, excessive caffeine/alcohol/stimulant intake or substance abuse, fractures or trauma, functional electrical stimulation, heterotopic bone, surgical or invasive procedures

Data from Consortium for Spinal Cord Medicine: *Acute management of autonomic dysreflexia: individuals with spinal cord injury presenting to health-care facilities*, ed 2, Washington, DC, 2001, Paralyzed Veterans of America.

impair seating and posture. It often develops near the large joints, such as the anterior area of the hip, knee, shoulder, and elbow. It is typically found below the level of the lesion and begins to develop within the first year after injury. The initial symptoms are soft tissue swelling, pain, redness, and increased temperature in the affected area. Asymmetric loss of ROM at the affected joint is a common sign of heterotopic ossification. Changes in bony alignment can develop secondary to muscle imbalances caused by unopposed contractions. Scoliosis can develop over time owing to lack of paraspinal support, as depicted in Fig. 34.11.

## Pain

Individuals with SCI must deal with a number of secondary complications in addition to disability caused by the injury itself. Pain, weakness, and fatigue appear to be most common and most closely linked to individual social and mental health functioning.[72] The number of reported pain sites increases over time, regardless of level or completeness of injury. While physical independence, mobility, and social integration remain relatively stable despite increasing numbers of pain sites, increases in depressive symptoms are associated with increased pain. Smokers with SCI report more pain sites than their nonsmoking counterparts.[106]

Pain caused by irritation of the nerve root is common, especially in cauda equina injury. Dysesthesia, impairment of sensation usually perceived as pain, can occur in areas with sensory loss and is often described as burning, pins and needles, or tingling. Disturbances of proprioception are related, where the person feels that a limb is in a different position than it is.

Musculoskeletal pain can result from faulty posture and overuse of limbs. Joint, ligament, and tendon deterioration is common, and secondary injuries from muscle imbalances are related to significant dependence on upper extremities for all activities of daily living (ADLs) and functional mobility—for example, frequent use of anterior shoulder muscles for wheelchair propulsion without equal use of shoulder extensors. Proper strength training can reduce these injuries and lead to more independence.

## Fatigue

Fatigue, noted to be higher than in the general population, may be associated with changes in several systems. ANS changes with inadequate sweating and thermoregulation can cause activity intolerance. Psychologic well-being is associated with fatigue; depression and decreased community mobility can be predicted by increasing reports of fatigue. The amount of effort it takes to accomplish even small tasks after an SCI, such as getting out of bed, showering, and dressing, may also contribute to increased levels of fatigue.

## Respiratory Complications

Respiratory complications associated with SCI can be life threatening. Paralysis of inspiratory muscles, thoracic injuries, and pain can reduce vital capacity.

Lesions above C4 result in paralysis of the diaphragm and generally necessitate artificial ventilation because of loss of phrenic nerve innervation. Pulmonary complications with lesions at C5 through T12 arise as a result of loss of innervation of the abdominal and intercostal muscles. Without the presence of abdominal muscles to provide anterior support to the abdominal cavity, the organs tend to sag forward and inferiorly, compromising the position of the diaphragm. In addition, the abdominal musculature is unable to exert pressure during forced expiration, impairing the ability to cough or create force necessary during loud vocalization or singing. Paralysis of the external oblique muscles also inhibits the person's ability to cough and expel secretions.

An altered breathing pattern, known as the paradoxical breathing pattern, develops in conjunction with the loss of the intercostal muscles and dependence solely on the diaphragm for inhalation. The upper chest wall flattens and the abdominal wall expands, leading to musculoskeletal changes in the trunk.

Aspiration and pneumonia occur frequently in individuals with SCI and are usually associated with high-level injuries, complete lesions, and advanced age. Pneumonia is the most common cause of death, especially in the period immediately after the injury. With no other

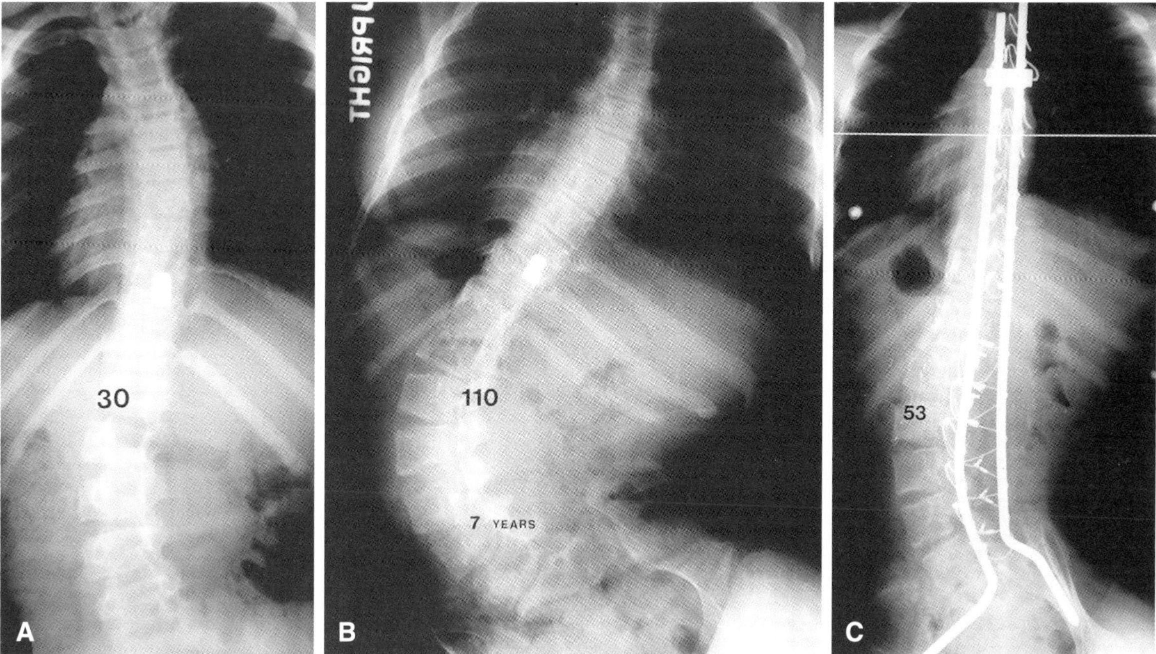


**Fig. 34.11**

**Progressive paralytic scoliosis after a gunshot wound.** (A) Initial curve of 30 degrees. (B) Curve is 110 degrees 7 years later. (C) Correction to 53 degrees after fusion and segmental instrumentation. (From Canale ST, ed: *Campbell's operative orthopaedics*, ed 10, St. Louis, 2003, Mosby.)

complications, proper rehabilitation, and stable respiration, the death rate from pneumonia matches that in the general population.[104]

Impaired ANS control affects the cardiovascular system and includes altered hormonal effects on the cardiovascular system, such as loss of the peripheral muscle pump causing decreased venous return, muscle weakness, and atrophy. Decreased size of cardiac chamber along with greater use of type II over type I muscle fibers and a sedentary lifestyle also compromise cardiac status.[100]

Deep vein thrombosis and pulmonary embolism are associated with SCI because of increased coagulability of blood and decreased venous return. This may be associated with sympathetic dysfunction and unopposed vagal action. Risk of cardiovascular involvement is due to a greater prevalence of obesity, lipid disorders, metabolic syndrome, and diabetes. Daily energy expenditure is significantly lower in individuals with SCI, not only because of a lack of motor function but also because of a lack of accessibility and fewer opportunities to engage in physical activity.[94]

### Metabolic Conditions

Persons with SCI are prone to abnormal carbohydrate metabolism and are found to develop hyperinsulinemia and insulin resistance. During the acute phase of SCI, there is significant weight loss, especially with tetraplegia, associated with increased metabolic demands, muscle atrophy, and a negative nitrogen and calcium balance. Hypoproteinemia can be caused by pressure ulcers. Over time, there is usually an increase in body fat in proportion to lean tissue in persons with chronic SCI. A more sedentary lifestyle as a result of SCI may predispose a person to some of these conditions.

Soon after SCI, bones start losing minerals and become less dense. This may be due to alteration of the autonomic and circulatory systems. Inactivity and lack of weight bearing also foster the development of osteoporosis. It is thought that individuals with SCI may have an earlier onset and a greater extent of osteoporosis, with higher risk of fracture.

### Pressure Ulcers

Pressure ulcers are a frequent complication of SCI. They arise primarily because of persistent pressure in the area of a bony prominence. Moisture, poor nutrition, complete lesions, acute illness, and cigarette smoking predispose the skin to breakdown. Persons who do not follow through on self-care requirements because of their own choice, depression, lack of motivation, substance abuse, or alcoholism are also prone to develop more and deeper pressure ulcers. Initially the sacrum, heel, and scapula are the most common sites of ulcer formation because of time spent in bed. As the individual begins to use a chair for mobility, the trochanter and ischium become common sites of pressure ulcers.[128]

### Bowel and Bladder Control

Bowel and bladder control is commonly impaired in a person with SCI. The spinal center for urination is in the conus medullaris. Primary reflex control originates from the sacral segment. During the stage of spinal shock, the bladder is flaccid, with absence of muscle tone and bladder reflexes. Lesions above the conus medullaris will cause a reflex neurogenic bladder, demonstrated by spasticity, voiding difficulties, detrusor muscle hypertrophy, and urethral reflux. Lesions at the conus medullaris cause nonreflex bladders, resulting in flaccidity and decreased tone of the perineal muscles and urethral sphincter. These

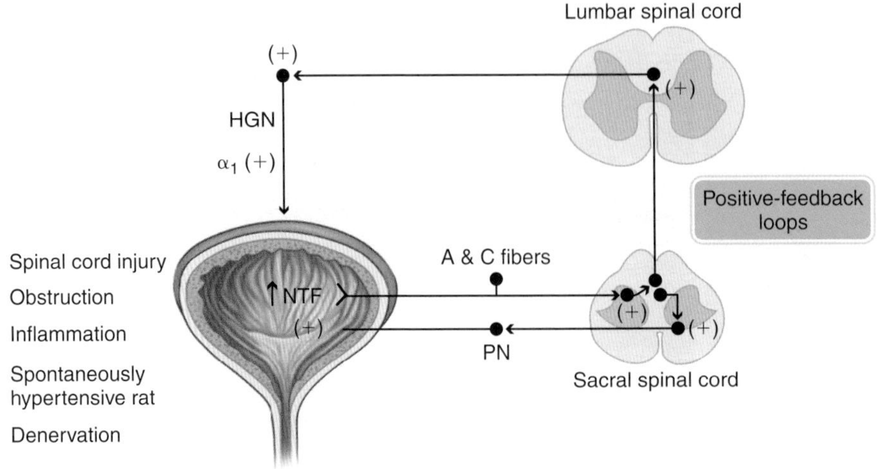


**Fig. 34.12**

**Possible mechanisms underlying spasticity in bladder reflex pathways induced by various pathologic conditions.** Bladders from rats with chronic spinal cord injury exhibit increased levels of neurotrophic factor *(NTF)* such as nerve growth factor. Neurotrophic factors can increase the excitability of C-fiber bladder afferent neurons and alter reflex mechanisms in parasympathetic excitatory pathways in the pelvic nerve *(PN)* as well as in sympathetic pathways in the hypogastric nerve *(HGN)*. These reflex circuits are organized in the spinal cord as positive-feedback loops that induce involuntary bladder activity. (From Wein AJ, et al: *Campbell-Walsh urology*, ed 9, Philadelphia, 2007, Saunders.)

are characterized as lower motor neuron lesions. Bowel patterns mimic bladder responses in their response to spinal shock; reflex bowel occurs in upper motor neuron lesions above the conus medullaris, and nonreflex bowel is caused by lower motor neuron damage to the conus and cauda equina.[82] Fig. 34.12 shows bladder reflex pathways in an animal model.

Urinary tract infection is the most frequent secondary medical complication seen in persons with SCI. This persists despite improved catheter materials and design and use of antibiotics. In concert with this is the increased concentration of calcium in the urinary system, which leads to formation of kidney stones. Calculi in the kidney are a complication found more frequently in individuals using an indwelling catheter.[19]

## Sexuality

Sexual response is directly related to the level and completeness of injury. Sexual function relies on pathways similar to those of the bladder and bowel and is altered as described earlier. There are two types of responses: reflexogenic, or a response to external stimulation seen in persons with upper motor neuron lesions, and psychogenic, a response that occurs through cognitive activity, such as fantasy, associated with lower motor neuron lesions. Men with higher-level lesions can often achieve a reflexive erection but typically do not ejaculate. With cauda equina lesions, erection and ejaculation are not usually possible. The primary reason for pursuing sexual activity is for intimacy needs, not fertility. Bladder and bowel concerns during sexual activity are not strong enough to deter the majority of the population from engaging in sexual activity. In addition, the occurrence of AD during typical bladder or bowel care is a significant variable predicting the occurrence and distress of AD during sexual activity.[5] Menses are typically interrupted for approximately 3 to 6 months after SCI; when restored, they can be another cause of AD. Fertility and pregnancy are not altered by SCI, but any pregnancy must be observed closely, especially in the last trimester. Labor may begin without the woman's knowledge because of loss of sensation, and labor may initiate AD.[109]

## Sleep Disorders

The prevalence of obstructive sleep apnea–hypopnea syndrome (OSAHS) is high after cervical cord injury. OSAHS is characterized by repeated oxygen desaturation. OSAHS should be suspected especially in individuals with daytime sleepiness, obesity, and frequent awakenings during sleep.[86] The changes in heart rhythm associated with OSAHS include sinusal arrhythmia, severe bradycardia, and ventricular and supraventricular tachycardia. The risk of sudden death, particularly of cardiovascular cause, is well known.[21]

# MEDICAL MANAGEMENT

**DIAGNOSIS.** Delayed recognition of SCI is a significant problem in emergent care of traumatic injuries, occurring in more than 20% of cases.

Lateral film studies with plain radiographs are a rapid and effective way of evaluating cervical SCI, with the ability to detect approximately 85% of such injuries. When the open-mouth odontoid view and supine anteroposterior view are added, the accuracy increases to almost 100%. Any area that is inadequately demonstrated in the three-view spinal series is examined by computed tomography (CT). Flexion-extension studies are used primarily to evaluate instability caused by occult ligamentous injury and should not be done if there is any neurologic, bony, or soft tissue injury. The sensitivity of CT scanning is much greater than plain x-rays in the detection of spinal injuries. CT is superior to other diagnostic procedures in demonstrating impingement on the neuronal canal.[37]

Magnetic resonance imaging (MRI) can show the extent of soft tissue damage when x-ray may not (Fig.

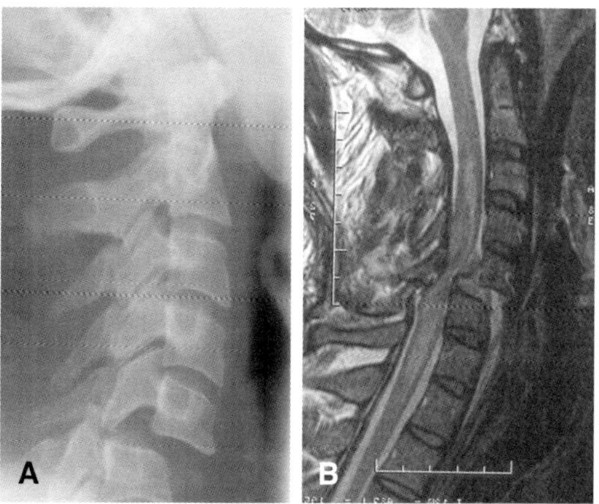

**Fig. 34.13**

(A) Plain lateral x-ray of the cervical spine showing a C5-6 dislocation. (B) T2-weighted magnetic resonance of the same patient showing severe spinal cord damage. (From Bersten AD, Soni N: *Oh's intensive care manual*, ed 6, Oxford, 2008, Butterworth-Heinemann.)

34.13). Fig. 34.14 shows a Jefferson fracture seen on x-ray and MRI. Fig. 34.15 compares fractures at time of injury and after stabilization. Myelography is indicated for optimal visualization of compression of the spinal cord after trauma. Myelography alone is rarely indicated; it is used in conjunction with CT in situations where MRI is not available or possible.

In acute SCI, MRI is sometimes contraindicated because of its limited use around ferromagnetic objects such as respirators, oxygen tanks, and traction devices. When these obstacles do not exist, the extent of spinal cord damage and the possibility of disk herniation can be more readily assessed by MRI. The presence of intradural or extradural hematoma can often be demonstrated on MRI. MRI is useful in excluding spinal cord contusion or hemorrhage in persons with neurologic deficits and normal CT scans and plain films.[41]

Advanced structural imaging techniques, such as diffusion tensor imaging and magnetization transfer, offer benefits over traditional structural imaging techniques. Diffusion tensor imaging provides a unique image contrast called diffusion anisotropy. This reveals tissue organization at the microscopic level based on the average motion of water molecules.[9,93]

Advanced MRI techniques are better than conventional MRI in visualizing chronic SCI. The development of functional MRI, currently useful in imaging the brain, and its application to the spinal cord could revolutionize the field of regeneration. Transplanted cells can now be tracked after they are placed in living organisms, using MRI. Neural stem cells are labeled with paramagnetic agents before they are transplanted, and MRI tracks their distribution and migration after they are placed in the damaged spinal cord.

In spinal trauma with severe neural malfunction, neurophysiologic studies help in determining which neural elements are involved; which spinal segment is responsible for mechanical or other irritation; and whether the lesion is chronic, acute progressing, or resolving. Neurophysiologic studies allow intraoperative monitoring and include somatosensory evoked potentials, motor evoked potentials, neurography, F-wave and H-reflex electromyography, and sympathetic skin response. Somatosensory evoked potentials and motor evoked potentials are useful in the investigation of the CNS. Electromyography, neurography, and F-wave and H-reflex studies are used for evaluation of the peripheral component of spinal injury.[129] The use of

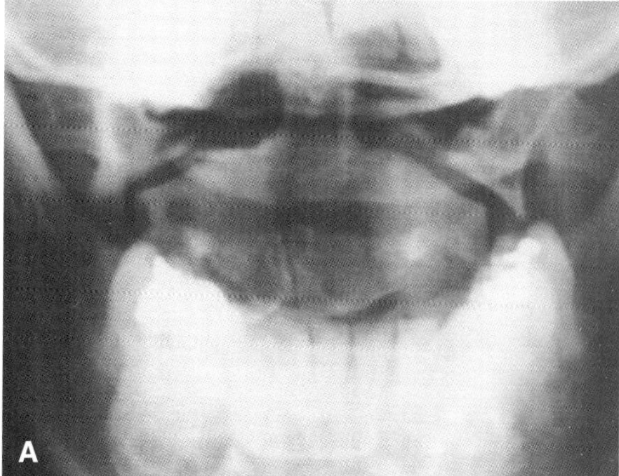

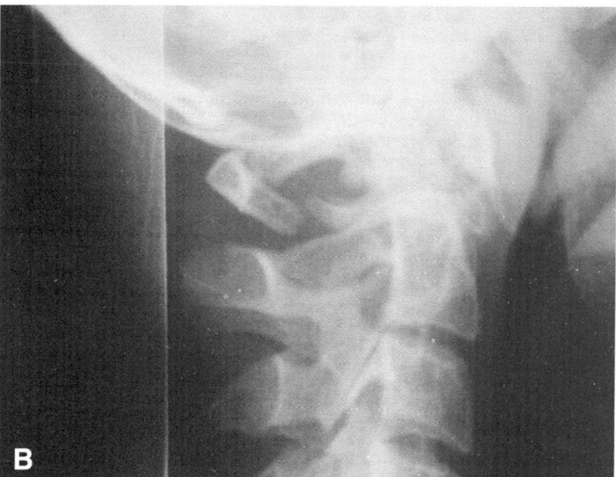

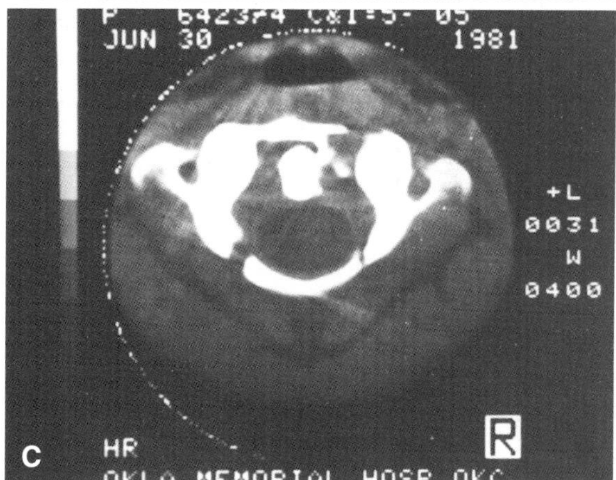


**Fig. 34.14**

**Fracture of C1 (Jefferson fracture).** (A) Anteroposterior view showing lateral displacement of the lateral mass and articulating facets of C1 on C2. (B) Oblique view illustrating disruption of the posterior aspect of the ring of C1. (C) Computed tomography scan revealing the true extent of the injury. (From Green NE, Swiotkowski MF, eds: *Skeletal trauma in children*, ed 3, Philadelphia, 2003, Saunders. Courtesy Dr. Teresa Stacy.)

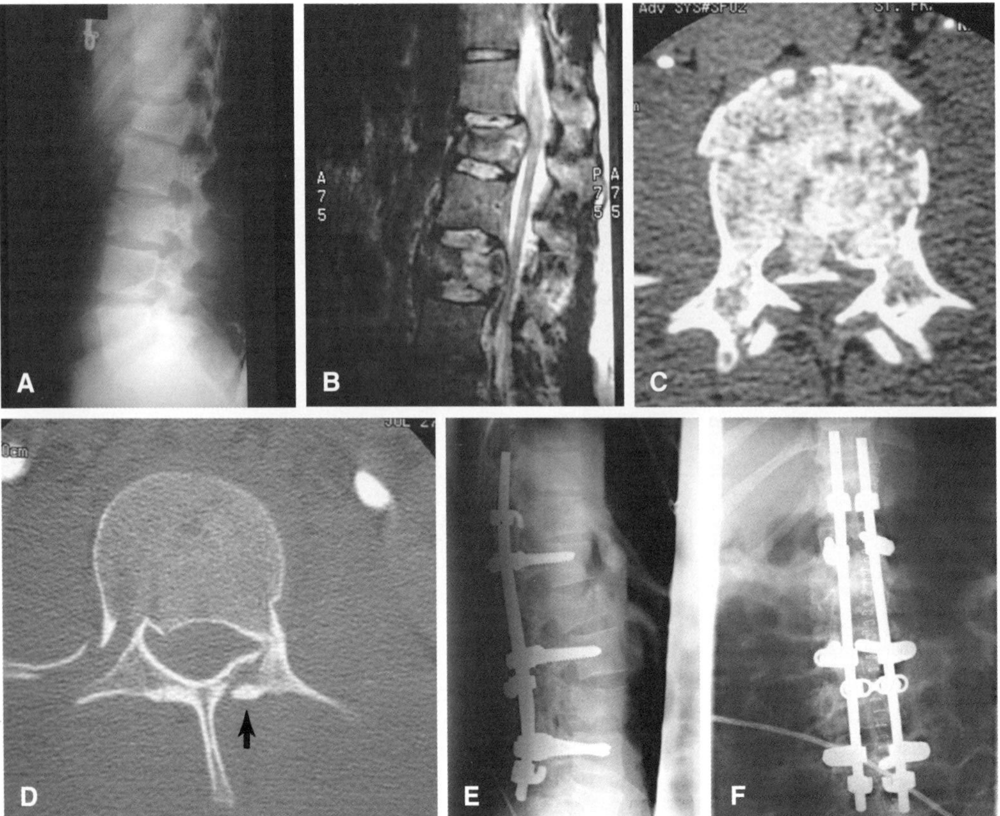

**Fig. 34.15**

A 21-year-old man involved in a motor vehicle accident sustained a burst fracture of L1 and L3. The patient had an incomplete spinal cord injury. (A) Preoperative lateral view shows loss of height predominantly at L1. (B) Sagittal-cut magnetic resonance imaging shows compression at both L1 and L3. (C) Axial-cut computed tomography (CT) scan at L3 shows a retropulsed fragment filling half the canal. (D) Axial CT scan at L1 shows a fracture of the lamina and retropulsion of a fragment into the canal. (E) This injury was stabilized with Isola instrumentation combining both pedicle screws and laminar hooks. Sagittal alignment was maintained. (F) Postoperative anteroposterior radiograph showing a cross-connection added for additional stability. (From Browner BD, et al: *Skeletal trauma: basic science, management, and reconstruction*, ed 3, Philadelphia, 2003, Saunders.)

neuromodulation and stimulation techniques is being actively studied in preclinical contexts, with increasing applications of these approaches to individuals with chronic SCI.

A unique SCI syndrome, burning hands syndrome, was first described in sports injury. This syndrome appears to be a variation of central cord syndrome associated with severe burning paresthesias and dysesthesias in the hands and/or the feet. Other signs of neurologic dysfunction are minimal or absent. More than 50% of the time there is an underlying spinal fracture-dislocation. It is important to differentiate this syndrome from the much more common and usually innocuous "burning" or "stinging" of brachial plexus origin.

Diagnosis of syringomyelia may be delayed because the early symptoms are so similar to symptoms of other, more common neurologic disorders. The accident that caused the initial damage may have occurred months to years before the onset of symptoms. MRI is the best imaging study for diagnosing this disorder in the beginning stages. MRI will show the syrinx number, size, and location and any other abnormalities of the spine and spinal cord. Functional MRI allows the surgeon to see the spinal fluid within the syrinx.

TREATMENT. Interventions at several levels are required to reduce mortality and morbidity while improving function and quality of life.

***Emergent Care.*** The emergent phase of care is crucial for the person with traumatic SCI. It can make the difference between living the rest of life with a disability or recovering with only temporary neurologic deficits. An incomplete injury can be made worse by mishandling and can be made better by prompt attention to critical procedures. Box 34.3 includes the guidelines endorsed by the International Association for Trauma Surgery and Intensive Care.

Assessment of the likelihood of SCI includes understanding the mechanics of the trauma and obtaining vital signs. In the case of a cervical injury, paradoxic respiration or abdominal breathing may be present, and immediate immobilization should be instituted. Use of a rigid collar and spinal board can help to prevent movement of the spinal column.

Monitoring in the critical care phase includes cardiac and neurologic status. Orthopedic management may begin at this phase and includes closed and open reduction of the vertebrae and decompression of the spinal cord. Surgery, including fusion and internal fixation, is

Box 34.3

**ESSENTIAL TRAUMA CARE SERVICES ENDORSED BY THE INTERNATIONAL ASSOCIATION FOR TRAUMA SURGERY AND INTENSIVE CARE AS THE RIGHTS OF THE INJURED**

- Obstructed airways are opened and maintained before hypoxia leads to death or permanent disability.
- Impaired breathing is supported until the injured person is able to breathe adequately without assistance.
- Pneumothorax and hemothorax are promptly recognized and relieved.
- Bleeding (external or internal) is promptly stopped.
- Shock is recognized and treated with intravenous fluid replacement before irreversible consequences occur.
- The consequences of traumatic brain injury are lessened by timely decompression of space-occupying lesions and by prevention of secondary brain injury.
- Intestinal and other abdominal injuries are promptly recognized and repaired.
- Potentially disabling extremity injuries are corrected.
- Potentially unstable spinal cord injuries are recognized and managed appropriately, including early immobilization.
- The consequences to the individual of injuries that result in physical impairment are minimized by appropriate rehabilitative services.
- Medications for these services and for the minimization of pain are readily available when needed.

From Mock C, et al: *Guidelines for essential trauma care*, Geneva, 2004, World Health Organization; with permission.

the most common procedure performed and typically requires use of an orthosis to stabilize the surgical site for 8 to 12 weeks. The goal is to restore spinal alignment, establish spinal stability, and prevent further neurologic deterioration, enhancing recovery. In this early phase of care, secondary injury to the spinal cord is minimized by surgical decompression and maintenance of perfusion by minimizing low blood pressure. Preclinical investigations are ongoing of various interventions with neuroprotective effects, with clinical trials in humans being conducted to investigate safety and efficacy for their use.[119] A systematic review of 16 clinical trials supports the use of methylprednisolone in some cases, with trends showing very modest benefits with the use of minocycline (antibiotic that crosses the blood-brain barrier), Sygen (GM-1 ganglioside, a component of CNS cell membranes), and progesterone with vitamin D (possible reduction of oxidative stress and apoptosis). Fig. 34.16 demonstrates the neuroprotective processes that may be integral within immunomodulation using minocycline. Human clinical trials are under way using riluzole, a medication used for amyotrophic lateral sclerosis that reduces excitotoxicity, and BA-210 (Cethrin), a medication applied directly to the dura after SCI, that may reduce inhibition of regeneration.[73]

The use of methylprednisolone sodium succinate (MPSS) after SCI has had a controversial course. Once used widely, revisions in clinical guidelines in 2002 and 2013 discouraged its use, but an American Association of Neurologic Surgeons clinical guideline[51] recommends MPSS as a treatment option if provided in a 24-hour dose (only if initiated in the first 8 hours after injury) regardless of level of SCI.[119] Loss of ANS control affects the function of the cardiovascular system.[52] The autonomic lesion predisposes persons with high spinal cord lesions to abnormal cardiovascular responses to vasoactive agents.

***Management of Complications.*** Management of complications of SCI is critical. High cervical injuries require immediate placement of ventilation equipment and maintenance of pulmonary hygiene. Therapy consists of intermittent positive-pressure breathing, bronchodilators, and mucolytics. Prevention of pulmonary infection is critical in SCI.

Bilateral diaphragmatic pacing can be considered as an alternative method of ventilatory support in a select group of patients who have high SCI and preserved function of the phrenic nerve–diaphragm unit. The most suitable candidates for pacing are patients with a preserved response to peripheral phrenic nerve stimulation but lacking a response to transcranial stimulation of the diaphragm motor area.[114]

Treatment of spasticity includes use of muscle relaxants and spasmolytic agents.[108] Peripheral nerve blocks, such as botulinum toxin (Botox) and phenol, provide a temporary reduction of spasticity. In cases where spasticity is severe and not managed well with oral and injected medications, intrathecal baclofen is also an alternative.[90] Intrathecal baclofen must be carefully monitored to avoid severe complications. Spasticity-related interventions need to be aimed at what matters most to the individual. It is critical for clinicians to understand individuals' experiences to make accurate assessments, effectively evaluate treatment interventions, and select appropriate management strategies.[87,88]

***Pain Management.*** Despite the fact that SCI causes loss of sensation, there is often significant pain that develops over time. Pain in SCI is classified in many different ways associated with intrinsic or neurogenic dysfunction, such as pain associated with syringomyelia and musculoskeletal or mechanical pain.

Management of neurogenic pain in SCI is by systemic or local drug therapy and by neuroaugmentative and neurodestructive intervention. The pharmacologic approach includes nonsteroidal analgesics, opioids, antidepressants, and anticonvulsants.[67] Pregabalin (Lyrica) is associated with relief of central neuropathic pain and with reduction in pain-related sleep interference and significant improvement in sleep problems. Action on centrally located calcium channels may be important in the effectiveness of pregabalin in managing central neuropathic pain.

Neurodestructive procedures include both chemical and surgical destruction of nervous structures. Procedures may include deafferentation, interruption of ascending pain systems, or destruction of cells in the dorsal horn.

Decompressive surgery is performed in individuals with spinal cord syringomyelia, depending on which area is affected. Surgery to create a pseudomeningomyelocele, an artificial CSF reservoir, performed to normalize the CSF flow may be effective. By draining the cyst, it is possible to prevent the cyst from reexpanding. Draining the fluid can relieve pain, headache, and a sensation of tightness in the head or neck. In a dural graft procedure, the

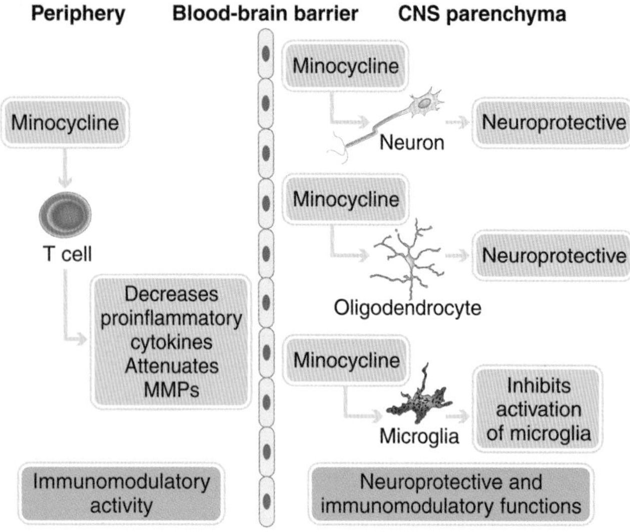


**Fig. 34.16**

**Peripheral and central functions of minocycline.** Minocycline has immunomodulatory activity in the periphery and both immunomodulatory and neuroprotective capacity within the central nervous system *(CNS)*. *MMPs,* Matrix metalloproteinases. (From Yong VW, Wells J, Giuliani F, et al: The promise of minocycline in neurology. *The Lancet Neurology* 3(12):744–751, 2004.)

space around the spinal cord is enlarged to allow free flow of fluid and reduce pressure.

***Strategies for Future Consideration.*** Transplantation of stem cells is being studied extensively in relation to the treatment of SCI. Processes include producing regenerative growth factors, expressing substances capable of breaking down scar tissue, and modulating the response of the immune system to injury. It appears that there will be potential for reprogramming the host microenvironment; for example, embryonic stem cell transplantation reduces macrophage influx by more than 50%. Table 34.1 describes different types of stem cells and how they may offer benefits after SCI; however, each cell type has different limitations that may include the development of tumors or immune system rejection. Currently clinical trials using stem cells have focused on safety, with no or very limited functional benefits in small cohort trials without controls.

Critical components of optimal care following SCI are protection of neural tissue and limitation of secondary damage, facilitation of axonal regrowth, and control of factors that inhibit intrinsic neural repair. Because the consequences of SCI are complex, it is most likely that a hierarchy of intervention strategies will be needed to restore suprasegmental control leading to the recovery of function in the spinal cord.[12,64] The phases of injury and the neurophysiologic events will create both limitations and advantages related to potential treatments administered during the different phases of injury. Preclinical studies using transplantation of activated autologous macrophages after experimental SCI have been performed, based on the premise that the relative inability of the CNS to regenerate may be a result of insufficient recruitment and activation of macrophages within the injured CNS. Studies from several laboratories have demonstrated the ability for peripheral macrophages to synthesize nerve growth factor and phagocytose myelin, providing an additional rationale for using hematogenous macrophages to repair the injured spinal cord. Human studies are under way; however, issues of cost and timing of application have limited outcomes.[2]

Embryonic stem cells are true stem cells that show unlimited capacity for self-renewal. In contrast, adult stem cells are progenitor cells or cells that are immature or undifferentiated. Numerous preclinical studies suggest that embryonic and adult stem cells, along with their lineage-specific progenitors, may improve outcome after experimental SCI. Transplanted stem cells may potentially act through several proposed mechanisms, which include providing trophic support to promote the survival and regrowth of host tissue, acting as a cellular scaffold to permit axonal elongation through the site of injury, and replacing lost or damaged cells. The demyelination of intact axons is a prominent feature of SCI and contributes to loss of function after injury, leading to potential therapeutic strategies that involve the replacement of myelin-producing cells through the transplantation of embryonic stem cells.[14]

Following tissue damage or injury, progenitor cells can be activated by growth factors or cytokines, leading to increased cell division important for the repair process. Progenitor cells participate in the normal maintenance of the CNS. These mechanisms include production and replacement of cells lost to normal aging and cell turnover. Human embryonic stem cells (hESCs) may offer a renewable source of a wide range of cell types for use in research and cell-based therapies to treat disease, but there are controversies associated with obtaining and using these cells. Researchers have successfully differentiated hESCs along the oligodendrocyte lineage, obtaining highly purified oligodendrocyte progenitor cells (OPCs). The transplantation of hESC-derived OPCs into adult rats after SCI has been shown to enhance remyelination and improve motor function. There may be potential to predifferentiate hESCs into functional OPCs offering therapeutic benefits. However, it remains unclear whether the improved functional recovery that has been seen in preclinical studies is due to enhanced remyelination, to the secretion of trophic factors by OPCs, or to other neuroprotective effects of OPC transplantation that have yet to be identified.[14]

Progenitor cells transplanted during the acute injury phase are vulnerable to the same set of cell death mechanisms predominant during the secondary phase of acute injury. Understanding the function of growth-inhibiting factors within the adult CNS may lead to control of the neural destruction after SCI.[16]

Astrocytes can express molecules that are both growth permissive and growth inhibitory at the same time. After SCI, reactive astrocytes form an astroglial scar that inhibits axonal regeneration that borders a nonneural lesion core.[101] Maintaining an environment to support the growth of axons may involve the selective removal of astrocytes from the site of injury.[39,115] In contrast, glial restricted precursor–derived astrocytes may promote axonal regeneration via suppression of astrogliosis, realignment of host tissues, and delay of expression of inhibitory proteoglycans. The glia, not the neurons, are the critical

**Table 34.1** Stem Cell Therapy for Spinal Cord Injury

| Stem Cell Type and Source | Possible Therapeutic Benefits in SCI | Advantages | Limitations |
|---|---|---|---|
| Mesenchymal stem cells—bone marrow, umbilical cord, amnion, placenta, fat tissue | Secretion of antiinflammatory factors, cytokines, growth factors to improve lesion environment; promotion of self-repair; immunomodulatory, neurotrophic, and antiapoptotic benefits | High differentiation, easily isolated and grafted, suitable for different postinjury stages, no ethical concerns, limited tumor risk, minimal immunoreactivity | Mechanisms still require research; results of clinical trials far from showing functional recovery or restoring neural circuits; effective way to deliver cells requires further research |
| Embryonic stem cells—obtained from fetal tissue, but can differentiate into different tissue cells | Differentiated neurons and glial cells used to address cell defects caused by SCI; secretion of active factors to inhibit further damage, supportive of nerve tissue regeneration | Long history of research, proven to have certain effects in various diseases, pluripotent cells can differentiate into all tissue cells | Difficulty with immune rejection; risk of tumor formation; ethical issues are significant |
| Neural stem cells—lateral ventricle of brain, dentate gyrus of hippocampus, central canal of spinal cord | Modulation of formation of glial scar, enhancement of oligodendrocyte and neuronal differentiation; replacement of necrotic cells and reconstruction of local loops that promote functional recovery; secretion of growth factors for damaged neurons; immunomodulatory effects | Reduced tumor risk for only glial and neuronal subtypes; can be harvested from adult or fetal spinal cord tissue | Additional study needed to confirm neurologic and functional benefits, safety, and appropriate doses and administration; determination of most promising cellular source is needed |
| Induced pluripotent stem cells (alternative to embryonic stem cells) | Cells induced to be neural progenitor cells, neurons, oligodendrocytes, and astrocytes; promotion of remyelination, axonal regeneration, and secretion of neurotrophic factors; reduction of inflammation | Can self-renew and differentiate into various neural cells; free of ethical issues associated with some transplant sources; can be performed autologously, so immune system suppression is not required | High risk of immune rejection and tumor development (teratoma and true tumors) |
| Spermatogonial stem cells | Potential to differentiate into various nervous system cells including functional GABAergic neurons, glutaminergic neurons, serotonergic neurons, and glial cells | Multidifferentiation potential; self-replication and self-renewal; avoid intermediate transition phase for embryonic stem cells and neural stem cells; can be produced throughout lifetime; lacks ethical issues, tumor risk, and immune rejection | Potential for differentiation is susceptible to environmental influences; use with neurologic diseases is designed to substitute for differentiation at present time; no reports of secretion of beneficial factors |
| Adult endogenous stem cells—located in adult nervous system | Activation and proliferation to produce glial cells with SCI; differentiation into astrocytes and oligodendrocytes | Noninvasive cell therapy that directly activates to function without need for traumatic cell transplantation | Limited ability to differentiate into neurons |

*SCI*, Spinal cord injury.
Adapted from Shao A, et al: Crosstalk between stem cell and spinal cord injury: pathophysiology and treatment strategies. *Stem Cell Res Ther* 10:238, 2019.

elements in preventing growth and in restoring it. Neurons retain the power to grow, and their sprouts await only the provision of a suitable glial pathway to be able to advance across the lesion core.

Inflammatory reactions in the CNS have a dual nature; they may be both neuroprotective and neurotoxic. Studies illustrate that the nervous and immune systems have overlapping rules of organization and intercellular communication. Schwann cells have been used to facilitate a permissive environment for the injured spinal cord to regenerate. The Schwann cell is one of the most widely studied cell types for repair of the spinal cord. These cells play a crucial role in endogenous repair of peripheral nerves because of their ability to dedifferentiate, migrate, proliferate, and express growth-promoting factors and extracellular matrix molecules and myelinate regenerating axons. Following SCI, Schwann cells migrate from the periphery into the injury site, where they participate in endogenous repair process. Previous experiments have shown compressive mechanical stress to be important in stimulating the regenerative behavior of Schwann cells. Transplantation of highly permissive Schwann cell–enriched peripheral nerve grafts may enhance regeneration in SCI.[43] For transplantation into the spinal cord, large numbers of Schwann cells are necessary to fill injury-induced cystic cavities. One of the problems encountered is the fact that axons do not regenerate beyond the transplant, owing to the inhibitory nature of the glial scar surrounding the injury. Although Schwann cells have great potential for repair, the process needs to be supplemented by using trophic factors and removing growth-inhibitory molecules associated with the astroglial scar and damaged myelin.

The use of olfactory ensheathing cells, harvested from the olfactory bulb and olfactory mucosa, have been extensively studied in animal models and applied in human studies, as these cells have the ability to improve axonal regeneration, naturally increase neurotrophic factors, and may reduce inhibitory factors in the microenvironment after an injury. Clinical trials in humans have demonstrated mixed effects that may relate to whether or not the cells harvested before use have been purified to ensure that the most effective cells are implanted. The development of consistent procedures in these treatment approaches may influence how widespread their use becomes.[127]

Peripheral nerves may be able to provide an axonal bridge across the longer areas of spinal cord damage by activating nerve impulses carried from the brain, through intercostal nerve axons grown from implanted nerve, into the isolated distal end of the transected spinal cord, bridging the transection and connecting with neurons in the gray matter of the isolated distal segment of the spinal cord. It is possible that inferior-to-superior nerve bridging can produce return of function, just as superior-to-inferior nerve bridging does. The methods used for peripheral nerve grafting continue to be explored and refined in preclinical studies. Peripheral nerve grafting techniques have been developed using segments of sciatic nerve, either placed directly between the damaged rostral and caudal ends of the injury site or used to form a bridge across the lesion to restore functional connectivity across the lesion site.[14]

The use of biomimetic neural scaffolds has also been a focus of extensive preclinical research with development of numerous applications approved by the Food and Drug Administration for use in peripheral nerve injury. Tubular conduits are created from collagen, using cross-species xenografts (e.g., porcine) or synthetic materials (e.g., silicone) with an architecture similar to the structures within peripheral nerves to guide nerve regrowth after injury, integrating methods to improve peripheral nerve regeneration such as growth factors and stem cells. These approaches have largely been tested in preclinical studies to bridge small gaps in peripheral nerves, but similar approaches may be applied to SCI in the future.[46]

***Neuromodulation.*** Increasingly there are studies using various forms of brain, spinal cord, and peripheral nerve stimulation to address the impairments that result from SCI that can be characterized as neuromodulation interventions.[38,64,70] Brain stimulation approaches include transcranial magnetic stimulation, transcranial direct current stimulation, deep brain stimulation, and epidural cortical stimulation. These applications target supraspinal input, often focusing on upper extremity control. Epidural spinal stimulation focuses on improving spinal circuitry and has primarily targeted locomotion or leg movements.[18] Brain–machine interfaces allow an individual to use brain activity to activate functional electrical stimulation (FES) of specific muscle groups or trigger epidural stimulation or in some instances to drive external devices, such as a robotic arm or an exoskeleton. More traditional FES is also used for peripheral nerve stimulation of particular muscle groups (to reach or grasp, for bladder voiding) or in multiple muscle groups required for stepping and locomotion or cycling. Electrical stimulation can be applied with surface electrodes or with implanted electrodes, depending on the target and intended use. While many of these interventions show promise, translation of their use to clinical practice is limited.

Preclinical and experimental studies in SCI have focused on single therapies but are beginning to combine interventions. It is likely that the complexity of SCI will not be addressed with a single intervention, but rather will require combined therapies that address various pathophysiologic factors after the injury. Specific methods, timing, dosing, and best therapy combinations are not simple questions to resolve in a research or clinical context.

**PROGNOSIS.** Prognosis related to ambulation is a concern to most persons with SCI. The prognosis for recovery depends on the level of the injury, muscle strength, and AIS at the initial injury.[78] The age of the individual is associated with recovery, with the best potential for recovery related to a younger age.[124]

For individuals with a complete lesion, outcomes can be anticipated using the Consortium for Spinal Cord Medicine clinical practice guideline. Most motor recovery occurs during the first 6 months,[31] and strength may continue to increase with appropriate facilitation. The muscles graded 1 to 3 in the zone of partial preservation have potential to recover motor function; however, less than 50% of the most cephalad muscle graded 0/5 at initial testing regained strength at 1 year. Overall, more than one-half of the SCI population will have return of some neurologic function. Compression fractures have the most favorable prognosis for return of function, with crush fractures having the least chance for return of function.[76] Preservation of axonal integrity and regrowth of neural tissue are anticipated to have a significant effect on the recovery of mobility after SCI. Turning this nervous system recovery into improved functional status is part of current and ongoing research in the rehabilitation field.

Morbidity and mortality during the first year following SCI are significantly higher than in subsequent years. Individuals with AIS scores of D at any level have higher life expectancy rates compared with individuals with AIS scores of A, B, or C. Clients with paraplegic injuries live longer than clients with low cervical and high cervical injuries. Clients who depend on ventilators have the shortest life expectancy. Long-term urinary tract infection continues to be a cause of death, but control of sepsis has improved markedly since 1970.[96] This is thought to be primarily a result of improvement in bladder training, antibiotic treatment, control of fluid intake, and surgery for obstruction of the lower urinary tract.

Another common cause of death is respiratory disease, specifically atelectasis and pneumonia. Pneumonia is the leading cause of death among clients with high cervical injury.[35] Pneumonia continues at a rate higher than in the general population, with pulmonary edema associated with injuries above T6. Heart disease is common, including myocardial infarction, cardiac arrest, myocarditis, and pulmonary embolism. However, the mortality rate is not much higher than that in the general population and is improving with increased pharmacologic control and improved medical knowledge of the cardiovascular changes accompanying SCI.

People with SCI experience significant problems in a number of areas of life, resulting in ongoing stress related to pain, lack of income and financial problems, spasticity, stress, and difficulty in their sex lives. These problems do not appear to be highly correlated with aging, suggesting that they will not necessarily become more problematic, but they are not likely to self-remediate.[80]

Age, employment status, motor level and completeness of injury, and ambulatory mode (use of hand-propelled or motorized wheelchair, use of crutches or canes, or walking independently) are independently associated with health-related quality-of-life scores. Chronic cough, chronic phlegm, persistent wheeze, dyspnea with ADLs, and lower forced expiratory volume and forced vital capacity are each associated with a lower health-related quality of life.[20,70,111] A recent study reported that 58% of visits to family physicians by individuals with SCI were the result of complications that accompany immobility, including bowel and bladder dysfunction, pathologic fractures, skin breakdown, pain, AD, and spasticity. Therefore exercise, prevention of secondary complications, injury prevention, good nutrition, and education are important components of health and wellness programs for individuals with SCI.[35,78,96,124]

Maintaining or increasing ROM, the beginning of a strength and endurance program, and education of both the client and the family are key components for preventing secondary complications of SCI and promoting optimal functional potential.[98] When possible, the client and/or family should be taught to maintain ROM of the extremities independently. Adequate hamstring length and shoulder flexibility are critical for performance of transfers, bed mobility, and independent dressing during later stages of rehabilitation.[112]

Proper padding and positioning in bed or while seated in a wheelchair are imperative for maintenance of skin integrity. A pressure-relieving cushion (filled with air, gel, or some combination) is engineered to disperse the pressure under the weight-bearing surface and should be used when sitting. Selection of a cushion is best made considering the pressure mapped while sitting on the cushion in the wheelchair to find the optimal pressure relief, while considering ease of transfer and maintenance for that individual. Weight shifts or pressure reliefs should be performed every 15 to 30 minutes for 2 to 3 minutes at a time. A pressure relief offloads the weight-bearing tissue, allowing blood flow to return to that area and preventing ischemia that leads to skin breakdown and pressure ulcers.[33,89,110]

**SPECIAL IMPLICATIONS FOR THE THERAPIST 34.1**

### *Traumatic Spinal Cord Injury*

Rehabilitation to enhance the function and lifestyle of clients with SCI has traditionally been aimed at helping clients to achieve the ability to perform ADLs and mobility-related ADLs.[112] This approach attempts to facilitate maximal independence with most daily tasks and allows clients to return to desired occupational and recreational activities.

Rehabilitation strategies address functional mobility skills, health maintenance, and vocational adjustments. Although the ideal goal is to reach the point where the disability is no longer the major focus of the client's life, the client often has to perform desired activities in a different way than before injury. Psychosocial adjustment can be a primary focus of rehabilitation as clients experience a mix of emotions and reactions to their injury. They may be thankful for their own survival yet grieving the loss of body function and their ability to fill their previous roles and social responsibilities. Clients should be involved in all aspects of rehabilitation and be provided the information and environment to foster independence. Most importantly, clinicians should "respect expressions of hope" and incorporate the client's goals into the rehabilitation plan.[28]

It is critical throughout the rehabilitation process that the therapist be prepared for secondary medical complications that could be life threatening, such as orthostatic hypotension, AD, deep vein thrombosis, pulmonary emboli, and pressure ulcers. Guidelines for management of these conditions can be found in the clinical practice guidelines published by the Paralyzed Veterans of America Consortium for Spinal Cord Medicine.[25,33,34,91] Guidelines are also available for secondary conditions that are critical for function and quality of life, including bowel and bladder management,[26,30] sexuality,[36] respiratory management,[35] upper extremity preservation,[32] depression,[27] and cardiometabolic risk.[29,102]

At minimum, in initial stages of rehabilitation, clinicians should monitor blood pressure, oxygen saturation, and pulse rate and be familiar with the signs and symptoms of common complications. In cases of AD, identification and elimination of the causal factor and notification of the occurrence to other team members are critical.[87] AD and pulmonary emboli require emergent medical attention. See Box 34.2 for symptoms and triggers of AD.[17,25]

In intensive care situations, physical therapists are concerned with preparation for and mobilization of the client. Emphasis is on respiratory management, adjusting to the upright position in sitting, increasing ROM, and prevention of pressure ulcers. Postural drainage and assisted coughing should be initiated for secretion clearance.[35,55,123]

Monitoring blood pressure and oxygen saturation at rest and during activity is critical. Use of an abdominal binder during upright activity has been found to assist with maintenance of blood pressure as well as promotion of optimal diaphragm efficiency.[15]

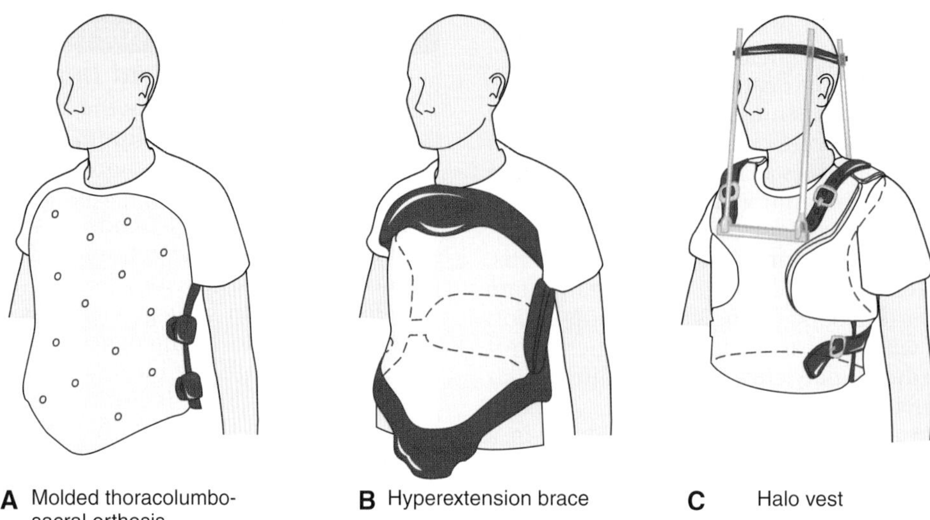


**Fig. 34.17**

(A) Molded thoracolumbosacral orthosis, designed to control extension and rotary movements. (B) Hyperextension brace, which restricts flexion in the thoracic area. (C) Halo vest, which restricts upper thoracic and cervical motion.

Orthotic management of the unstable and postoperative spinal column is often necessary, and the therapist should be familiar with the types of orthotic devices used. Fig. 34.17 illustrates several orthoses used with different levels of spinal cord lesions.[104,105]

As the client progresses through acute rehabilitation and into outpatient treatment phases, physical therapy focuses on achieving optimal functional independence. As Box 34.4 demonstrates, the level of the lesion will determine the degree to which independence can be expected in certain activities.[34] For clients with motor complete injuries, the therapeutic program must work toward developing the necessary ROM, strength, and appropriate mechanics and strategies for efficient performance of transfers and bed mobility using only the innervated muscles. Clients with thoracic and lumbar levels of injury will attain independence with bed mobility, transfers, and wheelchair mobility barring any significant medical complications or comorbidities, such as obesity, significant ROM restrictions, and persistent pain. Wheelchair mobility skills include propelling the manual or power wheelchair on indoor and outdoor surfaces, management of the wheelchair components, and, most important, pressure relief in the chair to prevent skin breakdown. Skills needed for mobility without assistive devices and adaptive equipment may be different from skills needed for mobility with equipment. In some cases, transfers into and out of bed can be done only with special equipment such as a transfer board or loop ladder.[79,112] Adaptations within the environment may be necessary for clients with weak upper extremities or poor hand control.

Depending on the motor level of the SCI, a client may require a significant amount of physical assistance after discharge from acute rehabilitation. More than 87% of persons admitted to an acute care hospital for treatment of SCI are ultimately discharged home. Among young adults with traumatic SCI, 50% are unmarried at the time of the incident.[96] Available caregiver support tends to be more limited, and external support systems may need to be established. For people with higher levels of injury, long-term care may be indicated if adequate caregiver support is not available. For older adults with SCI, there may be preexisting medical conditions and secondary complications necessitating need for long-term care.[58]

Rehabilitation traditionally focused on social reintegration is now giving way to inclusion of restoration of function by means of regeneration.[10] Activity-based rehabilitation (ABR) is a fundamental approach to rehabilitation, in which therapeutic interventions are provided that target activation of the neuromuscular system both above and below the injury level to facilitate restoration of function rather than teaching pure compensation for lost function.[107]

Evidence now indicates hope for more sparing of descending tracts at the level of the lesion, and even minimal sparing of white matter has been shown to have a profound impact on recovery of function.[8] ABR is based on the principles of activity-dependent plasticity, which assumes that neurons involved in appropriate task-specific training will reorganize both anatomic and functional connections to improve a motor behavior.[47]

ABR generally involves using intense practice and repetition of task-specific mobility training to promote neural recovery and elicit lasting changes in spinal cord function. Intensive therapy programs focused on recovery often utilize specialized rehabilitation interventions including, but not limited to, the following: locomotor training with body weight support (BWS)

Box 34.4

**DISABILITIES ASSOCIATED WITH LEVEL OF INJURY**

***C1-C5 Quadriplegia***

- Dressing
  Dependent in all dressing activities
- Bathing
  Dependent in all bathing activities
- Communication
  Independent with assistive devices for verbal communication (C1-C3)
  Independent verbal communication (C4-C5)
  Assistive devices necessary for keyboarding, writing, page turning, and use of telephone

***C6-C8 Quadriplegia***

- Dressing
  Independent with assistive device in bed (C7) or wheelchair (C8)
  Minimal assistance with lower body dressing in bed
  Moderate assistance undressing lower body in bed
  Able to dress and undress in wheelchair with assistive devices (C8)
- Bathing
  Minimal assistance for upper body bathing and drying
  Moderate assistance for lower body drying (C6)
  Independent with assistive devices (C7-C8)
  Assistive devices (tub chair necessary for tub or shower)
- Communication
  Independent in verbal communication
  Assistive devices necessary for keyboarding, writing, and use of telephone
  Setup required (C6)

***T1 and Below Paraplegia***

- Dressing
  Independent with use of assistive device
- Bathing
  Independent with use of assistive device (tub bench or cushion on bottom of tub)
- Communication
  Independent

Modified from Altrice MB, et al: Traumatic spinal cord injury. In Umphred DA, ed: *Neurological rehabilitation*, St. Louis, 1995, Mosby–Year Book, pp 502–506.

using robotic and manual assistance,[a] FES cycling,[b] FES neuroprosthetics designed to augment walking function,[7,83,84,117,118] and whole-body vibration.[72]

The recovery of walking is typically a priority for individuals who have sustained an SCI. Locomotor training using a treadmill with BWS is an activity-based therapy intervention that has gained popularity in recent years in the rehabilitation community. A growing body of evidence indicates that this type of intensive repetition of the walking pattern may be beneficial for individuals with incomplete SCIs to improve overground walking speed, endurance, and independence.[11,53,63,125,126] Locomotor training with BWS and manual assistance generally requires three to four therapists/trainers to deploy the intervention and can be very labor intensive for staff. Locomotor training devices using a robotic orthosis have been developed and are also being used to train walking function after individuals have sustained an incomplete SCI and require fewer staff members while also causing less physical stress on staff. Although evidence supports that locomotor training with BWS may be beneficial for improving walking function in individuals with motor incomplete SCI, there is insufficient evidence at the present time to demonstrate that one locomotor training strategy is superior over another.[44,53,84,92,99]

Robotic exoskeleton devices have recently become available for use in select rehabilitation centers. Many clinicians and consumers who have experience with this emerging technology agree that these devices need to be smaller and more adaptable to be considered community mobility devices used by a significant number of individuals with SCI. Multiple exoskeleton devices have been approved by the Food and Drug Administration for locomotor training, but the expense of these devices and the time required to learn how to use them have resulted in their use being primarily confined to outpatient rehabilitation facilities. Systematic reviews of exoskeleton use have been of lower quality and at times fail to recognize the nature of published studies that are often case series, not randomized clinical trials.[42] Nevertheless, these devices offer exciting future possibilities for individuals with both motor complete and motor incomplete SCIs.[116]

ABR may also include the use of numerous forms of electrical stimulation for individuals with SCI. Augmenting the force production of specific muscle groups of the trunk and upper and lower extremities, lower extremity FES cycling, upper extremity FES cycling, FES-assisted standing, and FES-assisted ambulation are commons ways that FES is used in spinal cord rehabilitation. The goals of using FES in the clinic may include to strengthen impaired or paralyzed muscle groups, to use as a neuroprosthesis for the upper and lower extremities, and to assist in the prevention of the secondary complications associated with immobility. When using FES in the clinic, it is important to remember that there are differences in the response of the neuromuscular system to electrical stimulation versus voluntary activation of a muscle group. During voluntary activation of a muscle group, the order of recruitment is generally from the smallest-diameter fibers to the larger-diameter fibers based on the load requirements of the muscle, whereas electrically stimulating a muscle group often leads to a reversed pattern of recruitment. This reversed pattern of recruitment is not as efficient as voluntary activation and may lead to premature fatigue of the muscle group. Attempts to minimize fatigue related to FES have led to use of units that are fired by feedback on voluntary muscle activity.

Lower extremity neuroprostheses designed to address footdrop as well as knee control are commercially available to augment walking in individuals with incomplete SCIs. Stimulation of the common peroneal

[a] References 11, 44, 53, 63, 84, 92, 99, 125, and 126.

[b] References 23, 40, 45, 54, 74, and 81.

nerve can facilitate swing phase activity, and stimulation of the hamstrings and quadriceps can support stance phase control and may assist with correction of knee hyperextension (genu recurvatum).[21] Improvements in gait speed, endurance, kinematics, and the physiologic cost of walking have been reported with the use of FES-assisted ambulation in individuals who have sustained incomplete SCIs.[7,83,84,117,118]

Neuroprostheses via surgically implanted FES devices are rehabilitative tools with the potential to increase independence. Studies assessing the efficacy and safety of implanted FES systems for standing and walking are under way, but there are no commercially available implantable systems at the present time. Therefore even though implanted FES systems may be promising for the future of SCI rehabilitation, they are not yet a feasible alternative to wheelchair use.

Cycling in combination with FES is an intervention often considered to be an ABR strategy. During FES cycling, software is used to stimulate lower extremity muscle groups including the quadriceps, hamstrings, gluteals, tibialis anterior, and gastroc/soleus at the appropriate intervals to allow an individual with little or no voluntary motor control to turn an ergometer using their own power. Improved cardiorespiratory fitness, improved lower extremity function, increased lower extremity circulation, muscle hypertrophy, decreased spasticity, decreased blood glucose and insulin levels, and improvements in bone mineral density have been reported by some authors.[23,40,45,54,74,81]

Deficits in upper extremity function in individuals with tetraplegia can significantly limit their functional independence. An intensive training intervention may induce both functional and neurophysiologic changes by driving cortical reorganization.[66] FES-assisted hand movement can enable clients with tetraplegia to perform many simple ADLs. Upper extremity FES cycling is also an available intervention for individuals with SCI. Multiple muscle groups of the arms and scapula may be stimulated to augment upper extremity ergometry with the goals of increasing upper extremity strength, limiting atrophy, and improving cardiovascular fitness. However, clinicians should be cautious when using this intervention with clients with high cervical injuries, as shoulder subluxation and instability are concerns.

Whole-body vibration is an intervention that has been studied in animals and humans with SCI. A systematic review suggests that the evidence for effectiveness is insufficient to support its use,[72] but several studies have documented improvement in spasticity and muscle activation with intermittent whole-body vibration (frequency 10 to 50 Hz, amplitude 0.6 to 4 mm) with individuals standing on the vibration platform with knees flexed 10 to 40 degrees.

Exercise is critical to individuals with SCI to maintain cardiac fitness levels. There are numerous reports of strategies to encourage regular exercise.[6] Circuit resistance exercise improves muscle strength, endurance, and anaerobic power in individuals with paraplegia while significantly reducing their shoulder pain.[95] Skeletal muscle atrophy is associated with accumulation of greater intramuscular fat in thigh muscle groups in SCI and continues to increase over time in incomplete SCI.[59] There is a link between adiposity (accumulation of fat in adipose tissue) and defining characteristics of metabolic syndrome. Adiposity is related to dyslipidemia, vascular inflammation, hypertension, and insulin resistance.[56] There is persistent adaptive capability within chronically paralyzed muscles. Preventing musculoskeletal adaptations after SCI may be more effective than reversing changes in the chronic condition.

Evidence supports that ABR may be beneficial for individuals who have sustained SCIs, promoting restoration of function and maximizing health and wellness, as well as limiting the impact of the secondary complications associated with immobility. Although this evidence is encouraging, compensatory strategies and ABR approaches must be used in parallel for individuals who have sustained SCIs to maximize functional independence while at the same time promoting recovery of the injured nervous system. Further research is needed in this area of rehabilitation to determine who benefits most from ABR approaches and at what phase of the recovery process these interventions can be most beneficial. As new modalities of treatment become available for individuals with SCIs, it is important that they are critically evaluated for their efficacy and used appropriately within the context of evidence-based practice.

## REFERENCES

To enhance this text and add value for the reader, all references are included in the enhanced ebook on Student Consult that accompanies this textbook. The reader can view the reference source and access it online whenever possible.

# CHAPTER 35

# Cerebral Palsy and Pediatric Stroke

HEATHER L. ATKINSON • ALLAN M. GLANZMAN (CEREBRAL PALSY)

## OVERVIEW

Cerebral palsy (CP) is an important childhood health condition that captures a variety of infant acquired brain injuries. The classic definition as described by Rosenbaum is

> *Cerebral palsy describes a group of permanent disorders of the development of movement and posture, causing activity limitation, that are attributed to non-progressive disturbances that occurred in the developing infant or fetal brain. The motor disorders of cerebral palsy are often accompanied by disturbances of sensation, perception, cognition, communication, and behavior, by epilepsy, and by secondary musculoskeletal problems.*[96]

CP is a diagnosis often given to children who experience an acquired brain injury under the age of 2, and is a large umbrella term that describes a variety of patterns of functional sequelae. Clinicians may learn to predict clinical manifestations, potential problems, and functional potential based on the neuropathophysiology. As will be discussed in the chapter, children born prematurely are vulnerable to different mechanisms of injury than children born at full term. In addition, stroke that occurs in childhood may result from different contributing factors than stroke that occurs in infants. Understanding the nuance of the timing, location, and type of injury can help physical therapists deepen their appreciation of how the child's pathology is affecting his or her ability to function and participate in meaningful activities. By recognizing and distinguishing patterns of the various forms of childhood acquired brain injury associated with cerebral palsy, clinicians can work to link pathophysiology to predicted patterns of functional movement problems and potential physical therapy plans of care.

The diagnosis of CP is often applied to any nonprogressive lesion of the brain occurring prior to 2 years of age resulting in a disorder of posture and movement. While the common mechanisms of injury and functional sequelae may differ between premature infants, full-term infants, and children, there are also similarities that are important to understand.

These nonprogressive lesions may fit within neuropathophysiology typically observed in CP, or could be a result of infant-acquired stroke or brain injury. A nonprogressive lesion in the developing brain can cause a range of dynamic issues throughout growth and development, which may span the musculoskeletal and neuromuscular systems, as well as cognition, language, and behavior.

This chapter will review the pathophysiology and clinical management of acquired brain injury in both preterm and full-term infants, as well as stroke that occurs in childhood.

## INCIDENCE AND ETIOLOGIC AND RISK FACTORS

The reported prevalence of CP ranges from 2.05 to 2.45 cases per 1000 births in most developed countries that have been surveyed.[49] Advances in perinatal care have improved the chances for survival of infants of extremely low birth weight and immature gestational age but it appears that the prevalence of children with CP has increased as well.[47,51,57]

Despite the increased use of fertility drugs, survival of infants in multiple births, and survival of extremely-low-birth-weight infants, the incidence (number of cases occurring over a certain period) of neurodisabilities, including CP, has remained constant among surviving premature infants.[67,82] In fact, incidence may have begun to show some recent decline,[50] most notably in premature infants, accompanied by a decline in the severity of disability.

**Table 35.1** Risk Factors for Cerebral Palsy

| Prenatal | Perinatal | Postnatal |
|---|---|---|
| Maternal infection<br>• Rubella<br>• Cytomegalovirus<br>• Herpes simplex<br>• Toxoplasmosis<br>Maternal diabetes<br>Rh incompatibility<br>Toxemia (undiagnosed or untreated)<br>Maternal malnutrition<br>Maternal thyroid disorders<br>Maternal seizures<br>Maternal radiation<br>Abnormal placental attachment<br>Congenital anomalies of the brain<br>Coagulation abnormalities<br>Antiphospholipid antibodies | Prematurity<br>Obstetric complications<br>• Mechanical birth trauma<br>• Breech delivery<br>• Forceps delivery<br>• Twin or multiple births<br>• Prolapsed umbilical cord or umbilical cord flow abnormalities<br>Low birth weight (<1750 g)<br>Small for gestational age (SGA)<br>Low Apgar scores (≤4 at 5 min)<br>Placenta previa (intrauterine bleeding)<br>Abruptio placentae | Neonatal infection (meningitis, encephalitis)<br>Environmental toxins<br>Trauma<br>Kernicterus<br>Brain tumor<br>Anoxia (e.g., near-drowning, assault)<br>Cerebrovascular accident<br>Neonatal hypoglycemia<br>Acidosis |

Pediatric stroke is also an important health issue, with an incidence of 2 to 13 per 100,000 children and 24 to 28 per 100,000 neonates.[45,46,64,68] This represents a small and phenotypically unique important subset of children with CP, at least 30% to 60% have persisting physical disability, 20% to 40% have persisting cognitive or neuropsychological disability, and 16% to 37% have behavioral problems.[53]

The specific cause of CP and childhood stroke may be unknown but is often multifactorial. It is thought that rather than a single causal factor, several predeterminants may interact to set the stage for injury to the developing brain.[70] In addition to known risk factors, ongoing work suggests that there may be a genetic predisposition for some children.[1,39,116]

In children of normal birth weight who have disabilities associated with CP, 80% of the disabilities are a result of factors occurring before birth and 10% to 28% are attributed to factors occurring around the birth in term or near-term infants.[27] In children of low birth weight who develop disabilities associated with CP (approximately 0.7 per 1000 live births), often uncertainty remains as to when the brain damage occurred (i.e., during fetal development or during or after birth). Any prenatal, perinatal, or postnatal condition that results in damage to the motor control systems of the brain can cause CP (Table 35.1). CP is the second most common neurologic impairment in childhood, intellectual disability being the first.[113]

## PATHOGENESIS

Although there is sometimes overlap in the use of terms regarding cerebral palsy and perinatal stroke, for the purposes of this chapter pathogenesis will be described based on typical mechanism of injury related to age of insult. It is well known that children born prematurely are vulnerable to certain risks, which differ from their counterparts born at full term. In addition, children who experience a stroke later in life typically have different mechanisms of injury.

### Mechanisms of Acquired Brain Injury in Preterm Infants

No consistent or uniform pathology is associated with CP. Several types of neuropathic lesions have been identified on the basis of autopsy: (1) hemorrhage below the lining of the ventricles (subependymal or interventricular), (2) hypoxia causing encephalopathy, and (3) malformations of the central nervous system (CNS).[122] In addition, preterm infants experience a range of vulnerabilities that can put them at risk for an event leading to CP, including anatomic and physiologic underdevelopment of the cerebral vasculature, immaturity of oligodendrocytes, cardiovascular underdevelopment, inflammation, and intravascular problems.[34]

Preterm infants are 30 times more likely than full-term infants to have an event resulting in CP.[34] This increased risk is due to several factors, including the underdevelopment and vulnerability of the anatomy and physiology of the cerebral vasculature. As the cerebral arteries grow inward toward the ventricles from the cortex from midgestation to term, they leave the germinal matrix area surrounding the ventricles more sparsely supplied and vulnerable to ischemia. Because the terminal branches of these developing arteries are fragile, these vessels increase the risk for hemorrhage.[34] Until recently, interventricular hemorrhage was the most common form of brain injury in the premature infant (Fig. 35.1). In recent years, the incidence of interventricular hemorrhage has declined from an incidence of 49% in very-low-birth-weight infants to 20% in the same population.[93] As a result, periventricular white matter injury has become the more common cause of long-lasting brain injury in this population.

Periventricular lesions can be either cystic, as in periventricular leukomalacia (PVL), or more diffuse and result in abnormal myelination (Fig. 35.2). Diffuse periventricular myelination abnormalities can be found in up to 65% of premature infants when they reach full term (9 months from conception). The incidence of PVL has declined somewhat, but when the mildest forms of PVL are included it can be seen in more than 20% of

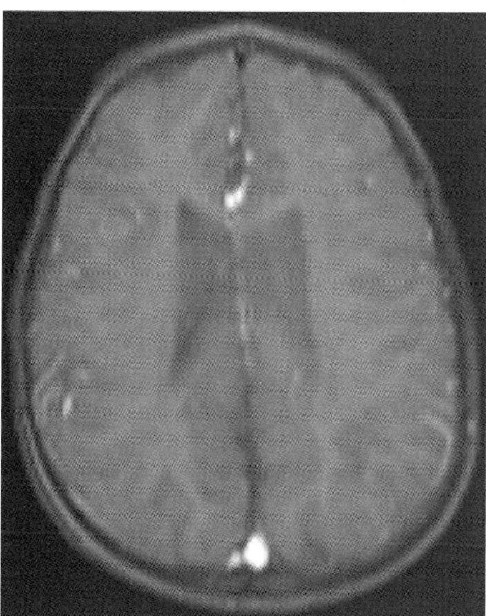

**Figure 35.1**

**Magnetic resonance image of an interventricular hemorrhage, with expansion of the lateral ventricles.** This child was born at 26 weeks' gestation and diagnosed with diplegic cerebral palsy. (Courtesy Allan Glanzman, Children's Seashore House of the Children's Hospital of Philadelphia, PA.)

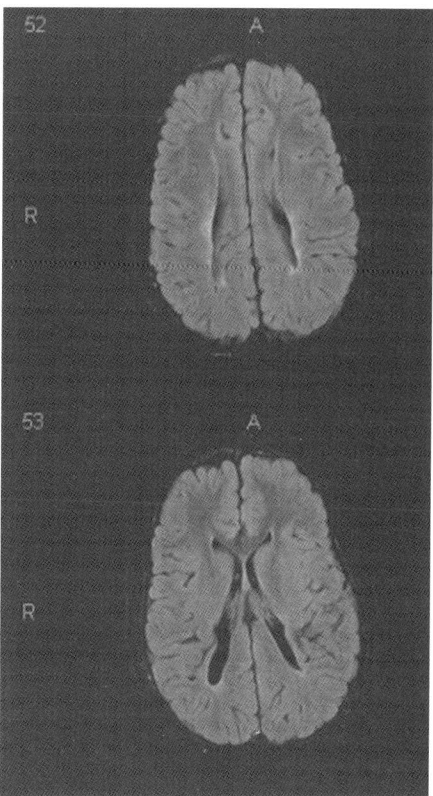


**Figure 35.2**

**Magnetic resonance image of a periventricular leukomalacia with cystic formation extending into the parenchyma in a child with quadriplegic cerebral palsy.** Top and bottom are serial sections in the same brain. In this child, the ventricles are a normal size. The abnormal finding is in the bottom slice where the cystic changes (black) extend into the brain tissue. (Courtesy Allan Glanzman, Children's Seashore House of the Children's Hospital of Philadelphia, PA.)

preterm infants. During the preterm period, infants are at heightened risk for ischemia in the periventricular areas. The heightened risk is the result of passive-pressure circulation in the premature infant. The autoregulation of CNS blood flow normally present in full-term infants is absent, making the CNS blood pressure more dependent on peripheral pressure. The premature infant between 23 and 32 weeks' gestation is at the highest risk of periventricular injury. As the periventricular white matter begins to myelinate and the vasculature matures, the risk of hypoxic injury declines.[26]

Hypoxic injury can also occur in the full-term infant; however, this represents only a small portion of infants with CP. Use of a more expansive definition of hypoxic events in all neonates, including those born prematurely with events beyond the antenatal period, increases the percentage with hypoxic injury. Causes for hypoxia include the presence of fetal bradycardia, intrauterine growth retardation, preeclampsia, placental abruption/impairment, and the presence of infection.[9,33]

Hypoxic-ischemic injury results from three possible underlying causes: (1) decreased perfusion resulting from systemic hypotension and poor autoregulation of cerebral blood flow; (2) emboli, which block distal perfusion, and (3) thrombosis; or clot formation from polycythemia or a hypercoagulable state.[92] Hypoxic-ischemic injury is known to disrupt normal metabolic processes, starving the cells of oxygen because of poor perfusion and poor oxygen delivery to the cells, resulting in a reliance on the cells' limited ability to maintain homeostasis through anaerobic energy metabolism.

Eventually, insufficient energy is available for powering the sodium-potassium pump in the cell membrane, and the ionic gradients across the cell membranes break down. The resulting influx of calcium begins a metabolic cascade that, along with the osmotic pressure gradient that has developed, ends in cell death. A second phase of cell damage occurs with reperfusion, when vasodilation allows increased blood flow and oxygen free radicals are released that trigger programmed cell death or apoptosis. The severity and topography of the damage depends on the gestational age at the time of the injury and the degree of injury sustained.[11,26]

The primary hypoxic-ischemic lesion found in the premature infant is PVL (bilateral necrosis of the white matter of the brain adjacent to the lateral ventricles), present in 42% of term and 87% of preterm infants with CP.[62,120] A portion of premature infants demonstrate impaired autoregulation of cerebral circulation and also demonstrate a passive-pressure cerebral circulation (i.e., blood pressure in the CNS is not able to remain constant with fluctuations in the peripheral circulation, placing them at risk of cerebral injury when fluctuations in peripheral pressure occur). The periventricular arterial border zones are at particular risk for hypoxic-ischemic injury in these children.[120] For preterm infants in the NICU, routine care such as diaper changes and heel sticks can create sharp spikes in systemic blood pressure, which can have direct adverse impact on the developing brain.[34]

Focal injury to the brain can also result from hemorrhage and ischemia, with the resulting collection of blood creating injury from direct mechanical pressure on the tissue and secondary ischemia. In the premature infant, hemorrhage of the germinal matrix (the cells from which the nervous system arises; in the adult, these cells, called ependymal cells, lie adjacent to the ventricular system) into the lateral ventricle (see Fig. 35.1) is a common cause of CP and can result in venous infarction of the periventricular area, with a resulting cystic lesion in that portion of the brain.[120]

Preterm infants also experience other vulnerabilities that place them at increased risk for these mechanisms of injury to unfold. Cardiovascular function is susceptible due to decreased and ineffective myocardial function, as well as delayed closure of patent ductus arteriosus and foramen ovale, all of which can lead to rapid decreases or spikes in heart rate and systemic blood pressure, which may adversely affect the vulnerable cerebral vasculature described above.[34] For babies born prematurely, developing oligodendrocytes are still in the premyelination phase at 24 to 32 weeks gestational age and are geographically close to areas at risk for hypoxic injury. Immature oligodendrocytes are vulnerable to oxidative stress, and injury often disrupts future myelination of critical motor pathways.[34] Children who develop CP fail to demonstrate normal CNS maturation after a CNS injury. Persistence of immature layers of the primary motor cortex is often present, and many of the other layers demonstrate abnormalities, particularly those with projections to the pyramidal tract.[4] Finally, infections or other systemic processes leading to inflammation can cause a cascading effect of releasing cytokines that are toxic to oligodendrocytes and can cause further ischemia [34]

## Mechanisms of Acquired Brain Injury in Full-Term Infants

Full-term infants can also experience acquired brain injury, but the pattern of insult differs from that in premature infants. Injuries include hypoxic ischemic encephalopathy (HIE), ischemic infarct/stroke, and hemorrhage. The cerebrovascular system is more mature, so areas of injury are typically those supplied by the anterior, posterior, and middle cerebral artery.[34] Developing oligodendrocytes are also more mature in the full-term infant, whereas neurons developing in the deep gray matter are more susceptible to ischemia due to their large demand for oxygen and glucose.[34] The fetus is equipped with a "brain sparing" mechanism of cerebral blood flow so that in the event of oxygen deprivation, blood flow is rerouted from the major internal organs to the areas of the brain most in need of oxygen, including the basal ganglia, thalamus, brainstem, and sensorimotor cortex.[34] Infants with a very brief episode of hypoxia may experience no ill effects, whereas infants with prolonged incomplete hypoxia will often experience parasagittal watershed and white matter injury, due to the fact that blood flow has been diverted to the deep gray matter for an extended pattern of time. Infants with a brief and complete loss of oxygen will experience injury to those deep gray matter areas that are sensitive to a hypoxic environment. In the small portion of infants who experience HIE, cooling treatments are effective in minimizing the CNS damage and improving functional outcomes.[16,52]

Hypoxic-ischemic injury in the mature neonate most commonly results in either selective neuronal cell damage or parasagittal brain damage. These HIE insults typically affect the border zones of the major cerebral arteries, either in the cerebral cortex, cerebellum, or the parietal or occipital regions. Focal or multifocal brain damage can result from either arterial embolism or venous thrombosis and is more common in the more mature neonate. The incidence of this mechanism of injury increases with gestational age greater than 28 weeks and typically presents as a unilateral injury.[11]

Full-term infants can also experience stroke due to infarct or hemorrhage. Perinatal stroke is defined as stroke in the fetus or infant before 28 days after birth.[48,65,76] Arterial ischemic stroke (AIS) most often affects the middle cerebral artery but can also occur in the anterior cerebral artery, posterior cerebral artery, or posterior circulation.[25] Causes of AIS include thrombus, embolus, clotting abnormality, arteriovenous malformation, or intravascular abnormalities.[25] Full-term infants can experience an array of stroke problems due to hemorrhage. Intracranial hemorrhage (ICH), which includes both intraventricular hemorrhage (IVH) and intraparenchymal hemorrhage (IPH), accounts for almost 50% of childhood stroke, but only about 12% of adult stroke.[12] Hemorrhage in children is not well understood and is thought to be caused predominantly from ischemic infarct transformation, bleeding from an arteriovenous malformation (AVM), or from an unknown cause.[25]

Infants can also experience cerebral sinovenous thrombosis (CSVT), which is clotting in the venous system or venous sinuses.[25] CSVT may be idiopathic or a result of clotting abnormalities, dehydration, infection, or trauma.[25] Venous occlusion caused by the clotting raises the pressure in surrounding tissues and can result in edema or hemorrhagic transformation.[25] Almost one third of infants with IVH have associated deep CSVT adjacent to the ventricles.

## Mechanisms of Stroke in Childhood

Similarly to full-term infants, children can experience ischemic infarct or hemorrhage in the cerebral vasculature, but present with different primary risk factors. Arteriopathy is perhaps one of the most important risk factors for childhood AIS, with 40% to 80% of children with diagnosed stroke demonstrating arterial abnormality upon imaging.[42] Infection, inflammation, and mechanical injury such as arterial dissection are important triggers that may initiate the pathogenesis leading to ischemic stroke in compromised vasculature.[42] Known disease to the cerebral vasculature, such as moya moya, is a risk for stroke, as are other conditions of childhood which can have secondary effects on the health of the cerebral vasculature, such as trisomy 21 and neurofibromatosis type I.[42] Children with cancer also have increased risk for stroke due to the complexity of effects from treatment and the disease process, including hypercoagulability, nonbacterial thrombotic endocarditis, and effects of cranial irradiation.[24,32,42] Cardiac disease in children is an important and well-known risk factor for developing

**Table 35.2** Classification of Cerebral Palsy

| | Category | Description |
|---|---|---|
| Topography | Monoplegia | Only one limb affected |
| | Diplegia | Involves trunk and lower extremities; upper extremities to a lesser degree |
| | Hemiplegia | Primarily one total side involved; upper extremity usually more than the lower extremity |
| | Quadriplegia (tetraplegia) | Involvement of all four limbs, head, and trunk; usually lower extremity more than upper extremity, but upper extremity with limitation of function. |
| Type of tone abnormality | Ataxia | Irregularity of muscular action manifested by dysmetria; may be pure or combined with other forms |
| | Dyskinesia (dystonic or choreoathetosis) | Presence of involuntary movement; poor control of proximal movement (chorea) alternating with repetitive, involuntary, slow, distal writhing movements (athetosis); or stereotypic sustained, intermittent involuntary muscle contractions resulting in end range posture (dystonic); movements increase with emotional stress and around adolescence |
| | Hypotonia | Abnormally reduced muscle tone characterized by decreased consistency of the muscle belly or decreased ability of the muscle to generate force as the result of diminished central drive. This is often associated with ligamentous laxity. |
| | Rigidity | Lead-pipe quality to the resistance to passive stretch |
| | Spasticity | Velocity-dependent resistance to stretch |

thromboembolism leading to AIS.[42,101] Children known to have sickle cell disease or thrombophilia are also at risk for forming a thrombus and occlusive stroke.[42] Hemorrhagic stroke in children is less understood than ischemic stroke, but can be caused by an AVM or vascular disease such as moya moya.[66,102]

## CLASSIFICATION

CP is often classified by the type of muscle tone, distribution of limb involvement, or functional skills. The types of muscle tone include hypotonia (low tone); hypertonia (high tone, spasticity); ataxia; and choreoathetosis, rigidity, or dystonia.[91]

*Dystonia* is characterized by involuntary sustained or intermittent muscle contraction, resulting in sustained end-range posture, sometimes including twisted postures and repetitive movements.[98]

*Choreoathetosis* is characterized by involuntary distal writhing movements (athetosis) and poorly graded proximal voluntary movement (chorea). *Rigidity* is characterized by a lead-pipe quality of resistance to passive movement that is independent of movement speed. *Spasticity* is characterized by a velocity-dependent resistance to passive stretch and is graded most commonly by using the modified Ashworth scale or by using Tardieu's R1 and R2.[15] *Ataxia* is characterized by incoordination of voluntary movement patterns with poor accuracy, targeting, and grading of movement as the target is approached. The patterns of motor involvement and distribution are described in Table 35.2.

Spastic CP, particularly quadriplegia and spastic diplegia, accounts for the majority of cases, with hemiplegia and triplegia being less common. The overwhelming majority of children have tone that is characterized by spasticity. Ataxia, dystonia, and choreoathetosis affect a relatively smaller number of children.[47] New cases of choreoathetoid CP have become rare in the United States and Canada as a result of improved prenatal care in the prevention of Rh incompatibility and hyperbilirubinemia, although this remains a problem in developing countries. In addition to these causes, the phenotypic improvement seen with cooling treatments in hypoxic ischemic encephalopathy now also contributes to a portion of those with choreoathetosis.

Functional skills are commonly used to classify individuals with CP. The Gross Motor Function Classification System provides a five-level system to classify motor involvement of children with CP on the basis of functional status and need for assistive technology and wheeled mobility (Box 35.1). The Gross Motor Function Classification System provides a means of grading age-related developmental skill.[80,81]

Level I includes children with neuromotor impairments whose functional limitations are less than what is typically associated with CP. It also includes children who have traditionally been diagnosed as having "minimal brain dysfunction" or "cerebral palsy of minimal severity." The distinctions between levels I and II therefore are not as pronounced as the distinctions between the other levels, particularly for infants less than 2 years of age.[80,81]

The descriptions of the five levels are broad and not intended to describe all aspects of the function of individual children. The focus is on determining which level best represents the child's present abilities and limitations in motor function. Emphasis is on the child's usual performance in home, school, and community settings (not best performance).[81]

The levels are described on a time line in categories as follows: before second birthday, between second and fourth

Box 35.1

**GROSS MOTOR FUNCTION CLASSIFICATION SYSTEM, EXPANDED AND REVISED, FOR CEREBRAL PALSY (GMFCS-E&R)**

***Before 2nd Birthday***

**LEVEL I:** Infants move in and out of sitting and floor sit with both hands free to manipulate objects. Infants crawl on hands and knees, pull to stand and take steps holding on to furniture. Infants walk between 18 months and 2 years of age without the need for any assistive mobility device.

**LEVEL II:** Infants maintain floor sitting but may need to use their hands for support to maintain balance. Infants creep on their stomach or crawl on hands and knees. Infants may pull to stand and take steps holding on to furniture.

**LEVEL III:** Infants maintain floor sitting when the low back is supported. Infants roll and creep forward on their stomachs.

**LEVEL IV:** Infants have head control but trunk support is required for floor sitting. Infants can roll to supine and may roll to prone.

**LEVEL V:** Physical impairments limit voluntary control of movement. Infants are unable to maintain antigravity head and trunk postures in prone and sitting. Infants require adult assistance to roll.

***Between 2nd and 4th Birthdays***

**LEVEL I:** Children floor sit with both hands free to manipulate objects. Movements in and out of floor sitting and standing are performed without adult assistance. Children walk as the preferred method of mobility, without the need for any assistive mobility device.

**LEVEL II:** Children floor sit but may have difficulty with balance when both hands are free to manipulate objects. Movements in and out of sitting are performed without adult assistance. Children pull to stand on a stable surface. Children crawl on hands and knees with a reciprocal pattern, cruise holding onto furniture and walk using an assistive mobility device as preferred methods of mobility.

**LEVEL III:** Children maintain floor sitting often by "W-sitting" (sitting between flexed and internally rotated hips and knees) and may require adult assistance to assume sitting. Children creep on their stomach or crawl on hands and knees (often without reciprocal leg movements) as their primary methods of self-mobility. Children may pull to stand on a stable surface and cruise short distances. Children may walk short distances indoors using a handheld mobility device (walker) and adult assistance for steering and turning.

**LEVEL IV:** Children floor sit when placed, but are unable to maintain alignment and balance without use of their hands for support. Children frequently require adaptive equipment for sitting and standing. Self-mobility for short distances (within a room) is achieved through rolling, creeping on stomach, or crawling on hands and knees without reciprocal leg movement.

**LEVEL V:** Physical impairments restrict voluntary control of movement and the ability to maintain antigravity head and trunk postures. All areas of motor function are limited. Functional limitations in sitting and standing are not fully compensated for through the use of adaptive equipment and assistive technology. At Level V, children have no means of independent movement and are transported. Some children achieve self-mobility using a powered wheelchair with extensive adaptations.

***Between 4th and 6th Birthdays***

**LEVEL I:** Children get into and out of, and sit in, a chair without the need for hand support. Children move from the floor and from chair sitting to standing without the need for objects for support. Children walk indoors and outdoors, and climb stairs. Emerging ability to run and jump.

**LEVEL II:** Children sit in a chair with both hands free to manipulate objects. Children move from the floor to standing and from chair sitting to standing but often require a stable surface to push or pull up on with their arms. Children walk without the need for a handheld mobility device indoors and for short distances on level surfaces outdoors. Children climb stairs holding onto a railing but are unable to run or jump.

**LEVEL III:** Children sit on a regular chair but may require pelvic or trunk support to maximize hand function. Children move in and out of chair sitting using a stable surface to push on or pull up with their arms. Children walk with a handheld mobility device on level surfaces and climb stairs with assistance from an adult. Children frequently are transported when traveling for long distances or outdoors on uneven terrain.

**LEVEL IV:** Children sit on a chair but need adaptive seating for trunk control and to maximize hand function. Children move in and out of chair sitting with assistance from an adult or a stable surface to push or pull up on with their arms. Children may at best walk short distances with a walker and adult supervision but have difficulty turning and maintaining balance on uneven surfaces. Children are transported in the community. Children may achieve self-mobility using a powered wheelchair.

**LEVEL V:** Physical impairments restrict voluntary control of movement and the ability to maintain antigravity head and trunk postures. All areas of motor function are limited. Functional limitations in sitting and standing are not fully compensated for through the use of adaptive equipment and assistive technology. At Level V, children have no means of independent movement and are transported. Some children achieve self-mobility using a powered wheelchair with extensive adaptations

***Between 6th and 12th Birthdays***

**Level I:** Children walk at home, school, outdoors, and in the community. Children are able to walk up and down curbs without physical assistance and stairs without the use of a railing. Children perform gross motor skills such as running and jumping but speed, balance, and coordination are limited. Children may participate in physical activities and sports depending on personal choices and environmental factors.

**Level II:** Children walk in most settings. Children may experience difficulty walking long distances and balancing on uneven terrain, inclines, in crowded areas, confined spaces or when carrying objects. Children walk up and down stairs holding onto a railing or with physical assistance if there is no railing. Outdoors and in the community, children may walk with physical assistance, a handheld mobility device, or use wheeled mobility when traveling long distances. Children have at best only minimal ability to perform gross motor skills such as running and jumping. Limitations in performance of gross motor skills may necessitate adaptations to enable participation in physical activities and sports.

**Level III:** Children walk using a handheld mobility device in most indoor settings. When seated, children may require a seat belt for pelvic alignment and balance. Sit-to-stand and floor-to-stand transfers require physical assistance of a person or support surface. When traveling long distances, children use some form of wheeled mobility. Children may walk up

Box 35.1

**GROSS MOTOR FUNCTION CLASSIFICATION SYSTEM, EXPANDED AND REVISED, FOR CEREBRAL PALSY (GMFCS-E&R)**

and down stairs holding onto a railing with supervision or physical assistance. Limitations in walking may necessitate adaptations to enable participation in physical activities and sports, including self-propelling a manual wheelchair or powered mobility.

**Level IV:** Children use methods of mobility that require physical assistance or powered mobility in most settings. Children require adaptive seating for trunk and pelvic control and physical assistance for most transfers. At home, children use floor mobility (roll, creep, or crawl), walk short distances with physical assistance, or use powered mobility. When positioned, children may use a body support walker at home or school. At school, outdoors, and in the community, children are transported in a manual wheelchair or use powered mobility. Limitations in mobility necessitate adaptations to enable participation in physical activities and sports, including physical assistance and/or powered mobility.

**Level V:** Children are transported in a manual wheelchair in all settings. Children are limited in their ability to maintain antigravity head and trunk postures and control arm and leg movements. Assistive technology is used to improve head alignment, seating, standing, and/or mobility but limitations are not fully compensated by equipment. Transfers require complete physical assistance of an adult. At home, children may move short distances on the floor or may be carried by an adult. Children may achieve self-mobility using powered mobility, with extensive adaptations for seating and control access. Limitations in mobility, necessitate adaptations to enable participation in physical activities and sports, including physical assistance and using powered mobility.

***Between 12th and 18th Birthdays***

**Level I:** Youth walk at home, school, outdoors, and in the community. Youth are able to walk up and down curbs without physical assistance and stairs without the use of a railing. Youth perform gross motor skills such as running and jumping but speed, balance, and coordination are limited. Youth may participate in physical activities and sports, depending on personal choices and environmental factors.

**Level II:** Youth walk in most settings. Environmental factors (such as uneven terrain, inclines, long distances, time demands, weather, and peer acceptability) and personal preference influence mobility choices. At school or work, youth may walk using a handheld mobility device for safety. Outdoors and in the community, youth may use wheeled mobility when traveling long distances. Youth walk up and down stairs holding a railing or with physical assistance if there is no railing. Limitations in performance of gross motor skills may necessitate adaptations to enable participation in physical activities and sports.

**Level III:** Youth are capable of walking using a hand-held mobility device. Compared to individuals in other levels, youth in Level III demonstrate more variability in methods of mobility, depending on physical ability and environmental and personal factors. When seated, youth may require a seat belt for pelvic alignment and balance. Sit-to-stand and floor-to-stand transfers require physical assistance from a person or support surface. At school, youth may self-propel a manual wheelchair or use powered mobility. Outdoors and in the community, youth are transported in a wheelchair or use powered mobility. Youth may walk up and down stairs holding onto a railing with supervision or physical assistance. Limitations in walking may necessitate adaptations to enable participation in physical activities and sports, including self-propelling a manual wheelchair or powered mobility.

**Level IV:** Youth use wheeled mobility in most settings. Youth require adaptive seating for pelvic and trunk control. Physical assistance from one or two persons is required for transfers. Youth may support weight with their legs to assist with standing transfers. Indoors, youth may walk short distances with physical assistance, use wheeled mobility, or, when positioned, use a body support walker. Youth are physically capable of operating a powered wheelchair. When a powered wheelchair is not feasible or available, youth are transported in a manual wheelchair. Limitations in mobility necessitate adaptations to enable participation in physical activities and sports, including physical assistance and/or powered mobility.

**Level V:** Youth are transported in a manual wheelchair in all settings. Youth are limited in their ability to maintain antigravity head and trunk postures and control arm and leg movements. Assistive technology is used to improve head alignment, seating, standing, and mobility, but limitations are not fully compensated by equipment. Physical assistance from one or two persons or a mechanical lift is required for transfers. Youth may achieve self-mobility, using powered mobility, with extensive adaptations for seating and control access. Limitations in mobility necessitate adaptations to enable participation in physical activities and sports, including physical assistance and using powered mobility.

***Distinctions Between Levels I and II***

Compared with children and youth in Level I, children and youth in Level II have limitations walking long distances and balancing; may need a handheld mobility device when first learning to walk; may use wheeled mobility when traveling long distances outdoors and in the community; require the use of a railing to walk up and down stairs; and are not as capable of running and jumping.

***Distinctions Between Levels II and III***

Children and youth in Level II are capable of walking without a handheld mobility device after age 4 (although they may choose to use one at times). Children and youth in Level III need a handheld mobility device to walk indoors and use wheeled mobility outdoors and in the community.

***Distinctions Between Levels III and IV***

Children and youth in Level III sit on their own or require at most limited external support to sit, are more independent in standing transfers, and walk with a handheld mobility device. Children and youth in Level IV function in sitting (usually supported) but self-mobility is limited. Children and youth in Level IV are more likely to be transported in a manual wheelchair or use powered mobility.

***Distinctions Between Levels IV and V***

Children and youth in Level V have severe limitations in head and trunk control and require extensive assisted technology and physical assistance. Self-mobility is achieved only if the child/youth can learn how to operate a powered wheelchair.

From Palisano R, Rosenbaum, P, and Bartlett D: *The Gross Motor Function Classification System (GMFCS), Expanded and Revised (E &R)* (2007). CanChild Centre for Childhood Disability Research, Institute for Applied Health Sciences, McMaster University, Hamilton, Ontario, Canada. User instructions and more information are available online at https://canchild.ca/en/resources/42-gross-motor-function-classification-system-expanded-revised-gmfcs-e-r. Used with permission.

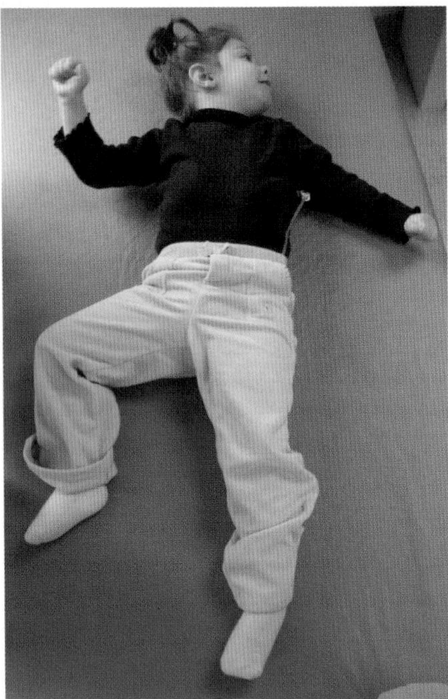

**Figure 35.3**

**Asymmetric tonic neck reflex.** Four-year-old with quadriplegic cerebral palsy demonstrating the asymmetric tonic neck reflex. This primitive reflex contributes to an obligatory change in body posture resulting from a change in head position. With head turning to one side, the arm and leg on the same side extend while the arm and leg on the opposite side flex. This posture resembles a fencing position and prevents the child from bringing the left hand to her mouth for exploration and self-feeding. (Courtesy Allan Glanzman, Children's Seashore House of the Children's Hospital of Philadelphia, PA.)

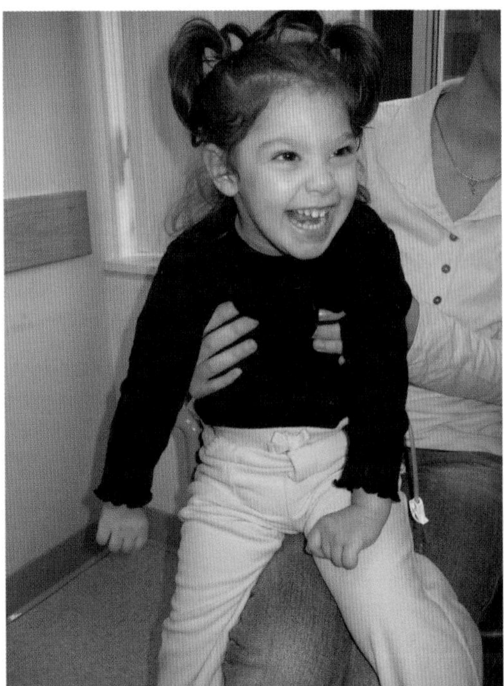

**Figure 35.4**

**Symmetric tonic neck reflex.** The same 4-year-old with quadriplegic cerebral palsy as in Figure 35.3 demonstrates another primitive reflex known as the symmetric tonic neck reflex (STNR). When the head and neck are extended, the arms extend; flexion usually predominates in the lower extremities. Flexion of the head and neck causes flexion in the upper extremities and extension in the lower extremities (not shown). In the normal infant the asymmetric tonic neck reflex and STNR are typically integrated by 6 to 8 months. Integration of the STNR allows voluntary flexion of both arms and legs, needed to sit comfortably. Prior to 6 to 8 months, these reflexes can be observed in developing infants, but when present are not obligatory (i.e., the person can voluntarily move out of the position). (Courtesy Allan Glanzman, Children's Seashore House of the Children's Hospital of Philadelphia, PA.)

birthdays, between fourth and sixth birthdays, between sixth and twelfth birthdays, and the expanded version now contains a category for children between their twelfth and eighteenth birthday, which is available at https://canchild.ca/en/resources/42-gross-motor-function-classification-system-expanded-revised-gmfcs-e-r. Distinctions between adjacent levels are outlined in Box 35.1.

For children with stroke, classification remains less well described. Depending on the location of insult, stroke may manifest motorically as hemiparesis, ataxia, or hypotonia, all of which are lacking in universally accepted terms regarding degree of severity. To help mitigate this lack of a universally accepted classification system, clinicians can select outcome measures that describe a child's ability to isolate and control specific movements, depending on the primary movement impairment such as the Selective Control Assessment of the Lower Extremity (SCALE)[43], as well as tests that measure the functional control of movement such as the Manual Ability Classification System (MACS) and/or Gross Motor Function Measure (GMFM).[3,36,63] A more detailed discussion of clinical evaluative tools and outcome measures for childhood stroke is available elsewhere.[7]

## CLINICAL MANIFESTATIONS

Although the neurologic manifestations of CP are nonprogressive, resulting motor impairments change with growth and maturation and may become more apparent as the child ages. Clinical manifestations of motor impairments associated with CP may include alterations of muscle tone, delayed postural reactions, persistence of primitive reflexes (Fig. 35.3), delayed motor development, and abnormal motor performance (e.g., delay in movement onset, poor timing of force generation, poor force production, inability to maintain antigravity postural control, decreased speed of movement, and increased cocontraction).[22]

Persistence of primitive reflexes and impaired motor function can affect the head, neck, trunk, and extremities, resulting in impaired sucking and swallowing, as well as delayed GI motility and gastroesophageal reflux, resulting in feeding and nutrition difficulties (Fig. 35.4).[103]

Associated disabilities may include cognitive impairments (e.g., intellectual disability, learning disabilities, seizure disorders); sensory impairments (in vision, hearing); feeding impairments, including oral motor dysfunction, constipation or bowel and bladder incontinence with their associated problems (e.g., poor hygiene, skin problems), and seizure disorders.[71,87] In individuals with spastic hemiplegic, spastic quadriplegic, or diplegic CP, these comorbidities occur relatively less frequently. The

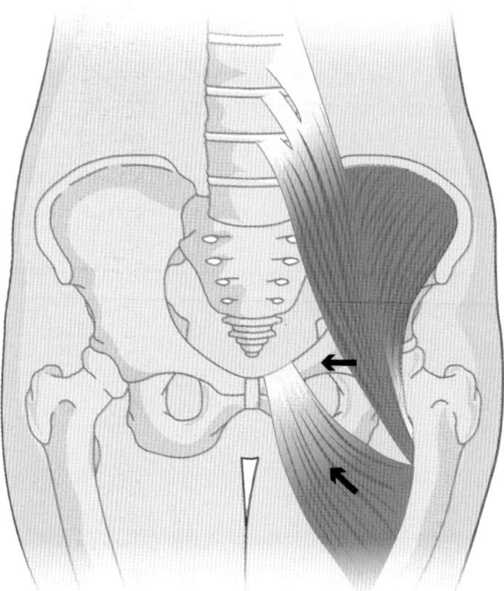

**Figure 35.5**

Spastic iliopsoas and adductor muscles are the initiating deforming force in acquired spastic hip dislocation.

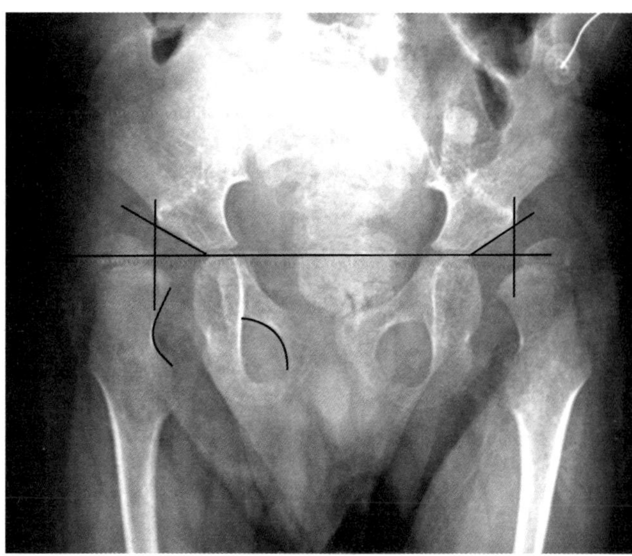

**Figure 35.6**

**Anteroposterior radiograph of a young child with spastic quadriplegia and subsequent hip dysplasia, with subluxation on the left.** Note that a line drawn vertically down from the outermost edge of the acetabulum would bisect the head of the femur. Failure of the acetabulum to deepen with weight bearing resulting in hip dysplasia and subluxation occur as a result of the inability to weight bear and abnormal muscular forces pulling on the bone. The standard measurement for hip dislocation is a migration percentage. This is done by drawing Hilgenreiner's line, which provides a horizontal reference to the pelvis and then drawing Perkin's line perpendicular to Hilgenreiner's line from the outermost edge of the acetabulum. (Courtesy Allan Glanzman, Children's Seashore House of the Children's Hospital of Philadelphia, PA.)

rate of comorbidity occurrence is significantly greater for individuals with dyskinetic, ataxic, or hypotonic CP.[100]

Microcephalus and hydrocephalus are also common findings, with the latter being the result of increased intracranial pressure. Behavioral signs of increased intracranial pressure accompanying hydrocephalus may include extreme irritability, resulting from headache and associated vomiting. Eventually delays in reaching developmental milestones are observed, resulting from pressure-induced damage.[86]

Musculoskeletal problems of altered muscle tone, muscle weakness, and joint restrictions are common and can result in functional and orthopedic impairments. For example, the abnormal pull of the spastic iliopsoas and adductor muscles are the initiating deforming force in hip dislocations (Fig. 35.5).[74] When spasticity and contracture of the iliopsoas occur, the medial joint capsule is compressed and the femoral head is pushed laterally. As lateral drift of the femoral head occurs, the iliopsoas insertion on the lesser trochanter becomes the center of rotation. Acetabular development ceases when the femoral head is completely displaced laterally, and further hip flexion pushes the head posteriorly, with progressive dislocation (Fig. 35.6).[14]

Abnormalities of the muscle, with a decrease in the number of sarcomeres[106] per muscle fiber, are associated with CP. Muscles also demonstrate increased variation in fiber size and type[95] with both hypertrophy and atrophy present, possibly representing an ongoing dynamic process. Increases in fat and fibrous tissue and a decrease in blood flow have been identified.[94] As the child ages, bone grows faster than muscle, resulting in a disadvantageous length-tension relationship of the muscle and an increased risk of subsequent contracture.[107] A characteristic decrease in muscle mass also results in decreased muscle power and endurance.

Changes in muscle tone affect a person's ability to control movement, resulting in poor selective control of muscles, poor regulation of activity and muscle groups, decreased ability to learn unique movements, inappropriate sequencing of movements, and delayed anticipatory postural response. Most often, the timing and sequence of muscle activity are also affected.

A significant number of children with a diagnosis of spastic CP present with low muscle tone in the first few months of life and later in the first year develop spasticity. Often flexor skills are delayed and antigravity skill for activities such as lifting the head, reaching, and kicking is limited. The child may attempt alternative strategies to complete these tasks, if control is not sufficient, that may allow completion of a particular sequence. Use of atypical movement strategies may prevent the progression of further development because foundational movements have not been mastered. For example, the use of a wide-based sitting posture may allow the child to maintain sitting but decreases the ability to turn and rotate in and out of the position, which is necessary for transitions to other positions. Likewise pulling to stand with increased reliance on the arms to assist the lower extremities may prevent learning how to move from squatting to standing. If practiced and repeated over time, these abnormal movements become habitual and are difficult to change.

Each type of CP is characterized by its own clinical picture, based on the presence and extent of clinical manifestations. The progression of motor development associated with each type of CP is beyond the scope of this chapter, but the reader should be familiar with the natural history of each as this will aid in the development of treatment goals. The reader is referred to other texts for a more detailed discussion.[21,108]

Clinical manifestations in childhood stroke are multifactorial and depend on the age, type, size, and location of insult. For example, if the stroke occurs perinatally and is diffuse or hemorrhagic in nature, clinical sequelae may appear very similar to those described for CP. If, however, the perinatal stroke is a focal ischemic stroke, infants may appear to be well, without overt clinical signs in the early days of life. Almost 50% of infants with stroke may be asymptomatic and go undiagnosed until they have a seizure, prompting a medical diagnostic workup, or the clinical motor sequelae may present around 4 months of age when hemiparesis or focal motor deficit may become more apparent.[25] Infants may also experience visual deficits, prompting head turn preference and the development of torticollis. Clinical manifestations of stroke in older children again depend on location and type of lesion, but often can be somewhat predictable depending on the vessel(s) or region(s) affected. For example, children with arterial ischemic stroke of the middle cerebral artery will have a comparable clinical presentation to that of an adult with a similar lesion—they may experience an initial period of flaccidity followed by the onset of spasticity and decreased selective motor control, which is well-described in the stroke literature.[56,114,124] Natural history of recovery from stroke in children is not well understood, but is thought to be related to experience-dependent practice and neuroplastic factors.[28,61] A full discussion of neuroplasticity and regenerative capabilities in the developing brain is beyond the scope of this chapter, but readers should understand that the natural course for children has the potential to be different from that of adults.[58,59,88]

## MEDICAL MANAGEMENT

**DIAGNOSIS AND ACUTE MANAGEMENT.** Children with acute stroke should be treated emergently and transferred to the intensive care unit for further management.[73] The medical team will evaluate the cause and extent of the stroke and determine if the child would benefit from anticoagulation therapy or other acute neurosurgical procedures. Adequate hydration and keeping the head of the bed flat are important standards of supportive care. Also, therapeutic hypothermia is being explored to help mitigate the secondary effects of neuronal cell death.[105] The critical team will evaluate any other physiologic needs to help gain medical stability.

For children with neurologic findings discovered subacutely, early diagnosis is important to ensure early intervention from both a medical and rehabilitative standpoint.[78] Observation, history, and a neurologic examination will provide the physician with the information necessary to make an accurate and early diagnosis. The diagnostic studies performed depend on clinical findings. For example, electroencephalography is indicated when seizures are present or suspected; hip radiographic films are indicated to rule out hip dislocations and should be followed over time, particularly in the presence of spasticity.

Blood or urine screening tests may be used to rule out certain metabolic or hematologic diseases, and a thorough workup should be undertaken if a history reveals a progressive course or positive family history. A CT or MRI scan can provide information on the location of the insult.

**TREATMENT.** Comprehensive and cooperative planning with an interdisciplinary team that may include physicians, therapists, nurses, special educators, psychologists, social workers, nutritionists, and family members is essential.

Some of the most common medical management strategies related to rehabilitative function include pharmacologic intervention, neurosurgical intervention, and orthopedic surgery. Skeletal muscle relaxants (e.g., baclofen, diazepam, dantrolene, tizanidine, and botulinum toxin) can be used to assist in controlling increased spasticity and can be administered orally (baclofen, dantrolene, tizanidine, and diazepam), intrathecally (baclofen), or directly to muscles through injection at the motor point (botulinum toxin).[84]

Intrathecal administration of baclofen (through the sheath of the spinal cord into the subarachnoid space) uses an implantable intrathecal infusion pump to deliver medication to the spinal cord without the associated CNS sedation found with oral administration. After the pump is implanted, the dosage can be titrated to the optimal level for each person. Any attempts to control excess muscle tone (pharmaceutically or otherwise) should always be paired with functional goals to take advantage of the modulated tone.[2,6]

Motor point blocks can also be used to control spasticity and can be paired with serial casting to increase muscle length. Muscles such as the gastrocnemius, hip adductors, or hamstrings are injected with a botulinum toxin (or phenol) to create a temporary denervation and to decrease tone and increase movement.[18,60,111]

The type A botulinum toxin (Botox) is injected directly into the muscle at the motor point and is used to blockade the neuromuscular junction by acting presynaptically to reduce the release of acetylcholine, resulting in partial denervation of the muscle. Muscle weakness and decrease in muscle spasm occur in 3 to 7 days and gradually reappear in 4 to 6 months.

Successful use of botulinum toxin type A in the upper extremity has been reported,[41,44,104] as has its use to control drooling in children with CP. The effects of these injections will wear off anywhere from several weeks to several months later, similar to the effect seen in lower extremity injections.[40,90]

Selective dorsal rhizotomy (surgically identifying the posterior roots of the spinal cord and selectively resecting some of them) to reduce spasticity has been used over the past decade. This is usually performed at the L2 to L5 spinal levels for clients with spastic diplegia who are independent or near independent ambulators but who have spasticity that results in abnormalities of posture and gait.[118] A rhizotomy may also be used effectively for clients with severe positioning difficulties, such as severe quadriplegia; however, in this population the relative benefit of rhizotomy versus intrathecal baclofen should be considered. In the population of children with quadriplegic CP, rhizotomy may reduce muscle tone enough to facilitate personal hygiene and provide improved sitting and comfort.[117]

Orthopedic surgery may include muscle lengthening or releases (e.g., adductors, iliopsoas, hamstrings, gastrocnemius) to address contracture, muscle transfers (e.g., rectus femoris or tibialis posterior) to increase

**Table 35.3** Predictors of Ambulation for Cerebral Palsy

| Predictors | Ambulation Potential |
|---|---|
| **By Diagnosis** | |
| Monoplegia | 100% |
| Hemiplegia | 100%[a] |
| Ataxia | 100% |
| Diplegia | 60%[a]-90% |
| Spastic quadriplegia | 0%-70% |
| **By Motor Function** | |
| Sits independently by age 2 | Good[b] |
| Sits independently by age 3-4 | 50% community ambulation |
| Presence of primitive reflexes beyond age 2 | Poor |
| Absence of postural reactions beyond age 2 | Poor |
| Independently crawled symmetrically or reciprocally by age 2.5 | Good[b] |

[a]From Pallas Alonso CR, de La Cruz Bértolo J, Medina López MC, et al: Cerebral palsy and age of sitting and walking in very low birth weight infants. *An Esp Pediatr* 53:48-52, 2000.
[b]From da Paz Jr AC, Burnett SM, Braga LW: Walking prognosis in cerebral palsy: a 22-year retrospective analysis. *Dev Med Child Neurol* 36:130-134, 1994.

control or decrease excessive muscle pull, or bone procedures (e.g., femoral derotational osteotomy; acetabular augmentation; triple arthrodesis; spinal fusions) to correct bony deformity, hip dislocation, scoliosis or patellar tendon advancement.[72]

Orthotic intervention may be used to maintain flexibility, support or stabilize a joint, or improve alignment. The ultimate goal is to delay the development of fixed contractures and improve function, with bracing based on both the impairment of gait deviation noted, along with the anticipated gait and impairment-based natural history of the disease taken into account.

For children with a gait marked by toe walking, an articulating molded ankle-foot orthosis will aid in maintaining the flexibility of the gastrocsoleus complex and a plantigrade gait pattern. Children with lever arm dysfunction who use a crouched pattern in standing may benefit from ground reaction force molded ankle-foot orthoses to restrain tibial progression through the stance phase of gait and improve the child's erect posture. Children with spasticity of the peroneal muscles and pronation, may be prescribed supramalleolar orthoses (SMOs) to maintain the integrity of the midfoot and help avoid an incompetent forefoot and rocker bottom posture if toe walking, drop foot, and crouch are not concerns.

**Prognosis.** Common causes of death in this population are related to infection, aspiration, respiratory compromise, and heart disease.[112]

Most children with mild to moderate CP have a normal life span, but there is some increased mortality in the early years (before age 4) and then again with advancing age (50 and older). In those individuals with quadriplegic CP, the excess death rate declines during childhood and adulthood only to climb again after the age of 50, as is noted in the more mildly involved population.[72] In one trial, mortality was highest under 15 years and then approached twice the general population rate by 35 years of age, with the nonambulatory population being at highest risk of death.

Ambulation potential may be predicted based on achievement of motor milestones (Table 35.3). Independent sitting before age 2 years is a positive indicator of future ambulation.[121] If ambulation is going to occur, it usually takes place by 8 years of age.[89]

**SPECIAL IMPLICATIONS FOR THE THERAPIST 35.1**

In addition to the treatment options discussed in the previous section, physical therapists are exploring a more focused and proactive approach of activity-based intervention through intense activity training protocols, lifestyle modifications, and mobility-enhancing devices. Increased motor activity may lead to better physical and mental health and improve various aspects of cognitive performance.[31]

Activity-based programs for individuals with CP and stroke focus on maximizing physical function while preventing secondary musculoskeletal impairments; foster cognitive, social, and emotional development; and potentially promote or enhance neural recovery.[30]

With new research information about the role of neural recovery in damaged nervous systems, therapists can expect to see continued changes in philosophy and intervention approaches with this unique population. Focus will continue with early intervention but include other phases throughout the life span. As attention is directed toward establishing, enhancing, and maintaining neural pathways, we may see changes in how CP is approached. For a more detailed discussion of traditional and emerging physical therapist practices for CP, the reader is referred to the seminal review paper by Novak and a commentary by Damiano.[31,77]

For rehabilitation of children with stroke, evidence is limited except for the wide array of studies examining intense upper extremity practice, either through constraint-induced therapy, bimanual intense therapy, or a combination approach.[5,35,38] Recent clinical guidelines on the subacute management of pediatric stroke[119] can be a helpful resource,as well as literature on cerebral palsy and adult stroke. Furthermore, because stroke may affect a wide array of functions (motor, cognitive, language, behavior, psychosocial), developing an understanding of common sequelae and how they affect the developing child is important in providing comprehensive and holistic care. For a detailed discussion of pediatric stroke rehabilitation, including physical therapy management and interprofessional collaboration, the reader is referred elsewhere.[7]

### Family-Centered Care

When designing a therapy program for a child with CP or stroke, the therapist should take a broad view of the child's needs and consider the interactive effects that the child's family environment has on the goals that have been developed. To provide family-centered care, the therapist must do the following[110]:

- Spend enough time with the family to understand their goals
- Listen carefully to the parents
- Make the parents feel like partners in the child's care
- Be sensitive to the family's values and customs
- Provide the specific information that the parents need

The strengths and weaknesses of each family need to be assessed and considered when designing a given child's program, and the therapist needs to consider what the impact of carrying out the physical therapy and multidisciplinary team program will be on the family and, as a result, on the child.

If the cost (emotional, social, financial) is too great, the family may choose to abandon the intervention. As a result, the child may lose ground in terms of altered musculoskeletal alignment and decreased function, and the family must bear the emotional impact.

If the therapist is able to match the program with the family's cultural expectations, ability to participate, and emotional and financial resources, then a partnership with the family can develop that will most benefit the child in the long run. Creation of the best therapeutic environment requires provision of support and education where it is needed and an expectation of only what is feasible within what the family's capabilities and environment will allow. This approach will help the family grow, and care for the child with special needs will create an environment to allow the child to thrive.

There is often a fine line between balancing the natural history of the condition with the family's commitment and understanding in maximizing the child's quality of life. In addition, families make choices in terms of providing for the child with CP. Often these choices must take into consideration other family members, expectations of themselves, expectations of the child, and, as mentioned, cultural and ethnic beliefs that may or may not be in line with the typical health care goals and plans for intervention.

### Early Intervention

A general review of intervention studies shows that children benefit from early intervention compared with those children not involved in specific programmed activities. Programming focused on cognitive outcomes has relatively stronger support[9] than programming aimed at solely motor outcomes.[55] The potential for improvement is better for children less than 9 months old but no greater than 2 years of age at a minimum frequency of intervention of two times per week.[13]

Early and accurate identification of CP provides the most likely opportunity for facilitation of optimal motor development.[71] Many motor milestone checklists are available to provide a reference for typical development.[40] In fact, the gross motor function of children with CP and outcomes of intervention have often been evaluated using measures on children without motor impairment.

It may prove more meaningful to make management decisions and evaluate intervention outcomes based on expectations for children with CP of the same age and gross motor function.[80] This type of evaluation can be made by using assessment tools specifically designed to evaluate the child with CP (e.g., Gross Motor Function Assessment[97]; Gross Motor Function Classification System[80,81]). An assessment of management practices with guidelines for the management of clients with CP is available,[23] as is a model for the acquisition of basic motor abilities and intervention implications.[10]

The therapist must carefully consider the effects of low muscle tone and later developing spasticity, because they influence habitual movement patterns a child uses to accomplish functional tasks. Therapy often encourages the use of more typical movement patterns in attempts to normalize postural control and reduce atypical strategies to accomplish tasks. The use of compensatory approaches may be necessary to optimize a child's independence in their daily life.

### Postoperative Concerns

After orthopedic surgery, the therapist can assist in reducing muscle spasms that increase postoperative pain by moving and turning the child carefully and slowly; however, adequate postoperative pain management should include medication (e.g., codeine and diazepam [Valium]) prescribed by the surgeon.

In the case of postoperative casting, the therapist can instruct the family to wash and dry the skin at the edge of the cast frequently, inspecting often for signs of skin breakdown. Repositioning and ventilation under the cast with a cool-air blow dryer can also assist in preventing skin breakdown. A flashlight can be used daily to inspect beneath the cast.

Surgical procedures (orthopedic or neurosurgical) may expose areas of underlying muscle weakness and instability. It is critical that an intensive therapy intervention program begin after surgery to assist with strengthening and improving functional performance.

### Assistive Technology

Properly prescribed assistive technology is vital in allowing the child with CP the least restrictive access to both the physical and social environment and is a critical part of the overall management of the child with CP. Assistive technology includes any device used to increase, maintain, or improve the functional ability of a person with a disability (Fig. 35.7).

This equipment can be either low tech (standers, positioning equipment, communication boards, or wheelchairs) or high tech (switch toys, power wheelchairs, or computer-based communication systems), as long as it is provided with a functional goal (Fig. 35.8).

Quality of life should be a focus in the management of all clients seeking health care services. Mobility impairment limits can negatively affect overall development, including social, cognitive, emotional, and physical development. A balanced approach to providing assistive technology as a compensation for functional limitations while focusing therapy on the impairment-based limitations that are affecting function, powered mobility is one example of assistive technology that can increase voluntary activity, function, and independence and has contributed to improved quality of life for many individuals with CP (Fig. 35.9).

For children who are dependent for mobility, power mobility can be an option and can be successful in

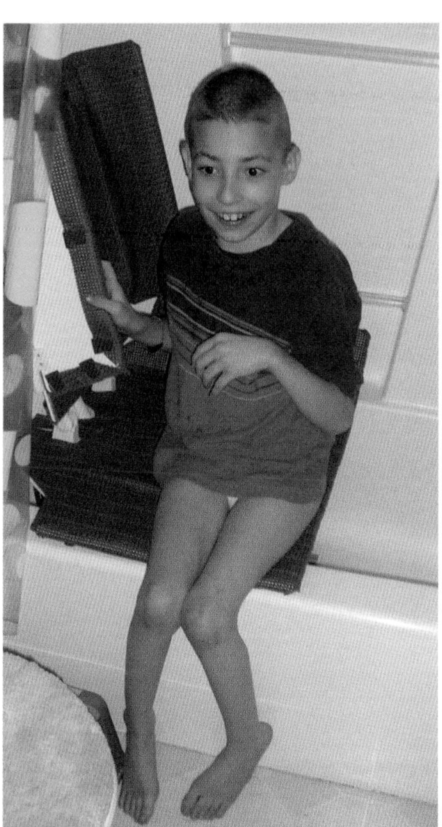

**Figure 35.7**

**Tub lift.** A battery-powered tub lift has been very successful with this child, who has spastic quadriplegic cerebral palsy. With help, he transfers from the toilet next to the tub to the tub seat. With assistance, he swings his legs into the tub, and then can independently operate the unit to lower (and later elevate) himself. (Courtesy Tamara Kittelson-Aldred, Access Therapy Services, Missoula, MT. Used with permission.)

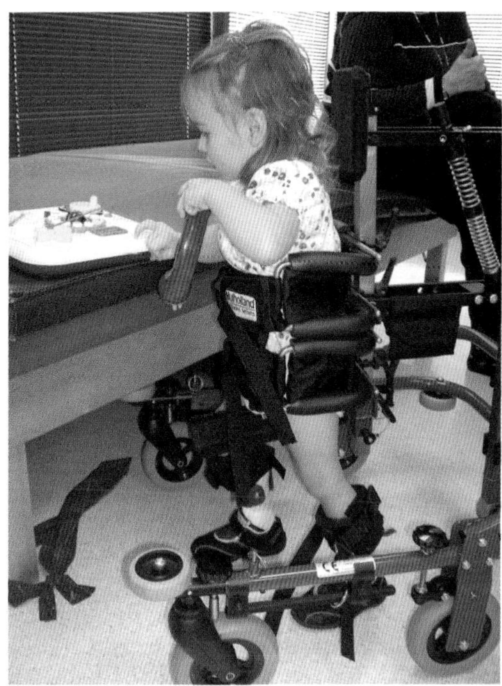

**Figure 35.8**

**Mulholland Walkabout.** This 3-year-old girl with spastic quadriplegia can propel this wheeled upright walker through space to explore her environment and play where she wants to. Although she may not become a functional ambulator, the use of this equipment is developmentally appropriate. She could be a candidate for independent wheelchair mobility, but her parents have deferred this decision for now. (Courtesy Tamara Kittelson-Aldred, Access Therapy Services, Missoula, MT. Used with permission.)

children as young as 2 years of age with corresponding cognitive skills.[19,20,109] These systems can be controlled with a standard joystick or adapted for control with a variety of switch systems and are available both as medical equipment and as adapted play equipment.[54,85]

These power wheelchair systems allow control with a switch array or by proportional control or control through the use of a single switch through a scanning program (Fig. 35.10). Access mode needs to be carefully assessed, as does switch or joystick location; hand use is obviously preferable, but if this is not possible, head placement is often a successful location for switches. When computer access is educationally appropriate, a team including OT and speech therapy can be assembled to assess the appropriate access for communication (if needed) and computer access. Often, the same wheelchair-based control system can be adapted through an infrared link and mouse emulator to operate the computer and communication system. The mouse emulator is an electronic link that allows use of the joystick to control the mouse, usually by infrared beam.

Use of mobility and speech-generating (communication) devices is encouraged with children at all levels of motor disability, including those with severe involvement, as is appropriate based on cognitive level.

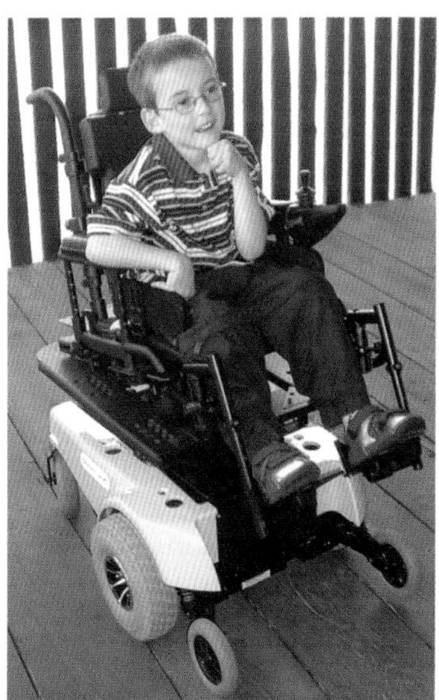

**Figure 35.9**

**New power wheelchair.** This 4-year-old child with cerebral palsy receives a new power wheelchair with a seat elevator to enable him to reach age-appropriate items on countertops and tabletops. Trunk supports and footplates help with alignment. The joystick on the left allows him to navigate independently. (Courtesy Tamara Kittelson-Aldred, Access Therapy Services, Missoula, MT. Used with permission.)

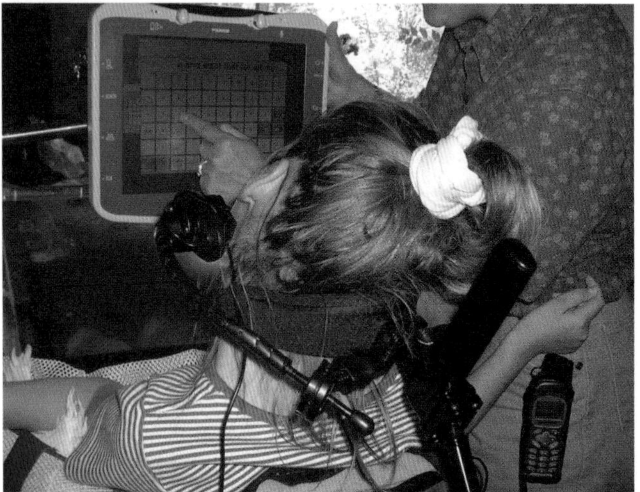

**Figure 35.10**

**This young lady with spastic quadriplegic cerebral palsy uses a DynaVox speech-generating device with a Tash Microlite switch on the left.** By moving her head, she is able to hit the switch with her cheek to stop the electronic scan where she wants it to create a message. Stealth neck rest provides suboccipital head support. (Courtesy Tamara Kittelson-Aldred, Access Therapy Services, Missoula, MT. Used with permission.)

Differences in clinical practice and debate continue over providing an external means of mobility in favor of promoting more voluntary activity. More definitive research guidance is needed in these areas.

Proper positioning is critical to the child with CP, both from a functional perspective and to help prevent the soft tissue limitations that can develop over time. Appropriate positioning has been shown to encourage smoother and faster reach, decrease extensor tone, increase vital capacity, and improve performance on cognitive testing.[75]

In addition to proper wheelchair position, time out of the chair to counteract the flexed posture of the body is necessary. A standing program can be initiated between 12 and 18 months of age in the child who is not pulling to stand independently to maintain flexibility and provide the normal weight-bearing forces across the hip joint.

Standing helps orient children to the upright position, assists with visual perception, and can aid in digestion and GI motility (Fig. 35.11). Standing can also be used for prolonged muscle stretching, especially in the older or larger child.

Positioning for feeding for the child with CP is often critical for his or her ultimate success and safety at this task. The child's head and neck posture is an important factor in the child's ability to protect their airway during the swallowing. Pelvic lumbar spinal postures contribute to intraabdominal volume and pressure, which can play a role in the development of gastroesophageal reflux. Inclination with respect to gravity is an important consideration when the speed of bolus progression in the mouth is considered and the child's ability to control its progression during swallowing is evaluated. A team approach using the skills of the physical and occupational therapist in conjunction with those of the speech therapist is essential in designing a program to optimize the child's oral motor skills (Fig. 35.12).

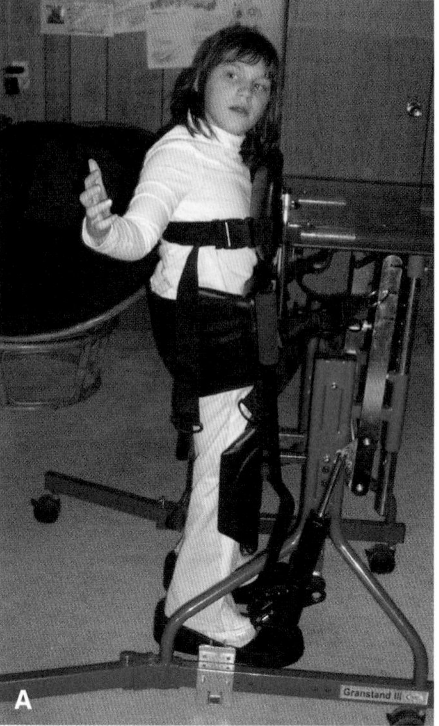


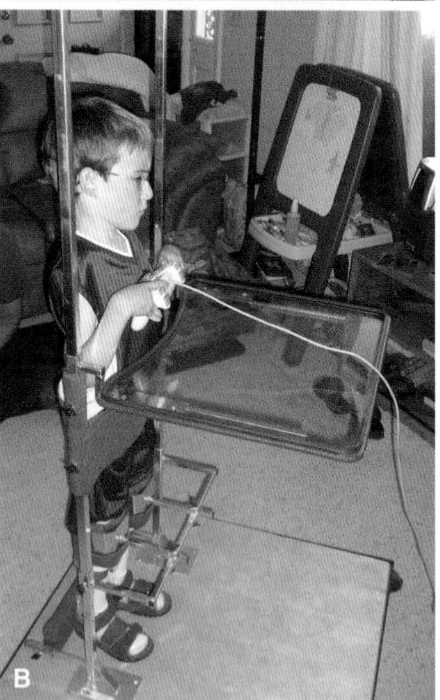


**Figure 35.11**

**Standing frame.** Many different types and styles of standers are available, with a variety of adaptive features. (A) Young girl with spastic hemiplegia from a birth injury/infection drives her power chair up to the stander. With assistance, she is able to get a seat sling under her buttocks to lift her up to standing. The sling is significant because it allows the parent to avoid lifting her into the stander. Shoe holders guide the placement of her feet. (B) This standing frame offers an additional fun feature: the ability to operate a PlayStation. (Courtesy Tamara Kittelson-Aldred, Access Therapy Services, Missoula, MT. Used with permission.)

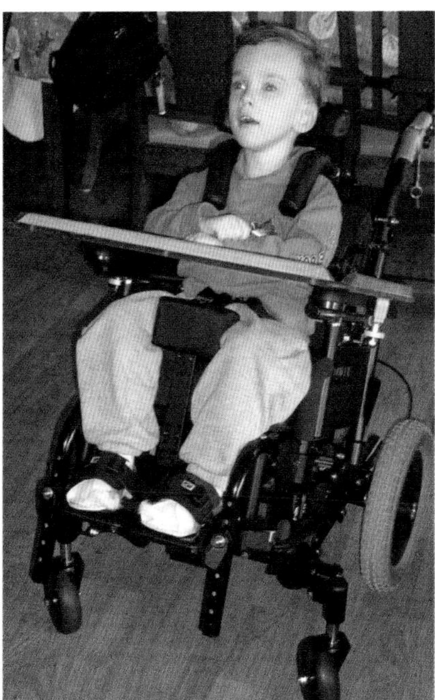

**Figure 35.12**

**Young boy with schizencephaly and cerebral palsy with severe involvement has a planar seating system with postural components.** A tilt-in-space feature and deep ischial ledge formed in the seat keep his pelvis aligned and hips back. Hip flexion is combined with the medial thigh support between his legs to keep his knees apart and allow him to relax. Shoulder pad retractors are a feature added when it was discovered that downward pressure and anterior support at the shoulders improved head control for this child. (Courtesy Tamara Kittelson-Aldred, Access Therapy Services, Missoula, MT. Used with permission.)

For children with expressive communication deficits, sign language, communication boards, and a variety of high-tech communication systems with voice synthesizers are available to augment spoken communication. These can also be linked with wheelchair-based control systems for the child using a power wheelchair.

When evaluating a person for assistive technology, consideration should be given both to the individual's unique abilities and challenges and to the environment in which the equipment will be used. The products should provide the person the greatest degree of functional independence in all the environmental situations encountered. The barriers in each environment may vary, and thus the solutions by necessity may be different in different environments.

### Manual Passive Range-of-Motion Exercise

Splinting or positioning that offers a low-load prolonged stretch that is used throughout the day (or night if tolerated) is recommended for children with CP at risk for contracture. Splints such as lower extremity ankle-foot orthoses (AFOs) to maintain ankle ROM or supported standing to control lower extremity flexion contractures and assist with weight bearing across the hip may be implemented. Manual passive ROM exercise is not without its applications and should be applied gently and to the person's tolerance. It is best combined with a well-thought-out positioning and splinting program.

Other interventions used by therapists to improve ROM and facilitate motor development or improve function include relaxation techniques such as neutral warmth or pressure to acupressure points; serial or tone casts (often in conjunction with botulinum toxin A injections); therapy ball activities; aquatic programs; and manual therapy techniques.[47,83,123]

### Orthoses

AFOs are probably the most commonly used orthoses for children with CP. A rigid polypropylene AFO is used to provide medial-lateral stability to the foot and ankle, while at the same time assisting with foot clearance during gait. The AFO can be set at +3 degrees of dorsiflexion to facilitate the increased ankle dorsiflexion necessary for the swing phase of gait or to decrease genu recurvatum (hyperextension at the knee) through ground reaction forces.

Hinged AFOs may be recommended once a child is moving in the upright position, especially when the child is beginning to walk, squat, or move up and down stairs, both to allow active ankle motion and to allow normal tibial progression during the stance phase of gait. A more flexible plastic such as copolymer or a thinner polypropylene may be used in the lighter child to provide more dynamic use of the foot musculature. In this case, the term *dynamic ankle-foot orthosis* is used.

In some cases, dorsiflexion assist hinges may be used, either with a plantar flexion stop or, in the more mild cases, with free plantar flexion. Care must be taken to choose the correct degree of hinge strength (or an adjustable hinge) so as not to create a crouched posture.

An SMO provides medial-lateral stability for the foot and ankle while allowing free plantar flexion and dorsiflexion. It is always helpful to have whatever plantar flexion is available, since this motion helps decelerate the limb during middle and late stances and facilitates the initial progression of the limb during late stance and early swing.

The SMO can be used when decreased active ankle dorsiflexion and excessive genu recurvatum are not problems. Extending the SMO proximally to the malleoli provides important support, whereas support distal to the malleoli usually shifts the deformity in a proximal direction. General guidelines and recommendations for foot and ankle splinting can be found in Table 35.4 (Fig. 35.13).

### Adolescents With Cerebral Palsy[79]

Therapists are encouraged to include older children and teens in problem solving to help them become more self-sufficient, assuming more responsibility during this developmental phase despite possible limitations in physical capability. Providing adolescents the opportunity to participate in planning and decision making is important for transition planning.

Adolescents may participate in decisions about assistive technology, environmental modifications, health and fitness, and prevention of secondary musculoskeletal impairments. Likewise, the therapist can work closely with those individuals interested in participating in recreation and sports activities. Client-centered assessment of strengths and needs identifying self-care, productivity, and leisure activities is possible and has been reported with this population.[79]

**Table 35.4** General Foot and Ankle Splinting Guidelines

| Splints | Status | Application |
|---|---|---|
| Adjustable dynamic response hinged AFO | Clients with some but limited, functional mobility who achieve foot flat in stance and demonstrate plantar flexion in swing | Independent standing and ambulation. Allows for both tibial progression in standing and eccentric plantar flexion loading on heel strike. |
| Solid AFO neutral to +3 degrees DF | Nonambulators | 1. Less than 3 degrees of DF<br>2. For use in stander<br>3. Need for medial-lateral stability<br>4. Nighttime/positional stretching |
| AFO with 90 degrees plantar flexion stop and free DF (hinged AFO) | Clients with some, but limited, functional mobility | Independent standing and ambulation. Allows for tibial progression for squatting, steps, ambulation and sit-to-stand |
| Floor reaction AFO (set dorsiflexion depending on weight line in standing) | Crouch gait<br>Full passive knee extension in standing (or set AFO to accommodate contracture) | For clients with crouch during standing and ambulation |
| SMO | Pronation in standing | 1. Individual needs medial-lateral ankle stability<br>2. Allows active plantar flexion |

*AFO*, Ankle-foot orthosis; *DF*, dorsiflexion; *SMO*, supramalleolar orthosis.

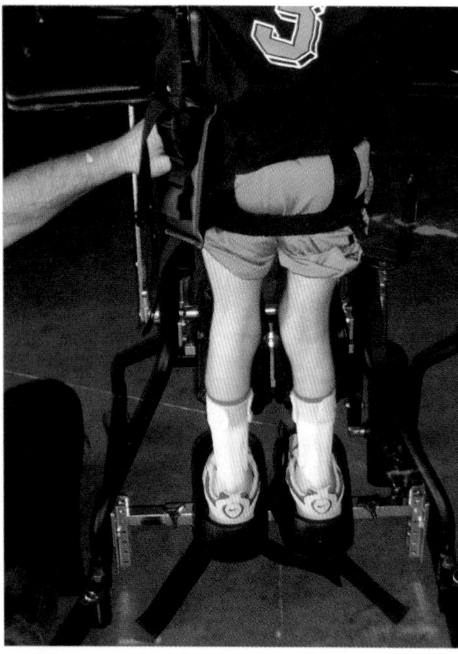

**Figure 35.13**

**Orthoses.** Ankle-foot orthoses (as seen from behind this client) in a standing frame are used for foot alignment and inhibition of tone associated with spastic quadriplegia. (Courtesy Tamara Kittelson-Aldred, Access Therapy Services, Missoula, MT. Used with permission.)

## Adults With Cerebral Palsy

Therapists must also recognize and address the ongoing and unique needs of adults with CP (Fig. 35.14). Improved understanding of CP and its associated long-term complications, combined with improved health care, has resulted in increased longevity. These factors have created a new area of concern for children with CP living into adulthood: managing the effects of the aging process. Years of walking with atypical patterns often result in pain. Decline of ambulation can lead to an enhanced fall risk, along with impaired muscle strength and elasticity, This loss of ambulatory status and other comorbidities affect how functional routines are carried out, reducing quality of life. Reduced bone density can also create a heightened risk of fracture with increased age, which can be accompanied by functional decline.[17]

Group homes, independent living centers, and sheltered workshops are now making it possible for many nonambulatory adults with disabilities to function independently or semi-independently. Regular daily living assistance is required by adults with spastic quadriplegia, especially in the area of lifts and transfers.

Degenerative arthritis, severe joint contractures, and other orthopedic deformities present the most common and challenging problems in this population (Fig. 35.15). Moderate to intense pain is a significant problem for the majority of adults with CP, accompanied by depressive symptoms that interfere with daily life. Further research is needed to determine the functional impact of this problem and appropriate interventions.[37,99]

Management strategies for older children and adults are different by virtue of their ability to participate in and understand the aims of therapy. Therapy is essential to maintain functional skills through the adolescent growth spurt, or when weight gain, weakness, and atrophy result in a decline in function. Aerobic training may prevent deterioration in body composition and muscle strength.[115]

Strengthening has become an integral part of therapy programs for individuals with CP and is especially helpful in this population. Isokinetic strength measurement is considered reliable in this population and should be used in rehabilitation protocols.[8] Isokinetic strengthening three times per week for 8 weeks can improve muscle strength and gross motor skills[69,115] and increase cadence[29] for those people who remain ambulatory into adulthood. A traditional upper extremity strengthening program of 6 to 10 repetitions three times per week for 8 weeks has also been useful in improving speed and endurance in independent wheelchair propulsion.

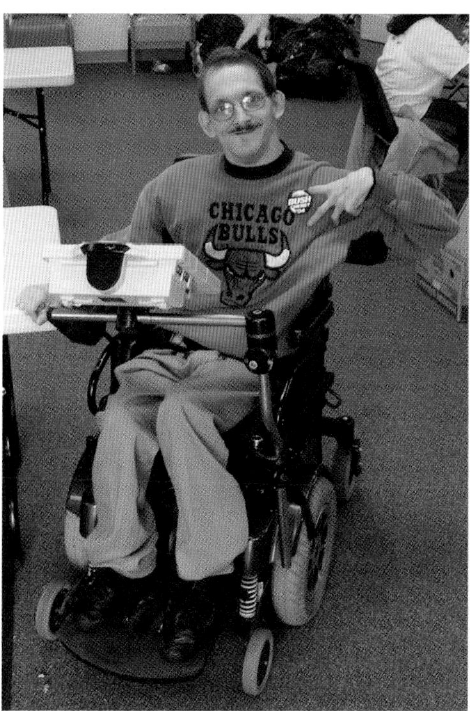


**Figure 35.14**

**Adult with cerebral palsy.** This 33-year-old man with athetoid cerebral palsy uses a speech-generating (communication) device and power chair; the joystick to operate the chair is under the client's right hand. The communication device can be folded and moved out to the side to allow for transfers. The chair has power tilt for independent position changes and pressure relief. Ankle huggers wrapped around the ankles keep his legs from flailing. A neoprene chest harness was added later to help provide external stability and increase control of his movements (not shown). This individual has clearly communicated how much he likes having the chest support, saying he feels much more in control of his body with it on. Straps and supports are fashioned with buckles, because Velcro is not strong enough to hold this client. The additional supports help reduce athetoid movements and improve function. (Courtesy Tamara Kittelson-Aldred, Access Therapy Services, Missoula, MT. Used with permission.)

## Lifelong Follow-Up

Physical therapists can anticipate the need for periodic reevaluation through the lifespan. Because the child is a dynamic system that constantly evolves due to growth and development, clinicians should plan to reevaluate the child's rehabilitation needs on a periodic basis, either through individual care at school, in an outpatient setting, or as part of a multidisciplinary clinic. Children with nonprogressive acquired brain injury due to cerebral palsy or stroke can have changing impairments due to growth, different equipment needs, or they may have increased capacity to participate in an intervention to achieve a specific goal. By understanding the child's neuropathophysiology, clinicians can contribute to the collective understanding of neuroplastic potential in children with acquired lesions and partner with patients and families to provide comprehensive and individualized family-centered care to maximize the child's ultimate functional potential.

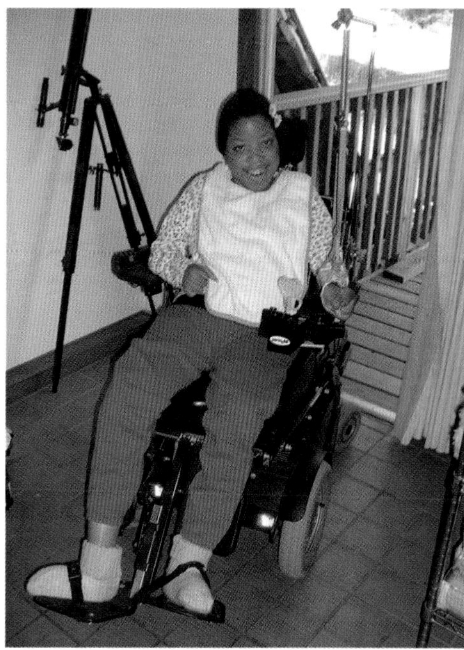

**Figure 35.15**

**Adult with cerebral palsy.** Adults with moderate to severe effects of cerebral palsy can face some difficult physical challenges. This 21-year-old woman has a power chair with seat elevator, power tilt in space, and power elevating leg rests she can operate herself. Each leg rest can be raised or lowered separately for her comfort. This client changes her lower extremity position frequently to manage pain related to spasticity and immobility. A spring upper extremity assist on the left helps keep her hand on a modified joystick to allow her to independently control her chair. (Courtesy Tamara Kittelson-Aldred, Access Therapy Services, Missoula, MT. Used with permission.)

## REFERENCES

To enhance this text and add value for the reader, all references are included in the enhanced ebook on Student Consult that accompanies this textbook. The reader can view the reference source and access it online whenever possible.

# CHAPTER 36

# Seizures and Epilepsy

KENDA S. FULLER • VICKI STEMMONS MERCER

## SEIZURES AND EPILEPSY

### Overview and Definition

*Epilepsy* comes from the Greek word meaning "possession." The Greek people believed that seizures were caused by demons. Stigma and prejudice surrounding epilepsy continue, and people living with epilepsy often are reluctant to admit it or to seek treatment.[11]

A fundamental difference exists between seizure and epilepsy. A seizure is a finite event; it has a beginning and an end. Seizures are a result of excessive hypersynchronous discharge of cerebral neurons resulting in paroxysmal alteration of neurologic function.[30] Seizures can be induced in any normal human brain by a variety of different electrical or chemical stimuli. The cerebral cortex in particular contains within its anatomic and physiologic structure a mechanism that is inherently unstable and capable of producing a seizure. Seizures are a relatively common symptom of brain dysfunction, and they may occur in many acute medical or neurologic illnesses if brain function is temporarily disrupted. These seizures are most often self-limited and do not persist after the underlying disorder has resolved. Seizures also can occur as a reaction of the brain to physiologic stress, sleep deprivation, fever, and alcohol or sedative drug withdrawal. Isolated seizures also occur sometimes for no discernible reason as unprovoked events in presumably healthy people. None of these kinds of seizures represents epilepsy.[9]

Epilepsy is the condition of recurrent, unprovoked seizures.[30] Epilepsy is diagnosed in an individual who has 1) at least two unprovoked or reflex seizures more than 24 hours apart, 2) one unprovoked or reflex seizure and a probability of having another seizure similar to the general recurrence risk after two unprovoked seizures (≥60%) over the next 10 years, or 3) an epilepsy syndrome.[9]

Epilepsy syndromes consist of clusters of clinical and electroencephalography (EEG) characteristics, imaging findings, age-dependent features, triggers, and sometimes prognostic features that occur together.[9] Although many epilepsy syndromes are well recognized, the International League Against Epilepsy (ILAE) has never created a formal classification or listing of these syndromes. New syndromes are constantly emerging.

### Incidence

Acute symptomatic seizures constitute 40% to 50% of all seizures but are not considered epilepsy.[25] The risk of acute symptomatic seizures is higher in males than females, a difference that may be attributable to the disparate incidence of predisposing factors, such as traumatic brain injury. Etiologic factors are varied and include infections, stroke, central nervous system (CNS) tumors, metabolic disorders, toxins, and arteriovenous malformations.

Unprovoked seizures occur in the absence of an inciting stimulus and raise concern for a predisposition to epileptic seizures. The incidence of unprovoked seizures is 50 to 70 per 100,000 and of epilepsy is 30 to 50 per 100,000.[25] After headache, epilepsy is the most frequent chronic neurologic condition seen in general practice worldwide. In developed countries the incidence is highest among young children and elderly adults. In comparison, incidence of epilepsy appears to peak in early adulthood in developing countries.[29]

### Etiologic and Risk Factors

The concept of genetic epilepsy is that epilepsy is the direct result of a known or presumed genetic defect in which seizures are the core symptom of the disorder. First-degree relatives with epilepsy account for 15% of cases, and of those, about 75% have just one affected relative. However, the risk is still higher in first-degree relatives of patients with epilepsy than in the general population. Heritable factors are important in children. Common features include a variable family history, generalized spike-wave abnormality on EEG, and onset in childhood or adolescence. Because there are no consistent, demonstrable pathologic changes in the brains of individuals with idiopathic generalized epilepsy, susceptibility to these seizures most likely results from inherited biochemical, membrane, or neurotransmitter defects that result in abnormal excitability within the involved circuits.

Box 36.1

**MUTATION OF GENES AND SEIZURE TYPE**

Benign familial neonatal seizures
- Potassium-channel *KCNQ2* and *KCNQ3*

Benign familial neonatal-infantile seizures
- Sodium-channel *SCN2A*

Generalized epilepsy with febrile seizures (+)
- Sodium-channel subunits *SCN1A, SCN1B,* and *SCN2A* and *GABRG2* subunit of $GABA_A$ receptor

Childhood absence epilepsy with febrile seizures
- *GABRG2* subunit of $GABA_A$ receptor

Autosomal dominant juvenile myoclonic epilepsy
- *GABRA1* subunit of $GABA_A$ receptor and in *EFHC1*, regulation of calcium currents

Autosomal dominant idiopathic generalized epilepsy
- Chloride-channel gene *CLCN2*

Autosomal dominant nocturnal frontal lobe epilepsy
- Nicotinic acetylcholine receptor subunits *CHRNA4* and *CHRNB2*

Autosomal dominant partial epilepsy with auditory features
- *LGI1* gene, involved in development of CNS

*CNS*, Central nervous system; *$GABA_A$*, γ-aminobutyric acid class A.

Data from Samuel Wiebe: The epilepsies. In Goldman L, Schafer AI, editors: *Goldman's Cecil medicine*, ed 24, St. Louis, 2011, Saunders.

Recent advances in epilepsy genetics are changing the conceptual boundaries between epilepsy phenotypes and the prospects for precision medicine and new drug discovery.[32] Next-generation sequencing (NGS) has led to substantial progress in the discovery of genes for monogenic epilepsy, in which a single variant of large effect is considered causative. NGS studies have revealed how mutations in the same gene can give rise to a spectrum of epilepsy phenotypes (or even different forms of neurodevelopmental disease) and have highlighted the genetic heterogeneity underlying some relatively well-defined epilepsy phenotypes. In some cases of epilepsy, data are most consistent with complex, polygenic influences.[4,23] Attempts to identify variants that confer susceptibility to complex epilepsy have been less successful than studies of single gene mutations. Box 36.1 describes relationships between mutations and type of epilepsy. Genetic predisposition to seizure activity may explain why one individual with brain damage develops epilepsy while another with similar damage does not .[32]

Structural/metabolic causes of seizures are multiple, and the symptoms may be transient, resolving after treatment of the primary disorder. Box 36.2 describes some of the causes of acute symptomatic seizures. In people older than age 50 years, cerebrovascular disease is the most common cause of seizures, which often accompany or follow a stroke. It is thought that perhaps even in the absence of stroke, cerebrovascular disease may predispose an individual to seizure activity.[10] Seizures may be the first symptom of an intracranial mass, and it is suggested that 10% to 15% of cases of older adult–onset epilepsy are a result of neoplasm. When the seizure is due to a permanent lesion or scar, the seizure activity may persist.

Head trauma is the most common preventable cause of epilepsy. Changes in estrogen and progesterone levels can alter seizure susceptibility.[12] Some women with epilepsy have a pattern of increased seizures at specific times in the menstrual cycle. Menopause tends to occur earlier in women with epilepsy, and this early menopause is associated with a history of high seizure frequency.[31] Fertility appears to be reduced by seizure activity when it is triggered by hormonal changes. Disruptions of reproductive function in women include anovulatory cycles that may increase the risk for infertility, migraine, emotional disorders, and reproductive cancers. Moreover, both epilepsy itself and use of antiepileptic medications have been implicated as causal or contributory factors that can

Box 36.2

**POTENTIAL CAUSES OF ACUTE SYMPTOMATIC SEIZURES**

***Medical Conditions***

*Metabolic Derangements*

- Hyponatremia (<120 mEq/L)—especially acute
- Hypernatremia (>150–155 mEq/L)—especially acute
- Hypoglycemia (<40 mg/dL)
- Hyperglycemia (>400 mg/dL)
- Hyperosmolality (>320 mOsm/L)
- Hypocalcemia (<7 mg/dL)
- Respiratory alkalosis—acute

*Drug-Induced Seizures*

- Isoniazid, penicillins
- Theophylline, aminophylline
- Lidocaine
- Meperidine
- Ketamine, halothane, enflurane, methohexital
- Amitriptyline, maprotiline, imipramine, doxepin, fluoxetine
- Haloperidol, trifluoperazine, chlorpromazine
- Ephedrine, phenylpropanolamine, terbutaline
- Methotrexate, BCNU (carmustine), asparaginase
- Cyclosporine
- Cocaine (crack), phencyclidine, amphetamines
- Alcohol (withdrawal)

*Illnesses*

- Eclampsia
- Hypertensive encephalopathy
- Liver failure
- Polyarteritis nodosa
- Porphyria
- Renal failure
- Sickle cell disease
- Syphilis
- Systemic lupus erythematosus
- Thrombotic thrombocytopenic purpura
- Whipple disease

***Neurologic Conditions***

- Angiitis of the nervous system
- Meningitis
- Encephalitis
- Acute head trauma (impact seizures)
- Stroke
- Brain abscess
- Brain tumor

Adapted from Pedley TA: The epilepsies. In Goldman L, editor: *Cecil textbook of medicine*, ed 22, Philadelphia, 2004, Saunders.

alter reproductive hormone levels and promote the development of reproductive endocrine disorders, especially polycystic ovarian syndrome. Gestational epilepsy results from hormonal and metabolic changes that exacerbate underlying epilepsy or adversely influence serum levels of anticonvulsants. Eclampsia or toxemia is a gestational hypertensive encephalopathy manifested by seizure, hypertension, coma, proteinuria, and edema. Convulsive generalized status epilepticus in pregnancy jeopardizes both the mother and the fetus.

The age-dependent appearance of spontaneous seizures in the primary epilepsies appears to depend on a critical period in cerebral maturation when the genetically determined defect is expressed clinically as a manifest change in behavior. Specific syndromes are typical at particular ages and are described at the end of this chapter.

Neonatal seizures, occurring within the first 30 days of life or before 44 weeks postconception in premature infants, merit special consideration because of their age-specific characteristics, varying etiologies, and unique pathophysiology.[30] Major causes of neonatal seizures include hypoxia-ischemia, hypoglycemia, hypocalcemia, hyponatremia, intracranial hemorrhage, infection, congenital malformations, genetic factors, inherited metabolic disorders, and drug withdrawal. Hypoxic-ischemic brain insult, resulting from compromise of oxygen to the brain before or during delivery, is the most common cause of neonatal seizures.. Hypoglycemia, most often seen in infants who are small for gestational age, produces neurologic symptoms of irritability, drowsiness, hypotonia, and apnea. Approximately 50% of infants with hypoglycemia develop neurologic symptoms, and about 25% of these infants subsequently develop seizures. Hypocalcemia (serum level below 7 mg/100 mL) may occur in the first 2 to 3 days of life in low-birth-weight infants or in association with the complications of birth asphyxia.

## Pathogenesis

A seizure occurs when there is distortion of the normal balance between excitation and inhibition in the brain.[30] This imbalance between excitation and inhibition can be caused by either a genetic or an acquired alteration at many levels of brain function. Genetic pathologies leading to epilepsy can occur anywhere from the circuit level to the receptor level to abnormal ionic channel function. Similarly, acquired cerebral insults can alter circuit function (e.g., structural alteration of hippocampal circuitry following prolonged febrile seizures or head trauma).[30] The original insult leads to a pathologic attempt at compensation by sprouting of the excitatory mossy fibers. Mossy fiber sprouting leads to increased excitability and to epilepsy.

Activation of the *N*-methyl-D-aspartate type of glutamate receptors potentiates cellular excitability and leads to sustained neuronal depolarization and calcium influx. Extracellular potassium and intracellular calcium concentrations increase and contribute to the overall excitability of the epileptic neuronal aggregate. Spread of bursting activity to other neurons is normally prevented by surrounding inhibitory mechanisms, such as hyperpolarization and inhibitory interneurons. The main inhibitory neurotransmitter of the CNS is γ-aminobutyric acid (GABA). When stimulated, GABA receptors modulate chloride ion flux, inhibiting membrane depolarization. GABA antagonists or functional depletion of GABA increases membrane depolarization and may result in seizures. GABA agonists (direct or indirect) therefore play a vital role in seizure termination. Loss of GABA-mediated inhibition results in seizures.[27]

During the seizure itself, neurons are tonically depolarized and fire continuously in a sustained, high-frequency discharge (tonic phase). The seizure ends as phasic repolarizations interrupt the continuous firing pattern (clonic phase) and gradually restore membrane potentials to normal or to a temporary hyperpolarized state (postictal depression). Prolonged *N*-methyl-D-aspartate receptor activation and excessive accumulation of intracellular calcium also result in neuronal toxicity and may lead to cell death. The thalamus plays a role in generating generalized seizures and the generalized spike-wave EEG patterns that accompany them. The substantia nigra also is crucial to the expression of generalized seizures, especially the tonic phase; GABAergic inhibitory transmission in the substantia nigra plays a regulatory role in the propagation of generalized seizure discharges. Generalized seizures and the rhythmic spike-wave discharges are dependent on ionic conductance of the neurons in the thalamic nucleus reticularis, allowing them to function as pacemaker control cells. In the focal epilepsies, abnormal neuronal behavior originates in and may remain confined to a restricted area of the cortex.[10]

Mesial temporal sclerosis, also called hippocampal sclerosis, is characterized by neuronal loss and gliosis; whether hippocampal sclerosis is the cause or the result of seizures (or both) is not known. The scarring is characterized by variable degrees of pyramidal cell loss and gliosis in the hippocampal subfields and dentate gyrus. This condition represents the most common pathologic substrate of focal epilepsy; postmortem studies identified mesial temporal sclerosis in 30.5% to 45% of all epilepsy syndromes and in 56% with mesial temporal lobe epilepsy.[33] Hippocampal atrophy and increased hippocampal signal are best seen on T2-weighted and fluid-attenuated inversion recovery coronal magnetic resonance imaging (MRI) sequences, and widespread interictal hypometabolism is seen in the temporal lobe on positron emission tomography. Fig. 36.1 shows mesial sclerosis identified on coronal MRI.

The hippocampus plays a critical role in both seizure activity and mood disorders. This suggests that pathology in this area of the brain might provide a link between epilepsy and depression. Remodeling of the hippocampal spine synapses may play a significant role in the neurobiology of depression and the effects of antidepressant therapy. Because the effects of estrogens on hippocampus parallel those of antidepressants, loss of estrogen appears to be a critical contributor to the etiology of depressive disorders. The increased incidence of depression observed in women with epilepsy might therefore reflect a hormonal deficiency state.[37] Shifts in levels of brain-derived neurotrophic factor in the brain may represent another common link between the distinctive patterns of epilepsy and depression seen in women. Dramatic fluctuations in

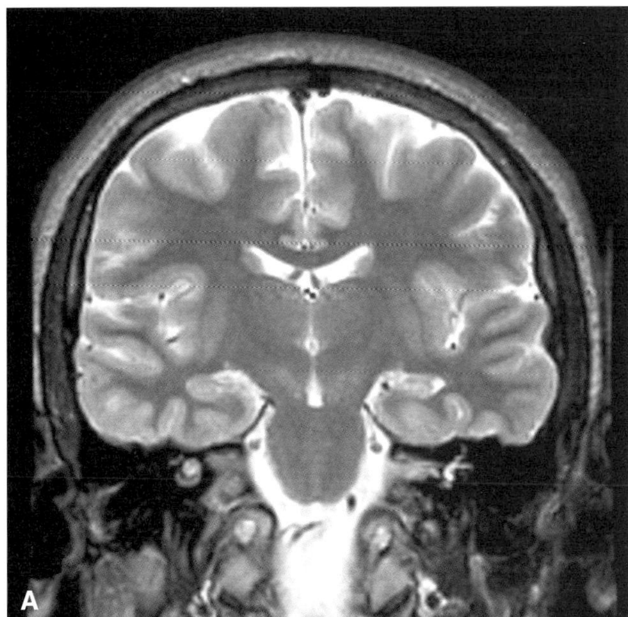


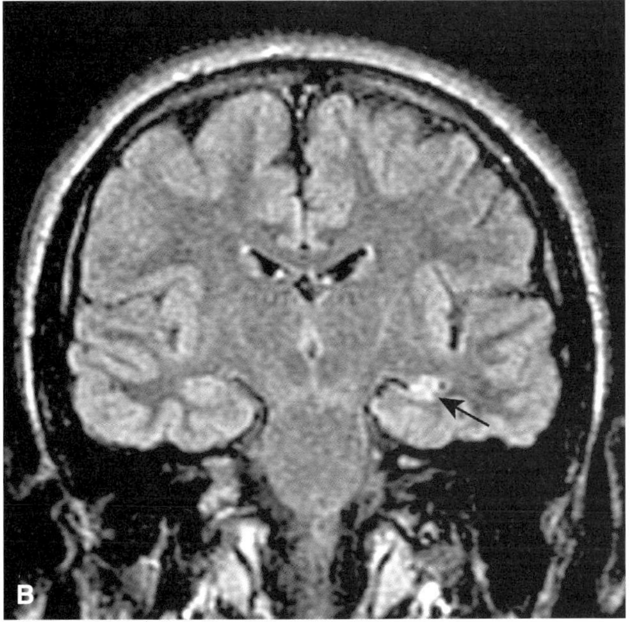


**Figure 36.1**

**Coronal magnetic resonance imaging (MRI) of temporal mesial sclerosis.** The coronal projection is essential to reveal hippocampal abnormalities. Fluid-attenuated inversion recovery MRI is superior to T2 weighting to show signal abnormalities because the saturation nullifies the signal from the cerebrospinal fluid. (A) T2-weighted scan shows volume reduction of the left hippocampus. (B) Fluid-attenuated inversion recovery sequence shows the abnormal high signal *(arrow)*, not seen on the T2 scan. (From Adam A, Dixon AK, Grainger RG, et al, eds: *Grainger and Allison's diagnostic radiology: a textbook of medical imaging*, ed 4, Philadelphia, 2001, Churchill Livingstone.)

estrogen levels in women may explain their greater vulnerability to depression, even as estrogen-related surges in brain-derived neurotrophic factor expression may lead to an increased propensity for seizures.

Another potential explanation of the facilitation of seizures is *kindling*. Kindling refers to the processes that mediate long-lasting changes in brain function in response to repeated, gradually augmented stimulation of the brain resulting in epileptiform activity. Kindling also refers to sensitization of neuronal tissue by the addition of a drug or electrical stimulus that renders it susceptible to subsequent seizure activity. This may explain why exposures to localized, repetitive, low-intensity electrical stimuli induce increasingly pathologic responses. This is a possible mechanism that exists during the latent period between the occurrence of a brain insult and the later onset of epilepsy. Among the many mechanisms of epileptogenesis, kindling-like processes may be critically involved in the progression from electrographic to clinically obvious seizures.[19] A state of abnormal focal (ictal) discharges may develop at the time of the initial injury, with the latent period involving a progressive process that gradually lowers the seizure threshold ("kindling") or the threshold to recruitment of other brain areas (maturation of epileptic networks).[19] Chronic focal epileptogenic lesions can cause distant areas to become capable of generating abnormal electrical discharges and seizures. This distant focus can continue to function independently after ablation of the primary lesion, with important implications for surgical treatment of epilepsy.

The concept of epileptic encephalopathy has grown in acceptance and use. Epileptic encephalopathy is the notion that the epileptic activity itself may contribute to severe cognitive and behavioral impairments above and beyond what might be expected from the underlying pathology (e.g., cortical malformation) alone and that these impairments can worsen over time. Cognitive and behavioral impairments may be global or more selective and may occur along a spectrum of severity. Although certain syndromes are often referred to as epileptic encephalopathies, the encephalopathic effects of seizures and epilepsy may potentially occur in association with any form of epilepsy.[2]

## Classification of Seizures

In the most recent ILAE classification system, seizures are defined by onset as focal, generalized, unknown, or unclassifiable.[9] Fig. 36.2 shows the expanded version of this classification system. *Focal seizure* describes activity either localized or more widely distributed within networks limited to one hemisphere. Focal seizures have clinical or EEG evidence of a local onset. *Generalized epileptic seizures* are conceptualized as originating at some point in one hemisphere, eventually activating distributed networks of both hemispheres. Generalized seizures can be asymmetric. "Unknown onset" refers to when the onset is unknown, but other manifestations of the seizure are known.

Focal seizures can be further classified as "aware" or "impaired awareness" seizures. "Impaired awareness" is not synonymous with loss of consciousness, but rather refers to the individual's awareness of the event and should be used if awareness is impaired at any time during a focal seizure. The next step after consideration of the level of awareness for a focal seizure involves defining the onset as motor or nonmotor. In distinguishing between motor and nonmotor, the initial sign or symptom defines the seizure type, even if more prominent features occur

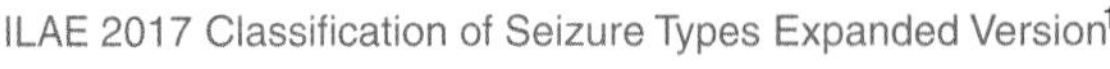


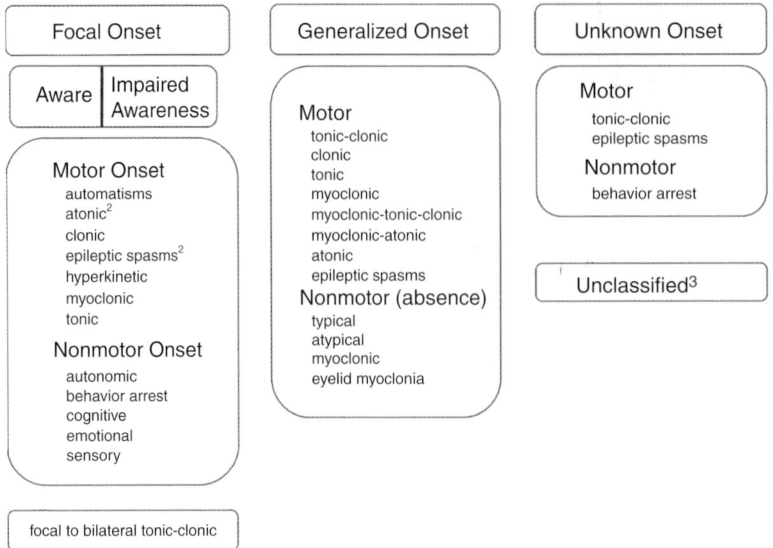


[1]Definitions, other seizure types and descriptors are listed in Fisher et al, Operational classification of seizure types by the International League Against Epilepsy: Position paper of the ILAE Commission for Classification and Terminology. Epilepsia, 2017

[2]Degree of awareness usually is not specified.

[3]Due to inadequate information or inability to place in other categories.

**Figure 36.2**

International League Against Epilepsy *(ILAE)* classification system defines seizures by onset as focal, generalized, unknown, or unclassifiable. (From Falco-Walter JJ, et al: The new definition and classification of seizures and epilepsy. *Epilepsy Res* 139:73–79, 2018.)

later in the course of the seizure. Focal onset seizures that spread to involve both hemispheres are called "focal to bilateral tonic-clonic seizures."[9]

Generalized seizures also are designated as motor or nonmotor (absence). Generalized motor seizures are further classified as tonic-clonic or other motor. Unknown onset seizures also can be classified as tonic-clonic or other motor.

## Clinical Manifestations

In most individuals, seizures occur unpredictably at any time and without any relationship to posture or ongoing activities.[16] In some individuals, seizures are provoked by specific stimuli, such as flashing lights or a flickering television. Box 36.3 lists the typical triggers to seizure. The presence of focal signs after the seizure suggests that the seizure may have a focal origin. Prodromal symptoms (premonitory symptoms that indicate an impending seizure) may include headache, mood alterations, lethargy, and myoclonic jerking. The initial events of a seizure, described either by the individual or by an observer, are usually the most reliable indicators of whether a seizure begins focally.[10]

### Focal Onset Seizures

Focal aware nonmotor seizures that begin in primary sensory areas can produce sensory symptoms, such as localized paresthesias, numbness, vertigo, auditory hallucinations, and unformed visual hallucinations. Focal seizures originating in the cortical area that represents sensation of the hand may begin with contralateral hand tingling and then progress to involve additional cortical regions ipsilaterally, producing more extensive sensory symptoms as well as clonic motor signs. The sensation seems to march from hand to arm to leg area ipsilaterally, a process referred to as a *Jacksonian march.* Note that despite the motor signs, this seizure would still be classified as nonmotor because the first sign or symptom was sensory. In focal aware seizures, consciousness is not depressed, and individuals can interact normally with their environment except for limitations imposed by the seizure.

Focal motor seizures may be characterized by various effects on muscles such as atonia, in which the involved part of the body suddenly goes limp; clonic activity, involving rhythmic contraction and relaxation of muscles; myoclonus, or brief, shocklike involuntary jerking of a muscle or group of muscles; tonic muscle contraction; or epileptic spasms, in which the body flexes and extends repeatedly.[24]

In focal impaired awareness seizures, alteration of cognition is the major feature. These seizures can originate from various brain regions but most often start in the temporal lobe or the frontal lobe. In temporal lobe seizures, loss of consciousness results when the discharge spreads bilaterally to involve areas of the hippocampus and amygdala. The person appears dazed and confused and may display strange, repetitious behaviors, such as mouth movements (often like chewing or swallowing),

Box 36.3
**EVENTS THAT MAY TRIGGER SEIZURE**

- Stress
- Poor nutrition
- Missed medication
- Skipping meals
- Flickering lights
- Illness
- Fever and allergies
- Lack of sleep
- Emotions such as anger, worry, fear
- Heat and humidity

pulling at clothing, or walking in a circle. These repetitious movements are called *automatisms*.[24] If the person is performing motor tasks, such as eating, drawing, or walking, when the seizure starts, the motor performance may continue in an awkward manner. These seizures usually last 1 to 2 minutes, followed by confusion and disorientation lasting several more minutes. Individuals are amnesic for details of the seizure that occurred after the aura. An olfactory relationship identifies an origin in or near the uncus of the medial temporal lobe and may have a higher association with brain tumors. Feelings of déjà vu and dreamy states, such as feelings of unreality and depersonalization, distortion of time, and depressed or fearful states, are common. Visual images with illusions of multiple images or distortions regarding size can occur, as well as hallucinatory phenomena. Autonomic symptoms reflect involvement of limbic structures that lie in the mesial temporal or frontal lobe and project to the hypothalamus and brainstem. Table 36.1 describes the symptoms and the associated area of activity in the brain.

### Generalized Onset Seizures

In generalized onset seizures, seizure activity starts throughout the brain or in groups of cells on both sides of the brain at the same time. Of the various types of generalized onset seizures, tonic-clonic seizures are the most common. Although this is the type of epilepsy that most people associate with the disorder, it is less common than focal seizures. The person has a sudden loss of consciousness at the start of a tonic-clonic seizure. In the tonic phase, the body becomes rigid and the person is at risk of falling. The person may grunt or scream as the respiratory muscles contract involuntarily and force air past the vocal cords.[24] Respiration may cease briefly, and the person may become cyanotic. In general, the person's jaw is fixed and hands are clenched. This phase usually lasts for 30 to 60 seconds. The clonic phase begins with rhythmic, jerky contraction and relaxation of all body muscles, especially in the extremities. Fig. 36.3 demonstrates the tonic and clonic phases of seizure. Biting of the tongue, lips, or inside of the mouth may occur. Saliva is blown from the mouth, with a froth appearing on the lips. Incontinence of bladder and bowel can occur.

Generalized tonic-clonic seizures result in many striking but transient physiologic changes, including hypoxia; lactic acidosis; elevated plasma catecholamine levels; and increased concentrations of serum creatine kinase, prolactin, corticotropin, cortisol, β-endorphin, and growth hormone. Recovery may be swift after a short seizure, but a prolonged seizure may induce a deep sleep. Altered speech and transient paralysis or ataxia may follow, as well as headache, disorientation, or muscle soreness. Another seizure may follow without recovery of consciousness, or after recovery of consciousness the person may experience seizure again. As recovery progresses, many individuals complain of headache, muscle soreness, mental dulling, lack of energy, or mood changes lasting 24 hours. Complications include oral trauma; vertebral compression fractures; shoulder dislocation; aspiration pneumonia; and sudden death, which may be related to acute pulmonary edema, cardiac arrhythmia, or suffocation. A person may also experience only the tonic phase. Tonic seizures, which typically last only about 20 seconds, are characterized by stiffening of the body. This stiffening can cause a fall if the seizure occurs when the person is standing. Clonic seizures, which involve only the jerking movements of the arms and legs, are rare, occurring most often in infants.[24]

Seizures with tonic and/or clonic manifestations involve brainstem, possibly prefrontal, and basal ganglia mechanisms. Ictal initiation of primarily bilateral events are predominantly disinhibitory, but other mechanisms are responsible for ictal evolution to the clonic phase, involving gradual periodic introduction of seizure-suppressing mechanisms.

Another type of generalized motor seizure, which may be difficult to distinguish from a clonic seizure, is a myoclonic seizure. Myoclonic seizures involve brief jerks of muscles on both sides of the body. The jerking is more irregular during a myoclonic seizure than a clonic one.[24] The myoclonic jerks may cause the individual to drop or fling objects. Myoclonic seizures are not associated with any obvious disturbance of consciousness.[30]

During a type of generalized motor seizure known as an atonic seizure, or a "drop attack," a person experiences a sudden loss of muscle tone. Atonic seizures occur without warning and often result in falls, with head or face injuries.[30] Sometimes the loss of muscle tone is limited or fragmentary, producing only a head drop. A person generally remains conscious during these seizures.

Generalized nonmotor (absence) seizures, formerly called petit mal seizures, consist of the sudden cessation of ongoing conscious activity, with only minor convulsive muscular activity or loss of postural control. The person often stares into space. Attacks start and end abruptly, usually lasting between 1 and 10 seconds. Absence seizures are not preceded by an aura and are followed by normal activity. If attacks occur during conversation, the person may miss a few words or may break off in midsentence for a few seconds. The person is unaware of the loss of conscious control. These seizures often occur in children and frequently disappear by adolescence. Atypical absence seizures are similar to absence seizures but may last more than 20 seconds.[24]

### Reflex Seizures

Reflex seizures are triggered by specific simple (e.g., flashing lights) or elaborate (e.g., reading) stimuli. Visual-sensitive seizures (triggered by light or visual patterns) are

**Table 36.1** Clinical Manifestations of Focal Seizures

| Seizure Type | Brain Activity | Clinical Expression |
|---|---|---|
| Somatosensory | Postcentral rolandic; parietal | Contralateral tingling, numbness, hot or cold, electric. Sensation of movement, sense of movement, or desire to move. "Marching" to other body segments |
| Parietal | | Contralateral agnosia of a limb, phantom limb, distortion of size or position of body part |
| | | Ipsilateral or bilateral facial, truncal, or limb tingling, numbness, or pain. Often involve lips, tongue, fingertips, feet |
| Motor | Precentral rolandic | Contralateral regional clonic jerking, usually rhythmic, may spread to other body segments in Jacksonian march. Often accompanied by sensory symptoms in same area |
| Supplementary sensory-motor | | Bilateral tonic contraction of limbs causing postural changes, may exhibit classic fencing posture, may have speech arrest or vocalization |
| Frontal | | Contralateral head and eye version, salivation, speech arrest or vocalization; may be combined with other motor signs (as above) depending on seizure spread |
| Auditory | Auditory cortex in superior temporal lobe | Bilateral or contralateral buzzing, drumming, single tones, muffled sounds |
| Olfactory | Orbitofrontal; mesial temporal cortex | Often described as unpleasant odor |
| Gustatory | Parietal; rolandic operculum; insula; temporal lobe | Often unpleasant taste, acidic, metallic, salty, sweet, smoky |
| Vertiginous | Occipitotemporal-parietal junction; frontal lobe | Sensation of body displacement in various directions |
| Visual | Occipital | Contralateral static, moving, or flashing colored or uncolored lights, shapes, or spots. Contralateral or bilateral partial or complete loss of vision |
| Temporal; occipitotemporal-parietal junction | Formed visual scenes, faces, people, objects, animals | |
| | | Autonomic: abdominal rising sensation, nausea, borborygmi, flushing, pallor, piloerection, perspiration, heart rate changes, chest pain, shortness of breath, cephalic sensation, lightheadedness, genital sensation, orgasm |
| Limbic | Limbic structures: amygdala, hippocampus, cingulum, olfactory cortex, hypothalamus | Psychic: déjà vu, jamais vu, depersonalization, derealization, dreamlike state, forced memory or forced thinking, fear, elation, sadness, sexual pleasure, hallucinations or illusions (visual, auditory, or olfactory) |
| Dyscognitive | Usually bilateral involvement of limbic structures (see above) | Previously known as complex partial seizures, characterized by a predominant alteration of consciousness or awareness. Current definition requires involvement of at least 2 of 5 components of cognition: perception, attention, emotion, memory, and executive function |

Adapted from Samuel Wiebe: The epilepsies. In Goldman L, Schafer AI, editors: *Goldman's Cecil medicine*, ed 24, St. Louis, 2011, Saunders.

the most common type of reflex seizures. They occur most commonly in females, and their incidence peaks around puberty, when they represent up to 10% of all new cases of epilepsy. Other triggers of reflex seizures include specific thoughts, actions, reading, tactile stimuli, adopting certain positions, eating, listening to music, startle, and contact with hot water. The triggered seizures can be myoclonic, tonic-clonic, atonic, or focal, depending on the triggering stimulus. The Epilepsy Foundation reports that 85% of people with reflex epilepsy experience generalized tonic-clonic seizures in response to their trigger.[24] Avoiding the offending stimulus is crucial to avoid seizures, emphasizing the importance of careful questioning about seizure triggers in patients with epilepsy.[3]

### Status Epilepticus

Status epilepticus is a condition in which seizures are so prolonged or so repeated that recovery does not occur between attacks. Status epilepticus can be convulsive (in which signs of a seizure can be seen by an observer) or nonconvulsive (which has no outward signs and is diagnosed on the basis of abnormal EEG). Convulsive status epilepticus occurs when the person has generalized tonic-clonic seizures, and no return to consciousness occurs between seizures. This is a medical emergency. The molecular events that cause death can occur with the first few seizures. Tonic-clonic status epilepticus is more common in people whose seizures have a known cause. Often it is the result of tumor, CNS infection, or drug abuse. Febrile

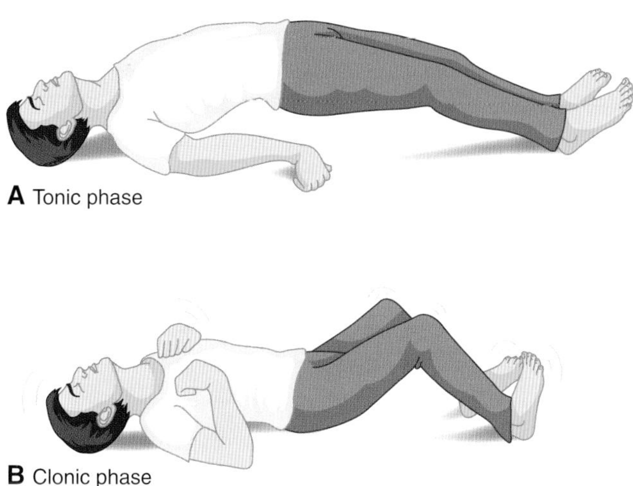


**Figure 36.3**

**Tonic and clonic phases of seizure activity.** (A) Posture typical of tonic phase. (B) Movement associated with clonic phase. (From Black JM: *Medical-surgical nursing: clinical management for positive outcomes*, ed 7, Philadelphia, 2004, Saunders.)

seizures are a common cause of status epilepticus in children younger than 3 years of age. Nonconvulsive status epilepticus is difficult to define, but it may be described as a syndrome in which the most fundamental feature is a change in the individual's behavior. A degree of clouding of mental processes occurs, ranging from drowsiness and confusion to disorientation and dysphagia. Nonconvulsive status epilepticus is seen in various neurologic diagnoses (i.e., trauma, stroke) in the acute intensive care unit setting. It also denotes a condition that can occur de novo in older adults without a precipitating cause and that is characterized by prolonged confusional episodes, which are caused by generalized slow spike-and-wave status epilepticus. There is evidence from surgically resected epileptic tissue that apoptotic pathways are activated in foci of intractable epilepsy.[3]

## MEDICAL MANAGEMENT

DIAGNOSIS. Diagnosis is not the same as a classification. An epilepsy syndrome diagnosis provides more sophisticated information than does an epilepsy type diagnosis for some patients. An epileptic syndrome is characterized with respect to many factors. Knowing a given patient's syndromic diagnosis provides key information about that patient's epilepsy, such as likely age at onset, EEG patterns, responses to medications, and cognitive and developmental status. Seizure etiology is a key consideration, with implications for management and prognostic counseling. The ILAE Task Force has defined six etiologic categories: structural, genetic, infectious, metabolic, immune, and unknown.[9] Not all epilepsies are recognized as electroclinical syndromes. For each seizure type, ictal onset is consistent from one seizure to another, with preferential propagation patterns that can involve the contralateral hemisphere.

The history obtained from the client and the observations of bystanders are important in establishing a diagnosis and classifying the seizure disorder correctly. To determine seizure type, a series of questions must be answered regarding the location of the seizure activity, the level of consciousness, the level of generalized motor activity, and the preceding level of seizure activity. The state of the client after the episode, including the level of confusion, sleepiness, or headache, must be determined. These data may be gathered from the paramedic or emergency personnel in the case of an individual who has been found on the floor.

It is important to recognize events that may mimic a seizure but are not related to the diagnosis of epilepsy. Early morning confusion and headache could be related to hypoglycemia in individuals on hypoglycemic medications. If the event is a transient ischemic attack, a loss of consciousness usually does not occur, and the neurologic insult is in the form of weakness or numbness. With a seizure, however, twitching or tingling is evident. Symptoms that are recurrent and stereotyped, with no evidence of infarct on brain imaging, suggest focal onset seizures rather than transient ischemic attack.[14] Behavioral disturbances seen in dementia can be difficult to distinguish from seizures. When nonconvulsive seizures are suspected in elderly persons, long-term EEG appears to be superior to standard EEG in detecting epileptiform activity.[6] Syncope, or a transient loss of consciousness, is related to an acute change in cerebral perfusion. The related transient cerebral anoxia may itself cause seizure activity.

Syncopal, vasodepressive, orthostatic, or arrhythmogenic states may be confused with ictal events when episodes are recurrent. In general, tonic-clonic movements are much more forceful and are more prolonged than the twitches sometimes associated with fainting. Most seizures are characterized by a postictal state, not seen with syncope except for atonic drop attack. The cause of an unwitnessed, unprovoked loss of consciousness resulting in a fall may be hard to classify. Retrograde amnesia suggests an ictal diagnosis.

Epileptic seizures manifesting as motor phenomena without concomitant change of consciousness may be confused with a paroxysmal movement disorder. Conversely, attacks of paroxysmal movement disorders may be thought to be epileptic owing to a number of factors, including their sudden, unpredictable, and transient nature; their response to anticonvulsants; and the premonitory sensations preceding attacks. These two conditions frequently co-occur. Increased understanding of the genetic underpinnings of the paroxysmal dyskinesias and epilepsy syndromes has provided insights concerning the shared mechanisms of these two conditions. A recently proposed pathophysiologic framework classifies the paroxysmal dyskinesias as representing dysfunction (caused by gene mutations) of ion channels (KCNMA1 and SCN8A) and of proteins associated with the vesical synaptic cycle (PRRT2 and MR1) or involved in energy metabolism (SLC2A1).[8]

Frontal lobe seizures arise predominantly during sleep and can have dramatic motor expression. They can be confused with nonepileptic psychogenic seizures, sleep disorders, or movement disorders. Video-EEG or video-polysomnography may be necessary for diagnosis.[34]

Psychogenic nonepileptic seizures (PNESs), are time-limited, paroxysmal changes in movements, sensations, behaviors, or consciousness that can resemble epileptic seizures, but are not associated with abnormal EEG

**Table 36.2** Behaviors to Distinguish Between Psychogenic Nonepileptic and Epileptic Seizures

| Observation | PNES | ES |
|---|---|---|
| Situational onset | Common | Rare |
| Gradual onset | Common | Rare |
| Precipitated by stimuli (noise, light) | Occasional | Rare |
| Purposeful movements | Occasional | Very rare |
| Opisthotonus (*arc de cercle*) | Occasional | Very rare |
| Tongue biting (tip) | Occasional | Rare |
| Tongue biting (side) | Very rare | Common |
| Prolonged ictal atonia | Occasional | Very rare |
| Vocalization during tonic-clonic phase | Occasional | Very rare |
| Reactivity during unconsciousness | Occasional | Very rare |
| Rapid postictal reorientation | Common | Unusual |
| Undulating motor activity | Common | Very rare |
| Asynchronous limb movements | Common | Rare |
| Rhythmic pelvic movements | Occasional | Rare |
| Side-to-side head shaking | Common | Rare |
| Ictal crying | Occasional | Very rare |
| Ictal stuttering | Occasional | Rare |
| Postictal whispering | Occasional | Not present |
| Closed mouth in tonic phase | Occasional | Very rare |
| Closed eyelids during seizure onset | Very common | Rare |
| Convulsion >2 min | Common | Very rare |
| Resisted lid opening | Common | Very rare |
| Pupillary light reflex | Usually retained | Commonly absent |
| Cyanosis | Rare | Common |
| Ictal grasping | Rare | Occurs in FLE and TLE |
| Postictal nose rubbing | Not present | Can occur in TLE |
| Stertorous breathing postictally | Not present | Common |
| Self-injury | May be present (especially excoriations) | May be present (especially lacerations) |
| Incontinence | May be present | May be present |

*ES*, Epileptic seizure; *FLE*, frontal lobe epilepsy; *PNES*, pyschogenic nonepileptic seizure; *TLE*, temporal lobe epilepsy.
From LaFrance WC: Differentiating frontal lobe epilepsy from psychogenic nonepileptic seizures. *Neurol Clin* 29:149–162, 2011.

activity. Psychogenic seizures can be difficult to diagnose because they can mimic almost any type of seizure, and they often coexist with epilepsy in the same patient. When there are variable clinical manifestations across episodes, frequent and prolonged episodes, out-of-phase upper and lower body movements, pelvic thrusting, and no rigidity, PNESs should be suspected. Individuals with PNESs often have a history of psychologic trauma, including sexual or physical abuse.[1] Neuropsychologic testing is not useful to differentiate PNES from epilepsy. However, psychologic testing may help to determine the psychiatric diagnosis after PNES is diagnosed. Table 36.2 presents behaviors that distinguish between PNESs and epilepsy.

Epileptic encephalopathy is an electroclinical syndrome associated with a high probability that features that manifest will worsen after the onset of epilepsy and tends to be pharmacoresistant. Pharmacoresponsiveness relates to the prediction that the seizures will rapidly come under control with appropriate medication. An encephalopathic course is identified by failure of an individual to develop as expected, relative to age-matched peers, or to actually regress. Epileptic encephalopathy can manifest along a continuum of severity and may occur at any age but is most common and severe in infancy and early childhood, when global and profound cognitive impairment may occur. However, adults can also experience cognitive losses over time from uncontrolled seizures.

Endocrine status is commonly abnormal in cases of epileptic encephalopathy, typically for the sex steroid hormones, manifesting as sexual dysfunction and lower fertility in men and women. Other signs and symptoms in women with epilepsy include menstrual irregularities, premature menopause, and polycystic ovarian syndrome. These concerns should be addressed in standard evaluations in individuals with epilepsy.[12]

***Electroencephalography.*** EEG has a central role in the diagnosis of epilepsy. EEG records the integrated electrical activity generated by synaptic potentials in neurons in the superficial layers of a localized area of cortex. In the epileptic focus, neurons in a small area of the cortex are activated for a brief period in a synchronized pattern and then inhibited. Interictal (between-seizure) activity on EEG provides strong presumptive evidence that the event was a seizure. The best way to diagnose the presence of seizures and to classify the seizure is to observe simultaneously the seizure and the associated EEG recording. A normal reading does not rule out the diagnosis, and in an older individual, it may be more difficult to distinguish normal from abnormal.[35] Prolonged EEG monitoring with simultaneous closed-circuit video recording is reserved for complicated cases of protracted and unresponsive seizures. It provides an invaluable method for recording ictal seizure events that are rarely captured during routine EEG studies. This technique is extremely helpful in the classification of seizures because it can accurately determine the location and frequency of seizure discharges while recording alterations in the level of consciousness and the presence of clinical signs.[15]

***Magnetoencephalography.*** Magnetoencephalography measures the small magnetic fields that are generated by electrical activity in the brain and approximates their location using mathematical models. Its use is largely restricted to evaluation of patients for epilepsy surgery, in whom it is used for mapping interictal discharges and the localization of brain function when superimposed on brain MRI.

***Metabolic Studies.*** Metabolic studies are ideally performed at the time of seizure occurrence, when values are most likely to be abnormal. Lumbar puncture should be considered for children with repeated seizures and other evidence of neurodevelopmental disability. It may be useful for detecting low cerebrospinal fluid glucose in glucose transporter disorder; alterations in amino acids, neurotransmitters, or cofactors in metabolic disorders; or evidence of chronic infection.

Aside from glucose determination, laboratory testing such as serum electrolyte levels and toxicology screening should be based on individual clinical circumstances, such as when dehydration is suspected. EEG is not warranted after a simple febrile seizure but may be useful for evaluating individuals with an atypical feature or with other risk factors for later epilepsy. Similarly, neuroimaging is also not useful for children with simple febrile convulsions but may be considered for children with atypical features, including focal neurologic signs or preexisting neurologic deficits.[9]

Specialized neuropsychologic testing is often needed in evaluating clients with seizures. These tests not only help determine general intelligence and state of brain functioning but also often help to localize lesions.

Imaging of the brain is indicated to rule out mass effect or vascular disease. MRI is the method of choice because the lesions that cause epilepsy are often subtle.

**TREATMENT.** Control of seizures, although paramount in the treatment of epilepsy, is only part of the treatment. Support and education provided by health care professionals is critical to manage the behavioral, social, and economic consequences of uncontrolled seizures. Reassurance should be given that, for most individuals, epilepsy does not indicate serious brain damage. The risk-to-benefit ratio for antiepileptic treatments is one of the biggest challenges in seizure management. Because antiepileptic drugs have various adverse effects, which may interfere with normal developmental processes and affect cognitive functions, the adverse effects of more aggressive treatments compared with the benefits of complete seizure control must be considered.[26,36] Table 36.3 describes common side effects of typical drugs. Antiepileptic drugs carry risks of side effects that are particularly important in children. The decision regarding whether or not to treat children and adolescents who have experienced a first unprovoked seizure must be based on a risk-benefit assessment that weighs the risk of having another seizure against the risks of long-term antiepileptic drug therapy. There appears to be no benefit of treatment with regard to the prognosis for long-term seizure remission.[26]

Antiepileptic drugs are used according to the type of seizure. In most people with seizures of a single type, satisfactory control can be achieved with a single anticonvulsant drug. Monotherapy with all indicated antiepileptic drugs should be attempted before starting combination therapy. Sometimes a trial of several different medications at different doses is needed to find the best fit. Routine monitoring of plasma drug levels is not correlated with reduction in adverse effects or improvement in effectiveness and is not recommended.[18] Clinical indications for monitoring drug levels include establishment of individual therapeutic concentrations when good seizure control has been established, diagnosing clinical toxicity, assessing adherence to the medication regimen, and guiding dosage adjustment in situations with increased pharmacokinetic variability.

Psychiatric comorbidities are extremely common in patients with epilepsy. Depression, anxiety disorders, panic disorder, psychosis, attention-deficit disorders, and autistic disorders are overrepresented in patients with epilepsy. Antiepileptic drugs can have significant psychotropic effects. Medications associated with a higher risk of psychiatric and behavioral side effects include levetiracetam and zonisamide.[5] Medications with decreased rates of psychiatric and behavioral side effects include carbamazepine, clobazam, gabapentin, lamotrigine, oxcarbazepine, phenytoin, and valproate. A slow titration and conservative maintenance doses are especially important in elderly patients.

The abundance of drugs makes decisions more complex, but can help manage the needs of more patients. The newer drugs have shown no better efficacy than the classic drugs, but they are easier to use, with much better pharmacokinetic profiles and fewer drug interactions. New drugs create broad-spectrum effects to control symptoms in patients with generalized epilepsies. Comorbidities can be managed using antiepileptic drugs; positive effects or at least no negative effects can increase tolerance to the drug. Fig. 36.4 diagrams the pharmacologic effects of some antiepileptic drugs at the GABA class A ($GABA_A$) receptor. The relationships among hormones, epilepsy, and the medications used to treat epilepsy are complex, with interactions that affect both men and women in different ways. Antiepileptic drugs and hormones have a bidirectional interaction that can impair the efficacy of contraceptive hormone treatments and the chosen epileptic drug.[12]

Anticonvulsive drugs are safe, but side effects do occur, especially at the start of drug therapy. Side effects of the medication may include ataxia, dysarthria, dizziness, and blurry or double vision. Fatigue is a common complaint.[18] When phenytoin is taken, osteomalacia may occur as a result of increased metabolism of vitamin D. Hyponatremia can occur at low doses of carbamazepine and can lead to serious nervous system and muscular disturbances.[20]

A ketogenic diet may be a helpful therapeutic approach for some individuals with epilepsy, especially children.

**Table 36.3** Side Effects of Commonly Used Antiepileptic Drugs

| Drug | Common Side Effects | Serious Side Effects |
|---|---|---|
| Acetazolamide | Anorexia, frequent urination, drowsiness, confusion, numbness of extremities, kidney stones | Metabolic acidosis, electrolyte imbalance, anaphylaxis, hematologic abnormalities, Stevens-Johnson syndrome |
| Brivaracetam | Dizziness, sleepiness, fatigue, mood changes | Suicidality, psychosis, hallucinations, hematologic abnormalities |
| Carbamazepine | Dizziness, diplopia, blurred vision, ataxia, sedation, nausea, neutropenia, rash, hyponatremia[a] | Hematologic abnormalities, hepatic failure, Stevens-Johnson syndrome |
| Clobazam | Fatigue, lethargy, insomnia, unsteadiness, changes in behavior, changes in appetite | Respiratory depression, suicidality, hematologic abnormalities, Stevens-Johnson syndrome |
| Clonazepam | Drowsiness, sleepiness, fatigue, poor coordination, unsteadiness, behavior changes | Respiratory depression, suicidality, tachycardia, blood dyscrasias |
| Ethosuximide | Loss of appetite, nausea, drowsiness, headache, dizziness, fatigue, rash | Hematologic abnormalities, lupus erythematosus, suicidality, Stevens-Johnson syndrome |
| Gabapentin | Sleepiness, dizziness, ataxia, fatigue, twitching, fluid retention, weight gain | Depression, suicidality, respiratory depression, Stevens-Johnson syndrome |
| Lacosamide | Dizziness, diplopia, blurred vision, headache, nausea, vomiting, fatigue, tremor | PR interval prolongation, atrial fibrillation, atrial flutter, Stevens-Johnson syndrome |
| Lamotrigine | Dizziness, diplopia, blurred vision, clumsiness, fatigue, tremor, insomnia, headache, rash | Stevens-Johnson syndrome, toxic epidermal necrolysis, multiorgan failure, hepatic failure |
| Levetiracetam | Fatigue, dizziness, somnolence, irritability, mood swings, headache | Psychosis, suicidality, hematologic abnormalities, Stevens-Johnson syndrome |
| Oxcarbazepine | Dizziness, diplopia, blurred vision, headache, nausea, hyponatremia | Anaphylaxis, Stevens-Johnson syndrome, toxic epidermal necrolysis |
| Phenytoin | Fatigue, dizziness, ataxia, nausea, confusion, gingival hyperplasia, hirsutism, osteopenia, rash | Stevens-Johnson syndrome, toxic epidermal necrolysis, blood dyscrasia, pseudolymphoma, lupus-like syndrome |
| Pregabalin | Fatigue, dizziness, ataxia, diplopia, weight gain, edema | Hypersensitivity reaction, angioedema, Stevens-Johnson syndrome |
| Primidone | Clumsiness, dizziness, appetite loss, fatigue, drowsiness, hyperirritability, insomnia, depression, hyperactivity (children) | Hematologic abnormalities, dyspnea, lupus erythematosus, suicidality |
| Rufinamide | Somnolence, headache, dizziness, diplopia, fatigue, nausea, vomiting | Shortened QT interval (no known clinical risk), multiorgan hypersensitivity, suicidality |
| Topiramate | Drowsiness, ataxia, word-finding difficulty, difficulty concentrating, anorexia, weight loss, paresthesias, metabolic acidosis, oligohidrosis, nephrolithiasis | Metabolic acidosis, nephrolithiasis, psychosis, suicidality, hematologic abnormalities, glaucoma |
| Valproic acid | Drowsiness, ataxia, tremor, weight gain, hair loss, thrombocytopenia, hyperammonemia | Hepatic failure, pancreatitis, aplastic anemia, blood dyscrasias, lupus-like syndrome, Stevens-Johnson syndrome, toxic epidermal necrolysis |
| Zonisamide | Drowsiness, ataxia, difficulty concentrating, anorexia, weight loss, nausea, nephrolithiasis, oligohidrosis | Aplastic anemia, rash, Stevens-Johnson syndrome, toxic epidermal necrolysis, heat stroke |

[a]HLA-B*1502 testing is recommended in patients of Asian descent (haplotype associated with higher risk of Stevens-Johnson syndrome).

Information compiled from Asconapé JJ: The selection of antiepileptic drugs for the treatment of epilepsy in children and adults. *Neurol Clin* 28:843–852, 2010; Epocrates, LLC. *Epocrates*. AthenaHealth; 2020. Available at: http://epocrates.com. Accessed July 20, 2020; Medication Guide—Epilepsy Foundation of Minnesota. Available at: https://www.epilepsyfoundationmn.org/resource/medication-guide-2/. Accessed July 20, 2020; and Liu G, Slater N, Perkins A: Epilepsy: treatment Options, *Am Fam Physician* 96(2):87–96, 2017.

It is a diet high in fats, with enough protein for normal growth and energy and a low threshold for carbohydrates. Although the mechanism by which the diet protects against seizures is unknown, some evidence suggests effects on intermediary metabolism that influence the dynamics of the major inhibitory and excitatory neurotransmitter systems in the brain. During consumption of the ketogenic diet, marked alterations in brain energy metabolism occur, with ketone bodies partly replacing glucose as fuel. Whether these metabolic changes contribute to acute seizure protection is unclear; however, the ketone body acetone has anticonvulsant activity and could play a role in the seizure protection afforded by the diet. In addition to acute seizure protection, the ketogenic diet provides protection against the development of spontaneous recurrent seizures in models of chronic epilepsy.

According to a Cochrane Review, the overall quality of evidence for use of the ketogenic diet in the treatment of epilepsy is poor.[21] Attrition rates were a problem across all studies reviewed. The ketogenic diet is not easy to maintain because it requires strict adherence to a limited range of foods. Consequently, nonacceptance of the diet is a common reason for participant dropout. In addition, adverse effects, including gastrointestinal symptoms, metabolic abnormalities, renal calculi, and cardiac disturbances have been reported.[18,21]

When drug therapy does not control the seizures or drugs become toxic at effective dosages, surgical treatment is indicated. Surgical resection of the seizure focus in appropriately selected patients often significantly reduces or halts seizures, with up to 76% of patients becoming seizure-free after resection.[18] Lobectomies,

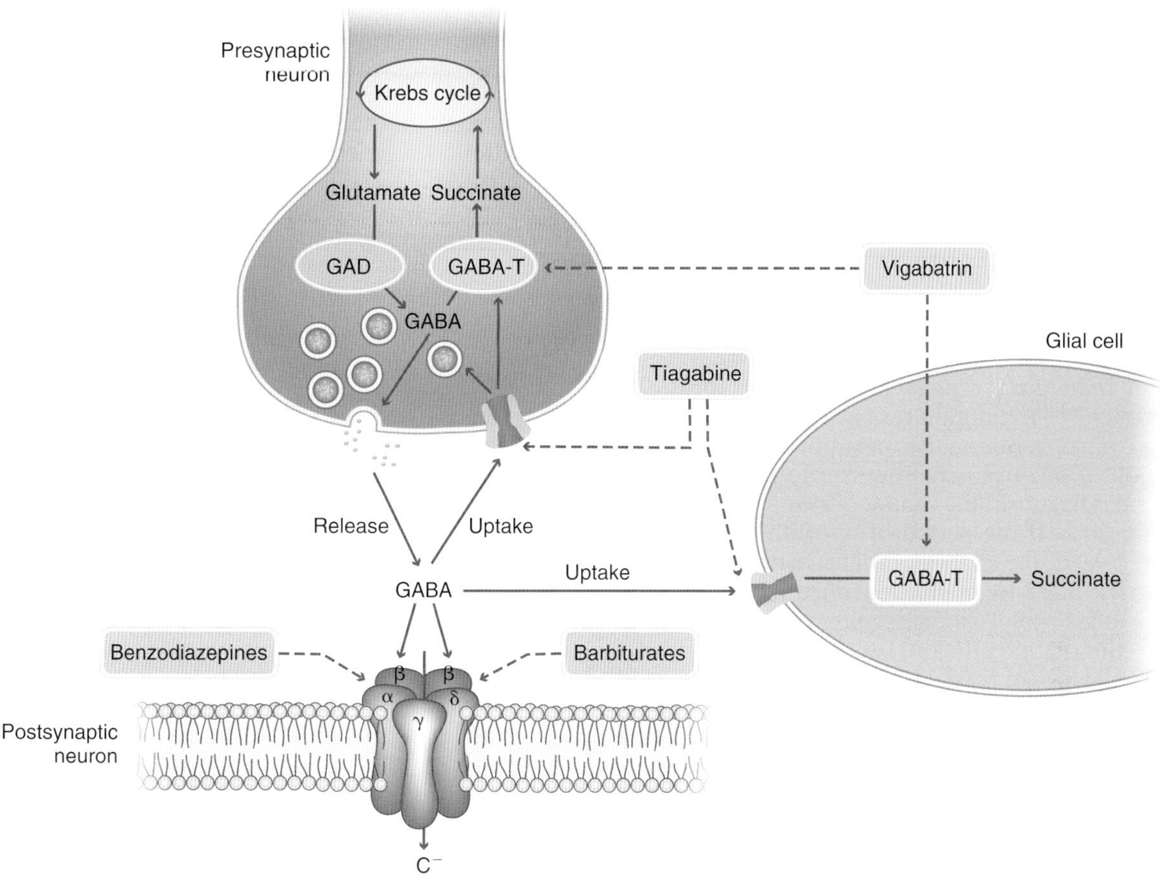


**Figure 36.4**

**Pharmacologic effects of antiepileptic drugs at the γ-aminobutyric acid class A ($GABA_A$) receptor.** Barbiturates bind to a β-subunit of the $GABA_A$ receptor to potentiate the action of the endogenous agonist γ-aminobutyric acid *(GABA)* and prolong the opening time of the chloride ion channel. Benzodiazepines bind to an α-subunit of $GABA_A$ to potentiate the action of GABA and increase the frequency of opening of the chloride ion channel. Vigabatrin irreversibly binds to γ-aminobutyric acid transaminase *(GABA-T)* to inhibit degradation of the inhibitory neurotransmitter GABA. Tiagabine blocks the uptake of synaptically released GABA into both presynaptic neurons and glial cells, allowing GABA to remain at the site of action for longer periods. *GAD,* Glutamic acid decarboxylase. (From Leach JP, Brodie MJ: Tiagabine. *Lancet* 351:203, 1998.)

cortical resections, and sectioning of the corpus callosum are the types of surgeries most often performed. Hemispherectomies, the removal of one of the hemispheres, can be effective for the severe, uncontrollable seizures usually found in children.

For individuals with medically refractory epilepsy who are not candidates for surgery or have not benefited from surgery, vagus nerve stimulation can be a safe adjunctive therapy. In this procedure, a stimulator is implanted, with the leads around the left vagus nerve and attached to a programmable pacemaker. The exact mechanism of action is unclear but likely involves suppression of electrical circuits in the brain by vagal afferent activity.[18]

Another approach to treating intractable focal onset seizures is responsive neurostimulation. This differs from vagus nerve stimulation in that the leads are implanted directly into the seizure-onset zone, which may be cortical or subcortical. In response to abnormal electrical activity, the neurostimulator delivers electrical stimulation to the target seizure focus.[3,18]

**PROGNOSIS.** Persons with epilepsy have increased mortality rates compared with the general population. Much of this increased risk occurs in individuals with symptomatic epilepsy in whom mortality relates to the underlying condition.

Death from asphyxia can occur when the individual has a seizure during eating or when breathing passages are compromised during the seizure or in the postictal phase. Drowning during a seizure has been documented and remains a serious consequence of swimming or bathing alone. Mortality also can be a consequence of uncontrolled status epilepticus. One of the greatest concerns is the risk of sudden unexpected death in epilepsy (SUDEP), in which a person with epilepsy dies without a clearly defined cause. SUDEP appears to be strongly related to the persistence of uncontrolled generalized tonic-clonic seizures; the risk of SUDEP can be decreased by optimizing seizure control.[18] Although researchers are unsure of why SUDEP occurs, some evidence points to abnormal cardioautonomic and respiratory function caused by gene abnormalities.[13]

The correlation between depression and epilepsy is strong, and attempted suicide is higher than the norm in those with epilepsy. People with epilepsy are more likely to be hospitalized for depression. Young people are at particular risk for development of depression and other psychiatric disorders and are less likely to be treated. Children with newly diagnosed epilepsy are more than three times more likely than control subjects to have a mood disorder.[30]

In people with epilepsy of no known cause and for whom a diagnosis is made before age 10, a 75% remission rate (defined as 5 seizure-free years) is seen. A child with epilepsy who has been free of seizures for more than 4 years while taking antiepileptic drugs has about a 70% chance of remaining in permanent remission when the drugs are withdrawn.

Chronic epilepsy is more likely when associated neurologic impairment is present at birth and when the seizures begin before 2 years of age. Individuals whose seizures have no identified etiology have a better outcome than individuals with a structural, metabolic, or genetic etiology.[30] The duration of active epilepsy before achieving control is one of the most powerful predictors of remission. If seizures remain uncontrolled during the first year after diagnosis, the chance of ever achieving control is only 60%. If the period of uncontrolled seizures extends to 4 years, the chance of ever achieving control is only 10%. The presence of multiple seizure types and frequent generalized tonic-clonic seizures is associated with a lower likelihood of remission. Less than 40% of patients with newly diagnosed mesial temporal lobe epilepsy will be controlled with medications, although familial cases are more easily managed medically. As noted earlier, the age of onset of epilepsy often reflects typical symptoms and these are reported as particular syndromes.

## Epilepsies of Infancy and Childhood

Epilepsy in infancy represents a nonspecific reaction on the part of the brain to a wide variety of insults. The condition is likely more age specific than disease specific. Infants who develop seizures often demonstrate a cessation of normal psychologic development and often show developmental deterioration that relates to the frequency of the spasms. Approximately 10% to 20% of infantile spasms develop after an uneventful pregnancy and birth history, as well as normal achievement of developmental milestones before the onset of seizures. The neurologic examination and CT and MRI scans of the head are normal, and there are no associated risk factors. In other situations the seizures can be related directly to several prenatal, perinatal, and postnatal factors. Prenatal and perinatal factors include hypoxia-ischemia, congenital infections, errors of metabolism, tuberous sclerosis, and prematurity. Postnatal conditions include CNS infections, head trauma (especially subdural hematoma and intraventricular hemorrhage), and hypoxic-ischemic encephalopathy. Dysfunction of the monoaminergic neurotransmitter system in the brainstem, derangement of neuronal structures in the brainstem, and an abnormality of the immune system may underlie the seizure activity. Stresses or injury to an infant during a critical period of neurodevelopment may cause corticotropin-releasing hormone overproduction, resulting in neuronal hyperexcitability. The number of corticotropin-releasing hormone receptors reaches a maximum in the infant brain, followed by spontaneous reduction with age, which may account for the high incidence of eventual resolution. Exogenous adrenocorticotropic hormone and glucocorticoids suppress corticotropin-releasing hormone synthesis, which may account for their effectiveness in treatment.

### Febrile Seizures

Febrile seizures, the most common seizure disorder during childhood, generally have an excellent prognosis but may also signify a serious underlying acute infectious disease such as sepsis or bacterial meningitis. They are rare before 6 months and after age 5 and are a result of fever. There is a genetic association, with febrile seizures occurring two to three times more frequently in affected families than in the general population.[30] The typical febrile seizure is brief, generalized, and tonic-clonic in sequence, and the body temperature is high. The seizures occur more often when the child is asleep. A seizure is often the first indication that the child is ill because 90% of all seizures occur in the first 24 hours of fever. Although most affected children have no long-term consequences, febrile seizures increase the risk of future epilepsy. This risk is low for most children but increases if the child has preexisting neurologic abnormalities; a family history of epilepsy; or a febrile seizure that is prolonged (>15 minutes), has focal components, or recurs within 24 hours.[30] Prophylactic treatment generally is not indicated because of the benign prognosis.

### Dravet Syndrome

Dravet syndrome, previously called severe myoclonic epilepsy of infancy, is a rare epilepsy syndrome in which children present with seizures before 18 months of age. They have early normal development followed by treatment-resistant seizures of various types and by developmental regression. Cognitive outcome typically is poor. About 70% to 80% of individuals with Dravet syndrome carry a mutation in the *SCN1A* gene, which causes seizures by affecting sodium ion channels.[30] Long-term outcome is dominated by premature mortality, affecting up to 21% of people with Dravet syndrome.[28]

### Myoclonic Epilepsy of Infancy

Myoclonic epilepsy of infancy is a rare syndrome characterized by brief, bilaterally synchronous myoclonic jerks. It typically manifests between the ages of 4 months and 3 years. Although most children have a benign course, some develop mild cognitive dysfunction and behavioral disturbances as well as other seizure types in adolescence.

### Lennox-Gastaut Syndrome

Lennox-Gastaut syndrome usually begins between 1 and 6 years of age. Children develop medically intractable seizures, constituting an epileptic encephalopathy. Characteristics of this syndrome include slow spike-wave EEG pattern, intellectual disability, and multiple seizure types. Children with Lennox-Gastaut syndrome have a poor neurologic prognosis.[30] The atonic, myoclonic, and atypical absence seizures that occur at early ages may decrease, but generalized tonic-clonic seizures increase, and focal seizures emerge over time. These seizures are notoriously refractory to antiepileptic drugs.

### Landau-Kleffner Syndrome

Landau-Kleffner syndrome is a rare epilepsy syndrome in which a child with no apparent neurologic abnormality

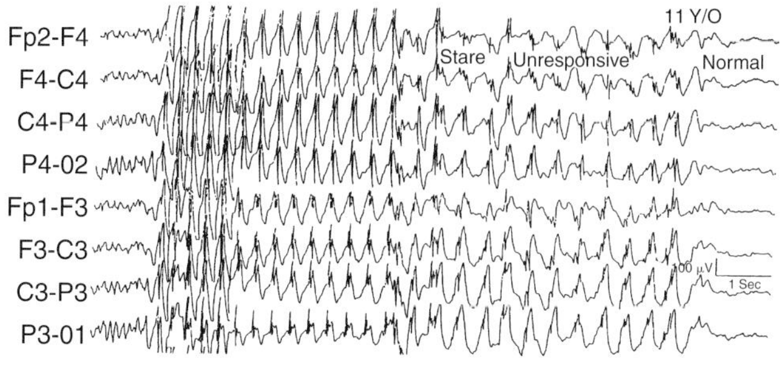


**Figure 36.5**

**Childhood absence epilepsy.** Electroencephalogram shows the typical pattern of generalized 3-Hz spike-wave complexes associated with a clinical absence seizure. (From Goldman L: *Cecil textbook of medicine*, ed 22, Philadelphia, 2004, Saunders.)

loses previously acquired language abilities. Often epileptic seizures and psychomotor disturbances develop at around the same time as the aphasia. The aphasia takes the form of an auditory agnosia, with an inability to understand spoken words. This disorder often begins between 2 and 8 years of age. The seizures in Landau-Kleffner syndrome are usually infrequent and easily controlled by antiepileptic drugs, and they remit by adolescence. The language deficits, however, can be much more severe than would be expected on the basis of the seizure frequency and the EEG abnormalities. The best evidence is for early treatment with corticosteroids.[22]

### Benign Childhood Epilepsy with Centrotemporal Spikes

Benign childhood epilepsy with centrotemporal spikes (BECTS) typically occurs between the ages of 3 and 13 and is characterized by brief, focal hemifacial motor seizures. Childhood epilepsy with occipital paroxysms is a syndrome similar to BECTS, but it includes visual symptoms at onset, and some children have associated migraine headache. Nearly 50% of affected children have a family history of epilepsy, and most have no known brain abnormality. EEG shows spiking in the centrotemporal region. BECTS has an excellent long-term prognosis, and relapse is rare when medications are stopped.

### Childhood Absence Epilepsy

Childhood absence epilepsy begins between ages 4 and 10 years. Note that "absence" refers to both a seizure type and an epilepsy syndrome. Absence seizures are characterized by a blank stare with unresponsiveness, typically lasting between 5 and 20 seconds.[30] Behavior and awareness return immediately to normal. There is no postictal period and usually no recollection that a seizure has occurred. Because absence seizures are brief and nonconvulsive, they are easily overlooked or misdiagnosed. When untreated, absence seizures can occur hundreds of times each day, a condition referred to as pyknolepsy. Fig. 36.5 shows EEG of a child with absence epilepsy.

Hyperventilation is a potent trigger for absence seizures and so can be used clinically for diagnosis and to assess treatment effectiveness.[30] Absence seizures can be controlled by drugs such as ethosuximide and valproic acid, which block low-threshold calcium currents in thalamic neurons. Childhood absence epilepsy, similar to other genetic generalized epilepsies, has a complex genetic basis, with only a few percent transmitted monogenically. This syndrome has a favorable prognosis, with most children becoming seizure-free on treatment. However, approximately 25% relapse when medications are withdrawn.[17]

### Juvenile Myoclonic Epilepsy

Juvenile myoclonic epilepsy (JME) has its onset in early adolescence, between 8 and 20 years of age, in otherwise healthy individuals with normal intelligence and a family history of similar seizures. JME consists of myoclonic or generalized tonic-clonic seizures. Myoclonic jerks of the head, neck, and upper limbs tend to occur early in the morning, soon after awakening, making hair combing and tooth brushing difficult. Generalized tonic-clonic seizures occur in as many as 90% of individuals with JME.[30] A gene locus has been identified on chromosome band 6p21. The seizures are especially linked to sleep deprivation and tend to appear often in college students. A proportion of these individuals have had absence seizures as well.

## Epilepsy Not Related to Age

### Posttraumatic Epilepsy

After penetrating wounds and other severe head injuries, about one-third of individuals have seizures within 1 year. Although most individuals experience seizures within 1 to 2 years of injury, new-onset seizures still may appear 5 or more years later. Two-thirds of individuals with posttraumatic epilepsy have generalized seizures. Mild head injuries (e.g., uncomplicated brief loss of consciousness, no skull fracture, absence of focal neurologic signs, no contusion or hematoma) do not increase the risk of seizures to a clinically significant degree.

Impact seizures (a generalized convulsion occurring at the time of, or immediately after, the injury) and early seizures (seizures occurring within the first 1 to 2 weeks) represent acute reactions of the brain to the trauma. Seizures beginning after 10 to 14 days reflect an increased risk of development of posttraumatic epilepsy. Early seizures should be treated with phenytoin. To minimize complications from seizures occurring during acute management, phenytoin also should be given prophylactically for 1 to 2 weeks to individuals who have had severe head injuries. In the absence of overt attacks, phenytoin use should be discontinued after 2 weeks because no data indicate that antiepileptic drugs prevent the development of later epilepsy.[18]

### Epilepsia Partialis Continua

Epilepsia partialis continua is characterized by continuous focal seizures that can involve part or all of one side of the body. In adults, epilepsia partialis continua occurs with severe strokes, primary or metastatic brain tumors, metabolic encephalopathies, encephalitis, and subacute or rare chronic inflammatory diseases of the brain. Antiepileptic drugs are usually ineffective, as are corticosteroids and antiviral agents. Seizures remit spontaneously in some cases. Rasmussen encephalitis is one cause of epilepsia partialis continua. The onset is usually before age 10. Sequelae include hemiplegia, hemianopia,

Box 36.4

### COMMON MISCONCEPTIONS ABOUT EPILEPSY

*Myth:* You can swallow your tongue during a seizure.
**Fact:** It is physically impossible to swallow your tongue.
*Myth:* You should restrain someone during a seizure.
**Fact:** Do not use restraint; the seizure will run its course and stop.
*Myth:* People with epilepsy should not be in jobs of responsibility and stress.
**Fact:** People with epilepsy hold many types of jobs; they often do not inform others of the disorder.
*Myth:* You cannot tell what a person may do during a seizure.
**Fact:** The characteristic form of seizure is consistent during each episode. Behavior may be inappropriate for the time and place but will most likely not cause harm.
*Myth:* You cannot die of epilepsy.
**Fact:** Status epilepticus can cause death. It should be treated as a medical emergency.

and aphasia. The disease is progressive and potentially lethal but more often becomes self-limited with significant neurologic deficits. Some experts believe that early surgery (hemispherectomy) affords a better prognosis in hemispheric epilepsy syndromes such as Rasmussen encephalitis.[30]

## SPECIAL IMPLICATIONS FOR THE THERAPIST 36.1

### *Epilepsy*

Understanding the facts about epilepsy is important for therapists who may encounter an individual with epilepsy or if a seizure occurs in the work environment. Box 36.4 presents basic information that separates fact from myth.

A client who is experiencing a seizure needs protection from injury in the environment. The therapist should make sure that no objects in the immediate area can be knocked onto the person and that during seizure activity the person is lying on a surface that will prevent a fall. Rolling the person onto his or her side may help to keep the airway clear. Observation of focal or generalized onset, physical manifestations, respiratory status, and duration of the seizure are important for ongoing medical management. When the seizure appears to be generalized, observation of frothing at the mouth, deviation of the eyes, and incontinence will add information for the health practitioners attempting to control the client's seizures medically.

If a seizure lasts more than 5 minutes, emergency measures must be taken. An individual who develops status epilepticus can develop irreversible brain damage as a result of hypoxia. Consequently, an airway must be established, possibly through endotracheal intubation. Medication given at this point to suppress the CNS usually includes intramuscular midazolam or intravenous lorazepam, and this often is effective in controlling the seizure.[7] If the seizure continues, a second-line antiepileptic drug such as phenytoin/fosphenytoin, phenobarbital, valproate sodium, or levetiracetam may be administered. If that is not successful, the person may require intubation, ventilatory assistance, and drug-induced coma.[7]

The psychologic consequences of seizure are of concern. Seizure activity can often cause severe loss of confidence and restriction of lifestyle. For the therapist treating a client with epilepsy, it is important to have an understanding of the triggering activities associated with seizure. Knowing the type and frequency of seizures helps the therapist make recommendations regarding activities that can be engaged in safely. If adherence to the medication regimen appears to be a problem, the therapist should give the family information regarding the need to maintain consistent dosages. The therapist may be able to help the client or family understand the relationship between epilepsy and depression and assist in the appropriate referral.

Evaluation of the home, work, and school environments should be performed so the therapist can make specific recommendations. The client sometimes needs to be encouraged to become part of a group activity. Too often, the client has been discouraged from engaging in sports or leisure activities even when seizures are controlled. When a potential safety hazard exists, the therapist is well suited to recommend adaptations to equipment or the environment to maintain safety. With direct supervision, clients usually can participate safely in swimming and other aquatic activities.

Seizures often occur after activity, and so safety measures should be considered even after the activity is finished. Loss of fluids from sweating during exercise can affect the serum blood levels of medication and increase the metabolism of liver enzymes. Decisions about whether to engage in vigorous activity should be based on whether seizures are controlled by medication and should be made only after close monitoring of blood levels of medication after exercise.

Side effects of medication can slow cognitive function or alter reaction time. Movement disorders including nystagmus, ataxia, and dysarthria may be related to medication. Lethargy, nausea, irritability, and skin rashes may be the result of intolerance to medication. When these symptoms are noted during intervention, the proper health care worker should be notified. The client and family should have a clear understanding of symptoms related to toxicity or nontherapeutic doses of medication.

Restriction of activity may be important in the first 2 to 3 months after the first seizure, after treatment is initiated and until it can be determined that further seizures are unlikely. When antiepileptic drugs are discontinued, activity should be limited initially. In the case of children for whom the epileptic syndrome progresses, limitations may change over time.

## REFERENCES

To enhance this text and add value for the reader, all references are included in the enhanced ebook on Student Consult that accompanies this textbook. The reader can view the reference source and access it online whenever possible.

# CHAPTER 37

# Headache

HEATHER CAMPBELL • NICOLE A. MIRANDA

## OVERVIEW

Headache is the most common pain complaint in the world, ranging in severity from mildly annoying to completely disabling. Although in rare cases headache may herald catastrophe, headache on its own is not contagious or fatal. However, the World Health Organization (WHO) labels headache disorders as "ubiquitous, prevalent, disabling and largely treatable, but under-recognized, under-diagnosed, and under treated" throughout the world.[219] The 2016 Global Burden of Disease (GBD) study [214] identified headache universally as second (tension-type headache; TTH), and sixth (migraine) of 328 disease states in prevalence. Migraine has consistently been ranked second for years lived with disability (YLD), after low back pain. In Europe, the Eurolight Study (8000 respondents, 11 countries) placed migraine as the leading cause of disability.[195] The most current GBD report apportioned medication overuse headache (MOH) as the third most commonly occurring headache type, rather than maintaining its independence as a distinct disease, suggesting greater prevalence of migraine and TTH.[195] Migraine and severe headache affect more than 15% of adults aged 18 to 65 in the United States, diminishing somewhat in the older adult population.[21,34,35] Children and adolescents experience a greater prevalence of up to 80%, affecting school participation, physical activity, social development, and emotional health.[112] These data represent a significant public health concern, at great cost in time, money, and well-being to society as well as to individuals who are affected. Despite new developments in treatment, the stability of statistics for several decades suggests that the impact of headache has not lessened. Lack of knowledge among health care providers is the principal clinical barrier to effective care.[214]

The International Classification of Headache Disorders 3rd Edition,[85] published in 2018, is the updated standard system used for both clinical diagnosis and research purposes. It is the most detailed classification in neurology, and represents a robust evidence-based clinical diagnostic instrument. In the absence of reliable and accessible biomarkers, the key word is "clinical," as understanding of the underlying pathophysiology remains unclear in many cases. The current investigative trajectory is revealing complex genetic influences potentially affecting both diagnosis and intervention, and the 4th edition will likely reflect enhanced understanding of the headache spectrum. Box 37.1 lists the major ICHD-3 categories and should be consulted for more detailed descriptions when needed. Conditions commonly encountered by physical therapists are explored with the goal of increasing understanding and awareness.

Headaches are described in ICHD-3 according to phenomenology of symptoms, including timing of onset, location, duration, nature of pain, associated symptoms and sensitivities. Frequency categories identify headaches as episodic, chronic or persistent. The status of "probable" applies when symptoms lead toward a diagnosis but do not fit all criteria.

Primary headaches (Part One) are those not caused by other diseases. Included are migraine, tension-type, trigeminal autonomic cephalgias, and other primary headaches (e.g., cough, cold exposure, and exercise headaches). Secondary headaches (Part Two) result from associated disease or trauma, categorized by etiology as well as symptoms, and can have diverse causes ranging from serious and life-threatening conditions to systemic illness, infectious diseases, and disorders of the head, face, and neck. The hallmark of secondary headaches is that they resolve when the underlying cause abates. Secondary headaches are further discussed in the chapters on the primary diagnoses (Stroke, Infectious Disease, Degenerative Disorders, Epilepsy and Vestibular Disorders, etc.). Part Three of the ICHD-3 addresses painful cranial neuropathies, other facial pains, and other headaches that do not meet the criteria of primary or secondary headaches.

A substantial Appendix follows the main categories, containing diagnoses that require further research validation before being incorporated into the ICHD. Vestibular migraine, infantile colic, menstrual migraines, visual snow, delayed onset acute or persistent headache attributed to traumatic head injury, headache attributed to space travel, and a more detailed list of psychiatric

Box 37.1

**INTERNATIONAL CLASSIFICATIONS OF HEADACHE DISORDERS III**

Classifications are hierarchical with diagnostic detail ranging from first-numeric primary categories to fifth-level subcategories.

***Part I: The Primary Headaches***

1. Migraine
   1.1. Migraine without aura
   1.2. Migraine with aura
   1.3. Chronic migraine
   1.4. Complications of migraine
   1.5. Probable migraine
   1.6. Episodic syndromes that may be associated with migraine
2. Tension-type headache
   2.1. Infrequent episodic tension-type headache
   2.2. Frequent episodic tension-type headache
   2.3. Chronic tension-type headache
   2.4. Probable tension-type headache
3. Trigeminal autonomic cephalalgias (TACs)
   3.1. Cluster headache
   3.2. Paroxysmal hemicrania
   3.3. Short-lasting unilateral neuralgiform headache attacks
4. Other primary headache disorders (10 subcategories)

***Part II: The Secondary Headaches***

5. Headache attributed to trauma or injury to the head and/or neck
   (Includes acute and persistent headache from head trauma, whiplash, and craniotomy)
6. Headache attributed to cranial and/or cervical vascular disorder
7. Headache attributed to nonvascular intracranial disorder
8. Headache attributed to a substance or its withdrawal (includes medication overuse)
9. Headache attributed to infection
10. Headache attributed to disorder of homoeostasis
11. Headache or facial pain attributed to disorder of cranium, neck, eyes, ears, nose, sinuses, teeth, mouth or other facial or cervical structures
12. Headache attributed to psychiatric disorder

***Part III: Painful Cranial Neuropathies, Other Facial Pain and Other Headaches***

13. Painful lesions of cranial nerves and other facial pain
14. Other headache disorders

Adapted from the International Headache Society, 2018.

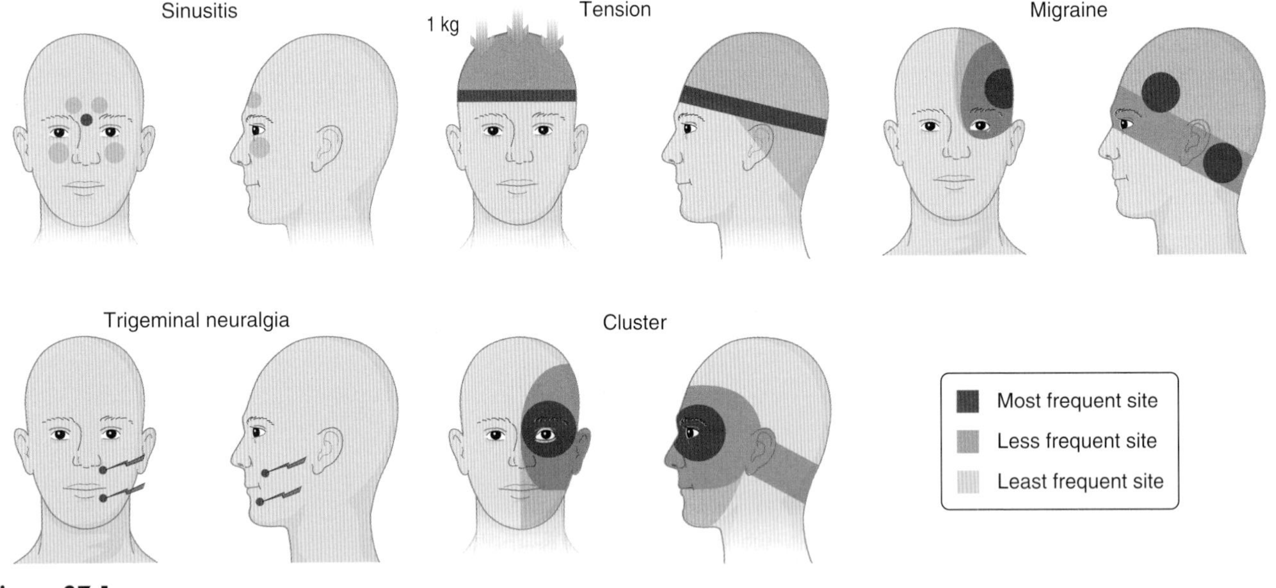


**Figure 37.1**

**Typical headache patterns.** Primary headaches include tension-type, migraine, and cluster. Acute rhinosinusitis headache, related to infection, is a common secondary headache. (From Weinstein JM: Headache and facial pain. In Yanoff M, Duker JS, Augsburger JJ, et al, eds: *Ophthalmology*, ed 2, St. Louis, 2004, Mosby.)

disorders causing headaches are among those being investigated for inclusion in the next edition.[85] Fig. 37.1 illustrates some pain patterns associated with typical complaints of headache and head pain.

## The Physical Therapist's Role

Whether presenting as the primary complaint, part of a patient history, or a coexisting issue, headache is a common concern among patients visiting physical therapists. Worldwide, physical therapy is the most frequently used service for complementary treatment for headache, with European countries reporting 68% and the Americas reporting 42% utilization.[219] Physical therapists should understand the cause, precipitating factors, and typical course of both episodic and chronic headache pain. A physical therapy evaluation must include headache history and assessments from screenings to detailed evaluations to help elucidate headache diagnoses. Identification of headache etiology and phenotype is of paramount importance, as some conditions benefit from physical therapy interventions, while others interfere with therapeutic response, such as headache related to psychiatric disorders. Appropriate referrals to other providers must be made where needed. The negative impact of headache on quality of life, cognition, attitude, and energy, as well as the influence of medications, may adversely affect a patient's ability to participate in a rehabilitation session, adhere to home programs, or learn new skills.

Although ICHD-3 is oriented toward physicians and physician extenders, physical therapists should be familiar with the classifications. Readers are encouraged to explore the International Headache Society (IHS) website https://www.ichd-3.org from which access to the entire classification system and supporting documentation is available. The *ATLAS of Headache Disorders and Resources in the World, by WHO & Lifting the Burden*, is also readily available online at http://www.who.int/mental_health/management/atlas_headache_disorders/en/. As practitioners committed to wellness, physical therapists participate in patient education regarding self-management, encourage adherence to prescribed interventions, and alert prescribing professionals to beneficial and adverse responses. Documenting interventions and results for specifically identified headache disorders will contribute to improved understanding of efficacious care.

# PRIMARY HEADACHES

## Migraine

### Overview

Migraine is a recurrent episodic neurovascular disorder of the brain characterized by dysfunction in areas of the brainstem and diencephalon that alters perception of sensory inputs and causes other transient neurologic deficits.[11,76,85] The characteristic of commonly unilateral throbbing moderate to severe head pain[85] may be accompanied by a variety of autonomic symptoms (nausea, vomiting, nasal/sinus congestion, rhinorrhea, lacrimation, ptosis, yawning, frequent urination, and diarrhea), affective symptoms (depression and irritability), cognitive symptoms (attention deficit, difficulty finding words, transient amnesia, and reduced ability to navigate in familiar environments), and sensory symptoms (photophobia, phonophobia, osmophobia, muscle tenderness, and cutaneous allodynia).[36,51] Whether increased central nervous system excitability or hyperresponsiveness is the underlying cause is debated by researchers. Attacks are widely variable in intensity, frequency, and duration.

### Prevalence

Migraines afflict 1 in 6 Americans, or about 15% overall.[34] During reproductive years, three times as many women experience migraine as men, and women report a higher level of disability. The number of headache days per month reported by adult men and women is about 2 for episodic migraine (defined as 15 days per month or less by ICHD) and 20 for chronic migraine (more than 15 days per month).[17,117] Mean onset age of pediatric migraine is 7 years 9 months, with an overall prevalence of nearly 8%.[71,146] About 50% of pediatric and adolescent migraineurs still report migraines at age 50.[23] Prevalence drops to 5.7% in Americans over 65 years of age.[21] The American Migraine Prevalence and Prevention (AMPP) longitudinal cohort study revealed peak prevalence in the mid to late 20s for both men and women.[146] Lost productivity in school and at work due to absenteeism and presenteeism (working while ill) is estimated in billions of dollars, far exceeding the cost of care.[139] There is also a higher burden of migraine headache and severe headache in historically disadvantaged populations, including Alaskan Natives, American Indians, the unemployed, disabled, and those with very low family income.[34] Barriers to effective management and prevention may include the high cost of medications and other health care, lack of access to practitioners educated in headache medicine, and a pervasive lack of patient-oriented treatment and goal setting.[37,57,116,219]

Psychosocial contributions to perceived disability are significant, including being poorly understood by friends and family, being viewed as drug-seeking by health care practitioners, lack of understanding by employers and educators of impaired performance and absence, and underfunding of research by policymakers who view migraine as a nonserious condition.[224] These psychosocial effects are particularly evident during childhood and adolescence, a crucial period for ego development and establishing social relationships. A higher frequency of suicidal ideation has been identified among adolescents suffering migraine with aura and more than 7 headache days/month.[162]

### Etiologic and Risk Factors

The etiology and pathophysiology of migraine remains largely ambiguous, creating controversy regarding the interplay between neurologic and vascular contributions to migraine headaches.[7] Some evidence suggests that the two most common forms of migraine, without aura (MO) and with aura (MA), may represent a spectrum disorder rather than separate diagnostic entities. Hereditary contribution to migraine is estimated at 42% from meta-analysis of linkage pedigree studies of large familial groups and twins.[157a]

A reliable method of establishing the diagnosis of migraine is critical to creating accurate pedigree studies to demonstrate hereditary patterns. Until reliable biomarkers become available, migraine is a clinical diagnosis determined by use of the most current ICHD criteria. The incidence in the general population is high enough that "control" subjects may be nonexpressive carriers who present with onset of migraine later in life, which challenges the validity and accuracy of inheritance patterns. Familial hemiplegic migraine (FHM), a severe and rare type of migraine, was the first migraine classification with evidence of monogenic hereditary contributions. There are three autosomal dominant forms of FHM (1.2.3.1) involving ion channel disturbances that impact glutamatergic neurotransmission leading to cortical hyperexcitability.[7,81,154]

1. In FHM1 a mutation of CACNA1A on chromosome 19 is associated with a calcium channelopathy in the presynaptic terminals of neurons associated with excessive neuronal release of glutamate.
2. FHM2 involves a disruption of the Na+/K+ ATPase pump in the astrocytic membrane affecting glutamate reuptake by glial cells related to a mutation of the ATP1A2 gene on chromosome 1.
3. FHM3 designates a variation of the SCN1A1 gene on chromosome 2, indicating a voltage-gated sodium channel alteration that enhances glutamatergic activity due to impaired GABAergic inhibition.

These single gene mutations do not fully explain the heterogenic clinical presentations of FHM, leading to further genetic research identifying candidate FHM genes with allele mutations that may reflect an abundance of aura phenotypes, such as transient ataxia, seizures, or basilar migraine features.[7] More recently, genome-wide association (GWA) studies of single nucleotide polymorphisms (SNPs) across large populations have permitted initial risk determination for comorbid diseases using a polygenic risk score (PRS). The majority of successful PRS research to date involves neuropsychiatric disorders, and provides a template for future studies in diagnoses such as migraine. This line of research may also improve pharmacogenomics to determine predicted response to migraine medications.[41] Initial GWA studies using PRS have investigated shared genetic risk between migraine and major depressive disorders, as well as migraine (MO) and stroke. Other disorders that are under GWA investigation or are anticipated to have a shared risk for comorbidity with migraine include autoimmune diseases, thyroid disorders, pain and chronic disorders, sleep disturbances, and endometriosis.

International collaborative research using linkage and GWA studies has confirmed previous studies and expanded the identification of 38 loci and 44 risk mutations for MA and MO.[77] Interestingly, the new loci discovered did not reveal robust ion channel involvement, but rather loci associated with vascular and gastrointestinal smooth muscle, involving nitric oxide and oxidative stress. In addition to GWA studies identifying genes responsible for certain traits, epigenetic GWA studies have begun to determine chemical influences upon the expression of those genes.[73] Ongoing interpretation of these findings and rapid future scientific discovery makes the validity of current findings and clarity regarding the role of neurovascular contributions to migraine pathophysiology beyond the scope of a textbook chapter.

A two-part publication by the American Migraine Prevalence and Prevention (AMPP) Study of a U.S. longitudinal database tracking the incidence of episodic and chronic migraine identified cardiovascular risk factors in men and women over the age of 22 with episodic migraine. A meta-analysis of 16 large cohort studies performed worldwide adds evidence that migraine (particularly migraine with aura) is an independent risk factor for stroke (ischemic and hemorrhagic) and myocardial events in men and women.[125a] Even with adjustment for age and other known cardiovascular risk factors such as hypertension, diabetes, and elevated cholesterol, individuals with migraine demonstrate an increased risk of sustaining a stroke or myocardial infarct based on longitudinal study over many years. A multicenter prospective study, the Women's Ischemia Syndrome Evaluation, was one of the four studies included in a meta-analysis on major adverse cardiovascular and cerebrovascular events. The hazard ratio of stroke in women with migraine was double that of women without a history of migraine.[166] The relevance of this work and application in physical therapy involves a role for primary care providers to identify individuals at risk for cardiovascular events, procedures, and condition. Providers should be mindful that the use of vasoconstrictors such as triptans and ergots to manage episodic migraine may increase CV risk and should be routinely monitored.[38,117]

Headache triggers are normally innocuous endogenous or exogenous mechanisms that may precipitate a headache episode by lowering the threshold of vulnerability. They are very heterogeneous among migraineurs, and should be inventoried individually via extensive headache diaries to help decode the interaction between environment and individual disease.[152,155] Many perceived triggers may in fact be premonitory symptoms. For instance, fatigue ranks third in the top 10 reported triggers, and is also the most common premonitory symptom.[155] It is interesting to note that there is no discussion in the literature of other primary or secondary headaches acting as triggers for migraine. Presumably the increased pain burden might lower the threshold of an already dysfunctional nociceptive modulation system. Developing an individual factor-attack profile is necessary to identify true triggers and to create trigger avoidance or desensitization strategies.

Stress is the most commonly reported headache trigger. Heightened activation of the hypothalamic-pituitary-adrenal axis may adversely affect an already dysfunctional hypothalamic modulation of nociception and autonomic functions, increasing vulnerability to migraine. Cognitive behavioral therapy (CBT) is very effective in "unlearning" many controllable triggers, more so than avoidance alone.[131]

The drop in estradiol during luteal phase of the menstrual cycle may trigger a menstrual migraine related to estrogen withdrawal. Nearly a quarter of female migraineurs report menses as a trigger.[125] The first and third trimesters of pregnancy may also exacerbate migraines. Migraine can be triggered during delivery and may be more prevalent in the weeks and months following childbirth.[49]

Many migraineurs report weather-related triggers. Hoffmann and colleagues analyzed attack prevalence and intensity with hourly meteorologic variables, including atmospheric pressure, temperature change, and relative humidity, for one year in a cohort of 100 and found a strong correlation in a small subset of 13 subjects. Their predictive values, however, were too small to justify preventative treatment based on weather data alone.[89]

There is a strong association of psychiatric symptoms, pain catastrophizing, and beliefs about headache locus of control with severe migraine-related disability. Depression and anxiety are highly comorbid with migraine, with greater prevalence in individuals with chronic versus episodic disease. Even small increases in depression and anxiety symptoms are associated with higher migraine frequency and headache-related disability.[182] There is also an increased risk of headache, migraine more than tension-type headache, in individuals with history of childhood maltreatment, including emotional neglect, sexual abuse, and emotional abuse.[203]

Modifiable migraine risks for adults include obesity, depression, ineffective acute migraine treatment, medication overuse headache, and high frequency headaches. Lifestyle risk factors in young people include obesity, inactivity, caffeine, and smoking.[71,146,217]

## Pathogenesis

Migraine involves multiple processes and complex interactions. Exact initiation mechanisms precipitating, sustaining, and resolving migraine attack are not yet completely clear. However, interictal studies have revealed many subtle differences between migraine brains and nonmigraine controls, including structure, functional connectivity, metabolism, neurochemistry, trigeminovascular system sensitivity, and the inability to habituate to noxious stimuli.[76] Triggered headache imaging studies using nitroglycerin (facilitates neuronal hyperexcitability), ammonia (pain stimulus), or calcium gene-related peptide (CGRP) as a neural inflammatory agent reveal stark differences in nociceptive processing between migraineurs and healthy control subjects.[128,179] Research attention is shifting away from vasodilation, suggesting that change in diameter of cranial vessels is more of an epiphenomenon rather than a causative mechanism in migraine pain. Greater interest has developed in the rich population of vascular nociceptors and endothelial cell expression of neurochemicals that contribute to abnormal pain and sensory processing thought to be the basis of migraine disease.[36,97,204]

Structural differences in gray matter volume (GMV) in brains of migraineurs compared to healthy controls have been recorded in pain modulating and processing areas of the brainstem, midbrain, cortex, and cerebellum. Interestingly, in people with chronic migraine, GMV differences are most associated with chronicity, psychological distress, and poor sleep quality. These structural brain factors are less apparent in those with effective pain self-efficacy behaviors and beliefs.[218] Increased thickness of the somatotopical head-face area on the somatosensory cortex has also been identified, but it is unknown whether these changes occur as a result of headache frequency or relate to disease etiology.[76] Differences in GMV between male and female migraineurs highlight emotional and perceptual pain processing differences, likely influenced by ovarian steroids on neuroendocrine receptors throughout the brain.[32] Positron emission tomography (PET) has demonstrated increased perfusion in the hypothalamus, dorsolateral pons, and several cortical areas during the prodromal stage, confirming a functional correlation between symptoms and imaging findings.[128] Most reported premonitory and postdromal symptoms are functions regulated by the hypothalamus, and implicate hypothalamic dysfunction as an initiating mechanism of migraine. Cortical disturbance locations relate to abnormal sensory phenomena, such as photophobia, phonophobia, and concentration difficulties.[105]

Resting state functional MRI studies reveal abnormal functional connections, or "cross-talk," between the periaqueductal gray (PAG), raphe nuclei, and pain modulating areas of the thalamus and cerebellum.[43,137] Resting state fMRI has differentiated migraine brains from healthy controls with 80% accuracy, specific to 6 regions of interest. Of those 6 areas, four are part of the limbic system, where sensory discriminative and emotional components of pain experience are processed.[43] This finding alone should alert health care providers to the importance of a cognitive emotional aspect to management.

Neurochemical differences in migraineurs involve immune response and oxidative stress, as well as factors associated with pain transmission and emotions.[108] In particular, when compared to nonmigraineurs, migraineurs demonstrate lower between-episode levels of serotonin 5-$HT_{1B/1D}$ from the brainstem raphe nucleus, with a sharp rise of serotonin 5-$HT_{1B/1D}$ at headache onset, and higher expressions of neural inflammatory calcium gene-related peptide (CGRP) during episodes.[96,149] Additionally, neuroendocrine factors influence the hypothalamus, forebrain, midbrain, limbic system and spinal cord function in areas associated with nociceptive modulation. Estrogen and progesterone have opposite effects on neural excitability and functional processing, whereas testosterone may improve migraine in both men and women and may suppress cortical spreading depression (CSD).[32] Men with migraine show higher levels of estradiol than male nonmigraineurs, with similar levels of testosterone, creating a lower androgen:estrogen ratio that may increase migraine susceptibility.[208]

Habituation is the ability to gradually reduce response to a constant stimulus of unchanging intensity. Numerous electrophysiological studies have demonstrated that those who experience migraine habituate poorly during the interheadache phase in all sensory domains, reflecting deficient serotonergic activity.[36,51,157,213] Although genetic influences are not fully understood, Di Clemente and colleagues' study of habituation to nociceptive blink reflex revealed significantly deficient habituation in subjects with personal migraine history, but also showed habituation deficiencies in those without migraine but with a close family history (e.g., sibling or parent with migraine).[54] Sensitivity to light is measurable in the interictal period and is not thought to be a function of insufficient habituation, but a sensitized retino-thalamo-cortical pathway.[120]

Current theories of the development of migraine head pain suggest hypothalamic and brainstem centers respond abnormally to changes in homeostasis and emotion at much lower thresholds than nonmigraineurs, possibly facilitated by a chronically low serotonin state, neuroendocrine influences and genetic susceptibility.[36] Hypothalamic influences on the autonomic system through the superior salivary nucleus and sphenopalatine ganglion may heighten parasympathetic tone, resulting in many of the symptoms of prodrome.[105] The resulting activation of nociceptive neurons originating in the trigeminal nucleus, depicted in Fig. 37.2, that richly innervate

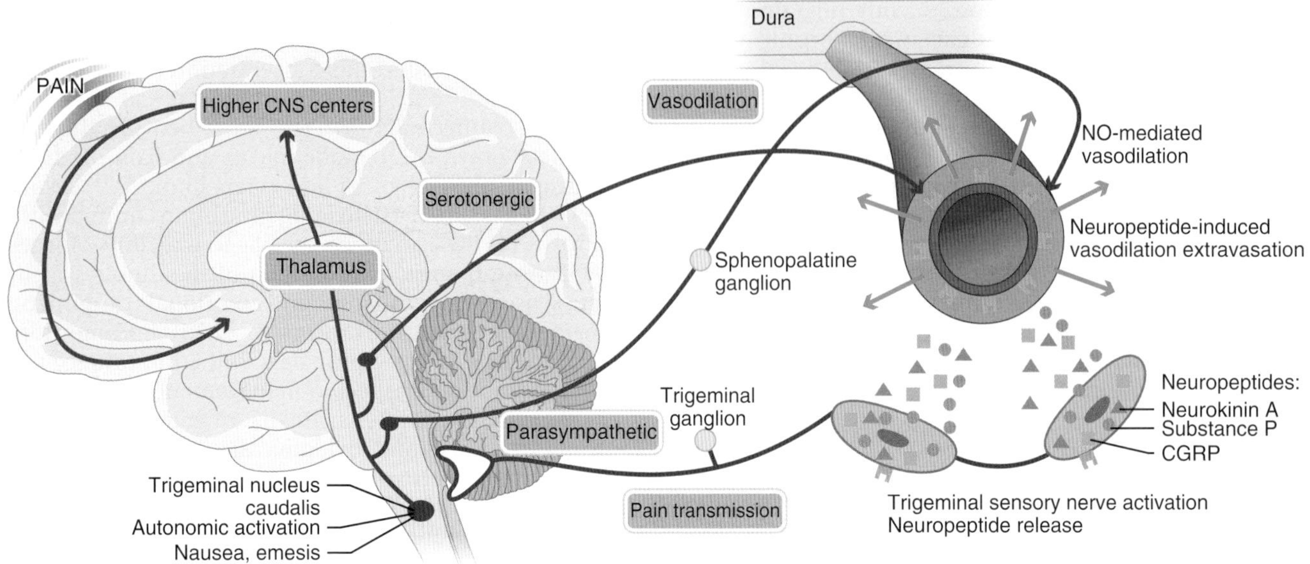


**Figure 37.2**

**Trigeminal vascular theory of migraine headaches.** Cortical hyperexcitable neurons, perhaps with an additional influence from brainstem structures, leads to activation of the trigeminovascular system. Signals reach the trigeminal nucleus caudalis in the brainstem, which in turn signals the thalamus, which innervates cortical regions, leading to the conscious sensation of headache and pain. Note that activation of the trigeminal nerve afferents leads to neuropeptide release and vasodilation of dural blood vessels, which in turn leads to release of more neuropeptides, perpetuating the cycle. (From Liu GT, Volpe, NJ, Galetta, SL: *Neuro-ophthalmology*, ed 2, Philadelphia, 2010, Saunders.)

meningeal and cerebral vascular networks may also be instigated by cortical spreading depression in migraineurs with aura. Second-order afferents from the deep dorsal horn of upper cervical levels also innervate the dura mater of the posterior fossa and converge on trigeminal neurons in the trigeminal caudate nucleus, creating the trigeminocervical complex. Trigeminal-vascular-cervical nociception is modulated in bidirectional pathways through brainstem and midbrain pain processing areas prior to being selected, amplified, and prioritized in the thalamus to cortices for sensibility and interpretation. Nociceptive nonmyelinated (C-fibers) and thinly myelinated (Aδ-fibers) axonal projections in the meninges release neuroinflammatory peptides (e.g., CGRP), perpetuating and increasing temporal and spatial nociceptive activity. If not inhibited or disregarded, the threshold is crossed to headache.[76]

Neural sensitization results in a decreased response threshold and increased response magnitude to a stimulus. Exposure to the described altered molecular environment sensitizes peripheral trigeminovascular neurons to non-noxious dural stimulation, developing a throbbing pain that intensifies with movements that increase intracranial pressure (bending, climbing stairs, coughing, sneezing) that are not typically painful.[108] When central trigeminovascular afferents in the trigeminal nucleus and ventral posterior medial thalamic nuclei become sensitized, their spontaneous activity and receptive fields expand. Mechanical and thermal stimulation to the skin of the face and neck is perceived as noxious, a response described as cutaneous allodynia.[36,76] Selective activation and sensitization of the retino-thalamic pathway during migraine may lead to photic allodynia, a perception of light as painful.[120] Auditory and olfactory sensitization may also occur, creating phonophobia and osmophobia. After peak sensitization is reached at about 120 minutes, abortive medications are not effective. Sensitization may play an important role in transforming high-frequency episodic migraine cycles into chronic migraine. Fig. 37.3 illustrates possible mechanisms related to migraine.

## Clinical Manifestations

**Migraine Stages.** Migraine episodes are divided into four stages—prodrome, aura, headache, and postdrome—and are classified as episodic or chronic based on number of headache-days per month. Nonheadache manifestations of migraine may include autonomic symptoms (nausea, vomiting, nasal/sinus congestion, rhinorrhea, lacrimation, ptosis, yawning, frequent urination, and diarrhea), affective symptoms (depression and irritability), cognitive symptoms (attention deficit, difficulty finding words, transient amnesia, and reduced ability to navigate in familiar environments), and sensory symptoms (photophobia, phonophobia, osmophobia, muscle tenderness, facial or tongue paraesthesias, and cutaneous allodynia).[36,51,76] Phases of migraine are not necessarily sequential, often overlap, or may not be expressed at all during a particular episode. The period between headaches (interictal) may also be considered a stage, because there are neurologic, biologic, and psychologic differences during that time compared to healthy nonmigraineurs.

The premonitory/prodrome phase may occur anytime up to 72 hours prior to headache. Hypothalamic-driven symptoms include fatigue, appetite changes, thirst, polyuria, cognitive deficits (reading, writing, speech, concentration), sleep disturbances, mood changes, repetitive yawning, sensory disturbances, and neck stiffness. Some

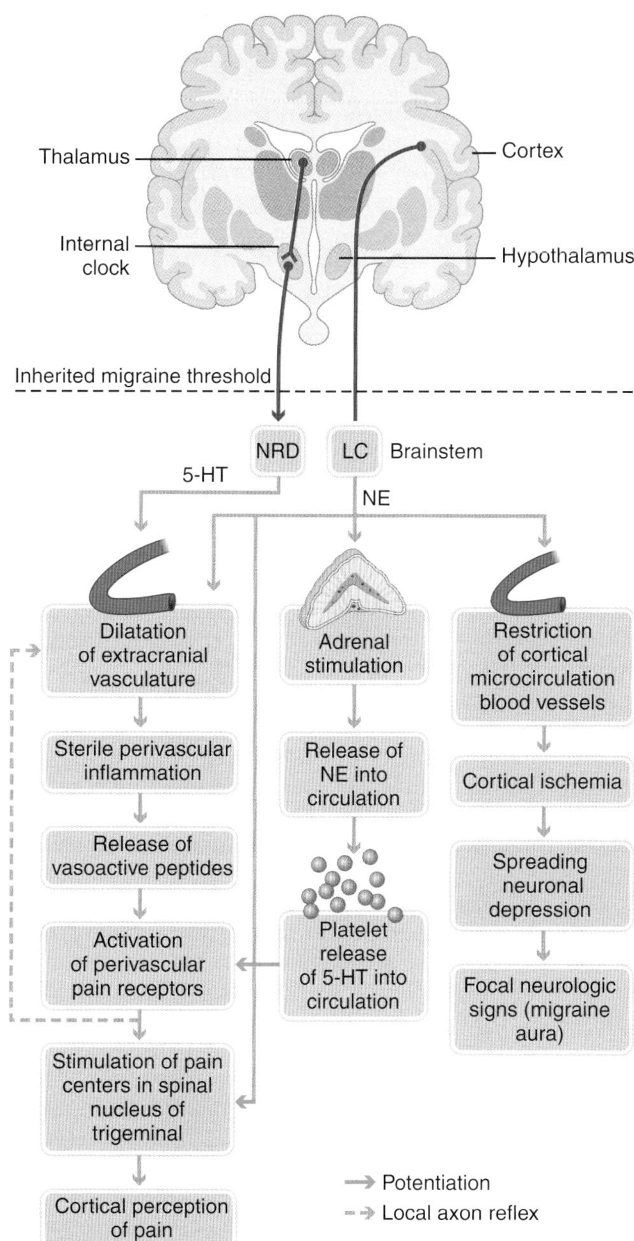


**Figure 37.3**

**Mechanisms that are related to the pathogenesis of migraine headache based on current proposals.** (From Weinstein JM: Headache and facial pain. In Yanoff M, Duker JS, Augsburger JJ, et al, eds: *Ophthalmology*, ed 2, St. Louis, 2004, Mosby.)

migraineurs are able to predict headache onset from prodromal symptoms. Cortical disturbances can manifest as cognition changes and visual, auditory or olfactory hypersensitivities. Many conditions thought to be triggers for migraine may in fact be part of premonitory hypothalamic dysfunction.[104,105,152]

Aura phase, experienced by one third of migraineurs, manifests as transient fully reversible focal neurologic deficits. Ninety percent of migraineurs with aura report visual symptoms. These may include loss of focus, spots of darkness, and zigzag flashing lights. Scintillating vision describes luminous, bright, flickering colors of

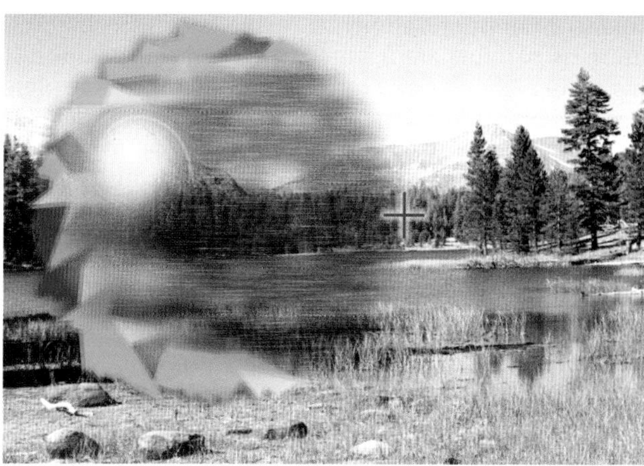

**Figure 37.4**

**Scintillating scotoma in migraine with aura.** The leading edge of the scotoma is "positive" (i.e., it consists of bright flickering imagery that obscures or replaces the normal visual field), whereas the trailing edge of the scotoma often is "negative" (i.e., it displays a relatively dark area that fully or partially obscures the visual surround). The illustration depicts a typical fortification scotoma with sharply angulated borders; many other variants of the migraine scotoma may occur. (From Weinstein JM: Headache and facial pain. In Yanoff M, Duker JS, Augsburger JJ, et al, eds: *Ophthalmology*, ed 2, St. Louis, 2004, Mosby.)

the spectrum, much like a prism catching light. It can be combined with a scotoma, an area of vision that appears to be obstructed or missing.[211] Fig. 37.4 shows the image as it would appear during a migraine. Paresthesias of the hand and face are the second most common aura symptom. Other aura symptoms may include disturbances in other sensory areas, speech, motor, brainstem, and retinal function, and are classified by symptoms.[85] Retinal aura involves repeated attacks of strictly monocular visual disturbance, including scintillations, scotomata, or blindness. Basilar aura (previously termed basilar migraine) presents with two or any combination of dysarthria, vertigo, tinnitus, hypacusis, diplopia, ataxia not attributable to sensory deficit, decreased level of consciousness (13 ≥GCS) and no motor or retinal symptoms.[85] Given how often vertigo, fluctuating hearing, and tinnitus occur together, basilar aura may be difficult to distinguish from peripheral vestibular disorders such as endolymphatic hydrops (see Chapter 38) and vertebrobasilar TIAs (see Chapter 32). The ICHD describes aura as lasting 5 to 60 minutes (per each type of disturbance), but a small percentage of migraineurs have reported individual sensory disturbances lasting longer than an hour.[211] Motor aura symptoms such as in hemiplegic migraine often last much longer. It is not clear whether aura triggers headache by increasing sensitization or is a comorbid condition.

Headache phase includes pulsating unilateral head pain of moderate to severe intensity made worse with normal activity or increased head pressure (bending, coughing, Valsalva maneuver) accompanied by nausea, phonophobia, and/or photophobia, building over 4 to 72 hours.[85] The trigeminal dermatome and high cervical dermatomes produce the typical migraine pain patterns via convergence within the trigeminal nucleus caudalis. Severe sensory sensitivity often promotes seeking dark, quiet locations for rest and avoidance of all movement.

Cutaneous or photic allodynia (experiencing normal sensation as painful) are features of central sensitization in this phase. As measured on a posturographic force plate, postural instability nearly doubles during attack compared to interictal measures and healthy controls, which may suggest a cerebellar dysfunction during the ictal phase.[5] For those individuals who are able to continue to function in a "normal" life context, energy and cognitive costs may promote irritability and severe fatigue.

The postdrome recovery phase is marked by hypothalamic-mediated symptoms, including remarkable "washed-out" fatigue, cognitive impairments, and stiff neck. It is often referred to as a headache hangover, and is not necessarily a side effect of medications taken to mitigate the headache. The prodrome and postdrome may be a single phase of migraine that is simply not apparent during the painful headache stage.[74]

The interictal (between headache) stage of migraine may be marked with hypersensitivities to light, sound or smell that nonmigraineurs do not experience. Trepidation about the next headache attack may promote avoidance behaviors and anxiety. These findings raise important considerations for practitioners regarding environment of clinics, as well as when planning treatment techniques that might aggravate visual, cutaneous, auditory or olfactory sensitivities (lighting options, manual techniques, perfume, cleaning agents, background music or television in the clinic).

**Typical Aura Without Headache.** Complaints of aura stage not followed by headache are more common in older individuals. Ruling out other neurologic conditions is especially important when the symptoms are very short or very long, or if they begin after the age of 40.[21]

**Chronic Migraine or Transformed Migraine.** The IHS definition for chronic migraine (CM) refers to migraine events with 15 or more headache days per month for more than 3 months.[85] The new definition only requires 8 headache days to be migrainous, resulting in a threefold increase in reported CM, which means newer studies do not compare directly to older study populations.[132] About 8% of migraineurs suffer chronic migraine, carrying a heavy disability burden because there may be very few if any days without headache or premonitory or recovery symptoms. The progression from episodic migraine to chronic migraine represents a failure of preventative strategies, and may be the result of central sensitization. As revealed in the Chronic Migraine Epidemiology and Outcomes (CaMEO) study, there is a high level of short-term variability across diagnostic boundaries of CM and episodic migraine.[183] Two thirds of medication overuse headache (MOH) occurs related to migraine medication for this group, the greatest risk for transformation from episodic to chronic status.

**Episodic Syndromes Associated with Migraine.** A number of episodic syndromes demonstrate a relationship to migraine, perhaps as precursors, with onset of specific syndromes occurring at different points across the lifespan. Pediatric syndromes associated with migraine include benign paroxysmal torticollis of infancy (BPTI), benign paroxysmal vertigo of childhood (BPVC), cyclic vomiting syndrome (CVS), abdominal migraine (AM), and vestibular migraine (VM). The high correlation of migraine behavior to abdominal pain in childhood is demonstrated by the shared diagnostic criteria between the ICHD migraine classification and the Rome IV classification of functional gastrointestinal disorders (FGIDs).[61] The recognition of these migraine equivalents in early childhood and adolescence is complicated by lack of expressive language and vocabulary to describe symptoms to parents or health care providers. Symptoms may manifest as colic, behavioral regression, withdrawal, attention seeking, or aggressive behaviors, as children may lack coping mechanisms for pain, vertigo and dizziness, altered perception of motion, balance disruption, or gastrointestinal upset. These conditions combined evoke a significant disease burden on the child and family, with the potential for large disruptions in school and age-appropriate activity participation.

Paroxysmal torticollis describes an episodic movement disorder that occurs in infancy and toddler years, and typically resolves between the ages of 3 and 5 years. BPTI has been shown to have a hereditary component and genetic correlation to the *CACNA1A* gene in familial hemiplegic migraine in some cases.[186] The diagnostic and clinical features of BPTI include recurrent episodes of cervical dystonia causing tilt and rotation of the head, combined with irritability, pallor, dizziness, and nausea or vomiting.[85] In a retrospective study some children reportedly experienced BPTI concurrent with acute otitis media, and 78% of children with BPTI experienced gross motor delay and balance impairments.[33] Abnormal rotary chair findings in those with BPTI were associated with transition to BPVC.

BPVC is diagnosed, typically in children between 2 and 12 years of age, when at least 5 spontaneous brief attacks of vertigo are accompanied by either nystagmus, ataxia, vomiting, pallor, or fearfulness.[85,165] As with BPTI, a subset of children with BPVC demonstrates gross motor delay, imbalance, and perhaps some correlation with acute otitis media during vertiginous episodes.[33] There are studies indicating a "vestibular march" from BPVC to migraine or vestibular migraine, and future research is likely to uncover further insight into the shared pathophysiology, as well as the prevalence of this developmental spectrum disorder.[129] One study in particular followed children with BPVC for 15 years; those with BPVC were three times more likely than the average population to develop migraine, but not necessarily vestibular migraine, in early adulthood.[14]

Cyclic vomiting syndrome involves intense recurrent attacks of nausea and vomiting occurring at least 4 times per hour and can last for 2 to 3 days, most often with onset between 4 to 8 years of age.[85] The severity of episodes results in pallor and lethargy, but full resolution should occur between attacks. Children experiencing recurrent vomiting require full gastrointestinal workup to rule out other primary causes, for medical support, and for pharmacologic management.[94] Those with a history CVS demonstrate an increased likelihood of developing migraine.

Onset of abdominal migraine (AM) most often occurs between the ages of 7 and 10 years. AM is an episodic syndrome involving moderate to severe, sharp or dull midline abdominal pain in an otherwise healthy child with normal physical exam, typical development, and a stable body mass index.[6,85] The abdominal pain may be accompanied by pallor, loss of appetite, nausea, or vomiting suggestive of symptoms related to dysautonomia. AM often does not include headache but may involve light or noise sensitivity.[50]

Although the pathophysiology of AM is largely unknown, proposed differences from other forms of migraine include alterations in the gut-brain axis, altered gastric emptying, and altered gut permeability.[127] A retrospective study of over 1000 children with headaches found migraine equivalent headaches in 70% of subjects, and identified an association between abdominal migraine, limb pain (growing pains), and motion sickness, suggesting a possible addition to the diagnostic criteria.[198] Newer areas of research have uncovered associations between abdominal pain and headache related to mast cell activation and mucosal inflammation, triggered by allergens or stress, particularly localized in the duodenum.[68] For more information on related gastrointestinal pathophysiology, the reader is directed to Chapter 16. Abdominal migraine has been shown to be a strong predictor of development of migraine in adulthood.

Typically, the above episodic syndromes of childhood resolve over time, though each condition can persist into adulthood. A family history of migraine appears to be a contributing factor to childhood migraine equivalents, and transition to migraine with or without aura or to episodic vestibular migraine is not uncommon.

**Vestibular Migraine.** The detailed diagnostic criteria for vestibular migraine and probable vestibular migraine have been established by collaboration between the Bárány Society and the International Headache Society.[115] Episodic VM must include recurrent vestibular symptoms, migraine headaches, and at least one migraine symptom during a vertigo attack lasting minutes to 72 hours or more. Migraine symptoms may include unilateral pulsating headache of moderate to severe intensity that increases with exertion, phonophobia or photophobia, and visual aura. The Bárány Society classification adds depth to the ICHD criteria with vertigo categorized as spontaneous vertigo (internal or external), positional vertigo, visually induced vertigo, head motion–induced vertigo or head motion–induced dizziness with nausea.[85]

Although largely unknown, the pathophysiology of VM is believed to involve cortical spreading depolarization and neurotransmitters common to migraine and vestibular pathways, such as calcitonin gene-related peptide, serotonin, noradrenaline, and dopamine.[114] Vestibular tests including video-oculography and visual evoked myogenic potentials (VEMP) are not currently reliable in elucidating a diagnosis of VM.[199] However, recent data suggest that unilateral abnormal findings on ocular VEMP in the presence of bilateral normal cervical VEMP may represent utricle involvement in unilateral VM.[126] Imaging studies are helping to determine pathway involvement in VM. Ipsilateral medio-dorsal thalamic activation viewed on blood-oxygen-level-dependent (BOLD) fMRI during unilateral caloric vestibular stimulation may contribute to pain modulation and cortical hyperexcitability, and PET images have demonstrated alterations in cerebellar metabolism during and between VM episodes.[175,185]

The clinical diagnosis remains complicated by the broad phenotypic presentations of VM and the need for clarification of nomenclature used to describe symptoms of vestibular aura. The differential diagnosis of vestibular migraine includes Meniere's disease, benign paroxysmal positional vertigo, and other neuro-vestibular disorders discussed in Chapter 38. The VM Phenotypes Project in Italy and Spain involves a collaborative effort to create a database to study individuals with vestibular migraine.[200] Initial data revealed that 75% of subjects experienced a sensation of internal vertigo, 25% described external vertigo, and 62% reported imbalance. Correlations were made between childhood motion sickness and the development of external vertigo, and the childhood precursors of migraine (BPTI, BPVC, and CVS), in addition to motion sickness, were associated with the onset of vertigo at a younger age than in those without a childhood history.

Unstable hormone fluctuations during perimenopause may trigger a change in migraine frequency and intensity. Dizziness is a common complaint of perimenopause, and should be differentially evaluated for evidence of vestibular migraine to avoid misdiagnosis as nonspecific climacteric or psychological symptoms.[150]

Similar to primary migraine, individuals with vestibular migraine often undergo trials of a combination of prophylaxis medication and acute abortive agents, and patient education is paramount in reducing triggers and assessing response to pharmaceutical therapies. Preliminary information indicates that VM is a common diagnosis seen in vestibular physical therapy and balance disorder clinics, with 38% of people in a single cohort demonstrating balance dysfunction on sensory organization testing.[158] Further studies should develop a clear role for physical therapy in the management of headache, dizziness, and imbalance related to VM.

### Complications of Migraine

**Status Migrainosus.** The unrelenting headache of status migrainosus (SM) lasts more than 72 hours, and may resemble the individual's usual severe migraine or a prolonged aura. Pain may spread to areas further afield, with significant allodynia. Overuse of analgesics and rebound withdrawal-type headache are the most common triggers. Risks include changes in hormone status in the premenstrual phase, pregnancy, miscarriage, or change in birth control pills. Upper respiratory or urinary tract infections can also trigger SM. Dehydration from prolonged vomiting is common and hospital admission may be necessary. Comorbid depression is frequently seen. Emergency department or inpatient treatment will include ample IV hydration, IV NSAIDs (ketorolac), and dopamine receptor antagonists to stop emesis. Antiepileptics may be considered, as well as regional anesthesia (nerve blocks). Inpatient care will include detoxification from medications.[172]

**Migraine Aura-Triggered Seizure.** There is very little evidence that migraine aura triggers seizure activity. Seizure aura is a focal paroxysmal depolarization shift, whereas migraine aura is a spreading cortical depolarization proceeding at about 3 mm/min. Seizure aura usually lasts less than 5 min, is not associated with onset of head pain or autonomic symptoms that occur as a result of a migraine, and may be lateralized. Both conditions share pathophysiologic similarities, including periodicity, higher concentration of extracellular glutamate, sodium

**Table 37.1** Migraine Disability Assessment (MIDAS) Questionnaire

Please answer the following questions about *all* your headaches you have had over the past 3 months. Write your answer in the box next to each question. Write zero if you did not perform the activity in the past 3 months.

1. How many days in the past 3 months did you miss work or school because of your headaches?
2. How many days in the past 3 months was your productivity at work or school reduced by half or more because of your headaches? (Do not include days you counted in question 1 when you missed work or school.)
3. How many days in the past 3 months did you not do household work because of your headaches?
4. How many days in the past 3 months was your productivity in household work reduced by half or more because of your headaches? (Do not include days you counted in question 3 when you did not do household work.)
5. How many days in the past 3 months did you miss family, social, or leisure activities because of your headaches?

TOTAL days

A. How many days in the past 3 months did you have a headache (if a headache lasted more than 1 day, count each day)?
B. On a scale of 0 to 10, on average how painful were these headaches (in which 0 = no pain at all, and 10 = pain as bad as it can be)?

Once you have filled in the questionnaire, add up the total number of days from questions 1 through 5 (ignore A and B).
Grading system for the MIDAS Questionnaire:

| Grade | Definition | Score |
|---|---|---|
| I | Little or no disability | 0-5 |
| II | Mild disability | 6-10 |
| III | Moderate disability | 11-20 |
| IV | Severe disability | 21+ |

From Stewart WF, Lipton RB, Dowson AJ, et al: Development and testing of the Migraine Disability Assessment (MIDAS) Questionnaire to assess headache-related disability, *Neurology* 56:S20–S28, 2001.

and potassium channelopathies, and higher incidences of affective disorders. "Migralepsy" is more likely comorbidity of both conditions.[84,225]

## MEDICAL MANAGEMENT

**DIAGNOSIS.** In most cases the diagnosis of migraine can be established by a careful history, and detailed headache diaries are useful in clarifying triggers, symptoms, strategies, and periodicity. There are patient-friendly electronic applications as well as handwritten tools available. Two common inventories used to measure the impact of headache are the Headache Impact Test (HIT-6) and the Migraine Disability Assessment (MIDAS), illustrated in Table 37.1. Determining severity, frequency, and disability is important in developing the best course of intervention, as well as identifying comorbidities. Additional patient inventories can be helpful, such as the Generalized Anxiety Disorder 7-item scale (GAD-7), the Pain Catastrophizing Scale, Beck Depression Scale, and any patient health scale with quality-of-life measures. A neurologic examination is typically normal and diagnostic procedures unnecessary in most cases. Magnetic resonance images (MRI) often show diffuse white matter hyperintensities (WMH) in the frontal subcortical and deep white matter at the level of the basal ganglia of migraine brains. Although WMH are commonly observed as a function of age and vascular disease, they are also more prevalent in migraineurs compared to age-matched healthy controls, possibly resulting from recurrent perfusion deficits, and appear to be related to length of disease and frequency of attacks.[170]

**TREATMENT.** There are multiple therapeutic options with proven efficacy for any of the primary headaches, but limited practitioner training, inaccurate diagnoses, and use of treatments with suboptimal evidence basis (including self-treatment choices) confound the outcomes.[57] Goals of treatment from a health care delivery perspective are to (1) abort and abate acute symptoms and (2) prevent escalation of a potentially chronic, progressive disease process by reducing or limiting severity, frequency, and duration of headache episodes and the associated disability. The medical model focuses on pharmacotherapeutics, for which there are evidence-based guidelines.[15,146,151,187] Outcome measures for pharmaceutical interventions are specific: acute pain free status within 2 hours with relief lasting at least 24 hours, and prevention measured by a 50% reduction in frequency and/or intensity of attacks over 3 months.[156,188] However, patients need more practical outcome measures (as in International Classifications of Function participation measures). Patient acceptance, adherence, preferences, and responses to treatment influence commitment to treatment plans. Patients also want (1) answers to questions about their condition, (2) education about their illness, and (3) education in self-treatment and prevention strategies.[57] Goals established for pediatric migraine management to reduce disability, develop adaptive pain-coping strategies, reduce risk of disease progression, and improve health-related quality of life also apply to adults, and to all headache sufferers.[146] In particular, children with migraine need to be carefully ushered into the adult care system after adolescence.[144]

Pharmaceutical migraine interventions in the medical model are outlined in Table 37.2. Medications target the headache and aura stages of migraine. Intervention aimed at the prodrome stage would seem an ideal attempt to keep abnormal neural activity under the threshold of pain, but that is not the current emphasis. While triptans are the most efficacious acute intervention, not all migraineurs can tolerate them. Too-frequent use of triptans leads to medication overuse headache (MOH) and indicates poor effectiveness.[76,187] Fig. 37.5 illustrates mode of delivery and

**Table 37.2** Migraine Interventions (Pharmacologic)

| Acute Intervention | Action | Risks and Benefits |
|---|---|---|
| Triptans[20,187,130] | Specific serotonin ($5\text{-}HT_{1B/1D}$) receptor agonist; abort progression | Auto-injectable or oral, time dependent; chest pain, vasoconstriction, CVD precautions; MOH, short-term use only for menstrual migraine prevention |
| Ergot alkaloids[188] | Nonspecific agonist for $5\text{-}HT_{1B/1D}$, dopamine D2, α-adrenergic antagonist | GI distress, vasoconstriction, peripheral vascular ischemia, CVD risk, not as effective as triptans; no longer recommended |
| NSAIDS and acetaminophen[148,130] | Oral or intravenous: inhibit prostaglandin synthesis, modulate serotonin turnover, inhibit trigeminovascular sensitization | Kidney injury, dyspepsia, rebound headache |
| Antidopaminergics[156,130] | Dopamine D2 receptor antagonists for acute headache pain and nausea | Akathisia (psychomotor restlessness), drowsiness, orthostatic hypotension |
| **Preventive Intervention** | | |
| CGRP monoclonal antibodies ("gepants")[96,201] Newest class of meds uniquely created for migraine prevention | CGRP receptor antagonist or direct molecular antagonist; repress cellular events contributing to central and peripheral sensitization from trigeminovascular nociceptive and trigeminal sensory systems. | Expensive, auto-injectable: no adverse interactions with other meds, bypasses GI tract, no vasoconstriction, reduces cortical sensitivities and nausea |
| Beta-blockers without sympathomimetic activity[188] | Vascular beta-adrenergic receptor antagonist; may inhibit platelets from expressing neuroinflammatory molecules | Behavioral, vascular, and respiratory adverse effects: 50% effective in reducing frequency by 50% |
| Antiepileptic drugs (primarily topiramate and valproate)[13] | Sodium channel blockers; target nociceptive trigeminovascular and trigeminothalamic dural pathways, CSD | GI distress, weight gain, cognitive effects, may interfere with oral contraception |
| Antidepressants: TCAs, SSRIs, SNRIs[221] | Increase availability of serotonin, reduce headache frequency, improve response to acute meds | Drowsiness, weight gain, anticholinergic adverse events |
| Onabotulinum toxin type A (Botox)[190] | Disrupts pain signaling in trigeminal nociceptive fields from pericranial musculature, used in chronic migraine only | Expensive, invasive, repeat Q12 wks; good for those with intolerance to other medications |
| Regional anesthesia: greater occipital nerve block[213] | May result in raised baseline serotonergic tone; thought to modulate brain excitability acting on input gate at the brainstem level | Localized; may be useful for patients who cannot tolerate systemic medications; anesthesia lasts 3 days, corticosteroids may last 2-3 months |
| Sphenopalatine ganglion block with lidocaine (intranasal catheterization)[24] | Blocks parasympathetic outflow to trigeminal nucleus and reduces central sensitization | Brief throat numbness, nausea, dizziness |

effects of triptans and ergot alkaloids. Abortive agents are most beneficial if administered at the first sign of attack; if migraine progresses to central sensitization in the form of cutaneous allodynia, effectiveness of all medications is very limited. Patients need to be encouraged to utilize abortive agents early rather that "toughing it out."

More than half of individuals experiencing migraine self-treat with over-the-counter NSAIDs or supplements, rather than or in addition to prescription medications. NSAIDs alone or in combination with triptans may improve acute abortive results. In addition to targeting specific inflammatory agents, NSAIDs may reinforce descending pain modulation pathways, and inhibit structures in the salience network that direct attention to pain.[76,146] A disconcerting trend was reported by Mazer-Amirshahi and colleagues, that despite recommendations against use of opioids due to lack of evidence-based efficacy and unfavorable risks, the decade of 2000 to 2010 saw a 70% increase in use of opioids for headache in U.S. emergency departments.[135]

Preventive strategies can be preemptive, short term, or maintenance. The first is to prevent response to a known trigger, such as taking indomethacin prior to exercise to dampen down inflammatory response and support nociceptive inhibition. The second involves planning for a limited trigger exposure time, such as during menses or a trip to high altitude. The third serves as ongoing treatment, as with chronic migraine, to reduce hyperexcitability. Topiramate is a common preventative agent, but can have a very unfavorable risk profile for some patients. Results of the AMPP study indicated that only 13% of individuals eligible for preventive care were utilizing a preventative protocol.[188] At best, preventive medications have only a 50% success rate.

Probyn and colleagues compared self-management programs of cognitive behavior therapy, mindfulness, and education (including in groups) to usual migraine care, measuring headache frequency, intensity, mood, disability, quality of life, and medication usage. Modest superior improvements were noted in all areas but frequency, confirming that patient self-efficacy and cognitive-emotional skills are powerful agents in managing migraine disease.[160] These strategies do not alter the biologic basis for migraine but may reduce susceptibility. Table 37.3 summarizes nonpharmaceutical interventions for migraine.

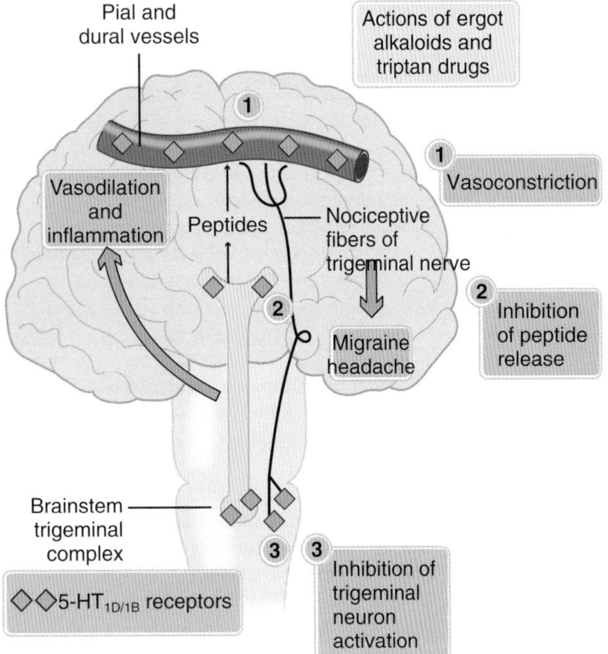


**Figure 37.5**

**Mechanisms of ergot alkaloids and triptan drugs used in the treatment of migraine headache disorder.** Ergot alkaloids and triptan drugs terminate the pain by activating serotonin 5-$HT_{1B/1D}$ receptors at several sites: (1) They activate receptors on pial and dural vessels and thereby cause vasoconstriction. (2) They activate presynaptic receptors to inhibit the release of peptides and other mediators from trigeminal neurons. (3) They activate receptors in the brainstem, which is thought to inhibit activation of trigeminal neurons responsible for migraine attacks. (From Brenner GM, Stevens, C: *Pharmacology*, ed 4, Philadelphia, 2012, Saunders.)

Despite positive anecdotal evidence, investigations of various supplements in treating migraine are generally considered of low quality, with inconclusive results. Nonetheless, headache societies give strong recommendations for magnesium and riboflavin ($B_2$), and somewhat less enthusiastic support for coenzyme Q10, melatonin, and feverfew. Due to evidence of hepatic toxicity, butterbur root extract (Petadolex) is no longer recommended, despite demonstrating a 50% reduction in headache frequency. Although believed to be essential for neural health, omega-3 polyunsaturated fats have not resulted in any difference in migraine behavior.[47,161,164,201] Magnesium is chronically deficient in the brains of many migraineurs, potentially affecting cell permeability, metabolism, and neural function. At sufficient dosages, regular supplementation may significantly reduce headache frequency.[161] Although not yet being examined in the migraine population, magnesium L-threonate (a smaller compound than typical oral supplements) is more effective in raising cerebrospinal fluid levels of $Mg^{++}$ and is currently being tested for effects in memory and learning, and in reducing neuropathic pain related to antineoplastic agents.[193,220]

Aerobic exercise is recommended by the American Academy of Neurology, American College of Physicians, American Headache Society, and the National Institute of Neurological Disorders and Stroke as means of managing migraine.[93] Control of symptoms with consistent exercise may be as effective topiramate.[210] Improvement in depression-related symptoms in neuroinflammatory, neurovascular, neurolimbic, and neuroendocrine domains may have similar biologic and psychologic mechanisms.[3,93]

**PROGNOSIS.** Frequency and intensity of headache determine the long-term impact of migraine. Specific aspects of headache as measured by the Migraine Disability Assessment (MIDAS) and the Headache Impact Test (HIT-6), can be used to help identify current status outcomes to help direct long-term management.[37] Patients with migraine are two to four times more likely to develop lifetime major depressive disorder, likely due to related underlying neuropathophysiology and genetic mechanisms.[4] Quality-of-life and health-related outcomes may be worse over a lifetime for those who suffer both conditions, making careful management and close follow-up imperative. Nearly 50% of children and adolescents will still report migraines in adulthood. Migraines tend to decrease in prevalence in the seventh decade of life, with an increase in aura without headache, and the gap between men and women narrowing when sex steroids are no longer as influential.[21] A transformation from episodic to chronic migraines darkens the prognosis with significant disability, no matter the individual's age.

## SPECIAL IMPLICATIONS FOR THE THERAPIST 37.1

### *Migraine*

After ensuring appropriate referral to a headache medicine specialist, physical therapists may still be involved in nonpharmacologic care of migraine through exercise prescription, lifestyle education and support, dietary guidelines, and support for identification and management of triggers. Pain self-efficacy behaviors for migraineurs are similar to those for any neuropathic and chronic pain condition, and should be promoted and coached at every opportunity. Biofeedback is the best known and most widely used nonpharmacologic procedure for the treatment of migraine, allowing the client to make intrinsic changes in both the autonomic and somatic nervous systems via thermal and surface EMG feedback. Noninvasive neuromodulating devices are demonstrating promising treatment effects, and may take a role in physical therapy practice.[161]

Migraineurs demonstrate more upper quarter myofascial trigger points than nonheadache patients, potentially introducing a secondary source of pain into the trigeminal-cervical nociceptive system.[56] Palliative relief of neck and head pain with cervical spine manipulation or other physical modalities may complement a medical treatment regimen; however, it is important to remember that neck pain during and after migraine is likely related to dural vascular nociception and the shared neural pathways of the trigeminal nucleus caudalis rather than pain from primary neck dysfunction. Those with chronic migraine or migraine with aura have been shown to have significant report of imbalance and higher risk of falls, indicating a need for a thorough neuro-vestibular balance assessment for complete evaluation of related impairments.[40]

**Table 37.3** Migraine Interventions (Nonpharmacologic)

| Intervention | Action | Risks and Benefits |
|---|---|---|
| Noninvasive neuromodulation[161] | Single-pulse transcranial magnetic stimulation<br>Transcutaneous vagus nerve stimulation<br>Transcutaneous supraorbital stimulation<br>Anodal transcranial direct current stimulation<br>Central or peripheral stimulation to modulate pain mechanisms | Paresthesia under area of stimulation; benefit: immediate response, may disrupt chronic pattern |
| Nutraceuticals/ supplements[118,161,164,201] | Magnesium, riboflavin, coenzyme Q10: may affect mitochondria metabolism, $Mg^{++}$ may reduce neural hyperexcitability | Muscle relaxant, diarrhea |
| | Melatonin: hormone plays an important role in modulating the activity of the suprachiasmatic nucleus (SCN) and the circadian system via the hypothalamic-pineal axis | may reduce frequency and duration of headache phase |
| | Caffeine: analgesic adjuvant, crosses blood-brain barrier, improves mood and alertness, speeds gastric motility | Nervousness, may interfere with other med effects |
| Behavioral therapies[160,161] | Relaxation, thermal and surface EMG biofeedback, coping strategies, stress response, pain management self-efficacy | Face-to-face time requirements |
| Exercise[3,210] | May have neuroinflammatory, neurovascular, neurolimbic, neuroendocrine, psychological and behavioral effects | Ideal parameters for frequency and intensity are unknown |
| Acupuncture[47] | Biologic mechanism poorly understood; promotes relaxation, may reduce neural hyperexcitability | Practitioner qualifications and knowledge |

## Tension-Type Headache

### Overview

TTHs are the most common type of primary headache; as many as 90% of adults have had or will have tension headaches, representing 25 million people in the United States. Infrequent episodic tension-type headaches are those that occur less than once per month and are usually self-managed, requiring little medical attention. Prevalence appears to peak in 30- to 40-year-olds slightly more often in women, increasing with level of education in both genders.[180] The socioeconomic burden increases in the individual with frequent episodic TTH, which occurs from 2 to 14 days per month. Chronic TTHs are those reported more than 15 days per month and have a different neurobiologic pathogenesis.[85] Chronic TTHs occur most often in women older than age 50 years and have usually evolved from episodic tension headaches.[196] Distinguishing chronic TTH from migraine and from medication-overuse headache is a diagnostic challenge, and the management is different.

### Etiologic and Risk Factors

Myofascial trigger point pain involving muscles of the head, neck, and shoulder regions demonstrates pain referral patterns consistent with pain descriptions and drawings of adults and children with TTH. Additionally, reduction in cervical motion and postural changes, such as forward head posture, may increase risk and incidence of episodic TTH.[56] A study of individuals with TTH found that subjects meeting prediction criteria related to lower frequency and duration of headache (frequent episodic) as well as pain and perceived disability on the SF-36 demonstrated localized and remote reduction in pressure point pain thresholds, indicating hypersensitivity and higher rates of anxiety that may be indicative of developing chronic TTH.[65] Focused visual attention has also been implicated in production of episodic TTH related to increased ocular muscle tension.[39] Studies report correlations between stress, altered sleep patterns, and headache activity in a variety of age populations worldwide, recognizing that lack of sleep and oversleep can promote headache activity.[140,163]

### Pathogenesis

Pericranial and myofascial trigger point nociception represents the pathophysiology of episodic TTH. Stimuli to skin, tendons, and muscle cause pain, resulting in peripheral sensory afferent activation and release of endogenous substances such as serotonin and bradykinin. Sensitization of central nociceptive pathways seems responsible for the conversion of episodic to chronic TTH.[19] The sensitization of second-order neurons and neurons at the level of the trigeminal nucleus alters nonpainful input so that it is perceived as noxious at the level of the cortex. This may be consistent with referred hyperalgesia, relating to the convergence of multiple peripheral sensory afferents onto sensitized spinal cord neurons, which project to central structures that have another level of sensitization.[18,70]

Sympathetic tone and autonomic dysregulation is evidenced by resting heart rate, which is higher in migraine and chronic TTH than in episodic TTH.[223] Compiled evidence demonstrates interplay between peripheral contributions to episodic TTH and central "top down" regulation, which could be associated with chronic TTH or overlap of mixed headache pathophysiology.[56] There are many similarities between the central pathophysiology of migraine and chronic TTH; however, recent findings in a voxel-based gray matter study indicate that changes in gray matter volume may be predictive of headache type.[42]

### Clinical Manifestations

Tension-type headaches (TTH) produce bilateral headache pain described as pressure or tightness (nonpulsing) of mild to moderate intensity that does not worsen with physical activity and most often does not elicit light or noise sensitivity, nausea or vomiting.[85] The frequency and duration and presence or absence of pericranial pressure further define the nature of TTH. There is increased tenderness to palpation of the tissues around the head. Both muscles and tendon insertions have been found to be excessively tender, and pressure pain sensitivity maps appear to be different in chronic TTH.[1,10] The level of tenderness correlates to the intensity of the headache. Fig. 37.1 provides an image representing the sensation of a band around the head and a weight upon the head that can occur with TTH.

## MEDICAL MANAGEMENT

**DIAGNOSIS.** The diagnosis of tension headache requires the exclusion of other causative disorders. The medical history should include the evolution of the headache, preferably utilizing a headache diary. A general physical and neurologic examination should be performed to rule out a disease process, including palpation of the pericranial muscles to identify tenderness and trigger points. Referred pain patterns should be recorded, specifically targeting the suboccipital, temporal, lateral pterygoid, masseter, sternocleidomastoid, and trapezius muscles. It should be noted whether the palpation is done during the headache or nonheadache phase, as there can be up to 25% increase in pain perception during headache.

Except for their frequency and intensity, chronic TTHs are similar to frequent episodic TTHs. Chronic TTH may be linked with medication overuse, addressed later in the chapter, and the diagnosis should be made only after there have been 15 days free of medication. It is important to recognize that individuals with confirmed migraine are prone to increased incidence of chronic TTHs between migraine attacks. The individual will usually describe a difference between the headache types.

**TREATMENT.** Analgesics and NSAIDs are the most typical medications used for control of acute episodic TTHs, and often the individual will self-select the dosage. Most randomized placebo-controlled trials have demonstrated that aspirin (in doses of 500 and 1000 mg) and acetaminophen (1000 mg) are effective in the acute therapy for TTH.[53] The combination of analgesics and NSAIDs with caffeine (64-200 mg) can be helpful but caffeine withdrawal can cause further headache.[17] Overuse of analgesics and NSAIDs may increase the frequency of TTH, and combination therapy with codeine or barbiturates is not recommended. Further, compiled evidence from the European Federation of Neurological Societies (EFNS) Guidelines does not support the use of triptans, muscle relaxants or opioids for management of acute TTH.

Tricyclic antidepressants such as amitriptyline (first choice), followed by mirtazapine (Remeron) and venlafaxine (Effexor), are useful prophylaxis agents in chronic TTH but do have side effects.[17] If depression is comorbid, tricyclics are generally regarded as more effective than selective serotonin reuptake inhibitors. Previously studied NMDA antagonists have been found ineffective in chronic TTH, and there is evidence presented in the EFNS Guidelines that botulinum toxin may be harmful in chronic TTH.

Physical therapy is the most utilized nonpharmacologic treatment of TTH and promotes improvement through of postural exercise and education, relaxation training, exercise programs, biofeedback, and electrical stimulation. Techniques to reduce trigger point pain through manual therapy, mobilization and exercise have been shown to be relatively low cost, low risk and effective in reduction of TTH intensity.[123] A systematic review of random control trials of manual therapy for those with TTH indicates that manual therapy can reduce headache frequency, increase cervical mobility, reduce pain pressure thresholds, and improve quality of life.[119] One particular RCT involving university students diagnosed with TTH in Spain found that motor control training of the deep craniocervical flexors and mid-lower cervical extensors, combined with stretching of hypertonic superficial prime movers, postural/ergonomic education, and relaxation training effectively reduced headache frequency and intensity significantly greater than relaxation training alone.[2]

Relaxation training allows patients to consciously reduce muscle tension and reduce autonomic arousal. SEMG biofeedback is used to change the amplitude of pericranial muscle tension, which is a way to establish central brain changes. The supraorbital transcutaneous electrical stimulator (SOES) is a more recently developed pericranial electrical stimulation device designed for pain relief in chronic TTH.[82]

**PROGNOSIS.** Over time, there is an increased risk of the episodic TTH developing into a chronic TTH. As discussed for those with migraine, patient education modules, cognitive behavior therapy, and mindfulness training promote self-management of mood, headache pain intensity, and perceived level of disability in TTH.[160] Multidisciplinary headache care produces the most positive results in long-term control of symptoms.

## Trigeminal Autonomic Cephalgias (TACs)

### Overview

Trigeminal autonomic cephalalgia (TAC) encompasses four unique primary headache types: cluster headache, paroxysmal hemicrania, hemicrania continua, short-lasting unilateral neuralgiform headache attacks with conjunctival injection and tearing (SUNCT) and short-lasting unilateral neuralgiform headache attacks with cranial autonomic symptoms (SUNA).[216]

Cluster headaches, the most common TAC, produce severe unilateral pain accompanied by at least one ipsilateral autonomic symptom: orbital redness, tearing, or swelling, sinus congestion or drainage, or facial sweating. Individual headaches last from 15 to 180 minutes and occur up to eight times in a single day, often eliciting a restless agitation.[85] Episodic cluster headaches involve at least 2 intervals of ongoing attacks lasting 7 days to one year that are separated by 3 months or greater of remission. Cluster headaches become chronic when remission is less than 3 months for at least one year.

Cluster headaches affect approximately 1% to 4% of the population and predominantly occur between ages 20 and 40, with a higher frequency in men. Headache severity is disabling to the individual as almost 20% of cluster headache patients have lost a job, while another 8% are out of work or on disability secondary to their headaches. Suicidal ideations are substantial, occurring in 55%.[173] The genetic contributions to cluster headache remain elusive though a low-frequency inheritance pattern is suspected. Genome-wide analysis studies are focused on correlation to the circadian rhythm due to the predictable onset of headaches in the predawn hours.

### Pathogenesis

The pathophysiology of cluster headaches remains under investigation though a prominent hypothesis involves hypothalamic activation due to the correlation with the circadian rhythm and seasonal changes.[87] During this vulnerable period, vasodilators such as histamine, alcohol, and nitroglycerine, combined with a genetic susceptibility, may trigger the onset of cluster headaches. Stimulation of the trigeminal nerve appears to elicit a unilateral cerebral vasodilator response and activation of the trigeminocervical complex, with an increase in the level of CGRP and substance P. Unilateral headache pain occurs in the ophthalmic distribution of the trigeminal nerve. Subsequently, trigeminal activation of the facial nerve, through the superior salivatory nucleus, is thought to induce a parasympathetic response of the sphenopalatine ganglion, resulting in ipsilateral ocular and nasal autonomic symptoms.

Findings from imaging studies support the suspected involvement of the hypothalamus during acute attacks.[222] Changes in the structural and functional connectivity of the hypothalamus to the frontal lobe, cerebellum, and occipital lobe may help elucidate the pathophysiology and clinical features for future diagnosis. Additionally, comparison of in-bout and out-of-bout voxel-based morphometry alongside DTI and fMRI may help unravel theories related to pain modulation of cluster headaches. As with most headaches, pharmacologic and intervention studies contribute to the understanding of pathophysiology by monitoring pharmacogenetics and patient response.[106]

### Clinical Manifestations

The onset is sudden, with excruciating pain that ranges from throbbing to sharp and stabbing. In the majority of cases, the headache remains on one side of the head in all recurrences throughout life, though a side shift can occur.[133] The headache is usually localized to one eye and the frontotemporal region (see Fig. 37.1). Autonomic changes occur on the same side as the headache but may be bilateral. Occasionally, Horner syndrome (constricted pupil, droopy eyelid) or forehead sweating will appear on the uninvolved side of the face.[27] Fig. 37.6 shows the interrelationship of pain and autonomic symptoms in cluster headache. Different from those with migraine who seek dark and sleep, people experiencing cluster headache may appear restless, with a need to rock, pace, or apply firm pressure to the area as they cope with up to eight attacks within one day.

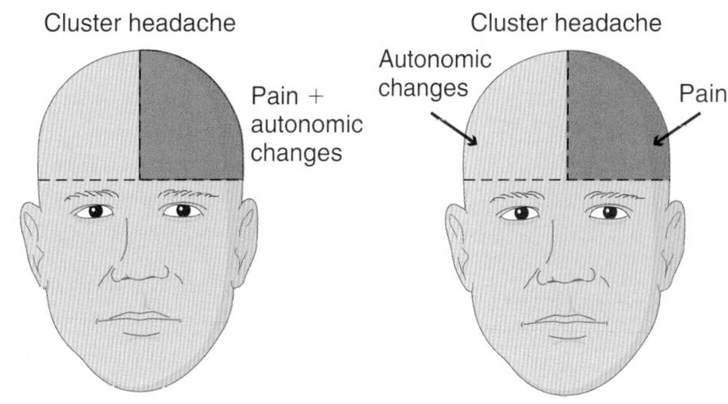


**Figure 37.6**

**The interrelationship of pain and autonomic symptoms and signs in cluster headache.** The usual pattern is pain and autonomic changes on the same side *(left)*. A less common pattern is pain on one side and autonomic changes on the opposite side *(right)*. (From Sjaastad O: *Cluster headache syndrome*, London, 1992, Saunders, p. 49.)

## MEDICAL MANAGEMENT

**DIAGNOSIS.** There remains a significant diagnostic delay for cluster headache patients, on average 5 or more years, with only 21% receiving a correct diagnosis at time of initial presentation.[173] Diagnosis is based on the symptoms and history. Paroxysmal hemicrania, trigeminal neuralgia, and temporal arteritis may have similar symptoms, but they are not episodic. Diagnostic criteria are strict unilaterality, severe intensity, orbital localization, and short duration. Differential diagnosis includes migraine, trigeminal neuralgia, chronic paroxysmal hemicrania, pericarotid syndrome, sinusitis, and glaucoma.[48] The overlap of shared complexity of pathway involvement and hypersensitivity patterns can contribute to the challenge in differentiating cluster from migraine headaches. It is important to note that trigeminal autonomic cephalgia and cluster headache can be classified as a secondary headache if there is a known causative factor, particularly in the event of head trauma or a condition affecting the nose or jaw. The sphenopalatine ganglion (SPG) has been implicated in headaches and cranial neuralgias, with a variety of interventions to block the SPG dating back to Sluder syndrome in 1908.[169]

**TREATMENT.** Management of acute cluster headaches involves abortive therapy that is most successfully reported with subcutaneous injection or nasal spray administration of sumatriptan.[87] Approximately 66% of patients report resolution of acute symptoms using 12 to 15L of high-flow mask oxygen therapy in an upright position.[46] Multiple studies have investigated the efficacy of 4% to 10% lidocaine nasal spray to reduce autonomic symptoms associated with the sphenopalatine ganglion with mixed success.[169]

Verapamil is the most widely used prophylactic medication, and requires monitoring of cardiac function due to the dosage required. At the start of a cluster, transitional preventive treatment such as corticosteroids or greater occipital nerve blockade can be helpful. In chronic and in long-standing clusters, lithium, methysergide, topiramate, valproic acid, and ergotamine tartrate can be used as add-on prophylactic treatment.[72] Central neuromodulation with deep brain stimulation of the hypothalamus or spinal cord stimulation with implanted electrodes are alternative treatment strategies.[111] Studies directed toward peripheral neuromodulation involve botulinum toxin injection into the SPG as well as electrical stimulation of the SPG, occipital nerve, and vagus nerve.

Education should be provided regarding precipitating factors, including alcohol, abrupt changes in sleeping patterns related to travel, and work shift changes. Lack of sleep or afternoon naps may precipitate a headache. Bursts of anger or prolonged anticipatory anxiety can provoke a headache during the cluster period. Avoiding these situations may reduce the frequency of cluster headache during a cluster period. Upright activities, including walking, appear to be of some relief. Few people choose to lie down during an attack.[58]

Chronic cluster headache, which accounts for about 10% to 15% of patients with cluster headache, is often resistant to pharmacologic management. The sphenopalatine ganglion has been a target for blocking catheter devices, chemical neurolysis, and percutaneous radiofrequency ablation procedure.[169]

**PROGNOSIS.** In the natural course of cluster headache, around 10% of those affected will transition from episodic to chronic, and that same number may change from chronic to episodic. One third will suffer for around 20 years and then experience a complete remission. In another one third, the attacks will be mild and no longer require medical intervention. The final one third of individuals continue to have attacks in the same pattern and to the same degree.

SPECIAL IMPLICATIONS FOR THE THERAPIST 37.2

### *Cluster Headache*

It is important for the therapist to be able to recognize the symptoms of cluster headache and to differentiate it from tension headache. Tension headache often is improved when drinking alcohol. Relaxation and stress reduction may be of benefit if the client has a history of episodes triggered by stress response. Use of thermal and EMG biofeedback may be of benefit (see "Migraine" above). Aggressive exercise appears to improve symptoms in cluster headache as it does in migraine.

**Table 37.4** Pathologic Conditions Causing Secondary Headache

| Pathologic Condition | Signs and Symptoms |
|---|---|
| Subdural hematoma | Mild to severe, intermittent headache; neurologic symptoms include fluctuating consciousness |
| Subarachnoid hemorrhage | Sudden onset, severe and constant headache; elevated blood pressure; can cause change in consciousness |
| Increased cranial pressure | Mild to severe headache; neurologic symptoms include hemiparesis, visual changes, and brainstem symptoms, including vomiting, altered consciousness |
| Meningitis, viral, and bacterial | Headache severe with radiation down neck; acutely ill and febrile; positive Kernig sign |
| Brain abscess | Mild to severe headache; local or distant infection; may be afebrile; neurologic signs consistent with local site of infection |
| Central nervous system | Localized headache and focal neurologic symptoms; often see cranial nerve symptoms |
| Central nervous system neoplasm | Localized headache and focal neurologic symptoms; often see cranial nerve symptoms |
| Toxicity | Generalized headache, pulsating; may show other signs of toxicity |
| Sinusitis | Frontal or dull headache, usually worse in morning; increased pain in cold damp air; nasal discharge |
| Otitis media, mastoiditis | Feeling of fullness in ear, stabbing pains in head, vertigo, and tinnitus |

## SECONDARY HEADACHES

A sudden onset of severe headache is usually related to an intracranial disorder such as subarachnoid hemorrhage, brain tumor, or meningitis (see Chapter 29). These headaches will most often be accompanied by other neurologic signs, such as weakness, visual disturbances, and possibly altered mental status or coma. A structural, or space-occupying, lesion is suspected in headaches that disrupt sleep, are triggered by exertion, or cause excessive drowsiness. Headaches secondary to brain tumors, endocrinopathies, and other medical problems are only a very small percentage of all headaches.[98] Even though pathologic conditions account for only a few cases of headache pain, it is critical for the therapist to understand what mechanisms may be responsible and when the client may need medical or emergent care. Table 37.4 lists some of the causes of headache that may require immediate medical attention.

### Headache Attributed to Disorder of the Neck: Cervicogenic Headache

#### Overview

Although theories about headache originating from the neck have circulated for more than a century, the term "cervicogenic headache" was coined by Sjaastad in 1983,[191] leading to establishment of the Craniocervical Headache International Study Group (CHISG) and the first diagnostic guidelines.[192] Updated in 2005, they remain far more detailed than the ICHD classifications.[66]

Cervicogenic headache (CGH) is perceived in the head but originates from a primary disorder of the cervical spine and its component bony, disc, and/or soft tissue elements, usually but not invariably accompanied by neck pain.[85,192] Those disorders include tumors, fractures, infections, and rheumatoid arthritis of the upper cervical spine, as well as musculoskeletal and vascular disorders.[30] Most often (but not always) there will be a history of neck pain preceding the headache, often with motion, and strength and functional limitations. Headache may be aggravated by specific movements or sustained postures of the head, neck, and shoulder girdle. The similarities of pain pattern with TTH, migraine without aura, and hemicrania continua can make diagnosis challenging, particularly in those infrequent cases where CGH is accompanied by nausea, vomiting, and photophobia.[66,174] Neck pain is also common in migraine and TTH, due to the convergence of bidirectional trigeminal neurons in the trigeminal nucleus caudalis, which may extend into the spinal cord as low as C5, and cervical afferents of C1 to C3 levels, but the causative disorder is not in the neck (see section on migraine). The biologic marker of fluctuations in CGRP that activate the trigeminocervical and trigeminovascular complexes in migraine is not present in CGH.[67]

## Prevalence

Approximately 20% of headaches are of cervical origin, affecting 2.5% of the general population.[209] Incidence in women is four times that of men, and while quality of life deterioration reflects that of migraine and tension-type headache, there is greater physical disability reported among cervicogenic headache sufferers.[25] Prevalence increases modestly with age, possibly linked to progressive degenerative changes leading to mechanical dysfunction and nerve entrapment. A sudden onset is usually linked to trauma, including but not limited to whiplash associated disorders (WAD). Although the IHS specifies an arbitrary temporal association of headache within 7 days of a trauma, delayed onset is being considered for the next edition of ICHD, based on emerging evidence of progressive changes occurring in neck and brain neurophysiology following trauma.[85] More than 80% of people experiencing WAD report headaches, as do more than 50% of persons under 50 years of age with all forms of neck pain.[209]

## Pathogenesis

Branching and comingling of the cervical nerves of C1-4 create the anterior and posterior neural plexuses, both superficial and deep, to supply sensory and motor innervation to all upper cervical and lower cranial structures from skin to periosteal bone. C1 also contributes to the vertebral nerve supplying afferents to the vertebral artery. C1, C2, and C3 sinuvertebral (recurrent) nerves, accompanied by an autonomic root, supply the upper cord dura, sheaths of the nerve roots themselves, as well as entering the foramen magnum to innervate the dura in the posterior cranial fossa and tentorial membrane. All spinal nerves other than C1 have ascending and descending branches to structures of neighboring segments, permitting multilevel innervation.[31,167] The posterior divisions of C1, C2, and C3 create the greater and lesser occipital nerves supplying the occipital and temporal-occipital scalp and all deep myofascial structures of the craniovertebral junction, traversing through soft tissues between the posterior arch of atlas and cranium, where they are vulnerable to compression. The anterior divisions give rise to the greater auricular and third occipital nerves, the latter looping around the C2 to C3 facet as it courses toward the ear and parieto-temporal scalp, vulnerable to injury during a whiplash event.[26]

When primary afferents from upper cervical dorsal root ganglia converge on second order trigeminal neurons in the spinal cord, connecting two topographically separate regions of the body, nociceptive signals in one of the afferents can be perceived as pain arising in the territory of the other.[31] The upper cervical nerves also directly innervate lower cranial structures, creating a scenario for direct head pain as well. Functional convergence of sensorimotor fibers of C2-4 with the spinal accessory nerve (CN XI) directly affects upper trapezius and sternocleidomastoid function and reactivity, as well as interfacing with descending trigeminal nerves leading to pain referral to head and face.[206] Anterior branches of the high cervical plexus also communicate with the vagus nerve (X) supplying the salivary glands, parts of the ear, pharynx, larynx, and viscera; the hypoglossal nerve (XII) supplies the tongue and the upper cervical sympathetic ganglia.[79]

Central sensitization (described under migraine) can both perpetuate and enlarge a field of perceived pain through maladaptation of cortical representation. Cervicogenic headache is episodic but not cyclic, and may last from hours to weeks, promoting neural response to constant exposure to nociception. Individuals experiencing such regional pain syndromes, particularly if coexistent with other centralized pain syndromes, including fibromyalgia, irritable bowel syndrome, migraine, and chronic fatigue syndrome, report fatigue, mood and sleep disorders, and poor quality of life.[62] Psychological factors combine with neurophysiologic, cognitive, and environmental influences in any chronic pain disorder.

Vascular disorders, primarily aneurysms, or dissection of the carotid or vertebral arteries (see Chapter 32) cause sudden and intense neck pain with headache. There may be progressive neurologic symptoms, and emergent care is required. Although dissection due to trauma is very rare, it can happen concurrently, and may be mistaken for concussion symptoms.[110]

Metabolic or neoplastic sources of cervical disorders may cause headache through the same neurologic mechanisms. Although pain may be produced by movement or pressure, in these disorders there is a hallmark of pain that is not relieved with rest and may be perceived as worse with rest associated with lack of large proprioceptive fibers capable of gating pain at the spinal cord level.

A little-reported potential cause of headache is foramen arcuale (FA), a partial or complete bony bridge across the transverse process of atlas over the groove for the vertebral artery and occipital nerves, observable on radiographs. Although literature reports are mixed on the causative relationship of FA with CGH, Pekela and colleagues analyzed several studies and concluded that there was a statistical trend toward higher prevalence of neurologic symptoms with any form of FA.[125a] Craniocervical flexion and extension may cause vertebral artery compression, entrapment of occipital nerves, and tension on the dura via the atlanto-occipital membrane attachment to the transverse process. Surgical decompression is a successful remedy.[147]

Musculoskeletal causes of cervicogenic headaches arising from the craniovertebral junction may include disruption of alar or transverse ligaments, burst of the C1 arch, fracture of the C2 dens, joint pain from atlanto-occipital or atlanto-axial facets, myofascial pain including trigger points, or nerve entrapment. Fracture sites will often produce inflammatory edema and extreme reflexive muscle guarding not relieved with support, potentially contributing ischemic muscle pain to headache. Acute exacerbations of systemic inflammatory diseases, particularly rheumatoid arthritis which has a predilection for atlanto-axial destruction, may cause regional guarding and stiffness, local edema, heat, and tenderness, as well as referred headache. Intractable headache from instability may require fusion, for neurologic safety more than pain.

Mechanical forces may promote dysfunction in the atlanto-occipital articulations and surrounding musculature, leading to referred headache pain. Activities, sustained postures, or injuries causing compression and extension of C0 to C1 compress soft tissues, including nerves and vessels, load joint cartilage and capsules, and may require sustained contraction and structural shortening of musculature to support the cranium. Narrowed space between the occiput and atlas can be easily visualized on flexion-extension films, where a lack of subcranial change might be observed in the transition from extension to flexion, replaced by excessive flexion in lower segments. The greater occipital nerve, composed of primarily C2 and C3 dorsal root fibers, supplies sensory pathways to the occiput and parietal areas. It exits to the scalp through all extensor attachments along the nuchal ridge and lies within the occipital groove, located one third posterior to the mastoid process and two thirds lateral to the midpoint of the occiput. The nerve sheath may become inflamed and edematous, and is easily palpated. Occiput-atlas hyperextension and chronic significantly tight short extensors may compress the nerve. Pain may be aching or sharp, with scalp paresthesia, from occiput to temple.

The atlas-axis (C1-2) articulation produces 40% of spine rotation from the head to T4. Loss of available range is highly associated with CGH. Normal mechanics of C1 to C2 rely on smaller but synchronized motions of C0 to C1. Pain referral patterns from C1-2 reach the periorbital area, vertex, occiput, and occipito-parietal areas.[8]

The C2 to C3 apophyseal joint is biomechanically vulnerable as a transition between subcranial biomechanical patterns and the lower cervical spine. It bears both vectors of stress, and introduces the first cervical disc, uncinate joints, and lateral foramen as potentially sensitized structures. Nociception from C2 to C3 may alter function in the sternocleidomastoid and trapezius muscles, contributing postural and timing abnormalities. In a recent study Ko and Son reported an unusual case of headache from a C3 nerve root radiculopathy. Pain distribution was chronic intermittent aching over the lesser occipital nerve distribution (temple), developing over 4 years. The source was lateral foraminal stenosis at C2 to C3, and was completely relieved by decompression surgery.[107]

While all innervated structures in the neck can refer pain, zygapophyseal joints are fairly common sources.[95] Traumatic damage to the capsule, including bleeding or bruising, has been found on postmortem examination. Fig. 37.7 illustrates composite results of hypertonic saline injections into z-joints, beginning at C2 to C3. It is interesting to note that the original study was conducted on healthy male volunteers with no histories of neck pain, resulting in pain patterns not affected by chronicity, sensitization, or maladaptation of response.[9]

Morphologic changes in cervical musculature have been registered in women with cervicogenic headache.[207] Cross-sectional area (CSA) changes and fatty infiltration have been demonstrated in past studies of traumatic and nontraumatic cervical spine dysfunction. In this cohort, reduced CSA of cervical extensors, specifically the rectus capitus posterior major and multifidus, and fatty infiltration of the rectus capitus posterior major and minor, and splenius capitus were identified using MRI. No changes were noted in anterior musculature. The involved muscles are most responsible for sustained head control and segmental stability.

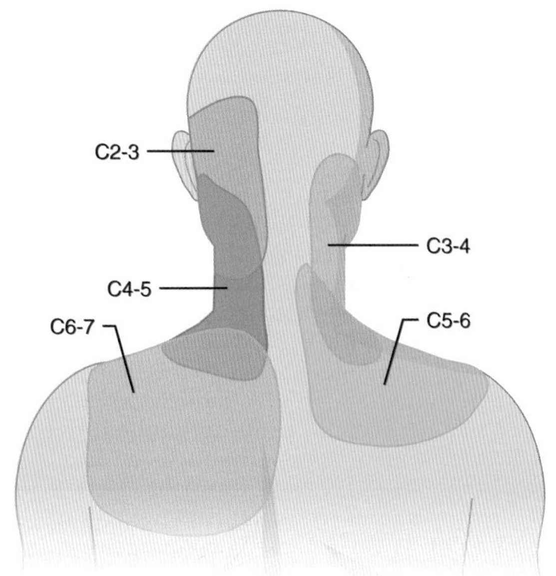


**Figure 37.7**

**Patterns of referred pain evoked from the cervical zygapophyseal joints and intervertebral discs.** (Based on Dwyer et al, Schellhas et al, and Grubb and Kelly. From Bogduk N, McGuirk B: *Management of acute and chronic neck pain: An evidence-based approach.* Pain Research and Clinical Management, Philadelphia, 2006, Elsevier.)

Trigger points are taut bands of localized contractions within muscles, or localized areas of hyperirritability in tissue that, when compressed, produce local tenderness and may refer in predictable patterns.[59] Trigger points are biochemically different from normal muscle, with higher concentrations of bradykinin, CGRP, substance P, TNF-α (tumor necrosis factor-alpha), IL-1β (interleukin 1-beta), serotonin, and NE (norepinephrine), as well as increased EMG activity in muscles with trigger points during rest and contraction.[56] The pain referral maps published by Janet Travel in 1986 are still used as reliable guides. Muscles of the subcranium refer pain similarly to high cervical joints, including periorbital, vertex, temporal, and occipital areas. The large superficial muscles of the neck are primary movers of the shoulder girdle (upper trapezius, sternocleidomastoid, and levator scapula) and can refer pain to the head and face. Their innervations are substantially contributed by upper cervical levels, and their cephalad attachments are the occiput, mastoid, and transverse processes of C1 to C4, respectively, giving them significant influence on head position, movement, and muscle tension in the subcranial area. Trigger points may be secondary to underlying causes, or may result from chronic muscular activity without sufficient relaxation to provide normal circulation.[56] Once established, trigger points may become self-perpetuating, furthering inefficient or abnormal muscular recruitment pattern and referring pain.

## MEDICAL MANAGEMENT

**CLINICAL MANIFESTATIONS.** Unilateral headache aggravated by neck posture and movement is the most consistent reported presentation of cervicogenic headache. Pain usually starts in the neck, though not always, spreading to the frontal-temporal area. It may be moderate to severe nonthrobbing, nonlancinating pain or pressure and is invariably unilateral. If bilateral pain is reported, there is likely some level of dysfunction on both sides of the neck. Usually pressure in the occipital region or onto a specific high cervical anatomic feature will reproduce or worsen the pain. Autonomic symptoms and signs, such as photophobia, phonophobia, nausea, vomiting, and ipsilateral periocular edema, are generally less frequent and less marked than in common migraine, but they can occur. Blurred vision resulting from oculomotor tension or fatigue that often accompanies suboccipital muscular dysfunction, and difficulty swallowing may be reported, associated with the upper cervical neural sharing with the hypoglossal nerve. Episodes last hours to weeks, and though constant may fluctuate in intensity. Diffuse shoulder and arm pain are included symptoms in the CHISG diagnostic guidelines.[192] If reproduction of symptoms is possible by provocative maneuvers that facilitate closure or narrowing of the neuroforamina, then nerve root involvement is of high probability. Such compression maneuvers also provoke the uncinate joints, which begin at C2 to C3, and are known to be enlarged by shear forces of injury, excess mobility, and aging. An altered neuromuscular strategy with inhibited deep neck flexors and excessive sternocleidomastoid contraction has been noted in neck pain cases. This dysfunctional movement pattern may also occur in the client with cervicogenic headache.[102]

**DIAGNOSIS.** It can be difficult to readily diagnose cervicogenic headache due to overlap in the symptoms with tension-type headache, migraine without aura, and hemicrania. ICHD criteria include demonstration of clinical signs that implicate a source of pain in the neck, reduced cervical range of motion, reproduction of pain with pressure or positioning, abolition of headache following diagnostic blockade of a cervical structure or its nerve supply, and pain that resolves within 3 months after successful treatment of the causative disorder or lesion (less than 5 on a 100-point visual analog scale).[85] The first requires careful assessment to identify the pain generator as accurately as possible to direct successful intervention. Anesthetic blockade is not obligatory and is not a cost-effective procedure in most cases. The last criterion (pain resolving within 3 months of treatment) can only be determined after successful intervention, making it of limited use for the initial diagnosis.

Obtaining an accurate history is the initial step in formulating a differential diagnosis, including neck or head trauma if there is a possible whiplash mechanism. However, a trauma history combined with headache does not immediately implicate the cervical spine (see section on posttraumatic headache). Perception of disability using the Neck Disability Index, HIT-6, and quality-of-life questionnaires (such as Short-Form Health Survey SP-36) helps elucidate the patient's global functional and psycho-emotional status, and while not clarifying specific diagnoses, serves as a valuable outcome measure of interventional success. The lack of complete response to indomethacin or sumatriptan may assist differential diagnosis away from primary headache. Medication overuse is common among individuals with all types of chronic headache, and MOH may also be coexistent.

Imaging identifies anatomic integrity, variants, pathology, and space-occupying lesions, but has no correlation to nociception, with the exception of evidence of instability. Movement abnormalities in flexion/extension, abnormal posture, fractures, congenital abnormalities, bone tumors, rheumatoid arthritis, or other distinct pathology (but not spondylosis or osteochondrosis, because these are conditions that are common incidental findings in asymptomatic individuals) may be identified. MRI studies of the head may include the craniovertebral junction in cross-sectional views, but unless specifically requested, cervical spine series routinely begin cross-sectional images at C2 to C3. Findings of disc abnormalities are common among asymptomatic adults and do not clearly identify a pain generator. However, disc disruption anywhere in the cervical spine has been linked to cervicogenic headache via immediate relief after surgical intervention.[26] It is not surprising that mid and lower cervical motion segments may contribute to cephalic pain when considering the multilevel innervation described above, and significant variation in radicular pain patterns.[136]

Recommendations for referral for medical consultation, referral for imaging, use of activity and participation measures, and impairment-based examination measures are outlined with evidence-based confidence levels in the 2017 Neck Pain Clinical Practice Guidelines Revision.[28] Box 37.2 presents current physical diagnostic procedures recommended for a physical therapy examination. Expected findings include positive cervical flexion-rotation test, headache reproduced with provocation of involved cervical segments, limited cervical range of motion, restricted segmental mobility, and deficits in strength, coordination, and endurance of cervical musculature.[28]

**TREATMENT.** Pharmacotherapeutic treatment may include analgesics or NSAIDs, tricyclic antidepressants, and muscle relaxants. Botulinum toxin or steroid mixed with anesthetic are used to inject specific dysfunctional muscles. Cervical epidural steroid injections may be indicated for multilevel disk or spine degeneration. Nerve blocks, trigger point injections, or radiofrequency thermal neurolysis may block the cascade of sensitization to central mechanisms. Surgical interventions, such as neurotomy, dorsal rhizotomy, and microvascular decompression of nerve roots to perform blocks or reduce pressure on a nerve, often also provide only temporary relief, with the possibility of later intensification of pain.

Strong evidence supports physical and manual therapies, including exercise for treatment of cervicogenic headache. Guidelines for treatment of neck pain with headache recommend guided and carefully graded exercise in the acute phase, including self-mobilization of the C1 to C2 segment and controlled nodding of the C0 to C1 articulation. Subacute interventions include mobilization and manipulation combined with specific exercise,

Box 37.2

**CLINICAL EXAMINATION AND MEASURES ASSOCIATED WITH CERVICOGENIC HEADACHE**

- Neck Pain and Disability Index (NDI)[45]
  - 0-4/50 = no disability
  - 5-14/50 = mild
  - 15-24/50 = moderate
  - 25-34/50 = severe
  - >34/50 = complete disability
- Alar and transverse ligament integrity testing[12,92]
- Vertebral artery dependency test: a negative test does not rule out caution
- Headache symptoms reproduced with mechanical pressure on myofascial trigger points, myotendinous insertions, or facet capsules.
- Headache symptoms reproduced with specific head/neck motions, within available range (denotes active inflammation) or at end range.
- Symptoms reproduced with Spurling test of lateral foraminal compression [22,215]
- Limited C1-2 range of motion using cervical flexion rotation test (significant limitation on ipsilateral side of headache)[81]
- Limited active range of motion[69]
- Limited passive cervical and thoracic range of motion[44,176]
- Manual muscle test of all cervical musculature, observing substitutions and cocontractions, as well as target muscle response[100,101]
- Craniocervical flexion test (CCFT) for assessment of deep cervical flexor strength and neuromotor pattern[64,103]
- Neck Flexor Muscle Endurance Test (NFMET) results have a negative or inverse association with cervical spine dysfunction and pain[83]
- Joint Position Error Test (JPE)[52]

(including self-mobilization of C1-2 rotation). Chronic care may include cervical manipulation for mobility but not pain control, cervico-thoracic manipulation, exercise for the cervical and scapulothoracic region, strengthening and endurance exercise with neuromuscular training, including motor control and biofeedback elements, and techniques that combine manual therapy with exercise.[28]

SPECIAL IMPLICATIONS FOR THE THERAPIST 37.3

*Cervicogenic Headaches*

Designing an effective treatment strategy is predicated on results of a careful and detailed evaluation using the elements specified above. As highlighted in previous sections, maintaining a biopsychosocial model yields the most satisfying results to patients. The most unique skill that physical therapists offer is movement analysis. Careful observation of posture and movement in normal and special activities can elucidate the mechanical stressors leading to identified impairments.

The rich presence of sensory receptors in subcranial tissues suggests the importance of sensory feedback for head/neck function. The interface between upper cervical and oculomotor systems for gaze stability, and among the upper cervical, vestibular, and visual systems for equilibrium and spatial orientation, may be disturbed by headache. Rehabilitation intervention for the upper cervical spine should therefore be based in a motor pattern and recruitment sequence approach.[205] Task-specific activities have the most reliable and lasting effects on recovering normal movement patterns.[91] Accurate sensation recognition and motor patterns are continuously influenced by use-related experience and progressive adaptation of motor behavior.[60] Intentionally incorporating vestibulo-colic, cervico-ocular, vestibulo-ocular reflexes, proprioception and kinesthesia, head righting, and postural responses in varying conditions supports recovery. Neural plasticity is continuous and relies on high repetition, sufficient intensity, variability, and feedback. Salience and attention are imperative to encourage adherence to self-management. Although inclusion of these components in treatment programs for cervicogenic headache has not been specifically addressed in the literature, the case can be made that neuromotor rehabilitation principles apply to the upper cervical spine.

## Posttraumatic Headache

### Overview

Headaches associated with known or suspected concussion or blast related injury are predominantly investigated through athlete and military populations, though can be associated with adverse events across the lifespan related to falls, recreational accidents, motor vehicle collisions, violence or abuse, and even childbirth related complications. Headache is the most common complaint following concussion. Historically onset of posttraumatic headaches (PTH), classified as secondary headaches in the ICHD, must occur within a 7-day timeframe after date of injury to establish a clinical diagnosis. In the ICHD-3 revisions, the appendix criteria acknowledge that delayed-onset persistent headache may develop as a result of mild to severe brain injury, with recognition of onset recognized outside of the first week post injury.[85] Acute PTH refers to identified headache symptoms lasting less than 3 months, while symptoms are considered persistent if duration exceeds 3 months. In many cases, especially related to competitive sports and active duty service members, repeated injuries and/or unrecognized lesser severe traumatic events may confound the diagnosis and timeframes for proper diagnostic classification. The risk of developing chronic posttraumatic headache is estimated at 57.8%, and is greater for mild head injury than for moderate or severe head injury.[143]

Hospital-based concussion clinics estimate the incidence of PTH following concussion and mild traumatic brain injury across all ages at approximately 70%.[16,86] The clinical presentations of PTH often mimic the primary headache types and appear to respond to management employed for primary headache patterns, though there is speculation that the 7-day timeframe for diagnosis may be too restrictive and initial diagnosis may be challenged by complex multisymptom overlay.[202] Studies repeatedly indicate that migraine and probable migraine represent the most frequent form of PTH, followed by TTH and

**Table 37.5** Clinical Presentation of Posttraumatic Headache Types

| Migraine Headache | Tension-Type Headache | Cervicogenic Headache |
|---|---|---|
| Unilateral/bilateral pain | Bilateral pain | Unilateral pain |
| Throbbing/pulsing pain | Pressure or band-like tightening pain | Starts in neck, often with a sense of locking or stiffness |
| Nausea/vomiting | No associated symptoms | Trigger points present |
| Photophobia/phonophobia | Lower pain intensity than migraine | Evidence of cervical dysfunction with manual examination |
| Worsened with physical activity | Lasts 30 minutes to several hours | Worsened with neck positions |
| Lasts 4-72 hours | | |
| Aura possible | | |

From Riechers RG, et al: Post-traumatic headaches. In Grafman J, Salazar AM: *Handbook of Clinical Neurology, vol. 128(36) Traumatic Brain Injury II*, Amsterdam, 2015, Elsevier; 2015, p 571. https://doi.org/10.1016/B978-0-444-63521-1.00036-4.

cervicogenic headache in both civilian and military populations.[121] The prevalence of headache can remain high over the first year.[88] A history of headache before a head injury occurs and female gender are risk factors for headache after TBI.[122] Preexisting episodic headaches, anxiety, depression, and a high number of other posttraumatic symptoms increase chance of headache.[116] While secondary headaches following injury to the head and neck correspond to primary headache classifications, hereditary, genetic, and pathophysiology findings specific to PTH demand further discussion and should be monitored for ongoing research developments.

### Pathogenesis

The pathophysiology associated with head trauma involves a neurometabolic cascade of events that can result in ion influx, glutamate release, hyperglycolysis, axonal degradation, impaired neurotransmission, and apoptosis.[75] Aspects of this process related to glutamate toxicity have been similarly described as related to cortical spreading depression associated with primary migraine. Individuals with a family history of migraine in a first-degree relative have been found to be 2.6 times more likely to develop posttraumatic migraine (PTM), a subcategory of PTH, within 2 weeks of injury compared to people without familial migraine.[197] Apolipoprotein (APOE) has been investigated for genetic contributions to PTH in athletes as the presence of the e4 allele may predispose one to development of PTH and promote headache severity by impeding neuronal regrowth and repair after injury.[138]

A transient dysautonomia has been described following mild traumatic brain injury, resulting in dysregulation of the autonomic nervous system, as well as endocrine and cardiovascular responses that may result in persistent autonomic dysregulation and systemic inflammatory processes.[63] A study comparing individuals with persistent PTH against individuals with migraine and healthy controls found that those with PTH had higher levels of dysautonomia measured with the Composite Autonomic Symptom Score 31 (COMPASS-31), which could have implications in headache management.[90] Persistent neuroinflammation may represent a maladaptive activation of glial cells causing release of proinflammatory substances involved in trigeminal sensitization that may develop into a chronic headache presentation.[134] The connection between the cervical nerves (C1 to C3) and the cervical portion of the trigeminal nucleus forming the trigeminocervical nucleus has been previously described in cervicogenic headache. Although there is no direct head trauma with some whiplash injuries, studies show that altered afferent signals from the cervical nerve roots, cervical spinal cord, and brainstem may contribute to headache.

### Clinical Manifestations

Posttraumatic headaches may present with similar clinical feature to primary tension-type, migraine, or cluster headache, or may be complex due to overlap of a multitude of symptoms. Table 37.5 describes the classic clinical presentations of posttraumatic headache. Depending on the injury severity there may be shear damage to the brain and musculoskeletal damage to the soft tissues in the neck, jaw, and scalp. Box 37.3 lists the typical complaints associated with posttraumatic headaches. When dizziness is triggered by physical exertion, the headache can worsen. Balance deficits may be a result of sensory organization deficits typically seen with sensory motor processing disorders and brain injury (see Chapter 33).

Visual dependency progressing to visual motion sensitivity, also common after vestibular disorders, may cause symptoms in environments with peripheral visual movement. In an effort to control the sensation of dizziness that comes with head movement or when there is excessive visual stimulation, the individual will cocontract the muscles of the neck to limit stimulation of the vestibular system, resulting in complaints of neck soreness and stiffness and increase in headache (addressed previously in "Cervicogenic Headaches"). Fig. 37.8 illustrates the areas of involvement and associated phenomenon. Psychological symptoms can be associated with this type of headache associated with the cycle of stress, anxiety, as well as related to the neurochemical changes occurring as a result of injury.

## MEDICAL MANAGEMENT

**DIAGNOSIS.** Diagnosis of PTH is complicated as there are many other physiologic and psychological symptoms associated with concussion and TBI, such as dizziness and nausea, imbalance, sleep disturbances, altered cognition, and mood changes.[189] A detailed history should include personal and family history of headache, mechanism of injury, and specific details related to the evolution of headache symptoms since the time of injury (location, quality, intensity, duration, and frequency of pain).[29]

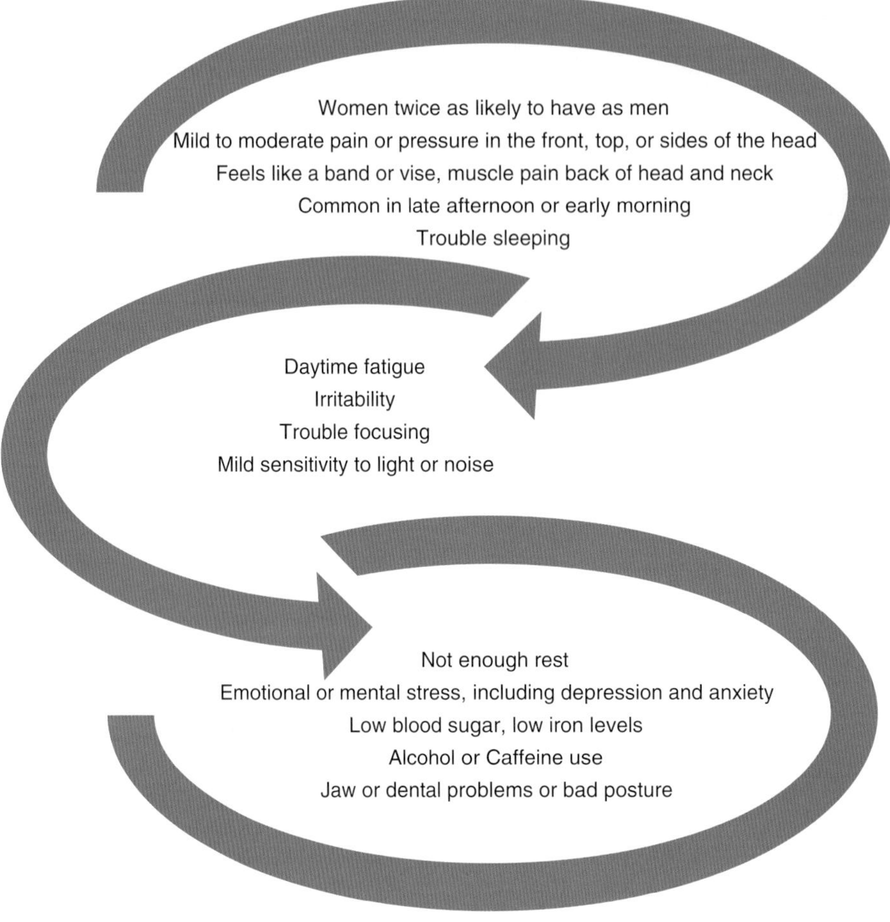


**Figure 37.8**

**Tension-type headache.**

Population specific tools available for the acute assessment of global symptoms when a concussion or brain injury is suspected include the Sport Concussion Assessment Tool, 5th Edition (SCAT 5) and the Military Acute Concussion Evaluation (MACE). More detailed questionnaires that are useful for qualifying and quantifying headache pain in the context of head and neck trauma include the Headache Disability Index, the MIDAS, the Neck Disability Index, and the Headache Impact Test (HIT-6).

Due to the complexity of pathophysiology associated with head and neck trauma, a full neurologic, vestibular, oculomotor, cervical, and somatosensory assessment must be conducted to ascertain the contributions of various systems to the expression of a secondary headache. The COMPASS 31 shows some utility in determining when autonomic dysfunction may be contributing to additional headache propagation and highlights the need for multidisciplinary care.[90] Emerging evidence demonstrates differing pathophysiology between persistent PTH and migraine on 3D-T1 weighted MRI; however, the development of diagnostic imaging and biomarkers specific to headache remain obscure.[181]

**TREATMENT.** Immediately following an acute injury to the head and neck individuals are advised to manage pain with acetaminophen instead of NSAIDs during the first 24 hours as a precaution against complications related to intracranial hemorrhage. Evidence to direct the pharmacologic management of PTH is poor. Many individuals self-medicate with NSAIDs or other agents and risk development of medication overuse headaches which further complicate the symptoms. Depending on the headache features, abortive and prophylaxis therapies targeting migraine and tension-type headaches most often include NSAIDs, triptans, combination drugs, antiemetic medications, tricyclic antidepressants, antihypertensives, and anti-seizure medications.[29,168]

Physical therapists have a primary role in the nonpharmacologic management of PTH, particularly in the diagnosis and management of comorbidities that may contribute to secondary headache, such as cervical, oculomotor, and vestibular contributions.[168] Cognitive behavioral therapy, biofeedback, massage, acupuncture, and other relaxation modalities may be relieving to some individuals. All providers must unite to provide patient education and create a multidisciplinary approach to monitoring headache patterns, determining response to all types of interventions. Physical therapists diagnose and manage a broad number of impairments related to head and neck injuries; headache must be regarded within the context of the injury sustained. See Chapter 33 on traumatic brain injury for further discussion of treatment related to mild traumatic brain injury.

Box 37.3

**TYPICAL COMPLAINTS ASSOCIATED WITH POSTTRAUMATIC HEADACHE SYNDROME**

***Head and Face Pain***

- Cervicogenic or tension-type headaches
- Cranial myofascial injury
- Secondary to neck injury (cervicogenic)
  - Myofascial injury
  - Intervertebral disks
  - Cervical spondylosis
  - C2-3 facet joint (third occipital headache)
- Temporomandibular joint injury
- Occipital neuralgia
- Migraine with and without aura
- Cluster
- Dysautonomic cephalalgia
- Supraorbital and infraorbital neuralgia
- Hemorrhagic cortical contusions
- Subdural or epidural hematomas
- Low cerebrospinal fluid pressure syndrome

***Brainstem Symptoms***

- Dizziness
- Vertigo
- Tinnitus
- Hearing loss
- Blurred vision
- Diplopia
- Convergence insufficiency
- Light and noise sensitivity
- Diminished taste and smell

***Psychological and Somatic Complaints***

- Irritability
- Anxiety
- Depression
- Personality change
- Posttraumatic stress disorder
- Fatigue
- Sleep disturbance
- Nausea/vomiting
- Decreased appetite

***Cognitive Impairment***

- Memory dysfunction
- Impaired concentration and attention
- Slowing of reaction time
- Slowing of information-processing speed

SPECIAL IMPLICATIONS FOR THE THERAPIST 37.4

### *Posttraumatic Headache Syndromes*

Individuals with posttraumatic complications are seen by physical therapists in many different settings. The differential diagnosis of symptoms related to posttraumatic headache can be complicated by vague complaints of pain and dizziness that are difficult to effectively localize or describe. With better understanding of the mechanisms of pain, and the autonomic and cognitive changes associated with these injuries, the therapist may be better able to address the specific issues.

Early detection of exertion intolerance can reveal ongoing central pathophysiology, perpetuating dysautonomia with new or increased headache and other symptoms.[141] Multidisciplinary care is warranted on an individualized basis to address a variety of impairments contributing to headache. In addition to multimodal physical therapy, this may include speech and cognitive therapy, occupational therapy, neuropsychiatry or psychology, neuro-optometry or ophthalmology, neuro-otology or ENT, neurology, and a variety of adjunctive therapies.

Headache is a common complaint reported to the therapist treating soft tissue dysfunction associated with trauma. Often there are complaints of excessive fatigue, eyestrain, inability to concentrate, depression, and dizziness in these same patients. The nature of headache(s) should be evaluated to help determine the appropriate intervention. Collaboration with medical providers can facilitate the selection of pharmacologic agents, and communication regarding response to medications can be instrumental in reducing recovery timeframes. Trigger-point treatment of the pericranial and cervical tissue has been used to help control the pain, which may be indicative of TTH post injury. As an understanding of the relationship of the pericranial structures and central modulation of pain emerges, combining treatment of soft tissue and use of CNS-mediating drugs may bring more relief from these disabling symptoms.

## 37.4 SPECIAL IMPLICATIONS FOR THE THERAPIST

### Medication Overuse Headaches

Medication overuse headaches (MOH) are secondary headaches that develop from excessive medication use, most often to manage chronic migraine. The updated ICHD-3 criteria for MOH require development of a new headache or significant worsening or a prior headache for greater than 15 days per month in response to regular use of one or more medications for greater than 3 months in an effort to control headache pain.[85] The pathophysiology of MOH is unknown, but current research points to genetic polymorphisms that may influence central sensitization and pain habituation, combined with direct overuse medication effects on neurotransmitters and neuronal hyperexcitability.[55]

Risk factors associated with MOH include individuals with chronic headache, musculoskeletal pain, or gastrointestinal disturbances. The increased likelihood in the female gender may correlate to the increased incidence of migraine headache in women. Lower education level, lower income, disorders of mood, and fear of pain behaviors show association with MOH and dependency patterns.[153] Patient education, guidance in the use of a headache diary, and increased frequency of follow-up may help prevent MOH though no definitive clinical practice guidelines exist. Treatment involves patient education, individualized withdrawal management, and subsequent headache reassessment. Medication prophylaxis, cognitive behavioral therapy, and mindfulness training may be implemented for improved underlying chronic headache management.[80]

## Headache Attributed to Arteritis

Individuals over the age of 50 experiencing new onset or alterations in headache patterns should be considered for risk of giant cell arteritis. Typically the headache is located over a branch of the superficial temporal artery and is described as a dull ache with scalp tenderness that persists throughout the day. Physical therapists should assess integrity of temporal pulses, inquire regarding presence of fever, and assess active ROM of the shoulders, neck, and hips to determine potential concurrent onset of polymyalgia rheumatica and refer to a medical provider.[159] Symptoms of vasculitis and vascular insufficiency are common, relating to extracranial carotid circulation. See Chapter 12 for the description and medical management.

Sedimentation rate should be measured in individuals older than age 60 years who have headache or facial pain, unless the pain obviously results from another cause.[99] Findings from a temporal artery biopsy can confirm the diagnosis. Unless otherwise contraindicated, corticosteroid therapy should be instituted, pending results of the biopsy, to avoid visual loss.

## Headache Attributed to Acute Rhinosinusitis (Formerly Sinus Headache)

Sinus headache is an outdated term no longer used in the medical literature. Headaches attributed to acute rhinosinusitis are very uncommon, but represent the most common misdiagnosis of migraine headache. Sinus abnormalities have been shown to be a normal finding on neuroimaging in children, and symptoms associated with autonomic nasal drainage or nasal congestion may reflect migraine activity in the absence of fever or abnormal discharge.[212] Acute rhinosinusitis (ARS), defined as symptomatic inflammation of the paranasal sinuses and nasal cavity lasting less than 4 weeks, can be viral or bacterial. Four or more acute episodes over one year without ongoing symptoms between constitute recurrent ARS, whereas chronic rhinosinusitis describes symptoms greater than 12 weeks in duration.[171] Clinical practice guidelines for the medical diagnosis of adult ARS require purulent nasal drainage along with complaint of facial pain, pressure, and fullness and/or nasal obstruction. Much of the controversy related to accuracy in the medical diagnosis surrounds the natural extended timeframe of acute symptoms (≥14 days) and the historical overuse of antibiotics leading to drug resistance. Headaches associated with ARS should develop in close temporal relationship to ARS, and headache symptoms should escalate and resolve in correlation with ARS symptoms.

## Headache Related to Increase or Decrease in Cerebral Spinal Fluid Pressure

Elevated cerebrospinal fluid pressure is most often associated with a neurologic process related to an intracranial tumor or hydrocephalus. Idiopathic intracranial hypertension (IIH) produces a rare daily headache caused by elevated cerebrospinal fluid (CSF) pressure of unknown etiology.[78] Papilledema is a cardinal feature with report of blind spots or visual field changes. Theories surrounding the cause of IIH include obesity-related increase in abdominal and thoracic pressure and altered blood volume, or altered production or absorption of CSF, resulting in elevated fluid pressure.

Low pressure CSF headaches are attributed to spontaneous CSF leaks most often related to trauma, particularly whiplash injury, and to a lesser extent postsurgically where the dura can be punctured.[78] Risk factors associated with CSF leaks include connective tissue disorder, such as Marfan syndrome and hypermobility spectrum disorders, including Ehlers-Danlos syndrome.[145,178] Spontaneous intracranial hypotension produces an orthostatic headache with bilateral occipital pain. Headaches can occur later in the day because lying in bed overnight can be restorative if a leak is very slow. Bending forward may elicit a rhinorrhea or nasal drip, and many individuals with CSF leak report tinnitus and altered hearing as if underwater, nausea, dizziness, and/or neck pain. Advanced imaging techniques allow improved localization of CSF leaks and improved options for repair.[177]

## Painful Neuralgias

### Overview

Trigeminal neuralgia is a disorder of the trigeminal (fifth cranial) nerve in which there are intense and brief paroxysms of electrical shock-like pain within the nerve distribution. The hallmark is no clinically evident neurologic deficit. The pain is always unilateral, and there is usually a refractory period after an episode in which the pain cannot be elicited. Trigeminal neuralgia is a rare disorder, approximately 10 cases per 100,000, affects more women than men, and is more common after the age of 50 years. Fig. 37.9 shows the trigeminal distribution pattern.

### Etiologic and Risk Factors

Classic trigeminal neuralgia is diagnosed in the presence of nerve root atrophy caused by compression or displacement of the nerve by neurovascular structures, as seen on MRI or during surgery.[85] Secondary trigeminal neuralgia is caused

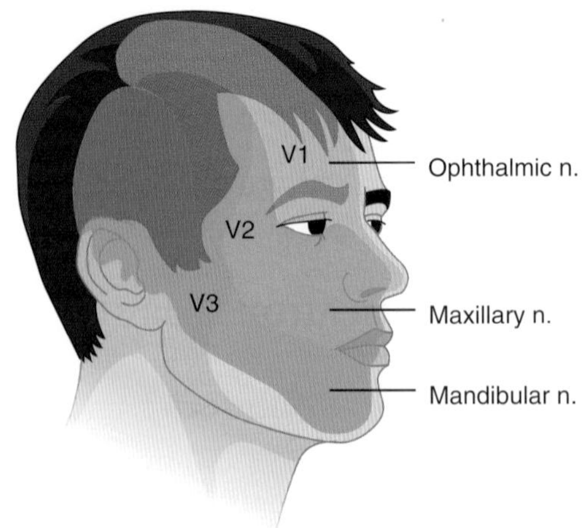


**Figure 37.9**

**Dermatomes for trigeminal nerve. *V1*, Ophthalmic nerve; *V2*, maxillary nerve; *V3*, mandibular nerve.** (From Waldman SD: Trigeminal nerve block: coronoid approach. In Waldman SD, ed: *Atlas of interventional pain management*, ed 3, Philadelphia, 2009, Saunders.)

by multiple sclerosis, vascular lesions, or tumors. When the cause is unknown it is described as idiopathic neuralgia; if related to trauma or an infection such as herpes zoster it is referred to as painful trigeminal neuralgia. It can be associated with an inflammatory process, typically occurring in women between the ages of 50 and 70 years.

### Pathogenesis

Results from experimental studies suggest that demyelinated axons are prone to ectopic impulses, which may transfer from light touch to pain fibers in proximity known as ephaptic conduction. Demyelination results from vascular compression of the nerve root by aberrant or tortuous vessels, usually the superior cerebellar artery. Demyelination has also been demonstrated in cases of trigeminal neuralgia associated with multiple sclerosis or tumors affecting the nerve root.

### Clinical Manifestations

The pain associated with trigeminal neuralgia has a sudden onset and has been described as sharp, knife-like, lancinating, and "like a lightning bolt inside the head that lasts for seconds to minutes." The sensation is typically restricted to the maxillary (V2) division of the nerve, but it may involve the maxillary and mandibular divisions together. Less likely is involvement of the ophthalmic (V1) division.

The painful sensation often occurs in clusters. Any mechanical stimulation, chewing, smiling, or even a breeze, can trigger an attack. Clients avoid stimulating the trigger zone. Remissions occur between attacks, but these remission periods shorten and attacks become more frequent over the course of the disorder. In a small number of the cases, the pain occurs bilaterally, but this typically is related to probable multiple sclerosis.

## MEDICAL MANAGEMENT

**DIAGNOSIS.** A careful neurologic examination of the head and neck is performed at initial contact. The ears, mouth, teeth, and temporomandibular joint should be examined for other problems that might cause facial pain. The finding of typical trigger zones verifies the diagnosis of trigeminal neuralgia. Sensory abnormalities in the trigeminal area, loss of corneal reflex, or evidence of any weakness in the facial muscles may indicate another cause of symptoms.[109]

MRI of the brain is used to look for multiple sclerosis, tumors, or other causes of secondary symptomatic trigeminal neuralgia and is typically performed early when the symptoms occur.[113]

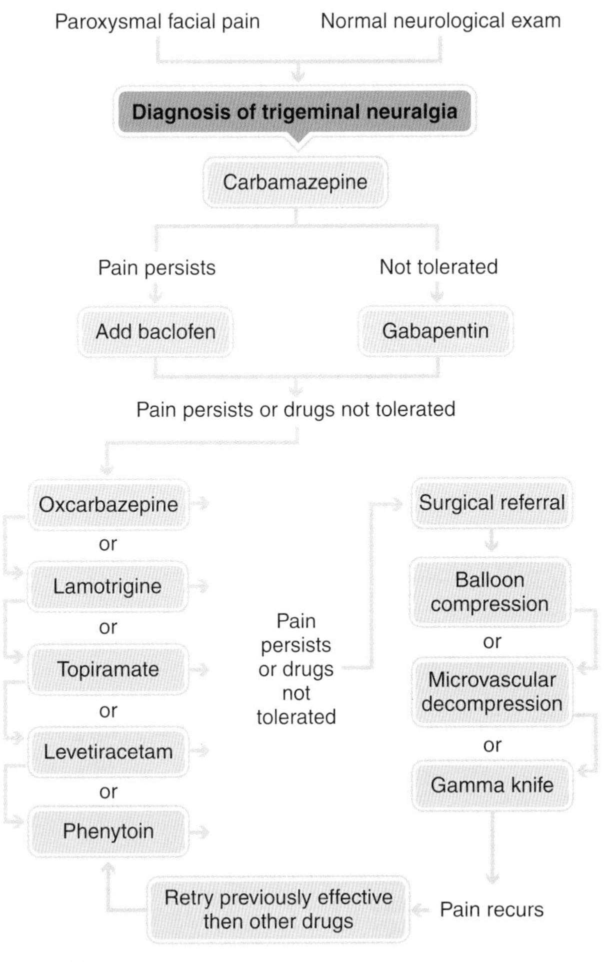


**Figure 37.10**

**Suggested scheme for treating trigeminal neuralgia.** The same pharmacologic strategy may be applied to the treatment of glossopharyngeal neuralgia. The order of choices differs for individual patients. (From Johnson RT, Griffin JW, McArthur JC: *Current therapy in neurologic disease*, ed 7, St Louis, 2008, Mosby.)

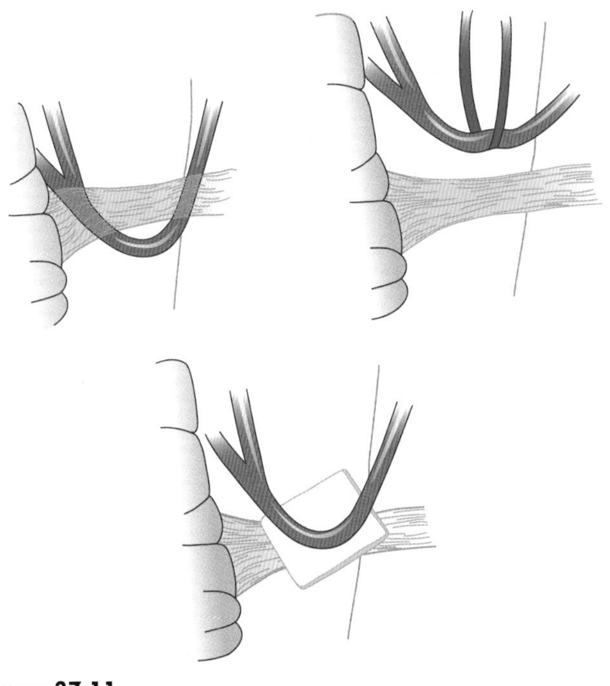

**Figure 37.11**

(Top left) Microscopic vascular decompression to alleviate trigeminal neuralgia represents a major neurosurgical advance. The aim is to place a barrier between the vessel and trigeminal nerve. As pictured through an operating microscope, the brainstem is on the left side of the field and the trigeminal nerve lies horizontally to the right. A large, aberrant artery compresses the nerve from below. (Top right) A surgical loop plucks the artery out from beneath the trigeminal nerve. (Bottom) The artery is then placed over a piece of muscle or artificial material that cushions the nerve. (From Kaufman DM, Milstein MJ: *Clinical neurology for psychiatrists*, ed 6, Philadelphia, 2006, Saunders.)

**TREATMENT.** The first line of treatment for trigeminal neuralgia is anticonvulsants; carbamazepine or Tegretol is usually tried first. Other medications are listed in Fig. 37.10. Pain can be controlled about 75% of the time with oral medications, but some older adults show less tolerance for these medications. A small number of randomized controlled trials demonstrate that subcutaneous botulinum neurotoxin type A is an effective and safe nonsurgical treatment option for TN.[142] Neurosurgical treatments include percutaneous procedures, stereotactic radiosurgery, and microvascular decompression.[184] Microvascular surgery is used when small blood vessels have been found to constrict the trigeminal nerve near its root. This procedure provides immediate pain relief; however, it is a major and difficult surgery. Minimal trigeminal nerve root trauma via nerve-combining technique demonstrated a beneficial impact.[124] Fig. 37.11 shows the mechanism to remove pressure from the nerve from the vascular loop. Management decisions are dependent on personal preference and clinical factors such as age and overall health.

**PROGNOSIS.** The efficacy of evaluating treatments is complicated by the fact that the disorder may remit spontaneously. Remissions that occur soon after onset may last for years. For those who do not remit, trigeminal neuralgia can be managed medically in most cases. The Trigeminal Neuralgia Association provides information and support for persons with this diagnosis. Ophthalmoplegic neuropathy results in pain around the eye and paralysis in the distribution of the third, fourth, or sixth cranial nerve and can produce diplopia, or double vision. One of the features of ophthalmoplegic migraine is that the headache always precedes the oculomotor deficit by several hours or days. The paralysis can progress from being transient to lasting several days, and in some persons it becomes permanent. People with ophthalmoplegic migraine typically give a history of many years' duration of migraine without oculomotor involvement before the ophthalmoplegia develops.[194]

## CHAPTER SUMMARY

Although the precise origin of head pain and the related pathophysiology is not always clearly understood, accurate diagnosis of headache disorders and an understanding of the individual's biopsychosocial context and resources are imperative to choosing the most efficacious intervention. It is often complicated by multiple types of headaches presenting comorbidly, and by recurrent headaches presenting with widely differing symptom phenotypes. Physical therapists are integral to the diagnostic process in many instances, and can provide effective treatments for several headache classifications.

### REFERENCES

To enhance this text and add value for the reader, all references are included in the enhanced ebook on Student Consult that accompanies this textbook. The reader can view the reference source and access it online whenever possible.

# CHAPTER 38

# Vestibular Disorders

KENDA S. FULLER • CHELSEA R. VAN ZYTVELD

## VESTIBULAR DISORDERS

### Overview

Most people are only familiar with the vestibular system when they experience momentary dizziness during activities such as riding carnival rides or standing at great heights. During these activities, the vestibular system is stimulated beyond normal. This sensation of dizziness is like the dizziness that occurs when the brain encounters sudden changes in input from the vestibular system due to pathology at the peripheral or central nervous system levels.

The role of the vestibular system is to maintain clear vision during head motion, to determine head position in space, and to determine the speed and direction of head movement. The brain interprets the force of gravity as well as the force of fluid movement through the peripheral vestibular system in order to generate appropriate postural reflexes.[71] The vestibular system is also critical for postural control because it uniquely identifies self-motion as different from motion in the environment.

Vestibular disorders, with the exception of aggressive forms of neoplasm, are not life-threatening but can cause significant disability, with a devastating sense of abnormal movement, visual instability, and loss of balance.[120] However, symptoms of dizziness and imbalance cannot always be assumed to be an actual loss of vestibular function as they may also reflect inadequate sensory integration appropriate for the environmental context. The vestibular system works as part of the sensory triad, in conjunction with vision and somatosensory inputs, for postural stability. Sensory information from all three systems is centrally integrated to determine appropriate postural strategies. Comorbid dysfunction can affect functional recovery from a vestibular condition, especially if it affects the visual or somatosensory inputs. Prior trauma, either physical or psychological, can also cause maladaptation, resulting in responses to intervention that are inconsistent with typical recovery patterns.

### Physiology of the Peripheral Vestibular System

At the most peripheral level, the end organ of the vestibular system is primarily a mechanical system designed to identify movement of the head. It consists of a fluid-filled membranous labyrinth, which is bordered laterally by the middle ear and medially by the petrous portion of the temporal bone. Figs. 38.1 and 38.2 show the anatomy of the vestibular system and the relationship of the vestibular system to the nearby structures of the brain and bony structures.

The semicircular canals of the membranous labyrinth are ring-shaped, fluid-filled structures oriented in three dimensions (Fig. 38.3). These canals provide sensory input about head velocity, or angular acceleration, through the movement of endolymphatic fluid or endolymph in the direction opposite of the head movement (Fig. 38.4). The movement of the endolymph deflects the ampulla and the stereocilia, or hair cells, within the ampulla, away from the direction of head movement (Fig. 38.5). The speed and direction of the deflection of the hair cells determine the rate of firing of the vestibular nerve. When the head is not moving, the tonic resting firing rate of the hair cells is symmetrical on both sides of the system at approximately 50 spikes per second. When the head is turned toward one side, the firing rate increases on the ipsilateral side and decreases on the contralateral side. The difference between the rate of firing of the left and right vestibular nerves is interpreted by the brain as the amount of angular acceleration of the head.[89]

Both ends of each fluid-filled semicircular duct open into the otolith, which contains the utricle and saccule. A portion of the floor of the utricle and saccule is thickened and contains hair cells covered with a gelatinous membrane known as the otolithic membrane. Calcium carbonate crystals, or otoconia, adhere to this membrane and sit above the hair cells (Fig. 38.6). The weight of the otoconia pulled by gravity produces a shear force on the hair cells, both when the head is still and when it moves. This shear force is transmitted to the vestibular nerve to provide information about linear acceleration (versus velocity), the tilt of the head, or the static position of the head with respect to gravity.

When the head is upright in the gravitational field, the saccule is oriented vertically and the utricle is oriented horizontally. Therefore, the saccule primarily detects linear acceleration in the saggital plane, such as when the head pitches forward, while the utricle detects acceleration in the horizontal plane, such as laterally tilting the head. When the head is upright and still, acceleration due to gravity, which is 9.8m/s$^2$, pulls the saccular otoconial mass straight toward the earth (Fig. 38.7 A). When the head is pitched forward or backward, shear force increases on the saccule and decreases on the utricle. Similarly, when the head is tilted laterally, shear force increases on the utricle (Fig. 38.7 B and C). The pull of the otoconia also creates a counter roll of the eyes in the opposite direction. This maintains focus of the eyes as the head tilts, a vestibular ocular reflex, that is is further described in the following section.

Disorders at the labyrinthine and otolithic level are directly related to the structures involved and are most often related to changes in endolymphatic fluid pressure, changes in the contents of the fluid, and inflammatory or infectious agents that affect the homeostasis of the system. Blows to the head or acceleration-related injuries can cause direct damage to the labyrinthine system. Ischemia in the surrounding vasculature can cause disrupted function. When there is disruption of the vestibular nerve on one side, causing loss of tonic firing, the resting symmetry that is perceived as the head being still is disrupted. The brain, as it compares input from both sides, interprets greater tonic firing on the intact side as a perception of the head rotating. This results in eye movement normally associated with rotation, nystagmus, and is described as spontaneous when it occurs when the head is still. This is the true phenomenon of vertigo, or the illusion of

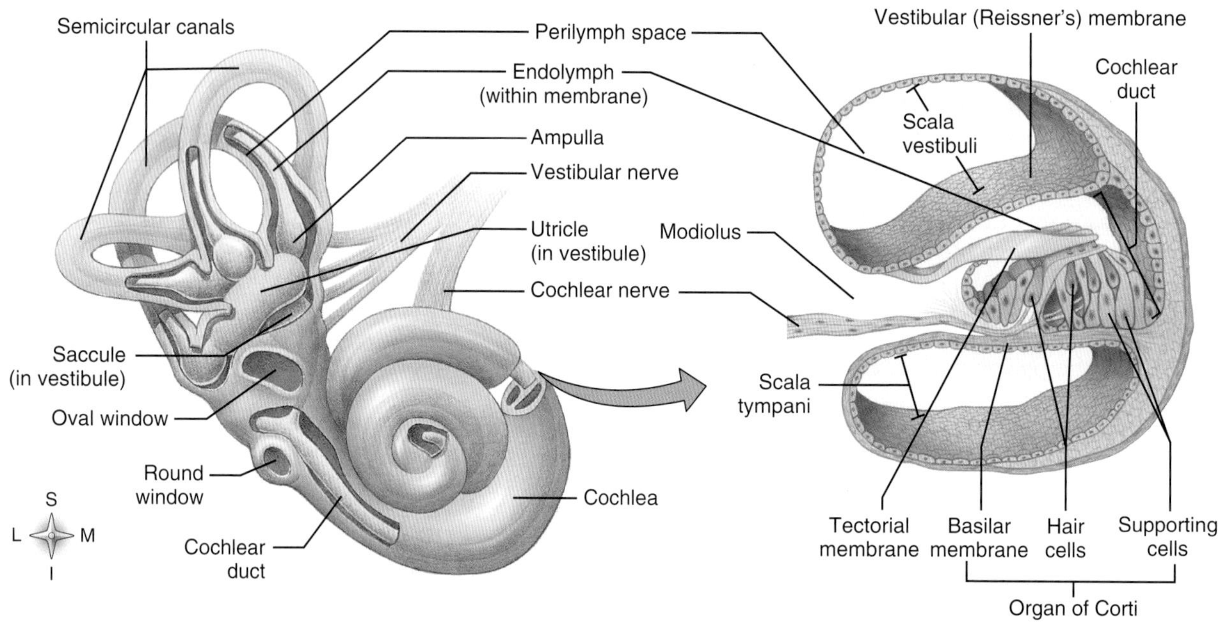


**Figure 38.1**

**Components of the vestibular system and cochlea, with distribution of neural connections.** (From Thibodeau GA: *Anatomy and physiology*, ed 8, St. Louis, 2013, Mosby.)

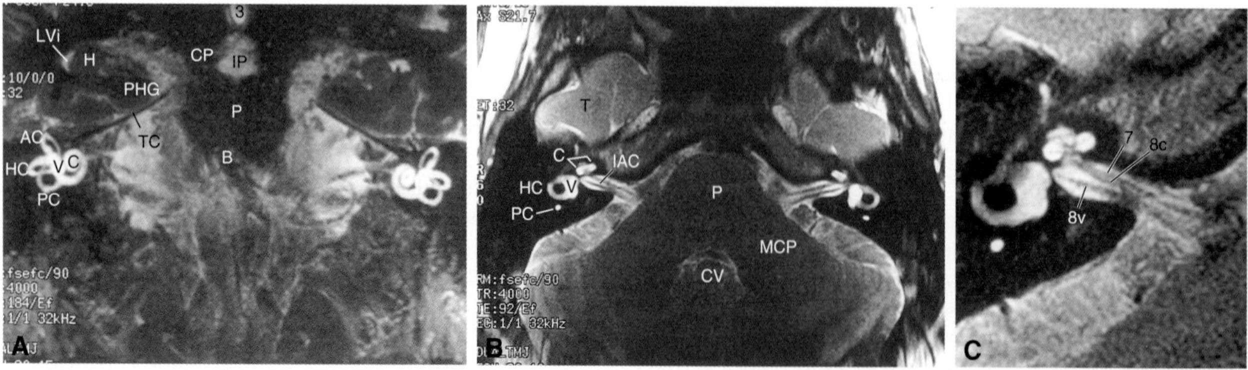


**Figure 38.2**

**MRIs of the labyrinth.** (A) Coronal view. (B) Axial view. (C) Enlarged view. *AC*, Anterior semicircular canal; *HC*, horizontal canal; *PC*, posterior semicircular canal; *C*, cochlea; *IAC*, internal auditory canal; *P*, pons; *8v*, eighth cranial nerve (vestibulocochlear nerve). (From Nolte J: *The human brain: An introduction to its functional anatomy*, ed 5, St. Louis, 2002, Mosby.)

turning or spinning. The individual will sense that the head is turning or the room is rotating.

The brain quickly identifies this sensation as an abnormal state and begins central nervous system (CNS) recalibration so that the vestibular system input from each side becomes calibrated to match the visual and somatosensory system input. Typically central adaptation adequate to stop the spontaneous nystagmus occurs in a lighted environment within 3 days. Spontaneous nystagmus may continue to be active in a dark room, and there may still be a sensation that the head is rotating when the eyes are closed for weeks after the onset.[12,23,42] When the otolith system is not working properly, there is loss of the ability to orient to gravity, and the person complains of bouncing or feels as if he or she were on a ship. This creates difficulty when encountering moving environments.[12,52]

### Central Processing of Vestibular Input

The vestibular nerve transmits afferent signals from the otoliths and labyrinths, extending through the internal auditory canal and entering the brainstem at the pontomedullary junction. The majority of the afferent fibers from the vestibular nerve terminate in the vestibular nuclear complex. This complex consists of four major nuclei (superior, medial, lateral, and descending) and is located primarily within the pons in the brainstem. All eight vestibular nuclei are connected to each other in a complex manner and process not only vestibular input, but also somatosensory, visual, tactile, and auditory information.[26,61] The vestibular nuclei serve as relays for the vestibular reflexes and the cerebellum. Therefore, the vestibular reflexes become uncalibrated and ineffective when the cerebellum is dysfunctional (see Chapter 28).

The cortex and other areas of the brain also receive projections from the vestibular nucleus. Connections between the vestibular nucleus and cortex provide information about spatial orientation and perceived verticality within the environmental context. The role of the vestibular cortical areas such as the parieto-insular vestibular cortex are the focus of research directed toward changing firing patterns within the brain to address a phenomenon called Mal de debarquement,[32] which is described later in this chapter. The thalamus also works as part of the sensory relay system. With connections between the vestibular cortex and reticular formation, the thalamus affects arousal and conscious awareness of the body to help determine self versus environmental movement. These connections to the autonomic nervous system, such as the locus coeruleus, amygdala, and parabrachial nucleus, are involved in the common symptoms of stress and panic, activation of the fight or flight sympathetic nervous system response, emotional memories, malaise, and nausea.[146] This can work in two ways, dizziness can cause additional symptoms of stress, and stress responses can create symptoms that can include dizziness.

The hippocampus is functionally linked to the vestibular system. Information from the vestibular nuclei[139] is transmitted to both the dorsal and ventral hippocampus. The hippocampus creates an inner map of our environment by using "place cells." These cells receive projections from entorhinal and thalamic areas to assist us in way finding, or spatial orientation. It also appears that place cells require input from the otoliths in order to develop and maintain stable function.[76] In peripheral vestibular loss, place cells become dysfunctional and lose their specificity for orientation in the environment,[139] and bilateral vestibular loss appears associated with atrophy of the hippocampus.[20]

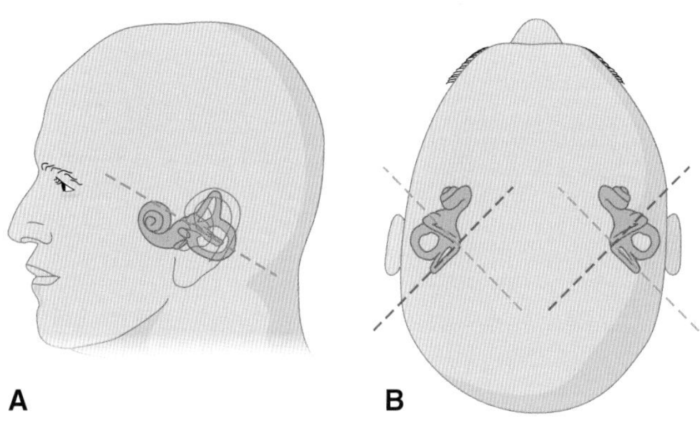


**Figure 38.3**

**Orientation of the labyrinth.** (A) Side view. (B) From the top. Labyrinth is enlarged relative to the head in this drawing for clarity. (From Nolte J: *The human brain: An introduction to its functional anatomy*, ed 5, St. Louis, 2002, Mosby.)

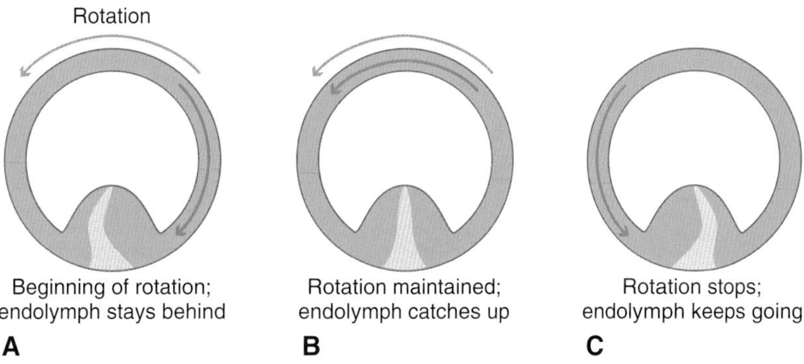


**Figure 38.4**

**Relative movement of semicircular canals.** (A) Beginning of rotation. (B) During rotation. (C) End of rotation. (From Nolte J: *The human brain: An introduction to its functional anatomy*, ed 5, St. Louis, 2002, Mosby.)

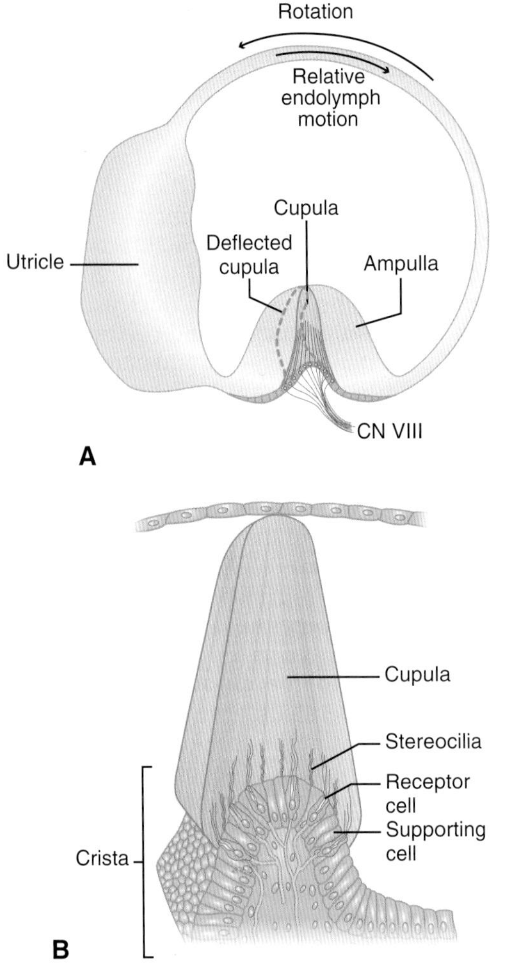


**Figure 38.5**

**Two views of the ampulla.** (A) View of the semicircular canal and movement of the endolymph and resulting deflection of the cupula within the ampulla relative to head motion. (B) Enlargement of the cupula showing its components. (From Nolte J: *The human brain: An introduction to its functional anatomy*, ed 5, St. Louis, 2002, Mosby.)

There is a further connection to the striatal component of the basal ganglia, which has an additional impact on both spatial orientation and cognition. This may be the reason that diseases affecting the basal ganglia, such as Parkinson disease, have components that may overlap. There appears to be a connection to vestibular dysfunction related to atrophy of the hippocampus and changes in the posterior parietal-temporal, medial temporal, and cingulate regions seen in persons with Alzheimer's Disease, mostly in the subset known to have spatial disorders that lead to wandering.[131]

### Vestibular Reflexes

The vestibular system drives eye movement through its connections in the vestibular nucleus through the oculomotor nuclei to the extraocular muscles. This connection is known as the vestibulo-ocular reflex (VOR). The extraocular muscles are arranged in pairs and connected to the vestibular system so that a pair of canals is connected to a pair of extraocular muscles. Through the complex connections of the vestibular and oculomotor nuclei, information regarding direction and speed of head movement is directed to the eye muscles so that they react and move in the opposite direction at the same speed as the head is moving, thus keeping the visual environment in focus during rapid head movement (Fig. 38.8). When one side of the system is damaged or stimulated abnormally, the intricate coupling of the vestibular system and eye movements becomes disturbed.[42,72] When there is imbalance in the firing rate between the two sides of the vestibular system, the brain perceives movement of the head, and the VOR mechanism causes subconscious eye movement or nystagmus in order to match the perception. As the eyes move, the person experiences the sensation of spinning and visually sees the room move.

For head rotations at frequencies below approximately 0.1 Hz, the vestibular nerve afferent firing rate gives a poor representation of head velocity. In response to a constant velocity rotation, the cupula initially deflects

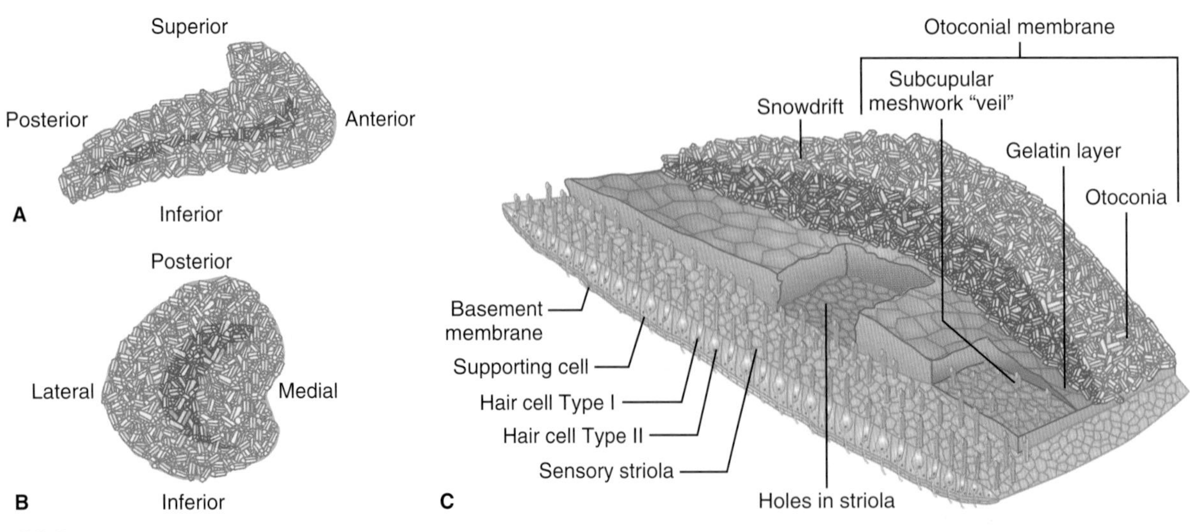


**Figure 38.6**

**Arrangement of otoliths in the two maculae.** (A) Saccule. (B) Utricle. (C) Composition of the saccular otoconial membrane in a section taken at the level shown in A. (From Paparella MM, Shumrick DA, eds: *Textbook of otolaryngology, vol 1*, Philadelphia, 1980, WB Saunders.)

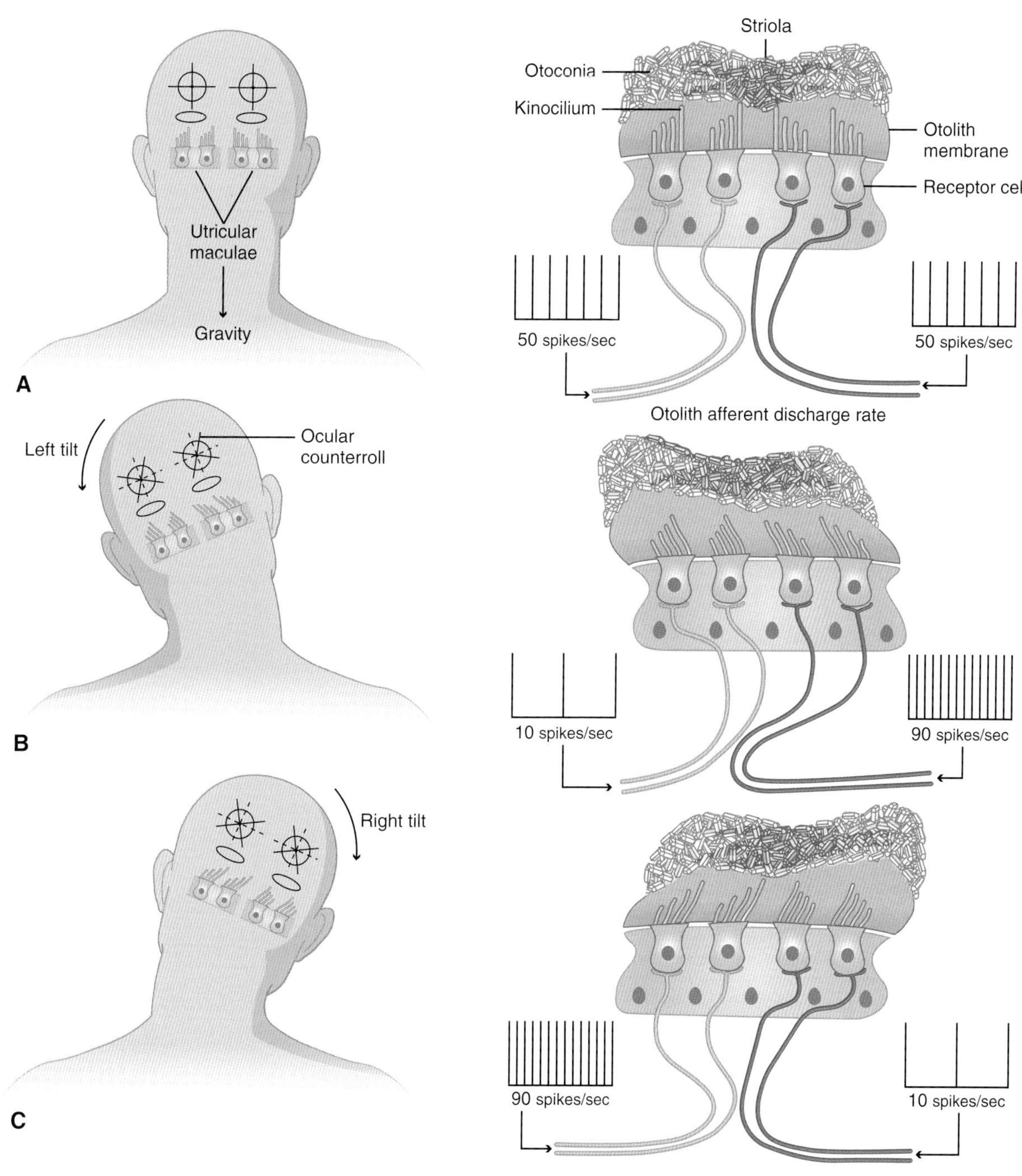


**Figure 38.7**

Patterns of excitation and inhibition for the left utricle and saccule when the head is tilted with the right ear 30 degrees down (A), upright (B), and tilted with the left ear 30 degrees down (C). The utricle is seen from above and the saccule from the left side. The background color represents baseline activity and black and white represent depolarization and hyperpolarization, respectively. (Modified from Haines DE: *Fundamental neuroscience for basic and clinical applications*, ed 3, Philadelphia, 2006, Churchill Livingstone.)

but then returns back to its resting position with a time constant of approximately 13 seconds. Neural circuits in the brainstem seem to maintain the canal signals, stretching them out in time. This effect is called *velocity storage* because it appears to "store" the head velocity information for a short time. It appears to allow the vestibular system to function better at lower frequencies, that is, down to 0.08 Hz. There is overlap between the VOR and lower-frequency gaze-stabilizing systems of smooth pursuit and optokinetic nystagmus to allow function at all frequencies.

Velocity storage creates the prolonged nystagmus that occurs after sustained constant-velocity rotation in one direction. Rotation to one side generates a positive change in afferent firing on the ipsilateral side and a negative change on the contralateral side. Because of the excitation-inhibition asymmetry inherent in the semicircular canal signals, the net result is not zero change

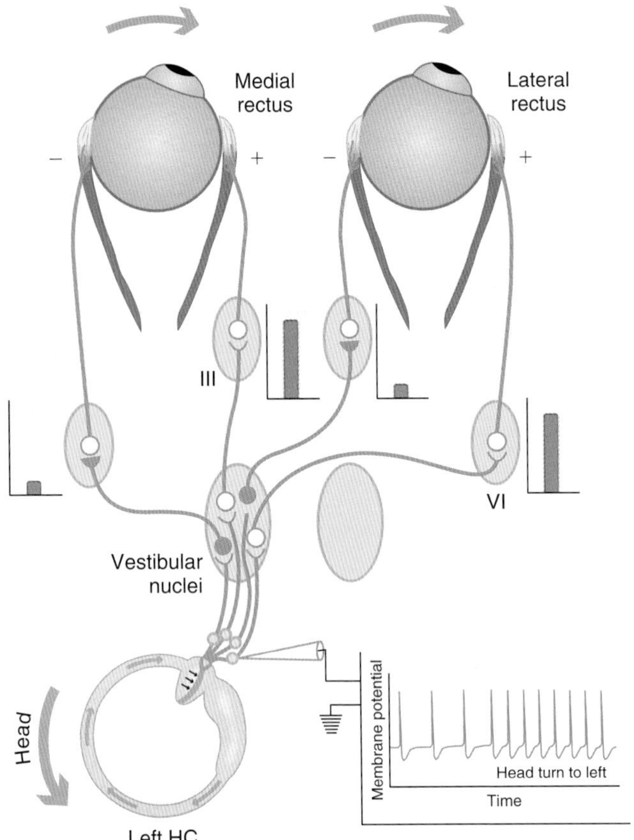


**Figure 38.8**

**Neural connections in the direct pathway for the vestibulo-ocular reflex (VOR) from excitation of the left horizontal canal (HC).** As seen from above, a leftward head rotation produces relative endolymph flow in the left HC that is clockwise and toward the utricle. The cupular deflection excites the hair cells in the left HC ampulla, and the firing rate in the afferents increases *(inset)*. Excitatory interneurons in the vestibular nuclei connect to motor neurons for the medial rectus muscle in the ipsilateral third nucleus (III) and lateral rectus muscle in the contralateral sixth nucleus (VI). Firing rates for these motor neurons increase *(mini bar graphs)*. The respective muscles contract and pull the eyes clockwise, opposite the head, during the slow phases of nystagmus. Inhibitory interneurons in the vestibular nuclei connect to motoneurons for the left lateral rectus and right medial rectus. Their firing rates decrease, and these antagonist muscles relax to facilitate the eye movement. (From Flint: Cummings otolaryngology: Head & neck surgery, ed 5, St. Louis, 2010, Mosby.)

in the afferent firing rate sensed by the brainstem, but rather a net excitation on the ipsilateral side. The excitation extends beyond the time that the cupula deflection has returned to resting state and causes the perception of rotation toward the same side. The perception and nystagmus decays with the time constant of approximately 20 seconds. The spatiotemporal properties of velocity storage, which are processed between the nodulus and uvula of the vestibulocerebellum and the vestibular nuclei, are likely to represent the source of the conflict responsible for producing motion sickness.[44]

The vestibular system is also responsible for motor output through the vestibulospinal reflexes (VSRs). The purpose of the VSR is to stabilize the body using the information provided by the vestibular system. Three pathways connect the vestibular nuclei to the anterior horn cells of the spinal cord. The lateral vestibulospinal tract, with its connection to the lateral vestibular nucleus, receives the majority of its input from the otoliths and the cerebellum. It is responsible for postural activity in the lower extremities in response to head position changes that occur with respect to gravity.[73] The medial vestibulospinal tract from the medial, superior, and descending vestibular nuclei gets its input from the semicircular canals and triggers postural responses with regard to angular head motion. The medial vestibulospinal tract descends only through the cervical spinal cord. The reticulospinal tract gets its input from all the vestibular nuclei in addition to other systems concerned with maintaining balance. These reflexes together provide automatic control of the activity of the postural muscles in the trunk and limb. Because these tracts are the output for the vestibular system, damage to any part of the system can result in abnormal postural responses to movement.[91]

## Blood Supply of Vestibular System

The vertebral-basilar artery supplies blood to the components of the vestibular system. The posterior and inferior cerebellar arteries feed this area of the CNS. Because there is redundant blood supply via the circle of Willis, ischemia in this area is rare. The anterior inferior cerebellar arteries supply the peripheral mechanism via the labyrinthine, common cochlear, and anterior vestibular arteries.[26] Disorders that affect the small vessels can cause direct damage to the peripheral vestibular system, or the ischemia can cause direct damage to the vestibular nuclei. Fig. 38.9 demonstrates the pathways associated with the end organ, vestibular nuclei, fibers of the cerebellum, and the extraocular muscles. This pathway involves inhibition in the process of modulating output to extraocular muscles.

## Incidence, Etiology, and Risk Factors

The vestibular system can be involved in many conditions, either directly or indirectly, and therefore, it is difficult to determine the incidence of disorders within the general population. Even the most common causes of vestibular lesions vary in incidence estimates.

Although dizziness is common in all age groups, the frequency of dizziness increases with age. Approximately 10% of people older than 45 years visit their physicians complaining of dizziness, with rates increasing further in those older than 75 years.[38] Aging has a significant direct effect on vestibular function. Hair cell loss occurs with aging, particularly in the ampulla. Demineralization and fragmentation of the otoconia, also increases with age, especially in those with osteoporosis and vitamin D deficiency.[9,165,168] Neuronal loss in the vestibular nuclei is also estimated to occur at a rate of approximately 3% per decade from the age of 40 years.[112]

However, while these changes happen during the normal aging process, dizziness reported to physicians is most likely caused by a pathologic process versus age-related structural changes. Similarly, less than 10% of falls in the elderly population are the result of an acute attack of vertigo or dizziness. Rather, most falls in the elderly population result from an accidental slip or trip, often

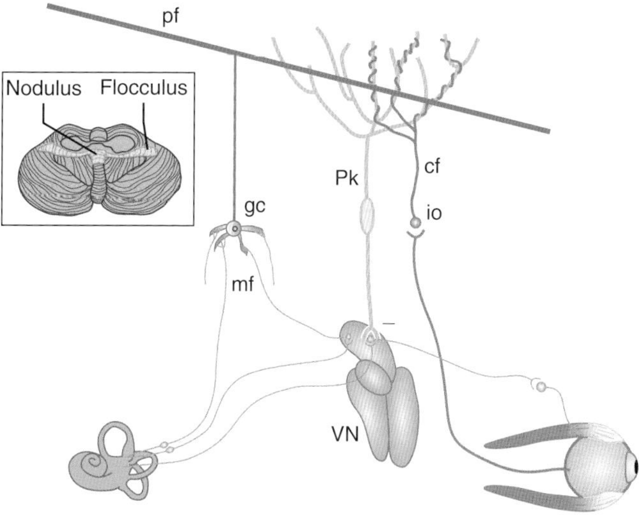


**Figure 38.9**

**Circuitry of the cerebellum involved in modifying the vestibulo-ocular reflex (VOR).** Inputs from primary vestibular afferents and secondary vestibular neurons (VN) form mossy fiber (mf) inputs to cerebellar granule cells (gc). Parallel fibers (pf) originating from these synapse weakly with Purkinje cells (Pk), causing a highly tonic inhibitory output of simple spikes from the Purkinje cells onto secondary vestibular neurons controlling the VOR. Climbing fiber (cf) input from the inferior olive (io) carries sensorimotor error information such as retinal slip. Climbing fibers make extensive and strong synapses onto Purkinje cells. Climbing fiber activity leads to complex spikes in the Purkinje cells, which can alter the efficacy of the parallel fibers' synapses onto the Purkinje cells—a form of learning. (From Flint: Cummings otolaryngology: Head & neck surgery, ed 5, St. Louis, 2010 Mosby.)

related to an unsteady gait. It appears that over time there is selective nonuse of vestibular cues during balance activities. Age-related increases in sway have been found for conditions that involved sway referencing of visual or somatosensory cues. Dizziness is reported more frequently by women than by men.[51]

Vestibular dysfunction can affect the system at any level. Disorders of the labyrinth can affect the sensory end organs, resulting in abnormal input into other levels of the vestibular system. Damage to the peripheral vestibular nerve can be from a neurologic pathology, mechanical deformation from a nonneurologic pathologic condition, or trauma to the structures surrounding the nerve. A central deficit can be the result of damage to the areas in the brainstem or cortex that process vestibular information. Pathologic processes in the brainstem can be direct, as in mechanical damage of the neurons in brain injury, bleeding disorders, and neoplasia. Hypoxic damage from a stroke or other conditions can cause decreased perfusion of oxygen into the brainstem. Degenerative diseases, such as multiple sclerosis (MS), Parkinson disease, and Alzheimer disease, can cause abnormal function in the brainstem and its connections.

## Medical Management

### Diagnosis

*History and Symptoms.* When there is disruption of information from the vestibular, visual, and/or somatosensory systems, dizziness is the most common symptom reported. Dizziness is a broad term that can describe various sensations. Therefore, the clinician should elicit additional descriptions of the client's dizziness to help determine the nature of the disorder and lead toward diagnosis. Often the client's history is complex, and much insight is gained by listening carefully and allowing the client to provide his or her own thoughts on the probable cause. The client's symptoms can reflect an abnormality in the vestibular system or may indicate some other general medical cause.

Often, the client describes a sensation of motion when the head is stable while sitting unsupported, giving initial cues about the vestibular system function and degree of adaptation. Because the visual system is required for adaptation following vestibular dysfunction, the brain will initially use the visual system as a substitute to determine movement of the head. The visual system can effectively determine head position in a visually stable environment. However, when the CNS fails to appropriately adapt and integrate vestibular inputs, this visual dependence can become chronic. Visual dependence results in a sense that the head is moving when vision is occluded or when the visual environment is not stable. A sensation of rotation may represent lack of adaptation to changed vestibular input on one side versus the other, reflecting a unilateral disorder. The client may also describe a sensation of floating, swimming, or tilt when seated with eyes closed. These sensations may represent abnormal otolith response, with the inability to determine head position relative to gravity. When the client describes feeling lightheaded, as opposed to sensation of rotation or tilt, the clinician should assess the accuracy of somatosensory input and consider several conditions. When the complaint of lightheadedness is accompanied by a lack of feeling grounded, the integration between the vestibular and somatosensory system may be disrupted, with impairment of the somatosensory reference mechanism likely being the cause. Presyncope can create a sensation of lightheadedness due to limited cerebral blood flow and may be related to orthostatic hypotension. Anxiety or panic can trigger sensation of lightheadedness, but usually, people also experience other sensations, such as paresthesia or shortness of breath. When the client's report of lightheadedness is accompanied by buzzing, disorientation, and fear or panic, maladaptation of all three systems (vestibular, visual, and somatosensory) is suspected.

Nausea is a frequent complaint associated with dizziness and reflects the stimulation of the medullary centers by abnormal sensory input. Direct damage to the medulla causes the most severe nausea, as in stroke or traumatic brain injury. Additionally, differences in white matter microstructure within tracts that connect visual motion and nausea-processing brain areas may contribute to nausea susceptibility.[116] Sudden-onset conditions often create a high level of nausea that decreases as the system recalibrates. Canal stimulation, especially during repositioning maneuvers for benign positional vertigo, can cause nausea. Horizontal canal stimulation typically provokes higher levels of nausea than the posterior or anterior canal.

Disorientation is often described as feeling out of sync with the environment and is usually associated with other deficits, such as short-term memory loss, lack of concentration, and irritability, reflecting the intricate integration with the limbic, hippocampal, and reticular systems throughout the brainstem.[19] Disequilibrium is reported as feeling unsteady or clumsy or as if one were swaying. History of falls is often associated. Fear of falling reduces balance safety and increases risk of falling during complex tasks.[47,169] Abnormal patterns such as wide-based gait, excessive use of touch, and lack of weight shift are seen in these clients.

The side effects associated with use of some medications, as well as other medical conditions, such as anemia, hypoperfusion of the brain from postural hypotension, cardiac arrhythmia, endocrine disorders, hypoglycemia, cranial and spinal cerebrospinal fluid leaks, and dysautonomia, may mimic symptoms of a vestibular disorder. If the cause of a client's dizziness is a medical condition or the use of medications, the symptoms should decrease when the appropriate condition is treated or when the medication is stopped.

***Examination.*** The visual-ocular system is examined when looking for a disorder of the vestibular system and, when abnormal, can provide clues about where the damage is located. If the motor component of the VOR is damaged, both visual and vestibular controlled eye movements are abnormal. If the sensory component of the vestibular system is damaged, visually controlled eye movements are usually normal, but vestibular-dependent eye movements are abnormal and can cause nystagmus. Nystagmus is involuntary, rhythmic oscillation of the eye, and when pathologic, can be spontaneous, gaze evoked, or positional (Box 38.1). Nystagmus may be caused by other brain dysfunction, as well as vestibular dysfunction. Therefore, pathologic nystagmus must be carefully observed, with consideration of the effects of fixation, eye position in the orbit, and head position.[82] Nystagmus related to vestibular disorders usually has a particular direction, intensity, and shape. Measurement of the interaction of the visual and vestibular systems can be accomplished by a variety of tests, with each test providing information that can be compared with the results of other tests to help determine the diagnosis.

**Medical Testing**

***Nystagmography.*** Video nystagmography (VNG) captures nystagmus and eye movements related to vestibular dysfunction, using video goggles by recording eye movements during various test conditions. During these tests, the angular velocity, amplitude, and frequency of nystagmus are quantified while the direction of the nystagmus reflects possible origin. Purely vertical or torsional spontaneous nystagmus suggests a central origin; however, nystagmus caused by a central nervous system lesion can be in any direction (vertical, oblique, horizontal, rotational). Central nystagmus may change direction as gaze direction changes and is not suppressed by fixation of gaze.[102] Nystagmus caused by acute unilateral loss of vestibular function is spontaneous, with a horizontal and torsional pattern, with the slow-phase of the nystagmus beating toward the affected ear. This nystagmus can be suppressed with visual fixation.[79,104] Nystagmus related to benign paroxysmal positional vertigo (BPPV) will be positional, fatiguing, and have specific direction and pattern, depending on the involved canal (see more in Special Implications for Therapist).

Oculomotor testing is included in the VNG to determine the status of saccades and smooth pursuits, as well as eye speed and optokinetic responses (Fig. 38.10 A). Table 38.1 describes different functions of eye movements. *Saccadic eye movement,* the ability to move the eyes quickly from one target to another intended target, is induced by presenting intermittent dots or lights as

**Box 38.1**

**THREE TYPES OF PHYSIOLOGIC NYSTAGMUS**

- Vestibular induced, or spontaneous
- Visually induced, or optokinetic
- Cerebellar, or end-gaze induced

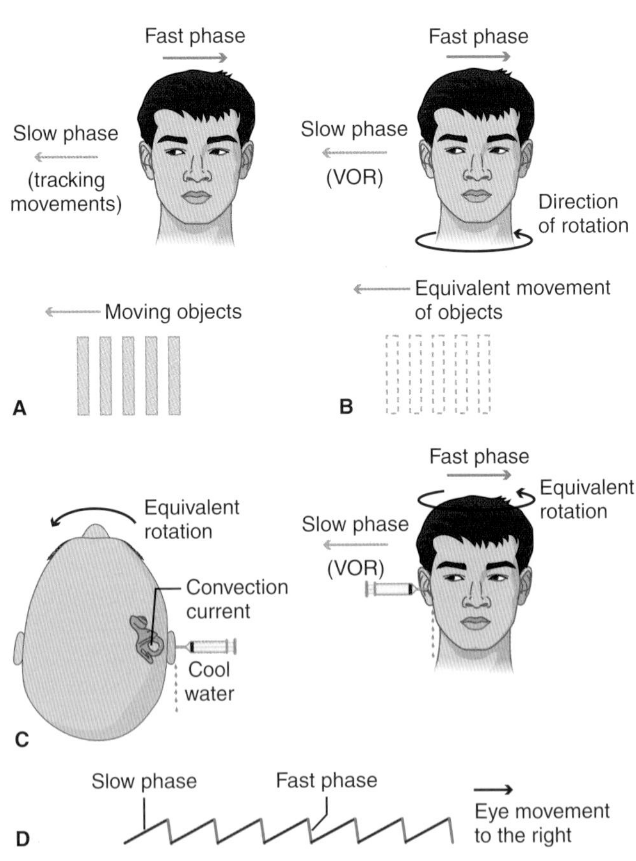


**Figure 38.10**

**Three different ways to cause nystagmus.** (A) Movement of a series of objects to the individual's right causes slow tracking eye movements to the right, followed by rapid movements to the left. (B) Rotation to the left is equivalent to the movement of objects to the right as perceived by the retina. (C) Cool water or air placed near the horizontal canal via the external ear canal causes the same movement of the endolymph as head rotation in B. (D) Electrical recording of horizontal nystagmus with its fast phase to the left. (From Nolte J: The human brain: An introduction to its functional anatomy, ed 5, St. Louis, 2002, Mosby.)

**Table 38.1** Different Functions of Eye Movements

| Class of Eye Movement | Main Function |
|---|---|
| Vestibular | Holds images steady on the retina during brief head rotations |
| Visual fixation | Holds the image of a stationary object on the fovea |
| Optokinetic | Holds images steady on the retina during sustained head rotation |
| Smooth pursuit | Holds the image of a small moving target on the fovea or holds the image of a small near target on the retina during linear self-motion; with optokinetic responses, aids gaze stabilization during sustained head rotation |
| Nystagmus quick phases | Reset the eyes during prolonged rotation and direct gaze toward an oncoming visual scene |
| Saccades | Bring objects of interest onto the fovea |
| Vergence | Moves the eyes in opposite directions so that images are placed or held simultaneously on both foveas |

targets at different amplitudes. If a target is missed on the first movement, there is a catch-up saccade used to move the eye directly to the target. Catch-up saccades are normal in some cases, such as when the targets are far enough apart that the eyes have to move greater than 20 degrees from one target to the other. At these distances, there will be consistent undershooting, and catch-up saccades will be performed to move the additional distance to the target. Slow saccadic eye movements can be related to lesions in the central pathways that control their movement. This may be an abnormal motor response of the VOR, or it can be a part of many other degenerative or static lesions that can affect the same part of the system, such as MS or parkinsonian disorders.

*Smooth pursuits*, or the ability to follow a target through a trajectory, are observed by recording the eye movement as the client attempts to follow targets at varying velocities. Use of a pendulum or computer-generated movement of lighted targets allows a sinusoidal tracking that can be measured by electro-oculographic recording. Two measures are usually applied to the recordings. Pursuit gain compares the velocity of the eye to the velocity of the target. Pursuit phase lag refers to the difference in time between waveforms of the target and the responsive eye movement. A person with normal tracking will predict the target motion and make the precise eye movements necessary to stay on target.[170] Normal smooth pursuits reflect an intact visual-ocular system and vestibulo-ocular output. An acute vestibular lesion will cause an impairment of smooth pursuit, but accuracy should eventually return. CNS conditions, such as cerebellar lesions, can also cause abnormalities of the smooth pursuit system.

*Optokinetic nystagmus* is the eye movement elicited by tracking a visual field instead of a target in order to stabilize visually an entire moving visual field. Optokinetic nystagmus is recorded by VNG when a striped drum surrounding the client is moved at a constant velocity at a slow speed of 30 degrees and a fast speed of 60 degrees. Abnormalities of slow components of optokinetic nystagmus parallel those of smooth pursuits and are related to disorders of the cortex, brainstem, diencephalon, or cerebellum.

Finally, VNG testing is used to measure eye movements caused by activation of the VOR and records spontaneous eye movements caused by alteration of the vestibular discharge rate (Fig. 38.10 B). The limitations of smooth pursuit and optokinetic nystagmus illustrate the important concept that reflexive sensorimotor systems have optimal operating ranges. Smooth visual pursuit functions are best for low-frequency slow head movements. The VOR is essential for gaze stabilization during higher-frequency, velocity, and acceleration head movements.[126]

The elderly show reduced VOR speeds, abnormal smooth pursuits and increases in saccade latencies. Such age-related alterations might interfere with appropriate responses to fast head movements. Initially, reduction of the inhibitory system mediated through the cerebellum can compensate for decreased sensitivity. Over time, the combination of reduced peripheral sensitivity and central inhibition decreases the range in which the system responds.[112]

***Bithermal Caloric Test.*** Manipulation of endolymphatic flow in the semicircular canals by creating a temperature gradient is known as *bithermal caloric stimulation*. When warm air is infused in the external auditory meatus, the skin of the horizontal canal is heated, resulting in a temperature change that is transmitted into the horizontal semicircular canal. The endolymph closest to the canal wall is heated, causing it to become relatively less dense than the surrounding endolymph. The fluid movement that results from the heating of the endolymph deflects the hair cells in the ampulla, simulating head movement (Fig. 38.10 C). The result is a nystagmus, with the fast component moving toward the canal that was stimulated. Cold air or water has created movement in the opposite direction. The mnemonic COWS (cold opposite, warm same) describes the movement of nystagmus related to the temperature of the stimulus used. The caloric examination allows the clinician to evaluate each horizontal semicircular canal separately.[87] VNG recordings during this stimulation can indicate abnormalities in different locations of the vestibular system and brain. Paresis can indicate damage anywhere from the end organ to the entry of the nerve root in the brainstem. A central disorder that affects the nerve root, such as MS or brainstem strokes, can cause paresis recording on caloric testing. Lesions of the cerebellum evoke heightened caloric responses and a suppression fixation deficit. Abnormalities in the characteristics of the nystagmus, such as vertical or oblique responses, are associated with CNS disorders.[102]

***Rotational Chair Testing.*** During rotational chair testing, horizontal semicircular canal function is assessed by controlling the angular acceleration of a motorized rotational chair and measuring the response of the horizontal canal. Persons who suddenly lose vestibular function on one side have asymmetric responses to rotational stimuli. Rotational stimuli are ideally suited for testing persons with bilateral peripheral vestibular lesions because both labyrinths are stimulated at the same time and the degree of function is accurately quantified. As with lesions of the peripheral vestibular structures, lesions of the central VOR patterns can lead to changes in the gain of rotational-induced nystagmus. Rotary chair testing may consist of either steps of constant-velocity rotation or sinusoidal harmonic oscillations, typically from 0.01 to 0.6 Hz. Velocity steps may be delivered by suddenly starting the rotation of the chair from zero velocity to a sustained constant velocity in one direction. The same stimulus may be obtained by braking the chair after a prolonged constant velocity rotation in the other direction. The horizontal canals' endolymph and cupula keep moving in the direction that the chair had been moving, so that the stimulus is equivalent to a velocity step in the direction opposite to that in which the chair had been turning.

Cerebellar dysfunction will result in abnormal amplitudes and arrhythmia on rotational chair testing. Cerebellar ataxia with bilateral vestibulopathy causes a high prevalence of subnormal function of both central and peripheral vestibular function. This is an easily missed clinical entity that is often associated with normal caloric investigations.[129] Dysfunction of the neural integrator and velocity storage can also be seen in the results of rotary chair testing.

***Electrocochleography.*** Electrocochleography is used to record elevation of endolymphatic fluid pressure. It is the recording of acoustically evoked electrical potentials arising from the cochlea and the eighth cranial nerve. An electrode is placed on the tympanic membrane or on the wall of the external ear canal near the tympanic membrane.[64]

***Subjective Visual Vertical.*** *Subjective visual vertical* (SVV) is the ability to recognize vertical or horizontal in a darkened room using the utricle to reference to gravity. During the acute phase of unilateral vestibular lesion, a nonparalytic ocular misalignment or skew can occur due to utricle-ocular pathway asymmetry.[22] SVV is tested in a darkened room to prevent visual referencing. The client is asked to orient a light bar to either a horizontal or vertical position. The degree of off-axis tilt of the light bar represents the torsion of the eye. The offset from the true horizontal or vertical is often up to 15 degrees during an acute phase of unilateral vestibular lesion. With a compensated lesion, accuracy typically improves to 4 degrees but often does not return to normal. Subjective visual testing will not detect bilateral utricular lesions.[71,163] The "bucket test," a clinical simulation of formal SVV testing, may identify spatial orientation deficits in clients with known vestibular disorders, but it is not useful for the diagnosis of vestibular impairment.[37] A variation of the bucket test uses a smartphone to determine the degree of off-axis tilt.[54,132] A nonparalytic ocular skew should not be confused with a paralytic skew as the result of a nerve palsy, intranuclear ophthalmoplegia (disruption of the medial longitudinal fasciculus), or a medullary lesion. A paralytic skew versus a nonparalytic skew can be determined using a Maddox rod or the cover-uncover and alternate cover tests that are typically addressed as part of ocular function testing

***Vestibular-Evoked Myogenic Potentials.*** The vestibular-evoked myogenic potential (VEMP) test applies the principle that the saccule is sensitive to sound and responds in a similar way to clicking sounds as it does to tilt of the head.[5] Click-sensitive neurons in the vestibular nerve are the same neurons that respond to tilt of the head. During the VEMP test, a click produced in the ear stimulates the saccule. Surface electromyography (EMG) is used to measure inhibition of the sternocleidomastoid (SCM) muscle on the same side during recorded sounds. It is thought that this inhibition developed to reflexively turn the head toward sounds, an action critical for the survival of early humans. During a VEMP test, the response of one ear is compared to the response of the other ear in the same person. VEMPs are abnormal when one side is more than 2 times smaller than the other side, is low in amplitude, or absent. An abnormal VEMP can represent ipsilateral lesion in the saccule, inferior vestibular nerve, lateral vestibular nucleus, or the medial vestibulospinal tract.[3,43,124]

***Computerized Dynamic Posturography.*** Computerized dynamic posturography (CDP) uses force plates to test the vestibulospinal reflex, vision, and somatosensory influences on posture and equilibrium by measuring the center of pressure under different conditions. The CDP test is comprised of both a motor control and a sensory organization portion. In the *motor control test,* the individual stands on a support surface that is suddenly displaced forward and backward. The force plates provide information about the individual's automatic postural reactions and the distribution of weight through the feet, while surface EMG recordings on the medial gastrocnemius and tibialis anterior muscles reflect the activation of the segmental (gastrocnemius to spinal cord), spinal (gastrocnemius to multiple spinal levels and cerebellum), and long-loop (gastrocnemius to cortex to tibialis anterior) response pathways. Special attention is given to the latency of movement to stabilize the center of pressure. Prolonged latencies are evidence for abnormality in any one or a combination of components making up the long-loop automatic system, and therefore, are strong indications for nonvestibular, spinal cord, brainstem, and subcortical involvement.[28,118,119]

The *sensory organization test,* the second component of the CDP, creates six different sensory conditions in which an individual's postural sway is measured (Fig. 38.11). These six conditions vary the amount and accuracy of the sensory information (somatosensation, vision, vestibular input) available to maintain balance. The SOT manipulates vision (eyes open or closed), somatosensory input from the feet (stable or sway referenced platform), and perceived body position in relation to the environment (stable or sway referenced visual surround).[117] Vestibular dysfunction patterns are seen in virtually all persons with bilateral peripheral vestibular deficits. These individuals are able to maintain balance when vision or somatosensation is available (conditions 1, 2, 3, 4), but they free fall repeatedly when conditions require dependence primarily on vestibular input (conditions 5, 6).[16] Similar vestibular dysfunction patterns are seen in people with peripheral vestibular lesions and CNS lesions affecting central pathways of the vestibular system. Persons who compensate after a unilateral lesion will have a normal sensory organization test result in 2 to 4 weeks after the initial insult.[62] Individuals with sensory dependency, such as many older adults, typically have an abnormal

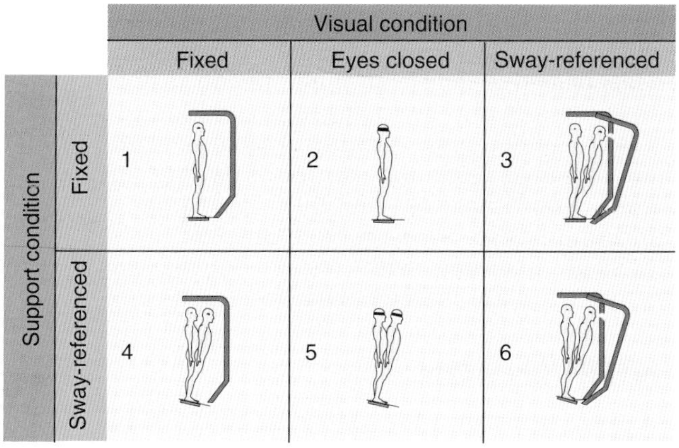

| Support condition | | Visual condition: Fixed | Visual condition: Eyes closed | Visual condition: Sway-referenced |
|---|---|---|---|---|
| Fixed | | 1 | 2 | 3 |
| Sway-referenced | | 4 | 5 | 6 |

**Figure 38.11**

**Diagram of the sensory conditions related to the sensory organization test, a component of posturography.** (Courtesy NeuroCom International, Clackamas, OR.)

preference for vision, with loss of balance on conditions where visual information is decreased or inaccurate (conditions 2, 3, 5, 6). In individuals with maladaptation, balance reactions may be preserved during isolated testing of conditions that primary rely on vestibular input (conditions 5 and 6), but use of the vestibular system may not be integrated during daily activity. The addition of head movement during the sensory portion of the CDP can increase the value of the measure.[106]

Observation and measurement of movement strategies (ankle, hip, stepping) used to maintain balance is the third component of the CDP. Abnormal strategy selection can represent poor adaptation of the vestibular spinal reflex. If the VSR is not providing appropriate top down input to maintain head stability, the maladapted client will maintain the ankle at 90 degrees in an attempt to use somatosensory input to maintain the head in relationship to the surface. This would be considered bottom up reference rather than the top down reference utilizing vestibular input. See "Special Implications for the Physical Therapist 38.1" for further discussion of strategy selection.[40,117]

***Imaging.*** When a central cause of dizziness and imbalance is suspected based on clinical findings and vestibular testing, magnetic resonance imaging (MRI) with contrast is indicated. Central brainstem lesions, such as stroke, trauma, or multiple sclerosis, can be identified. Neoplasms, including schwannomas, meningiomas, and metastases, can also be seen on imaging. A vascular loop or sling can be seen on MRI, as well as inflammatory conditions such as labyrinthitis and inflammatory lesions of the eighth cranial nerve. It is important to note that people may experience dizziness during an MRI due to magnetic vestibular stimulation occurring from an interaction between the magnetic field and naturally occurring ionic currents in the labyrinthine endolymph fluid. This interaction pushes on the semicircular canal cupula, leading to nystagmus and a sense of rotation or floating. Such effects could confound functional MRI studies of brain behavior, including resting-state brain activity.[135]

**Treatment.** Treatment of dizziness reflects the spectrum of etiologies and depends on the nature of the underlying vestibular disorder. The physical therapist plays a major role in the interdisciplinary approach to the management of symptoms.

When symptoms are due to a peripheral vestibular lesion, functional recovery will begin within 2 days to 4 weeks through adaptive mechanisms of the brain.[170] When a client's symptoms are severe, sedatives may be given, but ideally only for the first 24 hours. Rehabilitation should begin within the first 3 days if possible. The goal is to eliminate the frequency and duration of the abnormal sensation of motion and the symptoms of nausea, vomiting, and anxiety.[8] If the central adaptation process is inadequate, vestibular suppression medications can be helpful but must be used judiciously.

Surgical intervention is considered when the symptoms are unrelenting and the underlying condition is determined but is unresponsive to other medical measures. Local application of gentamicin to selectively destroy the end organ is often used rather than ablative surgery. Surgery may be indicated with neoplasia (see Chapter 30), perilymph fistula, persistent benign paroxysmal positional vertigo (BPPV), hydrops, and vascular loop. These conditions are covered later in this chapter.[98]

**Prognosis.** When a client has a unilateral peripheral vestibular system lesion, but the CNS is intact, recovery of functional mobility is possible. Recovery of static imbalance, or the differences in the tonic firing rate within the vestibular nuclei, is part of the adaptation process. When adaptation occurs, spontaneous nystagmus at rest resolves, and the client will no longer experience a sensation of movement at rest. Recovery of dynamic disturbances, reflecting the relationship of the coupling of the two sides of the system during movement, requires visual experience that requires use of the vestibular system. The visual experience allows the brain to recognize the error of the system through the retinal slip, causing oscillopsia, or loss of visual stability that occurs immediately after some lesions. It is this sensory mismatch provided by the visual system that allows the CNS to recognize the need for adaptation and drives the readjustment of motor reflexes.[92,111] The VOR should return to near normal within 2 to 6 weeks for slower movements, so that motion of the head during typical activities no longer disrupts vision or causes nausea. However, the client will continue to have an abnormal reaction to rapid head turns and will typically avoid these provoking head movements. Restriction of head movement will delay recovery because the CNS is never given the opportunity to adapt to the asymmetric firing patterns of the peripheral vestibular system.[100] Lack of head movement over time may also result in cervical musculoskeletal impairments.

Complete bilateral vestibular loss can occur as a result of use of ototoxic medications but is relatively rare; more often there is decreased function in both sides, often to a different degree on each side. Rehabilitation can provide adaptation to whatever degree possible and compensation for the remaining loss of function.[97] When a client has complete bilateral loss, substitution of the other intact sensory inputs for balance is required. The use of visual and somatosensory inputs to substitute for loss of vestibular function is possible when the environment provides adequate cues, as in well-lighted environments with firm, level surfaces. Substitution of small saccades in the direction opposite to head rotation can augment inadequate gain. Smooth pursuit accuracy can improve, and predictive strategies can improve gaze stability. More accurate use of spatial localization is reflected in the ability to imagine the location of stationary targets.[68,170] The VSRs are slower to return in both unilateral and bilateral vestibular loss, and the individual may continue to experience instability when turning quickly or walking on uneven surfaces or in the dark for weeks or months after the insult.

Prognosis for fluctuating conditions such as endolymphatic hydrops or Ménière disease is highly variable, depending on the frequency of vertigo episodes and severity of vestibular loss. Over time, there can be a gradual decline in the function of the vestibular system, and imbalance and symptoms related to a unilateral dysfunction become common. Rehabilitation can improve adaptation of the vestibular system between episodes and provide compensation as needed as the condition progresses.

Recovery rate in a central vestibular system disorder causing dizziness or disequilibrium depends on the nature of the lesion and the concomitant neurologic dysfunction. If vertigo is part of a progressive disease, it should be addressed as part of the overall rehabilitation. A disease such as multiple sclerosis can cause episodes of symptoms and progressive dysfunction with poor adaptation and compensation because of the other damage within the CNS.[19] Vestibular rehabilitation is critical in these individuals.[77,78] In a disorder of the central as well as the peripheral vestibular system, as in head injury or multisensory disorders, recovery is related to recognizing and treating the individual components and working on the reintegration process effectively.

Evaluation in the clinic also includes testing of the motor control of the visual-ocular component. VOR integrity is demonstrated by the client's ability to maintain visual focus during quick head turns. The therapist must be aware that other reflexive systems can compensate for the loss of vestibular reflexes and make it appear that there is no deficit. For example, a patient with well-compensated, longstanding bilateral loss of vestibular function may have no difficulty keeping vision fixed as the examiner rotates the client's head slowly from side to side. The client can maintain visual fixation at slower head speeds by using smooth pursuits, optokinetic nystagmus, and the cervico-ocular reflex to compensate for the vestibular deficit. This is an example of a head movement that *can* be sensed by the vestibular system, but that is not in the range of frequencies and accelerations sensed *exclusively* by the vestibular system. If the speed of the head movement is increased, rapid head rotation may pull the client's eyes off target and thus unmask a vestibular deficit.[59,158]

In order to determine if there is a central cause of the client's symptoms, the therapist must carefully examine the CNS by testing of function associated with cranial nerves, cerebellum, brainstem, and cortical connections. Often, both central and peripheral lesions can be identified. The therapist should also evaluate the musculoskeletal and neuromuscular systems because compensatory movements related to deficits in these systems may mimic vestibular dysfunction or impact recovery.

Many individuals awaiting discharge from hospital have impaired vestibular control of balance that is associated with impaired mobility. Evaluating vestibular function prior to discharge from hospital could improve discharge planning with respect to management of impairments that threaten balance and safe mobility.[67]

## INTERVENTION

Recovery from an acute vestibular injury requires both visual input and movement of the body and head to trigger vestibular adaptation. Input from the vision and body produces an error signal and indicates to the brain that adaptation is needed. For example, when the client is unable to maintain gaze stabilization and the image moves or slips on the retina, the nervous system will identify this error and try to adapt and modify the gain of the vestibular system. This process of adaptation is facilitated by vestibular rehabilitation.[59,65,70] Depending on the severity of the symptoms, exercises may begin in a supine or sitting position in order to decrease the vestibulospinal challenge. The system is progressively challenged by adding activities that incorporate movement of the eyes, head, and body, such as tracking a ball tossed from hand to hand.

Adaptation of the vestibular system is context specific. Treatment should therefore address the multitude of environments that the person will encounter. Exercises should stress the integration of all systems involved in balance, synthesizing the visual and somatosensory cues with the vestibular cues.[18] To stimulate use of somatosensory inputs, environments are designed to place less emphasis on vision, while providing reliable somatosensory inputs. To stimulate the use of visual inputs, environments are designed to place less emphasis on somatosensation, while providing reliable visual cues. The vestibular system is naturally stimulated when visual and somatosensory cues are distorted or decreased.[61]

Altered postural alignment is common with vestibular dysfunction. Sudden loss of vestibular function can result in both static lateral flexion of the head and an abnormal shift of the center of gravity to the side of the lesion. Vestibular pathologic conditions result in an inability to accurately determine one's limits of stability, resulting in maintaining the center of gravity outside of or on the edge of the actual limits of stability, which may cause loss of balance.[73] It is often noted that the person is unable (or unwilling because of fear of falling) to move the center of gravity far enough to perform a functional task, such as descending stairs.[155] When the balance disorder results in an inability to move the center of gravity through the ranges necessary to perform mobility tasks, the client will benefit from activities directed toward increasing the limits of stability.[87]

Center-of-pressure biofeedback provides input regarding control of center of gravity during weight shifts.[119] Lesions of the vestibular system can result in abnormal postural reactions to changes in head and body positions.

SPECIAL IMPLICATIONS FOR THE THERAPIST 38.1

### *Vestibular Dysfunction*

Vestibular rehabilitation is used extensively for individuals with vestibular dysfunction, with good evidence for effectiveness.[80,105,145] The 36-item Vestibular Rehabilitation Benefit Questionnaire (VRBQ) appears to be a concise and psychometrically robust questionnaire that addresses the main aspects of dizziness impact.[114] The Dizziness Handicap Inventory is another psychometrically robust self-report scale used to assess disability related to dizziness and imbalance.[153]

The appropriate choice and progression of exercises are critical for the outcome.[118,127,152] One of the greatest challenges in working with a client with symptoms of dizziness and imbalance is making the correct determination of precipitating factors and understanding concomitant disorders of the brain and musculoskeletal system.[108] Often health care providers stop short of the success that can be achieved because they do not fully understand the very complex mechanisms related to balance and dizziness. When the system recovers, typical activity should provide adequate stimulus to maintain vestibular function.[74] Individuals will often avoid situations on the edge of their tolerance, especially if there is additional brain dysfunction, as in concussion. These individuals may show some decline in function over time if the system does not continue to be challenged as it is during the rehabilitation process.

### *Examination*

During clinical evaluation of the client with vestibular dysfunction, the therapist integrates the history with objective evaluation findings. The history can guide the therapist regarding the mechanism of injury and location within the system. The nature of the symptoms and the precipitating, exacerbating, and relieving factors are also reviewed.[4,115,117] The therapist can structure the evaluation around clinical syndromes to identify sensory and movement impairments. Vestibular dysfunction is often referred to as a unilateral hypofunction; however, a unilateral vestibular dysfunction can result for any number of pathologies and conditions, and vestibular dysfunction can occur without direct injury to the peripheral vestibular structure. The therapist can use these clinical syndromes to evaluate patients with any diagnosis to make the connection between history, symptoms, evaluation, and intervention as seen in Box 38.2.

Identification of sensation of motion at rest points to basic lack of adaptation of tonic firing rate, whereas head motion–provoked dizziness occurs when the calibration between the two sides is inefficient during movement. Head-righting responses should be evaluated to determine if there is ability to use the otolith mechanism without override of the somatosensory system. Evaluation of balance strategies under altered sensory conditions that isolate vision, somatosensory, and vestibular inputs (see earlier discussion of the sensory organization test) will identify visual and somatosensory dependency patterns. Visual and somatosensory dependence develops early when the vestibular input is inadequate and can persist throughout the course of rehabilitation if not identified and treated. Visual motion sensitivity results from the inability to filter out movement in the peripheral visual fields and is related to, but not exactly the same as, visual dependency. With visual motion sensitivity, clients experience an abnormal perception of self-motion in relationship to movement in the environment. Therefore, conditions that increase optic flow, such as walking in a crowded environment, riding on an escalator, or walking in a grocery store may create increased symptoms of dizziness. Walking is often easier in an empty shopping mall than in a crowded one and walking with the crowd is less taxing than walking against the crowd.

When observing upright balance, evaluation of strategy selection is critical in identifying abnormal hip or stepping strategy, a common finding in clients with vestibular disorders.[4,75] When standing on a firm, flat surface, the client will use an ankle strategy. The torque for the motion is controlled at the ankle. Vestibular dysfunction does not appear to affect this strategy because the input to drive the response comes primarily from the somatosensory system. However, initially, a person with vestibular loss may have difficulty performing an ankle strategy without the use of vision as a second sensory system with which the brain can compare.[75] A hip strategy is used when the client is standing on a narrow (beamlike) surface or when the surface is soft. A hip strategy is used on a flat surface when the center of gravity moves beyond the base of support. In a hip strategy, the torque is controlled at the hip. Individuals with a vestibular loss have difficulty using the hip strategy, and therefore, have difficulty performing activities such as single-leg stance, heel-toe walk, and standing on a beam or a compliant surface. The individual with vestibular loss can generate a hip strategy but have difficulty maintaining control with perturbations of the surface and tend to use a stepping strategy to compensate for inability to maintain balance using the hip strategy.[4,73,75] Stepping strategy is used to bring the center of gravity over the base of support when it moves too far to control with an ankle or hip strategy.

When the individual relies on vestibular cues for the primary input for balance, the impaired system fails to provide the necessary input. Orientation to gravity or to support surface changes that include dorsiflexion or plantar flexion is inadequate to maintain upright position.[85] This is seen in the inability to maintain balance on a compliant surface or on a surface that rotates at the ankle. It becomes difficult to walk in the dark, on soft surfaces, and up and down ramps or stairs. Postural strategies, or postural control synergies, are triggered in preparation for movement and in response to changes in the environment.

Box 38.2

**FUNCTIONAL CLASSIFICATION GUIDELINES**

When there is lack of central mediated adaptation, symptoms can manifest and affect function. These categories can be identified during the examination. The symptoms will lead the clinician toward the most effective interventions.

***Sensation of Motion at Rest***

1. Test Position
   - Patient sits unsupported with feet on floor, hands on lap and closes eyes.
2. Test procedure
   - Examiner asks patient to report any sensation of motion inside head.
3. Responses
   - No motion reported: Symmetrical vestibular system function.
   - Rotation: Unequal signals coming from each side of the vestibular system.
   - Tilt: Inability to find vertical position from gravity sensors (i.e., otoliths).
   - Lightheadedness or Rocking: Mismatch of vestibular and somatosensory input.
4. Functional Implications
   - Difficulty with routine mental tasks (i.e., sequential tasking, simple mathematical calculations, memory lapses).
   - Report of persistent dizziness, loss of balance with movement, especially with head rotation or tilt.
5. Intervention Options
   - Settling-giving the somatosensory system added input by increasing weight through spine. Weights on patient's shoulders while sitting in a firm chair with eyes closed or using hands to create a compressive force through spine.

***Head Motion–Provoked Dizziness***

1. Test Position
   - Patient is seated unsupported on a mat table or chair.
   - NOTE: Head motion–provoked dizziness can also be determined with head turns during other testing procedures (i.e., during tests for blurred vision during head turns)
2. Test Procedure
   - Examiner asks the patient to turn their head side to side in the horizontal and/or the vertical plane at a speed of between 1-3 Hz. The patient is requested to report any increase in the level of their symptoms of dizziness. Dizziness is persistent when head turns are tested on a firm support surface or on a compliant (foam) support surface.
3. Responses
   - Dizziness associated with lack of vestibular system calibration to determine the speed that the head is turning.
   - Dizziness associated with abnormal interpretation of somatosensory inputs in the neck.
4. Functional Implications
   - Unable to identify speed of rotation and angular acceleration of head in space in relation to the body
   - Dizziness and/or imbalance in situations requiring head movement (i.e., reading, turning around, walking and looking around).
   - Avoids head movement during daily tasks.
5. Intervention
   - Rolling
   - Head turns, tilts, and nods
   - Spin in chair
   - Walking turns

***Head Position–Provoked Dizziness***

1. Test Position
   - Dix-Hallpike
2. Test Procedure
   - Posterior/anterior canal: Dix-Hallpike (head rotated 45 degrees in long sit, then patient brought to supine while maintaining head rotation, extended over edge of table to 30 degrees
   - Horizontal Canal: Head held in 30 degrees of neck flexion, then rotated
   - Tests done both right and left directions
3. Response
   - Normal response: No dizziness.
   - Abnormal response: Reported change in level of dizziness related to head position changes
   - Nystagmus
4. Functional Implications
   - Dizziness when getting out of bed, rolling over, bending over or looking up
   - Imbalance when looking up or bending forward
   - Dizziness when driving due to head movement
5. Intervention
   - If there is dizziness without nystagmus, perform head position exercise to adapt system to provoking head position
   - If there is latent torsional nystagmus that lasts less than 60 seconds, perform the appropriate repositioning procedure
   - If there is latent horizontal nystagmus that lasts less than 60 seconds, perform appropriate horizontal roll
   - Adaptation exercise if nystagmus is persistent

***Gaze Stability with Head Turns***

1. Test Position
   - Patient sitting
2. Test Procedure
   - Examiner instructs patient to maintain stable gaze (keep target in focus) while rotating head from side to side at 1-3 Hz speed
3. Response
   - Normal response: Target begins in focus and stays in focus during head turns
   - Abnormal response: Image is blurred as the head turns
4. Functional Implications
   - Avoids head movement during typical activities
   - Decreases speed of walking
   - Difficulty driving and reading street signs
   - Headache and neck pain associated with attempts to decelerate head during typical activities
5. Intervention Options
   - Patient moves head only as fast as they can to maintain visual focus
   - Progress this activity to perform with increasing speed, in more visually stimulating environments and during more challenging surface conditions

***Head Righting Responses***

1. Test Position
   - Patient is seated on a tilt board or a rocker board with feet on floor, hands on lap, and eyes closed.
2. Test Procedure
   - Examiner assumes a position behind the patient and tips patient side to side, observing patient's head position.

Box 38.2

**FUNCTIONAL CLASSIFICATION GUIDELINES—cont'd**

3. Responses
   - Normal head righting: Head remains in vertical midline orientation.
   - Abnormal head righting: Head remains in alignment with trunk indicative of otolith impairment or somatosensory dominance.
4. Functional Implications
   - Difficulty with climbing stairs.
   - Symptoms noted during riding elevators.
   - Postural instability standing on moving surfaces (i.e., escalator, moving walkways).
   - Mobility issues in compromised visual environments (i.e., walking in the dark).
   - Lack of postural stability going from sitting to standing.
   - Excessive use of upper extremity to stabilize trunk during functional tasks
   - Patient fails to use appropriate stepping strategy in response to speed and direction of head and body (i.e., foot is not placed in the correct position to prevent a fall).
5. Intervention
   - Head tilts
   - Side reaches
   - Sit on tilt board
   - Semi-tandem stance to tandem stance to tandem walking
   - All postural work done on foam
   - Single leg stance
   - Sit on ball (marching with eyes closed)
   - Perturbed surface with vision disrupted

Dependency patterns are the result of substitution or compensatory strategies used when an individual does not recover satisfactory adaptation and integration of the sensory systems required for normal balance responses in a variety of environmental conditions. Imbalance occurs when the patient uses this system instead of the most appropriate and efficient sensory system for the environmental situation.

***Visual Dependency***

1. Test Procedure
   - Examiner instructs patient to stand with a base of support that is more narrow than the hips
   - Ask patient to follow a target with their central visual field that includes movement in a diagonal direction such as a figure eight.
   - Compare sway pattern during eyes open activities to eyes closed activities.
2. Response
   - Normal response: Patient maintains upright posture
   - Abnormal response: Patient sways excessively as the physiologic visual field moves away from vertical, or when vision is absent.
3. Functional Implications
   - Imbalance in dark environments especially when the surface is uneven
   - Loss of balance when the visual environment moves around them
   - More fatigued than expected by daily activity, especially when in stimulating visual environments
4. Intervention Options
   - Perform smooth pursuit tracking in a progression of environments.
   - Standing on firm surface, progressed to compliant or narrow based foot placement, to single leg, to walk with eye movement or head movement that induces changes in peripheral visual field.
   - Work on balance activity with eyes closed.

***Somatosensory Dependency***

1. Test Position
   - Standing on compliant, narrow, unstable or perturbed surfaces.
2. Response
   - Client maintains persistent joint angles (i.e., joints do not adapt to surface variability, resulting in postural instability).
3. Functional Implications
   - Somatosensory dependency causes difficulty on compliant or unstable surfaces, i.e. grass, thick padded carpet, sand, etc.
   - NOTE: This leads to excess reliance on ankle, hip and spinal orientation to the surface during balance tasks.
   - Inability to switch from an ankle strategy to a hip strategy as the surface becomes less stable, (i.e., walking from sidewalk to grass)
4. Intervention
   - Training on compliant, narrow, unstable or perturbed surfaces, giving verbal cues to prevent patient from maintaining persistent joint angles.

Hypersensitivity patterns develop when compensatory strategies become so dominant that the patient is intolerant of provoking visual stimulation, especially in moving environments. This may represent an unstable or fluctuating vestibular system.

***Visual Motion Hypersensitivity***

1. Test Position
   - This is noted during any tests of eye movement.
   - Optokinetic stimulus
2. Test Procedure
   - Asking patient if there are increases in the sensation of dizziness or nausea during eye movement testing
   - Use of optokinetic stimulus to provide peripheral visual movement
3. Response
   - Normal: No complaint of dizziness or nausea during exam
   - Abnormal: Report of dizziness or nausea
4. Functional Implications
   - Avoids environments that have visual stimulation such as grocery stores, hardware stores, and airports
   - Dizziness and nausea when using computers, watching TV or movies
   - Dizziness and nausea in cars especially in the back seat, patient prefers to drive rather than be a passenger
   - Difficulty reading unless book is held steady
5. Intervention
   - Provide visual stimulus by having patient perform eye movement with head still in progressively stimulating environments; then progress to include head movements
   - Use of optokinetic stimulus with progressive surface challenges and with eye movement

(Permission for use granted by Kenda Fuller.)

It is important for the therapist to educate and support the individual during the natural course of the recovery. A program should be designed to facilitate the use of vestibular input for balance progressively so that the individual does not become overly dependent on vision or somatosensation for balance. It appears that many individuals who have been considered compensated show less natural use of the vestibular system compared with individuals who have never had a vestibular problem. Current research is oriented toward more novel and effective ways to reestablish vestibular function. For example, use of repetitive platform perturbations at vestibular-dependent velocities demonstrates improved postural stability and greater functional abilities when compared to other forms of rehabilitation.[167] Guided home-based vestibular rehabilitation programs (GHVR) will likely become more widely used with enhanced education and increased adherence.[138]

**A THERAPIST'S THOUGHTS[a]**

While this chapter demonstrates the tremendous complexity of the balance sensory and motor system, the key to successful rehabilitation of the greatest percentage of dizzy patients of all etiologies often lies in the basic understanding of the many components within the system. Simple yet critical things such as listening carefully to the patient's description of the detail in symptom onset and quality, validating the intensity of discomfort reflected in the high perception of disability, and addressing compassionately the anxiety that is often present are all important..

The individual with BPPV or unilateral vestibular hypofunction, in the absence of comorbidities, will respond quickly and completely to the interventions of vestibular rehabilitation. However, many patients who present for help to a dizziness specialist are dealing with complex comorbidities, such as migraine, unidentified postconcussive syndrome, cervical somatosensory dysfunction, or disorders of the visual system either in perception or in eye position or oculomotor control. Guidance of the patient into complete adaptation and resolution of symptoms requires careful assessment and treatment of visual, oculomotor, and somatosensory system integration.

[a]Julie Knoll, PT, NCS

## Benign Paroxysmal Positional Vertigo (BPPV)

Episodic, intense vertigo related to head position, such as bending forward, looking up, or lying down, is most often a benign disorder called benign paroxysmal pos–itional vertigo (BPPV), also known simply as benign positional vertigo (BPV). It is considered a benign condition, because it is not the sign of a disease process but a mechanical disorder of the labyrinths.

### Incidence and Risk Factors

BPPV is the most common cause of vertigo. The prevalence of BPPV has been reported by some studies to range from 10.7 to 140 per 100,000 people.[60,160] Other studies have estimated a prevalence of 900 per 10,000.[90,96,123] Lifetime prevalence is estimated to be 2.4%.[162] Women are affected more often than men at a ratio of 1.6 : 1.

Over 50% of people with BPPV have an idiopathic form, meaning the exact cause is unknown. Age may be a contributing factor to idiopathic BPPV, as the prevalence of BPPV is greater in people over age 60 compared to those aged 18 to 39.[162] This increase may be related to increased demineralization and fragmentation of the otoconia with increased age, especially in those with osteoporosis and vitamin D deficiency.[9,165,168] Increased dehydration with age may also contribute to increased BPPV. It is unusual for a child to have BPPV.[53]

The second most common cause of BPPV is head trauma, followed by viral neuronitis as the third leading cause. Head trauma or infectious disorders may precede the onset of BPPV by months or even years.

BPPV spontaneously resolves in 20% of people within one month and up to 50% by 3 months.[53,14] However, the disorder recurs in 40% to 60% of the cases. BPPV may trouble the individual intermittently for years, but in this condition, a close examination of potential causes will often identify an underlying medical disorder, and recurrences decline when the underlying disorder is managed. For example, increased fluid pressure within the labyrinth may dislodge otoconia (see discussion of endolymphatic hydrops below) and migraine-induced ischemia may be responsible for the release of otoconia.

### Clinical Manifestations

Despite the use of the term *benign*, the symptoms related to positional vertigo are intense and can cause significant disability. Clients often experience a strong sense of falling or spinning out of control, even when lying on a bed. Before the individual is aware of the mechanism, the condition seems uncontrollable because symptoms occur with changes of head position.

Typically, a person with BPPV will complain of brief episodes of vertigo precipitated by head movement in a specific direction such as bending over, looking up to take an object off a shelf, tilting the head back to shave, lying back to get a haircut, or turning the head rapidly while backing up a car. Vertigo often also occurs with getting into bed, lying down, sitting up, or rolling over. Often the client's report of first experiencing vertigo is when waking up suddenly in the night with the room spinning. In BPPV, these episodes of vertigo occur suddenly and typically last 20 seconds, but usually not more than a minute. The subjective impression of attack duration reported is frequently longer than the actual period of dizziness.[56,82] It is important to note that vertigo or the true sensation of the "room spinning" is not always present in BPPV. Some patients only report lightheadedness, sensation of floating, dizziness, imbalance, and/or nausea.[14,162] Box 38.3 gives typical complaints related to BPPV.

### Pathogenesis

In BPPV, the otoconia in the otolith can become loose, clump together, and form densities known as canaliths. Canaliths move through the endolymphatic fluid and become problematic when they float into the semicircular canals. Canaliths can potentially move into any of the three canals, but the posterior canal is most commonly involved (about 85-90% of cases)[125,140] because of the relationship of the posterior canal to the otolith. The

Box 38.3

**COMMON CHARACTERISTICS OF BENIGN PAROXYSMAL POSITIONAL VERTIGO**

- Episodic sensation of intense vertigo with head position changes
- Sensation stops after 20 to 30 seconds in static position
- Nausea with vertigo, with reports of spinning inside the head
- Autonomic changes such as sweating, feeling like passing out
- Sensation of movement of the environment and blurred vision
- Reports of disequilibrium during typical activities
- Waking up dizzy at night after rolling over in bed
- Symptoms during head movement or bending forward during typical activities

Box 38.4

**CANALITHIASIS OF BENIGN PAROXYSMAL POSITIONAL VERTIGO**

- The canalithiasis mechanism explains the latency of nystagmus as a result of the time needed for motion of the material within the posterior canal to be initiated by gravity.
- The nystagmus duration is correlated with the length of time required for the dense material to reach the lowest part of the canal.
- The vertical (upbeating of fast phase) and torsional (superior poles of the eyes beating toward the lower-most ear) components of the nystagmus are consistent with eye movements evoked by stimulation of the posterior canal nerve in experimental animals.
- The reversal of nystagmus when the patient returns to the sitting upright position is due to retrograde movement of material in the lumen of the posterior canal back toward the ampulla, with resulting ampullopetal deflection of the cupula.
- The fatigability of the nystagmus evoked by repeated Dix-Hallpike positional testing is explained by dispersion of material within the canal.

posterior canal is placed in the vertical position when the body is supine and the head is extended beyond neutral and rotated 45 degrees to the same side. The canaliths drift out of the otolith through the opening to the posterior canal.

In canalithiaisis BPPV, when the head is moved and the involved canal is placed in a gravity dependent position, the canaliths fall through the endolymphatic fluid to the lowest portion of the canal relative to head position. This movement of the fluid creates drag on the endolymph, which bends the cupula and causes excessive deflection of the hair cells. The increased firing of the hair cells creates a sensation of rotation of the head and stimulates the VOR in response to the abnormal perception that the head is rotating quickly. The eyes are activated to respond to the perceived movement, and as the VOR is attempting to establish the appropriate gain of the system, there is nystagmus. As soon as the head stops moving, otoconia come to rest at the lowest point in the canal, the pressure on the hair cell is relieved, and the nystagmus subsides. This takes about 20 to 60 seconds. There is no nystagmus or sensation of spinning until the head is moved into another gravity dependent position, causing the otoconia to roll once again through the canal.[133]

By observing the specific nature and pattern of the nystagmus relative to head position during positional testing, the clinician can identify the location of the canaliths, critical to determining and performing the appropriate intervention. Based on the VOR connections between pairs of extraocular muscles and semicircular canals, the direction and pattern of nystagmus will be different depending on the location of the canaliths. Due to the architecture of the canals in relationship to the otoliths, the otoconia can appear on either side of the cupula, in either the short arm or the long arm of the canal. The otoconia will either push or pull the hair cells depending on the head position, thus influencing direction of nystagmus. Additionally, the canaliths may fall through the center of the canal, creating a strong nystagmus, or it may roll along the wall of the canal, moving slower and causing less drag on the cupula, therefore, smaller amplitude nystagmus. The timing of the fall, or sedimentation, is dependent on how many otoconia have stuck together, which determines the canalith size. A single large canalith will fall faster and create more drag than several smaller canaliths falling at the same time in the canal.[122] Box 38.4 describes the phenomenon of canalithiasis.

A less common form of BPPV is cupulolithiasis, which occurs when the canalith is adhered to the cupula and causes a direct pull on the hair cells. Because movement of the cupula is not dependent on the drag of the endolymph, the nystagmus has immediate onset and longer duration. Symptoms will begin immediately with movement of the head in the provoking position and will persist as long as the head is held in the position. The symptoms may decrease slightly because of adaptation of the CNS, and therefore, may mimic the fatigue of canalithiasis. The otoconia can adhere to either side of the cupula, depending on whether it initially entered the long or short arm of the canal. The nystagmus pattern will reflect the direction of pressure on the cupula and the resulting bend of the kinocilium. Cupulolithiasis, either occurring independently or in combination with canalithiasis, is more likely to be involved in the etiology of horizontal canal BPPV than is the case for posterior canal BPPV.[81]

## MEDICAL MANAGEMENT

DIAGNOSIS. The diagnosis of BPPV is made based on a suggestive history and report of current clinical manifestations as described above. Classic patterns of nystagmus are seen with positional testing, confirming the diagnosis. Because BPPV is the most common cause of dizziness and should not require a hospital stay, emergency room personnel are being training to identify, rule out other causes, and provide the appropriate repositioning procedures.[25]

The Dix-Hallpike maneuver is the gold standard test to establish the diagnosis of posterior and anterior benign

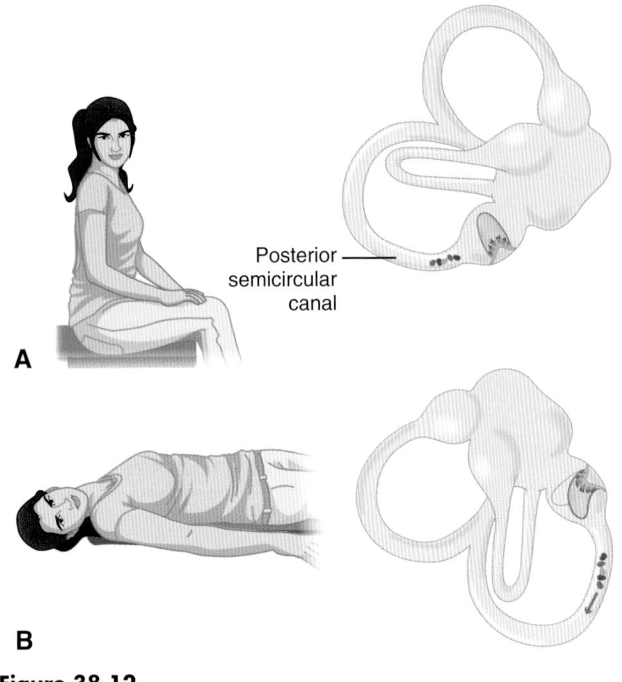


**Figure 38.12**

**The Dix-Hallpike maneuver.** (A) Starting position with head rotated toward the side to be tested. (B) Lowering the patient's head backward and to the side allows debris in the posterior canal to fall to its lowest position, activating the canal and causing eye movements and vertigo. (From Lundy-Ekman L: *Neuroscience: Fundamentals for rehabilitation*, ed 4, Philadelphia, 2013, Saunders.)

positional vertigo (BPPV).[14] With posterior or anterior canal BPPV, the client typically experiences symptoms with bending forward, looking up, and rolling in bed. These movements place the vertical canals in the plane of gravity, causing the canaliths to shift and stimulate the cupula.[107]

To perform the Dix-Hallpike maneuver, the client is brought from long sitting to supine with the head turned 45 degrees to one side and the neck extended 20 degrees (Fig. 38.12). The examiner holds the head in this position for 20 to 30 seconds while monitoring for symptoms of vertigo and observing the eyes for nystagmus.[79] A positive response for posterior canal BPPV is torsional, upbeating nystagmus with a latency of 3 to 15 seconds. The intensity of the nystagmus increases before decreasing until it completely resolves, typically fatiguing in less than 60 seconds.[11] The nystagmus occurs when the affected ear is placed down. If the anterior canal is involved, the nystagmus will appear torsional and downbeating. The nystagmus may reverse and beat in the opposite direction upon return of the head to the upright position. Although a positive test is pathognomonic for posterior BPPV, a negative test indicates only that BPPV is not active at that movement. If a brief period of dizziness is experienced during the Dix-Hallpike maneuver as the head is approaching the full supine position, and there is no evidence of posterior or anterior canal BPPV, there is a possibility of horizontal canal involvement, which should be further investigated.

When otoconia are present within the horizontal canal, the client will experience vertigo with rolling in either direction, especially when the head is elevated on a pillow, and may have vertigo with bending forward. Horizontal canal BPPV is usually associated with autonomic symptoms, such as lightheadedness, nausea, and vomiting.[11] The supine horizontal roll test is the most commonly used test to determine the presence of horizontal canal BPPV. During the roll test, the client lies in supine with the head held in 30 degrees flexion to keep the horizontal canal perpendicular to the ground. The head is then turned 90 degrees to one side while the eyes are observed for nystagmus. The head is returned to neutral and then rotated 90 degrees to the other side. A positive response is horizontal nystagmus that changes direction when head position is changed (e.g., right beating with the head turned right and left beating with the head turned left) and is stronger on one side than the other. The nystagmus can be either geotropic or apogeotropic. In geotropic horizontal canal BPPV, the more intense nystagmus beats toward the affected ear (toward the ground) when the client is lying on the affected side. This suggests the otoconia are located in the long or posterior arm of the horizontal canal. In the apogeotropic type, the more intense nystagmus beats away from the affected ear (away from the ground) when the client is lying on the affected side. Apogeotropic nystagmus indicates the otoconia is adhered to the ampulla on either the utricular or canal side (cupulolithiasis) or is located in the short arm or in the anterior portion of the long arm of the horizontal canal (canalithiasis).

The posterior arm of the canal opens to the otolith, which allows the otoconia to be moved back into place. It is the goal of repositioning maneuvers to shift the otoconia towards the otolith. When the otoconia is in the anterior portion of the horizontal canal, it must be moved into the posterior portion of the canal to be removed from the canal. Fig. 38.13 shows the movement of the debris in the horizontal canal.

Identification of the involved side is critical to treating horizontal canal BPPV. The bow and lean tests can be performed in addition to the horizontal roll test to provided increased certainty about the side of involvement. The bow test is performed by having the client bend the head forward by 90 to 120 degrees in sitting, while the lean test is performed by having the client lean the head backward by 45 to 60 degrees or by having the client lie in supine with the head supported on a pillow. The direction of nystagmus is noted. In geotropic BPPV, nystagmus will beat towards the affected ear in the bow test and away from the affected ear in the lean test. In apogeotropic BPPV, the reverse is true with nystagmus beating away from the affected ear in the bow test and towards the affected ear in the lean test.[36,101]

Another form of positional dizziness that must be ruled out in making the diagnosis of BPPV is central positional vertigo. Nystagmus that is sustained and not suppressed by visual fixation reflects a central lesion. These findings can be indicative of ischemia of the pontomedullary brainstem or another part of the central vestibular pathway. Cerebellar involvement will cause dizziness in positions of supine, head rotated left with

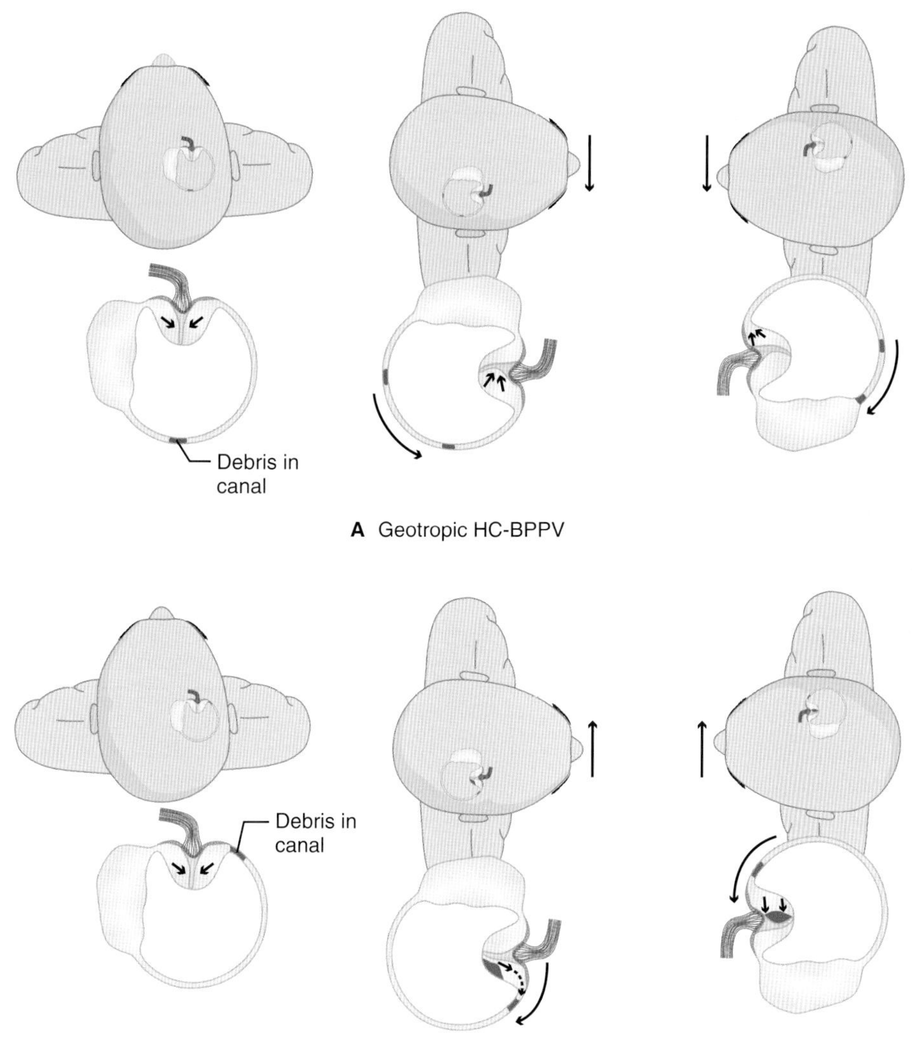


**Figure 38.13**

**Relative movement of the debris in the horizontal canal during changes of head position.** Note the position of the debris is in the back of the canal in relationship to the nose, representing geotropic movement of the nystagmus in A, in B the debris in in the front of the canal in relationship to the nose and the nystagmus would be apogeotropic. (From Flint: Cummings otolaryngology: head & neck surgery, ed 5, St. Louis, 2010, Mosby.)

extension, and head rotated right with extension. Pure downbeating nystagmus in either the sitting or supine position may indicate an infratentorial disorder. This can be related to vascular insults such as Arnold-Chiari malformation, stroke, or subdural hematoma. Multiple sclerosis lesions are common in this area and are associated with the progressive forms. Unilateral lesions, perilymphatic fistula, superior semicircular canal dehiscence, or middle ear problems can cause positional dizziness and are discussed later in this chapter. Intermittent dizziness that is made worse with position changes could also be part of the aura of migraine.

It should also be noted that it is typical to experience dizziness with the head pitched backward, as it puts the otoliths at an angle that is not a part of daily activity. Orthostatic hypotension can also create a brief episode of dizziness when going from supine to standing.

**Treatment.** Specific, highly effective procedures can be performed in the clinical setting to remediate the disorder. Canalith repositioning is a series of passive movements designed to move the canaliths through the canal and back into the otolith. Each canal requires specific movements and changes in head position to affectively move the canaliths. Typically 2 to 4 repeated procedures are necessary. The Epley maneuver is the procedure most typically used to move canaliths from the posterior canal (Fig. 38.14). An alternate maneuver for posterior canal BPPV is the Semont liberatory maneuver.[143] Even if the canalith-repositioning procedure clears the posterior canal, there is an elevated risk of reentry or canal conversion to the horizontal canal. In this case, additional maneuvers are required to clear the debris; the risk can be reduced by waiting at least 15 minutes between repetitions of a canalith-repositioning procedure.[58]

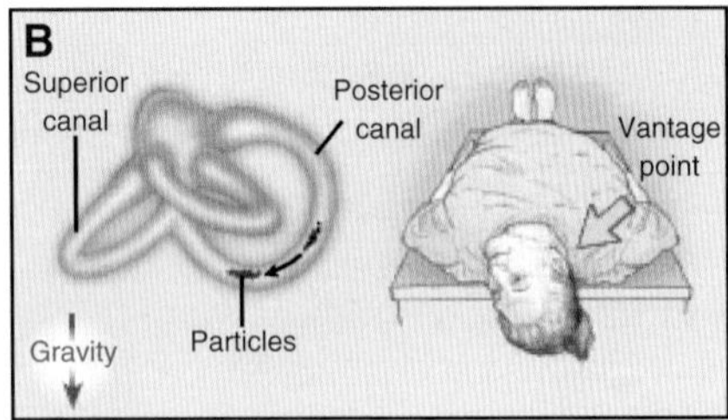


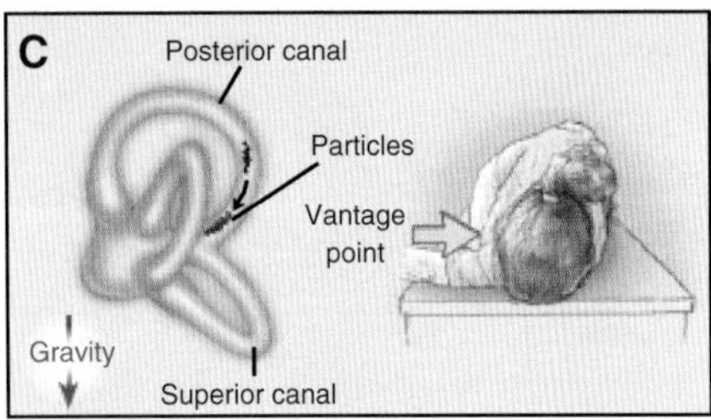


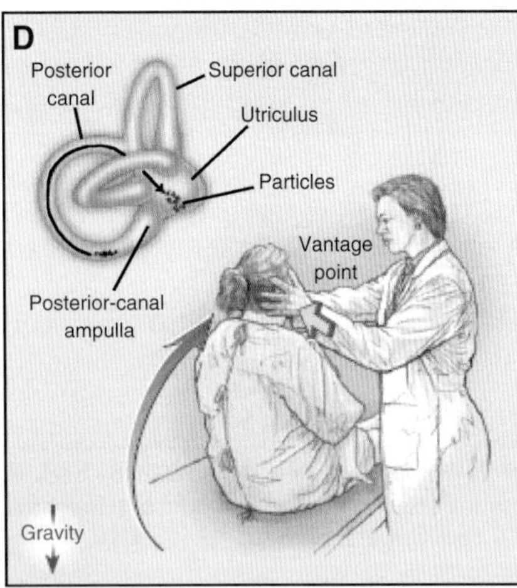


**Figure 38.14**

**Canalith repositioning maneuver for the patient with posterior canal benign positional vertigo (BPV).** Figure represents procedure for right-side BPV. Movement of particles through the canal is shown in each position. A shows the beginning position, B represents the rotation of the head in the opposite direction, C shows the position of the head that causes the particles to move into position to be moved out of the canal, and D is the final position.

Horizontal canalithiasis BPPV is most commonly treated using the barbecue roll maneuver. During the barbecue roll, the client lies in supine, and the head or full body is turned toward the affected ear. The head is then turned away from the affected ear before turning the head down towards the ground and then sitting up.[27] The Gufoni maneuver is an alternative procedure for horizontal canal BPPV, with positioning modified depending on if geotropic or apogeotropic nystagmus is present.[6,159] A final treatment that can be used in conjunction with the barbecue roll or the Gufoni manever is forced prolonged positioning during which the client lies on the unaffected side (for geotropic BPPV) or the affected side (for apogeotropic BPPV) for the entire night. The Kim maneuver and head-shaking maneuver are additional procedures effective in treating apogeotropic horizontal cupulolithiasis BPPV.[93]

Traditionally, the client was instructed to follow specific instructions for 24 hours following canalith repositioning to prevent displacement of the otoconia back into the treated canal. These instructions included sleeping with the head elevated to at least 30 degrees and avoiding head movement. More recent studies suggest there is insufficient evidence to support the recommendation of these restrictions following canalith repositioning for posterior canal BPPV.[50] However, some clients, such as those with frequent reoccurrence of BPPV, may still benefit from these restrictions.

## SPECIAL IMPLICATIONS FOR THE THERAPIST 38.3

### *BPPV*

Ability to perform repositioning maneuvers is the basis for treating BPPV. It is critical to be aware of the confounding nature of multiple canal involvement. Because of the high degree of recurrence, some individuals do best with a program they can perform at home. However, because the correct canal must be identified, return to the clinic is warranted in many cases. When a client has symptoms that they are unable to control, use of anti-nausea medication prior to repositioning to control symptoms can be helpful.

When the individual has had a period of dizziness, and especially when the BPPV has recurred or has been persistent over years, there is a high incidence of maladaptation of sensory integration for balance, resulting in somatosensory and visual dependence for balance. Although the individual no longer complains of dizziness, there may be imbalance in low light or when standing or walking on compliant surfaces. This maladaptation increases the individuals' risk of falling earlier compared to those who have not had BPPV.[14] Visual motion hypersensitivity is common and responds well to intervention. Evaluation for BPPV should include the balance system, and intervention for balance disorder should follow clearing of BPPV.[81,164]

## Infection

Acute unilateral vestibulopathy, or vestibular neuritis, is the second most common cause of vertigo. Viral infection is common and usually affects the vestibular nerve unilaterally. Vestibular neuritis can be a partial unilateral vestibular lesion, and this partial lesion can affect the superior division of the vestibular nerve, which includes the afferents from the horizontal and anterior semicircular canals.[55]

### Incidence and Etiology

The incidence of vestibular neuritis is 3.5 in 100,000. Viral infections are common between the ages of 30 and

60 years, with a peak for women in the fourth decade and men in the sixth decade.[56] The apparent etiology of the disease is multifactorial. Viral pathogens include mumps, rubella, herpes simplex virus type 1, cytomegalovirus, and Epstein-Barr virus. Enteroviruses are among the other rare viral causes. Onset is often preceded by a systemic viral illness, such as an upper respiratory tract infection or gastritis. The illness may precede the vestibular dysfunction by up to 2 weeks but can happen within the course of a bout of cold or flu. When illness such as measles, mumps, or infectious mononucleosis is the source, hearing loss may accompany the vestibular symptoms. Polyneuritis of the seventh and eighth cranial nerves, known as Ramsay Hunt syndrome, can be the result of herpes zoster and cause perivascular, perineural, and intraneural infiltration. The cortical vestibular projection fibers can be affected by herpes zoster encephalitis, which has a predilection for the temporal lobe. Other viruses are suspected but have yet to be positively identified.

The use of antibiotics in general has decreased the incidence of bacterial infections affecting the vestibular system. However, infections still do arise and can be introduced into the vestibular apparatus through the various fluid systems involved or through breakdown of the bony labyrinth.

### Pathogenesis

Histopathologic studies have suggested involvement of the superior vestibular nerve and vestibular ganglion, often with little or no involvement of the actual end organ. This is true of vestibular neuritis, in which there is no cochlear involvement. However, many viruses do damage throughout the labyrinth and cochlea. Typically, in vestibular neuritis, the end organ is filled with lymphocytes. Intracytoplasmic particles have been found in the vestibular ganglia and are thought to be dormant forms of a virus that may produce infection and result in inner ear disease.[12]

Persons with bacterial meningitis develop labyrinthitis when bacteria enter the perilymphatic space from the cerebrospinal fluid by way of the cochlear aqueduct or the internal auditory canal. Some bacterial infections result in biochemical irritation of the membranes through a toxic reaction. Both congenital and acquired syphilitic infections produce labyrinthitis as a latent manifestation.

### Clinical Manifestations

Acute unilateral vestibular neuronitis causes sudden onset of vertigo, spontaneous horizontal and torsional nystagmus, nausea, and vomiting. The person will immediately experience intense disequilibrium, and his or her ability to perceive position and motion will be profoundly disturbed. The person will have a false sense of angular motion (i.e., rotation). With the eyes closed, there is an illusion of spinning, or sense of motion of the body turning on its long axis toward the involved side. When the eyes are open, the illusion is of spinning of the environment in the opposite direction. The person will also have a tonic ocular tilt reaction consisting of head tilt, conjugate eye torsion, skew deviation, and lateropulsion, seen as an abnormal weight shift toward the side of the lesion.[39] This tilt reaction is due to the otolithic hypofunction on the side with the lesion.[117,118]

## MEDICAL MANAGEMENT

**DIAGNOSIS.** Unilateral hypofunction results in abnormal VOR, with loss of gaze stabilization with head movement. Therefore, movement of the head causes blurring of vision, resulting in dizziness and loss of ability to use visual cues to maintain balance. EMG testing reveals a unilateral hypofunction.

A spontaneous mixed torsional and horizontal nystagmus is often present immediately after unilateral hypofunction. The slow phases are directed toward the side of the lesion, and the quick phases are to the intact side. As the eyes are observed, it is the quick phases that are apparent, and therefore, the nystagmus appears to be moving away from the side with the lesion. The nystagmus is suppressed by gaze fixation or looking at a static object.[79,104,118]

**Treatment.** Medications are used for symptoms of acute vertigo and include antihistamines, anticholinergic agents, antidopaminergic agents, steroids, and antivirals such as acyclovir. Glucocorticoids administered within 3 days after onset of vestibular neuronitis improve long-time recovery of vestibular function and reduce length of hospital stay.[88]

Recovery of function and resolution of dizziness is accomplished through a program to facilitate the vestibular system. Recalibration, or adaptation of the system, comes by facilitating the integration of somatosensory input and recovery of normal postural responses. (See "Special Implications for the Therapist 38.1: Vestibular Dysfunction.")

**Prognosis.** The symptoms slowly resolve over 6 weeks to 3 months, but clients can complain of persistent imbalance, motion intolerance, and headache related to decrease in the natural motion of the head. In some cases, decreased functional use of the vestibular mechanism develops and is related to excess caution on uneven surfaces, dizziness that is more easily provoked, an overall decrease in activity level, or avoidance of activity that may cause dizziness. These individuals may complain of dizziness with quick head turns and imbalance in the dark. Often, visual motion sensitivity will develop. These conditions are justification for further rehabilitation. (See"Special Implications for the Therapist 38.1: Vestibular Dysfunction.")

## Endolymphatic Hydrops and Ménière Syndrome

### Definition and Overview

Endolymphatic hydrops is a disorder of the membranous inner ear, with overaccumulation of endolymph and resulting compromise of the perilymphatic space. The overaccumulation of the endolymph often occurs in an episodic manner as a result of either a sudden increase in the secretory function of the stria vascularis or spontaneous obstruction of the endolymphatic sac. Hydropic distension then causes mechanical deflection of the macula and crista of the otoliths and semicircular canals, respectively, resulting in vestibular hair cell depolarization and the sensation of vertigo. Long-term changes to the neurosensory function of the vestibular apparatus may be the consequence of increased hydrodynamic pressure, causing increased vascular resistance, compromised blood flow, and chronic ischemic injury.[2]

Ménière syndrome is thought by many to be a form of endolymphatic hydrops, but the relationship is not absolute and cannot be proven. The symptoms of Ménière syndrome, however, lead to this hypothesis, and treatments are directed toward the control of fluids. The diagnosis of Ménière syndrome is based on symptoms of characteristic episodic vertigo, fluctuating, sensorineural hearing loss, sensation of fullness in the ears, and tinnitus. Tinnitus is an abnormal sound in the ear usually described as a ringing, buzzing, clicking, or crackling sound. It is often associated with other abnormal sensations, such as fullness of the ear. Vertiginous attacks are the most debilitating symptom of Ménière syndrome, with intervals between attacks that can be hours or days. Acute attacks can be superimposed on a gradual deterioration in sensorineural hearing in the involved ear, typically in the low frequencies initially. Over time, a reduction in responsiveness of the involved peripheral vestibular system can occur.

### Incidence and Risk Factors

Caucasian women are most prone to Ménière syndrome. Diagnostic criteria have varied across epidemiologic studies, with prevalence rates from 157 per 100,000 persons in England to 46 per 100,000 in Sweden and 7.5 per 100,000 in France. The peak incidence of Ménière syndrome is in the 40- to 60-year-old age group, with a nearly equal female to male ratio (1.3:1). Estimates of symptoms arising in the opposite ear vary from 2% to 50%. Whether the variability in prevalence rates is caused by differences in environment, genetics, or diagnostic criteria is unclear.[161] Familial occurrence of Ménière syndrome has been reported in 10% to 20% of cases. Genetic inheritance plays a role. The mode of transmission appears variable; however, an autosomal-dominant mode of inheritance with increased penetrance has been documented. The incidence of Ménière syndrome is greater in individuals with certain genetically acquired major histocompatibility complexes. Specifically, human leukocyte antigens B8/DR3 and Cw7 have been associated with Ménière syndrome. The etiology for disease in these individuals may be autoimmune.[57]

### Etiology

The cause of endolymphatic hydrops is multifactorial and may be related to fibrosis, atrophy of the sac, obstruction of the endolymphatic duct, infection, or the vascularity in the region of the inner ear. It can also be caused by otosyphilis, or involvement of the inner ear in collagen vascular diseases. Immune responses are likely within the complex, including the endolymphatic sac, related to allergic reactions and histamine. There may be a predisposing viral infection that may cause the inner ear to be more susceptible to changes in thyroid, sodium, or hormone dysfunction. The deficit may also be related to overproduction of endolymph by the stria vascularis.[48] Posttraumatic endolymphatic hydrops can be observed following a blow to the head, a fall, or flexion or extension injury sustained in an automobile accident.

### Pathogenesis

Despite the variety within the etiologic factors, there is a consistent disruption of homeostasis of inner ear fluid. Endolymphatic hydrops may be an epiphenomenon rather than directly responsible for the symptoms. Animal models of endolymphatic hydrops have provided a basic scientific understanding of endolymphatic hydrops, including the mechanical characteristics and the influence of hydrops on inner ear anatomy and function. These studies have shown that endolymphatic hydrops is accompanied by a cascade of subtle biochemical and morphologic alterations, each of which may contribute to the dysfunction.

Pathologic studies of the human sac in the hydrops patient have recorded ischemia and fibrosis around the endolymphatic sac. Alterations in the size of the endolymphatic duct and sac, along with reductions in the lining of these structures, have also been noted in both the diseased and nondiseased inner ears. This supports the theory that an abnormal endolymph drainage system may predispose individuals to the future development of Ménière syndrome. Alterations in endolymph $Ca^{2+}$ has been shown to influence transduction in hair cells, and it is likely that endolymph $Ca^{2+}$ changes contribute to functional losses present in the hydropic cochlea of animals, and possibly in the ears of humans with Ménière disease. These ionic disturbances may be caused by ischemia resulting from changes in local vasculature. It has been suggested that the endolymphatic sacs of patients with Ménière disease have significantly higher vasopressin receptor levels, suggesting that the ears of these patients may be more sensitive to vasopressin.[2] A common vascular mechanism for migraine headaches and Ménière disease has also been proposed. A hydropic state may leave those persons sensitive to stresses to the inner ear.[161]

Deficits are related to the volume and pressure changes within closed fluid systems. The increase in the volume of endolymph causes the membranous labyrinth to progressively dilate until the wall makes contact with the stapes footplate and the cochlear duct fills the entire scala vestibuli, causing both vestibular and cochlear dysfunction. Distension of the otoliths can put pressure on the ampulla, creating the sensation of spinning that is characteristic of acute unilateral dysfunction.

### Clinical Manifestations

The typical attack of hydrops related to Ménière syndrome is experienced as an initial sensation of fullness of the ear, a reduction in hearing, and tinnitus followed by a rotational vertigo, postural imbalance, nystagmus, and nausea. The vertigo may last from 30 minutes to 24 hours. The symptoms abate over time, and the individual regains the ability to maintain balance. However, he or she may still experience a sense of disequilibrium. Hearing slowly returns, but over time there may be a permanent loss of hearing. Tinnitus is common in hydrops and is commonly described as a low-pitched roaring or similar to a seashell noise. Box 38.5 gives some of the characteristics consistent with the diagnosis of Ménière syndrome.

## MEDICAL MANAGEMENT

**DIAGNOSIS.** The complaints of vertigo, hearing loss, and tinnitus do not automatically confirm a diagnosis of endolymphatic hydrops or Ménière syndrome. The definitive vertiginous attack is sudden in onset with nausea and vomiting and lasts 20 minutes but abates by 24 hours. Typically, any movement during an attack aggravates the vertigo. The presence of neurologic signs or symptoms such as syncope, visual aura, and motor weakness suggest another diagnosis. Disorders that can present with similar symptoms include migraine, acoustic neuroma, perilymphatic fistula, dehiscence of the superior semicircular canal, labyrinthitis, autoimmune inner ear disorder, and MS.

An audiogram, or test of hearing, typically demonstrates low-frequency hearing loss on one side. Perceived hearing loss can be difficult to verify without audiometry, especially during an exacerbation of tinnitus or aural pressure. Improvement in audiograms can reflect better control of fluid, and decreases in hearing are suggestive of progressive disease.[161]

Electrocochleography may provide objective evidence of the presence of endolymphatic hydrops in the presence of large summating potentials. However, the diagnostic utility of the test is limited by the variability of the ratio both in individuals with hydrops and in normal individuals. The results should be used in the face of other subjective history. Fig. 38.15 shows typical ECoG responses. It is also important to note that elevation of SP/AP is not specific to Ménière syndrome. Similar ECoG abnormalities have been reported in patients with perilymph fistula and superior semicircular canal dehiscence. See section below.

**Treatment.** Acutely, treatment of endolymphatic hydrops is focused on symptom management. Although hospitalization is rarely required, intravenous fluids may be required in the emergency department. Vestibular suppressants can be used for symptomatic control, although they can delay patients' recovery by suppressing the adaptive response if used over a longer interval. Salt restriction and lifestyle modification are typically suggested as a first course. Levels of recommended salt restriction vary; but figures often quoted range from 2 g per 24 hours down to 1 g per 24 hours, with the suggestion to pay close attention to food labeling and to avoid processed foods.

Diuretics are used to reduce the amount of endolymphatic hydrops by reducing the extracellular fluids in the body. Hydrochlorothiazide is the most widely advocated, although furosemide and spironolactone have been used as well.

Betahistine has been used as a treatment because of its theoretic vasodilatory effects on the blood supply to the inner ear, as cochlear vascular insufficiency may result from autonomic dysfunction in hydrops. Steroid perfusion can influence sodium and fluid dynamics in the inner ear because of their mineralocorticoid properties. This effect may be particularly advantageous for those patients with bilateral involvement.

Box 38.5

**SOME CHARACTERISTICS CONSISTENT FOR THE DIAGNOSIS OF MÉNIÈRE SYNDROME**

The diagnosis of Ménière syndrome is primarily based on the medical history. According to established guidelines, a definite diagnosis requires the following:

- Two or more definitive episodes of spontaneous rotational vertigo lasting at least 20 minutes
- Low-frequency sensorineural hearing loss documented by audiometry
- Tinnitus or aural fullness in the affected ear
- Exclusion of other causes for the symptoms

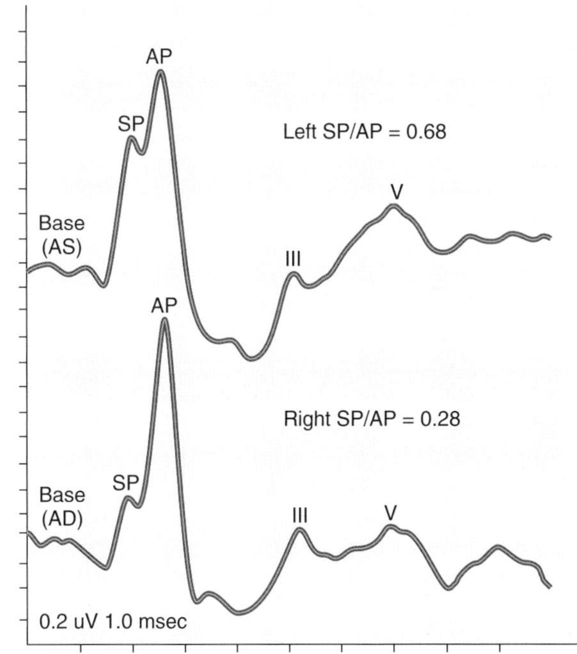


**Figure 38.15**

Click-evoked ECoG response recorded with a hydrogel tympanic membrane surface electrode in a patient with Ménière disease in the left ear. This response was elicited by an alternating click stimulus presented at 85 dB non-Hodgkin lymphoma. The SP and AP are measured from the prestimulus baseline. Note the increased SP in the diseased left ear. *SP,* Summating potential; *AP,* cochlear nerve action potential. (From Adams ME, Heidenreich KD, Kileny PR: Audiovestibular testing in patients with Meniere's disease, *Otolaryngol Clin North Am* 43(5):995-1009, 2010.)

The Meniett device[113] is minimally invasive and nondestructive, providing stimulation to the inner ear. It is based on the observation that pressure changes applied to the inner ear result in beneficial changes in the symptoms. The Meniett device applies pulses of pressure to the inner ear through a ventilation tube. A treatment cycle takes 5 minutes and is repeated 3 times a day.

When there are intractable symptoms, administration of an aminoglycoside such as gentamicin to the inner ear can control symptoms. Systemic administration, transtympanic injection, and the placement of Gelfoam soaked in aminoglycoside into the round window niche have been used. Surgical treatment to restore normal endolymph volume includes endolymphatic decompression procedures.[41]

**Prognosis.** The natural history of endolymphatic hydrops and Ménière syndrome is highly variable. Clusters of attacks may be separated by periods of long remission. Balance function between attacks can be normal. Over time, there is a gradual decline in the function of the vestibular system, and complaints of imbalance and mild symptoms related to a unilateral dysfunction become common. The attacks increase in frequency in the first years and then decrease. Ménière syndrome initially affects only one ear but can progress to a bilateral condition in some individuals. If bilateral involvement has not occurred within 5 years of onset of disease in the first ear, then there is less likelihood of developing bilateral involvement.

The hearing loss in Ménière syndrome is a fluctuating, low-frequency sensorineural loss early in the clinical course. Eventually, the loss becomes irreversible, often progressing in severity with involvement of higher frequencies and loss of speech discrimination.

An estimated 2% to 6% of patients with Ménière syndrome of long duration can experience "drop attacks" known as otolithic crisis of Tumarkin, characterized by being abruptly thrown to the ground without loss of consciousness and with little or no vertigo.[65]

SPECIAL IMPLICATIONS FOR THE THERAPIST 38.4

*Endolymphatic Hydrops*

Endolymphatic hydrops leads to great insecurity. If an acute attack occurs in social situations, it understandably can lead to social phobic reactions, even if no psychopathologic predisposition is present. Anxiety arises from the unpredictable pattern of endolymphatic hydrops, the feeling of being overcome by the attacks and having to stop all activity until the attacks subside. The concern over not finding a safe place during an acute attack and negative reactions from observers causing embarrassment can cause sufferers to withdraw from social life. When invasive treatments such as gentamicin injections or sac decompression are performed, it increases the complexity of the disorder. Severe cases of Ménière syndrome ultimately can lead to reactive depressive disorders. Antidepressant medications may be helpful. The therapists' role is critical to providing education, support, and the treatment of any progressive loss of vestibular function. Physical therapy is often halted when a patient begins a course of diuretics or steroids, then resumes as the system becomes more stable.

## Autoimmune Ear Disease

### Overview and Definition

Autoimmune ear disease (AIED) is rapidly progressive bilateral sensorineural hearing loss that responds to the administration of immunosuppressive therapy. The disease is typically characterized by symptoms of pressure and tinnitus in the ears, with or without dizziness. Autoimmune disease can affect the inner ear with resultant vertigo, sensorineural hearing loss, aural fullness, and tinnitus.

### Clinical Manifestations

AIED mimics Ménière disease, with fluctuating hearing loss and vestibular dysfunction. Symptoms usually progress over weeks or months, and there is often a known systemic immune disease, such as rheumatoid arthritis. The otologic symptoms may occur as a direct assault by the immune system or as the deposition of antibody-antigen complex in the capillaries or basement membranes of inner ear structures. Approximately 50% of those testing positively for AIED have positive serum antibody tests. The Western blot is currently the most widely reported diagnostic tool used in the diagnosis of AIED, with autoantibodies directed against the 68-kilodalton protein.[10]

### Treatment

Typical patients with AIED are managed medically with corticosteroids at the lowest dose that prevents fluctuating hearing. Most patients achieve mild recovery of sensorineural hearing loss on corticosteroids. Patients with AIED present with varied symptoms, and some have only vestibular symptoms.[46] In more severe cases, there is report of medical management with methotrexate.[44]

## Perilymph Fistula

### Definition and Overview

Perilymph fistula, an abnormal communication of the inner and middle ear spaces, can cause vertigo. Fistulas commonly occur at the round and oval windows of the middle ear. Attempts to identify the prevalence and characterize auditory and vestibular symptoms have been inconclusive. Some studies report vestibular symptoms as the major presenting complaint, whereas others indicate hearing loss equal to or more common than balance-related symptoms. It is thought that most fistulas result from congenital malformations or prior ear surgery. Damage can also result from pressure applied via the external ear, via the eustachian tube, or by an increase in the pressure of the cerebrospinal fluid.[21]

### Clinical Manifestations

Characteristics of perilymph fistula include easing of symptoms at rest and increases with activity, including the Valsalva maneuver. Barotrauma, violent exercise, heavy lifting, or even sneezing may cause a fistula. Other mechanisms include head trauma or explosive blast. Sensorineural hearing losses vary from an isolated high-frequency loss to a low-frequency or flat one. Speech discrimination test results are not characteristic. Both the pure-tone threshold and speech discrimination scores have been noted to fluctuate. Isolated mild conductive losses have been noted. Vestibular symptoms are also variable and include episodic incapacitating vertigo, equivalent to a Ménière attack, positional vertigo, motion intolerance, or occasional disequilibrium. Disequilibrium after increases in cerebrospinal fluid pressure (e.g., nose blowing, lifting), called *Hennebert sign,* has been noted, as has vertigo after exposure to loud noises, which is known as Tullio phenomenon.

## MEDICAL MANAGEMENT

**DIAGNOSIS.** The inability to reliably predict the presence of a fistula before surgical exploration, as well as the lack of standard criteria for recognizing a fistula intraoperatively, have resulted in confusion and even doubt as to the existence of symptomatic fistulas. Because fistulas have been identified intraoperatively and their repair has resulted in symptomatic and objective improvement, this diagnosis must be kept in mind in the evaluation of the vertiginous patient.

Audiologic tests considered to be helpful in the diagnosis, include electrocochleography. Electrocochleography can demonstrate a larger summating potential due to endolymph/perilymph disequilibrium. However, the test is not sensitive or specific for perilymph fistula. Results of vestibular testing are nondiagnostic, but the most consistent abnormality seen is a unilateral reduced caloric response in the affected ear.

A fistula test is done by introducing positive pressure into the suspected ear, either by rapid pressure on the tragus, compression of the external canal, or use of a pneumatic otoscope, while observing the eyes. A positive fistula sign consists of conjugate contralateral slow deviation of the eyes, followed by three to four beats of nystagmus. Vertigo is usually elicited at the same time. Measuring body sway during pressure on the tympanic eardrum can help make the diagnosis.

**TREATMENT.** Recommendations with suspected inner ear fistula include head elevation during bed rest, laxatives to reduce the risk of increased intracranial pressure, and monitoring of both hearing and vestibular function. In those instances in which hearing loss worsens or vestibular symptoms persist, surgical exploration is warranted.

Intraoperative identification of a fistula, regardless of criteria used, is reported in about 50% of individuals explored. At the time of surgery, the oval and round windows are patched with tissue, such as blood clot, fat, fascia, or absorbable gelatin sponge.[41]

**PROGNOSIS.** The outcome of surgical repair is variable. An appropriate surgical candidate is probably the most significant factor in outcome. Reduction in vestibular-related complaints has been reported in more than 50% of surgeries. Hearing is improved about 25% of the time.

SPECIAL IMPLICATIONS FOR THE THERAPIST 38.5

### *Perilymphatic Fistula*

The therapist can be instrumental in helping to determine the possibility of perilymph fistula. An individual who is compliant with prescribed exercise but lacks progress over time and reports or demonstrates fluctuating symptoms and status of balance may be suspect for possible fistula. It is important to maintain close contact with the physician, as these individuals become very frustrated and may not follow through with medical attention. Vestibular therapy should be continued after surgery, as good recovery is expected. Often the physician is uncertain whether the patient's complaints are because of stable vestibular disease with inadequate central compensation or by unstable labyrinthine function. In this setting, a trial of vestibular rehabilitation is appropriate and assists in the diagnosis by clarifying this important distinction. Failure to improve with vestibular rehabilitation lends further credibility to the diagnostic impression that the lesion is unstable or progressive. It is then suitable to proceed with appropriate surgical management if the symptoms are severe enough to warrant the procedure, and they emanate from the end organ.

## Superior Semicircular Canal Dehiscence Syndrome

### Definition and Overview

Superior semicircular canal dehiscence syndrome (SCDS) is a syndrome of vertigo and oscillopsia induced by loud noises or by stimuli that change middle ear or intracranial pressure in patients with a dehiscence of bone overlying the superior semicircular canal. As seen in fistulas, Tullio phenomenon (eye movements induced by loud noises) or Hennebert sign (eye movements induced by pressure in the external auditory canal) develop, and often there is chronic disequilibrium.

### Pathogenesis and Clinical Manifestations

The dehiscence creates a "third mobile window" into the inner ear, thereby allowing the superior canal to respond to sound and pressure stimuli. The evoked eye movements in this syndrome typically align with the affected superior canal. Loud sounds, positive pressure in the external auditory canal, and the Valsalva maneuver can cause characteristic eye movements. A larger length of dehiscence overlying the superior canal (5 mm or greater) can lead to dysfunction in the affected canal when evaluated by responses to rapid head movements in the plane of the superior canal. Visual fixation can suppress the evoked eye movements.[49] Fig. 38.16A shows the schematic representation of superior semicircular canal dehiscence; Fig. 38.16B shows the condition as seen on CT scan.

### Treatment

The window is repaired surgically, with good results. Bilateral superior canal (SC) dehiscence syndrome will result in some degree of oscillopsia after bilateral SCDS surgery, but surgery should provide relief from other SCDS symptoms.[1]

## Ototoxicity

### Overview

Aminoglycoside antibiotics can be ototoxic, with auditory toxicity estimated at 20% and vestibular toxicity affecting 15% of the individuals receiving the drug. There appears to be a genetic vulnerability to ototoxicity from aminoglycoside antibiotics, with a link between mitochondrial DNA mutations and ototoxic hearing loss.[63] Streptomycin and gentamicin specifically target the vestibular end organ. Other members of this group of drugs include kanamycin, tobramycin, amikacin, netilmicin, and sisomicin. Ototoxicity is usually seen in individuals who are given multiple doses over time or one large dose, usually aimed at managing a threatening infection. Damage to the hair cells in the inner ear can result in complete

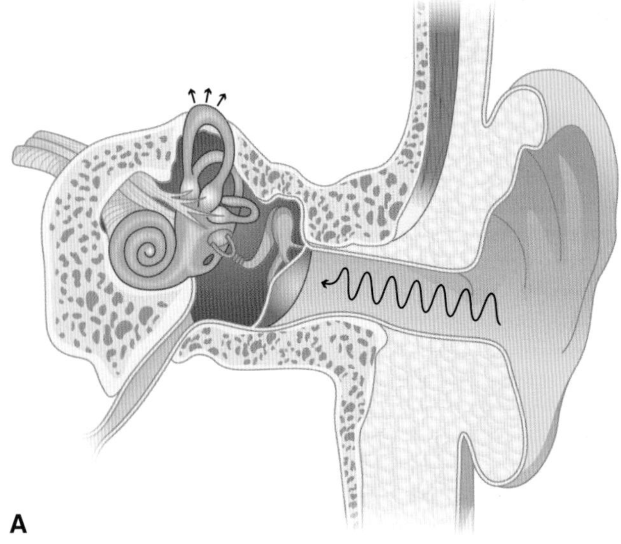


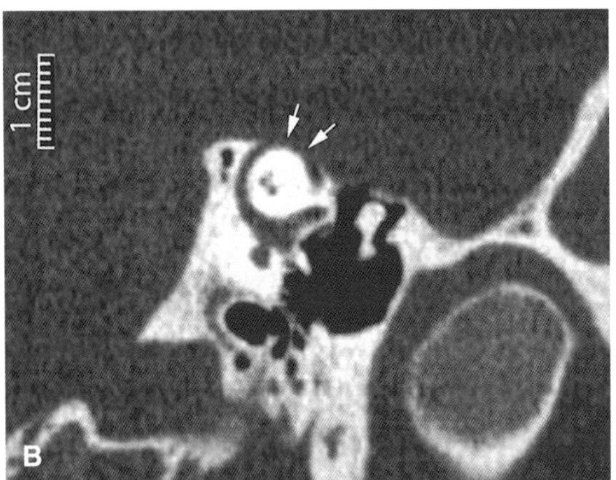


**Figure 38.16**

(A) In superior semicircular canal dehiscence syndrome, sound waves can excite the superior canal because the "third mobile window" created by the dehiscence allows some sound pressure to be dissipated along a route through the superior canal in addition to the conventional route through the cochlea. (B) CT scan demonstrating dehiscence *(arrows)* of the superior canal. (From Cummings CW, Haughey BH, Thomas R, et al: *Cummings otolaryngology: head and neck surgery*, ed 4, St. Louis, 2004, Mosby.)

loss of vestibular function within 2 to 4 weeks after these drugs are given.[73]

### Etiology and Risk Factors

Approximately 3% of an orally administered aminoglycoside is absorbed from the gastrointestinal tract. They are normally injected for severe systemic infections. Penetration of the blood-brain barrier is generally poor, so that aminoglycosides are injected intrathecally to treat meningitis. Aminoglycosides are excreted primarily by the kidney by glomerular filtration, and therefore, high concentrations of drug in the urine may be achieved. Impaired renal function reduces the rate of excretion. Therefore, renal failure is a risk factor for ototoxicity, and dosing of aminoglycosides must be modified to compensate for delayed renal excretion. Measurement of peak and trough serum levels of aminoglycosides provides rough guidelines for therapeutic efficacy but is not an absolute guarantee for prevention of ototoxicity, particularly vestibular ototoxicity.[41]

### Pathogenesis

The aminoglycoside reacts with inner ear tissues to form an active, ototoxic metabolite. The drug in its inactive form combines with iron to form an ototoxic complex. This complex reacts with oxygen to produce reactive oxygen species. These species can then react with various cell components—including the phospholipids in the cell membrane, proteins, and DNA—to disrupt the function, primarily in the outer hair cell. This process can then trigger programmed cell death, resulting in apoptosis. Histopathologic studies demonstrate that the cochlear and/or vestibular hair cells serve as primary targets for injury. Inner hair cells seem to be more resistant to injury than the outer hair cells. In some cases, spiral ganglion cells may be damaged directly by aminoglycosides, without injury to outer hair cells. The damage is primarily bilateral, although there may be a difference in severity of loss between the two inner ear systems.

### Clinical Manifestations and Treatment

One of the most debilitating early symptoms is oscillopsia. Oscillating vision is the illusion of environmental movement caused by excessive motion of images of stationary objects on the retina, known as retinal slip. Oscillopsia of vestibular origin is brought on or accentuated by head movement, due to insufficient VOR. When the vestibular system is unable to keep an image stationary by controlling the movement of the eyes, the visual slip occurs. Severe or complete bilateral loss of peripheral vestibular system function will result in inability to stabilize vision during head movement and produce oscillopsia.[66,69]

### MEDICAL MANAGEMENT

**PROGNOSIS.** It is generally considered that the damage is permanent and that the recovery of function of the vestibular mechanism is limited. Initially, the person will experience severe disability related to sensation of dizziness, oscillopsia, and imbalance. Compensatory strategies using visual references and somatosensory input can improve mobility, taking approximately 6 weeks to become effective. There are some circumstances that will always be problematic, such as walking in the dark, especially on uneven surfaces, or swimming. Night driving or driving in inclement weather should be avoided as vision is less available to provide stability.

## Mal de Debarquement

### Overview and Definition

Mal de debarquement is a syndrome that is named essentially for the symptoms related to "getting off the boat." Mal de debarquement is usually triggered by a long time spent on a ship, such as during a cruise, or by an extended train ride. The complaints occasionally occur after international or extended air travel, especially if there is turbulence. The symptoms of dizziness and disequilibrium that

SPECIAL IMPLICATIONS FOR THE THERAPIST 38.6

*Ototoxicity*

When there is bilateral vestibular loss secondary to ototoxicity or by any other means that is considered permanent, the individual must be "uptrained" in the use of vision and somatosensation. They will essentially be "hanging on" with their eyes. Exercises for individuals with bilateral peripheral vestibular loss must be aimed at substitution of visual and somatosensory cues for the lost vestibular function.[80,144] The ability to maintain stable gaze is critical. Gaze stability exercise incorporates the VOR, facilitating any possible remaining vestibular function. Modifications in eye movements can be used to improve gaze stability with head movement. No mechanism to improve gaze stability will fully compensate for the loss of the VOR, and clients will continue to have difficulty seeing during rapid head movements. Some persons can learn to close their eyes during a turn and then focus quickly on a stable object to regain stability. This technique increases stability because the disruptive visual input is temporarily eliminated.[42] Strategies must be developed when the environment provides less than optimal sensory information, such as the use of an assistive device on uneven surfaces and the use of night lights to provide light at night.

usually subside within hours after exiting a boat, train, or plane become persistent and can last for weeks, months, and even years. Mal de debarquement is also reported as rocking vertigo because the sensation is usually one of rocking back and forth and is experienced to a greater degree at rest than during movement.[24] The individual with Mal de debarquement syndrome (MdDS) would prefer to be moving in a car rather than standing still, which distinguishes it from other disorders that cause abnormal sense of movement. In addition to the rocking sensation, individuals also complain of fatigue, mental clouding, visual motion intolerance, anxiety, tinnitus, and headaches.

Women in their third and fourth decade represent the highest percentage of people reporting symptoms; there has not been a clear relationship established with hormone levels, however, migraine history appears to be more common in the affected group.

### Pathogenesis, Clinical Manifestations, and Treatment

The basis for MdDS is uncertain but seems to be related to abnormal adaptation from one sensory context to another. An association between resting state metabolic activity and functional connectivity between the entorhinal cortex and amygdala has been found in the human disorder of abnormal motion perception.[30]

During passive motion, there may be a mismatch between the vestibular inputs that encode head motion and other sensory and motor cues. The particular movements of a boat on the water, with both a rolling (side to side) and surging (forward) cause high activation and referencing of the vestibular system, and the brain must decrease the use of surface reference at the ankle. Central adaptation may minimize the symptoms provoked by this mismatch, but when the movement ends, the brain must readapt to the stationary environment using an ankle strategy for balance. It has been suggested that patients with MdDS undergo a physiologic adaptive process during passive motion, but for unknown reasons, they do not readily adapt back to the stable environment. This impaired return to baseline results in a perception of motion when the patient is stationary.[105] In other words, somatosensory input is no longer able to override vestibular input for stability. Providing cues outside the vestibular system is helpful, and using somatosensory weighting to provide cues about position in space appears to help the system to recalibrate. Vestibular suppressants or other medications directed at the vestibular system do not improve control of symptoms. Benzodiazepines, such as clonazepam, are of the most benefit.[33] There are some reports of MdDS following use or withdrawal from serotonergic medications. The connection here is that serotonin may inhibit glutamate, an excitatory transmitter in the vestibular nucleus.[148]

Studies are underway to determine the use of transcranial magnetic stimulation for the treatment of MdDS.[31] Use of transcranial stimulation may give some insight into the condition, as well as some potential intervention. The assumption that the brain is made up of oscillators, and MdDS occurs after exposure to oscillation (passive movement of the boat), is the basis of this approach.[95] It appears that the neural activity in the brain in individuals who develop MdDS is different from the control population in studies performed. The hypothesis of introducing oscillation through transmagnetic stimulation may be able to uncouple the abnormal functional connectivity associated with MdDS. Ongoing research is targeted toward the most appropriate area of the brain to stimulate.[29]

### Prognosis

This sensation of constant motion at rest can be debilitating in that the person has difficulty managing the symptoms and tends to limit activity or overmedicate to dampen the sensation.[91] Patients with MdDS reported a poor overall quality of life, especially related to role limitations due to physical problems, energy, and emotional problems. Indirect costs of lost wages during the time course add to the equation.[109]

## Neoplasia

### Overview

Primary carcinoma can directly involve the end organ, the middle ear, or the mastoid. Glomus tumors are the most common tumor of the middle ear, arising from the chemoreceptor system of the ninth through twelfth cranial nerves and producing focal symptoms. See Chapter 30 for more information on the type of tumor presented here and information regarding treatment.

Schwann cell tumors arise from the nerve sheath of the vestibular nerve. The term *acoustic neuroma* is commonly used to describe this tumor, especially with regard to surgery. The tumor usually arises from the vestibular component of the nerve rather than the cochlea. Schwannomas

SPECIAL IMPLICATIONS FOR THE THERAPIST 38.7

### *Mal de Debarquement*

Traditional vestibular therapy has not proven beneficial for the treatment of MdDS in most cases. Because the symptoms are related to the abnormal re-adaptation of the somatosensory and vestibular systems, interventions that target the somatosensory system are critical. Passive head motion during exposure to rotating full-field visual surround is a protocol that improved symptoms in some clients.[45]

The high degree of autonomic complaints may reflect an association of the amygdala as part of the processing deficit and may impact self-regulatory systems and disrupt homeostasis. Interventions that include addressing breath patterns, dorsal/ventral vagal integration, meditation, and mindfulness are appropriate. See Chapter 3 for further information on these topics.

are usually small, firm, encapsulated tumors that grow very slowly. They form in the internal auditory canal or cerebellopontine angle and produce symptoms by compressing the nerve. Initial symptoms are usually related to hearing loss. Eventually mild symptoms of dizziness or balance disorders can develop as the tumor increases in size and the ability to adapt to the loss of function is lost. Fig. 38.17 shows the resulting findings on audiogram and imaged with MRI.

Intravestibular lipoma and intravestibular schwannoma are rare tumors occupying the intravestibular space. Patients with intravestibular lipoma or schwannoma complain of hearing impairment, tinnitus, or recurrent rotatory vertigo. Therefore, the clinical practitioner could misdiagnose them with sudden sensorineural hearing loss or Ménière disease. Because delayed diagnosis and treatment could lead to more severe and refractory symptoms, clinicians should be suspicious early.

#### Diagnosis

Recent advancements in imaging diagnostic tools, such as computed tomography and magnetic resonance imaging have facilitated the correct diagnosis of these intravestibular tumors without surgical removal.[35] MRI with gadolinium contrast is used to diagnose these tumors. Surgical removal of schwannoma can be achieved by performing

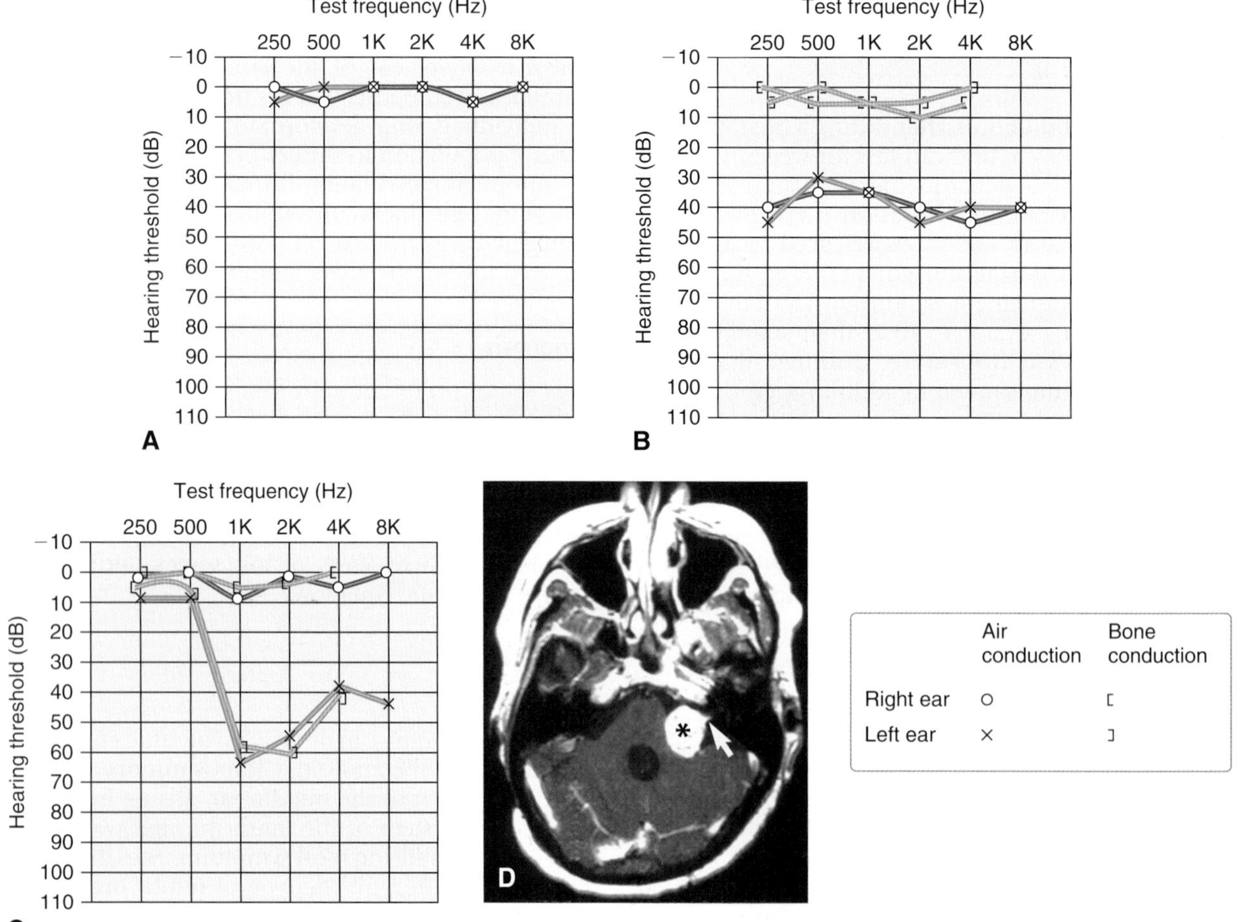


**Figure 38.17**

(A) Normal audiogram. (B) Abnormal audiogram in an individual with bilateral hearing loss. (C) Abnormal audiogram in left ear with loss of both air and bone conduction. (D) Vestibular schwannoma pressing against the left side of the brainstem and into the internal auditory canal. (A, B, and C redrawn from and D from Nolte J: *The human brain: an introduction to its functional anatomy*, ed 5, St Louis, 2002, Mosby.)

middle fossa craniotomy. The translabyrinthine approach is appropriate for tumors up to 3.0 cm. Radiosurgery (a single treatment of high-dose irradiation stereotactically administered) has been used successfully with fewer complications than surgery. There is a chance of progressive loss of hearing in the years following this procedure.

Meningiomas arise from the arachnoid layer in the area of the petrosal and sigmoid sinuses. The tumor is encapsulated and therefore does not invade the neural tissue. Displacement of the cranial nerves, brainstem, and cerebellum is common, causing complaints consistent with compressive damage.

Gliomas arising from the brainstem grow slowly and progressively disrupt the brainstem centers, invading the vestibular and auditory systems in 50% of cases.[38] Gliomas arising in the cerebellum are relatively silent until there is compression of the brainstem or obstruction of cerebrospinal fluid. Medulloblastomas, which occur primarily in children and adolescents, are rapidly growing tumors of the vermis and hemispheres of the cerebellum.

Metastatic neoplasms involve the vestibular and auditory functions primarily through involvement of the temporal bone. The internal auditory canal is a frequent site of metastatic tumor growth. Medical interventions to control growth can cause disruption of the neural tissue and trigger edema in the area of the vestibular system. This can cause acute symptoms; there is usually a good response to vestibular rehabilitation in that case.

## Traumatic Brain Injury and Concussion

### Risk Factors

Complaints of dizziness and imbalance are common after traumatic brain injury (TBI) and are associated with prolonged recovery. There may be direct injury to the vestibular system as a result of the forces encountered during the impact. The vestibular and cochlear nerve can be damaged in the trauma, producing peripheral vestibular disorders. Labyrinthine concussion can trigger BPPV.[112] Posttraumatic endolymphatic hydrops can cause intermittent dizziness (see endolymphatic hydrops above). Perilymphatic fistula is more common after head injury and can be difficult to assess given the fluctuating nature of brain injury. Blasts or explosions are the most common mechanisms of injury in modern warfare, and TBI is a frequent consequence of exposure to such attacks.[142] There is a greater incidence of peripheral vestibular hypofunction in dizzy service members with blast-related TBI relative to those who do not report dizziness.[10,141]

### Pathogenesis

Direct damage of the vestibular nuclei or cerebellar connections can cause persistent and disabling positional dizziness.[7,99] Brainstem or midbrain damage involving the vestibular nuclei can create inability to integrate somatosensation, visual, or vestibular input. In this case, the individual will often choose to decrease the use of the vestibular system by limiting head motion and using predominantly visual or somatosensory cues for balance. The ability of the vestibular system to perform is further decreased by general lack of challenge. Then when the vestibular system is stimulated during daily activity, there is a sensation of dizziness and loss of postural stability. (See Chapter 33, "Traumatic Brain Injury," for more complete information on the pathology of brain injury.)

**SPECIAL IMPLICATIONS FOR THE THERAPIST 38.8**

### *Vestibular Dysfunction in Traumatic Brain Injury and Concussion*

The individual with TBI may have more difficulty providing a clear history and may be plagued by other issues such as photophobia, hyperacusis, and visual hypersensitivity. Because of the damage to the central mechanisms that are necessary for the adaptation of vestibular impairment, recovery can take up to three times as long as would otherwise be expected.

Central nervous system adaptation for vestibular disorders requires the use of vision and somatosensory references to recover function. As the vestibular system becomes more efficient, the need for substitution of the other systems should decrease. In both moderate and mild brain injury, this return to normal reliance on the vestibular system is often limited. Persistent overdependence on vision or somatosensory information can create inefficient strategies and dependency patterns (see Box 38.2). The patient with visual dependence will rely on vision and will have abnormal increases in sway or instability when the eyes are closed. Instability or loss of balance can result in the presence of visual stimulation created by pursuits and optokinetic stimulation. There is often a complaint of dizziness when the eyes are closed, or when walking in the dark. Avoidance of activity during excessive visual stimulation is common.

Somatosensory dependence is often seen as overdependence on an ankle strategy when a hip strategy would be more appropriate. This locks the head to the body and reduces the normal trunk sway during balance on a compliant or narrow surface, or when tested on a tilting surface. This dependence will limit function on uneven surfaces, hills and ramps. Somatosensory dependence leads to excessive activity of the muscles of the neck and trunk, will limit mobility, and can contribute to neck and back pain.

Visual hypersensitivities are a very common complaint early in the recovery and may persist if the visual system is allowed to remain dominant. Intolerance to visual stimulation in the environment, especially with electronics, can be debilitating. Intervention to activate appropriate vestibular dominance in the face of visual dependency and visual hypersensitivity is critical throughout recovery.[4,110,112,144,147]

Cervical flexion-extension injury is a common comorbid condition with concussion and may limit the ability to perform therapy involving head motion. There is often a cervicogenic component to the dizziness that may be related to both cervical and ocular control. Proprioceptive disruption is thought to be the primary cervical spine contribution to disturbances of sensory conflict relating to vestibular and oculomotor function following concussion.[157]

With the onset of legislation regarding the determination of return to play after sports-related brain injury, the physical therapists' knowledge of the critical components of injury and recovery are paramount.[130]

## Persistent Postural-Perceptual Dizziness (PPPD)

### Overview

Persistent postural-perceptual dizziness (PPPD or 3PD) is a syndrome that unifies key features of what was known as chronic subjective dizziness, phobic postural vertigo, and related disorders. PPPD describes a common chronic dysfunction of the vestibular system and brain that produces persistent dizziness, nonspinning vertigo, and/or perceived unsteadiness. The disorder constitutes a long-term maladaptation to a neuro-otologic, medical, or psychological event that triggered vestibular symptoms and is believed to be a specific complication to healing following an inner ear crisis. Clients often develop secondary functional gait disorder, anxiety, avoidance behavior, and severe disability.

### Etiology and Risk Factors

Clients will usually describe an initial event of vertigo or unsteadiness related to a vestibular condition such as BPPV, vestibular neuritis, or vestibular migraine. PPPD has also been documented in association with migraine, concussion, primary anxiety, panic attacks, dysautonomia, or an acute medical crisis that disturbs postural stability orthostasis or syncope. Prior anxiety or neurotic personality types appear to increase the likelihood of developing PPPD following an acute vestibular condition.[13,150] Increased levels of distress measured using the Hospital Anxiety and Depression Scale (HADS) in clients with chronic symptoms suggest that the emotional status of clients may contribute to prolongation of dizziness symptoms from the acute phase. There is also interest in the possibility of inherited vulnerabilities in sensory processing that may underlie PPPD. Brain imaging research studies are showing some distinct areas of decreased functional connectivity during fMRI.[86,134] These findings may lead to a greater understanding of the changes in neuronal function and lead to new intervention strategies.

### Pathogenesis

In response to the initial event of vertigo or unsteadiness, the client develops appropriate acute adaptation responses including a stiff posture, high dependency on visual and somatosensory inputs, and high vigilance and awareness of environmental threats, surfaces changes, and vestibular sensations. However, when the acute phase of the vertigo event has resolved, the client's system fails to stop using these compensatory strategies, creating a cycle of maladaptation. As a result, the central cortical processing mechanisms fail to modulate postural reactions and vestibular sensations, creating distorted processing of afferent input and incorrect perception of imbalance. Clients become hyperaware of differences between predictive versus actual postural responses, which increases their conscious effort to hold themselves stable. These responses contribute to a sensation of dizziness, neck stiffness, functional gait disturbances, and fear and avoidance behaviors.[128]

Vestibular disorders have an influence on autonomic regulation. Following a vertigo episode, an individual may experience abnormal manifestations of arousal, with exaggerated startle response, hypervigilance, sleep disturbance, and irritability. On the opposite spectrum there is detachment, estrangement, and numbing of emotions. An individual may experience other autonomic symptoms, such as heart palpitations, fainting spells, and chronic fatigue. As central neurologic links are found to exist between the vestibular and autonomic systems, it is hypothesized that dizziness and panic symptoms may have a common neuroanatomic basis.

### Diagnosis

Diagnostic tests and conventional imaging are usually negative in PPPD. Therefore, the diagnosis of PPPD is made when the client meets all positive diagnostic criteria[128] based on their history and symptom description. The client must report dizziness, unsteadiness, and/or nonspinning vertigo on most days for greater than 3 months. These symptoms typically get worse when the person is standing upright, actively moving, or passively moving in a car. A client with PPPD also describes increased symptoms and poor tolerance in visually complex and moving environments such as crowds, grocery stores, airports, and theaters. Clients will additionally avoid activities that normally trigger dizziness, such as activities that involve head spins or sudden changes in motion.[149]

### MEDICAL MANAGEMENT

Once recognized, PPPD can be managed with effective communication and tailored treatment strategies, including specialized physical therapy, serotonergic medications, and cognitive-behavioral therapy.[84,94] Providers should educate clients about PPPD as a common, treatable condition. Medical[136] management of PPPD includes the use of low dose selective seratonin reuptake inhibitors (SSRI/SNRI)[151] to reduce dizziness and unsteadiness. A positive response to medication is typically seen in 8 to 12 weeks and is usually continued for at least one year, if effective.[128] Physical therapy interventions should include exposure to optokinetic and visual stimulation, motion desensitization, and recalibration of the somatosensory reference. Physical therapy exercises for individuals with PPPD should be started and progressed more slowly than for those with other vestibular conditions.[156] Management of the autonomic phenomenon through interventions that decrease the fight-or-flight response can increase tolerance to the adaptation process.

**PROGNOSIS.** Early diagnosis of PPPD and a systematic treatment plan that includes patient education, vestibular rehabilitation, cognitive and behavior therapies, and medication has been shown to reduce morbidity, prevent further chronicity, and improve potential for long-term remission.[137]

SPECIAL IMPLICATIONS FOR THE THERAPIST 38.9

*Persistent Postural-Perceptual Dizziness*

Individuals who are predisposed to anxiety and panic reactions can interpret a physical sensation, such as dizziness, or a physical symptom of illness as catastrophic or a sign of a severe and threatening illness. This can result in an escalated anxiety or panic reaction. This anxiety reaction leads to a further increase in the level of autonomic nervous system arousal, leading to panic and, in some, fear of death. When this symptom complex is joined by episodes of hyperventilation, with the corresponding physical consequences, such as paresthesia resulting from alkalosis, an increase in feeling of dizziness, and presyncope, this cycle can escalate further. Unexpected dizziness creates a feeling of helplessness and can trigger typical anticipation anxiety and phobic avoidance behavior. Avoidance behavior usually means avoiding body movements, thereby causing sensory integration deficits. The symptoms persist, made worse by the anxious introspection, ultimately becoming chronic. Identification and explanation to the client are the key components of providing the correct intervention. Recognizing how autonomic nervous system responses can be modified is critical. Mindfulness that incorporates breathing can be effective in managing the exacerbation of symptoms. As the autonomic nervous system moves toward normalization, physical therapists can be instrumental in reintegrating sensory references. Chapter 3 describes the phenomenon related to the dysfunction related to PPPD.

## Comorbid Disorders with Vestibular Consequences

### Congenital Vestibular Loss

Events before birth can cause loss of vestibular function and are related to genetics or intrauterine infection, intoxication, or anoxia. Rubella and cytomegalovirus are responsible for most cases. Thalidomide, no longer commonly used, can cause loss of vestibular function.[56]

### Vascular Disease

Vertebrobasilar insufficiency is a common cause of vertigo in persons older than 50 years. This is often due to atherosclerosis of the vertebral and basilar arteries. Ischemia confined to the labyrinthine artery distribution results in infarction of the vestibular labyrinth and cochlea. Ischemia can also cause vertigo without hearing loss. A vascular loop compressing the eighth cranial nerve can cause vertigo, tinnitus, and hearing loss. Spontaneous hemorrhage into the inner ear, resulting in vertigo and hearing loss, mainly occurs in persons with underlying bleeding disorders. Leukemia is the most common disorder associated with labyrinthine hemorrhage.

Cerebellar infarction simulating vestibular neuritis is more common than previously thought. Early recognition of the pseudo-vestibular neuritis of vascular cause may allow specific management. Infarcts located dorsolateral to the fourth ventricle can cause interruption of the vestibular nuclei-archicerebellar loop, which seems to be responsible for central paroxysmal positional vertigo.[83]

Vestibular dysfunction is a common component with brainstem stroke and may respond to intervention. See Chapter 32 for a more complete description of these stroke syndromes.[7]

### Vestibular Migraine

A type of migraine headache that results in symptoms of dizziness is associated with vascular changes in the area of the vestibular apparatus and is common in both children and adults. (See Chapter 37 for the full description of vestibular migraine.) Approximately 30% of the population with migraine report episodic vertigo, in some cases during the headache-free period.

The aura or even the primary symptom of migraine may be dizziness. Diagnosis of the vestibular variant of migraine is based on the episodic nature, with the specific reports of one or more of the following: spontaneous vertigo, visual motion hypersensitivity, sensation of disrupted spatial orientation, head motion dizziness often with nausea, and occasional head position dizziness without evidence of BPPV. Recognition of triggers, history of migraine, and combination of dizziness with the other typical prodromes of migraine, including photophobia, nausea, and vestibulo-cochlear symptoms of tinnitus and sensitivity to sound can help identify migraine.[166] Symptoms are of moderate or severe intensity. Duration of acute episodes is limited to a window of between 5 minutes and 72 hours.[103] Younger to middle-age females are affected most, often with a history of motion sickness, or family history of migraine.[15,34]

There seems to be more pathology in the VEMP circuitry in migraineurs than in healthy controls, causing more sensitivity for motion triggers.[17] VEMP asymmetry is more common in individuals with Ménière disease than vestibular migraine.[154]

### Metabolic Disorders

When vascular and nerve changes associated with diabetes mellitus occur in the area of the peripheral or central vestibular system, symptoms may develop. Loss of proprioceptive input and visual degeneration will further exacerbate the sense of disequilibrium. Metabolic disorders affecting the resorption of bone, such as *otosclerosis* and *Paget disease*, may develop to the point of causing degeneration of the labyrinths or nerves, resulting in vertigo and dizziness.

### Allergies

Adverse reactions to foods and chemicals have been recognized as important etiologic agents in allergy. Otolaryngologic allergists address the clinical aspects of food sensitivity and dizziness after exposure to specific chemicals. There is clinical evidence of the relationship of dizziness with food allergies.[102,121]

### Aural Cholesteatomas

Aural cholesteatomas are cysts of the middle ear or mastoid arising from squamous epithelial lining, containing keratin. Cholesteatomas erode the temporal bone and may be congenital or acquired. The cholesteatoma can cause resorption of the adjacent bone by a process of pressure erosion. This process can cause damage to the labyrinths and result in vestibular dysfunction. Annual incidence in children is 3 per 100,000 and 12.6 per 100,000 in adults. The diagnosis of aural cholesteatoma is made on otoscopic examination, including endoscopic and microscopic evaluation or surgical exploration. Special imaging procedures, such as high-resolution CT scanning and MRI, may suggest the presence of cholesteatoma within the temporal bone and may be used to complement the clinical examination. High-resolution CT scanning is useful for operative planning and is recommended for all revision mastoid operations. The symptoms of cholesteatoma vary; some cholesteatomas are asymptomatic, whereas others become infected and rapidly cause bone destruction.

### Malignant External Otitis

Malignant external otitis, an infection affecting older people with diabetes or immunosuppression, begins in the external auditory canal and spreads to the temporal bone, putting pressure on the facial nerve or the surrounding nerves.

The most common intracranial complication of otitic infections is *extradural abscess*, a collection of purulent fluid between the dura mater and bone of the middle or posterior fossa. Spread of the infection across the dura from the epidural space may result in thrombophlebitis of the lateral venous sinus, subdural abscess, meningitis, and brain abscess.

In some cases the damage is temporary, as in serous labyrinthitis, and vestibular and auditory function return to varying degrees. Permanent damage is possible when the infection causes damage to the structures of the labyrinth or the eighth cranial nerve. When the membranous labyrinth becomes permanently damaged, endolymphatic hydrops may result (see "Ménière Disease" above) and the symptoms can become episodic.

Malignant external otitis in the mastoid bone is a major clinical problem. It often occurs in persons with a chronic illness, such as diabetes, or a malignancy who are receiving broad-spectrum antibiotics. The infection enters the middle and inner ear via the nasal sinuses. The infection can spread into the intracranial cavity and create thrombosis of the cerebral arteries. The eighth cranial nerve can be affected along with surrounding cranial nerves in the presence of basilar meningitis.[12]

## REFERENCES

To enhance this text and add value for the reader, all references are included in the enhanced ebook on Student Consult that accompanies this textbook. The reader can view the reference source and access it online whenever possible.

# CHAPTER 39

# The Peripheral Nervous System

ROBYN GISBERT • KENDA S. FULLER

## OVERVIEW

The peripheral nervous system (PNS) is composed of 31 pairs of spinal nerves that attach to the spinal cord and 10 pairs of cranial nerves that attach to the brainstem. There are 12 pairs of cranial nerves, two of which (the optic and olfactory) attach to the telencephalon and are considered part of the central nervous system (CNS).[183] The PNS serves to link the CNS to muscles for movement, and provides information back to the CNS about both internal and external conditions. Disruption of PNS function can range from a localized response that disables a single segment of an extremity to conditions that progressively degrade a person's quality of life and limit ability to work. Both the somatic and autonomic nervous systems (ANS) can be affected by PNS pathology. Although sensory loss and weakness are easily recognized hallmarks of a peripheral lesion, autonomic symptoms in the same nerve distribution may also be noted, such as lack of normal skin wrinkling and cessation of sweating in the affected area. Furthermore, cardiac irregularities and circulatory problems may coexist with weakness and need to be identified properly in relationship to the PNS injury or disorder. The connections between the PNS and the CNS are complex, and in part responsible for conditions of central sensitization that result in changes to both systems that are both difficult to identify and challenging to determine appropriate interventions.

As a continuation of the description of the nervous system from Chapter 28, it is important to recall the pertinent anatomic components related to the PNS. Cell bodies of peripheral motor neurons are located within the spinal cord and brainstem, whereas those of peripheral sensory neurons reside in ganglia located outside the CNS in the periphery. Cell bodies of ANS neurons reside in the brainstem and spinal cord, and within ganglia that lie outside the CNS. Axons of PNS neurons extend from the cell bodies to form peripheral and cranial nerves (Fig. 39.1). The peripheral nerves are covered and protected by the extension of the meninges.

The *epineurium*, an extension of the dura mater, creates a substantial covering around the nerve trunks, providing tensile strength through the longest part of the nerve, and then becomes thinner around the smaller branches. It can continue to form encapsulated endings such as Meissner corpuscles.

The *perineurium* extends not only the form but also the function of the arachnoid covering, providing a blood–nerve barrier, and continues as the capsule of some nerve endings, such as Pacinian corpuscles, muscle spindles, and Golgi tendon organs. In some areas, the perineurium is open ended, and can allow toxins and viruses to gain access to the nervous system. The *endoneurium* surrounds individual fibers and may contribute to directing the regrowth of nerve fibers after injury.[178]

The diameter of a nerve is associated with function; larger fibers conduct faster than smaller fibers. The fiber type involved in the injury or dysfunction will contribute to the constellation of symptoms, such as weakness or the type of sensory deficit. The surface of an axon itself is formed by a phospholipid membrane called the *axolemma*. Lying between the axolemma and the endoneurium are specialized glial cells called Schwann cells. In large-diameter axons (greater than 1 cm), the Schwann cell receives a signal to wrap its membrane around the axon, thus creating myelin (see Fig. 28.3). Myelin not only provides electrical insulation essential for rapid conduction of the axon potential but also affects axonal properties. The presence of myelin causes sodium channels to cluster at the nodes of Ranvier, thus reinforcing efficient and fast conduction.[135] As in the CNS, myelination patterns affect speed of transmission (Table 39.1). Within a peripheral nerve, only approximately 25% of the individual fibers are myelinated.[80] Schwann cells maintain mitotic capacity, have a role in peripheral nerve regeneration, and are subject to injury both from mechanical and biologic mechanisms.[235]

Normal propagation of the action potential also requires sufficient energy, supplied by a vascular plexus interlaced between connective tissue layers. Each peripheral nerve receives an artery that penetrates the epineurium; this artery's branches extend into the perineurium as arterioles, and branches from the arterioles enter the endoneurium as capillaries. Vessels supplying peripheral nerves appear coiled when a limb is in a shortened position, but uncoiled after movement so that neural vascular supply is not impaired with a limb's normal excursion. This rich vascular supply makes peripheral nerves relatively resistant to ischemia.[207]

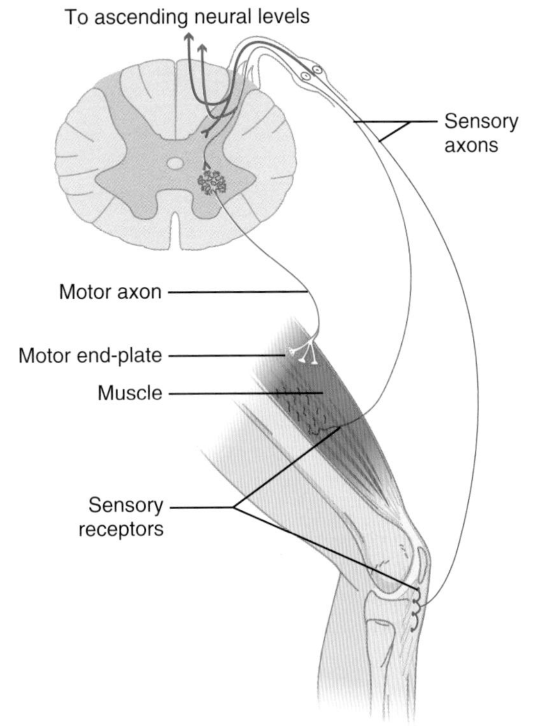


**Figure 39.1**

**Potential sites of involvement in the peripheral nervous system.** Motor: motor neuron cell body, axon, motor end plate, muscle fiber. Sensory: cell body in ganglion, axon, sensory receptor.

## PATHOGENESIS

Trauma, inherited disorders, environmental toxins, metabolic or nutritional disorders may affect the myelin, axon, or the adjacent motor units activated by the peripheral nerve. The severity of the involvement causes changes in the nerve and muscle response, so determines the amount of function lost (Table 39.2).[43] Table 39.3 describes common pathologies and level of involvement.

### Lower Motor Neuron

The cell bodies of lower motor neurons (LMNs) that carry a signal to move are located in the CNS—either in the anterior horn of the spinal cord or the cranial nerve nuclei of the brainstem. Their axons travel through the ventral root to the intended target as a spinal or cranial nerve. When damage occurs to the motor portion of a peripheral nerve, paresis or paralysis will occur in muscles innervated by that nerve distal to the lesion. When spinal motor nerves are impaired, weakness occurs in all the muscles receiving axons from that spinal level (see Fig. 34.9). Deep tendon reflexes (DTRs) are diminished or absent. This is most observable in the distal regions. In the presence of axonal degeneration, rapid atrophy occurs. Prolonged paralysis gives rise to potential secondary complications, such as contracture formation, deformity, and edema. In addition to the peripheral nerve, the motor end plate or muscle itself may be involved in a peripheral disorder. Involvement of muscle, termed *myopathy*, follows a different clinical pattern than nerve. When muscle is involved, the disorder typically is reflected by proximal weakness, wasting, and hypotonia without sensory impairments.

Damage to ANS motor fibers results in alterations of involuntary motor functions, such as heart rate, breathing, and gut motility. Preganglionic fibers are myelinated and can also be affected by segmental demyelination. Figure 28.[17] depicts the sympathetic and parasympathetic divisions of the ANS.

**Table 39.1** Relationship of Myelin Thickness, Conduction Velocity, and Sensory and Motor Fibers

| Myelin | Conduction Velocity | Sensory Fibers | Motor Fibers |
|---|---|---|---|
| Very thick | Very fast | Proprioception (muscle spindle and Golgi tendon organ) | To skeletal muscle fibers (alpha) |
| Thick | Fast | Touch, pressure | To muscle spindle (gamma) |
| Thin | Slow | Touch, temperature | To ANS ganglia |
| None | Very slow | Pain | From ANS ganglia to smooth muscle |

*ANS*, Autonomic nervous system.

**Table 39.2** Relationship of Nerve and Muscle Responses to Disease and Trauma

| Level of Severity | Response to Disease | Response to Trauma | Response of Muscle |
|---|---|---|---|
| Mild | Myelinopathy (segmental demyelination) | Neurapraxia (segmental demyelination) | Paresis/paralysis, no atrophy |
| Severe | Axonopathy (wallerian degeneration) | Axonotmesis (wallerian degeneration) | Paresis/paralysis with atrophy |
| Severe | – | Neurotmesis (wallerian degeneration) | Paresis/paralysis with atrophy |

**Table 39.3** Causes of Peripheral Neuropathies and Myopathies and Their Effects

| | INVOLVEMENT[a] | | | | | |
|---|---|---|---|---|---|---|
| **Cause** | **Axonal Degeneration** | **Demyelination** | **Motor End Plate** | **Muscle** | **Motor** | **Sensory** |
| Charcot-Marie-Tooth disease | X | X | | | X | X |
| Mechanical compression/ entrapment | | | | | | |
| Neurapraxia | | X | | | X | X |
| Axonotmesis | X | | | | X | X |
| Neurotmesis | X | | | | X | X |
| Postpolio syndrome | X | | | | X | |
| Diabetic mellitus | X | X | | | X | X |
| Alcohol | X | X | | | X | X |
| Guillain-Barré syndrome | X | X | | | X | X |
| Toxins | | | | | | |
| Lead | X | | | | X | X |
| Organophosphate | X | X | | | X | X |
| Myasthenia gravis | | | X | | X | |
| Botulism | | | X | | X | |
| Muscular dystrophy | | | | X | X | |
| Inflammatory myopathy | | | | X | X | |
| Steroid-induced myopathy | | | | X | X | |
| Overuse myopathy | | | | X | X | |
| Aging | X | X | X | X | X | X |
| AIDS/HIV (including associated vasculitis) | X | X | | | X | X |
| Vitamin $B_{12}$ deficiency | X | X | | | | X |
| Chronic renal failure | X | | | | X | X |

*AIDS*, Acquired immunodeficiency syndrome; *HIV*, human immunodeficiency virus.
[a]The Xs indicate the most common types of involvement for each cause.

### Sensory Neuron

Lesions of PNS sensory fibers may occur in the dorsal root ganglion or in the dorsal nerve root proximal to the ganglia. Damage can also be to distal fibers of the peripheral nerve. Loss of sensation will follow a peripheral nerve distribution if that is the anatomic region involved, or it will follow a dermatomal pattern when the spinal nerve, dorsal root ganglia, or cell body has been affected (Fig. 39.2). When sensory ANS fibers are affected there can be abnormal transmission into the CNS relayed from viscera, glands, or smooth muscle. Unconscious sensory functions, such as those mediated by baroreceptors signaling arterial pressure, receptors within organs signaling irritants, distention, or hypoxia, may be affected.

## PERIPHERAL NERVOUS SYSTEM CHANGES WITH AGING

Changes that occur in the PNS may be considered as one component of a continuum that relates to normal growth and development, or the changes may represent a combination of pathologic processes superimposed on the normal aging process. Because of the difficulty of studying human peripheral nerves in vivo, experimental animals have been used to assess the effects of aging.

Age does not affect the size or number of fascicles, but the perineurium and epineurium do thicken with age and the endoneurium often becomes fibrosed with increased collagen. Even with these changes, the cross-sectional area decreases slightly with age as a result of a reduced number of unmyelinated and myelinated fibers. Ventral root motor fibers are more affected than dorsal root sensory fibers. Recall that ventral roots are comprised of motor fibers, and dorsal roots are comprised of sensory fibers. Blood vessels to nerves may become atherosclerotic with aging, and occlusion may contribute to loss of nerve fibers. The prevalence of peripheral neuropathies seen in older people has been attributed to reduced microvascular caliber.[56]

Both the peripheral and central nervous systems are affected by aging. Centrally, there is a reduction in β-endorphin content and γ-aminobutyric acid synthesis in the lateral thalamus and a reduced concentration of γ-aminobutyric acid and serotonin receptors. Peripherally, speed of processing nociceptive stimuli and both C- and Aδ-fiber function also decrease with age, which can lead to corresponding reductions in older adults' ability to sense and respond to "first or initial pain." As a result, older adults may have greater susceptibility to burns and other injuries such as lacerations because they are not as likely to sense the initial nociceptive input.[17]

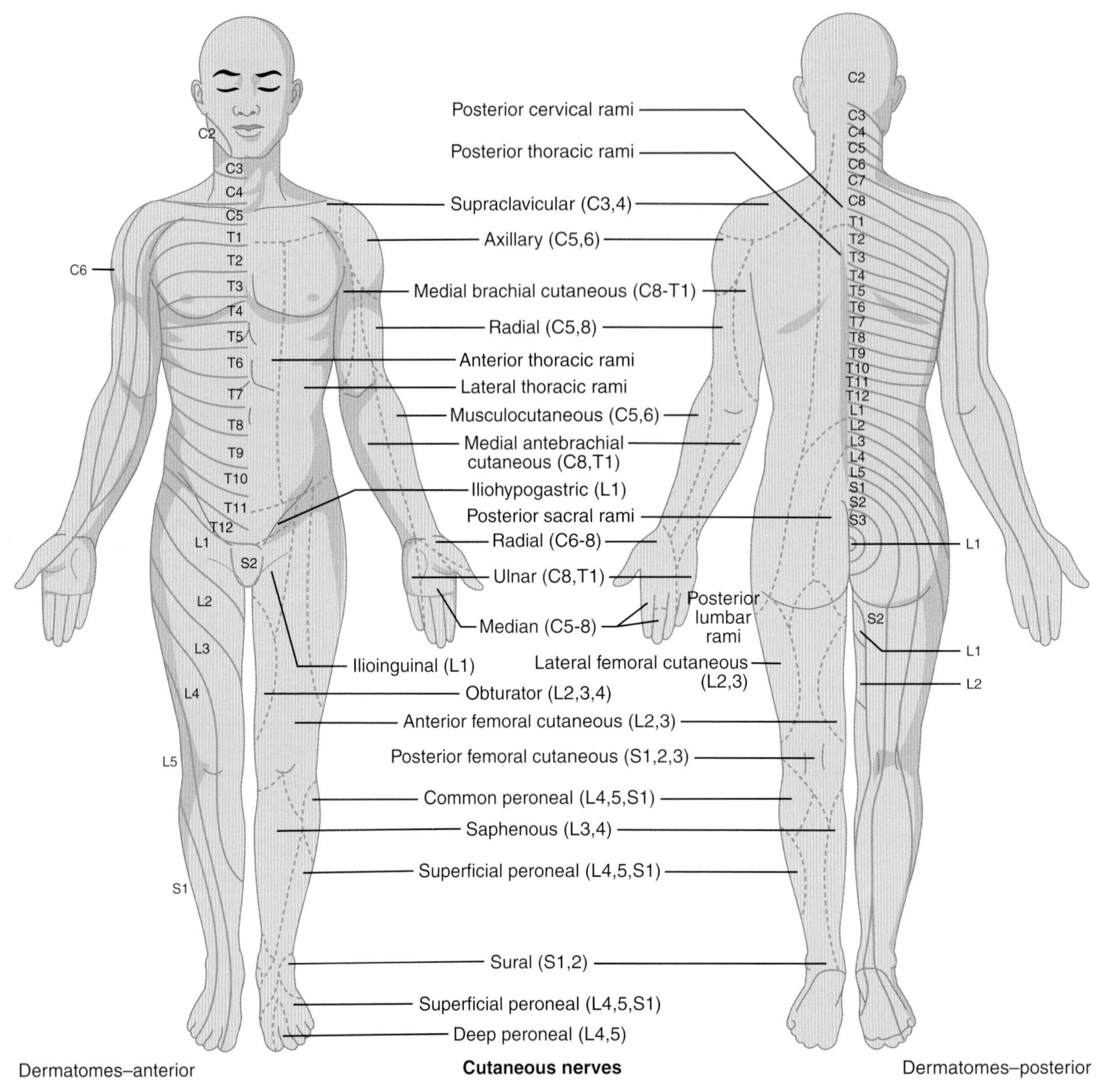


**Figure 39.2**

**Dermatomal (right side of body, anterior and posterior) and peripheral sensory nerve (left side of body, anterior and posterior) patterns.** (From Auerbach PS: *Wilderness medicine*, ed 5, St Louis, Mosby, 2007)

ANS dysfunction is more common in the elderly.[71] Cell bodies show chromatolysis, as well as an accumulation of lipofuscins, representing a diminished ability of the cell to rid itself of toxins. Loss of cell bodies has been observed in the sympathetic ganglia, along with a loss of unmyelinated fibers in peripheral nerves. Sympathetic control of dermal vasculature shows an age-related decline that leads to diminished wound repair efficiency.

When the motor end plate is examined, age-related changes have occurred, but these changes are seen as early as the third decade of life and are not observed in all muscles. When sensory receptors have been evaluated, density and morphology have been found to be altered in the elderly. Altered axonal myelination creates slowing of nerve conduction velocities (NCVs). In addition, the loss of fibers decreases the amplitude of the potential. Decreases in protein production are hypothesized to cause myelin deterioration.[219] When individual myelinated fibers are examined, shorter internodes are seen, suggesting that a demyelinating–remyelinating process occurs with aging. This structural alteration in peripheral nerve myelination may be reflected in diminished appreciation of vibratory sense.

Simultaneous with decreased protein production is a decrease in intraaxonal transport by cytoskeletal elements in the peripheral nerve. Electromyographic (EMG) studies of elderly people without evidence of neurologic disorders of the PNS show loss of motor units, as well as signs of reinnervation. Morphologic changes observed in people older than 60 years of age are manifested by decreased strength and sensory changes.[147] This can have consequences for movement, safety, and quality of life.

Healthy elderly people, with no evidence of neurologic disease, may provide a clinical history suggestive of peripheral neuropathy. This includes numbness and tingling in the hands and feet along with mild, diffuse weakness—especially in the distal muscles of the hand. Sensory alterations may lead to poor balance and gait instability. On examination, sensory thresholds are increased.

The cause of an aging neuropathy can be attributed to a combination of factors. First, loss of both motor and sensory cell bodies; second, a dying-back condition, suggesting neurons can metabolically support a limited number of fibers or receptors, similar to that seen in other systemic neuropathies; and last, over the course of a lifetime, chronic compression of the peripheral nerves or repetitive trauma may have damaged the nerves. All these factors, combined with coexisting medical conditions, atherosclerosis, and nutritional deficiencies, may create this neuropathy of aging. In animal studies, a repetitive task performed by aging rats caused sensorimotor declines that were associated with decreased nerve conduction, and increased proinflammatory cytokines.[58] When the aging PNS is damaged, wallerian degeneration is delayed and regeneration takes longer because secretion of trophic factors is slower than in younger individuals. Density of regenerating axons is less. In a partial nerve injury, collateral sprouting is reduced, further limiting recovery of function.[219]

## DIAGNOSIS OF PERIPHERAL NERVOUS SYSTEM DYSFUNCTION

### Electrodiagnostic Studies

Because the nervous system is the means of signaling from the CNS to the muscle, conduction of the action potential is affected in neuropathies and myopathies. In most disorders, electrophysiologic studies are used to determine where and how the nerve or muscle may be affected. Table 39.4 lists normal values. Although the phenotype of peripheral dysfunction (i.e., physical characteristics/traits) remains unchanged, much of the current research in peripheral nerve pathophysiology is concerned with genetic and molecular changes. Findings in these areas may allow development of treatments aimed at altering cellular function and thereby preserving conduction.

Electromyography (needle EMG) involves the recording of electrical activity within muscles by way of a needle electrode similar to having an electrical microphone at the tip of the needle. Three types of information can be obtained. Healthy muscle at rest should have no spontaneous electrical activity except at the neuromuscular junction. If the muscle is denervated, there will be positive sharp waves and fibrillation potentials. Myotonia, fasciculations, and cramps can also be identified in denervated muscle at rest. With slight exertion of the muscle, motor units around the needle should fire synchronously. Axon damage will result in asynchronous firing with multiphasic or complex patterns. Amplitude of the firing may also represent dysfunction. Muscle damage causes decreased firing; in nerve injury amplitudes in a nerve may be normal above the level of damage and in the case of regeneration after injury, the axon may have spread to other muscle fibers, causing the amplitude to be higher than normal. Increases in number and rate of motor unit firing reflect normal responses to maximum exertion. In muscle disease, the number of units may be increased (hyperrecruitment), whereas in nerve dysfunction, the response to maximum exertion is reduced recruitment.

Nerve conduction study involves placing two electrodes along the length of a nerve. One electrode stimulates the peripheral nerve greater than the threshold values required to cause firing. The second electrode records the characteristics of the generated action potential at a different point than the stimulation. Information is obtained about conduction velocity, wave forms, and amplitude.

Localization of injury can be confirmed, for example determining whether ulnar nerve damage is at the

**Table 39.4** Normal Nerve Conduction Velocities and Distal Latencies[a]

| Nerve | Motor Conduction Velocity (m/s) | Motor Distal Latency (ms) | Motor Amplitude (mV) | Sensory Conduction Velocity (m/s) | Sensory Distal Latency (ms) | Sensory Amplitude (μV) |
|---|---|---|---|---|---|---|
| Median | 63.5±6.2 | 3.49±0.34 | 7.0±2.7 | 56.2±5.8 | 2.84±0.34 | 38.5±15.6 |
| Ulnar | 61.0±5.5 | 2.59±0.39 | 5.5±1.9 | 54.8±5.3 | 2.54±0.29 | 35.0±14.7 |
| Tibial | 48.5±3.6 | 3.96±1.00 | 5.1±2.2 | | | |
| Peroneal | 52±6.2 | 3.77±0.86 | 5.1±2.3 | | | |

**Normal F Wave Values**

| Nerve | Stimulation Site | F Wave Latency to Recording Site (ms) |
|---|---|---|
| Median | Elbow | 22.8±1.9 |
| Ulnar | Above Elbow | 23.1±1.7 |
| Peroneal | Above Knee | 39.9±3.2 |
| Tibial | Knee | 39.6±4.4 |

[a]In general, in the upper extremities, nerve conduction velocity for motor fibers averages about 60 m/s. Investigators have reported values ranging from 45 to 75 m/s. In the lower extremity, the normal range for motor nerve conduction is in the 40 to 50 m/s range. Distal latency is a time value, reported in milliseconds, that it takes for an evoked potential to be propagated along the nerve and recorded from either the muscle (motor) or the skin (sensory).

From Dyck PJ, Thomas PK, eds: *Peripheral neuropathy*, ed 3, Philadelphia, 1993, WB Saunders.

location of the elbow or wrist. LMN versus upper motor neuron (UMN) lesions can be identified if the cause of a motor problem is not clear. The degree of damage (neurapraxia, axonotmesis, or neurotmesis) can be identified. While a clinical exam may not clearly determine the difference between myelin and axon damage, the EMG/nerve conduction study can help to clarify the state of damage. EMG/nerve conduction studies must be performed and considered in concert with the history and examination. Table 39.5 shows the relationship of findings to level of likely involvement.

## CLASSIFICATION OF NERVE INJURY AND NEUROPATHY

Traumatic injury to peripheral nerves from mechanical involvement secondary to compression, ischemia, and stretching can be classified based on the structural and functional changes that result. Seddon[188] divided nerve injury into three categories: neurapraxia, axonotmesis, and neurotmesis. Sunderland[202] divided this classification into five categories, based on the extent of tissue injury.[203] Table 39.6 compares the classification according to Seddon and Sunderland with MacKinnon's modifications. Peripheral nerve injuries are common, and healing potential is widely variable. Treatments range from nonsurgical to surgical and despite much research in this area, it remains unknown what treatments are ideal for full recovery.[38]

### Demyelination: Neurapraxia

Demyelination, or loss of myelin, typically in segments, leaves the axon intact but bare where the myelin is lost. This is called *segmental demyelination*. In this scenario, speed of transmission is decreased, with effects of weakness and loss of sensory conduction. *Neurapraxia* is the temporary failure of nerve conduction in the absence of structural changes, typically the result of blunt injury, compression, or ischemia. It is caused by segmental demyelination, which slows or blocks local conduction of the action potential while conduction of the action potential remains normal above and below the point of compression. Because the axon remains intact, muscle does not atrophy. The result is paresis without degeneration and is usually followed by slow and full recovery of function. When segmental demyelination occurs because of disease, the response may be termed a *myelinopathy*. If segmental demyelination has occurred, molecular signaling to remaining Schwann cells causes them to begin dividing mitotically. Newborn Schwann cells move to envelope the denuded segment of nerve and once these cells are in place they will begin to form myelin.

### Degeneration: Axonotmesis and Neurotmesis

Degeneration occurs in any peripheral nerve disorder that directly affects the axon, including physical injury (crush, stretch, or laceration), as well as disease. *Axonotmesis*

**Table 39.5** Relationship of Electromyographic Findings to Innervation

| Condition | Normal Innervation | Segmental Demyelination | Axonal/Wallerian Degeneration | Myopathy |
|---|---|---|---|---|
| Insertion | Normal insertional noise | Normal insertional noise | Increased insertional noise | Increased insertional noise |
| At rest | Quiet | Quiet | Spontaneous (abnormal) potentials: fibrillation potential, positive sharp wave potential | Quiet, except end stage: fibrillation potentials |
| Minimal contraction | Normal motor unit potential | Affected fibers: no motor unit potential | Affected fibers: no motor unit potential | Low amplitude, polyphasic potential |
| Maximal contraction | Complete interference pattern | Nerve partially affected: decreased interference pattern | Nerve partially affected: decreased interference pattern; nerve completely affected: no interference pattern | Low amplitude–full interference pattern, accomplished with increased frequency of firing and with moderate effort |

**Table 39.6** Nerve Trauma Classifications

| | CLASSIFICATION | | |
|---|---|---|---|
| **Injured Tissue(s)** | **Seddon** | **Sunderland** | **Modification (MacKinnon)** |
| Myelin | Neurapraxia | Grade I | — |
| Myelin, axon | Axonotmesis | Grade II | — |
| Myelin, axon, endoneurium | Neurotmesis | Grade III | — |
| Myelin, axon, endoneurium, perineurium | Neurotmesis | Grade IV | — |
| Myelin, axon, endoneurium, perineurium, epineurium | Neurotmesis | Grade V | — |
| Combination | | | Grade VI |

From Daroff RB: *Bradley's neurology in clinical practice*, ed 6, Philadelphia, 2012, WB Saunders.

occurs when the axon has been damaged, but the connective tissue coverings that support and protect the nerve remain intact. Prolonged compression producing an area of infarction and necrosis can cause axonotmesis. In the presence of disease, Wallerian degeneration creates an axonopathy, which is analogous to an axonotmesis. *Neurotmesis,* the most severe axonal loss, is the complete severance of the axon, as well as the disruption of its supporting connective tissue coverings (endoneurium, perineurium, and/or epineurium) at the site of injury. Neurotmesis can be caused by gunshot or stab wounds or avulsion injuries that disrupt a section of the nerve or entire nerve. When axonal continuity is lost (either axonotmesis or neurotmesis), axons degenerate distal to the lesion. Wallerian degeneration begins immediately after involvement and is completed over a period of a few weeks. The nerve cell swells and undergoes chromatolysis. Ribosomes that normally make protein for the cell disperse throughout the cytoplasm. *Chromatolysis* reflects a change in the metabolic priority of the cell as it switches from daily needs to a repair mode. Distally the axon begins to degenerate and myelin fragments within 12 hours of the lesion. This material is removed by macrophages responding to the inflammatory process. As long as the cell body remains viable, a regenerative process begins with sprouting of a growth cone as soon as new cytoplasm is synthesized and transported down the axon from the cell body. As the growth cone grows, it releases proteases that dissolve material and permit the axon to enter the tissue more easily. Filopodia, which are fingerlike projections extending from the growth cone, sample the environment searching for chemical and tactile cues to guide the regenerating axon; however, because the tactile cues provided by the endoneurium are absent, these fibers may become misguided and form a neuroma. The standard used to anticipate return of function is based on a growth rate of 1 mm a day or an inch a month. In reality, this is an average reflecting the delays that occur while the growth cone crosses the repair site and makes connection with sensory end organs or motor end plate. Growth occurs faster nearer the lesion site (3 mm/day) and slower as the length of the axon increases (1 mm/day).[157]

### Clinical Manifestations

Clinical presentation is correlated to the severity and location of the injury. In any case, flaccid paralysis occurs in muscles distal to the lesion. Rapid atrophy ensues because of loss of the trophic influences of the nerve that innervated the muscle fibers. Sensory function is also lost distal to the lesion.

## MEDICAL MANAGEMENT

**DIAGNOSIS.** History and clinical examination are used to diagnose neurotmesis. In addition, electrophysiologic studies may be performed. EMG will demonstrate the presence of fibrillation potentials and positive sharp waves, indicating denervation of muscle fiber. EMG can be used to determine whether the lesion is complete or partial.

**TREATMENT.** Surgical management is needed to suture the connective tissue bundles together to guide the regenerating growth cone. Various microsurgical techniques (cable and interfascicular grafts) are used to try and direct the axon into the appropriate fascicle by restoring connective tissue continuity. After complete axonal transection, the neuron undergoes a number of degenerative processes, followed by attempts at regeneration. A distal growth cone seeks out connections with the degenerated distal fiber. The current surgical standard is epineurial repair with nylon suture. To span gaps that primary repair cannot bridge without excessive tension, nerve-cable interfascicular autografts are employed. There is much ongoing research regarding pharmacologic agents, plant-derived and synthetic immune system modulators, enhancing factors, and entubulation chambers. Clinically applicable developments from these investigations will continue to improve the results of treatment of nerve injuries.[121] Ideally, a primary repair will be carried out; operative delays lead to shrinkage and fibrosis of the distal connective tissue support structures.[95] Nerve transfer surgery, performed outside the zone of nerve injury, has been suggested for penetrating upper extremity injuries. These procedures occur closer to the motor end plate, thus shortening the interval to reinnervation and optimizing recovery of functional strength.[106]

Other treatments are symptomatic. For the therapist this means splinting to support structures. Use of electrical stimulation to maintain muscle bulk is controversial; recent studies have shown that the chemical signal guiding the nerve (neural cell adhesion molecule) disappears when denervated muscle receives electrical stimulation.[180]

**PROGNOSIS.** Because muscle fibers innervated by the axon depend on the nerve cell body as a source of nourishment or trophic control, when axons degenerate, muscle fibers rapidly atrophy. The potential for regeneration after axonal degeneration is possible as long as the nerve cell body remains viable; new axons can sprout from the proximal end of damaged axons. However, successful functional regeneration requires that the proximal and distal ends of the connective tissue tube are aligned. This can occur in axonotmesis because the connective tissue covering remains intact. In a neurotmesis, without surgical intervention, recovery is less likely because the proximal end of the endoneurium is not approximated to the distal endoneurium. Without surgery, axonal sprouts often enter nearby soft tissue and form a neuroma, or axonal regrowth occurs down the incorrect endoneurial tube, rendering reinnervation nonfunctional.[219] Even with surgical intervention, prognosis for recovery is poor.

Once the axon has established a distal contact either with muscle or sensory receptor, remyelination will begin. When partial axonal degeneration occurs, adjacent noninvolved axons may produce collateral sprouts that will innervate muscle fibers before the damaged axons have time to grow and reinnervate those muscle fibers. This results in an enlarged motor unit for the neuron that has collateral sprouts. Numerous reports in the literature link various molecular factors to nerve regeneration and healing following repair.[159,206]

## Neuropathy

Neuropathies result from a wide variety of causes and can be classified in many ways, including the rate of onset, type and size of nerve fibers involved, distribution pattern, or pathology.[90] For example, when a single peripheral nerve is affected the result is a *mononeuropathy,* which is commonly a result of trauma. The term *polyneuropathy* indicates involvement of several peripheral nerves. A *radiculoneuropathy* indicates involvement of the nerve root as it emerges from the spinal cord, and *polyradiculitis* indicates involvement of several nerve roots and occurs when infections create an inflammatory response. Neuropathic diseases that affect the axon or its cell body causing axonal degeneration typically affect the longest nerve fibers first, with signs and symptoms beginning distally and spreading proximally as the disease progresses. Because nerves in the legs are longer, the feet and lower legs are often involved before the fingers and hands. Those conditions that affect only myelin cause segmental demyelination in both sensory and motor fibers.

The first noticeable features of neuropathies are often sensory in nature and consist of tingling, prickling, burning, or band-like *dysesthesias* and *paresthesias* in the feet. When more than one nerve is involved, the sensory loss follows a glove-and-stocking distribution that is attributed to the dying-back of the longest fibers in all nerves from distal to proximal (Fig. 39.3). The most common symptoms of motor neuropathy include distal weakness, decreases of tone (hypotonicity or flaccidity), and muscle tenderness or cramping. This can be evident when clients are asked to walk on their heels or toes, recruiting dorsiflexors or plantarflexors, respectively. It is important to recognize that the motor loss in a myopathy is opposite to that of a neuropathy. In a myopathy, the weakness tends to be proximal.

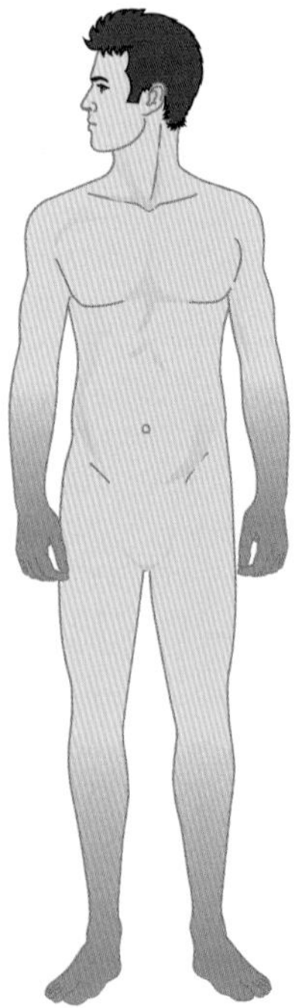

**Figure 39.3**

**A stocking-and-glove pattern of sensory loss occurs in polyneuropathy.** A gradient of greater distal loss tapering to less proximal involvement is seen.

## MECHANICAL INJURIES: COMPRESSION AND ENTRAPMENT SYNDROMES

Compressive neuropathies occur due to the proximity of peripheral nerves to bony, muscular, and vascular structures. Chronic nerve compression develops over time and reflects particular changes in the lining of the nerve. Mechanical injury occurs as a result of traction on a nerve, with damage occurring once tension exceeds 10% to 20% of the axon's resting length and the available slack is taken up.[14] Repetitive motion injuries affecting the hands can result from repeated grasping, typing, or playing a musical instrument.

### Median Neuropathy (Carpal Tunnel Syndrome)

Carpal tunnel syndrome (CTS) is not a single event, but more likely a cascade of dysfunction that causes symptoms when it reaches a critical state. Described in 1854 by Paget, CTS (tardy median palsy) is the result of compression of the median nerve within the carpal tunnel in the wrist. Chronic CTS is marked by pain, paresthesia, numbness, and weakness in the distribution of the median nerve (Fig. 39.4). Although there are many causative factors, chronic CTS is most commonly associated with performance of repetitive tasks determined by position of the hand and degree of load. Physical therapists have been involved in intensive study of the causes and treatments associated with this complex disorder. Animal models exhibit the features of human CTS, including impaired sensation, motor weakness, and decreased median NCV. It is well established that a causal relationship exists between performance of a repetitive task and development of CTS.[6]

Acute CTS is less common and directly associated with fractures, dislocation, and vascular disorders of the wrist. Rheumatologic disorders and anomalous anatomy may cause sudden symptoms. The acute form of CTS may require urgent surgical intervention to avoid serious and permanent damage.[185]

#### Incidence

Carpal tunnel is one of the top reasons for lost workdays, with the average being between 10 and 27 days and the cost of an occurrence at more than $30,000 in medical costs. The incidence of CTS in general populations is approximately 2.8 per 1000 in studies using nerve conduction study to confirm the diagnosis. The prevalence ranges from 1% to 10% among the general population, and up to 14.5% among specific occupational groups. Nearly 70% of all CTS cases occur in women. Conventional thinking is that the tunnel is relatively smaller in females compared to males.[158] The incidence of surgery for CTS peaks in the 45- to 55-year-old group in women and in the older-than-65-years group in men.[175] Prevalence is increased in tasks that require gripping, holding tools that vibrate, lifting more than 12 kg, or working in an extremely cold environment.[61]

#### Etiology

The carpal tunnel is basically a structure with four sides, three of which are defined by the carpal bones and the

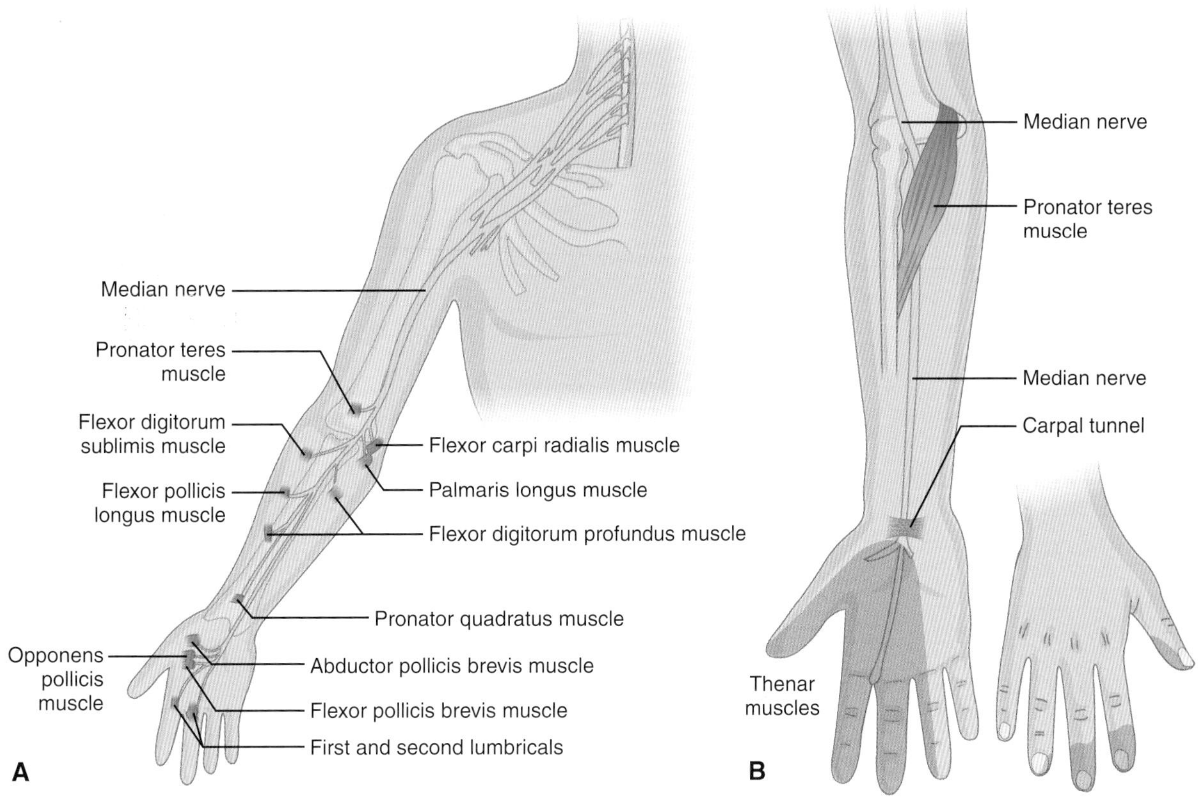


**Figure 39.4**

(A) Median nerve course and motor innervation. (B) The point of compression of the median nerve as it passes through the carpal tunnel. The lightly stippled area shows the sensory supply of the palmar cutaneous branch, which arises proximal to the carpal tunnel and thus is spared in the carpal tunnel syndrome. The densely stippled zone represents the cutaneous sensory area of the median nerve distal to the carpal tunnel. (A, From Canale ST: *Campbell's operative orthopaedics*, ed 10, St Louis, 2003, Mosby; B, from Noble J: *Textbook of primary care medicine*, ed 3, St Louis, 2001, Mosby.)

fourth, the "top" of the tunnel, by the transverse carpal ligament (Fig. 39.5). Tendons passing through the tunnel with their synovial sheaths include the flexor pollicis longus, the four flexor digitorum superficialis, and the four flexor digitorum profundus tendons. Closest to the surface and most vulnerable to changes of the palm in relation to the wrist is the median nerve. The hallmark of the carpal tunnel is that it is cylindrical and inelastic. None of the sides of the tunnel yields to expansion of the fluid or structures within. Change within the tunnel is the basis of study related to the etiology of carpal tunnel, but the matrix of possible causes proves to be complex and not fully understood at this time.[131] The primary problem is that pressures are increased, even at rest with the wrist held in neutral. When the individual flexes or extends the wrist, the pressure exerted on the structures can be double or triple. With sustained position of the wrist, the excessive pressure can cause neurapraxia of the median nerve.

## Risk Factors

Neuropathic conditions, including diabetes mellitus, alcoholism, and toxic exposure, can lead to carpel tunnel. Risk for developing CTS occurs in people with osteoarthritis of the carpometacarpal joint of the thumb, rheumatoid tenosynovitis, edema, pregnancy, hypothyroidism, and congestive heart failure. Physically inactive individuals are at greater risk for developing CTS over their lifetime. CTS is also 2.5 times more likely in obese individuals (body mass index >29).[63] Smoking cigarettes increases the likelihood of developing CTS, with changes in tissue common to the smoker juxtaposed to a typical extended position of the wrist while holding the cigarette. Anomalous structures within the carpal tunnel, such as variations in the branching pattern of the median nerve, range in length and width of the lumbricals, and extra tendinous slips from the long flexors within the tunnel, may contribute to development of CTS.15 Box 39.1 includes suggested causes of CTS.[110,161,200]

Although CTS has been reported in several occupations, the convincing link between work and CTS remains inconclusive.[63] In most cases, work acts as the "last straw" in CTS causation. Except in the case of work that involves very cold temperatures (possibly in conjunction with load and repetition) such as butchery, work is less likely than demographic and disease-related variables to cause CTS. It has been reported that computer use does not pose a severe occupational hazard for development of symptoms of CTS. The responsibility of addressing correctable lifestyle factors and treatable illnesses, such as obesity, diabetes, smoking, and increased alcohol intake, results in both avoidable long-term health effects and ongoing costs to the community.[63] Patients older than age 63 years have a different pattern of risk factors for CTS than do younger patients. This suggests that CTS in the elderly

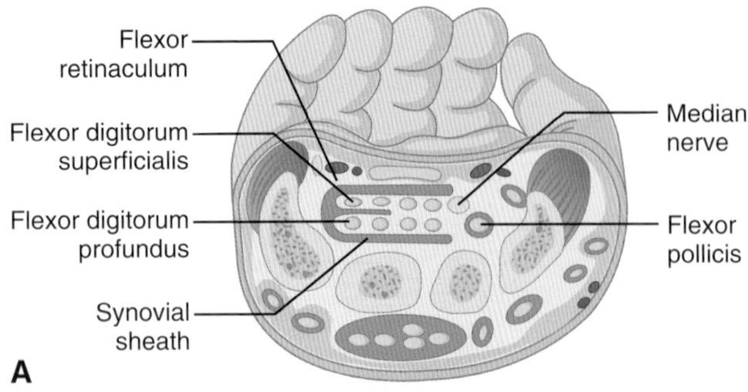


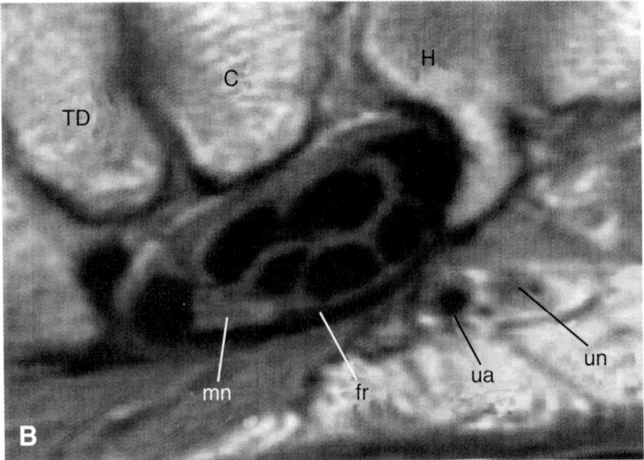


**Figure 39.5**

(A) Cross-section of the carpal tunnel at the wrist. Contents of the tunnel include the tendon of the flexor pollicis longus *(FPL)*, the four tendons of the flexor digitorum profundus *(FDP)*, the four tendons of the flexor digitorum superficialis *(FDS)*, and the median nerve. (B) Carpal tunnel. *C*, Capitate; *fr*, flexor retinaculum; *H*, hamate; *mn*, median nerve; *TD*, trapezoid; *ua*, ulnar artery; *un*, ulnar nerve. (A, From Noble J: *Textbook of primary care medicine*, ed 3, St Louis, 2001, Mosby; B, from Yu JS, Habib PA: Normal MR imaging anatomy of the wrist and hand, *Radiol Clin North Am* 44(4):569–581, 2006.)

population may have different underlying pathogenetic mechanisms.[20] Senile systemic amyloidosis, with deposition of transthyretin in the canal may be responsible for the increase in men at that age.[189]

### Pathogenesis

Schwann cell changes underlie the initial mechanism of CTS and are independent of axonal damage. Mechanical pressures induce Schwann cells to undergo apoptosis, or cell death, causing demyelination at the area of the nodes of Ranvier. At the same time, proliferation of myelin is triggered. This may be caused by cell membrane proteins, known as integrins, that migrate into the area because of increased nutritive demands and appear to be involved in regulating Schwann cell activation, resulting in remyelination. However, the remyelination is not the same as the original myelin. The result is that compressed nerve segments show thinner myelin sheaths. Cytokines are most likely involved in the pathophysiology of repetitive motion injuries in peripheral nerves.[6] Interleukin-1β and tumor necrosis factor-α increase in forearm flexor muscles and tendons in study animals involving reaching and grasping involving moderate repetitive reaching with negligible force. Increases in interleukin-1β and tumor necrosis factor-α negatively correlate with grip strength. Disorganization of receptive fields and alterations of neuronal properties suggest that both peripheral inflammation and cortical neuroplasticity jointly contribute to the development of chronic repetitive motion disorders. Patterns of movement degrade over time without intervention, thus illustrating both the link between central and peripheral processing and the importance of early and appropriate intervention.[35,59] Heat and cold hyperalgesia may reflect impairments in central nociceptive processing seen in patients with unilateral CTS. The bilateral thermal hyperalgesia associated with pain intensity and duration of pain history supports a role of generalized sensitization mechanisms in the initiation, maintenance and spread of pain in CTS.[69,184] Slowing of nerve conduction noted on EMG with CTS reflects changes in both myelin and axons.[205] If the mechanical pressures are high enough, compression can create an axonotmesis in which axon continuity is lost and wallerian degeneration occurs.

### Clinical Manifestations

CTS causes sensory symptoms in the median nerve distribution. Pain may be located distally in the forearm or wrist and radiate into the thumb, index, and middle fingers. It may also radiate into the arm, shoulder, and neck. Comparing self-reported symptoms recorded on the Katz hand diagram allows symptoms to be assessed as classic, probable, possible, or unlikely to be CTS.[39] Nocturnal pain is the hallmark of CTS. Even in the early stages of CTS most people will report being awakened by painful numbness in the middle of the night. Sensory symptoms usually precede motor symptoms. Diminished two-point discrimination, diminished ability to perceive vibration, and elevation of threshold in Semmes-Weinstein monofilament testing routinely occur. Thenar weakness is seen in advanced cases. In nearly half of all cases, symptoms occur bilaterally. If CTS goes untreated, symptoms escalate into persistent pain with atrophy of the thenar musculature and the person will have a loss of grip strength. The combined loss of grip strength, inability to pinch, and sensory loss causes clumsiness in the hands.[44]

## MEDICAL MANAGEMENT

**DIAGNOSIS.** CTS appears more often as a syndrome rather than a singular finding. Diagnosis can be determined in up to 90% of instances by careful history, physical examination, and provocation tests, which are considered positive when pain, numbness, and paresthesia are produced in the median nerve distribution. The *Phalen test* involves flexing the wrist to 90 degrees for 1 minute (Fig. 39.6A); the *Tinel test* is wrist percussion over the carpal tunnel (Fig. 39.6B); the *Durkan carpal compression test* involves compression applied to the median nerve for 30 seconds with the thumbs or an atomizer bulb attached to a manometer. The *lumbrical incursion* test is performed by asking the patient to make a fist with the wrist in the neutral position. The test is positive if pain and paresthesia occur within 30 to 40 seconds. A full fist results in approximately 3 cm of lumbrical muscle incursion into the carpal tunnel contributing to median nerve compression.[62]

It is often suggested that the "gold standard" test of CTS is electrodiagnostic testing, but debate exists as

Box 39.1

## CAUSES OF CARPAL TUNNEL SYNDROME

***Neuromusculoskeletal***

IDIOPATHIC
Cause unknown

*Anatomic (Compression)*

Small carpal canal, anomalous muscles/tendons
Basal joint (thumb) arthritis
Cervical disk lesions
Cervical spondylosis
Congenital anatomic differences or anatomic change in nerve or carpal tunnel (e.g., shape, size, volume of structures; presence of palmaris longus)
History of wrist surgery, especially previous carpal tunnel surgery
Injection: high pressure
Peripheral neuropathy
Poor posture (may also be associated with thoracic outlet syndrome)
Tendinitis
Trigger points
Tenosynovitis
Thoracic outlet syndrome

*Trauma/Exertional*

Swelling, hemorrhage, scar, wrist fracture, carpal dislocation
Cumulative trauma disorders
Repetitive strain injuries
Vibrational exposure (jackhammer or other manual labor equipment)

*Systemic*

Chronic kidney disease (fluid imbalance)
Congestive heart failure (fluid imbalance)
Hemochromatosis
Leukemia (tissue infiltration)
Liver disease
Medications
- Nonsteroidal antiinflammatory drugs
- Oral contraceptives
- Statins
- Alendronate (Fosamax)
- Lithium
- β Blocker

Obesity
Pregnancy (fluid retention)
Tumors (lipoma, hemangioma, ganglia, synovial sarcoma, fibroma, neuroma, neurofibroma)
Use of oral contraceptives
Vitamin deficiency

*Endocrine*

Acromegaly
Diabetes mellitus
Gout (deposits of tophi and calcium)
Hormonal imbalance (menopause; posthysterectomy)
Hyperparathyroidism
Hyperthyroidism (Graves disease)
Hypocalcemia
Hypothyroidism (myxedema)

*Infectious Disease*

Atypical mycobacterium
Histoplasmosis
Rubella
Sporotrichosis

*Inflammatory*

Amyloidosis
Arthritis (rheumatoid, gout, polymyalgia rheumatica)
Dermatomyositis
Gout/pseudogout
Scleroderma
Systemic lupus erythematosus

*Neuropathic*

Alcohol abuse
Chemotherapy (delayed, long-term effect)
Diabetes
Multiple myeloma (amyloidosis deposits)
Thyroid disease
Vitamin/nutritional deficiency (especially vitamin $B_6$, folic acid)
Vitamin toxicity

From Goodman CC, Snyder T: *Differential diagnosis for physical therapists: screening for referral*, ed 5, Philadelphia, 2013, WB Saunders.

to whether it is necessary to confirm CTS.[158] Electromyography and nerve conduction studies can confirm the diagnosis, determine the severity of nerve damage, guide and measure the effect of treatment, and rule out other conditions such as radiculopathy and brachial plexus damage. Distal motor and sensory latencies and sensory NCV across the carpal tunnel are most frequently administered.[191] Changes in the sensory conduction across the wrist are reportedly the most sensitive indicator of CTS.[231] Ultrasound studies, which reveal an enlarged median nerve, may assist with the diagnosis.[57,109,120] The injection of corticosteroids or bupivacaine into the carpal tunnel has been used to determine involvement, therefore when the injection is

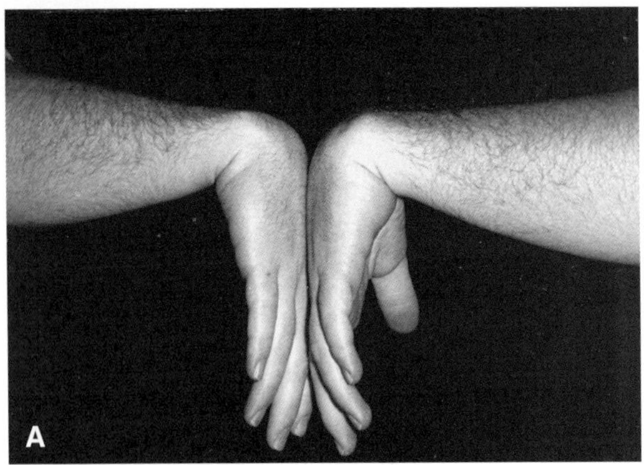


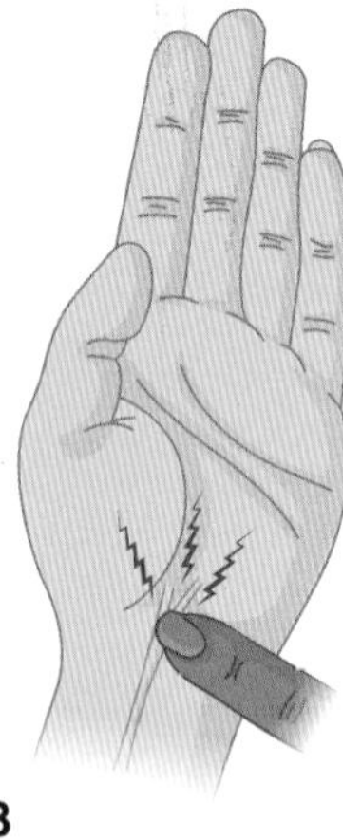


**Figure 39.6**

(A) The Phalen test. Patients maximally flex both wrists and hold the position for 1 to 2 minutes. If symptoms of numbness or paresthesia within the median nerve distribution are reproduced, the test is positive. (B) The Tinel sign in carpal tunnel syndrome. (A, From Frontera WR, Silver JK: *Essentials of physical medicine and rehabilitation*, Philadelphia, 2002, Hanley and Belfus; B, from Noble J: *Textbook of primary care medicine*, ed 3, St Louis, 2001, Mosby.)

accompanied by a relief of symptoms, it provides diagnostic evidence of CTS.

**TREATMENT.** Because causes appear to be multifactorial, treatment approaches address several components. Early management typically involves ergonomic modification of the client's environment and lifestyle changes. A current concept in treatment of CTS involves preventing inflammation, as well as minimizing cortical dedifferentiation.[35] Local neurostimulation and acupuncture treatments are showing promise to rewire cortical areas affected by CTS.[134] Long-term use of antiinflammatory medications leads to gastric complications without significant change in symptoms. Steroid injection into the carpal canal shows relief up to 1 year.[42]

Surgical release of the transverse carpal ligament is indicated when symptoms have lasted longer than 1 year and there is both motor and sensory NCV involvement, or denervation is evidenced by fibrillation potentials on EMG. Flexor tenosynovectomy with transverse carpal ligament division, endoscopic release of the ligament, and neurolysis of the median nerve are performed through limited incisions and require minimal exposure and manipulation of the nerve. Seventy-six percent of the surgical cases experience return of normal two-point discrimination and up to 70% have normal muscle strength return.[101] After surgery, nerve and tendon gliding techniques are advocated to reduce scarring, adhesions, and subsequent formation of fibrotic tissue.[214]

**PROGNOSIS.** Prognosis relates directly to the severity of the nerve entrapment at diagnosis, clinical cause, and mode of treatment.

**SPECIAL IMPLICATIONS FOR THE THERAPIST 39.1**

### *Carpal Tunnel Syndrome*

Overuse syndromes involve a degree of edema; consequently, icing after long periods of use is advocated to reduce the pain and swelling. Use of phonophoresis and iontophoresis can be effective to reduce local inflammation and swelling.[88] Because generalized deconditioning exacerbates the symptoms of CTS, exercise is encouraged; however, strengthening exercises in the involved wrist and hand should be avoided until symptom relief is nearly complete. Use of neutral splinting has been found to be beneficial in severe CTS when worn either at night or full time.[227] A combination of a cock-up splint with lumbrical intensive stretches appears to be the most effective combination for improvements in functional gains when measured at 24 weeks of intervention.[11] Therapists should not overlook the possibility that somatosensory and motor skill retraining may have to be included in treatment plans in order to regain function and to prevent further tissue damage when managing chronic repetitive motion injury. Proper biomechanics, frequent breaks, and strategic movement patterns may prevent the persistent changes seen in these individuals.[111]

## Thoracic Outlet Syndrome

Individuals with thoracic outlet syndrome (TOS) may have vague symptoms or symptoms that are difficult to interpret. Despite TOS being a common clinical disorder, conclusive evidence is lacking to support most currently used treatments.[118,166]

### Definition

TOS is an entrapment syndrome caused by pressure from structures in the thoracic outlet on fibers of the brachial plexus at some point between the interscalene triangle and the inferior border of the axilla. In addition, vascular symptoms can occur because of compression of the subclavian artery (Fig. 39.7).

### Etiology

The anatomy of the region of the thoracic outlet is extremely complex. Spinal nerve roots of the brachial plexus interact with surrounding bony ribs, muscles, tendons (subclavius, anterior and middle scalene, and pectoralis minor), and the vascular supply (subclavian artery and vein) to the region. In addition to neurologic structures becoming entrapped, arterial and venous structures also may be affected individually or in combination. Practically, TOS can be divided into three groups: neurogenic (compression of brachial plexus), vascular (compression of subclavian artery and/or vein), and disputed (nonspecific TOS with chronic pain and symptoms of brachial plexus involvement).[22,97]

## Risk Factors

Postural changes associated with growth and development, trauma to the shoulder girdle, and body composition have all been identified as contributing to the development of TOS. In human upright posture, gravity pulls on the shoulder girdle creating traction on the structures and may contribute to the development of TOS. Additionally, congenital factors that affect the bony structures, such as a cervical rib or fascial bands, also compress the neurovascular bundle. TOS is reported more commonly in women than in men, and rarely occurs in individuals younger than the age of 20 years.[70]

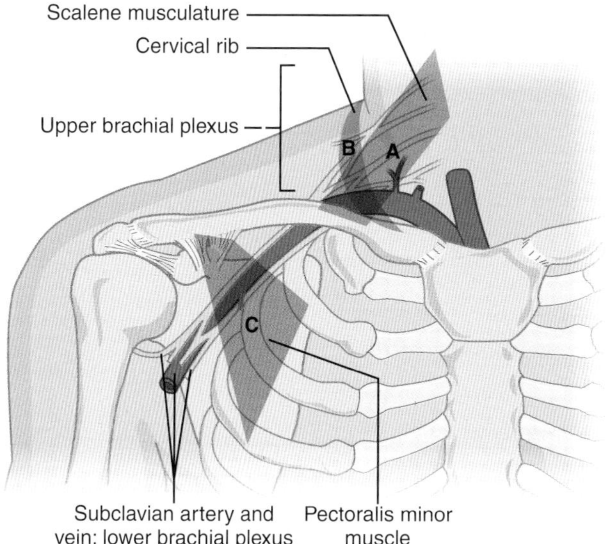


**Figure 39.7**

**Schematic relationship of structures in development of thoracic outlet syndrome.** Compression of the neurovascular bundle can occur with (A) hypertrophy of scalene musculature impinging on structures lying between middle and anterior scalene; (B) the presence of cervical rib or fibrous bands between the cervical and first rib; or (C) compression by pectoralis minor during hyperabduction. (From Rakel RE: *Textbook of medicine*, ed 7, Philadelphia, 2007, WB Saunders.)

**Pathogenesis.** Chronic compression of nerve roots or proximal plexus and arteries between the clavicle and first rib or impinging musculature results in edema and ischemia in the nerves (see Fig. 39.7). This compression initially creates a neurapraxia. After loss of myelin the axons are more vulnerable to unrelieved compression. The neurapraxia can progress to an axonotmesis in which axon continuity is lost and wallerian degeneration occurs.

**Clinical Manifestations.** The nerve compression in TOS results in paresthesias and pain in the arm, particularly at end of day. Other symptoms may include pain, tingling, and paresis. If the upper nerve plexus is involved (C5 to C7), pain is reported in the neck; this may radiate into the face (sometimes with ear pain) and anterior chest, as well as over the scapulae. Symptoms may also extend over the lateral aspect of the forearm into the hand. If the lower plexus is compromised (C7 to T1), pain and numbness occur in the posterior neck and shoulder, medial arm, and forearm, and radiate into the ulnarly innervated digits of the hand. Weakness occurs in the muscles corresponding to nerve root innervation, and atrophy follows in severe cases. Vascular symptoms may include coldness, edema in the hand or arm, Raynaud phenomenon (cyanosis), fatigue in hand and arm, and superficial vein distention in the hand (Fig. 39.8). Overhead and lifting activities, along with movements of the head, can aggravate symptoms in the upper plexus.

## MEDICAL MANAGEMENT

DIAGNOSIS. Provocative tests based on the belief that the anterior scalene can compress the neurovascular bundle are used to elicit symptoms of TOS.[215] However, these tests have a high false-positive response, and are of

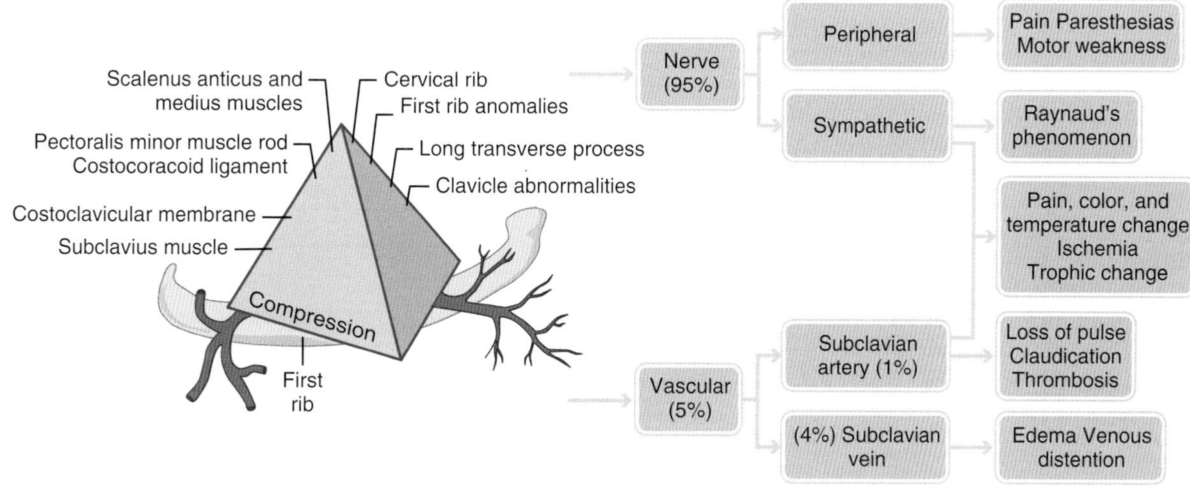


**Figure 39.8**

Relationship of thoracic outlet abnormalities and impairments. (From Marx RS, Hockberger RS, Walls RM: *Rosen's emergency medicine: concepts and clinical practice*, ed 6, St Louis, 2006, Mosby.)

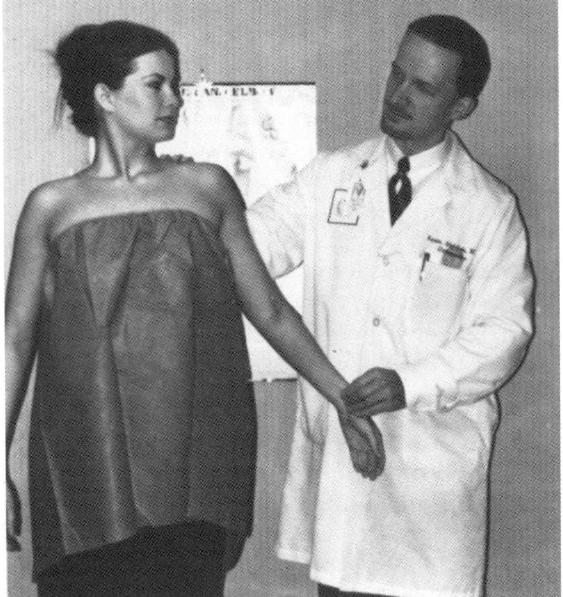

**Figure 39.9**

**The Adson test is one of many diagnostic tests used to examine the upper extremity to determine presence of thoracic outlet syndrome: arterial or neurologic.** Hold patient's arm in slight abduction while palpating the radial pulse. Ask the patient to inhale and hold the breath while extending the neck and rotating toward the affected side. The Adson test is positive if the patient reports paresthesia or if the pulse fades away. (From DeLee JC, Drez D, Miller MD: *DeLee and Drez's orthopaedic sports medicine*, ed 2, Philadelphia, 2003, WB Saunders.)

disputable diagnostic value.[70] Maneuvers are performed bilaterally, and the pulse is monitored to note a change in its quality. However, mere obliteration of the peripheral pulse does not necessarily mean that TOS exists as an entrapment problem; sensory symptoms must be reproduced. For persons with a vascular component, blood pressure may differ from side to side. Although there is no universally accepted reliable diagnostic test for TOS, the *Adson maneuver* (Fig. 39.9) appears among the most effective. Several other maneuvers with a positional component of the head, shoulder, or arm have been found to compress vascular or neural structures and thus evoke symptoms. These tests include the Allen, Wright, Halsted, costoclavicular, and Roos (or elevated arm stress test). Table 39.7 includes assessment of symptoms of TOS. The sensitivity and specificity of the Adson maneuver improve when used in combination with the hyperabduction test (symptom replication), the Wright test (symptom replication), or the Roos test (Table 39.8).[79]

**Radiographic Tests.** Radiographic procedures are used to identify bony abnormalities. Presence of a cervical rib may place the nerve at risk for compression; however, presence of the rib alone does not necessarily replicate symptoms. Plane films are used to distinguish between a C7-T1 discogenic lesion and TOS.

**Electrophysiologic Studies.** Because symptoms of TOS are related to neural compression, electrophysiologic studies are valuable in documenting the presence of neuropathy. NCV allows the examiner to pinpoint the lesion, either because of a change in amplitude or a slowing in conduction velocity (Box 39.2). Other, more refined

**Table 39.7 Assessing Symptoms of Thoracic Outlet Syndrome[a]**

| Component | Symptoms |
|---|---|
| Vascular | 3-Minute elevated test<br>Adson test<br>Swelling (arm/hand)<br>Discoloration of hand<br>Costoclavicular test<br>Hyperabduction test<br>Upper extremity claudication<br>Differences in blood pressure<br>Skin temperature changes<br>Cold intolerance |
| Neural | **Upper plexus**<br>Point tenderness of C5-C6<br>Pressure over lateral neck elicits pain and/or numbness.<br>Pain with head turned and/or tilted to opposite side<br>Weak biceps<br>Weak triceps<br>Weak wrist<br>Hypoesthesia in radial nerve distribution<br>3-Minute abduction stress test<br>**Lower plexus**<br>Pressure above clavicle elicits pain<br>Ulnar nerve tenderness when palpated under axilla or along inner arm<br>Tinel sign for ulnar nerve in axilla<br>Hypoesthesia in ulnar nerve distribution<br>Serratus anterior weakness<br>Weak hand grip |

[a]Although no specific testing for thoracic outlet has proven valid in detecting upper-extremity pain of a neurogenic origin, the use of these special tests may help identify patterns of positive objective findings to help characterize thoracic outlet syndrome.

From Table 17-5 in Goodman CC, Snyder T: *Differential diagnosis for physical therapists: screening for referral*, ed 5, Philadelphia, 2013, WB Saunders.

**Table 39.8 Diagnostic Utility of Tests for Thoracic Outlet Syndrome**

| Provocation Test | Sensitivity | Specificity |
|---|---|---|
| Adson | 0.79 | 0.76 |
| Hyperabduction (HA)—pulse abolition (HAp) | 0.84 | 0.4 |
| Adson + HAs (symptom replication) | 0.72 | 0.88 |
| Adson + Wright's | 0.54 | 0.94 |
| Adson + Roos | 0.72 | 0.82 |

electrophysiologic techniques, including somatosensory evoked potentials and F waves, are used to confirm a diagnosis of nerve root entrapment.

TOS should be distinguished from other disorders with similar symptoms. These include cervical radiculopathy, reflex sympathetic dystrophy, tumors of the apex of the lung, and ulnar nerve compression at either elbow or wrist. The sensory pattern of TOS distinguishes it from an ulnar neuropathy such as tardy ulnar palsy. Because the nerve roots are affected, the sensory changes extend above

Box 39.2

**TYPICAL ELECTROPHYSIOLOGIC FINDINGS IN THORACIC OUTLET SYNDROME**

***Upper Sensory***

- Decreased amplitude

***Median Sensory***

- Normal

***Ulnar Motor***

- Normal or decreased amplitude

***Median Motor***

- Decreased amplitude

***Electromyography***

- + Positive fibrillation potentials: first dorsal interosseus

Adapted from Huang JH, Zager EL: Thoracic outlet syndrome, *Neurosurgery* 55:897–903, 2004.

Box 39.3

**SURGICAL PROCEDURES AND APPROACHES FOR THORACIC OUTLET SYNDROME**

***Procedures***

- Scalenotomy
- Scalenectomy
- Clavicle resection
- Pectoralis minor release
- First rib resection
- Cervical rib resection

***Approaches***

- Axillary
- Supraclavicular
- Combined axillary and supraclavicular
- Posterior
- Subclavicular
- Transclavicular

the hand and wrist into the forearm in TOS and follow a dermatomal pattern. Myofascial pain patterns may also mimic TOS symptoms.

**TREATMENT.** Given that TOS is a complex disorder, management is best approached by a multidisciplinary team, which may include, but is not limited to, physicians, surgeons, work-related case managers, and physical and occupational therapists.[119] Management is divided into conservative and surgical approaches. The initial treatment of the person with TOS is conservative when symptoms are mild to moderate in severity. Postural and breathing exercises and gentle stretching are the cornerstones of the initial conservative program. This is followed by strengthening exercises for shoulder girdle musculature. Initially, overhead exercises should be avoided because they tend to evoke symptoms. Therapists are cautioned against forceful stretching to mobilize the first rib.[85]

Surgical management of TOS is reserved for cases that are refractory to postural and exercise correction and those with vascular compromise.[34,118] There are at least six different surgical procedures and six different anatomic approaches for TOS (Box 39.3). In scalenotomy, the muscle is detached from the first rib; unfortunately, with this approach a high percentage of people experience recurring symptoms. Scalenectomy, removal of the scalene muscle, is advocated for people who have had recurrence of their symptoms. Clavicle resection is indicated primarily when the clavicle is damaged. When scalenectomy, with or without first rib resection, is the surgical approach used, its 5-year success rate is approximately 70%.[179]

**PROGNOSIS.** After surgery, 70% of cases have a good or excellent response using a supraclavicular or transaxillary resection of the first rib. Improvement in pain symptoms ranges from 70% to 80%, some patients require occasional analgesics, and 10% note no improvement. In individuals with signs, symptoms, and electrophysiologic changes consistent with classic TOS, no improvement in strength is noted when atrophy was present before surgery.[34] Complications during surgery include pneumothorax, nerve compression, and transient winging of the scapula because the upper digitations of the serratus are detached.

A 4-year follow-up reported no significant difference in return to work or symptom severity when the first rib was resected compared to a conservative, nonoperative approach.[83] Factors that are associated with long-term disability include preoperative depression, single status, and less than high school education.[9]

**SPECIAL IMPLICATIONS FOR THE THERAPIST 39.2**

## *Thoracic Outlet Syndrome*

Physical therapy management alone has been shown to be successful in a third of patients with TOS.[12] Therapists need to consider using an upper-quarter screen to rule out cervical radiculopathy or shoulder dysfunction during their evaluation. If this screen is negative, range of motion and posture should be evaluated to identify soft tissue restrictions. The client's response to provocative maneuvers should be assessed along with a sensory evaluation, preferably using Semmes-Weinstein monofilaments. Manual muscle testing or other method of evaluating strength should be performed. Treatment is aimed at pain relief along with postural correction.[228]

One reason TOS has been difficult to diagnose relates to the client's subjective report. Frequently, signs and symptoms do not correspond to a single lesion, but to multifocal lesions, either of vascular and/or neurogenic origin. For clients who do not respond to treatment, some believe that compression at a proximal or distal source might increase the vulnerability of nerves, making them more susceptible to compression at another site. A functional tool such as the DASH (Disabilities of the Arm, Shoulder and Hand) outcome measure should be used to track objective and functional changes. This measure has proven to be a valid, reliable, and responsive test in evaluating people with a variety of upper extremity problems as has the shortened Quick DASH measure.[16,27]

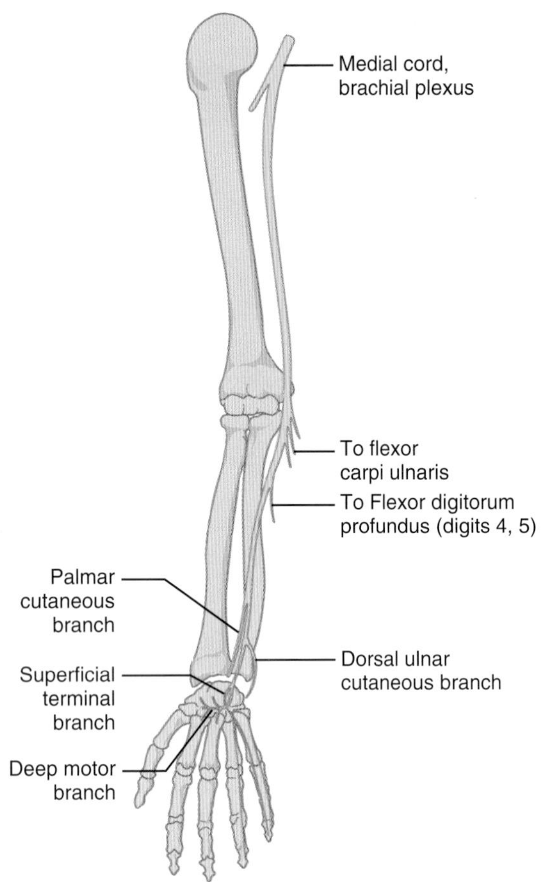


**Figure 39.10**

**Distribution of the ulnar nerve.** A tardy ulnar palsy impinges the ulnar nerve as it passes behind the medial epicondyle of the humerus. (From Steward JD: *Focal peripheral neuropathies*, ed 3, Philadelphia, 2000, Lippincott Williams & Wilkins.)

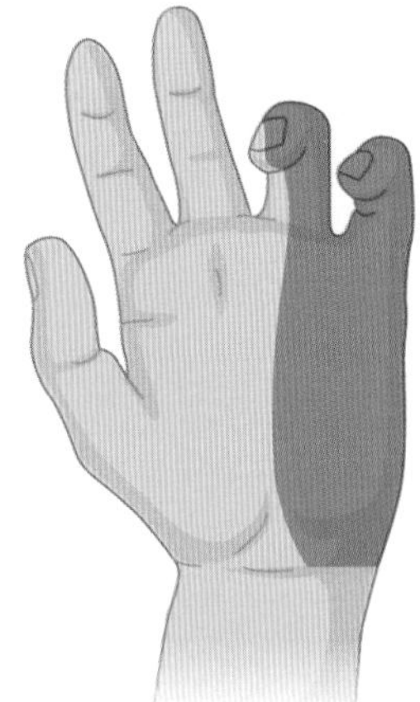

**Figure 39.11**

Clawing of the ring and little fingers (hyperextension of the metacarpophalangeal joint and flexion of the interphalangeal joints) from unopposed action of extensor musculature combined with paralysis of the intrinsic muscles of the hand occurs when there is involvement of the ulnar nerve. Shaded area represents ulnar nerve sensory distribution in the hand. (From Marx RS, Hockberger RS, Walls RM: *Rosen's emergency medicine: concepts and clinical practice*, ed 6, St Louis, 2006, Mosby.)

## Tardy Ulnar Palsy/Retroepicondylar Palsy

### Anatomy

The ulnar nerve arises from the lower trunk of the brachial plexus and carries fibers from C8 and T1 nerve roots. At the elbow, it passes behind the medial epicondyle and then passes between the two heads of the flexor carpi ulnaris through the forearm to the wrist. The distal portion of the nerve enters the palm by crossing the flexor retinaculum and divides into a superficial and deep branch in the hand (Fig. 39.10).

### Etiology

Ulnar nerve entrapment (also called tardy ulnar palsy, cubital tunnel syndrome, and ulnar nerve neuritis) at the elbow is one of the most common entrapment neuropathies encountered in clinical practice.[226] Because of its anatomic location, ulnar nerve palsy is a common complication of fractures in the region of the elbow. A late or tardy ulnar palsy may occur years after a fracture and is associated with callus formation or a valgus deformity of the elbow. These produce a gradual stretching of the nerve in the ulnar groove of the medial epicondyle.

### Risk Factors

A similar type of tardy ulnar palsy occurs with repeated trauma for relatively long periods of time in clients with a shallow ulnar groove at the elbow. Ulnar neuropathy from entrapment at the elbow is the second most frequent upper extremity neuropathy (after CTS).

### Pathogenesis

The mechanism of injury compressing the ulnar nerve has been attributed to recurrent microtrauma associated with fracture and fibrous bands or recurrent cubital subluxations, as well as entrapment at the entrance or exit of the cubital tunnel.[128] Elbow flexion aggravates symptoms. Compression will initially cause a neurapraxia with demyelination of the nerve; if the pressure goes unrelieved, this will progress to an axonotmesis, with denervation occurring below the level of the elbow.

### Clinical Manifestations

Tardy ulnar palsy can result in a clawhand deformity with metacarpophalangeal extension and interphalangeal flexion of the ring and little fingers because of the unopposed action of the extensor muscle group and paralysis of the third and fourth lumbricals that normally flex the metacarpophalangeals and extend the interphalangeals (Fig. 39.11). Flattening of the hypothenar eminence along with abduction of the little finger coincides with weakness of the palmaris brevis and abductor digiti minimi. Marked atrophy of the interossei on the dorsal surface of the hand with guttering between the extensor tendons indicates the presence of denervation. Abduction and adduction movements of the fingers are impaired. Paralysis of the flexor carpi ulnaris produces a radial deviation of the hand when wrist flexion is attempted. Sensory loss is variable, but impaired sensation may be expected involving the little finger and the ulnar aspect of the ring finger and along the ulnar aspect of the palm of the hand to the wrist. Occasionally, sensory symptoms extend proximally to the wrist.

### MEDICAL MANAGEMENT

**DIAGNOSIS.** Percussion of or bending the elbow can replicate symptoms.[128] NCV studies are helpful only when sufficient nerve damage has occurred to produce definite strength or sensory changes in the hand. NCVs are slowed through the involved region but are relatively normal above and below the epicondyle. Electromyography reports slowing of sensory or motor NCV across the elbow, prolonged conduction (termed a *latency*) to the flexor carpi ulnaris, along with changes in amplitude, duration, or shape of the sensory potential across the elbow. Detection of an abnormal latency requires accurate measurement of ulnar nerve segment length.[145]

**TREATMENT.** Mild entrapments are managed conservatively; moderate and severe compression require surgery. To relieve the compression, either decompression, the preferred method (medial epicondylectomy), or transposition of the ulnar nerve to the anterior aspect of the elbow is performed.[24,199] Symptomatically, the clawhand deformity should be treated with a splint that blocks metacarpophalangeal hyperextension (lumbrical bar) and allows the extensor digitorum to extend the interphalangeal joints.

**PROGNOSIS.** Results of surgery are normally good when the individual has not had a chronic tardy ulnar involvement. Decompression surgery should lead to complete restoration of function quickly, but recovery after transposition surgery may take up to 6 months. Surgery to treat chronic involvement (over 3 months) may have a less certain restoration of function.[199] After nerve transposition, most NCVs at follow-up are improved. However, the magnitude of change in the motor conduction velocity does not correlate well with clinical improvement. One factor that has been identified to affect outcome is body mass index; increased body weight is related slightly to patient's perception of poorer improvement.[152]

## Saturday Night Palsy/Sleep Palsy

### Definition and Etiology

*Saturday night palsy* is associated with radial nerve compression in the arm. It results from direct pressure against a firm object and typically follows deep sleep on the arm with compression of the radial nerve at the spiral groove of the humerus in a person who is sleeping after becoming intoxicated. Sleep palsy has also been associated with lipoma compressing the radial nerve.[68] If the radial nerve is compressed in the axilla, the damage is often referred to as a crutch palsy.

### Pathogenesis

Compression of the nerve causes segmental demyelination.

### Clinical Manifestations

Symptoms of radial nerve paralysis depend on the level of the lesion. The more proximal the involvement, the more extensive the paralysis. When involvement occurs in the axilla, weakness occurs in elbow extension (triceps), elbow flexion (brachioradialis), and supination (supinator). If the nerve is damaged in the upper arm, the triceps is spared. In addition, in both instances there will be weakness of wrist extensors and the extensors of the fingers and thumb, diminishing grip strength. Sensory loss with radial nerve involvement is variable. If present, it is typically confined to the dorsum of the hand but may extend to the dorsum of the forearm.

### MEDICAL MANAGEMENT

**DIAGNOSIS.** Diagnosis is by history, clinical examination, and electrophysiologic examination. This type of paralysis is usually classified as a neurapraxia or conduction block, signifying demyelination. There is slowing of nerve conduction in both motor and sensory fibers across the lesion site.

**TREATMENT.** Medical management is aimed at asymptomatic management. A cock-up splint is used to maintain the wrist in an extended position until return of function.

**PROGNOSIS.** Radial nerve injuries such as Saturday night palsy have a good prognosis. Recovery rate is approximately 67% to 100% within 3 months, with the main goal being return of hand function.[229] If a neurapraxia is reported, normal conduction can be anticipated within a few months because the paralysis is related to a focal demyelination.[87]

## Parsonage-Turner Syndrome

Parsonage-Turner syndrome, also known as *neuralgia amyotrophy* is a rare condition affecting the LMNs of the brachial plexus or individual nerves or nerve branches. Etiology and incidence are unknown. Clinical presentation can vary but usually involves sudden pain, muscle weakness, and eventual atrophy of affected muscles in the shoulder girdle/upper extremity. There may be a precipitating event such as a prolonged static posture or sustained or repetitive load to the arm or upper quadrant. Recovery is usually spontaneous over a period of months up to several years; some residual muscle weakness may persist. Physical therapy to assist with return of strength, motor function (including scapulohumeral rhythm), and proprioception may be needed. The therapist should assess for myofascial pain patterns, tendinitis, and other soft tissue impairments caused by compensatory movement patterns. The differential diagnosis includes cervical radiculopathy, rotator cuff disease, and TOS.[177]

## Sciatica

### Incidence and Etiology

Sciatica is a radiculopathy that occurs most often in individuals between the ages of 40 and 60 years in which the sciatic nerve root is affected, most typically by compression. Of those who develop lumbosacral radiculopathy, 10% to 25% develop symptoms that last more than 6 weeks. Less commonly, sciatica may occur in the presence of abscess, blood clots, or tumors. Sciatica may be mistaken for intermittent claudication or low back pain without discogenic involvement and is one of the most common conditions managed in primary care settings.

### Pathogenesis

The epidural space is innervated by a meningeal branch of the spinal nerve, the recurrent sinuvertebral nerve. Arising from the dorsal root ganglion, this nerve enters through the intervertebral foramen, divides into ascending and descending branches to blood vessels, and supplies the posterior longitudinal ligament, superficial anulus fibrosis, anterior dura mater, and dural sleeve.[97] In animal studies, the sinovertebral nerve responded to high threshold mechanical stimuli. Conduction velocity for fibers in the nerve corresponded to types III and IV, which lead researchers to correlate nerve function with nociception.[190] Herniation of the intervertebral disc can impinge on the nerve root or structures innervated by the recurrent sinuvertebral nerve to cause pain. Disc herniation, usually at the L4-5 and L5-S1 levels, is the most common cause of sciatica (i.e., pain radiating down the posterior leg from sciatic nerve root irritation).[140]

### Clinical Manifestations

In addition to low back pain, when sensory fibers are affected, pain may radiate into one or both legs. The motor and sensory nerves are affected easily in a radiculopathy because compression occurs in an area where CNS connective tissue coverings meet the protective tissue coverings of the peripheral nerve, leaving that region of the nerve "at risk."[104] Coughing, sitting, and sneezing worsens the pain. Both clinical and experimental studies show that adjacent nerve roots may be affected when a lumbar disc herniates. Inflammatory chemical mediators released into the epidural space affect nearby nerve roots, without any direct compression of those roots.[155]

## MEDICAL MANAGEMENT

**DIAGNOSIS.** Radiologic tests and electrophysiologic studies may be used in diagnosing sciatica. MRI is preferred to CT scanning for lumbar spine imaging; however, because 60% of people without back symptoms have disc bulging on MRI, protrusion and bulges may not correlate with symptoms.[13] A screening EMG examination of only four muscles in the leg identified more than 89% of surgically confirmed involvement of the nerve root.[32] Others have noted that the H-reflex has provided better predictive value of nerve root involvement than standard motor and sensory nerve conduction radiculopathies.[4] Just as radiologic studies are not sufficient alone to distinguish sciatica neither is electrophysiologic testing.

**TREATMENT.** Conservative efforts and rehabilitation are recommended. Selective epidural injection of steroids at target nerve roots through the intervertebral foramina has offered short-term benefit for pain relief, as has the use of nonsteroidal antiinflammatory drugs.[37] Also unclear are the long-term effects of chemonucleolysis, which is reported to be less effective than discectomy.[78]

**PROGNOSIS.** Subjects who were evaluated 1 year after discectomy had recovery in unmyelinated and small myelinated fibers; the function of larger myelinated fibers did not improve. This provides a physiologic rationale for residual motor and sensory involvement.[155]

**SPECIAL IMPLICATIONS FOR THE THERAPIST 39.3**

*Sciatica*

It has been recommended that physical therapy interventions emphasize the use of joint mobilizations and exercise for improvements in health in people with sciatica.[102]

For those physical therapists using the visual analogue scale (VAS) to assess pain in sciatica, a range of minimal clinically relevant change has been reported. Using a 100-mm VAS, Todd et al[213] reported that a 13-mm change is needed to discriminate a crude change in pain, whereas Farrar et al[66] estimated a 20-mm change was needed to discriminate a crude change in pain. More recently, Giraudeau et al[81] also reported that 30 mm reflected a crude change in pain. Outcome assessments such as the Oswestry Disability Index and the Patient-Specific Functional Scale should be used to quantify meaningful functional changes with intervention.

## Morton Neuroma

Morton neuroma is a common entrapment neuropathy in the forefoot, most often involving the third toe interspace. It is also called Morton metatarsalgia, interdigital neuritis, and *interdigital perineural fibroma*. The term *neuroma* is misleading, because the problem is degenerative, not proliferative as the term implies.[2]

### Definition and Etiology

No incidence or prevalence for Morton neuroma has been published in any study. However, the average age of individuals diagnosed with Morton neuroma is reported to be between 45 and 60 years, with women affected more than men, in a ratio of 5:1. Bilateral involvement is uncommon.[31]

### Pathogenesis

Three common digital nerves, two arising from the medial plantar nerve and the third from the lateral plantar nerve, pass between divisions of the plantar aponeurosis where each bifurcates into two interdigital nerves. The first common digital nerve supplies adjacent sides of the great and second toe, those of the second common digital nerve supply adjacent sides of the second and third toes, and the sides of the third and fourth toes are supplied by the third common digital nerve (Fig. 39.12). Mechanical irritation resulting from intrinsic factors, such as diminished intermetatarsal head distance[86] and poor foot mechanics (excessive pronation during gait) that pulls the nerve more medially than normal and taut as the toes extend during terminal stance, and extrinsic factors, such as high heels in which the weight is transferred onto the forefoot, maintaining the nerve in a taut condition; narrow toe box on shoe that creates a greater compression in the area; and thin-soled shoes where ground forces interact with the deep transverse metatarsal ligament, causing

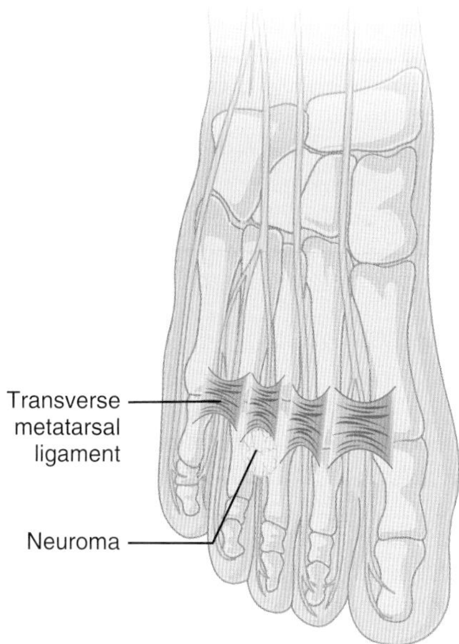


**Figure 39.12**

**Morton neuroma involves the common digital nerve.** The most frequent location is between third and fourth metatarsals. (From Frontera WR, Silver JK: *Essentials of physical medicine and rehabilitation*, Philadelphia, 2002, Hanley and Belfus.)

compression in this confined space, have been implicated as contributing to this condition. Additionally, inflammatory conditions, such as arthritis, and activities that involve application of repetitive forces to the plantar nerves, such as jogging on a hard surface, produce shear forces that can irritate the nerve.

Entrapment produces some or all of the following histopathology: thickening of the endoneurium, hyalinization of endoneurial vessels, thickened perineurium, and demyelination of nerve fibers.[31,181]

### Clinical Manifestations

Symptoms include burning, tingling, or sharp lancinating pain in one of the interspaces of the forefoot that occurs while walking. Pain may radiate into adjacent toes or proximally into the foot. Individuals may state that they must stop, remove their shoe, and massage their foot to relieve the symptoms. At its worst, the person may be apprehensive about stepping with the involved foot. Symptoms occur paroxysmally over many years and can limit participation in activities involving standing and walking.

## MEDICAL MANAGEMENT

**DIAGNOSIS.** In 2009, a practice guideline algorithm was published that aids the clinician in management of this common condition.[211] Typically, history and clinical examination have been used to diagnose this disorder. Two tests that provoke symptoms include plantar palpation of the involved space at the metatarsal heads as mediolateral compression is applied to the metatarsal heads (Mulder sign) and dorsiflexion of the involved toe producing symptoms and plantarflexion of the toe relieving them (Lasègue sign).[72] The reported positive predictive values of these clinical tests vary widely. Sonography and MRI have been used to assess the presence of Morton neuroma. Whereas the sensitivity for predicting the presence of Morton neuroma is reported at 0.79 and 0.86, respectively, the specificity of both sonography and MRI is 1.0194 and has been used to diagnose Morton neuromas.[168,209]

Differential diagnoses considered would include metatarsal stress fractures, metatarsalgia, and metatarsal phalangeal derangement. Radiographs may prove helpful in differential diagnosis.

**TREATMENT.** Conservative, nonoperative management is directed at pressure relief and involves use of a soft orthosis (insoles) or metatarsal pad. These may provide symptom relief as long as the shoes the person is wearing have a wider toe box and a lower heel. If symptoms continue, injection of a local anesthetic or corticosteroid from the dorsal direction may be helpful. Recent review suggests invasive treatments produce better outcomes in management of Morton neuromas.[217] Surgical treatment involves either neural decompression by releasing the intermetatarsal ligament or neurectomy proximal to the location of the neuroma to allow retraction of the plantar nerve away from the weight-bearing surface. Individuals undergoing surgical interventions have experienced complications such as postsurgical hammertoe deformity, keloid scar formation, and complex regional pain syndrome.[2]

**PROGNOSIS.** A systematic review of these interventions reports that for studies in which orthoses have been used, 45% to 50% of the participants reported pain relief of more than 50% up to 1 year postintervention. For various surgical approaches, pain relief of more than 50% occurred in 65% to 100% of patients up to 3 years postsurgery.[212]

## Idiopathic Facial Paralysis/Bell Palsy/ Facial Nerve Compression Damage

### Incidence

Bell palsy is a common clinical condition in which the facial nerve (cranial nerve [CN] VII) is unilaterally affected and is characterized by facial hemiparesis. Bell palsy affects 20 to 30 of 100,000 people each year. Although any age group can be affected, it is most common in persons between the ages of 15 and 45 years.[94]

### Etiology and Pathogenesis

A direct link between Bell palsy and viral infection has been difficult to establish. Serologic studies have found a lack of signs of an acute infection immediately preceding the onset of the Bell palsy. No seasonal predilection or epidemic clustering has been documented; it is much more likely that Bell palsy is caused by reactivation of a latent virus rather than direct, communicable viral infection, most likely a latent herpes virus (herpes simplex type 1/herpes zoster). Although it is likely that the underlying disease in Bell palsy is viral polyneuropathy, an unresolved question is why such a profound effect on the facial nerve occurs, in contrast with the relatively minor and transient changes in the other cranial nerves. The major anatomic difference between the facial and other cranial nerves is in its long bony canal and because the facial nerve lies in the auditory canal, any agent that causes inflammation and swelling creates a compression that could potentially cause demyelination, ischemia, and axonal degeneration.[73] In addition, centrally located structures, such as a schwannoma (acoustic neuroma) which is a slow growing tumor of the sheath of the nerve, can produce unilateral paralysis in the face by impinging on the facial nerve as it emerges from the brainstem. The weakness can appear similar; however there is slowly progressive paralysis and presence of auditory impairments.

### Risk Factors

Acute facial paralysis can occur as part of many viral illnesses, including mumps, rubella, herpes simplex, and Epstein-Barr virus. People with diabetes mellitus and pregnant women[33] have an increased incidence of Bell palsy.

### Clinical Manifestations

A unilateral facial paralysis develops rapidly, often overnight. Paralysis of the muscles of facial expression on one side creates an asymmetrical facial appearance (Fig. 39.13). The corner of the mouth droops, the nasolabial fold is flattened, and the palpebral fissure is widened because the eyelid does not close. In addition to the motor fibers providing innervation for facial musculature, the facial nerve also innervates the stapedius muscle of the middle ear and the sensory and autonomic fibers, which innervate for taste and lacrimation and salivation, respectively. Therefore involvement of these fibers may produce additional signs and symptoms to those of facial paralysis. If the lesion is proximal to where the fibers of the chorda tympani enter the facial nerve, the client will experience loss of taste on the affected side. In a similar fashion, if the autonomic fibers are involved, the client will experience dry eye (lack of tearing) and will produce less but thicker saliva. Some clients report that sounds are louder than normal (hyperacusis) because the stapes bone of the middle ear is less able to accommodate sound when the stapedius muscle's innervation is lost.

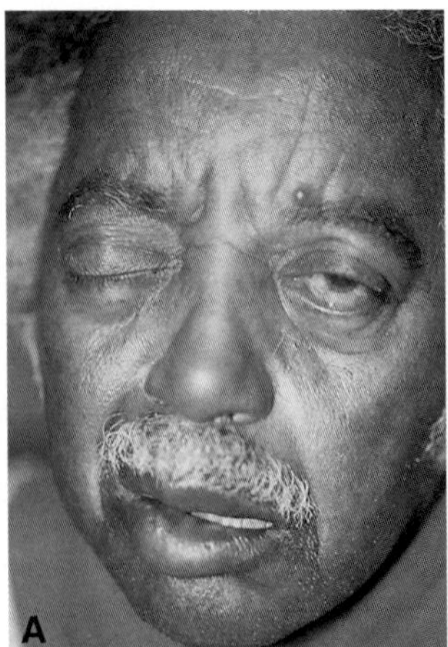


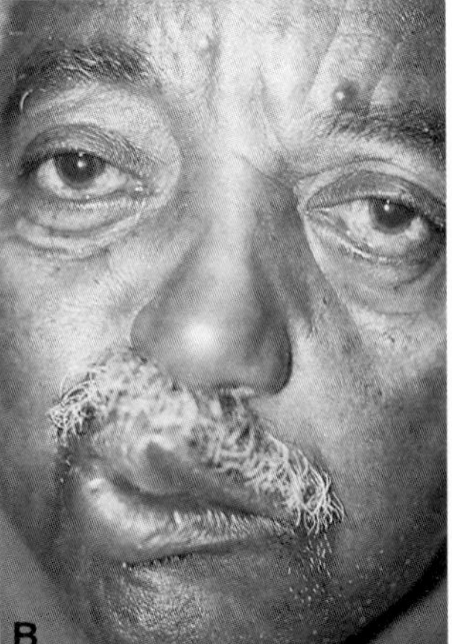


**Figure 39.13**

**A patient with a lesion of the facial nerve.** (A) The patient has difficulty in closing his left eye, and the left corner of his mouth droops. (B) The latter defect is especially evident when the patient attempts to purse his lips. (From Haines DE: *Fundamental neuroscience for basic and clinical applications,* ed 3, Philadelphia, 2006, Churchill Livingstone.)

## MEDICAL MANAGEMENT

**DIAGNOSIS.** Bell palsy is diagnosed in part by observation and in part by the physical examination. The individual is asked to wrinkle the forehead, close the eyes tightly, smile, and whistle while observed for facial asymmetry. In addition to the clinical presentation and history, electrodiagnostic tests can be used to demonstrate whether the lesion is one of demyelination or axonal degeneration. However, EMG as a diagnostic tool is only helpful after the nerve has degenerated; therefore testing is most accurate after 1 week. Tests of facial nerve excitability will also indicate whether the paralysis is complete.

LMN involvement of the facial nerve can be differentiated from an UMN involvement of this nerve because with UMN involvement, the client can close the eye and wrinkle the forehead but cannot smile voluntarily. With LMN involvement, the client is unable to close the eye, wrinkle the forehead, or smile voluntarily.

**TREATMENT.** The Quality Standards Subcommittee of the American Academy of Neurology recommends that early treatment with oral corticosteroids is probably effective in improving facial function outcomes in Bell palsy, and that the addition of acyclovir to prednisone is possibly effective; insufficient evidence exists to recommend facial nerve decompression.[103]

General medical care includes proper eye care. Reduced blinking and inability to completely close the eye increases the risk of corneal abrasion and ulceration. Artificial tears and ophthalmic ointments can prevent these complications. Patients should be instructed to use proper eye protection to prevent injuries. Facial muscle massage, facial nerve stimulation, and acupuncture have insufficient evidence to support their use.[124,148] Corticosteroids effectively reduce the risk of an unfavorable outcome. Antiviral agents, when administered concurrently with corticosteroids, may result in additional benefit.[208] However, patients offered antivirals should be counseled that a benefit from antivirals has not been established, and, if there is a benefit, it is likely that it is modest at best.[85]

**PROGNOSIS.** The overall prognosis of Bell palsy is favorable with most patients experiencing spontaneous resolution.[216] In one study of untreated patients, 85% showed signs of recovery within 3 weeks. Ultimately, 71% experienced complete recovery, and an additional 13% were thought to have only slight residual weakness. The degree of weakness at onset is an important prognostic indicator: 94% of patients with incomplete paralysis experienced complete recovery. At 3 to 4 months, the absence of any improvement, no matter how small, should raise concern regarding the diagnosis and lead to a search for alternative etiologies.

Motor nerve conduction studies, or electroneurography, can be used to help predict prognosis in selected patients. Patients with incomplete lesions that have an excellent prognosis do not require further evaluation. Motor nerve conduction studies involve stimulating the facial nerve electrically and recording muscle responses with surface electrodes over appropriate muscles. The amplitude of the evoked muscle response on the affected side at 10 days can be compared to the unaffected side, giving an estimate of the degree of axonal loss. A 90%

drop in amplitude predicts less than complete recovery, and loss greater than 98% predicts significant residual weakness and synkinesis.

During recovery from severe nerve injury, axonal regrowth may be misdirected, resulting in synkinesis. Voluntary activation of one muscle group can cause activation of other muscles, which is known as synkinesis. Attempts at blinking can result in twitching of the mouth, or smiling can cause involuntary blinking. Misdirection of autonomic fibers can result in the syndrome of "crocodile tears," involuntary lacrimation while eating.

Recurrent attacks of facial paralysis on the ipsilateral or contralateral side occur in up to 15% of patients, even after many years. Additional recurrences are quite rare, being reported at a rate between 1% and 3%.

SPECIAL IMPLICATIONS FOR THE THERAPIST 39.4

### *Bell Palsy/Facial Nerve Palsy*

Because experiments using animals have indicated that electrical stimulation suppresses neuronal sprouting, electrical stimulation is no longer routinely used. Motor control of facial musculature and recovery of function using neuromuscular reeducation can be enhanced by use of surface EMG feedback. Changes in the brain map associated with individual muscles result from prolonged inactivity of the facial muscles when the course of flaccidity is prolonged. Synkinesis, or the firing of more muscle groups than necessary for the movement, occurs over time, as a result of both cortical reorganization and sprouting of recovering nerve ending to adjacent muscles. Improvement in cortical reorganization through guided facial movement with surface EMG feedback contributes to isolation and control of specific muscle groups and reduction of synkinesis.

Initially, there is profound weakness of the face, with decreased firing at rest. As time passes, and neurologic recovery progresses, the resting tone tends to increase along with the synkinesis. Often, the focus of the intervention is on reducing tone at rest to improve ability to normalize facial expression and improve function during eating.[126] Bell reflex, the rolling up of the eye ball during closing of the eye, is the result of an unconscious attempt to occlude vision if the upper lid does not close far enough to meet the lower lid. The rolling of the eye is not controlled by CN VII, so the movement can be extinguished by conscious downward gaze during eye closure.

## HEREDITARY NEUROPATHIES

Hereditary neuropathies were once considered rare, genetically determined disorders; however, recent studies reflect, in some cases, that these represent 43% of undiagnosed neuropathies.[204] Hereditary neuropathies can be divided into two broad categories: those in which neuropathy is the primary disorder and those in which neuropathy is part of a greater multisystem disorder.[18] This section concentrates on the first group, which includes Charcot-Marie-Tooth disease and its related hereditary polyneuropathies.

### Charcot-Marie-Tooth Disease

Charcot-Marie-Tooth (CMT) disease, also known as hereditary motor and sensory neuropathy, progressive muscular atrophy, or peroneal muscular atrophy, is the most common inherited disorder affecting motor and sensory nerves. It was originally described by three neurologists, Jean Martin Charcot, Pierre Marie, and Howard Henry Tooth, in the 1880s.[171] Initially, the disorder involves the fibular (peroneal) nerve and affects muscles in the foot and lower leg. It later progresses to the muscles of the forearms and hands, making activities like buttoning or writing difficult. CMT is a genetically heterogeneous group of disorders with the same clinical phenotype, characterized by distal limb muscle wasting and weakness, usually with skeletal deformities, distal sensory loss, and abnormalities of DTRs.[162]

#### Incidence

Of the neuropathies, CMT is relatively common; it is estimated that 1 in 2500 persons in the United States has some form of CMT. Onset may occur in childhood or adulthood.[147]

#### Etiology

CMT is a genetically heterogeneous neuropathy that is most commonly inherited as autosomal dominant pattern with a genetic mutation on a chromosome other than X or Y with one normal gene and one CMT gene. Children of the affected individual will have a 50% chance of inheriting CMT. There is an autosomal recessive form of CMT in which the affected person's children have a 25% to 50% chance of inheriting the disease. It can also present as a first time occurrence in a family as a result of a spontaneous mutation.

More than 50 loci defects on chromosomes have been identified through deoxyribonucleic acid (DNA) testing.[18,154,195] These chromosomal defects create duplication, deletion, or point mutations in the genetic code for proteins that are involved in the process of myelination. CMT1 is the most common autosomal dominant pattern and is subdivided into three forms: CMT1A, -1B, and -1C. CMT1A accounts for 70% of all CMT1 cases and is caused by a DNA duplication on chromosome 17 for peripheral myelin protein 22 (PMP22), creating segmental demyelination of the fibular (peroneal) nerve.[121] A less-common form, CMT2, has had chromosomal abnormalities mapped to chromosomes 1, 8, and X. On chromosome 1, CMT2 is associated with a mutation in human myelin protein zero (P0), which is associated with axonal dysfunction. This second form of CMT is associated with axonal degeneration. CMT2 has an onset that varies between the second and seventh decades and has less involvement in the small muscles of the hands than CMT1.[42]

#### Pathology

Mutations in proteins (PMP, P0, and connexin) associated with Schwann cell myelination create extensive demyelination along with a hypertrophic onion bulb formation in which demyelinated axons are surrounded by Schwann cells and their processes as remyelination is attempted. The onion bulb formation creates palpable, enlarged peripheral nerves. CMT2 is associated with genetic mutations that disrupt neurofilament assembly and thus affect axonal transport, creating axonal involvement.[18]

### Clinical Manifestations

Although the two major types of CMT have differing chromosomal etiologies, it is nearly impossible to tell CMT1 from CMT2 clinically. In all autosomal dominant disorders, there are degrees of genetic dominance. The presence of symptoms are not all-or-none but are graded, with differing degrees of signs and symptoms among family members who have inherited the defective gene. This is termed *variable expressivity.* In CMT1 some members of a family with the genetic mutation may have greater signs of the disorder than others, who have only minor involvement.[132] In the X-linked form of CMT, men are affected and have signs of both demyelination and axonal degeneration are evident. CMT generally does not affect a person's intelligence, memory, or life span.

CMT is a slowly progressive disorder and although CMT1 begins in childhood, the actual onset may be difficult to determine. Clinical signs of CMT include distally symmetric muscle weakness, atrophy, and diminished DTRs. Because of the muscles affected, the client will have weakness of the dorsiflexors and evertors (peroneal musculature) and will ambulate with a footdrop (steppage) gait pattern. As CMT progresses, involvement will be seen distally in the upper extremities. Weakness and wasting of the intrinsic muscles of the hand occurs, followed by progressive wasting in the forearms. Because CMT1 demyelinates peripheral nerves, proprioception is lost in the feet and ankles, and cutaneous sensation is diminished in the foot and lower legs. Sensory loss is minimal in CMT2. Sensory symptoms can include tingling and burning in the feet and legs, as well as impaired proprioception.[233]

Feet have pes cavus (high arch) deformities and hammer toes (Fig. 39.14). As muscle atrophy progresses below the knee, the appearance of the client's legs takes on the shape of an inverted champagne bottle because normal muscle bulk is maintained above the knees.

## MEDICAL MANAGEMENT

**DIAGNOSIS.** CMT is diagnosed by history and clinical examination, hereditary picture, electrophysiologic studies, and nerve biopsy. Most recently, because of the sensitivity and specificity of genetic studies, the diagnosis of CMT can be confirmed using gel electrophoresis to detect duplication, deletions, or sequence variations in genes.[18] Although CMT1 produces demyelination, electrophysiologic testing reveals underlying axonal degeneration. Slowed motor nerve conduction does not have a linear correlation with the clinical severity of the disease.[117]

Both motor and sensory NCVs will be slowed in CMT1[130] but are normal or only slightly slowed in CMT2. Abnormalities of electrophysiologic studies in CMT2 include decreased amplitude of the potential, indicating axonal loss. The nerve biopsy is abnormal and will demonstrate either a demyelinating or axonal degenerative process.

**TREATMENT.** CMT is an inherited disorder, and there is no specific treatment to date to alter its course. Treatment is symptomatic to ensure that function is maintained in a safe manner. Footdrop and hand deformities can be helped by orthotic devices. Because the possibility of skin ulceration exists when discriminative touch and proprioception are affected, skin care precautions should be followed when total contact orthoses are used. To prevent contractures clients should be instructed in range-of-motion exercises. Whether strengthening exercises can be used to counteract the effects of CMT has not been addressed; however, the long-term effects would be of little benefit in the presence of ongoing axonal degeneration. In a study examining the effects of weakness in CMT, results have found that individuals with CMT tend to be obese and have poor exercise tolerance. It is unknown whether exercise interventions can improve body composition and function.[30]

Studies using animal models have reported that antiprogesterone therapy combined with ascorbic acid have a positive effect on CMT1A. Although stem cell and gene therapy have been considered, the most promising treatment is pharmacologic therapies targeting the genetic mutation.[154] Because specific treatments are currently lacking, and care is largely symptom based, the role of the clinician becomes increasingly important. Clinicians may contribute to accurate diagnosis based upon sensory, motor, and observational findings. Individuals with CMT need lifelong support through the disease process, as well as clinicians who can modify care based on the disease progression, and develop outcome measures to monitor the disease, its progression, and the impact of interventions.[173]

**PROGNOSIS.** CMT is a slowly progressive disorder that is currently considered incurable. However, the CMT Association has launched a research initiative called the Strategy to Accelerate Research (STAR) to look for more effective therapies and possibly a cure for the most common forms of CMT. If unmanaged, contracture formation resulting from weakness will create further gait

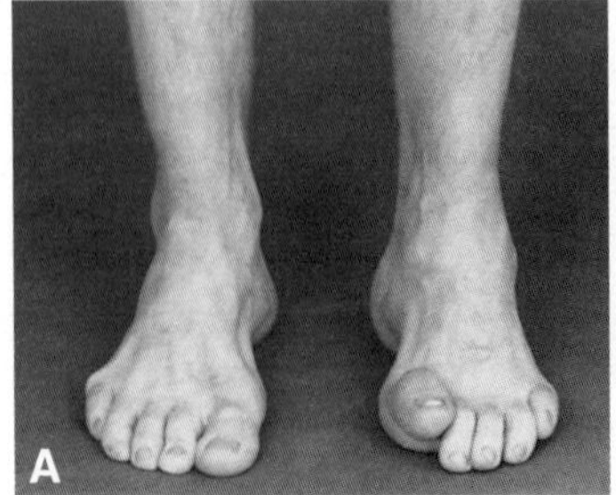

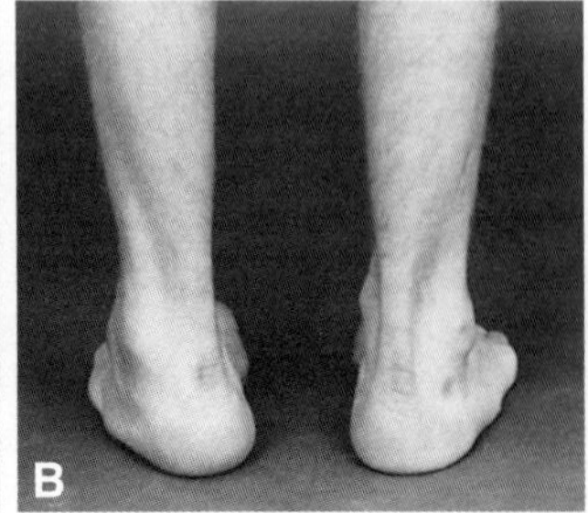

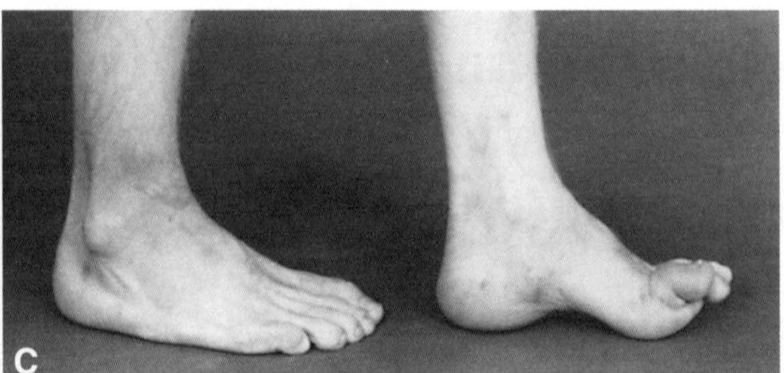


**Figure 39.14**

**Pes cavus foot deformity in Charcot-Marie-Tooth disease.** (A) Clawing of left great toe. (B) Left foot varus deformity. (C) Cavus deformity with hammer toes. (From Canale ST: *Campbell's operative orthopaedics*, ed 10, St Louis, 2003, Mosby.)

abnormalities, with clients reporting an increased number of falls. In the upper extremities, clients may develop problems with writing and handling objects. Individuals with CMT should be cautioned that some medications have been reported to cause an exacerbation of CMT. A database of the drugs that should be avoided is maintained by the CMT Association. Among the identified medications are several anticancer drugs, including vincristine, cisplatin, carboplatin, and taxoids.[230]

SPECIAL IMPLICATIONS FOR THE THERAPIST 39.5

*Charcot-Marie-Tooth Disease*

The goal in this progressive disorder is to minimize deformity and maximize function. As with other peripheral neuropathies in which muscle imbalances arise, for CMT management, the physical therapist should anticipate that deformities will arise from the imbalance between the tibialis anterior and peroneus longus and the tibialis posterior and peroneus brevis, which leads to a pes cavus and varus deformity, respectively. This weakness may be combined with diminished or lost proprioception and some degree of cutaneous involvement that can lead to an unsteady gait. These problems should be addressed with stretching, range-of-motion exercises, strengthening, endurance training, and bracing to improve ambulation.[36]A recent systematic review of randomized controlled trials raises question about the effectiveness of stretching programs for people with CMT and other neurologic conditions that place a person at risk for deformity and contracture. In fact, this review concluded that stretching programs have little or no effect when applied for less than 7 months. Effects of longer-duration stretching programs have not been elucidated.[107] An emphasis on compensation for safety with gait and function is recommended. Along with orthotic assessment and gait training, appropriate skin care should be taught to the client when total contact orthoses are used. When the individual has developed rigid deformities, a triple arthrodesis is the option to salvage remaining function.[156]

# METABOLIC NEUROPATHIES

## Diabetic Neuropathy

### Definition

A consensus conference has agreed that a detailed definition of diabetic neuropathy (DN) is "a descriptive term meaning a demonstrable disorder, either clinically evident or subclinical, that occurs in the setting of diabetes mellitus without other causes for peripheral neuropathy."[7,122] DN is a common complication associated with diabetes mellitus comprised of a heterogeneous group of progressive syndromes with diverse clinical manifestations. Neuropathies may be focal or diffuse and involve the autonomic or somatic PNS.[21,22,221] Typically, the involvement occurs in a distally, symmetric pattern, termed *diabetic polyneuropathy,* although single, focal nerve involvement may be seen.

### Incidence

In the United States, diabetes mellitus affects more than 34 million people, and this number is expected to increase by 5% every year. The prevalence of DN is greater (54%) in type 1 diabetes (insulin-dependent diabetes mellitus) than in type 2 diabetes (noninsulin-dependent diabetes mellitus), which is 30%. The most reliable estimates from clinical studies report that DN, although present in individuals with diabetes lasting longer than 25 years, is present in 7% of people within 1 year of diagnosis with diabetes.[196]

### Etiology

DN is likely caused by the chronic metabolic disturbances that affect nerve cells and Schwann cells in diabetes. For years, hyperglycemia was considered the sole cause of these secondary complications of diabetes. Although consequences of hyperglycemia include elevated levels of sorbitol and fructose, which coincides with deficiencies of sodium-potassium and adenosine triphosphate that alter the function of peripheral nerves, chronic hyperglycemia leads to abnormalities in microcirculation, creating endothelia capillary changes and local ischemia that affect the nerve. Excess sorbitol damages Schwann cells. Researchers have suggested that alterations in insulin levels appear to alter gene regulation of neurotrophic factors, adhesion molecules, and modification of proteins.[196]

### Risk Factors

Although hyperglycemia is not directly attributed to damaging nerve fibers causing DN, it is a contributing factor. Conversely, some people develop neuropathies even when glycemic control is good. A clear relationship does exist between duration of diabetes and development of DN. After the onset of the neuropathy, control of hyperglycemia is known to enhance the possibility of regeneration of fibers. Although studies have confirmed a genetic predisposition to diabetes, they have not confirmed such a predisposition to development of DN nor has a familial tendency been reported. Up to 50% of all people with diabetes never develop symptoms of neuropathy.

### Pathogenesis

Many hypotheses exist for the pathogenesis of this disorder. The metabolic effect of hyperglycemia exposes nerves and their associated Schwann cells to glucose. The most prominent change in DN is loss of both myelinated and unmyelinated axons. Nerves are affected distally more than proximally. Subtle changes have been reported at the nodes of Ranvier in nerves of people with DN. This is associated with slowing of the NCV.[220]

A number of studies suggest that vascular changes affect peripheral nerves in diabetes. Evidence demonstrates endoneurial microvascular thickening. In the sural nerve, this has resulted in increased numbers of closed capillaries, which are believed to cause multifocal regions of ischemia and hypoxia in the nerve, resulting in an axonal degeneration.

Another explanation for the development of DN proposes that the concentration of nerve growth factor, which has a structure molecularly and physiologically similar to insulin, is reduced. Because nerve growth factor acts as a trophic factor, its reduction also reduces nutrition to the nerve.

Box 39.4

**CLASSIFICATION OF DIABETIC NEUROPATHY**

*Rapidly Reversible*

- Hyperglycemic neuropathy

*Generalized Symmetric Polyneuropathies*

- Acute sensory
- Chronic sensorimotor
- Autonomic

*Focal Neuropathies*

- Cranial
- Focal limb

Adapted from Boulton AJ, Vinik AI, Arezzo JC, et al: Diabetic neuropathies. A statement by the American Diabetes Association, *Diabetes Care* 28:956–962, 2005.

## Clinical Manifestations

DN is classified in a number of ways: presumed etiology, pathologic features, anatomic location, and a mixture of these. Box 39.4 describes the disturbances that occur in DN.

**Rapidly Reversible Neuropathy**

*Hyperglycemic Neuropathy.* Hyperglycemic neuropathy occurs in individuals with poorly controlled diabetes, and rapidly reversible nerve conduction abnormalities are reported in those who have been newly diagnosed. These abnormalities are accompanied by distally symmetric sensory changes, such as burning, paresthesia, and tenderness in the feet and legs. Symptoms disappear when the individual's blood sugar is controlled, although abnormalities in nerve conduction may persist.[22]

**Generalized Symmetric Polyneuropathies**

*Acute Sensory Neuropathy.* Hallmarks of acute sensory neuropathy are the rapid onset of severe burning pain, deep aching pain, a sudden sharp "electric shock–like" sensation, and hypersensitivity of the feet that is often worse at night. Persons with this painful condition may have mild impairments in the physical exam, such as motor examinations in which the tendon reflexes are normal or reduced at the ankle and may have none or only mild symmetric sensory loss, with allodynia (painful sensation to nonnoxious stimuli). Testing procedures to confirm allodynia include application of a phasic stimulus (rub) to various parts of the body and asking the person whether burning occurs in a nearby region (application of a cotton ball or Semmes-Weinstein monofilament is not applied long enough for the slow summation required for allodynia). Another way of testing involves placing a towel on the body and waiting for a period of time before asking whether the cover creates pain. Nociceptive stimuli are perceived normally in acute sensory neuropathy. Electrophysiologic studies (NCV) may be normal or show minor changes. If the person can achieve and maintain stable blood glucose, recovery can occur within 1 year, even with severe symptoms.[22]

*Chronic Sensorimotor Neuropathy.* Chronic sensorimotor neuropathy, or diabetic polyneuropathy (DPN), is the most common type of DN and up to 50% of patients may develop this condition. Typically, its onset is insidious, but occasionally signs and symptoms appear acutely. The clinical features of DPN include sensory loss, occasionally with selective fiber-type involvement. Small fiber involvement leads to burning pain, and paresthesias, such as those described for acute sensory neuropathy, are more profound at night in the feet and lower legs (stocking pattern). Large fiber involvement results in painless paresthesia, with impaired vibration, proprioception, touch, and pressure, along with loss of ankle DTRs. Clients may report that they feel as if they were walking on cotton or clouds. In DPN, motor weakness is mild but can still cause hammer toes and/or pes cavus, with wasting of small muscles in the feet and hands in more advanced cases. The presence of pronounced motor involvement implies that this is not DPN. DPN may be accompanied by clinical or subclinical autonomic involvement that can include cardiovascular and sympathetic disturbances resulting in sweating, orthostatic hypotension, and resting tachycardia with greater than100 beats/min at rest.[22]

*Autonomic Neuropathy.* Sympathetic and parasympathetic involvement may occur in both type 1 and type 2 diabetes; however, in type 2 diabetes, parasympathetic functions are more affected. After 10 to 15 years, 30% of patients have subclinical manifestations of autonomic involvement. Box 39.5 shows the major manifestations associated with autonomic involvement.[172] Autonomic involvement is associated with significant morbidity and mortality in persons with DM.[76]

**Focal Neuropathies**

*Mononeuropathies.* Mononeuropathies in the limbs or cranial nerves may occur in diabetes less often than the generalized, symmetric patterns. The median, ulnar, and fibular (peroneal) nerves are most commonly affected in limb focal neuropathies. The somatic division of the oculomotor nerve is the most commonly involved cranial component.

## MEDICAL MANAGEMENT

**DIAGNOSIS.** The diagnosis is based on the history, clinical examination, electrodiagnostic studies, quantitative sensory evaluation, and autonomic function testing. Diagnosis of DN should not be based on a single symptom, sign, or test; a minimum of two abnormalities (signs and symptoms from NCV, sensory, or autonomic tests) has been recommended.[7] Tools required for the sensory examination include a 128-Hz tuning fork to assess vibration and a 1-g monofilament for touch. Autonomic functions can initially be assessed by blood pressure and heart rate response at rest, in standing, and with exercise. Because diabetes is a common disorder and because neuropathies may be related to other causes, mere association of neuropathic signs and symptoms in a person with diabetes is not sufficient to diagnose DN. Other causes must be excluded.[91]

Sensory, motor, and F-responses are important to assess nerve function at baseline and intermittently at follow-up visits. The most common electrical change is a reduced amplitude in the sensory nerve action potential, which

Box 39.5

**MANIFESTATIONS OF AUTONOMIC DIABETIC NEUROPATHY**

***Cardiovascular***

- Tachycardia
- Exercise intolerance
- Orthostatic hypotension
- Dizziness

***Gastrointestinal***

- Esophageal motility dysfunction
- Diarrhea
- Constipation

***Genitourinary***

- Neurogenic bladder
- Bladder urgency, incontinence
- Erectile dysfunction

***Other***

- Sweating, heat intolerance
- Dry skin
- Pupillary dysfunction, blurred vision

Adapted from Boulton AJ, Malik RA, Arezzo JC, et al: Diabetic somatic neuropathies, *Diabetes Care* 27:1458–1486, 2004.

suggests axonal degeneration. A recent report found that a high percentage of newly diagnosed patients with type 2 diabetes have reduced sensory nerve action potential in upper extremity nerves.[176] Slowing of sensory and/or motor NCV suggests a demyelinating neuropathy, and pronounced slowing suggests that an alternative diagnosis should be explored.[8] Sensory fibers are generally affected first before motor fibers.

**TREATMENT.** Management is divided into general and specific measures. General measures include control of hyperglycemia[222] and specific measures address the symptomatic management of the disorders. Because there is evidence that further complications can be reduced by maintaining control of the diabetes, this is a specific area addressed by health care professionals. In addition, specific drug therapies are being evaluated. Tricyclic antidepressants are used alone or in combination with fluphenazine to treat painful neuropathies and gabapentin or carbamazepine is used in the management of pain in focal neuropathies.[222] Angiotensin-converting enzyme inhibitors act on the vascular dysfunction and prevent the development and progression of DN.[138] In a systematic analysis of seven qualifying studies, researchers found vitamin $B_{12}$ (either as $B_{12}$ complex or as methylcobalamin, one of two coenzyme forms of $B_{12}$) had beneficial effects on pain and paresthesia rather than electrophysiologic changes. Methylcobalamin shows improvement in autonomic symptoms.[201]

If the person has a painful DN, an algorithm has been developed that begins with physical modalities to manage pain. This is combined with simple analgesics. Further management may include a trial of topical or benign drugs.[220] A myriad of treatments (various pharmacologic agents, topical agents, magnets, acupuncture, biofeedback, and exercise) have been suggested to manage painful DN. Of these the anticonvulsants pregabalin and gabapentin, and antidepressants duloxetine and amitriptyline have been shown to be safe and effective and have the strongest evidence according to recent guidelines.[25,197]

A common complication of DN is the development of neuropathic foot ulcers. When great toe and ankle joint mobility is limited, greater forefoot pressures occur during gait, which may place patients with diabetes (type 1 or 2) at risk for development of metatarsal ulceration.[236] In type 2 diabetes, early detection of DN along with prophylactic foot care regimens have led to fewer foot ulcerations and amputations.[192] Institution of foot care procedures is essential. With the development of a foot-drop gait, orthotic devices should be considered for the person's safety. The type of orthosis and shoe construction prescribed should be carefully considered based on the sensory status and the person's ability to demonstrate appropriate foot care.

**PROGNOSIS.** DN is a slowly progressive metabolic disorder that affects many body systems. Estimates are that more than 50% of nontraumatic amputations in the United States occur in people with diabetes. The presence of autonomic involvement is associated with an increased mortality risk.

SPECIAL IMPLICATIONS FOR THE THERAPIST 39.6

### *Diabetic Polyneuropathy*

Type 2 diabetes is established as an epidemic in developed countries such as the United States, and it is expected to increase in prevalence through the year 2050. Carrying risks and complications for many body systems, included but not limited to DN, physical therapists should focus treatments not just on the specific impairments targeting the problems of neuropathy, but also the overall health condition of the individual with diabetes. Beyond this, because there is such strong evidence that regular physical activity can prevent and delay the onset of the disease, it is suggested that the physical therapist may be ideal and uniquely trained to influence prevention programs for this population.[50] As impairments of DN can lead to problems with safety and mobility, therapists should work to maintain and improve function while preventing falls in this population. Furthermore, a 2010 randomized control trial demonstrated that gait and balance of patients with diabetes can be improved using a specific task-based exercise program.[5]

## Alcoholic Neuropathy

Peripheral neuropathies, typically with distally symmetric involvement, appear in persons with chronic alcoholism. This alcohol-related peripheral neuropathy is known to affect sensory, motor, and autonomic fibers and can be a debilitating problem in people with chronic alcoholism.

### Etiology and Risk Factors

Although the exact pathogenesis of alcoholic neuropathy remains unclear,[223] lesions affecting the peripheral nerves have been attributed to both the direct toxic effects of alcohol on nerve and nutritional deficiencies in thiamine and other B vitamins from poor dietary habits. However, there is more recent evidence that neither age nor nutritional status plays a part in development of alcoholic neuropathies. Rather, alcohol-related neuropathies appear to be a result of the total lifetime accumulation of ethanol.[60] Patients exhibiting alcoholic neuropathy were divided into those with and without a coexisting thiamine deficiency. Researchers reported that patients without thiamine deficiency tended to have a more slowly progressive disorder in which sensory symptoms were dominant, primarily pain or a burning sensation. Along with these symptoms, the nerve biopsy demonstrated greater small fiber axonal loss. Those with alcoholic neuropathy with thiamine deficiency had large fiber involvement with segmental demyelination, and an acutely progressive motor dominant pattern along with loss of superficial and deep sensation. These findings further support the view that alcohol directly and adversely affects nerve fibers.[115]

### Pathogenesis

The exact pathogenesis of alcoholic neuropathy remains unclear. Segmental demyelination and axonal degeneration have been described in persons with alcoholic polyneuropathy; these differences may relate to the presence of vitamin deficiencies, as noted above. Changes occur distally at first and become more marked and proximal.[82]

### Clinical Manifestations

Mild forms of alcoholic neuropathy exhibit minor loss of muscle bulk, diminished ankle reflexes, impaired sensation in the feet, and aching in the calves. Distal sensory changes include pain, paresthesia, and numbness in a symmetric stocking-and-glove pattern. In addition, vibratory perception is impaired. It begins insidiously and progresses slowly; occasionally the onset may occur acutely. In the most advanced cases, symptoms involve all four extremities. Weakness and atrophy of distal musculature occurs, with lower-extremity involvement greater than upper extremity. Bilateral footdrop is observed during gait, and a wristdrop contributes to diminished grip strength because of the person's inability to extend the wrist. Both of these features are often combined with varying amounts of peripheral weakness in other muscles.

### MEDICAL MANAGEMENT

**DIAGNOSIS AND TREATMENT.** The diagnosis is made by history, clinical examination, and electrodiagnostic testing showing loss of action potential amplitude (sensory and motor). Although diet is no longer implicated as a contributing factor in the development of alcoholic neuropathies, diet to improve nutritional status, along with vitamin supplements and abstinence from alcohol, is the treatment of choice.

It has been suggested that aerobic exercise may benefit individuals during alcohol recovery by decreasing stress and improving coping mechanisms.[26] Given that alcohol-related peripheral neuropathies have a toxic cause; treatments that either block or reverse the target of the attacking substances are being investigated.[143]

All other treatment is symptomatic. Orthotic devices, such as ankle-foot orthoses and cock-up splints, are used to manage weakness and improve function. Medications for sensory changes include carbamazepine, salicylates, and amitriptyline. Additional suggested therapeutic options include benfotiamine, α-lipoic acid, acetyl-L-carnitine, vitamin E, methylcobalamin, myoinositol, *N*-acetylcysteine, tricyclic antidepressants, gabapentin, and topical capsaicin. Further investigations are needed to make evidence-based recommendations for the treatment and prevention of alcoholic neuropathy.[32]

**PROGNOSIS.** If the client totally abstains from alcohol, mild improvement can be expected, but recovery is slow (months to years) and incomplete when axonal degeneration has occurred.[160] Therefore, to anticipate the outcome, review the client's electrophysiologic studies to determine whether demyelination or degeneration is present.

Compression neuropathies, such as Saturday night palsy or peroneal nerve compression, may result from a bout of chronic alcohol intoxication where prolonged pressure compromises nerve function. Excessive alcohol intake may also produce rhabdomyolysis which produces proximal muscle weakness, swelling, and pigmented urine. Rhabdomyolysis can occur as a product of renal failure after drinking.

## Chronic Renal Failure

Chronic renal failure results from a gradual and progressive loss of kidney function. Electrolytes and waste products accumulate and are toxic to body systems.

### Clinical Manifestations

Alteration of CNS and PNS function often occurs with chronic renal failure associated with uremia. CNS involvement (uremic encephalopathy) is manifested by recent memory loss, inability to concentrate, perceptual errors, and decreased alertness. Uremic toxins induce demyelination and atrophy, thus likewise are detrimental to both sensory and motor nerves of the PNS. The lower extremities are much more commonly affected than the upper extremities; neurologic changes are typically symmetric and can also be manifested as peripheral neuropathy or restless leg syndrome, which is more pronounced at rest.

## Anemia

CNS symptoms can develop in cases of severe pernicious anemia, whereas PNS symptoms of neuropathy are observed in early cases of vitamin $B_{12}$ deficiency. The findings typically consist of a symmetric sensory neuropathy that begins in the feet and lower legs, causing moderate pain or paresthesias, although it may sometimes involve the upper extremities, especially fine motor coordination of the hands. This upper extremity neuropathy may clinically manifest as problems with deteriorating handwriting. With a loss of proprioception, the person may interpret the neuropathy as difficulty with locomotion. The affected individual may need to hold on to the wall, countertops, or furniture at home as a result of difficulties maintaining balance. There may be an associated positive Romberg sign. Loss of motor function is a late manifestation of vitamin $B_{12}$ deficiency. Although a symmetric neuropathy is the usual pattern, vitamin $B_{12}$ deficiency occasionally presents as a unilateral neuropathy and/or bilateral but asymmetric neuropathy. Rarely, subacute degeneration of the spinal cord caused by vitamin $B_{12}$ deficiency can occur in pernicious anemia, characterized by pyramidal and posterior column deficits. CNS manifestations may include headache, drowsiness, dizziness, fainting, slow thought processes, decreased attention span, apathy, depression, and irritability.

# INFECTIONS/INFLAMMATIONS

## Guillain-Barré Syndrome

### Overview and Definition

Guillain-Barré syndrome (GBS) was originally described by and named for the French neurologists who published case reports describing a syndrome of flaccid paralysis, areflexia, and albuminocytologic dissociation. More recently, the syndrome has been viewed as having distinct subtypes with varying distributions worldwide. Since the virtual elimination of poliomyelitis in North America, GBS is the most common cause of rapidly evolving motor paresis and paralysis and sensory deficits. Individuals affected with GBS typically reach maximal weakness within 2 to 3 weeks, but spend weeks to months recovering. The most common form of GBS is also known as acute inflammatory demyelinating polyradiculoneuropathy.

### Incidence

Annual incidence varies from 1 to 2 cases per 100,000 people. Although GBS occurs at all ages, peaks in frequency can be seen in young adults and in the fifth through the eighth decades. Occurrence is slightly greater for men than women and for whites more than blacks. Some researchers have noted a seasonal relationship associated with infections.

### Etiology and Risk Factors

Evidence supports the view that GBS is an immune-mediated disorder. Bacterial *(Campylobacter jejuni)* and viral (*Haemophilus influenza*, Epstein-Barr virus, and cytomegalovirus) infections, surgery, and vaccinations have been associated with the development of GBS. Acute infection in one study preceded onset of GBS. In one study, 90% of persons with GBS had illnesses (e.g., respiratory or gastrointestinal) during the preceding 30 days.[163]

### Pathogenesis

Lesions occur throughout the PNS from spinal nerve roots to the distal termination of both motor and sensory fibers. Originally, GBS was classified as a single entity characterized by PNS demyelination. Now, however, it is defined as several heterogeneous forms (Table 39.9). *C. jejuni* is associated more commonly with the axonal form, whereas greater sensory involvement is seen following cytomegalovirus.[98] The axonal pattern of involvement can involve motor fibers only or in the more severely involved form, motor and sensory fiber degeneration. Miller-Fisher syndrome is characterized by an acute onset of extraocular muscle paralysis with sluggish pupillary light reflexes, a peripheral sensory ataxia, and loss of DTRs with relative sparing of strength in the extremities and trunk. Facial weakness and sensory loss in the limbs may also occur.

Molecular mimicry remains the primary theory for the cause of GBS because evidence exists for antibody-mediated demyelination. Myelin of the Schwann cell is

**Table 39.9** Guillain-Barré Syndrome and Its Variants

| Abbreviation | Name | Clinical Characteristics |
|---|---|---|
| AIDP | Acute inflammatory demyelinating polyneuropathy | Primary demyelination: progressive paralysis, areflexia |
| AMAN | Acute motor axonal neuropathy | Axonal variant, more severe: frequent respiratory involvement/ventilator dependence and significant residual impairments |
| ASAN | Acute sensory ascending neuropathy | Sensory changes more prominent than weakness |
| AMSAN | Acute motor and sensory axonal neuropathy | |
| | Acute autonomic neuropathy | Manifested by postural hypotension, impaired sweating, lacrimation, bowel and bladder function |
| | Fisher/Miller-Fisher syndrome | Ophthalmoplegia, ataxia, areflexia with significant weakness |
| CIDP | Chronic inflammatory demyelinating polyneuropathy | Slower onset, relapses and remissions or progressive course over year |

the primary target of attack. Circulating antibodies to gangliosides penetrate and bind to an antigen on the surface of the myelin and activate either complement or an antibody-dependent macrophage.[100] The earliest pathologic changes in the PNS take the form of a generalized inflammatory response. Lymphocytes (T cells) and macrophages are the inflammatory cells present. Demyelination, initiated at the node of Ranvier, occurs because macrophages, responding to inflammatory signals, strip myelin from the nerves. After the initial demyelination, the body initiates a repair process. Schwann cells divide and remyelinate nerves, resulting in shorter internodal distances than were present initially.

Axons are damaged during the inflammatory process, according to what has been called a "bystander effect." Products that are liberated by the macrophages as they strip myelin (e.g., free oxygen radicals and proteases) also damage axons.

Researchers have reported the presence of macrophages that invade periaxonal spaces, causing the axon to degenerate within the ventral roots. Recovery for this wallerian-like degeneration would require an extremely long period. Binding of antibodies to the nodes of Ranvier may cause blocking of nerve conduction by altering sodium channel conductance.

### Clinical Manifestations

Various subtypes of GBS exist; however, the classic picture is an acute form in which the time from onset to peak impairment is 4 weeks or less. A recurrent form of GBS is reported in up to 10% of cases. Acute relapses may occur in GBS making it difficult to differentiate the acute from the chronic form, called *chronic inflammatory demyelinating polyradiculoneuropathy*. Most cases of chronic inflammatory demyelinating polyradiculoneuropathy progress over a period of months instead of weeks.

GBS is characterized by a rapidly ascending bilateral symmetric motor weakness and distal sensory impairments. The first neurologic symptom is often paresthesia in the toes. This is followed within hours or days by weakness distally in the legs. Weakness spreads to involve arms, trunk, and facial muscles. Flaccid paralysis is accompanied by absence of DTRs. Occasionally, sensory and motor symptoms begin in the hands and arms instead of the feet and legs. Palatal and facial muscles become involved in about half of all cases; even the muscles of mastication may be affected, but nerves to extraocular muscles typically are not involved. Up to 30% of all cases require mechanical ventilation.

Because the preganglionic fibers of the ANS are myelinated, they, too, may be subject to demyelination. If this occurs, tachycardia, abnormalities in cardiac rhythm, blood pressure changes, and vasomotor symptoms occur.

In 50% of the cases, progression of symptoms generally ceases within 2 weeks and in 90% of the cases, progression ends by 4 weeks. After the progression stops, a static phase begins, lasting 2 to 4 weeks before recovery occurs in a proximal to distal progression. This recovery may take months or even years.

## MEDICAL MANAGEMENT

**DIAGNOSIS.** Careful clinical and neurophysiologic examinations and laboratory tests are needed to diagnosis GBS. Criteria have been developed by the National Institute of Neurologic and Communicative Disorders and Stroke (Box 39.6).[28]

To aid in diagnosis a lumbar puncture can be performed to withdraw cerebrospinal fluid. Albumin (a protein) is elevated in the cerebrospinal fluid with 10 or fewer mononuclear leukocytes present. Electrophysiologic tests will reveal slowed NCVs the entire length of the nerve when demyelination is present, as well as fibrillation potentials when axonal degeneration occurs. When both axonal involvement and demyelination occur, the amplitude of the evoked (NCV) potential will be reduced and the velocity is slowed, respectively.

These abnormalities may not be apparent during the first few weeks of the illness. In addition, to determine the extent of demyelination of the more proximal nerve roots, an F-wave electrophysiologic test may be performed; it is often prolonged or absent. As recovery occurs, slowed NCVs persist, even though the person has made a full clinical recovery. Although electrophysiologic studies are used for diagnosis, the distal compound motor action potential is a predictor of prognosis. If the compound

**Box 39.6**

**CRITERIA FOR DIAGNOSIS OF GUILLAIN-BARRÉ SYNDROME**

***Symptoms Required for Diagnosis***

- Progressive weakness in more than one extremity
- Loss of deep tendon reflexes

***Symptoms Supportive of Diagnosis (in Order of Importance)***

- Weakness developing rapidly that ceases to progress by 4 wk
- Symmetric weakness
- Mild sensory symptoms and signs
- Facial weakness common and symmetric; oral-bulbar musculature may also be involved
- Recovery usually begins 2 to 4 wk after GBS ceases to progress
- Tachycardia, cardiac arrhythmias, and labile blood pressure may occur
- Absence of fever

***CSF Features***

- CSF protein levels increased after 1 wk; continue to increase on serial examinations
- CSF contains 10 or fewer mononuclear leukocytes/mm3

***Electrodiagnostic Features***

- Nerve conduction velocity slowed

*CSF*, Cerebrospinal fluid; *GBS*, Guillain-Barré syndrome.
Adapted from Hund EF, Borel CO, Cornblath DR, et al: Intensive management and treatment of severe Guillain-Barré syndrome, *Crit Care Med* 21:435, 1993.

motor action potential amplitude is less than 20% of normal limits at 3 to 5 weeks, it predicts a prolonged or poor outcome.[167]

Conversion disorder is a differential misdiagnosis. Because of the speed of onset, a stroke involving the brainstem will also be considered. Less-common causes of acute neuropathies must also be considered, including tick paralysis, and metabolic disorders such as porphyria. Care should be taken to rule out other potential causes of weakness including toxic exposures.

**TREATMENT.** Because GBS is believed to be an autoimmune disease, treatment has been aimed at controlling the response. High-dose intravenous (IV) administration of immunoglobulin (Ig; a protein the immune system normally uses to attack foreign organisms) has been found safe and effective in the treatment of GBS.[218] Plasmapheresis, a technique (also called plasma exchange) that removes plasma from circulation and filters it to remove or dilute circulating antibodies, significantly improves the impairments in GBS. Plasmapheresis is instituted when respiratory function drops precipitously (to 1.0-1.5 L), and the person is placed on a respirator.[23] For children with severe GBS, either treatment approach is an option.[99]

**PROGNOSIS.** The primary methods of managing GBS have helped to improve mortality rates, which can exceed 5%. Factors that predict a poor outcome include onset at an older age, a protracted time before recovery begins, and the need for artificial respiration. An important objective evaluation finding that predicts a poor outcome is significantly reduced evoked motor potential amplitude, which correlates with the presence of axonal degeneration. A recent analysis of prognostic predictors in GBS concluded a younger age, absence of preceding diarrhea, lower levels of disability and admission, longer interval between symptoms and admission, and absence of ventilator support need are all favorable factors.[170] Although most persons recover, up to 20% can have remaining neurologic deficits. After 1 year, 67% of clients have complete recovery, but 20% remain with significant disability.[67] Even after 2 years, 8% have not recovered. Complications that can persist, even when function is recovered, include neuropathic pain, autonomic changes, and distal weakness in the extremities.

SPECIAL IMPLICATIONS FOR THE THERAPIST 39.7

## *Guillain-Barré Syndrome*

Physical therapy is initiated at an early stage in this condition to maintain joint range of motion within the client's pain tolerance and to monitor muscle strength until active exercises can be initiated. During the ascending phase, when the person is losing function and becoming weaker, the person can become easily fatigued and overwhelmed. Focus is toward prevention of complications associated with immobilization. Physical status and gains should be monitored with outcome measures such as the functional independence measure (FIM) or the activity measure for postacute care (AM-PAC).

Meticulous skin care is required by all staff members to prevent skin breakdown and contractures. A strict turning schedule should be established and followed by all health care providers. After each position change, skin should be inspected (especially the sacrum, heels, ankles, shoulders, and greater trochanter).

Deep muscular discomfort or pain in the proximal muscles may be reported by clients. Paresis or paralysis requires positioning and appropriate splinting, which can help alleviate muscle and joint pain. Bed cages may reduce dysesthesias that are present in the feet. Palliative modalities, such as hot packs and gentle massage, may also bring relief of musculoskeletal pain.

Care in the intensive care unit (ICU) requires observation of arterial blood gas measurements. Because the disease results in primary hypoventilation with hypoxemia and hypercapnia, watch for $PO_2$ below 70 mm Hg, which signals respiratory failure. Report any signs of rising $PCO_2$ (e.g., confusion, tachypnea). Pulse oximetry may be used to monitor peripheral oxygen saturation. Auscultate breath sounds, turn and position the person, and encourage coughing and deep breathing to maintain clear airways and prevent atelectasis. The therapist must also follow universal precautions to help prevent any respiratory infection for the client. Respiratory support is needed at the first sign of dyspnea (in adults, vital capacity less than 800 mL; in children, less than 12 mL/kg of body weight) or decreasing $PO_2$.

Ventilation is instituted when pulmonary function is compromised by loss of respiratory skeletal muscle control. Coughing and clearing of tracheal secretions becomes difficult. In addition, weakness of laryngeal and pharyngeal muscles makes swallowing difficult and increases the risk of aspiration. Early tracheostomy is indicated in people with clinical and EMG evidence of axonal involvement together with respiratory failure.

Clinical indications for weaning from the ventilator include improved forced vital capacity and improved inspiratory force concomitant with improved muscle stretch. Finally, the chest should be clear of atelectasis. Communication using a communication board or other method is needed during ventilatory support.

### Exercise and Guillain-Barré Syndrome

When the person's condition stabilizes, aqua therapy can be used to initiate movement in a controlled environment. A major precaution during the early treatment phase is to provide gentle stretching and active or active-assistive exercise at a level consistent with the person's muscle strength. During the descending phase, when the paralysis slowly recedes and physical function returns, neuromuscular facilitation techniques may be integrated into the active and resistive exercises. Evidence now suggests that higher intensity rehabilitation for people with GBS produces greater functional improvements and reduces disability than does lower-intensity rehabilitation.[174]

Longer length of stay is correlated with presence of muscle tenderness, extreme lower-limb weakness, and low functional independence measure scores at admission. Although the presence of axonal involvement was not significantly related to length of stay, it does affect severity of involvement and the need for ventilator and orthosis, which tended to require longer stays.[75] The length of time to maximum impairment (respiratory compromise and motor involvement) has not been found to correlate with outcome. Generally, the shorter the time it takes for recovery to begin after maximum impairment has been reached, the less likely it is that long-term disability will occur.[153] When the person is discharged from therapy, recovery may not be complete. Impaired function may require the continued use of assistive devices and possibly even mobility equipment such as a wheelchair or scooter. The home may require modifications, which should be evaluated and planned for before discharge.

## Postpolio Syndrome/Postpolio Muscular Atrophy

### Overview

Poliomyelitis (polio) virus infection was virtually eradicated in the United States with the advent of the Salk vaccine in the 1950s and the Sabin vaccine in the 1960s. However, it remains a global health concern. It is a highly infectious and potentially deadly disease that is transmitted through person-to-person contact. Much of what is known about its course is based upon the epidemics in the United States. Clinically, the disease is characterized as one of three patterns: (1) an asymptomatic or (2) nonparalytic infection that produced gastrointestinal, flu-like symptoms and muscular pain or (3) a paralytic infection that also began with flu-like symptoms. The paralytic form generally developed within a week after the onset of the symptoms and is caused by the virus invading anterior horn cell bodies. The extent of the asymmetric paresis and paralysis that ensued depended on the degree of anterior horn cell involvement. When cell bodies were killed, motor axons underwent wallerian degeneration and muscles rapidly atrophied. Of those persons developing acute paralysis, equal numbers (30%) recovered, had mild residual paralysis, or were left with moderate to severe paralysis. Ten percent died from respiratory involvement. Recovery was attributed to the recovery of some anterior horn cells, as well as collateral sprouting from intact peripheral nerves, and to hypertrophy of spared muscle fibers.[49]

Polio is a unique neuropathy that creates focal and asymmetric motor impairments, rather than the typical distal, symmetric motor and sensory losses associated with other neuropathies. For decades it was considered a static disease; after the initial episode there was no further progression of the disease. The last major epidemics of polio in the United States occurred in the early 1950s; thus most of the people who had paralytic polio are at least 70 years old today. Most people had significant recovery of function and went on to live very productive lives.

### Definition

Postpolio syndrome (PPS), or postpolio muscular atrophy, refers to new neuromuscular symptoms that occur decades (average postpolio interval is 25 years) after recovery from the acute paralytic episode.[164] It can be difficult to diagnose because symptoms may be nonspecific.[125] PPS is generally characterized by weakness, declines in functional mobility and reports of fatigue.

### Incidence and Risk Factors

It is estimated that there are 1.63 million polio survivors in the United States and that one fourth to one half of them will develop PPS.[89] A previous diagnosis of polio is essential for this diagnosis. As well, the degree of initial motor involvement as measured by weakness in the acute stage is a factor in the development of PPS. These combine with long-term overuse of muscle that places increased demands on joints, ligaments, and muscle.

### Etiology

PPS appears to be related to the initial disorder of the motor neuron cell body affected by the poliovirus. Much of the recovery of muscle strength that occurred after the axonal degeneration can be attributed to reinnervation of denervated muscle fibers by collateral sprouts from other nearby surviving axons. That is, surviving axons increased the size of their innervation ratio. For example, instead of one axon innervating 3000 muscle fibers in the quadriceps, one axon innervated 5000 fibers. Studies confirm that denervation progresses in persons with prior poliomyelitis in both clinically affected and unaffected muscles, and indicate that this progression is more rapid than that occurring in normal aging. Overall, there was a 13.4% reduction in motor-unit number and a 18.4% diminution in M-wave amplitude ($p < 0.001$). The rate of motor-unit loss was twice that occurring in healthy subjects older than age 60 years.[142]

### Pathogenesis

Muscle biopsy and EMG both indicate ongoing muscle denervation. PPS seems to be an evolution of the original motor neuron dysfunction that began after the poliovirus affected the alpha motor neuron. PPS is manifested when the compensated reinnervation that occurred cannot maintain that muscle fiber innervation. The nervous system is pruning back axonal sprouts in this enlarged motor unit that it no longer has the metabolic ability to support; thus new denervation results. Symptoms are related to an attrition of oversprouting motor neurons that can no longer support these axonal spouts.[40]

### Clinical Manifestations

Symptoms vary, but in general, muscle strength declines in all people, with periods of stability for 3 to 10 years in muscles that had previously been affected by polio and had fully or partially recovered. Administration of an index of postpolio sequelae has shown that pain, atrophy, and bulbar (respiratory and swallowing) problems are the three most prominent sequelae from poliomyelitis.[105]

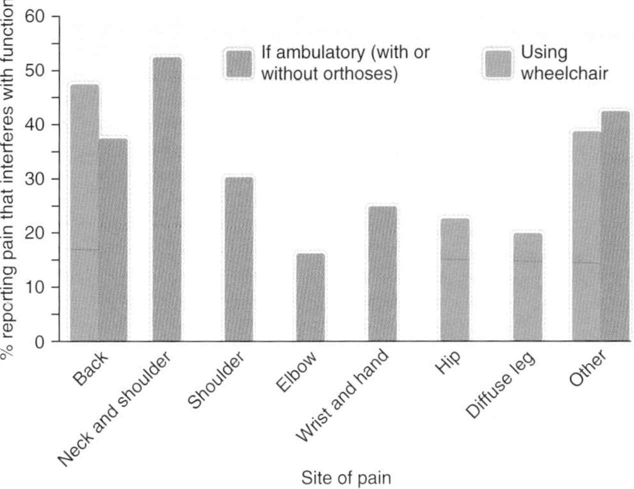


**Figure 39.15**

Location of pain reported in ambulatory and wheelchair-bound persons diagnosed with postpolio syndrome. (Data from Department of Physical Therapy, Institute for Rehabilitation and Research, Houston: *An instructional course on physical therapy management of post-poliomyelitis: new challenges*. Presented at the 65th American Physical Therapy Association Annual Conference, Chicago, June 1986.)

Affected persons have also reported myalgias, joint pain, increased muscle atrophy, and new weakness, as well as excessive fatigue with minimal activity, vasomotor abnormalities, and diminishing endurance. These all combine to contribute to a loss of function. Researchers report that the rate of strength deterioration is faster than would occur in normal aging. Deterioration in the lower extremity predisposes individuals to overuse of upper extremity musculature to compensate.[113]

Typically, symptoms are related to the individual's activities of daily living, such as crutch walking and wheelchair propulsion (Fig. 39.15). Pain is commonly located in the low back and joints of the upper extremity in women; it is worse at night and increases with physical activity and changes in climate.

## MEDICAL MANAGEMENT

**DIAGNOSIS.** PPS is a clinical diagnosis requiring the exclusion of other medical, neurologic, orthopedic, or psychiatric disorders that could explain the new symptoms. Routine EMG can be used to confirm any new denervation, as can muscle biopsies. Single-fiber EMG and spinal fluid studies are rarely needed to establish a diagnosis.[40]

**TREATMENT.** Medical management is aimed at symptomatic treatment and modification of lifestyle. Surgery for residual calcaneovalgus deformities at the ankle includes triple arthrodesis.[64] Perimalleolar tendon transfers have been performed to compensate for triceps surae insufficiency.[51] Small controlled studies investigating specific treatments with therapeutic agents such as steroids and amantadine report no definitive benefit.[65,129] It is recommended that the care of individuals with PPS be carried out by a multidisciplinary team, including specialists in rehabilitation. Treatments aimed at lifestyle intervention and activity modification are also recommended.[141]

**PROGNOSIS.** PPS is a slowly progressive disorder with stable periods that last 3 to 10 years. A decline in functional status is reported to correlate with a poorer quality of life in individuals affected by PPS.[114] Patients with PPS report concerns that health care providers often do not fully understand their condition.[54]

**SPECIAL IMPLICATIONS FOR THE THERAPIST 39.8**

### *Postpolio Syndrome*

Of importance to therapists is the ongoing question of the use of exercise in the management of PPS. Partially denervated muscle does not have the physiologic capacity to respond to a conventional strengthening program. Instead, programs aimed at nonexhaustive exercise and general body conditioning are preferable.[86] The client should never exercise to the point of fatigue, and vital signs are monitored before and after exercise to assess the client's response to even mild activity. Caution the client to stop if pain persists or weakness increases. Because individuals with PPS have decreased peak workloads and decreased oxygen uptake, functional exercises of submaximal intensity are stressed, with the goal of maintaining and improving endurance and functional capacity. For those with relatively good strength, a program to improve aerobic fitness is appropriate; for those with weaker leg musculature, a generalized fitness program should be aimed at endurance and improving work capacity.[232] Additionally, clients with PPS may also benefit from lifestyle modifications, including energy conservation techniques. Late-onset weakness, pain, and fatigue have been reported in individuals who had not developed the paralytic form of the disease.[89] Furthermore, as fatigue is identified as a common impairment that negatively impacts quality of life in people with motor neuron diseases such as PPS, it is recommended that a balance between exercise and rest be sought. Fatigue appears to have both a psychologic and physiologic component and manifestation, indicating that both physical and cognitive approaches may be of benefit.[1]

Posturally induced mechanical strain and overuse have led to degenerative changes and pain, as well as unstable joints. For these deformities to be mitigated, the therapist should explore the use of orthoses, especially for gait. Many clients who have developed PPS are former brace users and may have an aversion to orthoses, but the braces they formerly used were not the cosmetic lightweight braces that can be constructed today. Some clients may also be resistive to the idea of using an assistive device for ambulation. Individuals with PPS who report engaging in physical activity twice weekly demonstrate better gait characteristics than those who are less active. Likewise, those who use an assistive device can walk faster.[165] The physical therapist can consider these findings in developing an overall plan of care for function and health.

## Trigeminal Neuralgia/Tic Douloureux

Trigeminal neuralgia (TN), or tic douloureux, is a disorder of the trigeminal (fifth cranial) nerve in which there are intense paroxysms of lancinating pain within the nerve's distribution.

### Incidence

TN is not a common disorder (5 cases per 100,000 population). It typically occurs in women between the ages of 50 and 70 years. However, TN can occur at any age, and does affect both genders.

### Etiology

TN arises from many causes: herpes zoster, multiple sclerosis, vascular lesions, or tumors that affect the nerve to produce the painful sensations. Many times it will be referred to as idiopathic because the cause remains undetermined. Physical triggers can elicit paroxysms of pain.

### Pathogenesis

Researchers hypothesize the pain is caused by ectopic activity generated at the site of involvement. Demyelinated fibers become hyperexcitable. Light mechanical stimulation recruits nearby pain fibers, causing them to discharge and create the sensation of intense pain.

### Clinical Manifestations

The pain associated with TN has a sudden onset and has been described as sharp, knife-like, lancinating, and "like a lightning bolt inside my head that lasts for seconds to minutes." The sensation is typically restricted to the maxillary (V2) division of the nerve, but it may involve the maxillary and mandibular divisions together. Less common is involvement of the ophthalmic (V1) division.

The painful sensation often occurs in clusters. Any mechanical stimulation, chewing, smiling, or even a breeze can trigger an attack. Clients avoid stimulating the trigger zone. Remissions occur between attacks, but these remission periods shorten and attacks become more frequent over the course of the disorder. In approximately 10% of the cases, the pain occurs bilaterally.

### MEDICAL MANAGEMENT

**DIAGNOSIS.** Subjective reports of pain in the typical pattern are the basis for diagnosis. No impairment or loss of sensation or motor control is obvious on physical examination. The person can identify the trigger site. Skull radiographs, CT scans, and MRI are used to rule out tumors and vascular causes.

**TREATMENT.** Sodium channel blockers are the first line of medical interventions, followed by neurosurgery for those unresponsive to pharmacologic treatments.[133] The preferred treatment of TN is oral carbamazepine (Tegretol, an anticonvulsant). Pain can be controlled with appropriate dosage in approximately 75% of clients with TN. Side effects of this medication include blurred vision, dizziness, drowsiness, as well as hematologic changes (anemia) and altered liver function. In addition, because carbamazepine has teratogenic effects, it should not be used in the first trimester of pregnancy nor should it be used by nursing mothers.[80] Other medications, such as phenytoin (Dilantin), are less effective but should be tried in those who cannot tolerate carbamazepine. Promising new medications to manage TN include pimozide, tizanidine hydroxychloride, and topical capsaicin.[47]

In persons whose pain is refractory to medications, neurosurgical procedures are advised. Radiofrequency rhizotomy is preferred over trigeminal nerve section or alcohol ablation. Microvascular surgery has also been used when small blood vessels have been found to constrict the trigeminal nerve near its root. This procedure provides immediate pain relief; however, it is a major and difficult surgery. Individuals may also wish to consider alternative approaches to pain management. A recent review concluded that acupuncture for TN is equally effective to carbamazepine and with fewer side effects.[127]

**PROGNOSIS.** The efficacy of evaluating treatments for TN is complicated by the fact that the disorder may remit spontaneously. Remissions that occur soon after onset of TN may last for years. For those who do not remit, TN can be managed medically in most cases. The Facial Pain Association provides information and support for persons with this diagnosis.

## Human Immunodeficiency Virus Advanced Disease (Acquired Immunodeficiency Syndrome)

Peripheral neuropathy, disease- or drug-induced myopathy, and musculoskeletal pain syndromes occur most often in advanced stages of human immunodeficiency virus (HIV) disease but can occur at any stage of HIV infection and may be the presenting manifestation. During the early phases of HIV when the immune system has altered responsiveness, GBS can develop. When immunoincompetence is severe, distal symmetric peripheral neuropathies occur; however, other parts of the body may be affected, such as the face or trunk. The polyneuropathies are predominantly sensory. Painful dysesthesias characterized by burning, tingling, contact sensitivity and proprioceptive losses begin in the feet and ascend. Involvement of the upper extremities can occur, but this is less common and usually later in the disease progression.[35]

In severe cases, secondary motor deficits also occur. In the individual with HIV and newly acquired neuropathy with a strong major motor component, vasculitis may be the underlying etiology (see "Vasculitis" in Chapter 12). Successful treatment of HIV-related distal symmetric peripheral neuropathies is difficult. Topical analgesics and anticonvulsants are thought to be the most effective.[186] However, pregabalin failed to prove effectiveness over a placebo in a randomized control trial. Optimizing the environment for the nerves by assuring excellent nutrition is also important in the treatment of individuals with HIV-related neuropathy.[225]

## Vasculitic Neuropathy

### Overview, Incidence, and Risk Factors

Vasculitis can occur as a primary inflammation and necrosis of blood vessel walls (polyarteritis nodosa) or as a secondary process associated with autoimmune responses (rheumatoid vasculitis or systemic lupus erythematosus vasculitis), infections (hepatitis C with vasculitis), toxins, or drug exposure. Vasculitis can involve blood vessels of any size, type, or location and can affect any organ system, including blood vessels that supply the PNS, as well as the CNS. However, because watershed zones between major vascular supplies exist in the PNS, peripheral nerves are likely to sustain ischemia.[149] Vasculitis may range from acute to chronic. Distribution of lesions may be irregular and segmental rather than continuous. The reported annual incidence is 40 to 54 cases per 1 million persons, with variance according to age, geography, and seasonal challenges.[193]

#### Pathogenesis

Immune (antibody–antigen) complexes to each disorder are deposited in the blood vessels, resulting in varying symptoms, depending on the organs affected. In the case of vasculitic neuropathy, the formation of antibody–antigen complexes activates the complement cascade with generation of C3a and C5a (chemotactic agents that recruit polymorphonuclear leukocytes to the vessel walls). Phagocytosis of the immune complexes takes place, and release of free radicals and proteolytic enzymes disrupt cell membranes and damage blood vessel walls. The complement cascade generates the formation of a complement membrane attack complex that also contributes to endothelial damage. The resulting damage to endothelial cells results in thickening of the vessel wall, occlusion, and ischemia to the affected nerves, with axonal degeneration and the resultant neuropathy. Classification is usually according to the size of the predominant vessels involved. In either case, the resulting ischemia may affect peripheral nerves.

#### Clinical Manifestations

Symptoms of vascular neuropathy reflect the distribution of the peripheral nerve involved. Onset is generally acute, and individuals complain of burning pain in the nerve's distribution. In addition motor weakness can be anticipated. Although a single nerve may be involved (mononeuritis), overlapping asymmetric polyneuropathies are relatively common.[84]

Peripheral neuropathy is a well-known and frequently early manifestation of many vasculitis syndromes. The pattern of neuropathic involvement depends on the extent and temporal progression of the vasculitic process that produces ischemia. Severe, burning dysesthetic pain in the involved area is present in 70% to 80% of all cases. Other symptoms may include paresthesias and sensory deficit; severe proximal muscle weakness and muscular atrophy can occur secondary to the neuropathy. In the early phase, one nerve is affected and causes focal symptoms in one extremity (mononeuritis multiplex) but can involve other nerves as the disorder progresses. The therapist should watch for anyone with neuropathy who exhibits constitutional symptoms, such as fever, arthralgia, or skin involvement. This may herald a possible vasculitis syndrome and requires medical referral for accurate diagnosis. Early recognition of vasculitis can help prevent a poor outcome. Untreated or with a poor outcome to intervention, CNS involvement (e.g., encephalopathy, ischemic and hemorrhagic stroke, or cranial nerve palsy) can occur late in the course of vasculitis.

#### Treatment

When corticosteroids (e.g., prednisone alone or sometimes in combination with other medications) are used (such as in the case of vasculitic neuropathy), the therapist should be aware of the need for osteoporosis prevention and attend to the other potential side effects from the chronic use of these medications. Alternative methods of pain control may be offered in a rehabilitation setting, such as biofeedback, transcutaneous electrical nerve stimulation, and physiologic modulation.

## CANCER INDUCED

### Paraneoplastic Neuropathies

A little more than 50 years ago the symptoms of two individuals were reported whose autopsy revealed bronchial carcinoma. Both had developed a sensory neuropathy. Subsequent reports of similar sensory neuropathies associated with other carcinomas have been reported and it is clear that paraneoplastic syndromes can affect any portion of the nervous system (Table 39.10).

#### Etiology

In most individuals diagnosed with paraneoplastic neuropathy, the development of symptoms occurs subacutely or chronically over weeks to months and precedes the discovery of the tumor from months to years. The clinic features and electrophysiologic abnormalities indicate that the cell body is the primary site of involvement. Large-diameter neurons are preferentially affected.

#### Incidence

Numbers vary depending on how the disorder is defined, but estimates range from 10% to 50% that individuals with cancer will develop a paraneoplastic syndrome at some time during the course of their disease. Using a restrictive definition, paraneoplastic syndromes are rare.

#### Pathogenesis

The current theory is that an autoimmune response, initially directed against the cancer's antigen, subsequently attacks membrane receptors on or receptors within (antinuclear) neurons. See Chapter 30 for discussion of CNS neoplasms.

#### Clinical Manifestations

The most common symptoms are numbness and paresthesias, initially asymmetric, but progressing to involvement of all extremities. Burning and aching or lancinating pain is common. Although individuals exhibit symptoms of areflexia, weakness is not common and when it occurs, generally is related to an inability to sustain the contraction secondary to impaired proprioceptive feedback. Many individuals with paraneoplastic neuropathy develop additional symptoms demonstrating a progressive involvement of central neural structures. This includes dysarthria, cerebellar ataxia (limb and truncal), ocular nystagmus, memory loss, and ANS involvement. When these central structures are involved, the diagnosis is termed *paraneoplastic encephalomyeloneuritis*.[41]

**Table 39.10** Paraneoplastic Antibodies, Associated Carcinoma, and Symptoms That Develop

| Antibody | Associated Carcinoma | Paraneoplastic Syndrome | Antibody Reactions with Region Involved | Signs and Symptoms |
|---|---|---|---|---|
| Anti-Hu | SCLC (oat cell) | Paraneoplastic sensory/ sensorimotor neuropathy | Antibody affects neuronal nuclei in PNS: produces peripheral neuropathies: acute, subacute, or chronic | Sensory neuropathy<br>Encephalomyeloneuropathy |
| | SCLC | Paraneoplastic encephalomyeloneuritis | Multifocal disorder<br>Antibody affects all neuronal nuclei in PNS and CNS: produces both peripheral neuropathies and cerebellar, brainstem, cerebral, and spinal signs<br>Autonomic nervous system involvement may occur | Sensory neuropathy plus:<br>Cerebellar ataxia, dysarthria, nystagmus<br>Vertigo<br>Confusion<br>Areflexia |
| | SCLC lymphomas | Subacute motor neuropathy | Loss of anterior horn cells in spinal cord | Impaired motor function; sensation is spared |
| Anti-Yo | SCLC | LEMS | Antibodies directed against voltage-gated calcium channels that regulate ACh release in neuromuscular junction | Proximal muscle weakness |
| Anti-Tr | Ovarian, breast, uterine | Pancerebellar syndrome, dysarthria, and nystagmus | Purkinje cell cytoplasm and deep cerebellar neurons: subacute (weeks to months) cerebellar symptoms (limb and truncal ataxia, dysarthria, nystagmus) | Cerebellar ataxia |
| Anti-Ri | Hodgkin lymphoma | Slowing developing cerebellar syndrome | Purkinje cell cytoplasm | Cerebellar ataxia |
| Antiamphiphysin | Breast, SCLC | Opsoclonus–myoclonus | CNS nuclei: opsoclonus (involuntary conjugate multidirectional saccades) | Opsoclonus |
| Anti-VGC | Breast | Stiff person syndrome | | |
| Anti-T[a] | SCLC | LEMS | | Proximal weakness |
| | Testicular | Limbic encephalitis | Limbic and brainstem neuronal nuclei | |

*ACh*, Acetylcholine; *ANS*, autonomic nervous system; *CNS*, central nervous system; *LEMS*, Lambert-Eaton myasthenic syndrome; *PNS*, peripheral nervous system; *SCLC*, small cell lung carcinoma.
[a]Paraneoplastic syndromes are associated with a variety of tumors and the antibodies that are produced affect PNS, CNS, and ANS.

## MEDICAL MANAGEMENT

**DIAGNOSIS.** The differential diagnosis of paraneoplastic neuropathy is extensive and includes many disorders identified in this chapter that affect sensory nerve fibers or neurons. Recognition and diagnosis at earlier stages can expedite treatment and provides better outcomes.[116] In addition to electrophysiology findings of severely reduced amplitude or absence of sensory nerve potentials, with normal to slightly slowed sensory NCVs, nerve biopsies show nonspecific axonal degeneration and a reduction in myelinated fibers. Lumbar puncture and serum assays for antibodies may be included in the diagnostic workup. High serum titers for antibodies are suggestive of an occult tumor, but the sensitivity and specificity of these tests yield false positives and negatives. CT and MRI scanning are used to locate the tumor.[53]

**TREATMENT.** Typical treatments for autoimmune disorders, such as immunosuppression using prednisone, cyclophosphamide, IVIg, or plasmapheresis, generally do not work with antinuclear antibodies because receptors are located within the nucleus of the neuron.

**PROGNOSIS.** The course is fairly stereotypical. Individuals deteriorate over weeks or months and then stabilize at a level of severe disability; for example, sensory polyneuropathies progress proximally, then ataxias develop and become progressively greater. Neurologic improvement is rare.

**SPECIAL IMPLICATIONS FOR THE THERAPIST 39.9**

### *Polyneuropathy in Malignant Diseases*

Physical therapists will want to approach the care of individuals with paraneoplastic neuropathy holistically. It is important to address the symptoms of the neuropathy, the overall health condition of cancer, and the effects of immunosuppression. Recognizing and preventing problems of the integumentary system, preserving safety with mobility and gait, and prevention of falls are of great importance.

**Table 39.11** Medications Toxic to Peripheral Nerves

| Medication | Use |
|---|---|
| Doxorubicin (Adriamycin) | Cancer |
| Amiodarone | Irregular heartbeat |
| Chloramphenicol | Antibiotic |
| Cisplatin | Cancer |
| Dapsone | Skin diseases |
| Phenytoin (Dilantin) | Seizures and pain |
| Disulfiram (Antabuse) | Alcoholism |
| Ethionamide | Tuberculosis |
| Metronidazole (Flagyl) | *Trichomonas* infection |
| Gold | Rheumatoid arthritis |
| Isoniazid | Tuberculosis |
| Lithium | Manic depression and headache prevention |
| Nitrofurantoin (Furadantin) | Urinary tract infection |
| Nitrous oxide | Anesthetic |
| Penicillamine | Rheumatoid arthritis |
| Suramin | Cancer |
| Paclitaxel (Taxol) | Cancer |
| Vincristine | Cancer |

Adapted from Asbury AK: Disorders of peripheral nerve. In Asbury AK, McKhann GM, McDonald WI, editors: *Disease of the nervous system: clinical neurobiology*, Philadelphia, 1986, WB Saunders, 326–327.

# TOXINS

In addition to toxic substances in the environment, some medications prescribed to treat medical conditions can be toxic to the PNS (Table 39.11).[8] While DM remains cause of peripheral neuropathy, toxic exposures can instigate similar symptoms.[198]

## Lead Neuropathy

### Definition

Toxic substances, such as lead, affect peripheral myelin and/or axons.

### Etiology and Risk Factors

Although lead has been virtually eliminated in urban environments, it may exist in third world countries or in some industries such as ceramics. The leading cause of lead neuropathy is the ingestion of lead from paint by children who live in old homes that were built before 1925. However, lead exposure may also occur after inhaling fumes from car batteries, and after drinking contaminated water or moonshine whiskey. Lead neuropathies also occur in workers in industries that use materials containing lead or who live near lead smelters. The Consumer Product Safety Commission has identified inexpensive plastic miniblinds as a source of lead exposure. As the blind is exposed to sunlight, the plastic disintegrates and sheds dust that is high in lead. Interestingly, a case report describes a woman who presented with symptoms of weakness, cognitive loss, and declines in function, and who was using heated lead as part of an unbewitching ritual. Following treatment and cessation of exposure, she recovered well.[10]

### Pathogenesis

Both the CNS and PNS can be affected. In the PNS, lead exposure initially causes segmental demyelination, but with prolonged exposure damage to axon cell bodies causes axonal degeneration.[80]

### Clinical Manifestations

Unlike most neuropathies, lead neuropathies primarily affect neurons innervating muscles in the upper extremity. After months of exposure, persons with a lead peripheral neuropathy will develop wrist-drop, with consequences in grasping functions.

### MEDICAL MANAGEMENT

**DIAGNOSIS, TREATMENT, AND PROGNOSIS.** Diagnosis is based on the history, clinical examination, and motor NCVs, which will be slowed. If axonal degeneration has occurred, EMG will reveal fibrillation potentials, demonstrating loss of axonal innervation. Other tests to check for concentration of lead in the body are urine evaluation and radiographs to reveal a lead line at the metaphysis in the iliac creases, long bones, and tips of the scapula.

Treatment consists of the removal of the source of the lead toxin along with the introduction of the chelating agent, edetate calcium disodium (EDTA), administered twice daily, to rid the body of lead. Symptomatic management consists of cock-up splints for the wrist-drop. Recovery depends on the length of exposure and removal of the toxin.

## Pesticides and Organophosphates

### Etiology

Insecticides are used extensively worldwide in industry and agriculture. Some compounds have contaminated cooking oils, and outbreaks of organophosphate poisoning have been reported after ingestion. Parathion has been responsible for more accidental poisonings and deaths than any other organophosphate.

### Pathogenesis and Clinical Manifestations

All organophosphate compounds inhibit cholinesterase activity, thus creating an acute cholinergic crisis. Acutely, organophosphate toxins affect systemic functions throughout the body; they are also capable of producing a less acute, more chronic neuropathy. Nausea and vomiting, diarrhea, muscle fasciculations, weakness, and paralysis, including sudden paralysis of the respiratory musculature, can occur after overstimulation at the neuromuscular junction. Death can result from vasomotor collapse that coincides with respiratory paralysis. Symptoms of peripheral nerve involvement appear within 1 to 4 days and because they arise quickly, may resemble GBS. A chronic peripheral neuropathy may persist for months or years or a delayed neuropathy may have its onset weeks after exposure.[182]

### MEDICAL MANAGEMENT

**DIAGNOSIS.** Overexposure to organophosphates will reduce cholinesterase activity of erythrocytes to less than 25% of normal. History and clinical evaluation may be accompanied by electrophysiologic studies to indicate the severity of the neuropathy (e.g., segmental demyelination or axonal degeneration or both).

**TREATMENT.** Insecticides should be washed from the skin and hair; if toxins have been ingested, emesis or lavage should be carried out. Acutely, atropine is given in doses every 10 minutes until the pupils are dilated, the skin flushed and dry, and the pulse rate rises. Neuromuscular paralysis can be reversed by injection of pralidoxime, a cholinesterase reactivator. Endotracheal intubation and ventilation may be required in the presence of respiratory paralysis. Strictly neuropathic management is aimed at symptomatic management.

**PROGNOSIS.** Recovery is based on removal from the toxin and the degree of involvement. If only segmental demyelination occurs, recovery will occur in weeks to months, but if axonal degeneration is present, recovery will take months to years.

# MOTOR END PLATE DISORDERS

## Myasthenia Gravis

### Overview and Definition

Myasthenia gravis (MG) is the most common of the disorders of neuromuscular transmission. It is characterized by fluctuating weakness and fatigability of skeletal muscles.

### Incidence

The incidence of MG is estimated at 1:200,000. Estimates from the National Myasthenia Gravis Foundation are that there are more than 100,000 clients with MG and an additional 25,000 undiagnosed cases. MG can affect people in any age group, but peak incidences occur in women in their twenties and thirties and in men in their fifties and sixties. Overall, the ratio of women affected compared to men is 3:2.

### Etiology

MG is an autoimmune disorder whose action takes place at the site of the neuromuscular junction and motor end plate.

### Risk Factors

Disorders associated with an increased incidence of MG are thymic disorders such as hyperthyroidism, thymic tumor, or thyrotoxicosis. There is an association with diabetes and immune disorders, such as rheumatoid arthritis or lupus. Exacerbations may occur before the menstrual period or shortly after pregnancy. Chronic infections of any kind can exacerbate MG. Five percent to 7% appear to have a familial association.

### Pathogenesis

In MG, the fundamental defect is at the neuromuscular junction. Receptors at the motor end plate normally receive acetylcholine (ACh) from the motor nerve terminal. An action potential occurs that leads to a muscle contraction. In MG, the number of ACh receptors is decreased and those that remain are flattened, which results in decreased efficiency of neuromuscular transmission. The neuromuscular junction can normally transmit at high frequencies so that the muscle does not fatigue. With fewer active ACh receptors, the nerve impulses fail to pass across the neuromuscular junction to stimulate muscle contraction. The neuromuscular abnormalities in MG are brought about by an autoimmune response mediated by specific anti-ACh receptor antibodies. The antibodies may block the site that normally binds ACh, or the antibodies may damage the postsynaptic muscle membrane. There may be endocytosis (pinching off of regions of the cell's membrane) of the receptor site.

Although the cause of the autoimmune response in MG is not well understood, the thymus appears to play a role in the disease; 75% of persons with MG have abnormalities of the thymus (e.g., thymic hyperplasia or thymoma). Cells within the thymus bear ACh receptors on their surface, and may serve as a source of autoantigen to trigger the autoimmune reaction within the thymus gland when an immunologic abnormality causes a breakdown or an autoimmune attack on ACh receptors.[52]

### Clinical Manifestations

Although MG can be mild to severe, its cardinal features are skeletal muscle weakness and fatigability. Repetition of activity causes fatigue, whereas rest restores activity. Other than weakness, neurologic findings are normal. A system of four major categories is used to classify MG: ocular, mild generalized, acute fulminating, or late severe.

The distribution of muscle weakness has a dichotomous pattern affecting only the ocular muscles, or a more variable, generalized pattern occurs. In approximately 85% of persons with MG, the weakness is generalized and affects the limb musculature. This fluctuating weakness is often more noticeable in proximal muscles.

Cranial muscles, particularly the eyelids and the muscles controlling eye movements, are the first to show weakness. The weakness and imbalance in the muscles controlling eye movement results in diplopia (double vision) and ptosis (drooping eyelids) as common early signs. The person will tilt the head back to accommodate (Fig. 39.16). Weak neck muscles may cause head bobbing in this position.

Chewing of meat produces fatigue, and the facial expression is one that seems to be snarling because the lips do not close. Speech tends to be nasal. Difficulty in swallowing may occur as a result of palatal, pharyngeal, and tongue weakness. Nasal regurgitation or aspiration of food is common.

### MEDICAL MANAGEMENT

**DIAGNOSIS.** History and clinical observation of symptoms of weakness with continued use and improvement with rest are important in diagnosing MG. Several conditions that cause weakness of cranial, or somatic, muscles must also be considered. These include drug-induced myasthenia, hyperthyroidism, botulism, intracranial mass lesions, and progressive disorders of the eye. Lambert-Eaton syndrome is a presynaptic disorder of the neuromuscular junction that can cause symptoms similar to those of MG. Lambert-Eaton syndrome is an

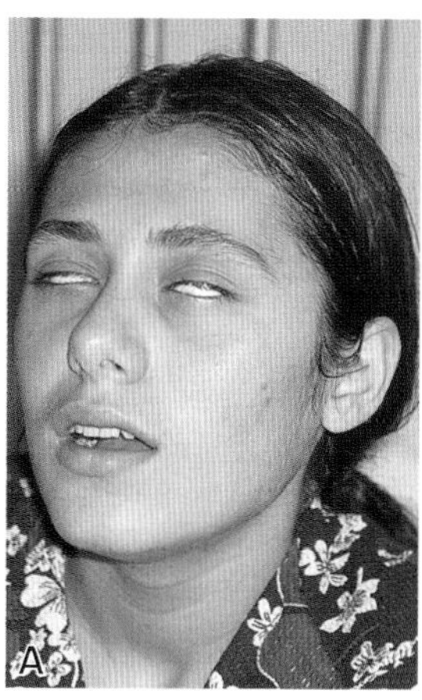
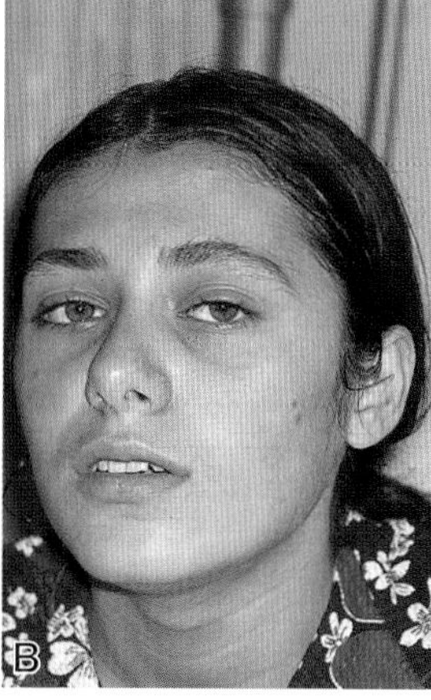


**Figure 39.16**

(A) Facial weakness with myasthenia gravis is easily identified when the patient is asked to perform repeated facial movement. Note inability to fully open eyelids and the open jaw. (B) Edrophonium (Tensilon) test can be used to confirm the diagnosis. Edrophonium chloride is a short-acting anticholinesterase that is injected intravenously. In myasthenia gravis, the facial weakness is rapidly relieved by this test. Similar responses occur elsewhere in the body. (From Goldman L, Ausiello D: *Cecil textbook of medicine*, ed 22, Philadelphia, 2004, WB Saunders.)

autoimmune disorder associated with neoplasm, most commonly small cell (oat cell) carcinoma of the lung, which is believed to trigger the autoimmune response.

The three methods used to diagnose MG are (1) immunologic, (2) pharmacologic, and (3) electrophysiologic testing.[144] Immunologic testing detects anti-ACh receptor antibodies in the serum. The presence of anti-ACh receptor antibodies is virtually diagnostic of MG, but a negative test does not exclude diagnosis of the disease. There is no correlation between the amount of anti-ACh receptor antibodies and the severity of the disease. However, in a person with MG a treatment-induced fall in the antibody level often correlates with clinical improvement. Current research in immunopathogenesis and antibody subtyping holds promise for specialized management of individuals with MG.[139]

The drug edrophonium (Tensilon) is used to demonstrate improvement in the myasthenic muscles by inhibiting acetylcholinesterase (AChE), an enzyme required for ACh uptake. Muscle strength and endurance are measured before and after administration of the drug. This test confirms that ACh uptake is part of the pathologic status; however, a control test of saline should also be used for comparison.

Electrophysiologic testing of myasthenic disorders demonstrates a normal EMG at rest. Specialized testing must be employed using repetitive stimulation to demonstrate a rapid decrement in the motor action potential's amplitude. Absence of sensory deficits and retention of tendon reflexes throughout the course of the disease also tend to confirm the diagnosis of MG. Because respiratory impairment is a serious complication of MG, measurements of ventilatory function should be performed.[210]

**TREATMENT.** AChE inhibitor medication provides for improvement of weakness but does not treat the underlying disease. Administration of this medication is tailored to the individual's requirements throughout the day. For example, a person with difficulty chewing and swallowing would take the medication before meals. Side effects of AChE inhibitors include gastrointestinal effects such as nausea and vomiting, abdominal cramping, and increased bronchial and oral secretions.

Surgical removal of the thymus is successful in 85% of persons with MG. Up to 35% of those undergoing thymectomy achieve a drug-free remission, although this may take years.

Immunosuppression using drugs, such as corticosteroids (prednisone) and azathioprine, are effective in nearly all persons with MG. Initially, high daily doses are begun and then followed by alternate-day high doses that are tapered slowly over a period of months. Unfortunately, adverse side effects are associated with high-dose steroids. These include cushingoid appearance, weight gain, hypertension, and osteoporosis.

Plasmapheresis is performed to remove substances that affect ACh receptors. However, plasmapheresis produces only short-term reduction in anti-AChE antibodies and is not effective for long-term symptom control.

**PROGNOSIS.** The course of MG is variable, typified by remissions and exacerbations, especially within the first year after onset. Symptoms often fluctuate in intensity during the day. This daily variability is superimposed on longer-term spontaneous relapses that may last for weeks. Remissions are rarely complete or permanent. This disorder follows a slowly progressive course. Onset of other systemic disorders and infections may precipitate an exacerbation of the disease and are the most common cause of a crisis. A myasthenic crisis is a medical emergency requiring attention to life-endangering weakening of the respiratory muscles and requires ventilatory assistance. Treatment of a crisis occurs in the ICU because the client requires careful, immediate control of medications for survival.[234]

When MG begins in children, it is important to establish the form it takes. Because AChE antibodies cross the placenta, 10% of newborns of mothers with MG develop a myasthenic reaction. Newborns with neonatal MG have a weak suck and cry and are hypotonic. Fortunately, this resolves in a few weeks.

**SPECIAL IMPLICATIONS FOR THE THERAPIST 39.10**

### *Myasthenia Gravis*

Physical and occupational therapy may be indicated as supportive care to assist the client with MG. In the acute care setting, the therapist must establish an accurate neurologic and respiratory baseline. Tidal volume, vital capacity, and inspiratory force should be monitored regularly during treatment. Deep breathing and coughing should be encouraged. When eating, the person should be instructed to sit upright and to swallow when the chin is tipped slightly downward toward the chest and never with the neck extended because of the risk of aspiration. Finally, the client should never speak with food in the mouth.

The therapist must also be alert to signs of an impending myasthenic crisis (increasing muscle weakness; respiratory distress; or difficulty while talking, chewing, or swallowing). Make sure the client recognizes the side effects and signs of toxicity of AChE inhibitor medications. For those receiving a prolonged course of corticosteroids, report adverse side effects to the physician.

Plan therapy and teach the client to plan activities to coincide with periods of maximum energy. The home should be arranged to help prevent unnecessary energy expenditure. Frequent rest periods help conserve energy and give muscles a chance to regain strength. The person with MG should avoid strenuous exercise, stress, and excessive exposure to the sun or cold weather. All of these can exacerbate signs and symptoms.

Researchers report that a strength training program eliciting maximal isometric contractions could be instituted in clients with mild-to-moderate MG.[146]

Because individuals diagnosed as having MG are placed on long-term corticosteroid medication, the treatment may induce a secondary condition: osteoporosis. These individuals should be encouraged to undergo dual energy x-ray absorptiometry (DXA scan) and to receive calcium supplements to counteract osteoporosis.123

Importantly, clinicians should monitor signs and symptoms and the impact on participation and quality of life. A preliminary version of a MG-specific, patient reported disability assessment instrument has been developed called the MG_DIS. It is based on the International Classification of Functioning, Disability, and Health (ICF) and is designed to monitor changes of functioning in people with MG, as well as serve as an outcome measure in clinical trials.[169]

# BOTULISM

## Definition and Incidence

Botulism is a rare, often fatal condition (20% mortality) caused by ingestion of a potent neurotoxin produced by *Clostridium botulinum,* which is found in improperly preserved or canned foods, as well as in contaminated wounds. The Centers for Disease Control and Prevention recognizes five categories of botulism: (1) foodborne, (2) wound, (3) infant, (4) adult intestinal toxemia, and (5) iatrogenic—when too much botulism is injected for cosmetic or medical reasons.[29,48] Approximately 10 adult cases and 100 cases of infant botulism are reported each year in the United States.

### Etiology and Pathogenesis

The anaerobic bacillus releases a protein neurotoxin that is heat labile; it is destroyed by boiling food for 10 minutes; inadequate food preparation allows the neurotoxin to be ingested.

Infant botulism affects babies ages 3 weeks to 9 months; the most common source of infant botulism arises from the ingestion of honey, which is why children younger than 1 year are not allowed to have honey.

Botulism is not always ingested orally. Some cases occur after wounds are contaminated with soil, in chronic drug abusers, after cesarean delivery, and may even occur when antibiotics are administered to prevent wound infection.

When the neurotoxin is ingested, digestive acids and proteolytic enzymes cannot destroy the molecules of the toxin and it is absorbed into the blood from the small intestine. Minute amounts of circulating toxin reach the cholinergic nerve endings at the motor end plate and bind to gangliosides of the presynaptic nerve terminals. Flaccid paralysis is caused by inhibition of ACh released from cholinergic terminals at the motor end plate. Inhibition of ACh release causes a symmetric paralysis with normal sensory and mental status.

### Clinical Manifestations

Onset of symptoms develops 12 to 36 hours after ingestion of food containing the toxin. Signs and symptoms include malaise, weakness, blurred and double vision (diplopia), dry mouth, and nausea and vomiting. Progression is variable, but respiratory failure can occur in 6 to 8 hours. People may also report difficulty swallowing (dysphagia), dysarthria (slurred speech), and photophobia. Because the motor end plate is involved, there are no direct sensory changes. Motor weakness of the face and neck muscles progresses to involve the diaphragm, accessory muscles of respiration, and muscles controlling the extremities. Secondary effects from the flaccid paralysis, such as severe muscle wasting, pressure sores, and aspiration pneumonia, may occur.

### MEDICAL MANAGEMENT

**DIAGNOSIS, TREATMENT, AND PROGNOSIS.** A history suggesting a food source, and toxin identification made by serum or stool analysis are used in the diagnosis. EMG testing demonstrates a decreasing amplitude and facilitation of muscle action potential after tetanic stimulation. Differential diagnosis includes disorders that also display a rapidly evolving flaccid paralysis, such as GBS, MG, and tick paralysis.

Immediate treatment is directed toward neutralizing the toxin using injectable trivalent ABE (botulism equine trivalent antitoxin) serum, an antitoxin. Antitoxin prevents further binding of free botulism toxin to the presynaptic endings. If paralysis occurs because of wound botulism, care should include débridement and antibiotics.

Removal of unabsorbed toxin from the gastrointestinal tract is accomplished by gastric lavage and induced emesis. Finally, supportive measures should be instituted in the hospital; intubation and mechanical ventilation are needed when the individual's vital capacity is compromised.

If untreated, this disorder can be fatal within 24 hours of ingestion. Respiratory failure leads to death. In mild-to-moderate cases, a gradual recovery of muscle strength can take as long as 12 months after onset. After hospitalization, graded rehabilitation is instituted to treat muscle wasting, deconditioning, and orthostatic hypotension.

# ABNORMAL RESPONSE IN PERIPHERAL NERVES

## Complex Regional Pain Syndrome/Reflex Sympathetic Dystrophy/Causalgia

Complex regional pain syndrome (CRPS), first described in 1864, is characterized by sensory, autonomic, motor, and dystrophic signs and symptoms. CRPS includes disorders of the sympathetic nervous system with or without known trauma. New insights into nervous system function and pain mechanisms have led to reclassification of the syndrome.

CRPS I (formerly reflex sympathetic dystrophy) is the label used to describe this syndrome when there is an absence of known traumatic nerve injury; however, there is usually an initiating noxious event. CRPS II (formerly causalgia) refers to a similar condition associated with known traumatic nerve injury. A third type (CRPS-NOS) (not otherwise specified) only partially meets CRPS criteria and cannot be explained by any other condition.

### Incidence

CRPS I may occur after 5% of all injuries, with a reported number of new cases each year of approximately 50,000 in the United States. Because the diagnosis is often missed or delayed, estimates on incidence may be underreported. Some very mild cases may resolve and others may progress to become a chronic, debilitating disorder. Although the average age of an individual with CRPS is in the mid-30s, it has been reported in all age groups, including children as young as 3 years. Women are three times more likely to develop CRPS than men.[46]

### Etiology

CRPS has its origin in a variety of conditions: it can follow medical procedures, including surgery, such as arthroscopy; it can occur after an UMN lesion arising from traumatic brain injury, cerebrovascular accidents (often in the presence of flaccidity), or destructive lesions of the CNS; or it can occur after LMN disorders from peripheral nerve injuries, neuropathies, and entrapments. CRPS has been reported following motor vehicle accidents, fractures, bites (human, animal), falls, assault, shoulder subluxation or dislocation, and even what seem like minor strains or sprains. Any event that causes traction of the brachial plexus and nerve roots resulting in constant nerve irritation may result in CRPS.

### Pathogenesis

CRPS is now regarded as a systemic condition that involves both central and peripheral components of the neuraxis and interactions between the immune and nervous systems. No one knows for sure what causes the cascade of neurogenic responses that leads to CRPS. Laboratory studies of blood and tissue samples appear normal, although there is some evidence of elevated systemic levels of inflammatory markers and catecholamines (mediators in sympathetic hyperactivity).[45] There is no apparent inflammation of the affected soft tissues (e.g., skin, muscles). There is some evidence that the cellular changes are occurring within the nerve fibers to the affected tissues.

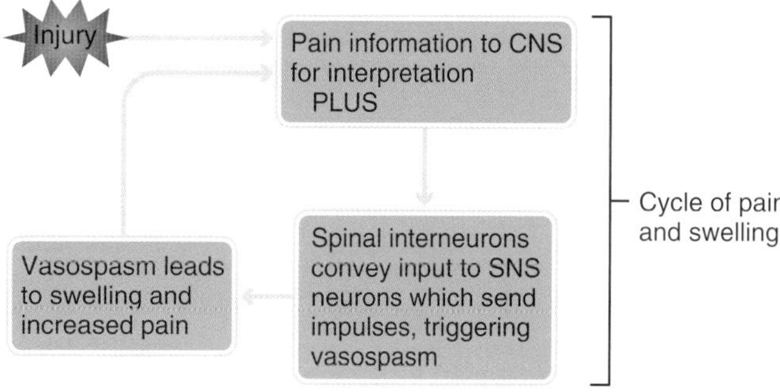


**Figure 39.17**

**The exaggerated pain associated with sympathetic over activity occurs after minor trauma.** Normally, the response of the sympathetic nervous system after injury causes cutaneous blood vessels to contract. This response shuts down appropriately within minutes to hours. In complex regional pain syndrome, the sympathetic nervous system functions abnormally and causes vasospasm, which creates cycles of swelling and pain. Initially, vasodilation occurs that increases skin temperature. Later in the course of the disorder, symptoms consist of cyanosis and coldness in the involved extremity.

An injury at one somatic level initiates sympathetic efferent activity that affects many segmental levels. CRPS is thought to represent a reflex neurogenic inflammation. Facilitation of the sympathetic nervous system (SNS) and its neurotransmitters and catecholamines activates primary afferent nociceptors to create the sensation of pain. Deterioration of the SNS function is common. Excess release of substance P from terminal sensory nerves is part of the overreaction of the neurogenic inflammatory process.

Migraine headaches appear to overlap with CRPS. The signaling neuropeptide CGRP (calcitonin gene-related peptide) appears to be linked to the hyperresponsiveness in both migraine headaches and CRPS. Loss of inhibition in the complex cascade of nerve-related inflammatory chemicals that can occur after major or minor trauma suggests it's not the trauma itself that exaggerates the process, but rather, the nervous system's response to injury.[19] It has been suggested that people with CRPS who lose their automatic nervous system reflex responses might have a faulty nervous system to begin with, which could explain why they develop CRPS when others with similar injuries recover normally.[224]

Thermal dysfunctions are related to either the inhibition of SNS vasoconstriction or facilitation of the SNS causing excessive vasoconstriction (Fig. 39.17). Clinical studies have shown abnormal SNS reflexes that indicate CNS dysfunction exists as well.[231]

### Clinical Manifestations

The natural history of CRPS is one of change over time. CRPS has overlapping but identifiable clinical stages (Table 39.12). The primary clinical features of CRPS fall into 4 distinct subgroups: (1) abnormalities in pain processing, (2) skin color and temperature changes, (3) edema, vasomotor, and sudomotor abnormalities, and (4) motor dysfunction and trophic changes. Intense, burning pain in a specific area, most often an extremity, is the most commonly reported symptom. Other clinical manifestations vary widely and can include headache,

**Table 39.12** Complex Regional Pain Syndrome: Progressive Clinical Stages

| Stage | | Classic Signs and Symptoms |
|---|---|---|
| Stage I: Acute inflammation: denervation and sympathetic hypoactivity | Begins up to 10 days following injury; lasts 3-6 months | **Pain**—more severe than expected; burning or aching character; increased by dependent position, physical contact or emotional disturbances<br>**Hyperalgesia** (lower pain threshold, increased sensitivity), **allodynia** (all stimuli are perceived as pain), and **hyperpathia** (threshold to pain is increased, once exceeded, sensation intensity increased more rapidly and greater than expected)<br>**Edema**—soft and localized<br>**Vasomotor/thermal changes**—affected limb is warmer<br>**Skin—Hyperthermia** and **dry**<br>Increased hair and nail growth |
| Stage II: Dystrophic: paradoxic sympathetic hyperactivity | Occurs 3-6 months after onset of pain, lasts about 6 months | **Pain**—worsens: constant, burning and aching<br>**Allodynia**, **hyperalgesia,** and **hyperpathia** almost always present<br>**Edema**—becomes thicker and more fibrotic, causing joint stiffness<br>**Vasomotor/thermal changes**—neither warm nor cold<br>**Skin**—thin, glossy, cool (vasoconstriction) and sweaty<br>Thin, ridged nails<br>X-rays reveal disuse **osteoporosis**, cystic and subchondral bone erosion |
| Stage III: Atrophic | Begins about 6-12 months after onset; may last for years, or may resolve and reoccur | **Pain**—spreads proximally, occasionally to entire skin surface or plateaus; joint stiffness progresses<br>**Edema**—continues to harden<br>**Vasomotor/thermal changes—s**ympathetic nervous system regulation is decreased on affected extremity, affected limb is cooler<br>**Skin**—thin, shiny, cyanotic, and dry<br>Fingertips and toes on involved extremity are atrophic<br>Fascia is thickened; contractures may occur<br>X-ray demonstrates bony **demineralization and ankylosis** |

difficulty sleeping, fatigue, difficulty concentrating, memory loss, edema, inability to initiate movement, weakness, tremor, muscle spasms, dystrophy, and atrophy.

The pain that occurs is disproportionate to what would be expected. The overall pain intensity increases with disease duration. Even tactile stimulation may be perceived as pain (allodynia).[77] The pain spreads from localized to a regional distribution, including to the same extremity on the contralateral side of the body in a mirror pattern (e.g., right arm to left arm), to the other extremity on the ipsilateral side (e.g., right arm to right leg), and to the other extremity on the opposite side (e.g., right arm to left leg).

Although sensory impairments are most often the hallmark of CRPS, movement disorders also occur. Motor symptoms may precede the appearance of other impairments by weeks or months or may appear on the contralateral extremity in a mirror fashion but most often they occur concomitantly, with autonomic changes and pain. All manifestations contribute to impairments of function and alter quality of life.

Despite the fact that three stages of CRPS were originally identified and are still referred to, the course of this disorder is more unpredictable than the stages imply.[112] Individuals typically remain in a specific stage for 6 to 8 months; however, some may progress rapidly to and through the next stage. As the condition progresses, symptoms may spread proximally and even spread to affect other extremities. In a few cases, the entire body may become involved.[137]

Three abnormal vasomotor patterns have been identified; these relate to the temperature and color (warmth or heat with redness, cool with bluish tint) of the extremity and the acuity of CRPS. Hypersensitivity and abnormal sweating may be followed by dry skin. Other vasomotor changes include changes in the nails in which they become thick, brittle, and ridged.

## MEDICAL MANAGEMENT

**DIAGNOSIS.** In the absence of a specific biomarker, the diagnosis of CRPS is based primarily on the clinical examination and history. Proposed diagnostic criteria for CRPS requires at least one symptom in each of the four subgroups, and one sign in at least two of the four subgroups. A combination of diagnostic tests aimed at assessing secondary changes (radiographic examinations, thermographic studies, sudomotor function tests, NCV or somatosensory evoked potentials, and laser Doppler flowmetry) may aid in establishing a diagnosis. Because of the evolutionary nature of CRPS, a correct diagnosis may be delayed, especially in children.[55,92]

**TREATMENT.** Treatment for CRPS tends to be multifactorial and prolonged. Successful treatment depends on early diagnosis, treatment of the underlying cause, and aggressive and sustained physical therapy.[96] Although stellate ganglion blocks or sympathectomy are used to alleviate pain and early symptoms, this approach is based on weak evidence.[136] All of the following treatments have limited evidence for their effectiveness.[74] Medications such as corticosteroids, nonsteroidal antiinflammatory drugs, antidepressants, antianxiety agents, and anticonvulsants may offer pain relief by normalizing overactive pain pathways but do not vary the duration of the disease. Amitriptyline has been used to facilitate sleep and relieve depression. Calcium channel blockers help to improve peripheral circulation through their effect on the SNS. Newer, more selective drugs (e.g., immunomodulators) are showing promising results.[187]

IV ketamine infusion has been used in severe cases unresponsive to other therapies. This drug works by shutting off the *N*-methyl-D-aspartate receptors in the brain but must be supported by a wide range of other management tools (e.g., good nutrition, physical and occupational therapy, exercise, cognitive behavioral counseling).[77]

Sympathetic, somatic, and trigger point blocks, spinal cord stimulators, and intrathecal pumps for the delivery of baclofen or morphine decrease pain intensity and perception of pain, but do not alter the disease progression. Hyperbaric oxygenation therapy is used to restore circulation, reduce inflammation, and eliminate swelling in affected limbs while also changing pain processing in the brain.[108]

Integrative medicine has a role in the treatment of chronic conditions like CRPS. Some people find relief from their symptoms (or at least an ability to cope better and improve function) when traditional allopathic medicine is augmented by acupuncture, craniosacral therapy, BodyTalk, Reiki, tai chi, yoga, or other forms of complementary care. Cognitive behavioral therapy, although not a cure for CRPS, can help improve pain, mood, and function.[92,93]

**Prognosis.** CRPS is a complex syndrome with varying severity and disability. In many cases, the pain continues for years or, less frequently, it may remit, then recur after another injury. Spontaneous remission is unusual; only modest improvements have been reported with most current therapies.[187]

In some cases, malingering for secondary gain has been documented.[237] Outcome measures for CRPS I typically concentrate on impairments, leaving measurement of disability, which is the most relevant to function, with few assessments.[182] Physical therapy is indicated, particularly as part of a program of pain control. Although the goal is to maintain function so that the individual can perform normal activities, a vigorous approach is not indicated. Current research is aimed at understanding physiologic processes and finding the most effective interventions.

SPECIAL IMPLICATIONS FOR THE THERAPIST 39.11

### *Complex Regional Pain Syndrome*

Goals for physical therapy include educating the client and encouraging normal positioning and use of the involved extremity while minimizing pain and normalizing sensation. Stress loading (loading and scrubbing) is a key part of the rehabilitation program. Weight bearing and compression through the affected extremity is followed by a distraction force (e.g., carrying weights or a bucket with weights inside. Scrubbing is performed on hands and knees or for just lower extremity involvement in the standing position. A scrub brush held in the hand or attached to the foot is held with constant pressure against the contact surface and a scrubbing motion applied in various directions. All scrubbing and loading activities are done daily with gradual progression to tolerance.

At first, there is often an increase in pain and swelling with this type of program, but these symptoms decrease after a few days. Desensitization techniques may also assist in normalizing sensation to the affected area. This consists of progressive stimulation with very soft material to more textured fabrics or materials. Sensory input is graded from light touch to deep pressure and from consistent to intermittent duration with each material.

There is evidence that graded motor imagery reduces pain and swelling in some people with CRPS. This approach involves recognizing pictured hands (or whatever body part is affected) as being right or left, imagining movements, and mirroring movements. The affected individual must practice hourly for several weeks to have an effect.[150,151]

Although modalities are used to provide pain relief, the greatest success occurs when they are administered during earlier stages of CRPS. External transcutaneous electrical nerve stimulator units are reported to be minimally effective.[34] When the lower extremity is involved, aquatic therapy is helpful for improving mobility when weight bearing on land is problematic.

The therapist should be aware of the potential for significant psychologic, emotional, social, and spiritual issues associated with any chronic condition, but especially one as painful and debilitating as CRPS can become. Furthermore, because the pain is often disproportionate to the incident, people with CRPS may be misunderstood by their loved ones and by clinicians. Attentive listening; acknowledging and validating feelings of anger, worthlessness, anxiety/depression, and hopelessness; referral to support groups; and communication with the physician about the individual's needs are essential during the long process of recovery.

A report of increased spontaneous falls throughout the course of the illness has been documented for more than a quarter of individuals with CRPS. It would be advisable to conduct a falls assessment and institute client safety education and falls prevention.[187]

## REFERENCES

To enhance this text and add value for the reader, all references are included in the enhanced ebook on Student Consult that accompanies this textbook. The reader can view the reference source and access it online whenever possible.

# CHAPTER 40

# Laboratory Tests and Values

JAMES TOMPKINS • TRACI NORRIS • KIMBERLY LEVENHAGEN

## INTRODUCTION[a]

Laboratory tests may be used for a variety of reasons. Tests can be used for screening to search for an occult disease process in an otherwise healthy person or risk stratification to assess need for preventative therapy or for diagnosis. In addition, once a disease has been diagnosed a laboratory test can monitor a patient's condition.[60] Specific tests may be used for any of these purposes, depending on what information is needed. For example, a glucose test or glycated hemoglobin may be used for screening a population, for diagnosis of diabetes mellitus, or to monitor the effectiveness of an individual's therapy.

Risk stratification and screening tests may be used on populations to identify individuals who are at risk for certain diseases, for example, those with high cholesterol who could benefit from treatment before disease manifestations become evident. Screening is also performed for genetic or metabolic diseases to find individuals before disease occurs. State laws generally require routine screening in newborns for several disorders, notably phenylketonuria, sickle cell disease, and hypothyroidism.

Lab values can be used in predictive scoring systems within intensive care units to measure severity, length of stay, and outcomes such as mortality. Predictive scoring systems such as the Acute Physiologic and Chronic Health Evaluation (APACHE III), Simplified Acute Physiologic Score (SAPS), Mortality Prediction Model (MPMO), and Sequential Organ Failure Assessment (SOFA)[26,76] review admission data, initial diagnosis, comorbidities, and lab values to assist in determining a plan of care and survival.

The different laboratory tests have differing sensitivity and specificity for varying pathological conditions. The lab finding may provide only one piece of evidence to suggest a certain diagnosis.[88] Laboratory values should guide intervention selection and safe mobility recommendations. The acute care environment rapidly evolves, and therefore therapists should be knowledgeable regarding critical laboratory values, as well as understand the clinical implications of values that are trending up or down. Therapists should not rely solely on a single lab value in the medical record but rather in collaboration with the health care team monitor for signs and symptoms to determine appropriateness of activity. The therapist must collaborate with other members of the health care team by assessing vitals and communicating symptoms to determine appropriateness for activity. Therapists should be knowledgeable regarding clinical presentation and implications for critical values.[88] For example, an individual undergoing hematopoietic stem cell transplant may develop refractoriness to platelet transfusion resulting in severe thrombocytopenia. Historically, therapists would not mobilize the patient until the platelet count was within an acceptable range. By collaborating with the health care team all can consider the risks and the benefits for mobilizing the patient and therefore use a symptom-based approach for progression of treatment.[75] Physicians or facilities may adopt criteria for deferring physical therapy that vary from those suggested in the text. In addition, lab values may not always reflect an individual's current physiologic status. Other members of the health care team may be aware of a person's medical situation and provide recommendations on that individual's current physiologic status. Other reasons for not relying solely on a single lab value are discussed below under limitations of lab testing.

### Limitations of Lab Testing

The reference intervals for a given test associated with defined states of health is known as the *reference range.* The reference range depends on many factors, including the demographics of the healthy population and the methods used for the test. Each laboratory must establish and validate its reference range specific to each laboratory test.[6] How well that reference range depicts homeostasis may vary with sex, age, weight, physiologic changes (such as pregnancy), and fluid status. Therapists should be aware that some diseases are more prevalent in specific races and ethnicities. Racial differences in laboratory

[a] Note to Reader: This chapter contains content that does not fall strictly within the Lab Values material (for example, vascular pressures and pulmonary function tests) so that the material can be easily accessed with other similar information.

Box 40.1

**UNITS FOR CLINICAL LABORATORY DATA[a]**

| | |
|---|---|
| g | gram |
| ng | nanogram |
| mg | milligram |
| mL | milliliter |
| L | liter |
| dL | deciliter (100 mL) |
| pg | picogram |
| $mm^3$ | cubic millimeter |
| mmol | millimole |
| U | unit |
| IU | international unit |
| mU | milliunit |
| µg | microgram |
| µU | microunit |
| µm | micron |
| mEq | milliequivalent |

[a]Note: Some of the items in this box are on the official Do Not Use List (see Table 40.1) but are still commonly used and thus listed.

values may be genetic or related to lifestyle preferences. In addition, therapists should consider the patient's biologic sex, gender, and gender identity to determine appropriate normative reference ranges.[88]

Each laboratory will include a means of assessing the results—sometimes by placing *L* for low or *H* for high after a test result, or by providing the reference range for the tests performed, or documenting the lab value in red when it is outside the range. Although lab tests are generally reliable, a test may fail to produce a result that should indicate an abnormal condition that truly exists (false negative) or the results may falsely indicate that an abnormal condition exists (false positive). Laboratory tests are frequently "rechecked" to ensure a higher degree of diagnostic accuracy.

Some tests may have less predictive value regarding the individual's physiology than we would expect. The positive predictive value of a test depends on the prevalence of the disease in a population. The less prevalent the disease, the less accurate laboratory results may be. Statistically, as the number of tests performed on a single individual increase, the possibility of an incorrect conclusion also increases, regardless of whether the individual is sick.[51] This phenomenon is purely related to chance because a significant margin of error arises from the arbitrary setting of limits for normal or reference values at a given facility.

Results may be inaccurate, outdated, or the abnormality indicated by the test may not have the expected impact on a person. Inaccurate values may be obtained if samples used for lab analysis are contaminated, mishandled, or mislabeled, or testing materials and techniques are flawed. Results may not accurately portray a person's physiologic status because of medications, diet, activity, or change with intravenous infusions. There are several considerations in the elderly population such as polypharmacy, diminished homeostatic mechanisms, biologic variability due to hormones and slowed metabolism.[44]

In some cases, the condition of the individual may have changed between the time obtaining the sample and when receiving physical therapy. Therefore, the values recorded in the medical record may not reflect a person's current condition, resulting in a false-positive or false-negative result. Alternately, the person may have recovered spontaneously or received treatment that has restored normal physiology. For example, a lab report may indicate that a person is anemic, but the individual may have received a blood transfusion since the initial report was generated. Therefore, communication with other members of the health care team is essential because interventions to correct a person's condition may not have been noted in the medical record.

People may have vastly different tolerances for the alterations in homeostasis implied by abnormal lab test results. In particular, the chronicity of the condition may affect an individual's tolerance. For example, a person with chronic anemia may be able to ambulate without symptoms, and another person with similar lab values, but with acute anemia may be symptomatic while sitting upright. Often a discussion with the patient and the health care team in addition to monitoring vital signs may help guide recommendations made regarding safe mobility.

In summary, reference values or "normal" ranges provided in this chapter are not meant to be memorized and applied as a standard to every case. Instead, therapists should consider all the clinical factors. Interpretation of specific individual refence ranges must be done using trends in the laboratory values over time, as well as clinical implications. Based on emerging evidence regarding early mobilization, the Academy of Acute Care Physical Therapy revised the Laboratory Values Interpretation Resource in 2017. This document provides therapists an overview of trending values and clinical implications which are important in clinical decision making.[88]

### Abbreviations

Box 40.1 provides recommended units for clinical laboratory data. Table 40.1 lists The Joint Commission's official "do not use" list of abbreviations. The list was originally created in 2004 by The Joint Commission as part of the requirements for meeting a National Patient Safety Goal and then integrated into the Information Management Standards in 2010 to standardize abbreviations, acronyms, and symbols that are not to be used throughout the organization.

## BASIC METABOLIC PANEL

The most common lab tests constitute what are known as the *basic metabolic panel* (BMP),[36] *comprehensive metabolic panel* (CMP), and *hepatic function panel*. These three terms are based on current procedural terminology (CPT) codes.[11] These replace a variety of other outdated panel names, such as SMA-6, SMA-7, SMA-12, SMA-20, Chemistry Panel, Chem Screen, Chem-6, Chem-7, Chem-12, Chem-20, SMAC-6, SMAC-7, SMAC-12, and SMAC-20.

The BMP is a group of seven to eight specific tests for electrolyte level, acid–base balance, blood glucose, and kidney function. The tests consist of serum concentrations of sodium, potassium, chloride, carbon dioxide, blood urea nitrogen (BUN), creatinine, glucose, and calcium. The BMP may be done as part of a routine

**Table 40.1** Official "Do Not Use" List[a]

| Do Not Use | Potential Problem | Use Instead |
|---|---|---|
| U, u (unit) | Mistaken for "0" (zero), the number "4" (four) or "cc" | Write "unit" |
| IU (International Unit) | Mistaken for IV (intravenous) or the number 10 (ten) | Write "International Unit" |
| Q.D., QD, q.d., qd (daily) | Mistaken for each other | Write "daily" |
| Q.O.D., QOD, q.o.d., qod (every other day) | Period after the Q mistaken for "1" and the "O" mistaken for "I" | Write "every other day" |
| Trailing zero (X.0 mg)[b] | Decimal point is missed | Write X mg |
| Lack of leading zero (.X mg) | | Write 0.X mg |
| MS | Can mean morphine sulfate or magnesium sulfate | Write "morphine sulfate" |
| $MSO_4$ and $MgSO_4$ | Confused for one another | Write "magnesium sulfate" |

[a]Applies to all orders and all medication-related documentation that is handwritten (including free-text computer entry) or on preprinted forms.
[b]**Exception:** A "trailing zero" may be used where required to demonstrate the level of precision of the value being reported, such as for laboratory results, imaging studies that report size of lesions, or catheter/tube sizes. It may not be used in medication orders or other medication-related documentation.
To prevent misunderstandings and potential risks to patient safety The Joint Commission publishes an Official "Do Not Use" List of Abbreviations which is available at: https://www.jointcommission.org/-/media/tjc/documents/fact-sheets/do-not-use-list-fact-sheet-06-28-19.pdf.

**Table 40.2** Reference Values for Basic Metabolic Profile and Magnesium

| Test | Reference Value | Possible Critical Value |
|---|---|---|
| Sodium | Newborn: 134–144 mEq/L<br>Infant: 134–150 mEq/L<br>Child: 136–145 mEq/L<br>Adult/elderly: 136–145 mEq/L | Adult: <120 or >160 mEq/L |
| Potassium | Newborn: 3.9–5.9 mEq/L<br>Infant: 4.1–5.3 mEq/L<br>Child: 3.4–4.7 mEq/L<br>Adult/elderly: 3.5–5.0 mEq/L | Newborn: <2.5 or >8mEq/L<br>Adult: < 2.5 or >6.5 mEq/L |
| Chloride | Premature infant: 95–110 mEq/L<br>Newborn: 96–106 mEq/L<br>Child: 90–110 mEq/L<br>Adult/elderly: 98–106 mEq/L | Adult: <80 or >115 mEq/L |
| Calcium | Newborn <10 days: 7.6–10.4 mg/dL<br>Infant 10 days to 2 years: 9–10.6 mg/dL<br>Child: 8.8–10.8 mg/dL<br>Adult, older: 9–10.5 mg/dL | <6 or >13 mg/dL |
| Blood urea nitrogen (BUN) | Newborn: 3–12 mg/dL<br>Infant: 5–18 mg/dL<br>Child: 5–18 mg/dL<br>Adult: 10–20 mg/dL<br>Elderly is slightly higher than those of adult. | >100 mg/dL (indicates serious impairment of renal function) |
| Creatinine | Newborn: 0.3–1.2 mg/dL<br>Infant: 0.2–0.4 mg/dL<br>Child: 0.3–0.7 mg/dL<br>Adolescent: 0.5–1.0 mg/dL<br>Adult female: 0.5–1.1 mg/dL<br>Adult male: 0.6–1.2 mg/dL | >4 mg/dL (indicates serious impairment in renal function) |
| Magnesium | Newborn: 1.4–2.0 mEq/L<br>Child: 1.4–1.7 mEq/L<br>Adult, older: 1.3–2.1 mEq/L | <0.5 or >3.0 mEq/L |

Creatinine for older adult decreases with decreased muscle mass. The BUN/creatinine ratio is a good measurement of kidney and liver function. Normal BUN/Creatinine is 10:1 to 20:1. A ratio > 20:1 may indicate prerenal causes; while a ratio < 10:1 could infer renal causes
Data from Pagana RN, Pagana TJ, Pagana, TN: *Mosby's diagnostic and laboratory test reference*, ed 14, St Louis, 2018, Elsevier.

physical examination as an outpatient, routine testing of inpatients, or when a physician suspects an abnormality that may be detected by one or more components of the BMP.

Normal values for BMP are given in Table 40.2, along with possible causes and consequences of abnormal values. BMP may be used as a screening tool, especially for diabetes and kidney disease. The sample is obtained by venipuncture, preferably after 10 to 12 hours of fasting.[1]

As an indicator of current status of electrolytes, acid–base balance, renal function, and blood glucose, significant changes in BMP values may indicate a number of acute problems, such as kidney failure, insulin shock, diabetic coma, and respiratory distress.[1] Changes in sodium, potassium, and calcium alter the excitability of neurons as well as cardiac and skeletal muscle. This can produce weakness, spasms, altered sensation, cardiac arrhythmias, and potentially death.[19] Each component of the BMP is described below.

## Sodium

Sodium is a critical determinant of fluid volume in the body. Under normal circumstances, increases in the amount of sodium in the body leads to retention of water and a loss of sodium leads to loss of water in the body. Normally, small increases in sodium concentration increase thirst, which corrects sodium quantities. Derangement of homeostatic mechanisms may impair the linkage between thirst and sodium concentration. Sodium concentration may be decreased (hyponatremia) by excessive infusion or ingestion of water, excessive production of antidiuretic hormone, or by diseases that cause retention of water, such as heart failure, cirrhosis, nephrotic syndrome, and syndrome of inappropriate antidiuretic hormone release (SIADH). Some medications such as diuretics or corticosteroids can contribute to hyponatremia. Increased fluid volume elevates blood pressure and may contribute to cell swelling. Neurons are especially vulnerable to cell swelling, leading to neurologic dysfunction, possibly progressing to coma or death.

Sodium concentration may increase (hypernatremia) when excessive water is lost from the body, such as in profuse sweating or a decrease in antidiuretic hormone (ADH) production (such as diabetes insipidus). Changes in sodium concentration may lead to visible changes in body fluid volume, such as pitting edema or clinical manifestations associated with dehydration. Rapid changes to the serum sodium concentrations in either direction can cause temporary symptoms or permanent injury.[83] Guidelines have been established in the United States and Europe[82,87] to assist providers in diagnosing and managing hyponatremia.

## Potassium

Potassium is particularly important for function of excitable cells—nerves, muscles, and heart. Therefore, the normal range for potassium is very narrow. Excitable cells remove the vast majority of potassium from surrounding fluids to maintain their resting potentials. Small alterations in extracellular potassium have profound effects on these cells. The heart muscle is very susceptible to potassium disturbances. Arrhythmias and cardiac arrest can result from hypokalemia (low potassium levels) or hyperkalemia (high potassium levels). Unique electrocardiogram findings can be found if either condition is suspected,[88] therefore therapists should monitor for arrhythmias. Abnormal values in either direction can also lead to muscle weakness or irritability. Potassium measurements provide useful information about renal and adrenal disorders and about water and acid–base imbalances.

Use of loop diuretics in particular can lead to compensatory reabsorption of sodium at the expense of losing potassium in the urine. In addition to cardiac arrhythmias, signs of hypokalemia may include mental status changes, dizziness, weakness, myalgia, muscle twitches, nausea, vomiting, clammy skin, and potentially respiratory failure caused by weakness of muscles of inspiration.

Hyperkalemia may result from excessive potassium replacement, consumption of foods such as many fruits with high potassium content, excessive alcohol use, and several drugs such as angiotensin-converting enzyme inhibitors. Hyperkalemia can also produce numbness, tingling, flaccid paralysis, nausea, vomiting, diarrhea, and anorexia. Any abnormal value should lead to consultation before treatment due to the potential for severe consequences.

## Chloride

Chloride levels tend to change along with changes in sodium and water. It may also change in response to alterations in cellular pH and bicarbonate levels. Carbon dioxide that diffuses into cells, especially red blood cells, generates carbonic acid that must be managed by exchanging bicarbonate ions for chloride ions. As carbon dioxide is added to the blood, chloride moves into red cells and bicarbonate moves out. In the lungs, the process is reversed. Hyperchloremia is usually found with hypernatremia because they usually have the same causes, but hyperchloremia can occur as a result of hyperventilation. Conversely, hypochloremia can occur with hypoventilation, which is usually caused by chronic respiratory disease resulting from the chloride shift in response to changes in pH. Additional signs of hypochloremia include hyperexcitability of the muscles, tetany, and hypotension.

## Calcium

Calcium is tested most commonly to rule in or rule out kidney or bone disease and to rule out changes in ionized calcium as a cause of neuromuscular dysfunction. It is commonly tested along with phosphorus and vitamin D because of kidney disease and osteoporosis and with parathyroid hormone, as serum calcium concentration can be altered by various forms of parathyroid disorders.

Hypercalcemia may also be present with kidney stones and certain forms of cancer, especially multiple myeloma. Arrhythmias may result from the role of calcium in some specific forms of electrical potentials of the heart. Calcium is also responsible for neuronal excitability. Hypercalcemia decreases the firing of neurons, resulting in muscle weakness, fatigability, and decreased muscle tone and reflexes. Decreased ionized calcium can cause numbness around the mouth and in the fingers and toes, and muscle spasms, often secondary to respiratory alkalosis that may result from hyperventilation.

## Magnesium

Magnesium, like calcium, is involved in regulation of excitable cells but is not part of the BMP and must be ordered separately. Low magnesium also results in arrhythmias, weakness, muscle spasms, and numbness. Magnesium (see Table 40.2) may be reduced in diabetes, with the use of diuretics, as a result of chronic vomiting or diarrhea, and may be increased by renal failure, hyperparathyroidism, excessive consumption of magnesium containing antacids, or hypothyroidism.

## Blood Urea Nitrogen and Creatinine

BUN and creatinine (see Table 40.2) are used to evaluate kidney function in individuals with kidney failure, for differential diagnosis if kidney disease is suspected, to monitor treatment of kidney disease, and to monitor kidney function while individuals are using certain drugs.[1] Creatinine is a normal waste product related to creatine phosphate, a mechanism of regenerating adenosine triphosphate in skeletal muscle. Normally, the amount of creatinine in the blood is kept at a normal level by clearance in the kidneys. Because release of creatinine into the blood from muscle remains constant, a rise in serum creatinine usually represents a decline in the kidney's capacity for excreting wastes.

The rise in creatinine levels is directly correlated with the amount of loss of nephron function. With aging, and in diseases with progressive muscle weakness, such as muscular dystrophy, a decrease in lean body mass (muscle tissue) may result in decreasing creatinine values. However, serum creatinine may remain normal in an older person, even with significant declines in creatinine clearance and renal function because of the decline in lean body mass.

Causes for elevated creatinine may include glomerulonephritis, pyelonephritis, acute tubular necrosis, urinary obstruction by prostate disease or kidney stones, or decreased renal blood flow. Creatinine may also be elevated as a result of excessive release of creatine caused by muscle injury.

BUN also rises with decreased renal function, caused by decreased renal blood flow, as opposed to decreased glomerular filtration rate (creatinine). Because BUN reflects a balance of nitrogen added to the blood and excreted by the kidney, BUN may be elevated by increased protein catabolism or dietary intake of protein.

Gastrointestinal bleeding will increase BUN because of the breakdown of protein from the blood within the gastrointestinal tract. The synthesis of urea also depends on the liver. People with severe primary liver disease will have a decreased BUN. With combined liver and renal disease (as occurs in hepatorenal syndrome), the BUN can be normal, not because renal excretory function is good, but because poor hepatic functioning resulted in decreased formation of urea. Failure of the liver to convert nitrogen from amino acids to urea results in accumulation of ammonia, which is discussed in the "Comprehensive Metabolic Panel: Blood Ammonia" section.

## Blood Glucose

In addition to being part of the BMP, blood glucose may be measured under particular conditions to diagnose a suspected alteration in glucose homeostasis. Table 40.3 lists reference values for glucose testing. There are several guidelines and reference ranges for glucose testing, including the World Health Organization,[15,17,25,90] American Association of Endocrinologists, and American Diabetes Association (ADA).[2] BMP glucose testing only reflects the blood glucose at the time the sample is obtained. Random testing may be performed to understand how well a person with diabetes manages the body's ability to clear glucose from the blood over time. Whereas a blood draw for BMP may be performed at random times with respect to eating. Testing can occur after a period of fasting (fasting blood sugar), two hours after consuming a large meal, and with one or more draws taken after fasting within a few hours of each other. The glycated hemoglobin test (A1c also written as HgA1c), denotes the patient's glycemic control over the past three months by providing an average level of blood glucose.

**Table 40.3** Blood Glucose Tests

| | Adults Prediabetes | Adults With Diabetes | Children With Type I Diabetes | Pregnancy |
|---|---|---|---|---|
| Fasting | 100–125 mg/dL (5.6–6.9 mmol/L) | 80–130 mg/dL (4.4–7.2 mmol/L) | Before Meals: 90–130 mg/dL (5.0–7.2 mmol/L)<br>Bedtime/overnight: 90–150 ng/dL (5.0–8.3 mmol/L) | <95 mg/dL (5.3 mmol/L) |
| 1-hour postprandial | | | | 140 mg/dL (7.8mmol/L) |
| 2-hour postprandial | 140–199 mg/dL (7.8–11.0 mmol/L) | <180 mg/dL (10.0 mmol/L) | | <120 mg/dL (6.7 mmol/L) |
| A1c | 5.7%–6.4% | <7.0% (53 mmol/mol)[a] | <7.0% (53 mmol/mol)[b] | 6%–6.5% (42–48 mmol/mol)<br>6% (42 mmol/mol) can be relaxed to <7% (53 mmol/mol if necessary to prevent hypoglycemia)[b] |

[a]Individualized based on age, comorbidities, and known microvascular and macrovascular complications.
[b]Updated guidelines from 2020 Standard of Medical Care in Diabetes. Available at: https://care.diabetesjournals.org/content/43/Supplement_1.
From American Diabetes Association: Glycemic targets: standards of medical care in diabetes-2018, *Diabetes Care* 41(Suppl 1):S55–S64, 2018. https://doi.org/10.2337/dc18-S006.

Fasting blood glucose, as the name implies, is done after fasting (at least 8 hours). Not eating overnight should allow the blood glucose to fall to normal, whereas a random measurement as part of the BMP may be elevated from eating close to the time of the test. The *2-hour postprandial blood glucose test* assesses a person's response after eating a meal as 2 hours should be sufficient time for blood glucose to return to normal following eating. A more rigorous test to determine the body's ability to clear glucose from the blood is the *oral glucose tolerance test*. This test involves consumption of a fixed amount of glucose and measurement of a person's blood glucose at specified time intervals to determine how quickly the body reaches homeostasis. A person with a normal response will have a modest elevation in blood glucose after 1 hour and a return to normal by 2 hours. Blood glucose in an individual with either a lack of insulin or lack of insulin response will remain elevated after more than 2 hours.

A test for long-term glycemic control (ability to maintain a steady blood glucose concentration over a period of many days) is A1c. The amount of A1c measured in the red blood cells (RBCs) depends on the amount of glucose available in the bloodstream over the 120-day life span of the RBC, thereby reflecting the average blood glucose level for the 100 to 120-day period before the test.

The A1c test determines the fraction of hemoglobin containing bound glucose. The A1c value reflects the average blood glucose concentration over several weeks to months, as opposed to the snapshot view provided by blood glucose monitoring. The more glucose the RBC was exposed to, the greater the A1c percentage. An important advantage of this test is that the sample is not affected by short-term variations, such as food intake, exercise, stress, hypoglycemic agents, or compliance. The A1c measurement is now used more frequently than the 2-hour postprandial blood glucose in monitoring people with known diabetes. It is recommended that the A1c test be performed at least twice a year in patients with stable glycemic control (meeting therapy goals) and at least quarterly in those who are not meeting glycemic goals (or whose medical therapy has changed).[2]

The A1c goal for most nonpregnant adults is less than 5.7%. In addition, the ADA provides guidelines for children and adults with diabetes and women who are pregnant (refer to Table 40.3). Several studies have shown that significantly reducing one's A1c decreases the risk for development and progression of macrovascular and microvascular complications of diabetes (i.e., neuropathy, retinopathy).[16,33,37,50,61,95] The recommendation is to prevent hypoglycemia in all patients but to achieve optimization without increasing morbidity and mortality. Individuals who present with severe or frequent hypoglycemic episodes, a long history of diabetes, advanced age/frailty, or advanced atherosclerosis may require modification to A1c reference ranges.[2,95]

Fructosamine is an alternative to using A1c to identify persons at risk for diabetes[69,78] and/or to monitor long-term control of diabetes mellitus.[69,78] Fructosamine is formed by the glycosylation of proteins by excessive serum glucose. Whereas A1c reflects average blood glucose of 2 to 3 months, fructosamine indicates the average over a 2- to 3-week period because of the shorter life span of individual protein molecules as opposed to RBC life span. Measurement of fructosamine may be preferred in circumstances in which A1c measurement is unavailable or unreliable (such as in the case of disorders of RBCs, hemolytic anemia or chronic blood loss).[77]

Diabetes-related antibodies can be measured to distinguish type 1 from 2 upon diagnosis of diabetes mellitus. Several different antibodies may be responsible for type 1 diabetes mellitus. The ability to determine whether a person has type 1 or 2 diabetes can aid in the treatment protocol and prognosis of the disease, particularly because of the greater risk of ketoacidosis in type 1.

Individuals may be allowed to have a blood glucose concentration above normal for exercise (up to 240 mg/dL), but blood glucose below 100 mg/dL is considered unsafe because of hypoglycemia. A value below 60 mg/dL may cause diabetic shock and a value above 300 mg/dL may lead to ketoacidosis with strenuous exercise. Release of glucose from the liver during exercise in the presence of already elevated blood glucose (above 240 mg/dL) may lead to further increases and therefore, exercise should be monitored to avoid adverse effects.

Signs of hypoglycemia are related to activation of the sympathetic nervous system as a compensation for low blood sugar and signs of decreased neural function. These signs include diaphoresis, tachycardia, increased respiratory rate, hypotension, inability to follow commands, tingling, visual changes, shakiness, irritability, and hunger, and can progress to unresponsiveness, seizure, coma, or death. Signs of diabetic ketoacidosis are related to dehydration and acidosis. They include lethargy, acetone or fruity odor to the breath, dehydration, polyuria, thirst, confusion, nausea and vomiting, weak rapid pulse, and Kussmaul breathing, which is a deep, rapid, labored breathing pattern unique to ketoacidosis.

## Carbon Dioxide

Carbon dioxide is a byproduct of aerobic metabolism and is intimately involved in the regulation of acid–base balance. Bicarbonate ion ($HCO_3-$) is produced in a reaction between carbon dioxide and water, producing bicarbonate and hydrogen ions. Therefore, each bicarbonate ion available to fluids negates the effect of a single hydrogen ion on a fluid's pH. As such, bicarbonate ion acts as a buffer, preventing changes in plasma pH. Low $HCO_3-$ occurs in conditions that produce metabolic acidosis, such as diabetic ketoacidosis and compensation for hypoventilation (respiratory acidosis) in chronic respiratory disease.

Respiratory compensation for metabolic acidosis results in the loss of carbon dioxide from the plasma, which in return reduces the amount of $HCO_3-$ in the plasma. The renal system also contributes to pH regulation by altering the amount of $H+$ that passes in the urine and by synthesizing $HCO_3-$. Renal compensation is slower to correct pH, requiring several days, as opposed to the more rapid respiratory response. The ability to regulate pH can be compromised by either respiratory or renal disease. Hypoventilation allows carbon dioxide, and thereby acid, to accumulate. Renal disease decreases

**Table 40.4** Laboratory Values in Acid–Base Disorders[a]

| | ARTERIAL BLOOD | | | |
|---|---|---|---|---|
| | **pH (7.35-7.45)** | **$PCO_2$ (35-45 mm Hg)** | **$HCO_3$– (22-26 mEq/L)** | **Signs** |
| **Metabolic Acidosis** | | | | |
| Uncompensated | <7.35 | Normal | <22 | Headache, fatigue; nausea, vomiting, diarrhea, muscular twitching; convulsions; coma, hyperventilation |
| Compensated | Normal | <35 | <22 | Increased respiratory rate |
| **Metabolic Alkalosis** | | | | |
| Uncompensated | >7.45 | Normal | >26 | Nausea, vomiting, diarrhea, confusion, irritability, agitation; muscle twitching, muscle cramping, muscle weakness, paresthesias, convulsions, slow breathing |
| Compensated | Normal | >45 | >26 | Decreased respiratory rate |
| **Respiratory Acidosis** | | | | |
| Uncompensated | <7.35 | >45 | Normal | Headache, diaphoresis, tachycardia, disorientation, agitation, cyanosis, lethargy, ↓ deep tendon reflex |
| Compensated | Normal | >45 | >26 | – |
| **Respiratory Alkalosis** | | | | |
| Uncompensated | >7.45 | <35 | Normal | Rapid, deep respirations, light headedness, muscle twitching, anxiety and fears; paresthesias, cardiac arrhythmia |
| Compensated | Normal | <35 | <22 | – |

*$PCO_2$*, Partial pressure of carbon dioxide.
Data from Pagana RN, Pagana TJ, Pagana, TN: *Mosby's diagnostic and laboratory test reference*, ed 14, St Louis, 2018, Elsevier.

the ability of the kidney to selectively alter fluid concentration, usually resulting in acidosis. Table 40.4 provides lab values that indicate whether acidosis or alkalosis is metabolic or respiratory and whether it is compensated or uncompensated.

Blood lactate is a result of metabolism exceeding what can be supplied by aerobic metabolism. Although this is usually associated with athletes performing anaerobic exercise, blood lactate can increase significantly in critically ill patients. Lack of cardiac output, anemia, and low hemoglobin saturation may lead to inadequate oxygen transport and promote anaerobic metabolism and lactate accumulation in a resting critically ill patient. Elevated lactate is associated with poor outcomes.

## COMPREHENSIVE METABOLIC PANEL

The comprehensive metabolic panel is composed of the BMP, and may be accompanied by tests related to liver and other organ functions. These additional tests may be conducted separately as the liver panel. The liver has an important role in the production of albumin, as well as molecules involved in regulating coagulation. Impaired liver function and hypoalbuminemia is frequently associated with systemic infection.

The liver panel consists of bilirubin, total protein, albumin, and serum enzymes that are altered when liver function is compromised. These tests are aspartate aminotransferase (AST, formerly called serum glutamic-oxaloacetic transaminase), alanine aminotransferase (ALT, formerly called serum glutamic-pyruvic transaminase), lactate dehydrogenase (LDH), γ-glutamyl transferase (GGT), and alkaline phosphatase (ALP).

The Model for End-Stage Liver Disease (MELD)[20,59,99] is a prognostic model that uses laboratory values such as serum bilirubin, serum creatinine, and international normalized ratio (INR) to predict a three-month survival among adults with liver disease such as cirrhosis. An increasing score is associated with severity of hepatic dysfunction and mortality. Variations in the MELD include the MELD-Na which incorporates the serum sodium lab value for individuals with an initial MELD score greater than 11,[20,43,48,59,99] and the Pediatric End Stage Liver Disease (PELD) which uses albumin, bilirubin, and INR lab values.[12] In 2016, the United Network for Organ Sharing began using the MELD-Na in prioritizing allocation for people awaiting liver transplantation.[53,62]

> **Note to Reader:** Please note that even though these tests are collectively known as the liver panel, diseases of other tissues or organs may cause deviations from the reference values.

**Table 40.5** Laboratory Tests for Liver and Biliary Tract Disease

| | Normal Range | Comment |
|---|---|---|
| **Serum Bilirubin** | | |
| Direct (conjugated) | Adult/elderly/child:<br>0.1–0.3mg/dL | Increased with obstruction |
| Indirect (unconjugated) | Adult/elderly/child:<br>0.2–0.8 mg/dL | Increased with cirrhosis; hepatitis, hemolytic anemia, jaundice, transfusion reaction |
| Total | Adult/elderly/child:<br>0.3–1.0 mg/dL AND<br>Newborn: 1.0–12.0 mg/dL | Possible critical values:<br>Total bilirubin<br>Adult: >12 mg/dL<br>Newborn: >15 mg/dL |
| **Serum Proteins** | | |
| Albumin (A) | Adult elderly: 3.5–5.0 g/dL | Decreased in liver damage, burns, Crohn disease, SLE, malnutrition (e.g., anorexia nervosa), digoxin (digitalis) toxicity |
| Globulin (G) | Adult/elderly: 2.3–3.4 g/dL | Increased in hepatitis |
| Total | Adult/elderly: 6.4–8.3 g/dL | Decreased in liver damage (synthesis is impaired) |
| A/G ratio | 1.5:1 to 2.5:1 | Ratio reverses with chronic hepatitis or other chronic liver disease |
| Transferrin (iron levels) | Newborn: 130–275 mg/dL<br>Child: 203–360 mg/dL<br>Adult male: 215–365 mg/dL<br>Adult female: 250–380 mg/dL | Decreased in liver damage, increased in iron deficiency |
| α-Fetoprotein | Child (<1 yr.): <30ng/mL<br>Adult: <40 ng/mL | Cancer associated antigen; made by fetus but not by healthy adults. Increased levels could indicate hepatocellular carcinoma |
| **Serum Enzymes** | | |
| AST | 0–5 days: 35–140 units/L<br><3 years: 15–60 units/L<br>3–6 years: 15–50 units/L<br>6–12 years: 10–50 units/L<br>12–18 years: 10–40 units/L<br>Adult: 0–35 units/L<br>Infant may be twice as high as adult. | Increased in liver damage, released by liver when damage occurs to liver cells; increased with primary muscle diseases (e.g., myopathy) |
| ALT | Adult/Child: 4–36 units/L | Same as above |
| LDH | Newborn: 160–450 units/L<br>Infant: 100–250 units/L<br>Child: 60–170 units/L<br>Adult/elderly: 100–190 units/L | Same as above; increased with metastatic disease osteosarcoma |
| GGT | Newborn: five times higher than adult level<br>Child: similar to adult level<br>Female younger than age 45 years: 5–27 units/L<br>Male and Female age 45 years and older: 8–38 units/L | Age- and gender-dependent elevated with significant liver disorder |
| ALP | Child/adolescent:<br><2 years: 85–235 units/L<br>2–8 years: 65–210 units/L<br>9–15 years: 60–300 units/L<br>16–21 years: 30–200 units/L<br>Adults: 30–120 U/L | Increased with liver tumor, biliary obstruction, rheumatoid arthritis, hyperparathyroidism, Paget disease of bone |
| Blood Ammonia | Newborn: 90–150 mcg/dL<br>Child: 40–80 mcg/dL<br>Adult: 10–80 mcg/dL | Increased in severe liver damage, high levels of ammonia can be associated with coma and encephalopathy. |

*AST*, Aspartate aminotransferase; *ALT*, alanine aminotransferase; *LDH*, lactate dehydrogenase; *GGT*, γ-glutamyl transferase; *INR*, *ALP*, Alkaline phosphatase; *SLE*, systemic lupus erythematosus.
Data from Pagana RN, Pagana TJ, Pagana, TN: *Mosby's diagnostic and laboratory test reference*, ed 14, St Louis, 2018, Elsevier.

## Hepatic Function Panel

These tests consist of enzymes that are abundant in hepatocytes (AST, ALT, LDH, GGT, ALP), a substance that indicates the effectiveness of the liver in clearing a product from the blood (bilirubin), and products of the liver (total protein and albumin). Therefore, injury to cells of the liver (hepatocytes) may cause AST, ALT, LDH, GGT, and ALP concentrations in the blood to increase. However, these enzymes are not unique to the liver and individual abnormal values are usually not sufficient to diagnose a particular liver dysfunction. Consequently, physicians rely on various tests and measures in conjunction with clinical observations and other diagnostic tests (Table 40.5).

Measuring transaminases (enzymes) released into the blood from liver cells when they are damaged provides information about liver function and, in particular, the amount of inflammation in the liver. ALT, AST, GGT, and LDH are elevated with injury to hepatocytes. For example, ALT is an enzyme that serves as a sensitive indicator of hepatocellular damage; it is the primary test for detecting hepatitis. GGT has been found to be the most sensitive enzyme for identifying biliary obstruction or cholecystitis; it is a test used to detect chronic alcohol ingestion.[23]

ALP is related to the bile ducts and is increased when they are blocked and may indicate gallbladder, liver, and bile duct disease,[1] but may also be elevated from increased bone turnover in chronic renal failure.[94] Increased levels of this enzyme may be caused by hyperparathyroidism, Paget disease, osteoblastic metastatic tumors, or rheumatoid arthritis. It is also elevated in biliary obstruction or with hepatocytic carcinoma.

AST is also abundant in kidney cells. It is used in conjunction with ALT to determine the possible cause of liver injury. Total LDH is composed of five separate isoenzymes. Each isoenzyme comes from different parts of the body, including the heart, lungs, reticuloendothelial system, skeletal muscle, kidney, pancreas, and the liver. It is used for differential diagnosis of chest pain and may be elevated by injury to cancer cells. Therefore, elevated LDH may raise the suspicion of metastatic disease, particularly osteosarcoma.

Elevated bilirubin indicates the inability to clear sufficient bilirubin from the blood, similar to the way BUN and creatinine are instrumental in clearing the kidneys. Bilirubin is measured as either total bilirubin, or direct and indirect bilirubin separately, to determine the cause of elevated bilirubin. Total bilirubin can be elevated by liver disease or other causes, such as bile duct occlusion and hemolytic anemia in which the amount of bilirubin to be cleared is elevated by excessive destruction of RBCs. Levels of albumin and total protein reflect the ability of the liver to synthesize proteins.[1]

Total protein and albumin may be decreased because of their excretion in the urine as a result of kidney disease. Therefore, the results of multiple tests must be combined with other clinical data to determine the causes of changes in total protein and albumin. Decreased albumin causes edema, including ascites and pulmonary edema. It also alters the serum concentration of drugs that would normally bind to albumin. Lack of albumin also impairs wound healing and leads to muscle atrophy. Because albumin has a half-life of 18 to 20 days, production of proteins by the liver may be impaired for several days before showing up in a comprehensive metabolic panel. If malnutrition is suspected, prealbumin with a half-life of 24 to 48 hours may be measured to give an indication of the direction that albumin concentration is heading.

The albumin-to-globulin ratio (A/G) may provide additional information to the comprehensive metabolic panel. The ratio of albumin to globulin is normally slightly greater than 1.0. The ratio may change either from an increase or decrease in albumin or globulin. A/G may be decreased due to an underproduction of albumin as a result of liver disease, loss of albumin as a result of nephrotic syndrome, or excessive production of globulins in multiple myeloma and autoimmune disorders. The ratio can be increased by diminished immunoglobulin production caused by either genetic disorders or some forms of leukemia. Abnormal A/G requires further investigation into the cause.[3]

### Blood Ammonia

Ammonia is an intermediate product of breaking down amino acids. Severe liver injury results in the inability to convert ammonia into urea to be excreted by the kidneys and leads to accumulation of ammonia. Ammonia accumulation because of hepatic disease may result in hepatic encephalopathy, including confusion, lethargy, dementia, daytime sleepiness, tremors, deterioration of fine motor skills, and speech impairment. Ammonia level may be tested if hepatic encephalopathy or Reye syndrome is suspected as a cause of unexplained mental status or coma. A combination of elevated ammonia and decreased glucose in a child is indicative of Reye syndrome.

Other causes of elevated ammonia may include gastrointestinal bleeding, portal hypertension, and genetic defects in the enzymes of the urea cycle.[1] Table 40.5 lists reference values and interpretations for the hepatic function panel and ammonia. When liver dysfunction results in increased serum ammonia and urea levels, peripheral nerve function can also be impaired. Asterixis and numbness or tingling (misinterpreted as carpal or tarsal tunnel syndrome) can occur as a result of this ammonia abnormality causing intrinsic nerve pathologic findings.

## COMPLETE BLOOD COUNT

The complete blood count (CBC) is a common laboratory test performed routinely in many clinical settings. The CBC measures the components (cells) that make up the blood. Although the term *complete* is commonly used, different degrees of detail are available. The CBC is an automated test that provides details from a sample of blood regarding the concentration of RBCs (erythrocytes), WBCs (leukocytes), and platelets (thrombocytes). From this sample of blood, a clinician may be able to assess for anemia or responses to blood following administration of medications or chemotherapeutic agents. Additionally, the CBC test helps with differential diagnoses of symptoms, including fatigue, bruising, and fever.

Table 40.6 lists normal and abnormal values related to blood testing, with a number of potential causes and the consequences of abnormal values. A simple count of RBCs, WBCs, and platelets may be sufficient for determining the appropriate level of mobilization and exercise. Table 40.7 lists reference values for the CBC. Table 40.8 includes CBC guidelines as related to exercise in adults.

### Red Blood Cells

RBCs are important, as they help transport oxygen and carbon dioxide throughout the body. Oxygen binds to the hemoglobin protein within the RBC, while carbon dioxide is carried by the hemoglobin and does not compete with oxygen molecules. Therefore it is important to understand the total count of RBCs and concentration of hemoglobin (Hb), as well as the percentage of the blood that is comprised of RBCs. This percentage to RBC within the

**Table 40.6** Complete Blood Count

| Abbreviation | Measure of | Significance |
|---|---|---|
| Leukocytes (WBCs) | Total number of WBCs; fight infection and react against foreign bodies or tissues | *Decreased:* infection, bone marrow suppression or failure (e.g., following neoplastic chemotherapy/radiotherapy, bone marrow infiltrative diseases), AIDS, alcoholism, diabetes, autoimmune diseases; lowest in morning<br>*Increased:* indicates infection, inflammation, tissue necrosis, leukemia, tissue trauma or stress (physical or emotional), burns, thyroid storm, dehydration |
| Red blood cells (RBCs) | Erythrocyte (red cell count) | *Decreased:* anemia, hemorrhage, hemolysis, dietary insufficiency of iron and vitamins essential in RBC production, chemotherapy, various disorders/disease (e.g., Hodgkin disease, multiple myeloma, leukemia, SLE, rheumatic fever, endocarditis)<br>*Increased:* COPD, dehydration (hemoconcentration), polycythemia vera, severe diarrhea, poisoning, pulmonary fibroses, high altitude, chronic heart disease |
| | Hematocrit (Hct) is percentage of whole blood occupied by RBCs | *Decreased:* anemia caused by blood loss (e.g., hemorrhage, trauma, surgery, gastrointestinal bleeding), nutritional deficiency (e.g., folate, iron, vitamin $B_{12}$), leukemia, hyperthyroidism cirrhosis, hemolytic reaction (e.g., blood transfusion, chemicals or drugs, severe burns, prosthetic heart valve)<br>*Increased:* erythrocytosis, polycythemia, severe dehydration, shock caused by severe dehydration or burns, cor pulmonale |
| | Hemoglobin (Hb) measures $O_2$-carrying capacity of RBCs | *Decreased:* hemoglobinopathy (e.g., sickle cell disease), pregnancy, hyperthyroidism, some medications (e.g., antibiotics, antineoplastic drugs, aspirin, rifampin, sulfonamides), cirrhosis, severe hemorrhage, severe burns, systemic disease (e.g., Hodgkin disease, leukemia, lymphoma, SLE, sarcoidosis)<br>*Increased:* living in high altitudes, some medications (e.g., gentamicin, methyldopa [Aldomet]), COPD, congestive heart failure, dehydration, polycythemia vera |
| Platelets (thrombocytes) | Clotting potential | *Decreased:* bone marrow failure or infiltration (tumor, fibrosis), hemorrhage, antiplatelet therapy, use of antibiotics, toxic effect of many drugs (e.g., antiinflammatories, steroids), pneumonia and other infections, HIV infection, cancer chemotherapy<br>*Increased:* inflammation, infection, cancer, postsplenectomy syndrome, trauma, rheumatoid arthritis |

*AIDS*, Acquired immunodeficiency syndrome; *COPD*, chronic obstructive pulmonary disease; *HIV*, human immunodeficiency virus; *SLE*, systemic lupus erythematosus.

unit of blood is defined as hematocrit (Hct). Both the Hb and Hct refer to oxygen carrying capacity and therefore correlate with a person's endurance and orthostatic tolerance. A relative decrease in the capacity of blood to carry oxygen is termed *anemia*. Several additional tests may be required to determine the cause of anemia, including intrinsic factor, and vitamin $B_{12}$ and folic acid, which are necessary for erythropoiesis. Mean cell volume, mean cell Hb, red cell distribution width (variation in RBC size), presence of immature cells (reticulocytes), and ferritin may be necessary to diagnose the cause of anemia.

Ferritin is an intracellular store of iron. Its value declines in anemia caused by chronic iron deficiency and severe protein depletion that may occur in conditions such as burns or malnutrition. Elevation of ferritin is also used as an indicator of states of chronic iron excess, such as hemochromatosis.[1]

Men with essential hypertension may have a syndrome known as insulin-resistance–associated hepatic iron overload syndrome, which is characterized by increased iron stores and metabolic abnormalities.[65] In general, individuals with elevated ferritin are at increased risk for insulin-resistance syndrome.[24,101] Ferritin can also be elevated in conditions that do not reflect iron stores, such as acute inflammatory diseases, infections, and metastatic malignancies.

## White Blood Cells

WBCs are cells of the immune system which help protect the body from foreign and infectious agents. The quantity of individual WBCs within the blood can provide insight to the severity of the disease. Number of leukocytes in the blood is often an indicator of disease. WBCs may either increase or decrease in disease. In general, an increase suggests infection or other inflammatory response. WBC count may decrease as a result of bone marrow disease, radiation, or medications, including chemotherapy.

The primary therapy implications are related to the presence of infection with elevated leukocyte count (leukocytosis) or risk of patients becoming infected with a low WBC count (leukopenia). The most abundant WBC type is the neutrophil which protects against bacterial and fungal infections. A reduction of the neutrophil

**Table 40.7** Complete Blood Count Reference Values

| Age | WBCs (/mm³) | RBCs (/mm³) | Erythrocyte Sedimentation Rate (ESR; mm/hr)[a] | Hematocrit (Hct; %) | Hemoglobin (Hb; g/dL) | Platelet Count (/mm³) |
|---|---|---|---|---|---|---|
| Newborn | 9,000–30,000 (drops to adult levels in 2–3 wk) | 4.8–6.1 | 0–2 mm/hr | 44–64 | 14–24 | 150,000–300,000<br>100,000–300,000 (Premature infant)<br>200,000–475,000 (infant) |
| Children | 6,200–17,000 (varies with age) | 4.5–5.0 (varies with age) | ≤10 mm/hr | 1–6 years: 30–40<br>6–18 years: 32–44 (varies with age) | 1–6 years: 9.5–14 g/dL<br>6–18 years: 10–15.5 g/dL (varies with age) | 150,000–400,000 |
| Adult men | 5000–10,000 | 4.7–6.1 | Child: ≤15 mm/hr | 42–52 | 14–18 | 150,000–400,000 |
| Adult women | 5000–10,000 | 4.2–5.4 | ≤20 mm/hr | 37–47 | 12–16 | 150,000–400,000 |
| Pregnant women | 4500–16,000 | Slightly lower | | > 33 | >11 | 150,000–400,000 |

[a]Westergren method.
Data from Pagana RN, Pagana TJ, Pagana, TN: *Mosby's diagnostic and laboratory test reference*, ed 14, St Louis, 2018, Elsevier.

count in a blood test is termed *neutropenia* and increases the risk for nosocomial infections. Facility policy may require supply of individual equipment, air filtration systems, gowning, gloving, and face masks.[98] Physical therapists treating immunocompromised patients should educate patients and their caregivers on the importance of basic hygiene and to avoid exposure to others with contagious illnesses.

## Platelets

The primary role of platelets is to aid in blood clotting and prevent bleeding. Indications for platelet count include unexplained bruising and prolonged coagulation time. Increased platelet count is termed *thrombocytosis*. Although uncommon, it may be caused by splenectomy, some forms of leukemia, other forms of cancer, and iron-deficiency anemia. Decreases in platelet count (*thrombocytopenia*) are much more common in clinical situations. A reduction of the platelet count may be due to hemorrhage, coagulation disorders, autoimmune disorders, histocompatibility problems caused by transfusion of incompatible platelets, or bone marrow diseases such as aplastic anemia, leukemia, and multiple myeloma. Furthermore, autoimmune disease, cancer, chemotherapy, antiplatelet therapy, or drugs that suppress cell production in the bone marrow may cause thrombocytopenia.[38,86]

Thrombocytopenia increases the risk of bleeding into muscles and joints with activity. Caution should be taken with manual therapy, wound débridement, physical therapy modalities, and equipment that may cause minor trauma, such as blood pressure cuffs, pneumatic therapies, compression hose, elastic or resistive bands, cuff weights, and heavy lifting in general. A person's cognition, safety awareness, strength, balance, and coordination become more important considerations with low platelet counts.

# BLOOD TESTS

Tests may be conducted on characteristics and subpopulations of different cells to determine the causes of altered blood counts. Bone marrow disease may be suspected for a number of reasons, particularly a global decrease of blood cells (pancytopenia).

Aspiration of bone marrow may also be required when cancer involving the bone marrow is suspected.[74] Bone marrow aspiration or biopsy allows evaluation of blood formation (hematopoiesis) by quantifying blood elements and precursor blood cells, as well as any abnormal or malignant cells.

## Tests of Red Blood Cells

Symptoms of anemia may be present in spite of normal RBC count, or the cause of anemia may need to be identified. Therefore more specific testing of RBCs may be needed. These include tests of RBC size, shape, maturity, and the type and concentration of Hb inside them.

### Hematocrit

Hct is a simple blood test that measures how much of the blood is made up of red blood cells. A blood sample is drawn into an airtight vial and placed into a centrifuge to determine the relative volume of RBCs expressed as the percentage of the total volume of the blood sample. This test is a quick screen for anemia. A low Hct is indicative

**Table 40.8** Complete Blood Count: Exercise Guidelines (Adult)[a88]

| Complete Blood Count (CBC)[b] | | Causes | Presentation | Clinical Implications |
|---|---|---|---|---|
| **White Blood Cells**<br>Routine test to identify the presence of infection, inflammation, allergens<br>Reference Values<br>5000–10,000/mm$^3$ | Trending Upward *(leukocytosis)* >10,000/mm$^3$ | Infection<br>Leukemia<br>Neoplasm<br>Trauma<br>Surgery<br>Sickle-cell disease<br>Stress/pain<br>Medication-induced<br>Smoking<br>Obesity<br>Congenital<br>Chronic inflammation<br>Connective tissue disease | Fever<br>Malaise<br>Lethargy<br>Dizziness<br>Bleeding<br>Bruising<br>Weight loss (unintentional)<br>Lymphadenopathy<br>Painful inflamed joints | Symptoms-based approach when determining appropriateness for activity, especially in the presence of fever.<br>Consider timing of therapy session due to early-morning low level and late-afternoon high peak. |
| | Trending Downward *(leukopenia)* <4,000/mm$^3$ | Viral infections<br>Chemotherapy<br>Aplastic anemia<br>Autoimmune disease<br>Hepatitis | Anemia<br>Weakness<br>Fatigue<br>Fever<br>Headache<br>Shortness of breath | Symptoms-based approach when determining appropriateness for activity, especially in the presence of fever. |
| | Trending Downward *(neutropenia)* <1500/mm$^3$ = neutropenia<br>500–1000/mm$^3$ = moderate neutropenia;<br><500/mm$^3$ = severe neutropenia<br>500–1000/mm$^3$ = severe neutropenia | Stem cell disorder<br>Bacterial infection<br>Viral infection<br>Radiation | Low-grade fever<br>Skin abscesses<br>Sore mouth<br>Symptoms of pneumonia | Neutropenic precautions (dependent on facility guidelines).<br>Symptoms-based approach when determining appropriateness for activity, especially in the presence of fever. |
| **Platelets**<br>Reference Values<br>Adult/elderly: 150,000–400,000/mm$^3$ or 150–400 × 109/L (SI units) | Trending Upward *(thrombocytosis)* >450,000/mm$^3$ | Splenectomy<br>Inflammation<br>Neoplasm/cancer<br>Stress<br>Iron deficiency<br>Infection<br>Hemorrhage<br>Hemolysis<br>High altitudes<br>Strenuous exercise<br>Trauma | Weakness<br>Bleeding<br>Headache<br>Dizziness<br>Chest pain<br>Tingling in hands/feet | Symptoms-based approach when determining appropriateness for activity; monitor symptoms; collaborate with heath care team<br>Elevated levels can lead to venous thromboembolism. |
| | Trending Downward *(thrombocytopenia)* <150,000/mm$^3$ | Viral infection<br>Nutrition deficiency<br>Leukemia<br>Radiation<br>Chemotherapy<br>Malignant cancer<br>Liver disease<br>Aplastic anemia<br>Premenstrual and postpartum | Petechiae<br>Ecchymosis<br>Fatigue<br>Jaundice<br>Splenomegaly | In presence of severe thrombocytopenia (<20,000/m$^3$): Symptoms-based approach when determining appropriateness for activity; collaborate with heath care team (regarding possible need for/timing of transfusion prior to mobilization)<br>Fall risk awareness (risk of spontaneous hemorrhage). |
| **Hemoglobin**<br>Assess anemia, blood loss, bone marrow suppression<br>Reference Values<br>Male: 14–18 g/dL<br>Female: 12–16 g/dL<br>Pregnant female: >11 g/dL<br>***Note:*** *Values are slightly decreased in elderly.* | Trending Upwards *(polycythemia)* | Congenital heart disease<br>Severe dehydration (or hemoconcentration)<br>Chronic obstructive pulmonary disease (COPD)<br>Congestive heart failure (CHF)<br>Severe burns<br>High altitude | Orthostasis<br>Presyncope<br>Dizziness<br>Arrhythmias<br>CHF onset/exacerbation<br>Seizure<br>Symptoms of transient ischemic attack (TIA)<br>Symptoms of MI<br>Angina | Low critical values (<5–7 g/dL) can lead to heart failure or death.<br>High critical values (>20 g/dL) can lead to clogging of capillaries as a result of hemoconcentration.<br>Symptoms-based approach when determining appropriateness for activity, monitor symptoms, collaborate with heath care team. |

**Table 40.8** Complete Blood Count: Exercise Guidelines (Adult)[a][88]—cont'd

| Complete Blood Count (CBC)[b] | | Causes | Presentation | Clinical Implications |
|---|---|---|---|---|
| **Hemoglobin—cont'd**<br>Assess anemia, blood loss, bone marrow suppression<br>Reference Values<br>Male: 14–18 g/dL<br>Female: 12–16 g/dL<br>***Note:*** *Values are slightly decreased in elderly.* | Trending Downward *(anemia)* | Hemorrhage<br>Nutritional deficiency<br>Neoplasia<br>Lymphoma<br>Systemic lupus erythematosus<br>Sarcoidosis<br>Renal disease<br>Splenomegaly<br>Sickle cell anemia<br>Stress to bone marrow<br>RBC destruction | Decreased endurance<br>Decreased activity tolerance<br>Pallor<br>Tachycardia | Monitor vitals including $SpO_2$ to predict tissue perfusion. May present with tachycardia and/or orthostatic hypotension.<br>Medical team might monitor patients with preexisting cerebrovascular, cardiac, or renal conditions for ineffective tissue perfusion related to decreased hemoglobin.<br>If <8 g/dL: Symptoms-based approach when determining appropriateness for activity; collaborate with heath care team (regarding possible need for/timing of transfusion prior to mobilization) |
| **Hematocrit**<br>Assess blood loss and fluid balance.<br>Reference Values<br>***Note:*** *Values are slightly decreased in the elderly.* | Trending Upward *(polycythemia)* | Burns<br>Eclampsia<br>Severe dehydration<br>Erythrocytosis<br>Tend to be elevated with those living in higher altitude<br>Hypoxia due to chronic pulmonary conditions (COPD, CHF) | Fever<br>Headache<br>Dizziness<br>Weakness<br>Fatigue<br>Easy bruising or bleeding | Low critical value (<15–20%) cardiac failure or death.<br>High critical value (>60%) spontaneous blood clotting.<br>Symptoms-based approach when determining appropriateness for activity; monitor symptoms; collaborate with heath care team. |
| Assess blood loss and fluid balance.<br>Reference Values<br>Male: 42–52%<br>Female: 37–47%<br>***Note:*** *Values are slightly decreased in the elderly.* | Trending Downward *(anemia)* | Leukemia<br>Bone marrow failure<br>Multiple myeloma<br>Dietary deficiency<br>Pregnancy<br>Hyperthyroidism<br>Cirrhosis<br>Rheumatoid arthritis<br>Hemorrhage<br>High altitude | Pale skin<br>Headache<br>Dizziness<br>Cold hands/feet<br>Chest pain<br>Arrhythmia<br>Shortness of breath | Patient might have impaired endurance; progress slowly with activity.<br>Monitor vitals including $SpO_2$ to predict tissue perfusion. Might present with tachycardia and/or orthostatic hypotension.<br>Medical team might monitor patients with preexisting cerebrovascular, cardiac, or renal conditions for ineffective tissue perfusion related to decreased hematocrit.<br>If <25%: Symptoms-based approach when determining appropriateness for activity; collaborate with heath care team (regarding possible need for/timing of transfusion prior to mobilization) |

[a]Therapists should make individual determinations depending on the total picture taking into consideration the consequences of treatment versus no treatment, patient's age, general health status, and disease or condition present. For example, someone with an acute episode of urinary tract infection with altered WBC count and fever would be treated differently from someone with a chronic condition, such as diabetes mellitus. An important question to ask yourself is: Will a person fare better or worse with physical therapy intervention? Consult with the physician and other members of the team for guidance and restrictions when needed.

[b]Reference values included in this table are from: Pagana RN, Pagana TJ, Pagana, TN: *Mosby's diagnostic and laboratory test reference*, ed 14, St Louis, 2018, Elsevier.

*INR*, International normalized ratio.

The definition of exercise is not standard when applying these lab values. The therapist must keep in mind that what constitutes "aerobic exercise" for one individual (e.g., getting on and off the toilet) may not elevate the heart rate of someone else who is in good physical health. The recommendation for "no exercise" must be interpreted carefully as well, and does not necessarily mean "no physical therapy." Practicing safe bed-to-commode transfers, gait in room or hallway, and activities of daily living may be appropriate and indicated when lab values fall into the "no exercise" category.

From Tompkins J: Academy of Acute Care Physical Therapy Laboratory Values Interpretation Resource Updated 2017. https://c.ymcdn.com/sites/acutept.site-ym.com/resource/resmgr/docs/2017-Lab-Values-Resource.pdf. Accessed 9/12/18. Reprinted with permission, APTA Acute Care.

of anemia, but anemia could still exist in the presence of a normal *relative* volume of RBCs. A condition of excessive numbers of RBCs is termed *polycythemia*. It may be present with dehydration (relative loss of water from the blood) or as a secondary response to persistent hypoxemia caused by chronic pulmonary disease or living at a high altitude. Polycythemia vera is a disease in which Hct is elevated and is discussed in Chapter 14. Hct values that are even slightly out of the normal range put older adults at increased risk for heart problems and even death when undergoing major surgery.[102] Note that the Wu 2007 study[102] demonstrated increased mortality with both anemia and polycythemia.

### Hemoglobin

Hemoglobins (Hb) are red proteins responsible for transporting and delivering oxygen to target organs. Because Hb is packaged in RBCs, the relative volume of red cells (Hct) and the concentration of molecules carrying oxygen in the blood are usually correlated. However, certain disease states may allow normal numbers of RBCs, but result in reduced concentration of Hb within individual cells. Therefore a person with normal Hct may have reduced Hb concentration. Hct and Hb concentration are frequently tested simultaneously. When done this way, the term *H&H* is generally used.

Hb levels of 12 to 18 g/dL are considered normal, however studies show that older adults with a low-normal value of 12 g/dL are more likely to have difficulty performing daily tasks. It is not uncommon for mild anemia to cause significant functional challenges. Difficulty walking, climbing stairs, or doing house or yard work may be an early sign of low-normal Hb levels.[13]

In individuals with anemia, it would be anticipated to identify decreased tolerance of activity and upright positioning, dyspnea, tachycardia, and subjective complaints of fatigue/feeling weak. With severe anemia, there will be far less oxygenated blood supply to the heart. This may also produce angina in some individuals. H&H alone may not be sufficient predictors of a person's tolerance of activity. In some instances, individuals with chronic anemia may exhibit much better tolerance than those with more acute anemia.

In most people with anemia, exercise and upright positioning will need to be progressed gradually, with close monitoring of vital signs to identify physiologic stressors. In some cases of anemia, Borg's Rating of Perceived Exertion may be a better predictor of exercise tolerance than heart rate alone.

In hospitalized patients, a decrease in Hb to 8 g/dL or below should trigger discussion with the patient's nurse and physician concerning activity level and need for transfusion or other interventions to improve Hb. However, note that the number of transfusions received by a patient is an independent predictor of patient outcome. As the number of transfusions received by a patient increases, patients have longer ICU stays, longer hospital stays, increased mortality, and more complications.[14] Anemia is common in patients with complex medical conditions. Although trauma and bleeding may produce anemia in many patients, most cases of anemia in ICUs are not a result of hemorrhagic conditions, but are the effects of inflammatory cytokines associated with poor health suppressing RBC production.

### Red Blood Cell Shape

The normal biconcave disc of RBCs may be altered by genetic or acquired diseases. A number of rare genetic diseases may also alter the shape of RBCs. For example, hereditary spherocytosis, as the name implies, allows red cells to take on a spherical shape. The crescent shape of RBCs with an abnormal form of hemoglobin may be seen microscopically to confirm the diagnosis of sickle cell disease.

### Iron

Iron is required for the synthesis of Hb. The lack of iron results in small, hypochromic (pale) RBCs that have difficulty binding as much oxygen as normal. Iron status is determined by serum transferrin. Iron-deficiency anemia is discussed further in Chapter 14.

### Vitamin $B_{12}$ and Folic Acid

Both of these vitamins are critical to the production of RBCs. Deficiencies of these vitamins may result in the release of large immature RBCs from the bone marrow. Vitamin $B_{12}$ is obtained from ingesting animal proteins, including meats, fish, poultry, eggs, and dairy. When absorption of vitamin $B_{12}$ is inadequate due to diet or a malabsorption syndrome, pernicious anemia may develop.

Vitamin $B_{12}$ shots may be prescribed when serum levels are deficient. Folic acid (folate), one of the B vitamins, is also necessary for normal formation of RBCs and WBCs and for the adequate synthesis of certain purines and pyrimidines, which are precursors to deoxyribonucleic acid (DNA). As with vitamin $B_{12}$, folate depends on normal absorption in the intestinal mucosa.

### Erythrocyte Sedimentation Rate

Although not related to anemia, erythrocyte sedimentation rate (ESR) is clustered with other tests of RBCs and is presented in Table 40.7. ESR is a nonspecific test for inflammatory disorders, which is associated with a number of potential disorders, including cancer, autoimmune diseases, and infection. As the name implies, the test is based on how quickly RBCs sink to the bottom of a test solution containing anticoagulated (unclotted) blood. ESR is increased in the sense that sedimentation is more rapid (more cells sink to the bottom per time) when they clump together.

Clumping is caused by a change in blood proteins brought on by inflammation, specifically the presence of globulins or fibrinogen in the blood. The more severe the inflammation, the faster the sedimentation rate or settling of cells and the higher the ESR; a significant increase in the ESR warrants closer investigation.

By itself, this test is nonspecific and therefore not diagnostic for any particular organ disease or injury, but the ESR may be used as a screening test to rule out certain diseases or to monitor treatment in specific diseases such as juvenile rheumatoid arthritis, Kawasaki disease, temporal arteritis, gout, and polymyalgia rheumatica. It can be used as an index of musculoskeletal dysfunction, such as tissue injury or inflammation or bone infections.

ESR is a fairly reliable indicator of the course of many diseases and, therefore, may be used to monitor the course of such diseases or responses to treatment of these diseases. In general, as the disease worsens, the ESR increases and as the disease improves, the ESR decreases. ESR also increases with age.[84]

## White Blood Cell Tests

Various disease states are characterized by their effects on specific types of WBCs. The elevation or depression of these cells may be useful in the differential diagnosis. A simple CBC test can demonstrate a normal level, a decreased level (*leukopenia*), or an elevated level (*leukocytosis*). Leukopenia can result from cancer, cancer chemotherapy, aplastic anemia, and other causes. Leukocytosis is frequently a result of an inflammatory response, resulting from an infection, as well as some forms of leukemia. Both the absolute numbers and the numbers of white cells relative to each other can be useful in diagnosis. An analysis of the relative numbers of different types of white cells is known as a white cell differential.

### Neutrophils

Neutrophils are a type of WBC that protects against infections. They represent the majority of WBCs present in the blood. A decreased number is termed *neutropenia* and an increased number is termed *neutrophilia*. Neutropenia is clinically significant as a risk factor for infection and may result from a large number of causes. In general, neutrophilia suggests the presence of infection or a proliferative disorder seen with cancers, such as acute myelocytic leukemia.

Because of their appearance, neutrophils are also called polymorphonuclear (PMN) cells. Mature cells are segmented (called segs), whereas immature cells appear to be banded (bands). Bands make up approximately 3% to 5% of WBCs and circulate for about 6 hours before they mature into segmented neutrophils. During counting, PMNs are divided into bands and segs. The presence of relatively high numbers of immature PMNs (bands) indicates rapid production of neutrophils in response to events such as acute infection, necrosis, or autoimmune disease. This may be referred to as a left shift because of the historic method of hand counting the white cell differential.

Absolute neutrophil count (ANC) is determined by multiplying the WBC count by the percentage of cells that are neutrophils. ANC is an indication of a person's ability to prevent infection. This measurement is particularly important for individuals receiving cancer chemotherapy and those who have received bone marrow transplants. Individuals with low ANC may be placed on neutropenic precautions. These precautions include protective isolation and either not allowing the individuals to leave their rooms or requiring them to wear masks. Neutropenic precautions may be put into effect with a WBC count less than 1000 or an ANC less than 500/μL.[46]

### Basophils, Eosinophils, and Monocytes

Basophils are implicated in immune responses, particularly those that cause allergies. Eosinophils are commonly elevated (*eosinophilia*) in the presence of parasitic conditions or allergies. Monocytes are blood cells that migrate into tissues as needed during injury or infection. After migration they are referred to as macrophages.

**Table 40.9** T- and B-Cell Lymphocyte Surface Markers

| Surface Markers | Normal Findings |
|---|---|
| T-cells (CD2) | 60%–95% |
| Helper T-cells (CD4) | 60%–75% |
| CD8 T-cells | 25%–30% |
| B-cells | 4%–25% |
| Natural killer cells | 4%–30% |

From: Pagana RN, Pagana TJ, Pagana, TN: *Mosby's diagnostic and laboratory test reference*, ed 14, St Louis, 2018, Elsevier.

### Lymphocytes

Lymphocytes are divided into B cells (capable of producing antibodies) and T cells that either produce toxic granules containing powerful enzymes to destroy pathogen-infected or otherwise damaged cells (cytotoxic or killer T cells), produce direct injury to cells carrying foreign markers (helper T cells), or assist in modulating B- and T-cell function (regulator T cells). A third type of lymphocyte called natural killer (NK) cells, is part of the innate immune system. NK cells provide rapid responses to viral infected cells to minimize tumor formation.

Interest in lymphocyte subtypes is primarily a result of the effect of acquired immunodeficiency syndrome (AIDS) on particular subtypes of WBCs. In particular, helper T cells are vulnerable to human immunodeficiency virus (HIV) destruction, resulting in immunosuppression. The relative populations of each are determined by the presence of cell markers denoted CD2, CD4, CD8, and CD19. Cytotoxic (killer) T cells have CD2; helper T cells have CD4; regulatory T cells have CD8; and B cells are detected by CD19. Table 40.9 lists the relative numbers of these cells. Table 40.10 lists the potential indications of varying proportions in the WBC differential.

## BLEEDING RATIO/VISCOSITY

Bleeding disorders are characterized by impairments in the hemostasis process which involves interaction between blood vessel wall and platelets, blood coagulation, and fibrinolysis. Tests relevant to bleeding viscosity involve platelets; enzymes required to initiate, promote, or inhibit hemostasis; binding of coagulation factors; and calcium. Platelets are discussed in the previous section on CBC. Lab values related to tests of bleeding ratios and viscosity, listed in Table 40.11, are referred to as the coagulation profile. Coagulation tests are important to determine whether a person clots too easily or does not clot sufficiently to prevent excessive bleeding.

In addition to thrombocytopenia, disorders such as hemophilia, von Willebrand disease, and bone marrow suppression may lead to excessive bleeding. Therefore, coagulation status should be known before performing therapy that might cause bleeding. This might include resistance exercise, activities with risk of falling, or sharp débridement.

**Table 40.10** Differential White Blood Cell Count Reference Values

| Cell | Function | Absolute Count (cells/mm³) | Differential Count (%) |
|---|---|---|---|
| Neutrophils | Neutrophils are WBCs that constitute a defense against foreign substances (usually bacterial infections). | 2500–8000 | 55–70 |
| Lymphocytes | Produce antibodies, fight tumor cells, and respond to viral infection | 1000–4000 | 20–40 |
| Monocytes | Clean up debris after neutrophils have done their job | 100–700 | 2–8 |
| Eosinophils | Attack parasites and play a role in asthma and allergy | 50–500 | 1–4 |
| Basophils | Release histamines during allergic reactions | 25–100 | 0.5–1 |

From Pagana RN, Pagana TJ, Pagana, TN: *Mosby's diagnostic and laboratory test reference*, ed 14, St Louis, 2018, Elsevier.

**Table 40.11** Coagulation Profile (Platelets)

| International Normalized Ratio (INR) | Prothrombin Time (PT) | Activated Partial Thromboplastin Time (aPTT) | Anti-factor Xa Heparin Assay |
|---|---|---|---|
| Normal range: 0.8–1.1 (ratio)<br>Therapeutic range DVT prophylaxis: 1.5–2<br>Orthopedic surgery, DVT, Atrial fibrillation: 2.0–3.0<br>Pulmonary embolism: 2.5–3.5<br>Prosthetic valve prophylaxis: 3.0–4.0<br>Possible critical value: >5.5 | 11–12.5 sec<br>Possible critical value: >20 sec | 30–40 sec<br>Possible critical value: >70 sec | Therapeutic ranges (adults and children > 8 weeks):<br>LMWH: 0.5–1.2 IU/mL<br>UH: 0.3–0.7 IU/mL<br>Prophylactic ranges:<br>LMWH: 0.2–0.5 IU/mL<br>UH: 0.1–0.4 IU/mL<br>Therapeutic ranges (children <8 weeks):<br>LMWH: 0.5–1.0 IU/mL<br>UH: 0.3–0.7 IU/mL<br>Prophylactic ranges:<br>LMWH: 0.1–0.3 IU/mL |

From Pagana RN, Pagana TJ, Pagana, TN: *Mosby's diagnostic and laboratory test reference*, ed 14, St Louis, 2018, Elsevier.

Individuals may be anticoagulated for a number of reasons. When individuals are treated for venous thrombosis, atrial fibrillation, or coronary artery disease they may become overly anticoagulated and bleed excessively. Tests for coagulation involve the function of the terminal products of the coagulation cascade. Coagulation factors interact and result in the production of thrombin, which activates the reaction to convert fibrinogen to fibrin. The tests in the next section evaluate bleeding time. Because of how the tests are performed, they indicate the effectiveness of different mechanisms within the coagulation cascade.

## Tests of Coagulation

The coagulation cascade involves a homeostatic relationship between the intrinsic and extrinsic pathways. These pathways join to form the common pathway resulting in the conversion of factor X to Xa, converting prothrombin to thrombin and leading to the aggregation of platelets to form a stable fibrin clot. Historically, prothrombin time (PT) and activated partial thromboplastin time (aPTT) have been used to determine coagulability, either diagnostically or to monitor anticoagulant therapy with vitamin K antagonists, such as warfarin and heparins. In an effort to create safer anticoagulants as well as reduce frequency of strict drug monitoring, newer anticoagulants (factor Xa inhibitors and direct thrombin inhibitors) were developed to target different aspects of the coagulation cascade.[27] These medications are used for many conditions, including atrial fibrillation; prevention of acute myocardial infarction (MI) in people with peripheral arterial disease; prevention of stroke, recurrent MI, or death in people who have had an MI; valvular heart disease (native and prosthetic); and venous thromboembolism (prevention or treatment).[39,42,49] Because the various anticoagulation drug therapies target different points in the coagulation cascade, the laboratory monitoring varies. Therefore physical therapists must be aware of the tests as well as the ranges given the patients' diagnoses and comorbidities to determine safe application of interventions.

The international normalized ratio (INR) was developed to provide PT results that would not vary between laboratories. Individuals receiving anticoagulation therapy because of coronary artery disease, cerebrovascular disease, atrial fibrillation, history of deep venous thrombosis, and other reasons are anticoagulated to an INR of 2 to 3.[29,39,49]

As INR increases, however, the risk of bleeding with minor trauma increases and excessive bleeding may occur during surgery, as well as spontaneous bleeding. Note, however, that INR and other tests of coagulation report how quickly a person will coagulate with a standardized stimulus; they are not tests of whether a person will bleed with trauma. Therefore, some people may experience excessive bleeding with minor injury at a therapeutic INR and others with supratherapeutic INR may not experience significant bleeding episodes with trauma.

Although INR has been an effective test for anticoagulation produced by unfractionated heparin (an historically manufactured heparin consists of a wide range of sizes of individual heparin molecules as opposed to LMWH) and warfarin, aPTT is used to monitor the effectiveness of LMWH. Therapeutic INR takes days to reach with unfractionated heparin or warfarin and is related more to extrinsic coagulation pathway, whereas LMWH can reduce coagulability much more rapidly as measured by aPTT, which is a better measure of intrinsic coagulation pathway.

Heparin anti-Xa is an alternative test that can be used to assess the effectiveness of both unfractionated and LMWH. Heparin impairs the coagulation sequence primarily through inhibiting coagulation factors Xa and thrombin. Whereas unfractionated heparin exerts its effect through both factors Xa and thrombin and has more variable effects on coagulation, LMWH acts primarily on factor Xa and produces a more predictable anticoagulant effect. Although routine monitoring of LMWH is not needed to the extent that it is needed for unfractionated heparin, heparin anti-Xa is preferred for special circumstances, such as during pregnancy, in the presence of kidney disease, or other populations.

Heparin anti-Xa may also be used for some individuals who do not respond as expected to heparin because of an underlying disorder such as systemic lupus erythematosus (SLE), which affects partial thromboplastin time.[30]

Side effects of heparin in addition to excessive bleeding include hypersensitivity reaction, osteopenia in elderly or bed-bound patients, and heparin-induced thrombocytopenia. Heparin-induced thrombocytopenia is caused by heparin-dependent platelet activating antibodies that cause a paradoxical thrombosis as a result of release of microparticles from platelet surfaces and is potentially fatal. It is more common with unfractionated heparin than with LMWH. Thrombosis occurs prior to the decrease in platelet count. Consequences of heparin-induced thrombocytopenia include deep venous thrombosis, pulmonary embolism, gangrene, MI, cardiovascular accident, skin lesions at injection sites, and disseminated intravascular coagulation. Nonheparin anticoagulants are needed to reduce the risk of thrombosis.

Platelet function tests are separate tests run on specialized devices to determine how well platelets aggregate and initiate the coagulation sequence.[64] These tests may be run either because of increased risk of excessive coagulation or because of deficient coagulation. The tests consist of the time to form a clot (closure time assay), the strength of the clot (viscoelastometry), and the rate of platelet aggregation (end point platelet aggregation assay). Different disorders of coagulation can be determined by the combination of results from these assays.

## Components of Coagulation

Specific components of coagulation may be tested on suspicion of their involvement in bleeding disorders. These include specific coagulation factors that produce hemophilia and von Willebrand factor.

### Coagulation Factors

Individual factor testing may also be performed as a follow-up to abnormal PT, aPTT, or because of suspected coagulation factor deficiencies. Deficiencies may be genetic, such as hemophilias A and B, or acquired in conditions such as disseminated intravascular coagulation, liver disease, or vitamin K deficiency.[1,10,63]

Of particular interest are factors VIII and IX. Genetic defects in the production of these factors produce hemophilia A and B, respectively. Hemophilia B is also known as Christmas disease. Genetic defects may also occur in coagulation factors other than VIII and IX, but are very rare. Abnormal aPTT (intrinsic pathway) with normal PT indicates involvement of factors VIII, IX, XI, or XII, whereas normal aPTT with prolonged PT (extrinsic pathway) suggests factor I, II, V, VII, or X.[1]

von Willebrand disease, a genetic disease like hemophilia, impairs coagulation because of a lack of effective von Willebrand factor, which along with factor VIII, is necessary for binding of platelets to collagen.

Antiphospholipid antibodies are associated with inappropriate coagulation and autoimmune diseases, especially SLE. Cardiolipin antibodies are the most common, along with lupus anticoagulant and anti-$\beta_2$ glycoprotein I. Cardiolipins are a class of phospholipid molecules found on the membranes of a number of cells, notably platelets.

Antibodies to cardiolipin increase the risk of inappropriate coagulation and are associated with thrombocytopenia, premature labor, and preeclampsia. Antiphospholipid syndrome is the term used for the clinical syndrome associated with elevated antiphospholipid antibodies and morbidity resulting from inappropriate clotting and recurrent spontaneous abortion. Secondary antiphospholipid syndrome is secondary to an autoimmune disease such as SLE, whereas primary disease is not.[21]

## Regulation of Coagulation

Either excessive or deficient clotting may occur as a consequence of deficiencies or defective components of the system to regulate coagulation. Antithrombin is naturally produced as a means of counterbalancing the coagulation sequence. The balance of thrombin produced by the coagulation cascade and antithrombin produced by the liver determines the likelihood of coagulation/thrombosis.

Antithrombin inhibits both thrombin itself and several of the factors involved in the coagulation cascade that culminates in thrombin production. Antithrombin deficiency can be inherited or acquired. Heterozygous individuals experience episodes of excessive coagulation in early adulthood, whereas homozygous individuals develop excessive coagulation early in life. Antithrombin deficiency can result in either normally functional, but insufficient quantities of antithrombin or in sufficient quantities, but dysfunctional antithrombin. Testing can determine which is the case. Acquired antithrombin deficiency can result from liver disease, disseminated intravascular coagulation, cancer, and nephrotic syndrome.

Proteins C and S are measured in the routine work-up for unexplained excessive coagulation. Deficiencies of proteins C and S are both associated with excessive coagulation. These proteins, along with thrombin, are responsible for preventing dysfunction of the coagulation cascade. As the coagulation cascade is activated, the mechanism for halting it is also activated. Thrombin is activated by the coagulation cascade resulting in clotting, but it also combines with thrombomodulin to activate protein C. Activated protein C combines with protein S to degrade factors VIIIa and Va, the factors that are responsible for the production of thrombin itself. When functioning normally, the production of thrombin with an appropriate stimulus leads to coagulation sufficient to stop bleeding and then halting of the coagulation process.

Genetic defects may result in insufficient quantities of either protein C or S, abnormal function of either protein C or S, or increased clearance of protein S, with the result that these proteins are not capable of halting thrombin production in a timely manner and either excessive or inappropriate coagulation/thrombosis may occur. The excessive clotting usually occurs in veins, increasing the risk of pulmonary embolism, but can also occur in arteries.[40]

Factor V Leiden mutation and Prothrombin 20210A are genetic mutations associated with increased risk of venous thromboembolism.[92] Tests for these genetic mutations may be performed in the presence of unexplained excessive coagulation or a family history of thrombotic disease. Factor V Leiden is a mutation that results in a form of factor V that degrades more slowly following coagulation and therefore promotes extended coagulation. Factor V Leiden is fairly common (5% of the white population). The risk of thromboembolic events is increased three to eight times in heterozygous individuals and 50 to 80 times in those who are homozygous for this gene.

Those who are heterozygous for the Prothrombin 20210A gene produce excess thrombin and have approximately three times the risk of thromboembolic events of those without the gene. This gene is less prevalent and being homozygous for this gene is extremely rare.[22]

### D-Dimer

D-dimer is a specific type of fragment produced by lysis of products of coagulation by plasmin. These fragments of crosslinked fibrin are not detectable under normal circumstances, but in the presence of clotting or coagulation, these fibrin degradation products will be released in proportion to the quantities of fibrin and plasmin in the circulation. Before a D-dimer test is ordered the individual's clinical probability for venous thomboembolism is determined. Individuals with high clinical probability will not be tested with a D-dimer because the test has poor positive predictive value for a venous thromboembolism. A negative test for D-dimer suggests a low likelihood of a large thrombus or clot. Elevated D-dimer suggests the possibility of a number of unfavorable coagulation conditions, including age, pregnancy, cancer, pulmonary embolism, and intravascular coagulation in addition to thromboembolism associated with surgery, immobilization, and atherosclerosis. Further testing is required to determine the cause of elevated D-dimer.[66,93]

### Warfarin Sensitivity Testing

Two genotypes, CYP2C9 and VKORC1, are associated with abnormal sensitivity to warfarin (Coumadin). These genetic variations alter the doses necessary to produce optimum anticoagulation with warfarin. Warfarin prevents the recycling of vitamin K, which, in turn, reduces the production of a number of factors in the coagulation cascade, and thereby decreases the risk of coagulation.

Vitamin K epoxide reductase (VKOR) is the protein responsible for the production of clotting factors II, VII, IX, and X. Variations in the gene VKORC1 alter the sensitivity of VKOR to warfarin, requiring either an increase or decrease in the normal dose of warfarin to produce the desired anticoagulation response.

Another protein, cytochrome P450 2C9 (CYP2C9) is important because of its role in degrading warfarin. Genetic variations in this gene lead to slower breakdown and greater accumulation of warfarin, which then leads to excessive anticoagulation. Individuals with this gene mutation require a lower dose of warfarin or risk excessive bleeding.[85]

## CARDIOVASCULAR LAB TESTS

Tests in this section are related to the diagnosis of heart failure, MI, and assessing the risk of coronary artery disease.

### Congestive Heart Failure

Atrial natriuretic peptide (ANP) was discovered many years ago and found to provide a minor contribution to regulation of extracellular fluid volume by regulating renal sodium excretion.[8] ANP is synthesized and secreted by cardiac muscle cells. As blood volume increases, stretching the atria, ANP secretion is increased, resulting in renal sodium and fluid excretion, which subsequently lowers fluid volume.

A similar peptide, brain natriuretic peptide (BNP), was discovered in the brain. Subsequent research showed that BNP was also secreted by muscle cells of the heart, but the name was retained. Similar to ANP, BNP is excreted from the heart ventricles in response to stretching caused by excessive blood volume. The physiologic actions of both ANP and BNP is an increase in sodium excretion in urine, which results in a decrease in blood pressure, primarily due to decreases in vascular resistance and afterload. The tests for these peptides are used for differential diagnosis of shortness of breath because BNP is elevated in congestive heart failure.[18,29,54] A value of greater than 100 pg/mL is considered positive for congestive heart failure. Levels of BNP rise with disease severity, so levels from 100 to 300 pg/mL generally indicate mild heart failure; 300 to 700 pg/mL indicates moderate heart failure; and levels above 700 pg/mL indicate severe heart failure.[79] Even smaller elevations of BNP above normal are indicative of impaired cardiac pump function[32] and future mortality.[96,97] The BNP test can also be used to monitor disease progression in individuals with left-sided heart failure.

Table 40.12 Serum Isoenzymes and Markers

| Isoenzyme | Where Found | Increased in |
|---|---|---|
| CK-BB | Brain | Central nervous system surgery, cardiac arrest, Reye syndrome, cerebral contusion, cerebrovascular accident, malignant hyperthermia, bowel infarction, renal failure |
| CK-MB | Myocardium | Myocardial injury, ischemia, MI, cardiac contusion, cardiac trauma, congestive heart failure, tachyarrhythmias with underlying coronary artery disease, cardiac surgery, myocarditis |
| CK-MM | Skeletal muscle | Intramuscular injections, skeletal muscle trauma, extreme muscle exertion, tonic clonic seizures, surgery, excess alcohol (toxic effect on muscle), alcohol withdrawal syndrome, seizures, electric countershock, muscular dystrophy, severe hypokalemia, hypothyroidism, extreme hypothermia or hyperthermia |
| LDH-1 | Primarily from the heart | Myocardial injury (MI), myocarditis |
| LDH-2 | Primarily reticuloendothelial system | Injury to any tissue except skeletal muscle |
| Troponins (I, T) | Contractile proteins found primarily in cardiac tissue | MI (specific isoforms or troponin I and T) |
| Myoglobin | Skeletal and cardiac muscle | Immediate rise when cardiac or skeletal muscle is damaged |

*CK-BB, -MB, -MM,* Creatinine kinase subunits; *LDH,* lactate dehydrogenase.

## Cardiac Enzymes and Markers

As described with the liver panel, upon injury cells release some of their intracellular enzymes and ultimately are cleared via renal and hepatic metabolism. The more cells that are damaged, the higher the concentration of these enzymes that will be found in the circulation of blood. The release and clearance of different enzymes after cell injury varies widely. In some cases, enzymes rise rapidly, but also are cleared rapidly. For this reason, more than one enzyme is generally measured for diagnostic purposes, and evaluated in conjunction with clinical signs and symptoms. Table 40.12 lists some of the enzymes released into plasma with injury and which cells (and therefore which organs) are damaged.

### Creatine Kinase

Creatine kinase (CK) is a major cytoplasmic enzyme of muscle present in three major isoenzymatic forms: skeletal muscle (MM), brain (BB), and cardiac muscle (MB). CK-MM constitutes more than 90% of serum total CK. Trauma to skeletal muscle can cause CK release, and elevation of total serum CK levels is associated with muscle soreness. Increase in serum CK occurs within 6 to 24 hours of direct muscle injury.[81] Although CK-MB is found almost exclusively in myocardial muscle, CK-MB may not reach the threshold required to diagnose MI for several hours.[1] Other tests that provide results of myocardial cell wall injury more rapidly include troponin and myoglobin.

### Myoglobin

Myoglobin is a small protein involved in the transport and storage of oxygen in muscle cells. It is only found in the bloodstream of humans following muscle injury. Myoglobin is released from damaged muscle soon after injury. The molecule leaks out of cells and into the bloodstream. Levels of myoglobin can be measured and are noted to begin to rise within 2 to 3 hours of a MI and reach their peak in 8 to 12 hours.[1] However, levels fall rapidly back to normal within 1 to 2 days after the MI. Myoglobin is present in large quantities of skeletal muscle and although helpful in ruling out MI, it is not utilized as a sole test for diagnosis. Myoglobin may also be elevated by trauma to muscle, including by the use of defibrillators, and drugs administered in the field to degrade thrombi responsible for chest pain.

### Troponin

Three types of troponin proteins which are integral to muscle contraction and are found in skeletal and cardiac muscle. Proteins troponin subtypes I (TnI) and T (TnT) are measured in the blood and the presence of the proteins is sensitive and specific to myocardial injury.[68] Normally, these troponin subunits are found at very low to undetectable levels in the blood. Elevations suggestive of cardiac muscle injury are detectible within 3 to 4 hours and can remain sufficiently elevated for diagnosis up to 14 days, depending on the extent of the cardiac muscle injury.

Slight elevations are indicative of unstable angina or MI and may be predictive of a person's risk of having a future coronary event, or the potential benefit from early revascularization.[57] Studies have indicated that individuals with elevated troponin are at increased risk for mortality for the next few months.[35,41]

**Table 40.13** Cardiac Enzymes and Markers (Serum)

| Enzyme | Normal Range | Appears (hr) | Peaks (hr) | Normalizes |
|---|---|---|---|---|
| CK-MB | 0% | 3–6 | 12–24 | 12–48 hours |
| Myoglobin | <90 μg/L | 3 | | |
| Troponin I | <0.03 ng/mL | 2–3 | remain elevated from 7–10 days | |
| Troponin T | <0.10 ng/mL | 2–3 | remain elevated up to 14 days | |

*CK-MB*, Creatine kinase submit; *LDH*, lactate dehydrogenase.
Data from Pagana RN, Pagana TJ, Pagana, TN: *Mosby's diagnostic and laboratory test reference*, ed 14, St Louis, 2018, Elsevier.

Although cardiac troponins are more specific than CK-MB and myoglobin, troponin levels may be elevated for reasons other than myocardial tissue injury. These proteins may be elevated with vigorous exercise (e.g., marathon, high-intensity training), traumatic injury (including defibrillation, ablation, cardiac surgery), inflammatory disease involving the heart, high-dose chemotherapy, sepsis, or accumulation in the blood secondary to kidney disease. Although in itself troponin may not be an independent tool for an evolving MI, an elevated troponin level remains predictive of compromised cardiac function and must be evaluated in context of the whole picture (i.e., patient's medical status and physiology, trend or pattern of serial troponin values). Table 40.13 lists reference values for the cardiac subunits and isozymes.

## Risk Factors for Atherosclerotic Disease

Lipids are important molecules involved in the storage of energy, production of steroids and bile acids, and maintenance of cell membranes. Inappropriate serum levels of certain lipids are associated with atherosclerotic vascular disease. Those of particular interest include triglycerides, cholesterol, and lipoproteins. Review of several blood lipids levels are utilized for cardiovascular risk stratification.

### Lipids

The liver metabolizes cholesterol to its free form, which is then transported in the bloodstream by lipoproteins. Lipid measurements are important in detecting genetically determined disorders of lipid metabolism and in assessing the risk of coronary artery disease and other diseases caused by atherosclerosis. In particular, elevation of low-density lipoprotein (LDL) is a strong predictor of cardiovascular disease. Lower-than-normal levels of high-density lipoprotein (HDL) also increase the risk. In addition to genetic defects associated with elevated LDL, other factors, such as smoking, diet, certain drugs (oral contraceptives, sulfonamides, aspirin, and steroids), hypothyroidism, exercise, and alcohol, alter one or both. A full lipid profile includes total cholesterol, LDL, HDL, and triglycerides (Table 40.14). The tests may also be used to assess the need for and the efficacy of treatment.

**Table 40.14** Full Lipid Profile

| Lipids, Lipoprotein | Value | Comments | |
|---|---|---|---|
| LDL | | **Adult** | **Children** |
| | Normal | >130 mg/dL | >110 mg/dL |
| | <70 mg/dL | Recommended in patients at high risk for heart disease | |
| | ≤100 mg/dL | Recommended in patients at moderate risk for heart disease | |
| HDL | | **Male** | **Female** |
| | Normal | >45 mg/dL | >55 mg/dL |
| | <35mg/dL | Increased risk for Coronary Artery Disease | |
| | >60mg/dL | Protective against CAD | |
| | <200 mg/dL | Adult (normal) | |
| Total Cholesterol | | | |
| | 120–200 mg/dL | Child (normal) | |
| | 70–175 mg/dL | Infant (normal) | |
| | 52–135 mg/dL | Newborn (normal) | |
| | 200–239 mg/dL | Borderline high | |
| | ≥240 mg/dL | Higher risk (twice the risk of heart disease than normal cholesterol) | |
| Triglycerides | | **Male** | **Female** |
| | 0–5 years | 30–86 mg/dL | 32–99 mg/dL |
| | 6–11 years | 31–108 mg/dL | 35–114 mg/dL |
| | 12–15 years | 36–138 mg/dL | 41–138 mg/dL |
| | 16–19 years | 40–163 mg/dL | 40–128 mg/dL |
| | Normal adult | 40–160 mg/dL | 35–135 mg/dL |
| | >400 mg/dL | Possible Critical Value | |

Data from Pagana RN, Pagana TJ, Pagana, TN: *Mosby's diagnostic and laboratory test reference*, ed 14, St Louis, 2018, Elsevier.

For screening purposes, total cholesterol may be used. Unlike HDL, LDL, and triglycerides, total cholesterol does not need to be measured after fasting. Approximately 75% of cholesterol is bound to LDL and 25% to HDL. LDL can accumulate in the blood as a result of genetic defects in its metabolism by the liver and become incorporated into atherosclerotic plaques, thereby increasing the risk of coronary artery disease, stroke, and other vascular disease. The predictive accuracy of lipoprotein testing is improved by measuring specific subtypes of LDL, especially the very-low-density forms. HDL is associated with removing excess cholesterol from the blood, and the risk of coronary artery disease is decreased as HDL concentration increases. Therefore, the combination of high LDL and low HDL indicates a greater risk of coronary artery disease.

Triglycerides are a component of fat and are converted between glycerol, free fatty acids, and monoglycerides

**Table 40.15** Homocysteine and C-Reactive Protein

| | | |
|---|---|---|
| Homocysteine | 4–14 (levels may increase with age) μmol/L | Normal |
| CRP | 1.0 mg/dL | Low risk |
| | 1–3 mg/dL | Average risk |
| | >3 mg/dL | High risk |

*hs-CRP*, High-sensitivity C-reactive protein.
Data from Pagana RN, Pagana TJ, Pagana, TN: *Mosby's diagnostic and laboratory test reference*, ed 14, St Louis, 2018, Elsevier.

**Table 40.16** Vascular Pressures

| Pressure | Reference Range |
|---|---|
| Pulmonary artery systolic | 15–28 mmHg |
| Pulmonary artery diastolic | 5–16 mmHg |
| Pulmonary artery wedge pressure | 6–15 mmHg |
| Central venous pressure | 2–14 cm $H_2O$ |

Data from Pagana RN, Pagana TJ, Pagana, TN: *Mosby's diagnostic and laboratory test reference*, ed 14, St Louis, 2018, Elsevier.

within the liver and adipose tissue as the need to either store or release energy arises. The liver can convert glycerol, fatty acids, and monoglycerides back to triglycerides in adipose tissue when the body requires an additional source of energy.

Elevated serum triglyceride will usually occur in conjunction with elevated cholesterol and is a risk factor for atherosclerotic disease. Because cholesterol and triglycerides can vary independently, measurement of both values is more meaningful than the measurement of either substance alone. Elevated levels of triglyceride may require treatment with lipid-lowering medications. Poor glycemic control can also elevate triglycerides. A very high level of triglycerides (1000 mg/dL) is also a risk factor for pancreatitis.[1]

Direct LDL cholesterol (direct LDL-C), as the name implies, measures LDL directly rather than calculating it from measures of total cholesterol, HDL, and cholesterol. In standard serum cholesterol testing, LDL cannot be computed accurately in the presence of high triglyceride concentration either because of a recent meal or a metabolic disorder. Measurement of lipoprotein-associated phospholipase $A_2$ may also be used to determine risk of heart disease. This substance is produced by macrophages. Lipoprotein-associated phospholipase $A_2$ in the blood is largely bound to LDL and is speculated to promote the inflammation of blood vessels responsible for atherosclerosis. Table 40.14 lists reference values for the lipid profile.

### Homocysteine

Other cardiac markers include homocysteine and C-reactive protein (CRP), which are both risk factors and cardiac markers. Homocysteine is a naturally occurring amino acid in the blood produced by the breakdown of various proteins in the body. It is related to free radicals, which may be involved in the oxidation of LDL and plaque formation in arteries. Homocysteine levels increase with age; high levels have a significant effect in accelerating the aging process of the arteries caused by atherosclerosis (Table 40.15).

Homocysteine is also linked to the development of early arterial changes characteristic of development of Alzheimer disease, hypertension, and the risk of stroke. An elevated homocysteine level is also an independent risk factor for osteoporotic fractures in older adults.[4] The magnitude of the effect of homocysteine level on fracture risk is similar to its observed effect on the risk of cardiovascular disease and dementia.

### C-Reactive Protein

CRP is produced by the liver in response to the presence of inflammation anywhere in the body. Systemic inflammation has been implicated in the pathogenesis of atherosclerosis and in particular an association with high-sensitivity CRP (hs-CRP). CRP is an indicator of systemic inflammation[70] and may be directly involved in the atherothrombotic process itself.[73]

Clinically, levels of hs-CRP above 3 mg/L indicate elevated risk for MI and stroke, even among apparently healthy individuals with low-to-normal lipid levels.[77] Elevated CRP is an independent predictor of future cardiovascular events that also predicts the risk of hypertension, diabetes, and restenosis after angioplasty.[34,72] Table 40.15 lists the values for these tests.

Half of all heart attacks and strokes in the United States occur in people with normal cholesterol levels, and 20% of all cardiac-related events occur in people with no major risk factors. People with low LDL and high CRP have more cardiovascular events than people with high LDL and low CRP. Using hs-CRP along with traditional methods of measuring risk may help prevent morbidity and mortality associated with vascular disease.[73]

CRP is associated with elevated blood sugar and triglycerides, poor diet, and sedentary lifestyle.

CRP levels are also measured in secondary prevention (individuals already diagnosed at high risk for coronary events) toward dual-goal therapy of LDL reduction and reduction of CRP levels, because CRP levels correlate with progression of atherosclerosis and clinical outcomes in individuals with coronary artery disease who are treated with statins. This reflects a change from previous policies in which it was assumed CRP levels did not provide additional information for at-risk individuals.[58,67]

Elevated levels of CRP have been identified as a predictive factor in HIV disease progression, independent of CD4 T-cell count and HIV ribonucleic acid (RNA) level. Levels of CRP above 2.3 mg/L may signal faster progression of HIV to AIDS and may provide additional prognostic information.[47]

## Cardiovascular Pressures

A number of physiologic measurements are made in the ICU or coronary care unit to monitor cardiovascular health and response to treatment. These include central venous pressure (CVP), pulmonary artery wedge pressure (PAWP), and pulmonary artery pressure. CVP is measured from a catheter introduced from a peripheral vein such as the subclavian or jugular into the right atrium. CVP indicates the working pressure of the right ventricle, which can either indicate the effectiveness of the right ventricle as a pump or the fluid status of the individual. Increased

CVP indicates either poor pumping function of the right ventricle or fluid overload. Dehydration, on the other hand, causes CVP to decrease.

PAWP provides an indirect measure of the right arterial pressure and the effectiveness of the left ventricle as a pump. A balloon-tipped catheter is inserted from a central vein, through the right side of the heart, through the pulmonary artery, and is advanced into progressively smaller branches of pulmonary arterial vessels. The balloon tip is then forced or wedged into a small arterial vessel, and the balloon is inflated. With the balloon inflated, the catheter is exposed only to the pressure present in the fluid between the catheter tip and the left atrium. Poor pumping function of the left ventricle leads to increased pressure as determined by PAWP. PAWP is considered the gold standard for determining the cause of pulmonary edema.

Pulmonary artery pressure is also determined by a catheter inserted through a central vein, through the right side of the heart, and into the pulmonary arterial circulation. However, no balloon is inflated. The catheter is exposed to the fluctuations in pressure that occur with the cardiac cycle as blood fills and is emptied from the pulmonary arterial vessels. Generally, one is interested in whether pulmonary hypertension exists. Pulmonary artery pressure can be measured by the same catheter used for PAWP by deflating the balloon and withdrawing the tip so it is no longer wedged. Manipulating this catheter is not considered part of physical therapy practice. Table 40.16 lists reference values for vascular pressures.

## PULMONARY FUNCTION TESTS

Pulmonary function tests evaluate respiratory function for diagnosing and assessing severity of obstructive and restrictive abnormalities. These tests may reveal abnormalities in the airways, alveoli, and pulmonary vascular bed early in the course of disease when physical examinations and x-ray studies are still normal. Although useful, the U.S. Preventative Services Task Force does not recommend screening for chronic obstructive pulmonary disease prior to symptoms since it does not alter morbidity, mortality, or quality life.[89] Indications for pulmonary function tests include preoperative evaluation, monitoring progression and response to treatment, surveillance following lung transplantation, investigation of signs/symptoms that suggest pulmonary disease, or investigation of diseases that may have respiratory complications (neuromuscular or connective tissue disorders). In addition, the location of an airway abnormality can be determined (i.e., upper airway, large airway, or small airway) to assist in directing treatment.

Tests include static lung volumes, dynamic breathing tests, and physiologic tests. Imaging may also be used to augment these tests. Normal or predicted values are obtained from population norms and matched for age, height, sex, and ethnicity. Pulmonary function tests are performed three times to ensure data are reproducible. These tests can provide additional information for the physical examination of a person with compromised respiratory function, such as distinguishing obstructive from restrictive disease, separating airway disease from issues with elasticity, and determining central from peripheral causes of breathing disorders.

Tidal volume (TV) is one component of the static lung volume tests and measures the normal amount of air ventilated at rest. The amount that can be inspired beyond normal inspiration with a maximal inspiratory effort is the inspiratory reserve volume (IRV). The name implies that it is a reserve for increasing the volume of air inspired if needed during exercise or other stress. The amount of air that can be expired beyond the normal expiration using maximal expiratory effort is the expiratory reserve volume (ERV). Vital capacity (VC) represents the maximal volume that can be moved. Mathematically, VC is the sum of the IRV + TV + ERV tapping the total reserves of both inspiration and expiration. Table 40.17 lists the names given to these lung volumes.

Spirometry is a dynamic study used to measure lung volume against time. Lung volumes are measured from a reference point of the muscles of inspiration being relaxed. The test is performed by taking a maximal inspiration and then forcefully expelling the air for as long and as quickly as possible (forced vital capacity). A simple, but powerful diagnostic test is the computation of the ratio of forced expiratory volume in 1 second ($FEV_1$) to forced vital capacity (FVC). The $FEV_1$ can be expressed as a percentage to predict severity of airflow obstruction. With normal lung function, a person will have expired 80% of FVC in 1 second with maximal effort. This is expressed as $FEV_1/FVC = 0.8$. With obstructive disease (COPD and asthma), a person will be unable to expire 80% within 1 second and the $FEV_1/FVC$ will continue to decline as severity of the obstructive disease increases. Restrictive disease (pulmonary fibrosis and chest wall abnormalities) is characterized by diminished volumes of all types as well as difficulty taking a deep breath, although $FEV_1/FVC$ may be normal or greater than normal because of decreased elasticity of the lungs. Further information can be obtained by computing the slope of the middle 50% of the maximum VC as an index of small airway resistance.

The volumes measured with a spirometer are only the changes that occur with breathing and not the actual volume contained in the lungs. Additional volumes are determined by dilution techniques that can be used to compute the volume of air present in the lungs. Residual volume (RV) is the volume of air present in the lungs at the end of maximal expiration as a result of anatomic and physiologic properties of the lungs and airways. RV is increased in obstructive diseases and decreased in restrictive diseases. It is determined by use of helium or nitrogen dilution techniques in pulmonary function labs. An amount of helium or nitrogen is added from a known volume after maximal expiration occurs. The subject breathes in and out of the closed system until the helium or nitrogen concentration equilibrates. Then the unknown volume of the lungs (RV) is computed. When this volume is determined, both functional residual capacity (FRC) and total lung capacity can be determined. FRC represents the actual volume of the lungs when the muscles of inspiration are relaxed. It is the volume of the lungs before normal tidal inspiration and after normal tidal expiration. FRC, like RV is increased in obstructive

**Table 40.17** Pulmonary Function Test Components

| | | |
|---|---|---|
| **Lung Volumes and Capacities** | | |
| VC | Vital capacity | Volume of air that is measured during a slow, maximal expiration after a maximal inspiration; normal range varies with age, gender, and body size |
| IC | Inspiratory capacity | Largest volume of air that can be inhaled from resting expiratory volume |
| IRV | Inspiratory reserve volume | Maximal volume of air that can be expired after a normal inspiration |
| ERV | Expiratory reserve volume | Largest volume of air exhaled from resting end-expiratory level |
| FRC | Functional residual capacity | Volume of air remaining in lungs at resting end-expiratory level |
| RV | Residual volume | Volume of air remaining in lungs at end of maximal expiration |
| TLC | Total lung capacity | Volume of air contained in lungs after maximal inspiration |
| $V_T$ | Tidal volume | Volume of air inhaled or exhaled during each respiratory cycle; normal range: 400–700 mL |
| *f* | Respiratory rate | Frequency of breathing is number of breaths per minute; normal range: 10–20 |
| **Lung Mechanics** | | |
| FVC | Forced vital capacity | Maximal volume of air that can be forcefully expired after a maximal inspiration to total lung capacity |
| $FEV_t$ | Forced expiratory volume (in 1 sec) | Volume of air expired during a given time interval (*t* in sec) from the beginning of an FVC maneuver; and indication of how open the respiratory channels are and how much air can get pushed out |
| $FEF_{25–75\%}$ | Forced expiratory flow 25%–75% | Average of flow during middle of an FVC maneuver |
| PEFR | Peak expiratory flow rate | Maximal flow rate attained during an FVC maneuver |
| MVV | Maximal voluntary ventilation | Largest volume that can be breathed during a 10- to 15-second interval with voluntary effort |
| MIP | Maximal inspiratory pressure | Greatest negative or subatmospheric pressure that can be generated during inspiration against an occluded airway |
| MEP | Maximal expiratory pressure | Highest positive pressure that can be generated during a forceful expiratory effort against an occluded airway |
| **Diffusing Capacity** | | |
| $D_LCO$ | Diffusing capacity for carbon monoxide | Reflects ability of lung to transfer gas across the alveolar/capillary interface (assists in diagnosis of diffuse infiltrative lung disease and emphysema) |

Data from Pagana RN, Pagana TJ, Pagana, TN: *Mosby's diagnostic and laboratory test reference*, ed 14, St Louis, 2018, Elsevier.

disease and decreased in restrictive diseases. FRC is computed by adding RV to ERV. Total lung capacity is computed as TLC = TV + IRV + ERV + RV (see Table 40.17).

Physiologic testing may also include maximum inspiratory pressure, which is measured with a manometer attached to a mouthpiece. Maximum inspiratory pressure is an index of the strength of the muscles of inspiration. Other functional testing includes the maximum voluntary ventilation, which tests physiologic components of strength and endurance of breathing.

A simple device frequently used for monitoring airway resistance in persons with asthma is the peak flow meter. An individual expires, as forcefully as possible, for one breath. The device is individualized for a given person with areas of the scale marked with colors to indicate whether function is adequate (green), some intervention is needed (yellow), or emergency care should be sought (red).

Measurement of the quantity of serum α1-antitrypsin (AAT) is used for the diagnosis of early onset emphysema or liver disease. Physiologically, AAT protects against the effect of elastase in the lungs. Genetic mutation in the gene for AAT decreases the amount of AAT produced. AAT production less than 30% of normal results in AAT deficiency increasing the risk of developing emphysema. Those with AAT deficiency may develop emphysema without smoking and those who smoke develop emphysema earlier and have more severe disease. A genetic mutation that produces abnormal AAT may lead to liver disease as a result of the accumulation of AAT in the liver cells that produce it. Signs of liver disease, such as jaundice, may appear at birth and may require liver transplantation, depending on the AAT mutation. Because of the large number of possible mutations, lab testing to determine the mutation is necessary to predict the extent of liver or lung injury.

## Oxygenation of the Blood

Assessing the cardiopulmonary system's ability to deliver oxygen may be done simply and noninvasively with pulse oximetry, which provides an estimate of the

**Table 40.18** Arterial Blood Gas Values

| Term | Definition | Reference Value |
|---|---|---|
| pH | Measure of blood acidity; ratio of acids to bases | Newborn: 7.32–7.49<br>2 months-2 years: 7.34–7.46<br>Adult/Child: 7.35–7.45 |
| $PCO_2$ | Pressure or tension exerted by $CO_2$ dissolved in arterial blood; measures effectiveness of alveolar ventilation (i.e., how well air is exchanging with blood in the lungs) | Child <2 years: 26–41 mm Hg<br>Adult/child: 35–45 mm Hg |
| $HCO_3-$ | Amount of bicarbonate or alkaline substance dissolved in blood; influenced mainly by metabolic changes | Newborn/infant: 16–24 mEqL<br>Adult/Child: 21–28 mEq/L |
| $PO_2$ | Pressure exerted by $O_2$ dissolved in arterial blood in attempting to diffuse through pulmonary membrane | Newborn: 60–70 mm Hg<br>Adult/child: 80–100 mm Hg |
| $O_2$ saturation | Oxyhemoglobin saturation: percentage of $O_2$ carried by hemoglobin | Newborn: 40–90%<br>Adult/child: 95–100%<br>Elderly: 95% |
| **Possible Critical Values** | | |
| pH | <7.25 or >7.55 | |
| $PCO_2$ | <20 or >60 mm Hg | |
| $HCO_3-$ | <15 or >40 mEq/L | |
| $PO_2$ | <40 mm Hg | |
| $O_2$ saturation | 75% or lower | |

*$CO_2$*, Carbon dioxide; *$HCO_3-$*, bicarbonate ion; *$O_2$*, oxygen; *$PaCO_2$*, partial pressure of arterial carbon dioxide; *$PaO_2$*, partial pressure of arterial oxygen; *$PO_2$*, partial pressure of oxygen; *$PCO_2$*, partial pressure of carbon dioxide.
Data from Pagana RN, Pagana TJ, Pagana, TN: *Mosby's diagnostic and laboratory test reference*, ed 14, St Louis, 2018, Elsevier.

relative concentrations of saturated and unsaturated Hb by passing different wavelengths of red light through tissue and determining the absorption at these different wavelengths. This device displays percentage of Hb saturation, pulse rate, and an indication of the quality of the signal. Because this device's accuracy declines when arterial blood flow becomes decreased or with movement, the signal quality indicator must be used to determine the trustworthiness of the percent saturation reading. Pulse oximetry also does not give information about the ability to rid the body of carbon dioxide ($CO_2$) and regulate acid–base balance, and its accuracy is limited to about ±2%.[80]

## Arterial Blood Gases

A more accurate means of assessing cardiopulmonary function and the effectiveness of ventilation and oxygen transport is by analyzing the oxygen ($O_2$) and carbon dioxide ($CO_2$) levels dissolved in the blood and related chemical components. The measurements are used primarily to analyze the effectiveness of the respiratory system.

Under normal circumstances, regulation of pH by the respiratory system provides near maximal saturation of Hb by oxygen, as well as maintaining the partial pressure of $CO_2$ and arterial pH. Arterial samples provide information on the ability of the lungs to regulate acid–base balance through retention or release of $CO_2$ and the effectiveness of the kidneys in maintaining appropriate bicarbonate ($HCO_3-$) levels.

Arterial blood gas results are dependent on other systems of the body to function, including ventilation of the lungs which add oxygen and remove $CO_2$ from the alveoli before transporting these gases from the alveoli to and from the blood. These results also rely on the heart's ability to distribute blood flow as well as metabolic and renal functions. Arterial pH is determined by the amount of acid added to the blood by metabolism and removed by breathing and disposal of $H^+$ in the urine. Other factors involve the amounts of acid or base added or removed by the gastrointestinal and renal systems, and the amount of buffer available. Because of the complex interactions of $O_2$, $CO_2$, and buffering, measurements associated with arterial blood gases include serum pH, partial pressure of $CO_2$, $HCO_3-$, partial pressure of $O_2$, $O_2$ saturation, and base excess (Table 40.18). A detailed explanation of these measures and how they interrelate is included in Chapter 5. Measurements are performed on a sample of arterial blood, usually drawn from a radial artery.

Bicarbonate and base excess measurements are used to determine whether compensations for metabolic or respiratory shortfalls in pH regulation are occurring. In addition to the typical radial artery sample site, samples from other vessels can be taken to determine the performance of the cardiac and ventilatory pumps in their roles of gas exchange. For example, a person with poor cardiac pump performance but normal gas exchange in the lungs may initially demonstrate good arterial blood gases, but low venous $O_2$ and high venous $CO_2$.

# SERUM HORMONES

Several hormones are frequently affected in populations seen in physical therapy and may impact systems relevant to the provision of therapy. Most common is hypothyroidism. Alterations in parathyroid hormone, cortisol, and adrenocorticotropic hormone may also occur.

Table 40.19 Thyroid Function Reference Values

| Age | Thyroxine ($T_4$) (μg/dL) | Triiodothyronine ($T_3$) (ng/dL) | Free $T_4$ Index (ng/dL) | Thyroid-Stimulating Hormone (TSH) (μIU/L) |
|---|---|---|---|---|
| Adolescent, adult, older adult | 5–10 years: 6–13 mcg/dL or 83–172 nmol/L (SI units)<br>10–15 years: 5–12 mcg/dL or 72–151 nmol/L (SI units)<br>Adult male: 4–12 mcg/dL or 59–135 nmol/L (SI units)<br>Adult female: 5–12 mcg/dL or 71–142 nmol/L (SI units)<br>Adult > 60 years: 5–11 mcg/dL or 64–142 nmol/L (SI units)<br>Pregnancy: 9–14 mcg/dL or 117–181 nmol/L (SI units) | 6–10 years: 95–240 ng/dL<br>11–15 years: 80–215 ng/dL<br>16–20 years: 80–210 ng/dL<br>20–50 years: 70–205 ng/dL or 1.2–3.4 nmol/L (SI units)<br>>50 years: 40–180 ng/dL or 0.6–2.8 nmol/L (SI units) | Adult: 0.8–2.8 ng/dL or 10–36 pmol/L (SI units) | Adult: 2–10 μU/mL or 2–10 mU/L (SI units) |

Data from Pagana RN, Pagana TJ, Pagana, TN: *Mosby's diagnostic and laboratory test reference*, ed 14, St Louis, 2018, Elsevier.

Thyroid hormone is necessary initially for normal growth and development. It is routinely tested in newborns to detect hypothyroidism, a potential cause of cognitive delays or developmental disability when left untreated or when treatment is delayed.

In adults, a slowing of metabolism with hypothyroidism may cause sensitivity to cold; brittle, coarse skin and nails; bradycardia; constipation; and slower cognitive processing. Hypothyroidism has also been linked to musculoskeletal injuries and affective changes, including depression and anxiety.

Severe chronic hypothyroidism may progress to a condition known as myxedemic coma. Hypothyroidism may be caused by either pituitary dysfunction or thyroid dysfunction. Thyroid testing includes both thyroid-stimulating hormone (TSH) and thyroxine ($T_4$). TSH (produced in the pituitary) stimulates the thyroid to produce thyroid hormones ($T_3$ and $T_4$). Elevated TSH with decreased $T_4$ indicates thyroid disease, whereas depressed TSH indicates pituitary disease. Hyperthyroidism, most notably from Graves disease, may produce atrial fibrillation and exophthalmos, which is a protrusion of the eyes.

Parathyroid hormone regulates calcium metabolism. In the face of hypocalcemia, release of parathyroid hormone causes bones to release calcium into the blood. Cortisol and adrenocorticotropic hormone are related to adrenal cortex function. Adrenocorticotropic hormone is released by the anterior pituitary to stimulate release of cortisol by cells of the adrenal cortex. Cortisol, a glucocorticoid, is released in response to stress and provides glucose to circulate in the blood. In particular, protein reservoirs are made available for conversion of amino acids into fuel sources, which can damage musculoskeletal structures. Cortisol also inhibits the immune system.

Fluid volume and composition may be altered by changes in the release of several hormones. ADH may be either elevated or depressed as a result of injury to or disease of the posterior pituitary. ADH is increased in what is termed SIADH, causing fluid retention and hyponatremia.

The potentially life-threatening disease diabetes insipidus results in decreased ADH with extreme loss of water in the urine and hypernatremia. Tests may also be performed for renin, angiotensin, and aldosterone as part of a work-up for low potassium (hypokalemia), muscle weakness, hypertension, or hypotension. Table 40.19 lists reference values for serum thyroid hormones.

## IMMUNOLOGIC

Diagnostic immunology or serodiagnostic testing uses blood tests to aid in the diagnosis of infectious disease, immune disorders, allergic reactions, neoplastic disease (e.g., genetic changes and tumor-related antigens), and in blood grouping and typing (not discussed further here). Blood tests can be used to determine whether particular antigens are present (bacteria, viruses, parasites, fungi, or enzymes).

Immunoglobulins, the general term for antibodies that are produced in response to antigens, are divided into five subclasses (IgA, IgD, IgE, IgG, and IgM). These classes of immunoglobulins can be differentiated by morphology and by their roles in the immune system. During lab testing, the globulins are separated by electrophoresis into different fractions. Different fractions are indicative of different diseases. For example, α-globulin is elevated in rheumatoid arthritis and β- and γ-globulins are elevated in multiple myeloma.

Ideally, serum is collected at the beginning of the illness during the acute phase and again 3 to 4 weeks later during the convalescent phase. An increase in the quantity (titer) of a specific antibody between these two phases is diagnostically significant. The specific antibody tests for individual antigens are beyond the scope of this chapter.

**Table 40.20** Diseases Associated with Increased Levels of HLA-B Antigen[a]

| Disease |
|---|
| Ankylosing spondylitis |
| Multiple sclerosis |
| Myasthenia gravis |
| Psoriasis |
| Reiter syndrome |
| Juvenile diabetes |
| Graves' disease |
| Rheumatoid arthritis |
| Celiac disease or gluten enteropathy |
| Hemochromatosis |

[a]HLA testing is used as a differential diagnosis in addition to a careful history and physical examination.

Data from Pagana RN, Pagana TJ, Pagana, TN: *Mosby's diagnostic and laboratory test reference*, ed 14, St Louis, 2018, Elsevier.

*HLA*, Human leukocyte antigen.

The reader is referred to more comprehensive laboratory and diagnostic manuals.

## Tumor-Associated Antigens

Knowledge of the interactions between tumor cells and the immune system has made identification of tumor-associated antigens possible. Tumor-associated antigens discovered by these methods are being used to develop passive (humoral), as well as active immunotherapy strategies to stimulate the immune system. Development of biomarkers is ongoing in hopes of developing better screening techniques for early detection,[31,55] along with identifying strategies for personalized cancer immunotherapy (targeted therapies),[28] and even better, prevention with antitumor vaccines.[91,100]

Investigations and identification of gene expression profiles and prognostic markers for different types of cancer (e.g., breast, prostate, ovarian, or lung) are ongoing. Efforts to find molecular methods to detect disease recurrence and micrometastases using biomarkers are also underway. Although not completely reliable, tumor-antigen markers such as prostate-specific antigen and CA-125 for ovarian cancer are already in use.

## Rheumatoid Factor

Rheumatoid factor (RF), an anti–γ-globulin antibody, is elevated in rheumatoid arthritis and Sjögren syndrome. However, a negative test does not rule out either disease. Approximately 20% of those diagnosed with these diseases are negative for RF. A positive RF test may also occur with chronic diseases such as SLE, endocarditis, syphilis, tuberculosis, sarcoidosis, cancer, and viral infections, as well as other diseases.[1,45]

Cyclic citrullinated peptide antibody is also used to assist in the diagnosis of rheumatoid arthritis. Excessive conversion of the amino acid arginine to citrulline leads to the production of abnormal structures called cyclic citrullinated peptides. Cyclic citrullinated peptide antibodies are produced against these abnormal protein products that are associated with the disease process of rheumatoid arthritis. Both RF and cyclic citrullinated peptide antibody testing are requirements of the American College of Rheumatology Rheumatoid Arthritis Classification Criteria.[7]

## Human Leukocyte Antigen

Human leukocyte antigen (HLA) refers to inherited components of the immune system. Inheritance of certain HLA proteins increases the risk of specific diseases, especially spondyloarthropathies such as ankylosing spondylitis, reactive arthropathy, Reiter syndrome, and psoriatic arthropathy (arthritis). Not all persons with a certain HLA pattern will develop the disease, but those who do have that HLA pattern have a greater probability for its development than the general population. As an example, Table 40.20 lists diseases associated with increased HLA-B27 antigens.

## Antinuclear Antibodies

Measurement of serum antinuclear antibodies is used in the diagnosis of autoimmune diseases, such as polymyositis, scleroderma, mixed connective tissue disease, Sjögren syndrome, and SLE. Exacerbations of SLE are related to elevations in antinuclear antibody (ANA), which may occur with events such as exposure to sunlight.

Individuals with signs suggestive of these diseases may have a blood sample examined for the presence of a number of ANAs for diagnosis and prognosis of these diseases. Different patterns of ANA assist in the diagnosis of different diseases and subtypes of them. Other indicators of systemic inflammation, such as CRP and ESR, are likely to be ordered at the same time. A generalized test of ANA may be followed up by tests of subsets of ANA for diagnosis and prognosis. The pattern of ANA is used along with clinical signs and symptoms for diagnosis and prognosis.[56]

# URINALYSIS

Urine is composed of 95% water and 5% solids, although its composition may vary from almost 100% water. It is the end product of metabolic processes carried out in the body. Although urine contains thousands of dissolved substances, the three main components are water, urea, and sodium chloride.

Urine is created through the processes available to the kidney. With a large number of nephrons and long, coiled tubules, healthy kidneys have the opportunity to maintain the composition of body fluids by the filtration of blood and both passive and active mechanisms that result in its final composition. Many substances dissolved in the blood are reabsorbed, including glucose. However, the ability of the kidneys to reabsorb some of them is limited. If the concentration of glucose in the blood becomes great enough, it will exceed the kidney's ability to reabsorb what was filtered and it will begin to appear in the urine.

**Table 40.21** Routine Urinalysis and Related Tests

| General Characteristics and Measurements | Chemical Determinations | Microscopic Examination of Sediment |
|---|---|---|
| Appearance: clear; Color: amber yellow<br>Turbidity: clear to slightly hazy<br>Specific gravity (with a normal fluid intake):<br>Newborn: 1.001–1.020<br>Adult: 1.005–1.030 (usually 1.010–1.025)<br>Elderly: values decrease with age<br>pH: 4.6–8.0 (average pH: 6)<br>Protein:<br>0–8 mg/dL<br>50–80 mg/24 hr (at rest)<br><250 mg/24 hr (exercise) | Glucose (fresh specimen): negative<br>Ketones: negative<br>Blood: negative<br>Bilirubin: negative<br>Nitrate for bacteria: negative<br>Leukocyte esterase: negative | Casts: none present, occasional hyaline casts especially after exercise or dehydration.<br>Red blood cells: negative or rare<br>Crystals: negative<br>White blood cells: negative or rare<br>Epithelial cells: few |

Data from Pagana RN, Pagana TJ, Pagana, TN: *Mosby's diagnostic and laboratory test reference*, ed 14, St Louis, 2018, Elsevier.

The kidney has a remarkable ability to rid the body of a number of substances, especially urea. Urea, for example, is present in the blood but at a much lower concentration than in the excreted urine. A simple yet important screening test is performed by placing a small patch of urine on a dipstick to quickly assess for proteinuria or hematuria. Important components of urinalysis include color, odor, specific gravity, glucose, ketone, WBCs, RBCs (occult blood), electrolytes, and drug screens.

## Color and Appearance

The color of urine is related to a number of factors and the most important is its concentration. A pale yellow color is considered normal. Dilution of solute by increased volume of water in the urine decreases its color, whereas reduced volume caused by dehydration increases its yellow appearance. The presence of blood with intact RBCs produces a more purple-to-red color, and hemolyzed blood produces a smoky appearance.

Color may also be altered by medications, including antibiotics, antimalarials, anticonvulsants, some laxatives, phenazopyridine (a muscle relaxant), and Pyridium. Pyridium is an anesthetic used for treating the burning pain of urinary tract infection that colors the urine orange. The ingestion of certain foods, such as rhubarb, carrots, and beets, and some vitamins and herbal supplements can cause a change in the color of urine. For example, asparagus can cause a characteristic odor to the urine and vitamin C can cause the urine to turn a bright yellow or orange.

Dark brown urine may occur with liver disease or with disseminated intravascular coagulation. Highly concentrated urine (e.g., decreased hydration or renal dysfunction) is also colored differently depending on the individual and may appear dark yellow, gold, or orange, often accompanied by a strong odor.

Bleeding from the upper urinary tract (kidney and ureters) may produce dark red urine, whereas bleeding in the lower urinary tract (bladder and urethra) produces bright red urine. Occult blood, meaning hidden blood, represents a more subtle change in urine color than the red, purple, or smoky-appearing urine and is tested as part of urinalysis. Bleeding can indicate a number of disorders such as kidney stones, infection, or cancer. Frank purulence (visible pus in the urine) or a cloudy appearance is indicative of infection of the urinary tract.

When urine gives a positive result for occult blood but no RBCs are seen on a microscopic examination, myoglobinuria is suspected. Myoglobinuria is the excretion of myoglobin, a muscle protein, into the urine as a result of traumatic muscle injury (e.g., automobile accident, football injury, or electric shock), muscle disorder (e.g., muscular dystrophy, arterial occlusion to a muscle), certain kinds of poisoning (e.g., carbon monoxide) or heat stroke. Odor is part of the urinalysis. Acids create a fresh aromatic odor to urine which can be altered during an episode of disease. Patients in diabetic ketoacidosis have a urine odor that is strong, sweet, and could smell of acetone. Patients with a foul odor may have a urinary tract infection (UTI) or a fecal odor in the urine could be indicative of an enterovesical fistula.

## Specific Gravity

Specific gravity is a test performed to assess the kidneys' ability to vary the concentration of solute in the urine appropriately. The specific gravity measured is determined by the amount of solute present. Urine with no solute has a specific gravity of 1.0; specific gravity increases with the concentration of solute present in urine. A high specific gravity indicates concentrated urine, whereas a low specific gravity indicates dilute urine. Renal dysfunction is suspected when the kidney is unable to concentrate or dilute the urine as needed for homeostasis. Dilute urine has a specific gravity approaching 1.0, whereas the specific gravity caused by dehydration may reach 1.2 or greater. Specific gravity correlates with color. Urine with a specific gravity close to 1.0 will be clear, whereas specific gravity closer to 1.2 produces dark yellow urine.

## Glucose and Ketones

Glucose and ketones present in the urine represent alterations in glucose metabolism. Glucose present in the urine indicates saturation of the active transport mechanism for glucose from the filtered urine. Under normal circumstances, virtually all glucose that filters from the blood can be reabsorbed from the urine.

When the blood glucose level exceeds the reabsorption capacity of the renal tubules, glucose will be spilled into the urine. Failure to absorb all of the glucose indicates a very high plasma glucose concentration and most likely diabetes mellitus. Metabolism of triglycerides by the Krebs cycle requires glucose. When intracellular glucose becomes low from starvation or insufficient insulin, excess fatty acids that cannot be metabolized by the Krebs cycle are converted to ketones.

In healthy individuals, the quantity of ketone bodies formed in the liver is completely metabolized so that only negligible amounts (if any) appear in the urine. However, excessive production of ketones caused by either diabetes mellitus or starvation (including eating disorders) results in detectible concentrations of ketones in the urine. Table 40.21 lists reference values for urinalysis.

## DRUG SCREENING

Employees of health care facilities may be subjected to preemployment screening, random tests, postaccident testing, or reasonable suspicion testing if the employee is under the influence based on objective and observable factors. Laws and policies vary between facilities and may include screening of students on clinical affiliations. Also, drug screening may be part of the diagnostic process. False-positive tests are a concern as cross reactions with other medications can occur. For example, over-the-counter decongestants may test positive for amphetamines. Tests may be performed for several substances, including alcohol, amphetamines, methamphetamines, barbiturates, cocaine, LSD, marijuana, opiates, phencyclidine, and other drugs that might impair employee performance or confound an individual's diagnosis, including analgesics, tranquilizers, sedatives, and stimulants. The Americans with Disability Act provides protection to individuals using prescription drugs taken under the supervision of a prescribing physician. Blanket drug testing programs that are applied inconsistently or target certain individuals without reasonable suspicion can form the basis of an unlawful discrimination claim. Awareness of current federal, state, and local laws is imperative due to a number of states legalizing medicinal and/or recreational use of marijuana.

## MICROBIOLOGIC STUDIES

Many microbiologic studies are available to identify potential causes of infection. Infections may be caused by bacteria, viruses, fungi, and parasites. Microbiologic studies are selected based on signs and symptoms and should be collected prior to the administration of the antimicrobial agents. Identification of the pathogen aids in the prognosis and treatment of infectious disease. In particular, individuals with microorganisms that are resistant to antimicrobial agents require transmission-based isolation procedures, as well as special attention to their therapy and the most effective antimicrobial agents for a person's condition. Gram stains and cultures are the most commonly encountered microbiologic studies in confirming a clinical diagnosis of an infectious disease.

### Cultures

Cultures are obtained to detect the presence of bacteria in the blood (e.g., bacteremia), sputum (e.g., pneumonia or tuberculosis), pleural fluid (e.g., empyema), throat (e.g., streptococci, meningococci, or gonococci), urine (e.g., urinary tract infection), skin (e.g., staphylococci, streptococci, or *Pseudomonas*), and wounds (e.g., staphylococci, streptococci, or *Pseudomonas*).

Other cultures may include stool and anal, cerebrospinal fluid (CSF), cervical, and urethral cultures. Cultures are usually performed when clinical presentation is suggestive of infection (e.g., chills, fever, or pus). This can be performed with qualitative (bacterial presence/absence), semiquantitative (some form of bacterial count), or quantitative (full bacterial count) microbiological methods. Cultures should be performed before antibiotic therapy is initiated; otherwise, the antibiotic may interrupt the organism's growth in the laboratory.

Samples of tissue or body fluids are used to determine the species or quantity of microbes present. A quantitative culture by tissue biopsy or fluid obtained by needle aspiration is best to determine the number of organisms present. Infection, delayed wound healing, and failure of skin grafts are associated with cultures numbering 100,000 or more organisms per gram.

Blood cultures are taken when systemic infection is suspected. These may be done when individuals have indwelling catheters, localized infection, and other risk factors in the presence of fever, malaise, or anorexia. Skin, even in healthy individuals, is expected to have a number of organisms on its surface. In particular, species of *Streptococcus*, *Staphylococcus*, and various fungi are commonly present. In some cases, virulent strains may become present and lead to infection. Infection may take the form of a crusty, honey-colored area (impetigo), spread through follicles (folliculitis), cause abscess formation (furuncles), spread through fascial planes (carbuncles), or appear as fungal manifestations such as ringworm or athlete's foot.

Wounds are frequently cultured for a number of reasons. Both quantitative and qualitative cultures may be taken to determine the appropriate medical treatment. Swab cultures with culturettes are still used frequently, but only represent surface bacteria, which may not be the source of the infection. Biopsy of the wound or removal of fluid deep in the wound is more likely to identify the problematic microbes than a swab.

### Tests for Rapid Identification

Rapid identification and susceptibility testing of fungal and bacterial pathogens enables earlier identification and improved antimicrobial stewardship. Standard techniques for identification of a pathogen may take 48 to 72 hours.[5] To optimize outcomes and decrease hospital lengths of stays, rapid microbiologic tests have found their importance in early identification of *Clostridium difficile* and multidrug-resistant organisms. Rapid molecular assays are selected based on the organism, such as gram positive, gram negative, or fungal. Gram stain is used to distinguish organisms that take up the stain (gram positive) from those that do not (gram negative). A number of

Box 40.2

**DIAGNOSTIC LUMBAR PUNCTURE IN ADULTS**

Diseases detected with high sensitivity and high specificity
- Bacterial meningitis
- Tuberculous meningitis
- Fungal meningitis

Diseases detected with high sensitivity and moderate specificity
- Viral meningitis
- Subarachnoid hemorrhage
- Multiple sclerosis
- Neurosyphilis
- Infectious polyneuritis
- Paraspinal abscess

Disease detected with moderate sensitivity and high specificity
- Meningeal malignancy

Diseases detected with moderate sensitivity and moderate specificity
- Intracranial hemorrhage
- Viral encephalitis

Other recognized indications for lumbar puncture
- Toxoplasmosis
- Amebic infections
- Aseptic meningitis
- Inflammatory neuropathies
- Metastatic brain tumors
- Normal-pressure hydrocephalus
- Hepatic encephalopathy
- Systemic lupus erythematosus

Modified from McConnell H: Current and future clinical utility of cerebrospinal fluid in neurology and psychiatry. In McConnell H, Bianchine J, editors: *Cerebrospinal fluid in neurology and psychiatry*, London, 1998, Chapman & Hall; and Irani DN: *Cerebrospinal fluid in clinical practice*, Philadelphia, WB Saunders, 2008.

common pathogens are gram positive, including *Staphylococcus* and *Streptococcus* species. Gram-negative organisms frequently require different antimicrobial drugs.

# FLUID ANALYSIS

Samples of fluid may be drawn from a number of body compartments. Tests are performed for a variety of reasons, including determining the cause of fluid accumulation in these spaces, determining whether these compartments are infected, or whether cancer or other cells or substances are present. Compartments may include the area around the brain and spinal cord, joints, the spaces around the lungs or heart, and in the abdomen.

## Cerebrospinal Fluid

This fluid surrounds the brain and spinal cord and also exists in cavities within the brain called ventricles and within the central canal of the spinal cord. CSF is typically collected by a *lumbar puncture* (or *spinal tap*). At this site distal to the end of the spinal cord, a needle can be introduced without risk of injuring the spinal cord.

Both the composition and pressure of CSF may be analyzed. Infections (meningitis) may be determined by both presence of bacteria and by alterations in the normal the composition of CSF. Pressure within the CSF space may be altered through blockage of the normal flow and reabsorption mechanisms of the brain, which may alter cerebral function or even cause death.

Box 40.3

**FACTORS EVALUATED IN CEREBROSPINAL FLUID**

- Appearance (color, clarity)
- Cells
- Inorganic compounds
- Acid–base status
- Organic compounds
  - Lactate
  - Glucose
  - Proteins
  - Immunoglobulins
  - Enzymes
  - Amino acids
  - Peptides, neuropeptides

The presence of immunoglobulins may be indicative of other disorders, especially the presence of IgG with multiple sclerosis. Box 40.2 includes other indications for lumbar puncture.

### Appearance

Testing of CSF involves measurement of a variety of substances and states. Box 40.3 lists standard pathologic levels of substances found in the CSF. Appearance is normally clear; cloudiness indicates a disease state, graded from 0 to 4+ (indicating progressive levels of cloudiness)—0 denotes a clear fluid, and 4 indicates inability to see newsprint through the fluid.[9] Bilirubin accumulating in the body (jaundice) can give the CSF a yellow tinge, increases in WBC or protein may cause cloudiness, and blood in the fluid will cause it to turn pink.

Cells found in the CSF usually indicate an abnormality in the central nervous system, as the CSF is normally virtually free of cells. Cell types found in disease or trauma include WBCs, macrophages, cartilage cells, glial cells, bone marrow, and various tumor cells.

Levels of inorganic compounds in the CSF can reflect disorders of the nervous system. Calcium can alter the activation of various neurotransmitters, and low levels are implicated in seizure disorders. Low levels of calcium are also associated with tetany and tumors of the diencephalon. Increased levels of calcium are seen in meningitis.

Magnesium levels will drop in cases of meningitis and ischemic brain disorders. Increased levels of magnesium are seen after intracranial hemorrhage. CSF sodium levels normally change as the plasma levels change. Sodium levels can be out of proportion in the CSF in encephalomalacia and tuberculous meningitis. Elevated potassium levels are seen in neonatal hemorrhage, aspiration pneumonia, seizure disorders, and cardiac arrest.

Glucose is present in CSF due to active transport by endothelial cells and diffusion along a concentration gradient between CSF and blood plasma. Due to these transport delays, glucose concentrations in CSF usually parallel plasma levels but can have a several hour lag period for glucose in CSF to be accurately interpreted. Spinal fluid glucose concentration should be approximately 60% of the plasma/serum concentration. Decreased[9] glucose levels are seen as a result of subarachnoid hemorrhage, hypoglycemia, neoplastic or inflammatory infiltration of the meninges, and many forms of meningitis. LDH is increased in meningitis. Amino acids acting as neurotransmitters in CSF represent an important regulatory mechanism. Levels are increased in meningitis and in CSF blockages and are decreased in multiple sclerosis. Abnormalities are found in Parkinson's disease and depression.

The CSF plays an important role in the transport of peptides to target areas of the brain. Neuropeptides (e.g., endorphins) are related to higher brain functions, such as learning, memory, posture, and movement, as well as to emotions[52] and pain mechanisms. Persons with phantom and neurogenic pain have been found to have low CSF endorphin levels.

## Synovial Fluid Analysis

Arthrocentesis, the surgical puncture of a joint cavity for aspiration (withdrawal) of synovial fluid, is performed by inserting a sterile needle into the joint space. Although the knee is the most commonly aspirated joint, arthrocentesis can be done on any major joint (e.g., shoulder, hip, elbow, wrist, ankle). This test is performed for many different reasons, such as to establish the presence of infection, crystal-induced arthritis (gout), synovitis, neoplasms or to inject medication (corticosteroids).

Fluid may be aspirated from joints to determine the cause of joint effusion, or simply to relieve pressure caused by effusion due to acute trauma. Joint aspiration also offers the potential benefit of removing WBCs, a source of destructive enzymes, from the joint. Joint effusions may increase intraarticular pressure, impairing synovial capillary perfusion. Removing synovial fluid via arthrocentesis could potentially improve the delivery of nutrients to cartilage and surrounding tissues.

Once the fluid sample is obtained, it is examined microscopically and chemically. Normal joint fluid is clear, colorless or straw-colored, and viscous because of hyaluronic acid in the absence of inflammation. A small amount of blood may be caused by needle trauma; true hemarthrosis gives the fluid a homogeneous pink or red appearance. Viscosity is reduced in people with inflammatory arthritis, and the synovial fluid tends to drip like water; fluid of high viscosity forms a string several inches long.

The mucin clot test correlates with the viscosity and is performed by adding acetic acid to joint fluid. Poor appearance of mucin clots can be found in the presence of inflammatory conditions like rheumatoid arthritis. Cell counts are also performed, including a WBC count (normal joint fluid contains fewer than 150/mm$^3$) and neutrophils (PMNs). The concentration of WBCs determines cloudiness.

Although a low WBC count usually indicates a noninflammatory condition, a higher count does not exclude traumatic effusion. Synovial fluid WBC counts may approach 100,000/μL immediately after joint surgery. Normal synovial fluid contains 25% or fewer neutrophils. A very high percentage of PMNs (>75%) is found in most people with acute bacterial infectious arthritis).

Fluid containing 70% or more of PMNs may indicate an inflammatory process, even if the total WBC count is low. The presence of crystals, which is usually associated with an inflammatory process, can be determined by examining the synovial fluid under polarized light. This test is used to differentiate between gout and pseudogout and other crystal-induced arthropathies. Finding characteristic crystals does not rule out concomitant infection.

## Pleural and Pericardial Fluid Analysis

Accumulations of fluid around the lungs and heart may result from inflammatory diseases, neoplastic disease, infection, or altered lymphatic drainage. Either of these compartments may be affected in isolation or both may be affected, particularly in systemic inflammatory diseases such as amyloidosis, sarcoidosis, rheumatoid arthritis, or SLE. Accumulation of fluid in the pleural space may impair inspiration, increase the work of breathing, and in severe cases, cause respiratory failure.

The pericardial space may be filled with inflammatory fluid or blood. Pericarditis may produce audible changes (friction rub) and electrocardiographic changes and other symptoms. Filling of the pericardium with blood, however, is a potentially life-threatening condition called *hemopericardium*.

When the right side of the heart cannot fill sufficiently to maintain cardiac output, the condition is known as *cardiac tamponade*, resulting in acute heart failure. Fluid can be drawn from either the pleural (pleurocentesis) or pericardial spaces (pericardiocentesis) with a needle for either analysis or to relieve pressure within these spaces.

Peritoneal fluid may accumulate for a large number of reasons, including hepatic failure and cancer metastasizing to the peritoneum. Fluid drawn from the peritoneum will be analyzed for infectious agents, cancer cells, electrolytes, and other fluid components to investigate the reason for ascites, the term used to describe peritoneal fluid accumulation. Withdrawal of fluid from the peritoneum is paracentesis.

## REFERENCES

To enhance this text and add value for the reader, all references are included in the enhanced ebook on Student Consult that accompanies this textbook. The reader can view the reference source and access it online whenever possible.

# APPENDIX A

# Guidelines for Activity and Exercise

LORI THEIN BRODY

## PHYSICAL ACTIVITY

The benefits of physical activity have been recognized since the time of Hippocrates, as evidenced by the following quote attributed to Hippocrates (460–377 BCE): "All parts of the body which have a function, if used in moderation and exercised in labours in which each is accustomed, become thereby healthy, well-developed and age more slowly; but if unused and left idle they become liable to disease, defective in growth, and age quickly."[18a] The importance of physical activity is as relevant today as it was then.

*Physical activity* is defined as any bodily movement produced by skeletal muscles that results in an expenditure of energy.[89] Physical activity contributes both directly and indirectly to health status and outcomes. Physical activity levels appear to contribute directly to disease mortality and morbidity, as well as indirectly by the influence of physical activity on conditions such as obesity, diabetes, cardiovascular disease, and osteoporosis.[58]

*Physical fitness* may be defined as "a set of attributes a person has in regards to a person's ability to perform physical activities that require aerobic fitness, endurance, strength, or flexibility and is determined by a combination of regular activity and genetically inherited ability."[89] Physical fitness and physical activity are related, as increased physical activity is required to improve physical fitness, although one can perform a modest amount of physical activity without seeing improvements in fitness.

### Effects of Physical Activity on Morbidity and Mortality

Much has been learned in the last decade about the adaptability of various biologic systems and the ways that regular physical activity and exercise can influence them. Participation in regular physical activity (both aerobic and strength training) is an effective intervention modality to reduce and/or prevent a number of functional declines associated with aging and to elicit a number of favorable responses that contribute to healthy aging (Box A.1).[12] Additionally, as people with disabilities live longer, the need for addressing long-term health issues, assessing the risk for secondary disability, and prescribing exercise from the perspective of disease prevention and reducing the risk for age-related decline becomes apparent (Table A.1).

Aging adults with or without disabilities face additional problems of deconditioning or impaired balance and stability as a result of disuse, disease, or illness. The effect of training dosage, psychosocial variables, and the breadth of emotional benefit from physical activity and exercise is a source of ongoing research.[60,94] The most successful exercise programs take into consideration the person's functional capacity, medical status, and personal interests. Some helpful strategies for facilitating an exercise program are listed in Box A.2.

#### Morbidity

Physical inactivity contributes to the onset and progression of some chronic diseases.[47,74,84,85] According to the World Health Organization, there is convincing evidence that physical inactivity increases the risk of obesity and type 2 diabetes. In other words, regular physical activity decreases the risk of cardiovascular disease, type 2 diabetes, obesity, and osteoporosis and decreases the risk of some types of cancers (e.g., colorectal).[26,54,58]

Regular physical activity appears to modify or reverse cardiovascular disease severity in individuals with known cardiovascular disease.[58] These effects include decreased risk of death from cardiovascular causes, decreased hospital admissions (and resultant decreased health care costs), and improved health-related quality of life.[2]

Aerobic and resistive exercise appear to be associated with a decreased risk for type 2 diabetes, even among people at high risk for the disease.[6] In a meta-analysis of 10 prospective cohort studies, individuals who were regularly engaged in moderate-intensity physical activity had 31% lower risk of type 2 diabetes compared with sedentary individuals.[32] Activity for up to 5 to 7 hours per week showed reductions in risk for type 2 diabetes, whether the activity was leisure, low intensity, or vigorous intensity.[6] In addition, moderate physical activity was shown to be more effective than one type of diabetes medication (metformin) in increasing insulin sensitivity in people considered to be prediabetic.[57]

Osteoporosis is associated with increased disability and frequency of some types of fractures. The greatest benefits to bone mineral density and the incidence of osteoporosis appear to come from resistance training.[70] Exercise training programs have been found to prevent the bone loss observed in the hips and lumbar spine in premenopausal and postmenopausal women.[42,99]

Box A.1

**BENEFITS OF REGULAR PHYSICAL ACTIVITY AND EXERCISE**

- Reduces/prevents functional declines associated with aging
- Maintains/improves cardiovascular function; enhances submaximal exercise performance; reduces risk for high blood pressure; decreases myocardial oxygen demand
- Aids in weight loss and weight control
- Improves the functioning of hormonal, metabolic, neurologic, respiratory, and hemodynamic systems
- Alters carbohydrate/lipid metabolism, resulting in favorable increase in high-density lipoproteins
- Strength training helps to maintain muscle mass and strength, especially in the aging group
- Reduces age-related bone loss; reduction is risk for osteoporosis
- Improves flexibility, postural stability, and balance; reduces risk of falling and associated injuries
- Psychologic benefits (e.g., lowers risk of cognitive decline and dementia, prevents and alleviates symptoms/behavior of depression and anxiety, improves self-awareness, promotes sense of well-being)
- Reduces disease risk factors for stroke, type 2 diabetes, coronary heart disease, and some forms of cancer (colon, breast)
- Improves functional capacity
- Improves immune function (excessive exercise can inhibit immune function)
- Reduces age-related insulin resistance
- Contributes to social integration
- Improves sleep pattern

An association has been found between physical activity and preventing some types of cancers.[64] Mortality (all cause) is reduced by 33% in physically active cancer survivors.[22] It is unclear how much physical activity is necessary to achieve these benefits, and it may vary by tumor type.[54] Research suggests that moderate activity (>4.5 metabolic equivalents [METs]) has greater benefit than light activity (<4.5 METs).[88] One MET is the amount of oxygen consumed while sitting at rest and is approximately equivalent to 3.5 mL of oxygen per kilogram of body weight per minute.

### Mortality

Physical activity patterns have a direct effect on all-cause and disease-specific mortality.[4,49,51] Data from the National Health and Nutrition Examination Survey (NHANES) demonstrate that individuals in the highest tertile of total activity had one-fifth the risk of death of individuals in the lowest tertile, while controlling for multiple confounders.[27] Increased levels of physical activity appear to reduce the relative risk of death in both men and women by up to 39%.[4] Further research into the dose-response relationship between physical activity and mortality shows that compared with individuals performing *no* leisure-time activity, those performing less than the minimum (7.5 MET/week) showed a 20% decreased risk in mortality, those performing the recommended minimum showed a 31% decreased risk, and those performing above the minimum had a 39% decreased risk of mortality.[4] There was no upper limit, with no harm observed with performing at levels 10 times or more the minimum. Other research shows that an individual's perception of their activity level is associated with mortality.[102] Individuals who perceived their activity level was lower than their peers were up to 71% more likely to die (all-cause mortality) in the follow-up period than individuals who perceived themselves as more active.

In a culture where sitting is a part of the workday for many individuals, physical activity becomes even more important. It is unclear if or how much physical activity can attenuate the detrimental effects of prolonged sitting

**Table A.1** Centers for Disease Control and Prevention 2018 Key Guidelines for Physical Activity in Older Adults and Adults With Disabilities

| Key Guidelines for Older Adults | Key Guidelines for Adults With Disabilities |
|---|---|
| Key Guidelines for All Adults also apply to older adults. In addition, when older adults cannot do 150 minutes of moderate-intensity aerobic activity a week because of chronic conditions, they should be as physically active as their abilities and conditions allow. | Adults with disabilities who are able to should get at least 150 minutes a week of moderate-intensity or 75 minutes a week of vigorous-intensity aerobic activity, or an equivalent combination of moderate- and vigorous-intensity aerobic activity. Activity should be performed in episodes of at least 10 minutes, preferably spread throughout the week. |
| Older adults should do exercises that maintain or improve balance if they are at risk of falling. | Adults with disabilities who are able to should also do muscle-strengthening activities of moderate or high intensity that involve all major muscle groups on 2 or more days a week. |
| Older adults should determine their level of effort for physical activity relative to their level of fitness. | When adults with disabilities are unable to meet the Guidelines, they should engage in regular physical activity according to their abilities and should avoid inactivity. |
| Older adults with chronic conditions should understand whether and how their conditions affect their ability to do regular physical activity safely. | Adults with disabilities should consult their health care provider about the amounts and types of physical activity appropriate for their abilities. |

From U.S. Department of Health and Human Services. *Physical activity guidelines for Americans*, ed 2, Washington, DC: U.S. Department of Health and Human Services; 2018. Available at: https://health.gov/paguidelines/.

Box A.2

**STRATEGIES TO FACILITATE SUCCESSFUL EXERCISE PROGRAMS**

- Ask the client if he or she is currently exercising regularly (or was before illness or injury). Provide a brief description of benefits that the person could achieve from such a program.
- Stress exercise benefits of improving health rather than achieving weight loss.
- Allow the person to respond to the recommendation for an exercise program. Encourage the person to verbalize any thoughts or reactions to your suggestions.
- Determine whether the person believes that an exercise program will benefit him or her personally. Help the person to set personal goals for exercise.
- Establish a patient/client self-charge contract and plan to monitor his or her own success.
- Be aware of any cultural or philosophical beliefs the person may have regarding exercise.
- If resistance to the idea of an exercise program is encountered, give the person an opportunity to list potential barriers to exercise. Ask the person to suggest ways to overcome potential barriers.
- Whenever possible, provide a written (preferably just pictures because of the potential of undisclosed illiteracy) of the proposed exercise program. Review progress and reward attempts, successes, and progression of the exercise program.
- Make it fun to foster a lifestyle approach characterized by long-term adherence.

during the day. For individuals who sat for more than 8 h/day but also achieved >35.5 MET h/week (60 to 75 min/day), there was no increase in mortality.[26] However, this high activity level attenuates, but does not eliminate, the increased mortality risk associated with high television watching time (≥5 h/day). In contrast, individuals sitting for >8 h/day and with the lowest activity levels demonstrated a significantly increased risk of mortality.

Physical fitness and physical activity, while related, both serve as confounders in assessing mortality risk factors. The relationship among cardiorespiratory fitness, strength, physical activity, and mortality is complicated with ongoing research in this area.[11] Additionally the relationship among these variables appears to be modified by multiple factors, including body weight and age.[35] Overall death rates are highest in the lowest quartile of fitness. The greatest improvement in mortality occurs between the lowest and next lowest category of fitness, suggesting there is a graded effect of improved fitness on mortality. This is consistent with other research that demonstrates that small improvements in fitness are associated with significant reduction in risk of cardiovascular events and death, especially as people age.[50]

The association of improved health with increased physical activity requires defining how much physical activity is beneficial. There is debate over the optimal amount of exercise needed for health benefits, although the general agreement is that more is better.[95] Given that moderate exercise appears to provide significant health benefits and that vigorous exercise is difficult for individuals to achieve, public health policy has emphasized regular moderate exercise as an achievable goal for the greatest number of individuals. Data from NHANES provide further information on light activity and mortality. For every 60-minute increase in light-intensity activity, a 16% decrease in all-cause mortality was found.[55]

The current recommendation of the U.S. Surgeon General[89] indicates that adults gain substantial benefits from 2 hours 30 minutes a week of moderate-intensity aerobic physical activity or 1 hour 15 minutes of vigorous-intensity aerobic physical activity; each person is encouraged to accumulate 30 minutes of moderate exercise on most days of the week. Minimum increments of 10 minutes are advised. Additional wording indicates that people who are already active may benefit from more intense levels of physical activity.[89]

## Occupational Versus Leisure-Time Physical Activity

Not all physical activity is the same, and researchers should clearly define the type of activity their subjects are undertaking. Most notably, occupational physical activity must be distinguished from leisure-time physical activity. Much of the literature, including the Surgeon General's report, has investigated leisure-time physical activity. More time spent in leisure activities compared with occupational physical activity is associated with improved markers of morbidity and mortality.[82]

Despite being physically active in some occupations, research shows that employees who performed moderate-to-hard occupational physical activity and no leisure-time physical activity had the greatest risk for all-cause mortality.[38] This suggests that occupational physical activity is not a substitute for leisure-time physical activity. The difference in temporal patterns between occupational and leisure activity (occupational walking was performed in brief periods <5 minutes) may play a role in this finding.[37] However, the variability in time spent in leisure activity between blue-collar and white-collar workers cannot be explained by the number of hours worked.[10] Additionally, self-reported health was lower in people with active and strenuous jobs.[90]

In a study of industrial workers over a 28-year period, vigorous leisure-time activity was associated with low risk of poor physical function, but strenuous work activity, smoking, and being overweight increased the risk of poor physical function.[53] However, even low-intensity leisure-time activity showed a beneficial effect. A systematic review of 12 studies was completed in 2011. One study reported a significant relationship between increased leisure-time activity and improved low back pain, and one study found that lower levels of physical activity were associated with higher levels of pain and disability. All other studies found no relationship between measures of activity levels and either pain or disability, thus coming to the conclusion that validated activity measurement in future research is required to better evaluate the relationships between physical activity and low back pain.[39]

## Aerobic Capacity Versus Musculoskeletal Fitness

Physical activity, regardless of aerobic capacity level, appears to provide health benefits. Musculoskeletal performance is increasingly linked to improved physical function and prevents or modifies disability.[19,52] Many activities of daily living (ADLs) require more musculoskeletal performance and rely less on aerobic capacity. Furthermore, a decline in physical performance, defined by activities such as rising from a chair, getting up and down from the floor, and climbing stairs, is associated with frailty, dependence in ADLs, and assisted living placement.[3]

## Prevalence of Physical Activity Behaviors

Two behavioral strategies for reducing the risk for chronic disease have been identified: (1) consuming fruits and vegetables five or more times per day and (2) engaging in regular physical activity. Despite the importance of physical activity, only a minority of Americans are meeting physical activity guidelines.

Data for the prevalence of physical activity behaviors are available from a variety of population surveys. One common source of information is the Behavioral Risk Factor Surveillance System,[13] a population-based, random digit-dialed telephone survey of the U.S. population older than age 18 years conducted by the Centers for Disease Control and Prevention.[14] Information regarding health risk behaviors, clinical preventive health practices, and health care access primarily related to chronic disease and injury is obtained from a representative sample of adults in each state.[62] Respondents are asked to recall the overall frequency and time spent in a variety of leisure-time activities, as well as in moderate and vigorous physical activity.

The current Behavioral Risk Factor Surveillance System indicates that less than half (48%) of U.S. adults meet the physical activity guidelines; less than 30% of high school students get at least 60 minutes of daily physical activity.[14] Rates of activity and inactivity vary across states and regions: for example, individuals living in the South are less physically active than any other region. Reports of adults who participated in no leisure-time activity in the past month averaged 25.5% with ranges of 17.6% in Colorado and 47% in Puerto Rico.[14] Adults with higher education and socioeconomic status are more likely to remain physically active.[12]

There is also great concern about activity levels of children. Based on the Youth Risk Behavior Surveillance System published in 2018, most children and youths are not meeting current physical activity guidelines.[15] Approximately 15% of children had not been physically active for at least 60 minutes at least 1 day in the last 7. Nationwide, 46.5% of students had been physically active for at least 60 minutes per day on 5 or more days during the 7 days before the survey, while 26% had been this active on all 7 days.[15] This number was higher among boys than girls. Approximately 25% of youths reported no vigorous physical activity; however, 25% also reported walking or biking nearly every day (equivalent to light or moderate activity). Participation in physical activity decreases significantly as age or grade in school increases. Additionally the Youth Risk Behavior Surveillance System reports that one-third of all students in grades 9 to 12 did not meet national guidelines for physical activity in 2010; only 31% attended physical education class daily.[16]

Regular physical activity is beneficial in improving both physical and mental health outcomes. There is evidence that physical activity decreases blood pressure, improves lipid profile by decreasing triglycerides and total cholesterol while increasing high-density lipoprotein, improves insulin sensitivity, and enhances endothelial function, all of which contribute to decreasing cardiovascular risk.[51] Regular physical activity helps build and maintain healthy bones and muscles. In addition, regular physical activity is associated with an increased sense of well-being, can modify the symptoms of depression, and increase self-efficacy (the ability or confidence of a person to implement an effective behavior).[16]

## Interventions for Increasing Physical Activity

Given the benefits of physical activity, it is helpful to know what type of interventions are successful in changing health behaviors, including increasing physical activity. A variety of strategies are used to encourage physical activity, including self-directed behavior, exercise referral schemes,[72] supervised programs, online interventions, specific reminders (including electronically generated), or combined approaches. A multitude of factors contribute to an individual's decision to participate in ongoing physical activity. Adherence is affected by personal and environmental factors, all of which must be addressed on an individual basis.[75,76,93] Issues with the physical environment include availability, access, and convenience of resources for ongoing activity. Along with this, social support from people close to the individual can have an impact, particularly in the continuation of a health behavior change.[65]

Theories of behavior change can be applied to persons who are encouraged to begin or increase a physical activity program.[65,67,59] Barriers to physical activity participation must be identified, and the individual must be willing to actively participate. Individual mental models of adherence to routines can be used to support ongoing physical activity.[75] Other personal factors such as age, gender, social and educational status, psychologic status, and overall character, also contribute to initiating and sustaining physical activity.[98] Understanding the many factors that are barriers or support systems for physical activity is essential for improving physical activity participation (Box A.3; Table A.2).

**Note to Reader** For full details of Physical Activity Guidelines for Americans by age group (life stage) with a review of the strength of the scientific evidence, go to http://www.health.gov/paguidelines/guidelines/default.aspx. These are general guidelines and provide a starting point to help people of all ages engage in more physical activity. The complete publication can be accessed at http://journals.lww.com/acsm-msse/Fulltext/2011/07000/Quantity_and_Quality_of_Exercise_for_Developing.26.aspx.

There are additional health benefits from increasing activity levels beyond these initial guidelines. Physical therapists' understanding of pathophysiology and ability to consider patient/client goals and individual factors (age, general health, lifestyle, comorbidities) position them as the health professionals best suited to prescribe exercise programs for all ages and all groups (e.g., pregnant or postpartum women, individuals with disabilities, athletes, centenarians, individuals with chronic conditions, and so on).

Box A.3

**PROMOTING PHYSICAL ACTIVITY**

Healthful exercise and eating behaviors have been shown unequivocally to reduce the risk for health compromise and chronic disease. Physical therapists are in an ideal position to promote healthy behaviors and reduce the risk of chronic disease in all individuals by including each of the following steps.

- Assess physical activity along with other health indicators and risk factors, such as smoking, heart disease, and hypertension
- Work with other public health groups to address the importance of increasing physical activity
- Recommend physical activity as part of a physical therapy plan of care

***Physical Activity Recommendations***[1]

- Accumulating 30 minutes of daily physical activity for adults and 60 minutes daily for children and adolescents (ages 6–17) has been shown to have health benefits; however, the minimum amount of time to be spent in physical activity is 10 minutes. Most of this time should be either moderate- or vigorous-intensity aerobic activity.
- Adults are advised to complete a total of 2½ hours of moderate-intensity physical activity each week or 75 minutes (1 hour 15 minutes) each week of vigorous-intensity aerobic physical activity.
- Moderate exercise is defined as reaching a certain threshold of energy expenditure. Energy expenditure estimated in METs gives a guideline for energy expenditure. By definition, 1 MET is equivalent to the amount of oxygen consumed at rest, averaged at 3.5 mL/kg$^{-1}$/min$^{-1}$. Moderate activity ranges from 3 to 6 METs, or 10.5 to 21.0 mL of oxygen consumed for each kilogram of body weight per minute. This leads to approximately 100 calories burned for 30 minutes of exercise in an individual who weighs 150 lb.
- Muscle- and bone-strengthening exercises should be performed at least 3 days a week for children and teens and a minimum of twice a week (more often is preferable) for adults of all ages.
- Older adults should do exercises that maintain or improve balance.
- How can physical therapists estimate energy expenditure? Table A.2 provides some estimates of energy expenditure for the average person that can be used in physical therapy settings.

*METs*, Metabolic equivalents.

## GUIDELINES FOR ACTIVITY AND EXERCISE

Frequently, older adults with physical therapy needs are inactive, are hypertensive, and have multiple risk factors for comorbidities. These factors often are not documented, and the client is treated for a specific condition without regard for the past medical history or current cardiopulmonary (or other) condition.

For these reasons, the health care provider must view the effect of other systems on the client's current condition and rehabilitation outcome. A thorough evaluation may be necessary, and monitoring cardiopulmonary responses to exercise may be required. Postoperative considerations for various conditions are important when planning a rehabilitation program; these guidelines are listed in each section throughout this text whenever possible.

Exercise should be specific to the functional and medical needs of each individual. Whenever possible, physical activity and exercise should be at a level that causes minimal to no symptoms, and progression should be built into the program. For aging adults, physiologic homeostasis may be altered by stress, medications, illness, and exercise. To assist in balancing and maintaining homeostasis, some period of rest between each exercise session may be recommended for some individuals.

Interval training, consisting of short-term periods of large muscle group activity such as walking followed by a period of rest is well tolerated by many patients. Such a program activates the oxygen transport to skeletal and circulatory systems for improving cardiorespiratory and musculoskeletal endurance. Progress slowly by increasing duration to 30 minutes before increasing intensity. Encourage the individual to keep an exercise diary that includes any symptoms that may occur during or after exercise. Review the diary and compare this report with the client's verbal report because the person may forget or deny important information.

**Table A.2** Estimates of Energy Expenditure

| METs | Oxygen Consumption | Kcal/min | Kcal for 30-min Exercise | Walk Speed |
|---|---|---|---|---|
| 3 | 10.5 mL/kg$^{-1}$/min$^{-1}$ | 3.5 | 100 | 2.6 mph |
| 4 | 14 mL/kg$^{-1}$/min$^{-1}$ | 4.5 | 135 | 3.9 |
| 5 | 17.5 mL/kg$^{-1}$/min$^{-1}$ | 5.75 | 175 | 3.0 mph 4.2% grade |
| 6 | 21 mL/kg$^{-1}$/min$^{-1}$ | 7 | 210 | 3.0 mph 9.2% grade |

*Kcal*, Kilocalories; *METs*, metabolic equivalents; *mph*, miles per hour.

## MEDICATIONS AND EXERCISE

Some clients may be taking medications that can have considerable side effects and interactions when combined with other medications, including effects on exercise parameters such as heart rate, blood pressure, or respiratory rate. Medications can also affect balance, posture, motor control, sleep, and mood, which may affect the individual's performance in rehabilitation. Common drugs with side effects that may affect an exercise program are listed in Table A.3.

People who are taking drugs that can cause volume depletion or orthostatic hypotension should have their blood pressure and pulse checked in both reclining and standing positions. Avoiding sudden postural changes or activities, limiting activities that promote vasodilation, and providing an adequate warm-up and cooldown period are essential. Therapeutic intervention, especially

**Table A.3** Common Drugs That May Affect an Exercise Program[a]

| Drugs | Effects |
|---|---|
| Anticoagulants | Bleeding into tissues |
| Antidepressants, antipsychotics | Sedation, lethargy, muscle weakness, orthostasis and falls, arrhythmias<br>Antipsychotics only: extrapyramidal motor effects (change in posture, balance, and involuntary movements) |
| Antihypertensive agents | Hypotension, orthostasis and falls<br>Reduced exercise capacity (β-blockers) |
| β-Adrenergic blockers | Decreased heart rate (resting and exercise), fatigue, masking of hypoglycemic symptoms |
| Corticosteroids | See Table 5.4 |
| Immunosuppressants | See Table 5.3 |
| NSAIDs | See Table 5.2 |
| Diuretics | Hypokalemia—arrhythmias, muscle cramps (see Chapter 5)<br>Dehydration—orthostasis and falls, thermoregulatory disturbance<br>Elevated heart rate with all activity |
| Insulin, oral hypoglycemics | Hypoglycemia |
| Pain medication, narcotics, opioids | Blunted respiratory response, sedation, lethargy, muscle weakness, incoordination |
| Thyroid medication | Altered metabolic state (see Chapter 5)<br>Impaired cardiopulmonary function<br>Myalgias, stiffness, trigger points<br>See further discussion in Chapter 11 |
| Tranquilizers, sedatives | Relaxation, reduced coordination, orthostasis and falls |

[a]See also Table 12.5 and Box 5.2.
*NSAIDs,* Nonsteroidal antiinflammatory drugs.

exercise, should be scheduled according to medication peak blood levels to minimize effects on participation and to enhance rehabilitation performance.

## GUIDELINES FOR MONITORING VITAL SIGNS

It is important to know normal responses to movement and activity (including exercise) to be able to identify abnormal responses in a client with a medical diagnosis. Safe and effective exercise can be measured in part by monitoring vital sign responses (temperature, heart rate, respiratory rate, blood pressure, oxygen saturation, pain levels). Such data can be used as specific outcome measures to substantiate decision making. For example, how quickly the heart rate returns to normal after exercise or activity is an outcome measurement of fitness and conditioning.

The use of walking velocity has been proposed as the "sixth vital sign."30 Walking speed is a general indicator of function and, as such, a reflection of many variables, such as health status, motor control, muscle strength, and endurance.[63] It is a reliable, valid, and sensitive measure of functional ability with additional predictive value in assessing future health status, functional decline, potential for hospitalization, and even mortality.[18]

The test is conducted using a timed 10-m walk test on a 20-m-long straight path. Complete descriptions of the test and expected results are available.[9,18,30] As specialists in human movement and function, therapists can use walking speed as a practical and predictive "vital sign" of general health that can be used to monitor change (improvement or decline) in health and function.

A person with a significant past medical history of cardiovascular or pulmonary disease requires monitoring of vital signs and perceived exertion during exercise. The more coronary risk factors present (see Table 12.3), the greater the need for monitoring. For any client with known coronary artery disease and/or previous history of myocardial infarction, exercise testing should be performed before an exercise program is undertaken.

If this testing has not been accomplished and baseline measurements are unavailable for use in planning exercise, the therapist must monitor the client's heart rate and blood pressure and note any accompanying symptoms during exercise. Too rapid a rise in heart rate, respiratory rate, or blood pressure for the workload is a general indication for modifying the activity or exercise program (see Abnormal Heart Rate Response and Abnormal Respiratory Rate Response later).

The type of exercise may make a difference in the changes observed in vital signs in older adults. Measurement of heart rate and blood pressure responses to typical isometric, isokinetic, and eccentric resistance-training protocols in older adults showed that changes in blood pressure, arterial pressure, and rate-pressure product were significantly greater during isometric exercise than during eccentric exercise. Clinically an isokinetic eccentric exercise program enables older adults to work at the same torque output with less cardiovascular stress than isometric exercise.[43]

### Temperature

Normal body temperature is not a specific number but a range of values that depends on factors such as the time of day, age, medical status, and presence or absence of

**Table A.4** Body Temperature Conversions

| Celsius (°C) | Fahrenheit (°F) |
|---|---|
| 34.0 | 93.2 |
| 35.0 | 95.0 |
| 35.6 | 96.1 |
| 35.8 | 96.4 |
| 36.0 | 96.8 |
| 36.2 | 97.2 |
| 36.4 | 97.5 |
| 36.6 | 97.9 |
| 36.8 | 98.2 |
| **37.0** | **98.6** |
| 37.2 | 99.0 |
| 37.4 | 99.3 |
| 37.6 | 99.7 |
| 37.8 | 100.0 |
| 38.0 | 100.4 |
| 38.2 | 100.8 |
| 38.4 | 101.1 |
| 38.6 | 101.5 |
| 38.8 | 101.8 |
| 39.0 | 102.2 |
| 39.2 | 102.6 |
| 39.4 | 102.9 |
| 39.6 | 103.3 |
| 39.8 | 103.6 |
| 40.0 | 104.0 |
| 40.2 | 104.4 |
| 40.4 | 104.7 |
| 40.6 | 105.2 |
| 40.8 | 105.4 |
| 41.0 | 105.9 |
| 41.2 | 106.1 |
| 41.4 | 106.5 |
| 42.0 | 107.6 |
| 42.4 | 108.3 |
| 43.0 | 109.4 |

infection. Oral body temperature ranges from 96.8°F to 99.5°F (36°C to 37.5°C) with an average of 98.6°F (37°C) (Table A.4).

The clinical implications of fever and approach to fever vary considerably from person to person, institution to institution, and physician to physician. For example, there is a tendency among the aging population to develop an increase in temperature on hospital admission or in response to any change in homeostasis. Alternatively, fever in older adults residing in extended care facilities may suggest an infectious process, whereas postoperative fever can indicate a surgical complication, such as intraabdominal abscess, leaking anastomosis with peritonitis, or an infected surgical site or prosthesis (e.g., valve, joint, graft). Fever response in adults older than 75 years is often blunted and sometimes even absent.

Other people who may remain afebrile in the presence of significant infectious pathology include people who are immunocompromised (e.g., transplant recipients, patients taking corticosteroids, patients with cancer undergoing treatment), alcoholics, individuals with chronic renal insufficiency, and individuals taking excessive antipyretic medications. Establishing a basal body temperature and monitoring for changes in temperature (of more than 2.4°F [1.3°C]) can assist in early detection of infection (see Box 8.1 for other manifestations of infection).[33]

Single temperature spikes (sudden elevation that returns to normal without intervention) is usually of no diagnostic significance unless it occurs in an immunocompromised individual.[20] Common causes of sustained fever are listed in Box 8.2 and Table 8.1. Unexplained fever in adolescents may be a manifestation of drug abuse or endocarditis.[21]

The therapist should use discretionary caution with a client who has a fever. Exercise with a fever stresses the cardiopulmonary and immune systems, which may be further complicated by dehydration.

## Heart Rate (Pulse Rate)

Measuring the heart rate by taking the pulse is really a measurement of the pulse rate. A true measure of the heart rate requires measurement of the electrical impulses of the heart. Resting heart rate is age dependent, with minimal variation for each individual within the normal ranges.

The normal range for the resting pulse rate is 60 to 100 beats/min. A rate above 100 beats/min indicates tachycardia; a rate below 60 beats/min indicates bradycardia. Some variations occur with age and training (Table A.5). For example, a well-trained athlete whose heart muscle develops along with the skeletal muscle may have a resting heart rate of less than 60 beats/min.

The force of the pulse represents the strength of the heart's stroke volume. A weak, thready pulse reflects a decreased stroke volume such as occurs with hemorrhagic shock. A full, bounding pulse indicates an increased stroke volume, possibly associated with anxiety, exercise, or some pathologic condition. The pulse force (pulse amplitude) is recorded using the following 3-point scale (some physicians/nurses use a 4-point scale):

| | |
|---|---|
| 3+ | Full, bounding |
| 2+ | Normal |
| 1+ | Weak, thready |
| 0 | Absent |

The pulse should be measured before and during the activity, using the same position both times. Count for 6 seconds and add a 0 to that number for a beats/min count or count for 10 seconds and multiply by 6. Palpating for a full minute may reveal an irregular heart rate. Heart rate response should increase gradually with an increase in the workload of the heart. Once a steady state has been achieved, little change should occur in heart rate during sustained endurance activities (e.g., water aerobics, riding a stationary bicycle). Factors affecting heart rate responses are listed in Box A.4.

### Effect of Deconditioning

Heart rate responses are different in a deconditioned person because the resting heart rate is higher to begin with. The heart rate increases more rapidly for the same workload compared with the change in a healthy individual. A rapid heart rate may occur during activity in response to

**Table A.5** Normal Resting Pulse Rates Across Age Groups

| Age | Average (beats/min) | Normal Limits (beats/min) |
|---|---|---|
| Newborn | 125 | 70–190 |
| 1 y | 120 | 80–160 |
| 2 y | 110 | 80–130 |
| 4 y | 100 | 80–120 |
| 6 y | 100 | 70–110 |
| 8–10 y | 90 | 70–110 |
| 12 y | | |
| Female | 90 | 70–110 |
| Male | 85 | 65–105 |
| 14 y | | |
| Female | 85 | 65–105 |
| Male | 80 | 60–100 |
| 16 y | | |
| Female | 80 | 60–100 |
| Male | 75 | 55–95 |
| 18 y | | |
| Female | 75 | 55–95 |
| Male | 70 | 50–90 |
| Well-conditioned athlete | May be 50–60 | 50–100 |
| Adult | — | 60–80 |
| Aging adult | — | 60–100 |

From Kliegman RM, et al: *Nelson textbook of pediatrics*, ed 20, Philadelphia, 2016, Elsevier.

**Box A.4**

**FACTORS AFFECTING HEART RATE**

- Age
- Anemia
- Anxiety, panic
- Autonomic dysfunction (e.g., diabetes, spinal cord injury)
- Caffeine
- Cardiac muscle dysfunction
- Deconditioned state
- Dehydration (decreased blood volume causes increased heart rate)
- Drugs (e.g., blood pressure medication, asthma inhalants, antihistamines such as over-the-counter cold medications, narcotics)
- Emotional or psychologic stress
- Exercise
- Fear
- Fever
- Hyperthyroidism
- Infection
- Pain
- Potassium level
- Sleep disturbances/sleep deprivation
- Stress

dehydration because the decreased plasma volume results in decreased blood volume and subsequent decreased blood to the heart.

A decreased stroke volume (volume ejected per heartbeat) is compensated for by a higher heart rate to match the demands for oxygen caused by the activity. The term *cardiac muscle dysfunction* is used when a decreased stroke volume occurs as a result of diseased cardiac muscle that can no longer contract and pump blood out of the heart normally. Decreased stroke volume results in a more rapid rise in heart rate unless the person is taking a β-blocker medication. When exercising in chest-deep water or deeper, the exercising heart rate will be approximately 20 beats/min lower than during comparable land-based exercise, owing to the Frank-Starling mechanism.[7] This will be accompanied by an increase in stroke volume resulting in a cardiac output that is similar to land-based exercise.[73,100]

## Effect of Age

Aging is accompanied by a decreasing maximum heart rate. The age-predicted method for calculating the predicted maximal (target) heart rate (PMHR) is 220 – age. For example, for a 70-year-old adult the PMHR = 220 – 70, or 150 beats/min. This principle is based on the fact that the heart's maximal rate is 220 beats/min and that this maximal rate declines by one beat each year (probably as a result of the heart's stiffening and becoming less compliant).[44,69] Target heart rate is the first number calculated in determining the *training zone*—that is, keeping the heart rate during exercise between 65% and 85% of the estimated peak heart rate. The lower end of the range is for strengthening the heart, lungs, and circulatory system; the upper end builds endurance. Lower targets are used for individuals who are just beginning an exercise program, individuals who are deconditioned, and individuals with known heart disease.

Concern about the use of this formula has been raised; some clinicians consider it inaccurate because it was based on early research that examined only sedentary men younger than age 60. The formula does not take into account female gender, older age, diagnosis, fitness level, or the presence of comorbidities. It has been suggested that the standard formula overestimates maximum heart rate in older adults. This would have the effect of underestimating the true level of physical stress imposed during exercise testing and the appropriate intensity of prescribed exercise programs.[5,31,66]

There are a number of revised age-adjusted formulas to calculate target heart rate that may be more accurate, particularly for persons older than age 40, such as 208 – (age × 0.70) with an error range of ±7 to 11 beats/min.[7] Gellish et al.[31] found that the formula $HR_{max}$ = 207 – (0.7 × age), where $HR_{max}$ is maximum heart rate, fit objective measures taken during graded exercise testing. Nes et al.[66] found the formula $HR_{max}$ = 211 – (0.64 × age) to fit their population (standard error [] = 10.8 beats/min). There is a revised gender-adjusted formula for women based on the St. James Women Take Heart Project launched in 1992 with published recommendations in 2010.[34] The new formula for estimating peak heart rate in women is 206 – (age × 0.88). Under the old formula (220 – age), the estimated peak heart rate for women was higher, so it could lead to overdiagnosis of heart disease and less conclusive results of stress tests. The 220 – age formula sets a higher-than-necessary heart rate target that may discourage some women from exercising at an appropriately vigorous rate. This is an especially important point, as many pieces of exercise equipment (in the home and at gyms) use the 220 – age formula, thus misleading women to exercise at an uncomfortable level to achieve an artificially determined goal for peak heart rate.[87] The therapist should be aware of any alternative formulas recommended for people of different ages or medical conditions.[8,29,56,66,91]

The standard method should not be applied to individuals with peripheral neuropathies, individuals with chronotropic incompetence (irregular contraction of the heart), or clients taking β-blockers for hypertension and angina. β-blockers are medications that block input of the sympathetic nervous system to the $\beta_1$-receptors in the heart, thus affecting heart rate and contractility. The net effect is a decrease in the resting heart rate, exercise heart rate (drug-induced bradycardia), and blood pressure.[29]

The most accurate way to determine maximum heart rate is a stress test in consultation with a cardiologist. As this may not be practical or cost-effective, the therapist can teach the client how to use rate of perceived exertion (RPE) as a more user-friendly method. For most clients, it is best to wait until the person has exercised for at least 5 minutes before applying the formula. When using the 6-to-20 scale (very, very light effort to very, very hard effort), multiply the RPE number that matches the client's effort by 10 (or simply add a zero after the number). This figure gives a close estimate of the expected heart rate in a healthy individual; cardiovascular (aerobic) exercise should be in the 11-to-14 RPE range depending on the individual's level of fitness.[81]

Keep in mind that clients taking cardiac medications may not be able to achieve a target heart rate above 90 beats/min. Therefore symptoms of shortness of breath, the use of RPE, or the "talk test" may be much better ways to determine exercise intensity. According to the talk test, an individual is exercising at a moderate intensity if able to talk (or sing) out loud while exercising. Anyone having trouble finishing a sentence should slow down. Many individuals who are compromised need more time to work up to the exercise load and to cool down. Using RPE still requires close monitoring of heart rate and blood pressure.

Other methods for prescribing exercise intensity by target heart rate include (1) the heart rate reserve (Karvonen) method, which takes into account the person's resting heart rate; (2) the rate-pressure product method (valid indicator of myocardial oxygen uptake); (3) maximal oxygen consumption ($VO_{2max}$ or maximal functional capacity); and (4) the systolic blood pressure method. Information on each of these methods and their recommended applications and known limitations is available.[1]

Most methods for determining exercise intensity are based on target heart rates that are 40% to 85% of $VO_{2max}$. However, there are some people for whom exercise intensity should not be prescribed by a target heart rate method, such as individuals who are deconditioned. In such cases, exercise should be prescribed at the lower end of the intensity continuum. In this situation, avoid increases of more than 20 beats/min over resting heart rate. (See Exercise and Antihypertensive Medications in Chapter 12.)

A safe rate of exercise will allow the heart rate to return to the resting level within 5 minutes after stopping exercise (blood pressure returns to resting levels after heart rate). Do not remove telemetry immediately after exercise (wait 5 to 10 minutes); in the case of cardiac transplantation, cooldown may take up to 1 hour (warm-up should last 30 to 45 minutes).

## ABNORMAL HEART RATE RESPONSE

Heart rate should increase commensurately with exercise; as the intensity of exercise increases, the heart rate increases.[97] Similar to systolic blood pressure, heart rate also increases according to MET; only a minimal increase in heart rate would be expected with a low-MET activity. Heart rate is a simple method for determining cardiac response to the exercise load.

If the pulse is irregular, count the pulse for a full minute and document the number of beats per minute as well as the number of irregular beats (see next section). Abnormal heart rate responses include a rapid rate of rise in heart rate (judging from the activity, age, and training history) or a decreased heart rate with activity (e.g., arrhythmias or pauses in pulse). For example, a doubling of the heart rate with walking on a flat surface (no incline) would be considered outside normal parameters.

A decreased heart rate with activity may occur as a normal response when the person is sympathetically overloaded before treatment. For example, a person who takes inhalants for asthma just before therapy or who drinks more than three cups of coffee within 2 hours of the therapy appointment may have an artificially elevated baseline heart rate. Over the course of therapy, without further stimulation, this person's heart rate may decrease, especially if the therapy session has no exercise component. Factors such as these require individual evaluation of abnormal responses for each person.

Pulse amplitude (weak or bounding quality of the pulse) that fades with inspiration and strengthens with expiration is paradoxic (paradoxical pulse) and should be reported to the physician. When there is compression or constriction around the heart (e.g., pericardial effusion, tension pneumothorax, pericarditis with fluid, pericardial tamponade) and the person inhales, the increased mechanical pressure of inspiration added to the physiologic compression from the underlying disease prevents the heart from contracting fully and results in reduced pulse. When the individual exhales, the pressure from chest expansion is reduced and the pulse increases. A pulse increase of more than 20 beats/min lasting for more than 3 minutes after rest or changing position should also be reported.

If ischemia occurs as evidenced by angina or (on visual readout) depression of ST segment on electrocardiography, the person should rest and then return to an activity level below ischemic level. For example, if the ST segment drops below baseline with activity or the client experiences angina when the heart rate is at 140 beats/min, the activity level should be reduced so that the heart rate remains below 140 beats/min.

## HEART RHYTHM

For a person with an abnormal heart rhythm, the pulse should be palpated throughout the activity if no electrocardiography or Holter monitor reading is available

**Table A.6** Normal Resting Respiratory Rates

| Age | Breaths/min |
|---|---|
| Premature | 40–70 |
| Birth–3 mo | 35–55 |
| 3–6 mo | 30–45 |
| 6–12 mo | 25–40 |
| 1–3 y | 20–30 |
| 3–6 y | 20–25 |
| 6–10 y | 15–25 |
| 10–16 y | 12–30 |
| 18 y | 12–20 |
| Adult | 10–12[a] |

[a]Typical for average, healthy adult; low for older adult.
From Kliegman RM, et al: *Nelson textbook of pediatrics*, ed 20, Philadelphia, 2016, Elsevier.

during exercise. If any abnormal pulse beats are noted (e.g., absent, irregular), the number of pauses per minute should be counted at rest and during activity. There should be no more than six abnormal or absent beats per minute. The normal heart rhythm should not change, and individuals with arrhythmias at rest should not show an increase in number of irregular heartbeats with increased activity.[28]

## RESPIRATORY RATE

Normal resting respiratory rates are presented in Table A.6. The ratio of pulse rate to respiratory rate is fairly constant (4:1). The respirations can be counted at the same time that the pulse is counted. If an abnormality is suspected, these measurements should be taken for a full minute. A normal pulmonary response to exercise is an increase in breathing rate and depth based on body type and disease present. Factors that can affect respiratory rate include the following:

- Altered lung compliance (chronic obstructive pulmonary disease [COPD], hyaline membrane disease) or any other restrictive condition
- Airway resistance (asthma)
- Alterations in lung volumes/lung capacity (smokers, persons with emphysema or occupational lung disease)
- Body position (diaphragm cannot drop down enough to expand the lungs in the fully supine position in pregnant, obese, or spinal cord–injured clients)

## ABNORMAL RESPIRATORY RATE RESPONSE

An abnormal respiratory rate response is usually characterized by too rapid a rise in respiratory rate for the activity and medical condition of the client. Increases in respiratory rate greater than 10 respirations/min must be monitored carefully. Measuring the respiratory rate may be difficult. The client must be observed for how much work is required to breathe, and whenever possible a pulse oximeter should be used to measure arterial oxygen saturation noninvasively (Fig. A.1).

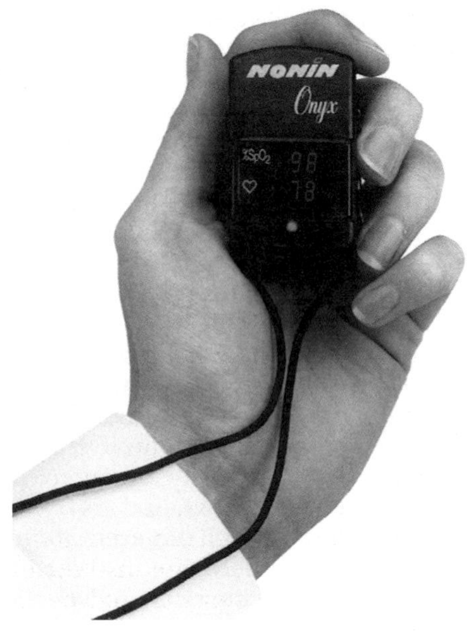


**Fig. A.1**

**Noninvasive monitoring of oxygen saturation ($Sao_2$), sometimes referred to as the fifth vital sign, can be done with a pulse oximeter.** A finger probe is used most frequently during stationary activities. This compact unit (Onyx) is small enough to carry and ideal for spot checks anytime. The person slips this digital pulse oximeter onto a finger for an immediate pulse rate and oxygen saturation percentage. An ear probe (not shown) can be used to measure oxygen saturation continuously during exercise. (Courtesy Nonin, Inc., Plymouth, MN.)

### Pulse Oximetry

The saturation of hemoglobin with oxygen can be measured via pulse oximetry ($Spo_2$) or arterial blood gas (ABG) analysis ($Sao_2$). A normal $Spo_2$ or $Sao_2$ value is 95% or higher. An $Sao_2$ or $Sao_2$ value below 90% means the $Pao_2$ is below 60 mm Hg, indicating the person is not adequately oxygenated ($Pao_2$ is a measure of the pressure of oxygen dissolved in plasma as measured by ABG analysis).

The $Pao_2$ at rest may decline with age because of a loss of surface respiratory space for ventilatory exchange, especially in adults 70 years old or older. The $Pao_2$ increases with activity in older adults as blood volume and respiratory volume increase.[17,96]

Using a pulse oximeter with clients with pulmonary conditions can provide an outcome measure with exercise for documentation. Oxygen saturation values must be interpreted within the context of the person's medical status as well as respiratory and metabolic status (as determined by ABG measurements). Respiratory and metabolic status are taken into consideration because shifts in the oxyhemoglobin curve caused by factors such as temperature fluctuations or acidosis will change the affinity of oxygen to the hemoglobin.

Normal oxygen saturation is 98%, with no change in this measurement during activity or exercise. Clients with chronic respiratory disease may experience a drop in oxygen saturation that is considered normal for them, but this represents a normal response to pathology and is not truly normal.

There has been some question as to whether nail polish can affect the accuracy of pulse oximetry readings.

Studies to date have shown mixed results, with some research reporting statistically and clinically significant differences in readings, particularly with dark-colored polish (i.e., purple, black) and with acrylic nails.[36,40,41,86] Other research has shown no statistically different measures with nail polish in mildly hypoxic patients.[101] For a full review of pulse oximetry and the factors that affect its validity, the reader is referred to a review by Jubran.[46]

Activity should be terminated if oxygen saturation drops to 90% or less in an acutely ill individual or 86% in a person with chronic lung disease. Individuals with decreased oxygen saturation may require more time to accomplish tasks and often experience fatigue and/or shortness of breath. Panic values (critical values or the values that must be reported immediately) may vary according to institution and physician. Increased oxygen during activity may prevent such drops but should be discussed with the physician before it is instituted.

At all times, other vital signs should be monitored (heart rate, respiratory rate, and blood pressure) to assess how well the person is tolerating the activity and oxygen desaturation. If pulse oximetry measures large changes in oxygen saturation with no changes in vital signs, the pulse oximetry may be inaccurate and requires a mechanical check.

Use caution when using a finger probe on an individual with cold, discolored hands (blue or white); this is an indication that blood has already been shunted from the fingers. Pulse oximetry as a measure of oxygen saturation would be inaccurate in such a situation.[46] Peripheral arterial vasoconstriction during the early phases of treadmill exercise has been documented in individuals with vascular pathology secondary to atherosclerosis.[61]

### Supplemental Oxygen

Supplemental oxygen is given if an individual has documented or suspected hypoxemia or deficient oxygenation of the blood, defined as a $Pa{O_2}$ below 60 mm Hg, an $Sa{O_2}$ or $Sp{O_2}$ below 90%, or either value below the desirable range for the clinical situation.[68]

Supplemental oxygen may be needed in cases of severe trauma or acute myocardial infarction, during or after labor and delivery, or as part of procedural sedation or general anesthesia. The therapist should be alert for any signs of increasing hypoxia (reduced tissue oxygenation despite adequate perfusion) indicating a possible need for supplemental oxygen. These include increasing tachypnea and dyspnea, skin color changes (pale, cyanotic), increasing tachycardia, hypertension, restlessness, and disorientation.[68]

Oxygen supplementation in clients with COPD must be prescribed and monitored very carefully to avoid oxygen toxicity and absorption atelectasis. The therapist should watch for blunting of the respiratory drive. Too much oxygen can depress the respiratory drive of a person with COPD. For example, in a person with emphysema, low arterial oxygen levels are the respiratory drive triggers. For this reason, too much oxygen delivered as an intervention can depress the respiratory drive, which is now reliant on lower levels of arterial oxygen.

**Table A.7** Normal Blood Pressures for Children[a]

| Age | Blood Pressure (mm Hg)[b] |
|---|---|
| Premature | 55–75/35–45 |
| 0–3 mo | 65–85/45–55 |
| 3–6 mo | 70–90/50–65 |
| 6–12 mo | 80–100/55–65 |
| 1–3 y | 90–105/55–70 |
| 3–6 y | 95–110/60–75 |
| 6–12 y | 100–120/60–75 |
| 12 y | 110–135/65–85 |

[a]Normal blood pressure values for children and adolescents of various ethnic groups are under investigation.
[b]Systolic range/diastolic range.
From Kliegman RM, et al: *Nelson textbook of pediatrics*, ed 20, Philadelphia, 2016, Elsevier.

The drive to breathe in a healthy person results from an increase in the arterial carbon dioxide level ($P{CO_2}$). Because an individual with COPD chronically retains excessive amounts of carbon dioxide, an increased arterial $P{CO_2}$ is no longer an effective respiratory drive mechanism.[24,71]

If oxygen flow rate must be increased during exercise for individuals with chronic lung disease, it must be returned promptly to its set value at the end of exercise. Failure to return flow rate to the value determined by the physician may result in hypoventilation, retention of carbon dioxide, and respiratory acidosis.

## BLOOD PRESSURE

To monitor blood pressure effectively, the therapist must be familiar with normal (Table A.7; see Table 12.8) and abnormal blood pressure responses to exercise and must keep in mind that arterial blood pressure is a general indicator of the function of the heart as a pump and a measure of the peripheral arterial resistance. Systolic pressure measures the force exerted against the arteries during the ejection cycle, and diastolic pressure measures the force exerted against the arteries during rest or against peripheral resistance.

Systolic blood pressure normally rises with increased exertion in proportion to the workload (approximately 7 to 10 mm Hg/MET) with little or no change in diastolic blood pressure, and it rises more quickly in men than in women.[97] For example, during endurance activities, the systolic blood pressure gradually increases, but with sustained activity no further change should occur. Exercise involving a small total muscle mass, such as a single extremity, typically elicits minimal incremental changes in systolic blood pressure and greater increases in diastolic blood pressure.[23,45]

Diastolic blood pressure may increase or decrease a maximum of 10 mm Hg owing to adaptive dilation of peripheral vasculature. A highly trained athlete may exhibit a drop in diastolic blood pressure of more than 10 mm Hg as a result of increased vasodilation, but this would be considered an abnormal response in an older or untrained adult. A sustained elevation of the diastolic blood pressure during the recovery phase of activity is also considered abnormal. More specific abnormal responses to activity are discussed in detail elsewhere.[83]

If the resting blood pressure is excessively high (systolic blood pressure 200 mm Hg or diastolic blood pressure 105 to 110 mm Hg), physician clearance should be obtained before continuing with evaluation or treatment. Exercise should be terminated if blood pressure becomes excessively high (systolic blood pressure higher than 250 mm Hg or diastolic blood pressure higher than 110 mm Hg). Systolic blood pressure increase during exercise (19.7 mm Hg/min of exercise duration) and a relatively slow recovery in systolic pressure after exercise are associated with the risk of any stroke and of ischemic stroke.[48]

Blood pressure should always be measured in the same position because it can drop quickly with cessation of activity (e.g., do not measure blood pressure while the client is sitting, then have the client ambulate, and recheck blood pressure in the standing position; measure in the standing position, have the client ambulate, and remeasure while standing). In fact, because blood pressure changes can occur within 10 seconds, a truly accurate postexercise blood pressure may be difficult to obtain. Always observe for associated symptoms such as shortness of breath, dizziness, palpitations, or increase in heart rate.

### Blood Pressure After Stroke

Patients in the acute care setting after stroke may have orders for permissive hypertension (e.g., up to 220 mm Hg systolic and up to 120 mm Hg diastolic). This is important to facilitate brain tissue perfusion with ischemic strokes. The therapist may find that even basic bed mobility (e.g., moving from supine to sitting) can increase blood pressure beyond acceptable limits. Concern for complications such as hemorrhagic conversion may dictate the need to return the individual to a resting position and notify a nurse or physician before proceeding further.

Some therapists do not immediately return the patient to a supine resting position, but rather try to obtain blood pressure measurements in sitting, standing, and return to supine positions. This gives the physician a better idea of what is needed to control blood pressure with daily activities. For example, if the diastolic blood pressure is 180 mm Hg when sitting but increases to 200 mm Hg when standing, then medicating for a diastolic measurement of 160 mm Hg while resting in supine is not likely going to provide adequate (functional) control needed for daily activities.

### Blood Pressure in Children

Blood pressure is usually much lower in children than in adults. Children are at risk for developing high blood pressure if they exceed the guidelines listed in Table A.6. The overall prevalence of hypertension in children and adolescents is 3%, an increase over previous national survey data.[77,79] The cause is often unknown. When a child's high blood pressure is severe, it is often because of another serious condition, such as kidney disease or heart disease.

Children can inherit high blood pressure from their parents. Overweight children are also at higher risk. Children who both have a family history of hypertension and are overweight should be screened for aberrant blood pressure. The American Heart Association recommends that all children 3 years of age and older have their blood pressure checked once a year.

A child's sex, age, and height are used to determine age-, sex-, and height-specific systolic and diastolic blood pressure percentiles (see Table 12.8).[92] This approach provides information that lets researchers consider different levels of growth in evaluating blood pressure. It also demonstrates the blood pressure standards that are based on sex, age, and height and allows a more precise classification of blood pressure according to body size.[92] More importantly, the approach avoids misclassifying children at the extremes of normal growth.

The therapist can provide an important service by including this type of assessment. In children, even a mild elevation of blood pressure can lead to serious medical conditions, such as cardiomyopathy and kidney or visual impairments. Medical evaluation and monitoring for signs of early organ damage are needed for any child or adolescent with high blood pressure.[78]

Current guidelines for children may not be very accurate. Normal blood pressure values may be different for children and adolescents of various ethnic groups.[25,78,80] Previously, values have been established without consideration of ethnicity and/or culture and were based mostly on normal values for white children. Investigation to establish more accurate norms and to verify standards for current blood pressure guidelines set by national committees are under way.[77,79]

## ABNORMAL BLOOD PRESSURE RESPONSE

An abnormal blood pressure response may result in hypotension or hypertension as reflected by any of the following responses:

- Too rapid a rise in systolic blood pressure for the workload; in a healthy adult the systolic blood pressure should increase by 20 mm Hg with minimal to moderate exercise and 40 to 50 mm Hg with intensive exercise. These values are less likely with cardiac clients.
- Very little change in systolic blood pressure with excessive workload in an unfit or deconditioned person.
- Progressive rise of diastolic blood pressure.
- Diastolic blood pressure should remain the same or change slightly (less than 5 mm Hg increase/decrease should be noted); a drop of more than 10 mm Hg in diastolic blood pressure is considered abnormal.
- Drop in systolic pressure (or both systolic and diastolic pressure) of 10 to 20 mm Hg or more associated with an increase in pulse rate of more than 15 beats/min (depleted intravascular volume).
- Narrowing of pulse pressure (systolic blood pressure – diastolic blood pressure).

An increase in diastolic blood pressure of 20 mm Hg or more may be a sign that the person has exceeded cardiac reserve capacity and that blood flow to the liver, kidneys, and digestive tract has been critically reduced. A

Box A.5

**FACTORS AFFECTING BLOOD PRESSURE**

- Age
- Blood vessel size
- Blood viscosity
- Force of heart contraction
- Medications
  - Angiotensin-converting enzyme inhibitors
  - Adrenergic inhibitors
  - β-Blockers
  - Diuretics
  - Narcotic analgesics
- Diet and exercise
- Obesity
- Time of recent meal (eating increases systolic pressure)
- Caffeine
- Nicotine
- Alcohol and other drugs
- Cocaine
- Anxiety, panic
- Presence or perceived degree of pain
- Living at higher altitudes
- Distended urinary bladder
- Sleep apnea
- Pregnancy
- Pain

decrease in diastolic blood pressure may occur as a result of rapid vasodilation, an effect of training in an athletic individual.

A drop in diastolic blood pressure may also indicate normalization in a hypertensive individual as a result of vasodilation and decreased peripheral resistance. For example, this may occur if a hypertensive person experiences a calming effect as a result of participating in a regular routine of exercise after driving in heavy traffic to get to the clinic on time. Other factors that affect blood pressure are listed in Box A.5.

## REFERENCES

To enhance this text and add value for the reader, all references are included in the enhanced ebook on Student Consult that accompanies this textbook. The reader can view the reference source and access it online whenever possible.

# INDEX



*Note:* Page numbers followed by "f" indicate figures and "t" indicate tables "b" indicate boxes.

## B

## C

## D

## E

## F

## G

## H

## I

## J



## K

## L

## M

## O

## P

## S

## T

## V

## W



## X



## Y



## Z

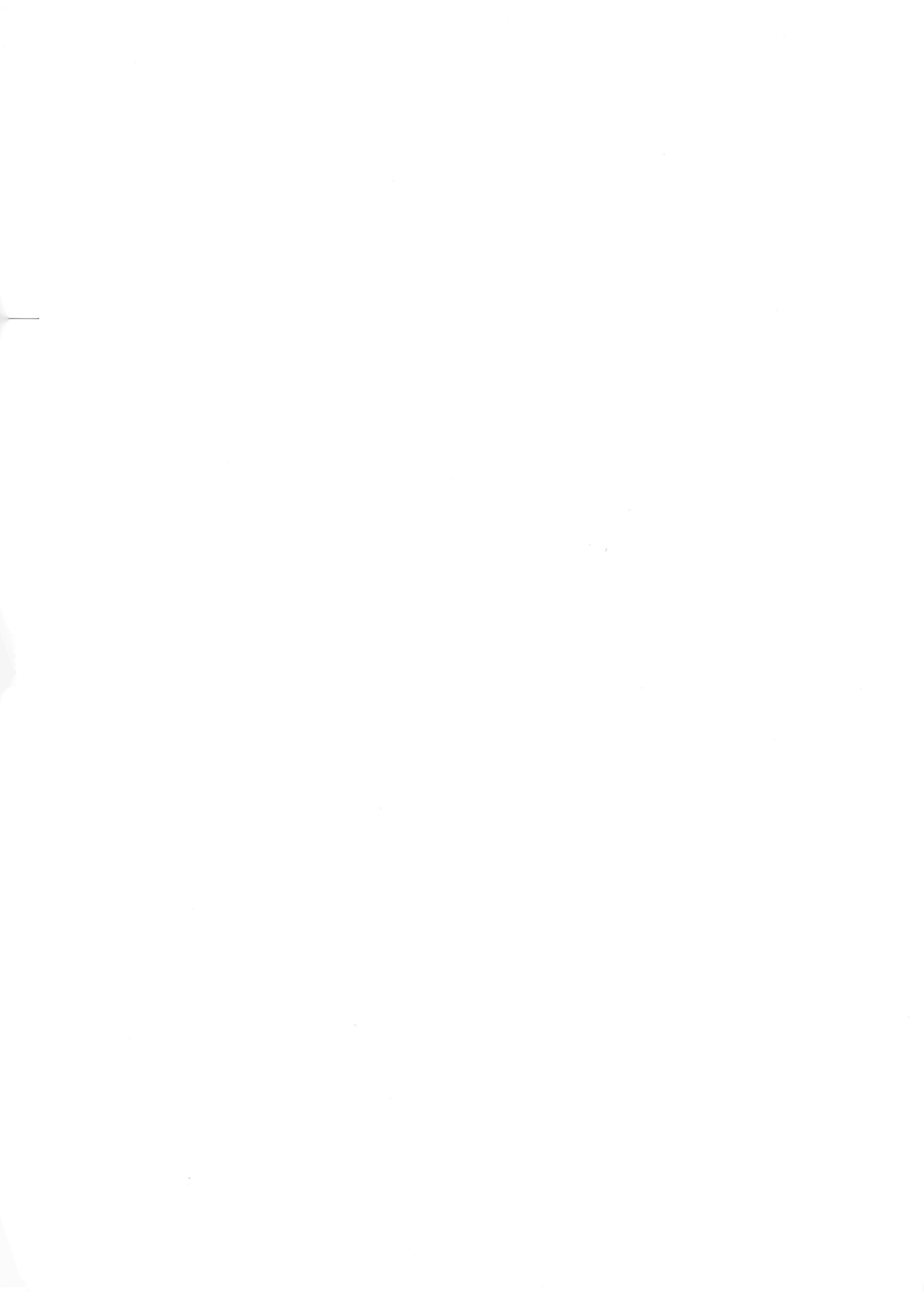

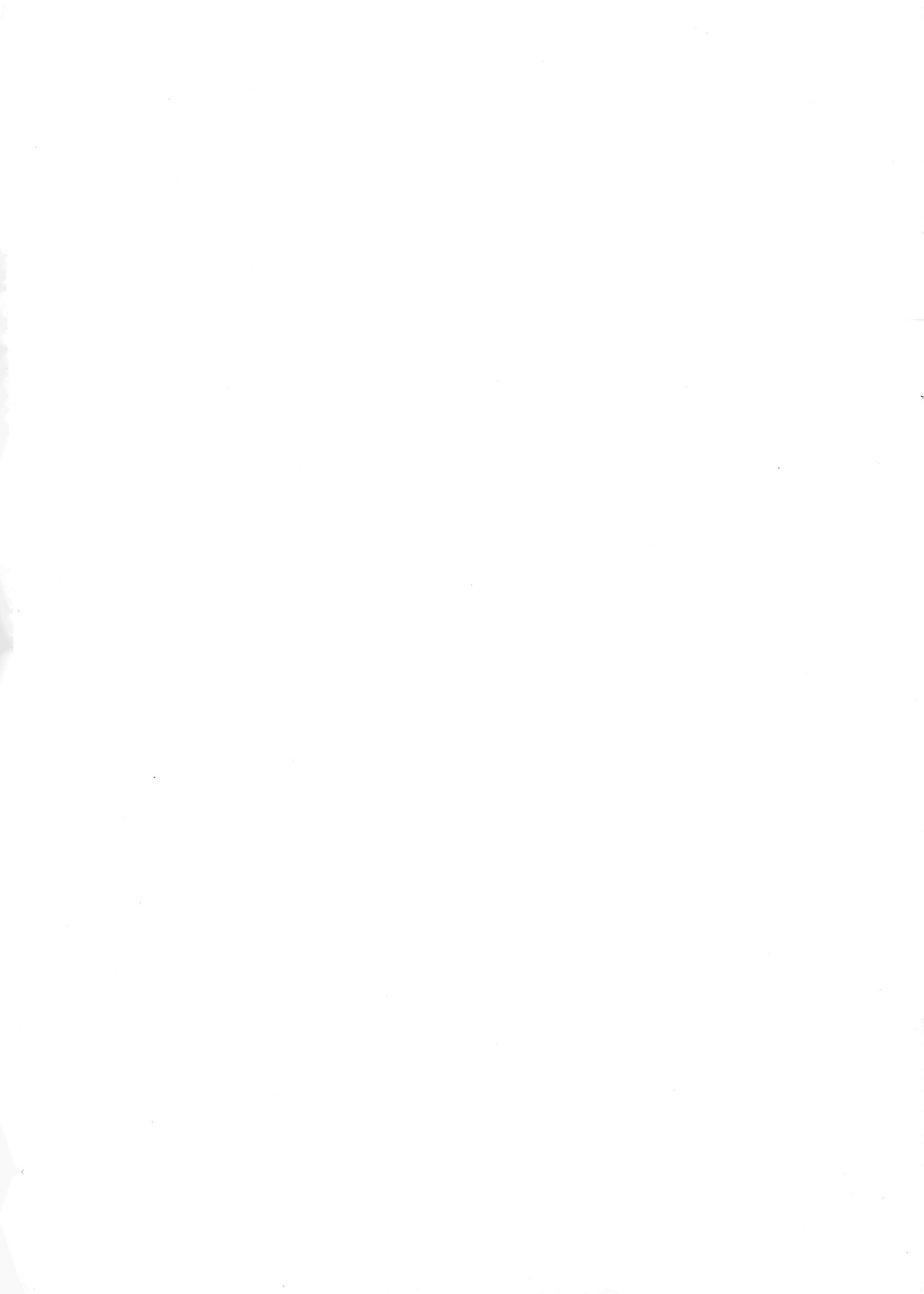